Topley & Wilson's

MICROBIOLOGY
AND MICROBIAL
INFECTIONS

First published in Great Britain 1929
Second edition 1936
Third edition 1946
Fourth edition 1955
Fifth edition 1964
Sixth edition 1975
Seventh edition 1983 and 1984
Eighth edition 1990
Ninth edition published as a complete set in Great Britain 1998
by Arnold, a member of the Hodder Headline group,
338 Euston Road, London NW1 3BH
Ninth edition published as single volumes in Great Britain 1999

Co-published in the United States of America by
Oxford University Press, Inc.,
198 Madison Avenue, New York, NY 10016
Oxford is a registered trademark of Oxford University Press

Whilst the advice and information in this book is believed to be true and
accurate at the date of going to press, neither the authors nor the publisher
can accept any legal responsibility or liability for any errors or omissions
that may be made. In particular (but without limiting the generality of the
preceding disclaimer) every effort has been made to check drug dosages;
however it is still possible that errors have been missed. Furthermore,
dosage schedules are constantly being revised and new side-effects
recognized. For these reasons the reader is strongly urged to consult the
drug companies' printed instructions before administering any of the drugs
recommended in this book.

British Library Cataloguing in Publication Data
A catalogue record for this book is available from the British Library

Library of Congress Cataloging-in-Publication Data
A catalog record for this book is available from the Library of Congress

ISBN 0 340 663170 (Volume 2)
ISBN 0 340 614706 (Set)

Publisher:	Georgina Bentliff
Project Editor:	Sophie Oliver
Project Coordinator:	Melissa Morton
Production Controller:	Helen Whitehorn
Copy Editor:	Kathryn Bayly
Proofreader:	Elizabeth Weaver
Indexer:	Jan Ross; Roderick Gibb; Michael Heary

Typeset in 9.5/11pt New Baskerville by Photo·graphics
Printed and bound in Great Britain at The Bath Press, Avon

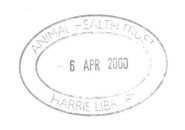
Topley & Wilson's

MICROBIOLOGY AND MICROBIAL INFECTIONS

NINTH EDITION

Leslie Collier
Albert Balows ● Max Sussman

VOLUME 2

SYSTEMATIC BACTERIOLOGY

VOLUME EDITORS
Albert Balows ● Brian I Duerden

ARNOLD

A member of the Hodder Headline Group
LONDON ● SYDNEY ● AUCKLAND
Co-published in the USA by Oxford University Press, Inc., New York

Editor-in-Chief

Leslie Collier MD, DSc, FRCP, FRCPath

Professor Emeritus of Virology, The London Hospital Medical College, London; formerly Director, Vaccines and Sera Laboratories, The Lister Institute of Preventive Medicine, Elstree, Hertfordshire, UK

General Editors

Albert Balows AB, MS, PhD, ABMM

Professor Emeritus, Emory University School of Medicine and Georgia State University; Former Director at The Center for Infectious Diseases, Centers for Disease Control and Prevention, Atlanta, Georgia, USA

Max Sussman BSc, PhD, CBiol, FIBiol, FRCPath

Professor Emeritus of Bacteriology, Department of Microbiology, The Medical School, Newcastle upon Tyne, UK

Volume Editors

Albert Balows AB, MS, PhD, ABMM

Professor Emeritus and Director Emeritus, National Center for Infectious Diseases, Centers for Disease Control and Prevention, Atlanta, Georgia, USA

Brian I Duerden BSc, MD, FRCPath

Professor and Head of Department of Medical Microbiology, University of Wales College of Medicine; Deputy Director (Programmes), Public Health Laboratory Service, London, UK

CONTENTS OF VOLUME 2
SYSTEMATIC BACTERIOLOGY

Contents of Volumes 1, 3, 4 and 5

CONTRIBUTORS

Masamichi Aikawa MD, PhD
Professor, The Research Institute of Medical Sciences, Tokai University, Boseidai, Isehara, Kanagawa, Japan

Libero Ajello PhD
Adjunct Professor, Department of Ophthalmology, Emory University Eye Center, Atlanta, Georgia, USA

RP Allaker BSc, PhD
Lecturer in Oral Microbiology, Department of Oral Microbiology, St Bartholomew's and the Royal London School of Medicine and Dentistry, London, UK

Stephen D Allen MA, MD
Director, Division of Clinical Microbiology, Director of Laboratories, Department of Pathology and Laboratory Medicine, Indiana University School of Medicine, and Director, Disease Control Laboratories, Indiana State Department of Health, Indianapolis, Indiana, USA

Martin Altwegg PhD
Professor of Medical Microbiology, Head of Molecular Diagnostics Unit, Department of Medical Microbiology, University of Zurich, Zurich, Switzerland

Daniel Amsterdam PhD
Professor of Microbiology and Pathology, Associate Professor of Medicine, Director of Clinical Microbiology and Immunology, Director, Department of Laboratory Medicine, Erie County Medical Center, University of Buffalo Medical School, Buffalo, New York, USA

Larry J Anderson MD
Chief, Respiratory and Enteric Viruses Branch, Centers for Disease Control and Prevention, Atlanta, Georgia, USA

Roy M Anderson BSc, PhD, FRS
Director, Wellcome Trust Centre for the Epidemiology of Infectious Disease; Linacre Professor and Head, Department of Zoology, University of Oxford, Oxford, UK

Jørn Andreassen PhD
Assistant Professor, Department of Population Biology, Zoological Institute, University of Copenhagen, Copenhagen, Denmark

Masanori Aoki MS
Professor of Physics, School of Health Sciences, Faculty of Medicine, Kanazawa University, Kanazawa, Ishikawa, Japan

Sarath N Arseculeratne MB BS, DipBact, DPhil
Professor of Microbiology, Faculty of Medicine, University of Peradeniya, Sri Lanka

RW Ashford PhD, DSc
Professor of Medical Zoology, The Liverpool School of Tropical Medicine, Liverpool, UK

Hazel M Aucken MA, PhD
Clinical Microbiologist, Laboratory of Hospital Infection, Central Public Health Laboratory, Colindale, London, UK

L Andrew Ball D Phil
Professor of Microbiology, Department of Microbiology, University of Alabama at Birmingham, Birmingham, Alabama, USA

Albert Balows AB, MS, PhD, ABMM
Professor Emeritus, Emory University School of Medicine and Georgia State University; Former Director at The Center for Infectious Diseases, Centers for Disease Control and Prevention, Atlanta, Georgia, USA

Jangu E Banatvala MA, MD, FRCP, FRCPath, DCH, DPH
Professor of Clinical Virology, Department of Virology, United Medical and Dental Schools of Guy's and St Thomas's, St Thomas's Hospital, London, UK

PA Bates BA, PhD
Lecturer in Medical Parasitology, The Liverpool School of Tropical Medicine, Liverpool, UK

Derrick Baxby BSc, PhD, FRCPath, FRSA
Senior Lecturer in Medical Microbiology, Department
of Medical Microbiology and Genitourinary Medicine,
Liverpool University, Liverpool, UK

Norman T Begg MBCLB, DTM&H, FFPHH
Consultant Epidemiologist, Public Health Laboratory
Service Communicable Diseases Surveillance Centre,
London, UK

William J Bellini PhD
Chief, Measles Virus Section, Respiratory and
Enterovirus Branch, Centers for Disease Control and
Prevention, Atlanta, Georgia, USA

PM Bennett BSc, PhD
Reader in Bacteriology, Department of Pathology and
Microbiology, School of Medical Sciences, University of
Bristol, Bristol, UK

Ruth L Berkelman MD
Deputy Director, National Center for Infectious
Diseases, Centers for Disease Control and Prevention,
Atlanta, Georgia, USA

Jennifer M Best PhD, FRCPath
Reader in Virology, Department of Virology, United
Medical and Dental Schools of Guy's and St Thomas's,
St Thomas's Hospital, London, UK

Jochen Bockemühl MD, PhD
Head, Division of Bacteriology, Institute of Hygiene,
Hamburg, Germany

SP Borriello BSc, PhD, FRCPath
Director, Central Public Health Laboratory, Colindale,
London, UK

Edward J Bottone PhD
Director, Consultative Microbiology, Division of
Infectious Diseases, Department of Medicine, Mount
Sinai Hospital, Mount Sinai School of Medicine, New
York, New York, USA

George HW Bowden PhD
Professor, Department of Oral Biology, Faculty of
Dentistry, University of Manitoba, Winnipeg, Manitoba,
Canada

Janet M Bradbury BSc, MSc, PhD
Reader, Department of Veterinary Pathology, University
of Liverpool, Leahurst, Neston, South Wirral, UK

William J Britt MD
Professor, Department of Pediatrics, University of
Alabama at Birmingham, Birmingham, Alabama, USA

B Kay Buchanan PhD
Microbiology and Immunology Director, Microbiology
Laboratory, Sarasota Memorial Hospital, Sarasota,
Florida, USA

Donald E Burgess PhD
Associate Professor, Veterinary Molecular Biology
Laboratory, College of Agriculture, Agricultural
Experiment Station, Montana State University,
Bozeman, Montana, USA

James P Burnie MD, PhD, MSc, MA, MRCP,
FRCPath
Head of Department, Department of Medical
Microbiology, Manchester Royal Infirmary, Manchester,
UK

Colin K Campbell BSc, MSc, PhD
Clinical Scientist, Mycology Reference Laboratory,
Bristol, UK

Richard Campbell BSc, MSc, PhD
Senior Lecturer, School of Biological Sciences, Bristol,
UK

Michael Cappello MD
Assistant Professor, Pediatric Infectious Diseases,
Laboratory of Epidemiology and Public Health, Yale
University School of Medicine, New Haven,
Connecticut, USA

Keith AV Cartwright MA, BM, FRCPath
Group Director, Public Health Laboratory Service,
South West, Gloucester Royal Hospital, Gloucester, UK

Pascal Cassinotti PhD
Deputy Head, Molecular Biology Division, Institute for
Clinical Microbiology and Immunology, St Gallen,
Switzerland

E Owen Caul FIBMS, PhD, FRCPath
Deputy Director, Head of Virology, Regional Virus
Laboratory, Public Health Laboratory, Bristol, UK

Glenn H Chambliss BSc, MSc, PhD
Professor and Chair, Department of Bacteriology,
Madison, Wisconsin, USA

Francis W Chandler DVM, PhD
Professor of Pathology, Department of Pathology,
Medical College of Georgia, Augusta, Georgia, USA

Ken Charlton DVM, PhD
Formerly Research Scientist, Animal Diseases Research
Institute, Nepean, Ontario, Canada

T Cheasty BSc
Head, *E. coli* and *Shigella* Reference Unit, Laboratory of
Enteric Pathogens, Central Public Health Laboratory,
Colindale, London, UK

Ian L Chrystie TD, PhD
Lecturer, Department of Virology, United Medical and
Dental Hospitals of Guy's and St Thomas's, St
Thomas's Hospital, London, UK

Ian N Clarke BSc, PhD
Senior Lecturer in Microbiology, Molecular
Microbiology, University Medical School, Southampton
General Hospital, Southampton, UK

Jill E Clarridge PhD, ABMM
Chief, Microbiology Section, Veterans Administration
Medical Center; Associate Professor, Baylor College of
Medicine, Houston, Texas, USA

Timothy J Cleary PhD
Director of Clinical Microbiology, Department of
Pathology, University of Miami, Jackson Memorial
Hospital, Miami, Florida, USA

J Barklie Clements BSc, PhD, FRSE
Professor of Virology, Department of Virology, Institute
of Virology, University of Glasgow, Glasgow, UK

Leslie Collier MD, DSc, FRCP, FRCPath
Professor Emeritus of Virology, The London Hospital
Medical College, London; formerly Director, Vaccines
and Sera Laboratories, The Lister Institute of
Preventive Medicine, Elstree, Hertfordshire, UK

Michael J Corbel PhD, DSc, MRCPath, CBiol,
FIBiol
Head, Division of Bacteriology, National Institute for
Biological Standards and Control, Potters Bar,
Hertfordshire, UK

CS Cox BSc, PhD
Research Leader, DERA, Chemical and Biological
Defence, Porton Down, Salisbury, Wiltshire, UK

Francis EG Cox PhD, DSc
Professor of Parasite Immunology, School of Life, Basic
Medical and Health Sciences, King's College London,
London, UK

Gary M Cox MD
Assistant Professor of Medicine, Duke University
Medical Center, Durham, North Carolina, USA

Nancy J Cox PhD
Chief, Influenza Branch, Division of Viral and
Rickettsial Disease, Centers for Disease Control and
Prevention, Atlanta, Georgia, USA

Marie B Coyle PhD
Professor of Laboratory Medicine and Microbiology,
Department of Laboratory Medicine, Harbor View
Medical Center, University of Washington, Seattle,
Washington, USA

Dorothy H Crawford PhD, MD, MRCPath, DSc
Professor of Microbiology, Department of Medical
Microbiology, University of Edinburgh, Medical School,
Edinburgh, UK

DWT Crompton MA, PhD, ScD, FRSE
John Graham Kerr Professor of Zoology, Division of
Environmental and Evolutionary Biology, Institute of
Biomedical and Life Sciences, University of Glasgow,
Glasgow, UK

William L Current BS, MS, PhD
Senior Research Scientist, Infectious Diseases Research,
Lilly Research Laboratories, Eli Lilly and Company,
Indianapolis, Indiana, USA

A Curry BSc, PhD
Top Grade Clinical Scientist, Public Health Laboratory,
Withington Hospital, Manchester, UK

Melanie T Cushion PhD
Associate Professor of Medicine, Division of Infectious
Diseases, Department of Internal Medicine, University
of Cincinnati College of Medicine, Cincinnati, Ohio,
USA

William Cushley BSc, PhD
Senior Lecturer, Division of Biochemistry and
Molecular Biology, Institute of Biomedical and Life
Sciences, University of Glasgow, Glasgow, UK

David AB Dance MB ChB, MSc, FRCPath,
DTM&H
Director/Consultant Microbiologist, Public Health
Laboratory Service, Derriford Hospital, Plymouth, UK

Gregory A Dasch BA, PhD
Senior Microbiologist, Viral and Rickettsial Diseases
Program, Infectious Diseases Department, Naval
Medical Research Institute, Bethesda, Maryland, USA

AJ Davison MA, PhD
Senior Scientist, MRC Virology Unit, Institute of
Virology, Glasgow, UK

Martin Day BSc, PhD
Reader in Microbial Genetics, School of Pure and
Applied Biology, University College Wales, Cardiff, UK

DD Despommier BS, MS, PhD
Professor of Public Health and Microbiology, Division
of Environmental Health Sciences, Faculty of Medicine,
School of Public Health, Columbia University, New
York, New York, USA

Ulrich Desselberger MD, FRCPath, FRCP
Director, Clinical Microbiology and Public Health
Laboratory, Addenbrooke's Hospital, Cambridge, UK

Arthur F DiSalvo MD
Director, Nevada State Health Laboratory, Reno,
Nevada, USA

Edouard Drouhet MD
Professor of Mycology, Pasteur Institute, Mycology Unit,
Pasteur Institute, Paris, France

JP Dubey MVSC, PhD
Senior Scientist/Microbiologist, Parasite Biology and
Epidemiology Laboratory, US Department of
Agriculture, Beltsville, Maryland, USA

Brian I Duerden BSc, MD, FRCPath
Professor and Head, Department of Medical
Microbiology, University of Wales College of Medicine,
Cardiff; Deputy Director, Public Health Laboratory
Service, London, UK

Lee M Dunster PhD
Co-ordinator, Viral Haemorrhagic Fever/Arbovirus
Surveillance, Kenya Medical Research Institute, Virus
Research Centre, Nairobi, Kenya

Daniel Elad DVM, PhD
Head, General Bacteriologic and Mycologic Diagnostics
Division, Kimron Veterinary Institute, Beit Dagan, Israel

David B Elkins MSPH, PhD
Senior Research Fellow, Australian Centre for
International and Tropical Medicine and Nutrition,
Queensland Institute of Medical Research, Brisbane,
Queensland, Australia

David H Ellis BSc, MSc, PhD
Associate Professor, Department of Microbiology and
Immunology, University of Adelaide and Head,
Mycology Unit, Women's and Children's Hospital,
North Adelaide, Australia

Gisela Enders MD
Professor Dr, Institut für Virologie und Epidemiologie,
Stuttgart, Germany

Sir MA Epstein CBE, MA, MD, PhD, DSc, FRCPath,
FRS
Professor, Nuffield Department of Clinical Medicine,
University of Oxford, John Radcliffe Hospital, Oxford,
UK

Martha Espinosa Cantellano MD, DSc
Associate Professor, Department of Experimental
Pathology, Center for Research and Advanced Studies,
Mexico City, Mexico

SJ Eykyn FRCP, FRCS, FRCPath
Reader (Hon Consultant) in Clinical Microbiology,
Division of Infection, United Medical and Dental
School of Guy's and St Thomas's, St Thomas's Hospital,
London, UK

Richard R Facklam PhD
Chief, Streptococcus Laboratory, Centers for Disease
Control and Prevention, Atlanta, Georgia, USA

S Faine MD, DPhil, FRCPA, FASM
Emeritus Professor, Department of Microbiology,
Monash University, Melbourne; Armadale, Victoria,
Australia

Heinz Feldmann MD
Assistant Professor, Institut für Virologie, Philipps
University Marburg, Marburg, Germany

Hugh J Field ScD, FRCPath
Lecturer in Virology, Centre for Veterinary Science,
University of Cambridge, Cambridge, UK

Roger G Finch FRCP, FRCPath, FFPM
Professor of Infectious Diseases, Department of
Microbiology and Infectious Diseases, Nottingham City
Hospital, University of Nottingham, Nottingham, UK

Sydney M Finegold MD
Professor of Medicine; Professor of Microbiology and
Immunology, UCLA School of Medicine; Staff
Physician, Infectious Diseases Section, Veteran Affairs
Medical Center, Los Angeles, California, USA

Michelle Nett Fiordalisi PhD
Fellow, William W McLendon Clinical Immunology
Laboratory, University of North Carolina Hospitals,
Chapel Hill, North Carolina, USA

Ana Flisser BS, PhD
Director, National Institute for Epidemiological
Diagnosis and Reference, Ministry of Health, Carpio,
Mexico City, Mexico

James D Folds PhD
Professor, Pathology and Laboratory Medicine;
Director, McLendon Clinical Laboratories, University of
North Carolina Hospitals, Chapel Hill, North Carolina,
USA

Thomas M Folks BA, MS, PhD
Chief, HIV/Retrovirus Diseases Branch, DASTLR,
Centers for Disease Control and Prevention, Atlanta,
Georgia, USA

Edward AC Follett BSc, PhD, FRCPath
Adviser in Microbiology, Scottish National Blood
Transfusion Service, Regional Virus Laboratory, Ruchill
Hospital, Glasgow, UK

Jocelyn RL Forsyth MB ChB, Dip Bact, MD,
FRCPA
Senior Associate, Department of Microbiology, The
University of Melbourne, Parkville, Victoria, Australia

Hisashi Fujioka PhD
Assistant Professor of Pathology, Institute of Pathology,
Case Western Reserve University, Cleveland, Ohio, USA

Guido Funke MD, FAMH
Consultant in Medical Microbiology, Department of
Medical Microbiology, University of Zurich, Zurich,
Switzerland

Kenneth L Gage PhD
Plague Section Chief, Bacterial Zoonoses Branch,
Division of Vector-Borne Infectious Diseases, Centers
for Disease Control and Prevention, Fort Collins,
Colorado, USA

N Spence Galbraith CBE, MB, FRCP, FFPHM,
DPH
Formerly Director, Public Health Laboratory Service,
Communicable Disease Surveillance Centre, Colindale,
London, UK

Lynne S Garcia MS, F(AAM)
Manager, UCLA Brentwood Facility Laboratory,
Pathology and Laboratory Medicine, University of
California at Los Angeles Medical Center, Los Angeles,
California, USA

Nigel J Gay MA, MSc
Mathematical Modeller, Immunisation Division, Public
Health Laboratory Service, Communicable Disease
Surveillance Centre, London, UK

Edwin E Geldreich AB, MS
Microbiology Consultant in Drinking Water, Cincinnati,
Ohio, USA

Caroline Attardo Genco PhD
Associate Professor, Department of Microbiology and
Immunology, Morehouse School of Medicine, Atlanta,
Georgia, USA

Wolfram H Gerlich PhD
Professor, Institute of Medical Virology, Giessen, Germany

Saheer E Gharbia BSc, PhD
Research Fellow (Hon), National Collection of Type Cultures, Public Health Laboratory Service, Colindale, London, UK

David I Gibson PhD, DSc
Head, Parasitic Worms Division, Department of Zoology, The Natural History Museum, London, UK

RJ Gilbert MPharm, PhD, DipBact, FRCPath
Director, Food Hygiene Laboratory, Central Public Health Laboratory, London, UK

Herbert M Gilles MSc, MD, DSc, DMedSc, FRCP, FFPHM
Emeritus Professor, Liverpool School of Tropical Medicine, Liverpool, UK

Youri Glupczynski MD, PhD
Head, Department of Clinical Microbiology, Centre Hospitalier Universitaire André Vésale, Montigny-le-Tilleul, Belgium

Robert C Good BA, MS, PhD
Guest Researcher, TB/Mycobacteriology Branch, Division of AIDS, STD and TB Laboratory Research, Centers for Disease Control and Prevention, Atlanta, Georgia, USA

Michael Goodfellow PhD, DSc, CBiol, FIBiol
Professor of Microbial Systematics, Department of Microbiology, The Medical School, Newcastle upon Tyne, UK

Norman L Goodman PhD
Professor and Director of Clinical Microbiology Laboratory, Department of Pathology, College of Medicine, University of Kentucky, Lexington, Kentucky, USA

Michael C Goodnough PhD
Assistant Scientist, Department of Food Microbiology and Toxicology, University of Wisconsin, Madison, Wisconsin, USA

Alexander WC von Graevenitz MD
Professor of Medical Microbiology; Director, Department of Medical Microbiology, Department of Medical Microbiology, Zurich University, Zurich, Switzerland

JM Grange MD, MSc
Reader in Clinical Microbiology, Imperial College School of Medicine, National Heart and Lung Institute, London, UK

John R Graybill MD
Chief, Infectious Diseases Division, Audie Murphy Veterans, Administration Hospital; and University of Texas Health Science Center, San Antonio, Texas, USA

David Greenwood PhD, DSc, FRCPath
Professor of Antimicrobial Science, Division of Microbiology and Infectious Diseases, Department of Clinical Laboratory Sciences, University Hospital, Queen's Medical Centre, Nottingham, UK

Duane J Gubler ScD, MS
Director, Division of Vector-Borne Infectious Diseases, Centers for Disease Control and Prevention, Fort Collins, Colorado, USA

Eveline Guého PhD
Researcher at INSERM, Unité de Mycologie, Institut Pasteur, Paris, France

Jacques Guillot DVM, PhD
Assistant Professor of Parasitology-Mycology, Unité de Parasitologie-Mycologie, URA-INRA Immunopathologie Cellulaire et Moleculaire, Ecole National Vétérinaire d'Alfort, Maisons-Alfort, France

Stephen C Hadler MD
Director, Epidemiology and Surveillance Division, National Immunization Program, Centers for Disease Control and Prevention, Atlanta, Georgia, USA

Thomas L Hale PhD
Department Chief, Department of Enteric Infections, Walter Reed Army Institute of Research, Washington DC, USA

Pekka E Halonen MD
Emeritus Professor of Virology, Department of Virology, University of Turku; MediCity, Turku, Finland

JM Hardie BDS, PhD, DipBact, FRCPath
Professor of Oral Microbiology, Department of Oral Microbiology, St Bartholomew's and the Royal London School of Medicine and Dentistry, London, UK

Melissa R Haswell-Elkins BA, MSc, PhD
Senior Research Fellow, Indigenous Health Programme, Australian Centre for International and Tropical Health and Nutrition, University of Queensland, Royal Brisbane Hospital, Brisbane, Queensland, Australia

Charles L Hatheway PhD
Chief, Botulism Laboratory, Centers for Disease Control and Prevention, Atlanta, Georgia, USA

Harald zur Hausen MD, DSc
Managing Director, Deutsches Krebsforschungszentrum, Heidelberg, Germany

Sir David L Hawksworth CBE, DSc, FDhc, CBiol, FIBiol, FLS
President, International Union of Biological Sciences; Visiting Professor, Universities of Kent, London and Reading; Director, International Mycological Institute, Egham, Surrey, UK

Roderick J Hay DM, FRCP, FRCPath
Mary Dunhill Professor of Cutaneous Medicine, St John's Institute of Dermatology, United Medical and Dental Schools of Guy's and St Thomas's, Guy's Hospital, London, UK

John C Hierholzer PhD
Former Supervisory Research Microbiologist, Centers
for Disease Control and Prevention, Atlanta, Georgia,
USA

Tor Hofstad MD, PhD
Professor of Medical Microbiology, Department of
Microbiology and Immunology, The Gade Institute,
University of Bergen, Bergen, Norway

John J Holland PhD
Professor Emeritus, Biology Department, University of
California at San Diego, La Jolla, California, USA

Barry Holmes PhD, DSc, FIBiol
Clinical Scientist, National Collection of Type Cultures,
Central Public Health Laboratory, Colindale, London,
UK

Stanley C Holt PhD
Professor of Microbiology, Department of Microbiology,
University of Texas Health Science Center at San
Antonio, San Antonio, Texas, USA

Marcel Hommel MD, PhD
Alfred Jones and Warrington Yorke Professor of
Tropical Medicine, Liverpool School of Tropical
Medicine, Liverpool, UK

GS de Hoog PhD
Professor of Mycology, Centraalbureau voor
Schimmelcultures, Baarn, The Netherlands

Douglas B Hornick MD
Associate Professor of Pulmonary and Critical Care
Medicine, Department of Medicine, University of Iowa
School of Medicine, Iowa City, Iowa, USA

Peter J Hotez MD, PhD
Associate Professor, Department of Pediatrics and
Epidemiology, Yale University School of Medicine, New
Haven, Connecticut, USA

TGB Howe MD, PhD
Senior Lecturer in Bacteriology, Department of
Pathology and Microbiology, School of Medical
Sciences, University of Bristol, Bristol, UK

TJ Humphrey BSc, PhD, MRCPath
Professor; Head of Public Health Laboratory Service
Food Microbiology Research Unit, Heavitree, Exeter,
Devon, UK

Hilary Humphreys MD, FRCPI, FRCPath
Consultant Microbiologist, Federated Dublin Voluntary
Hospitals, Dublin, Ireland

Charles J Hunter MD
Fellow, Department of Pathology, Division of Infectious
Diseases, University of Virginia Health Science Center,
Charlottesville, Virginia, USA

Thomas J Inzana PhD
Professor of Microbiology, Department of Biomedical
Sciences and Pathobiology, Virginia-Maryland Regional
College of Veterinary Medicine, Blacksburg, Virginia,
USA

J Michael Janda BSc, MS, PhD
Chief, Enterics and Special Pathogens Section,
Microbial Diseases Laboratory, California Department
of Health Services, Berkeley, California, USA

AE Jephcott MA, MD, FRCPath, DipBact
Director, Public Health Laboratory, Bristol, UK

Robert C Jerris PhD
Assistant Professor, Department of Pathology and
Laboratory Medicine, Emory University School of
Medicine, Atlanta, Georgia, USA

David T John MSPH, PhD
Professor of Microbiology/Parasitology; Associate Dean
for Basic Sciences, Department of Biochemistry and
Microbiology, Oklahoma State University, College of
Osteopathic Medicine, Tulsa, Oklahoma, USA

Elizabeth M Johnson BSc, PhD
Clinical Scientist, Mycology Reference Laboratory,
Bristol, UK

Eric A Johnson ScD
Professor of Food Microbiology and Toxicology, Food
Research Institute, College of Agricultural and Life
Sciences, University of Wisconsin, Madison, Wisconsin,
USA

Russell C Johnson PhD
Professor of Microbiology, Department of Microbiology,
University of Minnesota, Minneapolis, Minnesota, USA

Dorothy Jones BSc, MSc, PhD, DipBact
Honorary Fellow, Department of Microbiology and
Immunology, University of Leicester, Leicester, UK

J Zoe Jordens BSc, PhD
Clinical Scientist/Honorary Senior Lecturer,
Haemophilus Reference Laboratory, Oxford Public
Health Laboratory and Nuffield Department of
Pathology & Bacteriology, John Radcliffe Hospital,
Headington, Oxford, UK

Stephen L Josephson PhD
Director, Microbiology/Virology, APC 1136, Rhode
Island Hospital, Providence, Rhode Island, USA

Kimberly L Kane BSc, PhD
Postdoctoral Fellow, Clinical Microbiology–Immunology
Laboratories, University of North Carolina Hospitals,
Chapel Hill, North Carolina, USA

Michael Kann MD
Research Fellow, Institute of Medical Virology, Justus-
Liebig-Universität Giessen, Giessen, Germany

SHE Kaufmann PhD
Professor and Head of Immunology, Department of
Immunology, University of Ulm, Ulm, Germany

Yoshihiro Kawaoka PhD
Professor, Department of Pathobiological Science,
School of Veterinary Medicine, University of Wisconsin-
Madison, Madison, Wisconsin, USA

Masako Kawasaki PhD
Instructor, Department of Dermatology, Kanazawa
Medical University, Uchinada, Ishikawa, Japan

Rima F Khabbaz MD
Associate Director for Medical Science, Division of Viral
and Rickettsial Diseases, National Center for Infectious
Diseases, Centers for Disease Control and Prevention,
Atlanta, Georgia, USA

Michael P Kiley BS, MS, PhD
Senior Scientific Adviser, Federal Laboratories for
Health Canada and Agriculture and Agri-Food Canada,
Winnipeg, Manitoba, Canada

Mogens Kilian DMD, DSc
Professor of Microbiology, Head, Department of
Medical Microbiology and Immunology, University of
Aarhus, Aarhus, Denmark

Hans-Dieter Klenk MD
Professor of Virology, Head, Department of Hygiene
and Medical Microbiology, Institute for Virology,
Philipps-University Marburg, Marburg, Germany

Wesley E Kloos PhD
Professor of Genetics and Microbiology, Department of
Genetics, North Carolina State University, Raleigh,
North Carolina, USA

Somei Kojima MD, PhD
Professor of Parasitology, Department of Parasitology,
University of Tokyo, Minato-ku, Tokyo, Japan

Paul E Kolenbrander PhD
Research Microbiologist, National Institute of Dental
Research, National Institutes of Health, Bethesda,
Maryland, USA

Myriam S Künzi PhD
Postdoctoral Fellow, John Hopkins Oncology Center,
Baltimore, Maryland, USA

Ralph Lainson OBE, FRS, AFTWAS, DSc
Professor (Honoris Causa), Federal University of Pará,
ex Director, The Wellcome Belém Leishmaniasis Unit,
Departamento de Parasitologia, Instituto Evandro
Chagas, Belém, Pará, Brazil

Paul R Lambden BSc, PhD
Senior Research Fellow, Molecular Microbiology,
University Medical School, Southampton General
Hospital, Southampton, UK

Sandra A Larsen MS, PhD
Guest Researcher, Bacterial STD Branch, Division of
AIDS, Sexually Transmitted Diseases and Tuberculosis
Laboratory Research, National Center for Infectious
Diseases, Centers for Disease Control and Prevention,
Atlanta, Georgia, USA

Edward R Leadbetter PhD
Professor of Microbiology, Department of Molecular
and Cell Biology, University of Connecticut, Storrs,
Connecticut, USA

James W LeDuc PhD
Associate Director, Global Health, National Center for
Infectious Diseases, Centers for Disease Control and
Prevention, Atlanta, Georgia, USA

Paul F Lehmann PhD
Professor of Microbiology and Immunology,
Microbiology Department, Medical College of Ohio,
Toledo, Ohio, USA

Stanley M Lemon MD
Professor of Microbiology and Immunology and
Internal Medicine, Chairman, Department of
Microbiology and Immunology, University of Texas
Medical Branch at Galveston, Galveston, Texas, USA

Lony Chong-Leong Lim PhD
Fellow, William W McLendon Clinical Immunology
Laboratory, University of North Carolina Hospitals,
Chapel Hill, North Carolina, USA

Graham Lloyd BSc, MSc, PhD
Head of Diagnosis, Centre for Applied Microbiology
and Research, Porton Down, Salisbury, Wiltshire, UK

Alberto T Londero MD
Emeritus Professor, Department of Microbiology,
Session Medical Mycology, School of Medicine, Federal
University of Santa Maria, Santa Maria, RS, Brazil

Francisco J López-Antuñano MD, MPH
Consultant, Instituto Nacional de Salud, Morelos,
Mexico

Mario Lozano Chiu PhD
Postdoctoral Fellow, University of Texas Medical
School, Houston, Texas, USA

David M MacLaren MA, MD, FRCP, FRCPath
Emeritus Professor of Medical Bacteriology, Moidart
House, Bodicote, Banbury, Oxford, UK

Alastair P MacMillan BVSc, MSc, MRCVS
Head, FAO/WHO Collaborating Centre for Reference
and Research on Brucellosis, Central Veterinary
Laboratory, Addlestone, Surrey, UK

CR Madeley MD, FRCPath
Consultant Virologist, Public Health Laboratory Service,
Institute of Pathology, Newcastle General Hospital,
Newcastle upon Tyne, UK

John T Magee PhD, MSc, FIMLS
Top Grade Scientific Officer, Department of Medical
Microbiology and Public Health Laboratory, University
of Wales College of Medicine, Cardiff, UK

Brian WJ Mahy PhD, ScD
Director, Division of Viral and Rickettsial Diseases,
Centers for Disease Control and Prevention, Atlanta,
Georgia, USA; formerly Director, The Animal Virus
Research Institute, Pirbright, Surrey, UK

Scott A Martin BS, MS, PhD
Professor, Department of Animal and Dairy Science,
College of Agriculture, Livestock and Poultry,
University of Georgia, Athens, Georgia, USA

William J Martin PhD
Director, Scientific Resources Program, National Center for Infectious Diseases, Centers for Disease Control and Prevention, Atlanta, Georgia, USA

Adolfo Martínez-Palomo MD, DSc
Director General, Centro de Investigación y de Estudios Avanzados, Mexico City, Mexico

Tadahiko Matsumoto MD, DMSc
Director, Department of Dermatology, Toshiba Hospital, Higashi-oi, Shinagawa-ku, Tokyo, Japan

Ruth Matthews MD, PhD, MSc, FRCPath
Reader in Medical Microbiology, Department of Medical Microbiology, Manchester Royal Infirmary, Manchester, UK

Joseph E McDade PhD
Associate Director for Laboratory Science, National Center for Infectious Diseases, Centers for Disease Control and Prevention, Atlanta, Georgia, USA

Michael R McGinnis PhD
Director, Medical Mycology Research Center, Associate Director, University of Texas at Galveston-WHO Collaborating Center for Tropical Diseases, and Professor, Department of Pathology, University of Texas Medical Branch at Galveston, Galveston, Texas, USA

Jim McLauchlin PhD
Clinical Scientist, Central Public Health Laboratory, Colindale, London, UK

Heinz Mehlhorn PhD
Professor of Parasitologie, Institut für Zoomorphologie, Zellbiologie und Parasitologie, Heinrich-Heine-Universität, Düsseldorf, Germany

A Leonel Mendoza MS, PhD
Assistant Professor, Department of Microbiology, Medical Technology Program, Michigan State University, East Lansing, Michigan, USA

Volker ter Meulen MD
Chairman, Institute for Virology and Immunobiology, University of Würzburg, Würzburg, Germany

Gillian Midgley BSc, PhD
Lecturer in Medical Mycology, Department of Medical Mycology, St John's Institute of Dermatology, United Medical and Dental School of Guy's and St Thomas's, St Thomas's Hospital, London, UK

Michael A Miles MSc, PhD, DSc
Professor of Medical Parasitology and Head, Applied Molecular Biology Unit, Department of Medical Parasitology, London School of Hygiene and Tropical Medicine, London, UK

J Michael Miller PhD, ABMM
Chief, Diagnostic Microbiology Section, Hospital Infections Program, National Center for Infectious Diseases, Centers for Disease Control and Prevention, Atlanta, Georgia, USA

P Minor BA, PhD
Head, Division of Virology, National Institute for Biological Standard and Control, Potters Bar, Hertfordshire, UK

AC Minson BSc, PhD
Professor of Virology, Virology Division, Department of Pathology, University of Cambridge, Cambridge, UK

DH Molyneux MA, PhD, DSc
Director, Professor of Tropical Health Sciences, Liverpool School of Tropical Medicine, Liverpool, UK

Arnold S Monto MD
Professor of Epidemiology, School of Public Health, University of Michigan, Ann Arbor, Michigan, USA

Stephen A Morse MSPH, PhD
Associate Director for Science, Division of AIDS, STD and Tuberculosis Laboratory Research, Centers for Disease Control and Prevention, Atlanta, Georgia, USA

RP Mortlock BS, PhD
Professor of Microbiology, Section of Microbiology, Cornell University, Ithaca, New York, USA

Ralph Muller DSc, PhD, BSc, FIBiol
Formerly Director, International Institute of Parasitology, St Albans, Hertfordshire, UK

David A Murdoch MA, MBBS, MSc, MD, MRCPath
Honorary Clinical Research Fellow, Department of Microbiology, Southmead Health Services NHS Trust, Westbury-on-Trym, Bristol, UK

Frederick A Murphy DVM, PhD
Professor, School of Veterinary Medicine, University of California, Davis, California, USA

PR Murray PhD
Professor, Division of Laboratory Medicine, Departments of Pathology and Medicine, Washington University School of Medicine, St Louis, Missouri, USA

David Mutimer MBBS
Senior Lecturer, Birmingham University Department of Medicine; Honorary Consultant Physician, Liver and Hepatobiliary Unit, Queen Elizabeth Hospital, Edgbaston, Birmingham, UK

Irving I Nachamkin PhD
Professor of Pathology and Laboratory Medicine, Department of Pathology and Laboratory Medicine, University of Pennsylvania School of Medicine, Philadelphia, Pennsylvania, USA

Francis E Nano PhD
Associate Professor, Department of Biochemistry and Microbiology, University of Victoria, Victoria, British Columbia, Canada

AA Nash BSc, MSc, PhD
Professor, Department of Veterinary Pathology, University of Edinburgh, Edinburgh, UK

Neal Nathanson MD
Professor and Chair Emeritus, Department of
Microbiology, University of Pennsylvania Medical
Center, Philadelphia, Pennsylvania, USA

James C Neil BSc, PhD
Professor of Virology and Molecular Oncology,
Department of Veterinary Pathology, University of
Glasgow, Glasgow, UK

WC Noble DSc, FRCPath
Professor of Microbiology, Department of Microbial
Diseases, St John's Institute of Dermatology, United
Medical and Dental Schools of Guy's and St Thomas's,
St Thomas's Hospital, London, UK

Steven J Norris PhD
Professor of Pathology and Laboratory Medicine,
Microbiology and Molecular Genetics, Department of
Pathology, University of Texas Health Science Center,
Houston, Texas, USA

David C Old PhD, DSc, FIBiol, FRCPath
Reader in Medical Microbiology, Department of
Medical Microbiology, Ninewells Hospital and Medical
School, Dundee, UK

Arvind A Padhye PhD
Chief, Fungus Reference Laboratory, Emerging
Bacterial and Mycotic Diseases Branch, Division of
Bacterial and Mycotic Diseases, Centers for Disease
Control and Prevention, Atlanta, Georgia, USA

Norberto J Palleroni PhD
Professor of Microbiology, Center for Agricultural
Molecular Biology, Cooke College, Rutgers University,
New Brunswick, New Jersey, USA

Stephen R Palmer MA, MB, BChir, FFPHM
Professor & Director, Welsh Combined Centres for
Public Health, University of Wales College of Medicine;
Head, Communicable Disease Surveillance Centre
Welsh Unit, Cardiff, UK

Demosthenes Pappagianis PhD, MD
Professor of Medical Biology and Immunology,
Department of Medical Microbiology and Immunology,
University of California, Davis, California, USA

M Thomas Parker MD, FRCPath, DipBact
Formerly Director, Cross-Infection Reference
Laboratory, Central Public Health Laboratory,
Colindale, London, UK

D Parratt MD, FRCPath
Senior Lecturer, Department of Medical Microbiology,
Ninewells Hospital, Dundee, UK

Roger Parton BSc, PhD
Senior Lecturer, Division of Infection and Immunity,
Institute of Biomedical and Life Sciences, University of
Glasgow, Glasgow, UK

Thomas F Patterson MD
Associate Professor of Medicine, Division of Infectious
Diseases, Department of Medicine, University of Texas
Health Science Center, San Antonio, Texas, USA

Charles W Penn BSc, PhD
Reader in Microbiology, School of Biological Sciences,
University of Birmingham, Edgbaston, Birmingham, UK

T Hugh Pennington MB, BS, PhD, FRCPath, FRSE
Professor of Bacteriology, Department of Medical
Microbiology, University of Aberdeen, Aberdeen, UK

John R Perfect MD
Professor of Medicine, Duke University Medical Center,
Durham, North Carolina, USA

William A Petri Jnr MD, PhD
Professor, Department of Infectious Diseases, University
of Virginia Health Sciences Center, Charlottesville,
Virginia, USA

Paula M Pitha BS, MS, PhD
Professor of Oncology, Oncology Center and
Department of Molecular Biology and Genetics,
Baltimore, Maryland, USA

Tyrone L Pitt MPhil, PhD
Deputy Director, Laboratory of Hospital Infection,
Central Public Health Laboratory, Colindale, London,
UK

Tanja Popovic MD, PhD
Principal Investigator, Diphtheria Research Project,
Childhood and Respiratory Diseases Branch, Division of
Bacterial and Mycotic Diseases, National Center for
Infectious Diseases, Centers for Disease Control and
Prevention, Atlanta, Georgia, USA

R Scott Pore PhD
Professor of Microbiology and Immunology,
Department of Microbiology and Immunology, West
Virginia University School of Medicine, Morgantown,
West Virginia, USA

Roger Pradinaud MD
Directeur, Service de Dermato-Vénéreo-Leprologie,
Centre Hospitalier de Cayenne, Guyane Française

Craig R Pringle BSc, PhD
Professor of Biological Sciences, Biological Sciences
Department, University of Warwick, Coventry,
Warwickshire, UK

Stanley B Prusiner AB, MD
Professor of Neurology, Biochemistry and Biophysics,
Department of Neurology, University of California, San
Francisco, California, USA

Thomas J Quan PhD, MPH
Microbiologist, Imu-Tek Animal Health Inc, Fort
Collins, Colorado, USA

CP Quinn BSc, PhD
Head, Biotherapy Unit, Centre for Applied
Microbiology and Research, Porton Down, Salisbury,
Wiltshire, UK

Sharath K Rai PhD
Postdoctoral Fellow, Department of Molecular
Immunology, Bristol Myers Squibb PRI, Seattle,
Washington, USA

Anita Rampling MA, PhD, MB ChB, FRCPath
Director, Public Health Laboratory, Department of
Pathology, West Dorset Hospital, Dorchester, UK

Robert C Read MD, MRCP
Senior Clinical Lecturer in Infectious Diseases,
Department of Medical Microbiology, University of
Sheffield Medical School, Sheffield, UK

Stephen C Redd MD
Chief, Measles Elimination Activity, Epidemiology and
Surveillance Division, Centers for Disease Control and
Prevention, Atlanta, Georgia, USA

Sanjay G Revankar MD
Infectious Diseases Fellow, Department of Medicine,
Division of Infectious Diseases, University of Texas
Health Science Center, San Antonio, Texas, USA

John H Rex MD
Associate Professor, University of Texas Medical School,
Houston, Texas, USA

Malcolm D Richardson BSc, PhD, CBiol, MIBiol,
FRCPath
Director, Regional Mycology Reference Laboratory,
Department of Dermatology, Glasgow, UK

Geoffrey L Ridgway MD, BSc, MRCP, FRCPath
Consultant Microbiologist, Department of Clinical
Microbiology, University College London Hospitals;
Honorary Senior Lecturer, University College Hospital,
London, UK

Glenn D Roberts PhD
Director, Clinical Mycology and Mycobacteriology
Laboratories; Professor of Microbiology and Laboratory
Medicine, Mayo Medical School, Division of Clinical
Microbiology, Mayo Clinic, Rochester, Minnesota, USA

Betty H Robertson PhD
Chief, Virology Section, Hepatitis Branch, Division of
Viral and Rickettsial Diseases, Centers for Disease
Control and Prevention, Hepatitis Branch, Atlanta,
Georgia, USA

Frank G Rodgers PhD
Professor of Microbiology; Editor, Journal of Clinical
Microbiology, Department of Microbiology, Rudman
Hall, University of New Hampshire, Durham, New
Hampshire, USA

John T Roehrig PhD
Chief, Arbovirus Diseases Branch, Division of Vector-
Borne Infectious Diseases, National Center for
Infectious Diseases, Centers for Disease Control and
Prevention, Fort Collins, Colorado, USA

MJ Rosovitz BSc
Research Assistant, Department of Bacteriology,
University of Wisconsin-Madison, Madison, Wisconsin,
USA

Paul A Rota PhD
Research Microbiologist, Measles Virus Section, Centers
for Disease Control and Prevention, Atlanta, Georgia,
USA

Andrew H Rudolph MD
Clinical Professor of Dermatology, Dermatology
Department, Baylor College of Medicine, Houston
Texas, USA

Kathryn L Ruoff PhD
Assistant Professor of Pathology, Harvard Medical
School; Assistant Director, Microbiology Laboratories,
Massachusetts General Hospital, Boston, Massachusetts,
USA

A Denver Russell BPharm, PhD, DSc, FRCPath,
FRPharmS
Professor, Welsh School of Pharmacy, University of
Wales at Cardiff, Cardiff, UK

WC Russell BSc, PhD, FRSE
Emeritus Research Professor, School of Biological and
Medical Sciences, University of St Andrews, St Andrews,
Fife, UK

Maria S Salvato PhD
Assistant Professor, Department of Pathology and
Laboratory Medicine, Services Memorial Institute,
University of Wisconsin Medical School, Madison,
Wisconsin, USA

Anthony Sanchez PhD
Special Pathogens Branch, Division of Viral and
Rickettsial Diseases, National Center for Infectious
Diseases, Centers for Disease Control and Prevention,
Atlanta, Georgia, USA

Klaus P Schaal MD
Director, Professor of Medical Microbiology, Institute
for Medical Microbiology and Immunology, University
of Bonn, Bonn, Germany

Julius Schachter PhD
Professor of Laboratory Medicine, World Health
Organization Collaborating Centre for References and
Research on Chlamydia, Chlamydia Research
Laboratory, Department of Laboratory Medicine, San
Francisco General Hospital, San Francisco, California,
USA

Wiley A Schell MSc
Research Associate, Department of Medicine, Duke
University Medical Center, Durham, North Carolina,
USA

Walter F Schlech III MD
Professor of Medicine, Faculty of Medicine, Dalhousie
University, QE II HSC, Halifax, Nova Scotia, Canada

L Schlesinger MD
Associate Professor of Medicine, Department of
Medicine, Division of Infectious Diseases, University of
Iowa, Iowa City, Iowa, USA

Connie S Schmaljohn PhD
Chief, Department of Molecular Virology, US Army
Medical Research Institute of Infectious Diseases, Fort
Detrick, Maryland, USA

Gabriel A Schmunis MD, PhD
Coordinator, Communicable Diseases Program, Pan American Health Organization, Washington, DC, USA

Sibylle Schneider-Schaulies PhD
Lecturer, Institut für Virologie und Immunbiologie, Universität Würzburg, Würzburg, Germany

John Richard Seed PhD
Professor, Department of Epidemiology, School of Public Health, University of North Carolina, Chapel Hill, North Carolina, USA

Esther Segal PhD
Professor of Microbiology/Mycology, Department of Human Microbiology, Sackler School of Medicine, Tel Aviv University, Ramat Aviv, Tel Aviv, Israel

Bernard W Senior BSc, PhD, FRCPath
Lecturer in Medical Microbiology, Department of Medical Microbiology, Dundee University Medical School, Ninewells Hospital and Medical School, Dundee, UK

Haroun N Shah BSc, PhD, FRCPath
Head, Identification Services Unit, National Collection of Type Cultures, Central Public Health Laboratory, Colindale, London, UK

Jeffrey J Shaw PhD, DSc
Professor, Departamento de Parasitologia, Instituto de Ciências Biomédicas, Universidade de São Paulo, São Paulo, Brazil

Thomas M Shinnick PhD
Chief, Tuberculosis/Mycobacteriology Branch, Centers for Disease Control and Prevention, Atlanta, Georgia, USA

Stuart G Siddell BSc, PhD
Professor of Virology, Institute of Virology, University of Würzburg, Würzburg, Germany

Gunter O Siegl PhD
Professor and Head, Institute for Clinical Microbiology and Immunology, St Gallen, Switzerland

Lynne Sigler MSc
Curator and Associate Professor, University of Alberta Microfungus Collection and Herbarium, Devonian Botanic Garden, Edmonton, Alberta, Canada

RB Sim BSc, DPhil
MRC Scientific Staff, MRC Immunochemistry Unit, Department of Biochemistry, University of Oxford, Oxford, UK

Peter Simmonds BM, PhD, MRCPath
Senior Lecturer, Department of Medical Microbiology, University of Edinburgh Medical School, Edinburgh, UK

Anthony Simmons MA, MB, BChir, PhD, FRCPath
Senior Medical Specialist, Infectious Diseases Laboratories, Institute of Medical and Veterinary Science, Adelaide, Australia

Martin B Skirrow MB, ChB, PhD, FRCPath, DTM&H
Consultant Medical Microbiologist, Public Health Laboratory, Gloucestershire Royal Hospital, Gloucester, UK

Mary PE Slack MA, MB, FRCPath
Lecturer (Honorary Consultant) in Bacteriology, Haemophilus Reference Laboratory, Oxford Public Health Laboratory and Nuffield Department of Pathology and Bacteriology, John Radcliffe Hospital, Oxford, UK

Henry R Smith MA, PhD
Deputy Director, Laboratory of Enteric Pathogens, Central Public Health Laboratory, Colindale, London, UK

Eric J Snijder PhD
Assistant Professor, Department of Virology, Institute of Medical Microbiology, Leiden University, Leiden, The Netherlands

Phyllis H Sparling DVM, MS
Liaison, Centers for Disease Control and Prevention, Atlanta, Georgia, USA

David CE Speller MA, BM, BCh, FRCP, FRCPath
Emeritus Professor of Clinical Microbiology, University of Bristol, Bristol, UK

Carol A Spiegel PhD
Associate Professor, Department of Pathology and Laboratory Medicine, University of Wisconsin, Madison, Wisconsin, USA

Andrew Spielman ScD
Professor of Tropical Public Health, Department of Tropical Public Health, Harvard School of Public Health, Boston, Massachusetts, USA

Bret M Steiner PhD
Chief, Treponemal Pathogenesis, Division of Sexually Transmitted Diseases, Centers for Disease Control and Prevention, Atlanta, Georgia, USA

Scott J Stewart BS
Formerly of National Institute of Allergies and Infectious Diseases; 344 Roaring Lion Road, Hamilton, Montana, USA

Max Sussman BSc, PhD, CBiol, FIBiol, FRCPath
Emeritus Professor of Bacteriology, Department of Microbiology, The Medical School, Newcastle upon Tyne, UK

Roland W Sutter MD, MPH, TM
Deputy Chief for Technical Affairs, Polio Eradication Activity, National Immunization Program, Centers for Disease Control and Prevention, Atlanta, Georgia, USA

Bala Swaminathan PhD
Chief, Foodborne and Diarrhoeal Diseases Laboratory 333 Section, Foodborne and Diarrhoeal Diseases Branch, Centers for Disease Control and Prevention, Atlanta, Georgia, USA

Robert V Tauxe MD, MPH
Chief, Foodborne and Diarrhoeal Diseases Branch,
Division of Bacterial and Mycotic Diseases, Centers for
Disease Control and Prevention, Atlanta, Georgia, USA

David J Taylor MA, VetMB, PhD, MRCVS
Reader in Veterinary Microbiology, Department of
Veterinary Pathology, University of Glasgow, School of
Veterinary Medicine, Bearsden, Glasgow, UK

John M Taylor PhD
Senior Member, Fox Chase Cancer Center,
Philadelphia, Pennsylvania, USA

David Taylor-Robinson MD, MRCP, FRCPath
Emeritus Professor of Microbiology and Genitourinary
Medicine, Department of Genitourinary Medicine, St
Mary's Hospital, London, UK

Lucia Martins Teixeira PhD
Associate Professor, Universidade Federal do Rio de
Janeiro, Instituto de Microbiologia, Rio de Janeiro,
Brazil

Sam Rountree Telford III DSc
Lecturer in Tropical Health, Department of Tropical
Public Health, Harvard University, Boston,
Massachusetts, USA

Ram P Tewari PhD
Professor of Microbiology, Department of Medical
Microbiology and Immunology, Southern Illinois
University, Springfield, Illinois School of Medicine,
Springfield, Illinois, USA

E John Threlfall BSc, PhD
Grade C Clinical Scientist, Laboratory of Enteric
Pathogens, Central Public Health Laboratory,
Colindale, London, UK

Richard C Tilton BS, MS, PhD
Senior Vice President, Chief Scientific Director, BBI
Clinical Laboratories, New Britain, Connecticut, USA

Noel Tordo PhD
Head, Laboratoire de Lyssavirus, Institut Pasteur, Paris,
France

Anna Maria Tortorano PhD
Associate Professor of Hygiene, Laboratory of Medical
Microbiology, Institute of Hygiene and Preventive
Medicine, School of Medicine, Università degli Studi di
Milano, Milano, Italy

Kevin J Towner BSc, PhD
Consultant Clinical Scientist, Public Health Laboratory,
University Hospital, Queen's Medical Centre,
Nottingham, UK

JG Tully BS, MS, PhD
Chief, Mycoplasma Section, Laboratory of Molecular
Microbiology, National Institute of Allergy and
Infectious Diseases, National Institutes of Health,
Frederick, Maryland, USA

Peter C B Turnbull BSc, MS, PhD
Head, Anthrax Section, Centre for Applied
Microbiology and Research, Porton Down, Salisbury,
Wiltshire, UK

Kenneth L Tyler MD
Professor of Neurology, Medicine, Microbiology and
Immunology, Department of Neurology, University of
Colorado Health Sciences Center, and Chief,
Neurology Service Denver Veteran Affairs Medical
Center, Denver, Colorado, USA

Edward J Usherwood MA, PhD
Research Fellow, Department of Veterinary Pathology,
Edinburgh, UK

Maria Anna Viviani MD
Associate Professor of Hygiene, Laboratory of Medical
Microbiology, Institute of Hygiene and Preventive
Medicine, School of Medicine, Università degli Studi di
Milano, Milano, Italy

Martin I Voskuil BA
Research Scientist, Department of Bacteriology,
University of Wisconsin-Madison, Madison, Wisconsin,
USA

William G Wade BSc, PhD
Richard Dickinson Professor of Oral Microbiology,
Head of Oral Biology Unit, Department of Oral
Medicine and Pathology, United Medical and Dental
Schools of Guy's and St Thomas's, Guy's Hospital,
London, UK

Derek Wakelin BSc, PhD, DSc, FRCPath
Professor of Zoology, Department of Life Science,
University of Nottingham, Nottingham, UK

Alexander Wandeler MSc, PhD
Head of Rabies Unit, Animal Diseases Research
Institute, Nepean, Ontario, Canada

Audrey R Wanger PhD
Assistant Professor, Department of Pathology and
Laboratory Medicine, University of Texas Medical
School at Houston, Houston, Texas, USA

Bodo Wanke PhD, MD
Head of Laboratório de Micologia Médica, Laboratório
de Micologia, Hospital Evandro Chagas, Rio de Janeiro,
Brazil

ME Ward BSc, PhD
Professor of Medical Microbiology, Molecular
Microbiology, Southampton University School of
Medicine, Southampton General Hospital,
Southampton, UK

MFR Waters OBE, MB, FRCP, FRCPath
Formerly Consultant Leprologist and Physician,
Hospital for Tropical Diseases, London, UK

Emilio Weiss BS, MS, PhD
Emeritus Chair of Science, Naval Medical Research
Institute, Bethesda, Maryland, USA

Irene Weitzman PhD
Assistant Director, Clinical Microbiology Service, and
Associate Professor of Clinical Pathology in Medicine,
Columbia Presbyterian Medical Center, New York, New
York, USA

Lawrence J Wheat MD
Professor of Medicine, Infectious Disease Division,
Wishard Memorial Hospital, Indianapolis, Indiana, USA

Richard J Whitley MD
Professor of Pediatrics, Microbiology and Medicine,
Department of Pediatrics, University of Alabama at
Birmingham, Birmingham, Alabama, USA

James Whitworth MD, FRCP, DTM&H
Team Leader, MRC Programme on AIDS, Entebbe,
Uganda

Louis A Wilson BS, MSc, MD, FACS
Professor of Ophthalmology, Emory University School
of Medicine and Adjunct Professor of Microbiology,
Georgia State University, Atlanta, Georgia, USA

John A Wyke MA, VetMB, PhD, MRCVS, FRSE
Director of Research, Beatson Institute, Honorary
Professor at University of Glasgow, Beatson Institute for
Cancer Research, Glasgow, UK

Kentaro Yoshimura BVM, DVM, PhD
Professor of Parasitology, Chairman, Department of
Parasitology, Akita University School of Medicine, Akita,
Japan

Viqar Zaman MBBS, DSc, DTM&H, FRCPath
Professor, Department of Microbiology, The Aga Khan
University, Karachi, Pakistan

Stephen H Zinder BA, MS, PhD
Professor of Microbiology, Section of Microbiology,
Cornell University, Ithaca, New York, USA

EDITOR-IN-CHIEF'S PREFACE

The period since publication of the first edition in 1929 has seen various modifications in the form and content of *Topley and Wilson*, perhaps the most important of which was the change with the 7th edition to a multi-author work in four volumes. This, the 9th edition, marks three spectacular departures from past policy.

First, and most obviously, the work now covers every class of pathogen: viruses, bacteria, fungi and parasites, including the helminths. The arrangement is in order of complexity, ranging from *Virology* in Volume 1 through *Systematic Bacteriology* and *Bacterial Infections* in Volumes 2 and 3, *Medical Mycology* in Volume 4 and *Parasitology* in Volume 5. Each has its own index, and a general index to the entire work is provided in Volume 6.

This major expansion called for a change in authorship, which previously was almost entirely British. Clearly, the range of expertise now needed to cover every aspect of medical microbiology, including mycology and parasitology, can no longer be provided from any one country and we have been fortunate in recruiting leading experts from many parts of the world for this expanded edition. In all, there are 234 chapters, of which the USA has provided 45% and the UK 35%; the remainder come from 20 other countries.

The third important new feature is the appearance of an electronic version alongside the printed work, which will facilitate information retrieval, cross-referencing and, most important, a continual programme of revision and updating.

During the planning phase, surveys of known and potential readers indicated a majority demand for more detailed referencing than hitherto, and the provision of factual material rather than the more speculative and discursive treatment characteristic of the early editions. This trend has become increasingly apparent with successive editions, and there is now no justification for retaining the word 'Principles' in the title. Despite this change in emphasis, the readership

for whom the work is intended remains the same; it comprises primarily microbiologists working in research, diagnostic and public health laboratories and those teaching both undergraduates and postgraduates. Although it is first and foremost a treatise on microbiology, the comprehensive coverage of the clinical and pathological features of infection makes it also an invaluable source of reference for physicians dealing with infective disease.

The 8th edition comprised four volumes of text, of which the first covered *General Bacteriology and Immunity*, and was intended to service those dealing with the more specialized topics. This arrangement did not, however, prove satisfactory; the 9th edition is therefore designed to make the volumes more self-contained, and descriptions of the immune response as it relates respectively to viruses, bacteria and the eukaryotic parasites are provided in the appropriate volumes.

The arrangement of the *Virology* volume is similar to that in the 8th edition, except that it is divided into five rather than two parts. Accounts of the general characteristics of bacteria and of bacteria in the environment will now be found in Volume 2 (*Systematic Bacteriology*). Both this and Volume 3 (*Bacterial Infections*) can be read individually, but, as in past editions, they obviously complement each other. The quantity of information now available has meant a further increase in size of Volumes 1, 2 and 3, which now contain about 30% more material than did the whole of the 8th edition. The two new volumes, dealing respectively with *Medical Mycology* and *Parasitology*, greatly enhance the value of the work as a whole. Whether to include the helminths under the title *Microbiology and Microbial Infections* was a debatable point, which succeeded on the grounds that to omit them would impair coverage of the entire gamut of infection, and that a separate mention in the title would have made it unwieldy.

Some points of editorial policy deserve mention. As in previous editions, the emphasis throughout is on infections of humans; animal diseases are given much less prominence, usually receiving mention only when they cause zoonoses, serve as models of pathogenesis or are of economic importance. Sections likely to be of interest only to the more specialized reader are indicated by the use of a small typeface, and the location and cross-referencing of specific sections are now made easier by numbering them.

The standard of the illustrations, many of which are now in colour, is considerably higher than in previous editions; in particular, there is a wealth of excellent drawings and photographs in Volumes 4 and 5. The quality of the references has been greatly improved by providing the titles of papers and both first and last pages; and the international provenance of the contributors has resulted in broader surveys of the world literature than is usual in predominantly British or American texts.

In conclusion, I take this opportunity of saying how much I appreciate the efforts of all those concerned with bringing this large and complex work to fruition. Almost by definition, the more distinguished the author, the more he or she will have other pressing commitments, a consideration that applies to most of our contributors. Sincere thanks are due to them for their participation and for providing the huge fund of learning and expertise that is apparent throughout the edition. I gladly take this opportunity of expressing my gratitude to all my colleagues on the editorial team for the intensive and sustained effort they have devoted to bringing this large and complex publication to fruition. It would be invidious to single out individuals among the copy-editors and the staff at Arnold who have laboured so devotedly behind the scenes, but to each of them my gratitude is also due for their competent help and unfailing support during the preparation of this edition.

LC

VOLUME EDITORS' PREFACE

Change in a work of this nature is inevitable and this edition of the volume on Systematic Bacteriology is a dramatic departure from its predecessors in many ways. Each chapter has been rewritten in its entirety to present new information on the biotechnical and molecular aspects of bacteria while retaining the fundamentals of bacteriology. Students of medical microbiology and infectious diseases should benefit from this fresh approach in presenting the basic facts of bacteriology and in describing the various genera of bacteria responsible for infectious diseases. Each of the five volumes of the 9th edition can be used as a 'stand alone' text, but Volume 2 and its companion Volume 3 on *Bacterial Infections* differ from the others in that they are also intended to complement one another, thus enhancing their value to the reader.

Volume 2 consists of 64 chapters. These reflect a combination of the chapters dealing with general bacteriology and with specific genera of pathogens in Volumes 1 and 2 of the 8th edition respectively.

The first 19 chapters cover fundamentals of bacteriology with a strong leaning to those topics that are of interest to students, research workers and teachers of microbiology. Following an historical introduction by M.T. Parker, the next 6 chapters deal with how bacteria are built, grow and become part of the biosphere, and comprise topics such as structure, morphology, metabolism and diversity. The next 4 chapters address the ways in which bacteria compete in their environment: viz., bacteriocins and bacteriophages, the effects of antibiotics, bacterial genetics, human microflora and bacterial diversity. These are followed by chapters covering the role of bacteria in our environment: soil, air, water, dairy products and foodstuffs. An additional segment of fundamentals is contained in 4 chapters dealing with classification and taxonomy, isolation and identification, and immunoserology. The last 45 chapters contain comprehensive descriptions and discussions of bacterial genera or groups of bacterial pathogens with coverage extending to new, emerging or re-emerging pathogens as well as current information on established pathogens.

We are confident that, particularly in association with Volume 3, *Systematic Bacteriology* will continue to provide a comprehensive *vade mecum* of medical bacteriology.

AB
BD

ABBREVIATIONS

5-BU	5-bromouracil
AAF/I, II	aggregative adherence fimbriae I, II
AB	*Adalia bipunctata* (bacterium)
ABC	ATP-binding cassette
ABS	Animal Biosafety Level
AC	adenylate cyclase
ACES	N-2-acetamido-2-amino-ethanesulphonic acid
ACIP	Advisory Committee on Immunization Practices
ACP	acyl carrier protein
ACT	adenylate cyclase toxin
ADA	adenosine deaminase
ADCC	antibody-dependent cellular cytotoxicity
ADH	arginine decarboxylase
ADP	adenosine diphosphate
AE	attaching and effacing (lesions)
AFA	afimbrial adhesin
AFB	acid-fast bacilli
AFIP	Armed Forces Institute of Pathology
Ag-EIA	antigen capture enzyme immunoassay
AGE	agarose gel electrophoresis
AGG	agglutinogen
AI	artificial insemination
AIDS	acquired immune deficiency syndrome
AMAN	acute motor axonal neuropathy
AMES	aminoglycoside-modifying enzymes
ANF	absolute non-fermenting
ANUG	acute necrotizing ulcerating gingivitis; acute necrotizing ulcerating gingivostomatitis
AOAC	Association of Official Analytical Chemists
AP	alkaline protease
APC	antigen-presenting cells; antigen-processing cells
APD	average pore diameter
APPCR	arbitrarily primed PCR
APS	adenosine 5′-phosphosulphate; adenyl sulphate
ARC	AIDS-related complex
ARDS	acute respiratory distress syndrome; adult respiratory distress syndrome
ASH test	antihyaluronidase test
ASK test	antistreptokinase test
ASO test	antistreptolysin O test
ASTPHLD	Association of State and Territorial Public Health Directors
ATCC	American Type Culture Collection
ATF	ambient temperature fimbriae
ATPase	adenosine 5′-triphosphatase
ATS	American Thoracic Society
BA	bacillary angiomatosis
BB	mid-borderline (leprosy)
BCG	bacille Calmette–Guérin
BCYE	buffered charcoal yeast extract
BFP	bundle-forming pilus
BG	Bordet–Gengou
BHI	brain–heart infusion
BI	bacterial index; biological indicator
BIG	botulism immune globulin
BL	borderline lepromatous (leprosy)
BLIS	bacteriocin-like inhibitory substances
BMT	bone marrow transplant
BOD	biochemical oxygen demand
BoNT	botulinum neurotoxin
BP	bacillary peliosis
BPASU	British Paediatric Association Surveillance Unit
BPI	bactericidal/permeability increasing protein
BPL	β-propiolactone
BSA	bovine serum albumin
BSK	Barbour–Stoenner–Kelly (medium)
BT	borderline tuberculoid (leprosy)
C1-inh	C1-inhibitor
CA	chorioallantoic
CAM	cell adhesion molecule
CAMP	Christie–Atkins–Munch-Petersen (test)
cAMP	cyclic adenosine 5′-monophosphate
CAP	catabolite gene activator protein (see also CRP)
CAPD	continuous ambulatory peritoneal dialysis
CBPP	contagious bovine pleuropneumonia
CCC DNA	covalently closed circular DNA
CCDC	Consultant in Communicable Disease Control
CCFA	cycloserine-cefoxitin-egg yolk-fructose agar
CCP	critical control point
CCPP	contagious caprine pleuropneumonia
CDC	Centers for Disease Control

CDP	cytidine 5′-diphosphonate
CDSC	Communicable Disease Surveillance Centre
CE	Chief Executive
CF	complement fixation; cystic fibrosis
CFA	complete Freund's adjuvant
CFA	cycloserine–egg yolk–fructose agar
CFA/I, II	colonization factor antigen I, II
cfu	colony-forming unit
CGD	chronic granulomatous disease
CHEF	contour-clamped homogeneous electric field electrophoresis
CHO	Chinese hamster ovary
CIE	countercurrent immunoelectrophoresis
CIN	cefsulodin–Irgasan–novobiocin
CLED	cysteine lactose electrolyte-deficient
CMA	cycloserine-mannitol agar
CMBA	cycloserine-mannitol blood agar
CMC	critical micelle concentration
CMGS	cooked meat medium containing glucose and starch
CMI	cell mediated immunity
CMP-NANA	cytidine-5′-monophospho-*N*-acetylneuraminic acid
CMR	chloroform–methanol residue
CMRNG	chromosomally resistant *Neisseria gonorrhoeae*
CMV	cytomegalovirus
CNA	Columbia colistin–nalidixic acid agar
CNS	central nervous system; coagulase-negative staphylococcus
CNW	catalase-negative or weakly reacting
COPD	chronic obstructive pulmonary disease
COVER	Cover of Vaccination Evaluated Rapidly
CP	capsular polysaccharides
CPHL	Central Public Health Laboratory
CR1	complement receptor type 1
CR2	complement receptor type 2
CRA	chlorine-releasing agent
CRD	chronic respiratory disease
CRE	catabolite responsive elements
CRF	coagulase-reacting factor
CRMOX	Congo red magnesium oxalate
CRP	cAMP receptor protein or catabolite gene activator protein (see also CAP); C-reactive protein
CRS	congenital rubella syndrome
CS1, 2, etc.	coli surface associated antigen 1, 2, etc.
CSD	cat scratch disease
CSF	cerebrospinal fluid
CT	cholera toxin
CTL	cytotoxic lymphocytes
CVD	Center of Vaccine Development
CWDF	cell wall deficient forms
DAEC	diffusely adherent *Escherichia coli*
DAF	decay-accelerating factor
DAP	diaminopimelic acid
DCA	deoxycholate–citrate agar
DCCD	*N,N′*-dicyclohexylcarbodiimide
DFA-TP	direct fluorescent antibody test for *Treponema pallidum*
DFAT-TP	direct fluorescent antibody tissue test for *Treponema pallidum*
DFD	dark, firm and dry
DGI	disseminated gonococcal infection
DHEA	dehydroepiandrosterone
DHFR	dihydrofolate reductase
DIF	direct immunofluorescence
dmfs	decayed, missing and filled surfaces (deciduous teeth)
DMFS	decayed, missing and filled surfaces (permanent teeth)
dmft	decayed, missing and filled teeth (deciduous teeth)
DMFT	decayed, missing and filled teeth (permanent teeth)
DN	double-negative
DNA	deoxyribonucleic acid
DNAase	deoxyribonuclease
DNP	2,4-dinitrophenol
DNT	dermonecrotic toxin
DoH	Department of Health
DOTS	directly observed therapy, short course
Dp	electrochemical potential
DRT	decimal reduction time; D value
DS	double-staining
DSB	double-strand break
DSO	double-strand origin
DST	Diagnostic Sensitivity Test
DT	definitive phage type
DTaP	diphtheria and tetanus toxoids and acellular pertussis vaccine
DTH	delayed-type hypersensitivity
DTP	diphtheria, tetanus, pertussis
dUMP	deoxyuridine 5′-monophosphate
E-Hly	enterohaemolysin
EAE	erythema arthriticum epidemicum
EAF	EPEC adherence factor
EAggEC	enteroaggregative *Escherichia coli*
EAST	enteroaggregative *Escherichia coli* heat-stable enterotoxin
EB	ethidium bromide
EBSS	Earle's balanced salt solution
EBV	Epstein–Barr virus
ECF-A	eosinophil chemotactic factor of anaphylaxis
ECP	extracellular products
ED	Entner–Doudoroff
EDTA	ethylenediaminetetraacetic acid
EF	oedema factor
EF-2	elongation factor 2
EGF	epidermal growth factor
EGTA	ethyleneglycol-bis(β-aminoethylether)-*N,N,N′,N′*-tetraacetic acid
EHEC	enterohaemorrhagic pathovar of *Escherichia coli*
EI, EII	enzyme I, enzyme II
EIA	enzyme immunoassay
EIEC	enteroinvasive *Escherichia coli*
ELISA	enzyme-linked immunosorbent assay
EM	environmental mycobacteria
EMB	eosin–methylene blue; ethambutol
EMC	encephalomyocarditis
EMJH	Ellinghausen, McCullough, Johnson, Harris (medium)
EMP	Embden–Meyerhof–Parnas
EMRSA	epidemic methicillin-resistant *Staphylococcus aureus*
EMS	ethylmethane sulphonate
ENL	erythema nodosum leprosum
EOP	efficiency of plating
EPEC	enteropathogenic *Escherichia coli*
EPHLS	Emergency Public Health Laboratory Service
EPS	expressed prostatic secretions; extracellular polysaccharides

ERCP	endoscopic retrograde cholangiopancreatography	**HEPA**	high efficiency particulate air
ERIC	enterobacterial repetitive intergenic consensus	**HETES**	monohydroxyeicosatetraeonic acid
		Hfr	high-frequency recombination
ERIC-PCR	enterobacterial repetitive intergenic consensus typing	**HFT**	high-frequency transduction
		HG	hybridization group
ERL	Epidemiological Research Laboratory	**Hib**	*Haemophilus influenzae* type b
ESM	extended spectrum macrolide	**HiPIP**	high potential iron protein
ESR	erythrocyte sedimentation rate	**HIV**	human immunodeficiency virus
ET	electrophoretic type; enzyme type; epidermolytic toxin; erythrogenic toxin	**HLA**	human major histocompatibility antigen
		HLT	heat-labile toxin
		HLY	haemolysin
ETA	exfoliatin A; exotoxin A	**HMP**	hexose monophosphate pathway
ETB	exfoliatin B	**HMWP**	high molecular weight protein
ETEC-ST	*Escherichia coli* producing heat-stable enterotoxin; enterotoxigenic *Escherichia coli*	**HNIG**	human normal immunoglobulin
		HPLC	high performance liquid chromatography
		HRF	homologous restriction factor
ETO	ethylene oxide	**HSP, hsp**	heat shock protein
ETS	exotoxin S	**HSV**	herpes simplex virus
ETZ	electron transparent zone	**HT**	haemorrhagic toxin
Ext-A	exfoliative toxin A	**HTE**	hamster trachea epithelial
FA	fluorescent antibody	**HTIG**	human tetanus immunoglobulin
FAD	flavin adenine dinucleotide	**HTST**	high temperature, short time
FAME	fatty acid methyl ester	**HUS**	haemolytic–uraemic syndrome
FAS	fluorescence actin-staining	**IATS**	International Antigenic Typing Scheme
FBP	ferrous sulphate, sodium metabisulphite and sodium pyruvate; fructose-1,6-biphosphate	**IBK**	infectious bovine keratoconjunctivitis
		ICAM	intercellular adhesion molecules
		ICC	Infection Control Committee
FD	ferredoxin	**ICD**	Infection Control Doctor
FDC	follicular dendritic cells	**ICDDR,B**	International Centre for Diarrhoeal Disease, Bangladesh
FHA	filamentous haemagglutinin		
FIGE	field inversion gel electrophoresis	**ICMSF**	International Committee on Microbiological Specifications for Food
FIRN	fimbriation-, inositol- and rhamnose-negative		
		ICN	Infection Control Nurse
FITC	fluorescein-isothiocyanate	**ICS**	intercellular spread
Fla	polar flagellum	**ICSB**	International Committee for Systematic Bacteriology
FMN	flavin adenine mononucleotide		
FnBP	fibronectin-binding protein	**ICT**	Infection Control Team
FP	flavoprotein	**ICTV**	International Committee for Taxonomy of Viruses
FPH2, FPH$_2$	reduced flavoprotein		
FT-IR	Fourier transform infrared	**idt**	indeterminate (leprosy)
FTA	fluorescent treponemal antibody	**IE**	infective endocarditis
FTA-ABS	fluorescent treponemal antibody-absorption (test)	**IF**	inactivation factor
		IFA	indirect fluorescent antibodies
GBS	Guillain–Barré syndrome	**IFAT**	indirect fluorescent antibody test
GDP	guanidine diphosphate	**IFN**	interferon
GLC	gas-liquid chromatography	**IG**	immune globulin
GLP	glycolipoprotein	**Ig**	immunoglobulin
GMCSF	granulocyte-macrophage colony-stimulating factor	**IHF**	integration host factor
		IJSB	International Journal of Systematic Bacteriology
GMP	guanosine 5′-monophosphate		
GMS	Gomori's methenamine silver nitrate	**IL**	interleukin
GPAC	gram-positive anaerobic cocci	**IMIG**	immune globulin intramuscular injection
GPIC	guinea pig eye inoculation with *Chlamydia psittaci*	**IMP**	inosine 5′-monophosphate
		IMS	immunomagnetic separation
GPL	glycopeptidolipid	**INH**	isoniazid
GTP	guanosine 5′-triphosphate	**Ipa**	invasion plasmid antigen
GUM	genitourinary medicine	**IPS**	intracellular polysaccharides
GVHD	graft-versus-host disease	**IPV**	inactivated poliovirus vaccine
HACCP	hazard analysis of critical control points	**IR**	intercept ratio; inverted repeat
HAP	haemagglutinin/protease	**IS**	insertion sequence
HAV	hepatitis A virus	**ISCOM**	immune stimulating complexes
HBIG	hepatitis B immunoglobulin	**ISG**	immune serum globulin
HBT	human blood bilayer Tween	**ITU**	intensive therapy unit
HBV	hepatitis B virus	**IUCD**	intrauterine contraceptive device
HCV	hepatitis C virus	**IVD**	intravascular device
HDP	hexose diphosphate (pathway)	**IVDU**	intravenous drug user
HE	haematoxylin–eosin	**IVIG**	immune globulin intravenous injection
HEA	Hektoen enteric agar		

IWGMT	International Working Group on Mycobacterial Taxonomy		**MEM**	minimum essential medium
JH	Jarisch–Herxheimer (reaction)		**MGRSA**	methicillin–gentamicin resistant *Staphylococcus aureus*
KDO	2-keto-3-deoxyoctonate; 2-keto-3-deoxyoctonic acid		**MHA-TP**	microhaemagglutination assay for antibodies to *Treponema pallidum*
KDPG	2-keto-3-deoxy-6-phosphogluconate		**MHC**	major histocompatibility complex
KIA	Kligler's iron agar		**MI**	morphological index
KID50	50% kidney infecting dose		**MIC**	minimum inhibitory concentration
KP	Kanagawa phenomenon		**MICP**	major iron-containing protein
L–J	Lowenstein–Jensen		**MIF**	microimmunofluorescence
LAB	lactic acid bacteria		**MIP**	macrophage infectivity potentiator
LAF	laminar air flow		**MK**	menaquinone
Laf	lateral flagellum		**MLEE**	multilocus enzyme electrophoresis; syn. MEE
LAL	*Limulus* amoebocyte lysate		**MLO**	*Mycoplasma*-like organisms
LAM	lipoarabinomannan		**MLP**	mitral leaflet prolapse
LAMP	lipid-associated membrane proteins		**MLS**	macrolides, lincosamides and streptogramin B
LAO	lysine–arginine–ornithine		**MMO**	methane mono-oxygenase
LAP	leucine aminopeptidase		**MMR**	mass miniature radiology; measles, mumps and rubella
Laz	lipid-associated azurin			
LC	large colony		**MNNG**	*N*-methyl-*N*′-nitro-*N*-nitrosoguanidine; syn. NTG
LCR	ligase chain reaction			
LDC	lysine decarboxylase		**MOEH**	Medical Officer for Environmental Health
LF	lactoferrin; lethal factor		**MOH**	Medical Officer of Health
Lf	lines of flocculation or flocculation units		**MOI**	multiplicity of infection
			MOMP	major outer-membrane protein
LGV	lymphogranuloma venereum		**MOTT**	mycobacteria other than tubercle
LJP	localized juvenile periodontitis		**MP**	mononuclear phagocyte
LL	lepromatous (leprosy)		**MPD**	maximum pore diameter
LLS	lipopolysaccharide-like substance		**MPL**	monophosphoryl lipid A
LOH	large, opaque, hazy edge		**MR**	mannose-resistant; methyl red
LOS	lipo-oligosaccharide		**MR/K**	mannose-resistant *Klebsiella*-like
LP	lactoperoxidase		**MR/P**	mannose-resistant *Proteus*-like
LPS	lipopolysaccharide		**MREHA**	mannose-resistant and eluting haemagglutinin
LT	*Escherichia coli* heat-labile toxin; lethal toxin; leukotriene			
			MRM	murine respiratory mycoplasmosis
LTA	lipoteichoic acid		**MRSA**	methicillin-resistant *Staphylococcus aureus*
LTSF	low temperature steam with formaldehyde			
			MRSE	methicillin-resistant *Staphylococcus epidermidis*
LTT	lymphocyte transformation test			
mA₂pm	*meso*-diaminopimelic acid (see also m-Dpm)		**MRSP**	mapped restriction site polymorphism
			MRT	milk ring test
mAb	monoclonal antibody		**MS**	mannose-sensitive; mutans streptococci
MAC	membrane attack complex; *Mycobacterium avium* complex; *Mycobacterium avium–intracellulare* complex		**MSCRAMMs**	microbial surface components recognizing adhesive matrix molecules
			MSSA	methicillin-sensitive *Staphylococcus aureus*
MAFF	Ministry of Agriculture, Fisheries and Food		**MUG**	methylumbelliferyl-β-D-glucuronidase
MAI	*Mycobacterium avium-intracellulare*		**MuLV**	murine leukaemia virus
MALT	mucosa-associated lymphoid tissue		**MW**	molecular weight
MAM	*Mycoplasma arthritidis* mitogen		**NAB**	nucleic acid-binding
MAP	major antigenic protein		**NAD**	nicotinamide adenine dinucleotide
MASPs	MBL-associated proteases		**NADase**	nicotinamide adenine dinucleotidase
MAT	microscopic agglutination test		**NaDCC**	sodium dichloroisocyanuric acid
MBC	minimum bactericidal concentration		**NADPH**	nicotinamide adenine dinucleotide phosphate (reduced) oxidase
MBL	mannose-binding lectin; syn. MBP			
MBP	mannose- or mannan-binding protein; syn. MBL		**NANAT**	nalidixic acid, novobiocin, cycloheximide and potassium tellurite
MCA	Medicines Control Authority		**NAP**	*p*-nitro-α-acetylamino-β-propiophenone
MCLO	*Mycobacterium chelonae*-like organisms		**NCCLS**	National Committee for Clinical Laboratory Standards
MCMP	major cytoplasmic membrane protein			
MCP	membrane cofactor protein; monocytic chemotactic protein		**NCHI**	non-capsulate *Haemophilus influenzae*
			NFA	non-fimbrial adhesins
MDP	muramyl dipeptide		**NGU**	non-gonococcal urethritis
m-Dpm	*meso*-diaminopimelic acid (see also mA₂pm)		**NHS**	National Health Service; normal human serum
MDR	multidrug resistance		**NIBSC**	National Institute of Biological Standards and Control
MDR-TB	multidrug-resistant tuberculosis			
MDT	multidrug therapy			
MEE	multilocus enzyme electrophoresis; syn. MLEE		**NIH**	National Institutes of Health

NITU	neonatal intensive therapy unit
NK	natural killer
NMO	non-mobile
NNIS	National Nosocomial Infection Surveillance
NPPC	*p*-nitrophenylphosphorylcholine
Nramp	natural-resistance-associated macrophage protein
NSAID	non-steroidal anti-inflammatory drug
NTG	*N*-methyl-*N'*-nitro-*N*-nitrosoguanidine; syn. MNNG
NTM	non-tuberculous mycobacteria
NVS	nutritionally variant streptococci
O-SP	O-specific polysaccharide
O–R	oxidation–reduction
OA	oleic acid–albumin
OC	Outbreak Committee
ODC	ornithine decarboxylase
OE	outer envelope
OF	oxidation–fermentation
OM	outer membrane
OMP	outer-membrane protein
ONPG	*o*-nitrophenyl-β-D-galactopyranoside
ONS	Office for National Statistics
OPCS	Office of Population Censuses and Surveys
OPV	oral polio vaccine
ORF	open reading frame
ORT	oral rehydration treatment
P-EI	phosphorylated enzyme I
P–V	Panton–Valentine (leucocidin)
PA	protective antigen
PAF	platelet-activating factor
PAGE	polyacrylamide gel electrophoresis
PAI	*Pseudomonas aeruginosa* autoinducer
PALCAM	polymyxin–acriflavine–lithium chloride–ceftazidime–aesculin–mannitol
PANTA	polymyxin, amphotericin, nalidixic acid, trimethoprim and azlocillin
Pap	pili associated with pyelonephritis
PAP	primary atypical pneumonia
PAS	*p*-aminosalicylic acid; periodic acid–Schiff
PBP	penicillin-binding protein
PCF	putative colonization factor
PCP	*Pneumocystis carinii* pneumonia
PCR	polymerase chain reaction
PCV	proportion of cases in the vaccinated
PDH	pyruvate dehydrogenation complex
PE	elastase
PEA	phenylethyl alcohol agar
PEP	phosphoenolpyruvate
PFGE	pulse field gel electrophoresis
Pfk	phosphofructokinase
pfu	plaque-forming unit
PG	prostaglandin
PGI$_2$	prostacyclin
PGL-I	phenolic glycolipid I
PGP	polyglycerophosphate
PGU	post-gonococcal urethritis
PHA	passive haemagglutination assay; poly-β-hydroxyalkanoate
PHB	poly-β-hydroxybutyrate
PHLS	Public Health Laboratory Service
PHMB	polyhexamethylene biguanide
PI	gonococcal protein; propamidine isethionate; protein I
PID	pelvic inflammatory disease
PK-TP	PK-*Treponema pallidum*
Pla	plasminogen activator protease

PLC	phospholipase C
PLD	phospholipase D
PLET	polymyxin–lysozyme–EDTA–thallous acetate
PLGA	polylactic and polyglycolic acids
PMC	pseudomembranous colitis
PMF	*Proteus mirabilis* fimbriae
pmf	proton-motive force
PMN	polymorphonuclear leucocyte
PMS	pyrolysis mass spectrometry
PNG	polymorphonuclear neutrophilic granulocyte
PNH	paroxysmal nocturnal haemoglobinuria
PNS	purple non-sulphur (bacteria)
POL	physician's office laboratory
PPD	Purified Protein Derivative of Tuberculin
PPE	porcine proliferative enteropathy
PPEM	potentially pathogenic environmental mycobacteria
ppGpp	guanosine 5′-diphosphate 3′-diphosphate
PPLO	pleuropneumonia-like organisms
PPNG	penicillinase-producing *Neisseria gonorrhoeae*
pppGpp	guanosine 5′-triphosphate 3′-diphosphate
PPV	proportion of population vaccinated
PRAS	pre-reduced anaerobically stabilized (media)
PRN	pertactin
PROS	pathogen-related oral spirochaete
PRP	polyribosephosphate
PS	purple sulphur (bacteria)
PS/A	polysaccharide adhesin
PSE	pale, soft exudative
PSI	photosystem I
PSII	photosystem II
PSP	paralytic shellfish poisoning
PT	pertussis toxin
Ptd	pertussis toxoid
PTS	phosphoenolpyruvate phosphotransferase system
Pva	polyvinyl alcohol
PVE	prosthetic valve endocarditis
PYG	peptone–yeast extract–glucose
PYR	pyrrolidonyl-β-naphthylamide
PZA	pyrazinamide
QAC	quaternary ammonium compound
r-det	resistance determinant
RAG	recombinant activating gene
RAPD	random amplified polymorphic DNA fingerprinting
RaRF	Ra reactive factor
RAS	Ribi Adjuvant System
RBP	rose bengal plate
RC	rolling circle
RCA	regulation of complement activation
RCCS	random cloned chromosomal sequence
rDNA	DNA coding for RNA
REA	restriction endonuclease analysis
REAC	restriction endonuclease digestion of chromosome DNA
REAP	restriction endonuclease digestion of plasmid DNA
rep-PCR	repetitive element polymerase chain reaction
REP-PCR	repetitive extragenic palindromic element typing
rEPA	*Pseudomonas aeruginosa* exoprotein A
RFLP	restriction fragment length polymorphism

RGM	rapidly growing mycobacteria
RH	relative humidity
RIM	Rapid Identification Method
RIT	rabbit infectivity testing
RMAT	rapid microagglutination test
RMSF	Rocky Mountain spotted fever
RNA	ribonucleic acid
RNAase	ribonuclease
RNI	reactive nitrogen intermediate
ROI	reactive oxygen intermediate
RPLA	reversed passive latex agglutination
RPP	rapid progressive periodontitis
RPR	rapid plasma reagin
rRNA	ribosomal RNA
RSS	recurrent non-typhoidal salmonella septicaemia
RST	reagin screen test
RSV	respiratory syncytial virus
RT	ribotyping
RTD	routine test dilution
RTF	Reduced Transport Fluid; resistance transfer factor
RTX	repeats in toxin
SAF	sodium acetate–acetic acid–formalin; Syntex Adjuvant Formulation
SAK	staphylokinase
SAL	sterility assurance level
SARA	sexually acquired reactive arthritis
SASP	small acid-soluble protein
SAT	standard tube-agglutination test
SBA	sheep blood agar
SC	secretory component; small colony
SCID	severe combined immunodeficiency
SCIEH	Scottish Centre for Infection and Environmental Health
SDA	strand displacement amplification
SDH	succinate dehydrogenase
SDS	sodium dodecyl sulphate
SDS-PAGE	sodium dodecyl sulphate polyacrylamide gel electrophoresis
SE	staphylococcus enterotoxin
SE-A	staphylococcus enterotoxin A
SE-C	staphylococcus enterotoxin C
SFG	spotted fever group
ShET	*Shigella* enterotoxin
SHHD	Scottish Home and Health Department
SIDS	sudden infant death syndrome
SIM	sulphide–indole–motility
SIRS	systemic inflammatory response syndrome
SLE	systemic lupus erythematosus
SLT	Shiga-like toxin; syn. VT
SMAC	sorbitol MacConkey
SMD	smooth domed (colony morphology)
SMG	'*Streptococcus milleri* group'
SMT	smooth transparent (colony morphology)
SNAP	synaptosomal-associated protein
SOD	small, opaque, defined border; superoxide dismutase
SPA	species-specific surface protein antigen
SPE	streptococcal pyrogenic exotoxin
SPEA	streptococcal pyrogenic exotoxin A
SPG	sucrose phosphate glutamate
SPS	sodium polyanethol sulphonate
SRS	slow-reacting substance
SRS-A	slow-reacting substance of anaphylaxis
SRSV	small, round structured virus
SS	salmonella–shigella (agar); Stainer–Scholte (medium)

SSB	single-strand break
SSSS	staphylococcal scalded skin syndrome
SSU	small subunit
ST	*Escherichia coli* heat-stable toxin
STD	sexually transmitted disease
STM	signature tagged mutagenesis
STP	standard plate count
SXT	co-trimoxazole; sulphamethoxazole–trimethoprim (see also TMP–SMX)
TA	transaldolase
TAP	transporters associated with antigen processing
TBW	tracheobronchial washings
TCA	tricarboxylic acid; trichloroacetic acid
TCBS	thiosulphate–citrate–bile salts–sucrose
TCF	tracheal colonization factor
TCH	thiophen-2-carboxylic acid hydrazide
TCID	tissue culture infective dose
TCR	T cell receptor
TCT	tracheal cytotoxin
Td	diphtheria toxoid
TDE	transmissible degenerative encephalopathy
TDH	thermostable direct haemolysin
TDHT	5-thyminyl-5,6-dihydrothymine
TDM	trehalose dimycolate
TDP	thermal death point
TDT	thermal death time
TeTx	tetanus toxin
TF	transferrin
THF	termination host factor
TK	transketolase
TMP–SMX	trimethoprim–sulphamethoxazole (see also SXT)
TNase	thermonuclease
TNF	tumour necrosis factor
TOC	total organic carbon
TPGY	trypticase–peptone–glucose–yeast extract
TPHA	*Treponema pallidum* haemagglutination
TPI	*Treponema pallidum* immobilization
TPP	thiamine pyrophosphate
TRH	thermostable related toxin
TRUST	toluidine red unheated serum test
TSB	trypticase–soy broth
TSI	triple sugar iron (agar)
TSST-1	staphylococcal toxic shock toxin-1; toxic shock syndrome toxin-1
TT	tetanus toxoid; tuberculoid
TTP	thrombotic thrombocytopenic purpura
TWAR	Taiwan acute respiratory
UCA	uroepithelial cell adhesin
UCNC	unclassified catalase-negative coryneform
UHT	ultra-heat-treated
UMP	uridine 5′-monophosphate; uridylic acid
UNDP	undecaprenol phosphate
UPGMA	unweighted pair-group method with arithmetic averages
UPTC	urease-positive subgroup
USR	unheated serum reagin
UTI	urinary tract infection
VAMP	vesicle-associated membrane protein; vesicle-associated protein
VB	voided bladder urine
VD	venereal disease
VDRL	Venereal Disease Research Laboratory
VE	vaccine efficacy
VEE	Venezuelan equine encephalomyelitis
VFA	volatile fatty acid
VOMP	variable outer-membrane protein

VP	Voges–Proskauer		**VZV**	varicella zoster virus
VPI	Virginia Polytechnic Institute		**WC-BS**	whole cell B subunit
VSC	volatile sulphur compounds		**XLD**	xylose–lysine–deoxycholate
VT	verotoxin; syn. SLT		**XMP**	xanthosine 5′-monophosphate
VTEC	Vero cytotoxin-producing *Escherichia coli*; verotoxigenic *Escherichia coli*		**YPM**	*Yersinia pseudotuberculosis*-derived mitogen

Chapter 1

THE BACTERIA: HISTORICAL INTRODUCTION

M T Parker

1 MICROBIOLOGY

Microbiology is the study of living organisms ('micro-organisms' or 'microbes'), simple in structure and usually small in size, that are generally considered to be neither plants nor animals; they include bacteria, algae, fungi, protozoa and viruses. 'Pure' microbiology concerns the organisms themselves and 'applied' microbiology their effects on other living beings, when they act as pathogens or commensals, or on their inanimate environment, when they bring about chemical changes in it. Thus microbiology has applications in human and veterinary medicine, in agriculture and animal husbandry and in industrial technology.

Micro-organisms were first seen and described by the Dutch lens-maker Antonie van Leeuwenhoek (1632–1723) who devised simple microscopes capable of giving magnifications of c. ×200. In a number of letters to the Royal Society of London between 1673 and his death he gave clear and accurate descriptions and drawings of a variety of living things that undoubtedly included protozoa, yeasts and bacteria (Dobell 1932). These striking observations did not lead immediately to great advances in the knowledge of microbes. These were delayed for nearly 2 centuries, until essential technical advances had been made by workers who nowadays would be described as industrial or medical microbiologists.

2 COMMUNICABLE DISEASES

Long before microbes had been seen, observations on communicable diseases had given rise to the concept of contagion: the spread of disease by contact, direct or indirect. This idea was implicit in the laws enacted in early biblical times to prevent the spread of leprosy. It became less influential in the classical era, when supernatural and miasmatic causes were favoured. In the later Middle Ages there was renewed interest in contagion, reinforced at the end of the fifteenth century by the spread of syphilis in Europe, which was obviously associated with a specific form of contact. Fracastorius (Girolamo Fracastoro), a physician of Verona, published in 1546 an influential analysis of contagion:

1 by physical contact alone
2 by formites and
3 at a distance.

He was led to conclude that communicable diseases were caused by living agents; these he spoke of as 'seminaria' or 'seeds', but he was unable to give a more definite opinion about their nature.

In the subsequent 250 years several authors speculated that the agents of contagious diseases were animate, but little evidence for this was produced. Even the recognition of parasitism by animals, e.g. scabies, some forms of helminthiasis (see Foster 1965), appears to have had little impact on thinking about the role of micro-organisms as pathogens. Early in the nineteenth century improvements had been made in the design of microscopes and between 1834 and 1850 numerous accounts were published of morphologically recognizable micro-organisms in material from diseased animals or human subjects: of fungi subsequently called *Botrytis* in the silkworm disease 'calcino' by Bassi; of trichomonads in human vaginal discharges by Donné; of ringworm fungi by Schönlein and by Groby; of vibrios in cholera stools by Pouchet; and of large rod-shaped bacteria in anthrax blood by Rayer and Davaine (for references see Bulloch 1938). In 1840, Henle affirmed his belief in what came to be called the 'germ theory of disease', which asserted that certain diseases were caused by the multiplication of micro-organisms in the body, but he advanced little supporting evidence for this and his view was hotly disputed.

3 FERMENTATION AND PUTREFACTION

In the first half of the nineteenth century, chemists became interested in fermentation: industrial processes in which organic substances underwent changes that yielded useful compounds, such as alcohol and acetic acid. A similar process, termed putrefaction, led to the decay of organic matter, usually with the production of an unpleasant odour and taste. In the 1830s several observers, notably Cagniard-Latour and Schwann, saw yeasts in liquors undergoing alcoholic fermentation and concluded that these were living organisms and the cause of the process. This view was resisted by leading authorities of the day (Berzelius, Liebig, Wohler) who considered that fermentation was a purely chemical process and that the yeasts were a consequence rather than the cause of it. Between 1836 and 1860 controversy raged but without a clear outcome.

3.1 The work of Louis Pasteur

Louis Pasteur (1822–1895) (Fig. 1.1) produced strong experimental evidence that micro-organisms were the cause of fermentation and in so doing laid the foundations of microbiology as a science. He was a chemist whose early studies of fermentation aroused his interest in the molecular asymmetry of some of the compounds formed. He concluded that optically active chemical compounds, such as the stereoisomeric forms of tartaric acid and amyl alcohol, never arose from the purely chemical decomposition of sugars but were formed from them by the action of micro-organisms; these were always present in fermenting liquors and increased in number as the process continued. Different fermentation processes (e.g. alcoholic, acetic, butyric) were each associated with particular organisms which were often recognizable by their morphology or requirements for growth.

To maintain that micro-organisms caused fermentation it was necessary to establish that they did not arise de novo. This was contrary to the widely held belief in the spontaneous generation of living things from dead animal or vegetable material ('heterogenesis'). Controversy about this in the eighteenth century had centred around the conditions under which putrefaction developed in organic matter that had been subjected to supposedly sterilizing temperatures in closed containers. This matter was unresolved in 1860. In a series of admirable experiments reported

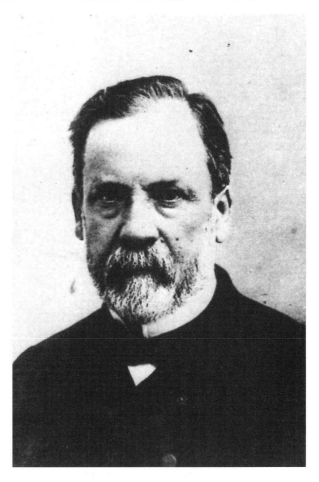

Fig. 1.1 Louis Pasteur (1822–1895).

in the next 4 years (see Vallery-Radot 1922–33), Pasteur disposed of many purported instances of heterogenesis by showing that they could be attributed to failure of the intitial sterilization or to subsequent recontamination. He emphasized the need for scrupulous sterilization of everything coming into contact with the material under examination and demonstrated numerous sources of contamination from air, dust and water. He showed that some organisms were not destroyed by boiling. For the sterilization of fluids he advocated heating to 120°C under pressure and for glassware the use of dry heat at 170°C; he showed the value of the cotton-wool plug for protecting material from aerial recontamination.

In the course of these experiments Pasteur used various forms of nutrient fluid to grow micro-organisms and showed that a medium suitable for one might be unsuitable for another, so for successful cultivation it was necessary to discover a suitable growth medium and to establish optimal conditions of temperature, acidity or alkalinity, and oxygen tension.

The mass of experimental data produced by Pasteur carried general conviction, but a minority of adherents of heterogenesis continued to maintain their position, often supporting this by experiments in which inadequate heating had failed to destroy very heat-resistant bacteria. The observations of Tyndall in the early 1870s that all actively multiplying bacteria were easily destroyed by boiling led to the introduction of a method of sterilization by repeated cycles of heating interspersed with periods of incubation. This method of 'tyndallization' served to eliminate many of the anomalies reported by the advocates of heterogenesis (see Bulloch 1938).

Pasteur devoted much effort to investigating the troubles of French winemakers, brewers and vinegarmakers. These studies often led him to perform experiments of fundamental scientific importance, as when his involvement in the problems of vinegarmaking led to valuable observations on the constancy of microbial characters in culture. His general conclusion was that fermentations owed their diversity to the characters of the several organisms responsible for them, but final proof of this was not obtainable until methods of obtaining pure cultures had been discovered.

4 PATHOGENIC MICRO-ORGANISMS

About 1865 Pasteur responded to an appeal to investigate a formidable disease of silkworms in southern France (pébrine) and by 1869 his experiments had led him to the conclusion that this was a communicable disease transmitted by direct contact or faecal contamination. This, according to his biographer Vallery-Radot (1919), engendered in his mind the idea that communicable diseases of animals and man, like the 'diseases' of wine and beer, might be a consequence of microbial multiplication.

From 1857 onward there had been reports, notably by Brauell and Davaine, of the transmission of anthrax between animals by the injection of blood. At that time there was also much interest in the septic and pyaemic diseases of man, including 'surgical fever' (see Bulloch 1938). In 1865, Coze and Felty began to publish a series of papers reporting the presence of bacteria in the blood of dogs and rabbits that had received injections of purulent material from human patients. In 1872, Davaine, starting with blood from patients suffering from 'putrid' infections, performed serial passage in experimental animals and demonstrated enhancement of virulence.

Joseph Lister (1827–1912) was aware of Pasteur's demonstration that both fermentation and putrefaction might be initiated by air-borne organisms. On the assumption that 'putrefying' wounds might be similarly caused, he attempted to prevent surgical sepsis by denying access to wounds of microbes from the patient's surroundings, particularly from the air. His 'antiseptic' regimen, first described in 1867, was strikingly successful and transformed the prognosis of major surgical operations. Lister did not prove that this was due to the destruction of potentially pathogenic microbes, but this was rendered highly probable by the contemporary work of French and German bacteriologists.

4.1 The work of Robert Koch

In 1876, while a country physician at Wollstein in eastern Germany, Robert Koch (1843–1910) (Fig. 1.2) published his first scientific work, a study of the anthrax bacillus in experimental animals, of its growth in vitro and of the formation and germination of its spores. This opened up a new era in bacteriology. Next year he described the fixing and staining of bacteria with the newly introduced aniline dyes. In 1878 his study of wound infections explored the role of animal experimentation in establishing the cause of bacterial infections. Then, in 1881, he described means of cultivating bacteria on solid media, thus making it possible to obtain pure cultures by transferring material from a single colony. First he used as his growth medium pieces of potato, then nutrient gelatin and later agar-gel media. In 1882 and 1884 he published classic papers on the tubercle bacillus and in 1883 described the cholera vibrio.

Koch had now assembled the techniques needed to investigate the bacterial causes of many communicable diseases. He had moved to Berlin where Loeffler and Gaffky were already his assistants; later came Pfeiffer, Kitasato, Welch and many others. Koch began to gather round him the group of followers who were destined to introduce his methods into many laboratories throughout the world. The fruits of this technical revolution appeared with remarkable speed; during the years 1876–90, the period described by Bulloch (1938) as 'the heyday of bacterial aetiological discovery' most of the important groups of bacterial pathogens for man and animals were recognized.

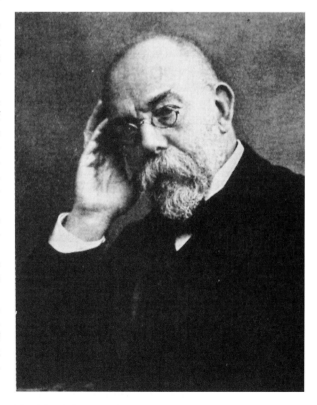

Fig. 1.2 Robert Koch (1843–1910).

4.2 Differential staining

In 1878 Paul Ehrlich had noted differences in the affinity for aniline dyes of various types of living cells, an observation that started him on his long search for chemotherapeutic agents (see Volume 3, Chapter 1). In 1882 he reported that tubercle bacilli stained with fuchsin retained the dye when subsequently treated with a mineral acid; this property of 'acid-fastness' formed the basis for methods later developed to detect mycobacteria in tissue sections, in sputum and other secretions and in cultures.

A differential staining method of even wider applicability arose from the observation, reported in 1884 by the young Danish physician Christian Gram, that certain bacteria, when stained with methyl violet and treated with an iodine solution as a mordant, retained the violet dye when washed briefly with ethyl alcohol. The 'gram reaction' proved to be a useful means of dividing bacteria into 2 categories: 'gram-positive' organisms that were stained violet and 'gram-negative' organisms that lost the violet dye and were stained red by a counterstain applied after washing with alcohol. This property was later found to reflect differences in cell-wall composition and to be correlated with a number of other characters; organisms that retained the violet stain were in general less susceptible, than those that did not, to various chemical substances and to lysis by complement in the presence of specific antibody.

4.3 Establishing the pathogenicity of bacteria

As the number of different bacteria found in constant association with human and animal diseases grew, the question of how to establish their aetiological role assumed importance. Already, in the 1880s it was being recognized that, though the internal organs were normally sterile or nearly so, many surface sites and body cavities communicating with the outside had a rich bacterial flora, so the presence of an organism here was of little significance. When inflammatory lesions appeared in such places it was often difficult to decide which, if any, of the organisms present was responsible.

Koch's experience with anthrax, wound infection and tuberculosis led him to place much reliance on the evidence of animal experimentation in establishing relationships between disease and isolate. A set of conditions, all of which must be fulfilled to justify such a conclusion, has been called Koch's postulates. They are as follows (see Topley and Wilson 1931), though Koch did not state them in precisely this form:

1 the organism is regularly found in the lesions of the disease
2 it can be grown in pure culture outside the body of the host, for several generations and
3 such a culture will reproduce the disease in question when administered to a susceptible experimental animal.

It subsequently proved difficult or impossible to fulfil all these criteria in respect of many microbial diseases.

4.4 Immunity

Folk medicine had long established that exposure to certain infective agents might engender immunity to them (see Volume 3, Chapter 1) and experience with Jennerian vaccination against smallpox had indicated the value of selecting a strain of the agent with low virulence for use as an inducer of immunity. While Koch and his pupils were continuing to characterize more and more pathogens, Pasteur turned his attention to the possibility of inducing prophylactic immunity by injections of live cultures of organisms the virulence of which had been attenuated by prolonged culture or by growth under suboptimal conditions. Success was reported in 1877 with a live vaccine against the pasteurella of chicken cholera and in 1881 with one against anthrax in animals. In 1886 Pasteur reported on the use of an attenuated live vaccine against rabies. This consisted of a dried suspension of spinal cord from an infected rabbit. Its use was an extension of the original principle of vaccination in that the material was given after infection had taken place. It was used with apparent success to prevent disease in human subjects who had been bitten by a rabid animal. Most of the early attenuated living vaccines caused appreciable morbidity and even some deaths, but in 1886 Salmon and Smith showed that it was possible to protect pigeons against salmonella infection by the injection of heat-killed organisms. Pfeiffer demonstrated in 1889 that immunity conferred by vaccination was usually highly specific, but there were exceptions to this (see p. 8).

At a somewhat earlier date, Metchnikoff had observed the engulfment of bacteria and other microbes by phagocytes; in 1891 he expressed the view that immunity was primarily cellular. This conflicted with growing evidence for the importance of serum factors; the alternative humoral view of immunity was that 'antibodies' appeared in the serum of vaccinated or infected animals and that their specificity corresponded to that of the 'antigens' that elicited them.

Strong evidence for humoral immunity emerged after Roux and Yersin in Paris had demonstrated in 1888 the characteristic lethal effects of broth cultures of diphtheria bacilli on guinea-pigs and shown that these were caused by the liberation of a soluble toxin, an 'exotoxin'. In the following year, Behring in Koch's laboratory observed that chemically sterilized broth cultures of diphtheria bacilli retained their toxicity for guinea-pigs but animals given sublethal doses of them were subsequently immune to diphtheria. He also showed that the pleural fluid of animals dead of diphtheria was toxic but yielded no diphtheria bacilli on culture; however, injections of it rendered other guinea-pigs immune. By 1890 Behring had demonstrated that the blood of immunized guinea-pigs neutralized diphtheria toxin in vitro. Faber demonstrated tetanus toxin in 1889; next year, Behring and Kitasato immunized rabbits against it and showed that their serum protected mice against tetanus.

These closely spaced events are summarized in Table 1.1. By the end of the century the importance of humoral immunity was firmly established. Subsequent developments, which included a reinstatement of cellular factors in the immune process, are recorded in Volume 3 (see Volume 3, Chapter 1). Figure 1.3 shows the Bacteriological Section of the Congress of Hygiene and Demography, London 1891.

4.5 Bacterial filters

An important technical advance in the latter part of the nineteenth century was the development of filters that held back bacteria but allowed the passage of smaller micro-organisms and biologically important macromolecules: Chamberland in 1884 introduced filters made of unglazed porcelain and Nordtmeyer in 1891 the Berkefeld type of filter composed of kieselguhr. There were several important consequences of these innovations as follows.

Filtration provided a convenient means of producing bacteria-free preparations of soluble toxins and thus greatly simplified the task of producing reagents for passive and active immunization against diphtheria and tetanus. It was also an essential preliminary to the purification of toxins and to chemical studies of their constitution.

It soon became apparent that some disease agents passed through bacteria-retaining filters; thus the first viral pathogens were recognized. In 1892 Iwanowski

Table 1.1 Bacteriology in the 19th century

1834–50	Fungi, protozoa and bacteria seen in diseased tissues or secretions (see text)
1836–37	Yeasts seen in liquors undergoing alcoholic fermentation
1840	Henle: 'germ theory of disease'
1844–57	Pasteur studies optically active compounds from fermented fluids
1857–63	Reports that anthrax is transmitted by injections of blood from diseased animals
1860–64	Pasteur: experimental evidence that fermentation and putrefaction are effects of microbial growth
1865–67	Pasteur studies 'pébrine' of silkworms; concludes that it is caused by microbial action
1867	Lister: success of 'antiseptic surgery' supports view that microbes cause postoperative sepsis
1876	Koch demonstrates pathogenicity and sporulation of anthrax bacilli
1877	Koch: staining of bacteria by aniline dyes
1877	Tyndall: heat-resistant bacteria destroyed by repeated cycles of moderate heating and incubation
1877	Pasteur: chicken cholera prevented by injections of live, attenuated culture
1877	Soil nitrates replenished by microbial action
1878	Koch: studies of wound infection; use of experiments on animals to establish aetiology
1879	Ehrlich: differences in affinity of chemical substances for various sorts of living cells
1881	Koch: use of solid media to obtain pure cultures of bacteria
1881	Pasteur: anthrax prevented by live attenuated vaccine
1882	Ehrlich: acid fastness of the tubercle bacillus
1882–84	Koch: aetiological role of the tubercle bacillus; 'Koch's postulates'
1883	Koch describes the cholera vibrio
1883–91	Metchnikoff studies cellular defence mechanisms
1884	Chamberland filters
1884	Gram's stain
1886	Pasteur's rabies vaccine
1886	Salmon and Smith: killed bacterial vaccines effective
1888	Roux and Yersin: diphtheria bacillus forms exotoxin
1888	Nuttall: serum killing of bacteria
1889	Behring: antitoxic immunity to diphtheria
1889	Pfeiffer: specificity of immunity conferred by vaccines
1889	Faber: tetanus bacillus forms exotoxin
1889	Buchner: serum killing of bacteria inhibited by heating the serum
1890	Behring: diphtheria antitoxin neutralizes toxin in vitro
1890	Behring and Kitasato: antitoxic immunity to tetanus
1890	Winogradsky: nitrite- and nitrate-forming bacteria in soil
1892	Tobacco-mosaic disease transmitted by filtered material
1894	Pfeiffer's phenomenon: lysis of vibrios in peritoneal cavity
1895	Bordet: heat-stable and heat-labile factors (respectively antibody and complement) in immune lysis
1897	Ehrlich: 'side chain theory' of antibody production
1898	Foot-and-mouth disease transmitted by filtered material

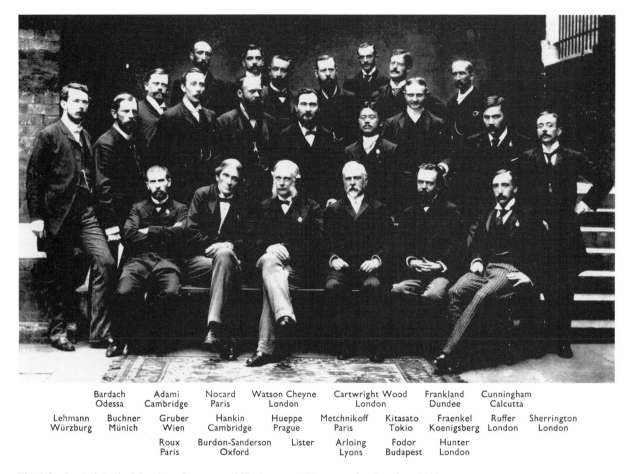

Bardach Odessa	Adami Cambridge	Nocard Paris	Watson Cheyne London	Cartwright Wood London	Frankland Dundee	Cunningham Calcutta		
Lehmann Würzburg	Buchner Münich	Gruber Wien	Hankin Cambridge	Hueppe Prague	Metchnikoff Paris	Kitasato Tokio	Fraenkel Koenigsberg	Ruffer London	Sherrington London
		Roux Paris	Burdon-Sanderson Oxford	Lister	Arloing Lyons	Fodor Budapest	Hunter London		

Fig. 1.3 Bacteriological Section, Congress of Hygiene and Demography, London 1891.

described the transmission of mosaic disease to tobacco plants and in 1898 Loeffler and Frosch described the transmission of foot-and-mouth disease in bovines by the injection of filtrates of infective material.

A later consequence of the use of bacterial filters was the discovery, independently by Twort in 1915 and d'Herelle in 1917, of bacteriophages, subsequently shown to be viruses that multiply in bacterial cells. Intensive study of the interaction of bacteriophage and bacterium by Delbrück and Hershey in the early 1940s contributed much to the knowledge of viral infections and also led to important developments in bacterial genetics (see section 7.4, p. 9).

5 NON-MEDICAL APPLICATIONS OF BACTERIOLOGY

The discoveries of Pasteur and Koch had important applications for agriculture and industry. The replacement of nitrates lost from the soil by the washing action of rain had long been a mystery but it seemed in some way to be connected with the decomposition of organic matter. In 1877 Schloesing and Muntz, acting on a suggestion from Pasteur, showed by experiment that the formation of nitrates was due to the action of living organisms; Warington confirmed this in 1878 and 1879 and demonstrated that the process took place in 2 stages: first, the conversion of

ammonia to nitrites, then the oxidation of nitrites to nitrates. He believed that these 2 stages were performed by different organisms but failed to prove this. In 1890 Winogradsky isolated and described the nitrogen-fixing bacteria that caused the formation of nodules on the roots of leguminous plants. Later Winogradsky described a free-living anaerobic organism that fixed atmospheric nitrogen and Beijerinck, some 10 years afterwards, a large free-living nitrogen-fixing aerobe that he named *Azotobacter*.

The importance of bacteria in maintaining the fertility of the soil has thus been recognized for over a century. A more recent concept is that the chemical activities of primitive ancestral microbial forms may have created the atmospheric conditions essential for the appearance of plants and animals on earth (see Schlegel 1984).

Bacteria cause diseases of plants as well as animals. In 1878 Burrill described the organism responsible for pear blight and in 1883 Wakker the bacterial cause of 'yellows' of hyacinths. Recognition of the role of bacteria in the spoilage of foodstuffs and in the production of organic chemicals useful to man led to the entrance of the bacteriologist into numerous industrial fields.

6 THE DEVELOPMENT OF 'PURE' BACTERIOLOGY

Pasteur's studies of fermentation in the early 1860s revealed the physiological diversity of microbes and may be looked upon as the starting-point of 'pure' bacteriological studies. During the 1870s he became more concerned with the role of microbes as pathogens, but he continued to be interested in their basic properties. For example, in 1878 he described under the name 'Vibrion septique' a pathogenic clostridium responsible for gangrenous conditions in animals and demonstrated that it was an obligate anaerobe. Within a few years it became possible to obtain pure cultures of many sorts of bacteria by colony selection on solid media and then to collect reliable data about their phenotypic characters. Accounts of their growth on various media under different physical conditions were soon supplemented by information about the range of their fermentative action on organic compounds and the products of fermentation and by the identification of chemical requirements for growth. Thus the raw materials for systematic bacteriology began to be accumulated and basic studies of bacterial metabolism could begin.

For more detailed accounts of the early history of bacteriology, and for references, see Bulloch (1938), Clark (1961), Lechevalier and Slotorovsky (1965) and Foster (1970).

7 SYSTEMATIC BACTERIOLOGY

7.1 Definition of the bacteria

The applied microbiologists of the time of Pasteur and Koch were not much interested in the classification of the micro-organisms they considered responsible for fermentation or for communicable diseases. Contemporary biologists recognized 2 kingdoms of living things, plants and animals, but were uncertain in which to place the bacteria. In 1838, Ehrenberg had used the term 'bacteria' to describe rod-shaped organisms visible only with a microscope and considered them animals, but F Cohn in 1854 claimed them for the botanists and Haeckel in 1866 thought that they should be placed, along with fungi, algae and protozoa, in a third kingdom, distinct from plants and animals, the Monera or Protista. Haeckel's view did not receive wide acceptance and for the next 50 years and more the bacteria were in a taxonomic limbo. Then, technical advances, notably the introduction of the electron microscope in 1932 and of the phase-contrast microscope in 1935, led to the recognition, usually associated with the names of Stanier and van Niel (1941), that the bacteria and certain bacteria-like blue-green algae differed from most other microbes in that their genetic material was not separated from the cytoplasm by a nuclear membrane.

This view was later formalized into the concept that there were 2 sorts of living things differing fundamentally in cellular structure (Murray 1962, Gibbons and Murray 1978):

1 the Prokaryotae, comprising the bacteria (Eubacteria) and the blue-green algae, which were now recognized to be phototrophic bacteria and
2 the Eukaryotae, which included fungi, algae, protozoa and all the metazoa of the plant and animal kingdoms.

The prokaryotes were characterized by the absence of a membrane-bounded nucleus and also of cellular organelles such as mitochondria and chloroplasts. As pointed out by Woese, the definition of bacteria as non-phototrophic prokaryotes is based entirely on negative characters and provides no grounds for distinguishing the conventional bacteria from the so-called Archaebacteria. These are organisms that inhabit environmentally 'hostile' habitats and include methanogens, extreme halophiles and thermoacidophiles; they are said to form a coherent group of organisms with characteristic isoprenoid lipids and cell wall components (see Woese and Wolfe 1985) and to be survivals from an earlier geological era. Woese (1994) considers that genetic evidence (see section 7.4, p. 9) should take precedence over cellular anatomy in defining the relationships of the prokaryotes and eukaryotes to each other and to these primitive forms.

7.2 Classification of bacteria

Linnaeus (1707–1778) classified plants and animals according to a hierarchical system based on Aristotle's theory of logical division (see Cain 1962) by placing individuals that were alike in 'essential' characters in the same species and then constructing genera and other higher taxa on the basis of progressively greater differences in characters. The selection of essential characters ('weighting') was at first made according to the intuition of the classifier, but post-Darwinian biologists used the fossil record, often supplemented by embryological evidence, to construct classifications of plants and animals that were wholly or in part phylogenetic. This sort of evidence was not available to microbiologists and the apparent absence of sexual reproduction in bacteria meant that the biologists' favoured criterion for the definition of the species, self-fertility, was denied them.

After 1880 the ability to study bacteria in pure culture led to the rapid accumulation of vast amounts of data about their phenotypic characters: colonial appearance, growth on various media, nutritional requirements, biochemical activities, serological relationships, pathogenicity for laboratory animals, and so on. Practical bacteriologists selected sets of key tests that seemed useful in identifying organisms of interest to them and in many cases attached Linnaean binomial epithets to species so characterized. What resulted was not a general classification of bacteria but a series of mini-classifications used by workers in laboratories studying medical, agricultural or various sorts of industrial problems. There was a great deal of duplication in the naming of species and the intuitional handling of complex collections of data led to some uncertainties in classification and identification.

NUMERICAL TAXONOMY

An alternative to seeking 'key' characters had been proposed in 1763 by Adanson, a contemporary of Linnaeus, who considered that biological classification should be based on general similarity in phenotypic characters. He rejected 'weighting' and determined, for each possible pair of individuals in a collection, the proportion of all ascertainable characters that were in accord: the so-called 'overall' similarity. Adanson found the manual computation of similarities between large numbers of pairs excessively laborious and his method could not be employed on a large scale until electronic computers became available. Then, the new discipline of numerical taxonomy was developed (Sneath 1957a, 1957b, Sneath and Sokal 1974) and applied to collections of bacterial cultures that had been studied extensively. This made great contributions to bacterial classification at the levels of species and genus by providing an objective measure of the degree of similarity between large numbers of cultures. However, it is remarkable how often numerical-taxonomic studies supported earlier conclusions arrived at by the intuitional recognition of a 'good' classification as one that placed like organisms in the same taxon. Some taxonomists, for example, Cowan (1962), expressed the view that the bacterial species was simply a man-made artefact, albeit a useful one, designed to put phenotypic data into manageable form. Numerical taxonomy provided a powerful impetus to the 'anti-essentialist' view of bacterial classification, but the practitioners of 2 other disciplines, chemotaxonomy and bacterial genetics, continue to search for 'key characters' that might form a basis for a broad classification of micro-organisms (see Chapter 3).

7.3 Antigenic specificity and chemotaxonomy

In the early years of the twentieth century the antibody response to bacterial antigens had been studied intensively in vitro (see Volume 3, Chapter 1). In the 1920s evidence began to appear of the chemical nature of some of these antigens. This was investigated eagerly by medical bacteriologists because the antigens in question appeared to have some association with pathogenicity. Thus a great deal of information accumulated about certain classes of antigenic macromolecules and some of this was of significance for bacterial classification.

From 1923 onwards, Avery and Heidelberger at the Rockefeller Institute in New York studied the type-specific capsular polysaccharides of pneumococci and showed that antibodies to them conferred type-specific immunity on experimental animals. Rebecca Lancefield, in the same laboratory, described in 1933 the so-called group polysaccharides from the cell walls of haemolytic streptococci; some of these characterized streptococcal groups that caused disease only in certain species of mammals. These polysaccharides had several characters in common:

1 Though determining the specificity of the antibody response they were unable to elicit it when separated from the bacterial body and purified; in 1921 Landsteiner coined the term 'hapten' for such molecules.
2 The specificity of the antibody response to them was relatively limited. Pneumococcal polysaccharides, for example, though defining clear-cut serotypes among pneumococci, cross-reacted widely with polysaccharides of otherwise dissimilar bacteria and even with non-bacterial polysaccharides, as shown by Heidelberger, Austrian and their colleagues. This was explained by the limited repertoire of specificities provided by the sequence of sugars in the terminal part of the polysaccharide chain. The role of the terminal sugars as antigenic determinants was further illuminated by the work of McCarty and Krause on the cross-reactions between streptococcal group antigens.
3 Though sometimes clearly associated with virulence, the polysaccharides were not toxic for experimental animals.

In 1943 Rebecca Lancefield described a class of type-specific cell wall protein antigens in *Streptococcus pyogenes*. Like other proteins they were fully antigenic when extracted and purified. Antibodies to them were highly specific and conferred type-specific immunity. Though non-toxic, these M proteins determined pathogenicity by interfering with phagocytosis.

Certain other cell-bound bacterial constituents proved to have toxic properties when injected into animals. These included the endotoxins of gram-negative bacteria, first described by Boivin and his associates at the Institut Pasteur in Paris in 1932–35. These were complex macromolecules in the cell envelope comprising:

1 a polysaccharide responsible for antigenic specificity
2 a lipid conferring toxicity and
3 a protein that, when linked to the polysachharide, rendered it antigenic.

Studies of the amino-acid composition of the cell walls of gram-positive bacteria by Cummins and Harris in 1956 led to the recognition by Ghysen in 1965 of the structure of their main component, the peptidoglycan or mucopeptide. Schleifer and Kandler in 1972 showed that similarities in the cross-linking of the main components of the peptidoglycan molecule were of value in establishing relationships between bacterial genera that would have been difficult to ascertain by conventional serological means. It has since been noted that all eubacterial peptidoglycans contain *N*-acetyl muramic acid but that this is absent from the cell walls of archaebacteria.

Since 1970 the chemical study of bacterial macromolecules has advanced rapidly. New information about the distribution of particular classes of lipids and isoprenoid quinones has provided grounds for establishing relationships between higher taxa of gram-positive bacteria and for distinguishing eubacteria from archaebacteria (for references see Jones and Krieg 1984).

Protein antigens, when studied by conventional serological methods, showed such a narrow specificity as to limit their value to the identification of species or serotypes. Recent studies of the chemistry of some widely distributed classes of protein, e.g. the cytochromes (Jones 1980) have revealed differences relevant to the general classification of bacteria. The increasing ability to determine the sequence of amino acids in individual proteins will add information to that provided by antigenic analysis. If a constant rate of mutation is assumed, this might be thought to provide evidence of the evolutionary 'distance' between taxa. Such considerations may be attractive to those who favour a phylogenetic approach to bacterial classification.

7.4 Bacterial genetics

At the beginning of the twentieth century it was generally recognized that the characters of bacterial strains in culture might vary, either temporarily, in response to changes in the environment ('adaptation'), or permanently, independent of environmental conditions ('mutation'). The latter phenomenon suggested the possession by bacteria of a genetic system analogous to that of larger organisms, but proof of this was lacking in the absence of a distinct nuclear apparatus.

In 1928 F Griffith demonstrated 'transformation' among pneumococci, that is to say, transfer to a non-capsulate strain of the ability to form capsular polysaccharide of a particular type by contact with a heat-killed culture of a capsulate strain of that type. This indicated a permanent modification of the genetic apparatus of one organism by inanimate material from another. The nature of the transforming material remained unknown until 1944, when Avery, Macleod and McCarty showed that it was deoxyribonucleic acid (DNA).

In 1946 Lederberg and Tatum demonstrated 'recombination' between 2 biochemical mutants of a strain of *Escherichia coli*, each lacking different characters of the wild strain; when placed in cell-to-cell contact a strain with all the parental characters was formed. In this process, 'conjugation' had resulted in the transfer of genetic material between cells. Hayes in 1953 discovered that this was a one-way process in which a small amount of genetic material passed from a donor ('male') to a recipient ('female') cell and was thus different from sexual reproduction in plants and animals. The capacity to donate genetic material in this way depended on possession by the donor of an F (for fertility) factor.

Increasing interest in bacteriophages in the 1940s had revealed that their genetic material became incorporated into that of the bacteria they infected, and in 1952 Zinder and Lederberg showed that on occasion they might take a part of the bacterial genome with them when they left one organism and entered another, a process called transduction. Thus, by the early 1950s it was possible to study the genetics of bacteria by exploiting the phenomena of transformation, recombination and transduction.

Information gained from these genetic studies, together with physicochemical work on the constitution of nucleic acids, played a major role in Watson and Crick's formulation in 1953 of their hypothesis of the genetic code; according to this the information that determines the phenotypic characters of an organism is embodied in paired linear strands of deoxyribonucleotides whose sequence in a particular region constitutes a gene. Most bacterial genes form part of a single, circular chromosome but some are on smaller extrachromosomal closed circles of DNA called plasmids. Plasmid DNA may determine the inheritance of a single character or a few characters; examples are resistance to certain antimicrobial agents or heavy metals, individual biochemical properties, toxin production and virulence. Hayes's F factor, too, is a plasmid, one of a class of plasmids that mediate cell-to-cell transfer of genetic material, usually by means of conjugative pili.

The fact that the code is a sequence of 4 bases, guanine (G), cytosine (C), adenine (A) and thymine (T), had considerable significance for bacterial classification. In 1950 Chargaff had observed that, whatever the source of DNA, it contained equal amounts (in mol) of G and C, and of A and T. However, the ratio of G to A and C to T varied widely. Thus, the mol percentage of G + C came to be used as a measure of the genetic unrelatedness of groups of bacterial taxa. This was of most use in drawing attention to groups that were not easily distinguished by their phenotypic characters, for example, the staphylococci and the micrococci, but had widely differing base compositions. Of course, the converse did not hold: similar base compositions did not necessarily indicate genetic 'nearness'.

Recognition that the base sequence of the DNA determines phenotypic characters suggested that it might provide the ultimate criterion for bacterial classification. At first such sequences could be determined only in small lengths of genome. But in 1961 Schildkraut and coworkers showed that it was possible to measure the total similarity in the sequences of the 2 organisms without knowing the actual sequence in either. This was done by denaturing their DNA into the single-stranded form, mixing preparations from the 2 organisms under appropriate conditions and then measuring the amount of reassociation of the 2 strands. The amount of complementary base-pairing is taken as a measure of the relatedness of the organisms. DNA–DNA pairing provided a great deal of information about the relations between organisms at or around the level of species but gave no grounds for relating the degree of homology to a definition of the species or genus. Indeed, the degree of homology within species previously defined on phenotypic grounds proved to be highly variable and proposals have been made to conflate a number of long-recognized species on the grounds of close genetic similarity.

Studies of DNA–DNA homology proved of little value in revealing broader groups among the bacteria. However, some parts of the genome, notably those coding for the production of ribosomal and transfer RNA, have come to be regarded as more 'conserved' than the rest, that is to say, to have evolved more slowly. Thus, taxonomists with a phylogenetic bent consider that studies of the homology of ribosomal RNA or of the oligonucleotide sequence on the RNA cistrons would be decisive evidence of the evolutionary 'distance' between the higher taxa of bacteria and bacteria-like organisms and thus provide a firm basis for classification (Johnson 1984).

The debate between rival concepts of the pheno-species and genospecies (Hill 1990) is unresolved and perhaps unresolvable. The difference between the 2 schools of thought – the Lockean view that classification is a man-made device for handling information and the Aristotelian concept that the 'essence' of classification is the genetic code – is perhaps better looked upon as a philosophical than a scientific question.

The history of some other aspects of bacteriology – the mechanisms of pathogenicity and of immunity to infection, the antibacterial agents and resistance to them, and laboratory methods of investigating bacterial infections – is summarized briefly in Volume 3 (Volume 3, Chapter 1).

REFERENCES

Bulloch W, 1938, *The History of Bacteriology*, Oxford University Press, London.

Cain AJ, 1962, The evolution of taxonomic principles, *Microbial Classification*, eds Ainsworth GC, Sneath PHA, The University Press, Cambridge, 1–13.

Clark PF, 1961, *Pioneer Microbiologists of America*, University of Wisconsin Press, Madison.

Cowan ST, 1962, The bacterial species – a macromyth?, *Microbial Classification*, eds Ainsworth GC, Sneath PHA, The University Press, Cambridge, 433–55.

Dobell C, 1932, *Antony van Leeuwenhoek and his 'Little Animals'*, John Bale, Sons and Danielson, London.

Foster WD, 1965, *A History of Parasitology*, Livingstone, London and Edinburgh.

Foster WD, 1970, *A History of Medical Microbiology and Immunology*, Heinemann, London.

Gibbons NE, Murray RGE, 1978, Proposals concerning the higher taxa of bacteria, *Int J Syst Bacteriol*, **28**: 1–6.

Hill LR, 1990, Classification and nomenclature of bacteria, *Topley and Wilson's Principles of Bacteriology, Virology and Immunity*, vol. 2, 8th edn, eds Parker MT, Duerden BI, Edward Arnold, London, 20–9.

Johnson DL, 1984, Nucleic acids in bacterial classification, *Bergey's Manual of Systematic Bacteriology*, vol. 1, eds Krieg NR, Holt JG, Williams and Wilkins, Baltimore, 8–11.

Jones CW, 1980, Cytochrome patterns in classification and identification, including their relevance in the oxidase test, *Microbiological Classification and Identification*, Goodfellow M, Board RG, Academic Press, London and New York, 127–38.

Jones D, Krieg NR, 1984, Serology and chemotaxonomy, *Bergey's Manual of Systematic Bacteriology*, vol. 1, eds Krieg NR, Holt JG, Williams and Wilkins, Baltimore, 15–18.

Lechevalier HA, Slotorovsky M, 1965, *Three Centuries of Microbiology*, McGraw-Hill, New York.

Murray RGE, 1962, Fine structure and taxonomy of bacteria, *Microbial Classification*, eds Ainsworth GC, Sneath PHA, The University Press, Cambridge, 119–44.

Schlegel HG, 1984, Global impacts of prokaryocytes and eukaryocytes, *The Microbe*, eds Kelly DP, Carr NG, The University Press, Cambridge, 1–32.

Sneath PHA, 1957a, Some thoughts on bacterial classification, *J Gen Microbiol*, **17**: 184–200.

Sneath PHA, 1957b, The application of computers to taxonomy, *J Gen Microbiol*, **17**: 201–26.

Sneath PHA, Sokal RR, 1974, *Numerical Taxonomy: the Principles and Practice of Numerical Classification*, WH Freeman, San Francisco.

Stanier RY, van Niel CB, 1941, The main outlines of bacterial classification, *J Bacteriol*, **42**: 437–66.

Topley WWC, Wilson GS, 1931, *The Principles of Bacteriology and Immunity*, vol. 2, 1st edn, Edward Arnold, London, 591–4.

Vallery-Radot R, 1919, *The Life of Pasteur*, English translation by Mrs RL Devonshire, Constable, London.

Vallery-Radot R, 1922–33, *Oeuvres de Pasteur*, 6 vols, Masson, Paris.

Woese CR, 1994, There must be a prokaryote somewhere: microbiology's search for itself, *Microbiol Rev*, **58**: 1–9.

Woese CR, Wolfe RS, eds, 1985, *The Bacteria, a Treatise on Structure and Function: vol. 8 Archaebacteria*, eds Gunsalus IC, Stanier RY, Academic Press, London and New York.

Chapter 2

STRUCTURE–FUNCTION RELATIONSHIPS IN PROKARYOTIC CELLS

S C Holt and E R Leadbetter

1 INTRODUCTION

According to a current widely accepted interpretation, cells that are themselves unicellular organisms or exist as a group to constitute a multicellular organism are categorized as Archaea (formerly: archaeo- or archaebacteria), bacteria or Eukarya. Perhaps the most significant characteristic of Archaea and bacteria that distinguishes them from the Eukarya is the absence of a membrane surrounding the nuclear region; the presence of such a membrane is a defining trait of cells of Eukarya. The structure of archaeal and bacterial cells is termed **prokaryotic**, whereas those with a membrane-bounded nucleus are termed **eukaryotic**. Prokaryotic cells have, generally, much smaller dimensions than most eukaryotic cells, lack the subcellular organelles (e.g. chloroplasts, mitochondria) typical of most eukaryotes, and contain ribosomes smaller in size than those of eukaryotes.

Biologists have long recognized that the greater the surface-to-volume ratio of a cell the greater is the metabolic activity of the cell and, usually, the rate of cell division. If one assumes that the diameter of a typical prokaryotic cell is 1 μm and that of a eukaryotic cell 10 μm, the volume of the former cell is some 8000 times less than the latter; that smaller cell, however, has a surface area approximately 20 times greater than the larger cell. A consequence, then, of the small dimensions of prokaryotic cells is that they have the potential to consume their sources of energy for growth, and produce metabolic end products at rates far greater than do eukaryotic cells; accordingly, in a finite period of time they have a far greater impact on the environment in which they are functioning. As a group the prokaryotes are far more versatile, in the metabolic sense, than are eukaryotes and are able to thrive in a range of environments that seem unusual, if not extreme, by comparison to those inhabited by animals and plants. This combination of traits – high metabolic rate, short generation time, and ability to use an infinite array of energy sources both chemical (i.e. inorganic as well as organic) and physical (e.g. radiant energy) and a wide variety of oxidants other than molecular oxygen (e.g. carbonate, ferric iron, nitrate, sulphate, various organic molecules) – enables prokaryotic cells to compete very effectively with those of eukaryotes not only in the natural environment in which animals and plants thrive, but also on or within these animals and plants, i.e. when host-associated (Stanier et al. 1986, Schlegel 1993, White 1995).

Another consequence of the small size of prokaryotes is the restriction placed on the number of molecules that can be present in a cell at any given time. Apart from water, which constitutes 70–80% of the cell mass, the major organic components are proteins (approximately 50% of the cell dry weight). A 1 μm diameter cell is estimated to contain in the order of 100 000 protein molecules, but a much smaller number of polysaccharide, lipid and nucleic acid molecules. The synthesis of cellular components is, energetically speaking, an expensive process and in the course of their long evolution on the planet, prokaryotic cells have come to regulate (by processes termed **induction, repression or end product inhibition**) these syntheses to produce only those enzymes and other cellular components required for metabolism and growth in a particular environment. Although prokaryotes are constrained by size as to the number of enzyme molecules they contain, they none the less are able to adapt for survival in different environments by altering the number, nature, or type of the proteins they synthesize. On the other hand, those cellular components that must be present at all times in the life of a cell and are concerned with energy conservation and protein and nucleic acid synthesis are usually not subject to induction or repression; these syntheses are termed **constitutive**. However, not all prokaryotes are endowed with equally enormous physiological flexibility (Brock et al. 1993, Schlegel 1993); some organisms are able to thrive in only a few habitats, or by a single type of physiology (e.g. are obligately chemolithotrophic or phototrophic or are obligately dependent upon growth within a particular type of host cell). No other biota appear to be so diverse in their traits and the habitats they occupy as are the prokaryotes (Leadbetter 1997).

Thus, the ability to adapt and alter cellular traits is not without limits, and is a direct consequence of the genetic composition of the particular organism. The recent mapping of the complete nucleotide sequence of *Haemophilus influenzae* and *Mycoplasma genitalium* (Fleischmann et al. 1995, Fraser et al. 1995) has provided the first firm indication of the number of genes on any prokaryotic chromosome, and vindicates earlier suggestions that the chromosome of the well studied *Escherichia coli* contains c. 3000 genes (Krawiec and Riley 1990). Additional physical and genetic maps of genomes of prokaryotes are certain to become abundant in the near future (e.g. Gaeher et al. 1996).

This chapter will discuss general as well as some specialized features of prokaryotic cell size, shape and architecture and will integrate consideration of structural features of selected bacteria with a discussion of the synthesis of these components and the ability of the organisms to survive and function.

2 MORPHOLOGICAL EXAMINATION OF PROKARYOTIC CELLS: MICROSCOPY

The visual observation of structural detail requires the use of a specific type of radiation. This radiation, or wavelength, is the limiting factor in the visualization of any structural detail in that a specific radiation is not capable of visualizing structure smaller than its own wavelength. Therefore, as discussed below, the limiting resolving power of the light microscope, that is, the ability to distinguish clearly 2 points as individual points, is a function of the wavelength of visible light; in the case of the light microscope these wavelengths are between 400 nm (violet light) and 700 nm (red light). The small size of most known prokaryotes limits the study of their morphology to microscopic techniques. The fact that the unaided human eye cannot resolve objects less than 0.1 mm apart mandates the use of microscopes for the visualization of prokaryotic cells. The light microscope has long been an excellent instrument for the examination of many bac-

terial properties. Shapes are readily discernible, motility easily determined and some internal cell features (e.g. endospores, granules) noted. The light microscope employs visible light and glass lenses to form the image of the object. The best light microscopes, using the most advanced optics, are capable of magnifications of 1000–2000 ×. In addition to the quality of the lenses (optics), the ability to resolve cells and to discern their shape and detail is also a function of the wavelength of light employed; the standard laboratory microscope, which uses visible light of wavelengths 400–600 nm and an objective lens with a numerical aperture of 1.3, is capable of resolving objects as small as 0.21 µm (Fig. 2.1).

The electron microscope employs electromagnetic lenses and electrons for the formation of an image. These instruments provide superb resolving power, and their ability to magnify images is limited only by their capability to generate high and stable voltages (higher voltage and shorter wavelength permits higher resolving power and magnification).

2.1 Light microscopy

There are 6 main techniques of light microscopy: brightfield, phase contrast, darkfield, interference, fluorescence and confocal (laser) microscopy. The reader is referred to any basic consideration of microscope optics (e.g. Kapitza 1994) for a complete discussion of the various instruments and their light paths.

Brightfield microscopy is the most common of the light microscopic techniques. The microscopic optics are such that the bacteria, usually stained, appear dark against a brightly illuminated field. The bacteria appear this way since they do not absorb light at the wavelengths of visible light employed. Enhancement of the contrast between the bacterial cells and surrounding background usually necessitates

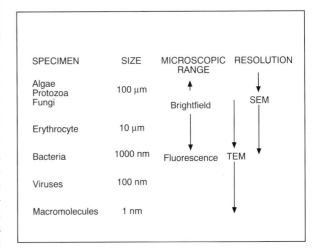

Fig. 2.1 Comparison of cell sizes of representative biological specimens and the different forms of microscopy often used for their visualization. The ability of the different microscopes to resolve objects is indicated by the vertical arrows. (Modified from Slots and Taubman 1992).

application of one or several stains, using standardized procedures.

Phase contrast microscopy is used routinely for the examination of wet-mount preparations (i.e. unstained cells). The human eye is constructed such that although it can discern differences in light intensity, it cannot detect differences in phases. Phase contrast microscopy has as its basis the artificial transfer of phase differences into brightness or intensity differences and is superior to brightfield microscopy in that living, unstained specimens are observed clearly because of slight differences in their thickness and density, i.e. differences in refractive index (see below). These slight differences in refractive index are amplified such that they are translated into intensity differences, producing an image of much greater contrast. The major optical differences between the brightfield microscope and the phase contrast microscope are the substitution of a specialized substage condenser and different objective lenses. To intensify the phase differences, an optical component, a **phase annulus**, is added to the objective lens. Corresponding to the objective annulus is a **fixed annular phase ring** present in the substage condenser. Light entering the condenser is separated into 2 components: one which passes through the periphery of the field, and one which passes directly through the specimen. Light leaving the surface of the specimen enters the objective lens where it encounters a **phase ring** of the same geometry as that found in the condenser. The objective lens phase ring optically shifts the light emerging from the top of the specimen at least one-quarter wavelength (i.e. it becomes one-quarter wavelength out of phase). Since this incident light is both refracted and diffracted because of differences in the density and thickness of the specimen (refractive index), specimen brightness will appear either greater (in phase) or lower (out of phase). Bacteria examined by phase contrast microscopy appear dark against a light background.

Darkfield microscopy produces images that are reversed from those of brightfield and phase contrast microscopy. The images appear bright against a dark background and the specimen appears to be illuminated against the dark background. The major modification of the microscope for darkfield microscopy is the incorporation of a large central opaque 'stop' in the substage condenser; this prevents the direct axial illumination of the specimen. Thus, light rays reach the specimen only from the periphery and at an angle that exceeds the light collecting angle of the objective lens. Accordingly, only light that is scattered by the specimen will enter the objective lens, producing the high contrast of the specimen. Darkfield microscopy is particularly useful for examining very thin, living specimens (e.g. many spirochaetes) which, because of their slender diameter, would be nearly invisible by brightfield and phase contrast microscopy.

2.2 Fluorescent microscopy

As discussed above, the visualization of biological structural detail requires well constructed lenses, and suitable wavelengths of light. These 2 factors, lens construction and wavelength, limit the resolution of the microscope. However, even with this limitation, it is possible to increase specimen detail. Since the majority of a cell's content is water (70–80% or greater), various cellular substructures are virtually invisible to the eye, even when the best lenses are employed. The introduction of stains has provided a technique for the visualization of cell structure. So, for example, malachite green is useful for the visualization of bacterial spores, Sudan black B reveals cellular lipids, whereas Feulgen stains are capable of revealing the nucleoid. Haematoxylin, used for many years as a general stain of mammalian cells, is excellent for the visualization of negatively charged molecules such as acidic proteins, and RNA and DNA. Coomassie brilliant blue, an organic dye used almost universally in staining proteins after polyacrylamide electrophoresis, has also been used for detecting cellular proteins in prokaryotes. However, although several of the organic stains are specific for a particular chemical compound, the majority of them are non-specific. This lack of specificity has resulted in the development of specific probes such as the fluorescent dyes.

Fluorescence and **interference microscopy** take advantage of the fact that many organic compounds fluoresce when illuminated with ultraviolet radiation. These organic dyes (**fluorochromes**) have the ability to absorb light at one wavelength and to emit this light as a different colour at another wavelength. Therefore, illumination of these fluorescent dyes at one wavelength (i.e. its absorbing wavelength), and viewing through a specific filter which specifically absorbs this wavelength but passes the light of the emitted wavelength (emission wavelength), results in fluorescence against a dark background. The fact that the background is dark permits detection of even very dim fluorescence so very small numbers of fluorescent cells can be detected (Kepner and Pratt 1994).

The optics of this microscopy include the use of 2 optical filters: an **exciter filter** functions to remove all light except that of a specific wavelength desired (e.g. blue light), and a **barrier filter** removes the 'exciting' light and permits the emergence of emitted light of a different wavelength (e.g. green light) that can be visualized. The fluorescence approach permits identification and enumeration of specific cell types, localization of specific reactive molecules and the measurement of membrane potentials. The methanogenic archaeans, for example, contain a unique cofactor that fluoresces when excited, thus permitting the rapid and specific detection of methanogens when they are present, even in a mixed bacterial population. The fluorescence microscope has been used very successfully to localize specific antibodies to intact cells as well as to cell components (Manafi, Kneifel and Bascomb 1991, Pogiliano, Harry and Losick 1995). A fluorochrome such as fluorescein or rhodamine can be chemically linked (tagged) to an antibody formed to a specific antigenic cell component (e.g. a protein) and used to localize the component in or on a living cell. The fluorescein dye emits an intense green fluorescence when excited in blue light, and rhodamine emits a red fluorescence when excited in green-yellow light. Thus, not only can these dyes be used separately, but they can be used together with 2 antibodies to tag 2 different molecules in the same cell. In addition, the specific antibody-fluorescent tag can be used to assess changes, kinetically, in the localization of the antibody (hence to the cell antigen to which it was formed) in response to external stimuli and/or changes in environment. Another useful feature of many fluorochromes is that they are able to function in a manner analogous to that of pH indicators with colour changes of the dye being reflective of physiological changes within the cell.

2.3 Confocal microscopy

The entire specimen is uniformly and simultaneously illuminated in addition to its focus within the focal plane of the objective. The result of this optical path is the formation of out-of-focus images both above and below the focal plane of the specimen. These out-of-focus images result in a reduction in contrast and in resolution, which decreases the ability to discern fine detail and structure. The basis of the confocal microscope is such that the illumination produced by the light source is focused as a spot at specific specimen planes. As the illuminating spot is focused above and below the plane of focus, specimen components farther away from the focal plane receive less light and therefore less illumination, which results in a reduction in the amount of out-of-focus information available. To remedy this both the illumination and detection systems are simultaneously focused on a single area of the specimen in such a way that the specimen image signals in the focal plane are detected, and signals outside or away from the specimen are removed by a filter. Thus, the basic concept of confocal microscopy is that the illumination, the specimen and the detection system are all at the same focus – they are confocal.

The original design of the confocal microscope was that of Minsky at Harvard University. The most significant advantage and novel feature of this microscope is its extended dynamic range such that an almost infinite number of aperture planes are available; this permits studies of the optical properties of a specimen, and the relationship between one component (e.g. an invading bacterium) and its host. The use of specific antibodies to selected bacterial components, to viruses and to specific antimicrobial agents permits the real-time visualization of the organization within a cell. The design of the confocal microscope includes replacement of the condenser lens with a lens identical to the objective lens. The major goal of confocal microscopy is to reduce the field of illumination to a very small point-light source such that a pinhole of light is obtained. The basis of the optics is to form images of a very thin plane of a specimen and to limit peripheral and out-of-focus light. This is achieved by limiting the field of illumination by introducing a pinhole at the level of the microscope axis. In this way a reduced image of the pinhole of illumination is projected onto a specimen screen by the condenser lens. A second pinhole is also introduced at the level of the image plane which is placed confocally to the illuminated spot of the specimen and the first pinhole. Thus, the ideal confocal optics are those that employ perfectly matched condenser and objective lenses with infinitely small apertures. It is the apertures that are scanned relative to the specimen to image the field of view.

The image of the specimen is captured by scanning its surface with the point light source in a raster pattern similar to that for scanning electron microscopy. However, in confocal microscopy, the light passing the specimen is modulated by the thickness of the specimen and a second pinhole. The light differences that are generated produce the final image. A major component in the formation of the confocal image of the specimen is the **Nipkow disc**, which functions to scan the light beam. This disc functions to transfer a 2-dimensional optical image into an electrical signal which is transferred as a one-dimensional time-dependent signal over an electrical wire. This is achieved by the use of 2 tandemly placed discs consisting of a series of matching holes arranged around the periphery of the circle at a constant angle from its centre. The holes are such that the pinhole of light produced matches the pinhole in the viewing aperture. When placed at the level of the specimen, and rotated at a constant speed, raster scanning of the specimen surface results in the separation of individual brightness patterns of the specimen. It is these brightness differences, which are separated by the holes in the disc, that are transmitted to a photoelectric cell. The individual differences represent the brightness of the sequentially scanned image. This output of the photoelectric cell drives a neon bulb, which when viewed through another part of the Nipkow disc produces the final picture of the individual images.

During the past several years, considerable emphasis has been placed on developing confocal instrumentation with improved light scanning designs. The major outcome of these advances was the scanning laser design. The laser replaces the pinholes of the rotating Nipkow discs with a beam of coherent laser light. The scanning function of the discs is replaced by scanning the laser beam across the specimen with either mirrors or acoustic–optic couplers. The light generated is detected with a photomultiplier and visualized on an oscilloscope.

2.4   Electron microscopy

The **transmission electron microscope** (electrons are transmitted through the specimen) was the invention of Ruska and Marton in 1934. As seen in Fig. 2.2, the electron microscope is basically identical in its lens configurations to that of the basic light microscope (Fig. 2.2), but whereas this employs glass lenses, electron microscopes utilize circular electromagnetic lenses. Glass lenses have a fixed focal point, whereas in the electromagnetic lens this feature varies as a function of the voltage applied to the magnetic lens. The lenses are the condenser coil, an objective and a projector lens, the latter comparable to the eyepiece in a brightfield microscope.

Since the wavelength of light is a function of the speed with which an electron travels, applying significantly high voltages permits the electrons to move with considerable speed through the various electromagnetic lenses. Wavelengths of 10^{-5}–10^{-6}, that of visible light, are achieved in modern electron microscopes, and produce magnifications capable of discerning atomic structure.

Because water absorbs electrons, dehydrated specimens are routinely examined in these microscopes. Whole cells are also often examined after negative staining (with phosphotungstate, for example). Quite often very thin specimen sections are examined, and these ultrathin sections are examined either directly or first stained with heavy metals (lead, uranium) to increase their electron density. Aside from results obtained by the use of specialized techniques (freeze-fracture etching, shadow-casting), the transmission electron microscope produces a one-dimensional image of the specimen. Newer techniques of freeze-substitution and other low-temperature procedures are replacing the standard chemical fixation and organic dehydration procedures in the study of biological structure (Graham 1992).

The **scanning electron microscope** (Fig. 2.2), which provides a 3-dimensional image of the specimen, employs the principle of a demagnified electron beam which is focused to an electron point (probe) of c. 0.1 mm. The beam is projected and moves over the surface of the specimen in a raster motion, and a picture is formed, in a way not unlike that on a television screen. Probing the specimen surface with the concentrated electron beam results in the emission of secondary electrons as a result of electron–electron interactions in the specimen surface. These secondary, or 'back-scattered' electrons are then collected by a positively charged collector and transferred to a scintillator. The scintillator generates protons which are visualized on a fluorescent screen. The resolution provided by the scanning electron microscope is of the order of 5–10 μm.

Use of these different microscopic approaches has played a significant role in the elucidation of the structure of both eukaryotic and prokaryotic cells and extended our analysis and understanding of cell functions. Standard light microscopy, although permitting the examination of living cells and providing some understanding of the dynamic processes of cell movement and interaction, is limited in its ability to discern ultrastructural features of cell interiors and exteriors because of its inherent limit in resolution. Fluor-

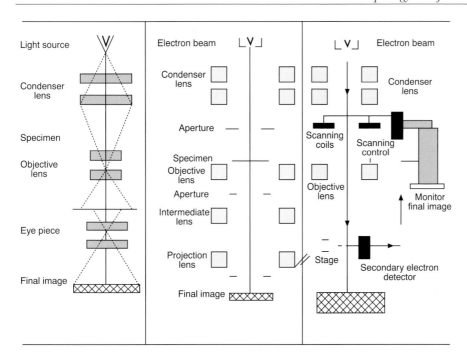

Fig. 2.2 Comparison of the optical paths of the light (left), transmission (centre) and scanning electron microscopes (right). (From Holt and Beveridge 1982).

escence and interference light microscopy provide some additional increase in resolution and additional details of structure, but this increase is also significantly limited in scope. Electron microscopy extends the study of biological structure and function to the realm of atomic dimensions. It permits analysis of internal as well as external structural cell details, including the distribution of selected atoms within and on cells. However, the preparative techniques required for transmission and scanning electron microscopic analyses result in significant specimen modification. Transmission electron microscopy provides significant resolution, but it provides only a static, 2-dimensional image. Particularly for prokaryotic cells, these images are difficult (but not impossible) to reconstruct to provide a 3-dimensional perspective. The introduction of confocal microscopy has brought significant advances in the examination of cells, especially in dynamic terms: how cells interact with other cells, and with their environment (Matsumoto 1993).

3 MORPHOLOGY AND FUNCTION OF THE PROKARYOTIC CELL

Three fundamental characteristics are often considered to distinguish prokaryotes from the eukaryotes typified by animals and plants: small size, absence of a complex, organelle-containing cytoplasm, and the absence of a nuclear membrane (Table 2.1). The vast majority of prokaryotic cells are quite small, having diameters of 1 μm and less, with the bacteria often said to range in size between the larger viruses (e.g. 'pox') and erythrocytes, but there are many exceptions; many bacteria are less than 1 μm in diameter, and many species have diameters much greater (*Thiovulum* 5–15 μm; *Thiospirillum* 2.5–4 μm), and lengths many times (*Oscillatoria* 100 μm; *Beggiatoa* 50–100 μm) that of *E. coli* (2–6 μm). Although not yet cultivated, one prokaryote, *Epulopiscium fishelsoni*, obtained from the gut of a fish, has dimensions of 80 × 600 μm. The wall-less *Mycoplasma* represent some of the smallest cultivable prokaryotes, ranging as they do in diameter from 0.12 to 0.25 μm. However, some eukaryotes have size dimensions that overlap with even the smaller prokaryotes (Courties et al. 1994).

Prokaryotes not only vary greatly in size but they also exist in different shapes. Examples of the more common bacterial shapes are sketched in Fig. 2.3. Many are spherical and exist as single cells (cocci), whereas other cocci regularly exist as chains of cells (streptococci, as in the genus *Streptococcus*); other cocci divide in 2 planes and exist as tetrads, others divide in 3 planes and form regular aggregates of 8 or more cells (sarcinae, genus *Sarcina*); still others as irregular clusters of spherical cells (staphylococci, genus *Staphylococcus*). A rod-shaped cell is often termed a bacillus, as in *Bacillus* and *Lactobacillus*; some rods are partially curved (vibrioid, genus *Vibrio*) whereas others form nearly a closed circle (cyclobacilli, genus *Cyclobacillus*). A cell with several pronounced curvatures, as in a spiral, is termed a spirillum (as in the genus *Spirillum*) whereas those with even more helical aspects (spirochaetes) are given generic designations such as *Leptospira*, *Spirochaeta*, *Borrelia*, *Treponema*, *Cristispira*. Cells that have the shape of rectangles and triangles are also known, as are some that are square. Not all cells of prokaryotes have uniform surfaces (as *Caulobacter*, a cell with 'stalks'; *Hyphomicrobium*, with 'buds' and hypha-like connections; *Sulpholobus*, more or less a coccus but with an uneven, or lobed surface). Some have a sheath surrounding the cell (*Sphaerotilus*) whereas others have a loose-fitting coat (*Thermotoga*).

Figure 2.4 describes diagrammatically the basic differences between the ultrastructure of eukaryotes (Fig. 2.4a) and prokaryotes (Fig. 2.4b). Immediately apparent in Fig. 2.4b is the stark simplicity of the prokaryotic cytoplasm – its absence of unit membrane-limited organelles and a nuclear membrane surrounding the nuclear material (Beveridge 1989). For ease of presen-

Table 2.1 Major characteristics of eukaryotes and prokaryotes

	Eukaryotes	Prokaryotes
Major groups	Algae, fungi, protozoa, plants, animals	Bacteria
Size (approx.)	>5 μm	1×3 μm
Nuclear structure	Nuclear membrane	None
Chromosome type	Strands of DNA	Single, closed, linear DNA
Cytoplasmic structures		
Mitochondria	+	–
Golgi apparatus	+	–
Endoplasmic reticulum	+	–
Ribosomes	80S	70S
Cytoplasmic membrane	+; sterols	+; no sterols[a]
Cell wall	–; or + with cellulose/chitin	Complex peptidoglycan:
Reproduction	Sexual/asexual	Binary fission
Movement	Flagella complex when present	Flagella simple when present

[a]See text.

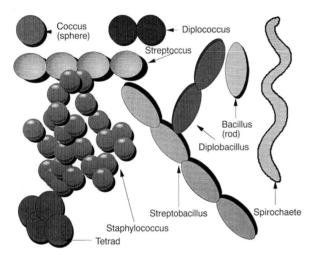

Fig. 2.3 Diagrammatic representation of some different shapes of prokaryotic cells.

tation, the morphology of typical prokaryotic cells, both gram-negative and gram-positive, is discussed, beginning with their most internal anatomy (nuclear region) to their most external surfaces (walls, capsules, fimbriae, flagella). Where appropriate, the synthesis and assembly of the major prokaryotic cell structures are also described.

3.1 Cytoplasmic region

The cytoplasmic (or, cell) membrane encloses the extensive electron-dense region, termed the **cytoplasm**, or **cytoplasmic region** (Fig. 2.5a, b). The cytoplasm consists of the nuclear region (nucleoid) and a large number of **ribosomes** and **polysomes** that surround and intercalate the nucleoid, as well as an array of low molecular weight (MW) organic molecules and inorganic ions, in addition to water. The cytoplasm may contain granules or inclusions such as starch, glycogen, poly-β-hydroxyalkanoates, sulphur globules, magnetosomes, parasporal bodies, gas vesicles and endospores. All these components are bathed in the aqueous portion of the cytoplasm (cytosol), which also contains non-ribosomal proteins, some transfer RNA (tRNA), and the array of organic and inorganic molecules required for biosynthesis; this array includes low MW organic compounds such as coenzymes, fatty and organic acids, nucleotides and nucleosides, inorganic ions, etc. The commingling of these molecules with the cell's biosynthetic apparatus for macromolecular syntheses (polysomes, RNA, DNA) in the cytoplasm permits the rapid synthesis of essential bacterial anatomical components (cell wall, lipopolysaccharide, other membrane lipids, membrane proteins) and it helps account for the very high metabolic rates and reproduction characteristics of most bacteria.

Mycoplasma genitalium is considered to have the smallest genome known for free-living bacteria, being approximately one-fifth (580 kb) the size estimated for *E. coli*. Depending upon the bacterial growth rate, cells contain from one to several nucleoids, with each nucleoid containing an entire chromosome. In addition to DNA, the chromosome has associated with it a small amount of RNA (in the form of RNA polymerase) and some histone-like proteins.

3.2 Nucleus (nucleoid)

The absence of a nuclear membrane in cells defines them as prokaryotes and different from eukaryotic cells, all the latter of which have a unit nuclear membrane which encloses a multi-chromosomal nucleus. The nuclear material (Robinow and Kellenberger 1994) of prokaryotic cells occupies a great deal of the central, core region of the cell (Figs 2.4b, 2.5a, b). In most bacteria studied (Cole and Saint Girons 1994), the chromosome(s) consists of a single, naked, closed circular DNA molecule (see Fig. 2.6a). Linear, as well as circular plasmids have been found in some bacteria (see below) (Fig. 2.6b). The genes carried on plasmid DNA encode contrasting functions as diverse as resistance to antibiotics and the ability to degrade a hydrocarbon as a source of carbon and energy for growth, and genes which encode major outer-membrane proteins. Some plasmids are notable because they are

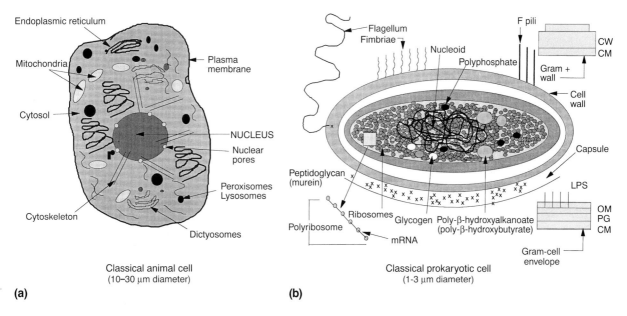

Fig. 2.4 Diagrammatic comparison of structural features of (a) eukaryotic and (b) prokaryotic cells. A typical eukaryotic cell contains numerous membrane-limited organelles (e.g. nucleus, mitochondria) whereas prokaryotic cells are devoid of these. Depicted in (b) are subcellular entities commonly found in prokaryotic cells and a comparison of the different layers associated with gram-positive and gram-negative cells. CM, cytoplasmic membrane; CW, cell wall; OM, outer membrane; PG, peptidoglycan.

involved in transfer of genetic material from one cell to another; some may exist in multiple copies, in contrast to the chromosome, which ordinarily is considered to exist in a single copy (except during its replication).

Electron micrographs of thin sections reveal the electron-dense fibrils (Fig. 2.5a, b) of the nucleoid. Chemical and physical studies established these fibrils to be DNA, with a MW of c. 10^6 kDa. The DNA is not only present as a single circular and closed molecule (Fig. 2.6), but unfolded it has been estimated to span a distance of about 1 mm; it occupies as much as 10% of the cell volume. It is no small feat, then, to have such a length of material duplicated and packaged in a cell that is perhaps only c. 3 µm in length. Although the majority of the best-studied prokaryotes have chromosomes that are circular closed molecules, more recent studies employing newer analytical techniques such as pulse field electrophoresis reveal that some cells (e.g. *Borrelia burgdorferi*, several streptomycetes) have linear DNA elements (Fig. 2.6b).

The formation of a cell and its component parts requires the complex interaction between the cell's DNA and RNA. The end products of these interactions (DNA replication, transcription and translation), are the cell's proteins. In DNA replication, parent DNA is duplicated, and transferred to the daughter cells. With only minor errors (or mutations) the DNA molecule is routinely and faithfully replicated. In many prokaryotic cells, the DNA is a circular chromosome (see Fig. 2.6a) and in the process of replication one end of the mother DNA molecule is attached to cytoplasmic membrane, and remains with the mother cell, while the replicated molecule is transferred to the daughter cell. As seen in Fig. 2.7, this process of replication provides for the equal transfer of the DNA molecule.

DNA REPLICATION

The faithful replication of the prokaryotic DNA molecule requires that it first be unwound at a specific point on the chromosome, the origin, and the formation of the new DNA strand occurs along the unwound linear molecule (Fig. 2.7). The enzyme, **DNA polymerase**, is essential for this initial duplication. Synthesis of the new DNA strands occurs from both ends of the unwound DNA strand until 2 replication forks, which are formed during synthesis, meet at a specific point, or terminus 180° from the origin. Since the DNA strands are exact complementary sequences of each other, each of the newly synthesized strands will therefore be an exact complementary copy itself.

PROTEIN SYNTHESIS, RIBOSOMES AND POLYSOMES

As shown in Fig. 2.5b (see p. 18), the cytoplasmic region of a well studied bacterium (i.e. *E. coli*) consists predominantly of small, electron-dense particles. These particles, the ribosomes, are the location for all bacterial protein synthesis. The functioning ribosome translates (**translation**) the information encoded in messenger RNAs (mRNA) into the amino acid sequences of proteins. Ribosomes are complex units comprised of ribonucleoproteins (Fig. 2.8). They are c. 25 nm in their longest dimension, and comprise c. 20% of the dry weight of a typical bacterium. Physical analyses reveal the ribosome to have a sedimentation rate of 70 Svedberg (S) units, and are different in size due to the number of nucleotides found in the prokaryotic ribosome, as well as several other important properties (see Fig. 2.8 and Table 2.2).

Chemical analysis reveals the ribosome to be composed of 50 different proteins associated with 3 types of RNA. **Ribosomal (r)RNA** is composed of 3 subunits of sizes 23S, 16S and 5S. rRNA is the most abundant of the RNAs, accounting for almost 80% of the total; **tRNA** amounts to about 15% of the

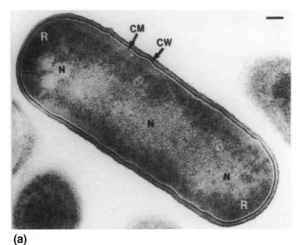

(a)

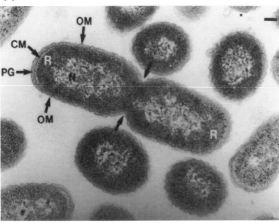

(b)

Fig. 2.5 Transmission electron photomicrographs of the prokaryotic cells (a) *Bacillus subtilis* (gram-positive) and (b) *Escherichia coli* (gram-negative). CM, cytoplasmic membrane; CW, cell wall; N, nuclear region; OM, outer membrane; PG, peptidoglycan; R, ribosomes. Note in (b) that the nuclear material is nearly equally distributed between cells in the process of dividing. The arrows point to the region of transverse cell division. (From Slots and Taubman 1992).

RNA, and **messenger (m)RNA** accounts for only 4% of the total cellular RNA. The prokaryotic ribosomes differ from their eukaryotic counterparts in that the latter are heavier and categorized as '80S'.

Close examination of ribosome structure reveals that many of them exist not as single, or individual units, but rather that they are joined together in a way similar to 'beads on a string' (see Fig. 2.4b, p. 17). Chemical analysis revealed that the 'string' is mRNA, and the term used for ribosomes physically connected by the mRNA is **polysome**. During active growth and rapid protein synthesis almost all (80–90%) ribosomes exist as polysomes. Figure 2.9 provides a diagrammatic representation of the basic elements of prokaryotic protein synthesis.

In the translation of a gene into its protein, polysomes are attached to a specific gene (i.e. DNA) encoded on the mRNA. The polysomes increase in length during the interaction, a characteristic of the transcription of the gene into mRNA. Evidence indicates that RNA polymerase is associated at the junction of the gene and the mRNA; it has been hypothesized further that the individual ribosomes of the polysome unit move along the mRNA strand, synthesizing pro-

tein in the process. The completed protein is then transported by specific transport mechanisms to specific locations in the cell.

TRANSCRIPTION

The genetic information contained in the bacterial DNA is only useful to the cell if it can be used for the formation of new cellular material. This translation of the genetic information into specific proteins takes place in the cell's ribosomes. mRNA serves as a template for the formation of the primary protein structure, and functions to transfer the genetic information contained in the DNA molecule to the ribosome, where protein synthesis occurs. Thus the mRNA molecule functions to link the information content of DNA with the information needed for synthesis of the appropriate polypeptide by the ribosome. The mRNA is a single-stranded molecule which is synthesized on the transcriptional DNA strand – thus it is a complementary copy of the information in that DNA strand.

DNA transcription is representative of RNA synthesis and involves the synthesis of the 3 cellular RNAs, mRNA, tRNA and rRNA. Whereas the transcription of the DNA molecule to RNA is essentially identical to that of DNA replication, RNA synthesis requires a **DNA-dependent RNA polymerase**, and occurs in 3 distinct phases. The first is **initiation**, in which the polymerase with the aid of a specific protein (σ factor), attaches to a specific DNA sequence, or promoter, and the formation of a stable **RNA polymerase–DNA initiation complex**. **Elongation** of the RNA molecule then follows, in which the RNA polymerase moves along the DNA template strand. RNA synthesis ends with a **termination** event and the dissolution of the polymerase complex.

TRANSLATION

Translation is the final event in the synthesis of a protein. It represents the interaction between mRNA (which carries the codon for the synthesis of a specific amino acid), and the anticodon (tRNA). tRNA specifically transfers the genetic information carried in the mRNA into functional protein.

The amino acids formed from the information carried in the mRNA codon is transferred to a tRNA specific for that particular amino acid. Interaction of the tRNA–amino acid, ribosome, ATP, and specific cofactors on the ribosome results in the formation of a specific polypeptide chain (i.e. protein). The tRNA–amino acid complex (charged tRNA) is situated on the ribosome such that it can form a peptide bond with an adjacent tRNA–amino acid.

The functional protein is the result of its primary (amino acid sequence), secondary (folding), and tertiary (coiling) structure. Protein export then transports the protein to specific cellular locations. In the majority of cases of protein export, the N-terminal end of the protein contains a specific sequence of 15–30 amino acids. These **signal sequence proteins**, which are of similar charge or hydrophobicity, function to mediate the attachment of the new polypeptide to the cytoplasmic membrane. After binding, the signal sequence is released, and moves back into the cytoplasm, degraded back to single amino acids, to be used again in protein synthesis.

3.3 Intracellular storage materials

The synthesis and accumulation of intracellular inclusions in different prokaryotes is usually dependent upon both nutrient availability and environmental growth conditions (e.g. pH, redox potential). The insoluble inclusions or granules deposited in the cytoplasm are osmotically inert, neutral polymers.

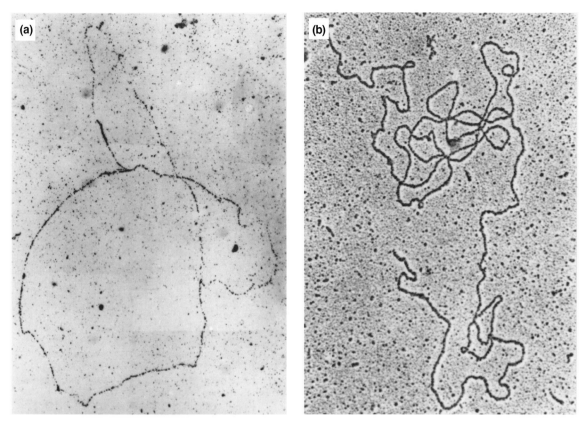

Fig. 2.6 Electron micrograph of circular bacterial chromosome (a) isolated from *E. coli* and a linear plasmid and (b) from *Borrelia burgdorferi*. In (a), the chromosome was obtained by osmotic lysis directly on to the surface of a grid used in electron microscopy and the preparation then shadow-cast using a heavy metal so as to reveal the chromosome. In (b) the 49 kb plasmid is seen prior to treatment with a nuclease which prevents rapid renaturation of the plasmid DNA after alkaline denaturation. [(a), from Cairns 1963; (b), from Barbour and Garon 1987].

Although most are organic in character, several are inorganic. Limitation in nutrients such as nitrogen, sulphur, phosphorus, acetate, or the existence of other unfavourable growth conditions often results in assimilation of excess available carbon into 'storage' granules. These include polysaccharides (starch, glycogen) and lipids – commonly poly-β-hydroxyalkanoic acids (PHA), of which poly-β-hydroxybutyrate (PHB) is one of the best known. Inorganic phosphate is polymerized into polyphosphate (volutin) granules, and sulphide can be oxidized to form globules of elemental sulphur. In most instances these storage products disappear when they are degraded to products used in metabolism and growth.

POLYSACCHARIDE

Starch and glycogen, the most commonly recognized polysaccharide inclusions formed in bacteria, are polymers of D-glucose linked in helical chains by 1,4-glycosidic bonds (Fig. 2.10a). *Clostridium*, *Acetobacter* and *Neisseria* spp. are examples known to store starch. Members of the genera *Bacillus*, *Escherichia*, *Micrococcus* and *Salmonella* are known to form glycogen when under growth stress in the presence of excess D-glucose. Glycogen and starch appear as electron-dark bodies when viewed in the electron microscope (Fig. 2.10b).

LIPID

The lipid storage granules in prokaryotic cells often are polymers of β-hydroxy, short-chain fatty acids. The fatty acids are ester-linked to form PHA chains that in turn take the form of granules. Neutral lipid inclusions are, however, becoming increasingly known (Olukoshi and Packter 1995) (Fig. 2.11a). Under conditions of either oxygen or nitrogen limitation, PHA accumulates as granules that can not only be seen by selective stains (Fig. 2.11b) but can also be seen in phase contrast microscopy of living cells. The lipid vaporizes in the beam of the electron microscope and appears as an electron-transparent single-membrane limited structure (Fig. 2.11c). *Bacillus*, *Clostridium*, *Pseudomonas* and *Rhodobacter* spp. are among those noted for PHA synthesis.

POLYPHOSPHATE

Many bacteria form polyphosphate inclusions during generalized nutrient limitation (cells deprived of almost any nutrient except phosphate). Chemically, the polymers consist of long chains of orthophosphate linked by phosphoanhydride bonds (Fig. 2.12a). These electron-dense bodies are formed by the sequential addition of phosphate residues to one end of the elongating chain. They are also referred to as **volutin** or **metachromatic granules** (reflecting the fact

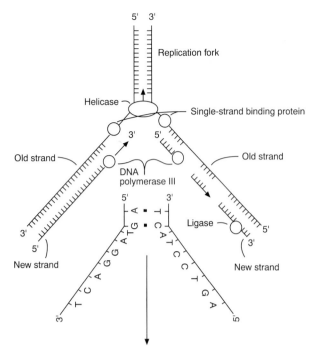

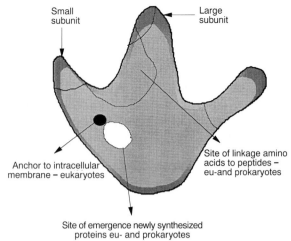

Fig. 2.8 Diagrammatic representation of a ribosome typical of eukaryotic and prokaryotic cells; the 3-lobed structure consists of a large and a smaller subunit. Table 2.2 lists similarities and differences in ribosomes from the 2 cell types.

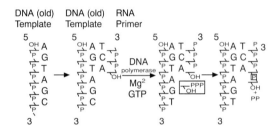

Fig. 2.7 Diagrammatic representation of DNA replication in a prokaryote. Replication initially involves the enzymes helicase and DNA polymerase, and single-strand binding proteins, all acting near the replication fork where replication of each of the DNA strands occurs. Replication of one strand occurs in a 5′ to 3′ direction, whereas in the other it is from 3′ to 5′. (From Slots and Taubman 1992).

that they take on a red appearance when stained with a blue dye). As seen in Fig. 2.12b, these inclusions are formed in close association with the nucleoid.

SULPHUR

Several different species whose metabolism involves sulphur compounds accumulate elemental sulphur as globules in their cytoplasm. Among these are the purple sulphur (*Chromatium*) phototrophic bacteria and several filamentous chemolithotrophs (*Thiothrix, Beggiatoa*). The granules are highly refractile and can be seen easily with light or phase contrast microscopy. It is in the presence of elevated concentrations of sulphide that its oxidation leads to the formation and storage of elemental sulphur; when environmental sulphide concentrations lower, or become limiting, the stored sulphur is oxidized to sulphate; the electrons released may be used via the electron transport chain for energy conservation.

MORE COMPLEX INTRACYTOPLASMIC INCLUSIONS

Many different bacterial species are able to form complex intracytoplasmic single- or unit membrane limited inclusions. Among these are the **magnetosomes** (composed of iron in various chemical forms) of the magnetotactic bacteria (Fig. 2.13a, b); these granules apparently permit a magnetic taxis (an orientation of the bacteria with respect to the earth's magnetic axis) that permits these micro-aerophiles to migrate to suitable growth conditions. **Gas vesicles** (or vacuoles) (Fig. 2.13e, f) are found (Walsby 1994) in several phototrophic bacteria (including some cyanobacteria) as well as in Archaea such as *Halobacterium* spp.; these vesicles permit the organisms to be positioned vertically in a water column and to maintain their buoyancy at specific levels in the column as they are filled with, or emptied of, gas in response to chemical or physical stimuli or both. Chemical analysis of the vesicle membrane reveals it to consist primarily of protein; lipid has not been detected. The stability of the membrane, especially its resistance to chemical solubilization, has limited investigations into the chemical composition of the enclosed gas, and the mechanism by which the vesicles provide buoyancy and promote movement in a vertical plane. Only 2 membrane-associated proteins have been found in the gas vesicle membrane, GvpA and GvpC. **Carboxysomes** (Fig. 2.13c, d) are essentially pure crystals of the enzyme ribulose bisphosphate carboxylase and are present in different autotrophic organisms that utilize this enzyme in the assimilation of carbon dioxide for growth. These polyhedral inclusions have been isolated from most of the ammonia-, nitrate- and sulphur-oxidizing bacteria, as well as from several thermophilic bacteria. They have also been isolated from all the cyanobacteria examined to date. *Bacillus thuringiensis* synthesizes a paracrystalline protein (parasporal body)

Table 2.2 Comparison of prokaryotic and eukaryotic ribosomes

	Prokaryotic ribosome		Eukaryotic ribosome	
Sedimentation constant	70S		80S	
Molecular weight (intact molecule)	2.8×10^6		4.5×10^6	
Number of subunits	2		2	
Subunit structure	30S	50S	40S	80S
Molecular weight (subunits)	1.5×10^6	3×10^6	1.5×10^6	3.0×10^6
Sedimentation rate	16S	5.8S; 28S; 5S	18S	5.8S; 28S; 5S
Number of nucleotides	2000	160, 5000, 120	2000	160, 200, 120
Protein coding number	21	45	33	45

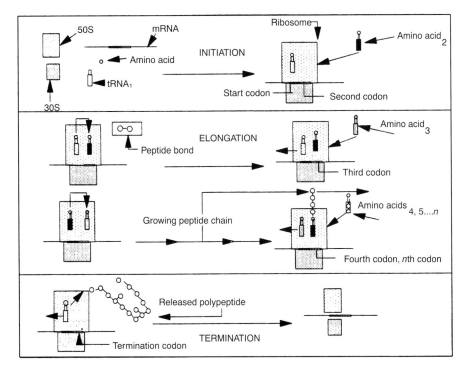

Fig. 2.9 Diagrammatic representation of events of (polypeptide) protein synthesis in a prokaryotic cell. The information for determining the sequential arrangement of amino acids in a protein are encoded in the cell's DNA; this information is then transcribed into the mRNA. Upon interacting with ribosomes, the mRNA codons bind specific tRNA molecules which bear specific amino acids (initiation). As peptide bonds are formed, additional amino acyl–tRNA molecules bind to sites on mRNA and the peptide chain becomes elongated. At a specific codon, the termination signal causes the polypeptide to be released, after which it may fold and coil to become a functional protein. (Modified from Schlegel 1993).

during endospore formation; the protein is a very potent toxin against lepidopteran insects.

3.4 Periplasm

Considerable controversy exists as to the physical and chemical consistency of the **periplasmic space** (**periplasm**) (see Figs 2.5b, 2.13a) in gram-negative bacteria. Classical chemical fixation of gram-positive bacteria reveals a continuous cell wall structure (Fig. 2.14c), whereas in gram-negative bacteria a space between the inner face of the outer membrane and the outer face of the cytoplasmic membrane is seen (Fig. 2.14d). This enclosed compartment, termed the periplasmic space (or periplasm), was thought to consist of a simple solution of low viscosity that contained a variety of enzymes (see below) involved in the degradation of macromolecules required for the growth and metabolism of the cell. Analysis of this region after chemical fixation revealed that it accounted for c. 20–40% of the cell volume. It has now been estimated that the periplasm contains at least 50 different proteins. In addition to the degradative enzymes, several proteins that function to bind specific amino acids, vitamins, or ions, for transport into the cell were also considered to be part of the periplasm. The degradative enzymes included alkaline phosphatase and 5-nucleotidase, and proteolytic enzymes that function to break down non-transportable large molecules into smaller transportable ones. β-Lactamase and aminoglycoside phosphorylase are also found in the periplasm and function to inactivate certain antibiotics. Gram-positive bacteria cannot contain a periplasm of the same physical arrangement as in gram-negative cells, but a functional equivalent of the periplasm may be present (Beveridge 1995, Merchante, Pooley and Karamata 1995).

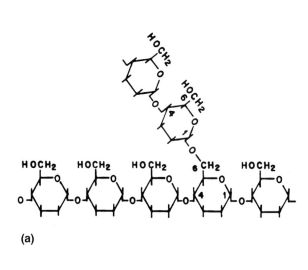

(a)

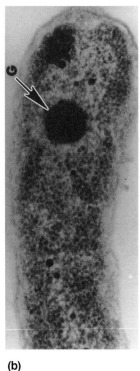

(b)

Fig. 2.10 Bacterial storage materials: (a) chemical structure of glycogen (branched amylopectin) and starch; (b) transmission electron micrograph of a gram-negative bacterium containing a glycogen granule (G). The smaller, electron-dense granules present in the cytoplasm, but in close association with the nuclear region, are probably granules of polyphosphate (see Fig. 2.13). [(b) from Holt, Shively and Greenawalt 1974].

A variety of evidence has called into question the physical description of the periplasm as a simple low viscosity medium. The application of new procedures for the preservation of bacterial structure (cryofixation and cryosubstitution) led to the conclusion that the periplasm probably consists of a high viscosity gel (compare Fig. 2.14a, b). This conclusion was founded on several observations: after cryofixation

$$(CH_3CHOHCH_2COOH)_n$$

Poly-β-hydroxybutyric acid (PHB)

(a)

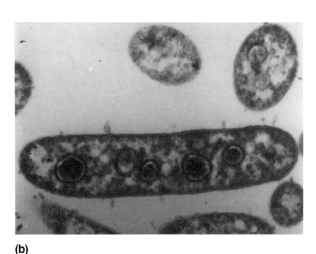

(b)

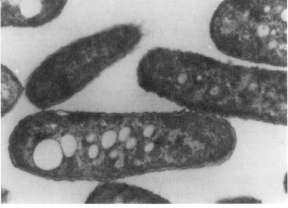

(c)

Fig. 2.11 Bacterial storage materials: (a) chemical structure of PHB; (b) transmission electron micrograph of PHB granule in *Vibrio harveyi* stained with malachite green, and (c) without stain. The stain stabilizes the granules and reveals them as membrane-limited and sponge-like, whereas without malachite green, the granules appear as empty areas, due to the vaporization of the lipid by the electron beam. [(b, c) from Sun et al. 1995].

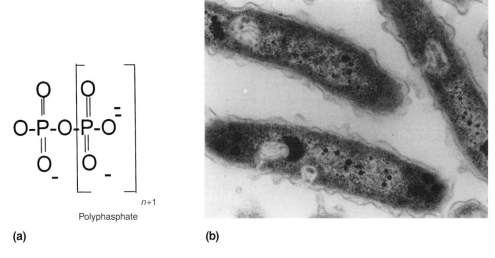

Fig. 2.12 Bacterial storage materials: (a) chemical structure of polyphosphate; (b) transmission electron micrograph of a gram-negative bacterium containing polyphosphate granules. These are in close apposition to the nuclear region. In this preparation the cells' outer membrane is uneven (wavy). (Courtesy J Shively).

and cryosubstitution (which involves cell suspension in organic solutions in which there is no biological turgor pressure) the periplasm was maintained as a space of uniform diameter; studies of the speed of lateral diffusion of selected periplasmic proteins revealed that the diffusion rates observed were consistent with a solution of high, rather than low, viscosity; and staining of this region to reveal proteins did not result in electron densities expected for a region supposedly filled with large amounts of proteins. Finally, combining conventional staining of the peptidoglycan with cryofixation and cryosubstitution revealed the periplasm to consist of a continuous sacculus more than likely filled with a gel, the outer part of which was stable, and composed entirely of layers of peptidoglycan. The inner portion of the gel appeared much more fragile, and subject to significant autolytic events upon cell death. Therefore, the supposition that numerous enzymes are present within the confines of the periplasmic area remains somewhat equivocal.

CYTOPLASMIC MEMBRANE

The prokaryotic cytoplasmic (or cell) membrane encloses the cytoplasm (see, for example, Fig. 2.5a, b). Electron micrographs of bacterial cell sections reveals this membrane to be structurally identical to the long-standing notion of the classical unit membrane (Fig. 2.15) of eukaryotic cells, composed of a phospholipid bilayer enclosed by, and associated with, several low and high MW proteins. Chemically, the best studied prokaryotic cytoplasmic membrane consists of phospholipids and many (200?) different proteins. On a dry weight basis, almost 70% of the membrane is protein, the remainder lipid. The prokaryotic cytoplasmic membrane is often distinguished from that of eukaryotes by the absence of sterols. However, prokaryotes such as *Mycoplasma* and many methane-oxidizing bacteria also contain sterols (i.e. cholesterol) in their membrane (which in the wall-less organisms serves as the outermost layer). It seems likely that other excep-

tions to the 'no sterol' generalization will become established as more and more different bacteria are studied in detail.

Early electron microscopic observations of thin sections of chemically fixed bacteria, especially gram-positive ones, revealed the apparent differentiation of the inner leaflet of the cytoplasmic membrane into a complex convoluted membrane that intruded into the cytoplasmic region (Figs 2.12, 2.16). These 'structures' became known as **mesosomes** and were associated with the cytoplasmic membrane at sites of cross-wall formation (hence, **septal mesosome**) or associated with the cytoplasmic membrane in a more random fashion (**lateral mesosomes**). Although it was not possible to isolate a 'mesosomal unit' into pure form, various functions were attributed to them, including participation in cell division and association with the DNA molecule during cell division. Some investigators also postulated that in very metabolically active cells there was a significant increase in the number of mesosomes associated with the lateral portion of the cytoplasmic membrane. When these results of classical methods of bacterial fixation for electron microscopy were compared with results obtained with newer fixation techniques, an original argument that the mesosome was a chemical (or fixation) artefact gained additional support.

Functionally, the prokaryotic cytoplasmic membrane, like that of the eukaryotic plasma membrane, is involved in **selective permeability** and transport of molecules into and out of the cell. The membrane is also the site for **specific receptors**. However, in contrast to the energy-conserving system of eukaryotic cells, which is limited to the mitochondrion and the chloroplast, the prokaryotic cytoplasmic membrane houses the complete electron transport and phosphorylation systems involved in respiration and, for the phototrophs, early events associated with light harvesting. In addition, enzymes and carrier molecules that function in DNA synthesis, in the synthesis of cell

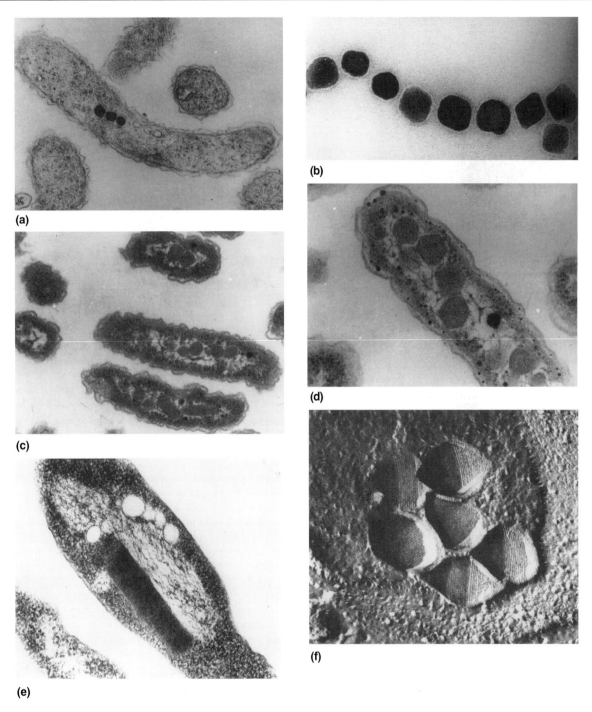

Fig. 2.13 Inclusion bodies: magnetosomes. (a, b) Transmission electron photomicrographs of thin sections of *Aquaspirillum magnetotacticum*; in (a), 3 electron-dense (dark) granules are visible; (b) a chain-like array of particles. (c, d) Carboxysomes: granules formed largely of the protein ribulose-1,5-bisphosphate carboxylase in a thin section of a *Thiobacillus* species. The granules often appear as 6-sided regular structures (d) which do not appear to be membrane-limited. The smaller electron-dense granules are likely to be polyphosphate. (e) Gas vesicles: transmission electron micrograph of thin section of the halophile *Halobacterium halobium* where several vesicles are apparent in the cytoplasm. (f) Freeze-fracture preparation revealing ultrastructural features of the vesicle surfaces. [(a, d) courtesy of Y Gorby; (b) courtesy of R and N Blakemore; (c) courtesy of J Shively; (e) from DasSarma et al. 1994; (f), courtesy of S DasSarma].

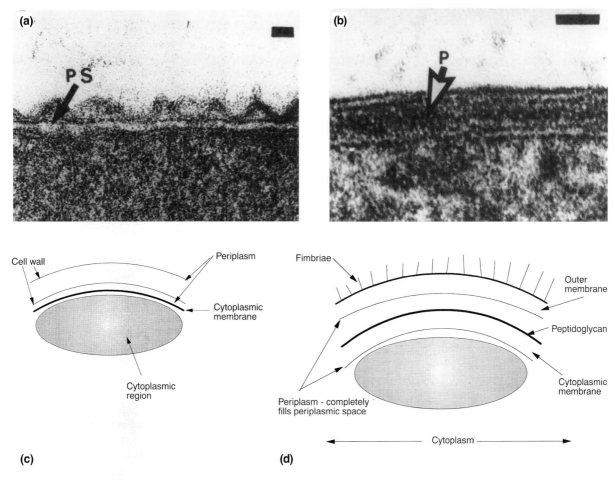

Fig. 2.14 Results of use of different fixation techniques for electron microscopy of thin sections of gram-negative bacteria. In (a) *Aquaspirillum serpens* cells were prepared by standard glutaraldehyde–osmium tetroxide fixation whereas in (b) freeze-substitution of *E. coli* was employed. In (a), note the cell envelope consists of a loosely fitting outer membrane which encloses an apparently empty periplasmic region (PS), except for the thin peptidoglycan layer marked by the tip of the arrow. In (b) the outer portion of the envelope fits tightly and is juxtaposed to a well preserved, rather electron-dense 'periplasmic gel' (P) in the periplasmic space. Diagrammatic interpretations of (a) and (b) are shown in (c) and (d). [(a, b) from Beveridge 1995].

wall polymers (including the lipopolysaccharide) and membrane lipids are membrane-associated. Many sensory and chemotaxis proteins are also associated with the cytoplasmic membrane. At least 20 different chemoreceptors have been localized in the *E. coli* cytoplasmic membrane.

3.5 Permeability and transport

A major function of the cytoplasmic membrane is its role as a permeability barrier. **Permeases** housed in the membrane facilitate the passive diffusion of specific solutes, or catalyse energy-dependent active transport.

ACTIVE TRANSPORT

In the active transport of a molecule across a cell membrane, energy in the form of ATP must be supplied in order for the molecule to traverse the membrane. There are at least 3 forms of transport of solutes into a bacterial cell: **primary** and **secondary** active transport, and **group translocation**. In **primary active transport**, an energy pump is employed to assist the

movement of a specific solute across the cytoplasmic membrane. In primary transport, this movement occurs against a concentration gradient. Thus, for example in bacteria living by respiration, the primary system employed for energy conservation is the electron transport system (cytochrome system) housed in the cytoplasmic membrane. The flow of proteins to the cell exterior, as electrons move along the electron transport chain, establishes a protein gradient across the membrane; as protons re-enter the cell via ATP syntheses located in the membrane, the ATP used in active transport is produced. By contrast, bacteria (usually anaerobic), employing fermentation, lack a complete electron transport system and ATP synthesis occurs by substrate/level phosphorylation.

Secondary active transport takes advantage of the storage of the energy formed in the electron transport system for the transport of selected solutes, primarily amino acids and sugars. Secondary active transport routinely involves specific carrier molecules, primarily proteins. Gram-negative bacteria have a large number of specific carrier or binding proteins located in the

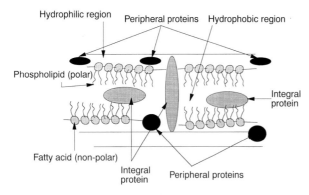

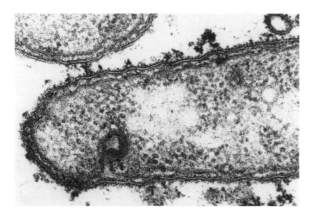

Fig. 2.15 Diagrammatic representation of the structure of the unit membrane common to eukaryotic and prokaryotic cells. The hydrophilic portion of the membrane consists of hydrophilic proteins ('peripheral') in close apposition to the polar 'head-groups' of lipid (often phospholipid) molecules; the polar portion (largely the fatty acyl portion) of the lipid molecules extend into the membrane interior where they may interact not only with other lipid molecules, but with hydrophobic portions of entire proteins or membrane-spanning regions.

Fig. 2.16 Transmission electron photomicrograph of thin section of a gram-negative prokaryote showing a 'whorl' of membrane invaginated from the inner (cytoplasmic) membrane; such structures have been assigned the name 'mesosome', but current views suggest that these may be an artefact of fixation or preparative procedures (see text). The electron-dense material exterior to the cell envelope may be a capsule.

periplasmic space for the transport of specific nutrients into the cell for growth and metabolism. In this co-transport, the specific carrier protein binds to the solute (i.e. amino acid) as well as to a proton or cation, and both are transported simultaneously across the cytoplasmic membrane into the cell.

Group translocation involves the alteration of the solute prior to its transport, in contrast to active transport in which the solute is not changed in structure. Group translocation routinely involves the transport of sugars (i.e. glucose, galactose, mannose), and is mediated by a **phosphotransferase**. A specific membrane carrier protein is initially phosphorylated while it is located at the cytoplasmic face of the cell membrane. The phosphorylated carrier then moves to the external face of the cytoplasmic membrane where it binds the sugar to be transported via a phosphate bond, and moves it across the cytoplasmic membrane into the cytoplasm. The carrier is then enzymatically cleaved from the phosphorylated sugar, and the free sugar phosphate is then utilized in growth and metabolism.

ELECTRON TRANSPORT AND OXIDATIVE PHOSPHORYLATION

In prokaryotes, the cytoplasmic membrane contains the apparatus for the generation of energy in the form of ATP. This membrane is functionally similar to the eukaryotic mitochondrion. Prokaryotic respiration and energy conservation are discussed in Chapter 5.

3.6 Cell wall

With the exception of members of the wall-less mycoplasmas and thermoplasmas, prokaryotes are surrounded by a layer(s) external to the cytoplasmic membrane, commonly referred to as a **cell wall** or **cell envelope** (Figs 2.5a, b, 2.12b, 2.13a, c, d, 2.14, 2.16). Gram-positive bacteria are routinely surrounded by a cell wall that is 200–300 nm thick. This cell wall consists predominantly of peptidoglycan and teichoic acid (see below), whereas the wall (or envelope) of gram-negative prokaryotes is more complex in both the anatomical and chemical sense. In addition to a thinner peptidoglycan layer, these cells have an outer membrane external to the peptidoglycan. A primary function of the cell wall is to impart shape and rigidity to the cell (Fig. 2.17) (Ghuysen and Hakenbaeck 1994). However, in addition to determining cell shape, the walls of several prokaryotes also function in interactions (e.g. adhesion) with other bacteria and with mammalian cells, and also provide specific protein and carbohydrate receptors for the attachment of some bacterial viruses.

A macromolecule unique to the cell walls of many bacteria is the **peptidoglycan** (murein, mucopeptide) (Fig. 2.18). Isolation and purification of peptidoglycan from bacteria of different shapes and sizes makes clear the fact that it is this component of the cell wall that is responsible for shape determination and maintenance as a coccus, rod, spirillum, or a spirochaete. Most bacteria are known to concentrate solutes in their cytoplasm against a concentration gradient (see below), such that the resultant hydrostatic (turgor) pressure within the cytoplasm is as much as 5–20 times atmospheric pressure. This is sufficient to cause a cell to burst under most circumstances unless it is surrounded by a girdle of sufficient strength. The peptidoglycan provides the tensile strength to maintain the structural integrity of those bacteria that possess a wall of this composition, as has been demonstrated by removal, or weakening, of the peptidoglycan; unless such an altered cell is in an environment of iso-osmotic pressure, the cell bursts (Fig. 2.19)

Chemically (Fig. 2.18), peptidoglycan is unique to prokaryotes and not known to occur in any other biota except where it may be present around organelles pre-

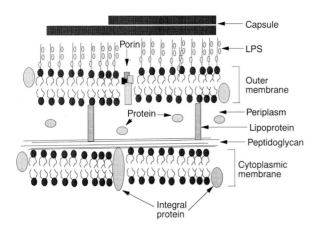

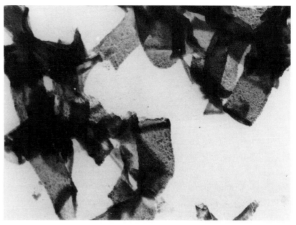

Fig. 2.17 Diagrammatic representation of the cell envelope of a gram-negative bacterial cell. From the cell interior, moving to the exterior, one sees the cell (cytoplasmic) membrane; the thin peptidoglycan layer; the periplasm (in which are found different proteins, some often with enzymatic properties, as well as the lipoproteins that anchor the peptidoglycan to the outer membrane; the outer membrane with porins (which form specific channels) and lipopolysaccharide (LPS) depicted; the cell capsule. (From Slots and Taubman 1992).

Fig. 2.19 Transmission electron micrograph of phosphotungstate stained peptidoglycan fragments isolated from the gram-positive rod-shaped *Bacillus macroides*. Note that the fragments have maintained a rod-like appearance. (From Barnard and Holt 1985).

sumed to be of prokaryotic origins (Pfanzagl et al. 1996). It is a heteropolymeric macromolecule consisting of alternating residues of *N*-acetylglucosamine (GlcNAc) and *N*-acetylmuramic acid (MurNAc) linked by β-1,4-glycosidic bonds. These glycan chains are in turn linked one to another by short (tetra-) peptides covalently attached to the lactyl moiety of muramic acid and usually composed sequentially of residues of D-alanine, D-glutamic acid, *meso*-diaminopimelic acid (or lysine) and a second D-alanine. A 3-dimensional

network, sometimes called a 'bag-shaped macromolecule', results from the cross-linking of glycan chains by the tetrapeptides, either directly or by means of an **interpeptide bridge** (see below).

In **gram-positive** cells, the wall also contains several teichoic and teichuronic acids (Figs 2.20, 2.21), water-soluble polymers of ribitol or glycerol phosphates that can account for as much as 50% of the wall dry weight. These chemicals occur only in gram-positive cells. At least 2 types of teichoic acids have been reported: **cell wall teichoic acids** (which are covalently linked to peptidoglycan) and **membrane teichoic acids** (or **lipoteichoic acids**) that are covalently linked to the cell membrane by glycolipids present there.

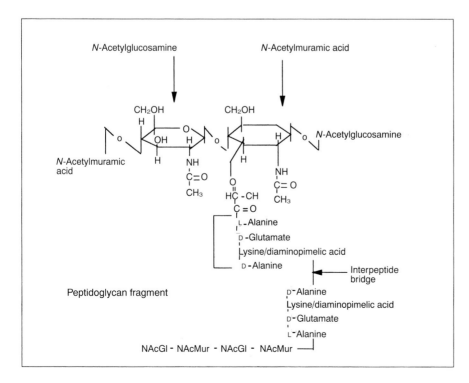

Fig. 2.18 Peptidoglycan fragment. Chemical structure. The glycan portion of the molecule is composed of repeating units of *N*-acetylglucosamine and *N*-acetylmuramic acid; one glycan chain is joined to other glycan chains by a peptide. Often the latter is a rather simple tetrapeptide composed of L-alanine, D-glutamic acid, lysine (or diaminopimelic acid) and D-alanine. In other instances a variety of different amino acids compose an interpeptide bridge interposed between the tetrapeptides of one glycan chain and another.

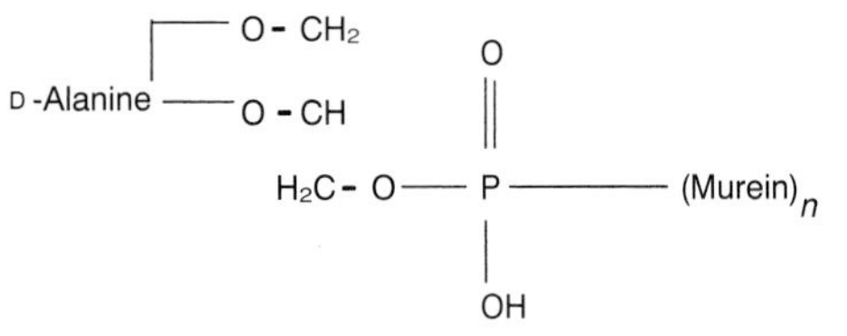

Fig. 2.20 Chemical structure of glycerol teichoic acid.

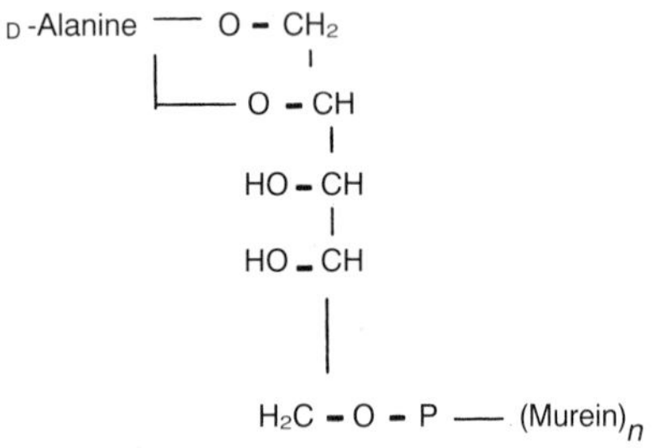

Fig. 2.21 Chemical structure of ribitol teichoic acid.

A major functional aspect of the teichoic acids is their role as a **major surface antigen** of gram-positive bacteria; these antigens are involved in the serological categorization of such bacteria. The **M protein** of *Streptococcus pyogenes*, for example, is associated with a lipoteichoic acid and both the protein and the teichoate traverse the thick peptidoglycan layer to emerge on the cell surface to form microfibrils, which play a role in the attachment of the bacterium to mammalian cells. These acids are also considered to stabilize and strengthen the wall, and are also known to bind magnesium ions; thus they may also play a role in transport of this cation into the cell or its wall.

Other components of walls of gram-positive cells are **teichuronic acids**, so named because of their content of uronic acids, and neutral polysaccharides, which are antigenic and are the basis for categorizing some bacteria, in particular lactobacilli and streptococci, into different serological groupings. An increasing number of gram-positive cells are recognized for their content of **glycolipids** (or **lipoglycans**), often associated with the cell surface where they seemingly substitute for lipoteichoic acids.

The **gram-negative** cell wall (or cell envelope; see Fig. 2.17) is structurally quite different from that of gram-positive cells (compare Figs 2.5a, b and 2.14c, d with Fig. 2.16). The peptidoglycan in such cells is one or a very few layers thick and accounts for only 5–15% of the entire cell envelope. Since there are far fewer peptide bridges (compared to gram-positive cells), the gram-negative wall is less rigid and lacks the strength of the gram- positive wall. In gram-negative cells these peptide bridges are 'direct', i.e. the tetrapeptide of a muramyl residue on one galactan chain is linked by a peptide bond, to the tetrapeptide of a muramyl resi-

due of a different chain. This contrasts with what is often the 'indirect' case in gram-positive bacteria – an interpeptide bridge (of a variable number and type of amino acid residues) connects the tetrapeptide of one galactan chain with the tetrapeptide on another chain.

External to the peptidoglycan, and attached to it by lipoproteins is the **outer membrane** (Fig. 2.20). The lipoproteins, or murein lipoproteins (approximately 7.2 kDa) seemingly attach (both covalently and non-covalently) to the peptidoglycan by their protein portion, and to the outer membrane by their lipid component. The outer membrane, in contrast to the cytoplasmic cell membrane, is not of classic phospholipid bilayer construction; rather, whereas the inner leaflet of the outer membrane is composed of phospholipid, the outer leaflet differs in very significant ways. In the outer leaflet is found another molecule unique to the bacterial wall, the **lipopolysaccharide** (LPS; Figs 2.17, 2.23) in place of phospholipids characteristic of the inner leaflet; thus the outer membrane has a pronounced asymmetry.

Synthesis of peptidoglycan

As shown in Fig. 2.18, the peptidoglycan consists of an amino sugar polysaccharide backbone comprised of alternating residues of **N-acetylglucosamine** and **N-acetylmuramic acid**. The amino sugars are joined together by glycosidic linkage and are connected together into a tight 3-dimensional network by interpeptide amino acids. The size and 3-dimensional complexity of the peptidoglycan precludes it being completely synthesized and assembled within the confines of the cytoplasmic region. Instead, it is made in separate subunits within the cytoplasm and the subunits are transported across the cytoplasmic membrane to the cell surface where they are assembled into the peptidoglycan.

Peptidoglycan synthesis can be separated into 4 integrated events (Fig. 2.22):

1   Phases 1 and 2. These steps are carried out in the cytoplasm with the formation of the uridine diphosphate-N-acetylglucosamine-N-acetylmuramic acid pentapeptide precursor (UDP-N-acetyl-Glu-Mur). The 2 sugars are linked together via the pyridine nucleotide carrier, uridine triphosphate (UTP). The activated sugars are then able to react with specific amino acids found in peptidoglycan. Both the initial linkage of the sugars to the carrier UDP, and the chemical addition of the specific amino acids (alanine, glutamic acid, diaminopimelic acid or lysine) occur on the inner surface of the cytoplasmic membrane. The biosynthesis of the basic peptidoglycan backbone is completed within the cytoplasm with the formation of a pentapeptide. The amino acids are sequentially added to the UDP-MurNAc and UDP-GluNAc to form a UDP-sugar-pentapeptide.

2   Phase 3. Both the MurNAc-peptide unit and the GluNAc must be transported across the cytoplasmic membrane for their final assembly on the outer surface of the cytoplasmic membrane. This transport is accomplished with the assistance of a specific carrier lipid, a C55 bactoprenol (undecaprenylphosphate). Because of the hydrophobic nature of the C55 carrier lipid, attachment of the MurNAc-peptide unit and the GluNAc occurs within the hydrophobic domain of the cytoplasmic membrane. With attachment to the carrier, the entire complex is transported through the cytoplasmic membrane to the 'periplasmic space', where it is chemically linked to one end

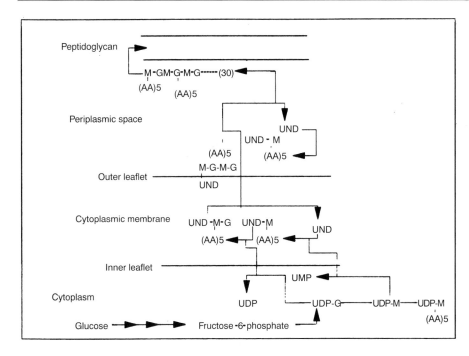

Peptidoglycan

Periplasmic space

Outer leaflet

Cytoplasmic membrane

Inner leaflet

Cytoplasm

Glucose → Fructose-6-phosphate

Fig. 2.22 Synthesis and translocation of peptidoglycan; schematic representation. See text for description of sequential events. (From Slots and Taubman 1992).

of a nascent peptidoglycan by glycosidic bonding between the GluNAc and MurNAc sugars. A transpeptidase on the outer face of the cytoplasmic membrane catalyses the formation of the interpeptide cross-links. The C55 carrier is cleaved from UDP complex by specific phosphatases, making the lipid available for continued transport of other peptidoglycan subunits.

3 Phase 4. The final phase in the synthesis of the peptidoglycan occurs with the cross-linking of the polypeptide in the nascent peptidoglycan to pre-existing cell wall. The cross-bridge is formed either directly as a bond between diaminopimelic acid (or lysine) of one tetrapeptide and the penultimate D-alanine of another, or by the addition of a peptide bridge (of variable composition) between the dibasic amino acid and the D-alanine of a different tetrapeptide. The synthesis is completed with the release of the terminal D-alanine and the formation of the characteristic 'direct' or 'indirect' bridge.

LIPOPOLYSACCHARIDE

Generalizations deriving from the characteristics found in the enteric bacteria (particularly *E. coli* and *Salmonella* Typhimurium) are that LPS is a large molecule, 10 kDa or greater (Hitchcock et al. 1986). It consists of 3 components and is **amphipathic** in character in that one end of the molecule is hydrophilic and the other hydrophobic (Fig. 2.23). The hydrophilic end is the **polysaccharide** or **O-specific (somatic) antigen** that is on the exterior surface of the outer membrane and, accordingly, exposed to the environment external to the cell. A **core region** chemically links the polysaccharide to the hydrophobic portion of the LPS, termed **lipid A**. The lipid A is embedded in the lipid portion of the outer membrane, whereas the core region, which like the polysaccharide portion is hydrophilic, extends more towards the cell surface, away from the lipid bilayer aspect of the membrane.

Chemically, lipid A consists of a glucosamine disaccharide, whose hydroxyl groups are esterified at the C3 and C3′ positions. The disaccharide is linked to a variety of long-chain fatty acids through mono- and diphosphate groups. The C14 fatty acid, β-hydroxymyristic acid, is uniquely and regularly present in lipid A, whereas a variety of other fatty acids, and substituent groups on the phosphate groups, are variably present in different gram-negative bacteria. In some rare instances, the lipid A backbone is formed of a dimer of dideoxyglucose or dideoxyglucose plus a glucosamine. However, these are very rare structures.

The **core region** consists of an inner and an outer segment. The inner segment joins the unique 8-carbon compound, **3-deoxy-D-mannooctulosonate** (often referred to as **KDO** from an older name, **2-keto-3-deoxyoctonoic acid**), and the 7-carbon sugar, heptose. The KDOs present in the core form covalent connections between the lipid A and the heptoses of the core. The outer core, which consists of a branched chain of several other sugars, including glucose, galactose and N-acetylglucosamine, connects the inner segment with the polysaccharide (O-antigen) portion of LPS.

The **polysaccharide** or **O antigen** consists of repeating units of oligosaccharides. This region is the most external component of the LPS, and extends beyond the outer membrane and is thus exposed at the cell surface. The polysaccharide chain can vary in length from several sugars to as many as 40. Identical to the hydrophilic character of the gram-positive cell wall, the O antigen provides significant hydrophilicity to the surface of gram-negative bacteria, and is therefore highly effective in the selective transport of solutes. The antigenic specificity of many gram-negative bacteria is determined by the sequence and composition of the oligosaccharide units.

A very significant aspect of many, but not all, LPSs is the toxicity to animals, including humans. This toxicity, and its strong associations with cells, led to the use of the term **endotoxin** for this material, since it

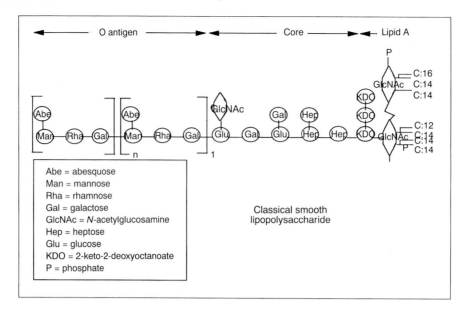

Fig. 2.23 Schematic diagram of the smooth LPS of *Salmonella* Typhimurium. The backbone of lipid A is composed of β,1–6 linked *N*-acetylated glucosamine residues (GlcNAc). The 7 fatty acyl moieties are indicated by C, with numerals indicating the carbon-chain length; OH indicates a hydroxylated moiety. The chemical composition of the fatty acyl moieties varies between different bacterial species. In addition, esterified phosphate (P), amino groups (not shown), or both may be substituted at the 1 and 4′ positions of the non-reducing and reducing glucosamines, respectively. The C8 keto sugar known as KDO (see text) links, via the 6′ carbon atom, the lipid A and polysaccharide components of the LPS molecule. The number of KDO residues varies between species. Other sugars of the 'core' region include heptose, glucose, galactose and *N*-acetylglucosamine; some of these sugars may be modified by either phosphate or amino groups, or both. The antigenic region (O antigen) of *S.* Typhimurium is composed of the sugars abequose, galactose, mannose and rhamnose; galactose may bear glucose substituents in a significant fraction (c. 30%) of the LPS molecules. (From Hitchcock et al. 1986).

was seemingly released from cells only when they were lysed; this contrasted endotoxin with the properties of exotoxins (Schletter et al. 1995). Essentially all of the toxicity is based in the lipid A portion of LPS.

Not all gram-negative bacteria have identical LPS composition, and thus not all display the same biological activity (Fig. 2.24). Several gram-negative bacteria associated with mucosal surfaces (*Neisseria meningitidis, Neisseria gonorrhoeae, H. influenzae*), possess only very short, branched glycans. The colonies formed by such cells are not glistening and smooth in appearance but instead appear as dry and rough. The LPS of these organisms is often termed 'R-type' (for 'rough'); characteristically these LPS have either very short O-antigenic polysaccharides, or lack the O antigen completely. Their structure is similar to that of the glycosphingolipids found in mammalian cell membranes, and are referred to as **lipo-oligosaccharides** (**LOS**). LOS possess significant virulence activity, in that epitopes of the molecule have been found that mimic host structures and therefore might permit the LOS-containing bacteria to evade host immune mechanisms by appearing more as 'self' than 'not self'. For example, the LOS from *N. gonorrhoeae* and *N. meningitidis* contain terminal *N*-acetyllactosamine (GalB1–4-GluNAc) residues that are similar to a human erythrocyte antigen, the erythrocyte **i antigen**. *N. gonorrhoeae* and *N. meningitidis* are able to synthesize the enzyme sialyltransferase, which acts on cytidine monophospho-*N*-acetylneuraminic acid to produce the sialylated residue, *N*-acetyllactoamine. The sialylations provide

the bacterium with a molecular mimicry of the host antigen and a biological 'masking'. Accordingly, it is clear that variations in carbohydrate surface antigen composition is related to the pathogenesis of an organism (see Roche and Maxon 1995).

In addition to LPS, the outer membrane also contains several important proteins that function in the selective transport of nutrients into the cell (see Fig. 2.17, p. 27). Again, based on the models developed from studies of *E. coli* membranes, **porins**, or trans-

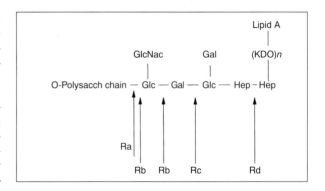

Fig. 2.24 Representation of some variations in LPS composition reflecting mutations affecting biosynthesis of the molecule. The classic, complete or smooth molecule consists (see Fig. 2.23) of the O antigen (O-polysaccharide chain), inner core sugars, heptose (Hep), KDO and lipid A regions. Arrows and letters (e.g. Ra) indicate the sites of change (shortening of the LPS) in some altered LPSs.

membrane proteins, traverse the outer membrane and form trimeric channels that permit the non-specific transport of low MW hydrophilic molecules such as amino acids, sugars and ions (mainly of c. 0.6 kDa or less) into the cell. The porins and membrane lipids also limit the entrance of many antibiotics into the cell. Accordingly, gram-negative bacteria are significantly more resistant to many antibiotics than are gram-positive bacteria. **Integral proteins** are embedded in the membrane and function to maintain the integrity of the outer membrane. The major proteins comprising the porins are routinely named by the genes that code for them. For example, OmpC, OmpD, OmpF, PhoE, characteristic of *E. coli* and *S.* Typhimurium, function to transport specific proteins into the cell, whereas other porins function to transport specific sugars across the outer membrane. Many nutrients required for biosynthesis are larger than 0.6 kDa and are unable to be transported through the porin channels. To accommodate such essential nutrients the outer membrane also contains a variety of surface proteins (**peripheral proteins**) that function in specific permeation mechanisms in which a specific peripheral protein (i.e. iron siderophore for the transport of iron) transports the molecule across the outer membrane. These peripheral proteins show a very high affinity for their substrates and transport their substrates in a classical carrier transport mechanism.

Synthesis of lipopolysaccharide

The synthesis of LPS is similar to that of peptidoglycan (Fig. 2.25). Because of its size, it is formed in subunits in the cell cytoplasm and the subunits are transported across the cytoplasmic membrane into the periplasmic space where major subunits of the LPS are formed. These subunits are then transported to the outer membrane where the LPS synthesis is completed.

1   Phase 1. Within the cytoplasm, UTP-dependent reactions similar to those described for the peptidoglycan.
2   Phase 2. The UTP sugars formed are linked to a fatty

acid acyl carrier protein and transported across the cytoplasmic membrane into the periplasmic space where a large portion of the LPS biosynthesis occurs. Within the periplasm, the chemical constituents are formed into a large subunit in a temporal fashion. Lipid A synthesis is completed in the periplasm by the addition of KDO, and specific fatty acids to the *N*-acetylglucosamine dimer. When completed, the lipid A functions as a primer for the sequential addition of nucleotide sugars to form the inner core. The O-antigen polysaccharide is formed coincident with the formation of the lipid A. Sugars found in the cytoplasm are activated with UTP and are polymerized on a second lipid carrier, an undecaprenol phosphate (UNDP), as short oligosaccharides (3–6 sugar residues). These short oligosaccharide subunits are then polymerized into longer polysaccharide units, which comprise the final O-specific antigen polysaccharide. The longer subunits are then enzymatically transferred to the distal portion of previously synthesized polysaccharides. The length of the O antigen is genetically determined and provides the individual species with their own unique antigenicity. When the correct O-antigen size is reached, it is enzymatically transferred to the distal sugar of the completed lipid A core subunit. These subunits are then linked together by phosphodiester bonds.

3   Phase 3. The completed LPS molecule (lipid A core polysaccharide–O-antigen polysaccharide) is transferred to the outer membrane through specific outer-membrane pores (the putative 'Bayer's junctions') where it is assembled into the outer leaflet of the outer membrane.

INTERACTION BETWEEN THE INNER (CYTOPLASMIC) AND OUTER MEMBRANE

Some 30 years ago it was noted that when strongly plasmolysed *E. coli* was fixed in glutaraldehyde and formaldehyde after plasmolytic shock for 7–10 min and post-fixed in osmium tetroxide, the outer membrane appeared to be linked to the cytoplasmic membrane by what were regarded as local zones of adhesion. These adhesion sites, or **Bayer's junctions**, numbered approximately 200 per cell (Fig. 2.26). These sites were postulated to function in linking the outer membrane to the cytoplasmic membrane, and to provide a

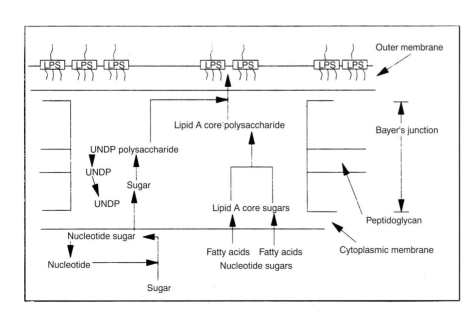

Fig. 2.25 Schematic representation of biosynthesis of LPS. See text for description. (From Slots and Taubman 1992).

channel for protein transport, and for transport of LPS subunits to the outer leaflet of the outer membrane for final assembly into the complete LPS structure. After comparing the chemical fixation approach with cryofixation, and considering the fact that these adhesion sites have never been adequately isolated and purified, one concludes that these 'junctions' do not actually occur in living cells, but that they may be artefacts of the fixation procedures carried out for electron microscopy.

DIVERSITY IN CELL WALL AND ENVELOPE COMPOSITION

Many of the characteristics of the *E. coli* membrane are not generalizable to membranes of other bacteria, let alone the Archaea. The so-called ornithine-aminolipids are significant components of membranes of some pseudomonads, for example, and are major components of the outer membrane of several *Cytophaga, Flexibacter* and *Flavobacterium* spp.; this may also be the case for intestinal *Bacteroides* isolates. Cytophagas, flexibacters, and some flavobacters are known to contain very large quantities of another unusual lipid type, the sulphonolipids, in their outer membranes. In these organisms, both the ornithine-aminolipids and the sulphonolipids contain very large amounts of branched, fatty acyl moieties of carbon chains with odd numbers. In some instances only a single phospholipid is present, and then in the inner membrane only. This chemical composition is quite different from that of membranes of enteric bacteria where fatty acyl moieties are usually unbranched and usually of even-number carbon chain length, and where the membrane lipids are primarily phospholipids. The membrane protein composition of the cytophagas, flexibacters and flavobacters appears to be markedly different, at least in size range, from the profile seen for enteric bacteria and many other gram-negative bacteria, as judged by polyacrylamide gel electrophoretic analyses of membrane preparations. The influence of membrane composition on the lives

of prokaryotes can be exemplified in terms of the susceptibility, or lack of it, of gram-negative cells to the antibiotic actinomycin D. Ordinarily this antibiotic is not inhibitory for gram-negative cells, except for the simple gliding bacteria (cytophagas, flexibacters) noted above, and for the more complex gliding bacteria (e.g. *Myxococcus*); the myxobacter cell envelope is also characterized by its content of branched, fatty acyl moieties of odd-number carbon chain length. Apparently the characteristics of these membranes allow entry of actinomycin D into these cells where it exerts its inhibitory action, whereas cells of enteric and other gram-negative bacteria are unaffected because the antibiotic does not gain entry. Careful removal of the outer membrane from the cells of some pseudomonads also rendered them susceptible to the effects of this antibiotic.

Other differences in cell wall and membrane composition are noted in the Archaea where peptidoglycan is either absent or of a modified structure, **pseudopeptidoglycan** or '**pseudomurein**'. This pseudoglycan wall complex is constructed of protein, glycerol ethers (instead of the ester-linked lipids characteristic of bacteria), and the acetylated uronic acid, *N*-acetyltalosaminuronic acid. MurNAc and diaminopimelic acid have not been found in the Archaea. Those archaeans that lack even a pseudomurein contain a protein layer(s), or sulphated polysaccharides, which serve the function of the peptidoglycan-based wall of bacteria. The lack of peptidoglycan synthesis as an effective inhibitory site for some antibiotics renders the archaeans insensitive to some antibiotics, whereas the differences in lipid composition may also contribute to the lack of sensitivity to other antibiotics.

Members of the genera *Mycoplasma* and *Thermoplasma* represent some of the smallest prokaryotes capable of saprophytic growth. They are unique among the known prokaryotes in that they lack either peptidoglycan or a substitute for it; thus the exterior of these cells is not rigid, but 'plastic'. This plasticity provides the *Mycoplasma* (predominantly host-associated organisms) with the ability to assume many different shapes. At least 3 *Mycoplasma* spp. are known to cause human disease: *Mycoplasma pneumoniae* (primary atypical pneumoniae), *Mycoplasma hominis* and *Ureaplasma urealyticum* (non-gonococcal urethritis). A newly described species, *Mycoplasma penetrans*, has been frequently isolated from HIV-positive individuals, although, the role of this bacterium in HIV infection remains to be determined. *Mycoplasma genitalium* has an aetiological role in genital tract diseases of humans. The absence of a cell wall in these organisms means that many antibiotics, especially those active in the inhibition of cell wall synthesis, are of no use in the control of infections. Fortunately, most of the pathogenic mycoplasmas (except *M. penetrans*) are sensitive to tetracycline and erythromycin.

Bacteria of at least one group possess a cell wall that is not peptidoglycan-based but rather is constructed of protein; these organisms, budding bacteria of genera such as *Planctomyces, Pirellula, Gemmata* and *Isosphaera* are presently known only as non-host-associated iso-

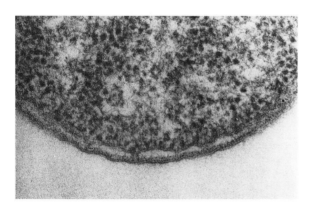

Fig. 2.26 Transmission electron photomicrographs of *E. coli* cells prepared by use of glutaraldehyde–osmic acid fixative. In the apparently empty area ('periplasmic space') between the inner and outer membrane can be seen connections or junctions that have been termed Bayer's junctions. See text for discussion. (Courtesy of T Beveridge).

lates, but their mention here is designed to re-emphasize the diversity in chemical features of anatomical traits, even among bacteria. The host-associated chlamydiae lack peptidoglycan and in these organisms cross-linked envelope proteins may be the functional equivalent (Hatch 1996).

CELL WALL CHARACTERISTICS AND GRAM'S STAIN

The differences in chemical composition between those cells that resist decolorization when treated with ethanol (retain the crystal violet initially applied in the staining reaction; 'gram-positive') and those from which the crystal violet is readily extracted ('gram-negative') have been noted above and this differential behaviour is often, but not always, correlated with dramatic chemical differences.

Some bacteria stain as gram-positive when cells are young, but gram-negative when cells are older. Other bacteria that stain gram-negative have, none the less, walls that appear more akin to gram-positive cells when examined by electron microscopy; they may, in addition be devoid of detectable lipopolysaccharide. The gram stain, then, may have significant use in indicating when more than one cell type is present in a mixed culture, but considerable caution must be taken in inferring likely chemical and ultrastructural features of a cell's surface features from the gram-staining characteristics alone.

THE ACID-FAST (STAINING) CELL WALL

Complex lipids are not routinely found associated with the gram-positive cell wall, and only occur in gram-negative cell walls as part of the LPS; however, several bacterial species, some associated with animal hosts, others not (e.g. *Mycobacterium tuberculosis, Cornybacterium diphtheriae, Nocardia asteroides*) contain complex lipids in their walls. These organisms are termed **acid-fast** because of notable staining characteristics particular to them – they stain poorly with usual Gram's stain protocols and are resistant to decolorization by acid and alcohol (thus the term 'acid-fast'). This resistance to decolorization has its basis in the chemistry of the walls (referred to as **chemotype IV walls**) of these cells in the mycobacteria–nocardia group. The chemical structure of the mycobacterial peptidoglycan is shown in Fig. 2.27; the major diamino acid present is diaminopimelate; the mycobacterial muramate residue is N-glycolyated, not N-acetylated (as in other peptidoglycans). A high MW polysaccharide, termed an **arabinogalactan** (or **arabinan**, **galactan**) is another major wall component. This polymer bears long-chain fatty acids (mycolic acids) that in the mycobacteria often contain 70–90 carbon atoms, whereas in corynebacteria and nocardia they are somewhat shorter (40–60 carbon atoms) (Brennan and Nikaido 1995). In an analogy to the toxicity aspects of LPS, it has been noted that the reaction of humans to exposure to mycolic acid–muramyl dipeptide (peptidoglycan) complexes resulted in the formation of granulomas, whereas the mycobacterial phospholipids have been reported to lead to caseation necrosis.

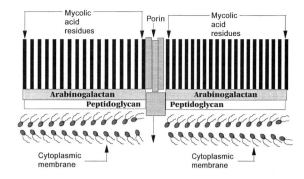

Fig. 2.27 Diagrammatic representation of the acid-fast cell envelope common to many members of the mycobacterium–nocardia group. The outer portion of this envelope characteristically contains long units of mycolic acid linked to arabinogalactan residues.

In addition to these unique mycolic acids and polysaccharides, several other 'free' (as opposed to combined) lipids have been noted in mycobacterial walls. These include lipo-oligosaccharides that contain the sugar trehalose as well as **lipoarabinomannans**.

3.7 Capsules, slimes and the crystalline S layer

Many prokaryotes produce a variety of hydrophobic extracellular polysaccharides or protein polymers. These polymers, the majority of which are polysaccharide, are tightly associated with the cell wall and are referred to as **capsules** (Fig. 2.28a, b). **Slime layers** are represented as large amounts of extracellular polymer that appear to entrap the bacterial cells within it. Slime layers do not appear to be attached directly to the cell wall. Many investigators now term any polysaccharide associated with the surface of bacterial cells as a **glycocalyx**. On the other hand, a crystalline surface layer (S layer) is intimately associated with the surface of selected gram-positive and negative bacteria (see Fig. 2.29a, b).

EXTRACELLULAR POLYMERS: CAPSULES AND SLIMES

The presumed function of these extracellular, accessory structures (they are not required for survival, at least in the artificial environment of the laboratory), is to protect the cell from harsh environmental stresses, including increases in temperature, changes in pH, etc. (Cross 1990, Roberts 1995). Several capsules also are known to function to protect the cells from phagocytic activity (unless coated with anticapsular antibody) by polymorphonuclear leucocytes (PMNs). Recent observations indicate that the capsules in several bacterial species assist the cell to adhere to both mammalian cells (Fig. 2.30) and other bacteria (i.e. coaggregation; Fig. 2.31). The capsules of oral streptococci such as *Streptococcus mutans* and *Steptococcus salivarius* function to attach these bacteria to both hard (i.e. tooth) and soft tissue (i.e. mucosal surfaces). In some instances, bacterial capsules have been observed

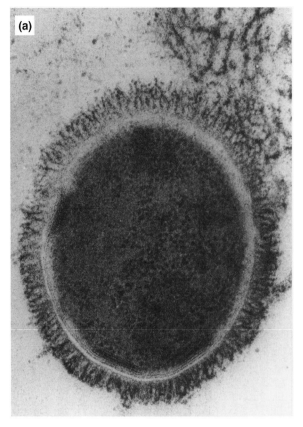

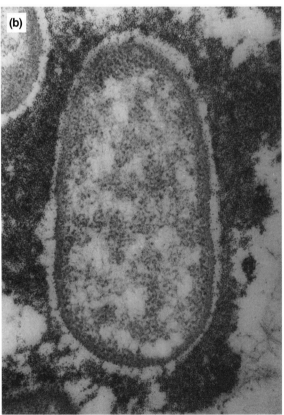

Fig. 2.28 Capsules of prokaryotic cells: (a) transmission electron photomicrograph of *Neisseria gonorrhoeae* prepared by freeze-substitution. The thick capsule, seemingly composed of hair-like projections, surrounds the cell. (b) The capsule of *Klebsiella pneumoniae* is evident around this cell which had been prepared by cationized ferritin staining. (Courtesy of T Beveridge).

to increase virulence. With·*S. mutans*, for example, the capsule immobilizes the cells to tooth surfaces, and in the presence of high sucrose concentrations produces large amounts of lactic acid, which accumulate at the attachment site and result in the destruction of tooth enamel and the formation of a carious lesion.

The best studied of the bacterial capsules are those of the genus *Streptococcus*. The polysaccharide polymers are synthesized by specific enzymes located in the streptococcal cell wall. In the oral streptococcus, *S. mutans*, 2 cell wall associated enzymes, **glucosyl transferase** and **fructosyl transferase**, catalyse the synthesis of 2 long-chain polymers, one a **dextran**, poly-D-glucose (β-glucan), the other a **levan**, poly-D-fructose (polyfructan).

Acetobacter xylinum synthesizes a cellulose (β-1,4-linked glucose) layer on its external surface (Ross, Mayer and Benziman 1991). The cellulose accumulates on the cell surface as crystalline microfibrillar aggregates. Although the entire biosynthetic pathway for cellulose synthesis has not been elucidated in this bacterium, radioactive carbon labelling indicates that it occurs through glucose phosphates and UDP intermediates: glucose → glu-6-P → UDPG → cellulose.

Although the majority of prokaryotic capsules and slimes are polysaccharide, some bacteria synthesize high MW peptides as capsules; *Bacillus anthracis* and *Yersinia pestis* are 2 examples. *B. anthracis* forms a γ-glutamyl-polypeptide capsule both in vivo and in vitro. The formation of the *B. anthracis* capsule in vitro is regulated by carbon dioxide or bicarbonate in the medium. The presence of these compounds (or of DL-isoleucine, DL-phenylalanine, or glutamic acid) results in capsule formation. *Bacillus subtilis* synthesizes a heteropolypeptide capsule composed of D- and L-glutamic acids.

S LAYERS

The regularly structured S layer has been observed external to the cell walls (or envelopes) of many bacteria and Archaea. The most studied of the S layers are those of *Aeromonas* (sometimes referred to as an A layer) and *Campylobacter* spp. These are highly structured, paracrystalline protein multimers composed of identical protein or glycoprotein subunits (Fig. 2.29a, b). Their MW is 50–200 kDa. In those bacteria which have them, an S layer comprises a major portion of total cell protein, with amounts approaching 20% of the total. Characteristic of these layers is their crystalline substructure, with forms ranging from square, hexagonal, to oblique (Fig. 2.29b). Their relatively high abundance and their physical location suggests that the S layer plays an important role in bacterial survival. In fact, these layers are routinely found associated with bacteria that live in stressful or harsh microenvironments, i.e. high temperature, extremes of pH, restricted metabolic niches (methane, limiting iron, high sulphur), and wide variations in redox potential. S layers have been found to be protective from bacteriophage infection, to be antiphagocytic, to function as a protective barrier against host destructive proteins (i.e. protease, complement,

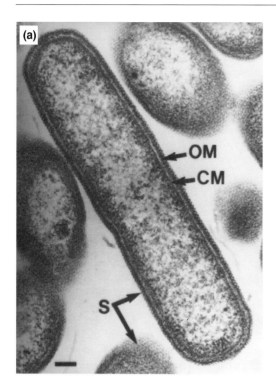

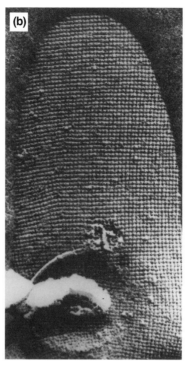

Fig. 2.29 S layers. Transmission electron photomicrograph of these layers in (a) *Campylobacter rectus* and (b) freeze-fracture preparation of *Desulfotomaculum nigrificans*. CM, cytoplasmic membrane; OM, outer membrane; S, S layer. The view in (b) displays the lattice-arrangement of the S layer. [(a) from Borinski and Holt (1990); (b) courtesy of UB Sleytr].

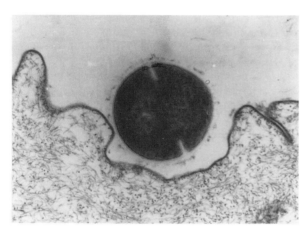

Fig. 2.30 Prokaryotic–epithelial cell interaction. Apparently dividing cell of *Streptococcus pyogenes* with a 'fuzzy' surface M protein loosely associated with the surface of a rat tongue epithelial cell. (From Ellen and Gibbons 1972).

immunoglobulins), and to be involved in the binding of such molecules as iron, porphyrins, immunoglobulins, and numerous extracellular matrix proteins. Recent observations have revealed that the S layer from *Aeromonas salmonicida* is associated with the LPS O antigen. Several experiments suggest that the O antigen functions as the surface receptor for the organism's A layer, and that it is co-assembled with the A layer. Other experiments also suggest that the A layer of this species might also be associated with a major outer-membrane porin, and also be structurally co-assembled. Functionally then, it is not unreasonable to conclude that S layers function in an analogous manner as capsules (see above) – to protect the bacterium from harsh environments.

3.8 Prokaryotic motility: swimming and gliding

FLAGELLA

Bacterial flagella are appendages responsible for the ability of bacteria to swim through liquids and, for some bacteria, to 'swarm' over solid surfaces. The number and arrangement of these thin, thread-like structures on the bacterial cell surface is characteristic of an organism (Fig. 2.32), and these traits have been used in bacterial categorization (Table 2.3). Flagella exist in 2 forms – sheathed and unsheathed (naked). The typical diameter of a naked flagellum is 20 nm; thus it is not visible with simple light microscopy even after simple staining procedures (Fig. 2.33). A motile cell may swim at rates of 1–5 mm min^{-1}. It is the rotation of the flagellum that imparts the ability of the organism to swim.

Chemically, the bacterial flagellum is composed of multiple copies of subunits consisting of a single protein, termed **flagellin**. Several bacteria are now known to synthesize more than one type of flagellin (e.g. *Bacillus* and *Rhizobium*) whereas some *Caulobacter* strains synthesize 3 chemically different flagellins. Flagellins of different bacteria are not necessarily identical, either in size or amino acid sequence, although considerable homology of the latter exists in the 2 terminal portions of many, but not all flagellins. Flagella are highly antigenic, and several of the immune responses mounted by host systems are directed against these flagellar H antigens.

A prokaryotic flagellum consists of 3 major components: a long, semi-rigid, helical shaft or **filament** which rotates and propels the bacterium, a connecting **hook** region which in turn is connected to the **basal**

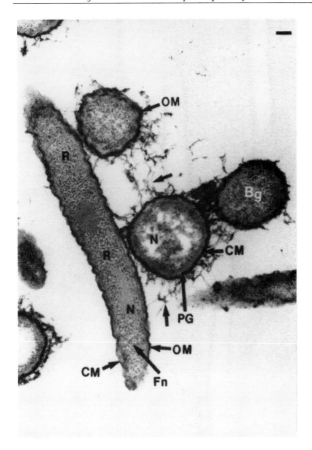

Fig. 2.31 Prokaryotic cell interaction. Coaggregation between *Bacterioides gingivalis* (*Porphyromonas gingivalis*) (Bg) and the longer, thinner filament of another 'oral' bacterium, *Fusobacterium nucleatum* (Fn). The aggregation is mediated by thin electron-dense fibrils (arrows). CM, cell (cytoplasmic) membrane; N, nuclear region; OM, outer membrane; PG, peptidoglycan layers; R, ribosomes. (From Kinder and Holt 1989).

Table 2.3 Taxonomic descriptions of prokaryotic flagella arrangements

Descriptive term	Flagellum arrangement
Atrichous	No flagella
Monotrichous	One flagellum, each end
Amphitrichous	One/several flagella each end
Lophotrichous	Two/several flagella each end
Peritrichous	Flagella surrounding cell

body which is embedded in the cytoplasmic membrane (Fig. 2.34). Stabilization of the flagellum in the bacterial surface structures occurs by means of flagellar **rings** (one pair in gram-positive cells; 2 or more in gram-negative cells). The flagellar **hook** functions as a universal joint between the basal body and the filament. The 'motor', which provides the energy required for flagellar rotation, is located in the membrane, near the basal body. Chemical analysis of the basal body reveals it to contain at least 15 proteins,

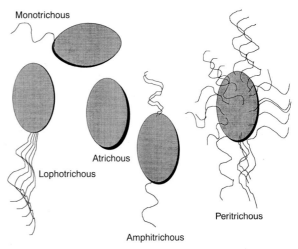

Fig. 2.32 Diagrammatic representation of different flagellar arrangements on bacterial cells. Atrichous organisms have no flagella.

some of which aggregate to form the stabilization rings that anchor the basal body to the cytoplasmic membrane. In gram-negative cells, the additional rings are thought to act, in the outer membrane, in the manner of a bushing to enable rotation of the central rod while at the same time providing additional stability. Flagellar rotation results from the flow of protons into the cell as a result of the existence of a proton gradient in many bacteria, although a sodium gradient is the effective source of energy in a few bacteria. In contrast to the case of the anatomically quite different flagellum of eukaryotes, ATP is not the immediate source of energy for flagellar function in prokaryotes.

Flagella assembly

The formation of a functional flagellum is a complex process, and some estimate that at least 40 different genes are required for synthesis and orderly assembly of the final structure (Aizawa 1996). Assembly begins in the cytoplasmic region where flagellin synthesis occurs, and proceeds from the proximal to the distal (growing) end of the flagellum; the protein subunits travel in the central hole or channel of the flagellum to the tip where they are assembled. The basal body is the first component to be synthesized (near the cytoplasmic membrane), the hook is next formed (within the periplasm), and the filament formed last. The filament extends beyond the cell membrane into the environment surrounding the cell. The entire flagellar apparatus is needed for swimming to occur.

Some bacteria (e.g. *Bdellovibrio*, *Vibrio*) have flagella in which the flagellin is surrounded by a sheath, seemingly derived from the outer membrane. Another significant difference in flagella is seen in spirochaetes in which the flagella do not protrude into the extracellular environment, but rather are located within the outermost layer of these cells; these are sometimes termed **endoflagella** or, more often, **axial filaments** (Fig. 2.35).

The environment for cell growth has an effect on

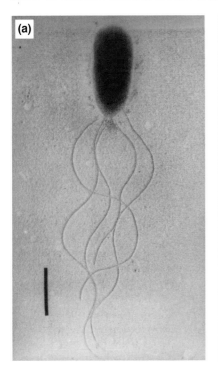

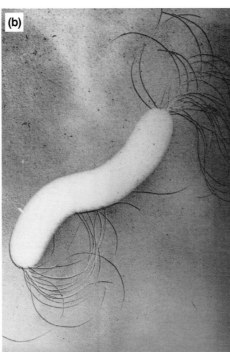

Fig. 2.33 Two types of flagellar arrangements seen in transmission electron microscope photomicrographs: (a) *Pseudomonas putida* strain PRS2000; in this negatively stained preparation, 5 flagella are seen to emerge from one pole of the cell. Bar = 1 μm. (b) In this heavy-metal shadow-casting of *Aquaspirillum bengal* several flagella are seen attached to both poles of the cell. [(a) from Harwood, Fausnaugh and Dispensa 1989; (b) courtesy of NR Kreig].

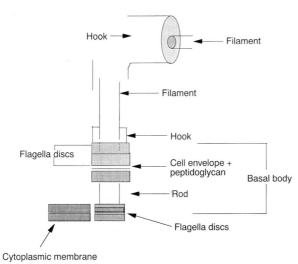

Fig. 2.34 Diagrammatic representation of the apical portion of the prokaryotic flagellum and component and associated structures. (From Newman and Niesengard 1988).

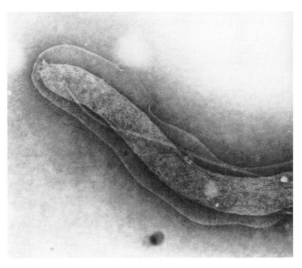

Fig. 2.35 Endoflagellum or axial filament of a spirochaete. Transmission electron photomicrograph of a negatively stained preparation. A thin sheath is exterior to the protoplasmic cylinder of this free-living spirochaete; the thin axial filament (endoflagellum) emerges from one pole of the cell and extends along the protoplasmic cylinder's length, internal to the sheath.

flagella formation, at least in some organisms. Growth in a liquid medium results in different numbers, types (sheathed, unsheathed) and cellular localization (lateral; peritrichous) than does growth on a solid medium; *Vibrio parahaemolyticus* is one of the better studied examples of this influence of environment on flagella formation.

Gliding motility

Many gram-negative bacteria, and at least one gram-positive bacterium, move over the surface of solid substrates by a mechanism referred to as **gliding motility**. Among the best known prokaryotic species that 'glide' are filamentous and unicellular cyanobacteria, at least

one green, non-sulphur phototrophic bacterium, *Beggiatoa* spp., cytophagas, flexibacters and myxobacters, for example. At least one host-associated species, *Capnocytophaga*, also glides and is a frequently found pathogen in oral diseases and brain abscesses (Fig. 2.36a, b). It appears to be a major cause of systemic infections in immunocompromised patients.

Locomotor organelles have never been visualized in the gliding bacteria and so the precise mechanism involved in gliding motility remains unclear. Although many explanations for this motility have been offered,

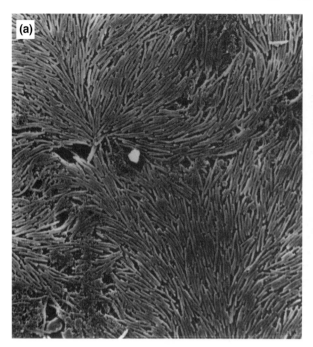
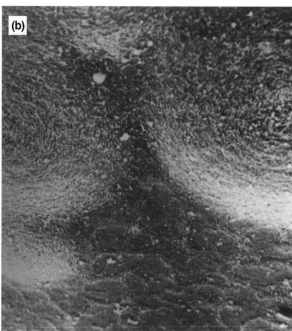

Fig. 2.36 Examples of spreading colony formation resulting from gliding motility of an oral isolate of a *Capnocytophaga*. (a) Individual cells that have moved from different directions are seen to have coalesced to form multicellular arrays. (b) Cells in a colony compose several layers; at colony edges, rafts of cells are seen to have moved away from the colony, resulting in trails of cells. (From Leadbetter, Holt and Socransky 1979).

none is established; among these are the secretion of a surface active agent, formation of an extracellular slime, and the flow of a changing charge on the cell surface. The sole known molecular correlate of the ability or inability for cells to glide, or not, has been noted in *Cytophaga johnsonae* where the absence of a sulphonolipid in a mutant renders the bacterium non-gliding, whereas restoration of the lipid content, by provision of a specific lipid precursor, restores gliding ability.

ADHERENCE AND CONJUGATION: THE ROLE OF FIMBRIAE AND PILI

Many bacteria, among them many gram-negative host-associated species, are covered by thin, straight appendages (in contrast to the thicker helical flagella), which emerge from the cell envelope or cell wall; these appendages are often referred to as **fim-briae** ('fringes') or **pili** ('hairs'), depending on their functions (Fig. 2.37a, b). Well studied representatives of these fimbria-containing species include *Escherichia*, *Salmonella*, *Neisseria*, *Proteus*, *Caulobacter*, *Vibrio* and *Bacteroides* spp. The term **fimbriae** describes the thin rod-like adhesins that emerge from the cell wall (Fig. 2.37a, b), and **pili** is routinely used to describe the very long, flexible, rod-like structures that also emerge from the cell wall and are involved in bacterial conjugation (Fig. 2.38). Fimbriae may be c. 3–25 nm in diameter; they may be very long, often reaching lengths of 20 μm. Single cells have been seen to be covered with as few as 10 fimbriae to as many as 1000. Those fimbriae involved in adherence to other bacteria or to hard and soft mammalian cell surfaces are referred to as **type-specific fimbriae**. The pilus tip, instrumental in attachment, attaches to specific receptors on the surface of host cells; many of these receptors are either glycoproteins or glycolipids. The specificity of the pilus–receptor interaction is important, since the location of the specific host pilus receptor will determine which host site is susceptible to infection. There is also a specificity in attachment to host surfaces (certain sugars exposed on the host surface appear essential for pilus attachment). Type-specific fimbriae (e.g. type 1) are also involved in adherence to erythrocytes, characteristic of erythrocyte agglutination. Similar to bacterial flagella, fimbriae and pili are composed of a single protein subunit, **pilin**, of c. 20 kDa. The pilin subunits are packed in a helical array (similar to flagellin) and, when completed, form long, helical structures. Although the majority of fimbriae and pili are comprised of only one pilin type, several bacteria have at least a second protein distributed along the length of the pilus. The **sex pili** are involved in the formation of conjugation bridges between donor and recipient bacteria during conjugation (Fig. 2.38). The sex pili originate from the donor cells.

The type-specific fimbriae play an important role in the virulence of several pathogenic bacteria. In addition to the production of major virulence factors (i.e. toxins), the type-specific fimbriae function as colonization antigens, providing the pathogen with specific adherence characteristics. In enteropathogenic *E. coli* both the production of enterotoxin and type-specific fimbriae are essential for virulence. Both are genetically determined by transmissible plasmids.

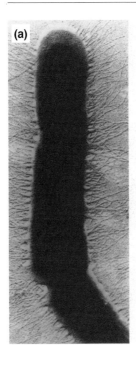
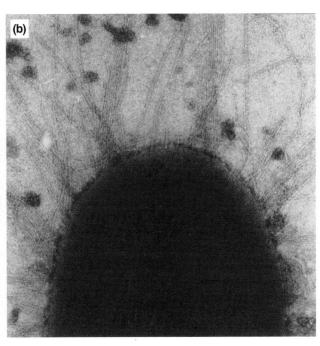

Fig. 2.37 Transmission electron photomicrographs of bacterial fimbriae: (a) heavy-metal shadow-cast preparation of an oral bacterium (*Actinomyces naeslundii*); (b) negatively stained preparation of *E. coli*. Numerous of the thin fimbriae of differing lengths are seen to emerge from the edges of both cells. (b) reveals the structural features of the fimbriae as seen in higher magnification. [(a) from R Ellen in Genco and Mergenhagen 1982; (b) from Beveridge and Graham 1991].

In the genus *Streptococcus* (specifically *S. pyogenes*), the type-specific fimbriae represent the major surface antigen of the genus and is referred to as the **M protein**. This M protein comprises the long, thin fibrils that cover the *S. pyogenes* surface. The M protein was considered to be a major *S. pyogenes* adhesin (Fig. 2.39). However, recent observations employing M protein-negative mutants revealed the mutants to still be capable of adherence to host cells, primarily through fibronectin interaction. Therefore, it is likely that the M protein is not functioning as a bacterial adhesin. *S. pyogenes* also possesses a non-fibrillar adhesin, **protein F**, which mediates the attachment of the cells to fibronectin, a ubiquitous protein covering the surface of most host cells.

Notions of pilus function are being expanded by the demonstration of their function in the 'twitching' motility (Darzins 1994) and their sequence similarity to chemotaxis proteins of some enteric bacteria, as well as those of the gliding bacterium *Myxococcus xanthus*.

Pilus assembly

Pili are assembled in a different fashion from that of flagella. Whereas flagella assembly occurs by protein addition at the distal growing end of the structure, pili (specifically the sex pili) are assembled by the insertion of preformed proteins at the pilus base. It has been hypothesized that pilus assembly occurs at the base because the subunit proteins are too large to traverse the small pilus channel, in contrast to the larger channel in the flagellar filament.

ADHERENCE (ADHESION) AND THE SURVIVAL OF BACTERIA IN THE ENVIRONMENT

For the majority of prokaryotes to survive in the environment, either associated within animal or plant hosts, or even to exist 'free' in a stream or in the

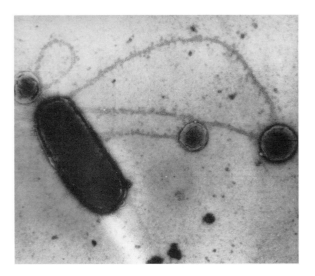

Fig. 2.38 Interaction of 2 *E. coli* cells during exchange of genetic information. The larger, rod-shaped cell with numerous fimbrial appendages (type 1 pili) is the genetic donor to the cells, lacking appendages, that are seen in a more spherical orientation. Along each F-pilus can be seen numerous small, spherical virus particles that infect cells through the F-pilus. (Courtesy of CC Brinton and J Carahan).

ocean, they must associate in some way with a receptor molecule or surface. Without this association, the environment will eventually 'wash' the organism out. Free-living bacteria appear to have a difficult time competing in the environment for essential nutrients, and surviving simple predation from host tissue and host cell functions (e.g. respiratory cilia, PMN pseudopodia). Interaction with a receptive host, or with a compatible substrate, results in colonization.

For colonization to be successful, several factors are required: the presence of hydrophobic or electrostatic interacting molecules; the presence of specific recep-

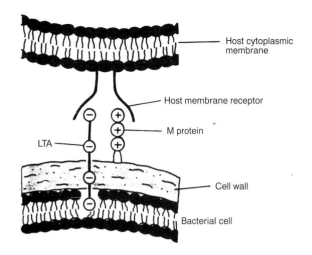

Fig. 2.39 Diagrammatic representation of the probable interaction of lipoteichoic acid (LTA) and the M protein of *Streptococcus pyogenes* with an epithelial cell of a host-cell membrane. The negatively charged LTA interacts with the positively charged M protein with the result that exposed lipids are then able to bind to receptors on the host cell.

tor macromolecules (i.e. adhesins) on that surface; and complementarity between the bacterium's adhesin and the host (or substrate) receptor. Adhesins are either proteinaceous molecules or lipoteichoic acid molecules associated with the bacterial surface, which bind in a stereospecific manner to complementary molecules or receptors on the host surface. For the most part, adhesins are considered to be lectins and the receptors to be saccharides, or glycoproteins. Some bacteria (e.g. *Vibrio cholerae*), are capable of utilizing their flagella to locate and attach to a selected surface. There is some evidence that specific receptors located in the cytoplasmic membrane function as sensing devices to locate specific chemical (oxygen, specific amino acids, sugars) and/or physical (light, heat) signals in the environment. Formation of these chemical complexes, or sensing a favourable or unfavourable environment results either in a positive movement (taxis) towards or away from the specific signal.

Bacterial adhesins are found associated either with the surface of the cell wall (or cell envelope), or with the fimbriae (Bullett and Makowski 1995). Although specific surface-associated surface molecules and fimbriae predominate as bacterial adhesins, capsules have also been reported to function as adhesins. The majority of studies of the interaction of bacteria with a host have been carried out with *N. gonorrhoeae*, *S. pyogenes*, *S.* Typhimurium and *E. coli*. In *N. gonorrhoeae*, at least 2 surface components have been identified that appear to be associated with attachment to epithelial cells in the genitourinary tract. These 2 are referred to as **protein II** (PII) and **type-specific pili**. It is clear that piliated strains of *N. gonorrhoeae* attach to host cells better than do non-piliated mutants of the same strain.

Non-piliated strains of *N. gonorrhoeae* attach to host surfaces better than commensal strains, indicating that surface molecules other than pili are involved in

adherence of the *Neisseria* to host tissue. Protein II appears to function to attach these non-piliated strains to non-ciliated host surfaces. There is some evidence that protein II might also function in the aggregation of the bacteria at the initial site of attachment. *S. pyogenes* is localized to the nasopharynx and skin. Lipoteichoic acid (see p. 27) functions in the attachment of *S. pyogenes* strains to host tissues (Fig. 2.39). As seen in Fig. 2.39, the lipoteichoic acid molecules traverse the cell wall of the gram-positive bacterium, where they attach to the M protein (see p. 28). In the process of this interaction, some of the lipid ends of the lipoteichoic acid remain exposed, and bind to the host receptor glycoprotein (usually fibronectin). In *E. coli*, which functions aetiologically in diarrhoeal and urinary tract diseases, interaction with host tissue occurs through the type I specific pili (see pp. 38–39), or through another pilus, referred to as colonization factor antigen types I and II (CFA/I, CFA/II). Binding of the type I pili occurs through interaction with mannose receptors on the host surface. The type-specific pili appear to be essential for the interaction of specific bacterial species with specific host tissues, but they do not themselves appear to be mediators of disease. Their primary function is to provide the mechanism for the adherence of the pathogen to the host for colonization and eventual emergence of the strain in the host.

4 GROWTH IN A SPECIALIZED HOST ENVIRONMENT AND HUMAN DISEASE

4.1 *Helicobacter pylori*

For many years the association between gastric ulcers and a microbial aetiological agent was unknown. However, examination of gastric biopsies revealed that patients with gastric cancer and peptic ulcer disease essentially always had several types of spirochaetes and spirilla associated with the tissue lesion. As early as 1975, it was revealed that these gram-negative spirilla and spirochaetes were associated with 80% of patients presenting gastric ulcers. In 1983, a *Campylobacter*-like bacterium was isolated from these specimens, and in 1994 it was reported that this bacterium, renamed *Helicobacter pylori* (originally *Campylobacter pylori*) was the causative agent of gastroduodenal ulcerations. In fact, *H. pylori* plays a causal role in the chain of events leading to cancer. The discovery that *H. pylori* was capable not only of surviving but also of growing in the human stomach was astonishing to many, and numerous experiments which followed the presentation by the Cancer Working Group confirmed the central role of *H. pylori* in gastric and duodenal ulcer development and cancer. As with other bacteria-mediated infections, elimination of *H. pylori* by antibiotic therapy results in the resolution of the disease.

H. pylori is a gram-negative curved, spiral, or gull-shaped bacterium. It is characterized by the presence of 1–6 polar flagella (Fig. 2.40a). *H. pylori* appears to

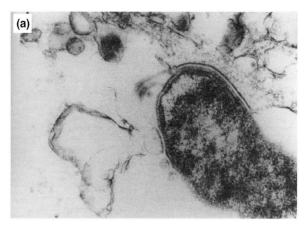
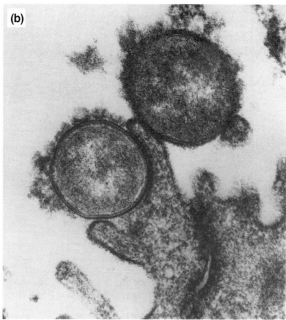

Fig. 2.40 *Helicobacter pylori* interactions with cells of the human stomach. (a) Transmission electron photomicrograph of a thin section at the level of the stomach antrum; the bacterial cell is shown quite close to, and possibly attached to the epithelial cell. (b) The tannic-acid fixed preparation reveals the adhesion of the bacterial cell to the host cell, as a result of the stabilization of the bacterial cell's capsule, or glycocalyx. (Courtesy of CS Goodwin and JA Armstrong).

colonize only gastric epithelia, specifically the non-acid-secreting mucosa (Fig. 2.40a, b). Although there is little biochemical or genetic evidence, *H. pylori* appears to remain associated with the epithelial surface by several adhesins, including those that bind to **Lewis antigens** (an erythrocyte antigen) with terminal fucose residues, some that bind to phosphatidylethanolamine, adhesins that bind to sialic acid–lactose residues, and a laminin-binding protein. Much of the evidence of the pathogenic nature of *H. pylori* is attributed to the fact that its presence is always associated with chronic active gastritis.

Although *H. pylori* survives very nicely in the hostile environment of the stomach, it does not grow well, or survive, in the gastric lumen. Large numbers of *H. pylori* are found under the mucous layer, and attached to gastric epithelial cells where the pH is between 4 and 7. Associated with bacterial growth and division is the production of a large amount of ammonia and carbon dioxide as end products of urea degradation by the bacterium's urease. There is some evidence that an 'ammonia layer' either surrounds the bacterium or is located in close proximity. The presence of this base results in the neutralization of the high stomach acidity and aids in the survival of the bacterium. Urease in the host environment thus functions to permit the growth and emergence of *H. pylori*, as well as functioning as a virulence factor in the destruction of the epithelial lining of the stomach. The large number of polar flagella may function to enable the bacterium to survive gastric flushing. *H. pylori* also contains several enzymes, which may serve as significant virulence factors. These include catalase, oxidase, protease and phospholipase. Finally, *H. pylori* contains a vacuolating

cytotoxin, the product of the *vacA* gene. The production of this cytotoxin is co-ordinated with the production of a high MW (120–128 kDa) major protein, a cytotoxin-associated protein antigen.

4.2 *Legionella pneumophila*

Legionella pneumophila is the causative agent of **Legionnaires' disease**, an acute respiratory disease first discovered in 1976 in Philadelphia. It is an aerobic, gram-negative bacterium. Ecologically, *L. pneumophila* is found primarily in water, including streams, creeks, lakes and in thermal effluent water cooling towers, as in the initial Legionnaires' disease outbreak (Barbaree, Breiman and Dufour 1993).

It appears that *L. pneumophila* survives in human hosts as an intracellular parasite within mononuclear phagocytes, but not in neutrophils or lymphocytes. It survives within the monocyte by preventing fusion of the phagosome with the lysosome.

Although the exact mechanism by which *L. pneumophila* invades monocytes is uncertain, it does contain a 24 kDa outer-membrane protein, which has been designated as a **macrophage invasion protein, Mip**. Whereas normal phagocytic uptake involves the internalization of the particle (or bacterium) inside a spherical vacuole (Fig. 2.41a), uptake of *L. pneumophila* occurs by a novel mechanism, **coiling phagocytosis** (Fig. 2.41b). This mode of phagocytosis involves the formation of a long, thin pseudopod that appears to engulf the bacterium in a coiled vesicle. The vesicle does not acidify and phagolysosome fusion does not occur, and there is intracellular growth of *L. pneumophila*.

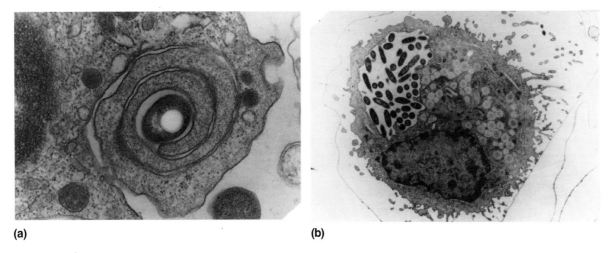

(a)   **(b)**

Fig. 2.41   Interaction of *Legionella pneumophila* with guinea pig monocytes. (a) The host cell's long monocyte pseudopods are seen coiled around *L. pneumophila*, which contains a large lipid granule. (b) A later stage in phagocytosis in which numerous bacterial cells are enclosed in a large vacuole contained by an apparent membrane. Several cells in the vacuole were apparently in the process of dividing at the time of fixation. [(a) from Horwitz 1984a; (b) from Horwitz 1984b].

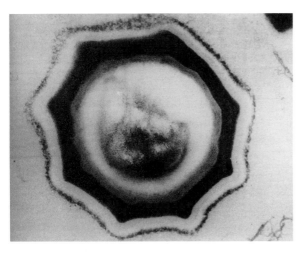

Fig. 2.42   Ultrastructural features of the endospore of a *Bacillus* after liberation from the sporangium in which the spore was formed. Transmission electron micrograph of a thin section. A thin, loosely fitting, outermost exosporium (darkly stained) can be seen to surround several layers of spore coat, some layers more darkly stained than others. Interior to this laminated structure is the essentially unstained spore cortex which in turn surrounds the spore body; the latter is composed of the genetic and physiological components which will be involved in enabling the dormant spore to become an active vegetative cell during the germination and outgrowth events.

5   BACTERIAL ENDOSPORES

Members of genera such as *Bacillus, Clostridium, Sporosarcina, Thermoactinomyces* and perhaps *Coxiella* produce unique structures, termed **endospores**, within a vegetative cell. These highly refractile bodies are formed in response to environmental stresses, notably nutrient deprivation, by a complex series of biochemical and structural events (Fig. 2.42). The terminal event in spore formation (sporulation), is the freeing of the endospore from the vegetative cell into the environ-

ment as a 'free spore' (Fig. 2.42). These spores are resistant to heating (some even at 100°C, for hours), desiccation, radiation and harsh chemicals. Spores have also been recovered from ancient artefacts; whether the organisms and the spores they formed are as ancient as at first asserted (Cano and Borucki 1995) is arguable (Beckenbach 1995, Priest 1995). Providing the free spores with a suitable growth environment results in another complex series of biochemical and structural changes (germination and outgrowth), which results in the formation of a new vegetative cell capable of growth and division.

Figure 2.43 shows a simple diagram of the morphological events in sporulation. In *B. subtilis*, for example, the initial sporulation event involves the modification of the nucleoid into a thin filamentous form. Soon after the formation of this special aspect of the nucleus, an ingrowth of the cytoplasmic membrane at one pole of the cell occurs to result in what has been termed an unequal or asymmetric cell division (Hitchens and Slepecky 1969). The infolding of the cytoplasmic membrane during these events results in the formation of a double membrane whose surfaces correspond to the peptidoglycan-synthesizing surfaces. With the continued infolding of the membrane to form a completed septum, the forespore is the result; in essence a new cell has begun to be formed inside another one. The vegetative cell cytoplasm and membranes provide the significant building blocks for the series of complex events (Errington 1993) in the formation of the free spore. Immediately after the formation of the complete forespore, there is the active synthesis of a thick wall, consisting of the spore wall, and the cortex between the forespore facing membranes. The terminal events in spore formation involve the formation of a series of spore coats and exosporium which surround the cortex. With endospore maturation and vegetative cell lysis, the free spore is released into the environment where it may begin its life cycle anew.

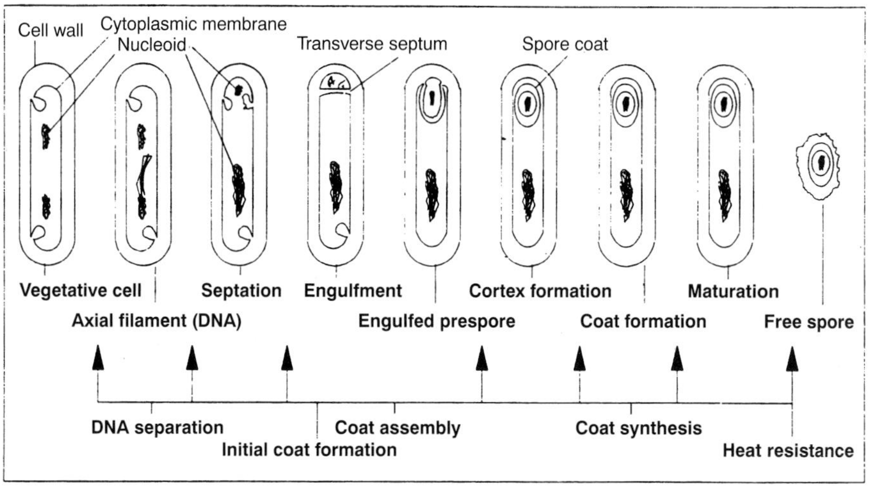

Fig. 2.43 Diagrammatic representation of the events of endospore formation. Upon nutrient depletion the vegetative cell begins an alternative, asymmetric form of cell division. This involves DNA separation, transverse septum formation, engulfment of that portion of the cell genome destined for the endospore, and then other biochemical events leading to synthesis of cortex materials, those of the spore coats and, often, the exosporium. Sporangium lysis results in liberation of the mature, dormant spore. (From Slots and Taubman 1992).

6 SUMMARY

This chapter presents a broad, but not all-inclusive, survey of some morphological, anatomical and chemical features of a diverse array of prokaryotes, some of which are, and some of which are not, known to be of clinical significance. If, from the lessons of the past some confident predictions can be made of progress in these areas in the next decade, as newer, more refined methods become available for the analysis and examination of prokaryotic cells, the present understanding of their chemical composition and ultrastructural features will become significantly enlarged.

One set of remarkable examples already emerging are those permitting novel insights into subcellular localization of specific proteins that affect such fundamental traits as cell division and cell symmetry or polarity (Shapiro 1993, Arigoni et al. 1995, Rothfield and Zhao 1996).

In addition, as an ever-increasing variety of prokaryotes are brought into culture and their interesting, probably often novel, traits are deciphered, it seems quite certain that now current perceptions of prokaryotic properties will in the future appear limited, when compared with those that will by then have been elucidated.

REFERENCES

Aizawa S-I, 1996, Flagellar assembly in *Salmonella typhimurium*, *Mol Microbiol*, **19**: 1–5.

Arigoni F, Pogliano K et al., 1995, Localization of protein implicated in establishment of cell type to sites of asymmetric division, *Science*, **270**: 637–40.

Barbaree JM, Breiman RD, Dufour AP (eds), 1993, Legionella: *Current Status and Emerging Perspectives*, ASM Press, Washington DC.

Barbour AG, Garon CF, 1987, Linear plasmids of the bacterium *Borrelia burgdorferi* have covalently closed ends, *Science*, **237**: 409–11.

Barnard MR, Holt SC, 1985, Isolation and characterization of the peptidoglycans from selected gram-positive and gram-negative peridontal pathogens, *Can J Microbiol*, **31**: 154–60.

Beckenbach AT, 1995, Age of bacteria from amber, *Science*, **270**: 2015–16.

Beveridge TJ, 1989, The structure of bacteria, *Bacteria in Nature*, vol. 3, Plenum, New York, 1–65.

Beveridge TJ, 1995, The periplasmic space and the periplasm in gram-positive and gram-negative bacteria, *ASM News*, **61**: 125–30.

Beveridge TJ, Graham LL, 1991, Surface layers of bacteria, *Microbiol Rev*, **55**: 684–705.

Borinksi R, Holt SC, 1990, Surface characteristics of *Wolinella recta* ATCC 33238 and human clinical isolates: correlation of structure with function, *Infect Immun*, **58**: 2770–6.

Brennan PJ, Nikaido H, 1995, The envelope of mycobacteria, *Annu Rev Biochem*, **64**: 29–63.

Brock TD, Madigan MM et al., 1993, *Biology of Microorganisms*, 7th edn, Prentice-Hall, Englewood Cliffs NJ.

Bullitt E, Makowski L, 1995, Structural polymorphism of bacterial adhesion pili, *Nature (London)*, **373**: 164–7.

Cairns J, 1963, The bacterial chromosome and its manner of replication as seen by autoradiography, *J Mol Biol*, **6**: 208–16.

Cano RJ, Borucki MK, 1995, Revival and identification of bacterial spores in 25- to 40-million-year-old Dominican amber, *Science*, **268**: 1060–4.

Cole ST, Saint Girons I, 1994, Bacterial genomics, *FEMS Microbiol Rev*, **14**: 139–60.

Courties C, Vaquer A et al., 1994, Smallest eukaryotic organism, *Nature (London)*, **370**: 255.

Cross A, 1990, The biological significance of bacterial encapsulation, *Curr Top Microbiol Immunol*, **150**: 87–95.

DasSarma S, Arora P et al., 1994, Wild-type gas vesicle formation requires at least ten genes in the *gvp* cluster of *Halobacterium halobium* plasmid pNRC100, *J Bacteriol*, **176**: 7646–52.

Darzins A, 1994, Characterization of a *Pseudomonas aeruginosa* gene cluster involved in pilus biosynthesis and twitching motility: sequence similarity to the chemotaxis proteins of enterics and the gliding bacterium *Myxococcus xanthus*, *Mol Microbiol*, **11**: 137–53.

Ellen RP, Gibbons RJ, 1972, M-protein-associated adherence of

Steptococcus pyogenes to epithelial surfaces: prerequisite for virulence, *Infect Immun*, **5:** 826–30.

Errington J, 1993, *Bacillus subtilis* sporulation: regulation of gene expression and control of morphogenesis, *Microbiol Rev*, **57:** 1–33.

Fleischmann RD, Adams MD et al., 1995, Whole genome random sequencing and assembly of *Haemophilus influenzae* Rd, *Science*, **269:** 496–512.

Fraser CM, Gocayne JD et al., 1995, The minimal gene complement of *Mycoplasma genitalium*, *Science*, **270:** 397–403.

Gaeher M, Einsiedler K et al., 1996, A physical and genetic map of *Neisseria meningitidis*, *Mol Microbiol*, **19:** 249–59.

Genco R, Mergenhagen S (eds), 1982, *Host–Parasite Interactions in Periodontal Diseases*, ASM Press, Washington, DC.

Ghuysen JM, Hakenbaeck R, 1994, *Bacterial Cell Wall*, Elsevier, Amsterdam.

Graham LL, 1992, Freeze-substitution studies of bacteria, *Electron Microsc Rev*, **5:** 77–103.

Harwood CS, Fosnaugh K, Dispensa M, 1989, Flagellation of *Pseudomonas putida* and analysis of its motile behavior, *J Bacteriol*, **171:** 4063–6.

Hatch TP, 1996, Disulfide cross-linked envelope proteins: the functional equivalent of peptidoglycan in chlamydiae?, *J Bacteriol*, **178:** 1–5.

Hitchcock PJ, Leive L et al., 1986, Lipopolysaccharide nomenclature – past, present, future, *J Bacteriol*, **166:** 699–705.

Hitchens AD, Slepecky RA, 1969, Bacterial spore formation as a modified procaryotic cell division, *Nature (London)*, **223:** 804–7.

Holt SC, Beveridge TJ, 1982, Electron microscopy: its development and application to microbiology, *Can J Microbiol*, **28:** 1–53.

Holt SC, Shively JM, Greenawalt JW, 1974, Fine structure of selected species of the genus *Thiobacillus* as revealed by chemical fixation and freeze-etching, *Can J Microbiol*, **20:** 1347–51.

Horwitz MA, 1984a, Phagocytosis of the Legionnaires' disease bacterium (*Legionella pneumophila*) occurs by a novel mechanism: engulfment with a pseudopod coil, *Cell*, **36:** 27–33.

Horwitz MA, 1984b, State of the Art Lecture: Interactions between *Legionella pneumophila* and human mononuclear phagocytes, *Legionella: Proceedings of the Second International Symposium*, Eds Thornsberry C, Balows A et al., American Society for Microbiology, Washington, DC, 156–66.

Kapitza HG, 1994, *Microscopy From the Very Beginning*, Carl Zeiss, Oberkochen.

Kepner RL, Pratt JR, 1994, Use of flurochromes for direct enumeration of total bacteria in environmental samples: past and present, *Microbiol Rev*, **58:** 603–15.

Kinder S, Holt SC, 1989, Characterization of coaggregation between *Bacteroides gingivalis* T22 and *Fusobacterium nucleatum* T18, *Infect Immun*, **57:** 3425–33.

Krawiec S, Riley MR, 1990, Organization of the bacterial chromosome, *Microbiol Rev*, **54:** 502–39.

Leadbetter ER, 1997, Prokaryotic diversity: form, ecophysiology, habitat, *Manual for Environmental Microbiology*, ASM Press, Washington, DC, 14–24.

Leadbetter ER, Holt SC, Socransky SS, 1979, *Capnocytophaga*: new genus of gram-negative gliding bacteria. I. General characteristics, taxonomic considerations, and significance, *Arch Microbiol*, **122:** 9–16.

Manafi M, Kneifel W, Bascomb S, 1991, Fluorogenic and chromogenic substrates used in bacterial diagnostics, *Microbiol Rev*, **55:** 335–48.

Matsumoto B, 1993, Cell biological applications of confocal microscopy, *Methods Cell Biol*, **38:** 1–380.

Merchante R, Pooley HM, Karamata D, 1995, A periplasm in *Bacillus subtilis*, *J Bacteriol*, **177:** 6176–83.

Newman MG, Nisengard R, 1988, *Oral Microbiology and Immunology*, WB Saunders, Philadelphia.

Olukoshi ER, Packter NM, 1995, Importance of stored triacylglycerols in *Streptomyces*: possible carbon source for antibiotics, *Microbiology*, **140:** 931–3.

Pfanzagl B, Zenker A et al., 1996, Primary structure of cyanelle peptidoglycan of *Cyanophora paradoxa*: a prokaryotic cell wall as part of an organelle envelope, *J Bacteriol*, **178:** 332–9.

Pogiliano K, Harry E, Losick R, 1995, Visualization of the subcellular location of sporulation proteins in *Bacillus subtilis* using immunofluorescence microscopy, *Mol Microbiol*, **18:** 459–70.

Priest FG, 1995, Age of bacteria from amber, *Science*, **270:** 2015.

Roberts IS, 1995, Bacterial polysaccharides in sickness and in health, *Microbiol Rev*, **141:** 2023–31.

Robinow C, Kellenberger E, 1994, The bacterial nucleoid revisited, *Microbiol Rev*, **58:** 211–32.

Roche RJ, Moxon ER, 1995, Phenotypic variation of carbohydrate surface antigens and the pathogenesis of *Haemophilus influenzae* infections, *Trends Microbiol*, **3:** 304–9.

Ross P, Mayer R, Benziman M, 1991, Cellulose biosynthesis and function in bacteria, *Microbiol Rev*, **55:** 35–58.

Rothfield LI, Zhao C-R, 1996, How do bacteria decide where to divide?, *Cell*, **84:** 183–6.

Schlegel HG, 1993, *General Microbiology*, 7th edn, Cambridge University Press, Cambridge.

Schletter J, Heine H et al., 1995, Molecular mechanisms of endotoxin activity, *Arch Microbiol*, **164:** 383–9.

Shapiro L, 1993, Protein localization and assymetry in the bacterial cell, *Cell*, **73:** 841–5.

Slots J, Taubman A, 1992, *Contemporary Oral Microbiology and Immunology*, 2nd edn, Mosby, St Louis, MO, 3–43.

Stanier RY, Ingraham JL et al., 1986, *The Microbial World*, 5th edn, Prentice-Hall, Englewood Cliffs, NJ.

Sun W, Teng K, Meighen E, 1995, Detection of poly(3-hydroxybutyrate) granules by electron microscopy of *Vibrio harveyi* stained with malachite green, *Can J Microbiol*, **41, Suppl. 1:** 131–7.

Walsby AE, 1994, Gas vesicles, *Microbiol Rev*, **58:** 94–144.

White DC, 1995, *The Physiology and Biochemistry of Prokaryotes*, Oxford University Press, New York.

Chapter 3

Taxonomy and nomenclature of Bacteria

J T Magee

This chapter is intended as a brief introduction to the strange mixture of science, philosophy and formal regulation that guides the division of bacteria into named groups. This is not an unbiased account. In the Alice in Wonderland of taxonomy, nothing is quite what it seems and, as in politics and theology, opinion is an indispensable ingredient. Anyone who reads this set of volumes has reached some viewpoint on bacterial taxonomy, consciously or subconsciously. There is a considerable breadth of opinion in key arguments: utilitarian versus 'natural' classification, genomic versus phenotypic versus polyphasic classification, 'splitting' or 'lumping' of taxa (Cowan 1968) and so on. This range guarantees that each microbiologist will have found some unique position in the spectrum of opinion, and so will disagree with at least some opinions expressed here. Constructive, logical criticism and discussion are essential for the subject to progress.

1 AN INTRODUCTORY PERSPECTIVE

The practice of medical bacteriology is founded upon the ability to distinguish between the bacteria that are isolated and to predict their pathogenicity and epidemiology from in vitro characteristics. This predictive capability is essential and flows from the work of many microbiologists over 2 centuries. Their cumulative

efforts have provided the current formal species nomenclature under the aegis of the International Committee for Systematic Bacteriology (ICSB), reviewed regularly in successive editions of *Bergey's Manual of Systematic Bacteriology* (*Bergey's Manual*), and a wealth of vernacular schemes. Together, these schemes provide much of the technical vocabulary of microbiology and are the basis of interpretation and prediction from laboratory tests.

In a laboratory deprived of all knowledge of the classification of bacteria, their morphological and biochemical characteristics and the relevance of individual characterization tests, each isolate would have to be regarded as unique. It would be impossible to distinguish between pathogens and commensals, or to assess the cross-infection potential of an isolate, from in vitro tests. All available antibiotics would have to be tested for each isolate. How long would it take, for example, to untangle the characteristics of the enteric pathogens from those of gut commensals, or to rediscover the link between diphtheria and toxin-producing corynebacteria? Clearly, it would be impossible to operate under such conditions. The laboratory would be forced to search for links between in vitro characteristics and effects on patients, to divide isolates into named groups, and so to re-invent the science of taxonomy.

Despite this key role, many diagnostic microbiologists profess a disregard for taxonomy (Magee 1993a). This attitude may derive from early specialist education, where the subject is often presented as an apparently endless list of genus and species names for rote learning, along with associated laboratory and medical characteristics. The underlying science, philosophy and history of the subject are rarely taught; when they are, the students are often so inundated by the nomenclature and lacking in a context for their brief contact with taxonomy *per se* that these are soon forgotten. Further conscious contact with the subject is usually when rote learning is overturned by changes in the names of bacteria, for reasons that may appear obscure and irrelevant. Therefore it is not surprising that most medical microbiologists regard taxonomy as an unimportant, dull and arcane science practised by academics in isolation for their own edification.

This common view is grossly inaccurate, but is also a self-fulfilling proposition. It builds barriers between routine microbiologists and taxonomists that limit communication and co-operation. This breaks the feedback process that is essential to the production of relevant, sensible classifications of the bacteria. Taxonomy and classifications are fundamental to all microbiological work and an appreciation of the concepts involved is an absolute requirement for all practitioners of microbiology. Equally, taxonomists require the input of other microbiologists to direct them to areas of taxonomic confusion, supply cultures, moderate wilder taxonomic excursions and, more importantly, to supply knowledge of the characteristics of the organisms in the broader context outside the laboratory.

2 ONE CLASSIFICATION OR MANY? THE IMPORTANCE OF CONTEXT

Cowan (1962) illustrated the range of possible classifications with the example of objects intended to join materials. He divided them first into animal (glues), vegetable (wooden pegs) and mineral (metal nails, bolts or screws, or plastic adhesives, screws and pins), then presented an alternative classification into solid devices, and liquid glues. A dealer in scrap metals might classify these objects as ferrous, non-ferrous, or non-metal in the context of work, but quite differently in the context of repairing a broken china ornament or a broken chair. Humans have little difficulty in employing a multiplicity of overlapping, but distinct and context-specific, classifications for everyday objects. Microbiologists differ only in that most are trained to acknowledge a single formal scheme and so feel constrained to argue about its minutiae to the exclusion of other possibilities.

However, when presented with a set of clinical isolates, workers revert to practicality, happily employing classifications that have little in common with that embodied in the current edition of *Bergey's Manual.* At the faeces bench, isolates are divided into lactose fermenters and non-fermenters, faecal pathogens and non-pathogens, aerobes, anaerobes and micro-aerophiles. Staphylococci are divided in 3 distinct ways

when dealing with blood cultures, skin swabs or urines, reflecting experience of potential pathogenicity and the importance of further identification in the context of the specimen type, the sex of the patient and catheterization status. Diverse gram-negative and gram-positive species are lumped together under the heading of respiratory pathogens, recognizing the need to extend this definition in the context of special cases: cystic fibrosis patients, or those on ventilators. These vernacular or 'trivial' classifications even intrude into reports in phrases such as 'coagulase-negative staphylococcus' or as multi-valued context-specific phrases such as 'commensals only'.

Trivial classifications are as real and valid as those described in the successive editions of *Bergey's Manual.* They exist because some worker perceived a new way of dividing bacteria that had practical use or significance, and many other microbiologists recognized the utilitarian value of the division. They reflect unavoidable deficiencies in the flexibility of nomenclature in the formal ICSB scheme, and the fact that a single classification cannot cater for all the myriad ways in which bacteria can be usefully grouped.

These trivial classifications have, by their nature, consensus acceptance and are strongly utilitarian. However, they lack mechanisms for definition and regulation of any nomenclature involved, and so are open to degradation by misuse. Terms such as 'faecal streptococcus' or 'enterobacteria' lack clear definition and are used in any of a range of senses from the all-inclusive to the restricted. Equally, these classifications tend to be restricted by their utilitarian nature to specific branches of applied microbiology.

By contrast, the formal scheme has a strictly defined, regulated nomenclature recognizable by the italicization of the formal genus and species names. It is less robust on consensus acceptance, but is broadly applicable in all branches of microbiology. The defined nomenclature makes this the vocabulary of choice for international and interdisciplinary communication. However, the rigidity of a defined nomenclature causes problems when changes become necessary (see section 12, p. 60). A second context for the formal system is as a scheme supplying descriptions of the minimum sized groups of bacteria about which one can make useful generalizations. These species definitions are the building blocks that can be assembled into larger groups in as many ways as utility demands. The Bacteriological Code provides a formal system of nomenclature (Sneath 1992); by contrast, the classifications into higher taxa outlined in successive editions of *Bergey's Manual* are not official (Staley and Krieg 1984) and tend to change markedly between editions.

However, the formal scheme serves many interest groups. Those who wish the scheme to supply a phylogeny of the bacteria, a 'natural' classification, or to be bent to conform with the results of a specific characterization test, or to suit the requirements of some specialist branch of microbiology would all disagree.

3 STACK OR FLAT: THE PRACTICAL RELEVANCE OF HIERARCHICAL CLASSIFICATIONS

Classification embraces not only the division into named species, but also the further grouping of species into genera, genera into families and so on through orders, classes and phyla to kingdoms. This hierarchical approach has much to commend it in the classification of higher organisms. The many morphological and developmental features allow division into higher groupings in agreement with fossil evidence of evolutionary development; for the most part, these groups can be neatly packaged into specialist areas relevant to the applied science. However, hierarchical classification has had a more chequered history in bacteriology. Successive editions of *Bergey's Manual* have portrayed gross changes in the arrangement and membership of higher taxa. Equally, each of the major applied specialist areas of bacteriology – medical, veterinary and industrial – deals with a host of diverse bacteria whose membership could not conceivably be grouped into any exclusive 'natural' or phylogenetic higher taxon, but rather form a diverse portion of the all-inclusive group of 'the bacteria'.

One major difficulty is the lack of non-arbitrary definitions of the taxon concept at any division from species upwards. The definition of a species concept for the bacteria has been in dispute for more than a century, and definitions of the genus, order and higher taxonomic ranks are successively more elusive. The value judgements that set these divisions are likely to be as controversial in the new era of phylogenetic classification as they were in the days of van Niel's physiological classifications (van Niel 1946). However, despite these difficulties, the search for a phylogenetic classification of the bacteria and other prokaryotes is of enormous importance to biology. Results from this search are likely to shape our future views on the origins of life and of the eukaryote and prokaryote forms.

For medical microbiologists, much of the turmoil in the upper reaches of hierarchical classification has remained unnoticed. Changes at genus level have affected the naming of species in laboratory reports, causing considerable inconvenience. However, the higher taxonomic divisions form a province that academics may re-map with little fear of criticism from applied microbiologists, who are more interested in nomenclature and divisions at species level than in higher taxonomic ranks.

This highlights an important, but rarely discussed, contrast of attitude between academic taxonomy and applied bacteriology. The applied bacteriologist is almost solely interested in divisions at species level, and particularly in those species where identification yields an associated prediction of properties, such as pathogenicity or cross-infection potential, that cannot be examined readily or economically in the laboratory. His requirements are for a division of the bacteria into readily identified species, each with clear and distinct properties significant to his application, and a stable, widely accepted species nomenclature, to allow concise communication of his findings. In contrast to the taxonomist, who attempts to group species in a hierarchy determined by phylogeny or similarity, the applied bacteriologist assembles species in a multitude of distinct classifications of convenience.

The single-tier classification of species nomenclature is common ground for the taxonomist and applied bacteriologist, and deserves a distinguishing name, such as the agnostic, agnarchic (by contrast to hierarchic, from the Greek root *hieros*, sacred, and *arche*, rule) or monadic (Gr. *monados*, unity) classification because of this unique unifying position. Adoption of one of these terms might eliminate the misunderstanding inherent in use of the term 'classification' to cover both the untiered division of bacteria into species, the sense in which many applied microbiologists instinctively interpret the term, and hierarchical schemes.

4 HISTORY AND OPERATION OF THE FORMAL CLASSIFICATION

In the early days of biology, Linnaeus recognized that biologists required a concise, precise and internationally recognized scheme of species nomenclature. He proposed a scheme of latinized binomials comprising a genus and species epithet, referring to a formal description of the species. This was universally accepted, replacing the babel of trivial, poorly defined synonyms individual to each language with a defined vocabulary common to all biologists. This technical vocabulary now bridges language and speciality, providing an essential method of communication. Whatever other gulfs of language and misunderstanding may exist, biologists can guarantee that a species name will communicate a complex detailed description of an organism with precision, and in a remarkably concise form.

Microbes, observed earlier by van Leeuwenhoek, were assigned to 6 species in the class *Chaos* by Linnaeus. Work in the late nineteenth century led to the description of many bacterial pathogens, and the first recognizable attempt to classify bacteria by the botanist Cohn (1872). The rapid growth in species descriptions required regulation and individual international committees were eventually set up to govern the nomenclature of animals and plants, including bacteria. Important landmarks in the advance of bacterial taxonomy were the classifications of Chester (1901), Orla-Jensen (1919) and the work of Buchanan (1918, 1925). Committees for bacterial and viral taxonomy (Murphy et al. 1995) came later, with a breakaway group covering the blue-green algae, claimed originally by the botanists, and now by the bacteriologists. Regulations covering validation of new names and changes in nomenclature are embodied in Codes for each of these groups and are supervised by the appropriate International Committee.

The ICSB is responsible for the Bacteriological

Code (Buchanan, St John-Brooks and Breed 1948, Buchanan et al. 1958, Lapage et al. 1973, Sneath 1992), providing lists of recent validly published species names and proposed changes in nomenclature regularly in the *International Journal of Systematic Bacteriology* (IJSB). In an effort to rationalize nomenclature, remove the burden of early errors and synonyms and simplify access to the nomenclature, a list of the c. 2300 historical bacterial species names considered to be valid was published as the Approved Lists of Bacterial Names (Skerman, McGowan and Sneath 1980, 1989). This, supplemented by the subsequent IJSB validation lists, defines the current, formal nomenclature of bacterial species.

The status of this scheme is reviewed every c. 10 years in successive editions of *Bergey's Manual*; the current classification for each group of bacteria is summarized by experts and the various genera and species are described. Although there is no formal link between the ICSB and *Bergey's Manual*, both clearly draw upon the same pool of expertise and the nomenclature of the Validation and Approved Lists tends to be closely conserved in *Bergey's Manual*.

There are numerous subcommittees of the ICSB, most of which deal with specific groups of bacteria and give recommendations and advice on their area. Meetings of the ICSB and of the subcommittees occur regularly, usually associated with symposia organized by the International Union of Microbiological Societies. Most of the subcommittee meetings are open, allowing participation by any interested parties.

Those wishing to propose new species or changes in systematic nomenclature must follow the rules of the Bacteriological Code if their proposal is to be considered valid. Briefly, the proposal must be published in the IJSB or, if it is published elsewhere, a copy of the paper must be submitted to the IJSB for inclusion of the proposal in the Validation Lists. If a new, culturable species is proposed, then a type culture should be designated and deposited with a recognized service culture collection. There are further detailed rules, particularly on nomenclature, and it is advisable to read the latest version of the Bacteriological Code (Sneath 1992) in detail before submission of a proposal. In addition, minimal acceptable standards for species descriptions are being formulated for specific groups of bacteria (Lévy-Frébault and Portaels 1992, Ursing, Lior and Owen 1994, ICSB Subcommittee on the Taxonomy of Mollicutes 1995) and the standards for the appropriate group should be consulted. Provisions for proposed species that are (currently) non-culturable but have been characterized by DNA sequencing have been clarified (Murray and Schleifer 1994, Murray and Stackebrandt 1995).

5 THE PROCESS OF CLASSIFICATION

This begins with the selection of a limited series of isolates that appear to show restricted diversity (Fig. 3.1). This is simplification by selection and requires an intuitive recognition of probable groups. Inclusion of a range of reference and type cultures and of many strains isolated from a broad range of sources is advisable. The strains are then characterized in a large number of selected tests, producing descriptions for each. These descriptions are compared, either by calculation of a coefficient of similarity for each pair of isolates in numerical taxonomy (Sokal and Sneath 1963, Sneath and Sokal 1973), or intuitively. From these similarities, the existence of sets of isolates, or taxa is postulated. It is desirable that the taxa should be cohesive and differentiable, i.e. that the differences between taxa should be greater than the variation within a taxon.

The taxa are then described and named, according to the rules of nomenclature (Bousfield 1993, MacAdoo 1993), allowing the cohesive (least variable) portions of the description to be communicated in the shorthand form of a name. There are some minor, but irritating, problems with the current nomenclatural system. There is no maximum length in characters for a species binomial, but long species names can tax those installing computerized reporting systems, and occupy inordinate space in journals. In the absence of an ICSB recommendation on this, authors proposing new names should recognize the problem and avoid imposition of this inconvenience on their colleagues. Also, there is no universally accepted guidance on standards for abbreviation of generic names, e.g. *Str.* for *Streptococcus* or *Streptomyces*, and this is a problem in wide ranging papers, or general texts.

Finally, new isolates can be identified, i.e. named as being members of one of the postulated taxa, on the basis of their similarity to the taxon description, or to exemplar members of the taxon (type and reference strains). The taxon description will often have been enlarged by this stage. In particular, evidence on

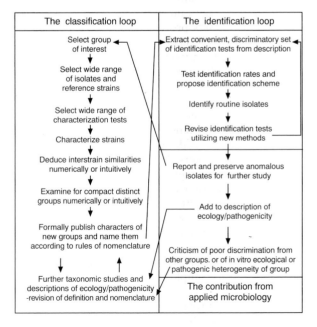

Fig. 3.1 The taxonomic process represented as a flow diagram.

properties too difficult, time consuming or costly to assess in initial tests may have accumulated. In microbiology, this will often include a mass of anecdotal evidence ascribing particular pathogenic, ecological or spoilage properties to a species. This evidence is a key ingredient in the prediction of significant pathogenic (and other) properties from identification, transforming a new taxon from the arena of solely academic interest to that of significance in applied bacteriology. New tests that are more convenient, reliable or rapid may have been shown to differentiate the species. Usually, fewer tests are applied in identification than in classification; only those that have proved reproducible, discriminatory, convenient and inexpensive are used. Note the crucial distinction between classification, which seeks to elucidate a group structure, and identification, which seeks to assign new isolates to an appropriate group within an existing classification.

6 IDENTIFICATION

There are 3 broad approaches to identification in general use. The first, and most important, is recognition of colony morphology (and its variation over a range of isolation media) by an experienced microbiologist, sometimes with confirmation by a few rapid, simple tests. This is the basis on which most clinical isolates are divided into commensals or contaminants of no interest, possible pathogens and probable pathogens. Without this rapid triage of isolates, most diagnostic laboratories would be faced with an overwhelming workload of formal identification. However, the apparent simplicity of the process conceals much complexity and has far-reaching consequences upon the practice of medical microbiology.

Intuitive human pattern recognition is notoriously difficult to document, impossible to teach in a formal setting, and requires prolonged training, strong perceptive and intuitive talents and considerable intelligence. This shapes a long training process of one-to-one teaching at the bench, with either tight selection or a high failure rate. Equally, the triage of isolates must be performed or checked by those with great expertise and experience. The screening process is an art, rather than a science; however, it is difficult to justify the expense of the costly but essential training in this art to paymasters. As in the production of hand crafted furniture, the quality of the reports that a laboratory generates depends heavily on the expertise, skill and time that staff can devote to each specimen. Surprisingly, there appears to be no published study that documents the error rate of this process; whether this reflects an unquestionable accuracy, overweening ego, a profound fear of the consequences of documenting errors, or simple omission is difficult to ascertain.

The second approach is the 'key', exemplified by the identification scheme for coagulase-negative staphylococci proposed by Kloos and Schleifer (1975). This was the favoured approach in the early editions of *Bergey's Manual* and in the various earlier schemes (Chester 1901, Orla-Jensen 1919), reflecting the lasting botanical influence on early bacterial taxonomy. Keys depend heavily upon invariant characteristic reactions, although the later efforts, particularly the Kloos and Schleifer scheme, make some allowance for test variation. However, the work of numerical taxonomists brought general acknowledgement that bacterial species are polythetic, i.e. any individual property may vary within a species. Only the most sophisticated and complex keys could cope with this variation and, with the introduction of numerical identification, formal keys have declined greatly in importance.

Numerical identification is based on surveys of the properties of species that define tables of the expected frequency of positivity in a series of tests for each species. The reaction pattern of an 'unknown' isolate is compared to this table, and its 'goodness of fit' with each species is determined. This comparison may be intuitive, as in the early schemes (Castellani and Chalmers 1919, Cowan 1956, Enterobacteriaceae Subcommittee 1958) and in the tables of the various editions of Cowan and Steel's classic identification manual (Cowan and Steel 1965), or by formal mathematical comparisons. The latter may be calculated concurrently by computer programs, or the calculations may be performed earlier, giving lists of common reaction patterns with the best-fit identification for each, as in the various identification listings for API identification systems. The underlying mathematical principles are described in the classic paper of Willcox, Lapage and Holmes (1980) on numerical identification.

In contrast to classification, where a host of ill-defined mathematical assumptions must be made during data processing, the mathematical identification strategies described by Willcox, Lapage and Holmes (1980) rely on only 6 clear prior assumptions. These are that:

1 the isolate under study cannot be a member of more than one taxon
2 the isolate is a member of a known taxon
3 each of the tests employed yields a result that varies independently of all others
4 the tests have roughly equal within-strain reproducibility
5 reproducibility does not vary significantly between species or strains and
6 the tests yield clear negative or positive results.

Two important parameters in assessing numerical identifications are the 'strangeness' or absolute likelihood of obtaining the observed pattern, often assessed as the estimated frequency of occurrence, logarithmic probability or modal likelihood fraction, and the 'equivocality' or relative likelihood of the fit with known result patterns, often assessed as a percentage relative likelihood or 'identification score'. The 'strangeness' index is calculated for each known species (Table 3.1) and the species with the highest index is chosen as the best-fit identification. Caution is required if the strangeness index is low. This indicates that the observed pattern of reactions is most unusual, even for the best-fit species, and the isolate may well be a 'stranger' – a member of a species not listed in the table. The equivocality index indicates the level of uncertainty in ascribing the isolate to the best-fit species if it is not a 'stranger'. Again, if this index is low, the identification is uncertain, split finely between 2 or more species, and it would be wise to check the fit for the second best-fit species.

A common reason for unusual reaction patterns is that the culture is impure; close examination of prolonged subcultures on a wide variety of media, incubated under a range of conditions, will often reveal cryptic contaminants in these cases. Equally, isolates of *Bacillus* or *Clostridium* that are asporogenous and show a negative gram-staining reaction present an insidious trap for the unwary, who may waste considerable effort under the false assumption that these organisms are true gram-negative bacilli. Conclusive proof of the true nature of such isolates may be difficult to obtain, although colony morphology often provides an indication of the problem.

Ascribing a species name to an isolate should be a carefully considered action. The name will usually communicate an implicit description of many properties that have not been, or cannot be, examined in the laboratory. Once identified, the isolate will be assumed to possess all these implied properties, whether these describe biochemistry, pathogenicity, capability of cross-infection, etc. A poor identification, arrived at with much equivocation, can acquire an undeserved aura of precision during the reporting process. In these cases it might well be more accurate to state that the isolate is unusual and, although most similar to the best-fit species, may well not share all the species properties.

Further, the perception of the properties implied in the species name will vary between individuals, according to their knowledge of systematics and the biases imbued in training and specialization. This is a problem of the 'shorthand' communication of data via a species name, which requires good-to-perfect agreement between the communicating parties on the definition implied in the species name. Clearly, the level of agreement on the implied description may well be unsatisfactory if one side is employing a current nomenclature and description while the other has little contact or interest in microbiology and is struggling to remember information from a minor part of a syllabus learned decades before. The laboratory cannot assume that clinicians will understand the full implications of a species name for any but the most frequently encountered species, and should take every opportunity to expand upon the properties that are intended to be communicated. The possibilities of gross distortion of important clinical implications in this communication have become ever greater with reductions in resources, increasing time constraints, and the increasing speed of change in species nomenclature.

7   CHARACTERIZATION TESTS

The lack of a non-arbitrary, generally accepted definition of the species concept in bacteria (see section 10, p. 59) inevitably, but probably wrongly, directs bacteriologists to definitions based on some particular characterization technology. A broad description of the various technologies is given below and in Table 3.2. It is important to recognize that none of these methods yields results that can be considered to give invariably the isologous comparisons of truly independent variables required in taxonomy.

7.1   Microscopic morphology

These characters comprise: cell shape, size, arrangement, staining, motility and capsule characteristics, spore morphology and flagellar arrangement. Electron microscopy extends these somewhat to fimbriation, wall and cytoplasmic structures. Early microbiologists of the van Leeuwenhoek era were limited to describing the cell morphology and ecological occurrence of those few groups of bacteria distinguishable on the basis of light microscopy. Macroscopic organisms show a massive range of readily observed distinct morphological characters, sufficient to distinguish a huge number of groups. However, bacteria, at the limit of resolution in light microscopy, can be divided into few groups on the basis of cell morphology.

This may have been a major factor in forming a sharp difference of attitude between bacteriologists and macrobiologists. While eighteenth and nineteenth century biologists sought to document the diversity of macro-organisms, ranging throughout the world in their search for specimens and describing hundreds of thousands of species, bacteriologists centred their work on groups that were involved in disease or had industrial importance. With few exceptions, bacteriologists did not participate in the eighteenth and nineteenth century 'collection fever' phase of biology because bacterial characterization was still primitive. By 1989, only c. 2300 bacterial species were cited in the Approved Lists, indicating the low level of interest in discovery and documentation of new taxa during the prior century.

This omission is reflected in the often cited histogram (Fig. 3.2) of the number of known biological species versus adult size. The diagram shows a maximum number of species at a size corresponding to the limit of resolution of the human eye. This may well be an artefact of limited endeavour. The c. 4000 currently described species of bacteria probably represent a tiny fraction of bacterial diversity, a contention supported by recent studies of 16S rRNA diversity in natural environments (Liesak and Stackebrandt 1992, Stackebrandt, Liesak and Goebel 1993).

7.2   Colonial morphology

With the invention of solid media and pure culture techniques came colonial morphological characters. For an experienced bacteriologist, the wealth of data

Table 3.1 Mathematical identification: a worked example

(a) Unknown isolate reaction pattern:

	T1	T2	T3	T4	T5	T6	T7
	+	+	−	+	−	+	+

(b) Identification table:

Taxon	Known frequency of positive reactions in test:							Maximum likelihood
	T1	T2	T3	T4	T5	T6	T7	
A	0.99	0.01	0.99	0.01	0.99	0.99	0.99	0.932
B	0.99	0.75	0.01	0.90	0.75	0.90	0.10	0.442
C	0.90	0.85	0.10	0.95	0.05	0.99	0.99	0.609
D	0.95	0.99	0.99	0.99	0.95	0.01	0.01	0.858
E	0.01	0.01	0.05	0.01	0.99	0.01	0.99	0.894

For each taxon, multiply frequencies for each test together, substituting (1− frequency) for the frequency if it is <0.5, to obtain the maximum likelihood, i.e. the likelihood for the reaction pattern showing the best possible fit for that taxon.

(c) Calculate likelihood of obtaining isolate pattern:

Taxon	Likelihood
A	$0.99 \times 0.01 \times (1-0.99) \times 0.01 \times (1-0.99) \times 0.99 \times 0.99 = 9.70 \times 10^{-9}$
B	$0.99 \times 0.75 \times (1-0.01) \times 0.90 \times (1-0.75) \times 0.90 \times 0.10 = \mathbf{0.147}$
C	$0.90 \times 0.85 \times (1-0.10) \times 0.95 \times (1-0.05) \times 0.99 \times 0.99 = \mathbf{0.609}$
D	$0.95 \times 0.99 \times (1-0.99) \times 0.99 \times (1-0.95) \times 0.01 \times 0.01 = 4.66 \times 10^{-9}$
E	$0.01 \times 0.01 \times (1-0.05) \times 0.01 \times (1-0.99) \times 0.01 \times 0.99 = 9.41 \times 10^{-11}$
	Sum = 0.756

For each taxon, multiply the frequencies for each test together, substituting (1− frequency) for the frequency if the reaction of the unknown isolate is negative. This yields the likelihood of the pattern shown by the unknown being obtained from a member of that taxon.

(d) Calculate identification parameters:

'Strangeness' parameters

Taxon	Log probability	Modal likelihood fraction
A	$-\log(9.70 \times 10^{-9}) = 8.01$	$9.70 \times 10^{-9}/0.932 = 1.04 \times 10^{-8}$
B	$-\log(0.147) = \mathbf{0.83}$	$0.147/0.442 = \mathbf{0.333}$
C	$-\log(0.609) = \mathbf{0.22}$	$0.609/0.609 = \mathbf{1.00}$
D	$-\log(4.65 \times 10^{-9}) = 8.33$	$4.66 \times 10^{-9}/0.858 = 5.42 \times 10^{-9}$
E	$-\log(9.41 \times 10^{-11}) = 10.03$	$9.41 \times 10^{-11}/0.894 = 1.06 \times 10^{-10}$
		Sum = 0.756

'Equivocality' parameters

Taxon	Identification score	Relative likelihood
A	$9.70 \times 10^{-9}/0.756 = 1.24 \times 10^{-10}$	$9.70 \times 10^{-9}/0.609 = 1.59 \times 10^{-6}$
B	$0.147/0.756 = \mathbf{0.194}$	$0.147/0.609 = \mathbf{24.1}$
C	$0.609/0.756 = \mathbf{0.806}$	$0.609/0.609 = \mathbf{100}$
D	$4.65 \times 10^{-9}/0.756 = 6.16 \times 10^{-9}$	$4.66 \times 10^{-9}/0.609 = 5.42 \times 10^{-9}$
E	$9.41 \times 10^{-11}/0.756 = 1.24 \times 10^{-10}$	$9.41 \times 10^{-11}/0.609 = 1.06 \times 10^{-10}$

(e) Conclusion: A poor and equivocal identification as taxon B or C. Further tests should be performed.

from this source is often sufficient for identification at genus or finer taxonomic levels. Most isolates that are discarded in routine diagnostic work as not clinically significant are identified solely on this basis. However, although often highly discriminatory, particularly after prolonged incubation, the many subtle characters involved are often medium- and incu-

bation-dependent and are notoriously difficult to document. Taxonomists should not ignore this elementary investigation, which will often delineate important divisions within a collection of strains and is crucial to exclusion of impure cultures.

Table 3.2 Characterization methods: features dictating their practical utility

Method	High-speed	Good throughput	Low skill	Automated	Low costs		Differentiation level
					Capital	Running	<Genus Species Type>
Ecological	–	–	–	– – –	++	–	<‹– – – – – – – ›
Morphological	++	++	–	– – –	++	++	<‹– – – – ›
Colonial	+++	+++	+	– – –	+++	+	<‹– – – – – – – ›
'Biochemical'	+	+++	+++	p	+++	++	<‹– – – – – – – ›
Enzyme detection	+++	+++	+++	p	+++	++	<‹– – – – – – – ›
Serology	+++	++	++	p	++	–	<– – – – ››
Chemotaxonomy	– –	– –	– –	– –	–	–	<‹– – – – – ›
Fingerprinting	+++	+++	+	s	–	++	<‹– – – – – ››
DNA Base ratios	–	–	–	– –	++	++	<‹– – – ›
DNA Hybridization	– –	– –	– –	– – –	++	++	<– – – ›
16S sRNA sequencing	–	+	+	– – –	++	–	<– – – – ››
Polyphasic studies	– –	++	– –	– – –	++	+	<– – – – – – ››

Key: –, – –, – – –, increasingly less favourable; +, ++, +++ increasingly more favourable; p, possible; s, some.

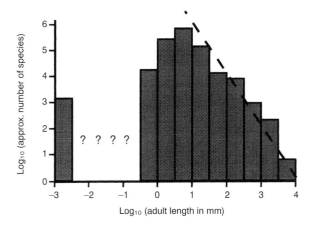

Fig. 3.2 A histogram representing the number of known species versus adult size. The dotted line indicates proportionality of the number of species with the inverse square of adult body length. (Modified from May 1988).

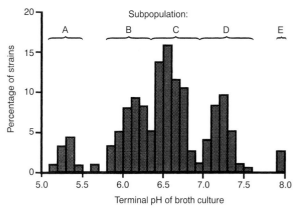

Fig. 3.3 Terminal pH of sugar containing media: a histogram for 420 strains of anaerobic gram-negative bacilli showing multiple distinct populations. (Unpublished data provided by Professor BI Duerden).

7.3 Biochemical tests

Early experiments on optimization of medium composition and incubation conditions led naturally to assessment of nutritional characteristics. The so-called 'biochemical tests' that evolved became an essential tool in bacterial classification and identification. These include tests for: fermentation or oxidation of sugars; waste products; metabolism of organic acids, proteins, amino acids and lipids; temperature, pH and redox range for growth or survival; and tolerance of various chemical agents. In short, they collectively define the nutritional and physiological interactions of the organism with its environment.

These tests are usually technically simple, inexpensive and have high throughput when adapted to multi-point inoculation, commercial test strip, or micro-titration plate formats. Most yield bi-state, i.e. positive or negative, results that are convenient to read. However, it should be recognized that these bi-state results usually represent a simplification of a more complex situation.

As an example, the test for production of acid from sugars measures a fall in pH, separating as 'positive' those strains that produce sufficient excreted acidic metabolites to reduce the pH below a threshold where the indicator dye changes colour. Measuring the pH of the culture (Fig. 3.3) may reveal more complexity, with distinct groups that produce a large, moderate or small fall in pH, no change, or even a rise in pH. On further examination, the results of the test depend upon many factors: the threshold at which the indicator changes colour; the buffering capacity of the medium; the concentration of the sugar; the amount of acidic products excreted; the strength (pKa) and hence molecular structure of the acidic products; the parallel production of alkaline products (e.g. production of ammonia from amino acids or peptides in *Bacillus* and *Clostridium* spp.); the further metabolism of the acids; and the loss of volatile acids from the medium.

Clearly, the technical simplicity of this test conceals far-reaching complexity. Strains that produce small amounts of acetic acid and others that produce large amounts of caproic acid may both yield positive results, because the quantitative difference is balanced by the qualitative difference in the nature and therefore strength of the acids. Equally, organisms with identical glycolytic pathways, but differing in the presence of a tricarboxylic acid cycle and electron transport chain would differ in their acidification of aerobic glucose-containing media. Strains with similar biochemistry may differ in ability to acidify glucose-containing media and strains with distinct biochemistry and end products may yield identical results. In taxonomic studies comparisons are assumed to be of isologous characters, yet acidification tests may reflect anything from a remote ecological similarity in acidification of sugar-containing environments to truly isologous biochemistry.

A further problem results from this 'thresholding' of biochemical tests. Equivocal results and test irreproducibility are likely to be a problem if the test threshold does not coincide with a population minimum. In Fig. 3.3, a detection threshold pH of 5.5 coincides with a minimum in the population distribution. A threshold at this level would give few equivocal results. However, a threshold at pH 6.2 would coincide with a subpopulation maximum, giving many equivocal results, and a division into positive and negative groups that would not reflect real underlying similarities in the biochemistry for subpopulation B.

Formal proof of adequate thresholding is rare in biochemical tests, but the range of genus-specific basal medium and indicator system formats of, for example, sugar acidification tests, clearly indicates intuitive recognition of the problem. Finally, strains that give delayed metabolism of acid products, or produce highly volatile acids, may yield an early positive result, but revert to negative on prolonged incubation.

Morphological, colonial, biochemical and enzyme detection tests are the basis of current routine identification technology. For routine bacteriologists, it is essential that any species or genus name reaching the Validation Lists should have a description of these characters that allows clear identification and discrimination from similar taxa. Applied microbiologists have a clear interest in ensuring that this principle is a central feature of the minimal descriptions formulated by the ICSB committees to direct taxonomists on a line that is compatible with the current requirements of routine laboratories.

7.4 Tests for enzyme activity

Further characterization strategies were investigated. Research showed that some pathogenic effects of bacteria were due to toxins. These toxins included exoenzymes and an offshoot of this work was a clear lineage of characterization tests based on detection of individual enzymes, from the early tests for proteolytic and lipolytic activity, to the modern preformed enzyme tests (Manafi, Kneifal and Bascomb 1991, James 1994). This line produced major advances in biology. Monod's work on the lactose fermentation system of *Escherichia coli* laid the foundations of our understanding of underlying control mechanisms of the cell biochemistry of all living things.

The trend in bacteriology from morphological to physiological and biochemical characterization contrasted with that in macrobiology. Here, morphology still retained practical precedence, but phylogeny, classification based on the postulated evolutionary history of organisms, was becoming a target for academic biologists. Bacteriologists, driven by a paucity of morphological characterization tests, and lacking the fossil material required for phylogeny, resorted to ever more biochemically oriented characterization technology. It is ironic that this technology ultimately led to the precedence of bacteriology in the discovery of DNA as the substance governing inheritance, and in much of the molecular biology that flowed from that event. Bacteriology, which had largely turned its back on phylogeny, provided the basis for the nucleic acid sequencing methods so essential to modern molecular phylogeny.

7.5 Chemotaxonomy

Early work on immunology produced serological characterization tests (Bowden 1993). Interest in the chemical basis of these tests, and work on the mode of action of β-lactam antibiotics, gave a detailed understanding of the chemical structure of bacterial cell walls. The remarkably diverse structures that were found correlated with other properties. Crucially, this clarified grouping of genera into families and laid the foundations of chemotaxonomy, the examination and comparison of cell macromolecules. This approach to characterization has become steadily more important in classification (Goodfellow and O'Donnell 1994).

Methods include comparison of: cell envelope macromolecular structure, particularly the murein polypeptide links, teichoic and teichuronic acids, polar and non-polar lipids (Embley and Wait 1994, Hancock 1994); electron transport chain components of oxidative and photosynthetic metabolism, the quinones, cytochromes and bacteriochlorophylls (Collins 1994, Poole 1994, Richards 1994); and overall base ratios of DNA (Tamaoka 1994). For the most part these are costly, slow, low throughput methods requiring considerable expertise, but provide detailed chemical information relevant to classification at species, genus and suprageneric levels.

7.6 Fingerprinting

Another characterization technology related to chemotaxonomy is termed fingerprinting. The methods include SDS-PAGE analysis of proteins (Vauterin, Swings and Kersters 1993, Pot, Vandamme and Kersters 1994), pyrolysis mass spectrometry (Hindmarch et al. 1990, Goodfellow et al. 1994) and others of less familiar nature (Nelson 1991, Magee 1993b, 1994). These investigations yield results that reflect the chemical composition of the cell, but in comparative terms rather than by elucidation of detailed chemical structure. Fingerprinting methods utilize rapid physicochemical separation methods which produce profiles that can be compared to detect similarities between strains. The profiles are often complex; the underlying nature of differences can not be deduced from fingerprinting alone; and the methods are often based on costly instrumentation. However, these methods usually have a high throughput, automated processing, low running costs, and produce large amounts of data relevant to cell composition, a facet that is otherwise difficult, slow and costly to investigate. These data are pertinent at taxonomic levels from subspecies to supragenus.

7.7 Molecular genetics

The first inroads into DNA-based bacterial classification came with assays for the ratio of guanine–cytosine (GC) to adenine–thymidine (AT) pairs in DNA (Tamaoka 1994), detecting the frequency of usage for GC-rich codons. The G + C content of bacterial DNA varies widely across the genera (Tamaoka 1994), but less so within a genus. This is a useful tool to detect inhomogeneity at genus level. Although significant differences clearly indicate dissimilarity, close similarity of G + C content does not necessarily indicate close similarity in other properties. Clearly, although the proportion of base pairs may be similar, the base sequence of the DNA may differ widely, and code for a distinct metabolic pattern.

Later, DNA–DNA hybridization techniques allowed comparison of base sequence compatibility between strains (Krieg 1988, Johnson 1991, Stackebrandt and Goebel 1994). In this, DNA from a marker strain is annealed with DNA from the strain to be compared, and unbound DNA is removed. The extent of heterologous duplex formation indicates the extent of matching base sequences between the marker and test strain. As a control, 100% sequence compatibility is assessed by hybridization of marker and test DNA from the same strain. Annealing is performed under stringent conditions, at a high temperature, ensuring that only fragments with close sequence similarity remain bound, and at a lower, non-stringent temperature, where fragments may bind despite deletions and point base differences.

Hybridization is currently recognized as the definitive test for similarity at species level. Strains showing >70–75% binding with <5% difference between binding under stringent and non-stringent conditions are considered to belong to the same species (Wayne et al. 1987). Binding at this level indicates c. 96% sequence identity (Stackebrandt and Goebel 1994). Anomalies between hybridization results and biochemical classifications occur in *Xanthomonas* (Hildebrandt, Palleroni and Schroth 1989), *Pseudomonas* (Roselló et al. 1991), the Enterobacteriaceae (Gavini et al. 1989) and *Bacillus* (Priest 1993).

However, hybridization is a prolonged, low throughput approach requiring considerable expertise, hampered by technical difficulties (Sneath 1983, Hartford and Sneath 1988, Johnson 1991) and potential distortion where repetitive sequences occur. Heteroduplex formation decreases markedly at supraspecies levels and no inferences can be drawn on similarities at genus or further levels. Schleifer, Ludwig and Amann (1993) have developed a rapid lysis blotting hybridization system suited to identification.

Comparison of the base sequence for specific genes, usually that coding for the 16S rRNA of the small ribosome subunit, has become a fashionable approach. Various methods are available, including the original technique of direct sequencing of the 16S rRNA (Donis-Keller, Maxam and Gilbert 1977, Peattie 1979, Stackebrandt and Liesack 1993), but most groups currently utilize the polymerase chain reaction (PCR) and DNA sequencing. DNA is extracted from the strain and purified. Two primers, short oligonucleotides corresponding in sequence to 2 highly conserved regions at either end of the 16S rRNA gene, are added, along with Taq polymerase and nucleoside triphosphates. The primers are annealed to the strain DNA, the polymerase attaches to the lead (3′) primer and copies the sequence between the primers. The reaction mixture is heated to denature the copied duplex, releasing single strand DNA. Then the mixture is cooled, re-annealed with the primers, and copied again in multiple cycles. The product DNA contains many copies of the sequence between the 2 priming points.

The product DNA is then extracted, purified and subjected to a second amplification, in the presence of trace amounts of fluorescent base analogues for each of the 4 natural nucleoside triphosphates, with each of the 4 analogue bases tagged with a distinct fluorogen. The infrequent incorporation of a base analogue into the copied DNA terminates the polymerase copying of the template, releasing a copy of the sequence to that point, tagged with a fluorogen. The product comprises copies of portions of the sequence of varying length, but all starting from the same point and each tagged with a fluorogen that identifies the last base incorporated. Electrophoresis of the products separates them according to the length of sequence copied. When the gel is scanned, the smallest fluorescent fragment will be the primer plus the next base in the sequence, tagged with an identifying fluorogen, giving the first base of the sequence. The next fragment will be the primer plus 2 bases, with the last identified by the attached fluorogen, and so on. This process can determine the base sequence of fragments up to c. 400 bases in size. For complete sequences above this size PCR must be performed on several overlapping sections of the gene with primers designed from known portions of the sequence, and copying from the original products, or a copy of the gene ligated into a plasmid.

The 16S rRNA gene is eminently suited to sequencing by this approach, as it contains 3′ and 5′ sequences that are virtually identical in all bacteria, are a suitable size for priming, and are separated by a sequence of a size (c. 1.5 kb) that is readily copied by the polymerase. Furthermore, it is suggested that much of the sequence is highly conserved and so is unlikely to be subject to strain variation. Databases of known 16S rRNA sequences are available on the world-wide web, notably on http:/www.bdt.org.br/structure/molecular.html. Strains of the same species show sequence similarities >97%. However, strains showing similarity at or above this level may belong to distinct species as defined by DNA hybridization (Ash et al. 1991, Fry et al. 1991, Fox, Wisotskey and Jurtshuk 1992, Martinez-Murcia, Benlock and Collins 1992, Stackebrandt and Goebel 1994). This is a slow, costly, low throughput technique requiring expertise, but considerably less demanding in all these aspects than hybridization.

Despite its current popularity, there may be several problems with 16S rRNA sequencing. Flawless transcription of a sequence of c. 1500 base abbreviations to paper or computer file is no mean feat and the inevitable errors in proofreading these transcripts become embedded in the literature. This is no small source of inaccuracy, as noted elsewhere (Bernard et al. 1995, Meissner 1995). Sequences determined for the same species, or even the same strain, by different groups can differ significantly (Clayton et al. 1995). The source of these differences could be sequencing errors, intraspecies variation or, as many species contain multiple copies of the rRNA operon, interoperon differences. Several methods have been used in sequencing and the copy error level with different enzyme preparations is known to differ. Small differences in error rates or bias in the types of error from either source could lead to significant sequence differences. A level of c. 3% sequence difference is suggested as a species cutoff, yet 18% of sequence pairs determined independently for the same strain differed by >1% in the study of Clayton et al. (1995) and 8% differed by >2%. Clearly, the overall error level in deposited sequences is close to the natural variation between closely similar species.

The sequence of individual product DNA molecules copied in PCR may differ slightly from that of the original template, or the operon copied may be atypical. With low error rate polymerase, these erroneous products are unlikely to affect direct sequencing of the pooled product. However, some groups select a single product molecule by cloning into a plasmid for later sequencing and there is a possibility that an atypical product may be selected in cloning. A large blind-coded interlaboratory study to define the accuracy of sequence determination for the various methods and modifications might help convert the doubters, as would an effort to weed out or confirm any possibly inaccurate sequences in the databases.

The 'black box' approach to numerical analysis that is evident in many papers on 16S rRNA sequencing has also been criticized. Goodfellow, Manfio and Chun (1997), reviewing a single issue of IJSB, found clear deficiencies in the numerical methods section of 6 papers on sequencing. Numerical analysis of similarity data is a complex subject unsuited to black box processing. The deficiencies are highlighted by comparison with work on other characterization techniques, in which data are often analysed with 4 or more distinct numerical approaches, and the homogeneity of the proposed consensus groups is then examined to verify the conclusions. Sequence data present greater difficulties in numerical analysis than most other characterization data. There are problems of alignment around deletions and insertions and in the interdependency of base sequences in distinct regions that hydrogen-bond together to form a functional tertiary structure. Sequence data require a greater effort in numerical analysis, and greater caution in interpretation, rather than less. Unfortunately, the rise in availability of numerical taxonomic computer programs has encouraged cursory analysis, without the underlying understanding and caution required in interpretation.

Nevertheless, gene sequencing has opened the possibility that the evolutionary descent (phylogeny) of the current range of bacterial species may be determined. A phylogeny based on the 16S rRNA gene is now well advanced (Woese 1987, 1992). This is likely to be a major influence on the classification presented in the next edition of *Bergey's Manual* and the few studies based on sequences of other conserved genes seem to verify this phylogeny.

7.8   Polyphasic taxonomy

Each of these individual characterization approaches has been hailed in its time as the last great advance in taxonomy, the discovery that would put every bacterium in its proper place in a 'natural classification'. Having seen 4 such definitive advances in one professional lifetime, a more sanguine approach is engendered. Each approach has its individual advantages and disadvantages. Each gives a different, and sometimes contrasting, insight into the differences between bacteria. Each has its place in taxonomic research, classification and identification. Together, the results of all these approaches should give a robust general classification. The deficiencies of low throughput,

high cost methods can be offset by testing the typical members of clusters detected in high throughput, low cost techniques. High throughput techniques are suited to the search of large strain collections for potential new species.

Taxa that are distinct and cohesive in the large range of current techniques should stand the test of time. Colwell (1970) first suggested this polyphasic approach. However, despite its unarguable logic and repetition of the simple message by many experienced bacterial taxonomists, papers suggesting major taxonomic revisions based on a single technique continue to appear, often to be debunked later. The increasing instability of nomenclature at genus level in some areas of bacterial classification may well reflect the failure of workers to implement this polyphasic approach. A craftsman uses many tools to fashion a useful object; taxonomists should recognize that the many approaches to characterization each has an individual appropriate use in the construction of classifications. Although a classification can be based on a single characterization method, it is as unlikely to be of general use as a car built solely with a chisel.

8   VISUALIZING THE RESULTS OF A CLASSIFICATION STUDY

The presentation of results is one of the greatest problems in taxonomy. Most authors choose diagrammatic representations: dendrograms, rooted or unrooted trees, or occasionally 2- or pseudo-3-dimensional ordination diagrams (Fig. 3.4). Each has advantages and disadvantages, but none can represent the full complexity of the data. The alternative tabular presentations (Fig. 3.4) – full or shaded similarity matrices – show the full data, but are unwieldy and difficult to interpret. Many applied microbiologists do not have the knowledge to interpret the subtleties of these diagrams and many would-be taxonomists use the programs that generate these diagrams as black boxes, in ignorance of the principles and shortcomings of the calculations involved (Goodfellow, Manfio and Chun 1997).

The dendrogram (Fig. 3.4a) has a single axis indicating similarity between strains or between groups. The tree-like structure represents fusions of strains or groups, stretching from the multiple tips, each representing a single strain, to the root, a single line representing the fusion of all strains into a single group. Each branch point in the dendrogram represents the formation of a group with the level of intragroup similarity indicated by the position of the join relative to the axis. Where the join is between 2 single strains, the similarity of the strains is represented without distortion, but fusions between groups of strains become successively less representative of similarities between individual strains in the groups. In the unweighted pair-group method with arithmetic averages (UPGMA; Sneath and Sokal 1973), the most common method for constructing these figures, the mean group properties, are compared at these group fusions; the

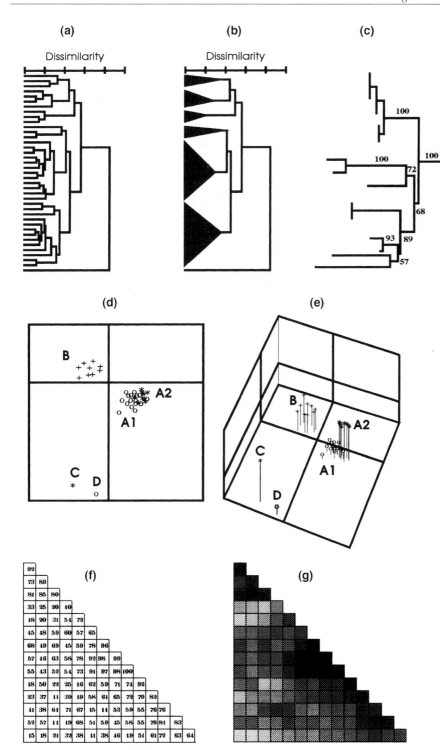

Fig. 3.4 (a–g) Representations of taxonomic data: (a, b) dendrograms; (c) tree (phenogram); (d) 2-dimensional ordination; (e) pseudo-3-dimensional ordination; (f) similarity matrix; (g) shaded, ordered similarity matrix. (Data simplified from various biochemical and pyrolysis mass spectrometry studies by the author and colleagues).

groups formed at low levels of similarity may contain such diverse organisms that the mean group properties have little relevance to the properties of individual members.

Rooted and unrooted trees (Fig 3.4c) are essentially dendrograms that radiate from a central fusion out to radial tips representing individual strains. In this case the distance from the tip to a group fusion point represents the level of dissimilarity between the strain and the group mean. Often, each fusion point is annotated with a number showing the number (or proportion) of independent 'bootstrap' analyses that produced a similar fusion, indicating the degree of certainty that the fusion reflects a clear discontinuity in the original data.

Ordination diagrams represent interstrain dissimilarity as a distance. In Fig. 3.4(d), each strain is represented as a point; the distance between pairs of points indicates the dissimilarity between the appropriate strains. However, the distance structure is only partially represented; clusters of points may contain individual strains or small groups that are distant from the main cluster. This is illustrated in Fig. 3.4(e), where the data for Fig 3.4(d) is re-plotted on 3 axes, showing that group A1 is clearly resolved when a larger proportion of the distance structure is represented. The full distance structure from a large taxonomic study cannot usually be represented on <8 axes.

Ordinations represent the distances between major groups well, but distances for some smaller groups and between individual strains are often poorly represented. This is the converse of tree representations and comparison of the 2 types of diagram can highlight defects in the representations. The axes of ordination diagrams are usually complex, statistically derived functions termed canonical discriminant variates or principal components. For the mathematically inclined, Manly (1994) gives an excellent explanation of these functions. For those averse to mathematics, each function is a composite measure of many properties that collectively distinguish between groups. These are similar to intuitively derived composite measures that are used in descriptions of stature – ectomorphic, mesomorphic or endomorphic – where the relative measurements of a complex set of features, rather than any single measurable feature, divides the groups. Composite measures are a common feature of languages; 'fair' complexion describes a composite of pigmentation features and 'gangly' describes a combined measure of limb length, posture and 'slimness', itself a composite measure.

Similarity matrices and shaded, ordered similarity matrices are represented in Fig. 3.4(f) and 3.4(g), respectively. These represent the interstrain similarities as numbers or graded shading in a tabular form, similar to the tables of intercity distances that can be found in roadmap atlases. The shaded tables are particularly useful in highlighting intermingling at the edges of clusters, and intergroup similarities that may not be apparent in the topology of a dendrogram. It should be noted, however, that the order of strains markedly influences the clarity of these matrices.

The diagrammatic representations face the fundamental difficulty that it is usually impossible to represent fully the distance structure determined in a taxonomic study in a 2-dimensional diagram. Mathematically, it can be shown that if n strains are examined in t discriminatory tests and $n < t$, then the distance structure may require up to $n - 1$ dimensions for accurate representation, and can only rarely be fully represented in $<(n - 1)^{1/2}$ dimensions. For a taxonomic study involving c. 100 strains, this would mean that the data would only be fully representable in 10 or more dimensions. Clearly, pictorial 2-dimensional representations of similarity data are likely to be deficient or misleading in some aspects. Failure to reveal differences may occur when clusters overlap in ordinations because the axes on which they separate are not plotted, or when isolates 'chain' into unsuitable groups in dendrograms.

9 THE 'TYPE' CONCEPT AND SERVICE CULTURE COLLECTIONS

The type concept originated from botany, where a single typical dead specimen can supply a wealth of morphological data sufficient to define the species, and to identify further examples. Sneath (1995) has suggested that, with modern characterization methods, preserved dead bacterial specimens might eventually prove equally useful. However, for more than a century bacteriologists have preserved cultures of bacteria as viable organisms. Private collections exist in most departments, but the national service collections, which supply preserved viable cultures, are the prime source of reference and type cultures. Each valid culturable species has a type culture, considered by Buchanan (1955) to be the reference point for the species.

These service collections are of paramount importance to bacteriology. They provide reference cultures for comparative identification, quality control of characterization tests, teaching and taxonomic studies. They often also provide focal expertise in taxonomy and identification and an essential service for identification of the more unusual organisms isolated in routine laboratories. Individual routine laboratories have insufficient time and see insufficient material to register rare, unrecognized pathogens as anything other than unusual. The long-standing high throughput of 'unusual' isolates for identification at national centres has repeatedly allowed identification of previously unnamed groups of bacterial pathogens as new species.

The CDC laboratories in Atlanta have a notable record for the detection of such groups, recognized in the genus epithet *Cedecea*. It is particularly important that routine laboratories continue to send unusual isolates to such units, along with definitive information on their source and pathogenic effects, despite budgetary constraints. Equally, these units must continue to provide the identification service and maintain and review their collections of unnamed strains if new and rare pathogens are to be adequately monitored.

However, there are problems with these type and reference cultures. Live cultures maintained by serial subculture inevitably undergo selection and adaptation. Experimental evidence in chemostat (Helling, Vargas and Adams 1987) and batch culture (Atwood, Scheider and Ryan 1951) strongly suggest that pure cultures undergo virtually complete clonal replacement with mutated variants after every c. 100 divisions. Many older type strains were maintained by serial culture in early collections and it is likely that most collection strains have undergone multiple predeposition culture cycles. Equally, the methods used to avoid continued subculture, freeze-drying and freezing in cryoprotectants are highly selective. It is rare to recover >1% of the initial population from these preserved specimens; such high kill rates must exert some selective pressure. This selection may be particularly severe for obligate anaerobes exposed to air during subculture. Early microbiologists recognized that biological variation was an inescapable consequence of the culture and storage of strains (Rahn 1929) and used the effect in attenuation of the pathogenicity of anthrax and tubercle bacilli. Modern microbiologists would do well to remember their conclusions.

Equally, reference cultures must be treated with the utmost care outside central collections. There have been several incidents of mislabelled reference strains being passed between research laboratories, with consequent errors in published work, notably with *Candida albicans* (Mackenzie and Odds 1991). All reference cultures should be obtained directly from a recognized culture collection and replaced regularly from the same source.

10 THE SPECIES CONCEPT

The definition of the species concept in bacteriology continues to be a favourite topic of debate where those of a philosophical bent can argue free from the constraint of experimental data. A criticism of this debate is of the lack of enterprise in obtaining data that might elucidate a solution, rather than of the discussion of this central problem in classification.

In general biology, the best known species definition is that of a sexual interbreeding capability with production of offspring capable of further interbreeding. This definition clearly is not applicable to asexual organisms and is extremely difficult to test in the wild. Indeed, there are many examples where interspecies hybrids are viable, particularly in plants (Eckenwalder 1984), but also in animals (Hall 1978). Clearly, the capability of promiscuous genetic exchange in bacteria invalidates these definitions based on interfertility (Jones 1989). Interspecies exchange of chromosomal DNA has been demonstrated repeatedly (Maynard-Smith, Dowson and Spratt 1991); transposons and promiscuous plasmids can transfer large genetic elements across massive taxonomic gulfs (Arthur, Brisson and Courvalin 1987, Kirby 1990, Natarajan and Oriel 1991). Other species definitions of more general applicability exist (Simpson 1961, Hutchinson 1965, Van Valen 1976, Templeton 1989), but are not helpful in practical delineation of species.

In practice, identification and most classification work in general biology still relies almost exclusively on comparison of phenotypic characters. The various fine shadings of sexual species definitions are discussed with vigour, but their impact on practical aspects is small. Bacteriologists are probably further advanced on the species concept, with reasonable consensus agreement on a practically applicable, though arbitrary, definition based on DNA hybridization (Wayne et al. 1987).

However, even this consensus has been confused by the adoption of a series of terms that fragment the species concept into variants. Ravin (1963) proposed the terms genospecies, encompassing mutually inter-

fertile organisms, nomenspecies, encompassing organisms 'similar' to the type strain, and taxospecies, encompassing groups that share a high proportion of common properties. The term genomic species, readily confused with genospecies, encompasses organisms showing high DNA sequence similarity. These concepts have pragmatic merit (Ursing et al. 1995), but offer a dangerous attraction to an explosive diversification of concepts of convenience, each with its own classification and nomenclature. Medical microbiologists could easily find the concept of a medicospecies, encompassing a classification that they found particularly convenient, irresistible in the current milieu of rapid nomenclatural change.

The species concept that seems most universally accepted in practice, if not in theoretical discussion, is the taxospecies: a group of organisms that show high similarity in a broad range of characterization approaches and are delimited from other organisms by an area of character combinations that are rarely found in nature. This definition is implicit in the numerical taxonomic approach and naturally entrains the concept of polyphasic taxonomy. It does not imply any arbitrary breakpoint of similarity in a specific test, but requires proof of a discontinuity of variation at the species boundary.

Dividing organisms into species is an unavoidable necessity in biology; routine work invariably requires inference of more general properties from a limited number of observed characters. However, the organisms have no knowledge of, nor obligation to obey, the divisions that are drawn. The boundaries between species can often be diffuse, particularly in bacteriology. However, biologists often give the impression that the natural world can be segmented with absolute clarity into the divisions that we desire. Propagation of this erroneous impression in the general population may well encourage the view that humanity itself can be divided with equal clarity, with all the unsavoury consequences that ensue. A definition of the species concept that denies the diffuse uncertainty of biological divisions is as undesirable politically as it is scientifically.

11 SPECIATION AND EVOLUTION

This is a much neglected area of research, but one in which bacteriology could make a considerable contribution to our understanding. In contrast to higher organisms, bacteria reproduce rapidly. It is possible to produce populations comparable to the entire worldwide population of man within a few days in a fermenter of modest size. Furthermore, bacteriologists have evolved sophisticated techniques for the detection and selection of variants forming a tiny proportion of a population. This offers the capability to observe evolution in action over short periods and in a level of detail that cannot be approached in macrobiology. It is unfortunate that the potential for useful work in this area has lain fallow for so long. The few studies to date (Atwood, Scheider and Ryan 1951, Helling, Vargas and Adams 1987, Lenski and Travisano 1994) have been largely ignored, possibly because they emphasize a level of variability during successive culture cycles that many modern bacteriologists would prefer to ignore.

Equally, bacteriologists have observed evolution in the wild for many years, but ignored its implications for evolutionary science. This is particularly true in medical microbiology. The introduction of antibiotics unintentionally produced the largest experiment in evolution ever undertaken by man, but its results have never been analysed from an evolutionary viewpoint and the period in which a control population could be observed has long passed. What is obvious from this experiment is that bacteria are eminently suited to evolutionary studies. The high selective pressure of antibiotics and the rapid reproduction of bacteria has spawned, for example, at least 5 distinct successive races of *Staphylococcus aureus* suited to spread within 50 years in the ecological niche offered by hospitals. Fortunately, much material has been stored in culture collections and this could provide an invaluable resource should sufficient funding and interest become available.

It is singularly unfortunate that the unique combination of the capabilities of bacteriological techniques and the highly selective environments found in hospitals, particularly intensive care units, have not been brought to the attention of evolutionary scientists, population geneticists and microbial ecologists. The potential for mutual advantage from such a combination of expertise is enormous. However, the beginnings of interest are now obvious in studies of the genetics of evolutionary change in, for example, the acquisition of resistance to penicillin in commensal *Neisseria* (Bowler et al. 1994). Population geneticists are beginning to study variation in bacteria (Baumberg et al. 1995) and the impetus provided by the rapidly decreasing effectiveness of antibiotics against hospital-evolved pathogens may lead to funding of such projects.

12 WHAT'S IN A NAME?

Extrapolation of current trends is notoriously unreliable in science, but it is likely that bacterial systematics will have to cope with a major increase in the rate of description of new taxa. The background trend is already well established and may well be magnified by new influences. Automated acquisition of characterization data is becoming well established for an ever wider range of characterization approaches, speeding experimental work, and changing the emphasis of problem-solving effort to data handling. The international agreements on biodiversity may well increase funding for taxonomic studies, hitherto poorly funded by industry and public sources. The prospect that species may be patented will clearly lead to increased discovery efforts and provide a financial incentive to the 'splitter' faction. Pending patents have already caused difficulties in the deposition of type strains of

commercial significance (Labeda, Kurtzman and Swezey 1995). New technology may well redouble productivity from the molecular biology faction and DNA sequencing studies of natural environments have already revealed an astounding diversity of non-culturable bacteria.

However, the speed of change in nomenclature has become a problem in applied bacteriology; those who deal with cystic fibrosis patients are, hopefully, aware of the multiple changes in the nomenclature of 2 major pseudomonad pathogens in recent years (Hugh 1981, Swings et al. 1983, Yabuuchi et al. 1992, Palleroni and Bradbury 1993). Changes in the nomenclature of pathogens generates considerable criticism among medical microbiologists. They are not merely inconvenient; they increase the problems of communication and may well have unforeseen implications in the complex legislation that touches on microbiology in each of the various countries of the world. A further increase in the rate of change could generate a major rift between those who use and those who produce classifications (Magee 1993a).

Key issues for clarification are the date from which proposed changes in nomenclature are to be regarded as active, in the sense that legal proceedings might judge a microbiologist to have erred by using an older nomenclature, and the process of consensus acceptance of change. Most taxonomists and many users regard the date of publication in the IJSB as the date of active change, but many may postpone judgement until the first date of inclusion in an edition of *Bergey's Manual*. The latter includes sufficient time to judge the consensus acceptability of the change, the former clearly does not. However, neither solution seems completely acceptable, even at the present rate of change in nomenclature.

If changes in nomenclature are active from their appearance in the IJSB, each change is governed by a group comprising the authors of the paper, an editor and a few referees. Is the judgement of so small a group invariably so reliable, and their insight into the ramifying consequences so broad, that the general community of microbiologists will find the change acceptable? Notwithstanding respect for fellow microbiologists, it is frightening that any unselected group this small can institute changes that may have considerable legal and other consequences on the whole of bacteriology and that these changes become active, without prior notice, on publication in a journal subscribed to by a minority of applied bacteriologists.

Equally, if active change coincides with mention in *Bergey's Manual*, the interval between editions, c. 10 years, is too long and the number of concurrent changes to be made is too large. Even here, there is no defined mechanism for judging consensus acceptance of change. One, or at most a few, experts on each major group write on their subject. There is no guarantee that their interests are so all-inclusive that some change crucial to one branch of the applied science is missed, or that their own biases reflect a consensus view of bacteriologists.

The ICSB has a pivotal role in guiding developments in bacterial systematics, including nomenclature, and its members face a new century that is likely to tax their powers of mediation. Negotiating satisfactory compromise between the wishes of applied microbiologists and taxonomists, 2 groups with widely differing views and requirements, could well require considerable diplomacy. However, the alternative to compromise and co-operation between taxonomists and users is to discard our only internationally accepted scheme of bacterial nomenclature and this is clearly unacceptable. The solutions to these problems can not be coercive; the nomenclatural code does not, and can not, dictate the nomenclature used by individuals. The wisdom of preserving general acceptance of the formal nomenclature must be convincingly explained to a silent majority, who would much prefer to remain with the nomenclature they were taught years before.

Many of these communication problems could be solved by computerized communication of changes and opinions on the world-wide web. One major advance is the availability of lists of all validated names on the world-wide web (http://www.bdt.org.br/cgi-bin/ bdtnet/bacteri1name). In the interim, efforts are being made to disseminate notification of proposed changes more widely (Frederiksen and Ursing 1995a, 1995b) and this should be supported and encouraged by the community of applied bacteriologists.

An associated problem is the growing gap between the characterization methods used by taxonomists and those available for identification in the routine laboratory. Base ratio determinations, DNA–DNA hybridization, 16S rRNA sequence determination and chemotaxonomic methods are only available in a minority of routine laboratories and are, as yet, too specialized, tortuous and slow to have major relevance to identification in routine bacteriology. However, an increasing number of taxonomic papers neglect any mention of characters that can be determined in routine laboratories. The bench microbiologist whose skills lie in identification from colony morphology, pure culture and biochemical tests could be excused for regarding this change with horror. This generates a backlash, which is now regularly heard as detrimental comments on the probable capabilities of taxonomists to perform conventional tests or to examine plate cultures adequately. Clearly, this is an area where medical microbiological input to the formulation of minimal standards for the description of new species is essential to our interests. Taxonomists and applied microbiologists must seek mixes of characterization methods that fulfil the requirements of both research and routine work and revise these as technology advances.

However, medical microbiologists must recognize that they live in a time of great change in bacterial systematics. As in all science, taxonomic truth is approached by successive revision in the light of new facts and the current turmoil in nomenclature is a reflection of growing interest in a subject that forms the basis of routine laboratory work. Nomenclatural change is inevitable and can not be ignored. Many of the changes may increase the capability to predict important properties from identification results. However, applied microbiologists must also ensure that, when the changes cause problems, these are voiced to the ICSB with sufficiently convincing force, clarity and representation. The widespread tradition of ignoring nomenclatural change and restricting critical comment to colleagues in the same field is not helpful either to medical microbiology or to taxonomy.

13 THE FUTURE

The future course of bacterial taxonomy is likely to be interesting and turbulent. The attitudes and assumptions stemming from the late nineteenth century that have shackled progress for the greater part of the twentieth century are beginning to be discarded. The introduction of numerical taxonomy marked the first major break with the early botanical influence, allowing recognition of the true nature of variation within bacterial species and disposing of the baggage of monothetic groups and invariant diagnostic characters. Characterization tests now allow comparison of features other than the physiological and nutritional interactions with the environment. Together, these have encouraged the beginnings of exploration of the true diversity of bacteria, which may well produce many unforeseen discoveries of economic significance. Molecular methods are beginning to be used to explore diversification in bacteria; there is now a possibility that the enormous potential of bacteria in the study of evolutionary processes may be recognized. The phylogeny of bacteria, or at least that of the 16S rRNA gene, is now becoming apparent.

These changes are bringing a host of problems. Non-taxonomists are increasingly bewildered by sudden changes in nomenclature and the alienation that this produces must be tackled. The tendency of workers to adopt uniformly a single characterization technique, rather than a polyphasic approach, must be actively discouraged, for it will certainly lead to large, unsupportable swings in nomenclature as techniques fall in and out of favour. A major problem of the polyphasic approach is that the full range of characterization techniques cannot be supported in a single laboratory. The consequences of this are that several groups must be involved in each study and the paper produced must acknowledge a host of workers in the authorship. The non-scientific problems of contact, co-operation, precedence of discovery and adequate acknowledgement must be tackled if the polyphasic approach is to become the accepted method of taxonomic advance. Bacterial taxonomy is advancing into the next century in the midst of change. Hopefully, solutions to these problems will be found in a newly matured science that will continue to produce spin-off discoveries of enormous importance in general biology.

REFERENCES

Arthur M, Brisson NA, Courvalin P, 1987, Origin and evolution of genes specifying resistance to macrolide, lincosamide and streptogramin antibiotics: data and hypotheses, *Antimicrob Chemother*, **20:** 783–802.

Ash C, Farrow JAE et al., 1991, Phylogenetic heterogeneity of the genus *Bacillus* revealed by comparative analysis of small subunit-ribosomal RNA sequences, *Lett Appl Microbiol*, **13:** 202–6.

Atwood KC, Scheider LK, Ryan FJ, 1951, Periodic selection in *Escherichia coli*, *Genetics*, **37:** 146–55.

Baumberg S, Young JPW et al., 1995, *Population Genetics of Bacteria*, Cambridge University Press, Cambridge.

Bernard H-U, Chan S-Y et al., 1995, Reply to 'On the nature of papillomavirus hell', *J Infect Dis*, **172:** 895–6.

Bousfield IJ, 1993, Bacterial nomenclature and its role in systematics, *Handbook of New Bacterial Systematics*, eds Goodfellow M, O'Donnell AG, Academic Press, London, 318–38.

Bowden GHW, 1993, Serological identification, *Handbook of New Bacterial Systematics*, eds Goodfellow M, O'Donnell AG, Academic Press, London, 429–62.

Bowler LD, Zhang QY et al., 1994, Interspecies recombination between the PenA genes of *Neisseria meningitidis* and commensal *Neisseria* species during the emergence of penicillin resistance in *N. meningitidis*: natural events and laboratory simulation, *J Bacteriol*, **176:** 333–7.

Buchanan RE, 1918, Studies in the nomenclature and classification of the bacteria. V. Subgroups and genera of the Bacteriaceae, *J Bacteriol*, **3:** 27.

Buchanan RE, 1925, *General Systematic Bacteriology. History, Nomenclature, Groups of Bacteria*, Williams & Wilkins, Baltimore.

Buchanan RE, 1955, Taxonomy, *Annu Rev Microbiol*, **9:** 1–20.

Buchanan RE, St John-Brooks R, Breed RS, 1948, International bacteriological code of nomenclature, *J Bacteriol*, **55:** 287 and *J Gen Microbiol*, **3:** 44.

Buchanan RE, Cowan ST et al., 1958, *International Code of Nomenclature of Bacteria and Viruses*, State College Press, Ames, Iowa. Reprinted with corrections 1959: Iowa State University Press, Ames, Iowa.

Castellani A, Chalmers AJ, 1919, *Manual of Tropical Medicine*, 3rd edn, Baillière, Tindall & Cox, London.

Chester FD, 1901, *A Manual of Determinative Bacteriology*, Macmillan, New York.

Clayton RA, Sutton G et al., 1995, Intraspecific variation in small-subunit rRNA sequences in GenBank: why single sequences may not adequately represent prokaryotic taxa, *Int J Syst Bacteriol*, **45:** 595–6.

Cohn F, 1872, Untersuchungen über Bacterien, *Beitr Biol Pfl 1 Heft*, **2:** 127.

Collins MD, 1994, Isoprenoid quinones, *Chemical Methods in Procaryotic Systematics*, eds Goodfellow M, O'Donnell AG, John Wiley & Sons, Chichester, 265–309.

Colwell RR, 1970, Polyphasic taxonomy of bacteria, *Culture Collections of Microorganisms*, eds Iizuka H, Hasegawa T, University of Tokyo Press, Tokyo, 421–36.

Cowan ST, 1956, Taxonomic rank of the Enterobacteriaceae 'groups', *J Gen Microbiol*, **15:** 345–9.

Cowan ST, 1968, *A Dictionary of Microbial Taxonomic Usage*, Oliver & Boyd, Edinburgh.

Cowan ST, 1962, The microbial species – a macromyth?, *Microbial Classification*, eds Ainsworth GC, Sneath PHA, Cambridge University Press, Cambridge, 433–55.

Cowan ST, Steel KJ, 1965, *Manual for the Identification of Medical Bacteria*, Cambridge University Press, Cambridge.

Donis-Keller H, Maxam AM, Gilbert W, 1977, Mapping adenines, guanines, and pyrimidines in RNA, *Nucleic Acids Res*, **4:** 2527–37.

Eckenwalder JE, 1984, Natural intersectional hybridisation between North American species of *Populus* (*Salicaceae*) in sections *Aigeiros* and *Tacamahaca*. III, Paleobotany and evolution, *Can J Bot*, **62:** 336–42.

Embley TM, Wait R, 1994, Structural lipids of eubacteria, *Chemical Methods in Procaryotic Systematics*, eds Goodfellow M, O'Donnell AG, John Wiley & Sons, Chichester, 121–61.

Enterobacteriaceae Subcommittee, 1958, Report of the Enterobacteriaceae Subcommittee of the Nomenclature Committee of the International Association of Microbiological Societies, *Int Bull Bacteriol Nomencl Taxon*, **8:** 25–33.

Fox GE, Wisotskey JD, Jurtshuk P Jr, 1992, How close is close: 16S rRNA sequence identity may not be sufficient to guarantee species identity, *Int J Syst Bacteriol*, **42:** 166–70.

Frederiksen W, Ursing J, 1995a, Proposed new bacterial taxa and proposed changes of bacterial names published during 1994 and considered to be of interest to medical or veterinary bacteriology, *J Med Microbiol*, **43:** 315–17.

Frederiksen W, Ursing J, 1995b, Proposed new bacterial taxa and proposed changes of bacterial names published during 1994 and considered to be of interest to medical and veterinary bacteriology, *APMIS*, **103:** 651–4.

Fry NK, Saunders NA et al., 1991, The use of 16S ribosomal RNA analyses to investigate the phylogeny of the family Legionellaceae, *J Gen Microbiol*, **137:** 1215–22.

Gavini F, Mergaert J et al., 1989, Transfer of *Enterobacter agglomerans* (Beijerinck 1888) Ewing & Fife 1972 to *Pantoea* gen. nov. as *Pantoea agglomerans* comb. nov. and description of *Pantoea dispersa*, *Int J Syst Bacteriol*, **39:** 337–45.

Goodfellow M, Manfio GP, Chun J, 1997, Towards a practical species concept for cultivable bacteria, *Species: the Units of Biodiversity*, eds Claridge MS, Dawah HA, Wilson MR, Chapman & Hall, London, in press.

Goodfellow M, O'Donnell AG, 1994, Chemosystematics: current state and future prospects, *Chemical Methods in Procaryotic Systematics*, eds Goodfellow M, O'Donnell AG, John Wiley & Sons, Chichester, 1–20.

Goodfellow M, Chun J et al., 1994, Curie-point pyrolysis mass spectrometry and its practical application to bacterial systematics, *Bacterial Diversity and Systematics*, eds Priest FG, Ramos-Cormenzana A, Tindall BJ, Plenum Press, New York, 87–104.

Hall RL, 1978, Variability and speciation in canids and hominids, *Wolf and Man, Evolution in Parallel*, eds Hall RL, Sharp SH, Academic Press, New York, 153–77.

Hancock IC, 1994, Analysis of cell wall constituents of Gram-positive bacteria, *Chemical Methods in Procaryotic Systematics*, eds Goodfellow M, O'Donnell AG, John Wiley & Sons, Chichester, 63–84.

Hartford T, Sneath PHA, 1988, Distortion of taxonomic structure from DNA relationships due to different choice of reference strains, *Syst Appl Microbiol*, **10:** 241–50.

Helling RB, Vargas CN, Adams J, 1987, Evolution of *Escherichia coli* during growth in a constant environment, *Genetics*, **116:** 349–58.

Hildebrandt DC, Palleroni NJ, Schroth MN, 1990, Deoxyribonucleic acid relatedness of 24 xanthomonad strains representing 23 *Xanthomonas campestris* pathovars and *Xanthomonas fragariae*, *J Appl Bacteriol*, **68:** 263–9.

Hindmarch JM, Magee JT et al., 1990, A pyrolysis mass spectrometry study of *Corynebacterium* spp., *J Med Microbiol*, **30:** 137–49.

Hugh R, 1981, *Pseudomonas maltophilia* sp. nov. nom. rev., *Int J Syst Bacteriol*, **31:** 195.

Hutchinson GE, 1965, The niche: an abstractly inhabited hypervolume, *The Ecological Theatre and Evolutionary Play*, Yale University Press, New Haven, CT, 26–78.

ICSB Subcommittee on the Taxonomy of Mollicutes, 1995, Revised minimal standards for description of new species of the class Mollicutes, *Int J Syst Bacteriol*, **45:** 605–12.

James AL, 1994, Enzymes in taxonomy and diagnostic bacteriology, *Chemical Methods in Procaryotic Systematics*, eds Goodfellow M, O'Donnell AG, John Wiley & Sons, Chichester, 471–92.

Johnson JL, 1991, DNA reassociation experiments, *Nucleic Acid Techniques in Bacterial Systematics*, eds Stackebrandt E, Goodfellow M, John Wiley & Sons, Chichester, 21–44.

Jones D, 1989, Genetic methods, *Bergey's Manual of Systematic Bacteriology*, vol. 4, eds Williams ST, Sharpe ME, Holt JG, Williams & Wilkins, Baltimore, 2310–12.

Kirby R, 1990, Evolutionary origin of aminoglycoside phosphotransferase resistance genes, *J Mol Evol*, **30:** 489–92.

Kloos WE, Schleifer KH, 1975, Simplified scheme for routine identification of human staphylococci, *J Clin Microbiol*, **1:** 82–91.

Krieg NR, 1988, Bacterial classification: an overview, *Can J Microbiol*, **34:** 536–40.

Labeda DP, Kurtzman CP, Swezey JL, 1995, Taxonomic note: use of patent strains as type strains in the valid description of new bacterial taxa, *Int J Syst Bacteriol*, **45:** 868.

Lapage SP, Clark WA et al., 1973, Proposed revision of the International Code of Nomenclature of Bacteria, *Int J Syst Bacteriol*, **23:** 83.

Lenski RE, Travisano M, 1994, Dynamics of adaptation and diversification: a 10,000-generation experiment with bacterial populations, *Proc Natl Acad Sci USA*, **91:** 6808–14.

Lévy-Frébault VV, Portaels F, 1992, Proposed minimal standards for the genus *Mycobacterium* and for description of new slowly growing *Mycobacterium* species, *Int J Syst Bacteriol*, **42:** 315–23.

Liesack W, Stackebrandt E, 1992, Occurrence of novel groups of the domain bacteria as revealed by analysis of genetic material isolated from an Australian terrestrial environment, *J Bacteriol*, **174:** 5072–8.

MacAdoo TO, 1993, Nomenclatural literacy, *Handbook of New Bacterial Systematics*, eds Goodfellow M, O'Donnell AG, Academic Press, London, 339–58.

Mackenzie DWR, Odds FC, 1991, Nonidentity and authentication of 2 major reference strains of *Candida albicans*, *J Med Vet Microbiol*, **29:** 225–61.

Magee JT, 1993a, Forsaking the tome – a worm's eye view of taxonomy, *J Med Microbiol*, **39:** 401–2.

Magee JT, 1993b, Whole organism fingerprinting, *Handbook of New Bacterial Systematics*, eds Goodfellow M, O'Donnell AG, Academic Press, London, 383–427.

Magee JT, 1994, Analytical fingerprinting methods, *Chemical Methods in the Classification of Prokaryotes*, eds Goodfellow M, O'Donnell AG, John Wiley & Sons, Chichester, 523–53.

Manafi M, Kneifel W, Bascomb S, 1991, Fluorogenic and chromogenic substrates used in bacterial diagnostics, *Microbiol Rev*, **55:** 335–48.

Manly BFJ, 1994, *Multivariate Statistical Methods: A Primer*, 2nd edn, Chapman & Hall, London.

Martinez-Murcia AJ, Benlock S, Collins MD, 1992, Phylogenetic interrelationships of members of the genera *Aeromonas* and *Plesiomonas* as determined by 16S ribosomal DNA sequencing: lack of congruence with results of DNA:DNA hybridisation, *Int J Syst Bacteriol*, **42:** 412–21.

May RH, 1988, How many species are there on Earth?, *Science*, **241:** 1441–9.

Maynard-Smith J, Dowson CG, Spratt BG, 1991, Localised sex in bacteria, *Nature (London)*, **343:** 418–19.

Meissner JD, 1995, On the nature of papillomavirus hell, *J Infect Dis*, **72:** 95.

Murphy F, Fouquet CM, et al. (eds), 1995, *Virus Taxonomy. Sixth Report of the International Committee on Taxonomy of Viruses, Supplement 10*, Springer-Verlag, Berlin.

Murray RGE, Schleifer KH, 1994, Taxonomic notes: a proposal for recording the properties of putative taxa of procaryotes, *Int J Syst Bacteriol*, **44:** 174–6.

Murray RGE, Stackebrandt E, 1995, Taxonomic note: implementation of the provisional status *Candidatus* for incompletely described prokaryotes, *Int J Syst Bacteriol*, **45:** 186.

Natarajan MR, Oriel P, 1991, Conjugal transfer of recombinant transposon Tn*916* from *Escherichia coli* to *Bacillus stearothermophilus*, *Plasmid*, **26:** 67–73.

Nelson WH (ed.), 1991, *Modern Techniques for Rapid Microbiological Analysis*, VCH Publishers, New York.

van Niel CB, 1946, The classification and natural relationships of bacteria, *Cold Spring Harbour Symp Quant Biol*, **11:** 285–301.

Orla-Jensen S, 1919, *The Lactic Acid Bacteria*, Høst & Son, Copenhagen.

Palleroni NJ, Bradbury JF, 1993, *Stenotrophomonas*, a new bacterial genus for *Xanthomonas maltophilia* (Hugh 1980) Swings *et al.* 1983, *Int J Syst Bacteriol*, **43:** 606–9.

Peattie DA, 1979, Direct chemical method for sequencing RNA, *Proc Natl Acad Sci USA*, **76:** 1760–4.

Poole RK, 1994, Analysis of cytochromes, *Chemical Methods in Prokaryotic Systematics*, eds Goodfellow M, O'Donnell AG, John Wiley & Sons, Chichester, 311–44.

Pot B, Vandamme P, Kersters K, 1994, Analysis of electrophoretic whole-organism protein fingerprints, *Chemical Methods in Prokaryotic Systematics*, eds Goodfellow M, O'Donnell AG, John Wiley & Sons, Chichester, 493–521.

Priest FG, 1993, Systematics and ecology of *Bacillus*, Bacillus subtilis *and Other Gram-positive Bacteria: Biochemistry, Physiology and Molecular Genetics*, eds Sonnenheim AL, Hoch JA, Losick R, American Society for Microbiology, Washington, DC, 3–16.

Rahn O, 1929, Contributions to the classification of bacteria, *Zentralbl Bakteriol Parasitenkd Abt II*, **78:** 8–27.

Ravin AW, 1963, Experimental approaches to the study of bacterial phylogeny, *Am Nat*, **97:** 307–18.

Richards WR, 1994, Analysis of pigments: bacteriochlorophylls, *Chemical Methods in Prokaryotic Systematics*, eds Goodfellow M, O'Donnell AG, John Wiley & Sons, Chichester, 345–401.

Rosselló R, Garcia-Valdés J et al., 1991, Genotypic and phenotypic diversity of *Pseudomonas stutzeri*, *Syst Appl Microbiol*, **8:** 124–7.

Schleifer KH, Ludwig W, Amann R, 1993, Nucleic acid probes, *Handbook of New Bacterial Systematics*, eds Goodfellow M, O'Donnell AG, Academic Press, London, 463–510.

Simpson GG, 1961, *Principles of Animal Taxonomy*, Columbia University Press, New York.

Skerman VBD, McGowan V, Sneath PHA, 1980, Approved lists of bacterial names, *Int J Syst Bacteriol*, **30:** 225–420.

Skerman VBD, McGowan V, Sneath PHA, 1989, *Approved Lists of Bacterial Names (amended edition)*, American Society for Microbiology, Washington, DC.

Sneath PHA, 1983, Distortions of taxonomic structure from incomplete data on a restricted set of reference strains, *J Gen Microbiol*, **129:** 1045–73.

Sneath PHA, 1992, *International Code of Nomenclature of Bacteria, 1990 revision*, American Society for Microbiology, Washington, DC.

Sneath PHA, 1995, Taxonomic note: the potential of dead bacterial specimens for systematic studies, *Int J Syst Bacteriol*, **45:** 188.

Sneath PHA, Sokal RR, 1973, *Numerical Taxonomy: the Principles and Practice of Numerical Classification*, Freeman, San Francisco.

Sokal RR, Sneath PHA, 1963, *Principles of Numerical Taxonomy*, Freeman, San Francisco.

Stackebrandt E, Goebel BM, 1994, Taxonomic note: a place for DNA:DNA reassociation and 16S rRNA sequence analysis in the present species definition in bacteriology, *Int J Syst Bacteriol*, **44:** 846–9.

Stackebrandt E, Liesack W, 1993, Nucleic acids and classification, *Handbook of New Bacterial Systematics*, eds Goodfellow M, O'Donnell AG, Academic Press, London, 152–94.

Stackebrandt E, Liesack W, Goebel BM, 1993, Bacterial diversity in a soil sample from a subtropical Australian environment as determined by 16S rDNA analysis, *FASEB J*, **7:** 232–6.

Staley JT, Krieg NR, 1984, Classification of prokaryotic organisms: an overview, *Bergey's Manual of Systematic Bacteriology*, vol. 1, eds Krieg NR et al., Williams & Wilkins, Baltimore.

Swings J, De Vos P et al., 1983, Transfer of *Pseudomonas maltophi-*

lia Hugh 1981 to the genus *Xanthomonas* as *Xanthomonas maltophilia* (Hugh 1981) comb. nov., *Int J Syst Bacteriol*, **33**: 409–13.

Tamaoka J, 1994, Determination of DNA base composition, *Chemical Methods in Prokaryotic Systematics*, eds Goodfellow M, O'Donnell AG, John Wiley & Sons, Chichester, 463–9.

Templeton AR, 1989, The meaning of species and speciation: a genetic perspective, *Speciation and its Consequences*, eds Otte D, Endler JA, Sinaeur Associates Inc., Sunderland, MA, 3–27.

Ursing JB, Lior H, Owen RJ, 1994, Proposal for minimal standards for describing new species of the family Campylobacteriaceae, *Int J Syst Bacteriol*, **44**: 842–5.

Ursing JB, Rosselló-Mora RA et al., 1995, Taxonomic note: a pragmatic approach to the nomenclature of phenotypically similar genomic groups, *Int J Syst Bacteriol*, **45**: 604.

Van Valen L, 1976, Ecological species, multispecies and oaks, *Taxon*, **25**: 233–9.

Vauterin L, Swings J, Kersters K, 1993, Protein electrophoresis and classification, *Handbook of New Bacterial Systematics*, eds Goodfellow M, O'Donnell AG, Academic Press, London, 251–80.

Wayne LG, Brenner DJ et al., 1987, Report of the *ad hoc* committee on reconciliation of approaches to bacterial systematics, *Int J Syst Bacteriol*, **37**: 463–4.

Willcox WR, Lapage SP, Holmes B, 1980, A review of numerical methods in bacterial identification, *Antonie van Leeuwenhoek*, **46**: 233–99.

Woese CR, 1987, Bacterial evolution, *Microbiol Rev*, **51**: 221–71.

Woese CR, 1992, There must be a prokaryote somewhere: microbiology's search for itself, *Microbiol Rev*, **58**: 1–9.

Yabuuchi E, Kosako Y et al., 1992, Proposal of *Burkholderia* gen. nov. and transfer of seven species of the genus *Pseudomonas* homology group II to the new genus, with the type species *Burkholderia cepacia* (Palleroni and Holmes 1981) comb. nov., *Microbiol Immunol*, **36**: 1251–75.

Chapter 4

Isolation, description and identification of bacteria

B I Duerden, K J Towner and J T Magee

1 Obtaining pure cultures of bacteria	2 Identification of bacteria

1 OBTAINING PURE CULTURES OF BACTERIA

For the first 150 years of microbiology, the essential first step in the study of bacteria was to obtain them in pure culture. This is still a basic principle of most microbiological work but detection and identification by modern molecular techniques of DNA amplification means that this is not an absolute requirement in all instances. During the 1860s and 1870s, only liquid media were available for the cultivation of micro-organisms, and the preparation of pure cultures was difficult. The only method available was to dilute the cultures with a sterile fluid until there was only about one organism in each 2 drops and to seed a number of tubes of liquid medium each with one drop (Lister 1878); but even this afforded no certainty that the cultures so obtained were pure. The introduction of solid media by Robert Koch in 1881 enabled the easy separation of different organisms, because most of them formed discrete colonies, and serial subculture could be made from single colonies. Originally the medium was spread in the melted state on glass slides and allowed to set. Later, the petri dish was introduced and agar replaced gelatin as the solidifying agent; the resultant technique has since remained virtually unchanged.

1.1 Collecting suitable samples

To isolate the desired organisms, a suitable sample of the material to be examined must be provided. This is generally not collected by a laboratory worker and microbiologists need to spend time educating clinicians, environmental health officers, etc., in the appropriate methods of obtaining samples and transmitting them to the laboratory. These methods depend to some extent on the materials sampled, the bacteria being sought and the practicability of rapid transport to the laboratory. In many instances the laboratory is seeking to isolate pathogenic bacteria which may not be present in large numbers and which may be mixed with many other commensal bacteria. The site sampled must be appropriate, i.e. one at which the pathogen may be harboured, and the sample should be of adequate size. In general, a quantity of exudate, transudate, or a piece of tissue, when obtainable, is preferable to a swab. When swabbing a dry surface such as the anterior nares or the skin, it may help first to moisten the swab. The swab should be rubbed firmly over the site to be sampled but care should be taken to avoid contact with adjacent areas likely to yield large numbers of irrelevant organisms; for example, when swabbing the throat, contact with the buccal mucosa and tongue should be avoided.

SAMPLES FOR QUANTITATIVE CULTURE

For liquids or solid material that can be emulsified in liquids, the number of viable bacteria can be measured by plating measured dilutions onto a solid medium and counting the colonies (Miles, Misra and Irwin 1938), or when the number of colonies is small, by filtering a known volume through a membrane filter that is then placed upon a suitable medium for incubation. Quantitative sampling of surfaces by means of swabs does not give results in absolute numbers because only a proportion of the organisms is picked up and many of these remain attached to the fibres of the swab on plating or elution; nevertheless, comparative results can be obtained if the method is carefully standardized. Alternatively, surfaces can be sampled by applying a measured volume of fluid, detaching the organisms into it by a standard procedure, and performing colony counts. In a different method of sampling surfaces, by making impression preparations, agar medium is applied directly to the surface, or a moistened carrier, such as velvet, is used to transfer the inoculum to an agar surface (Holt 1966). The resultant colony counts bear no relation to those obtained by swabbing or elution; they give some indication of the distribution of organisms on the surface but none about the numbers present at each point at which a colony appears.

None of these cultural methods measures the number of viable bacterial cells, because bacteria tend to form clumps or chains; they measure the significant viable unit, which for colony-counting methods is the colony-forming unit. Attempts should therefore be made to standardize the degree of bacterial aggregation by using a constant method of shaking and a dispersing agent such as Triton X100.

1.2 Transport to the laboratory

Every effort should be made to ensure that the organism sought is viable when it reaches the laboratory. Organisms may die out in specimens for various reasons: bacterial multiplication may cause an adverse change in pH; growth of one species may inhibit another; some organisms are very sensitive to oxygen and some to drying. Thus, no one set of conditions is likely to be optimal for all pathogens. Rapid transport of samples to the laboratory is always desirable and in a few instances even that is inadequate and media should be inoculated directly from the sampling site. Swabs, whether made of cotton or synthetic fibres, tend to contain inhibitory material (Dadd et al. 1970); these may be removed or neutralized by boiling in phosphate buffer, by impregnating with horse serum (Rubbo and Benjamin 1951) or bovine albumin when viruses are also being sought (Bartlett and Hughes 1969), or by coating the swab with powdered charcoal.

Several general purpose transport media have been designed in which most pathogens will survive without being overgrown by more robust organisms. The most successful are semi-solid media containing thioglycollate but little nutrient (Stuart 1959, Amies 1967, Gästrin, Kallings and Marcetic 1968); powdered charcoal may be added to neutralize inhibitors. For the survival of the more fastidious anaerobes, swabs should be submerged deeply into semi-solid thioglycollate medium. Samples of fluid or tissue may be placed in a variety of small containers that either contain an oxygen-free gaseous atmosphere or from which oxygen is removed by chemical reaction. Material from transport media is seldom suitable for direct microscopic examination. Virus transport media often contain antibiotics and are thus unsuitable for the isolation of bacteria, rickettsiae and chlamydiae. It may be necessary to refrigerate specimens during transit to the laboratory, but this is less to attempt to preserve viable organisms than to prevent growth when quantitative culture is to be performed.

1.3 Plating on solid medium

This is usually the first step in obtaining a pure culture. The media chosen will depend upon what bacteria are sought; guidance on this is given in the appropriate chapters of this book. After the inoculum has been seeded onto a plate, careful streaking with a loop or bent glass rod to spread it in an even gradient of decreasing concentration is essential if well spaced colonies are to be obtained.

The optimal temperature and gaseous atmosphere for growth of any pathogen that might be present must be provided. Most pathogens will grow at 37°C but some do rather better at slightly lower temperatures; 35–36°C is therefore preferable for routine diagnostic bacteriology. Some organisms that grow in the presence of oxygen do so only when CO_2 is added and routine primary cultures from many specimens such as respiratory tract samples, pus, etc. are made in air with 5–10% CO_2. For anaerobic organisms, cultures must be incubated in an atmosphere from which oxygen has been removed. Sealed anaerobic jars equipped with catalysts active at room temperature can be used very effectively and reliably for relatively small numbers of plates. Most of the air can be evacuated and replaced with an oxygen-free gas (usually H_2 10%, CO_2 10%, N_2 80%), with remaining oxygen removed by reaction with the H_2; or sachets containing water-activated chemicals can be used to generate H_2 and remove all the O_2 by reduction to water. Jars must be well maintained and the system should incorporate checks of anaerobiosis and catalyst activity. When larger numbers of anaerobic cultures need to be handled, sealed anaerobic cabinets or work stations allow all processing and examining of cultures to be done in an oxygen-free atmosphere. Freshly poured media or media that have been held in anaerobic conditions should be used for anaerobic cultures. Atmospheres for culture of anaerobes should contain 10% CO_2 and cultures should not be exposed to oxygen, e.g. through opening jars, until they have been incubated for 48 h.

After the primary plate has been incubated, it is inspected – under magnification if necessary – and a representative of each colonial type is subcultured. The ideal means of subculture is with a straight wire. Careful subculture usually results in pure cultures, but this cannot be guaranteed. In critical circumstances, it is advisable to replate supposedly pure cultures at least once and to inspect the resultant colonies for homogeneity. Culture plates should be fairly dry before inoculation; if there is a layer of moisture on the medium, organisms may form a film of confluent growth over the whole surface. This may lead to difficulties in obtaining pure cultures of organisms, such as many clostridia, that tend to spread unless the surface of the medium is very dry. The pour plate method is, generally, of less value than surface cultures. Deep colonies are not usually as characteristic as surface colonies, and subculture from them carries greater risks of contamination.

1.4 Isolating organisms from mixtures

In only a minority of clinical settings is one specific pathogen sought from the outset; more commonly the causative organism may be one of a range of organisms. In other instances, more than one species may contribute to the pathology. In both instances, sufficiently varied conditions must be provided to ensure no pathogen is missed. In many instances, clinical specimens yield a mixed flora, whether from true mixed infections, contamination with extraneous commensal flora (as in contamination of sputum or throat swabs with salivary flora), or because the pathogen infects a site with intrinsic commensal flora (e.g. lower gastrointestinal tract). Numerous methods have been devised to isolate organisms that form a minority of a bacterial population in a sample. These methods seldom yield pure cultures in the first instance; their use must be followed by subculture from a single well spaced colony.

First, the material itself may be treated to destroy unwanted organisms or separate them physically from the organisms to be cultured. **Heating** a mixture to 80°C for 10 min destroys vegetative bacteria but not spores. This method is used in the purification of clostridia. **Chemicals** can be used to destroy susceptible organisms while leaving the more resistant unaffected. For example, tubercle bacilli are more resistant than most other vegetative organisms to chemical disinfectants. They may be isolated by treating sputum with acid or alkali strong enough to kill the accompanying bacteria. **Filtration** may be used to separate viruses from bacteria. Also, L forms and small bacteria such as *Campylobacter* can grow slowly through a membrane filter and so be separated from larger organisms. The membrane is placed on the surface of a suitable medium and a drop of fluid containing the organisms to be isolated is placed on it; after incubation, the membrane is removed and the plate reincubated.

Various methods have been devised for separating motile from non-motile or less motile organisms. One device used is that described by Craigie (1931). A test tube of semi-solid agar medium contains a piece of glass tubing that projects above the agar surface. The medium in the inner tube is seeded with the culture under test. Motile organisms pass down the inner tube and up the outer tube, from the top of which they may be subcultured after incubation (see also Tulloch 1939). By incorporating a specific antiserum in the agar, flagella agglutination may be used to inhibit the motility of one organism in the presence of another, as in separating the phases of diphasic salmonellae (see Chapter 41). Although strict aerobes will not migrate through semi-solid agar, these methods can be applied to pseudomonads if nitrate is added to the medium (see Chapter 47). Swarming organisms such as *Proteus* spp. can be prevented from swarming by increasing the agar concentration of solid media to 3%, thus enabling the separation of other organisms in a mixture.

Second, growth conditions may be arranged to favour the desired organism. It is sometimes possible to make use of the **optimum temperature for growth** of an organism. Thermophilic bacteria may be separated from others by growth at 60°C. Certain other bacteria can grow at low temperatures; thus *Yersinia enterocolitica* may be more readily isolated from faeces after 'cold enrichment' in a broth culture held at 4–10°C for several days (Kontiainin, Sivonen and Renkonen 1994). **Aerobic and anaerobic** culture may be used to

separate some groups of bacteria. Incubated aerobically, the strict anaerobes will not grow; incubated anaerobically, most strict aerobes will not grow, although some (see Chapter 47) can obtain oxygen by denitrification and may grow unless the nitrate content of the medium is very low. Many facultative species do not grow as well in anaerobic as aerobic conditions.

The addition of **chemical substances** to a medium may facilitate the isolation of an organism by stimulating its growth or by inhibiting the growth of other organisms that may be present in larger numbers. In either case, in a liquid medium, the desired organism increases in numbers both absolutely and relative to other organisms; this is known as an **enrichment medium**. If a substance that inhibits the growth of some organisms is added to a solid medium, the colonies that form will be mainly of organisms that are resistant to it. Such a solid medium is known as a **selective medium**. It is common to use the 2 types of media in conjunction, inoculating material first into enrichment medium and later subculturing from this onto a selective medium. The colonies on a selective medium are, however, not necessarily pure. At the base of the colony other organisms may be present which, though unable to develop on the selective medium, will grow when transferred to a non-selective medium. Therefore, it is wise to replate organisms from a selective medium onto a plain medium before beginning to study them. Enrichment media containing substances that are a source of energy only for some organisms have been widely used by soil microbiologists. The same principle is applied in the use of tetrathionate broth for the enrichment of salmonellae, which obtain energy by means of a tetrathionate reductase (Pollock, Knox and Gell 1942); but some other enterobacteria, including *Proteus* and *Citrobacter*, also form this enzyme (Le Minor and Pichinoty 1963), so it is advisable also to include selective chemicals in tetrathionate broth.

Another selective procedure is to add to the medium a substance that is not harmful to bacteria but may be metabolized by some strains with the production intracellularly of a toxic substance. Thus *Escherichia coli* and other organisms that form β-galactosidase will hydrolyse phenylethyl β-D-galactopyranoside with the release of phenylethyl alcohol; organisms such as salmonellae of subspecies I, which lack this enzyme, are unaffected (Johnston and Thatcher 1967, Johnston and Pivnik 1970).

Selective substances used either in enrichment broths or in solid selective media include aniline dyes, metallic salts and bile salts. Antibiotics are also useful selective agents, e.g. aminoglycosides or nalidixic acid for the isolation of anaerobes (resistant) from mixtures with aerobic gram-negative bacilli (generally inhibited).

Third, **an indicator** may be added to the medium, which changes colour when there is growth of a certain organism or group of organisms. Thus the diphtheria bacillus reduces sodium tellurite, whereas most other organisms likely to be present in a throat swab do not. The colonies of the diphtheria bacillus and some other corynebacteria are coloured black; those of the streptococci and numerous other organisms are colourless. Indicators are frequently used to detect the production of acid from a carbohydrate incorporated in the medium. Blood is a very useful indicator; some organisms produce no alteration in it, others form from it a green pigment ('partial haemolysis'), and others lyse it completely.

Selective agents and indicators are frequently included in the same medium. Thus in MacConkey's medium, bile salts inhibit the growth of non-intestinal organisms and lactose and neutral red are added to distinguish the lactose-fermenting enterobacteria from the non-fermenting group.

MAINTENANCE OF PURE CULTURES

Having obtained an organism in pure culture, its viability and purity need to be maintained while it is being studied. With good technical standards, this should seldom prove difficult but the possibility of contamination, or the inadvertent substitution of one culture by another, should always be kept in mind. When an unexpected result is obtained, this should be an indication for replating the culture and comparing the appearances of the colonies with that recorded earlier.

Protracted chemical and genetic studies are particularly liable to be marred by contamination. Before they are begun, therefore, freeze-dried stocks of the cultures to be used should be prepared, samples of them should be checked for purity, and a full cultural and biochemical examination of the organisms should be made. When possible, they should be typed, e.g. serologically or by means of phage or other methods. These tests should be repeated at intervals during the experiments. Particular care should be taken to avoid errors due to contamination or substitution when organisms are re-isolated after injection into animals and when they are being repeatedly selected on plates containing inhibitory agents. Suspicion should be aroused when 'variants' are isolated that appear to differ from the parent organism in several phenotypic characters.

2 IDENTIFICATION OF BACTERIA

This is performed within the framework of **bacterial classification**, in which species and genera have been carefully defined and comprehensively described, and each is represented by a type culture; order is preserved by the use of an agreed system of **bacterial nomenclature** (see Chapter 3). The properties of an unknown organism can be compared with those of type cultures of the organisms it appears to resemble to determine its identity, but it must always be remembered that no 2 bacterial strains are identical in all respects, although the members of a species show much greater similarity to one another than to members of other species.

Ideally, the characters of the unknown organism should be compared with those of all recognized groups of bacteria, but this is impracticable. Most microbiologists work with material from limited sources; the medical bacteriologist is familiar with organisms isolated from humans and other mammals and from their immediate surroundings, but plant pathologists and marine bacteriologists, for example, work with quite different ranges of organisms. Therefore, several distinct systems of bacterial identification are used in practice. This is generally satisfactory, but occasionally an 'intrusion' from an unfamiliar environment may not be recognized, such as soil and water organisms that can cause serious infection in compromised patients.

Classification of bacteria into species is generally based upon similarity in a broad range of characters, the so-called polyphasic approach (see Chapter 3). Identification to known species can employ far fewer tests, and the number and types of tests chosen represent a compromise between economy, speed and the desired level of confidence in the identification. For some species, most strains are presumptively identified on colony morphology and a single highly discriminatory test is available, sufficient to give a high confidence of identification, e.g. *Staphylococcus aureus* and the coagulase test. Other species are less readily identifiable from morphology, or require considerably more tests to distinguish strains from other similar species. For some pathogens, isolation has such an impact that the laboratory may wish to employ extensive or elaborate confirmatory tests. Equally, one might require a rapid presumptive identification of, for example, salmonellae, for early reporting followed up by more rigorous identification. These compromises depend upon many factors, including the discriminatory capabilities of the available identification tests.

In the worst case, an isolate shows unfamiliar morphology and must be processed through a comprehensive identification protocol. An initial set of tests to determine the genus or family of genera that best fits the properties of the isolate might comprise: gram, spore and acid-fast stains; determination of motility and atmospheric requirements for growth; oxidase and catalase tests; and a test for oxidation or fermentation of glucose. With this information the organism can be allocated tentatively to one of the main groups of organisms of medical importance and a series of secondary tests appropriate for the group in question can be addressed (see Barrow and Feltham 1993).

In the following discussion of tests that may be used for the identification of bacteria, it is not practicable to include technical details of the tests and reference should be made to the books devoted to the identification of bacteria, for example, those of Skerman (1969), Cowan and Steel (Barrow and Feltham 1993) and Weyant et al. (1996). Only widely applied tests are mentioned; others for the identification of particular organisms are described in the appropriate chapters in this volume.

An alternative approach to identification involves the application of modern, rapid molecular methods. Recent developments have seen a major shift from phenotypic to molecular techniques for the identification of bacteria (Towner and Cockayne 1993). The application of these methods has challenged some long-established taxonomic groupings based on phenotypic properties and has resulted in a re-evaluation of the whole process of bacterial identification and classification. The major advantages of these techniques are their speed and the fact that they do not necessarily require the isolation and growth of pure cultures, or even viable bacterial cells. They are particularly useful for the rapid identification of bacteria that are slow-growing or otherwise difficult to cultivate in the laboratory.

2.1 Conventional identification methods

MORPHOLOGY

The description of a micro-organism includes the shape and size of the cells, their arrangement and staining behaviour; motility; the number, distribution and shape of flagella; the presence of fimbriae (pili); the shape and position of spores; and capsule formation. It is impossible to study all these properties on a single medium. The shape and size of organisms vary and are often influenced by the type of medium on which they are grown. With a few exceptions, such as the corynebacteria, organisms are larger in young than in old cultures (Henrici 1926, Wilson 1926); and some organisms, for example, *Acinetobacter*, are bacillary in young cultures but may be mistaken for diplococci in stationary cultures. Even in one preparation the individual cells may vary so much in size and shape to justify the term 'pleomorphic'. The arrangement of the organisms may be characteristic; cocci may be arranged singly, in pairs, tetrads, packets, clusters or chains; bacilli may be arranged singly, in pairs end to end, in bundles, chains, clusters, or in Chinese-letter forms in which the individual bacilli lie more or less at right angles to each other; vibrios may be arranged singly, in S forms, semicircles or wavy chains composed of S forms. Chain formation in cocci may be more evident in liquid media than on solid. Motility should be looked for in a young, rapidly growing broth culture, and in some species is evident only at temperatures at the lower end of the growth range; flagella are best seen from young agar cultures, fimbriae after several subcultures in liquid medium, spores in old cultures, and so on.

The size and shape of the organisms may be studied best in preparations that have been stained lightly with a weak dye, such as methylene blue or safranin. Heavy staining (e.g. with crystal violet) tends to increase the apparent size of the organism and may obscure fine detail. Phase-contrast microscopy shows some of the internal structure of bacteria and electron microscopy reveals many more differences in morphology. It is not used regularly in bacterial identification, but may be necessary to detect whether flagella are attached at the pole or at the side of an organism. Fimbriae can be demonstrated only by electron microscopy, but their presence can often be inferred by other means (see Chapter 40). Gram's stain divides bacteria into 2 classes, the gram-positive and the gram-negative, reflecting major differences in cell wall structure (see

Chapter 2). Ziehl–Neelsen's stain divides them into acid fast and non-acid fast. Numerous other stains are used for special purposes, such as the demonstration of flagella, capsules, spores, nuclei and metachromatic granules. *Mycobacterium tuberculosis* fluoresces when stained with auramine (see Chapter 26). Among the organisms that take up the ordinary aniline dyes irregularly are some that contain granules of poly-β-hydroxybutyrate, which stain with Sudan black (Forsyth, Hayward and Roberts 1958). For technical details of the main staining processes, see Barrow and Feltham (1993).

A scheme for the systematic recording of the morphological appearances of bacteria is given at the end of this chapter (see Appendix 1, p. 80).

CULTURAL APPEARANCES

The appearances of colonies formed on various solid media and the type of growth in liquid media are important in the recognition and identification of bacterial isolates. Observations are often made after incubation for 24 h under optimal conditions for growth but some organisms require longer for colonies to develop. The colonial forms of many groups of bacteria are fairly distinctive, and within a group there may be important differences between members. For bacteriologists, colonial morphology is often the only means available of selecting clones for further investigation, but the appearances of colonies may be influenced by quite small differences in the composition of media.

The appearances of colonies on special media – including indicator media that give evidence of biochemical characters – are of great assistance in arriving at a preliminary identification. Changes produced in blood agar help in the recognition of many organisms, but the animal species of origin of the blood, the composition of the basal medium and growth in the presence or absence of oxygen all affect the results. No one type of blood agar medium is suitable for all purposes.

Pigmentation The production of coloured colonies or the secretion of pigments into the surrounding medium is often of value in the recognition of bacterial species, but non-pigmented strains occur in most pigmented species. Bacterial pigments are of many different colours. Optimal conditions for their production vary widely, many being formed only under certain conditions of temperature or atmosphere, or in media of a particular composition.

REQUIREMENTS FOR GROWTH

Growth of any bacteria requires an appropriate temperature, gaseous atmosphere and nutritional provision. Bacteria are divided into 3 classes according to their oxygen requirements:

1 **strict aerobes** grow only in the presence of oxygen
2 **strict anaerobes** grow only in the absence of oxygen and
3 **facultative organisms** (or **facultative anaerobes**) grow under aerobic and anaerobic conditions, though usually better in the presence of oxygen.

A fourth class, the **micro-aerophiles**, grow best under a pressure of oxygen less than that of the atmosphere. The distinction between micro-aerophiles and strict anaerobes is one of degree. Among the strict anaerobes there are wide differences in the maximum oxidation–reduction potential at which growth may occur. Because some strict aerobes can obtain oxygen from nitrate, tests for their inability to grow anaerobically should be made in nitrate-free media. Both facultative and strict anaerobes may require CO_2. In temperature requirements, bacteria may be divided into:

1 **psychrotrophic** organisms that can grow at low temperatures, e.g. 2–5°C, and usually have a temperature optimum in the range 20–30°C
2 **mesophilic** organisms, that grow within the range 10–45°C and have a temperature optimum between 30 and 40°C and
3 **thermophilic** organisms, that grow poorly or not at all at 37°C and have a temperature optimum between 50 and 60°C.

A detailed study of the nutrients required for growth seldom forms part of the identification process, but individual characters are often used. These include the ability to grow on a basic nutrient medium, and the effect of adding blood, serum or glucose. Requirement for some nutrients, such as the X and V factors required by *Haemophilus* spp., can be tested in a complex medium known not to contain them (see Chapter 50), but with other more widely distributed substances a synthetic or chemically defined basal medium must be used. Tests for the ability to grow in mineral salts medium with ammonium ions and a range of single organic compounds play a considerable part in the identification of gram-negative bacilli with simple requirements for nutrients.

METABOLISM AND BIOCHEMICAL ACTIVITIES

Among the numerous tests for the chemical activities of bacteria, some indicate important metabolic characters common to members of a species, genus or even family of bacteria and others that are irregularly distributed and so have less significance in identification. The methods employed to test for biochemical activity are often empirical. In many cases bacteria are grown with a substrate in an undefined medium; the results of the test may therefore be complicated by secondary chemical reactions. A positive result may be the final outcome of a series of linked enzymic reactions, and if any one of these enzymes is missing the results may be negative. In other cases, several different tests may be influenced by a single enzymic reaction. Some of the reactions traditionally recorded as 'biochemical characters' are in reality evidence of nutritional requirements, e.g. Koser's citrate test, or of resistance to single chemicals, e.g. the KCN test.

Respiratory function

The **catalase test** for the ability to release oxygen from H_2O_2 gives evidence of a functioning cytochrome system. The results are usually easy to interpret, but some

species, e.g. lactobacilli and pediococci, give weakly positive results that are not due to a true catalase (Whittenbury 1964). A test for iron porphyrins by flooding an agar plate culture first with benzidine dihydrochloride and then with H_2O_2, producing a blue colour, confirms the presence of catalase (Deibel and Evans 1960). Most anaerobic bacteria and lactobacilli are catalase-negative. Some catalase-negative organisms form H_2O_2; tests for this are of value in the identification of some streptococci (Whittenbury 1964, Marshall 1979).

The **oxidase test** (Gordon and McLeod 1928) is believed to detect a cytochrome oxidase that catalyses the oxidation of reduced cytochrome by molecular oxygen; it is usually performed by the simplified method of Kovács (1956).

Nitrate reduction is usually tested for by a modification of the Greiss–Ilosvay method. The test determines whether nitrite is formed from nitrate, and whether all the nitrate is reduced beyond nitrite. The inclusion of a Durham's tube detects the formation of gaseous nitrogen.

The term **denitrification** is applied in soil bacteriology to the reduction of nitrate to molecular nitrogen or nitrous oxide, in which nitrate is used as an electron acceptor alternative to oxygen. Strictly aerobic denitrifiers can grow anaerobically in the presence of nitrate, usually, but not invariably, forming gaseous nitrogen.

The reduction of various dyes, tetrazolium salts, tellurites and selenites forms the basis of various empirical tests used in bacterial identification.

Action on carbohydrates and related compounds

Tests on 'sugars' are of 2 sorts: those that reveal the general method of action on these substances (usually exemplified by glucose); and those that determine the range of sugars from which the organism will produce acid. Some tests in the first category are useful for making broad distinctions between groups of bacteria; others, and tests in the second category, are used mainly to characterize species and biotypes.

Method of attack on sugars The oxidation–fermentation (OF) test (Hugh and Leifson 1953) distinguishes between fermentation, for which oxygen is not necessary, and oxidation, for which it is essential. Two narrow tubes of semi-solid agar medium containing only 0.2% of peptone, together with a sugar and an indicator, are seeded with the organism and the surface of the medium in one tube is covered with a thick layer of soft paraffin. In fermentation, acid is formed in both tubes; in oxidation, only in the open tube. OF tests are usually performed with glucose, but a few organisms oxidize maltose but not glucose. OF tests in Hugh and Leifson's medium usually give clear-cut results with gram-negative aerobes, but are less successful with some other groups of organisms, such as staphylococci.

Sugars may be fermented by one of 2 main pathways: **homofermentative organisms**, such as streptococci, convert glucose almost entirely to lactic acid; **heterofermentative organisms,** such as the enterobacteria and the staphylococci, form other organic acids and alcohols, together with varying amounts of CO_2 and H_2. Large amounts of gas can be detected by means of a Durham's tube, but some heterofermentative organisms do not form sufficient gas for a bubble to appear in peptone–water sugars.

Analysis of the products of fermentation by gas chromatography, first used by Moore, Cato and Holdeman (1966) to characterize the species of clostridia by their production of volatile fatty acids and alcohols, is used for the classification of many groups of organisms, mainly but not exclusively anaerobes (Holdeman, Cato and Moore 1977, Larsson and Mårdh 1977). These methods may be used to identify strains to appropriate large groups, even to the level of species in the case of some clostridia, but have not replaced traditional methods generally for species identification (Wren 1991).

The methyl red (MR) and Voges–Proskauer (VP) tests Some coliform organisms produce considerable amounts of acid from glucose, but the pH change is partially reversed on incubation when pyruvic acid, mainly responsible for the initial acidity, is further degraded to neutral substances. In the MR test (Clark and Lubs 1915), strains that produce and maintain a high concentration of hydrogen ions give a red colour when the indicator is added to a culture in glucose phosphate peptone medium after incubation for 5 days at 30°C (MR+) and those in which reversion of pH occurs give a yellow colour (MR−).

The VP test (Voges and Proskauer 1898) detects acetylmethylcarbinol, an intermediate in the conversion of pyruvic acid to 2,3-butylene glycol. This reaction takes place only at an acid pH and results in the formation of one molecule of a neutral substance from 2 molecules of acid. If a glucose phosphate peptone culture incubated for 2 days at 30°C is treated with strong alkali and exposed to air, the acetylmethylcarbinol is oxidized to diacetyl, which reacts with a constituent of the peptone to form a pink fluorescent substance (see Barrow and Feltham 1993).

Among the enterobacteria, the expected negative correlation between the results of the 2 tests is fairly consistent, but in other bacterial groups many strains give a negative or a positive result in both tests.

Acidification of sugars Traditional tests for the production of acid from sugars are made in tubes of a nutrient medium containing a sugar, usually at 1% concentration, and an indicator of pH – a method devised early in the twentieth century for the examination of enterobacteria. With bacteria of many groups (but not the enterobacteria) the results are influenced by the composition of the medium, especially when little acid is formed and the organism also forms alkali from nitrogenous compounds. If the organism has simple nutrient requirements, more consistent results are obtained in appropriate synthetic media, but care must be taken to distinguish between failure to attack the sugar and failure to grow.

For tests with some groups of bacteria it may be necessary to add extra nutrients. If natural products such as yeast extract, serum or ascitic fluid are added, these must be heated to inactivate enzymes.

Acidification of sugars may be the end result of the action of several enzymes, and a negative or delayed reaction may be due to the absence of any one of these. A single enzyme may be concerned with action on several sugars. Enzymes responsible for the acidification of sugars may be genetically determined by plasmids. For all these reasons, individual sugar reactions, particularly when performed in different laboratories and by different methods, should not be regarded as definitive in bacterial identification.

β-Galactosidase To ferment lactose, an organism must possess not only a β-galactosidase to split it into monosaccharides but also a permease to enable it to enter the cell. In the absence of the permease, acidification of lactose peptone water may be delayed or absent. The galactosidase can be detected by release of *o*-nitrophenol from *o*-nitrophenyl-β-D-galactopyranoside (ONPG), producing a yellow colour (Lederberg 1950); either the organism is incubated overnight in peptone water containing 0.15% ONPG (Lowe 1962) or a suspension of the organism in buffered saline is treated with toluene to release the enzyme and the ONPG is added (Le Minor and Ben Hamida 1962).

Oxidation of potassium gluconate Oxidation of potassium gluconate to a reducing substance, presumed to be potassium 2-keto-gluconate, detected by heating with Benedict's solution, is useful for the differentiation of organisms in the pseudomonas and coliform groups.

Fermentation of organic acids The fermentation of organic acids is distinct from their simple utilization as the sole source of carbon. In fermentation, the salt of the organic acid is broken down with the release of free sodium ions and the production of an alkaline pH, which can be detected by means of a suitable indicator. The salts usually employed are D-, L- and i-tartrate, citrate, mucate (Kauffmann and Peterson 1956) and malonate (Leifson 1933).

Action on nitrogenous compounds

Bacteria break down nitrogenous compounds by various metabolic pathways, including deamination and decarboxylation. The patterns of reactions for decarboxylation of lysine, arginine and ornithine are particularly useful in distinguishing species of the Enterobacteriaceae.

Decarboxylation of amino acids The simplified methods introduced by Møller (1954, 1955) for the detection of lysine, arginine, ornithine and glutamic acid decarboxylases by a pH fall, and of arginine dihydrolase (or deaminase) by the addition of Nessler's reagent, are useful in the identification of enterobacteria and many other groups of gram-negative bacteria. For tests on streptococci, the arginine-containing medium of Niven, Smiley and Sherman (1942) should be used.

Deamination of amino acids   This may be tested for by the conversion of phenylalanine to phenylpyruvic acid (Henriksen 1950, Ewing, Davis and Reavis 1957).

Indole production   The ability to form 'indole', which includes indole and several related substances (Isenberg and Sundheim 1958), from a tryptophan-rich peptone may be detected by the appearance of a red colour when Ehrlich's reagent (*p*-dimethylamino-benzaldehyde in acid-ethanol) is added to an ether, petroleum or preferably amylalcohol extract of the culture. Alternative methods are:

1   a paper impregnated with oxalic acid is suspended over a peptone–water culture during incubation and observed for the appearance of a pink colour or
2   growth from an agar culture may be smeared on filter paper soaked in 1% *p*-dimethylaminocinnam-aldehyde in 10% HCl and observed for a blue-black colour (Sutter, Citron and Finegold 1980).

Hydrogen sulphide   Several methods are available for detecting the production of H_2S from sulphur-containing amino acids. The most sensitive are those in which a rich source of a suitable sulphur compound is provided, and the H_2S is detected by suspending a strip of lead acetate paper over a culture in a test tube. Alternatively, a metallic salt, such as lead acetate, ferric ammonium citrate or ferrous acetate, may be included in the medium (Levine, Epstein and Vaughan 1934, Zobell and Feltham 1934). Similar results are given by Kligler's iron sugar agar or ferrous chloride gelatin (Kauffmann 1954), both of which have been used with the enterobacteria.

Urea hydrolysis   The hydrolysis of urea is detected either by an alkaline reaction or by a chemical test for ammonia. A simple buffered medium containing urea as the sole source of nitrogen and a pH indicator are suitable for tests with the Proteeae (Ferguson and Hook 1942, Stuart, van Stratum and Rustigian 1945), but other organisms hydrolyse urea only when provided with an additional source of nitrogen. Christensen's (1946) agar medium contains peptone as well as urea and a small amount of glucose, with phenol red as indicator; this gives reliable results with many groups of bacteria. If organisms produce alkali without attacking urea and there is doubt about the results, a urease method should be used in which ammonia is detected by means of Nessler's reagent (Elek 1948).

Hydrolysis of hippurate   The ability to hydrolyse hippurate to benzoate is important in the classification of streptococci (Ayers and Rupp 1922). The organism is grown in hippurate broth and ferric chloride is then added. Both hippurate and benzoate are precipitated but the hippurate is soluble in excess ferric chloride. The amount of ferric chloride to add is just sufficient to redissolve the precipitate in uninoculated broth. In the test, a precipitate indicates hippurate hydrolysis (Hare and Colebrook 1934). A different test has been used with enterobacteria (Hajna and Damon 1934); a

mineral salts medium is employed so that it examines both ability to hydrolyse hippurate and to use it as the sole carbon source. Rapid methods applicable to the identification of streptococci are described by Hwang and Ederer (1975) and Edberg and Samuels (1976).

Hydrolysis of complex biological substances

The ability to break down complex polymers present in host tissues is part of the pathogenic attributes of many bacteria. It was recognized that the ability to break down structural macromolecules in host tissues was important in pathogenesis in early investigations of bacterial disease. Nucleases, proteolytic and lipolytic enzymes are key factors in host tissue and cell destruction, and it was natural that tests for these and other enzymes acting on biological polymers were devised. These have proved to be of considerable value in discrimination between bacterial species.

Proteinases   Classical tests for the liquefaction of gelatin and coagulated serum or egg, and for the coagulation and peptonization of milk, are now used only rarely. Gelatinase is conveniently detected in gelatin agar plates; after flooding with a protein precipitant, a clear zone around the inoculated area indicates hydrolysis (Frazier 1926). Discs of formalin-denatured gelatin containing powdered charcoal may be incubated in growing cultures or with washed suspensions of bacteria; the release of charcoal particles by hydrolysis of the gelatin is a sensitive method of detecting gelatinase activity. Numerous plate tests for the hydrolysis of other proteins are available.

Deoxyribonucleases   Organisms may be incubated on plates of DNA agar which is then flooded with acid to precipitate unchanged DNA. This test is made more sensitive by using methyl green DNA agar (Smith, Hancock and Rhoden 1969) on which DNAase activity is indicated by a colourless zone around the growth.

Lipases   Natural fats may be used as substrate with hydrolysis detected by the disappearance of fat globules, by pH change or by the use of specific fat stains, but the results are often indefinite. Tests with the related Tween compounds, with which hydrolysis gives products that are precipitated in the presence or calcium ions (Sierra 1957) are easier to interpret. The production of opacity in serum or egg-yolk media are empirical tests that may be due to the action of lecithinases, lipoproteinases or lipases.

Diastases   The production of enzymes that hydrolyse starch by organisms that ferment glucose can be inferred from the production of acid in a conventional 'sugar' tube. A more sensitive and widely applicable test is to grow the organism on a plate of starch agar and flood this with a solution of iodine.

NEWER METHODS OF BIOCHEMICAL TESTING

The imprecision of conventional biochemical tests and the time taken to obtain results, together with the demands on the laboratory of preparing and standardizing special media, have resulted in the development of several rapid and automated procedures.

Many reactions can be speeded up by adding very large inocula to small volumes of substrate and determining the activity of 'pre-formed' enzymes in the heavy inoculum on the substrate, without depending on bacterial growth. Early approaches to mechanization made use of batch-testing in which a multiple-point inoculator transferred a large number of different organisms simultaneously to clusters of small tubes, to wells in microtitration plates or to segments of a petri dish. These methods were laborious for testing many strains and were of little help to the clinical microbiology laboratory which required procedures by which smaller numbers of strains could be subjected to a battery of tests. Numerous attempts to meet this need have been made by commercial manufacturers who have devised sets of papers, discs or tablets impregnated with substrate or medium, or plastic cupules containing substrates. The company bioMérieux produces a comprehensive system for the identification of medically important bacteria (the API system), comprising a series of galleries of cupules mounted in plastic strips. These enable a wide range of tests of the usual types to be performed and also enable tests for a number of single enzymes. The results of these tests, although generally consistent within the system, do not always conform with those obtained by conventional test methods and must be interpreted according to the information provided from the company's analysis. The use of these and similar systems has greatly increased the range of tests that can be performed in many laboratories. A disadvantage is that laboratory workers are encouraged to set up identification tests from primary cultures before the purity of the isolate has been established; therefore it is essential to inoculate a 'purity plate' in parallel with the identification tests and to examine it carefully for uniformity of colonial type.

SUSCEPTIBILITY TO PHYSICAL AND CHEMICAL AGENTS

Gross resistance to heat occurs only in spore-bearing bacteria; most vegetative bacteria are destroyed by moist heat at 60°C in 1 h. However, spores vary greatly in their susceptibility to heat; spores of some strains of *Clostridium perfringens* are destroyed by boiling for a few minutes whereas those of *Clostridium botulinum* may withstand boiling for hours. Some clostridia rarely spore on laboratory media and may appear to be sensitive to heat. Small degrees of heat resistance may be useful in the identification of some species, e.g. enterococci survive 60°C for 30 min. Resistance to other extreme conditions, e.g. of pH and salt concentration, are also useful characters. Mycobacteria are characteristically resistant to disinfectants. Resistance to KCN (Braun and Guggenheim 1932) helps distinguish between enterobacteria; resistance to the pteridine compound O/129 separates the genera of polar-flagellate gram-negative bacilli. Other useful tests for sensitivity or resistance include ethylhydrocupreine (optochin) sensitivity in pneumococci, tellurite resistance in corynebacteria and group D streptococci, and dye sensitivity in brucellae and some gram-negative, non-sporing anaerobes.

Antibiotic susceptibility tests may be of some value in identification although resistance to many antibiotics in common use is a character of individual strains rather than species and may be mediated by genetic determinants that are easily lost or gained. However, sensitivity or resistance of certain groups of bacteria to individual antibiotics is sufficiently stable to be useful in identification, e.g. the sensitivity of group A streptococci to bacitracin. Only strict anaerobes are sensitive to metronidazole and this is a useful means of distinguishing them from micro-aerophilic and CO_2-dependent organisms, provided that cultures have been incubated under strictly anaerobic conditions. The general pattern of susceptibility of gram-negative, non-sporing anaerobes to antibiotics may be a useful aid to their identification.

2.2 Molecular identification methods

Conventional identification methods suffer from the basic drawback that tests designed for one group of organisms are not always useful for identifying other groups. Thus, for example, many tests used for identifying different members of the Enterobacteriaceae are unsuitable for identifying non-fermentative gram-negative bacteria. In some cases, reliance on a small number of phenotypic properties for identification purposes can lead to serious errors. Indeed, some taxonomic groupings based on phenotypic properties have been shown to contain a wide range of heterogeneous organisms. The application of molecular methods offers the possibility of a 'universal' approach to identification that is applicable to all bacterial groups.

Of the various molecules in a bacterial cell, only nucleic acids, proteins and lipopolysaccharides (LPS) carry sufficient information in their sequences to offer the possibility of a simple uniform approach to the identification of bacteria. Historically, methods used to isolate and characterize such macromolecules have involved complex and time-consuming procedures that have prevented their introduction into routine microbiology laboratories. Modern developments have now made the isolation of these macromolecules increasingly rapid and simple, so that they can be studied with relative ease by most trained microbiologists. However, although the analysis of proteins and LPS has been used successfully to type a variety of different bacteria (see section 2.3, p. 76), expression of these molecules may also reflect the phenotype rather than the genotype of a particular organism. For this reason, most molecular methods for the rapid identification of bacteria have concentrated on the analysis of nucleic acids. It has been stated that the ultimate goal of such methods is 'to eliminate routine cultures, whether they be bacterial, viral or fungal'. Although this goal will certainly be difficult to attain in the near future, the rapid evolution and commercial development of identification methods based on nucleic acid analysis suggests that they will displace or supplant at least some of the more cumbersome or inconvenient conventional identification procedures that are used currently by many laboratories.

Specific nucleic acid probes

Hybridization tests involving specific nucleic acid probes are now used increasingly by many laboratories for the direct identification of bacteria in a wide variety of samples. Such tests take advantage of the ability of nucleic acid molecules to form double strands in which nucleotides on opposing strands are held together by hydrogen bonds. When these hydrogen bonds are broken, normally by treatment with alkali or heating, the opposing strands separate and the nucleic acid molecule is said to be denatured. If a specific nucleic acid probe molecule carrying a recognizable label (either radioactive or non-radioactive) is introduced at this stage, subsequent neutralization or cooling will allow the probe to form hydrogen bonds with any complementary sequence that is present in the original denatured target molecule. A positive hybridization reaction is then recognized by detecting the residual (hybridized) probe label after washing to remove excess unbound probe.

The basic requirement for a nucleic acid probe is that it should hybridize with the target nucleic acid sequence, but fail to hybridize with any other nucleic acid molecules that may be present in the sample being examined (Stahl and Amann 1991). By definition, each bacterial species contains at least one sequence of DNA that serves to distinguish it from all other organisms and can therefore function as a probe. The entire sequence can be cloned and used as a probe, but once this unique sequence has been defined, it is also then possible to synthesize artificially a very small stretch of DNA (termed an oligonucleotide) from within the overall sequence for use as a probe. Such oligonucleotide probes are stable, simple to prepare, and hybridize to their target sequence extremely rapidly, often with reaction times of <30 min.

Various kits based upon the use of specific nucleic acid probes are now available commercially for identifying the presence of specific bacteria in a sample. The latest versions of these kits combine the advantages of high specificity and speed (1–2 h) with the convenience of non-radioactive labelling and detection systems. A major consideration to be borne in mind when using such methods is that hybridization procedures do not distinguish between viable and non-viable bacteria (a fact which may be either advantageous or disadvantageous, depending upon the precise circumstances of the test and the bacterial species involved). Furthermore, specific nucleic acid probes will yield a positive result only if a reasonable number of bacteria (generally $\geq 10^5$ cfu) are present in the sample being examined, although this problem can be overcome by the use of nucleic acid amplification procedures (see section on 'Nucleic acid amplification').

Ribotyping

An alternative to the use of specific nucleic acid probes for identifying particular bacteria is to use a broad spectrum (or 'universal') probe. The best example of this type of approach is termed ribotyping and involves the use of probes capable of detecting genes coding for ribosomal RNA (rRNA). Since its first description (Grimont and Grimont 1986), ribotyping has emerged as one of the most powerful of the 'universal' methods available currently for identifying and typing bacteria. The rationale for using rRNA genes as the basis for an identification method has its origin in the high degree of conservation found in certain regions of such nucleic acid sequences (Woese 1987). rRNA genes in bacteria are organized into operons, within which the individual genes are often separated by non-coding spacer DNA. Many of the rRNA sequences found in bacteria appear to have changed little during the course of evolution, and this high degree of conservation of certain regions of the rRNA genes means that a probe consisting of labelled rRNA or rDNA from one bacterial species will still hybridize (albeit to varying regions of the chromosome) with the DNA of unrelated bacterial species. The technique of ribotyping involves isolating total chromosomal DNA from the bacterium being examined, and then using a suitable restriction endonuclease to generate a collection of DNA fragments with an even distribution of sizes. These fragments are separated by agarose gel electrophoresis and transferred to a blotting membrane (Towner and Cockayne 1993). Following transfer, the fragments are hybridized with a labelled 'universal' probe for rRNA genes (commercially available rRNA from *E. coli* is often used). Hybridization occurs only with those chromosomal fragments that contain portions of conserved rRNA genes. The resulting 'fingerprint' can then be compared with a computerized database to identify the unknown organism being investigated.

Ribotyping has several advantages over other molecular identification methods. In particular, rRNA genes appear to be extremely stable and most bacteria contain multiple copies of the rRNA operons. This means that a single protocol involving hybridization with a labelled 'universal' probe can be used to generate a ribotyping fingerprint pattern of acceptable complexity, no matter which organism is being investigated. Precise determination of the size of fragments that hybridize with the probe is essential. It is also important to note that the discriminatory ability of ribotyping will depend on the precise probe and restriction enzyme(s) being used to generate the ribotyping fingerprint, and these variables should be standardized if results are to be compared with a database.

For further information about ribotyping, see Grimont and Grimont (1991).

Nucleic acid amplification

The main problem with identification procedures involving either specific or 'universal' nucleic acid probes is one of sensitivity, in that the target nucleic acid is available only in very limited quantities unless the organism is first cultivated. This problem can be overcome by amplifying artificially the amount of target nucleic acid available for detection. Various strategies have been developed for amplifying specific nucleic acid sequences (see Towner and Cockayne 1993), and these methods are revolutionizing many procedures in molecular biology, including those used for identifying specific bacteria. To date, the most widely accepted of the various amplification methods is the polymerase chain reaction (see below). The availability of nucleic amplification techniques has revolutionized many microbiological procedures, especially in the field of rapid identification of micro-organisms, and such techniques are now used routinely in many laboratories to detect the presence of particular bacteria in unpurified samples by selectively amplifying a specific diagnostic segment of the genome.

Polymerase chain reaction

The polymerase chain reaction (PCR) uses a thermostable DNA polymerase, 2 synthetic oligonucleotide primers and the 4 standard deoxyribonucleosides found in DNA to produce multiple copies of specific nucleic acid regions quickly and exponentially, including non-coding regions of DNA as well as particular genes. Each PCR amplification consists of 3 steps that are repeated in cycles:

1 strand separation (denaturing) of the double-stranded sample DNA
2 hybridization (annealing) of the 2 primers to opposite DNA strands and
3 extension of the primers by polymerase mediated nucleotide additions to produce 2 copies of the original sequence.

The repeated cycles result in an exponential reaction in which the original target sequence is amplified a million-fold or more within a few hours.

The specificity of a PCR is controlled by the synthetic oligonucleotide primers, which are normally designed by reference to DNA sequence databases. Each pair of primers must be relatively specific for their binding sites, since if one or both of the primers fails to hybridize at its designated site, there will be no specific amplification products. It has been found that primers that are 20–30 nucleotides long usually provide a good balance between efficiency and specificity. Non-specific amplification of DNA fragments is sometimes observed, but this can be eliminated in most cases by careful adjustment of the reaction conditions. The visualization of a specific amplification product by electrophoresis on an agarose or polyacrylamide gel is often sufficiently diagnostic for most amplification purposes, but PCR amplification is sometimes combined with a hybridization assay to confirm the specificity of the reaction.

Apart from the need for specific primers to direct the amplification reaction, the main problem with the use of PCR is identifying bacteria for diagnostic purposes from the exquisite sensitivity of the technique. Since even a single molecule of target DNA can, in theory, be amplified to give a positive reaction, the slightest contamination of glassware, pipettes or reagents can result in the production of false positive results unless appropriate stringent laboratory procedures are followed carefully. As an additional consequence, quantification of the number of specific bacteria in a sample is not possible, and it is also important to remember that the technique will detect dead as well as viable bacterial cells.

For more information on PCR amplification of nucleic acids, see Erlich (1989) and Innis et al. (1990). Methods for DNA amplification by PCR are covered by patents held or pending by Hoffmann-La Roche Inc.

Amplification of 16S-23S rDNA

Most PCR systems involve the use of genus- or species-specific primers to identify particular bacteria present in a sample. A more universal method combines ribotyping and PCR by using conserved rDNA primers to amplify the 16S-23S rDNA spacer regions from the bacterial chromosome (Jensen, Webster and Straus 1993). Most bacteria have multiple copies of the rRNA operon, with the length and sequence of the 16S-23S intergenic spacer regions within the operons differing both between operons on the same genome and between operons within a bacterial species. This normally results in the generation of multiple PCR products, with size distribution profiles (sometimes analysed only following restriction endonuclease digestion) that can be used for the direct identification and differentiation of bacterial species by comparison with a database of band patterns obtained from standard strains. Although advanced procedures of this type are, as yet, still in the early stages of development, they offer the eventual possibility of being able to identify bacteria present in clinical and environmental samples rapidly without any need for isolation and cultivation.

NUCLEIC ACID SEQUENCING

The most precise (and ultimate 'gold standard') method for identifying particular micro-organisms is to determine the nucleotide sequence of definitive regions of the chromosome. This is not a method for routine use, but sequencing methods have developed so rapidly in recent years that comparative sequencing of homologous genes is now a standard technique in molecular systematics and phylogenetic studies (Ludwig 1991). PCR now provides a rapid method for producing relatively large quantities of template material for sequencing purposes from a selected locus in genomic DNA, thereby allowing work that would previously have taken weeks to be performed in a few hours. Coupled with the availability of equipment for automated DNA sequencing, such developments mean that a rapid automated sequencing procedure for determining sequence variations between different micro-organisms for identification purposes is now a realistic goal.

2.3 Molecular typing methods

Although the molecular identification methods referred to above have resulted in some real advances in the rapid identification of specific bacteria, particularly those that are difficult to cultivate by conventional procedures, it is the area of epidemiological typing which has seen some of the most productive applications of molecular biology to routine microbiology. Whereas conventional phenotypic typing schemes (such as biotyping, phage typing and serotyping) are time-consuming to develop and suffer from instability caused by environmental influences, molecular techniques can be performed in such a manner as to generate stable and reproducible results. They also offer the possibility of a 'uniform approach' to bacterial typing that can be applied immediately to any new epidemiological problem.

Of the methods based on nucleic acid content, analysis of plasmid profiles and restriction endonuclease fingerprints have been applied successfully for typing purposes to many different gram-positive and gram-negative bacteria. These techniques can provide information on the degree of relatedness of bacterial isolates within a single day. Plasmid content variations can occur between closely related bacteria, but this problem can be overcome by generating DNA fingerprints based on restriction endonuclease digestion of the entire chromosome and analysing these by pulsed field gel electrophoresis (PFGE); however, this is a relatively time-consuming and skill-intensive process that is unsuitable for routine diagnostic laboratories. A different approach involves examining particular defined regions of the chromosome in fine detail, either by means of hybridization techniques with nucleic acid probes or by employing an amplification technique such as PCR. Hybridization analysis is also relatively complex and time-consuming, but has been used with some success for typing particularly 'difficult' organisms. However, currently it is the use of amplification procedures that offers the most powerful DNA-based method for typing bacteria. By means of specific primers it is possible to amplify defined regions of the chromosome for direct analysis of restriction fragment length polymorphisms (RFLPs). Only a few cells are required for the amplification procedure and the whole analysis process can be completed within a single working day. Alternatively, fingerprints can be generated by random amplification of chromosomal DNA from a variety of sites by means of a single primer chosen arbitrarily. This process can be completed within 2–3 h, does not require any restriction endonuclease digestion to generate the RFLPs, requires no previous knowledge of the bacteria being investigated, and can be used to study any organism from which DNA can be extracted.

Proteins or LPS can also be used to generate fingerprint data for molecular typing purposes. Typing schemes based on sodium dodecyl sulphate polyacrylamide gel electrophoresis (SDS-PAGE) protein profiles have been used extensively for both gram-positive and gram-negative bacteria, and this technique is both relatively simple and applicable to any organism for which sufficient biomass can be obtained in a pure form. Whole cell analysis provides most information for detailed comparisons of strains, but fingerprints of subcellular fractions, including outer-membrane proteins or LPS, may provide sufficient information for typing many gram-negative bacteria. Immunoblotting with polypeptide antigens or LPS separated by SDS-PAGE provides an additional method of typing bacteria that is akin to the DNA-based hybridization methods described above. Such immunoblotting techniques are extremely powerful and offer an additional level of discrimination to that obtained by simple analysis of stained polypeptide or LPS fingerprint profiles. However, it should be noted that organisms sharing similar protein, LPS or immunoblotting profiles may be quite dissimilar on a genetic basis. Finally, the technique of multilocus enzyme electrophoresis (MLEE), in which organisms are differentiated by analysis of the electrophoretic mobility of a range of metabolic enzymes, has proved to be extremely useful for tracing bacteria in epidemiological studies, and for differentiating organisms in cases where other methods of phenotypic or serological analysis have lacked reproducibility or been ineffective.

Conventional methods for typing bacteria have filled a need for many years and will probably remain the methods of choice in cases where extensive and well recognized typing schemes have been developed over a long period. Molecular fingerprinting methods offer a new 'universal' approach to bacterial typing and are particularly useful for species that lack established or suitably discriminating typing schemes, or in cases where it is simply necessary to obtain a rapid answer to questions about the relatedness or identity of individual isolates.

For more information on molecular identification and typing methods, see Towner and Cockayne (1993).

2.4 Chemical composition

Analysis of whole cell composition, or of specific chemical components, has proved a valuable aid in the classification of bacteria (Goodfellow and O'Donnell 1994), particularly those groups that are unreactive in conventional biochemical tests. Initially, there seemed little application for this chemosystematic approach in routine identification; such techniques as peptidoglycan, isoprenoid quinone and lipid analysis (Suzuki, Goodfellow and O'Donnell 1993) required expertise in chemistry and prolonged, complex analyses. However, a wide variety of promising 'fingerprinting' techniques that reflect chemical composition have become available (Nelson 1991, Magee 1993; see Chapter 3), but remain largely unexploited.

Peptidoglycan analysis

The peptidoglycan polymer confers strength to the eubacterial cell wall, but is absent in the Archaea, mycoplasmas and planctomycetes (Kandler 1982,

König, Schlesner and Hirsch 1984). The backbone comprises repeating β-1,4-linked *N*-acetylglucosamine, *N*-acetyl (or, in some actinomycetes, *N*-glycolyl) muramic acid units (see Chapter 2, Fig. 2.18). Cummins and Harris (1956) noted that the amino acid cross-bridges that link these glycan strands into a complex mesh often differ in composition between genera among the gram-positive bacteria. By contrast, the amino acid composition in gram-negative species is remarkably uniform, with the exception of the spirochaetes where L-ornithine substitutes for *meso*-diaminopimelate. Further details of methods and bibliographies can be found in Schleifer and Kandler (1972), Schleifer and Seidl (1985) and Suzuki, Goodfellow and O'Donnell (1993). Teichoic and teichuronic acids are often found covalently linked to peptidoglycan in gram-positive organisms, forming the hot-acid-extractable 'group' antigens important in the characterization of the streptococci and lactobacilli and in the taxonomy of staphylococci (Easmon and Goodfellow 1990).

LIPID ANALYSIS

The mycolic acids and polar lipids are important in the classification of the actinomycetes, and in the identification of 'atypical' mycobacteria (Jenkins, Marks and Schaefer 1972). Membrane isoprenoid quinones are important components of electron transport systems and are found in facultative and obligate aerobes and some obligate anaerobes. Variation occurs in the nature of the quinone nucleus, the length of the polyprenyl side chain, and the saturation of the side chain. Initial studies by Yamada, Aida and Uemura (1968) and Jeffries et al. (1968) showed that the isoprenoid quinones were useful markers and their use is now established in taxonomic studies. Further details can be found in Suzuki, Goodfellow and O'Donnell (1993). The lipopolysaccharide endotoxin of gram-negative bacteria contains polysaccharide side chains that form the O antigen of smooth strains. This is important in the antigenic subtyping of species (see Chapter 41). Cellular fatty acids are amenable to rapid analysis by gas-liquid chromatography after methylation, a fingerprinting technique discussed below (see section on 'Physicochemical fingerprinting', p. 78).

PROTEIN ELECTROPHORESIS

Electrophoretic separation of bacterial proteins forms the basis of several useful characterization techniques. Undenatured proteins may be separated by conventional electrophoresis or isoelectric focusing, and then stained with a variety of chromogenic substrates to visualize specific enzymes. Differences between organisms are often found, revealing the differing isoelectric points, or electrophoretic mobility, of enzymes fulfilling the same function in distinct organisms. This has proved a useful approach in typing, in the study of population genetics in bacteria, and in distinguishing enzymes involved in antibiotic inactivation. However, most electrophoretic approaches involve protein denaturation. Urea or non-ionic detergents are denaturing agents that preserve the specific charge of proteins and are sometimes applied in isoelectric focusing or 2-dimensional polyacrylamide gel electrophoresis (PAGE) (Miner and Heston 1972, O'Farrell 1975). Denaturation in sodium dodecyl sulphate (SDS) solution is a more frequently utilized, and distinct approach. This anionic detergent destroys inter- and intrapeptide hydrogen and charge bonds to produce soluble linear peptides, hydrophobically bound to the detergent. The charge-to-peptide mass ratio of these complexes is nearly constant (Maizel 1969), and so the electrophoretic mobility of each peptide complex is proportional to the molecular weight of the peptide. SDS denaturation usually also involves concurrent reduction of disulphide bridges. This is achieved by adding 2-mercaptoethanol to the SDS buffer and heating at 100°C for a few minutes, which ensures linearization of peptides with intrapeptide disulphide bonds, and separation of peptides joined by interpeptide disulphide bonds. The peptides are then separated by electrophoresis and visualized by staining, usually with Coomassie blue. Radiometric visualization involves labelling the culture with [^{35}S]methionine and scanning the gel with a detector for methionine-containing peptides (Andersen et al. 1987), or by autoradiography. The most favoured electrophoresis method is the discontinuous polyacrylamide gel system of Laemmli (1970).

This SDS-PAGE system has been applied to whole cell proteins, but the banding patterns are complex and can be difficult to interpret. Alternatively, protein fractions extracted from purified cell envelopes, or the proteins detached by EDTA or EDTA and lysozyme treatment of bacteria in isotonic buffer, often referred to as outer-membrane proteins (OMPs), can be analysed. Another approach is to electrophorese whole cell proteins, blot the bands onto a protein-binding membrane, add antiserum raised against whole cell extracts of a single strain and visualize the bound antibody by immunoperoxidase staining. These modifications produce simple banding patterns, but the difficulties in interpreting whole cell proteins must be balanced against the more demanding preparations involved. Although discrimination may potentially be less, in practice these simpler patterns are usually as discriminatory as whole cell patterns.

Most applications of protein electrophoresis are in typing rather than species identification. It is difficult to standardize SDS-PAGE at a level that allows valid comparisons of banding patterns between gels, and the number of isolates that can be analysed on a single gel is limited. However, SDS-PAGE of whole cell proteins is a useful general-purpose 'fingerprint' typing method within the reach of most routine laboratories. Vauterin, Swings and Kersters (1993) give a comprehensive discussion and bibliography of these approaches. With strict standardization, protein electrophoresis may also be useful in classification studies.

ANTIGEN DETECTION

This approach is important in routine identification of β-haemolytic streptococci and leptospires, and is the basis for the typing of salmonellae, shigellae, pneumococci and *Streptococcus pyogenes*, and to a lesser extent, meningococci and *Haemophilus influenzae*. However, the reaction of an impure antigen with a polyclonal antibody must be interpreted with caution. The possibility of cross-reactions with an unrelated organism is an ever-present hazard, and results from these classical rapid serological methods must be regarded with suspicion until the organism has been conclusively identified to species level by other methods. Newer technology may reduce these problems, notably the use of monoclonal antibodies which is now reaching routine use in reference laboratories, for example in the typing of gonococci (Tam et al. 1982).

PHYSICOCHEMICAL FINGERPRINTING

Many physicochemical analytical techniques are applicable to bacterial characterization (Nelson 1991, Magee 1993). Most were developed initially for the analysis of pure chemicals. However, with the introduction of sophisticated pattern-analysis strategies, and the availability of cheap powerful computers, several of these approaches have been applied successfully to complex organic mixtures. Their increasing use in the quality control of raw materials has encouraged the development of robust, automated instruments, for example, the modern Fourier-transform near infrared spectrometers, and exploration of the wider applications for further similar approaches.

For most of these techniques, the potential for microbiological applications remains untapped. The few that have been investigated have proved to be applicable in the characterization of bacteria at all taxonomic levels, from subspecies discrimination to differentiation at generic and higher taxonomic levels. Examples include: pyrolysis mass spectrometry (Magee 1993), analysis of cell fatty acids (Moss, Samuels and Weaver 1972, Moss and Dees 1975), infrared spectrometry (Naumann et al. 1991), electrophoresis of cell proteins (discussed above, p. 77) and flow cytometry (Lloyd 1993).

Broadly, these approaches tend to be instrument-based, with simple, rapid, specimen preparation, short automated analysis, high throughput, and automated data acquisition. These techniques produce complex pattern data ('fingerprints') that often reflect cell composition. Data analysis usually requires knowledge of sophisticated mathematical or statistical techniques at the development stage, but these can be reduced to simpler, objective 'black box' computerized analyses thereafter. Disadvantages tend to be the high initial cost of the instrument and problems with long-term reproducibility. Rigid standardization of growth conditions is normally required, but these techniques are not species-specific; a single standard method can usually be applied for any organism that can be grown in pure culture. Further information and bibliographies

on these approaches can be found in Nelson (1991), Lloyd (1993) and Magee (1993).

2.5 Bacteriophages and bacteriocins

The host specificity of phage- and bacteriocin-induced lysis (see Chapter 8) is often exploited in typing, and less frequently in species identification.

Phages vary greatly in their range of lytic activity. Some lyse all members of a particular species (e.g. *Brucella abortus* or *Bacillus anthracis*), others only specific serotypes or biotypes (e.g. in *Vibrio cholerae*). Phages used in the infraspecific typing systems, such as those for *Pseudomonas aeruginosa* and *Staphylococcus aureus*, have narrow lytic spectra. These usually give patterns of lysis that are strain- or type-specific, and seldom attack organisms outside the species; thus, typability may be good evidence that an organism belongs to the species, but untypability does not exclude this possibility.

The range of activity of bacteriocins also varies widely. Many of those formed by gram-positive bacteria have a wide range of activity on members of other genera but some, e.g. those of haemolytic streptococci, are serotype- or serogroup-specific. Bacteriocins of gram-negative bacilli generally show narrow specificity within individual species, genera or groups of genera. Bacteriocin typing systems are useful within species and may be:

1 'active', in which a strain is characterized by the range of activity of its bacteriocins against a set of indicator strains, or
2 'passive', in which it is characterized by the pattern of its susceptibility to the bacteriocins of a set of indicator strains, or
3 a combined active–passive system.

In each case, strains being typed and the indicator strains are usually, but not invariably, members of the same species. Pyocins, although active on *P. aeruginosa* but not usually on other pseudomonads or enterobacteria, also attack gonococci and meningococci. Colicins attack a wide range of enterobacteria.

2.6 Pathogenicity

Tests for pathogenicity are used in the final stages of identification for a new species, particularly when the ability of an isolate to produce a known biologically active toxin is crucial to diagnosis. A particular example is the mouse test for active botulinum toxin, produced by some but not all isolates identified as *C. botulinum*. Similarly, a laboratory may well feel it is necessary to confirm that isolates of *Clostridium tetani* or *Corynebacterium diphtheriae* are toxigenic in laboratory animals. Diagnosis of the diseases caused by these organisms has such impact that toxin detection by immunological methods alone may be regarded as insufficient, because of the possibility that an immunologically reactive but biologically inactive toxin is produced. Similarly, detection of an enterotoxin in the ileal loop model may be the only reliable method for distinguishing enterotoxigenic strains of some species. The high costs and the ethical considerations involved in animal tests have limited their application to a few specific applications. Earlier, routine use in identification of, for example, *M. tuberculosis*, has generally been superseded by less costly in vitro tests.

2.7 Identification

The various approaches to identification from a set of characterization results are discussed in detail in Chapter 3. Formal identification at species level in the routine laboratory usually occurs in 2 stages, reflecting the progression from first to second stage tests in Cowan and Steel's Manual (Barrow and Feltham 1993). In the first, the organism is identified to genus or slightly broader level on the basis of a restricted set of tests. In the routine laboratory these will usually include gram-staining reaction, cellular morphology, catalase and cytochrome oxidase production, and atmospheric requirements, and possibly acid-fast staining, spore production and morphology, a Hugh and Liefson OF test and motility. These tests, together with expert interpretation of colony morphology, are sufficiently powerful to assign most clinical isolates to a broad generic group.

However, an error in the results obtained at this stage will often result in much futile, wasteful effort to identify an isolate to an inappropriate group. Asporogenous variants and gram-variable organisms (or the frank gram-negative reaction of some *Bacillus* and *Clostridium* spp.) often overcome all efforts of the inexperienced worker, and their unequivocal identification can often tax the expert.

Equally, impure cultures are probably the most frequent cause of puzzling result patterns at this and later stages of identification. The answer is often obvious from the purity plate, but some mixed cultures can be difficult to detect, particularly when a large-colony, rapidly growing organism is associated with a slow-growing, small-colony organism that obtains an essential growth factor from its comparison. This and other modes of cryptic contamination can cause much difficulty. The most essential components of any identification test are the single, well separated colony, carefully picked from a rich non-selective plate for the inoculum suspension, and the purity plate, carefully spread for the growth of single colonies on a rich non-selective medium, to assess the purity of this inoculum. If the identification tests yield an unusual pattern, the purity plate should be inspected for contaminants. If no contaminants are visible, then it is a wise precaution to further incubate the purity plate at room temperature for 48 h, and to culture from the identification media under a variety of conditions to ensure the absence of contaminating organisms.

The second stage of formal identification is now usually performed with miniaturized kits, rather than the locally made identification media that were the mainstay of identification when Cowan and Steel's classic identification tables first appeared in 1965. These kits offer many advantages to the busy labora-

tory. The costs are probably less than local preparation of the host of identification media required for a comprehensive identification service. The media probably undergo a more comprehensive quality control process than would be possible in most routine laboratories and, given careful adherence to the manufacturer's instructions, probably show greater interlaboratory reproducibility than was possible in earlier times. The identification process is probably also more objective. Precalculated tables of identification probabilities for common reaction patterns are often issued with the kits, and computer programs, or a computerized identification service, are often available to cope with less common patterns.

On the debit side, expertise in the preparation of identification media and interpretation of result patterns is often lost with the introduction of kits. This affects the service that can be offered for the minority of isolates that cannot be identified with the available kits. A third stage option for these, and the more refractory isolates from common genera is a centralized identification service. Reference laboratories, service culture collections, and some identification kit manufacturers may provide this service.

It is important to refer isolates that reach this third stage without a firm identification. These may represent species that are only rarely involved in infection, or species that are in the early stages of becoming problem opportunist pathogens. One of the reference laboratories' functions is to monitor and publish information on new and rare pathogens, and the throughput of cultures from routine laboratories is essential to this task. Without this service, there is little opportunity to accumulate the pool of information on pathogenicity, susceptibility, cross-infection potential and sources of these species, that is so essential when the clinicians request advice.

THE USE OF SPECIES NOMENCLATURE

Species names should be ascribed with due caution. Names carry a host of implied information, and there is an unavoidable tendency to assume that an isolate shows all the properties typical of the species to which it has been assigned. For some isolates, it may well be appropriate to note that this organism is atypical of the species in laboratory tests, and may show other atypical properties in vivo. For other, more difficult isolates, a frank admission that no species name can be ascribed with any certainty may be appropriate. These options are not admissions of incompetence, but rather an acknowledgement that bacteria show variation that cannot always be separated into discrete species compartments, and that we are only beginning to catalogue the enormous diversity of species in the bacterial kingdom.

Species names are italicized because they have a highly specific meaning – that the organism named has sufficient similarity in laboratory tests to the current formal description of the species, and so is likely to share many other properties ascribed to the species, but which have not been investigated for this particular isolate. Misuse of species names can cause misunderstanding and confusion to a stage where a name carries little useful information. *Staphylococcus epidermidis*, for instance, has a definition which does not include all coagulase-negative staphylococci, but is still often used in this wider sense. Similarly, one occasionally sees the name *Staphylococcus albus* in reports, although it has long been discarded and carries no current taxonomic definition. This misuse of names has made the literature on coagulase-negative staphylococcal infections very confusing. The formal species nomenclature exists to prevent such confusion; its abuse is an admission of ignorance.

Vernacular names are even more prone to confusion. For instance, the Enterobacteriaceae are a formally defined taxonomic group, but 'the enterobacteria' is a term that may include or exclude *P.*

aeruginosa and other organisms because it has been used in a such a wide variety of senses. Many of these terms describe groupings of bacterial species with no formal taxonomic definition, but the vernacular name conveys a concept of practical significance in everyday use. Degradation by misuse removes any meaning from these terms and effectively removes a useful concept from the technical language of microbiology.

APPENDIX 1

SYSTEMATIC DESCRIPTION OF MORPHOLOGICAL AND CULTURAL CHARACTERS OF BACTERIA

Table 4.1 Checklist of the morphological characters of bacteria

Shape Cocci, spherical, oval or lanceolate; short rods, long rods, filaments, commas or spirals
Axis Straight or curved
Size Length and breadth
Sides Parallel, bulging, concave or irregular
Ends Rounded, truncate, concave or pointed
Arrangement Singly, in pairs, in chains, in fours, in groups, in grape-like clusters, in cubical packets, in bundles or in Chinese letters
Irregular forms Variations in shape and size; club, filamentous, branched, navicular, citron, fusiform, giant swollen forms and shadow forms
Motility Motile or non-motile
Flagella Polar (monotrichate, amphitrichate, lophotrichate) or peritrichate, or both (Fig. 4.1). (In electron micrographs, length, breadth, wavelength and amplitude)
Fimbriae In electron micrographs, approximate number and size, polar or peritrichate
Spores Spherical, oval, or ellipsoidal; equatorial, subterminal or terminal; single or multiple; causing bulging of bacillus or not (Fig. 4.2)
Capsules Present or absent, indefinite mucoid sheath or envelope
Staining Even, irregular, unipolar, bipolar, beaded, barred; and variations in depth between different organisms; presence of metachromatic granules; reaction to gram and to Ziehl–Neelsen stains

Table 4.2 Check-list for description of the appearances of growth on solid or in liquid medium[a]

Surface colonies on solid media (see Fig. 4.3)
Shape Circular, irregular, radiate rhizoid
Size In millimetres
Elevation Effuse, raised, low convex, convex or dome-shaped, umbonate, umbilicate; with or without bevelled margin
Structure Amorphous; fine, medium or coarsely granular; filamentous, curled
Surface Smooth; contoured; beaten-copper; rough; fine, medium or coarsely granular; ringed; striated; papillate; dull or glistening
Edge Entire, undulate, lobate, crenated, erose, fimbriate, curled, effuse, spreading
Colour Colour by reflected and transmitted light; fluorescent, iridescent, opalescent, self-luminous
Opacity Transparent, translucent or opaque
Consistency Butyrous, viscid, friable, cohesive, membranous, 'corroding'; growth down into medium
Emulsifiability Easy or difficult; forms homogeneous or granular suspension or remains membranous when rubbed up in a drop of water with a loop
Differentiation Differentiated into a central and a peripheral portion
Growth in fluid medium
Degree None, scanty, moderate, abundant or profuse
Turbidity Present or absent; if present, slight, moderate or dense; uniform, granular or flocculent
Deposit Present or absent; if present, slight, moderate or abundant; powdery, granular, flocculent, membranous or viscid; disintegrating completely or incompletely on shaking
Surface growth Present or absent; if present, ring growth around wall of tube; or surface pellicle, which is thin or thick, with a smooth, granular or rough surface, and which disintegrates completely or incompletely on shaking
Odour Absent, decided, resembling ——

[a]On nutrient agar and in nutrient broth (if the organism will grow) under stated conditions of time, temperature and atmosphere. Record appearances also on special media that reveal characters of the group of organisms under investigation.

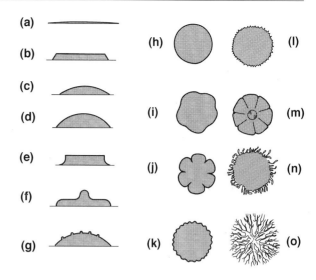

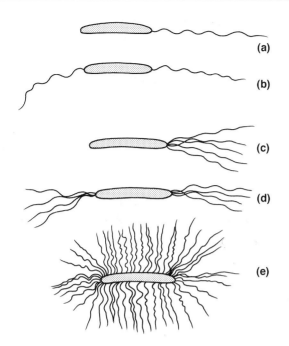

Fig. 4.1 (a–d) Polar distribution of flagella: a, monotrichate; b, amphitrichate; c and d, lophotrichate; e, peritrichate.

Fig. 4.3 Description of colonies. (a–g) Elevation of colonies: a, flat or effuse; b, raised; c, low convex; d, convex or dome-shaped; e, raised with concave bevelled edge; f, umbonate; g, convex with papillate surface. (h–o) Edge of colonies: h, entire; i, undulate; j, lobate; k, crenated; l, erose or dentate; m, radially striated periphery with lobate edge; n, fimbriate; o, rhizoid or arborescent.

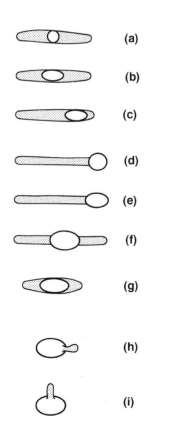

Fig. 4.2 Spores (a–c) without distortion of bacterial cell: a, spherical equatorial; b, oval equatorial; c, oval subterminal. (d–g) With distortion of bacterial cell: d, spherical terminal; e, oval terminal; f, oval equatorial; g, oval equatorial. (h and i) Germination of spores: h, polar germination; i, equatorial germination.

APPENDIX 2

GLOSSARY OF TERMS USED TO DESCRIBE THE MORPHOLOGICAL AND CULTURAL APPEARANCES OF BACTERIA

Amorphous (colonies): without visible differentiation in structure

Amphitrichate: having one (or two) flagella at each pole

Beaded (stained bacteria): deeply staining granules arranged at regular intervals along the course of the rod. (In stab or stroke culture): disjointed or semi-confluent colonies along the line of inoculation

Beaten-copper: multiple small crateriform depressions on the surface of a growth, resembling beaten copper

Bipolar: at both ends or poles of the bacterial cell

Butyrous: growth of butter-like consistency

Chains: 4 or more organisms attached end to end

Citron: shaped like a lemon, having a small knob at each end

Clavate: club-shaped

Contoured: an irregular, smoothly undulating surface, or like a relief map

Convex: the segment of a sphere of short radius; **low convex**, the segment of a sphere of long radius

'Corroding': causes depressions in the medium under colonies

Crenated: small, shallow indentations of the edge, which has a scalloped appearance

Cuneate: wedge-shaped

Curled: composed of parallel chains in wavy strands, as in anthrax colonies

Effuse: growth thin, hardly raised at all from the medium

Endospores: thick-walled spores formed within the bacterial cell

Entire: with an even margin

Equatorial: situated about equidistant from each end

Erose: border showing fine, pointed, tooth-like projections

Filaments: applied to morphology of bacteria, refers to thread-like forms, generally unsegmented; if segmented, to be distinguished from chains (q.v.) by the absence of constrictions between the segments

Filamentous: growth composed of long, often interwoven threads

Filiform in stroke or stab cultures, a uniform growth confined to the line of inoculation

Fimbriate: fine, sometimes recurved, processes projecting from the edge of the colony or growth. Also used to denote the presence of fimbriae

Flocculent: containing small adherent masses of bacteria of various shapes floating in the culture fluid, or deposited at the bottom

Fluorescent: having one colour by transmitted light and another by reflected light

Friable: growth dry and brittle, when touched with a needle

Granular: composed of granules; fine, medium or coarse

Haemolysis: on blood agar plate; α-haemolysis: colonies surrounded by a greenish ring; β-haemolysis: colonies surrounded by an area of clearing, which is transparent (see Chapter 28)

Heaped-up: irregular, coarse processes projecting considerably above the level of the rest of the growth

Iridescent: exhibiting changing rainbow colours in reflected light

Lenticular: surface colony, which is convex and translucent, and which acts like a planoconvex lens, giving an inverted image of an object viewed through it. Deep colony, which is shaped like a lentil

Lobate: having the margin deeply undulate, producing lobes (see **Undulate**)

Lophotrichate: having a tuft of flagella at one or both poles

Luminous: glowing in the dark, phosphorescent

Membranous: growth thin, coherent, like a membrane

Mirror-like: having a smooth glistening surface, in which reflections of surrounding objects, e.g. window bars, can be seen

Monotrichate: having a single flagellum at one pole

Navicular: shaped like a boat

Opalescent: coarsely iridescent, like an opal

Opaque: objects, e.g. window bars, cannot be seen through growth

Papillate: growth beset with small nipple-like processes

Pellicle: bacterial growth forming either a continuous or an interrupted sheet on the surface of the culture fluid

Petritrichate: having flagella disposed around the organism

Punctiform: very small, but visible to naked eye; under 0.5 mm in diameter

Radiate: showing fissures or ridges arranged in a radial manner

Raised: growth thick, with a comparatively flat surface, and with abrupt or terraced edges

Rhizoid: growth of an irregular branched or root-like character, as in *Bacillus mycoides*

Ring: growth at the upper margin of a liquid culture, adhering to the glass

Ringed: having one or more circular depressions or elevations on the surface, sometimes giving a draughtsman-like appearance

Rough: general term for an irregular surface, the irregularity being of a coarsely granulated type, or resembling morocco leather

Spreading: growth extending much beyond the line of inoculation, i.e. several millimetres or more; sometimes over an entire slope or plate

Subterminal: situated towards the end

Terminal: situated at the extreme end

Translucent: objects, e.g. window bars, are visible through growth, but growth is not water-clear

Transparent: growth is water-clear

Truncate: ends abrupt, square

Turbid: cloudy; may be a uniform flocculent, or granular turbidity

Umbonate: having a button-like, raised centre

Undulate: border wavy, with shallow sinuses

Unipolar: at one end only of the bacterial cell

Viscid: sticky, semifluid; on withdrawal of the needle, the growth follows it in the form of a thread; sediment on shaking rises as a coherent swirl

REFERENCES

Amies CRF, 1967, A modified formula for the preparation of Stuart's transport medium, *Can J Public Health*, **58:** 296–300.

Andersen H, Birkelund S et al., 1987, Electrophoretic analysis of proteins from *Mycoplasma hominis* strains detected by SDS-PAGE, two-dimensional gel electrophoresis and immunoblotting, *J Gen Microbiol*, **133:** 181–91.

Ayers SH, Rupp P, 1922, Differentiation of hemolytic streptococci from human and bovine sources by the hydrolysis of sodium hippurate, *J Infect Dis*, **30:** 388–99.

Barrow GI, Feltham RKA (eds), 1993, *Cowan and Steel's Manual for the Identification of Medical Bacteria*, 3rd edn, Cambridge University Press, Cambridge.

Bartlett DI, Hughes MH, 1969, Bacteriological swabs, *Br Med J*, **3:** 450–1.

Braun H, Guggenheim K, 1932, Ueber Atmungstypen bei fakultativ aeroben pathogenen Bacterien, *Zentralbl Bakteriol Parasitenkd Infektionskr Hyg*, **127:** 97–104.

Christensen WB, 1946, Urea decomposition as a means of differentiating *Proteus* and paracolon cultures from each other and from *Salmonella* and *Shigella* types, *J Bacteriol*, **52:** 461–6.

Clark WM, Lubs HA, 1915, The differentiation of bacteria of the colon-aerogenes family by the use of indicators, *J Infect Dis*, **17:** 160–73.

Craigie J, 1931, Studies on the serological reactions of the flagella of *B. typhosus*, *J Immunol*, **21:** 417–511.

Cummins CS, Harris H, 1956, The chemical composition of the cell wall in some Gram-positive bacteria and its possible value as a taxonomic character, *J Gen Microbiol*, **14:** 583–600.

Dadd AH, Dagnall VP et al., 1970, The survival of *Streptococcus pyogenes* on bacteriological swabs made from various fibres, *J Med Microbiol*, **3**: 561–72.

Deibel RH, Evans JB, 1960, Modified benzidine test for the detection of cytochrome-containing respiratory systems in microorganisms, *J Bacteriol*, **79**: 356–60.

Easmon CSF, Goodfellow M, 1990, *Staphylococcus* and *Micrococcus*, *Topley & Wilson's Principles of Bacteriology, Virology and Immunity*, vol. 2, 8th edn, eds Parker MT, Collier LH, Edward Arnold, London, 161–86.

Edberg SC, Samuels S, 1976, Rapid, colorimetric test for the determination of hippurate hydrolysis by group B streptococcus, *J Clin Microbiol*, **3**: 49–50.

Elek SD, 1948, Rapid identification of *Proteus*, *J Pathol Bacteriol*, **60**: 183–92.

Erlich HA, 1989, *PCR Technology – Principles and Applications for DNA Amplification*, Stockton Press, New York.

Ewing WH, Davis BR, Reavis RW, 1957, Phenylalanine and malonate media and their use in enteric bacteriology, *Public Health Lab*, **15**: 153–67.

Ferguson WW, Hook AE, 1942, Urease activity of *Proteus* and *Salmonella* organisms, *J Lab Clin Med*, **28**: 1715–20.

Forsyth WGC, Hayward AC, Roberts JB, 1958, Occurrence of poly-β-hydroxybutyric acid in aerobic gram-negative bacteria, *Nature* (London), **182**: 800–1.

Frazier WC, 1926, A method for the detection of changes in gelatin due to bacteria, *J Infect Dis*, **39**: 302–9.

Gästrin B, Kallings LO, Marcetic A, 1968, The survival time for different bacteria in various transport media, *Acta Pathol Microbiol Scand*, **74**: 371–80.

Goodfellow M, O'Donnell AG, 1994, Chemosystematics: current state and future prospects, *Chemical Methods in Procaryotic Systematics*, eds Goodfellow M, O'Donnell AG, John Wiley & Sons, Chichester, 1–20.

Gordon J, McLeod JW, 1928, The practical application of the direct oxidase reaction in bacteriology, *J Pathol Bacteriol*, **31**: 185–90.

Grimont F, Grimont PAD, 1986, Ribosomal ribonucleic acid gene restriction patterns as potential taxonomic tools, *Ann Inst Pasteur Microbiol*, **137B**: 165–75.

Grimont PAD, Grimont F, 1991, rRNA probes as tools for molecular epidemiology of microbial infections, *Rapid Methods and Automation in Microbiology and Immunology*, eds Vaheri A, Tilton RC, Balows A, Springer-Verlag, Berlin, 47–53.

Hajna AA, Damon SR, 1934, Differentiation of *A. aerogenes* and *A. cloacae* on the basis of the hydrolysis of sodium hippurate, *Am J Hyg*, **19**: 545–8.

Hare R, Colebrook L, 1934, The biochemical reactions of haemolytic streptococci from the vagina of febrile and afebrile parturient women, *J Pathol Bacteriol*, **39**: 429–42.

Henrici AT, 1926, Morphologic variations of bacteria in the lag phase, *J Infect Dis*, **38**: 54–65.

Henriksen SD, 1950, A comparison of the phenylpyruvic acid reaction and the urease test in the differentiation of *Proteus* from other enteric organisms, *J Bacteriol*, **60**: 225–31.

Holdeman LV, Cato EP, Moore WEC (eds), 1977, *Anaerobe Laboratory Manual*, 4th edn, Anaerobe Laboratory, Virginia Polytechnic and State University, Blacksburg, VA.

Holt RJ, 1966, Pad culture studies on skin surfaces, *J Appl Bacteriol*, **29**: 625–30.

Hugh R, Leifson E, 1953, The taxonomic significance of fermentative versus oxidative metabolism of carbohydrates by various gram negative bacteria, *J Bacteriol*, **66**: 24–6.

Hwang M, Ederer GM, 1975, Rapid hippurate hydrolysis method for presumptive identification of group B streptococci, *J Clin Microbiol*, **1**: 114–15.

Innis MA, Gelfand DH et al., 1990, *PCR Protocols – a Guide to Methods and Applications*, Academic Press, San Diego.

Isenberg HD, Sundheim LH, 1958, Indole reactions in bacteria, *J Bacteriol*, **75**: 682–90.

Jeffries L, Cawthorne MA et al., 1968, Menaquinone determination in the taxonomy of Micrococcaceae, *J Gen Microbiol*, **54**: 365–80.

Jenkins PA, Marks J, Schaefer WB, 1972, Thin layer chromotography of mycobacterial lipids an aid to classification: the scotochromogenic mycobacteria, including *Mycobacterium scrofulaceum*, *M. xenopi*, *M. aquae*, *M. gordonae*, *M. flavescens*, *Tubercle*, **53**: 118–27.

Jensen MA, Webster JA, Straus N, 1993, Rapid identification of bacteria on the basis of polymerase chain reaction-amplified ribosomal DNA spacer polymorphisms, *Appl Environ Microbiol*, **59**: 945–52.

Johnston MA, Pivnick H, 1970, Use of autocytotoxic β-D-galactosides for selective growth of *Salmonella typhimurium* in the presence of coliforms, *Can J Microbiol*, **16**: 83–9.

Johnston MA, Thatcher FS, 1967, Selective inhibition of *Escherichia coli* in the presence of *Salmonella typhimurium* by phenethyl β-D-galactopyranoside, *Appl Microbiol*, **15**: 1223–8.

Kandler O, 1982, Cell wall structures and their phylogenetic applications, *Zentralbl Bakteriol C*, **3**: 149–60.

Kauffmann F, 1954, *Enterobacteriaceae*, 2nd edn, Einar Munksgaard, Copenhagen.

Kauffmann F, Peterson A, 1956, The biochemical group and type differentiation of Enterobacteriaceae by organic acids, *Acta Pathol Microbiol Scand*, **38**: 481–91.

Koch R, 1881, Investigations into the aetiology of the traumatic infective diseases. New Sydenham Society, London 1881, *Mitteilungen aus dem Reichsgesundheitsante*, **1**: 1.

König E, Schlesner H, Hirsch P, 1984, Cell wall studies on budding bacteria of the *Planctomyces/Pasteuria* group and a *Prosthecomicrobium* sp., *Arch Microbiol*, **138**: 200–5.

Kontiainen S, Sivonen A, Renkonen OV, 1994, Increased yields of pathogenic *Yersinia enterocolitica* strains by cold enrichment, *Scand J Infect Dis*, **26**: 685–91.

Kováks N, 1956, Identification of *Pseudomonas pyocyanea* by the oxidase reaction, *Nature* (London), **178**: 703.

Laemmli UK, 1970, Cleavage of the structural proteins durihg the assembly of the head of bacteriophage T4, *Nature* (London), **227**: 680–5.

Larsson L, Mårdh P-A, 1977, Application of gas chromatography to diagnosis of microorganisms and infectious diseases, *Acta Pathol Microbiol Scand Suppl Sect B*, **259**: 5–15.

Lederberg J, 1950, The β-D-galactosidase of *Escherichia coli*, strain K-12, *J Bacteriol*, **60**: 381–92.

Leifson E, 1933, The fermentation of sodium malonate as a means of differentiating *Aerobacter* and *Escherichia*, *J Bacteriol*, **26**: 329–30.

Le Minor L, Ben Hamida F, 1962, Avantages de la recherche de la β-galactosidase sur celle de la fermentation du lactose en milieu complexe dans le diagnostic bacteriologique, en particulier des Enterobacteriaceae, *Ann Inst Pasteur (Paris)*, **102**: 267–77.

Le Minor L, Pichinoty F, 1963, Recherche de la tetrathionate-reductase chez les bactéries gram négatives anaerobies facultatives (Enterobacteriaceae, *Aeromonas* et *Pasteurella*) méthode et valeur diagnostique, *Ann Inst Pasteur (Paris)*, **104**: 384–93.

Levine M, Epstein SS, Vaughan RH, 1934, Differential reactions in the colon group of bacteria, *Am J Public Health*, **24**: 505–10.

Lister J, 1878, On the nature of fermentation, *Q J Microsc Soc*, **18**: 177.

Lloyd D (ed.), 1993, *Flow Cytometry in Microbiology*, Springer-Verlag, London.

Lowe GH, 1962, The rapid detection of lactose fermentation in paracolon organisms by the demonstration of β-D-galactosidase, *J Med Lab Technol*, **19**: 21–5.

Ludwig W, 1991, DNA sequencing in bacterial systematics, *Nucleic Acid Techniques in Bacterial Systematics*, eds Stackebrandt E, Goodfellow M, John Wiley & Sons, Chichester, 69–94.

Magee JT, 1993, Whole organism fingerprinting, *Handbook of New Bacterial Systematics*, eds Goodfellow M, O'Donnell AG, Academic Press, London, 383–427.

Maizel JV, 1969, Acrylamide gel electrophoresis of proteins and nucleic acids, *Fundamental Techniques in Virology*, eds Habel K, Salzman PP, Academic Press, London, 334–62.

Marshall VM, 1979, A note on screening hydrogen peroxide-producing lactic acid bacteria using a non-toxic chromogen, *J Appl Bacteriol*, **47:** 327–8.

Miles AA, Misra SS, Irwin JD, 1938, The estimation of the bactericidal power of the blood, *J Hyg (Lond)*, **38:** 732–49.

Miner GD, Heston LL, 1972, Method for acrylamide gel isoelectric focusing of insoluble brain proteins, *Anal Biochem*, **50:** 313–16.

Møller V, 1954, Activity determination of amino acid decarboxylases in Enterobacteriaceae, *Acta Pathol Microbiol Scand*, **34:** 102–14.

Møller V, 1955, Simplified tests for some amino acid decarboxylases and for the arginine dihydrolase system, *Acta Pathol Microbiol Scand*, **36:** 158.

Moore WEC, Cato EP, Holdeman LV, 1966, Fermentation patterns of some *Clostridium* species, *Int J Syst Bacteriol*, **16:** 383–415.

Moss CW, Dees SB, 1975, Identification of micro-organisms by gas chromatographic-mass spectrometric analysis of cellular fatty acids, *J Chromatogr*, **112:** 595–604.

Moss CW, Samuels SB, Weaver RE, 1972, Cellular fatty acid composition of selected *Pseudomonas* species, *Appl Microbiol*, **24:** 596–8.

Naumann D, Helm D et al., 1991, The characterization of micro-organisms by Fourier-transform infrared spectroscopy (FT-IR), *Modern Techniques for Rapid Microbiological Analysis*, ed. Nelson WH, VCH Publishers Inc., New York, 19–42.

Nelson WH (ed.), 1991, *Modern Techniques for Rapid Microbiological Analysis*, VCH Publishers Inc., New York.

Niven CF, Smiley KL, Sherman JM, 1942, The hydrolysis of arginine by streptococci, *J Bacteriol*, **43:** 651–60.

O'Farrell PH, 1975, High resolution two-dimensional electrophoresis of proteins, *J Biol Chem*, **250:** 4007–21.

Pollock MR, Knox R, Gell PGH, 1942, Bacterial reduction of tetrathionate, *Nature* (London), **150:** 94.

Rubbo SD, Benjamin M, 1951, Some observations on survival of pathogenic bacteria on cotton-wool swabs: development of a new type of swab, *Br Med J*, **1:** 983–7.

Schleifer KH, Kandler O, 1972, Peptidoglycan types of bacterial cell walls and their taxonomic implications, *Bacteriol Rev*, **34:** 407–77.

Schleifer KH, Seidl PH, 1985, Chemical composition and structure of murein, *Chemical Methods in Bacterial Systematics*, eds Goodfellow M, Minnikin DE, Academic Press, London, 201–19.

Sierra G, 1957, A simple method for the detection of lipolytic activity of micro-organisms and some observations on the influence of the contact between cells and fatty substrates, *Antonie van Leeuwenhoek Ned Tidschr Hyg Microbiol Serol*, **23:** 15–22.

Skerman VBD, 1969, *Abstracts of Microbiological Methods*, John Wiley & Sons, New York.

Smith PB, Hancock GA, Rhoden DL, 1969, Improved medium for detecting deoxyribonuclease-producing bacteria, *Appl Microbiol*, **18:** 991–3.

Stahl DA, Amann R, 1991, Development and application of nucleic acid probes, *Nucleic Acid Techniques in Bacterial Systematics*, eds Stackebrandt E, Goodfellow M, John Wiley & Sons, Chichester, 205–48.

Stuart CA, van Stratum E, Rustigian R, 1945, Further studies on urease production by *Proteus* and related organisms, *J Bacteriol*, **49:** 437–44.

Stuart RD, 1959, Transport medium for specimens in public health bacteriology, *Public Health Rep*, **74:** 431–8.

Sutter VL, Citron DM, Finegold SM, 1980, *Wadsworth Anaerobic Bacteriology Manual*, 3rd edn, Mosby, St Louis.

Suzuki K, Goodfellow M, O'Donnell AG, 1993, Cell envelopes and classification, *Handbook of New Bacterial Systematics*, eds Goodfellow M, O'Donnell AG, Academic Press, London, 195–250.

Tam MR, Buchanan TM et al., 1982, Serological classification of *Neisseria gonorrhoea* with monoclonal antibodies, *Infect Immun*, **36:** 1042–53.

Towner KJ, Cockayne A, 1993, *Molecular Methods for Microbial Identification and Typing*, Chapman and Hall, London.

Tulloch WJ, 1939, Observations concerning bacillary food infection in Dundee during the period 1923–38, *J Hyg*, **39:** 324–33.

Vauterin L, Swings J, Kersters K, 1993, Protein electrophoresis and classification, *Handbook of New Bacterial Systematics*, eds Goodfellow M, O'Donnell AG, Academic Press, London, 251–80.

Voges O, Proskauer B, 1898, Beitrag zur Ernahrungphysiologie und zur Differential-diagnose der Bakterien der hamarrhagischen Septicamie, *Z Hyg Infektionskr*, **28:** 20–32.

Weyant RS, Weaver RE et al., 1996, *Identification of Unusual Pathogenic Gram-negative Aerobic and Facultatively Anaerobic Bacteria*, Williams & Wilkins, Baltimore and London.

Whittenbury R, 1964, Hydrogen peroxide formation and catalase activity in the lactic acid bacteria, *J Gen Microbiol*, **35:** 13–26.

Wilson GS, 1926, The proportion of viable bacilli in agar cultures of *B. aertrycke* (mutton), with special reference to the change in size of the organisms during growth, and in the opacity to which they give rise, *J Hyg*, **25:** 150–9.

Wilson GS, 1959, Faults and fallacies in microbiology: the Fourth Marjory Stephenson Memorial Lecture, *J Gen Microbiol*, **21:** 1–15.

Woese CR, 1987, Bacterial evolution, *Microbiol Rev*, **51:** 221–71.

Wren MWD, 1991, Laboratory diagnosis of anaerobic infections, *Anaerobes in Human Disease*, eds Duerden BI, Drasar BS, Arnold, London, 180–96.

Yamada Y, Aida K, Uemura T, 1968, Distribution of ubiquinone 10 and 9 in acetic acid bacteria and its relation to the classification of the genera *Gluconobacter* and *Acetobacter*, especially of so-called intermediate strains, *Agric Biol Chem*, **32:** 786–8.

Zobell CE, Feltham CB, 1934, A comparison of lead, bismuth, and iron as detectors of hydrogen sulphide produced by bacteria, *J Bacteriol*, **28:** 169–76.

BACTERIAL GROWTH AND METABOLISM

R P Mortlock

1   REGULATORY MECHANISMS IN METABOLISM

1.1   Introduction

GENERAL COMPOSITION OF BACTERIA

In order for bacterial cells to grow, they must be provided with all of the chemical elements needed for the synthesis of new cellular material. Once, organisms that could use simple molecules to satisfy their nutritional requirements, such as carbon dioxide as the sole carbon source, were thought of as 'simple' organisms. We now understand that the simpler the nutrients, the more complex the biochemical reactions required by the cell to convert those nutrients into complex cellular material.

The water content of bacterial cells can vary from 75 to 90% of the total weight. The dry weight, after removal of water, is composed of about 50% carbon, about 10% hydrogen and about 20% oxygen. The nitrogen content of the dry weight can vary from 8 to 15%, sulphur from 0.1 to 1.0% and phosphorus may vary in the range from 1 to 6% of the dry weight. The iron content is also variable and is highest in cells with haem proteins. Other elements found are potassium, calcium, magnesium, chlorine, sodium, zinc, cobalt, molybdenum, manganese and copper. These and other trace elements total about 0.3% of the dry weight.

CELLULAR POLYMERS

Most of the organic material in the bacterial cell is in the form of large polymers. However, the cell cytoplasm also contains a 'soluble pool' of smaller, unpolymerized organic molecules such as amino acids, nucleotides, carbohydrates, fatty acid precursors of these molecules, as well as degradation products from the breakdown of any compounds providing carbon and energy sources for growth. Large organic polymers of the cell include those made of amino acids (proteins), those made of ribonucleotides (RNA), those made of deoxyribonucleic acid (DNA), and those composed of carbohydrates and lipids. Protein represents about 50% of the dry weight of a typical bacterial cell and *Escherichia coli* has been reported to synthesize about 1850 different protein molecules with an average molecular weight of about 40 kDa (Neidhardt 1987a).

RNA represents about 20% of the dry weight of a bacterial cell but can vary depending upon growth conditions. About 90% of the RNA is the ribosomal RNA (rRNA) which consists of 3 species, the 23S rRNA, the 16S rRNA and the 5S rRNA. The transfer RNA (tRNA) represents about 9% of the total RNA with 60 types of tRNA and about 198 000 molecules per cell. The messenger RNA (mRNA) represents about 0.2–1% of the total RNA. There may be 1–4 molecules of DNA, depending upon the growth rate, representing about 3.3% of the dry weight (Neidhardt 1987a). Carbohydrate polymers can be present in the cell wall and may be stored in the cytoplasm as food materials such as glycogen. Lipid material can vary from 1 to 8% of the cell dry weight, depending upon growth conditions, and can be found in the cell membrane and wall or as reserve food material, often in the form of polyhydroxybutyric acid granules in the cytoplasm. For the synthesis of this storage material, 2 acetyl-CoAs are converted to acetoacetyl-CoA, this is changed to D-(-)-3-hydroxybutyryl-CoA which is polymerized to form polyhydroxybutyric acid (Steinbuchel and Schlegel 1991).

Capsules

Capsule or slime layers may exist as polymers outside the cell wall. They are usually made of amino acids, carbohydrates or both. As a rough rule, these extra-cellular polymers of bacteria in the genus *Bacillus* tend to be made of amino acids whereas the polymers of enteric bacteria tend to be made of carbohydrates. As examples, the polypeptide capsule of *Bacillus anthracis* is mostly D-glutamic acid whereas the *E. coli* K-12 capsule consists of D-glucose, L-fucose, galactose, hexuronic acid, acetate and pyruvate. Capsule polymers are rarely linked to one another by strong bonding forces although highly acetic types can be cross-linked by divergent metals such as Mg^{2+} or Ca^{2+}.

External appendages

The bacterial flagella move bacteria in directions favourable for survival and growth. Flagella function as rotating propellers and consist of a long helical filament composed of the protein flagellin, a short hook, and a basal structure of 2–5 rings mounted on a rod. The rotation of the flagella is driven by a transmembrane ion gradient that usually involves protons but in some cases may involve sodium ions. The concentration of chemicals in the external environment is detected in *E. coli* by the use of transmembrane chemoreceptors which use a series of intracellular protein phosphorylation reactions to 'signal' the flagella motors. Counterclockwise rotation of the flagella produces forward movement termed 'runs' whereas clockwise rotation causes cellular 'tumbling'. Stimuli that prolong runs are called attractants and stimuli that shorten the length of a swimming interval are called repellents. Changes in attractant or repellent levels cause changes in flagella rotation and result in movement in favourable directions. The cell may also possess external protein fibres known as pili or fimbriae composed of protein (pilin). Pili may be involved in bacterial conjugation or the adherence of the cells to surfaces. The pili of pathogenic bacteria may contain adhesions that allow the bacteria to attach to and colonize host tissues.

EUBACTERIAL CELL WALLS

Peptidoglycan material

The backbone structure of the eubacterial cell wall is the peptidoglycan material. The 'backbone' of the peptidoglycan is a polymer of the disaccharides N-acetylglucosamine and N-acetylmuramic acid, joined together by β-1,4 or 1,6 alternating units and about 12 carbohydrates long. The disaccharide chains are linked together by polypeptide chains, usually from 3 to 8 amino acids long and containing some D-amino acids such as D-alanine and D-glutamic acid. The polypeptide chain is attached by a peptide bond to the carboxyl group of the muramic acid. It normally contains one diamino acid, such as lysine or diaminopimelic acid, but not both, and a short peptide bridge joining the free amino group of the diamino acid to the terminal carboxyl group of a similar polypeptide branch from a different disaccharide strand. In such a manner the backbone disaccharide strands are joined

together. The cross-links in the peptidoglycan material form a 'web' capable of supporting stress in any direction. During synthesis of the peptidoglycan material, a disaccharide of N-acetylglucosamine and N-acetylmuramic acid is first formed and the amino acid bridges then are attached with an extra D-alanine on the end of the peptide chain. Teichoic acid and peptide bridge material may also be added to the unit. To build new wall material, this disaccharide–peptide unit is inserted into the existing cell wall in the space between the cytoplasmic membrane and the cell wall. A membrane-linked transpeptidase removes the final D-alanine unit, from one peptide chain or peptide bridge, and instals in its place the extra amino group on the diamino acid of another chain. The presence of D-amino acids in the cell wall is believed to give protection to external proteolytic enzymes. Enzymes that attack the bacteria cell wall are termed lysins and autolysins are lysins produced by the bacterium itself. Some lysins attack the peptidoglycan backbone whereas others attack the peptide portion or the point where the peptide chain joins the glycan strand. Lysozyme is a lysin that cleaves a the β-1,4 linkage of N-acetylglucosamine.

Gram-positive cell walls

Gram-positive cell walls may also contain some teichoic acid, which are polymers of glycerol or ribitol, usually about 10–50 units long, and linked together through phosphate bonds. Side groups on the teichoic acids can be carbohydrates such as glucose and N-acetylglucosamine, amino acids such as D-alanine, or a combination of carbohydrates and amino acids. Teichuronic acid, a polymer consisting of alternating glucuronic acid and N-acetylgalactosamine, is sometimes found in the cell walls, especially when phosphate is limiting. The lipoteichoic acids are polymers of glycerophosphate covalently linked to the cytoplasmic membrane.

Gram-negative cell walls

The gram-negative outer cell envelope, such as that of *E. coli*, consists of 3 layers. The inner layer is the cell cytoplasmic membrane, there is a middle layer containing peptidoglycan material, and a convoluted outer membrane consisting of protein and at least 2 types of lipids – lipopolysaccharides (LPS) and phospholipids. The peptidoglycan material only makes up about 12% of the total cell wall material in *E. coli* and the 4 amino acids usually found in the peptidoglycan material of gram-negative cells are L-alanine, D-glutamic acid, *meso*-diaminopimelic acid, and D-alanine. LPS consists of 3 parts: an inner hydrophobic lipid A, region; an outer hydrophilic O antigen polysaccharide region; and a core polysaccharide region that connects the 2 others. Included among the outer-membrane proteins of *E. coli* are murine lipoproteins, whose main function may be to stabilize the outer membrane–peptidoglycan complex, and porins, major outer-membrane proteins which form channels to allow the diffusion of hydrophilic molecules. Other proteins in the outer membrane are those involved in specific diffusion processes.

Between the outer and cytoplasmic membrane of gram-negative organisms is located the periplasmic space which contains many proteins, including transport binding proteins, scavenging enzymes, detoxifying enzymes and others. Periplasmic enzymes are synthesized in the cytoplasm and are constructed with a hydrophobic core region and a signal sequence peptide of from 20 to 40 amino acid residues long. The signal sequence affects the protein secretion through the cell membrane and, once transport is completed it is cleaved off (Oliver 1987). Many bacteria, including eubacteria and archaea, possess an outermost crystalline surface layer of regular closely packed protein subunits known as S layers that can be found in both eubacteria and archaea and may make up to 1% of the total cell protein.

Archaea cell walls

The third domain of life, the archaea, have distinctively different cell wall polymers from the eubacteria. They do not possess the peptidoglycan polymer but may posses a slightly different polymer termed pseudopeptidoglycan. In the species *Methanobacterium thermoautotrophicum*, this polymer contains *N*-acetyltalosaminuronic acid and only L-amino acids, such as L-lysine, L-alanine and L-glutamate. The cell wall of *Methanobrevibacter ruminantium* has L-threonine in place of L-alanine, and *N*-acetylglactosamine in place of *N*-acetylglucosamine. The cell walls in the genus *Methanosarcina* are made of an acid heteropolysaccharide which contains galactosamine, neutral sugars and uronic acids. No muramic acid, glucosamine, glutamic acid or other amino acids typical of peptidoglycan are found. A new pathway of peptide biosynthesis, consisting of 7 steps, has been found in some pseudopeptidoglycan-containing methanogens. In contrast, archaea in the genus *Methanospirillum* have 18 amino acids in the cell wall but no muramic acid, diaminopimelic acid or amino sugars have been found. For the archaea bacterium *Methanocorpusculum sinense*, the cell envelope consists of a cytoplasmic membrane and an S layer, composed of hexagonal arranged subunits. The crystalline surface S layers have been found to represent an almost universal feature of archaebacterial cell envelopes.

Cytoplasmic membrane

The cytoplasmic membrane contains about 30–40% lipid and 60–70% protein and makes up about 10% of the dry weight of the bacterial cell. The lipids include phospholipids that total about 75% of the total lipid of the membrane, as well as fatty acids and branched chain C-15 acids. At least 200 different kinds of protein representing about 6–9% of all the cellular proteins are located in the cytoplasmic membrane. Some of these proteins are cytochromes, dehydrogenases, NADH-oxidases, enzymes involved in cell wall synthesis, enzymes involved in electron transport and oxidative phosphorylation, and proteins involved in the transport of specific molecules through the membrane.

Enzymes and chemical pathways

A bacterial cell has the capability to synthesize over several thousand different enzymes to catalyse the many chemical reactions needed for cell growth. Catabolic pathways provide the cell with the energy for growth whereas anabolic reactions are the biosynthetic reactions whose purpose is the formation new cellular material. Although a bacterial cell may possess the ability to synthesize thousands of different enzymes, its regulatory systems are evolved to control the synthesis of such proteins and the exact type and quantity of enzyme may be carefully regulated.

Enzymes function as catalysts and rapidly cause the equilibrium of thermodynamically feasible, chemical reactions to be reached. Although an enzyme must participate in the reaction it catalyses, binding substrates and releasing products, it is normally regenerated and can be reused when the reaction is completed. The activity of many enzymes is associated with a relatively low molecular weight compound termed a coenzyme (or prosthetic group or cofactor). The catalytic site of the enzyme binds the substrate and the enzyme–substrate complex changes to an enzyme–product complex with the release of the product. The specificity of enzyme action results from the specific recognition of the substrate by the catalytic site. Many enzymes will act upon compounds related in chemical structure to the natural substrate but usually with lower binding affinities. Sometimes such compounds are converted to products and released but some can bind to the enzyme and block activity. Enzyme activity can also be destroyed or inhibited by a variety of chemicals or conditions, including those that alter the structure of proteins in a non-specific manner.

As increasing concentrations of a substrate are presented to an enzyme, the velocity of the enzyme-catalysed reaction will increase until, at substrate concentrations sufficient to saturate the available catalytic sites, the rate of reaction will be sustained at some maximum value (V_{max}). Thus, a plot of reaction rate (v) versus substrate concentration [S] frequently approximates to a rectangular hyperbola. An enzyme displaying these kinetic properties is said to demonstrate Michaelis–Menten kinetics and the reaction relation between the reaction rate and substrate concentration can be described by the maximum velocity (V_{max}) constant and the Michaelis constant (K_m), which is the substrate concentration that limits the rate of the enzyme-catalysed reaction to be one-half that of V_{max}. Studies of how V_{max} and K_m change under different chemical and physical conditions can provide information on the nature of the substrate–enzyme complex. Enzyme activity will usually be destroyed by treatments that denature proteins, such as treatment with heat or acids.

The regulatory mechanisms of bacterial metabolism are designed to permit a controlled synthesis of cellular polymers, usually as rapid as possible under the existing environmental conditions. Bacterial cells are not simply a 'bag of enzymes', as was once suggested. Indeed, there is careful organization of many proteins within the bacterial cell. Multienzyme complexes can be found within the cytoplasm and many enzymes and transport proteins are incorporated in the cell membrane or, in the case of gram-negative bacteria, within the periplasmic space. In addition to the substrate–product binding site, allosteric proteins possess a site, termed an effector, for binding a low molecular weight molecule. If the protein is an enzyme, the effector molecule may be quite different from the substrate molecule, but its binding to the enzyme results in a conformational change at the active site with a change in the affinity of the active site for the normal enzyme substrate. A positive effector will increase the binding capability of the enzyme for its substrate whereas a negative effector will decrease the binding capability. With normal intercellular substrate concentrations, a positive effector will increase the rate of reaction whereas a negative effector will decrease the rate of reaction. Proteins with nucleic acid binding sites can also have their binding ability increased or decreased by effector molecules.

1.2   Regulation of catabolic operons

THE OPERON HYPOTHESIS

In order to grow using the disaccharide lactose as a carbon and energy source, *E. coli* requires the presence of the enzyme β-galactosidase (once termed lactase) to cleave lactose into the monosaccharides, D-glucose and D-galactose. This enzyme is **inducible**, meaning that without the presence of lactose in the growth medium, there is only a very low basal or endogenous level of the enzyme in the cells. However, if lactose is added, then within minutes the differential rate of synthesis of the enzyme (the rate of enzyme synthesis as compared to the rate of total cell protein synthesis) increases until the amount of enzyme in the cells is 10 000 times higher than previously. If the lactose is removed from the medium, the rate of β-galactosidase synthesis decreases to the previous basal level as the concentration of enzyme in the cell is diluted by the synthesis of new proteins during cell growth. When cells are provided with lactose, several proteins are induced at the same time, a phenomenon known as **co-ordinate induction**. These proteins include β-galactosidase, lactose permease (the protein responsible for the transport of lactose through the cell membrane), and a protein catalysing the acetylation of certain disaccharides. **Gratuitous inducers**, which differ slightly in structure from the normal inducer and can not be metabolized by the cells, can still cause induction, showing that the chemical inducer does not always have to be the substrate of the pathway or even a compound that can be catabolized.

During studies on lactose catabolism by *E. coli*, mutants were obtained that changed the regulation of these 3 enzymes and permitted them to be produced at high levels in the absence of lactose. Such mutants were termed **constitutive mutants** and, since a single mutation affected the regulation synthesis of all 3 pro-

teins at once, the expression of the genes coding for those proteins had to be under the control of a common regulatory gene. Such enzymes are said to be **co-ordinately controlled**. The analysis of structural gene and regulatory gene mutations that affected lactose catabolism in *E. coli* led Jacob and Monod (1961) to postulate the operon hypothesis. The nucleotide sequence of the 3 genes coding for the enzymes was copied or **transcribed**, using ribonucleotides, into a single strand of RNA termed messenger RNA or mRNA. The mRNA carried the information of the sequence of amino acids in the proteins, from the DNA structural genes to the cell ribosomes where amino acid polymerization actually occurred. The region of the DNA transcribed into this single strand of mRNA was termed the operon.

Further studies provided evidence that the regulatory gene produced a product that normally blocked the formation of the enzymes involved in lactose catabolism. This product was termed the **repressor** and was later shown to be a protein. When the lactose operon was induced, an RNA polymerase would bind to the DNA at a site named the **promoter** region. Using the DNA as a template, this RNA polymerase would transcribe the DNA sequence of the 3 genes into mRNA, a process known as **transcription**. In the absence of the inducer, however, the repressor protein bound to a DNA site named the operator region and prevented transcription by the RNA polymerase. Thus, the regulation was a **negative control system** in that the normal function of the regulator gene was to prevent the formation of mRNA for the operon. Any mutation resulting in the loss of function of the repressor (the product of the *lacI* gene) would result in the loss of repression and the **constitutive** expression of the enzymes of the lactose operon (Jacob and Monod 1961).

The lactose operon of *E. coli*

The arangement of the genes of the lactose operon of *E. coli* is shown in Fig. 5.1. The order of the 3 **structural genes** of the *lac* operon is *lacZ*, *lacY* and *lacA*, encoding the sequence of amino acids for β-galactosidase, lactose permease and thiogalactoside transacetylase, respectively. The promoter (*lacP*) and operator

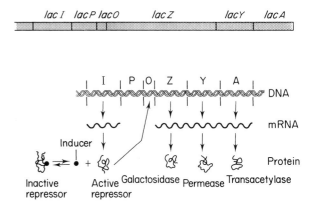

Fig. 5.1   The lactose operon of *E. coli*.

(*lacO*) regions are adjacent to the *lacZ* gene and actually overlap. The regulator gene (*lacI*) is situated next to the operon. When the operon is induced, RNA polymerase binds to the promoter region and transcribes the operon into mRNA by copying the order of nucleotides of the structural genes into ribonucleotides. This mRNA is then **translated** into proteins by the ribosomes of the cell. The regulator gene (*lacI*) is the structural gene for a protein that is termed the **lactose repressor**, an allosteric protein that is expressed constitutively and has a DNA binding site at the **operator** region of the operon. Even though the RNA polymerase can bind to the promoter, the DNA-bound repressor physically blocks transcription of the operon by the RNA polymerase. The repressor is an allosteric protein and it also possesses a second binding site for the inducer of the lactose operon. The inducer serves as a negative effector and when bound to the repressor it decreases the binding efficiency of the repressor to the DNA. With the removal of the repressor from the operator region, RNA polymerase can transcribe the operon into mRNA which can be translated into the proper proteins. The actual inducer molecule is not lactose but an isomer of lactose, allolactose, which is a disaccharide formed by a side reaction of β-galactosidase. Lactose is a D-glucose-D-galactose dimer with a β-1,4 linkage whereas allolactose differs from this in that it possesses a β-1,6 linkage.

The nature of inducers

The inducer of a catabolic enzyme pathway need not be the initial substrate of the pathway. It may be an intermediate of the pathway, an end product, or even a compound formed by a side reaction, as for the lactose operon of *E. coli* where allolactose in the inducer. If the inducer is produced by the action of the enzyme it induces, some small basal or endogenous level of the enzyme must always be present for the inducer to be quickly synthesized once the pathway substrate becomes available. For the lactose operon of *E. coli*, in addition to the normal promoter site for binding RNA polymerase, there is a second site that permits the synthesis of small levels of permease and β-galactosidase even in the absence of inducer. Enough of these proteins is present in uninduced cells to permit the rapid synthesis of allolactose when lactose becomes available.

The purpose of the thiogalactoside transacetylase, coded by the *lacA* gene, remained a mystery for a number of years. This enzyme is now believed to be associated with the lactose operon for purposes of detoxification. The enzyme possesses the ability to acetylate a variety of different disaccharides, but lactose is one of the poorest substrates. The lactose permease is able to transport a number of disaccharides other than lactose into the cell and if these disaccharides can not be further metabolized they accumulate and may be toxic for cell growth. Upon acetylation of these disaccharides by the thiogalactoside transacetylase, they are rapidly excreted by the cells and not transported back into the organism.

The lactose operon of *Staphylococcus aureus*

Staphylococcus aureus possesses a different pathway of catabolism for lactose, using enzyme II^{Lac} and enzyme III^{Lac} of the phosphoenolpyruvate phosphotransferase (PTS) system to transport lactose through the cell membrane (see section 2.2, p. 97). During transport, lactose is phosphorylated to phospholactose which is cleaved by a phosphogalactosidase enzyme to form D-glucose and D-galactose-6-phosphate. The genes coding for these 3 enzymes are designated *lacF*, *lacE* and *lacG*, respectively, and are located on a common operon which appears to be under the negative control of a repressor gene (*lacR*). Galactose-6-phosphate is the inducer of the galactose operon and is also the inducer of the enzymes for the further degradation of galactose-6-phosphate.

The L-arabinose operon of *E. coli*

While studying the catabolism of the pentose L-arabinose by *E. coli* strain B/r, Englesberg and his co-workers found differences from the regulation of the lactose operon (Sheppard and Englesberg 1967). After the transport of L-arabinose into the cells it is isomerized by the enzyme L-arabinose isomerase to the 2-ketopentose, L-ribulose. The enzyme L-ribulokinase phosphorylates L-ribulose to form L-ribulose-5-phosphate which is epimerized to D-xylulose-5-phosphate by L-ribulose-5-phosphate 4-epimerase. The latter compound is further degraded by other cellular enzyme systems. These 3 enzymes are all co-ordinately induced when L-arabinose is present and the genes encoding for the 3 enzymes are termed *araA*, *araB* and *araD*, respectively. These genes are located on a common operon with a regulatory gene, *araC*, located next to the operon. However, deletions of the *araC* gene do not lead to constitutive expression of the enzymes. By contrast, deletion of the *araC* gene results in mutants in which the L-arabinose catabolic enzymes can never be induced. Since the function of the regulator gene is essential for gene expression, this is termed a **positive control** system.

The repressor protein, encoded by the *araC* gene, can bind to 4 different operator regions, O_1, O_2, I_1 and I_2, all connected to the L-arabinose operon. When it binds to both the O_2 and I_1 sites, a loop is formed in the DNA, preventing transcription of the operon. When the inducer, L-arabinose, binds to the allosteric repressor protein, the protein's DNA binding affinity changes and it now binds to operator sites O_1 and O_2, permitting transcription of the operon into mRNA. Since the repressor–inducer complex is required for transcription of the operon, mutants unable to synthesize the repressor protein are unable to utilize L-arabinose as a growth substrate.

AUTOINDUCTION

Certain genes are only expressed when the concentration of bacterial cells reaches a critical level. This process is called **autoinduction.** The bacteria release a compound (the autoinducer) into the surrounding environment and the external concentration of autoinducer increases as the cell population increases.

When the concentration of autoinducer surrounding the cells reaches the proper level, it signals for genes to be expressed. The autoinduction of gene expression was first found in *Vibro fischeri*, when light production in this photobacterium was found to be dependent upon cell concentration. However, autoinduction has now been described in a variety of other gram-negative bacteria. Regulatory systems that are autoinducible have been termed 'quorum-sensing' systems (Gray et al. 1995).

1.3 Regulation of biosynthetic operons

END PRODUCT OR FEEDBACK REPRESSION

The synthesis of the enzymes involved in biosynthetic or anabolic pathways is controlled to prevent their synthesis when the end product of the pathway is present in the cells in sufficient concentration to meet biosynthetic needs. In the case of a biosynthetic operon, the normal product of the regulator gene is usually an inactive repressor. When it combines with the proper effector molecule its binding affinity for the operator region of the operon increases, resulting in repression of transcription of the operon. This process is referred to as **enzyme repression** or **feedback repression**. The effector is usually the product of the biochemical pathway or a metabolite derived from the product of the pathway. Thus, the concentration of the internal pool of the end product of a biosynthetic pathway will control the rate of synthesis of the biosynthetic enzymes leading to the end product. For example, if *E. coli* is growing on a minimal salts medium, and an amino acid is added to the medium, the rate of synthesis of the enzymes specifically involved in synthesis of that amino acid may be repressed to a few per cent of the fully expressed level. On some branched biosynthetic pathways, such as those leading to the synthesis of L-leucine, L-valine and L-isoleucine in *E. coli*, there is no repression of synthesis of the common enzymes until each of the end products is present in excess concentrations. This type of feedback repression, requiring more than one effector, has been termed **multivalent repression**.

REGULATION BY ATTENUATION

Another means of regulating the expression of biosynthetic pathways is by attenuation. An operon, such as the tryptophan operon which encodes genes for the biosynthesis of L-tryptophan, may be regulated by both feedback repression and attenuation. In *E. coli*, the gene encoding for the repressor of the operon is some distance from the operon. Between the location where transcription of the operon actually begins and the beginning of the first structural gene of the operon, there is an attenuator site or termination site. If internal L-tryptophan levels are high, then the level of tRNA charged with L-tryptophan will also be high and 9 out of every 10 transcriptions forming mRNA will be stopped at this site. Regions of the RNA synthesized at this site base pair with each other, loops are formed and transcription is terminated. This termination is controlled by interactions between the RNA transcript, ribosomes translating the short leader transcript, tRNA and other termination factors. In cells starved for tryptophan this termination site does not stop mRNA formation.

A different type of attenuation control for the tryptophan operon has been reported in *Bacillus subtilis* where there is a leader sequence of 204 nucleotides prior to the structural genes of the operon. There is also a *trp* RNA-binding attenuation protein and in the absence of L-tryptophan the operon is expressed but in the presence of L-tryptophan, this attenuator protein is activated and binds to the leader sequence, blocking transcription of the operon (Antson et al. 1995).

Reports of bacterial operons regulated by transcriptional attenuation mechanisms have been increasing. The *ilv* and *leu* genes in enteric bacteria are regulated mostly by a translational-dependent attenuation but the *ilv-leu* operon of *B. subtilis* is reported to be regulated, at least in part, by transcriptional attenuation (Lu, Turner and Switzer 1995). Regulation by attenuation has also been reported for the *E. coli* threonine and histidine operons. The *B. subtilis* operon encoding enzymes responsible for pyrimidine nucleotide biosynthesis may possess 3 tandem attenuators.

1.4 Global control networks

INTRODUCTION

If more than one operon is under the control of a regulatory factor, those operons are said to constitute a **regulon**. The word **modulon** has been used to describe units of operons and regulons under the control of a regulatory protein and the term **alarmone** has been used to describe a chemical regulator compound which is produced by the cell under conditions of sudden stress. A number of **global** regulatory systems exist to control the expression of many different catabolic operons. By having such master control systems, cells can quickly respond to sudden changes in the environment by increasing or decreasing the rate of synthesis of entire systems of proteins.

Since the synthesis of cellular RNA requires a DNA-dependent RNA polymerase, to transcribe the nucleotide sequence of the DNA into a polymer of ribonucleotides, regulation of transcription of operons can result not only from the effects of DNA binding proteins, such as repressors and activators, and attenuation sequences, but also from changes in the binding efficiency of RNA polymerase to various promoter regions.

The concept of catabolite repression

It is not uncommon for an organism to utilize preferentially those catabolites most common in its natural environment. Therefore, a bacterium, given 2 possible carbon and energy sources simultaneously, may not use them at the same time but may use one before beginning catabolism of the other. An example is the 'glucose effect' first reported in 1942 by Gale and Epps. They found the synthesis of certain enzymes by *E. coli* was inhibited by the presence of D-glucose in the medium. In 1947, Monod reported that the presence of glucose prevented the induction of many other sugar catabolic pathways in *E. coli*, especially those sugars catabolized by inducible pathways. If 2 carbohydrates, such as glucose and lactose, were both present in the growth medium, the growth curve showed 2 successive growth cycles separated by a lag period (Monod 1947). This was termed a diauxic growth curve and it is possible to classify carbohydrates as to whether or not a diauxic growth curve results when they are incubated with glucose.

In 1961, the word 'catabolite repression' was used to describe this type of repression of enzyme pathways. It was later shown that catabolite repression by glucose of the synthesis of β-galactosidase involves a block in the synthesis of mRNA for the enzyme. Mutants with a *lacI* deletion and, therefore, constitutive for β-galactosidase production, are still subject to catabolite repression by glucose (Magasanik 1961). When a culture of *E. coli* is induced for the lactose operon by a gratuitous inducer, one that does not require the lactose transport system, the addition of glucose produces 2 effects. The first is a severe but transient repression of β-galactosidase synthesis, lasting about 0.5 h or half a generation. The second is a less severe but permanent repression of synthesis of the enzyme.

The role of cyclic AMP (cAMP)

In enteric bacteria, the rate of transcription of genes that are subject to regulation by catabolite repression was found to be controlled by the intracellular concentration of a nucleotide, cyclic adenosine 5′-monophosphate (**cAMP**). The internal level of cAMP in *E. coli* is very low in cultures grown on glucose and addition of cAMP to the medium results in partially overcoming the glucose catabolite. Mutants deficient in adenylate cyclase, the enzyme responsible for the synthesis of cAMP from ATP, can synthesize β-galactosidase only when cAMP is added to the medium (Pastan and Adhya 1976).

The catabolite gene activator protein

Mutants were obtained that could not make β-galactosidase or similar catabolite-repressible enzymes, even when cAMP was added to the medium. These mutants were found to be deficient in the synthesis of a protein named the **catabolite gene activator protein** (**CAP**) and sometimes the cAMP receptor protein (CRP). This protein was found to be a dimer having 2 identical subunits, each capable of binding one molecule of cAMP. The cAMP–CAP complex binds to DNA at the operator-distal part of the promoter region of the lactose operon and increases RNA polymerase binding efficiency. Thus, the rate of transcription of the operon is dependent upon the presence of both the CAP protein and the intracellular level of cAMP. In the presence of glucose the internal concentration of cAMP is low and the transcription of those operons requiring the cAMP–CAP complex is repressed.

The enzyme **adenylate cyclase** converts ATP to cAMP and the intracellular level of cAMP appears to be at least partially regulated in growing cells by the rate of activity of this enzyme. Under conditions of catabolite repression, adenylate cyclase activity is inhibited and the cellular level of cAMP decreases and, as a result, the activity of the cAMP–CAP-dependent promoters also decreases. It has been proposed that activation of transcription occurs through direct contact between cAMP–CAP and RNA polymerase. The CAP protein is a global regulator of gene expression and has been found to activate transcription at more than 50 promoters. The cAMP–CAP complex has different affinity for promoters so the response of separate operons may differ at any concentration of cAMP. The genes controlled by CAP are sometimes referred to as members of the carbon–energy regulon.

The activity of adenylate cyclase appears to be regulated by interactions with components of the cytoplasmic membrane transport system. In the presence of carbohydrates being brought through the membrane by the PTS, adenylate cyclase is almost inactive and the level of cAMP in the cells is very low.

Inducer exclusion is a separate regulatory process where the transportation of sugars into the cells by the PTS mechanism selectively inhibits other types of transport systems. Even in cells constitutive for a transport system, the phenomenon of inducer exclusion can still inhibit that activity of that transport system and that inhibition is not overcome by addition of cAMP. It has been shown that unphosphorylated III^{glu} directly acts upon transport systems to inhibit their activity.

Other mechanisms of catabolite repression

Catabolite repression also exists in strict aerobes such as those in the genus *Pseudomonas*. However, several studies have shown that in *Pseudomonas aeruginosa* and *Pseudomonas putida*, cAMP is not involved with catabolite repression. Since these bacteria receive most of their energy by oxidative phosphorylation with electrons obtained from the oxidation of acetate by the tricarboxylic acid (TCA) cycle, it is catabolites such as acetate and TCA cycle intermediates that cause repression of other catabolic pathways including those for glucose (MacGregor et al. 1991).

Catabolite repression in gram-positive bacteria may be controlled by a number of different mechanisms. No cAMP has been detected in *B. subtilis* under aerobic conditions (the addition of cAMP does not affect catabolite repression in that organism) and no CAP-like protein has been identified in any gram-positive bacteria. *Cis*-acting sequences named catabolite-responsive elements or CRE seem to be responsible for catabolite repression in *B. subtilis* and these CREs also have been found to function in *Bacillus megaterium* and *Staphylococcus xylosus*. A catabolite control protein (CcpA) has been identified and mutations in this gene have been found to prevent CRE-dependent catabolite repression in both *B. subtilis* and *B. megaterium*. However, the exact mechanism of action of CcpA is still not understood.

In addition to the CRE–CcpA regulation of *B. sub-*

tilis, catabolite repression in this organism is also linked to the PTS system, but in a different manner than in gram-negative bacteria. During the normal function of the PTS system, the HPr protein is phosphorylated at His-15. However, in a reaction that might be unique to gram-positive bacteria, the HPr protein is phosphorylated at seryl residue 46 by an ATP-dependent kinase, a reaction that is required for catabolite repression (Deutscher et al. 1994). HPr(Ser-P) also regulates non-PTS transporters in *Lactobacillus brevis* and a sugar-phosphate phosphatase in *Lactococcus lactis* by direct interactions between HPr(Ser-P) and the enzymes (Hueck and Hillen 1995).

σ FACTORS

RNA polymerases

Bacterial RNA polymerases consists of at least 4 polypeptides termed a, b, b′ and σ. The core RNA polymerase consists of the various a and b subunits and this core unit will bind randomly to DNA. If the σ subunit is also present, the enzyme is termed a holoenzyme and the presence of the subunit directs the holoenzyme to bind at specific promoter regions and transcribe specific operons. By changing σ factors, the cell can initiate the transcription of different regulons, thereby synthesizing new families of enzymes in response to changing environmental conditions. The RNA polymerase holoenzymes have been designated as E-σ^x, with E representing the core polymerase and σ^x the particular σ factor attached. After the first few nucleotides have been placed into the new RNA polymer, the σ factor is released and the core enzyme continues the polymerization of the ribonucleotides.

Alternative σ factors in *E. coli*

Lonetto, Gribskov and Gross (1992) studied the amino acid sequence of bacterial σ factors and classified them into 3 broad groups. Group 1 proteins are the **primary σ factors.** Primary σ factors from different organisms are very similar and the regions involved in promoter recognition are especially highly conserved. These primary σ factors are required for the survival of bacterial cells and are responsible for most RNA synthesis in exponentially growing cells. The primary σ factor in *E. coli* is σ^{70} which is responsible for transcription of most of the genes expressed during exponential growth. A second group of σ factors are very similar to group 1 but are not essential for cell growth. The third group consists of the **alternative σ factors** that are responsible for the transcription of specific regulons. Apparently these σ factors all compete for RNA polymerase.

The ability of the cell to produce a variety of alternative σ factors with different promoter specificity permits 'global' regulatory systems and control of the activation of large numbers of different regulons. Bacteria have evolved mechanisms that permit them to resist a variety of different environmental stresses, such as heat or cold shock, acid pH, lack of oxygen, and starvation. Bacterial response to stress is to change the expression of groups of genes known under the general term of 'stress genes'. Alternative σ factors direct

sets of genes whose products are needed for specific functions and the proteins encoded by these genes give the cells some protection from damaging conditions. Although σ factors were once identified by a number that corresponded to their apparent mass, some of the initial mass determinations were found to be in error and the tendency now is to replace the numbers with letters.

The response of micro-organisms to elevated temperatures has been termed **heat shock response**. Heat shock response is a rapid, transient increase in the rate of synthesis of certain proteins (heat shock proteins or HSPs) within seconds of a shift of the culture to higher temperatures. If the growth temperature of *E. coli* is shifted up, for example from 37°C to 46°C, the rate of synthesis of proteins concerned with transcription and translation is decreased. However, the synthesis of heat shock proteins is increased, some as much as 100-fold. If the growth temperature is returned to normal, the rate of synthesis of these proteins returns to normal. Heat shock seems to provide the cells with some resistance to lethal high temperatures such as 55°C and *E. coli* cells heat shocked at 42°C have a slower death rate at 55°C than cells that had not been previously exposed to the 42°C temperature (Moat and Foster 1995).

Heat shock-induced transcription in *E. coli* is associated with the heat shock-specific σ factor, σ^{32}. The heat shock regulon consists of over 20 genes and at least 13 promoters are known to be specifically transcribed by the holoenzyme containing σ^{32} ($E\sigma^{32}$). The actual amount of gene transcription depends upon the cellular concentration of σ^{32} and, under heat shock conditions, σ^{32} levels increase by enhanced synthesis, elevated stability and increased activity of the σ factor. During normal growth conditions, the σ^{32} polypeptide is very unstable in vivo with a half-life of about 1 min and mutants lacking σ^{32} are deficient or lacking in most HSPs. When the temperature is shifted from 30 to 42°C, the polypeptide rapidly becomes stabilized and has an 8-fold longer half-life (Mager and De Kruijff 1995). The gene encoding another σ factor, σ^E, also appears to be essential for growth of *E. coli* at temperatures above 43.5°C. The functions of most of these HSPs are to bind to cytoplasmic proteins and protect them from stress. Many proteins require aid in obtaining their tertiary structures and proteins that give this assistance but are not components of the final product are termed **chaperones**. Chaperones are normally constitutive proteins that increase in amount following stress such as heat shock. For *E. coli*, HSPs are known to regulate interactions between other proteins, regulate HSP synthesis and aid in moving some proteins across the cytoplasmic membrane.

The heat shock response is also initiated by placing the cells under a variety of other stresses such as exposure to H_2O_2, UV radiation, some heavy metals (i.e. Cd^{2+}), canaverine, puromycin, extremes of pH, nalidixic acid and ethanol. One explanation for a common response is that the heat shock response may be triggered by the accumulation of denatured or damaged proteins. The heat shock response has been observed in thermophilic, mesophilic and psychrophilic eubacteria and in the archaea (Neidhardt and VanBogelen 1987). Similarities are found between HSPs from different organisms. *E. coli* is known to be able to synthesize 17 proteins in response to heat shock whereas *B. subtilis* has been reported to synthesize 66. The heat shock response in *P. aeruginosa* is similar in many ways to that of *E. coli.* and 17 HSPs have been observed, 5 of them major proteins.

If the temperature is dropped to 10°C, many bacterial cells synthesize a group of proteins known as **cold shock proteins**. In *E. coli*, a sudden drop in the growth temperature results in a growth lag of several hours while the cells adapt to the new temperature. Although at least 14 cold shock proteins are synthesized during this lag period, overall protein synthesis is decreased. At least some of these cold shock proteins are involved in restoring the cell's ability to transcribe DNA and translate the information into polypeptides.

If a culture of *E. coli* is subjected to conditions that either damage the DNA or block DNA replication, the result is the **SOS response**, an increased expression of genes for DNA repair. Activation of the SOS regulatory network stops cell division while many genes involved in DNA repair are activated. More than 17 different types of protein are induced and many of them give protection to cells with damaged DNA, such as the repair of breaks in double stranded DNA (Walker 1987).

The starvation of bacteria can result in increased resistance to a variety of different stresses. This **starvation effect** also depends upon alternative σ factors and involves the expression of starvation genes that code for special resistance factors. This starvation-induced resistance depends upon expression of the regulons controlled by the alternative σ factors, σ^{32} and, a major regulator of the general starvation response in *E. coli*, σ^{38} (σ^{s}). Starvation causes a general response with the synthesis of 30–50 proteins. If cells of *E. coli* in the stationary growth phase are starved for glucose they also gain an increased resistance to heat, to oxidizing agents such as hydrogen peroxide and to sodium chloride. The 'starvation proteins' of *E. coli* are also induced by exposure to heat shock or oxidative stresses.

Alternative σ factors in *B. subtilis*

The *B. subtilis* σ factor termed σ^{A} (formally σ^{55}) is a primary σ factor present in vegetatively growing cells (Haldenwang 1995) whereas the secondary σ factor σ^{B} (σ^{37}) controls general stress response. It is normally present inactivated in a complex but is released from the complex when *B. subtilis* is subjected to different environmental stresses, such as heat, salt, ethanol or peroxide, or if cells reach stationary phase in a medium that will not permit sporulation. Another known σ factor not essential for sporulation is σ^{D}, which controls the chemotaxis-motility regulon. The major cold shock protein from *B. subtilis* is a single stranded DNA binding protein with about 67 amino acid residues. This protein possesses sequence identity

(about 60%) with the major cold shock proteins from other bacteria, including *E. coli* (Makhatadze and Marahiel 1994). About 53 polypeptides are induced in *B. subtilis* in response to cold shock, some of these proteins unique in that they are only synthesized in response to cold shock.

Under conditions of starvation, *B. subtilis* begins the differentiation process that results in the formation of an endospore. After the initiation of sporulation, there is an asymmetrical cell division forming 2 cells of different sizes. In the smaller or prespore cell, σ factor σ^{F} is activated whereas in the larger cell, a different σ factor, σ^{E}, is activated. This secondary σ factor is not required for growth but is required for the sporulation of *B. subtilis* (Haldenwang 1995). It has been suggested that σ^{F} is activated first, it somehow activates σ^{E}, and then σ factors σ^{F}, σ^{G} and σ^{K} are activated.

TWO-COMPONENT SIGNAL TRANSDUCTION SYSTEMS

External environmental changes are often detected by bacteria using a 2-component transduction system, a system involving 2 sets of proteins. Despite the name, different systems may have more than 2 components and may be very complicated (Bourret, Borkovich and Simon 1991). The first protein to detect the external signal is usually a transmembrane phosphorylating protein which transmits the signal by means of its cytoplasmic domain to a cytoplasmic component that can be termed the regulator protein. The mechanism of action of this system appears to be similar in different bacteria and often involves the transfer of a phosphate group to a cytoplasmic regulator protein, altering the regulator's activity. A phosphatase may later remove the phosphate, restoring the system to its original state.

1.5 Altering the catalytic activity of existing enzymes

FEEDBACK INHIBITION

The regulatory processes described previously affect the rate of synthesis of enzymes. The process named **feedback inhibition** acts to halt the activity of previously synthesized enzymatic pathways. The mechanism of feedback inhibition usually functions by the end product of a pathway inhibiting the activity of the first enzyme in the pathway that is specific for the synthesis of that particular end product. The enzyme will be allosteric with separate binding sites for substrate and effector molecules. The product of the pathway acts as a negative effector and, when bound to the enzyme, decreases the affinity of the enzyme for its substrate. To stop the entire pathway from functioning it is only necessary to inhibit the activity of the first enzyme in the pathway specific for the end product. With the inhibition of that enzyme, the latter enzymes in the pathway will have no substrates and production of the end product must cease.

Feedback inhibition in branching biosynthetic pathways

In many biosynthetic pathways a single reaction might produce a product whose further metabolism leads to the synthesis of 2 or more different end products. Four types of mechanism have been described that can regulate such a key reaction by feedback inhibition. With **cumulative inhibition** the end product of each pathway will not only feedback inhibit the first enzyme specific for the formation of that particular end product, but will also partially inhibit the activity of the shared enzyme. The accumulation in the cell of both end products will have a cumulative effect, resulting in additive inhibition of the shared enzyme activity. **Concerted inhibition** differs from cumulative in that neither end product alone will affect the activity of the enzyme. The presence of both end products, however, results in inhibition of the enzyme activity. Thus, when both end products accumulate, and only when both end products are present, the enzyme activity is inhibited.

If 2 or more pathways use the same initial substrate produced by a shared enzyme, and the pathways are subjected to feedback inhibition, the common substrate will accumulate. If that substrate causes feedback inhibition of the enzyme producing it, then feedback inhibition of the pathways will result in feedback inhibition of the common enzyme. This is termed **sequential inhibition**.

An alternative but very common method for a bacterium to regulate the activity of an enzymatic reaction shared by several pathways is for the organism to possess different enzymes to catalyse the same reaction. These isozymes (or isofunctional enzymes) are encoded by different genes and, therefore, can be both repressed and inhibited separately. Regulation by means of isozymes permits each structural gene coding for an isozyme to be part of a different regulon controlled for a separate end product. The possible disadvantage of the organism having to possess genes to code for 2 different enzymes catalysing similar reactions may be offset by the efficiency of regulation.

Enzyme inhibition and activation in catabolic pathways

The regulation of the activity of allosteric enzymes by effectors also functions in catabolic pathways. The effectors may be negative, inhibiting enzyme activity, or positive, activating enzyme activity. An example is the regulation of the activity of lactic dehydrogenase in homolactic acid bacteria (see section 3.2, p. 102). In these bacteria, the reduction of pyruvate to lactate by lactic dehydrogenase permits the rapid oxidation of NADH that has been reduced by the hexose diphosphate (HDP) pathway. If the rate of NADH oxidation is insufficient to maintain a pool of NAD^+, there will be an increase in the internal pool of fructose-1,6-diphosphate. Lactic dehydrogenase from these organisms is an allosteric enzyme that has an absolute requirement for fructose-1,6-diphosphate as a positive effector. The increase in the internal pool of this diphosphate results in the activation of more lactic dehydrogenase enzymes and an increase in the rate of NADH oxidation.

1.6   Biosynthetic of DNA, RNA and protein molecules

The bacterial chromosome and DNA replication

The DNA of the chromosome in a typical bacterial cell is compacted into a strand about 1000 times as long as the cell itself. If the chromosome is over-wound or under-wound, the DNA can twist upon itself, forming supercoils. The unwinding of DNA is caused by topoisomerase type I which breaks phosphodiester bonds in the double stranded DNA (Krawiec and Riley 1990).

The initiation of chromosomal replication occurs at fairly constant intervals since a certain cell mass must accumulate before initiation of replication will begin. Replication of the chromosome proceeds bidirectionally from the *oriC* locus (83.5 min on the *E. coli* map). The *dnaA* gene encodes for a DNA binding protein (DnaA) that binds to specific 9 bp sequences in the *oriC* region and is active in initiating replication. The 3 DNA polymerases of *E. coli* synthesize DNA in the 5′–3′ direction using a 3′-hydroxyl primer. Since these polymerases need a primer to begin DNA polymerization on a single stranded template, a polymerase is needed first to form an RNA primer. After these primers have been used for the elongation of the DNA by DNA polymerase, they are replaced by DNA. In the 3′–5′ prime direction, RNA primers are formed and, after the formation of 1000–2000 long DNA strands termed 'Okazaki' fragments, destroyed. The nicks in the DNA are repaired by DNA ligase (Bremer and Churchward 1991).

The DNA-directed DNA polymerases have been classified on the basis of their amino acid sequences into 4 major groups or families, DNA polymerase I, DNA polymerase II, DNA polymerase III and a family X representing other DNA polymerases.

Some strains of bacteria have been reported to have more than one chromosome. A strain of *Rhodobacter sphaeroides* (strain 2.4.1) has been reported to contain 2 circular chromosomes as well as 5 plasmids. This strain was found to be more resistant to ultraviolet radiation than *E. coli* and it has been speculated that the reason for the evolution of 2 chromosomes was to provide this photosynthetic organism with this increased resistance (Mackenzie et al. 1995).

Protein synthesis

Whereas the DNA contains the information for the structure of the various proteins of the cell, the RNA is the machinery that translates that information into the polypeptide chains. The genetic code is triplet, meaning that 3 nucleotides determine the code 'word' for each amino acid. Since there are 4 nucleotide 'letters' (A, T, G and C in the DNA alphabet and A, U, G and C in the RNA alphabet) it is possible to have 64 different 'words' or codons for the 20 amino acids normally found in proteins. The genetic code is degenerate, in that there may be more than one codon for any one amino acid but no nucleotide triplet will code for more than one amino acid. For example, there are 4 mRNA codons for serine: UCU, UCC, UCA and UCG. It has been speculated that the code was once a doublet rather than a triplet and, therefore, the original doublet code for serine might have been UC. Three codons called nonsense codons usually do not code for any amino acid and signal when to end synthesis of a polypeptide chain.

Amino acids are activated before being added to a polypeptide chain by being placed on specific transfer RNA molecules (tRNA). An enzyme specific for each amino acid (aminoacyl tRNA synthetase) transfers the amino acid to the tRNA specific for the transfer of that amino acid. These tRNA molecules are about 80 nucleotides in length and each has a site recognized by its tRNA synthetase. The amino acid is activated with the use of ATP, resulting in the formation of an aminoacyl–AMP complex. This complex is transferred to the tRNA molecule and the tRNA molecule is said to be 'charged'. In such a manner, each tRNA can become 'charged' at its amino acid attachment sites with the proper amino acid. The tRNA also possesses a ribosomal recognition site as well as a codon recognition site that will recognize the mRNA codon for that amino acid.

Polymerization of the amino acids takes place with the aid of the ribosome. A ribosome consists of 2 subunits, designated 30S and 50S, which combine to form the 70S ribosome. The complete ribosome is made of 3 different ribosomal rRNAs and 52 different proteins (r-proteins). The smaller 30S subunit contains 21 proteins and a 16S rRNA; the larger subunit has 21 proteins and 2 species of rRNA, 23S and 5S. Eubacteria, eukaryotes, most archaebacteria and the sulphur-dependent archaebacteria have differences in their ribosomal structures.

The rRNA is cotranscribed from the DNA as single 30S precursors that are then broken into the 3 components. *E. coli* K-12, as an example, has 7 rRNA operons. The ribosomal protein (r-protein) L7/L12 is present in 4 copies per ribosome, whereas other ribosomal proteins are present in one copy per ribosome. The genes responsible for the synthesis of the 52 r-proteins are organized into at least 20 translational units (operons) containing 1–11 r-protein genes. At least 6 of the tRNA species are cotranscribed with rRNA species. The rates of synthesis of the 52 ribosomal proteins of *E. coli* and the 3 rRNA components are balanced so there is normally very little excess ribosomal protein (r-protein) or rRNA in the cells. The translation of ribosomal proteins from an operon can be inhibited by the proteins coded in that operon. These proteins normally bind to rRNAs but if their concentration is higher than required they will bind to their own mRNA, blocking translation. In addition, if sufficient r-proteins are not present, rRNA will combine with other proteins but the complex formed will not function as ribosome (Nomura, Gourse and Baughman 1984).

The mRNA represents only 2–3% of the total cellular RNA and its synthesis is controlled at the operon level. In translation of the mRNA into protein, a complex is formed between the 30S ribosomal subunit and certain protein initiation factors. The mRNA binds to the 30S subunit as does the first charged tRNA, the 'initiator' tRNA. The eubacterial initiator tRNA is *N*-formylmethionyl-tRNA, which binds to a site termed the P site. The initiator tRNA appears to be methionine-tRNA for the archaebacteria. The ribosome also contains a binding site for the other charged tRNAs (the A site) and the codons found in the mRNA determine the order of alignment of the charged tRNAs. Once the charged tRNA binds at the A site, a peptide bond is formed between its amino group and the amino acid on the tRNA at the P site. The polypeptide chain is attached to the tRNA at the A site and the now uncharged tRNA at the P site is released. The tRNA at the A site and its polypeptide chain move to the P site (translocation) as the ribosome moves to the next codon on the mRNA. The charged tRNA with the proper anticodon binds to the A site and the process of polypeptide chain elongation continues. The termination codons (UAA, UGA and UAG) are not charged with any amino acid. When such codons appear on the mRNA, the polypeptide chain is released from the P site. Either the formyl group is removed from the first amino acid or the entire formylmethionine is removed.

Chaperones

The completed polypeptide chain must fold into a proper 3-dimensional structure. Since many proteins require aid in obtaining their tertiary structures, this folding may be assisted by special proteins known as 'chaperones'. Chaperones may also be used in the secretion of proteins into or through the cell membrane and in aiding the cells to recover from environmental stresses, such as high temperature. Molecular chaperones have been defined as 'a family of unrelated classes of protein that mediate the correct assembly of other polypeptides, but are not themselves components of the final structures' (Ellis 1991). The word 'chaperonin' describes one class of chaperones that have related sequences and are found in all bacteria that have been examined.

Protein trafficking

Some proteins that are synthesized in the cytoplasm must find their way through the cytoplasmic membrane to the outer membrane or periplasm of the cell. Most of these proteins are synthesized in a precursor form with a signal sequence of 15–30 amino acids at the N-terminus. This signal sequence aids the binding of the polypeptide chain to the membrane or gives it a conformation that facilitates transport through the membrane. During or after the peptide is translocated across or into the membrane of the cell, the signal peptide is cleaved off by a membrane protease termed the signal peptidase.

THE REGULATION OF SYNTHESIS OF MACROMOLECULES

The regulation of protein synthesis

In order for a protein to be synthesized, the cell must possess the mRNA encoded for that protein, all the amino acids needed for the structure of the protein, the respective tRNAs must be charged with those amino acids, and the cell ribosomes must be present and functioning. For bacteria growing at fairly rapid rates, with doubling times of 90 min or less, the rate of protein synthesis is controlled by the amount of RNA present. Since ribosomes usually function at a relatively constant rate and they make up most of the cell's RNA, for a shift up or down in the rate of protein synthesis and the growth rate of the cells there must be an increase or decrease in the rate of RNA synthesis.

The regulation of RNA synthesis

Early experiments found that if bacteria were lacking in just one amino acid needed to make protein, then not only protein synthesis stopped but the synthesis of most of the cellular RNA also stopped. Thus the lack of only one amino acid exerted a **stringent control** on RNA synthesis and resulted in a decrease in the rate of synthesis of not only rRNA and tRNA, but also the ribosomal proteins. The lack of a single amino acid required for protein synthesis also resulted in a reduction in the rate of biosynthesis of nucleotides and lipids as well as the inhibition of the biosynthesis of a wide variety of intermediate metabolites and the transport of many molecules into the cell.

A lack of any charged species of tRNA was found to result in the stringent response. Mutants, termed **relaxed** mutants, could be isolated where RNA synthesis was released from this dependency on the availability of all amino acids. The mutation mapped in a gene called the *relA* gene and the gene product (the stringent factor) was found to be a protein. In 1969, 2 spots were found on a chromatogram of extracts from cells undergoing the stringent response, spots that were not present in extracts from relaxed mutants. These were named 'magic spots' and were identified as guanosine 5′-diphosphate 3′-diphosphate, (ppGpp) and guanosine 5′-triphosphate 3′-diphosphate (pppGpp). It is ppGpp that causes the stringent response and the accumulation of ppGpp has been shown to occur in many bacteria when amino acid limitation occurs. The stringent factor protein (RelA) is a ribosome-bound phosphotransferase (ppGpp synthetase I). When a ribosome containing the stringent factor protein binds to an mRNA and an uncharged tRNA, then guanosine 5′-triphosphate 3′-diphosphate (pppGpp) is synthesized from guanine triphosphate (GTP). The pppGpp is converted to ppGpp which is directly responsible for the stringent effect. There is an alternative route for ppGpp synthesis involving a ppGpp synthetase II.

The ppGpp may initiate the stringent response in a variety of ways. The attachment of ppGpp to RNA polymerase may decrease the ability of the polymerase to bind to certain promoter regions and lower the rate of synthesis of tRNA, rRNA and r-proteins (Pao, Chia and Dyess 1981). It may inhibit translation by blocking the binding of the initiator tRNA complex to the ribosome. Using plasmids, Herman and Wegrzyn (1995) were able to increase the ppGpp concentration in *E. coli* cells without starvation and directly investigate the effect of ppGpp on DNA replication. They found evidence that most, but not all, DNA replication was also sensitive to ppGpp concentration and thus under stringent control.

The regulation of DNA synthesis

The replication of bacterial DNA has been divided into 3 stages: initiation, elongation and termination. Replication is initiated at the *oriC* site and proceeds approximately at the same rate in both directions by a semiconservative mechanism until the replication forks collide at a termination site (*terC*) located opposite the *oriC* site. Protein and RNA synthesis is required for DNA replication to be initiated but once replication is initiated it usually continues to completion, even if protein synthesis is prevented. Under normal conditions, it takes about 40 min for the *E. coli* chromosome to replicate and, therefore, the initiation of replication must begin 40 min before cell division is to take place. As the rate of cell growth slows, chromosomal replication occupies a smaller fraction of the division cycle and the number of chromosomes per cell is reduced. At very slow growth rates there tends to be only one chromosome per cell (Bremer and Churchward 1991).

Bernander, Akerlund and Nordstrom (1995) obtained a strain of *E. coli* in which the initiation of chromosomal replication could be turned off by a reduction in growth temperature of only 3°C. When the initiation of chromosomal replication was blocked in this gentle manner, chromosomal replication in progress continued to completion and cell division took place. After this, cell growth continued but no further cell division took place and long, filamentous cells were formed. An hour after the growth temperature was returned to a permissive level, normal growth with cell division resumed.

2 TRANSPORT OF SOLUTES INTO THE CELL

2.1 Simple and facilitated diffusion

Most small solutes can diffuse through the peptidoglycan material and many hydrophilic compounds can pass through the porins of the outer membrane of gram-negative bacteria. However, the cytoplasmic membrane of both gram-negative and gram-positive bacteria is a barrier to hydrophilic compounds and special arrangements must be made to allow nutrients to pass through this membrane fast enough to allow competitive growth rates. The unassisted movement of compounds through the cytoplasmic membrane and into the cytoplasm is termed **simple** or **passive** diffusion. With the exception of certain hydrophobic compounds, such diffusion will be very slow. The rate of entry of a compound into the cytoplasm by simple diffusion will often be dependent upon its concentration in the medium and a linear relationship can exist between the substrate concentration and the cell growth rate. To increase growth rates in the presence of low levels of nutrients, bacteria have evolved a number of different types of transport systems to speed the transport of solutes through the membrane and into the cell.

Facilitated diffusion results when the cell possess a protein (the facilitator protein) to aid or facilitate the transport of a compound through the membrane. This facilitator protein permits the compound to be transferred down a concentration gradient from one side of the membrane to the other. The process is not directly coupled to metabolic energy and the compound can not be accumulated against a concentration gradient but it may be altered and trapped to prevent it from leaving once it enters the cell. Transport across the cytoplasmic membrane by the process of facilitated diffusion is common for glycerol. Once inside the bacterial cell, glycerol is phosphorylated by glycerol kinase and glycerol phosphate can accumulate within the cells. The phosphorylation is essential to trap glycerol in the cells and mutants lacking glycerol kinase are not able to accumulate glycerol. Facilitated diffusion is most common in the case of glycerol but facilitator transport systems do exist for other compounds. An unusual case of the transport of glucose by facilitated diffusion has been reported in *Zymomonas mobilis*. The facilitator protein in this organism is a low-affinity, high-velocity carrier which has also been reported to transport fructose and xylose (Weisser et al. 1995).

2.2 Active transport systems

Most solutes are brought into the cell by means of active transport systems which involve the use of metabolic energy. Since energy is used, these active transport systems can accumulate the compound within the cell at a concentration 1000 times greater than the concentration in the surrounding medium, greatly increasing the growth rate of the cell when nutrients are limited.

Substrates can be transported in various bacteria by several different active transport systems. Included among these are the ATP-binding cassette (ABC)-type carriers. These are also known as periplasmic-binding protein-dependent transport systems or osmotic shock-sensitive transport systems, since one of the protein components of the system is released from the cell periplasm by cold osmotic shock. Another type of active transport system are the chemiosmotic-driven, ion gradient-linked permeases, that use proton- or sodium-motive force to transport nutrients into the cell. The ATP and the proton-motive force (pmf) systems are interconvertible via ATP synthase but can be differentiated by the use of inhibitors that prevent ATP from accumulating or by using proton iono-phores, such as dinitrophenol (DNP), that collapse the proton gradient. A third type of transport, primarily associated with fermenting bacteria, is the phosphoenolpyruvate phosphotransferase system (PTS system) in which the compound is phosphorylated during transport through the cytoplasmic membrane.

ATP-BINDING CASSETTE, PERIPLASMIC-BINDING PROTEIN-DEPENDENT TRANSPORT SYSTEMS

These transport systems in gram-negative bacteria are composed of a substrate-binding receptor protein associated with the cell periplasm plus several membrane-bound components. Sometimes these are termed primary transport systems and they are often referred to as osmotic shock-sensitive permeases, since a cold osmotic shock causes the loss of the substrate-binding protein which is loosely attached in the periplasmic space. In gram-positive bacteria, the substrate-binding receptor protein is represented by a lipoprotein fastened to the membrane. After binding to the substrate, it changes configuration and transfers the substrate to a membrane-bound complex of proteins or domains, the ATP-binding cassette (ABC) proteins, that are often fused with one another. A subset of these transport systems are known as 'traffic ATPases'. The transfer of the substrate to the membrane-bound protein complex results in ATP hydrolysis and the substrate passes through the membrane to enter the cytoplasm. In different situations, the membrane components might be 2, 3 or 4 proteins and in some cases the membrane-bound complex may be used by more than one binding protein for the transport of different substrates (Ames, Mimura and Shyamala 1990). Substrates reported to be transported by this system in *E. coli* include carbohydrates such as L-arabinose, maltose, D-ribose, D-xylose, succinate, malate, and amino acids such as leucine, isoleucine, valine, histidine, lysine and ornithine.

ION GRADIENT-LINKED OR CHEMIOSMOTIC-DRIVEN TRANSPORT SYSTEMS

Chemiosmotic-driven transport systems, sometimes termed secondary transport systems, use an ion gradient, such as proton-motive force or sodium-motive force, as the energy to drive the transport of the substrate through the membrane. The 3 basic types are the symport, the antiport and the uniport. With symport, a single carrier simultaneously transports 2 substances in the same direction. Antiport involves a common carrier transporting 2 substances at the same time but in opposite directions. Uniport is the situation where movement is independent of any coupled ion (Moat and Foster 1995).

Electrochemical ion gradient permeases are usually composed of a single, very hydrophobic, membrane protein that can undergo reversible oxidation–reduction reactions. The oxidized state binds the sugar or compound to be transported and the reduced state has a conformational change and releases the compound in the cell cytoplasm.

Many of these bacterial transport systems are exogenously induced, in that only external substrates cause their induction. *E. coli* and many other enteric bacteria have inducible transport systems to bring certain phosphorylated sugars such as glucose-6-phosphate and glycerol-3-phosphate into the cells, but these sugar phosphates do not induce their transport systems when they are produced internally. In *E. coli*, the *uhpT* gene product, UhpT, is responsible for the entry of a number of organic phosphate compounds, including the phosphate esters of a variety of sugars (Kadner, Murphy and Stephens 1992).

In some of the thermophilic *Bacillus* species, such as *B. stearothermophilus*, Na^+ is used for the coupling ion for amino acid transport. The transport of glutamate and aspartate is driven by the proton-motive force as well as an inward directed Na^+ gradient. Sodium/proton glutamate transporters have been found in a number of thermophilic *Bacillus* spp. However, in *B. subtilis*, glutamate uptake was coupled to proton-motive force (Tolner et al. 1995). In *E. coli* and *Salmonella* Typhimurium, carbohydrate–sodium cotransport systems have been reported for melibiose and proline. Carbohydrate–sodium cotransport systems are common in halophilic bacteria.

THE PHOSPHOENOLPYRUVATE PHOSPHOTRANSFERASE SYSTEM

The **phosphoenolpyruvate phosphotransferase system** (PTS) uses the phosphate from phosphoenolpyruvate (PEP) for the transport and phosphorylation of incoming sugars. The phosphate group is first transferred from PEP to a non-specific enzyme component termed enzyme I or EI. The phosphorylated EI (P-EI) transfers the phosphate to histidine residue 15 on a small, heat-stable protein, designated HPr. The phosphate is then transferred from phospho-HPr to a sugar-specific, membrane-bound, enzyme II (EII) complex, which catalyses the transport of the carbohydrate through the membrane as well as its phosphorylation.

The EII complex consists of domains termed IIA, IIB, IIC (and sometimes IID) that may exist as separate proteins or components of the same protein. The IIA and IIB protein domains are associated with the cytoplasmic side of the membrane and are involved in phosphate transfer. If these domains are located in separate proteins, the IIA domain will have the first phosphorylation site and the IIB domain will have the second phosphorylation site. The IIC protein or domain is located in the cytoplasmic membrane, possesses the carbohydrate-binding site and is responsible for the transport of the carbohydrate through the membrane. The overall effect of the PTS system is both to phosphorylate the carbohydrate and to transport it into the cytoplasm of the cell. In the family Enterobacteriaceae, the regulatory functions of the PTS have been chiefly assigned to the protein IIA^{Glc} specifically associated with the transport of glucose.

The EI and HPr components are the non-specific portions of the PTS system. The other, carbohydrate-specific components of the PTS transport system can be indicated by placing the name of the transported sugar after the enzyme designation. The EII protein or domain that is specific for the transport of D-glucose into the cells as glucose-6-phosphate can be designated as enzyme EII^{Glucose} or EII^{Glc}. Some EII PTS transport systems may have activity upon more than one carbohydrate. For example, *E. coli* enzyme II^{Man} has activity for the transport and phosphorylation of glucose, mannose, 2-deoxyglucose, glucosamine and fructose, in that order (Saier Jr and Reizer 1994).

Since the PTS transport system requires phosphoenolpyruvate as the initial phosphate donor, it tends to be found in facultative or anaerobic bacteria that utilize the hexose diphosphate pathway and produce 2 PEP molecules for each hexose catabolized. The PTS system is common in such bacteria as *E. coli* and other enteric bacteria, *Bacillus*, *Clostridium*, *Bacteroides*, *Staphylococcus*, *Lactobacillus* and *Streptococcus*. It is not common in aerobic bacteria employing other catabolic pathways, such as *Arthrobacter*, *Azotobacter*, *Micrococcus*, *Pseudomonas*, *Nocardia*, or *Caulobacter*. In *E. coli*, the PTS transport system is used for the transport of such carbohydrates as mannitol, sorbitol, galactitol, glucose, glucose–mannose, fructose and N-acetylglucosamine. Many gram-positive bacteria transport lactose, sucrose, maltose and pentitols via the PTS system. Alternative, non-PTS transport systems for glucose may also be present (Cvitkovitch et al. 1995).

The role of the PTS system in catabolite repression

As mentioned previously (see p. 90), in enteric bacteria catabolite repression results from a decrease in the internal cAMP concentration. When D-glucose is being transported through the membrane by the PTS system, adenylate cyclase is almost inactive and, as a result, the level of cAMP in the cells is very low. The metabolite responsible for catabolite repression in many bacteria appears to be enzyme IIA^{Glc}. When glucose and other sugars transported by the PTS system are not present, the HPr protein remains phosphorylated and enzyme IIA^{Glc} is also phosphorylated. The phosphorylated form of enzyme IIA^{Glc} activates adenylate cyclase, resulting in the activation of adenylate cyclase and the synthesis of cAMP. When cells are growing upon glucose or other sugars transported by the PTS system, IIA^{Glc} will be donating its phosphate group to the incoming sugar and will be unphosphorylated. Unphosphorylated IIA^{Glc} inhibits the activity of adenylate cyclase, leading to a decrease in cAMP levels (Saier and Roseman 1976). When glucose is being transported by the PTS system, many other catabolite transport systems are shut down, a separate regulatory phenomenon known as **inducer exclusion**. At least some forms of inducer exclusion are the result of the direct inhibition of other transport systems by the non-phosphorylated form of IIA^{Glc}.

The HPr of *Streptococcus pyogenes* can also be phosphorylated on a serine residue (Ser-46) using ATP, by a specific HPr kinase. This reaction has been found to be widespread among gram-positive bacteria but not gram-negative bacteria and even has been shown to occur in some species lacking a functional PTS. It has some regulatory roles, regulating glucose and lactose permease activity in *L. brevis*, inducer exclusion in *L. lactis*, and is involved in catabolite repression in *B. subtilis* (Thevenot et al. 1995).

2.3 Siderophores

The presence of oxygen results in the oxidation of ferrous iron to highly insoluble ferric compounds. For this reason, bacteria have had to develop special methods for obtaining iron and many synthesize and secrete small iron-chelating compounds termed siderophores. The siderophores carrying ferric iron are all taken up by specific high-affinity outer-membrane receptor proteins (Touati et al. 1995). *E. coli* has been reported to be able to synthesize at least 5 different siderophore–ferric iron transport systems.

3 BACTERIAL CATABOLIC PATHWAYS

3.1 The hexose diphosphate pathway

INTRODUCTION

A very efficient pathway for the production of ATP during the catabolism of d-glucose and similar carbohydrates is often referred to as the **EMP** pathway to honour 3 scientists who contributed greatly to its elucidation, Embden, Meyerhof and Parnas. One of the unique things about this pathway, however, is the formation of a hexose diphosphate as an intermediate. Therefore an alternative and descriptive name is the **hexose diphosphate** or **HDP** pathway (Fig. 5.2).

THE PHOSPHORYLATION OF GLUCOSE

The catabolism of glucose by the HDP pathway begins by phosphorylation at the 6-carbon position. Various different mechanisms have been reported for this reaction. If glucose is transported into the cells via the PTS system, this efficient transport system will convert glucose to the 6-phosphate upon passage through the cell membrane. If glucose enters the cell by a different transport system or is produced within the cell, it must be phosphorylated by other means.

Hexokinase is a non-specific kinase found in a variety of micro-organisms. It can catalyse the phosphorylate of hexoses such as D-glucose, D-fructose, D-mannose and D-glucosamine to the 6-phosphate with ATP as the phosphate donor. Some bacteria, such as those in the genera *Staphylococcus*, *Streptococcus*, *Clostridium* and *Lactobacillus*, possess a glucokinase specific for the phosphorylation of glucose to glucose-6-phosphate. At least some bacteria in the genus *Propionibacterium* can phosphorylate glucose using inorganic pyrophosphate as the phosphate donor. Transfer enzymes have been reported that can transfer the phosphate group from a different hexose phosphate to glucose.

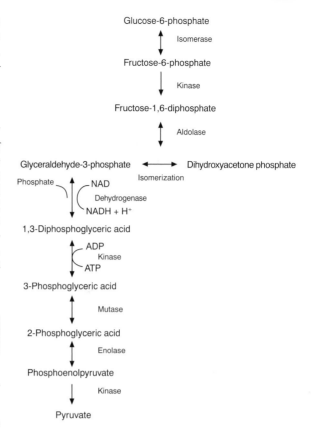

Fig. 5.2 The hexose diphosphate (HDP) or EMP pathway. Glucose-6-phosphate is converted to fructose-1,6-diphosphate which is cleaved to produce the 3-carbon, triose phosphates. Glyceraldehyde-3-phosphate is oxidized and the product of the oxidation converted to pyruvate.

CONVERSION OF GLUCOSE-6-PHOSPHATE TO GLYCERALDEHYDE-3-PHOSPHATE

The reactions of the HDP resulting in the conversion of glucose-6-phosphate to the 2 triose phosphates, glyceraldehyde-3-phosphate and dihydroxyacetone phosphate, are illustrated in Fig. 5.2. The first step is the isomerization of glucose-6-phosphate to the 2-keto sugar, fructose-6-phosphate. The enzyme catalysing the reaction is glucose-6-phosphate (fructose-6-phosphate) isomerase, an enzyme with the older name of hexose phosphate isomerase. The equilibrium of this reaction is back towards glucose-6-phosphate. However, the equilibrium of the next reaction, the conversion of fructose-6-phosphate to fructose-1,6-diphosphate, is strongly towards product formation. The phosphorylating enzyme is fructose-6-phosphokinase (also known as phosphofructokinase or Pfk) and ATP normally is the phosphate donor. Two isozymes for Pfk have been found in *E. coli*. Most of the activity (90%) is provided by Pfk-1, an enzyme activated by nucleotide diphosphates such as ADP, and inhibited by PEP. Several nucleotide triphosphates such as ATP, UTP (uridine triphosphate) and ITP (inosine triphosphate), can serve as phosphate donors. However, excess ATP and PEP are negative effectors of the enzyme and inhibit activity. Thus, the activity of the enzyme (and the HDP pathway) will be inhibited in cells with high energy charges (high levels of nucleotide triphosphates). The second enzyme, Pfk-2, is inhibited by ATP and the product of the reaction, fructose-1,6-diphosphate.

Aldolase catalyses the cleavage of fructose-1,6-diphosphate to the 2 triose phosphates, glyceraldehyde-3-phosphate and dihydroxyacetone phosphate, as shown in Fig. 5.2. The equilibrium of the reaction is back towards fructose-1,6-diphosphate so that an accumulation of triose phosphates will lead to an accumulation of fructose-1,6-diphosphate. The accumulation of this hexose diphosphate often serves as a regulatory signal that the oxidation of glyceraldehyde-3-phosphate is not functioning properly. The 2 triose phosphates, glyceraldehyde-3-phosphate and dihydroxyacetone phosphate, are interconvertible by the enzyme triose phosphate isomerase.

CONVERSION OF GLYCERALDEHYDE-3-PHOSPHATE TO PYRUVATE

The energy yielding reaction of the hexose diphosphate pathway involves the oxidation of glyceraldehyde-3-phosphate to 1,3-diphosphoglyceric acid. This oxidation is catalysed by glyceraldehyde-3-phosphate dehydrogenase and the energy released is conserved in an energy-rich bond between phosphoglyceric acid and phosphate to yield 1,3-diphosphoglyceric acid. This reaction is reversible and NAD is usually (not always) the electron acceptor. Phosphate esterification in this manner, with the phosphate group eventually being transferred to ADP to form ATP, is termed **substrate level phosphorylation**.

ATP-phosphoglyceric transphosphorylase, also known as phosphoglycerate kinase, catalyses the reversible transfer of the phosphate from carbon-1 of 1,3-diphosphoglyceric acid to ADP, to form ATP and 3-phosphoglyceric acid. Another enzyme, phosphoglycerate mutase, catalyses the transfer of phosphate from the 3 to the 2 position of glyceric acid, producing 2-phosphoglyceric acid. Then 2-phosphoglyceric acid dehydrase, also known as enolase, removes water to form PEP. Pyruvate kinase transfers the phosphate to ADP to form ATP and pyruvic acid.

Two isozymes of pyruvate kinase have been reported in *E. coli*. They are Pyk-F, activated by fructose-1,6-diphosphate, and Pyk-A, activated by AMP. Mutants lacking one of these 2 enzymes can still grow on glucose but mutants lacking both enzymes grow poorly on glucose, except aerobically on substrates transported into the cells by the PTS system. In the latter case, pyruvate is generated from PEP during substrate transport. The net gain of energy from the HDP pathway is 2 ATP for each glucose catabolized. This pathway is an efficient pathway for the fermentation of hexoses and is common in fermenting bacteria. If the HDP pathway is used to convert glucose to 2 pyruvate, the carboxyl groups of the pyruvate must originate from carbons 3 and 4 of the glucose.

3.2 The glucose fermentations

THE HOMOLACTIC ACID FERMENTATION

The electron carrier reduced by the oxidation of glyceraldehyde-3-phosphate during the HDP pathway, usually NAD, must be reoxidized if the pathway is to continue functioning. In industry the term fermentation is used to denote many metabolic reactions caused by micro-organisms. However, in microbial physiology and metabolism the term **fermentation** has a very specific meaning. A fermentation is the condition where the **final electron acceptor** of a catabolic pathway is an **organic compound**.

Pyruvate, produced as a result of the HDP pathway, is an excellent acceptor for the electrons produced by the oxidation of glyceraldehyde-3-phosphate and most bacteria possess the metabolic capability of reducing pyruvate to lactic acid (see Fig. 5.3). For some bacteria, however, the reduction of pyruvate to lactate is the most important method of reoxidizing NADH and such bacteria produce large amounts of lactic acid as final products of glucose fermentation. For this reason, such bacteria are termed **lactic acid bacteria**. If glucose is the only carbon source provided to the cells, some of the products of glucose degradation by the HDP must be used for biosynthetic purposes to make new cell material. However, since the energy gained as the result of fermentation is relatively low, most of the carbon from the glucose must be converted to fermentation products. The term **homolactic acid fermentation** means that significantly more than half the carbon from the glucose fermented is in the form of lactic acid. It is apparent that any bacterium that carries out a homolactic acid fermentation must be able to survive in the presence of large amounts of lactic acid and at low pH.

Lactic acid is the major product of the homolactic acid fermentation but other products may be formed in lesser amounts. Many homolactic acid bacteria produce such fermentation products as acetate, ethanol and formate, in addition to lactate. The conversion of pyruvate to formic acid, ethanol and acetic acid, rather than lactose, actually increases the energy gained by the fermentation, but it also increases the

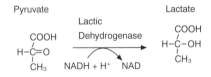

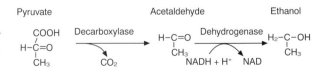

Fig. 5.3 Formation of lactate and ethanol from pyruvate. Pyruvate can be directly reduced to lactate or decarboxylated to acetaldehyde which can be reduced to ethanol.

amount of acid formed. Regulatory systems of homolactic acid bacteria tend to shift the fermentation to larger amounts of these compounds at higher pH values, at which acid production would be less likely to inhibit growth.

The purification of lactic dehydrogenase from a homolactic acid bacterium led to the discovery that this enzyme was an allosteric enzyme with an absolute requirement of a positive effector for enzyme activation. If the reduction of pyruvate to lactic acid does not proceed efficiently enough to reoxidize the NADH formed from the oxidation of glyceraldehyde-3-phosphate, the oxidation of the triose phosphate is inhibited. Because of the reversibility of the aldolase-catalysed reaction, the internal pool of the positive effector of lactic dehydrogenase, fructose-1,6-diphosphate, increases. This results in the activation of more molecules of lactic dehydrogenase and the more rapid reduction of pyruvate.

Some of these lactic acid bacteria can slowly transport electrons to oxygen if oxygen is available. After a lactic acid fermentation is complete, exposure of the culture to air may result in the slow oxidation of lactose with the production of acetate and CO_2. One mechanism for this effect is the passage of electrons from NADH to flavoproteins with the reduced flavoproteins (FPH2) becoming autoxidized by oxygen. The oxygen is reduced to hydrogen peroxide which must be eliminated by catalase or other means. The oxidation of NADH and FPH2 permits lactate to be oxidized back to pyruvate and the pyruvate oxidized and decarboxylated with the production of acetyl phosphate and additional ATP. Energy calculations have shown that some lactic acid bacteria also obtain energy from the transport of electrons directly to oxygen. They can produce at least a partial system of membrane electron transport when incubated or grown under aerobic conditions and oxidative phosphorylation takes place with ATP formation (Moat and Foster 1995).

Lactic acid bacteria can transport lactose into the cells by a variety of different methods, including the phosphotransferase system, ATP-dependent osmotic shock-sensitive proteins, proton symport and lactose–galactose antiport systems. The most efficient system is the lactose-specific PTS, since transport is coupled with lactose phosphorylation. Translocation of lactose by lactic acid bacteria can also be coupled to ions or other solutes. *L. lactis* has a proton-coupled translocation of lactose with a permease similar to the LacY of *E. coli*. *Streptococcus thermophilus* has a transport system for lactose (LacS) that can function as a proton symport system or as a lactose–galactose antiporter (Poolman 1993, deVos and Vaughan 1994).

THE DIRECT ALCOHOL FERMENTATION

The direct **alcohol fermentation** or 'yeast type' of alcohol fermentation, permits the oxidation of NADH from the HDP pathway without the formation of large amounts of lactic acid. Pyruvate is directly decarboxylated by **pyruvate decarboxylase** to yield acetaldehyde and CO_2. The enzyme **alcohol dehydrogenase** catalyses the reduction of acetaldehyde to ethyl alcohol with electrons from NADH and the major products of the fermentation are ethanol and CO_2 (see Fig. 5.3). This mechanism of ethanol formation is common in yeast but, although many bacteria are capable of ethanol production, only a few do so by this pathway. Some of those bacteria using this 'yeast type' of pathway for ethanol formation include those in the genera *Zymomonas*, *Acetomonas* and *Sarcina ventriculi*.

THE FORMIC ACID FERMENTATION

Some bacteria have evolved the ability to obtain extra energy from pyruvate. In one mechanism for pyruvate fermentation, the enzyme **formate–pyruvate lyase** cleaves pyruvate to formic acid and a 2-carbon fragment that becomes acetyl-CoA. This enzyme can be present in an inactive form (Ej) which is converted to an active form (Ea) by an 'activase' enzyme which requires pyruvate as a positive allosteric effector. The cleavage of *S*-adenosylmethionine into methionine and 5′-deoxyadenosine is also required for enzyme activation. The active form of the enzyme normally functions only under anaerobic conditions and is rapidly and irreversibly inactivated by oxygen (Sawer and Bock 1988). This enzyme is common in enteric bacteria and also accounts for the formic acid produced during some homolactic acid fermentations.

For every pyruvate converted to formate and acetyl-CoA, the NADH produced by the HDP pathways must be reoxidized by a different mechanism. For this purpose, some of the acetyl group on the acetyl-CoA is reduced twice, first to acetaldehyde and then to ethanol. This reduction is catalysed by a special alcohol dehydrogenase, a **CoA-linked alcohol dehydrogenase**. The energy of the acetyl-CoA bond is sacrificed in the reaction but 2 NADH can be oxidized for each ethanol produced. Facultative bacteria, such as *E. coli*, have a single large polypeptide responsible for both activities. The *adhE* gene of *E. coli* K-12 encodes a polypeptide of 891 amino acids, equivalent in size to a combined alcohol dehydrogenase and an acetaldehyde dehydrogenase, and may represent an evolutionary fusion product of separate genes. Some obligate anaerobes, such as *Clostridium*, have 2 proteins to catalyse the reduction of acetyl-CoA to ethanol, a Co-linked acetaldehyde dehydrogenase and an alcohol dehydrogenase. These 2 separate polypeptides form a complex so that free acetaldehyde is not released.

The acetyl-CoA that is not needed for the oxidation of NADH can be used for the generation of additional ATP. The enzyme phosphotransacetylase catalyses the reversible transfer of acetate from acetyl-CoA to phosphate with the formation of acetyl phosphate. The enzyme acetokinase, in a reaction that is also reversible, transfers the phosphate from acetyl phosphate to ADP, to form ATP and liberate acetate. Therefore, 2 pyruvate and 2 NADH can result in 2 formate, one ethanol and one acetate, with the gain of one ATP. This fermentation is also known as the **mixed acid fermentation** and the metabolic reactions leading to these products are illustrated in Fig. 5.4.

Some of these bacteria possess the ability to oxidize

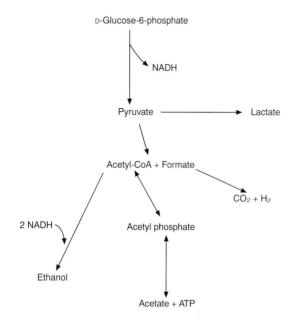

D-Glucose-6-phosphate

NADH

Pyruvate ——————→ Lactate

Acetyl-CoA + Formate

$CO_2 + H_2$

2 NADH

Acetyl phosphate

Ethanol

Acetate + ATP

Fig. 5.4 Possible products of the formic acid or mixed acid fermentation. Pyruvate can be cleaved to yield acetyl-CoA and formate. The acetyl-CoA can be converted to acetate yielding a high energy phosphate bond or reduced to ethanol. If the proper enzymes are present the formate can be oxidized to yield carbon dioxide and hydrogen gases.

formic acid and lower the amount of acid produced as a result of this fermentation. Formic dehydrogenase, an anaerobic, inducible enzyme, catalyses the oxidation of formate to carbon dioxide. Formate is required for induction of the enzyme (Ferry 1990) and a special electron carrier is needed, often a cytochrome *e* type of carrier. The electron carrier transfers electrons to a hydrogenase which reduces protons to form hydrogen gas. This hydrogenase is inducible, is inactivated by air and is not present when the cells are grown in the presence of oxygen. This complete system, consisting of formic dehydrogenase, an electron carrier and hydrogenase, was once known as the hydrogen lyase system. It results in the conversion of formic acid to carbon dioxide and hydrogen gases and its function is to reduce the production of acid during fermentation. The enzymes are synthesized under anaerobic conditions, when formate is present, and when the pH is acid.

E. coli normally produces some lactic acid as a result of glucose fermentation as do many fermenting bacteria. Mutants of *E. coli* lacking lactic dehydrogenase grow normally under anaerobic conditions, but if also lacking pyruvate–formate lyase they cannot grow by fermenting glucose or other sugars (Mat-Jan, Alam and Clark 1989). If mutants of *E. coli* lack the ability to produce ethanol from acetyl-CoA they can not grow anaerobically on glucose unless provided with some alternative electron acceptor such as nitrate. However, an additional mutation also eliminating the pyruvate–formate lyase enzyme will restore the ability to grow on glucose anaerobically with the cells now producing lactic acid.

BUTANEDIOL FORMATION

Some bacteria have developed an enzyme pathway for the degradation of pyruvate that produces less acid. An α-acetolactate synthesizing enzyme, with a pH optimum at 6.0, converts 2 pyruvates to α-acetolactate and CO_2. This enzyme is sometimes named the **pH 6.0 α-acetolactate synthesizing** enzyme to distinguish it from a biosynthetic enzyme that carries out the same reaction but possesses a pH optimum of 8.0. During the fermentative pathway the α-acetolactate is decarboxylated by α-acetolactate decarboxylase to produce another CO_2 and acetoin. The acetoin produced can be reduced to 2,3-butanediol by the action of butanediol dehydrogenase and the oxidation of NADH. This system of enzymes appears to be induced by acetate and at high pH values it is inhibited from operating (Zeng and Deckwer 1991). Since this pathway utilizes 2 pyruvate and only results in the oxidation of one NADH, it can not be the sole fermentation route of glucose by a micro-organism. The advantage of this pathway is the production of neutral products. There have also been reports of diacetyl, formed from acetyl-CoA, being reduced to acetoin.

PYRUVATE:FERREDOXIN OXIDOREDUCTASE

In many strictly anaerobic bacteria and archaea, the oxidation and decarboxylation of pyruvate is catalysed by **pyruvate:ferredoxin oxidoreductase**, an enzyme that catalyses the oxidation of pyruvate to form acetyl-CoA and carbon dioxide. The electrons are placed on the electron carrier ferredoxin which may donate them to a hydrogenase with the eventual formation of hydrogen gas. The class of electron carriers known as ferredoxins are small (6–13 kDa), iron–sulphur proteins that function in a variety of reactions, including nitrogen fixation and photosynthesis. Bacterial ferredoxins are classified on the basis of their iron–sulphur clusters and their peptide sequences.

Pyruvate:ferredoxin oxidoreductase is noted for catalysing a rapid exchange reaction between the carbon dioxide and the carboxyl group of the pyruvate, an exchange reaction that can be used to differentiate pyruvate:ferredoxin oxidoreductase from other pyruvate cleavage enzymes. Under proper reducing conditions, the reaction can be reversed, permitting the synthesis of pyruvate from acetate and CO_2. Three types of pyruvate:ferredoxin oxidoreductase have been characterized. One type, found in clostridia and certain other bacteria, is composed of only one polypeptide. A second type, the enzyme from *Halobacterium halobium*, is composed of 2 different subunits of 86 and 42 kDa. The third type, found in such organisms as *Pyrococcus furiosus*, *Thermotoga maritima*, *Methanococcus maripaludis* and *Archaeoglobus fulgidus*, has been shown to possess 4 different subunits of apparent molecular masses of about 47, 32, 25 and 13 kDa (Kunow, Linder and Thauer 1995).

The butanol fermentation pathway

The acetyl group from the acetyl-CoA obtained by the oxidative decarboxylation of pyruvate can be used for the production of acetate and ATP, via phosphotransacetylase and acetokinase, or utilized to generate electron acceptors for the NADH formed by the HDP pathway. In some bacteria, such as those in the genus *Clostridium*, an enzyme named acetyl coenzyme A acetyltransferase condenses 2 molecules of acetyl-CoA to produce one molecule of acetoacetyl-CoA. This compound can be reduced with β-hydroxybutyryl coenzyme A dehydrogenase and NADH to produce β-hydroxybutyryl-CoA. This latter compound can be dehydrated by 3-hydroxyacyl coenzyme A hydrolase (crotonase) to form crotonyl-CoA. The double bond in crotonyl-CoA is further reduced by butyl coenzyme A dehydrogenase to butyryl coenzyme A with electrons again coming from NADH. Thus, the overall series of reactions decarboxylates 2 pyruvates with the acetyl groups becoming condensed into a 4-carbon compound which undergoes 2 reduction steps to form butyryl-CoA.

The butyryl-CoA can have different fates. Acetyltransferase may transfer a free acetate onto the CoA group, producing acetyl-CoA and yielding free butyric acid. A second possibility is for phosphotransbutyrylase to transfer the butyryl group to phosphate to form butyryl phosphate. The phosphate can be donated to ADP to form ATP. Some clostridia produce free acetoacetate from acetoacetyl-CoA by replacing the acetoacetate with acetate. The free acetoacetate can be decarboxylated by acetoacetyl decarboxylase, producing acetone and CO_2 and the acetone may be reduced by isopropyl dehydrogenase, yielding isopropyl alcohol.

The pyruvate:ferredoxin oxidoreductase type of metabolism can also be found in some of the anaerobic spirochaetes, such as *Spirochaeta aurantia* and *Spirochaeta stenostrepta*. With these bacteria, the HDP pathway is involved in converting glucose to pyruvate and some of the electrons are used to convert acetyl-CoA to ethanol. Fermentation products from glucose include CO_2 and H_2 gases as well as acetate and ethanol. A thermophilic spirochaete has been described that appears to possess similar metabolism in that lactate, acetate and hydrogen gas are formed as products from glucose fermentation (Rainey et al. 1991, Janssen and Morgan 1992).

Sarcina maxima possesses a pyruvate:ferredoxin oxidoreductase enzyme and ferments glucose by the HDP pathway to produce carbon dioxide, hydrogen, acetate and butyrate as a result of glucose fermentation. *S. ventriculi*, on the other hand, possesses 2 enzyme systems for cleaving pyruvate: a pyruvate decarboxylase that produces acetaldehyde and carbon dioxide and a formate–pyruvate lyase enzyme system (Canale-Parola 1970, Lowe and Zeikus 1992).

The fermentation of ethanol

Some bacteria such as *Clostridium kluyveri* are able to gain energy by the fermentation of ethanol. Ethanol is oxidized and activated to form acetyl-CoA and the electrons obtained by this oxidation are eliminated by the production of hydrogen gas and the formation of fatty acids. Two acetyl-CoA molecules are condensed to form acetoacetyl-CoA and this compound proceeds through the metabolic pathways described previously with 2 reduction steps giving butyryl-CoA. Additional acetyl molecules may be added with the production of larger fatty acids as final products. Pyruvate is synthesized by reversal of pyruvate:ferredoxin oxidoreductase.

THE PROPIONIC ACID FERMENTATIONS

Some bacteria, for example those in the genera *Propionibacterium*, *Veillonella* and *Bacteroides*, produce propionic acid as a fermentation product. Some of the pyruvate formed as a result of fermentation is usually decarboxylated to yield acetate and CO_2. Other major products of fermentation are succinic and propionic acids. These bacteria can ferment lactic acid since reducing reactions involved in the production of these latter compounds permits the oxidation of lactic acid to pyruvic acid.

Oxaloacetate is an intermediate in the formation of succinate and propionate. Carbon dioxide is activated using ATP and is placed on a biotin coenzyme to form a enzyme biotin–ADP–CO_2 complex. The activated CO_2 is transferred to phosphoenolpyruvate, which is formed from either pyruvate or the HDP pathway catabolism of glucose. The enzyme is carboxytransphosphorylase and the products of the reaction are oxaloacetate and inorganic pyrophosphate. The reduction of the oxaloacetate to malate, its conversion to fumarate and the reduction of the fumarate to succinate, can be used to dispose of electrons, such as those obtained from the HDP pathway or the oxidation of lactic acid. A transferase enzyme exchanges the succinate with the propionyl group on a molecule of propionyl-CoA to form free propionic acid and succinyl-CoA. An isomerase then converts the succinyl-CoA to methylmalonyl-CoA, which donates a carboxyl group to the enzyme–biotin complex to form a biotin–ADP–CO_2 complex and a molecule of propionyl-CoA. The activated CO_2 is used to convert another PEP to oxaloacetate while propionic acid is liberated during the activation of another succinate. By these reactions, a typical propionic acid bacterium such as *Propionibacterium pentosaccium* will produce carbon dioxide gas, acetic acid, propionic acid and succinic acid as a result of glucose or lactic acid fermentation.

When there are high transmembrane differences in the electrochemical potentials of Na^+, the Na^+-oxaloacetate decarboxylase of certain bacteria begins to operate as a Na^+ channel (carrier) and some of these decarboxylases are able to use the free energy of decarboxylation to transport sodium ions across the cell membrane. This process requires carboxylation–decarboxylation of the biotin group. Enzymes included as sodium ion pump decarboxylating enzymes are methylmalonyl coenzyme A (CoA) decarboxylase, oxaloacetate decarboxylase and glutaconyl-CoA decarboxylase (Skulachev 1994, Huder and Dimroth 1995).

Propionibacterium modestum, a strict anaerobe isolated from salt water, fermented succinate stoichiometrically to produce propionate and carbon dioxide. The key enzyme of succinate fermentation was methylmalonyl coenzyme A decarboxylase and ATP synthesis during succinate fermentation was driven directly by a sodium ion gradient generated upon decarboxylation of methylmalonyl-CoA.

Bacteroides fragilis is an obligate anaerobic, gram-negative bacterium that uses the HDP pathway but lacks phosphofructokinase. Instead, it has a pyrophosphate-dependent 6-phosphofructo-phosphorylating enzyme. It produces propionic acid, acetic acid, lactic acid and succinic acid, from glucose fermentation with traces of ethanol, fumaric acid and pyruvic acid. Bacteria in the genus *Veillonella* also produce propionic acid but differ from the other propionic acid bacteria by possessing the pyruvate:ferredoxin oxidoreductase enzyme for the decarboxylation of pyruvate. *Selenomonas ruminantium* catabolizes glucose by the HDP pathway, possesses a pyruvate:ferredoxin oxidoreductase, and produces lactate, acetate, succinate and propionate as fermentation products. Acetyl-CoA is converted to acetate, coenzyme A and ATP using acetate thiokinase but acetyl phosphate is not an intermediate (Melville, Michel and Macy 1988).

Clostridium propionicum also produces propionic acid as a fermentation product but the pathway differs from those above. Pyruvate is converted to propionic acid by a direct reduction route, involving reduction to lactate which is used to form lactyl-CoA. This latter compound is dehydrated and reduced to propionyl-CoA.

Glycerol fermentation

Some micro-organisms with high levels of NADH will dispose of electrons by reducing dihydroxyacetone phosphate and forming glycerol as a fermentation product. *E. coli* can grow on glycerol either anaerobically or aerobically, producing 2 different glycerol-3-phosphate dehydrogenases in each case. Aerobically, the *glpD* gene is expressed, whereas anaerobically, the *glpA* gene product is synthesized. The anaerobic enzyme is a flavoenzyme that often occurs associated with fumarate reductase. Electrons can be transferred from glycerol-3-phosphate to fumarate by a short electron transport chain. Certain *Klebsiella* and *Citrobacter* strains can ferment glycerol by dehydrating it to 3-hydroxypropionaldehyde which is reduced to 1,3-propanediol.

3.3 The fermentation of pentoses

CONVERSION OF PENTOSES TO THE HDP PATHWAY

Some bacteria are able to ferment certain 5-carbon sugars such as D-xylose and L-arabinose. The fermentation route of these pentoses by enteric bacteria generally involves isomerization of the aldopentose to the 2-keto isomer or pentulose. A pentulose kinase then catalyses phosphorylation to form the pentulose-5-phosphate. In such a manner, D-xylose is isomerized to D-xylulose and then phosphorylated to D-xylulose-5-phosphate whereas L-arabinose is isomerized to L-ribulose and then phosphorylated to L-ribulose-5-phosphate. Epimerization reactions convert the

pentulose-5-phosphates to D-xylulose-5-phosphate which represents the common intermediate in the catabolism of these sugars. The exception is D-ribose which is usually phosphorylated first and then isomerized to D-ribulose-5-phosphate.

The pentulose phosphates are converted to intermediates of the HDP pathway by a series of reactions known as the transketolase–transaldolase rearrangements. The enzyme transketolase (TK) cleaves 2-keto sugars such as D-xylulose-5-phosphate between the 2- and 3-carbons and transfers the 2-carbon group to a proper aldehyde receptor, such as D-ribulose-5-phosphate, forming glyceraldehyde-3-phosphate and the 7-carbon carbohydrate sedoheptulose-7-phosphate. Transaldolase (TA) cleaves similar carbohydrates between the 3- and 4-carbons, transferring the top moiety to an appropriate acceptor such as glyceraldehyde-3-phosphate. These rearrangements convert the 5-carbon sugar phosphate to intermediates of the HDP pathway such as glyceraldehyde-3-phosphate and fructose-6-phosphate with 4- and 7-carbon carbohydrates as intermediates. The structures of some substrates and products of the TK–TA rearrangements are shown in Fig. 5.5.

The conventional HDP pathway enzymes will convert glyceraldehyde-3-phosphate to pyruvate with the production of normal fermentation products. Since these enzyme-catalysed reactions are reversible,

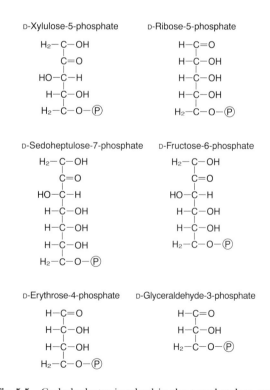

Fig. 5.5 Carbohydrates involved in the transketolase–transaldolase reactions. D-Xylulose-5-phosphate, D-fructose-6-phosphate and D-sedoheptulose-7-phosphate can serve as substrates to be cleaved by transketolase or transaldolase. D-Glyceraldehyde-3-phosphate, D-erythrose-4-phosphate and D-ribose-5-phosphate can serve as acceptors for the 2- or 3-carbon moiety being transferred.

pentose can also be synthesized from HDP pathway intermediates.

The hexose monophosphate or pentose phosphate pathway

Many bacteria, including *E. coli*, can oxidize glucose-6-phosphate at the 1-carbon to form 6-phosphogluconic acid. The enzyme, glucose-6-phosphate dehydrogenase, normally uses NADP, rather than NAD, as the electron acceptor. The 6-phosphogluconolactone formed by this reaction is converted to 6-phosphogluconate by a lactamase. The 6-phosphogluconate can be further oxidized and decarboxylated by 6-phosphogluconate dehydrogenase to produce CO_2, D-ribulose-5-phosphate and, usually, NADPH. In many bacteria, such as the enterics, this is primarily a biosynthetic route, providing the cells with pentose for RNA and DNA synthesis and NADPH for biosynthetic reducing power, and in aerobically growing *E. coli*, about 15% of the glucose is diverted to pentoses by this route. However, the pathway can be used for glucose catabolism with the pentose phosphates converted to HDP intermediates via the TK–TA rearrangements. This route of glucose catabolism does not involve a sugar diphosphate as an intermediate and is known as the hexose monophosphate pathway (HMP) or sometimes the pentose phosphate pathway. With an *E. coli* mutant unable to use the HDP, such as a glucose-6-phosphate isomerase-negative mutant, the cells can still grow on glucose using the HMP pathway, but at a slower rate than when the HDP pathway is employed.

Since fructose-6-phosphate can be one of the products produced from pentulose phosphate by the TK–TA reactions, the potential exists for some organisms to convert fructose-6-phosphate to glucose-6-phosphate and oxidize this compound to 6-phosphogluconate and then to ribulose-5-phosphate. In such a manner a HMP cycle may exist, with the oxidation of hexoses not requiring the oxidation of glyceraldehyde-3-phosphate.

THE HETEROLACTIC ACID FERMENTATION PATHWAY

A bacterium using the HDP pathway to ferment glucose to pyruvate can gain 2 ATP per glucose used by substrate level phosphorylation, but the energy yield is less for the fermentation of a pentose. Theoretically, a homolactic acid fermenter using the HDP pathway could gain 6 ATP by the fermentation of 3 glucose to 6 lactate. However, it could only gain 5 ATP by the fermentation of 3 pentose to 5 lactate using the pentose phosphate route and the TK–TA rearrangements.

Some lactic acid bacteria have evolved a more efficient pathway for the fermentation of 5-carbon sugars. Instead of the D-xylulose-5-phosphate being cleaved by transketolase, it is cleaved by an enzyme termed phosphoketolase in a reaction that results in the esterification of inorganic phosphate and the formation of glyceraldehyde-3-phosphate and acetyl phosphate as products. The glyceraldehyde-3-phosphate can be converted to pyruvate by normal HDP pathway enzymes, yielding a gain of 2 ATP. The

acetyl phosphate can be used to phosphorylate ADP to generate an ATP through the action of acetokinase. Since one ATP is used to form the pentulose phosphate, the result is a net gain of 2 high energy phosphate bonds for each pentose fermented. Bacteria that possess this fermentation route for pentoses normally possess high activity for lactic dehydrogenase and reduce most of the pyruvic acid to lactic acid. Therefore, the fermentation products from 5-carbon sugars are primarily lactate and acetate in equal amounts.

Bacteria possessing phosphoketolase are often lacking key enzymes of the hexose diphosphate pathway such as fructose-6-phosphokinase and aldolase and are unable to use the complete HDP pathway for the catabolism of glucose. If provided with D-glucose as a carbon and energy source, they use the enzymes glucose-6-phosphate dehydrogenase and 6-phosphogluconate dehydrogenase to form D-ribulose-5-phosphate and CO_2. The ribulose-5-phosphate can be epimerized to D-xylulose-5-phosphate which is cleaved by phosphoketolase to produce glyceraldehyde-3-phosphate and acetyl phosphate. The glyceraldehyde-3-phosphate is converted to pyruvate and lactate in a normal manner for a homolactic acid fermentation. However, in order to dispose of all the electrons from the oxidation of the 6-carbon sugar to the pentulose, the acetyl phosphate must be reduced to ethanol in 2 reduction steps. Thus, the products of the fermentation of glucose by this route are CO_2, ethanol and lactic acid and the energy yield is only one ATP per hexose fermented. This fermentation of glucose is termed a **heterolactic acid fermentation** since the 3 major products are produced in approximately equal amounts. The CO_2 is derived from the 1-carbon of the hexose, the ethanol from the 2- and 3-carbons and the lactic acid from the 4-, 5- and 6-carbons.

A variation of this fermentation is carried out by bacteria in the genus *Bifidobacterium*. These bacteria also lack the aldolase of the HDP pathway but possess a fructose-6-phosphate phosphoketolase that converts fructose-6-phosphate to acetyl phosphate and erythrose-4-phosphate. The acetyl phosphate can be used for the production of ATP with acetate being liberated. The transketolase and transaldolase enzymes can act upon the erythrose-4-phosphate and fructose-6-phosphate, producing 7- and 5-carbon carbohydrates and eventually forming some glyceraldehyde-3-phosphate that can be converted to pyruvate. Thus, these bacteria ferment glucose to large amounts of acetic acid with smaller amounts of lactic acid, ethanol and formic acid. The lactic dehydrogenase of *Bifidobacterium* has a requirement for fructose-1,6-diphosphate as a positive effector, as do the homolactic acid fermenters.

GLUCOSE FERMENTATION BY *ZYMOMONAS*

Bacteria in the genus *Zymomonas* are obligate fermentative bacteria with substrate-level phosphorylation as the only source of energy but it is not a strict anaerobe and can grow in the presence of oxygen. The fermentation of glucose produces ethanol, carbon dioxide and lactic acid as primary products. The pathway of glucose catabolism is unusual in that it is the 2-keto-3-deoxy-6-phosphogluconate (KDPG) route, a pathway usually associated with strict aerobes. The KDPG route is not an efficient route for the fermentation of glucose since only one ATP can be gained per glucose fermented. The pyruvate formed from glucose is oxidized to acetaldehyde and CO_2 by a pyruvate decarboxylase similar to the enzyme common in yeast and the acetaldehyde is directly reduced to ethanol by alcohol dehydrogenase. The pyruvate decarboxylase has an especially efficient promoter and represents about 4% of the total cellular protein (Neale et al. 1987). *Z. mobilis* has no TCA cycle and only remnants of a respiratory chain. The KDPG pathway is constitutive and the glucose-6-phosphate dehydrogenase can use either NAD or NADP as electron acceptor, so reducing power for biosynthetic reactions can be provided.

4   ANAEROBIC RESPIRATION

4.1   Nitrate reduction

As mentioned previously, fermentation is the condition in which the final electron is an organic compound. In respiration, oxygen is the final electron acceptor but in **anaerobic respiration** the final electron acceptor is an **inorganic compound other than oxygen**. Many bacteria can use nitrate as a terminal electron acceptor if oxygen is not available. However, 2 different types of nitrate reduction pathways may be found in bacteria. In addition to the use of nitrate for anaerobic respiration, there are also enzyme systems to use nitrate for biosynthetic purposes. This biosynthetic enzyme system is regulated differently, is not sensitive to oxygen and is not coupled to ATP formation.

ENERGY-YIELDING NITRATE REDUCTION

Bacteria that can use nitrate as a terminal electron acceptor for energy production normally will not do so in the presence of oxygen, since respiration can yield more energy. Possible electron donors for nitrate reduction include NADH formed from a variety of catabolic pathways, formate, hydrogen, glycerol-3-phosphate, succinate and lactate. The electron flow is from NAD, through flavoproteins, to cytochromes, and finally to nitrate. Special types of cytochromes and membrane enzymes are required for nitrate reduction and up to 3 ATP can be obtained for each nitrate reduced, although *E. coli* probably gets less.

The first step in nitrate reduction involves a membrane-bound nitrate reductase which reduces nitrate to nitrite. The enzyme is composed of 3 subunits, a, b, and g (cytochrome b_{NR}) and also contains a molybdopterin cofactor, several iron–sulphur centres and haem groups. Quinols are the apparent natural electron donor and menaquinone-9 has been reported to be bound to the ab dimer (Brito, DeMoss and Dubourdieu 1995). The nitrite produced in this

reaction is reduced to nitric oxide by a soluble nitrite reductase. The nitric oxide is further reduced to nitrous oxide by a soluble nitric oxide reductase. Finally, the nitrous oxide is reduced to nitrogen gas by a membrane-bound nitrous oxide reductase. Each step uses a pair of electrons. When nitrate concentrations are low and nitrite concentration are high, nitrite can be reduced to ammonia by an alternative route. In such cases, an NADH-linked, soluble nitrite reductase may be used to detoxify some of the nitrite and produce ammonia and NAD⁺. Although different enzymes are involved, no additional energy is obtained.

REGULATION OF NITRATE REDUCTION IN *E. COLI*

The presence of nitrate not only induces the synthesis of the respiratory chain components for nitrate but represses synthesis of other anaerobic respiratory chains and fermentation pathways. The regulation of the nitrate anaerobic respiration pathway in *E. coli* has different levels of regulation at a global level. The control system requires a protein (FNR) that has sequence similarity to the CRP protein of catabolite repression. In the presence of nitrate, 2 membrane-bound sensor proteins, NARX and NARQ, phosphorylate 2 other proteins, NARL and NARP, respectively. The phosphorylated forms of these latter proteins activate transcription of operons important for nitrate reduction and inhibit the expression of operons for alternate respiration pathways (Stewart 1993).

4.2   Sulphate reduction

Some bacteria can use sulphate as the electron acceptor during anaerobic respiration. The first step in the use of sulphur as electron acceptor is its activation on an AMP molecule. The enzyme adenyltransferase (ATP-sulphurylase) uses ATP and sulphate as substrates to form adenyl sulphate (APS) and inorganic pyrophosphate. The pyrophosphate may be hydrolysed by inorganic pyrophosphatase with the energy in the pyrophosphate bond lost to the cells. Bacteria in one genus, however, *Desulfotomaculum*, conserve the bond energy in the pyrophosphate by using acetate–pyrophosphate phosphotransferase and acetate to form acetyl phosphate (Moat and Foster 1995).

The enzyme APS reductase adds 2 electrons to APS to reduce the sulphate to sulphite with the liberation of AMP. Next, sulphide reductase reduces sulphide to form trithionate ($S_3O_6^{2-}$). This latter compound is reduced to thiosulphate ($S_2O_3^{2-}$) which is then reduced to sulphide (S_2). Energy is gained by oxidative phosphorylation as the electrons flow from NADH to sulphate. Two ATP may be gained for each sulphide formed.

Desulfovibrio desulfuricans is a strict anaerobe that can ferment glucose and pyruvate and can also grow using lactate if sulphate is present to serve as an electron acceptor. Pyruvate, formed by either the HDP pathway or by lactate oxidation, is cleaved by pyruvate:ferredoxin oxidoreductase, yielding CO_2, H_2 and acetyl coenzyme A. The acetyl-CoA can be converted to acetyl phosphate and then acetate with ATP formation. *D. desulfuricans* can also grow using CO_2, H_2 and acetate if sulphate is present. In this case, electrons are transferred from H_2 to sulphate to gain energy and the pyruvate:ferredoxin oxidoreductase reaction is reversed to make pyruvate for biosynthetic reactions.

Cell suspensions of *Desulfovibrio vulgaris* were found to catalyse, in the absence of sulphate, the complete conversion of one lactate to one acetate, one CO_2 and $2 H_2$. It has been suggested that the ATP gained from acetyl phosphate is used to drive the oxidation of lactate to pyruvate and the electrons from the oxidation of lactate can be used to make hydrogen gas (Pankhania et al. 1988).

5 AEROBIC CATABOLISM

5.1 The pyruvate dehydrogenation complex

The pyruvate dehydrogenation complex (PDH) is a multienzyme complex catalysing the decarboxylation of pyruvic acid with an acetyl transfer from pyruvate to coenzyme A. The complex has a structural core of dihydrolipoic reductase transacetylase (E2) components surrounded by independently bound pyruvate dehydrogenase (E1) and dihydrolipoic dehydrogenase (E3). The cofactor requirements of the complex include dithiooctanoic acid (lipoic acid), coenzyme A, NAD, FAD (flavin adenine dinucleotide) and TPP (thiamine pyrophosphate). The complex catalyses the oxidation and decarboxylation of pyruvate, producing CO_2, acetyl coenzyme A and NADH.

The complex isolated from *E. coli* possesses a chain ratio of E1:E2:E3 or 1.6:1.0:0.8 with a core of 24 E2 chains. The genes encoding for the E1 and E2 enzymes (*aceE* and *aceF*) are part of the same operon. The gene encoding for E3 (*ipd*) is linked to the *aceF* gene. The E3, the *ipd* gene product, is also produced and used during metabolism of the α-ketoglutarate dehydrogenase complex of the TCA cycle. The E1 and E2 subunits are assembled around an icosahedral core composed of E2 polypeptides and form the complex with its molecular size of about 10 000 kDa (Hiromasa, Aso and Yamashita 1994).

This pyruvate dehydrogenase from *E. coli* is stimulated by HDP intermediates such as fructose-6-phosphate. It is inhibited by a high adenylate energy charge but such inhibition is overcome by fructose-1,6-diphosphate. The ratio of NADH:NAD seems to influence the flow of pyruvate between pyruvate–formate lyase and the PDH. The activity of the complex increases with increased NAD^+ concentration within the cells but is inhibited when intracellular NADH levels are high, such high levels indicating a problem in the disposal of electrons (Snoep et al. 1991). For these reasons, utilization of the system tends to increase under aerobic conditions or when the oxidation of NADH is not a problem for the cells.

5.2 The tricarboxylic acid cycle or citric acid cycle

ACETATE AS A CARBON AND ENERGY SOURCE

E. coli has 2 pathways that can be used to convert acetate to acetyl-CoA. One pathway uses acetate kinase and ATP to produce acetyl phosphate while phosphotransacetylase transfers the acetyl moiety to CoA to form acetyl-CoA. However, this route is believed to function primarily in a catabolic role, generating ATP when acetate is being excreted. This system would be used to activate acetate only when acetate was present in large amounts outside the cells. The second pathway is believed to function to use extracellular acetate that is present in low concentrations. It uses the enzyme acetyl-CoA synthetase to convert acetate and ATP to acetyl-AMP and inorganic pyrophosphate. The acetyl-AMP can react with CoA to release inorganic phosphate and form acetyl-CoA. Although wild-type *E. coli* cells grow well on acetate at concentrations ranging from 2.5 to 50 mM, mutants lacking acetyl-CoA synthetase grow poorly on low acetate concentrations. Mutants lacking acetate kinase and phosphotransacetylase grow poorly on high concentrations of acetate and mutants lacking all 3 enzymes did not grow on acetate at any concentration tested (Kumari et al. 1995).

THE OXIDATION OF ACETATE

The tricarboxylic acid (TCA) cycle, also known as the citric acid cycle or the Krebs cycle, is a means of oxidizing acetate to CO_2 and electrons but these reactions have both anabolic and catabolic functions in many bacteria. The acetyl group from acetyl-CoA is transferred by citrate synthase to the α-keto, 4-carbon, dicarboxylic acid, oxaloacetate, to form citric acid. The methyl carbon of the acetyl moiety is attached to the 2- or α-carbon of the oxaloacetate with the keto group of oxaloacetate becoming a hydroxyl group. This hydroxyl group is transferred to a different carbon by isocitrate isomerase (aconitase) with the formation of isocitric acid. This hydroxyl group is then oxidized to an α-keto group by isocitrate dehydrogenase with the formation of oxalosuccinic acid. Oxalosuccinic acid is further oxidized with decarboxylation by isocitrate dehydrogenase to form α-ketoglutaric acid, a compound that is important in anabolic pathways. Reactions of the TCA cycle are shown in Fig. 5.6.

In the catabolic TCA cycle, α-ketoglutaric acid is oxidized and decarboxylated by an α-ketoglutarate enzyme complex, involving coenzyme A and lipoic acid. This complex is similar to the pyruvate dehydrogenation complex described previously, with CO_2 produced and a lipoic succinyl intermediate formed. The succinyl group is transferred to coenzyme A to give succinyl-CoA which can be converted to succinic acid with the formation of a high energy bond (ATP) in a manner similar to the formation of acetate from acetyl-CoA. Succinic acid is then oxidized to fumarate by succinate dehydrogenase with the reduction of a flavoprotein.

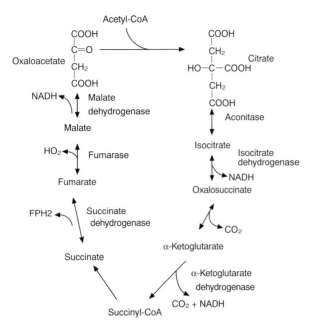

Fig. 5.6 The tricarboxylic acid (TCA) cycle, showing the reactions resulting in the oxidation of acetate to carbon dioxide.

Succinate dehydrogenase (SDH) is a membrane-bound enzyme which is part of the respiratory chain and appears to be present in all aerobic cells. It is composed of 2 subunits, a flavoprotein (FP) and an iron–sulphur protein and, in prokaryotic cells, SDH is fastened to the inner side of the cytoplasmic membrane by a cytochrome. Fumaric acid is hydrated by malate dehydrase (fumarase) to form malate, malate is oxidized by malate dehydrogenase to produce oxaloacetic acid, and the cycle is complete. For each acetate oxidized, provided as acetyl-CoA, 2 molecules of CO_2 and 8 pairs of electrons are obtained. Two of these electrons are transported to flavoproteins and 6 to NAD. An ATP can be obtained from the succinyl-CoA.

Succinate and oxaloacetate, as well as α-ketoglutarate, are important compounds in biosynthetic reactions. Even anaerobic bacteria, which do not utilize the TCA cycle for complete oxidation of acetate, may need TCA cycle enzymes for biosynthetic reactions. However, it would not be efficient for anaerobic bacteria to completely oxidize acetate since they would have difficulty in disposing of the electrons. Such bacteria often lack the α-ketoglutarate enzyme complex. This complex, usually missing in anaerobes, is known as the 'anaerobic lesion' of the TCA cycle.

5.3 Respiration

Respiration is the condition in which **oxygen is the final electron acceptor** of catabolism. In bacteria that can utilize respiration, the presence of oxygen will result in the repression of any fermentation pathways or anaerobic respiration pathways. When oxygen is limiting, a global transcription factor in *E. coli*, termed FNR, related to the CAP protein, activates the tran-

scription of genes for anaerobic energy-generating pathways and represses transcription of genes required for aerobic respiration.

A number of different electron carriers are involved in bacterial respiration, including NAD and NADP, flavoproteins, quinones, iron–sulphur proteins and cytochromes. Flavoproteins are oxidation–reduction enzymes that contain FMN (flavin adenine mononucleotide) or FAD. Flavins are synthesized from riboflavin and, when reduced, transport 2 protons and 2 electrons and are usually written as FPH_2 or FPH2. The actual redox potential of the oxidation–reduction reaction of flavoproteins can vary depending upon the protein group, although a range of 0–0.2 is normal. Quinones are lipids that can carry 2 protons when reduced and can carry electrons to fixed electron carriers. Bacteria have several kinds of quinone: ubiquinone (coenzyme Q), and menaquinone (vitamin K or MK). Bacteria may also possess non-haem iron and sulphur proteins, such as ferredoxin, rubredoxin, and a high potential iron protein (HiPIP) found in some photosynthetic bacteria. These proteins carry only one electron and cover a range of potentials from −0.40 to + 0.35 V. Cytochromes are redox proteins that contain haem and transport a single electron. When cytochromes are reduced, they have characteristic light absorption bands in the visible range and they are usually named for those bands.

Dehydrogenases are enzymes that take electrons from substrates to NAD, to flavoproteins, iron–sulphide proteins and quinones. Oxidases transfer electrons to the final electron acceptor, oxygen in respiration or nitrate in anaerobic respiration. The enzymes transferring electrons to oxygen are called cytochrome oxidases and these oxidases are often inhibited by such chemicals as cyanide, azide or carbon monoxide.

Bacteria may differ greatly in the exact composition of their respiratory chains. Even in individual bacteria, variations can result from changes in growth conditions, such as the amount of oxygen available, especially in the quinones and terminal oxidases. Both *E. coli* and *S. typhimurium* contain branches at the beginning and end of their respiratory pathways and each have 2 NADH dehydrogenases at the beginning of the respiratory chain. Type I NADH dehydrogenase is a large multi-subunit complex, partly integrated in the cell membrane that contributes protons to the electrochemical gradient as it transfers electrons to ubiquinone. The type II NADH dehydrogenases are soluble enzymes, composed of a single subunit, which do not translocate protons.

More than one cytochrome oxidase may be present at the end of the respiratory chain. As an example, *E. coli* can transport electrons through 2 different cytochrome routes depending on whether or not conditions are fully aerobic. With higher levels of oxygen present, a cytochrome *o* oxidase is expressed. Under micro-aerophilic conditions, however, the *cyd* operon is expressed, producing an alternative cytochrome *d* terminal oxidase.

OXIDATIVE PHOSPHORYLATION

It has been known for many years that aerobes gained ATP from the transport of electrons in the cell membrane, a phenomenon called oxidative phosphorylation. During respiration, oxidation–reduction reactions take place in the membrane of the cells so that an electrochemical potential (Dp) or proton-motive force is created with protons on the exterior side of the membrane. Since the respiratory chain consists of hydrogen carriers and electron carriers in alternating sequences across the cytoplasmic membrane and since the cell membrane is impermeable to OH^- and H^+ as oxidation reactions transfer protons from one side of the membrane to the other, a pH gradient and an electrical potential are established across the membrane (Mitchell 1961).

The membrane contains an ATP synthase which is a complex multiprotein system and has been compared to a small organelle. When protons pass from the outside to the inside of the membrane, their passage through the ATP synthase causes inorganic phosphate to be esterified and ADP is converted to ATP. When cell free extracts are prepared, a portion of this ATP synthase complex often becomes solubilized and acts as an ATPase.

ATP synthase is composed of several subunits termed F_0 and F_1. The structure named F_1 consists of 6 different protein subunits that are arranged into 6 knobs reaching to the interior of the cell. The F_1 structure is attached to another set of proteins (F_0) in the cell membrane. The F_0 complex usually consists of 3 different subunits in bacteria and acts as a H^+ channel to translocate H^+ across the cytoplasmic membrane. It has been proposed that a phosphate ion binds to an active site in F_1 and when the 2 protons pass through the F_0 portion of the complex they remove an oxygen atom from the phosphate. The unattached phosphorus bond then binds directly to ADP. This translocation activity is blocked by compounds such as N,N'-dicyclohexylcarbodiimide (DCCD) 1 and antibiotics such as venturicidin and oligomycin. One ATP appears to be produced for every pair of proteins passing through the F_1–F_0 complex.

All bacteria, even strict anaerobes, must maintain an electrochemical gradient of protons across the membrane of the cell. This is needed to support the integrity of the cell membrane, to provide energy for motility and to transport nutrients into the cell. Under anaerobic conditions, the F_1–F_0 complex can function in the reverse direction, hydrolysing ATP by means of an ATP hydrolase associated with the cell membrane to generate an electrochemical gradient. Some fermenting bacteria are also able to use the excretion of fermentation products through the cell membrane to generate a proton gradient.

In some bacteria, Na^+ substitutes for H^+ as the coupling ion and ATP-driven Na^+ pumps have been described in several genera. All cells appear to transfer energy obtained from external sources to energy stored as either ATP, proton- or sodium-motive force. These energy sources may be interconvertible and it appears that any one can satisfy all the energy sources of the cell (Skulachev 1994).

OXYGEN TOXICITY

Cells growing in the presence of molecular oxygen produce some very reactive and toxic oxygen species, such as the superoxide radical, the hydroxyl radical and hydrogen peroxide. In order to protect themselves against such compounds, bacteria have evolved special enzymes. Oxidative stress that results in an increase in the toxic superoxide anion (O_2^-), leads to the induction of superoxide dismutase (SOD) which eliminates the superoxide anion and converts it to hydrogen peroxide. *E. coli* is known to possess 3 species of superoxide dismutase, a Mn-SOD, a Fe-SOD and a Cu,Zn-SOD (Benov and Fridovich 1994).

Hydrogen peroxide is destroyed by catalase and a class of enzymes named peroxidases. Catalase converts hydrogen peroxide to O_2 and water. The synthesis of catalase is normally regulated and the level of activity kept low until needed. *E. coli* has been reported to produce 2 different catalases, hydroperoxidase I and hydroperoxidase II. The synthesis of the first enzyme is increased upon exposure of the cells to hydrogen peroxide whereas the level of the second catalase is controlled by a σ factor (σ^s) that is synthesized at high levels during stationary phase growth and may control as many as 50 genes.

E. coli has 2 separate stress regulons that are triggered by either hydrogen peroxide or redox-cycling agents such as paraquat. Exposure causes the cells to induce the synthesis of about 40 proteins, including a Mn-superoxide dismutase, endonuclease IV, fumarase C, aconitase, NADPH–ferredoxin and glucose-6-phosphate dehydrogenase. In addition to its normal function in providing cells with NADPH and pentoses, glucose-6-phosphate dehydrogenase also appears to be controlled by other regulons, including ones protecting against oxidative stress.

6   CARBOHYDRATE CATABOLISM BY THE STRICT AEROBES

6.1   The KDPG pathway

An alternative route for the conversion of glucose to pyruvate is known as the Entner–Doudoroff pathway or the 2-keto-3-deoxy-6-phosphogluconate (KDPG) pathway, since this latter compound is an intermediate unique for this metabolic route. This catabolic pathway is often a major route for glucose catabolism in strictly aerobic bacteria since such bacteria obtain most of their metabolic energy by oxidative phosphorylation. Most of the electrons transported during oxidative phosphorylation are obtained by the oxidation of acetate via the TCA cycle and the KDPG pathway can convert glucose-6-phosphate to pyruvate in 4 reactions. The 2 enzymes unique to the KDPG route are **glucose-6-phosphate dehydratase** and **KDPG aldolase**.

Glucose-6-phosphate is oxidized to 6-phosphogluconate by the action of glucose-6-phosphate dehydrogenase. The 6-phosphogluconate is dehydrated by **6-phosphogluconate dehydrase**, to form 2-keto-3-deoxy-6-phosphogluconate or KDPG. This latter compound is cleaved by **KDPG aldolase**, producing pyruvate from the first 3 carbons and glyceraldehyde-3-phosphate from the 4-, 5- and 6- carbons. These 2 reactions are shown in Fig. 5.7. The pyruvate can be oxidized and decarboxylated to form acetyl-CoA and the acetyl group can be oxidized via the TCA cycle whereas the glyceraldehyde-3-phosphate produced by the action of KDPG aldolase can be converted to pyruvate by the normal enzymes of the HDP pathway.

The KDPG route in enteric bacteria

The KDPG route is not normally used by *E. coli* cells catabolizing glucose but can be used when gluconic acid is the substrate. *E. coli* catabolizes gluconate by first using gluconokinase to phosphorylate it to 6-phosphogluconate. Some of the 6-phosphogluconate may be oxidized to D-ribulose-5-phosphate and CO_2 and degraded by the HMP pentose route. About half, however, is dehydrated by 6-phosphogluconate dehydrase to KDPG, which is cleaved by KDPG aldolase.

KDPG aldolase is believed to be induced by KDPG (Fradkin and Fraenkel 1972) but gluconokinase and 6-phosphogluconate dehydrase are induced in *E. coli* by gluconate but not glucose. Since *E. coli* is unable to oxidize glucose to gluconate, the KDPG route is not induced when D-glucose is the substrate. With mutants of *E. coli* deficient in KDPG dehydrase, all gluconate must be metabolized through the pentose phosphate route. If another mutation occurs so that the organism also loses 6-phosphogluconate dehydrogenase activity, the cells can not grow on gluconate at all.

6.2   Glucose catabolism by strict aerobes

Glucose catabolism in the genus *Pseudomonas*

The phosphorylated routes for glucose catabolism

In addition to catabolizing D-glucose through phosphorylated intermediates, bacteria in the genus *Pseudomonas* can obtain energy from glucose by an oxidative route, in which phosphorylated compounds are not involved. The phosphorylated route involves the phosphorylation of glucose to glucose-6-phosphate

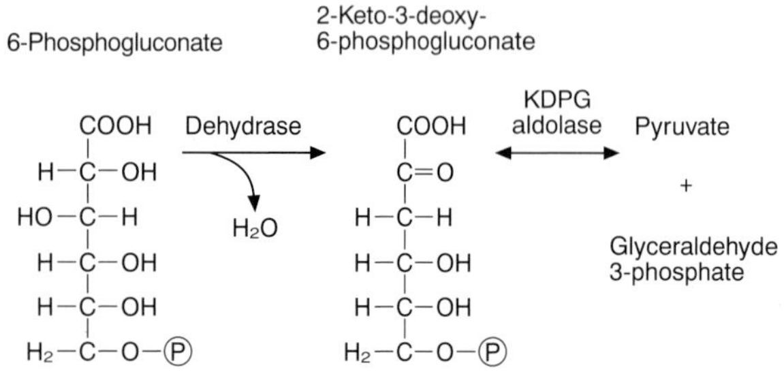

and its oxidation to 6-phosphogluconate. Much of the 6-phosphogluconate formed will be degraded through the KDPG route although some may be diverted to the HMP route. Glucose-6-phosphate isomerase is usually present, and aldolase may also be present, but fructose-6-phosphokinase is often lacking or very weak, so the HDP route usually does not function.

Since aldolase can be present to form fructose-1,6-diphosphate from triose phosphates, some of these organisms may have the ability to convert the glyceraldehyde-3-phosphate, formed by KDPG aldolase, back to fructose-1,6-diphosphate. Phosphatase activity can cleave phosphate to form fructose-6-phosphate and this can be isomerized to glucose-6-phosphate, which can be oxidized and converted to KDPG. This route, from hexose phosphate to KDPG, to triose phosphate, and back to hexose phosphate, can be considered as a KDPG–hexose cycle. Some mutants blocked in the conversion of glyceraldehyde-3-phosphate to pyruvate can still grow on glucose by using this cycle (Lessie and Phibbs 1984).

In many bacteria, the oxidation of glucose-6-phosphate to 6-phosphogluconate also serves an anabolic or biosynthetic function, producing pentoses and reducing power (NADPH) for biosynthetic reactions. In aerobes where glucose-6-phosphate dehydrogenase is also an important catabolic enzyme, the reaction may need to serve both catabolic and biosynthetic purposes. In some cases, either NAD or NADP may serve as the electron acceptor for glucose-6-phosphate dehydrogenase, depending upon the needs of the cell. In other cases, isozymes may be involved in the reaction, one isozyme reducing NAD and another reducing NADP. Two different 6-phosphogluconate dehydrogenases were found in *Pseudomonas putida*, one enzyme constitutive and using NADP as the electron acceptor and one inducible using either NADP or NAD. This latter enzyme was regulated coordinately with the enzymes of the oxidative route and was important in producing the NADH and NADPH needed to reduce 2-ketogluconate to gluconate. It was not found in cells growing on substrates metabolized via the phosphorylated route alone (Lessie and Phibbs 1984). Evidence has been presented that gluconate is often the inducer of both gluconokinase and KDPG dehydrase in *Pseudomonas*. KDPG is the apparent inducer of the KDPG aldolase, but, since the reaction catalysed by KDPG aldolase is reversible, the presence of the products of the reaction can result in its induction.

The route of catabolism for 5-carbon carbohydrates by pseudomonads can be similar in many ways to the KDPG route of glucose catabolism. The aldopentose substrate can be oxidized directly to a pentonic acid and a dehydration reaction can follow to form the 2-keto-3-deoxypentonic acid. This may be cleaved by an aldolase to yield pyruvate and glycolaldehyde with the glycolaldehyde oxidized to glycolic acid. In this manner D-xylose can be oxidized to D-xylonic acid which can be dehydrated to 2-keto-3-deoxyxylonic acid. In a similar manner, D-ribose can be oxidized to ribonic

Fig. 5.7   Reactions of the KDPG route to pyruvate. Two reactions convert 6-phosphogluconic acid to pyruvate and glyceraldehyde-3-phosphate.

acid which can be dehydrated to 2-keto-3-deoxyribonic acid.

THE OXIDATIVE PATHWAY FOR HEXOSES

In addition to the phosphorylated pathways for the catabolism of sugars described above, many pseudomonads also possess oxidative pathways. In this case, flavin or cytochrome-linked, membrane-bound oxidase enzymes, located in the periplasmic space, oxidize the sugars with electrons passing from the electron acceptor directly to O_2. Glucose oxidase oxidizes glucose to form gluconate whereas other oxidases can convert the gluconate to keto sugars such as 2-ketogluconate and 2,6-diketogluconate. The glucose oxidase (sometimes called dehydrogenase) of *Pseudomonas fluorescens* was found to be a quinoprotein whereas the gluconate oxidase was found to be a flavoprotein. Such oxidation reactions, associated with the cell membrane, provide the cells with rapid energy. Pseudomonads lacking glucose oxidase are unable to produce gluconate and can not induce the KDPG pathway enzymes.

The keto sugars formed by the oxidative reactions may be later transported into the cells, phosphorylated and further degraded by phosphorylated routes. Pseudomonads lacking gluconokinase can not form glucose-6-phosphate from glucose but may utilize the oxidized products from the periplasm. Some pseudomonads can grow in the absence of oxygen by using nitrate as an electron acceptor. However, then they must use the direct phosphorylated pathways for catabolism since nitrate will not replace oxygen in the oxidative pathways.

If the oxygen concentration is low, the catabolism of glucose in *P. aeruginosa* is decreased from the extracellular, direct oxidative route to the intracellular, phosphorylative route. The change results in a decrease in the concentrations of glucose dehydrogenase and gluconate dehydrogenase activities and decreases the transport systems for gluconate and 2-ketogluconate, but there is increased activity for glucose transport (Mitchell and Dawes 1982). Global regulatory controls of these strict aerobes differ from the enteric bacteria. The major energy supply comes from oxidative phosphorylation reactions and substrates that can be quickly oxidized, such as acetate or TCA cycle intermediates, cause catabolite repression of glucose catabolism enzymes (MacGregor et al. 1991).

OTHER AEROBIC BACTERIA

The metabolism of bacteria in the genus *Acetobacter* is characterized by a weak HDP pathway, an active KDPG route and an active hexose monophosphate pathway. These bacteria may utilize a hexose cycle with triose phosphate, originating either from the KDPG route or the pentose phosphate route, going to fructose-6-phosphate, glucose-6-phosphate and 6-phosphogluconate. The oxidation of ethanol produces acetate, which is only slowly degraded by a weak or slow TCA cycle. Bacteria classified as *Gluconobacter* do not possess a complete TCA cycle, a complete HDP pathway or a KDPG pathway. They can use glucose either by a terminal oxidative route or a pentose phosphate cycle. Since there is no TCA cycle, acetate is the final product of the oxidation of ethanol.

Other strictly aerobic bacteria tend to favour the degradation of glucose by the KDPG route and the HDP pathway is rarely used, although some glucose carbon may pass through the pentose phosphate pathway. As examples, bacteria in the genus *Agrobacterium* have been reported to catabolize glucose 55% by the KDPG pathway and 44% by the pentose route. For bacteria in the genus *Azotobacter* there is no HDP pathway, the pentose pathway is of minor importance, but the KDPG route is the major pathway for glucose degradation. Bacteria in the genus *Sphaerotilus* have also been reported to metabolize glucose via the KDPG and pentose phosphate pathways as have bacteria in the genus *Rhizobium*. For bacteria in the genus *Arthrobacter*, however, both a HDP pathway and a pentose pathway have been reported. For *Neisseria gonorrhoeae*, about 80–87% of glucose goes through the KDPG pathway whereas 13–20% has been reported to pass through the HMP route.

7 PHOTOSYNTHETIC ELECTRON TRANSPORT

7.1 Purple photosynthetic bacteria

The purple photosynthetic bacteria possess bacteriochlorophyll *a* or *b*, with reaction centres, associated with pigment–protein complexes that absorb light at wavelengths of 400–500 nm and 700–1000 nm. As light energy is transmitted to the reaction centre chlorophyll, an electron becomes energized and leaves the reaction centre, flowing through a series of electron carriers in the membrane and creating a proton-motive force that can be used for the synthesis of ATP in the membrane. One photon of light is believed to result in the synthesis of between 0.66 and one molecule of ATP in the photosynthetic bacteria. During photosynthesis, the purple photosynthetic bacteria use cyclic electron flow where the electron is recycled and reused. However, when reducing power is needed for biosynthesis, NAD and NADP must be reduced and the electrons can not return to the reaction centre. Under these conditions, an external electron donor is required and the green and purple sulphur bacteria, using hydrogen sulphide as a source of electrons, have sulphur as a waste product of photosynthesis.

Two different types of purple bacteria that oxidized ferrous iron to ferric iron in the light have been reported (Ehrenreich and Widdel 1994). These bacteria also used a variety of other substrates as electron sources, including organic compounds, but they did not use free sulphide. Ferrous iron oxidation was dependent upon the presence of both light and carbon dioxide.

7.2 Non-sulphur purple photosynthetic bacteria

Purple non-sulphur bacteria, such as *R. sphaeroides*, are photoheterotrophic and at high oxygen concentration can grow using organic compounds as carbon and energy sources. They contain bacteriochlorophyll *c*, *d* or small amounts of *a*. The photosynthetic apparatus is controlled by oxygen as well as light intensity and can be induced in the absence of light if the oxygen tension should drop below a certain level. Pigment synthesis in *Rhodobacter capsulatus* is repressed by both oxygen and high light intensity. The organism synthesizes its photosynthetic apparatus only under anaerobic growth conditions but cells grown under high light intensity have lower photopigment levels than cells grown under low levels of light.

7.3 The cyanobacteria

Cyanobacteria differ from other photosynthetic bacteria by using water as the source of electrons for photosynthesis. Since there is not sufficient energy in a quantum of light of the wavelength used in photosynthesis to move an electron from H_2O, reduce NADP and still make ATP, 2 light reactions are required to raise electrons to the desired potential. The conversion of light energy into chemical energy (ATP) and reducing power (NADPH) requires light harvesting antenna pigments and electron transport components, as well as the activity of photosystem I (PSI) and photosystem II (PSII). NADPH is produced by linear electron flow through both PSI and PSII, but ATP can be produced by linear electron flow or by cyclic electron flow around PSI alone. PSI is excited by light absorbed by chlorophyll *a* whereas PSII obtains most of its excitation energy from light absorbed by the phycobilisomes. Electrons can be diverted from ferredoxin (FD) to NAD and NADP for CO_2 fixation and non-cyclic photophosphorylation. When electrons are diverted for biosynthetic purposes, oxygen is a waste product of photosynthesis.

Some cyanobacteria can fix N_2 as a nitrogen source, but in all cyanobacteria, the use of nitrogen sources is tightly regulated and the presence of ammonia will result in the repression of the synthesis of enzymes for the use of other nitrogen sources. If ammonia is not present, nitrate or nitrite may be used or, if there are no alternative sources of nitrogen, molecular nitrogen may be fixed into ammonia. If the cells do not possess nitrogenase and have no external sources of nitrogen, they may degrade their phycobiliproteins by a process called chlorosis.

8 METABOLISM AMONG THE ARCHAEBACTERIA

Archaebacteria (domain archaea) encompass 3 basic types: the methanogenic, the halophilic and the sulphur-dependent. The methanogens are strict anaerobes producing methane gas as their final fermentation project. The sulphur-dependent archaebacteria are found in thermophilic environments and either reduce or oxidize sulphur to gain energy. Both aerobic and anaerobic species are known. Many archaebacteria are thermoacidophiles and all seem to have the ability to synthesize D-glucose (gluconeogenesis) from 3-carbon or 4-carbon compounds.

8.1 The methane fermentation

All known methanogens are members of the domain archaea and represent the largest group in that domain with thermophiles, mesophiles and halophiles included in the group. Methanogens are obligatory anaerobic bacteria that reduce CO_2 to produce the most reduced organic compound, methane. Most methanogens are autotrophs and the reduction of CO_2 is their only energy-yielding pathway. However, some methanogens can use other one-carbon compounds such as formate, methanol, methylamines or acetate.

Bacteria in the genus *Methanosarcina* are among the most versatile methanogens in that they can also reduce the methyl groups of methanol or acetate to methane. *Methanosarcina barkeri* can grow on hydrogen and carbon dioxide, but can also use methanol, methylamines and acetate as carbon and energy sources. Such bacteria tend to use the methanol first since it provides more energy. Both phosphotransacetylase and acetate kinase have been found in *Methanosarcina thermophila* and have been shown to convert acetate to acetyl-CoA which activates the pathway for reduction of acetyl-CoA to methane. It has been reported that acetate-grown cells contained nearly 100 polypeptides that are not present in cells grown on methanol (Singh-Wissmann and Ferry 1995). A mutant of *M. barkeri* has been isolated that is capable of growing on pyruvate as the sole carbon and energy source. Apparently, pyruvate:ferredoxin oxidoreductase is used to convert pyruvate to acetyl-CoA whereas CO_2 and methane are products of the fermentation.

In methanogens, ATP formation is coupled to a chemiosmotic ion gradient generated through the translocation of protons, sodium or both. The first step is catalysed by either a tungsten- or molybdenum-containing formyl-methanofuran dehydrogenase. Carbon dioxide is activated on methanofuran and reduction converts it to an aldehyde as tetrahydromethanopterin. This is further reduced to the hydroxyl with hydrogen as the electron donor. Another reduction forms a methyl group which is transferred to coenzyme M to form methyl coenzyme M. The fourth reaction, the reduction of N^5,N^{10}-methenyl-H_4MPT to N^5,N^{10}-methylene-H_4MPT, can be catalysed by either an H_2-dependent (cofactor F_{420}-independent) methylene dehydrogenase (MTH) or a F_{420}-dependent methylene- H_4MPT dehydrogenase (MTD). Finally, 2 methyl-CoM reductases (MRI) and MRII) catalyse the final methane-releasing step. Most of the energy is obtained in the last step which is coupled to the generation of a proton-motive force at the membrane.

Methanogens must synthesize all cellular organic compounds from simple starting material and some methanogens can grow on a completely minimal medium and convert CO_2 to all required organic material. Carbon dioxide is converted to acetyl-CoA which is used for the synthesis of pyruvate. Pyruvate, in turn, is converted to phosphoenolpyruvate, then to oxaloacetate, and other organic compounds by reversal of the citric acid cycle. However, bacteria such as *Methanobacterium* and *Methanosarcina* both assimilate CO_2 but have an incomplete TCA cycle. In *Methanobacterium*, succinate apparently is converted to succinyl coenzyme A and then to α-ketoglutarate. In *Methanosarcina*, oxaloacetate appears to be converted to citrate which is converted to isocitrate and then α-ketoglutarate. Although glucose is not a carbon or energy source for growth, there are some reports of methanogens taking up and metabolizing glucose and the distribution of radioactive label that suggests the presence of the HDP pathway. However, there is no report of the presence of fructose-6-phosphokinase, a key enzyme of the catabolic HDP pathway.

8.2 Halophilic and thermoacidophilic archaebacteria

Many of the halophilic and thermophilic archaea use proteins and amino acids as carbon and energy sources but a few have been shown to use carbohydrates. Some are extreme thermophiles, such as *Thermoplasma* and *Sulfolobus*, and some are extremely halophilic, such as *Halobacterium* and *Halococcus*. *Halobacterium saccharovorum* has been shown to possess a modified KDPG (Entner–Doudoroff) pathway (compare with Fig. 5.7) in which unphosphorylated glucose is oxidized to gluconate by a NAD-dependent dehydrogenase and a gluconate dehydrogenase converts the gluconate into 2-keto-3-deoxygluconate. Next a kinase, using ATP as the phosphate source, phosphorylates the 2-keto-3-deoxygluconate to form 2-keto-3-deoxy-6-phosphogluconate (KDPG). KDPG aldolase cleaves this to form glyceraldehyde-3-phosphate and pyruvate as in the normal KDPG pathway, and glyceraldehyde-3-phosphate is converted to pyruvate by the usual HDP pathway enzymes. Pyruvate is converted to acetyl-CoA using pyruvate:ferredoxin oxidoreductase.

Some halobacteria protect themselves against photochemical damage by possessing a red membrane with purple areas containing carotenoids. These bacteria are obligate aerobes that are able to utilize amino acids and organic acids as carbon and energy sources. At low concentrations of oxygen, ATP is not only generated by oxidative phosphorylation, but also by a type of photosynthesis. The purple areas of the membrane contain bacteriorhodopsin and, in a light-dependent reaction, a proton is released to the outside, establishing an electrochemical gradient across the membrane. During the dark, the proton can return to the inside of the membrane with the formation of ATP.

Thermoacidophilic archaebacteria such as *Sulfolobus solfataricus* and *Thermoplasma acidophilum* have no phosphofructokinase and, therefore, no HDP pathway. Instead, they have been shown to use another variation of the KDPG pathway, a completely nonphosphorylated pathway. Glucose is oxidized to gluconic acid which is dehydrated to 2-keto-3-deoxygluconate. This is cleaved by an aldolase to yield pyruvate and glyceraldehyde. The glyceraldehyde is oxidized to glyceric acid which is phosphorylated to 2-phosphoglyceric acid and converted to phosphoenolpyruvate. The latter compound is cleaved by pyruvate:ferredoxin oxidoreductase. There is no evidence for acetyl phosphate formation as a precursor to acetyl-CoA formation (Danson 1988).

8.3 Sulphate reduction by archaebacteria

D. desulfuricans possesses a strictly anaerobic, clostridial-type of fermentation of glucose and pyruvate. Pyruvate is decarboxylated by pyruvate:ferredoxin oxidoreductase to form acetyl-CoA, carbon dioxide and reduced ferredoxin. *D. desulfuricans* can also grow using lactate if sulphate is present to serve as an electron acceptor. It can also grow using CO_2, H_2 and acetate, if sulphate is present to accept the electrons from the oxidation of hydrogen. Under these conditions, the pyruvate:ferredoxin oxidoreductase reaction is reversed to make pyruvate.

The first reaction in the reduction of sulphate is activation of the sulphate on the end of an AMP molecule, as described previously (p. 107). The enzyme adenyltransferase uses ATP and sulphate to produce adenosine 5′-phosphosulphate (APS) and pyrophosphate. The APS is reduced by APS reductase to sulphite. The sulphite is reduced by reductase to trithionate, which is reduced to thiosulphate and then to sulphide. Energy is gained from oxidative phosphorylation as the electrons flow from ferredoxin to NADH, to flavoproteins, to cytochromes and finally, to sulphate. Two ATP may be obtained for each sulphide formed (Pankhania et al. 1988).

9 BIOSYNTHETIC REACTIONS

9.1 Small molecule biosynthesis

AMINO ACIDS

In general, the normal routes of synthesis for amino acids produce the α-oxoacid and a transamination reaction then adds the amino group. The amino acids may be grouped into 6 families based upon their routes of synthesis (Moat and Foster 1995). Aspartate, threonine, methionine, isoleucine and lysine make up the aspartic group which originates from an intermediate in the TCA cycle, oxaloacetate. Another TCA cycle intermediate, α-ketoglutarate (α-oxoglutarate), is converted to glutamic acid. The triose, 3-phosphoglycerate, is an intermediate in the formation of serine, glycine, cysteine and cystine. Histidine is produced from ATP and phosphoribosylpyrophosphate whereas erythrose-4-phosphate forms shikimate which in turn leads to phenylalanine, tyrosine and tryptophan.

PURINES AND PYRIMIDINES

The cells must have a supply of phosphorylated ribonucleotides and deoxyribonucleotides for the synthesis of RNA and DNA. Purines and pyrimidines are synthesized by quite different routes. The purine ring has as its starting material ribose-5-phosphate whereas the pyrimidine ring originates in aspartate plus carbamoyl phosphate. The pathways of biosynthesis, yielding inosine-5′-phosphate (IMP) and uridylic acid (UMP) respectively, are complex. In bacteria such as *E. coli*, deoxyribonucleoside diphosphates are produced by the reduction of the corresponding ribonucleotide diphosphates in a reaction catalysed by a ribonucleotide reductase. In a few species of bacteria, vitamin B12 is required for the reduction which takes place at the nucleoside triphosphate level. Methylation of the uracil ring to produce thymine occurs at the level of dUMP (deoxyuridine 5′-monophosphate) with methylene tetrahydrofolate usually the donor of the C1 group and the reductant.

FATTY ACIDS AND LIPIDS

Lipids may serve as reserve food materials or as constituents of bacterial membranes, including phospholipids, lipoproteins, glycolipids and the lipopolysaccharide of gram-negative bacteria. Bacteria synthesize fatty acids from acetyl-CoA using an acyl carrier protein (ACP) with a prosthetic group of 4′-phosphopantetheine. Synthesis is accomplished by the addition of C2 units to the growing acyl chain attached to ACP. Introduction of a double bond into a fatty acid molecule to yield a monounsaturated fatty acid can be accomplished in one of 2 ways. Under anaerobic conditions, the β-hydroxydecanoyl-ACP is acted upon by a special dehydratase to yield a *cis* double bond between carbon atoms 3 and 4. Two-carbon units are added until the proper length is obtained. Under aerobic conditions, molecular oxygen is used to introduce hydroxyl groups which can be removed by dehydration reactions to produce double bonds.

9.2 Nitrogen fixation

Some bacteria, such as those in the genera *Clostridium, Klebsiella, Rhizobium, Rhodospirillum, Azotobacter, Mycobacterium, Chromatium* and *Cyanobacterium*, are capable of utilizing nitrogen gas as the sole source of nitrogen for biosynthetic reactions. The reduction of N_2 to ammonia takes place at an enzyme complex termed nitrogenase. The nitrogenase of *Clostridium pasteurianum*, one of the first to be studied, is composed of 2 proteins, azoferredoxin and molybdoferredoxin, with a ratio of 2 molecules of azoferredoxin to one molecule of molybdoferredoxin. Neither protein is active by itself and both contain iron sulphate. The hydrolysis of ATP is used to form H′, a super reduced proton capable of breaking the nitrogen–nitrogen triple bond and reducing N_2.

Azotobacter vinelandii contains 3 different nitrogenases, each able to reduce nitrogen gas to ammonia. If the growth medium contains molybdenum, the molybdenum-containing nitrogenase 1 is synthesized. Nitrogenase 1 has 2 components, dinitrogenase reductase 1 and dinitrogenase 1. If the medium contains vanadium, nitrogenase 2 containing vanadium is produced. This is composed of dinitrogenase reductase 2 and dinitrogenase 2. If the medium does not contain sufficient amounts of either of these 2 metals, nitrogenase 3 is synthesized, composed of dinitrogenase reductase 3 and dinitrogenase 3.

Nitrogenase activity is normally repressed when other nitrogen compounds are available and its activity is inhibited by ADP, destroyed by O_2 and repressed by ammonia. In aerobes the enzyme must be protected from oxygen. A post-translational regulation of nitrogenase activity has been found in many different nitrogen-fixing bacteria. It involves the transfer of the ADP-ribose from NAD to the Arg-101 residue of one subunit of the dinitrogenase reductase dimer, inactivating the enzyme. This group can be removed by another enzyme which restores nitrogenase activity.

9.3 Five-carbon sugars and reducing power

The oxidation of glucose-6-phosphate to 6-phosphogluconate by glucose-6-phosphate dehydrogenase is an important reaction for the biosynthesis of 5-carbon compounds as well as the generation of NADPH for biosynthetic reduction reactions. Mutants of *E. coli* lacking glucose-6-phosphate dehydrogenase can still make 5-carbon sugars for biosynthetic purposes by utilizing intermediates of the HDP pathway and reversing the TK–TA reactions. Cells deficient in reduced NADPH may transfer electrons from NADH by use of an oxidoreductase enzyme (transhydrogenase), that can transfer electrons between these electron carriers.

Some strains of *Streptococcus mutans*, which lack both glucose-6-phosphate dehydrogenase and 6-phosphogluconate dehydrogenase, have 2 glyceraldehyde-3-phosphate dehydrogenases, one specific for the reduction of NAD^+ and the other reducing $NADP^+$, and this provides NADPH for biosynthetic reactions. The $NADP^+$-associated dehydrogenase is not dependent upon the presence of phosphate, carries out the irreversible oxidation of glyceraldehyde-3-phosphate with the formation of 3-phosphoglycerate, and can provide the NADPH required for biosynthetic reactions. A similar enzyme has been shown to exist in *Streptococcus salivarius* (Boyd, Cvitkvitch and Hamilton 1995).

9.4 TCA cycle intermediates as biosynthetic compounds

Bacterial cells need many intermediates for biosynthetic purposes, including 6-carbon sugars for synthesis of cell walls, triose phosphates to make glycerol and lipids, and acetyl-CoA for the synthesis of fatty acids. In aerobic bacteria, the TCA cycle functions to oxidize acetate and provide energy. However, another major function of the TCA cycle enzymes is to produce intermediates such as α-ketoglutaric acid and oxaloacetic acid for biosynthetic reactions. During the TCA cycle, one oxaloacetate combines with the acetyl group from an acetyl-CoA to yield citric acid which eventually is converted back to oxaloacetate and there is no net gain in di- or tricarboxylic acid TCA intermediates. Since some of these intermediates are being used for biosynthetic reactions, mechanisms must exist for their net synthesis.

A very important biosynthetic enzyme, especially in enteric bacteria, is **phosphoenolpyruvate carboxylase**, which forms oxaloacetate from phosphoenolpyruvate and carbon dioxide. Once formed, oxaloacetate can be converted to aspartic acid or reduced to malate by malate dehydrogenase with the oxidation of NADH. Malate dehydrase (fumarase) removes water from malate to form fumarate and fumarate reductase can reduce the fumarate to form succinate. Oxaloacetate and aceyl-CoA can also yield citric acid which can be converted to α-ketoglutaric acid by normal TCA cycle enzymes. These reactions regenerate TCA intermediates and replace those used for biosynthesis. The enzyme phosphoenolpyruvate carboxylase is biosynthetic in its regulation and is inhibited by aspartate. Mutants of enteric bacteria that lack the enzyme are unable to grow on a glucose-salts minimal medium unless the medium is supplemented with a compound capable of providing a TCA cycle intermediate.

The glyoxylate bypass

Some bacteria can grow aerobically using acetate, pyruvate or lactate as carbon and energy sources. These bacteria must have the enzyme capability to reverse the HDP pathway and form pentoses and hexoses from these simple 2- and 3-carbon compounds. If pyruvate or lactate are substrates, *E. coli* can use the enzyme phosphoenolpyruvate synthase and ATP to convert pyruvate back to PEP with AMP and inorganic phosphate as products. The HDP pathway can then be reversed (glucogenesis) to fructose-1,6-diphosphate and a phosphatase can cleave phosphate from the 1-carbon position to yield fructose-6-phosphate. The PEP also can be combined with CO_2 (phosphoenolpyruvate carboxylase) to form oxaloacetate which can be converted to other TCA cycle intermediates.

However, if a bacterium, such as *E. coli*, is growing aerobically with acetate and CO_2 as the sole carbon sources, the cells must still be able to synthesize pyruvate and TCA cycle intermediates. Whereas some strict anaerobes are able to reverse the pyruvate:ferredoxin oxidoreductase reaction to form pyruvate from CO_2 and acetate, most bacteria that can grow with only acetate as the carbon source incorporate it into TCA cycle intermediates (see Fig. 5.6) by a series of reactions known as the **glyoxylate bypass or glyoxylate cycle**.

This metabolic route first phosphorylates acetate to form acetyl phosphate which is converted to acetyl-CoA. The acetyl-CoA is combined with a molecule of existing oxaloacetic acid to form citrate and the citrate is isomerized to isocitrate by normal TCA cycle enzymes. A unique enzyme, however, **isocitrate lyase**, cleaves the isocitrate to produce succinate and glyoxylate. The glyoxylate is condensed with acetyl-CoA by the enzyme **malate synthase** to form malate as shown in Fig. 5.8. In this manner, one oxaloacetate and 2 acetyl groups have been converted to malate and succinate. These latter 2 compounds can be oxidized and converted to 2 oxaloacetates so the overall series of reactions form 2 oxaloacetates from one oxaloacetate and two acetates. Oxaloacetate can be used to form other TCA intermediates for biosynthetic purposes and some can be decarboxylated to PEP by the enzyme phosphoenolpyruvate carboxykinase.

Data suggest that only one isocitrate lyase exists in *E. coli* regardless of the carbon source used for growth (Ikeda, Houtz and LaPorte 1992). The genes coding for isocitrate lyase and malate synthase are located in the same operon and the synthesis of the enzymes is regulated so they are formed when 2-carbon intermediates are the sole source of carbon other than CO_2. The enzymes of the bypass are induced by acetate and repressed by most other carbon compounds. The flow of isocitrate through the glyoxylate bypass, rather than the TCA cycle, is controlled by activation and deactivation of isocitrate dehydrogenase. When bacteria are grown on glucose, isocitrate dehydrogenase is fully operational but when cells are grown on acetate, the activity of the enzyme is decreased by 70% (Chung, Klumpp and LaPorte 1988). This decrease is the result of the enzyme being phosphorylated at multiple sites by isocitrate dehydrogenase kinase/phosphatase. Some strains of *E. coli* can not grow upon acetate without the expression of this regulatory enzyme (Cortay et al. 1988).

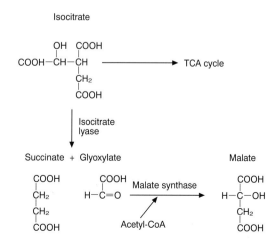

Fig. 5.8 Reactions of the glyoxylate bypass. Oxaloacetate and acetate are converted to citrate and then isocitrate. The isocitrate is cleaved to succinate and glyoxylate and the glyoxylate is combined with another acetate to yield malate.

9.5 Methods for incorporation of one-carbon compounds into cellular material

THE CALVIN CYCLE FOR CO_2 FIXATION

Various different pathways exist among micro-organisms for the conversion of carbon dioxide into organic compounds. As mentioned previously (p. 115), phosphoenolpyruvate carboxylase and phosphoenolpyruvate carboxykinase can convert carbon dioxide into oxaloacetate. Strict anaerobes that possess pyruvate:ferredoxin oxidoreductase can, with proper reducing potential, reverse the normal reaction to convert acetyl-CoA and CO_2 to pyruvate.

The Calvin cycle, sometimes termed the reductive pentose phosphate pathway, is found in some photosynthetic bacteria and many chemoautotrophs and involves the conversion of a 5-carbon sugar and CO_2 to form 2 molecules of 3-phosphoglyceric acid. The unique enzymes of the Calvin cycle are **phosphoribulokinase**, converting ribulose-5-phosphate to ribulose-1,5-biphosphate, and **ribulose biphosphate carboxylase** (sometimes called ribulose-1,5-biphosphate carboxylase/oxygenase). Ribulose-1,5-biphosphate carboxylase converts ribulose biphosphate and CO_2 to 2 3-phosphoglyceric acids. The enzyme is strongly inhibited by 6-phosphogluconate, which can act as a signal to the cells that organic substrates are present and CO_2 fixation is not required.

To form additional organic compounds, the 3-phosphoglyceric acid is phosphorylated with the use of ATP and phosphoglycerate kinase, to 1,3-diphosphoglyceric acid. This latter compound is reduced by glyceraldehyde-3-phosphate dehydrogenase to glyceraldehyde-3-phosphate, which can be converted to dihydroxyacetone phosphate by triose phosphate isomerase. Aldolase can catalyse the synthesis of fructose-1,6-diphosphate from the triose phosphates and fructose-1,6-diphosphate phosphatase can cleave the phosphate from the 1-carbon position to produce fructose-6-phosphate. A variety of enzyme pathways exist to regenerate the pentose phosphates from hexose phosphates.

THE ARNON CYCLE FOR CO_2 FIXATION

Bacteria such as cyanobacteria, Rhodospirillaceae, Chromatiaceae and Chloroflexaceae will use the Calvin cycle for CO_2 fixation when growing with CO_2 as the only carbon source. Organisms such as the Chlorobiaceae, however, do not possess the enzymes of the Calvin cycle. This family of organisms uses the Arnon cycle, also known as the reductive TCA cycle or the reductive C_4 dicarboxylic acid CO_2 fixation pathway.

The fixation of CO_2 begins with the reversal of the pyruvate:ferredoxin oxidoreductase reaction and the formation of pyruvate from acetyl-CoA and CO_2. To convert the pyruvate to PEP the enzyme pyruvate orthophosphate dikinase and ATP are used to form PEP, AMP and inorganic pyrophosphate. The PEP is carboxylated to oxaloacetate and the normal TCA cycle is reversed, with the oxaloacetate reduced to malate and the malate dehydrated to fumarate. The fumarate is reduced to succinate by NADH and a special enzyme, fumarate reductase, and the succinate is phosphorylated and changed to succinyl coenzyme A. The enzyme reaction producing succinyl-CoA during the normal TCA cycle is irreversible, so a special enzyme is employed during the Arnon cycle, an α-ketoglutarate–ferredoxin oxidoreductase. The α-ketoglutarate is changed to citrate by normal enzymes of the TCA cycle and an ATP-citrate lyase cleaves citrate to form oxaloacetate and acetyl-CoA. Through these reactions, 4 molecules of CO_2 have been converted to one molecule of oxaloacetate which can be used for other biosynthetic purposes.

OTHER PATHWAYS FOR INCORPORATION OF ONE-CARBON COMPOUNDS INTO CELLULAR MATERIAL

Methanotrophs are gram-negative bacteria that use methane as their sole source of carbon and energy. To obtain energy, methane is converted to methanol by methane mono-oxygenase (MMO). The methanol is then oxidized to formaldehyde which can be further oxidized to carbon dioxide to provide energy or converted into cellular material. The MMO exists in either of 2 forms, a cytoplasmic (soluble) form and a membrane-bound (particulate) form.

Methylotrophic bacteria can use methanol as the only source of carbon for biosynthetic reactions. Such bacteria include those in the genus *Methylomonas* as well as the newly isolated *Mycobacterium gastri* MB19. Methanol is oxidized to formaldehyde by alcohol oxidase and the formaldehyde is added to D-ribulose monophosphate by the enzyme hexulose phosphate synthase. The product is D-fructose-6-phosphate which can be converted to other carbohydrates such as glucose-6-phosphate and glyceraldehyde-3-phosphate, or converted back to ribulose-5-phosphate by means of the transketolase and transaldolase rearrangements. The enzyme is specific for D-ribulose-5-phosphate as a substrate but can use other aldehydes, such as glycolaldehyde, in place of formaldehyde (Kato et al. 1988, Beisswenger and Kula 1991).

The methane-producing bacteria have the ability to synthesize acetate from one-carbon compounds. The methyl group of acetate comes from methyltetrahydromethanopterin which is a folate analogue and an intermediate in the reduction of CO_2 to methane. Another molecule of CO_2 is reduced to a bound carbon monoxide by carbon monoxide dehydrogenase and the molecules are condensed to form acetyl-CoA.

10 GROWTH OF BACTERIA

10.1 Bacterial nutrition and culture media

A minimal medium is one that contains the simplest chemical composition needed to support the growth of an organism. Some bacteria can grow quite well on a minimal medium consisting of distilled water, a carbon and energy source such as D-glucose, and some inorganic salts, for example sodium and potassium phosphates, ammonium sulphate, magnesium sulphate and ferrous sulphate. Bacteria able to grow in such a medium must be able to gain metabolic energy by the catabolism of glucose, and to synthesize all organic molecules needed for growth from carbon degradation products of the glucose and the inorganic salts. This carbohydrate-salts medium is **chemically defined**, in that the exact chemical composition is known and can be reproduced. Stating that such a medium is defined ignores the requirement for trace elements such as copper, zinc, cobalt, etc., that are required in only minute amounts and are provided as contaminants in the other ingredients.

If an organism lacks the enzymatic capability to synthesize any organic biosynthetic compounds from such a medium, then growth of that organism can not occur using that medium unless such compounds are provided. If a mutant of *E. coli* loses that ability to synthesize an amino acid, then that amino acid has become a required growth factor and must be added to the medium for growth of that mutant to occur. Many bacteria, especially those whose natural environment contains many complex organic compounds, such as pathogens, are unable to synthesize a wide range of biosynthetic intermediates, such as amino acids, nucleosides, vitamins, etc., and these must be supplied to permit growth. Such a growth medium may be complicated and difficult to assemble, but it is still chemically defined in that the exact chemical composition is known. Because a chemically defined growth medium is reproducible, it is often preferred for studies on the metabolism of bacteria.

Complex and rich bacterial growth media such as those made from nutrient broth (beef extract and peptone) or L-broth (peptone and yeast extract) will support the growth of many bacteria and are convenient to use, but such media are undefined in that the exact chemical composition is not known. Complex and undefined media of these types are often used for the isolation and growth of bacteria but it should be realized that the exact composition of such media may vary from batch to batch.

Microbiologists have been ingenious in devising selective media that are designed for the isolation from natural sources of a particular type of micro-organism. Such media are designed to facilitate the growth of organisms possessing the properties of the one to be isolated while discouraging, as far as possible, growth of contaminating organisms. **Enrichment cultures** are not only designed to possess the proper media for isolation of a desired organism, but growth conditions such as temperature can also be designed to aid in the isolation. A wide variety of media have also been designed to aid in the rapid isolation and identification of micro-organisms, especially pathogens.

10.2 Growth in liquid culture

A growing bacterial cell increases in size until it separates into 2 daughter cells. If growth is balanced and the replication of the macromolecules has been carefully controlled, all the macromolecules of the mother cell must have doubled in mass and each daughter cell is a duplicate of the mother cell. At that time, a cell generation or division cycle has taken place. The growth of bacterial cells may become temporarily unbalanced, due to environmental stress, but regulatory systems will normally adjust growth rates so that synthesis of macromolecules once again becomes balanced. Continued unbalanced growth can lead to cell death.

Measurement of cell number is often done by viable cell count. With the pour plate method, various dilutions of cells are mixed into tubes of a melted agar-growth medium that has been cooled to just above the temperature of solidification. The tubes are poured into petri dishes and, after incubation, the number of colonies is taken as the number of viable cells in the original dilution. An alternative method is the spread plate method, where samples of 0.1 or 0.2 ml of the appropriate cell dilutions are spread over the surface of a solidified agar-growth medium plate. The spread plate method is reported to give slightly higher colony counts and has the advantage that individual colonies can be easily sampled for further testing.

Such information as the viable cell count or number is valuable to many microbiologists, especially those concerned with infectious diseases or food poisoning, since it counts cells capable of growth. However, such techniques really measure colony-forming units, not necessarily individual cells, as clusters of cells in packets or chains will give a single colony. Also, it takes many generations of growth for a single cell to produce a colony visible to the unaided human eye. By this technique, a bacterial cell could produce hundreds of thousands of descendants and still be classified as non-viable. A direct cell count measures all the cells present, including those not capable of growth. It is possible to count the total number of cells per unit volume, both living and dead, microscopically, using a special slide. Cell count and mass can also be determined by impedance counting in which cells pass through a narrow chamber and disrupt the flow of an electrical current.

A problem with using viable or total cell counts to measure bacterial growth is the inability to detect increases in cell mass during the division cycle. Growing bacterial cells must increase their mass before division and an increase in cell mass must be considered as growth, even though the cell number may not have increased. Cell mass can be determined directly by measurement of cell weight after drying a sample of cells in an oven. Cell mass is often estimated by determining the light scattering of a suspension of bacterial cells with a standard curve to relate light scattering to mass.

The amount of bacterial growth that has taken place

in a culture can be estimated by a variety of methods that measure a result of growth rather than cell number. The disappearance of a substrate such as glucose, or the utilization of oxygen during respiration, can be determined. A product of growth such as cell DNA, RNA or protein can be determined, or, during fermentation, the amount of acid produced might be used as an estimate of cell growth.

The time for a division cycle to be completed is the time for a generation of growth to take place and is known as the **generation time**. If growth of a bacterial culture is **synchronized**, all cells are in exactly the same phase of the division cycle and all will divide simultaneously. With synchronized cell division, the total cell number immediately increases from the initial number (N_0) to $2 \times N_0$. If the cells remain synchronized, another generation will simultaneously raise the cell number to $2 \times 2N_0$. Techniques that have been used for synchronizing cell cultures involve the germination of spores, filtration or centrifugation of cells to obtain a constant size cell, and preventing initiation of DNA replication by amino acid starvation. Special mutants have also been used, such as those with temperature-sensitive mutations in genes required for initiation of DNA replication, to prevent cell growth at the restrictive temperature. Upon change to permissive temperature, DNA replication in all cells in the culture will begin simultaneously and all cells will enter the same phase of the division cycle. Synchronization of cell growth can be useful in studying cell chemistry at different phases of the division cycle, but synchronization usually only lasts for a few generations.

CELL GENERATIONS AND GROWTH RATES

Since the total cell number doubles each division cycle or generation (g), the number of cells produced by growth (N) will be equal to the original number (N_0) times 2 to the power g. Therefore:

$$N = N_0 \times 2^g$$

It is normal to use logarithms to the base 10 to solve this equation and calculate the value of g.
Since $\log_{10}2$ is equal to 0.301, the equation becomes:

$$\frac{\text{Log}_{10}N - \text{Log}_{10}N_0}{0.301} = g$$

If cell mass (M) is being determined rather than cell number, then M could be substituted for N. Once the number of generations is known, the average generation time (t) can be calculated by dividing the time for growth (T) by the number of generations that have taken place during that time period.

The rate of increase of bacterial number (or mass) is exponential since the population doubles with each generation. If the bacteria are growing at a constant rate, then a plot of cell number or mass against time results in an exponential curve as shown in Fig. 5.9(a). The plot of the $\log_{10}$ of bacterial number / mass

against time will give a linear relationship, as shown in Fig. 5.9(b), provided the cells are growing at a constant rate. This is the conventional method of plotting bacterial growth.

The rate of increase in total cell number during growth is the initial cell number times the specific growth rate constant (μ):

$$\frac{\text{d}M}{\text{d}T} = \mu M$$

The value of the specific growth rate constant can be derived from the plot of log N versus t where its value will be given by the slope of the linear plot.

THE GROWTH PHASES AND THE GROWTH CURVE

The lag phase

When an inoculum of cells are transferred to a growth medium, a delay may take place before measurable growth occurs. This lag time is a period where cells are adjusting to new growth conditions and growth may be temporarily unbalanced during this growth phase. The greater the change in growth conditions experienced by the cells, the longer the predicted lag

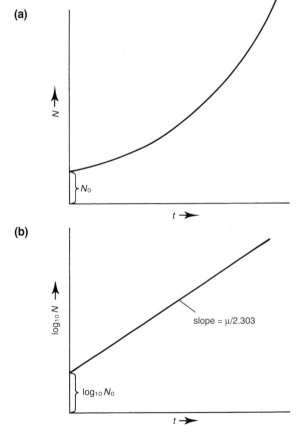

Fig. 5.9 Theoretical growth curves illustrating instantaneous exponential growth in a bacterial batch culture. Total cell number (N, i.e. number of bacterial cells per ml) plotted against time (t). N_0, inoculum cell concentration; μ, specific growth rate.

phase. Since cells must increase their size before cell division can take place, their exact length of the lag period may depend upon whether cell number or cell mass is being measured. A typical bacterial growth curve, with lag, exponential and stationary and phases, is shown in Fig. 5.10.

The exponential (logarithmic) growth phase

Once the cells have adjusted their regulatory systems to produce maximum growth under the new conditions, the culture enters the exponential or logarithmic growth phase where cells have approximately the same generation time. Growth is normally not synchronized and, at any moment, cells will be in different stages of the division cycle. In batch culture the growth rate eventually must begin to decrease as the availability of some essential nutrient becomes limiting or the accumulation of some produce becomes toxic.

The stationary phase

Eventually the stationary phase is reached, a period when measurable growth ceases. Note that if a new viable cell was formed for each cell that lost viability or if loss and increase in cell mass were balanced, there would be no measurable increase in cell growth.

If *E. coli* cells are growing on a minimal salts medium containing a carbon and energy source and the energy source becomes exhausted, the pH will remain constant and growth and nitrogen utilization will both stop. However, under conditions in which the nitrogen becomes depleted and the energy source is in excess, the cells will continue to use the energy source, even if the energy gained from catabolism is discarded. If possible, the bacteria will increase their internal supply of reserve food material under these conditions, while denying surrounding microorganisms a potential energy source. Traditionally, 'resting cells' of bacteria are those incubated without any added nitrogen source. Such cells are still able to induce enzymes and catabolize carbohydrates and these types of resting cells have been used for many metabolic studies.

The death phase

Some bacteria retain viability upon reaching the stationary phase whereas others rapidly lose viability and enter a death phase. A variety of reasons may cause bacteria to lose viability. Some bacteria produce autolysins under these conditions and cause their own lysis. Reserve food sources that may be accumulated by bacteria, such as poly-β-hydroxybutyric acid and glycogen, are usually used quickly when the cells are starving but once such reserve food materials are exhausted, cellular RNA may serve as its major source of energy. Ribosomal RNA degradation may increase 208-fold during starvation conditions and within 4 h of starvation *E. coli* can degrade 20–30% of its RNA. The degradation of ribosomes will lead to the eventual death of the cell since cells lacking ribosomes are incapable of synthesizing protein. Starvation also increases the rate of protein degradation and peptidase-deficient mutants of *E. coli* have been shown

to have poor survival during starvation for carbon and nitrogen. Nine soluble endoproteolytic activities that degrade protein substrates have been described in that organism. The amino acids produced by protein degradation can be used for the synthesis of new proteins to aid in survival under stress conditions.

A drop in internal energy levels may prevent the cells from proper transport functions of the cytoplasmic membrane so that, upon transfer to recovery medium, the cell is unable to take up nutrients. The energy charge of a cell has been reported as the total ATP plus half the ADP over the totals of the cellular ATP, ADP and AMP. Since 2 ADP are capable of forming one ATP and one AMP, the amount of ATP that can be obtained from ADP is equal to one-half the ADP present. The equation:

$$\text{Energy charge} = \frac{\text{ATP} + \frac{1}{2}\text{ADP}}{\text{ATP} + \text{ADP} + \text{AMP}}$$

gives the ratio of available ATP to the total adenine nucleotides present. If all of these nucleotides were in the form of the triphosphate, the energy charge would be one. For the normal growth and metabolism of bacterial cells, the energy charge must be maintained in the range of 0.8–0.95. *E. coli* has been reported to grow only when the energy charge is over 0.8, it will maintain its viability when the energy charge is between 0.5 and 0.8, but it will die when the value is under 0.5. There is a certain amount of maintenance energy required just for cells to repair continuing damage but this may vary for different organisms. In experiments with *E. coli*, it was found that once the glucose was exhausted the organism maintained its energy charge at 0.8 by using acetate that had been excreted during growth on glucose. If no other substrates were present then the capacity for protein synthesis and enzyme induction was lost along with cell viability.

Since a starving cell must maintain a certain level of metabolism and energy to remain viable, many bacteria activate special regulatory systems in response to· starvation, regulatory systems that allow them to express 'starvation' genes (Matin 1992). These new proteins improve the cell's ability to use low levels of nutrients, regulate the degradation of their own polymers for carbon and energy, and aid the cells in surviving. Many of these genes encoding for these proteins require cAMP for their induction. The starvation stress regulatory system may overlap with other stress regulatory systems since starved *E. coli* cells have been shown to acquire resistance to heat stress.

A nucleotide involved in the stringent response, ppGpp, has an essential role in the regulatory adjustments made by cells starved for amino acids. In cells with an insufficient carbon source, the stringent response will cause a rapid reduction in the rates of synthesis of protein and RNA. Apparently ppGpp can be synthesized by 2 different methods. The one described previously requires ribosomes binding to both mRNA and an uncharged tRNA. Another method, however, appears to be ribosome-independent since mutants unable to synthesize the stringent factor protein still have a slow increase in the concentration of ppGpp when starved for carbon (Matin et al. 1989).

CHANGING GROWTH RATES

The rate of growth of a bacterial strain may be shifted up or down with changes in growth conditions, such as medium composition or temperature. Shift-up experiments refer to a change in growth conditions with an increase in the growth rate of a bacterium. As an example, an improvement in nutrient conditions can lead to an increase in the internal amino acid concentration, thus resulting in an increase in rate of RNA synthesis, an increase in rate of protein synthesis, and a more frequent initiation of DNA synthesis. Faster growing cells tend to be larger, with an increase in the amount of the protein synthesizing machinery, the RNA. While the regulatory systems are adjusting to the new conditions, the cell length may continue to increase and the cell may become unusually long. Eventually, the cell length decreases to reach the proper size for the new growth rate (Cooper 1991).

By contrast, a transfer of cells from a complex undefined medium, such as a nutrient broth, to a minimal salts medium can result in a shift-down or decrease in growth rate caused by a sudden decrease in internal concentration of nutrients, such as amino acids. A decrease in the internal concentration of amino acids leads to a stringent response with a decline in the rate of RNA synthesis, a decline in the rate of protein synthesis, and a less frequent initiation of DNA replication. In fact, DNA synthesis may halt altogether, until activation of biosynthetic pathways can produce the required building block compounds to permit cell growth.

10.3 Continuous culture of bacterial cells

Chemostat is a name given to devices that maintain the growth of bacteria in a constant exponential growth rate. A typical chemostat possesses a container containing sterile growth medium that is transferred into the growth chamber at a controlled rate. The growth chamber has an overflow device so that the entrance of new medium results in the overflow and exit of an equal volume of used medium as shown in Fig. 5.10.

CHEMOSTAT GROWTH RATES

The medium in the growth chamber of a chemostat can be inoculated with a bacterium to give an initial cell concentration of N. If growth takes place, the rate of increase in cell mass against time can be represented by $\Delta N / \Delta t = \mu N$, where N is the cell number per unit volume and μ stands for the growth rate constant. The rate of increase in cell number can be represented as μN. If the growth rate constant is a positive number, the cell mass in the chemostat will be increasing. However, new media is introduced into the chemostat at a constant flow rate and old media is overflowing out of the chemostat at the same rate,

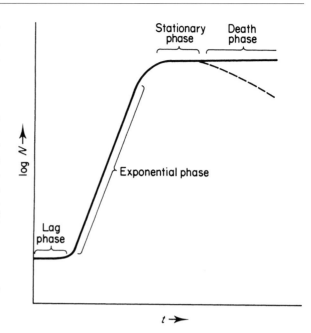

Fig. 5.10 Idealized growth curve of a bacterial batch culture. ——, total cell count; ·····, viable cell count.

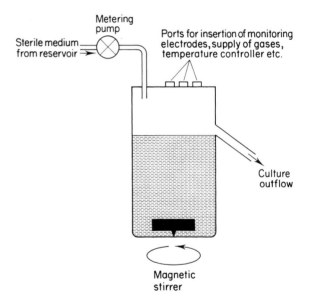

Fig. 5.11 Principal features of a continuous flow culture apparatus.

removing cells. If the flow rate into the chamber is F volumes per unit time period, and the volume of the growth chamber is V, then the fraction of the culture media that overflows and is replaced each unit time period is represented by F / V. Therefore, the total amount of cells lost each time period by overflow would be $N \times F / V$. The real rate of change of cell number in the chemostat is the rate of increase due to growth (μN), minus the rate of decrease due to washout which is $N \times F / V$. Therefore, the rate of change in the chemostat is $\mu \times N - N \times F / V$, or $N(\mu - F / V)$.

If F / V is greater than μ, the cells are being washed out of the chemostat faster than they can grow and eventually all the cells will leave the chemostat. If F / V is smaller than μ, the number of cells will increase. However, as the cell mass increases, there are more cells competing for a constant food supply, since the flow rate into the growth chamber is constant and this competition causes a decrease in the growth rate constant. Eventually μ will decrease until it equals F / V and then a steady state will exist, with μ held constant. In such a manner, by controlling the rate of flow of new medium into the chemostat, the experimenter can control the growth rate of the cells in the chemostat.

Chemostats are usually established with the growth rate limited by a single known factor, such as a limiting supply of a required growth factor or the carbon and energy source. Chemostats are very useful for obtaining mutants, since once a growth rate is established there is strong evolutionary pressure for the selection of mutants that have increased their growth rates under the competitive chemostat conditions. However, chemostat experiments must often be terminated because of the selection of 'sticky' mutants that cling to the culture vessel surface and are not washed out.

Chemostat cell populations

If the concentration of the limiting nutrient in the reserve chamber is designated as S_r and the unused amount of that nutrient that washes out of the chemostat is S, then the amount of nutrient used by the cells in the growth chamber is $S_r - S$. If Q represents the amount of that limiting nutrient needed to make one bacterial cell, then the total population of cells will be equal to $S_r / Q - S / Q$. However, S is usually close to zero and then the equation becomes S_r / Q, which represents the total population of cells. The growth rate in the chemostat is controlled by the rate of flow of new media into the chemostat, but the total population of cells present is determined by the concentration of the limiting substrate.

10.4   Growth on solid surfaces

Good growth for a bacterium such as *E. coli*, on rich medium, under aerobic conditions, may range from 10^{10} to 5×10^{10} cells per ml. The final yield of cells per ml in liquid culture can be considerably increased if the cells are placed within a dialysis sack that is suspended in a large vessel of growth medium. The dialysis sack permits waste products to diffuse out of the sack, away from the cells, while fresh nutrients can diffuse into the sac. Cells growing on an agar surface can form colonies with high concentrations of cells per unit volume for a similar reason. The agar permits nutrients to diffuse toward the colony while waste products diffuse away.

The nutritional state of bacteria may also influence their adhesion to solid surfaces. Many bacteria have increased adhesion under starvation conditions but some bacteria actually display the opposite effect. Colonization of surfaces by bacteria may be influenced by motility and cell surface hydrophobicity as well as nutritional status (James et al. 1995).

10.5   Growth of bacteria under extreme conditions

Extreme thermophiles

Organisms that grow in extreme environments have been termed extremophiles. In recent years extreme thermophilic bacteria have been isolated whose very existence would have been doubted only a few years ago. Bacteria in the domain archaea seem to be more common under natural growth conditions of extreme temperature and pressure. Especially interesting are the organisms isolated from then deep abyssal vents. Although glass plates placed in such vents have shown the attachment of micro-organisms at temperatures of 120–130°C, it can not be proved that the organisms are living when they became attached.

A number of studies have attempted to correlate growth at high temperatures with temperature resistance of enzymes. The enzyme adenylate kinase has been studied from one mesophilic and 3 thermophilic archaea bacteria in the genus *Methanococcus*. The mesophilic bacterium grew at an optimum temperature of 30°C whereas the thermophilic bacteria grew at optimum temperatures of 70, 80 and 80–90°C, respectively. The optimum temperature for activity for each enzyme was similar to the optimum temperature of growth from the bacterium from which it was isolated, but no correlation could be found between amino acid compositions and the enzyme's optimal temperature for activity (Rusnak, Haney and Konisky 1995).

The extreme thermophilic archaea bacterium *S. solfataricus*, in the bacteria family Sulfolobaceae, can grow using sulphur or organic compounds as electron sources. The enzyme maltase, isolated from this organism, was found to have a temperature optimum of 105°C, the highest temperature optimum so far reported for an enzyme from this bacterial family. The half-life of the enzyme was 2.75 h at 100°C and the pH optimum at 85°C was 4.5. The native enzyme was resistant to proteases but, when denatured, the enzyme was degraded by trypsin, chymotrypsin and proteinase K. The purified enzyme from *S. solfataricus* did not appear to be structurally related to maltases from eubacteria (Rolfsmeier and Blum 1995).

Another enzyme that has been isolated and characterized from a hypothermophilic archaea bacterium is the tungsten-containing, aldehyde ferredoxin oxidoreductase which catalyses the oxidation of aldehydes to acids with reduction of the ferredoxin. The source of the enzyme was *Pyrococcus furiosus* which has an optimal growth rate of 100°C. The enzyme had an optimal temperature for activity of more than 95°C but its amino acid composition was not unusual. The enzyme does have a reduced rate of surface area to volume, as compared to other enzymes, and it was suggested that this might be related to the enzyme's thermostability (Chan et al. 1995).

BAROPHILES

Bacteria that have an increased growth rate at pressures above one atmosphere are termed barophiles (also known as piezophiles). For example, the deep-sea, thermophilic archaea *Methanococcus jannaschii*, has been grown in a high-pressure, high-temperature bioreactor at 86°C and 500 atmospheres of hyperbaric pressure. Eubacteria are known to adapt to changes in temperature by changing the fatty acids in the cell membranes and it has been suggested that archaea may have an advantage in survival under such extreme conditions because the membrane lipids of archaea differ from those of eubacteria (Kaneshiro and Clark 1995). The lipid chains of archaea are based on saturated isoprenoid alcohols containing 20 or 40 carbon atoms, often connected to a glycerol by ether bonds. Shifts in temperature or pressure of some archaea have been shown to result in changes in the distribution of their core lipids. Therefore, the ability of micro-organisms to survive at high pressures may result not only from changes in enzyme stability but also from shifts in the organism's membrane lipid composition.

REFERENCES

Ames GF, Mimura CS, Shyamala V, 1990, Bacterial periplasmic permeases belong to a family of transport proteins operating from *Escherichia coli* to human traffic ATPases, *FEMS Microbiol Rev*, **75:** 429–46.

Antson AA, Otridge J et al., 1995, The structure of *try* RNA-binding attenuation protein, *Nature (London)*, **374:** 693–9.

Beisswenger R, Kula MR, 1991, Catalytic properties and substrate specificity of 3 hexulose phosphate synthase from *Methylomonas* M15, *Appl Microbiol Biotechnol*, **34:** 604–7.

Benov LT, Fridovich I, 1994, *Escherichia coli* expresses a copper-and-zinc-containing superoxide dismutase, *J Biol Chem*, **269:** 25310–14.

Bernander R, Akerlund T, Nordstrom K, 1995, Inhibition and restart of initiation of chromosome replication: effects on exponentially growing *Escherichia coli* cells, *J Bacteriol*, **177:** 1670–82.

Bourret RB, Borovich KA, Simon MI, 1991, Signal transduction pathways involving protein phosphorylation in prokaryotes, *Annu Rev Biochem*, **60:** 401–41.

Boyd DA, Cvitkovitch DG, Hamilton IR, 1995, Sequence, expression, and function of the gene for the nonphosphorylating, NADP-dependent glyceraldehyde-3-phosphate dehydrogenase of *Streptococcus mutans*, *J Bacteriol*, **177:** 2622–7.

Bremer H, Churchward G, 1991, Control of cyclic chromosomal replication in *Escherichia coli*, *Microbiol Rev*, **55:** 459–75.

Brito F, DeMoss JA, Dubourdieu M, 1995, Isolation and identification of menaquinone-9 from purified nitrate reductase of *Escherichia coli*, *J Bacteriol*, **177:** 3728–35.

Canale-Parola E, 1970, Biology of the sugar fermenting *Sarcina*, *Bacteriol Rev*, **34:** 82–97.

Chan MK, Mukund S et al., 1995, Structure of a hyperthermophilic tungsten enzyme, aldehyde ferredoxin oxidoreductase, *Science*, **267:** 1463–9.

Chung T, Klumpp DJ, LaPorte DC, 1988, Glyoxylate bypass operon of *Escherichia coli*: cloning and determination of the functional map, *J Bacteriol*, **170:** 386–92.

Cooper S, 1991, Synthesis of the cell surface during the division cycle of rod-shaped, gram-negative bacteria, *Microbiol Rev*, **55:** 649–74.

Cortay JC, Bleicher F et al., 1988, Nucleotide sequence and expression of the *aceK* gene coding for isocitrate dehydrogenase kinase/phosphatase in *Escherichia coli*, *J Bacteriol*, **170:** 89–97.

Cvitkovitch DG, Boyd DA et al., 1995, Glucose transport by a mutant of *Streptococcus mutans* unable to accumulate sugars via the phosphoenolpyruvate phosphotransferase system, *J Bacteriol*, **177:** 2251–8.

Danson MJ, 1988, Archaebacteria, *Adv Microb Physiol*, **29:** 166–231.

Deutscher J, Reizer J et al., 1994, Loss of protein kinase-catalyzed phosphorylation of HPr, a phosphocarrier protein of the phosphotransferase system, by mutation of the *ptsH* gene confers catabolite repression resistance to several catabolite genes of *Bacillus subtilis*, *J Bacteriol*, **176:** 3336–44.

deVos WM, Vaughan EE, 1994, Genetics of lactose utilization in lactic acid bacteria, *FEMS Microbiol Rev*, **15:** 217–37.

Ehrenreich A, Widdel F, 1994, Anaerobic oxidation of ferrous iron by purple bacteria, a new type of phototrophic metabolism, *Appl Environ Microbiol*, **60:** 4517–26.

Ellis RJ, 1991, Molecular chaperones, *Annu Rev Biochem*, **60:** 321–47.

Ferry JG, 1990, Formate dehydrogenase, *FEMS Microbiol Rev*, **87:** 377–82.

Fradkin JE, Fraenkel DG, 1972, 2-Keto-3-deoxygluconate 6-phosphate aldolase mutants of *Escherichia coli*, *J Bacteriol*, **108:** 1277–83.

Gale EF, Epps HMR, 1942, The effect of the pH of the medium during growth on the enzymatic activities of bacteria (*Escherichia coli* and *Micrococcus lysodeikticus*) and the biological significance of the changes produced, *Biochem J*, **36:** 600–23.

Gray CM, Passodor L et al., 1995, Interchangeability and specificity of components from the quorum sensing regulatory systems of *Vibrio fischeri* and *Pseudomonas aeruginosa*, *J Bacteriol*, **176:** 3076–80.

Haldenwang WG, 1995, The sigma factors of *Bacillus subtilis*, *Microbiol Rev*, **59:** 1–30.

Herman A, Wegrzyn G, 1995, Effect of increased ppGpp concentration on DNA replication of different replicons in *Escherichia coli*, *J Basic Microbiol*, **35:** 33–9.

Hiromasa Y, Aso Y, Yamashita S, 1994, Thermal disassembly of pyruvate dehydrogenase multienzyme complex from *Bacillus stearothermophilus*, *Biosci Biotech Biochem*, **58:** 1904–5.

Huder JB, Dimroth P, 1995, Expression of the sodium ion pump methylmalonyl-coenzyme A-decarboxylase from *Veillonella parvula* and of mutated enzyme specimens in *Escherichia coli*, *J Bacteriol*, **177:** 3623–30.

Hueck CJ, Hillen W, 1995, Catabolite repression in *Bacillus subtilis*: a global regulatory mechanism for the Gram-positive bacteria, *Mol Microbiol*, **15:** 395–401.

Ikeda TP, Houtz E, LaPorte D, 1992, Isocitrate dehydrogenase kinase/phosphate: identification of mutations which selectively inhibit phosphate activity, *J Bacteriol*, **174:** 1414–16.

Jacob F, Monod J, 1961, *On the Regulation of Gene Activity*, vol. 26, Waverly Press, Baltimore, MD, 193–211.

James GA, Korber DR et al., 1995, Digital image analysis of growth and starvation responses of a surface-colonizing *Acinetobacter* sp., *J Bacteriol*, **177:** 907–15.

Janssen PH, Morgan HW, 1992, Glucose catabolism by *Spirochaeta thermophila* RI 19.B1, *J Bacteriol*, **174:** 2449–53, **54:** 502–39.

Kadner RJ, Murphy GP, Stephens CM, 1992, Two mechanisms for growth inhibition by elevated transport of sugar phosphates in *Escherichia coli*, *J Gen Microbiol*, **138:** 2007–14.

Kaneshiro SM, Clark DS, 1995, Pressure effects on the composition and thermal behavior of lipids from the deep-sea thermophile *Methanococcus jannaschii*, *J Bacteriol*, **177:** 3668–72.

Kato N, Miyamoto N et al., 1988, Hexulose phosphate synthase from a new facultative methylotroph *Mycobacterium gastri* MB19, *Agric Biol Chem*, **52:** 2659–62.

Krawiec S, Riley M, 1990, Organisation of the bacterial chromosome, *Microbiol Rev*, **54:** 502–39.

Kumari S, Tishel R et al., 1995, Cloning, characterization, and functional expression of *acs*, the gene which encodes acetyl coenzyme A synthetase in *Escherichia coli*, *J Bacteriol*, **177:** 2878–86.

Kunow J, Linder D, Thauer RK, 1995, Pyruvate:ferredoxin oxidoreductase from the sulfate-reducing *Archaeoglobus fulgidus*, *Arch Microbiol*, **163:** 21–8.

Lessie TG, Phibbs Jr PV, 1984, Alternate pathways of carbohydrate utilization in pseudomonads, *Annu Rev Microbiol*, **38:** 359–87.

Lonetto M, Gribskov M, Gross CA, 1992, The σ^{70} family: sequence conservation and evolutionary relationships, *J Bacteriol*, **174:** 3843–9.

Lowe SE, Zeikus JG, 1992, Purification and characterization of pyruvate decarboxylase from *Sarcina ventriculi*, *J Gen Microbiol*, **138:** 803–7.

Lu Y, Turner RT, Switzer RL, 1995, Roles of the three transcriptional attenuators of the *Bacillus subtilis* pyrimidine biosynthetic operon in the regulation of its expression, *J Bacteriol*, **177:** 1315–25.

MacGregor CH, Wolff JA et al., 1991, Cloning of a catabolite repressor control (*crc*) gene from *Pseudomonas aeruginosa*, expression of the gene in *Escherichia coli*, and identification of the gene product in *Pseudomonas aeruginosa*, *J Bacteriol*, **173:** 7204–12.

Mackenzie C, Chidambaram M et al., 1995, DNA repair mutants of *Rhodobacter sphaeroides*, *J Bacteriol*, **177:** 3027–35.

Magasanik B, 1961, Catabolic repression, *Cold Spring Harbor Symp Quant Biol*, **26:** 249–56.

Mager WH, De Kruijff AJJ, 1995, Stress induced transcriptional activation, *Microbiol Rev*, **59:** 506–31.

Makhatadze GI, Marahiel M, 1994, Effect of pH and phosphate ions on self-association properties of the major cold-shock protein from *Bacillus subtilis*, *Protein Sci*, **3:** 2144–7.

Matin A, 1992, Physiology, molecular biology and applications of the bacterial starvation response, *J Appl Bacteriol Symp Suppl*, **73:** 49S–57S.

Matin A, Auger A et al., 1989, Genetic basis of starvation survival in nondifferentiating bacteria, *Annu Rev Microbiol*, **43:** 293–316.

Mat-Jan F, Alam KY, Clark DP, 1989, Mutants of *Escherichia coli* deficient in the fermentative lactic dehydrogenase, *J Bacteriol*, **171:** 342–8.

Melville SB, Michel TA, Macy JM, 1988, Pathway and sites for energy conversion in the metabolism of glucose by *Selenomonas ruminantium*, *J Bacteriol*, **170:** 5298–304.

Mitchell CG, Dawes EA, 1982, The role of oxygen in the regulation of glucose metabolism, transport and the tricarboxylic acid cycle in *Pseudomonas aeruginosa*, *J Gen Microbiol*, **128:** 49–59.

Mitchell P, 1961, Coupling of phosphorylation to electron and hydrogen transfer by a chemi-osmotic type of mechanism, *Nature (London)*, **191:** 144–8.

Moat AG, Foster JW, 1995, *Microbial Physiology 3*, Wiley-Liss, New York, 1–580.

Monod J, 1947, The phenomenon of enzymatic adaptation and its bearings on problems of genetics and cellular differentiation, *Growth Symp*, **11:** 192–289.

Neale AD, Scopes RK et al., 1987, Pyruvate decarboxylase of *Zymomonas mobilis*: isolation, properties and genetic expression in *Escherichia coli*, *J Bacteriol*, **169:** 1024–8.

Neidhardt FJ (ed.), 1987a, *Escherichia coli* and *Salmonella typhimurium*: Cellular and Molecular Biology, vol. 1, American Society for Microbiology, Washington, DC, 3–6, 56–69.

Neidhardt FJ (ed.), 1987b, Escherichia coli *and* Salmonella typhimurium: Cellular and Molecular Biology, vol. 2, American Society for Microbiology, Washington, DC, 1358–85.

Neidhardt FC, VanBogelen RA, 1987, Heat shock response, Escherichia coli *and* Salmonella typhimurium: Cellular and Molecular Biology, American Society for Microbiology, Washington DC, 1334–45.

Nomura M, Gourse R, Baughma G, 1984, Regulation of the synthesis of ribosomes and ribosomal components, *Annu Rev Biochem*, **53:** 75–117.

Pankhania IP, Spormann AM et al., 1988, Lactate conversion to acetate, CO_2 and H_2 in cell suspensions of *Desulfovibrio vulgaris* (Marburg): indications for the involvement of an energy driven reaction, *Arch Microbiol*, **150:** 26–31.

Pao A, Chia C, Dyess BT, 1981, The effect of unusual guanosine nucleotides on the activities of some *Escherichia coli* cellular enzymes, *Biochem Biophys Acta*, **677:** 358–62.

Pastan I, Adhya S, 1976, Cyclic adenosine 5′-monophosphate in *Escherichia coli*, *Bacteriol Rev*, **40:** 527–51.

Poolman B, 1993, Energy transduction in lactic acid bacteria, *FEMS Microbiol Rev*, **12:** 125–47.

Rainey FA, Janssen PH et al., 1991, Isolation and characterization of an obligately anaerobic, polysaccharolytic, extremely thermophilic member of the genus *Spirochaeta*, *Arch Microbiol*, **155:** 396–401.

Rolfsmeier M, Blum P, 1995, Purification and characterization of a maltase from the extremely thermophilic crenarchaeot *Sulfolobus solfataricus*, *J Bacteriol*, **177:** 482–5.

Rusnak P, Haney P, Konisky J, 1995, The adenylate kinases from a mesophilic and three thermophilic methanogenic members of the Archaea, *J Bacteriol*, **177:** 2977–81.

Saier Jr MH, Reizer J, 1994, The bacterial phosphotransferase system: new frontiers 30 years later, *Mol Microbiol*, **13:** 755–64.

Saier Jr MH, Roseman S, 1976, Sugar transport. The *crr* mutation: its effect on the repression of enzyme synthesis, *J Biol Chem*, **251:** 6598–605.

Sawer G, Bock A, 1988, Anaerobic regulation of pyruvate formate-lyase from *Escherichia coli* K-12, *J Bacteriol*, **170:** 5330–6.

Sheppard DE, Englesberg E, 1967, Further evidence for positive control of the L-arabinose system by gene *araC*, *J Mol Biol*, **25:** 443–54.

Singh-Wissmann K, Ferry JG, 1995, Transcriptional regulation of the phosphotransacetylase-encoding and acetate-encoding genes (*pta* and *ack*) from *Methanosarcina thermophila*, *J Bacteriol*, **177:** 1699–702.

Skulachev VP, 1994, Chemiosmotic concept of the membrane bioenergetics: what is already clear and what is still waiting for elucidation?, *J Bioenerg Biomembr*, **26:** 589–98.

Snoep JL, Joost M et al., 1991, Effect of the energy source on the NADH/NAD ratio and on pyruvate catabolism in anaerobic chemostat cultures of *Enterococcus faecalis* NCTC 775, *FEMS Microbiol Lett*, **81:** 63–6.

Steinbuchel A, Schlegel HG, 1991, Physiology and molecular genetics of poly(β-hydroxyalkanoic acid) synthesis in *Alcaligenes eutrophus*, *Mol Microbiol*, **5:** 535–42.

Stewart V, 1993, Nitrate regulation of anaerobic respiratory gene expression in *Escherichia coli*, *Mol Microbiol*, **9:** 425–34.

Thevenot T, Brochu D et al., 1995, Regulation of ATP-dependent P-(Ser)-HPr formation in *Streptococcus mutans* and *Streptococcus salivarius*, *J Bacteriol*, **177:** 2751–9.

Tolner B, Ubbink-Kok T et al., 1995, Characterization of the proton/glutamate symport protein of *Bacillus subtilis* and its functional expression in *Escherichia coli*, *J Bacteriol*, **177:** 2863–9.

Touati D, Jacques M et al., 1995, Lethal oxidative damage and mutations are generated by iron in Dfur mutants of *Escherichia coli*; protective role of superoxide dismutase, *J Bacteriol*, **177:** 2305–14.

Walker GC, 1987, Escherichia coli *and* Salmonella typhimurium: Cellular and Molecular Biology, American Society for Microbiology, Washington, DC, 1346–57.

Weisser P, Kramer WR et al., 1995, Functional expression of the glucose transporter of *Zymomonas mobilis* leads to restoration of glucose and fructose uptake in *Escherichia coli* mutants and provides evidence for its facilitator action, *J Bacteriol*, **177:** 3351–4.

Zeng A. Deckwer W, 1991, A model for multiproduct-inhibited growth of *Enterobacter aerogenes* in 2,3-butanol fermentation, *Appl Microbiol Biotechnol*, **35:** 1–3.

BACTERIAL DIVERSITY

S H Zinder

1 INTRODUCTION

Since the studies of Pasteur and Koch, the pathogenic bacteria have taken the centre stage in bacteriological research. The exploits of the 'microbe hunters' captivated the public attention in the early twentieth century and to this day the main public perception of bacteria is as 'germs' to be killed. Indeed, the process of elimination of microbial diseases through the development of vaccines, chemotherapy and improved sanitation is one of the great scientific achievements of this century, although, as readers are surely aware, several bacterial diseases are re-emerging as significant world-wide health threats and further research into the basic biology of the causative organisms is urgently needed. Part of that basic information is the place of pathogens in the natural order of bacteria, i.e. how they are related to other pathogens and non-pathogens.

Most informed people know that pathogens represent only a small fraction of the total bacterial species. Most of the bacteria that live in soils and waters and even on the surfaces of the human body have not developed the capacity to invade the animal body; if fortuitously allowed entrance into tissues, they cannot evade the immune and other protective systems present and cannot produce virulence factors such as toxins. Indeed, the activities of most of these organisms can be considered beneficial to mankind. Not only do bacteria play crucial roles in the general decomposition of organic matter and biodegradation of pollutants, but if one accepts that mitochondria and chloroplasts are derived from bacteria and cyanobacteria respectively, then essentially all photosynthesis and respiration on earth is carried out by bacteria. Moreover, until the development of the Haber process for chemical nitrogen fixation in 1913, essentially all nitrogen in living matter was originally derived by bac-

terial nitrogen fixation. Fixed nitrogen in eukaryotes is obtained from bacteria, either directly, as in the *Rhizobium*-legume symbiosis, or indirectly, usually through the breakdown of cell components of nitrogen-fixing bacteria in soils. Similarly, until its chemical synthesis, all vitamin B_{12} on earth was derived from bacteria.

Eukaryotes outclass bacteria in their ability to form multicellular differentiated structures, at least partly due to their internal cytoskeleton, and the process of mitosis which allows for a larger genome size. Although many bacteria have interesting life cycles, the most complex differentiated structures formed by bacteria, such as the fruiting bodies of myxobacteria, are primitive when compared to those of eukaryotes. However, bacteria surpass eukaryotes in their metabolic diversity and in their abilities to colonize many extreme habitats.

Examples of the diversity of metabolic modes in bacteria is shown in Table 6.1. Eukaryotes are only capable of 3 basic modes of metabolism, aerobic respiration, oxygenic photosynthesis and a limited number of fermentations. Even in these metabolic modes, bacteria usually show much greater versatility than do eukaryotes. Respiring bacteria are capable of oxidizing an enormous range of organic molecules and are evolving capabilities to utilize synthetic chemicals never encountered previously by nature, such as the herbicide 2,4,5-T (Agent Orange) (Haugland et al. 1990). An exception is lignin, which is degraded much more rapidly by fungi producing peroxidase enzymes than by bacteria. Respiration in bacteria is not limited to using oxygen as an electron acceptor. Many other electron acceptors can be used, including nitrate, sulphate, Fe^{3+} and CO_2, as well as some organic electron acceptors tied to electron transport phosphorylation, such as fumarate. Cyanobacteria carry out 'plant-type' oxygenic photosynthesis, but purple and green photosynthetic bacterial groups can use other electron

Table 6.1 Metabolic modes in bacteria

Process	Representative equation	Comments
Aerobic respiration	$DH_2 + \frac{1}{2}O_2 \rightarrow D + H_2O$	Electron donor (D) can be essentially any organic and many inorganic compounds. Usually associated with electron-transport phosphorylation
Fermentation	$R_1H_2 + R_2 \rightarrow R_1 + R_2H_2$	R_1 and R_2 are a variety of organic compounds, often the same one. Examples are fermentation of sugars to lactate and fermentation of amino acids to fatty acids and amines. Usually tied to substrate-level phosphorylation
Anaerobic respiration	$DH_2 + A \rightarrow D + AH_2$	Electron acceptor (A) can be a variety of inorganic and some organic compounds. Examples for A are: CO_2 ($\rightarrow CH_4$ methanogenesis); SO_4^{2-} ($\rightarrow H_2S$ sulphate reduction); NO_3^- ($\rightarrow N_2$, denitrification). Usually tied to electron-transport phosphorylation
Lithotrophy	$IH_2 + A \rightarrow I + H_2A$	I is an inorganic electron donor; A is an electron acceptor, often O_2. Examples for I are: S^0 ($\rightarrow SO_4^{2-}$, colourless sulphur bacteria; NH_3 ($\rightarrow NO_2^- \rightarrow NO_3^-$, nitrifiers). Many lithotrophs are also autotrophs, i.e. fix CO_2
Oxygenic photosynthesis	$CO_2 + H_2O + light \rightarrow CH_2O + O_2$	Carried out by cyanobacteria and chloroplasts. CH_2O represents cell organic carbon. Requires more energy than anoxygenic photosynthesis
Anoxygenic photosynthesis	$CO_2 + 2DH_2 + light \rightarrow CH_2O + H_2O$	Carried out by purple and green photosynthetic bacteria and heliobacteria. Examples for DH_2 are: S compounds, H_2, Fe^{2+} and organic compounds
Nitrogen fixation	$N_2 + 8H + 16ATP \rightarrow 2NH_3 + H_2 + 16ADP$	Carried out by diverse Eubacteria and Archaea. Nitrogenase is oxygen-labile, so that aerobes that fix N_2, such as *Azotobacter* and cyanobacteria, must protect their nitrogenase from oxygen

See also Volume 2, Chapter 5.

donors for CO_2 reduction to cell material, including sulphur compounds, Fe^{2+} and organic molecules. In terms of fermentation, a much wider variety of organic molecules can be degraded anaerobically by bacteria, including amino acids, nucleotides, fatty acids and even many aromatic molecules when H_2 is consumed by other organisms such as methanogens (Zinder 1993).

Bacteria can also colonize extreme habitats, many of which are inhospitable to eukaryotes. The best example of this phenomenon is high-temperature habitats, with Eubacteria being able to grow at temperatures as high as 95°C and Archaea capable of growth at temperatures greater than 110°C (Stetter 1995). The highest known growth temperature for a eukaryote is near 60°C, presumably because of their complex structure. Only Archaea are capable of growing in salinities near saturation, but eukaryotic algae and fungi are capable of growth at salinities nearly that high and fungi excel at growing at extremely low water potentials (such as in maple syrup). Similarly, while there are some acidophilic Eubacteria and Archaea that can grow to pH values below 1.0, there are fungi and algae which can grow at pH values near 2.0.

Although it was clear that bacteria presented con-

siderable ecophysiological diversity, it was not clear how great was their phylogenetic diversity until the recent advent of molecular phylogenetic techniques. These have allowed us to determine natural relationships among bacteria. This chapter will survey the diversity of bacteria, using their molecular phylogeny as an organizing principle, and will discuss their ecophysiology as different organisms are encountered. Many of the important animal pathogens will be included in the discussion, so that their place in the overall phylogenetic scheme will be shown. More detail about important pathogenic bacterial groups are discussed in other chapters in this volume.

2 DEVELOPMENT OF A PHYLOGENETIC CLASSIFICATION FOR BACTERIA

When it was clear that bacteria could not be classified as plant or animal, they were given their own 'kingdom' called Schizomycetes, or Monera, typically one of the 5 kingdoms. In 1962, Stanier and van Niel (1962) challenged this view with a proposal that there was really a dichotomy in living organisms and resurrected the terms prokaryotes and eukaryotes, originally coined in the 1930s by the French protozoologist E. Chatton. They went on to describe the salient features of prokaryotes including:

1 the lack of an organized nucleus, mitosis, or meiosis
2 a single circular chromosome
3 respiration and photosynthesis carried out by the cell membrane and its extensions rather than in membrane-bound organelles
4 presence of a muramic acid containing cell wall in most bacteria.

The hierarchical classification of bacteria has always been problematic, since there was no useful fossil record to base it on, nor was there a richly complex morphology as in plants and animals. Moreover, there is no objective definition of a bacterial species. Classification on the basis of phenotypic characteristics (morphology, gram reaction, growth characteristics, substrate utilization, biochemical reactions, etc.) provided useful determinative keys that sorted out relatively closely related organisms and allowed rapid identification of pathogens, but really provided no natural order to the bacteria. For example, one did not know whether to place the purple and green photosynthetic bacteria with other gram-negative bacteria, or to classify them as a separate group based on their physiology, as was done in many classification schemes.

Molecular biology provided extremely useful phylogenetic tools when methods were developed to obtain sequences of proteins and nucleic acids, which Zuckerkandl and Pauling (1965) in a seminal paper termed semantides. The closer the semantide sequences of 2 different organisms are to each other, the more likely that they shared a common ancestor more recently than organisms harbouring more divergent sequences. This assumes that there is no horizontal transfer of the genes involved. The first information-containing macromolecules used with success in the early 1970s were small proteins, such as cytochrome *c*, that provided a phylogeny for animals similar to that in the fossil record.

In bacteria, because of their great physiological diversity, most proteins were unsuitable either because they were not universally distributed in bacteria, or they were difficult to sequence using the technologies that were available then. For example, most anaerobes lack cytochrome *c*, as do some aerobes such as *Escherichia coli*, whereas other organisms may have several distinct copies of cytochrome *c*. Early use of molecular biological methods with bacteria focused on nucleic acids and used the crude technology that was available at that time. This included determining the G + C % of the organisms' DNA. This test is exclusionary since if the G + C % in 2 organisms differs by several per cent, then their DNA sequences should be distinctly different, while 2 organisms with differing DNA sequences can have similar G + C %. For example, it was found that the DNA of the gram-positive cocci *Staphylococcus* and *Micrococcus* had greatly different G + C % and therefore they were not closely related to

each other. The G + C % is considered a necessary test when characterizing a new organism (Johnson 1994a).

The next molecular test that was used for bacterial phylogeny was DNA–DNA hybridization, which tested the ability of single-stranded DNA from one organism to form a heteroduplex with single-stranded DNA from another. This test had many drawbacks for providing an overall phylogeny. Results were sensitive to slight variations in technique (Johnson 1994a) and sequences with greater than approximately 15% sequence mismatch will not usually form heteroduplexes, so that distantly related organisms gave no reaction (DNA–rRNA hybridization was more suitable). Thus, DNA–DNA hybridization was most useful at the species level and one of the most robust definitions of a bacterial species is a group of organisms showing ≥70% DNA–DNA hybridization (Stackebrandt and Goebel 1994). Moreover, neither DNA–DNA nor DNA–rRNA hybrdization provides a predictive database, since knowing the similarity between organisms A and B and between A and C does not allow one to predict the similarity between B and C; the pairwise hybridization of a new organism must be determined for essentially every other organism in the database.

In the mid-1970s Carl Woese at the University of Illinois began investigating ribosomal RNA sequences as a potential phylogenetic marker. The molecule used was the 16S rRNA, which is between 1500 and 1600 nucleotides long in most prokaryotes (it is18S in eukaryotes). It is part of the smaller 30S subunit of the ribosome and it is useful to call it SSU (small subunit) rRNA and the DNA encoding it SSU rDNA, a more general term which does not presuppose the Svedberg constant of the rRNA. The technique involved the prevailing technology of the time, to isolate the rRNA and digest it with the enzyme T_1 ribonuclease, which cleaves after each guanine (G), thereby producing a variety of oligonucleotide fragments 1–25 ribonucleotides long, each ending with G. These were then separated and identified using 2-dimensional electrophoresis. The oligonucleotides of length 6 or greater (typically 25–50 per SSU rRNA molecule) were recorded as a catalogue that could then be compared with the catalogue from another organism and a similarity coefficient (called S_{AB}), varying between 0 for no similarity and 1 for complete identity, would be assigned. Among Woese's rationales for using SSU rRNA are that:

1 it is found in all cells and serves the same function in them
2 it is relatively easily isolated
3 its sequence changes slowly compared to most proteins (although it has both slow and fast-changing regions which could be used with both close and distantly related organisms)
4 because it is part of complex in which it specifically interacts with several ribosomal proteins, it is unlikely that horizontal transfer of rRNA genes would occur.

In early studies using these methods, it was shown that

enterics, the *Vibrio* group and the purple non-sulphur bacterium *Rhodopseudomonas sphaeroides* grouped together and were distinct from gram-positive organisms and cyanobacteria (Zablen and Woese 1975), that chloroplasts were closely related to cyanobacteria (Zablen et al. 1975) and that eukaryotes (excluding the organelles) showed little similarity to prokaryotes. It was also noted that some oligonucleotides were conserved in all organisms, some were group specific and others were organism specific. These findings helped bring credibility to the method.

A subsequent finding was more unexpected. The SSU rRNA from methanogenic bacteria was examined and their oligonucleotide catalogues were found to be completely divergent from both other bacteria and eukaryotes (Balch et al. 1977), suggesting that methanogens were a third form of life, dubbed the Archaebacteria, since methanogens were considered to be an ancient form of life likely to be present on the early earth and because the divergence between them and other organisms was ancient. As more diverse bacteria were studied, the halobacteria and some thermoacidophilic bacteria were added (Woese, Magrum and Fox 1978). On the basis of this work, the cell walls of the Archaebacteria were investigated (Kandler and König 1978) and most were found to consist of protein. A few methanogens had a peptidoglycan cell wall resembling those of gram-positive bacteria but lacking muramic acid and D-alanine; this cell wall was therefore called pseudomurein. It had been known that both halobacteria and the thermoacidophiles had ether-linked isoprenoid lipids rather than the ester-linked fatty acids typically found and these were considered to be an adaptation to extreme environments. It was found that methanogens, many of which inhabit relatively non-extreme environments, also contained these unusual lipids (Tornabene and Langworty 1978). The cell wall and lipid data supported the proposition that the Archaebacteria should be a separate group.

Oligonucleotide catalogues were obtained for many more diverse bacteria and by 1980 more than 170 organisms were characterized and the general outlines of the bacterial groups became apparent (Fox et al. 1980). Several eubacterial lines were defined, many of which had photosynthetic representatives, making it likely that photosynthesis was an ancient phenotype in the Eubacteria. Obtaining oligonucleotide sequence catalogues for SSU rRNA molecules was a difficult and tedious process that only a few laboratories in the world developed the capability to perform. Moreover, the oligonucleotide methods provided only a fraction of the information present in the entire molecule and the relationship between the S_{AB} coefficient and overall sequence similarity was not linear (Woese 1987). Techniques for DNA sequencing were developed in the late 1970s. This provided opportunities to sequence DNA obtained from the cloned gene for SSU rRNA or from fragments a few hundred nucleotides long derived from reverse transcriptase. These methods were rapidly superseded by the development of the polymerase chain reaction (PCR) in the mid-

1980s, allowing the amplification of almost the entire SSU rDNA using primers to sequences conveniently located near the 5' and 3' ends of the gene (Johnson 1994b). Thus, any laboratory outfitted for standard molecular biological techniques can readily determine an SSU rDNA sequence. It should be pointed out that for taxonomy at the species level, SSU rRNA methods are often not sensitive enough, since strains showing 70% DNA–DNA reassociation have SSU rRNA sequences that are nearly indistinguishable (Stackebrandt and Goebel 1994). It should also be pointed out that while molecular phylogenetic analysis helps place bacteria in a natural order, this information can only be used wisely if the phenotypic characteristics of the organisms are understood (Palleroni 1994).

The PCR method has led to an explosion of numbers of SSU rDNA sequences obtained from diverse bacteria, more than 2000 of which are presently compiled at the rRNA database project at the University of Illinois (Maidak et al. 1994). These sequences, as well as phylogenetic trees containing them, can be obtained readily through the Internet (email: server'@ rdp.life.uiuc.edu; WWW: http://rdp.life.uiuc.edu/). The phylogenetic trees in this chapter were downloaded from this database. Although the SSU rDNA sequences of an enormous number of organisms, including most important pathogens, are present in this database, a considerable number of common organisms, such as *Klebsiella* and *Azotobacter*, are not yet present in it so that there are gaps in our knowledge, but these are becoming fewer with time. Extensive reviews on prokaryote phylogeny are available (Woese 1987, 1994, Olsen, Woese and Overbeek 1994).

Since one can obtain rDNA sequences directly from natural habitats without the need to culture organisms, rDNA techniques provide a powerful tool for studying microbial ecology. Indeed, one can even stain individual cells with a specific fluorescently labelled oligonucleotide probe and identify them in natural populations (DeLong, Wickham and Pace 1989). There are now numerous sequences derived from natural habitats, representing presently uncultured organisms, some of which are free-living and others which are endosymbionts of other organisms. These studies show that only a fraction of the microbial species present in most environments is known and this has been especially well demonstrated for the Archaea (Barns et al. 1994, Olsen 1994), but holds true for many other bacterial groups. A major challenge to microbiologists in the future will be to identify and culture these organisms (Amann, Ludwig and Schleifer 1994). Molecular phylogenetic tools also hold great promise in rapidly identifying bacteria in a clinical setting.

3 THE 3 DOMAINS

Figure 6.1 is a dendrogram showing the 3 primary domains: Eubacteria, Archaea and Eukaryota (Woese,

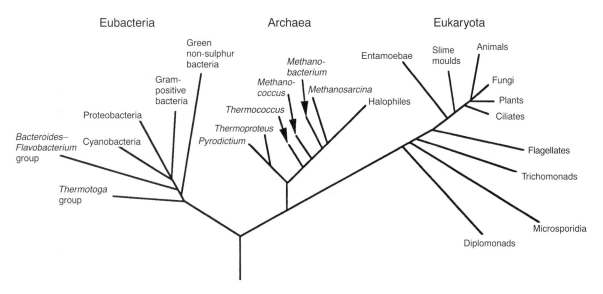

Fig. 6.1 Universal phylogenetic tree (after Woese 1994) based on SSU rDNA sequence showing the 3 domains.

Kandler and Wheelis 1990). Two of the domains are what Stanier and van Niel would call prokaryotes and the generic term bacteria will be used in this chapter for them; Eubacteria will be used to denote the 'common' bacteria. Woese renamed the Archaebacteria the Archaea to emphasize their unrelatedness to the Eubacteria. Woese also used the term Eucarya for eukaryotes, but the more traditional Eukaryota will be used here. The term 'domain' is a wise choice, distinct from the term 'kingdom' which in its classical sense is clearly a lower taxon. The root of this tree, representing the position of the ancestral organism, has been placed between the Eubacteria and the Archaea based on studies of sequences of other macromolecules including ATPases and elongation factors (Woese, Kandler and Wheelis 1990), but there is still controversy about this assignment. So far, all known organisms are members of the 3 domains. The deepest branches in the eukaryotic domain are protists lacking mitochondria, such as the diplomonad *Giardia*.

Table 6.2 compares the properties of the 3 domains. The overall architecture of archaeal cells clearly resembles the Eubacteria; however, their molecular details resemble the Eubacteria in some respects, the eukaryotes in others, whereas still others are unique. For example, their ribosomes are 70S in size, yet are resistant to the classical eubacterial protein synthesis inhibitors streptomycin and chloramphenicol, as well as the eukaryotic inhibitor cycloheximide; however, peptide elongation can be inhibited by diphtheria toxin as in eukaryotes. Archaeal genes are generally arranged in polycistronic operons resembling eubacterial ones, whereas their RNA polymerases most closely resemble RNA polymerase II in eukaryotes and transcription is initiated using TATA box-type proteins rather than eubacterial σ factors (Keeling, Charlebois and Doolittle 1994).

4 THE EUBACTERIA

Figure 6.2 shows 16 of the major lines of descent in the Eubacteria. The taxonomic status of these lines is unclear. They have been called phyla and if one examines Fig. 6.1, they are clearly the equivalent of kingdoms. They also might be compared to orders in classical bacterial taxonomy and they have also been called classes (Stackebrandt, Murray and Truper 1988). At this point, it is simplest to call them divisions. Some of them essentially correspond to classically defined groups such as spirochaetes, cyanobacteria and gram-positive bacteria, whereas others represent relationships which were not suspected previously.

The 3 earliest-branching divisions contain mainly thermophiles, making it likely that the original ancestor of the Eubacteria was a thermophile. When the interior branches are examined using different phylogenetic techniques, or using different representatives of the branches, their branching order readily changes (Vandepeer et al. 1994), indicating that the order of the branching may not be resolved by these techniques. In fact, it is not clear that the high G + C gram-positive and the low G + C gram-positive bacteria cluster together, although the analysis in Fig. 6.2 suggests that they do. This inability to resolve the branching order suggests that there was a rapid radiation of the lines, resembling the Cambrian explosion of animals. The factor involved may have been the 'invention' of photosynthesis, present in 5 of the major eubacterial divisions (green non-sulphur, low G + C gram-positive, Proteobacteria, green sulphur and cyanobacteria). The eubacterial divisions themselves have proven robust, i.e. differing phylogenetic techniques do not generally cause organisms to shift from one line to the other (Vandepeer et al. 1994).

Table 6.2 The three primary domains

Characteristic	Eubacteria	Archaea	Eukaryota
Cell diameter	Typically ~1 μm	Typically ~1 μm	Typically ≥10 μm
Nucleus, mitosis, meiosis	−	−	+
Chromsomes	Typically one: usually circular (+ plasmids)	Typically one: usually circular (+ plasmids)	Usually more than one, linear (+ plasmids)
Genome size (base pairs)	$0.6–12 \times 10^6$	$1–4 \times 10^6$	17×10^6 (yeast) 3×10^9 (human)
DNA containing organelles	−	−	+ (mitochrondria and chloroplasts)
Cytoskeleton	−	−	+
Flagella	Simple submicroscopic, rotate, powered by ion gradients across cell membrane	Simple, submicroscopic, rotate, powered by ion gradients across cell membrane	Complex (9 + 2), visible under light microscope, whip, powered by ATP
Cell wall	Murein peptidoglycan, gram +ve or gram −ve, nearly always contain muramic acid (no cell wall in mycoplasmas)	Protein or pseudomurein, no muramic acid (no cell wall in *Thermoplasma*)	None, cellulose or chitin, etc. No muramic acid
Inhibition of cell wall synthesis by penicillin	+	−	−
Membrane lipids	Ester linked, branching rare, sterols rare	Ether-linked isoprenoids, sterols?	Ester-linked, branching rare, sterols common
Maximum known growth temperature	95°C	110°C	60°C
Ribosome size	70S	70S	80S (70S in mitos and chloros)
Ribosome sensitivity to streptomycin or chloramphenicol	+	−	−
Ribosome sensitivity to cycloheximide	−	−	+
Ribosome sensitivity to diphtheria toxin	−	+	+
Initiator amino acid	*n*-Formylmethionine	Methionine	Methionine
RNA polymerase structure	Simple	Complex	Complex
Operons	+	+	−
Transcription initiator	Sigma factors	TATA-binding protein	TATA-binding protein

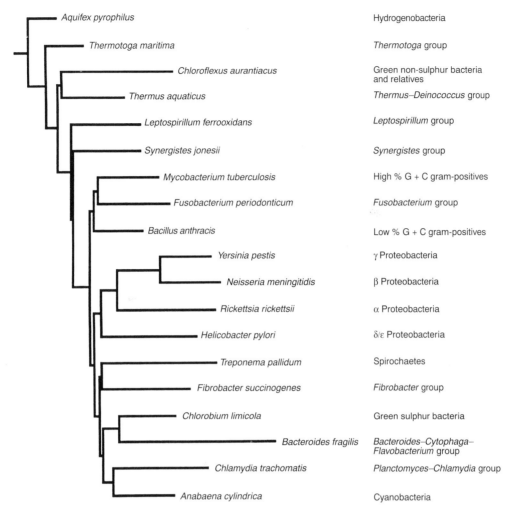

Aquifex pyrophilus — Hydrogenobacteria

Thermotoga maritima — *Thermotoga* group

Chloroflexus aurantiacus — Green non-sulphur bacteria and relatives

Thermus aquaticus — *Thermus–Deinococcus* group

Leptospirillum ferrooxidans — *Leptospirillum* group

Synergistes jonesii — *Synergistes* group

Mycobacterium tuberculosis — High % G + C gram-positives

Fusobacterium periodonticum — *Fusobacterium* group

Bacillus anthracis — Low % G + C gram-positives

Yersinia pestis — γ Proteobacteria

Neisseria meningitidis — β Proteobacteria

Rickettsia rickettsii — α Proteobacteria

Helicobacter pylori — δ/ε Proteobacteria

Treponema pallidum — Spirochaetes

Fibrobacter succinogenes — *Fibrobacter* group

Chlorobium limicola — Green sulphur bacteria

Bacteroides fragilis — *Bacteroides–Cytophaga–Flavobacterium* group

Chlamydia trachomatis — *Planctomyces–Chlamydia* group

Anabaena cylindrica — Cyanobacteria

Fig. 6.2 The major eubacterial groups. When possible, each group was represented by a pathogen.

The Proteobacteria (which include most of the common gram-negative bacteria) and the gram-positive bacteria account for approximately 90% of the known bacterial species and a clear majority of the pathogens. To some extent, this dominance represents the bias of researchers studying bacteria. Members of these groups are often readily cultured using standard heterotrophic media. Certainly more study of members of the other groups is leading to a greater appreciation of their diversity and speciation. Having said this, the diversity of the Proteobacteria and gram-positives is enormous and will occupy the most space in this chapter.

4.1 The Proteobacteria

The Proteobacteria is the name given to a group previously called 'purple bacteria and relatives' (Stackebrandt, Murray and Truper 1988); this group includes most of the common gram-negative bacteria (Fig. 6.3). The purple photosynthetic bacteria carry out anoxygenic (non-oxygen evolving) photosynthesis using bacteriochlorophyll *a* or *b* that absorbs light maximally in the infrared near 870 and 1000 nm, respectively. They are purple or other colours (pink,

orange, brown, etc.), due to the presence of carotenoid pigments.

The purple bacteria were classically subdivided into sulphur and non-sulphur bacteria. Purple sulphur (PS) bacteria favour sulphur compounds such as H_2S, as their electron donors for CO_2 reduction, so that their generalized equation for photosynthesis ($2H_2S + CO_2 \rightarrow CH_2O + H_2O$) resembles that for cyanobacteria and plants that use H_2O rather than H_2S as an electron donor for CO_2 reduction (see Table 6.1 and section 4.5, p. 141). Some PS bacteria have limited abilities to use organic compounds photosynthetically and can sometimes grow micro-aerophilically in the dark. The purple non-sulphur (PNS) bacteria favour organic electron donors and can use them for CO_2 reduction in photosynthesis so that a generalized equation is $2RH_2 + CO_2 \rightarrow 2R + CH_2O + H_2O$. When growing in this manner (photoheterotrophically) the PNS bacteria often incorporate the organic carbon directly into their cell material rather than use it to fix CO_2 in a complex process called photoassimilation. Many purple bacteria can use H_2 as an electron donor for CO_2 reduction and thereby grow as autotrophs fixing all their own CO_2; some can use Fe^{2+} (Widdel et al. 1993) or low concentrations of H_2S as electron

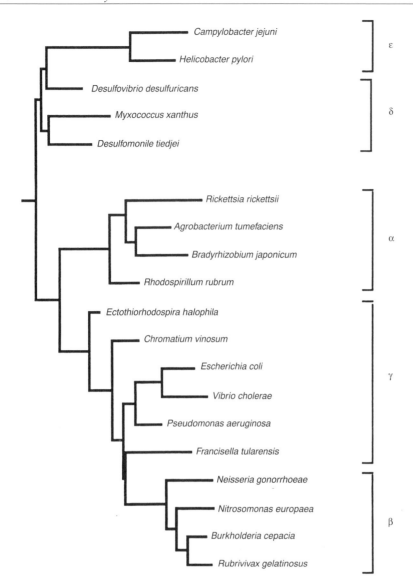

Fig. 6.3 The Proteobacteria.

donors. Most PNS bacteria are very metabolically versatile and can grow as aerobic heterotrophs, with oxygen typically repressing bacteriochlorophyll synthesis; some can use electron acceptors other than oxygen, such as nitrate, and grow via anaerobic respiration. Because the photosynthetic reactions carried out by purple bacteria require less free energy input than those of organisms using H_2O, they require only one photosystem instead of the 2 required by cyanobacteria and plants. This relative simplicity led to the determination of the crystal structure of the photosystem of a PNS bacterium (Diesenhofer and Michel 1989).

When purple photosynthetic bacteria were first studied using SSU rRNA oligonucleotide cataloguing techniques, it was found that there were 2 groups of PNS bacteria, named the α and β subdivisions, and one group of purple sulphur bacteria, named the γ subdivision. However, a surprising discovery was that many common gram-negative bacteria were also associated with these groups (Fox et al. 1980) and that the purple photosynthetic bacteria were widespread

within the groups. The simplest explanation for these results was that the ancestor of all the common gram-negative bacteria was a purple photosynthetic bacterium and that most of the common heterotrophic bacteria are descended from photosynthetic organisms that had lost their ability to carry out photosynthesis. This is not completely surprising in retrospect, since many PNS bacteria are capable of non-photosynthetic modes of metabolism and one can readily obtain non-photosynthetic mutants of these organisms that would be indistinguishable from common aerobic heterotrophs. Still, until the advent of SSU rRNA studies, the relationship between the purple photosynthetic bacteria and other gram-negative bacteria was not clear and this finding caused a major reappraisal of the origins of these organisms.

Clustering with the purple bacteria were many gram-negative sulphate-reducing bacteria along with some micro-aerophiles and these were originally called the δ subdivision; later, the micro-aerophiles were placed in the ε subdivision. No photosynthetic organisms have been found in these subdivisions. It should also be pointed out that subsequent analyses, using complete sequences rather than cataloguing of oligonucleotides, have shown that β and γ divisions form a supercluster with the purple sulphur bacteria, such as *Chromatium* and *Ectothiorhodospira*, considered part of the γ cluster, lying on the periphery of the cluster and the β and γ groups clustered within (Fig. 6.3).

Several genera within the Proteobacteria have been subdivided into new genera. For example, any rod-shaped PNS bacterium was given the genus name *Rhodopseudomonas*, but even by classical taxonomic criteria it was realized that the genus needed to be split up and other genus names developed were *Rhodobacter* and *Rubrivivax*; this is supported by the 16S rRNA trees shown in Figs 6.4 and 6.5. The familiar genus *Pseudomonas* was classically defined as non-fermentative polarly flagellated oxidase-positive rods. Standard taxonomic techniques and DNA–DNA and DNA–rRNA hybridization studies have showed that this diverse genus could be subdivided into 5 assemblages: the fluorescent, pseudomallei, acidivorans, diminuta and xanthomonas groups. These groups have been given the genus names *Pseudomonas*, *Burkholderia*, *Comamonas*, *Sphingomonas* and *Xanthomonas*, respectively.

Each subdivision of the Proteobacteria is rather large and will therefore be discussed separately. Unless described otherwise, the organisms described are aerobic heterotrophic rods.

THE α SUBDIVISION

The α subdivision (Fig. 6.4) contains many well known gram-negative species. PNS bacteria are widely distributed in this subdivision. It is also noted for containing the plant-associated bacteria *Rhizobium*, *Bradyrhizobium* and *Agrobacterium* and several intracellular animal parasites and pathogens, which are the closest known relatives of mitochondria.

One large cluster contains the rhizobia and related bacteria. *Rhodopseudomonas palustris* is the type species for its genus and is very versatile, able to metabolize a wide variety of organic compounds, including aromatics. Closely related to *R. palustris* are the slow-growing rhizobia (doubling time ≥ 8 h), represented by *Bradyrhizobium* (formerly *Rhizobium*) *japonicum*, which produces nitrogen-fixing root nodules in soy plants. An organism from nitrogen-fixing nodules in the stems of certain tropical plants was found to produce bacteriochlorophyll and has been named '*Photorhizobium thompsonianum*' (Eaglesham et al. 1990), although it is closely enough related to *Bradyrhizobium* to include it in this genus. This photosynthetic ability is less surprising considering its close relationship to *R. palustris* and retaining the ability to carry out photosynthesis is reasonable considering that light is available in the stem nodules, but not usually in underground root nodules.

Another closely related organism is *Nitrobacter winogradskyi*, an aerobic lithotroph which derives energy from oxidizing nitrite to nitrate by the equation: $NO_2^- + \frac{1}{2}O_2 \rightarrow NO_3^-$. More distantly related to these organisms is *Methylobacterium extorquens*, an aerobic methylo-troph, an organism that can use one-carbon compounds such as methanol or methylamines but not necessarily methane for energy generation. *Methylosinus trichosporium* is a methanotroph, an aerobe able to oxidize methane and other one-carbon compounds, but no other organic substrates. Distantly related is *Rhodopseudomonas viridis*, one of the few PNS bacteria that contains bacteriochlorophyll *b*, and the organism that had the crystal structure of its reaction centre determined (Diesenhofer and Michel 1989). Two organisms that divide by forming daughter cells as buds on the end of hyphae, long cellular appendages, are the PNS bacterium *Rhodomicrobium vannielii* and the aerobic heterotroph *Hyphomicrobium vulgare*.

The rest of the cluster is dominated by members of the genus *Rhizobium*, the so-called fast-growing rhizobia (doubling time ≈ 4 h), that form nitrogen-fixing nodules in a variety of agriculturally important legumes including beans and peas (*R. leguminosarum*), alfalfa (*R. meliloti*), clover (*R. trifolii*) and lotus (*R. loti*). Genes for nitrogen fixation (*nif*) and nodulation (*nod*) are found on large (200–1500 kb) plasmids called Sym plasmids. Nodule formation involves a complex interchange of chemical signals between the plant host and the bacterium, a subject of recent intensive study (Fisher and Long 1992). Closely related to *Rhizobium* is the genus *Agrobacterium*, which forms tumours in plants by transfer of a piece of oncogenic DNA into the plant cells, causing tumours which then produce a large amount of compounds called opines, which can be used as a growth substrate by the *Agrobacterium*. The transferred genes, as well as other genes important in virulence and opine utilization, are found on c. 200 kb plasmids called a Ti plasmids. Substances in plant wounds activate a *virA/virG* 2-component regulatory system analogous to those found in many animal pathogens (Winans 1992). Interestingly, closely related to these plant symbionts or pathogens are the animal pathogens *Brucella abortus* and *Bartonella bacilliformis*.

Caulobacter crescentus is an aerobic heterotroph that attaches to surfaces using a stalk at one end and forming swarmer cells at its other end. Its life cycle has been studied as a model developmental system with asymmetric distribution of cell components (Shapiro 1993). *Caulobacter* seems to form a separate line in this analysis and directly below it is a diverse and interesting cluster. *Sphingomonas paucimobilis* was once called *Pseudomonas* and represents the 'diminuta' group. *Zymomonas mobilis*, a micro-aerophile, under anaerobic conditions ferments sugars to high concentrations of ethanol using the Entner–Doudoroff pathway for sugar metabolism and uses the pyruvate decarboxylase pathway (the same pathway as in yeasts) for pyruvate metabolism. The pyruvate decarboxylase and alcohol dehydrogenase genes from *Z. mobilis* have been cloned into *E. coli* and related bacteria (Ohta et al. 1991), which can use a much wider variety of sugars than can *Z. mobilis*. These genes turned the recipient bacteria into vigorous ethanol producers, but the maximum ethanol concentration tolerated by *E. coli* was near 5%, about half that tolerated by *Z. mobilis*. *Erythrobacter*

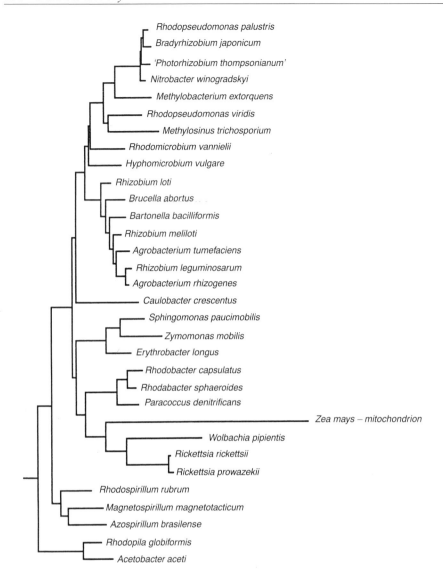

Rhodopseudomonas palustris
Bradyrhizobium japonicum
'Photorhizobium thompsonianum'
Nitrobacter winogradskyi
Methylobacterium extorquens
Rhodopseudomonas viridis
Methylosinus trichosporium
Rhodomicrobium vannielii
Hyphomicrobium vulgare
Rhizobium loti
Brucella abortus
Bartonella bacilliformis
Rhizobium meliloti
Agrobacterium tumefaciens
Rhizobium leguminosarum
Agrobacterium rhizogenes
Caulobacter crescentus
Sphingomonas paucimobilis
Zymomonas mobilis
Erythrobacter longus
Rhodobacter capsulatus
Rhodabacter sphaeroides
Paracoccus denitrificans
Zea mays – mitochondrion
Wolbachia pipientis
Rickettsia rickettsii
Rickettsia prowazekii
Rhodospirillum rubrum
Magnetospirillum magnetotacticum
Azospirillum brasilense
Rhodopila globiformis
Acetobacter aceti

Fig. 6.4 The α subdivision of the Proteobacteria.

longus is an example of a recently discovered group of PNS bacteria that can produce bacteriochlorophyll and other photopigments and use them to generate energy in the presence of oxygen, as opposed to typical PNS bacteria in which oxygen represses photopigment production.

The next cluster contains the PNS bacteria in the genus *Rhodobacter*, used extensively in genetic studies of photosynthesis. An interesting finding in *R. sphaeroides* is that it has 2 chromosomes, one 3050 kb in size and a smaller one of 914 kb (Suwanto and Kaplan 1989). Closely related is *Paracoccus denitrificans*, which, when grown aerobically, contains a respiratory electron transport chain essentially identical to that in mitochondria.

Even more interesting is the final subcluster within this cluster, containing members of the intracellular parasitic genus *Rickettsia*, the cause of Rocky Mountain spotted fever and typhus, *Ehrlichia* (not shown) and *Wolbachia*, an intracellular parasite infecting insects. Related to these intracellular parasites are the mitochondria, represented by ones from corn. The mitochondrial SSU rRNA sequences have apparently

undergone rapid evolution, represented by the length of the line leading to the *Zea mays* mitochondrion. Many other mitochondrial sequences have gone through even greater changes, such as the human mitochondrion SSU rRNA, which has been pared down to just 1100 bases. Despite these changes, sequence comparisons indicate that the mitochondria had a single origin within this group. The close relationships with present-day intracellular parasites and the relatively close similarity of cytochromes with those of *P. denitrificans* suggest that mitochondria were derived from an endosymbiotic bacterium related to the ancestors of these present-day organisms.

A more divergent cluster contains some spiral-shaped bacteria, including the PNS bacterium *Rhodospirillum rubrum*. The micro-aerophile *Magnetospirillum magnetotacticum* forms intracellular magnetite granules which allows it to orient itself along the earth's magnetic field causing cells to swim north in the northern hemisphere (while cultures from the southern hemisphere swim south). Although the function of magnetotaxis remains obscure, a plausible hypothesis (Bazylinski 1995) is that the earth's magnetic field lines are directed downward, so that the bacteria following them can find aerobic or anaerobic interfaces in muds. Once they find these interfaces, they can then fine-tune their positions using chemotaxis. *Azospirillum*, a soil bacterium, fixes nitrogen under microaerophilic conditions and associates with plant roots, although not in the tight intracellular manner of the rhizobia. The most divergent cluster in the α subdivision shown here contains the PNS bacterium *Rhodopila globiformis* and *Acetobacter aceti*, an aerobe that incompletely oxidizes ethanol to acetic acid, and used for vinegar production.

THE β SUBDIVISION

The β subdivision (Fig. 6.5) does not have as many known members as the α or γ subdivisions. PNS bacteria are fairly widely distributed within it and it also contains several lithotrophs. The pathogens *Bordetella pertussis* and *Neisseria* spp. are members of the β subdivision.

Leptothrix and the closely related genus *Sphaerotilis* form sheathed trichomes, are common in fresh waters and sometimes deposit ferric iron or manganese dioxide on their sheaths. *Rubrivivax gelatinosis* is a PNS bacterium and was originally given the genus name *Rhodopseudomonas*. The 'acidivorans' group of the genus *Pseudomonas* had been given the name *Comamonas* and is represented by *Comamonas testosteroni*. *Zoogloea* forms large microbial aggregates and is believed to play an important role in aggregate formation in the activated sludge process at sewage plants. What was originally the 'pseudomallei' group of the genus *Pseudomonas* has now been given the genus name *Burkholderia*. *Burkholderia cepacia* is a plant pathogen and soil organism with versatile biodegradative abilities which can also

be an opportunistic human pathogen in a manner similar to *Pseudomonas aeruginosa*. *Burkholderia mallei* cause glanders in horses. *Alcaligenes faecalis* is usually a common saprophyte but can be an opportunistic pathogen, while *Bordetella pertussis* is the causative agent of whooping cough and does not typically survive outside the human body.

*Spirillum volutan*s is a large spiral aquatic microaerophile which often contains large granules of the reserve material poly-ß-hydroxybutyrate. *Thiobacillus thioparus* is a sulphur-oxidizing lithotroph which grows at neutral pH and oxidizes sulphur compounds such as elemental sulphur by the equation: $S^0 + 1\frac{1}{2}O_2 + H_2O \rightarrow H_2SO_4$. It is common in soils and waters. *Rhodocyclus tenuis* is a spiral-shaped PNS bacterium, once named *Rhodospirillum*. *Gallionella ferruginea* is a bean-shaped organism that forms large spiral stalks with ferric iron precipitated on them and is typically found in iron seeps. *Nitrosomonas europaea* is a rod-shaped ammonia-oxidizing lithotroph common in soils and waters; it oxidizes ammonia to nitrite by the equation $NH_4^+ + 1\frac{1}{2}O_2 \rightarrow NO_2^- + H_2O + 2H^+$). It and organisms like the previously mentioned *Nitrobacter winogradskyi* (α subdivision) are responsible for nitrification, the process of aerobically converting ammonia to nitrate in soils and waters.

Probably the most prominent pathogens in the β subdivision belong to the genus *Neisseria*, here represented by *Neisseria gonorrhoeae* and *Neisseria meningitidis*, which form a relatively deep branch in the β subdivision. Another member of this cluster is *Eikenella corrodens*, a facultative anaerobe often associated with a variety of infectious diseases.

THE γ SUBDIVISION

The γ subdivision of the Proteobacteria (Fig. 6.6), as originally defined, contains the purple sulphur (PS) photosynthetic bacteria although in presently constituted trees, most of the other members of the γ subdivision cluster together with the members of the β subdivision to the exclusion of the PS bacteria and relatives. There are no known photosynthetic members of the interior cluster of the γ subdivision. The γ subdivision contains many familiar bacteria, including the enteric/*Vibrio* group, the fluorescent pseudomonads and *Legionella pneumophila*.

The exterior cluster contains PS bacteria including *Chromatium*, which deposits elemental sulphur granules inside the cell, and *Ectothiorhodospira*, which deposits elemental sulphur outside the cell. There are also some lithotrophs in this cluster including the ammonia oxidizing *Nitrosococcus* and *Thiobacillus ferrooxidans*, an acidophile which can grow by oxidizing ferrous iron to ferric iron according to the equation $4Fe^{2+} + 4H^+ + O_2 \rightarrow 4Fe^{3+} + 2H_2O$, and can also oxidize iron pyrite (FeS_2) and other sulphidic minerals according to the equation: $4FeS_2 + 15O_2 + 2H_2O \rightarrow 2Fe_2(SO_4)_3 + 2H_2SO_4$. When sulphidic minerals are exposed to oxygen during coal mining, *T. ferrooxidans* is afforded a chance to oxidize them and the sulphuric acid released causes acid mine drainage. A beneficial activity of these organisms is that they can oxidize

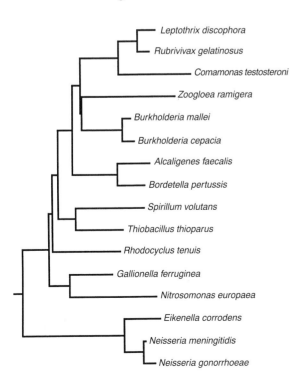

Fig. 6.5 The β subdivision of the Proteobacteria.

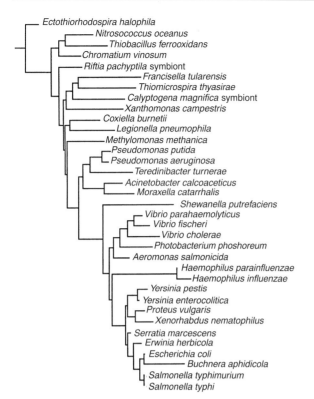

Ectothiorhodospira halophila
Nitrosococcus oceanus
Thiobacillus ferrooxidans
Chromatium vinosum
Riftia pachyptila symbiont
Francisella tularensis
Thiomicrospira thyasirae
Calyptogena magnifica symbiont
Xanthomonas campestris
Coxiella burnetii
Legionella pneumophila
Methylomonas methanica
Pseudomonas putida
Pseudomonas aeruginosa
Teredinibacter turnerae
Acinetobacter calcoaceticus
Moraxella catarrhalis
Shewanella putrefaciens
Vibrio parahaemolyticus
Vibrio fischeri
Vibrio cholerae
Photobacterium phoshoreum
Aeromonas salmonicida
Haemophilus parainfluenzae
Haemophilus influenzae
Yersinia pestis
Yersinia enterocolitica
Proteus vulgaris
Xenorhabdus nematophilus
Serratia marcescens
Erwinia herbicola
Escherichia coli
Buchnera aphidicola
Salmonella typhimurium
Salmonella typhi

Fig. 6.6 The γ subdivision of the Proteobacteria.

other sulphidic minerals such as CuS and CuFeS$_2$ to soluble sulphate forms. *T. ferrooxidans* and other metal-leaching bacteria are used in the western United States for the recovery of copper, uranium, gold and molybdenum low-grade ores (Rawlings and Silver 1995). Another member of this cluster is an uncultured bacterial symbiont (Distel et al. 1988) found inside cells in a tissue called the trophosome in the tubeworms *Riftia pachyptila.* These tubeworms reside near undersea spreading centres, which are essentially underwater hot springs releasing large amounts of reduced sulphur compounds into the surrounding waters. These bacteria oxidize sulphur compounds derived from the hot spring waters and use that energy to fix CO$_2$ by the Calvin cycle (the key enzyme ribulose diphosphate carboxylase has been found in tissues containing these symbionts). Somehow energy, cell carbon, or a combination of both is transferred to the tubeworm host, a reaction analogous to that of the chloroplast, except that the process is the result of chemosynthesis rather than photosynthesis.

Starting with interior clusters in the γ subdivision, one contains the plant pathogen *Xanthomonas* and related organisms. The sulphur-oxidizing lithotroph *Thiomicrospira* is also present, as is a sulphur-oxidizing endosymbiont in tissues of *Calyptogena magnifica,* a large clam found in the same undersea spreading centres as *Riftia.* Finally, *Francisella tularensis,* an animal pathogen, is also found within this cluster. The pathogens *Legionella pneumophila* and *Coxiella burnetii* cluster together. *Legionella* spp. are capable of living saprophytically in environments such as water tanks and

may gain entry to the lungs when water is aerosolized in showers, air conditioning systems, etc.

The methanotroph *Methylomonas methanica* and other related methanotrophic genera (not shown) form a distinct cluster. An important cluster in the γ subdivision includes the fluorescent pseudomonads. They have maintained their genus name *Pseudomonas* and are represented by the opportunistic pathogen *Pseudomonas aeruginosa* and the metabolically versatile *Pseudomonas putida.* An interesting relative of these pseudomonads is *Teredinibacter turnerae,* a symbiont of wood-eating shipworms (Greene 1994). The shipworm was a major problem when ships were made out of wood and is actually a bivalve which uses its shells to burrow through and ingest wood. The bacterial symbiont has been isolated and not only can it break down cellulose, but it can also fix nitrogen under micro-aerophilic conditions, which probably plays a role in allowing the shipworm to survive on wood that is poor in combined nitrogen. Also in this cluster are the diplococci *Acinetobacter calcoaceticus* and *Moraxella catarrhalis,* once considered to be in the genus *Neisseria,* but clearly unrelated according to this analysis, supporting the classical taxonomic criteria used to separate the 2 genera.

The enteric and *Vibrio* groups are classic taxonomic groupings which are supported by SSU rRNA analysis. *Shewanella putrefaciens* is distinguished by its ability to use an enormous number of electron acceptors besides oxygen to support energy conservation by anaerobic respiration (Nealson and Saffarini 1994). The *Vibrio* group contains the pathogens *Vibrio cholerae* and *Vibrio parahaemolyticus,* as well as the fish pathogen *Aeromonas salmonicida.* Also within this group are the luminous marine bacteria, represented by *Vibrio fischeri* and *Photobacterium phoshoreum.* These bacteria can be found free-living in seawater, but many of them are found in light organs of fish and invertebrates. The basis of host and symbiont specificity is being investigated in a squid/*Vibrio* system (Ruby and McFall-Ngai 1992). One interesting aspect of luminous bacteria is their ability to sense their own density by producing an autoinducer that must build up to a sufficient concentration in their environment before bioluminescence is derepressed. It has now been found that several other bacteria have similar density-sensing mechanisms, including ones involving conjugation in *Agrobacterium* and production of elastase, an enzyme important in pathogenesis, by *P. aeruginosa* (Fuqua, Winans and Greenberg 1994).

The genus *Haemophilus* forms a separate cluster within the enteric/*Vibrio* group and includes several pathogens. *Haemophilus influenzae* has the distinction of being the first free-living organism to have its entire genome (c. 1.8 million bp) sequenced (Nowak 1995).

One subcluster of the enteric group includes *Yersinia,* as well as the opportunistic pathogen *Proteus vulgaris.* Another interesting member of this cluster is *Xenorhabdus nematophilus.* This insect pathogen is typically found associated with nematode worms that prey on the insects killed by *X. nematophilus.* An interesting aspect of *X. nematophilus* is that it is bioluminescent with a system homologous to the marine *Vibrio* and *Photobacterium* spp. It is likely that it obtained this system by horizontal genetic transfer, since it is not closely related to those organisms. *Xenorhabdus luminescens* has been isolated from human wounds (Colepicolo et al. 1989).

Serratia marcescens is an opportunistic pathogen known for the production of the red pigment prodigiosin. Colonies of this organism growing on host wafers are believed to be the explanation for such phenomena as the miracle of Bolsena, their red colour interpreted as the blood of Christ (Cullen 1994). The genus *Erwinia* includes many plant pathogens and plant-associated bacteria. *E. coli* is found in the human gut and in most molecular biology laboratories, and some strains are enteropathogenic. The closely related pathogen *Shigella* has not had its SSU rRNA sequenced, but is likely to be extremely closely related, if not identical. The pathogens *Salmonella typhi* and *Salmonella typhimurium* are indistinguishable from each other by SSU rDNA analysis and are closely related to *E. coli*, as would be expected from extensive genetic analysis. Somewhat distantly related to *E. coli* is *Buchnera aphidicola*, an uncultured endosymbiont of aphids. When the branching pattern of SSU rDNA sequence strains of *B. aphidicola* found in different aphid species (not shown) was compared to the pattern for their aphid hosts, based on the fossil record and other taxonomic criteria, they were nearly identical (Moran et al. 1993). Using the fossil record for aphids as a calibration, it was determined that the mutation rate for the SSU rDNA in *B. aphidicola* was c. 0.05 per position per million years. Whether this rate applies to other organisms is not known.

THE δ AND ε SUBDIVISIONS

The δ subdivision (Fig. 6.7) contains no known photosynthetic bacteria and is dominated by organisms that use oxidized sulphur compounds, such as sulphate or elemental sulphur, as electron acceptors, reducing them to H_2S. These bacteria have been called sulphidogens or sulphate reducers; typically their genus names begin with *Desulfo-*. A representative equation for sulphate is: $2 \text{ lactate}^- + SO_4^{2-} \rightarrow 2 \text{ acetate}^- + 2CO_2 + H_2S + 3H_2O$. Most sulphidogens are obligate anaerobes; they have limited abilities to use other electron acceptors such as nitrite and fumarate. *Desulfomonile tiedjei* can also use the carbon–chlorine bond of 3-chlorobenzoate and a few related compounds as an electron acceptor for growth by a process called reductive dechlorination (Mohn and Tiedje 1992) which has the general equation $R\text{-}Cl + 2H \rightarrow R\text{-}H + HCl$. There has been considerable interest in organisms carrying out reductive dechlorination, mainly anaerobes, since they can detoxify many highly chlorinated organics that are not attacked by aerobes, such as highly chlorinated ethylenes and polychlorinated biphenyls (Mohn and Tiedje 1992). *Geobacter metalireducens* is capable of using Fe^{3+} as an electron acceptor for the oxidation of acetate, toluene and other organic molecules by the generalized equation $RH_2 + 2Fe^{3+} \rightarrow R + 2Fe^{2+} + 2H^+$ (Nealson and Saffarini 1994). *Syntrophobacter* can oxid-

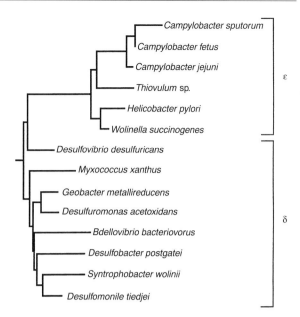

Fig. 6.7 The δ and ε subdivisions of the Proteobacteria.

ize propionic acid by the equation: $\text{propionate}^- + H_2O \rightarrow \text{acetate}^- + 3H_2 + CO_2$. This reaction is important in anaerobic habitats and its free energy is favourable only if the H_2 partial pressure is kept below 10^{-4} atm by being consumed by an organism such as a methanogen (Zinder 1993).

There are no animal pathogens in the δ subdivision, but there are some bacterial cannibals. *Bdellovibrio bacteriovorus* is an obligate aerobe consisting of small highly motile comma-shaped cells that attack other gram-negative bacteria by burrowing into their periplasm, killing the host cell inside and digesting the contents of that cell for its own nutrition. *Myxococcus xanthus*, a representative of the myxobacteria, is a long rod which typically travels in multicellular aggregates (likened to wolf packs) gliding along a surface; it produces enzymes which lyse other bacteria, providing them with a growth substrate. When food is scarce, the myxobacteria form intricate fruiting bodies, making them an interesting system for studying developmental biology in prokaryotes. Why these 2 aerobic genera are related to the anaerobic sulphidogens is unclear.

The ε division is dominated by micro-aerophiles, including the genus *Campylobacter*, some species of which, such as *C. fetus* and *C. jejuni*, are enteric pathogens whereas others are saprophytic. *Helicobacter* (previously *Camplylobacter*) *pylori* has received considerable attention for its role in gastric ulcers and potentially in gastric cancer. *Wolinella succinogenes* is a micro-aerophile found in the animal rumen; it is capable of using several different electron acceptors. Also found in this group is the genus *Thiovulum*, a micro-aerophilic sulphur-oxidizing lithotroph.

4.2   The low % G + C gram-positive bacteria

The low % G + C gram-positive group, sometimes called *Clostridium* and relatives, is an extremely diverse group (Fig. 6.8); it includes mycoplasmas, some truly gram-negative bacteria and even a photosynthetic member. The % G + C in members of this group is not necessarily low; although some mycoplasmas and clostridia have % G + C values of <30, in other members, the % G + C can be >50. This distinction is between these organisms and the high % G + C gram-positive bacteria or actinomycetes, which typically have % G + C values >60.

The wide distribution of endospore-forming clostridia in the group suggests that the original ancestor of the group was an endospore-former and also indicates that the genus *Clostridium* needs to be subdivided into several genera. A recent and extensive analysis of this group (Collins et al. 1994) retains the name *Clostridium* for the butyric acid group, since *Clostridium butyricum* is the type species, and proposes 4 new generic names for other organisms previously called *Clostridium*. A large number of other strains still require reclassification after this analysis. Several lines of clostridia contain moderate thermophiles and it is unclear whether the ancestor of this group was thermophilic, or whether several groups adapted to higher temperature independently.

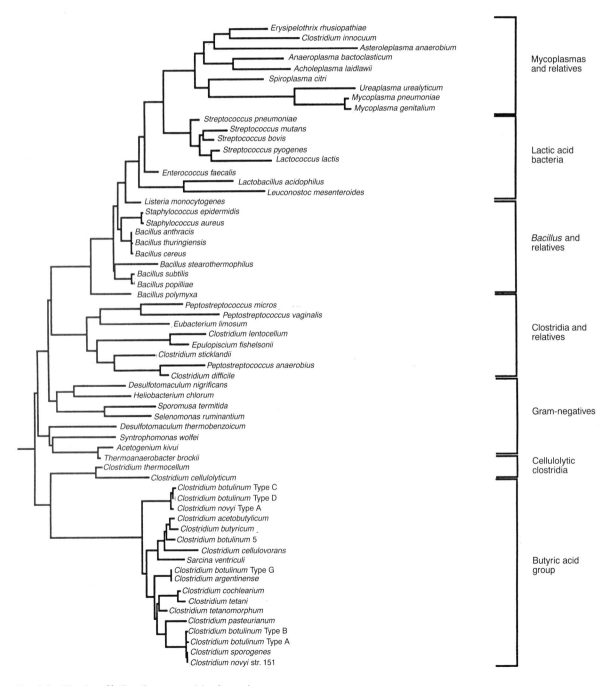

Fig. 6.8   The low % G + C gram-positive bacteria.

Early phylogenetic studies using SSU rRNA oligonucleotide cataloguing (Fox et al. 1980) first showed the definite relationship between mycoplasmas, which lack a cell wall, and gram-positive bacteria. This finding was not completely unexpected since their metabolism in many ways resembled that of lactic acid bacteria, carrying out simple fermentations and having only a flavin-linked peroxidase-type aerobic metabolism. The mycoplasmas often have genome sizes of < 1000 kb and lack many biosynthetic pathways, leading to their having a complex nutrition. Some strains even use a slightly altered genetic code. An early interpretation was that mycoplasmas represent primitive cells, a still-extant early stage of evolution. Their close relationship to clostridia by SSU rDNA analysis suggests that instead they represent de-evolved cells which lost the ability to synthesize peptidoglycan cell walls and many other cell components. That they are a rapidly evolving group is evident from their distance from the root of the group relative to other members (Woese 1987).

Most pathogenic mycoplasmas require sterols to strengthen their cell membranes and are associated with animal or plant hosts, including the pathogens *Mycoplasma pneumoniae*, *Mycoplasma genitalium*, *Ureaplasma urealyticum* and *Spiroplasma citri*. Spiroplasmas are associated with either plant or insect hosts, have a spiral morphology, due to the presence of filaments running down the centre of the cell, and show motility even though they lack a structure resembling a true bacterial flagellum. *Acholeplasma*, *Asteroleplasma* and *Anaeroplasma* do not require sterols and can be found living outside animal or plant tissues. *Anaeroplasma*, for example, has been isolated from the bovine rumen. There are cell wall-containing strains of clostridia which cluster within the mycoplasma group, as does the pathogen *Erysipelothrix*.

The lactic acid bacteria are a classically defined bacterial group which cluster together according to SSU rDNA analysis; they include the significant pathogens *Streptococcus pyogenes* and *Streptococcus pneumoniae*. This group has a fermentative metabolism in which only sugars are used. Homofermentative lactic acid bacteria, such as members of the genus *Streptococcus*, produce only lactic acid as a primary product of sugar fermentation (hexose → 2 lactic acid), whereas heterofermentative strains, such as *Leuconostoc*, also produce ethanol and carbon dioxide (hexose → lactic acid + ethanol + CO_2). Members of the group typically have complex nutrition, requiring amino acids, vitamins and nucleotide precursors. Most lactic acid bacteria are resistant to high acid concentrations. This ability allows *Streptococcus mutans* (and other lactic acid bacteria living in dental plaque) to produce enough acid from ingested sugars to dissolve tooth enamel, thereby causing cavities. A more innocuous activity associated with many non-pathogenic lactic acid bacteria is the production of fermented foods such as cheese, yogurt, sauerkraut and pickles. These foods are preserved by their high acid content and were especially important before refrigeration was available for food preservation. These so-called lactic streptococci have been reclassified as *Lactococcus*; the enteric or faecal streptococci, occasional pathogens living in gastrointestinal tracts, have been reclassified as *Enterococcus*.

Another fairly diverse cluster contains *Bacillus* and relatives, essentially all the respiratory aerobes in the low % G + C gram-positives. Loosely affiliated with this group and the lactic acid bacteria is the pathogen *Listeria monocytogenes*. Also within this group are the staphylococci. It is interesting that the potent animal pathogen *Bacillus anthracis* and the insect pathogen *Bacillus thuringiensis* are closely related to each other and to the saprophyte *Bacillus cereus*; the insect pathogen *Bacillus popilliae* is closely related to *Bacillus subtilis*.

The next cluster contains various morphologies of anaerobes. It contains members of the genus *Peptostreptococcus*, anaerobic chain-forming cocci, some of which cause wound infections, and the intestinal pathogen *Clostridium difficile*. Also present is a member of the genus *Eubacterium* which has been the name given to any non-spore-forming anaerobic rod; some members of this genus will need reassignment. One of the most interesting members of this assemblage is *Epulopiscium fishelsonii*. This is the name given to giant bacteria (up to 600 μm in length) that were found in the gastrointestinal contents of the surgeonfish. This organism, which has not been cultured, was once believed to be a protozoan, but electron micrographs show an essentially prokaryotic cell structure with extensive membrane invaginations to overcome its low surface area to volume ratio. The prokaryotic nature of the cell was confirmed when a specific fluorescently labelled SSU rDNA probe derived from a sequence obtained from the mixed population was shown to hybridize with rRNA in cells of this organism (Angert, Clements and Pace 1993). Curiously, *E. fishelsonii* is fairly closely related to the ordinary cellulose-utilizing *Clostridium lentocellum*.

The next cluster consists of truly gram-negative organisms; these organisms not only stain gram-negative, but thin sections show a typical gram-negative ultrastructure, including a thin peptidoglycan layer, and usually even an outer membrane. The genus *Sporomusa* forms a true endospore, as does *Desulfotomaculum*. Members of the genus *Desulfotomaculum* are sulphate reducers. *Selenomonas ruminantium* is an important member of the microbial population in the animal rumen and was traditionally considered a gram-negative bacterium.

Probably the most surprising member of the gram-positive division is *Heliobacterium chlorum*, an anoxygenic photosynthetic bacterium that metabolizes organic compounds in a manner similar to the purple non-sulphur bacteria. Its primary photopigment is bacteriochlorophyll *g*, which spontaneously reacts with oxygen to form chlorophyll *a*. It was surprising that this recently discovered organism and its relatives grouped within the gram-positives, but the gram-positive nature of these organisms was confirmed by the more recent finding that some strains produce true endospores! The presence of this deep branching assemblage of gram-negatives within the gram-positives suggests that perhaps the ancestor of this group was actually gram-negative and that the simpler gram-positive cell wall architecture is the result of loss of the outer membrane. Moreover, it also suggests that the original ancestor of the group was photosynthetic.

Another deep branching assemblage also contains some gram-negative members, such as *Syntrophomonas wolfei*, which oxidizes butyrate to acetate (butyrate$^-$ → 2 acetate$^-$ + 2H$_2$ + H$^+$) when grown together with a hydrogen-consuming organism, such as a methanogen, which will keep the H$_2$ partial pressure low enough to allow the reaction to be thermodynamically favourable. Also included in this group is the thermophile *Acetogenium kivui* (which may be renamed *Thermoanaerobacter kivui* (Collins et al. 1994). *A. kivui* is an acetogen, an organism which is capable of reducing CO$_2$ to acetate, a form of anaerobic respiration, using reducing power derived from either fermentation of sugars and other compounds or from H$_2$ directly according to the equation: 8H + 2CO$_2$ → CH$_3$COO$^-$ + 2H$_2$O + H$^+$. Acetyl-CoA is synthesized *de novo* in a fascinating process involving the nickel-containing carbon monoxide dehydrogenase–corrinoid protein complex (Drake 1994). This pathway is widespread in the anaerobic gram-positives, being found in members of the genera *Sporomusa*, *Desulfotomaculum*, *Peptostreptococcus*, *Eubacterium* and several clostridia (Drake 1994).

A cluster of mainly cellulolytic clostridia is represented by the thermophile *Clostridium thermocellum* and the mesophile *Clostridium cellulolyticum*. The ability to use cellulose is found in several of the clostridial clusters and this is not surprising, since this plant polymer is the most abundant source of carbon and energy available to anaerobes in many habitats.

The final large cluster includes *C. butyricum*, which produces butyric acid from sugars as a major product, as well as *Clostridium acetobutylicum*, which produces the solvents acetone and butanol and was an important source of these chemicals earlier in the century. Several pathogens producing potent exotoxins are present in this cluster, including *Clostridium tetani* and many strains of *Clostridium botulinum*. The wide distribution of production of the various botulism toxin types within this group is suggestive of genetic exchange; at least some of these toxins have been found to be associated with bacteriophage causing lysogenic conversion.

4.3   The high % G + C gram-positive bacteria

This group has also been called the actinomycetes; it is characterized by generally having % G + C values >60 and its phylogeny has recently been reviewed (Embley, Hirt and Williams 1994). It has traditionally been considered a sister group to the low % G + C gram-positive bacteria and some analyses support this. Other methods show no particular relationships between the 2 groups (Vandepeer et al. 1994), even when % G + C bias is taken into account in the analysis. Many of the members of this group undergo life cycles and many form branched filaments. Although

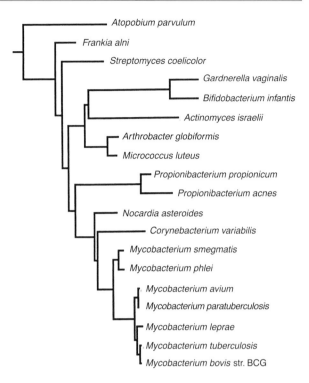

Fig. 6.9   The high % G + C gram-positive bacteria.

various spore types can be formed by members of this group, none is a true endospore (the genus *Thermoactinomyces*, which does form a true endospore, was shown by early analysis (Fox et al. 1980) to belong to the low % G + C gram-positive bacteria). The deepest branch in the group is represented by *Atopobium* (Fig. 6.9), an obligate anaerobe with DNA containing only 44% G + C. *Atopobium* was thought to be a divergent member of the low % G + C gram-positive bacteria, but was shown by more careful analysis to be a member of this group (Stackebrandt and Ludwig 1994).

The typical streptomycetes are soil organisms that form branched filaments resembling fungi. Many undergo life cycles in which they form exospores. One genus, *Frankia*, forms nitrogen-fixing nodules considerably different from those formed by rhizobia, in the alder tree, and a variety of other trees and shrubs (Benson and Silvester 1993). Nitrogen fixation occurs in specialized cell packets called vesicles in which the nitrogenase is protected from oxygen by a thick glycolipid layer. The genus *Streptomyces* is a diverse genus containing organisms important in soils (among other things, they produce substances which give soil its smell). Various *Streptomyces* strains produce many of the important antibiotics used today.

Bifidobacterium is an important organism colonizing the gut of breast-fed infants. Although it carries out a fermentation resembling that of lactic acid bacteria, it uses a different glycolytic pathway and SSU rRNA analysis confirms that it is unrelated to the typical lactics. Related to *Bifidobacterium* is the sometime pathogen *Gardnerella vaginalis*.

Members of the genus *Actinomyces* are typically found in soils, but *Actinomyces israelii*, *Actinomyces viscosus* and *Actinomyces naeslundii* are inhabitants of the oral mucosa and are frequently found in oral and systemic infections. *Micrococcus luteus* is a common inhabitant of skin and dust particles in the air. This organism was once considered to be an obligately aerobic relative of the facultative anaerobe *Staphylococcus* because of their morphological similarity, but first % G + C analysis, and now SSU rRNA analysis, does not support any specific relationship between these organisms. Members of the genus *Arthrobacter* are numerous in soil and this organism is noted by going through a life cycle in which it is a rod when growing, and a coccus when in stationary phase. *Arthrobacter* spp. are also extremely starvation-resistant, with some strains capable of surviving for years in the absence of substrate.

Members of the genus *Propionibacterium* are aerotolerant anaerobes producing propionic acid from sugars. By virtue of the CO_2 produced in its fermentation, *Propionibacterium propionicum* is responsible for the holes (actually thin sections through bubbles) in Swiss cheese, whereas *Propionibacterium acnes* is an inhabitant of skin which may cause infections. Finally, there is the *Nocardia, Corynebacterium, Mycobacterium* cluster, which contains several pathogens of note. It is likely that *Corynebacterium diphtheriae* is related to *Corynebacterium variabilis*, but its SSU rDNA sequence is not presently in the database. The pathogenic mycobacteria group closely together and separately from the saprophytic ones.

4.4 The spirochaetes

The spirochaetes are corkscrew-shaped bacteria which have their flagella located inside the periplasmic space, which is why they are called endoflagella (they were formerly called axial filaments). Because of their shape, spirochaetes are capable of moving through highly viscous environments, including animal tissues. Members of this classically defined group also form a robust cluster according to SSU rRNA analysis (Fig. 6.10).

The leptospiras are aerobes, many of which are saprophytic, but some of which, such as *Leptospira interrogans*, cause leptospirosis. Many spirochaetes are either facultative or obligate anaerobes; they are found in many habitats including hot springs (*Spirochaeta thermophila*) and hypersaline waters (*Spirochaeta halophila*). Most free-living spirochaetes do not degrade cellulose, but are capable of using sugars derived from cellulose, and are found closely associated with cellulolytic bacteria. Spirochaetes are also found in gingival plaque and large numbers of spirochaetes are considered indicators of periodontal disease. *Treponema pallidum*, the causal agent of syphilis, resisted culture until it was realized that it was a microaerophile. Also included in this group are the pathogens *Serpulina* (formerly *Treponema*) *hyodysenteriae* and *Borrelia burgdorferi*, the causative agent of Lyme disease.

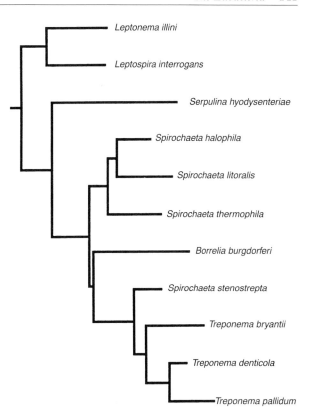

Fig. 6.10 The spirochaetes.

4.5 The cyanobacteria

Cyanobacteria, formerly called blue-green algae, are prokaryotes that carry out oxygenic (oxygen-evolving) photosynthesis, deriving electrons from water to reduce carbon dioxide to cellular material by the general equation: $H_2O + CO_2 \rightarrow CH_2O + O_2$. Water is a much poorer electron donor than are the donors used

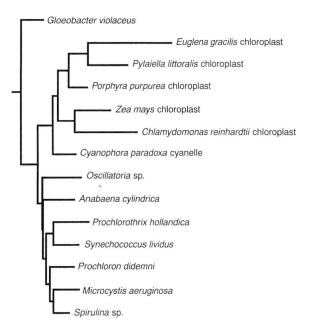

Fig. 6.11 The cyanobacteria.

by purple and green photosynthetic bacteria, such as H_2S or organic material. Consequently, this reaction requires an enormous input of energy to proceed and this energy is derived from light using 2 sequential photosystems, rather than the single one in the anoxygenic organisms. At present, the cyanobacteria group does not contain any non-photosynthetic members (Fig. 6.11).

Cyanobacteria are widespread, found in diverse freshwater and marine environments receiving light, as well as in some soils. In these habitats, they compete with eukaryotic algae. One advantage many cyanobacteria have over eukaryotes is that they can fix nitrogen, often a limiting nutrient. None of the cyanobacteria is a pathogen, but certain freshwater strains, such as *Anabaena* and *Microcystis*, produce saxitoxin-like neurotoxins in the waters in which they grow. This is usually not a problem for humans, but farm animals can be poisoned by drinking water from ponds containing dense cyanobacterial blooms. It has been hypothesized that these toxins are produced to kill fish, thereby releasing nutrients.

The cyanobacteria were originally classified into groups on the basis or morphology, such that unicellular cyanobacteria were grouped with each other as were filamentous forms. This taxonomic principle was not upheld by SSU rDNA studies. One classically defined group that has withstood SSU rDNA analysis is the filamentous cyanobacteria with heterocysts, specialized cells that fix nitrogen, represented by *Anabaena cylindrica*. Heterocysts protect the oxygen-labile enzyme nitrogenase, since, unlike vegetative cells, heterocysts do not carry out oxygen-evolving photosynthesis and further protect the nitrogenase by having an oxygen-impermeable glycolipid layer and a suite of respiratory enzymes.

Within the cyanobacteria group are the chloroplasts of algae and plants, consistent with their being derived from a cyanobacterium engulfed by a eukaryotic host. Chloroplasts have a genome size of 100–200 kb and therefore have lost most of their genetic material. Among the chloroplasts represented here are those of green plants (*Zea*), green algae (*Chlamydomonas*), red algae (*Porphyra*), diatoms (*Pylaiella*) and *Euglena*. Also represented is the cyanelle of *Cyanophora paradoxa*, an organelle which has a peptidoglycan cell wall and was thought to be closer to a free-living cyanobacterium; however, it has a genome size of only 135 kb. Despite the diversity in chloroplast pigmentation, thus far SSU rDNA analysis indicates that there was a single origin for the chloroplast line.

Most cyanobacteria use pigmented proteins called phycobilins as their accessory pigments, as do the chloroplasts of red algae and cyanelles. When cyanobacteria containing chlorophyll *b* instead of phycobilins were found, such as *Prochloron* and *Prochlorothrix*, it was concluded by some that they represent the ancestors of the green plant and green algal chloroplasts. However, SSU rDNA analysis does not show any specific relationship between these so-called prochlorophytes and the appropriate chloroplasts (Fig. 6.11) and one must conclude that chlorophyll *b* was

invented several times in the cyanobacteria and chloroplasts. Finally, chloroplasts and nearly all cyanobacteria contain several layers of thylakoid membranes, or lamellae, within them. An exception to this is *Gloeobacter*, which carries out its photosynthesis in a single cell membrane. This is the deepest branch in the cyanobacteria, suggesting that it represents a form of cyanobacteria extant before the development of lamellae.

4.6 The other eubacterial groups

Figure 6.12 shows representatives of the remaining eubacterial groups along with some of the groups previously discussed as points of reference. Only 2 of these groups contain pathogens of note, the *Bacteroides–Cytophaga–Flavobacterium* group and the *Planctomyces–Chlamydia* group.

The *Bacteroides–Cytophaga–Flavobacterium* group consists mainly of long rods, which may be aerobic or anaerobic. *Cytophaga*, an aerobe found in waters and soils, uses complex substrates such as cellulose, chitin, or agar and moves by gliding along surfaces, as does *Capnocytophaga*, a long facultatively anaerobic rod which is a member of the oral microbiota and which requires high CO_2 concentrations. *Flavobacterium* is an aerobic long rod, which can be yellow due to carotenoid pigments. The genus name *Bacteroides* was once given to practically any obligately gram-negative anaerobic rod; more recently the genus has been divided (many members were in the Proteobacteria), with members of this group retaining the genus name (Paster et al. 1994). Many members are common inhabitants of animal gastrointestinal tracts and some, such as *Bacteroides fragilis*, can cause infections. *Prevotella denticola* was once named *Bacteroides* and is a common member of the oral microbiota.

The *Planctomyces–Chlamydia* group has the interesting property that its members have cell walls lacking muramic acid-containing peptidoglycan. *Planctomyces* and its relatives are spherical organisms often containing stalks; they are common in waters and soils. The cell wall of *Planctomyces* consists of protein and they are resistant to β-lactam antibiotics. *Chlamydia* are obligate intracellular pathogens causing a variety of animal diseases. *Chlamydia trachomatis* is a human pathogen which can cause the eye infection trachoma and nongonoccocal urethritis, a common venereal disease. Although they lack the typical murein cell wall, *Chlamydia* contain penicillin-binding proteins.

The green sulphur photosynthetic bacteria are represented by *Chlorobium limicola*. All members of this group are photosynthetic, using sulphur compounds as electron donors in a manner similar to the purple sulphur bacteria. They have little ability to use organic compounds and are obligate anaerobes. Their primary reaction centre chlorophyll is bacteriochlorophyll *a* and their accessory bacteriochlorophylls are usually *c* and *e*, present in proteinaceous structures associated with the cell membrane called chlorosomes. They are green (or brown) due to carotenoids. They do not fix CO_2 using the Calvin cycle, instead using a reversal of

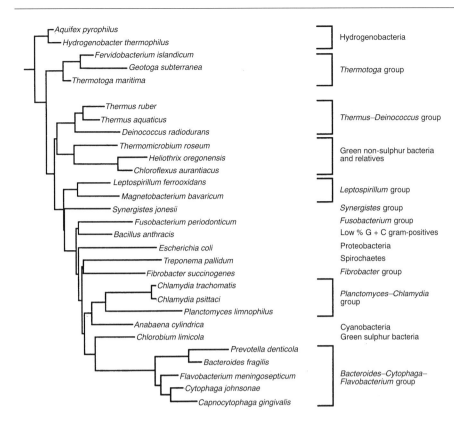

Fig. 6.12 Other eubacterial groups not represented in Figs 6.3–6.11.

the tricarboxylic acid cycle. Green sulphur bacteria are found in anaerobic waters and muds receiving light.

Certain genera appear to form clusters separate enough from others to deserve group status; 3 examples of this are *Fibrobacter*, *Fusobacterium* and *Synergistes*. *Fibrobacter succinogenes* was once called *Bacteroides*, is a gram-negative anaerobic rod and is considered one of the most important bacteria in the animal rumen responsible for degrading plant cellulose. The fusobacteria are long anaerobic rods with blunt ends; they are among the common oral flora and can cause periodontal disease. *Synergistes jonesii* is an amino acid-fermenting anaerobe which was isolated from the rumen of animals by virtue of its ability to detoxify products of mimosine, a compound found in the tropical legume *Leucaena*. This organism and others capable of detoxifying mimosine products are often not found in ruminants fed *Leucaena*, but which have not grazed extensively on this legume; however, inoculation with *S. jonesii* alleviates toxicity problems (Hammond 1995).

Leptospirillum ferrooxidans is an acidophilic aerobe which oxidizes ferrous iron in a manner similar to *Thiobacillus ferrooxidans* (Rawlings and Silver 1995); it can play an important role in the leaching of sulphidic minerals (Sand et al. 1992). *Magnetobacterium bavaricum* is an uncultured magnetotactic rod with sulphur granules; it is found in the micro-areobic zone of lake sediments (Spring et al. 1993) and shows no relationship to *Magnetospirillum*, which is in the β subdivision of the Proteobacteria. *Leptospirillum* and *Magnetospirillum* are united by iron metabolism, but it would have been unclear from phenotypic analysis that they were

not related to proteobacteria with similar metabolisms.

The green non-sulphur photosynthetic bacteria group contains *Chloroflexus*, a gliding thermophilic long rod abundant in hot spring photosynthetic mats. *Chloroflexus* has chlorosomes and pigmentation similar to that of the green sulphur bacteria. However, its metabolism is considerably different; it resembles the purple non-sulphur photosynthetic bacteria, since it uses a wide variety of organic compounds and low concentrations of sulphide. *Chloroflexus* is also capable of growing as an aerobic heterotroph in the absence of light. It fixes CO_2 by a novel pathway involving hydroxypropionate. Another thermophilic phototroph in this group is *Heliothrix*, which does not contain chlorosomes. *Thermomicrobium* is a thermophilic non-photosynthetic aerobic heterotroph.

Thermus aquaticus is a thermophilic aerobic heterotroph readily isolated from hot springs; its claim to fame is that its heat-stable DNA polymerase (Taq polymerase) allowed the polymerase chain reaction (PCR) to be automated. Previously, fresh DNA polymerase needed to be added after each time the DNA strands were denatured at 90–95°C. The DNA polymerases from other thermophiles, such as the archaeon *Pyrococcus furiosus*, are now also used for PCR. A curious relative of *Thermus* is *Deinococcus*, a mesophilic aerobic heterotrophic coccus that stains gram-positive, but has an outer membrane. This organism was discovered as the last survivor during trials of food sterilization by irradiation. It is about a 1000-fold more resistant to radiation than is *E. coli* and its mechanisms for radiation resistance have been studied (Udupa et al. 1994).

The *Thermotoga* group is one of the most divergent of the Eubacteria. *Thermotoga maritima* is a fermentative anaerobic heterotroph whose growth is stimulated by elemental sulphur; it has a maximum growth temperature near 90°C. It is rod shaped with a peptidoglycan cell wall and a loose outer layer which has been called the 'toga'. Its lipids have ether linkages like archaeal lipids, but the hydrocarbon chains are not isoprenoid. *Fervidobacterium* has metabolism similar to *Thermotoga* and grows at temperatures up to 80°C whereas *Geotoga* is a more moderate thermophile with an optimum growth temperature near 50°C (Davey et al. 1993). The *Thermotoga* group has many properties resembling the Archaea and until recently, it was considered the most deeply branching eubacterial group, leading to the proposition that it is most similar to the original ancestor of the Eubacteria.

More recently, the organism *Aquifex pyrophilus* took from *Thermotoga* the title of most thermophilic eubacterium (95°C) and perhaps the most divergent (Huber et al. 1992). *A. pyrophilus* also has a respiratory metabolism, using H_2 as an electron donor and using as electron acceptors oxygen (micro-aerophilically) or nitrate. Also clustering with *Aquifex* is the more moderate thermophile *Hydrogenobacter* (Pitulle et al. 1994). Since this branch may be deeper than the *Thermotoga* branch (there is some controversy over the branching order) it is less clear what type of metabolism the ancestor of the Eubacteria had.

5 THE ARCHAEA

The Archaea divide into 2 major branches (Fig. 6.13): the Euryarchaeota, which has been called methanogens and relatives, and the Crenarchaeota, which has been called the sulphur-dependent thermophiles. The

Euryarchaeota are a diverse group containing a wide variety of methanogens, sulphate-reducing bacteria, aerobic halophiles, aerobic thermoacidophiles and anaerobic hyperthermophiles. The few genera of Crenarchaeota that are known are all thermophiles and their metabolism is described as being either sulphur-reducing heterotrophs, or as aerobes capable of oxidizing sulphur compounds, some other inorganic compounds, or organic compounds. However, recent ecological studies on hot springs (Barns et al. 1994) and open ocean waters (Olsen 1994) have shown that there is considerably greater diversity present in natural habitats than there is in culture collections. None of the Archaea is known to be pathogenic, unless flatulence caused by methanogens is considered a pathological condition.

The methanogens are stringent anaerobes which have a limited metabolic repertoire, generally only growing by producing methane from a limited number of simple substrates. The 2 most important substrates in nature are H_2/CO_2 ($4H_2 + CO_2 \rightarrow CH_4 + 2H_2O$) and acetate ($CH_3COOH \rightarrow CH_4 + CO_2$). Nearly all methanogens can grow by the former reaction; for some it is the only catabolic reaction they are capable of carrying out. Elucidating the pathway to methane led to the discovery of 6 new cofactors (DiMarco, Bobik and Wolfe 1990) and several novel enzymes (Ferry 1993). Many methanogens are autotrophs and fix their own CO_2 by forming acetyl-CoA by a reaction resembling that carried out by acetogens. The taxonomy of the methanogens is based on SSU rDNA sequences and they can be divided into 5 orders (Boone, Whitman and Rouvière 1993).

The Methanosarcinales is the most metabolically versatile of the orders and *Methanosarcina* is the most versatile methanogen genus, with strains being able to

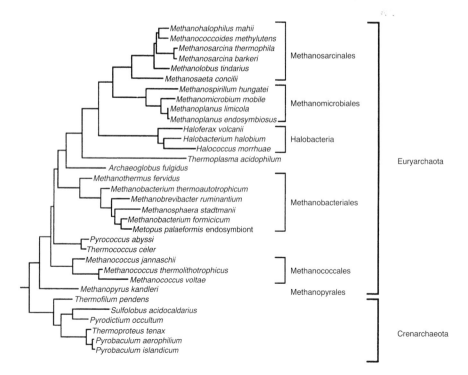

Fig. 6.13 The Archaea.

use H_2/CO_2, acetate, methanol ($4CH_3OH \rightarrow 3CH_4 + CO_2 + 2H_2O$), and methylamines by reactions analogous to methanol. The latter substrates can be important in some habitats where they are the breakdown products of choline and the osmolytes glycine-betaine and trimethylamine-*N*-oxide. *Methanosarcina*, when grown in media with freshwater-like osmolarity, grows as coccoid cells in large aggregates surrounded by a thick acidic polysaccharide sacculus. In marine medium, most *Methanosarcina* strains lose the outer sacculus (they also have a protein cell wall) and grow as individual coccoid cells. The outer sacculus apparently serves as a corset to prevent lysis under conditions of low osmotic strength. *Methanolobus*, *Methanococcoides* and *Methanohalophilus* are all coccoid organisms growing on methylated compounds with the former 2 being marine organisms and the latter being a halophile. *Methanosaeta concilii* (also called *Methanothrix soehngenii*) is a sheathed filamentous rod which only grows on acetate. It and *Methanosarcina* are the only methanogen genera which can use this important fermentation product.

The Methanomicrobiales all grow on H_2/CO_2 or formate ($4HCOOH \rightarrow CH_4 + 3CO_2 + 2H_2O$). They all have protein cell walls, and *Methanospirillum hungatei* and *Methanomicrobium mobile* are motile by polar flagella. *Methanoplanus endosymbiosus* is found inside the anaerobic protozoan *Metopus contortus*. There are several other examples of this phenomenon in the methanogens, including one in the Methanobacteriales in Fig. 6.13, of methanogens residing inside protozoans where they presumably consume H_2 produced by the host (Zinder 1993).

The Methanobacteriales all have cell walls made of pseudomurein and resmble gram-positive bacteria in thin-section electron micrographs (Ferry 1993). All can use H_2/CO_2 and most can use formate, except for *Methanosphaera stadtmanii*, which only grows by the reaction ($H_2 + CH_3OH \rightarrow CH_4 + H_2O$). *Methanobacterium thermoautotrophicum* can grow in temperatures up to 75°C while *Methanothermus fervidus* can grow at temperatures up to 97°C. *Methanobrevibacter ruminantium* and the closely related *Methanobrevibacter smithii* are both common in animal gastrointestinal tracts including those of humans. About one-third of humans produce considerable amounts of methane and in these individuals numbers of methanogens can range from 10^8 to more than 10^{10} per gram dry weight of faeces, whereas numbers in non-producers are fewer than 10^7 (Miller and Wolin 1982). Hereditary and dietary factors and age can all influence the amount of methane produced in the gastrointestinal tract; there has been some evidence for correlation with the amount of bile acids secreted into the gut (Florin and Jabbar 1994).

The Methanococcales are motile marine cocci, all of which can use H_2/CO_2 and most formate. *Methanococcus voltae* is a mesophile, *Methanococcus thermolithotrophicus* can grow at temperatures up to 70°C, whereas *Methanococcus jannaschii* can grow at temperatures up to 92°C. Many methanogens are slow-growing, with doubling times of the order of several hours or days, but *M. jannaschii* can grow in a mineral medium on

H_2/CO_2 with a doubling time near 20 min! Because of their divergence from the mesophilic cocci and from each other, *M. thermolithotrophicus* and *M. jannaschii* will probably be reassigned to the novel genera *Methanothermococcus* and *Methanocaldococcus* respectively (Boone, Whitman and Rouvière 1993). *Methanopyrus* is the only genus representing the Methanopyrales. This rod-shaped organism has a pseudomurein cell wall and can grow on H_2/CO_2 at temperatures up to 110°C.

Other members of the Euryarchaeota are quite diverse. The halobacteria are aerobic heterotrophs which typically grow in waters with NaCl concentrations greater than 1 m, such as in the Great Salt Lake in Utah, the Dead Sea in Israel and in salt evaporation ponds. Halobacteria, especially *Halococcus*, which has a thick polysaccharide sacculus allowing it to withstand lower NaCl concentrations, can cause spoilage of salted fish. The membranes of some halobacteria contain bacteriorhodopsin, a protein which has a retinal prosthetic group identical to that in rhodopsin found in animal eyes. Bacteriorhodopsin serves as a light-driven proton pump, which allows generation of a proton-motive force. Animal rhodopsins do not pump ions; rather they activate G proteins in a sensory cascade. Also found in some halobacteria are halorhodopsin, a light-driven chloride pump, and sensory rhodopsin, which plays a role in phototaxis (Spudich 1993).

Thermoplasma acidophilum lacks a cell wall and is an aerobic heterotroph which grows at temperatures up to 60°C; it is an acidophile, preferring pH values near 2.0. It forms fried egg-like colonies and was classified with the mycoplasmas until its archaeal nature was discovered. It does not require sterols for growth and was originally discovered in self-heating acidic piles of coal refuse; it has been found in acidic hot springs. *Archaeoglobus* is a thermophilic sulphate reducer which grows at temperatures up to 85°C. It contains coenzyme F_{420} and methanopterin, which are also found in methanogens, but does not contain coenzyme M, which is the immediate precursor of methane in methanogens. Thus, its metabolism shows some similarities to the methanogens to which it is closely related. *Thermococcus* and *Pyrococcus* are 2 highly thermophilic anaerobic heterotrophs whose growth is stimulated by addition of elemental sulphur. *Pyrococcus abyssi* and *Pyrococcus furiosus* grow optimally near 100°C and the latter is the source of some extremely themostable enzymes, including an amylase which has optimal activity at 120°C (Koch et al. 1990) and a DNA polymerase which is used for the PCR which is more thermostable and shows better proofreading ability than the *Thermus aquaticus* enzyme. It has been found that only subtle changes in amino acid composition are responsible for the remarkable thermostability of proteins from these organisms.

The known Crenarchaeota are not as diverse as the Euryarchaeota. Most of the Crenarchaeota are obligate anaerobes that use organic electron donors or H_2 to reduce elemental sulphur to H_2S by the equation: $H_2 + S^0 \rightarrow H_2S$. One of these, the genus *Pyrodictium*, can grow at temperatures up to 110°C, the melting point of elemental sulphur. *Sulfolobus* and its relatives can grow at temperatures up to 85°C and at pH values as low as 1.0; they are metabolically versatile, able to grow aerobically on a variety of organic molecules, as well as sulphur compounds and Fe^{2+}. Some strains can grow aerobically on metal sulphide minerals in a manner similar to *T. ferrooxidans* and some strains can grow anaerobically, reducing S^0. *Pyrobaculum aerophilum* can grow micro-aerophilically and can reduce nitrate, in a manner similar to the eubacterium *Aquifex pyrophilus*.

6 SUMMARY AND CONCLUSIONS

It is hoped that this chapter has convinced the reader that there is an enormous diversity of bacteria, only a small fraction of which have evolved mechanisms of pathogenesis. Several of the divisions of the Eubacteria, which presumably diverged well before animals existed, have developed pathogenic mechanisms. Four out of the 5 proteobacterial subdivisions contain pathogens, as have both gram-positive lines, and most of the important bacterial pathogens (as well as most of the known bacterial species) are found in these groups. Other groups that have developed mechanisms of pathogenesis are the spirochaetes, the *Planctomyces–Chlamydia* group and the *Bacteroides–Cytophaga–Flavobacterium* group. The cyanobacteria do not invade the animal body, but some produce potent neurotoxins.

Phylogenetic analysis helps place pathogenesis in a broader evolutionary perspective. A deeper understanding of the mechanisms of pathogenesis may be obtained by examining relatives of pathogens, both pathogenic and non-pathogenic. In this respect, the clustering of *Rickettsia*, *Wolbachia* and mitochondria points to fundamental aspects that make these organisms so successful inside eukaryotic cells. Such increased understanding may help us in the future to determine mechanisms for the prevention and treatment of bacterial infections.

REFERENCES

Amann R, Ludwig W, Schleifer H-H, 1994, Identification of uncultured bacteria: a challenging task for molecular taxonomists, *Am Soc Microbiol News*, **60**: 360–5.

Angert ER, Clements KD, Pace NR, 1993, The largest bacterium, *Nature (London)*, **362**: 239–41.

Balch WE, Magrum LJ et al., 1977, An ancient divergence among the bacteria, *J Mol Evol*, **9**: 305–11.

Barns SM, Fundyga RE et al., 1994, Remarkable archaeal diversity detected in a Yellowstone National Park hot spring environment, *Proc Natl Acad Sci USA*, **91**: 1609–13.

Bazylinski DA, 1995, Structure and function of the bacterial magnetosome, *Am Soc Microbiol News*, **61**: 337–43.

Benson DR, Silvester WB, 1993, Biology of *Frankia* strains, actinomycete symbionts of actinorhizal plants, *Microbiol Rev*, **57**: 293–319.

Boone DR, Whitman WB, Rouvière P, 1993, Diversity and taxonomy of methanogens, *Methanogenesis* , ed. Ferry JG, Chapman Hall Routledge, New York, 36–80.

Colepicolo P, Cho KW et al., 1989, Growth and luminescence of the bacterium *Xenorhabdus luminescens* from a human wound, *Appl Environ Microbiol*, **55**: 2601–6.

Collins MD, Lawson PA et al., 1994, The phylogeny of the genus *Clostridium*: proposal of five new genera and eleven new species combinations, *Int J Syst Bacteriol*, **44**: 812–26.

Cullen JC, 1994, The miracle of Bolsena, *Am Soc Microbiol News*, **60**: 187–91.

Davey M-E, Wood WA et al., 1993, Isolation of three species of *Geotoga* new-genus and *Petrotoga* new-genus: two new genera representing a new lineage in the bacterial line of descent distantly related to the Thermotogales, *Syst Appl Microbiol*, **16**: 191–200.

DeLong EF, Wickham GS, Pace NR, 1989, Phylogenetic stains: ribosomal RNA-based probes for the identification of single microbial cells, *Science*, **243**: 1360–3.

Diesenhofer J, Michel H, 1989, The photosynthetic reaction center from the purple bacterium *Rhodopseudomonas viridis*, *Science*, **245**: 1463–73.

DiMarco AA, Bobik TA, Wolfe RS, 1990, Unusual coenzymes of methanogenesis, *Annu Rev Biochem*, **59**: 355–94.

Distel DL, Lane DJ et al., 1988, Sulfur-oxidizing bacterial endosymbionts: analysis of phylogeny and specificity by 16S rRNA sequences, *J Bacteriol*, **170**: 2506–10.

Drake HA, 1994, *Acetogenesis*, Chapman and Hall, New York, 647 pp.

Eaglesham ARJ, Ellis JM et al., 1990, The first photosynthetic N_2-fixing *Rhizobium*: characteristics, *Nitrogen Fixation: Achievements and Objectives*, eds Grasshoff PM, Roth LE et al., Chapman and Hall, New York, 805–12.

Embley TM, Hirt RP, Williams DM, 1994, Biodiversity at the molecular level: the domains, kingdoms and phyla of life, *Philos Trans R Soc Lond [Biol]*, **345**: 21–33.

Ferry JG, ed., 1993, *Methanogenesis*, Chapman and Hall, New York, 536.

Fisher RF, Long SR, 1992, *Rhizobium*-plant signal exchange, *Nature (London)*, **357**: 655–9.

Florin THJ, Jabbar IA, 1994, A possible role for bile acid in the control of methanogenesis and the accumulation of hydrogen gas in the human colon, *J Gastroenterol Hepatol*, **9**: 112–17.

Fox GE, Stackebrandt E et al., 1980, The phylogeny of procaryotes, *Science*, **209**: 457–63.

Fuqua WC, Winans SC, Greenberg EP, 1994, Quorum sensing in bacteria: the *luxR-luxI* family of cell density-rs.eponsive transcriptional regulators, *J Bacteriol*, **176**: 269–75.

Greene RB, 1994, Challenges from the sea. Marine shipworms and their symbiotic bacterium, *Soc Indust Microbiol News*, **44**: 51–9.

Hammond AC, 1995, *Leucaena* toxicosis and its control in ruminants, *J Anim Sci*, **73**: 1487–92.

Haugland RA, Schlemm DJ et al., 1990, Degradation of the chlorinated phenoxyacetate herbicides 2,4-dichlorophenoxyacetic acid and 2,4,5,-thrichlorophenoxyacetic acid in pure and mixed bacterial cultures, *Appl Environ Microbiol*, **56**: 1357–62.

Huber R, Wilharm T et al., 1992, *Aquifex pyrophilus* new-genus new-species represents a novel group of marine hyperthermophilic hydrogen-oxidizing bacteria, *Syst Appl Microbiol*, **15**: 340–51.

Johnson JL, 1994a, Similarity analysis of DNAs, *Methods for General and Molecular Bacteriology*, ed. Gerhardt P, American Society for Microbiology, Washington, DC, 655–82.

Johnson JL, 1994b, Similarity analysis of rRNAs, *Methods for General and Molecular Bacteriology*, ed. Gerhardt P, American Society for Microbiology, Washington, DC, 683–700.

Kandler O, König H, 1978, Chemical structures of the peptidoglycan-free cell walls of methanogenic bacteria, *Arch Microbiol*, **118**: 141–52.

Keeling PJ, Charlebois RL, Doolittle WF, 1994, Archaebacterial genomes: eubacterial form and eukaryotic content, *Curr Opin Gen Devel*, **4**: 816–22.

Koch R, Zablowski P et al., 1990, Extremely thermostable amylolytic enzyme from the archaebacterium *Pyrococcus furiosis*, *FEMS Microbiol Lett*, **71**: 21–6.

Maidak BL, Larsen N et al., 1994, The ribosomal database project, *Nucleic Acids Res*, **22**: 3485–7.

Miller TL, Wolin MJ, 1982, Enumeration of *Methanobrevibacter smithii* in human feces, *Arch Microbiol*, **131**: 14–18.

Mohn WW, Tiedje JM, 1992, Microbial reductive dehalogenation, *Microbiol Rev*, **56**: 482–507.

Moran NA, Munson MA et al., 1993, A molecular clock in the endosymbiotic bacteria is calibrated using the insect hosts, *Proc R Soc Lond [Biol]*, **253**: 167–71.

Nealson KH, Saffarini D, 1994, Iron and manganese in anaerobic respiration: environmental significance, physiology, and regulation, *Annu Rev Microbiol*, **48**: 311–43.

Nowak R, 1995, Bacterial genome sequence bagged, *Science*, **269**: 468–70.

Ohta K, Beall DS et al., 1991, Genetic improvement of *Escherichia coli* for ethanol production: chromosomal integration of *Zymomonas mobilis* genes encoding pyruvate decarboxylase and alcohol dehydrogenase II, *Appl Environ Microbiol*, **57**: 893–900.

Olsen GJ, 1994, Microbial ecology. Archaea, Archaea, everywhere, *Nature (London)*, **371**: 657–8.

Olsen GJ, Woese CR, Overbeek R, 1994, The winds of (evolutionary) change – breathing new life into microbiology, *J Bacteriol*, **176**: 1.

Palleroni NJ, 1994, Some reflections on bacterial diversity, *Am Soc Microbiol News*, **60**: 537–40.

Paster BJ, Dewhirst F et al., 1994, Phylogeny of *Bacteroides*, *Prevotella*, and *Porphyromonas* spp. and related bacteria, *J Bacteriol*, **176**: 725–32.

Pitulle C, Yang YQ et al., 1994, Phylogenetic position of the genus *Hydrogenobacter*, *Int J Syst Bactetiol*, **44**: 620–6.

Rawlings DE, Silver S, 1995, Mining with microbes, *Bio/Technology*, **13**: 773–8.

Ruby EG, McFall-Ngai MJ, 1992, A squid that glows in the night: development of an animal-bacterial mutualism, *J Bacteriol*, **174**: 4865–70.

Sand W, Rohde K et al., 1992, Evaluation of *Leptospirillum ferrooxidans* for leaching, *Appl Environ Microbiol*, **58**: 85–92.

Shapiro L, 1993, Protein localization and asymmetry in the bacterial cell, *Cell*, **73**: 841–55.

Spring S, Amann R et al., 1993, Dominating role of an unusual magnetotactic bacterium in the microaerobic zone of a freshwater sediment, *Appl Environ Microbiol*, **59**: 2397–403.

Spudich JL, 1993, Color sensing in the archaea – a eukaryotic-like receptor coupled to a prokaryotic transducer, *J Bacteriol*, **175**: 7755–61.

Stackebrandt E, Goebel BM, 1994, Taxonomic note: a place for DNA–DNA reassociation and 16S rRNA sequence analysis in the present species definition in bacteriology, *Int J Syst Bacteriol*, **44**: 846–9.

Stackebrandt E, Ludwig W, 1994, The importance of using outgroup reference organisms in phylogenetic studies – the *Atopobium* case, *Syst Appl Microbiol*, **17**: 39–43.

Stackebrandt E, Murray RGE, Truper HG, 1988, Proteobacteria classis nov., a name for phylogenetic taxon that includes 'purple bacteria and their relatives', *Int J Syst Bacteriol*, **38**: 321–5.

Stanier RY, van Niel CB, 1962, The concept of a bacterium, *Arch Mikrobiol*, **42**: 17–35.

Stetter KO, 1995, Microbial life in hyperthermal environments, *Am Soc Microbiol News*, **61**: 285–90.

Suwanto A, Kaplan S, 1989, Physical and genetic mapping of the *Rhodobacter sphaeroides* 241 genome: presence of two unique circular chromosomes, *J Bacteriol*, **171**: 5850–9.

Tornabene TG, Langworty TA, 1978, Diphytanyl and dibiphytanyl glycerol ether lipids of methanogenic archaebacteria, *Science*, **203**: 51–3.

Udupa KS, Ocain PA et al., 1994, Novel ionizing radiation-sensitive mutants of *Deinococcus radiodurans*, *J Bacteriol*, **176**: 7439–46.

Vandepeer Y, Neefs JM et al., 1994, About the order of divergence of the major bacterial taxa during evolution, *Syst Appl Microbiol*, **17**: 32–8.

Widdel F, Schnell S et al., 1993, Ferrous iron oxidation by anoxygenic phototrophic bacteria, *Nature (London)*, **362**: 834–6.

Winans SC, 1992, Two-way chemical signalling in *Agrobacterium*–plant interactions, *Microbiol Rev*, **56**: 12–31.

Woese CR, 1987, Bacterial evolution, *Microbiol Rev*, **51**: 221–71.

Woese CR, 1994, There must be a prokaryote somewhere – microbiology's search for itself, *Microbiol Rev*, **58**: 1–9.

Woese CR, Kandler O, Wheelis ML, 1990, Towards a natural system of organisms: proposal for the domains Archaea, Bacteria, and Eucarya, *Proc Natl Acad Sci USA*, **87**: 4576–9,

Woese CR, Magrum LJ, Fox GE, 1978, Archaebacteria, *J Mol Evol*, **11**: 245–52.

Zablen L, Woese CR, 1975, Procaryote phylogeny IV: concerning the phylogenetic status of a photosynthetic bacterium, *J Mol Evol*, **5**: 25–34.

Zablen LB, Kissil MS et al., 1975, Phylogenetic origin of the chloroplast and the procaryotic nature of its ribosomal RNA, *Proc Natl Acad Sci USA*, **72**: 2418–22.

Zinder SH, 1993, Physiological ecology of methanogens, *Methanogenesis*, ed. Ferry JG, Chapman Hall Routledge, New York, 128–206.

Zuckerkandl E, Pauling L, 1965, Molecules as documents of evolutionary history, *J Theor Biol*, **8**: 357–66.

Chapter 7

MICROBIAL SUSCEPTIBILITY AND RESISTANCE TO CHEMICAL AND PHYSICAL AGENTS

A D Russell

---

1 Introduction	3 Physical agents
2 Chemical agents	

1 INTRODUCTION

Chemical and physical agents have, in one form or another, been used for many centuries to destroy micro-organisms. In ancient times, methods were empirical and it is only within the last 150 years or so that a scientific basis for them has been developed and their applications expanded. Alexander the Great realized the importance of boiling drinking water, of burying dung and of treating timber for bridge-building with olive oil. Mummification, involving desiccation and balsams, was practised in early Egyptian civilization. The preservation of foods by various means, including salting, smoking, acidifying and the later development of canning, the brilliant studies on contagion by Fracostoro in the fourteenth and fifteenth centuries, the use by Semmelweiss of chloride of lime to counteract the agent of puerperal fever, the development of antiseptic surgery in the 1850s–1870s by Le Beuf, Lemair, Küchenmeister and Lister, and the work of Pasteur and Koch, all provided a slow but steady increase in knowledge about micro-organisms and their inhibition or inactivation. Other studies too, notably the development of methods by Pringle, Koch and Geppert for evaluating bactericidal activity, the classic work on the dynamics of disinfection by Krönig and Paul in 1897 and the studies by William Henry on the inactivation of cowpox virus vaccine by heat provided the beginnings of the microbiological evaluation of chemical and physical processes. These early studies, considered in part by Hugo (1991), form the basis of the scientific consideration of antisepsis, disinfection, preservation and sterilization.

This chapter will consider various types of chemical and physical agents, their medical and other uses and the mechanisms of both microbial inactivation and microbial resistance. Because the subject area is so vast, appropriate review articles will be cited frequently together with salient research papers when necessary.

2 CHEMICAL AGENTS

There are several types of chemical antimicrobial agents (for chemical structures, see Hugo and Russell 1992). They have a variety of uses, both medical and otherwise; their activity is influenced by many factors – physical, chemical and biological; their efficacy may be evaluated by various techniques; and their mechanism of action varies from one type of chemical to another. These and other aspects will be considered in this section. However, it must be pointed out that chemical disinfectants are less efficient than physical agents and are used only when heat, radiation, etc., cannot be employed.

2.1 Terminology

The terminology used throughout this chapter is that provided by the British Standards Institute (1976). The following terms are the most important:

1 **Sterilization**, the destruction or removal (by filtration) of all micro-organisms.
2 **Disinfection**, the destruction of many micro-organisms, but not usually bacterial spores. Usually applied to the treatment of inanimate objects, it can also refer to the disinfection of the skin, e.g. before an operation. In some countries, a disinfectant is considered to be a substance that will also kill bacterial spores.

3 **Antisepsis**, the destruction or inhibition of micro-organisms on living tissues, thereby limiting or preventing the harmful effects of infection.
4 **Preservation**, the prevention of multiplication of micro-organisms in formulated products (e.g. food, pharmaceuticals, cosmetics), thereby preventing spoilage or contamination which could render the product a possible hazard.

Other terms are more specific, e.g. those having the suffix 'stat' or 'cide'. A static agent, e.g. bacteriostat, fungistat, sporistat, inhibits the growth of bacteria, fungi or spores, respectively, whereas a cidal agent, e.g. bactericide, fungicide, sporicide, virucide, kills bacteria, fungi, spores or viruses, respectively. A general term increasingly used is 'biocide' which refers to a chemical agent that inactivates microbes.

2.2 Types and uses of chemical agents

Antimicrobial agents are widely used for many purposes (Table 7.1). In this section the various types and their antimicrobial and, where necessary, chemical and physical properties, are considered. Comprehensive data are provided by Maurer (1985), Block (1991), Gardner and Peel (1991), Russell, Hugo and Ayliffe (1992), Ayliffe, Coates and Hoffman (1993), Gould (1994) and Rutala (1990, 1995).

Phenols and cresol

Most phenols used as disinfectants are obtained from tar, a byproduct in the destructive distillation of coal. Fractionation of the tar yields a group of products including phenols (tar acids). A coal tar produced in a low temperature carbonization process contains (in parentheses, boiling range in °C) phenol (182), cresols (189–205), xylenols (210–230) and high-boiling tar acids (230–310). The combined fraction of cresols plus xylenols is also available commercially as cresylic acid. Non-coal tar phenols are also available, e.g. 2-phenylphenol (*o*-phenylphenol). Phenol itself is now made in large quantities synthetically, as are some of its derivatives.

Para(4)-substitutions in phenols of an alkyl chain up to 6 carbon atoms in length increase antimicrobial activity. Activity is also improved by halogenation and by a combination of alkyl and halogen substitution; greatest activity is achieved when the alkyl group is in the *ortho*(2) and the halogen *para*(4) positions in relation to the phenolic group. Nitration also increases antimicrobial potency, but unfortunately also enhances systemic toxicity; nitrophenols act as uncoupling agents and interfere with oxidative phosphorylation. Phenols are more active in the undissociated forms at acid than at alkaline pH.

As a group, phenols and cresols are bactericidal to gram-positive and gram-negative bacteria, but bacterial spores are resistant at ambient temperatures. 2-Phenylphenol and the black fluids are particularly effective against mycobacteria, but bisphenols are ineffective. Phenols and cresols, especially when halogenated, possess antifungal activity. Lipid-enveloped viruses may be sensitive to phenolics whereas non-enveloped viruses are more resistant: 2-phenylphenol is active against both types.

Black fluids consist of a solubilized crude phenol fraction prepared from tar acids (boiling range 250–310°C). On dilution with water, black fluids give either clear solutions or emulsions. White fluids consist of emulsified phenolic compounds. On dilution with water, they form weaker emulsions and are more stable in the presence of electrolytes than are black fluids. Black and white fluids are the subject of a British Standard (British Standards Institute 1986a).

Acids, acidulants and esters

Many aliphatic and aromatic acids are employed as preservatives, especially in the food industry, and to some extent in pharmaceutical and cosmetic products. They include acetic, benzoic, propionic and sorbic acids and the methyl, ethyl, propyl and butyl esters (the parabens) of *para*(4)-hydroxybenzoic acids. They are not sporicidal and the activity of the acids, but not the esters, is very pH dependent, since activity is associated mainly with the undissociated form. Acids may be added to various foods as acidulants, notably the organic lipophilic acids (benzoic, sorbic, propionic) referred to above. Organic acids of chain length greater than C_{10} or C_{11} are highly effective against gram-positive but not against gram-negative bacteria (Russell and Gould 1988) but their low solubility restricts their use (Sofos and Busta 1992). Lactic acid, an acidulant exhibiting preservative activity, is the main product of many food fermentations.

Citric acid is an approved disinfectant against foot-and-mouth virus. Lactic acid, CH_3-CH(OH)COOH, has been employed as an aerial disinfectant against non-sporing bacteria. Formic acid, HCOOH, and propionic acid are useful in controlling salmonellae in feedstuffs (Hinton, Linton and Perry 1985), an important finding because the ingestion by animals of contaminated feeds often results in subsequent contamination at slaughter of meat, which, unless properly cooked, might infect humans.

Two mineral acids employed in veterinary work are hydrochloric and sulphuric acids. The former, but not the latter, is sporicidal and has been used at a concentration of 2.5% for disinfecting hides and skin contaminated with anthrax spores. In some countries, a 5% solution of sulphuric acid has been used, usually in combination with phenol, for decontaminating floors, feed boxes and troughs (Russell and Hugo 1987).

Alkalis

The antimicrobial action of alkalis is related to hydroxyl ion concentration. Sodium hydroxide (caustic soda, lye, soda lye, NaOH) possesses strong alkali properties. It kills most common vegetative bacteria and high concentrations (5% and above) are lethal to anthrax spores. Calcium hydroxide (hydrated lime, air-slaked lime, $Ca(OH_2)$) is produced and heat is generated when calcium oxide (lime, quicklime, CaO) is moistened with water. As a 20% suspension, calcium hydroxide is effective for whitewashing surfaces, which kills most types of non-sporing bacteria. Sodium carbonate (Na_2CO_3) is used primarily as a cleaning agent, a 4% w/v solution being used for washing vehicles before disinfecting them after a shipment of animals. It has also been used extensively as a cleaning agent in outbreaks of foot-and-mouth disease. Trisodium phosphate (Na_3PO_4) has similar properties and uses.

More comprehensive data about the veterinary uses of alkalis are provided by Huber (1982) and Linton, Hugo and Russell (1987).

CHLORINE-RELEASING AGENTS (CRAs)

The stability of free available chlorine in solution depends upon a number of factors, in particular chlorine concentration, pH, presence of organic matter and light (Dychdala 1991).

Hypochlorites and organic *N*-chloro compounds are the 2 most widely used types of CRAs. The hypochlorites have a wide antimicrobial spectrum and are among the most potent sporicidal agents. They are active against enveloped and non-enveloped viruses (Springthorpe and Sattar 1990, Sattar et al. 1994) but were considered to be rather ineffective against mycobacteria (Croshaw 1971). More recent studies demonstrate, however, that they are mycobactericidal (Favero and Bond 1993).

Two factors with pronounced effects on their antimicrobial action are the presence of organic matter, chlorine being highly reactive, and pH, the hypochlorites being more active in acid than in alkaline conditions: the active factor is undissociated hypochlorous acid, HClO. Hypochlorite solutions gradually lose strength on storage, so fresh solutions must be prepared before use. Methanolic solutions buffered to pH 7.6–8.1 appear to show maximal stability and sporicidal activity and are worthy of further investigation. In addition to their medical uses, hypochlorites are used widely in the dairy industry and as disinfectants of farm buildings, e.g. for concrete floors, walls and ceilings. Sodium hypochlorite is normally used for the disinfection of swimming pools.

N-chloro compounds, containing the =N–Cl group, possess microbicidal activity; they include chloramine T, dichloramine, halazone and the sodium salts of dichloroisocyanuric (NaDCC) and trichloroisocyanuric acids. All appear to hydrolyse in water to produce an imino (=NH) group. Their action is slower than that of the hypochlorites, but can be increased under acidic conditions. The disinfecting action of chloramine decreases less significantly than that of the other compounds in the presence of organic matter, and it has been used in veterinary practice for washing and spraying surfaces and for soaking items to be decontaminated. The uses of chlorine compounds are summarized in Table 7.1. NaDCC has been recommended as a disinfectant for use against various body spillages from AIDS patients (Bloomfield, Smith-Burchnell and Dalgleish 1990).

IODINE AND IODOPHORS

Iodine was first employed for the treatment of wounds nearly 150 years ago. Normally it is used in aqueous or alcoholic solution but it is only sparingly soluble in cold water; solutions can be made with potassium iodide. Iodine is an efficient microbicidal agent rapidly lethal to bacteria and their spores, moulds, yeasts and viruses. Antiseptic strength iodine solutions are not sporicidal (Russell 1990a, 1990b, Favero and Bond 1993). Iodine is less reactive than chlorine but, whereas the activity of high iodine concentrations is little affected by the presence of organic material, that of low concentrations is significantly reduced. The activity of iodine is greater at acid than at alkaline pH; the most active form is diatomic iodine (I_2). At acid and neutral pH, hypoiodous acid (HIO) is less bactericidal. At alkaline pH, hypoiodite ion (HIO^-) is even less active and iodate (IO_3^-), iodide (I^-) and triiodide (I_3^-) ions are all inactive (Trueman 1971, Dychdala 1991).

Because iodine has certain limitations in use, viz. toxicity and staining of fabrics, attention has been turned towards the iodophors (literally, 'iodine carriers'), solutions in which iodine is solubilized by surface-active agents and which retain the microbicidal, but not the undesirable, properties of iodine. In most iodophor preparations the carrier is usually a non-ionic surfactant, whereas in poloxamer iodine formulations the carriers are poloxamers, a series of non-ionic polyoxethylene–polyoxypropylene polymers. When an iodophor is diluted with water, dispersion of the micellar aggregates of iodine occurs and most of the iodine is liberated slowly (Gottardi 1985). Dilutions of commercial povidone-iodine solutions may be more bactericidal (Berkelman, Holland and Anderson 1982) or sporicidal (Williams and Russell 1993) than undiluted stock solutions. The reasons are complex but iodine complexation is involved since the concentration of free iodine (I_2) determines activity (Gottardi 1985).

The iodophors are microbicidal with activity over a wide pH range. Provided that the pH does not rise above about 4, iodophors retain their antimicrobial potency in the presence of organic matter. There is a pronounced decrease in activity if solutions are diluted excessively with water that has a high alkaline hardness. The presence of a surface-active agent as carrier improves the wetting capacity. Iodophors are used in the dairy industry; when employed in the cleansing of dairy plant, it is important to keep the pH acidic with phosphoric acid, to ensure adequate removal of milkstone (dried residue of milk). They are also used for skin and wound disinfection. In some countries, alcoholic solutions of iodophors are widely used for disinfection of operation sites. In the veterinary context, iodophors formulated with phosphoric acid are employed as antiseptics, disinfectants and teat dips (Huber 1982, Russell and Hugo 1987).

Table 7.1 Summary of uses of some antimicrobial agents

Group	Use(s)	Example(s)
Acids and esters	Preservation	Organic acids, parabens
	Aerial disinfection	Lactic acid
	Veterinary disinfection	Hydrochloric, sulphuric, citric acids
	Salmonella control in feedstuffs	Formic acid, propionic acid
Alcohols	Working surfaces, equipment, gloved hands (rapid action)	Ethanol, isopropanol
Aldehydes	Preservation	Bronopol, ethanol
	Disinfection/sterilization of thermolabile medical equipment	Glutaraldehyde, succinaldehyde-based products, orthophthalaldehyde (?)
	Virucide in preparation of some human and veterinary vaccines; removal of warts; antiseptic mouthwash	Formaldehyde solution
	Topically; irrigation solutions; treatment of peritonitis	Formaldehyde-releasing agents, e.g. noxythiolin, taurolin[a]
	Cosmetic preservatives	Formaldehyde-releasing agents, e.g. imidazole derivatives
Alkalis	Vehicle disinfection	Sodium carbonate, trisodium phosphate
	Whitewashing surfaces	Calcium hydroxide
Alkylating agents	See vapour-phase disinfection	Ethylene oxide, propylene oxide, β-propiolactone
Amphoteric surfactants	Skin 'disinfection'; disinfection of surgical instruments; sanitizers and disinfectants in food industry	Dodecyl-di(aminoethyl)-glycine derivatives
Antibiotic	Food preservative	Nisin
Biguanides	Antiseptic, disinfectant, preservative in some ophthalmic products; antiplaque agent; veterinary teat dip	Chlorhexidine, alexidine
	Swimming pool disinfection; application to surfaces in food industry; preservation of leather	Polyhexamethylenebiguanide (PHMB), a polymeric biguanide
Bisphenols	Surgical scrubs; medicated soaps; limited uses as preservative in cosmetics	Hexachlorophane
	Surgical scrubs; soaps; deodorants; hand-cleansing gels	Triclosan

Diamidines	Topical application to wounds	Propamidine, dibromopropamidine, as isethionates
Halogen-releasing agents	Disinfection of blood spillages containing HIV or HBV; industrial sanitizing compounds (food, dairy, restaurant, swimming pool); veterinary disinfection	Hypochlorites, dichloro- and trichloro-isocyanuric acids
	Disinfection of hands preoperatively; antiseptics; cleansing of dairy plant; veterinary teat dip	Iodophors (including povidone-iodine)
Heavy metal derivatives	Algicides; fungicides; wood, paint, cellulose and fabric preservation	Copper derivatives
	Fungicides; bactericides; textile and wood preservation	Organotin compounds
	Pharmaceutical preservation	Organomercurials
	Prevention of infection in burns	Silver nitrate, silver sulphadiazine
Isothiazolones	Preservatives for cosmetics, toiletries and pharmaceuticals, fabrics	Mixture of chloromethyl and methyl derivatives
Phenols and cresols	Preservation	Phenol, cresol, chlorocresol
	Disinfection	Black fluids, white fluids
	Aerial disinfection	Hexylresorcinol
	Food preservatives	Phenolic antioxidants, e.g. butylated hydroxyanisole, butylated hydroxytoluene
Quaternary ammonium compounds	Preoperative disinfection, bladder and urethra irrigation, ophthalmic preservation, skin disinfection, oral and pharyngeal antisepsis, cosmetic preservation, of emulsions	Cetrimide, benzalkonium chloride, cetylpyridinium chloride (as appropriate)
Sulphites and nitrites	Food preservation	Sodium metabisulphite, sodium nitrite (carcinogenic?)
Vapour-phase disinfections	Medical and pharmaceutical sterilization	Ethylene oxide
	Disinfection/sterilization of heat-sensitive materials	Low temperature steam with formaldehyde
	Veterinary fumigation	Formaldehyde
	Decontamination	β-Propiolactone (carcinogenic?)
	Surface sterilization	Hydrogen peroxide (vapour phase)

[a]There is some doubt as to whether taurolin acts as a formaldehyde releaser.

SURFACE-ACTIVE AGENTS

Surface-active agents (surfactants) have hydrophobic and hydrophilic regions in their molecular structure. On the basis of the charge or the absence of ionization of the hydrophilic group, these surfactants are classified into anionic, cationic, non-ionic and ampholytic (amphoteric) compounds.

Non-ionic surfactants are not antimicrobial, but low concentrations of polysorbates (Tweens) are claimed to affect the permeability of the outer membrane of gram-negative bacteria (Brown 1975). High concentrations, however, neutralize the activity of some types of antimicrobial agents (Russell, Ahonkhai and Rogers 1979, Russell 1992a).

Anionic surfactants usually have strong detergent but weak antimicrobial properties, except at high concentrations which induce lysis of gram-negative bacteria (Salton 1968). Fatty acids are considerably more active against gram-positive than gram-negative organisms (Russell and Gould 1988).

Amphoteric agents combine the detergent properties of anionic with the antimicrobial properties of the cationic compounds. Activity remains virtually constant over a wide pH range and they are inactivated less readily than cationic surfactants by proteins. Examples of amphoteric surfactants are the Tego series of compounds (Hugo and Russell 1992).

For microbiological use, most important surface-active agents are quaternary ammonium compounds (QACs) which are cationic. They possess strong bactericidal but, at normal in-use concentrations, weak detergent properties. QACs may be considered as organically substituted ammonium compounds in which the nitrogen atom has a valency of 5; 4 of the substituent radicals (R^1–R^4) are alkyl or heterocyclic and the fifth is a small anion. The sum of the carbon atoms in the 4 R groups is >10. For a QAC to have high antimicrobial activity, at least one of the R groups must have a chain length in the range C_8–C_{18}. Further details are provided by Hugo and Russell (1992). The QACs are primarily active against gram-positive, non-sporing bacteria; at high concentrations they are lethal to gram-negative organisms, although *Pseudomonas aeruginosa* tends to be particularly resistant (Russell 1992a). They are sporostatic but not sporicidal, and fungistatic rather than fungicidal. They are active against viruses with lipid envelopes, e.g. herpes and influenza, but are much less so against non-enveloped viruses, e.g. enteroviruses (Narang and Codd 1983, Resnick et al. 1986).

The QACs are incompatible with a wide range of chemical agents, including non-ionic and anionic surfactants and phospholipids such as lecithin; use is made of this property in evaluating the lethal effects of QACs by employing a combination of lecithin and a non-ionic surfactant as a neutralizing agent (Russell, Ahonkhai and Rogers 1979). Antimicrobial activity is affected greatly by organic matter and by pH, activity being greater in alkaline conditions because of an increase in the degree of ionization of bacterial surface groups so that the cell surface becomes more negatively charged.

Organosilicon-substituted quaternary ammonium salts, organic amines or amine salts with antimicrobial activity in solution are also highly effective on surfaces. One such, 3-(trimethoxysilyl)propyloctadecyldimethyl ammonium chloride, exhibits powerful antimicrobial activity while chemically bonded to a variety of surfaces (Malek and Speier 1982, Speier and Malek 1982). Uses of the QACs are summarized in Table 7.1.

BIGUANIDES AND POLYMERIC BIGUANAIDES

The most important member of the family of N^1,N^5-substitued biguanides is chlorhexidine, which is available as dihydrochloride, diacetate and gluconate, the last-named being the most water soluble. Chlorhexidine has a wide spectrum of activity against gram-positive and gram-negative bacteria, but is not sporicidal or mycobactericidal; it is also generally considered as having a low activity against fungal spores and viruses (Hugo and Russell 1992, Russell 1992a, Russell and Day 1993). Potency is reduced in the presence of serum, blood, pus and other organic matter. Because of its cationic nature, activity is also reduced in the presence of soaps and other anionic compounds. Chlorhexidine is more active at alkaline pH because an increase in the degree of ionization of bacterial surface groups renders the cell surface more negatively charged (Hugo 1992). The main uses of chlorhexidine are as a medical, dental and veterinary antiseptic, as a disinfectant and as a preservative in some types of pharmaceutical products (Russell and Day 1993).

Alexidine differs from chlorhexidine in that it posesses ethylhexyl end groups (Russell and Chopra 1996); it is also more rapidly bactericidal and produces a significantly faster alteration in bacterial permeability (Chawner and Gilbert 1989a, 1989b).

Vantocil® is a heterodispersed mixture of polyhexamethylene biguanides (PHMB) with a molecular weight of approximately 3 kDa. It is active against gram-positive and negative bacteria (*P. aeruginosa* and *Proteus vulgaris* are less sensitive) but is not sporicidal. Because of the residual positive charges on the polymer, PHMB is precipitated from aqueous solutions by anionic compounds.

DIAMIDINES

The aromatic diamidines are organic cationic agents that show antimicrobial activity (Hugo 1971). The 2 most important members are propamidine (4,4'-diamidinophenoxypropane) and the more active dibromopropamidine, both used as the soluble isethionate salts. Gram-positive bacteria are considerably more sensitive than gram-negative organisms and activity decreases at acid pH and in the presence of organic matter. Bacteria cultured in the presence of increasing doses of a given diamidine rapidly acquire resistance to it and to other diamidines (Hugo 1971). The last decade or so has seen the isolation of multiple antibiotic-resistant strains of *Staphylococcus aureus* (Townsend et al. 1984) and *Staphylococcus epidermidis*

(Leelaporn et al. 1994) that possess plasmid mediated resistance to cationic agents, including propamidine.

ALDEHYDES

Two aldehydes are of considerable importance, i.e. glutaraldehyde (pentane-1,5-dial) and formaldehyde (methanal), although others also possess antimicrobial activity, e.g. succinaldehyde, orthophthalaldehyde.

Glutaraldehyde

Glutaraldehyde is a saturated 5-carbon dialdehyde with an empirical formula of $C_5H_8O_2$ and a molecular weight of 100.12. The aldehyde is highly active, reacting with enzymes and proteins, but only slightly with nucleic acids; it prevents dissociation of free ribosomes. Probably because of increased interaction with -NH_2 groups, such activities increase with increasing pH, a factor of considerable importance to microbicidal activity (Russell 1994).

Glutaraldehyde possesses high microbicidal activity against bacteria and their spores, mycelial and spore forms of fungi and various types of viruses, including HIV and enteroviruses (Hanson et al. 1994, Russell 1994). Despite earlier reports to the contrary, glutaraldehyde is now considered to be mycobactericidal (Russell 1992b), although *Mycobacterium avium–intracellulare* might be of above-average resistance (Hanson 1988) and highly resistant strains of *Mycobacterium chelonae* have been isolated (van Klingeren and Pullen 1993). In solution, glutaraldehyde is more stable at acid than at alkaline pH, whereas the converse is true for its antimicrobial activity. In practice, 2% solutions of glutaraldehyde are alkalinated when required and are used within a stipulated period. Some formulations are available which appear to have overcome the problem of stability (Babb, Bradley and Ayliffe 1980).

The dialdehyde is an important fixative in leather tanning, in electron microscopy and in biochemistry. It is employed widely for the disinfection or sterilization of medical equipment liable to damage by heat, in particular endoscopes. Nevertheless, there is the possibility of severe toxic reactions arising in personnel and the replacement of glutaraldehyde by other equally microbiologically active agents is being actively pursued.

Formaldehyde

Formaldehyde (CH_2O) is employed in the liquid and vapour states; use of the latter is described below (see section on 'Vapour-phase disinfectants', p. 157).

Formaldehyde solution (formalin) is an aqueous solution containing 34–38% w/w of formaldehyde (CH_2O). The presence of methyl alcohol (methanol, CH_3OH) delays polymerization. Formaldehyde is lethal to bacteria and their spores (but less so than glutaraldehyde), fungi and viruses. It combines readily with proteins and is less effective in the presence of organic matter. Formaldehyde is employed as a virucidal agent in the preparation of many human and veterinary vaccines (Russell and Hugo 1987), as an antiseptic mouthwash, for the disinfection of membranes in dialysis equipment and as a preservative in hair shampoos.

Formaldehyde is often employed in the form of formaldehyde-releasing agents. Examples of these are: noxythiolin (hydroxymethylenethiourea), a bactericidal agent widely used both topically and in accessible body cavities, e.g. as an irrigation solution in the treatment of peritonitis (Browne and Stoller 1970); taurolin, in which the amino acid taurine acts as a formaldehyde carrier (Browne, Leslie and Pfirrman 1976; cf. Myers et al. 1980); others, including hexamine (methenamine), imidazole derivatives, triazines and oxazolo-oxazoles. For further information see Hugo and Russell (1992).

Alcohols

Several alcohols possess antimicrobial properties. Generally, they kill bacteria (Morton 1983), including acid-fast bacilli, rapidly but are not sporicidal and have poor activity against some viruses, although HIV type 1 is susceptible to ethanol and isopropanol in the absence of organic matter (van Bueren, Larkin and Simpson 1994). The presence of water is essential to the antimicrobial action of ethanol, which is most effective at concentrations of 60–70% (Price 1950). Isopropanol (propan-2-ol) is a more effective bactericide. Benzyl alcohol (phenylmethanol) is a weak local anaesthetic and also possesses antimicrobial properties. Phenylethanol (phenylethyl alcohol) is selectively active against gram-negative bacteria in mixed flora and is sometimes used as a preservative in ophthalmic solutions. Phenoxyethanol (phenoxetol) has significant activity against *P. aeruginosa* but less against other bacteria. Bronopol (2-bromo-2-nitropropane-1,3-diol) has a broad spectrum of activity, which is reduced in the presence of serum and especially of sulphydryl compounds. The effect of pH on its activity is complex (Croshaw and Holland 1984). Bronopol is widely used as a cosmetic preservative. Chlorbutanol (chlorbutol, trichloro-*t*-butanol) has been used as a bactericide in solutions for injection but its instability presents a problem.

Isothiazolones

Three isothiazolones have been studied comprehensively: 1,2-benzisothiazol-3-one (BIT), 5-chloro-*N*-methylisothiazol-3-one (CMIT) and *N*-methylisothiazol-3-one (MIT). They are widely used as industrial preservatives. Their activity is rapidly quenched by thiol-containing compounds and by valine and histidine, non-thiol amino acids (Collier et al. 1990).

DYES

Three groups of dyes find application as antimicrobial compounds:

1   The acridines, which are heterocyclic compounds and which have been studied extensively. Albert (1979) showed that small changes in their chemical structure cause significant changes in biocidal properties, the most important factor being ionization, which must be cationic in nature. Acridines

compete with H^+ ions for anionic sites on the bacterial cell and are more effective at alkaline than at acid pH.

2 The triphenylmethane dyes (e.g. crystal violet, brilliant green and malachite green), which were used as topical antiseptics. However, their uses were limited because they are effective only against gram-positive bacteria (Hugo and Russell 1992). This property does, however, have a practical application in the formulation of selective media for diagnostic purposes. Like the acridines, these dyes are more active at alkaline pH.

3 The quinones, which are natural dyes imparting colour to many forms of plant and animal life. Some members are important agricultural fungicides, notably chloranil and dichlone (Owens 1969, D'Arcy 1971).

HEAVY METAL DERIVATIVES

The salts of heavy metals are sometimes employed as antimicrobial agents. The main antimicrobial use of copper derivatives is as algicides and fungicides; some copper compounds are used as preservatives in wood, cellulosics, paints and fabrics (Hilditch 1992, Springle and Briggs 1992).

Mercury compounds, in the form of organic derivatives (e.g. phenylmercuric nitrate and acetate), are often used as preservatives for parenteral and ophthalmic solutions; thiomersal serves this purpose for various immunological products. They are active against both gram-positive and gram-negative bacteria but are sporistatic, not sporicidal, at ambient temperatures (Hugo and Russell 1992, Russell 1992a).

Organotin compounds are used as biocides (e.g. fungicides, bactericides), and textile and wood preservatives (Hilditch 1992, McCarthy 1992).

Silver and its salts have long been used as antimicrobials. In recent years, silver nitrate has been employed to prevent infection of burns. Lowbury (1992) has reviewed the use of this compound, at a concentration of 0.5%, for topical antimicrobial prophylaxis, and as a more satisfactory topical prophylactic, silver sulphadiazine (which, however, has the disadvantage that many bacteria are sulphonamide-resistant). Russell and Hugo (1994) have described the antimicrobial properties and actions of various silver compounds.

CHELATING AGENTS

Chelating agents are not usually considered as being antimicrobial in their own right. However, ethylenediamine tetraacetic acid (EDTA) is important because it enhances the activity of many antiseptics and disinfectants. In medicine, EDTA is used to treat chronic lead poisoning, and pharmaceutically as a stabilizer in certain parenteral and ophthalmic preparations (Russell 1992a). In the context of disinfection, EDTA potentiates the effects of many antibacterial agents against gram-negative, but not gram-positive, bacteria (Brown 1975, Russell and Furr 1977, Ayres, Furr and Russell 1993).

ANILIDES

Anilides have the general structure C_6H_5NHCOR. In salicylanilide, R is C_6H_4OH and in carbanilide (diphenylurea) it is C_6H_5NH. Salicylanilide was introduced in 1930 as a fungistat for use in textiles and has also been used in ointment form for treating ringworm. Of the many substituted salicylanilides tested, the tribromo- and tetrachlorosalicylanilides have been the most widely used as antimicrobial agents. Their photosensitizing properties have, however, restricted their use in situations in which they come into contact with human skin. Trichlorocarbanilide, although one of the most potent members of the substituted carbanilides, has the same disadvantage.

QUINOLINE AND ISOQUINOLINE DERIVATIVES

There are 3 main groups: 8-hydroxyquinoline, 4-aminoquinaldinium and isoquinoline derivatives. 8-Hydroxyquinoline (oxine) is a chelating agent active only in the presence of certain metal ions (Albert 1979). The 4-aminoquinaldinium derivatives are QACs that contain one or more quinoline ring systems; examples are laurolinium acetate and dequalinium chloride (a bis-QAC), both of which are active against gram-positive bacteria and many species of yeast and fungi (D'Arcy 1971). The most important isoquinoline derivative is hedaquinium chloride, another bisquaternary salt, which possesses antibacterial and antifungal properties.

PEROXYGENS

A peroxygen is a compound containing an –O–O– group. Hydrogen peroxide and peracetic acid are important peroxygens.

Hydrogen peroxide

Hydrogen peroxide, H_2O_2, is active against gram-positive and gram-negative bacteria and at high concentrations is sporicidal (Bloomfield 1992). It is environmentally friendly because its decomposition products are oxygen and water.

Peracetic acid

Peracids can be considered as derivatives of H_2O_2 in which a hydrogen atom is replaced by another group. The best known example is peracetic acid, CH_3COOOH, which is lethal for a wide range of microbes, including bacterial spores (Baldry 1983). It is currently of considerable interest because it is being considered as a possible replacement for glutaraldehyde in endoscope disinfection (Bradley, Babb and Ayliffe 1995).

OZONE

Ozone, O_3, is an allotropic form of oxygen. Because of its powerful oxidizing properties, ozone is bactericidal, virucidal and sporicidal, although spores are some 10–15 times more resistant than vegetative cells. Gaseous ozone reacts with amino acids, especially those containing sulphur, and with RNA and DNA. In water, ozone is unstable chemically but activity persists because of the production of free radicals, including ●OH.

SULPHITES AND NITRITES

Traditional chemical food preservatives include common salt, sucrose, spices and smoke and its components. Sulphur dioxide has for centuries been used as a fumigant and as a wine preservative. Metabisulphites have been widely used as antioxidants in foods (and in some pharmaceutical products), and sulphur dioxide and sulphites are used to preserve a variety of food products (Gould and Russell 1991, Sofos and Busta 1992).

Nitrite (NO_2^-) and nitrate (NO_3^-) have been used for centuries in meat processing. By reaction with haem proteins, nitrites are responsible for colour formation in cured meat. They are antimicrobial, especially against outgrowing *Clostridium botulinum* spores. Nitrates function solely as a source of nitrite. The antimicrobial activity of nitrite is affected by many factors (Roberts et al. 1991). Carcinogenic nitrosamines are formed in some cured meat products cooked under certain conditions.

VAPOUR-PHASE DISINFECTANTS

Gas- or vapour-phase chemical agents have long been used to achieve disinfection or sterilization. Sulphur dioxide (obtained by burning sulphur) or chlorine found early application for fumigating sickrooms, but the scientific basis for their use was established only comparatively recently. A brief historical account is provided by Richards, Furr and Russell (1984); Kaye and Phillips (1949) reviewed early studies on ethylene oxide (ETO).

The 2 most important vapour-phase agents are ethylene oxide (ETO) and formaldehyde.

Ethylene oxide, $(CH_2)_2O$, is a colourless gas that is soluble in water, most organic solvents and oils and diffuses into rubber in a manner similar to entering a solution. It is inflammable when more than 3% is present in air, but this hazard can be overcome by mixing it with carbon dioxide or an appropriate fluorocarbon compound. The antimicrobial activity of ETO depends upon several factors, notably relative humidity (RH), temperature, concentration and time and especially on the presence of water vapour (Ernst 1974). Its high toxicity must be borne in mind when devising safe sterilization procedures. Furthermore, porous materials absorb the gas to various degrees during the sterilization cycle, so various periods of time after sterilization must be allowed for desorption of residual ETO. ETO is used as a decontaminating agent, for sterilizing ophthalmic and anaesthetic equipment, crude drugs and powders and in veterinary practice for fumigating eggshells.

Formaldehyde gas can be generated by various means, viz. evaporation of commercial formaldehyde solution (formalin), addition of formalin to potassium permanganate, or volatilization of paraformaldehyde, $HO(CH_2)_nH$, where n = 8–100. Its antimicrobial activity depends upon several factors, including RH; it increases with RH up to a figure of 50%, but higher RH values confer little further advantage (Nordgren 1939). Formaldehyde is toxic, and inhalation of the vapour may pose a risk of carcinogenesis; adequate precautions should be taken to protect personnel. Low temperature steam with formaldehyde (LTSF) is useful for disinfecting or sterilizing heat-sensitive materials (Alder and Simpson 1992). In the veterinary field, formaldehyde vapour is an important fumigant of animal buildings (Russell and Hugo 1987).

Other gases include the following:

1 β-Propiolactone (BPL). Its activity depends primarily on RH, concentration and temperature. BPL may be carcinogenic, but it has been claimed to have a use in decontamination of animal premises. Liquid BPL is used widely in the preparation of many veterinary viral vaccines.
2 Methyl bromide, CH_3Br. This is less active than ETO and is highly toxic but has been used as a fumigant.
3 Propylene oxide, C_3H_6O. This is also less active than ETO. It has been used as a decontaminating agent, e.g. for animal feeds.
4 Ozone. This was considered earlier (see section on 'Ozone', p. 156).
5 Carbon dioxide, CO_2. This inhibits the growth of bacteria, including slime-producing ones, in soft drinks. Its activity depends upon low temperatures, its addition at an early stage and its concentration.

Aerial disinfectants

An effective aerial disinfectant should be capable of being dispersed so as to ensure its complete and rapid mixing with infected air. An effective concentration should be maintained in the air and the disinfectant must be highly and rapidly active against air-borne micro-organisms at different relative humidities. In addition, it should be non-toxic and non-irritant.

Early samples of aerial disinfectants were fumigants, such as sulphur dioxide and chlorine, employed in sickrooms. However, aerosols – which consist of a very fine dispersed liquid phase in a gaseous (air) disperse phase – are the most important form of aerial disinfectant.

Examples of aerial disinfectants are: hexylresorcinol, which is vaporized from a thermostatically controlled hotplate; lactic acid, which is effective but unfortunately an irritant at high concentrations; propylene glycol, which may be used as a solvent for dissolving a solid disinfectant prior to atomization, but which is also a fairly effective and non-irritating antimicrobial agent in its own right; and fumigants such as formaldehyde.

NATURAL ANTIMICROBIAL SYSTEMS

Natural antimicrobial systems (reviewed by Wilkins and Board 1989) occur in animals, plants and micro-organisms. Major components of natural defence systems are classified broadly into inducible, e.g. complement, and constitutive. Principal representatives of the latter are enzymes, for example lysozyme (a cell wall lytic agent, see section 2.6, p. 163) and lactoperoxidase (LP) which mediates the production of compounds toxic to foreign, but not to host, cells. LP is most abundant in bovine cells. With a halide or thiocyanate and hydrogen peroxide, LP forms a potent antimicrobial lactoperoxidase system.

Additionally, transferrin in mammalian blood cells and milk, and lactoferrin in milk may show antibacterial activity.

2.3 Factors influencing activity

The activity of antimicrobial compounds may be influenced by various extraneous factors, including concentration, pH, time, temperature and the type, number and location of micro-organisms, and the presence of other agents that may reduce or increase their potency. A sound knowledge of these factors is essential to their most effective deployment, e.g. in the design of hospital disinfection policies (Coates and Hutchinson 1994).

CONCENTRATION OF ANTIMICROBIAL AGENT

The effect of concentration, or dilution, on the activity of an antimicrobial compound is not a simple arithmetic one. As was first pointed out by Krönig and Paul (1897), microbial death is not an all-or-nothing response but depends greatly on the period of contact and concentration (Fig. 7.1).

In kinetic studies, η, the concentration exponent (dilution coefficient), is used to express the effect of changes in concentration (or dilution) on cell death rate. Its value may be determined by measuring the times necessary to kill the same number of bacteria in a suspension exposed to 2 concentrations of the antimicrobial agent. If C_1 and C_2 represent the 2 concentrations and t_1 and t_2 the respective times to reduce the viable population to the same end point, then

$$C_1^{\eta} t_1 = C_2^{\eta} t_2 \qquad (1)$$

from which

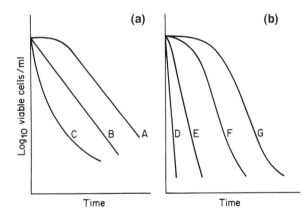

$$\eta = (\log t_2 - \log t_1) / (\log C_1 - \log C_2) \qquad (2)$$

Alternatively, η may be calculated from the slope of the straight line resulting when $\log_{10}$ death time ($\log t$) is plotted against $\log_{10}$ concentrations ($\log C$) (see Russell 1992a). Examples of η values are provided in Table 7.2.

A decrease in concentration of compounds with high η values results in a pronounced increase in the time necessary to achieve a comparable kill, other conditions remaining constant. By contrast, agents with low η values are much less affected (Table 7.2).

Knowledge of the effect of concentration on antimicrobial potency is essential:

1 in evaluating activity
2 in testing medical and pharmaceutical products for sterility
3 in ensuring adequate concentrations of preservative in pharmaceutical, cosmetic and food products and
4 in providing adequate concentrations of antiseptics and disinfectants for practical purposes (Russell 1992a).

TEMPERATURE

The activity of a disinfectant or preservative is usually increased when the temperature at which it acts is raised, although compounds vary considerably in response to temperature changes (Table 7.2).

Useful formulae for measuring the effect of temperature on activity are given by

$$\theta^{T2-T1} = k_2/k_1 = t_1/t_2 \qquad (3)$$

in which θ is the temperature coefficient, k_2 and k_1 the rate (velocity) constants at temperatures T_2 and T_1, respectively, and t_2 and t_1 are the respective times to bring about a complete kill at T_2 and T_1.

The velocity constant (k) can itself be obtained from a knowledge of the time (t) taken to reduce the initial viable number of cells (N_0) to a value N_t at time t, thus:

$$k = \frac{1}{t} \log_e \frac{N_0}{N_t} = \frac{1}{t} 2.303 \log_{10} \frac{N_0}{N_t} \qquad (4)$$

The temperature coefficient, θ, refers to the effect on activity per 1° rise and is nearly always between 1.0 and 1.5 (Bean 1967). It is more meaningful to specify the θ^{10} (also known as Q^{10}) value, which is the change in activity per 10° rise in temperature (Table 7.2). At temperatures above about 40°C, there is little, if any, difference in activity between acid and alkaline glutaraldehyde, although the latter formulation is less stable (Gorman, Scott and Russell 1980).

ENVIRONMENTAL pH

pH can influence the activity of antimicrobial agents in the following ways:

1 Changes may occur in the molecule. Phenols and benzoic, sorbic and dehydroacetic acids are effec-

Fig. 7.1 Examples of time–survivor curves of bacterial suspensions exposed to disinfectants. (a) Bacterial responses: A, initial 'shoulder' followed by exponential death; B, exponential death; C, exponential death followed by 'tailing'. (b) Effects of different concentrations (D, highest; G, lowest) of phenol acting on *Escherichia coli*. At the lowest concentration, a sigmoidal curve is produced. This becomes less pronounced as the concentration increases, leading to an apparent straight-line response at the highest concentration.

Table 7.2 Effects of concentration and temperature on activity of some antimicrobial agents

Concentration exponents (η)*	Temperature coefficients [Q$_{10}$ (or θ^{10}) values]†
Group A (η <2) Hydrogen peroxide, mercurials, chlorhexidine, formaldehyde, QACs	θ^{10} 1.5–5 Phenolics, ethylene oxide, β-propiolactone, phenols and cresols
Group B (η 2–4) Parabens, sorbic acid	θ^{10} 30–50 Aliphatic alcohols
Group C (η >4) Aliphatic alcohols, phenolics, benzyl alcohol, phenethanol	

*Based on Hugo and Denyer (1987).
†Based on Bean (1967).

tive predominantly in the unionized form and, as pH rises, their degree of dissociation increases. It is claimed that the dissociated form of sorbic acid may make a small contribution to activity.

2 Changes may occur in the microbial cell surface. As pH increases, the number of negatively charged groups on the cell surface increases, causing enhanced binding of positively charged molecules, e.g. QACs (Hugo 1992), dyes (Moats and Maddox 1978), acridines (Albert 1979) and chlorhexidine (Hugo 1992).

It must also be pointed out that the sporicidal activity of sodium hypochlorite is potentiated in the presence of methanol, although there is no simple relationship between activity, stability and change of pH of the mixture (Coates and Death 1978). Maximal sporicidal activity and stability are achieved by buffering hypochlorite alone or a hypochlorite–methanol mixture to within a pH range of 7.6–8.1 (Death and Coates 1979).

INTERFERING SUBSTANCES

Organic matter

Organic soiling matter may be present as, for example, serum, blood, pus, soil, food residues, dried milk (milkstone) or faecal material; it can interfere with the action of an antimicrobial agent, usually because an interaction results in a reduced effective concentration of the latter (Russell 1992a).

Such reduction in activity is most noticeable with highly reactive compounds such as chlorine disinfectants. Iodine and iodophors, because of their lower chemical reactivity, are influenced to a rather lesser extent. Cationic agents such as QACs and chlorhexidine show a considerable reduction in activity, whereas the efficacy of phenols depends upon the actual phenolic compound; lysol, for example, retains much of its activity in the presence of faeces and sputum (Russell 1992a).

Adequate precleaning before employment of a disinfectant, or a combination of disinfectant with a suitable detergent, may overcome the problem caused by the presence of organic soil. However, it should be noted that the activity of disinfectants may suffer considerably in the presence of certain detergents.

Surface-active agents

Cationic bactericides and anionic surfactants are incompatible. Low concentrations of non-ionic surfactants such as polysorbates, tritons and tergitols increase the activity of cationic agents and of parabens (Allwood 1973), whereas at higher concentrations of the non-ionic detergents, significantly greater concentrations of the antimicrobial substances are necessary to inhibit or kill microbes. It is believed that below the critical micelle concentration (CMC) of the non-ionic compound, potentiation occurs by action on the surface layers of the bacterial cell, resulting in enhanced permeability to the antimicrobial agent; above the CMC, it either forms a complex with the antimicrobial compound or the latter is partitioned between the aqueous and micellar phases, only the concentration in the aqueous phase being available for microbial attack.

Because of their ability to inactivate various types of antimicrobial compounds, non-ionic surfactants are frequently employed as neutralizing agents in sterility testing and in antimicrobial evaluation (Russell, Ahonkhai and Rogers 1979).

Oils

A problem encountered in the formulation of pharmaceutical and cosmetic creams and emulsions is that the antimicrobial activity of a preservative may be high in aqueous conditions, but much less so when an oil is present. The reason for this is that the preservative is partitioned between the oily and aqueous phases (Bean 1972).

Other factors

The hardness of water with which disinfectants are prepared or diluted is a contributory factor in reducing the effectiveness of QACs and iodophors; black (but not white) fluids are incompatible with hard waters. Partitioning into rubber may cause problems in the preservation of multiple dose parenteral and ophthalmic solutions. Relative humidity has a profound influence on the activity of gaseous disinfectants (see section on 'Vapour-phase disinfectants', p. 157).

CONDITION AND SIZE OF MICROBIAL POPULATION

It is clearly easier for an antimicrobial agent to be effective when there are few micro-organisms against which to act. Adequate and thorough precleaning is usually an important prerequisite to a disinfection process.

The association of bacteria (or other micro-organisms) with solid surfaces leads to the production of a biofilm, a consortium of bacteria organized within an extensive exopolymer (glycocalyx). Within the depths of the biofilm, growth rates are likely to be reduced as a consequence of nutrient limtation (Poxton 1993) which can alter the bacterial cell surface and hence be responsible for modified sensitivity to antibacterial agents (Costerton et al. 1987, Brown and Gilbert 1993, Carpentier and Cerf 1993). This is one reason for the reduced sensitivity of the sessile cells found in biofilms; other reasons are chemical reaction with glycocalyx and prevention by the glycocalyx of access of biocide to the underlying cells.

2.4 Types of micro-organism

The activity of antimicrobial agents depends greatly upon the type of micro-organism present. Because antimicrobial compounds may be called on to act in specific ways (e.g. as bactericides, fungicides, sporicides, virucides), it is pertinent to examine the sensitivity of various types of microbes which, for convenience, have been classified into the following groups.

GRAM-POSITIVE BACTERIA (COCCI)

As well as including important pathogens, gram-positive bacteria may be associated with spoilage of pharmaceutical and cosmetic products. Generally, they are more sensitive to antimicrobial agents than are gram-negative bacteria (Russell and Gould 1988). The effects of various disinfectants, antiseptics and preservatives on them are well documented (Baird-Parker and Holbrook 1971). Cocci are readily killed by halogens, phenols, especially bisphenols, and QACs. However, multiple antibiotic-resistant *S. aureus* and *S. epidermidis* may show reduced sensitivity to cationic-type agents (see section 2.2, p. 150). Clinical isolates of enterococci (*Enterococcus faecium* and *Enterococcus faecalis*) are often antibiotic-resistant but do not appear to be more resistant to chlorhexidine than staphylococci (Baillie, Wade and Casewell 1992).

MYCOBACTERIA

The sensitivity of acid-fast bacteria to disinfectants is intermediate between that of other non-sporulating bacteria and bacterial spores (Ayliffe, Coates and Hoffman 1993, Favero and Bond 1993). QACs and dyes inhibit tubercle bacilli but do not kill them. *Mycobacterium tuberculosis* is also insensitive to chlorhexidine, acids and alkalis, but moderately sensitive to amphoteric surface-active agents, including the Tego compounds. Of the phenols, 2-phenylphenol is particu-

larly effective, but the bisphenols are inactive. Alcohols, liquid and vapour-phase formaldehyde, formaldehyde–alcohol, iodine–alcohol and ethylene oxide are all tuberculocidal; despite earlier doubts to the contrary, so is glutaraldehyde (Favero and Bond 1993). However, *M. avium–intracellulare* (Hanson 1988) and *M. chelonae* (van Klingeren and Pullen 1993) may be resistant to the dialdehyde.

GRAM-NEGATIVE BACTERIA

Many types of gram-negative bacteria, especially *Escherichia coli*, *Klebsiella* spp., *Proteus* spp., *P. aeruginosa* and *Serratia marcescens* are increasingly implicated as hospital pathogens. In the veterinary context, bacteria causing zoonotic diseases include *Campylobacter* spp., salmonellae and brucellae (see Linton 1983, Russell, Yarnych and Koulikovskii 1984). Gram-negative bacteria are usually less sensitive than gram-positive bacteria and *P. aeruginosa* and *Proteus* spp. often contaminate solutions of QACs (Russell, Hammond and Morgan 1986). These bacteria and others such as *Providencia stuartii* are also more resistant to chlorhexidine than is *E. coli* (Ismaeel et al. 1986).

Legionella pneumophila is frequently found in domestic water and cooling water systems of large buildings, although outbreaks of Legionnaire's disease are uncommon. Nevertheless, adequate control measures should be taken. Neither raising the temperature of hot water systems nor continuous chlorination alone is completely effective. Control of the organism in recirculating water systems has also been studied, but extrapolation from laboratory conditions to such systems is often unrealistic because of possible interaction between the biocide and other water treatment chemicals as well as slime (Elsmore 1992). Wang et al. (1979) found hypochlorite to be effective against *L. pneumophila*, but Kurtz et al. (1982) showed a chlorinated phenol to be more effective than a QAC–tributyl tin oxide mixture or sodium dichloroisocyanurate. Bronopol is effective both under laboratory conditions and in cooling towers (Elsmore 1992).

BACTERIAL SPORES

In general, bacterial spores are killed only slowly or not at all by many antibacterial compounds. Nevertheless, these are not entirely without effect on spores because they can prevent germination or outgrowth, or both. Chemicals that are sporistatic rather than sporicidal include phenols and cresols, parabens, QACs, biguanides, alcohols, dyes and mercury compounds. Comparatively few substances are sporicidal and even then the process may be comparatively slow. Examples of sporicides are hydrogen peroxide, hypochlorites, glutaraldehyde, formaldehyde, iodine compounds, ethylene oxide, peracetic acid and β-propiolactone (Russell 1990a, Bloomfield 1992, Bloomfield and Arthur 1994).

MOULDS AND YEASTS

Several species of moulds and yeasts are pathogenic. Others are important in spoiling foods, pharmaceutical and cosmetic products.

Many compounds show both antibacterial and antifungal activity, although the latter may be fungistatic rather than fungicidal (Russell 1992c). These include phenolics (notably the halogenated members and hexachlorophane), QACs, oxine (8-hydroxyquinoline), diamidines, organic mercury derivatives and the parabens. Sorbic acid shows significant antifungal activity at low pH values when it occurs in solution mainly in the undissociated form. At higher pH values, activity is lost. Fungal spores are often resistant to chemical disinfectants (Russell 1992c).

Protozoa

Several distinctly different types of protozoa, including *Giardia, Cryptosporidium, Naegleria, Entamoeba* and *Acanthamoeba*, are potentially pathogenic and may be acquired from water. Furthermore, their life cycles may contain a resistant cyst stage (Jarroll 1992). Agents, in ascending order of efficacy, that are cysticidal towards *Giardia muris* cysts are monochloramine, free chlorine, iodine, chlorine dioxide and ozone (Jarroll 1988, 1992). Chlorine dioxide is more effective against *Cryptosporidium* oocysts than is either free chlorine or monochloramine; these cysts are also sensitive to ozone (Korich et al. 1990).

Acanthamoeba spp. are responsible for corneal keratitis, sometimes associated with the use of contaminated contact lenses or contact lens solutions. Whereas trophozoites are readily inactivated by contact lens disinfecting solutions, cysts are more refractory and the presence of proteinaceous matter is an additional hazard (Seal and Hay 1992).

Viruses

Several bactericidal agents are virucidal, but antibacterial activity does not necessarily imply antiviral potency. An excellent comprehensive treatise of virus disinfection is that by Grossgebauer (1970). Viruses are classified primarily as to whether they contain DNA or RNA, but the presence or absence of a lipid envelope is in general more important in relation to disinfection. An important hypothesis was put forward in 1963 and modified some 20 years later by Klein and Deforest (1983) who classified viruses into 3 groups:

1. lipid enveloped viruses, e.g. herpes simplex virus (HSV), human immunodeficiency virus (HIV), hepatitis B virus (HBV)
2. small, non-enveloped viruses, e.g. picornaviruses, parvoviruses
3. larger non-enveloped viruses, e.g. rotaviruses.

In terms of biocide sensitivity, 1>3>2.

A knowledge of the inactivation of viruses has, in the past, been important in the preparation of vaccines such as inactivated (Salk) poliomyelitis vaccine, in which formaldehyde was used as the virucidal agent. Nowadays, with the current importance of HIV, HBV and hepatitis A virus (HAV), plus the need to prevent the transmission of viral infection, it is essential to have a sound knowledge of viral inactivation. Important virucidal agents include chlorine-releasing agents, formaldehyde (in inactivated vaccine production), glutaraldehyde at alkaline pH and peracetic acid (Springthorpe and Sattar 1990, Sattar et al. 1994). Bacteriophages are currently being considered as indicator 'organisms' for assessing the virucidal activity of biocides (Davies et al. 1993, Maillard et al. 1995; see also section 2.5).

Viruses also cause many diseases of animals. For veterinary use, lists of approved dilutions of approved disinfectants are frequently published in the UK by the Ministry of Agriculture, Fisheries and Foods for general use and in connection with certain statutory Orders applying to viral infections (foot-and-mouth disease, swine vesicular disease) and bacterial disease (tuberculosis). Porcine parvovirus, which causes reproductive failure in swine, is quite resistant to disinfectants, only sodium hypochlorite and sodium hydroxide being rapidly virucidal; by contrast, 2 enveloped swine viruses (pseudorabies and transmissible gastroenteritis viruses) are highly sensitive to a wide range of disinfectants.

Russell (1990b) has provided a comprehensive list of the susceptibility of different types of viruses to heat and chemical biocides, as well as considering acid stability and sensitivity to the organic solvent, ether, which inactivates most lipid-enveloped viruses.

Prions

Prions are responsible for a distinct group of unusual neurological diseases, the transmissible degenerative or spongiform encephalopathies (TDEs or TSEs) and are sometimes referred to as unconventional transmissible agents. Examples of TDEs are Creutzfeldt–Jakob disease (CJD), scrapie in sheep, bovine spongiform encephalitis (BSE) and kuru.

Prions are composed of an altered protein and are inordinately resistant to most chemical and physical agents, including glutaraldehyde, formaldehyde, organic solvents, chlorine dioxide, iodine, strong acids, autoclaving, dry heat and ionizing and ultraviolet radiations (Taylor 1992). However, as prions have yet to be purified, it is difficult to state whether this is an intrinsic property or to what extent it is influenced by the protective effect of host tissue. They are inactivated by strong alkali.

2.5 Evaluation of antimicrobial activity

No attempt has been made here to review the numerous published methods for evaluating antimicrobial activity. A summary is provided in Table 7.3 and the following should be consulted for additional information: Cremieux and Fleurette (1991), Quinn (1992) and Reybrouck (1992).

Preliminary tests

The determination of the minimum inhibitory concentration (MIC) of a substance as determined by a liquid or solid method is often a useful basis on which to undertake further tests. Experiments should also be made to find suitable neutralizing agents (Russell 1992a).

Table 7.3 Examples of methods used for evaluating antimicrobial activity

Test/evaluation	Examples of methods available*†	Comments
Bacteriostatic/fungistatic potency (MIC determination)	Broth/agar serial dilution methods; agar diffusion methods	Provide preliminary information only
Bactericidal/fungicidal activity	1 Suspension tests with determination of numbers of survivors. Include sporicidal and mycobactericidal estimations (AFNOR 1989) 2 European Suspension Test	1 Neutralization of agent essential to prevent 'carryover' into recovery medium. Rapid methods increasingly being studied 2 5 Log reduction in specified period
Phenol coefficient tests	RW, CM, AOAC methods	
Capacity-type tests	Kelsey–Sykes test	See Kelsey and Maurer (1974)
Carrier tests	AOAC use-dilution confirmatory test; DGHM test	
Virucidal tests	Tissue culture, eggs, plaque counting; animal models; enzyme activity	Bacteriophages suggested as model systems
Skin disinfection	MIC and lethal effects (presence of serum or blood). Skin test at 37°C	
Aerial disinfection	Closed-chamber evaluation of microbial population before and after exposure to aerial disinfectant	
Preservative activity	MIC evaluation, lethal activity; challenge testing of preserved pharmaceutical and cosmetic products	See, e.g. *British Pharmacopoeia* (1993)

*For further information, see Quinn (1987), Cremieux and Fleurette (1991) and Reybrouck (1992). (The paper by Quinn is particularly useful as it presents a detailed appraisal of the evaluation of disinfectants in veterinary practice.)
†Suitable tests must be done where relevant to demonstrate adequate neutralization of antimicrobial agents.
AFNOR, Association Française de Normalisation; AOAC, Association of Official Analytical Chemists; CM, Chick–Martin; DGHM, Deutsche Gesellschaft für Hygiene und Mikrobiologie; MIC, minimum inhibitory concentration; RW, Rideal–Walker.

DETERMINATION OF LETHAL ACTIVITY

Suspension tests may be employed for determining bactericidal, fungicidal or virucidal activity. Other methods include carrier and capacity tests.

Suspension tests

Bactericidal (including sporicidal) and fungicidal activity may be determined qualitatively and quantitatively by means of suspension tests. Quantitative measurements yield information about the rate of microbial inactivation at a given concentration of antimicrobial agent.

Phenol coefficient procedures are special types of suspension tests that compare the activity of a phenolic disinfectant against a standard (phenol) on a specified test organism. In the UK this is *Salmonella typhi* in both the Rideal–Walker (British Standards Institute 1985) and Chick–Martin (British Standards Institute 1986b) methods; in the latter, a source of organic matter is present to stimulate practical situations. In the USA, the Association of Official Analytical Chemists (AOAC 1984) permits the use of *S. typhi*, *S. aureus* and *P. aeruginosa*.

Carrier tests

Organisms are dried on appropriate carriers, such as pieces of cotton or porcelain cylinders, that are then placed in an appropriate dilution of test disinfectant for a specified period, after which they are transferred to a nutrient medium, e.g. DGHM (1981) and AOAC (1984). The latter also has a specific carrier test for evaluating sporicidal activity.

Capacity tests

These measure the capacity of a disinfectant to retain its activity when repeatedly used microbiologically, e.g. in the Kelsey–Sykes test (Kelsey and Maurer 1974). On the basis of this technique, use of dilutions of the disinfectant under both clean and dirty conditions can be recommended to hospitals, which should check their efficacy under their own working conditions, using porcelain cylinders or silk suture loops, for evaluating sporicidal activity.

Virucidal tests

The evaluation of virucidal activity is not an easy matter. Viruses are unable to grow in artificial laboratory culture media and some other system, usually involving living cells, must be employed. In essence, the principles of testing follow methods of evaluating bactericidal or fungicidal activity in that the virus is exposed to appropriate concentrations of disinfectant in suspension, or on a carrier, e.g. glass cover-slips, as used with herpes virus and poliovirus (Tyler and Ayliffe 1987). Inactivation is then tested in an appropriate manner, care being taken to ensure that residual disinfectant is neutralized and that the antimicrobial agent has no toxic effects on host cells.

Estimation of virucidal activity can be made using the following systems:

1   Tissue culture or fertile eggs, which after incubation are examined for signs of viral infection.
2   Plaque-counting procedures, which have been used for various viruses, e.g. herpes and poliovirus (Tyler and Ayliffe 1987) and human rotaviruses (Lloyd-Evans, Springthorpe and Sattar 1986, Springthorpe et al. 1986).
3   Use of an 'acceptable' animal model, e.g. the chimpanzee, for studying survival of hepatitis B virus. The discovery of hepadnaviruses that infect ducks and small animals might provide a suitable alternative (Tsiquaye and Barnard 1993).
4   Immunological reactions: tests for the inactivation of the hepatitis B surface antigen (HBsAg) were at one time used to assess the efficacy of disinfection procedures for this virus; however, since this component is much more stable to chemical and physical agents than those conferring infectivity, the method is no longer used.
5   Endogenous reverse transcriptase: human immunodeficiency viruses (HIVs) are enveloped RNA retroviruses. After HIV enters a cell, RNA is converted to DNA under the influence of an enzyme, reverse transcriptase. HIVs replicate in certain T lymphocytes and in the assay reverse transcriptase activity is not a satisfactory alternative to tests in which infectious HIV can be detected in systems employing fresh human peripheral blood mononuclear cells (Resnick et al. 1986).
6   Use of bacteriophages as model systems: bacteriophages have been suggested as model systems for human viruses (Davies et al. 1993). Certainly, they have several advantages such as ease of handling and fairly rapid and reproducible results. Their resistance to biocides should, of course, mimic a particular virus (or viruses), e.g. coliphage MS2 has the same order of response to some biocides as poliovirus.

2.6   Mechanisms of action of antimicrobial agents

Considerable progress has been made in understanding the mechanisms of action of many antibacterial agents. The same is not always true when the target organisms are yeasts, fungi, bacterial spores or viruses. However, this section will summarize current knowledge about target sites in, and inactivation of, different types of microbes.

The initial reaction between an antimicrobial agent and a microbial cell takes place at the cell surface. This is followed by penetration of the chemical to reach its site(s) of action, usually within the cell itself. Unlike most antibiotics, however, many biocides have more than one site of action and it is thus often difficult to elucidate the exact mechanism whereby cellular inactivation is achieved. Furthermore, secondary effects may make a significant contribution to the overall process.

ACTION ON NON-SPORULATING BACTERIA

Uptake of an antibacterial agent by bacteria represents an early manifestation of its effect, although there is little information available about uptake by mycobacteria (Russell 1996).

Different agents have different sites and modes of action. Data are presented below, and summarized in Table 7.4, of the ways in which they act (Russell and Russell 1995, Russell and Chopra 1996). It must again be emphasized, however, that little is known about the mechanisms of inhibition and inactivation of mycobacteria (Russell 1996).

Cell wall or cell envelope effects

Ethylenediamine tetraacetic acid (EDTA) is not a powerful bactericide in its own right. Generally, it has little effect on gram-positive bacteria or fungi and some effect on certain gram-negative bacteria, especially *P. aeruginosa* (Hugo and Russell 1992). Its usefulness resides in the fact that it is a chelating agent that combines with cations associated with the outer membrane (OM) of gram-negative bacteria with the release of some 30–50% of OM lipopolysaccharide (LPS). These changes in the OM render the cells more sensitive to many chemically unrelated compounds such as lysozyme, QACs, dyes and phenols (Hugo 1992).

EDTA thus increases the permeability of gram-negative bacteria and is thereby known as a permeabilizing agent. Other chemicals that act in a similar manner include sodium hexametaphosphate, gluconic acid, citric acid and malic acid (Vaara 1992, Ayres, Furr and Russell 1993).

The important biocide, glutaraldehyde, has several effects on non-sporulating bacteria (Russell 1994). It causes cross-linking of the peptidoglycan in gram-positive bacteria so that lysis of this component is reduced on subsequent treatment with lysozyme (*Bacillus subtilis*) or lysostaphin (*S. aureus*). Glutaraldehyde interacts with protein in the cell envelope of gram-negative bacteria, with consequent reduction of lysis by sodium lauryl sulphate or EDTA–lysozyme. The dialdehyde increases resistance to lysis of protoplasts and spheroplasts, by stabilizing the cytoplasmic membrane.

Membrane-active agents

Perturbation of homoeostatic mechanisms in bacteria may be achieved by various chemical agents in 2 ways

Table 7.4 Mechanisms of antibacterial action*

Target site	Example(s)†	Mechanism(s)
Outer cell layers (cell wall/outer membrane)	Glutaraldehyde	Interaction with $-NH_2$ groups, e.g. proteins, peptidoglycan
	EDTA	Chelation of divalent cations, especially Mg^{2+}
	Lysozyme	$\beta,1-4$ links in peptidoglycan
	Cationic biocides e.g. CHA, QACs, DBPI, PHMB	Outer-membrane damage, thereby promoting own entry postulated
Cytoplasmic (inner) membrane	Phenols, QACs	Generalized membrane damage
	CHA	Low concentrations affect membrane integrity, high ones congeal protoplasm
	Alexidine, PHMB	Phase separation and domain formation of acidic phospholipids
	Hexachlorophane	Inhibits membrane-bound electron transport chain
	Phenoxyethanol	Proton-conducting uncoupler
	Sorbic acid	Transport inhibitor (effect on pmf); another unidentified mechanism?
	Parabens	Low concentrations inhibit transport, high ones affect membrane integrity
	Metallic compounds‡ (mercury, silver, copper)	Interaction with $-SH$ groups in proteins and enzymes
	Isothiazolones‡	Interaction with $-SH$ groups in proteins and enzymes
	Bronopol‡	Oxidizes thiol groups to disulphides
Cytoplasmic constituents	Alkylating agents (ETO, BPL, PO, formaldehyde)	Combination with amino, carboxyl, sulphydryl and hydroxyl groups in protein. ETO also interactions at N-7 guanine moieties in DNA
	Cross-linking agents (glutaraldehyde, formaldehyde)	Intermolecular protein cross-links
	Intercalating agents	Acridines intercalate between 2 layers of base pairs in DNA
	Oxidizing agents	
	1 Hypochlorites‡	Progressively oxidize thiol groups to disulphides, sulphoxides or disulphoxides
	2 Hydrogen peroxide‡	Formation of free hydroxyl radicals ($\bullet OH$) causes oxidation of thiol groups in enzymes and proteins
	3 Peracetic acid‡	Possibly disrupts thiol groups in proteins and enzymes
	Iodine	Interaction with cytoplasmic protein

*For further information, see Russell and Chopra (1996).
†Some agents affect more than one target site. EDTA, ethylenediamine tetraacetate; CHA, chlorhexidine diacetate; QACs, quaternary ammonium compounds; DBPI, dibromopropamidine isethionate; PHMB, polyhexamethylene biguanide; ETO, ethylene oxide; BPL, β-propiolactone; PO, propylene oxide; pmf, proton-motive force.
‡These compounds might affect enzymes and proteins in both the cytoplasmic (inner) membrane and cytoplasm.

(Gould 1988, Russell and Hugo 1988). In the first, leakage of intracellular materials is promoted by their physical interaction with the cytoplasmic membrane. In the second there is a specific attack on the insulatory function of the membrane such that the proton-motive force across it is either discharged or prevented from forming.

Leakage   Leakage is usually measured by the release of K^+ (which is the first index of membrane damage; Lambert and Hammond 1973), inorganic phosphates, 260 nm absorbing material and pool amino acids. In addition, the release of pentoses, diphenylamine-positive material and folin-positive material (indicative of RNA, DNA and protein, respectively) can be determined. Leakage can be considered as being a measure of the generalized loss of function of the cytoplasmic membrane as a permeability barrier, the rate and extent of leakage usually depending on the concentration of the inhibitor and the time and temperature of exposure. Leakage may be related to bacteriostasis but not necessarily to cell death. Examples of antibacterial agents that induce leakage are cationic, anionic and polypeptide surface-active agents, phenol, chlorhexidine, parabens, hexachlorophane (hexachlorophene), phenoxyethanol and salicylanilides. These effects are not, however, necessarily responsible for cell death.

Chlorhexidine has a biphasic effect on membrane permeability:

1   an initial high rate of leakage occurs as the biguanide concentration increases
2   a progressive decrease in leakage takes place at higher chlorhexidine concentrations as a consequence of coagulation or precipitation of the cytosol (Hugo 1992).

Both alexidine and the polymeric biguanide PHMB produce lipid phase separation and domain formation of the acidic phospholipids in the cytoplasmic membrane (Broxton, Woodcock and Gilbert 1984, Chawner and Gilbert 1989a, 1989b). Chlorhexidine and QACs also combine with membrane phospholipids but do not bring about lipid phase separation and domain formation.

Ethanol and isopropanol are membrane disrupters, inducing a rapid leakage of intracellular constituents; disorganization of the membrane probably results from their penetration into the hydrocarbon core of the membrane (Seiler and Russell 1991).

Effects on proton-motive force (pmf)   Mitchell's (1961) chemiosmotic theory seeks to explain active transport, synthesis of adenosine triphosphate (ATP) and flagellar movement. During metabolism, protons are extruded to the exterior of the bacterial cell, resulting in acidification of the exterior and positivity in charge relative to the cell interior.

Several chemicals that are antiseptics, disinfectants or preservatives behave in a manner similar to 2,4-dinitrophenol (DNP), i.e. they act as uncouplers of oxidative phosphorylation. Examples include 2-phenoxyethanol, bisphenols and pentachlorophenol. Tetra-chlorosalicylanilide discharges the membrane potential, $\Delta\Psi$, in *E. faecalis*. The thiobisphenol, fentichlor, behaves very much like DNP, having a direct action on the collapse of a proton potential (Bloomfield 1974). Phenoxyethanol and the alkyl phenols act as proton-conducting uncoupling agents. Pharmaceutical and food preservatives such as the parabens and lipophilic acids (propionic, sorbic, 4-hydroxybenzoic) inhibit the active uptake of some amino and oxo acids in *E. coli* and *B. subtilis*. Sorbic acid affects the pmf in *E. coli* and accelerates the movement of H^+ ions from low pH media into the cytoplasm. Sorbic acid appears to dissipate ΔpH, having a much smaller effect on $\Delta\Psi$ (Eklund 1983, 1985a, 1985b, Salmond, Kroll and Booth 1984).

Agents acting on nucleic acids and proteins

Intercalation   The antimicrobial activity of the acridines increases with degree of ionization (Albert 1979). Ionization is the most important factor governing their activity, but it must be cationic in nature, because acridine derivatives that are ionized to form anions or zwitterions are only poorly antibacterial by comparison. The acridines induce filamentous forms in gram-negative bacteria, inhibit DNA synthesis and combine strongly with DNA, although binding to other sites such as RNA, cell envelopes and ribosomes has also been reported. Binding to DNA has been studied extensively. The classic studies of Lerman (1961) suggested that the planar drug molecules become intercalated between adjacent base pairs in DNA. Binding to DNA occurs by 2 distinct mechanisms (Peacocke and Skerrett 1956): in the first, there is a first order reaction with one proflavine molecule binding to every 4 or 5 nucleotides, whereas in the second there is a slower, higher order of reaction with one molecule per single nucleotide.

Alkylation   Alkylation is defined as the conversion of

$$H—X \rightarrow R—X$$

where R is an alkyl group. Biological activity of alkylating agents is indicated by reaction with nucleophilic groups.

Epoxides, of which ethylene oxide is an example, interact with amino acids and proteins. Ethylene oxide causes hydroxyethylation of amino acids and combines with the amino, carboxyl, sulphydryl and hydroxyl groups of proteins (Russell 1976). Alkylation of phosphated guanine in non-sporing bacteria has been proposed as the primary reason for the lethal effect of ethylene oxide (Michael and Stumbo 1970, Russell 1976).

It has been suggested that formaldehyde also acts by its alkylating effect. Binding to RNA is reversible up to a point (Staehelin 1958). Interaction of formaldehyde with T2 bacteriophage DNA and with protein has been described (Grossman, Levine and Allison 1961).

The reaction of glutaraldehyde with nucleic acids follows pseudo-first order kinetics at high temperatures but there is little evidence for the formation of intermolecular cross-links. Glutaraldehyde inhibits synthesis of protein, DNA and RNA in *E. coli*, but this is believed to arise from an inhibition of precursor uptake as a consequence of protein–dialdehyde interaction in the outer structures of the cell.

Interaction with enzymes Metals such as mercury and silver interact with thiol (–SH) groups on enzymes to form mercaptides (Hugo 1992). This reaction may be reversed by excess of an –SH compound such as sodium thioglycollate or cysteine, an important finding since such agents are used to inactivate metals in microbicidal testing (Russell, Ahonkhai and Rogers 1979, Russell 1992a). The mode of action of silver salts resides in the Ag$^+$ ion (Russell and Hugo 1994). Bronopol also interacts with –SH groups (Hugo 1992).

Other effects Silver salts also produce structural changes in the cell envelope of *P. aeruginosa* and the Ag$^+$ ion reacts preferentially with the bases rather than the phosphate groups in DNA (Russell and Hugo 1994).

ACTION ON BACTERIAL SPORES

Comparatively few chemicals are sporicidal (Russell 1990a, 1990b). The mechanism of action of those that are is often poorly understood, although progress continues to be made. The reasons for this comparative lack of knowledge are not hard to find. Bacterial spores are more complex than vegetative cells; furthermore, extensive chemical and structural changes occur during the processes of sporulation, germination and outgrowth. Although it is possible to correlate these changes with the development of resistance (sporulation) or sensitivity (germination and outgrowth), it is rather more difficult to identify the mechanism whereby cell death is brought about.

Bacterial spores are not inactivated rapidly or readily at ambient temperatures (Bloomfield 1992, Bloomfield and Arthur 1994). Low concentrations (0.01%) of alkaline glutaraldehyde inhibit germination and outgrowth, whereas much higher concentrations must be used for long periods to kill spores (Russell 1990a). In fact, as with formaldehyde (Spicher and Peters 1981), it has been shown (Power, Dancer and Russell 1989, Williams and Russell 1993) that it is possible to revive some glutaraldehyde-treated spores by means of a sublethal heat shock. It is thus possible that the dialdehyde is a less effective sporicide than orginally thought, but that its cross-linking effect on bacterial spores will, under ordinary circumstances, be sufficient to prevent spore germination and subsequent vegetative development.

The enzyme lysozyme hydrolyses β1–4-linkages between *N*-acetylmuramic acid and *N*-acetylglucosamine in spore peptidoglycan in coatless spores. Sodium nitrite breaks the peptidoglycan chain at the muramic lactam residues unique to spores. Hypochlorites interact strongly with spore coats, but their major site of sporicidal action is believed to be on the cortex (Bloomfield and Arthur 1994). The alkylating agents ethylene and propylene oxides are considered to inactivate bacteria and their spores by combining with amino, carboxyl, sulphydryl and hydroxyl groups of proteins, as mentioned earlier.

The general antimicrobial activity of ethylene oxide (CH_2CH_2O) and related substances parallels their activity as alkylating agents (Phillips 1952). Thus, cyclopropane ($CH_2CH_2CH_2$), which is not an alkylating agent, is devoid of antimicrobial activity, whereas ethylene sulphide (CH_2CH_2S) and ethylene imine (CH_2CH_2NH) are potent alkylating compounds that demonstrate antimicrobial properties.

ACTION ON FUNGI

It is often assumed that the same effects as those in non-sporulating bacteria are responsible for fungal inactivation but in view of the considerable structural and biochemical differences between these microbes this is undoubtedly an oversimplification. However, as with bacteria, it is likely that an initial interaction at the cell surface is followed by passage of a biocide across the fungal cell wall to reach its target site(s), but little information is available about the ways uptake into fungal cells is achieved despite long-standing studies of biocide adsorption to yeasts and moulds (Lyr 1987, Gadd and White 1989, Russell 1992c).

Although the fungal cell wall may be a prime target for developing new antifungal antibiotics (Hector 1993), few biocides are likely to have the wall as a sole target. Chitin has been suggested as a potentially reactive site for glutaraldehyde action in yeasts (Gorman and Scott 1977). Glutaraldehyde is also known to cause agglutination of yeast cells (Navarro and Monsen 1976).

Chlorhexidine induces K$^+$ release from bakers' yeast (Elferink and Booji 1974) and affects the ultrastructure of budding *Candida albicans* with the loss of cytoplasmic constituents (Bobichon and Bouchet 1987). QACs also affect membrane integrity. Heavy metals probably bind to key functional groups of enzymes (Lyr 1987).

Very few relevant studies have been made on other target sites, but DNA and RNA would be expected to be targets for a number of biocides, such as cationic agents that interact strongly with nucleic acids (Hugo 1992).

ACTION ON VIRUSES

The mechanisms whereby viruses are inactivated by biocidal agents are still poorly understood although recent progress has been encouraging. In an excellent paper over 25 years ago, Grossgebauer (1970) discussed the possible effects of biocides on viruses and proposed that water-saturated phenol caused separation of protein from infectious RNA in poliovirus, that low formaldehyde concentrations produced an antigenic but non-infectious particle (for use in a vaccine) whereas higher aldehyde concentrations gave a non-infectious destroyed particle. Thurman and Gerba (1988, 1989) considered the possible interactions between viruses and biocides as being:

1 adsorption to capsid receptors
2 conformational changes in virus
3 destruction of capsid leading to release of infectious nucleic acid
4 as for 3 but nucleic acid rendered non-infectious
5 capsid remaining intact, but nucleic acid rendered non-infectious.

They pointed out that CRAs could inactivate viruses by attacking either capsid proteins or nucleic acid.

Glutaraldehyde reduces the activity of hepatitis B surface antigen and especially core antigen in hepatitis B virus (Adler-Storthz et al. 1983) and interacts with lysine residues on the surface of hepatitis A virus (Passagot et al. 1987). Low concentrations (<0.1%) of alkaline glutaraldehyde act against purified poliovirus whereas poliovirus RNA is highly resistant to higher concentrations (Bailly et al. 1991). From this, it may be inferred that changes to the capsid are responsible for loss of infectivity. Support for this contention has been obtained by demonstrating that the capsid proteins of poliovirus and echovirus react with low concentrations (0.05 and 0.005%, respectively) of the dialdehyde, the 10-fold difference in aldehyde concentration probably reflecting major structural alterations in the 2 viruses (Chambon, Bailly and Peigue-Lafeuille 1992). Some biocides (hypochlorite, 70% ethanol and cetrimide) induce a rapid loss of the outer capsid layer, whereas chlorhexidine and phenol affect morphology only after extended periods of exposure (Rodgers et al. 1985).

Recently, mechanistic studies of the effects of biocides on bacteriophages have been undertaken. These investigations (Maillard et al. 1995) have provided useful information about the interaction of biocides with phage protein and nucleic acid and on the inhibition of transduction, but much remains to be done to understand fully the mechanisms of inactivation.

ACTION ON PROTOZOA

Virtually nothing is known about the mechanisms of antiprotozoal action of biocides, a disappointing gap in our knowledge and one that needs to be rectified.

2.7 Mechanisms of microbial resistance to antimicrobial agents

By contrast with antibiotics, mechanisms of microbial resistance to antiseptics, disinfectants and preservatives have been little studied. Three levels of biocidal activity have been recognized (Favero and Bond 1993):

1 high level, involving the inactivation of bacterial spores, fungi, mycobacteria and viruses
2 intermediate level, in which mycobacteria, fungi and viruses are inactivated and
3 low level, in which only non-sporulating bacteria (not including mycobacteria) and enveloped (lipid) viruses are rendered non-viable.

Thus, different organisms show different responses (see also section 2.4, p. 160) and possible reasons will be provided below.

In general terms, resistance mechanisms are either intrinsic (innate, natural) or acquired (one specific bacterial type of mechanism).

RESISTANCE OF NON-SPORULATING BACTERIA

These will be considered (see also Table 7.5) by reference to mycobacteria, other gram-positive organisms and gram-negative bacteria.

Mycobacterial resistance

The mycobacterial cell wall is highly hydrophobic with a mycoylarabinogalactanpeptidoglycan skeleton. Thus, hydrophilic agents have difficulty in penetrating the wall in sufficiently high concentrations to achieve a mycobactericidal effect. However, it is clear that low concentrations must traverse the wall because inhibitory concentrations of non-mycobactericidal agents such as chlorhexidine are generally of the same order as those against other, non-mycobacterial, organisms (Russell 1996). The component(s) of the mycobacterial wall responsible for the high level of biocide resistance is (are) unknown, but both the mycolic acids and arabinogalactan appear to be inhibited (Russell 1996). Acquired mycobacterial resistance by repeated exposure to a biocide is a possibility but there appears to be no evidence that plasmids are involved.

Resistance of other gram-positive bacteria

The cell wall of gram-positive bacteria is a thick, fibrous layer pressed against the cytoplasmic membrane; the wall consists mainly of an inelastic peptidoglycan interspersed with which may be lipids and teichoic and teichuronic acids. The peptidoglycan comprises at least 50% of the dry weight of the walls. Mechanisms whereby antimicrobial agents enter gram-positive bacteria have been little studied but passive diffusion across the wall is probably a major factor. Thus, organisms such as staphylococci and streptococci are usually highly susceptible to biocides (Russell 1992a, 1995, Russell and Russell 1995, Russell and Chopra 1996). However, bacteria grown under different conditions may show a wide response to biocides. For instance, fattened cells of *S. aureus* produced by repeated subculturing in glycerol-containing media are more resistant to benzylpenicillin and higher phenols (Hugo 1992). Additionally, nutrient limitation and reduced growth rates (Brown and Gilbert 1993, Poxton 1993) can alter sensitivity to biocides by changes in peptidoglycan thickness and cross-linking. Such changes in these 2 examples can be regarded as the expression of intrinsic resistance brought about in response to a phenotypic (physiological) adaptation.

Acquired resistance is also known in some strains of *S. aureus*. Inorganic mercury (Hg^{2+}) resistance is a common property of clinical isolates of *S. aureus* containing penicillinase plasmids. These plasmids are either narrow spectrum, specifying resistance to Hg^{2+} and some organomercurials, or broad spectrum, encoding additional resistance to other organomercurials. The enzymes involved are mercuric reductase (Hg^{2+}) and lyase (hydrolase) and reductase (organo-com-

Table 7.5   Mechanisms of bacterial resistance to biocides*

Bacteria	Mechanism(s) of	
	Intrinsic resistance	**Acquired resistance**
Mycobacteria	Permeability barrier associated with mycolate of arabinogalactan	Not described, unlikely
Other non-sporulating gram-positive bacteria	Cell wall modulation 1 Peptidoglycan changes 2 Lipid increase	Plasmid mediated efflux of cationic biocides in multiple antibiotic-resistant *S. aureus*; enzymatic inactivation of Hg compounds
Bacterial spores	Permeability barrier associated with outer membrane	Not described, unlikely
Gram-negative bacteria	1 Permeability barrier associated with outer membrane 2 Constitutive biocide-degrading enzymes?	Enzymatic inactivation of Hg compounds; efflux of cationic biocides?

*For further information, see Russell and Russell (1995) and Russell and Chopra (1996).

pounds) (Foster 1983). Resistance to other metals has been described (Silver et al. 1989) and often involves efflux mechanisms. Silver (Ag^+) reduction may not form the basis of silver or silver sulphadiazine (AgSD) resistance (Belly and Kydd 1982, Foster 1983, Silver et al. 1989) but may be associated with accumulation (Trevor 1987, Russell and Hugo 1994).

Some methicillin-resistant strains of *S. aureus* (MRSA) containing plasmids encoding gentamicin resistance (MGRSA) also have increased MIC values towards such biocides as QACs, chlorhexidine, ethidium bromide (EB), acridines and propamidine isethionate (PI) (Lyon and Skurray 1987, Cookson and Phillips 1990). At least 3 genetic determinants are responsible for cationic biocide resistance in clinical isolates of *S. aureus*: these are *qac*A, which specifies resistance to QACs, acridines, EB, propamidine isethionate and low level chlorhexidine resistance; *qac*B, which is similar; and the genetically unrelated *qac*C encoding QAC and low level EB resistance.

These cationic biocides bind strongly to DNA and have been termed nucleic acid-binding (NAB) compounds. Those MGRSA strains without NAB plasmids are more sensitive to chlorhexidine than are methicillin-sensitive *S. aureus* (MSSA) strains, whereas MRSA with such plasmids (termed GNAB) encoding resistance to gentamicin and NAB compounds are more resistant to chlorhexidine (Cookson, Bolton and Platt 1991). Curing of methicillin resistance does not produce changes in chlorhexidine sensitivity in MRSA strains with or without NAB plasmids, whereas curing of GNAB plasmids produces a reduced MIC of chlorhexidine (Cookson, Bolton and Platt 1991). From this, it is clear that GNAB is related to chlorhexidine resistance. There is evidence that there is an efflux of cationic agents (including chlorhexidine?) from such antibiotic-resistant strains (Midgley 1986, 1987).

Resistance of gram-negative bacteria

Gram-negative bacteria such as pseudomonads and Enterobacteriaceae are usually less sensitive to a variety of chemically unrelated inhibitors than are gram-positive cocci. One reason for this lies in the different structural and chemical composition of the outer layers of the organisms, thereby conferring an intrinsic resistance mechanism on gram-negative bacteria. The cell envelope of gram-negative bacteria is more complex: the inner (cytoplasmic) membrane is adherent to the peptidoglycan which is covalently linked to Braun's elongated lipoprotein. The peptidoglycan–lipoprotein complex partly occupies the periplasmic space that exists between the outer and inner hydrophobic membranes. Chemically, the outer membrane (OM) consists of lipopolysaccharide (LPS), phospholipids and proteins. The major OM protein with the fastest electrophoretic mobility is the lipoprotein. Other major proteins in *E. coli* K12 are outer-membrane proteins (Omp) A, C and F and protein *a* (Hammond, Lambert and Rycroft 1984). Lipoprotein stabilizes the OM, OmpA has a role in conjugation. Protein *a* is a protease involved in capsular biosynthesis, and OmpC and OmpF are matrix proteins, tightly bound to peptidoglycan and known as porins because they act as general pores for the passage of hydrophilic solutes of low molecular weight (<c. 650) across the OM. Minor OM proteins of *E. coli* include PhoE and LamB. In *Salmonella typhimurium*, OmpC and OmpF are also present, but there is also a third major OM protein, OmpD, which has no counterpart in *E. coli*.

The OM acts as a permeability barrier in limiting or preventing the entry of many chemically unrelated types of antibacterial compounds into gram-negative bacteria. Some antibacterial agents, e.g. polymyxins and possibly chlorhexidine, damage the OM and could thus promote their own entry into the cell (Hancock 1984).

Acquired resistance of gram-negative bacteria to biocides may occur as a result of mutation or by the acquisition of plasmids or transposons (Russell 1985, Russell and Chopra 1996). Acquired chromosomal resistance by mutation has been described for chlorhexidine resistance with *P. stuartii* (Chopra, Johnson and Bennett 1987) and *S. marcescens* (Lannigran and Bryan 1985), alcohols with *E. coli* (Fried and Novick 1973) and cationic bactericides with various organisms (Chopra 1987). Resistance is not always stable. Temporary resistance by phenotypic adaptation to alcohols is described by Chopra (1987), who also considers that, in general, a non-genetic adaptive type of resistance is unlikely to play an important part in determining the long-term survival of bacteria to antiseptics and disinfectants.

Strains of *P. stuartii* isolated from paraplegic patients often harbour plasmids conferring resistance to Hg^{2+} and several antibiotics and the organisms may also express resistance to cationic biocides. However, attempts to transfer chlorhexidine and QAC resistance to suitable recipients have failed and the occurrence of a plasmid-linked association between antibiotic and antiseptic resistance has not been substantiated.

High level resistance to biocides has been observed in hospital isolates of other gram-negative bacteria but no clear role for plasmid mediated biocide resistance has emerged in the following:

1 chlorhexidine-, antibiotic-resistant *P. mirabilis*
2 chlorhexidine-resistant strains of *Burkholderia cepacia* and *Alcaligenes denitrificans*
3 chlorhexidine- and QAC-resistant *P. aeruginosa* and several members of the Enterobacteriaceae (Russell and Chopra 1996).

BACTERIAL SPORE RESISTANCE

Bacterial spores differ fundamentally in both structure and composition from vegetative cells. In essence, a spore usually consists of a central core (protoplast, germ cell) and germ cell wall surrounded by a cortex, external to which are an inner and an outer spore coat. Under certain circumstances, spores can germinate and outgrow to produce vegetative cells which have the typical form and composition of non-sporulating bacteria (Russell 1990a). Bacterial spores are amongst the most resistant of all microbial forms to inactivation by chemical or physical agents. The outer spore layers (coats: Russell 1990a) and to some extent the cortex (Bloomfield and Arthur 1994) present a barrier to the intracellular penetration of many biocides. Several studies (Power, Dancer and Russell 1988, Shaker et al. 1988, Knott, Russell and Dancer 1995) have been undertaken to examine the stage of sporulation associated with development of resistance to a particular biocide. An early resistance develops to formaldehyde, whereas resistance to chlorhexidine and QACs is an intermediate event and to glutaraldehyde a late event. Susceptibility to an antibacterial agent is regained during germination or outgrowth (Russell 1990a).

FUNGAL RESISTANCE

Two basic mechanisms of fungal resistance to biocides can be envisaged: intrinsic and acquired (Dekker 1987, Russell 1992c). The fungal cell wall contains various types of polymers, including chitin and chitosan (Zygomycetes), chitin and glucan (mycelial forms of ascomycetes and deuteromycetes), glucan and mannan (yeast forms of ascomocytes and deuteromycetes). Thus, there is ample opportunity for a cell to exclude biocide molecules. Studies on the sensitivity of *C. albicans* to the polyene antibiotic, amphotericin, suggests that glucan may have a role to play in limiting drug uptake (Gale 1986). Comparable studies with biocides are sparse but there is tentative evidence that glucan, but not mannan, in yeast cell walls could have a role to play in limiting chlorhexidine uptake (Hiom et al. 1993).

There is no evidence linking the presence of plasmids in fungal cells and the ability of the organisms to acquire resistance to fungistatic or fungicidal agents, although acquired resistance of yeasts to organic acids is known (Warth 1986, 1989).

BIOFILMS AND RESISTANCE

A biofilm is a consortium of bacteria or other microbes organized within an extensive exopolysaccharide exopolymer (glycocalyx: Costerston et al. 1987, 1994, Denyer, Gorman and Sussman 1993). Biofilms may consist of monocultures, diverse species or mixed phenotypes of a given species. Bacteria in different parts of a biofilm experience different nutrient environments and varying oxygen tensions and growth rates are likely to be reduced within the depths of the biofilm as a consequence of nutrient limitation (Brown and Gilbert 1993, Carpentier and Cerf 1993, Poxton 1993). Bacteria within a biofilm may be much less sensitive to antibiotics and biocides. Possible reasons for this increased intrinsic resistance are:

1 prevention by the glycocalyx of access of the agent to underlying cells
2 chemical reaction between the agent and glycocalyx
3 modulation of the microenvironment to produce changes in the chemical composition of the cell envelope, growth rate or both
4 increased production of enzymes that degrade antibacterial agents (Brown and Gilbert 1993).

Some strains of *M. chelonae* that are highly resistant to glutaraldehyde have been isolated (van Klingeren and Pullen 1993). The mechanism(s) of this resistance is (are) unknown but might be associated with biofilm production.

VIRAL RESISTANCE

Conflicting results have been reported about the action of biocides on different types of viruses. In part, this can probably be explained on the basis of different methodologies. However, the penetration of biocides into viruses and phages of different types has not been examined in depth, nor has interaction with viral protein and nucleic acid. It is, therefore, difficult to provide adequate reasons to explain the relative response, or resistance, of different virus types to biocides. Nevertheless, some progress has been made on the basis of the scheme of Klein and Deforest (1983), as described in section 2.4 (p. 160). Thurman and Gerba (1988) have suggested that the structural integrity of a virus is altered by an agent that reacts with viral capsids to increase viral permeability, so that a '2-stage disinfection' could offer an efficient means of viral inactivation whilst overcoming the possibility of multiplicity reactivation first put forward in 1947 to explain an initial reduction and then an increase in titre of biocide-treated bacteriophage.

RESISTANCE OF PROTOZOA

The cyst form represents the stage in life cycle which is resistant to biocides. No significant studies appear to have been undertaken about biocide sensitivity or resistance during encystment and excystment or about the relative uptake of biocides into cysts and trophozoites. It must be concluded tentatively that the outer regions of cysts limit entry of biocides, thus providing one mechanism of intrinsic resistance.

3 PHYSICAL AGENTS

Physical agents are normally used in preference to chemical agents for sterilization, either by microbial destruction or by removal of micro-organisms (Dewhurst and Hoxey 1990, Soper and Davies 1990, Kowalski 1993). It is also practicable, however, to employ cold, desiccation and freeze-drying as methods of preservation. Traditionally, heat in one form or another has been employed as a sterilization procedure. It still occupies a key role and is the method of choice whenever possible. Filtration is also based on ancient knowledge, but suffers several limitations. The most recent modern process uses ionizing radiation. This section deals with the types of processes available, the principles involved and their medical and other uses, process validation, the mechanisms of microbial inactivation or removal, and the reasons for the above-average resistance of certain types of micro-organism. Some uses of physical processes are provided in Table 7.6.

3.1 Moist heat

Heating in the presence of water has been used for many years as a method of sterilization, or sometimes of disinfection. It can be employed in different ways, e.g. at temperatures below, at or above 100°C.

TERMINOLOGY

Thermal death time (TDT) Thermal death time is the time (in min) required to kill all cells in a suspension at a given temperature. TDT is highly dependent on the inoculum size.

Thermal death point (TDP) Thermal death point is the temperature needed to kill all cells in suspension

after a fixed exposure time, e.g. 10 min. There are many variables associated with this term, notably inoculum size, and as such it is of little value.

D Value The D value (decimal reduction time, DRT), is the time (in min) needed at a particular temperature to reduce the viable organisms by 90%, i.e. to 10% or by 1 $\log_{10}$ unit. D value is independent of inoculum size and is inversely related to temperature. Examples are given in Table 7.7.

The D value can be calculated in several ways (Russell 1982). The usual method is to plot the $\log_{10}$ number, or fraction, of surviving cells against time. When a straight line response is obtained (A in Fig. 7.2), D can be read easily from the graph. With an initial shoulder response (B in Fig. 7.2), or when there is a decreasing death curve (C in Fig. 7.2), it is usual to calculate the D value from the straight line portion of the curve provided that this is clearly stated and that the extent of the shoulder (B in Fig. 7.2) or tail (C in Fig. 7.2) is also expressed. Heat activation is demonstrated in the initial portion of curve D in Fig. 7.2.

Inactivation factor (IF) Inactivation factor (IF) is the degree of reduction in the number of viable cells and is obtained by dividing the initial viable count (N_0) by the final viable count (N_u), i.e. IF = N_0/N_u.

An alternative procedure is to use the D value approach; IF = $10^{t/D}$ (in which t represents the treatment dose, i.e. time). There are, however, pitfalls with this method (Russell 1982).

z Value The z value, defined as the number of degrees (°C) to bring about a 10-fold reduction in TDT or D value, is obtained from the slope of the curve in which temperature is plotted against time (see Russell 1982). An alternative method is based on a knowledge of the temperature coefficient (Q_{10}) per 10-fold rise in temperature, i.e. $Q_{10} = 10^{10/z}$ from which z = 10/log Q_{10}.

F and F_0 values The F value is the time in minutes to destroy an organism in a specified medium at 121°C (250°F). F_0 is the F value when z = 10°C (18°F). Calculations employing F_0 values are used in validating thermal sterilization processes (Soper and Davies 1990).

***Y* intercept and Y_0/N_0 values** Deviations from exponential rates of inactivation occur frequently (Fig. 7.2 B, C, D) (Cerf 1977). With convex- or concave-type curves, extrapolation of the line to cut the *Y*-axis gives the *Y*-intercept value (Y_0). If N_0 represents the initial number of cells, then

1 when $Y_0 = N_0$, there is a straight line response
2 when $Y_0 > N_0$, there is an initial shoulder
3 when $Y_0 < N_0$, a decreasing death rate is obtained.

The intercept ratio (IR) is a ratio of the 2 values, i.e.

$$IR = \log Y_0/\log N_0$$

and is thus useful in characterizing time-survivor curves.

Table 7.6 Some applications of sterilization processes

Process	Application(s)
Moist heat (autoclave)	Sterilization of many ophthalmic and parenteral products, surgical dressings, rubber gloves (high-vacuum autoclave)
Dry heat	Sterilization of glassware, glass syringes, oils and oily injections, metal instruments; depyrogenation at high temperatures
Ionizing radiation	Sterilization of single-use disposable medical items
Ultraviolet radiation	Poor sterilizing agent; use restricted to air sterilization (in conjunction with air filtration) and water disinfection
Ethylene oxide	Sterilization of fragile, heat-sensitive equipment, powders, components of spacecraft
Low temperature steam with formaldehyde (LTSF)	Disinfection/sterilization of some heat-sensitive materials
Filtration	Air sterilization; sterilization of thermolabile ophthalmic and parenteral solutions, and of sera

Table 7.7 Responses* of some bacterial spores to heat and to ionizing radiation

Bacterial spore	Moist heat		Dry heat		Ionizing radiation (D)	
	D (min) at 121°C	z	D (min) at 160°C	z	Mrad	kGy
B. stearothermophilus	4–5	8–10	<1	15–25	...	...
B. subtilis	<1	5.5–9.5	1–5	20	0.15	1.5
B. cereus	<1	...	...	20	0.1	1
B. pumilus	...	...	...	25	0.2	2
C. sporogenes	<1	10	2	20	0.15–0.2	1.5–2
C. botulinum type A	<1	9.5	...	...	0.1	1

*Values are approximate responses to a particular process. The actual response will depend upon several parameters (see text and Russell 1982, where comprehensive details are provided).
D, time (min) at a specified temperature or radiation dose needed to reduce the viable population by one $\log_{10}$ unit.
z, temperature (°C) needed to reduce the D value by 90%.

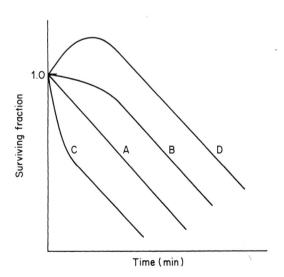

Fig. 7.2 Thermal inactivation curves of bacterial spores. A, exponential death; B, increasing death rate; C, decreasing death rate; D, heat activation.

MICROBIAL SENSITIVITY TO MOIST HEAT

Non-sporulating bacteria are heat-sensitive and are usually destroyed at temperatures of 50–60°C. Thermal death times of fungi and protozoa are similar and most viruses are inactivated at 60°C for 20 min (Alder and Simpson 1992). D and z values for some bacterial spores are listed in Table 7.7.

Bacterial spores are considerably more resistant to moist heat. Among *Bacillus* spp., *Bacillus stearothermophilus* is the most heat-resistant. There is a considerable variation in sensitivity among *Clostridium* spp., *Clostridium botulinium* type E being far more sensitive than types A, B or C (Russell 1982).

Sensitivity to moist heat depends on the conditions of exposure and recovery. Alder and Simpson (1992) point out that in medical, surgical and veterinary practice micro-organisms are often embedded in organic debris which may to some extent insulate them from the effect of heat; these authors emphasize the need for thorough cleaning prior to sterilization.

TYPES OF MOIST HEAT PROCESSES

Temperatures below 100°C

A temperature of 60°C was employed by Pasteur during his studies on spoilage of French wines. Subsequently, his process (60°C for 30 min) was used for the pasteurization of milk; a 'flash' method (71.1°C for 15 s) was introduced later. A procedure similar to pasteurization is employed in the production of certain bacterial vaccines, e.g. typhoid vaccine, the aim being to kill the organisms while preserving their immunogenicity.

Although some types of spore are killed by moist heat at about 80°C, temperatures below 100°C cannot be relied upon to achieve sterilization.

Temperatures around 100°C

These temperatures also cannot be relied upon to kill bacterial spores, and steaming is thus of limited use. Two variations have been used. The first (tyndallization) involves steaming for 30 min (originally 80°C for 60 min) on each of 3 consecutive days, the principle being that spores that survived the heating process would germinate before the next thermal exposure and would then be killed. Spores will not, however, germinate in a non-nutrient medium and, although tyndallization was originally an official method for sterilizing injections, it is no longer used. The second variation involves heating to 98–100°C in the presence of a specified antimicrobial agent (the activity of which is considerably potentiated at the high temperature; see temperature coefficient, section 2.3, p. 158). This method is no longer permitted in the *British Pharmacopoeia* (1988, 1993) for sterilizing any injectable and eyedrop formulations.

Temperatures above 100°C (autoclaving)

Sterilization by steam under pressure depends upon 4 properties of dry saturated steam: high temperature, wealth of latent heat, ability to form water of condensation, and instantaneous contraction in volume that occurs during condensations. These properties are optimal only in steam on the phase boundary between itself and condensate at the same temperature (Fig. 7.3). The process has been described more fully by Bowie (1955).

Steam formed at any point on the phase boundary has the same temperature as the boiling water from which it was derived but holds an extra and relatively heavy load of latent heat which, without drop in temperature, is available instantly and entirely as soon as it wets a cooler surface.

Superheated steam must be avoided; this is hotter than dry, saturated steam at the same pressure, the process becoming akin to dry heat which is much less efficient. Superheated steam behaves as a gas and only slowly yields its heat to cooler objects. In Fig. 7.3, steam at any point A on the phase boundary is saturated: if, however, the temperature is raised to B (keeping pressure constant) then superheated steam is generated. A small amount (5°C) of superheat may be tolerated in practice.

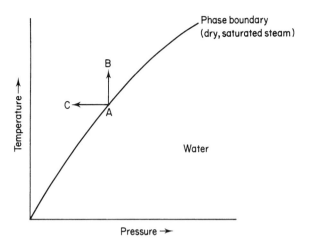

Fig. 7.3 Phase diagrams for water vapour, depicting the phase boundary for dry saturated steam and the production of superheated steam (points B and C). A, any point on the phase boundary; B, pressure kept constant, temperature increased; C, temperature kept constant, pressure increased.

When air is present in a space with steam, the air will carry part of the load so that the pressure of the steam is reduced, creating a condition equivalent to that defined by the horizontal line AC in Fig. 7.3. This can also be deduced from Dalton's law of partial pressures which, applied to the present context, can be written as $P_{total} = P_{steam} + P_{air}$. The removal of air is, in fact, important in ensuring efficient autoclaving and can be achieved in various ways. In downward displacement sterilizers, air is displaced downwards, being heavier than steam; this process may, however, be wasteful of steam and time-consuming. Its widest application is in the sterilization of bottled fluids (Owens 1993). Bulky packages of, for example, surgical dressings are, however, air retentive and the downward displacement method of removing air is not efficient. Removal of air before admission of steam is far more effective and can be achieved by the use of high prevacuum autoclaves or by means of a pulsed evacuation and steam admission. Thermal processing is also widely employed in the food industry (Gould 1992, Brown 1994). Table 7.8 lists the time–temperature relationships provided by the *British Pharmacopoeia* (1993). Sterilizers designed for bottled fluids generally employ temperatures of 121°C and those for porous loads 126–134°C.

Low temperature steam with formaldehyde (LTSF)

Low temperature steam (LTS) at subatmospheric pressure was developed originally for disinfecting heat-sensitive materials. LTS at 80°C was found to be much more effective than water at the same temperature. The addition of formaldehyde to LTS to produce LTSF achieved a sporicidal effect (Dewhurst and Hoxey 1990, Soper and Davies 1990), and LTSF is thus suitable for sterilizing thermolabile equipment although there are now doubts about this process.

Details of sterilizer design and mode of operation are provided by Alder and Simpson (1992).

Table 7.8 Permitted time–temperature relationships in moist heat and dry heat sterilization processes*

Process	Temperature (°C)		Holding period (min)	
Moist heat (autoclave)		121		15
		126		10
		134		3
Dry heat		160		120
	Minimum of	170	Not less than	60
		180		30

*Based on recommendations in *British Pharmacopoeia* (1993).

MECHANISMS OF MICROBIAL INACTIVATION BY MOIST HEAT

Heat induces a multiplicity of injuries in sporing and non-sporing bacteria.

In bacterial spores, thermal injury has been attributed to denaturation of vital spore enzymes, impairment of germination or outgrowth or both, membrane damage (leading to leakage of calcium dipicolinate), increased sensitivity to inhibitory agents, structural damage (as observed by electron microscopy) and damage to the spore chromosome (as evinced by mutations or DNA strand breaks). Effects on DNA are much more pronounced during dry heating (see section 3.2, p. 174) which generates a high level of mutants in spore populations (Gould 1989). DNA is, however, an important target, although the exact mechanism of spore inactivation is unknown. Deficiencies in DNA repair mechanisms are known to render spores more heat-sensitive (Hanlin, Lombardi and Slepecky 1985). Spore proteins have also been implicated (Belliveau et al. 1992, Setlow 1994) although the nature of these proteins is unclear.

In non-sporulating bacteria, mild heat treatment (c. 45–50°C) damages the outer membrane of *E. coli*, rendering cells more sensitive to hydrophobic inhibitors (Hitchener and Egan 1977, Mackey 1983). Extensive studies have demonstrated lethal damage to the cytoplasmic membrane, RNA breakdown and protein coagulation (Tomlins and Ordal 1976) and damage to the bacterial chromosome (Pellon and Sinskey 1984; these authors point out that virtually all structures and functions can be damaged by heat but repair to non-DNA structures can occur only if DNA remains functional, thereby providing the necessary genetic information). There is now a wealth of evidence, both biochemical and genetic, implicating the involvement of DNA in heat damage, probably as a result of enzymatic action after thermal injury (Pellon and Sinskey 1984). Using repair-deficient *E. coli* mutants, Mackey and Seymour (1987) proposed that heat-induced DNA damage occurred indirectly via an oxidation mediated by hydrogen peroxide (or free radicals derived from it) in peroxide-generating complex recovery media. Their results also provide a satisfactory explanation for the 'minimal medium recovery' phenomenon which appears to involve protection from this peroxide-induced effect.

MECHANISMS OF RESISTANCE OF BACTERIAL SPORES TO MOIST HEAT

The exact mechanism whereby bacterial spores are heat-resistant remains arguable. Several theories have been put forward, the most important of which will now be considered briefly.

The resistance of spores to heat can be manipulated over several orders of magnitude by exposure to extreme pH values and cationic exchange treatment (H-form and Ca-form, respectively: Alderton and Snell 1963, Alderton, Chen and Ito 1980). The content and location of water in spores play important roles in their heat resistance. Spores have a low water content (see below) and this is an essential factor in resistance. Spore coats do not contribute to thermal resistance since coatless spores are not more heat-sensitive than ordinary spores. Gould and his colleagues (reviewed by Gould 1989) found that resuspension of newly germinated spores in high concentrations of sucrose or sodium chloride (but not of glycerol) restored resistance to heat and ionizing radiation. In such an osmoregulatory mechanism the cortical structure would have to maintain a uniform pressure upon, and thereby control, the water content of the spore core. Warth (1985) considered 3 types of mechanism which could contribute to the stability of proteins in the spore: they could be intrinsically stable; substances might be present which help stabilize them (there is no strong evidence to support this notion but calcium dipicolinate may play a role); and the removal of water could alter their stability.

Several spore properties are, in fact, important for heat resistance, notably protein thermotolerance, dehydration, mineralization, thermal adaptation and cortex function (Murrell 1981, Beaman and Gerhardt 1986, Beaman, Pankratz and Gerhardt 1988, 1989, Gerhardt and Marquis 1989, Marquis, Sim and Shin 1994). In addition, small acid-soluble spore proteins (SASPs) found in the spore core have some role to play. SASPs are of 2 types, α/β-type associated with spore DNA, and γ-type, not associated with any spore macromolecule. Spores lacking α/β-type SASPs are more sensitive than wild-type spores and it is likely that heat-induced DNA damage is the mechanism involved (Setlow 1994). However, these SASPs are not a major determinant of spore resistance to moist heat because heat resistance during sporulation is attained well after their synthesis (Setlow 1994).

3.2 Dry heat

Dry heat is a less efficient sterilization process than moist heat. The terminology used in describing moist heat sterilization is also employed here. Bacterial spores are the most resistant organisms to dry heat and D and z values are much higher than for moist heat (Table 7.7; Molin 1992, Wood 1993).

TYPES OF DRY HEAT PROCESSES

Normally, dry heat sterilization processes are in hot-air ovens, a number of combinations of temperature and time being permitted (Table 7.8). It is essential that the hot air can circulate between objects being sterilized, which must therefore be loosely packed with adequate air spaces, to ensure optimum heat transfer. A fan is essential to prevent the wide variation in temperature that would otherwise occur. Industrially, sterilization equipment can consist also of forced convection ovens, rapid heat transfer sterilizers and continuous-belt sterilizers (Wood 1993). Dry heat sterilization (Table 7.6) is the method of choice in the pharmaceutical industry for many heat-stable objects and materials (Dewhurst and Hoxey 1990) and at higher temperatures it can also destroy pyrogens (depyrogenation; Wood 1993).

MECHANISMS OF MICROBIAL INACTIVATION BY DRY HEAT

Microbial inactivation by dry heat has been considered primarily an oxidation process. Spores heated in oxygen would thus be expected to be more sensitive than when heated in the presence of other gases, but this is not necessarily true (Pheil et al. 1967). Thus, although oxidation may play an important part, other possibilities must be considered.

An effect on DNA is one possibility, sublethal temperatures inducing mutants in *B. subtilis* spores (Zamenhof 1960) as a consequence of depurination (Northrop and Slepecky 1967). The water content of spores is an important factor in determining inactivation by dry heat. Rowe and Silverman (1970) postulated that only a relatively small amount of water is needed to protect the heat-sensitive site in spores and that resistance to dry heat depends mainly on the location, rather than on the amount, of water in the spore, and on its association with other molecules.

3.3 Inactivation by cold

Growth of micro-organisms is retarded and eventually ceases if they are held at reduced temperatures. Some can grow at temperatures approaching 0°C and these psychrophiles may be important food-spoilage organisms. Environmental factors such as nutrient status, pH, salt concentration and a_w (water activity or moisture content) can alter the minimum growth temperature (Herbert 1989).

Freeze-drying involves rapid freezing with subsequent drying in a vaccum and is used widely for preserving microbial cultures and certain foodstuffs, but its use subjects micro-organisms to stresses such as freezing, drying, storage and eventual rehydration (Mackey 1984). Single-strand breaks in DNA and an increase in the frequency of mutation may be caused by freeze-drying (Asada, Takano and Shibasaki 1979).

Freezing and thawing can inactivate bacteria. Membrane damage may ensue, as evidenced by the loss of intracellular materials and the penetration into cells of certain compounds that are normally excluded. Damage to the outer membrane of the cell envelope has also been shown in frozen and thawed *E. coli* (Mackey 1983, 1984). For comprehensive accounts, the papers by MacLeod and Calcott (1976) and Mackey (1984) should be consulted.

Cold shock is a process in which organisms are suddenly chilled without freezing. Gram-positive and gram-negative bacteria may be killed, but not yeasts (MacLeod and Calcott 1976, Rose 1976). Several factors influence the response of cells, notably the age of the culture (since exponential phase, but not stationary phase, cells are susceptible) and the composition of the medium. Divalent cations can protect cells against chilling. Low molecular weight materials are released from chilled cells as a consequence of increased membrane permeability caused by a phase transition in membrane lipids (Rose 1976). A modification of this treatment is cold osmotic shock, in which bacteria are suspended in a hypertonic sucrose solution containing EDTA and are then suspended in ice-cold magnesium chloride solution. This treatment does not kill the cells but does induce the release of periplasmic enzymes, including β-lactamases, from gram-negative bacteria.

3.4 Hydrostatic pressure

Some organisms can exist at the bottom of deep oceans where they are subjected to high pressure (Dring 1976). Bacterial spores are more resistant to hydrostatic pressure than are germinated spores or non-sporulating bacteria. Temperature profoundly affects bacterial sensitivity to hydrostatic pressure, the rate of inactivation increasing as the temperature rises. This combined effect can be potentiated if an additional heat treatment is given after pressurization (Gould 1970, Gould and Jones 1989) (see also section 3.8, p. 178). The application of hydrostatic pressure is a useful technique because it enables investigations to be made of germination in the absence of physiological germinants. In view, however, of the occurrence of 'superdormant' spores (Gould, Jones and Wrighton 1968) which are resistant to hydrostatic pressure, it is unlikely that this process will find use as a sterilization procedure.

3.5 Ionizing radiation

Ionizing radiations such as x-rays, γ-rays and high speed electrons (β-rays) strip electrons from the atoms of the material through which the radiations pass; essentially all the chemical changes produced in the microbial cell are due to these stripped-off electrons, which initiate a chain of chemical reactions. Ionizations occur principally in water, resulting in the formation of short-lived but highly reactive radicals (hydroxyl, •OH) and protons (H$^+$). Single-strand, and sometimes double-strand, breakage in DNA ensues.

By contrast, ultraviolet (UV) radiation does not possess enough energy to eject an electron to produce an ion, although there is an alteration of electrons within their orbits. It is not therefore an ionizing radiation. Infrared radiations rapidly raise the temperature of objects which they strike and are thus employed for their heating effect.

x-Rays and γ-rays are of very short wavelengths, and are generated by machines or radioactive sources (e.g. ^{60}Co). High-speed electrons were originally produced from radioactive isotopes, but had little penetration; various machines have been developed that accelerate atomic particles to give them the energies for penetrating deeply. x-Rays and γ-rays have considerable penetrating power. By contrast, α-particles which consist of helium nuclei ($^4_2$He) have little penetration and thus are not used for sterilization. Industrially, radioisotopes in the form of ^{60}Co (Herring and Saylor 1993) and accelerated electrons (Cleland, O'Neill and Thompson 1993) are the main sources of ionizing radiation.

The unit of radiation most widely used in microbiology was the rad, a measurement of the energy absorbed from ionizing radiation by the matter through which the radiation passes. The newer, more modern (SI) unit is the gray (Gy) which is defined as the deposition of 1 J kg^{-1} energy in tissue, whereas 1 rad is the deposition of 10^{-2} J kg^{-1} (or 100 erg g^{-1}) of energy. Thus, 1 Gy = 100 rad or 10 000 Gy (10 kGy) = 1 Mrad.

MICROBIAL SENSITIVITY TO IONIZING RADIATIONS

Bacterial spores are generally more resistant than non-sporulating bacteria, although *Deinococcus radiodurans* is the most resistant organism known (Moseley 1989). Among the clostridia, *C. botulinum* types A and B are the most resistant, type E being highly sensitive. Among *Bacillus* spp., *Bacillus pumilus* E601 is probably the most resistant (see Table 7.7). During bacterial sporulation, resistance to γ-radiation develops about 2 h before the onset of heat resistance (Durban, Goodnow and Grecz 1970). Although spore coat disulphide bonds were believed to be radioprotective, it is now clear that the –S–S rich protein structure does not afford resistance, since coatless spores are as resistant as normal spores (Hitchins, King and Gould 1966, Gould and Sale 1970, Farkas 1994).

MECHANISMS OF MICROBIAL INACTIVATION BY IONIZING RADIATIONS

Ionizing radiations induce structural defects in microbial DNA which, unless repaired, are likely to inhibit DNA synthesis, leading to cell death (Hutchinson 1985). DNA is not the only target relevant to inactivation, although it is undoubtedly the principal one (Lindahl 1982), with single-strand breaks (SSB) and double-strand breaks (DSB) depending on the intensity of the radiation dose (Moseley 1989).

The state of DNA in the cell is important in relation to bacterial inactivation. Spores are generally more resistant to ionizing radiation than are non-sporing organisms. There are several possible reasons, notably that:

1 spores contain a radioprotective substance (but there is no evidence to support this supposition)
2 spore coats confer protection, but coatless spores are not less resistant and
3 DNA is in a different state in spores.

DNA in bacterial spores exists in the A form, associated with a low a_w value, and it is certainly true that DNA in the intact spore is more resistant to SSB and DSB than DNA in the intact vegetative cell. However, DNA extracted from spores shows the same response in vitro to ionizing radiation as DNA extracted from non-sporulating bacteria. Furthermore, newly germinated spores exposed to ionizing radiation in an environment of high osmotic pressure again become radiation-resistant (Gould 1983, 1984, 1985). Damage to DNA is less extensive under such circumstances.

α/β-type SASPs have some role to play in conferring heat resistance on spores, presumably by stabilizing DNA (see section 3.1, p. 170); however, neither they nor γ-type SASPs are involved in ionizing radiation resistance (Setlow 1994).

MECHANISMS OF MICROBIAL REPAIR FOLLOWING IONIZING RADIATION

Several micro-organisms show above-average resistance to ionizing radiation (and to UV radiation, see section 3.6, p. 176) because they possess enzymes capable of repairing damage to DNA (Bridges 1976, Moseley 1984, 1989). Repair has been widely studied in *D. radiodurans* and in *E. coli* mutants in which sensitivity to ionizing radiations is conferred by genes such as *rec* (*A, B, C*), *polA* and *lon*.

Single-strand breaks in bacterial spores can be repaired during post-irradiation germination (Terano, Tanooka and Kadota 1966, 1971). In *C. botulinum* 33A, which is highly radiation-resistant, direct repair (rejoining) of SSB takes place during or after radiation in spores existing under non-physiological conditions at 0°C and in the absence of germination (Durban, Grecz and Farkas 1974). Such repair of single-strand breaks within these dormant, ungerminated spores may result from DNA ligase activity (Gould 1984).

USES OF IONIZING RADIATION

Ionizing radiation has found particular use as a means of sterilizing single-use medical devices (Christensen, Kristensen and Miller 1992). Food irradiation has long been considered as a means of sterilizing or preserving food (Christensen, Kristensen and Miller 1992) but has met with considerable consumer resistance.

3.6 Ultraviolet radiation

Ultraviolet (UV) radiation has a wavelength of c.328–210 nm. Its maximum bactericidal effect is documented at 240–280 nm (Sykes 1965). Modern mercury-vapour lamps emit more than 95% of their radiation at 253.7 nm, which is at or near the maximum for microbicidal activity. The quantum of energy liberated is low, and consequently UV radiation has less penetrating ability and is less effective than other types of radiation. It is not, therefore, considered as being an effective method of sterilization (Russell 1992d, 1993).

Microbial sensitivity to UV radiation

Bacterial spores are generally more resistant to UV light than are vegetative cells, although mould spores may be even more resistant. Viruses are also inactivated; they tend to be more sensitive than bacterial spores but are often more resistant than non-sporulating bacteria (Morris and Darlow 1971). HIV is not inactivated by UV radiation (Report 1986).

Mechanisms of microbial inactivation by UV radiation

Exposure of non-sporulating bacteria results in the formation of purine and pyrimidine dimers between adjacent molecules in the same strand of DNA (e.g. the forward reaction in Fig. 7.4a). Another type of photoproduct (5,6-hydroxydihydrothymine) is also found in *D. radiodurans* exposed to ionizing and UV radiation (Fig. 7.4b). In bacterial spores, yet another type of photoproduct, 5-thyminyl-5,6-dihydrothymine (TDHT) (Fig. 7.4c) accumulates in DNA. The photoproducts, unless removed, form non-coding lesions in DNA and bacterial death results.

Mechanisms of microbial repair: non-sporulating bacteria

There are 3 major repair mechanisms:

1 Photoreactivation (light repair), in which the exposure of UV-irradiated cells to light of a higher wavelength but below 510 nm results in the induction of a photoreactivating enzyme that monomerizes thymine dimers in situ (Fig. 7.4a, reverse direction) and results in the recovery of a large proportion of cells that would otherwise have been inactivated (Moseley 1989, Russell 1992d).

2 Dark repair (excision), in which the stages are, first the action of a dimer-specific endonuclease which 'nicks' the DNA, second a dimer-specific exonuclease which excises the damaged portion together with a number of nucleotides on each side, followed by the action of DNA polymerase I, and, finally DNA ligase which is responsible for the final joining together.

3 Dark repair (post-replication recombination), in which replication proceeds normally until it reaches an unexcised dimer, which is a non-coding lesion. A gap is left opposite the dimer and replication recommences at a new initiation site some 800–1000 bases downstream. Because dimers occur in both parental strands of DNA, both daughter strands contain gaps, which are repaired by recombinational insertion of parental DNA from the sister duplex. The process requires a functional *recA* gene product. Recombination-deficient mutants are abnormally sensitive to UV and ionizing radiations.

For additional information on repair, mutants and error-prone repair, see Bridges (1976), Moseley (1984, 1989) and Sancar and Sancar (1988).

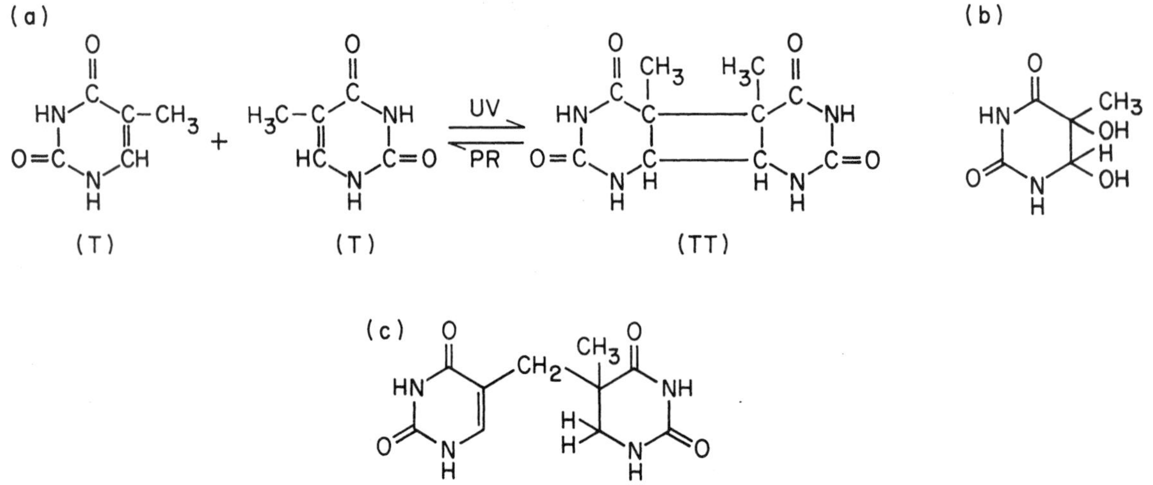

Fig. 7.4 UV-induced changes in DNA: (a) pyrimidine dimer formation and reversal (photoreactivation, PR); (b) 5,6-dihydroxydihydrothymine; (c) 5-thyminyl-5,6-dihydrothymine (TDHT). T, thymine; TT, thymine dimer.

MECHANISMS OF MICROBIAL REPAIR: BACTERIAL SPORES

The spore photoproduct 5-thyminyl-5,6-dihydrothymine (TDHT) is identical to one that accumulates in hydrolysates of DNA exposed dry, or as a frozen solution, to UV radiation (Rahn and Hosszu 1968, Varghese 1970). With the exception of *D. radiodurans*, vegetative cells in the frozen state are supersensitive to UV and a photoproduct (presumably TDHT) other than thymine dimers accumulates which is less susceptible to repair. UV-sensitive mutants of UV-resistant *B. subtilis* spores form the same photoproduct (TDHT) and to the same extent for a given dose of radiation, as do the resistant spores; UV resistance is thus linked to the ability to remove TDHT (Munakata and Rupert 1972). Two genetically controlled mechanisms have been described for this removal (Munakata and Rupert 1972, 1974):

1 'spore repair' involving the elimination of TDHT during germination, although vegetative growth is not required and
2 excision repair, in which TDHT disappears slowly from the large molecular weight trichloracetic acid (TCA-insoluble) fraction and appears in the TCA-soluble fraction.

PRACTICAL USES OF UV RADIATION

UV radiation has little penetrative power through solids and is extensively absorbed by glass and plastics. Sterilization is achieved only by doses of radiation beyond the limits of practicability. It does, however, have some use as a disinfection procedure. It has been used to disinfect drinking water (Sykes 1965); as a possible means of obtaining pyrogen-free water; and especially for air disinfection, notably in hospital wards and operating theatres, in aseptic laboratories and in ventilated safety cabinets in which dangerous micro-organisms are being handled (Morris and Darlow 1971).

Sunlight also has disinfecting properties, rays of wavelengths 254–257 nm possessing the greatest bactericidal activity. It has been claimed that sunlight can inactivate *Bacillus anthracis* spores on wooden and metal surfaces, although only after prolonged exposure. Infectivity of viruses may be reduced on exposure to direct sunlight (Russell, Yarnych and Koulikovskii 1984).

3.7 Sterilization by filtration

Filtration in various forms was used in ancient times, e.g. in attempts to purify water and sewage by allowing it to percolate through beds of sand, gravel or cinders. These and other applications are considered by Denyer (1992) who also describes the development of modern filtration devices.

TYPES OF FILTER

Several types of filters are used, including the following.

Unglazed ceramic filters, e.g. the Chamberland and Doulton filters, are manufactured in several different grades of porosity and have been used industrially for the large-scale clarification of water. After use, they can be cleaned with sodium hypochlorite solutions and will withstand scrubbing.

Compressed diatomaceous earth filters, examples of which are the Berkefeld and Mandler filters, are manufactured in different grades of porosity. They have been used industrially for the large-scale clarification of water. After use, they can be cleaned with sodium hypochlorite but without scrubbing.

Asbestos filters include Seitz, Carlson and Sterimat filters. They have high adsorbing capacities and tend to alkalinate solutions being filtered. There is also a possibility of toxic effects (including carcinogenesis) in handling these filters and they are now practically obsolete.

Sintered glass filters are prepared by size-grading finely powdered glass followed by heating. The pore size can be controlled by the general particle size of the glass powder. The filters are easily cleaned, have low adsorption properties and do not shed particles, but they are fragile and relatively expensive.

Membrane filters consist of cellulose esters and are used routinely in water analysis and purification, sterilization and sterility testing. They are the most suitable for preparing sterile solutions for parenteral use. Membrane filters are available in a range of pore sizes from c. 12 μm down to 0.5 μm, sterilizing filters usually having an average pore diameter (APD) of 0.2–0.22 μm. The ratio of maximum pore diameter (MPD) to APD is in general 3.5–5. Membrane filters have several advantages over conventional depth filters (Denyer 1992).

High efficiency particulate air (HEPA) filters remove particles of 0.3 μm or larger (and probably particles <0.1 μm; Denyer 1992) and are widely used in air filtration especially that type incorporating laminar air flow (LAF; White 1990). LAF units are of 2 types, horizontal and vertical, depending upon the direction of the air flow.

MECHANISMS OF STERILE FILTRATION

Membrane filters are often described as 'screen' filters in contrast to media such as sintered glass, asbestos fibre and ceramic which are believed to retain organisms and particles by a 'depth' process in which particles are trapped or adsorbed within the interstices of the filter matrix. Screen filtration, on the other hand, has been considered to exclude (sieve out) all particles larger than the rated pore size. However, it is now apparent that the filtration characteristics of many membrane filters cannot be accounted for in terms of the sieve retention theory alone, but that other factors are involved including van der Waals' forces and electrostatic interactions.

Additional information is provided by Lukaszewicz and Melzer (1979), Tanny et al. (1979) and Denyer (1992).

APPLICATIONS OF FILTRATION

Filtration can be used for sterilization of thermolabile parenteral and ophthalmic solutions; for sterility testing of pharmaceutical products; for clarification of water supplies; for microbiological evaluation of water purity; for viable counting procedures, including estimation of survivors following exposure to antibiotics or disinfectants; and for determination of viral particle size (see also Table 7.6). For most of these applications, membrane filters are usually employed.

Additionally, filters are used in air sterilization, including LAF cabinets as described above.

3.8 Combined treatments

Enhanced antimicrobial efficacy is often achieved by combining 2 or more processes, chemical or physical. There are various types of combined treatment (Gould and Jones 1989).

THERMOCHEMICAL TREATMENT

The antibacterial activity of a compound usually increases as the temperature rises (see section 2.3, p. 158). This was exemplified by using certain preservatives at high temperatures in the sterilization of certain injectable and ophthalmic products (Russell 1992a), although this process is no longer approved. The gaseous sterilant ethylene oxide is also employed at higher temperatures (c. 60°C) and low temperature steam with formaldehyde (LTSF) is proving a useful sterilization procedure (Alder and Simpson 1992). In the food industry, acid–heat treatment is an important method of sterilization (Gould and Jones 1989).

CHEMICAL TREATMENT AND IRRADIATION

The presence of various chemicals during irradiation may either sensitize bacterial spores to, or protect them from, the consequences of ionizing radiation. Spores are more sensitive under oxic than under anoxic conditions. Ketonic agents of widely differing electron affinities sensitize spores suspended in anoxic buffers to subsequent radiation although the maximum sensitization achieved is only about 40% of that in oxygen alone (Tallentire and Jacobs 1972). Sensitizing agents appear to act by removing electrons from the conversion of •OH to OH⁻ which is harmless to the spore. These findings have not, as yet, been exploited for practical use.

THERMORADIATION

Thermoradiaton is the simultaneous use of heat and ionizing radiation. Careful selection of temperature is, however, important because a 'paradoxical inversion' or 'thermorestoration' occurs at certain temperatures; e.g. with *C. botulinum* 33A spores there is an increase in sensitivity above 80°C (Grecz 1965).

Despite convincing evidence of the synergy between heat and radiation, the process has yet to be widely employed for sterilization.

OTHER COMBINATIONS

Other combined processes that have been examined include hydrostatic pressure combined with heat or radiation (Wills 1974), ultrasonic waves with glutaraldehyde (Boucher 1979) and combinations of chemicals (Russell 1982).

3.9 Process validation, monitoring and parametric release

It is important that strict control measures are employed to validate and monitor the efficacy of sterilization processes. In addition, sterility tests on samples of a batch of treated product are necessary (*British Pharmacopoeia* 1993), although undue reliance should not be placed on such tests alone.

Process validation is a means of demonstrating that a process actually works, i.e. that it kills (or removes) micro-organisms, thereby achieving what it purports to do (achieve sterilization). For this reason the choice of a test organism is important: it must possess above-average resistance to the process in question although it need not necessarily be the most resistant organism known. Bacterial spores are usually chosen as what are termed biological indicators (BIs) to validate those processes designed to inactivate microbes. Although *D. radiodurans* is even more resistant to ionizing radiation than spores (see section 3.5, p. 174) it is not used as a BI for this process because it is not a normal contaminant (bioburden) on pharmaceutical or medical products and its inactivation would require unacceptably high radiation doses that could damage many such products. Examples of BIs are provided in Table 7.9.

Table 7.9 Validation and monitoring of sterilization processes

Process	Validation*	Monitoring†‡
Moist heat	*B. stearothermophilus*	Temperature recording charts; thermocouples; CI
Dry heat	*B. subtilis* var. *niger*	Temperature recording charts; thermocouples; CI
Ionizing radiation	*B. pumilus*	Dosimeters; CI
Ethylene oxide	*B. subtilis* var. *niger*	Temperature probes; relative humidity; *B. subtilis* var. *niger*
Filtration	*S. marcescens*; *P. diminuta*	Bubble point pressure test

*In addition to BIs listed, the desired physical and chemical conditions to achieve sterilization must also be validated, e.g. measuring devices for heat, dosimeters for radiation, physical methods for determining filter integrity and temperature and relative humidity for gaseous sterilization.
†CI, chemical indicator (used as a visual check that a sterilization process has been undertaken: a colour change does not necessarily mean that sterilization has been achieved).
‡Samples taken at random from a batch may also be subjected to sterility testing.

The principle involved in validating sterile filtration is to use a smaller-than-average organism. If this is retained by the filter then larger organisms also will not pass through the filter.

In addition to validating a process with BIs, it is also necessary to measure and record the required physical or chemical conditions reached throughout the sterilization cycle within every part of the load (Haberer and Wallhaeusser 1990).

Routine monitoring of a process is carried out by appropriate physical methods, except for ethylene oxide where difficulties still persist (Table 7.9). Sterility can then be assessed, except with ethylene oxide, by monitoring only the physical conditions of the process. Such a system (parametric release) is defined as the release of sterile products based on process compliance to physical specification (Dewhurst and Hoxey 1990).

Sterility assurance level (SAL) is a term employed to provide an expected level of safety with a sterilization process. It is generally accepted that terminally sterilized products, i.e. those sterilized in their final containers, have a safety level (SAL) of not more than one unsterile article per 10^6 items processed (Haberer and Wallhaeusser 1990, Bruch 1993, Graham and Boris 1993). SAL is thus based upon a sound knowledge of microbial inactivation kinetics rather than upon sterility testing which can only detect gross contamination.

REFERENCES

Adler-Storthz K, Schultster LM et al., 1983, Effect of alkaline glutaraldehyde on hepatitis B virus antigens, *Eur J Clin Microbiol,* **2:** 316–20.

AFNOR, 1989, *Association Française de Normalisation – Official French Standards,* T72-301, AFNOR, Paris.

Albert A, 1979, *Selective Toxicity: The Physiochemical Basis of Therapy,* 6th edn, Chapman and Hall, London.

Alder VG, Simpson RA, 1992, Heat sterilization. A. Sterilization and disinfection by heat methods, *Principles and Practice of Disinfection, Preservation and Sterilization,* 2nd edn, eds Russell AD, Hugo WB, Ayliffe GAJ, Blackwell Science, Oxford, 483–98.

Alderton G, Chen JK, Ito KA, 1980, Heat resistance of the chemical resistance forms of *Clostridium botulinum* 62A spores over the water activity range 0 to 0.9, *Appl Environ Microbiol,* **40:** 511–15.

Alderton G, Snell NS, 1963, Base exchange and heat resistance in bacterial spores, *Biochem Biophys Res Commun,* **10:** 139–43.

Allwood MC, 1973, Inhibition of *Staphylococcus aureus* by combinations of non-ionic surface-active agents and antibacterial substances, *Microbios,* **7:** 209–14.

AOAC, 1984, *Disinfectants – Official Methods of Analysis of the Association of Agricultural Chemists,* 14th edn, AOAC, Arlington, VA.

Asada S, Takano M, Shibasaki I, 1979, Deoxyribonucleic acid strand breaks during drying of *Escherichia coli* on a hydrophobic filter membrane, *Appl Environ Microbiol,* **37:** 266–73.

Ayliffe GAJ, Coates D, Hoffman PN, 1993, *Chemical Disinfection in Hospitals,* 2nd edn, Public Health Laboratory Service, London.

Ayres H, Furr JR, Russell AD, 1993, A rapid method of evaluating permeabilizing activity against *Pseudomonas aeruginosa, Lett Appl Microbiol,* **17:** 149–51.

Babb JR, Bradley CR, Ayliffe GAJ, 1980, Sporicidal activity of glutaraldehydes and hypochlorites and other factors influencing their selection for the treatment of medical equipment, *J Hosp Infect,* **1:** 63–75.

Baillie LWJ, Wade JJ, Casewell MW, 1992, Chlorhexidine sensitivity of *Enterococcus faecium* resistant to vancomycin, high levels of gentamicin, or both, *J Hosp Infect,* **20:** 127–8.

Bailly J-L, Chambon M et al., 1991, Activity of glutaraldehyde at low concentrations (<2%) against poliovirus and its relevance to gastrointestinal endoscope disinfection procedures, *Appl Environ Microbiol,* **57:** 1156–60.

Baird-Parker AC, Holbrook R, 1971, The inhibition and destruction of cocci, *Inhibition and Destruction of the Microbial Cell,* ed. Hugo WB, Academic Press, London, 369–98.

Baldry MGC, 1983, The bactericidal, fungicidal and sporicidal properties of hydrogen peroxide and peracetic acid, *J Appl Bacteriol,* **54:** 417–23.

Beaman TC, Gerhardt P, 1986, Heat resistance of bacterial spores correlated with protoplast dehydration, mineralization and thermal adaptation, *Appl Environ Microbiol,* **52:** 1242–6.

Beaman TC, Pankratz HS, Gerhardt P, 1989, Heat shock affects permeability and resistance of *Bacillus stearothermophilus* spores, *Appl Environ Microbiol,* **54:** 2515–20.

Beaman TC, Pankratz HS, Gerhardt P, 1989, Low heat resistance of *Bacillus sphaericus* spores correlated with high protoplast water content, *FEMS Microbiol Lett,* **58:** 1–4.

Bean HS, 1967, Types and characteristics of disinfectants, *J Appl Bacteriol,* **30:** 6–16.

Bean HS, 1972, Preservatives for pharmaceuticals, *J Soc Cosmet Chem,* **23:** 703–20.

Belliveau BH, Beaman TC et al., 1992, Heat killing of bacterial spores analyzed by differential scanning calorimetry, *J Bacteriol,* **174:** 4463–74.

Belly RT, Kydd GC, 1982, Silver resistance in microorganisms, *Dev Ind Microbiol,* **34:** 751–6.

Berkelman RL, Holland BW, Anderson RL, 1982, Increased bactericidal activity of dilute preparations of povidone-iodine solutions, *J Clin Microbiol,* **15:** 635–9.

Block SS (ed.), 1991, *Disinfection, Sterilization and Preservation,* 4th edn, Lea and Febiger, Philadelphia.

Bloomfield SF, 1974, The effect of the phenolic antibacterial agent fentichlor on energy coupling in *Staphylococcus aureus, J Appl Bacteriol,* **37:** 117–34.

Bloomfield SF, 1992, Bacterial sensitivity and resistance. C. Resistance of bacterial spores to chemical agents, *Principles and Practice of Disinfection, Preservation and Sterilization,* 2nd edn, eds Russell AD, Hugo WB, Ayliffe GAJ, Blackwell Science, Oxford, 230–45.

Bloomfield SF, Arthur M, 1994, Mechanisms of inactivation and resistance of spores to chemical biocides, *J Appl Bacteriol Symp Suppl,* **76:** 91S–104S.

Bloomfield SF, Smith-Burchnell CA, Dalgleish AG, 1990, Evaluation of hypochlorite-releasing agents against the human immunodeficiency virus (HIV), *J Hosp Infect,* **15:** 273–8.

Bobichon H, Bouchet P, 1987, Action of chlorhexidine on budding *Candida albicans*: scanning and transmission electron microscopic study, *Mycopathologia,* **100:** 27–35.

Boucher RMG, 1979, Ultrasonics. A tool to improve biocidal efficacy of sterilants or disinfectants in hospital and dental practice, *Can J Pharm Sci,* **14:** 1–12.

Bowie JH, 1955, Modern apparatus for sterilisation, *Pharm J,* **174:** 473–7.

Bradley CR, Babb JR, Ayliffe GAJ, 1995, Evaluation of the Steris System 1 peracetic acid endoscope processor, *J Hosp Infect,* **29:** 143–51.

Bridges BA, 1976, Survival of bacteria following exposure to ultraviolet and ionizing radiations, *The Survival of Vegetative Microbes. 26th Symposium of the Society for General Microbiology,* eds Gray TGR, Postgate JR, Cambridge University Press, Cambridge, 183–208.

British Pharmacopoeia, 1988, HMSO, London.

British Pharmacopoeia, 1993, HMSO, London.

British Standards Institute, 1976 , BS5283, *Glossary of Terms Relating to Disinfectants*, BSI, London.

British Standards Institute, 1985, BS541, *Method for Determination of the Rideal–Walker Coefficient of Disinfectants*, BSI, London.

British Standards Institute, 1986a, BS2462, *Specification for Black and White Disinfectant Fluids*, BSI, London.

British Standards Institute, 1986b, BS808, *Method for Assessing the Efficacy of Disinfectants by the Modified Chick–Martin Test*, BSI, London.

Brown KL, 1994, Spore resistance and ultra heat treatment processes, *J Appl Bacteriol Symp Suppl*, **76**: 67S–80S.

Brown MRW, 1975, The role of the cell envelope in resistance, *Resistance of* Pseudomonas aeruginosa, ed. Brown MRW, John Wiley, London, 71–99.

Brown MRW, Gilbert P, 1993, Sensitivity of biofilms to antimicrobial agents, *J Appl Bacteriol Symp Suppl*, **74**: 87S–97S.

Browne MK, Leslie GB, Pfirrman RW, 1976, Taurolin, a new chemotherapeutic agent, *J Appl Bacteriol*, **41**: 363–8.

Browne MK, Stoller JL, 1970, Intraperitoneal noxythiolin in faecal peritonitis, *Br J Surg*, **57**: 525–9.

Broxton P, Woodcock PM, Gilbert P, 1984, Interaction of some polyhexamethylene biguanides and membrane phospholipids in *Escherichia coli*, *J Appl Bacteriol*, **57**: 115–24.

Bruch CW, 1993, The philosophy of sterilization validation, *Sterilization Technology. A Practical Guide for Manufacturers and Users of Health Care Products*, eds Morrissey RF, Phillips GB, Van Nostrand Reinhold, New York, 17–35.

van Bueren J, Larkin DP, Simpson RA, 1994, Inactivation of human immunodeficiency virus type 1 by alcohols, *J Hosp Infect*, **28**: 137–48.

Carpentier B, Cerf O, 1993, Biofilms and their consequences, with particular reference to hygiene in the food industry, *J Appl Bacteriol*, **75**: 499–511.

Cerf O, 1977, Tailing of survival curves of bacterial spores, *J Appl Bacteriol*, **42**: 1–19.

Chambon M, Bailly J-L, Peigue-Lafeuille H, 1992, Activity of glutaraldehyde at low concentrations against capsid proteins of poliovirus type 1 and echovirus type 25, *Appl Environ Microbiol*, **58**: 3517–21.

Chawner JA, Gilbert P, 1989a, A comparative study of the bactericidal and growth inhibitory activities of the bisbiguanides alexidine and chlorhexidine, *J Appl Bacteriol*, **66**: 243–52.

Chawner JA, Gilbert P, 1989b, Interaction of the bisbiguanides chlorhexidine and alexidine with phospholipid vesicles: evidence for separate modes of action, *J Appl Bacteriol*, **66**: 253–8.

Chopra I, 1987, Microbial resistance to veterinary disinfectants and antiseptics, *Disinfection in Veterinary and Farm Animal Practice*, eds Linton AH, Hugo WB, Russell AD, Blackwell Science, Oxford, 43–65.

Christensen EA, Kristensen H, Miller A, 1992, Radiation sterilization. A. Ionizing radiation, *Principles and Practice of Disinfection, Preservation and Sterilization*, 2nd edn, eds Russell AD, Hugo WB, Ayliffe GAJ, Blackwell Science, Oxford, 528–43.

Cleland MR, O'Neill MT, Thompson CC, 1993, Sterilization with accelerated electrons, *Sterilization Technology. A Practical Guide for Manufacturers and Users of Health Care Products*, eds Morrissey RF, Phillips GB, Van Nostrand Reinhold, New York, 218–53.

Coates D, Death DE, 1978, Sporicidal activity of mixtures of alcohol and hypochlorite, *J Clin Pathol*, **31**: 148–52.

Coates D, Hutchinson DN, 1994, How to produce a hospital disinfection policy, *J Hosp Infect*, **26**: 57–68.

Collier PJ, Ramsey AJ et al., 1990, Growth inhibitory and biocidal activity of some isothiazolone biocides, *J Appl Bacteriol*, **69**: 569–77.

Cookson BD, Bolton MC, Platt JH, 1991, Chlorhexidine resistance in *Staphyloccus aureus* or just an elevated MIC? An *in vitro* and *in vivo* assessment, *Antimicrob Agents Chemother*, **35**: 1997–2002.

Cookson BD, Phillips I, 1990, Methicillin-resistant staphylococci, *J Appl Bacteriol Symp Suppl*, **69**: 55S–70S.

Costerton JW, Chang K-J et al., 1987, Bacterial biofilms in nature and disease, *Annu Rev Microbiol*, **41**: 435–64.

Costerton JW, Lewandowsik Z et al., 1994, Biofilms, the customized niche, *J Bacteriol*, **176**: 2137–42.

Cremieux A, Fleurette J, 1991, Methods of testing disinfectants, *Disinfection, Sterilization and Preservation*, 4th edn, ed. Block SS, Lea and Febiger, Philadelphia, 1009–27.

Croshaw B, 1971, The destruction of mycobacteria, *Inhibition and Destruction of the Microbial Cell*, ed. Hugo WB, Academic Press, London, 420–49.

Croshaw B, Holland VR, 1984, Chemical preservatives: use of bronopol as a cosmetic preservative, *Cosmetic and Drug Preservation. Principles and Practice*, ed. Kabara JJ, Marcel Dekker, New York, 31–62.

D'Arcy PF, 1971, Inhibition and destruction of moulds and yeasts, *Inhibition and Destruction of the Microbial Cell*, ed. Hugo WB, Academic Press, London, 614–86.

Davies JG, Babb JR et al., 1993, Preliminary study of test methods to assess the virucidal activity of skin disinfectants using poliovirus and bacteriophages, *J Hosp Infect*, **25**: 125–31.

Death JE, Coates D, 1979, Effect of pH on sporicidal and microbicidal activity of buffered mixtures of alcohol and sodium hypochlorite, *J Clin Pathol*, **32**: 148–52.

Dekker J, 1987, Development of resistance to modern fungicides and strategies for its avoidance, *Modern Selective Fungicides*, ed. Lyr H, Longman, Harlow, 39–52.

Denyer SP, 1992, Filtration sterilization, *Principles and Practice of Disinfection, Preservation and Sterilization*, 2nd edn, eds Russell AD, Hugo WB, Ayliffe GAJ, Blackwell Science, Oxford, 573–604.

Denyer SP, Gorman SP, Sussman M, 1993, *Microbial Biofilms: Formation and Control*, Society for Applied Bacteriology Technical Series No. 30, Blackwell, Oxford.

Dewhurst E, Hoxey EV, 1990, Sterilization methods, *Guide to Microbiological Control in Pharmaceuticals*, eds Denyer S, Baird R, Ellis Horwood, Chichester, 182–218.

DGHM, 1981, *Richtlinien für die Prüfung und Bewertung Chemische Desinfectionverfarhen*, Fisher Verlag, Stuttgart.

Dring GJ, 1976, Some aspects of the effects of hydrostatic pressure on micro-organisms, *Inhibition and Inactivation of Vegetative Microbes*, eds Skinner FA, Hugo WB, Society for Applied Bacteriology Symposium Series No. 5, Academic Press, London, 257–78.

Durban E, Grecz N, Farkas J, 1974, Direct enzymatic repair of DNA single strand breaks in dormant spores, *J Bacteriol*, **118**: 129–38.

Durban E, Goodnow R, Grecz N, 1970, Changes in resistance to radiation and heat during sporulation and germination of *Clostridium botulinum* 33A, *J Bacteriol*, **102**: 590–2.

Dychdala GR, 1991, Chlorine and chlorine compounds, *Disinfection, Sterilization and Preservation*, 4th edn, ed. Block SS, Lea and Febiger, Philadelphia, 131–51.

Eklund T, 1983, The antimicrobial effect of dissociated and undissociated sorbic acid at different pH levels, *J Appl Bacteriol*, **54**: 383–9.

Eklund T, 1985a, The effect of sorbic acid and esters of *p*-hydroxybenzoic acid on the protonmotive force in *Escherichia coli* membrane vesicles, *J Gen Microbiol*, **131**: 73–6.

Eklund T, 1985b, Inhibition of microbial growth at different pH levels by benzoic and propionic acids and esters of *p*-hydroxybenzoic acid, *Int J Food Microbiol*, **2**: 159–67.

Elferink JGR, Booij HL, 1974, Interaction of chlorhexidine with yeast cells, *Biochem Pharmacol*, **23**: 1413–19.

Elsmore R, 1992, Bacterial sensitivity and resistance. E. *Legionella*, *Principles and Practice of Disinfection, Preservation and Sterilization*, 2nd edn, eds Russell AD, Hugo WB, Ayliffe GAJ, Blackwell Science, Oxford, 254–63.

Ernst RR, 1974, Ethylene oxide sterilization kinetics, *Biotechnol Bioeng Symp*, **No. 44, Suppl.**: 865–78.

Farkas J, 1994, Tolerance of spores to ionizing radiation: mechanisms of inactivation, injury and repair, *J Appl Bacteriol Symp Suppl*, **76:** 81S–90S.

Favero MS, Bond WW, 1993, The use of liquid chemical germicides, *Sterilization Technology. A Practical Guide for Manufacturers and Users of Health Care Products*, eds Morrissey RF, Phillips GB, Van Nostrand Reinhold, New York, 309–34.

Foster TJ, 1983, Plasmid-determined resistance to antimicrobial drugs and toxic metal ions in bacteria, *Microbiol Rev*, **47:** 361–409.

Fried VA, Novick A, 1973, Organic solvents as probes for the structure and function of the bacterial membrane; effects of ethanol on the wild type and on an ethanol-resistant mutant of *Escherichia coli* K-12, *J Bacteriol*, **114:** 239–48.

Gadd GM, White C, 1989, Heavy metal and radionuclide accumulation and toxicity in fungi and yeasts, *Metal–Microbe Interactions*, eds Poole RK, Gadd GM, Special Publications of the Society for General Microbiology No. 26, Oxford University Press, Oxford, 19–38.

Gale EF, 1986, Nature and development of phenotypic resistance to amphotericin B in *Candida albicans*, *Adv Microb Physiol*, **27:** 277–320.

Gardner JF, Peel MM, 1991, *Introduction to Sterilization and Disinfection*, Churchill Livingstone, Edinburgh.

Gerhardt P, Marquis RE, 1989, Spore thermoresistance mechanisms, *Regulation of Procaryotic Development*, eds Smith I, Slepecky R, Setlow P, American Society for Microbiology, Washington, DC, 17–63.

Gorman SP, Scott EM, 1977, Uptake and media reactivity of glutaraldehyde solutions related to structure and biocidal activity, *Microbios Lett*, **5:** 163–9.

Gorman SP, Scott EM, Russell AD, 1980, Antimicrobial activity, uses and mechanism of action of glutaraldehyde, *J Appl Bacteriol*, **48:** 161–90.

Gottardi W, 1985, The influence of the chemical behaviour of iodine on the germicidal action of disinfectant solutions containing iodine, *J Hosp Infect*, **6, Suppl. A:** 1–11.

Gould GW, 1970, Potentiation by halogen compounds of the lethal action of γ-radiation on spores of *Bacillus cereus*, *J Gen Microbiol*, **64:** 289–300.

Gould GW, 1983, Mechanisms of resistance and dormancy, *The Bacterial Spore*, vol. 2, eds Hurst A, Gould GW, Academic Press, London, 173–209.

Gould GW, 1984, Injury and repair mechanisms in bacterial spores, *The Revival of Injured Microbes*, eds Andrew MHE, Russell AD, Society for Applied Bacteriology Symposium Series No. 12, Academic Press, London, 199–220.

Gould GW, 1985, Modifications of resistance and dormancy, *Fundamental and Applied Aspects of Bacterial Spores*, eds Dring GJ, Ellar DJ, Gould GW, Academic Press, London, 371–82.

Gould GW, 1988, Interference with homeostasis: food, *Homeostatic Mechanisms in Microorganisms*, eds Whittenbury R, Gould GW et al., Bath University Press, Bath, 200–28.

Gould GW (ed.), 1989, Heat-induced injury and inactivation, *Mechanisms of Action of Food Preservation Procedures*, Elsevier Applied Science, London, 11–42.

Gould GW, 1992, Heat sterilization. D. Applications of thermal processing in the food industry, *Principles and Practice of Disinfection, Preservation and Sterilization*, 2nd edn, eds Russell AD, Hugo WB, Ayliffe GAJ, Blackwell Science, Oxford, 519–29.

Gould GW, 1994, *New Methods of Food Preservation*, Chapman and Hall, London.

Gould GW, Jones MV, 1989, Combination and synergisitic effects, *Mechanisms of Action of Food Preservation Procedures*, ed. Gould GW, Elsevier Applied Science, London, 401–22.

Gould GW, Jones A, Wrighton C, 1968, Limitations of the initiation of germination of bacterial spores as a spore control procedure, *J Appl Bacteriol*, **31:** 357–66.

Gould GW, Russell NJ, 1991, Sulphite, *Food Preservatives*, eds Russell NJ, Gould GW, Blackie, Glasgow and London, 72–88.

Gould GW, Sale AJH, 1970, Initiation of germination of bacterial spores by hydrostatic pressure, *J Gen Microbiol*, **60:** 335–46.

Graham GS, Boris CA, 1993, Chemical and biological indicators, *Sterilization Technology. A Practical Guide for Manufacturers and Users of Health Care Products*, eds Morrissey RF, Phillips GB, Van Nostrand Reinhold, New York, 36–69.

Grecz N, 1965, Biophysical aspects of clostridia, *J Appl Bacteriol*, **28:** 7–35.

Grossgebauer K, 1970, Virus disinfection, *Disinfection*, ed. Benarde MA, Marcel Dekker, New York, 103–48.

Grossman L, Levine SS, Allison WS, 1961, The reaction of formaldehyde with nulceotides and T2 bacteriophage DNA, *J Mol Biol*, **3:** 47–60.

Habarer J, Wallhaeusser K-H, 1990, Assurance of sterility by validation of the sterilization process, *Guide to Microbiological Control in Pharmaceuticals*, eds Denyer S, Baird R, Ellis Horwood, Chichester, 219–40.

Hammond SM, Lambert PA, Rycroft AN, 1984, *The Bacterial Cell Surface*, Croom, Helm, London.

Hancock REW, 1984, Alterations in membrane permeability, *Annu Rev Microbiol*, **38:** 237–64.

Hanlin JH, Lombardi SJ, Slepecky RA, 1985, Heat and UV light resistance of vegetative cells and spores of *Bacillus subtilis* Rec⁻ mutants, *J Bacteriol*, **163:** 774–7.

Hanson PJV, 1988, Mycobacteria and AIDS, *Br J Hosp Med*, **40:** 149.

Hanson PJV, Bennett J et al., 1994, Enteroviruses, endoscopy and infection control: an applied study, *J Hosp Infect*, **27:** 61–7.

Hector RF, 1993, Compounds active against cell walls of medically important fungi, *Clin Microbiol Rev*, **6:** 1–21.

Herbert RA, 1989, Microbial growth at low temperature, *Mechanisms of Action of Food Preservation Procedures*, ed. Gould GW, Elsevier Applied Science, London, 71–96.

Herring CM, Saylor MC, 1993, Sterilization with radioisotopes, *Sterilization Technology. A Practical Guide for Manufacturers and Users of Health Care Products*, eds Morrissey RF, Phillips GB, Van Nostrand Reinhold, New York, 196–217.

Hilditch EA, 1992, Preservation in specialized areas. G. Wood preservation, *Principles and Practice of Disinfection, Preservation and Sterilization*, 2nd edn, eds Russell AD, Hugo WB, Ayliffe GAJ, Blackwell Science, Oxford, 459–73.

Hinton M , Linton AH, Perry FG, 1985, Control of salmonella by acid disinfection of chick's food, *Vet Rec*, **116:** 502.

Hiom SJ, Furr JR et al., 1993, Effects of chlorhexidine diacetate and cetylpyridinium chloride on whole cells and protoplasts of *Saccharomyces cerevisiae*, *Microbios*, **74:** 111–20.

Hitchener BJ, Egan AF, 1977, Outer membrane damage to sublethally heated *Escherichia coli* K-12, *Can J Microbiol*, **23:** 311–18.

Hitchins AD, King WL, Gould GW, 1966, Role of disulphide bonds in the resistance of *Bacillus cereus* spores to gamma irradiation and heat, *J Appl Bacteriol*, **29:** 505–11.

Huber WB, 1982, Antiseptics and disinfectants, *Veterinary Pharmacology and Therapeutics*, eds Booth NH, McDonald LE, Iowa State University Press, Ames, Iowa, 693–716.

Hugo WB, 1971, Amidines, *Inhibition and Destruction of the Microbial Cell*, ed. Hugo WB, Academic Press, London, 121–36.

Hugo WB, 1991, A brief history of heat and chemical preservation and disinfection, *J Appl Bacteriol*, **71:** 9–18.

Hugo WB, 1992, Disinfection mechanisms, *Principles and Practice of Disinfection, Preservation and Sterilization*, 2nd edn, eds Russell AD, Hugo WB, Ayliffe GAJ, Blackwell Science, Oxford, 187–210.

Hugo WB, Denyer SP, 1987, The concentration exponent of disinfectants and preservatives (biocides), *Preservation in the Food, Pharmaceutical and Environmental Industries*, eds Board RG, Allwood MC, Banks JG, Society for Applied Bacteriology Technical Series No. 22, Blackwell Science, Oxford, 281–91.

Hugo WB, Russell AD, 1992, Types of antimicrobial agents, *Principles and Practice of Disinfection, Preservation and Sterilization*,

2nd edn, eds Russell AD, Hugo WB, Ayliffe GAJ, Blackwell Science, Oxford, 7–88.

Hutchinson F, 1985, Chemical changes induced in DNA by ionizing radiation, *Prog Nucleic Acid Res Mol Biol*, **32:** 115–54.

Ismaeel N, El-Moug T et al., 1986, Resistance of *Providencia stuartii* to chlorhexidine: a consideration of the role of the inner membrane, *J Appl Bacteriol*, **60:** 361–7.

Jarroll EL, 1988, Effect of disinfectants on *Giardia* cysts, *CRC Rev Environ Control*, **18:** 1–28.

Jarroll EL, 1992, Sensitivity of protozoa to disinfectants, *Principles and Practice of Disinfection, Preservation and Sterilization*, 2nd edn, eds Russell AD, Hugo WB, Ayliffe GAJ, Blackwell Science, Oxford, 180–6.

Kaye S, Phillips CR, 1949, The sterilizing action of gaseous ethylene oxide. IV. The effect of moisture, *Am J Hyg*, **50:** 296–306.

Kelsey JC, Maurer IM, 1974, An improved (1974) Kelsey–Sykes test for disinfectants, *Pharm J*, **207:** 528–30.

Klein M, Deforest A, 1983, Principles of viral inactivation, *Disinfection, Sterilization and Preservation*, 3rd edn, ed. Block SS, 422–34.

van Klingeren B, Pullen W, 1993, Glutaraldehyde-resistant mycobacteria from endoscope washers, *J Hosp Infect*, **25:** 147–9.

Knott AG, Russell AD, Dancer BN, 1995, Development of resistance to biocides during sporulation of *Bacillus subtilis*, *J Appl Bacteriol*, **79:** 492–8.

Korich DG, Mead JR et al., 1990, Effects of ozone, chlorine dioxide, chlorine and monochloramine on *Cryptosporidium parvum* oocyst viability, *Appl Environ Microbiol*, **56:** 1423–8.

Kowalski JB, 1993, Selecting a sterilization method, *Sterilization Technology. A Practical Guide for Manufacturers and Users of Health Care Products*, eds Morrissey RF, Phillips GB, Van Nostrand Reinhold, New York, 70–8.

Krönig B, Paul T, 1897, Die chemischen Grundlagen der Lehre von der Giftwirkung und Desinfektion, *Z Hyg Infektionskr*, **25:** 1–112.

Kurtz JB, Bartlett CLR et al., 1982, *Legionella pneumophila* in cooling water systems, *J Hyg Camb*, **88:** 369–81.

Lambert PA, Hammond SM, 1973, Potassium fluxes. First indications of membrane damage in microorganisms, *Biochem Biophys Res Commun*, **54:** 796–9.

Lannigan R, Bryan LE, 1985, Decreased susceptibility of *Serratia marcescens* to chlorhexidine related to the inner membrane, *J Antimicrob Chemother*, **15:** 559–65.

Leelaporn A, Paulsen IT et al., 1994, Multidrug resistance to antiseptics and disinfectants in coagulase-negative staphylococci, *J Med Microbiol*, **40:** 214–20.

Lerman LS, 1961, Structural considerations in the interaction of DNA and acridines, *J Mol Biol*, **3:** 18–30.

Lindahl T, 1982, DNA repair enzymes, *Annu Rev Biochem*, **51:** 61–87.

Linton AH, 1983, *Guidelines on Prevention and Control of Salmonellosis*, World Health Organization, Geneva. VPH/83.42.

Linton AH, Hugo WB, Russell AD, 1987, *Disinfection in Veterinary and Farm Animal Practice*, Blackwell Scientific, Oxford.

Lloyd-Evans N, Springthorpe VS, Sattar SA, 1986, Chemical disinfection of human rotavirus-contaminated inanimate surfaces, *J Hyg Camb*, **97:** 163–73.

Lowbury EJL, 1992, Special problems in hospital antisepsis, *Principles and Practice of Disinfection, Preservation and Sterilization*, 2nd edn, eds Russell AD, Hugo WB, Ayliffe GAJ, Blackwell Science, Oxford, 310–29.

Lukaszewicz RC, Melzer TH, 1979, Concerning filter validation, *J Parent Drug Ass*, **33:** 187–94.

Lyon BR, Skurray RA, 1987, Antimicrobial resistance of *Staphylococcus aureus*: genetic basis, *Microbiol Rev*, **51:** 88–134.

Lyr H, 1987, Selectivity in modern fungicides and its basis, *Modern Selective Fungicides*, ed. Lyr H, Longman, Harlow, 31–58.

McCarthy BJ, 1992, Textile and leather preservation, *Principles and Practice of Disinfection, Preservation and Sterilization*, 2nd edn, eds Russell AD, Hugo WB, Ayliffe GAJ, Blackwell Science, Oxford, 418–30.

Mackey BM, 1983, Changes in antibiotic and cell surface hydrophobicity in *Escherichia coli* injured by heating, freezing, drying or gamma radiation, *FEMS Microbiol Lett*, **20:** 395–9.

Mackey BM, 1984, Lethal and sublethal effects of refrigeration, freezing and freeze-drying on micro-organisms, *The Revival of Injured Microbes*, eds Andrew MHE, Russell AD, Society for Applied Bacteriology Symposium Series No. 12, Academic Press, London, 45–76.

Mackey BM, Seymour DA, 1987, The effect of catalase on recovery of heat-injured DNA-repair mutants of *Escherichia coli*, *J Gen Microbiol*, **133:** 1601–10.

MacLeod RA, Calcott PH, 1976, Cold shock and freezing damage to microbes. *The Survival of Vegetative Microbes*, eds Gray TRG, Postgate JR, 26th Symposium of the Society for General Microbiology, Cambridge University Press, Cambridge, 81–109.

Maillard J-Y, Beggs TS et al., 1995, Electronmicroscopic investigation of the effects of biocides on *Pseudomonas aeruginosa* PAO bacteriophage F116, *J Med Microbiol*, **42:** 415–20.

Malek JR, Speier JL, 1982, Development of an organosilicone antimicrobial agent for the treatment of surfaces, *J Coated Fabrics*, **12:** 38–45.

Marquis RE, Sim J, Shin SY, 1994, Molecular mechanisms of resistance to heat and oxidative damage, *J Appl Bacteriol Symp Suppl*, **76:** 40S–48S.

Maurer IM, 1985, *Hospital Hygiene*, 3rd edn, Edward Arnold, London.

Michael GI, Stumbo CR, 1970, Ethylene oxide sterilization of *Salmonella senftenberg* and *Escherichia coli*; death kinetics and mode of action, *J Food Sci*, **35:** 631–4.

Midgley M, 1986, The phosphonium ion efflux system of *Escherichia coli*: relationship to the ethidium efflux system and energetic studies, *J Gen Microbiol*, **132:** 1387–93.

Midgley M, 1987, An efflux system for cationic dyes and related compounds in *Escherichia coli*, *Microbiol Sci*, **14:** 125–7.

Mitchell P, 1961, Coupling of phosphorylation to electron and hydrogen transfer by a chemiosmotic type of mechanism, *Nature (London)*, **191:** 144–8.

Moats WA, Maddox SE Jr, 1978, Effect of pH on the antimicrobial activity of some triphenylmethane dyes, *Can J Microbiol*, **24:** 658–61.

Molin G, 1992, Heat sterilization. B. Destruction of bacterial spores by thermal methods, *Principles and Practice of Disinfection, Preservation and Sterilization*, 2nd edn, eds Russell AD, Hugo WB, Ayliffe GAJ, Blackwell Science, Oxford, 499–511.

Morris EJ, Darlow HM, 1971, Inactivation of viruses, *Inhibition and Destruction of the Microbial Cell*, ed. Hugo WB, Academic Press, London, 687–702.

Morton HE, 1983, Alcohols, *Disinfection, Sterilization and Preservation*, 3rd edn, ed. Block SS, Lea and Febiger, Philadelphia, 225–39.

Moseley BEB, 1984, *Radiation damage and its repair in non-sporulating bacteria*, The Revival of Injured Microbes, eds Andrew MHE, Russell AD, Society for Applied Bacteriology Symposium Series No. 12, Elsevier Applied Science, London, 43–70.

Moseley BEB, 1989, Ionizing radiation: action and repair, *Mechanisms of Action of Food Preservation Procedures*, ed. Gould GW, Elsevier Applied Science, London, 43–70.

Munakata N, Rupert CS, 1972, Genetically controlled removal of 'spore photoproduct' from deoxyribonucleic acid of ultraviolet-irradiated *Bacillus subtilis* spores, *J Bacteriol*, **111:** 192–8.

Munakata N, Rupert CS, 1974, Dark repair of DNA containing 'spore photoproduct' in *Bacillus subtilis*, *Mol Gen Genet*, **130:** 239–50.

Murrell WG, 1981, Biophysical studies on the molecular mechanisms of spore heat resistance and dormancy, *Sporulation and Germination*, eds Levinson HS, Sonenshein AL, Tipper DJ, American Society for Microbiology, Washington, DC, 64–77.

Myers JA, Allwood MC et al., 1980, The relationship between structure and activity of taurolin, *J Appl Bacteriol*, **48:** 89–96.

Narang HJ, Codd AA, 1983, Action of commonly used disinfectants against enteroviruses, *J Hosp Infect*, **4:** 209–12.

Navarro JM, Monsen P, 1976, Étude du mécanismes d'interaction du glutaraldéhyde avec les micro-organismes, *Ann Microbiol (Paris)*, **127B:** 295–307.

Nordgren C, 1939, Investigations on the sterilising efficacy of gaseous formaldehyde, *Acta Pathol Microbiol Scand*, **Suppl. XL:** 1–165.

Northrop J, Slepecky RA, 1967, Sporulation mutations induced by heat in *Bacillus subtilis*, *Science*, **155:** 838–9.

Owens JE, 1993, Sterilization of LVPs and SVPs, *Sterilization Technology. A Practical Guide for Manufacturers and Users of Health Care Products*, eds Morrissey RF, Phillips GB, Van Nostrand Reinhold, New York, 254–85.

Owens RG, 1969, Organic sulphur compounds, *Fungicides*, vol. 2, ed. Torgeson DC, Academic Press, New York, 147–301.

Passagot J, Crance JM et al., 1987, Effect of glutaraldehyde on the antigenicity and infectivity of hepatitis A virus, *J Virol Methods*, **16:** 21–8.

Peacocke AR, Skerrett JNH, 1956, The interaction of aminoacridines with nucleic acids, *Trans Faraday Soc*, **52:** 261–79.

Pellon JR, Sinskey AJ, 1984, Heat-induced damage to the bacterial chromosome and its repair, *The Revival of Injured Microbes*, eds Andrew MHE, Russell AD, Society for Applied Bacteriology Symposium Series No. 12, Academic Press, London, 105–26.

Pheil CG, Pflug IJ et al., 1967, Effect of various gas atmospheres on destruction of microorganisms in dry heat, *Appl Microbiol*, **15:** 120–4.

Phillips CR, 1952, Relative resistance of bacterial spores and vegetative bacteria to disinfectants, *Bacteriol Rev*, **16:** 135–8.

Power EGM, Dancer BN, Russell AD, 1988, Emergence of resistance to glutaraldehyde in spores of *Bacillus subtilis* 168, *FEMS Microbiol Lett*, **50:** 223–6.

Poxton IR, 1993, Prokaryote envelope diversity, *J Appl Bacteriol Symp Suppl*, **67:** 91–8.

Price PB, 1950, Re-evaluation of ethyl alcohol as a germicide, *Arch Surg*, **60:** 492–502.

Quinn PJ, 1987, Evaluation of veterinary disinfectants and disinfection processes, *Disinfection in Veterinary and Farm Animal Practice*, eds Linton AH, Hugo WB, Russell AD, Blackwell Science, Oxford, 66–116.

Quinn PJ, 1992, Virucidal activity of disinfectants, *Principles and Practice of Disinfection, Preservation and Sterilization*, 2nd edn, eds Russell AD, Hugo WB, Ayliffe GAJ, Blackwell Science, Oxford, 150–70.

Rahn RO, Hosszu JL, 1968, Photoproduct formation in DNA at low temperatures, *Photochem Photobiol*, **8:** 53–63.

Report, 1986, *LAV/HTLV III – The Causative Agent of AIDS and Related Conditions – Revised Outlines*, Advisory Committee of Dangerous Pathogens, DHSS, London.

Resnick L, Veren K et al., 1986, Stability and inactivation of HTLV-III/LAV under clinical and laboratory environments, *JAMA*, **255:** 1887–91.

Reybrouck G, 1992, Evaluation of the antibacterial and antifungal activity of disinfectants, *Principles and Practice of Disinfection, Preservation and Sterilization*, 2nd edn, eds Russell AD, Hugo WB, Ayliffe GAJ, Blackwell Science, Oxford, 114–33.

Richards C, Furr JR, Russell AD, 1984, Inactivation of microorganisms by lethal gases, *Cosmetic and Drug Preservation. Principles and Practice*, ed. Kabara JJ, Marcel Dekker, New York, 209–22.

Roberts TA, Woods LFJ et al., 1991, Nitrite, *Food Preservatives*, eds Russell NJ, Gould GW, Blackie, Glasgow and London, 89–110.

Rodgers FG, Hufton P et al., 1985, Morphological response of human rotavirus to ultraviolet radiation, heat and disinfectants, *J Med Microbiol*, **20:** 123–30.

Rose AH, 1976, Osmotic stress and microbial survival, *The Survival of Vegetative Microbes*, eds Gray TRG, Postgate JR, 26th Symposium of the Society for General Microbiology, Cambridge University Press, 155–82.

Rowe AJ, Silverman GJ, 1970, The absorption–desorption of water by bacterial spores and its relation to dry heat resistance, *Dev Ind Microbiol*, **11:** 311–26.

Russell AD, 1976, Inactivation of non-sporing bacteria by gases, *Inhibition and Inactivation of Vegetative Microbes*, eds Skinner FA, Hugo WB, Society for Applied Bacteriology Symposium Series No. 5, Academic Press, London, 61–88.

Russell AD, 1982, *The Destruction of Bacterial Spores*, Academic Press, London.

Russell AD, 1990a, The bacterial spore and chemical sporicides, *Clin Microbiol Rev*, **3:** 99–119.

Russell AD, 1990b, The effects of chemical and physical agents on microbes: disinfection and sterilization, *Topley & Wilson's Principles of Bacteriology, Virology and Immunity*, 8th edn, vol. 1, eds Parker MT, Collier LH, Edward Arnold, London, 71–103.

Russell AD, 1992a, Factors influencing the efficacy of antimicrobial agents, *Principles and Practice of Disinfection, Preservation and Sterilization*, 2nd edn, eds Russell AD, Hugo WB, Ayliffe GAJ, Blackwell Scientific, Oxford, 89–113.

Russell AD, 1992b, Bacterial sensitivity and resistance. D. Mycobactericidal agents, *Principles and Practice of Disinfection, Sterilization and Preservation*, 2nd edn, eds Russell AD, Hugo WB, Ayliffe GAJ, Blackwell Scientific, Oxford, 246–53.

Russell AD, 1992c, Antifungal activity of biocides, *Principles and Practice of Disinfection, Sterilization and Preservation*, 2nd edn, eds Russell AD, Hugo WB, Ayliffe GAJ, Blackwell Scientific, Oxford, 139–49.

Russell AD, 1992d, Radiation sterilization. B. Ultraviolet radiation, *Principles and Practice of Disinfection, Sterilization and Preservation*, 2nd edn, eds Russell AD, Hugo WB, Ayliffe GAJ, Blackwell Scientific, Oxford, 544–6.

Russell AD, 1993, Theoretical aspects of microbial inactivation, *Sterilization Technology. A Practical Guide for Manufacturers and Users of Health Care Products*, eds Morrissey RF, Phillips GB, Van Nostrand Reinhold, New York, 3–16.

Russell AD, 1994, Glutaraldehyde: current status and uses, *Infect Control Hosp Epidemiol*, **15:** 724–33.

Russell AD, 1995, Mechanisms of bacterial resistance to biocides, *Int Biodet Biodeg*, **36:** 247–65.

Russell AD, 1996, Activity of biocides against mycobacteria, *J Appl Bacteriol Symp Suppl*, **81:** 87S–101S.

Russell AD, Ahonkhai I, Rogers DT, 1979, Microbiological applications of the inactivation of antibiotics and other antimicrobial agents, *J Appl Bacteriol*, **46:** 207–45.

Russell AD, Chopra I, 1996, *Understanding Antibacterial Action and Resistance*, 2nd edn, Chapman and Hall, London.

Russell AD, Day MJ, 1993, Antibacterial activity of chlorhexidine, *J Hosp Infect*, **25:** 229–38.

Russell AD, Furr JR, 1977, The antibacterial activity of a new chloroxylenol preparation containing ethylenediamine tetraacetic acid, *J Appl Bacteriol*, **43:** 253–60.

Russell AD, Gould GW, 1988, Resistance of Enterobacteriaceae to preservatives and disinfectants, *J Appl Bacteriol Symp Suppl*, **65:** 167S–195S.

Russell AD, Hammond SA, Morgan JR, 1986, Bacterial resistance to antiseptics and disinfectants, *J Hosp Infect*, **7:** 213–25.

Russell AD, Hugo WB, 1987, Chemical disinfectants, *Disinfectants in Veterinary and Farm Animal Practice*, eds Linton AH, Hugo WB, Russell AD, Blackwell Science, Oxford, 12–42.

Russell AD, Hugo WB, 1988, Perturbation of homeostatic mechanisms in bacteria by pharmaceuticals, *Homeostatic Mechanisms in Microorganisms*, eds Whittenbury R, Gould GW et al., Bath University Press, Bath, 206–19.

Russell AD, Hugo WB, 1994, Antimicrobial activity and action of silver, *Prog Med Chem*, **31:** 351–71.

Russell AD, Hugo WB, Ayliffe GAJ (eds), 1992, *Principles and Practice of Disinfection, Preservation and Sterilization*, 2nd edn, Blackwell Science, Oxford.

Russell AD, Russell NJ, 1995, Biocides: activity, action and resistance, *Fifty Years of Antimicrobials: Past Perspectives and Future Trends (53rd Symposium of the Society for General Microbiology)*, eds Hunter PA, Darby GK, Russell NJ, Cambridge University Press, Cambridge, 328–65.

Russell AD, Yarnych VS, Koulikovskii AV, 1984, *Guidelines on Disinfection in Animal Husbandry for Prevention and Control of Zoonotic Diseases*, World Health Organization, Geneva. VPH/84.4.

Rutala WA, 1990, APIC guidelines for selection and use of disinfectants, *Am J Infect Control*, **18:** 99–117.

Rutala WA, 1995, *Chemical Germicides in Health Care*, Polyscience, Morin Heights, PQ, Canada.

Salmond CV, Kroll RG, Booth IR, 1984, The effect of food preservatives on pH homeostasis in *Escherichia coli*, *J Gen Microbiol*, **130:** 2845–50.

Salton MRJ, 1968, Lytic agents, cell permeability and monolayer penetrability, *J Gen Physiol*, **52:** 227S–252S.

Sancar A, Sancar GB, 1988, DNA repair enzymes, *Annu Rev Biochem*, **57:** 29–67.

Sattar SA, Springthorpe VS et al., 1994, Inactivation of the human immunodeficiency virus: an update, *Rev Med Microbiol*, **5:** 139–50.

Seal DV, Hay J, 1992, Contact lens disinfection and Acanthamoeba: problems and practicalities, *Pharm J*, **248:** 717–19.

Seiler DAL, Russell NJ, 1991, Ethanol as a food preservative, *Food Preservatives*, eds Russell NJ, Gould GW, Blackie, Glasgow and London, 153–71.

Setlow P, 1994, Mechanisms which contribute to the long-term survival of spores of *Bacillus* species, *J Appl Bacteriol Symp Suppl*, **76:** 49S–60S.

Shaker LA, Dancer BN et al., 1988, Emergence and development of chlorhexidine resistance during sporulation of *Bacillus subtilis* 168, *FEMS Microbiol Lett*, **51:** 73–6.

Silver S, Nucifora G et al., 1989, Bacterial ATPases: primary pumps for exporting toxic cations and anions, *Trends Biochem Sci*, **14:** 76–80.

Sofos JN, Busta FF, 1992, Chemical food preservatives, *Principles and Practice of Disinfection, Preservation and Sterilization*, 2nd edn, eds Russell AD, Hugo WB, Ayliffe GAJ, Blackwell Science, Oxford, 351–97.

Soper CJ, Davies DJG, 1990, Principles of sterilization, *Guide to Microbiological Control in Pharmaceuticals*, eds Denyer S, Baird R, Ellis Horwood, Chichester, 157–81.

Speier JL, Malek JR, 1982, Destruction of micro-organisms by contact with solid surfaces, *J Coll Int Sci*, **89:** 68–76.

Spicher G, Peters J, 1981, Heat activation of bacterial spores after inactivation by formaldehyde. Dependance of heat activation on temperature and duration of action, *Zentralbl Bakteriol Mikrobiol [B]*, **173:** 188–96.

Springle WR, Briggs MA, 1992, Preservation in specialized areas. E. Paint and paint films, *Principles and Practice of Disinfection, Preservation and Sterilization*, 2nd edn, eds Russell AD, Hugo WB, Ayliffe GAJ, Blackwell Science, Oxford, 431–6.

Springthorpe VS, Sattar SA, 1990, Chemical disinfection of virus-contaminated surfaces, *Clin Rev Environ Control*, **20:** 169–229.

Springthorpe VS, Grenier JL et al., 1986, Chemical disinfection of human rotaviruses: efficacy of commercially available products in suspension tests, *J Hyg Camb*, **97:** 139–61.

Staehelin M, 1958, Reactions of tobacco mosaic virus nucleic acid with formaldehyde, *Biochim Biophys Acta*, **29:** 410.

Sykes G, 1965, *Disinfection and Sterilization*, 2nd edn, E & F N Spon, London.

Tallentire A, Jacobs GP, 1972, Radiosensitization of bacterial spores by ketonic agents of differing electron affinities, *Int J Radiat Biol*, **21:** 205–13.

Tanny GB, Strong DK et al., 1979, Adsorptive retention of *Pseudomonas diminuta* by membrane filters, *J Parent Drug Ass*, **33:** 40–51.

Taylor DM, 1992, Inactivation of unconventional agents of the transmissible degenerative encephalopathies, *Principles and Practice of Disinfection, Preservation and Sterilization*, 2nd edn, eds Russell AD, Hugo WB, Ayliffe GAJ, Blackwell Science, Oxford, 171–9.

Terano H, Tanooka H, Kadota H, 1969, Germination induced repair of single strand breaks of DNA in irradiated *Bacillus subtilis* spores, *Biochem Biophys Res Commun*, **37:** 66–71.

Terano H, Tanooka H, Kadota H, 1971, Repair of radiation damage to deoxyribonucleic acid in germinating spores of *Bacillus subtilis*, *J Bacteriol*, **106:** 925–30.

Thurmann RB, Gerba CP, 1988, Molecular mechanisms of viral inactivation by water disinfectants, *Adv Appl Microbiol*, **33:** 75–105.

Thurmann RB, Gerba CP, 1989, The molecular mechanisms of copper and silver ion disinfection of bacteria and viruses, *CRC Crit Rev Environ Control*, **18:** 295–315.

Tomlins RI, Ordal ZJ, 1976, Thermal injury and inactivation in vegetative bacteria, *Inhibition and Inactivation of Vegetative Microbes*, eds Skinner FA, Hugo WB, Society for Applied Bacteriology Symposium Series No. 5, Academic Press, London, 153–90.

Townsend DE, Ashdown N et al., 1984, Transposition of gentamicin resistance to staphylococcal plasmids encoding resistance to cationic agents, *J Antimicrob Chemother*, **14:** 115–34.

Trevor JT, 1987, Silver resistance and accumulation in bacteria, *Enzyme Microb Technol*, **9:** 331–3.

Trueman JR, 1971, The halogens, *Inhibition and Destruction of the Microbial Cell*, ed. Hugo WB, Academic Press, London, 137–84.

Tsiquaye KN, Barnard J, 1993, Chemical disinfection of duck hepatitis B virus: a model for inactivation of infectivity of hepatitis B virus, *J Antimicrob Chemother*, **32:** 313–23.

Tyler R, Ayliff GAJ, 1987, A surface test for virucidal activity: preliminary study with herpes virus, *J Hosp Infect*, **9:** 22–9.

Vaara M, 1992, Agents that increase the permeability of the outer membrane, *Microbiol Rev*, **56:** 395–411.

Varghese AJ, 1970, 5-Thyminyl-5,6-dihydrothymine from DNA irradiated with ultraviolet light, *Biochem Biophys Res Commun*, **38:** 484–90.

Wang WLL, Blaser MJ et al., 1979, Growth, survival and resistance of the Legionnaires' disease bacterium, *Ann Intern Med*, **90:** 614–18.

Warth AD, 1985, Mechanisms of heat resistance, *Fundamental and Applied Aspects of Bacterial Spores*, eds Dring GJ, Gould GW, Ellar DJ, Academic Press, London, 209–25.

Warth AD, 1986, Effect of benzoic acid on growth yield of yeasts differing in their resistance to preservatives, *Int J Food Microbiol*, **3:** 263–71.

Warth AD, 1989, Relationships among cell size, membrane permeability and preservative resistance in yeast species, *Appl Environ Microbiol*, **55:** 2995–9.

White PJP, 1990, The design of controlled environments, *Guide to Microbiological Control in Pharmaceuticals*, eds Denyer S, Baird R, Ellis Horwood, Chichester, 87–124.

Wilkins KM, Board RG, 1989, Natural antimicrobial systems, *Mechanisms of Action of Food Preservation Procedures*, ed. Gould GW, Elsevier Applied Science, London, 285–362.

Williams ND, Russell AD, 1993, Injury and repair in biocide-treated spores of *Bacillus subtilis*, *FEMS Microbiol Lett*, **106:** 183–6.

Wills PA, 1974, Effects of hydrostatic pressure and ionising radiation on bacterial spores, *Atomic Energy Aust*, **17:** 2–10.

Wood RT, 1993, Sterilization with dry heat, *Sterilization Technology. A Practical Guide for Manufacturers and Users of Health Care Products*, eds Morrissey RF, Phillips GB, Van Nostrand Reinhold, New York, 81–119.

Zamenhof S, 1960, Effects of heating dry bacteria and spores on their phenotype and genotype, *Proc Natl Acad Sci USA*, **46:** 101–5.

Chapter 8

BACTERIOCINS AND BACTERIOPHAGES

M Day

1 Introduction	3 Bacteriophages
2 Bacteriocins	4 Conclusions

1 INTRODUCTION

Bacteriocins are a group of proteins secreted by bacteria that kill or inhibit competing strains. Bacteriophages are viruses that infect bacteria. Both agents have antimicrobial activity and they share some features, such as the uptake site on their host bacterium. However, examination of their modes of action, reproduction and genetics reveals differences. The major difference is that only bacteriophages carry a genome (DNA or RNA) enabling them to reproduce in the cells they infect; bacteriocins are only proteins and cannot reproduce. Irradiating a phage will irreparably damage its genome; this irradiated lysate will have no killing activity. Bacteriocins have no genome and are thus insensitive to this level of irradiation. Both bacteriocins and phages can kill susceptible cells. However, it is now clear that, in some instances, some bacterial strains will only show some degree of growth inhibition from their action.

2 BACTERIOCINS

Micro-organisms naturally produce a range of protein components from simple polypeptides to very complex macromolecules such as toxins, pili, adhesins, siderophores, flagella, etc. Bacteriocins are grouped under the term toxins and provide a means of defence against, or a growth advantage over, other micro-organisms in the same environment. The term colicin is used to describe those antagonistic compounds produced by *Escherichia coli* (Frederique 1957). It was coined by Gratia and Fredericq (1946) for these substances, the effects of which had been described by Gratia in 1925. Jacob and Woolman (1953) introduced the general term bacteriocin to describe substances with similar activity produced by a wide range of bacteria. Tagg, Dajani and Wannamaker (1976) defined bacteriocins, a subgroup of bacterial toxins,

as proteinaceous compounds that kill closely related bacteria. Although this is true for most bacteriocins it is evident that these molecules take many forms and may have bactericidal actions beyond closely related species. Individual bacteriocins are named by attaching 'cin' to the root of the genus or species name. For example, *Pseudomonas aeruginosa* produces aeruginocins and *Bacillus megaterium* produces megacins. The synthesis of most colicins (and this will probably be true of bacteriocins in general) are SOS inducible (Pugsley 1984a, 1984b). Frequently bacterial species carry genes that encode both the production of one or more bacteriocins and immunity to them on the chromosome or on plasmids (Frank 1994). The significance of the latter location is that the distribution of individual plasmid types in bacterial communities fluctuates under selection, for and against the plasmid and host cell, which provides opportunities for closely related and competing populations to gain and lose advantage. Loss and acquisition of bacteriocins is a consequence of plasmid stability, incompatibility and transfer. Thus a great diversity of bacteriocins can be produced within a single species. Bacteriocins have a spectrum of sizes; generally proteinaceous agents, they are sometimes complexed with lipids, carbohydrates or other distinctive proteins (Lewus, Kiaser and Montville 1991, Nissen-Meyer et al. 1992, Jiminez-Diaz et al. 1993). There are 3 general classes:

1 the microcins, small molecules produced in stationary phase by gram-negative bacteria
2 the lantibiotics, small molecules produced by gram-positive bacteria and
3 bacteriocins, a group encompassing medium to large phage-like structures, whose synthesis generally appears to be induced by the SOS response.

These proteins share many characteristics. Many have a low molecular weight, are cationic, amphiphilic, tend to aggregate and are benign to the producing organism. They kill their target cells in one of 3 distinct ways – via a ribonuclease or deoxyribonuclease activity or by forming pores in the target cell's membrane. Since their sites of synthesis and modes of action are frequently intracellular, they must also be able to enter susceptible cells to exert their effects. Many are capable of killing activity at extremely low concentrations (one to a few molecules per susceptible cell) and target specific cellular pathways. Death of the cell is a consequence of transport collapse at membrane level, depleting proton-motive force (pmf) and resulting in a rapid reduction in indispensable metabolites or ions, or blocking of macromolecule synthesis (protein or DNA). There is a further and historical complication in this analysis as bacteriocins are effectively antibiotics. Thus there is an activity, structural and biochemical overlap between these molecules. Historically, some were initially regarded as antibiotics and have now been recognized as bacteriocins, and vice versa for others.

2.1 Assay

A simple method for assaying bacteriocin activity is to take the supernate of an overnight culture of the putative bacteriocinogenic strain grown in broth culture, dilute this as a series of doubling dilutions, and place 10 μl drops on the surface of a dry nutrient agar plate pre-spread with a lawn of the indicator bacterium. After overnight incubation the lawn will have grown and the area containing bacteriocin will show a circular zone of clearing. The further down the dilution series the inhibition zones are found, the more bacteriocin is produced by the strain (Benkerroum et al. 1993). This demonstration of the inhibitory effect is also the basis of bacteriocin typing methods (see p. 187).

2.2 Modes of action

A neat and satisfying taxonomy of bacteriocins remains to evolve. Bacteriocins have been described variously in terms of size, types of activity and chemical nature. As there is no consistent theme it is difficult to obtain a proper grasp of their relationships. It seems sensible to categorize them through their modes of action, but the problem with this approach is that for most the mechanisms of activity are unknown. However, the general strategies employed by these antimicrobial agents are illustrated by the examples that follow.

Destruction of membrane potential

The membrane is composed of many different molecules in complex functional associations. Bacteriocins that target individual proteins, in associations concerned with membrane potential, lead directly to a loss in pmf. Bacteriocins produced by lactic acid bacteria commonly act by this mechanism, but the role of receptor proteins and the mechanism by which pmf is depleted remain unresolved. Many that act in this way are lantibiotics and are produced only by gram-

positive bacteria. The most striking feature of lantibiotics is the occurrence of intramolecular rings, introduced by the thioether amino acids lanthionine and 3-methyllanthionine, and unusual amino acids such as didehydroalanine and didehydrobutyrine (Bierbaum and Sahl 1993). These smaller bioactive molecules, which in gram-positive strains are 30–60 amino acids in size (Jack, Tagg and Ray 1995), as a group have both broad and narrow spectra of activity. Some are phospholipases that cause susceptible cells to leak intracellular contents through the damaged cell membranes. In gram-negative bacteria some of the colicins destroy the membrane potential by forming pores in the membrane (Lau, Parsons and Uchimura 1992). Colicin A is an example of a water-soluble protein that inserts into lipid bilayers and produces this effect (Lakey et al. 1992, Lakey, Vandergoot and Pattus 1994).

Nucleolytic activity

Sano et al. (1993) examined pyocins S1 and S2, S-type bacteriocins of *P. aeruginosa* which have different receptor recognition specificities. The sequence homology suggests that pyocins S1 and S2 originated from a common ancestor of the E2 group colicins. Purified pyocins S1 and S2 make up a complex of the 2 proteins. Both pyocins cause breakdown of chromosomal DNA and complete inhibition of lipid synthesis in sensitive cells. Colicin E2 inhibits protein synthesis through endonucleolytic activity (Lau, Parsons and Uchimura 1992). Colicin E3 has endonucleolytic activity cleaving the 16S RNA moiety of the 30S ribosome subunit. Microcin B17 inhibits DNA gyrase (Vizan et al. 1991).

Inhibition of protein synthesis

The large particulate bacteriocins, e.g. the pyocin-R (aeruginocins) produced by *P. aeruginosa* (Hayashi et al. 1994), are derived from defective phage particles; they contain the phage component capable of attaching to the cell surface. This class of agent generally shows a narrow spectrum of specificity, inhibits protein synthesis, but does not lyse the cell. The genes specifying this type of bacteriocin are chromosomally encoded.

2.3 Synthesis

The physiological state of the cell affects all cellular metabolism. The biosynthesis of bacteriocins is no exception and thus the yields of bacteriocin depend on local environmental influences on the producer cell physiology and the regulatory mechanisms governing the expression of the bacteriocin. For example, Malkhosyan, Panchenko and Relesh (1991) showed that levels of DNA supercoiling are influenced by anaerobic metabolism and that this regulates the level of expression of the colicin genes. The expression of the *cea* gene, which encodes colicin El, on the ColE1 plasmid was greatly increased when the cells were grown anaerobically (Eraso and Weinstock 1992). By using *cea–lacZ* fusions to quantitate expression, levels of β-galactosidase produced under aerobic conditions from the fusion were found to be only a few % of the anaerobic levels. The gene is also induced by the SOS response and subject to catabolite repression.

The majority of bacteriocins, such as colicins, aeruginocins, megacins, etc., are produced as the result of normal gene expression. Their synthesis starts with gene transcription, producing an mRNA, which is then translated into an active protein. This synthetic sequence is mediated by ribosomes (Pugsley 1984a, 1984b). The lantibiotics class of bacteriocins (Hansen 1993) frequently contains unusual amino acids that contribute to their properties and functions. Most are synthesized as peptides by non-ribosomal mechanisms (Klienkauf and von Dohren 1990), but some are synthesized by pathways that involve post-translational modification of ribosomally synthesized precursor peptides. Examples of the latter are nicin and subtilisin (Nishio, Komura and Kurahashi 1983).

2.4 Release from cells

The microcins, e.g. colV, are small (6 kDa) and are not induced by the SOS system; their release coincides with the stationary phase. They do not utilize a lysis protein for release, but have a dedicated pathway (Gilson, Mahanty and Kotter 1990, Van der Wal, Luirick and Oudega 1995). The lantibiotics generally use a dedicated secretion pathway (Fath and Kolter 1993).

2.5 Uptake sites

It has long been recognized that only a few molecules (perhaps only one) are necessary to kill a susceptible cell and the receptor targets are known for several bacteriocins, in particular some of the colicins. Susceptible cells bear specific protein receptors in their outer membranes, which explains why colicins attach only certain strains of bacteria.

Tolerance and resistance are 2 terms that are often incorrectly and synonymously used in medical microbiology. The term tolerance describes a state in which the bacteriocin fails to gain access to the target site within the cell because the receptor is absent or altered and the colicin remains unattached to the cell; thus it cannot exert a lethal effect. Tolerance may also be produced by mutations (e.g. of *tolA*, *tolB* or *tolC* genes) that affect the outer-membrane proteins and the interactions between the cytoplasmic and outer membranes, which can prevent the uptake of the bacteriocin into the cell. Resistance occurs when the bacteriocin can be taken up but either it cannot reach the target site or the site is lost or altered by mutation and thus the cell remains unaffected. There is often a commonality in receptors, which also have a cellular functional role, utilized by phage and bacteriocins. For example, the site used by colicin K and bacteriophage T6 is implicated in nucleoside uptake. The colicins E1, E2 and E3, phage BF2 (phage T5-like) use a glycoprotein receptor involved in vitamin B12 uptake. TonB is a membrane transport protein utilized by

many substances and *tonB⁻* membrane mutants are tolerant to colV (Pugsley and Schwartz 1985).

2.6 Host range

Although the general statement that most bacteriocins have a narrow host range (Jack, Tagg and Ray 1995) is true for many, work on bacteriocins produced by *B. megaterium* (megacins), for example, shows that some have a broad spectrum and attack most strains of this species. These megacins are phospholipases and cause susceptible cells to leak intracellular contents by attacking the membrane phospholipids. The bacteriocins produced by lactic acid bacteria exhibit a relatively broad antimicrobial spectrum and are active against several food-spoilage and health-threatening micro-organisms (Kim 1993).

2.7 Immunity

The production of bacteriocins is the result of deregulation of one or more genes and in many instances the release is by a dedicated export mechanism and not cell lysis (Lakey, Vandergoot and Pattus 1994). Strains harbouring plasmid or chromosomally encoded colicins, e.g. colicin E3, have immunity to the lethal activity of the colicin (Riley 1993, Frank 1994).

2.8 Clinical, technological and ecological importance

Applications of bacteriocinogeny have been used as epidemiological tools through bacteriocin typing of clinical strains to aid in the identification or discrimination of opportunist and pathogenic bacterial strains. Bacteriocins that show narrow specificity within individual species or genera, such as the bacteriocins of gram-negative bacilli, have been particularly useful in bacteriocin typing. A strain may be characterized actively by the range of activity of its bacteriocins against a set of indicator strains of the same or closely related species, or passively in which it is characterized by the pattern of its susceptibility to the bacteriocins of a set of indicator strains. The former approach has proved particularly useful in typing isolates of *Shigella sonnei* (see Chapter 40) and *P. aeruginosa* (see Chapter 47), and a combination of the 2 approaches has been used for *Proteus* spp. (see Chapter 43). In colicin and pyocin typing, strains to be typed are streaked across an agar plate and grown overnight so that their bacteriocins diffuse into the agar. Growth is removed from the surface and remaining viable bacteria are killed by exposure to chloroform, and then the indicator strains are streaked across the original line of growth and again incubated overnight. The bacteriocin type is indicated by the pattern of inhibition of the indicator strains (Gillis 1964).

Bacteriocins have been used in the food industry for a long time. There is a potential for this to increase as more food is required to have a longer shelf-life. Applications stem from their lack of mammalian toxicity and the spectrum of activities available. For example, bacteriocins produced by lactic acid bacteria exhibit a relatively broad antimicrobial spectrum and are active against several food-spoilage and health-threatening micro-organisms (Kim 1993) and some produce bacteriocins active against *Listeria monocytogenes*, a food-borne pathogen (Hechard et al. 1993). Nisin, produced by some strains of *Lactococcus lactis* subsp. *lactis*, was originally described in 1928 and is the most highly characterized bacteriocin produced by lactic acid bacteria. Nisin has been permitted as a food additive in the UK since the early 1960s and is currently an accepted food additive in at least 45 other countries (Harris, Fleming and Klaenhammer 1992). One example of its use is in the preservation of liquid egg (Delvesbroughton, Williams and Williamson 1992).

The activity or role of colicins in vivo is not clear. Pugsley (1984a) suggested that high proteolytic activity in the intestinal tract (an anaerobic environment) would degrade colicins and thus lead to an effective loss of their activity. Later Luria and Suit (1987) stated that 'colicinogeny appears an unnecessary complication in the life of coliform bacteria'. It seems a little premature to write off a group of proteins which are expressed from highly organized genetic systems, released from cells by specialized export processes and which selectively target specific pathways in selected species. It appears more likely that they do have an ecological role to promote the growth of the producer against its immediate competitors. These are likely to be strains with a similar metabolism (biochemistry and physiology) and will be related strains and species. As the particular and immediate requirement for bacteriocin activity is to inhibit cells adjacent to the one producing the bacteriocin, it is local spatial activity that is required. An agent that diffuses into larger volumes will help other competitors. This argument is supported by Frank (1994) whose hypothesis was that bacteriocin diversity in species could not occur if the organisms mixed freely. Spatial variation and poor habitats favoured both susceptibility and bacteriocin diversity in strains. Bacteriocin producers are favoured in good habitats where competition is likely to be high.

3 BACTERIOPHAGES

Bacteriophages (phages) are viruses that grow in bacterial cells utilizing their biosynthetic systems for reproduction. Their effects were first observed by Twort (1915) who described an infectious agent that distorted the morphology of staphylococcal colonies. D'Herelle (1917) found a filterable agent that sterilized broth cultures of *Shigella* sp. and he believed such agents might be useful in combating bacterial diseases, as they had no infectivity towards eukaryotic cells.

Phages are extremely common in the environment and can be found wherever their host bacteria are present. They are readily detected for most bacterial species. It is probable that all bacteria are sensitive to one or more phages which thus prey on their specific host strain or strains; it is rare to find one that infects a large number of species. The population density of their host cells is a major component determining the density and distribution of phage (Ogunseitan, Sayler and Miller 1990, Proctor and Fuhrman 1990). For example, high counts of phage occur in biofilms ($>10^8$ cm^{-2}; Ewert and Paynter 1980) where bacterial density is high, but are far lower in bulk waters (10^{3-4} cfu ml^{-1}; Saye and Miller 1989) where bacterial density is also low. In sewage, enumeration by electron microscopy (Ewert and Paynter 1980) revealed 10^{8-10} phages ml^{-1}, compared to c. 10^8 ml^{-1} in freshwater and the open ocean (Bergh et al. 1989).

3.1 Phage morphology

As an overall group of viruses, phages show considerable morphological diversity (Ackermann 1983). Some are filamentous, isometric and superficially resemble animal viruses, whereas others show complex morphologies. The capsid or the phage head is the structure containing the genome; this can be single or double stranded DNA or RNA. Some phages are virulent, killing each cell they infect, whereas others are temperate. In the latter case the phage resides, as a prophage, in a cell termed a lysogen and replicates synchronously with the cell. When phage replication is completed the particles are released from the cell. They usually contain a phage genome. The phage capsid recognizes an adsorption site on the outside of a susceptible cell, binds to it and injects the genome, held within the capsid, into the cell. The genome then redirects the cellular metabolism to synthesize more phage. In the lysogenic state the phage genome does not disrupt bacterial metabolism and replication, but may contribute specific characteristics to its host, e.g. toxin production by *Corynebacterium diphtheriae* (see Chapter 25) and *Streptococcus pyogenes* (see Chapter 28).

3.2 Single stranded RNA phages

These are the simplest of phages in terms of their genomic size and morphology. This is not to imply that the organization of their replicative cycle or their economy in genome size, relative to other phages, makes their biological activities simple, but reflects an evolutionary adaptation. They rely on the host cell for all metabolic activities except for certain replicative functions to complete their life cycle. The RNA coliphage MS2, termed male specific, utilizes the pilus of an F$^+$ *E. coli* cell as an infection site. The MS2 capsid is icosohedral, largely composed of a single protein species, which encloses a phage genome of 3569 nucleotides (nt) of linear plus strand (sense) RNA. The capsid binds to the side of the F pilus and the phage genome is transferred into the cell. Once internalized, the phage RNA genome acts as messenger RNA and is translated by the ribosomes. There is no transcriptional control, as promoters and RNA polymerase are not involved, and yet there is temporal control over the expression of proteins. This is achieved by changes in conformation of the RNA genome. Relatively large numbers of coat protein molecules (Van Duin 1988) are needed per virion. The RNA-directed RNA polymerase, a lysin gene and an absorption protein are synthesized in smaller amounts and their expression is regulated by secondary structures formed in the phage genome (Kastelein et al. 1982, Berkhout et al. 1987).

On average, 20 000 phage particles are produced from one cell infected by one phage and this can be achieved in as little as 22 min. To achieve this efficiency, replication proceeds alongside expression and the phage polymerase acts in concert with some host accessory functions. The polymerase initiates repeatedly, at the 3′ end of the RNA (Haruna and Spiegelman 1965), enabling multiple copies (of the minus strand) to be made. Concurrently these full length minus strands are then copied to yield the plus strands, which are used initially for the expression of phage proteins. Later in the infection cycle the plus strands are individually packaged into a capsid. Cell lysis is induced by the final product, the lysis protein.

3.3 Single stranded DNA phages

The isomeric phage φX174 was the first single stranded DNA phage to be identified (Hayashi et al. 1988). It has a circular genome (5387 nt) that codes for 10 proteins. Four different monomers are present in the capsid, one of which is an internal protein and is surrounded by a second (60 copies) which forms the icosahedral capsid. The other 2 monomers form 'spike' proteins, which are essential for infectivity. The phage receptor is a lipopolysaccharide that allows entry of the phage genome. This DNA is used as a template for single minus-strand synthesis and is entirely dependent upon the host cell to create a biologically active phage genome (Goulian, Kornberg and Sinsheimer 1967). Once established as a duplex, the phage genome reproduces by rolling circle replication (Lewin 1987). This is initiated by a phage replication enzyme expressed from the newly formed duplex. Transcription proceeds in the same direction as replication. As the pools of capsid precursors and replicated genomes increases, the plus strands become encapsulated (Aoyama and Hayashi 1986). The reproductive cycle can be complete within 13 min, resulting in cell lysis yielding up to 180 phage particles.

Although the replication cycles of the filamentous phages are similar to that of φX174, their structure, attachment and the absence of cell lysis on phage release are different (Lindquist, Dehó and Calendar 1993). The genome of phage M13 is circular (6407 nt) and encapsulated as a single strand by a flexible helical capsid composed largely of a single protein species (Model and Russell 1988). At the ends of this tube-like filamentous phage capsid are the 'minor' proteins. Those at one end are responsible for phage attachment to the F plasmid pilus via which, it

appears, the phage genome is internalized. Replication proceeds in the same manner as for φX174. The host cell continues to grow and divide and as the phage particles become 'mature' they are released through an intact cell envelope. Thus phages are continually released after a latent period of 30 min, resulting in very high phage yields. The filamentous phages are good cloning vectors because foreign DNA can be spliced into the genome at appropriate sites and transformed into a host bacterial cell to give high yields of cloned material. The splicing of novel genes with the coat protein gives protein chimeras in which the novel peptide component may be exposed on the capsid surface (Barbas et al. 1991). As methods for purifying phages are well established, this provides an easy method for screening for protein activities.

3.4 Double stranded DNA phages

The double stranded DNA phages are divided into 2 groups, based on their virulent or temperate nature. Phage T4 is a virulent and morphologically complex phage; it has an elongated icosahedral capsid composed of one major and several minor (in terms of percentage) proteins (Mathews et al. 1983). The capsid is placed upon a tail comprising a core and contractile sheath on a base plate with 6 kinked tail fibres. In the capsid the c. 170 kb DNA is linear and double stranded, with about a 5 kb terminal repeat. Free phage particles recognize a lipopolysaccharide receptor on the cell surface and become anchored to it. The proteins in the baseplate then reorientate to allow the core to be driven onto and through the cell surface as the sheath contracts. The DNA is then extruded from the head into the cell's cytoplasm. Phage replication uses the host polymerase and normal vegetative σ factor (σ_{70}). The phage reproductive cycle, from infection to lysis, is highly organized and complex. For example, transcription is temporally organized such that some genes are expressed early and in the middle of the replicative cycle (Mosig and Eiserling 1988). The late genes are transcribed by a phage-encoded σ factor and also govern DNA synthesis. Immediately after infection this phage degrades the host genome and inhibits host transcription. After replication, the concatomeric DNA is injected into the preformed heads and cut, and then the tail structures are added (Bhattacharyya and Rao 1993). Expression of the late phage genes results in cell lysis and release of ≥200 mature phage particles 23 min after infection.

3.5 Experimental analysis

Phages may be investigated by a variety of molecular and standard laboratory techniques. Three terms describe key points in the analysis of phages; a plaque-forming unit (pfu) is a phage particle which is capable of forming a plaque; the efficiency of plating (EOP) is the proportion of pfu to total phage particles (enumerated by electron microscopy) in a lysate (Adams 1959); the multiplicity of infection (MOI) is the ratio of host cells to phage in a mixture.

ASSAY

It is a simple procedure to estimate the number of phage particles in a lysate. As titres are frequently 10^6–10^{11} pfu ml^{-1}, 10-fold dilution series of phage lysate is prepared to obtain 10–100 pfu ml^{-1}. A small volume (e.g. 100 μl) of diluted lysate is mixed with an equal volume of host bacterial cells in about 3.0 ml of 0.6% molten nutrient agar, held at 46°C. This is vortex mixed and poured onto the surface of a standard nutrient agar plate. After overnight incubation, to allow the plaques to develop in the growing bacterial lawn, the number of plaques formed will reflect the original phage concentration and the dilution of the lysate. At high dilutions no phage will be present and no plaques will develop; at a lower dilution a few plaques (zones of lysis a few mm in diameter) will be present in the lawn and at the next dilution, the plaque count will be high, the plaques may even merge in places. At the next dilution, the MOI will be about 1:1 and confluent lysis will occur, although it is likely that a few bacterial colonies, resistant to the phage, will grow (at a frequency of 10^{-8}). This may be due to phenotypic variation (the lack of expression of a phage uptake site) or to a resistant mutation (leading to a loss of the target site), or the cell may become infected by a normally lytic phage and yet become lysogenized. In each case, the cell remains unaffected by the phage and continues to grow. The titre of phage is calculated by dividing the dilution assayed into the plaque count from the plate with the highest number of countable plaques.

PLAQUE MORPHOLOGY

Phages can replicate only in an actively metabolizing host cell. A poor nutritional environment will reduce the plaque size and probably also reduce the phage yield. The morphology of the plaque is due to repeated cycles of infection, replication and lysis of the phage; from the point of infection of a single cell, phages released by lysis infect adjacent cells. This process repeats itself while the bacteria in the lawn are growing, causing a circular plaque to form. Thus the titre and plaque morphology remain consistent provided the media, incubation conditions and host are constant. Changes in environmental conditions, the genetic status of the host bacterium or the phage can all influence both plaque morphology and the reproductive success of the phage.

TRANSDUCTION

Transduction is achievable with only some phages. For gene transfer, a proportion of the phage particles generated in a lysate have to package some host chromosomal DNA instead of a phage genome. The phage particle acts as a vector for host chromosomal genes, transferring the packaged sequence into the cytoplasm of a recipient cell. Providing the DNA sequence has homology with a recipient sequence (chromosomal or plasmid), recombination can then occur. This is mediated by the host-specified RecA protein, replacing the host sequence by the transferred sequence. The process is termed transduction.

If any gene on the bacterial chromosome may be transferred by the phage, this is termed generalized transduction (Margolin 1987), but if the phage will only transfer a few genes from one site on the genome, this is termed specialized or restricted transduction (Weisberg 1987).

About 2% of the phage particles produced by the *Salmonella typhimurium* phage P22 contain host DNA (Ebel-Tsipis, Botsyein and Fox 1972), as do c. 0.3% of *E. coli* phage P1 in a lysate (Lennox 1955). The frequencies of transfer of auxotrophic markers varies between 10^{-5} and 10^{-7} per pfu (Harriman 1971) for both of these phages. However, Schmeiger (1972) has shown that with different genes and hosts the frequencies can vary over 1000-fold.

There are various fates for DNA transduced into a recipient cell. The DNA that is recombined is stably inherited, giving rise to a stable transductant. The displaced strand is degraded and the nucleotides are reutilized. If the DNA sequence fails to become integrated then it may persist for several generations, producing what is termed abortive transductants (Ozeki 1959). These transductants show unilinear inheritance of the character transferred. This is explained by using a cell which is an auxotroph (carries a mutation in the gene coding for an enzyme required for the synthesis of an amino acid), so it cannot synthesize a particular amino acid as a recipient. This is transduced to prototrophy by an 'abortive fragment' which contains the prototrophic gene so the cell is able to synthesize the amino acid. When the cell divides, one daughter inherits the wild-type gene and continues to express the enzyme and consequently synthesizes the amino acid and grows. The other cell now has the mutant genotype but is phenotypically wild-type; it retains an active biosynthetic pathway while the enzyme retains its activity. This is lost gradually as it becomes diluted out through growth and cell division; the cell grows, but increasingly slowly. Hence abortive transductants generate very small colonies which appear some time after the wild-type has fully grown. The condition is relatively stable as less than 1% of cells go on to become complete transductants (Ozeki and Ikeda 1968). Schmeiger (1982) has shown that abortive transduction by P22 is a common phenomenon and varies over a range of 50% to <1% for different loci.

Specialized transduction occurs with *E. coli* phage λ. In this type of transduction the phage enters the chromosome by site-specific recombination at *attB*, using a homologous sequence on the phage termed *attP* (Weisberg and Landy 1983), to form a lysogen. Transducing particles are formed by the illegitimate excision of the phage genome, in which part of the phage sequence remains in the chromosome to be replaced by an adjacent host chromosomal sequence. Thus genes to one side or the other of the *attB* site may be packaged in the capsid (hence the term specialized). The transducing phage genome is defective and cannot reproduce in the recipient cell. These transducing phages occur at a frequency of about 10^{-6}. If these defective phages co-infect a new recipient with a wild-type phage, 50% of the phage in the lysate produced from that cell will be capable of transducing the host gene. The frequency of transduction now is far greater; it can be 100% (Lewin 1987). Transducing phages of both types are common in other genera.

3.6 Environmental role

The role of phages in natural bacterial populations remains largely a point of conjecture. They seem to have a dramatic influence on population densities of bacteria in natural habitats (Ogunseitan, Sayler and Miller 1990, Proctor and Fuhrman 1990). Host range has been established by the observation of plaques on putative host strains and on this basis most phages have a narrow host range. There is a widespread assumption that the plating range (i.e. the ability of the phage to form plaques) is a direct reflection of the transduction range. The ambiguity of this has been illustrated with *E. coli* phage P1. Productive infections with phage P1 can be made from *Citrobacter freundii*, *Shigella* spp., *Salmonella* spp., *Serratia* spp., *Enterobacter liquefaciens*, *Erwinia* spp., *Proteus* spp., *Pseudomonas* spp. and *Klebsiella* spp. (Yarmolinsky and Sternberg 1988). In addition, phage P1 can naturally transduce DNA into *Yersina* spp., *Flavobacterium* sp. M46, *Agrobacterium tumefaciens*, *Alcaligenes faecalis* and *Myxococcus xanthus*. Goldberg, Bender and Streicher (1974) have reported transduction by phage P1 into *S. typhimurium* even though they were unable to isolate stable lysogens and *Enterobacter amylovora* lysogens did not produce P1 phage. This provides evidence to support the proposal that the transduction and titration ranges for a phage are not unambiguously equivalent and the associations between phage and their host bacteria are not clear cut. Thus the contribution of phages to gene exchange remains an open and unanswered question. In addition, the host range can be influenced by the presence or absence of adsorption sites and the mechanism of phage replication. The restriction enzymes possessed by the new host target the phage genome (Roberts 1985). If the phage fortuitously evades the restriction enzymes and becomes modified, to shield the restriction sites, or if these sites are absent, then the phage may be able to replicate.

3.7 Phage identification and typing

The specificity and variety of phages that can infect many bacterial species have enabled phages to be used both for the identification of species when all strains of the species are susceptible to one phage, or for detailed typing within a species when various phages will attack only a proportion of strains. Phages that lyse all members of a particular species have been used in the identification of *Brucella abortus* and *Bacillus anthracis*. The phages active on *Vibrio cholerae* are specific in their action on serotypes or biotypes. Phage typing within species has been most widely developed and most effectively used in the epidemiological investigation of *Staphylococcus aureus* infection and for strain identification within several *Salmonella* serotypes, including Typhi. Typing phages are propagated on a susceptible host strain of the test species to give a high-titre phage suspension, which is then diluted to a concentration (the routine test dilution, RTD) that gives barely confluent lysis of the propagating culture growing on a solid medium. In phage typing, a set of phages active on only some strains within a species is applied to a lawn of the isolate in question on an agar medium. After incubation, susceptibility is seen as lysis (i.e. plaques) produced by particular phages. The pattern of activity gives the phage type of the organism (Parker 1972).

4 CONCLUSIONS

Both bacteriocins and bacteriophages are universally present in microbial populations, affecting growth and biochemical relationships within and between bacterial populations. Frank (1994) has suggested that the great diversity of bacteriocins produced by a single species cannot occur if the organisms mix freely. His analysis suggests that spatial variation and poor habitats favour susceptible and polymorphic strains, populations with a variety of bacteriocin types. Toxin producers are favoured in good habitats since the rate of competition for resources is lower. Although most bacteriocins inhibit the growth of closely related bacteria, some, typified by those produced by lactic acid bacteria (LAB), exhibit a relatively broad antimicrobial spectrum and are active against several food-spoilage and health-threatening micro-organisms. Thus there is circumstantial evidence for a role in the regulation of competing bacteria.

The most general use of bacteriophages in the medical sphere has been to phage type bacterial strains of clinical importance. They have been studied since the 1940s and have provided basic information on how DNA and RNA genomes replicate and express genes. Because of the relative ease with which they can be grown, purified and now manipulated, they have become of primary importance (with plasmids) in the development of the molecular biological techniques used to clone and analyse genes and their products. Thus they have provided a basis for the development of the biotechnological era.

Those debating the risks of recombinant genes being transferred from genetically manipulated bacteria into indigenous bacterial populations now accept that transfer will occur. Although bacteriophages may be one class of the mediators of such gene exchange, it is still an open question as to how efficient they might be as mechanisms for exchange in situ or in vivo. It will be an interesting step in our ecological appreciation of these genetic determinants when their true ecological value to microbial populations can be demonstrated.

REFERENCES

Ackermann HW, 1983, Current problems in bacterial virus taxonomy, *A Critical Appraisal of Viral Taxonomy*, ed. Mathews REF, CRC Press, Boca Raton, FL, 105–22.

Adams MH, 1959, *The Bacteriophages*, Interscience Publishers Inc., New York.

Aoyama A, Hayashi M, 1986, Synthesis of bacteriophage ϕX174 *in vitro* mechanism of switch from DNA replication to DNA packaging, *Cell*, **47:** 99–106.

Barbas CF, Kang AS et al., 1991, Assembly of combinatorial antibody libraries on phage surfaces. The gene IV site, *Proc Natl Acad Sci USA*, **88:** 7978–82.

Benkerroum N, Ghouati Y et al., 1993, Methods to demonstrate the bacteriocidal activity of bacteriocins, *Lett Appl Microbiol*, **17:** 78–81.

Bergh O, Borsheim KY et al., 1989, High abundance of viruses found in aquatic environments, *Nature (London)*, **340:** 467–8.

Berkhout B, Schmidt BF et al., 1987, Lysis gene of bacteriophage MS2 is activated by translation termination at the overlapping coat gene, *J Mol Biol*, **195:** 517–24.

Bhattacharyya SP, Rao VB, 1993, A novel terminase activity associate with the DNA packaging protein gp17 of bacteriophage T4, *Virology*, **196:** 34–44.

Bierbaum G, Sahl HG, 1993, Lantibiotics – unusually modified bacteriocin-like peptides from gram-positive bacteria, *Int J Med Microbiol Virol Parasitol Infect Dis*, **278:** 1–22.

Delvesbroughton J, Williams GC, Williamson S, 1992, The use of bacteriocin, nisin, as a preservative in pasteurised liquid whole egg, *Lett Appl Microbiol*, **15:** 133–6.

D'Herelle R, 1917, Sur un microbe invisible antagoniste des bacilles dysentériques, *C R Acad Sci*, **165:** 373–5.

van Duin J, 1988, The single-stranded RNA bacteriophages, *The Bacteriophages*, vol. 1, ed. Calendar R, Plenum Publishing Corp., New York, 117–68.

Ebel-Tsipis J, Botsyein D, Fox MS, 1972, Generalised transduction by phage P22 in *Salmonella typhimurium*. 1 Molecular origin of transducing DNA, *J Mol Biol*, **71:** 433–48.

Eraso JM, Weinstock GM, 1992, Anaerobic control of colicin E1 production, *J Bacteriol*, **174:** 5101–9.

Ewert DL, Paynter MJB, 1980, Enumeration of bacteriophage and host bacteria in sewage and activated sludge treatment processes, *Appl Environ Microbiol*, **39:** 576–83.

Fath MJ, Kolter R, 1993, ABC transporters – bacterial exporters, *Microbiol Rev*, **57:** 995–1017.

Frank SA, 1994, Spatial polymorphism of bacteriocins and other allelopathic traits, *Evol Ecol*, **8:** 369–86.

Frederique P, 1957, Colicins, *Annu Rev Microbiol*, **11:** 7–22.

Gillis RR, 1964, Colicine production as an epidemiological marker of *Shigella sonnei*, *J Hyg*, **62:** 1–9.

Gilson L, Mahanty HR, Kotter R, 1990, Genetic analysis of an MDR-like export system: the secretion of ColV, *EMBO J*, **9:** 3875–84.

Goldberg RB, Bender RA, Streicher SL, 1974, Direct selection for P1-sensitive mutants of enteric bacteria, *J Bacteriol*, **118:** 810–14.

Goulian M, Kornberg A, Sinsheimer RL, 1967, Enzymatic synthesis of DNA XXIV. Synthesis of infectious phage ϕX174 DNA, *Proc Natl Acad Sci USA*, **58:** 2321–8.

Gratia A, 1925, Sur un remarquable example d'antagonisme entre deux souches de colibacille, *C R Soc Biol*, **93:** 1040.

Gratia A, Fredericq P, 1946, Diversité des souches antibiotiques de B coli et étendue variable de leur champ d'action, *C R Soc Biol*, **140:** 1032–3.

Hansen JN, 1993, Antibiotics synthesised by posttranslational modification, *Annu Rev Microbiol*, **47:** 535–64.

Harriman P, 1971, Appearance of transducing activity in P1 infected *Escherichia coli*, *Virology*, **45:** 324–5.

Harris LJ, Fleming HP, Klaenhammer TR, 1992, Developments in nisin research, *Food Res Int*, **25:** 57–66.

Haruna I, Spiegelman S, 1965, Specific template requirements of RNA replicases, *Proc Natl Acad Sci USA*, **54:** 579–87.

Hayashi M, Aoyama A et al., 1988, Biology of the bacteriophage ϕX174, *The Bacteriophages*, vol. 2, ed. Calendar R, Plenum Publishing Corp., New York, 1–72.

Hayashi M, Matsumoto H et al., 1994, Cytotoxin converting phage, Phi-ctx and PS21 are R-pyocin related phages, *FEMS Microbiol Lett*, **122:** 239–44.

Hechard Y, Renault D et al., 1993, Anti-listeria bacteriocins – a new family of proteins, *Lait*, **73:** 207–13.

Jack RW, Tagg JR, Ray MR, 1995, Bacteriocins of Gram-positive bacteria, *Microbiol Rev*, **59:** 171–200.

Jacob F, Woolman EL, 1953, Induction of phage development in lysogenic bacteria, *Cold Spring Harb Symp Quant Biol*, **18:** 101–21.

Jiminez-Diaz R, Rios-Sanchez RM et al., 1993, Plantaricins S and T, two new bacteriocins produced by *Lactobacillus plantarum* LPCO10 isolated from green olive fermentation, *Appl Environ Microbiol*, **59:** 1416–24.

Kastelein RA, Remaut E et al., 1982, Lysis gene expression of RNA phage MS2 depends on a frameshift during translation of the overlapping coat protein gene, *Nature (London)*, **285:** 35–41.

Kim WJ, 1993, Bacteriocins of lactic-acid bacteria – their potentials as food, *Food Rev Int*, **9:** 299–313.

Klienkauf H, von Dohren H, 1990, Nonribosomal biosynthesis of peptide antibiotics, *Eur J Biochem*, **192:** 1–15.

Lakey JH, Vandergoot FG, Pattus F, 1994, All in the family – the toxic activity of pore-forming colicins, *Toxicology*, **87:** 85–108.

Lakey JH, Gonzalezmanas JM et al., 1992, The membrane insertion of colicins, *FEBS Lett*, **307:** 26–9.

Lau PCK, Parsons M, Uchimura T, 1992, Molecular evolution of colicin plasmids with emphasis on the endonuclease types, *Bacteriocins and Lanbiotics*, ed. James R, NATO series, Springer-Verlag, Berlin–Heidelberg–New York.

Lennox ES, 1955, Transduction of linked genetic characters of the host by bacteriophage P1, *Virology*, **1:** 190–206.

Lewin BJ, 1987, *Genes III*, John Wiley & Sons, New York.

Lewus CB, Kiaser A, Montville TJ, 1991, Inhibition of food-borne bacteriocins by bacteriocins from lactic acid bacteria isolated from meat, *Appl Environ Microbiol*, **5:** 1683–8.

Lindquist BH, Dehó G, Calendar R, 1993, Mechanisms of genome propagation and helper exploitation by satellite phage P4, *Microbiol Rev*, **57:** 683–702.

Luria SE, Suit JL, 1987, Colicins and col plasmids, Escherichia coli *and* Salmonella typhimurium, *cellular and molecular biology*, ed. Neidhardt FC, American Society for Microbiology, Washington, DC, 1615–24.

Malkhosyan SR, Panchenko YA, Relesh AN, 1991, A physiological role for the DNA supercoiling in the anaerobic regulation of colicin gene expression, *Mol Gen Genet*, **225:** 342–5.

Margolin P, 1987, Generalized transduction, Escherichia coli *and* Salmonella typhimurium, *cellular and molecular biology*, ed. Neidhardt FC, American Society for Microbiology, Washington, DC, 1154–68.

Mathews CK, Kutter EM et al., 1983, *Bacteriophage T4*, American Society for Microbiology, Washington, DC.

Model P, Russell M, 1988, Filamentous bacteriophage, *The Bacteriophages*, vol. 2, ed. Calendar R, Plenum Publishing Corp., New York, 375–456.

Mosig G, Eiserling F, 1988, Phage T4 structure and metabolism, *The bacteriophage*, vol 2, ed. Calendar R, Plenum Publishing Corp., New York, 521–606.

Nishio C, Komura S, Kurahashi K, 1983, Peptide antibiotic subtilin is synthesised via precursor proteins, *Biochim Biophys Res Commun*, **116:** 751–8.

Nissen-Meyer J, Holo H et al., 1992, A novel lactococcal bacteriocin whose activity depends on the complimentary action of two peptides, *J Bacteriol*, **174:** 5686–92.

Ogunseitan OA, Sayler GS, Miller RV, 1990, Dynamic interactions of *Pseudomonas aeruginosa* and bacteriophages in lake water, *Microb Ecol*, **19:** 171–85.

Ozeki H, 1959, Chromosome fragments participating in transduction in *Salmonella typhimurium*, *Genetics*, **44:** 457–70.

Ozeki H, Ikeda H, 1968, Transduction mechanisms, *Annu Rev Genet*, **135:** 175–84.

Parker MT, 1972, Phage typing of *Staphyloccus aureus*, *Methods in Microbiology*, vol. 7b, eds Norris JR, Ribbons DW, Academic Press, London, 1–28.

Proctor LM, Fuhrman JA, 1990, Viral mortality of marine bacteria and cyanobacteria, *Nature (London)*, **343:** 60–2.

Pugsley AP, 1984a, The ins and outs of colicins. Part 1: production and translocation across membranes, *Microbiol Sci*, **1:** 168–75.

Pugsley AP, 1984b, The ins and outs of colicins. Part 2: lethal action, immunity and ecological implications, *Microbiol Sci*, **1:** 203–5.

Pugsley AP, Schwartz M, 1985, Export and secretion of proteins by bacteria, *FEMS Microbiol Rev*, **32:** 3–38.

Riley MA, 1993, Positive selection for colicin diversity in bacteria, *Mol Biol Evol*, **10:** 1048–59.

Roberts RJ, 1985, Restriction and modification enzymes and their recognition sequences, *Nucleic Acids Res*, **13, Suppl.:** r165–200.

Sano Y, Matsui H et al., 1993, Molecular-structures and functions of pyocin-s1 and pyocin-s2 in *Pseudomonas aeruginosa*, *J Bacteriol*, **175:** 2907–16.

Saye DJ, Miller RV, 1989, The aquatic environment: consider-ation of horizontal gene transmission in a diversified environment, *Gene Transfer in the Environment*, eds Levy SB, Miller RV, McGraw-Hill, New York, 223–59.

Schmeiger H, 1972, Phage P22 mutants with increased or decreased transduction abilities, *Mol Gen Genet*, **119:** 75–88.

Schmeiger H, 1982, Packaging signals for phage P22 on the chromosome of *Salmonella typhimurium*, *Mol Gen Genet*, **187:** 516–18.

Tagg JR, Dajani AS, Wannamaker LW, 1976, Bacteriocins of Gram-positive bacteria, *Bacteriol Rev*, **40:** 722–56.

Twort FW, 1915, An investigation on the nature of ultramicroscopic viruses, *Lancet*, **189:** 1241–3.

Van der Wal FJ, Luirick J, Oudega B, 1995, Bacteriocin release proteins: mode of action, structure and biotechnological application, *FEMS Microbiol Rev*, **17:** 381–99.

Vizan JL, Hernadez-chico C et al., 1991, The peptide antibiotic microcin B17 induces double stranded cleavage of DNA mediated by DNA gyrase, *EMBO J*, **10:** 467–76.

Weisberg RA, 1987, Specialized transduction, Escherichia coli *and* Samonella typhimurium*: Cellular and Molecular Biology*, vol. 2, eds Neidhardt FC, Ingraham JL et al., American Society for Microbiology, Washington, DC, Chapter 69.

Weisberg R, Landy A, 1983, Site specific recombination, *Llambda II*, eds Hendrix R, Roberts J et al., Cold Spring Harbor Laboratory, Cold Spring Harbor, New York.

Yarmolinsky MB, Sternberg N, 1988, Bacteriophage P1, *The Bacteriophages*, vol.1, ed. Calendar R, Plenum Publishing Corp., New York, 291–438.

Chapter 9

Antibiotics and Chemotherapeutic Agents Used in the Therapy of Bacterial Infection

D Greenwood

1 Historical background	6 Agents that act on the bacterial cell membrane
2 Classification of antibacterial agents in clinical use	7 Laboratory control of antimicrobial chemotherapy
3 Agents acting on bacterial cell wall synthesis	8 General aspects of the use of antimicrobial agents
4 Inhibitors of bacterial protein synthesis	
5 Inhibitors of bacterial nucleic acid synthesis	

1 HISTORICAL BACKGROUND

Strangely, the first really effective treatments for infectious diseases, quinine (from the bark of the cinchona tree) and emetine (from ipecacuanha root) were (and are) active, not against bacteria, but protozoa. Certain anthelminthic agents, including male fern (*Dryopteris filix-mas*) for tapeworm and various forms of 'wormwood' for intestinal roundworms, have also been known for centuries, probably because their ability to expel worms is evident to the naked eye.

By contrast, the development of potent antibacterial agents is a modern phenomenon. Since use of medicinal drugs is a universal human trait, natural remedies have, no doubt, been applied successfully to the treatment of bacterial infection among most, if not all, cultures throughout the world. There are, however, very few examples of antibacterial agents of proven efficacy in systemic disease before the twentieth century: chaulmoogra oil (a product obtained from the seeds of *Hydnocarpus* spp.) was used with some success in leprosy in India, and heavy metals (notably mercury in the treatment of syphilis) had been widely used in Europe since the sixteenth century by followers of the doctrines of the Swiss physician, Theophrastus Bombastus von Hohenheim (Paracelsus). At the end of the nineteenth century, the first report of the successful use of Urotropin (hexamine; methenamine) in cystitis was published (Nicolaier 1895). Apart from these examples, virtually all other traditional remedies were used only for topical application as antiseptics in skin diseases (Selwyn 1983).

During the early part of the twentieth century, progress was slow. Paul Ehrlich, the 'father of chemotherapy' had originally focused his attention on the possibility of using, first aniline dyes, then arsenicals, in malaria and trypanosomiasis, protozoan diseases that were of great importance to colonial powers, particularly those with territories in Africa. Ehrlich and his colleagues, Alfred Bertheim and Sahachiro Hata, tested many arsenical derivatives in an attempt to separate the toxic from the antimicrobial effects and the spirochaetes of chicken spirillosis and syphilis were included in their animal screening tests. In 1909 compound '606', arsphenamine, later marketed as Salvarsan, was shown to exhibit acceptable toxicity without loss of activity against *Treponema pallidum*. Neoarsphenamine (Neosalvarsan) followed in 1912.

1.1 Synthetic chemotherapeutic agents

SULPHONAMIDES

Paul Ehrlich had established his reputation with aniline dyes. He reasoned that, since parasites and tissues can be stained differentially, they must possess different receptors for the dyes, and this was the basis for his search for compounds that were 'parasitotrophic' rather than 'organotrophic' (Ehrlich and Hata 1911). This principle, **selective toxicity**, is fundamental to all antimicrobial chemotherapy.

The dyestuffs industry was particularly strong in Germany in the early years of the twentieth century and the dye companies, notably Friedrich Bayer, were expanding into pharmaceuticals (Beer 1958). Several antimalarial and other compounds were the among first fruits of this development (Dünschede 1971). In 1932, Gerhard Domagk, a bacteriologist in the Elberfeld laboratories of Bayer (by then part of the I G Farbenindustrie group), tested a red dye, provided by the firm's chemists, in mice experimentally infected with a virulent strain of *Streptococcus pyogenes*. The results, which were not made public until 1935 (Domagk 1935), showed unequivocally that the dye, Prontosil red, cured the mice of the otherwise lethal infection. Proof of the dye's efficacy in human infection quickly followed, notably from Leonard Colebrook's work on puerperal fever in young mothers (Colebrook and Kenny 1936).

Inexplicably, Prontosil had no effect against streptococci when tested in vitro. The solution to this mystery was solved by the Tréfouëls and their colleagues in France, who showed that the active substance was the colourless sulphanilamide group which was enzymically released from the dye complex in the body (Tréfouël et al. 1935).

OTHER SYNTHETIC ANTIBACTERIAL AGENTS

Despite much effort, no clinically useful antibacterial agent has yet emerged from any systematic programme of research aimed at designing compounds that would disable a defined vulnerable target within the bacterial cell.

Among the first synthetic agents to appear were the antituberculosis drugs, *p*-aminosalicylic acid (PAS) and isoniazid. Isoniazid and some other synthetic chemicals used in tuberculosis, including ethambutol and pyrazinamide, arose from research on thiosemicarbazones carried out in the course of investigations intended to improve the feeble tuberculostatic activity of sulphonamides (Fox 1953). Curiously, PAS, which is most closely related to the sulphonamides, arose from independent investigations on the physiology of tubercle bacilli (Lehmann 1946).

Among other synthetic agents, nalidixic acid, forerunner of the quinolone group of compounds, emerged from research on related antimalarial drugs (Siporin 1989); nitrofurans appear to have been investigated originally for their disinfectant properties (Dodd and Stillman 1944). Metronidazole, the first of the nitroimidazoles, was discovered by chemical synthesis of analogues of a naturally occurring antibiotic, azomycin, which exhibited activity against *Trichomonas* spp. (Cosar and Julou 1959, Editorial 1978). Efficacy of the compound against anaerobic bacteria was fortuitously recognized when a woman being treated for trichomonal vaginitis noticed that her ulcerative gingivitis had also been cured (Shinn 1962). Trimethoprim followed from work on the related antimalarial compound, pyrimethamine, which had itself been recognized among a group of folate antagonists originally investigated as anticancer compounds (Falco et al. 1951, Hitchins 1969).

1.2 Antibiotics

PENICILLIN AND OTHER β-LACTAM ANTIBIOTICS

Who discovered penicillin? Alexander Fleming is generally credited with the discovery; he certainly published the first clear description of the antibacterial activity of a substance produced by a *Penicillium* mould and gave it the name penicillin (Fleming 1929). However, the phenomenon of antibiosis was already well known at this time and there is good evidence that various predecessors of Fleming, the surgeon, Joseph Lister, and the physicist, John Tyndall, among them, were aware of the antibacterial properties of *Penicillium* (Selwyn 1979). The first documented use of penicillin dates from 1930, when C G Paine, a young doctor who had been a pupil of Fleming, successfully used a crude extract of *Penicillium* to treat ophthalmia neonatorum. The patients' notes are still extant (Wainwright and Swan 1986).

Whatever the truth of the matter of precedence for the discovery, the development of penicillin as a 'miracle drug' can be confidently attributed to Howard Florey, Ernst Chain and their colleagues at the Sir William Dunn School of Pathology in Oxford. Chain, a refugee biochemist from Germany, had been set the task of investigating bacteriolytic substances (including lysozyme, another of Fleming's discoveries), but the therapeutic potential of penicillin was rapidly revealed in a small but convincing series of tests in mice and men (Chain et al. 1940, Abraham et al. 1941).

The cephalosporins followed in the 1950s. Guiseppe Brotzu, of the Institute of Hygiene in Cagliari, Sardinia, isolated an antibiotic-producing mould from a local sewage outfall, and the discovery was brought, by a circuitous route, to the attention of Florey's team in Oxford. Edward Abraham and his colleagues found that most of the antibiotic activity was attributable to 2 compounds, neither of which was a cephalosporin. Cephalosporin C, the parent molecule of the cephalosporin family, was later detected as a minor product of the mould. It attracted attention chiefly because of its stability to staphylococcal penicillinase, which was at that time beginning to cause serious problems in hospitals (Abraham 1990).

The development of semi-synthetic penicillins was given a major boost by the demonstration that the phenylacetamido side chain of benzylpenicillin could be removed enzymically to provide the basic 6-aminopenicillanic acid nucleus to which other chemical groupings could be easily attached (Rolinson 1979); semi-synthetic cephalosporins were similarly produced from 7-aminocephalosporanic acid. Related compounds that shared the characteristic β-lactam ring structure of the penicillins and cephalosporins, including the cephamycins, clavams, carbapenems and monobactams, were discovered at regular intervals as naturally occurring molecules that could also be developed into clinically useful drugs, usually after chemical manipulation to improve their pharmacological properties. By the mid-1990s, about 80 different β-lactam antibiotics were in use around the world.

OTHER ANTIBIOTICS

In 1939 René Dubos, working at the Rockefeller Institute, New York, isolated an antibiotic complex, tyrothricin (later shown to be a mixture of 2 cyclic peptides, gramicidin and tyrocidine) from the soil organism *Bacillus brevis* (Dubos 1939, Hotchkiss 1990). Dubos had been a student of the Ukrainian émigré, Selman Waksman, a soil microbiologist at Rutgers University, who was interested in microbial antagonism. Stimulated by Dubos' success, he initiated a systematic search for naturally occurring inhibitory substances among soil micro-organisms, which achieved its greatest success when his research assistant, Albert Schatz, discovered streptomycin in 1943 (Schatz, Bugie and Waksman 1944, Wainwright 1990).

Streptomycin, with its activity against gram-negative bacilli and *Mycobacterium tuberculosis*, neatly complemented the spectrum of penicillin. The pharmaceutical industry, realizing the potential of these naturally occurring molecules, launched massive screening programmes, which rapidly yielded chloramphenicol (1947), chlortetracycline (1948), erythromycin (1952) and vancomycin (1956), among others. By the mid-1960s, most of the natural compounds now used in bacterial infection had been discovered.

1.3 Prospects for the future

At the close of the twentieth century, more than 250 antibacterial agents are in use throughout the world. With such an abundance at the prescribers' disposal it might be imagined that bacterial infection has become a minor problem and that bacterial drug resistance would be unable to keep pace with resources available to counteract it. Nothing could be further from the truth. Bacteria appear to possess a limitless ingenuity in avoiding the effects of antimicrobial agents, as well as in finding new ways to invade the compromised host. Moreover, mutations conferring resistance to one antibiotic can, at a stroke, render a whole drug family impotent. Bacteria resistant to one sulphonamide or one tetracycline are usually resistant to all sulphonamides, or all tetracyclines; 'methicillin-resistant' staphylococci are resistant to all β-lactam antibiotics. Even worse, bacteria can assemble resistance genes for unrelated classes of agents on plasmids that can be readily transmitted between bacterial species or, sometimes, genera (see Chapter 10).

For these reasons it is unwise to be complacent about our ability to control infection. Resistance is a serious global problem that must be countered by discriminating use of antimicrobial agents by all prescribers, by vigorous application of control of infection measures in hospitals, and at government level by effective regulation of drug production, distribution and use (Kunin 1993).

2 CLASSIFICATION OF ANTIBACTERIAL AGENTS IN CLINICAL USE

Since antibacterial agents exhibit a very wide variety of properties, the simplest way to categorize them is according to their site of action in the bacterial cell: agents acting on the bacterial cell wall; agents acting on bacterial protein synthesis; agents acting on nucleic acid synthesis; and agents acting on the bacterial cell membrane (Table 9.1).

3 AGENTS ACTING ON BACTERIAL CELL WALL SYNTHESIS

The bacterial cell wall is a structurally unique feature that is absent from mammalian cells and is thus a prime target for selectively toxic agents. The cell wall of gram-negative organisms is very different from that of gram-positive bacteria (see Chapter 2) and the complex of lipopolysaccharide and lipoprotein that forms the gram-negative outer-membrane confers properties of differential permeability that has a profound effect on the susceptibility to antibacterial agents of all kinds (Nikaido and Vaara 1985, Hancock and Bellido 1992). Within the gram-negative outer membrane are hydrophilic channels (porins) that allow the differential passage of many agents whose target is the underlying peptidoglycan. Permeation of these porin channels by β-lactam antibiotics depends on molecular size and ionic charge and these factors may strongly influence the spectrum of activity and potency (Nikaido 1985). Glycopeptides are too large to penetrate the gram-negative outer membrane, and consequently their spectrum of activity is virtually restricted to gram-positive organisms.

3.1 β-Lactam antibiotics

Structure

Antibacterial agents that share the structural feature of a β-lactam ring are now known to be very diverse. The classic penicillins are penams, characterized by a fused heterocyclic structure composed of a β-lactam ring and a 5-membered sulphur-containing thiazolidine ring. In the cephalosporins the fused dihydrothiazine ring has an extra carbon with an unsaturated bond between C-3 and C-4, giving a cephem structure. The cephamycins are similar, but the β-lactam ring is substituted with a methoxy group which confers stability to many β-lactamase enzymes. Other structural variants represented among clinically useful compounds are: carbapenems, carbacephems, oxacephems, clavams, sulphones and monocyclic monobactams (Fig. 9.1).

Mode of action

All β-lactam antibiotics interfere with bacterial cell wall synthesis, but the effect on gram-positive and gram-negative bacteria is very different because of the

Table 9.1 Classification of antibacterial agents according to their site of action

Cell wall synthesis	Protein synthesis	Nucleic acid synthesis	Cell membrane
Penicillins	Aminoglycosides	Sulphonamides[a]	Polymyxins
Cephalosporins	Chloramphenicol	Diaminopyrimidines[a]	Gramicidin
Other β-lactams	Tetracyclines	Quinolones	Tyrocidine
Glycopeptides	Macrolides	Rifamycins	Valinomycin[b]
Bacitracin	Lincosamides	Nitroimidazoles	Monensin[b]
Cycloserine	Fusidic acid	Nitrofurans	
Fosfomycin	Streptogramins	Novobiocin	
Isoniazid	Mupirocin		

[a]Indirect action on nucleic acid synthesis.
[b]Not used in human medicine.

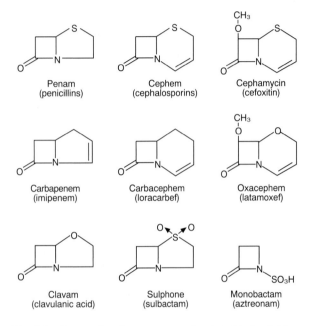

Fig. 9.1 Core molecular structures of various kinds of β-lactam antibiotics (examples in parentheses). (From Greenwood D (ed.), 1995a, *Antimicrobial Chemotherapy*, 3rd edn, Oxford University Press, Oxford).

differing nature of their cell walls. In the simplest terms, β-lactam antibiotics interfere with the final transpeptidation reaction that forms the cross-link between adjacent peptidoglycan strands and gives the cell wall its essential rigidity. Various forms of transpeptidase exist depending on whether cell wall structure is engaged in extension of the cylinder of rod-shaped cells, forming the poles of the cell, or separating the 2 daughter cells during the division process. Realization that β-lactam antibiotics affected all of these processes came from studies that showed concentration-dependent effects on the morphological response of gram-negative bacilli (Greenwood and O'Grady 1973a); by observation that certain β-lactam agents were anomalous in the morphological effects they produced (Greenwood and O'Grady 1973b); and by the demonstration of differential affinity of β-lactam agents for penicillin-binding proteins (PBPs) in isolated cell membranes (Spratt 1975). The morphological consequences of binding to various PBPs of

Escherichia coli are shown in Fig. 9.2. PBPs have been investigated in many gram-positive and gram-negative bacteria. Although their number and molecular size vary considerably, they are always present in multiple forms.

β-Lactam antibiotics are normally bactericidal drugs, but the mechanism of bactericidal activity seems to be different in gram-negative and gram-positive bacteria. In gram-negative rods, cell death can be quantitatively prevented by provision of adequate osmotic protection (Greenwood and O'Grady 1972), so that the mechanism appears to be simple osmotic lysis of bacteria deprived of their normal cell wall. In gram-positive cocci the situation is more complicated: exposure to β-lactam agents causes a loss of lipoteichoic acid from the wall and this seems to remove control from normal autolytic processes that dismantle the peptidoglycan (Tomasz 1979).

Certain strains of gram-positive cocci succumb to the bactericidal effects of penicillin and other β-lactam agents more slowly than usual. Such strains have been dubbed **tolerant** to penicillin (Sabath et al. 1977, Handwerger and Tomasz 1985). Penicillin tolerance may have some relevance in the treatment of bacterial endocarditis or in other situations in which a bactericidal effect is crucial to therapeutic success.

Other in vitro phenomena that have been described with β-lactam antibiotics include: **persistence** (Bigger 1944, Greenwood 1972), in which a small proportion of the bacterial population escapes the lethal effects of penicillin; **Eagle's paradoxical effect** (Eagle and Musselman 1948) in which high concentrations of penicillins may have a lesser bactericidal effect on gram-positive cocci than lower concentrations; and the **post-antibiotic effect** (Bundtzen et al. 1981, Craig and Gudmundsson 1991) in which the inhibitory effect may persist for a short period (usually about 1 h) after the antibiotic is removed. The clinical significance, if any, of these effects remains to be defined.

Resistance to β-lactam antibiotics

The most common form of resistance to β-lactam agents is caused by enzymes that render the molecules inactive by opening the β-lactam ring. In staphylococci the enzymes involved are inducible exoenzymes that conform to a small number of related types. In contrast, the β-lactamases of gram-negative bacilli vary

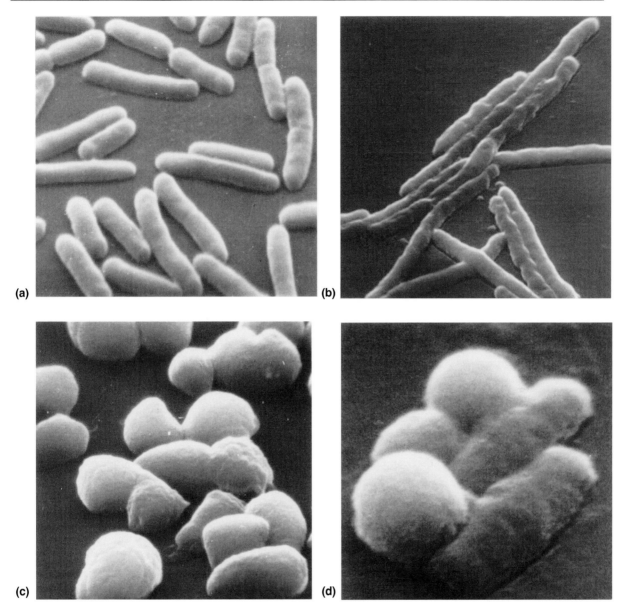

Fig. 9.2 Morphological effects of β-lactam antibiotics in *Escherichia coli*: (a) normal cells (no antibiotic); (b) filamentation caused by cephalexin (binding to PBP-3); (c) generalized effect on cell wall caused by mecillinam (binding to PBP-2); (d) formation of osmotically fragile spheroplasts caused by cephalexin and mecillinam in combination (binding to PBP-2 and PBP-3). Most β-lactam antibiotics, in sufficient concentration, also bind to the PBP-1 complex and cause rapid lysis of susceptible gram-negative bacilli.

greatly in their physicochemical characteristics. Indeed, all gram-negative bacilli appear to exhibit some β-lactamase activity as a chromosomally encoded genetic feature. These inherent β-lactamases may be inducible and certain β-lactam antibiotics, notably cefoxitin, are particularly efficient inducers.

There have been various attempts to classify β-lactamases, particularly the many types found in gram-negative rods (Ambler 1980, Richmond and Sykes 1973, Bush 1989). The latest comprehensive classification scheme recognizes 4 separate molecular types and several functional groupings (Bush, Jacoby and Medeiros 1995).

Although these classification schemes attempt to include all the known types of β-lactamases, and are

therefore quite complex, most of the enzymes that commonly cause problems in clinical isolates of gram-negative bacilli belong to a few related types that share the feature of having serine at the active site and are susceptible to inhibition by clavulanic acid and other β-lactamase inhibitors. Most common of all are the TEM-l and TEM-2 enzymes found widely among enterobacteria and elsewhere, and SHV-l, found predominantly in *Klebsiella pneumoniae*. Many variants of the TEM enzymes have arisen, often by single amino acid substitutions, and these may exhibit extended, or idiosyncratic, substrate ranges. TEM-1 itself, and some other β-lactamases, have found their way onto transposons and this has aided their transmission and spread. Bacterial β-lactamases that are able to hydrolyse carbapenems like imipenem are unusual in that they are zinc-requiring metalloenzymes that are not susceptible to β-lactamase inhibitors (Payne 1993). They are presently found most commonly in *Bacteroides fragilis* and in *Stenotrophomonas* (*Xanthomonas*) *maltophilia*, and are classified by Bush et al. (1995) as a separate molecular class B (group 3).

Resistance to β-lactam antibiotics can arise by means other than β-lactamases. Alterations in porins in the outer membrane of gram-negative bacilli can affect transport of β-lactam antibiotics to their site of action (Nikaido 1985). More importantly, mutations affecting the structure of PBPs can alter their affinity to β-lactam compounds so that inhibitory effects become much less efficient. This, for example, is the mechanism of resistance in 'methicillin-resistant' *Staphylococcus aureus* and in strains of *Streptococcus pneumoniae* that display reduced susceptibility to penicillin (Klugman 1990, Jacoby and Archer 1991).

Toxicity and side effects

Since the β-lactam antibiotics act on a target (bacterial peptidoglycan) that is absent from mammalian cells, they are among the least toxic of all antimicrobial agents. The most troublesome side effect is hypersensitivity, which can range from relatively trivial rashes to life-threatening anaphylactic reactions. Only about 10% of patients hypersensitive to penicillins are cross-allergic to cephalosporins. Ampicillin and amoxycillin commonly give rise to a maculopapular rash when given to patients with glandular fever; this is not a true hypersensitivity reaction and is not a contraindication to subsequent use of a penicillin. Various other side effects are occasionally encountered. A fuller discussion is provided in the standard texts (Kucers and Bennett 1987, Dollery 1991, O'Grady et al. 1997).

PENICILLINS

Classification and spectrum of activity

The various penicillins differ in the nature of the side chain at the C-6 position of the molecule. All except mecillinam (amdinocillin), in which the side chain is joined in an amidino linkage, are acyl derivatives of 6-aminopenicillanic acid (Fig. 9.3).

The original penicillin, benzylpenicillin (penicillin G), has a phenylacetamido group at the 6-amino position. It exhibits exceptionally good activity against the classic pyogenic cocci: staphylococci, streptococci (including pneumococci and enterococci), meningococci and gonococci. It is also very active against spirochaetes, most anaerobes (but not *Bacteroides* spp.) and many gram-positive bacilli. Enterobacteria, *Haemophilus influenzae*, *Pseudomonas aeruginosa* and obligate intracellular bacteria are mostly insensitive.

The chief imperfections of penicillin are: lability to gastric acid, so that it cannot be given orally; an exceptionally short plasma half-life; susceptibility to staphylococcal β-lactamase; and a restricted spectrum of activity. Subsequent developments of penicillin have sought to overcome these shortcomings and presently available compounds can be categorized

into several groups with distinctive properties (Table 9.2).

The long-acting salts of penicillin are poorly soluble depot preparations that are injected intramuscularly and release benzylpenicillin slowly from the injection site. In this way, procaine penicillin can maintain a concentration of penicillin inhibitory to many sensitive organisms for up to 24 h. Benzathine and benethamine penicillin are even less soluble and liberate small amounts of penicillin over several days. An alternative way of sustaining penicillin levels in plasma is by the concurrent administration of probenecid, which competes for the active tubular secretion sites in the kidneys.

Oral derivatives of penicillin, notably phenoxymethylpenicillin (penicillin V), have antibacterial properties very similar to those of benzylpenicillin.

The antistaphylococcal penicillins, of which the isoxazolyl derivatives, oxacillin, cloxacillin, dicloxacillin and flucloxacillin, are most widely used, were designed to overcome the problem of enzymic resistance in staphylococci. They are intrinsically less active than benzylpenicillin and, although they retain adequate antistreptococcal activity, their use is largely restricted to infections with penicillinase-producing staphylococci, which now account for more than 80% of all isolates.

The first successful extension of the spectrum of benzylpenicillin was achieved in 1961 with the α-amino derivative, ampicillin (Rolinson and Stevens 1961). Unlike the parent compound, ampicillin exhibited useful activity against some gram-negative bacilli, including *H. influenzae*, *E. coli*, *Salmonella* spp. and *Shigella* spp., but not *Klebsiella* spp. or *P. aeruginosa*. Amoxycillin, which is better absorbed when administered orally, followed in 1970. In the meantime, the first penicillin to exhibit (albeit weak) antipseudomonal activity, carbenicillin, the α-carboxy derivative of benzylpenicillin, was described (Knudsen, Rolinson and Sutherland 1967). The thienyl variant of carbenicillin, ticarcillin, and a series of acylureido derivatives of ampicillin (azlocillin, mezlocillin, piperacillin and apalcillin), all of which display improved antipseudomonal activity, were developed later. None of these compounds is stable to staphylococcal β-lactamase.

Among penicillins that possess an idiosyncratic spectrum of activity that excludes gram-positive cocci and anaerobes are the amidinopenicillin, mecillinam, and temocillin, a compound structurally similar to ticarcillin, but rendered stable to enterobacterial β-lactamases by incorporation of a methoxy group onto the β-lactam ring (cf. cefoxitin and other cephamycins). Neither mecillinam nor temocillin has any useful activity against *P. aeruginosa*.

Pharmacological properties

Most penicillins are absorbed erratically when given orally, often because of hydrolysis by gastric acid. Phenoxymethylpenicillin and related compounds are acid stable, and are used as oral substitutes for benzylpenicillin. Among isoxazolyl penicillins, flucloxacillin achieves the highest plasma concentrations after

PENICILLINS

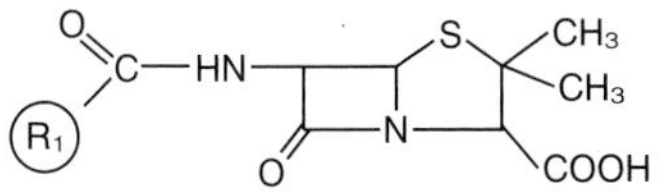

UREIDO PENICILLINS

Benzylpenicillin
(Penicillin G)

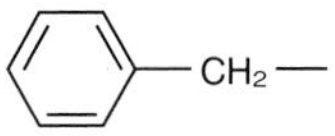

Phenoxymethylpenicillin
(Penicillin V)

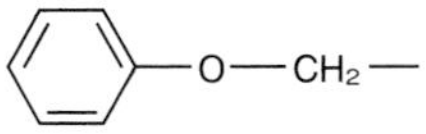

Phenethicillin

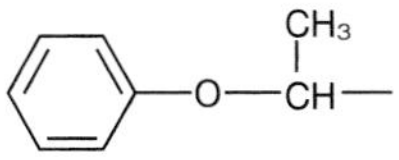

Azlocillin

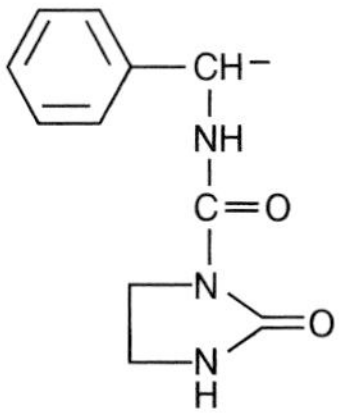

Mezlocillin

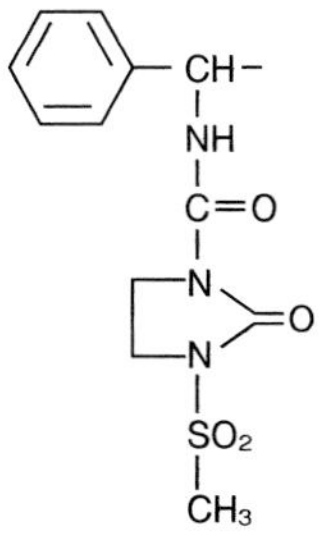

Piperacillin

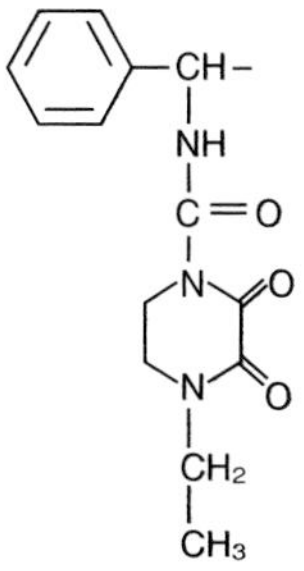

AMINO PENICILLINS

Ampicillin

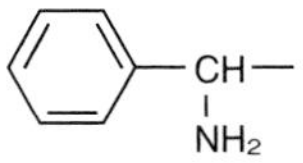

Amoxycillin

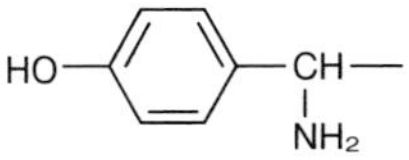

CARBOXY PENICILLINS

Carbenicillin

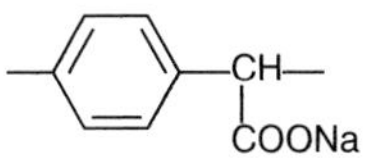

Ticarcillin

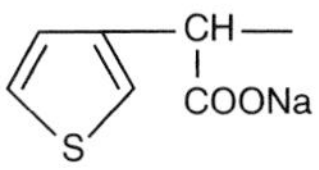

OTHER PENICILLINS (FULL STRUCTURES)

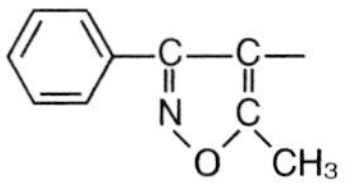

Temocillin

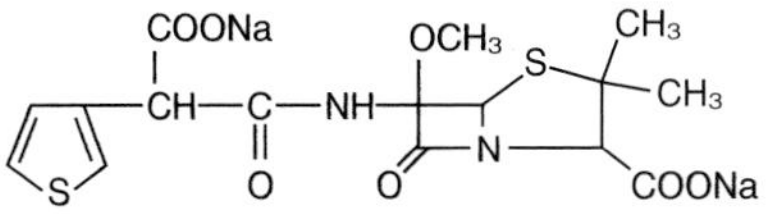

ANTISTAPHYLOCOCCAL PENICILLINS

Methicillin

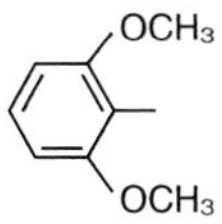

Cloxacillin

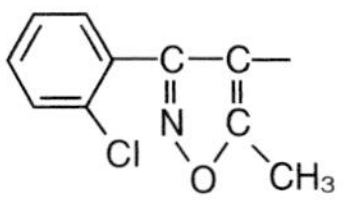

Flucloxacillin

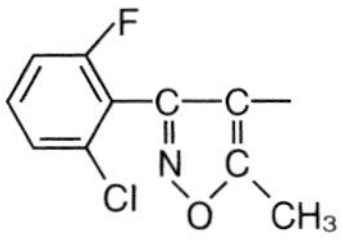

Mecillinam

Oxacillin

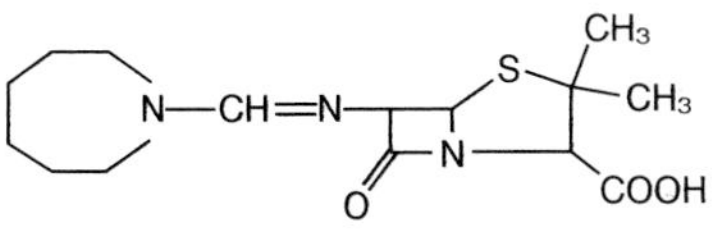

Fig. 9.3 Structures of the most important penicillins.

Table 9.2 Categorization of the most important penicillins in clinical use

Benzylpenicillin (penicillin G)
Long-acting salts (depot preparations)
Procaine penicillin
Benzathine penicillin
Benethamine penicillin
Acid-stable (oral) derivatives
Phenoxymethylpenicillin (penicillin V)
Azidocillin
Phenethicillin
Propicillin
Antistaphylococcal penicillins (stable to staphylococcal β-lactamase)
Methicillin
Cloxacillin
Flucloxacillin
Oxacillin
Dicloxacillin
Nafcillin
Penicillins with activity against enterobacteria
Ampicillin (and esters)
Amoxycillin
Mecillinam (and ester)
Ciclacillin
Epicillin
Penicillins that are stable to enterobacterial β-lactamases[a]
Temocillin
Penicillins with activity against *Pseudomonas aeruginosa*
Carbenicillin (and esters)
Ticarcillin
Azlocillin
Mezlocillin
Piperacillin
Apalcillin

[a]Ampicillin, amoxycillin, ticarcillin and piperacillin are also formulated with β-lactamase inhibitors that confer the property of stability to enterobacterial β-lactamases.

oral administration. About 30% of an oral dose of ampicillin is absorbed, but this can be much improved by esterification of the carboxyl group. These ampicillin esters, talampicillin, pivampicillin, bacampicillin and lenampicillin, are inactive prodrugs that are de-esterified during passage through the intestinal mucosa with liberation of ampicillin into the bloodstream. Prodrug esters of carbenicillin and mecillinam have also been produced as oral formulations.

Benzylpenicillin and phenoxymethylpenicillin are extremely rapidly excreted, with a plasma half-life of about 30 min. Most other penicillins exhibit elimination half-lives of around 30 min to 1.5 h. Temocillin has an unusually extended half-life of c. 4–5 h. Protein binding is generally less than 50%; the isoxazolylpenicillins are extensively (>90%) protein-bound in plasma, but this does not seem to adversely affect their therapeutic activity.

Penicillins do not penetrate the intact blood–brain barrier well, but in the presence of meningeal inflammation concentrations are sufficient to treat pyogenic meningitis and benzylpenicillin (meningococcal and pneumococcal meningitis) and ampicillin (haemophilus meningitis) have been widely used for this purpose.

CEPHALOSPORINS

Classification and spectrum of activity

Since they first became available in the mid-1960s, the cephalosporins have developed more diversely than any other group of antimicrobial agents. They have overlapping properties that defy any rigid classification, but can usefully be divided into 6 broad classes (Table 9.3). In the cephalosporins, the extra carbon of the dihydrothiazine ring carries an additional side chain, the nature of which often affects the pharmacokinetic behaviour of the molecule and, in some cases, the toxicity. Structures of some of the commonly used cephalosporins are shown in Fig. 9.4. As a group the cephalosporins have certain properties in common: relative stability to staphylococcal β-lactamase; broad spectrum activity that encompasses most enterobacteria, including *Klebsiella* spp.; and lack of activity against enterococci.

Like the penicillins, cephalosporins interfere with bacterial cell wall synthesis through binding to PBPs. Some cephalosporins, notably cephalexin and cephradine, bind almost exclusively to PBP-3, which has the effect of halting division, but not growth, of susceptible gram-negative bacilli. Consequently, these cephalosporins are much more slowly bactericidal than the others.

Parenteral cephalosporins

The first cephalosporins, cephalothin and cephaloridine, modestly expanded the spectrum of ampicillin (e.g. to include *Klebsiella* spp.) and possessed relative stability to staphylococcal β-lactamase. Some later derivatives offered little, if any, improvement, but cephazolin exhibited the unusual characteristic of achieving enhanced concentrations in bile and cephamandole offered partial resistance to some enterobacterial β-lactamases.

The first major improvement in cephalosporins came with the introduction of compounds that displayed stability to a wide range of enterobacterial β-lactamases. One such compound, cefoxitin, is a semi-synthetic derivative of a naturally occurring compound in which the β-lactam ring is substituted with a methoxy grouping that confers stability to the structure. Such compounds are called **cephamycins**; various examples, including cefotetan, cefbuperazone, cefmetazole and cefminox, are in use around the world. They are unusual among cephalosporins in their activity against *B. fragilis*.

β-Lactamase stability was achieved in a different way by pharmaceutical chemists who found that addition of a methoximino group to the side chain on 7-amino-cephalosporanic acid also protected the β-lactam ring from enzymic attack. The first cephalosporin of this

Table 9.3 Categorization of cephalosporins in clinical use

Cephalosporins					
Parenteral compounds			**Oral compounds**		
Cephalothin	Cephacetrile	Ceforanide	Cephalexin		Cephaloglycin
Cephaloridine	Cefapirin	Cefonicid	Cephradine		Cefatrizine
Cephazolin	Cefazedone		Cefaclor		Cefroxadine
Cephamandole	Ceftezole		Cefadroxil		Cefprozil
Compounds with improved β-lactamase stability			**Compounds with improved β-lactamase stability**		
				Non-esterified	**Esterified**
Cefuroxime	Cefmetazole[a]	Cefotiam		Cefixime	Cefuroxime axetil
Cefoxitin[a]	Cefbuperazone[a]			Ceftibuten	Cefpodoxime proxetil
Cefotetan[a]	Cefminox[a]			Cefdinir	Cefetamet pivoxil
					Cefteram pivoxil
Compounds with improved intrinsic activity and β-lactamase stability					
Cefotaxime	Cefmenoxime				
Ceftizoxime	Cefodizime				
Ceftriaxone	Latamoxef[b]				
Compounds distinguished by activity against *Pseudomonas aeruginosa*					
Broad spectrum		**Medium spectrum**		**Narrow spectrum**	
Ceftazidime		Cefoperazone		Cefsulodin	
Cefpirome		Cefpimazole			
Cefepime		Cefpiramide			

[a]Cephamycins.
[b]Oxacephem.
Adapted from Greenwood (1995).

type was cefuroxime, but this was quickly followed by a family of compounds, of which cefotaxime was the forerunner, in which the side chain carried an amino-thiazole group as well as the methoximino substitution. The effect of this was not only to provide β-lactamase stability, but also to much improve the intrinsic antibacterial activity, particularly against enterobacteria. Activity of these compounds against *P. aeruginosa* is, however, poor, but some later derivatives, notably ceftazidime, include this organism in the spectrum. Cefsulodin is unique in exhibiting good anti-pseudomonal activity, but little or no useful activity against other organisms.

Oral cephalosporins

Few cephalosporins are absorbed when administered by the oral route. Cephalexin was the first of those that are well absorbed; it exhibits modest antibacterial activity against a wide spectrum of gram-positive and gram-negative bacteria, but is slowly bactericidal to enterobacteria because of its preferential affinity for penicillin-binding protein 3 (see above). It has no useful activity against *P. aeruginosa*, *H. influenzae* or *B. fragilis*. Most other oral cephalosporins are structurally similar to cephalexin and, not surprisingly, share its limitations. Cefaclor is unusual in displaying useful activity against *H. influenzae*. Attempts have been made

to improve the intrinsic activity of oral cephalosporins, or to esterify parenteral compounds to enhance their absorption. Cefixime and ceftibuten display much improved activity against enterobacteria, but have some important weaknesses in their gram-positive spectrum, in particular in their poor activity against staphylococci, enterococci and some streptococci.

Pharmacological properties

Cephalosporins, like penicillins, are generally excreted rapidly by the kidneys with elimination half-lives that usually range from 1 to 2 h. The expanded spectrum compound, ceftriaxone, is unusual in that its plasma half-life is about 6–8 h. Cephazolin, cefoperazone and ceftriaxone are notable in achieving significant concentrations in bile. Those cephalosporins that carry an acetoxymethyl group at C-3 (including cephalothin and cefotaxime) are susceptible to hepatic enzymes which deacetylate the molecule to the corresponding hydroxymethyl derivative. This reduces the inherent antibacterial activity, but there is little evidence that this affects the therapeutic potency. Some other cephalosporins, cephamandole, cefotetan and cefoperazone among them, have a nitrogen-rich tetramethylthiomethyl substituent at C-3. Compounds with this feature have been implicated in hypo-

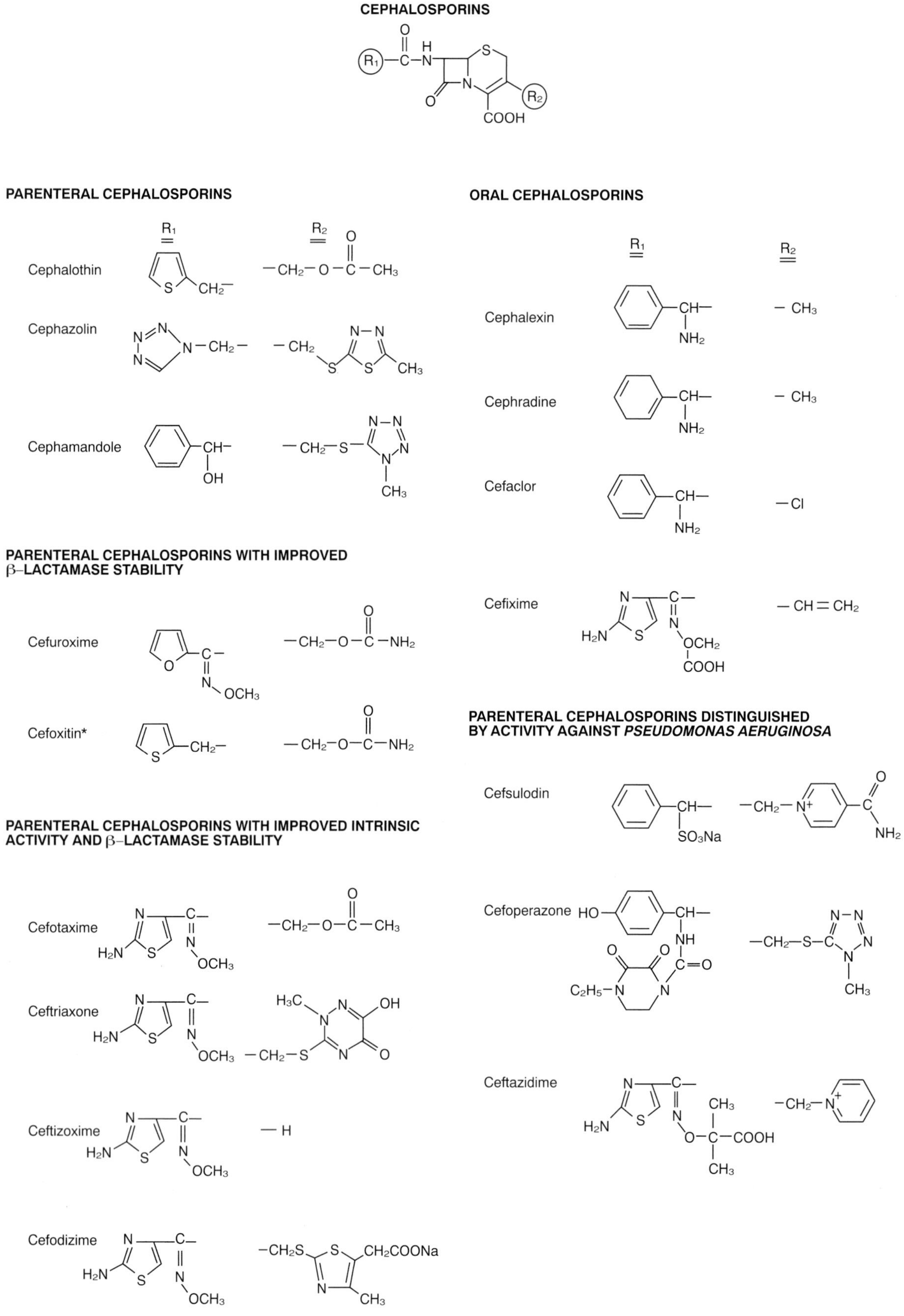
CEPHALOSPORINS
PARENTERAL CEPHALOSPORINS
Cephalothin
Cephazolin
Cephamandole
PARENTERAL CEPHALOSPORINS WITH IMPROVED β-LACTAMASE STABILITY
Cefuroxime
Cefoxitin*
PARENTERAL CEPHALOSPORINS WITH IMPROVED INTRINSIC ACTIVITY AND β-LACTAMASE STABILITY
Cefotaxime
Ceftriaxone
Ceftizoxime
Cefodizime
ORAL CEPHALOSPORINS
Cephalexin
Cephradine
Cefaclor
Cefixime
PARENTERAL CEPHALOSPORINS DISTINGUISHED BY ACTIVITY AGAINST PSEUDOMONAS AERUGINOSA
Cefsulodin
Cefoperazone
Ceftazidime

* Cefoxitin (a cephamycin) also has a methoxy group on the β-lactam ring.

Fig. 9.4 Structures of the most important cephalosporins.

prothrombinaemia that is reversible by administration of vitamin K (Lipsky 1988).

Cephalosporins penetrate poorly into cerebrospinal fluid after intravenous administration, but some, notably cefotaxime, ceftriaxone and cefuroxime, achieve sufficient concentration in the CSF in the presence of inflammation for them to be useful for intravenous treatment in bacterial meningitis.

OTHER β-LACTAM ANTIBIOTICS

Several variants on the β-lactam theme other than penams (penicillins) and cephems (cephalosporins and cephamycins) are in therapeutic use (Fig. 9.5).

β-Lactamase inhibitors

Certain molecules that possess a β-lactam ring, including the naturally occurring antibiotic, clavulanic acid, and the penicillanic acid sulphones, sulbactam and tazobactam, are noteworthy not for their intrinsic antibacterial activity, but because they have a high affinity for, and stability to, bacterial β-lactamases. These agents are formulated with β-lactamase labile partner compounds to secure their activity against otherwise resistant organisms: clavulanic acid with amoxycillin (co-amoxiclav) or ticarcillin; sulbactam with ampicillin (or with cefoperazone in some countries); tazobactam with piperacillin.

Carbapenems, carbacephems, oxacephems

In the mid-1970s, a potent, broad spectrum β-lactam compound, thienamycin, was found as a naturally occurring product of *Streptomyces cattleya* (Kahan et al. 1979). The substance, which was found to possess an unusual carbapenem ring structure, was, unfortunately, inherently unstable, but this was overcome by synthesis of the *N*-formimidoyl derivative, imipenem (Kahan et al. 1983) (see Fig. 9.5). Imipenem has exceptionally good activity against most gram-positive and gram-negative bacteria, including organisms like enterococci, *P. aeruginosa* and *B. fragilis* that are resistant to most cephalosporins. It is very stable in the presence of bacterial β-lactamases, but by a strange trick of nature it is hydrolysed by a dehydropeptidase located in the brush border of the mammalian kidney and has to be given with a dehydropeptidase inhibitor, cilastatin (Kahan et al. 1983). A related carbapenem, meropenem, is not susceptible to dehydropeptidase and is therefore administered alone. These compounds are not absorbed when given by mouth and are administered parenterally. Resistance to carbapenems is uncommon, but they are hydrolysed by metallo-β-lactamases produced by strains of *S. maltophilia* and some *B. fragilis*. Methicillin-resistant staphylococci and penicillin-resistant enterococci are usually refractory to carbapenems.

The possibility of synthesizing carbacephems and oxacephems has also been explored. Two such compounds, loracarbef (a carbacephem) and latamoxef (an oxacephem), have been developed (Fig. 9.5). Loracarbef can be given orally, but does not have the breadth of spectrum or the β-lactamase stability of the carbapenems; its activity and use are similar to those of cefaclor, to which it is related structurally. Latamoxef (also known as moxalactam) is a parenteral compound that exhibits properties similar to those of the expanded spectrum cephalosporins such as cefotaxime, but including *B. fragilis* within the spectrum. It has a methyltetrazole group at C-3 and the associated bleeding problems (see above) have restricted its popularity.

Monobactams

The idea of developing therapeutically useful compounds in which the β-lactam ring was not fused with another cyclic structure was once thought to be unlikely, if not impossible. Therefore, it came as a surprise when naturally occurring compounds with this feature were described. Only one such compound is in therapeutic use, the semi-synthetic monobactam, aztreonam (Fig. 9.5). In marked contrast to the ultrabroad spectrum of the carbapenems, aztreonam is a narrow spectrum agent, the useful activity of which is restricted to enterobacteria and *P. aeruginosa*. It is administered parenterally. Aztreonam specifically inhibits penicillin-binding protein 3 in *E. coli* and causes filamentation of susceptible gram-negative bacilli, which are killed slowly.

3.2 Glycopeptide antibiotics

STRUCTURE AND SPECTRUM OF ACTIVITY

Two glycopeptides, vancomycin and teicoplanin, are in clinical use. A related compound, avoparcin, is used as a growth promoter in animal husbandry. They are complex heterocyclic compounds composed of a heptapeptide substituted with certain sugars, one of which, in teicoplanin, carries a fatty acid chain (Fig. 9.6). The molecule is too large to penetrate the outer membrane of gram-negative bacilli, although some gram-negative anaerobic bacilli are anomalously sensitive, particularly to teicoplanin (Greenwood et al. 1988). Nearly all gram-positive organisms are susceptible, although some genera, including *Lactobacillus*, *Pediococcus* and *Leuconostoc*, are intrinsically resistant (Ruoff et al. 1988). They are mainly used in serious infection with staphylococci and enterococci that are resistant to other drugs. Oral vancomycin has been used in antibiotic-associated colitis in which *Clostridium difficile* is implicated, but this is no longer recommended.

MODE OF ACTION

Glycopeptides prevent the transfer of peptidoglycan building blocks to the growing cell wall by binding to the acyl-D-alanyl-D-alanine terminus of the pentapeptide side chain (Reynolds 1989).

RESISTANCE

Acquired resistance in normally susceptible gram-positive species is uncommon, but there are many reports of resistance in enterococci (Johnson et al. 1990), and coagulase-negative staphylococci (Sanyal et al. 1993). In enterococci, resistance is associated with enzymic

β-LACTAMASE INHIBITORS

Clavulanic acid

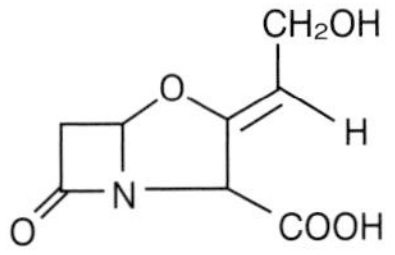

Sulbactam

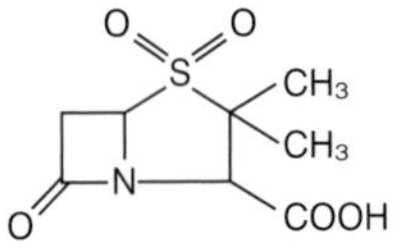

Tazobactam

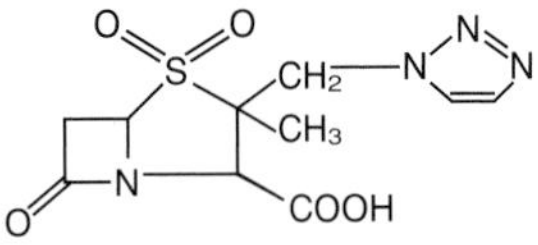

OXACEPHEM

Latamoxef

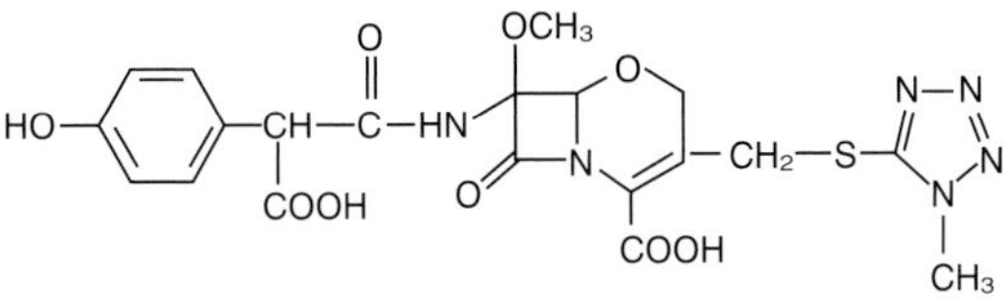

CARBACEPHEM

Loracarbef

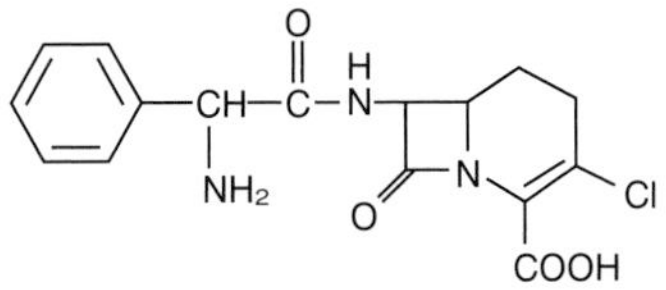

CARBAPENEMS

Imipenem

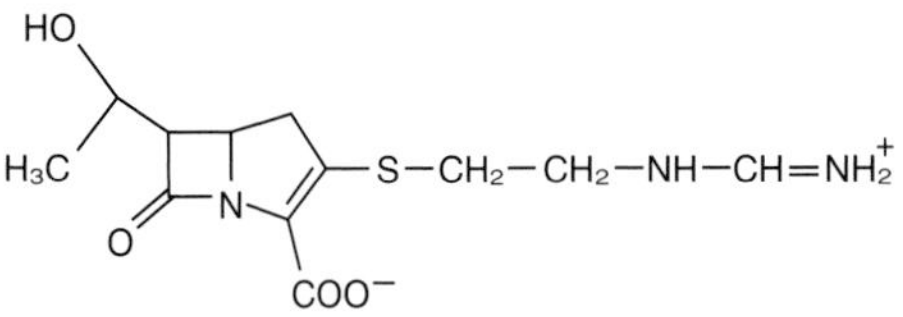

Meropenem

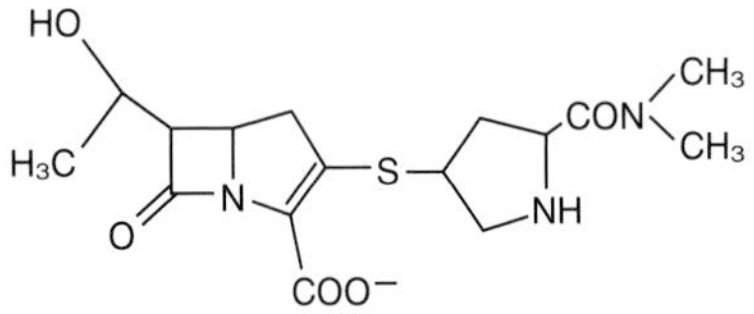

MONOBACTAM

Aztreonam

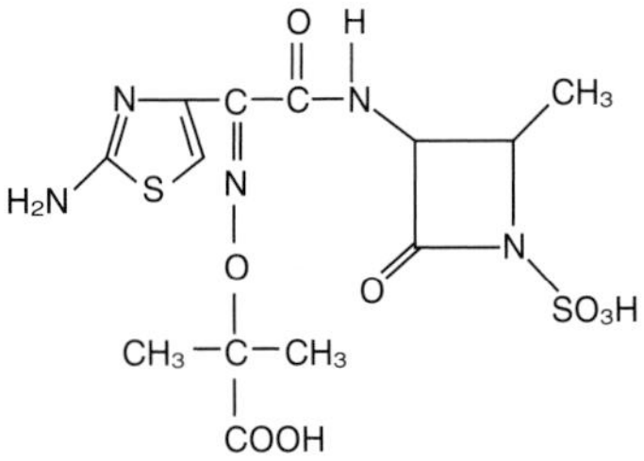

DEHYDROPEPTIDASE INHIBITOR (USED WITH IMIPENEM)

Cilastatin

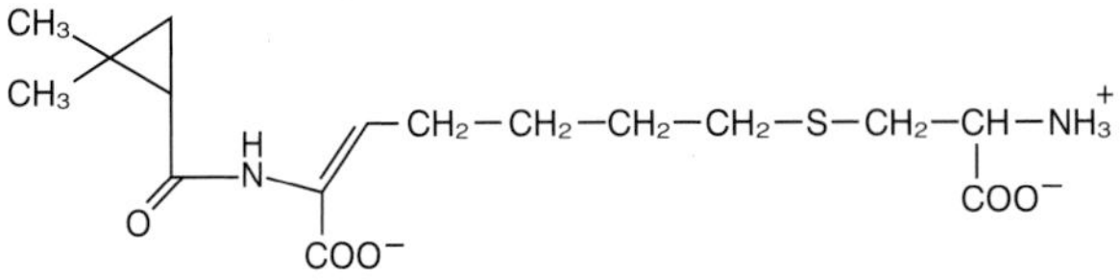

Fig. 9.5 Structures of important β-lactam compounds other than penicillins and cephalosporins, and of the dehydropeptidase inhibitor cilastatin.

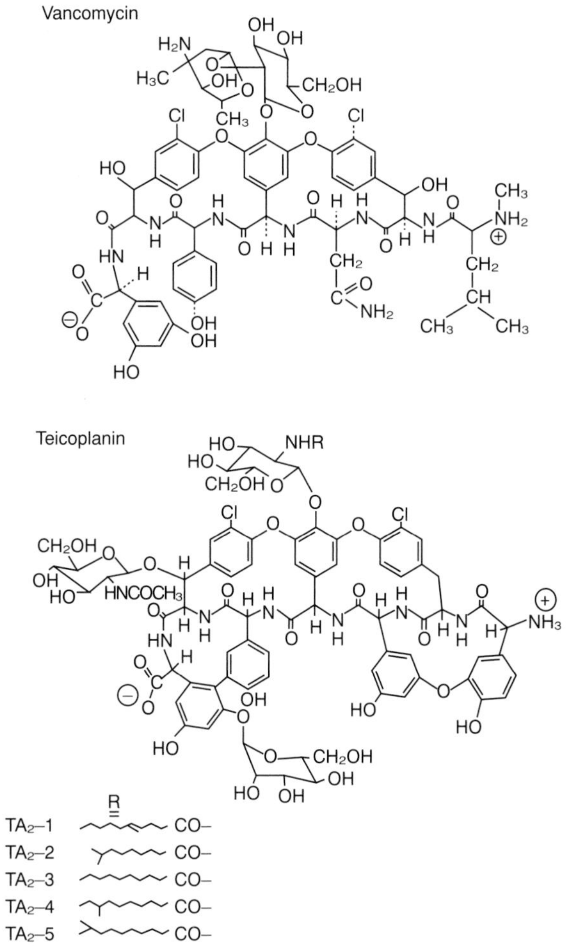

Vancomycin

Teicoplanin

	R	
TA₂–1		CO–
TA₂–2		CO–
TA₂–3		CO–
TA₂–4		CO–
TA₂–5		CO–

Fig. 9.6 Structures of the glycopeptide antibiotics, vancomycin and teicoplanin.

alteration of the D-alanyl-D-alanine target to D-alanyl-D-lactate (Walsh 1993), but other mechanisms are found in coagulase-negative staphylococci. The commonest type of resistance in enterococci is inducible and transferable (Shlaes et al. 1989, Healy and Zervos 1995); high level resistance to both vancomycin and teicoplanin is conferred. Transfer to *S. aureus* has been reported (Noble, Virani and Cree 1992) but at the time of writing no clinical isolate of glycopeptide-resistant *S. aureus* has yet been described. Some vancomycin-resistant isolates of enterococci retain susceptibility to teicoplanin, but *Staphylococcus haemolyticus* isolates are often more resistant to teicoplanin than to vancomycin.

PHARMACOLOGICAL PROPERTIES AND TOXICITY

Vancomycin has to be administered by slow intravenous infusion, since bolus injection is apt to cause 'red-man syndrome' owing to the release of histamine. Teicoplanin is less likely to cause this complication (Sahai et al. 1990). In addition, teicoplanin does not cause tissue necrosis that is associated with intramuscular injection of vancomycin and it can be safely given by this route. The elimination half-life of teico-

planin (c. 40 h) is much longer than that of vancomycin (c. 7 h), and it is much more extensively protein bound (90% versus 50%). Renal and ototoxicity are more common with vancomycin.

3.3 Other cell wall active agents

BACITRACIN

This is a cyclic peptide that prevents the dephosphorylation of the lipid carrier molecule that transfers newly formed peptidoglycan across the cell membrane during cell wall synthesis. It is too toxic for systemic use, but is found in several topical preparations. It is mainly active against gram-positive cocci. The exquisite sensitivity of *S. pyogenes* is exploited in a laboratory screening test for that organism (see Chapter 28).

CYCLOSERINE

This is an analogue of D-alanine, which prevents the racemization of L-alanine and the ligation of D-alanyl-D-alanine. It is quite toxic and is used only as a reserve agent for drug-resistant *M. tuberculosis*.

FOSFOMYCIN

Fosfomycin (epoxypropylphosphonic acid) is a broad spectrum antibiotic that blocks the formation of *N*-acetylmuramic acid from *N*-acetylglucosamine by inhibition of pyruvyltransferase. In vitro activity against *E. coli* and some other gram-negative rods is potentiated by glucose-6-phosphate, which induces a hexose phosphate transport pathway. The sodium salt is used for parenteral administration; for oral use, the earlier calcium salt has been superseded by the much more soluble trometamol formulation, which is particularly suitable for the treatment of urinary tract infection (Reeves 1994). Resistance to fosfomycin emerges readily in vitro, but the drug has been extensively used in some countries without apparent problem. Plasmid mediated resistance has been reported (Suárez and Mendoza 1991), but is as yet uncommon. A somewhat similar phosphonic acid derivative, fosmidomycin, is available in Japan.

ETHAMBUTOL, ISONIAZID AND PYRAZINAMIDE

These are agents used specifically in mycobacterial disease; they have no useful activity against other bacteria. Although the mode of action has not been definitely established, it is likely that they act on the mycobacterial cell wall, which is unusual in its composition (see Chapter 26). Isoniazid is most active against *M. tuberculosis* against which it exerts bactericidal activity. It is well absorbed when given orally and is eliminated in the urine, largely in an acetylated form. In persons with a genetically determined ability to acetylate the drug rapidly, excretion is hastened and plasma concentrations correspondingly low. Pyrazinamide is also mycobactericidal, but only at an acid pH and after intracellular conversion by a bacterial amidase to pyrazinoic acid (Mitchison 1992). Ethambutol, by contrast, is predominantly mycobacteristatic, but it has a wider spectrum of activity within the myco-bacteria, including activity against organisms of the *Mycobacterium avium* complex.

4 INHIBITORS OF BACTERIAL PROTEIN SYNTHESIS

Many of the naturally occurring antibiotic families that were discovered by mass screening of soil samples in the 1940s and 1950s turned out to achieve their antibacterial effect by interfering with various stages of the process of protein synthesis. Some, but not all, owe their selective toxicity to the difference in structure between bacterial and mammalian ribosomes.

4.1 Aminoglycosides

STRUCTURE AND SPECTRUM OF ACTIVITY

Aminoglycosides are complex heterocyclic compounds that usually possess an aminocyclitol group in addition to one or more amino sugars. Spectinomycin is unusual in being a pure aminocyclitol and has properties, including predominantly bacteristatic activity, that separate it from the aminoglycosides proper. It is used only as a reserve agent in gonorrhoea. The remaining aminoglycosides can be divided into 2 main types depending on the structure of the amino-cyclitol ring: those (of which streptomycin and dihyd-rostreptomycin are the only surviving examples) in which the aminocyclitol is streptidine; and those in which the aminocyclitol moiety is deoxystreptamine. The deoxystreptamine-containing aminoglycosides can, in their turn, be divided into neomycin derivatives, kanamycin derivatives and gentamicin derivatives (Fig. 9.7).

The neomycins (including framycetin; neomycin B), are mainly used in topical preparations because of their toxicity, but one member of the group, paromo-mycin, is more conspicuous for its activity against the protozoa *Entamoeba histolytica* and *Leishmania* spp. Most of the remaining aminoglycosides in common therapeutic use, including gentamicin, tobramycin (deoxykanamycin B), netilmicin and the semi-synthetic antibiotic, amikacin, share a common spectrum of activity that encompasses staphylococci and enterobacteria, but excludes streptococci, entero-cocci, anaerobes and intracellular bacteria. Certain aminoglycosides exhibit activity against *M. tuberculosis* (streptomycin, kanamycin and amikacin) or against *P. aeruginosa* (gentamicin, tobramycin, netilmicin, amikacin). Members of this last group have been widely used in the management of serious infection, often in combination with a β-lactam agent with which they may interact synergically. Bactericidal synergy with penicillin is also exploited in the therapy of strep-tococcal and enterococcal endocarditis.

MODE OF ACTION

Aminoglycosides bind to bacterial ribosomes. A single amino acid change in a protein of the 30S ribosomal subunit renders the cells completely resistant to strep-tomycin, but not to deoxystreptamine-containing aminoglycosides, which bind to both subunits. The mechanism of action is uncertain. Binding induces misreading of messenger RNA so that defective pro-teins are produced, but it is likely that aminoglycosides also interfere with the formation of functional initiation complexes. Neither of these mechanisms sat-isfactorily explains the potent bactericidal activity of these compounds and this may follow from mem-brane-related effects (Tai and Davis 1985, Davis 1988).

RESISTANCE

Aminoglycosides are taken up by bacterial cells by an active transport process that involves respiratory pro-cesses. The absence of such a transport mechanism in anaerobes, streptococci and enterococci accounts for the relative resistance of these organisms.

Alterations in permeability characteristics of sensi-tive bacteria may lead to relative resistance to amino-glycosides and such bacteria are usually resistant to all members of the group. However, acquired resistance in otherwise sensitive species is most commonly due to the production of enzymes that adenylate or phos-phorylate hydroxyl groups on the aminoglycoside mol-ecule, or acetylate exposed amino groups. Since these antibiotics vary in the availability of vulnerable group-ings on the molecule, they exhibit variable suscepti-bility to the many aminoglycoside-modifying enzymes that have been described. Some examples are shown in Table 9.4.

PHARMACOLOGICAL PROPERTIES

Aminoglycosides are very poorly absorbed by the oral route and are administered by intramuscular injection or intravenous infusion. They do not penetrate into cells or cross the blood–brain barrier to enter the cerebrospinal fluid. They are excreted almost entirely in the urine via the glomerular filtrate with an elimin-ation half-life of about 2–4 h. Protein binding is gener-ally low (<25%).

TOXICITY AND SIDE EFFECTS

All members of this antibiotic family are nephrotoxic and ototoxic, but they vary in their propensity to cause these adverse effects. For example, gentamicin and tobramycin are less likely to cause vestibular toxicity than is streptomycin, but are somewhat more likely to cause renal damage. Because of the risk of toxicity, it is common practice to assay aminoglycoside levels about 1 h after intramuscular injection or intravenous infusion ('peak' level) and immediately before the next dose ('trough' level). If single large daily doses of aminoglycosides are used, as is sometimes advocated (Levison 1992), peak levels become difficult to inter-pret, but trough levels still need to be monitored.

4.2 Chloramphenicol

STRUCTURE AND SPECTRUM OF ACTIVITY

Chloramphenicol is a relatively simple antibiotic (Fig. 9.8) that is nowadays synthesized rather than being

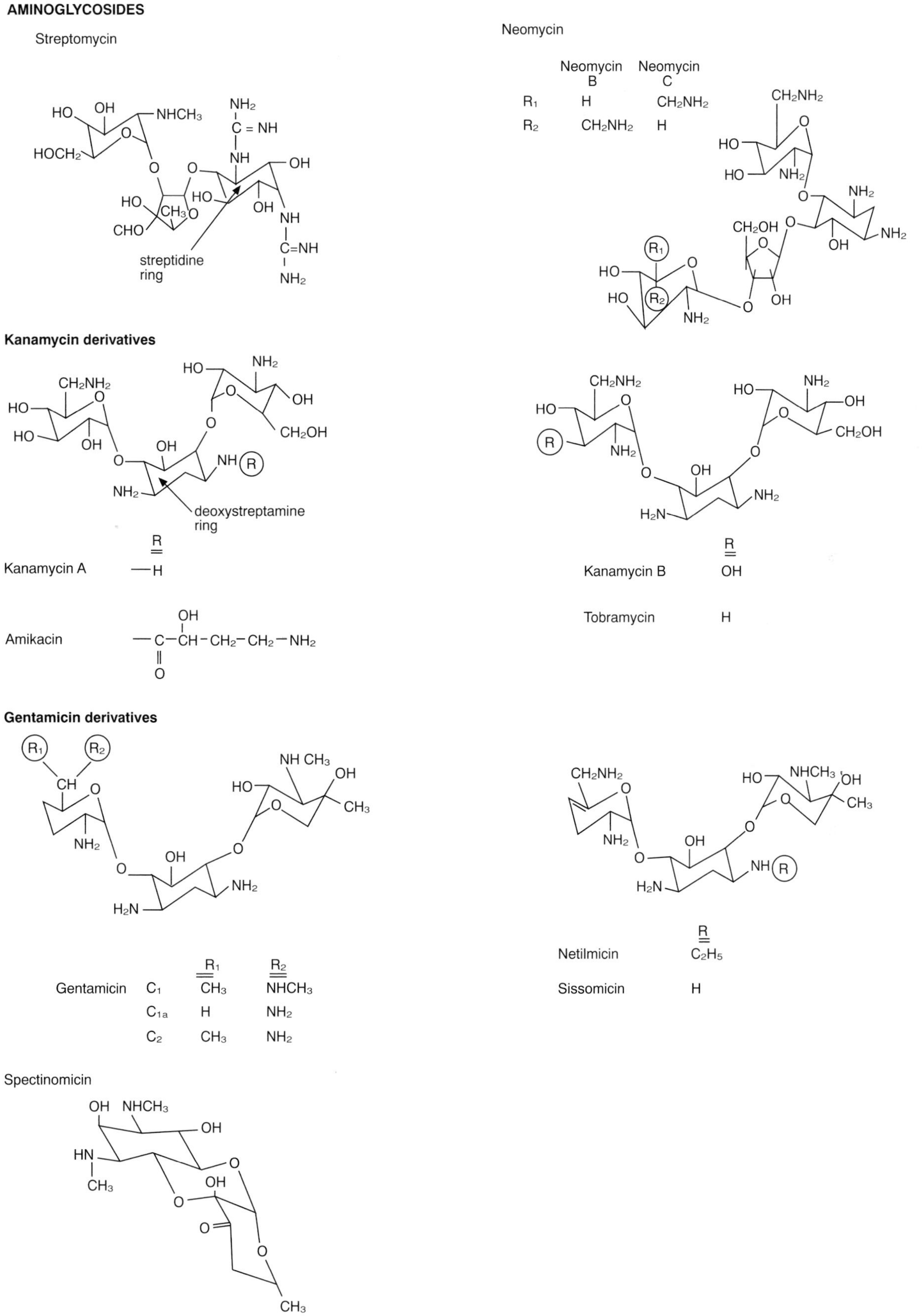

AMINOGLYCOSIDES

Streptomycin

Neomycin

Fig. 9.7 Structures of the most important aminoglycosides.

Table 9.4 Some common aminoglycoside modifying enzymes

Enzyme	Preferred substrates	Typical bacterial distribution	
		Gram-positive	Gram-negative
Acetyltransferases			
AAC(3)-I	Gen, Sis	−	+
AAC(3)-II	Gen, Kan, Net, Sis, Tob	−	+
AAC(2′)	Gen, Neo, Net, Sis, Tob	−	+
AAC(6′)-I	Amk, Net, Tob	+	+
AAC(6′)-II	Gen, Kan, Net, Sis, Tob	−	+
Nucleotidyltransferases (adenylyltransferases)			
AAD(6)	Str	+	−
AAD(4′)(4″)	Amk, Kan, Neo, Tob	+	−
AAD(2″)	Gen, Kan, Sis, Tob	−	+
AAD(3″)(9)	Spc, Str	−	+
AAD(9)	Spc	+	−
Phosphotransferases			
APH(6)	Str	−	+
APH(3′)	Kan, Neo	+	+
APH(2″)	Gen, Net, Sis, Tob	+	−
APH(3″)	Str	+	+

Amk, amikacin; Gen, gentamicin; Kan, kanamycin; Neo, neomycin; Net, netilmicin; Sis, sissomicin; Spc, spectinomycin; Str, streptomycin.
The figures in parentheses indicate the sites of modification of exposed amino or hydroxyl groups according to the international numbering system for the heterocyclic ring structure of the aminoglycosides. Bifunctional enzymes that act at more than one site have two such numbers. Roman numerals indicate different forms of the enzyme acting at that site.

obtained by fermentation from the producer organism. Modification of the molecule has not been very productive, although thiamphenicol, in which a sulphomethyl substituent replaces the nitro group, is available in some countries. Fluorinated derivatives, such as florphenicol, have also been made, but are not used in human medicine.

The spectrum is very broad and includes intracellular pathogens such as chlamydiae and rickettsiae as well as most conventional gram-positive and gram-negative bacteria. *P. aeruginosa* and *M. tuberculosis* are usually resistant.

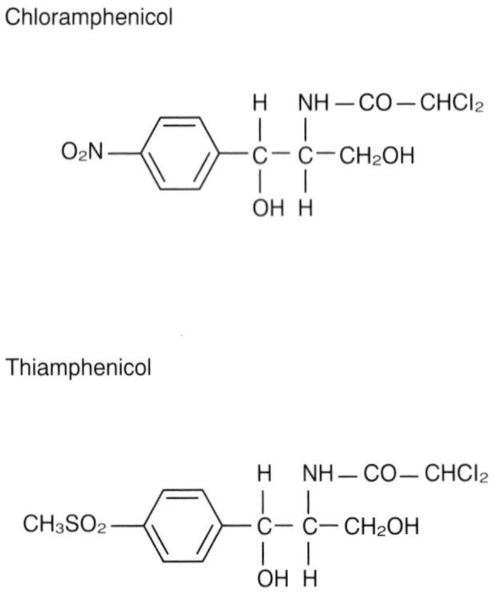

Chloramphenicol

Thiamphenicol

Fig. 9.8 Structures of chloramphenicol and thiamphenicol.

MODE OF ACTION

Chloramphenicol inhibits the enzyme peptidyltransferase which links new amino acids from aminoacyl transfer RNA to the growing peptide chain. It does not bind to mammalian ribosomes except, perhaps, those within mitochondria.

RESISTANCE

Target site alterations and reduction in drug uptake have been described, but the most common form of resistance is due to the production of chloramphenicol acetyltransferases. These enzymes acetylate the C-3 hydroxyl group preferentially, but also attack the C-1 hydroxyl; interest in the fluorinated derivatives centres on their resistance to these enzymes. Inactivation of chloramphenicol by a nitroreductase has also been described in *B. fragilis* (Tally and Malamy 1984).

PHARMACOLOGICAL PROPERTIES

Because chloramphenicol is poorly soluble and tastes very bitter, prodrugs are used in therapy: water-soluble chloramphenicol succinate is used for injection and the more palatable chloramphenicol palmitate or stearate for oral administration. These salts release chloramphenicol in the body, but are themselves inactive and unsuitable for laboratory tests. The oral route of administration is very efficient and is generally preferred. The drug is well distributed, with excellent penetration into cerebrospinal fluid. It is excreted into urine, largely as inactive glucuronide conjugates, with a half-life of about 2–5 h in adults. Plasma protein binding is c. 50%.

TOXICITY AND SIDE EFFECTS

The popularity of this excellent antibiotic suffered a severe setback when it was realized that it occasionally caused an irreversible aplastic anaemia. The overall incidence of this lethal side effect is about 1 in 40 000 courses of therapy, but there may be a genetic component that makes it more likely in some patients. There is concern that sufficient chloramphenicol may be absorbed systemically after topical use, e.g. in eye ointments, for aplastic anaemia to be a hazard (Doona and Walsh 1995), but the degree of risk is disputed (Mulla et al. 1995). Thiamphenicol appears to be free of this side effect, but is more likely to cause reversible depression of the bone marrow.

Young infants have a limited capacity to conjugate and excrete chloramphenicol; accumulation of the drug may lead to 'grey baby' syndrome, with circulatory collapse. For this reason chloramphenicol levels should be assayed if the drug is used in neonatal meningitis or other life-threatening conditions in young infants.

4.3 Tetracyclines

STRUCTURE AND SPECTRUM OF ACTIVITY

The tetracyclines are a closely related group of naturally occurring and semi-synthetic antibiotics that differ according to the nature of chemical substituents on the basic tetracyclic skeleton (Fig. 9.9). They are distinguished more for differences in pharmacokinetic behaviour than for variations in antimicrobial activity. The spectrum of activity is broad. They have been widely and successfully used in many types of infection including those in which chlamydiae, rickettsiae and mycoplasmas are involved. They have some antiprotozoal activity and are sometimes used in drug-resistant malaria.

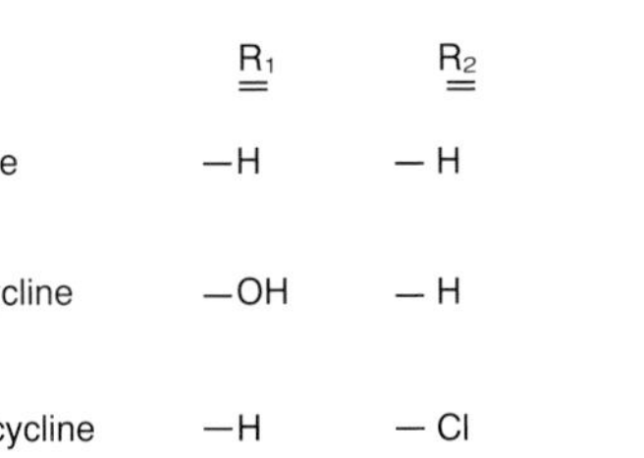

MODE OF ACTION

Tetracyclines enter bacterial cells by an active uptake process. They bind to the 30S ribosomal subunit and prevent access of aminoacyl transfer RNA to the acceptor site by a mechanism that has not been fully elucidated (Chopra, Hawkey and Hinton 1992). Mammalian cells do not concentrate tetracyclines in the way that bacteria do and the ribosomes (other than mitochondrial ribosomes) are relatively insusceptible.

RESISTANCE

The emergence of resistance in gram-positive and gram-negative bacteria has seriously undermined the value of tetracyclines. Resistance is generally plasmid mediated and is commonly found on transposons. Several mechanisms of resistance have been described, but the most prevalent appears to be due to production of a novel cytoplasmic membrane protein that mediates active efflux of the drug so that inhibitory levels are not maintained within the cell (Chopra, Hawkey and Hinton 1992, Speer, Shoemaker and Salyers 1992).

Resistance usually affects all tetracyclines equally, although minocycline may retain activity against some strains. Efforts have been made to devise tetracyclines that overcome resistance mechanisms. Several candidate molecules have been described, including the glycylcyclines which are under investigation (Tally, Ellestad and Testa 1995).

PHARMACOLOGICAL PROPERTIES

The tetracyclines are usually given orally, but since they form non-absorbable chelates with divalent cations, administration with milk or other food may interfere with absorption. Doxycycline and minocycline are among the best absorbed; these compounds also have a longer plasma half-life (c. 16–18 h) than other congeners (generally c. 6–12 h), but are more extensively (minocycline 75%; doxycycline 90%) protein bound. They penetrate well into tissues, but not into cerebrospinal fluid. They are excreted by glomerular filtration into the urine and into faeces via the bile.

TOXICITY AND SIDE EFFECTS

Diarrhoea and other forms of gastrointestinal intolerance are common. Renal failure may occur in patients who already have impaired renal function, but doxycycline, which is predominantly excreted by the hepatobiliary route, may be safely given to such patients. Since tetracyclines are yellow compounds that chelate calcium, the pigment is deposited in growing bone and teeth. For this reason tetracyclines should not be given to young children when the dentition is being formed as permanent discoloration of teeth may occur.

4.4 Macrolides

STRUCTURE AND SPECTRUM OF ACTIVITY

The macrolides are a family of related compounds that feature a large macrocyclic lactone structure sub-

	R₁	R₂	R₃
Tetracycline	—H	—H	$\genfrac{}{}{0pt}{}{CH_3}{OH}$
Oxytetracycline	—OH	—H	$\genfrac{}{}{0pt}{}{CH_3}{OH}$
Chlortetracycline	—H	—Cl	$\genfrac{}{}{0pt}{}{CH_3}{OH}$
Minocycline	—H	—N(CH₃)₂	$\genfrac{}{}{0pt}{}{H}{H}$
Doxycycline	—OH	—H	$\genfrac{}{}{0pt}{}{CH_3}{H}$

Fig. 9.9 Structures of the most important tetracyclines.

stituted with various unusual sugars (Fig. 9.10). Erythromycin (the oldest and best known member of the group), oleandomycin, clarithromycin (6-*O*-methyl erythromycin), dirithromycin and roxithromycin have a 14-membered lactone ring. Some others that are used in various parts of the world, including spiramycin, josamycin, midecamycin, kitasamycin and rokitamycin, possess a 16-membered lactone structure. In azithromycin, the 14-membered structure of erythromycin has been expanded by insertion of a methyl-substituted nitrogen atom; the 15-membered ring thus produced is sometimes referred to as an **azalide** structure.

Erythromycin and other macrolides are unable to penetrate easily through the outer membrane of enteric gram-negative bacilli, although they exhibit a variable degree of activity against *H. influenzae*, *Legionella pneumophila* and *Campylobacter jejuni*. They exhibit good activity against staphylococci and streptococci, and useful activity against *M. pneumoniae* (but not *Mycoplasma hominis*) and some environmental mycobacteria. Chlamydiae are susceptible and azithromycin is effective in the single-dose treatment of genital infections (Martin et al. 1992, Stamm et al. 1995) and trachoma (Bailey et al. 1993). Spiramycin has been successfully used in toxoplasmosis, and clarithromycin may have a place in regimens for the eradication of *Helicobacter pylori*.

MODE OF ACTION

Erythromycin, and by implication other macrolides, bind to 50S ribosomal subunits in bacteria and interfere with the translocation process during synthesis of polypeptides, probably by causing dissociation of peptidyl transfer RNA from the ribosome (Mazzei et al. 1993).

RESISTANCE

Resistance to macrolides is quite commonly encountered in staphylococci and streptococci but the prevalence varies considerably from country to country. Resistance may arise from alterations in ribosomal proteins, but is more commonly due to an inducible, plasmid mediated enzyme that methylates an adenine residue in ribosomal RNA (Weisblum 1995a). The methylase also confers resistance to lincosamides and streptogramins, but these antibiotics do not act as inducers, so the organisms appear sensitive in laboratory tests unless erythromycin is also present to induce the enzyme. However, variants exhibiting constitutive resistance readily emerge on exposure to lincosamides or streptogramins (Weisblum 1995b).

PHARMACOLOGICAL PROPERTIES

Macrolides are mostly irregularly absorbed when given orally; in the case of erythromycin this is because it is unstable at gastric pH. Newer macrolides, such as

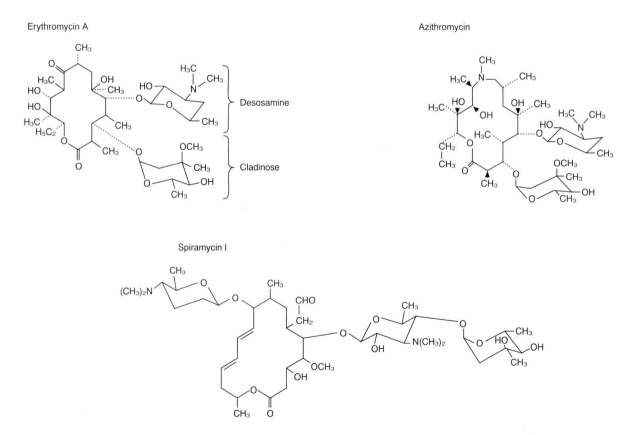

Fig. 9.10 Structures of erythromycin A (a 14-membered macrolide); azithromycin (a 15-membered macrolide and an azalide); and spiramycin I (a 16-membered macrolide).

azithromycin and clarithromycin, are more acid stable and their oral absorption is consequently much improved. Oral formulations of erythromycin are either coated to avoid destruction in the stomach, or are presented as prodrug salts or esters (estolate, stearate or ethylsuccinate). The lactobionate or gluceptate salts are used for parenteral administration.

All these drugs are well distributed in the body, but azithromycin and clarithromycin are said to achieve particularly good tissue levels, especially in the lung (Honeybourne and Baldwin 1992). Penetration into cerebrospinal fluid is poor. They are extensively metabolized (except azithromycin) and excreted largely by the hepatobiliary route. The plasma half-life is variable and may be dose-dependent. Azithromycin is unusual in that it has a much extended terminal half-life.

TOXICITY AND SIDE EFFECTS

Nausea and other gastrointestinal side effects are common, but newer derivatives, including azithromycin and clarithromycin, are better tolerated. Cholestatic jaundice is described as an uncommon complication, particularly with erythromycin formulations.

4.5 Lincosamides

STRUCTURE AND SPECTRUM OF ACTIVITY

The original lincosamide antibiotic, lincomycin, has been largely superseded by the 7-deoxy-7-chloro derivative, clindamycin (Fig. 9.11), which is more active and better absorbed by the oral route. The most potent activity is against staphylococci, streptococci and anaerobes, including *B. fragilis*. Enterobacteria and *P. aeruginosa* are resistant. Activity against *Propionibacterium acnes* and corynebacteria has led to the use of clindamycin in acne, but its success in this condition may be equally due to the anti-inflammatory and antiphagocytic activity that it is known to possess (Oleske and Phillips 1983) or to effects on skin lipids. Clindamycin possesses some antiprotozoal activity and has been used in malaria and toxoplasmosis.

MODE OF ACTION

The mechanism of action of lincosamides is not known for certain. Early work suggested that these drugs, like chloramphenicol, interfere with the peptidyltransferase reaction (Weisblum and Davies 1968), but later evidence pointed to effects on peptide chain initiation (Pestka 1971, Reusser 1975). Although the structure of lincosamides is completely different from that of macrolides, the site of action appears to be similar since methylation of an adenine residue in ribosomal RNA confers resistance to both types of antibiotic.

RESISTANCE

As well as resistance caused by ribosomal methylase, described above, resistance may also arise by enzymic modification by nucleotidylation (Russell and Chopra 1996). Resistance emerges readily and is common among methicillin-resistant *S. aureus* (Maple, Hamilton-Miller and Brumfitt 1989).

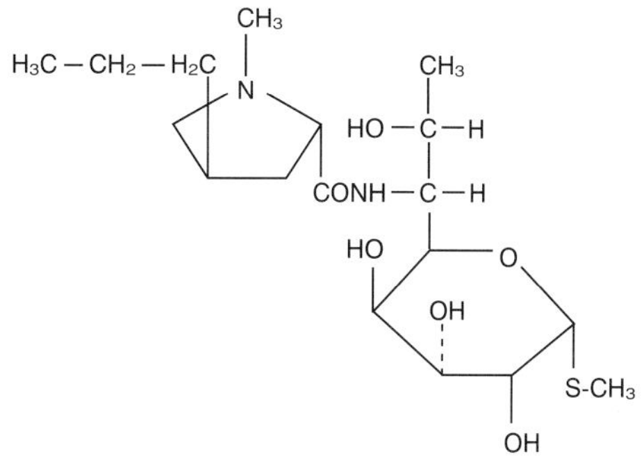

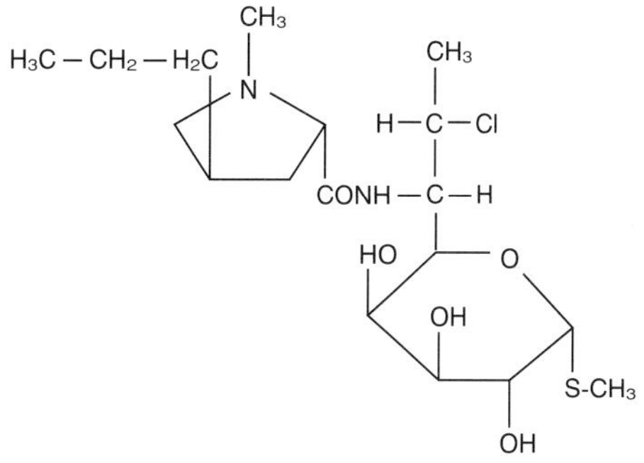

Fig. 9.11 Structures of the lincosamides, lincomycin and clindamycin.

PHARMACOLOGICAL PROPERTIES

Like chloramphenicol, clindamycin is poorly soluble and very bitter, so that it has to be administered as inactive prodrugs, clindamycin palmitate (for oral use) and clindamycin phosphate (for injection). It is well absorbed when given orally and, after hydrolysis, achieves good concentrations in tissues, but not in the cerebrospinal fluid. It is metabolized in the liver and excreted mainly in bile with a half-life of about 2–3 h. Plasma protein binding is 94%.

TOXICITY AND SIDE EFFECTS

Rashes and other occasional adverse events have been overshadowed by the reputation of clindamycin for inducing diarrhoea associated with *C. difficile* toxins, which may progress to a life-threatening pseudomembraneous colitis. Other antibiotics, including β-lactam agents, have been implicated in this side effect, but it seems to be more common with clindamycin (Tedesco, Barton and Alpers 1974, Aronsson, Möllby and Nord 1984).

4.6 Fusidic acid

STRUCTURE AND SPECTRUM OF ACTIVITY

Fusidic acid is an antibiotic with a steroid-like structure (Fig. 9.12) that does not possess steroid-like activity. It exhibits modest activity against streptococci, gram-positive and gram-negative anaerobes, *Nocardia asteroides* and *M. tuberculosis*, and good activity against *Corynebacterium diphtheriae*, but its place in therapy hinges on its excellent activity against staphylococci (Greenwood 1988, Verbist 1990). Various interactions with penicillins (synergy, antagonism and indifference) have been described (O'Grady and Greenwood 1973). Activity against the protozoa, *Giardia lamblia* (Farthing and Inge 1986) and *Plasmodium falciparum* (Black, Wildfang and Borgbjerg 1985), have been reported. Enterobacteria and pseudomonads are resistant.

MODE OF ACTION

Unlike other inhibitors of bacterial protein synthesis, fusidic acid does not bind directly to the ribosome. It forms a stable complex with guanosine triphosphate and 'factor G', an elongation factor involved in the translocation of the growing peptide chain (Cundliffe 1972).

RESISTANCE

Resistance may be plasmid mediated, but is more commonly due to chromosomal mutation resulting in alteration in the factor G target. This type of resistance emerges readily in vitro, but the general prevalence of resistance in staphylococci has remained low (Shanson 1990). This may have been helped by the fact that fusidic acid is usually given in combination (often with a penicillin) to avoid the emergence of resistance during therapy, but topical preparations are normally given alone.

PHARMACOLOGICAL PROPERTIES

Fusidic acid is very well absorbed by the oral route and penetrates well into tissue, including bone. It is excreted via the bile, mostly as inactive metabolites, with a half-life of about 9 h (Reeves 1987, MacGowan et al. 1989). More than 95% is bound to plasma protein.

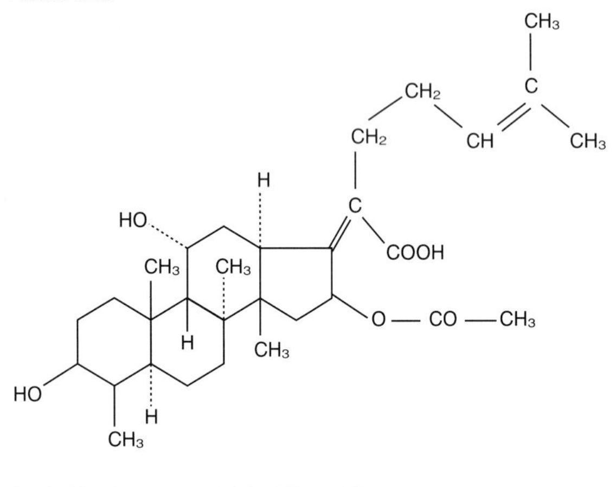

TOXICITY AND SIDE EFFECTS

A small proportion of patients develop transient jaundice by interference with the metabolism and excretion of bilirubin. It is more common in patients receiving intravenous fusidic acid (Humble, Eykyn and Phillips 1980). Mild gastrointestinal upsets and rashes are occasionally experienced.

4.7 Other inhibitors of bacterial protein synthesis

STREPTOGRAMINS

The streptogramins are a family of antibiotics that consist of 2 synergically interacting macrolactone components: a polyunsaturated peptolide and a hexadepsipeptide. The bactericidal synergy that results from the combined action of the 2 components of streptogramins is thought to arise through binding to adjacent sites on the bacterial ribosome (Aumercier et al. 1992). The best known members of the group are pristinamycin and virginiamycin, which are used as antistaphylococcal agents in animal husbandry and, in some countries, in human medicine. Lack of aqueous solubility and poor oral absorption have limited their value, but water-soluble derivatives of the 2 components of pristinamycin (known respectively as quinopristin and dalfopristin) have been synthesized to allow parenteral administration and these are under investigation (Barrière et al. 1992, Etienne et al. 1992). Macrolide–lincosamide resistance associated with an adenine methylase also extends to streptogramins (see section on macrolide resistance, p. 212).

MUPIROCIN

Mupirocin is a naturally occurring antibiotic product of *Pseudomonas fluorescens*. It was formerly known as pseudomonic acid. The structure (Fig. 9.13) is unrelated to other antibiotics and consists of 'monic acid', the distal portion of which is a structural analogue of isoleucine, and a short fatty acid (nonanoic acid). The useful activity is restricted to gram-positive cocci, in which it presumably halts protein synthesis by binding to isoleucyl transfer RNA synthetase as it does in *E. coli* (Hughes and Mellows 1980).

Although it displays low toxicity, systemic use of mupirocin is precluded by the fact that it is rapidly inactivated in the body. Consequently, it is used only for topical application in skin infections and to eradicate staphylococci from nasal carriers. For the latter purpose, which has been of particular value in carriers

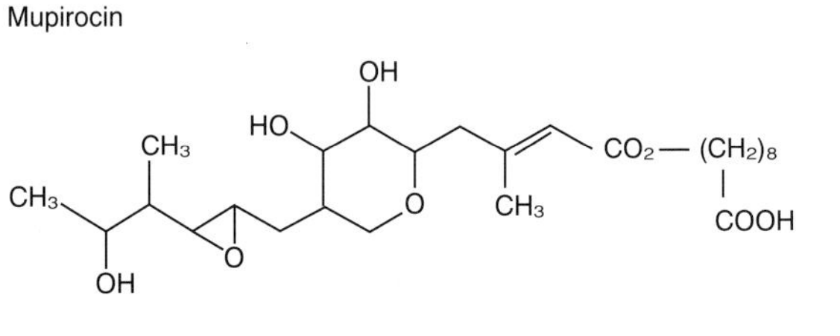

Fusidic acid

Fig. 9.12 Structure of fusidic acid.

Mupirocin

Fig. 9.13 Structure of mupirocin.

of methicillin-resistant *S. aureus*, a paraffin-based formulation is used, not the polyethylene glycol-based ointment applied to skin.

5 INHIBITORS OF BACTERIAL NUCLEIC ACID SYNTHESIS

A surprising number of antibacterial agents achieve their effect by interacting with bacterial DNA in various ways. Sulphonamides and trimethoprim have an indirect effect on other cellular functions as well as DNA through their effect on folic acid synthesis, but for convenience are dealt with under this heading.

5.1 Sulphonamides

STRUCTURE AND SPECTRUM OF ACTIVITY

The sulphonamides are a large family of compounds, all of which are derived from the original hydrolysis product of Prontosil red, sulphanilamide (see section 1, p. 195). They differ in the nature of the substitution on the amino group of the sulphonamide (SO_2NH_2) moiety (Fig. 9.14). The antileprosy drug, dapsone (diaminodiphenylsulphone) and the tuberculostatic *p*-aminosalicylic acid are related substances that are thought to act in a similar way.

They are broad spectrum, predominantly bacteristatic compounds that have a relatively slow effect in halting bacterial growth. They have some activity against protozoa, including *Plasmodium* spp. and *Toxoplasma gondii*. The various sulphonamides do not differ greatly in their intrinsic activity, but sulphadiazine, sulphafurazole and sulphamethoxazole appear to be somewhat more active than others. Activity in vitro is profoundly affected by the composition of the culture medium, because of the possible presence of interfering substances such as folic acid, *p*-aminobenzoic acid and thymidine. Lysed horse blood, which contains the enzyme thymidine phosphorylase, is commonly added to remove thymidine (Waterworth 1978) and media recommended for sensitivity testing have low levels of this and other sulphonamide antagonists (Report 1991). Inoculum density also has a marked effect on the apparent sensitivity of bacteria to sulphonamides in vitro, but this is likely to be a laboratory artefact arising from the delayed effect of these drugs (Greenwood and O'Grady 1976).

MODE OF ACTION

Sulphonamides are analogues of *p*-aminobenzoic acid. They inhibit folic acid synthesis by competitive inhibition of dihydropteroic acid synthetase, the enzyme that brings about the condensation of dihydropteridine with *p*-aminobenzoic acid in the early stage of folate production. Since folic acid is conserved in bacterial cells, the inhibitory effects of sulphonamides become apparent only after several generations of growth when the folate pool has been progressively diluted to below a functional level by distribution to the bacterial progeny.

The selective toxicity of sulphonamides arises

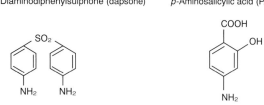

Fig. 9.14 Structures of some sulphonamides and related compounds.

because bacteria synthesize folic acid de novo, whereas humans absorb the vitamin preformed. Since they block an early stage of the same metabolic pathway as diaminopyrimidines, sulphonamides interact synergically with those compounds (see section 5.2, p. 216).

RESISTANCE

Resistance to sulphonamides occurs readily and was soon apparent in the early life of these agents. There is complete cross-resistance among different members of this drug class. Resistance is commonly plasmid mediated and is usually caused by alterations in dihydropteroate synthetase, leading to less efficient binding of sulphonamides, or bypass of the effects of the agents by a duplicate, insensitive version of the enzyme (Huovinen et al. 1995). Chromosomal resistance due to hyperproduction of *p*-aminobenzoic acid is also recognized (Towner 1992a).

PHARMACOLOGICAL PROPERTIES

Differences in pharmacokinetic behaviour are the chief distinguishing characteristics of the various members of the sulphonamide family. In particular, they vary in oral absorption (e.g. phthalylsulphathiazole is very poorly absorbed), protein binding (e.g. sulphadimidine and sulfadoxine are more than 90% protein bound) and, above all, plasma half-life, which can vary from about 2.5 h (sulphamethizole) to >100 h (sulfadoxine). The most commonly used sulphonamides, sulphadiazine and sulphamethoxazole (as co-trimoxazole) are well absorbed by the oral route and are excreted into urine, partly as inactive *N*-acetylated metabolites and glucuronide conjugates, with a half-life of about 8–10 h. They are well distributed and penetrate into the cerebrospinal fluid in effective concentrations.

TOXICITY AND SIDE EFFECTS

Crystalluria, with renal blockage, is a problem with some of the less soluble compounds, including sulphadiazine and sulphathiazole, especially if excessive dosage is used. Rashes are common and erythema multiforme (Stevens–Johnson syndrome) is a rare, but potentially life-threatening complication. Serious haematological effects are also seen occasionally.

5.2 Diaminopyrimidines

STRUCTURE AND SPECTRUM OF ACTIVITY

This family of synthetic pyrimidine derivatives includes trimethoprim, the most familiar member of the group (Fig. 9.15), and the closely related antibacterial agents, tetroxoprim and brodimoprim which are in use in some countries, but offer little, if any, advantage over trimethoprim. Also related are the antimalarial agents pyrimethamine and cycloguanil (the in vivo metabolite of proguanil), the antipneumocystis agent, trimetrexate, and the anticancer drug, methotrexate.

Trimethoprim and its congeners are active against many gram-positive and gram-negative bacteria, but *P. aeruginosa*, *B. fragilis*, chlamydiae, rickettsiae, myco-

plasmas and mycobacteria are outside the spectrum. Although they exhibit excellent activity in their own right, they are often formulated with sulphonamides, with which they interact synergically, at least in vitro. Among such combination products are: co-trimoxazole (trimethoprim + sulphamethoxazole); co-trimazine (trimethoprim + sulphadiazine); co-trifamole (trimethoprim + sulphamoxole) and co-tetroxazine (tetroxoprim + sulphadiazine).

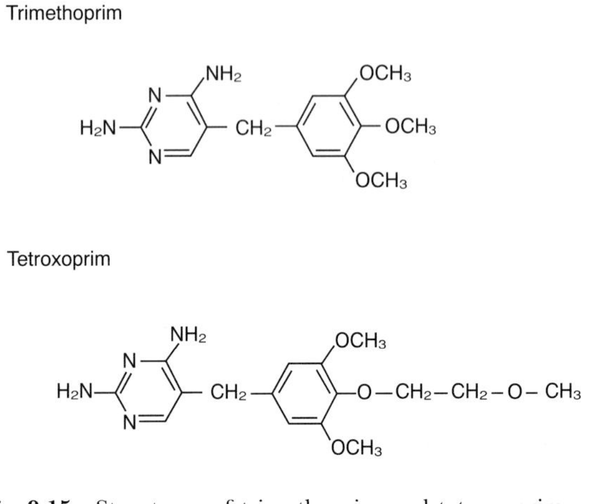

MODE OF ACTION

Diaminopyrimidines act on the same metabolic pathway as sulphonamides, but at a later stage. They inhibit dihydrofolate reductase, the enzyme that converts the precursor form of folic acid, dihydrofolate, to the active cofactor, tetrahydrofolic acid. The human form of the enzyme is much less susceptible: the affinity of trimethoprim for bacterial dihydrofolate reductase is several thousand times greater than for the corresponding human enzyme (Hitchins 1969). Tetrahydrofolic acid is an essential carrier molecule in many single-carbon transactions within cells and is usually regenerated unchanged. However, in one such transfer, the production of thymidylic acid from deoxyuridylic acid, diaminopyrimidines act as hydrogen donors as well as methyl-group carriers, and emerge from the reaction in the oxidized form, dihydrofolate. Trimethoprim and its relatives prevent regeneration of tetrahydrofolic acid and thus trap the vitamin in the unusable precursor form. Consequently, these drugs influence bacterial growth more quickly than sulphonamides, which rely on dilution of the folate pool to achieve their bacteristatic effect. In the presence of sufficient diaminopyrimidine to completely halt folate activity, the sulphonamides in combined formulations get no opportunity to interfere with bacterial growth, although they still contribute substantially to the overall toxicity of the mixtures.

RESISTANCE

The prevalence of resistance to trimethoprim has steadily increased since its introduction in 1969. Several mechanisms are recognized, the most common of which is attributable to mutations that lead to the production of altered dihydrofolate reductases (Towner 1992a, Huovinen et al. 1995).

PHARMACOLOGICAL PROPERTIES

Trimethoprim can be given by the oral and parenteral routes. It is widely distributed in tissues, including bronchial secretions. Concentrations achieved in cerebrospinal fluid are about 30–50% of the corresponding plasma level. Excretion is almost entirely renal, partly as metabolites, some of which retain antibacterial activity. The plasma half-life is about 10 h and it is less than 50% protein bound.

TOXICITY AND SIDE EFFECTS

Trimethoprim is well tolerated and most of the side effects of co-trimoxazole are usually attributable to the sulphonamide component. Nevertheless, trimethoprim itself may give rise to idiosyncratic reactions. The

Trimethoprim

Tetroxoprim

Fig. 9.15 Structures of trimethoprim and tetroxoprim.

potential for exacerbating folate deficiency can normally be countered with folate supplements, but the drug is not recommended in pregnancy.

5.3 Quinolones

STRUCTURE AND SPECTRUM OF ACTIVITY

The quinolones are a large family of compounds, the molecular similarity of which is based on the quinolone nucleus, or related naphthyridine, cinnoline or pyridopyrimidine structures (Smith and Lewin 1988) (Fig. 9.l6). The first member of the group to be used in therapy, nalidixic acid, is a naphthyridine derivative with a narrow spectrum of activity directed almost exclusively against enterobacteria. Later congeners, including the cinnoline, cinoxacin, and the quinolones, oxolinic acid and acrosoxacin, exhibited essentially similar properties. Addition of a fluorine atom at C-6 (flumequine) or a piperazine substituent at C-7 (pipemidic acid) improved the activity against enterobacteria and *P. aeruginosa*, respectively, but it was not until these features were combined in the quinolone derivative, norfloxacin, that the intrinsic activity and spectrum were substantially altered. Norfloxacin is about 50 times more active than nalidixic acid against sensitive enterobacteria and also exhibits some activity against gram-positive cocci and *P. aeruginosa*. Other derivatives with the 6-fluoro-7-piperazinyl substitutions (now collectively called fluoroquinolones) followed. The naphthyridine, enoxacin, and the quinolones, pefloxacin and lomefloxacin, display activity similar to that of norfloxacin; other quinolones, such as ciprofloxacin and ofloxacin, offer further improved activity. Certain closely related compounds, including enrofloxacin and sarafloxacin are used in veterinary practice.

Some of the more active quinolones, including ciprofloxacin and ofloxacin, exhibit activity against chlamydiae (Oriel 1989) and mycobacteria (Garcia-Rodriguez and Gomez Garcia 1993), but this does not always translate into therapeutic success (Oriel 1989, Young 1993). Many other quinolones are under development, some with further interesting properties of spectrum, activity or pharmacology (Domagala 1994, Hooper 1995).

Quinolones are bactericidal drugs, although the killing effect is paradoxically reduced as the concentration is raised. The activity is variably affected by pH (the activity usually being reduced at acid pH values) and by the presence of magnesium and other cations (Smith and Lewin 1988).

MODE OF ACTION

The primary site of action of quinolones is DNA gyrase (topoisomerase II), the remarkable enzyme that engineers the breaking and rejoining of supercoiled DNA. The action mainly involves the DNA gyrase A subunit, although alterations in the B subunit also affect some quinolones (Hooper and Wolfson 1989).

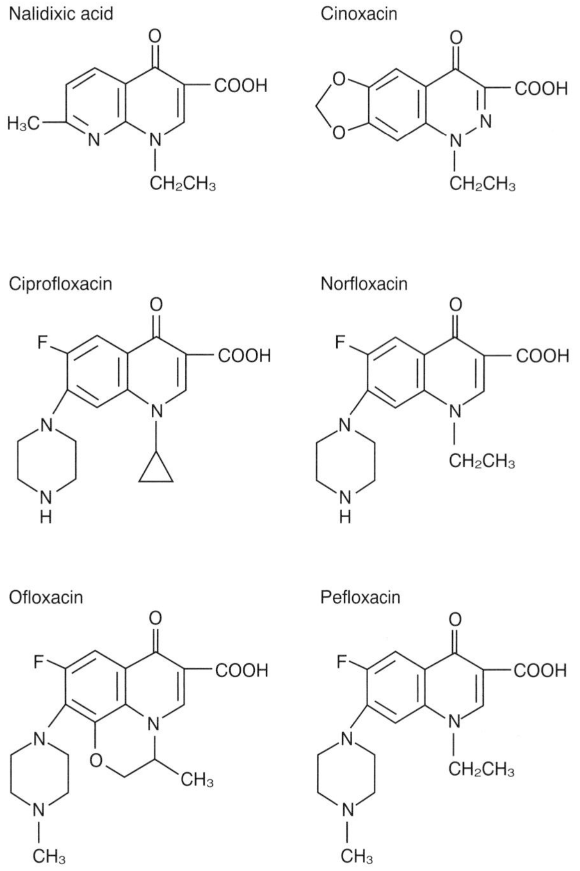

Fig. 9.16 Structures of some quinolones.

RESISTANCE

Resistance to earlier quinolones of the nalidixic acid type occurs readily by chromosomal mutation and restricts the value of these compounds in the treatment of complicated urinary tract infection (Greenwood and O'Grady 1977). Such resistance also affects newer fluoroquinolones, but the reduction of activity is such that variants resistant to nalidixic acid are still inhibited by concentrations achievable therapeutically. Early optimism that this, together with the absence of convincing reports of plasmid mediated resistance, would reduce the likelihood of resistance to fluoroquinolones becoming widespread, have not been realized. As might be expected, the emergence of resistance is particularly common in bacteria, such as *P. aeruginosa* and *S. aureus*, for which the minimum inhibitory concentration of fluoroquinolones does not greatly exceed therapeutically achievable concentrations (Wolfson and Hooper 1989, Peterson 1994, Wiedemann and Heisig 1994). Resistance is usually due to mutations in genes for DNA gyrase, but may also follow from alterations in drug accumulation, sometimes associated with alterations in outer-membrane proteins of gram-negative bacilli (Wolfson and Hooper 1989).

PHARMACOLOGICAL PROPERTIES

Quinolones are quite well absorbed when given orally, but some fluoroquinolones, including ciprofloxacin and ofloxacin, are also available in parenteral formulations. Nalidixic acid and the early congeners are extensively metabolized in vivo and sufficient unchanged drug to achieve an antibacterial effect is found only in urine. Fluoroquinolones are, in general, less susceptible to metabolic changes and, since they are well distributed in the body, they may be of value in systemic infection. Concentrations achievable in cerebrospinal fluid are generally subtherapeutic. Plasma elimination half-lives of the fluoroquinolones presently available vary from c. 3–4 h (ciprofloxacin and norfloxacin) to c. 6–7 h (enoxacin, ofloxacin and lomefloxacin). Protein binding is low.

TOXICITY AND SIDE EFFECTS

They are generally well tolerated, though rashes, gastrointestinal upsets and photosensitivity may occur and there are persistent reports of occasional neurotoxic side effects (Hooper and Wolfson 1991, Midtvedt and Greenwood 1994). The observation that fluoroquinolones can cause arthropathy in young experimental animals has led to a recommendation that these drugs should be avoided in young children and in women of child-bearing age. Cases of Achilles tendinitis, sometimes with rupture of the tendon, have been reported (Ribard et al. 1992).

5.4 Rifamycins

STRUCTURE AND SPECTRUM OF ACTIVITY

The rifamycins that are most widely used clinically, rifampicin (Fig. 9.17; known in the USA as rifampin) and rifabutin (also known as ansamycin), are semi-synthetic derivatives of the naturally occurring antibiotic, rifamycin B. Rifampicin exhibits good activity against gram-positive and gram-negative cocci, particularly staphylococci, but is more noted for its antimycobacterial activity. Gram-negative bacilli are much less susceptible. Rifabutin has been introduced specifically because of its activity against organisms of the *M. avium* complex.

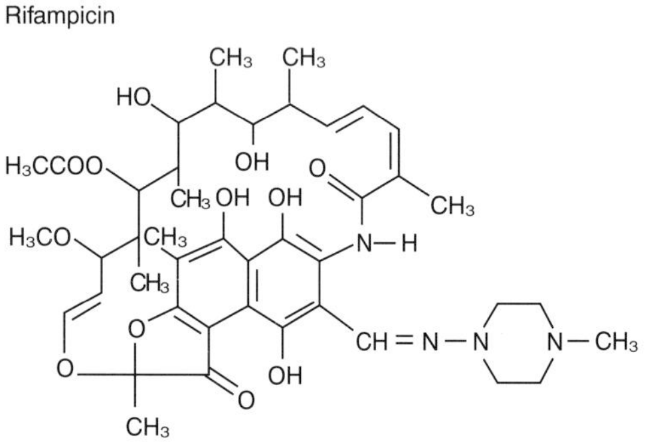

Rifampicin

Fig. 9.17 Structure of rifampicin.

MODE OF ACTION

Rifampicin and other rifamycins bind to the β-subunit of DNA-dependent RNA polymerase and prevent initiation of RNA synthesis (Wehrli and Staehelin 1971).

RESISTANCE

Resistance caused by mutational alterations in the target enzyme arises readily and may be a cause of treatment failure if rifampicin is used alone. In tuberculosis and leprosy, in which rifampicin is normally used in combination with other drugs, resistance is presently uncommon, though by no means unknown; indeed, multiply-resistant strains of *M. tuberculosis* have caused concern in some places (Young 1993). Surprisingly, resistance to rifabutin was not observed in a trial of prophylaxis in AIDS patients, for unexplained reasons (Böttger and Wallace 1994).

PHARMACOLOGICAL PROPERTIES

Rifampicin is very well absorbed when given by mouth, but the bioavailability of oral rifabutin is variable (Skinner et al. 1989). Both drugs are well distributed and excreted primarily by the hepatobiliary route, but also renally. They impart a red colour to the urine and to tears, so that they may discolour soft contact lenses. They are potent inducers of liver enzymes, which promote self-metabolism of the antibiotics as well as that of other drugs, including oral contraceptives and warfarin. There is significant binding to plasma proteins (c. 70%). The terminal half-life of rifabutin (c. 36 h) is much longer than that of rifampicin (c. 3.5 h).

TOXICITY AND SIDE EFFECTS

Rifampicin may cause sensitization when used intermittently, as in some recommended regimens for the treatment of tuberculosis. Gastrointestinal upsets, jaundice and (particularly with rifabutin) haematological effects are recognized. Induction of microsomal liver enzymes may lead to important interactions with other drugs, including failure of oral contraception.

5.5 Nitroimidazoles

STRUCTURE AND SPECTRUM OF ACTIVITY

Azole derivatives of various kinds have wide-ranging antimicrobial activities against fungi, protozoa and helminths, as well as bacteria. Some may have a role as radiosensitizing agents in cancer therapy. Those that exhibit useful antibacterial activity are 5-nitroimidazoles. Only 2, metronidazole and tinidazole (Fig. 9.18), are used in human medicine in the UK, but others, such as nimorazole, ornidazole and secnidazole, are available elsewhere and yet more are used in veterinary practice. They are primarily antiprotozoal agents, but also exhibit potent activity against anaerobic bacteria. Metronidazole offers a useful alternative to vancomycin (p. 205) in the treatment of *C. difficile*-associated colitis.

Micro-aerophiles and oxygen-tolerant species, such as *Actinomyces* spp. and *Propionibacterium* spp., are

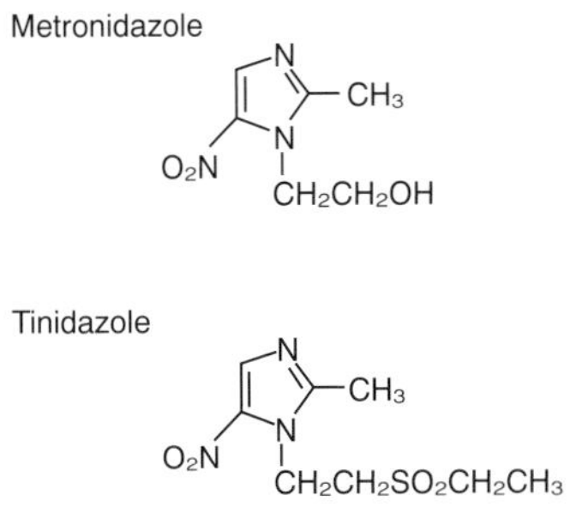

Metronidazole

Tinidazole

Fig. 9.18 Structures of metronidazole and tinidazole.

mostly insensitive (Greenwood, Watt and Duerden 1991), though they have been successfully used in infections with *H. pylori* and *Gardnerella vaginalis*.

MODE OF ACTION

The narrow spectrum of activity of 5-nitroimidazoles arises because the antibacterial effect is dependent on reduction of the nitro group under anaerobic conditions. The compounds capture electrons from reduced ferredoxin generated in the course of the decarboxylation of pyruvate by the pyruvate–ferredoxin oxidoreductase complex. The short-lived reduction product kills the cell, probably by inducing breaks in the DNA strands (Edwards 1993a). The anomalous susceptibility of certain micro-aerophiles remains unexplained, although there is evidence that it is related to unusual metabolic pathways in these organisms (Smith and Edwards 1995).

RESISTANCE

Resistance to metronidazole and other 5-nitroimidazoles remains very uncommon despite the widespread use of these compounds. Some reports have subsequently been shown to have been erroneous because sensitivity tests were carried out under inadequately anaerobic conditions. There are, nevertheless, well documented accounts of resistance in clinical isolates of *B. fragilis* and other anaerobes, usually associated with a decreased ability to reduce the drug (Edwards 1993b).

PHARMACOLOGICAL PROPERTIES

Metronidazole is usually administered by mouth, though intravenous, suppository and topical preparations are also available for various purposes. Tinidazole is available in the UK only in tablet form. They are virtually completely absorbed by the oral route and are widely distributed, including into cerebrospinal fluid. Plasma protein binding is negligible. Tinidazole has a somewhat longer half-life than metronidazole (12–14 h versus 8–10 h). Both are metabolized and excreted chiefly into urine, partly as glucuronide conjugates.

TOXICITY AND SIDE EFFECTS

Nausea and abdominal cramps occur quite frequently; various other side effects have been reported occasionally. Patients often complain of dryness in the mouth and a metallic taste. Alcohol should be avoided

because of a disulfiram-like reaction. Fears that the effect of metronidazole on DNA might lead to mutagenic or teratogenic effects in humans have not been borne out in practice (Morgan 1978, Beard et al. 1979); clinical evidence for tinidazole is lacking. It is none the less considered prudent to avoid using these drugs during pregnancy, particularly during the first trimester.

5.6 Nitrofurans

STRUCTURE AND SPECTRUM OF ACTIVITY

Various nitrofuran derivatives are in use around the world as antibacterial agents, including furazolidone and nifuratel (which are said to possess antiprotozoal as well as antibacterial activity) and nitrofurazone. However, the most widely used agent of this type, and the only one available in the UK, is nitrofurantoin (Fig. 9.19), which is used as a urinary antiseptic. Nitrofurantoin is bactericidal to most urinary pathogens at concentrations achievable in urine, although activity against *Proteus* spp. is unreliable, partly because the drug is less active in the alkaline conditions produced by urea-splitting organisms.

MODE OF ACTION

Like the nitroimidazoles, the nitrofurans are susceptible to nitroreductases, though in this case reduction takes place in an aerobic environment. The most likely explanation for the bactericidal action of these drugs is, therefore, that a reduced intermediate causes DNA strand breakage in a manner analogous to that of nitroimidazoles. This suggestion has the attraction of accounting for the known mutagenic effects of these compounds in vitro (McCalla 1977). However, more recently it has been suggested that reactive nitrofurantoin metabolites interfere not with DNA but with protein synthesis (McOsker and Fitzpatrick 1994). These authors also suggest an alternative mechanism of action that does not depend on bacterial nitroreductases.

Nitrofurantoin antagonizes the antibacterial effect of nalidixic acid and other quinolones against *Proteus mirabilis* and certain other enterobacteria (Shah and Greenwood 1988) by an unknown mechanism.

RESISTANCE

Acquired resistance in susceptible bacterial species is uncommon and, even when it does occur, is rarely plasmid mediated. For this reason multiresistant strains of enterobacteria usually remain susceptible to nitrofurantoin.

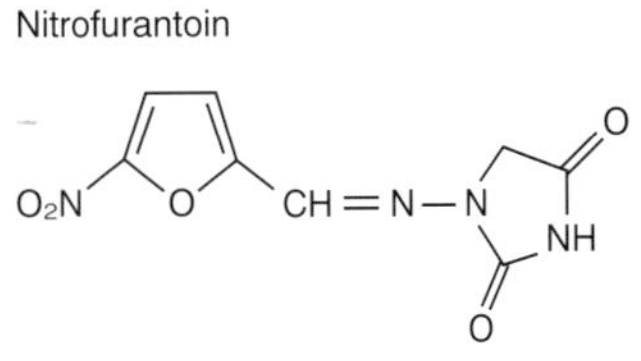

Nitrofurantoin

Fig. 9.19 Structure of nitrofurantoin.

PHARMACOLOGICAL PROPERTIES

Nitrofurantoin is administered by mouth and is rapidly and almost completely absorbed. It is excreted extremely rapidly into urine (half-life 20–60 min) and such drug as finds its way into body tissues is metabolized to the inactive derivative, aminofurantoin.

TOXICITY AND SIDE EFFECTS

Nausea is the most frequent complaint of patients receiving nitrofurantoin, but this is less common with a microcrystalline formulation. Among less common side effects, pulmonary complications are prominent, but even these are rarely seen. The mutagenic potential of nitrofurans has not prevented their widespread and evidently safe use, even in pregnancy.

5.7 Novobiocin

Novobiocin is a naturally occurring antibiotic related to the coumarin anticoagulants. It acts on the B subunit of bacterial DNA gyrase. It is quite active against staphylococci and streptococci, but not Enterobacteriaceae or pseudomonads. It was formerly used principally as an antistaphylococcal agent, but toxicity has limited its value. Multiresistant staphylococci may remain susceptible to novobiocin, but mutations to resistance occur readily.

6 AGENTS THAT ACT ON THE BACTERIAL CELL MEMBRANE

In contrast to antifungal agents, in which the cell membrane is the most common target (see Volume 4, Chapter 9), few antibacterial agents act at this level, and those that do are quite toxic. Among membrane-active agents used in human medicine, only the polymyxins have been regularly used systemically.

6.1 Polymyxins

STRUCTURE AND SPECTRUM OF ACTIVITY

The polymyxins are a family of antibiotics produced by species of *Bacillus*. They are made up of a polypeptide portion, much of which is arranged in a cyclic fashion, with a hydrophobic octanoic acid tail (Fig. 9.20). Two members of the family are in therapeutic use: polymyxin B and colistin (polymyxin E). Derivatives in which the diaminobutyric acid residues are sulphomethylated are also available. These sulphomethyl polymyxins exhibit reduced antibacterial activity, but they spontaneously break down to the more active parent compounds. Most gram-negative bacilli (with the exception of *Proteus* spp.) are sensitive to polymyxins, but their chief attraction is their activity against *P. aeruginosa*. Gram-positive organisms are much less susceptible.

MODE OF ACTION

The polymyxins act like cationic detergents to destabilize the cytoplasmic membrane. They also act on the outer membrane of gram-negative bacilli by binding to lipopolysaccharide. Polymyxin B nonapeptide, a derivative in which the fatty acid tail has been removed, binds to lipid A of lipopolysaccharide (but not to the cytoplasmic membrane) and has attracted some attention because of its anti-endotoxin properties (Danner et al. 1989).

RESISTANCE

Primary resistance in sensitive species is uncommon. However, adaptation to resistance readily occurs when dense bacterial populations are exposed to the drug (Greenwood 1975). This type of resistance is readily reversible and is apparently due to phenotypic changes in the membrane structure (Gilleland, Champlin and Conrad 1984).

PHARMACOLOGICAL PROPERTIES

Polymyxins are nowadays more widely used as topical than as systemic agents. Polymyxin B in particular features as an ingredient of a number of topical preparations. They are not absorbed when given by mouth, but oral suspensions of colistin are used in several selective digestive tract decontamination regimens in neutropenic patients (Donnelly 1993). After injection of parenteral preparations, the polymyxins bind to tissue cells, but sulphomethyl derivatives are less readily bound and are excreted more rapidly. They do not penetrate into cerebrospinal fluid. They are excreted renally with a half-life of about 6 h, but tissue binding ensures that much of the dose is retained for much longer periods. Protein binding is low.

TOXICITY AND SIDE EFFECTS

The major toxicity problems of the polymyxins relate to their affinity for cell membranes, including those of mammalian cells. Nephrotoxicty and neurotoxicity occur, but are usually reversible. Sulphomethyl polymyxins are somewhat less toxic than the sulphates. Topical preparations are generally well tolerated.

6.2 Other agents acting on bacterial membranes

Several antibiotics that are found in topical formulations, including gramicidin and tyrocidine, interfere with the integrity of bacterial cell membranes. Similarly, a number of agents used in animal husbandry, including valinomycin and monensin, achieve their effect at the membrane level. These agents act as ionophores: compounds that form transmembrane channels with consequent leakage of cellular potassium and other cations (Pressman 1973).

In addition, many antiseptics and disinfectants disrupt bacterial membranes (see Chapter 7). Naturally occurring antimicrobial peptides that are widespread in nature, such as the magainins, cecropins, defensins and the lanthionine-containing lantibiotics, also act selectively on cell membranes (Boman, Marsh and Goode 1994). There has been much interest in these and related synthetic oligopeptides, but any possible

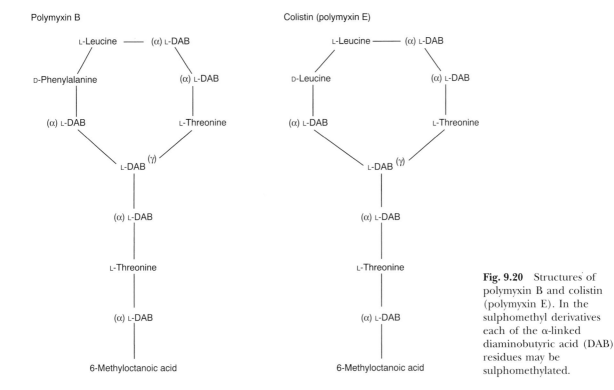

Polymyxin B

Colistin (polymyxin E)

Fig. 9.20 Structures of polymyxin B and colistin (polymyxin E). In the sulphomethyl derivatives each of the α-linked diaminobutyric acid (DAB) residues may be sulphomethylated.

future for these compounds as therapeutic agents is still some way off.

7 LABORATORY CONTROL OF ANTIMICROBIAL CHEMOTHERAPY

The performance of antimicrobial sensitivity tests and antibiotic assays are among the most important functions of medical microbiology service laboratories. Similarly, the provision of advice to clinicians and to hospital therapeutics committees on the use of antimicrobial agents forms a crucial part of the role of the clinical microbiologist. Indeed, it is essential that this role is preserved if rational antibiotic use is to be encouraged and the threat of multidrug resistance is to be kept at bay. In addition, the microbiology laboratory provides an important service in monitoring local trends of antibiotic drug resistance and in disseminating this information to prescribers (Greenwood 1993).

7.1 Sensitivity test methods

ANTIBIOTIC TITRATIONS

The intrinsic activity of antimicrobial drugs in vitro is usually expressed in terms of the **minimum inhibitory concentration** (MIC); less commonly by the **minimum bactericidal concentration** (MBC). These values are derived by titration of the drug against a standard inoculum of a pure culture of an isolated bacterial species in broth or on agar plates. The MIC is the lowest concentration that prevents the development of visible growth after a period of incubation that is usually 16–20 h for most common pathogens, but may be longer for slow-growing organisms. The MBC is assessed from broth titrations by subculture of those dilutions of antibiotic that are above the MIC. The lowest concentration of antibiotic that achieves a 1000-fold or greater reduction in the original bacterial inoculum (i.e. a fall in viable count of at least 3 $\log_{10}$ colony-forming units) is generally taken as the MBC. The rate of killing may be more important than the overnight MBC value. In this case it is necessary to count the number of viable organisms at regular intervals after exposure to appropriate concentrations of the antimicrobial agent. In assessing viablity it is good practice to specify **colony-forming units** rather than bacterial numbers, since bacteria may grow in clumps or chains that give rise to single colonies on solid media.

Although MIC titrations provide figures that are widely used in comparing the activity of different antimicrobial agents, the results may be extremely variable depending on the test conditions and on the bacterial inoculum (Amsterdam 1991). Moreover, the factors determining the end point of MIC titrations vary from drug to drug and from organism to organism (Greenwood 1981). Selected MIC values shown in Table 9.5 should be interpreted in the light of these provisos.

MIC titrations are generally too time-consuming for routine purposes, although prepared microtitration trays containing suitable dilutions of lyophilized antibiotic can be used to simplify the procedure. Alternatively, the E test, in which a linear gradient of antibiotic is carried on a special strip applied to a plate inoculum of the test organism, can be used. This method is very simple and appears to correlate well

Table 9.5 Activity in vitro of some representative antibacterial agents against selected micro-organisms

Antibacterial agent	Minimum inhibitory concentration (mg l^{-1})									
	Staphylococcus aureus	*Streptococcus pyogenes*	*Streptococcus pneumoniae*	*Neisseria meningitidis*	*Haemophilus influenzae*	*Escherichia coli*	*Klebsiella pneumoniae*	*Pseudomonas aeruginosa*	*Bacteroides fragilis*	*Chlamydia trachomatis*
Benzylpenicillin	0.1	0.01	0.02	0.02	1	64	R	R	16	R
Amoxycillin	0.1	0.01	0.03	0.06	0.25	2	R	R	16	R
Cephalexin	2	1	2	2	16	8	8	R	R	R
Cefuroxime	1	0.02	0.02	0.06	0.5	2	4	R	R	R
Cefotaxime	1	0.02	0.02	<0.01	0.01	0.06	0.03	16	R	R
Imipenem	0.03	0.01	0.01	0.03	0.25	0.25	0.25	1	0.1	R
Gentamicin	0.25	8	16	2	0.5	0.5	0.5	1	R	R
Chloramphenicol	4	4	2	1	0.5	4	1	R	2	2
Doxycycline	0.5	0.25	0.25	2	1	2	4	R	0.25	0.02
Erythromycin	0.25	0.06	0.06	1	1	R	R	R	1	0.25
Fusidic acid	0.06	8	8	0.25	R	R	R	R	2	...
Sulphamethoxazole	8	2	16	0.25	2	4	8	R	R	R
Trimethoprim	0.25	0.25	1	8	0.25	0.25	0.5	R	4	R
Nalidixic acid	64	R	R	0.5	1	4	4	R	R	R
Ciprofloxacin	0.5	0.5	1	<0.01	0.01	0.06	0.06	0.25	8	0.5
Rifampicin	0.03	0.06	0.06	0.01	0.5	8	16	32	0.25	<0.01
Metronidazole	R	R	R	R	R	R	R	R	0.5	R
Nitrofurantoin	4	4	...	...	...	4	32	R	8	R
Polymyxin B	R	R	R	...	0.03	0.03	0.03	0.03	...	...

These minimum inhibitory concentrations refer to approximate modal values for fully susceptible strains without acquired resistance traits. In using this table it should be borne in mind that inhibitory concentrations may vary considerably depending on the conditions of the test and the bacterial inoculum used.
R, intrinsically resistant (agent has no useful activity).

with more traditional methods (Baker et al. 1991, Brown and Brown 1991).

DISC DIFFUSION METHODS

Most medical microbiology laboratories use one of the disc diffusion techniques in which antibiotics incorporated into absorbent discs are applied to the surface of culture plates seeded with the test organism (Acar and Goldstein 1991, Brown 1994). Antibiotic diffuses rapidly from the disc into the surrounding medium, setting up a concentration gradient of the drug. The edge of a zone of inhibition is formed where the concentration is able to prevent visible growth of the micro-organism (Barry 1991).

In the USA, a highly standardized disc method based on the technique originally described by Bauer et al. (1966), and consequently known as the **Bauer–Kirby** (or **Kirby–Bauer**) **test** is widely used. In the UK it is more usual to use Stokes' comparative disc method, in which the test and control organism are both exposed to the gradient of antibiotic under identical conditions on the same plate (Stokes, Ridgway and Wren 1993). Stokes' method is particularly useful in conditions such as exist in many developing countries in which refrigeration facilities are unreliable, so that discs are kept in unsatisfactory, often humid conditions.

By comparing disc zone sizes and MIC values for many different organisms, a relationship between the 2 is evident and this can be formalized by regression analysis. However, since the factors that determine the end point of MIC titrations differ considerably from those that operate in the conditions of the disc diffusion test, the relationship is less than perfect. This is particularly true for those organisms that are of intermediate susceptibility, for which there may be wide discrepancies between the 2 methods.

BREAKPOINT METHOD

Many laboratories with large workloads find it convenient to use the **breakpoint** method of sensitivity testing, since this allows many isolates of bacteria to be tested together. In this method antibiotics are incorporated into agar plates at predetermined 'breakpoint' concentrations based on therapeutically meaningful levels. Plates are spot-inoculated with a multipoint inoculation device and incubated overnight. If no growth occurs at the breakpoint concentration, the organism is scored as sensitive; if growth occurs, the organism is regarded as resistant. Sometimes a second, higher breakpoint is also used in order to establish a category of 'reduced susceptibility'. By use of a plate scanner to read the result, the whole method can be semi-automated.

OTHER METHODS OF SENSITIVITY TESTING

Many different mechanized or semi-automated methods have been devised for determining MICs or otherwise estimating the sensitivity status of bacteria (Tilton 1991). Some of these machines produce results much more rapidly than traditional methods, but the correlation is often less than perfect, partly

because of the requirement for reading the end point turbidimetrically (Greenwood 1985).

DNA probes that are able to detect the genetic potential for resistance have also received much attention in recent years. These methods need to be refined if they are to be of use as routine methods, since most probes are too specific to detect the wide range of resistance mechanisms that may be present. Moreover, the presence of a resistance gene does not guarantee that it will necessarily be expressed (Towner 1992b). None the less, DNA probes offer an attractive solution to the problem of detecting specific resistance mechanisms, particularly in organisms that are difficult to grow.

CHOICE OF METHOD

All methods of sensitivity testing have their advantages and disadvantages and none can satisfy the requirements of all types of micro-organism and antimicrobial drug. Even the type of culture medium to use is problematical. Mueller–Hinton medium has been widely used, especially in the USA, but it is difficult to standardize and media that have been specially formulated for sensitivity testing purposes, such as Iso-Sensitest medium, or Diagnostic Sensitivity Test medium, may be more appropriate as general purpose media (Report 1991).

In the USA and some other countries, prescribed methods of susceptibility testing carried out under closely defined conditions are formulated by the National Committee for Clinical Laboratory Standards (NCCLS 1992, 1993) and endorsed by official approval. This policy has the advantage of fostering reproducibility among different laboratories, but is inflexible and does not guarantee that the agreed procedure is therapeutically meaningful. In the UK, a more permissive approach is favoured, in which laboratories are free to use whatever method is considered appropriate for their particular circumstances (Report 1991). Performance is monitored by participation in an external quality assurance scheme. Other countries have their own variants of these recommendations.

CLINICAL RELEVANCE OF ANTIBIOTIC SENSITIVITY TESTS

A laboratory report indicating in vitro susceptibility of a micro-organism to a particular agent by no means ensures that a therapeutic response will be achieved if that drug is used in treatment. Much will depend on the type of infection, the condition of the patient, and the pharmacological properties of the drug. A statement about in vitro resistance is more likely to indicate that treatment with that agent will not influence the course of infection, although the patient may recover for other reasons: for example, through the influence of normal host defence mechanisms, by the surgical drainage of a collection of pus, or by the removal of a catheter.

In vitro susceptibility tests by their very nature offer only a crude approximation to the complex situation that exists in the infected patient. Laboratory reports merely provide information that needs to be interpreted thoughtfully in the light of the limitations of the tests and the condition of the individual patient (Slack 1995a).

7.2 Antibiotic assays

INDICATIONS FOR ANTIBIOTIC ASSAY

Aside from the need to establish the pharmacokinetic behaviour of antimicrobial drugs in the early stages of their development, indications for the assay of antimicrobial agents in clinical practice are few. The most common grounds for antibiotic assay are provided by those agents, pre-eminently the aminoglycosides, in which the therapeutic range (the difference between an effective concentration and a toxic concentration) is relatively narrow. With such agents, dosage is often initated by use of a nomogram that takes account of the sex-related creatinine concentration (a measure of renal function), body weight and age of the patient (Mawer et al. 1974). Assays are subsequently performed 1 h after the dose, to establish that an adequate peak concentration of the drug has been achieved, and just before the next dose ('trough' concentration) to check that drug accummulation has not occurred (Humphreys and Reeves 1991).

Other antibiotics that may require laboratory assay during drug therapy include vancomycin (though the need for this has been disputed: Ackerman 1994, Cantú, Yamanaka-Yuen and Lietman 1994) and chloramphenicol in young infants who may be in danger of the 'grey baby' syndrome through an immature capacity to metabolize the drug.

ASSAY METHODS

Traditional plate diffusion methods of antibiotic assay have largely been superseded by automated immunoassay procedures that are more specific, more accurate and much more rapid. High pressure liquid chromatography methods are also available for most antimicrobial agents. They are useful for certain purposes, since metabolites can often be identified and quantified by this means, but they are too cumbersome for routine use. The various assay methods that are in use are described in detail by Reeves et al. (1978) and Chapin-Robertson and Edberg (1991).

SERUM BACTERICIDAL TEST

A type of antibiotic assay commonly called **back-titration**, in which the bactericidal activity of the patient's serum is titrated against the organism responsible for the infection, is sometimes used in conditions in which it is important to achieve a bactericidal effect. The test is commonly used in the management of infective endocarditis and is also sometimes recommended in other types of infection, including osteomyelitis and sepsis in immunocompromised patients. Peak (usually 1 h after administration of the dose) and trough (immediately before the next dose) concentrations are assayed. The bactericidal end point is measured by subculture of dilutions of patient's serum that inhibit growth of the organism during overnight incubation. The result may reflect the activity of more than one agent if combination therapy is being used.

The value of the serum bactericidal test has been questioned, not least because of the many technical variables that may affect the result (Peterson and Shanholtzer 1992). Moreover, clinical correlates with successful therapy have been hard to come by, although a peak serum bactericidal titre ≥ 32, and a trough ≥ 16 are usually associated with a bacteriological cure.

8 GENERAL ASPECTS OF THE USE OF ANTIMICROBIAL AGENTS

8.1 The rational use of antimicrobial agents

Antimicrobial agents are widely used in human and veterinary medicine for the prevention and treatment of infection. In addition, they are exploited for growth promotion in animal husbandry. As will be evident from this chapter, we possess an abundance of antibacterial agents, but the seemingly endless ability of micro-organisms to develop and spread resistance determinants poses a constant threat to the efficacy of these valuable drugs (Cohen 1992, Greenwood 1995b).

Although large amounts of antibiotics are used in animals, with the consequent emergence of resistant strains of bacteria that undoubtedly enter the food chain, the impact of this on the efficacy of drugs used in human medicine is thought to be overshadowed by the selective pressures imposed by human use (Linton 1985, Walton 1992). Certainly, the regulation and use of antimicrobial agents in human medicine throughout the world leaves much to be desired (Chetley 1995).

In most countries of the industrially developed world, antibiotics used in human and veterinary practice are presently available only on prescription. It is most important that this status is maintained if resistance problems are to be kept under control. Most hospitals now have some sort of antibiotic usage policy and this is also a valuable means of controlling the use of these drugs. Equally important is the strict implementation of infection control procedures, so that hospital-acquired infection and the attendant need for broad spectrum therapy is kept to a minimum.

In developing countries where regulation of pharmaceutical products is generally more lax, more responsible national drug policies need to be enforced (Kunin 1993). The World Health Organization is actively engaged in promoting rational policies of drug use, but much remains to be done. One important initiative has been the formulation of an essential drug list which is updated at regular intervals (World Health Organization 1995). Only a handful of antibacterial agents appear on this list (Table 9.6); significantly, there are no cephalosporins or quinolones on the main list, emphasizing the restricted need for these extensively promoted and commonly prescribed drugs.

Indeed, a great deal of antibiotic usage is unnecessary. Attention has been drawn many times, for example, to the inappropriate use of antibacterial drugs in acute diarrhoea and upper respiratory tract infection, much of which is viral in origin. Several surveys have noted a trend towards the more frequent use of antibiotics (particularly newer, more expensive agents) in general practice (Wyatt et al. 1990, Anon. 1994, McCaig and Hughes 1995).

8.2 General principles of use of antimicrobial agents for treatment and prophylaxis

The general principles underlying the choice of antimicrobial agents in infection are discussed by Lambert and O'Grady (1996) and Finch (1995). In brief, antibiotics should be used therapeutically only after thorough clinical assessment of the need, whenever possible on the basis of laboratory evidence of infection. Factors to be considered should include: the type of infection; the age and condition of the patient; the local prevalence of resistance (in the absence of specific laboratory guidance); the pharmacological properties of the agent in its various formulations; the likelihood of adverse reactions; possible interactions with other medications; and cost. Antimicrobial agents should be used for chemoprophylaxis only in individuals in whom the risk of infection is high. The agents chosen should be reliably active against the organisms likely to be encountered and use should be confined to the period of greatest risk (Slack 1995b).

ANTIMICROBIAL DRUG COMBINATIONS

The use of combinations of antimicrobial agents is seldom necessary and increases the risk of adverse reactions from the antibiotics themselves and from interactions with other drugs that the patient may be receiving. Exceptions include: use of combination therapy in tuberculosis and leprosy; use of compounds that interact synergically to achieve improved bactericidal activity in certain serious infections, notably infective endocarditis; use of combinations to achieve adequate cover of mixed infections or in the 'blind' therapy of serious undiagnosed sepsis; use of certain β-lactam agents with β-lactamase inhibitors; and use of co-trimoxazole in circumstances in which the benefits of the combination outweigh the risks.

The twentieth century has seen unprecedented advances in the treatment of infection. More than 250 individual compounds are now on the world market for the systemic treatment of bacterial infection. However, the process of drug discovery and development is now so costly and the return so uncertain that it is unlikely that this abundance will be matched in the next century (Billstein 1994). Already pharmaceutical companies are turning their attention from antibacterial agents to the potentially more profitable areas of antiviral and antifungal compounds.

The ability of the drug houses to come up with new and ever more potent agents has, until now, blunted the impact of bacterial resistance and weakened our resolve to preserve the value of antibiotics by circumscribing their use. Such wastefulness can no longer be afforded. The second half of the twentieth century has truly been a golden age of antibiotics. The future is largely in the hands of the prescriber.

Table 9.6 Antibacterial agents (excluding topical agents) on the World Health Organization's list of essential drugs (WHO 1995)

Main list			Complementary list[a]
Penicillins	**Other antibacterial agents**	**Antimycobacterial agents**	
Amoxycillin[b]	Chloramphenicol[b]	Clofazimine	Chloramphenicol (oily suspension)
Ampicillin	Co-trimoxazole[b]	Dapsone	Ciprofloxacin
Benzathine penicillin	Doxycycline	Ethambutol	Clindamycin
Benzylpenicillin	Erythromycin[b]	Isoniazid	Nalidixic acid
Cloxacillin[b]	Gentamicin[b]	Pyrazinamide	Nitrofurantoin
Phenoxymethylpenicillin	Metronidazole[b]	Rifampicin	Trimethoprim
Piperacillin[b]	Spectinomycin	Rifampicin + isoniazid	Thioacetazone + isoniazid (antimycobacterial)
Procaine penicillin	Sulphadimidine[b]	Streptomycin	
	Tetracycline[b]		

[a]For use when drugs on the main list are known to be ineffective or inappropriate for a given individual, or for use in exceptional circumstances (e.g. chloramphenicol oily suspension in epidemics of meningitis) when the health services are overwhelmed. The need for additional reserve agents, e.g. a cephalosporin or vancomycin, is acknowledged.
[b]Example of a therapeutic group for which acceptable alternatives exist.

REFERENCES

Abraham EP, 1990, Oxford, Howard Florey, and World War II, *Launching the antibiotic era*, eds Moberg CL, Cohn ZA, Rockefeller University Press, New York, 19–30.

Abraham EP, Chain E et al., 1941, Further observations on penicillin, *Lancet*, **2**: 177–89.

Acar JF, Goldstein FW, 1991, Disk susceptibility test, *Antibiotics in Laboratory Medicine*, 3rd edn, ed. Lorian V, Williams & Wilkins, Baltimore, 17–52.

Ackerman BH, 1994, Clinical value of monitoring serum vancomycin concentrations, *Clin Infect Dis*, **19**: 1180–1.

Ambler RP, 1980, The structure of β-lactamases, *Philos Trans R Soc Lond [Biol]*, **289**: 321–31.

Amsterdam D, 1991, Susceptibility testing of antimicrobials in liquid media, *Antibiotics in Laboratory Medicine*, 3rd edn, Lorian V, Williams & Wilkins, Baltimore, 53–105.

Anon., 1994, *Diseases Fighting Back – the Growing Resistance of TB and Other Bacterial Diseases to Treatment*, Parliamentary Office of Science and Technology, London.

Aronsson B, Möllby R, Nord CE, 1984, Diagnosis and epidemiology of *Clostridium difficile* enterocolitis in Sweden, *J Antimicrob Chemother*, **14, Suppl. D:** 85–95.

Aumercier M, Bouhallab S et al., 1992, RP 59500: a proposed mechanism for its bactericidal activity, *J Antimicrob Chemother*, **30, Suppl. A:** 9–14.

Bailey RL, Arullendran P et al., 1993, Randomised controlled trial of single-dose azithromycin in treatment of trachoma, *Lancet*, **342**: 453–6.

Baker CN, Stocker SA et al., 1991, Comparison of the E test to agar dilution, broth microdilution, and agar diffusion susceptibility test techniques using a special challenge set of bacteria, *J Clin Microbiol*, **29**: 533–8.

Barrière JC, Bouanchaud DH et al., 1992, Antimicrobial activity against *Staphylococcus aureus* of semisynthetic injectable streptogramins: RP 59500 and related compounds, *J Antimicrob Chemother*, **30, Suppl. A:** 1–8.

Barry AL, 1991, Procedures and theoretical considerations for testing antimicrobial agents in agar media, *Antibiotics in Laboratory Medicine*, 3rd edn, ed. Lorian V, Williams & Wilkins, Baltimore, 1–16.

Bauer AW, Kirby WMM et al., 1966, Antibiotic susceptibility testing by a standardized single disk method, *Am J Clin Pathol*, **45**: 493–6.

Beard C, Noller KL et al., 1979, Lack of evidence for cancer due to use of metronidazole, *N Engl J Med*, **301**: 519–22.

Beer JJ, 1958, Coal-tar dye manufacture and the origins of the modern industrial research laboratory, *Isis*, **49**: 123–31.

Bigger JW, 1944, Treatment of staphylococcal infections with penicillin by intermittent sterilization, *Lancet*, **1**: 497–500.

Billstein SA, 1994, How the pharmaceutical industry brings an antibiotic drug to market in the United States, *Antimicrob Agents Chemother*, **38**: 2679–82.

Black FT, Wildfang IL, Borgbjerg K, 1985, Activity of fusidic acid against *Plasmodium falciparum* in vitro, *Lancet*, **1**: 578–9.

Boman HG, Marsh J, Goode JA (eds), 1994, *Antimicrobial Peptides. Ciba Foundation Symposium 186*, John Wiley & Sons, Chichester.

Böttger EC, Wallace RJ, 1994, Lack of rifabutin resistance with prophylaxis for disseminated *Mycobacterium avium* complex, *Lancet*, **344**: 1506–7.

Brown DFJ, 1994, Developments in antimicrobial susceptibility testing, *Rev Med Microbiol*, **5**: 65–75.

Brown DFJ, Brown L, 1991, Evaluation of the E test, a novel method for quantifying antimicrobial activity, *J Antimicrob Chemother*, **27**: 185–90.

Bundtzen RW, Gerber AU et al., 1981, Postantibiotic suppression of bacterial growth, *Rev Infect Dis*, **3**: 28–37.

Bush K, 1989, Characterization of β-lactamases, *Antimicrob Agents Chemother*, **33**: 259–76.

Bush K, Jacoby GA, Medeiros AA, 1995, A functional classification scheme for β-lactamases and its correlation with molecular structure, *Antimicrob Agents Chemother*, **39**: 1211–33.

Cantú TG, Yamanaka-Yuen NA, Lietman PS, 1994, Serum vancomycin concentrations: reappraisal of their clinical value, *Clin Infect Dis*, **18**: 533–43.

Chain E, Florey HW et al., 1940, Penicillin as a chemotherapeutic agent, *Lancet*, **2**: 226–8.

Chapin-Robertson K, Edberg SC, 1991, Measurement of antibiotics in human body fluids: techniques and significance, *Antibiotics in Laboratory Medicine*, 3rd edn, ed. Lorian V, Williams & Wilkins, Baltimore, 295–366.

Chetley A, 1995, *Problem Drugs*, Zed Books, London.

Chopra I, Hawkey PM, Hinton M, 1992, Tetracyclines, molecular and clinical aspects, *J Antimicrob Chemother*, **29**: 245–77.

Cohen ML, 1992, Epidemiology of drug resistance: implications for a post-antimicrobial era, *Science*, **257**: 1050–5.

Colebrook L, Kenny M, 1936, Treatment of human puerperal infections, and of experimental infections in mice, with prontosil, *Lancet*, **1**: 1279–86.

Cosar C, Julou L, 1959, Activity of 1-(2^1-hydroxyethyl)-2-methyl-5-nitroimidazole (8823 RP) against experimental *Trichomonas vaginalis* infection, *Ann Inst Pasteur*, **96**: 238–41.

Craig WA, Gudmundsson S, 1991, The post-antibiotic effect, *Antibiotics in Laboratory Medicine*, 3rd edn, ed. Lorian V, Williams & Wilkins, Baltimore, 403–31.

Cundliffe E, 1972, The mode of action of fusidic acid, *Biochem Biophys Res Commun*, **46**: 1794–801.

Danner RL, Joiner KA et al., 1989, Purification, toxicity, and antiendotoxin activity of polymyxin B nonapeptide, *Antimicrob Agents Chemother*, **33**: 1428–34.

Davis BD, 1988, The lethal action of aminoglycosides, *J Antimicrob Chemother*, **22**: 1–3.

Dodd MC, Stillman WB, 1944, The in vitro bacteristatic action of some simple furan derivatives, *J Pharmacol Exp Ther*, **82**: 11–18.

Dollery C (ed.), 1991, *Therapeutic Drugs*, 2 volumes + supplements, Churchill Livingstone, Edinburgh.

Domagala JM, 1994, Structure–activity and structure–side-effect relationships for the quinolone antibacterials, *J Antimicrob Chemother*, **33**: 685–706.

Domagk G, 1935, Ein Beitrag zur Chemotherapie der bakteriellen Infektionen, *Dtsch Med Wochenschr*, **61**: 250–3.

Donnelly JP, 1993, Selective decontamination of the digestive tract and its role in antimicrobial prophylaxis, *J Antimicrob Chemother*, **31**: 813–29.

Doona M, Walsh JB, 1995, Use of chloramphenicol as topical eye medication: time to cry halt? *Br Med J*, **310**: 1217–18.

Dubos RJ, 1939, Bactericidal effect of an extract of a soil bacillus on Gram-positive cocci, *Proc Soc Exp Biol Med*, **40**: 311–12.

Dünschede H-B, 1971, *Tropenmedizinische Forschung bei Bayer*, Michael Triltsch Verlag, Düsseldorf.

Eagle H, Musselman AD, 1948, The rate of bactericidal action of penicillin *in vitro* as a function of its concentration, and its paradoxically reduced activity at high concentrations against certain organisms, *J Exp Med*, **88**: 99–131.

Editorial, 1978, The nitroimidazole family of drugs, *Br J Vener Dis*, **54**: 69–71.

Edwards DI, 1993a, Nitroimidazole drugs – action and resistance mechanisms. I. Mechanisms of action, *J Antimicrob Chemother*, **31**: 9–20.

Edwards DI, 1993b, Nitroimidazole drugs – action and resistance mechanisms. II. Mechanisms of resistance, *J Antimicrob Chemother*, **31**: 201–10.

Ehrlich P, Hata S, 1911, *The Experimental Chemotherapy of Spirilloses*, Rebman Ltd, London.

Etienne SD, Montay G et al., 1992, A phase I, double-blind, placebo-controlled study of the tolerance and pharmacokinetic behaviour of RP 59500, *J Antimicrob Chemother*, **30, Suppl. A:** 123–31.

Falco EA, Goodwin LG et al., 1951, 2:4-diaminopyrimidines – a new series of antimalarials, *Br J Pharmacol*, **6:** 185–200.

Farthing MJG, Inge PMG, 1986, Antigiardial activity of the bile salt-like antibiotic sodium fusidate, *J Antimicrob Chemother*, **17:** 165–71.

Finch RG, 1995, General principles of the treatment of infection, *Antimicrobial Chemotherapy*, 3rd edn, ed. Greenwood D, Oxford University Press, Oxford, 179–87.

Fleming A, 1929, On the antibacterial action of cultures of a penicillium, with special reference to their use in the isolation of *B. influenzae*, *Br J Exp Pathol*, **10:** 226–36.

Fox HH, 1953, The chemical attack on tuberculosis, *Trans NY Acad Sci*, **15:** 234–42.

Garcia-Rodriguez JA, Gomez Garcia AC, 1993, In-vitro activities of quinolones against mycobacteria, *J Antimicrob Chemother*, **32:** 797–808.

Gilleland HE, Champlin FR, Conrad RS, 1984, Chemical alterations in cell envelopes of *Pseudomonas aeruginosa* upon exposure to polymyxin: a possible mechanism to explain adaptive resistance, *Can J Microbiol*, **20:** 869–73.

Greenwood D, 1972, Mucopeptide hydrolases and bacterial 'persisters', *Lancet*, **2:** 465–6.

Greenwood D, 1975, The activity of polymyxins against dense populations of *Escherichia coli*, *J Gen Microbiol*, **91:** 110–18.

Greenwood D, 1981, *In vitro veritas*? Antimicrobial susceptibility tests and their clinical relevance, *J Infect Dis*, **144:** 380–5.

Greenwood D, 1985, The alteration of microbial growth curves by antibiotics, *Rapid Methods and Automation in Microbiology and Immunology*, ed. Habermehl K-O, Springer-Verlag, Berlin, 497–503.

Greenwood D, 1988, Fusidic acid, *The Antimicrobial Agents Annual 3*, eds Peterson PK, Verhoef J, Elsevier, Amsterdam, 106–12.

Greenwood D, 1993, Antimicrobial susceptibility testing: are we wasting our time? *Br J Biomed Sci*, **50:** 31–4.

Greenwood D (ed.), 1995a, *Antimicrobial Chemotherapy*, 3rd edn, Oxford University Press, Oxford.

Greenwood D, 1995b, Tarnished gold: sixty years of antimicrobial drug use and misuse, *J Med Microbiol*, **43:** 395–6.

Greenwood D, O'Grady F, 1972, The effect of osmolality on the response of *Escherichia coli* and *Proteus mirabilis* to penicillins, *Br J Exp Pathol*, **53:** 457–64.

Greenwood D, O'Grady F, 1973a, Comparison of the responses of *Escherichia coli* and *Proteus mirabilis* to seven β-lactam antibiotics, *J Infect Dis*, **128:** 211–22.

Greenwood D, O'Grady F, 1973b, The two sites of penicillin action in *Escherichia coli*, *J Infect Dis*, **128:** 791–4.

Greenwood D, O'Grady F, 1976, Activity and interaction of trimethoprim and sulphamethoxazole against *Escherichia coli*, *J Clin Pathol*, **29:** 162–6.

Greenwood D, O'Grady F, 1977, Factors governing the emergence of resistance to nalidixic acid in the treatment of urinary tract infection, *Antimicrob Agents Chemother*, **12:** 678–81.

Greenwood D, Watt B, Duerden BI, 1991, Antibiotics and anerobes, *Anaerobes in Human Disease*, eds Duerden BI, Drasar BS, Edward Arnold, London, 415–29.

Greenwood D, Palfreyman J et al., 1988, Activity of teicoplanin against Gram-negative anaerobes, *J Antimicrob Chemother*, **21:** 500–1.

Hancock REW, Bellido F, 1992, Antibiotic uptake: unusual results for unusual molecules, *J Antimicrob Chemother*, **29:** 235–43.

Handwerger S, Tomasz A, 1985, Antibiotic tolerance among clinical isolates of bacteria, *Rev Infect Dis*, **7:** 368–86.

Healy SP, Zervos MJ, 1995, Mechanisms of resistance of enterococci to antimicrobial agents, *Rev Med Microbiol*, **6:** 70–6.

Hitchins GH, 1969, Species differences among dihydrofolate reductases as a basis for chemotherapy, *Postgrad Med J*, **45, Suppl.:** 7–10.

Honeybourne D, Baldwin DR, 1992, The site concentrations of antimicrobial agents in the lung, *J Antimicrob Chemother*, **30:** 249–60.

Hooper DC, 1995, From fluoroquinolones to 2-pyridones, *Lancet*, **345:** 1192–3.

Hooper DC, Wolfson JS, 1989, Mode of action of the quinolone antimicrobial agents: review of recent information, *Rev Infect Dis*, **11, Suppl. 5:** S902–11.

Hooper DC, Wolfson JS, 1991, Fluoroquinolone antimicrobial agents, *N Engl J Med*, **324:** 384–94.

Hotchkiss RD, 1990, From microbes to medicine: gramicidin, René Dubos, and the Rockefeller, *Launching the Antibiotic Era*, eds Moberg CL, Cohn ZA, Rockefeller University Press, New York, 1–18.

Hughes J, Mellows G, 1980, Interaction of pseudomonic acid A with *Escherichia coli* B isoleucyl-tRNA synthetase, *Biochem J*, **191:** 209–19.

Humble MW, Eykyn S, Phillips I, 1980, Staphylococcal bacteraemia, fusidic acid, and jaundice, *Br Med J*, **280:** 1495–8.

Humphreys H, Reeves D, 1991, Aminoglycoside assays, *Rev Med Microbiol*, **2:** 13–21.

Huovinen P, Sundström L et al., 1995, Trimethoprim and sulphonamide resistance, *Antimicrob Agents Chemother*, **39:** 279–89.

Jacoby GA, Archer GL, 1991, New mechanisms of bacterial resistance to antimicrobial agents, *N Engl J Med*, **324:** 601–12.

Johnson AP, Uttley AHC et al., 1990, Resistance to vancomycin and teicoplanin: an emerging clinical problem, *Clin Microbiol Rev*, **3:** 280–91.

Kahan JS, Kahan FM et al., 1979, Thienamycin, a new beta-lactam antibiotic: I. Discovery, taxonomy, isolation and physical properties, *J Antibiot*, **32:** 1–12.

Kahan FM, Kropp H et al., 1983, Thienamycin: development of imipenem-cilastatin, *J Antimicrob Chemother*, **12:** 1–35.

Klugman KP, 1990, Pneumococcal resistance to antibiotics, *Clin Microbiol Rev*, **3:** 171–96.

Knudsen ET, Rolinson GN, Sutherland R, 1967, Carbenicillin: a new semisynthetic penicillin active against *Pseudomonas aeruginosa*, *Br Med J*, **3:** 75–8.

Kucers A, Bennett NMcK, 1987, *The Use of Antibiotics*, 4th edn, Heinemann, London.

Kunin CM, 1993, Resistance to antimicrobial drugs – a worldwide calamity, *Ann Intern Med*, **118:** 557–61.

Lambert HP, O'Grady FW, 1997, General principles of chemotherapy, *Antibiotic and Chemotherapy*, 7th edn, eds O'Grady F, Lambert HP, Finch RG, Greenwood D, Churchill Livingstone, Edinburgh, 131–35.

Lehmann J, 1946, *Para*-aminosalicylic acid in the treatment of tuberculosis, *Lancet*, **1:** 15–16.

Levison ME, 1992, New dosing regimens for aminoglycoside antibiotics, *Ann Intern Med*, **117:** 693–4.

Linton AH, 1985, Antibiotic resistance in bacteria associated with animals and their importance to man, *J Antimicrob Chemother*, **15:** 385–6.

Lipsky JJ, 1988, Antibiotic-associated hypoprothrombinaemia, *J Antimicrob Chemother*, **21:** 281–300.

McCaig LF, Hughes JM, 1995, Trends in antimicrobial drug prescribing among office-based physicians in the United States, *JAMA*, **273:** 214–19.

McCalla DR, 1977, Biological effects of nitrofurans, *J Antimicrob Chemother*, **3:** 517–20.

MacGowan AP, Greig MA et al., 1989, Pharmacokinetics and tolerance of a new film-coated tablet of sodium fusidate administered as a single oral dose to healthy volunteers, *J Antimicrob Chemother*, **23:** 409–15.

McOsker CC, Fitzpatrick PM, 1994, Nitrofurantoin: mechanism of action and implications for resistance development in common uropathogens, *J Antimicrob Chemother*, **33, Suppl. A:** 23–30.

Maple PAC, Hamilton-Miller JMT, Brumfitt W, 1989, World-wide antibiotic resistance in methicillin-resistant *Staphylococcus aureus*, *Lancet*, **1:** 537–40.

Martin DH, Mroczkowski TF et al., 1992, A controlled trial of a single dose of azithromycin for the treatment of chlamydial urethritis and cervicitis, *N Engl J Med*, **327**: 921–5.

Mawer GE, Ahmad R et al., 1974, Prescribing aids for gentamicin, *Br J Clin Pharmacol*, **1**: 45–50.

Mazzei T, Mini E et al., 1993, Chemistry and mode of action of macrolides, *J Antimicrob Chemother*, **31, Suppl. C**: 1–9.

Midtvedt T, Greenwood D, 1994, Miscellaneous antibacterial drugs, *Side Effects of Drugs Annual 17*, eds Aronson JK, van Boxtel CJ, Elsevier Science BV, Amsterdam, 303–18.

Mitchison DA, 1992, Understanding the chemotherapy of tuberculosis – current problems, *J Antimicrob Chemother*, **29**: 477–93.

Morgan I, 1978, Metronidazole treatment in pregnancy, *Int J Gynaecol Obstet*, **15**: 501–2.

Mulla RJ, Barnes E et al., 1995, Is it time to stop using chloramphenicol on the eye? *Br Med J*, **311**: 450–1.

National Committee for Clinical Laboratory Standards, 1992, 1993, Performance standards for antimicrobial disk susceptibility tests, *Approved Standard*, 5th edn, Documents No. M2-A5; M100-S4, NCCLS, Villanova, PA.

Nicolaier A, 1895, Ueber die therapeutische Verwendung des Urotropin (hexamethylentetramin), *Dtsch Med Wochenschr*, **21**: 541–3.

Nikaido H, 1985, Role of permeability barriers in resistance to β-lactam antibiotics, *Pharmacol Ther*, **27**: 197–231.

Nikaido H, Vaara M, 1985, Molecular basis of bacterial outer membrane permeability, *Microbiol Rev*, **49**: 1–32.

Noble WC, Virani Z, Cree RGA, 1992, Co-transfer of vancomycin and other resistance genes from *Enterococcus faecalis* NCTC 12201 to *Staphylococcus aureus*, *FEMS Microbiol Lett*, **93**: 195–8.

O'Grady F, Greenwood D, 1973, Interactions between fusidic acid and penicillins, *J Med Microbiol*, **6**: 441–50.

O'Grady F, Lambert H, Finch RG, Greenwood D, (eds) 1997, *Antibiotic and Chemotherapy*, 7th edn, Churchill Livingstone, Edinburgh.

Oleske JM, Phillips I (eds), 1983, Clindamycin: bacterial virulence and host defence, *J Antimicrob Chemother*, **12, Suppl. C**: 1–124.

Oriel JD, 1989, Use of quinolones in chlamydial infection, *Rev Infect Dis*, **11, Suppl. 5**: S1273–6.

Payne DJ, 1993, Metallo-β-lactamases – a new therapeutic challenge, *J Med Microbiol*, **39**: 93–9.

Pestka S, 1971, Inhibitors of ribosome functions, *Annu Rev Microbiol*, **25**: 487–562.

Peterson LR, 1994, Quinolone resistance in Gram-positive bacteria, *Infect Dis Clin Pract*, **3, Suppl. 3**: S127–37.

Peterson LR, Shanholtzer CJ, 1992, Tests for bactericidal effects of antimicrobial agents: technical performance and clinical relevance, *Clin Microbiol Rev*, **5**: 420–32.

Pressman BC, 1973, Properties of ionophores with broad range cation selectivity, *Fed Proc*, **32**: 1698–703.

Reeves DS, 1987, The pharmacokinetics of fusidic acid, *J Antimicrob Chemother*, **20**: 467–76.

Reeves DS, 1994, Fosfomycin trometamol, *J Antimicrob Chemother*, **34**: 853–8.

Reeves DS, Phillips I et al., 1978, *Laboratory Methods in Antimicrobial Chemotherapy*, Churchill Livingstone, Edinburgh.

Report, 1991, A guide to sensitivity testing, *J Antimicrob Chemother*, **27, Suppl. D**: 1–50.

Reusser F, 1975, Effect of lincomycin and clindamycin on peptide chain initiation, *Antimicrob Agents Chemother*, **7**: 32–7.

Reynolds PE, 1989, Structure, biochemistry and mechanism of action of glycopeptide antibiotics, *Eur J Clin Microbiol Infect Dis*, **8**: 943–50.

Ribard P, Audisio F et al., 1992, Seven achilles tendinitis including 3 complicated by rupture during fluoroquinolone therapy, *J Rheumatol*, **19**: 1479–81.

Richmond MH, Sykes RB, 1973, The β-lactamases of Gram-negative bacteria and their possible physiological role, *Adv Microb Physiol*, **9**: 31–88.

Rolinson GN, 1979, 6-APA and the development of the β-lactam antibiotics, *J Antimicrob Chemother*, **5**: 7–14.

Rolinson GN, Stevens S, 1961, Microbiological studies on a new broad-spectrum penicillin 'Penbritin', *Br Med J*, **2**: 191–6.

Ruoff KL, Kuritzkes DR et al., 1988, Vancomycin-resistant gram-positive bacteria isolated from human sources, *J Clin Microbiol*, **26**: 2064–8.

Russell AD, Chopra I, 1996, *Understanding Antibacterial Action and Resistance*, 2nd edn, Ellis Horwood, London, 191.

Sabath LD, Wheeler N et al., 1977, A new type of penicillin resistance of *Staphylococcus aureus*, *Lancet*, **1**: 443–7.

Sahai J, Healy DP et al., 1990, Comparison of vancomycin- and teicoplanin-induced histamine release and 'red man syndrome', *Antimicrob Agents Chemother*, **34**: 765–9.

Sanyal D, Johnson AP et al., 1993, In-vitro characteristics of glycopeptide resistant strains of *Staphylococcus epidermidis* isolated from patients on CAPD, *J Antimicrob Chemother*, **32**: 267–78.

Schatz A, Bugie E, Waksman SA, 1944, Streptomycin, a substance exhibiting antibiotic activity against gram-positive and gram-negative bacteria, *Proc Soc Exp Biol Med*, **55**: 66–9.

Selwyn S, 1979, Pioneer work on the 'penicillin phenomenon' 1870–1876, *J Antimicrob Chemother*, **5**: 249–55.

Selwyn S, 1983, The history of antimicrobial agents, *Clinical Chemotherapy*, vol. I, eds Grassi C, Lorian V, Williams JD, Thieme-Stratton Inc., New York, 1–38.

Shah S, Greenwood D, 1988, Interactions between antibacterial agents of the quinolone group and nitrofurantoin, *J Antimicrob Chemother*, **21**: 41–8.

Shanson DC, 1990, Clinical relevance of resistance to fusidic acid in *Staphylococcus aureus*, *J Antimicrob Chemother*, **25, Suppl. B**: 15–21.

Shinn DLS, 1962, Metronidazole in acute ulcerative gingivitis, *Lancet*, **1**: 1191.

Shlaes DN, Bouvet A et al., 1989, Inducible, transferable resistance to vancomycin in *Enterococcus faecalis* A256, *Antimicrob Agents Chemother*, **33**: 198–203.

Siporon C, 1989, The evolution of fluorinated quinolones: pharmacology, microbiological activity, clinical uses, and toxicities, *Annu Rev Microbiol*, **43**: 601–27.

Skinner MH, Hsieh M et al., 1989, Pharmacokinetics of rifabutin, *Antimicrob Agents Chemother*, **33**: 1237–41.

Slack RCB, 1995a, Use of the laboratory, *Antimicrobial Chemotherapy*, 3rd edn, ed. Greenwood D, Oxford University Press, Oxford, 128–36.

Slack RCB, 1995b, Chemoprophylaxis, *Antimicrobial Chemotherapy*, 3rd edn, ed. Greenwood D, Oxford University Press, Oxford, 219–30.

Smith MA, Edwards DI, 1995, Redox potential and oxygen concentration as factors in the susceptibility of *Helicobacter pylori* to nitroheterocyclic drugs, *J Antimicrob Chemother*, **35**: 751–64.

Smith JT, Lewin CS, 1988, Chemistry and mechanisms of action of the quinolone antibacterials, *The Quinolones*, ed. Andriole VT, Academic Press, London, 23–82.

Speer BS, Shoemaker NB, Salyers AA, 1992, Bacterial resistance to tetracycline: mechanisms, transfer, and clinical significance, *Clin Microbiol Rev*, **5**: 387–99.

Spratt BG, 1975, Distinct penicillin-binding proteins involved in the division, elongation and shape of *Escherichia coli* K12, *Proc Natl Acad Sci USA*, **72**: 2999–3003.

Stamm W, Hicks CB et al., 1995, Azithromycin for empirical treatment of the nongonococcal urethritis syndrome in men, *JAMA*, **274**: 545–9.

Stokes EJ, Ridgway GL, Wren MWD, 1993, *Clinical Microbiology*, 7th edn, Edward Arnold, London.

Suárez JE, Mendoza MC, 1991, Plasmid-encoded fosfomycin resistance, *Antimicrob Agents Chemother*, **35**: 791–5.

Tai PC, Davis BD, 1985, The actions of antibiotics on the ribosome, *The Scientific Basis of Antimicrobial Chemotherapy*, eds Greenwood D, O'Grady F, Cambridge University Press, Cambridge, 41–68.

Tally FT, Ellestad GA, Testa RT, 1995, Glycylcyclines: a new generation of tetracyclines, *J Antimicrob Chemother*, **35:** 449–52.

Tally FP, Malamy MH, 1984, Antimicrobial resistance and resistance transfer in anaerobic bacteria. A review, *Scand J Gastroenterol*, **19, Suppl. 91:** 21–30.

Tedesco FJ, Barton RW, Alpers DH, 1974, Clindamycin-associated colitis. A prospective study, *Ann Intern Med*, **81:** 429–33.

Tilton RC, 1991, Automation and mechanization in antimicrobial susceptibility testing, *Antibiotics in Laboratory Medicine*, 3rd edn, ed. Lorian V, Williams & Wilkins, Baltimore, 106–19.

Tomasz A, 1979, The mechanism of the irreversible antimicrobial effects of penicillins: how the beta-lactam antibiotics kill and lyse bacteria, *Annu Rev Microbiol*, **33:** 113–37.

Towner KJ, 1992a, *Resistance to antifolate antibacterial agents*, *J Med Microbiol*, **36:** 4–6.

Towner KJ, 1992b, Detection of antibiotic resistance genes with DNA probes, *J Antimicrob Chemother*, **30:** 1–2.

Tréfouël J, Tréfouël J et al., 1935, Activité du *p*-aminophénylsulfamide sur les infections streptococciques expérimentales de la souris et du lapin, *C R Soc Biol*, **120:** 756–8.

Verbist L, 1990, The antimicrobial activity of fusidic acid, *J Antimicrob Chemother*, **25, Suppl. B:** 1–5.

Wainwright M, 1990, *Miracle Cure. The Story of Antibiotics*, Blackwell, Oxford.

Wainwright M, Swan HT, 1986, CG Paine and the earliest surviving records of penicillin therapy, *Med Hist*, **30:** 42–56.

Walsh CT, 1993, Vancomycin resistance: decoding the molecular logic, *Science*, **261:** 308–9.

Walton JR, 1992, Use of antibiotics in veterinary practice, *J Med Microbiol*, **36:** 69–70.

Waterworth PM, 1978, Sulphonamides and trimethoprim, *Laboratory Methods in Antimicrobial Chemotherapy*, eds Reeves DS, Phillips I et al., Churchill Livingstone, Edinburgh, 82–4.

Wehrli W, Staehelin M, 1971, Actions of the rifamycins, *Bacteriol Rev*, **35:** 290–309.

Weisblum B, 1995a, Erythromycin resistance by ribosome modification, *Antimicrob Agents Chemother*, **39:** 577–85.

Weisblum B, 1995b, Insights into erythromycin action from studies of its activity as inducer of resistance, *Antimicrob Agents Chemother*, **39:** 797–805.

Weisblum B, Davies J, 1968, Antibiotic inhibitors of the bacterial ribosome, *Bacteriol Rev*, **32:** 493–528.

Wiedemann B, Heisig P, 1994, Quinolone resistance in Gram-negative bacteria, *Infect Dis Clin Pract*, **3, Suppl. 3:** S115–26.

Wolfson JS, Hooper DC, 1989, Bacterial resistance to quinolones: mechanisms and clinical importance, *Rev Infect Dis*, **11, Suppl. 5:** S960–8.

World Health Organization, 1995, The use of essential drugs. Sixth report of the WHO Expert Committee, *WHO Tech Rep Ser*, **850:** WHO, Geneva.

Wyatt TD, Passmore CM et al., 1990, Antibiotic prescribing: the need for a policy in general practice, *Br Med J*, **300:** 441–4.

Young LS, 1993, Mycobacterial diseases in the 1990s, *J Antimicrob Chemother*, **32:** 179–94.

Chapter 10

BACTERIAL AND BACTERIOPHAGE GENETICS

P M Bennett and T G B Howe

BACTERIAL GENETICS

1 INTRODUCTION

The similarities displayed among bacteria and the differences that distinguish one from another reflect the content and expression of the genes possessed by each individual cell. The genes control every property of a cell or virus, including morphology, physiology, biochemistry and, in general, an exact copy of each one is inherited by the cell's progeny. Genetics is the study of genes, their structures, organizations and expression.

With the exception of some bacteriophages (see p. 264), the genetic information of bacterial systems is encoded in DNA (see Chapter 5). The characteristics expressed by a cell are referred to as its phenotype. The set of genes found in any particular cell constitutes its genome, which consists of a large circular DNA molecule, the bacterial chromosome, and possibly one or more smaller circular DNA molecules called plasmids (see p. 251).

Bacteria are, in general, very adaptable and may alter their phenotype in response to environmental change while the genotype remains unchanged. The ability to adapt the phenotype to the prevailing environmental conditions is determined genetically, i.e. not all the genes of a bacterial cell are expressed all the time. For example, β-galactosidase, an enzyme

that hydrolyses lactose to its constituent sugars glucose and galactose, is required by *Escherichia coli* only when lactose is its main source of carbon and energy and normally it is produced only under such circumstances. The gene and associated sequences that control the expression of β-galactosidase are, together with the gene for β-galactosidase itself and 2 other associated genes, encoded in a single DNA sequence, the *lac* operon (Chapter 5). This is just one example of the many complex systems that can be switched on or off to allow bacteria to make best use of the nutrients available to them and to adjust their biochemical makeup rapidly in response to changes in their environments. Such switches are termed phenotypic variation; the phenotype of the cell changes while the genotype remains unaltered. By contrast, genotypic variation involves a change in the genetic information that determines the phenotype. This type of change occurs by mutation, an alteration of the nucleotide sequence of DNA of which there are several types.

In general, all the cells in a bacterial culture respond phenotypically in the same way to a change (often nutritional) in their environment. The change in phenotype is normally rapid and reversible, e.g. synthesis of the enzyme β-galactosidase starts within seconds of the addition of lactose to a suitable culture medium and ceases just as rapidly when lactose is withdrawn (or exhausted). Genotypic change (mutation) affects the individual cell and is, effectively, irreversible. There are, however, exceptions to these generalizations and it is sometimes difficult to determine into which category a particular variation fits. For example, lysozyme treatment of a culture of *Bacillus subtilis* converts the cells to protoplasts by removing the cell wall. Removal of lysozyme, however, does not always result in a return to normal cell physiology; the cells either continue to grow as protoplasts or show mass reversion to the bacillary form depending upon the conditions of culture. This is an example of a phenotypic change that, in some circumstances, could appear as heritable and permanent. By contrast, physiological changes resulting from mutation may give the impression of being phenotypic because bacteria can multiply so rapidly; a mutant cell, with a temporary selective advantage, can overgrow a population of unaltered cells within a few hours. When the conditions are reversed the mutant may be at a selective disadvantage and, in turn, may be overgrown by cells of the original type. If cells are examined on time scales that permit many generations, what is in reality genotypic variation may appear to be phenotypic variation.

Bacteria are haploid organisms with no true nucleus or sexual reproductive cycle. The great expansion of knowledge of bacterial genetics followed the discovery that genes (DNA) can be passed from one bacterial cell to another by several mechanisms. The bacterium about which most is known is *E. coli* K12, whose single chromosome is a circular DNA molecule of approximately 2 mm, about 1000 times longer than the bacterial cell in which it is contained. The DNA molecule contains c. 4 700 000 base pairs (bp) or 4700 kilobases (kb), which is sufficient capacity to accommodate approximately 4000 average sized genes. Other bacteria whose genetics have been studied also have single circular chromosomes; this is true both of bacteria related to *E. coli*, such as *Shigella* and *Salmonella* spp. (Sanderson 1976), and of unrelated ones such as *Pseudomonas aeruginosa* (Holloway, Krishnapillai and Morgan 1979) and *B. subtilis* (Henner and Hoch 1980). Circularity has usually been established by gene linkage experiments. In the case of *E. coli* K12 its chromosome has also been extracted and visualized (by autoradiography) and shown unequivocally to be circular (Cairns 1963), so confirming the genetic data. In some bacteria of medical importance, such as streptococci, staphylococci and clostridia, molecular genetic studies are in hand; in others, however, genetic information is rudimentary or non-existent, often because no easy and reliable genetic technology is available for the particular organism.

Bacterial chromosomes must replicate before cell division and be distributed (partitioned) so that each daughter cell has its own copy. A complex organization exists to ensure that this happens. Plasmids also encode replication functions that allow them to replicate independently of the bacterial chromosome and many also encode partition functions, as well as other stabilization mechanisms. DNA molecules that are able to replicate are called replicons (Jacob, Brenner and Cuzin 1963), and most bacterial replicons are circular. The chromosome is the replicon(s) in which are encoded those genes that are essential for the cell's survival. It is also the largest replicon in the cell.

2 MUTATION

Mutation can be defined as any permanent change in the sequence of bases of DNA, irrespective of a detectable change in the cell phenotype. In practice, of course, most mutations are detected by virtue of the change in phenotype generated, although now, with many DNA sequences being determined, it is seen that silent mutation is very common, i.e. a change in the nucleotide sequence that has no detectable phenotypic effect. A given gene can exist in a variety of different forms – some functional, some not – as a result of mutation. These different forms are called alleles. The form in which a gene exists in a bacterium as it is first isolated from nature is defined as the **wild-type allele** of the gene; all other forms resulting from mutation are, by definition, **mutant alleles**.

Mutations may occur spontaneously, i.e. in the absence of a specific treatment to generate them, or they may be induced deliberately (the cells of the bacterial culture may be treated in one of several ways so as to provoke changes in the base sequence of the DNA). Classically, induction of mutations has been achieved by chemical treatment with known mutagens such as ethylmethane sulphonate (EMS, $CH_3CH_2.O.SO_2.CH_3$) and N-methyl-N'-nitro-N-nitrosoguanidine (MNNG, NTG) or by irradiation with ultraviolet or γ rays. These treatments generate DNA lesions at random and the particular mutation desired is selected by judicious manipulation of the subsequent growth conditions of the culture. It has become possible to target mutations, i.e. to introduce specific changes into a particular nucleotide sequence, using recombinant DNA technology, a procedure termed site-specific mutagenesis.

The spontaneous nature of mutation was demonstrated by Luria and Delbrück (1943) by an experiment known as the **fluctuation test**. The experiment exploited the observation that in a large enough population of cells sensitive to a particular bacteriophage (phage) there will be a few cells resistant to the phage. When equal volumes of a broth culture, each containing approximately 10^9 *E. coli*, were spread on plates seeded with the phage the number of colonies arising from resistant cells showed a small fluctuation from plate to plate (Fig. 10.1). In a parallel experiment, small inocula (c. 10^3 cells) of the same culture were used to produce a series of 50 separate broth cultures. When the same volumes of these (i.e. containing approximately 10^9 bacteria) were spread on agar seeded with the phage, much larger fluctuations were seen in the number of colonies obtained per plate (Fig. 10.1). The results reflected the random nature of the mutations that had occurred in each culture, i.e. mutations arose at different times in different cultures (the earlier the mutation the greater is the proportion of resistant cells in that population). The experiment is depicted in Fig. 10.1.

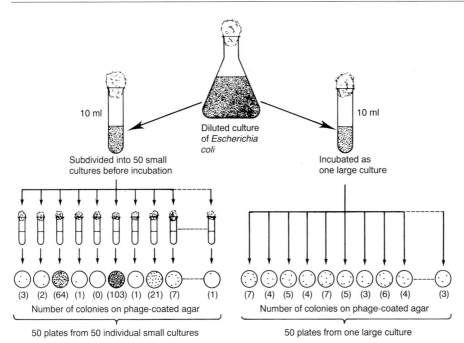

(3) (2) (64) (1) (0) (103) (1) (21) (7) — (1)
Number of colonies on phage-coated agar

50 plates from 50 individual small cultures

(7) (4) (5) (4) (7) (5) (3) (6) (4) — (3)
Number of colonies on phage-coated agar

50 plates from one large culture

Fig. 10.1 Proof of the non-directed (spontaneous) nature of bacterial mutation by the 'fluctuation test'.

That mutations can arise spontaneously in a population of cells was demonstrated directly by Ester and Joshua Lederberg in 1952. Approximately 10^8 phage-sensitive *E. coli* cells were inoculated onto nutrient agar and the plate was incubated. The resulting colonial growth was replica-plated to nutrient agar and nutrient agar seeded with the phage, where only phage-resistant cells grew to form colonies. Each colony that developed came from an inoculum of a phage-resistant cell (or cells) on the master plate. The locations of these were determined, and approximately 10^5 cells from the phage-free nutrient agar were transferred into tubes of broth. From each of the resulting cultures 10^5 cells were spread on individual nutrient agar plates. The colonies that developed were again replica-plated to nutrient agar and nutrient agar seeded with phage and the entire process was repeated several times. By picking only phage-resistant colonies (identified by growth on the replica plate containing nutrient agar seeded with phage) from the phage-free nutrient agar to generate cultures for further testing, it was possible eventually to obtain a pure culture of a phage-resistant mutant. During the entire procedure the populations of cells used in the purification steps were never exposed to the phage, demonstrating unequivocally that resistant variants (i.e. mutants) emerged in the complete absence of the selective agent.

2.1 **Mutagenesis**

Much of our understanding of the mechanisms of mutation derives from experiments in which mutations have been induced by chemical agents that react with DNA in a known manner. Experiments designed to study the chemical basis of mutation have been carried out extensively with *E. coli* and several bacteriophages for which *E. coli* is a normal host. The protocols of mutation experiments vary according to the particular mutagen to be tested. For those reagents that react chemically with the constituent bases of DNA, bacteria are mixed with the mutagen and the suspension is incubated. The concentration of mutagen used and the time of incubation are determined pragmatically as those conditions under which approximately 5% of the input cells survive the treatment. The survivors are then permitted to grow in normal culture. Among the population that results the proportion of mutants is high; in practice, however, the abundance of a particular mutation, although considerably enhanced with respect to the untreated starting culture, may still be below the level at which a screen of individual cells in the population would readily detect it. Hence, populations of cells obtained after mutagenic treatment may be subject to culture on selective growth medium, constituted to favour the growth of the desired mutant.

Some chemicals cause mutation because they mimic one of the constituent bases of DNA and may be incorporated into DNA during replication when present in the growth medium. 5-Bromouracil (5-BU), an analogue of thymine with a bromine atom at the C-5 position instead of a methyl (CH_3) group, is one such compound. Once part of DNA, such substitutions cause misincorporation of normal bases in subsequent rounds of replication, e.g. 5-BU causes misincorporation of guanine. For these mutagens the cells must necessarily grow during treatment because DNA replication is essential for the effect. The concentration of the reagent has to be chosen so that the level of incorporation is high enough to raise the frequency of mutation but not so high as to kill the majority of cells in the treated population. Again, the conditions of treatment are determined pragmatically.

Often the easiest way to decide if the mutagenic treatment has been successful is to determine the percentage of **auxotrophs** generated, i.e. mutants that have acquired a nutritional requirement. For example, samples of a suitable dilution of a mutagenized culture of *E. coli* are spread onto nutrient agar, so as to give 100–150 colonies per plate after a suitable period of incubation. These colonies are then tested individually to determine if they can grow on a minimal-salts agar that supports growth of the parent bacterium. A satisfactory mutagenic treatment will generate 5–10% auxotrophs that will be unable to grow on the minimal agar. Alternatively, the increase in the proportion of cells resistant to certain antibiotics, e.g. rifampicin or nalidixic acid, to which the cells in the treated culture were susceptible before treatment, can be monitored.

Various experimental 'tricks' can be used to enhance the chances of success in finding a particular mutant. Two are worthy of mention. The abundance of particular auxotrophic mutations in a population can be increased by **penicillin enrichment** to the point where they form the majority. Penicillin kills only growing bacterial cells. Non-growing cells survive the treatment, provided the medium is osmotically buffered. Hence, a whole mutagen-treated culture is inoculated into liquid medium lacking the particular growth factor (amino acid, vitamin, purine or pyrimidine) needed by the desired auxotroph. After a short incubation (15–20 min), during which time the growth of the mutant type required is arrested, penicillin is added to the culture. The cells that do not need an exogenous supply of the growth factor grow and are killed by the penicillin. The auxotrophs survive. On removal of the penicillin and inoculation into a growth medium supplemented with the growth requirement, these proliferate, together with any other survivors, to generate a new population of cells, among which the desired auxotrophs constitute a much increased proportion. In practice, the procedure is not an all-or-none effect and a single round of treatment rarely increases the proportion of mutants sought by more than 100-fold. However, 4 or 5 cycles of treatment can usually enhance the proportion of the auxotroph required to greater than 10% of the surviving population of cells (Miller 1972), at which point mutants are easily identified.

The second technique that has been indispensable in the search for bacterial mutants is **replica-plating.** Velvet is pressed gently onto the surface of agar on which bacterial colonies of interest have grown, leaving a sample of each colony imprinted on the velvet, which is then used to inoculate plates of sterile agar differing in composition from that on which the colonies originally appeared. After incubation, the ability of individual colonies to grow under the new conditions can be assessed; e.g. a population of cells can be screened for auxotrophs of a particular type by replica-plating from a medium supplemented with the growth factor in question to a medium that lacks the growth factor but which is otherwise the same. The desired auxotrophs will fail to grow. An experienced person can easily screen 200–300 colonies per plate.

Mutations can be divided into 2 groups, micro- and macrolesions, depending on the extent of the alteration to the base pair sequence of DNA. Microlesions are also known as point mutations.

2.2   Microlesions

Point mutations are of 2 classes: **base pair substitutions** and **frame-shift mutations**. The first class comprises those mutants in which a single base pair has been altered, and can be subdivided into **transitions** and **transversions**. Such changes may be expressed (i.e. are detected as an altered phenotype) or silent. Frame-shift mutations are those in which one or a few base pairs have been added to or removed from the DNA with the consequence that the translational reading frame of the transcript, i.e. of messenger RNA (mRNA), of the mutated gene is altered. Point mutations are, in general, **revertible**, i.e. a second mutational event at the same site can precisely reverse the first mutation and restore the original base sequence.

A transition occurs when one purine is replaced by another purine and a pyrimidine is replaced by a different pyrimidine, e.g. a change from a guanine–cytosine (GC) base pair to an adenine–thymine (AT) base pair, or vice versa; in this situation the purine–pyrimidine axis of the double helix at the point of mutation is preserved. Most chemically induced base substitutions are transitions. Transversions are those base pair substitutions in which the purine–pyrimidine axis is changed as a result of the mutation, e.g. a change from GC to CG or to TA. Such changes are much less common than transitions and probably arise as a consequence of occasional mistakes made during DNA replication and by one or more of the cell's DNA repair systems.

All 4 of the bases in DNA can exist in different tautomeric forms which are related to each other by single proton shifts. The tautomeric forms arise when the keto (C=O) group of a base is changed to the enol (C–OH) form or when the amino (–NH$_2$) group is changed to an imino (=NH) group. The enol and imino groups exist in equilibrium with the keto and amino forms, respectively, but the latter predominate under normal conditions, i.e. at ambient temperatures and at pH values near neutrality. Such tautomeric shifts are important because they can relax the normally strict Watson and Crick complementary base pairing conventions, permitting, for example, G to pair with T instead of with C, while retaining purine–pyrimidine base pairing. If these occasional mispairings are not corrected, on replication one daughter chromosome will have an AT base pair at a particular location instead of a GC base pair and mutation will have occurred. These different forms are illustrated in Fig. 10.2.

As well as occurring naturally, transitions may be formed by the incorporation of base analogues into the DNA. Among the most important analogues are the halogenated pyrimidines, particularly 5-BU. This compound can be incorporated into DNA in place of thymine. The halogen atom is strongly electronegative and can pull electrons from the oxygen of the keto group of 5-BU, converting it to an enol group. 5-BU and similar analogues, therefore, tautomerize much more readily than the natural base under normal physiological conditions. In its keto form 5-BU can pair with A and be incorporated into DNA to form a pseudo-AT base pair. If 5-BU then undergoes a tautomeric shift to the enol form, at the next round of replication it will direct the incorporation of G rather than A into the newly synthesized strand of DNA. A further round of replication will establish an AT to GC transition. Because they are incorporated into DNA by replication, base analogues are effective only in growing cells. By contrast, other chemicals such as nitrous acid and

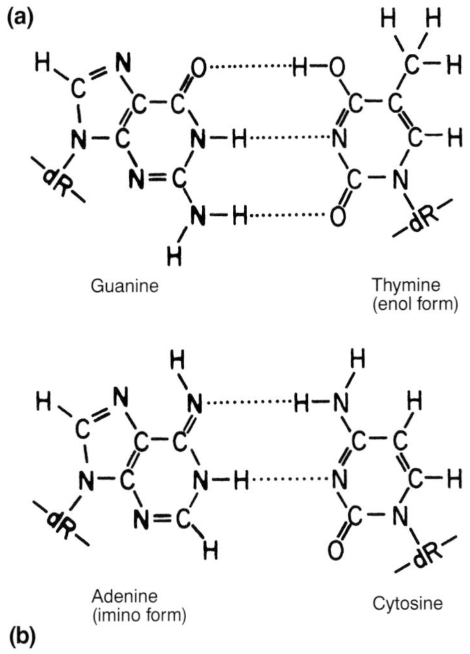

(a)

Guanine

Thymine
(enol form)

(b)

Adenine
(imino form)

Cytosine

Fig. 10.2 Changes in base pairing as the result of tautomeric shifts. In the enol form (a), thymine forms hydrogen bonds with guanine, instead of with adenine. In the imino form (b), adenine forms hydrogen bonds with cytosine, instead of with thymine. Similar shifts in guanine and cytosine will also cause changes in base pairing.

various alkylating agents interact with non-replicating as well as replicating DNA.

Transitions can be generated by the action of nitrous acid. This chemical reacts with amine groups, converting them to hydroxyl groups (oxidative deamination). Deamination of the adenine converts it to hypoxanthine which can base pair with cytosine. Therefore, upon replication, hypoxanthine may cause misincorporation of C. A further round of replication will then establish the AT to GC transition. In similar reactions thymine is converted to uracil and guanine is converted to xanthine. The first of these changes can be detected by a dedicated repair system and reversed, whereas the latter appears to be lethal rather than mutagenic.

Alkylating agents are powerful mutagens that predominantly generate transition mutations, although some have been reported to generate transversions and frameshifts as well; the mechanisms by which the latter changes are achieved are not fully understood. Alkylating agents all carry one, 2 or more reactive alkyl groups. An example, widely used to generate bacterial mutants, is EMS. The action of alkylating agents on DNA is complex. They are known to react with purine bases, predominantly guanine, and the alkylated bases can cause base misincorporation if the damage is not corrected before replication. Bifunctional alkylating agents, i.e. those with 2 or more reactive alkyl groups, bring about cross-linking of the 2 strands of the double helix. This reaction is not, of itself, mutagenic but is lethal because cross-linking the strands of the double helix inhibits replication. However, attempts by the cell to repair the damage may result in mutation.

Transversions may arise spontaneously or may be induced at low frequency by some mutagenic treatments. However, no known chemical or irradiation treatment generates transversion exclusively, or even predominantly. Less is known about the mechanisms that generate transversions than about those that generate transitions, but many are probably due to replication or repair errors, rather than to the direct consequence of mutagenic treatment.

Acridine dyes induce frameshift mutations. The properties of these mutations are accounted for by the insertion or deletion of one, or a few, base pair(s) in DNA. Because the message encoded in mRNA is read as a sequence of triplets, insertion or deletion of bases (other than multiples of 3) causes a shift in the reading frame with the result that all codons (triplets) beyond the site of mutation are changed; a second frameshift, of similar magnitude but opposite sign, will correct the reading frame beyond the second mutation. If the amino acid sequence encoded by the base sequence between the 2 sites of mutation is not critical to the function of the gene product, the 2 mutations may cancel each other out and an altered but functional peptide may be produced. When this occurs, the second mutation is said to be a **suppressor** of the first and, because it is within the same gene, the phenomenon is termed **intragenic suppression**. When separated from the primary mutation by recombination, an intragenic frameshift suppressor mutation acts exactly like a primary frameshift mutation. Although they revert to the wild-type phenotype spontaneously and can be induced to revert at a higher rate by acridine dyes, frameshift mutations are never induced to revert by base analogues, nitrous acid or hydroxylamine.

One of the best known acridine dyes is proflavine. Because it is a planar (flat) molecule with dimensions similar to that of a purine–pyrimidine base pair, it can intercalate between the stacked bases of DNA. It has been proposed that proflavine exerts its mutagenic effect on DNA undergoing recombination. This idea arose from the observation that proflavine is a relatively poor mutagen for normal cells of *E. coli* but that its mutagenic effect is considerably increased, (1) in the case of *E. coli* bacteriophage T4 which indulges in a considerable degree of recombination during the course of its development; and (2) with partial diploids of *E. coli* formed during bacterial conjugation as the result of incomplete transfer of the chromosome of one bacterium to another. In the latter system frameshifts are generated at a higher frequency in that region of the genome that is temporarily duplicated than in the remainder. **Recombination** of DNA involves breakage and reformation of phosphodiester bonds and it has been proposed that frameshift mutagens act by temporarily stabilizing mispaired sequences that may form following strand cleavage and transient strand separation. All frameshift mutagens are intercalating agents, but not all intercalating agents are frameshift mutagens. Another common intercalating agent, widely used in molecular genetics as a frameshift mutagen, is ethidium bromide.

In practice, when studying a mutagen or suspected mutagen it is easier to gauge its effects on the frequency of reversion of a set of known point mutants than to analyse its ability to generate 'knock out' mutations in a particular gene(s). Although reversion frequencies are generally somewhat lower, analysing reversion offers considerably more sensitivity and convenience. This is the basis of the well known Ames test, used to test chemicals to determine if they are mutagenic (and so, potentially carcinogenic) (Ames et al. 1973, Ames 1979).

Transition, transversion and frameshift mutations generate alterations in the sense of the mRNA transcript. A **mis-sense mutation** gives rise to a codon that specifies an amino acid different from that originally encoded. The effect on the polypeptide product depends on the position of the altered amino acid and the precise nature of the change. In some cases, the polypeptide may show no obvious change in its properties; in others, all protein function may be lost. The change may generate a protein with altered thermal stability such that at a relatively low (permissive) temperature the protein functions more or less normally, whereas at higher (non-permissive) temperatures the protein is non-functional; if this results in cell death the mutation is said to be a **conditional-lethal mutation**, i.e. the mutation is lethal, but only at the elevated temperature. In the case of most enteric bacteria, such as *E. coli*, the permissive temperature would normally be 30°C and the non-permissive 42°C. There are many other examples of conditional-lethal mutants in which a normally lethal mutation can be tolerated under particular physiological conditions. Such mutations can be invaluable when studying a vital component of the cell.

Point mutations may change a codon from one specifying an amino acid to one specifying termination of protein synthesis, namely UAG, UAA or UGA, when a truncated polypeptide is produced instead of the full length protein. Such mutant codons, when they appear within a gene, are called **nonsense codons** because they do not code for an amino acid. The introduction of a nonsense codon into an early gene of an operon may produce an effect known as **polarity**. An **operon** consists of a set of genes that are transcribed as a single mRNA. A **polar mutation** is one that results not only in the loss of expression of the mutated gene but also in loss or significantly lower expression of those genes in the operon located **distal** to (or **downstream** from) the nonsense mutation, i.e. located on the opposite side of the mutation to that of the operon promoter. Translation of mRNA ceases at a nonsense mutation, the nascent peptide is released and ribosomes are discharged. Some may re-attach to the mRNA downstream of the mutation at an appropriate ribosome binding sites preceding the next translation start signal. When fewer than normal re-attach, polarity results. In some instances the polar effect is so strong that genes distal to the nonsense mutation are barely expressed, if at all. Transcription of most genes is coupled to translation of the transcript. If these processes are uncoupled, transcription may also be terminated prematurely as a consequence of what is termed rho-dependent transcription termin-

ation (Landick, Turnbough and Yanofsky 1996). Severe polar effects are often related to the location of the mutation close to the start of the mutated gene, when translation is uncoupled from transcription for a prolonged distance. In such instances, mRNA distal to the point mutation is either not synthesized, due to premature transcription termination (attenuation), or is synthesized in considerably reduced quantities. This coupling of mRNA synthesis to its translation has evolved in some systems to provide a sensitive mechanism of control of enzyme synthesis termed **attenuation** (for further details, see Yanofsky 1987, Landick. Turnbough and Yanofsky 1996).

2.3 Suppression of base substitution mutations

As in the example of frameshift mutations, it is sometimes possible to have a second mutation at a site different from the first, the result of which is to restore the lost phenotype. Secondary mutations of this type are referred to as suppressors. The phenomenon is called **suppression** and the double mutants are referred to as **pseudorevertants**. Suppressor mutations may be either **intragenic**, as in the case of some frameshift suppressors, or **intergenic**, i.e. the second mutation is in an entirely different gene. Mutations due to base substitutions may be suppressed either intragenically or intergenically. In the former case, the suppressor mutation alters a second amino acid in the polypeptide; the second substitution neutralizes the effect of the first and restores protein activity. Again, if the second mutation is separated from the first by recombination, it may also be recognized as a fully fledged mutation in its own right. Such suppressors are quite specific for the original mutation. Intergenic suppression operates at the level of protein synthesis. Mutations of this type mostly give rise to altered transfer RNA (tRNA) molecules, although alterations in ribosome components, the so-called *ram* alleles of ribosomal protein genes, have been reported. The altered tRNA molecules are able to read one, or sometimes 2, of the 3 nonsense codons (UAG, UAA and UGA) as an amino acid codon (Engelberg-Kulka and Schoulaker-Schwarz 1996). The change in specificity is, in many cases, the result of a base pair substitution in the DNA sequence that determines the anticodon of the tRNA species generating an anticodon to one of the terminating codons. Such suppressors will recognize the cognate codon, i.e. a particular nonsense mutation, wherever it occurs and will translate it. The efficiency with which a nonsense codon is translated by an appropriate suppressor tRNA will be determined by how effectively the mutant tRNA competes with the normal translation termination factors, which will also react to the nonsense codon, and the influence of the nucleotide context, i.e. the surrounding sequences within which the terminating codon appears (Bossi 1983). The affinities of both factors for the nonsense codon are known to alter with the context of the codon.

It was thought initially that suppression must be highly inefficient if the cell is to survive. This is now known not to be true and individual suppressors can translate nonsense codons with efficiencies of 60–75%. By contrast, some suppressors are relatively inefficient but, for many enzymes, even a small level of production, say 5% of the wild-type level, is sufficient to permit growth of the cell.

The generation of a suppressor, i.e. mutation of a tRNA gene, can be tolerated only if the cell produces an alternative tRNA with which it can translate the codons that the mutant tRNA would have recognized before its mutation. In many cases this is possible because there is a redundancy of tRNA species for a number of codons. Hence, one of them can be mutated to recognize a different, but related, codon with little or no damage to the protein synthetic apparatus of the cell.

Since tRNA suppressors may be generated by mutation of the anticodon sequence, it should, in principle, be possible to isolate mis-sense suppressors as well. Several of these have indeed been isolated. They tend to involve minor species of tRNA and their efficiency of suppression is low but effective for the reasons given above. In addition, tRNA frameshift suppressors have also been isolated where the mutations are insertions in the anticodon sequences that increase their sizes from 3 to 4 bases (Engelberg-Kulka and Schoulaker-Schwarz 1996).

The importance of tRNA suppressors rests in the fact that they have been used extensively, particularly before gene cloning and sequencing was more or less routine, to demonstrate that mutations were located within nucleotide sequences that encode peptide products, since the effectiveness of such suppressors depends on their abilities to decode mutant codons and restore function to the protein affected by the mutation. Their existence also helped to establish the current model of protein synthesis.

2.4 Macrolesions

Alterations of DNA involving large numbers of base pairs are of 4 types: **deletions**, **duplications**, **inversions** and **additions**. Deletion mutations are recognized by their inability to revert and by their failure to recombine with 2 or more distinct point mutations. A number of mechanisms can be proposed to explain the generation of deletions, including errors in replication, in recombination and in DNA repair. In addition, the activities of transposable elements (see p. 241) can and do generate deletions.

Errors in DNA replication (copy errors) involve sequence duplications and slippage of one strand of the replicating DNA in relation to the other. A disruption in the pairing between the parental template strand, DNA polymerase and the newly synthesized daughter strand could lead to either of the 2 results outlined in Fig. 10.3. After having separated transiently, the 2 strands re-anneal, but misalign because of the sequence duplication. The misalignment is accommodated by one of the strands looping out part of its sequence. A 'jump ahead' in copying produces a deletion in the daughter strand; a 'jump back' produces a duplication.

Deletions and inversions may be produced as the results of intra- and inter-replicon recombination, as outlined in Fig. 10.4. These events also require sequence duplications. Recombination between homologous sequences carried in the same orientation on the same DNA molecule results in the loss of one copy of the duplicated sequence and of the sequence between the duplication. Recombination between homologous but inverted sequences results in the inversion of the intervening sequence. Inter-replicon recombination between regions that have sequence duplications may result in sequence duplication in one of the DNA molecules involved and

deletion in the other (what is lost by one molecule is gained by the other) (Fig. 10.4).

2.5 UV-induced mutations

Mutations may be induced by ultraviolet (UV) light. DNA strongly absorbs UV light at an absorption maximum of c. 260 nm. Cells are killed by UV light and there is a high proportion of mutants among the survivors. The most frequent lesion introduced into DNA by UV irradiation is the formation of **pyrimidine dimers**; covalent bonds are formed between adjacent pyrimidines on the same DNA strand so that the 2 pyrimidine residues are joined by a cyclobutane ring. The most common are thymine dimers, but cytosine dimers and thymine–cytosine dimers are also generated. The appearance of these dimers distorts the shape of the DNA molecule (i.e. distorts the double helix) by interfering with normal base pairing.

DNA replication stalls at thymine dimers. Replication may be reinitiated some distance away from the lesion, so generating a gap in the daughter strand. Therefore, unless repaired, the generation of a pyrimidine dimer is a lethal event. Not surprisingly, cells have evolved a number of mechanisms to repair pyrimidine dimers and restore the normal base sequence. If UV-treated cells are immediately exposed to visible light of wavelength 300–400 nm, both mutation frequency and lethality are greatly reduced, a phenomenon called **photoreactivation**. The visible light treatment activates an enzyme, **photolyase**, that hydrolyses the cyclobutane ring, precisely reversing the reaction mediated by exposure to UV. The mechanism is accurate and error free. In addition, the cell has various repair systems that do not need light stimulation: the dark repair processes. One or more of these systems is error prone and it is the activity of this system (or systems) that can result in mutation. DNA replication is involved because inhibiting DNA synthesis under post-irradiation conditions that favour repair processes causes a decline in the number of mutants recovered among the surviving population of cells.

2.6 Other types of mutation

Spontaneous mutations may occur in the absence of known mutagenic treatment. There are probably many reasons for this. Various products or intermediates of the cell's own metabolism are demonstrably mutagenic; these include peroxides, nitrous acid, formaldehyde and purine analogues. Some spontaneous mutations may, therefore, be induced by endogenously generated mutagens. Alkaline pH and elevated temperature have also been implicated in mutation.

Finally, it has been discovered that certain mutations of bacteria themselves predispose the mutant cell to further mutation. Several loci are now known to be involved. They include functions connected with DNA replication and, particularly, with a process termed mismatch repair. In these cases the initial mutation diminishes the reliability of either those

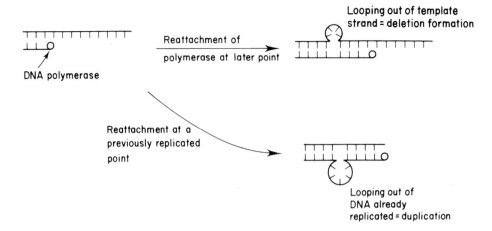

Fig. 10.3 Errors in DNA replication.

functions that ensure the fidelity of replication (i.e. the error rate is increased) or one of the repair mechanisms, the purpose of which is constantly to scan the DNA for damage and correct it when found. These mutations generate alleles called **mutator** (*mut*) genes because they enhance the frequency of mutation (Hutchinson 1996). There is a similar mutator gene in coliphage T4, whose product has been identified as a DNA polymerase. Mutator genes have been reported to induce transversions at relatively high frequencies, consistent with a partial breakdown in the mechanisms that maintain DNA fidelity.

SITE-DIRECTED MUTATION

Until the advent of gene cloning, the introduction of mutations into a particular gene was a strictly random process; mutant alleles could be selected or identified, but the location of the mutation could not be con-

trolled. Now, by exploiting DNA synthesis in vitro, mutations can be targeted precisely to any base pair that is desired. DNA synthesis requires DNA polymerase, a template, deoxyribonucleotide triphosphates and a priming sequence. In the cell this is usually a short RNA sequence but, in vitro, synthetic oligodeoxyribonucleotide primers of approximately 20 nucleotides (nt) are used instead. The gene to be mutated is cloned into a suitable cloning vector. This will constitute the template DNA for the in vitro synthesis. Vectors based on the genome of bacteriophage M13, which is a circular, single-stranded DNA molecule, are commonly used, because the recovery of single-stranded DNA for the reaction is greatly facilitated. The primer used is complementary to the sequence at the prospective site of mutation. By deliberately incorporating a mismatch into the primer, a targeted mutation can be engineered into the gene of

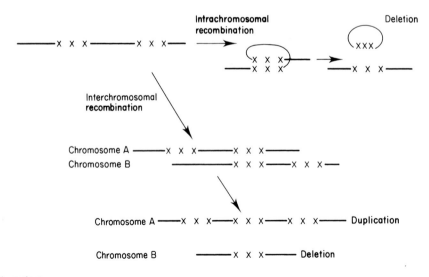

Fig. 10.4 Inter- and intrachromosomal recombination.

interest. The primer is extended by the DNA polymerase, using the circular single-stranded DNA molecule as template until the $5'$ end of the primer is encountered, when the newly synthesized DNA circle is closed by DNA ligase. The genetically engineered molecule can then be recovered by transforming a suitable bacterial host. The gene is then resequenced, to ensure that the desired mutation is the only one that has been introduced. By using a set of primers, each with a different, but deliberately designed, mismatch in the reaction, a set of mutants with site-directed mutations can be generated. This allows a region of a gene, or indeed the entire gene if so desired, to be subjected to systematic mutation for structure–function studies of the gene product or for analysis of the sequences controlling gene expression.

FLIP-FLOP MECHANISMS

Some functions expressed by bacteria and bacteriophages undergo changes that at first sight appear to be mutations. However, the basis of the changes is more like the operation of a switch than a random change in the DNA. Such changes occur as a result of **site-specific recombination** mechanisms that invert specific DNA sequences, the consequence of which is to turn off expression of one gene(s) and activate that of an alternative gene(s) (Craig 1988, Nash 1996). Two particularly well characterized systems, encoded by bacteriophages Mu and P1, operate to control the bacterial host ranges of the phages by controlling the production of alternative tail fibres for the phages (Giphart-Gassler, Plasterk and van de Putte 1982). In *Salmonella* Typhimurium **flagellar antigen phase variation**, which allows the bacterium to evade the immune response of an infected host, is controlled by a very similar DNA inversion mechanism. Two genes, *H1* and *H2*, code for alternative subunits of the flagellar protein, flagellin. The cell can alternate between expression of these 2 genes by inverting a short segment of the chromosome (Zieg et al. 1977). In phase I, flagellin encoded by *H1* is produced. In phase II, *H2*-encoded flagellin is synthesized; in addition, a gene called *rhI* is activated, the product of which is a transcriptional repressor of *H1*, so that production of flagellin encoded by *H1* is switched off. The recombination inverts an approximate 1 kb sequence that in phase II orientation provides a promoter for *H2* and *rhI*. The sequence also encodes a gene called *hin*, the product of which mediates the inversion. The *hin* gene shows considerable homology with both *gin* and *cin*, the site-specific recombinase genes of bacteriophages Mu and P1, respectively, that determine host specificity. The products of these 3 genes are functionally interchangeable.

Each of these 3 systems operates infrequently, the probability of inversion being about 10^{-8} per cell per generation. However, this low frequency is sufficient, within a population of cells or bacteriophages, to extend significantly the versatility of the organism. The ability of *S.* Typhimurium to switch flagellin production confers some protection against the immune response, whereas the ability to produce 2 sets of tail fibres broadens the host ranges of both Mu and P1, each set of tail fibres permitting infection of particular bacterial strains.

Other examples of phase variation, controlled by invertible DNA segments are *E. coli* type I fimbriae (pili) (Abraham et al. 1985) and the fimbriae of *Moraxella bovis* (Marrs et al. 1988).

3 MOBILE GENETIC ELEMENTS

3.1 Insertion sequences and transposons

In the 1960s evidence accumulated for the existence of a hitherto undescribed form of mutation. The first of these to be recognized in bacteria was found by Lederberg who in 1960 described an unusual class of Gal⁻ mutants in *E. coli*. They reverted to Gal⁺ at frequencies of 10^{-6}–10^{-8}, but the reversion frequency was not enhanced by mutagenic treatments, results suggesting that these mutations were neither deletions nor classical point mutations. When the mutation was in one of the first genes of a set it exerted an unusually strong polarity on expression of subsequent genes in the operon, virtually eliminating expression from them (unlike polar nonsense mutations that merely reduce expression of the distal genes). The new type of mutation was described as a strong polar mutation (Jordan et al. 1968). Molecular genetic analysis of these mutations, using λ*gal* transducing phages (see p. 282), demonstrated that the *gal* operons of the mutants contained extra DNA sequences; revertants to Gal⁺ had lost the additional sequences. The conclusion from these studies was that the mutations were generated by the insertion of extra pieces of DNA, called **insertion sequences** or **IS elements** (Jordan, Saedler and Starlinger 1968), at the point of mutation. IS elements are now known to be but one type of a class of genetic elements called **transposable elements**. The one characteristic that all such elements possess is the ability to transpose, i.e. they can insert into different sites, usually unrelated, on the same or on different DNA molecules. Unlike host-mediated homologous recombination, transposition requires no homology between the transposable element and its sites of insertion, and the mechanisms are independent of the *recA⁺* gene product of the bacterial host.

Since the initial discovery of IS*1*, IS*2* and IS*3* (Fiant, Szybalski and Malamy 1972) in *E. coli*, many IS elements have been described from a wide variety of bacteria (Galas and Chandler 1989). They are common in bacterial plasmids and are normal components of many, if not all, bacterial chromosomes. They are also cryptic in the sense that they do not confer on the host bacterium a predictable phenotype. Their presence is usually first indicated by mutation, i.e. the genetic damage they cause, although modern molecular genetic techniques, such as Southern blotting and polymerase chain reaction (PCR), can detect silent copies of a known IS element on both plasmids and the bacterial chromosome.

In 1974, the discovery of a new type of transposable element that encoded a recognizable gene product, the TEM-2 β-lactamase determining resistance to several β-lactam antibiotics, including ampicillin (see Chapter 9), was reported by Hedges and Jacob (1974). It was termed a **transposon**, and many others carrying various resistance and other genes have been identified and analysed (see Berg and Howe 1989). Because of the ability of transposable elements to insert into a large number of sites, both on the bacterial chromosome and on plasmids, they assumed the popular name of 'jumping genes'. A few of these elements are described in Table 10.1.

It is now clear that there are several types of transposable element. IS elements are generally small (1–2 kb) and encode only those functions needed for their own transposition, whereas transposons are larger, usually 4–25 kb (although considerably larger elements have been described), and they encode at least one function unconnected to transposition that alters the cell phenotype predictably (e.g. by conferring a particular antibiotic resistance). In addition, there are the transposing bacteriophages, such as Mu and D108 (Toussaint and Résibois 1983) (see also p. 275).

Bacteriophage Mu, mentioned earlier in relation to its site-specific recombination system, resembles a transposable element in that it inserts more or less at random into many different sites in the *E. coli* chromosome, as a consequence of its mode of replication. Indeed, it is this ability that gave rise to its name, Mu (for mutator phage). It is now known that phage Mu is a large transposable element that uses a form of transposition for replication (see p. 275).

Table 10.1   Some transposable elements in bacteria

Transposable element	Size (kb)	Terminal[a] repeats (bp)	Target size[b] (bp)	Phenotype[c] conferred	Origin
Insertion sequences					
IS*1*	0.768	18/23	9	None	Gram −ve
IS*2*	1.327	32/41	5	None	Gram −ve
IS*3*	1.3	32/38	3/4	None	Gram −ve
IS*4*	1.426	16/18	11/12	None	Gram −ve
IS*10*	1.329	17/22	9	None	Gram −ve
IS*50*	1.531	12/18	9	None	Gram −ve
IS*903*	1.05	18/18	9	None	Gram −ve
IS*256*	1.35	nd	nd	None	Gram +ve
Composite transposons					
Tn*5*	5.7	IS*50*(IR)	9	Km	Gram −ve
Tn*9*	2.5	IS*1*(DR)	9	Cm	Gram −ve
Tn*10*	9.3	IS*10*(IR)	9	Tc	Gram −ve
Tn*903*	3.1	IS*903*(IR)	9	Km	Gram −ve
Tn*1681*	2.1	IS*1*(IR)	9	Heat-stable toxin[d]	Gram −ve
Tn*4001*	4.7	IS*256*(IR)	nd	Gm Tb Km	Gram +ve
Complex transposons					
Tn*1* family					
Tn*1*, Tn*3*	4.957	38/38	5	Ap	Gram −ve
Tn*21*	19.5	35/38	5	Hg Sm/Sp Su	Gram −ve
Tn*501*	8.2	35/38	5	Hg	Gram −ve
Tn*1721*	11.4	35/38	5	Tc	Gram −ve
Tn*951*	16.5		5	Lac	Gram −ve
Tn*551*	5.3	35/35	5	Ery	Gram +ve
γδ(Tn*1000*)	5.8	36/37	5	None	Gram −ve
Others					
Tn*7*	14	22/28	5	Tp Sm/Sp	Gram −ve
Tn*554*	6.2	None	0	Sp Ery	Gram +ve
Tn*916*	15	20/26	10	Tc, conjugal transfer[e]	Gram −ve
Tn*4291*	nd	nd	nd	Mec	Gram +ve

[a]The number of identical base pairs in both terminal repeats/size of terminal repeats. DR, direct repeat; inverted repeat.
[b]The size of the direct duplications which are found to flank the transposon in situ.
[c]Entries which relate to an antibiotic(s) refer to resistance to that drug(s). Abbreviations used: Ap, ampicillin; Cm, chloramphenicol; Ery, erythromycin; Gm, gentamicin; Hg, mercuric ions; Km, kanamycin; Mec, methicillin; Sm, streptomycin; Sp, spectinomycin; Su, sulphonamide; Lac, lactose metabolism; Tb, tobramycin; Tc, tetracycline; Tp, trimethoprim. Sm/Sp indicates resistance to both antibiotics conferred by the same modifying enzyme.
[d]Heat-stable toxin produced by some enterotoxigenic strains of *Escherichia coli.*
[e]See text p. 239.
nd, not determined.

Because transposition involves the movement of DNA sequences from one site to another, it is clear that whatever the mechanism, it is, by definition, a recombination event, often referred to as illegitimate recombination to indicate that it proceeds independently of a classical recombination system dependent on extensive sequence homology.

The majority of known IS elements have a similar structure, namely a unique central sequence comprising most of the element flanked by short perfect or near-perfect inverted repeat (IR) sequences. These differ in sequence and size from one element to another (c. 10–40 bp) (Table 10.1). For those elements that have been analysed in detail, the unique central section encodes an element-specific transposition function(s). The IR sequences delineate the element, serving as specific sites for recombination mediated by the transposition enzyme(s). The inverted character of the terminal repeats ensures that both are retained in the transposed structure, i.e. the same sequence is recognized at both ends and the DNA is cleaved at the same end of this sequence in both cases.

Most transposons can be assigned to one of 2 broad groups, called **composite transposons** and **complex transposons**. Composite transposons, as their name implies, are constructed from simpler units. Their overall form comprises a unique central sequence that encodes the function(s) by which the element is recognized and which lacks transposition functions, flanked by long sequence repeats (1–2 kb) which are arranged as direct repeats or, more commonly, as IRs. These terminal repeats provide transposition functions and, in all cases examined so far, comprise a pair of IS elements. The more common inverted arrangement possibly reflects the fact that it confers greater stability (coherence) on the composite structure than direct repeats where deletion of the transposon's distinguishing feature(s) as the result of recombination between the terminal IS elements, mediated by the host's homologous recombination machinery, is an ever-present threat (Fig. 10.4).

Complex transposons do not have a modular structure. Rather, both transposition and non-transposition functions are usually flanked by short (c. 40 bp) terminal IRs (as are IS elements). The first transposon identified, Tn*1* (formerly Tn*A*; Hedges and Jacob 1974), typifies this type of element. Its structure is illustrated in Fig. 10.5. Tn*1* is one of a family of transposons that are ancestrally related with respect to their transposition functions. This was first recognized because of a striking similarity in sequences of their IRs. Subsequently, more extensive sequence analysis of several of these elements has demonstrated that the entire transposition mechanism of one is related to that of the others. In some cases the evolutionary divergence is small, so that the transposition functions are interchangeable. In other instances, elements are more distant in terms of evolution and analogous functions cannot be interchanged (Sherratt 1989, Grinsted, de la Cruz and Schmitt 1990).

IS elements and composite transposons are called **class 1 transposable elements,** whereas Tn*1* and related tranposons are called **class 2 transposable** elements. **Class 3** accommodates the transposing bacteriophages such as Mu. Finally, **class 4** at present accommodates those elements that do not naturally fall within classes 1–3. Perhaps 2 of the best known are Tn*7*, a compound transposon encoding resistance to trimethoprim and streptomycin prevalent in gram-negative bacteria, particularly the Enterobacteriaceae, and Tn*916*, an unusual transposon from *Enterococcus faecalis* that encodes resistance to tetracycline and which is conjugative, i.e. can

mediate its transfer not only from one replicon to another by transposition but also from one bacterial cell to another by a form of conjugation (Salyers et al. 1995). Transposons with similar conjugative properties have also been found in *Bacteroides* spp. (Salyers and Shoemaker 1995).

It has become clear that transposable elements are instrumental in bringing about important rearrangements in DNA molecules. Not only do they add extra sequences and useful genes, but their transposition activities can generate other macrolesions such as deletions, duplications and inversions. Because many of them insert into DNA molecules more or less at random, they can generate mutation by disrupting the sequence continuity of genes. That the insertions are often polar has been noted for IS elements; this is also true for transposons. In addition, they can, in some instances, activate previously silent genes by inserting upstream and adjacent to the gene to provide a functional promoter. The polar effects arise because transposable elements are, in general, self-contained and often encode both translational and transcriptional terminators, so that transcription proceeding into the element rarely goes very far. Unless there is a terminal promoter at the other end directing transcription out of the element (which in a few cases there is), the remaining genes of the operon, downstream of the insertion, will be silent.

IS*2* exerts strong polar effects when in one of its 2 possible orientations (this was how it was discovered). In this orientation (designated orientation I) a rho-dependent transcription termination site prevents transcription proceeding through the element into adjacent sequences. In the opposite orientation (orientation II) it can provide a promoter sequence that can switch on downstream genes. Mutations in wild-type IS*2* that create promoters have also been described. It is of interest to note that cloned genes (see p. 262), either not expressed or expressed poorly, may be activated by insertion of a transposable element upstream from them. However, it should be noted that this aspect of transposable element activity appears to be restricted to a minority of specific elements, of which IS*2* is one.

SPECIFICITY AND MECHANISM OF INSERTION

When transposable elements insert into new sites, short duplications of recipient DNA sequence are usually generated. These flank the transposable sequence. The size of the duplication is specific to the element, but is commonly 5 or 9 bp (Table 10.1). The duplications arise because the recipient DNA at the target site is cleaved across both its strands as a short staggered cut into which the transposon is inserted by joining it to the single-strand extensions. The short single-stranded regions of recipient DNA that result from the ligation are then filled in to generate the short duplication.

A wide range of insertion specificities has been found for different transposons and some display different characteristics with different DNA molecules. Some (e.g. Tn*1*) insert at many places on different

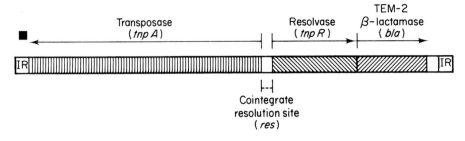

Fig. 10.5 Map of Tn*1* showing the location of its 3 genes. The arrows indicate the direction of transcription. The cointegrate resolution site (*res*) is necessary for resolution of cointegrates, by resolvase, during transposition (see Fig. 10.6). IR, perfect 38 bp inverted repeats.

plasmids and into the bacterial chromosome with little recognizable specificity save, perhaps, a preference for AT-rich regions; others appear to be rather more specific, e.g. IS*4* has been found to insert into only one position in the *gal* region of the *E. coli* chromosome. Although Tn*10* inserts at many different sites, they are all related to the 9 bp consensus sequence, NGCTNAGCN (where N denotes any base). The more closely a site approximates to this sequence the more readily it is used as a site of Tn*10* insertion. The preference for AT-rich regions shown by some transposons suggests that the transposition mechanism used may involve a degree of strand separation at the target, since AT bps are inherently more easily disrupted than GC bps.

Initially, research workers sought to describe transposition in terms of a single mechanism. It is now clear that this notion was misconceived and that there are several different mechanisms. One, used by several IS elements and their composite transposons, is called **conservative**, or **cut-and-paste**, **transposition** (Fig. 10.6a). In this the transposable element is cut from the donor DNA as a discrete double-stranded section of DNA with flush ends. The free ends are ligated to the target site using the single strand extensions generated by the staggered cut at the target site. The small gaps that remain are filled in, probably by repair synthesis, generating the direct repeats. In this mechanism the entire transposable sequence on one DNA molecule is moved to another DNA molecule (Bolland and Kleckner 1996). It is believed that the donor molecule minus the transposon is degraded (Berg 1989, Kleckner 1989). Some transposons, e.g. Tn*7*, also use a cut-and-paste transposition system (Sarnovsky, May and Craig 1996). Conjugative transposons also use a cut-and-paste mechanism of transposition, although the details differ from the simple description given above (Salyers et al. 1995).

A second mechanism of transposition involves semi-conservative DNA replication. This was appreciated when it was found that certain mutants of Tn*1* generated end products somewhat different from those of the parental transposon. With these mutants the products of transposition were **cointegrates** – recombinant DNA molecules comprising both the donor and the recipient replicons with directly repeated copies of Tn*1* at the plasmid junctions, i.e. the transposon had been replicated (Fig. 10.6b). These recombinants could then break down in a *rec*+ host, via normal

recombination, to yield a replicon indistinguishable from the original plasmid donor and a transposon-carrying derivative of the recipient plasmid, i.e. a product indistinguishable from that generated by the parental transposon. Shapiro (1979) and Arthur and Sherratt (1979) synthesized these observations, and others involving bacteriophage Mu, into the now generally accepted model of **replicative transposition** (Fig. 10.6b).

For some IS elements a small proportion of transposition events appear to occur via replicative rather than conservative transposition. This observation has been taken to imply that the 2 forms represent a split pathway proceeding from a common start (Ohtsubo et al. 1981). Consistent with this interpretation is the observation that c. 5% of transpositions of Tn*1* appear to be by a direct pathway rather than by replicative transposition (Bennett, de la Cruz and Grinsted 1983).

More recently, it has been discovered that a novel class of IS elements, of which IS*91* is the type element (Mendiola, Jubete and de la Cruz 1992), that lack terminal IR sequences transpose by a mechanism that involves a form of rolling circle transposition. Insertion is also site-specific. The transposases of these elements are related to the initiator proteins of certain plasmids of *Staphylococcus aureus* (although the IS elements were isolated from gram-negative bacteria) (Mendiola and de la Cruz 1992). The plasmids replicate via a rolling circle mechanism that generates a single-strand version of the plasmid which is then converted to the double-stranded form (see p. 252). It is conceivable that this family of IS elements transposes by a mechanism that also involves a single-stranded intermediate.

Deletions, duplications and insertions

Deletion induced by a transposable element was first seen for IS*1*. In the *E. coli* chromosome, the frequency of deletions near a copy of IS*1* was 100- to 1000-fold higher than that observed elsewhere. Subsequently, other elements and transposons were also shown to stimulate the frequency of deletions in their vicinity. Several studies have demonstrated that the deletions always extend precisely from one end of the particular transposable element, leaving the element itself intact but removing one copy of the direct repeats that originally flanked it. Deletions such as these can, in principle, be formed in one of 2 ways. First, a second copy of the transposable element can insert into a different position on the same replicon, but in the same orientation as the

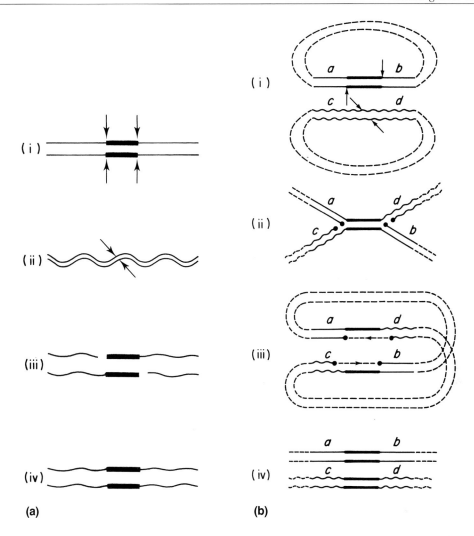

Fig. 10.6 Models for transposition. (a) **Conservative transposition**. (i) Flush double-stranded cuts (vertical arrows) are made at the ends of the transposable element (bold lines) and a staggered cut (diagonal arrows) is made at the target site. (ii) One end of the transposable element is attached by a single strand to each protruding strand at the staggered cut to insert the transposable element into the target site. (iii) Two small gaps, generated as the consequence of the staggered cut, are left on opposite strands, one at each end of the element. (iv) The gaps are filled in by DNA repair synthesis to produce short direct repeats that flank the transposable element. (b) **Replicative transposition**. (i) Single-stranded cuts are made at the ends of the transposable element, and a staggered cut of opposite polarity is made in the target DNA. (ii) One end of the transposable element is attached by a single strand to each protruding end of the staggered cut. Two replication forks are thus created, and replication may proceed to copy the transposable element. (iii) Semi-conservative replication has generated 2 new transposable elements from the original element and a short direct repeat of the target site. If *ab* and *cd* were circles, *a*, *b*, *c* and *d* would now be covalently connected and transposable elements would form the joint regions of a fused replicon. (iv) A site-specific crossover between the transposable elements would resolve the cointegrate into the starting replicon *ab* and the target replicon *cd*, which now has a copy of the transposable element flanked by short direct repeats of the site of insertion (Shapiro 1979).

first. Host mediated recombination can then occur between the copies, effectively deleting one copy and the intervening DNA sequence (see Fig. 10.4, p. 238). Second, an element may transpose to a nearby site on the same DNA molecule by replicative transposition. If the insertion at the new site assumes the same orientation as that at the first site the result is an automatic deletion of one of the copies of the element and the DNA sequences between the original and new sites of insertion (Arthur and Sherratt 1979).

DNA inversions may also arise by one of 2 mechanisms. Following insertion of a second copy of a transposable element into a DNA sequence to generate an inverted repeat, a single host mediated recombination event across the repeated sequences will invert the intervening sequence (see Fig. 10.4, p. 238). Alternatively, when an element transposes by replicative transposition to a new site on the same DNA molecule in such a manner as to generate inverted repeats of the element, the intervening sequence is automatically inverted, again as a consequence of the mechanics of the transposition (Arthur and Sherratt 1979). In practice, after the event, it is impossible to determine which mechanism generated a particular inversion because extended IRs act as recombination loci periodically to invert and reinvert the intervening sequence. As noted earlier, this property is exploited in the site-specific recombination systems that control P1 and Mu phage host range and *S.* Typhimurium flagellar type.

Transposition functions

Several transposons have now been studied in detail and, with very few exceptions, each element encodes its own transposition functions (see Berg and Howe 1989). Perhaps the best studied to date is Tn*3* (which is virtually identical to Tn*1*), the class II element that confers resistance to a range of penicillins, including ampicillin and carbenicillin. The element is 5 kb and encodes 3 proteins: a TEM β-lactamase and 2 proteins that are necessary for transposition (see Fig. 10.5, p. 242). The larger of these, called **transposase**, is encoded by *tnpA* and is indispensable; it mediates **cointegrate** formation (Fig. 10.6b). The second transposition enzyme, **resolvase** (encoded by *tnpR*), is normally responsible for **resolution** of the cointegrate to release the final transposition product. The promoters for both genes are located in the length of c. 100 bp that separates them. The site at which resolvase acts is called the *res* site, also located in the intergenic region between *tnpA* and *tnpR* (Sherratt 1989). A consequence of mutations in *tnpR* is that the frequency of transposition increases by approximately 2 orders of magnitude, i.e. resolvase functions not only as a site-specific recombination enzyme but also as a transcriptional repressor. This duality indicates a more general feature of prokaryotes that seems to be emerging, namely optimization of the genome. It is not uncommon to find the same DNA sequence performing more than one function.

In a *rec⁺* host (Watson et al. 1987), cointegrate resolution can be effected by the host's own recombination system, since the 2 copies of the element in the cointegrate are direct repeats and provide extensive sequence homology. Hence, *tnpR* mutants of Tn*3* generate cointegrates that are relatively stable in a recombination-deficient host, e.g. one which is *recA*, whereas normal transposition products are generated in a recombination-proficient host. Analyses of other class II transposons, e.g. γδ (Tn*1000*), Tn*21*, Tn*501* and Tn*1721* (see Table 10.1, p. 240), have shown that each encodes a transposase and a resolvase of approximately the same sizes as those of Tn*3*. Some of these analogous enzymes are functionally interchangeable but others are not, indicating different degrees of evolutionary proximity (Grinsted, de la Cruz and Schmitt 1990).

Well studied class I elements are IS*1*, IS*10* (Tn*10*), IS*50* (Tn*5*) and IS*903* (Tn*903*) (see Table 10.1, p. 240). Each is genetically distinct and encodes its own unique transposition functions. The transposition of each is also regulated, but the strategies of regulation differ from one element to another. Thus IS*10* regulates both transcription and translation of its single transposition gene, whereas IS*50* regulates transcription of its transposition gene and modulates the activity of the enzyme with another IS*50*-encoded protein (Berg 1989, Kleckner 1989). Bacteriophage Mu, as might be expected of a lysogenic phage, has a variety of control systems to regulate its transposition (i.e. replication) activity (Toussaint and Résibois 1983), which is essentially dependent on a single phage gene designated *A*.

Not all transposition systems have so few element-encoded transposition functions. Tn*7*, for example, has 5 transposition genes, 3 of which are needed for all transposition events. Tn*7* displays 2 types of transpositional behaviour. It can insert more or less at random into many different sites on plasmids at a relatively low frequency but it can also insert into one specific site on the *E. coli* chromosome at high frequency. Which transposition event occurs is determined by which one of the other 2 functions is used in the reaction (Craig 1989, Sarnovsky, May and Craig 1996).

In addition to element-encoded functions and irrespective of the transposition mechanism, host functions are also required, such as DNA polymerase and DNA ligase activities. Others have been implicated.

Ubiquity of insertion sequences

The importance of insertion sequences and transposons in mediating bacterial variation cannot be overstated. Not only can they add useful genes to an organism directly (e.g. antibiotic resistance) but also, because of their ability to operate in pairs to transpose otherwise non-transposable genes (e.g. the unique central sequences of class I transposons), they can, in principle, effect the transposition of any bacterial DNA sequence from one DNA molecule to another. These types of elements are not restricted to prokaryotes; indeed, the first reports of transposable elements in higher organisms, specifically maize, preceded description of those in *E. coli* by 10–15 years (McClintock 1953). Transposable elements are now known to exist in a number of eukaryotes, including yeast and *Drosophila* (see Shapiro 1983, Berg and Howe 1989).

MUTATION BY TRANSPOSON INSERTION

Because of their ability to insert into replicons almost at random, transposons have been exploited as mutagens. They possess the advantage over other random forms of mutation that the site of mutation is grossly altered by the addition of new DNA sequences, which can be physically mapped by restriction enzyme analysis. Because of this, artificial transposons with a range of properties have been created from natural ones. These characteristics have been designed to facilitate molecular genetic investigations (Berg, Berg and Groisman 1989, de Lorenzo et al. 1990).

Transposon mutagenesis has been adapted in an ingenious way to generate mutations in bacterial virulence genes (Hensel et al. 1995) and to allow negative selection. This technique, signature tagged mutagenesis (STM), is a negative selection method for bacterial virulence gene identification based on the ability to follow simultaneously the fates of many different mutants within a single animal. Individual copies of a transposon (mini-Tn*5*, de Lorenzo et al. 1990) were tagged with small, unique nucleotide sequences. The identity of any particular copy of the transposon could then be determined readily by hybridization techniques. These tagged transposons were then used to generate a bank of 1510 random transposon mutants in a strain of *S.* Typhimurium. Each isolate in the bank was checked to confirm that it had acquired a uniquely tagged copy of the mini-Tn*5*, yielding a slightly smaller bank of 1152 mutants. Cultures of each isolate were grown in the wells of microtitration trays and 12 mixtures, each with 96 strains, were prepared and used to inoculate BALB/c mice by intraperitoneal injection. Three days later the mice were killed and the bacteria were recovered from each mouse by plating spleen homogenates onto a suitable medium. Approximately 10 000 colonies recovered from each mouse were pooled and the total DNA was extracted. The transposon tags were amplified and labelled by PCR and colony blots of the original 96 mutants in the subset were probed. The results were compared with the hybridization pattern obtained with a 'tag probe' obtained with DNA from the mixed inoculum of 96 mutants. Colonies which probed positive in the control but not with the probe prepared from DNA from cells post-passage through mice were shown to have had a virulence gene inactivated by the mini-Tn5. Because these strains were less virulent they survived less well in the mouse and so were poorly recovered from the spleen of the infected animals, in turn giving a much reduced yield of that particular transposon tag in the DNA used to prepare the 'tag probe'. Forty virulence mutants were identified in the bank of 1152. Among these mutants, approximately half were in genes known to be involved in virulence. The remainder constituted a set of new virulence genes. These results accord well with an estimate of approximately 150 virulence genes in *S.* Typhimurium (Groisman and Saier 1990), of which about 75 have been identified.

Integrons and gene cassettes

In addition to plasmids and transposable elements, bacteria have yet other systems for gene dissemination, namely, **integrons** (Stokes and Hall 1989). Integrons are essentially site-specific recombination systems that mediate the movement of small DNA elements called **gene cassettes**. Most of the gene cassettes described carry a single resistance gene. About 40 antibiotic resistance genes, including those for resistance to aminoglycosides, β-lactams, chloramphenicol, erythromycin, sulphonamides, tetracycline and trimethoprim have been identified as being on gene cassettes (Recchia and Hall 1995).

Integrons were first identified on Tn*21* and closely related transposons (Grinsted, de la Cruz and Schmitt 1990), but are now known to be more widely distributed (Hall and Collis 1995). Molecular analysis of the resistance genes of Tn*21* and related elements revealed that although different transposons carried different complements of resistance genes, most appeared to be accommodated at a single point on the basic structure, i.e. irrespective of the identity of the resistance gene(s) carried on a particular transposon, the sequences flanking the gene or gene cluster were the same, called the 3′- and 5′-conserved regions. Analysis of the 5′-conserved region revealed a gene, *int*, encoding a protein of the 'integrase' family. The *int* gene product, called integrase, is a site-specific recombinase. Beside *int* is *attI*, a site that is recognized and utilized by the integrase to capture gene cassettes. The essential components of an integron, located in the 5′-conserved region, are an *int* gene, an *attI* site and a promoter in the correct orientation to express the genes on captured cassettes, because these resistance genes lack their own promoters. Within the 3′-conserved region is often found the *sul1* gene, encoding resistance to sulphonamides. Most, but not all, integrons carry the *sul1* gene (Hall and Collis 1995).

A gene cassette can exist in 2 forms:

1   as a linear insert within an integron or
2   transiently as a small double-stranded circle of DNA carrying one (or occasionally 2) resistance genes and a recombination site called a 59-base element (Hall, Brookes and Stokes 1991).

Integrase mediated recombination between a 59-base element on a cassette and the *attI* site inserts the cassette gene(s) into the integron and orients it so that it is expressed from the integron promoter (Collis et al. 1993). Several cassettes may be captured in this way to form a resistance gene array in which each gene is separated from the next by a 59-base element. Arrays of 5 and 6 resistance genes have been found; 59-base pair elements do not have a unique sequence, but all conform to a consensus, which may be longer than 59 bases.

Movement of gene cassettes is possible because the integration of a cassette into an integron is a reversible process, so what has been captured by one integron can subsequently be released and captured by another (Collis and Hall 1992). In this way the complement of resistance genes can be constantly rearranged and moved from one DNA molecule to another, providing it carries an integron or a suitable integration site.

4   ACQUISITION OF NEW GENES

Genetic diversity in bacteria growing in monoculture in the laboratory can occur only by mutation, as described above. In mixed cultures, as are found in nature, diversity can be provided by the transfer of DNA from one cell to another, provided that the new genes can be stably inherited by the progeny of the transcipient cell. Four mechanisms of gene transfer have been described for bacteria, although not all necessarily apply to a particular bacterial species or strain; these are **transformation**, **transduction**, **conjugation** and **cell–cell fusion**.

Genetic information (i.e. DNA) acquired by one of these 4 mechanisms is inherited provided that one of 2 situations pertains; either the newly acquired DNA is incorporated into one of the replicons in the recipient cell by some form of recombination, or the newly introduced DNA is self-maintaining, i.e. is a replicon in its own right. In the former case newly incorporated sequences are substituted for existing ones. The 'invading' DNA is usually linear and homologous to only part of the rescue replicon and is itself not a replicon. Homologous sequences on the acquired DNA and on the appropriate resident replicon (chromosome or plasmid) are efficiently paired and exchanged by recombination (Fig. 10.7). DNA sequences not rescued by recombination are ultimately degraded. The mechanism is one of general recombination and requires that the host be recombination-proficient (Rec⁺) (Smith 1988, 1989). In particular, the host must have a *recA*⁺ gene (Smith 1988), the product of which is essential for homologous recombination. In laboratory studies of this type, gene exchange often involves wild-type genes and their mutant alleles. For example, a length of DNA that includes the lactose fermention genes (*lac*⁺) from *E. coli* K12 is introduced into a strain that cannot ferment lactose because of mutation in its *lac* operon. Recombination between the newly acquired chromosomal segment of DNA and the equivalent region on the chromosome of the recipient cell results in the substitution of the wild-type allele for the mutant allele and restoration the recipient cell's ability to ferment lactose. Allelic variation is seen in naturally occurring bacteria, e.g. the genes that determine the antigens of *Salmonella*. When that part of the chromosome of *Salmonella* Paratyphi B that encodes antigen b is transferred into *S.* Typhimurium, recombination can lead to the substitution of the sequence encoding antigen b for the chromosomal sequence that encodes antigen i. In this way new *Salmonella* serotypes are created. Phylogenetic relationships among Enterobacteriaceae have been reviewed by Sanderson (1976) (see also Chapter 39).

DNA may also be added to the genome of the recipient cell. **Plasmids** (see section 5, p. 251) are autonomous DNA molecules and to survive transfer do not need to be rescued by recombination. Transposable elements, as discussed above, although not replicons, may insert into other DNA sequences with no requirement for homology nor any loss of recipient DNA (although the insertion may result in loss of a particular function).

It is now known that all 4 mechanisms of gene transfer apply to both gram-positive and gram-negative bacteria, although not necessarily with any one particular bacterial strain. However, some transfer systems that are widely used in the laboratory (e.g. transformation of *E. coli*) are likely to be laboratory artefacts rather than naturally occurring transfer systems, whereas others (e.g. transformation of *Neisseria* spp. and *Streptococcus pneumoniae*) are likely to play an important role in gene dissemination in nature (Dowson, Coffey and Spratt 1994). For more information, see Grinsted and Bennett (1988).

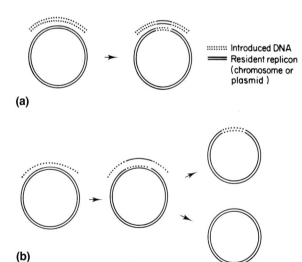

(a)

::::::: Introduced DNA
═══ Resident replicon (chromosome or plasmid)

(b)

Fig. 10.7 General recombination. The figure shows 2 crossovers in homologous DNA having occurred between (a) 2 duplex molecules and (b) a single-stranded and a duplex molecule. Multiple crossovers (not illustrated) usually occur between homologous regions of DNA. The figure does not illustrate the mechanism of crossover. The RecA protein is required and some understanding of the mechanism is emerging (see text).

4.1 Transformation

The first observation of bacterial transformation was by Griffith (1928) when studying pneumococcal infection in mice. The virulence of pneumococci depends on the capsular polysaccharide that gives the colonies a smooth appearance (S phenotype). Colonies of nonvirulent strains, without capsules, have a rough appearance (R phenotype). Griffith observed that when a mixture of living avirulent R cells and heat-killed virulent S cells was injected into mice, some of them died, whereas injection of either live R cells or heat-killed S cells was not lethal. From the dead animals Griffith isolated virulent S cells whose capsular type was the same as that of the injected dead S cells. Griffith concluded that the heat-killed S cells had released something that had been taken up by the live R cells and had transformed them to the virulent S cell type. It was not until 1944 that Avery, MacLeod and McCarty, using fractionated cell components, demonstrated that the transforming factor was DNA.

Cells that are able to take up DNA from their environment and incorporate it into the genome are said to be **competent**. In the case of some bacteria (e.g. *E. coli*), a state of competence can be developed by washing the cells with certain salt solutions (see p. 247) but is otherwise absent. In others, competence is a natural feature of the life cycle as, for example, in the pneumococcus. Furthermore, some bacteria are competent at all times, whereas others display competence only at a particular phase of the growth cycle. In the latter case competence commonly develops towards the end of logarithmic growth in batch culture. Species that display natural, rather than laboratory-induced competence include *Acinetobacter calcoaceticus, Azotobacter vinelandii, B. subtilis, Haemophilus influenzae, Moraxella* spp., *Neisseria* spp., *Pasteurella novicida*, some *Pseudomonas* spp., *Rhizobium, S. pneumoniae* and *Xanthomonas phaseoli*. Species that can be made competent artificially, by one means or another, include *E. coli, Pseudomonas* spp., *S.* Typhimurium and *S. aureus*.

NATURAL COMPETENCE

Competence involves the ability to bind DNA to the cell surface and then transport it through the cell envelope into the cytoplasm prior to incorporation into the genome. The first of these activities, particularly in cases of natural competence, may involve specific cell receptors; this idea is supported by studies of interaction of competent pneumococci with DNA, in which the kinetics have been found to follow those of a classic enzyme–substrate reaction, and by the finding that new envelope proteins are synthesized as competence is acquired.

The best characterized naturally occurring transformation systems are those of *S. pneumoniae, B. subtilis* and *H. influenzae*. In all 3 systems, double-stranded donor DNA binds to the cell surface and is cut into discrete lengths giving fragments of 15–30 kb in the case of *B. subtilis*, 8–9 kb for *S. pneumoniae* and c. 18 kb for *H. influenzae*. The transforming activity of chromosomal DNA is better with large DNA fragments than with small, and there is a minimum size requirement for the donor DNA below which no transformation activity is seen. With *B. subtilis* and *S. pneumoniae* there is a period after DNA uptake during which the acquired DNA is incorporated into the genome. This period has been termed the **eclipse phase**.

B. subtilis and *S. pneumoniae* take up DNA from unrelated (heterospecific) bacteria as well as from closely related (homospecific) bacteria, whereas *H. influenzae* takes up efficiently only homospecific DNA. The first 2 bacteria have endonucleases located on the cell surface that degrade one strand of the bound DNA while the complementary strand is taken into the cell. By contrast, no endonuclease has been found on the surface of *H. influenzae* and it is the bound double-stranded DNA that is taken up. A membrane protein, detectable only in competent *H. influenzae*, capable of binding DNA, has been reported and Sisco and Smith (1979) found that a specific nucleotide sequence of 8–12 bp mediates binding to the protein. It has been estimated that there are approximately 600 copies of this sequence on the *H. influenzae* chromosome, but it is rarely encountered on heterologous DNA. Such a specific mechanism is unlikely to have been preserved by chance, which implies that transformation plays an important role in the life-style of *H. influenzae*. Similar 'transformation sequences' have not yet been identified for any other bacterial species, although the possibility has been investigated in *Neisseria gonorrhoeae* (Burnstein, Dyer and Sparling 1988).

The fate of transformed donor DNA depends largely on its source. If the DNA is linear and homospecific, it is incorporated into the chromosome of the recipient cell by recombination. If the linear DNA is heterospecific, its rescue will depend on whether there is sufficient homology with a resident replicon to permit recombination. Recombination with a resident replicon is not necessary when the donor DNA is itself a replicon, i.e. bacteriophage DNA (in which case the phenomenon is called transfection) or plasmid DNA. In these cases, however, successful transformation appears to require the uptake of more than one copy of the replicon, although complete duplication of sequence is not necessary. This finding indicates that replicon establishment, also involves recombination. In systems that rely on natural competence, transformation with homospecific chromosomal DNA is usually much more efficient than with intact heterospecific replicons, probably because of the requirement for sequence duplication. Consistent with this interpretation is the finding that transformation with plasmid dimers (i.e. duplicate copies of the same plasmid joined head to tail in the same DNA molecule) is as efficient as transformation with homospecific chromosomal DNA.

Artificial competence

The ability to transform bacteria is a valuable experimental tool but several commonly used laboratory bacteria (e.g. *E. coli*, *Pseudomonas putida*, *S.* Typhimurium and *S. aureus*) do not display transformation competence at any stage of their life cycles. Therefore, methods have been devised that can induce artificial competence. The common feature of these methods is the treatment of bacteria with salt solutions at 0°C. The most commonly used salt is calcium chloride. The method was first developed to enable *E. coli* to take up non-infective phage DNA, and has since been used extensively to introduce plasmid DNA.

These transformation systems appear to work best with plasmid or bacteriophage DNA, rather than with chromosomal DNA. Indeed, *E. coli* does not transform efficiently with chromosomal DNA unless it is deficient in exonuclease V (encoded by the *recBCD* genes), since this enzyme degrades invading linear DNA; in addition, the cell must also be mutated at another locus, *sbcB*. This mutation restores recombination proficiency which is lost by mutations at *recB*

and *recC*. Recombination is necessary to rescue linear homospecific DNA sequences.

Transformation with artificial competence works most efficiently with covalently closed circular (ccc) DNA, i.e. intact replicons such as bacteriophage genomes and plasmids (Cohen, Chang and Hsu 1972). These double-stranded DNA molecules are taken up intact and incorporated efficiently into the genome as autonomous replicating units. Any damage to the ccc form reduces the efficiency of transformation. It should be noted that induction of artificial competence is bacterial species-specific. Although very efficient systems have been developed for particular laboratory strains of a particular organism, these systems often do not work efficiently with other types of bacteria, or even with natural isolates of the same bacterium.

DNA may also be induced to enter bacterial cells when cell suspensions are subject to electrical discharge through the suspension, a procedure termed **electroporation** (or electrotransformation). This is now a commonly used method to introduce DNA molecules into many different bacterial species and electroporation apparatus is readily available commercially.

4.2 Conjugation

Conjugation is the term used to describe the transfer of DNA directly from one bacterial cell to another by a mechanism that requires cell-to-cell contact. DNA is transferred in a nuclease-resistant form that distinguishes the mechanism from transformation and without the aid of a bacteriophage, which distinguishes the mechanism from transduction.

Bacterial conjugation was discovered by Lederberg and Tatum (1946) when testing pairs of mutant strains of *E. coli* K12 for evidence for DNA transfer and recombination. From a mixture of a strain that required phenylalanine, cysteine and biotin (a triple auxotroph) and another that required threonine, leucine and thiamine, they obtained some clones that were **prototrophs**, i.e. they required none of the nutrients required by the 2 parental strains, and other clones with various combinations of these requirements. These recombinant clones could only have arisen as the result of acquisition of chromosomal DNA from one bacterial cell by the other. Further studies, over several years, showed that the recombination was not the result of sexual reproduction in the normal sense of equal participation of both parents in zygote formation. Rather, it appeared that only a small amount of DNA from the 'male' (**donor**) parent was incorporated into the offspring (**recombinants**) which otherwise showed all the characteristics of the 'female' (**recipient**) parent. The capacity to donate genetic information (DNA) in these experiments was shown to depend upon possession of the **F (fertility) factor**. Strains were found that had become infertile, having lost their F factor, but they could regain fertility by contact with an F-carrying (F^+) strain (Hayes 1953a). At the time of these experiments, the role of DNA and the nature of the F factor were unknown; the F factor is now known to be a conjugative plasmid (see below).

In the first conjugation experiments the bacterial characters transferred were encoded by chromosomal genes. The F factor mediated transfer of part of the donor (F⁺) cell's chromosome and this was rescued by homologous recombination into the chromosome of the recipient (F⁻) cell, resulting in recombinant clones of bacteria with new assortments of characters. The recombinants remained F⁻, i.e. they did not also acquire the F factor.

Conjugation is not a normal function of bacteria but determined by a variety of plasmids of which the F factor is just one. Conjugal transfer of chromosomal DNA is a relatively infrequent event, but many different plasmids are able to mobilize chromosomal genes with various degrees of efficiency. **Chromosome-mobilizing ability** (*cma*) is a byproduct that arises from certain interactions of the plasmids concerned with the bacterial chromosome, just as transduction of chromosomal genes is a byproduct of phage particle production (see p. 282). The main result of conjugation is transfer of the plasmid concerned to another bacterial cell; but plasmid transfer systems can also mobilize other DNA molecules present in the donor cells, including the chromosome.

For many years conjugation was thought to be the prerogative of plasmids found in gram-negative cells, and most of our knowledge derives from these systems. However, conjugation systems have been reported in gram-positive bacteria, notably strains of *E. faecalis*. The mechanics of these systems appear to differ somewhat from those found in gram-negative bacteria (Clewell et al. 1986).

Conjugation determined by F

F was the first conjugative plasmid to be discovered and the functions that enable conjugation to occur have been analysed in detail. The genes that determine these functions are arranged as a continuous array, mostly in a single operon on the F factor in a region c. 30 kb in length, called the transfer (*tra*) region (Firth, Ippen-Ihler and Skurray 1996). This cluster, comprising approximately 24 genes, is found not only on the F factor but also on several resistance (R) plasmids, e.g. Rl and R100. Other plasmids encode unrelated but analogous Tra functions. Several different conjugation systems have now been described.

Conjugative pili

For conjugation to occur, donor and recipient cells must contact each other. This contact is not random but is directed by thin protein filaments on the donor cell, called **conjugative** or 'sex' **pili**. These can be visualized by electron microscopy (Fig. 10.8). Cells that lack conjugative pili cannot transfer DNA. Precisely how 'sex' pili work is not known, but the current view is that they make the initial contact between the donor and recipient cells and then are retracted into the donor to draw the 2 cells together until direct contact is made. The protein, **pilin**, of which F pili are made, exists as a pool of unpolymerized molecules in the outer membrane of the cell.

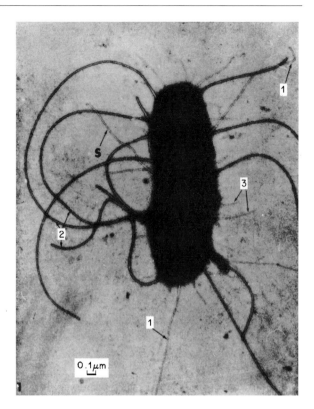

Fig. 10.8   *E. coli* K12 F⁺. The electron micrograph shows 3 kinds of appendage to the cell: 1, F pili; 2, flagella; and 3, common pili or fimbriae. (From Meynell, Meynell and Datta 1968).

Conjugative pili may act as receptors for bacteriophages. F⁺ cells are therefore susceptible to certain phages that cannot infect F⁻ bacteria whereas some other phages will infect only cells that carry one of another class of conjugative plasmid. Because these phages are specific for particular pili, they can be used as indicators for the presence of particular types of plasmids (Willetts 1988).

Mating pair formation

Random collision of bacteria is the first stage in conjugation or **mating**; accordingly, plasmid transfer is rarely detected at low cell densities (Broda 1979). Initial contact between donor and recipient cells is fragile and easily disrupted (e.g. by pipetting), so not all encounters are productive. Before any DNA is transferred, mating pairs are stabilized in the sense that much greater force than simple pipetting is then needed to separate them; they can, however, be separated by vigorous vortex mixing or in an electric blender.

High frequency of recombination (Hfr) and F′ formation

The first bacterial conjugation experiments involved transfer of chromosomal genes mediated by F. For this to occur, F must first fuse with the bacterial chromosome to form one large circular molecule. F, like many other plasmids, carries several transposable elements, specifically IS2, IS3 and γδ (Tn1000). Copies of the

IS sequences are also to be found on the chromosome of *E. coli* and so can serve as loci for recombination between F and the chromosome (Brooks Low 1996, Deonier 1996). A single crossover between copies of the same element on F and the chromosome inserts one replicon into the other to form one large conjugative DNA molecule, transfer of which can proceed from the **origin of transfer** (*oriT*) of the integrated plasmid. Plasmid integration into the chromosome can also be by transposition (by, for example, γδ) with the formation of a transposition cointegrate. Either of these mechanisms can generate integration events that may be transient or relatively stable. Clones with the F factor stably integrated into the chromosome are called **Hfr** (high frequency of recombination) strains because, in matings in which these are donors, chromosomal genes are carried into all recipient cells and high numbers of recombinants can be recovered (Hayes 1953b). Transfer of F DNA is rapid once a stable mating pair is formed; but the chromosome is about 50 times as long as F, and complete transfer takes about 100 min. In practice, mating pairs usually separate before this, so the chromosome is rarely transferred in its entirety.

F can be inserted into the bacterial chromosome at numerous loci and in either orientation. For each Hfr strain the chromosome is transferred to recipients unidirectionally from the *oriT* of F. Genes nearest the transferring end of F enter the recipient first (Fig. 10.9). As a consequence, these donor alleles are recovered in greatest numbers in recombinants. The further a gene is from the leading end of F, the lower the probability that it will be transferred because, as noted above, it is rare that the entire chromosome is transferred; i.e. the longer a mating proceeds, the greater the probability that the participating cells will separate. One consequence is that chromosomal genes are transferred as a gradient from the point in the chromosome where F is inserted. Accordingly, these gradients can be plotted to show the positions of the genes in relation to the *oriT* of the integrated F. The same gradient, more directly related to the time of entry of each gene into recipient cells, can be determined from the results of interrupted matings. In these experiments, samples of a mating mixture are removed at intervals, diluted so as to prevent further mating pair formation, sheared in a blender or mixer to separate stabilized pairs and then plated onto selective media to detect recombinants (Fig. 10.9). When such experiments are performed with several different Hfr strains, the results indicate that the chromosome of *E. coli* is a circular molecule, because linear permutations of the same circular gene array are always obtained. As a consequence, the map of the *E. coli* chromosome is depicted as a circle with 100 min as reference points (Berlyn, Brooks Low and Rudd 1996). Similar experiments with other bacteria, notably *S.* Typhimurium, *Proteus mirabilis*, *P. aeruginosa* and *P. putida*, using F or a suitable analogue have shown that the chromosomes of these are also circular and of a similar size (see O'Brien 1987).

When a plasmid integrates into the chromosome,

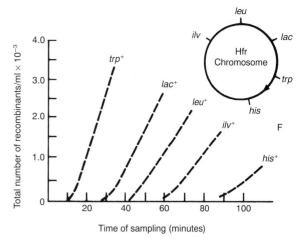

Fig. 10.9 Interrupted mating experiment. An Hfr strain of *E. coli*, with F inserted at the position shown, was mixed with an F⁻ strain that was *lac* (lactose non-fermenting), *trp*, *leu*, *ilv*, *his* (required tryptophan, leucine, isoleucine–valine and histidine for growth), *str* (streptomycin-resistant). Samples removed from the mixture at times shown were 'whirl-mixed' and plated on medium selective for the respective recombinants and containing streptomycin (to inhibit the Hfr donor).

either by transposition or by recombination between copies of a common sequence (e.g. an IS element), the overall result is the same, namely, formation of a cointegrate in which the plasmid is flanked by direct repeats of the transposable element (see p. 241) or of the common sequence. Recombination across these direct repeats will restore the plasmid to its autonomous state. The integrated F of an Hfr strain can be excised from the chromosome in this way. Sometimes, however, excision is not precise and chromosomal DNA adjacent to one side or to both sides of the integrated plasmid is also removed and becomes part of the plasmid; sometimes a remnant of F is left in the chromosome. The derivative plasmids generated by the imprecise excision events are called **plasmid primes**; e.g. F′*lac is* F with the *lac* operon of *E. coli* incorporated into it (see also p. 282 to compare λ specialized transduction). In this case the operon is functional so that when an F′*lac is* transferred to a lactose non-fermenting strain the transconjugants (i.e. the progeny of the cross) are *lac*⁺ (i.e. are able to ferment lactose).

E. coli K12 strains that carry an F′ plasmid are normally diploid for the chromosomal sequence carried on the plasmid. Recombination between these homologous sequences may be frequent and results in re-entry of the F sequence into the chromosome to generate an Hfr strain with the same origin and direction of chromosome transfer as the Hfr from which the F′ originated. In practice, F′ cultures transfer chromosomal DNA at frequencies between that of a normal F⁺ culture (with autonomous F) and that of the originating Hfr strain, because the cells in the culture are a mixture of those with the F′ integrated into the chromosome and others in which the plasmid is autonomous, i.e. the integrated and free plasmid forms in these cell lines will be in dynamic equilibrium. This phenomenon is not, in principle, restricted to F. Any plasmid can be integrated into the bacterial chromosome by a suitable transposition with subsequent imprecise excision generating plasmid primes that, in turn, can be used in mapping studies, provided that the original plasmid mediates its own transfer.

F or F′ plasmids can be transferred to species other than *E. coli*, including ones belonging to different genera, such as *Yersinia* and *Vibrio* and the *E. coli* genes are expressed in these organisms. In the main, incorporation of chromosomal DNA from *E. coli* into the chromosomes of bacteria of other genera is not observed, unless there is a close phylogenetic relationship as, for example, between *E. coli* and *Shigella* spp., because there is insufficient homology to permit recombination. Even between *E. coli* and *Salmonella*, chromosomal recombination is rare. As might be expected, however, F can insert into the chromosomes of those bacteria in which it can be established to generate Hfr strains, so furnishing a tool for genetic analysis.

CONJUGATION IN OTHER GENERA

Conjugative plasmids have been identified in many different bacteria including all gram-negative enterobacteria, in species of *Pasteurella*, *Yersinia* and many non-fermenting gram-negative aerobes such as *Pseudomonas* and *Acinetobacter*, as well as in *Haemophilus*, *Neisseria*, *Campylobacter* and *Bacteroides* spp., and grampositive organisms such as *Streptomyces*, *Streptococcus* and *Clostridium*. Demonstration of conjugation in all these species does not necessarily imply that the mechanisms are the same; e.g. conjugative pili have not been identified in all the genera listed above. However, conjugative plasmids in *Pseudomonas* (Holloway, Krishnapillai and Morgan 1979), *Streptomyces* (Hopwood et al. 1973) and *Acinetobacter* (Towner and Vivian 1976) spp. mediate chromosomal DNA transfer in ways that appear to be analogous to that of F in *E. coli*.

In some genera, conjugation and transfer of antibiotic resistance determinants have been observed although no plasmid DNA could be identified (Stuy 1980). The mobile DNA seems to be incorporated into the bacterial chromosome, but the strains do not behave as Hfr strains. Rather, transfer appears to involve a discrete DNA sequence, i.e. genetically the element behaves like a plasmid, but it cannot be isolated by conventional plasmid isolation procedures. One example is typified by the transposon Tn*916* which originated in the chromosome of a strain of *E. faecalis*. Tn*916* encodes resistance to tetracycline and accommodates conjugation functions that mediate transfer of the transposon alone, even between Rec⁻ hosts (Franke and Clewell 1981, Clewell et al. 1988). No plasmid is involved and the element transposes from the chromosome in the donor cell into the chromosome in the recipient (Salyers et al. 1995).

The conjugative functions of F are naturally derepressed, so that F transfers at high frequency. By contrast, most natural plasmids transfer at rather low frequencies. In some cases mutant plasmids can be isolated that transfer at greatly increased frequencies, indicating that expression of the *tra* genes is normally genetically repressed. In other cases genetic derepression has not been found, although the transfer frequency is relatively low; an example is the R plasmid RP4, which originated in a strain of *P. aeruginosa* but which can be transferred to virtually all gram-negative bacteria (Thomas and Smith 1987).

One consequence of regulating the expression of a set of transfer genes negatively, i.e. with a repressor, is that immediately after plasmid transfer expression of the transfer system is transiently derepressed in the recipient and remains so until sufficient repressor has been synthesized to re-establish control. During this time the recipient temporarily becomes capable of high-frequency plasmid transfer. If there are sufficient potential recipient cells available, the plasmid will spread from one to the other like a chain reaction (epidemic spread) until the system is saturated, as was seen in early studies on the transfer kinetics of R plasmids such as Rl and R100. This finding has practical significance in the design of experiments to test for plasmid transfer (Broda 1979, Willetts 1988).

Conjugative plasmids in genera other than those of the Enterobacteriaceae may also repress expression of their transfer genes. In *E. coli* the only mechanism known to lift repression, other than mutation, is transfer to a new host. In other genera, however, induction of the conjugation functions has been reported, e.g. conjugation mediated by a tetracycline resistance plasmid in *Bacteroides fragilis* is induced by low concentrations of tetracycline together with induction of resistance to tetracycline (Privitera, Sebald and Fayolle 1981). This phenomenon does not appear to be widespread.

Conjugation in gram-positive bacteria appears to differ somewhat from that in gram-negative bacteria in the manner in which the donor and recipient cells are brought together. In *E. faecalis*, conjugation is mediated via **sex pheromones** excreted by potential recipient cells (Clewell 1993). These compounds cause donor and recipient cells to clump to form mating aggregates, a necessary prerequisite to plasmid transfer. Upon acquisition of the plasmid the recipient promptly ceases to produce the particular pheromone that triggered plasmid transfer. Different plasmids respond to different pheromones and potential recipient cells produce several.

An unusual form of plasmid transfer, called **phage mediated conjugation**, has been reported to occur with some strains of *S. aureus*. Lacey (1980) described the carriage of penicillin and cadmium resistance genes by elements with some of the characters of defective phages. Not only were these genetic elements themselves transmissible between nonlysogenic staphylococci but they could also mediate transfer of unlinked resistance plasmids in mixed culture (but not in conventional transduction experiments).

4.3 Transduction

Gene transfer between bacteria can also be mediated by some bacteriophages in a process known as **transduction**. Two forms have been described: **generalized transduction** and **specialized transduction**. In the first, any part of the donor genome can be transduced; in the second, specific sequences are transduced. Phages and transduction are considered in more detail later (see p. 282; see also Masters 1996, Weisberg 1996).

4.4 Protoplast fusion

When the cell wall of a bacterial cell is removed, an osmotically fragile form called a **protoplast** is generated (see Chapter 2). This remains intact as long as the growth medium is osmotically buffered. Bacterial protoplasts can fuse with one another, a process called **protoplast fusion**. This generates cytoplasmic bridges that allow mixing of the cytoplasms of the fused cells and exchange of genetic material. **Fusions** can be obtained between unrelated cells, even between members of different kingdoms, and gene transfer by this mechanism has been termed **genetic transfusion**.

As in the other forms of gene transfer, plasmid or phage DNA can be transferred interspecifically or intergenerically, but for recombination between chromosomal DNAs a close relationship between the participating cells is necessary in practice. In this case, 2 complete chromosomes are brought together to generate an artificial diploid and from such fusions haploid recombinants with many permutations of the traits of the parent cells can be recovered. Protoplast fusion is an artificial system of gene transfer that has little or no relevance to gene transfer in nature. However, protoplast (or spheroplast) fusion has proved to be a valuable experimental tool that is likely to find even more uses in the advance of molecular genetics.

5 PLASMIDS

Plasmids are extrachromosomal, autonomous DNA molecules (i.e. **replicons**) found in many bacterial cells. Plasmids have also been found in lower eukaryotes, e.g. the 2 μm plasmid of yeast. The term 'plasmid' was proposed by Lederberg (1952) for all extrachromosomal genetic structures that can replicate autonomously. The adjective 'autonomous' here means self-governing and separate from the chromosome of the host, rather than an entity capable of separate existence, in that plasmids are obligate **endosymbionts** of bacteria, using the replication enzymes of their host to ensure their own propagation, but retaining control over replication. They differ from bacteriophages in having no independent, extracellular form. Most plasmids, whether from gram-negative or gram-positive bacteria, are circular elements, but linear plasmids have been reported in *Streptomyces* spp. and in *Rhodococcus* spp. (Hinnebusch and Tilly 1993).

The term 'episome' has, in the past, been used as a synonym for plasmid. Episomes were defined as genetic elements that could exist and be replicated in either of 2 modes, autonomously or as part of a cointegrate with the bacterial chromosome. As it came to be realized that almost any plasmid can be integrated into the bacterial chromosome, the term lost its usefulness as the definition of a particular class of replicon (Novick et al. 1976). However, the adjective 'episomal' may be useful when applied in particular circumstances, e.g. to describe the state of F in an Hfr strain.

Plasmids are widespread (Stanisich 1988), but the practical importance of bacterial plasmids was first recognized in the early 1960s when transferable drug resistance was discovered (Watanabe 1963). Although plasmids represent only a fraction of the prokaryotic gene pool, they have attracted and continue to attract a disproportionate degree of research interest because the genes they carry determine many of the more interesting features displayed by bacteria, e.g. resistance to antibiotics and heavy metals, virulence, symbiosis and nitrogen fixation, exotic metabolic capacity and many more (Stanisich 1988). They also serve as convenient models, particularly of replication and partition mechanisms.

The extrachromosomal natures of F and of the first R plasmids discovered were deduced from their genetic behaviours. One feature is the tendency for clones in the culture to lose the plasmid, the set of plasmid-determined characters thus being lost simultaneously and irreversibly. The stability of inheritance of plasmids varies from one to another; some are lost very easily, at rates much higher than the rate of mutation, e.g. 1% or more of cell progeny may not have inherited the plasmid, compared with normal mutation frequencies in the range 1 in 10^6–10^8. Others are very stable indeed and are rarely, if ever, lost. Some plasmids can be eliminated from the host artificially (**cured**) by treatment with one of a variety of chemicals (**curing agents**). The quinolone drugs seem to be particularly effective (Weisser and Wiedemann 1985). However, no single curing agent or treatment can be relied upon; finding an appropriate agent or treatment for a specific plasmid is an empirical exercise that may well fail (Caro, Churchward and Chandler 1984). The F plasmid is readily eliminated by treatment with acridine orange (Hirota 1960), but few others succumb to this agent. Some plasmids have temperature-sensitive replication systems and so are eliminated by growth of the cell at the non-permissive temperature (May, Houghton and Perret 1964, Yokota et al. 1969), but this feature is not widespread. It has also been reported that the conversion of some bacteria to protoplasts (spheroplasts), e.g. *B. subtilis* and *S. aureus*, can result in plasmid loss. Again this is not a universal finding. Irreversible loss of a particular character, or set of characters, either spontaneously or after treatment, is still powerful genetic evidence for the existence of a plasmid but the inability to cure a specific feature, for the reasons given above, does not necessarily indicate that the gene(s) responsible is chromosomal.

With the development of methods for isolating plasmid DNA the presence of a plasmid can be determined directly. Modern small-scale preparative procedures (Sambrook, Fritsch and Maniatis 1989) and the use of agarose gel electrophoresis allow plasmids to be detected in very small culture volumes (0.5–1.0 ml of a stationary phase culture). Plasmid DNA can be purified and reintroduced into bacterial cells by transformation (or electroporation) to establish definitively the connection between the phenotype of interest and the plasmid. However, this is still not always possible, particularly with large plasmids (≥100 kb), or when investigating a poorly characterized bacterium, in which case it may be necessary to fall back on classical genetic techniques (conjugation, transduction, curing).

5.1 Plasmid genes

The only genes that are formally necessary to a plasmid are those needed for its replication. The amount of DNA devoted to this task is surprisingly small (Scott 1984, Thomas and Smith 1987) and rarely, if ever, exceeds a few kb. The minimum requirement is an origin sequence, *oriV* (**origin of vegetative replication**), at which replication can start, all enzyme functions being provided by the host. Several small plasmids have this arrangement, e.g. ColEI from *E. coli* and the related plasmid, CloDF13 from *Enterobacter cloacae*. In addition to an *oriV*, such plasmids also encode functions that control the extent of plasmid replication, i.e. ensure that the plasmid copy number per cell is maintained within fairly narrow limits specific to the particular plasmid (Sherratt 1986). In these plasmids no more than 1–2 kb is devoted to plasmid replication and its control. In others more complex arrangements have evolved both to execute replication and to regulate it.

There are basically 2 modes of replication for circular plasmids: θ replication and RC (rolling circle) replication (Helinski, Toukdarian and Novick 1996). In the former, replication proceeds from a fixed origin in a unidirectional or bidirectional manner round the plasmid circle and both strands of the plasmid are replicated simultaneously, in a manner precisely equivalent to chromosome replication. Both strands of the parent plasmid remain intact during the replication process. The type of replication gets its name from the fact that a part replicated plasmid/chromosome would resemble the Greek letter theta, θ, if opened out. For most of the gram-negative plasmids studied this is the mode of replication utilized.

A few plasmids from gram-negative bacteria and the single-stranded coliphages (Baas and Jansz 1988) have been shown to use the alternative, RC replication mode, as does a family of highly related plasmids in gram-positive bacteria (del Solar, Moscoso and Espinosa 1993). These plasmids always encode an initiator protein which introduces a site-specific nick at the DSO (double-strand origin) to generate a 3′-OH group, which serves as a priming terminus. In some cases it has been shown that the initiator is covalently attached to the 5′-phosphate exposed by the cut. Replication proceeds by extension from the 3′-OH primer site, using the complementary strand (designated the plus-strand) as template. The old complementary strand (called the minus-strand) is displaced as replication proceeds. Once replication has travelled right round the circle (hence the designation RC) the minus-strand is circularized. Consequently, one double-stranded DNA molecule and one single-stranded molecule result. The circular single-stranded minus-strand is then converted to a double-stranded molecule using a second origin of replication that is specific to the minus-strand. Replication of plasmids, including linear plasmids, has been reviewed by Helinski, Toukdarian and Novick (1996).

Plasmids range in size from c. 1 kb to >400 kb (equivalent to c. 10% of the *E. coli* chromosome). The smallest have only enough DNA to accommodate 2

or 3 small genes (e.g. Pl5A; Chang and Cohen 1978). Nevertheless, small plasmids are relatively abundant (Fig. 10.10); many confer no obvious phenotype on their host. Such plasmids (large or small) are said to be cryptic, a description that is largely an acknowledgement of ignorance.

Plasmids capable of mediating conjugation have a minimum size of c. 30 kb. Several have now been analysed extensively with respect to the plasmid-encoded information needed for replication. Here again it is found that relatively little genetic content is devoted to replication. In addition to *oriV*, these plasmids encode one or 2 specific proteins necessary for their own replication, together with one or more replication-control functions (Scott 1984, Thomas and Smith 1987). These functions define the essential replicon of the plasmid and can be encoded in 4–5 kb.

The relatively small amount of plasmid-encoded information needed for plasmid replication is a reflection of the fact that most of the replication apparatus is provided by the host. Most of the panoply of functions used to replicate the bacterial chromosome is borrowed to replicate the plasmid. Although not all plasmids have exactly the same requirements, they all use a common core of enzymes, e.g. either all or the bulk of the DNA synthesis is carried out by DNA polymerase III. A number of small plasmids (e.g. ColE1 and related plasmids) require DNA polymerase I (product of the

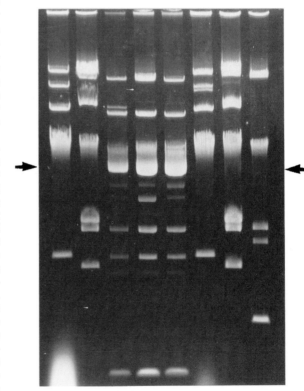

Fig. 10.10 Plasmid profiles from isolates of *E. coli* obtained from slurry waste from a calf-rearing unit. The diffuse band (arrows) in each track represents DNA fragments (chromosome and plasmid) that arose during the course of the preparation. Plasmid size decreases from top to bottom. The smallest plasmids seen in these preparations have sizes of 1–2 kb.

polA gene) in the early stages of replication, before switching to DNA polymerase III for the bulk of the synthesis. Consequently, such plasmids cannot be established in a *polA* mutant strain of *E. coli*. Most plasmids described to date, however, do not show this requirement.

F and many other plasmids maintain themselves at a low **copy number**, i.e. 1–4 copies of the plasmid per bacterial chromosome. These plasmids have been described as being under **stringent replication control**. By contrast, other plasmids, usually small ones such as ColEI, maintain themselves at a relatively high plasmid:chromosome ratio (15–20). Plasmids of this type are said to be subject to **relaxed replication control** because initially it was thought that replication control of these latter elements was less rigorous than for low copy number plasmids. This is now known not to be true; rather, the threshold value at which inhibition of replication operates is set higher. Once activated it is just as efficient.

For each plasmid there is a charactenstic copy number, although this can be altered by mutation. Some plasmids also show changes in copy number in response to the prevailing culture conditions; e.g. some plasmids continue to replicate when the cells enter stationary phase (when chromosomal replication stops) with the accumulation of large numbers of plasmid molecules per cell. Treatment of a culture of *E. coli* carrying ColE1, or a related plasmid, with chloramphenicol (at a concentration sufficient to inhibit protein synthesis) has the same effect; whereas the initiation of new rounds of replication of the bacterial chromosome (and many plasmids) requires *de novo* protein synthesis, that of ColE1 does not.

The genes that control plasmid replication include functions that act repressively, i.e. inhibit replication. One consequence is **plasmid incompatibility**. It was discovered early that 2 variants of the same plasmid cannot be maintained stably in the same bacterial cell, i.e. they are incompatible. This arises because each directs the production of replication inhibitors that act on the other replicon, as well as on themselves. The consequence is that the content of plasmid molecules in the cell is set to a lower level than the sum of the 2 individual copy numbers. If the plasmids involved are unit, or low copy number plasmids, plasmid segregation at cell division is a likely result, i.e. clones emerge in which one or other of the plasmids has not been inherited (Novick 1987). Plasmids with unrelated replication control systems do not, in general, interact in this way and so do not destabilize each other; they are said to be compatible. Plasmids that are incompatible are said to belong to the same **incompatibility (Inc) group**; plasmids that are compatible necessarily belong to different incompatibility groups.

5.2 Plasmid partition systems

To be stably inherited, plasmid DNA not only has to be replicated but also at each cell division both progeny cells must obtain at least one copy of the plasmid (which will be replicated until the appropriate copy number has been achieved). For low copy number plasmids such as F and some common R plasmids (Rl, R100), plasmid distribution at cell division – namely, **plasmid partition –** is an active process involving both plasmid- and host-specified products (Hiraga 1992).

The former are designated *par* functions. The mechanism of partition is still poorly understood. The components comprise a small sequence of a few hundred base pairs, carried on the plasmid, and is believed to function like a primitive centromere to pair plasmids prior to cell division. This sequence, together with one or more proteins that interact with it, and which may be plasmid- or host chromosome-encoded, constitute the partition system. The system may direct plasmid DNA membrane association at or near the point of septum formation. If 2 different plasmids have related partition systems, to the extent that each is unable to distinguish the 2 plasmids, incompatibility will result. This will reinforce any incompatibility between the 2 plasmids that arises as a consequence of 'common' replication systems. However, the replication and partition functions on a plasmid act independently, as can be demonstrated by creating synthetic replicons with the replication system of one plasmid and the partition system of an unrelated plasmid. These hybrids are stably maintained, i.e. they are efficiently replicated and partitioned (Austin and Abeles 1983).

In contrast to the active partition described above, small plasmids with high copy number do not encode specific *par* functions. They rely on the random distribution of units to daughter cells. When the copy number is 15–20, the plasmid content of a cell immediately before cell division will be at least 30–40. Assuming random distribution of plasmids throughout the cell, the probability of one daughter cell inheriting the entire complement of plasmid molecules while the other inherits none is negligible (this would not be true for low copy number plasmids). Nevertheless, and somewhat paradoxically, some small, very high copy number cloning vectors generated in the laboratory are not efficiently inherited, in contrast to the plasmid from which they were derived.

If low copy number plasmids, in particular, are to be partitioned accurately, it is desirable, if not essential in all cases, that the molecules be in the form of monomers. Cells in a natural environment are recombination proficient. Hence they will actively pair and recombine homologous sequences, including plasmid DNA. A single crossover between 2 plasmid molecules will fuse them to form a dimer. If this were to happen with a unit copy number plasmid immediately after it had replicated and no steps were taken to reverse the event, at cell division one daughter cell would inherit both copies of the plasmid. The accumulation of plasmid dimers (and higher multimers) is prevented by plasmid-encoded, site-specific recombination systems (Austin, Ziese and Sternberg 1981, Lane et al. 1986, Dodd and Bennett 1987, Garnier, Saurin and Cole 1987, Krause and Guiney 1991, Eberl et al. 1994, Guhathakurta, Viney and Summers 1996). These are specialized recombination systems that comprise a specific DNA sequence and a recombination enzyme that acts at the sequence (Smith 1988). The site must be part of the plasmid, but the enzyme can be either a plasmid-encoded function or a host function (Sherratt 1986, Dodd and Bennett 1987). These recombination systems rapidly convert plasmid multimers to their momomeric units.

5.3 Post-segregational killing

Some plasmids have a third type of mechanism that acts to maintain their stability. These systems act after segregational loss of the plasmid to kill the plasmidless cell (Jensen and Gerdes 1995, Yarmolinsky 1995). These systems comprise 2 genes; one encodes a toxin, the other an antidote. The toxin is more stable than than the antidote, which means that to neutralize the toxin the antidote must be produced continuously. This is possible so long as the cell carries a copy of the plasmid. However, in those unfortunate progeny that fail to acquire a copy of the plasmid at cell division, the toxin activity is unmasked as the antidote decays and the cell is killed.

A variation on the theme is encoded by the resistance plasmid R1. In this instance the control exerted over the toxin is at the point of production, rather than inhibition of activity. The control locus, *sok*, overlaps the toxin gene, *hok*, which is encoded on the opposite strand of the DNA duplex. Both genes are transcribed, but translation of the *hok* mRNA is prevented as a consequence of the 2 mRNA molecules annealing to one another over the region of overlap, where they are complementary. This prevents ribosome binding. However, the *sok* mRNA decays faster than the *hok* mRNA, so if the R1 plasmid is lost then the *hok* mRNA is translated and the toxin produced causes the collapse of the transmembrane potential and the cell dies (Gerdes, Rasmussen and Molin 1986, Gerdes et al. 1988).

Plasmid replication functions together with **stability functions** (*par* and site-specific recombination functions) comprise the minimum requirements of a stable, low copy number replicon, i.e. one that will be inherited efficiently despite there being very few copies of the plasmid. The whole can be accommodated in a sequence of <10 kb (a stable miniplasmid derived from F, which is 94 kb in size, carries just 9.2 kb of F, in addition to a selectable marker).

5.4 Genes determining conjugation

Conjugation determined by F and by many other plasmids is a complex process requiring many genes. Accordingly, conjugative plasmids cannot be very small. The smallest conjugative plasmids in the Enterobacteriaceae are about 30 kb (of which 15–20 kb are devoted to transfer compared with F which devotes approximately 30 kb to transfer functions) (Avila and de la Cruz 1988, Thomas 1989).

Most natural plasmids that are unable to mediate their own transfer can, nevertheless, be transferred conjugally by co-opting the transfer functions of a conjugative plasmid. Such plasmids, e.g. ColEI, have their own origin of transfer (*oriT*) and encode functions specific to it (**mob genes**) but require a helper plasmid to provide the missing transfer functions; e.g. F can serve as a helper plasmid for ColE1 (Dougan and

Sherratt 1977). Some other plasmids possess only an origin of transfer, and transfer only when the other necessary transfer functions are provided by helper plasmids; e.g. the small plasmid Pl5A has its own *oriT*, but to transfer it requires both Mob and Tra functions provided by ColEI and F (or equivalents), respectively.

5.5 Other plasmid genes

Replication and its control, maintenance and transfer functions may be considered as inherent plasmid characteristics. Together they direct both vertical (inheritance) and horizontal (transfer) transmission in bacterial populations. However, these features alone, no matter how intrinsically interesting, would have been insufficient to attract the degree of interest that bacterial plasmids have engendered. Indeed, until the discovery of **transmissible multiple drug resistance** (Watanabe 1963) the study of plasmids and their activities was a minority interest. The veritable explosion of interest shown since then reflects the variety of other genes carried on plasmids.

Antibiotic resistance determined by plasmids was first discovered in Japan in the late 1950s. Until then it had been assumed that antibiotic resistance in bacteria, which had already become a clinical problem, resulted from the selection of chromosomal mutants, multiple resistance resulting from the sequential accumulation of mutations. Then, unexpectedly, epidemiological analysis of drug resistance in *Shigella flexneri* indicated that resistance could be transmitted between bacteria. Bacillary dysentery was common in Japan after the second world war. By the mid-1950s, most Japanese infections with *S. flexneri* involved bacteria that were resistant to sulphonamides, so antibiotic treatment (now known to be inappropriate) was switched to streptomycin, tetracycline or chloramphenicol (much of it self-prescribed). In due course a few strains resistant to the 4 unrelated drugs were isolated; thereafter such strains became progressively more common (Table 10.2). Isolates resistant to 2 drugs, which one would expect to see if sulphonamide-resistant clones mutated to resistance to another drug, were rare. Instead, in outbreaks of infection with a single *S. flexneri* serotype, strains from some patients had the multiple-resistance pattern, whereas others did not. Furthermore, *E. coli* strains with the same pattern of resistance were found in the faeces of patients with dysentery. Given these observations, Akiba and, independently, Ochiai in 1959 (cited by Watanabe 1963) tested the hypothesis that multiple resistance might be carried by an infective agent analogous to the F factor of *E. coli*. Mixed culture experiments proved this idea correct: multiple drug resistance could be transferred from *S. flexneri* to *E. coli*. The infective agents are now called **resistance (R) plasmids**.

The increasing frequency of drug resistance in *S. flexneri* in Japan was not an isolated phenomenon. The emergence of resistance was recorded in diverse strains world wide: in *Shigella sonnei* in the London area, in *Salmonella* strains in the Netherlands and in *S.* Typhimurium in England (see Datta and Nugent 1983). These cases differed to some extent from the Japanese experience in that there was a stepwise accumulation of resistance, first to sulphonamides and streptomycin, then to tetracycline and subsequently (and infrequently) to chloramphenicol (Anderson 1968). Nevertheless, the resistance was primarily plasmid mediated and transmissible; ampicillin resistance then emerged, and within a decade had

Table 10.2 Multiple drug resistance in *Shigella flexneri* isolated in Japan

Year	No. of isolates tested	Percentage multiresistant
1956	4399	0.02
1958	6563	2.9
1960	497	15
1962	6853	23
1964	5388	45
1966	4292	75
1968	1237	64
1970	562	74
1972	824	76

Multiresistant strains were resistant to chloramphenicol, tetracycline, streptomycin and sulphonamide. Figures from Mitsuhashi (1977).

become common in *Salmonella* and *Shigella* strains throughout Europe (although it remained uncommon in Japan).

At the time of the discovery of R plasmids in the Enterobacteriaceae, multiresistant strains of *S. aureus* were a cause of concern in hospital infection. Penicillinase-producing strains of *S. aureus*, first recognized in the 1940s, had become common and had acquired resistance to new antibiotics as each was introduced into clinical practice. In 1963 it was shown that penicillinase synthesis by *S. aureus* was a plasmid-determined characteristic (Novick 1963), as are many other antibiotic resistances in that species (Lacey 1975). Penicillin-resistance plasmids in *S. aureus* have been studied extensively. They encode not only the penicillinase, but also the means to regulate its production which is induced when the cells are exposed to penicillin and other β-lactam agents. The mechanism involves a form of signal transduction, because the inducers (β-lactams) do not penetrate the cytoplasmic membrane, but the details are poorly understood (Everett, Chopra and Bennett 1990, Bennett and Chopra 1993). These plasmids often also encode resistance to mercury or cadmium salts, or both, and sometimes to erythromycin or fusidic acid. Resistance to tetracycline, chloramphenicol and neomycin is also extrachromosomal in *S. aureus*, but these markers are usually found on separate plasmids.

Not only are many resistance determinants in *S. aureus* encoded by plasmids, but several are also carried on transposons (Murphy 1989). Tn*551*, encoding resistance to erythromycin, was the first to be discovered in *S. aureus* (Novick et al. 1979). More recently, a transposon encoding resistance to gentamicin, kanamycin, tobramycin, trimethoprim, ethidium bromide and quaternary ammonium compounds, designated Tn*4001*, has been reported (Lyon, May and Skurray 1984). This element was found in a multiresistant **MRSA** (methicillin-resistant *S. aureus*; see Chapter 27 and Volume 3, Chapter 14) strain isolated in Melbourne. Strains of this type have been causing concern in several parts of the world because they are resistant to all β-lactam agents and many other antibiotics that might be used against them. The methicil-

lin-resistance gene, *mecA* is part of a 30–40 kb element of unknown origin that integrates into the chromosome of *S. aureus* between the *spa* and *purA* genes. The *mecA* gene encodes a penicillin-binding protein (PBP-2a or PBP-2′, Utsui and Yokota 1985, Reynolds and Fuller 1986) that is not inhibited by β-lactam agents at clinically achievable concentrations and can substitute for the cell's normal PBPs at concentrations of β-lactam agents that would normally be lethal to the cell (Archer and Niemeyer 1994, Berger-Bächi 1994). A drug of last resort is the glycopeptide antibiotic vancomycin. This inhibits peptidoglycan synthesis by binding to the terminal pair of D-Ala residues in the pentapeptide chain of the sugar–peptide cell wall precursor. Resistance to vancomycin has now appeared in the enterococci and the mechanism involves remodelling the pentapeptide precursor. The terminal D-Ala residue of the pentapeptide is changed to D-lactate. The loss of the amino group significantly reduces the affinity for vancomycin. Because the D-lactate is cleaved from the precursor in the terminal stages of peptidoglycan synthesis, as the short peptide chains are joined together, the finished product is largely unaffected, although synthesis is slower. Remarkably, expression of vancomycin resistance can be inducible and the mechanism also involves signal transduction, using what is known as a **2-component regulatory system**. Two genes are involved, *vanS* and *vanR*. The former encodes a membrane protein, VanS, that senses the effect of the drug (Ulijasz, Grenader and Weisblum 1996), records the fact by phosphorylating itself, when it can then phosphorylate the second component, VanR. This converts VanR to an activator specific for expression of the vancomycin resistance genes (Arthur and Courvalin 1993). A similar mechanism is used to regulate expression of virulence genes in *S.* Typhimurium and many other types of virulence gene (see Salyers and Whitt 1994). As if this degree of complexity were not sufficient, the whole system is carried on a bacterial transposon, Tn*1546* (Arthur and Courvalin 1993). Although this form of vancomycin resistance has not yet been detected in clinical strains of MRSA, it is likely to be only a matter of time before it is, because it has been demonstrated in the laboratory that plasmids encoding vancomycin resistance transfer readily between enteroccocal strains and *S. aureus*.

Many new antibacterial drugs have been introduced into clinical medicine in the last 25 years and plasmids conferring resistance to most of them have appeared within a relatively short time. Not only has the range of plasmid-determined resistance broadened but also more and more bacterial genera that carry resistance plasmids are being found (Tables 10.3 and 10.4). The appearance in the mid-1970s of plasmid-determined β-lactamase production, first in *H. influenzae* and then in *N. gonorrhoeae*, was of prime importance, not only to clinical medicine where the strains presented a significant public health problem, but also to the study of plasmid evolution (Saunders, Hart and Saunders 1986; see also Volume 3, Chapter 33) because some of the plasmids in both species were found to be closely

Table 10.3 Some antibacterial drugs to which plasmids determine resistance

Penicillins and cephalosporins	
Erythromycin, lincomycin and streptogramin B	
Streptomycin	Tetracyclines
Neomycin	Chloramphenicol
Kanamycin	Fusidic acid
Gentamicin	Sulphonamides
Tobramycin	Trimethoprim
Amikacin	

related (Laufs et al. 1979). The TEM β-lactamase produced in both these organisms is encoded by a gene, bla_{TEM}, carried on various transposons, among them Tn*1* and Tn*3* (Fig. 10.5), which are predominantly found on plasmids. The production of a TEM β-lactamase by clinical isolates of a wide variety of gram-negative bacteria, particularly among the Enterobacteriaceae, of both human and veterinary origin, is common. Undoubtedly, the presence of this gene on a transposon and its ability to transpose readily to many different plasmids facilitated its rapid intergeneric spread. The route taken by such a resistance determinant, before it enters a particular bacterial species, may be circuitous, but if acquisition is desirable (i.e. of advantage to the survival of the organism), it is almost certainly inevitable. Indeed, reports indicate that transfer of resistance genes is not restricted to gram-positive–gram-positive and gram-negative–gram-negative exchanges but can take place between gram-positive and gram-negative bacteria (Mazodier and Davies 1991) and even between bacteria and mammalian cells (Courvalin, Goussard and Grillot-Courvalin 1995), although such events seem to be rare. Trieu-Cuot and Courvalin (1986) reported a kanamycin-resistance determinant encoding an APH(3')III aminoglycoside phosphotransferase in a strain of *Campylobacter coli* identical to that previously found in streptococcal strains. For an account of antibiotic resistance in clinical practice, see Chapter 9.

Table 10.4 Some genera in which R plasmids have been found

Enterobacteriaceae, i.e. *Escherichia, Salmonella, Shigella, Proteus, Providencia, Klebsiella, Serratia,* etc.	
Pseudomonas	
Acinetobacter	*Staphylococcus*
Vibrio	*Streptococcus*
Yersinia	*Bacillus*
Pasteurella	*Clostridium*
Campylobacter	*Corynebacterium*
Haemophilus	
Neisseria	
Bacteroides	

ORIGIN OF RESISTANCE GENES

The origin of resistance genes has been a puzzle for many years. Before the introduction of antibiotics these genes were rare, although plasmids similar to those now carrying resistance determinants were relatively common (Hughes and Datta 1983). Perhaps the most persistent and logical suggestion is that they originated in the antibiotic-producing organisms themselves, since these organisms, mostly streptomycetes, are sensitive to the antibiotics and so must necessarily protect themselves. This suggestion has been given credence by the finding that the amino acid sequences of several classes of the APH(3') aminoglycoside phosphotransferases, which confer resistance to kanamycin and neomycin, from both gram-positive and gram-negative bacteria, are evolutionarily related to another from the neomycin-producing *Streptomyces fradiae*. An interesting variation on this theme is that in the production of antibiotics small amounts of DNA from the producing organism remain as a contaminant and this may be the source of some resistance genes seen in clinical strains (Webb and Davies 1993). Clearly, if true, this has considerable significance for future antibiotic production, particularly in terms of quality control measures.

Some, if not all, β-lactamases have probably evolved from the same ancestral gene(s) that produced the penicillin–cephalosporin targets, the PBPs. Recent work has clearly shown the evolutionary relationship between the class A β-lactamase of *Bacillus cereus* and a PBP from *Streptomyces* (Samraoui et al. 1986, Joris et al. 1988, 1991). Furthermore, Ghuysen and his colleagues have shown that the protein structures of several β-lactamases and some PBPs are highly conserved, strongly indicating an evolutionary link (Ghuysen 1991, 1994, Frère 1995). The branches from the ancestral gene that yielded present-day β-lactamases, on the one hand, and PBPs, on the other, almost certainly diverged a long time before the discovery of penicillin, let alone its use in clinical medicine. Furthermore, the evolution of β-lactamase genes continues to the present day (Dubois, Marriott and Amyes 1995, Galleni et al. 1995, Bush and Jacoby 1997). Although most clinically significant β-lactamases are plasmid-encoded and constitutively expressed (particularly in gram-negative bacteria), β-lactamases are also relatively common chromosome-encoded enzymes in many types of bacteria, not only those causing disease, and their expression can be elaborately controlled; some species even have multiple, co-ordinately controlled β-lactamases (Hayes, Thomson and Amyes 1994, Paton, Miles and Amyes 1994, Walsh et al. 1995, Yang and Bush 1996). These findings suggest that protection against β-lactam antibiotics is a common and desirable property in nature, although high concentrations of β-lactam agents in the soil, or in other natural habitats, have not been detected. So it is not at all clear from where the selection pressure for the evolution, particularly of the inducible β-lactamases, comes.

An equally intriguing case is that of trimethoprim.

This is a purely synthetic compound that has no known natural analogue. Its mode of action is to inhibit dihydrofolate reductase, which catalyses one of the steps in folic acid synthesis (see Chapter 9). The enzymes in many bacteria are quite sensitive to this antibiotic. Resistance to trimethoprim, e.g. as encoded by Tn7 (Craig 1989), arises because of the acquisition of a gene encoding a dihydrofolate reductase that is much less sensitive to trimethoprim. The source of the gene is unknown. It may be one that naturally encodes a resistant enzyme; alternatively, it may be a mutant form of a naturally sensitive one. Several trimethoprim-resistance alleles, each encoding a dihydrofolate reductase, are now known (Amyes 1986, Amyes and Towner 1990). The speed with which resistance emerged, approximately 10 years after the introduction of the drug into clinical practice, is impressive and gives considerable cause for thought, because on an evolutionary time scale 10 years is but a blink.

The case of trimethoprim is not an isolated example. The emergence of resistance somewhere in the bacterial kingdom, following widespread use of a new antibiotic, and its subsequent dissemination among many bacterial species appears to be the norm rather than the exception, attesting to highly efficient gene transfer processes within populations of bacterial cells (Bennett, 1995). The frequency of transfer does not need to be high to achieve efficient spread of a particular gene. Even rare transfer events can be effective if the environmental conditions impose a strong selection pressure on those few progeny cells that do acquire the gene in question, which they do because antibiotics either inhibit the growth of, or kill, sensitive cells. These few resistant cells will then rapidly reproduce, whereas the majority of their bacterial relatives are unable to do so, to become the dominant bacterial species. There is no reason to believe that the extensive interspecific gene transfer highlighted by resistance genes is confined to them. Rather, the view that perhaps all bacterial genes are potentially available to all bacteria is gaining more general acceptance.

RESISTANCE GENE CREATION BY MUTATION

Resistance to an antibiotic may be the result of acquiring new genetic information in the form of a plasmid or transposon, or it may be due to a mutation in the gene for the antibiotic target that renders it less susceptible to the drug. This form of resistance is often readily selected in the laboratory; however, it is much less common in clinical experience, probably due to the success of plasmid–transposon systems. Nevertheless, there is one instance where acquisition of resistance by mutation is clinically significant and that is in *Mycobacterium tuberculosis* in which plasmids have little or no role to play (Cole and Telenti 1995).

ANTIBIOTIC SYNTHESIS

Plasmids determine the production of **bacteriocins** and **microcins** (Pugsley and Oudega 1987; see also Chapter 8). They also play a part in the production of a variety of antibiotics, including some of those used in medicine (Hopwood 1978, Chater and Hopwood 1989). Plasmid SCP1, in *Streptomyces coelicolor* determines production of the antibiotic methylenomycin. The same plasmid confers resistance to the antibiotic. Plasmids can carry structural or control genes determining production by *Streptomyces* of oxytetracycline, chloramphenicol and perhaps other antibiotics. The genetics of antibiotic-producing microorganisms is of great interest and of enormous potential importance in the pharmaceutical industry, and rapid progress is now being made in this area (see, for example, McDaniel et al. 1995).

RESISTANCE TO OTHER AGENTS

Plasmids may also confer resistance to antibacterial compounds other than clinically useful antibiotics, such as a variety of metal ions and organometallic compounds. Plasmid-determined resistance to mercuric ions (Hg^{2+}) is very common in bacteria found in soil and water (Bale, Fry and Day 1987) such as *Pseudomonas* spp., in members of the Enterobacteriaceae and in *Staphylococcus* spp.; this is frequently linked to antibiotic resistance. In different surveys, 25–60% of R plasmids determined Hg^{2+} resistance. In general, high frequencies of antibiotic resistance are found in environments where antibiotic concentrations are high, e.g. hospitals and farms on which livestock are reared intensively. The apparent linkage of Hg^{2+} resistance stems, in part at least, from the finding that a family of large transposable elements encoding clinically significant antibiotic resistance appears to have evolved from an ancestral element that encoded Hg^{2+} resistance. These transposable sequences seem now to be widespread, particularly among the Enterobacteriaceae (Grinsted, de la Cruz and Schmitt 1990). Mercury resistance linked to antibiotic resistance may also be perpetuated by the use of dental amalgams that incorporate mercury (Summers et al. 1993).

Mercury resistance is effected by reducing ionic mercury to the pure metal and releasing it in gaseous form (volatilization). The mechanism also involves active concentration of mercuric ions prior to reduction. The complexity of the system suggests one of some antiquity rather than one of recent evolution.

Resistance to cadmium, lead, antimony, arsenic, tellurium and silver compounds are plasmid-determined in staphylococci and gram-negative bacteria (Summers and Jacoby 1977, Summers and Silver 1978, Foster 1983, Silver and Phung 1996). Resistance to silver salts was first reported after the use in burns units of silver sulphonamide compounds (McHugh et al. 1975). Resistance to copper salts in bacteria isolated on pig farms where copper is used as a feed additive has also been reported (Tetaz and Luke 1983, Brown et al. 1995). In these cases, the immediate selective conditions are obvious; however, when and where the resistance mechanisms evolved is another question.

Plasmids may also change the sensitivity of their bacterial host to UV light and other mutagens (Mortelmans and Stocker 1976) and to bacteriocins (Pugsley and Oudega 1987).

The degradation of several toxic organic compounds, such as camphor, naphthalene, octane and toluene, may be determined by plasmids, particularly in soil bacteria. These bacteria, often *Pseudomonas* or *Flavobacterium* spp., have evolved the ability to use these toxic compounds as nutrients. The use of these and similar bacteria to effect biological detoxification and reverse environmental pollution has been attempted, with some success, but this area of bacterial exploitation is still very much in its infancy (Shannon and Unterman 1993, Janssen et al. 1994, Spain 1995).

Virulence factors

Virulence determinants are genes, the expression of which is necessary for bacteria to establish and maintain an infection (see Chapter 12 and Roth 1988, Dorman 1994, Salyers and Whitt 1994). They include colonization mechanisms, mechanisms to overcome host defence systems and the production of toxins. All these functions may be encoded by plasmids (Brubaker 1985). For example, enterotoxin production in *E. coli* and *S. aureus* (Betley, Miller and Mekalonos 1986) and production of surface antigens by *E. coli* that allow colonization of the small intestine in specific mammals, including humans, can both be plasmid-determined (Brubaker 1985). At least one enterotoxin gene found in *E. coli* has been found on a transposon (Tn*1681*) (So and McCarthy 1980).

Strains of *E. coli* isolated from systemic infections in humans and pigs are more frequently haemolytic and more frequently produce colicin V than comparable faecal strains and both characteristics are plasmid-determined. Carriage of a ColV plasmid increases the virulence of *E. coli* strains for calves, chickens and mice (Smith and Huggins 1976); however, the effect is not due to the colicin itself, but to other determinants encoded by the plasmid. The ColV plasmid encodes functions that facilitate the uptake of iron by the bacterial host (Williams 1979) and others that increase bacterial resistance to serum (Binns, Davies and Hardy 1979). Plasmids other than ColV also confer serum resistance on *E. coli* (Taylor 1983). In one instance this seems to involve the acquisition of an additional outer-membrane protein, which is a component of the plasmid transfer system (Moll, Manning and Timmis 1980). A plasmid that confers serum resistance on *Salmonella* Dublin has also been described (Terakado, Hamaoka and Danbara 1988, Foster and Spector 1995).

The smooth to rough (S→R) variation in *S. sonnei* is accompanied by loss of the form I (S) antigen and loss of virulence. Kopecko, Washington and Formal (1980) demonstrated that this conversion is determined by a large plasmid, loss of which results in the S→R change. Transfer of the plasmid to *S. flexneri* 2a or *Salmonella* Typhi generated derivatives that were agglutinable both by their own specific antisera and by antiserum specific to *S. sonnei* form I antigen. In *S. sonnei* the form I antigen, and hence the plasmid that encodes it, is one of the requirements for virulence (Chapter 12), as demonstrated in the Serény test.

Strains of *S. aureus* responsible for scalded-skin syndrome produce exfoliating toxins that, in some cases, are encoded by plasmids (Wiley and Rogolsky 1977). Some *Staphylococcus* spp. produce enterotoxins that cause the syndrome known as intoxicating staphylococcal food poisoning. Some of the toxin genes responsible for this syndrome are encoded by plasmids (Couch, Soltis and Betley 1988). Other examples of pathogenic properties determined by or associated with plasmids have been described and reviewed elsewhere (Elwell and Shipley 1980, Brubaker 1985) (see also Chapter 12, Dorman 1994, Salyers and Whitt 1994).

The role of R plasmids as possible virulence factors has been discussed by Elwell and Shipley (1980). Resistant bacteria, such as chloramphenicol-resistant *S.* Typhi, penicillin-resistant *N. gonorrhoeae* or multiresistant *S. aureus* may sometimes appear to be of unusual virulence simply because the infections they cause do not respond to the first line of antibacterial therapy. This property certainly may facilitate dissemination, but does not necessarily imply increased virulence. Particular R plasmids may well have specific effects upon virulence, either increasing or decreasing it, depending on how expression of plasmid-encoded functions affects other virulence determinants. Indeed, Lacey and Kruczenyk (1986) have argued that the plasmid-carrying MRSA, although posing an undeniable clinical problem, are not as virulent as their predecessors. However, generalizations in this area without rigorous experimental evidence are inappropriate.

In plants, *Agrobacterium tumefaciens* has long been known as the causative agent of crown gall, a tumorous disease that affects many plants and causes serious losses in fruit growing. The transformation to a tumour-like growth requires transfer from the bacterium to the plant cell of genetic information, part of which is incorporated permanently into the genome of the plant cell. The requisite information is encoded on large tumour-inducing (Ti) plasmids which mediate the transfer. This process is an elegant example of natural genetic engineering since the transformed plant cells produce compounds that can be used as nutrients by the *Agrobacterium* responsible for the transformation (Hooykaas 1989, Hooykaas and Beijersbergen 1994).

Metabolic characters

The metabolic diversity of the pseudomonads is due, in part, to the carriage of plasmids that specify degradation of unusual, often toxic, organic compounds, as already noted (see Harayama and Timmis 1989). 'Metabolic' plasmids have also been reported in other genera. When they are present in clinical isolates, such plasmids can initially complicate strain identification in the diagnostic laboratory. Lactose fermentation by strains of *Salmonella* (including Typhi) is usually plasmid-determined. Plasmids encoding lactose catabolism have also been found in isolates of *Proteus* and *Yersinia enterocolitica* (Falkow et al. 1964, Cornelis, Bennett and Grinsted 1976) and appear to be relatively common in *Klebsiella* (Reeve and Braithwaite 1973), although in *Klebsiella* they are not prominent because the chromosome has a *lac* operon. In the study involving *Y. enterocolitica*, the particular genes were not only carried on a plasmid but were also transposable (Cornelis, Ghosal and Saedler 1978).

Genes for the utilization of other sugars, especially sucrose (*suc*) and raffinose (*raf*) may be plasmid-borne. Plasmids with both *lac* and *suc* genes have been found in *Salmonella* (Johnson et al. 1976), and *raf* genes are associated with those determining the K88 antigen adhesion factor which has been shown to be important in porcine *E. coli* enteritis (Shipley, Gyles and Falkow 1978; see also Chapter 12). Plasmids determining H_2S production (Ørskov and Ørskov 1973), urease production (Farmer et al. 1977,

Wachsmuth, Davis and Allen 1979) or citrate utilization (Smith, Parsell and Green 1978) have also been found in clinical isolates. Their preponderance is difficult to assess from phenotypic observation. However, modern molecular genetic techniques such as DNA probing, or possibly PCR analysis, could supply an answer, if needed. Such plasmids are not restricted to clinically important bacteria. Lac plasmids in *Lactobacillus lactis* cheese starter strains are of major importance to the dairy industry (Farrow 1980; see also Chapter 16).

PHAGE INHIBITION

Carriage of certain plasmids can alter the susceptibility of the host to certain bacteriophages, thus changing the phage type of that particular isolate, which may be important in diagnostic and epidemiological investigations. Usually the molecular basis for the change is unknown; however, some plasmids encode one of a class of DNA-degrading enzymes known as **restriction endonucleases** that fragment foreign DNA as it enters the bacterial cell. Such plasmids also encode the means to protect the host cell DNA, including the plasmid itself, from similar attack. This usually involves methylation of particular bases within specific short sequences which are also the sites recognized by the restriction endonuclease (Old and Primrose 1989).

5.6 Mapping of plasmids

Because plasmids are small, relative to bacterial chromosomes, they are popular molecules with which to investigate numerous aspects of DNA metabolism, including replication mechanisms (Scott 1984), recombination (Dressler and Potter 1982, Hsu and Landy 1984) and gene expression (Old and Primrose 1989). This interest has led to the development of an impressive range of techniques designed to study DNA in general and plasmid DNA in particular (see Grinsted and Bennett 1988, Sambrook, Fritsch and Maniatis 1989). Electron microscopy has been employed extensively to analyse DNA molecules, both as a simple tool to estimate plasmid size and, by means of **heteroduplex analysis** (Burkardt and Puhler 1988), to examine DNA rearrangements such as insertions, deletions and inversions. Electron microscopy has, however, been largely replaced by **restriction enzyme analysis** and **DNA sequencing**. In the former technique DNA molecules are cut at selective sites (**restriction sites**) by one or more restriction endonucleases. Each enzyme recognizes a specific nucleotide sequence and cleaves the DNA only at that sequence to generate a specific and reproducible pattern of fragments from a particular DNA molecule. By a judicious choice of enzyme combinations the relative positions of the restriction sites on the DNA molecule can be deduced to construct a restriction map of the plasmid (Fig. 10.11). By a similar analysis of derivatives of the plasmid that have lost a particular function(s), because of deletion (natural or generated in vitro) or transposon insertion, and comparison of these maps with that of the parent plasmid, coincident physical and genetic maps can be constructed. Once genes of interest have been located on the plasmid, they can be cut out and inserted into another DNA replicon (cloned) that is more suitable for further investigations, such as DNA sequencing and gene transcription analysis (Grinsted and Bennett 1988, Old and Primrose 1989, Brown 1995). This technology has now evolved to the point where DNA sequencing of very large DNA molecules (e.g. human chromosomes) has been undertaken. The complete sequences of several bacterial chromosomes (e.g. *E. coli, H. influenzae, Mycobacterium genitalium* and *Methanococcus jannaschii*) are now available. The techniques of gene cloning and DNA sequencing bring mapping to the ultimate point of accuracy. Furthermore, by means of mutagenesis in vitro, genes can be systematically altered by the introduction into the DNA sequence of quite specific base changes (Brown 1995, Old and Primrose 1989). These mutations can then be analysed for their effects in the same way as if they had occurred naturally.

5.7 Evolution and classification of plasmids

Plasmids are found in most, perhaps all, bacterial genera. Their origins are a matter for speculation. Each bacterial genus or group of genera appears to have its set of plasmids. Host specificities of plasmids have not been much studied, with one or 2 notable exceptions such as RK2 (RP4) (Thomas and Smith 1987) and RSF1010 (Barth, Tobin and Sharpe 1981, Buchanan-Wollaston, Passiator and Cannon 1987). In general, plasmids resident in gram-positive bacteria appear not to be able to establish themselves in gram-negative bacteria and vice versa. However, R plasmids of *S. aureus* can replicate in *B. subtilis* (Ehrlich 1977) and some R plasmids in *E. faecalis* can transfer by conjugation to *S. aureus* (Engel, Soedirman and Rost 1980) and to lactobacilli (Gibson et al. 1979). Plasmids found in the Enterobacteriaceae can usually be transferred between many, if not all, the genera. Some transfer more widely.

In classifying plasmids, host range might be expected to be an important criterion but in practice it is not a very convenient one. When a newly discovered plasmid is not transferred to a new host in laboratory experiments it may be for any one of a variety of reasons, of which an inability to replicate in the new host is one. In practice, a much more convenient criterion is available. As stated above, it was discovered relatively early that certain pairs of plasmids cannot coexist stably in the same bacterial cell, a phenomenon termed **incompatibility** (see p. 253) (Novick and Richmond 1965), which is expressed when 2 plasmids have the same, or very closely related, replication systems or partition systems, or both (Novick 1987). A strong incompatibility reaction generally indicates similarity in the former.

Replication systems and partition systems are not mutually dependent, and perfectly stable replicons having the replication system of one plasmid and the partition system of another can be constructed in the laboratory. In nature, however, it is likely that a particular replication system and a particular partition system will be found in association.

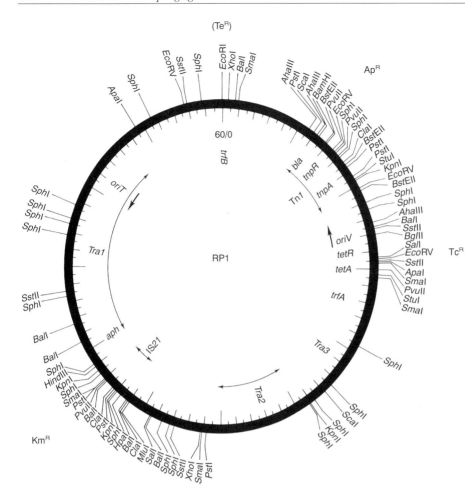

Fig. 10.11 Restriction and genetic maps of RP1. Plasmid RP1 is a 60 kb IncP conjugative resistance plasmid conferring resistance to ampicillin (Ap), kanamycin (Km) and tetracycline (Tc) that was isolated from a strain of *P. aeruginosa*. Genetic loci: *aph*, aminoglycoside phosphotransferase (resistance to kanamycin and neomycin); *bla*, TEM-2 β-lactamase (resistance to β-lactams including ampicillin and carbenicillin); *tet*, tetracycline resistance genes; *oriT*, origin of conjugative transfer; *Tra*, genes required for conjugative transfer; *oriV*, origin of replication; *trf*, plasmid replication genes; *tnp*, transposition genes of Tn*1* (Fig. 10.5). Te[R] indicates the position of a cryptic gene that confers resistance to tellurite when active. The scale indicates plasmid co-ordinates in kb. The map is redrawn, with permission, from that of Thomas and Smith (1987).

When each plasmid in a collection is tested, in turn, against all others in the set, those which are incompatible can be identified and so the collection can be ordered into **incompatibility (Inc) groups**. This means of classification has been applied to plasmids in the Enterobacteriaceae, particularly *E. coli* (Jacob et al. 1977), in *Pseudomonas* spp. (Jacoby 1977) and in *S. aureus* (Novick et al. 1977). Plasmids that can replicate in both *E. coli* and *Pseudomonas* spp. are included in both classifications (Hedges and Jacoby 1980), e.g. RP4 is IncP when in the Enterobacteriaceae but IncPI when in *Pseudomonas* spp.

Because it principally reflects the primary plasmid maintenance systems (replication and partition), incompatibility is a sound basis for grouping plasmids, and there is good evidence that it reflects evolutionary relationships. Within any one Inc group, plasmids, in general, show extensive DNA homology, i.e. common sequences are not restricted simply to replication and partition functions. By contrast, plasmids of different Inc groups rarely show extensive homology (Table 10.5). Exceptions are plasmids of the IncF complex, which can be grouped into at least 5 Inc groups but which nevertheless display extensive homology because their transfer systems are closely related.

Plasmids that belong to the same incompatibility group in general encode the same or similar sex pili. By contrast, plasmids belonging to different Inc groups are more likely to encode sex pili that differ morphologically and serologically (Table 10.6). Sex pili can act as receptors for bacteriophages. One practical consequence of this is that pili can often be detected as the consequence of specific bacteriophage adsorption (Fig. 10.12). However, because of the normally repressed nature of a number of plasmid transfer systems it may be necessary transiently to derepress a specific system before its identity can be established by the use of specific bacteriophages (Willetts 1988). In electron microscopy studies of their morphology and serology, Bradley (1980b) identified pili determined by conjugative plasmids of many known Inc groups of *E. coli* and several of *P. aeruginosa* (Table 10.6). His work shows that, with very few exceptions, all conjugative plasmids within an incompatibility group determine the same type of pilus, a finding consistent with conclusions from DNA homology studies.

The converse is not true. A collection of plasmids, all of which determine related pili (as determined serologically), will not necessarily be incompatible one with the other; e.g. the fi[+] R plasmids that were first identified in Japan have F-like pili yet are compatible with F. For historical reasons, the incompatibility group that includes F is called IncFI; many R plasmids, including Rl, R6 and R100 (alternatively, NRI), which have been studied intensively in several laboratories, are classified as IncFII. Other plasmids with F-like pili have been placed in other incompatibility groups such as IncFIII, IncFIV, etc. These groups are often referred to as the F incompatibility complex. A number of groups outside the F complex have thick flexible pili morphologically similar but serologically unrelated to those of F (Bradley 1980b, 1981).

Rigid pili of various serological types are determined by plasmids of several incompatibility groups. Such plasmids generally are poorly transferred, if at all, in liquid culture, but transfer efficiently on solid surfaces such as agar or membrane filters (Willetts 1988). Rigid pili are, in all examples studied, produced constitutively; by contrast, the production

Table 10.5 Incompatibility grouping of plasmids related to their molecular sizes and DNA homologies

Unlabelled DNA of:			Percentage hybridization with ^{3}H-labelled DNA of:								
Plasmid	Inc gp	Size (kb)	R1	R144	R724	TP114	N3	RP4	S-a	R27	TP116
F	FI	166	43	...	...	...	...	...	...	...	...
R1	FII	104	100	6	...	...	6	9	14	5	1
CoIb-P9	I_1	104	...	...	...	2	...	...	...	...	...
R144	I_1	100	...	100	28	...	5	<1	2	0	3
R64	I_1	115	...	78	...	6	...	...	...	...	...
R621a	I_2	103	...	...	...	40	...	...	...	...	...
R724	B	93	...	...	100	...	...	...	...	...	...
TP113	B	91	...	...	96	3	...	...	...	2	4
TP114	I_2	66	...	...	...	100	...	...	...	0	1
N3	N	51	8	2	...	...	100	1	10	2	5
R15	N	64	...	...	...	...	75	...	...	...	...
RP4	P	54	...	3	...	...	4	100	3	...	...
R702	P	74	...	...	...	...	...	80	...	...	...
S-a	W	40	4	5	...	...	8	4	100	...	...
R388	W	34	...	...	...	...	...	...	79	...	...
R27	H	180	...	...	...	1	...	...	...	100	3
TP124	H	192	...	...	...	...	...	...	...	97	2
TP116	H	230	...	...	...	...	...	...	...	2	100

The figures are adapted from Grindley et al. (1973) and Falkow et al. (1974). Three dots indicates experiment not done. In general, plasmids within a group have similar molecular weights. There is a high degree of homology between plasmids within a group (i.e. incompatible plasmids), a significant degree between compatible plasmids whose conjunctive pili are antigenically related (see Table 10.6), and little between other pairs of plasmids. An exception is among plasmids of IncH: these are incompatible with one another, have antigenically related pili and high molecular weights but by DNA hybridization tests fall into 2 distinct groups, designated H1 and H2 (Smith et al. 1973).

of flexible conjugative pili, thick or thin, is frequently repressed under normal growth conditions (Firth, Ippen-Ihler and Skurray 1996).

Plasmids of the same incompatibility group often share a similar host range, show considerable DNA homology, are of similar molecular sizes and, with conjugative plasmids, possess related transfer systems. By contrast, other plasmid-encoded properties, in particular antibiotic resistance, are not indicative of a particular incompatibility group. Most antibiotic resistance genes, which can be identified either as DNA sequences or as their protein products, are found on a wide variety of otherwise unrelated plasmids. It seems that present-day plasmids have evolved and continue to evolve by the accretion of DNA sequences of transient or lasting value to bacterial cells. These sequences are often components of bacterial transposons and integrons (Wiedemann, Meyer and Zuhlsdorf 1986, Hall and Collis 1995; see also Levy and Novick 1986, Berg and Howe 1989).

It is often stated that R plasmids consist of a resistance transfer factor (RTF) (a conjugative plasmid component) linked to a resistance determinant (r-det). The reason is historical (see Novick 1969, Helinski 1973) because the earliest studies of R plasmids involved members of one incompatibility group, IncFII, which display precisely this form. In the light of more diverse studies it can be seen that the description is specific rather than general and many R plasmids have structures that do not conform to this simple compartmentalized scheme, e.g. RP1 (Fig. 10.11) (Gorai et al. 1979, Villarroel et al. 1983, Thomas 1989).

6 BACTERIAL VARIATION AND EPIDEMIOLOGY

In epidemiological studies the aim is to identify a particular clone within a bacterial species in order to trace its spread and, if possible, to determine its origin. Biochemical and serological characters, phage sensitivities and lysogeny, production of or sensitivity to bacteriocins, sensitivity or resistance to antibiotics and other antibacterial agents, and plasmid profiles may all be exploited to this end. These characters are usually sufficiently stable to be useful when tracing a bacterial strain, but it should be remembered that none of them is immutable and several are encoded by extrachromosomal elements which may be lost over a period of time. Furthermore, new characters can be acquired by acquisition of a plasmid or a transposon. In epidemiological studies, therefore, as many characters of the strain under study as possible should be used in its identification. The isolation of variants indicates either genetic change in an epidemic strain or the discovery of a different strain of the same species. It is not always possible to distinguish between these alternatives (Seal et al. 1981), but the more characters used to identify the strain, the greater the chance that these alternatives can be distinguished.

7 GENETIC MANIPULATION IN VITRO

Molecular genetics, especially **recombinant DNA** technology (or genetic engineering), provides powerful tools with which to analyse any genetic system. These techniques make it possible, in principle, to isolate any gene from any cell type and manipulate it so that it can be expressed in a bacterial cell such as *E. coli* and then return it, perhaps in a modified form, to the cell line of origin.

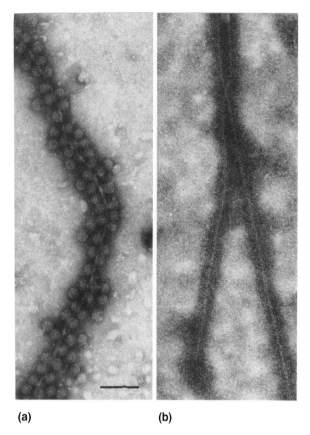

(a)   **(b)**

Fig. 10.12 Conjugative pili labelled with phage or antibody. (a) F pilus labelled with particles of phage R17. (Reproduced with permission from Bradley 1977). (b) D pilus labelled with specific antiserum (D E Bradley, unpublished). Bar = 100 μm.

The bacterial chromosomes of *E. coli* and similar bacteria contain almost 5×10^6 bp. In a human cell the DNA is packed into 46 chromosomes, each containing about 3000×10^6 bp. The problem is, therefore, how one gene a few thousand bp in length can be recovered from such a mass of DNA. Until the mid-1970s such a feat was not possible. This situation was changed by the discovery of the class of DNA endonucleases (type II restriction enzymes, Old and Primrose 1989) that cleave double-stranded DNA at specific nucleotide sequences, cutting it into much smaller linear pieces that can then be recovered and identified. The target sites for these enzymes normally comprise 4, 5 or 6 bp of specific sequence and are usually rotationally symmetrical, often termed palindromic because the sequence of the site read in the 5′ to 3′ direction on one strand is the same as that read in the 5′ to 3′ direction on the opposite strand (Fig. 10.13). There are 2 ways in which these enzymes cut double-stranded DNA. Some cut at positions on the DNA strands opposite each other, giving 'blunt' or flush ends. Others give a staggered cut, producing short single-stranded extensions (Fig. 10.13) that, because they are generated from palindromic sites, are the same. Fragments generated by type II restriction enzymes (restriction fragments) can be joined

together in vitro by DNA ligase. Ligation of fragments with single-stranded extensions generated by the same restriction enzyme proceeds more efficiently than ligation of fragments with flush ends because the complementary nature of single-strand extensions, sometimes called 'sticky ends', encourages fragments to align end to end, so facilitating the ligation reaction. The most commonly used ligase commercially available is that encoded by phage T4. After manipulation in the test tube, desired recombinant DNA molecules are recovered by transformation of a suitable bacterial host. The formation of novel hybrid DNA molecules in vitro, coupled with their recovery and amplification in bacteria, is termed cloning (for a more detailed exposition, see Old and Primrose 1989, Brown 1995).

7.1   Gene cloning

To be perpetuated, cloned genes must become part of a DNA molecule that is replicated in each division cycle. There are 2 convenient types of genome that can be used for cloning – plasmids and bacteriophages. The latter will be discussed later (see p. 284).

In bacterial genetics the most commonly used **plasmid cloning vectors** are small, multicopy plasmids. Many are derivatives of 2 early vectors, pBR322 and pACYC184 (see, for example, Thompson 1988), constructed in the laboratory from small natural plasmids, pMBI and pl5, respectively. They have been manipulated to possess several desirable features not present on the original elements, such as a choice of suitable cloning sites (preferably associated with insertional inactivation) and a convenient and reliable marker for selection (usually a drug resistance gene); for example, one of the first cloning vectors, pBR322, has approximately 4200 bp and single sites for a number of restriction enzymes, including *Bam*HI, *Hin*dIII, *Pst*I and *Sal*I. The single *Pst*I site is within the ampicillin resistance gene which encodes a β-lactamase. Cloning into this site results in loss of the ability to confer resistance to several β-lactam antibiotics, including ampicillin, i.e. cloning into this site causes **insertional inactivation** of the Amp resistance determinant. Hence, clones containing recombinant plasmids are recognized because they acquire resistance to tetracycline but not to ampicillin. Similarly, cloning into the single *Bam*HI, *Hin*dIII or *Sal*I sites creates hybrid plasmids that confer resistance to ampicillin but not to tetracycline. Foreign DNA is inserted into the plasmid vector by linearizing the circular plasmid molecule with a particular restriction enzyme. The DNA fragment to be cloned – usually generated by the same restriction enzyme used to cut the cloning vector – is joined (ligated) at both ends to the linearized vector to form a circular molecule. The hybrid DNA is then introduced into a suitable bacterial cell by transformation. The desired recombinant clones then have to be identified. This may be done by selection if the gene of interest confers a selectable phenotype; otherwise, a set of recombinants called a gene bank is collected and the individual members of the set are screened to identify those with the relevant gene.

Table 10.6 Incompatibility groups of plasmids in Enterobacteriaceae

| Plasmid incompatibility (Inc) group[a] | Conjugative pili | | Receptors for phages[c] | | Expression repressed (R) or constitutive (C)[d] | Mating type[e] |
	Morphology	Serological specificity[b]	pilus sides	pilus tips		
B	Thin flexible	I_1	...	...	C or R	Universal
C	Thick flexible	C	C-1	...	C or R	Surface preferred
D	Thick flexible	D	...	fd	C	Surface preferred
FI	Thick flexible	F	R17	fd	C or R	Universal
FII	Thick flexible	F	R17	fd	R	Universal
H	Thick flexible	H	...	...	R	Universal
I_1	Thin flexible	I_1	...	Ifl	R	Universal
I_2	Thin flexible	I_1	...	Ifl	R	Universal
$I\gamma$	Thin flexible	$I\alpha$	...	Ifl	R	Universal
J	Thick flexible	C	C-1	...	R	Universal
K	Thin flexible	$I\alpha$	...	...	R	Universal
M	Rigid	M	...	X	C	Surface obligatory
N	Rigid	N	...	Ike, PP4	C	Surface obligatory
P	Rigid	P	PRR1	PR4, X	C	Surface obligatory
T	Thick flexible	T	t	...	C	Surface preferred
U	Rigid	U	...	X	C	Surface obligatory
V	Thick flexible	nd	...	...	R	Universal
W	Rigid	W	...	PR4, X	C	Surface obligatory
X	Thick flexible	X	...	X	C	Surface preferred

The table indicates the pilus for plasmids within each incompatibility group and summarizes work by Bradley and his colleagues (Bradley 1980a, 1980b, Bradley, Taylor and Cohen 1980, Bradley et al, 1981a, 1981b). Although generally plasmids within an incompatibility group determine pili of uniform type, an exception has been reported, a plasmid of IncM determining F pili (Taylor, Levine and Bradley, 1981).

[a] Incompatibility grouping (Novick et al, 1976). I_1 is synonymous with $I\alpha$, and I_2 with $I\delta$. IncFIII, FIV, FVI are similar to FI and FII in their pilus type. Plasmid Folac (not listed) determines pili antigenically unrelated to F pili that act as receptors to phage fd.

[b] Serological specificity: antibody adsorbed to pili seen by electron microscopy. Antiserum of each specificity, prepared by immunizing rabbits with appropriate pili, showed no reaction with heterologous pili except where listed. The only unexpected cross-reaction (not shown) was with pili of plasmid R805a that reacted with anti-I, and anti-I_2 (Bradley 1980a).

[c] Examples are given for phages that attach to conjugative pilus; e.g. numerous F-pilus specific phages have been described, but only 2 are listed here. It can be seen that phages that attach to the sides of pili reflect the serological type, but attachment to the tips tends to be less specific.

[d] Pilus synthesis listed as constitutive when large numbers of pili were seen in pure cultures by electron microscopy and repressed when none, or very few, was seen in pure cultures but only in 'high-frequency transfer' mixtures of donor and recipient strains (see text).

[e] Mating type was designated universal when frequencies of transfer were similar in broth and on solid medium, surface preferred when frequencies were 50–500 times higher on surfaces and surface obligatory when they were >2000 times higher on surfaces. Rigid pili are associated with obligatory surface mating.

... not determined.

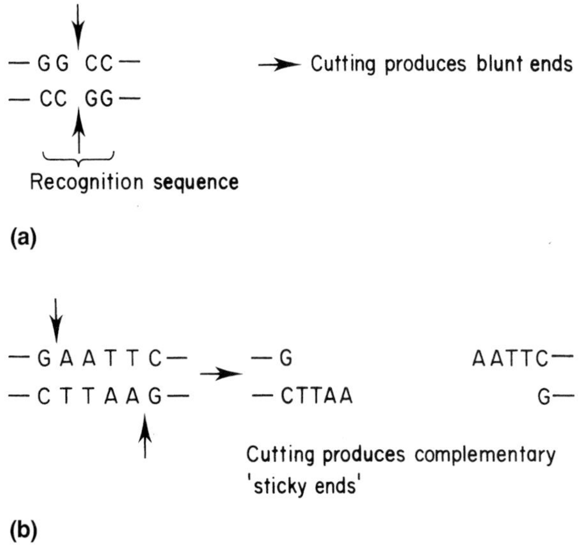

```
        ↓
  — G G  C C —              ──→  Cutting produces blunt ends
  — C C  G G —
         ↑
    ‿‿‿‿‿‿‿
  Recognition sequence
```

(a)

```
        ↓
  — G A A T T C —      — G            A A T T C —
  — C T T A A G —  ──→  — C T T A A            G —
          ↑
              Cutting produces complementary
              'sticky ends'
```

(b)

Fig. 10.13 Type II restriction enzymes. (a) *Hae*III from *Haemophilus aegyptius*. (b) *Eco*RI from *E. coli* RY13.

Eukaryotic genes are not transcribed in bacteria from their own promoters because these promoters are not recognized by bacterial RNA polymerases. Hence, to express a eukaryotic gene in a bacterial cell it is necessary to join the gene to a suitable bacterial promoter sequence. A number of cloning vectors with cloning sites close to and downstream from active promoters are now available for this purpose (see Thompson 1988).

A fundamental problem that arises when genes are cloned on a fragment generated by a restriction endonuclease is that what is recovered is not only the gene(s) of interest, but also unwanted sequences that flank it. It is often desirable that these unwanted sequences are removed prior to analysis. This can be achieved by **subcloning**, i.e. the fragment recovered in the primary cloning is cut into smaller pieces by a different restriction enzyme and these, in turn, are recovered in the same or in a different cloning vector. The desired transconjugant is again detected by screening. If the fragment is still considered to be too large, the reducing process is repeated with another restriction enzyme until the smallest fragment that still encodes the intact gene(s) is recovered. An alternative approach that bypasses the problem completely, and which is suitable for small peptides, is to synthesize the gene chemically and then insert it into a suitable cloning vector. This was first achieved with the gene for somatostatin – a pituitary hormone of 14 amino acids, the sequence of which was known. The genes for human growth hormone, thymosin and insulin have also been synthesized.

A second problem, that does not arise with bacterial genes, is encountered with many eukaryotic genes. Not only are they too large to synthesize with existing techniques but, unlike the genes of bacteria, they may also be discontinuous ('split' genes), the continuity of the coding sequence being disrupted by one or more unrelated sequences (introns) (see, for example,

Lewin 1994). Such sequences are removed after transcript synthesis but before translation, a process referred to as RNA splicing, i.e. a functional mRNA is produced by splicing together those sequences necessary for the production of the particular peptide. Another approach must therefore be used. This involves isolating the functional mRNA (already processed), which is used as a template to synthesize a complementary DNA (cDNA) sequence using reverse transcriptase (an enzyme that synthesizes single-stranded DNA from an RNA template). The single-stranded DNA is then converted to double-stranded DNA, inserted into a suitable cloning vector and the reconstructed, uninterrupted gene recovered by transformation of an appropriate bacterial cell line. The necessary mRNA can be prepared by one of a number of techniques; which one is chosen depends largely on the task in hand (Old and Primrose 1989).

Several mammalian proteins are now being made in bacteria as the result of gene cloning. They include somatostatin, human growth hormone, insulin, several interferons and tissue plasminogen activator. Many more can be expected in the future.

Genetic engineering is also likely to make a major impact in the field of vaccines. By making only the antigen against which antibody response is required, the risk associated with the intact pathogen is minimized. This technique is being pursued with respect to many pathogens, notably rabies and hepatitis B viruses, malaria and *Bordetella pertussis* to name but 4. The techniques of molecular biology that have been developed are so powerful, both with respect to unlocking the molecular biology of genetic systems and in furnishing the potential to allow specific manipulation of genes, that they offer the promise of major advances in our understanding of many diseases and of better informed positive intervention.

BACTERIOPHAGE GENETICS

8 VIRUSES ACTIVE ON BACTERIA

The notion of viruses as pathogens of bacteria has been with us for some 80 years, and is responsible for the name bacteriophage, from the Greek 'eater of bacteria' (usually abbreviated to phage). Early observations by Twort (1915) on lysis of staphylococcal colonies and d'Herelle (1917) on clearance of cultures of *Shigella* led initially to the name Twort–d'Herelle phenomenon, but it rapidly became clear that the causative agents were viruses with strong similarities to those active on mammalian and other cells, with the important difference of the need for specialized means of penetrating and being released from the tough outer layers of the bacterial cell. A section on the genetics of phage could as easily fit in Volume 1 (*Virology*) of this publication as in that on general bacteriology; insofar as our emphasis as a whole is on the role of micro-organisms in medicine, there is clear justification for treating bacterial viruses in their bacterial context.

Much of the published literature on phages has centred on genetic systems. This is not by chance; many phages have a developmental cycle within their host bacteria of 30 min or less and an efficiency of plating of near 100%. Many bacteria also have a doubling time of this order so that it is possible to obtain phage lysates of $\geq 10^{10}$ particles per ml in a few hours, and since mutant frequencies are of the order of 10^{-8} to 10^{-9} per cell generation it is feasible to screen for mutations in a range of phage genes in overnight experiments. The methods by which such mutants can be recognized is described below (p. 266). This simplicity of handling has meant that phages have been used in some of the most fundamental experiments in the science of genetics, such as Benzer's (1955) definition of the unit of gene function and Watson and Crick's demonstration of the triplet nature of the genetic code (Crick et al. 1961). Many of these classic experiments predate the modern molecular era in genetic research. More recently, however, many phages have proved ideal for modification as cloning vectors (p. 285), and research continues to reveal new biological principles of wide and general importance.

The importance of phage extends beyond molecular genetics. Classically, phage typing schemes have been used to differentiate variants of pathogens, especially *Salmonella* spp. and *S. aureus*, responsible for epidemic spread in susceptible populations. These schemes have been especially useful when serological or conventional biochemical tests could not achieve sufficient discrimination. Although typing methods based on molecular techniques such as plasmid profiling and DNA sequencing have in some cases supplanted phage-based approaches as the techniques of choice, phage typing retains its importance in some key areas. Some other instances of the practical importance of the study of phage are shown in section 15 (see p. 284).

Ritchie (1983) summarized many of the fundamental aspects of phage biology in the seventh edition of Topley & Wilson, and in the eighth edition Bennett and Howe (1990) gave an account based on a limited number of illustrative examples concentrating on the well studied T-even and λ phages. In this chapter it is intended to consolidate and update the text of the eighth edition and also to focus on some new areas that have become important since publication of the eighth edition.

9 THE STUDY OF PHAGES

The lytic cycle of phages (see section 11, p. 270) is the series of events that occurs between attachment of a phage particle to a cell and the subsequent release of daughter phage particles by the cell. When this takes place in liquid medium the daughter phage particles are themselves available to infect further cells in the culture. The rate of production of phage particles in these circumstances depends on the number released from each infected cell (the **mean burst size**) and the time taken to complete the cycle; if cells are lysed faster than fresh cells arise by cell division, the culture becomes clear except for the outgrowth of phage-resistant mutant cells (p. 282). Hence, for many phages, the production of a high-titre lysate requires only the addition of a suitable number of phage particles to a growing culture of the host, the proportion of particles to cells being termed the **multiplicity of infection** (MOI). A MOI of around 1:10 is often desirable for optimum lysate production; a MOI >10 can result in premature lysis of the cells without production of daughter phage particles ('lysis-from-without').

When this sequence of events occurs on solid medium the released phage particles are necessarily restricted to the region around the initially infected cell on the plate, resulting in a small circular zone of clearing or plaque. Each particle capable of initiating a lytic cycle is hence known as a **plaque-forming unit** (pfu), and the proportion of pfu to the total count of morphologically normal particles is the **efficiency of plating** (EOP).

The extreme simplicity of these 2 methods of phage production, in liquid and on solid medium, accounts for the ease of production of high-titre suspensions and of counting phage plaques. The addition of a specific cofactor may be needed for optimum adsorption of phage particle to host cell; of the phages active on *E. coli*, T2 requires monovalent cations, λ requires Mg^{2+}, and some strains of T4 are Ca^{2+}-dependent (see Adams 1959, for details of these and other technical factors affecting the growth of phage).

9.1 Bacteriophage plaques

Under standard conditions, the size and appearance of phage plaques is characteristic of the combination of phage and bacterial host. Small phages tend to form large plaques and vice versa, and the size of the plaque is reduced in poor nutritional conditions that increase the length of the latent period and reduce the mean burst size (see p. 270). A proportion of the host cells may fail to undergo lysis; some may have lost surface receptors as a result of mutation, some may contain restriction endonucleases to which the phage genetic material is sensitive (p. 284), and some may have become lysogenized (p. 278) by the genome of the same or a related phage. Such cells are able to grow and form colonies within the plaque, obscuring its appearance; where lysogeny is the reason, the immune cells form a colony with greatest density at the centre of the plaque, giving a characteristic turbid-centred appearance.

Several types of mutant affecting plaque appearance are known. The rapid lysis (*r*) mutants of phage T4 form plaques larger than normal; these lie in one of a group of genes, 2 of which (*rIIA*, *rIIB*) have been of particular value in studies of mutation, genetic coding and definition of the unit of gene function or **cistron**. Host range mutants (*h*) result in a change of adsorption specificity of the type outlined in the preceding paragraph, and can be recognized by plating the phage suspension on 2 or more potential host strains.

The most useful mutants for the delineation of morphogenetic pathways in phages are known as **conditional lethal** or **conditional defective** mutants. These are of 2 types: in the first a phage gene is mutated to form a product of greater temperature sensitivity than the parent. At normal temperatures such a phage stock fails to form plaques as a result of loss of function of the mutated product, but if the temperature is lowered the product again becomes active and plaques are formed. These mutants are genetically **mis-sense** (p. 236). The second type is non-functional because of a chain terminator mutation, but if the phage stock is grown on a host carrying a suitable **suppressor gene** (p. 236) a plaque again forms. The value of these mutants, both of which form plaques only on a suitable permissive host, is that they can lie in almost any phage gene, unlike those affecting plaque appearance or host range, thus allowing the experimenter to relate the mutated gene to the gene product (see p. 268 for the assembly pathway for phage T4).

9.2   **Bacteriophage particles**

Lysates prepared as above are freed from cellular debris and media components by low speed centrifugation (3000 **g**, 30 min), resuspension in buffer, and deposited as a pellet by high speed centrifugation (50 000 **g** or higher, 6 h). The deposited phage particles can be purified by washing and treatment with nucleases. Phages prepared in this manner can be made ready for electron microscopy by the technique of negative staining in which the phage suspension is mixed with a 2% solution of phosphotungstate or uranyl acetate and dried on a microscope grid. The regions penetrated by the stain appear electron-dense in contrast to those from which the stain is excluded.

Phages, like other viruses, have a head (capsid) which may contain DNA or RNA that may in turn be single- or double-stranded. The Fifth Report of the International Committee for Taxonomy of Viruses in 1991 (ICTV; see discussion in Maniloff, Ackermann and Jarvis 1994) includes 4007 phage descriptions, of which 3853 have a chacteristic tailed morphology differing from that found in animal or plant viruses. An earlier classification by Bradley (1967) defined 6 morphological groups. Group A has a head approximating in appearance to an elongated hexagon, to which is attached a tail with a contractile sheath; tail fibres and whiskers (Fig. 10.14) are attached. The head contains double-stranded DNA. This group includes the complex and well studied 'T-even' phages of *E. coli* (T2, T4, T6). Group B resembles group A except that the tail is non-contractile and includes phages T1, T5 and λ of *E. coli*. Group C resembles A and B, but the tail is very short (and non-contractile); members include phages T3 and T7 of *E. coli*, P22 of *Salmonella* and phage 29 of *Bacillus*. Group D phages have a tail-less head consisting of large subunits (capsomeres) containing single-stranded DNA; they include phage φX174 and S13 of *E. coli*. Group E resembles D but the heads have small capsomeres and contain single-stranded RNA; *E. coli* phages in this group include MS2 and Mu2. Group F phages are flexible filaments containing single-stranded DNA and contain *E. coli*

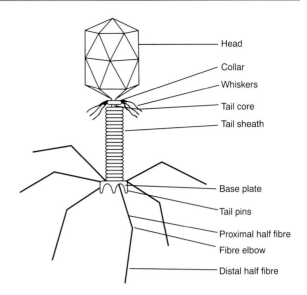

Fig. 10.14 The T4 phage particle. The particle is represented with the tail sheath in the uncontracted position.

phages M13 and fd. The last 2 groups most closely resemble the isometric and filamentous forms found among the animal viruses. Two additions were subsequently made to Bradley's scheme: first, phages such as φ6 of *Pseudomonas syringae* pv *phaseolicola*, otherwise placed in group E, contain 3 pieces of double-stranded RNA and have a lipid-containing envelope; second, enveloped double-stranded DNA-containing particles without a rigid head are assigned to a new group, G. Table 10.7 lists the dimensions of some representative phage particles.

Table 10.7   Dimensions of representative phage particles

Type	Phage	Head	Tail	Host genus
A	T2	100 × 70	110 × 25	*Escherichia*
	PST	126 × 95	115 × 25	*Pasteurella*
	PBS1	120	200 × 22	*Bacillus*
	P1	90	220 × 20	*Shigella*
B	T1	60	140 × 10	*Escherichia*
	λ	54	140 × 7	*Escherichia*
	B3	55	163 × 8	*Pseudomonas*
	MSP8	70 × 55	150 × 10	*Streptomyces*
C	T3	55	15 × 8	*Escherichia*
	P22	60	7 × 7	*Salmonella*
	φ29	42 × 32	13 × 6	*Bacillus*
	AA-1	65	18 × 13	*Acinetobacter*
D	φX174	25	…	*Escherichia*
	S13	26	…	*Escherichia*
	M20	30	…	*Escherichia*
E	MS2	25	…	*Escherichia*
	μ2	24	…	*Escherichia*
	φcb23	22	…	*Caulobacter*
	7s	25	…	*Pseudomonas*
F	M13	…	800 × 8	*Escherichia*
	fd	…	700 × 5	*Escherichia*
	f1	…	850 × 5	*Escherichia*

Dimensions are given in nm. Where the length and width of the head are the same only a single dimension is given.

9.3 Phage classification

The ICTV classification (see Maniloff, Ackermann and Jarvis 1994) groups all phages known in 1991 into 12 families, of which 11 are named (Table 10.8). Among the double-stranded DNA group the *Plasmaviridae* include a group of pleomorphic enveloped phages growing on *Acholeplasma laidlawii*; infection leads to an infectious cycle in which progeny particles are released by budding from the cell membrane, the host surviving as a lysogen in which the phage genome is integrated at a unique site in the host chromosome. The SSV1-type phages grow on the archaebacterium *Sulfolobus shibatae* B12, the phage genome being present in the cells as a plasmid or integrated into specific sites; large numbers of particles are released by UV induction but without lysis. The *Lipothrixviridae* grow on *Thermoproteus tenax*, infection resulting in lytic production or formation of a carrier state in which pieces of viral genome are integrated into the host chromosome. The *Tectiviridae* grow on several bacterial genera carrying drug-resistance plasmids (p. 254) that specify the appropriate pili as receptors: the best known example is phage PRD1 which establishes lytic infection. The *Corticoviridae* establish lytic infection in *Alteromonas*. The *Myoviridae* include the well known virulent T-even phages of *E. coli* together with phages infecting several other gram-positive and gram-negative genera. The *Siphoviridae* include the important λ group of coliphages that provide the paradigm of lysogeny by phage genome integration into the host chromosome. The *Podoviridae* comprise the coliphage T7 group and some similar phages of Enterobacteriaceae and perhaps other bacterial groups. Among the single-stranded DNA phages the *Microviridae* are typified by the coliphage φX174 group and the *Inoviridae* by the coliphage fd group which adsorb to pili and are released by extrusion through the host cell membranes without lysis.

The RNA phages fall into 2 groups. The *Cystoviridae* are represented solely by the *Pseudomonas* phage φ6, an enveloped double-stranded RNA-containing particle that adsorbs to the sides of pili and establishes lytic infection. The *Leviviridae* comprise single-stranded RNA-containing particles, including the coliphage MS2 group, that adsorb to the sides of sex pili determined by several different plasmids, also establishing lytic infection.

This classification does not imply phylogenetic relationships within each group. The early literature (Adams 1959) contains various proposals for establishing a taxonomy on Linnean principles, but it is clear that phages as a group are susceptible to continuous changes of host range, as indeed are other viruses, and such attempts are now only of historical interest; phages continue to be described by the type of symbol used in this chapter. Some groups (*Myoviridae*, *Siphoviridae*) have received intensive interest since almost the earliest days of bacterial virology, whereas little is known of some others and morphological descriptions may be incomplete, a situation reminiscent of early schemes for the classification of bacteria. The ICTV classification is useful, however, in providing a framework in which newly described phages may be accommodated; a full phylogenetic tree will have to await detailed nucleic acid comparisons, which may themselves be difficult because of the presence of sections of host cell genomes.

10 MOLECULAR STRUCTURE OF PHAGES

10.1 Phage proteins

If T-even phages are transferred from high salt concentrations to distilled water they rapidly lose their infectivity and the DNA dissociates from the structural components (osmotic shocking). The latter appear to be anatomically undamaged except that the heads are collapsed and empty ('ghosts') and consist almost entirely of protein; the double-stranded DNA appears as a mass of threads outside, 2 nm in diameter and 49 μm long. Osmotically shocked particles also release about 2% of the phage protein with a little acid-soluble peptide, spermidine and putrescine.

Further dissociation of phage T4, chosen here as the best studied example of a complex phage particle, shows that many proteins are present. More than 40% of the genetic information is devoted to synthesis and assembly of the structural protein components (Mosig 1994); 24 genes are involved in head morphogenesis, more than 25 are needed for the tails and tail fibres, and 5 others are needed for assembly. The head is composed of a number of identical capsomeres consisting predominantly of a single protein, P23*, with 2 minor components *hoc* and *soc* (see Fig. 10.15); these are thought to be assembled as a capsid resembling a prolate icosahedron of approximate dimensions 125 nm length and 81 nm width, accounting for the 'elongated hexagon' appearance in electron micrographs. The midpiece consists of a hollow cylinder, 95 × 7.5 nm, with a central channel of 2 nm diameter; this is surrounded by a sheath composed of about 200 helically arranged subunits of 50 kDa. The sheath is 95 nm long but contracts to 38 nm on infection of a host cell (see section 11.2, p. 273). At the top of the central cylinder is an adaptor, apparently to accommodate the 5-fold symmetry of the head to the 6-fold symmetry of the midpiece, a collar, and 6 whiskers; at the bottom is a base plate 22 nm deep carrying 6 tail pins or spikes. The tail consists of 6 fibres, each 140 × 2 nm, attached to the top of the base plate with 2 subunits of 100 kDa joined endwise by the products of 2 genes, *38* and *57*, that are not present in the mature particle. The outer (distal) of these 2 subunits differs from those of the other T-even phages and form the basis for distinction of the different T-even phages by their host range (Mosig 1994).

The morphogenetic pathway of phage T4 has been elucidated by the study of conditional lethal mutants which can be isolated in any of the various phage genes, and the missing function can in each instance be identified by electron microscopic examination of

Table 10.8 The 1991 ICTV Classification of Bacteriophage

	DNA	RNA
2-stranded	*Plasmaviridae* (enveloped, pleomorphic) SSV-1-type phages (non-enveloped, lemon-shaped) *Lipothrixviridae* (enveloped, rod-shaped) *Tectiviridae* (non-enveloped, double capsids) *Corticoviridae* (non-enveloped, lipid-containing) *Myoviridae* (non-enveloped, contractile tails) *Siphoviridae* (non-enveloped, long non-contractile tails) *Podoviridae* (non-enveloped, short tails)	*Cystoviridae* (segmented, enveloped)
1-stranded	*Microviridae* (non-enveloped, isometric) *Inoviridae* (non-enveloped, rod-shaped)	*Leviviridae* (non-segmented, non-enveloped)

Adapted from Maniloff, Ackermann and Jarvis (1994).

premature lysates grown under restrictive conditions. This anaylsis reveals 3 pathways – for assembly of head, midpiece, and tail – and these 3 subunits are then assembled into mature particles in the host.

Among the other groups, φX174 (see McKenna, Ilag and Rossmann 1994) is of interest in that spikes are present at each of the 12 apices of the icosahedron and any of these is able to act as the organelle by which the particle adsorbs to the host and injects its nucleic acid. The single-stranded RNA phages, the simplest of all isometric viruses, have a capsid consisting of 180 identical protein subunits and a single molecule of a maturation (A) protein to enable adsorption. Phage φ6, the single known example of a double-stranded RNA phage, has a flexible lipid-containing envelope and dodacehedral capsid (see Bamford 1994 for details). Phage PRD1, another membrane-enveloped phage, infects both *E. coli* and *S.* Typhimurium and translocates its membrane from the host to virus particles (Bamford and Bamford 1990).

Another approach to the examination of phage particles and their components is the use of antibody neutralization techniques. Antibody raised specifically against head protein does not neutralize infectivity. The T-even phages all cross-react serologically with each other but not with the other T phages, emphasizing the close relationship implied by their structural similarity. When cells are infected with 2 closely related phages such as T2 and T4 some T2 daughter DNA becomes wrapped in T4 heads, as judged by antigenic specificity, and vice versa; this is called **phenotypic mixing**. By contrast, antibody to tail protein is highly effective in abolishing infectivity; phage particles neutralized in this way can still adsorb to their hosts without injecting DNA, thus discriminating between adsorption and injection functions. Antibodies highly specific to one particular phage component can thus be used to identify the defects in premature lysates of conditional lethal mutants.

10.2 Phage nucleic acids

Phages may contain either DNA or RNA as genetic material, and both single- and double-stranded forms of each are known. The structure, with a few exceptions, is the same as that found universally among living organisms: a polynucleotide chain consisting of a deoxyribose (or ribose)-phosphate backbone to which are attached specific sequences of the 4 nucleotides adenine, thymine (or uracil), guanine and cytosine; in all except the single-stranded phages 2 such complementary chains are paired together in a Watson–Crick double helix (Watson and Crick 1953). Many phage nucleic acids have now been sequenced and much is known about coding regions and open reading frames. A few unusual features of phage nucleic acids and of their chromosomal organization should be noted:

1 The T-even phages contain 5-hydroxymethylcytosine in place of cytosine and some *B. subtilis* phages have 5-hydroxymethyluracil or uracil in place of thymine (Kornberg 1980). The GC:AT ratio of some phage nucleic acids also differs considerably from that of the host. These findings suggest that at least some phages may have an evolutionary origin quite different from that of their hosts rather than having evolved from an intracellular particle.

2 The 5-hydroxymethyl residues have attached glucose groupings that differ between T2, T4 and T6 both in their distribution and in the type of bonding (Stent 1963). These patterns of glucosylation may be analogous to the distribution of methyl residues acquired when DNA enters a new host cell

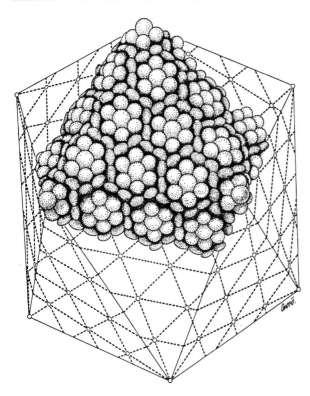

Fig. 10.15 Components of the head of phage T4. Six molecules of P23* and one molecule of *hoc* protein form a hexamer and a centre unit; these units are located around the 6-fold axes and are bridged by molecules of *soc* protein, as either 2 trimers or 3 dimers. The P23* subunits of neighbouring hexamers may be connected to each other beneath the *soc* protein. The capsid lattice is based on the left-handed T = 13 icosahedron with one extra equatorial band. (Reproduced, with permission, from Yanagida 1977).

and becomes adapted so as to resist the restriction endonucleases of the host (DNA modification).

3 Some bacteriophages carry introns, short DNA sequences interposed within coding regions that mediate splicing of RNA transcripts and hence do not themselves contribute to the gene product. The first was discovered within the phage T4 *td* gene encoding thymidylate synthase (Chu et al. 1984). Phage introns are all similar to one another and also to several introns identified in eukaryotes, raising questions both of phylogenetic origin and of the selective advantage seemingly conferred on phage genomes by their presence (Belfort 1989, 1990).

The genome of phage T4 contains about 168 000 nt within which about 130 genes with known functions have been defined together with about 100 unidentified open reading frames (Mosig 1994). The single-stranded DNA phage φX174 has 5386 nt coding for 11 known gene products (Denhardt 1994). Phage φ6 contains 3 double-stranded RNA species of 2948, 4057 and 6374 nt, each fragment coding for 4 proteins (Bamford 1994), and the single-stranded RNA phage MS2 contains a single 3569 nt fragment coding for 4 proteins (see p. 270 for **overlapping genes**): phage

GA, within this last group, has an even smaller (3466 nt) genome (van Duin 1994).

With some exceptions (see φ6 above) the genetic material is organized as a single molecule of DNA or RNA, the chromosome. This may be visualized by electron microscopy and further information about its structure can be gained by examining the distribution of restriction endonuclease cleavage sites, giving a physical map. Another approach is to study the distribution of mutational sites by genetic crosses to obtain a genetic map. Genetic markers on a single chromosome are described as being in a single linkage group but, since genetic experiments usually rely on scoring recombinants between large numbers of phages, the diagrammatic representation of a linkage group may differ from that of a chromosome. This point is made clear in the description of phage T4 below.

Phage nucleic acids range from 3 to c. 200 000 kDa. The DNA of single-stranded phages such as φX174 can be isolated from the phage head as a continuous loop although during vegetative replication this assumes a double-stranded form (see p. 274). RNA phage genomes are linear. The greatest variety is seen among the double-stranded DNA phages:

1 The T-even phages have a circular genetic map, but the chromosomes are linear and non-identical, each beginning at an almost random point on the map (circular permutation). In addition to this, each chromosome has a sequence of 3–5% of its bases at one end that is an exact repetition of that at the other (terminal redundancy). The chromosomes of some other phages such as P22 are likewise permutated, but here each chromosome origin lies within a limited region of the genetic map. These 2 features (Fig. 10.16) have a quite simple explanation when the mode of replication and maturation of the DNA are considered: treatment of the chromosome population with an enzyme such as exonuclease III which removes nucleotides from the 3' end of a double helix will, because of the terminal redundancy, expose self-complementary regions that allow the projecting 5' ends to anneal to one another and result in each chromosome forming a double-stranded ring (see p. 273 for a discussion of the processing of this structure into mature daughter chromosomes).

2 The chromosomes of phages such as λ are all linear and identical to one another, i.e. there is no circular permutation. Neither is there terminal redundancy of the kind found among the T-even phages, but λ chromosomes have a 12-base single-stranded extension at each 5' end of the double-stranded molecule; the 2 single-stranded regions are complementary to each other (cohesive ends, *cos* site), again allowing circularization of the chromosome as a prerequisite to replication.

3 Phage T5 has 3 discontinuities at specific points in one of the 2 strands of the double-stranded molecule, and some other phages have similar discontinuities but apparently at random points.

Some small phages achieve a surprising degree of

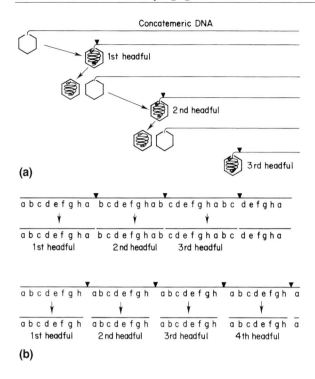

(a)

(b)

Fig. 10.16 Packaging of phage DNA from a concatemeric intermediate; a–h inclusive represents one complete genome. Empty head structures (proheads) are filled with DNA (double-stranded) from a concatemeric precursor. After completion of one headful, the remaining DNA is cleaved through both strands (▼) and proceeds to fill subsequent proheads. (a) T-even phage: each headful equals one complete genome plus a terminal redundancy (= 'a' for the first headful). Note that each subsequent headful begins at a different point in the genome, leading to a series of headfuls that are circular permutations of the sequence a–h. (b) λ phage: the point of cleavage is always between sequences h and a. Hence there is neither terminal redundancy nor circular permutation. (Each headful, however, has a 12 base single-stranded cohesive end at the 5′ ends of the double-stranded molecule – not shown in the diagram.)

economy in the use of their genetic material by virtue of the phenomenon of overlapping genes. The single-stranded DNA phage φX174 has 10 genes (Fig. 10.17). Genes *A* and *A** are in the same reading frame, but *A** is read from an internal codon within the *A* sequence. The nucleotide sequence of gene *E* lies within that of *D*, in a different frame (+1), which in turn overlaps the beginning of gene *J* by one base. Furthermore, genes *A* and *C* overlap by 2 bases that lie within the coding sequence for *K*; 4 bases in this overlap region are used in all 3 possible reading frames to contribute to the coding of distinct products. Some (but not all) members of the very small single-stranded RNA *Leviviridae* group code for a lysis gene that overlaps and is out of frame with respect to the other 3 genes present (for maturation, coat protein and RNA replicase). It remains to be seen whether overlaps of this kind are common in organisms with larger genomes.

11 THE LYTIC CYCLE

The lytic cycle is the sequence of events between infection of a cell and its subsequent release of daughter phage particles. Some phages (*Plasmaviridae*, *Inoviridae*) infect their host cells and are then released without death of the host, as do some animal viruses; for them it is not strictly correct to refer to a lytic cycle although the term has come to be applied universally. It is also necessary to distinguish infective events that result in the phage genome becoming latent within the host and continuing to divide with it, i.e. the **lysogenic cycle** (see section 12, p. 278).

It is convenient to regard the lytic cycle as consisting of 4 phases: adsorption of phage to host cell, penetration of phage nucleic acid, intracellular development, and release. The classic type of investigation for determining the outline of these events is the **one-step growth cycle** (Ellis and Delbrück 1939) in which phage at an MOI of about 0.1 is added to an early log phase suspension of host cells; the mixture is left for a few minutes to allow phage particles to adsorb and then any unadsorbed particles are either counted or neutralized with anti-phage serum. Samples are then removed every few minutes and the pfus are counted.

An example of the result to be expected with a lytic phage is shown in Fig. 10.18, in which the numbers of pfus of phage T4 are plotted against time. When the phage suspension is added, its count initially drops as particles adsorb to host cells (the **adsorption period**) and then remains constant while the injected phage genomes replicate and daughter phage particles are made; this is the **latent period**. The cells lyse once their complement of daughter particles is complete, so the plaque-forming particle count now rises steeply (the **rise period**) until all the cells have reached a plateau, or step, which gives this type of experiment its name. The lengths of the adsorption, latent and rise periods can be read off from the graph; it is also possible to measure the number of particles released per infected cell – the **mean burst size**. For phage T2 and *E. coli* B the adsorption period is quite short (c. 5–8 min), the latent period is around 25 min under optimal conditions, the rise period is similar in length to the adsorption period (reflecting asynchrony of infection of host cells), and the mean burst size is about 200 pfu per infected cell.

The course of the one-step growth experiment is modified in poor nutritional conditions when, in general, the latent period is lengthened and the mean burst size reduced. It is possible, however, for a longer latent period to be correlated with an increase in burst size which occurs, for instance, when T2-infected cells are deliberately infected with further T2 particles just before lysis; the latter repress late gene expression of the developing particles (**lysis inhibition**) but do not inhibit particle assembly, a process which is essentially independent of protein synthesis. The same effect is observed when inhibitors of protein synthesis, such as 5-methyltryptophan or chloramphenicol, are added and this can be of value in increasing the particle yield in genetic modification experiments (see section 15.2, p. 285). It is also possible to modify the one-step growth experiment to yield additional information. When samples are removed for counting, they may be split into 2 aliquots of which one is counted as above and the other counted after cellular disruption, e.g. with chloroform, which lyses the cells and releases any mature intracellular particles; during approximately the

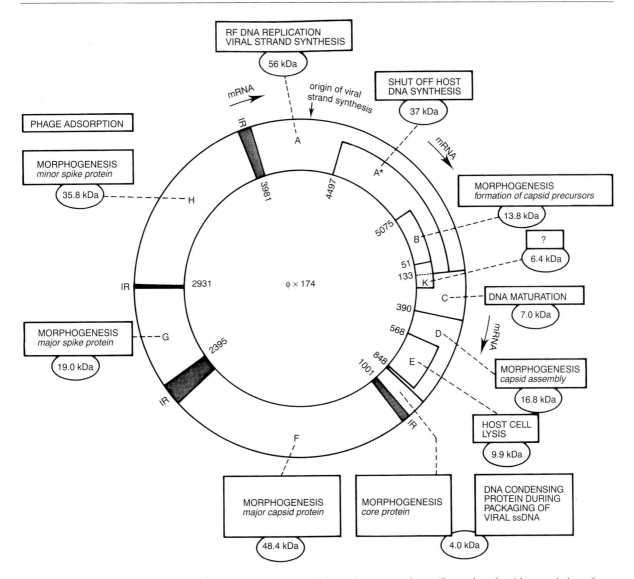

Fig. 10.17   Gene map of phage φX174. See text for description of gene overlaps. (Reproduced, with permission, from O'Brien 1987).

first half of the latent period no intracellular particles can be found in the premature lysate (the **eclipse phase**), and intracellular particles then increase in number (the **post-eclipse phase**) until they reach the burst size and normal lysis occurs. In the single-burst experiment (Burnet 1929, developed by Ellis and Delbrück 1939), a sample is taken during the latent period and then greatly diluted so that small subsamples have a low probability of containing a single infected bacterium. The subsamples are dispensed to broth at 37°C, the bacteria are allowed to lyse, and the phage particles are then counted. From the number of tubes found to contain no phage particles, the proportion of the remainder receiving only one infected cell can be calculated by the Poisson distribution, and hence the range of individual burst sizes contributing to the mean burst size can be ascertained.

11.1   Adsorption to the host cell

The primary encounter between a complex phage particle such as T4 and its host entails random collision, resulting in an irreversible interaction between the adsorption apparatus of the phage (the base plate and

tail fibres) and the cell envelope. Each of these is considered in turn, followed by a brief examination of the role of environmental factors.

PHAGE STRUCTURES PARTICIPATING IN ADSORPTION

The initial contact of the T-even phages appears to be established by the distal ends of the tail fibres, after which the spikes on the base plate make contact (Furukawa and Mizushima 1982). The tips of the T4 fibres (gp37) interact with the diglucosyl residues of a lipopolysaccharide of *E. coli* B or with the OmpC protein of *E. coli* K12, whereas those of the T2 fibres (gp38) interact with OmpF and those of the related phage K3 with OmpA (Mosig 1994). A detailed study of these fibre proteins has been reported by Henning's research group (Montag et al. 1987, Riede et al. 1987a, 1987b); all closely resemble each other and have further similarities to the outer-membrane proteins with which they interact. In each there is a

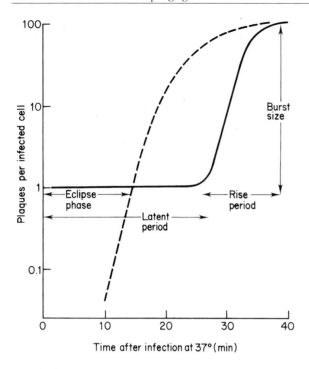

Fig. 10.18 One-step growth curve of phage T4. The solid line represents the one-step growth curve obtained by the spontaneous lysis of infected cells. The dashed line is the curve for prematurely lysed cells and shows the kinetics of intracellular phage production.

constant amino-terminal and carboxy-terminal region spanning a hypervariable region; changes in the latter are likely to reflect the successive evolutionary steps of the phage and its host strain. The product of gene *38* in phage T4 serves a different function to that in phage T2, being required for the dimerization of the fibre itself and not found in the mature particle. Following this fibre–cell encounter there is an interaction between the spikes of the base plate and the cell surface, accompanied by extension of gene *12* proteins from the base plate as short fibrils (Crowther et al. 1977). The association of these structures becomes irreversible within 10 s (Wright, McConnell and Kanegasaki 1980).

The 12 apices of the ϕX174 icosahedron are each composed of 5 molecules of protein G and one molecule of protein H; mutations in the genes for these structures, and also gene *F*, affect host specificity, and all 12 apices appear to be used for adsorption with equal probability. Among the RNA phages protein P3 of ϕ6 and the maturation (A) protein of the single-stranded phages are responsible for adsorption to the host receptor, which in both cases is a pilus. Filamentous single-stranded phages such as M13 bind to the tip of the sex pilus elaborated by the F (fertility) factor (p. 247; see Willetts 1984 for a comprehensive list). Phage coat protein enters the cytoplasmic membrane and M13 receptor sites can be detected in extracts of F⁺ cells; details of the mode of entry are unknown. A match of symmetry has been detected between the filamentous phage fd and its F pilus tip receptor (Marvin and Folkhard 1986) and between phage Pf1 and the PAK pilus of *P. aeruginosa* (Folkhard et al. 1981). An analysis of the fd attachment protein by deletion mutation has

allowed discrimination of a receptor recognition region and a penetration region (Stengele et al. 1990).

The single-stranded RNA-containing phages such as R17 and Qβ are also 'F-specific' and can be seen microscopically to bind to lateral receptors on the F pilus; they are then drawn down to a receptor in the cell surface proper by a retraction of the sex pilus analogous to that which occurs during F mediated conjugation. The double-stranded DNA phage ϕ6 also attaches to a pilus receptor, pilus retraction being followed by fusion between the phage envelope and the host outer membrane (Romantschuk and Bamford 1985). The flagellotropic phage χ1 of the Enterobacteriaceae appears to encounter a primary receptor on a flagellum and to travel down to the base, where an encounter with a second receptor triggers DNA release and injection (Meynell 1961, Schade, Adler and Ris 1967); 2 flagellotropic phages of the genus *Bacillus* (PBS1 in *B. subtilis*; PBP in *Bacillus pumilus*) follow a similar pattern. It is therefore likely that all phages which primarily recognize a site on an extracellular appendage do not proceed to the further stage of nucleic acid penetration until they interact with a second receptor at the cell surface. The papers in Randall and Philipson (1980) should be consulted for further details of these and other systems.

HOST CELL ADSORPTION FUNCTIONS

The bacterial cell presents to the environment a surface consisting of capsular, outer-membrane and cell wall structures, possibly with flagella and sex or common pili in addition (see Chapter 2). Many of these structures have been exploited as receptor sites by phages and bacteriocins, as well in some cases as sex pilus receptors. Environments such as sewage in which phages and sensitive bacteria are constantly present show a rapid and complementary evolution between phage structures on the one hand and cellular adsorption sites on the other (p. 283). Many cell surface structures can be shown by mutational studies to be dispensable to the cell, and it would appear that almost all of these can be exploited by phages as receptors; adsorption of virulent phages to structures that cannot be changed mutationally without concomitant loss of cell viability would presumably result in extinction of the cell line by lytic infection, and hence ultimately of the phage concerned. It remains to be seen, however, whether phages that establish a carrier state might make use of such indispensable receptors.

Cell surface structures can be separated by, for example, lysozyme and EDTA treatment followed by an appropriate regimen of differential centrifugation; individual fractions can then be tested for their ability to neutralize phage suspensions. Several phages active on *E. coli* and *Salmonella* attach to different parts of the lipopolysaccharide (LPS) component of the outer membrane (Wright, McConnell and Kanegesaki 1980). Phages specific for the R core region may have wide host ranges because of the low degree of variability in this structure in the Enterobacteriaceae. More than one molecular species may be needed for successful infection: mutants lacking L-gala-D-mannoheptose are concomitantly resistant to phages T3, T4 and T7, whereas those lacking OmpC protein are resistant to T4 alone. The conformational interdependence of surface structures is emphasized by another study on T4 (Yu and Mizushima 1982); in the presence of OmpC protein the essential region of the LPS for adsorption is the core-lipid A region that includes heptose, whereas in the absence of OmpC a glucose residue exposed by removal of the distal end of the LPS is needed. Phage K20 requires both OmpF protein and LPS (Silverman and Benson 1987).

Phages specific for gram-positive cells may recognize receptors in the cell wall or cytoplasmic membrane, and some utilize flagella (see Randall and Philipson 1980, Lugtenberg and Van Alphen 1983).

ENVIRONMENTAL FACTORS IN ADSORPTION

Phages do not generally adsorb to their hosts in distilled water: cations are needed to neutralize the net negative charge on phage and bacterium. The rate of adsorption is also dependent on temperature. Some phage–bacterium interactions require specific cofactors: T2 requires monovalent cations, λ requires Mg^{2+}, and some T4 strains are Ca^{2+}-dependent. Some T4 and T6 strains must be sensitized by L-tryptophan prior to adsorption.

11.2 Penetration of nucleic acid

The classic double labelling experiment of Hershey and Chase (1952) shows that adsorption of phage T2 to its host is followed by ejection of DNA from the phage head into the interior of the cell; this requires the tip of the central core of the tail to be brought into apposition with the inner (cytoplasmic) membrane, probably at a site of fusion between inner and outer membrane. It is also accompanied by contraction of the sheath (Fig. 10.19), but contraction can be induced physically without DNA ejection; the existence of several phages (morphological groups B and C) with non-contractile tails shows that there must be some other means of energizing the ejection process (see discussion in Goldberg 1980).

It is evident from kinetic studies that T-even phage DNA must be transmitted from phage head to host cell through the 2 nm diameter core at a rate of at least 3 kb s^{-1}; a DNA nicking and repair system may be involved (Goldberg 1980). Transport of DNA across the inner membrane requires proton motive force but not ATP.

Phage T5 DNA is injected in 2 steps, the first comprising about 8% of the chromosome; neither step requires proton motive force or ATP. Penetration of the DNA of the isometric phage φX174 entails uncoating and exposure of the DNA on the cell surface in a DNAase-sensitive form, a process resembling bacterial transformation (p. 246), in contrast to that of the large T-even phages. The factors involved in translocation of DNA across bacterial membranes have been reviewed by Dreiseikelmann (1994).

11.3 Intracellular development

Although there are now examples of phages that are propagated by a process of progressive release from a carrier-like state in their host cells, resembling the lysogenic cycle entered into by some temperate phages as an alternative to lysis, the latent period of the classic lytic cycle has received most attention in the study of intracellular development of phage. In this the entire metabolic activity of a bacterial cell, which has been infected by a single molecule of nucleic acid perhaps less than one-thousandth the size of its own chromosome, is subverted into making and packaging 200 or more copies of the invading molecule within the time taken for a single normal cell division. The extent to which phages depend on host functions for this process is broadly related to their own size: large complex phages such as T4 possess more than 150 genes and can thus code for a range of enzymes and structural proteins, whereas the minute single-stranded RNA phages have only 4 gene activities. This section will first consider the best studied patterns of replication of DNA and RNA phages (**vegetative replication**) and then examine the appearance of new proteins and RNA species during the latent period, concluding by describing 3 other important events – recombination between phage DNA molecules, gene expression and its control, and the packaging of the nucleic acid and assembly of the mature particle.

DNA REPLICATION

The replication systems of phages T4 and λ can be viewed as paradigms for DNA phage replication in general. Study of the appearance of new DNA during the latent period of the T-even phages is greatly aided by the presence of 5-hydroxymethylcytosine, which serves as a marker to distinguish phage from bacterial DNA. New phage DNA can be detected about 6 min after infection and the amount then rises sharply until at the end of the eclipse phase some 50–80 phage equivalents of DNA are present. The size of the DNA pool so formed continues to rise during the post-eclipse phase, together with the newly formed daughter particles, until lysis. Labelling experiments show that about one-third of the nucleotides in the phage DNA originate from the host DNA which is being broken down during the latent period, but the remaining two-thirds are not derived from pre-existing polynucleotides.

Circular forms of the length of a single chromosome can be seen shortly after T4 infection (Mosig, Bowden and Bock 1972, Bernstein and Bernstein 1973). As described earlier, the terminally redundant region of each linear T4 chromosome is a ready substrate for exonuclease activity and hence for annealing of complementary single strands and circularization. Origins of replication near genes 41 and 5, and elsewhere, serve as sites for new DNA synthesis; from these the initial circularized chromosome builds up into a large expanding loop with linear branches attached, such that the final replicating structure is complex and may contain up to 60 replication forks. Both host functions and general recombination are responsible for generating the long DNA strands which can be shown by hybridization studies to consist of serial repetitions of the T4 genome (concatemers). Kornberg (1980, 1982) described the enzymology of the process. DNA is now packaged from the concatemers into the assembling protein heads so that each head contains

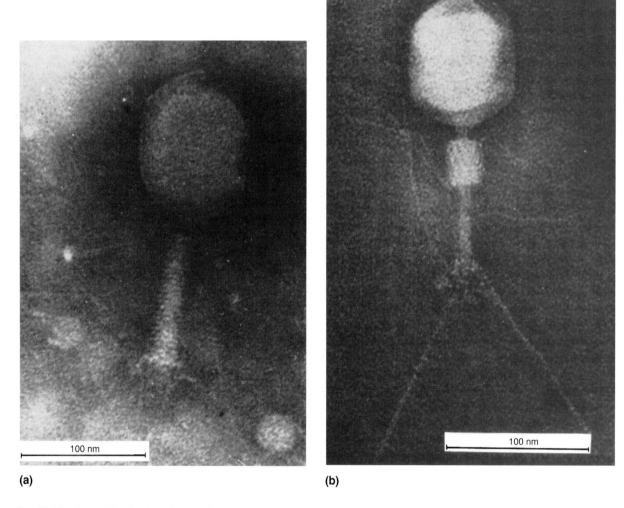

(a)   **(b)**

Fig. 10.19 Phage T2, showing the sheath (a) uncontracted and (b) contracted. See Fig. 10.14 for identification of morphological structures present. (Reproduced, with permission, from Brenner et al. 1959).

a little more than the equivalent of a single genome (see Fig. 10.16, p. 270), explaining both the terminal redundancy in each daughter chromosome and the circular permutation of the chromosome population as a whole.

A rather different mechanism for the production of new phage genomes is exhibited by phage λ in which each chromosome is identical and carries a cohesive end of 12 bases (*cos*). Immediately after infection the single-stranded sequence at each end of the chromosome anneals, and the hydrogen-bonded open circular molecule so formed is then converted into a fully double-stranded closed circle by ligation. Two replicative intermediates are now seen: bidirectional replication from an origin (*ori*) within the λ gene *O* produces 'θ' forms, analogous to the replicative intermediate of the bacterial chromosome itself, and nicking of a single strand allows synthesis of new DNA complementary to one of the 2 strands of the closed circle, the other remaining as a closed monomer ('σ' form). The λ gene P product interacts with the host replication apparatus and initiates the production of θ forms, and *O* product binds to sites with *ori*⁺ and stabilizes σ forms. Both θ and σ forms are made early during the infective process, but θ formation ceases about

16 min after infection and the σ forms continue to replicate and thereby form concatemers (the 'rolling circle' model of replication). A further contrast to T4 chromosome production is the manner in which the concatemers are converted into single chromosomes: a phage-coded **terminase** (Ter) together with host functions cleaves the concatemers at a staggered site between genes *Nu1* and *R*, thus generating identical chromosomes with single-stranded ends (see below). For further reading see Herskowitz and Hagen (1980) and Feiss (1986).

The λ scheme of replication resembles that of single-stranded DNA phages such as φX174 which are injected into the cell as closed circular chromosomes. The first event after infection is acquisition by the chromosome of a complementary strand of DNA, synthesized by host functions, to generate a double-stranded replicative form. The latter now replicates by a rolling circle mechanism, but instead of formation of a concatemer the replication cycle terminates after each daughter chromosome is produced (Fig. 10.20). After about 25 min the single-stranded products of this replication reaction, instead of acting as precursors of further rolling circles, are now packaged into phage heads (see Arai et al. 1981 and Denhardt 1994 for further details). Phage M13 also replicates via a double-stranded intermediate, a feature which has been exploited in its use as a cloning vector (p. 285).

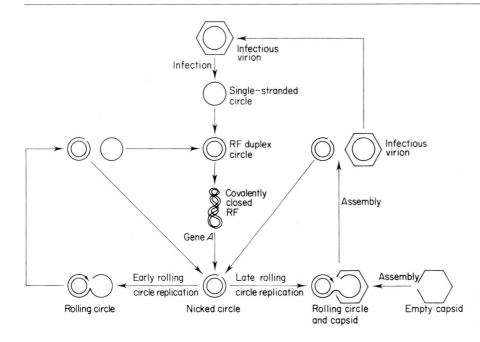

Fig. 10.20 The stages of φX174 replication. See text for details.

One system of special interest is that of the *E. coli* phage Mu which, because of its ability to integrate at perhaps any site in the bacterial chromosome, behaves as a transposon (p. 239). Mu has c. 38 kb of linear double-stranded DNA, which replicates by repeated transposition events in each of which a phage genome at one insertion site is copied at a new site, thus increasing the number of overall copies in the host chromosome by one each time. On maturation, phage DNA copies from each chromosomal site, together with short host sequences, are excised and packaged (Daniell, Kohne and Abelson 1975; see DuBow 1994b).

RNA REPLICATION

Whereas the genomes of RNA animal retroviruses replicate by reverse transcription of their RNA into DNA, which itself replicates and is then transcribed into RNA molecules that are packaged as daughter viruses, RNA phage molecules replicate directly. The single-stranded RNA of the closely related coliphages R17, f2 and MS2, and also of Qβ, itself codes for the gene products and is conventionally known as the '+' (plus) strand. How is it determined, therefore, whether this RNA molecule is to be replicated or translated into phage gene products? The first step is for the '+' strand to act as a template for the formation of a complementary '−' (minus) strand. This is mediated by the phage RNA replicase which binds at the start of the coat cistron: the 3′ end of the viral RNA now also binds at this point and the new '−' strand begins to be synthesized (Fig. 10.21). The '−' strands so synthesized then themselves act as templates for the synthesis of daughter '+' strands. This strategy ensures that the coat cistron itself cannot be translated; for translation to occur the '+' strand must assume a different conformation. A general account of the single-stranded RNA phages is given by van Duin (1994). φR73 of *E. coli* is unusual in behaving as a retroelement and integrates into a tRNA gene (Inouye et al. 1991).

DNA RECOMBINATION

One other activity of phage DNA during the period of intracellular development is genetic recombination, in which 2 molecules of phage DNA can break and rejoin in new combinations. This has the consequence that if a cell is infected simultaneously with 2 phage particles of different genotype, say A−B+ and A+B− , the lysate can be expected to contain some daughter phages of genotype A+B+ and A−B−.

Phages differ greatly in the number of rounds of breakage and rejoining that they can undergo during a single lytic cycle: phage T4 can undergo on average 5 rounds but λ less than one (Wollman and Jacob 1954). The immediate products of recombination of the single-stranded DNA phage f1 are one molecule of parental and one of recombinant genotype, for which a model has been proposed by Boon and Zinder (1969). Ritchie (1983) gave a detailed account of phage recombination and its use in genetic mapping. Phage chromosomes, and in particular the closed circular replicative forms of single-stranded phages such as φX174, have proved to be of great value in elucidating by electron microscopy the steps catalysed by individual enzymes in vitro (Dressler and Potter 1982).

Phage T4 has a recombination gene, *uvsX*, which codes for a product of 43 kDa. This gene has some sequence similarity to the *E. coli recA* gene to which it appears to be analogous (Fujisawa, Yonesaki and Minagawa 1985). The minimum degree of homology between the 2 recombining pieces of DNA must be about 50 bp but there is also a second, less efficient, pathway (Singer et al. 1982). Damage to an infecting molecule of T4 DNA stimulates the recombination process, allowing an increased likelihood of rescue of genes by another phage (Bernstein 1987). The genetics of recombination is particularly well understood in phage λ, which codes for 2 independent systems, *red* (recombination-deficient) which determines general recombination between λ chromosomes and is formally similar to the *E. coli rec* system, and *int* (integrase), which is primarily responsible for integration of λ prophage into its host chromosome during

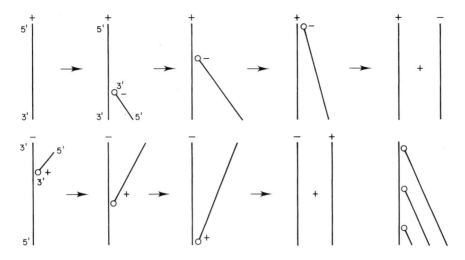

Fig. 10.21 Replication of RNA phage. The infecting viral strand (+) is used as a template for synthesis of a complementary '–' strand in a reaction catalysed by RNA replicase (○). Further '+' strands are then synthesized on '–' strands. All new strands are synthesized in the 5' to 3' direction. The diagram at bottom right shows how several progeny strands may be replicated simultaneously.

lysogeny, although *int* will also mediate recombination between 2 λ chromosomes by allowing crossing over specifically at their chromosomal attachment sites (see Fig. 10.22 for map). There are 3 *red* genes: *exo* determines an exonuclease; *bet* determines β protein, which binds to exonuclease and promotes DNA renaturation; and *gam* (γ) determines a protein that inactivates the exonuclease activity of the host RecBCD protein. This interaction between phage and host recombination systems is of special interest because there are several chi sites (χ) in the λ chromosome that react either with RecBCD itself or with another protein in its recombination pathway and act as 'hot spots' for generalized recombination (Smith 1983). An example of the reverse type of interaction is given by prophage P1 which has a function that stimulates generalized recombination of the *E. coli* chromosome.

Recombination has not been reported in the minute single-stranded RNA phages. There is no reason to believe, however, that the double-stranded RNA phage φ6, the genome of which is split into 3 'chromosomes', might not undergo a process analogous to the chromosome reassortment found in higher organisms.

PHAGE MAPS

Phage genetic maps can be prepared by co-infecting a host cell with 2 parental phage stocks carrying different mutational sites (**2-factor crosses**); sites that are very close to each other on the 2 chromosomes (**closely linked**) will give rise to fewer recombinants than those further apart. Maps derived from such crosses are liable to several sources of error: the first phage chromosome to enter the cell may inhibit the second with which it is intended that recombination should occur (**exclusion**), and the number of recombinants between distant markers may be lower than expected because of multiple crossovers and other effects (**negative interference**). These problems can be partly offset by including a third marker in the cross (**3-factor crosses**) but unequivocal ordering of sites can be achieved only by **deletion mapping**. Using such techniques, it is possible to deduce the order of both the genes on the chromosome and of individual mutational sites within them. T2 and T4 phages have circular maps because of the circular permutation of their chromosome populations, and λ has a linear genetic map because it has a unique linear chromo-

some; the gene order of the latter becomes altered, however, on transition to the integrated prophage state during lysogeny (p. 279).

An alternative approach to analysis of the phage chromosome is to make use of the sensitivity of specific sites to restriction endonucleases (**physical mapping**). Treatment with one or a combination of type II endonucleases yields a series of fragments of specific length, thus locating the position of the cleavage sites within the DNA, and the genes carried by the individual fragments can then be identified. Physical mapping has the great advantage over genetic mapping of being carried out entirely in vitro and therefore of being insusceptible to the various sources of biological error associated with the latter. Detailed correlations between genetic and physical maps are now available for several phages (O'Brien 1987).

GENE EXPRESSION

After host cells are infected with DNA, phages such as T4 production of bacterial RNA ceases: phage messenger RNA begins to be made and can be shown to hybridize to the phage DNA (Mathews 1977, Rabussay and Geiduschek 1977). The enzymes already present in the host cell remain active, however, and the host's own ribosomes are available for translation of the phage mRNA. The timing of expression of the functions for which this mRNA codes is strictly controlled: 2 broad classes are distinguished – genes coding for **early proteins** (enzymes involved in subsequent steps in phage production) and those coding for **late proteins**, which are structural components of the phage itself. Genes determining lysis are expressed last of all.

The most important factor controlling gene expression is the structure of the DNA-dependent RNA polymerase that transcribes the phage DNA. The general structure of this enzyme is $\alpha_2\beta\beta'\sigma$, in which α, β and σ are component polypeptide chains. The role of the σ polypeptide is to confer specificity of recognition of the appropriate promoters in the DNA to be transcribed: that of the uninfected host is the product of the *rpoD*+ gene and is written σ_h to indicate that it recognizes promoters in host (bacterial) DNA. RNA polymerase containing this subunit is capable of reading the promoters for the earliest expressed phage genes (**immediate**

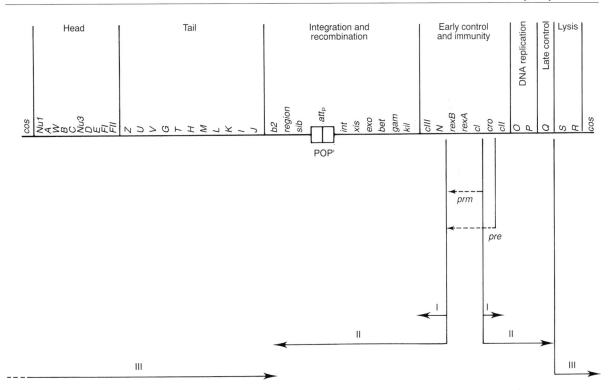

Fig. 10.22 Gene map of phage λ. Broken arrows: mode of transcription of gene *cI* during establishment (lower arrow) and maintenance (upper arrow) of lysogeny. Solid arrows: groupings of genes ('sets') during transcription in the lytic cycle; note that the DNA is circularized by joining of the 2 cohesive ends (*cos*), so that genes *R* and *Nu1* are contiguous and set III is transcribed as a single grouping. (After Herskowitz 1974, with permission). Map not to scale, and some genes are omitted. See O'Brien (1987) for comprehensive map.

early). Further genes (**delayed early**) are transcribed from the same promoters but are not expressed until the immediate early genes have been read; among these are sequences coding for a new factor, σ_e (the product of the T4 *motA*[+], *motB*[+] and *motC*[+] genes), which associates with the α and β RNA polymerase polypeptides to form a new polymerase, $\alpha_2\beta\beta'\sigma_e$; this modified polymerase no longer recognizes promoters in the host DNA, but it allows transcription of a different set of phage genes whose protein products are known as **quasi-late**. Among the quasi-late products is yet another subunit, σ_1: this is gene 55[+] product in phage T4 (Kassavetis and Geiduschek 1984) which further modifies the RNA polymerase and allows expression of the **true late** genes. Hence the production of altered σ subunits governs the range of genes that can be transcribed, and are thus available for translation, throughout the latent period. The structure and function of bacterial σ factors has been reviewed by Helmann and Chamberlin (1988); see Geiduschek (1991) for a review of regulation of phage T4 late genes.

The early functions are involved in turning off host protein synthesis and their mRNA molecules can be detected at the beginning of the latent period. The quasi-late functions, for which mRNA is found at about 2 min into the latent period, code for DNA replication (see p. 272). The true late functions, which constitute the structural components of the phage particle, are coded for by genes that lie in the genetic map in discrete clusters corresponding to operons, indicating that they are subject to a secondary type of genetic control allowing distinct expression of each individual operon (see Chapter 5 for the lactose operon, etc.). The isolation of conditional lethal mutations in these late genes has revealed the morphogenetic pathway for the assembly of phages such as T4.

The double-stranded DNA phage λ has fewer genes than T4 and the morphology of the phage particle is correspondingly simpler, but one additional feature is the controlling switch which determines whether the infecting DNA will enter a lytic or a lysogenic mode. The nature of this switch is considered below (p. 280). Expression of λ genes in the lytic mode, however, broadly resembles that of T4 in that the genes are grouped into 3 'sets' which are expressed sequentially (Fig. 10.22). Set I comprises 2 genes, *N* and *cro*, which are transcribed divergently from promoters that recognize host RNA polymerase. Set II is transcribed from the same 2 promoters but requires the gene *N* product (made as a result of set I transcription) which acts as an antiterminator at the 2 sites at which set I transcription is arrested (see Friedman and Court 1995). The set III genes, analogous to the late structural genes of T4, require the product of the set II gene *Q* for transcription, possibly again as an antiterminator. As with T4 there are subsidiary levels of control within the sets, but λ does not form modified RNA polymerase subunits (Herskowitz 1974, Herskowitz and Hagen 1980).

The genome of single-stranded RNA phages not only acts as messenger for translation into gene products but is also replicated directly into daughter RNA molecules; the latter process entails blocking of the start region of the coat cistron by the phage RNA replicase. Regions of intrastrand base complementarity in the RNA molecule also allow it to assume a partially duplex secondary structure, in which the ribosome-binding site at the start of the coat cistron lies in an exposed position although the start regions of the maturation and replicase genes are occluded. As translation of the coat gene proceeds, the duplex regions are opened up and the other genes can now be translated, but the coat protein molecules can themselves bind to the RNA specifically at the replicase gene start site, thus repressing replicase production late in the infective cycle. Hence the single-stranded RNA phages regulate their expression according to the conformation assumed by the genome, and both coat protein and replicase can bind to the start of the cistron for each other.

11.4   Packaging of the genome and particle assembly

Both T4 and λ form a long strand of DNA (concatemer) consisting of repeated genomes. The DNA of phage T4 is run into the head linearly and unidirectionally from one end such that each head contains slightly more than one complete genome (the 'headful' hypothesis), hence the finding that each chromosome has a terminal redundancy in its DNA (p. 269; Fig. 10.16). Once the first head is filled the concatemer is cut and the second head begins to be filled, beginning at the new leading end of the concatemer, which in turn explains the circular permutation of the chromosome population as a whole. It is probable that the DNA that enters the head first is anchored to the proximal apex of the head at protein p20 and is then deposited at the centre of the capsid, being pumped in enzymically by proteins p20 and p17, which induce torsion in the DNA; this same end is ejected first when the daughter phage subsequently infects a host cell itself (Black and Silverman 1978).

This method of head filling differs from that of λ where all the chromosomes are identical. Mature chromosomes are generated by the terminase (Ter) function (see p. 274), which cleaves sites known as *cos* (for 'cohesive end') in the concatemer to leave 12 base single-stranded complementary ends; *cos* lies between genes *R* and *Nu1* so that each chromosome has these genes at either end. Terminase is coded for by the phage genes *A* and *Nu1*; **termination host factor** (THF) and **integration host factor** (IHF) are also required and the binding sites for these products in the cleaved region have been defined (Feiss 1986, Gold and Parris 1986, Murialdo et al. 1987, Higgins, Lucko and Becker 1988, Murialdo 1991). The mode of packaging the chromosome inside the λ head seems to vary from one particle to another (Harrison 1983, Widom and Baldwin 1983).

It is appropriate to conclude with a comment about the filamentous single-stranded DNA phages because their head structure so evidently differs from the other phages discussed here. The DNA and the capsid protein both assemble on the inner membrane of the host cell, and the hydrophobic protein then forms an α-helical tube around the helical DNA (Marvin and Wachtel 1975). See Black (1989) for a general review of DNA packaging.

11.5   Release of daughter particles

The final stage in the infective cycle of a phage is often the release by lysis of particles to the environment. This is achieved by disruption of the cell envelope by one or more late-expressed phage functions. The genetic activities responsible for lysis have been identified in several phages. Many T phages code for an endolysin (*e*+ gene product) and T4 (Poteete and Hardy 1994) has a further gene (*t*+) that blocks energy coupling in the inner membrane, apparently allowing the endolysin to make contact with the cell wall peptidoglycan (Josslin 1971, Ritchie 1983). Phage λ has 3 genes: *S*+ codes for a polypeptide of 85 kDa that causes cell death and renders the inner membrane permeable; *R*+ codes for a transglycosylase that is also required for lysis; and *Rz*+ facilitates lysis by acting on the outer membrane. φX174 has a single gene, *E*+, that is necessary and sufficient for lysis and whose product resembles that of λ gene *S*+ (Altman et al. 1985). The L protein of the single-stranded RNA phage f2, which is read in the same phase as maturation protein but in a phase different from coat protein and RNA replicase, is implicated in lysis (Beremand and Blumenthal 1979). The mechanism and regulation of phage lysis have been reviewed by Young (1992).

Cells infected with an excessively large number of particles may undergo immediate killing and lysis without production of daughter phage particles, a process ascribed to rapid digestion of the cell envelope by the attached particles that is known as **lysis from without**. The filamentous DNA phages emerge through the cell envelope by budding, entailing release from the infected cell over a period of time and in this respect resembling the viruses of eukaryotes.

12   THE LYSOGENIC CYCLE

12.1   Temperate bacteriophage and prophage

Phages undergo several possible fates following host infection. These frequently entail self-propagation by means of nucleic acid replication and lysis, but some can establish, at low frequency, a latent mode of infection in which the injected nucleic acid replicates together with the host genes for several generations without major metabolic consequences for the cell. Such cells show few, if any, differences from uninfected cells (their cell division frequency, for instance, is identical or similar) but the phage genes in this state may occasionally revert to the lytic cycle, leading to the release of phage particles. This property is known as **lysogeny**, and phages that can develop both lytically and lysogenically are said to be **temperate** (cf. **virulent** phages such as T4 which develop only lytically). When in the latent state the phage genome is known as **prophage**.

The property of lysogeny was originally detected

when cultures of lysogenic bacteria (**lysogens**) were cross-plated with sensitive uninfected cells; occasional plaques were formed by phage particles released from lysogens that had reverted to the lytic cycle. Such sensitive cultures are sometimes termed **indicator bacteria**. Many wild-type strains can be shown to be lysogenic in this way and some may be found to contain the latent genomes of several temperate phages. The best studied examples are phages λ and P1 in *E. coli* and P22 in *S.* Typhimurium; a strain lysogenized with P22, for example, is represented as *S.* Typhimurium (P22). The frequency with which a phage in the lysogenic state can revert to the lytic cycle is in some cases greatly increased by induction with UV light, mitomycin C, or other agents.

In addition to the occasional acquisition of new properties by a lysogenized cell that can be ascribed to the presence of prophage (see section 12.6, p. 281), all lysogens are immune to further productive infection by phage of the type that has already lysogenized them (**superinfection immunity**). This important property has the consequence that plaques formed by temperate phages (Fig. 10.23) have turbid centres; the edge of each plaque is clear because most cells undergo lytic infection, but among the cells infected in the centre, earlier in the life of the plaque, a few cells will have been lysogenized and will form visible microcolonies.

12.2 The relation between prophage and its host cell

Phages that establish lysogeny are in all respects identical to those that may be released many cell generations later by spontaneous lysis or by induction: the genetic information in prophage is the same as that of the parent phage. Prophages differ, however, in their mode of association with the host; 2 types of association are known:

1 The prophage is a low copy number plasmid (p. 250), replicating independently of the bacterial chromosome. This is illustrated by phage P1 (Ikeda and Tomizawa 1968).

2 The prophage integrates into the bacterial chromosome by reciprocal crossing over, replicating passively with the chromosome. Phage λ can integrate in this manner into a preferred site between the genes for galactose and biotin metabolism, although if this site is deleted a number of secondary sites may be used at a lower frequency. Mutants of λ that form plasmid-like prophage of type 1, above, have been isolated (Matsubara and Kaiser 1968), and a number of phages showing strong similarities to λ are known as 'lambdoid' (Campbell and Botstein 1983). The *E. coli* phage P2 can integrate at several sites although a single one is preferred. Phage Mu can probably integrate into any site within DNA; it replicates by accumulating copies of its own genome in the bacterial chromosome (p. 240). There is therefore a spectrum of rigour in requirement for the site of inser-

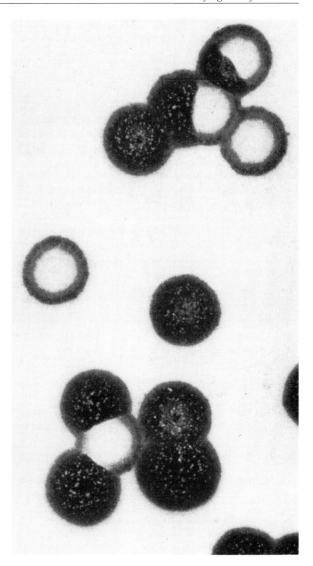

Fig. 10.23 Plaques formed by phage λ and 2 of its mutants. Wild-type λ forms turbid-centred plaques; one of the clear-plaque mutants allows no bacterial growth in the centre of its plaque, and the other does so. (Reproduced, with permission, from Weigle 1953).

tion by such phages that resembles that of transposons.

The mechanism by which the phage λ genome integrates into the *E. coli* chromosome has been investigated intensively. The first event after injection of λ DNA into the cell is that the 12 base single-stranded complementary ends of the phage chromosome anneal with one another, and the open circle so formed is ligated into closed circular DNA. Reciprocal crossing over can now occur between a region within the prophage DNA and one within the bacterial chromosome (Campbell 1962; the 'Campbell model' of integration, Fig. 10.24). Reversion of a cell from the lysogenic to the lytic state requires excision, a process in which the integration event is essentially reversed. The process differs from the normal type of genetic recombination event in 2 respects. First, it is catalysed by the product of the phage *int*⁺ gene, integrase, a 40.3 kDa polypeptide with topoisomerase (nicking and closing) activity on DNA, and also by a host product, IHF (see Nash 1990 for a review of topological events at the attachment site). The excision reaction also requires integrase and a further phage-coded product, excisase, formed by the λ *xis⁺* gene. Second, the degree of homology between the prophage and the bacterial chromosome attachment site extends to only 15 bases; to either side of this lie 2 larger but non-homologous regions. Bauer et al. (1986) identified several distinct binding sites for integrase, IHF and excisase by site-directed mutagenesis, and Kitts and Nash (1987) analysed in detail the location of the sites of crossing over. The secondary integration sites that λ can use with low efficiency if its primary site is deleted are, as might be expected, partly homologous with the primary site; see Campbell (1992) for a discussion of prophage insertion sites.

A site-specific recombination system designated Cre, which catalyses recombination between 2 sites of 34 bases (*lox*), has been described in phage P1 (Abremski, Hoess and Sternberg 1983, Hoess, Wierzbicki and Abremski 1987). Kilby, Snaith and Murray (1993) give an account of site-specific recombination enzymes.

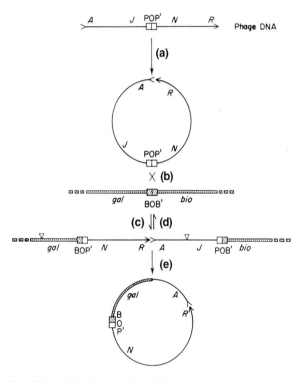

Fig. 10.24 The Campbell model for prophage λ integration into the bacterial chromosome. (a) Circularization of λ DNA by attachment of cohesive ends (arrows) followed by ligation. (b and c) Integration by site-specific recombination between phage (POP′) and host (BOB′) attachment regions; 4 phage genes (*A, J, N, R*) and 2 host gene clusters (*gal, bio*) are shown for reference, and phage integrase (*int⁺* product) and integration host factor (IHF) are required. Note that the prophage genes are permuted relative to those in the phage DNA. (d) Normal excision: integrase and excisase (*xis⁺* product) are required. (e) Abnormal excision, by recombination between 2 points (▽) other than the attachment regions, generating a defective λ particle carrying host *gal* genes (see p. 282 of text for specialized transducing particles); a particle carrying *bio* genes can be formed similarly.

12.3 Superinfection immunity

Temperate phages form plaques that are characteristically turbid-centred because of the immunity of lysogenized cells to lytic infection by further adsorbing particles; such cells grow to form microcolonies within the plaque. Early in the study of λ lysogeny it was noticed that a few plaques lacked this central zone of turbidity (Weigle 1953) (see Fig. 10.23); mutants forming such plaques were designed *c* (for clear plaque) and the *c* mutations were found to lie in one of 3 phage genes, *cI, cII, cIII*. Of these 3, the *cI* gene has the most clearly understood role. *cI⁺* codes for an acidic protein of 30 kDa known as the **immunity substance** or **immunity repressor**; it recognizes and binds to sites within 2 operator regions, o_L and o_R, that govern expression of the leftward- and rightward-transcribed set I genes (Fig. 10.22), respectively; these include the *cro⁺* gene which is required for activation of the lytic cycle. Hence in a cell in which *cI⁺* product is expressed, the set I genes are repressed and the lytic cycle does not develop, Moreover, the *cI⁺* product can bind to the set I operator sites of any superinfecting λ, blocking their expression in the same manner.

cII⁺ product specifically activates 3 promoters – those for *cI* itself, for *int* (integrase), and for an RNA fragment which has the effect of reducing expression of the late gene *Q* – functions that all favour lysogenic development (Ho, Wulff and Rosenberg 1986). *cII⁺* is regulated by the *hfl* functions of the host (Banuett and Herskowitz 1987), which in turn are regulated by *cIII⁺* product. It will therefore be apparent that although the repression of lytic growth in lysogens is in one sense a simple matter of interaction between *cI⁺* product and 2 operator regions, its control involves several interacting factors. The importance of the latter will be seen when the mechanism that switches λ into one of its 2 pathways, lysis or lysogeny, is discussed.

12.4 Reversion to the lytic cycle

Lambda lysogens, once established, are stable; spontaneous reversion to the lytic state occurs only rarely, although with sufficient frequency for extracellular particles always to be detectable in broth cultures. The frequency of reversion to the lytic cycle can be greatly increased, however, by low doses of UV light (**induction**), which have the effect of raising the level of RecA protein 17-fold within 10 min of irradiation. RecA protein is not only a key enzyme in the process of generalized recombination; it is also a coprotease and can stimulate the self-cleavage of *cI⁺* product into 2 pieces, thus abolishing the ability of the latter to act as an immunity substance. It can likewise cleave the corresponding repressor of P22 prophage and also the product of the bacterial *lexA⁺* gene which is a repressor for *recA* itself, so *recA⁺* can be regarded as a self-repressing gene.

12.5 Switching between the lytic and lysogenic pathways

The amount of cI^+ product in the lysogenized cell, and hence the level of immunity, is set by a series of controls involving both phage (cII^+, $cIII^+$) and host (hfl) functions. An important step in the establishment of lysogeny by λ is the formation of sufficient cI^+ product to block the expression of the set I genes, thereby preventing the onset of a lytic cycle. cI^+ messenger RNA can be read from 2 promoters: a cell that is in the process of becoming a lysogen reads from a promoter known as *pre* (promoter for establishment) but once lysogeny is successfully established cI^+ is read from a second promoter, *prm* (promoter for maintenance). This has an interesting consequence (see Fig. 10.22) for the *cro* region: *cro* is read either from left to right from promoter p_R as part of set I, leading to development of a lytic cycle, or it is read in the opposite direction from *pre* as part of the cI^+ transcript required for lysogeny (the 'anti-*cro*' messenger RNA made during this latter process has no known biological function). When conditions in the cell are such that this region can be transcribed in either direction the RNA polymerase molecules moving towards one another collide and further transcription is blocked (Ward and Murray 1979). Hence one aspect of switching between lysis and lysogeny centres on which of the 2 possible directions of transcription of the *cro* region prevails.

Another aspect of switching – at first sight paradoxical – concerns the structure of the operator regions o_L and o_R that bind cI^+ product and hence govern set I transcription. These regions also bind cro^+ product which, nevertheless, influences gene expression in precisely the converse manner. The paradox is resolved when the structure of o_L and o_R is examined: each consists of 3 contiguous operator sequences with different affinities for the 2 proteins (Table 10.9). Depending on which of the 2 predominates, the phage will be switched into a mode in which further production of that same protein will be enhanced.

Finally, leftward transcription of the set II genes in the lytic mode continues into the *sib* region. The messenger RNA copy of *sib* forms an intrastranded hairpin structure that acts as a binding site for ribonuclease III which cleaves the hairpin and exposes the messenger to destruction by other enzymes. Hence *sib*-bearing messenger is sequentially destroyed, beginning at *sib* and proceeding back towards the *N* region, which has the consequence that information coding for *int*+ is destroyed before that encoding *xis*+ (retroregulation). The messenger therefore produces more *xis*+ than *int*+ product and lytic gene transcription, once it reaches set II, tends to become self-reinforcing (Ptashne 1992).

The switching between lytic and lysogenic cycles appears to occur by a similar mechanism in other temperate phages. It has been discussed at some length because of its considerable influence on thinking about switching in other areas of biology and because of the importance of understanding regulatory influences on DNA–DNA and DNA–protein interactions elsewhere where, however, the molecular mechanisms may be different. The reader is referred to Echols (1986) and Ptashne (1992) for lucid accounts of experimental work on this aspect of phage behaviour.

12.6 Lysogenic conversion

With the exception of superinfection immunity, prophage usually has no obvious phenotypic effect on its carrier cell. The immunity may sometimes extend to unrelated phages (prophage interference); thus, *E. coli* (P1) will not allow lytic development of T1, T3, T7 and P2, and the *rII* mutants of T4 cannot develop in *E. coli* (λ). Such events occasionally result in the loss of surface receptors for a phage rather than production of a cytoplasmic repressor, as exemplified by λ (Schnaitman, Smith and de Salsas 1975). Sometimes, however, a lysogen shows a striking difference in comparison to its uninfected parent (**lysogenic** or **phage conversion**). Thus, it has been shown that prophage β of *Corynebacterium diphtheriae* (β) itself carries the gene for diphtheria toxin production, a situation that may be contrasted with that in which a phage transfers a bacterial gene from one cell to another (**transduction**). Toxin production by *Clostridium botulinum* strains C and D has also been ascribed to the presence of prophage. The filamentous M13-related phage φCTX of *Vibrio cholerae* codes for at least 6 genes involved in formation and expression of cholera toxin; this phage transmits the toxin gene efficiently in vivo (Waldor and Mekalanos 1996). About one-third of the phage λ genome is dispensable for normal lytic growth, yet it has been found to code for 2 virulence-associated factors expressed in the lysogenic state (*lom*,

Table 10.9 Loading of the three O_R sites of phage λ by cro^+ and cI^+ gene products

Binding of cro^+ or cI^+ product			Gene transcribed		State of cell
o_{R3}	o_{R2}	o_{R1}	cro^+	cI^+	
…	…	cI	Repressed	Stimulated	
…	cI	cI	Repressed	Stimulated	Immune;
cI	cI	cI	Repressed	Repressed	→ lysogeny
cro	…	…	Stimulated	Repressed	
cro	cro	…	Stimulated	Repressed	Anti-immune;
cro	cro	cro	Repressed	Repressed	→ lysis

The three o_R sites are designated o_{R1}, o_{R2} and o_{R3}. cI^+ product binds preferentially at o_{R1}, stimulating further cI^+ production and repressing cro^+ transcription. cro^+ product, conversely, binds preferentially at o_{R3}, stimulating further cro^+ production and repressing cI^+ transcription. A similar hierarchy of binding can be demonstrated at the 3 o_L sites.
After Takeda (1979), with permission.

homologous to some virulence proteins, and *bor*, which increases survival of the host cell in animal serum (Barondess and Beckwith 1990). Some *Salmonella* serotypes owe their O-antigenic specificities to the presence of resident prophages that convert lipopolysaccharide residues into antigenically different types (Mäkelä and Stocker 1969) so that the large number of types in this particular genus reflects phage as well as bacterial diversity. *Bacillus megaterium* undergoes a change from smooth to rough colonial form on lysogeny. Formally, the appearance of a new character as a result of lysogenic conversion is no different from that arising in consequence of acquisition of a plasmid (p. 250). Not all phage conversion events necessarily entail lysogeny; filamentous phage infection generates pIV, an integral membrane protein of *E. coli* that induces high levels of the bacterial shock protein Psp (Brissette et al. 1990).

13   TRANSDUCTION

Transduction is the transmission of a piece of host DNA from one cell (the **donor**) to another (the recipient) by a phage particle. The process has been examined chiefly in 3 phage–host systems: *S.* Typhimurium–P22, *E. coli*–P1 and *E. coli*–λ. In the first 2 of these almost any piece of host DNA can be transduced and the transduction event may be followed by crossing over in the recipient cell to yield a recombinant (**generalized transduction**). The third, however, exemplifies a quite different process in which the phage transduces only those genetic markers that are close to its prophage attachment site on the bacterial chromosome (**specialized transduction**). Generalized transducing particles are formed because of errors in the process by which phages package their DNA during replication, host genes being occasionally packaged by accident instead of phage chromosomes (see section 13.1), whereas specialized transducing particles arise because of unusual excision events in the recombination region between phage and bacterial DNA on induction of the lytic pathway. It is possible to detect instances in which generalized transducing phages themselves undergo the second type of event and form specialized transducing particles.

13.1   Generalized transduction: phage heads as carrier of bacterial genes

Phage P1 replicates during infection of its *E. coli* host cell in a manner similar to T4, i.e. by building up in the cell long concatemers of DNA that are subsequently cut into new phage chromosomes by the assembling phage particles (the 'headful' hypothesis; Fig. 10.16). Transducing particles of P1 contain a short length of the host chromosome and no detectable phage DNA at all, suggesting that some heads erroneously take in a section of bacterial rather than phage DNA during the later stages of intracellular development. Such particles are morphologically normal and are released in the lysate along with ordinary

phage particles; they can then infect fresh cells, injecting the contents of the head into the cell in the usual manner. The length of bacterial DNA transduced is similar to that of a normal phage chromosome but there is conflicting evidence as to whether particular regions of the host chromosome are preferentially transduced. A phage-infected cell has a roughly similar amount of phage DNA at the end of the latent period as there was bacterial DNA at the outset, yet only a minority of phage particles contain bacterial DNA, indicating that the head-filling process must operate more efficiently when packaging phage rather than host DNA. There may be a subsequent homologous recombination event between the transduced DNA and the recipient cell's chromosome although it is common for the transduced DNA to persist extrachromosomally in the cell without the ability to participate in later cell divisions, thus forming an abortive transductant. The frequency of transduction of any one bacterial genetic marker is around 10^{-6} per surviving recipient cell.

Insofar as generalized (and specialized) transduction depends on infection by a phage, it is usual to find that bacterial genes can be transduced only to a recipient of the same species, or perhaps even strain, as the donor; the host range of a phage is generally delimited by the presence of specific surface receptors (p. 272). Generalized transduction is not, however, a property of temperate phages alone. The lysates of even highly virulent phages such as those in the T series in *E. coli* are found to include some particles containing host DNA (Borchert and Drexler 1980, Young and Edlin 1983), but if such particles infect a recipient and establish a transductant the latter is usually killed by superinfection with other lytic particles.

Phages can also transduce plasmids, as well as fragments of the donor chromosome, provided these are sufficiently small to be contained within the phage head; where plasmids are too large for this to occur variants with partial deletions may still be transducible, a useful technique for the isolation of plasmid deletion mutants (**transductional shortening**). The transduction of antibiotic resistance plasmids in staphylococci is of great medical importance (see Chapter 27). The frequency of cotransduction of 2 plasmids in *S. aureus* is often much higher than would be expected from the likelihood of transduction of each plasmid separately, probably as a result of cointegrate formation between the 2 (Novick et al. 1981, Novick, Edelman and Lofdahl 1986).

13.2   Specialized transduction: hybrids between bacterial and phage DNA

Phage λ integrates at a specific site in the chromosome of *E. coli* by means of a recombination event mediated by *int*[+] and IHF. On induction of the lytic cycle the integration event can be reversed in the presence of an additional function, *xis*[+]. Both integration and excision are therefore highly specific with respect to the site in the DNA in which they can occur. Occasionally, however, recombination during the excision process occurs between 2 sites other than the normal attachment regions of phage and host DNA; these sites lie one within the prophage and one just outside (see Fig. 10.24, p. 280). The consequence is that a ring of DNA is excised that consists partly of λ genes and partly of host genes from one side of the attachment region. In the presence of other λ DNA molecules undergoing normal lytic replication in the cell, this hybrid DNA ring can be packaged in a λ head and released in the lysate where it is available to infect a further cell and inject into it DNA that contains some host genes. The word 'hybrid' here refers to double-stranded DNA that by virtue of a recombination event has 2 separate origins, not to DNA in which the 2 complementary polynucleotide chains come from different sources (heteroduplex DNA).

The gene clusters on the bacterial chromosome that lie closest to the λ integration site and are most easily selectable in genetic crosses are *gal* and *bio* (Fig. 10.24), and hence it is these genes that are readily found in specialized transducing particles represented as λ*gal* and λ*bio*. Lambdoid phages (Campbell 1994) are closely related to λ but many have a different host integration site and are therefore able to transduce correspondingly different genes; thus, φ80 acts as a specialized transducing phage for the tryptophan genes in *E. coli*. Less closely related phages are exemplified by P22 in *S.* Typhimurium, the prophage of which integrates within the proline genes; hence P22, which is a generalized transducing phage in *Salmonella*, is also a specialized transducing phage for the *pro* region.

The positions of the 2 sites that undergo recombination to form a specialized transducing particle differ in different isolates; the recombination event itself may be controlled by insertion sequences (p. 239) nearby. There are 2 constraints on the ability of a λ particle to form a specialized transducing particle: the recombination event must not exclude the cohesive end (*cos*) site and the total length of DNA in the particle must not significantly exceed that of wild-type λ itself to allow for packaging in the head. A consequence of the second point is that, because the particle acquires some host genes, it must lose some phage genes and hence it is often defective in formation of a particle capable of self-replication; but with the exception of this limitation on particle size, specialized transducing phage formation is closely similar to the process by which substituted plasmid such as F-primes are formed (p. 248).

Specialized transduction differs from generalized transduction in many respects: the transducible genes are limited to those near the prophage integration site and the transducing particle is a hybrid of phage and bacterial DNA rather than consisting entirely of the latter. A further distinction is that the transduced DNA is added to the genome of the recipient cell rather than replacing recipient genes as in generalized transduction of chromosomal markers; it can itself integrate into the prophage attachment site of the recipient's DNA. This has an important consequence if the transductant is subsequently induced to enter a lytic cycle. The transduced particle will then form a large number of copies (a process which may require the presence of superinfecting normal particles to supply any missing phage functions), each of which carries bacterial genes; thus if this lysate is allowed to infect a further population of sensitive cells the transduction frequency will increase about 1000-fold – **high-frequency transduction** (HFT).

14 PHAGE HOST RANGES

It is probable that all bacterial groups can be infected by phages that are adapted to them, but individual phages in general have very limited host ranges; often a phage is capable of propagation in just a single strain of a bacterial species. This is perhaps not surprising in view of the degree of dependence of any virus on its host for several metabolic functions but, despite this, phages show a ready ability to alter or extend their host range under appropriate selective conditions. It is convenient to consider the limitations that are imposed on host range under 2 headings, surface receptors and intracellular factors.

14.1 Surface receptors as host range determinants

Because the surface receptors used by phages for adsorption are dispensable structures for the host (p. 271), bacteria can easily mutate to resistance by losing the receptor concerned. This can be seen when a suspension of sensitive *E. coli* cells is infected with a virulent phage such as T2; under ideal conditions the suspension clears within a few hours because of lysis of the infected cells, but this is followed by a further phase of turbidity as resistant cells continue to multiply in the presence of the phage. A second phase of clearing may now follow owing to the selection of phage mutants able to utilize a receptor not used by the parent stock; these are designated host range mutants. It is sometimes claimed that yet further phases of turbidity and clearing may follow as resistant cells and subsequent host range mutants are selected, a process that is likely to occur continuously in an environment such as sewage (see Chapter 15) from which phages may easily be isolated and where phage and potential hosts are repeatedly interacting.

In some instances acquisition of one receptor may be associated with loss of another, either by physical masking of a cell surface grouping by one newly acquired or by a conformational change induced in the latter. Thus Burnet (1930) noted that acquisition of an O antigen resulted in loss of susceptibility of *Salmonella* to rough-specific phages, and mucoid variants may become phage-resistant by occlusion of surface factors. LPS carrying O antigen prevents the access of a number of phages to their receptors in the outer membrane (van der Ley, de Graaff and Tommassen 1986). Lysogenization with one (temperate) phage may affect the sensitivity of the host to others; it has been noted that lysogenic conversion in *Salmonella* may lead to the appearance of new O antigens. Schnaitman, Smith and de Salsas (1975) found that phage PA2 causes insertion of a new protein in the *E. coli* K12 outer membrane that apparently blocks the receptor for PA2 itself – an unusual kind of superinfection immunity. Other lysogenic conversion events by lambdoid phages in *E. coli* K12 may also be associated with new outer-membrane proteins (Poon and Dhillon 1986).

Some phages have an unusually broad host range. The rough-specific phages of the Enterobacteriaceae recognize a receptor that is widespread in the family and the pilus-specific phages can utilize as host any strain carrying the plasmid that produces the pilus concerned; conspicuous examples are phages such as PRD1 and PR4 (Bradley and Cohen 1977), which adsorb to bacteria harbouring the broad host range plasmids of incompatibility group P1. Phage Mu can alternate between 2 different hosts as a result of inversion of a genetic segment in a manner analogous to *Salmonella* flagellar phase variation. The G region of phage Mu in one orientation allows growth on *E. coli* K12; in the reverse orientation the phage propagates on *E. coli* C and *Citrobacter freundii* (van de Putte, Cramer and Giphart-Gassler 1980). The orientation of the C region of phage P1 likewise affects the ability to propagate on *E. coli* (Iida 1984).

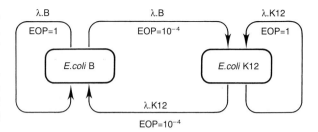

Fig. 10.25   Host-controlled restriction and modification of phage λ growing in *E. coli* strains B and K12. EOP, efficiency of plating.

14.2   Intracellular factors in host range determination

One of the intracellular factors that affects phage host range is superinfection immunity (p. 279): a host cell carrying a prophage cannot be lytically infected by a further particle responsive to the immunity repression system of the prophage. Related phages such as the lambdoid series may differ in chromosomal integration site but share the operators responding to a single repressor; these are therefore affected by each other's immunity system and are described as **homo-immune** or **co-immune**.

A second intracellular factor is related to the presence of specific endonucleases, commonly known as restriction enzymes, in the host cell. When phage λ is propagated on *E. coli* K12, the resulting lysate plates on another strain such as *E. coli* B with an efficiency of only about 0.01%, but the few plaques that form on B contain particles that plate with about 100% efficiency on that strain. Exactly the converse phenomenon occurs when particles from B are plated back on K12; the efficiency of plating again falls to around 0.01% but the particles now formed plate with high efficiency on K12 (Fig. 10.25). Hence λ evidently adapts to its host strain: it can propagate with high efficiency on K12 or B, but not on both. The reason is that K12 and B specify different restriction endonucleases that cleave the incoming λ DNA at specific sites and thereby restrict its host range. Both the DNA of the host and that of the minority of particles that succeed in establishing infection are protected by the presence of methyl groupings at sites on the DNA that inhibit the cleavage reaction of the endonuclease, a process known as **modification**. Hence the phage's host range is altered by a mechanism that is independent of mutational changes in the base sequence of its DNA.

Restriction and modification may be regarded as complementary processes whereby a host cell on the one hand protects itself against invading DNA and, on the other, the invading DNA evades the defence. Some restriction and modification activities (type I) are subunits of a single enzyme that recognizes DNA at a specific site and, if that site is not already methylated, either adds a methyl group or (more frequently) cleaves the DNA at a distinct site nearby. Other activities (type II) are mediated by independent proteins, each of which recognizes and cuts or methylates the

same DNA sequence. A considerable number of type II restriction nucleases have now been isolated from different bacterial groups and are exploited for specific DNA cleavage reactions employed in genetic modification procedures. The reader is referred to Old and Primrose (1989) for a full account.

Some prophages such as P1 themselves code for restriction and modification systems which are thus superimposed on the cellular system of the host they lysogenize. Furthermore, phage T2 can undergo a type of modification dependent on glucosylation rather than methylation (Adams 1959). Phage Mu has a modification (*mom*[+]) function that converts adenine to acetoadenine, when in a specific sequence, thereby protecting the DNA against several type I and II systems (Toussaint 1976). Other host genes that inhibit the development of particular phages have been described (see Guarneros et al. 1987). Several elements, including some prophages, kill their host cell after infection by other phages, hence blocking propagation of the latter (Snyder 1995).

A consequence of host range variation is that phage lines may be derived that grow specifically on a single strain of a host species. Phages may be used in this way (**phage typing**) to discriminate between bacterial strains that would be difficult to distinguish by other means for epidemiological purposes. The use of phage for this purpose is examined in section 15.

15   **PRACTICAL IMPORTANCE**

15.1   **Use as research tools**

The importance of phage in basic biological studies is very great. The deduction of the triplet nature of the genetic code (Crick et al. 1961) might have been delayed for many years without the availability of frameshift mutants in the *r*II region of phage T4 and the resulting simplicity of observation of recombinant phenotypes. The *r*II region was also used by Benzer (1955) for fine structure analysis and development of the complementation (*cis–trans*) test. Such work was so fundamental to present-day genetic studies that its importance is easily overlooked. The integration mechanism whereby prophage λ inserts into the *E. coli* chromosome is a model for DNA–DNA and DNA–protein interactions generally and has also stimulated thinking on the intracellular state of eukaryotic retroviruses.

15.2 Phages as vectors for genetic modification

Phages and genetically modified variants are used extensively as vectors in genetic modification (cloning) experiments in *E. coli* and other organisms. Genetic modification is undertaken for 2 primary purposes: to allow the isolation of a desired fragment of DNA in quantities suitable for sequencing or related studies, and to enable the experimenter to insert a known gene into a cellular environment suitable for formation of its product in large amounts. The 2 phages that have proved the most useful in this respect are the single-stranded DNA phage M13 and the double-stranded DNA phage λ.

Phage M13 has a 6.4 kb genome in which a 507 base intergenic region can be used for the introduction of up to 1.5 kb of cloned material. The great value of this particular phage is that, although it replicates as a double-stranded element that can be introduced by transfection into a host cell in the same manner as in plasmid transformation (p. 246), its DNA when packaged is single-stranded – an ideal element for DNA sequencing and some mutagenesis procedures in vitro. It is beyond the scope of this chapter to discuss the design of cloning vectors in detail but the procedure entails:

1. introducing a functional *lacZ* gene into the 507 base region available for cloning, thus forming the derivative M13mp1, which forms blue plaques on a suitable indicator medium (X-gal agar)
2. introducing an *Eco*RI site at one end of the *lacZ* gene into which the desired DNA will be cloned (derivative M13mp2) and
3. introducing into this *Eco*RI site a polylinker, a short DNA sequence consisting of additional endonuclease-sensitive cloning sites arranged symmetrically.

Depending on the complexity of the polylinker the DNA to be cloned into the phage vector can have 2 different 'cohesive ends' (p. 273); vectors are often available in pairs, each member of the pair having the polylinker in reverse orientation, a useful feature that facilitates the sequencing of a cloned fragment of DNA from both ends. Hybrid plasmid–M13 vectors ('phagemids') are also available that allow for cloning of DNA fragments of increased size. For a fuller account see Brown (1995).

Phage λ has a much larger genome (52 kb) than does M13 and, by deleting the inessential integration functions and also material in the b2 region (see Fig. 10.22, p. 277), it is possible to accommodate up to 25 kb of cloned DNA. One consequence of the large genome size is that there are several copies of all the common restriction endonuclease cut sites, so a further step in the design of a cloning vector is to remove all but one or 2 of each; this is accomplished by in vitro mutagenesis and also by selection of variants grown in a host that forms the endonuclease concerned. Two types of λ vector are in common use. **Insertion** vectors have a unique site (usually *Eco*RI) into which the DNA is cloned, thus inactivating the gene in which the site lies and allowing detection of the vector whose gene is inactivated; λ NM607 has such a site within the *cI*⁺ gene which, when inactivated, eliminates the immunity function and gives clear plaques, and λ Charon 16 has a functional *lacZ* gene (see above for the use of this detection system in M13). In replacement vectors there are 2 endonuclease-sensitive sites and the region lying between

them is replaced by the material to be cloned (e.g. λWES. λB′, λEMBL4). The efficiency of the subsequent transfection step can be improved by utilizing a packaging procedure in vitro rather than introducing the entire vector molecule into its host. The ultimate development of λ as a cloning agent is the **cosmid**: this is a hybrid between λ and a plasmid in which λ contributes the region containing its cohesive ends and the plasmid supplies an origin of DNA replication together with a gene suited to allowing selection of the desired clone. Cosmids do not contain the λ material needed for DNA replication and particle maturation and hence there is room for far more DNA to be cloned (up to about 40 kb); they have been used to construct **genomic libraries** of several organisms, a set of recombinant clones that between them contain all the DNA present in an individual organism.

Among the phages specific to other organisms the λ-like φC31 of *Streptomyces* has been used as the progenitor of several cloning vectors (see Pritchard and Holland 1985, Brown 1995b).

15.3 Phages in industrial processes and the environment

Douglas (1975) and Sanders (1994) have noted a number of instances in which phage infection of bacteria used in economically important processes is sufficiently troublesome to call for preventive measures. Thus, starter cultures of lactic streptococci in cheese-making (see also Chapter 16) are susceptible to phage attack (Relano et al. 1987), requiring the use either of mixed starter cultures or of calcium-free medium (most of the phages involved are calcium-dependent). Some actinomycetes used in the production of antibiotics are also reported as liable to phage attack. It has been suggested that treatment with phage might on occasion be a useful adjunct in water purification.

Proctor and Fuhrman (1990) have reported high counts of phage in marine studies and have found that up to 7% of heterotrophic bacteria and 5% of cyanobacteria from diverse marine locations contained mature phage, suggesting that phage may be a significant cause of mortality and perhaps of gene transfer in the ocean (see also Bergh et al. 1989).

15.4 Phages as therapeutic agents

The suggestion that pathogenic bacteria might be susceptible to a lytic agent was an important motive for the pioneering experiments of Twort (1915) and d'Herelle (1917) that led to the discovery of bacteriophage. Much research was done in the early years on the possibility of using phages in antibacterial therapy but the results were disappointing, either because of the high immunogenicity of the phage particles or their lability in physiological conditions such as low stomach pH, and interest subsided with the introduction of antibiotics (see Wilson and Miles 1975 for a discussion). Nevertheless, the problems associated with antibiotic therapy have directed the thoughts of some workers once again towards the possibility of an inexpensive and non-toxic approach to bacterial infections. Smith and Huggins (1983) found that calves inoculated with a potentially lethal strain of *E. coli*, B44, were protected by ingestion of a mixture of 2 phages (B44/1 and B44/2); phage-resistant mutants arising during the course of the infection were less virulent than B44, probably because of mutational loss of K antigens, and these observations have been extended to other enteropathogenic strains and to the factors influencing phage survival in vivo (Smith, Huggins and Shaw 1987a, 1987b).

15.5   Phage typing: the use of phage in epidemiological studies

Although the value of phages in controlling bacterial infections did not fulfil early expectations their use in epidemiological typing of bacteria (phage typing) has been highly successful. The principle of phage typing is that the limited host range of many phages enables them to be used to discriminate between bacterial strains that are serologically or biochemically distinguishable with difficulty or not at all, so that the distribution and spread of a pathogen within the community can be studied. The technique, which has been applied especially to *Salmonella* and to *S. aureus*, entails lawning a petri dish with the bacterial strain to be tested (or, in the case of more dangerous organisms, placing single droplets on the dish) and adding spots of each member of a set of typing phages. The pattern of lysis after incubation establishes the phage type of the bacterial strain.

An advantage of phage typing over other methods of subdividing bacterial species is its great simplicity: it is necessary to note only the presence or absence of phage plaques. Nevertheless, the organism must be divisible into an adequate number of types and several criteria must be observed in order to ensure reproducibility of results. The phages and any other reagents to be used should be stable; phages are used at concentrations that best reveal their specificity (the **routine test dilution**, RTD), and the titre of each is measured shortly before the test is carried out. Typing is frequently carried out in national centres where several strains can be typed in a single standard screening to improve comparability.

The typing phages used for *S.* Typhi are all derivatives of Vi phage II which use the Vi antigen as receptor and are adapted to replicate in different strains. One strain (type A) is sensitive to all the adapted phage preparations; the adaptations may reflect host-controlled variation, host range mutation, or both. The original scheme of Craigie and Yen (1938) has since been extended to several strains, and similar typing schemes have been devised for *Salmonella* serotypes Enteritidis, Paratyphi B, Typhimurium, Dublin and other salmonellae, allowing, for instance, discrimination between strains that may have caused infection as a result of breakdown of sanitation in the patient's country of residence and those brought in as a result of infection while travelling abroad. Schemes for coagulase-positive staphylococci, which require typing because of their propensity to cause cross-infection in hospitals, utilize a set of independently isolated phages and the staphylococcal strains are designated according to the spectrum of phages to which they are sensitive: as strains encountered in clinical practice develop resistance to a particular phage, that phage is replaced in the set used for typing by another which gives better discrimination. A random sample of 221 epidemiologically distinct strains of *S. aureus* isolated from humans (Adams 1959) yielded 169 different patterns of lysis. Isolates of *S. aureus* from bovine mastitis or septic lesions in dogs require other sets of phages distinct from each other and also from those used for typing human isolates. Adams (1959) discusses the theoretical and practical background to early schemes and Kasatiya and Nicolle (1978) give a comprehensive list of bacteria for which schemes have been devised, noting those for which international agreement has been obtained (see also DuBow 1994a).

REFERENCES

Abraham JM, Freitag CS et al., 1985, An invertible element of DNA controls phase variation of type 1 fimbriae of *Escherichia coli*, *Proc Natl Acad Sci USA*, **82**: 5724–7.

Abremski K, Hoess R, Sternberg N, 1983, Studies on the properties of P1 site-specific recombination: evidence for topologically unlinked products following recombination, *Cell*, **32**: 1301–11.

Adams MH, 1959, *Bacteriophages*, Interscience, New York.

Altman E, Young K et al., 1985, Subcellular localization of lethal lysis proteins of bacteriophages lambda and φX174, *J Virol*, **53**: 1008–11.

Ames BW, 1979, Identifying environmental chemicals causing mutations and cancer, *Science*, **204**: 587–93.

Ames BW et al., 1973, Carcinogens are mutagens: a simple test system combining liver homogenates for inactivation and bacteria for detection, *Proc Natl Acad Sci USA*, **70**: 2281–5.

Amyes SGB, 1986, Epidemiology of trimethoprim resistance, *J Antimicrob Chemother*, **18, Suppl. C**: 215–21.

Amyes SGB, Towner KJ, 1990, Trimethoprim resistance – epidemiology and molecular aspects, *J Med Microbiol*, **31**: 1–19.

Anderson ES, 1968, The ecology of transferable drug resistance in the Enterobacteria, *Annu Rev Microbiol*, **22**: 131–80.

Arai K-I, Arai N et al., 1981, Enzyme studies of φX175 recombination, *Prog Nucleic Acid Res Mol Biol*, **26**: 9–32.

Archer GL, Niemeyer DM, 1994, Origin and evolution of DNA associated with resistance to methicillin in staphylococci, *Trends Microbiol*, **2**: 343–7.

Arthur A, Sherratt D, 1979, Dissection of the transposition process: a transposon-encoded site-specific recombination system, *Mol Gen Genet*, **175**: 267–74.

Arthur M, Courvalin P, 1993, Genetics and mechanisms of glycopeptide resistance in enterococci, *Antimicrob Agents Chemother*, **37**: 1563–71.

Austin S, Abeles A, 1983, Partion of unit-copy miniplasmids to daughter cells 1. P1 and F miniplasmids contain discrete, interchangeable sequences sufficient to promote equipartition, *J Mol Biol*, **169**: 353–72.

Austin S, Ziese M, Sternberg N, 1981, A novel role for site-specific recombination in maintenance of bacterial replicons, *Cell*, **25**: 729–36.

Avery OT, MacLeod CM, McCarty M, 1944, Studies on the chemical nature of the substance inducing transformation of pneumococcal types, *J Exp Med*, **79**: 137–57.

Avila P, de la Cruz F, 1988, Physical and genetic map of the IncW plasmid R388, *Plasmid*, **20**: 155–7.

Baas P, Jansz H, 1988, Single-stranded DNA phage origins, *Curr Topics Microbiol Immunol*, **136**: 31–70.

Bale MJ, Fry JC, Day MJ, 1987, Plasmid transfer between strains of *Pseudomonas aeruginosa* on membrane filters attached to river stones, *J Gen Microbiol*, **133**: 3099–107.

Bamford DH, 1994, φ6 Bacteriophage, *Encyclopedia of Virology*, eds Webster RG, Granoff A, Academic Press, London, 978–80.

Bamford JKH, Bamford DH, 1990, Capsomer proteins of bacteriophage PRD1, a bacterial virus with a membrane, *Virology*, **177**: 445–51.

Banuett F, Herskowitz I, 1987, Identification of polypeptides encoded by an *Escherichia coli* locus (*hflA*) that governs the lysis-lysogeny decision of bacteriophage lambda, *J Bacteriol*, **169**: 4076–85.

Barondess JJ, Beckwith J, 1990, A bacterial virulence determinant encoded by lysogenic coliphage lambda, *Nature (London)*, **346**: 871–4.

Barth PT, Tobin L, Sharpe GS, 1981, Development of broad host-range vectors, *Molecular Biology, Pathogenicity, and Ecology of Bacterial Plasmids*, eds Levy SB, Clowes RC, Koenig EL, Plenum Press, New York and London, 439–48.

Bauer CE, Hesse SD et al., 1986, Mutational analysis of integrase arm-type binding sites of bacteriophage lambda, *J Mol Biol*, **192**: 513–27.

Belfort M, 1989, Bacteriophage introns: parasites within parasites?, *Trends Genet*, **5**: 209–13.

Belfort M, 1990, Phage T4 introns: self-splicing and mobility, *Annu Rev Genet*, **24**: 363–85.

Bennett PM, 1995, The spread of drug resistance, *Population Genetics of Bacteria*, eds Baumberg S, Young JPW, Wellington EMH, Saunders JR, Cambridge University Press, Cambridge, 317–44.

Bennett PM, Chopra I, 1993, Molecular basis of beta-lactamase induction in bacteria, *Antimicrob Agents Chemother*, **37**: 153–8.

Bennett PM, de la Cruz F, Grinsted I, 1983, Cointegrates are not obligatory intermediates in transposition of Tn*3* and Tn*21*, *Nature (London)*, **305**: 743–4.

Bennett PM, Howe TGB, 1990, Bacterial and bacteriophage genetics, *Topley and Wilson's Principles of Bacteriology, Virology and Immunity*, vol. 1, 8th edn, eds Linton AH, Dick HM, Edward Arnold, London, 153–210.

Benzer S, 1955, Fine structure of a genetic region in bacteriophage, *Proc Natl Acad Sci USA*, **41**: 344–54.

Beremand MN, Blumenthal T, 1979, Overlapping genes in RNA phage: a new protein implicated in lysis, *Cell*, **18**: 257–66.

Berg CM, Berg DE, Groisman EA, 1989, Transposable elements and the genetic engineering of bacteria, *Mobile DNA*, eds Berg DE, Howe MM, ASM Press, Washington, DC, 879–925.

Berg DE, 1989, Transposon Tn*5*, *Mobile DNA*, eds Berg DE, Howe MM, ASM Press, Washington, DC, 185–210.

Berg DE, Howe MM (eds), 1989, *Mobile DNA*, American Society for Microbiology, Washington, DC.

Berger-Bächi B, 1994, Expression of resistance to methicillin, *Trends Microbiol*, **2**: 389–93.

Bergh O, Yngve Børsheim K et al., 1989, High abundance of viruses found in aquatic environments, *Nature (London)*, **340**: 467–8.

Berlyn MKB, Brooks Low K, Rudd KE, 1996, Linkage map of *Escherichia coli* K-12, edition 9, Escherichia coli *and* Salmonella: *Cellular and Molecular Biology*, 2nd edn, ed. Neidhardt FC, American Society for Microbiology, Washington, DC, 1715–902.

Bernstein C, 1987, Damage in DNA of an infecting phage T4 shifts reproduction from asexual to sexual allowing rescue of its genes, *Genet Res*, **49**: 183–9.

Bernstein H, Bernstein C, 1973, Circular and branched circular concatenates as possible intermediates in bacteriophage T4 DNA replication, *J Mol Biol*, **77**: 355–61.

Betley MJ, Miller VL, Mekalanos JJ, 1986, Genetics of bacterial enterotoxins, *Annu Rev Microbiol*, **40**: 577–605.

Binns MM, Davies DL, Hardy KG, 1979, Cloned fragments of the plasmid ColV,I-K94 specifying virulence and serum resistance, *Nature (London)*, **279**: 778–81.

Black LW, 1989, DNA packaging in ds DNA bacteriophages, *Annu Rev Microbiol*, **43**: 267–92.

Black LW, Silverman DJ, 1978, Model for DNA packaging into bacteriophage T4 heads, *J Virol*, **28**: 643–55.

Bolland S, Kleckner N, 1996, The chemical steps of Tn*10*/IS*10* transposition involve repeated utilization of a single active-site, *Cell*, **84**: 223–33.

Boon T, Zinder ND, 1969, A mechanism for genetic recombination generating one parent and one recombinant, *Proc Natl Acad Sci USA*, **64**: 573–7.

Borchert LD, Drexler H, 1980, T1 genes which affect transduction, *J Virol*, **33**: 1122–8.

Bossi L, 1983, Context effects: translation of UAG codon by suppressor transfer-RNA is affected by the sequence following UAG in the message, *J Mol Biol*, **164**: 73–87.

Bradley DE, 1967, Ultrastructure of bacteriophages and bacteriocins, *Bacteriol Rev*, **31**: 230–314.

Bradley DE, 1977, Characterization of pili determined by drug resistance plasmids R711b and R778b, *J Gen Microbiol*, **102**: 349–63.

Bradley DE, 1980a, Morphological and serological relationships of conjugative pili, *Plasmid*, **4**: 155–69.

Bradley DE, 1980b, Determination of pili by conjugative bacterial drug resistance plasmids of incompatibility groups B, C, H, J, K, M, V and X, *J Bacteriol*, **141**: 828–37.

Bradley DE, 1981, Conjugative pili of plasmids in *Escherichia coli* K-12 and *Pseudomonas* species, *Molecular Biology, Pathogenicity, and Ecology of Bacterial Plasmids*, eds Levy SB, Clowes RC, Koenig EL, Plenum Press, New York and London, 217–26.

Bradley DE, Cohen DR, 1977, Adsorption of lipid-containing bacteriophages PR4 and PRD1 to pili determined by a P-1 incompatibility group plasmid, *J Gen Microbiol*, **98**: 619–23.

Bradley DE, Taylor DE, Cohen DR, 1980, Specification of surface mating systems among conjugative drug resistance plasmids in *Escherichia coli* K-12, *J Bacteriol*, **143**: 1466–70.

Bradley DE, Coetzee JN et al., 1981a, Phage X: a plasmid-dependent, broad host range, filamentous bacterial virus, *J Gen Microbiol*, **126**: 389–96.

Bradley DE, Coetzee JN et al., 1981b, Phage t: a group T plasmid-dependent bacteriophage, *J Gen Microbiol*, **126**: 397–403.

Brenner S, Streisinger G et al., 1959, Structural components of bacteriophage, *J Mol Biol*, **1**: 281.

Brissette JL, Russel M et al., 1990, Phage shock protein, a stress protein of *Escherichia coli*, *Proc Natl Acad Sci USA*, **87**: 862–6.

Broda P, 1979, *Plasmids*, W H Freeman, San Francisco.

Brooks Low K, 1996, Hfr strains of *Escherichia coli* K-12, Escherichia coli *and* Salmonella: *Cellular and Molecular Biology*, ed. Neidhardt FC, ASM Press, Washington, DC, 2402–5.

Brown, Barrett SR et al., 1995, Molecular genetics and transport analysis of the copper-resistance determinant (PCO) from *Escherichia coli* plasmid pRJ1004, *Molec Microbiol*, **17**: 1153–66.

Brown TA, 1995, *Gene Cloning: an Introduction*, 3rd edn, Chapman and Hall, London.

Brubaker RR, 1985, Mechanisms of bacterial virulence, *Annu Rev Microbiol*, **39**: 21–50.

Buchanan-Wollaston V, Passiator JE, Cannon F, 1987, The mob and oriT mobilization functions of a bacterial plasmid promote its transfer to plants, *Nature (London)*, **328**: 172–5.

Burkardt HJ, Puhler A, 1988, Electron microscopy of plasmid DNA, *Methods in Microbiology*, vol. 21, eds Grinsted J, Bennett PM, Academic Press, London, 155–77.

Burnet FM, 1929, A method for the study of bacteriophage multiplication in broth, *Br J Exp Pathol*, **10**: 109–15.

Burnet FM, 1930, Bacteriophage activity and the antigenic structure of bacteria, *J Pathol Bacteriol*, **33**: 647–64.

Burnstein KL, Dyer DW, Sparling PF, 1988, Preferential uptake of restriction fragments from a gonococcal cryptic plasmid by competent *Neisseria gonorrhoeae*, *J Gen Microbiol*, **134**: 547–57.

Bush K, Jacoby G, 1997, Nomenclature of TEM β-lactamases, *J Antimicrob Chemother*, **39**: 1–3.

Cairns J, 1963, The bacterial chromosome and its manner of replication as seen by autoradiography, *J Mol Biol*, **6**: 208–13.

Campbell A, 1994, Comparative molecular biology of lambdoid phages, *Annu Rev Microbiol*, **48**: 193–222.

Campbell A, Botstein D, 1983, Evolution of the lambdoid phages, *Lambda II*, eds Hendrix RW, Roberts JW et al., Cold Spring Harbor Laboratory, New York, 365–80.

Campbell AM, 1962, Episomes, *Adv Genet*, **11**: 101–45.

Campbell AM, 1992, Chromosomal insertion sites for phages and plasmids, *J Bacteriol*, **174**: 7495–9.

Caro L, Churchward G, Chandler M, 1984, Study of plasmid replication *in vivo*, *Methods in Microbiology*, vol. 17, eds Bennett PM, Grinsted J, Academic Press, London, 97–122.

Chang ACY, Cohen SN, 1978, Construction and characterization of amplifiable multicopy DNA cloning vehicles derived from the P15A cryptic miniplasmid, *J Bacteriol*, **134**: 1141–56.

Chater KF, Hopwood DA, 1989, Antibiotic synthesis in *Streptomyces*, *Genetics of Bacterial Diversity*, eds Hopwood DA, Chater KF, Academic Press, New York, 129–50.

Chu FK, Maley GF et al., 1984, Intervening sequence in the thymidylate synthase gene of bacteriophage T4, *Proc Natl Acad Sci USA*, **81**: 3049–53.

Clewell DB, 1993, Bacterial sex pheromone-induced plasmid transfer, *Cell*, **73**: 9–12.

Clewell DB, Flannagan SE, 1993, The conjugative transposons of Gram-positive bacteria, *Bacterial Conjugation*, ed. Clewell DB, Plenum Press, New York, 369–93.

Clewell DB, Ehrenfeld EE et al., 1986, Sex-pheromone systems in *Streptococcus faecalis*, *Antibiotic Resistance Genes: Ecology, Transfer and Expression*, eds Levy SB, Novick RP, Cold Spring Harbor Laboratory, New York, 131–42.

Clewell DB, Senghas E et al., 1988, Transposition in *Streptococcus*: structural and genetic properties of the conjugative transposon Tn*916*, *Transposition. Symposium 43 of the Society for General Microbiology*, eds Kingsman AJ, Chater KF, Kingsman SM, Cambridge University Press, Cambridge, 43–58.

Cohen SN, Chang ACY, Hsu L, 1972, Nonchromosomal antibiotic resistance in bacteria: genetic transformation of *Escherichia coli* by R-facter DNA, *Proc Natl Acad Sci USA*, **69**: 2110–14.

Cole ST, Telenti A, 1995, Drug-resistance in *Mycobacterium tuberculosis*, *Eur Respir J Suppl*, **20**: 701s–13s.

Collis CM, Hall RM, 1992, Gene cassettes from the insert region of integrons are excised as covalently closed circles, *Mol Microbiol*, **6**: 2875–85.

Collis CM, Grammaticopoulos G et al., 1993, Site-specific insertion of gene cassettes into integrons, *Mol Microbiol*, **9**: 41–52.

Cornelis G, Bennett PM, Grinsted J, 1976, Properties of pGC1, a *lac* plasmid originating in *Yersinia enterocolitica* 842, *J Bacteriol*, **127**: 1058–62.

Cornelis G, Ghosal D, Saedler H, 1978, Tn*951*: a new transposon carrying a lactose operon, *Mol Gen Genet*, **160**: 215–24.

Couch JL, Soltis MT, Betley MJ, 1988, Cloning and nucleotide sequence of the type E staphylococcal enterotoxin gene, *J Bacteriol*, **170**: 2954–60.

Courvalin P, Goussard S, Grillot-Courvalin C, 1995, Gene transfer from bacteria to mammalian cells, *C R Acad Sci III*, **318**: 1207–12.

Craig NL, 1988, The mechanism of conservative site-specific recombination, *Annu Rev Genet*, **22**: 77–105.

Craig NL, 1989, Transposon Tn*7*, *Mobile DNA*, eds Berg DE, Howe MM, ASM Press, Washington, DC, 211–25.

Craigie J, Yen CH, 1938, Demonstration of types of *B. typhosus* by means of preparations of type II Vi phage; principles and technique, *Can Public Health J*, **29**: 448–63.

Crick FHC, Barnett L et al., 1961, General nature of the genetic code for proteins, *Nature (London)*, **192**: 1227–32.

Crowther RA, Lenk EV et al., 1977, Molecular reorganization in the hexagon to star transition of the baseplate of bacteriophage T4, *J Mol Biol*, **116**: 489–523.

Daniell E, Kohne DE, Abelson J, 1975, Characterization of the inhomogeneous DNA in virions of bacteriophage mu by DNA reannealing kinetics, *J Virol*, **15**: 739–43.

Datta N, Nugent ME, 1983, Bacterial variation, *Topley and Wilson's Principles of Bacteriology, Virology and Immunity*, vol. 1, 7th edn, eds Wilson G, Dick HM, Edward Arnold, London, 145–76.

Denhardt DT, 1994, φX174 bacteriophage and related bacteriophages, *Encyclopedia of Virology*, eds Webster RG, Granoff A, Academic Press, London, 989–96.

Deonier RC, 1996, Native insertion sequence elements: locations, distributions, and sequence relationships, *Escherichia coli and Salmonella: Cellular and Molecular Biology*, ed. Neidhardt FC, ASM Press, Washington, DC, 2000–11.

Dodd HM, Bennett PM, 1987, The R46 site-specific recombination system is a homologue of the Tn*3* and γδ (Tn*1000*) cointegrate resolution system, *J Gen Microbiol*, **133**: 2031–9.

Dorman CJ, 1994, *Genetics of Bacterial Virulence*, Blackwell Scientific Publications, Oxford.

Dougan G, Sherratt DS, 1977, The transposon Tn*1* as a probe for studying ColE1 structure and function, *Mol Gen Genet*, **151**: 151–60.

Douglas J, 1975, *Bacteriophages*, Chapman and Hall, London, 119–26.

Dowson CG, Coffey TJ, Spratt BG, 1994, Origin and molecular epidemiology of penicillin-binding-protein-mediated resistance to β-lactam antibiotics, *Trends Microbiol*, **2**: 361–6.

Dreiseikelmann B, 1994, Translocation of DNA across bacterial membranes, *Microbiol Rev*, **58**: 293–316.

Dressler D, Potter H, 1982, Molecular mechanisms of genetic recombination, *Annu Rev Biochem*, **51**: 727–61.

Dubois SK, Marriott MS, Amyes SGB, 1995, TEM-derived and SHV-derived extended-spectrum β-lactamases: relationship between selection, structure and function, *J Antimicrob Chemother*, **35**: 7–22.

DuBow MS, 1994a, Bacterial identification – use of bacteriophages, *Encyclopedia of Virology*, eds Webster RG, Granoff A, Academic Press, London, 78–81.

DuBow MS, 1994b, Mu and related bacteriophages, *Encyclopedia of Virology*, eds Webster RG, Granoff A, Academic Press, London, 868–76.

van Duin J, 1994, Single-stranded RNA bacteriophages, *Encyclopedia of Virology*, eds Webster RG, Granoff A, Academic Press, London, 1334–9.

Eberl L, Kristensen CS et al., 1994, Analysis of the multimer resolution system encoded by the parCBA operon of broad-host-range plasmid RP4, *Mol Microbiol*, **12**: 131–41.

Echols H, 1986, Bacteriophage lambda development: temporal switches and the choice of lysis or lysogeny, *Trends Genet*, **2**: 26–30.

Ehrlich SD, 1977, Replication and expression of plasmids from *Staphylococcus aureus* in *Bacillus subtilis*, *Proc Natl Acad Sci USA*, **74**: 1680–2.

Ellis EL, Delbrück M, 1939, The growth of bacteriophage, *J Gen Physiol*, **22**: 365–84.

Elwell LP, Shipley PL, 1980, Plasmid-mediated factors associated with virulence of bacteria to animals, *Annu Rev Microbiol*, **34**: 465–96.

Engel H, Soedirman N, Rost J, 1980, Transferability of macrolide, lincomycin, and streptogramin resistances between Group A, B, and D Streptococci, *Streptococcus pneumoniae*, and *Staphylococcus aureus*, *J Bacteriol*, **142**: 407–13.

Engelberg-Kulka H, Schoulaker-Schwarz R, 1996, Suppression of termination codons, *Escherichia coli and Salmonella: Cellular and Molecular Biology*, ed. Neidhardt FC, ASM Press, Washington, DC, 909–21.

Everett MJ, Chopra I, Bennett PM, 1990, Induction of the *Citrobacter freundii* group I β-lactamase in *Escherichia coli* is not dependent on entry of β-lactam into the cytoplasm, *Antimicrob Agents Chemother*, **34**: 2429–30.

Falkow S, Wohlhieter JA et al., 1964, Transfer of episomic

elements to *Proteus*. II Nature of *lac⁺ Proteus* strains isolated from clinical specimens, *J Bacteriol*, **88:** 1598–601.

Falkow S, Guerry P et al., 1974, Polynucleotide sequence relationships among plasmids of the I compatibility complex, *J Gen Microbiol*, **85:** 65–76.

Farmer JJ, Hickman FW et al., 1977, Unusual Enterobacteriaceae: '*Proteus rettgeri*' that 'change' into *Providencia stuartii, J Clin Microbiol*, **6:** 373–8.

Farrow JAE, 1980, Lactose hydrolysing enzymes in *Streptococcus lactis* and *Streptococcus cremoris* and also in some other species of streptococci, *J Appl Bacteriol*, **49:** 493–503.

Feiss M, 1986, Terminase and the recognition, cutting and packaging of lambda chromosomes, *Trends Genet*, **2:** 100–4.

Fiant M, Szybalski W, Malamy M, 1972, Polar mutations in *lac, gal* and phage λ consist of a few IS-DNA sequences inserted with either orientation, *Mol Gen Genet*, **119:** 223–31.

Firth N, Ippen-Ihler K, Skurray RA, 1996, Structure and function of the F factor and mechanism of conjugation, Escherichia coli *and* Salmonella: *Cellular and Molecular Biology*, ed. Neidhardt FC, ASM Press, Washington, DC, 2377–401.

Folkhard W, Marvin DA et al., 1981, Structure of polar pili from *Pseudomonas aeruginosa* strains K and O, *J Mol Biol*, **149:** 79–93.

Foster JW, Spector MP, 1995, How *Salmonella* survive against the odds, *Annu Rev Microbiol*, **49:** 145–74.

Foster TJ, 1983, Plasmid determined resistance to antimicrobial drugs and toxic metal ions in bacteria, *Microbiol Rev*, **47:** 361–409.

Franke AK, Clewell DB, 1981, Evidence for a chromosomal-borne resistance transposon (Tn*916*) in *Streptococcus faecalis* that is capable of 'conjugal' transfer in the absence of a conjugative plasmid, *J Bacteriol*, **145:** 494–502.

Frère J-M, 1995, β-Lactamases and bacterial resistance to antibiotics, *Mol Microbiol*, **16:** 385–95.

Friedman DI, Court DL, 1995, Transcription antitermination: the lambda paradigm updated, *Mol Microbiol*, **18:** 191–200.

Fujisawa H, Yonesaki T, Minagawa T, 1985, Sequence of the T4 recombination gene, *uvsX*, and its comparison with that of the *recA* gene of *Escherichia coli, Nucleic Acids Res*, **13:** 7473–81.

Furukawa H, Mizushima S, 1982, Roles of cell surface components of *Escherichia coli* K-12 in bacteriophage T4 infection: interaction of tail core with phospholipids, *J Bacteriol*, **150:** 916–24.

Galas DJ, Chandler M, 1989, Bacterial insertion sequences, *Mobile DNA*, eds Berg DE, Howe MM, ASM Press, Washington, DC, 109–62.

Galleni M, Raquet X et al., 1995, DD-peptidases and β-lactamases: catalytic mechanisms and specificities, *J Chemother*, **7:** 3–7.

Garnier T, Saurin W, Cole ST, 1987, Molecular characterization of the resolvase gene, *res*, carried by a multicopy plasmid from *Clostridium perfringens*: common evolutionary origin for prokaryotic site-specific recombinases, *Mol Microbiol*, **1:** 371–6.

Geiduschek EP, 1991, Regulation of expression of the late genes of bacteriophage T4, *Annu Rev Genet*, **25:** 437–60.

Gerdes K, Rasmussen PB, Molin S, 1986, Unique type of plasmid maintenance function: postsegregational killing of plasmid-free cells, *Proc Natl Acad Sci USA*, **83:** 3116–20.

Gerdes K, Helin K et al., 1988, Translational control and differential RNA decay are key elements regulating postsegregational expression of the killer protein encoded by the *parB* locus of plasmid R1, *J Mol Biol*, **203:** 119–29.

Ghuysen J-M, 1991, Serine β-lactamases and penicillin-binding proteins, *Annu Rev Microbiol*, **45:** 37–67.

Ghuysen J-M, 1994, Molecular structures of penicillin-binding proteins and β-lactamases, *Trends Microbiol*, **2:** 373–80.

Gibson EM, Chace NM et al., 1979, Transfer of plasmid-mediated antibiotic resistance from streptococci to lactobacilli, *J Bacteriol*, **137:** 614–19.

Giphart-Gassler M, Plasterk RHA, van de Putte P, 1982, G inversion in bacteriophage Mu: a novel way of gene splicing, *Nature (London)*, **297:** 339–42.

Gold M, Parris W, 1986, A bacterial protein requirement for the bacteriophage lambda terminase reaction, *Nucleic Acids Res*, **14:** 9797–809.

Goldberg E, 1980, Bacteriophage nucleic acid penetration, *Virus Receptors, Part I, Bacterial Viruses: Receptors and Recognition, B7*, eds Randall LL, Philipson L, Chapman and Hall, London, 115–41.

Gorai AP, Heffron F et al., 1979, Electron microscope heteroduplex studies of sequence relationships among plasmids of the W incompatibility group, *Plasmid*, **2:** 485–92.

Griffith F, 1928, The significance of pneumococcal types, *J Hyg*, **27:** 113–59.

Grindley NDF, Humphreys GO, Anderson ES, 1973, Molecular studies of R factor compatibility groups, *J Bacteriol*, **115:** 387–98.

Grinsted J, Bennett PM (eds), 1988, *Methods in Microbiology*, vol. 21, Academic Press, London.

Grinsted J, de al Cruz F, Schmitt R, 1990, The Tn*21* subgroup of bacterial transposable elements, *Plasmid*, **24:** 163–89.

Groisman EA, Saier Jr MH, 1990, Salmonella virulence – new clues to intramacrophage survival, *Trends Biochem Sci*, **15:** 30–3.

Guarneros G, Machado G et al., 1987, Genetic and physical location of the *Escherichia coli rap* locus, which is essential for growth of bacteriophage lambda, *J Bacteriol*, **169:** 5188–92.

Guhathakurta A, Viney I, Summers D, 1996, Accessory proteins impose site selectivity during ColE1 dimer resolution, *Mol Microbiol*, **20:** 613–20.

Hall RM, Brookes DE, Stokes HW, 1991, Site-specific insertion of genes into integrons: role of the 59-base element and determination of the recombination cross-over point, *Mol Microbiol*, **5:** 1941–59.

Hall RM, Collis CM, 1995, Mobile gene cassettes and integrons: capture and spread of genes by site-specific recombination, *Mol Microbiol*, **15:** 593–600.

Harayama S, Timmis KN, 1989, Catabolism of aromatic hydrocarbons by *Pseudomonas, Genetics of Bacterial Diversity*, eds Hopwood DA, Chater KF, Academic Press, New York, 151–74.

Harrison SC, 1983, Packaging of DNA into bacteriophage heads: a model, *J Mol Biol*, **171:** 577–80.

Hayes MV, Thomson CJ, Amyes SGB, 1994, Three beta-lactamases isolated from *Aeromonas salmonicida*, including a carbapenemase not detectable by conventional methods, *Eur J Clin Microbiol Infect Dis*, **13:** 805–11.

Hayes W, 1953a, Observations on a transmissible agent determining sexual differentiation in *Bacterium coli, J Gen Microbiol*, **8:** 72–88.

Hayes W, 1953b, The mechanism of genetic recombination in *Escherichia coli, Cold Spring Harb Symp Quant Biol*, **18:** 75–93.

Hedges RW, Jacob AE, 1974, Transposition of ampicillin resistance from RP4 to other replicons, *Mol Gen Genet*, **132:** 31–40.

Hedges RW, Jacoby GA, 1980, Compatibility and molecular properties of plasmid Rms 149 in *Pseudomonas aeruginosa* and *Escherichia coli, Plasmid*, **3:** 1–6.

Helinski DR, 1973, Plasmid determined resistance to antibiotics: molecular properties of R factors, *Annu Rev Microbiol*, **27:** 437–70.

Helinski DR, Toukdarian AE, Novick RP, 1996, Replication control and other stable maintenance mechanisms of plasmids, Escherichia coli *and* Salmonella: *Cellular and Molecular Biology*, ed. Neidhardt FC, ASM Press, Washington, DC, 2295–324.

Helmann JD, Chamberlin MJ, 1988, Structure and function of bacterial sigma factors, *Annu Rev Biochem*, **57:** 839–72.

Henner DJ, Hoch JA, 1980, The *Bacillus subtilis* chromosome, *Microbiol Rev*, **44:** 57–82.

Hensel M, Shea JE et al., 1995, Simultaneous identification of bacterial virulence genes by negative selection, *Science*, **269:** 400–3.

d'Herelle F, 1917, Sur un microbe invisible antagonistic des bacilles dysenteriques, *C R Acad Sci*, **165:** 373.

Hershey AD, Chase M, 1952, Independent functions of viral protein and nucleic acid in growth of bacteriophage, *J Gen Physiol*, **36**: 39–46.

Herskowitz I, 1974, Control of gene expression in bacteriophage lambda, *Annu Rev Genet*, **7**: 289–324.

Herskowitz I, Hagen D, 1980, The lysis-lysogeny decision of phage lambda: explicit programming and responsiveness, *Annu Rev Genet*, **14**: 399–445.

Higgins RR, Lucko HJ, Becker A, 1988, Mechanism of *cos* DNA cleavage by bacteriophage lambda terminase: multiple roles of ATP, *Cell*, **54**: 765–75.

Hinnebusch J, Tilly K, 1993, Linear plasmids and chromosomes in bacteria, *Mol Microbiol*, **10**: 917–22.

Hiraga S, 1992, Chromosome and plasmid partition in *Escherichia coli*, *Annu Rev Biochem*, **61**: 283–306.

Hirota Y, 1960, The effect of acridine dyes on mating type factors in *Escherichia coli*, *Proc Natl Acad Sci USA*, **46**: 57–64.

Ho Y-S, Wulff D, Rosenberg M, 1986, Protein–nucleic acid interactions involved in transcription activation by the phage lambda regulatory protein cII, *Symp Soc Gen Microbiol*, **39**: 79–103.

Hoess R, Wierzbicki A, Abremski K, 1987, Isolation and characterization of intermediates in site-specific recombination, *Proc Natl Acad Sci USA*, **84**: 6840–4.

Holloway BW, Krishnapillai V, Morgan AF, 1979, Chromosomal genetics of *Pseudomonas*, *Microbiol Rev*, **43**: 73–102.

Hooykaas PJJ, 1989, Tumorigenicity of *Agrobacterium* on plants, *Genetics of Bacterial Diversity*, eds Hopwood DA, Chater KF, Academic Press, New York, 373–91.

Hooykaas PJJ, Beijersbergen AGM, 1994, The virulence system of *Agrobacterium tumefaciens*, *Annu Rev Phytopathol*, **32**: 157–79.

Hopwood DA, 1978, Extrachromosomally determined antibiotic production, *Annu Rev Microbiol*, **32**: 373–405.

Hopwood DA, Chater KF et al., 1973, Advances in *Streptomyces coelicolor* genetics, *Bacteriol Rev*, **37**: 371–92.

Hsu PL, Landy A, 1984, Resolution of synthetic att-site Holliday structures by the integrase protein of bacteriophage λ, *Nature (London)*, **311**: 721–6.

Hughes VM, Datta N, 1983, Conjugative plasmids in bacteria of the 'pre-antibiotic' era, *Nature (London)*, **302**: 725–6.

Hutchinson F, 1996, Mutagenesis, Escherichia coli *and* Salmonella*: Cellular and Molecular Biology*, ed. Neidhardt FC, ASM Press, Washington, DC, 2218–35.

Iida S, 1984, Bacteriophage P1 carries two related sets of genes determining its host range in the invertible C segment of its genome, *Virology*, **134**: 421–34.

Ikeda H, Tomizawa J-I, 1968, Prophage P1, an extrachromosomal replication unit, *Cold Spring Harb Symp Quant Biol*, **33**: 791–8.

Inouye S, Sunshine MG et al., 1991, Retrophage φR73: an *E. coli* phage that carries a retroelement and integrates into a tRNA gene, *Science*, **252**: 969–71.

Jacob AE, Shapiro JA et al., 1977, Plasmids studied in *Escherichia coli* and other enteric bacteria, *DNA Insertion Elements, Plasmids and Episomes*, eds Bukhari AI, Shapiro JA, Adhya SL, Cold Spring Harbor Laboratory, New York, 607–38.

Jacob F, Brenner S, Cuzin F, 1963, On the regulation of DNA replication in bacteria, *Cold Spring Harb Symp Quant Biol*, **28**: 329–48.

Jacoby GA, 1977, Plasmids studied in *Pseudomonas aeruginosa* and other pseudomonads, *DNA Insertion Elements, Plasmids and Episomes*, eds Bukhari AI, Shapiro JA, Adhya SL, Cold Spring Harbor Laboratory, New York, 639–56.

Janssen DB, Pries F, van der Ploeg JR, 1994, Genetics and biochemistry of dehalogenating enzymes, *Annu Rev Microbiol*, **48**: 163–91.

Jensen RB, Gerdes K, 1995, Programmed cell death in bacteria: proteic plasmid stabilization systems, *Mol Microbiol*, **17**: 205–10.

Johnson EM, Wohlhieter JA et al., 1976, Plasmid-determined ability of a *Salmonella tennessee* strain to ferment lactose and sucrose, *J Bacteriol*, **125**: 385–6.

Jordan E, Saedler H, Starlinger P, 1968, 0° and strong-polar mutations in the *gal* operon are insertions, *Mol Gen Genet*, **102**: 353–63.

Joris B, Ghuysen J-M et al., 1988, The active-site-serine penicillin-recognising enzymes as members of the *Streptomyces* R61 DD-peptidase family, *Biochem J*, **250**: 313–24.

Joris B, Ledent P et al., 1991, Comparison of the sequences of class A β-lactamases and of the secondary structure elements of penicillin-recognising proteins, *Antimicrob Agents Chemother*, **35**: 2294–301.

Josslin R, 1971, Physiological studies on the *t* gene defect in T4 infected *Escherichia coli*, *Virology*, **44**: 101–7.

Kasatiya SS, Nicolle P, 1978, Phage typing, *CRC Handbook of Microbiology*, 2nd edn, vol. 2. *Fungi, Algae, Protozoa and Viruses*, eds Laskin AI, Lechevalier HA, CRC Press, Boca Raton, FL, 699–715.

Kassavetis GA, Geiduschek EP, 1984, Defining a bacteriophage T4 late promoter: bacteriophage T4 gene 55 protein suffices for directing late promoter recognition, *Proc Natl Acad Sci USA*, **81**: 5101–5.

Kilby NJ, Snaith MR, Murray JAH, 1993, Site-specific recombinases: tools for genome engineering, *Trends Genet*, **9**: 413–21.

Kitts PA, Nash HA, 1987, Homology-dependent interactions in phage lambda site-specific recombination, *Nature (London)*, **329**: 346–8.

Kleckner N, 1989, Transposon Tn*10*, *Mobile DNA*, eds Berg DE, Howe MM, ASM Press, Washington, DC, 227–68.

Kopecko DJ, Washington O, Formal SB, 1980, Genetic and physical evidence for plasmid control of *Shigella sonnei* form I cell surface antigen, *Infect Immun*, **29**: 207–14.

Kornberg A, 1980, *DNA Replication*, Freeman, San Francisco.

Kornberg A, 1982, *1982 Supplement to DNA Replication*, Freeman, San Francisco.

Krause M, Guiney DG, 1991, Identification of a multimer resolution system involved in stabilization of the *Salmonella dublin* virulence plasmid pSDL2, *J Bacteriol*, **173**: 5754–62.

Lacey RW, 1975, Antibiotic resistance plasmids in *Staphylococcus aureus* and their clinical importance, *Bacteriol Rev*, **39**: 1–32.

Lacey RW, 1980, Evidence for two mechanisms of plasmid transfer in mixed cultures of *Staphylococcus aureus*, *J Gen Microbiol*, **119**: 423–35.

Lacey RW, Kruczenyk SC, 1986, Epidemiology of antibiotic resistance in *Staphylococcus aureus*, *J Antimicrob Chemother*, **18, Suppl. C**: 207–14.

Landick R, Turnbough Jr CL, Yanofsky C, 1996, Transcription attenuation, Escherichia coli *and* Salmonella*: Cellular and Molecular Biology*, ed. Neidhardt FC, ASM Press, Washington, DC, 1263–86.

Lane D, de Feyter R et al., 1986, D protein of mini F plasmid acts as a repressor of transcription and as a site-specific resolvase, *Nucleic Acids Res*, **14**: 9713–28.

Laufs R, Kaulfers P-M et al., 1979, Molecular characterization of a small *Haemophilus influenzae* plasmid specifying β-lactamase and its relationship to R factors from *Neisseria gonorrhoeae*, *J Gen Microbiol*, **111**: 223–31.

Lederberg EM, 1960, Genetic and functional aspects of galactose metabolism, 10th Symposium on General Microbiology, Cambridge University Press, Cambridge, UK, 115.

Lederberg J, 1952, Cell genetics and hereditary symbiosis, *Physiol Rev*, **32**: 403–30.

Lederberg J, Lederberg EM, 1952, Replica plating and indirect selection of bacterial mutants, *J Bacteriol*, **63**: 399–406.

Lederberg J, Tatum EL, 1946, Genetic recombination in *Escherichia coli*, *Nature (London)*, **158**: 558.

Levy SB, Novick RP (eds), 1986, *Banbury Report 24: Antibiotic Resistance Genes: Ecology, Transfer and Expression*, Cold Spring Harbor Laboratory, New York.

Lewin B, 1994, *Genes V*, Oxford University Press, Oxford, 127–59.

van der Ley P, de Graaff P, Tommassen J, 1986, Shielding of *Escherichia coli* outer membrane proteins as receptors for bacteriophages and colicins by O-antigenic chains of lipopolysaccharide, *J Bacteriol*, **168**: 449–51.

de Lorenzo V, Herrero M et al., 1990, Mini-Tn5 transposon derivatives for insertion mutagenesis, promoter probing, and chromosomal insertion of cloned DNA in Gram-negative eubacteria, *J Bacteriol*, **172**: 6568–72.

Lugtenberg B, van Alphen L, 1983, Molecular architecture and functioning of the outer membrane of *Escherichia coli* and other gram-negative bacteria, *Biochim Biophys Acta*, **737**: 51–115.

Luria SE, Delbruck M, 1943, Mutations of bacteria from virus sensitivity to virus resistance, *Genetics*, **28**: 491–511.

Lyon BR, May JW, Skurray RA, 1984, Tn4001: a gentamicin and kanamycin resistance transposon in *Staphylococcus aureus*, *Mol Gen Genet*, **193**: 554–6.

McClintock B, 1953, Induction of instability at selected loci in maize, *Genetics*, **38**: 579–99.

McDaniel R, Ebertkhosla S et al., 1995, Rational design of aromatic polyketide natural-products by recombinant assembly of enzymatic subunits, *Nature (London)*, **375**: 549–54.

McHugh GL, Moellering RC et al., 1975, *Salmonella* Typhimurium resistant to silver nitrate, chloramphenicol and ampicillin, *Lancet*, **1**: 235–40.

McKenna R, Ilag LL, Rossmann MG, 1994, Analysis of the single-stranded DNA bacteriophage φX174, refined at a resolution of 3.0 Å, *J Mol Biol*, **237**: 517–43.

Mäkelä PH, Stocker BAD, 1969, Genetics of polysaccharide biosynthesis, *Annu Rev Genet*, **3**: 291–322.

Maniloff J, Ackermann H-W, Jarvis A, 1994, Bacteriophage taxonomy and classification, *Encyclopedia of Virology*, eds Webster RG, Granoff A, Academic Press, London, 93–100.

Marrs CF, Ruehl WW et al., 1988, Pilin gene phase variation of *Moraxella bovis* is caused by an inversion of the pilin genes, *J Bacteriol*, **170**: 3032–9.

Marvin DA, Folkhard W, 1986, Structure of F-pili: reassessment of the symmetry, *J Mol Biol*, **191**: 299–300.

Marvin DA, Wachtel EJ, 1975, Structure and assembly of filamentous bacterial viruses, *Nature (London)*, **253**: 19–23.

Masters M, 1996, Generalized transduction, Escherichia coli *and* Salmonella: *Cellular and Molecular Biology*, ed. Neidhardt FC, ASM Press, Washington, DC, 2421–41.

Mathews CK, 1977, Reproduction of large virulent bacteriophages, *Comprehensive Virology*, vol. 7, eds Fraenkel-Conrat H, Wagner RR, Plenum, New York, 179–294.

Matsubara K, Kaiser AD, 1968, Lambda dv: an autonomously replicating DNA fragment, *Cold Spring Harb Symp Quant Biol*, **33**: 769–75.

May JM, Houghton RH, Perret CJ, 1964, The effect of growth at elevated temperatures on some heritable properties of *Staphylococcus aureus*, *J Gen Microbiol*, **37**: 157–69.

Mazodier P, Davies J, 1991, Gene transfer between distantly related bacteria, *Annu Rev Genet*, **25**: 147–71.

Mendiola MV, de la Cruz F, 1992, IS91 transposase is related to the rolling-circle-type replication proteins of the pUB110 family of plasmids, *Nucleic Acids Res*, **20**: 3521.

Mendiola MV, Jubete Y, de la Cruz F, 1992, DNA sequence of IS91 and identification of the transposase gene, *J Bacteriol*, **174**: 1345–51.

Meynell E, Meynell G, Datta N, 1968, Phylogenetic relationships of drug-resistance factors and other transmissible bacterial plasmids, *Bacteriol Rev*, **32**: 55–83.

Meynell EW, 1961, A phage, φ chi, which attacks motile bacteria, *J Gen Microbiol*, **25**: 253–90.

Miller JH, 1972, *Experiments in Molecular Genetics*, Cold Spring Harbor Laboratory, New York.

Mitsuhashi S, 1977, Epidemiology of bacterial drug resistance, *R Factor: Drug Resistance Plasmid*, ed. Mitsuhashi S, University Park Press, Baltimore, 1–24.

Moll A, Manning PA, Timmis KN, 1980, Plasmid-determined resistance to serum bactericidal activity: a major outer membrane protein, the *traT* gene product, is responsible for plasmid-specified serum resistance in *Escherichia coli*, *Infect Immun*, **28**: 359–67.

Montag D, Riede I et al., 1987, Receptor-recognizing proteins of T-even type bacteriophages, *J Mol Biol*, **196**: 165–74.

Mortelmans KE, Stocker BAD, 1976, Ultraviolet light protection, enhancement of ultraviolet light mutagenesis, and mutator effect of plasmid R46 in *Salmonella typhimurium*, *J Bacteriol*, **128**: 271–82.

Mosig G, 1994, T4 bacteriophage and related bacteriophages, *Encyclopedia of Virology*, eds Webster RG, Granoff A, Academic Press, London, 1376–83.

Mosig G, Bowden DW, Bock S, 1972, *E. coli* DNA polymerase I and other host functions participate in T4 DNA replication and recombination, *Nature New Biol*, **240**: 12–16.

Murialdo H, 1991, Bacteriophage lambda DNA maturation and packaging, *Annu Rev Biochem*, **60**: 125–53.

Murialdo H, Davidson A et al., 1987, The control of lambda DNA terminase synthesis, *Nucleic Acids Res*, **15**: 119–40.

Murphy E, 1989, Transposable elements in Gram-positive bacteria, *Mobile DNA*, eds Berg DE, Howe MM, ASM Press, Washington, DC, 269–88.

Nash HA, 1990, Bending and supercoiling of DNA at the attachment site of bacteriophage lambda, *Trends Biochem Sci*, **15**: 222–7.

Nash HA, 1996, Site-specific recombination: integration, excision, resolution, and inversion of defined DNA segments, Escherichia coli *and* Salmonella: *Cellular and Molecular Biology*, ed. Neidhardt FC, ASM Press, Washington, DC, 2363–76.

Novick RP, 1963, Analysis by transduction of mutations affecting penicillinase formation in *Staphylococcus aureus*, *J Gen Microbiol*, **33**: 121–36.

Novick RP, 1969, Extrachromosomal inheritance in bacteria, *Bacteriol Rev*, **33**: 210–35.

Novick RP, 1987, Plasmid incompatibility, *Microbiol Rev*, **51**: 381–95.

Novick RP, Edelman I, Lofdahl S, 1986, Small *Staphylococcus aureus* plasmids are transduced as linear multimers that are formed and resolved by replicative processes, *J Mol Biol*, **192**: 209–20.

Novick RP, Richmond MH, 1965, Nature and interactions of the genetic elements governing penicillinase synthesis in *Staphylococcus aureus*, *J Bacteriol*, **90**: 467–80.

Novick RP, Clowes RC et al., 1976, Uniform nomenclature for bacterial plasmids: a proposal, *Bacteriol Rev*, **40**: 168–89.

Novick RP, Cohen S et al., 1977, Plasmids of *Staphylococcus aureus*, *DNA insertion elements, plasmids and episomes*, eds Bukhari AI, Shapiro JA, Adhya SL, Cold Spring Harbor Laboratory, New York, 657–62.

Novick RP, Edelman I et al., 1979, Genetic translocation in *Staphylococcus aureus*, *Proc Natl Acad Sci USA*, **76**: 400–4.

Novick RP, Iordanescu S et al., 1981, Transduction-related cointegrate formation between staphylococcal plasmids: a new type of site-specific recombination, *Plasmid*, **6**: 159–72.

O'Brien SJ (ed.), 1987, *Genetic Maps 1987*, vol. 4, Cold Spring Harbor Laboratory, New York.

Ohtsubo E, Zenilman M et al., 1981, Mechanisms of insertion and cointegration mediated by IS1 and Tn3, *Cold Spring Harb Symp Quant Biol*, **45**: 283–95.

Old RW, Primrose SB, 1989, *Principles of Gene Manipulation*, 4th edn, Blackwell Scientific, Oxford.

Ørskov I, Ørskov F, 1973, Plasmid-determined H₂S character in *Escherichia coli* and its relation to plasmid-carried raffinose fermentation and tetracycline resistance characters, *J Gen Microbiol*, **77**: 487–99.

Paton R, Miles RS, Aymes SGB, 1994, Biochemical properties of inducible β-lactamases produced from *Xanthomonas maltophilia*, *Antimicrobial Agents Chemother*, **38**: 2143–9.

Poon APW, Dhillon TS, 1986, Lambdoid coliphages conferring a novel pattern of phage sensitivity on *Escherichia coli* K12, *J Gen Virol*, **67**: 2781–4.

Poteete AR, Hardy LW, 1994, Genetic analysis of bacteriophage T4 lysozyme structure and function, *J Bacteriol*, **176**: 6783–8.

Pritchard RH, Holland IB, 1985, *Basic Cloning Techniques: a Manual of Experimental Procedures*, Blackwell Scientific, Oxford.

Privitera G, Sebald M, Fayolle F, 1981, Common regulatory mechanism of expression and conjugative ability of a tetracycline resistance plasmid in *Bacteroides fragilis*, *Nature (London)*, **278**: 657–8.

Proctor LM, Fuhrman JA, 1990, Viral mortality of marine bacteria and cyanobacteria, *Nature (London)*, **343**: 60–2.

Ptashne M, 1992, *A Genetic Switch*, 2nd edn, Cell Press & Blackwell, Cambridge, MA.

Pugsley AP, Oudega B, 1987, Methods for studying colicins and their plasmids, *Plasmids, a Practical Approach*, ed. Hardy K, IRL Press, Oxford and Washington, DC, 105–61.

van de Putte P, Cramer S, Giphart-Gassler M, 1980, Invertible DNA determines host specificity of bacteriophage mu, *Nature (London)*, **286**: 218–22.

Rabussay D, Geiduschek EP, 1977, Regulation of gene action in the development of lytic bacteriophages, *Comprehensive Virology*, vol. 8, eds Fraenkel-Conrat H, Wagner RR, Plenum, New York, 1–196.

Randall LL, Philipson L (eds), 1980, *Virus Receptors, Part I, Bacterial Viruses: Receptors and Recognition, B7*, Chapman and Hall, London.

Recchia GD, Hall RM, 1995, Gene cassettes: a new class of mobile element, *Microbiology UK*, **141**: 3015–27.

Reeve ECR, Braithwaite JA, 1973, Lac-plus plasmids are responsible for the strong lactose-positive phenotype found in many strains of *Klebsiella* species, *Genet Res*, **22**: 329–33.

Relano P, Mata M et al., 1987, Molecular characterization and comparison of 38 virulent and temperate bacteriophages of *Streptococcus lactis*, *J Gen Microbiol*, **133**: 3053–63.

Reynolds PE, Fuller C, 1986, Methicillin-resistant strains of *Staphylococcus aureus*: presence of identical additional penicillin-binding protein in all strains examined, *FEMS Microbiol Lett*, **33**: 251–4.

Riede I, Drexler K et al., 1987a, DNA sequence of genes 38 encoding a receptor-recognizing protein of bacteriophages T2, K3 and of K3 host range mutants, *J Mol Biol*, **194**: 31–9.

Riede I, Drexler K et al., 1987b, T-even-type bacteriophages use an adhesin for recognition of cellular receptors, *J Mol Biol*, **194**: 23–30.

Ritchie DA, 1983, Bacteriophages, *Topley and Wilson's Principles of Bacteriology, Virology and Immunity*, vol. 1, 7th edn, eds Wilson G, Dick HM, Edward Arnold, London, 177–219.

Romantschuk M, Bamford DH, 1985, Function of pili in bacteriophage φ6 penetration, *J Gen Virol*, **66**: 2461–9.

Roth JA (ed.), 1988, *Virulence Mechanisms of Bacterial Pathogens*, American Society for Microbiology, Washington, DC.

Salyers AA, Shoemaker NB, 1995, Conjugative transposons: the force behind the spread of antibiotic resistance genes among *Bacteroides* clinical isolates, *Anaerobe*, **1**: 143–50.

Salyers AA, Whitt DD, 1994, *Bacterial Pathogenesis*, ASM Press, Washington, DC.

Salyers AA, Shoemaker NB et al., 1995, Conjugative transposons: an unusual and diverse set of integrated gene transfer elements, *Microbiol Rev*, **59**: 579–90.

Sambrook J, Fritsch EF, Maniatis T, 1989, *Molecular Cloning: a Laboratory Manual*, 2nd edn, Cold Spring Harbor Press, Cold Spring Harbor.

Samraoui B, Sutton BJ et al., 1986, Tertiary structural similarity between a class A β-lactamase and a penicillin-sensitive D-alanyl carboxypeptidase-transpeptidase, *Nature (London)*, **320**: 378–80.

Sanders ME, 1994, Bacteriophages in industrial fermentations, *Encyclopedia of Virology*, eds Webster RG, Granoff A, Academic Press, London, 116–21.

Sanderson KE, 1976, Genetic relatedness in the family Enterobacteriaceae, *Annu Rev Microbiol*, **30**: 327–49.

Sarnovsky RJ, May EW, Craig NL, 1996, The Tn 7 transposase is a heteromeric complex in which DNA breakage and joining activities are distributed between different gene products, *EMBO J*, **15**: 6348–61.

Saunders JR, Hart CA, Saunders VA, 1986, Plasmid-mediated resistance to β-lactam antibiotics in Gram-negative bacteria: the role of in-vivo recyclization reactions in plasmid evolution, *J Antimicrob Chemother*, **18, Suppl. C**: 57–66.

Schade SZ, Adler J, Ris H, 1967, How bacteriophage chi attacks motile bacteria, *J Virol*, **1**: 599–609.

Schnaitman C, Smith D, de Salsas MF, 1975, Temperate bacteriophage which causes the production of a new major outer membrane protein by *Escherichia coli*, *J Virol*, **15**: 1121–30.

Scott JR, 1984, Regulation of plasmid replication, *Microbiol Rev*, **48**: 1–23.

Seal DV, McSwiggan DA et al., 1981, Characterisation of an epidemic strain of *Klebsiella* and its variants by computer analysis, *J Med Microbiol*, **14**: 295–305.

Shannon MJR, Unterman R, 1993, Evaluating bioremediation: distinguishing fact from fiction, *Annu Rev Microbiol*, **47**: 715–38.

Shapiro JA, 1979, Molecular model for the transposition and replication of bacteriophage Mu and other transposable elements, *Proc Natl Acad Sci USA*, **76**: 1933–7.

Shapiro JA (ed.), 1983, *Mobile Genetic Elements*, Academic Press, Orlando, FL.

Sherratt DS, 1986, Control of plasmid maintenance, *Regulation of Gene Expression, 25 years on*, Symposium 39 of the Society for General Microbiology, eds Booth IR, Higgins CF, Cambridge University Press, Cambridge, 239–50.

Sherratt DS, 1989, Tn 3 and related transposable elements: site-specific recombination and transposition, *Mobile DNA*, eds Berg DE, Howe MM, ASM Press, Washington, DC, 163–84.

Shipley PL, Gyles CL, Falkow S, 1978, Characterization of plasmids that encode for the K88 colonization antigen, *Infect Immun*, **20**: 559–66.

Silver S, Phung LT, 1996, Bacterial heavy metal resistance: new surprises, *Annu Rev Microbiol*, **49**: 145–74.

Silverman JA, Benson SA, 1987, Bacteriophage K20 requires both the OmpF porin and lipolysaccharide for receptor function, *J Bacteriol*, **169**: 4830–3.

Singer BS, Gold L et al., 1982, Determination of the amount of homology required for recombination in bacteriophage T4, *Cell*, **31**: 25–33.

Sisco KL, Smith HO, 1979, Sequence-specific DNA uptake in *Haemophilus* transformation, *Proc Natl Acad Sci USA*, **76**: 972–6.

Smith GR, 1983, Chi hotspots of generalized recombination, *Cell*, **34**: 709–10.

Smith GR, 1988, Homologous recombination in procaryotes, *Microbiol Rev*, **52**: 1–28.

Smith GR, 1989, Homologous recombination in *E. coli*: multiple pathways for multiple reasons, *Cell*, **58**: 807–9.

Smith HR, Grindley NDF et al., 1973, Interactions of group H resistance factors with the F factor, *J Bacteriol*, **115**: 623–8.

Smith HW, Huggins MB, 1976, Further observations on the association of the colicine V plasmid of *Escherichia coli* with pathogenicity and with survival in the alimentary tract, *J Gen Microbiol*, **92**: 335–50.

Smith HW, Huggins MB, 1983, Effectiveness of phages in treating experimental *Escherichia coli* diarrhoea in calves, piglets and lambs, *J Gen Microbiol*, **129**: 2659–75.

Smith HW, Huggins MB, Shaw KM, 1987a, The control of experimental *Escherichia coli* diarrhoea in calves by means of bacteriophages, *J Gen Microbiol*, **133**: 1111–26.

Smith HW, Huggins MB, Shaw KM, 1987b, Factors influencing the survival and multiplication of bacteriophages in calves and in their environment, *J Gen Microbiol*, **133**: 1127–35.

Smith HW, Parsell Z, Green P, 1978, Thermosensitive H1 plasmids determining citrate utilization, *J Gen Microbiol*, **109**: 305–11.

Snyder L, 1995, Phage-exclusion enzymes: a bonanza of biochemical and cell biology reagents? *Mol Microbiol*, **15**: 415–20.

So M, McCarthy BJ, 1980, Nucleotide sequence of the bacterial transposon Tn*1681* encoding a heat-stable (ST) toxin and its identification in enterotoxigenic *Escherichia coli* strains, *Proc Natl Acad Sci USA*, **77**: 4011–15.

del Solar G, Moscoso M, Espinosa M, 1993, Rolling circle-replicating plasmids from Gram-positive and Gram-negative bacteria: a wall falls, *Mol Microbiol*, **8**: 789–96.

Spain JC, 1995, Biodegradation of nitroaromatic compounds, *Annu Rev Microbiol*, **49**: 523–55.

Stanisich VA, 1988, Identification and analysis of plasmids at the genetic level, *Methods in Microbiology*, vol. 21, eds Grinsted J, Bennett PM, Academic Press, Orlando FL, 11–47.

Stengele I, Bross P et al., 1990, Dissection of functional domains in phage fd adsorption protein, *J Mol Biol*, **212**: 143–9.

Stent GS, 1963, *Molecular Biology of Bacterial Viruses*, Freeman, San Francisco.

Stokes HW, Hall RM, 1989, A novel family of potentially mobile DNA elements encoding site-specific gene-integration functions: integrons, *Mol Microbiol*, **3**: 1669–83.

Stuy JH, 1980, Chromosomally integrated conjugative plasmids are common in antibiotic-resistant *Haemophilus influenzae*, *J Bacteriol*, **142**: 925–30.

Summers AO, Jacoby GA, 1977, Plasmid-determined resistance to tellurium compounds, *J Bacteriol*, **129**: 276–81.

Summers AO, Silver S, 1978, Microbial transformations of metals, *Annu Rev Microbiol*, **32**: 637–72.

Summers AO, Wireman J et al., 1993, Mercury released from dental 'silver' fillings provokes an increase in mercury- and antibiotic-resistant bacteria in oral and intestinal floras of primates, *Antimicrob agents Chemother*, **37**: 825–34.

Takeda Y, 1979, Specific repression of in vitro transcription by the Cro repressor of bacteriophage lambda, *J Mol Biol*, **127**: 177–89.

Taylor DE, Levine JG, Bradley DE, 1981, In vivo formation of a plasmid cointegrate expressing two incompatibility phenotypes, *Plasmid*, **5**: 233–44.

Taylor PW, 1983, Bactericidal and bacteriolytic activity of serum against Gram-negative bacteria, *Microbiol Rev*, **47**: 46–83.

Terakado N, Hamaoka T, Danbara H, 1988, Plasmid-mediated serum resistance and alterations in the composition of lipopolysaccharides in *Salmonella dublin*, *J Gen Microbiol*, **134**: 2089–93.

Tetaz TJ, Luke RKJ, 1983, Plasmid-controlled resistance to copper in *Escherichia coli*, *J Bacteriol*, **154**: 1263–8.

Thomas CM, ed., 1989, *Promiscuous Plasmids of Gram-negative Bacteria*, Academic Press, London.

Thomas CM, Smith CA, 1987, Incompatibility group P plasmids: genetics, evolution, and use in genetic manipulation, *Annu Rev Microbiol*, **41**: 77–101.

Thompson R, 1988, Plasmid cloning vectors, *Methods in Microbiology*, vol. 21, eds Grinsted J, Bennett PM, Academic Press, Orlando, FL, 179–204.

Toussaint A, 1976, The DNA modification function of temperate phage mu-1, *Virology*, **70**: 17–27.

Toussaint A, Résibois A, 1983, Phage Mu: transposition as a lifestyle, *Mobile Genetic Elements*, ed. Shapiro JA, Academic Press, Orlando, FL, 105–58.

Towner KJ, Vivian A, 1976, RP4-mediated conjugation in *Acinetobacter calcoaceticus*, *J Gen Microbiol*, **93**: 355–60.

Trieu-Cuot P, Courvalin P, 1986, Evolution and transfer of aminoglycoside resistance genes under natural conditions, *J Antimicrob Chemother*, **18, Suppl. C**: 93–102.

Twort FW, 1915, An investigation on the nature of ultra-microscopic viruses, *Lancet*, **2**: 1241–3.

Ulijasz AT, Grenader A, Weisblum B, 1996, A vancomycin-inducible LacZ reporter system in *Bacillus subtilis*: induction by antibiotics that inhibit cell wall synthesis and by lysozyme, *J Bacteriol*, **178**: 6305–9.

Utsui Y, Yokota T, 1985, Role of an altered penicillin-binding protein in methicillin-resistant and cephem-resistant *Staphylococcus aureus*, *Antimicrob Agents Chemother*, **28**: 397–403.

Villarroel R, Hedges RW et al., 1983, Heteroduplex analysis of P-plasmid evolution: the role of insertion and deletion of transposable elements, *Mol Gen Genet*, **189**: 390–9.

Wachsmuth IK, Davis BR, Allen SD, 1979, Ureolytic *Escherichia coli* of human origin: serological, epidemiological, and genetic analysis, *J Clin Microbiol*, **10**: 897–902.

Waldor MK, Mekalanos JJ, 1996, Lysogenic conversion by a filamentous phage encoding cholera toxin, *Science*, **272**: 1910–14.

Walsh TR, Payne DJ et al., 1995, A clinical isolate of *Aeromonas sobria* with three chromosomally mediated inducible β-lactamases: a cephalosporinase, a penicillinase and a third enzyme, displaying carbapenemase activity, *J Antimicrob Chemother*, **35**: 271–9.

Ward DF, Murray NE, 1979, Convergent transcription in bacteriophage lambda: interference with gene expression, *J Mol Biol*, **133**: 249–66.

Watanabe T, 1963, Infective heredity of multiple drug resistance in bacteria, *Bacteriol Rev*, **27**: 87–115.

Watson JD, Crick FHC, 1953, The structure of DNA, *Cold Spring Harb Symp Quant Biol*, **18**: 123–31.

Watson JD, Hopkins NH et al., 1987, *Molecular Biology of the Gene*, vol. 1, 4th edn, Benjamin/Cummings, Menlo Park, CA.

Webb V, Davies J, 1993, Antibiotic preparations contain DNA – a source of drug resistance genes? *Antimicrob Agents Chemother*, **37**: 2379–84.

Weigle JJ, 1953, Induction of mutations in a bacterial virus, *Proc Natl Acad Sci USA*, **39**: 628–36.

Weisberg RA, 1996, Specialized transduction, Escherichia coli *and* Salmonella*: Cellular and Molecular Biology*, ed. Neidhardt FC, ASM Press, Washington, DC, 2442–8.

Weisser J, Wiedemann B, 1985, Elimination of plasmids by new 4-quinolones, *Antimicrob Agents Chemother*, **28**: 700–2.

Widom J, Baldwin RL, 1983, Tests of spool models for DNA packaging in phage lambda, *J Mol Biol*, **171**: 419–37.

Wiedemann B, Meyer JF, Zuhlsdorf MT, 1986, Insertions of resistance genes into Tn*21*-like transposons, *J Antimicrob Chemother*, **18, Suppl. C**: 85–92.

Wiley BB, Rogolsky M, 1977, Molecular and serological differentiation of staphylococcal exfoliative toxin synthesized under chromosomal and plasmid control, *Infect Immun*, **18**: 487–94.

Willetts N, 1984, Conjugation, *Methods Microbiol*, **17**: 33–59.

Willetts N, 1988, Conjugation, *Methods in Microbiology*, vol. 21, eds Grinsted J, Bennett PM, Academic Press, Orlando, FL, 49–77.

Williams PH, 1979, Novel iron uptake system specified by ColV plasmids: an important component in the virulence of invasive strains of *Escherichia coli*, *Infect Immun*, **26**: 925–32.

Wilson GS, Miles AA (eds), 1975, *Topley and Wilson's Principles of Bacteriology, Virology and Immunity*, 6th edn, Edward Arnold, London, 1634–6.

Wollman E-L, Jacob F, 1954, Etude génétique d'un bactériophage tempéré d'*Escherichia coli*. II. Mécanisme de la recombinaison génétique, *Ann Inst Pasteur (Paris)*, **87**: 674–90.

Wright A, McConnell M, Kanegasaki S, 1980, Lipopolysaccharide as a bacteriophage receptor, *Virus Receptors, Part I, Bacterial Viruses: Receptors and Recognition*, B7, eds Randall LL, Philipson L, Chapman and Hall, London, 27–57.

Yanagida M, 1977, Molecular organization of the shell of T-even bacteriophage head. II. Arrangement of subunits in the head shells of giant phages, *J Mol Biol*, **109**: 515–37.

Yang Y, Bush K, 1996, Biochemical characterization of the carbapenem-hydrolysing β-lactamase AsbM1 from *Aeromonas sobria* AER 14M: a member of a novel subgroup of metallo-β-lactamases, *FEMS Microbiol Lett*, **137**: 193–200.

Yarmolinsky MB, 1995, Programmed cell death in bacterial populations, *Science*, **267**: 836–7.

Yanofsky C, 1987, Operon-specific control by transcription attenuation, *Trends Genet*, **3**: 356–60.

Yokota T, Kanamaru Y et al., 1969, Recombination between a thermosensitive kanamycin resistance factor and a nonthermosensitive multiple-drug resistance factor, *J Bacteriol*, **98**: 863–73.

Young KKY, Edlin G, 1983, Physical and genetical analysis of bacteriophage T4 generalized transduction, *Mol Gen Genet*, **192:** 241–6.

Young RY, 1992, Bacteriophage lysis: mechanism and regulation, *Microbiol Rev*, **56:** 430–81.

Yu F, Mizushima S, 1982, Roles of lipopolysaccharide and outer membrane protein OmpC of *Escherichia coli* K-12 in the receptor function for bacteriophage T4, *J Bacteriol*, **151:** 718–22.

Zieg J, Silverman M et al., 1977, Recombinational switch for gene expression, *Science*, **196:** 170–2.

Chapter 11

HUMAN MICROBIOTA

P R Murray

1   GENERAL COMMENTS

For the first 9 months of life, the human fetus lives in a sterile environment protected from microbes except when pathogens such as cytomegalovirus, rubella virus, or *Toxoplasma* are able to infect the child transplacentally. This state of sterility comes to an abrupt end, however, at the time of birth when the newborn is confronted with the mother's vaginal microbes and environmental organisms. The infant's skin surface is initially colonized and then the oropharynx, gastrointestinal tract and other mucosal surfaces rapidly become populated. Through the duration of the individual's life, the microbial population evolves with many organisms, transient colonizers and others becoming well established, permanent residents. It is important to recognize that this is a normal phenomenon. Even those microbes with the well recognized ability to cause serious disease are normally found in and on the human body. Indeed, one hallmark of pathogenesis is not the recovery of a specific organism, but rather the recovery of the organism in a normally sterile site. For example, *Escherichia coli* is a normal resident in the gastrointestinal tract. To find it there would be anticipated. However, *Escherichia coli* should remain confined to the gastrointestinal tract. If it is found in the abdominal cavity or the patient's bloodstream, this would be considered abnormal. Likewise, organisms such as *Streptococcus pneumoniae*, *Staphylococcus aureus*, *Neisseria meningitidis* and *Haemophilus influenzae* are all capable of causing lower respiratory tract infection. Recovery of these organisms in lower airway secretions would be consistent with their role in disease; however, isolation of the same organisms in a throat washing should be considered insignificant. Naturally, there are certain organisms whose recovery in humans is always associated with clinically

significant disease (e.g. *Bacillus anthracis*, *Brucella* spp., *Francisella tularensis* and *Histoplasma capsulatum*, to name just a few). However, the majority of microbes responsible for human disease are commonly part of the normal microbiota which are able to invade normally sterile tissues and spaces. For that reason it is important to know the normal habitats of the organisms associated with humans and to understand their capacity for producing disease.

It should also be appreciated that microbes serve a useful purpose in their human hosts. The normal microbiota maintain a protected environment that prevents colonization with potentially pathogenic organisms. For example, *Clostridium difficile* is able to produce gastrointestinal disease ranging from diarrhoea to pseudomembranous colitis only when the normal intestinal flora have been reduced or eliminated by antibiotics. The production of proteolytic enzymes by microbes augments host factors in the digestion of foods. Likewise, the disruption of the normal microbial flora can interfere with this process. For example, when the bacteria in the small intestine are replaced by colonic bacteria following small bowel stasis (blind loop syndrome), bile salts that are secreted into the intestines are metabolized by *Bacteroides* spp. with a resultant malabsorption syndrome. Intestinal bacteria can also synthesize vitamins (e.g. biotin, pantothenic acid, pyridoxine, riboflavin, vitamin K), many of which are required for the growth of other bacteria. For example, strains of *Escherichia coli* can produce vitamin K which is utilized as a required growth factor by *Porphyromonas melaninogenica*, which in turn produces penicillinases that protect other bacteria from penicillin. Thus, a complex relationship among the microbial species can be established for the mutual benefit of each organism.

It is important to define certain terms. The interaction between microbes and humans can result in 3 general outcomes: disease, transient colonization and prolonged colonization. Another term for colonization is infection, which does not imply disease but rather the association of the microbe with the human host for a time. Disease results when the interaction between microbe (e.g. bacterium, fungus, virus, or parasite) and human host results in a pathological process. This process can be due to microbial factors (e.g. hydrolytic enzymes, toxins) or the host's immune response to the presence of the organism. A few organisms have a high virulence potential and are always associated with disease, whereas most organisms are opportunistic pathogens and cause disease only when the host's immunity is suppressed or when the organisms are introduced into tissues in which they are able to express their virulence potential. The other 2 outcomes of microbe and host interaction result in colonization, either transiently or prolonged. It should be noted that transient and prolonged colonization implies a distinction based on the duration of the interaction. Although no specific time limit can be used to define prolonged colonization, it may extend to weeks, months, even years. The complex population of microbes that become established in a host are called a variety of names, including natural, indigenous, resident, and normal flora. In the previous edition of this text, they were referred to as normal microbiota, a term that has been retained here.

An individual is exposed to numerous organisms that colonize other human hosts and animals or are present in the air that is breathed and food and liquids that are consumed. Factors that determine whether exposure to a microbe results in transient passage through a human host or prolonged colonization are complex, involving environmental factors, host characteristics and microbial properties. Nutrients and environmental conditions must favour the survival of microbes. For example, vegetative forms of *Bacillus* and *Clostridium* cannot survive prolonged exposure to desiccation or heat. However, spores of these bacteria can exist in nature for months to years. The trophozoite forms of pathogenic amoeba are extremely susceptible to environmental factors and to stomach acid. Thus, trophozoites are found in the protected environment of the host (e.g. intestines) and are not considered infectious. By contrast, the cyst forms of these parasites are much more resilient, able to survive in the hostile environment and during passage through the stomach, and are responsible for disease transmission. Gram-positive bacteria have a thick peptidoglycan layer in their cell wall, which promotes osmotic stability and enables these organisms to exist on dry surfaces (e.g. household articles, hospital bed linens, skin surfaces). By contrast, gram-negative bacteria have a relatively thin peptidoglycan layer and a lipoprotein outer membrane. These structures reduce gram-negative bacteria to a more fragile state, restricting their survival to moist, protected areas (e.g. standing water, vegetation, sinks and showers). Thus, exposure to gram-positive bacteria is frequently by person-to-person contact or exposure to contaminated

fomites, whereas gram-negative bacteria are usually acquired following consumption of contaminated food or drink or exposure to a contaminated water source.

Various host factors determine the success of colonization with a microbe. Although the skin forms a barrier, preventing penetration of microbes into the deeper tissues, colonization of the surface is accomplished by organisms that can tolerate the dry surface and that are resistant to fatty acids produced by anaerobic bacteria and from the metabolism of sebum triglycerides. Some organisms are adapted to grow in skin areas with a high moisture content (e.g. axilla, skin folds, perianal area), whereas other organisms survive in hair follicles. The presence of lysozyme in tears and other secretions is highly toxic for many bacteria and restricts the organisms that can colonize these areas. Inhaled organisms can be rapidly trapped in the nasal passages, engulfed with secreted mucus, and either expelled or swallowed. Organisms ingested with food or drinks are frequently eliminated when exposed to the acidic environment of the gastric system or simply passed through the digestive tract. Other organisms fail to survive interaction with locally secreted antibodies, exposure to bacteriocins produced by the normal microbiota, or the localized environment (e.g. acidic pH of the vagina). The age of the host influences microbial colonization. The presence or absence of teeth, hormone secretions that are initiated at the time of puberty or altered in menopause, sexual activity, person-to-person interactions in day care facilities, the military, or nursing homes, alteration of dietary habits, and many other age-related factors determine which organisms an individual is exposed to and which ones will become successfully established as a part of the normal microbiota.

The final factors that determine the success of an organism to colonize on or in the human body are properties of the specific organism. For example, the terrain of the oropharynx is diverse with opportunities for organisms to colonize saliva, the mucosal surface, the tongue, gingiva above and below the tooth line, and teeth. Extremely oxygen-sensitive bacteria are able to proliferate in the gingival crevices where the *E*h is appropriately low. Organisms such as *Streptococcus mutans* and *Streptococcus sanguis* adhere to the hard, smooth surface of teeth by producing extracellular polysaccharides (e.g. glucans, dextrans, fructans) from dietary carbohydrates (Linton and Hinton 1990). A pellicle consisting of proteins from saliva and crevicular fluids initially forms on the enamel surface, which forms the anchor for the streptococcal polysaccharides. Subsequent layering of proteins, bacterial polysaccharides and mixed populations of bacteria leads to the formation of plaque on the tooth surface. Bacteria can also bind to cells lining the oropharynx, intestine and vagina via specific receptors for the bacterial pili. This ability to adhere can prevent the mechanical elimination of organisms when saliva washes the oropharynx and food and drink pass through the intestines.

With the complex environmental, host and

microbial factors that shape the normal microbiota, it should be appreciated that this population of organisms is constantly changing in an individual. For example, performing tests to determine which microbes colonize an individual's oropharynx provides data for that individual at a discrete point in time. Surveys that estimate the prevalence of colonization with microbes are at best an approximation for the individuals sampled. The ability to apply microbial colonization data from the individual studied to another person is dependent on the similarities between the 2 individuals. The data collected become more useful if the number of individuals studied is increased and the host factors minimized (e.g. study individuals with a broad age range, include immunocompetent and immunosuppressed patients, etc.). Furthermore, the utility of the data is determined by the thoroughness of the microbiological procedures. Adequate types and volume of specimens must be collected and transported to the laboratory in a manner that preserves the viability of the microbial population; isolation, detection and identification procedures that will permit recognition of all significant organisms must be used. Unfortunately, studies of the normal microbiota are limited by the numbers of individuals that can be studied using comprehensive microbiological techniques. In addition, refinements in microbiology procedures and changes in the taxonomic classification of microbes make it difficult to compare results of recent studies with those published in the older literature. Despite this caution, extensive literature exists that estimates the prevalence of organisms in different body sites. Table 11.1 is a summary of this literature for the 4 major body sites that are populated with microbes: respiratory tract, gastrointestinal tract, genitourinary tract and the body surface. The table indicates whether the organisms (bacteria, fungi, protozoa) are commonly present or not present in healthy individuals. The frequency with which these organisms are recovered is discussed in the following text. The source of this information is from the review articles and reference works that are listed in the bibliography section at the end of this chapter. The taxonomic classification of the organisms listed herein is consistent with *Bergey's Manual of Determinative Bacteriology* (Holt et al. 1994) and the *Manual of Clinical Microbiology* (Murray et al. 1995).

2 NORMAL MICROBIOTA OF THE RESPIRATORY TRACT

In the previous edition of this chapter, Linton and Hinton (1990) subdivided the respiratory tract anatomically into the upper airways which includes the anterior and posterior nares and the nasopharynx, the middle airways comprised of the oropharynx and tonsils, and the lower airways with the larynx, trachea, bronchi and lungs. This classification serves as a useful foundation for examining the dynamics of airway colonization. The structural and physiological differences at each site provides an environment compatible for some organisms and hostile for others.

2.1 Nares and nasopharynx

Relatively small numbers of organisms are present in the nares with *Staphylococcus*, including *S. aureus* and coagulase-negative species, *Corynebacterium*, *Peptostreptococcus* and *Fusobacterium* species the most numerous. The recovery of other organisms in the nares is common but they are usually present transiently and in small numbers. The microbial population in the nasopharynx is more complex with a predominance of streptococci and *Neisseria* species. The α-haemolytic (viridans) streptococci can be readily recovered in the nasopharynx, with *Streptococcus salivarius* and *Streptococcus parasanguis* most commonly isolated, as well as *Streptococcus pneumoniae*. Twelve species of *Neisseria*, including *N. meningitidis*, have been recovered in nasopharyngeal cultures. Colonization with *N. meningitidis* varies from less than 10% to as great as 95% with the highest incidence in young adults confined to institutions or in the military where focal epidemics of meningococcal disease are observed. The most commonly isolated species of *Neisseria* are *Neisseria subflava*, *Neisseria sicca*, *Neisseria cinerea*, *Neisseria mucosa* and *Neisseria lactamica*. Multiple species coexist in more than half of all individuals. Related gram-negative coccobacilli that colonize the nasopharynx include *Moraxella catarrhalis*, now recognized as a common cause of respiratory tract infections (e.g. sinusitis, bronchitis), and *Kingella* spp. Unencapsulated strains, as well as occasional encapsulated strains, of *H. influenzae* are commonly found in the nasopharynx, as is *Cardiobacterium hominis*, an organism associated with infections of previously damaged cardiac tissues.

2.2 Oropharynx and tonsils

The oropharynx is a complex mixture of ecosystems, each with a distinctive microbial population. Thus, predictable differences in organisms will be found in saliva, gingival crevices, surfaces of teeth, the tongue and the mucosal lining. Gram-positive and gram-negative cocci predominate in the oropharynx. Overall, anaerobes outnumber aerobic bacteria 100 to 1. The most common anaerobic bacteria are *Peptostreptococcus*, *Veillonella*, *Actinomyces* and *Fusobacterium;* the most common aerobic bacteria are *Streptococcus* and *Neisseria*.

Relatively small numbers of staphylococci are present, although it has been estimated that as many as 20% of individuals are colonized with *S. aureus*. Streptococcal species are more numerous, particularly members of the viridans group. *S. salivarius* is present in high numbers in saliva (as the name implies) and on the surface of the tongue. Tooth surfaces are colonized with *S. sanguis* and *S. mutans*, whereas the oral mucosa is populated with *Streptococcus vestibularis* and *S. sanguis*. Other streptococci that colonize the oropharynx include *S. pneumoniae*, commonly present in children and adults with children, and β-haemolytic streptococci, including groups A, C, F and G. Group A *Streptococcus* (*Streptococcus pyogenes*, the organism responsible for streptococcal pharyngitis) can trans-

Table 11.1   Human microbiota

Organism	Prevalence of carriage			
	Resp. tract	GI tract	GU tract	Skin, Ear, Eye
Abiotrophia adiacens	+	0	0	0
Abiotrophia defectiva	+	0	0	0
Acholeplasma laidlawii	+	0	0	0
Acidaminococcus fermentans	+	+	0	0
Acinetobacter spp.	+	+	+	+
Actinobacillus actinomycetemcomitans	+	0	0	0
Actinobacillus ureae	+	0	0	0
Actinomyces israelii	+	+	+	0
Actinomyces meyeri	+	+	+	0
Actinomyces naeslundii	+	+	+	0
Actinomyces odontolyticus	+	+	+	0
Actinomyces viscosus	+	+	+	0
Aerococcus viridans	0	0	0	+
Aeromonas spp.	0	+	0	0
Anaerorhabdus furcosus	0	+	0	0
Arcanobacterium haemolyticum	+	0	0	0
Bacillus spp.	0	+	0	+
Bacteroides caccae	0	+	0	0
Bacteroides capillosus	+	+	0	0
Bacteroides coagulans	0	+	+	0
Bacteroides distasonis	0	+	0	0
Bacteroides eggerthii	0	+	0	0
Bacteroides forsythus	+	0	0	0
Bacteroides fragilis	0	+	+	0
Bacteroides gracilis	+	0	0	0
Bacteroides ovatus	0	+	0	0
Bacteroides pneumosintes	+	0	0	0
Bacteroides putredinis	0	+	0	0
Bacteroides thetaiotaomicron	0	+	0	0
Bacteroides ureolyticus	+	+	+	0
Bacteroides vulgatus	0	+	0	0
Bacteroides, other spp.	+	+	+	0
Bifidobacterium adolescentis	0	+	0	0
Bifidobacterium angulatum	0	+	0	0
Bifidobacterium bifidum	0	+	+	0
Bifidobacterium catenulatum	0	+	+	0
Bifidobacterium dentium	+	+	+	0
Bifidobacterium longum	0	+	+	0
Bifidobacterium infantis	0	+	+	0
Bifidobacterium breve	0	+	+	0
Bifidobacterium pseudocatenulatum	0	+	0	0
Bilophila wadsworthia	+	+	+	0
Blastocystis hominis	0	+	0	0
Blastoschizomyces capitatus	0	0	0	+
Brachyspira aalborgii	0	+	0	0
Brevibacterium epidermidis	0	0	0	+
Burkholderia cepacia	+	0	0	+
Butyrivibrio crossatus	0	+	0	0
Campylobacter concisus	+	0	0	0
Campylobacter curvus	+	0	0	0
Campylobacter rectus	+	0	0	0
Campylobacter sputorum	+	+	0	0
Candida albicans	+	+	+	+
Candida (Torulopsis) glabrata	+	+	+	0
Candida guilliermondii	+	+	+	0
Candida kefyr	+	+	+	0
Candida krusei	+	+	+	0

Table 11.1   Continued

| Organism | Prevalence of carriage | | | |
	Resp. tract	GI tract	GU tract	Skin, Ear, Eye
Candida parapsilosis	+	+	0	0
Candida tropicalis	+	+	+	0
Capnocytophaga spp.	+	0	+	0
Cardiobacterium hominis	+	+	+	0
Chilomastix mesnili	0	+	0	0
Citrobacter spp.	0	+	0	0
Clostridium difficile	0	+	+	0
Clostridium perfringens	0	+	+	+
Clostridium, other spp.	0	+	+	0
Corynebacterium jeikeium	0	0	0	+
Corynebacterium matruchotii	+	0	0	0
Corynebacterium minutissimum	0	0	0	+
Corynebacterium pseudodiphtheriticum	+	0	+	0
Corynebacterium striatum	+	0	0	0
Corynebacterium ulcerans	+	0	0	0
Corynebacterium xerosis	+	0	0	+
Corynebacterium, other spp.	+	+	+	+
Cryptococcus albidus	+	0	0	0
Dermabacter hominis	0	0	0	+
Desulfomonas pigra	0	+	0	0
Desulfovibrio spp.	0	+	0	0
Eikenella corrodens	+	+	+	0
Endolimax nana	0	+	0	0
Entamoeba coli	0	+	0	0
Entamoeba hartmanni	0	+	0	0
Entamoeba gingivalis	+	0	0	0
Entamoeba polecki	0	+	0	0
Enterobacter spp.	+	+	0	0
Enterococcus spp.	0	+	+	0
Enteromonas hominis	0	+	0	0
Epidermophyton floccosum	0	0	0	+
Escherichia coli	0	+	+	0
Eubacterium spp.	+	+	+	0
Flavobacterium meningosepticum	+	0	0	0
Fusobacterium alocis	+	0	0	0
Fusobacterium mortiferum	0	+	0	0
Fusobacterium necrophorum	+	+	0	0
Fusobacterium naviforme	+	0	0	0
Fusobacterium nucleatum	+	+	+	0
Fusobacterium periodonticum	+	0	0	0
Fusobacterium sulci	+	0	0	0
Fusobacterium varium	0	+	0	0
Gardnerella vaginalis	0	0	+	0
Gemella haemolysans	+	0	0	0
Gemella morbillorum	+	+	0	0
Haemophilus aphrophilus	+	0	0	0
Haemophilus haemolyticus	+	0	0	0
Haemophilus influenzae	+	+	+	0
Haemophilus parahaemolyticus	+	+	0	0
Haemophilus parainfluenzae	+	0	+	0
Haemophilus paraphrophilus	+	+	0	0
Haemophilus segnis	+	+	0	0
Hafnia alvei	+	+	0	0
Helicobacter pylori	+	+	0	0
Iodamoeba butschlii	0	+	0	0
Kingella denitrificans	+	0	0	0
Kingella kingae	+	0	0	0

Continued

Table 11.1 Continued

Organism	Prevalence of carriage			
	Resp. tract	GI tract	GU tract	Skin, Ear, Eye
Klebsiella spp.	+	+	0	0
Lactobacillus acidophilus	+	+	+	0
Lactobacillus casei	+	0	+	0
Lactobacillus cellobiosus	0	0	+	0
Lactobacillus fermentum	+	+	+	0
Lactobacillus reuteri	0	+	0	0
Lactobacillus salivarius	+	+	0	0
Leptotrichia buccalis	+	+	+	0
Listeria monocytogenes	0	+	0	0
Malassezia furfur	0	0	0	+
Malassezia sympodialis	0	0	0	+
Megasphaera elsdenii	+	+	0	0
Micrococcus agilis	0	0	0	+
Micrococcus kristinae	0	0	0	+
Micrococcus luteus	0	0	0	+
Micrococcus lylae	0	0	0	+
Micrococcus nishinomiyaensis	0	0	0	+
Micrococcus roseus	0	0	0	+
Micrococcus sedentarius	0	0	0	+
Micrococcus varians	0	0	0	+
Microsporum audouinii	0	0	0	+
Microsporum ferrugineum	0	0	0	+
Miksuokella multiacidus	0	+	0	0
Mobiluncus curtisii	0	+	+	0
Mobiluncus mulieris	0	+	+	0
Moraxella atlantae	+	0	0	0
Moraxella catarrhalis	+	0	0	0
Moraxella lacunata	+	0	0	0
Moraxella nonliquefaciens	+	0	0	0
Moraxella osloensis	+	0	0	0
Moraxella phenylpyruvica	+	0	0	0
Morganella morganii	0	+	0	0
Mycoplasma spp.	+	0	+	0
Neisseria cinerea	+	0	0	0
Neisseria flavescens	+	0	0	0
Neisseria lactamica	+	0	0	0
Neisseria meningitidis	+	0	+	0
Neisseria mucosa	+	0	0	0
Neisseria polysaccharea	+	0	0	0
Neisseria sicca	+	0	0	0
Neisseria subflava	+	0	0	0
Oligella ureolytica	0	0	+	0
Oligella urethralis	0	0	+	0
Pasteurella multocida	+	0	0	0
Peptostreptococcus spp.	+	+	+	+
Porphyromonas spp.	+	+	+	0
Porphyromonas asaccharolytica	+	+	+	0
Porphyromonas endodontalis	+	0	0	0
Porphyromonas gingivalis	+	0	0	0
Prevotella bivia	0	0	+	0
Prevotella buccae	+	0	0	0
Prevotella buccalis	+	0	0	0
Prevotella corporis	+	0	0	0
Prevotella denticola	+	0	0	0
Prevotella disiens	+	0	+	0
Prevotella intermedia	+	0	0	0
Prevotella loescheii	+	0	0	0
Prevotella melaninogenica	+	0	0	0

Table 11.1 Continued

Organism	Prevalence of carriage Resp. tract	GI tract	GU tract	Skin, Ear, Eye
Prevotella nigrescens	+	0	0	0
Prevotella oris	+	0	0	0
Prevotella, other spp.	+	+	+	0
Propionibacterium acnes	+	+	+	+
Propionibacterium avidum	+	+	+	+
Propionibacterium granulosum	+	+	+	+
Propionibacterium propionicus	+	+	+	+
Proteus spp.	0	+	+	0
Providencia spp.	0	+	+	0
Pseudomonas aeruginosa	+	+	0	0
Pseudomonas, other spp.	0	+	0	0
Retortamonas intestinalis	0	+	0	0
Rhodotorula spp.	0	0	0	+
Rothia dentocariosa	+	0	0	0
Ruminococcus spp.	0	+	0	0
Selenomonas spp.	+	+	0	0
Serpulina spp.	0	+	0	0
Staphylococcus aureus	+	+	+	+
Staphylococcus, coagulase-negative	+	+	+	+
Stomatococcus mucilaginosus	+	0	0	0
Streptococcus agalactiae	+	+	+	0
Streptococcus bovis	0	+	0	0
Streptococcus pneumoniae	+	0	0	0
Streptococcus pyogenes	+	+	0	+
Streptococcus, group C, F, or G	+	+	+	0
Streptococcus, viridans group	+	+	+	0
Succinivibrio dextrinosolvens	0	+	0	0
Tissierella praeacuta	0	+	0	0
Treponema denticola	+	0	0	0
Treponema minutum	0	0	+	0
Treponema pectinovorum	+	0	0	0
Treponema phagedenis	0	0	+	0
Treponema refringens	0	0	+	0
Treponema skoliodontum	+	0	0	0
Treponema socranskii	+	0	0	0
Treponema vincentii	+	0	0	0
Trichomonas hominis	0	+	0	0
Trichomonas tenax	+	0	0	0
Trichophyton concentricum	0	0	0	+
Trichophyton gourvilii	0	0	0	+
Trichophyton kanei	0	0	0	+
Trichophyton megninii	0	0	0	+
Trichophyton mentagrophytes	0	0	0	+
Trichophyton raubitschekii	0	0	0	+
Trichophyton rubrum	0	0	0	+
Trichophyton schoenleinii	0	0	0	+
Trichophyton soudanense	0	0	0	+
Trichophyton tonsurans	0	0	0	+
Trichophyton violaceum	0	0	0	+
Trichophyton yaoundei	0	0	0	+
Turicella otitidis	0	0	0	+
Ureaplasma urealyticum	0	0	+	0
Veillonella atypica	+	0	0	0
Veillonella dispar	+	0	0	0
Veillonella parvula	+	+	0	0
Weeksella virosa	0	0	+	0

Incidence of carriage in respiratory (resp.) tract, gastrointestinal (GI) tract, genitourinary (GU) tract, and skin, ears and eyes; +, commonly present; 0, not typically isolated in healthy individuals.

iently colonize healthy individuals or become a more permanent member of the oral microflora. Other gram-positive cocci that are present in the oropharynx include *Stomatococcus mucilaginosus*, *Gemella* species, and *Peptostreptococcus* species. Both *Stomatococcus* and *Peptostreptococcus* are found in virtually all individuals.

As in the nasopharynx, gram-negative cocci and coccobacilli can colonize the oropharynx. *Veillonella* species, anaerobic gram-negative cocci, are the most numerous gram-negative cocci found in the oropharynx, representing as much as 15% of the total bacterial population. *Veillonella atypica* and *Veillonella dispar* are present on the tongue, oral mucosa and in saliva. *Veillonella parvula* is present in subgingival spaces and in dental plaque, in higher numbers in dental caries. Other gram-negative cocci include *Neisseria*, *Moraxella*, *Kingella*, *Cardiobacterium* and *Eikenella*. *Eikenella corrodens* can establish residence in the oropharynx by adhering to buccal epithelial cells.

Gram-positive bacilli are also prominent members of the oropharyngeal flora. *Actinomyces* are present in large numbers, comprising 20% of the bacterial flora in saliva and on the tongue, 35% in gingival crevices, and 40% of the bacteria in dental plaque. The *Actinomyces* spp. present in the oropharynx are *Actinomyces israelii*, *Actinomyces naeslundii*, *Actinomyces viscosus*, *Actinomyces odontolyticus* and *Actinomyces meyeri*. *A. israelii* and *A. naeslundii* also colonize the surface of the tonsils. The ability of *Actinomyces* spp. to colonize the various surfaces is mediated by the presence of fimbriae that can adhere to mucosal cells and the production of extracellular polysaccharides that form a slime over tooth surfaces, entrapping the organism and preventing its removal by the flow of saliva and food through the oropharynx. Other genera of gram-positive bacilli present in the oropharynx include *Actinobacillus*, *Corynebacterium*, *Eubacterium*, *Lactobacillus*, *Propionibacterium* and *Rothia*. *Actinobacillus actinomycetemcomitans* is an important cause of juvenile periodontitis and species of *Lactobacillus* are prominently associated with carious teeth, thriving in the acid environment produced by the streptococci responsible for the development of caries. *Eubacterium* spp. are isolated from subgingival crevices, dental plaques and calculus. Another group of bacteria commonly found in the oropharynx, particularly in the gingival crevices, and associated with periodontal disease are *Treponema* spp.

The predominant gram-negative bacilli in the oropharynx are anaerobes, including *Fusobacterium*, *Bacteroides*, *Porphyromonas*, *Prevotella* and *Selenomonas*. *Fusobacterium nucleatum* is the most common fusobacterium in the mouth, *Fusobacterium alocis* and *Fusobacterium sulci* are isolated in the gingival crevices, and the other species are present in smaller numbers throughout the mouth. Many of the anaerobic gram-negative bacilli in the mouth that were formerly classified as *Bacteroides* are now *Prevotella* and *Porphyromonas* spp. However, at least 5 species found in the mouth have been retained in the genus *Bacteroides*, while 9 *Prevotella* spp. and 3 *Porphyromonas* spp. colonize the mouth. At least 6 species of *Selenomonas* are present in the oropharynx, primarily in gingival crevices.

Haemophilus spp. are present in almost all individuals although in small numbers (<5% of the microbial population). The majority of the isolates (>50%) are non-encapsulated *H. influenzae*, with encapsulated species uncommonly found. *Haemophilus parainfluenzae* can comprise 10% of the bacterial flora in saliva and other species can be found associated with dental plaque and periodontal disease.

Members of the Enterobacteriaceae and non-fermentative gram-negative bacilli such as *Pseudomonas* spp. and *Acinetobacter* are present in the oropharynx of healthy individuals but usually only in small numbers or transiently. This changes in debilitated or hospitalized patients in whom these organisms can become the predominant bacteria in the oropharynx and are frequently responsible for lower respiratory tract disease.

Fungal colonization of the oropharynx is restricted to yeasts; *Candida albicans* is present in almost all individuals. Other *Candida* spp. are commonly detected, as are *Cryptococcus albidus*, although these organisms are generally present in small numbers and may require selective culture techniques for their detection. Protozoa present in the oropharynx are *Entamoeba gingivalis* and *Trichomonas tenax*. Neither is associated with disease.

2.3 Trachea, larynx, bronchi and lungs

Colonization of the lower airways is generally transient, with relatively few organisms present at any one time. The only time long-term colonization occurs is when the ciliated epithelial cells are damaged through infection (e.g. with influenza virus) or disease (e.g. chronic obstructive pulmonary disease). This permits drainage of respiratory secretions into the bronchials and lower airways, with subsequent proliferation of the microbes.

3 NORMAL MICROBIOTA OF THE GASTROINTESTINAL TRACT

As with the respiratory tract, the gastrointestinal tract can be subdivided into distinct anatomical areas, each harbouring its own indigenous microbiotica. These would include the oesophagus, stomach, jejunum and upper ileum, distal small intestine and large intestine. It should be obvious that within each of these areas, the microbial flora on the mucosa, within crypts, and in the lumen can also be different. Unfortunately, the ability to sample each area without contamination from other sites in healthy individuals is limited. The most complete information has been obtained for the stomach and the large intestine; the microbial flora at other sites is estimated by studying the microbial composition of faeces or the specimens collected at the time of intra-abdominal surgery.

3.1 Oesophagus

Insufficient information is available about the microbial flora of the oesophagus. However, oropharyngeal bacteria and yeast can be isolated from this site, as can the organisms that colonize the stomach; transient colonization occurs with these organisms in healthy individuals. In the diseased state, *Candida* is a prominent cause of oesophagitis and oesophageal infections with viruses such as herpes simplex and cytomegalovirus.

3.2 Stomach

The stomach is an inhospitable organ, containing hydrochloric acid and pepsinogen (precursor of pepsin) secreted by parietal and chief cells, respectively, that line the gastric mucosa. For this reason the normal microbial microbiota are sparse, primarily associated with the surface epithelium, and protected by secretions of mucus and bicarbonate. The organisms present in the stomach are acid-tolerant *Lactobacillus* spp., *Streptococcus* spp. and *Helicobacter pylori*. Whereas the first 2 organisms are not associated with gastric disease, *H. pylori* causes gastritis, gastric (peptic) and duodenal ulcers, and is associated with gastric malignancies. Other organisms may be isolated in the stomach, particularly a few hours after a meal, but are believed to represent transient passage through the stomach.

3.3 Jejunum and upper ileum

The number of microbes in the upper portion of the small intestine is low (generally much less than 10^5 organisms per ml fluid) and predominantly anaerobic, consisting primarily of *Lactobacillus*, *Streptococcus*, *Peptostreptococcus*, *Porphyromonas* and *Prevotella*. If upper tract obstruction and stasis occur (e.g. blind loop syndrome), then the microbial flora can shift to resemble colonic bacteria (e.g. *Bifidobacterium*, *Bacteroides*, *Clostridium*, *Escherichia*, *Enterococcus*) and lead to a malabsorption syndrome.

3.4 Distal small intestine

This is the transition area between the relatively sparse numbers of acid-tolerant bacteria that occupy the upper portion of the intestinal tract and the plethora of microbes that exist in the large intestine. Although it is unclear which organisms permanently colonize this portion of the gastrointestinal tract, it is known that the microbial population is large (approximately 10^{8-9} organisms per gram of faeces) and diverse, with a distinct predominance of strict anaerobes.

3.5 Large intestine

This is the most densely populated organ in the human body with more than 10^8 aerobic bacteria and 10^{11} anaerobic bacteria per gram of faeces. Various

yeasts and non-pathogenic parasites also establish residence in this area. The most numerous bacteria in the large intestine are *Bifidobacterium* spp., *Bacteroides fragilis* group, *Eubacterium* spp., *Enterococcus* spp. and *Escherichia coli*. It has been estimated that faeces consist of 10^{11} bacteroides per g with *B. fragilis* group species most numerous. Although *B. fragilis* is the most virulent species, *Bacteroides thetaiotaomicron* is more numerous in the colon. Other *Bacteroides* spp. in the colon include *Bacteroides capillosus*, *Bacteroides coagulans*, *Bacteroides putredinis* and *Bacteroides ureolyticus*. *Eubacterium* spp. are the second most commonly isolated bacteria in the intestine with more than 10^{10} organisms per g of faeces and 19 distinct species described. The most commonly isolated species are *Eubacterium aerofaciens*, *Eubacterium contortum*, *Eubacterium cylindroides*, *Eubacterium lentum* and *Eubacterium rectale*. Nine species of *Bifidobacterium* have been isolated in faeces, some species preferentially isolated from infants and others from adults. The most commonly isolated species are *B. bifidum*, *B. longum* and *B. adolescentis*. Ten species of *Enterococcus* have been described, all of which are present in the intestines. *Enterococcus faecalis* and *Enterococcus faecium* are most frequently isolated. *Escherichia coli* inhabits the intestine of virtually all humans, establishing intestinal colonization soon after an infant is born. Although it represents a relatively minor position quantitatively (approximately 1% of the total bacterial population), it is the most common facultative organism responsible for intra-abdominal infections.

A large number of other organisms have been demonstrated to colonize the large intestine. *Actinomyces* are frequently isolated in faecal specimens even though intestinal colonization has not been clearly demonstrated. *Streptococcus* spp., including *Streptococcus bovis* which is associated with intestinal malignancies, have been isolated from faecal specimens.

Gemella morbillorum is a member of the normal intestinal flora, as are a variety of *Peptostreptococcus* spp. (e.g. *Peptostreptococcus magnus*, *Peptostreptococcus prevotii*, *Peptostreptococcus asaccharolyticus*). The spore-forming *Bacillus* spp. and *Clostridium* spp. are isolated in faecal specimens. Although this may represent simple transit through the gastrointestinal tract following ingestion with food or drink, most believe *Clostridium* spp. are part of the permanent intestinal population. *V. parvula* can colonize the intestinal tract of humans, although it is generally present in small numbers. Like *Escherichia coli*, other members of the Enterobacteriaceae can establish residence in the intestines. *Citrobacter* spp., *Klebsiella* spp., *Enterobacter* spp., *Proteus* spp. and various other genera can be consistently isolated in faecal specimens. *Haemophilus* spp. can be recovered in faecal specimens if selective media are used. Other organisms commonly isolated but in small numbers include species of *Fusobacterium*, *Porphyromonas* and *Prevotella*. Uncultivable species of *Treponema* have been observed in faecal specimens.

Various species of yeast colonize the large intestine; *Candida albicans*, *Candida tropicalis*, *Candida para-*

psilosis, *Candida krusei* and *Candida glabrata* are the most numerous. Protozoa can also be recovered in the intestine although their presence is markedly influenced by the individual's diet and general hygienic condition of the environment. *Blastocystis hominis*, *Chilomastix mesnili*, *Endolimax nana*, *Entamoeba coli*, *Entamoeba hartmanni*, *Entamoeba polecki*, *Enteromonas hominis*, *Iodamoeba butschlii*, *Retortamonas intestinalis* and *Trichomonas hominis* have been most consistently isolated from healthy individuals living in underdeveloped countries.

4 NORMAL MICROBIOTA OF THE GENITOURINARY TRACT

The genitourinary tract is relatively sterile with the exception of the female urethra and vagina. Microbes can migrate up the urethra into the bladder but these are rapidly cleared in healthy individuals by the action of localized antibodies, microbicidal activity of the epithelial cells lining the bladder, and the flushing action of voided urine. The ureters, kidneys, prostate and cervix normally are sterile. The female urethra is colonized with large numbers of lactobacilli, streptococcal species and coagulase-negative staphylococci. Faecal organisms such as *Escherichia coli*, *Enterococcus* spp., *C. albicans* and *T. glabrata* can also colonize the female urethra but generally are transient and present in small numbers. When these latter organisms migrate up into the bladder, they are able to proliferate in urine and can establish an urinary tract infection.

The microbial flora in the vagina are more numerous and diverse. Lactobacilli are the predominant organisms because they are able to proliferate in the acidic environment. The most commonly isolated species include *Lactobacillus acidophilus*, *Lactobacillus fermentum*, *Lactobacillus casei* and *Lactobacillus cellobiosus*. Other anaerobes commonly isolated in vaginal secretions are *Bifidobacterium*, *Peptostreptococcus*, *Porphyromonas* and *Prevotella*. Six species of *Bifidobacterium* have been recovered in the vagina; *B. bifidum* and *B. longum* are the most numerous. Likewise, 6 species of *Peptostreptococcus* (i.e. *P. magnus*, *P. asaccharolyticus*, *P. prevotii*, *Peptostreptococcus anaerobius*, *Peptostreptococcus tetradius* and *Peptostreptococcus micros*) reside in the vagina. *Porphyromonas asaccharolytica*, *Prevotella bivia* and *Prevotella disiens* are also important residents of the vagina. *Actinomyces* spp. are believed to be present in the vagina because they are associated with vaginal infections; however, demonstration of their presence is controversial. *A. israelii* is most commonly associated with genital actinomycotic infections. *Propionibacterium*, particularly *Propionibacterium propionicus*, is also present in the vagina. Finally, *Mobiluncus* spp. are relatively uncommon in healthy women, but a significant cause of bacterial vaginosis. Thus, it is likely that this anaerobe is present in the vaginal microbial flora in small numbers.

Common aerobic bacteria present in the vagina include *Staphylococcus* (primarily coagulase-negative species), *Streptococcus* and *Corynebacterium* spp. The viridans group and β-haemolytic strains (e.g. groups B, C and G) of streptococci are present in the vagina. *Gardnerella vaginalis* can also colonize the human genital and urinary tract, although it is only present in high numbers in women with vaginosis and their male partners. *Neisseria* spp., including *N. meningitidis*, are recovered in vaginal secretions, as are species of *Haemophilus* (including *H. influenzae* and *H. parainfluenzae*). Although these organisms can be recovered from a large proportion of individuals, they are generally part of the minor bacterial population. Members of the Enterobacteriaceae, particularly *Escherichia coli*, can be found in the vaginal flora although generally in small numbers. *Weeksella virosa* is almost exclusively isolated in genital specimens, particularly from sexually active women. Three species of non-pathogenic *Treponema* (*Treponema phagedenis*, *Treponema refringens* and *Treponema minutum*) are isolated in vaginal specimens.

Six species of *Mycoplasma* (e.g. *Mycoplasma hominis*, *Mycoplasma genitalium*, *Mycoplasma fermentans*, *Mycoplasma primatum*, *Mycoplasma spermatophilum* and *Mycoplasma penetrans*) primarily colonize the genitourinary tract. In addition, the related organism *U. urealyticum* is a common inhabitant of this site. The role of these organisms in disease is controversial, but clearly *M. hominis* and *U. urealyticum* have pathogenic potential.

As with the gastrointestinal tract, *Candida* spp. (particularly *C. albicans*) and *T. glabrata* are common members of the microbial flora. The flagellate, *Trichomonas vaginalis*, is present in small numbers in healthy women, but can also proliferate and cause vaginitis.

5 NORMAL MICROBIOTA OF THE BODY SURFACE

The surface of the skin is relatively inhospitable in comparison with other body sites. It is exposed to extremes in temperature and moisture, and to chemical disinfectants such as soaps and shampoos. It is not surprising, therefore, that the microbial population is less numerous and complex than at other body sites. Despite this observation, many organisms, particularly gram-positive bacteria, are able to establish permanent residence on the skin surface; transient colonization with a diverse array of environmental and endogenous microbes can also occur.

As with other areas of the body, the skin should not be considered a homogeneous surface but rather a landscape of mountains and valleys, each with a specific environment and microbial population. Thus, there are relatively dry, hairless areas such as palms and soles, areas with a proliferation of apocrine glands such as the axillae, inguinal, and perineal areas, and areas rich with sebaceous glands such as the forehead and nasolabial folds. Each area is associated with distinct microbes. Most micro-organisms proliferate in a moist environment; hence, higher densities of microbes are present in areas rich with sweat glands or on occluded surfaces. The skin proximal to the oral cavity (face), gastrointestinal tract (perirectal area), or genitourinary tract (groin) has a more complex microbial flora than at other surface sites, although most of these organisms result from surface contamination and only transiently colonize the skin surface.

Anaerobic bacteria are 10- to 100-fold more numerous on the skin surface compared with aerobic bacteria; gram-positive bacteria predominate over gram-negative bacteria and bacteria far outnumber yeast. The bacteria most commonly recovered on the skin surface are members of the genera *Staphylococcus*, *Micrococcus*, *Corynebacterium*, *Peptostreptococcus* and *Propionibacterium*. *Staphylococcus epidermidis* is the most frequently isolated bacterium, present on surfaces where the moisture is highest. Other coagulase-negative staphylococci that are found on the skin include *Staphylococcus hominis*, *Staphylococcus haemolyticus*, *Staphylococcus warneri*, *Staphylococcus capitis* (particularly on the forehead and face after puberty), *Staphylococcus saprophyticus*, *Staphylococcus caprae*, *Staphylococcus saccharolyticus*, *Staphylococcus pasteuri*, *Staphylococcus lugdunensis*, *Staphylococcus simulans* and *Staphylococcus xylosus*. *Staphylococcus auricularis* is the most common species found colonizing the exterior auditory canal. The coagulase-positive *S. aureus* can colonize the skin adjacent to the nares and in moist folds, and less frequently at other sites.

Micrococcus luteus is the most common *Micrococcus* sp. present on the skin, found in virtually all adults and representing as much as 20% of the bacterial population on the head, legs and arms. However, relatively few micrococci are present in areas with a high moisture content and other competitive bacteria (e.g. axillae, nares). Additional *Micrococcus* spp. that colonize the skin surface include *Micrococcus varians*, *Micrococcus lylae*, *Micrococcus nishinomiyaensis*, *Micrococcus kristinae* and *Micrococcus roseus*.

Aerococcus viridans, *S. pyogenes* and various anaerobic *Peptostreptococcus* spp. can also establish residence on the skin surface. *Aerococcus* is an air-borne bacterium so the incidence of true colonization versus contamination and transient colonization is unknown. *S. pyogenes* differ from other streptococci in their tolerance to the dry surfaces of the skin and to the bactericidal fatty acids from sebum and also produced by the anaerobic cocci and bacilli. Thus, they are particularly well suited for dry skin surfaces. Anaerobic cocci (e.g. *Peptostreptococcus* spp.) survive in the anaerobic niches of hair follicles and skin glands.

Corynebacterium spp. present on the skin surface include *Corynebacterium striatum*, *Corynebacterium minutissimum*, *Corynebacterium pseudodiphtheriticum*, *Corynebacterium xerosis*, *Corynebacterium urealyticum* (especially in the groin area), and *Corynebacterium jeikeium* (on moist surfaces rich in apocrine glands in hospitalized patients). The anaerobic counterpart to these aerobic gram-positive bacilli are the *Propionibacterium*. *Propionibacterium acnes* is found in high concentrations in areas rich in sebaceous glands, as is *Propionibacterium granulosum*. *P. acnes* is the predominant species, found on virtually all individuals in high numbers, whereas *P.*

granulosum is recovered in small numbers and on fewer than 20% of individuals sampled.

Propionibacterium avidum, by contrast, requires an area high in moisture for survival and is most commonly found in axilla and perineum. Other resident gram-positive bacilli include *Dermabacter hominis*, *Brevibacterium epidermidis*, *Brevibacterium casei* and poorly defined *Brevibacterium* spp. *Turicella otitidis* colonizes the external ear. Some species of *Bacillus* and *Clostridium*, particularly *Clostridium perfringens*, can colonize the skin surface due to their ability to form spores and withstand desiccation and detergents. However, they are generally present in small numbers and only transiently.

Gram-negative bacteria are generally not recovered from the surface of the skin, except during transient colonization. The outer portion of the cell wall of gram-negative bacilli consists of a lipid membrane that is unable to survive exposure to detergents or the dry surfaces of the skin. However, *Acinetobacter* spp. have adapted to survive in moist areas such as toe webs, the groin and axillae. *Burkholderia cepacia* can also colonize the skin surface but generally is found only transiently.

Fungal colonization of the skin surface is commonly transient, following contamination with environmental moulds. This is significant only when the organisms are introduced into the subcutaneous or deeper tissues. The exceptions to this are few, but include colonization with selected yeasts (i.e. *Blastoschizomyces capitatus*, *C. albicans*, *Malassezia furfur*, *Malassezia sympodialis* and *Rhodotorula*) and dermatophytes (i.e. species of *Epidermophyton*, *Microsporum* and *Trichophyton*). Only *M. furfur* is present consistently in the majority of individuals and in high density.

6 NORMAL MICROBIOTA OF BLOOD, CEREBROSPINAL FLUID AND OTHER BODY FLUIDS

The human body is bathed in a variety of fluids including blood, cerebrospinal, synovial, pleural, pericardial, peritoneal and other exudates and transudates. All of these fluids are normally sterile or only transiently infected. Whereas microbes from the mouth or gastrointestinal tract can invade the bloodstream in healthy individuals (e.g. during tooth brushing or a bowel movement), these organisms are rapidly removed and generally of little or no significance. Thus, the isolation of an organism from a body fluid should be considered significant unless the specimen is contaminated during the process of collection.

7 NORMAL MICROBIOTA OF BODY TISSUES

As with body fluids, organ tissues are generally sterile unless they are infected following the systemic spread of an organism in the bloodstream. Some organisms (e.g. *Mycobacterium tuberculosis*) may be disseminated to tissues such as the lungs, liver, or kidneys at the time of initial infection and remain dormant for many years. In this situation it is possible that the organism could be recovered from tissue samples but even that would be unlikely unless the disease process was active. Likewise, long-term colonization with organisms such as *Pneumocystis carinii* or with latent viruses such as herpes simplex or cytomegalovirus commonly occur. Again, these organisms are not typically isolated unless the organisms are actively replicating and tissue pathology is observed.

8 Concluding comments

From the moment of birth until the terminal breath, the human body serves as a home for qualitatively and quantitatively numerous microbes. They cover the skin and mucosal surfaces of the body, occasionally invade into sterile tissues and fluids to produce disease, but more typically coexist with each other and their human host. These microbiota function as a microbial barrier to more virulent micro-organisms, supplement the human host's mechanical and enzymatic digestion of food, provide vitamins and other required growth factors for their host, or simply exist as a commensal inhabitant on their host. The complexity of the microbiota is shaped over time by environmental, host and microbial factors, but is remarkably predictable for a general population. Certainly the dominant microbial species at each of the major body sites (e.g. respiratory tract, gastrointestinal tract, genitourinary tract and body surface) are now well known. Variations from the expected population can predictably lead to disease (e.g. replacement of the microbial population of the small intestine with bacteria from the large intestine leading to a malabsorption syndrome). Likewise, spread of bacteria from their normal habitat into sterile tissues and fluids can initiate well characterized disease (e.g. colonic perforation leads to a polymicrobic peritonitis and intra-abdominal abscess formation by *B. fragilis*). Thus, knowledge of the human microbiota forms a fundamental building block for our knowledge of the normal physiological processes in the human body and our understanding of infectious diseases.

References

Balows A, Hausler WJ et al., 1988, *Laboratory Diagnosis of Infectious Diseases: Principles and Practice*, Springer-Verlag, New York.

Balows A, Truper HG et al., 1992, *The Prokaryotes*, 2nd edn, Springer-Verlag, New York.

Clarke RTJ, Bauchop T, 1977, *Microbiol Ecology of the Gut*, Academic Press, London.

Drasar BS, Hill MJ, 1974, *Human Intestinal Flora*, Academic Press, London.

Holt JG, Krieg NR et al., 1994, *Bergey's Manual of Determinative Bacteriology*, 9th edn, Williams & Wilkins, Baltimore.

Krieg NR, Holt JG, 1984, *Bergey's Manual of Systematic Bacteriology*, Williams & Wilkins, Baltimore.

Linton AH, Hinton MH, 1990, *Topley and Wilson's Principles of Bacteriology, Virology and Immunity*, 8th edn, Edward Arnold, London, 312, 329.

Maibach HI, Hildick-Smith G, 1965, *Skin Bacteria and Their Role in Infection*, McGraw-Hill, New York.

Mandell GL, Bennett JE, Dolin R, 1995, *Principles and Practice of Infectious Diseases*, 4th edn, Churchill Livingstone, New York.

Murray PR, Baron EJ et al., 1995, *Manual of Clinical Microbiology*, 6th edn, ASM Press, Washington, DC.

Noble WC, Sommerville JA, 1974, *Microbiology of Human Skin*, Lloyd Luke, London.

Rosebury T, 1961, *Microorganisms Indigenous to Man*, McGraw-Hill, New York.

Skinner RA, Carr JG, 1974, *The Normal Microflora of Man*, Academic Press, London.

Summanen P, Baron EJ et al., 1993, *Wadsworth Anaerobic Bacteriology Manual*, 5th edn, Star Publishing Co, Belmont, California.

ENVIRONMENTAL SENSING MECHANISMS AND VIRULENCE FACTORS OF BACTERIAL PATHOGENS

P E Kolenbrander

1 **Environmental sensors**	3 **Communication signals between pathogen and host**
2 **Virulence factors**	4 **Summary**

Perhaps the most important feature of a pathogen is its ability to sense continually its environment and coordinate its responsive genes. Most pathogens live in several distinct ecological niches. Food- and water-borne pathogens, for example, have to adapt to environments both outside and inside the human body. The ability to activate and repress genes encoding virulence factors is a key supplement to possessing virulence genes. A rapid response to environmental signals ensures success in the new econiche. A pathogen's success may simply be residence in the host with an occasional expression of virulence in concert with the appropriate environmental stimulus. Correctly sensing signals is a communication balancing act in which both pathogen and host cell participate. By definition, the pathogen occasionally asserts more influence in this act than the host. The pathogen then changes the communication balance from colonization to infection of the host.

Colonization of a eukaryotic host is itself a major accomplishment for a bacterial cell and it involves its own set of signals and responses that permit residence in or on the host. Infection, however, reflects the ability of a pathogen to cause a disease of the host. Bacteria that colonize a host generally persist and are transferred vertically from one generation to the next. Infections elicit a response by the host and the causative organisms are removed. Or, the pathogens may be reduced to a manageable number and convert the host to an asymptomatic carrier. The carrier state may be temporary and it may be recurring. Thus, the carrier may be a significant reservoir for reinfection of a population whose majority is susceptible to the infectious agent.

Pathogens are adaptable: they adapt to existing and to previously unexperienced environments. One example is the adaptation of *Pseudomonas aeruginosa* from a soil and fresh water habitat to human surfaces. It has few nutritional requirements and is able to utilize a broad spectrum of metabolic substrates. This organism is a serious problem in hospitals where it can survive in many different solutions including those of disinfectants. Under normal conditions human defences prevent the pseudomonad from becoming established in the body; it is recognized as an opportunistic pathogen in immunocompromised persons, in burn sites and in wounds. It is nearly always found in the lungs of persons with cystic fibrosis, who produce thick mucin coatings and impaired phagocytic capability. This species exemplifies a pathogen's capability to respond at the opportune moment with the expression of its virulence genes, which encode extracellular products such as proteases and exotoxins. The organism sparsely populates the fresh water ecological niche, in which these extracellular products would be diluted and wasted. However, when the organism colonizes susceptible humans, it becomes densely packed and signals itself to express a cluster of virulence genes. This mechanism of environmental sensing is called quorum sensing and centres on the regulation of gene expression in response to the increased concentration of diffusible small N-acylhomoserine lactone derivatives called autoinducers (see section 1.3, p. 309).

Bacterial virulence factors can be defined as the components and products of the bacterial cell which confer on the bacterium the potential to harm the host. Virulence involves cross-talk between the bacterial and host cells and cannot be attributed to a single virulence factor. Even the classic bacterial intoxications (e.g. botulism, where powerful exotoxins are produced) occur because the spores of *Clostridium botulinum* protect the species in harsh environments and virulence genes respond to environmental signals. In most cases the damage suffered by the host is multifactorial; the factors involved include those of host origin as well as bacterial factors. For example, in certain *Escherichia coli*-induced diarrhoeas in piglets, the organism requires at least 2 virulence factors such as surface fimbriae (that mediate adherence to the mucosa or underlying epithelial cells) and the ability to secrete enterotoxins. Other conditions favouring successful pathogenesis involve the animal host which must be of a certain genotype to express the receptors for the adherence factor and its age is often important. Examples of these, together with many others illustrating the complexity of bacterial virulence, are described in more detail later in this chapter.

The virulence factors of bacteria are conveniently divided into those that are **cell associated** (i.e. cell surface components) and those that are **extracellular** (i.e. the classic exotoxins and extracellular enzymes). It should be stressed that many of the virulence factors described here have functions other than those of damaging the host. Most have a role, which is often primary, in the anatomy or physiology of the bacterial cell, and that of a virulence factor is purely coincidental. Several surface components serve as **colonization factors** and others as **environmental sensors** that trigger transcriptional activation of virulence genes as well as genes that enhance the ecological adaptability of the organism. This chapter is organized to integrate descriptions of communication signals and virulence factors as both are critical for pathogenesis.

1 ENVIRONMENTAL SENSORS

1.1 Sensing nutrients

A pathogen encounters external stimuli whether it is stationary and sensing physical and chemical signals or passing from one environment to the next. Regulation of expression of genes for lactose metabolism in *E. coli* is an example of how a bacterium senses its environment. The essential elements of bacterial responses to their surroundings illustrate the biological and chemical complexities involved in this paradigm of gene regulation (Jacob and Monod 1961). In its most basic form, the communication consists of a bacterium sensing the lactose in the environment and responding by synthesizing β-galactosidase. The central element is the *lac* repressor which forms a tetramer comprised of identical subunits with a molecular mass of 154.52 kDa. In the absence of lactose, the tetramer complexes with the operator region of the *lac* operon and prevents transcription. There are 3 *lac* repressor recognition sites within a stretch of 500 base pairs around the 5′-coding sequence of the *lacZ*

gene, which encodes β-galactosidase. Examination of the crystal structure of the *lac* repressor and its complex with DNA suggests that the tetrameric repressor functions synergistically with a cyclic AMP-dependent catabolite gene activator protein (CAP), and a homotetramer interacts simultaneously with 2 sites on the DNA (Lewis et al. 1996). In the presence of lactose, the *lac* repressor is released from the operator region and transcription is initiated. Positive activation of the *lac* operon involves CAP, which increases transcription through binding to a region near the transcription start site and causing increased affinity of RNA polymerase for the promoter region. Considering the sophisticated communications involved in simply responding to a sugar in the environment points out the fact that constant sensing of the environmental signals elicits appropriate respective responses and the levels of communication are multiple and interactive.

Human pathogens employ sensing and response mechanisms. Some are variations of the lactose operon; they are called house-keeping because they involve normal growth and maintainence of cell viability. Other sensing and response mechanisms involve synthesis of toxins and colonization factors which characterize the organism as a pathogen. For example, the transcription of many toxin genes is regulated by iron. Iron binds to the repressor and the repressor–iron complex binds to the operator site, resulting in inhibition of transcription. Likewise, in an environment of low iron, as is the environment for most pathogenic ecological niches, the repressor is unable to complex with iron and thus unable to bind to the operator, which permits the virulence gene to be transcribed. Under low iron conditions, for example, genes encoding Shiga toxin from *Shigella dysenteriae* and diphtheria toxin from *Corynebacterium diphtheriae* are transcribed.

1.2 Two-component signal transduction

To communicate with its environment a pathogen's sensory response system must be tuned to effect an internal change in accord with the change it has detected in its environment. One of these systems is the bacterial 2-component regulatory system, which has been found in bacteria from a wide variety of econiches (Table 12.1) (Dziejman and Mekalanos 1995, Hoch and Silhavy 1995). Basically, this regulatory system consists of 2 central protein elements (Fig. 12.1). One senses the environment and the other conducts or effects the cell's internal response. The sensor and response regulator proteins exchange information by transferring a phosphate group from the sensor to the response regulator through evolutionarily conserved domains within the 2 proteins. Histidine phosphorylation of the sensor (a histidine protein kinase) occurs in a bimolecular reaction involving a sensor homodimer; each kinase monomer catalyses the phosphorylation of a histidine residue in the juxtapositioned paired monomer. By regulating the phosphorylation state of the response regulator and thus the strength of the response, the cell interior accurately reflects the status of the environment as detected by the sensor.

The sensor modulates the rate of the response regulator phosphorylation in 2 ways:

1   regulating the rate of autophosphorylation of its histidine residues and hence the availability of phosphorylated sensor and
2   the specificity of recognition between the protein–protein contacts on the cognate sensor–response regulator pair (Stock et al. 1995).

Cognate sensor–response regulator pairs catalyse the histidine–aspartate phosphotransfer at least 100-fold more rapidly than between non-cognate pairs. Because of this high specificity for its cognate, the protein–protein interaction is likely to occur at respective recognition sites in non-conserved regions on the 2 molecules. This is in sharp contrast to the highly conserved regions containing the phosphorylation sites of the respective histidine and aspartate residues. It also channels an environmental signal through the correct response regulator to its specific DNA binding site in the regulatory region of the intended virulence gene.

The phosphorylation–dephosphorylation state of the response regulator is achieved by balancing the kinase (phosphorylating) and phosphatase (dephosphorylating) activities. The sensor (kinase) must bind to the dephosphorylated form of the response regulator (phosphatase) and release the phosphorylated form (Stock et al. 1995). Assuming no auxiliary proteins participate, then binding between sensor and response regulator cognate pair occurs only when one or the other is phosphorylated but not between unphosphorylated cognates or phosphorylated cognates. When the rate of histidine phosphorylation is high, the phosphotransfer to the aspartate residue of the response regulator predominates; when the rate of histidine phosphorylation is low, dephosphorylation of the response regulator aspartate residue is favoured. Assuming that the phosphatase reaction occurs with monomers of response regulator molecules, the balance between phosphorylation and dephosphorylation could be controlled simply by the state of the sensor dimerization. Since the sensor is the component in contact with the environment, this sensing mechanism can respond quickly as the pathogen goes from one environment to the next.

1.3   Quorum sensing

With some gram-negative human pathogens, expression of virulence genes may be the indirect result of bacterial growth and an increase of cell density to reach a quorum of cells. The opportunistic pathogen *P. aeruginosa* expresses virulence factors in response to sensing its own cell density. The fundamental basis of this quorum sensing is the concentration of diffusible autoinducer molecules used for intercellular communication in the population

Table 12.1   Two-component regulatory proteins of human pathogens

Pathogen	Environmental signal	Adaptive response	Sensor/response regulator
Bacteroides fragilis	Tetracycline	Self-transfer of DNA	tetQ promoter (RteA?)/RteB
Bordetella pertussis	Temperature, SO$_4$, nicotinic acid	Activation and repression of virulence factors, including HA and toxin	BvgS/BvgA
Citrobacter freundii	Unknown	Vi antigen expression	ViaA/ViaB
Clostridium perfringens	Unknown	Perfringolysin-O, HA and collagenase expression	VirS/VirR
Enterococcus faecium	Vancomycin	Vancomycin resistance	VanS/VanR
Klebsiella pneumoniae	N$_2$	Urease production	NtrA/NtrC
	N$_2$, O$_2$	Nitrogen fixation	NifL/NifA
Neisseria gonorrhoeae	Stress	Pilin production	PilB/PilA
Mycobacterium tuberculosis	Macrophage entry	Intracellular survival?	MtrB/MtrA
Pseudomonas aeruginosa	Unknown	Pilin expression	PilR/PilS
	Enterobactin, iron	Ferric enterobactin receptor	PfeR/PfeS
	Osmolarity	Alginate synthesis	AlgR1/AlgR2
Salmonella typhimurium	pH, starvation	Outer-membrane protein expression	PhoQ/PhoP
Shigella flexneri	Osmolarity	Porin expression	EnvZ/OmpR
Vibrio cholerae	pH, osmolarity, temperature	Virulence factor expression including toxin and pili	ToxR/ToxT
Vibrio parahaemolyticus	pH	Thermostable direct haemolysin production	ToxR, (ToxS)

From Dziejman and Mekalanos (1995), Ba-Thein et al. (1996), Via et al. (1996).

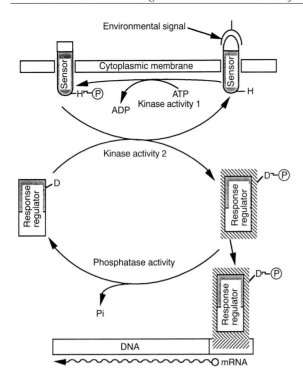

Fig. 12.1 Two-component signal transduction system. The sensor has access to the environment and is a histidine protein kinase. It responds to an environmental signal by binding ATP and phosphorylating a histidine residue (H~P) (kinase activity 1) in a conserved domain (shaded region). The phosphorylated sensor (squared-off top) transfers the phosphoryl group from phosphohistidine to an aspartate side chain in a conserved domain (shaded region) of the response regulator molecule (kinase activity 2). The activated response regulator (fuzzy rectangle) either binds to a site in the regulatory region of a target virulence gene to initiate gene expression or dephosphorylates (phosphatase activity).

(Fuqua et al. 1994). During normal growth cells continually secrete specific *N*-acylhomoserine lactones that act as autoinducers of expression of certain virulence genes. At low cell densities and correspondingly low concentrations of these signalling molecules, little or no expression of the responsive virulence genes occurs. When a quorum is reached, the autoinducer concentration is sufficiently high and virulence genes are transcribed (Fuqua et al. 1994, Swift et al. 1994). Population-density monitoring by diffusible molecules enables rapid adjustment of cellular metabolism in response to a new environment. It also conserves the energy required for synthesis of autoinducible gene products until the gene products can be most useful to the cell.

Quorum sensing always requires at least one additional factor, an intracellular transcriptional activator, which binds to the autoinducer to co-ordinate expression of the responsive genes. Bacteria from diverse ecological niches such as plant tumours (*Agrobacterium tumefaciens*) and the light organ of marine fish (*Vibrio fischeri*) exhibit quorum sensing. The primary structures of transcriptional activators from *P. aeruginosa*, *V. fischeri* and *A. tumefaciens* show

significant sequence homology, indicating that quorum sensing is a broad-based ecologically significant mechanism of environmental signalling. A family of transcriptional activator proteins and their cognate *N*-acylhomoserine lactones is emerging from studies of gram-negative bacteria and is based on the molecular pair, LuxR–LuxI, of the luminescent marine bacterium, *V. fischeri* (Fuqua et al. 1994). Members of the LuxR family share about 25–30% identity (Fuqua et al. 1994, Throup et al. 1995). The autoinducer products of the LuxI family are homoserine lactones with an *N*-linked acyl side chain of varying chain length and oxidation state (Fuqua et al. 1994).

P. aeruginosa secretes many extracellular virulence factors including exotoxin A, alkaline protease and elastase. Elastase is capable of degrading or inactivating several biologically significant proteins including elastin, collagen, fibrin, human immunoglobulins G and A, and serum complement factors. Elastase, the product of the *lasB* gene, is maximally expressed in response to *P. aeruginosa* autoinducer (PAI) (Gambello and Iglewski 1991, Passador et al. 1993) and transcriptional activator protein LasR, which is encoded by the *lasR* gene. PAI is *N*-(3-oxododecanoyl)homoserine lactone and is a product of the putative autoinducer synthase, LasI, encoded by the *lasI* gene. An autoinduction regulatory hierarchy was discovered when half-maximal expression of *lasI* required only 0.1 nM PAI, whereas a 10-fold higher concentration of PAI was needed for half-maximal expression of *lasB* (Seed et al. 1995). In this hierarchy, low PAI concentration plus LasR activates *lasI* expression, which in turn increases the PAI concentration and subsequent activation of *lasB* with the resultant secretion of elastase. This kind of positive regulation of *lasI* delineates a feedback loop that responds quickly to a change in cell density. For example, a small number of responding cells senses a quorum and excretes higher levels of PAI, which triggers neighbouring cells to do the same. The immediate result is that the entire population is now in the higher responding level of PAI synthesis completing the regulatory loop and excreting virulence factors such as elastase.

A second autoinducer, *N*-butyrylhomoserine lactone, was found to activate *lasB* when expression of *lasR* is controlled by its own promoter (Pearson et al. 1995). The synthesis of this second autoinducer is directed by the product of the *rhlI* gene (Winson et al. 1995), which acts in co-ordination with RhlR, the transcriptional activator gene product of *rhlR*, to synthesize extracellular rhamnolipid biosurfactants (Ochsner et al. 1994, Ochsner and Reiser 1995). Notably, multiple copies of the *lasR* gene in an *rhlR* mutant promoted a low level of rhamnolipids; multiple copies of the *rhlR* gene in a *lasR* mutant produced high levels of elastase (Ochsner and Reiser 1995). These results suggest that cross-communication between the RhlR–RhlI rhamnolipid regulatory system and the LasR–LasI elastase regulatory system is operational in *P. aeruginosa*. Quorum sensing may indeed be a cascade of events that constitute a network of interacting LuxR–LuxI homologues in certain gram-negative pathogenic bacteria.

Continued studies with *P. aeruginosa* and other human pathogens are uncovering more of the complex regulatory circuitry involving homologues of LuxR–LuxI. LasR and PAI activate *lasB* by reacting with 2 putative operator sequences located directly upstream from the *lasB* transcriptional start site (Rust et al. 1996). LasR also controls the expression of certain potentially pathogenic extracellular factors such as alkaline protease and exotoxin A (Gambello et al. 1993) and a second elastase, LasA (Toder et al. 1991). The RhlR–RhlI circuit does not appear to regulate exotoxin A but does modulate production of haemolysin, pyocyanin and cyanide (Latifi et al. 1995). Homologues YenR–YenI were found in *Yersinia enterocolitica*, a food- and water-borne pathogen causing gastroenteritis in humans (Throup et al. 1995). Insertional mutation in the *yenI* gene abolished synthesis of 2 autoinducer molecules, *N*-hexanoyl-L-homoserine lactone and *N*-(3-oxohexanoyl)-L-homoserine lactone. The target of the YenR–YenI putative regulatory circuit in *Yersinia enterocolitica* remains to be determined.

2 VIRULENCE FACTORS

Before discussing the various surface virulence factors, it is appropriate to describe the stages of the pathogenic processes, particularly those at which colonization factors may be important.

2.1 Colonization factors and pathogenesis

Once a pathogenic bacterium is in or on a susceptible host, it must become established at a suitable site. For example, at mucous membranes it is usual for the pathogen to penetrate the mucous blanket and subsequently to adhere to the epithelium. Movement through the mucus to the epithelial cells may be dependent on chemoattractants in host tissue, and the bacterium may require flagella and possibly mucus-degrading enzymes. Adherence to the tissue is then usual to avoid the mechanical action of the cilia or the flushing action of the body fluids. Colonization factors involved in adherence include fimbriae (pili), lipoteichoic acids, exopolysaccharides (capsules and glycocalyxes) and outer-membrane proteins. These factors may act in conjunction with host-derived polymers and those from other bacteria to produce a community or biofilm, e.g. in dental plaque. The binding of the receptor on the host cell surface and the bacterial adhesin is often highly specific and accomplished by complementary molecules. For example, the host cell surface protein, fibronectin, is a receptor for some pathogens but not others.

Once the organism is located in the host, subsequent factors in the pathogenic process include evasion of the host defence system and the ability of the pathogen to compete with the commensal flora for nutrients and space. Bacterial factors for the former step include possession of a capsule, which can be

both antiphagocytic and a camouflaging mechanism if it mimics host tissue. The long polysaccharide chains of 'smooth' lipopolysaccharide and of capsular polysaccharide allow the fixation of complement at a site distant from the bacterial cell membrane, thus making the bacterium resistant to the lethal lytic effect of normal serum. Some bacteria are classically intracellular and thus evade the defence mechanisms by their internal location. Factors that confer virulence on pathogens by allowing them to compete with the normal flora include the ability to secrete **antibacterial substances** (e.g. bacteriocins, organic acids, alcohols) and their ability to express **scavenging mechanisms** such as iron-binding proteins.

Subsequent steps in pathogenesis involve the mechanisms by which the host is harmed. It is at this stage that toxins – both the classic exotoxins and, in the case of gram-negative bacteria, the lipopolysaccharide (endotoxin) – exert their main influence. Their effects can be either local or systemic. The actions of the toxins are described in detail later (see section on 'Bacterial exotoxins', p. 318). Tissue damage can also result from direct invasion of tissue, from inflammation or from harmful immune responses, which include anaphylaxis, complement mediated cytolysis, immune complex reactions and cell mediated reactions.

Finally, to complete the cyclic process of pathogenesis, the organism is released from the host and is disseminated to other susceptible hosts. The ability to survive outside the host is indeed a virulence factor for many food- and water-borne pathogens. The waxy coat of the mycobacteria, the ability to form spores and the possession of a highly hydrated capsule are obvious examples of survival mechanisms but are not considered further in this chapter.

From this brief description of pathogenesis it is apparent that virulence factors are involved at all stages of the disease process and often the same component can be involved in more than one stage. Furthermore, the virulence determinants encompass the whole range of surface components. Table 12.2 summarizes the role of surface components as virulence factors.

2.2 Polysaccharide virulence factors

STRUCTURE

Exopolysaccharides include the discrete capsules of many pathogenic bacteria and the loosely associated slime produced by mucoid bacteria. They are the classic K antigens of the enterobacteria. Capsules were among the first known bacterial virulence factors. The first demonstration of bacterial transformation by Griffiths (1928) involved the transformation of rough (non-capsulate, non-virulent) pneumococci to the smooth (capsulate, virulent) form.

Exopolysaccharides form highly hydrated, water-insoluble gels. They can be readily demonstrated in the electron microscope with ruthenium red stain, which binds to negatively charged polymers. The chemical composition of exopolysaccharides can be of

Table 12.2   Bacterial cell surface components as virulence factors

Surface component	Contribution to virulence
Capsule/exopolysaccharide	Adhesion; antiphagocytic; camouflage from immune system/mimicry of host tissue; resistance to complement; invasiveness
Lipopolysaccharide	Resistance to complement; invasiveness; endotoxic: stimulation of many harmful immune responses; adhesion
Teichoic acid/lipoteichoic acid	Adhesion; sequestration of divalent ions; stimulation of many harmful immune responses
Fimbriae/pili/fibrillae/non-fimbrial adhesins	Adhesion; antiphagocytic; colonization factors
Flagella/axial filaments	Chemotaxis; penetration of mucus; adhesion; intracellular survival
Outer-membrane proteins	Adhesins; sequestration of iron; invasiveness; intracellular survival; resistance to complement
Surface proteins of gram-positive bacteria	Adhesion; binding to Fc region of immunoglobulins
Molecules that cross-talk with the host cells	Triggers actin rearrangement in host; bacteria adhere to host cells; some bacteria invade host cells

2 types: homo- and heteropolysaccharides, consisting respectively of a single sugar monomer (e.g. the levans and dextrans of many oral streptococci) or of repeating oligosaccharide units of more than one monomer. Many exopolysaccharides are acidic due to the possession of carboxyl groups, either from acidic sugars such as uronic acids or neuraminic acid, or from non-sugar substitutents such as pyruvyl, acetyl and formyl groups. Their acidic nature is reflected in many of their properties. A few of the bacilli (e.g. *Bacillus anthracis*) have a capsule made up of a single amino acid, poly-D-glutamic acid. In physical chemistry and function, however, it is similar to the polysaccharide capsules. Examples of the basic structures of the exopolysaccharides of several pathogenic bacteria are shown in Table 12.3, and the appearance of a capsulate bacterium is shown in Fig. 12.2.

BIOLOGICAL ACTIVITIES

As virulence factors, exopolysaccharides have 2 major roles. The first is in adhesion and is particularly obvious in *Streptococcus mutans*, the cariogenic organism. The bacterium can synthesize, from dietary sucrose, a branched, water-insoluble homopolymer of glucose which is dextran-like. It forms a glutinous layer on the surface of the tooth and contributes to the matrix of dental plaque. It also forms a metabolic substrate for acid formation. Other examples of polysaccharide mediated attachment are coagulase-negative staphylococci, which bind to indwelling catheters and prosthetic devices.

The second main role of capsular polysaccharide in virulence is **protection of the organism** from the host defence systems. Since the classic work on the pneumococcus it has been recognized that capsules prevent bacteria from being engulfed by phagocytes. There are several possible reasons. Capsulate or slime-producing bacteria usually grow in microcolonies in vivo and engulfment is difficult on purely steric con-

siderations. Furthermore, complement (see below) and opsonic antibodies cannot get access to the cell envelope. Another general observation is that the more hydrophilic the surface of a bacterium – and this can be related to the amount of polysaccharide – the less readily it can be phagocytosed. A good example of a potential virulence factor with some of the above properties is the alginate slime of mucoid *P. aeruginosa* in the lungs of children with cystic fibrosis.

Several species of bacteria produce a capsule with a chemical structure that mimics host tissue. This camouflages the organism from the immune system by appearing to the host as 'self'. Perhaps the best known examples are the K1 capsule of *E. coli* and the immunologically and structurally identical capsule of *Neisseria meningitidis* group B. These organisms have capsules of α-2,8-linked *N*-acetylneuraminic acid which is partially O-acetylated. It cross-reacts immunologically with neonatal neural cell adhesion molecules. Capsules of similar composition are found in the important sheep pathogen *Pasteurella haemolytica* type A2. Another example of a capsule mimicking host tissue is provided by the hyaluronic acid capsules of *Streptococcus pyogenes* and of *Pasteurella multocida* type A. Many of these capsules also confer resistance to the bactericidal effect of serum, and this is discussed further below.

As mentioned earlier, the capsule allows the bacterium to evade the immune system by making it resistant to the lytic action of complement. It is well known that, for lipopolysaccharide (LPS), which is described later (see section 2.3, p. 314), the longer the chains of O-polysaccharide, the more resistant they are to complement. This is thought to be because the complement cascade is activated at a distance from the bacterial membrane so that no lysis occurs. It has been recognized for many years that the capsular polysaccharide also confers this property of serum resistance, especially the K1 antigen of *E. coli*. Thus, the

Table 12.3 Examples of repeating unit structures for some capsular polysaccharides

Species	Group/type	Structure
Streptococcus pneumoniae	Type 1[a]	$- - -$ GalUA $\xrightarrow{1,3}$ GlcNAc $\xrightarrow{1,3}$ GalUA $- - -$
	Type 6	$\xrightarrow{2}$ Gal $\xrightarrow[1,3]{\alpha}$ Glc $\xrightarrow[1,3]{\alpha}$ Rha $\xrightarrow[1,3]{\alpha}$ Rib $-$ P $\xrightarrow[1]{}$ $\xrightarrow{1}$
	Type 8	$\xrightarrow{4}$ Glc $\xrightarrow[1,3]{\beta}$ Glc $\xrightarrow[1,4]{\alpha}$ Gal $\xrightarrow[1,4]{\alpha}$ GlcUA $\xrightarrow[1]{\beta}$
Neisseria meningitidis	Group A[b]	$\xrightarrow{6}$ ManNAc-1–P $\xrightarrow[1]{\alpha}$ $\vert$ 3 O-Ac
	Group B	$\xrightarrow{8}$ NeuNAc $\xrightarrow[2]{\alpha}$
	Group C[b]	$\xrightarrow{9}$ NeuNAc $\xrightarrow[2]{\alpha}$ $\vert$ 7/8 O-Ac
Haemophilus influenzae	Type b[c]	$\xrightarrow{3}$ Rib $\xrightarrow[1,1]{\beta}$ Rib $-$ P $\xrightarrow{5}$
Escherichia coli	K1[b,d]	$\xrightarrow{8}$ NeuNAc $\xrightarrow[2]{\alpha}$ $\vert$ O-Ac
Salmonella typhi	Vi[b]	$\xrightarrow{4}$ GalNAcUA $\xrightarrow[1]{\alpha}$ $\vert$ 3 O-Ac

Abbreviations: Ac, acetyl; Gal, galactose; GalNAcUA, *N*-acetylgalactosaminuronic acid; GalU, galacturonic acid; Glc, glucose; GlcNAc, *N*-acetylglucosamine; ManNAc-l-P, *N*-acetylmannosamine phosphate; NeuNAc, *N*-acetylneuraminic acid; Rha, rhamnose, Rib, ribose; Rib-P, ribitol phosphate.
[a]Partial structure only.
[b]Not all the sugar residues are O-acetylated.
[c]An example of a teichoic acid polymer in a gram-negative organism.
[d]Internal ester bridges are also present.

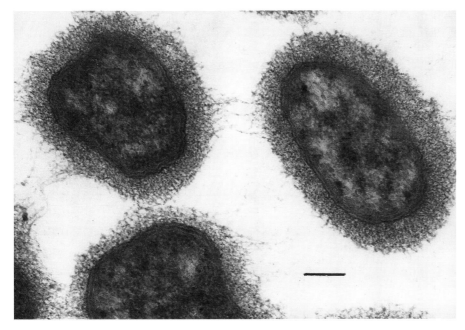

Fig. 12.2 Electron micrograph of a capsulate *Klebsiella* sp. stained with ruthenium red. Bar marker = 0.2 μm. (Photograph kindly supplied by Dr J R W Govan).

property of serum resistance is multifactorial. The LPS of some *E. coli* serotypes is incapable of protecting against serum lysis. For these strains the capsule, which is most commonly K1, confers protection. For other serotypes of *E. coli* (e.g. O6) the capsule is much less important. This serotype often possesses the K5 capsule, which is as non-immunogenic as K1, but does not confer resistance to serum on the bacterium. Finally, it should be noted that the anticomplementary and antiphagocytic effects of capsules of *E. coli* and many other species are usually overcome by opsonization of the bacterium with capsule-specific antibodies.

There is a possible connection between the ability of the organism to resist the action of complement and its ability to invade the host; again, in *E. coli* the K1 antigen is important. Most bacterial pathogens found outside the gut and inside functional barriers, e.g. those causing bacteraemia, meningitis and urinary tract infections – especially pyelonephritis – are capsulate. One of the most invasive of bacteria is *Salmonella typhi*. In this species the most important virulence determinant is the Vi antigen. This capsular antigen, which has a unit structure of partially O-acetylated, α-1,4-linked *N*-acetylgalactosaminuronic acid monomers, is important in invasion. The invasive, but noncapsulate, shigellae and enteroinvasive *E. coli* (EIEC) have unusual acidic O-polysaccharides which are proposed as functional analogues of the acidic capsule and as being important in the mechanism of invasion.

The capsule of *Bacteroides fragilis* and possibly of other *Bacteroides* spp. is said to have a role in inhibiting the phagocytosis and intracellular killing of facultative anaerobes (predominantly *E. coli*) in mixed anaerobic and aerobic infections. The mixed infection involves synergistic interactions between anaerobes and aerobes and a multifactorial mechanism, with LPS, protein, metabolites, chemotaxis of neutrophils and the redox potential of the system all possibly having an influence.

2.3 Lipopolysaccharides

Lipopolysaccharides (LPS, endotoxin) are the immunodominant antigens of most gram-negative bacteria and are considered intimately associated with the virulence properties of the pathogen. This amphipathic molecule, which is anchored in the outer membrane of the gram-negative bacterium and forms an essential constituent of the cell envelope, confers on the organism a wide range of biological properties involved in host–parasite interactions. Comprehensive summaries of current knowledge of the genetics and structure–function of LPS are recommended reading (Holst and Brade 1992, Schnaitman and Klena 1993).

STRUCTURE

LPS consists of 2 main regions: a **hydrophobic glycolipid** (the lipid A) and a **hydrophilic polysaccharide**. In many bacteria with a smooth form LPS the polysaccharide can be subdivided into the core oligosaccharide and the O-polysaccharide or O antigen. Rough mutants lack the O-polysaccharide. Some bacteria (e.g. *Neisseria* spp.) possess a naturally rough form LPS which is sometimes referred to as the lipooligosaccharide. The smooth–rough structure of LPS is summarized diagrammatically in Fig. 12.3.

The lipid A part is embedded in the outer membrane and is the toxic part of the molecule. It becomes exposed when cells lyse as a consequence of complement activation, engulfment by phagocytes or antibiotic-induced lysis. Lipid A can stimulate release of cytokines, which are part of the host defence system. In *E. coli* lipid A consists of a β-1,6-linked glucosaminyl–glucosamine disaccharide backbone which is

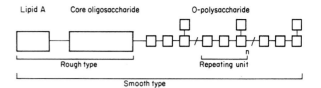

Fig. 12.3 Diagrammatic representation of lipopolysaccharide.

substituted with phosphate groups at the 1-position of the reducing end and at the 4-position of the nonreducing sugar. Each sugar monomer is substituted at the 2- and 3-positions with 3-hydroxymyristic acid residues through amide and ester linkages, respectively. The fatty acids on the non-reducing sugar are themselves substituted with lauric and myristic acid. Figure 12.4 shows the structure of the lipid A molecule of *E. coli*. This structure is more or less common to all LPS molecules that are endotoxic, the variations being in the length of the substituted fatty acid residues, the type and distribution of the substitutents of the fatty acids, and the additional substituents of the phosphoryl residues.

The structure of the core oligosaccharide consists of 11 or so monosaccharide units. The inner region of the core (i.e. the part proximal to the lipid A) is characterized by being made up of the unusual sugars 3-deoxy-D-manno-2-octulosonic acid (KDO) and L-glycero- or D-glycero-D-mannoheptose (heptose) together with phosphate and ethanolamine. This inner region of the core is largely conserved in a wide range of species. The outer part, consisting typically of glucose, galactose and glucosamine, is where a limited

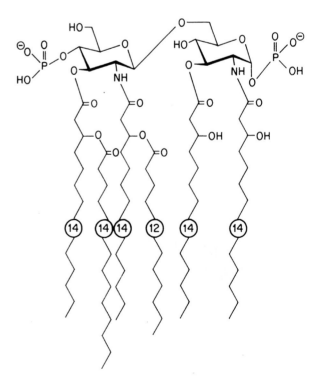

Fig. 12.4 The structure of lipid A from *Escherichia coli*.

amount of variation between and within species occurs. Some examples of core types are shown in Table 12.4.

It is in the O-polysaccharide where variation can be almost infinite. This is the part of the molecule which gives the O serogroup identity to a strain. The serological classification of an *E. coli* strain includes its serotype which is based on the flagellar H antigen. For example, an *E. coli* strain labelled O157:H7 (a known enterohaemorrhagic strain) is in the same serogroup as one labelled O157:H1 but is a different serotype. The O-polysaccharide consists typically of long chains of repeating units of oligosaccharides, usually made up of 3 or 4 monomers. There are over 160 serogroups in *E. coli*; some examples of the repeating unit structure of some O-polysaccharides from *E. coli* and other genera are shown in Table 12.5.

BIOLOGICAL ACTIVITY

The endotoxin or lipid A portion of LPS exerts its toxic activity by activating complement and by stimulating host cells to release cytokines. Cytokines initiate a cascade of events that may cause septic shock. The cytokines IL-1, IL-6 and IL-8 along with TNF-α and platelet-activating factor stimulate production of prostaglandins and leukotrienes. The main features of septic shock are hypotension, a fall in cardiac output and disseminated intravascular coagulation, which lead to death.

2.4 Teichoic acids and related polymers

STRUCTURE

The surface of the gram-positive bacterium typically has 2 structurally related, negatively charged components. Teichoic acid is covalently linked to the peptidoglycan and is defined as a polymer containing ribitol phosphate or glycerol phosphate with phosphodiester linkages, usually with hexose and D-alanine substituents. The second component, lipoteichoic acid, is anchored in the cytoplasmic membrane and protrudes through the peptidoglycan layer. It is usually composed of glycerol phosphate repeating units with a glycolipid at the terminus and often substituted

Table 12.4 Lipopolysaccharide core oligosaccharides

Abbreviations: Ac, acetyl; Ala, alanine; Gal, galactose; GalNAcUA, *N*-acetylgalactosaminuronic acid; GalN, galactosamine; GalU, galacturonic acid; Glc, glucose; GlcNAc, *N*-acetylglucosamine; Hep, heptose; KDO, 3-deoxy-D-*manno*-2-octulosonic acid; ManNAc-l-P, *N*-acetylmannosamine phosphate; NeuNAc, *N*-acetylneuraminic acid; Rha, rhamnose; Rib, ribose; Rib-P, ribitol phosphate.

Table 12.5   Examples of O-polysaccharide repeating units

Species (serotype)	Structure

Escherichia coli (O4)

$$\text{Glc} \xrightarrow[\alpha]{1,6} \text{Glc}$$
$$\alpha \downarrow 1,3$$
$$-4\ \text{GlcNAc} \xrightarrow[\beta]{1,2} \text{Rha} \xrightarrow[\alpha]{1,3} \text{FucNAc} \xrightarrow[\alpha]{1} -$$

E. coli (O86)

$$\text{Fuc}$$
$$\downarrow$$
$$-\text{Gal} - \text{GalNAc} - \text{GalNAc}$$

E. coli (O111)

$$\text{Col}$$
$$\alpha \downarrow 1,3$$
$$-4\ \text{Glc} \xrightarrow[\alpha]{1,4} \text{Gal} \xrightarrow[\alpha]{1,3} \text{GlcNAc} \xrightarrow[\beta]{1} -$$
$$\alpha \uparrow 1,6$$
$$\text{Col}$$

Salmonella typhi

$$\text{Tyv} \qquad\qquad \text{Glc-2OAc}$$
$$\alpha \downarrow 1,3 \qquad\qquad \alpha \downarrow 1,4$$
$$-2\ \text{Man} \xrightarrow[\alpha]{1,4} \text{Rha} \xrightarrow[\alpha]{1,3} \text{Gal} -$$

Salm. paratyphi A

$$\text{Par} \qquad\qquad \text{Glc}$$
$$\alpha \downarrow 1,3 \qquad\qquad \alpha \downarrow 1,6$$
$$-2\ \text{Man} \xrightarrow[\alpha]{1,4} \text{Rha} \xrightarrow[\alpha]{1,3} \text{Gal} \xrightarrow{1} -$$
$$\text{OAc}$$

Salm. typhimurium

$$\text{2OAc-Abe} \qquad\qquad \text{Glc}$$
$$\alpha \downarrow 1.3 \qquad\qquad \alpha \downarrow 1,4$$
$$-2\ \text{Man} \xrightarrow[\beta]{1,4} \text{Rha} \xrightarrow[\beta]{1,3} \text{Gal} \xrightarrow[\alpha]{1} -$$

Klebsiella (O3)

$$\xrightarrow{1,3} \text{Man} \xrightarrow[\alpha]{1,3} \text{Man} \xrightarrow[\alpha]{1,2} \text{Man} \xrightarrow[\alpha]{1,2} \text{Man} \xrightarrow[\alpha]{1} \text{Man} \xrightarrow[\alpha]{1} -$$

Klebsiella (O10)

$$\xrightarrow{3} \text{Rha} \xrightarrow[\alpha]{1,3} \text{Rib} \xrightarrow[\beta]{1,4} \text{Rha} \xrightarrow[\alpha]{1,3} \text{Rib} \xrightarrow[\beta]{1,4} \text{Rha} \xrightarrow[\alpha]{1} -$$

Abbreviations: Abe, abequose-(3,6-dideoxy-D-galactose); Ac, acetyl; Ala, alanine; Col. colitose (3,6-dideoxy-D-galactose); Gal, galactose; Fuc, fucose; FucN, fucosamine; GalNacUA, N-acetylgalactosaminuronic acid; GalN, galactosamine; GalU, galacturonic acid; Glc, glucose; GlcNAc, N-acetylglucosamine; Hep, heptose; KDO, 3-deoxy-D-*manno*-2-octulosonic acid; Man, mannose; ManNAc-l-P, N-acetylmannosamine phosphate; Par, paratose (3,6-dideoxy-D-glucose); NeuNAc, N-acetylneuraminic acid; Rha, rhamnose; Rib, ribose; Rib-P, ribitol phosphate; Tyv, tyvelose (3,6-dideoxy-D-mannose).

with D-alanine residues. Teichoic acids and lipoteichoic acids are not found on all gram-positive bacteria, but most gram-positive bacteria produce a functionally analogous negatively charged polymer. Examples of this family of molecules is shown in Fig. 12.5. Further reading of teichoic acid synthesis and genetic organization (Pooley and Karamata 1994) and of lipoteichoic acids (Fischer 1994) is encouraged.

BIOLOGICAL ACTIVITIES

Although gram-positive bacteria do not possess endotoxins, it is known that gram-positive cells elicit an inflammatory response that is identical to that triggered by gram-negative lipopolysaccharides. Teichoic acids and peptidoglycan polymers cause release of cytokines and the same kind of septic shock symptoms observed with gram-negative bacteria. Lipoteichoic acids have been implicated in adherence of group A streptococci to fibronectin, a protein widely found in the human host. Mating among enterococci is thought to involve lipoteichoic acid, and this activity may have large implications in the dissemination of multiple drug resistance markers among endocarditis-causing enterococci. Lipoteichoic acid may alter the structure of microbial communities comprising dental plaque because it contributes to the cell-to-cell interactions between oral bacteria. Lipoteichoic acids bind calcium and have a role in channelling divalent cations to the cytoplasmic membrane. They are involved in cell division; mutations in genes encoding biosynthetic enzymes of teichoic acids are lethal, indicating the central importance of these molecules to the bacteria.

2.5   Protein virulence factors

Proteins associated with the bacterial cell surface are in 2 main forms: those that form appendages discernible in the electron microscope – the **fimbriae** (or pili) and flagella – and those present on the surface as a layer, e.g. the S layer, a highly organized thin surface

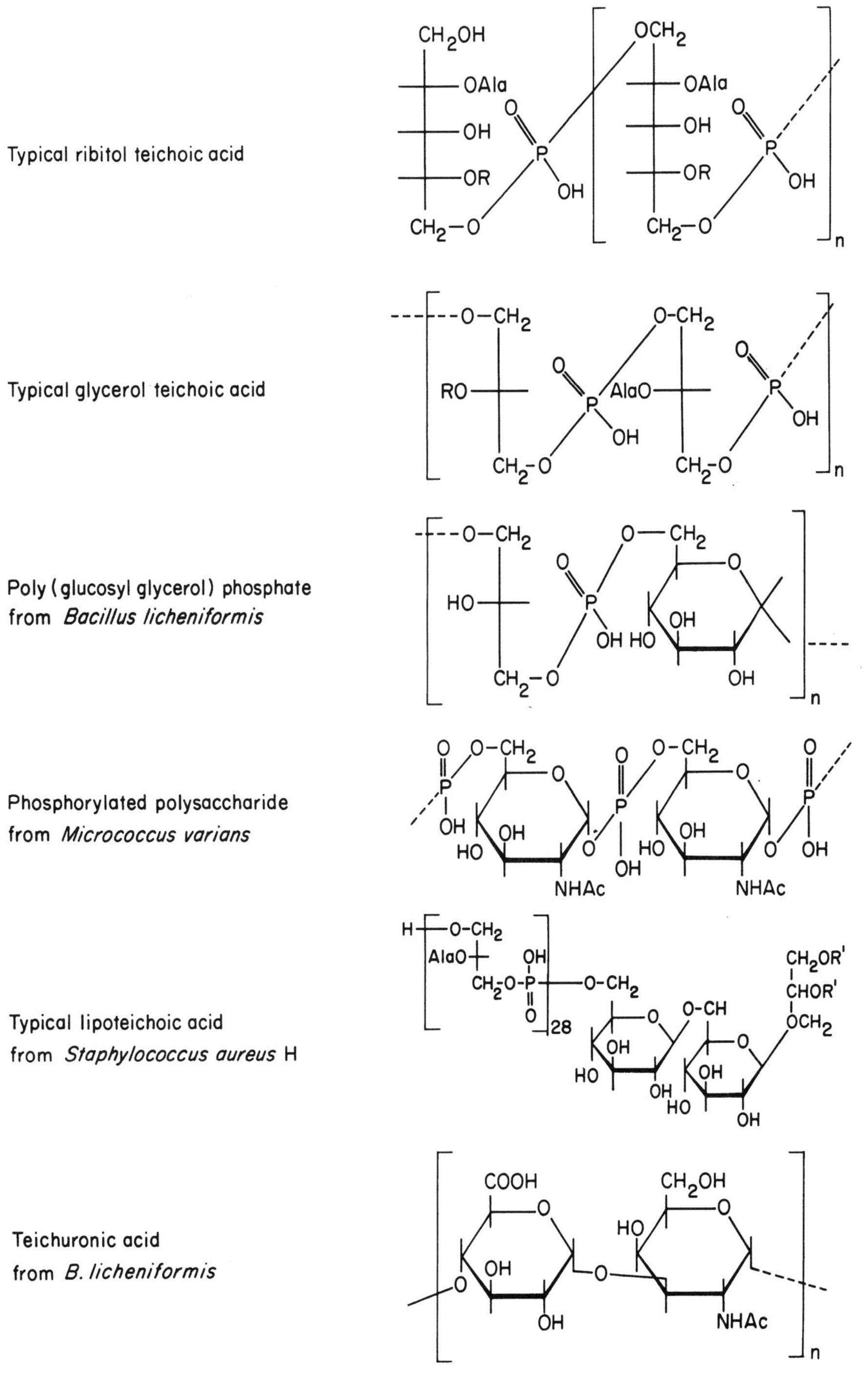

Fig. 12.5 Structures of some teichoic acids and related polymers: n, 30–40; R, sugar substitute; R′, fatty acid.

layer (Messner and Sleytr 1992). Flagella are the organs of motility and confer an obvious advantage on bacteria such as *Helicobacter pylori*, which must traverse a viscous layer of mucus to reach the stomach wall. The S layer is found on many oral bacteria and on fish pathogens such as *Aeromonas salmonicida*.

FIMBRIAE

It is in the Enterobacteriaceae that fimbriae are best characterized. The pioneering work of Duguid more than 40 years ago established the presence of fimbriae by agglutination of red blood cells from a range of species. This fimbria mediated haemagglutination could be resistant or sensitive to blocking by D-mannose (Duguid et al. 1955, Duguid, Anderson and Campbell 1966). The mannose-specific fimbriae are named type 1 fimbriae and are widespread in most species of enterobacteria. Structurally, they are composed of about 1000 protein subunits of 17 kDa called FimA, which are polymerized into a right-handed helical fibril of about 1 μm in length and 7–8 nm in diameter with a central hole. The assembly of the FimA subunits involves chaperone proteins to maintain the FimA protein in proper conformation while passing through the periplasmic space and outer membrane. The tip of the fimbriae consists of a specialized 28 kDa minor subunit called FimH which confers the adhesive function to the cell. Several kinds of fimbriae on *E. coli* are actively studied and include the Pap fimbriae (P fimbriae) associated with urogenital infections and the S fimbriae that recognize an α-sialyl-(2-3)-β-gal containing receptor on host cells. Although many uropathogenic *E. coli* strains bear S fimbriae, most S-fimbriated strains are isolated from cases of newborn meningitis. The Pap fimbriae (P pili) are probably the most completely studied to date (Hultgren et al. 1993). They are also composed of the primary structural subunit PapA and a fimbrial tip assembly containing PapE, PapF, PapK and PapG which has the adhesive function of binding to receptors containing the α-D-galactopyranosyl-(1-4)-β-D-galactopyranoside (Gal α1-4 Gal) disaccharide. Such receptors are part of the globoseries of glycolipids on cells lining the upper urinary tract. Up to 90% of the *E. coli* strains isolated from the urinary tract of children with acute pyelonephritis express the Pap fimbriae.

There are at least 8 kinds of fimbriae found on various isolates of *E. coli*. Among the type 1 mannose-specific fimbrial family, the FimA subunit is variable, but FimH is highly conserved antigenically and genetically among enterobacteria. A single amino acid substitution in FimH can confer a distinct adhesive phenotype, e.g. binding to yeast mannan and to human plasma fibronectin (Sokurenko et al. 1994). The minor subunits of these different fimbriae can be reciprocally exchanged as was shown with type 1 and F1C fimbriae resulting in hybrid organelles with changed receptor specificity and indicating the possibility of fimbrial promiscuity (Klemm et al. 1994). Some uropathogenic strains possess large, unstable DNA regions on the chromosome that are called pathogenicity islands. Deletion of these regions occur frequently and cause the strain to become avirulent. Genetic determinants for some fimbriae are located on a pathogenicity island, and deletion of this island both removes the genetic determinant and represses synthesis of S fimbriae, although the *sfa* genes encoding the S-fimbrial subunits are not located on the pathogenicity island (Morschhäuser et al. 1994). These observations have led the authors to propose

that cross-talk occurs between different adhesin gene clusters. Such cross-regulation of unlinked gene clusters can greatly influence the type of fimbriae presented on the enterobacterial surface and thus the virulence phenotype expressed.

Another well known group of fimbriae and fimbria-like structures is found on *E. coli* strains causing diarrhoea in man and domestic animals. The types of *E. coli* recognized as causing diarrhoea are listed in Table 12.6. However, not all these types produce fimbrial adhesins. Classically, fimbriae are associated with the enterotoxigenic *E. coli* and the adhesins are aften referred to as colonization factors. They include the mannose-resistant K88, K99, 987P and F41 antigens that cause diarrhoea in animals, and CFA/I, CFA/II and E8775 found in human strains. In structure, some (e.g. CFA/I and 987P) resemble common fimbriae, whereas others (e.g. K88 and K99) appear as more flexible and much thinner fibrils with a diameter of 2–3 nm.

Of other human *E. coli* strains that cause diarrhoea, only the uncommon enterohaemorrhagic strains possess fimbriae. For example, *E. coli* O157:H7 is the serotype associated with the bloody diarrhoea of haemorrhagic colitis. This syndrome is distinguished from dysentery by the lack of fever and by the copious volumes of stool. The strain is also associated with haemolytic–uraemic syndrome which, together with haemorrhagic colitis, is being increasingly reported. The strains are characterized as possessing a plasmid of molecular weight 60 000 kDa which codes for the fimbriae involved in binding the bacteria to cells.

BACTERIAL EXOTOXINS

Bacterial pathogenesis requires that the pathogen is able to colonize the human or animal host, to multiply on or in host tissues and to avoid antibacterial defences. These events lead to the establishment of a focus of infection and often culminate in significant damage to the tissues; such damage, which is often mediated by exotoxins, may be localized at the site of infection or generalized at distant sites. Bacterial protein exotoxins are thus important determinants of bacterial virulence. However, the galaxy of putative virulence determinants includes cell-associated factors discussed earlier, such as polysaccharide capsules,

Table 12.6 Strains of *Escherichia coli* that cause diarrhoea

Category of *E. coli*	Common O serogroups	Virulence factors
Enterotoxigenic (ETEC)	O6, O8, O11, O15, O20, O25, O27, O63, O78, O80, O85, O115, O128, O139, O148, O149, O153, O159, O167	Heat-labile (LT) and heat-stable (ST) toxins Fimbrial adhesion
Enteropathogenic (EPEC)	O20, O44, O55, O86, O111, O114, O119, O125, O126, O127, O128, O142, O158	Shiga-like toxin Outer-membrane protein adhesins
Enteroinvasive (EIEC)	O28, O29, O112, O124, O136, O143, O144, O152, O164, O167	Invasion of epithelium Shiga-like toxin
Enterohaemorrhagic (EHEC)	O26, O111, O157	Shiga-like toxin Fimbrial adhesins

Table 12.7 Toxins that affect the intestine

Pathogen	Disease	Toxin	Molecular structure	Mode of action
Vibrio cholerae	Cholera	Cholera toxin (CT)	MW 82 000 (A = 28 000; B = 11 500) Subunit structure A:5B	Binds to receptor (GM1 ganglioside) Enzymatic ADP ribosylation of GTP-binding regulator of adenylate cyclase causes activation of adenylate cyclase
Escherichia coli (enterotoxigenic *E. coli*; ETEC)	Travellers' diarrhoea	*E. coli* heat-labile (LT) toxin	MW 88 000 Subunit structure A:5B, as for CT. LT-B subunit shows 80% homology with CT-B	Activation of adenylate cyclase as for CT
		E. coli STa (human type)	Small peptide 17–19 amino acids long; 3 disulphide bonds	Activation of particulate guanylate cyclase in intestinal cells following binding to specific receptor
E. coli (enteropathogenic *E. coli*; EPEC)	Infant diarrhoea	Moderate levels of shiga-like toxin (SLT)	At least 2 forms exist, SLT_1, SLT_2 Shiga-like toxin is an A-B toxin with a sub-unit structure (A:5B) similar to Shiga toxin	Cytotoxic, neurotoxic and enterotoxic; like Shiga toxin. SLT is immunologically related but not identical to Shiga toxin
E. coli (entero-invasive *E. coli*; EIEC)	Dysentery-like illness	Multiple SLTs		
E. coli (entero-haemorrhagic *E. coli*; EHEC)	Haemorrhagic colitis with copious diarrhoea Haemolytic anaemia syndrome	High level production of SLT		
Shigella dysenteriae	Dysentery	Shiga toxin	MW 70 000 (A = 32 000; B = 7700) Subunit structure A:5B	A subunit inhibits protein synthesis by inactivation of 60S ribosomes. Toxin is enterotoxic, cytotoxic and neurotoxic
Clostridium perfringens	Food poisoning with diarrhoea	Cytotoxic enterotoxin	MW 34 000 single polypeptide chain	Causes cytotoxic damage to intestinal epithelial cells
Clostridium difficile	Pseudomembranous colitis	Toxin A	MW 440 000 Subunits (230 000, 47 000 and 16 000)	Enterotoxic; lethal; causes fluid accumulation; causes haemorrhagic diarrhoea
		Toxin B	MW 500 000	Lethal, highly cytotoxic for cultured mammalian cells; acts intracellularly
Staphylococcus aureus	Food poisoning with vomiting and diarrhoea	Seven enterotoxins (A, B, C_1, C_2, C_3, D, E)	Toxin A, MW 27 500; Toxin B, MW 28 500; Toxin C_1, MW 27 500; Toxin C_2, MW 26 900; Toxin C_3, MW 27 100; Toxin D, MW 27 200; Toxin E, MW 26 100	Exterotoxins cause fluid imbalance in colon but molecular mode of action on intestine unknown. Thought to stimulate vomiting centre through action on vagus nerve. Also causes systemic effects
Bacillus cereus	Food poisoning with vomiting and diarrhoea	Diarrhoeagenic toxin/lethal toxin	MW c. 50 000	Causes fluid accumulation, increased vascular permeability, necrosis and lethality; mode of action unknown

Table 12.8 Toxins that cause subepithelial or systemic damage

Species	Disease	Toxin	Molecular structure	Mode of action
Staphylococcus aureus	Wide range of infections, including wound infections, septicaemia, boils, and other primary and metastatic pyogenic lesions	α-toxin	Single chain, MW 33 000	Forms transmembrane channels consisting of hexameric ring structures Cytotoxic damage can result in death, necrosis, paralysis, or neurotoxicity depending on dose and target tissue
		β-toxin	Single chain, MW 30 000	Phospholipase with specificity for sphingomyelin Cytolytic for RBC and for macrophages and platelets
		γ-toxin	A, 2-component toxin γ_1-single chain, MW 32 000 γ_2-single chain, MW 36 000	The mechanism of cytolysis not known. It lyses RBC and certain other cell types
		δ-toxin	Small amphiphilic peptide, MW 3000	Causes detergent-like lysis of many cell types
		Leucocidin	A, 2-component toxin F, single chain, MW 32 000 S, single chain, MW 31 000	Binding of S followed by F leads to activation of endogenous phospholipase 2, initiation of arachidonic cascade and subsequent cytolysis. Acts on polymorphs and macrophages
	Scalded skin syndrome and bullous impetigo	Epidermolytic toxins	ET_A, single chain, MW 27 000 ET_B, single chain, MW 27 500	Acts on the stratum granulosum of the epidermis to cause cell separation and subsequent blister formation. Probably disrupts normal cytoskeletal structure through binding and effect on flaggrin
	Toxic shock syndrome	Toxic shock syndrome toxin-1 (TSST-1)	Single chain, MW 22 000	Induces the symptoms of toxic shock syndrome in animals, i.e. fever, muscle damage, hypotension, lethargy and shock Releases mediators, i.e. TNF and interleukin-1 from macrophages. Molecular mechanism unknown
Streptococcus pyogenes (group A streptococci)	Streptococcal sore throat, wound infection, pyogenic lesions, impetigo Complications: rheumatic fever, glomerulonephritis	Streptolysin O	Single chain, oxygen-labile haemolysin, MW 67 000	One of a group of O-labile cytolysins that polymerize in the form of rings and arcs on susceptible membranes to cause lysis. Haemolytic, lethal; acts on human leucocytes and attacks many other cell types
		Streptolysin S	Small polypeptide, MW 1800 that is active only when bound to carrier	A lethal cytolysin active on a wide range of cell types, including human leucocytes

Organism	Disease	Toxin	Structure (MW)	Description
			molecules such as serum albumin, lipoprotein and RNA	A lethal cytolysin active on a wide range of cell types, including human leucocytes
	Scarlet fever	Erythrogenic toxins (A, B and C)	A, single chain, MW 26 900 B, single chain, MW 17 500 C, single chain, MW 13 200	Toxins are pyrogenic, mitogenic and erythrogenic. Responsible for rash of scarlet fever
Clostridium perfringens	Wound infections, cellulitis and gas gangrene in man. Many toxaemic conditions in animals	α-toxin	Single chain, MW 43 000	Ca^{2+}-dependent phospholipase C that hydrolyses membrane phospholipids and is cytolytic for many cell types. Lethal and necrotizing
	Pig-bel, necrotic enteritis	β-toxin	Single chain, MW 28 000	Lethal, necrotizing and paralytic. Does not act as a general cytolysin. Necrosis of villi in the intestine causes symptoms of necrotic enteritis
		δ-toxin	Single chain, MW 42 000	A lethal cytolytic toxin that affects RBCs, leucocytes and platelets
		ε-toxin	Single chain, MW 35 600 Activated by tryptic cleavage of N-terminal peptide (14 residues)	A lethal and necrotizing toxin responsible for pulpy kidney disease (overeating disease) in sheep
		ι-toxin	Two component toxin ι_A MW 48 000 ι_B MW 70 000	Lethal and necrotizing toxin causing fatal enterotoxaemia in calves and lambs
		θ-toxin	Single chain O-labile toxin. MW 60 000	Potent cytolysin active against a wide range of cell types. Polymerization of the toxin on cholesterol-containing membranes leads to lysis
Bacillus anthracis	Anthrax	Anthrax toxin	Multicomponent toxin I, oedema factor (EF); MW 89 000 II, protective antigen (PA); MW 85 000 III, lethal factor (LF); MW 83 000	PA binds to receptor on target cell. Proteolytic nicking of PA creates receptor for either EF or LF with formation of toxic complexes which are internalized EF is an active adenylate cyclase which, when internalized, causes an increase in cAMP. Mode of action of LF not understood
Bordetella pertussis	Whooping cough	Petussis toxin	MW 105 700 A:B bipartite toxin Subunit structure: $A:S_1 \diagdown \begin{array}{c} S_2\text{–}S_4 \\ S_3\text{–}S_4 \end{array}$ S_2–S_4 and S_3–S_4 dimers act as B region	Binding occurs through B region, allows entry of A subunit. This causes ADP ribosylation of an inhibitory membrane-bound GTP-binding protein, with activation of adenylate cyclase Systemic effects include fever, lymphocytosis, leucocytosis, and impaired regulation of blood glucose

Table 12.9 Toxins that attack internal organs

Species	Disease	Toxin	Molecular structure	Mode of action
Clostridium botulinum	Botulism	Series of neurotoxins A, B, C_1, D, E, F, G	Toxin A, MW 145 000 Toxin B, MW 155 000 Toxin C_1, MW 141 000 Toxin D, MW 170 000 Toxin E, MW 147 000 Toxin F, MW 155 000 All are single chains activated by proteolytic cleavage to yield heavy (B) fragment and light (A) fragment	Toxins act presynaptically at neuromuscular junctions causing flaccid paralysis. They inhibit Ca^{2+}-dependent exocytosis of vesicles containing acetylcholine
		C_2	An A-B toxin containing 2 components: $C_{2.1}$ = A component, MW 51 000 $C_{2.2}$ = B component, MW 90 000	C_2 toxin acts as an ADP ribosylating toxin; its role in disease is unknown
C. tetani	Tetanus	Tetanospasmin	MW 150 000 Single chain activated by proteolytic cleavage to yield a heavy fragment and a light fragment. These probably function as A and B components	Toxin causes spastic paralysis due to inhibition of release of inhibitory neurotransmitter from inhibitory neurons. Heavy component binds to membranes but detailed mechanism still not clear
Corynebacterium diphtheriae	Diphtheria	Diphtheria toxin	Single chain, MW 62 000 Activated by proteolytic nicking and thiol reduction to give 2 fragments: A (active) MW 24 000 B (binding) MW 38 000	Binding of B region to receptor followed by nicking leads to entry of A fragment. This causes ADP ribosylation of elongation factor 2 and inhibition of protein synthesis Damages heart, kidney, liver and adrenals

lipopolysaccharide endotoxins, teichoic acids and fimbrial adhesins.

The targets for toxic action are:

1 mucosal epithelial cells, e.g. epithelial cells of the gastrointestinal tract
2 subepithelial tissues such as blood vessels, connective tissue and leucocytes (systemic effects are often triggered by toxins that act in this way) and
3 internal organs such as the heart, liver, kidney, central nervous system and neuromuscular junctions.

In classic toxinoses such as diphtheria, tetanus and botulism, the exotoxin produced by the causative organism is of paramount importance in pathogenesis. More commonly, pathogenesis depends on complex interactions, cell-associated factors and extracellular enzymes combining with exotoxins to produce infection and the clinical signs of disease. Indeed, as a result of recent advances in molecular biology, the roles of indiviual virulence factors have been determined for certain multifactorial pathogens.

The damaging effect of a toxin may result from direct impairment of an essential metabolic function of the target cell or it may be mediated indirectly through release of mediators such as interferons, interleukins, leukotrienes and prostaglandins. Moreover, toxicity does not always involve death or lysis of the target cell; selective impairment of physiological and metabolic functions can result from subtle non-lethal damage at the site of action.

In terms of mode of action, bacterial toxins fall into 2 main classes:

1 **cytolytic toxins** that damage cell membranes and
2 **A-B (bipartite) toxins** that bind to a specific receptor through the B (binding) subunit and then release the toxic A subunit which causes cell damage, usually at a site within the target cell.

In order to deal with this large topic economically, the properties of a number of toxins produced by bacteria pathogenic for man are summarized in Tables 12.7, 12.8 and 12.9 in which toxins are arranged according to the target tissue affected in the disease process.

The purification and molecular characterization of bacterial toxins has advanced rapidly in recent years such that the molecular properties of many important toxins are now well established. Knowledge of the mode of toxin action at the molecular level has also progressed rapidly. These advances have given impetus to researchers to study communication signals between pathogens and their hosts.

3 COMMUNICATION SIGNALS BETWEEN PATHOGEN AND HOST

3.1 Cellular microbiology: a new discipline

Cellular microbiology is a rapidly developing field that encompasses the mechanisms and outcomes of communication between pathogenic prokaryotes and their eukaryotic hosts (Cossart et al. 1996). A central role is played by actin polymerization triggered by binding of the pathogen to its host cell. Pathogens that prey on actin polymerization and depolymerization pathways can be genetically manipulated and used to probe the lines of communication newly initiated by the pathogen with the host cell. The critical control points of invasion and pathogen multiplication can be identified and modulated.

Consider that a bacterium binds to a host cell, triggers polymerization of actin, and communicates a signal that may be translated by tyrosine phosphorylation of specific host cell proteins, which in turn sets in motion a cascade of events. Each host cell type may respond with its own cell-specific set of physiological events that may involve hormones. Several pathogens are being intensely studied to unravel some of the control mechanisms responsible for these lines of communication.

Many of the host cells that are contacted by bacteria are the epithelial cells which form tight junctions and act as a barrier to the pathogens and to the flow of soluble toxins into deeper tissues. Epithelial cells may respond to bacterial adherence or binding of toxin molecules by secreting cytokines and by so doing, the epithelial cells are an active part of the mucosal immune system. Cellular microbiology is the discipline described, in part, by these events and it is nourished by understanding the co-evolutionary relationship of pathogens and their hosts. Cross-talk between the 2 cell types accompanying evolutionary changes in the respective cell types has assured that virulence factors of the pathogen should be in balance with host cell responses. In this way, well balanced pathogens such as *H. pylori* can go unnoticed for a lifetime of the host.

3.2 Adherence and invasion

The intrusion by a prokaryotic organism into a eukaryotic cell starts with adherence of the 2 cell types and causes a major cytoskeletal rearrangement. For many of these pathogens a single bacterium encountering the host cell may be sufficient for entry. For others several bacteria may be needed to promote invasion of the host cell. A general feature of many enteroinvasive bacteria including enteropathogenic *E. coli* (EPEC), *Listeria*, *Salmonella*, *Shigella* and *Yersinia* is an absolute requirement of actin polymerization in the host cell. The route that these pathogens take to accomplish invasion of and replication in host cells has several variations. Some bind to host cell receptors such as β1 integrin recognized by invasin, an outer-membrane protein of *Yersinia*; others such as *Salmonella* bind to epidermal growth factor receptor, whereas *Shigella* has no known cellular receptor. *Shigella* entry is facilitated by host cellular protrusions arising around the bacterium and contain very tightly packed F-actin parallel orientation and associated with plastin, the actin-bundling protein (Adam et al. 1995).

A stellar example of using actin polymerization to

advance intracellular life is the pathogen, *Listeria monocytogenes* (Tilney and Portnoy 1989, Theriot et al. 1994). Within 30 min after entry, *L. monocytogenes* lyses the vacuole that surrounds it and becomes cytosolic. Actin filaments coat the bacteria which grow and divide. Actin is rearranged into a tail that extends up to 40 μm. The bacterium moves about the cytoplasm, trailing the actin tail. Intercellular movement also occurs by utilizing the actin tail, which moves the bacterium to the front of protuberances up to 25 μm long that force their way into a neighbouring cell. A double membrane is formed around the bacterium and soon lysed to complete the transfer of the pathogen from one cell to another. Intracellular motility requires bacterial surface protein ActA that localizes in the older pole of dividing cells in direct contact with the actin tail but is not released from the cell. The protein, which consists of 639 amino acids with an N-terminal signal peptide and a hydrophobic C-terminal region, becomes phosphorylated only after the cell enters its host. Mutations in *actA* abolish actin assembly, tail formation and motility. Such communication between parasite and host are essential for maintenance of this pathogen in balance with its host.

3.3 Adherence in a caustic environment

An econiche seemingly inhospitable to bacterial growth is the acidic environment of the human stomach. Although the pH of the stomach is about 2, the spiral-shaped, gram-negative bacterium *H. pylori* naturally colonizes the gastric mucosa (pH about 6) of humans and primates (Marshall and Warren 1984). It is the main cause of chronic superficial gastritis and is closely associated with both gastric and duodenal ulcers. Mounting evidence also implicates it as a causative agent in gastric cancer. About 40% and 80% of the adult population in developed and developing countries, respectively, are infected with *H. pylori* which makes *H. pylori* one of the most common bacterial infections of humans (Borén et al. 1994).

A successful helicobacter colonization of the host may persist as an infection for the lifetime of the host. Several binding specificities have been reported including *N*-acetylneuraminyllactose-binding fibrillar haemagglutinin (Evans et al. 1988), binding to sulphatide (SO$_3$-Galβ1-1Cer) (Saitoh et al. 1991) and to phosphatidylethanolamine (Lingwood et al. 1992), lipopolysaccharide binding to basement membrane protein laminin (Valkonen et al. 1994) and binding to the Lewis[b] (Le[b]) blood group antigen (Borén et al. 1993). For example, the bacterium binds to fucosylated glycoproteins of the Le[b] antigen that are expressed on gastric surface mucous cells in stomach epithelium (Borén et al. 1993). The Le[b] antigen is associated with blood group O phenotype, which may be relevant to the higher incidence of ulcerative disease in persons of this blood group.

H. pylori adheres specifically to gastric epithelial cells lining the antrum of the stomach. The highly specific adherence properties of helicobacters are presumably a manifestation of tightly controlled expression of bacterial surface adhesive molecules. Expression requires that available metabolic energy be used to supply demands for synthesis of the surface adhesins.

Attachment of *H. pylori* to gastric epithelial cells closely resembles that of enteropathogenic *E. coli*, which involves effacement of microvilli at the point of attachment, cytoskeletal rearrangement to form a pedestal beneath the adherent cell, and activity of host tyrosine protein kinase at the attachment site (Segal et al. 1996). Such localized activity suggests direct communication exchanges between prokaryote and eukaryote. Although helicobacters have been observed inside host cells, they do not seem to grow and divide inside the host cell.

Most of the clinical isolates of *H. pylori* produce an 87 kDa vacuolating cytotoxin, VacA, that appears to be processed from a 139 kDa protoxin by removing a 33 amino acid leader from the N-terminus as well as a C-terminal peptide (Cover and Blaser 1995). VacA induces acidic vacuoles coated with Rab7, a small guanosine triphosphate-binding protein that may participate in vesicle trafficking within host cells.

Gastric epithelial cells from infected persons express enhanced levels of interleukin (IL-6), tumour necrosis factor (TNF) and IL-8 (Crabtree et al. 1993, 1994). The lipopolysaccharide (LPS) molecules have about a 1000-fold lower biological activity compared to Enterobacteriaceae and it has been suggested that this lower activity gives advantage to the helicobacter in preventing an exaggerated host response, which could lead to reducing the bacterial cell number through neutrophil infiltration of helicobacter-infected sites (Blaser 1993).

3.4 Cytokine response to bacterial attachment

The interactions of bacteria with eukaryotic cells are more than simple adherence and entry. The host cell responds to adherence in a variety of ways. One of these is the production of cytokines upon adherence of bacterial cells. A critical line of defence is the epithelial cell layer that forms a boundary between the external environment and deeper tissue. An important role for epithelial cells in mucosal immune responses is emerging (Hedges et al. 1995). By binding to and activating epithelial cells, bacteria participate in the stimulation or suppression of mucosal inflammation and immunity. Cytokines are known to be essential in modulating a variety of immune mucosal functions and the activation of epithelial cells by bacteria to secrete cytokines is an important part of the pathogenesis of mucosal infections.

A mucosal cytokine response after urinary tract colonization by *E. coli* was first observed as the secretion of IL-6 and IL-8 into the urine within 30 min of administering *E. coli*. P-fimbriated *E. coli* bind to receptors of the globoseries of glycosphingolipids, which contain Galα1→4Galβ-containing oligosaccharides bound to ceramide in the outer leaflet of the host cell lipid bilayer (Bock et al. 1985). Binding of

P-fimbriated *E. coli* to a human kidney cell line causes the release of ceramide, increases ceramide phosphorylation and secretion of high levels of IL-6 (Hedlund et al. 1996). Phosphorylation of ceramide involves serine- and threonine-specific protein kinases and inhibitors of these kinases reduces the IL-6 response. Inhibitors of tyrosine-specific protein kinases were ineffective. This ceramide-signalling pathway does not seem to respond to LPS of the bacterium and thus encourages thinking of a direct induction of cytokine release after P-fimbriated *E. coli* bind to host cells.

4 SUMMARY

Pathogenic bacteria have many responses to stimuli received from the external environment and from the internal corridors of human cells. They hold many answers to questions that are being explored experimentally in the emerging field of cellular microbiology. Some pathogens are invasive of human cells and others appear only to adhere to the cell surface. Some produce exotoxins that inactivate or destroy host cell functions, whereas others use the machinery already in place within the host cell to advance their pathogenic potential. Pathogens cross-talk with their host cells by sending molecular signals; the identification of these signalling molecules and their mode of action are active research areas (Galán 1996). With at least 2 of these invasive pathogens, *Salmonella* and *Shigella*, the proteins that mediate entry into host cells are markedly homologous. Studies with the classical protein toxins (Singh and Tu 1996), endotoxins (Levin et al. 1995), ADP-ribosylating toxins (Moss and Vaughan 1990) continue to uncover exciting surprises as evidenced by the discovery of a filamentous phage encoding cholera toxin (Waldor and Mekalanos 1996).

REFERENCES

Adam T, Arpin M et al., 1995, Cytoskeletal rearrangements and the functional role of T-plastin during entry of *Shigella flexneri* into HeLa cells, *J Cell Biol*, **129**: 367–81.

Ba-Thein W, Lyristis M et al., 1996, The *virR/virS* locus regulates the transcription of genes encoding extracellular toxin production in *Clostridium perfringens*, *J Bacteriol*, **178**: 2514–20.

Blaser MJ, 1993, *Helicobacter pylori*: microbiology of a 'slow' bacterial infection, *Trends Microbiol*, **1**: 255–60.

Bock K, Breimer ME et al., 1985, Specificity of binding of a strain of uropathogenic *Escherichia coli* to Galα1→4Gal-containing glycosphingolipids, *J Biol Chem*, **260**: 8545–51.

Borén T, Falk P et al., 1993, Attachment of *Helicobacter pylori* to human gastric epithelium mediated by blood group antigens, *Science*, **262**: 1892–5.

Borén T, Normark S et al., 1994, *Helicobacter pylori*: molecular basis for host recognition and bacterial adherence, *Trends Microbiol*, **2**: 221–8.

Cossart P, Boquet P et al., 1996, Cellular microbiology emerging, *Science*, **271**: 315–16.

Cover TL, Blaser MJ, 1995, *Helicobacter pylori*: a bacterial cause of gastritis, peptic ulcer disease, and gastric cancer, *ASM News*, **61**: 21–6.

Crabtree JE, Peichl P et al., 1993, Gastric interleukin-8 and IgA IL-8 autoantibodies in *Helicobacter pylori* infection, *Scand J Immunol*, **37**: 65–70.

Crabtree JE, Wyatt JI et al., 1994, Interleukin-8 expression in *Helicobacter pylori* infected, normal, and neoplastic gastroduodenal mucosa, *J Clin Pathol*, **47**: 61–6.

Duguid JP, Anderson ES, Campbell I, 1966, Fimbriae and adhesive properties in Salmonellae, *J Pathol Bacteriol*, **92**: 107–38.

Duguid JP, Smith IW et al., 1955, Non-flagellar filamentous appendages ('fimbriae') and haemagglutinating activity in *Bacterium coli*, *J Pathol Bacteriol*, **70**: 335–48.

Dziejman M, Mekalanos JJ, 1995, Two-component signal transduction and its role in the expression of bacterial virulence factors, *Two-component signal transduction*, American Society for Microbiology, Washington, DC, 305–17.

Evans DG, Evans JDJ et al., 1988, *N*-Acetylneuraminyllactose-binding fibrillar hemagglutinin of *Campylobacter pylori*: a putative colonization factor antigen, *Infect Immun*, **56**: 2896–906.

Fischer W, 1994, Lipoteichoic acids and lipoglycans, *Bacterial Cell Wall*, eds Ghuysen J-M, Hackenbeck R, Elsevier Science BV, Amsterdam, 199–215.

Fuqua WC, Winans SC et al., 1994, Quorum sensing in bacteria: the LuxR–LuxI family of cell density-responsive transcriptional regulators, *J Bacteriol*, **176**: 269–75.

Galán JE, 1996, Molecular genetic bases of *Salmonella* entry into host cells, *Mol Microbiol*, **20**: 263–71.

Gambello MJ, Iglewski BH, 1991, Cloning and characterization of the *Pseudomonas aeruginosa lasR* gene, a transcriptional activator of elastase expression, *J Bacteriol*, **173**: 3000–9.

Gambello MJ, Kaye S et al., 1993, LasR of *Pseudomonas aeruginosa* is a transcriptional activator of the alkaline protease gene (*apr*) and an enhancer of exotoxin A expression, *Infect Immun*, **61**: 1180–4.

Griffiths F, 1928, The significance of pneumococcal types, *J Hyg*, **27**: 113–59.

Hedges SR, Agace WW et al., 1995, Epithelial cytokine responses and mucosal cytokine networks, *Trends Microbiol*, **3**: 266–70.

Hedlund M, Svensson M et al., 1996, Role of the ceramide-signaling pathway in cytokine responses to P-fimbriated *Escherichia coli*, *J Exp Med*, **183**: 1037–44.

Hoch JA, Silhavy TJ, 1995, *Two-component Signal Transduction*, American Society for Microbiology, Washington DC.

Holst O, Brade H, 1992, Chemical structure of the core region of lipopolysaccharides, *Bacterial Endotoxic Lipopolysaccharides. Vol. 1. Molecular Biochemistry and Cellular Biology of Lipopolysaccharides*, eds Morrison DC, Ryan JL, CRC Press, Boca Raton, FL, 135–70.

Hultgren SJ, Abraham S et al., 1993, Pilus and nonpilus bacterial adhesins: assembly and function in cell recognition, *Cell*, **73**: 887–901.

Jacob F, Monod J, 1961, Genetic regulatory mechanisms in the synthesis of proteins, *J Mol Biol*, **3**: 318–56.

Klemm P, Christiansen G et al., 1994, Reciprocal exchange of minor components of type 1 and F1C fimbriae results in hybrid organelles with changed receptor specificities, *J Bacteriol*, **176**: 2227–34.

Latifi A, Winson MK et al., 1995, Multiple homologues of LuxR and LuxI control expression of virulence determinants and secondary metabolites through quorum sensing in *Pseudomonas aeruginosa* PAO1, *Mol Microbiol*, **17**: 333–43.

Levin J, Alving CR et al., 1995, *Bacterial Endotoxins: Lipopolysaccharides from Genes to Therapy*, Wiley-Liss Inc., New York.

Lewis M, Chang G et al., 1996, Crystal structure of the lactose operon repressor and its complexes with DNA and inducer, *Science*, **271**: 1247–54.

Lingwood CA, Huesca M et al., 1992, The glycerolipid receptor for *Helicobacter pylori* (and exoenzyme S) is phosphatidylethanolamine, *Infect Immun*, **60**: 2470–4.

Marshall BJ, Warren JR, 1984, Unidentified curved bacilli in the stomach of patients with gastritis and peptic ulceration, *Lancet*, **1**: 1311–15.

Messner P, Sleytr UB, 1992, Crystalline bacterial cell-surface layers, *Adv Microb Physiol*, **33**: 213–75.

Morschhäuser J, Vetter V et al., 1994, Adhesin regulatory genes within large, unstable DNA regions of pathogenic *Escherichia coli*: cross-talk between different adhesin gene clusters, *Mol Microbiol*, **11**: 555–66.

Moss J, Vaughan M, 1990, *ADP-ribosylating Toxins and G Proteins: Insights into Signal Transduction*, American Society for Microbiology, Washington DC.

Ochsner UA, Reiser J, 1995, Autoinducer-mediated regulation of rhamnolipid biosurfactant synthesis in *Pseudomonas aeruginosa*, *Proc Natl Acad Sci USA*, **92**: 6424–8.

Ochsner UA, Koch AK et al., 1994, Isolation and characterization of a regulatory gene affecting rhamnolipid biosurfactant synthesis in *Pseudomonas aeruginosa*, *J Bacteriol*, **176**: 2044–54.

Passador L, Cook JM et al., 1993, Expression of *Pseudomonas aeruginosa* virulence genes requires cell-to-cell communication, *Science*, **260**: 1127–30.

Pearson JP, Passador L et al., 1995, A second *N*-acylhomoserine lactone signal produced by *Pseudomonas aeruginosa*, *Proc Natl Acad Sci USA*, **92**: 1490–4.

Pooley HM, Karamata D, 1994, Teichoic acid synthesis in *Bacillus subtilis*: genetic organization and biological roles, *Bacterial Cell Wall*, eds Ghuysen J-M, Hackenbeck R, Elsevier Science BV, Amsterdam, 187–98.

Rust L, Pesci EC et al., 1996, Analysis of the *Pseudomonas aeruginosa* elastase (*lasB*) regulatory region, *J Bacteriol*, **178**: 1134–40.

Saitoh T, Natomi H et al., 1991, Identification of glycolipid receptors for *Helicobacter pylori* by TLC-immunostaining, *FEBS Lett*, **282**: 385–7.

Schnaitman CA, Klena JD, 1993, Genetics of lipopolysaccharide biosynthesis in enteric bacteria, *Microbiol Rev*, **57**: 655–82.

Seed PC, Passador L et al., 1995, Activation of the *Pseudomonas aeruginosa lasI* gene by LasR and the *Pseudomonas* autoinducer PAI: an autoinduction regulatory hierarchy, *J Bacteriol*, **177**: 654–9.

Segal ED, Falkow S et al., 1996, *Helicobacter pylori* attachment to gastric cells induces cytoskeletal rearrangements and tyrosine phosphorylation of host cell proteins, *Proc Natl Acad Sci USA*, **93**: 1259–64.

Singh BR, Tu AT, 1996, *Natural Toxins 2: Structure, Mechanism of Action, and Detection*, Plenum Press, New York.

Sokurenko EV, Courtney HS et al., 1994, FimH family of type 1 fimbrial adhesins: functional heterogeneity due to minor sequence variations among *fimH* genes, *J Bacteriol*, **176**: 748–55.

Stock JB, Surette MG et al., 1995, Two-component signal transduction systems: structure–function relationships and mechanisms of catalysis, *Two-component Signal Transduction*, ASM Press, Washington DC, 25–51.

Swift S, Bainton NJ et al., 1994, Gram-negative bacterial communication by *N*-acyl homoserine lactones: a universal language?, *Trends Microbiol*, **2**: 193–8.

Theriot JA, Rosenblatt J et al., 1994, Involvement of profilin in the actin-based motility of *L. monocytogenes* in cells and in cell-free extracts, *Cell*, **76**: 505–17.

Throup JP, Camara M et al., 1995, Characterisation of the *yenI/yenR* locus from *Yersinia enterocolitica* mediating the synthesis of two *N*-acylhomoserine lactone signal molecules, *Mol Microbiol*, **17**: 345–56.

Tilney LG, Portnoy DA, 1989, Actin filaments and the growth, movement and spread of the intracellular bacterial parasite *Listeria monocytogenes*, *J Cell Biol*, **109**: 1597–608.

Toder DS, Gambello MJ et al., 1991, *Pseudomonas aeruginosa* LasA: a second elastase under the transcriptional control of *lasR*, *Mol Microbiol*, **5**: 2003–10.

Valkonen KH, Wadström T et al., 1994, Interaction of lipopolysaccharides of *Helicobacter pylori* with basement membrane protein laminin, *Infect Immun*, **62**: 3640–8.

Via LE, Curcic R et al., 1996, Elements of signal transduction in *Mycobacterium tuberculosis*: in vitro phosphorylation and in vivo expression of the response regulator MtrA, *J Bacteriol*, **178**: 3314–21.

Waldor MK, Mekalanos JJ, 1996, Lysogenic conversion by a filamentous phage encoding cholera toxin, *Science*, **272**: 1910–14.

Winson MK, Camara M et al., 1995, Multiple *N*-acyl-L-homoserine lactone signal molecules regulate production of virulence determinants and secondary metabolites in *Pseudomonas aeruginosa*, *Proc Natl Acad Sci USA*, **92**: 9427–31.

Chapter 13

THE ECOLOGY OF BACTERIA IN SOIL AND IN PLANT ASSOCIATIONS

R Campbell

1 INTRODUCTION

Microbial ecology is the study of how bacteria and other micro-organisms interact with their natural environment and, contrary to popular opinion, man and other animals play only a very minor role as habitats for micro-organisms. The vast majority of micro-organisms do not have temperature optima at 37°C, many are not heterotrophs and even those that are will not grow on the rich media such as nutrient agar, commonly used in medical laboratories. Most bacteria in soil are nutrient limited and, therefore, are dormant either in the vegetative state or as spores. In many parts of the world, soil bacteria may also be short of water. The soil temperature may fluctuate depending on the time of day, the season of the year or the depth in the soil; the soil may be frozen for months at a time, or alternatively, in the tropics, the sun may heat the surface layers to 60 or 70°C.

There is great variation in soil environments. Different soils in the different biomes of the world have different vegetation types and therefore different microbiology. A single soil usually consists of a number of layers, called horizons, which are mostly caused by downward leaching of humic materials and minerals. The horizons vary in the physical structure (size and stability of mineral particles or composite crumbs), in their chemical characteristics (minerals, pH) and in the quality and the quantity of the organic matter which is the nutrient source for heterotrophic bacteria. There may be much greater differences between the microbiology of different horizons in a single soil than there are between the same horizons of soils on different continents, just as the gut flora of humans has similarities the world over, but is very different from the skin flora of the same individual.

On a much smaller scale there are many microhabitats in a single soil horizon or even within a single crumb of soil. If the bacterium is a heterotroph, the sort of soil particles affect the nutrition; most bacteria in soil occur on the surfaces of organic matter rather than sand particles. It matters to a bacterium just where it is, to within a few micrometres. Most active bacteria are adsorbed onto surfaces of particles or onto gas–liquid interfaces in the soil and they usually have colloidal organic matter and clay particles adsorbed onto their own surfaces (Savage and Fletcher 1985) (Fig. 13.1). This has many advantages and disadvantages; being adsorbed makes predation by protozoa less likely, it can increase nutrient availability and the extracellular enzymes produced by the bacterium will be adsorbed close by, and hence the products of those enzymes will be available to the bacterium rather than diffusing into the soil solution and being used by other organisms. On the other hand, toxic substances, such as antibiotics, can be adsorbed and hydrogen ions are usually 10 or 100 times more concentrated on surfaces than in free solution, and this reduction in pH has effects on mineral solubility, etc. (Burns 1986). Apart from these adsorption effects, the other main determining factor in a microhabitat is likely to be the availability of oxygen. Oxygen is poorly soluble in water and diffuses slowly; since many soil particles are covered in water films (Fig. 13.1) there can be very steep gradients of oxygen and many parts of the soil in water-sealed voids and in the centre of soil particles may be anaerobic or at least micro-aerophilic (Sexstone et al. 1985). The situation is made worse by aerobic heterotrophs using oxygen faster than it can diffuse into the system. Since there are environmental differences on a small scale, there are different populations of bacteria in different microhabitats; for example, the inside of a soil crumb tends to have anaerobic, desiccation-sensitive bacteria while the crumb surfaces have aerobic bacteria which have structures such as spores to allow them to overcome desiccation.

Because of this great variability within a small region of soil the methods of studying soil bacteria are time consuming and somewhat laborious, but they are extensively described (Grigorova and Norris 1990). Many methods depend on culturing the bacteria, but it is impossible to find culture conditions, media, etc. to suit all the possible organisms and recovery rates of the general bacterial population can be as low as 1–10% of the 'total' number estimated by direct counting methods. The main use of these viable counting methods is in the enumeration of particular organisms or groups of organisms for which there are specific media that are known to enable the recovery and growth of the bacterium under investigation; viable counts may be used, for example, to study *Pseudomonas* spp. or particular strains of bacteria that have been released into the environment (Levin, Seidler and Rogul 1992). However, many microbial ecologists have abandoned general culture methods altogether (Brock 1987). Direct counts are difficult in an opaque medium such as soil but epifluorescence microscopy can be used and, with the correct selection of fluorochromes, can distinguish between live and dead organisms. Measurements of general soil respiration rates, the levels of enzymes thought to be important in soil processes or the amounts of key metabolites such as ATP and ADP give an idea of net activity but do not, of course, distinguish between different micro-organisms.

Most identification and classification of soil organisms depends on a culture, though methods now exist to extract DNA direct from soil and use this in identification schemes, especially for particular strains of bacteria (Levin, Seidler and Rogul 1992). Even if there is a culture the bacteria are often gram variable and pleomorphic, and since most soil bacteria are nutrient limited, they are often smaller in the soil than in culture. This can make identification by traditional methods difficult. There is the added complication that there are relatively few cultures of bacteria from natural habitats in the type-culture collections so comparison is difficult. It has been estimated that only 12% of bacterial species (including all the well known medically important ones) have been described (Bull, Goodfellow and Slater 1992); it is clear that we do not have names for most bacteria in natural environments. Nevertheless, those that are known have been described and discussed extensively (Balows et al. 1992).

Many soil bacteria have a direct influence on medical practice, since many of the antibiotics that have revolutionized the treatment of infections in man and other animals are derived from micro-organisms from soil (for example, the fungi *Penicillium*, *Cephalosporium* and the bacterium *Streptomyces*; see Chapter 9). Until recently there was no positive evidence that antibiotics were part of the competition between micro-organisms in soil, though it was always assumed that they were important since they were such common metabolic products of soil micro-organisms (Williams 1986). Genetic engineering has shown that *Pseudomonas* with the ability to produce antibiotics deleted are no longer able to compete with other micro-organisms and that this competitive ability is restored when the antibiotic production is reintroduced. Antibiotics have now been detected in soils (Thomashow and Weller 1991), though the level of free antibiotics is very low because of adsorption.

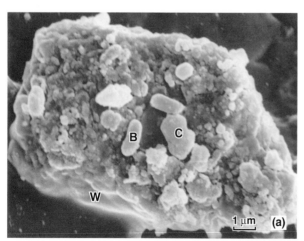
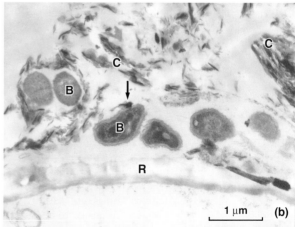

Fig. 13.1   (a) Low temperature scanning electron micrograph of a fully hydrated soil crumb. There are bacteria (B) on the dry surface together with clay particles (C). Note the water film (W) covering most of the surface; there will be bacteria within the film which are not visible. (b) Transmission electron micrograph of the surface of a wheat root (R) with bacteria of several morphological types surrounded by clay particles (C) adsorbed to the mucilage around the colonies. In some cases bacteria have clay directly adsorbed onto their surface (↓).

There is a potentially harmful side to soil bacteria for they can cause diseases of animals and be a reservoir of human pathogens. For example, *Clostridium tetani* (Chapter 32) and the gas gangrene group of organisms (Chapter 32) are common inhabitants of soil, especially that which has been manured. *Clostridium botulinum* (Chapter 32) occurs on fruits and other foods. Other genera of soil origin, especially gram-negative bacteria such as *Pseudomonas, Enterobacter* and *Acinetobacter*, can be medically important.

2   TYPES, NUMBERS AND DISTRIBUTION OF VIABLE BACTERIA IN THE SOIL

There is great variation in the numbers and sorts of micro-organisms that occur in soils. In most cases the bacteria recorded are heterotrophs, so the numbers or biomass are usually correlated with the organic matter in the soil on which the heterotrophs depend. There are comparatively short-term successions of bacteria on organic material which arrives on the soil (see p. 330), and longer-term changes in the population as the vegetation changes in higher plant and habitat successions or in different agricultural systems. The distribution of bacteria is therefore discontinuous in space and time and all that any method of assessing the population can do is to record numbers, activity or biomass for that soil at the time of sampling; it is very difficult to make generalizations or predictions from such data.

Estimates of the general numbers and biomass of bacteria and other micro-organisms to be found in soils show that bacteria are often the dominant part of the population (Table 13.1). The fungi are less numerous by several orders of magnitude (though it is often not clear what numbers of filamentous organisms like fungi mean, especially if derived from studies dependent on cultural methods), but the biomass is similar to that of bacteria. Bacterial biomass may exceed the total biomass of micro-organisms other than fungi and may also exceed the obvious biomass of the crop plants growing in the field.

Table 13.1   Relative numbers and the approximate biomass of microbiota in a fertile soil

Organisms	Numbers per m^2	per g	Biomass wet kg ha^{-1}
Bacteria	10^{13}–10^{14}	10^8–10^9	300–3000
Actinomycetes	10^{12}–10^{13}	10^7–10^8	300–3000
Fungi	10^{10}–10^{11}	10^5–10^6	500–5000
Microalgae	10^9–10^{10}	10^3–10^6	10–1500
Protozoa	10^9–10^{10}	10^3–10^5	5–200
Nematodes	10^6–10^7	10^1–10^2	1–100
Earthworms	30–300		10–1000
Other invertebrates	10^3–10^5		1–200

The numbers are based on the culture of heterotrophs. Data from a compilation by Metting 1993.

In natural soils which are not disturbed by agriculture, the biomass of bacteria is generally highest in the surface horizons where there are available nutrients in the form of organic matter and also oxygen from the soil surface (Fig. 13.2). However, it is also usual to have the highest numbers of anaerobes close to the soil surface, for their numbers are determined by the presence of anaerobic microhabitats created by the respiration of aerobes when the diffusion rate of oxygen is limiting. Bacteria in agricultural soils are affected by farming practices including the crops grown, the level of fertilizer applied or organic versus conventional farming systems. Numbers also vary from year to year (Table 13.2). The presence of any crop (as opposed to fallow) increases bacterial biomass and this is probably an effect of plant roots (see section 5.1, p. 335). Fertilizer differences also probably reflect increases in plant growth when fertilizers are used, and this affects microbial numbers, rather than any direct effects of the fertilizer on the bacteria.

All bacteria are limited at depth by the lack of available nutrients (Fig. 13.2), but there are bacteria much deeper in the soil and rock. These have largely been investigated in connection with the contamination of deep aquifers by pollutants, but bacteria exist even in virgin rocks of uncontaminated sites. Up to 10^4 or 10^5 bacteria per gram of rock are recorded from clean sediments 150 m below ground level (Chapelle et al. 1987).

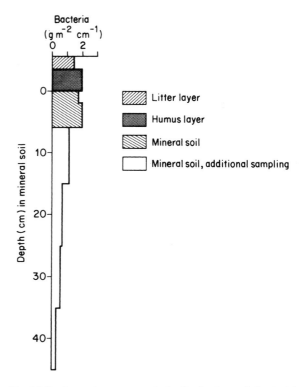

Fig. 13.2   Annual mean vertical distribution of bacterial biomass in a northern coniferous forest. These soils are very poor in nutrients and the climate is extreme, hence the low biomass compared with agricultural soils in temperate regions. These data are based on direct examination, by fluorescence microscopy. (Adapted from Persson et al. 1980).

Table 13.2 Compilation of data on annual variation in bacterial numbers and biomass in different crops vs fallow and with crops under different fertilizer and manure regimes

(a) Agricultural crop	Bacterial numbers 10^9 g^{-1} DW (mean ± *SEM*)	Bacterial biomass mg g^{-1} DW (mean ± *SEM*)
Grass meadow		
1981	5.3 ± 0.1	0.43 ± 0.02
1982	6.3 ± 0.4	0.53 ± 0.04
Lucerne		
1981	3.5 ± 0.2	0.29 − 0.02
1982	6.4 ± 0.5	0.51 ± 0.03
Barley, no nitrogen		
1981	4.4 ± 0.2	0.34 ± 0.02
1982	4.8 ± 0	0.42 ± 0.03
(b) Treatment		
Fallow	3.02 ± 0.21	
Cropped, no additions	3.50 ± 0.13	
Cropped +80 kg ha^{-1} year^{-1} N	4.26 ± 0.45	
Cropped +80 kg ha^{-1} year^{-1} N + 1800 kg C as straw	6.56 ± 0.51	

Compiled from: (a) Schnürer 1985 and (b) Schnürer, Clarholm and Rosswall 1985. Data are based on direct examination by fluorescence microscopy.
DW, dry weight.

The seasonal variation of microbial abundance follows factors such as temperature in northern coniferous forests (Fig. 13.3). The activity is greatest in late summer and autumn when the soil is warm, but drops during the winter as the ground freezes, and takes some time to become active again as the soil warms up in spring, though there is then activity as the nutrients released by the spring freeze–thaw cycles become available. In this example the low biomass during the middle of the summer could be caused by drought, which frequently limits the growth of soil bacteria, especially in the tropics.

Any organic matter which reaches the soil is rapidly colonized by micro-organisms including bacteria. The growing tips of fungi can penetrate organic matter either mechanically or by enzyme action, or a combination of both. However, bacteria are generally limited to surfaces and the size of the particle of organic matter (its surface:volume ratio) is, therefore, of great importance in their exploitation of the resource. Soil arthropods, though they decrease microbial populations by grazing, also comminute the plant litter,

expose it to bacterial attack and increase the nitrogen content by excreting uric acid; nitrogen availability generally limits decay rates. As the quality of the resource changes during decomposition, and there are variations in pH, etc., the populations of bacteria able to utilize the different components also alter (Struwe and Kjøller 1986), leading to successions of micro-organisms on substrates. The first bacteria to colonize the resource are those that can utilize the simple sugars and proteins. These are ruderal organisms (also called r-selected; Andrews and Harris 1986) that exist in the soil as dormant spores or vegetative structures for most of the time, but they have rapid germination and growth rates and colonize new materials; ruderal groups of organisms include *Pseudomonas* and *Bacillus*. The resource is then invaded by stress-tolerant or combative organisms (K-selected organisms). The stress may be environmental, such as low pH, or may be lack of available nutrients; stress tolerant organisms may have cellulases or lignin-degrading enzymes, for example, and so can colonize materials high in these complex polymers (e.g. wood) and they avoid competition by tolerating nutrient stress. Combative organisms can survive in crowded environments by tolerating the antibiotics produced by others; they grow slowly and do not reproduce so widely as ruderal organisms. Actinomycetes may be both stress tolerant (e.g. thermotolerant) and combative antibiotic producers and they are components of the successions of micro-organisms involved in the composting of organic material. There may also be secondary successions as the ruderal species become active again in colonizing the remains of the bacteria, fungi and arthropods which had been important in the early successional stages.

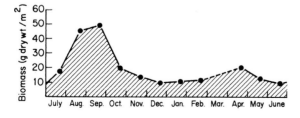

Fig. 13.3 Seasonal fluctuations in the biomass of bacteria in a northern coniferous forest, based on direct examination, by fluorescence microscopy. (Adapted from Persson et al. 1980).

Seres are long-term successions and these affect micro-organisms because of the changes in plant cover, but bacteria are important in determining the sere in the early stages of soil formation from bare rock or eroded surfaces (Campbell 1983). Cyanobacteria, especially, can fix both carbon and nitrogen in nutrient-deficient environments. Mutualistic symbiotic associations of cyanobacteria with fungi, to form lichens, are also very important in these early stages in soil formation. Heterotrophic bacteria become important only when the soil has formed and becomes relatively stable.

3 NUTRIENT CYCLING IN SOIL

3.1 Cycling of nutrients and organic matter breakdown

The recycling of nutrients is essential to life on earth. Energy is supplied from the sun and passes through an environment but, in contrast, there are finite amounts of minerals and nutrients which are continuously relocated and whose oxidation states are altered by biogeochemical processes. The decomposition of organic matter by micro-organisms (1 in Fig. 13.4) releases inorganic forms of plant nutrients and, despite the comparatively recent use of chemical fertilizers in intensive agriculture, this is still the main source of minerals for the growth of plants in all natural and many agro-ecosystems. There are four main groups of reactions in the cycling of nutrients.

First, all sorts of heterotrophic micro-organisms are involved in the oxidation of organic matter to yield energy, and this releases carbon, nitrogen, sulphur, phosphorus and other elements or compounds for re-use by both heterotrophs and autotrophs. Bacteria are especially important in the changes in oxidation states of elements and in the second group of reactions they can oxidize inorganic compounds to obtain energy (they are chemo-autotrophs). Thus, reduced forms of iron and manganese, reduced sulphur, and ammonium and nitrite can be oxidized, usually in aerobic conditions (3, 7, 8 in Fig. 13.4). However, by using terminal electron acceptors other than oxygen, some bacteria, e.g. *Thiobacillus denitrificans*, can carry out inorganic oxidations under anaerobic conditions. The third group of reactions is of various reductions; if the terminal electron acceptor is organic they are fermentations and they result in the production of ethyl alcohol, lactic acid, volatile fatty acids, etc. Inorganic terminal electron acceptors (other than oxygen) may also be used in these reductions and they include sulphate, tetrathionate or elemental sulphur, and nitrate and nitrite, so that hydrogen sulphide, and ammonium or nitrogen gas, respectively, are produced (6, 9, 12 in Fig. 13.4). The fourth group of reactions is carried out by bacterial photo-autotrophs which may use light energy to split hydrogen sulphide under anaerobic conditions, using the hydrogen to reduce carbon dioxide and releasing sulphur; this is anoxygenic photosynthesis (2b in Fig. 13.4). Cyano-bacteria carry out oxygenic photosynthesis, like higher plants, splitting H_2O instead of H_2S (2a in Fig. 13.4).

It may seem that the production of methane from carbon dioxide (4 in Fig. 13.4) is the use of the latter as a terminal electron acceptor, but the situation is more complex in these archaebacteria which do not have a cytochrome electron transport chain or the Calvin cycle. Molecular hydrogen and various simple organic molecules (formate, methanol) can be oxidized while the carbon dioxide is reduced, but some methanogens produce methane by the simultaneous oxidation and reduction of methanol or acetate to form carbon dioxide as well as the methane (Brock et al. 1994).

The overall control of the rate of organic matter breakdown (1 in Fig. 13.4) is climatic, especially temperature and water levels. Very low temperatures at high latitudes reduce decay and organic matter builds up faster than it is decayed and forms peat deposits. This is made worse by the drop in pH which may further reduce decay rates. Conversely, high temperature combined with high levels of available water in the humid tropics leads to vary rapid decay of organic matter. Water availability affects aeration, and anaerobic breakdown by bacteria, though possible, is much slower than aerobic processes which involve other organisms as well as bacteria. Organic matter has much more carbon than nitrogen, so the latter is often limiting; any nitrogen released by the decay is immediately immobilized in the micro-organisms, but as carbon is respired the carbon:nitrogen ratio drops and at about 20:1 release of mineral nitrogen occurs. This is why it is important to compost farmyard manure and other organic material before applying it to the land; if the C:N ratio is too high the applied material, though it contains nitrogen, may take up nitrogen from the soil and cause deficiency to plants until decay has become more advanced.

Phosphorus is usually present in organic matter in sufficient quantities not to have these problems and is normally released as phosphate (Fig. 13.4) and is not subject to oxidation state changes by micro-organisms. However, phosphate is very immobile in soil and it may need micro-organisms, especially fungi which form mycorrhizae, to assist in plant uptake.

There are two forms of decay of organic matter where bacteria are especially important. Herbivorous animals, the start of all the major terrestrial food chains, are unable to degrade cellulose which is a major component of the vegetation which they eat; only plants and micro-organisms have cellulases. The breakdown of the plant material is done in the rumen, or equivalent structure in non-ruminants such as the caecum of horses and rabbits, by bacteria and the protozoa which graze them. The animal absorbs the volatile fatty acids produced by the breakdown in this anaerobic environment and subsequently digests the micro-organisms. This symbiotic association is generally considered to be mutualism (Hobson 1988).

The other special case of organic matter breakdown by bacteria is in the production of silage where the environmental conditions are arranged to favour

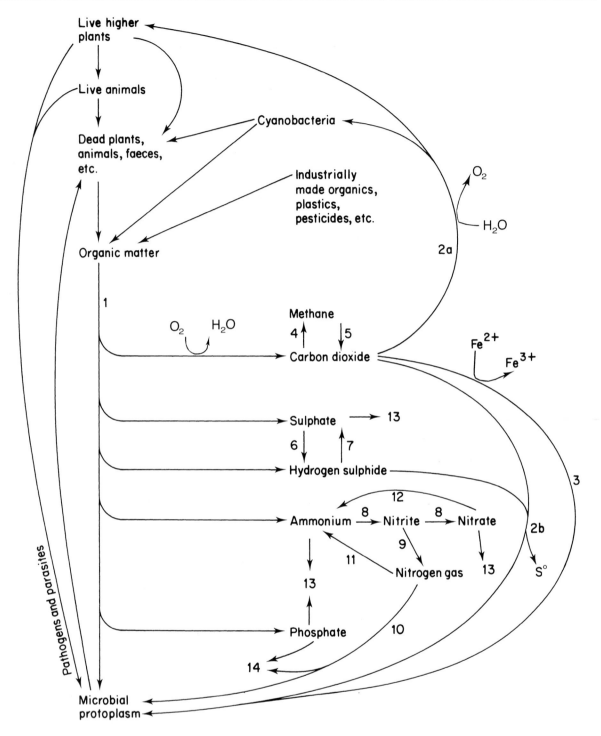

Fig. 13.4 The cycling of carbon, nitrogen, sulphur and phosphorus in soil with examples of the bacteria involved. The numbers refer to the following processes. 1. Decay by heterotrophs (many fungi and bacteria). 2a. Oxygenic photosynthesis (cyanobacteria and higher plants). 2b. Anoxygenic photosynthesis (*Chromatium, Chlorobium, Rhodopseudomonas*). 3. Oxidation of iron and other metals (*Siderocapsa, Gallionella, Pedomicrobium*), chemo-autotrophic carbon fixation, see also 7 and 8. 4. Use of carbon dioxide in methane formation (*Methanobacillus*). 5. Methane oxidation in aerobic conditions (*Methylomonas methanica, Methylomonas methano-oxidans*). 6. Use of sulphate as the terminal electron acceptor, hydrogen sulphide formation (*Desulfovibrio*). 7. Oxidation of hydrogen sulphide under aerobic conditions (*Thiobacillus*), chemo-autotrophic carbon fixation. 8. Nitrification (*Nitrosomonas, Nitrobacter*), chemo-autotrophic carbon fixation. 9. Denitrification, the reduction of nitrite to nitrogen gas which is then lost to the atmosphere (*Pseudomonas*). 10. Biological nitrogen fixation (*Azotobacter, Azospirillum, Rhizobium, Frankia*). 11. Industrial fixation of nitrogen to ammonium for fertilizers. 12. Nitrate and nitrite reduction, use of nitrate and nitrite as terminal electron acceptors (many genera, e.g. *Alcaligenes, Bacillus, Klebsiella, Pseudomonas*). 13. Higher plant uptake. 14. Higher plant uptake via microbial symbionts.

particular groups of micro-organisms so that the minimum breakdown of the plant material takes place. Anaerobic conditions are created by packing the grass tightly into the silo to exclude air and if sufficient sugar and protein are present in the grass the rapid growth of the *Lactobacillus* and *Streptococcus* spp. reduces pH. *Lactobacillus* spp., and also some *Streptococcus* and *Pediococcus* spp., are naturally present on plants in low numbers. Homofermentative species are preferred since they produce twice as much acid per molecule of glucose and the pH drops more quickly. If the system is merely anaerobic and not acidic then *Clostridium* spp. grow and reduce the cut grass to an evil-smelling, useless mess. Commercial inoculants containing selected strains of the bacteria are available and are used widely. Sometimes acids (sulphuric or formic) and additional sugars (as molasses, for example) are sold in commercial preparations to improve the fermentation, with or without the bacterial inoculant.

3.2 Carbon fixation

In soil the main primary producers (photoautotrophs) are higher plants, except in eroded or forming soils and in rice paddies where cyanobacteria and algae may be important (2a in Fig. 13.4). The contributions from anoxygenic photosynthesis and from chemo-autotrophic fixation (2b, 3, 7 and 8 in Fig. 13.4) is very small in soil, although it may be important in other ways: the deposition of iron III by *Pedomicrobium* is thought to contribute to the deposition of iron pans in some podsolic soils and such impermeable layers inhibit drainage, lead to waterlogged and therefore anaerobic conditions and alter the general microbiology. *Pedomicrobium* is also associated with the deposition of manganese nodules in marine situations.

3.3 Nitrogen conversions

Most of the nitrogen needed by plants is provided by the decay of organic matter. Biological nitrogen fixation (10 in Fig. 13.4), deposition of dust, lightening, etc. merely serve to top up the minerals lost by leaching. This is illustrated dramatically in the tropical rain forests which are very productive ecosystems but are actually not usually based on fertile soils. If the trees are removed and burnt during clearance for agriculture, it becomes all too obvious that the soils are not intrinsically fertile and that, without rapid nutrient cycling by micro-organisms, there is very poor plant growth. This picture has been distorted in western intensive agriculture by the addition of industrially fixed nitrogen (11 in Fig. 13.4) and, to a lesser extent, other elements as fertilizers. There is a considerable energy and environmental cost for this because much of the applied fertilizer is denitrified by bacteria and there is more leaching than would occur if nitrogen were supplied by biological fixation or the decomposition of organic matter. The balance of nitrogen compounds in the soil is mostly determined by the effects of aeration on the bacterial population. Ammonium is adsorbed to clay and organic matter colloids and this helps to prevent leaching, but in aerated soils ammonium will be converted to nitrate (8 in Fig. 13.4) in a process called nitrification which is carried out by various genera, of which the most important in soils are *Nitrosomonas* and *Nitrobacter*. Nitrate is usually the preferred form of nitrogen for higher plant uptake but, being negatively charged, is not adsorbed and is leached. Under conditions of poor aeration (less than 5 µM oxygen), brought about by waterlogging and compaction of the soil, the nitrate and nitrite can be used as a terminal electron acceptor and ammonium is formed (12 in Fig. 13.4). However, under similar conditions of poor aeration there can also be denitrification (9 in Fig. 13.4) in which the available nitrogen is converted to nitrous oxides or dinitrogen gas and lost to the soil and the plants. It is quite possible to cause a net loss of nitrogen by using heavy machinery on clay soils, even if the machines are being used to spread fertilizer!

Biological nitrogen fixation in soils, and anywhere else, is entirely done by prokaryotes (Bothe, de Bruijn and Newton 1988, Metting 1993, Brock et al. 1994). Fixation by symbionts (10 in Fig. 13.4) makes by far the most important contribution to the nitrogen economy of soil since the free-living heterotrophic genera are carbon limited, except perhaps genera such as *Azospirillum* around roots (in the rhizosphere, see section 5.1, p. 335), and so cannot fix appreciable quantities. Fixation by free-living autotrophs, especially cyanobacteria, may be significant in some situations such as at the beginning of seral successions mentioned above. There are symbiotic associations between cyanobacteria and various plants (*Gunnera*, cycads, etc.) although in most cases the contribution to the nitrogen nutrition must be small in view of the quantity of *Nostoc* in relation to the plant. The association with the aquatic fern *Azolla* is the only one of economic and social importance; it is responsible for feeding a considerable part of the population of South East Asia. The fern is grown in special ponds and let into the rice paddies when they are flooded and then trampled into the mud where it decomposes and gives nitrogen to the growing rice crop (Giller and Wilson 1991).

The main biological nitrogen fixation is by the mutualistic symbiosis of legumes (herbaceous plants, shrubs and trees) with *Rhizobium*, or other plants with *Frankia* (Bothe, de Bruijn and Newton 1988). *Rhizobium* is produced on a commercial scale and used for the field inoculation of crops, especially where a new legume crop is being grown (such as soybean) for the first time and for which the correct strain of *Rhizobium* is not present in the soil. Within the soil there is competition between strains of *Rhizobium*, so strains introduced into the soil for commercial use must be carefully selected for the crop to be grown and must be good competitors with resident strains and also good at fixing nitrogen, though all these attributes do not necessarily go together. The growth of the bacteria in the soil is specifically stimulated by the legume roots and the bacteria bind to adsorption sites on the root hair surface. After invading the root hair and crossing the root cortex in an infection thread formed by the invagination of the root hair wall, the bacteria, which have no cell walls at this stage, enter membrane-bound vesicles in polyploid cells of the cortex. The bacteria contain all the necessary enzymes for nitrogen fixation. Although the overall reduction of nitrogen gas to ammonium should yield energy, the initial breaking of the triple bond requires a high energy of activation which is supplied from the host's photosynthate, and up to 25% of the plant's primary production may go to feed the bacteria and their nitrogen fixation. Legumes with effective root nodules will fix considerable quantities of nitrogen (up to 400 kg of nitrogen per hectare per year) and they are vital in maintaining the productivity of many natural soils and agricultural soils where nitrogen fertilizers are not available or are too expensive for the farmers to use.

Frankia is an actinomycete which forms nodules with a wide variety of plants, usually woody shrubs and small trees (*Alnus, Casuarina, Myrica, Hippophae*) which grow on the fringes of deserts and on glacial moraines and other nitrogen-deficient soils (Skinner, Boddey and Fendrik 1989). *Frankia* does not grow easily in culture and is not available as a commercial inoculum, but the plants are widely used in afforestation and in the recovery of eroded soils and in slowing the advance of deserts. The *Frankia* grows in the cortical cells of the roots and, as in the *Rhizobium* association, the bacteria get carbohydrate from the host and the latter gets fixed, available nitrogen (up to 180 kg per hectare per year) which is significant in the very nitrogen-limited environments.

The biochemistry and molecular genetics of nitrogen fixation are well known (Bothe, de Bruijn and Newton 1988, Brock et al. 1994). The main problem is that the reaction requires a large amount of energy in the form of ATP and the enzyme nitrogenase reductase, which is part of the complex, is exceedingly oxygen sensitive. Various methods are used by the organisms to keep the site of fixation anaerobic while allowing aerobic respiration to produce the required ATP and the reduced cofactor, ferredoxin. In cyanobacteria the nitrogenase is in special cells called heterocysts, which exclude oxygen so that the organism can carry out oxygenic photosynthesis at the same time as anaerobic nitrogen fixation. Legumes carry oxygen to the nodules by leghaemoglobin so there is no free oxygen to denature the enzyme.

3.4 Sulphur conversions

The production of hydrogen sulphide during decay is uncommon in soils as they are usually too well aerated, but it can occur in some microhabitats and in soils such as rice paddies and waterlogged natural soils. Plants growing in such soils usually have special tissues, aerenchyma, to conduct oxygen down to their roots and this tissue is produced in response to microbially generated ethene under conditions of poor aeration. In most soils the sulphur is released from the organic matter as sulphate and this is the usual form taken up by plants. Similarly, the reduction of sulphur compounds (6 in Fig. 13.4) should not occur in most soils. In soils reclaimed from aquatic sediments, such as the Dutch polders, or other previously waterlogged soils which are drained, the initial oxidation of reduced sulphur compounds by *Thiobacillus* (7 in Fig. 13.4) can give problems as the pH drops.

4 POLLUTION CONTROL

As well as being responsible for the recycling of natural organic matter, the micro-organisms, and bacteria in particular, also degrade many man-made substances such as pesticides, plastics and other waste and also materials such as petroleum products spilt on land and in marine situations (Fry et al. 1992, Alexander 1994).

Much of the pesticide which is sprayed on crops reaches the soil either because it missed the target plant or the plant or insect dies and falls onto the soil. There is some chemical breakdown associated with UV light and also catalysis by adsorption on clays, but the great majority of the pesticide is broken down by microbial action; indeed, pesticides now cleared for use are required to be biodegradable (Fry et al. 1992). Much is now known as part of the registration procedures about the chemistry of the breakdown and the products produced. Pesticides, applied at the recommended rates, rarely have detrimental effects on the soil bacteria. This is partly because no bactericides are cleared for agricultural use in the UK, but antibiotics are used as livestock feed additives and arrive in the soil as slurry from animal houses. The use of pesticides often leads to an increase in bacterial activity in the soil because of the provision of organic substrates from the dead organism, rather than the degradation of the pesticide itself since the quantities of the latter are usually small.

Bioremediation is the in situ breakdown, by microorganisms, of pollutants in the soil (Fry et al. 1992, Metting 1993). These may be long-term accumulations on industrial sites and mines of such things as phenols, or one-off accidents such as the spillage of oil. There is usually no shortage of bacterial strains naturally present in the soil which can carry out the breakdown, usually an oxidation. There are, however, commercially available strains of bacteria and fungi, which have been specially selected or genetically engineered to degrade particular substances or to degrade them faster than natural populations. Usually all that is needed is to supply oxygen to the soil and probably mineral nutrients since many substrates, such as oil, are short of nitrogen. The supply of oxygen is needed to support the increased respiration rate of the soil organisms (Table 13.3) and this may be done by cultivating the soil or by injecting air. The cost of bioremediation procedures is usually less than the removal of the polluted material to landfill or incineration.

Table 13.3 Oxygen consumption of different soils polluted with hydrocarbon material

Soil		Hydrocarbon		Oxygen consumption (μl h^{-1} g^{-1} FW soil)	
Location	Type	Type	Origin	Polluted	Unpolluted
Strasbourg	Hydromull	Crude oil	Oil well	15.0	2.0
Rouen	Rendzina	Fuel oil[a]	Storage spill	15.7	1.0
Fontainebleau	Podsol	Crude oil	Oil well	19.0	4.0
Dunkirk	Dune sand	Sludge[b]	Cleaning oil	7.7	0.8
Dunkirk[c]	Dune sand	Sludge	Cleaning oil	18.3	0.8

Data from Gudin and Syratt 1975.
[a]Mixed spills of light and heavy gas oils from different crude oils occurring over a 4-year period.
[b]An emulsion of water and oil (9%) containing 7% by weight clay derived from a process to remove sulphur from the oil.
[c]As the previous sample but 0.1 M ammonium nitrate added 1 day before measurement.

5 BACTERIA ASSOCIATED WITH PLANTS

5.1 Root associations

Most of the heterotrophic bacteria in soil are nutrient limited, but this restriction is removed close to plant roots that supply the soil with sloughed off root cells, mucilage and soluble organic exudates (simple sugars, amino and organic acids) which together may amount to as much as 15–20% of their net primary production (Lynch 1990). The root also uses oxygen, produces carbon dioxide and alters the balance of water and minerals. The volume of soil influenced by the root is called the rhizosphere, and the effect on the microorganisms is to increase their numbers, diversity and activity, usually expressed as the R:S ratio (Table 13.4). The dimensions of the rhizosphere vary with the species of plant, the soil type, plant physiological status and age. If the soil is very poor, as in the sand dune plants (Table 13.4), then the addition of any organic matter has a great effect and the R:S ratio is high, even if the total numbers of bacteria are not as great as in agricultural soils.

Gram-negative bacteria, especially *Pseudomonas* spp., increase around the young parts of roots (near the tip) while coryneform bacteria are the main part of the population near older parts of the root. The host plant influences the rhizosphere population, presumably by affecting the quality and the quantity of ex-

udates, so that bacteria in the rhizosphere show specificity to species, cultivars or breeding lines. Indeed, this specificity may be so great that particular strains of bacteria are limited to one plant (Lambert et al. 1987).

There are bacterial pathogens of roots and below-ground stems, such as *Erwinia carotovora* and *Streptomyces scabies*, which cause soft rots and potato scab, respectively. Other bacteria growing on or near the plant root may have no effects on the plant (neutralism) but they can be deleterious by producing toxins such as cyanide, or they can increase plant growth by improving mineral uptake or altering the hormone balance of the plant. Because of the specificity outlined above, a bacterial species may be neutral on one crop species or cultivar, beneficial on another and harmful on a third. The manipulation of these bacteria, by genetically engineering either the host or the bacterium, or by altering the environmental conditions, may be another way of controlling plant production. Symbiotic root-colonizing bacteria that fix nitrogen have already been mentioned above, and there are also many beneficial symbiotic fungal associations which improve nutrient uptake (mycorrhizae).

5.2 Associations with stems and leaves

Some strains of *Frankia* and *Rhizobium* form their nodules on stems, especially in host genera which grow in

Table 13.4 Viable counts of bacteria in root-free soil and in the rhizosphere of crop plants and wild species

Species	Colony counts of bacteria (10^6 g^{-1} soil)		R:S ratio
	Rhizosphere (R)	Root-free soil (S)	
Trifolium pratense	3260	134	24
Avena sativa	1090	184	6
Linum usitatissimum	1015	184	5
Zea mays	614	184	3
Atriplex glabriuscula	23.3	0.016	1455
Ammophila arenaria	3.6	0.016	223
Elytrigia juncea	3.6	0.016	222

Data from Woldendorp 1978.
The last 3 species are sand dune plants and so there are very low numbers in the poor soil but a very pronounced rhizosphere effect because the low organic matter content makes any addition very significant.

waterlogged soils (Giller and Wilson 1991). There are also leaf nodules formed by bacteria of various genera; these are thought to alter the plant growth hormone balance and to affect plant growth patterns.

Apart from these special cases, bacteria are normal inhabitants of stems, leaves and flowers, though the numbers are often low because of low nutrient and water availability on many temperate plants. In the tropical and temperate rain forest areas high populations can develop. There is very little information on the species present on leaves, though a few pathogens have been studied in detail and there is information on *Pseudomonas syringae* derived from studies necessary for the release of genetically engineered organisms (see section 6). Most bacteria on leaves are gram negative (*Xanthomonas, Pseudomonas, Erwinia, Flavobacterium*; Blakeman 1982) and they are concentrated in the microhabitats giving some protection from the extreme environment such as epistomatal cavities and in the grooves between the epidermal cells of the leaf. There are more bacteria on the undersides of the leaf where again there is protection from UV and high temperatures; leaves are designed to trap visible light energy for photosynthesis, but they inevitably get UV and IR as well. Bacterial numbers rise during the growing season in temperate conditions and peak as the leaf senesces.

Some bacteria growing on leaves cause plant diseases (*P. syringae*, for example) and though these can be serious on particular crops they do not in general compare with fungi as disease-causing organisms for plants.

Some bacteria live in flowers, and of these *Erwinia amylovora*, the cause of fire blight in fruit trees, has been especially studied. It is carried and dispersed by bees and enters the shoot of the tree during the short time when the flower is open, causing death of the branch.

6 RELEASE OF GENETICALLY ENGINEERED BACTERIA IN SOIL AND ON PLANTS

The release of genetically engineered bacteria into the environment has been done with nitrogen-fixing symbionts, such as *Rhizobium*, and organisms to improve plant growth and control plant diseases (Keister and Cregan 1991, Jones 1993, Metting 1993). Some are commercially available and others are in various stages of development (Wilson and Lindow 1993). Bacterial genes, such as those responsible for the production of *Bacillus thuringiensis* toxins, have been transferred to plants to give protection from insect pests. There is little experience of risk assessment in these situations (Alexander 1992) and cases are being considered on an individual basis. The risk involved in release is thought by some to be high because most of these organisms are designed to be free living in the environment, as opposed to being used in industrial situations where they might be contained to some extent. Furthermore, the bacteria are designed or selected to survive and grow in the environment so that they may colonize plants, and this means the new genes or new genetic combinations which they contain could spread into other bacteria. In general, the regulations on release are strict and there are fears that this is discouraging the exploitation of organisms which could reduce pesticide and fertilizer use, especially in the developing world (Miller 1995). One of the main problems is a methodological one of re-isolating and identifying the released organisms so that they can be tracked; various reporter genes are being used, such as *LacZY* and *lux*, so that the organisms can be detected in the soil. One of the inconsistencies is that genetically engineered bacteria are subject to special consideration but traditionally mutated and selected strains are much less controlled, even though they may have been subjected to general mutagens and changed in unknown ways.

One of the examples extensively studied is *P. syringae*, a common inhabitant of plant leaves (Wilson and Lindow 1993). Frost-sensitive plants, such as potatoes, citrus, strawberry, etc., suffer frost damage because ice crystal formation either removes water from the cells or mechanically damages the walls and membranes. Ice crystals form about ice nuclei and *P. syringae* produces a protein which acts as such a nucleus. If the protein is eliminated from leaves they do not suffer ice damage down to $-10°C$; the water supercools without freezing. A strain of the bacterium without the protein, *P. syringae ice-* , has been produced and it competes successfully with the natural bacterial population and does not form the protein, and so protects the plants from ice crystal damage at low temperatures. There have been great problems in clearing this organism for release. Ironically, the wild-type strain, with the ice-nucleating protein, is not subject to restrictions; selected strains are widely used commercially in snow machines to encourage ice crystal formation (snow) at temperatures close to freezing point at ski resorts!

A better result has been obtained with release of the biocontrol agent *Agrobacterium* strain K84 which protects against *Agrobacterium tumifaciens*, the cause of crown gall in plants. This bacterium is extensively used in molecular genetics in general because it can transfer DNA from a prokaryote to a eukaryote. The control agent produces a specific antibiotic, a bacteriocin, against the pathogen but is, of course, resistant to its own bacteriocin. Since this resistance is plasmid-borne, there were worries that it could be transferred to the pathogenic bacterium and control would break down. A strain has now been produced that is incapable of transferring the plasmid, it is *tra-* , and this has been cleared for commercial use in Australia, but not in the USA or Europe at the time of writing. Different countries have their own regulations, further complicating matters.

Genetically engineered bacteria will continue to be released into the soil and plant environment and this may become easier and less expensive as experience is gained, so that this form of biotechnology can be used to reduce the damaging effects of fertilizers and pesticides.

7 FUTURE PROSPECTS

The main thrust of present research is to develop the potential of laboratory-selected and genetically engineered bacteria for the promotion of plant growth and the control of soil-borne plant diseases. There will be a continued development of commercially available inocula of organisms such as *Rhizobium* and *Pseudomonas*. The rhizosphere is seen as the main part of the plant–soil system that can be manipulated to the benefit of the plant. Reduction in the use of chemical fertilizers and pesticides is also possible by the microbiological manipulation of nutrient availability and uptake. It is possible that commercial packages could eventually be designed of particular varieties of plants, with bacteria that are specific to them for plant-growth promotion, disease control and for the utilization of fertilizers designed to complement the other components; the package will work only if complete so that the commercial firm corners the market and competitors' products will not be compatible. There is now comparatively little research on the bacteriology of natural soil environments, except in as much as it is necessary for understanding the risks of release of commercial organisms. However, we still lack understanding of adsorption phenomena which will greatly affect general ecology and the specific host interactions. Methods are needed for understanding phenomena at the microhabitat level so that isolation, identification and an understanding of the physiology of bacteria are possible on this scale.

REFERENCES

Alexander M, 1992, A microbial ecologist looks again at risk analysis, *Risk Assessment for Deliberate Release* , ed. Klingmuller W, Springer Verlag, Berlin, 1–9.

Alexander M, 1994, *Biodegradation and Bioremediation*, Academic Press, San Diego, California, 1–302.

Andrews JH, Harris RF, 1986, r- and K-selection in microbial ecology, *Adv Microb Ecol*, **9**: 99–147.

Balows A, Trüper HG et al., eds, 1992, *The Prokaryotes: a Handbook on the Biology of Bacteria, Ecophysiology, Identification, Applications*, 2nd edn, Springer-Verlag, New York, 1–4126.

Blakeman JP, 1982, Phylloplane interactions, *Phytopathogenic Prokaryotes*, eds Mount MS, Lacey GH, Academic Press, New York, 307–33.

Bothe H, de Bruijn FJ, Newton WE, 1988, *Nitrogen Fixation: Hundred Years After*, Gustav Fischer, Stuttgart, 1–878.

Brock TD, 1987, The study of micro-organisms *in situ*: progress and problems, *Ecology of Microbial Communities, 41st Symposium of the Society of General Microbiology*, eds Fletcher M, Gray TRG, Jones JG, Cambridge University Press, Cambridge, 1–17.

Brock TD, Madigan MT et al., 1994, *Biology of Micro-organisms*, 7th edn, Prentice-Hall, Englewood Cliffs, NJ, USA, 1–909.

Bull AT, Goodfellow M, Slater JH, 1992, Biodiversity as a source of innovation in technology, *Annu Rev Microbiol*, **46**: 219–52.

Burns R, 1986, Interaction of enzymes with soil mineral and organic colloids, *Interactions of Soil Minerals with Natural Organics and Microbes, Special Publ.17*, Soil Science Society of America, Madison, Wisconsin, 429–51.

Campbell R, 1983, *Microbial Ecology*, Blackwell Scientific, Oxford.

Chapelle FH, Zelibor JL et al., 1987, Bacteria in deep coastal plain sediments of Maryland: a possible source of CO_2 in ground water, *Water Resources Res*, **23**: 1625–32.

Fry JC, Gadd GM et al., eds, 1992, *Microbial Control of Pollution, Society for General Microbiology Symposium 48*, Cambridge University Press, Cambridge, 1–343.

Giller KE, Wilson KJ, 1991, *Nitrogen Fixation in Tropical Cropping Systems*, CAB International, Wallingford, UK, 1–313.

Grigorova R, Norris JR, eds, 1990, *Methods in Microbiology, vol. 22, Techniques in Microbial Ecology*, Academic Press, London, 1–627.

Gudin C, Syratt WJ, 1975, Biological aspects of land rehabilitation following hydrocarbon contamination, *Environ Pollut*, **8**: 107–12.

Hobson PN, 1988, *The Rumen Microbial Ecosystem*, Elsevier Scientific Publishers, Barking, Essex, 1–527.

Jones DG, ed., 1993, *The Exploitation of Micro-organisms*, Chapman and Hall, London, 1–488.

Keister DL, Cregan PB, eds, 1991, *The Rhizosphere and Plant Growth*, Kluwer Academic Publishers, Dordrecht, 1–386.

Lambert B, Leyns F et al., 1987, Rhizobacteria of maize and their antifungal activities, *Appl Environ Microbiol*, **53**: 1866–71.

Levin MA, Seidler RJ, Rogul M, 1992, *Microbial Ecology: Principles, Methods and Applications*, McGraw-Hill, New York, 1–945.

Lynch JM, 1990, *The Rhizosphere*, John Wiley & Sons, Chichester, UK, 1–458.

Metting FB, ed., 1993, *Soil Microbial Ecology*, Marcel Dekker, New York, 1–646.

Miller H, 1995, Biodiversity treaty misguided, *Nature*, **373**: 278.

Persson T, Bååth E et al., 1980, Trophic structure, biomass dynamics and carbon metabolism of soil organisms in a Scots pine forest, *Structure and Function of Northern Coniferous Forests, an Ecosystem Study, Ecology Bulletin (Stockholm)*, vol 32, ed. Persson T, Swedish National Science Research Council (NFR), 419–59.

Savage DW, Fletcher M, 1985, *Bacterial Adhesion, Mechanisms and Physiological Significance*, Plenum Press, New York, 1–476.

Schnürer J, 1985, *Fungi in Arable Soil*, Dissertation, Swedish University of Agricultural Sciences, Department of Microbiology, Uppsala, Sweden.

Schnürer J, Clarholm M, Rosswall T, 1985, Microbial biomass and activity in agricultural soil with different organic matter contents, *Soil Biol Biochem*, **17**: 611–18.

Sexstone AJ, Revsbech NP et al., 1985, Direct measurement of oxygen profiles and denitrification rates in soil aggregates, *Soil Sci Soc Am J*, **49**: 645–51.

Skinner FA, Boddey RM, Fendrik I, 1989, *Nitrogen Fixation with Non-legumes*, Kluwer Academic Publishers, Dordrecht, 1–366.

Struwe S, Kjøller A, 1986, Changes in population structure during decomposition, *Microbial Communities in Soil*, eds Jensen V, Kjøller A, Sørensen LH, Elsevier, London, 149–62.

Thomashow L, Weller D, 1991, Role of antibiotics and siderophores in biocontrol of take-all disease of wheat, *The Rhizosphere and Plant Growth*, eds Keister DL, Cregan PB, Kluwer, Dordrecht, 245–51.

Williams ST, 1986, The ecology of antibiotic production, *Microb Ecol*, **12**: 43–52.

Wilson M, Lindow SE, 1993, Release of recombinant organisms, *Annu Rev Microbiol*, 913–44.

Woldendorp JW, 1978, The rhizosphere as part of the plant-soil system, *Verh K Ned Akad Wet Ald Natuurkde Reeks*, **70**: 237–67.

Chapter 14

THE MICROBIOLOGY OF AIR[1]

C S Cox

1 INTRODUCTION

Lidwell (1990) in the eighth edition pointed out that previous interest in the microbiology of air (i.e. aerobiology) 'has progressed by fits and starts ... largely because of failure to appreciate the quantitative aspects; for example, it is often held that, because a pathogen is present only in small numbers in the air, this route of infection must be insignificant'. Nowadays, the situation is somewhat different as exemplified by recent publication of such titles as *Atmospheric Microbial Aerosols* (Lighthart and Mohr 1994), *Bioaerosols* (Burge 1995b) and *Bioaerosol Handbook* (Cox and Wathes 1995), concerned directly with quantitative aspects of characterising bioaerosols and their health hazards to man, animals and plants.

The contents of these monographs clearly demonstrate the wide range of disciplines involved in aerobiological studies and the increasing realization of the importance of aerobiology in an expanding range of aspects of life.

2 AEROBIOLOGY

Air movements readily transport particulate matter over considerable distances, e.g. spread of foot-and-mouth disease virus from Oswestry (Lidwell 1990), pollen deposits at the earth's poles and carriage of stem rust disease from the Mississippi valley (where it is endemic) to the northern regions of Canada. Such ubiquitous fine biological particles of diameter c. 0.05–100 μm are termed 'bioaerosols'. However, the

abilities of air-borne microbes to cause diseases also depend on their surviving and remaining infective for susceptible hosts. These functions, like allergenicity, depend on environmental parameters of relative humidity (RH), temperature, radiation intensity and wavelength, oxygen tension and pollutant levels.

Humans and their activities provide major sources of bioaerosols. For example, respiratory pathogens are liberated during talking, sneezing and coughing in particles small enough to remain air-borne for considerable periods, whereas others are large enough to fall rapidly on to the ground and other nearby surfaces (Lidwell 1990), but these, on drying, can become re-aerosolized through physical activity. As described below, differences in aerosol survival and infectivity are to be anticipated for the 2 sets of conditions that represent wet and dry dissemination.

People act as microbial reservoirs and amplifiers as well as disseminators, and represent the dominant sources of bacteria and viruses in indoor environments including residences (Burge 1995a). Indoor bioaerosols also include skin squames, dust mite fragments and faeces, fungal spores, hyphae and products and yeasts. Buildings, depending on use, e.g. homes (Burge 1995a), schools, hospitals and laboratories (Clark 1995, Macher, Stretfel and Vesley 1995), workplaces (Crook and Olenchock 1995), animal houses (Wathes 1995) and transport vehicles contain sources of infectious and allergenic materials and readily become contaminated via bioaerosols that, through diffusion and air currents, can reach the most inaccessible places (Cox 1987). In the process, viability, infectivity and allergenicity can be modified (Cox 1995a).

Outdoors rain action, air turbulence and diffusion, spray irrigation, sewage treatment, breaking of waves, bursting of bubbles, crop spraying, etc. ensure that multicomponent bioaerosols (Lighthart and Stetzenbach 1994, Lacey and Venette 1995) are formed continuously and travel downwind (Lighthart 1994). Nowadays, too, there are deliberate air-borne releases (hundreds of tonnes per year) of biological pesticides and genetically engineered micro-organisms. Consequently, increasing human exposure to bioaerosols in most environments seems inevitable with associated hazards arising primarily from high concentrations or unfamiliar micro-organisms. Respiratory distress, microbial infections, sensitization and allergenic reactions and toxicological reactions are some of these outcomes (Salem and Gardener 1994, Burge 1995a, 1995b, Cox and Wathes 1995). In addition, there are diseases and associated microbes of animals and crops (Lacey and Venette 1995, Madelin and Madelin 1995, Wathes 1995).

Potential and actual costs to society of bioaerosol hazards are great (Brosseau, Kuehn and Goyal 1994). For example, estimates from the 1981 National Health Survey (US Department HEW 1982) indicate that, in the USA alone, 200 million episodes of respiratory infection occur each year, or 75 million physician visits per year, 150 million days lost from work with costs of c. $10 billion plus medical care costs of c. $10 billion. From the corresponding 1991 survey the number of episodes increased to c. 250 million. To such burdens can be added those due to animal and crop diseases. World wide, bioaerosol hazards represent an enormous human problem with an associated large economic burden.

Understanding the nature of bioaerosols is an essential part of any remedial action and the first steps in studying bioaerosols include their sampling in a representative and quantitative manner to determine particle size and shape distributions and measure properties such as viability, infectivity, toxicity and allergenicity. As these represent subjects covered in depth in the monographs listed above, the remainder of this chapter is concerned mainly with the more recent aspects of survival and infectivity studies of air-borne microbes, and the stability of aeroallergens.

3 AIR-BORNE SURVIVAL

After take-off (generation), aerial transport (storage) and landing (collection), the ability of infectious microbes to initiate disease depends on how they survive (replicate) and maintain infectivity (cause infection). Although survival is a prerequisite for transmission, infectivity involves additional attributes that can be lost more readily.

Microbes and allergens comprise 'building blocks' of unequal inherent thermodynamic stability and most probably target molecules may be related to energies associated with stress factors operating in the air-borne state (Table 14.1). Effects of RH will be considered first because, being of low energy, they may be expected primarily to affect least stable entities.

Table 14.1 Summary of most probable target molecules

Air-borne stress	Most probable target
RH and temperature	Phospholipids, proteins
Oxygen	Phospholipids, proteins
Ozone	Phospholipids, proteins
Open air factor (ozone + olefins)	Phospholipids, proteins, nucleic acids
γ-rays, x-rays, UV	Phospholipids, proteins, nucleic acids

3.1 Dehydration and rehydration

When disseminated from liquid suspensions (e.g. in saliva), microbes desiccate, whereas they partially rehydrate when disseminated as dusts or freeze-dried powders. Thus, changes in water content occur for all aerosolized microbes and represent the most fundamental stress. Microbes and their constituent nucleic acids, proteins, carbohydrates and phospholipids are hygroscopic and demonstrate hysteresis in their water sorption isotherms. Consequently, at a given storage RH, equilibrium water contents of microbes are slightly higher in dehydrating than in rehydrating states.

COLIPHAGES

That changes can occur in microbial surface components is clearly demonstrated by the fragility of coliphage head–tail complexes that follow desiccation (Cox 1987, 1989), in that tails are easily sheared from coliphage heads (Fig. 14.1) by the action of aerosol samplers that impose high degrees of shear, e.g. all glass impingers such as AGI-30. This weakness of coliphage may be related to the morphological mismatch of tails and heads in that they have different rotational symmetries (Harris and Horne 1986).

The coliphage example is important for several reasons. It indicates how sampling rather than the intrinsic state of the phage can be responsible for observed loss of viability and, therefore, can be a source of serious experimental artefact. The relative fragility of some surface structures following desiccation also means that, after dehydration, biomaterials can demonstrate different allergenicity from the native material, i.e. some allergens are generated only following desiccation, whereas others active in the hydrated state are no longer allergenic.

VIRUSES

Viruses without structural lipids, such as mengovirus 37A, poliovirus, foot-and-mouth disease virus and encephalomyocarditis (EMC) virus, are unstable when wet disseminated and held at RH values below c. 70% because their surface structures are denatured (Cox 1987). The approach to establish this for poliovirus was to compare infectivity of whole virus with that of isolated infectious RNA (Akers and Hatch 1968) (Fig. 14.2). For EMC virus the approach was similar,

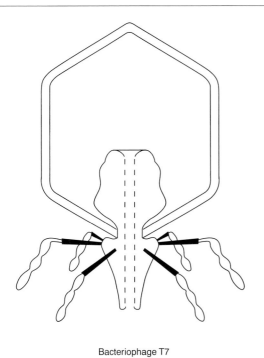

Bacteriophage T7

Fig. 14.1 T coliphage showing head–tail complex.

together with measurement of concomitant loss of haemagglutination activity and affinity for haemagglutination inhibiting antibodies.

By contrast, viruses that contain structural lipids, such as Langat, Semliki Forest, vesicular stomatitis, vaccinia, Venezuelan equine encephalomyelitis (VEE)

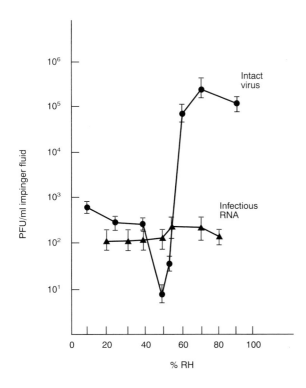

Fig. 14.2 Effect of RH on the survival of air-borne mengovirus 37A and isolated mengovirus 37A infectious RNA following storage for 2 h at 37°C.

and influenza viruses are least stable at RH values above c. 70%. Even so, loss of infectivity occurs, at least for Semliki Forest virus, in the same way as for lipid-free viruses, i.e. primarily through damage to the viral coat rather than to nucleic acid. By contrast, at ambient temperatures bioaerosols of DNA-containing pigeon pox and Simian 40 viruses maintain infectivity at high levels irrespective of RH, presumably because they have a more robust outer coat.

These observations are in keeping with the general findings that phospholipid–protein complexes denature most readily at mid to high RH, whereas proteins themselves denature most readily at low RH (Cox 1989, 1995a). As integrity and biological activity of phospholipid–protein complexes, e.g. membranes, depends on temperature as well as water content, virus survival may be enhanced at certain temperatures with little RH dependency. Under these conditions, there is usually a higher incidence of influenza (a lipid-containing virus) during winter than in summer, in both northern and southern hemispheres, whereas for polio (lipid-free) there is a higher incidence in summer than winter. This becomes more understandable if prevailing temperature is as important as, or more important than, RH for air-borne survival and transmission of diseases.

BACTERIA

Bacteria are more complex than phages and viruses (see Chapter 2) and may be expected to demonstrate more complex inactivation mechanisms. Hence, conflicts of opinion and contradictions in results of early work were unavoidable. Some of the difficulties arose because some gram-negative bacteria, after dehydration, are inactivated by oxygen, unlike phages and viruses (so far tested). Difficulties in assessing viability were increased by other problems associated with the collection of undamaged samples of air-borne microbes and the role in this of hypertonic collecting fluids, and of rehumidification before sampling, as well as the effects of sublethal injury.

Hess (1965) was the first to demonstrate systematically and unequivocally that bioaerosols of *Serratia marcescens* 8UK stored at below c. 70% RH become oxygen-sensitive, as do freeze-dried powders. Having once established oxygen toxicity, experiments in inert atmospheres (e.g. nitrogen, argon, helium) led to some surprising patterns of results and, eventually, to a partial understanding of the effects of desiccation. Aerosol experiments conducted in the late 1960s indicated that there are critical narrow RH bands above c. 80% RH where loss of viability of several strains of *Escherichia coli* sprayed from suspensions in triple glass-distilled water is rapid (Fig. 14.3). Also, in inert atmospheres, unlike in air, stability is greatest at low RH; previously, poor survival of these strains at low RH in air had been attributed, mistakenly, to desiccation rather than to oxygen toxicity.

Similar experiments with bacteria sprayed, for example, from suspensions in raffinose solutions, demonstrated a phenomenon associated with collection in that use of a sampling fluid of 1 M sucrose, or

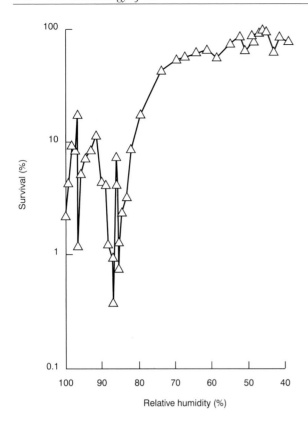

Fig. 14.3 Aerosol survival of *E. coli* B sprayed from suspension in distilled water into nitrogen as a function of RH at an aerosol age of 30 min at 26.5°C.

rehumidification in a warm atmosphere of 100% RH before sampling (as during inhalation), enhances survival (Figs 14.4 and 14.5). These effects are not additive but rather represent alternative techniques for producing the same effect (see also Bolister and Madelin 1992).

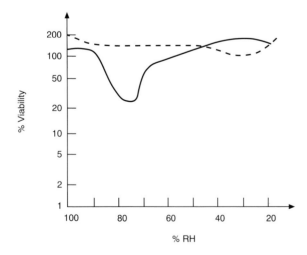

Fig. 14.4 Aerosol survival of *E. coli* commune sprayed from suspension in 0.3 M raffinose into nitrogen as a function of RH at an aerosol age of 30 min at 26.5°C. Collected into: ————, phosphate buffer; - - - - -, phosphate buffer + 1 M sucrose.

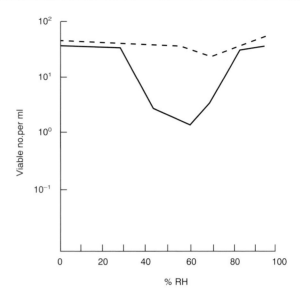

Fig. 14.5 Aerosol survival of *K. pneumoniae* into nitrogen as a function of RH: ————, direct sampling; - - - - -, rehumidified before sampling.

The use of wet or dry dissemination can, for some bacteria, e.g. *Francisella tularensis* LVS (Fig. 14.6), have a profound effect on survival at a given RH that is not due to the drying process. The observed survival level for microbes stored at a given RH can be markedly different depending on whether the bioaerosol was generated from a wet suspension or as a dry powder. For these experiments, the atmosphere was air but for *F. tularensis* oxygen toxicity is minimal. Hysteresis in water sorption isotherms is an unlikely cause because of the extent of the effect. Other possible causes, such as membrane phase changes, are discussed later (see section 5.2, p. 346) and whereas there is now potential understanding of why such differences arise, the initial observations remained unexplained for several years.

Such marked differences in the survival behaviour of the same microbe, whether disseminated wet or dry, are rarely considered important parameters that for the air-borne spread of disease that may be more important than RH.

In summary, for gram-negative bacteria (with their lipid-containing outer membrane) such as *E. coli, Klebsiella pneumoniae*, the primary effects of desiccation seem analogous to those for lipid-containing viruses, i.e. they are least stable at RH values above c. 80%, with the outermost layer a primary site of damage.

ANHYDROBIOTIC ORGANISMS

Higher organisms such as yeasts, fungi, seaweeds and nematodes can withstand the stresses associated with partial dehydration and rehydration that are traumatic for other organisms. For instance, dried yeast, when added to a weak nutrient solution, starts to metabolize and produce CO_2 quite rapidly. Such anhydrobiotic organisms share the property of containing quantities of trehalose, a very stable non-reducing disaccharide of glucose. Experiments have shown that trehalose is involved in the ability of these organisms to withstand

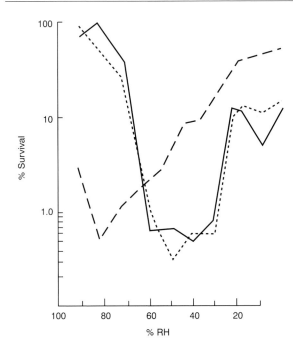

Fig. 14.6 Aerosol survival of *F. tularensis* LVS in air as a function of RH at an aerosol age of 15 min at 26.5°C when disseminated: ————, wet state; - - - - -, dry state; ...., wet state when suspension prepared by reconstituting the freeze-dried powder with distilled water.

desiccation and this point is discussed further (see section 5.3, p. 346). Consequently, anhydrobiotic organisms may be expected to be relatively aerostable.

SPORES

Gram-positive bacteria such as *Bacillus subtilis*, *Bacillus thuringiensis* and fungi have evolved an alternative strategy for withstanding desiccation, high temperatures and radiation. These species form spores with a thick outer coat that contains c. 20% by weight of calcium dipicolinate; they are relatively aerostable.

ALLERGENS

Bioaerosols that cause hypersensitivity or allergic responses include pollens, vegetable matter, house and paper dust mite parts and excreta, insect parts and excreta, proteins, and a wide range of microbes. Such entities can be effective whether 'alive' or 'dead' and their viability seems less important than their molecular nature. As indicated above, a molecular species can be modified by aerosolization. For example, a globular protein can partially lose its helical structure after desiccation, thereby exposing groups previously hidden in molecular interstices, to generate new antigenic sites. Furthermore, on collection, osmotic cell lysis can occur and collected samples may as a result be different allergenically both from native parent materials before aerosolization and from materials in the bioaerosol state. The allergenicity of a given material may depend critically on its fate in the air-borne state.

3.2 Temperature

Little has been published about air-borne survival as a function of temperature and most has been provided by Ehrlich and colleagues (see Cox 1987). Generally, optimum survival is at about +10°C with rate of viability loss increasing progressively both above and below that temperature. As discussed in more detail below (see section 5.1, p. 344), this situation is probably due to different mechanisms with positive and negative temperature coefficients operating, respectively, above and below the optimum. For disease spread via the air-borne pathway, air temperature may represent an environmental parameter with a greater importance than usually considered.

3.3 Oxygen

There are no reports of oxygen toxicity for phages and viruses whereas certain dehydrated pollen membranes and the Ca^{2+}-transporting activity of synthetic membranes are affected adversely. In addition, survival of aerosolized and freeze-dried gram-negative bacteria, e.g. *S. marcescens*, *E. coli*, *K. pneumoniae*, is impaired by oxygen (Cox 1987). Most laboratory studies have been carried out with *S. marcescens* for which oxygen toxicity is observed only at RH values less than c. 70% and with an effect that increases with degree of desiccation, time and oxygen concentration up to c. 30% when oxygen toxicity is maximum. Dry *E. coli* cells also suffer oxygen toxicity at low RH, but they are protected at high RH. Little is known for other organisms, but unless protected (e.g. by trehalose), dehydrated phospholipid membranes generally are likely to be inactivated by oxygen.

3.4 Open air factor and other pollutants

SO_2 and NO are less toxic than ozone whereas the reaction of the latter with olefins generates products, termed 'the open air factor' (OAF), that are toxic at the parts per hundred million (pphm) level. OAF high toxicity is considered to be due to its ready condensation on surfaces rather than to any particular chemical toxicity. However, this feature makes it difficult to maintain OAF concentrations in pipes or vessels unless they are rapidly ventilated – hence the term 'open air factor'. Because of the oxidizing nature of OAF, bioaerosol survival outdoors is generally lower than that indoors in otherwise similar conditions.

Sites of action for OAF have been little studied but nucleic acids and coat proteins are identified targets for vegetative organisms. Spores tend to be resistant as are *Micrococcus radiodurans*, foot-and-mouth disease and swine vesicular disease viruses (Cox 1987). Resistance to OAF may prove to be an important feature for the long distance transmission of the viruses (see section 2, p. 339).

3.5 Radiation

Radiation effects tend to follow those observed for microbes in aqueous environments or exposed on surfaces but they are enhanced by dehydration and oxygen (see Chapter 7). Longer wavelength radiations (infrared, microwave) with relatively low energies are considered to be limited in their effect mainly to inducing heating and dehydration. Shorter wavelength radiations (γ-rays, x-rays, UV) are more energetic and induce free radical mediated reactions, thereby damaging nucleic acids, proteins, sugars, lipids and membranes, including production of thymine dimers, DNA-strand breaks, protein–DNA complexes and protein–protein cross-links, as well as fragmentation and polymerizing Maillard reactions (Cox 1987, 1991). A specific target is the cytoplasmic membrane because it contains respiratory porphyrins that absorb strongly in the UV. Another target is nucleic acid with resulting enhanced mutation frequency to an extent depending on degree of repair. Spores tend to be relatively radiation resistant, at least partly because of their specialized coat.

As the result of photoreactivation, exposure to non-damaging UV wavelengths can result in the repair of damage. Outdoors, observed viable fractions can decrease during the early part of the day, then increase later, possibly because the prevailing UV flux and wavelength changes from the damaging to the repair part of the spectrum (Lighthart and Stetzenbach 1994).

4 INFECTIVITY

Survival is a prerequisite to infectivity and all factors that affect survival influence infectivity, but other factors can modify infectivity itself (see Chapter 12).

4.1 Particle size and host susceptibility

The respiratory tract may be considered in terms of 3 regions:

1 upper respiratory tract of the nasopharynx, mouth or both
2 conducting passages of larynx, trachea and large bronchi
3 respiratory gaseous exchange area of bronchi, alveolar sacs and alveoli.

Infectivity depends markedly on inhaled particle size (Cox 1987) because survival is affected by the landing (deposition) site and the efficiency of retention. Particles of about 0.5 μm are least retained in the alveoli whereas below that size retention increases through diffusion processes; above 0.5 μm and up to c. 5 μm, inertial impaction predominates. Larger particles are increasingly impacted in the upper respiratory tract.

Inhaled particles that are hygroscopic increase in size on passing into the respiratory tract at c. 100% RH and 37°C as a result of condensation and water absorption, a process referred to as vapour phase re-

hydration, or rehumidification. Microbes may also be carried on skin squames or other larger particles and this also modifies the point of their deposition.

Macrophages, ciliary action and the mucociliary escalator prevent particles from remaining at that initial landing site. After inhalation, microbes deposited in the bronchioles are subjected to the clearance mechanisms of the mucociliary escalator and antimicrobial components of mucus (e.g. immunoglobulins, interferon, circulating antibodies). Finer particles deposited in the alveoli are subject to the action of leucocytes and alveolar macrophages. However, the effectiveness of host clearance processes can be reduced by tobacco smoke, air pollutants, hypothermia, barbiturates, hypoxia, alcohol, endotoxins, etc. (Cox 1987). The simultaneous presence of inert particles also impairs microbial clearance (Gilmour, Taylor and Wathes 1989). Consequently, there are 2 basic and opposing processes for organisms such as *K. pneumoniae*, i.e. the growth and clearance of deposited bacteria and the outcome for the host depends on their relative rates (Cox 1995b).

4.2 Virulence

Infection can result from the inhalation of one bacterium of *F. tularensis* or a larger number of anthrax spores. Such differences are attributed to bacterial virulence factors. In the case of *F. tularensis* it depends on whether a capsule is present. Few papers have been directly concerned with the infectivity and virulence of air-borne micro-organisms and these are reviewed by Cox (1987).

5 MECHANISMS OF AIR-BORNE VIABILITY LOSS

Recent books and review articles include Cox (1987, 1989, 1991, 1993, 1995a), Israeli, Gitelman and Lighthart (1994), Marthi (1994) and Hensel and Petzoldt (1995).

5.1 Dehydration and temperature

To account for viability decay curves, mathematical models have been developed and based on second order denaturation kinetics and probability or catastrophe theory (Cox 1987, 1989, 1995a). It is supposed that on desiccation an essential moiety B forms a dimer:

$$B + B \rightarrow 2B$$

with the dimer being inactive. When coupled with catastrophe theory to link concentrations of species B to percentage viability, the following equation can be derived (Cox 1987):

$$V/100 = \{(K[B]_0 / (1 + K[B]_0 \, kt)) - K[B]_{min}\}^{\frac{1}{2}}$$

where V is the viability (%) at time t, $K[B]_0$ is a constant, k is the second order denaturation constant and $K[B]_{min}$ is a constant that can be zero. Examples of

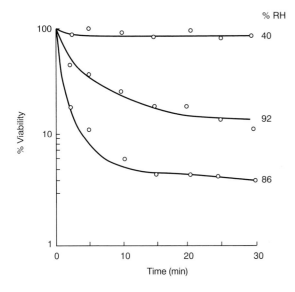

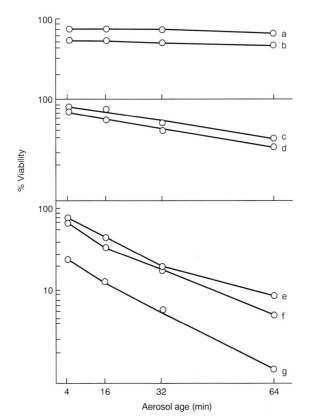

Fig. 14.7 Aerosol survival of *E. coli* Jepp sprayed from suspension in distilled water into nitrogen. Points are experimental data, lines calculated.

degree of fit to experimental data are given in Figs 14.7 and 14.8.

By fitting this equation to the data of Ehrlich and coworkers for decay curves obtained at different temperatures (e.g. Fig. 14.8), values for the constants

$K[B]_0$ and k (the second order denaturation constant) were derived as a function of temperature. On the basis of the Arrhenius equation,

$$k = A \exp - E/RT$$

where A is the frequency factor, E is the activation energy, R is the universal gas constant, T is the absolute temperature and k is the rate constant, a plot of their natural logarithms against the reciprocal of absolute temperature should give a straight line, the slope being related to the activation energy for the decay process.

Estimates of activation energies and optimum survival temperatures provide not only important indicators of possible underlying mechanisms but also clues to the nature of species B, if they exist. An example of this plot is given in Fig. 14.9 for wet disseminated *F. tularensis*. This demonstrates that the optimum survival temperature is c. +11°C. At higher temperatures the activation energy is positive (+43 kcal mol^{-1}), whereas below the optimum the activation energy is negative (−22 kcal mol^{-1}). Similar findings (see Cox 1987) apply to *Flavobacterium* (Fig. 14.10, optimum c. +8°C, +29 and −21 kcal mol^{-1}) and to VEE virus (optimum c. +24°C, +18 and 0 kcal mol^{-1}).

Consequently, 2 different mechanisms seem to cause desiccation damage, one occurring predominantly above the optimum temperature, the other predominantly below it. The former increases in rate with increasing temperature whereas the latter increases in rate with decreasing temperature.

Positive activation energies are lower than those associated with heat denaturation of proteins (c. 100 kcal mol^{-1}) and comparable to those for enzyme reactions and for non-enzymatic Maillard reactions (see section 5.3, p. 346) between amino groups and carbonyl groups.

Fig. 14.8 Effect of temperature on the aerosol survival of *Flavobacterium* sp. Points are experimental, lines are calculated for a second order denaturation process: a, − 18°C; b, − 40°C; c, 24°C; d, − 2°C; e, 29°C; f, 38°C; g, 49°C.

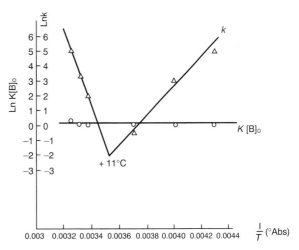

Fig. 14.9 Values of the constants derived by fitting catastrophe theory equation to wet disseminated *F. tularensis* viability–time curves as a function of reciprocal absolute air temperature.

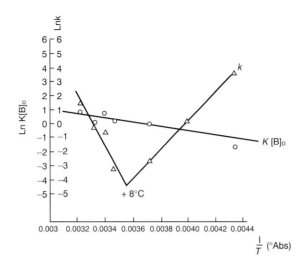

Fig. 14.10 As for Fig. 14.9 except for wet disseminated *Flavobacterium*.

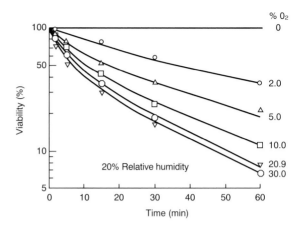

Fig. 14.11 Aerosol survival of *S. marcescens* 8UK sprayed from suspension in distilled water into nitrogen + oxygen mixtures at 25°C. Points are experimental data; lines calculated (see text).

5.2 Oxygen and OAF

As far as is known, data on effects on air-borne survival of oxygen concentration, RH and time are available in detail only for *S. marcescens* (Cox 1987). A model (see Cox 1987, 1989, 1995a) that fits these data well is based on an approach analogous to that for desiccation damage, i.e. a key moiety A, essential for viability, forms a series of hydrates that react with an oxidized carrier XO_2:

$$X + O_2 \leftrightarrow XO_2$$

without formation of ternary complex $A.XO_2$ to give AO_2 and free carrier X. Integration of the derived differential equations and use of probability theory to relate concentration of A to percentage viability leads to the following simplified equation:

$$\ln V\% = K[A]_0 \{\exp - (kt[X]_0[O_2]/(K_x + [O_2])) - 1\} + \ln 100$$

where V is the viability (%) at time t, $K[A]_0$ is a constant, k is the rate constant, $[X]_0$ is the concentration of carrier X, $[O_2]$ is the concentration of the oxygen environment and K_x is the equilibrium constant for the reaction between X and O_2.

Examples of experimental results and calculated lines are presented in Fig. 14.11. As discussed by Cox (1987), the species A, if it existed, would be expected to be inside the bacterial cell, unlike species B for purely desiccation damage which may be expected to reside on the outermost surface of the cell. The possibility of free radical involvement has been discussed by Cox (1987, 1989, 1991, 1995a).

A model for the action of OAF is similar except that the equilibrium reaction between carrier and OAF is established more slowly, thereby leading to a lag in onset of viability loss. Corresponding physical explanations are a slow condensation of OAF on to aerosol particles or an autocatalytic free radical mediated reaction mechanism, or both. Because of the ephemeral nature of OAF and its predicted relatively low con-

centrations (pphm) in the atmosphere, there are no known analytical techniques for the direct measurement of atmospheric OAF concentrations. Instead, its highly variable concentration is estimated from the rate of decay of viability of a hardy standardized *E. coli* strain. Measured decay curves for *E. coli* are compared with published calculated decay curves to give an arbitrary value for OAF concentration (approximately pphm) (Fig. 14.12). This technique is described in more detail by Cox (1987) and by de Mik (1976). It played a part in the 'identification' that OAF comprised, predominantly, reaction products of ozone and olefins derived in the main from unburnt hydrocarbon fuels.

5.3 Maillard reactions

As originally described by Louis-Carmille Maillard between 1912 and 1917, Maillard reactions are amino-carbonyl reactions of reducing sugars with amino groups of proteins. Their condensation with the elimination of a water molecule reversibly forms a Schiff base that can undergo slower Amadori rearrangements followed by numerous other rearrangements, fragmentations and subsequent reactions to give a wide range of products, e.g. reaction of glucose with a single amino acid gives rise to over 300 identified products. These non-enzymatic reactions can be of relatively low activation energy comparable to that of a strong H bond and are common (Cox 1991).

A typical Maillard reaction (analogous to the dimerization described above) is:

$$R_1-CHO + H_2N-R_2 \leftrightarrow R_1-HC=N-R_2 + H_2O \rightarrow$$
Free reactants   Schiff base

The Schiff base then undergoes slow Amadori rearrangement and subsequent reactions. The initial forward reaction involves the elimination of a water molecule and according to the law of mass action it will be accelerated by desiccation. Usually the rate of reaction is optimum in the RH range 60–80% with

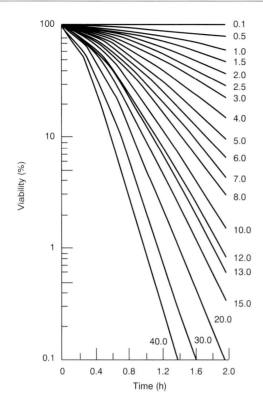

Fig. 14.12 Calculated percentage viability of *E. coli* commune as a function of OAF concentration and time (see text).

slowing below 60% attributed to decreased diffusion of products and reactants owing to increasing viscosity. Reactions with activation energies of c. +20 kcal mol^{-1} (see also section 5.1, p. 344) are generally characterized by being controlled by diffusion characteristics, whereas other properties described above for dehydrated gram-negative bacteria and for lipid-containing viruses are those frequently associated with Maillard reactions (Cox 1991). The Maillard reaction is referred to as the 'browning reaction' because of the colour of many of its products. A familiar example is the discoloration of apples after they have been cut. This colour also develops when a creamy paste of *E. coli* dries in a vacuum desiccator.

The protective action of raffinose is consistent with the conclusion that species B, if it exists, should be on the surface of gram-negative bacteria since raffinose and other substances protect under conditions in which they are confined to the outside of the cell wall (Cox 1987). Israeli, Gitelman and Lighthart (1994) reported a similar action for added trehalose. Raffinose, in common with many other sugars including trehalose and related compounds, rather than crystallizing forms an extremely viscous glass (supercooled liquid) on drying. Furthermore, since it is non-reducing it does not undergo Maillard reactions. Trehalose is similar but seems to have greater long-term stability, e.g. whereas other sugars hydrolyse slowly in the glass state, it does not. Consequently, compounds like raffinose and trehalose, through H bonding and the control of diffusion, are well suited for slowing Maillard

reactions of, for example, protein components (e.g. enzymes, Broadhead et al. 1994), associated with the membranes of gram-negative bacteria and lipid-containing viruses. In addition, such non-reducing sugars directly stabilize dehydrated phospholipid membranes and inhibit membrane fusion. The mechanisms probably involve hydrogen bond formation between sugar $-OH$ groups and phospholipid polar head groups, plus control of diffusion. The usual lesser effectiveness of reducing sugars (e.g. glucose) as stabilizers may be due to their high activity in Maillard reactions.

The rate of a chemical reaction depends on the speed at which reacting species move (or diffuse), which depends on the temperature and viscosity of the surrounding medium. At high viscosity, the speed of diffusion of reacting species is slowed, i.e. the rate of reaction becomes diffusion controlled. On dehydration, solutions of sugars like raffinose and trehalose form glasses of extremely high viscosity rather than crystallize. Rates of reactions (including Maillard reactions) in high viscosity media then are diffusion controlled, becoming much slower than those in low viscosity media such as water.

Vapour phase rehydration (rehumidification) after release of aerosols and before sampling could be effective, due partly to the reversibility of the initial stage of the Maillard reaction. For instance, the fragility on desiccation of the T3 phage head–tail complex, described above, could be through formation of a Schiff base cross-linking with relatively inflexible double bonds. In this state, head–tail complexes become sensitive to shearing on sampling with resulting loss of viability; however, on prior vapour phase rehydration, the Schiff base would convert back to free reactants, to release the double bond cross-links and so restore the original flexibility or strength of the head–tail complex, with preservation of viability. Many other similar phenomena are known to affect airborne microbes and Maillard reactions.

An overall conclusion about the survival of gram-negative bacteria (in the absence of oxygen), mycoplasmas and lipid-containing viruses, is that the lowest survival occurs at mid to high RH. Structurally, these microbes are similar in that they have outer lipid membranes of low inherent thermodynamic stability that are held together by weak non-covalent bonds, e.g. H and ionic bonds, van der Waals forces, hydrophobic interactions. Consequently, quite small perturbations can lead to drastic structural reorganizations, including membrane fusion, vesicle formation and altered membrane configurations, i.e. phases that can interconvert with small energy expenditure.

Toxicity to microbes of oxygen and other oxidizing agents (e.g. OAF) may also involve membranes and Maillard reactions. Phosphoglycerides when isolated are waxy materials that readily oxidize on exposure to air and darken through peroxidation in oxygen-dependent, free radical mediated Maillard reactions of phospholipids. These reactions have similar kinetics to viability loss, namely, a carrier mediated oxygen toxicity saturating at higher concentrations, and acceleration through desiccation (Cox 1991). A membrane site of action of oxygen is also considered likely, but on entirely different grounds (Israeli, Gitelman and Lighthart 1994). Hence, for gram-negative bacteria at higher temperatures there appears to be both an oxygen-independent and an oxygen-dependent mechanism of membrane damage as for synthetic Ca^{2+}-transporting phospholipid vesicles. It is possible that the former predominantly affects the outer membrane whereas the latter predominantly affects the cytoplasmic membrane. By contrast, at lower temperatures a different exothermic mechanism predominates.

5.4 Membrane phase changes

One exothermic reaction is a change of state (phase) from liquid to solid, thereby liberating heat of fusion. A change in the state of water is an unlikely cause of this in biological membranes as the optimum survival temperatures described above are c. +10°C. This observation is much more in keeping with phase changes in membrane phospholipids and their complexes. As described by Cox (1989, 1995a), optimum survival temperatures seem to match those for the gel $\leftrightarrow$ liquid crystal phase transitions of the predominant unsaturated fatty acid of the membranes, i.e. optimum survival temperature corresponds to a membrane of reduced fluidity. In turn, such low fluidity would be expected to reduce Maillard reactions by diffusion control, as it does for supersaturating non-reducing sugars such as trehalose and raffinose.

Membrane structures depend on water content as well as temperature because of their hydrophilic polar groups (Cox 1989, 1995a). Consequently, because of such complex membrane behaviour, findings reported above of comparatively narrow RH bands (see Fig. 14.3) in which gram-negative bacteria become particularly unstable, become less surprising. The involvement of membranes in the survival of desiccated microbes was discussed by Israeli, Gitelman and Lighthart (1994), Marthi (1994) and Hensel and Petzoldt (1995). Furthermore, Israeli, Gitelman and Lighthart (1994) indicated that for *E. coli*, trehalose stabilizes best under conditions when it saturates all the interphospholipid spaces. However, at least for liposomes, such beneficial action of trehalose involves both H bonding between sugar and polar head groups and the formation of a glass for diffusion control (Crowe, Leslie and Crowe 1994).

At least in model systems, membrane transitions tend to be reversible and of lower activation energy (e.g. <+10 kcal mol^{-1}) than the activation energies derived for desiccation-induced loss of viability (c. +30 kcal mol^{-1}). On the other hand, concomitant with loss of viability on desiccation is loss of permeability function and of the ability to generate energy (e.g. Cox 1987, 1989, 1995a), both being membrane functions. Such observations may be explained along the following lines. On dehydration of a gram-negative bacterium held at temperatures above c. +10°C, membranes undergo phase changes with rearrangement of

phospholipids and proteins, including perhaps the porin trimer proteins. These normally form water-filled pores required for the specific transport of water-soluble materials through hydrophobic membrane bilayers, and are stabilized in vivo by Maillard reactions. In the changed environment caused by desiccation and phase changes, newly juxtaposed proteins may undergo cross-linking Maillard reactions, resulting in loss of the permeability barrier function. Similarly, carbohydrates, other proteins and nucleic acids located in membranes and other cell regions may undergo Maillard reactions, accelerated by water loss and raised temperatures. Thus Maillard reactions are the rate-limiting steps in desiccation-induced loss of viability, and not membrane phase changes.

At temperatures less than c. +10°C, phospholipid gel $\leftrightarrow$ liquid crystal phase transitions are expected and, being exothermic, are accelerated by reduction in temperature. In addition to this change, on cooling some protein molecules may form subunits as do, e.g., chymotrypsin, cyctochrome *c*, myoglobin and lactate dehydrogenase. Such cryoinactivation subunit formation seems to be a general property of protein molecules and is followed by slow 'conformational drift' to conformationally different monomers. On warming, their reaggregation gives reassociated forms different from the original native states. A tentative estimate of the associated free energy change is −20 kcal mol^{-1} (Bowler and Fuller 1987) which is in keeping with that reported above for loss of viability at lower temperatures.

In summary, a primary cause of loss of viability of, for example, gram-negative bacteria at warmer temperatures, may arise at mid to high RH because of membrane phase changes coupled with concomitant rate-limiting and inactivating cross-linking Maillard reactions, e.g. association of proteins such as cross-linking of porin protein molecules. In contrast, at cooler temperatures, membrane phospholipid crystallization and dissociation of protein molecules into subunits followed by their conformational drift may result in biologically inactive forms on rehydration and warming. Consequently, there may be an optimum air-borne survival temperature possibly corresponding with the onset of a primary gel $\leftrightarrow$ liquid crystal transition leading to reduced membrane fluidity and diffusion control of potentially harmful Maillard cross-linking reactions of membrane proteins. The additional action of oxygen, oxidizing pollutants and radiation seems likely to exacerbate damage, possibly through the generation of additional free radicals, including hydroperoxide and hydroxyl, by reaction with phospholipids. Similar arguments seem likely to apply to other microbes.

6 REPAIR AND SUBLETHAL INJURY

Inflicted damage may or may not cause loss of viability, depending upon the extent and degree of repair. Sublethal injury may be thought of as damage that does not result necessarily in loss of viability but does lead to some impairment of function, e.g. causes bacteria to exhibit an extended lag phase through impaired permeability barrier function. Growth may not occur on a selective medium containing, for example, an antibiotic, but may still occur on a non-selective medium; this is a well recognized phenomenon with stressed bacteria. Other examples are the need to include catalase or pyruvate in growth media to remove traces of hydrogen peroxide that would inhibit the growth of sublethally injured bacteria but do not affect their unstressed counterparts.

The beneficial effects of rehumidification, or of a collecting fluid of 1 M sucrose described above, provide other examples of recovery from sublethal injury. The effect of sucrose may be due to osmotic factors as may the beneficial action of adding betaines to media described by Marthi (1994) and Hensel and Petzoldt (1995). On the other hand, they may represent stimulation of repair mechanisms. There are at least 2 types of repair process:

1 physicochemical, non-enzymatic
2 energy-dependent, enzyme-catalysed reactions.

Physicochemical repair includes vapour phase rehydration, e.g. restoration of flexibility and strength of phage head–tail bonding; induced membrane phase changes by, e.g. sucrose; water vapour or warming (annealing); and conversions of non-native Schiff bases back to native states through rehumidification, e.g. in vitro in artificial samplers and in vivo in animal respiratory systems (Cox 1995a).

Examples of enzyme-catalysed repair include excision of thymine dimers, repair of membranes and transport activity (Leopold 1986, Marthi 1994), repair of DNA strand breaks, or scission of desiccation-induced covalent DNA–protein cross-links (Dose et al. 1991, 1992). However, because of the fastidious nature of repair processes, microbes may appear non-viable under some growth conditions and viable under others (Andrews and Russell 1984, Mackey 1984, Cox 1987).

7 THE REPAIR PROBLEM

Repair can involve the action of enzymes and therefore requires energy; but, as indicated above, membranes and their associated energy-generating assemblages provide likely primary targets for desiccation and oxygen-induced damage because of their low inherent thermodynamic stability through non-covalent bondings. Consequently, desiccation may lead to loss of viability because of membrane damage, resulting in a lack of energy for repair enzymes to operate. Good correlations are observed between energy production, ATP levels and viability (Cox 1987). It is pertinent, too, in this context that many anhydrobiotic organisms synthesize quantities of trehalose that stabilizes polymers, including proteins and membranes, while also acting as an immediately available intracellular carbohydrate reserve. Anhydrobiotic organisms also maintain good reserves of energy-rich compounds such as ATP. This strategy for withstanding the traumas associated with desiccation seems to fit well with the findings presented above concerning mechanisms of viability loss caused by desiccation. In turn, they provide some understanding of why the strategy adopted by anhydrobiotic organisms works so well in nature.

8 CONTROL OF AIR-BORNE INFECTION

There are basically 4 approaches to controlling air-borne infection:

1 prevent dispersal
2 ventilation and filtration
3 inactivation by physical means, e.g. heat, radiation
4 inactivation by chemical means.

The varied nature of sources means that prevention of dispersal of microbes in many cases is impractical. In the laboratory and in industry, use of containment facilities can protect workers from infection, as described by Lidwell (1990), Hambleton, Melling and Salusbury (1994) and by Clark (1995). The main source of human infection by the air-borne route is other people but the strictest 'air space' isolation is impractical except for containing patients with the most hazardous of organisms. However, significant reductions in the air-borne bacterial load and the consequent risk of infection can be achieved with laminar flow systems used for surgery where air-borne infection is of particular concern, e.g. hip replacement, cardiac surgery and neurosurgery.

Patients known or suspected of being infected with highly pathogenic organisms, e.g. Lassa fever, may be nursed in protecting enclosures to prevent dispersal (source isolation). After use by an infected patient, contaminated rooms and equipment can be decontaminated with chemical and physical agents. However, for reducing the infection risk in public places and transport systems there is little alternative other than to utilize ventilation, thereby reducing air-borne concentrations of potentially pathogenic organisms by dilution. Currently, the costs to society of air-borne contagion are high and such procedures seem inadequate, especially when there are high rates of 'space occupancy' and ventilation rates are reduced to conserve energy. As pointed out by Burge (1995a), '...the efficacy of existing methods as well as the development of new methods of preventing exposure to bioaerosols needs investigation. These efforts will require multi-national and multi-disciplinary cooperation'.

REFERENCES

Akers TG, Hatch MT, 1968, Survival of a picornavirus and its infectious ribonucleic acid after aerosolisation, *Appl Microbiol*, 1811–13.

Andrew MHE, Russell AD (eds), 1984, *The Revival of Injured Microbes*, Academic Press, London.

Bolister NJ, Madelin TM, 1992, The influence of rehumidification and collection into fluids containing sucrose upon the viability of aerosolised *Klebsiella pneumoniae*, as determined using a novel rehumidification chamber, *J Aerosol Sci*, **23**, **Suppl. 1:** S539–42.

Bowler K, Fuller BJ (eds), 1987, *Temperature and Animal Cells. Symposia of the Society for Experimental Biology*, Number 41, The Company of Biologists Ltd, University of Cambridge, Cambridge.

Broadhead J, Rouen SK et al., 1994, The effect of process and formulation variables on the properties of spray-dried beta-galactosidase, *J Pharm Pharmacol*, **46:** 458–67.

Brosseau LA, Kuehn TH, Goyal SM, 1994, Investigate and identify means of controlling virus in indoor air by ventilation, filtration or source removal, *Final Report 776-RP*, American Society of Heating, Refrigeration and Air Conditioning Engineers, Inc., Atlanta, Georgia.

Burge HA, 1995a, Bioaerosols in the residential home, *Bioaerosols Handbook*, eds Cox CS, Wathes CM, CRC Press, Boca Raton, FL, 575–93.

Burge HA (ed.), 1995b, *Bioaerosols*, CRC Press, Boca Raton, FL.

Clark RP, 1995, Safety cabinets, fume cupboards and other containment systems, *Bioaerosols Handbook*, eds Cox CS, Wathes CM, CRC Press, Boca Raton, FL, 469–500.

Cox CS, 1987, *The Aerobiological Pathway of Microorganisms*, John Wiley & Sons, Chichester.

Cox CS, 1989, Airborne bacteria and viruses, *Sci Prog*, **73:** 469–500.

Cox CS, 1991, *Roles of Maillard Reactions in Diseases*, HMSO, London.

Cox CS, 1993, Roles of water molecules in bacteria and viruses, *Orig Life Evol Biosph*, **23:** 29–36.

Cox CS, 1995a, Stability of airborne microbes and allergens, *Bioaerosols Handbook*, eds Cox CS, Wathes CM, CRC Press, Boca Raton, FL, 69–92.

Cox CS, 1995b, Model of aerosol infectivity of *Klebsiella pneumoniae*, *Proceedings of the Scientific Conference on Chemical and Biological Defense Research, 15–18 November 1994*, ERDEC, Edgewood Area Conference Center, Aberdeen Proving Ground, MD.

Cox CS, Wathes CM (eds), 1995, *Bioaerosols Handbook*, CRC Press, Boca Raton, FL.

Crook B, Olenchock SA, 1995, Industrial workplaces, *Bioaerosols Handbook*, eds Cox CS, Wathes CM, CRC Press, Boca Raton, FL, 527–41.

Crowe JH, Leslie SB, Crowe LM, 1994, Is vitrification sufficient to preserve liposomes during freeze-drying?, *Cryobiology*, **31:** 355–66.

Dose K, Bieger-Dose A et al., 1991, DNA-strand breaks limit survival in extreme dryness, *Orig Life Evol Biosph*, **21:** 177–87.

Dose K, Bieger-Dose A et al., 1992, Survival in extreme dryness and DNA-single-strand breaks, *Adv Space Res*, **12:** 221–9.

Gilmour MI, Taylor FGR, Wathes CM, 1989, Pulmonary clearance of *Pasteurella haemolytica* and immune responses in mice following exposure to titanium dioxide, *Environ Res*, **50:** 184–94.

Hambleton P, Melling J, Salusbury TT, 1994, *Biosafety in Industrial Biotechnology*, Blackie Academic & Professional, Glasgow.

Harris JR, Horne RW (eds), 1986, *Electron Microscopy of Proteins. Volume 5. Viral Structure*, Academic Press, London.

Hensel A, the late Petzoldt K, 1995, Biological and biochemical analysis of bacteria and viruses, *Bioaerosols Handbook*, eds Cox CS, Wathes CM, CRC Press, Boca Raton, FL, 335–60.

Hess GE, 1965, Effects of oxygen on aerosolised *Serratia marcescens*, *Appl Microbiol*, **13:** 781–8.

Israeli E, Gitelman J, Lighthart B, 1994, Death mechanisms in microbial bioaerosols with special reference to the freeze-drying analogue, *Atmospheric Microbial Aerosols*, eds Lighthart B, Mohr AJ, Chapman & Hall, New York and London, 166–91.

Lacey J, Venette J, 1995, Outdoor sampling techniques, *Bioaerosols Handbook*, eds Cox CS, Wathes CM, CRC Press, Boca Raton, FL, 403–60.

Leopold AC (ed.), 1986, *Membranes, Metabolism and Dry Organisms*, Cornell University Press, Ithaca, NY.

Lidwell OM, 1990, The microbiology of air, *Topley & Wilson's Principles of Bacteriology, Virology and Immunity. Volume 1. General Bacteriology and Immunity*, 8th edn, eds Collier LH, Parker MT, Edward Arnold, London, 225–41.

Lighthart B, 1994, Dispersion models of microbial bioaerosols, *Atmospheric Microbial Aerosols*, eds Lighthart B, Mohr AJ, Chapman & Hall, New York and London, 285–303.

Lighthart B, Mohr AJ (eds), 1994, *Atmospheric Microbial Aerosols*, Chapman & Hall, New York and London.

Lighthart B, Stetzenbach LD, 1994, Distribution of microbial aerosol, *Atmospheric Microbial Aerosols*, eds Lighthart B, Mohr AJ, Chapman & Hall, New York and London, 68–98.

Macher JM, Stretfel AJ, Vesley D, 1995, Problem buildings, laboratories and hospitals, *Bioaerosols Handbook*, eds Cox CS, Wathes CM, CRC Press, Boca Raton, FL, 501–26.

Mackey BM, 1984, Lethal and sub-lethal effects of refrigeration, freezing and freeze-drying on microorganisms, *The Revival of Injured Microbes*, eds Andrew MHE, Russell AD, Academic Press, London.

Madelin TM, Madelin MF, 1995, Biological analysis of fungi and associated molds, *Bioaerosols Handbook*, eds Cox CS, Wathes CM, CRC Press, Boca Raton, FL, 357–82.

Marthi B, 1994, Resuscitation of microbial bioaerosols, *Atmospheric Microbial Aerosols*, eds Lighthart B, Mohr AJ, Chapman & Hall, New York and London, 192–225.

de Mik G, 1976, *The Open Air Factor*, PhD thesis, University of Utrecht, The Netherlands.

Salem H, Gardener DE, 1994, Health aspects of bioaerosols, *Atmospheric Microbial Aerosols*, eds Lighthart B, Mohr AJ, Chapman & Hall, New York and London, 304–30.

US Department HEW, 1982, *Current estimates from the National Health Interview Survey, 1981. Vital and Health Statistics*, US Department HEW, Washington, DC.

Wathes CM, 1995, Bioaerosols in animal houses, *Bioaerosols Handbook*, eds Cox CS, Wathes CM, CRC Press, Boca Raton, FL, 543–74.

Chapter 15

THE BACTERIOLOGY OF WATER

E E Geldreich

1 Characterizing the bacterial flora in the aquatic environment	5 Water quality criteria
2 Natural waters	6 Bacteriological analysis
3 Pathogenic bacteria in aquatic environments	7 Principles of pathogen detection
4 Natural self-purification factors	8 Strategies for rapid methods

Bacteriology of water continues to be an important component in defining the quality of public health. In recent years, expanding methodology has led to the discovery of additional pathogens as the cause of water-borne outbreaks. As a consequence of these new discoveries, the focus on water quality is being redirected towards better characterization of the microbial risks associated with this vital resource. It is important to note that although water is essential to sustain life, it can be a hostile environment to humans when grossly polluted.

1 CHARACTERIZING THE BACTERIAL FLORA IN THE AQUATIC ENVIRONMENT

The bacterial flora of water is a composite of organisms indigenous to high quality water or pristine waters plus all of the contributions from life's many controlled and uncontrolled uses or consumption of water.

1.1 Indigenous bacteria

These are naturally occurring bacteria found in waters that are remote from the activities of modern civilization. They are largely saprophytic organisms, some of which belong to the genera *Micrococcus, Pseudomonas, Serratia, Flavobacterium, Chromobacterium, Acinetobacter* and *Alcaligenes*. There are indigenous bacteria that are difficult to detect in routine laboratory techniques because of their slow growth or fastidiousness. In the past, these organisms received little attention but this attitude is changing because of problems with biofilm development in stream, ground water extraction, water pipe networks and industrial processes. An

additional threat is that some opportunistic pathogens such as *Legionella* may be ubiquitous in the water environment.

1.2 Contributed bacteria

Rainfall runoff is a major contributor to changes in the bacterial flora found in water. Whereas rain or snow falling over the watershed contains only occasional bacteria acquired from air-borne particles (Table 15.1), the microbial and chemical qualities of rain water drastically degrade upon contact with the soil (Geldreich et al. 1968). Various soil and faecal organisms are immediately accumulated into the drainage and merge as the bacterial flora. These organisms, though not normal inhabitants of high quality water, either adapt to the aquatic environment or die out over time because of various environmental adversities. Predominant among these soil and vegetation organisms are the aerobic spore-forming bacilli, such as *Bacillus subtilis, Bacillus megaterium* and *Bacillus mycoides*. Others, such as *Klebsiella pneumoniae, Enterobacter aerogenes* and *Enterobacter cloacae*, may be found growing in the water- and food-conducting tissue of trees (Knittel et al. 1977), on crops and other vegetation. By use of special media, a variety of other specialized bacterial groups can be isolated. In the bottom sediments of streams and lakes where oxygen is restricted, nitrate, sulphate-reducing and methanogenic bacteria can be detected and impart disagreeable earthy odours and tastes during summer periods of low stream flow.

The microbial flora of sewage is predominantly from faecal wastes including pathogens shed from individuals in the community. These would include species of *Salmonella, Shigella, Campylobacter, Yersinia, Leptospira, Streptococcus, Clostridium* and *Vibrio cholerae* and patho-

Table 15.1 Seasonal variations (median values) for bacterial discharges in rain water and storm water from suburban areas, Cincinnati, Ohio

Source	Period	Total samples	Season	Organisms per 100 ml			Ratios FC:FS	FC/TC × 100
				Total coliforms (TIC)	Faecal coliforms (FC)	Faecal streptococci (FS)		
Rain water	June 1965– February 1967	49	Spring	<1.0	<0.3	<1.0	–	–
			Summer	<1.0	<0.7	<1.0	–	–
			Autumn	<0.4	<0.4	<0.4	–	–
			Winter	<0.8	<0.5	<0.5	–	–
Wooded hillside	February 1962– December 1964	278	Spring	2400	190	940	0.20	7.9
			Summer	79 000	1900	27 000	0.70	2.4
			Autumn	180 000	430	13 000	0.30	0.2
			Winter	260	20	950	0.02	7.7
Street gutters	January 1962– January 1964	177	Spring	1400	230	3100	0.07	16.4
			Summer	90 000	6400	150 000	0.04	7.1
			Autumn	290 000	47 000	140 000	0.34	16.2
			Winter	1600	50	2200	0.02	3.1
Business district	April 1962– July 1966	294	Spring	22 000	2500	13 000	0.19	11.4
			Summer	172 000	13 000	51 000	0.26	7.6
			Autumn	190 000	40 000	56 000	0.71	21.6
			Winter	46 000	4300	28 000	0.15	9.4

Data from Geldreich et al. 1968.

genic types of *Escherichia coli*. Urban storm runoff, street flushings, automatic car washing operations and the processing of garden produce in markets, homes and restaurants contribute to the microbial flora.

Within the complex sewage flora contained in sewage sludge processes are organisms that are responsible for much of the biological breakdown of degradable waste products. Some of these beneficial organisms include the filamentous bacteria: *Sphaerotilus natans, Haliscomenobacter hydrossis, Nostocoida limicola, Microthrix parvicella, Flexibacter, Microscilla, Nocardia* (Eikelboom 1975) and the important floc-forming bacteria (*Zoogloea ramigera*), along with *Proteus* and the anaerobe *Clostridium sporogenes*.

Animal feedlot operations that require the confinement of cattle in small areas create a faecal waste removal problem equal to the domestic waste discharges of small cities (Geldreich 1972b). If the animal waste is not discharged to a lagoon or landfill, storm water runoff over the animal feedlots will bring massive loads of faecal pollution to the drainage basin. Poultry farm faecal wastes, perhaps with associated *Salmonella*, may contribute similar problems.

Beet, vegetable processing and sugar cane production have a drastic impact on the bacterial flora and the self-purification capacity of receiving waters. Elevated concentrations of nutrient wastes lead to oxygen depletion of the receiving waters plus an increase in environmental coliforms and faecal streptococci, particularly streptococci variants on biotypes (Mundt 1963, Mundt, Larsen and McCarty 1966). Most troubling is the extended persistence of *Salmonella* under these conditions (Geldreich 1972a).

Discharges of poorly treated paper mill waste to

receiving streams or lakes can also have a severe impact on the microbial quality of surface waters. The association of environmental *Klebsiella* with paper manufacturing and the excessive nutrients in paper mill waste cause a tremendous regrowth of this coliform in downstream waters. Environmental *Klebsiella* spp. colonize plants at flower pollination. As the seed germinates, *Klebsiella* spp. establish a coexistence with wood sugars (cyclitols) in the nutrient- and water-conducting tissues during the life of the tree (Seidler, Morrow and Bagley 1977). Another byproduct of paper processing is waste water sulphites which encourage the growth of biofilm mats of the nuisance organism *Sphaerotilus natans* along the shoreline of receiving streams.

Solid waste, generally referred to as garbage or rubbish, contains a multitude of items such as food discards, garden rubbish, manufactured products (paper, plastic, rubber, leather, textile, wool, metals, glass, ceramics), rock, dirt and ash residues and also faecal material (Table 15.2). Much of the faecal material in urban areas is derived from disposable nappies (diapers), pet litter material and faeces of rodents foraging for food in these waste collections (Geldreich 1978). Therefore, it is not surprising that solid wastes contain a large varied microbial population that includes a wide spectrum of bacteria (aerobes, anaerobes, thermophiles), actinomycetes and fungi (Cook, Cromwell and Wilson 1967). If properly disposed of through sanitary landfills, many of the problems (foraging wildlife, odours, unsightliness) common to open dumping are avoided; however, poor placement of landfill sites may result in the migration of leachates into nearby surface waters and ground water resources.

Table 15.2 Microbial characterization of solid wastes from various cities

Waste Collection site[b]	Number of samples	Organisms per g wet wt[a]			
		Total viable bacteria[c]	Spores	Total coliforms	Faecal coliforms
A	4	110 000 000	270 000	3 000 000	260 000
B	3	450 000 000	110 000	6 700 000	510 000
C	6	78 000 000	38 000	1 600 000	1 200 000
D	3	480 000 000	31 000	1 100 000	630 000
E	4	680 000 000	1 900 000	51 000 000	8 100 000
F	2	54 000 000	35 000	13 000 000	5 600 000
G	2	4 000 000	25 000	340 000	15 000
H	3	300 000 000	160 000	8 600 000	3 000 000

[a]Average moisture content was 41%.
[b]Waste collection sites in Cincinnati, Chicago, Memphis, Atlanta, and New Orleans.
[c]Spread plates (trypticase soy agar + blood) at 35°C for 48 h.
Data from Peterson ML (1971).

2 NATURAL WATERS

Natural waters occur either at or near the surface of the earth. Surface waters are frequently exposed to contamination from soil, storm water runoff, domestic sewage, agricultural and industrial wastes and decomposing organic matter. On the other hand, ground waters can be expected to be of excellent bacteriological quality due to the beneficial percolation into underground strata (aquifers). During downward passage to an aquifer, perhaps several hundred metres below the surface, most of the surface contaminants are entrapped in the soil or porous rock layers. One exception is a rock stratum composed of limestone which is very porous and often results in sink holes and caverns through which surface water passes without effective entrapment of contaminants. In other situations, excessive application of minimally treated surface waste waters may overwhelm the natural soil barrier (Kowal 1982). Once the aquifer becomes contaminated, restoration of water purity is very slow, even with accelerated intervention such as pumping the water to a treatment site and then returning it to the aquifer.

2.1 Surface waters

Natural water resources are replenished through rain, snow and hail. This atmospheric moisture comes in contact with particles of suspended dust and smog that immediately contaminate the moisture as it falls to the earth. The more dust encountered, the greater is the bacterial contamination. In remote areas away from the plumes of air pollutants, the total number of organisms may not exceed 10–20 l[-1]. Springtime dust storms originating in large farming areas may mix with atmospheric vapour to transport 1–2 total coliforms per litre of rain over great distances. Snow tends to be less pure than rain, probably because the snowflakes have greater surface area on which to collect suspended particles in the atmosphere, and also because their low temperature is conducive to the survival of bacteria. However, in snow on the tops of remote mountains, where the air is clean, very few organisms are present. Apparently hail contains more bacteria than either rain or snow. Hail examined from a storm over Padua during July, 1901 was found to contain 140 000 micro-organisms belonging to 9 different types (Belli 1902). This surprising finding was probably caused by air currents that cycle the raindrops through periods of freezing and thawing as they repeatedly traverse plumes of dust in the air before falling to the ground. The number of organisms in ice depends on the nature of the water from which the ice was formed. With the exception of ice from glaciers, it is generally impure. Various heterotrophic bacteria, including coliforms and pathogens, have been found in ice made with contaminated water.

In remote areas where human and farm animal populations are sparse, most organisms in water originate from soil with little evidence of contamination except for a few faecal coliforms (<100 organisms per 100 ml) originating from occasional wildlife inhabiting the immediate vicinity. Beaver and muskrats on the river banks, and significant concentrations of deer, elk and other game animals in grazing plains and forest reserves, are responsible for a residual level of faecal micro-organisms in water.

As these waters travel down a watershed, contact with agricultural and industrial activities increase and the river becomes laden with a variety of domestic and industrial wastes. As a consequence, rivers in most countries are heavily contaminated. Some measure of the potential occurrence of *Salmonella* in Hungarian ambient waters grouped at various average densities for several indicator groups is presented in Table 15.3. These data support the position that the greater the magnitude of faecal pollution, the greater the chance that some bacterial pathogens may also be present. Absence of any detectable faecal coliforms does not mean that there is no risk from *Giardia*, *Cryptosporidium* or a virus. These pathogenic agents frequently occur in small densities requiring the testing of larger volume samples. For this reason, a surrogate indicator examination at only one sample volume is not going to provide sufficient precision to ascertain the potential for extremely low density microbial occurrences.

Table 15.3   Indicator correlations with *Salmonella* occurrences in ambient waters*

Salmonella (%)	Clostridium	Faecal streptococcus	Faecal coliform	Total coliform
		←———————Densities per 100 ml———————→		
0	0	0	0	0
0	13	5	10	100
11	25	50	50	500
21	50	100	100	1000
33	125	300	1000	10 000
66	200	1500	5000	50 000
99	250	3000	10 000	100 000
100	2500	30 000	100 000	1 million
100	6250	250 000	850 000	2.5 million

*Data modified from Nemedi (1984).

In a study of surface water supplies used by 20 cities in the USA serving a total population of 7 million people, it was estimated that the minimum waste water component of the raw source water ranged from 2.3 to 16% and increased to predominantly waste water for several cities during low flow periods (Swayne, Boone and Baur 1980). This public health risk was verified by the finding of various serotypes of *Salmonella* at each water plant intake. Bacteriological examination of raw water quality at the water treatment plant intakes of Omaha, Nebraska, St Joseph, Missouri and Kansas City, Missouri on the Mississippi River (Table 15.4) frequently revealed faecal coliform densities in excess of 2000 organisms per 100 ml (Report 1971). This faecal pollution load resulted from inputs of raw sewage, effluents from primary and secondary waste water treatment plants of differing efficiencies, cattle feedlot runoff and discharges from meat and poultry processing plants. Faecal discharges entrapped on soil also entered the drainage basin by the flushing action of storm events. The major raw water quality concern is that human pathogens also may be present in surface waters.

Similarly high elevation lakes in remote portions of a watershed will contain high quality water (unless inhabited by flocks of aquatic birds) whereas those in the lower part of the watershed are fed with surface drainage from metropolitan areas and intense agricultural activity. For large lakes such as the North American Great Lakes, long retention time and vast volumes of water serve to buffer these magnificent water resources from the impact of storm water runoff. Unfortunately, pollution plumes around waste water discharges may spread to new areas by wind-driven currents. At greatest risk are the many small lakes surrounded by residential development that ultimately result in sporadic drainage from septic systems, and runoff from neighbourhood lawns.

Retention of surface water in lakes, impoundments and streams is an important contribution to water quality enhancement. Storage and sedimentation of surface water often improves the microbial quality. Many organisms are inactivated by natural self-purification processes whereas others are removed from the water through natural siltation (Romaninko 1971, Dzyuban 1975, Geldreich et al. 1980). These water quality improvements are variable and are directly proportional to retention time, dilution and the number of contributing sources (Geldreich 1990). In temperate zones with pronounced seasonal temperature changes, many lakes and impoundments are subject to periods of thermal stratification in the summer and winter and destratification (water turnover) periods in spring and autumn. During stratification, water movement in the deeper portion of raw water reservoirs becomes restricted, generally creating a zone of maximum bacterial contamination in the water layer above the thermocline (Weiss and Oglesby 1960, Collins 1963, Niewolak 1974, Drury and Gerheart 1975). With destratification, water from the bottom and top layers mix and develop a more uniform water quality. This mixing process causes decaying vegetation and entrapped organisms in settled particulates to re-enter the water (Weiss and Oglesby 1960, Niewolak 1987). Heterotrophic bacterial populations (including coliform bacteria), turbidity and humics from partially decomposed vegetation will temporarily increase in the water.

2.2   Ground waters

Ground water resources are the major source of water supply for many communities, farms and individual families world wide. In rural areas, many water supplies consist of dug wells less than 10 m deep. In these wells, source water is influenced by surface water runoff that percolates through the soil. Since there is no protective bedrock perched on top to seal off surface contaminants, water quality is erratic. Bore holes are often of better quality because casings are driven to depths of at least 30 m and soil depth does provide a barrier to much of the surface contamination. In general, public water supplies that use ground water attempt to reach productive aquifers at greater depths, often 300 m or more, to satisfy a greater water demand and reliable source of bacteriologically safe drinking water.

The quality of water flowing from springs depends

Table 15.4 Faecal coliform densities and pathogen occurrence at Missouri River public water supply intakes

Raw water intake	River mile	Date	Faecal coliforms (per 100 ml)[a]	Pathogen occurrence
Omaha, NB	626.2	7–18 Oct 1968	8300	NT
		20 Jan–2 Feb 1969	4900	NT
		8–12 Sep 1969	2000	*Salmonella enteritidis*
		9–14 Oct 1969	3500	*Salmonella anatum*
		3–7 Nov 1969	1950	NT
St. Joseph, MO	452.3	7–18 Oct 1968	6500	NT
		20 Jan–2 Feb 1969	2800	NT
		18–22 Sep 1969	4300	NT
		9–14 Oct 1969	NT	*Salmonella montevideo*
		22 Jan 1970	NT	19 virus PFU[b]
				Polio types 2, 3
				Eco types 7, 33
				3 virus PFU[b], not typed
Kansas City, MO	370.5	28 Oct–8 Nov 1968	6500	NT
		20 Jan–2 Feb 1969	8300	NT
		18–22 Sep 1969	3800	NT
				Salmonella newport
				Salmonella give
				Salmonella infantis
				Salmonella poona

[a]Geometric mean.
[b]PFU, plaque-forming units.
NT, No test for pathogens done.
Data from Report (1971).

mainly on their source and surroundings. Unfortunately, in many instances the source is unknown and could be under the influence of surface water, so quality may vary as a result of rainfall events and other activities on the watershed.

2.3 Cisterns

This source of water is generally rainfall from some catchment surface which often is a residential roof or paved hillside for water to drain down into a storage tank. Bacteriological quality is not only a reflection of rain water and dust particles but also of faecal contamination from birds perched on the catchment surface. Table 15.5 illustrates the varying densities of several indicator bacteria groups, the standard plate count and *Pseudomonas aeruginosa* that may be encountered in tropical cistern waters. In some areas of the world, cisterns have become a blend of rain water augmented by purchased water during the dry season.

2.4 Swimming pools and therapeutic baths

Swimming pools most often use treated municipal supplies for filling but the water may also be derived from thermal springs, mineral springs or ocean. Pool operation and construction materials (cement, plastic and redwood) have a definite effect on microbial growth (Castle 1985, Davis 1985) as does variability in water temperature in both indoor and outdoor pools (Schiemann 1985). Outdoor pools can be contaminated through storm water drainage, soil, vegetation debris and by pets and wildlife. Micro-organisms of major concern are those from the bather's body and mucosa and include those causing infections of the ear, eyes, upper respiratory tract, skin and intestinal tract (Favero and Drake 1966). Obviously the number of bathers is another serious contributor to the deterioration of water quality. Major microbial contributions are from saliva and sinus drainage as well as faecal contamination from the defaecation of infant bathers. Pool water disinfection can suppress many micro-organisms but effectiveness is limited by short contact time, disinfectant demand on bather body oils, particulates and sunlight exposure.

2.5 Bottled water

This water is generally an acceptable alternative drinking water supply. Bottled water sources are most often ground water or springs but in recent years reprocessed public water supply (carbon filtration, deionization or reverse osmosis) has also become available. Quality of the source water is dependent upon watershed protection, limited access to the area of extraction, and protected housing around well heads and spring outflows. Bottling operations follow prescribed sanitary codes for dispensing a food product and disposable plastic containers are commonly used to avoid possible contamination introduced from returnable glass bottles. As might be anticipated, microbial quality of freshly bottled water (within 48 h of bottling) is usually excellent. The rate of microbial change is related to a variety of factors including assimilable

Table 15.5 Microbial quality of cistern water, public housing, Virgin Islands[a]

Cistern site	No. samples	Range of counts per 100 ml			Range of counts per 1 ml	
		Total coliforms	Faecal coliform	Faecal streptococcus	Standard plate count[b]	*Pseudomonas aeruginosa*
1	9	<1–50	<1–3	<1–2	11–2400	<1–151
2	8	<1–340	<1–8	<1–160	10–5300	<1–72
3	8	<1–4	<1	<1–14	<1–14 000	<1–112
4	9	<1–11	<1–8	<1–640	2–12 000	<1–799
5	8	<1–100	<1–9	<1	6–2500	<1–1
6	6	<1–1	<1–1	<1	1–650	<1
7	10	<1–220	<1–27	<1–412	763–30 000	<1–91
8	5	<1–103	<1–20	<1–40	420–3000	<1–617
9	9	3–1700	3–570	<1–475	400–30 000	1–207
10	9	<1–29	<1–8	<1–972	210–4400	1–22

[a]Data adapted from Ruskin, Knudsen and Rinehart (1989).
[b]SPC agar spread plates, 35°C for 48 h.

organic nutrients in the water, organisms competing for dominance in the microbial flora, water pH and storage temperature. High quality bottled waters undergo a slow rate of change because growth of the indigenous organisms may take hours, not minutes, and the available nutrients are in trace amounts. Waters bottled from sources that have fluctuating water quality with an occasional coliform quickly deteriorate. These latter bottled waters are of concern because the general population of bacteria (heterotrophic bacteria) may have increased to densities that mask the laboratory's ability to detect faecal pollution and pathogens that might be present. Table 15.6 illustrates the variability in bacterial density and frequency of coliform-positive samples among bottled waters of unknown age purchased from retail outlets.

Although reported disease outbreaks due to contaminated bottled water are rare, the lack of documentation does not lessen the concern posed by use of this alternative. Any contaminated bottled water supply presents a unique hazard because of the widespread distribution of the product that is not necessarily confined to a single community. In April to November 1974, Portugal had a cholera epidemic that caused 2467 confirmed cases and 48 deaths (Blake et al. 1977). Most of the country was affected and the source of the infections was traced to the consumption of a brand of commercially bottled water as well as poorly cooked shellfish. The source water may have become contaminated from cholera-infected individuals living on the watershed or involved in the bottling operation. This outbreak clearly illustrates the importance of watershed protection for ground waters and springs.

2.6 Estuarine areas

These are the areas where fresh water mixes with the salt water environment either through direct discharge to the sea or by tidal flooding of fresh water pools near the ocean. Water quality protection and enhancement of estuarine waters are particularly important for shellfish cultivation. Release of wastes to shellfish growing waters bring a variety of organisms to the water, some of which may remain in suspension for varying periods before becoming entrapped in water turbidity. Most of the organisms reaching the area are either in aggregates or adsorbed to faecal cell debris and quickly accumulate in the bottom sediments, aided by the settling action of recirculating bottom silts. This natural deposition process concentrates much of the contaminants at the water–sediment interface where hard and soft shell clams browse for food. For these reasons, it is essential that shellfish harvesting areas be given a degree of protection from pollution that almost parallels the requirements for drinking water supplies. A zero tolerance for faecal pollution is not achievable in most shellfish growing waters, but there needs to be a maximum permissible contaminant level established for harvesting shellfish to ensure a minimal health risk from raw food consumption.

2.7 Coastal waters

Coastal marine waters receive much attention because of their use as recreational bathing waters, fishing resource and as disposal zones for rubbish dumping. Major sources of pollution are storm water runoff along the beach areas, release of sewage off shore, sanitary wastes from ships in harbour and improper disposal of rubbish outside designated ocean dumping areas. In the sea, off heavily polluted bathing beaches, the coliform content may rise to 200 000 or more per 100 ml and salmonellae are frequently present (Report 1959). Organic enrichment of the sea by pollution enhances the activities of sulphate-reducing bacteria in sediments near the water interface and methanogenesis in the sediments below. After discharge from a sewage outfall, faecal and enteric bacteria rapidly disperse if there is good diffuser design and high tidal energy. At Sidmouth, Devon, which has an outfall discharging 460 m from the high water mark, the median coliform count at the shore near

Table 15.6 Comparison of standard plate-count variability among brands of bottled water

Brand	Sample type[a]	No. of samples	Count range[b] (SPC ml^{-1})	Coliform positive samples[c]
A	Fresh	91	<10–25 000	3/91
	Retail	16	<10–28 000	0/16
B	Retail	6	<10–260 000	0/4
C	Fresh	1	<10	0/1
	Retail	11	1200–160 000	0/11
D	Retail	5	31–650	0/5
E	Fresh	1	<10	0/1
	Retail	2	10 000–390 000	2/2
F	Retail	2	<10–12 000	0/2
G	Fresh	2	<10	0/2
	Retail	1	<10	0/1
H	Retail	9	<10–390	1/9
I	Retail	2	<10	0/2
J	Retail	2	<10–2000	1/2
K	Retail	2	<10–12	1/2
L	Retail	4	13–4300	0/4
M	Retail	1	<10	0/1
N	Retail	1	<10	0/1
O	Retail	1	1×10^6	1/1
P	Retail	1	8600	0/1
Q	Retail	1	<10	0/1
R[d]	Retail	1	<10	0/1
R[d]	Retail	1	12	0/1

[a]Fresh, samples direct from bottler, examined within 24 h; Retail, samples of unknown age purchased from retail outlets.
[b]Standard plate count (SPC) range values represent average count of bacteria per ml calculated from 5 replicate plates incubated for 72 h at 35°C using plate-count agar.
[c]One or more coliforms per 100 ml.
[d]Imported bottled water, carbonated.
Data from Geldreich et al. (1975).

the outfall was 73 organisms per 100 ml in 1965, equivalent to dilution of the sewage by a factor of 400 000 (Gameson, Bufton and Gould 1967). Fresh seawater brings about a fairly rapid decline in faecal bacteria, salmonellae and viruses. The main inactivating agent is solar radiation at wavelengths less than 400 nm (Gameson and Saxon 1967, Gameson and Gould 1975, Chamberlin and Mitchell 1978, Fujioka et al. 1981).

3 PATHOGENIC BACTERIA IN AQUATIC ENVIRONMENTS

Numerous pathogenic agents have been isolated from ambient waters used for water supply, recreational bathing and irrigation of garden salad crops (Geldreich and Bordner 1971, Geldreich 1972a, Rosenberg et al. 1976, Cordano and Vergilio 1990, Rose 1990). The list of water-borne pathogens in polluted temperate and tropical drinking waters (Table 15.7) includes many of the same bacterial and viral agents but differs by the involvement of parasitic life cycles in many tropical waters. This list of water-borne agents will increase as new methodologies evolve to detect the more elusive organisms that cause gastroenteritis or other human illnesses.

The degree and frequency of pathogen reservoirs in the environment is exacerbated by expanding human populations world wide. Population crowding and the unregulated development of satellite communities places undue pressures on sanitation infrastructural barriers (sewage collection and treatment, solid waste disposal, potable water supply processing and its distribution). Add to these problems the mobility of people throughout the world and it becomes apparent that an outbreak can quickly reach epidemic proportions.

3.1 Pathogen pathways

Although sewage collection systems have decreased public health risk in urban centres, this practice only serves to transport the collected wastes to some selected destination, hopefully, where treatment is applied prior to release into a watercourse. Raw sewage discharges to receiving waters have often been shown to contain a variety of pathogens. The density and variety of human pathogens released is related to the population served by the sewage collection system, seasonal patterns for certain diseases and the extent of community infections at a given time. Some indication of the relative occurrences of various pathogens in raw

Table 15.7   Major infectious agents found in contaminated drinking waters world wide[a]

Bacteria	Viruses	Protozoa	Helminths
Campylobacter jejuni	Adenovirus (31 types)	*Balantidium coli*	*Ancylostoma duodenale*
Enteropathogenic *E. coli*	Enteroviruses (71 types)	*Entamoeba histolytica*	*Ascaris lumbricoides*
Salmonella (1700 spp.)	Hepatitis A	*Giardia lamblia*	*Echinococcus granulosus*
Shigella (4 spp.)	Norwalk agent	*Cryptosporidium*	*Necator americanus*
Vibrio cholerae	Reovirus		*Strongyloides stercoralis*
Yersinia enterocolitica	Rotavirus		*Taenia solium*
	Coxsackie virus		*Trichuris trichiura*

[a]Data from Geldreich (1990).

sewage is given in Table 15.8 for 2 cities in South Africa (Grabow and Nupen 1972).

In major river systems receiving discharges of meat processing wastes, raw sewage and effluents from ineffective sewage treatment plants, the densities of *Salmonella* spp. may be substantial. It has been calculated that the Rhine and Meuse rivers carry approximately 50 million and 7 million *Salmonella* bacilli per second, respectively (Kampelmacher and Van Noorle Jansen 1973). The Missouri River represents another example of a pollution conduit, transporting a faecal pollution load from raw sewage, effluents from primary and secondary treatment plants of differing efficiencies, runoff from numerous cattle feedlots and waste discharges from meat and poultry processing plants. As a consequence, it is not surprising that various *Salmonella* serotypes and viruses have been detected at the public water supply treatment plant intakes (see Table 15.4, p. 355).

Cattle feedlots and poultry operations result in an unusual concentration of farm animals and their faecal wastes in a confined space. In cattle feedlot operations, the density of beef cattle per square mile may approach 10 000 animals. Under such restrictions, removal of faecal wastes is a major disposal operation. The closeness of farm animals in confined feed-

ing operations invites the spread of disease in a healthy herd or poultry flock. Some farm animal pathogens (*Salmonella*, *E. coli* O157:H7, *Giardia* and *Cryptosporidium*) are also major human pathogens. Unless careful application of treated animal manures is practised, faecal material in storm water runoff from feedlots and poultry farms becomes a major source of contamination in rural watersheds, polluting streams and lakes in its drainage path. Recycling untreated farm animal wastes by application to fields may become an intensive contributor of pathogens to streams unless contour cultivation is undertaken to reduce runoff.

Wildlife refuges are also a significant source of faecal contamination, often on a seasonal basis, since many of these animals migrate seasonally in their search for food. The largest threat to wildlife pathogens is from those warm-blooded animals such as beaver, deer, coyote, pigeons and seagulls that are permanent residents of a watershed. These animals and others serve as reservoirs for *Salmonella*, *Campylobacter*, *Yersinia*, *Giardia* and *Cryptosporidium*. Wildlife is also attracted to protected watershed areas (forest reserves, private lands) where human activities are more restricted (Water and Bottam 1967). Protected nearshore water environments are often the location of large

Table 15.8   Microbial densities in municipal raw sewage from 2 cities in South Africa

Organism or microbial group	Average count per 100 ml	
	Worcester sewage	Pietermaritzburg sewage
Aerobic plate count (37°C, 48 h)	1 110 000 000	1 370 000 000
Total coliforms	10 000 000	–
E. coli, type 1	930 000	1 470 000
Faecal streptococci	2 080 000	–
C. perfringens	89 000	–
Staphylococci (coagulase-positive)	41 400	28 100
P. aeruginosa	800 000	400 000
Salmonella	31	32
Acid-fast bacteria	410	530
Ascaris ova	16	12
Taenia ova	2	9
Trichuris ova	2	1
Enteroviruses and reoviruses (TCID50)[a]	2890	9500

[a]TCID, Tissue culture infective dose.
Source: Grabow and Nupen (1972).

beaver colonies, including individual animals infected with *Giardia*. Infected coyotes, muskrats and voles are other wild animals that may be involved in the shedding of *Giardia* cysts and other pathogens into the aquatic environment. Terrestrial birds and waterfowl can be sources of bacterial pathogens. Songbird populations include individuals that may be infected with *Salmonella*. Seagulls are scavengers that frequent open rubbish dumps, eat contaminated food wastes, and contribute *Salmonella* in their faecal droppings to coastal lakes (Alter 1954, Fennel, James and Morris 1974). In one instance, seagulls were the contributors of *Salmonella* to an untreated surface supply in an Alaskan community, causing several cases of salmonellosis (Anonymous 1954). Pigeons colonizing 2 water storage towers in Gideon, Missouri, were considered the source of *Salmonella typhimurium* that contaminated the water supply, causing 600 illnesses and 4 deaths (Clark et al. 1996). Wildlife is also believed to be the source of *Campylobacter* that contaminated untreated or poorly treated streams and reservoirs of low turbidity in Vermont (Vogt et al. 1982) and British Columbia (Report 1981). Vacationers to national parks in Wyoming became ill after drinking water from mountain streams, resulting in a 25% increase state wide in *Campylobacter* enteritis (Taylor, McDermott and Little 1983).

3.2 Pathogen persistence

Upon discharge into the aquatic environment, the persistence of pathogens becomes a variable determined by many factors. For example, *Salmonella* strains were detected with regularity in surface water up to 250 m downstream from a waste water treatment plant but never at sample sites 1.5–4 km upstream (Kampelmacher and Van Noorle Jansen 1976). Various *Salmonella* serotypes transported by storm water through a residential storm sewer and a wash water drain at the University of Wisconsin experiment farm were isolated with regularity at a swimming beach approximately 800 m downstream (Claudon et al. 1971). Salmonellae were also detected in coastal waters from several Staten Island beaches and from shellfish harvested in New York harbour (Brezenski and Russomanno 1969).

Excessive BOD (biochemical oxygen demand) or TOC (total organic carbon) in a poor quality waste water effluent combined with low stream temperatures can also affect pathogen persistence. For example, *Salmonella* were isolated in the Red River of the North (North Dakota, Minnesota), 35 km downstream of sewage discharges from Fargo, North Dakota, and Moorhead, Minnesota, during September (Report 1965, Spino 1966). By November, *Salmonella* strains were found 99 km downstream of these 2 sites. In January, with the beginning of the sugar beet processing season, wastes reaching the stream under cover of ice brought high levels of bacterial nutrients. *Salmonella* were then detected 117 km downstream – a flow time of 4 days from the nearest point source discharges of warm-blooded animal pollution.

4 NATURAL SELF-PURIFICATION FACTORS

Natural waters provide a fragile purification buffer from limited amounts of raw wastes and storm water runoff entering the drainage basin. Every stream, lake, estuary and water aquifer has some limited capacity to self-purify; surface waters generally have greater capacity than ground waters. Stream self-purification is a complex and ill-defined process that involves bacterial adsorption with sedimentation, nutrients, predation, competitive microbial populations, dilution, aeration, water temperature, water pH and solar radiation (Geldreich 1986).

5 WATER QUALITY CRITERIA

Bacterial criteria for determining water quality have been directed primarily towards concern for microbial hazards to human health although some thought has been given to health hazards to farm animals, aqua cultures of fish stocks, shellfish and turtles (Report 1968, 1985). Indicators of faecal pollution have long been the predominant microbiological tool used to define the microbial quality of a water supply. However, there is growing evidence that water may not only transport intestinal pathogens via ingestion but also respiratory agents by inhalation and skin diseases through body contact. Thus the microbial risks in water quality may require not only traditional criteria (heterotrophic bacteria, total coliforms, faecal coliforms, *E. coli*, faecal streptococcus, enterococcus), but also special surrogates such as *Clostridium* or bacteriophages and species-specific pathogens, to evaluate status related to water use.

6 BACTERIOLOGICAL ANALYSIS

Standard methods for the analysis of a variety of waters are described in specific detail by the World Health Organization (Report 1984, 1992a), American Public Health Association (Report 1992b) and United Kingdom Report on Public Health and Medical Subjects (Report 1994) among other national documents world wide. These methods relate to drinking water, recreational waters, swimming pool waters, shellfish-growing waters, waste water discharges, recharge waters to aquifers and other re-use applications.

For monitoring purposes these indicators and various bacterial pathogens are detected by methods based on 3 principal procedures: pour or spread plates, selective cultivation in broth (multiple tube tests) and membrane filter techniques. More specific identification of selected heterotrophic organisms may be done by speciation of culture isolates.

Sample integrity is essential. Care must be exercised to collect samples representative of the water to be tested and to ensure that the sample does not become contaminated at the time of collection or before examination. Samples should be refrigerated or placed on ice and promptly transported to the laboratory. Sample transit time limits for total coliform analysis of drinking water have been established at 24 h only because these samples are free of the antagonistic factors found in polluted natural waters.

6.1 Heterotrophic plate count

Since the beginnings of bacteriology, the heterotrophic plate count has been used in an attempt to characterize water quality. Obviously, an excellent water was thought to have few bacteria per ml whereas water with more than 1000 bacteria was considered of poor quality. In time it was concluded that the general density of bacteria in water often had little specific relationship to organisms of sanitary significance and should be replaced by a search for organisms more specific to faecal contamination.

There has been a resurgence in the use of heterotrophic plate counts in the water supply to identify changes in the microbial quality of distribution water caused by accumulating pipe line sediments and subsequent loss of a protective disinfection residue. Most often these organisms are not of immediate public health significance but upon amplification in a protected pipe habitat become the source of customer complaints or emerge as an opportunistic pathogen threat to some segment of the population.

Traditionally, most water plant laboratories have been using standard plate count (SPC) agar or equivalent formulations for years and can produce an extensive database on heterotrophic bacterial densities in various water treatment processes. This approach to cultivation is beginning to be reconsidered in favour of a dilute nutrient medium such as R-2A agar which contains a diverse variety of biodegradable materials (peptone, casamino acids, glucose, soluble starch and sodium pyruvate). Colony densities are many times greater and a more diverse variety of organisms, including pigmented bacteria, are recovered (Reasoner and Geldreich 1985). To achieve this improvement, incubation for 5–7 days at a temperature of 28°C is preferred rather than the more conventional time of 48 h at 35°C. This change in cultivation provides more opportunities for the growth of slow-generating bacteria, stressed organisms and those species that have unique nutrient requirements.

Since pour plates limit the growth of obligate aerobes in agar and introduce the risk of heat shock from melted agar (Klein and Wu 1974), attention has turned to surface cultivation of bacteria by spread plate.

The membrane filter procedure provides another approach to surface cultivation of organisms. The unique advantage of this technique is that it permits the analysis of larger sample volumes of high quality water containing too few organisms to be detected by a 1 ml sample. The only restrictions to the size of sample analysed are turbidity and colony growth on the filter surface.

Some indication of the impact of membrane filter surface cultivation in comparison with pour plates and spread plates can be seen in Table 15.9. Recovery densities are significantly better on spread plates than by the traditional pour plate method because of agar temperature (Stapert, Sokolski and Northam 1962). Limited surface area on the membrane filter for discrete colony formation without developing confluence with the other colonies thereby restricts extended incubation time and is the major drawback for achieving results equivalent to the spread plate technique.

6.2 Total coliform bacteria

In an effort to obtain a better focus on the sanitary quality of water, coliform bacteria soon supplanted the heterotrophic plate count as the most widely used indicator for routine analysis. Coliform bacteria consist of an artificial grouping of organisms believed to be associated with faecal pollution but in reality may also include environmental organisms from soil, vegetation and decaying organic matter (Randall 1956, Geldreich et al. 1962, Schubert and Mann 1968). In the aquatic environment, environmental coliforms persist longer than do *E. coli*, the coliform constantly present in large numbers in faeces from humans and other warm-blooded animals (wildlife, farm animals, cats and dogs). Major members of these environmental coliforms include *Klebsiella*, *Enterobacter* and *Citrobacter*. Although not perfect, the coliform concept has been a practical tool for providing basic microbial information on water quality.

6.3 Faecal coliforms

Interest in further refining the total coliform group to exclude environmental coliforms, which are of no sanitary significance, led to the development of the faecal coliform (thermotolerant coliform) test based on lactose fermentation within 24 h at 44–44.5°C. The faecal coliform test proved to be a breakthrough with positive correlations of 93–99% to coliforms found in the faeces of warm-blooded animals (Geldreich 1966).

In polluted waters, faecal coliform measurements relate more precisely to faecal contamination than total coliforms and are significantly less susceptible to distortions caused by the regrowth characteristics of environmental strains in receiving waters. Essential factors that stimulate bacterial regrowth in polluted waters are nitrogen, carbon and a warm water temperature (above 15°C). The regrowth phenomenon for faecal coliforms requires excessive nutrient discharges generally associated with poor treatment practices, particularly those used on some food processing and paper mill wastes.

Confusion on the status of faecal *Klebsiella* and growth of the environmental component in the aquatic environment has led to attempts to search only for *E. coli*. Commercial biochemical kits for the identification of *E. coli* by detection of 4-methylumbelliferyl-β-D-glucuronidase (MUG) in either an amended medium or a chemically defined medium are now being used to further narrow the coliform group to one specific faecal organism.

Table 15.9 Effect of incubation temperature and time to recover heterotrophic bacteria from water supply samples by different methods[a]

Temp.	Medium	Method	Incubation time (days)			
			2	4	6	7
20°C	SPC-PP	Pour plate	22	130	570	900
	R2A-SP	Spread plate	90	1100	4700	6100
	R2A-MF	Membrane filter	75	650	3000	4900
	M-HPC-MF	Membrane filter	48	400	1600	2000
28°C	SPC-PP	Pour plate	90	640	950	1000
	R2A-SP	Spread plate	360	2800	6700	7200
	R2A-MF	Membrane filter	160	2200	3500	4000
	M-HPC-MF	Membrane filter	140	1000	1700	1900
35°C	SPC-PP	Pour plate	22	100	110	115
	R2A-SP	Spread plate	200	340	500	510
	R2A-MF	Membrane filter	41	200	270	280
	M-HPC-MF	Membrane filter	32	140	150	150

[a]Data revised from Reasoner (1990).

VERIFICATION OF COLIFORM BACTERIA

Verification of every positive coliform result is good laboratory practice that eliminates all doubts that the test results are perhaps caused by some analogous false reaction. Coliform analysis of drinking waters have revealed that as much as 30% of the samples having positive presumptive test results may also contain *Aeromonas* (Ptak, Ginsburg and Willey 1974, Leclerc et al. 1977). A few *Aeromonas* strains have been the cause of water-borne gastroenteritis (Moyer 1989), but most are saprophytic organisms in the aquatic environment. This situation illustrates the reason test results must be confirmed to eliminate false positive results in all methods even though this delay partly nullifies the rapidity of the results.

Rapid verification of coliform bacteria can be achieved in the demonstration of cytochrome oxidase and β-galactosidase activity. All coliform bacteria are positive for cytochrome oxidase while the enzyme β-glucuronidase appears to be highly specific for *E. coli*. This latter metabolic response has formed the basis of a rapid confirmatory test using the 4-nitrophenyl-β-D-glucuronide (Perez, Berrocal and Berrocal 1986) or 4-methylumbelliferyl-β-D-glucuronide (Report 1992b).

Coliform speciation is a more in-depth verification process that has been used to demonstrate the equivalence of methods to detect all coliforms. Speciation as a verification tool has its greatest use in the identification of a coliform biofilm event and in further confirmation of the existence of a microbial problem in the water supply. In either case, further exploration of the original sample may provide information on faecal contamination that might not be present in a repeat sample collected the next day. Most often, repeat samples are negative because the contaminating event is of short duration (Geldreich 1996).

6.4 Faecal streptococci

The occurrence of faecal streptococci in water generally indicates faecal pollution (Geldreich and Kenner 1969). Although faecal streptococci rarely multiply in polluted waters, they may persist for extended periods in irrigation waters with high electrolyte contents and favourable temperatures (Geldreich 1973). There is also some evidence that *Streptococcus faecalis* multiplies in water from vegetable processing plants (Mundt, Anandam and McCarty 1966). The reason for such contrasting responses is that the faecal streptococcus group includes a wide spectrum of strains that have specific faecal origins and diverse survival rates and includes several environmental biotypes (Mundt, Coggin and Johnson 1962, Mundt and Graham 1968). Within the faecal streptococcus group, *Streptococcus bovis* and *Streptococcus equinus* are specific indicators of farm animal pollution. This differential characteristic is particularly useful in pollution investigations involving cattle feedlot runoff, farm land drainage, discharge from meat and poultry processing operations and dairy plant wastes (Geldreich 1972b). In addition, *S. bovis* and *S. equinus* are the faecal streptococci that die off most rapidly outside the animal intestinal tract. Therefore, the detection of these strains in water indicates very recent farm animal contamination. By contrast, the ubiquitous *S. faecalis* var. *liquifaciens* may affect precision of this indicator system at counts below 100 faecal streptococci per 100 ml, because at these low population levels this biotype generally predominates. Faecal streptococcus counts greater than 100 per 100 ml, however, indicate significant faecal pollution derived from some warm-blooded animal source. The densities for this indicator group in polluted waters approach the magnitude observed for coliforms, or at times exceed it by a factor of 10, depending upon the source of faecal pollution.

The density difference between faecal coliforms and faecal streptococci in faecal material is a unique relationship that can be useful in defining sources of pollution. The ratio of faecal coliform to faecal streptococcus in human faeces and domestic wastes is greater than 4.0. The ratio of faecal coliforms to faecal streptococci in the faeces of farm animals, cats, dogs and rodents is less than 0.7. Such relationships between faecal coliform and faecal streptococci can only be developed from a faecal coliform medium (not an *E. coli* test) and from a faecal streptococcus medium such as KF agar or Pfizer Selective *Enterococcus* (PSE) agar (not from a medium dedicated to enterococcus).

Faecal streptococci are distinguished by their ability to grow at 45°C in the presence of 40% bile, and in the concentrations of sodium azide or potassium tellurite that are inhibitory to most coliform organisms. Methods are available using agar pour plates (KF agar, PSE agar), multiple tube (azide dextrose broth) and membrane filter (KF agar). If cultivation of the more restrictive enterococcus subgroup is desired, mE agar or m-enterococcus agar may be used.

6.5 *Clostridium perfringens*

The genus *Clostridium*, in particular *C. perfringens*, merits some attention as an indicator of faecal pollution because of its significant occurrence in faeces (Bishop and Allcock 1960). *Clostridium* spp. spores are resistant to waste water treatment practices, extremes in temperature and environmental stress. *C. perfringens* is an indicator of present faecal contamination as well as a conservative tracer of past faecal pollution (Wilson and Blair 1925). *C. perfringens* has been used in the UK to monitor the quality of ground water supplies that are examined infrequently at intervals of 4–6 months (Wilson 1931). When *C. perfringens* is found in these well waters, sampling is repeated, possibly weekly, using total coliform or faecal coli measurements to verify a faecal contamination problem and to demonstrate the need for appropriate corrective measures around the well head. The use of *C. perfringens* as a supplemental indicator to measure the efficiency of various water treatment processes has been proposed but the greater abundance of total aerobic spore formers in raw water may be a more effective system in providing evidence of treatment barrier performance (Rice et al. 1996).

The longer persistence of *C. perfringens* in the water environment creates a residual density of this organism which can obscure the detection of low densities of recent polluting discharges to receiving waters. However, Bonde reported that *C. perfringens* densities in the sediment of marine waters were proportional to pollution discharges and the ratios of spores to vegetative cells of this bacterial species increased with distance from the pollution source (Bonde 1962, 1967, 1968). Thus, vegetative cells of *C. perfringens* may be expected to predominate in raw sewage.

Although *C. perfringens* is an anaerobic organism, it can tolerate up to 5% oxygen without significant loss in quantitative recovery (Fulton and Richardson 1971). Therefore, methodology has not been complicated by the restrictions of complete anaerobiosis. On sulphite–alum agar (to reduce available oxygen) incubated at 48°C, 79–100% of the black sulphite-reducing colonies recovered from a variety of waters were verified as *C. perfringens* (Bonde 1962). The other black colonies on this medium may be *Salmonella*, *Proteus*, *Bacteroides* and sometimes *E. coli* (Johnston et al. 1964). This practical procedure has frequently been used to obtain a presumptive quantitation of *C. perfringens* in various fresh and marine waters and sediments. Another approach is to filter an appropriate volume of water sample through a membrane filter, place the membrane filter on a modified m-CP agar (Armon and Payment 1988) and incubate anaerobically for 24 h at 44.5°C. Upon exposure to ammonium hydroxide, the yellow to straw-coloured *C. perfringens* colonies turn dark pink to magenta. Confirmation may be done by anaerobic growth in thioglycollate, a positive gram stain reaction and stormy fermentation of iron milk.

PSEUDOMONAS SPP.

Pseudomonads are ubiquitous bacteria that are able to flourish in a wide variety of habitats (surface waters, aquifers, seawater, soil and vegetation). Some pseudomonads are among the prominent denitrifiers while others grow prodigiously in and on tertiary treatment devices such as reverse osmosis and electrodialysis membranes and in sand or carbon filtration beds. Pseudomonads reported in some drinking water supplies include: *Pseudomonas aeruginosa*, *Pseudomonas cepacia*, *Pseudomonas fluorescens*, *Pseudomonas mallei*, *Pseudomonas maltophila*, *Pseudomonas putida* and *Pseudomonas testosteroni* (Geldreich 1990, 1996, Gambassini et al. 1990). To this list can be added: *Pseudomonas stutzeri*, *Pseudomonas diminuta* and *Pseudomonas acidovorans* which have been found in bottled waters at densities ranging from 10^3 to 10^5 organisms per ml (Gavin and Leclerc 1974, Hernandez Duquino and Rosenberg 1987). These organisms metabolically adapt to survival on minimal nutrient concentrations typical of protected aquifers and treated drinking water. Enumeration of pseudomonads is not recommended routinely but may be of value in certain industries, such as those manufacturing foods, drink and pharmaceutical products, where high quality water is desirable. *P. aeruginosa* is an opportunistic pathogen and its presence in hospital water is a matter for concern.

7 PRINCIPLES OF PATHOGEN DETECTION

Detection of pathogens in the aquatic environment requires techniques to concentrate a few organisms from large samples and reduce the interfering flora of many heterotrophic bacteria that are certain to be a factor in contaminated water. For bacterial pathogens, this is generally accomplished through filtration of large volumes of water (1–2 litres) followed by cultivation in selective media for suppression of coliforms and other heterotrophic organisms. Another approach is to place gauze pads in the polluted stream for 3–5 days to entrap the pathogenic agent, then express the water from the pad to selective enrichment media (Moore 1948, 1950). A third approach is to filter samples of 1–2 litres through diatomaceous earth held in a MF (membrane filter) funnel by an absorbent pad, the placing sections of the plug in appropriate media.

8 STRATEGIES FOR RAPID METHODS

Rapid laboratory methods to better characterize water supply quality are an urgent research priority. The inability of microbiology to provide data within a few hours of sample processing has been a major deterrent to greater utilization of the science in water plant operations. With the discovery that disinfection byproducts may contribute carcinogens and possible other toxins to the water supply, treatment schemes are being modified to minimize these undesirable formations. In so doing the effectiveness of treatment barriers required to avoid microbial contaminant passages becomes a matter of greater concern. Consequently, the need for rapid assessment of water quality is more urgent than ever before. Such information would also be of singular value as an aid in restoring the quality of drinking water after contamination caused by treatment failures, distribution line breaks, poor practices in disinfection line repair and sudden occurrence of cross-connections.

Any breakthrough in the development of rapid tests must involve specificity, sensitivity and precision with achievement of a test result within a few hours. Searching for rapid methods in environmental microbiology has revealed a variety of candidate methods that have potential in real time monitoring (Geldreich and Reasoner 1985). As might be anticipated, rapid tests that can be performed in less than 1 h have little specificity and may possibly include non-viable cells. These limitations are being solved but the trade-off is in the need for more costly materials and instrumentation sensitive to trace concentrations of specific metabolic products produced by organisms of interest. One exception to this trend may be seen in a direct membrane filter method incorporating MUG in a modified medium (M-7h agar) which provides detection of as few as one faecal coliform per 100 ml in 6 h (Berg and Fiksdal 1988).

Efforts to shorten the time required to detect bacterial indicator systems or individual pathogen species in a water sample flora to less than 5 h will require instrumentation capable of detecting viable organisms directly or after a brief period of amplification in a selective enrichment medium. Instrumentation and test materials for these methods will become more readily available to the laboratory in the near future.

Of the rapid test candidates currently in development, gene probes appear to be the most promising (Richardson, Stewart and Wolfe 1991). Research into microbial genetics has led to techniques that can detect minute quantities of nucleotide sequences unique to a single species of organism, whether bacteria, fungi, virus or invertebrates. For example, 10 enterotoxigenic *E. coli* per ml of canal water were detected in the grossly polluted canals in Bangkok, Thailand, by using gene probe technology (Mosely et al. 1982).

The use of gene probes and automated microbiological techniques will become a major activity in the water plant laboratories of the future (Geldreich 1991). Perhaps development of multiplex probes to detect bacterial pathogens or enteroviruses will become sensitive enough to detect one organism per litre of sample within an hour. At the present time, some probe tests can be completed in 0.5–2 h, but may require 28–32 h for amplification to achieve acceptable sensitivities (Tenover 1988).

REFERENCES

Alter AJ, 1954, Appearance of intestinal wastes in surface water supplies at Ketchikan, Alaska, *Proceedings Fifth Alaska Science Conference*, Amer. Assoc. Adv. Sci., Anchorage, Alaska.

Anonymous, 1954, Ketchikan laboratory studies disclose gulls are implicated in spread of disease, *Alaska's Health*, **11**: 1–2.

Armon R, Payment P, 1988, A modified M-CP medium for the enumeration of *Clostridium perfringens* from water samples, *Can J Microbiol*, **34**: 78–9.

Belli CM, 1902, *Zentralbl Bakteriol 11 Abt*, **8**: 445.

Berg DJ, Fiksdal L, 1988, Rapid detection of total and fecal coliforms in water by enzymatic hydrolysis of 4-methylumbelliferone-β-D-galactoside, *Appl Environ Microbiol*, **54**: 2112–18.

Bishop RF, Allcock EA, 1960, Bacterial flora of the small intestine in acute intestinal obstruction, *Br Med J*, **5175**: 766–70.

Blake PA, Rosenberg ML et al., 1977, Cholera in Portugal, *Am J Epidemiol*, **105**: 337–43.

Bonde GJ, 1962, *Bacterial Indicators of Water Pollution*, Teknisk Forlag, Copenhagen, 422.

Bonde GJ, 1967, Pollution of a marine environment, *J Water Poll Control Fed*, **39**: R45–63.

Bonde GJ, 1968, Studies on the dispersion and disappearance phenomena of enteric bacteria in the marine environment, *Rev Int Oceanogr Med*, **9**: 17–44.

Brezenski FT, Russomanno R, 1969, The detection and use of *Salmonella* in studying polluted tidal estuaries, *J Water Poll Control Fed*, **40**: 725–37.

Castle S, 1985, Public health implications regarding the epidemiology and microbiology of public whirlpools, *Infect Control*, **6**: 418–19.

Chamberlin E, Mitchell R, 1978, A decay model for enteric bacteria in natural waters, *Water Pollution Microbiology*, John Wiley, New York, 325–48.

Clark RM, Geldreich EE et al., 1996, Tracking a *Salmonella* serovar *typhimurium* outbreak in Gideon, Missouri: Role of contaminant propagation modelling, *J Water SRT–Aqua*, **45**: 171–83.

Claudon DG, Thompson DI et al., 1971, Prolonged *Salmonella* contamination of a recreational lake by runoff waters, *Appl Microbiol*, **21**: 875–7.

Collins VG, 1963, The distribution and ecology of bacteria, *Proc Soc Water Treat Exam*, **12**: 40–73.

Cook HA, Cromwell DL, Wilson HA, 1967, Microorganisms in

household refuse and seepage water from sanitary landfills, *West Virginia Acad Sci*, **39:** 107–12.

Cordano AM, Vergilio R, 1990, Salmonella contamination on surface waters, *Proc Second Biennial Water Quality Symposium Microbiological Aspects*, University of Chile, Santiago.

Davis BJ, 1985, Whirlpool operation and the prevention of infection, *Infect Control*, **6:** 394–7.

Drury DD, Gearheart RA, 1975, Bacterial population dynamics and dissolved oxygen minimum, *J Am Water Works Assoc*, **67:** 154–8.

Dzyuban AN, 1975, The number and generation time of bacteria and production of bacterial biomass in water of the Saratov reservoir, *Gidrobiolog-icheskii Zh*, **11:** 14–19.

Eikelboom DH, 1975, Filamentous organisms observed in activated sludge, *Water Res*, **9:** 365–88.

Favero MS, Drake CH, 1966, Factors influencing the occurrence of high numbers of iodine-resistant bacteria in iodinated swimming pools, *Appl Microbiol*, **14:** 627–35.

Fennel H, James DB, Morris J, 1974, Pollution of a storage reservoir by roosting gulls, *J Soc Water Treat Exam*, **23:** 5–24.

Fujioka RS, Hashimoto HH et al., 1981, Effect of sunlight on survival of indicator bacteria in seawater, *Appl Environ Microbiol*, **41:** 690–6.

Fulton BV, Richardson G, 1971, Isolation of Anaerobes, Academic Press, London, 270.

Gambassini L, Sacco C et al., 1990, Microbial quality of the water in the distribution system of Florence, *Aqua*, **39:** 258–64.

Gameson ALH, Bufton AWJ, Gould DJ, 1967, Studies of the coastal distribution of coliform bacteria in the vicinity of a sea outfall, *Water Poll Control*, **66:** 501–24.

Gameson ALH, Gould DJ, 1975, Effects of solar radiation on the mortality of some terrestrial bacteria in sea water, *Discharge of Sewage from Sea Outfalls*, Pergamon Press, Oxford, 209–19.

Gameson ALH, Saxon JR, 1967, Field studies on effect of daylight on mortality of coliform bacteria, *Water Res*, **1:** 279–95.

Gavin F, LeClerc H, 1974, Etude des bacilles gram-pigmentés en joune isolés de l'eau, *Int Oceanogr Med*, **37:** 17–68.

Geldreich EE, 1966, *Sanitary Significance of Fecal Coliforms in the Environment*, Federal Water Pollution Control Administration, Cincinnati. WP-20-3, 122.

Geldreich EE, 1972a, Water-borne pathogens, *Water Pollution Microbiology*, John Wiley & Sons, New York, 207–41.

Geldreich EE, 1972b, Buffalo Lake recreational water quality: a study of bacteriological data interpretation, *Water Res*, **6:** 913–24.

Geldreich EE, 1973, The use and abuse of fecal streptococci in water quality measurements, *Proc First Microbiological Seminar on Standardization of Methods*, Environmental Protection Agency, Washington DC. EPA-R4-73-022.

Geldreich EE, 1978, Bacterial populations and indicator concepts in feces, sewage, stormwater and solid wastes, *Indicators of Viruses in Water and Food*, Ann Arbor Science Publishers, Ann Arbor, Michigan, 51–97.

Geldreich EE, 1986, Control of microorganisms of public health concern in water, *J Environ Sci*, **29:** 34–7.

Geldreich EE, 1990, Microbiological quality control in distribution systems, *Water Quality and Treatment*, McGraw-Hill, New York, 1113–58.

Geldreich EE, 1991, Visions of the future in drinking water microbiology, *J N Engl Water Works Assoc*, **106:** 1–8.

Geldreich EE, 1996, *Microbial Quality of Water Supply in Distribution Systems*, Lewis Publishers, Boca Raton, FL, 504.

Geldreich EE, Bordner RH, 1971, Fecal contamination of fruits and vegetables during cultivation and processing for market: a review, *J Milk Food*, **34:** 184–95.

Geldreich EE, Kenner BA, 1969, Concepts of fecal streptococci in stream pollution, *J Water Poll Control Fed*, **41, Part II:** R336–52.

Geldreich EE, Reasoner DJ, 1985, Searching for rapid methods in environmental bacteriology, *Rapid Methods and Automation and Immunology*, Springer-Verlag, Berlin, 696–707.

Geldreich EE, Bordner RH et al., 1962, Type distribution of coliform bacteria in the feces of warm-blooded animals, *J Water Poll Control Fed*, **34:** 295–301.

Geldreich EE, Best LC et al., 1968, The bacteriological aspects of stormwater pollution, *J Water Poll Control Fed*, **40, Part I:** 1861–72.

Geldreich EE, Nash HD et al., 1975, The necessity of controlling bacterial populations in potable waters – bottled water and emergency water supplies, *J Am Water Works Assoc*, **67:** 117–24.

Geldreich EE, Nash HD et al., 1980, Bacterial dynamics in a water supply reservoir: case study, *J Am Water Works Assoc*, **72:** 31–40.

Grabow WOK, Nupen EM, 1972, The load of infectious microorganisms in the waste water of two South African hospitals, *Water Res*, **6:** 1557–63.

Hernandez Duquino H, Rosenberg FA, 1987, Antibiotic-resistant *Pseudomonas* in bottled drinking water, *Can J Microbiol*, **33:** 286–9.

Johnston R, Harmon S et al., 1964, Method to facilitate the isolation of *Clostridium botulinum* Type E, *J Bacteriol*, **88:** 1521–2.

Kampelmacher EH, Van Noorle Jansen LM, 1973, *Legionella* and thermotolerant *E. coli* in the Rhine and Meuse at their point of entry into the Netherlands, *H₂0*, **6:** 199–200.

Kampelmacher EH, Van Noorle Jansen LM, 1976, *Salmonella* effluent from sewage treatment plants, wastepipes of butchers' shops and surface water in Walcheren, *Zentralbl Bakteriol Hyg Abt 1 Orig B*, **162:** 307–19.

Klein DA, Wu S, 1974, A factor to be considered in heterotrophic microorganisms enumeration from aquatic environments, *Appl Microbiol*, **27:** 429–31.

Knittel MD, Seidler RJ et al., 1977, Colonization of the botanical environment by *Klebsiella* isolates of pathogenic origin, *Appl Environ Microbiol*, **34:** 557–63.

Kowal NE, 1982, *Health Effects of Land Treatment: Microbiological*, US Environmental Protection Agency, Cincinnati. EPA-600/1-82-007, 58.

Leclerc H, Buttiaux R et al., 1977, *Microbiologie Appliquée*, Doin Editeurs, Paris.

Moore B, 1948, The detection of paratyphoid carriers in towns by means of sewage examination, *Monthly Bull Ministry Health, Public Health Lab Serv*, **7:** 241–8.

Moore B, 1950, The detection of typhoid carriers in towns by means of sewage examination, *Monthly Bull Ministry Health, Public Health Lab Serv*, **9:** 72–8.

Mosely SL, Echevaria P et al., 1982, Identification of enterotoxigenic *Escherichia coli* by colony hybridization using three enterotoxin gene probes, *J Infect Dis*, **145:** 863–9.

Moyer NP, 1989, *Aeromonas* gastroenteritis: another waterborne disease?, *Proc Water Qual Tech Conf*, Am Water Works Assoc, Denver, 239–61.

Mundt JO, 1963, Occurrence of enterococci on plants in a wild environment, *Appl Microbiol*, **11:** 141–4.

Mundt JO, Anandam EJ, McCarty IE, 1966, Streptococcease in the atmosphere of plants processing vegetables for freezing, *Health Lab Sci*, **3:** 207–13.

Mundt JO, Coggin JH, Johnson LF, 1962, Growth of *Streptococcus faecalis* var. *liquefaciens* on plants, *Appl Microbiol*, **10:** 552–5.

Mundt JO, Graham WF, 1968, *Streptococcus faecium* var. *casseliflavus*, nov. var., *J Bacteriol*, **95:** 2005–9.

Mundt JO, Larsen SA, McCarty IE, 1966, Growth of lactic acid bacteria in waste waters of vegetable processing plants, *Appl Microbiol*, **14:** 115–18.

Nemedi L, Borbala T et al., 1984, Hydrobiological evaluation of water samples from 'standing waters' (lakes, reservoirs and ponds) near Budapest, *Budapest Kozegeszsegugy*, **2:** 40–8.

Niewolak S, 1974, The occurrence of microorganisms in the waters of the Kortowskie Lake, *Pol Arch Hydrobiol*, **21:** 315–33.

Niewolak S, 1987, Bacteriological water quality of an artificially destratified lake, *Rocz Nauk Rol Hig*, **101:** 115–54.

Perez JL, Berrocal CI, Berrocal L, 1986, Evaluation of a commercial β-glucuronidase test for the rapid and economical identification of *Escherichia coli*, *J Appl Bacteriol*, **61:** 541–5.

Peterson ML, 1971, *Pathogens associated with Solid Waste Processing: a Progress Report*, SW-49r, US Environmental Protection Agency, Cincinnati, Ohio.

Ptak DJ, Ginsburg W, Willey BF, 1974, *Aeromonas, the great masquerader*, *Water Qual Tech Conf Dec 2–3*, Am Water Works Assoc, Denver.

Randall JS, 1956, The sanitary significance of coliform bacteria in soil, *J Hyg*, **54:** 365–77.

Reasoner DJ, 1990, Monitoring heterotrophic bacteria in potable water, *Drinking Water Microbiology*, Springer-Verlag, Berlin, 452–77.

Reasoner DJ, Geldreich EE, 1985, A new medium for the enumeration and subculturing of bacteria from potable water, *Appl Environ Microbiol*, **49:** 1–7.

Report, 1959, *Sewage Contamination of Bathing Beaches in England and Wales*, Medical Research Council, Memorandum no. 37, HMSO, London.

Report, 1965, *Pollution of Interstate Waters of the Red River of the North (Minnesota, North Dakota)*, Public Health Service, Cincinnati.

Report, 1968, *Water Quality Criteria, National Technical Advisory Committee to the Secretary of the Interior*, Federal Water Pollution Control Administration.

Report, 1971, *Report on the Missouri River Water Quality Studies*, USEPA, Kansas City.

Report, 1981, Possible waterborne *Campylobacter* outbreak – British Columbia, *Can Dis Weekly Rep*, **7:** 223.

Report, 1984, *Guidelines for Drinking Water Quality*, World Health Organization, Geneva, 1–3.

Report, 1985, *Microbiological Water Quality Criteria: a Review for Australia*, Australian Water Resources Council.

Report, 1992a, *Revision of the WHO Guidelines for Drinking Water Quality*, World Health Organization, Geneva.

Report, 1992b, *Standard Methods for the Examination of Water and Wastewater*, American Public Health Association, Washington, DC.

Report, 1994, Drinking water methods for the examination of waters and associated materials, *Rep Public Health Md Subj*, **No. 1, Part 1**.

Rice EW, Fox KR et al., 1996, Evaluating plant performance with endospores, *J Am Water Works Assoc*, **88:** 122–30.

Richardson KJ, Stewart MH, Wolfe RL, 1991, Application of gene probe technology for the water industry, *J Am Water Works Assoc*, **83:** 71–81.

Romaninko VI, 1971, Total bacterial numbers in Rybinsk reservoir, *Mikrobiologiya*, **40:** 707–13.

Rose JB, 1990, Emerging issues for the microbiology of drinking water, *Water/Eng Mgt*, **137:** 23–9.

Rosenberg ML, Hazelt KK et al., 1976, Shigellosis from swimming, *JAMA*, **236:** 1849–52.

Ruskin RH, Knudsen AN, Rinehart FP, 1989, *Water Quality of Public Housing Cisterns in the U. S. Virgin Islands*, Technical Report, Caribbean Research Institute, University of the Virgin Islands, St Thomas, VI.

Schiemann DA, 1985, Experiences with bacteriological monitoring of pool water, *Infect Control*, **6:** 413–17.

Schubert RHW, Mann SW, 1968, Zum derzeitigen stand der identifierungsmoglichkeiten von *Escherichia coli* als faekal indikator bei der trinkwasseruntersuchung, *Zentralbl Bakteriol*, **208:** 498–506.

Seidler RJ, Morrow JE, Bagley ST, 1977, *Klebsiella* in drinking water emanating from redwood tanks, *Appl Environ Microbiol*, **33:** 893–900.

Spino DF, 1966, Elevated temperature technique for the isolation of *Salmonella* from streams, *Appl Microbiol*, **14:** 591–6.

Stapert EM, Sokolski WT, Northam JI, 1962, The factor of temperature in the better recovery of bacteria from water by filtration, *Can J Microbiol*, **8:** 809–10.

Swayne MD, Boone GM, Bauer D, 1980, *Wastewater in receiving waters at water supply abstraction points*, US Environmental Protection Agency, Cincinnati. EPA-600/2-80-044, 189.

Taylor DN, McDermott KT, Little JR, 1983, *Campylobacter* enteritis associated with drinking water in back country areas of the Rocky Mountain, *Ann Intern Med*, **99:** 38–40.

Tenover FC, 1988, Diagnostic deoxyribonucleic acid probes for infectious disease, *Clin Microbiol Rev*, **1:** 82–101.

Vogt RL, Sours HE et al., 1982, *Campylobacter* enteritis associated with contaminated water, *Ann Intern Med*, **96:** 292–6.

Weiss CM, Oglesby RT, 1960, Limnology and water quality of raw water in impoundments, *Public Works*, **91:** 97–101.

Wilson WJ, 1931, *Official Circular 96*, British Waterworks Association.

Wilson WJ, Blair EMMcV, 1925, Correlation of the sulphite reduction test with other tests in the bacteriological examination of water, *J Hyg*, **24:** 111–19.

Chapter 16

THE MICROBIOLOGY OF MILK AND MILK PRODUCTS

A Rampling

1 **Milk**	5	**Butter**
2 **Milk powder**	6	**Ice cream**
3 **Cream**	7	**Cheese**
4 **Yoghurt**		

The milk of cows, buffaloes, sheep, goats, donkeys, horses and camels has been an important item of human food for centuries. Pathogenic microorganisms often contaminate milk, which has been recognized as a vehicle for disease since the late nineteenth century (Department of Public Health 1886). Strategies such as improved hygiene, eradication of tuberculosis and brucellosis from cattle, and heat treatment are now employed in most developed countries to reduce the risk to human health. Liquid milk and milk products such as cheese, yoghurt and fermented milks are often stored for days, weeks or months and finally consumed without cooking. It is not surprising, therefore, that these items are still implicated in major outbreaks of food poisoning and other communicable diseases (Sharp 1987, Sockett 1991).

Because milk and milk products are such universal items of food, sporadic infections caused by them may go unnoticed. Wilson (1942) discussed the difficulties of ascertaining the frequency of milk-borne disease. At that time pasteurization was not widely practised, and both milk-associated tuberculosis and undulant fever were major public health problems. Both diseases had long incubation periods, gradual onset and variable infectivity. It was therefore difficult to prove their relationship with the consumption of milk; moreover, if, in large explosive outbreaks of disease such as typhoid fever, scarlet fever or food poisoning, cases were scattered over a wide area, other sources of infection were often suspected. Thus, unless careful epidemiological investigations were made, the association with contaminated milk might be overlooked. Even nowadays in developing countries Wilson's observations remain true and where hygiene is poor

and animal disease uncontrolled, milk is an important vehicle for various human diseases.

Most developed countries have sophisticated disease surveillance systems in place and resources to investigate outbreaks. In addition, the pathogenic microorganisms likely to contaminate milk differ from those prevalent in 1942 (Bell and Palmer 1983, Milner 1995); some have decreased as a result of animal disease eradication programmes and changes in patterns of human disease but others have taken their place. It is clear that, although rare, public health problems with milk and milk products remain and where milk products are produced by large commercial establishments there is potential for a major outbreak should anything go wrong.

1 MILK

1.1 Microbiology of cows' milk

The major milk-producing animal is the cow and most of the available information and research into microbiology of milk relates to cows' milk. Micro-organisms in raw milk are derived from various sources, including the commensal or pathogenic flora of the udder, teat canals and skin, which varies depending on whether cattle are housed under cover or in yards or are out in pasture; faecal contamination; and environmental sources such as milking equipment, storage vessels or the water supply. Commensal or pathogenic organisms from the milkers may also contribute.

The importance of particular organisms depends on whether the milk is to be consumed raw or after heat processing, and on the temperature and duration of storage. In developed countries the commercial production of milk is subject to strict regulations regarding hygiene and refrigeration during transport and storage. The keeping quality and flavour of the heat-treated product is adversely affected by psychrotrophic bacteria (capable of growing at between 2 and 7°C), by thermoduric organisms and by postpasteurization contamination. Some of the enzymes produced by psychrotrophs are heat-tolerant and cause spoilage both before and after pasteurization. Postpasteurization contamination is the most important factor influencing the quality of pasteurized milk but the quality and hygiene of raw milk also have important effects on the quality of the heat-treated product.

No matter how good the health of the dairy herd, the milking hygiene and the storage conditions, the safety of raw milk cannot be guaranteed (Sharp, Paterson and Barrett 1985, Maguire 1993). Detailed reviews of the microbiology of raw milk are to be found in specialist publications (Bramley and McKinnon 1990, Gilmour and Rowe 1990). Most of the micro-organisms in hygienically produced raw milk with low bacterial counts are derived from the normal flora of the cow's teat canals and skin, and comprise coagulase-negative staphylococci, micrococci and streptococci. Streptococci belonging to Lancefield group N cause natural souring of raw milk. Commercially cultured strains of these organisms are used as cheese starters in the dairy industry.

The skin of the teats and udder inevitably becomes contaminated by faecal and environmental bacteria, viruses, yeasts and moulds. Cows housed inside during winter have very heavily soiled udders and the bacterial counts in milk are high even after washing the teats. The most effective way of removing contamination is careful washing followed by drying with paper towels or with a disinfectant impregnated cloth. When the cattle are turned out to pasture there is a pronounced decline in the total bacterial count in bulk milk, even compared with milk from carefully washed cows (Bramley and McKinnon 1990). Inadequately disinfected milking machines, pipes and tanks are also important sources of postmilking contamination with bacteria, which are mainly derived from milk previously in the system. In the UK, the water supply to all areas concerned with milking and milk collection must be potable, but in many countries farms obtain water from boreholes or springs which may at times be contaminated with pathogenic species such as *Campylobacter jejuni* or *Salmonella* serotypes or with psychrotrophic organisms such as *Pseudomonas* spp., which cause spoilage of refrigerated milk. Under modern systems of dairy management and marketing, milk is stored in refrigerated farm tanks for up to 48 h prior to collection. Once at the creamery it may again be stored overnight in large insulated or refrigerated silos. During this time there is considerable scope for multiplication of psychrotrophic organisms.

The bacterial count of raw milk increases significantly if the cow has mastitis and many of these organisms are potential causes of human infection or intoxication. The most common causes of mastitis are

Staphylococcus aureus (including enterotoxigenic strains); *Streptococcus agalactiae* (Lancefield group B); *Streptococcus uberis*; *Streptococcus dysgalactiae* (Lancefield group C); and *Escherichia coli*. Less common causes are *Leptospira interrogans* serovar. *hardjo, Streptococcus zooepidemicus* (Lancefield group C), *Listeria monocytogenes, Bacillus cereus, Pasteurella multocida, Clostridium perfringens, Nocardia* spp., *Cryptococcus neoformans, Actinomyces* spp. and *Corynebacterium ulcerans.*

At one time *Mycobacterium* spp. were an important cause of bovine mastitis in the UK and both *Mycobacterium bovis* and *Brucella abortus* were commonly present in milk even in the absence of mastitis (Galbraith and Pusey 1984). Both these pathogens are now virtually eradicated from cattle in most developed countries. Milk-borne scarlet fever due to *Streptococcus pyogenes* (Lancefield group A) was also common at one time (Eyler 1986). Group A streptococci are not natural pathogens of cattle but cows can develop teat lesions and mastitis if infected by a human carrier. Other pathogens such as *L. monocytogenes, Coxiella burnetii* and *S. zooepidemicus* may on occasions be excreted in milk in the absence of udder disease and *Salmonella* serotypes (Marth 1969) and *C. jejuni* occasionally cause clinical or subclinical mastitis (Morgan et al. 1985, Orr et al. 1995). Under natural conditions, faecal contamination is probably the most common source of salmonellae, *L. monocytogenes* or campylobacters and it is now becoming clear that in many countries cattle are an important reservoir for Vero cytotoxigenic *E. coli* O157 (Clarke et al. 1989, Chapman and Wright 1993, Chapman et al. 1993).

1.2 Microbiology of ewes' and goats' milk

Milk and in particular milk products made from ewes' and goats' milk have become very popular in recent years and the commercial market for cheese and yoghurt is expanding. Surveys of the microbiological quality of goats' milk have been performed in Scotland (Hunter and Cruickshank 1984) and in England and Wales (Roberts 1985). Both showed that high standards of hygiene were possible but that problems arose from inadequate disinfection of milking equipment or from inadequate control of storage temperatures at the point of sale.

Public Health Laboratory Service (PHLS) laboratories in England and Wales examined 2493 samples over 12 months (Roberts 1985). Total counts of $<10^5$ organisms per ml of raw milk at 37°C were given by 79% of samples, 71% contained <100 coliforms per ml; and 91% <10 *E. coli* per ml. However, 4% contained detectable numbers of *S. aureus*. Other pathogens isolated during this study were *Yersinia enterocolitica* from 2 samples and *C. jejuni* from one.

In the Scottish study, 483 freshly drawn samples and 154 packages of liquid or frozen milk were examined. Infection of the udder was a cause of high bacterial counts in 25% of samples drawn directly from the animal. Coagulase-negative staphylococci were the most common organisms and were associated with subclinical mastitis. *S. aureus* was present in 3%.

A study of goats' milk on 6 farms in Quebec over a 1 year period showed that total counts of aerobes, psychrotrophs, coliforms, yeasts and moulds increased during the summer months but that counts could be controlled by good hygiene, rapid cooling, refrigeration and frequent collections by refrigerated vehicles (Tirard-Collet et al. 1991). Somatic cell counts were also measured and these confirmed that in contrast to the finding with cows, counts varied with the season and the state of lactation and high counts were not necessarily an indication of mastitis (Hinkley 1991).

There are very few publications on the microbiology of sheep milk. Studies in Spain, Bulgaria and Norway have indicated that significant contamination with Enterobacteriaceae and coliforms may occur during milking and as a result of poor cleaning practices on the farm (Gaya, Medina and Nuñez 1987).

Even when hygiene is good, the risk of milk-borne infection from unpasteurized goats' or ewes' milk is similar to that for cows' milk. *Brucella melitensis* and *Brucella ovis* are still common in goats and sheep in the Mediterranean countries, Asia and Latin America and human infections are associated with the consumption of raw milk or cheese made from unpasteurized milk (Wallach et al. 1994, Report 1995). Other pathogenic micro-organisms such as *Salmonella* Typhimurium, *S. aureus*, *Y. enterocolitica*, *C. perfringens*, *B. cereus* and *C. jejuni* can survive in goats' milk under experimental conditions, and some of these pathogens multiply at temperatures of 22°C or more (Roberts 1985). Outbreaks and incidents of brucellosis, campylobacter infection, salmonellosis, viral tick-borne encephalitis, Q fever, staphylococcal food poisoning and *C. ulcerans* sore throat have been associated with consumption of untreated goats' milk or goat cheese in Canada, Britain and the USA in recent years (Hutchinson et al. 1985a, Sharp 1987, Fishbein and Raoult 1992, Report 1994a, 1995). There is also a high incidence of toxoplasma infection in goats (Skinner et al. 1987) and there is convincing evidence that consumption of unpasteurized goats' milk can transmit infection to man (Sacks, Roberto and Brooks 1982).

Sheep can also carry many micro-organisms pathogenic for man, such as *Salmonella* serotypes, *C. burnetii*, *Campylobacter* spp., *S. aureus*, *Toxoplasma gondii* and *L. monocytogenes*. *S. aureus* seems to be a common contaminant of both ewes' and goats' milk and more prevalent than in cows' milk (Valle et al. 1990). A high proportion of isolates produce enterotoxin. An outbreak of staphylococcal food poisoning in Scotland was traced to cheese made from unpasteurized sheep milk (Sharp 1987). Valle et al. (1990) examined 342 isolates of staphylococci from nasal mucosae, skin, udders, teats and milk of female goats from 11 Spanish flocks. They found that c. 20% of isolates were *S. aureus* of which 74% were enterotoxigenic. In addition, 22% of the coagulase-negative staphylococci produced enterotoxin. Most of the toxigenic isolates from goats produced staphylococcus enterotoxin C (SE-C). Staphylococcal counts of >600 per ml were detected in milk from 43 of 133 goats. Of these isolates

17 were enterotoxigenic *S. aureus* and 4 were enterotoxigenic coagulase-negative staphylococci (*Staphylococcus hyicus*, one; *Staphylococcus chromogenes*, 2; and *Staphylococcus epidermidis*, one).

Although *L. monocytogenes* is a cause of meningoencephalitis in sheep and may also be excreted in the milk and faeces of healthy sheep, the risk of contamination of ewes' milk on the farm does not seem to be any greater than for cows' milk. Rodriguez et al. (1994) sampled milk from 1052 farm bulk tanks on 283 Spanish farms throughout a 1 year period and found that *Listeria* spp. could be detected in 4.56% and *L. monocytogenes* in 2.19%. This compares with an overall incidence of 3.48% for *L. monocytogenes* in cows' raw milk calculated by pooling data from published surveys. A worrying finding in the Rodriguez study was the detection of *L. monocytogenes* in 25 of 136 samples of milk from transport tankers, suggesting that the tankers themselves were reservoirs of environmental contamination with *L. monocytogenes*.

1.3 Heat treatment of milk

PASTEURIZED MILK

The international definition of pasteurization (Report 1994b) is: 'A heat treatment process applied to a product with the aim of avoiding public health hazards arising from pathogenic micro-organisms associated with milk. Pasteurization as a heat treatment process is intended to result in only minimal chemical, physical and organoleptic changes.' The process was originally introduced by dairies to improve the keeping quality of milk (Wilson 1942). It soon became clear that heat treatment would also destroy pathogenic organisms such as tubercle bacilli and haemolytic streptococci. The public health aspects of the process then assumed the greater importance.

Several time–temperature combinations are effective. The Dairy Products (Hygiene) Regulations 1995 for England and Wales state that milk shall be pasteurized by means of a heat treatment involving a high temperature for a short time (at least 71.7°C for 15 s, or any equivalent combination) or a pasteurization process using different time and temperature combinations to obtain an equivalent effect. The product must give a negative phosphatase test immediately after heat treatment and be cooled as soon as practicable to a temperature of 6°C or lower and stored at or below that temperature until it leaves the treatment establishment.

The high temperature short time (HTST) method is most commonly used both in large commercial dairies and on farms. The HTST plant consists of a plate heat exchanger and a holding tube (Fig. 16.1). Raw milk enters the heat exchanger and is warmed by the hot milk leaving the hot section along the other side of the plates. The warmed milk is then heated to the statutory temperature before it runs through the holding tube for at least 15 s. The hot milk then re-enters the heat exchanger, being cooled initially by cold raw milk, then by tap water and finally by chilled water. The law requires that any HTST system has an automatic temperature control and a safety device that automatically diverts milk back for reheating if it has not been raised to the statutory temperature. In addition, there must be indicating and recording thermometers on the plant and an automatic recording device for the safety system.

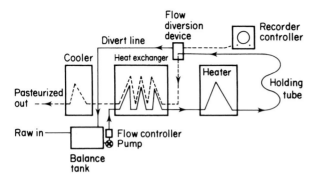

Fig. 16.1 Diagrammatic representation of milk flow through HTST pasteurizer.

An alternative method for small quantities of milk is the holder or batch heating process in which milk is heated to between 62.8 and 65.6°C and held at that temperature for 30 min, followed by rapid cooling to below 10°C. The heating vessel incorporates an insulated outer jacket through which the heating and cooling media can flow, an agitator to ensure uniform heating, thermometers, including a recording thermometer and a temperature control device that automatically regulates the heating of the milk to pasteurization temperature and the subsequent retention at this temperature for the holding period (Report 1994b). Nowadays the holder method is seldom practised even on farms.

The combinations of time and temperature used for the heat treatment of milk are designed to kill all pathogenic vegetative cells including *C. burnetii* which is relatively heat-resistant (Zall 1990). Bacterial spores and some preformed bacterial or fungal toxins, however, are not destroyed by pasteurization temperatures. The keeping quality of pasteurized milk depends both on the quality before heat treatment and on the amount of postpasteurization contamination. Thermoduric bacteria that survive pasteurization belong to the genera *Bacillus*, *Clostridium*, *Corynebacterium*, *Micrococcus*, *Streptococcus* and *Lactobacillus*. The importance of thermoduric organisms depends on the storage temperature. Some thermoduric faecal streptococci, *Bacillus* spp. and *Clostridium* spp. can grow below 7°C and are therefore also psychrotrophic. Most thermoduric organisms are mesophilic with optimum growth between 20 and 32°C. If pasteurized milk is allowed to remain at ambient temperature for several hours, as commonly happens with doorstep deliveries, growth of mesophilic bacteria such as *B. cereus* will soon cause bitterness, sweet curdling and 'bitty' cream. Contamination with *B. cereus* is very common and yet reports of bacillus food poisoning due to the consumption of milk or cream are rare (Gilbert 1979, Christiansson 1992). This is probably because enterotoxin is not usually produced by *B. cereus* until the bacterial counts are so high and consequent spoilage so great that the milk is unusable. The lactic acid-producing streptococci do not survive pasteurization and 'souring' does not therefore take place in pasteurized milk. Repasteurization of returned milk results in enrichment of the thermoduric organisms in the final product and so is bad practice.

The keeping quality and flavour of properly refrigerated pasteurized milk depends on the numbers of psychrotrophic organisms. The most important of these are species of *Pseudomonas*, *Flavobacterium*, *Alcaligenes*, *Acinetobacter*, yeasts and moulds. These organisms are not thermoduric but are derived from the postpasteurization environment. They outgrow any thermoduric psychrotrophs that may be present, and for this reason hygiene of the pipes, tanks and bottle fillers is the most important factor influencing the keeping quality of milk stored below 10°C (Schröder 1984). Psychrotrophic organisms are responsible for various 'off' flavours, ropiness and changes in colour.

Ultra-heat-treated (UHT) milk

According to the Regulations, the description 'UHT' may be applied to a continuous flow of milk that has been heated to a temperature of not less than 135°C and retained at that temperature for at least 1 s. The method of heating may be indirect or by direct injection of steam. After treatment, the milk must be packaged in sterile airtight containers that are filled and sealed with aseptic precautions. In practice the milk is usually heated to more than 140°C for 2–4 s to produce 'commercial sterility' – which means that it has a shelf-life of several weeks because, although small numbers of spores may survive, they are usually unable to grow under the conditions of storage (Lewis 1994).

Sterilized milk

The term 'sterilized' is applied to milk that has been filtered, clarified, homogenized and then heated to 100°C for long enough to denature all casein and whey proteins. Traditionally, sterilized milk is bottled and sealed before heating to 110–116°C for 20–30 min. The process inevitably results in a caramelized flavour and brownish colour but this is popular with some consumers, particularly in the industrial regions of the UK.

Thermized milk

In situations where raw milk has to be held under chilled conditions for some time, its keeping quality can be improved by a low temperature heat treatment called thermization. Thermized milk must conform to strict definitions according to European law. It must be obtained from raw milk which, if it is not treated within 36 h of acceptance by the establishment, has a plate count at 30°C prior to thermization which does not exceed 300 000 per ml in the case of cows' milk. The thermization treatment consists of heating raw milk for at least 15 s at between 57 and 68°C so that after such treatment the milk still shows a positive reaction in the phosphatase test. This treatment is not sufficient to eliminate pathogenic micro-organisms.

1.4 Legislation

In most developed countries the hygiene and composition of milk and milk products are subject to statutory controls, which specify general standards for production, transport and processing, and specific standards, which set microbiological and chemical limits for each product.

Council Directive 92/46/EEC (as amended) applies to milk from sheep, goats, buffaloes and cows and covers milk and milk products produced within the European Union. Detailed microbiological standards including absence of pathogenic micro-organisms are specified for raw milk, heat-treated milk and milk-based products, which must be sampled at the production or processing establishments. Non-microbiological tests are also specified, including somatic cell count, which is an indicator of mastitis in raw milk from cows and buffaloes (no such standard is specified for milk from sheep and goats because the counts are subject to wide natural fluctuations in these animals), and the phosphatase and peroxidase test for pasteurized milk. Greenwood and Rampling (1995) list the microbiological standards and guideline criteria specified in the Regulations for England and Wales based on the European Directive. Greenwood (1995) gives details of appropriate methods for the microbiological tests and the phosphatase and peroxidase tests.

Similar standards apply in the USA for milk and milk products from sheep, goats and cows. The US Food and Drug Administration produces a model code for grade A milk which is specified in the Pasteurized Milk Ordinance and the Dried Milk Ordinance. These cover production, transport and processing as well as microbiological and chemical tests. Grade A standards are applicable to all products that are produced in plants that produce milk for shipment between states (more than 95% of fluid milk products). Milk is produced on the farm as either 'Grade A' or 'Manufacturing Grade' but most milk for manufacture of dairy products is surplus grade A that has not been sold as liquid milk for drinking. The production of 'Manufacturing Grade' milk and of products such as cheese, butter and ice cream is subject to regulatory oversight by the US Department of Agriculture.

QUALITY CONTROL TESTS

The plate count at 30°C and the coliform count form the basis of microbiological quality control tests for milk and milk products in most countries, including the USA. In Europe the plate count at 21°C after pre-incubation at 6°C for 5 days has been adopted as the statutory test for pasteurized milk. This test was designed to assess the level of psychrotrophic bacteria and thus keeping quality, but it has been subject to much criticism because it is time-consuming, expensive to perform and has poor reproducibility (Scotter et al. 1993).

The coliform count is universally adopted as an indicator of poor hygiene and of postpasteurization contamination. High counts in pasteurized milk may also be due to faults in the pasteurizer or contamination of pasteurized milk with raw milk. Pasteurization plants that produce milk which fails this test repeatedly, in spite of attention to cleaning and disinfection routines, should be examined carefully for leaks in the pasteurizer or faulty operation of the plant.

Absence of detectable alkaline phosphatase is the most important test for adequate heat treatment of pasteurized milk or cream. Alkaline phosphatase is normally present in raw milk and is destroyed by heat treatment at a temperature slightly above that required to destroy *Mycobacterium tuberculosis* and slightly lower than those employed in the pasteurization of milk. Detection of phosphatase in pasteurized milk may therefore indicate inadequate heat treatment or contamination with raw milk. There are several internationally recognized methods of testing that may be used for enforcement purposes and which have a detection limit of as little as 0.006% of raw milk (Rocco 1990). It should be noted, however, that the test may not detect very small leaks in valves or pasteurizer plates. To monitor the process efficiently the test should be applied to samples taken from the cold milk exit side of the pasteurizer and immediately following an episode of flow diversion to check the integrity of the flow diversion valve.

Reactivation of phosphatase may occasionally occur, particularly with cream. Reactivation is mediated by a heat-stable activator in the presence of magnesium and β-lactoglobulin (Lyster and Aschaffenburg 1962). The degree of reactivation depends on the initial concentration of phosphatase and, since the enzyme is adsorbed to the phospholipid of the fat globule membrane, it varies with the amount of fat and is greatest in cream. Statutory phosphatase tests for cream include a test which distinguishes between native and reactivated phosphatase.

The peroxidase test is a test for excessive heat treatment. If milk is subjected to significantly higher temperatures than those used for standard pasteurization, inactivation of the enzyme will occur. Thus a positive peroxidase test indicates that milk has not been overheated.

RESTRICTIONS ON THE SALE OF UNPASTEURIZED MILK

Most milk for drinking and for the manufacture of milk products is pasteurized but few countries have formal restrictions on the sale of raw milk. In the USA, however, very few milk products can be sold in the unpasteurized state. Some states allow limited sale of raw fluid milk and some hard cheeses may be manufactured from raw milk (Childer RN, personal communication 1996). In England and Wales, legislation enacted in 1985 and 1986 limited sales of unpasteurized cows' milk to sales by farmhouse caterers, from farm gates and from local retail deliveries of milk bottled on the farm. In Scotland, legislation in 1983 and 1986 prohibited all sale of unpasteurized cows' milk and cream. There are no restrictions on the sale of raw liquid milk from goats, sheep or buffaloes or on any milk products made from raw milk anywhere in the UK and no restrictions on the sale of any unpasteurized milk or milk products elsewhere in Europe.

1.5 Outbreaks and incidents of infection associated with milk

Most outbreaks of infection due to the consumption of liquid milk have been caused by pathogens of animal origin (Editorial 1988). Salmonellae or campylobacters are most prevalent but there have also been incidents due to less common organisms such as *Y.*

enterocolitica, L. monocytogenes, S. zooepidemicus, Streptobacillus moniliformis, C. ulcerans, Cryptosporidium parvum and Vero cytotoxin-producing *E. coli* (VTEC).

Table 16.1 lists outbreaks of infection associated with milk and milk products in England and Wales from 1989 to 1994. The data for 1989–91 are not strictly comparable with those for 1992–94 because from 1992, the collection of data was more detailed and included the evidence for associating a food vehicle with an outbreak. In spite of legislation limiting sales, and even though less than 3% of the total milk production is unpasteurized in England and Wales, outbreaks are mostly due to raw milk. It is also clear that outbreaks due to milk products are usually due to those made from unpasteurized milk.

On the other hand, the situation is different in Scotland where, in the face of the epidemiological, microbiological and research evidence that heat treatment of all cows' milk would be cost-effective, the retail sale of untreated cows' milk was prohibited from August 1983. Thereafter incidents of infection related to milk were controlled in the general community but a small number persisted in the farming community where farm workers and their families received untreated milk as wage benefit. In September 1986 the requirement for heat treatment was extended to include benefits of that kind. In 1986, 2 small outbreaks occurred within farming communities but since the introduction of the policy there were no significant outbreaks of milk-borne infection in Scotland until 1994 when 2 outbreaks of *E. coli* O157 infection occurred due to pasteurized milk and farmhouse cheese.

A worrying trend everywhere is the increasing number of outbreaks associated with pasteurized milk (Sharp 1989). The organisms have often been isolated from the raw milk supplied to the plant and investigations have revealed faults in the plant or in its operation, or opportunity for post-treatment contamination with raw milk (Lecos 1986).

Table 16.1 Milk- and milk product-associated outbreaks and incidents of infection; reports to CDSC, England and Wales 1989–94

Year	Organism	Vehicle of infection	Number of outbreaks	Number of persons infected	Evidence
1989	*Salmonella* Dublin	Unpast. cheese	1	39	–
	Campylobacters	Milk[a]	1	14	–
	Clostridium botulinum	Hazelnut yoghurt	1	27	–
	Bacillus cereus	Cream	1	2	–
	Unknown aetiology	Unpast. cheese	1	155	–
1990[b]	*Salmonella* Typhimurium	Raw milk	1	5	–
	Campylobacters	Raw milk	2	11	–
1991[b]	*Salmonella*				
	Dublin	Raw milk	1	26	–
	Anatum	Raw milk	1	3	–
	Enteritidis	Ice Cream	3	7	–
	Escherichia coli O157	Unpast. yoghurt	1	16	–
	Campylobacters	Raw milk	1	4	–
	Campylobacters	Bird-pecked bottled milk	1	11	–
1992[b]	*Salmonella*				
	Enteritidis	Ice cream	1	25	D
	Enteritidis	School milk[a]	1	44	S
	Campylobacters	Past. milk	1	110	S
	Campylobacters	Raw milk	1	72	S
1993	*Salmonella*				
	Enteritidis	Ice cream	1	7	S
	Typhimurium	Raw milk	1	13	M, S
	Escherichia coli O157	Raw milk	1	11	M
	Campylobacters	Raw milk	1	22	D
1994	*Salmonella*				
	Typhimurium	Raw milk	1	11	M
	Typhimurium	Raw milk	1	4	M, S
	Typhimurium	Past. milk	1	26	M
	Campylobacters	Raw milk	1	23	S
	S. zooepidemicus	Raw milk	1	4	M

[a]Not known whether raw or pasteurized.
[b]Campylobacters: a number of incidents attributed to bird-pecked bottled milk were recorded.
M, Microbiological; S, statistical; D, descriptive.
Data supplied by the Public Health Laboratory Service, Communicable Disease Surveillance Centre, London.

In December 1985 the US Food and Drug Administration started a 3 year inspection and surveillance programme for all plants producing fluid milk and frozen desserts. The programme was designed to increase awareness of the microbiological hazards associated with dairy products and to improve the training of personnel (Report 1987a). Revised guidelines for controlling environmental contamination in dairy plants (Report 1987b) addressed the problems of detecting cross-connections and other routes for contamination of pasteurized products with raw milk and of preventing postpasteurization contamination with *Listeria* spp. and *Yersinia* spp. These efforts have resulted in a significant improvement in the quality of heat-treated milk and milk products in the USA. Most problems with pasteurized milk in Britain in recent years have been associated with pasteurization on farms and in small dairies. Now a British Standards code of practice for pasteurization of milk on farms and in small dairies (BS7771:1994) and guidelines for 'on farm' milk processors (ADAS 1996) have been published, which give guidance on process principles, design features and operation of equipment.

Evidence from a number of outbreak investigations has shown that it is not uncommon for operators to switch HTST pasteurizers to manual/clean mode during running, thereby removing the safety system and preventing flow diversion. This practice occurs most often with small producers who may be unaware of the exact sequence of events during flow diversion. In dairies that experience pasteurization failures, examination of thermograph records may show that soon after the milk temperature drops, initiating flow diversion, the plant has been switched to manual/clean mode, thus preventing the inevitable delay while the correct temperature is re-established. At the same time this has allowed inadequately heated milk to flow forward (Fig. 16.2).

The Dairy Products (Hygiene) Regulations 1995 for England and Wales state that HTST pasteurizers must have an automatic safety device to prevent insufficient heating and an automatic recording device that records operation of the safety system. The Regulations for Scotland also state that the record must include a record of when the cleaning mode is in operation. Some of the older designs of farm pasteurizers do not always incorporate chart recorders, which include a record of the operation of the safety system.

Process control in both large and small plants must include the whole plant. The hygiene of pipes, tanks, bottle or carton fillers and bottle washers should be monitored and the water supply must be of potable quality. Most dairies use mains tap water but occasionally the supply comes from another source. Whatever the source, water should be sampled regularly to check the microbiological quality. Where bottles are used, the final rinse consists of cold tap water and the bottles are not dried before filling with milk. This could potentially cause recontamination of milk and such a problem occurred many years ago when an outbreak of *Salmonella* Paratyphi B infections that continued for 2 years was eventually traced to river water supplying a pasteurization plant in South Wales (Thomas et al. 1948).

SALMONELLA OUTBREAKS

Cattle are the main reservoir of serotype Typhimurium and it is not surprising that this and other salmonella serotypes are frequently present in raw milk (Threlfall et al. 1980). Salmonellas and campylobacters are the pathogens most often associated with food poisoning outbreaks or incidents due to milk or milk products. Most of these are related to raw milk or raw milk products.

However, large processing dairies produce thousands of gallons of pasteurized milk daily and have the potential for causing major outbreaks if there is an unrecognized fault in the structure or operation of the plant. In 1985 such an outbreak occurred in Illinois, resulting in more than 16 000 confirmed cases of Typhimurium infection (Ryan et al. 1987, Report 1985). Investigations implicated 2% low fat milk, which had been processed at a dairy in Chicago. The fault seemed to be intermittent because batches of milk produced in August 1984 and in March and April 1985 caused infection. Subsequent investigations uncovered several contributing factors but the most likely explanation was postpasteurization contamination with raw milk that leaked through a valve from a pipe which linked the raw milk supply to another carrying pasteurized milk.

The plant had 400 miles of stainless steel pipes, hundreds of valves and many connections between pipes carrying raw and pasteurized milk. These connections were opened for in-place cleaning and closed by valves during milk processing. They provided opportunities for milk to bypass the pasteurization process through equipment failure or operator error (Lecos 1986). Other factors that probably contributed to the outbreak were the lack of proper training of dairy personnel and the absence of up-to-date diagrams of the plant and of plant inspection programmes (Kozak 1986).

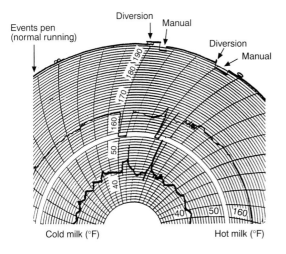

Fig. 16.2 Part of a pasteurizer thermograph chart demonstrating inappropriate use of manual/clean mode following flow diversion.

In March 1986 there was an outbreak of *Salmonella* Braenderup food poisoning due to pasteurized milk in East Anglia (Rampling, Taylor and Warren 1987); 54 patients, mostly children, were identified by culture and 8 were admitted to hospital. The epidemic serotype was isolated from the bulk raw milk of one of the farm suppliers. Examination of the pasteurizer thermograph charts showed that from time to time and, in particular, on the day that the production of contaminated milk was suspected, the pasteurizer was operated in the manual/clean mode with the automatic flow diversion mechanism switched off (Fig. 16.2). This could have allowed forward flow of inadequately heated milk into the pasteurized milk tank. There were also serious faults in the design of the associated plant which, as at Illinois, gave opportunities for milk to bypass the pasteurizer completely.

Numerous outbreaks of salmonellosis both in the UK and elsewhere have been traced to raw or improperly pasteurized milk and milk products (Schroeder 1967). On the other hand, there is no evidence that any milk-associated outbreak was due to asymptomatic carriage of a salmonella by a person. Both the dairy industry and those responsible for enforcing standards should concentrate attention on process control, particularly of pasteurization, instead of screening staff to detect harmless asymptomatic excreters of salmonellae (Editorial 1987).

The social and economic aspects of salmonellosis should not be underestimated. Infection ranges from symptomless excretion or mild nausea and diarrhoea to serious invasive illness that may result in admission to hospital or even, in a small proportion of cases, death. Costs affect the public sector and industry but those which are most difficult to quantify are borne by the infected individual and the family (Sockett and Roberts 1991). For further information on salmonella infections, see Chapter 41.

CAMPYLOBACTER

Faecal carriage of campylobacters is common in cattle and frequently results in contamination of milk. There is also good evidence that *C. jejuni* may cause clinical or subclinical mastitis resulting in the shedding of large numbers of organisms into the milk (Hudson et al. 1984, Hutchinson et al. 1985b, Orr et al. 1995). Several surveys have investigated the prevalence of campylobacters in milk from individual cows, farm bulk tanks and bottled unpasteurized milk. Results depend on the volume of milk analysed, the sensitivity of the method employed and on seasonal variations. Beumer, Cruysen and Birtantie (1988) examined 904 milk samples from individual cows on 13 farms in the Netherlands and showed that 4.5% were contaminated with *C. jejuni*. Humphrey and Hart (1988) examined 985 bottles or cartons of unpasteurized milk ready for sale and 153 samples from bulk milk tanks on 12 farms. *C. jejuni* was isolated from 5.9% of milk samples, from bottles or cartons and from bulk tanks. Rohrbach et al. (1992) surveyed bulk tank milk from 355 dairy producers in east Tennesee and southwest Virginia and showed that 12.3% contained *C. jejuni*.

The risk of infection following consumption of unpasteurized milk is substantial. Milk has been responsible for large numbers of outbreaks of campylobacter infection in many parts of the world (Skirrow 1991). Robinson (1981) demonstrated on himself that as few as 500 organisms mixed with 180 ml of pasteurized milk were sufficient to induce abdominal cramps, diarrhoea and an antibody response. Thus a low degree of contamination in a batch of milk could cause a large outbreak. Most outbreaks of campylobacter have been due to unpasteurized milk and more than one serotype may be incriminated in a single outbreak. Although *C. jejuni* does not multiply in milk, many strains survive for long periods and can be recovered from milk that has been stored for 14–21 days at 4°C. Pasteurization destroys even large numbers of organisms (Waterman 1982, D'Aoust et al. 1988) and properly controlled heat treatment is the most satisfactory way of ensuring that milk is free from campylobacters.

Wood, MacDonald and Osterholm (1992) conducted a 10 year retrospective survey in the USA and Puerto Rico and identified 20 outbreaks of campylobacter infection amongst children who had consumed raw milk during school field trips and organized youth activities. They identified 458 outbreak-associated cases from 1013 young persons who had drunk raw milk, an overall attack rate of 45%. They concluded that consumption of raw milk during these activities caused a significant but preventable public health problem in the USA.

Morgan et al. (1994) investigated an outbreak of campylobacter infections at a large music festival in southwest England where more than 70 000 people slept in tents and caravans and had very basic facilities for hygiene and sanitation. Two local farms had been issued with Temporary Producers Licences to enable them to sell raw milk at the festival and pasteurized milk was also available for sale. A case-control study based on 72 people with microbiologically confirmed *C. jejuni* infection investigated the possible association of infection with the consumption of various items of food, water or milk. Only the consumption of unpasteurized milk was shown to be associated with campylobacter infection with an odds ratio of 14.1 (95% confidence intervals 6.0–33.3). It was estimated that several hundred cases of campylobacter infection were linked with the festival. The supply of unpasteurized milk in this situation resulted in a significant but preventable public health problem.

Outbreaks of infection have also been associated with the consumption of milk from herds in which one or more animals have asymptomatic campylobacter mastitis. In this situation an outbreak could occur even though dairy hygiene is faultless and the milk achieves the microbiological standards for total plate count and coliforms. Orr et al. (1995) were alerted to a problem of milk-borne campylobacter infection when routine samples of bottled unpasteurized milk were culture-positive for the organism on 2 separate occasions 1 month apart. The milk came from a single dairy which supplied milk to a local village. Local general practitioners then identified 44 people who had had diarrhoea at about the time of the second positive finding. Faecal specimens were obtained from 16, 7 of which grew campylobacter.

Investigations on the farm revealed that although 6 of 10 cows that were sampled were excreting faecal campylobacters, another cow with negative faecal cultures and no clinical evidence of udder disease was excreting *C. jejuni* in milk. Improvements in general hygiene did not eliminate the problem of *C. jejuni* in bulk milk until the milk from the cow with subclinical mastitis was excluded from the tank. Typing of isolates by several methods showed that more than one strain was associated with the herd but that the source of infection for at least 2 of the patients was the cow that was excreting directly into the milk.

Outbreaks due to improperly pasteurized milk have also been documented on many occasions. In this circumstance large numbers of people may be put at risk. In 1979, 2500 children became ill after drinking free school milk supplied from a single milk processing plant in Luton. The campylobacter could not be isolated from the dairy or from raw milk but epidemiological studies strongly indicated milk as a source. A sample of milk taken 2 weeks after the outbreak failed the phosphatase test and inspection of the pasteurizer showed that raw milk could pass through the plant without treatment if the bypass system was operated incorrectly. Furthermore, there was evidence that the equipment had been used incorrectly on more than one occasion (Jones et al. 1981).

An outbreak of *C. jejuni* enteritis affecting schoolchildren and staff at a boarding school in Vermont in 1986 was traced to inadequate batch pasteurization of milk. Two serotypes of *C. jejuni* were isolated, from both the patients and the dairy cows. Samples of 'pasteurized' milk failed the phosphatase test (Birkhead and Vogt 1988).

During 1987, there were 2 more outbreaks of campylobacter infection in England and Wales, due to improperly pasteurized milk. More than 100 cases were confirmed by culture and serotyping following consumption of milk from a large dairy in East Anglia. A leaking valve and inappropriate use of the plant with the safeguards switched off were thought to be contributing factors (Rampling, Taylor and Warren 1987). Another outbreak in 1987 affected 346 students and staff at a field study centre in North Wales. Campylobacter was isolated from raw milk prior to pasteurization and once again investigations demonstrated deficiencies in pasteurization (Sockett 1991).

More recently in 1992 an outbreak in Northamptonshire affected at least 110 people of whom 41 had confirmed infection with *C. jejuni*. Consumption of pasteurized milk from a single farm dairy was implicated by case-control study. Investigation of the dairy showed that there were several problems with the pasteurizer, including an incorrectly wired element, and that the plant had been malfunctioning for some time (Fahey et al. 1995).

Finally, in recent years in England and Wales a new source of campylobacter contamination of pasteurized

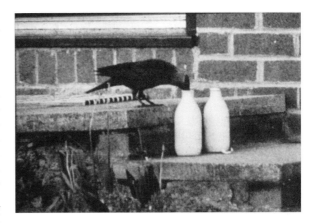

Fig. 16.3 Jackdaw attacking a milk bottle on a doorstep. (Courtesy of Dr NF Lightfoot, Director, PHLS North East).

milk, which may be responsible for many of the large numbers of sporadic infections that occur every year in the late spring, has been identified. During April, May, June 1989, during routine surveillance of campylobacter enteritis, a cluster of cases was identified in the western area of Gateshead. Many of those affected lived in newly developed housing adjacent to open countryside and most patients could remember that during the week prior to their illness they had consumed milk from bottles that had been pecked open by birds. In this area magpies and jackdaws commonly pecked at milk bottles on the doorstep and photographic evidence of this was obtained (Fig. 16.3). In addition, *C. jejuni* was isolated from milk in 2 of 5 damaged bottles but from none in intact bottles (Hudson et al. 1990, 1991). Further evidence was obtained by a case-control study of patients, a more detailed study of pecked milk bottles and by isolation of campylobacters from the bills of captured birds. These birds also eat carrion and animal dung, likely sources of campylobacters. Further evidence of this problem was obtained by studies in the Bridgend area of South Wales in May 1990 where a case-control study confirmed the association between campylobacter enteritis and consumption of bird-pecked milk (Southern, Smith and Palmer 1990). In May 1991 a point source outbreak in Exeter affected 11 children at a day nursery and was attributed to consumption of milk that had been pecked by magpies (Riordan, Humphrey and Fowles 1993). Evidence was obtained from a case-control study and by isolation of campylobacter from 2 bottles of milk that had been pecked. During 1990, 1991 and 1992, a number of other incidents of campylobacter infection attributed to bird-pecked milk were reported to CDSC and a publicity campaign was launched to warn the public to cover milk bottles to prevent such damage. It is likely, however, that this is a continuing cause of sporadic milk-associated infections. For further information on *Campylobacter* infections, see Chapter 54.

STREPTOCOCCUS ZOOEPIDEMICUS

S. zooepidemicus is an animal pathogen commonly associated with infection in horses but occasionally causing clinical or inapparent mastitis in cows. It has been associated with severe milk-borne illness in man. In 1968 there was an outbreak of infection among 74 adults and 11 children in a town in Romania, causing sore throat, fever and lymphadenitis, complicated by post-streptococcal glomerulonephritis in one-third of patients. Consumption of improperly pasteurized milk was implicated and *S. zooepidemicus* was isolated from cows with mastitis (Duca et al. 1969). In one week, 3 unrelated patients presented to the General Infirmary, Leeds, with *S. zooepidemicus* bacteraemia. One patient had meningitis, 2 had endocarditis and one subsequently died (Ghoneim and Cooke 1980). Investigations eventually confirmed that unpasteurized milk had been the source of infection in all 3 cases. In 1983, *S. zooepidemicus* infection was again associated with acute glomerulonephritis in 3 members of a north Yorkshire family who drank unpasteurized milk from their own cows (Barnham, Thornton and Lange 1983).

The most severe milk-associated outbreak of streptococcal infection in Britain in recent years was in West Yorkshire in 1984 (Edwards, Roulson and Ironside 1988): 12 people developed *S. zooepidemicus* septicaemia or meningitis, and 8 died following consumption of raw milk from a single supplier. Three cows in the herd were excreting the organism in the milk. In Australia a man developed septicaemia and glomerulonephritis due to *S. zooepidemicus* and 2 other members of the family were found to be asymptomatic throat carriers. The source of infection was unpasteurized milk from the house cow and typing demonstrated that the isolates from the 3 individuals and the cow's milk were indistinguishable from one another (Francis et al. 1993).

In England in 1994 an elderly couple who owned a dairy farm became ill and were admitted to hospital within days of one another (Report 1994c). The man developed fatal meningitis and *S. zooepidemicus* was isolated from his CSF. His wife had septic arthritis and the organism was isolated from pus from a knee joint aspirate. Another man who drank milk purchased at the farm gate became ill with empyema and subsequently died and a man who had eaten a chocolate cake made with cream from the farm developed endocarditis. *S. zooepidemicus* was also isolated from milk from the bulk tank and from one cow that appeared to have subclinical mastitis. Ribotyping of the isolates from the patients and the milk demonstrated that they were indistinguishable from one another (Burden, personal communication 1995).

It is clear that *S. zooepidemicus* is a rare but extremely serious cause of human illness. When it is diagnosed, milk should be suspected as the source of infection. For further information on streptococci, see Chapter 28.

CORYNEBACTERIUM ULCERANS

Although *C. ulcerans* usually causes only a mild sore throat, it can cause an illness indistinguishable from classic diphtheria. The organism is culturally similar to *Corynebacterium diphtheriae* var. *gravis* but is identified by the production of urease and of the exotoxins of both *C. diphtheriae* and *Corynebacterium ovis*. Cattle seem to be the main reservoir of infection and occasionally excrete the organism in milk. Isolated cases of human infection, including one of classic diphtheria, were identified by Meers (1979) in Devon and Cornwall. He postulated that some of the outbreaks of milk-borne diphtheria, which at one time were common in Britain, may have been caused by *C. ulcerans*. The organism does not seem to be prevalent in cattle nowadays but Hart (1984) isolated it from a patient with a sore throat and from one symptomless carrier, both of whom lived in a farming community. Of the 30 cattle on the farm, 8 were excreting toxigenic *C. ulcerans*. Hart also surveyed 52 other dairy herds in north Devon and found toxigenic *C. ulcerans* in milk from 4 of the herds.

STREPTOBACILLUS MONILIFORMIS

This organism causes a febrile septicaemic illness in man, characterized by an erythematous rash, most prominent on the hands and feet, arthralgia and sore throat. The disease was first described in Haverhill, Massachusetts, where an explosive outbreak affected 86 people and was termed 'erythema arthriticum epidemicum' (EAE). The outbreak was due to consumption of contaminated raw milk (Place and Sutton 1934). In February 1983 an outbreak of EAE affected 130 children attending a boarding school in Chelmsford, Essex. *S. moniliformis* was isolated from the blood of 4 of the children and unpasteurized milk from a local farm was again the suspected source of infection (Shanson et al. 1983).

YERSINIA ENTEROCOLITICA

The reported isolation rates of *Y. enterocolitica* from samples of raw milk vary from 14.3% to 48.1%. Most strains have the biochemical characteristics of environmental, non-pathogenic strains and are non-typable or belong to serotypes not associated with human illness; they presumably lack the specific resistance plasmid (Schiemann 1987). A few isolates from milk are pathogenic, however, and yersinia infection has been associated with consumption of raw milk in England and Wales and in the USA.

Case-control studies implicated pasteurized milk in a large multistate outbreak of yersiniosis in the USA in 1982 (Tacket et al. 1984); 172 infections were identified by culture. Enteritis occurred in 148 patients, mostly children, and extraintestinal infection in 24 adults. Appendicectomy was performed on 17 patients with intestinal infection. Investigations did not reveal any fault in the pasteurization process but indirect evidence that milk was the source was obtained by isolating the same unusual serotype (O:13,18) from the outside of a milk crate on a pig farm where outdated milk was used as pig feed. Another outbreak, in 1976 (Black et al. 1978), resulted in admission to hospital of 36 schoolchildren, 16 of whom had appendicectomies. Evidence from a case-control study implicated chocolate milk but chocolate syrup was added to the milk after pasteurization and this may also have been a source of the organism.

Y. enterocolitica can survive and replicate at refrigeration temperatures but although one strain of yersinia able to survive laboratory pasteurization has been reported, there is good evidence that HTST pasteurization will destroy all viable organisms (Francis, Spaulding and Lovett 1980). The presence of pathogenic yersiniae in pasteurized milk implies a fault during pasteurization or contamination afterwards (D'Aoust et al. 1988, Greenwood, Hooper and Rodhouse 1990).

LISTERIA MONOCYTOGENES

During the 1980s there was a world-wide rise in the number of outbreaks and sporadic cases of human listeriosis. The first conclusive evidence of acquisition of the infection from food was produced by Schlech et al. (1983) who described an outbreak in 1981 which was associated with contaminated coleslaw. Since then it has become clear that many foods, including milk and, in particular, soft cheese, may be contaminated with *L. monocytogenes* and may occasionally cause outbreaks or sporadic cases of human listeriosis (McLauchlin 1993).

L. monocytogenes is prevalent in farm environments, in the faeces of cattle and in raw milk (Slade, Fistrovici and Collins-Thompson 1989, Rampling et al. 1992, Sanaa et al. 1993, Fenlon, Stewart and Donachie 1995). In addition, the organism survives well in moist environments and multiplies slowly at refrigerator temperatures. Although it is killed by pasteurization, there may be opportunity for post-process contamination from plant or machinery. Food manufacturers, including manufacturers of dairy products, are very much aware of the problems of *L. monocytogenes* and are now very active in carrying out surveillance for this organism in environments and products.

Samples of milk from farm bulk tanks have shown that a high proportion (up to 16%) may be contaminated with *L. monocytogenes* at any one time. However, contamination is usually sporadic and persistent contamination seems to be rare. It can result from faecal contamination or from direct shedding by a cow with subclinical mastitis (Slade, Fistrovici and Collins-Thompson 1989, Fenlon, Stewart and Donachie 1995). Sanaa et al. (1993) carried out a detailed study of 128 selected dairy farms to assess the risk factors for contamination of milk with *L. monocytogenes*. They confirmed the findings of previous studies that poor quality silage (pH >4.0) was a major risk factor. Other predisposing conditions were infrequent cleaning of the cattle exercise area, obvious faecal soiling of udders, thighs and anal regions, insufficient lighting in milking barns or parlours, which presumably made it difficult to ensure optimal hygiene during milking, and inadequate disinfection of udder cloths between milkings.

Most of the isolates found in surveys of raw milk belong to serovar 1. More detailed subtyping by multi-enzyme electrophoresis (MEE) has indicated that many isolates belong to subtypes that are unique to milk or to the environment and are not associated with human or animal disease. However, Fenlon, Stewart and Donachie (1995) showed that whereas isolates from 25 of 160 milk producers could be subgrouped into 9 different electrophoresis types, most of which were unique to milk, some isolates belonged to a type that had been associated with human infection.

In most instances liquid milk is probably the original source of *L. monocytogenes* in a dairy product but the environment of dairy plants may also provide a reservoir of contamination from milk and other sources (Cotton and White 1992, Jacquet, Rocourt and Reynaud 1993, Peeler and Bunning 1994). In particular, processing plants that are adjacent to dairy farms are more likely to be contaminated with *Listeria* spp. than processing plants without on-site dairy farms (Pritchard et al. 1994).

The first evidence to suggest that raw milk could be a source of human infection came from Halle in Germany where Reiss, Potel and Krebs (1951) described a pathological condition of stillborn infants which they called **granulomatosis infantiseptica** on account of the distinctive focal necrosis found throughout the bodies. A series of outbreaks of this condition occurred over a long period from 1949 to 1957. Initially the organism responsible was identified as a new species of *Corynebacterium* but was later recognized as *L. monocytogenes*. These outbreaks were considered to be due to the ingestion of unpasteurized milk (Seeliger 1961).

In 1983 pasteurized milk was implicated in an outbreak in the USA: 49 patients were admitted to hospital in Massachusetts with meningitis, septicaemia or abortion due to *L. monocytogenes* serotype 4b (Fleming et al. 1985). Case-control studies demonstrated that infection was associated with consumption of a specific brand of whole or semiskimmed pasteurized milk; there had been an outbreak of encephalitis due to *L. monocytogenes* in one of the herds which supplied milk to the dairy. There was, however, no evidence of failure of pasteurization.

Recently, retrospective analysis of isolates of *L. monocytogenes* from 4 patients with invasive listeriosis demonstrated an unequivocal association with the consumption of chocolate milk from a dairy in Illinois. Luchansky (1995) reported an investigation in Wisconsin in 1994 which followed recall of 4 dairy products due to detection of contamination with *L. monocytogenes*. One of these products was a 1% low fat chocolate milk which had been stored at inappropriate temperatures and contained 10^9 cfu per ml of serovar 1/2b. It had been implicated in a small outbreak of fever and gastroenteritis in a group of picnickers. The Wisconsin Division of Health then identified 4 patients retrospectively who had suffered typical invasive listeriosis and had also drunk the recalled chocolate milk.

CRYPTOSPORIDIOSIS

An outbreak of acute gastroenteritis due to cryptosporidiosis occurred amongst children at a primary school in Yorkshire in September 1995. There were 52 cases of whom 50 were pupils at the school and 2 were secondary cases. Initially water was suspected as the likely source of infection but a case-control study implicated school milk supplied by a small producer with an on-farm pasteurizer. Subsequent investigation at the farm revealed that the pasteurizer had been failing intermittently and had not been working properly at the time of the outbreak (CDSC, unpublished information).

Vero cytotoxin-producing *Escherichia coli*

Certain strains of *E. coli* produce toxins that affect cultured Vero cells (African green monkey kidney cells). Some of these Vero cytotoxin-producing *E. coli* (VTEC) are pathogenic for man and cause disease which ranges from mild diarrhoea to haemorrhagic colitis. Illness is quite frequently complicated by haemolytic–uraemic syndrome (HUS) which most often affects children and is characterized by anaemia, thrombocytopenia and renal failure that may be permanent. Rarely, thrombotic thrombocytopenic purpura (TTP) develops in which, in addition to renal failure and severe thrombocytopenia, there is thrombus formation which may affect the brain.

Most outbreaks and sporadic cases of human VTEC infection in North America and Great Britain have been associated with one particular serovar, *E. coli* O157:H7 and with consumption of foods of bovine origin, in particular minced beef and raw cows' milk (Griffin and Tauxe 1993, Report of the Advisory Committee on the Microbiological Safety of Food 1995). Although many different VTEC are associated with clinical infection in farm animals, especially calves and pigs, *E. coli* O157:H7 does not seem to cause clinical infection of animals but has been isolated from healthy cattle and dairy calves (Wells et al. 1991, Chapman et al. 1993).

In April 1986 there was a large outbreak of colitis in 60 kindergarten children who had visited a dairy farm in southwest Ontario, where they drank unpasteurized milk (Borczyk et al. 1987); 48 children developed diarrhoea and abdominal cramps. Evidence of infection with *E. coli* serotype O157:H7 was demonstrated by isolating the organism or by detecting Vero cytotoxin in the faeces of 43 patients and by isolation of the organisms from the faeces of 2 cows. Later, Martin et al. (1986) investigated 2 cases of haemolytic–uraemic syndrome in young children. The first patient was a boy aged 13 months who regularly drank raw milk, and the second was a girl aged 5 months who drank raw milk just once, 10 days before becoming ill. *E. coli* serotype O157:H7 was isolated from a faecal specimen from the boy and also from cattle in both dairy herds which supplied the milk. In December 1992 there was a community outbreak in Oregon, USA, that was associated with the consumption of raw milk. Eight people were affected and 2 were hospitalized (Report of the Advisory Committee on the Microbiological Safety of Food 1995).

Three outbreaks in the UK have been convincingly associated with raw milk and with inadequately pasteurized milk, respectively. A community outbreak occurred in Sheffield in 1993 in which 11 patients, mostly children, were affected with *E. coli* O157:H7, PT2, VT2 and 3 developed HUS (Table 16.1). The organism was also isolated from farmyard slurry, 10 of 105 rectal swabs from dairy cattle and milk from one rectal culture-positive cow at the farm which supplied the milk. All isolates from patients, milk, cattle and slurry were *E. coli* O157:H7, PT2, VT2 and harboured a single 92 kb plasmid. This was the first incident of *E. coli* O157 infection in the UK in which a suspect food source was confirmed by culturing the outbreak organism (Chapman and Wright 1993). A longitudinal study of infection in the dairy commenced in 1993 and showed that although 29 of 130 cows secreted *E. coli* O157 on one or more occasions during the following year, there was no evidence of clinical disease (Report of the Advisory Committee on the Microbiological Safety of Food 1995).

In 1996, cases of infection with *E. coli* O157, PT1 in West Yorkshire were associated with the consumption of unpasteurized milk and the organism was isolated from a bottle of the milk (Report 1996). In May 1994 an outbreak of *E. coli* O157 infection involved a pasteurized milk supply in West Lothian, Scotland (Upton and Coia 1994). Over a 24 h period, 12 suspected and 7 confirmed cases of *E. coli* O157 infection were reported in the same local authority district. All had haemorrhagic colitis and 3 had HUS. Initial investigation suggested that milk from a local dairy could be the source. Milk production was suspended within 36 h of the report of the first cluster of cases. During the following 7 days it became clear that more than 100 people were affected. Sixty-nine had infection confirmed by culture and one was confirmed by serology. Forty-six were under 15 years of age and of these 32 were under 5 years. Almost one-third of patients required hospital admission and HUS developed in 9 children. Six required dialysis of whom 2 now have chronic renal failure. One child who did not have HUS died due to perforation of the large bowel. One elderly woman developed TTP. More than 90% of patients had consumed pasteurized milk from the local dairy and at least 7 cases resulted from secondary spread within households. Environmental investigation at the dairy and at the farms which supplied the dairy yielded isolates of *E. coli* O157 from faecal specimens from cattle, raw milk from the bulk tank at one of the farms, from a pipe which carried milk from the pasteurizer to the bottling machine, and from a discarded bottling machine rubber at the dairy. The isolates from the patients, the farm and the dairy were indistinguishable from one another by typing. All were *E. coli* O157:H7, PT2, VT2 and displayed identical restriction endonuclease digestion profiles as demonstrated by pulse field gel electrophoresis (PFGE) (Upton, personal communication 1995).

These 2 outbreaks, in addition to outbreaks incriminating yoghurt and cheese (see section 4, p. 382, and section 7, p. 385) confirm that raw milk or inadequately pasteurized milk may be an important source of human infection with *E. coli* O157 in the UK. In the light of this evidence the Advisory Committee on the Microbiological Safety of Food (Report of the Advisory Committee on the Microbiological Safety of Food 1995) has recommended that the Government should reconsider banning all sales of raw cows' milk in England and Wales and that raw cows' cream should be subject to the same regulations as raw cows' milk. They also recommend that the industry ensures that the pasteurization of milk and milk products is carefully controlled and that postpasteurization contamination is avoided.

There is evidence that other serotypes of VTEC that occasionally cause outbreaks of human illness may be derived from milk. In 1994, 4 persons in Helena, Montana, USA developed bloody diarrhoea due to *E. coli* O104:H21. Further case finding investigations revealed 11 confirmed and 7 suspected patients and a case-control study implicated one specific brand of pasteurized milk as the source of infection (Moore et al. 1995).

Selective culture techniques from *E. coli* non-O157 VTEC are not available and it is possible that sporadic cases or even outbreaks due to these organisms may be associated with milk, yet go undetected. For further information on VTEC, see Chapter 40.

Bacillus cereus and Bacillus anthracis

Spores of *B. cereus* are common in the farm environment and inevitably contaminate raw milk. The extent of contamination can be controlled by careful washing of the udder and teats prior to milking. Postpasteurization contamination may also contribute to the numbers of spores and the organism can grow readily and produce toxin in milk. *B. cereus* is a common cause of sweet curdling and bitty cream but documented cases of food poisoning due to *B. cereus* in milk are rare. However, in 1972 an outbreak of abdominal pain and diarrhoea of short duration affected 221 school-children in Romania after drinking contaminated milk. Two incidents documented in 1981 in Denmark involved a boy aged 12 months who drank curdled milk and a baby aged 6 months who developed diarrhoea and vomiting after drinking contaminated expressed breast milk (Christiansson 1992).

Milk-transmitted anthrax is more of a theoretical than a real danger but difficulties may arise regarding the action to be taken with milk that has been derived from a dairy herd in which anthrax infection is subsequently diagnosed. The chance that such milk could be contaminated is very remote because anthrax bacilli are not excreted in milk until bacteraemia develops. This occurs just prior to death at which stage it is likely that milk secretion will have ceased and, furthermore, the animal would be obviously ill and unsuitable for milking. Experiments have also shown that both spores and vegetative cells of *B. anthracis* (unlike those of *B. cereus*) disappear rapidly in milk (Bowen and Turnbull 1992) and infectivity of *B. anthracis* is low by the oral route.

Recent advice from the Department of Health (London, UK) (PL/CO(95)3 plus appendix and addendum) is that milk from animals known or suspected of being infected with anthrax at the time of milking must be excluded from the rest of the milk supply and sterilized (Anthrax Order 1991). The rest of the milk from the herd or flock must be pasteurized before being offered for sale. Where milk has already entered the public supply or where there is a suspicion that bulk milk may contain milk from an animal that could be suffering from anthrax or has died from the disease, pasteurization should suffice to protect the consumer against the risk of anthrax after consuming the milk.

2 Milk powder

Commercial drying of milk was introduced at the beginning of the twentieth century. The roller method was developed first followed by the spray method in the 1930s. Both were in operation until the 1950s when the spray method assumed popularity because it gave a more palatable product. For a detailed account of the various processes and designs of plant see Knipschildt and Anderson (1994).

The process is in 2 stages: preliminary concentration during which 90% of the water is removed by evaporation, followed by rapid drying. Before concentration, the milk must be preheated to pasteurization temperatures to kill vegetative pathogenic bacteria. The roller-drying process consists of feeding preconcentrated milk over rotating drums heated to 150°C by steam. The thin dry film of milk is scraped off by a sharp blade and falls into collecting troughs. The dry film attains a high temperature and has a low bacterial count. This method was favoured for the production of baby food for many years because of its exceptional safety record and was used in Britain for the manufacture of National Dried Milk during the war. Disadvantages of roller-drying are the cooked flavour and poor solubility of the product due to denaturation of protein. For the spray-drying process, concentrated milk is fed from vacuum evaporators to a balance tank and then through fine jets or rotary atomizers into the top of a large chamber supplied with filtered hot air. Dry powder is collected from the bottom of the chamber. Spray-drying is a mild process and the product has better physical properties than roller-dried powder. An extra process called 'instantization' is sometimes added to make the powder more rapidly soluble. The powder is rewetted with steam to about 14% moisture and dried again to form fine agglomerates. Lecithin may be added at this stage to increase wettability.

The microbiological quality of spray-dried milk is much less reliable than that of the roller-dried product. The development of processing conditions which minimize nutrient change and improve physical and organoleptic properties has increased the microbiological hazards (Lovell 1990). Spray-dried milk has been responsible for many outbreaks of food poisoning due to enterotoxigenic *S. aureus* and to salmonellae. The safety of the process relies on adequate preheating to destroy vegetative pathogenic organisms; if, however, they survive this stage, there is opportunity for them to multiply in the evaporators and the balance tank and thus for heavily contaminated milk to enter the spray-drier. Although hot air enters the spray-drier at over 160°C, cooling is rapid. There is good evidence that salmonellae can survive the drying process (McDonough and Hargrove 1968) and that the heat treatment is insufficient to inactivate *S. aureus* or its enterotoxin. Because of the complexity of the plant it is very difficult, if not impossible, to eradicate contamination once established in the plant or its environment.

In 1953, several outbreaks of staphylococcal food poisoning in schools near London were traced to powdered milk from the same source. Later that year, another outbreak in Yorkshire was traced to milk powder from a different source (Anderson and Stone 1955). Tests on batches of milk powder from the plant involved in the first outbreak demonstrated that on 2 days during May the total bacterial count was considerably higher than on other days and that there were approximately 10^4 *S. aureus* per gram. The organism was not detected in batches with low total counts. Other studies indicated that toxin was probably produced at some stage before the drying process. Investigations at another plant not implicated in the outbreaks showed that bacteria multiplied in the balance tank throughout the 12 h of continuous processing. There was also evidence that small amounts of contamination remained after cleaning and recontaminated the pasteurized concentrated milk as it passed through the tank (Hobbs 1955). Other studies have indicated that *S. aureus* contamination may occur during manufacture and that isolates from milk powder may not necessarily be the same as those in the raw milk (Lovell 1990). Harvey and Gilmour (1990) examined milk powders from 5 different processors in Northern Ireland for both *S. aureus* and coagulase-negative staphylococci. They found that low total viable counts were associated with low total staphylococcal counts but that 5 of 37 samples had high total counts and high counts of coagulase-negative staphylococci. The powders with high counts contained added fat which was mixed into the milk after pasteurization and concentration but prior to drying. No *S. aureus* or staphylococcal enterotoxins were detected but this study highlighted a potential source of contamination with micro-organisms which are able to survive the drying process. Even coagulase-negative staphylococci are undesirable as some strains can produce enterotoxins.

However, staphylococcal intoxication from dried milk does not seem to have caused many problems since the general introduction of refrigerated farm bulk milk tanks, which maintain raw milk at a temperature that inhibits multiplication and toxin production by staphylococci (Morgan-Jones 1987). There is one report from El-Dairouty (1989) that suggests that the problem has not disappeared entirely. He describes a series of food poisoning incidents involving 21 patients who consumed non-fat dried milk in Egypt in 1986.

Salmonella infection has been associated with the consumption of powdered milk on several occasions and its occurrence in dried milk is well documented. In 1966, an outbreak of *Salmonella* Newbrunswick

infection in the USA was associated with spray-dried milk (Collins et al. 1968). Following this episode the US Food and Drugs Administration instituted a large-scale testing programme (Marth 1969) and 156 milk plants in 56 states were examined. Of 2741 samples tested, 24 samples of non-fat dried milk and 27 environmental samples contained salmonellae. Later, in 1967, 200 factories in 19 states were surveyed: 1% of 3315 product samples and 8. 2% of 1475 environmental samples were positive for salmonellae. In total, 13% of the plants tested were manufacturing milk powder contaminated with salmonellae. These surveys also demonstrated the value of taking environmental rather than product samples to monitor for pathogenic bacteria.

Outbreaks have continued to occur in the USA. Pickett and Agate (1967) isolated a lactose-positive strain of *Salmonella* Newington from instant non-fat milk powder which had been responsible for 9 cases of salmonellosis. *Salmonella* Newport was isolated from dried skimmed milk and from 20 patients with diarrhoea and vomiting in Newfoundland (Marth 1969) and an outbreak of *Salmonella* Agona and *S.* Typhimurium infection was traced to powdered milk in Oregon (Furlong et al. 1979).

These episodes in North America are not unique. In England and Wales *S.* Typhimurium infection has been traced to spray-dried milk on several occasions (Galbraith, Forbes and Clifford 1982). In Australia, *Salmonella* Bredeney, harboured in the insulating material of a spray-drier, provided a continuing source of contamination for the milk powder via cracks in the stainless steel lining of the drier (Craven 1978). In Trinidad, approximately 3000 people, predominantly infants and small children, were infected with *Salmonella* Derby which was traced to contaminated powdered milk produced on the island (Weissman et al. 1977).

In November and December 1985, there was a cluster of *Salmonella* Ealing infections in infants in England and Wales (Rowe et al. 1987). Investigations showed that 76 people, including 48 babies, had been infected and that a smaller cluster of cases had occurred in May, June and July 1985. Seven of the babies were admitted to hospital and one died. A case-control study implicated dried milk from one manufacturer. *S.* Ealing was isolated from an unopened packet of baby food from the home of a patient and from 4 other packets from the same batch. Investigations at the factory revealed that the inside of the spray-drier had several minor pinholes and weld cracks and that there was an irregular hole 1×3 cm in the metal lining. Removal of the metal outer casing at the site of the hole showed stained insulation material and a large collection of discoloured milk powder. *S.* Ealing was isolated from the insulation material and the milk powder in continuity with the hole but not from the dry insulation material on the opposite side of the drier. It was thus likely that infected milk had gained access to the insulation material from the inside of the drier through the hole in the metal lining and had then remained within its wall as a continual source of contamination. *S.* Ealing was also found in the factory vacuum system and in a silo containing waste milk powder and sweepings. Examination of the pasteurizer revealed pinhole defects in the plate heat exchanger which could have been sufficient to allow contamination of the pasteurized milk with raw milk. *S.* Ealing was known to be present in one of the herds that supplied milk to the dairy in April 1985 and the organism may have gained access to the factory at that time.

The many incidents of infection associated with spray-dried milk have caused much concern among manufacturers and public health microbiologists. There has also been controversy about standards for total bacterial counts and the relevance of total counts as a method of monitoring quality and the frequency of sampling required. A standard for total count of no more than 50 000 per g after incubation for 3 days at 30°C is generally accepted (Lovell 1990) but in practice counts of less than 1000 per g can be achieved. It is customary to perform quality control tests on each batch of powder before releasing it for sale. As was clearly demonstrated by the surveys in the USA in 1966 and 1967, however, this practice is by no means as sensitive for detecting pathogens as testing the dust and waste powder in the factory environment. An obviously dangerous practice in some milk powder factories is the custom of blending powder with high bacterial counts into powder with low counts in order to give an apparently satisfactory final product (Rowe et al. 1987).

Mettler (1989) has reviewed the issues raised by the *S.* Ealing and other salmonella incidents. He points out that production of pathogen-free milk powder requires detailed committed attention to good manufacturing practice involving every aspect of the process, including design of equipment, management, staff training and discipline and control of the environment, including air quality. In addition, sampling programmes should be detailed and targeted and include the environment as well as the product; the test methodology should be assessed critically in relation to the detection of pathogens. Regular and thorough crack testing of the spray dryer should also be an essential part of the quality control programme. In the long term it should be possible to design spray-drying chambers that do not have this intrinsic fault and it should be possible to improve the processing equipment at all stages so that a buildup of micro-organisms does not occur.

More recently, guidelines for the hygienic manufacture of spray-dried milk powders have been issued by the International Dairy Federation (Report 1991a) but incidents continue to occur. In 1993 Louie et al. reported that 3 cases of *Salmonella* Tennessee infection in infants had been traced to the consumption of one particular brand of powdered infant formula and that this organism had also been isolated from production equipment at the spray-drying plant and from cans of powdered milk formula.

Salmonella spp. and *S. aureus* are the pathogens which have been associated with dried milk most often but other organisms have also caused public health problems. Three cases of neonatal meningitis due to *Enterobacter sakazakii* from infant milk formula were diagnosed in 1986 and 1987 at the National University Hospital, Reykjavik, Iceland (Biering et al. 1989). Two neonates who were normal at birth survived with severe brain damage and a third, who had Down's syndrome, died. *E. sakazakii* was isolated from cerebrospinal fluid from the 3 babies with meningitis and from urine of a fourth infant who had no signs of infection. It was also isolated by enrichment culture from 5 unopened packages of milk powder. All isolates from the babies and all but one of 23 isolates from the infant formula had identical biotypes, antibiograms and plasmid profiles. Other workers have isolated *E. sakazakii* from powdered milk (Muytjens, Roelofs-Willemse and Jaspar 1988) and powdered infant milk has been suspected in the past as a source of neonatal infection with this organism (Muytjens et al. 1983). These incidents confirm the importance of implementing the strictest possible measures for the control of microbiological quality during the manufacture of milk powder and in particular of infant milk. The Reykjavik outbreak demonstrated that even low numbers of *E. sakazakii* were significant perhaps because of the extreme susceptibility of the patients but also possibly because there was opportunity for multiplication in the reconstituted formula.

B. cereus is another contaminant of raw milk that is commonly present in milk powder (Becker et al. 1994, Crielly, Logan and Anderton 1994). The endospores are heat-resistant and able to survive the pasteurization and drying process. Indeed, replication may be encouraged at various stages of the production process and, in the case of infant formula, further contamination may be introduced with added ingredients. Once reconstituted there is opportunity for germination of spores, growth and enterotoxin production depending on the temperature of storage. In spite of this, *B. cereus* has rarely been documented as a cause of food poisoning associated with dried milk (Christiansson 1992, Becker et al. 1994). Finally, *C. perfringens* is another sporing organism which is a theoretical risk but has rarely been implicated in food poisoning due to powdered milk (Lovell 1990).

3 CREAM

Unless hygiene is strict, environmental contamination of cream may be considerable because of the many stages of handling during processing. When cream is separated by centrifugation most of the bacteria from the whole milk are separated with the cream. In addition, separation is often performed at 40–50°C which is a temperature that encourages the growth of many micro-organisms (Milner 1995). However, cream is normally subjected to higher pasteurization temperatures (up to 80°C) than milk and is expected to have a longer shelf-life (Davis and Wilbey 1990).

In 1970, a PHLS working party examined 4385 heat-treated, 282 clotted and 517 raw samples of cream

(Working Party to the Director of the Public Health Advisory Service 1971). Bacterial counts were frequently high and, although the unheated creams were the most unsatisfactory, many heat-treated creams also contained large numbers of bacteria including coliforms, thereby indicating either postpasteurization contamination or inadequate heat treatment. From 3417 samples examined, *S. aureus* was isolated from 59, 54 of which were unpasteurized. Other pathogens found in untreated samples were one isolation each of *S.* Typhimurium, *B. abortus* and *E. coli* serotype O126. *C. perfringens* was isolated from one heat-treated sample.

3.1 Infections and intoxications associated with cream

Raw cream is as likely as raw milk to contain pathogenic bacteria (Rothwell 1979). It is, however, surprising that few outbreaks have been attributed either to raw or to heat-treated cream. This may be because relatively small volumes are produced and sporadic infections are seldom reported. Furthermore, cream is usually incorporated into desserts, cakes, sauces, etc., and it may be difficult to incriminate the cream alone in the event of an outbreak. Food poisoning due to enterotoxigenic *S. aureus* was a well recognized hazard associated with cream before the introduction of farm refrigeration tanks and refrigerated storage in shops and homes. When detailed investigations have been made, the source of the organism has usually proved to be a cow or cows with symptomatic or asymptomatic *S. aureus* mastitis. Isolation of the same phage type of *S. aureus* from individual cows, from the cream and from patients with food poisoning has been reported (Steede and Smith 1954).

Raw and pasteurized cream have also been associated with many small incidents of salmonella food poisoning, often related to overt infections in cows or calves on the farms supplying the milk (Vernon and Tillett 1974, Sharp, Paterson and Barrett 1985). There have also been incidents of *B. cereus* food poisoning associated with cream (Galbraith, Forbes and Clifford 1982, Sockett 1991).

The potential risk associated with the consumption of raw cream was demonstrated in the recent outbreak of infections with *S. zooepidemicus* which occurred in the home counties of England in 1994. An elderly patient who developed endocarditis due to this organism acquired his infection by eating a chocolate cream cake made with contaminated raw cream (Burden, personal communication 1995). It is probable that he was unaware that the cream was unpasteurized.

4 YOGHURT

A wide variety of drinks and semi-solid foods are prepared by the fermentation of milk and yoghurt is by far the most popular. Nearly all yoghurt is made in large dairies under carefully controlled conditions but there is increasing interest in small-scale farm production, particularly from sheep and goat milks.

There are 2 systems for commercial manufacture (Robinson and Tamime 1993). In one, incubation and fermentation are performed in the retail container, resulting in **set yoghurt**. In the other, fermentation takes place in large tanks and the coagulum is stirred to produce a thick viscous fluid (**stirred yoghurt**) which is cooled and packaged by automatic fillers. Fruits or flavourings are added to stirred yoghurt after fermentation is completed and to set yoghurt before fermentation. Stirred yoghurt is sometimes pasteurized to give it an extended shelf-life.

The first stage of manufacture for both products is preparation and standardization of the milk mix. Fresh milk is preheated and separated through a centrifugal separator. The concentration of total solids in the skimmed milk is increased, either by evaporation to 15–16% or by adding milk powder. If a medium or full fat yoghurt is required, a monitored amount of cream and sugar is added. Stabilizers, such as pregelatinized starch or plant gums, may also be included at this stage. The mix must be homogenized if cream is added, otherwise separation will occur during incubation. Homogenization also increases the viscosity.

The mix is heat treated to kill pathogenic and spoilage organisms and to expel air in order to produce microaerophilic conditions for the fermentation. The optimum heat treatment for improving the physical state of the coagulum is a high temperature, long time treatment (85°C for 30 min). This is done in large tanks containing mechanical stirrers and heated by water jackets. The tanks are then cooled to 40–45°C, inoculated with the starter cultures and held at constant temperature until fermentation is complete after 3½–4½ h. Many dairies find this system too slow and prefer to treat the mix in a UHT pasteurizer (85°C for 2 s) before filling the fermentation tanks or the small volume containers used for set yoghurt.

Almost without exception, commercial producers use *Streptococcus thermophilus* and *Lactobacillus bulgaricus* in a ratio of 1:1 as a starter culture for fermenting yoghurt. The cultures are grown in milk in bulk starter vats and added to the basic mix to give a final concentration of 1–2% (v/v). An incubation temperature of 40–42°C is usually selected for the fermentation. This temperature lies between the optima for acid production by the 2 species (39°C for *S. thermophilus* and 45°C for *L. bulgaricus*). The 2 organisms grow symbiotically; *S. thermophilus* produces metabolites that encourage the growth of *L. bulgaricus*. *S. thermophilus* produces most of the lactic acid early in the fermentation, but later both organisms produce aldehydes and other fermentation products important for flavour. The final acidity is greater if the 2 cultures are grown together than if either is grown alone. A final concentration of 1% lactic acid (pH 4–4.2) should be achieved. Strict quality control is essential to ensure that starters are active and free from bacterial and bacteriophage contamination, and that the milk is free from antibiotics which would inhibit growth of the starter.

4.1 Microbiological quality of yoghurt

Yoghurt mix is heated to very high temperatures before fermentation. It should therefore be free from pathogenic and spoilage organisms but opportunities exist for contamination during fermentation and packaging. Additions such as fruit or flavourings may also carry contaminants. However, it is generally a very safe product because most potential pathogens are inactivated by the high level of acidity and antibiotic substances produced by the starter cultures (Robinson and Tamime 1990). *Campylobacter* spp. and *Salmonella* spp. are inactivated rapidly in yoghurt or fermented milks but under experimental conditions both *Y. enterocolitica* and *L. monocytogenes* can survive for several weeks in the refrigerated product (Schaack and Marth 1988, Ashenafi 1994, Aytac and Ozbas 1994). Between 1988 and 1991 a survey of the occurrence of *Listeria* spp. in milk and dairy products in England and Wales included 180 samples of yoghurt. *L. monocytogenes* was isolated from 4 yoghurt samples (one made from cows' milk, 2 from goats' milk and one from ewes' milk) (Greenwood, Roberts and Burden 1991). However, yoghurt does not seem to have been associated with any cases of human clinical infection due to *L. monocytogenes* or *Y. enterocolitica*.

Provided that yoghurt is produced under carefully controlled conditions with the correct starter cultures, pathogenic bacteria, but not their toxins or spores, should die out rapidly. The quality of added ingredients is equally important and these should be subject to the same quality control. An outbreak of staphylococcal food poisoning involving at least 67 people was traced to **dahi** (Indian yoghurt) made in a shop in Calcutta (Saha and Ganguli 1957). The suspected source was contaminated milk powder added to the mix just before incubation. It was clear that there was a fault in the fermentation process because it took 36 h to complete. The staphylococcal enterotoxin was presumably elaborated during this time.

Until 1989 there were no records of outbreaks of human infection associated with yoghurt in England or Wales or Europe (Galbraith, Forbes and Clifford 1982, Sharp 1987). In June 1989, however, yoghurt was associated with the biggest outbreak of botulism in Britain during this century (O'Mahony et al. 1990). Between 30 May and 13 June 1989, 27 cases of botulism, with one death, were traced to the consumption of low fat hazelnut yoghurt. *Clostridium botulinum* type B toxin was detected in the contents of an unopened can of the hazelnut purée used to flavour the yoghurts, and from unopened cartons of yoghurt. The yoghurt was made in the northwest of England, and the hazelnut purée was supplied in 6 lb cans by a factory in Folkestone. The hazelnut purée was sweetened with aspartamine, rather than sugar which might have prevented bacterial growth, and insufficient heat had been used in the manufacturing process to destroy spores of *C. botulinum*.

In the autumn of 1991 an unusual outbreak of *E. coli* O157:H7 PT 49 infections was associated with consumption of a brand of live yoghurt made specially for children by a farm producer in the northwest of England (Morgan et al. 1993). Sixteen cases of culture confirmed infection were identified from 1 September to 1 November 1991. Eleven of the children were age 10 years or less and 5 developed HUS. A formal case-control study confirmed a close association between consumption of the yoghurt and development of *E. coli* O157 infection. However, the organism was not isolated from raw or pasteurized milk on the farm nor from another batch of the implicated brand of yoghurt sampled at a later date.

5 BUTTER

Butter contains approximately 81% fat and, under commercial conditions, is prepared from pasteurized cream with or without the addition of starter cultures which increase the acidity and add flavour. Dairy spreads may be defined as products with more than half their ingredients derived from milk. They have a higher water content than butter and low fat spreads contain additional milk proteins which stabilize the product (Wilbey 1994).

Most of the bacteria that are present in raw milk separate with cream and potentially would contaminate butter so pasteurization is a very important part of the manufacturing process. The physicochemical characteristics of butter appear to inhibit the growth of many micro-organisms but it has been shown that under experimental conditions *Salmonella* spp. can grow in butter at room temperature and may survive for long periods at refrigeration temperatures (El-Gazzar and Marth 1992). It has also been demonstrated that *L. monocytogenes* can increase in numbers during refrigerated storage of butter made from contaminated cream and that both *L. monocytogenes* and *Y. enterocolitica* can grow in some refrigerated dairy spreads (Milner 1995).

Spoilage of butter and dairy spreads may occur due to surface growth of *Pseudomonas* spp. or yeasts and moulds (Milner 1995). There have been only a few incidents of food poisoning associated with butter and most of these have been due to *S. aureus* enterotoxin. In 1970, 24 customers and staff at a department store in Alabama became ill with acute gastroenteritis soon after consuming whipped butter in the restaurant. The butter had been prepared at the restaurant by whipping milk with softened butter but microbiological tests showed that the butter, not the milk, contained *S. aureus*. The same brand of butter was also implicated in a single case of typical staphylococcal food poisoning in Tennessee a few days later; tests on the butter demonstrated the presence of staphylococcal enterotoxin A (Wolf et al. 1970). A second outbreak of staphylococcal food poisoning, also associated with commercially produced whipped butter, occurred in Kentucky in 1977. More than 100 cases were diagnosed some of whom were admitted to hospital (Francis et al. 1977).

In 1991 an outbreak of food poisoning in California and Nevada involved more than 265 people and was traced to butter blend and margarine which was contaminated with enterotoxin-producing *Staphylococcus intermedius*. Isolates from patients and product produced staphylococcal enterotoxin A and PFGE analysis of restriction enzyme digests of DNA from 5 clinical and 10 food isolates provided evidence that all the isolates were derived from a single strain (Bennett, Khambaty and Shaw 1994).

Another very serious outbreak of gastroenteritis followed by HUS affected 9 children age 1–3 years at a nursery school in Germany (Tschäpe et al. 1995). All 9 children required admission to hospital and dialysis and one boy died shortly after the onset of illness. In addition, 6 children age 4–6 years developed gastro-enteritis without HUS. The children had eaten sandwiches prepared with 'green' butter which was made by mixing parsley with the butter. The parsley originated from a garden which had been manured with pig manure. The organism responsible for the infection was a Vero cytotoxin-producing isolate of *Citrobacter freundii* which was isolated from patients, some symptomless contacts and from the parsley. The isolates from the patients and the parsley were shown to be toxigenic by specific DNA probes and polymerase chain reaction (PCR) and to be genetically indistinguishable from one another. This outbreak again demonstrates that the quality and hygiene of added ingredients are as important as those of the dairy product.

6 ICE CREAM

Ice cream usually contains 8–18% fat, 9–12% milk solids-not-fat, sugar, small amounts of stabilizer and emulsifier. If the fat is entirely milk fat the product is known as dairy ice cream. When vegetable oils or other animal fats are used in manufacture the product cannot be described as 'dairy' ice cream.

Ice cream is a complex product and manufacture consists of several stages. Detailed descriptions of the process and plant are given by Rothwell (1990) and Mitten and Neirinckz (1993). Initially the mix is blended to give a homogenous product. Compositional and heat treatment legislation varies considerably around the world but most countries require pasteurization (Rothwell 1990). Following pasteurization the mix is homogenized and then cooled to 4°C or below and held in a tank for a variable time ranging from 4 to 12 or more hours to undergo ageing. During the ageing process protein is absorbed to fat globules, fat crystallization occurs and stabilizers increase in hydration. In large highly mechanized and sophisticated ice cream plants the ageing process is carefully controlled and relatively short. However, some processors use a longer ageing time of 24 h or more and at this stage there is opportunity for psychrotrophic micro-organisms to multiply unless careful attention is paid to hygiene and prevention of postpasteurization contamination.

Following ageing the mixture is frozen rapidly with agitation and air is incorporated into the mix. It is then extruded and may be dispensed as soft serve ice cream or packaged into bricks or large containers which are hardened at between −20 and −40°C and sold as hard ice cream. Flavourings are usually added to the mixing or ageing tanks but pieces of fruit, nuts, syrups or purées are added to the ice cream after extrusion from the freezer.

6.1 Microbiological quality of ice cream

There were many small and large outbreaks of food poisoning due to ice cream in the UK prior to the introduction of heat treatment legislation for commercial ice cream (Rothwell 1990, Nichols and de Louvois 1995). Outbreaks of both *S. aureus* and salmonella food poisoning are recorded. In 1946 a large outbreak of typhoid fever in Aberystwyth affected more than 100 people with 4 deaths and was due to

contamination of the ice cream by the manufacturer who was a typhoid carrier (Evans 1947). Following this incident heat treatment regulations were introduced but did not become effective immediately and between 1950 and 1955 there were 19 recorded outbreaks associated with consumption of ice cream and ice lollies (11 due to *Salmonella* spp., 2 due to *S. aureus* and 6 of unknown cause) (Rothwell 1990). Between 1955 and 1984 there were no outbreaks reported in the UK but since 1984 there have been a number due to home-made ice cream. In 1984 an outbreak of *Salmonella* serotype Enteritidis PT4 infection involving 12 people was attributed to home-made ice cream (Barrett 1986). In 1987, 6 members of a family were ill with *B. cereus* poisoning after eating home-made ice cream containing egg white and fresh cream. The product had >10^{10} *B. cereus* per ml (Sockett 1991).

Several outbreaks of Enteritidis PT4 infection have occurred due to the use of raw shell eggs in home-made ice cream. In 1988 an outbreak affected 18 of 75 people at a bridge party (Cowden et al. 1989). In 1991 there were 3 family outbreaks (Report 1991b, Morgan, Mawer and Harman 1994) and in 1993 another outbreak affected 7 staff at a hotel (CDSC 1993, unpublished data). In the UK it is illegal to use unpasteurized egg in commercial ice cream but it is clear that the continued use of raw egg in domestic homes and by commercial caterers poses a serious threat of food poisoning which may sometimes involve large numbers of people. A large number of outbreaks of salmonellosis in other countries have also been associated with unpasteurized ice cream and the use of contaminated eggs (Nichols and de Louvois 1995). A more recent very large outbreak involving more than 2000 people in the USA was attributed to use of eggs in nationally distributed ice cream products (Report 1994d).

Ice cream may also become contaminated with *L. monocytogenes*. In 1986 contamination of ice cream bars in the USA was thought to be responsible for a flu-like illness affecting at least 40 people in 4 states. This resulted in a recall of the product. Listeria contamination requiring recall of product has also been reported on other occasions in ice cream in the USA and France (Rothwell 1990).

Most countries have strict standards for hygiene and heat treatment requirements for commercial ice cream and it is clear that careful control of both ingredients and the production process is needed to produce a hygienic product and prevent postpasteurization contamination. In 1992 in the UK the Ice Cream Federation and the Ice Cream Alliance in collaboration with the Milk Marketing Board produced guidelines for the hygienic manufacture of ice cream and for the safe handling of products by retailers (Report of the Ice Cream Alliance and the Ice Cream Federation 1992a, 1992b). These outline the main principles of quality assurance and attention to premises, raw materials, equipment and finished products.

A survey of the microbiological quality of 2612 samples of ice cream, ice lollies and similar frozen products was performed in England and Wales in 1993 as part of the European Community Coordinated Food Control Programme (Nichols and de Louvois 1995). The results of this survey demonstrated wide variations in microbiological profile but concluded that generally ices were of good quality and unlikely to cause food poisoning. However, non-branded hard ice creams and soft ice creams were more likely to contain high aerobic counts, indicator organisms and potential pathogens than branded ice cream bars. *L. monocytogenes* was found in 4 of 1964 samples of non-branded hard ice cream and soft ice cream and Enteritidis PT4 was isolated from a sample of 'real fruit' ice cream.

7 CHEESE

Cheeses are a heterogeneous group of foods made by coagulating the solids from high or low fat milk by the action of lactic acid and rennet. The curds so formed are treated with varying degrees of heating ('scalding'), cutting, salting and pressing to produce greater or less acidity and moisture content. The resulting cheese can vary in size, softness, consistency and degree of ripening. Further modifications depend on the type of lactic acid bacteria used to initiate souring and on whether other bacteria or moulds are encouraged to grow within the cheese or on the surface. Survival of pathogens or development of spoilage organisms depends on the physical and chemical characteristics of the cheese and on the degree of maturation. Cheeses may be classified broadly into 3 main types: hard and semi-hard pressed cheeses, semi-soft cheeses which are usually not pressed, and soft cheeses. Hard cheeses include Parmesan, Gruyère, Cheddar, Derby, Leicester, Caerphilly, Edam, Gouda and Fynbo. Soft cheeses include Camembert, Brie, Livarot, Cambazola, Cambridge and Coulommiers and semi-soft include Munster, Stilton, Roquefort, Gorgonzola and Mozzarella. There are also a few unshaped curd cheeses such as cottage and lactic cheese which have high moisture content and acidity, and a very limited shelf-life (Shaw 1993, Tamime 1993).

Hard cheeses such as Cheddar or Swiss are typically large, with low moisture content (c. 39%) and a clear rind. The curds are scalded and then matted together while in the vats, 'milled', or chopped, salted and pressed into moulds under heavy weights. Ripening takes 3–9 months and proceeds evenly throughout the cheese. Flavour depends on enzymes from the starter culture and from rennet. The starter is usually a mixture of subspecies of *Lactococcus lactis*. Swiss cheeses such as Emmenthal and Gruyère are manufactured at high temperatures. Thermoduric starters such as *Streptococcus salivarius* subsp. *thermophilus* or *Lactobacillus* spp. are used. In addition, cultures of propionibacteria are added for development of the essential and characteristic flavours.

Semi-hard cheeses such as Caerphilly, Lancashire and the Dutch cheeses are lightly pressed cheeses with a moisture content of around 45–50%. The textures vary from smooth to crumbly. Most semi-hard cheeses are matured for 1–3 months but Caerphilly is usually eaten while quite fresh (around 2 weeks old) and Lancashire may be matured for as long as 12 months.

Soft cheeses have a high moisture content of 55–60%. The curds are not cut or scalded but are drained into small moulds without pressing. Cheeses such as Coulommiers or Cambridge are eaten fresh within a few days but surface-ripened cheeses such as Camembert or Port Salut are surface-ripened for 1–6 weeks by moulds (*Penicillium camemberti*) or bacteria (*Brevibacterium linens*).

Internally mould-ripened cheeses such as Gorgonzola or Stilton are semi-soft cheeses with a moisture content of 45–55%. They are made with high acid curd to which either *Penicillium glaucum* or *Penicillium roqueforti* is added. The curd is filled into tall moulds, which are turned frequently so that it is pressed down by its own weight. After a few weeks, the cheeses are pierced with skewers to admit air and encourage growth of moulds. Ripening is complete after 3–6 months, during which the pH rises to 6.0 or more, and lipolysis and proteolysis contribute to the flavour.

7.1 Defects and spoilage of cheese

Cheeses made from unpasteurized milk may develop numerous defects depending on the microbial quality of the raw milk and on subsequent contamination from vats and other equipment and from the curing rooms in which they are matured. The quality of cheese made with pasteurized milk depends mainly on the extent of contamination during manufacture and storage (Chapman and Sharpe 1990). Off flavours and gas production early in manufacture are usually due to lactose-fermenting Enterobacteriaceae or, sometimes, to lactose-fermenting yeasts. Swiss-type cheeses are liable to develop gas some weeks later due to clostridial contamination. Surface growth of yeasts, moulds or proteolytic bacteria can cause softening or discoloration of the rind and spoilage of the cheese. Blue vein cheeses are particularly susceptible to this defect. Growth of yeasts and moulds or slime production by psychrotrophic organisms is common in cottage cheese. Production requires a very high standard of plant hygiene.

FUNGAL TOXINS

Cheese-making experiments show that aflatoxin M_1 in milk will survive pasteurization and the cheese-making process, and will not deteriorate on storage. Growth of toxin-producing moulds in cheese is also possible. *Penicillium* spp. can produce toxins such as penicillic acid, patulin, cyclopiazonic acid and roquefortins both at room temperature and at temperatures below 10°C (Chapman and Sharpe 1990). Toxin-producing strains of *Penicillium* have been isolated from both Cheddar and Swiss cheese. There is concern that some of the strains of *P. camemberti* and *P. roqueforti* used for making blue cheese may be toxigenic but conditions in the cheese tend to be unfavourable for toxin production because of the low content of carbohydrate. Many countries, however, now screen for and select non-toxigenic strains for cheese production. The development of aflatoxin in cheese is probably of less concern because *Aspergillus flavus* and *Aspergillus parasiticus* do not produce toxins at temperatures below 10°C, at which most hard and semi-hard cheeses are ripened.

BACTERIAL TOXINS

Histamine poisoning associated with the consumption of cheese was first reported by Doeglas, Huisman and Nater in 1967. In 1980 a small outbreak occurred in New Hampshire. Specimens of suspect cheese contained 187 mg of histamine per 100 g and a strain of *Lactobacillus buchneri* isolated from the cheese was found to have very high histidine carboxylase activity (Sumner et al. 1985). Staphylococcal enterotoxin has also been the cause of many outbreaks of food poisoning associated with cheese.

7.2 Pathogenic bacteria in cheese

The efficient pasteurization of milk should eliminate the risk from all viable pathogenic organisms but many cheesemakers still use raw milk or add raw milk to the cheese milk, believing it essential for good flavour. Survival of pathogenic organisms in cheese depends on the method of manufacture, the competitive effect of the lactic acid-producing starter bacteria and on conditions of storage and length of maturation of the finished product. Safety cannot be guaranteed if cheese is made from raw milk.

There have been many outbreaks and sporadic cases of infection or food poisoning, including brucellosis and botulism, associated with the consumption of cheese. Most detailed investigations have demonstrated that the source of contamination was raw milk, inadequately pasteurized milk or postpasteurization contamination with organisms originally derived from raw milk. Tuberculosis in man has not been traced directly to the consumption of cheese but experimental work has shown that *M. tuberculosis* can survive in many varieties of cheese.

BRUCELLOSIS

Brucellosis is still an important cause of human and animal infection; 500 000 new cases of human infection are reported annually throughout the world. Many cases are associated with consumption of cheese made with raw milk. It has been shown that *B. abortus* and *B. melitensis* can survive and remain viable for many months even in hard cheese such as Cheddar (Chapman and Sharp 1990).

Wallach et al. (1994) described an outbreak affecting an Argentine family after eating unpasteurized goats' milk cheese. Nine of 14 became ill with *B. melitensis* and blood cultures were positive from 7 patients.

Human brucella infection is rare in England and Wales and with very few exceptions is acquired abroad after consumption of raw milk and cheese. Two cases of *B. melitensis* were reported in a family who stayed in Malta in April 1995 and ate a locally produced cheese pastry. They were among those affected in an outbreak involving at least 135 people (one death) which was linked to consumption of a soft cheese made with unpasteurized goats' and ewes' milk (Report 1995).

STREPTOCOCCUS ZOOEPIDEMICUS

In 1983, 16 cases of *S. zooepidemicus* occurred in New Mexico and were traced to a home-made cheese made with raw cows' milk which was sold at several stores. A case-control study confirmed the association between *S. zooepidemicus* infection and eating the suspect cheese. In addition, the organism was isolated from multiple samples of cheese and from milk from the cattle at the farm (Espinosa et al. 1983).

STAPHYLOCOCCUS AUREUS

Cheese is the milk product most often associated with food poisoning due to *S. aureus* enterotoxin. This organism is a common cause of mastitis in cattle and common in raw milk. Toxin may be present before pasteurization if the milk has been stored at ambient temperature. If sufficient numbers of *S. aureus* are present at the start of cheese-making, either because raw milk is used or because of postpasteurization contamination, they may multiply and produce toxin during the cheese-making process (Minor and Marth 1972). Experiments with cheddar cheese-making have shown that even heavily contaminated milk is unlikely to become toxic if the starter culture is working normally. If, however, development of acidity is slow because of the presence of bacteriophage, the numbers of *S. aureus* may attain values of 10^6–10^8 g^{-1} and produce toxin in the curd. During ripening, the numbers of *S. aureus* decline over the course of a few days or weeks in normally acidic cheese but may continue to multiply in cheese of low acidity during the first few weeks of ripening and survive for months thereafter.

Between 1951 and 1980 cheese was implicated in 16 recorded outbreaks of *S. aureus* food poisoning involving 507 people in England and Wales (Galbraith, Forbes and Clifford 1982). Cheddar, Stilton, homemade soft cheese and Romanian hard cheese were included. In 10 outbreaks it was suspected that contamination occurred during manufacture. In the 1950s and 1960s *S. aureus* intoxication was the most common cause of food poisoning in the USA, and numerous cases were traced to cheese (Hendricks, Belknap and Hausler 1959, Walker, Harmon and Stine 1961). Since the almost universal introduction of refrigerated storage for milk, there have been very few incidents. One small outbreak involving only 2 people occurred in 1983 (Barrett 1986) and in 1987 cheese was suspected as a source of *S. aureus* intoxication in an outbreak involving 28 of 350 people who attended a buffet lunch of a variety of food items (Communicable Disease Report 1987, unpublished). Sharp (1987), in his survey of infections associated with dairy products in Europe and North America from 1980 to 1985, found no other incidents associated with cheese made from cows' milk. Cheese made from contaminated sheep milk was, however, responsible for outbreaks in France and Scotland.

A series of 36 outbreaks of food poisoning in England from November 1988 to January 1989, affecting 155 people, were linked to consumption of Stilton cheese made from raw cows' milk. Although the microbiology and tests for toxin were negative, the clinical illness was typical of staphylococcal intoxication. Control measures included withdrawal of the implicated cheese from sale and subsequent change to use of pasteurized milk for cheese production (Maguire et al. 1991). For further information on *S. aureus* food poisoning, see Chapter 27.

SALMONELLA

Salmonellae can multiply rapidly during the cheese-making process and will survive in the curd unless a high degree of acidity is reached. During ripening, an initial rapid decline in numbers is followed by a relatively stationary phase. Small numbers have been detected even after storage for 6–10 months at refrigeration temperatures (Medina, Gaya and Nuñez 1982). It may be difficult to isolate the organisms because small numbers are slow to revive and are not distributed evenly through the cheese. Survival tends to be greater in the middle of the cheese and poor near the surface. The infective dose seems to be low. About 10^4 organisms can cause illness, presumably because the high lipid content of the cheese protects the bacteria from the acidity of the stomach (Ratnam and March 1986). Many outbreaks of salmonellosis have been traced to cheeses of all types. It is clear that effective pasteurization of the milk is the only dependable way of ensuring that salmonellae do not contaminate cheese (Fontaine et al. 1980). From 1980 to 1985 outbreaks were recorded in Italy, Canada, Finland and Switzerland (Sharp 1987).

In 1984 there was a huge outbreak of infection with serotype Typhimurium PT10 in the 4 Atlantic provinces of Canada and in Ontario (Ratnam and March 1986). The outbreak was the largest common source outbreak ever to occur in Canada and involved an estimated 10 000 persons. Typhimurium PT10 was isolated from the factory packed contaminated lots of Cheddar cheese as well as leftover cheese recovered from homes of human cases. Estimated numbers of Typhimurium in the cheese were low but the lots of cheese that were positive also contained high counts of coliforms and *E. coli*. Defective pasteurization was shown to be the underlying cause of contamination and the outbreak strain was isolated from milk from a cow on one of the farms supplying the factory. A careful investigation of the pasteurization process revealed that an employee manually overrode the controller and allowed unpasteurized milk to go through to the vats. The pasteurizer was shut down after filling 3 vats and later restarted to fill the next 3 vats so that the first and third vats contained Typhimurium when contaminated raw milk was being pasteurized (Johnson, Nelson and Johnson 1990).

In 1989, an outbreak of serotype Dublin affected 42 people in England and Wales and was traced to imported Irish soft cheese made with unpasteurized cows' milk. *S.* Dublin was isolated from samples of cheese and from the milk of 4 cows in the milking herd. The cheese was made on the dairy farm (Maguire et al. 1992).

In 1993, Paratyphi B infection in southwest France was traced to unpasteurized cheese made from goats'

milk. Serotype Paratyphi B was isolated from a batch of cheese and from milk from a goat in a herd which supplied the cheese makers (Desenclos et al. 1996).

LISTERIA MONOCYTOGENES

The fairly recent association of *L. monocytogenes* infections with soft cheese may be due to changes in marketing practices for dairy products. In recent years a wider range of dairy products, including many varieties of continental soft cheese, have become popular in Britain and North America and are available in most supermarkets. Many of these products are imported from the country of origin and all have been stored at refrigeration temperatures for days or weeks. *L. monocytogenes* multiplies at low temperatures and minor contamination may increase significantly during storage. *L. monocytogenes* appears to be common in raw milk and many soft cheeses are made from raw milk or have small amounts of raw milk added to them during manufacture. Post-process contamination with *Listeria* may also occur because of the wide environmental distribution of the organism; it can be prevented by strict attention to hygiene and the prevention of cross-contamination during handling and storage (Marfleet and Blood 1987).

In 1985, 86 cases of *L. monocytogenes* infection were identified in Los Angeles and Orange Counties, California (James et al. 1985); 58 cases were in mother–infant pairs. There were 8 neonatal deaths and 13 stillbirths out of a total of 29 deaths. Case-control studies implicated Mexican-style soft cheeses from one manufacturer. *L. monocytogenes* serotype 4b was isolated from patients and from packets of cheese. Although most of the cheese milk was pasteurized, about 10% was not.

Surveys in the USA and Europe (including the UK) have shown that *L. monocytogenes* may be found in a wide variety of soft cheeses (Gilbert 1987, Pini and Gilbert 1988, Greenwood, Roberts and Burden 1991). Experimental production of cottage cheese with artificially contaminated milk confirmed that a proportion of the inoculum survived manufacture (which included cooking at 57.2°C for 30 min). Organisms could be recovered from more than one-third of samples by direct plating after storage at 3°C (Ryser, Marth and Doyle 1985). Ryser, Marth and Doyle also showed that listeria survive during the manufacture of Cheddar cheese and that numbers increase during the first 14 days of ripening. Thereafter, numbers decrease but may persist for months.

Sporadic cases of listeria infection have been associated with the consumption of soft cheeses (Bannister 1987, Azadian, Finnerty and Pearson 1989, McLauchlin, Greenwood and Pini 1990). In 1987, cases of listeriosis in Switzerland were associated with Vacherins Mont d'Or soft cheese and investigations revealed that an outbreak lasting from 1983 to 1987 had involved 122 persons (with 34 deaths) (Bille 1990).

In an outbreak of listerosis reported in France (Goulet et al. 1995), 20 cases were identified between 2 April and 16 May 1995, including 11 in pregnant women, resulting in 2 spontaneous abortions, 4 premature births and 2 stillbirths. The source of infection was one specific chain of Brie de Meaux (a raw milk soft cheese) production. This is the first outbreak of listeriosis, documented in France, which has been linked to the consumption of a raw milk cheese.

ESCHERICHIA COLI

Outbreaks of illness due to pathogenic *E. coli* have been recorded in association with cheese and it has become clear that serious infection with both entero-invasive and Vero-toxinogenic *E. coli* (VTEC) may be acquired from contaminated cheese.

In 1971 there were 107 episodes of enteroinvasive *E. coli* illness involving 387 people in the USA (Marier et al. 1973). Imported French Brie, Camembert and Coulommiers cheeses made at a single factory over a period of 2 days were implicated. A slowly lactose-fermenting strain of *E. coli* serotype O124:B17 was isolated from samples of cheese and from the faeces of patients. Laboratory tests confirmed that the strain was invasive but not enterotoxigenic. There is no mention of whether the cheese milk had been pasteurized, but river water, used to wash the vats, was the suspected source of infection.

Epidemiological data incriminated French Brie and Camembert cheeses in a large outbreak of enterotoxigenic *E. coli* infection in 1983. This affected more than 3000 people in Washington, Illinois, Wisconsin and Georgia as well as in Denmark, Holland and Sweden (MacDonald et al. 1985, Nooitgedagt and Hartog 1988). *E. coli* serotype O25:H20 was isolated from faecal specimens and heat-stable (ST) toxin production was demonstrated. The plasmid profile of isolates from patients in Washington, Illinois, Georgia and Wisconsin were similar. The illness was associated with cheese from 2 separate batches made at the same factory 46 days apart. There was no information about pasteurization and the source of contamination was not discovered. Cultures of cheese samples did not grow *E. coli* serotype O27:H20 but organisms binding antiserum to *E. coli* O27 were detected in one cheese specimen by solid-phase radioimmunoassay at a concentration of 10^4 organisms per g.

Recently there have been 2 reports of outbreaks of *E. coli* O157:H7 infection due to the consumption of cheese. One cluster of 4 cases occurred in a rural community of France and was linked to 'fromage frais' made with unpasteurized goats' and cows' milk on a farm. Four children aged from 9 to 15 months were affected, 3 during the spring of 1992 and one during the spring of 1993. All children had diarrhoea and 3 developed renal failure. One child died. Samples taken from the farm yielded isolates of VTEC but not of *E. coli* O157 (Report 1994e). The second outbreak occurred in Scotland in 1994. Twenty cases of *E. coli* O157:H7 phage type 28 infection in the Grampian region were associated with a farm-produced cheese made with unpasteurized milk. Most of the patients had bloody diarrhoea and one had HUS. *E. coli* O157 PT28 was also isolated from a sample of the cheese and typing of the isolates from the patients and the cheese by PFGE demonstrated that they were indistinguishable from one another (Curnow 1994).

MICROBIOLOGICAL QUALITY CONTROL DURING MANUFACTURE OF CHEESE

In recent years there has been increasing concern about pathogens in cheese and particularly of the risk of contamination with *L. monocytogenes* and *E. coli* O157 (Report of the Committee on the Microbiological Safety of Food 1990, Report of the Advisory Committee on the Microbiological Safety of Food 1995). It is clear that soft and fresh cheeses which develop pH values in excess of 5.0 should be considered as high risk for *L. monocytogenes* whereas soft cheese which maintains a pH of less than 5.0 is of lower risk. Hard pressed cheese is also of low risk particularly if there is a long maturation time of 60 days or more, but no cheese is entirely without risk for contamination with *L. monocytogenes* or other pathogens if the hygiene during manufacture is poor or if the cheese has been manufactured from unpasteurized milk.

The industry has taken the problem of hygiene very seriously in the UK. The Creamery Proprietors' Association has published 'Guidelines for good hygienic practice in the manufacture of soft and fresh cheeses' (Report 1988) and the Milk Marketing Board has produced similar guidelines for the manufacture of soft and fresh cheeses in small and farm based units (Report 1989). In addition, the joint FAO/WHO Codex Alimentarius Commission is at present drafting a code of practice for hygienic practice for the manufacture of uncured, unripened and ripened soft cheeses (Alinorm 95/13). European Standards (Council Directive 92/46/EEC) and Dairy Products (Hygiene) Regulations 1995 reflect the current anxiety about *L. monocytogenes* and are very stringent for soft cheese whether it is made from raw or pasteurized milk. *L. monocytogenes* must be absent from 5 samples of 25 g taken at the manufacturing premises and each 25 g sample must consist of 5 pieces of 5 g from different parts of the same product. In the USA, *L. monocytogenes* must be absent from cheese and other milk products either home-produced or imported and this is monitored by testing performed by the States and Federal authorities.

In early 1995, 13 public health laboratories in England and Wales carried out a survey of the quality of a variety of imported and local soft and semi-soft cheeses purchased from retail outlets such as supermarkets, shops and delicatessens (Nichols, Greenwood and de Louvois 1996). The cheeses were examined by internationally accepted methods according to a standard protocol to see how they compared when tested for *Salmonella* spp., *L. monocytogenes*, *S. aureus*, coliforms and *E. coli*. Data obtained for 1437 samples showed that generally the standard was good and that most cheeses would satisfy the legal requirements.

Cheeses made from unpasteurized milk were of a lower microbiological quality than those prepared from pasteurized milk and it was of concern that for 67% of the cheeses sampled there was no information to enable the customer to determine whether the cheese was made from pasteurized milk or not. However, the isolation rate for *L. monocytogenes* was low for all cheeses (1.1% overall and 1.4% for cheese made from raw milk). This was significantly lower than that found during a previous survey in 1988–89 (Greenwood, Roberts and Burden 1991).

REFERENCES

ADAS, 1996, *Pasteurised Milk. Assured Hygienic Quality*, Issue 3, ADAS, Oxford, 1–21.

Anderson PHR, Stone DM, 1955, Staphylococcal food poisoning associated with spray-dried milk, *J Hyg Camb*, **53:** 387–97.

Ashenafi M, 1994, Fate of *Listeria monocytogenes* during the souring of Esgo, a traditional Ethiopian fermented milk, *J Dairy Sci*, **77:** 696–702.

Aytac SA, Ozbas ZY, 1994, Survey of the growth and survival of *Yersinia enterocolitica* and *Aeromonas hydrophila* in yoghurt, *Milchwissenschaft*, **49:** 322–5.

Azadian BS, Finnerty GT, Pearson AD, 1989, Cheese-borne listeria meningitis in immunocompetent patient, *Lancet*, **1:** 322–3.

Bannister BA, 1987, *Listeria monocytogenes* meningitis associated with eating soft cheese, *J Infect*, **15:** 165–8.

Barnham M, Thornton TJ, Lange K, 1983, Nephritis caused by *Streptococcus zooepidemicus* (Lancefield group C), *Lancet*, **1:** 945–7.

Barrett NJ, 1986, Communicable disease associated with milk and dairy products in England and Wales: 1983–1984, *J Infect*, **12:** 265–72.

Becker H, Schaller G et al., 1994, *Bacillus cereus* in infant foods and dried milk products, *Int J Food Microbiol*, **23:** 1–15.

Bell JC, Palmer SR, 1983, Control of zoonoses in Britain: past, present and future, *Br Med J*, **287:** 591–3.

Bennett R, Khambaty FM, Shah DB, 1994, *Staphylococcus intermedius*: etiologic association with foodborne intoxication from butter blend and margarine, *Dairy Food Environ Sanit*, **14:** 604.

Beumer RR, Cruysen JJM, Birtantie IRK, 1988, The occurrence of *Campylobacter jejuni* in raw cows' milk, *J Appl Bacteriol*, **65:** 93–6.

Biering G, Karlsson S et al., 1989, Three cases of neonatal meningitis caused by *Enterobacter sakazakii* in powdered milk, *J Clin Microbiol*, **27:** 2054–6.

Bille J, 1990, Epidemiology of human listeriosis in Europe with special reference to the Swiss outbreak, *Foodborne Listeriosis*, eds Miller AJ, Smith JL, Sumkuti GA, Elsevier, Amsterdam, 71–4.

Birkhead G, Vogt RL, 1988, A multiple-strain outbreak of *Campylobacter* enteritis due to consumption of inadequately pasteurized milk, *J Infect Dis*, **157:** 1095–7.

Black RE, Jackson RJ et al., 1978, Epidemic *Yersinia enterocolitica* infection due to contaminated chocolate milk, *N Engl J Med*, **298:** 76–9.

Borczyk AA, Karmali MA et al., 1987, Bovine reservoir for verotoxin-producing *Escherichia coli* O157:H7, *Lancet*, **1:** 98.

Bowen JE, Turnbull PCB, 1992, The fate of *Bacillus anthracis* in unpasteurised and pasteurised milk, *Lett Appl Microbiol*, **15:** 224–7.

Bramley AJ, McKinnon CH, 1990, The microbiology of raw milk, *Dairy Microbiology*, vol. 1, 2nd edn, ed. Robinson RK, Elsevier Applied Science, London and New York, 163–208.

Chapman HR, Sharpe ME, 1990, Microbiology of cheese, *Dairy Microbiology*, vol. 2, 2nd edn, ed. Robinson RK, Elsevier Applied Science, London and New York, 203–89.

Chapman PA, Wright DJ, 1993, Untreated milk as a source of verotoxigenic *E. coli* O157, *Vet Rec*, **133:** 171–2.

Chapman PA, Siddons CA et al., 1993, Cattle as a possible source of verocytotoxin-producing *Escherichia coli* O157 infections in man, *Epidemiol Infect*, **111:** 439–47.

Christiansson A, 1992, The toxicology of *Bacillus cereus*, Bacillus cereus *in Milk and Milk Products*, Internation Dairy Federation Bulletin 275, IDF, Brussels, 30–5.

Clarke RC, McEwen SA et al., 1989, Isolation of verocytotoxin-producing *Escherichia coli* from milk filters in south-western Ontario, *Epidemiol Infect*, **102:** 253–60.

Collins RN, Treger MD et al., 1968, Interstate outbreak of *Salmonella newbrunswick* infection traced to powdered milk, *JAMA*, **203:** 838–44.

Cotton LN, White CH, 1992, *Listeria monocytogenes*, *Yersinia enterocolitica* and *Salmonella* in dairy plant environments, *J Dairy Sci*, **75:** 51–7.

Cowden JM, Chisholm D et al., 1989, Two outbreaks of *Salmonella enteritidis* phage type 4 infection associated with consumption of fresh shell-egg products, *Epidemiol Infect*, **103:** 47–52.

Craven JA, 1978, Salmonella contamination of dried milk products, *Victorian Vet Proc*, **9:** 56–7.

Crielly EM, Logan NA, Anderton A, 1994, Studies on the bacillus flora of milk and milk products, *J Appl Bacteriol*, **77:** 256–63.

Curnow J, 1994, *E. coli* O157 phage type 28 infections in Grampian, *Commun Dis Environ Health Scot*, **28 (94/46):** 1.

D'Aoust JY, Park CE et al., 1988, Thermal inactivation of *Campylobacter* species, *Yersinia enterocolitica* and haemorrhagic *Escherichia coli* O157/H7 in fluid milk, *J Dairy Sci*, **71:** 3230–6.

Davis JG, Wilbey RA, 1990, Microbiology of cream and dairy desserts, *Dairy Microbiology*, vol. 2, 2nd edn, ed. Robinson RK, Elsevier Applied Science, London and New York, 41–108.

Department of Public Health, 1886, On the relation between milk-scarlatina in the human subject and disease in the cow, *Practitioner*, **37:** 61–80.

Desenclos JC, Bouvet P et al., 1996, *Salmonella enterica* serotype paratyphi B in goat milk cheese, France 1993: a case finding and epidemiological study, *Br Med J*, **312:** 91–4.

Doeglas HMG, Huisman J, Nater JP, 1967, Histamine intoxication after cheese, *Lancet*, **2:** 1361–2.

Duca E, Teodorovici G et al., 1969, A new nephritogenic streptococcus, *J Hyg Camb*, **67:** 691–8.

Editorial, 1987, Food handlers and salmonella food poisoning, *Lancet*, **2:** 606–7.

Editorial, 1988, Milk – with care, *Lancet*, **1:** 1086–7.

Edwards AT, Roulson M, Ironside MJ, 1988, A milk-borne outbreak of serious infection due to *Streptococcus zooepidemicus* (Lancefield group C), *Epidemiol Infect*, **101:** 43–51.

El-Dairouty KR, 1989, Staphylococcal intoxication traced to non-fat dried milk, *J Food Prot*, **52:** 901–2.

El-Gazzar FE, Marth EH, 1992, Salmonellae, salmonellosis and dairy foods: a review, *J Dairy Sci*, **75:** 2327–43.

Espinosa FM, Ryan WM et al., 1983, Group C streptococcal infections associated with eating home-made cheese – New Mexico, *Morbid Mortal Weekly Rep*, **32:** 510, 515–16.

Evans DI, 1947, An account of an outbreak of typhoid fever due to infected ice-cream in Aberystwyth Borough in 1946, *Med Officer*, **77:** 39–44.

Eyler JM, 1986, The epidemiology of milk-borne scarlet fever: the case of Edwardian Brighton, *Am J Public Health*, **76:** 573–84.

Fahey T, Morgan D et al., 1995, An outbreak of *Campylobacter jejuni* enteritis associated with failed milk pasteurisation, *J Infect*, **31:** 137–43.

Fenlon DR, Stewart T, Donachie W, 1995, The incidence, numbers and types of *Listeria monocytogenes* isolated from farm bulk tank milks, *Lett Appl Microbiol*, **20:** 57–60.

Fishbein DB, Raoult D, 1992, A cluster of *Coxiella burnetii* infections associated with exposure to vaccinated goats and their unpasteurised dairy products, *Am J Trop Med Hyg*, **47:** 35–40.

Fleming DW, Cochi SL et al., 1985, Pasteurised milk as a vehicle of infection in an outbreak of listeriosis, *N Engl J Med*, **312:** 404–7.

Fontaine RE, Cohen ML et al., 1980, Epidemic salmonellosis from cheddar cheese: surveillance and prevention, *Am J Epidemiol*, **111:** 247–53.

Francis AJ, Nimmo GR et al., 1993, Investigation of milk-borne *Streptococcus zooepidemicus* infection associated with glomerulonephritis in Australia, *J Infect*, **27:** 317–23.

Francis BJ, Langkop C et al., 1977, Presumed staphylococcal food poisoning associated with whipped butter, *Morbid Mortal Weekly Rep*, **26:** 268.

Francis DW, Spaulding PL, Lovett J, 1980, Enterotoxin production and thermal resistance of *Yersinia enterocolitica* in milk, *Appl Environ Microbiol*, **40:** 174–6.

Furlong JD, Lee W et al., 1979, Salmonellosis associated with consumption of nonfat powdered milk, Oregon, *Morbid Mortal Weekly Rep*, **18:** 129–30.

Galbraith NS, Forbes P, Clifford C, 1982, Communicable disease associated with milk and dairy products in England and Wales 1951–80, *Br Med J*, **284:** 1761–5.

Galbraith NS, Pusey JJ, 1984, Milkborne infectious disease in England and Wales 1938–1982, *Health Hazards of Milk*, ed. Freed DLG, Baillière Tindall, Eastbourne, 27–59.

Gaya P, Medina M, Nuñez M, 1987, Enterobacteriaceae, coliforms, faecal coliforms and salmonellas in raw ewes' milk, *J Appl Bacteriol*, **62:** 321–6.

Ghoneim ATM, Cooke M, 1980, Serious infection caused by group C streptococci, *J Clin Pathol*, **33:** 188–90.

Gilbert R, 1979, *Bacillus cereus* gastroenteritis, *Foodborne Infections and Intoxications*, eds Riemann H, Bryan FL, Academic Press, New York, 495–518.

Gilbert R, 1987, Foodborne infections and intoxications – recent problems and new organisms, *Microbiological and Environmental Health Problems relevant to the Food and Catering Industries*, Proceedings of a Joint Symposium (Campden Food Preservation Research Association and the Public Health Laboratory Service) 19–21 January, Stratford-upon-Avon, Campden Food Preservation Research Association, Chipping Campden, 1–22.

Gilmour A, Rowe MT, 1990, Micro-organisms associated with milk, *Dairy Microbiology*, vol. 1, 2nd edn, ed. Robinson RK, Elsevier Applied Science, London and New York, 37–75.

Goulet V, Jacquet C et al., 1995, Listeriosis from consumption of raw-milk cheese, *Lancet*, **345:** 1581–2.

Greenwood M, 1995, Microbiological methods for examination of milk and dairy products in accordance with the Dairy Products (Hygiene) Regulations 1995, *PHLS Microbiol Dig*, **12:** 74–82.

Greenwood MH, Hooper WL, Rodhouse JC, 1990, The source of *Yersinia* spp. in pasteurized milk: an investigation at a dairy, *Epidemiol Infect*, **104:** 351–60.

Greenwood M, Rampling A, 1995, A guide to the Dairy Products (Hygiene) Regulations 199[5] for Public Health Laboratory microbiologists, *PHLS Microbiol Dig*, **12:** 7–10.

Greenwood MH, Roberts D, Burden P, 1991, The occurrence of *Listeria* species in milk and dairy products: a national survey in England and Wales, *Int J Food Microbiol*, **12:** 197–206.

Griffin PM, Tauxe RV, 1993, *Escherichia coli* O157:H7 human illness in North America, food vehicles and animal reservoirs, *Int Food Safety News*, **2:** 15–17.

Hart RJC, 1984, *Corynebacterium ulcerans* in humans and cattle in north Devon, *J Hyg Camb*, **92:** 161–4.

Harvey J, Gilmour A, 1990, Isolation and identification of staphylococci from milk powders produced in Northern Ireland, *J Appl Bacteriol*, **68:** 433–8.

Hendricks SL, Belknap RA, Hausler WJ, 1959, Staphylococcal food intoxication due to cheddar cheese. 1. Epidemiology, *J Milk Food Technol*, **22:** 313–17.

Hinckley LS, 1991, Quality standards for goat milk, *Dairy Food Environ Sanit*, **11:** 511–12.

Hobbs BC, 1955, Public health problems associated with the manufacture of dried milk. 1. Staphylococcal food poisoning, *J Appl Bacteriol*, **18:** 484–92.

Hudson SJ, Sobo AO et al., 1990, Jackdaws as potential source of milk-borne *Campylobacter jejuni* infection, *Lancet*, **335:** 1160.

Hudson SJ, Lightfoot NF et al., 1991, Jackdaws and magpies as vectors of milkborne human campylobacter infection, *Epidemiol Infect*, **107:** 363–72.

Hudson PJ, Vogt RL et al., 1984, Isolation of *Campylobacter jejuni* from milk during an outbreak of campylobacteriosis, *J Infect Dis*, **150:** 789.

Humphrey TJ, Hart RJC, 1988, *Campylobacter* and *Salmonella* contamination of unpasteurised cows' milk on sale to the public, *J Appl Bacteriol*, **65:** 463–7.

Hunter AC, Cruickshank EG, 1984, Hygienic aspects of goat milk production in Scotland, *Dairy Food Sanit*, **4:** 212–15.

Hutchinson DN, Bolton FJ et al., 1985a, Campylobacter enteritis associated with consumption of raw goats' milk, *Lancet*, **1:** 1037–8.

Hutchinson DN, Bolton FJ et al., 1985b, Evidence of udder excretion of *Campylobacter jejuni* as the cause of a milk-borne campylobacter outbreak, *J Hyg Camb*, **94:** 205–15.

Jacquet CL, Rocourt J, Reynaud A, 1993, Study of *Listeria monocytogenes* contamination in a dairy plant and characterisation of the strains isolated, *Int J Food Microbiol*, **21:** 253–61.

James SM, Fannin SL et al., 1985, Listeriosis outbreak associated with Mexican-style cheese – California, *Morbid Mortal Weekly Rep*, **34:** 357–9.

Johnson EA, Nelson JH, Johnson M, 1990, Microbiological safety of cheese made from heat-treated milk. Part II Microbiology, *J Food Prot*, **53:** 519–40.

Jones PH, Willis AT et al., 1981, Campylobacter enteritis associated with the consumption of free school milk, *J Hyg Camb*, **87:** 155–62.

Kozak JJ, 1986, FDA's dairy program initiatives, *Dairy Food Sanit*, **6:** 184–5.

Knipschildt ME, Anderson GG, 1994, Drying of milk and milk products, *Modern Dairy Technology*, vol. 1, 2nd edn, ed. Robinson RK, Chapman and Hall, London, 159–254.

Lecos CW, 1986, A closer look at dairy safety, *Dairy Food Sanit*, **6:** 240–2.

Lewis MJ, 1994, Heat treatment of milk, *Modern Dairy Technology*, vol. 1, 2nd edn, ed. Robinson RK, Chapman and Hall, London, 1–60.

Louie KK, Paccagnella AM et al., 1993, *Salmonella* serotype Tennessee in powdered milk products and infant formula – Canada and United States 1993, *Morbid Mortal Weekly Rep*, **42:** 516–17.

Lovell HR, 1990, The microbiology of dried milk powders, *Dairy Microbiology*, vol. 1, 2nd edn, ed. Robinson RK, Elsevier Applied Science, London and New York, 245–69.

Luchansky JB, 1995, Use of pulsed-field gel electrophoresis to link sporadic cases of invasive listeriosis with recalled chocolate milk, *FRI Newslett*, **7 (2):** 1–2.

Lyster RLJ, Aschaffenburg R, 1962, The reactivation of milk alkaline phosphatase after heat treatment, *J Dairy Res*, **29:** 21–35.

MacDonald KL, Eidson M et al., 1985, A multistate outbreak of gastrointestinal illness caused by enterotoxigenic *Escherichia coli* in imported semisoft cheese, *J Infect Dis*, **151:** 716–20.

McDonough FE, Hargrove RE, 1968, Heat resistance of salmonella in dried milk, *J Dairy Sci*, **51:** 1587–91.

McLauchlin J, 1993, Listeriosis and *Listeria monocytogenes*, *Environ Policy Pract*, **3:** 201–14.

McLauchlin J, Greenwood MH, Pini PN, 1990, The occurrence of *Listeria monocytogenes* in cheese from a manufacturer associated with a case of listeriosis, *Int J Food Microbiol*, **10:** 255–62.

Maguire H, 1993, Continuing hazards from unpasteurised milk products in England and Wales, *Int Food Safety News*, **2:** 21–2.

Maguire H, Boyle M et al., 1991, A large outbreak of food poisoning of unknown aetiology associated with stilton cheese, *Epidemiol Infect*, **106:** 497–505.

Maguire H, Cowden J et al., 1992, An outbreak of *Salmonella dublin* infection in England and Wales associated with a soft unpasteurized cows' milk cheese, *Epidemiol Infect*, **109**: 389–96.

Marfleet JE, Blood RM, 1987, Listeria monocytogenes *as a Foodborne Pathogen*, British Food Manufacturing Industries Research Association Scientific and Technical Surveys no. 157, BFMIRA, Leatherhead, Surrey.

Marier R, Wells JG et al., 1973, An outbreak of enteropathogenic *Escherichia coli* foodborne disease traced to imported French cheese, *Lancet*, **2**: 1376–8.

Marth EH, 1969, Salmonellae and salmonellosis associated with milk and milk products. A review, *J Dairy Sci*, **52**: 283–315.

Martin ML, Shipman LD et al., 1986, Isolation of *Escherichia coli* O157:H7 from dairy cattle associated with two cases of haemolytic uraemic syndrome, *Lancet*, **2**: 1043.

Medina M, Gaya P, Nuñez M, 1982, Behaviour of salmonellae during manufacture and ripening of manchego cheese, *J Food Prot*, **45**: 1091–5.

Meers PD, 1979, A case of classical diphtheria, and other infections due to *Corynebacterium ulcerans*, *J Infect*, **1**: 139–42.

Mettler AE, 1989, Pathogens in milk powders – have we learned the lessons?, *J Soc Dairy Technol*, **42**: 48–55.

Milner J, 1995, *LFRA Microbiology Handbook, 1, Dairy Products*, Leatherhead Food RA, Leatherhead, Surrey.

Minor TE, Marth EH, 1972, *Staphylococcus aureus* and staphylococcal food intoxications. III Staphylococci in dairy foods, *J Milk Food Technol*, **35**: 77–82.

Mitten HL, Neirinckx JM, 1993, Developments in frozen-products manufacture, *Modern Dairy Technology*, vol. 2, 2nd edn, ed. Robinson RK, Elsevier Applied Science, London, 281–329.

Moore K, Damrow T et al., 1995, Outbreak of acute gastroenteritis attributable to *Escherichia coli* serotype O104:H21 – Helena, Montana, 1994, *Morbid Mortal Weekly Rep*, **44**: 501–3.

Morgan D, Mawer SL, Harman PL, 1994, The role of home-made ice cream as a vehicle of *Salmonella enteritidis* type 4 infection from fresh shell eggs, *Epidemiol Infect*, **113**: 21–9.

Morgan D, Newman CP et al., 1993, Verotoxin producing *Escherichia coli* O157 infections associated with consumption of yoghurt, *Epidemiol Infect*, **111**: 181–7.

Morgan D, Gunneberg C et al., 1994, An outbreak of *Campylobacter* infection associated with the consumption of unpasteurised milk at a large festival in England, *Eur J Epidemiol*, **10**: 581–5.

Morgan G, Chadwick P et al., 1985, *Campylobacter jejuni* mastitis in a cow: a zoonosis-related incident, *Vet Rec*, **116**: 111.

Morgan-Jones S, 1987, *Staphylococcus aureus* in milk and milk products, *Commun Dis Environ Health Scot*, **21 (87/43)**: 7–9.

Muytjens HL, Roelofs-Willemse H, Jaspar GHJ, 1988, Quality of powdered substitutes for breast milk with regard to members of the family Enterobacteriaceae, *J Clin Microbiol*, **26**: 743–6.

Muytjens HL, Zanen HC et al., 1983, Analysis of eight cases of neonatal meningitis and sepsis due to *Enterobacter sakazakii*, *J Clin Microbiol*, **18**: 115–20.

Nichols G, Greenwood M, de Louvois J, 1996, The microbiological quality of soft cheese, *PHLS Microbiol Dig*, **13**: 68–75.

Nichols G, de Louvois J, 1995, The microbiological quality of ice-cream and other edible ices, *PHLS Microbiol Dig*, **12**: 11–15.

Nooitgedagt AJ, Hartog BJ, 1988, A survey of the microbiological quality of Brie and Camembert cheese, *Neth Milk Dairy J*, **42**: 57–72.

O'Mahony M, Mitchell E et al., 1990, An outbreak of foodborne botulism associated with contaminated hazelnut yoghurt, *Epidemiol Infect*, **104**: 389–95.

Orr KE, Lightfoot NF et al., 1995, Direct milk excretion of *Campylobacter jejuni* in a dairy cow causing cases of human enteritis, *Epidemiol Infect*, **114**: 15–24.

Peeler JT, Bunning VK, 1994, Hazard assessment of *Listeria monocytogenes* in the processing of bovine milk, *J Food Prot*, **57**: 689–97.

Pickett G, Agate GH, 1967, Lactose-fermenting salmonella infection, *Morbid Mortal Weekly Rep*, **16**: 18.

Pini PN, Gilbert RJ, 1988, The occurrence in the UK of *Listeria* species in raw chickens and soft cheeses, *Int J Food Microbiol*, **6**: 317–26.

Place EH, Sutton LE, 1934, Erythema arthriticum epidemicum (Haverhill fever), *Arch Intern Med*, **54**: 659–84.

Pritchard TJ, Beliveau CM et al., 1994, Increased incidence of *Listeria* species in dairy processing plants having adjacent farm facilities, *J Food Prot*, **57**: 770–5.

Rampling A, Taylor CED, Warren RE, 1987, Safety of pasteurised milk, *Lancet*, **2**: 1209.

Rampling A, Mackintosh M et al., 1992, A microbiological hazard assessment of milk production on three dairy farms, *PHLS Microbiol Dig*, **9**: 116–19.

Ratnam S, March SB, 1986, Laboratory studies on salmonella-contaminated cheese involved in a major outbreak of gastroenteritis, *J Appl Bacteriol*, **61**: 51–6.

Reiss HJ, Potel J, Krebs A, 1951, Granulomatosis infantiseptica, *Z Gesamte Inn Med*, **6**: 451–7.

Report, 1985, *Salmonellosis Outbreak, Hillfarm Dairy, Melrose Park, Illinois*, Final Task Force report, US Food and Drugs Administration, Washington, DC.

Report, 1987a, *FDA's Dairy Product Safety Initiatives*, 2nd year status report, US Food and Drugs Administration, Washington, DC.

Report, 1987b, *Recommended Guidelines for Controlling Environmental Contamination in Dairy Plants*, US Food and Drugs Administration, Washington, DC, with Milk Industry Foundation, and International Ice Cream Association.

Report, 1988, *Guidelines for Good Hygienic Practice in the Manufacture of Soft and Fresh Cheeses – 1988*, Creamery Proprietors Association, 19 Cornwall Terrace, London NW1 4QP.

Report, 1989, *The Dairy Farmers Co-operative. Guidelines for Good Hygienic Practice for the Manufacture of Soft and Fresh Cheeses in Small and Farm Based Production Units*, Milk Marketing Board, Thames Ditton, Surrey.

Report, 1991a, *IDF Recommendations for the Hygienic Manufacture of Spray Dried Milk Powders*, International Dairy Federation Bulletin no. 267, IDF, Brussels.

Report, 1991b, *Salmonella enteritidis* associated with home-made ice cream, *Commun Dis Rep Weekly*, **1**: 175.

Report, 1994a, Outbreak of the tick-borne encephalitis; presumably milk borne, *Weekly Epidemiol Rec*, **69**: 140–1.

Report, 1994b, *Code of Practice for Pasteurisation of Milk on Farms and in Small Dairies*, BS 7771:1994.

Report, 1994c, Unpasteurised milk and *Streptococcus zooepidemicus*, *Commun Dis Rep Weekly*, **4**: 241.

Report, 1994d, Outbreak of *Salmonella enteritidis* associated with nationally distributed ice cream products – Minnesota, South Dakota, and Wisconsin 1994, *Morbid Mortal Weekly Rep*, **43**: 740–1.

Report, 1994e, Two clusters of haemolytic uraemic syndrome in France, *Commun Dis Rep Weekly*, **4**: 29.

Report, 1995, Brucellosis associated with unpasteurised milk products abroad, *Commun Dis Rep Weekly*, **5**: 151.

Report, 1996, VTEC O157 infection in West Yorkshire associated with the consumption of raw milk, *Commun Dis Rep Weekly*, **6**: 181.

Report of the Advisory Committee on the Microbiological Safety of Food, 1995, *Report on Verocytotoxin-producing* Escherichia coli, HMSO, London.

Report of the Committee on the Microbiological Safety of Food, 1990, *The Microbiological Safety of Food, Part 1*, London, HMSO.

Report of the Ice Cream Alliance and the Ice Cream Federation, 1992a, *Code of Practice for the Hygienic Manufacture of Ice Cream*, Milk Marketing Board, Thames Ditton, Surrey.

Report of the Ice Cream Alliance and the Ice Cream Federation, 1992b, *Code of Practice for the Safe Handling and Service of Scoop and Soft Serve Ice Cream*, Milk Marketing Board, Thames Ditton, Surrey.

Riordan T, Humphrey TJ, Fowles A, 1993, A point source outbreak of campylobacter infection related to bird-pecked milk, *Epidemiol Infect*, **10**: 261–5.

Roberts D, 1985, Microbiological aspects of goat's milk. A Public Health Laboratory Service survey, *J Hyg Camb*, **94**: 31–44.

Robinson DA, 1981, Infective dose of *Campylobacter jejuni* in milk, *Br Med J*, **282**: 1584.

Robinson RK, Tamime AY, 1990, Microbiology of fermented milks, *Dairy Microbiology*, vol. 2, 2nd edn, ed. Robinson RK, Elsevier Applied Science, London and New York, 291–343.

Robinson RK, Tamime AY, 1993, Manufacture of yoghurt and other fermented milks, *Modern Dairy Technology*, vol. 2, 2nd edn, ed. Robinson RK, Elsevier Applied Science, London and New York, 1–48.

Rocco RM, 1990, Fluorometric analysis of alkaline phosphatase in fluid dairy products, *J Food Prot*, **53**: 588–91.

Rodriguez JL, Gaya P et al., 1994, Incidence of *Listeria monocytogenes* and other listeria spp. in ewes' raw milk, *J Food Prot*, **57**: 571–5.

Rohrbach B, Draughon A et al., 1992, Prevalence of *Listeria monocytogenes*, *Campylobacter jejuni*, *Yersinia enterocolitica* and *Salmonella* in bulk tank milk: risk factors and risk of human exposure, *J Food Prot*, **55**: 93–7.

Rothwell J, 1979, Food poisoning risks associated with foods other than meat and poultry, *Health Hyg*, **3**: 3–10.

Rothwell J, 1990, Microbiology of ice cream and related products, *Dairy Microbiology*, vol. 2, 2nd edn, ed. Robinson RK, Elsevier Applied Science, London and New York, 1–39.

Rowe B, Begg NT et al., 1987, *Salmonella* Ealing infections associated with consumption of infant dried milk, *Lancet*, **2**: 900–3.

Ryan CA, Nickels MK et al., 1987, Massive outbreak of antimicrobial-resistant salmonellosis traced to pasteurized milk, *JAMA*, **258**: 3269–74.

Ryser ET, Marth EH, Doyle MP, 1985, Survival of *Listeria monocytogenes* during manufacture and storage of cottage cheese, *J Food Prot*, **48**: 746–50.

Sacks JJ, Roberto RR, Brooks NF, 1982, Toxoplasmosis infection associated with raw goat's milk, *JAMA*, **248**: 1728–32.

Saha AL, Ganguli NC, 1957, An outbreak of staphylococcal food poisoning from consumption of dahi, *Indian J Public Health*, **1**: 22–6.

Sanaa M, Poutrel B et al., 1993, Risk factors associated with contamination of raw milk by *Listeria monocytogenes* in dairy farms, *J Dairy Sci*, **76**: 2891–8.

Schaack MM, Marth EH, 1988, Survival of *Listeria monocytogenes* in refrigerated cultured milks and yoghurt, *J Food Prot*, **51**: 848–52.

Schiemann DA, 1987, *Yersinia enterocolitica* in milk and dairy products, *J Dairy Sci*, **70**: 383–91.

Schlech WF III, Lavigne PM et al., 1983, Epidemic listeriosis – evidence for transmission by food, *N Engl J Med*, **308**: 203–6.

Schröder MJA, 1984, Origins and levels of post pasteurisation contamination of milk in the dairy and their effects on keeping quality, *J Dairy Res*, **51**: 59–67.

Schroeder SA, 1967, What the sanitarian should know about salmonellae and staphylococci in milk and milk products, *J Milk Food Technol*, **30**: 376.

Scotter S, Aldridge M et al., 1993, Validation of European Community methods for microbiological and chemical analysis of raw and heat treated milk, *J Assoc Public Analysts*, **29**: 1–32.

Seeliger HPR, 1961, *Listeriosis*, 2nd edn, Hafner Publishing Co., New York.

Shanson DC, Gazzard BG et al., 1983, *Streptobacillus moniliformis* isolated from blood in four cases of Haverhill fever, *Lancet*, **2**: 92–4.

Sharp JCM, 1987, Infections associated with milk and dairy products in Europe and North America, 1980–85, *Bull W H O*, **65**: 397–406.

Sharp JCM, 1989, Milk-borne infection, *J Med Microbiol*, **29**: 239–42.

Sharp JCM, Paterson GM, Barrett NJ, 1985, Pasteurisation and

the control of milkborne infection in Britain, *Br Med J*, **291**: 463–4.

Shaw MB, 1993, Modern cheesemaking: soft cheeses, *Modern Dairy Technology*, vol. 2, 2nd edn, ed. Robinson RK, Elsevier Applied Science, London and New York, 221–80.

Skinner LJ, Chatterton JMW et al., 1987, Toxoplasmosis in the home and on the farm, *Commun Dis Environ Health Scot*, **21** (87/41): 5–7.

Skirrow MB, 1991, Epidemiology of *Campylobacter enteritis*, *Int J Food Microbiol*, **12**: 9–16.

Slade PJ, Fistrovici EC, Collins-Thompson DL, 1989, Persistence at source of *Listeria* spp. in raw milk, *Int J Food Microbiol*, **9**: 197–203.

Sockett PN, 1991, Communicable disease associated with milk and dairy products: England and Wales 1987–89, *Commun Dis Rep Rev*, **1**: R9–12.

Sockett PN, Roberts JA, 1991, The social and economic impact of salmonellosis. A report of a national survey in England and Wales of laboratory-confirmed salmonella infections, *Epidemiol Infect*, **107**: 335–47.

Southern JP, Smith RMM, Palmer SR, 1990, Bird attack on milk bottles: possible mode of transmission of *Campylobacter jejuni* to man, *Lancet*, **336**: 1425–7.

Steede FDW, Smith HW, 1954, Staphylococcal food-poisoning due to infected cow's milk, *Br Med J*, **2**: 576–8.

Sumner SS, Speckhard MW et al., 1985, Isolation of histamine-producing *Lactobacillus bucheri* from Swiss cheese implicated in a food poisoning outbreak, *Appl Environ Microbiol*, **50**: 1094–6.

Tacket CO, Narain JP et al., 1984, A multistate outbreak of infections caused by *Yersinia enterocolitica* transmitted by pasteurised milk, *JAMA*, **251**: 483–6.

Tamine AY, 1993, Modern cheesemaking: hard cheeses, *Modern Dairy Technology*, vol. 2, 2nd edn, ed. Robinson RK, Elsevier Applied Science, London and New York, 49–220.

Thomas WE, Stephens TH et al., 1948, Enteric fever (paratyphoid B) apparently spread by pasteurised milk, *Lancet*, **2**: 270–1.

Threlfall EJ, Ward LR et al., 1980, Plasmid-encoded trimethoprim resistance in multiresistant epidemic *Salmonella typhimurium* phage types 204 and 193 in Britain, *Br Med J*, **280**: 1210–11.

Tirard-Collet P, Zee JA et al., 1991, A study of the microbiological quality of goat milk in Quebec, *J Food Prot*, **54**: 263–6.

Tschäpe H, Prager R et al., 1995, Verotoxinogenic *Citrobacter freundii* associated with severe gastroenteritis and cases of haemolytic uraemic syndrome in a nursery school: green butter as the infection source, *Epidemiol Infect*, **114**: 441–50.

Upton P, Coia JE, 1994, Outbreak of *Escherichia coli* O157 infection associated with pasteurised milk supply, *Lancet*, **344**: 1015.

Valle J, Gomez-Lucia E et al., 1990, Enterotoxin production by staphylococci isolated from healthy goats, *Appl Environ Microbiol*, **56**: 1323–6.

Vernon E, Tillett HE, 1974, Food poisoning and salmonella infections in England and Wales 1969–1972, *Public Health*, **88**: 225–35.

Walker GC, Harmon LG, Stine CM, 1961, Staphylococci in Colby cheese, *J Dairy Sci*, **44**: 1272–82.

Wallach JC, Miguel SE et al., 1994, Urban outbreak of *Brucella melitensis* infection in an Argentine family: clinical and diagnostic aspects, *FEMS Immunol Med Microbiol*, **8**: 49–56.

Waterman SC, 1982, The heat-sensitivity of *Campylobacter jejuni* in milk, *J Hyg Camb*, **88**: 529–33.

Weissman JB, Deen RMAD et al., 1977, An island-wide epidemic of salmonellosis in Trinidad traced to contaminated powdered milk, *West Indian Med J*, **26**: 135–43.

Wells JG, Shipman LD et al., 1991, Isolation of *Escherichia coli* serotype O157:H7 and other shiga-like toxin producing *Escherichia coli* from dairy cattle, *J Clin Microbiol*, **29**: 985–9.

Wilbey RA, 1994, Production of butter and dairy based spreads,

Modern Dairy Technology, vol. 1, 2nd edn, ed. Robinson RK, Chapman and Hall, London, 107–58.

Wilson GS, 1942, *The Pasteurization of Milk*, Edward Arnold, London.

Wolf FS, Floyd C et al., 1970, Staphylococcal food poisoning traced to butter – Alabama, *Morbid Mortal Weekly Rep*, **19:** 271.

Wood RC, MacDonald KL, Osterholm MT, 1992, *Campylobacter* enteritis outbreaks associated with drinking raw milk during youth activities. A 10-year review of outbreaks in the United States, *JAMA*, **268:** 3228–30.

Working Party to the Director of the Public Health Laboratory Service, 1971, The hygiene and marketing of fresh cream as assessed by the methylene blue test, *J Hyg Camb*, **69:** 155–68.

Zall RR, 1990, Control and destruction of micro-organisms, *Dairy Microbiology*, vol. 1, 2nd edn, ed. Robinson RK, Elsevier Applied Science, London and New York, 115–61.

Chapter 17

THE BACTERIOLOGY OF FOODS EXCLUDING DAIRY PRODUCTS

B Swaminathan and P H Sparling

1 General principles of food microbiology	4 Bacteriology of specific food commodities
2 Factors influencing microbial growth in foods	5 New approach to assuring the safety of foods
3 Food processing and preservation	6 Conclusions

1 GENERAL PRINCIPLES OF FOOD MICROBIOLOGY

Food microbiology can be divided into 3 broad areas:

1 utilization of micro-organisms to enhance the nutritive value, organoleptic properties (colour, odour, flavour, texture, etc.) and the shelf-life of foods
2 control of food spoilage by reducing or eliminating the microbial content of foods or by making the food environment unsuitable for growth of spoilage micro-organisms and
3 food safety, the protection of the food supply from pathogenic bacteria that may be naturally present in foods or are introduced into foods during processing.

The food safety aspect of food microbiology is covered in other chapters of this treatise and will not be discussed in detail here. Local, national, and international laws and regulations are in place to protect the consumer from food-borne infections and intoxications of microbial and non-microbial origin. Because these are aimed at protecting the consumer from pathogenic micro-organisms, they will also not be the covered here.

Not all micro-organisms in foods are harmful. Without micro-organisms, we would not have the great variety of foods that we enjoy today. Examples of foods for which micro-organisms are essential include cheese, yogurt, fermented sausages, sauerkraut, and a whole array of fermented delicacies (tempeh, tofu, soy sauce). In addition, beer, wines, and other alcoholic beverages depend on the fermentation of appropriate substrates by yeasts. In order to produce a fermented food product that will have the desirable character-

istics mentioned earlier while preventing the spoilage organisms and pathogens from growing and causing problems requires an intimate knowledge of the micro-organisms involved in the 3 processes, particularly with respect to their behaviour in various food systems and their susceptibility to environmental conditions and chemicals. The branch of microbiology that deals with this specific area is called microbial ecology. The microbial ecology of foods is the central focus of this chapter. This topic is addressed in a concise manner with important references for additional information. The 2 volume treatise on *Microbial Ecology of Foods* developed by the International Commission on Microbiological Specifications for Foods (ICMSF) is highly recommended as an authoritative source for additional information on this subject (ICMSF 1980a, 1980b).

2 FACTORS INFLUENCING MICROBIAL GROWTH IN FOODS

Foods are very complex biological materials and they span a tremendous range in texture, fluidity and nutritional content, Nevertheless, several universal characteristics of foods influence the growth of micro-organisms in them. Among the major factors that must be considered are temperature, pH and water activity (a_w). In addition, the presence of organic acids, salts and other chemicals influences the growth of micro-organisms in foods.

2.1 Temperature

Although microbial growth can occur in the temperature range of $-8-90°C$, the range of temperature which must be considered in food microbiology is 1–50°C. Within this range, temperature affects the duration of lag phase, the rate of growth, the final population of cells, and the nutritional requirements. Temperatures immediately above and below the growth ranges of organisms may retard growth; if the temperature exceeds this upper limit, cell injury and cell death occur. The response of micro-organisms to freezing is more complex and depends on the cell wall composition of the organism, the final temperature and, more importantly, the rate of freezing.

Bacteria are classified into 4 groups based on their temperature ranges of growth: thermophiles, mesophiles, psychrophiles and psychrotrophs. Temperature optima for thermophiles are in the range of 55–75°C, for mesophiles 30–45°C, for psychrophiles 5–15°C, and for psychrotrophs 25–30°C. Most food spoilage and pathogenic bacteria are mesophiles. Psychrophiles are sensitive to temperatures higher than 20°C; therefore, they are not as important in foods as psychrotrophs which have temperature maxima in the range of 30–35°C. Because psychrotrophs are able to grow at refrigeration temperatures, they are important contributors to food spoilage. Bacteria in the genera *Acinetobacter*, *Alcaligenes*, *Bacillus*, *Chromobacterium*, *Enterobacter*, *Flavobacterium*, *Proteus*, *Pseudomonas* and *Serratia* are important causes of spoilage of foods, particularly those that are stored at refrigeration temperatures to increase their shelf-life. Some food-borne pathogenic bacteria (*Listeria monocytogenes*, *Yersinia enterocolitica*) are psychrotrophic and have caused disease outbreaks after contamination of a food product and its subsequent storage at refrigeration temperatures.

EFFECT OF CHILLING

As the temperature is lowered to the freezing point, the lag phase of bacterial growth increases rapidly. All except psychrotrophs stop growing; thus, psychrotrophs have a competitive advantage at low temperatures. Although generation times of psychrotrophs significantly increase at temperatures near freezing (for example, the generation time for *Pseudomonas fluorescens* at 0.5°C is 6.68 h), the refrigerated storage of foods for several days or weeks will allow their populations to reach several millions. As these bacteria grow using the food as the source of nutrients, they break down the lipids, proteins and carbohydrates in the food, producing degradation products of food components and their own metabolic byproducts which are associated with food spoilage.

EFFECTS OF FREEZING

The response of bacteria to freezing ranges from virtually no effect to injury and cell death. Most spores and some vegetative cells survive with nearly no effect whereas most non-spore-forming bacteria are affected to some extent. Generally, gram-negative bacteria are more sensitive to freezing than gram-positive bacteria. Among the bacteria sensitive to freezing, sublethal cell injury and cell death are the consequences. Sublethally injured cells are highly sensitive to selective agents used in selective enrichment and plating media; therefore, the use of these microbiological media to determine bacterial counts in frozen food products is most likely to underestimate the total microbial populations because of under-representation of sublethally injured bacteria. Because sublethally injured bacteria may repair their damage and become fully viable under appropriate environmental conditions, they remain a threat to the integrity of the food.

The rate of freezing and the final storage temperature influence bacterial injury and survival. The temperature range between −2 and −10°C is most detrimental for bacteria. Slow freezing of bacteria to approximately −10°C will cause maximum damage whereas rapid freezing of bacteria to −30°C or lower is likely to cause minimal damage. However, slow freezing also has a detrimental effect on the organoleptic characteristics of foods and is therefore not generally used as a means of bacterial inactivation.

The growth of bacteria in frozen foods after thawing depends on the numbers and types that survived the freezing process and the conditions used for thawing. Uncontrolled thawing may significantly increase the numbers of bacteria. When a large block of frozen food is thawed, the areas near the surface will thaw much faster than the core. Thus bacteria near the surface of the foods may initiate growth and go through several generations before the centre of the food is completely thawed. This is the reason for recommending that frozen foods (particularly large blocks such as frozen turkeys) should be thawed at refrigeration temperature or rapidly by microwave heating but not at room temperature.

EFFECTS OF HEATING

As the temperature is increased above the optimum growth range, growth of bacteria ceases, injury, and ultimately, cell death occur. As noted under freezing effects, mild exposures to heat cause sublethal injury in vegetative cells that is repairable; spores are much more refractile to heat. In fact, heat activates spores to germinate. An exposure of 5 min at 80°C is typically used to inactivate vegetative cells and induce spores to germinate. As the temperature is further increased, destruction of the bacterial population occurs at an exponential (logarithmic) rate. Figure 17.1 shows a typical survivor curve for bacteria. By plotting the logarithm of the number of survivors against the time of heating at a specific temperature, a straight line is obtained because the rate of death is constant at a given temperature and is independent of the initial population of cells. The decimal reduction time (time required to destroy 90% of the cells, D value) may be calculated from the survivor curve. The D value for the bacteria in Fig. 17.1 is 4.9 min at 121°C. Because the ordinate of the plot is on a logarithmic scale, it is evident that the population of bacteria would never be reduced to zero. Thus, if a known population of bacteria in each of several unit volumes or containers were exposed to lethal heat treatments, there will always remain a probability of a survivor in any one container. These calculations are used to determine the amount of heat treatment to be given to a specific type of food in a specific type of container so that the probability of survival is so low that it is acceptable. For example, a 12*D* process is generally used in commercial canning operations to assure that canned low-acid foods are free of botulism toxin hazard.

The survivor curve gives information on the time of heat treatment required to destroy a certain proportion of bacteria at a specific temperature. The thermal death time curve is used to determine the effect of heat treatment of bacteria suspended in a medium at several temperatures. A thermal death time curve is constructed by plotting the $\log_{10} D$ values against the treatment temperature. The slope of the curve is denoted by the term *z*, which is the temperature in °C

required for the thermal death curve to traverse one log cycle. *D* and *z* values are extensively used in determining the heating requirement for foods preserved by pasteurization and sterilization.

Many factors influence the heat resistance of bacteria. These may be divided into 3 broad types:

1 differences in heat resistance characteristics of different species within a genus
2 the environmental conditions to which the bacteria were previously exposed and
3 the properties of the food to which they are exposed during heat treatment.

If these factors are not considered in developing a thermal treatment process for foods, food spoilage and food-borne infection or intoxication may result.

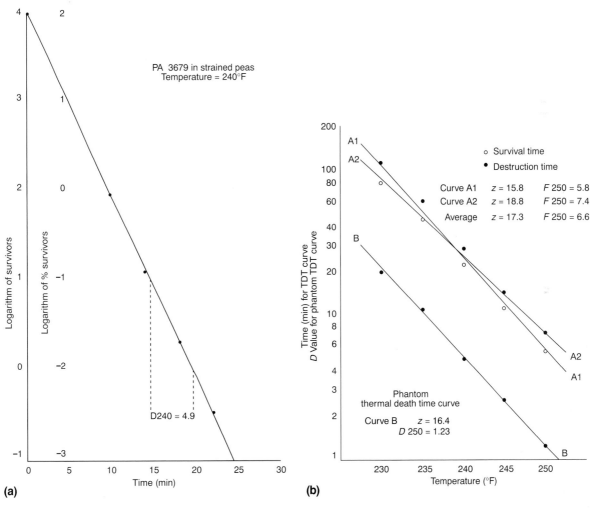

Fig. 17.1 (a) A typical survivor curve for bacteria. The test organism used to develop this curve is putrefactive anaerobe (PA) 3679 which is a non-toxigenic *Clostridium* species that has heat-resistance characteristics similar to that of *C. botulinum*. Therefore, PA 3679 is often used to determine or verify the thermal process conditions required to inactivate *C. botulinum* in specific foods. In this illustration, the *D* value for PA 3679 at 115°C (240°F) is 4.9 min. (b) An example of a thermal death time (TDT) curve. The *D* values are plotted on a logarithmic scale against the corresponding temperature on a linear scale to obtain the phantom TDT curves. These lines are described by the *D* value at a reference temperature (usually 60°C or 121°C) and the slope of the curve (denoted by *z*). '*z*' is defined as the temperature that is necessary to bring about a 10-fold change in the *D* value. '*F*' denotes the time of treatment necessary to destroy micro-organisms at a reference temperature, usually 60°C for vegetative cells and 121°C for spores. (Parts a and b based on Figures 7-7 and 7-8 from *Laboratory Manual for Food Canners and Processors*, vol. 1, National Canners Association Research Laboratories, 1968, AVI Publishing Company, Westport, CT with permission from National Food Processors Association, Washington, DC).

2.2   Water activity

Micro-organisms require water in an available form for growth and metabolism. The most useful measurement of available water is water activity (a_w). The a_w of a food or solution is the ratio of the water vapour pressure of the food (p) to that of pure water (p_0) at the same temperature. The a_w of pure water is assumed to be 1. When a solution becomes more concentrated with the addition of more solute (for example, salt, sugar, or other chemical), the vapour pressure decreases to a value less than 1. Most bacteria and fungi are unable to grow at a_w of less than 0.90. However, some bacteria and fungi are able to grow at a_w values below 0.90; these are the organisms to be considered in preventing food spoilage. These are variously referred to as halophiles, xerophiles and osmophiles. Gram-negative bacteria generally do not grow below a_w values of 0.97. Between a_w values of 0.98 and 0.93, gram-positive bacteria – Lactobacillaceae, Bacillaceae and Micrococcaceae – become important. Below 0.93, spoilage is primarily caused by yeasts and fungi. Xerophilic fungi and osmophilic yeasts cause spoilage at a_w values below 0.85. Below a_w of 0.60, micro-organisms are unable to grow.

2.3   pH

Bacteria have a minimum, optimum and maximum pH for growth. Because the cell membrane is only slightly permeable to hydrogen or hydroxyl ions, and the cytoplasmic contents have a buffering effect, the internal pH inside bacterial cells is usually close to 7.0. Bacteria differ in the minimum pH values at which they can initiate growth. In fact, some bacteria such as the lactic acid bacteria create an acid environment by producing acids as metabolic products and gain a selective advantage over bacteria that are less acid-tolerant. Most bacteria are unable to grow at pH levels less than 3.5. High pH values also inhibit micro-organisms. Egg white develops a pH of 9 because of the loss of CO_2 after the egg is laid; this protects the egg from bacterial invasion. Proteolytic organisms such as *Pseudomonas* spp. can grow in moderately alkaline substrates.

2.4   Redox potential

Redox potential (Eh) of a biological system is an index of its degree of oxidation and is an important selective factor in the food environment. Bacteria are classified as aerobic, anaerobic, facultative, or micro-aerobic based on the Eh required for their growth and metabolism. The Eh of a food is related to its chemical composition (pH, concentration of reducing substances such as ascorbic acid, mercapto groups in proteins, reducing sugars, etc.) and the oxygen partial pressures existing over the food during storage.

2.5   Nutrients

The nutritional composition of foods influences the type of bacteria that are likely to be present in them. The nutrient requirements of bacteria may change based on the environment in which they are grown. For example, bacteria generally become more fastidious at higher growth temperatures or lower a_w values. Generally, foods provide sufficient nutrients for most micro-organisms. However, there is a wide range in nutrient complexity and availability; meats are generally considered highly nutritious and vegetables are considered to provide minimal nutrients.

Spoilage of starchy foods like potatoes and cereal grains is primarily caused by bacteria that are able to break down the complex carbohydrates and thrive in a minimum nitrogen and salts environment. Fresh vegetables are spoiled primarily by cellulolytic organisms. Bacteria with high lipolytic activity are favoured in lipid-containing foods. Highly proteinaceous foods favour the growth of bacteria with complex nutritional needs.

2.6   Other factors

In addition to the factors discussed above, other factors that influence the growth of bacteria in foods are natural components of foods that have antibacterial properties (essential oils, tannins, and lectins). Animal foods contain many inhibitors of bacteria (lactenin in milk, lysozyme, conalbumin, ovomucoid, and avidin in eggs) but they usually have a narrow spectrum of activity and are quite labile. Therefore, they do not play a major role in preventing food spoilage.

Inhibitory factors may also be produced in foods as a result of processing. Sugar syrups undergo a browning reaction during storage, leading to the formation of furfural and its derivatives which have antimicrobial properties. Similarly, the oxidative chemical deterioration of foods during storage also leads to the formation of products with antimicrobial properties.

3   Food processing and preservation

Most agricultural products used for human food cannot be used directly without some processing. Even fresh produce like apples, potatoes, tomatoes, and beans must be washed, trimmed, sorted and packaged. Often, more extensive processing is needed to convert a raw agricultural commodity such as beef cattle, wheat kernels and sunflower seed into meat, flour, bread and cooking oil. Thus the primary objective of food processing is to convert raw agricultural commodities into processed foods or food ingredients. The food ingredients (flour, sugar, oil, etc.) may then be used in a secondary food processing operation to manufacture food ready for human consumption. Generally, food processing operations, particularly the secondary operations, integrate food processing with food preservation. The 2 objectives of preservation are to prolong the shelf-life of the processed food or food ingredient so that it can be stored for long periods of time and distributed efficiently over great distances, and to assure the safety of processed foods. Therefore, the food preservation aspect of food processing deals with the control of micro-organisms in foods to enhance the quality of foods, retard their spoilage, and eliminate pathogens. Strategies to achieve these objectives are developed on the basis of our knowledge of micro-organisms and their response to the various extrinsic and intrinsic environmental factors discussed earlier (see Table 17.1).

3.1 Food dehydration

Natural sun drying of foods is the oldest food preservation technique used by humans. Sun drying is still used to preserve large quantities of food in many developing countries, particularly those with tropical climates. In modern food processing, however, dehydration is accomplished in more controlled environments such as by using hot air (spray drying, fluidized bed drying, etc.), by contact with a hot surface (roller drying), or by sublimation of ice from frozen food (freeze drying). In addition to inhibiting the growth of micro-organisms, dehydration also reduces the bulkiness of foods, making them more economical to store and transport. Disadvantages of drying include the acceleration of undesirable chemical reactions that occur in foods during exposure to high temperatures. Some foods withstand dehydration better than others. Freeze drying has the least undesirable effects on the food quality but it is the most expensive and energy-intensive drying process.

It is important to control carefully the handling of foods before and after the drying operation to prevent microbial spoilage and food-borne illness. Ingredients for dried foods must be of good microbiological quality. They should be stored under conditions to minimize microbial growth before drying. Some foods, such as meats, require a heat treatment prior to drying. Cooking reduces the moisture content by approximately 20% and reduces the number of viable bacteria. Similarly, blanching of fruits and vegetables or the pasteurization of liquid eggs before dehydration reduces the total number of viable bacteria in the final product.

The total bacterial counts of dehydrated foods are usually lower than the counts in the food before drying on a per gram basis. This is due to the inactivation of some, but not all, the bacteria. Of the surviving bacteria, a proportion may be sublethally injured. The extent of cell death and cell injury depends on the type of food (fat content of the food, pH, presence of inhibitors, previous treatment history), the organism (species, strain, physiological age, state of the cells, and the concentration of cells), and the type of drying process.

Because freeze drying is the gentlest of freezing methods, it is likely to result in high survival of bacteria. The total bacterial counts of freeze-dried shrimps may be reduced only one or 2 logs; therefore, if one started with shrimp that had 10^6 bacteria per gram, one is likely to end up with 10^4 bacteria per gram after the freeze drying process, which is higher than the acceptable limit (10^2–10^3 cfu g^{-1}). Generally, gram-negative bacteria such as *Pseudomonas* spp., *Escherichia coli*, and *Vibrio* spp. do not survive freezing as well as gram-positive bacteria. Cells of *Lactobacillus acidophilus* that survived freeze drying revealed damage to cell membrane and cell wall (Brennan et al. 1986); cellular DNA may also be damaged.

Table 17.1 Preservation methods used in food processing

Process	How preservation is accomplished
Drying	Reduction of water activity below the level required for microbial growth
Chilling	Lowering of temperature to a point at which microbial growth is retarded or inhibited
Freezing	Changing of water to a form in which microbes are unable to utilize it; also, freezing temperatures inhibit enzymatic activity
Heat sterilization in hermetically sealed containers	Inactivation of all viable forms of bacteria followed by storage under conditions to prevent recontamination and chemical degradation
Pasteurization and other heat processes that do not completely eliminate micro-organisms	Reduction of spoilage bacteria to a significantly low level so that the shelf-life of the product is extended; also, pathogenic bacteria are eliminated
Irradiation	Inactivation of all viable bacteria
Pickling, salting and sugaring	Reducing the acidity and/or water activity to levels which inhibit the growth of micro-organisms
Fermentation	Controlling the environmental conditions to favour the growth of beneficial micro-organisms and retarding or inhibiting the growth of spoilage and harmful micro-organisms

During spray drying, finely aerosolized liquid food is brought into contact with hot air to remove the moisture. Bacteria are affected by the aerosolization, heating and drying. There may be changes in the outer layer of the cell envelope, cytoplasmic constituents may leak out, and they may lack control of ion transport (Banwart 1987). During the spray drying of liquid egg, a lower temperature during drying and rapid cooling of the product after drying enhance the qualities of the dried egg product; however, the same conditions are favourable for the survival of *Salmonella*. Over 99% of *Salmonella* cells are killed during spray drying if the inlet temperature is maintained at 121°C and the outlet temperature is maintained at 60°C (Banwart 1987). Although dried fish products can be produced with total bacterial loads as low as 10^2 cfu g^{-1}, commercial dried fish may have total bacterial counts as high as 10^7 cfu g^{-1}.

Because all bacteria in dried foods are not inactivated, the surviving viable and sublethally injured bacteria will initiate growth under appropriate environmental conditions. It is therefore critical to maintain product integrity by storing dried foods under appropriate storage conditions. Dried foods must be stored in moisture-impermeable containers under low humidity to prevent unacceptable increases in the a_w. Salmonellae that survive the drying of eggs are inactivated during the storage of the dried eggs even at low temperatures whereas salmonellae in dried albumen can be inactivated by storing the product at 50–60°C for up to 7 days. Generally, bacteria survive better in dried foods under vacuum than in the presence of oxygen.

3.2 Chilling and freezing

Clarence Birdseye in the USA and Bill Heeney in Canada pioneered the frozen foods industry in North America. The rapid expansion in frozen food technology paralleled the engineering developments in the refrigeration industry. Although frozen foods are expensive to process and store, food quality deterioration is greatly diminished by freezing compared with dehydration and heat sterilization.

The major difference between refrigerated food and frozen foods is the temperature at which the food is held. Because water in the refrigerated food is still available, psychrotrophic spoilage bacteria and pathogens can grow in it.

Freezing makes water unavailable to microorganisms by immobilizing it in the form of ice. The low temperature at which frozen food must be held deters the growth of micro-organisms. Freezing is not effective in inactivating bacteria, although some reduction in bacterial counts is achieved. Gram-negative bacteria are more susceptible than gram-positive bacteria to freezing-induced injury and death.

Several factors affect the effectiveness of freezing as a preservation technique. These include initial microbial load, the physical dimensions of the product being frozen, the packaging material, the freezing rate, the time and temperature of storage, the degree of fluctuation in the storage temperature, and the time–temperature conditions used for thawing. The freezing process can be divided into 3 stages:

1 cooling down from the initial temperature of the product to the temperature at which freezing begins
2 chilling at the latent heat plateau when there is no temperature change but phase change of water to ice occurs and
3 further cooling to the final storage temperature.

The initial cooling may inactivate a proportion of the micro-organisms due to cold shock; the decrease in temperature also reduces the growth rate of psychrotrophic bacteria. During the phase transition, bacteria may be killed due to mechanical injury to the cell wall and cell membrane during ice formation. Further cooling inhibits the growth of most cold-tolerant micro-organisms until it ceases at about –8°C. Slow freezing to a final temperature of –10°C is more lethal to bacteria than rapid freezing to –20°C; during slow freezing ice crystals form to concentrate soluble solids that affect the stability of cellular proteins. However, slow freezing also has adverse effects on the texture and structural integrity of foods.

Freezing may cause inactivation of 10–60% of the total bacterial populations depending on the food characteristics, the organism characteristics and the freezing conditions. Bacterial spores are not affected by freezing and bacterial toxins are not inactivated by freezing. Therefore, it is possible for food intoxication to occur from pre-formed toxin in frozen food.

3.3 Food preservation by heat treatment

Heat sterilization in hermetically sealed containers

The technology of conventional canning may be summarized as filling food into containers of metal, glass, thermostable plastic, or a multilayered flexible pouch, sealing the containers, and heat treating them. This process is sometimes called 'terminal sterilization' and is designed to destroy large numbers of *Clostridium botulinum* spores. The process also reduces the chances of survival of spores of spoilage organisms that are more heat-resistant that *C. botulinum* spores. After heating, the containers must be cooled and handled in such a manner as to assure container integrity and avoid contamination caused by leakage.

The sterilization parameters vary greatly and depend on the composition of the foods. One of the most important factors in determining the time–temperature combinations for foods is the pH of the food. Low-acid foods (pH >4.5) and a_w >0.85 are likely to support the germination of *C. botulinum* spores and the subsequent production of botulinal toxin. Therefore, specific regulations exist in most countries for processing low-acid foods in hermetically sealed containers. The minimum heat treatment process for these foods is a 12*D* reduction process based on the thermal death times determined for each specific food product. The 12*D* reduction process is sufficient to reduce the probability of survival of *C. botulinum* spores to no more than 1 in 10^{12} cans (containers) processed.

The manufacturing process must include appropriate good manufacturing practices before the heat sterilization step. The heat sterilization step will not inactivate pre-formed toxins that are heat-resistant. Therefore, the quality of the ingredients must be evaluated and their handling must be designed to prevent bacterial contamination and/or growth. If acidification of the product is possible, i.e. it does not adversely influence the organoleptic characteristics of the food, it should be included because acidified food products require much less heat treatment than low-acid foods to assure their safety. Examples of food products that are amenable to acidification include artichoke hearts, pimentos and many pickles.

The *D* and *z* values were described earlier in this chapter (see p. 397). Another term that figures in the calculation of heat treatment parameters for foods is the *F* value. *F* is defined as the time required to inactivate a given number of bacteria at a specified temperature, usually 121°C for spores and 60°C for vegetative cells. For example, *F*60 is the thermal death time (TDT) at 60°C and *F*121 is the TDT at 121°C. Esty and Meyer indicated in 1922 that *F* for *C. botulinum* spores was 2.78 min. Based on this, the generally accepted minimum treatment for achieving 12*D* reduction of *C. botulinum* spores is 3 min at 121°C. Commercially canned cured meat products receive thermal treatments well below this because their heat treatment is supplemented by the inhibitory effect of curing salts on the germination of spores of *C. botulinum*. Low-acid canned uncured meats are treated at an *F*121 of 6 min. Using the *D*, *F* and *z* values, the rate of heat penetration in a specific food, its pH, and the retort temperature, a thermal process for that specific food can be calculated. Experimental inoculated packs are processed at the calculated thermal process conditions to evaluate the adequacy of the process. *Clostridium sporogenes* PA3679 is usually used as the test organism in inoculated pack studies because the spores of this non-toxigenic strain have higher heat resistance than do those of *C. botulinum*.

Container integrity is essential for maintaining the safety of commercially sterilized food products and for preventing spoilage. If the cans develop leaks, air or water may enter, carrying spoilage bacteria; in some instances water may also carry pathogenic bacteria. Effective control measures to prevent post-processing contamination of cans are assuring proper function of sealing equipment, disinfection of the water used to cool the containers after heat treatment, keeping the containers dry in so far as possible, and avoidance of abuse of the containers.

Heat-sterilized foods in cans are subject to different kinds of spoilage. Spoilage may occur prior to processing or may be due to inadequate heat treatment or post-process contamination. Spoilage due to inadequate heat treatment is due to heat-resistant spores. Inadequate cooling or high storage temperature leads to spoilage by thermophilic bacteria. Spoilage due to water leakage usually involves non-spore-forming bacteria, yeasts and moulds. Spoilage may be indicated by bulging of the can at one or both ends. Spoilage due to flat sour organisms (*Bacillus coagulans* and *Bacillus stearothermophilus*) does not lead to bulging of cans.

ASEPTIC PACKAGING

In aseptic packaging, the food is sterilized, cooled and transported under aseptic conditions to the container, which has also been sterilized. The product is filled into the container and sealed under aseptic conditions. The end product is a hermetically sealed container that is holding a commercially sterile food, which can be stored at ambient temperature for prolonged periods.

PASTEURIZATION

The heat treatment of foods below the temperatures needed for sterilization is termed pasteurization. Generally, this type of heat treatment is used to prolong the shelf-life of foods that do not withstand sterilization. Pasteurization is usually used to inactivate specific groups of bacteria, particularly pathogenic bacteria, and to reduce the numbers of spoilage bacteria. In addition to milk and dairy products, pasteurization is used to control micro-organisms in liquid egg products, alcoholic beverages, smoked fish and high-acid products (fruit juices, pickles, sauerkraut and vinegar).

Food regulations in developed counties require that all liquid, frozen, and dried whole egg, yolk and white be pasteurized to destroy viable salmonellae. However, the temperature and time requirements vary from country to country, ranging from 62°C for 150 s to 68°C for 180 s.

3.4 Irradiation

The process of food irradiation uses γ-rays from radioactive isotopes such as caesium-137 or cobalt-60, or electrons from linear accelerators (Banwart 1987). Radiation treatment of foods can inhibit sprouting of vegetables (potatoes and onions), delay ripening of fruits and vegetables, destroy parasites and pathogenic bacteria in meats, poultry and fish, reduce viable bacteria in dried products such as spices and herbs, destroy spoilage organisms to extend the shelf-life of perishable and semi-perishable foods, and commercially sterilize various foods.

The ionizing radiation doses for the destruction of micro-organisms vary widely with the type and numbers of cells, type of substrate or suspending medium, oxygen tension, temperature, or the presence of protective compounds. Radiation causes cell death by directly attacking the DNA and causing single- or double-strand breaks. The resistance of an organism to ionizing radiation is, in part, dependent on the capacity of the organism to repair the damage to its DNA. Bacterial spores are highly resistant to ionizing radiations; reported *D* values for spores of *C. botulinum* type A are 2.18–2.35 kGy in cured ham. Generally, gram-positive bacteria are more resistant than gram-negative bacteria: *Pseudomonas* spp., *E. coli* and *Proteus* spp. are very sensitive to ionizing radiation.

Although ionizing radiation has the potential to enhance the quality of our food supply and to increase its safety, it has not gained wide acceptance for use in food processing because of the public's fear of anything 'nuclear'. Ionizing radiation treatment has been approved in the USA for fruits, vegetables, spices, poultry and pork but is not commercially used.

4   BACTERIOLOGY OF SPECIFIC FOOD COMMODITIES

4.1   Meats

Meat comprises the musculature of 'red meat' mammals, commonly bovines, ovines and porcines. Depending upon the country and its religion, the meat supply may be beef, pig, lamb, goat, camel or horse. Within a species, the proportions of muscle, fat and connective tissues vary from one breed to another, and with age and rearing conditions, particularly the energy content and quantity of feed. Young animals deposit mainly protein; fat deposition increases with physiological age at the expense of protein. The amount of connective tissue varies in different muscles, those with little being tender to eat even after mild cooking (e.g. grilling), whereas those containing larger amounts are considered tough unless subjected to more severe and prolonged cooking to gelatinize the collagen. With increasing age the collagen of the musculature becomes more heavily cross-linked. A proportion of cross-links are heat-stable, causing meat from older animals to be less tender unless cooked thoroughly (e.g. by cooking under pressure). Some fat is necessary for maximum eating quality, particularly succulence, and for the full development of cooked meat flavour, but there is sufficient intramuscular fat for these purposes in all but unusually lean animals.

The contractile elements of the muscle, the myofibrils, also contribute to meat texture. The ultimate pH of meat is proportional to the amount of lactic acid formed during postmortem glycolysis, which is dependent on the amount of glycogen in the muscles at death. In a muscle rested before slaughter almost all the glycogen is converted to lactic acid (a concentration of c. 1% lactic acid corresponds to pH 5.5), giving a muscle of normal appearance and texture. Low glycogen levels result in muscle of high ultimate pH. Such muscles often appear dark and, in addition, are firm and dry (DFD). In stress-susceptible animals, especially certain cross-bred pigs, excitement or stress before slaughter causes rapid conversion of muscle glycogen to lactic acid, resulting in a low pH before the muscles have cooled. This denatures sarcoplasmic protein and reduces the water-holding capacity of the tissue, giving a pale, soft, exudative (PSE) condition.

Meat comprises contractile myofibrillar elements and soluble sarcoplasmic proteins with up to one-quarter by weight connective tissue and as much as one-third fat. The presence of connective tissue seems unimportant microbiologically, but the relevant properties of the fat differ considerably from those of the muscle.

Intensive rearing of cattle, sheep and pigs has resulted in a large international trade in meat. International trade developed by transporting carcasses but, in transporting prime cuts, has become predominantly an intermediate stage between the carcass and the retail-sized portions. Muscle contains c. 75% water and a variety of substrates for microbial growth, including carbohydrates, amino acids, lactic acid (Dainty, Shaw and Roberts 1983, Lawrie 1985). The a_w of meat is high, c. 0.99, which is suitable for the growth of most microbes. Only by removing most of the water (e.g. by drying) will the a_w be reduced sufficiently to affect microbial growth.

Within the pH range of meat (c. 5.4–7.0), values approaching 5.4 are less favourable to the growth of many of the important bacteria; the lower pH values are particularly important in maintaining the microbiological stability and safety of cured meat products.

The redox potential of meat has been claimed to be important in determining the nature of microbial spoilage, but its exact role in permitting or preventing the growth of microbes has not been elucidated due to unresolved experimental problems of controlling and measuring redox potential. Tissue respiration of oxygen continues after death; because supply of oxygen via the blood has ceased, the oxygen content and the redox potential of muscle fall, leading to anaerobic conditions even a few millimetres below the surface. However, microbial growth in the deep musculature is rare except where refrigeration is inadequate (Gill 1979, Roberts and Mead 1986).

MICROBIOLOGY AT PRODUCTION

In industrially developed countries changed eating patterns and technological developments in animal husbandry, meat production, food processing and preservation have increased enormously the range of meat products available, and novel methods have been developed to maximize the recovery of meat from the carcass. Many meat products spend weeks, or even months, in distribution and storage before being offered for sale alongside the fresh product. The lower the number of microbes present initially, the longer will be the shelf-life of the perishable product.

Bacterial contamination of carcass surfaces can occur during slaughter and dressing procedures from a variety of sources, such as hides, intestinal contents, contact surfaces and handling by workers. Faecal contamination, routinely experienced during the normal slaughtering process contributes high levels of bacteria (typically >10 000 cfu cm^{-2}). Good sanitary practices during slaughter, trimming of visible faecal contamination, and washing of carcasses with or without sanitizers are the approaches usually employed to minimize the contamination of carcasses (Dickson and Anderson 1992). The addition of chlorine, acetic acid or lactic acid to the wash water reduces the bacterial load on the surface but does not significantly increase the shelf-life or completely eliminate pathogenic bacteria (Prasai et al. 1995). Higher water pressures (>13.8 bar) during spray washing are more effective in reducing bacterial loads on the surfaces of carcasses. Also, a 2-step washing procedure with a low pressure hot water (72°C) wash followed by a high pressure, low temperature (30°C) wash was reported to be effective in reducing surface bacterial contamination (Gorman et al. 1995, Dorsa et al. 1996).

The surface flora of freshly slaughtered carcasses, usually in the range of 10^1–10^3 cfu cm^{-2}, is primarily mesophilic, having originated in the alimentary tract and the external surfaces of the live animal. Contamination from the slaughtering environment is also predominantly by mesophiles; psychrotrophs originating from soil and water are also present, but at much lower levels. Usually carcasses are cut into smaller portions in refrigerated work rooms where most bacteria on the surfaces of processing equipment are psychrotrophic in nature. During refrigerated holding, the microflora of meats begins to shift towards psychrotrophs of the *Pseudomonas–Acinetobacter–Moraxella* group. These organisms are ultimately responsible for the spoilage of refrigerated meats. The spoilage is primarily a surface phenomenon resulting in the formation of slime and off-odour. The shelf-life of refrigerated meats is extended by controlling the factors contributing to the growth of psychrotrophs, namely, moisture levels at the surface of the meat, initial load of psychrotrophs, pH, oxygen tension, and temperature. Wrapping meat in oxygen-impermeable films retards surface growth and favours the growth of micro-aerophilic bacteria such as *Lactobacillus* and *Brochothrix thermosphacta* over the *Pseudomonas–Acinetobacter–Moraxella* group. The bacterial load of chilled meats at the retail market may bear no relationship to the load at the processing plant because of the continued growth of psychrotrophs during transportation and storage.

The microbiology of meat other than the musculature is relatively poorly researched, with few publications on the microbiology of edible offal such as heart, liver and kidney, despite their increasing use in meat products. The significance of microbial growth on fat and its role in spoilage have been evaluated only under a limited range of conditions.

Coliforms, *E. coli*, enterococci, *Campylobacter*, *Staphylococcus aureus*, *Clostridium perfringens*, *L. monocytogenes*, *Y. enterocolitica*, and *Salmonella* are often present on fresh tissues because the slaughtering process does not currently include a bactericidal step. *E. coli* O157:H7 is a newly emerged pathogen that has caused major food-borne disease outbreaks in which undercooked hamburgers were implicated. Enterohaemorrhagic *E. coli*, of which *E. coli* O157:H7 is the most frequently encountered serotype, have the ability to adhere intimately to human intestinal cells by an attaching and effacing mechanism and produce one or more phage-encoded Shiga-like toxins. In addition to haemorrhagic colitis, *E. coli* O157:H7 may cause serious life-threatening clinical diseases such as

haemolytic–uraemic syndrome and thrombotic thrombocytopenic purpura in children and the elderly. *E. coli* O157:H7 has a low infectious dose (estimated to be of the order of 10–100 cfu) and is spread by person-to-person contact in day care settings (Griffin 1995).

Cattle are the primary reservoirs of *E. coli* O157:H7. Carcasses may become contaminated during slaughter and dressing operations. Meat from a single carcass may contaminate large batches of ground beef because of the tendency to mix and blend meats of several animals from different farms during the production of ground meats. Withholding of feed, as is normally done before shipping or slaughter to reduce faecal contamination, can lead to intestinal outgrowth and colonization by *E. coli* O157:H7 and *Salmonella* due to the disruption of normal fermentation in the rumen (Rasmussen et al. 1993). Shedding of *Salmonella* and *E. coli* O157:H7 by feedlot cattle after shipping appears to be directly related to their length of stay in pens (National Animal Health Monitoring System 1995).

Few studies have been conducted on the prevalence of pathogenic bacteria at different locations on pork carcasses. Epling, Carpenter and Blankenship (1993) reported that the prevalence of *Salmonella* and *Campylobacter* spp. on shoulder and ham surfaces was as great or greater after 24 h of chilling at 4°C when compared with the numbers at slaughter. Swine are the main reservoir of *Y. enterocolitica*; the organism appears to have a predilection for the tonsils and tongue of swine. During the Christmas season in the southeastern USA, outbreaks of *Y. enterocolitica* infections have been caused by raw chitterlings (pork intestines); typically the organism is spread by adults who handle the chitterlings and then transmit the organisms to their infants and children (Lee et al. 1990).

Salmonella, motile aeromonads and *Y. enterocolitica* have been isolated from lamb carcasses sampled at commercial abattoirs (Sierra et al. 1995). Horizontal transmission of infection and persistent shedding (for 2 weeks) of *E. coli* O157:H7 were demonstrated after oral inoculations of lambs with 10^5–10^9 cfu of the organism. As observed in cattle, withholding of feed from lambs causes increased shedding of *E. coli* O157:H7 (Kudva, Hatfield and Hovde 1995). In nature, however, sheep appear to harbour *E. coli* O157:H7 and other enterohaemorrhagic *E. coli*.

Irradiation treatment has the potential to reduce pathogen contamination signficantly while prolonging the shelf-life of meats. Irradiation of ground beef in air with 1 kGy of γ-rays will reduce the numbers of *Salmonella*, *Y. enterocolitica* and *Campylobacter* spp. but may cause objectionable odour, colour and flavour changes. A 2 kGy treatment of vacuum-packaged beef at 25°C eliminates pseudomonads, enteric bacteria and enterococci and causes fewer odour and flavour problems (Lee et al. 1996).

SHELF-STABLE RAW SALTED AND SALT-CURED MEATS

Salting of meats was an extremely common practice used in the USA to preserve meats before the introduction of home refrigeration units. Raw salted products continue to be produced and sold in the USA, especially in predominantly agricultural areas. Salt pork, dry cured bacon, and country-cured hams continue to be sold in volume even today. The process of dry curing involves coating pieces of meat with salt and storing in bins at below 10°C. Water is released from the meat by the action of the salt. At intervals, the pieces of meat are recoated with salt. At the end of the salting period, the product contains high levels of salt and is racked and held at ambient temperature until the surface dries. Finally, then meat is rubbed with salt and spices, netted and sold. Because of the high salt content, the product does not require refrigeration. Products sold as country-cured hams or bacon are similarly processed except that sodium nitrite is used with a lower level of sodium chloride. The product is hung to dry at ambient temperature for 35–140 days before removal for sale as a shelf-stable product. During the curing process, the salts penetrate and equilibrate in the tissue. The combined action of reduced water activity and the preservative effect of nitrite inhibit or inactivate the bacteria that cause spoilage or human illness. During the subsequent drying period, salt-tolerant enterococci and micrococci begin to grow and predominate; they also suppress the growth of the undesirable bacteria.

PERISHABLE RAW SALTED AND SALT-CURED MEAT

Fresh sausages are the most commonly encountered perishable raw salted meat products. The method of packaging is the major factor that determines the predominant spoilage flora. Fresh sausage sold in bulk on trays or stuffed in casings is highly perishable with a shelf-life of just a few days; psychrotrophic pseudomonads are the primary spoilage organisms. The shelf-life of fresh sausage can be extended to one or more weeks by wrapping the sausage in oxygen-impermeable film. The restriction of oxygen favours the growth of lactic acid-producing bacteria which impart a tangy flavour to the product. Large quantities of perishable meat products are cured with salt, sodium nitrite and nitrate, ascorbic acid, and other flavouring materials. Most of these are cooked before shipping from the processing plants although some are sold with little or no heat treatment and must be cooked before eating. Some raw cured meats are heated or smoked to different degrees to produce dry surfaces and a smoked flavour; these procedures may also extend their shelf-life by reducing the numbers of bacteria.

PERISHABLE COOKED UNCURED MEATS

Most pork products are given a thorough heat treatment to destroy all non-spore-forming bacteria, with only spores at a level of approximately 10^2 g^{-1} surviving. Beef products are usually processed at a lower temperature sufficient to destroy non-spore-forming pathogens but not necessarily some of the thermoduric bacteria such as enterococci. Microbial levels depend on the initial microbial load and types of bacteria, the cooking time and temperature, and storage temperature and time. Freshly cooked meat products may have only about 10^2 cfu g^{-1} but contamination with spoilage bacteria and pathogens may occur during handling and packaging. Cooked uncured meat products are ideal substrates for microbial growth. They are highly nutritious, have favourable pH and a_w, and competing microflora have been reduced or destroyed. Many of these foods are frozen for shipment and distribution. However, if they are held at above freezing point for one to several days, spoilage will occur due to the growth of enterococci, pseudomonads, lactic acid bacteria, and other psychrotrophs.

PERISHABLE COOKED CURED MEATS

Precooked cured meats include a variety of popular luncheon meats including frankfurters, bologna and ham. The heating step destroys the normal meat microflora except for spores and possibly thermoduric bacteria. During chilling, holding and packaging, some contamination may occur to exposed surfaces. Salt and nitrite may inhibit the growth of survivors and contaminants. On prolonged storage at refrigeration temperatures, spoilage with slime formation occurs primarily due to enterococci, micrococci, lactic acid bacteria and yeasts. If oxygen-impermeable film is used for wrapping the product, spoilage is primarily due to lactic acid bacteria.

CANNED CURED MEATS

Canned cured meats may be shelf-stable or perishable. Examples of shelf-stable products include canned wieners, corned beef, frankfurters, meat spreads, luncheon meat, small canned hams, canned sausages covered with oil, and vinegar-pickled meats. The canned wieners and frankfurters are given a 'botulinal cook' under the regulations applicable for low-acid foods packed in hermetically sealed containers. Canned sausages covered in oil do not spoil unless the a_w is higher than recommended (ranging from 0.86 to 0.92, depending on the product) and the vacuum seal is broken. Pickled pigs' feet and pickled sausages are immersed in vinegar-brine and are preserved by low pH, acetic acid, little or no fermentable sugar remaining in the tissue, and/or an airtight package.

Perishable canned cured meats made from pork must be stored refrigerated. They contain nitrite and salt at levels used to prepare shelf-stable products but their heat treatment is inadequate to inactivate spores. Perishable canned cured meats may be shelf-stable for up to 3 years if properly processed and refrigerated. Spoilage is primarily due to psychrotrophic, thermoduric non-spore-forming bacteria (e.g. enterococci, *Lactobacillus viridescens*) that were present at abnormally high levels or survived an inadequate processing.

FERMENTED AND ACIDULATED SAUSAGES

Fermented products such as Thuringer, summer sausage, pepperoni, Lebanon bologna, Genoa salami and cervelat depend on lactic fermentation and low water activity for preservation. At the end of fermentation, lactics exceed 10^8 g^{-1}. Previously, the primary safety concern for these products was staphylococcal enterotoxins. Improved industry practices greatly reduced or eliminated the staphylococcal enterotoxin problem. However, these practices are not adequate to control acid-tolerant bacteria such as *E. coli* O157:H7 which can survive the fermentation and drying process (Glass et al. 1992) as evidenced by an outbreak (Anon 1995).

Spoilage of naturally fermented sausages is primarily due to fungi; *Penicillium* spp. are dominant but species belonging to *Aspergillus* and *Scopulariopsis* are also present (Anderson 1995). Acidulated products are produced by adding acidulants (citric acid, lactic acid, glucono-δ-lactone) to the meat. Because no fermentation is involved, the products require a higher heat treatment than fermented sausages.

DRIED MEATS

Commercial dried meat products such as beef jerky include a cooking step that destroys normal vegetative cells and a rapid drying step that reduces the water activity below the level at which micro-organisms of concern can grow.

4.2 Poultry and poultry products

Poultry production and processing range from small farm or yard operations in developing countries to almost exclusively large-scale, highly integrated and automated operations in developed countries. In the USA the per capita consumption of young chickens increased from 1.7 billion in 1961 to nearly 6.6 billion in 1993, surpassing even the consumption of beef (FSIS 1994). To meet this increased demand, production and processing operations have been integrated and centralized. Intensive production integrates breeding, hatching, rearing, feeding and slaughtering. The large numbers and close proximity of birds makes control of hygiene difficult, and introduction of pathogens into a flock has very serious consequences although it also provides the opportunity for preventive medicine, efficiencies of sale and genetic improvements.

In industrialized countries the microbiological condition of raw poultry at retail sale is a reflection of hygienic measures taken at the breeder farm, at the hatchery, through the growing period and throughout slaughtering and the subsequent handling and storage.

MICROBIOLOGY AT PRODUCTION

Although several pathogenic bacteria have been associated with outbreaks or sporadic disease caused by poultry products, *Salmonella*, *Campylobacter jejuni* and *Campylobacter coli* are considered predominant poultry-associated pathogens (Bryan and Doyle 1995). Microbial contamination of the egg can occur during its development or later by penetration of the shell. *Salmonella* serotype Enteritidis can infect the ovaries or oviduct of apparently healthy birds, leading to internal contamination of eggs (Coyle and Palmer 1988), but the frequency and extent of such infection is uncertain. Salmonellae are also present on the shell due to faecal contamination and may penetrate the shell during cooling after laying. Chicks and poults may become contaminated from the shell during or after hatching. In contrast, eggs derived from hens that were faecal excreters of *C. jejuni* failed to yield this organism from either the homogenates of yolks and albumen or shell surfaces (Bryan and Doyle 1995). Thus, *C. jejuni* is unlikely to be transmitted by eggs.

Poultry improvement programmes for *Salmonella* identify infected breeder flocks (USDA 1990). Infections may be controlled by treatment with antibiotics or by slaughter, particularly if serotype Typhimurium is identified. Breeder stock should be given feed made free from salmonellae by heating (Williams 1981a, 1981b) or by treatment with organic acids (Hinton and Linton 1988). Other sources of salmonellae, such as rodents and wild birds, should be excluded. New stock should be disease-free, and should be quarantined before being mixed with other birds. Contamination of the shell has been reduced by the use of cages and automated feeding systems, belt collection of eggs, and manure removal equipment. Other improvements include in-line washers, mass egg candling, and automated packing equipment (Bell 1995).

The development of the microflora of the live bird is reviewed by Grau (1986) and the origins and composition of the contamination of the carcass by ICMSF (1980b) and Mead (1980, 1982).

Within 24 h a single chick orally inoculated with *C. jejuni* can contaminate 70–100% of chicks held in transport boxes. *C. jejuni* colonizes primarily the lower intestinal tracts of chicks, principally the caeca, large intestine and cloaca. *C. jejuni* are chemotactically attracted to mucin; highly active flagella assist them to move into mucus-filled crypts where the organisms establish themselves. The colonization of poultry by *C. jejuni* and intervention strategies for prevention of the colonization have been described by Stern (1992).

Salmonellae have been isolated from yolk sacs of chicks, setters and chick belts sampled at hatcheries. The mechanism by which salmonellae colonize poultry is not fully understood; however, caeca are the principal sites of colonization. Chicks and poults are readily infected with salmonellae from contaminated feeds; infected chicks may shed as many as 10^8 cfu g^{-1} of faeces. As they mature, the birds tend to shed fewer salmonellae and fewer birds remain infected unless salmonellae are continuously reintroduced through contaminated feed or other environmental sources (Bryan and Doyle 1995).

Live poultry showing no symptoms of illness may carry low numbers of *Salmonella* and excrete them (symptomless excreters), thereby contaminating the environment. Litter becomes contaminated with droppings, feathers and soil; with time and use, the water activity, ammonia content and pH become unfavourable for the survival of *Salmonella*.

Transmission of micro-organisms continues during transportation from the farm to the slaughtering facilities. Intestinal colonization is the most important factor contributing to carcass contamination. Feed is usually withheld for several hours before transport to reduce the amount of faecal droppings; however, considerable defecation still occurs during transit. Birds stand, walk and fall on the faecal material present on crates and truck beds, thus allowing faecal bacteria including pathogens to be transferred to the feathers and skin. Stress caused by gathering, transporting, crowding and holding in crates greatly increases the bacterial load; the levels of *C. jejuni* on unprocessed chicken carcasses increase by 3–4 logs after transportation from the farm (Stern et al. 1995). Cleaning and disinfection of cages and truck beds after each use minimizes the transfer of contamination between flocks.

In countries where birds are killed at purchase by the consumer the hygienic conditions may be primitive but the brief time between slaughter and consumption of the cooked product usually prevents most microbiological problems.

Most modern poultry slaughter operations are largely automated with electrical stunning and mechanical severing of the blood vessels in the neck. Most dressing and processing steps are accomplished with minimal handling. Broilers entering the slaughtering plant are highly contaminated with *Salmonella*, *C. jejuni*, *C. coli* and *E. coli* (Kotula and Pandya 1995). Dressing procedures are designed to reduce contamination and controls such as chlorinated rinses of equipment minimize cross-contamination between carcasses.

Carcasses are scalded to facilitate the removal of feathers, most commonly by immersion scalding. Microbes from the exterior surface and from the intestinal and respiratory tracts are continually released into the scald water. Hot water sprays, steam and simultaneous hot water spray and plucking are alternatives to immersion scalding, but are rarely used. Build-up of contamination is prevented by controlled overflow and countercurrent replacement of scald water and by the lethal effects of the high temperature. High scalding temperatures (greater than 60°C) are more effective in eliminating vegetative microorganisms than are the lower temperatures commonly used (50°C) but the lower temperatures are sometimes preferred because they cause less damage to the appearance of the carcass (Slavik, Kim and Walker 1995).

Plucking (picking) to remove feathers is another operation that spreads contamination from one carcass to another. Effective cleaning of pluckers and plucking fingers is important to prevent transmission of contaminants from one carcass to the next. Spray washing of carcasses after plucking removes only loosely attached contaminating material along with a proportion of the microbial flora, many microbes remaining bound to the surface tissues. Evisceration may lead to further contamination of carcasses, particularly with intestinal organisms, commonly as a consequence of gut breakage. As bacteria become more firmly attached to the skin with time, washing

after evisceration should occur as soon as possible and should include both the body cavity and the outer surface of the carcass. The reduction of bacteria is usually limited to about 90%; the remaining bacteria are either entrapped within or adhere to skin and flesh surfaces.

Chilling delays the growth of spoilage bacteria and prevents the growth of food-borne pathogens. Continuous countercurrent immersion chilling, with or without ice, generally decreases counts on carcasses and minimizes cross-contamination if it is properly controlled and the water is properly chlorinated. Air chilling may be done with various combinations of temperature, humidity and time. During dry chilling there is less contact between carcasses; however, there is also less dilution of pathogens. Campylobacters are sensitive to drying; therefore, a reduction in the numbers of *C. jejuni* may be expected.

The number of microbes detected on the finished carcass varies with the site sampled and the method of sampling. Excised skin samples will yield a microflora of approximately 10^3–10^5 aerobic mesophiles cm^{-2}, 10^1–10^3 psychrotrophs cm^{-2} and 10^3–10^4 Enterobacteriaceae cm^{-2} (Grau 1986). The main causes of spoilage when carcasses are stored in air at approximately 1°C are pseudomonads, *Shewenella putrefaciens*, *Acinetobacter* and *Moraxella* spp. At higher temperatures atypical lactobacilli and *Serratia liquefaciens* (formerly *Enterobacter liquefaciens*) may predominate. *A. putrefaciens* and *Acinetobacter* grow better in leg muscle (pH 6–6.7) than in breast muscle (pH 5.7–5.9), whereas *Pseudomonas* spp. grow well in either. If carcasses are wrapped in oxygen-impermeable films, *Alteromonas*, *B. thermosphacta* and atypical lactobacilli are the principal causes of spoilage. Atmospheric concentrations of 10–25% carbon dioxide delay the growth of pseudomonads and other spoilage organisms when the product is held below c. 4°C. The increase in shelf-life is approximately proportional to the concentration of carbon dioxide up to 25%, at which point discoloration occurs.

Irradiation of poultry has been extensively investigated with respect to its effects on spoilage and pathogenic bacteria. Treatment of whole eviscerated chickens with 2.5 kGy of γ-rays increased the shelf-life from 10 to 40 days. The same dosage reduces the numbers of *Salmonella*, *Campylobacter* and *Y. enterocolitica* by 2.5–4 log units. The US Department of Agriculture issued regulations in 1992 permitting the irradiation of packaged, fresh or frozen poultry and poultry products, including ground and mechanically separated poultry products at a dosage level of 1.5–3.0 kGy (Lee et al. 1996).

4.3 Eggs and egg products

Since the pioneering study of egg microbiology in 1873 by Gayon, an associate of Louis Pasteur, several investigators have shown that the hen's egg is endowed with many chemical and physical defences against micro-organisms. The shell, shell membranes and bacterial inhibitors in the albumen protect the white and the yolk from bacterial contaminants. The shell membranes have bactericidal activity; they also act as physical barriers to bacterial penetration (Board et al. 1994). When the shell and the shell membrane are removed, this protection is gone. The yolk is an excellent medium for bacterial growth; either liquid whole egg or egg yolk permits rapid growth of bacteria if the temperature is appropriate.

Bacterial contamination of eggs can occur at different stages ranging from production to storage, processing, distribution and preparation (Board and Fuller 1994). Transovarian or 'vertical' transmission occurs when eggs are infected during their formation in the hen's ovaries. Horizontal transmission occurs when eggs are exposed to micro-organisms which subsequently penetrate the shell (Fajardo et al. 1995). *Salmonella* serotype Enteritidis (SE) emerged as a transovarian pathogen in 1985 (St Louis et al. 1988) and has caused several egg-related outbreaks in North America and Europe (Mishu et al. 1991). Phage types (PT) 4, 8 and 13a are 3 most frequently isolated phage types of SE. PT4 causes more severe disease than the other 2 phage types and has essentially displaced the other 2 phage types in Europe. PT4 is still rare in the USA but its recent isolation in California has caused major concern for the public health community. SE contamination of eggs may occur by both vertical and horizontal transmission.

Washing shell eggs does not assure removal of all bacteria. Whereas the temperature of the wash water is not high enough to effect any killing of bacteria, its pH may affect bacterial growth. Gram-negative bacteria on the egg shell can be resistant to detergents in the wash water; even chlorine rinses of shell eggs may not prevent contamination by salmonellae.

Success in preserving eggs depends on 3 steps:

1 preventing spoilage organisms from entering the egg
2 preventing pathogenic bacteria from entering the egg
3 maintaining egg quality by preventing loss of CO_2 and water.

Refrigeration is the most popular method of preserving egg quality. It retards CO_2 loss and slows the growth of pathogenic bacteria. Previously the recommended storage temperature for shell eggs in the USA was 13°C. However, *S.* Enteritidis grows in eggs stored at 13°C but not 7°C. Therefore, the 1995 Food Code currently requires the receipt of shell eggs at 5°C (Food Code 1995).

Liquid whole egg is a blend of egg albumen and yolk. It contains 23–25% solids. Liquid egg is used by bakeries, candy makers and many eating establishments. Contamination of liquid egg products is generally the result of contaminants within the shell egg, the cleanliness of the shells of eggs being broken, and the small egg shell particles that often drop into the liquid. At the time of laying, the egg temperature is over 41°C. The cooling and drying of the moist egg surface, especially the cuticle, and continued cooling of the contents causes a negative pressure inside the

egg. This pulls bacterial contaminants from the surface of the shell through its pores. Contaminants on the shell are therefore potential contaminants of the liquid egg; washing eggs in water is an effective method of removing the shell contaminants. Spoilage bacteria of liquid eggs are mostly gram-negative rods (*P. fluorescens*, *Alcaligenes bookeri*, *Paracolobacterium intermedium*, *Proteus melanovogenes*, *S. putrefaciens*, *Proteus vulgaris*, *Flavobacterium* spp.). *Salmonella* serotypes (Enteritidis, Gallinarum and Pullorum) are associated with egg products. Recent investigations suggest that *L. monocytogenes* and *Y. enterocolitica* may also be found in liquid eggs (Stadelman 1994).

In the USA, all liquid, frozen and dried whole egg, yolk and albumen must be pasteurized or otherwise treated to reduce the number of viable salmonellae to very low levels. The US regulations require that liquid whole egg be heated to at least 60°C and held for 3.5 min whereas UK regulations specify heat treatment at 64°C for 2.5 min. Either pasteurization process significantly reduces the number of spoilage bacteria and pathogens without affecting the functional properties of liquid egg. Because liquid egg white may have pH between 7.6 and 9.3, its pH should be stabilized by the addition of ammonium sulphate before heating. Processes using heat and hydrogen peroxide combinations are also acceptable (Baker 1994).

In 1993, a commercial mayonnaise was epidemiologically implicated as the source of *E. coli* O157:H7 in an outbreak of bloody diarrhoea. Subsequent studies have shown that *E. coli* O157:H7 is more acid-tolerant than other gram-negative enteric bacteria and can survive in refrigerated acidified foods, including mayonnaise. Interestingly, *E. coli* O157:H7 was rapidly inactivated in mayonnaise when it was stored at room temperature (Weagent, Bryant and Bark 1994, Zhao and Doyle 1994, Erickson et al. 1995).

4.4 Fish and fish products

In recent years, the consumption of seafood products has increased dramatically. This increased consumption of seafoods has focused greater attention on the quality and safety of these products and has led to the development of hazard analysis of critical control points (HACCP, see section 5, p. 413) systems and inspections.

Finfish are generally regarded as being much more perishable than other high-protein muscle foods. This high perishability is primarily due to the presence of high concentrations of non-protein nitrogenous compounds in fish muscle. These compounds (e.g. ammonia, triethylamine, creatine, taurine, etc.) are actively utilized by bacteria during spoilage (Jay 1986). In addition, the perishability of cold-water fish is not effectively reduced by refrigeration because they have a preponderance of psychrotrophs in their microflora.

It is generally accepted that the internal flesh of live, healthy fish is sterile, the natural bacterial flora reside primarily in the outer slime layer of the skin, on the gills, and in the intestines of feeding fish. Bacterial numbers range from 10^2–10^6 cfu cm^{-2} on the skin,

10^3–10^5 cfu g^{-1} on the gills, and very few in non-feeding fish to 10^7 cfu g^{-1} or greater in the intestines. These initial microflora are directly related to the environment, whereas the total microbial load is subject to seasonal variation. Warm-water fish tend to have a more mesophilic, gram-positive microflora (micrococci, bacilli, coryneforms) whereas cold-water fish harbour predominantly gram-negative psychrotrophs (*Moraxella, Acinetobacter, Pseudomonas, Flavobacterium, Vibrio*). Regardless of the initial microflora, spoilage of finfish during iced storage is primarily caused by *Pseudomonas* and *S. putrefaciens.*

Total bacterial counts of fish are not reliable indicators of their sensory qualities or shelf-life. Gram-negative bacteria are the major causes of fish spoilage; their metabolism produces the unpleasant odours and flavours associated with fish spoilage. *Shewanella putrefaciens* (previously classified in the genera *Alteromonas* and *Pseudomonas*) is the most important fish spoilage bacteria in marine fish stored at 0°C. *S. putrefaciens* produces H_2S and causes off-odours. Spoilage bacteria belonging to the family Vibrionaceae are important in spoilage of fish stored at temperatures higher than 0°C (Gram 1992).

CRUSTACEANS

Species of commercial importance include crabs, lobsters, shrimps and prawns. Crabs and lobsters are generally trapped, then transported live to the processing plant. Shrimps and prawns are usually captured by trawlers, then iced for transport to the processing plant. Because crustaceans may be caught close inshore, a proportion will be from polluted waters and will carry micro-organisms derived from sewage. Fortunately, these organisms are on the surfaces of the animals and are usually destroyed during cooking.

Shrimps and prawns are common causes of foodborne illness involving *S. aureus, Salmonella, Shigella* and *Vibrio parahaemolyticus.* They are harvested from coastal waters in many parts of the world, and are usually captured by fishing from boats or hand netted from the shore. To an increasing extent they are grown in ponds (aquaculture). Depending on where they are caught they may be contaminated with a variety of microbial pathogens originating from untreated sewage, such as *Salmonella* and *Shigella*, or with organisms that are part of the normal flora of the animal, such as *V. parahaemolyticus* or *Vibrio vulnificus.* Crustaceans should ideally be harvested from unpolluted water and, once harvested, cooled rapidly to a temperature of −1 to +2°C because they are extremely susceptible to microbial deterioration. The ice used for chilling should be of good microbiological quality, or clean refrigerated seawater may be used. If water quality is suspect, chlorinated or otherwise treated water should be used, but excessive use of chlorine or other biocidal agents should be avoided. On fishing vessels, holds and container boxes should be cleaned properly between catches to prevent build-up of contamination.

MOLLUSCS

Molluscan shellfish include bivalves, such as oysters, mussels, cockles, clams and scallops, and gastropods. With the exception of some oysters and scallops, which are harvested from deeper waters, most molluscs grow in estuarine and nearshore coastal waters where exposure to faecal contamination is possible. Clams and cockles are usually dug from the sand; oysters and scallops are either raked or trawled from the bottom; and mussels are hand picked. Oysters and mussels are often farmed. They are transported live in the shell, often with little refrigeration.

Vibrio spp. are important pathogens often associated with the consumption of clams and oysters. In 1989, a co-ordinated surveillance for human infections caused by *Vibrio* spp. in 4 Gulf Coast states (Alabama, Florida, Louisiana and Texas) revealed 121 cases of which 71 had gastroenteritis, 29 had wound infections, and 14 had primary septicaemia. *Vibrio cholerae* non-O1, *Vibrio hollisae, Vibrio alginolyticus, Vibrio fluvialis, V. parahaemolyticus* and *V. vulnificus* were isolated from the patients (Levine and Griffin 1993). *V. vulnificus* causes wound infections and primary septicaemia with high mortality in susceptible persons, particularly those with impaired liver function. Shellfish, particularly clams and oysters, taken from contaminated waters have also been incriminated as the source of outbreaks of infectious hepatitis A (Bryan 1980) and may serve to transmit other viruses, particularly enteroviruses (Cliver 1971).

The consumption of molluscs occasionally gives rise to a potentially serious disease, paralytic shellfish poisoning (PSP), resulting from particular environmental conditions that produce blooms of some species of marine dinoflagellates which synthesize a toxin during growth. Molluscs ingest these organisms and concentrate the toxin, which affects humans and other warm-blooded animals. The toxins are not denatured by cooking or eliminated by cleansing of shellfish in purification tanks. Hence the only available control measure is to prohibit collection of shellfish when, during periods of dinoflagellate blooms, the toxins in the shellfish approach dangerous concentrations.

4.5 Vegetables and fruits

Fresh vegetables and fruits are an essential part of the diet of people around the world. If land is available, families grow their own fruits and vegetables. Otherwise, produce is purchased from local farmers or retail establishments. In developed countries, the production, processing, storage and distribution of fruits and vegetables is highly integrated and consolidated in a few commercial companies. This has resulted in the year-round availability of a wide variety of fruits and vegetables. In addition, efficient production and processing of vegetables and fruits has enabled the industry to meet the increased demand for these items from a health- and nutrition-conscious public. However, the same practices have caused many new public health problems to be associated with vegetables and fruits.

VEGETABLES

Bacterial contamination of vegetables has been a public health concern because of the proximity of vegetables to soil and the possibility of contamination from water used for irrigation. Several studies have shown that bacteria of public health concern can be isolated from whole and prepared vegetables. The control of quality of plant foods begins at production with suitable geographical location; choice of seed, fertilizers and pesticides; effective use of irrigation or drainage systems; and crop rotation. In developed countries there is little obvious association between agricultural practices and food-borne illness. The relatively large scale of many agricultural operations results in minimal human or animal contact with crops and constitutes a useful safety factor. Practices such as prolonged cooking and rejection of bruised or rotted foods also minimize the consumption of potentially hazardous material. In developed countries the control measures for quality of plant foods and for minimizing product loss from bruising, browning, wilting or rot, result in foods with minimal microbiological hazards.

The nutrient content of vegetables is suitable for the growth of moulds, yeasts and bacteria (Jay 1986). Numbers of bacteria on vegetables upon arrival at a processing plant range from 4×10^5 to 3×10^7 g^{-1} (ICMSF 1980b); numbers of fungi on fresh vegetables at harvest ranged from 0 to 5×10^5, and at market from 5×10^3 to 2×10^6 (Brackett 1987). Fresh vegetables are inherently susceptible to spoilage because their a_w is above the minimum to support the growth of most micro-organisms, and the pH of most vegetables is within the range allowing multiplication. Washing can remove up to 90% of the surface micro-organisms but those trapped on the vegetable remain and any residual water facilitates their rapid multiplication. Micro-organisms multiply faster in cut produce because of the ready availability of nutrients and water. Further handling of the produce increases the likelihood of additional contamination from the handler, work surfaces or utensils which may have been contaminated previously by contact with other foods. Most fungal spoilage is caused by the genera *Penicillium*, *Sclerotinia*, *Botrytis* and *Rhizopus*. A more complete listing is given by Brackett (1987). Fungal spoilage of fresh vegetables is considered more an economic than a health threat because few spoilage fungi produce toxic metabolites. Exceptions include aspergilli, penicillia and *Alternaria*. Stress metabolites which are sometimes produced by plants in response to fungal infections can affect humans, e.g. furanocoumarin compounds, called psoralens, that are produced when *Sclerotinia sclerotiorum* produces 'pink rot' of celery. Its effects include blisters or lesions of the skin of consumers or those handling the diseased celery.

Bacteria cause a range of spoilage conditions known as rots, spots, blights and wilts. Soft rots, which occur during transport and storage, are usually caused by coliforms, *Erwinia carotovora* and certain pseudomonads. Bacteria causing spoilage other than soft rot include corynebacteria, xanthomonads and pseudomonads (Lund 1983). Soft rot of potatoes by *Clostridium* spp. has also been reported (Lund 1972, 1986). These organisms break down pectins, causing a soft consistency, sometimes with an objectionable odour and a watery appearance.

Storage

Harvested vegetables and fruits continue to respire actively and produce heat, so handling and storage procedures should minimize respiration and water loss and maintain an environment in which cells remain healthy. Rapid chilling is important for leafy vegetables. Proper temperature and humidity control are essential to promote wound healing and minimize spoilage of root crops. A weak link in the distribution chain for fruits and vegetables is the use of unsuitable containers or packaging material (e.g. large sacks, rough wooden boxes, bamboo baskets), which can cause crushing, bruising and puncturing. Long journeys, hot weather, unventilated trucks, heavy loads and unpaved roads in developing countries are responsible for huge losses of fruit and vegetables (Ryall and Lipton 1979, FAO 1981, Proctor, Goodliffe and Coursey 1981).

The only means of control of spoilage micro-organisms is by strict sanitation of equipment and control of the temperature, relative humidity and gas composition of the atmosphere in which the raw vegetable is stored. Further examples of vegetable spoilage are given in Jay (1986) and Dennis (1987).

Modified atmosphere packaging or vacuum packaging is used to suppress the proliferation of aerobic spoilage micro-organisms on vegetables. In addition, these processes reduce the rate of oxidative deterioration, enzymatic degradation and water loss. Modified atmosphere or vacuum packaging is used to market fresh-cut packaged vegetables including cabbage, lettuce, onions, green and red peppers, carrots, cauliflower, broccoli and other leafy salad vegetables. Spoilage of ready-to-use salads is frequently caused by pectinolytic pseudomonads such as *Pseudomonas marginalis*.

Freezing is a preferred means of preserving vegetables, because it retains the organoleptic and nutritional quality of vegetables better than other processes. Before freezing vegetables it is normal practice to blanch, usually at 86–98°C for several minutes to inactivate plant enzymes, thereby stabilizing the product during subsequent frozen storage. Blanching commonly reduces the microbial load 10^3–10^5 times. In most frozen vegetables lactic acid bacteria are numerically dominant although micrococci and gram-negative rods, including coliforms, comprise a considerable proportion of the total microflora of certain products. Microbial spoilage of frozen vegetables is rare, and frozen vegetables are rarely involved in food-borne illness because non-spore-forming pathogens do not survive blanching and most frozen vegetables are cooked before being consumed.

Dried vegetables are shelf-stable and rarely involved in food-borne illness. Modified atmospheres have been used to control fungal spoilage of vegetables, with mixed results. Increased carbon dioxide concentration is fungistatic for many fungi, including *Candida albicans*, *Botrytis cinerea*, *Botrytis parasiticus*, *Penicillium* spp., *Mucor* and *Aureobasidium pullulans*, but there are examples of vegetables being more or less sensitive to increased concentrations of carbon dioxide or off flavours developing.

Vegetables can be contaminated with pathogenic micro-organisms during growth in the fields, harvesting, post-harvesting handling and storage, and distribution. Beuchat (1996) has published a comprehensive review on this subject. Food-borne disease outbreaks of bacterial origin are most frequently associated with vegetables. Among bacterial pathogens of greatest concern in vegetables are *Shigella* spp., salmonellae, enterotoxigenic, enteropathogenic, enteroinvasive and enterohaemorrhagic *E. coli*, *Campylobacter* spp., *Y. enterocolitica*, *L. monocytogenes*, *Aeromonas* spp., *S. aureus*, *Bacillus cereus*, *C. perfringens* and *C. botulinum*.

Several large outbreaks of shigellosis have been traced to contaminated vegetables such as shredded or cut lettuce and fresh green onions. With the current popularity of fresh-cut packaged produce, there is a potential for causing large, geographically widespread outbreaks. *Shigella* spp. can survive on vegetables for several months at ambient and refrigerator temperatures.

Vegetables implicated as vehicles of *Salmonella* spp. in food-borne disease outbreaks include raw tomatoes and bean sprouts. *Salmonella* spp. can grow on raw tomatoes (pH 4.0) at 20–30°C. *L. monocytogenes* was established as a food-borne pathogen after a large outbreak of listeriosis in Nova Scotia in 1981 in which contaminated cole slaw was implicated (Schlech et al. 1983). The cabbage which was used to prepare the cole slaw had been grown on fields which were fertilized with contaminated sheep manure. In addition, the cabbage was stored at refrigeration temperatures over winter which probably allowed the psychrotrophic pathogen to multiply. Many cases of travellers' diarrhoea are attributed to enterotoxigenic *E. coli* acquired from contaminated salads eaten at restaurants.

Vegetables sold in modified atmosphere packages may pose a threat of botulism poisoning. *C. botulinum* type A spores have been isolated from shredded cabbage, chopped green pepper, and a salad mix. The presence of normal spoilage microflora in vegetables packaged under modified atmosphere may actually prevent the growth of *C. botulinum* and production of toxin. Packaging under modified atmosphere does not prevent the growth of *E. coli* O157:H7 on shredded lettuce or sliced cucumbers.

FRUITS

Losses due to rots and other defects of fresh fruit are usually caused by moulds. Some are able to invade and infect the intact healthy tissue whereas others can become established only after the fruit has been infected by a pathogen or has been damaged. Several diseases are named after the causative mould (e.g.

Alternaria, *Botrytis* and *Fusarium* rots) and others are derived from the appearance of the infected fruit (e.g. brown rot, stem-end rot). In some cases diseases of different fruits may have the same name despite the involvement of different moulds (e.g. black rot of apples is caused by *Physalospora obtusa*, whereas black rot of oranges is due to *Alternaria citri*). The market diseases of fruits, and the causative fungi, are tabulated by Splittstoesser (1987). Yeast spoilage of fresh fruits is usually from the fermentative action of, for example, *Hanseniaspora valbyensis*, *Candida* spp., *Candida* (*Torulopsis*) *stellata*, *Pichia kluyveri* and *Kloeckera apiculata*.

At the orchard or vineyard pruning, certain cultural practices and application of fungicides are the main ways by which infection and spoilage prior to harvest are minimized. After harvesting at optimum maturity, fruit should be handled gently to prevent physical injury and fruit contact surfaces should be cleaned regularly and treated to destroy fungal spores. Mouldy or bruised fruit are removed during sorting and grading. Fruit may be treated with hot water or with permitted fungicides to control, for example, *Phomopsis*, *Diplodia*, *Penicillium* and *Botrytis* (Salunkhe and Desai 1984).

Storage

Fruit are stored cooled but at temperatures that do not cause chill injury. The concentration of carbon dioxide in the atmosphere may be increased to inhibit *Alternaria*, *Botrytis* and *Rhizopus* spp. Fruit products can be preserved by heating to c. 80–90°C because most aciduric microbes are relatively sensitive to heating. Spoilage of canned soft drinks has occurred because ascospores of *Saccharomyces cerevisiae* or spores of *Kluyveromyces marxianus* survived the heat process. Spoilage of canned fruit products has been caused by the survival after heating of ascospores of moulds, e.g. *Penicillium vermiculatum*, *Byssochlamys* (Splittstoesser 1987).

Freezing is often used to preserve fruits and fruit products and causes some reduction in microbial numbers. Growth of yeasts and moulds does not occur if temperatures are maintained below −18°C, but exposure to automatic defrost cycles is undesirable in the long term because some multiplication may occur.

Reducing the water activity is a common means of preserving fruit, either by exposure to sun or by dehydration. Fungal spoilage of dried fruit does not take place when the water content is below 25%. Some high moisture dried fruits contain 30–35% moisture and are heated or treated with potassium sorbate to prevent mould growth. Many fruits are treated with sulphite before drying to prevent browning and this destroys a high proportion of the contaminating microbes. Yeasts and moulds able to grow on dried fruit include *Zygosaccharomyces bisporus*, *Zygosaccharomyces rouxii*, *Hanseniaspora*, *Candida*, *Penicillium* spp., *Aspergillus glaucus* and *Aspergillus niger*. *Monascus bisporus* is one of the most xerotolerant moulds and has spoiled dried prunes (Splittstoesser 1987). The relationship between water activity and fungal growth is reviewed thoroughly by Corry (1987).

Sliced fresh fruits support the growth of *Shigella* spp. and thus may serve as the vehicle of infection. Several outbreaks of salmonellosis have been associated with fresh fruits, particularly melons. *Salmonella* serotypes Oranienburg and Javiana have caused outbreaks traced to contaminated watermelons; serotypes Chester and Poona have been associated with outbreaks due to contamination of cantaloupes.

CANNED FRUIT AND VEGETABLE PRODUCTS

Preservation by canning is exploited to increase the shelf-life and availability of vegetables. The heat processing of fruits and vegetables and the importance of pH are discussed thoroughly elsewhere (Hersom and Hulland 1980, Lund 1986). Most vegetables intended for canning fall into the category of foods known as 'low-acid' because their pH is above 4.6. Low-acid foods must be heated sufficiently to destroy the spores of *C. botulinum* because, being derived from the soil, the spores are inevitable contaminants of agricultural products, including vegetables. The canning process is a good example of achieving a high margin of safety by control of the process rather than by microbiological tests on the raw material and final product. Dennis (1987) emphasizes the critical control points in the process, i.e. initial microbial contamination, time between filling and processing, cleanliness of equipment, heat process, cooling cycle and disinfection of cooling water, maintenance of container integrity by seam or seal control, and appropriate handling. Leaker spoilage is characterized by a mixture of microbial types, mainly bacteria, and underprocessing spoilage often by the presence of only one species.

Canned vegetables that have been heat processed to commercial sterility may still contain viable spores that are unable to grow under the normal temperature of storage, e.g. thermophilic spores of *B. stearothermophilus* and *B. coagulans* which cause flat sour spoilage with production of acid but not gas. Thermophilic anaerobic spoilage may be caused by obligately thermophilic spore-forming anaerobes such as *Clostridium thermosaccharolyticum*, which forms large quantities of hydrogen and carbon dioxide, or *Desulfotomaculum nigrificans*, which produces hydrogen sulphide, often with blackening of the food if iron is present. Thermophilic spoilage usually occurs after improper cooling of heat-processed vegetables (Hersom and Hulland 1980, ICMSF 1980b, Lund 1986, Dennis 1987).

4.6 Cereals

The microbiology of cereals is summarized by Pitt and Hocking (1986) and considered in greater detail in ICMSF (1980b). Microbial activity is controlled by drying the harvested cereals to a sufficiently low a_w (below 0.70) at which bacteria are unable to multiply, and growth of moulds is largely prevented in temperate zones. At the humidity levels common in tropical countries, mould growth is a serious problem. Historically, the moulds able to spoil cereals have been grouped into 'field' and 'storage' fungi, but some (e.g. *Aspergillus flavus*) grow in both situations. Field fungi are plant pathogens that invade the crop as a consequence of a combination of favourable circumstances. Particular moulds may cause problems in one geographical area but not another; e.g. in Japan an important disease of wheat and barley (red mould disease) is caused by *Fusarium* spp., predominantly *Fusarium graminearum*, whereas in Australia *Fusarium* spp. appear to cause little problem in wheat, probably because the climate is drier.

Fungi occurring commonly on wheat, barley and oats in Scotland include *Alternaria*, *Cladosporium*, *Epiccoccum* and *Penicillium* spp. Wheat in Egypt carries mainly *Aspergillus* and *Penicillium*, together with *Alternaria*, *Cladosporium* and *Fusarium*. Barley in Egypt also carries mainly *Aspergillus* and *Penicillium*, together with *Rhizopus*, *Alternaria*, *Fusarium* and *Drechslera* (Pitt and Hocking 1986).

WHEAT

Wheat grows best in fairly dry and mild climates. After harvesting it is dried and stored and may be transported long distances before final milling. Before consumption, milled wheat is cooked or baked. Because of the relatively low a_w, spoilage by bacteria is not usually a problem, but wheat may act as a passive carrier for bacterial pathogens (ICMSF 1980b). Mould growth, spoilage and the possible presence of mycotoxins are more important hazards. Mycotoxins can be produced under particular weather conditions while the wheat is growing (Saito and Ohtsubo 1974, Ichinoe et al. 1983) or during storage if the a_w becomes sufficiently high.

Microbiology at production

The diverse surface microflora of wheat in the field does no damage. The grain may, however, be infected by *F. graminearum* to produce wheat scab, red mould disease or fusarium head blight. Perithecia of *Gibberella zeae* (the perfect stage) maturing in the field liberate ascospores into the air which infect wheat at the heading stage. Under high relative humidity and low temperatures, *F. graminearum* grows and may produce trichothecenes (nivalenol or deoxynivalenol) and zearaleone (Saito and Ohtsubo 1974, Ichinoe et al. 1983, Hagler Jr, Tyczkowska and Hamilton 1984) although there are unresolved geographical differences in the occurrence of trichothecenes, perhaps related to the strains of *Fusarium* occurring (Osborne and Willis 1984). *A. flavus* and *A. parasiticus* are common contaminants of certain grains.

The crop is harvested as soon as possible after maturity, before rain can damage the grain (e.g. by causing sprouting). In one operation, combine harvesters reap, thresh, clean and load the wheat kernels into trucks for transport to storage. The rate and extent of subsequent drying of the crop depends on the moisture content at harvest (15–22%). It is important to harvest mature grain of known moisture content in dry weather without grain breakage and to separate kernels from hull and straw.

Harvested wheat can have a moisture content of up to 22% (a_w c. 0.95) and many temperatures reach near

40°C. The grain must be dried, and may need cooling, to prevent spoilage and mould growth, to lower the respiration rate of the wheat, and to prevent overheating and damage of the grain. Wheat is dried initially to about 13% moisture (Zeleny 1971) to an a_w less than 0.70, and later to 11–12% for long-term storage (ICMSF 1980b). The higher the moisture content of the grain, the lower the air temperature must be, to prevent heat damage (Kent 1966).

Storage

After drying and before primary storage, wheat is cleaned by screening and aspiration to remove dust, broken and light grain, and foreign material. Broken grain is more susceptible to mould and insect attack (Williams 1983).

When grain is moved from primary storage to long-term storage in terminal elevators by truck or railcar, the vehicles are sources of insects or storage moulds (Williams 1983) and may also be a source of contamination by salmonellae if the previous cargo was animals, meat scraps, or meat or fish meal (ICMSF 1980b). Cleaning and fumigation are used to keep transport vehicles clean and insect-free. Grain must be protected from rain. On grains at harvest time, mould propagules range from few to 10^5 g^{-1} and bacteria from 10^3 to 10^6 g^{-1}. Bacteria are usually from the families Pseudomonadaceae, Micrococcaceae, Lactobacillaceae and Bacillaceae. Indicators of faecal pollution are rare unless animals had access to fields. *Bacillus subtilis* and *B. cereus* have been demonstrated and other bacterial spores from the soil should be expected (e.g. *C. botulinum*, *C. perfringens*). Actinomycetes commonly exceed 10^6 g^{-1} and psychrotrophs 10^4 g^{-1}. Yeasts occur but do not cause problems during storage. During artificial drying, the temperatures achieved (40–80°C) destroy most mould spores. Sun drying is less effective in this respect.

Flour may be contaminated with spores of *B. subtilis* and *Bacillus licheniformis* that cause 'ropy' bread. There is increasing evidence associating large numbers of bacilli other than *B. cereus* with food-borne illness (Gilbert 1983).

RICE

Unlike wheat, much rice (*Oryza sativa*) is grown by relatively small production units without great benefit of mechanization. There is often much human and animal contact with the crop, but cooking destroys salmonellae and other vegetative pathogens. Rice is often harvested and stored under hot, humid conditions that increase the risk of fungal attack and present significant hazards from mycotoxins and spoilage losses. Because of its low a_w, bacterial spoilage is rarely a problem. Spores of *B. cereus* survive cooking and have caused food-borne illness (Gilbert and Taylor 1976, Gilbert 1983). The illness usually associated with the consumption of rice contaminated with *B. cereus* is referred to as the 'emetic syndrome'. It has a rapid onset (1–5 h) and the predominant symptoms are nausea, vomiting and malaise; occasionally diarrhoea may occur. Approximately 95% of the 'emetic syn-

drome' episodes have been associated with the consumption of Cantonese-style cooked rice served by Chinese restaurants (Kramer and Gilbert 1989). This is because the restaurants usually store cooked rice at room temperature for long periods. The chefs are reluctant to store cooked rice in the refrigerator because the grains become sticky and clump together.

Fungi can invade rice in the field and spoil developing grain (Fazli and Schroeder 1966, Bhat et al. 1982). Other fungi (storage fungi) can spoil rice during drying and storage (Mallick and Nandi 1981, Mossman 1983). A variety of mycotoxins have been found in rice (Jarvis 1976, ICMSF 1980b). It is crucial to reduce the a_w of rice quickly to c. 0.65 to prevent mould growth, and to maintain it at that level during storage even in unfavourable climates. Moulds can penetrate the endosperm and discolour the kernels. However, most of the mould growth and aflatoxin formation takes place in the bran layers that are removed during milling to produce white rice (Schroeder, Boller and Hein 1968). Milling also tends to break mouldy kernels which can then be removed, thereby improving the microbial quality of the rice (Ilag and Juliano 1982).

Losses from plant diseases and insects are reduced by planting resistant varieties and applying insecticides (Mikkelsen and DeDatta 1980). Provision of adequate drying and storage facilities for crops harvested in the wet season is critically important (Greeley 1983, Mossman 1983).

Microbiology at production

Rice is harvested when the moisture content is 18–23% (DeDatta 1981). Delaying harvest increases field losses (shattering and lodging) and causes subsequent milling losses due to sun-cracking (Chandler 1979, Mikkelsen and DeDatta 1980). Early harvesting gives a more moist grain, which is difficult to hand thresh and requires more drying.

In traditional tropical operations, rice stalks are pulled out by hand, bundled into sheaves for prethreshing drying, or threshed immediately (Mossman 1983). Manual harvesting causes less damage to the paddy, results in fewer weeds being incorporated into the crop, and allows the gathering of a higher percentage of mature grain. However, the longer that grain is left in the field for prethreshing drying, the greater is the risk of cracking and insect mould attack (Hall 1970). Drying is the most important step in production. Without it, or if it is delayed, a whole crop can spoil. Nevertheless, improper drying can cause grain breakage, partial spoilage or spoilage losses in storage.

Most rice is sun-dried, which, if done correctly, reduces the microbial population (Kuthubutheen 1984). The usual procedure in the tropics is to spread rice on a drying floor exposed to the sun for several days until the moisture is 14–16% (a_w c. 0.76–0.84). Since at this moisture content rice can not be stored safely, further drying during storage is needed. Traditional crops are harvested in the dry season at the time of maximum sun, but this process is often inadequate with increased yields and newer rice varieties that mature during the wet season. Artificial drying is then necessary, enabling harvests to be dried more uniformly with less loss from grain cracking, and to safe moisture levels (<13% moisture or a_w <0.70) regardless of vagaries of the weather.

Storage

Significant losses occur during storage if rice is not protected from rodents and insects, or if it is not dry enough to prevent mould growth. Mould attack is exacerbated by the high temperatures and humidities of tropical areas. At the start of storage, up to 85% of paddy rice kernels may be internally infected with field moulds. During storage, field moulds gradually disappear or are replaced by storage fungi (Mallick and Nandi 1981, Kuthubutheen 1984). The type and extent of growth of storage fungi depends on the initial load, temperature, a_w or relative humidity, and time (ICMSF 1980b). Paddy can be safely stored at 30°C with a constant moisture content of 12.5% (a_w 0.67) for 12 months with no fungal growth (Mallick and Nandi 1981). A moisture content of 14.3–14.5% (a_w c. 0.79) produces significant mould growth and deterioration within a few months.

Sacks or baskets give little protection from rodents or insects and may be a source of eggs, larvae and mould spores (Williams 1983). Some modern rice varieties have thinner husks than traditional cultivars and are more susceptible to insect attack (Greeley 1983). Storage in bins or solid-walled containers provides protection from ingress of rodents, insects and external moisture from rain or high humidity. However, failure to dry paddy to near 12% moisture (a_w 0.65) before, or soon after, bin storage causes considerable crop loss. Since rice insulates well, temperature gradients within the bin are readily established and lead to condensation and raised moisture contents in the cooler regions. The resultant increased metabolic activity and mould growth generate heat, carbon dioxide and more water, resulting in 'hot spots', which spread upwards and outwards. Bins made of metal are particularly susceptible to temperature gradients resulting from fluctuations in external temperatures.

Insect infestation is controlled by treating sacks, storage areas and stocks of stored rice with insecticides or fumigants, and by keeping storage areas free of dust, fines and spilt rice. Paddy rice is not generally transported long distances. Transportation should be regarded as an extension of storage, with the same principles of preventing exposure to rain, dew, insects and rodents. The transport vehicle should be clean, dry and provide cover and transport times should be minimized to limit absorption of moisture or insect infestation.

Milling can improve the microbiological quality of rice. Much of the bacterial and mould contamination and aflatoxin, if present, is on the husk and in the surface layers of the kernel which are removed by milling in the husk and bran fractions (Ilag and Juliano 1982). Grain heavily infested with mould will also break more readily during milling, yielding discol-oured, broken rice which is separated in the broken-grain fraction. Much dust is generated during milling; it may absorb enough moisture to allow microbial growth and can be a source of insects. It must be controlled by regular, sweeping, vacuuming or aspiration.

The absence of husk makes milled rice more susceptible to insect attack. During storage it must be protected from insects, rodents and from increases in moisture content. Thus the same principles of control apply to the milled rice as for paddy. Brown rice may also go rancid as a result of scratches in the bran, allowing lipases access to oils within it (Mossman 1983), possibly because of the presence and activity of a wide range of lipolytic bacteria and moulds (DeLucca, Plating and Ory 1978).

5 NEW APPROACH TO ASSURING THE SAFETY OF FOODS

Foods are essential to sustain life; therefore people expect safe foods and expect their governments to protect their food supply and assure the safety and wholesomeness of their foods. This is the basis for food laws, food regulations, the inspection programme which monitors compliance with the laws and the regulations, and the judicial system that punishes those who violate the laws. However, until recently, governments took the responsibility for inspections of foods, the food processing establishments and their environment. In several countries government inspectors are assigned to meat, fish and poultry processing plants. Inspectors of the US Food and Drug Administration carry out unannounced inspections of packaged or canned food processing plants and analyse finished products to monitor compliance; similar policies exist in other countries.

A new approach to assuring the safety of the food supply is being implemented in the USA and several other developed countries. The basis for this new approach is hazard analysis of critical control points (HACCP), a preventive approach designed in the 1950s to assure the safety of foods for the space programme (Pierson and Corlett Jr 1992).

HACCP is a systematic approach to assure safety in food production. It consists of a series of sequential steps. The first is hazard analysis, an assessment of risks associated with all aspects of food production from growing in the fields to consumption. The hazards may be physical, chemical or biological. The biological hazard category includes bacterial, viral, fungal or parasitic. Pathogenic bacteria are classified on the basis of severity of risk: those like *C. botulinum*, *Salmonella* serotype Typhi, and *V. cholerae* are classified as severe hazards; those like *L. monocytogenes*, *Salmonella* serotypes other than Typhi, and *E. coli* O157:H7 are classified as moderate hazards with potential for extensive spread; and those like *B. cereus* and *C. perfringens* are classified as moderate hazards with limited potential for spread.

The hazard analysis includes the ranking of food and its raw materials or ingredients according to 6 hazard characteristics followed by assigning risk categories to the food and its raw materials based on the hazard rankings. After the hazard analysis is completed, the next step is to determine the critical control points required to control the previously identified hazards. A critical control point (CCP) is defined as any point or procedure in a specific food system where a loss of control may result in an unacceptable risk. The third step is to establish the critical limits which must be met at each identified CCP. For example, the thermal treatment in a retort is a CCP in the production of low-acid canned foods and its components include pressure of the retort, retort temperature and time at the retort temperature. The fourth step is to establish procedures to monitor critical limits. One must then establish corrective action to be taken when a deviation is identified by monitoring critical components of a CCP. Finally, implementation of effective record-keeping systems that document the HACCP plan is also an essential requirement of HACCP.

HACCP-based regulations were published first in the USA for low-acid foods in hermetically sealed containers. HACCP regulations have also been issued for smoked fish products. In February 1995, the Food Safety and Inspection Service of the United States Department of Agriculture published proposed regulations (FSIS 1995) that will essentially overhaul the meat and poultry inspection system and change it from a reactive, federal inspection-based approach to a proactive HACCP approach in which the manufacturer or processor assumes greater responsibility for food safety than in the past.

6 CONCLUSIONS

As the year 2000 approaches, the processing and regulation of foods are poised to undergo significant changes that will have profound effects on the quality and safety of the food supply. The changes in food safety regulation are the driving force; changes in microbiological quality of foods will occur as a result of changes in the food safety approach, as an extension of the prevention-based HACCP implementation. In July 1996, the US Government published a sweeping reform of food safety rules for meat and poultry (FSIS 1996). The 4 major elements of the new rules are:

1   Every plant must develop and implement a system of preventive controls designed to improve the safety of their products, known as HACCP. The plant must demonstrate the effectiveness of the HACCP plan which federal inspectors will continually verify.
2   Every plant must regularly test carcasses for *E. coli* of faecal origin to verify the effectiveness of the plant's procedures for preventing and reducing faecal contamination, which is the major source of pathogenic bacteria.
3   All slaughter plants and plants producing raw ground meat and poultry products must ensure that the *Salmonella* contamination rate is below the current national baseline incidence.

4   Every plant must develop and implement written sanitation standard operating procedures as the foundation for its specific HACCP programme.

The entire plan must be implemented by large processing plants within 18 months; small and very small plants will have up to 42 months to comply with the new regulations. The federal regulatory agencies in the USA, in co-operation with state food regulatory agencies, also plan to set and enforce standards to minimize the growth of pathogenic bacteria in meat and poultry products during distribution (transportation and storage).

As this systematic programme to reduce and eliminate contamination of products of animal origin is implemented, food processing plants will critically review their processing operations as part of the hazard analysis component of HACCP. It is inevitable that they will identify steps in their processing that will affect the keeping quality (related to microbial spoilage) of their products and will implement appropriate control procedures to enhance the shelf-life and microbiological quality of foods.

Despite decades of effort by the food industry and the food regulatory agencies, it has not been possible to raise food animals free of pathogenic bacteria. In addition, many more problems of food-borne disease, caused by contaminated fresh fruits and vegetables, are being encountered, possibly as a result of increased world-wide production and movement of these commodities to meet consumer demands for year-round supplies. Because the growing conditions for fruits and vegetables vary widely, it may be very difficult to avoid their contamination by pathogenic bacteria. At the same time, populations in many developed countries are more susceptible to infectious diseases because of immune deficiencies caused by age, chronic diseases and emerging infectious diseases. How can consumers be assured of a safe food supply? At least for the foreseeable future, an effective approach seems to be the decontamination of the final raw product. The use of γ-irradiation or electron accelerators for terminal decontamination of food of plant and animal origin may be among the best available options (Corry et al. 1995). Unfortunately, the use of γ-irradiation has been very limited by public misconceptions about the radiation treatment of foods and the resulting reluctance of the food industry to utilize the process. There are other logistical problems with the use of radiation treatment for foods; these include the need for transporting foods from several processing plants to a central radiation treatment facility, safety problems associated with the use of radioactive materials, and problems associated with the disposal of radioactive wastes. Electron accelerators are more convenient; they do not have these problems because they do not use radioisotopes. However, their primary limitation is the inability to penetrate more than 1–2 cm below the surface. The ideal decontamination method for uncooked foods remains to be developed.

REFERENCES

Anderson SJ, 1995, Compositional changes in surface microflora during the ripening of naturally fermented sausages, *J Food Prot*, **58**: 426–9.

Anon, 1995, *Escherichia coli* O157:H7 outbreak linked to commercially distributed dry-cured salami – Washington and California, 1994, *Morbid Mortal Weekly Rep*, **44**: 157–60.

Baker RC, 1994, Effect of processing on the microbiology of eggs, *Microbiology of the Avian Egg*, eds Board RG, Fuller R, Chapman and Hall, London, 153–73.

Banwart GJ, 1987, *Basic Food Microbiology*, 2nd edn, AVI Publishing Co., Westport, CT.

Bell D, 1995, Forces that have helped shape the U.S. egg industry: the last 100 years, *Poult Trib*, 33–43.

Beuchat LR, 1996, Pathogenic microorganisms associated with fresh produce, *J Food Prot*, **59**: 204–16.

Bhat RV, Deosthale YG et al., 1982, Nutritional and toxicological evaluation of 'black tip' rice, *J Sci Food Agric*, **33**: 41–7.

Board RG, Fuller R, 1994, *Microbiology of the Avian Egg*, Chapman and Hall, London.

Board RG, Clay C et al., 1994, The egg: a compartmentalized aseptically packaged food, *Microbiology of the Avian Egg*, eds Board RG, Fuller R, Chapman and Hall, London, 43–61.

Brackett RE, 1987, Vegetables and related products, *Food and Beverage Mycology*, 2nd edn, ed. Beuchat LR, Von Nostrand Reinhold, New York, 129–54.

Bryan FL, 1980, Epidemiology of foodborne diseases transmitted by fish, shellfish and marine crustaceans, *J Food Prot*, **43**: 859–68, 873–6.

Bryan FL, Doyle MP, 1995, Health risks and consequences of *Salmonella* and *Campylobacter jejuni* in raw poultry, *J Food Prot*, **58**: 326–44.

Chandler RF, 1979, *Rice in the Tropics*, Westview Press, Boulder, CO.

Cliver DO, 1971, Transmission of viruses through foods, *Crit Rev Environ Control*, **1**: 551–79.

Corry JEL, 1987, Relationships of water activity to fungal growth, *Food and Beverage Mycology*, 2nd edn, ed. Beuchat LR, Van Nostrand Reinhold, New York, 51–100.

Corry JEL, James C et al., 1995, *Salmonella, Campylobacter* and *Escherichia coli* O157:H7 decontamination techniques for the future, *Int J Food Microbiol*, **28**: 187–96.

Coyle EF, Palmer SR, 1988, *Salmonella enteritidis* phage type 4 infection associated with hen's eggs, *Lancet*, **2**: 1295–6.

Dainty RH, Shaw BG, Roberts TA, 1983, Microbial and chemical changes in chill-stored red meats, *Food Microbiology: Advances and Prospects*, eds Roberts TA, Skinner FA, Academic Press, London, 151–78.

DeDatta SK, 1981, *Principles and Practice of Rice Production*, John Wiley & Sons, New York.

DeLucca AJ, Plating SJ, Ory RL, 1978, Isolation and identification of lipolytic microorganisms found on rough rice from two growing areas, *J Food Prot*, **41**: 28–30.

Dennis C, 1987, Microbiology of fruits and vegetables, *Essays in Agricultural and Food Microbiology*, eds Norris JR, Pettipher G, John Wiley & Sons, Chichester, 227–60.

Dickson JS, Anderson ME, 1992, Microbiological decontamination of food animal carcasses by washing and sanitizing systems: a review, *J Food Prot*, **55**: 133–40.

Dorsa WJ, Cutter CN et al., 1996, Microbial decontamination of beef and sheep carcasses by steam, hot water-spray washes, and a steam-vacuum sanitizer, *J Food Prot*, **59**: 127–35.

Epling LK, Carpenter JA, Blankenship LC, 1993, Prevalence of *Campylobacter* spp. and *Salmonella* spp. on pork carcasses and the reduction effected by spraying with lactic acid, *J Food Prot*, **56**: 537–40.

Erickson JP, Stamer JW et al., 1995, An assessment of *Escherichia coli* O157:H7 contamination risks in commercial mayonnaise from pasteurized eggs and environmental sources, and behavior in low-pH dressings, *J Food Prot*, **58**: 1059–64.

Esty JR, Meyer KF, 1922, The heat resistance of spores of *B. botulinus* and allied anaerobes XI, *J Infect Dis*, **31**: 650–63.

Fajardo TA, Anantheswaran RC et al., 1995, Penetration of *Salmonella enteritidis* into eggs subjected to rapid cooling, *J Food Prot*, **58**: 473–7.

FAO (United Nations Food and Agricultural Organization), 1981, *Food Loss Prevention in Perishable Crops*, FAO Agricultural Services Bulletin no. 43, FAO, Rome.

Fazli SFI, Schroeder HW, 1966, Effect of kernel infection of rice by *Helminthosporium oryzae* on yield and quality, *Phytopathology*, **56**: 1003–5.

Food Code, 1995, *1995 Recommendations of the United States Public Health Service, Food and Drug Administration*, US Department of Health and Human Services, Washington, DC.

FSIS (Food Safety and Inspection Service), 1994, *Statistical Summary, Federal Meat and Poultry Inspection for Fiscal Year 1993*, US Department of Agriculture, Food Safety and Inspection Service, Washington, DC.

FSIS (Food Safety and Inspection Service), 1995, Pathogen reduction; hazard analysis and critical control point (HACCP) systems, *Federal Register*, **60**: 6774.

FSIS (Food Safety and Inspection Service), 1996, Pathogen reduction; hazard analysis and critical control points (HACCP) systems, *Federal Register*, **61**: 38806.

Gilbert RJ, 1983, Foodborne infections and intoxications – recent trends and prospects for the future, *Food Microbiology: Advances and Prospects*, eds Roberts TA, Skinner FA, Academic Press, New York, 47–66.

Gilbert RJ, Taylor AJ, 1976, *Bacillus cereus* food poisoning, *Microbiology in Agriculture, Fisheries and Food*, eds Skinner FA, Carr JG, Academic Press, London, 197–213.

Gill CO, 1979, Intrinsic bacteria in meat, *J Appl Bacteriol*, **47**: 367–78.

Glass KA, Loeffelholz JM et al., 1992, Fate of *Escherichia coli* O157:H7 as affected by pH or sodium chloride in fermented dry sausage, *Appl Environ Microbiol*, **58**: 2513–16.

Gorman BM, Morgan JB et al., 1995, Microbiological and visual effects of trimming and/or spray washing for removal of fecal material from beef, *J Food Prot*, **58**: 984–9.

Gram L, 1992, Evaluation of the bacteriological quality of seafood, *Int J Food Microbiol*, **16**: 25–39.

Grau FH, 1986, Microbial ecology of meat and poultry, *Advances in Meat Research: Meat and Poultry Microbiology*, eds Pearson AM, Dutson TR, AVI Publishing/Macmillan, Westport, CT/London, 1–47.

Greeley M, 1983, Solving third world food problems: the role of post-harvest planning, *Post-harvest Physiology and Crop Protection*, ed. Lieberman M, Plenum Press, New York, 515–35.

Griffin PM, 1995, *Escherichia coli* O157:H7 and other enterohemorrhagic *Escherichia coli*, *Infections of the Gastrointestinal Tract*, eds Blaser MJ, Smith PD et al., Raven Press, New York, 739–61.

Hagler WM Jr, Tyczkowska K, Hamilton PB, 1984, Simultaneous occurrence of deoxynivalenol, zearalenone, and aflatoxin in 1982 scabby wheat from the midwestern United States, *Appl Environ Microbiol*, **47**: 151–4.

Hall DW, 1970, *Handling and Storage of Food Grains in Tropical and Sub-tropical Areas*, FAO Agriculture Development Paper no. 90, FAO, Rome.

Hersom AC, Hulland ED, 1980, *Canned Foods*, 7th edn, Churchill Livingstone, London.

Hinton M, Linton AH, 1988, Control of *Salmonella* infections in broiler chickens by the acid treatment of their feed, *Vet Rec*, **123**: 416–21.

Ichinoe M, Kurata H et al., 1983, Chemotaxonomy of *Gibberella zeae* with special reference to production of trichothecanes and zearalenone, *Appl Environ Microbiol*, **46**: 1364–9.

ICMSF (International Commission on Microbiological Specifications for Foods), 1980a, *Microbial Ecology of Foods*, vol. 1, Academic Press, New York.

ICMSF (International Commission on Microbiolological Specifications for Foods), 1980b, *Microbial Ecology of Foods*, vol. 2, Academic Press, New York.

Ilag LL, Juliano BO, 1982, Colonization and aflatoxin formation by *Aspergillus* spp. On brown rices differing in endosperm properties, *J Sci Food Agric*, **33**: 97–102.

Jarvis B, 1976, Mycotoxins in food, *Microbiology in Agriculture, Fisheries and Food*, eds Skinner FA, Carr JG, Academic Press, London, 251–67.

Jay JM, 1986, *Modern Food Microbiology*, 3rd edn, Van Nostrand Reinhold, New York.

Kent NL, 1966, *Technology of Cereals with Special Reference to Wheat*, Pergamon Press, London.

Kotula KL, Pandya Y, 1995, Bacterial contamination of broiler chickens before scalding, *J Food Prot*, **58**: 1326–9.

Kramer JM, Gilbert RJ, 1989, *Bacillus cereus* and other *Bacillus* species, *Foodborne Bacterial Pathogens*, ed. Doyle MP, Marcel Dekker, New York, 21–70.

Kudva IT, Hatfield PG, Hovde CJ, 1995, Effect of diet on the shedding of *Escherichia coli* O157:H7 in a sheep model, *Appl Environ Microbiol*, **61**: 1363–70.

Kuthubutheen AJ, 1984, Effect of pesticides on the seed-borne fungi and fungal succession on rice in Malaysia, *J Stored Prod Res*, **20**: 31–40.

Lawrie RA, 1985, *Meat Science*, 4th edn, Pergamon Press, Oxford.

Lee LA, Gerber AR et al., 1990, *Yersinia enterocolitica* O:3 infections in infants and children, associated with the household preparation of chitterlings, *N Engl J Med*, **322**: 984–7.

Lee M, Sebranek JG et al., 1996, Irradiation and packaging of fresh meat and poultry, *J Food Prot*, **59**: 62–72.

Levine WC, Griffin PM, 1993, *Vibrio* infections on the Gulf Coast: results of first year of regional surveillance, *J Infect Dis*, **167**: 479–83.

Lund BM, 1972, Isolation of pectolytic clostridia from potatoes, *J Appl Bacteriol*, **35**: 609–14.

Lund BM, 1983, Post-harvest pathology of fruits and vegetables, *Post-harvest Physiology of Fruits and Vegetables*, ed. Dennis C, Academic Press, London, 219–57.

Lund BM, 1986, Anaerobes in relation to foods of plant origin, *Anaerobic Bacteria in Habitats Other than Man*, eds Barnes EM, Mead GC, Academic Press, London, 351–72.

Mallick AK, Nandi B, 1981, Research: rice, *Rice J*, **84**: 8–13.

Mead GC, 1980, Microbiological control in the processing of chickens and turkeys, *Meat Quality in Poultry and Game Birds*, eds Mead GC, Freeman BM, British Poultry Science Ltd, Edinburgh, 99–104.

Mead GC, 1982, Microbiology of poultry and game birds (processed carcass), *Meat Microbiology*, ed. Brown MH, Applied Science Publishers, London, 67–101.

Mikkelsen DS, DeDatta SK, 1980, Rice culture, *Rice: Production and Utilization*, ed. Luh BS, AVI Publishing, Westport, CT, 147–234.

Mishu B, Griffin PM et al., 1991, *Salmonella enteritidis* gastroenteritis transmitted by intact chicken eggs, *Ann Intern Med*, **115**: 190–4.

Mossman AP, 1983, *Handbook of Tropical Foods*, ed. Chan HT, Marcel Dekker, New York, 489.

National Animal Health Monitoring System, 1995, Salmonella *Shedding by Feedlot Cattle*, US Department of Agriculture, Animal and Plant Health Inspection Service, Veterinary Services, Fort Collins, CO.

Osborne BG, Willis KH, 1984, The occurrence of some tricothecene mycotoxins in UK home grown wheat and in imported wheat, *J Sci Food Agric*, **35**: 579–83.

Pierson MD, Corlett DA Jr, 1992, *HACCP: Principles and Applications*, Van Nostrand Reinhold, New York.

Pitt JI, Hocking AD, 1986, *Fungi and Fungal Spoilage*, Academic Press, London.

Prasai RK, Phebus RK et al., 1995, Effectiveness of trimming and/or washing on microbiological quality of beef carcasses, *J Food Prot*, **58**: 1114–17.

Proctor FJ, Goodliffe JP, Coursey DG, 1981, *Vegetable Productivity*, ed. Spedding CRW, Macmillan, London, 139.

Rasmussen MA, Cray WC Jr et al., 1993, Rumen contents as a reservoir of enterohemorrhagic *Escherichia coli*, *FEMS Microbiol Lett*, **114**: 79–84.

Roberts TA, Mead GC, 1986, Involvement of intestinal anaerobes in the spoilage of red meats, poultry and fish, *Anaerobic Bacteria in Habitats Other than Man*, eds Barnes EM, Mead GC, Academic Press, London, 333–50.

Ryall AL, Lipton WJ, 1979, *Handling, Transportation and Storage of Fruits and Vegetables*, 2nd edn, AVI Publishing Co., Westport, CT.

Saito M, Ohtsubo K, 1974, Tricothecene toxins of *Fusarium*, *Mycotoxins*, ed. Purchase IFH, Elsevier Scientific, Amsterdam, 263–81.

Salunkhe DK, Desai BB, 1984, *Postharvest Biotechnology of Vegetables*, CRC Press, Boca Raton, FL.

Schlech WF, Lavigne PM et al., 1983, Epidemic listeriosis – evidence for transmission by food, *N Engl J Med*, **308**: 203–6.

Schroeder HW, Boller RA, Hein H, 1968, Reduction in aflatoxin contamination of rice by milling procedures, *Cereal Chem*, **45**: 574–80.

Sierra M-L, Gonzales-Fandos E et al., 1995, Prevalence of *Salmonella*, *Yersinia*, *Aeromonas*, *Campylobacter*, and cold-growing *Escherichia coli* on freshly dressed lamb carcasses, *J Food Prot*, **58**: 1183–5.

Slavik MF, Kim J-W, Walker JT, 1995, Reduction of *Salmonella* and *Campylobacter* on chicken carcasses by changing scalding temperature, *J Food Prot*, **58**: 689–91.

Splittstoesser DF, 1987, Fruits and fruit products, *Food and Beverage Mycology*, 2nd edn, ed. Beuchat LR, Van Nostrand Reinhold, New York, 101–28.

St Louis ME, Morse DL et al., 1988, The emergence of grade A eggs as a major source of *Salmonella enteritidis* infections: new implication for control of salmonellosis, *JAMA*, **259**: 2103–7.

Stadelman WJ, 1994, Contaminants of liquid egg products, *Microbiology of the Avian Egg*, eds Board RG, Fuller R, Chapman and Hall, London, 139–51.

Stern NJ, 1992, Reservoirs of *Campylobacter jejuni* and approaches for intervention in poultry, Campylobacter jejuni: *Current Status and Future Trends*, eds Nachamkin I, Blaser MJ, Tompkins LS, American Society for Microbiology, Washington, DC, 49–60.

Stern NJ, Clavero MR et al., 1995, *Campylobacter* spp. in broilers on the farm and after transport, *Poult Sci*, **74**: 937–41.

USDA (US Department of Agriculture), 1990, *National Poultry Improvement Plans and Auxillary Provisions*, Animal and Plant Health Inspection Service edn, US Government Printing Office, Washington, DC.

Weagent SD, Bryant JL, Bark DH, 1994, Survival of *Escherichia coli* O157:H7 in mayonnaise and mayonnaise-based sauces at room and refrigerator temperatures, *J Food Prot*, **57**: 629–31.

Williams JE, 1981a, Salmonella in poultry feeds – a worldwide review, *World Poult Sci J*, **37**: 6–25.

Williams JE, 1981b, Salmonella in poultry feeds – a worldwide review. Methods in control and elimination, *World Poult Sci J*, **37**: 97–105.

Williams PC, 1983, Maintaining nutritional and processing quality in grain crops during handling, storage and transportation, *Post-harvest Physiology and Crop Preservation*, ed. Liebermann M, Plenum Press, New York, 425–44.

Zeleny L, 1971, Criteria of wheat-m quality, *Wheat – Chemistry and Technology*, ed. Pomeranz Y, American Association of Cereal Chemists, St Paul, MN, 19–49.

Zhao T, Doyle MP, 1994, Fate of enterohemorrhagic *Escherichia coli* O157:H7 in commercial mayonnaise, *J Food Prot*, **57**: 780–3.

Chapter 18

BACTERIAL IMMUNOSEROLOGY

R C Tilton

1 Immunobiology	4 Applications of technology in bacterial serology
2 Immunochemistry and immunopathology	
3 Methods in bacterial serology	5 Seroepidemiology
	6 Summary

Immunological methods have long been a mainstay for the diagnosis of infectious diseases. The earliest methods for antibody detection included precipitation, agglutination and complement fixation. The last 2 decades have seen a proliferation in both antibody and antigen testing because of the availability of sensitive, automatable methods such as enzyme-linked immunosorbent assay (ELISA), radioimmunoassay (RIA) and fluorescence immunoassay (FIA) as well as the routine availability of high quality polyclonal and monoclonal antibodies and purified antigens.

Immunological methods in bacteriology are used not only for the detection of an immune response to a bacterial infection but also to detect bacterial antigens directly in body fluids and to type or otherwise identify bacterial isolates.

This chapter reviews the essential features of immunobiology, immunochemistry and immunopathology. Methods for immunological diagnosis are critically reviewed and their applications to the detection of specific bacterial diseases are presented. Basic concepts of seroepidemiology are discussed and applications of these techniques to practical epidemiology are featured.

1 IMMUNOBIOLOGY

Infection is a process by which a parasite enters into a relationship with its host and may cause a harmful event. Most host–parasite interactions do not result in disease, since the infection is eradicated or remains latent or subclinical. The outcome of this relationship is determined by the invasive and toxic characteristics of the parasite and the various host mechanisms that interact with these processes. If the parasite injures the host, disease will occur. Host defence systems include the first line of external defence (which is usually

physical), natural immunity and acquired immunity. These systems are modulated by a number of factors which can be separated into 2 groups.

The first group includes

1 non-specific anatomical barriers (e.g. skin and mucous membranes)
2 tissue products (e.g. lysozome, proteolytic enzymes, polypeptides, fatty acids, etc.)
3 physiological responses (e.g., fever, acid pH, etc.)
4 cellular components (e.g. phagocytes and natural killer cells)
5 acute proteins which mediate the inflammatory response (e.g. complement, C-reactive protein, interferon, cytokines, prostaglandins, leukotrienes and thromboxanes).

The second group consists of specific immune factors such as antibodies and T lymphocytes.

The issue of immunity to bacterial infection is not clear cut. Immunity is a relative term which ranges from susceptibility to total disease resistance and may be influenced not only by immunological factors but by gender, race, geographical and genetic origin and age. This is often termed **natural immunity**. As its name implies, this type of immune response has no specificity and shows no increase on subsequent exposure as specific immunity does. Non-specific immunity or natural immunity was probably the first defence mechanism to evolve and it is still the first line of defence in humans, ensuring relative freedom from infection (see Volume 3, Chapter 2).

The problems of infection arise initially either as a consequence of the ability of an organism to overcome the primary defences or as a result of a breach in these defences, allowing easy access to susceptible tissues or failure to phagocytose and remove offending micro-organisms. The skin and mucous membranes, the secretions of tears, saliva and gastric juices and the ciliary activity of the respiratory tract all combine to interpose a formidable barrier to the entry of disease-producing organisms. When any of these is abnormal, relatively easy access is afforded to deeper tissues where organisms can safely multiply before the second line of defence, the phagocytic cells, can engulf them. Any condition, whether hereditary or acquired, which affects the functions of these tissues and secretions predisposes to infection, and severe defects may even allow invasion by organisms otherwise not regarded as potential pathogens, the so-called **opportunistic** organisms. Many such infections are acquired in hospitals.

The non-specific mechanisms of immunity may also be impaired or absent as a result of congenital anomalies. Phagocytosis and intracellular killing of bacteria involve complex biochemical processes, and any step in these pathways may be interrupted by a genetically determined defect in one or more enzymes. Although some of these defects have been identified, it is likely that many others can occur, leading to defective phagocytosis or to ineffectual killing once the organism is inside the phagocyte, or both.

1.1   Phagocytic cells

The phagocytic cells of mammalian blood and tissues belong to the myeloid cell line. This originates from a common precursor population of stem cells which diverges to form 2 classes of cell – the neutrophilic leucocytes (or granulocytes) and the mononuclear phagocytes. Eosinophilic leucocytes resemble neutrophils morphologically but originate from a separate cell line. Neutrophils are often referred to as polymorphonuclear leucocytes (PMN) but, since the nuclei of other leucocytes may also be lobed, the term **neutrophil** is preferable. The mononuclear phagocyte system includes the blood monocytes and their marrow precursors, as well as the macrophage/histiocyte series found in many tissues, either as a resident population in the steady state or as a newly recruited population in inflamed tissues. It includes a variety of tissue-specific cells, including hepatic Kupffer cells, splenic macrophages and osteoclasts. Cells such as the Langerhans cells of the skin, the interdigitating cells of lymphoid tissue and other similar cells whose principal function is the presentation of antigen rather than direct disposal of pathogenic micro-organisms, are usually included in the mononuclear phagocyte system.

The process of phagocytosis of foreign bacteria or other particles can be subdivided into 3 phases: attachment, ingestion and intracellular killing.

Attachment requires that the phagocyte recognize the particle to be ingested. There are both non-immune and immune recognition; non-immune recognition is phylogenetically more primitive. There is a widely diverse collection of particles that may be phagocytosed in the absence of antibody or complement, of which polystyrene latex beads are probably in the widest experimental use. It is difficult to visualize specific receptors for such objects, and this is a poorly understood, but probably non-specific, form of phagocytic recognition. A more physiological example of non-immune phagocytosis is the recognition and ingestion of physically or chemically altered erythrocytes. Glutaraldehyde-treated erythrocytes are frequently used experimentally; this treatment may be analogous to the physiological mechanism for clearance of old erythrocytes from the body. Furthermore, many bacteria, particularly those of low virulence, may be cleared by non-immune phagocytic recognition. Immune phagocytosis, or immune recognition, suggests specific cell surface receptors on neutrophils, mononuclear phacocytes and eosinophils.

These phagocytic cells have plasma membrane receptors for the Fc region of IgG (the Fe receptors) and for the activated complement components C3b and C3bi. These receptors are known as CR1 (for C3b) and CR3 (for C3bi). During the course of an immunological response to a micro-organism or particulate antigen, the particle becomes coated with antibody bound to the surface antigens of the particle, so that the Fc region of the antibody is free, together with C'3b. The bound IgG and C3b can then interact with the appropriate receptors on the surface of the phagocytic cell and the opsonized particle becomes attached to the phagocyte. This event rapidly leads to activation of the ingestion process and, ultimately, the microbiocidal pathways of the phagocyte. It is probable that the majority of pyogenic bacteria are disposed of by opsonic phagocytosis.

Particle ingestion results from the formation of a cup-like process around the particle; the latter eventually becomes fully enclosed by the fusion of the edges of the advancing process. As the phagocyte encircles the particle, microfilamentous actin networks are actively formed in its advancing tip, the cytoplasm of which is probably gelated, while further back the networks are broken down and the cytoplasm is isolated. This breakdown is probably necessary to allow the next step once ingestion has been completed. The **phagosome** – the vesicle containing the ingested particle – is drawn through the cytoplasm towards the Golgi region, where fusion of cytoplasmic cranules with phagosome takes place.

NEUTROPHILS

Phagocytic cells probably have several mechanisms for killing bacteria and parasites. These include (1) oxidative microbicidal systems, (2) cationic proteins and (3) membrane-damaging enzymes including phospholipases. Of these, the first is probably the most important in the neutrophil. Normal neutrophils which are allowed to ingest a bacterium such as *Staphylococcus aureus* kill the majority of the bacteria within 20 min or so. In patients in whom a defect of the oxidative microbicidal system can be detected, for example children with chronic granulomatous disease, the bacteria are killed much more slowly and the children suffer from severe recurrent infections. Contact with phagocytosable particles or with chemotactic factors activates a rapid metabolic burst in neutrophils and monocytes with increased hexose monophosphate shunt activity and increased generation of superoxide anion and hydrogen peroxide. The latter molecules are believed to play an important role in the microbicidal pathway (Babior 1984, Roos and Balm 1980). Peroxide, in the presence of myeloperoxidase released from azurophil granules into the phagosome, together with halide, forms a rapidly acting microbicidal system (Klebanoff 1980).

EOSINOPHILS

Although resembling neutrophils morphologically and to some extent functionally, eosinophils are derived from a separate lineage of bone marrow precursors and perform specialized functions in 2 major immunological reactions, namely immediate hypersensitivity and the response to metazoan parasites. The most obvious immunological feature of the eosinophil is the presence of prominent specific cytoplasmic eosinophilic granules. These granules contain large quantities of cationic proteins, the major one being present in the crystalloid bar typically seen in transmission electron micrographs. These proteins are non-enzymatic with the exception of a cationic lysophospholipase (Charcot–Leyden crystal protein). Eosinophil granules also contain hydrolases, though in smaller quantities than in neutrophils. There is a peroxidase, which is different from the myeloperoxidase of neutrophils. A second series of small granules contains enzymes such as arylsulphatase. Like neutrophils, eosinophils can generate a strong metabolic burst of toxic products such as superoxide and hydrogen peroxide.

Eosinophils are phagocytic cells but are not as effective as neutrophils. Their primary function may be secretion and extracellular rather than intracellular killing.

1.2 Specific immunoreactive cells

The lymphocyte is the primary cell involved in the specific response to infection. Foreign material or antigen is initially recognized and processed. The ability to recognize foreign antigen, such as bacteria, is intrinsic to certain cells of the immune system, mainly (but not exclusively) cells of the macrophage/monocyte series, which are widely distributed in most tissues and organs, both as fixed and as mobile cells, moving in blood and tissue fluids and attracted to sites of inflammation. The subsequent response to antigen is the product of cellular interactions and is brought about primarily by lymphocytes. The characteristic features of this system are its specificity, i.e. the response is directed against the offending antigen, and the fact that the response increases with subsequent exposure to the same antigen.

There are 2 major populations of lymphocytes: B lymphocytes and T lymphocytes.

B LYMPHOCYTES

The principal function of B lymphocytes (B cells) is the production and secretion of antibody in response to stimulation by antigen. The 'B' is derived from the name of the organ which is the main site of production of this cell in chickens, the bursa of Fabricius. Although no similar organ has been identified in mammals, the original term has been extended to apply to all cells with the special characteristics of B cells. The antibody secreted by a B cell belongs to one of 9 different isotypes of immunoglobulin – IgM, IgD, IgGI, IgG2, IgG3, IgG4, IgAl, IgA2 and IgE – each of which has a different biological function. Before differentiating into a mature antibody-secreting form, the **plasma cell**, the B cell must first pass through a number of different stages, during which its immunoglobulin genes undergo rearrangement. Figure 18.1 presents human B cell differentiation.

T LYMPHOCYTES

T lymphocytes or T cells are characterized by a specific membrane-bound marker, the **T cell receptor** (Clevers et al. 1988). Their name derives from the central role played by the thymus in the maturation and eventual functional properties of these cells. The T cell receptor is not an immunoglobulin. It consists of a 90 kDa heterodimer, with 2 disulphide-linked polypeptide chains (α and β), and is found on the cell surface in close association with a second molecule, the CD3 antigen (formerly known as T3). Both the cell receptor and CD3 are transmembrane proteins and, like immunoglobulins, possess variable and constant regions. The antigen-binding site of the T cell receptor is formed by the interaction of the 2 variable regions, in a manner analogous to the antigen-binding site of immunoglobulins. Each T cell or clone formed by the expansion of a T cell after antigen exposure possesses an α–β receptor of unique antigen specificity. The associated invariant CD3 molecule probably acts as a signal transducer, conveying activation signal(s) to the interior of the cell. T cells can be further subdivided into 3 functional subpopulations.

T helper (Th) cells are immunoregulatory cells that, once activated by antigen, orchestrate the behaviour of the other types of cell involved in generating an immunological response by secreting a variety of cytokines (sometimes referred to as lymphokines). The cells can be recognized serologically by the expression of a surface glycoprotein, CD4 (formerly T4).

A second population of **cytotoxic T (Tc) cells** lyse specific target cells, including virus-infecting host cells, tumour cells and allogeneic graft cells in transplanted tissues. Tc cells possess the membrane glycoprotein CD8 (formerly T8).

A third population of **T suppressor (Ts) cells** with immunoregulatory function, this time to inhibit immunological responses, and also bearing the CD8 marker, has been postulated and it is claimed they can be distinguished from Tc cells in vitro (Gershon and Hondo 1971). Approximately two-thirds of circulating T cells in humans are CD4[+] and one-third CD8[+]. Figure 18.2 shows the differentiation of human T lymphocytes.

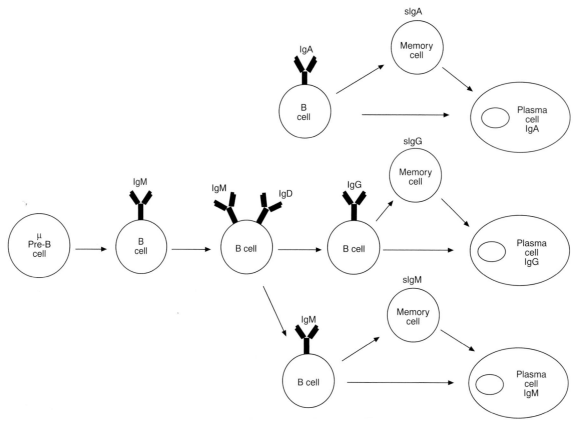

Fig. 18.1 Human B cell differentiation. sIg, surface immunoglobulin.

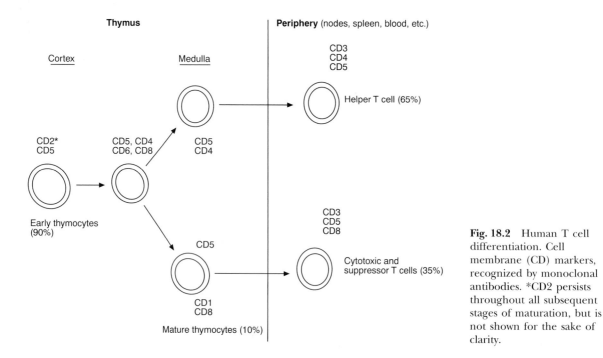

Fig. 18.2 Human T cell differentiation. Cell membrane (CD) markers, recognized by monoclonal antibodies. *CD2 persists throughout all subsequent stages of maturation, but is not shown for the sake of clarity.

1.3 Cytokines and T cell activation

Many of the interactions between cells of the immune response are mediated by soluble products, generally peptides of low molecular weight, originally called lymphokines but more correctly **cytokines** because they are produced by several cell types and not solely by activated lymphocytes. A summary of the best-defined cytokines and their functions is given in Table 18.1. The numerous cytokines secreted by activated cells affect both local cell division and the recruitment or activation (or both) of other cells involved in the response to antigen (Dinarello and Mier 1987).

Table 18.1   Cytokines and their actions

IL-1	Macrophage	Potent mediator of inflammation. Causes release of acute phase proteins. Activates endothelial cells. Activates resting T cells. Cofactor for haemopoietic growth factors
IL-2	T lymphocyte	Growth factor for activated T cells and B cells. Induces synthesis of other lymphokines
IL-3	T lymphocyte	Promotes proliferation of most haemopoietic stem cells
IL-4	T lymphocyte	Growth factor for activated B cells and resting T cells
IL-5	T lymphocyte	Promotes proliferation of eosinophils
IL-6	T lymphocyte/fibroblast	Promotes terminal differentiation of B cells into antibody-secreting plasma cells
Interferon-α	Macrophage	
Interferon-β	Fibroblast	Antiviral activity. Augments natural killer cell activity
Interferon-γ	T lymphocyte	Stimulates expression of class II MHC antigens on monocytes and other cells. Activates macrophages and endothelial cells. Augments natural killer cell activity. Antiviral activity
TNF-α TNF-β	Macrophage T lymphocyte	Induce fever and systemic acute phase response. Mediate inflammation and septic shock. Activate macrophages and endothelial cells

1.4   The role of the complement system in the immune response

The complement system, an integral component of the host's defences, has evolved primarily for protective functions, and is essential to maintaining health. The complement system offers 3 major functions in host defence:

1   coating pathogenic micro-organisms or immune complexes with opsonins, resulting in removal by phagocytes
2   activating inflammatory cells
3   killing target cells.

These 3 functions can be performed by the classical or alternative pathway. Both pathways have a similar molecular organization consisting of 3 operational phases: recognition, amplification and membrane attack. Understanding the modulating mechanisms operating in the 2 pathways which regulate the activation of the complement cascade and control the synthesis of biologically active split products is important for diagnosing and managing patients who present with recurrent allergic diseases and autoimmune disorders. The vital role of this system is illustrated by the onset of recurrent infections or immune complex diseases in patients with congenital defects of one or more of at least 20 proteins comprised by this system. (See Volume 3, Chapter 4 for further details of the complement system.)

2   IMMUNOCHEMISTRY AND IMMUNOPATHOLOGY

There are a variety of physical, chemical and bio-chemical barriers to bacterial antigens. These include skin and mucous membranes. Skin and mucosal surfaces are protected against offending micro-organisms by lactic acid, lysozyme, proteases, and pH. (See also Volume 3, Chapter 6 on the immunological basis of tissue damage.)

The non-specific immune system also consists of a variety of cellular products which respond to invasion by foreign antigenic substances. The end result is **inflammation**. Inflammation is initiated by trauma, tissue necrosis, infection or immune reactions. It can be induced, maintained or limited by signalling molecules or chemical mediators that act on smooth muscle, endothelial or white blood cells. The acute phase of inflammation spans a series of sequential events that begin with temporary vasoconstriction. Temporary vasoconstriction is believed to be mediated by the sympathetic nervous system. The first agents in the sequence affect smooth muscle cells of precapillary arterioles to produce dilatation and increased blood flow. Increased vascular permeability proceeds in 2 phases: an early phase, which occurs within minutes and is mediated by histamine and serotonin, and a late phase, which occurs in 6–12 h and is mediated by various molecules derived from different sources. These sources include arachidonic acid metabolites, breakdown products of the coagulation system (fibrin split products), peptides formed from blood or tissue proteins (bradykinin) and activated complement components, as well as factors released from bacteria, necrotic tissue, neutrophils (inflammatory peptides), lymphocytes (lymphokines) and monocytes (monokines). The cellular elements that play an important role in the acute inflammation process include mast cells, neutrophils, platelets and eosinophils, which act in sequence. They are activated by a variety of chemical processes and in turn produce and release a number of chemical mediators. Specific recognition of bacterial antigens is mediated by 2 types of molecules; immunoglobulins (antibodies) and T lymphocytes. There is much heterogenicity in both systems although they have a common ancestry.

Antibody molecules represent the functional products of the humoral arm of the mammalian immune system. Antibodies are glycoprotein molecules found mainly in the γ fraction of serum, and are members of the immunoglobulin family of serum proteins. The structural and functional properties of individual immunoglobulin molecules vary enormously but all have a common unit structure which forms the molecular basis for their immunobiological and immunochemical activities.

The site of antibody synthesis is the B lymphocyte. B cells are characterized by the presence of immunoglobulin on their plasma membranes, serving as the B cell receptor for antigen. Contact with complementary antigen results in expansion of the particular B cell clone and differentiation to plasma cells. Plasma cells represent the 'end cell' of the B lymphocyte lineage, and are therefore the terminal differentiation stage of the B cell. The humoral immune response displays characteristic features. After initial challenge with antigen, levels of antibody of the IgM class rise in 4–7 days. This is the primary humoral response. If antigenic challenge persists, IgG antibodies are produced. Levels of this secondary response begin to rise after 10–14 days or later. Subsequent challenge with the same antigen elicits a rapid increase in IgG antibody levels. The capacity to respond to rechallenge by a given antigen is long lived and resides in memory B cells. This secondary response also encompasses those antibody responses whose major component is of the IgA, IgE or IgD class.

2.1 Immunoglobulins

The 4-chain model describes the overall structure of IgG molecules (Porter 1962). Although immunoglobulin molecules exist as 5 classes, each with distinctive structural and functional properties, all are governed by the same rules of structure as those illustrated for the IgG molecule. (The immunoglobulins are discussed in detail in Chapter 3 of Volume 3.)

The general features of the 4-chain model are illustrated in Fig. 18.3, using human IgG1 as the example. Antibody molecules are composed of 2 identical light chains in such a way that the N-terminus of each heavy and light chain is juxtaposed in 3-dimensional terms to generate the antigen combining site. Interchain disulphide bonds not only link the heavy and light chains but also link the 2 heavy chains together. The IgG molecule is bivalent with respect to antigen binding. (Edelman and Poulik 1961, Porter 1962).

Human immunoglobulin molecules exist as 5 **classes**, or **isotypes**, each of which has characteristic structural features and particular immunobiological activities. The serological marker that defines immunoglobulin class or subclass is the isotype, and

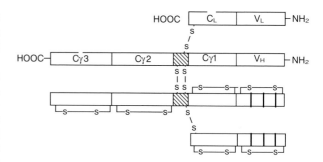

Fig. 18.3 Four-chain model of human IgG1. The left-hand side illustrates the nomenclature for individual domains of the IgG1 molecule and the approximate positioning of disulphide bonds.

the terms 'isotype', 'class' and 'subclass' are used interchangeably. All isotypes have a 4-chain unit as their fundamental structural feature, and each class is named for the γ heavy chain, IgM for the μ chain and IgA for the α chain. The principal molecular properties of the 5 human immunoglobulin classes are detailed in Table 18.2.

IgM

IgM is a pentameric structure comprising 5 4-chain units. The μ heavy chain has 5 domains, VH plus 4 C regions (Cμ1, Cμ2, Cμ3 and Cμ4), and lacks a hinge region. The pentameric structure is stabilized by disulphide bonding between adjacent Cμ3 domains, and by the presence of the J (joining) chain. A single J chain is disulphide-linked close to the C-terminus of the μ chain (Chapuis and Koshland 1974). The cysteine residue which participates in this bonding (Cys-575) is part of an 18 amino acid C-terminal peptide extension located immediately following the Cμ4 domain. The cysteine participates either in disulphide bonding to the J chain or to cysteines located in an identical position in other μ chains of the pentameric complex.

IgM is the principal component of the primary humoral response. Because of its large size (970 kDa, 19S), it is located mainly in the blood stream. It is decavalent, leading to highly avid binding of antigens (thus overcoming potential low affinity of the interaction), and is efficient in both opsonization and complement fixation.

IgG

IgG is the main class of immunoglobulin in serum. As will be obvious from the detailed discussion of the 4-chain model, it exists as a molecule of molecular weight 146–160 kDa (7S) in serum, and is the principal component of the secondary humoral immune response. This class of immunoglobulin is found not only in the blood stream itself but also in extravascular spaces. It is also transported across the placental membrane and is therfore responsible for passive immunity in the fetus and newborn infant.

There are 4 major subclasses of the IgG isotype in humans, each distinguished by the number and location of disulphide bridges and by minor variations

Table 18.2 Molecular properties of immunoglobulins

	Igm	IgG1	IgG2	IgG3	IgG4	IgA1	IgA2	sIgA	IgD	IgE
Heavy chain	μ	γ_1	γ_2	γ_3	γ_4	α_1	α_2	α_1/α_2	δ	ε
Mol. wt (kDa)	65	51	51	60	51	56	52	52 or 56	70	72.5
Assembled form	$(\mu_2 L_2)_5 J^a$	$\gamma_2 L_2{}^b$	$\gamma_2 L_2$	$\gamma_2 L_2$	$\gamma_2 L_2$	$\alpha_2 L_2$	$\alpha_2 L_2$	$(\alpha_2 L_2)_2 J.SC^c$	$\delta_2 L_2$	$\varepsilon_2 L_2$
Mol. wt (kDa)	970	146	146	160	146	160	160	385	188	184
Sedimentation coefficient (S)	19	7	7	7	7	7	7	11	7	8
Valency for antigen	5(10)	2	2	2	2	2	2	4	2	2
Serum concentration (mg/ml)	1.5	9	3	1	0.5	3	0.5	0.05	0.03	0.00005

[a]Molecular weight of J chain is 15 kDa.
[b]Written $\gamma_2 L_2$ for convenience formally $(\gamma 1)_2 L_2$.
[c]Molecular weight of secretory component is 70 kDa.

in amino acid sequence in the C region. The structural variations in amino acid has consequences for biological activity. Thus, the IgG1 and IgG3 isotypes are efficient in fixation of complement, whereas IgG2 and IgG4 subclasses are incapable of activating this effector function. Similarly, only IgG1 and IgG3 are capable of interacting with the Fc receptors on macrophages and therefore of acting as efficient opsonins.

IgA

IgA is found in 2 forms in the body. In serum it occurs as a monomer (160 kDa, 7S) but this isotype is found principally on secretory surfaces where it exists as a dimeric molecule (385 kDa, 11S). The dimeric form is known as secretory IgA (sIgA) and is found in association with J chain and with secretory component, the latter being involved in transport of the IgA to the secretory system.

IgD

IgD is present in serum at 0.2% of the concentration of IgG. It is found on the surface of B lymphocytes and functions as a cell surface receptor for antigen, probably involved in the differentiation of antibody secretory plasma cells.

IgE

IgE is present in serum in minute concentrations and is responsible for allergies to a wide variety of allergenic substances. IgE concentrations rise after infection with certain parasites, thus giving credence to the idea that IgE has a protective function at least for parasitic infections.

Antibody molecules participate in a variety of biological functions including complement fixation and binding to a variety of cells such as mononuclear cells, polymorphonuclear leucocytes, basophils, mast cells, T and B lymphocytes and platelets.

One of the most important functions of immunoglobulins is **complement fixation**. The complement system has 2 pathways of activation, the **classical** and the **alternative** pathways (Fig. 18.4). Activation of either leads to the generation of proteolytic enzymes termed C3 convertases, which are able to cleave and activate C3, the central protein of the system. It is this activation of C3 which results in the generation of the most of the biological activities of the system. Although the pathways are separate and involve different proteins, the mechanism by which they activate C3 is the same and the resultant biological activities (lysis, opsonization, etc.) are identical.

The 2 pathways have different mechanisms of activation. The proteins of the classical pathway as described in Table 18.3 are termed C1, C2 and C4. The proteins of the alternative pathways are termed factors D, B, P, H and I. Enzymes produced during the activation process are denoted by a bar placed over the precursor from which they are derived, e.g. $\bar{C1}$. The later-acting proteins of the system, termed C5, C6, C7, C8 and C9, which are involved in the lysis of susceptible micro-organisms, are common to both pathways.

2.2 Complement and bacterial killing

Complement is a major component of bacterial killing. The bacteriolytic potential of complement appears to be the same whether activation is by the classical or the alternative pathway. Gram-negative cocci such as *Neisseria* spp. appear to be particularly

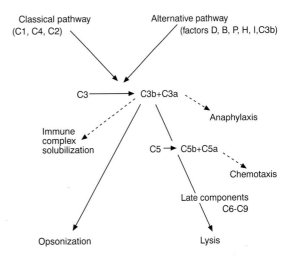

Fig. 18.4 The complement system.

Table 18.3 Complement components: proteins of the two pathways

Protein	Serum conc. (mg l^{-1})	Activation products	Function
A. The classical pathway			
C1q	150	–	Triggers activation of classical pathway on binding to antibody–antigen aggregates. Binds C1r2, C1s2, leading to activation
C1r	50	– C1r	Zymogen of serine protease. Binds C1q and C1s Autoactivated by binding to C1q, cleaves C1s
C1s	50	– C1s	Zymogen of serine protease activated by C1r When activated by C1r, cleaves C2 and C4 thus assembling C3 convertase
C4	300	– C4a C4b	Anaphylatoxin Binds covalently to immunoglobulin and cell surface Binds C2, allowing C3 convertase assembly
C2	15	– C2a C2b	Binds to C4b. Cleaved by C1s Contains active site of C3/C5 convertase; release from C4b results in delay in activity Contains Mg^{2+}-dependent binding site for C4b
B. The alternate pathway			
C3b		–	Multifunctional. Subunit of C3/CS convertase; binding site for activators, factor B, factor P, factor H
Factor D	5	–	Cleaves factor B which is complexed with C3b
Factor B	200	– Ba Bb	Binds to C3b, allowing cleavage by factor D Contains Mg^{2+}-dependent binding site for C3b Active site of C3/C5 convertase; release from C3b causes decay
Factor P (properdin)	25	–	Stabilizes C3/C5 convertase on activating surface
Factor I	25	–	Cleaves C3b under control of factor H or CR1. Limits fluid phase convertase activity
Factor H	700	–	Binds to C3b. Directs specificity of factor I to C3b

sensitive to lysis, accounting for recurrent gonorrhoea and meningococcal meningitis that may be associated with deficiencies, but the lysis of many other gram-negative organisms has also been documented.

The ability of bacterial cell surfaces to activate complement clearly depends on a variety of factors, including the chemical composition of the surface and the immune status of the host. Endotoxins from gram-negative bacteria are potent activators of the alternative pathway. The potency of activation depends on the polysaccharide composition of the lipopolysaccharide and certain virulent pathogens appear to have devised ways of limiting activation. The isolated lipid moiety of lipopolysaccharide from some species of *Klebsiella, Escherichia, Shigella* and *Salmonella* is able to activate the classical pathway but this process may also allow more rapid inactivation of the C1 proteases by C1 inhibitor. Gram-positive bacteria with their peptidoglycan coats also appear to be potent activators of the alternative pathway, although again the response varies (Joiner 1986, Clas and Loos 1987).

Polysaccharide capsules are generally assumed to be inefficient activators of either pathway, probably because of their sialic acid content (e.g. *Streptococcus pneumoniae*). Bacterial membranes may also contain proteins which limit complement activation, such as the M protein of group A streptococci which blocks C3 binding and the protein A of *Staphylococcus aureus* which binds to the Fc region of IgG. The complex carbohydrates of fungal cells are also potent activators of the alternative pathway.

Fragments of C3 deposited on the surface of bacteria and fungi trigger the rapid phagocytosis of the micro-organisms by neutrophils and macrophages. In the case of non-capsulate strains such as *S. pneumoniae, S. aureus, E. coli* and *Salmonella* spp. the C3b is covalently bound to the lipopolysaccharide and the rate of phagocytosis depends on the density of C3b, its ability to be cleaved to C3bi and the coexistence of immunoglobulin which can interact with Fc receptors on the phagocytes. Although the cell walls of capsulate strains of the same bacteria activate C3 by the alternative pathway, it appears that the C3b is inaccessible to the receptors and therefore these cells are not efficiently phagocytosed. By localizing the C3 products to the capsular surfaces, anticapsular antibodies may make an organism that would not be otherwise so, capable of being efficiently opsonized. The type III group B streptococcus is one example.

3 METHODS IN BACTERIAL SEROLOGY

A large variety of serological methods are in current laboratory use. Some, such as agglutination and precipitation, are old but still valuable techniques. Others such as ELISA and its variations are relatively new but now predominate, particularly as automated instruments become more widely available.

The measurement in vitro of the reaction between antigen and antibody may use a qualitative or a quantitative assay system; the former is chosen to achieve some degree of approximation to the expected functional properties designed to allow the 2 components to come together in controlled conditions so that a visible reaction is observed, either directly or indirectly. Qualitative assays do not always reflect what appears in vivo, although some are clearly intended to do so (e.g. toxin neutralization assays). Such tests may measure tissue-damaging potential only indirectly but this is less of a problem with antibody measurement than with tests designed to quantify lymphocyte function. In the context of quantitative assays, it should also be remembered that the antibody measured in the laboratory, however accurately, may not be the actual antibody which matters in the recovery from infection, or it may not have an opportunity to exercise its functional capabilities because of the nature of the infectious process – e.g. where there is a large collection of pus. In the presence of overwhelming numbers of rapidly multiplying organisms or in the absence of important additional factors such as complement (in deficiency disorders) or polymorphonuclear leucocytes (in leucopenia), what might seem to be adequate amounts of antibody may be relatively ineffective.

The microbiologist tends to make use of those techniques that rely for their endpoint on one of the 4 principal types of easily detected antigen–antibody reactions, which are listed in Table 18.4 together with the names of some of the most commonly used variations. The variations may employ either electrophoretic procedures (e.g. immunoelectrophoresis) to separate the components of a complex antigen or antibody mixture or inert carrier particles (latex or erythrocytes, sometimes rendered 'sticky' by treatment with tannic acid) to support soluble antigen or antibody molecules, thus making it possible to have a visible endpoint.

3.1 Precipitin tests

Serological precipitation occurs when an antigen in solution reacts with specific antibody. Many of the critical factors which influence the outcome were described by Landsteiner in a monograph devoted to the specificity of serological reactions and their quantification (Landsteiner 1942).

The appearance of a visible precipitate depends on the amount formed, which in turn is determined by several factors, including the relative amounts of antigen and antibody, the presence of electrolytes (particularly sodium chloride), and the time and temperature of incubation. The forces binding the complexes are relatively weak and derive mainly from attractions between oppositely charged ions in each molecule, as well as on the relative affinity of the antibody-combining site for the antigenic determinant. These intermolecular forces include van der Waals bonds, hydrogen bonds and hydrostatic forces as well as the hydrophobic properties of some protein aggregates. In vivo, the binding may also be affected by the sites of antigen or antibody, or both, e.g. whether immunoglobulin is bound to a cell by its Fc terminal end or whether the antigenic determinant is part of a cell or tissue. Both in vivo and in vitro, the complementary spatial relationship of antigen- and antibody-combining sites is crucial, contributing to the continuing exertion of the binding forces and being an important ingredient in determining whether dissociation of the complexes takes place sooner rather than later.

Precipitin tests are not widely used in most laboratories. However, modifications of the precipitation of antigen and antibodies diffusing in a solid medium with or without electric current have been popular. Examples include immunoelectrophoresis, immunodiffusion and counterimmunoelectrophoresis. Tests derived from the precipitin reaction are summarized in Table 18.5.

3.2 Agglutination

Agglutination may be regarded as a special case of the precipitin reaction, taking place at the surface of large particles such as bacteria, erythrocytes or artificial (e.g. carbon or latex) particles (Kabat and Mayer 1948). The antigenic determinants on the surface of the cell or of an inert particle coated with (soluble) antigen are linked together by the multivalent antibody. In principal, any type of cell may be agglutinated by an appropriate antibody. In practice, the test is most often applied to suspensions of bacteria or of erythrocytes. The latter may be agglutinated in their own right (e.g. by antibodies directed against blood group antigens) but are also frequently used as inert carriers of soluble antigens that provide a visible outcome in the form of 'indirect' haemagglutination when antibody reacts with the antigen. Numerous bacteria and plants also produce molecules (lectins) which are capable of agglutinating erythrocytes. Erythrocytes of many species are susceptible to these haemagglutinins: the phenomenon is not directly attributable to antigen–antibody interaction but depends on the presence of suitable receptors on the erythrocyte surface.

Agglutination is frequently used in tests for

Table 18.4 Antigen–antibody reactions

Reaction	Test(s)	Modifications
Precipitation	Oudin tube Ouchterlony test Single diffusion (Mancini)	Immunoelectrophoresis Immunoprecipitation –
Agglutination	Simple Mixed (cell type) Haemagglutination	Latex (and other inert particle) Indirect haemagglutination Coagglutination Antiglobulin (Coombs) test
Complement fixation	Haemolytic assay Cytotoxicity Cell lysis	Conglutination Plaque assay – –
Neutralization	Toxins, lysins etc. Viral cytopathic effect	Measurement of lethal dose (LD) –

Table 18.5 Tests derived from the precipitin reaction

Test	Reaction vessel	Antigen (Ag)	Antibody (Ab)	Diffusion	Examples of application
Ring	Test tube Capillary	In solution, layered over Ab	Whole serum, beneath Ag	Simple, $Ag \rightleftharpoons Ab$	Streptococcal grouping
Oudin	Test tube Capillary	In solution, layered over Ab	Serum, incorporated in agar, beneath Ag	Single, one dimension	–
Oakley–Fulthorpe variation of Oudin	Test tube Capillary	In solution over agar, which is layered over Ab	Serum, in agar	Double, one dimension	–
Ouchterlony	Petri dish Glass plate Microscope slide with thin layer of clear agar	In well cut in agar layer	In well cut in agar layer	Double, two dimensions	Aspergillosis, Farmer's lung
Immunoelectro-phoresis	Agar layer Agarose layer	In well or slot in agar layer	In trough in agar layer after electrophoresis	Electrophoresis (to separate components) followed by double diffusion of Ag and Ab	Characterization of Ag Detection of paraproteins

detecting and typing bacterial antigens, e.g. those of *Salmonella*. The test is adaptable to tube or slide techniques, the choice often depending on the volume of specific antiserum available. The bacterial suspension, in the presence of electrolytes, is clumped or agglutinated by the relevant antiserum. The reaction is complex, depending as it does on multiple antigenic determinants on the surface of the bacteria and on polyclonal antibodies. IgM antibodies are generally the most effective antibacterial agglutinins, but agglu-tinating properties are not confined to this class of immunoglobulin.

3.3 Coagglutination

An effective and adaptable modification of the principle of agglutination has been developed, making use of the separate binding sites on the IgG molecule. Immunoglobulin binds to the protein A of *Staphylococcus aureus* by the Fc terminal portion, leaving the antigen-combining Fab terminal free. Thus, *S. aureus* coated with IgG antiserum can be used in agglutination tests for bacterial antigens. The use of *S. aureus* as the 'carrier' allows the test to be adapted to detection of a wide range of bacterial antigens. It is economical in the amount of antibody required because the large surface area offered by the immunoglobulin-coated bacteria provides a distribution of antigen-combining sites ideal for the appropriate lattice formation. The test has been used for streptococcal grouping (Christensen et al. 1973), as well as for typing of *N. gonorrhoeae* (Shanker, Daley and Sorrell 1981), for mycobacterial grouping (Jublin and Winbald 1976) and for identifying antibacterial antibodies and antigens directly in body fluids (Tilton 1992).

Instead of whole organisms, extracts of antigen may be used, e.g. streptococcal antigens prepared by the use of enzymes. This technique seems to have the advantage, for streptococcal grouping at least, of reducing cross-reactivity which may be troublesome in tests with whole bacteria. Staphylococcal protein A may be obtained commercially for use in individual tests prepared in the laboratory and suited to the particular requirements of the work. Many commercial kits for rapid bacterial identification by serology now employ this method, but it may not be suitable for precise typing, because of the problems of cross-reactivity and false positivity.

3.4 Immunofluorescence

The binding of specific antibody to cellular antigen can be made visible if the antibody is tagged with a marker molecule or fluorochrome (e.g. fluorescein isothiocyanate or rhodamine) which can be rendered fluorescent by exposure to light of suitable wavelength, generally in the blue or ultraviolet wavelength zone of the spectrum (Coons, Creech and Jones 1941, Beutner, Nisengard and Albin 1983). The labelled antibody can be used to locate cellular products on the surface or even inside cells, either in tissues or in cultured material. The test is sensitive and highly specific when well-characterized reagents are used, but is subject to various pitfalls, some of which are peculiar to the fluorescence procedure. Non-specific staining can be a problem unless care is taken in the selection of the antiserum to be conjugated. The test may be used in direct or indirect form. Direct immunofluorescence uses fluorochrome conjugate of a selected specific antiserum (e.g. group-specific antistreptococcal antibody) and is useful for typing or for locating microbial antigen in tissues or on cells. Indirect immunofluorescence makes use of the antiglobulin reaction: instead of conjugating each individual specific serum, an antiglobulin serum is conjugated to the fluorochrome, providing a universal reagent for the detection of bound, unconjugated globulin. Thus, in the FTA test, the patient's serum is incubated with the treponemal suspension or layered over a smear and this is followed, after washing, by the fluorochrome-conjugated antiglobulin. Where specific treponemal antibody has bound, the fluorescent marker will in turn bind to the antibody and render it 'visible' when the smear is exposed to a suitable light source.

3.5 Enzyme immunoassay

There are 2 major types of enzyme immunoassay, homogeneous and heterogeneous. Heterogeneous immunoassays require physical separation of bound and unbound antigen, whereas homogeneous assays do not. Enzyme-multiplied immunoassays (EMIT) are homogeneous assays, and enzyme-linked immunoassays (ELISA) are heterogeneous. EMIT is a competitive assay. The substance to be tested, usually a low molecular weight antigen, is attached to an enzyme. This attachment occurs in such a way that binding of antibody to the antigen sterically blocks substrate binding. In the clinical test, a body fluid that purportedly contains free or unbound antigen is mixed with antibody and the enzyme-labelled or bound antigen. Both free and bound antigen compete for binding sites on the antibody. The more free antigen is present, the more enzyme remains unbound and catalytically active on the addition of a specific enzyme substrate. The reaction is read spectrophotometrically; the greater the enzyme activity, the greater the change in absorbance of the substrate. The absorbance change is directly correlated to the concentration of antigen in the patient's specimen.

Figure 18.5 depicts antigen measurement by the enzyme immunoassay (EIA) double sandwich technique. An antibody is bound to a solid support, such as a plastic tube, a tray or polystyrene beads. The antigen-containing body fluid is layered over the sensitized solid phase. An enzyme-labelled antibody is then added to form an antibody–antigen–antibody 'sandwich'. After separation of the bound and free enzyme-tagged antibody, a specific chromogenic enzyme substrate is added. The bound enzyme reacts with its substrate to produce a colour change, which indicates the presence of antigen. Enzyme substrate combinations commonly used include alkaline phosphatase and nitrophenyl phosphate or horseradish peroxidase and orthophylenediamine. A competitive ELISA (similar to the competitive RIA) may also be used to detect antigen.

In EIA, the amount of hydrolysis of the substrate is directly related to the amount of antigen or antibody present. The reaction may be read visually or spectrophotometrically. For screening tests, that is, simply determining positive or negative results, manual reading is acceptable. For most applications, however, quantitation of antigen content is desirable. Antigen/antibody can also be attached to a membrane. Diffusion of the specimen, enzyme conjugate and substrate through the membrane very rapidly produces a visual signal if positive. The signal can be a dot, a + sign, or any other type of mark.

Although EIA methodology is not conceptually difficult, in practice parameters such as the solid phase,

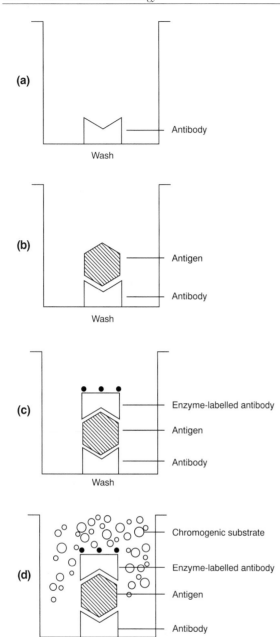

Fig. 18.5   The double sandwich enzyme immunoassay.

the washing process, enzymes, substrates and reaction termination must be strictly controlled.

3.6   Radioimmunoassay

Radioimmunoassay (RIA) techniqucs use a radioisotope, usually iodine-125, to detect antigen–antibody reactions. These techniques combine the specificity of immunology with the sensitivity of radiochemistry. Although the principal use of RIA is in endocrinology for the assay of hormones, all areas of laboratory medicine have found it to be a useful tool.

Radioimmunoassay has many variations, but in most clinical applications a competitive protein binding assay is used to measure antigen. In this assay, a known amount of radiolabelled antigen competes with an unknown quantity of antigen in a patient's serum for available binding sites on a specified amount of homologous antibody. If high concentrations of unlabelled antigen are present in the patient's serum, the amount of labelled antigen bound by antibody is reduced. After equilibrium between the bound and unbound antigen is reached, the bound fraction is separated from the unbound fraction by precipitation or centrifugation, and the radioactivity in the bound or free phase (or both) is measured in a scintillation counter. The counts are then related to concentration with the use of a standard curve.

3.7   Fluorescence immunoassay

The fluorescence immunoassay is similar to the RIA and EIA except that fluorescing compounds are used to tag antigens or antibodies instead of radioisotopes or enzymes. The assays may be competitive or non-competitive. Plastic beads, disks, tubes or paddles are coated with an antigen or antibody. If the tests are competitive, fluorescein-labelled compounds compete with non-labelled compounds for binding sites. As in the other systems, the bound and free components are separated by centrifugation, decanting, and most recently, by the use of magnetic beads.

The Abbott TDX instrument (Abbott Laboratories, Chicago) is based on fluorescence polarization immunoassay (FPIA) and is used in many laboratories. This assay is a non-separation immunoassay; that is, the bound and free complexes need not be separated before the test is read. FPIA is also a competitive assay in that bound and free antigen–antibody complexes generate different signals when fluorescent light is polarized in both horizontal and vertical planes. In FPIA, the specificity of an immunoassay is combined with the speed and convenience of a homogeneous method. Methods are currently available for the measurement of aminoglycosides and vancomycin in serum, as well as other low molecular weight substances such as digoxin, cortisol and illegal drugs or drugs of abuse. An updated version of the TDX is the Abbott IDX, which detects both high and low molecular weight antigens.

Time resolved fluoroimmunoassay (TRFIA) reduces background fluorescence by selective detection of long decay fluorescing molecules such as compounds of europium and terbium. These molecules, in the form of the lanthanide chelates, have a high quantum yield that enable emission peaks to be discerned from the background. A TRFIA instrument from Wallac (Turku, Finland) is used in Europe for viral antigen detection.

3.8   Automated immunoassays

A number of instruments are available which have automated the immunoassay for detection of both antigen and antibody. Examples of such instruments include (among others) those from Bio-Merieux (VIDAS), Bayer, Behring, Abbott and Sanofi. These instruments are not necessarily devoted to infectious disease diagnosis but may have applications for thera-peutic drugs and other assays available in clinical chemistry. Tests for antigens and antibodies to infec-tious agents usually include *Chlamydia* antigen detec-tion, *Clostridium difficile* toxin B, the TORCH complex, measles and varicella antibody.

The VIDAS instrument is pictured in Fig. 18.6.

4 APPLICATIONS OF TECHNOLOGY IN BACTERIAL SEROLOGY

The following account of specific immunological tech-niques used in bacterial serology is not meant to be exhaustive. Rather, critical descriptions are presented which will provide the reader with an appreciation of how the previously described methods are routinely used in the clinical laboratory.

Bacterial antigens detected by immunological methods consist primarily of cell envelope molecules ranging from polysaccharide capsular material to major outer membrane proteins. Few, if any, internal bacterial structures have been targeted for antigen detection tests. Some constituents, such as capsular polysaccharides, are not tightly cell-associated and are released in substantial quantity to the blood, urine, cerebrospinal fluid or other body fluids. Capsular anti-gen can be detected in the absence of whole bacteria. Other components such as major outer membrane proteins are more tightly cell-associated and cellular components in which bacteria are found, such as *Chla-mydia*, are necessary for a sensitive antigen detection test.

4.1 Group A β-haemolytic streptococci (*Streptococcus pyogenes*)

Rapid tests for group A β-haemolytic streptococci (GABS) were developed and initially marketed during the mid 1980s. The early kits were based on detection of antigen by latex agglutination following extraction of the C carbohydrate of the GABS. Within a few years, the number of commercially available test kits increased from 2 to over 50. These test kits are based on latex agglutination, coagglutination or enzyme immunoassay. A wide range of test sensitivity (55–95%) has been reported, although the specificity of most of the products is over 95%. Those kits that require extraction of the group antigen appear to be more sensitive. The kits were developed primarily for use in the physician's office or point-of-use testing. Although they can be used in the clinical laboratory, their value diminishes as the time between specimen collection and reporting increases.

Traditional culture for GABS, whether performed in the physician's office laboratory, private laboratory or hospital clinical laboratory, is time consuming (48–72 h). A test for GABS that requires 10 min or less has several advantages. If the rapid test is positive, then there is over 95% assurance that GABS are present. A number of studies now document the advantages of rapid treatment in children, including rapid improvement in clinical condition as well as reduction of the risk of transmission of the bacterium within the family unit (Gerber 1996). There are also studies indicating that rapid treatment abrogates anti-body formation which results in lack of immunity to the particular M-type (Gerber 1996). If the rapid test

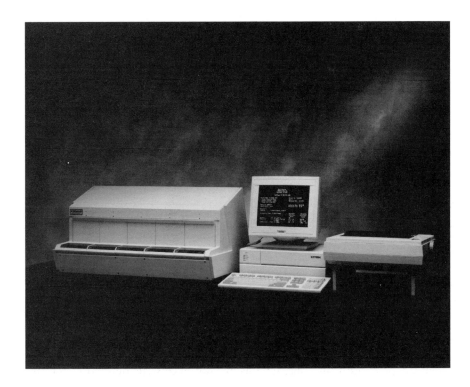

Fig. 18.6 The VIDAS automated immunoassay instrument (Biomerieux–Vitek).

is negative, then the physician may wish to perform a culture depending on the signs and symptoms observed. The recurrence of rheumatic fever in the USA again emphasizes the necessity of appropriate and prompt treatment of GABS pharyngitis. (See Chapter 28 of this volume and Volume 3, Chapter 15.)

4.2   Group B streptococci (*Streptococcus agalactiae*)

Group B streptococci (GBS) are leading causes of neonatal morbidity and mortality, with an incidence of between 1–4 per 1000 live births. However, approximately 20% of pregnant women are asymptomatic carriers of GBS. In the newborn, GBS disease may occur as an early onset disease, in which case the bacteria can be isolated from blood and gastric aspirates, or it may occur as a late onset disease in which the bacteria are usually isolated from the cerebrospinal fluid. A number of studies have indicated that intrapartum chemoprophylaxis reduces the incidence of GBS infection to nearly zero: hence the necessity of a rapid test. Latex agglutination, CA and EIA tests are available. A number of studies suggest that rapid tests on vaginal secretions can be used to identify women at high risk of delivering infants with GBS disease.

It is also possible to use the same tests to diagnose GBS in the newborn. A number of reports suggest that the antigen is more readily detected in urine than in blood or cerebrospinal fluid. Consequently, these tests should be used in conjunction with culture on women about to deliver as well as on infected infants. Sensitivity approaching 100% can be realized if urine and one other body fluid from infected infants are tested by latex agglutination, CA or EIA. (See Chapter 28 of this volume and Volume 3, Chapter 15.)

4.3   Detection of antigen in cerebrospinal fluid

A number of commercial LA and CA kits for detection of *Neisseria meningitidis*, *Haemophilus influenzae*, *Streptococcus pneumoniae* and group B streptococcal antigens are available (Tilton 1992). Most kits use polyclonal antibodies with the exception of a monoclonal antibody for group B *N. meningitidis*. The latex agglutination and coagglutination tests are rapid and the entire panel can be done in less than 30 min. The reagents are approved for cerebrospinal fluid, urine and serum although, in the author's experience, detection of capsular antigen in serum is rarely useful. All tests include directions for treatment of specimens in the event that non-specific agglutination occurs. Many reports document the broad range of sensitivity and specificity of these tests. Both of these statistical parameters are a function of the antigen detected and the body fluid analysed. Unfortunately, none is 100% sensitive and specific.

Two questions are asked when a child presents with signs and symptoms of meningitis. One is 'Does the child have meningitis?' and the other is, 'Is the aeti-ology bacterial, viral, or neither?' Non-microbiological parameters such as cerebrospinal fluid glucose and protein, cellular constituency and Gram's stain aid in the answers to these questions. Ninety-five per cent of cerebrospinal fluid specimens will show no abnormalities. Five per cent are potential candidates for cerebrospinal fluid antigen detection. However, the sensitivity of antigen detection is approximately the same as the Gram's stain, and false-positive agglutination does occur. Of the 5% of specimens that would suggest bacterial meningitis, 10–15% of these patients will have been partially treated. The cerebrospinal fluid will usually show a negative Gram's stain, i.e. no organism is observed. It is in these cases that antigen detection is worthwhile. Cerebrospinal fluid antigen detection is costly and should not be performed unless there are a significant number of white blood cells in the cerebrospinal fluid ($10->100$ mm $^{-3}$) or other constituents that point to bacterial meningitis. Thus, cerebrospinal fluid antigen detection should be reserved for partially treated patients or to confirm positive cerebrospinal fluid Gram's stain results. A number of investigators, however, have indicated that the sensitivity of meningitis diagnosis may be increased by testing concentrated urine specimens.

4.4   *Chlamydia trachomatis*

Other than culture, 4 methods are currently available to detect *Chlamydia trachomatis* in human specimens. They are enzyme immunoassay, direct fluorescence antibody microscopy (DFA), a nucleic acid probe (Gen-Probe, Pace II, San Diego, CA), and the polymerase chain reaction (PCR) or other nucleic acid amplification tests to detect *Chlamydia*-specific DNA or RNA.

The detection of *C. trachomatis* antigens has the potential to replace culture for the routine diagnosis of chlamydia cervicitis, urethritis, pneumonitis and conjunctivitis. Culture is technically difficult and time consuming, and requires a tissue culture facility. To date, however, because of sensitivity and specificity problems, antigen detection tests for *C. trachomatis* have not replaced culture but offer an acceptable alternative in populations at high risk for the disease. Enzyme immunoassay detects group antigens that are either genus- or species-specific for a variety of *C. trachomatis* serotypes, depending on the manufacturer. Both polyclonal and monoclonal antibodies directed to either the major outer-membrane protein or lipopolysaccharides are used. (See Chapter 59.)

Investigators have compared EIA methods to culture. One large study (Ryan and Kwasnik 1986) noted that Chlamydiazyme (Abbott Laboratories, North Chicago, IL) was a sensitive and specific test for a high risk population. However, when tested by Chlamydiazyme, both females at low to moderate risk and asymptomatic males revealed that the kit was less sensitive than for high-risk patients. False-positive results may also occur in both EIA and DFA. There are at least 3 bacteria that bind monoclonal antibodies against *C. trachomatis* major outer membrane protein to their surfaces. They include *Neisseria*, *Staphylococcus* and *Streptococcus* spp. It is also possible that false-positive antigens detection tests are, in fact, false-negative culture tests. Although this has been suspected in a number of patients, it is likely that neither EIA nor DFA tests are 100% specific. The true sensitivity of culture is not known, but if vials (not microdilution plates), one blind passage, and detection of inclusion bodies by FA are used, it is likely that culture is at least 80% sensitive.

One of the major disadvantages of EIA is that the cellular composition of the specimen, that is specimen quality, cannot be determined. The advantages include time (as little as 1–1.5 h for the result), the ability to batch specimens and the reading of the test by a spectrophotometer which reduces subjectivity. Enzyme immunoassay tests are more suitable to automated systems and, unlike culture, do not require a viable organism for a positive result. Transportation then becomes much less of a problem with the rapid test compared to culture.

A number of solid phase membrane EIAs such as the Abbott Testpak have been introduced. They are rapid (± 30 min) and potentially could be performed in a satellite clinic or a physician's office, although the performance characteristics are questionable.

Because of the nature of culture, non-cultural methods should be less expensive and much more applicable to the smaller laboratory. In order to be cost beneficial, however, testing should be reserved for groups of patients who might not be routinely treated for chlamydial infection or for those patients in whom the clinical outcome of infection is very serious. Because of the consequences of infection, such as salpingitis, and because of their epidemiological importance in transmitting the bacterium, women are the best candidates for specific *C. trachomatis* diagnosis. Children who are suspected of being sexually abused must be tested by culture.

4.5 *Clostridium difficile*

Pseudomembranous enterocolitis (PMC) is a life-threatening disease. The primary etiology is *Clostridium difficile*. Most patients are infected following antibiotic therapy, although various authors suggest that *C. difficile* colonization rates range from 2% to 24%, depending on the patient's environment and the administration of antibiotics (see chapter 32).

Pathogenic *C. difficile* secretes 2 toxins, A and B, and a motility factor (Onderdonk et al. 1995) There are non-toxigenic strains present, however, that produce neither toxin. Toxin A causes the intestinal pathology observed in animal models and toxin B is primarily responsible for the cytopathology observed in tissue cultures. Recent evidence suggests that toxin A is also cytotoxic. Enzyme immunoassays have been developed for both toxins A and B. Demonstration of *C. difficile* toxin(s) in stool filtrates has relied on the demonstration of characteristic cytopathology in a variety of cell lines, usually human diploid fibroblasts such as WI-38. Some feel that the sensitivity of cytotoxin detec-

tion compared to clinical disease may be low, and that toxin B titres do not necessarily correlate with the extent of the disease.

In 1986 Marion Scientific Company (Kansas City, MO) introduced a latex agglutination test for toxin A. Subsequently, it was shown that the protein detected by latex agglutination was not toxin A, but a structural protein of *C. difficile*. The latex agglutination reagent cross-reacts with *Clostridium sporogenes* and *Peptostreptococcus anaerobius*. The gene for production of this structural protein has been cloned. The gene product is not toxin A. The latex agglutination test, if positive, indicates the presence of C *difficile* or a cross-reacting bacterium: both toxigenic and non-toxigenic *C. difficile* will be detected.

A number of studies indicate that latex agglutination is an effective screening test for disease, However, if the latex agglutination test is positive, it has been suggested that a cytotoxin assay be performed on the stool filtrate. Although variations in sensitivity of latex agglutination tests have been reported, it is generally felt that a negative test correlates with the abscence of disease.

With few exceptions, no one laboratory test is definitive without supporting clinical information. Such is the case with *C. difficile*-associated disease (CAD). Many investigators have suggested that tissue detection of toxin B is the test by which all others should be judged. However, some claim that a 'suitably performed' culture of faeces for *C. difficile* must be included. It has been reported that up to 30% of patients with CAD are culture positive and cytotoxin negative, and that the majority of these cases have been associated with toxin-producing *C. difficile*. Thus, the 'gold standard' may be both direct cytotoxin detection in tissue culture and culture for the organism.

Compared to the cytotoxin assay (CTA), both the ELISA tests for toxins A/B and those for toxin A are highly specific. That is, if a test is positive, the probability of it being a true positive is very high. None of the ELISA tests is as sensitive as CTA. Sensitivity in past reports ranged from 63 to 96.6%. More recently, immunoassays for toxin A have been introduced with reported sensitivity of ± 90%. Specificity is excellent.

4.6 *Escherichia coli*

Escherichia coli K1 antigen has been detected in the cerebrospinal fluid and urine of neonates using *Neisseria meningitidis* group B antiserum. The antigens are immunologically identical. Commercial latex agglutination kits are available. This cross-reactivity must be carefully monitored so as not to confuse meningococcal disease diagnosis with *E. coli* K1 disease. Radioimmunoassay, latex agglutination and ELISA have been used to detect LT and ST toxins of enterotoxic *E. coli*. Kits are not commercially available, as demand for such assays has been minimal.

E. coli serotypes, predominantly 0157/H7, which produce shiga-like toxins (verotoxin) and have been associated with haemorrhagic diarrhoea and haemo-

Table 18.6 A summary of tests commonly used in bacterial serology

Antibody detected	Class(es)	Method(s)	Comments
Mycoplasma pneumoniae	IgG, IgM	ELISA, IFA, particle agglutination	Tests for specific Ab to *M. pneumoniae* are more specific than cold agglutinins. IgM specific assays available for acute infection are faster than culture but acute/convalescent specimens may be necessary
Bordetella pertussis	IgG, IgM, IgA	ELISA, agglutination, CF	Paired sera necessary for optimal sensitivity. Detects antibody to PT (pertussis toxin) or FHA (filamentous haemagglutinin). ELISA for FHA (IgA) shows promise as a sensitive diagnostic test. Antibody tests for pertussis should be used primarily for epidemiological purposes. IgA Ab to *B. pertussis* may be helpful to distinguish immune status.
Legionella pneumophila (serotypes 1–6)	IgG	IFA	Infection with *Legionella* causes a rise in specific antibody. Currently, indirect immunofluorescence (IFA) is used to detect total antibody to 6 serotypes of *L. pneumophila*. No IFA–IGM tests are currently available. A fourfold rise in titre to >1:128 over a period of 3–4 weeks is considered diagnostic for Legionnaire's disease. Many consider a single titre of >1:256 diagnostic, but such a conclusion must be made cautiously as elevated antibody titres may persist long after the infection has been eradicated
Helicobacter pylori	IgG, IgM, IgA	ELISA	ELISA tests for antibody have been shown to be comparable to, if not more sensitive, than invasive techniques. Quantitative IgG antibody tests are the 1st line of serological tests that should be ordered. IgG antibody tests are sensitive (>95%) and decrease within 6 months of eradication of the bacterium. The IgG antibody test is primarily useful for initial diagnosis. In one study, *H. pylori* IgG had a sensitivity of 100% and specificity of 98% when compared to the urea breath test. IgM and IgA antibody titres are less useful for diagnosis of *H. pylori* infections
Treponema pallidum	IgG, IgM	Agglutination, flocculation, ELISA, FTA-Abs, microhaemag-glutination (MHA), TPHA, *T. pallidum* immobilization (TPI)	Two types of tests available; 1) non-treponemal (NT) tests based on cross reacting cardiolipin Ag, 2) treponemal tests (TT) using whole inactivated treponemes. NT tests are sensitive but lack specificity. NT tests must be confirmed by specific treponemal tests such as the FTA-Abs or TPHA. The Reiter Protein Reagin (RPR) is the most commonly used NT test and the FTA, MHA or TPHA the most common confirmatory test for syphilis

Table 18.6 Continued

Antibody detected	Class(es)	Method(s)	Comments
Borrelia burgdorferi (Tilton 1994)	IgG, IgM, IgA	ELISA, FA, immunoblot, borreliacidal tests	IgG, IgM tests are commonly used for the detection of antibody in patients with Lyme disease. IgA is less useful. Antibody to *B. burgdorferi* may appear, disappear, and reappear as a function of antibiotic treatment and disease state. Therefore, Lyme disease remains a clinical diagnosis. It has been recommended that all Lyme screening tests that are equivocal or reactive be confirmed with western immunoblotting using separate IgG and IgM nitrocellulose strips. Borreliacidal antibody tests are available but their utility is limited to vaccine efficacy studies as there appear to be factors, including antibiotics in serum that affect viability of the *Borrelia* preparation
Human granulocytic *Ehrlichia* (HGE), *E. chafeensis* (HME)	IgG, IgM	IFA, Western immunoblotting	HGE is a newly recognized rickettsia. It is transmitted by *Ixodes* ticks as is *B. burdorferi*. Patients with HGE have high titres of both IgG and IgM. Because the antigen used is from an equine source (*E. equi*), all reactive IFA tests should be confirmed by Western blotting. A 44 kDa band on the immunoblot appears to confirm the presence, of the HGE antibody. There is little or no cross-reaction with the other species of *Ehrlichia* (*E. chaffeensis*) that cause human disease and is transmitted by *Ambylomma*, the Lone Star tick.

lytic uraemia syndrome, can be detected in stool filtrates using tissue culture. Although EIA for *E. coli* shiga-like toxin detection has been reported and the assays are now commercially available from Meridian Diagnostics, Cincinnati, Ohio, USA. A latex agglutination test is available for identification of 0157/H7 serotypes of *E. coli*.

(See Volume 3, Chapters 16, 25, 27, 32 for details of infections caused by *E. coli*.)

4.7 Detection of *Legionella* antigen in urine

The methods available for *Legionella* antigen detection are ELISA and RIA. The specimen of choice is urine. Kohler (1981) reported that *Legionella* antigen could be detected by RIA in the urine of patients shortly after infection. Ideally, the urine should be collected prior to antibiotic therapy. The sensitivity of RIA is ±95%. ELISA tests for urine antigen are not as sensitive as RIA. RIA for antigen detects only *L. pneumophila* Type 1. Patients with serogroups other than I or species other than *L. pneumophila* will be non-reactive. Sathapatayavongs, Kohler and Wheat (1983) reported on the use of the latex agglutination test for detection of *Legionella* antigen. Although it was 16-fold less sensitive than ELISA or RIA, it was much more rapid and

easier to perform. The reagents for these assays are not yet commercially available.

Muro and Tilton (1995) recently evaluated a commercially available ELISA kit for detection of *Legionella* urinary antigen. They observed little difference between ELISA and RIA, both being over 95% sensitive and specific.

(See Chapter 49 and Volume 3, Chapter 18 for further information on *Legionella* infection.)

4.8 Application of antibody detection methods

Methods applicable to bacterial antigen detection are equally applicable to antibody detection. IgG antibody tests do not provide a rapid diagnosis as acute and convalescent specimens are required 2–3 weeks apart. However, IgM antibody tests have become popular during the past decade primarily because of the potential for rapid detection of disease. Table 18.6 summarizes antibody tests commonly used for bacterial disease diagnoses.

5 SEROEPIDEMIOLOGY

The use of antibody tests to determine the epidemiology of bacterial disease is a valuable tool. The premise behind seroepidemiology is that the prevalence of disease or disease exposure in the community can be accurately assessed by determining specific antibody levels. Seroepidemiology is hampered by cross-reactions between organism groups, loss of antibody over a period of time, and differences in antibody expression between people. Not withstanding these limitations, serosurveys are still valuable especially in those situations such as syphilis when large populations are screened prior to marriage or childbirth or through blood banks.

Seroepidemiology is widely used to determine vaccination status, particularly for viral diseases. Recent outbreaks of measles and rubella have led to widespread antibody screening with the finding that portions of the population had either not been vaccinated or had lost their immunity and needed a booster immunization.

Much of the population based seroepidemiology is done in blood banks, particularly those of the American Red Cross and their UK counterparts. A Red Cross study on babesiosis, a disease caused by the periplasm *Babesia* (see Volume 5, Chapter 19), noted by serosurveys that people had been exposed to *Babesia* in the north-east but not in most other parts of the USA. Because the disease is transmitted by the same tick that harbours the causative agent of Lyme disease and ehrlichiosis, exposure to 2 and sometimes all 3 diseases was observed (Dumler and Bakken 1995). A baseline serosurvey of *Babesia* antibodies will enable epidemiologists to track the spread of disease via the tick vector.

See also Volume 3, Chapter 10.

6   SUMMARY

Immunological methods for detection and identification of bacterial disease are useful and commonly used. Both antigens and antibodies may be detected by a variety of methods as outlined in this chapter. The traditional growth-dependent culture techniques have in many cases been replaced by sensitive and specific antigen detection methods such as the detection of *Legionella* urinary antigen. Conversely, agglutination methods for serotyping of *Salmonella, Shigella and E. coli* have been used for over 60 years and are still the method of choice. Just as reliance on growth-dependent methods in bacteriology has contributed to the retrospective nature of bacterial disease diagnosis, so too has the requirement for paired acute and convalescent sera from patients suspected of bacterial disease detection produced a 'built in' 3–4 week delay in the provision of relevant results. However, the increased use of acute phase antibodies such as IgM and IgA has provided clinically relevant alternatives to the traditional serologic methods.

Contemporary microbiology and immunology laboratories use a variety of cultural, molecular and immunological methods to provide results rapidly in a time frame that is relevant to the care and treatment of the patient.

REFERENCES

Babior BM, 1984, The respiratory burst of phagocytes, *J Clin Invest*, **73:** 599–601.

Beutner EH, Nisengard RJ, Albin B, 1983, Defined immunofluorescence and related cytochemical methods, *Annals NY Acad Sci*, **420:** 434.

Chapuis RM, Koshland ME, 1974, Mechanism of IgM polymerization, *Proc Nat Acad Sci USA*, **71:** 657–61.

Christensen P, Kahlmeter G et al., 1973, New method for the serological grouping of streptococci with specific antibodies absorbed to protein A-containing staphylococci, *Infect Immun*, **7:** 881–6.

Clas F, Loos M, 1987, *Complement in Health and Disease*, ed. Whaley K, MTP Press, Lancaster, 201–25.

Clevers H, Alarcon BE et al., 1988, The T-cell receptor/CD3 complex: a dynamic protein ensemble, *Ann Rev Immunol*, **6:** 629–62.

Coons AH, Creech HJ, Jones RW, 1941, Immunological properties of an antibody containing a fluorescent group, *Proc Soc Exp Biol Med*, **47:** 200–7.

Dinarello CA, Mier JW, 1987, The lymphokines, *N Engl J Med*, **317:** 940–5.

Dumler JS, Bakken JS, 1995, Human granulocytic ehrlichiosis in the Upper Midwest United States, *Clin Infect Dis*, **20:** 1102–10.

Edelman GM, Poulik MD, 1961, Studies on structural units of the gamma globulins, *J Exp Med*, **113:** 861–84.

Gerber MA, 1986, Diagnosis of group A beta haemolytic streptococcal pharyngitis, *Diagnost Microbiol Infect Dis*, **4:** 5S–15S.

Gershon RK, Hondo K, 1971, Infectious immunological tolerance, *Immunology*, **21:** 903–14.

Joiner KA, 1986, *Immunobiology of the Complement System*, Ross GD (ed.), Academic Press, Orlando, FL, 186–201.

Jublin J, Winbald S, 1976, Serotyping of mycobacteria by a new technique using antibody globulin absorbed to staphylococcal protein A, *Acta Pathol Microbiol Scand B*, **81:** 179–80.

Kabat EA, Mayer MM, 1948, *Experimental Immunochemistry*, Charles C. Thomas, Springfield, IL, 105–31.

Klebanoff SJ, 1980, Oxygen metabolism and the toxic properties of phagocytes, *Ann Intern Med*, **93:** 480–9.

Kohler RB, Zimmerman SE, 1981, Rapid radioimmunoassay diagnosis of legionnaires disease, *Ann Intern Med*, **94:** 601–5.

Landsteiner K, Chase MW, 1942, The specificity of serological reactions, *Proc Soc Exp Biol*, **49:** 688–715.

Muro V, Tilton RC, 1995, Comparison of RIA and EIA for *Legionella* urinary antigen (abstract), *American Society for Microbiology Annual Meeting*, Washington, DC, 94.

Onderdonk AB, Allen SD et al., 1995, Clostridium, *Manual of Clinical Microbiology*, 6th edn, ed. Murray PJ et al., ASM Press, Washington DC, 574–86.

Porter RR, 1962, *Symposium on Basic Problems in Neoplastic Disease*, eds Gelhom A, Hirschberg E, Columbia University Press, New York, 177–88.

Roos D, Balm AJM, 1980, *The Reticuloendothelial System, Vol. 11, Biochemistry and Metabolism*, eds Strauss R, Sbarra A, Plenum Press, New York, 189–207.

Ryan RW, Kwasnik I, 1986, Rapid detection of *Chlamydia trachomatis* by an enzyme immunoassay method, *Diagnost Microbiol and Infect Dis*, **5:** 225–34.

Sathapatayavongs B, Kohler RB, Wheat JL, 1983, Rapid diagnosis of Legionnaire's disease by latex agglutination, *Am Rev Resp Dis*, **127:** 559–62.

Shanker S, Daley DA, Sorrell TC, 1981, Detection of *Neisseria gonorrhoeae* by coagglutination, *J Clin Pathol*, **34:** 429–33.

Tilton RC, 1987, Immunoserology in the clinical microbiology laboratory, *Clinical and Diagnostic Microbiology*, eds Howard BJ et al., CV Mosby, St. Louis, MO, 105–20.

Tilton RC, 1992, Microbial antigen detection, *Clinical Laboratory Medicine*, ed Tilton RC et al., CV Mosby, St. Louis, MO, 565–71.

Tilton RC, Ryan RW, 1993, The laboratory diagnosis of Lyme disease, *J Clin Immunoassay*, **16:** 208–12.

Chapter 19

Safety in the Microbiology Laboratory

A Balows

Although difficult to substantiate, our present knowledge of the infectivity of micro-organisms suggests that several, if not many, of the early investigators of infectious diseases became infected with a microbial agent while working with it in their laboratories. During the last 50 years, laboratory-acquired infections and their prevention and control have received considerable attention and this is even greater today. However, this was not always the case. Laboratory safety was not considered, or was poorly known, when the concept of contagion and the microbial aetiology for infectious diseases was advanced.

There is no way to determine accurately the incidence or estimate the number of laboratory personnel who have had laboratory-acquired infections. Reporting such infections has until recently been largely voluntary at best and glossed over or kept confidential at worst. Numerous attempts have been made to define the extent of laboratory-acquired infections. Surveys of the problem conducted at various times clearly indicate that the incidence of laboratory-acquired infections increases as new agents are discovered and as more people are involved in handling infectious material or agents. Only within the past decade or so have surveillance activities and reporting mechanisms for laboratory-acquired infections been established in most countries. This concern for the safety and protection of medical personnel involved in medical and related scientific activity has resulted in the development of guidelines by specific government bodies for implementation in each country. The World Health Organization (WHO) also fulfils an important role in this area with an ongoing laboratory improvement programme.

1 HISTORY

The contagious nature of some diseases was recognized in ancient times. A well known example is the Plague of Athens described by Thucydides in his *History*. Thucydides described how people caught the disease by caring for others (Thucydides 1972); he is the first writer to identify contagion clearly as the essential factor in the transmission of disease. In the Middle Ages writers were much more inclined to write about contagion due to personal contact or to touching objects used by diseased people (e.g. *The Decameron* of Giovanni Boccaccio in 1358). Fracastorius wrote in 1546 about contagion by fomites and spoke of the **seminaria** or 'seeds' or 'germs' of disease. Not until the latter part of the seventeenth century, when Leeuwenhoek described in detail the small animalcules that he viewed with his microscope, did we learn of the existence of bacteria and other microscopic forms of life in teeth and gum scrapings. The Golden Age of microbiology occurred during the latter part of the eighteenth and through the nineteenth centuries when the role of micro-organisms in many processes in nature was defined. Finally, the germ theory of disease was firmly established (see Chapter 1). The number of investigators and laboratories increased logarithmically. Technological advances for culturing, isolating and identifying bacteria and fungi also increased; we can be certain that with this growth of scientific pursuit laboratory-acquired infections occurred with increasing frequency. It is, however, difficult to find convincing documentation of these acquisitions.

One of the first fatal cases of laboratory-acquired infections was that of a pathologist who cut and infected his hand while performing an autopsy on a female patient who died after childbirth (Pike 1979). In 1873 cholera was responsible for the death of a laboratory worker who infected himself as a result of careless handling of excreta from cholera patients. Another cholera death occurred in 1894 in a laboratory technician, aged 29 years, who swallowed live *Vibrio cholerae* while pipetting (Pike 1979). Significant historical reports of laboratory rickettsial infections occurred in 1910 and in 1915, when HT Ricketts and S von Prowazek, respectively, accidentally infected themselves while independently working with the typhus agent.

Laboratory viral infections began to be reported in the early 1920s and a review of 222 viral infections was published in 1949 (Sulkin and Pike 1949) and now appear to represent a frequently encountered group of agents responsible for laboratory-acquired infections. Scientific journals began to publish reports of laboratory-acquired infections; slowly, but surely, the reluctance to inform on one's own laboratory or institution began to wane. Laboratory scientists also began to develop new and better methods and equipment to perform laboratory tests or research experiments. Better biological safety cabinets, safe and protected centrifuges, autoclaves with uniformly distributed temperature and pressure, and foolproof pipetting devices have been developed and brought into use and a long and continuing list of instruments, methods and laboratory protective clothing has been introduced to improve safety and reduce risk. In 1983, with the isolation of human immunodeficiency virus (HIV), the associated AIDS pandemic, coupled with the rise in tuberculosis and a host of other emerging or re-emerging infectious diseases stimulated a renewal of interest in an elaborate safety programme for all laboratory and health care workers. This reaffirmation, purpose and goal have led to the development of programmes that create a safer workplace for all health care workers while protecting the public through the safe disposal of infectious or hazardous wastes. The implementation of such objectives has generally been delegated to the public health agency of the ministries of health of each country with the close co-operation of the United Nations (UN), through WHO serving as the central focus for guidance and assistance. Each country must develop guidelines that meet its specific needs for the safety of health care workers and the public at large. At varying times and in different conditions health care workers may be exposed to a variety of occupational hazards that include infectious materials, cultures, toxic chemicals and their fumes, radiation and exposure to other elements that carry a risk. To meet these needs most, if not all, member nations of WHO have established within their respective governments agencies, centres, or other units to develop and disseminate guidelines for achieving a realistic and attainable set of safety procedures. Absolute safety in the laboratory or elsewhere is not possible. There is risk associated with every occupation involving health care workers. The major focus of this chapter is centred on the broad aspects of an active microbiological safety programme within the laboratory for and by its staff.

2 AETIOLOGY OF LABORATORY-ACQUIRED INFECTIONS

Generally, any microbial agent may be involved in a laboratory infection. Initially, publishing information on such infections was done primarily because the author wanted to call the attention of others to the circumstances involved in the infection and to describe the clinical aspects of the case. There was not a great deal of interest in the manner in which the disease was acquired. However, over time, interest in the infectious agent, its epidemiology, and the prevention of laboratory-acquired infections increased. Information on laboratory-acquired infections incidents has been obtained by questionnaires, surveys and reviews of oral and published reports. From these reports it is apparent that a wide and increasing spectrum of aetiological agents has been involved in laboratory-acquired infections. It also became evident that those agents that possess the greatest levels of infectivity and virulence were most frequently involved in laboratory-acquired infections. Brucellae, salmonellae, mycobacteria and chlamydiae are among bacteria with the highest occurrence of laboratory-acquired infections in European and American laboratories (Harrington and Shannon 1976, Pike 1978, 1979, Muller 1988, Sewell 1995) (Table 19.1).

Viral infections gained prominence as knowledge and diagnostic skills increased. Arboviruses and hepatitis viruses (HBV and HCV) are among the most frequent laboratory-acquired infections. Accidental exposure to HBV and HCV are not limited to laboratory personnel; all health care workers are at risk of infection with these viruses and safety precautions are necessary. Once HIV was isolated from patients with AIDS, the list of viruses was increased with another serious hazard to the laboratory staff and other health care workers (Hunt 1995). Although the number of reported cases of laboratory-acquired infections with HIV is not great, it is likely that there are additional unreported cases; in addition, many other viruses have been involved in laboratory-acquired infections (Sulkin and Pike 1949, Collins 1993, Richmond and McKinney 1993) (Table 19.2).

Among the fungi pathogenic to humans, *Coccidioides immitis* laboratory infections have been documented; *Histoplasma capsulatum* infections have also occurred in laboratory personnel, due primarily to the inhalation of conidia from cultures grown at room temperature. Other fungi, including many dermatophytes and other systemic fungi, have been incriminated in laboratory-acquired infections (Segretain 1959, Collins 1993, Richmond and McKinney 1993).

A surprising number of parasitic agents are associated with laboratory-acquired infections. The most frequently encountered are blood-borne agents such as *Toxoplasma gondii*, *Plasmodium* spp., *Trypanosoma* spp. and *Leishmania* spp. (Collins 1993, Herwaldt and

Table 19.1 Most frequently reported laboratory-acquired infections in the USA and UK (1969–89)

Infection	Total no. (%) of cases reported from			
	USA	USA and world	UK	NADC*
Brucellosis	274 (9.4)	423 (10.8)	2 (2.1)	18 (52.9)
Q Fever	184 (6.3)	278 (7.1)	0	
Typhoid fever	292 (10.0)	256 (6.5)	3 (3.2)	
Hepatitis	126 (4.3)	234 (6.0)	19 (20.0)	
Tularaemia	129 (4.4)	225 (5.7)	0	
Tuberculosis	174 (6.0)	176 (4.5)	24 (25.3)	4 (11.8)
Dermatomycosis	84 (2.9)	161 (4.1)	0	2 (5.9)
Venezuelan equine encephalitis	118 (4.1)	141 (3.6)	0	
Typhus	82 (2.8)	124 (3.2)	0	
Psittacosis	70 (2.4)	116 (3.0)	0	4 (11.8)
Coccidioidomycosis	108 (3.7)	93 (2.4)	0	
Streptococcal infections	67 (2.3)	78 (2.0)	3 (3.2)	
Histoplasmosis	81 (2.8)	71 (1.8)	0	
Leptospirosis	43 (1.5)	87 (2.2)	0	3 (8.8)
Salmonellosis	54 (1.9)	48 (1.2)	11 (11.6)	1 (2.9)
Shigellosis	54 (1.9)	58 (1.5)	26 (27.4)	
All reported infections	2912	3921	95	34

*NADC National Animal Disease Center, 1975–85.
Reprinted with permission from Sewell (1995).

Table 19.2 Occupationally acquired HIV infection or AIDS reported to CDC to end of 1992

Occupation	No. (%) of occupational transmissions[a]
Laboratory technician	25 (24.8)
Nurse	26 (25.7)
Physician	13 (12.8)
Medical technician/paramedic	7 (6.9)
Dentist/dental technician	6 (5.9)
Health aide/attendant	6 (5.9)
Housekeeper/maintenance worker	6 (5.9)
Mortuary technician	3 (3.0)
Technician/therapist	3 (3.0)
Respiratory therapist	2 (2.0)
Surgical technician	2 (2.0)
Other health care workers	2 (2.0)
Total	101

[a]HCW who had documented seroconversion after occupational exposure to HIV and HCW in whom occupational transmission was possible but HIV seroconversion was not documented.
Reprinted with permission from Sewell (1995).

Juranek 1993, Richmond and McKinney 1993, Advisory Committee on Dangerous Pathogens 1995, Fleming et al. 1995).

3 EPIDEMIOLOGY OF LABORATORY-ACQUIRED INFECTIONS

Several over-riding circumstances hamper efforts to develop an accurate evaluation of laboratory-acquired infections. Laboratory bench workers are obviously at the highest risk for acquiring these infections, but non-technical personnel who work in various parts of the laboratory are also at risk (e.g. clerical and custodial staff and animal caretakers). The incidence of laboratory-acquired infections and the distribution of the aetiological agents are not always well defined or understood. Generally, laboratory staff are responsible for practically all laboratory-acquired infections. Notable exceptions would be an unknown breakdown of protective equipment or unreported change in the circulating airflow within the laboratory and the biosafety cabinets. The health status of the laboratory staff also may be a contributing factor to laboratory-acquired infections.

Various laboratory techniques and microbiological procedures contribute to the exposure of laboratory personnel to microbial agents. Usually laboratory accidents set the scene for laboratory-acquired infections. Some of the more frequently occurring incidents are the production of aerosols, splashes or sprays, sticks or cuts with contaminated needles or sharp objects, mouth pipetting, bite or ectoparasite, or animal bite or scratch. Laboratory procedures that require shaking, sonicating, blending, lyophilizing or centrifuging liquids, or flaming an inoculating loop, opening tightly closed cultures, pouring and decanting cultures carry a risk of infection to the worker and, in some instances, to others not directly involved (Pike 1978, Sulkin and Pike 1981, Williams 1981, Fleming et al. 1995, Sewell 1995). Although exact data are not available, it is generally held that aerosols, regardless of how created, are the principal cause of laboratory-acquired infections. Not too surprising is the fact that most of these aerosol infections occur in research laboratories due to the indifference of researchers and a false sense of some inherent immunity to the agent(s) with which they are working. The second most common cause of laboratory-acquired infections is the broad category of accidents: splashes and sprays, 27%; needlesticks, 25%; cuts with sharp objects (sharps), 16%; bite or scratch, 14%; mouth pipetting, 13%; and other, 6% (Pike 1978, Sewell 1995) (Table 19.3).

The major focus of laboratory-acquired infections is the laboratory bench worker. Researchers, clinical microbiologists and technical support staff handle the specimens or cultures, design and conduct the bench experiments or tests, operate the equipment, and in general are responsible for the scientific and technical integrity of the laboratory. Behaviour patterns, attitudes and work habits become important factors in the personal profile of laboratory workers and should be considered when individuals are employed or elect to work in the laboratory (Martin 1980). Also to be considered in the profile of laboratory employees, because of enhanced susceptibility to some infections, are sex, age, pregnancy, major medical history (splenectomy, gastrectomy, diabetes, autoimmune diseases) and immunizations. The institution may require from the personal physician of new employees a pre-employment physical or health status statement that includes, among other information, the status of prophylactic immunizations.

4 RISK AND HAZARD ASSESSMENT: LEVELS OF BIOSAFETY FOR MICROBIOLOGY LABORATORIES

An essential segment of laboratory biosafety is the assessment of risk and hazard. Quantitative data on the risk associated with laboratory procedures with specific micro-organisms are not generally available. The variables are too great; standardized methods of assessing the risk of a laboratory task with a given organism do not exist. Four of the important variables are:

1 the virulence of the organism
2 the health status of the worker
3 the nature of the laboratory work and
4 the availability of a well equipped laboratory environment.

Risk is the probability that exposure to a micro-organism will occur. Hazard, another term that is difficult to quantify, is regarded as the potential of a given organism to cause an infection. The more serious the infection that may result, the greater is the hazard and the higher the risk. Zero risk and no hazard do not exist. It is, therefore, necessary for microbiologists (and others who work with micro-organisms) to be aware of the hazard (danger) and risk (chance) that working with a given organism carries. The desire to provide a safe work environment has prompted the ministries of health in virtually every country, in close

collaboration with WHO, to establish guidelines, recommendations and, in many instances, laws and regulations for laboratory workers to follow (Brunton 1993).

Four biosafety or containment levels for working with infectious micro-organisms have been established and accepted universally. Table 19.4 summarizes these levels as adopted in most countries. All laboratory personnel must become thoroughly familiar with the safety recommendations and regulations of their work environment. All laboratory personnel should receive training in the fundamentals of biosafety and participate in periodic review sessions for new information on all aspects of laboratory biosafety. The same applies to all animal handlers and health care workers who come in contact with patients or their tissues or excreta (Table 19.4).

In addition to the meticulously developed standards and regulations for biomedical laboratories, there are published lists of micro-organisms in which the organisms are grouped and classified according to a known or presumed level of risk. Public health organizations have assumed the responsibility to develop and publish such lists: the World Health Organization (1983) and Centers for Disease Control and Prevention (Richmond and McKinney 1993) in the USA and the UK Health and Safety Executive (Advisory Committee on Dangerous Pathogens 1995) in the UK.

Other countries have published similar lists and laboratory workers are enjoined to obtain and follow these recommendations. It is beyond the scope of this chapter to reproduce the long lists of agents, their risk group category and biosafety levels for working with each. Generally, the risk group parallels the biosafety laboratory level, e.g. work with an organism at risk group 3 demands biosafety level 3. The minimum level for any work with agents that cause human infection is level 2. If the required biosafety level facilities are not available in a given laboratory, work should not be done with agents of risk group 3 or higher.

5 PREVENTION AND CONTROL OF LABORATORY-ACQUIRED INFECTIONS

The recognition of hazardous micro-organisms and the assessment of their risk makes it possible to develop both general and specific programmes to prevent and control laboratory-acquired infections. Guidelines and regulations are published and available from professional scientific societies, academic institutions, industries and government agencies. The thrust of these publications is to assist laboratories to establish prudent biosafety practices. The prevention and control of laboratory-acquired infections are directed to protect all laboratory personnel, the environment and local community from contamination or infection with hazardous pathogens.

A litany of biosafety practices that are readily available from the sources listed above and elsewhere will not be reproduced here (Barkley and Richardson

Table 19.3 Route of laboratory-associated infections

Organism	Route of infection			
	Non-intact skin or mucosa contact	Inhalation	Ingestion	Animal contact
Bacteria				
Bacillus anthracis	X	X		X
Bordetella pertussis	X	X		
Borellia spp.	X			X
Brucella spp.	X	X		X
Campylobacter spp.	X		X	X
Chlamydia spp.	X	X		
Coxiella burnetii	X	X		X
Francisella tularensis	X	X	X	X
Leptospira spp.	X	X	X	
Mycobacterium tuberculosis	X	X		
Burkholderia (Pseudomonas) pseudomallei		X		
Rickettsia spp.	X	X		X
Salmonella typhi	X		X	
Other *Salmonella* spp.	X		X	X
Treponema pallidum	X	X		
Vibrio cholerae	X		X	
Other *Vibrio* spp.	X		X	X
Yersinia pestis	X	X	X	X
Fungi				
Blastomyces dermatitidis	X	?		
Coccidioides immitis	X	X		
Cryptococcus neoformans	X	?		X
Histoplasma capsulatum	X	X		
Sporothrix schenckii	X			X
Dermatophytes				X
Viruses				
Hantavirus	X	X	X	X
Hepatitis viruses (B,C)	X			
Herpes simplex virus	X			
Herpesvirus simiae	X			X
HIV	X			
Lassa virus	X	X	X	X
Lymphocytic choriomeningitis virus	X	X	X	X
Marburg and Ebola viruses	X			X
Parvovirus		X		
Rabies virus	X	X		X
Venezuelan equine encephalitis virus	X	X		X
Vesicular stomatitis virus	X	X		X
Parasites				
Leishmania spp.	X			X
Plasmodium spp.	X			
Toxoplasma gondii	X		X	X
Trypanosoma spp.	X	X		

Reprinted with permission from Sewell (1995).

1994). However, it is appropriate to list 4 common laboratory practices that must be established in clinical and biomedical laboratories of all sizes and which will serve as a nucleus for the development of a laboratory safety manual:

1   The clinical microbiology laboratory must not be located in or near areas of the general laboratory that have the heaviest traffic patterns; the microbiology laboratory should not be a gathering place and should be in a quiet or secluded area with signs on the doorways that limit entry to laboratory staff or others who have business with the laboratory.

Table 19.4 Recommended biosafety or containment levels (BSL) for micro-organisms

Containment level	Hazard of agent	Recommended level of microbiological practice	Safety equipment required	Laboratory facilities
1	Agent unlikely to cause disease in healthy adult	Basic level of standard microbiological practices BSL-1	Standard equipment for microbiology laboratory	Open bench top sink and cleanable bench top surfaces
2	Those agents assigned to biohazard group II: ingestion, mucous membrane, accidental needlestick risks	BSL-2, includes BSL-1 plus: restricted access, biohazard signs posted, needle and sharps precaution, safety manual for all, decontamination, and surveillance procedures	Physical containment devices or biosafety cabinets as required to contain aerosols, splashes, etc. Bench surface impervious to water, easy to clean, resistent to corrosives. Protective clothing as needed	BSL-1 plus available autoclave, access to incinerator, proper ventilation control
3	Any indigenous or exotic agent with potential for aerosolization; infection likely to cause serious illness or death but treatment and/or vaccination available	BSL-3 includes BSL-1 and 2 plus: separate laboratory and restricted access, control and decontamination of all laboratory waste, decontamination of all laboratory clothing, discard or laundry. Baseline serum taken from all employees and stored at −70°C	Class I or II biological safety cabinets and other physical containment for all procedures that may create aerosol or splash. Protective clothing and respiratory protection	BSL-2 plus negative air pressure to atmosphere HEPA filters in air exchange. Laboratory should contain its own equipment so far as practicable. Safe storage of agents
4	Dangerous or unknown suspect agents that have or are suspected of carrying a high risk for very serious or life-threatening disease Agents suspected to be related to these groups and whose risk of transmission is unknown	BSL-4 includes BSL-1, 2, and 3 plus access only to authorized personnel, with entry restricted to those assigned to work in laboratory. DO NOT work alone or unsupervised. Laboratory maintained at air pressure negative to atmosphere. All material must be autoclaved before removal from facility	All work conducted in Class III safety cabinet or class I or II cabinet in combination with full body positive pressure personal protective suit with individual air supply to suit. Laboratory is sealable and has full storage for biological materials	BSL-3 plus a separate building or totally isolated area. Contains all its own equipment. Incineration available on site for disposal of all carcasses and tissues. Dedicated air supply, exhaust and decontaminating systems

2 Work procedures should be established to protect eyes, nose, mouth, mucous membranes or abraded skin from contact with infected tissues or other clinical samples, or with cultures.

3 The single most important procedure is the need to wash hands with soap and warm water, before and after handling specimens or cultures, after dealing with any spillages, when leaving the microbiology laboratory, and when the day's work is complete.

4 Pipetting is the usual method of transferring liquids or suspensions. This must **never** be done by mouth. A wide range of hand manipulated pipettes are available and must be used for transferring all liquids and especially infectious or toxic materials. Similarly, careful attention is required in handling pipettes after use to prevent splashes, spills or sprays.

Clearly, a well developed and thorough safety plan is needed for any laboratory that handles potentially infectious materials or hazardous substances. The laboratory director with the support of the institutional administration must be charged with this responsibility. Among other things, this includes the development of a laboratory safety manual and an institutional commitment to control and prevention policies. The laboratory manual should cover safety in the workplace and provide a prudent approach to the handling of accidents within the laboratory and accidental exposure of laboratory staff to needlesticks, cuts, aerosols, etc. Employees must be trained to report immediately all incidents involving exposure to an infectious agent. Medical care should be provided for the employee involved and thorough investigation of the incident should be undertaken. This investigation should be extensive and, if necessary, the laboratory employee and source patient should be monitored for any delayed response. If needed, the family of the employee should be monitored and, if indicated, prophylaxis or therapy should be instituted. Review of the incident to determine corrective actions

to eliminate or prevent any repeat are necessary (Anonymous 1993).

The need for better delivery of medical care is an international concern and medical laboratories are being pressed for better and more rapid diagnostic tests. In many parts of the world an increasing amount of laboratory work is being done in small laboratories within physicians' offices. In the USA the number of physician's office laboratories (POL) has increased dramatically along with the ever-increasing number of rapid, kit-type microbiological procedures. At the other extreme is the consolidation and merging of hospitals, clinics and medical centres with the concomitant development of large, centralized laboratories designed to perform thousands of mostly automated tests on clinical specimens that are delivered to these laboratories from a wide range of clinical facilities by rapid courier services. Here, too, rapid, automated microbiological procedures are in demand, ranging from urinary screens to blood cultures to immunoserology for HIV antibody or antigen, etc. What is unclear at the present is what impact these 'non-traditional' laboratories are having in terms of biosafety. The guidelines and principles of biosafety that are presented here, coupled with a continuing review of regulatory issues, are the required preparation for these new laboratory activities (McGowan and MacLowry 1995).

The changing patterns of health care delivery, with the increasing growth in medical technology, are important signs of the technology-driven era. These changes and others to come clearly indicate that the strongest voice in the laboratory safety programme of any institution must be that of the chief of microbiology. By virtue of training, knowledge and experience, microbiologists are the best equipped members of hospital or laboratory staff to be in charge of the laboratory safety programme. Attempts to cut corners in the provision of proper equipment and appropriate training for staff cannot be tolerated. Exposure to hazards and associated risk are ever-present problems and cannot be disregarded for administrative convenience or economy.

REFERENCES

Advisory Committee on Dangerous Pathogens, 1995, *Categorization of Biological Agents according to Hazard and Categories of Containment*, 4th edn, Health and Safety Enquiries, HSE Centre, Sudbury, Suffolk, UK.

Anonymous, 1993, *Code of Safety Practice*, Centre for Applied Microbiology and Research, Public Health Laboratory Service, Porton Down, UK.

Barkley WE, Richardson JH, 1994, Laboratory safety, *General and Molecular Bacteriology*, eds Gerhardt P, Murray RGE et al., American Society for Microbiology, Washington, DC, 716–33.

Brunton WAT (ed.), 1993, *Safety Precautions. Notes for Guidance*, 4th edn, Public Health Laboratory Service, London.

Collins CH, 1993, *Laboratory Acquired Infections: History, Incidence, Causes and Prevention*, 3rd edn, Butterworth–Heinemann, Oxford.

Fleming DO, Richardson JH et al. (eds), 1995, *Laboratory Safety: Principles and Practice*, 2nd edn, American Society for Microbiology, Washington, DC.

Harrington JM, Shannon HS, 1976, Incidence of tuberculosis, hepatitis, brucellosis and shigellosis in British medical laboratory workers, *Br Med J*, 1: 759–62.

Herwaldt BL, Juranek DD, 1993, Laboratory-acquired malaria, leishmaniasis, trypanosomiasis, and toxoplasmosis, *Am J Trop Med Hyg*, 48: 313–23.

Hunt DL, 1995, Human immunodeficiency virus type 1 and other blood borne pathogens, *Laboratory Safety: Principles and Practice*, eds Fleming DO, Richardson JH et al., American Society for Microbiology, Washington, DC, 33–66.

McGowan JE Jr, MacLowry JD, 1995, Addressing regulatory issues in the clinical microbiology laboratory, *Manual of Clinical Microbiology*, 6th edn, eds Murray PR, Baron EJ et al., American Society for Microbiology, Washington, DC, 67–74.

Martin JC, 1980, Behavior factors in laboratory safety: personnel characteristics, *Laboratory Safety: Theory and Practice*, eds Fuscaldo AA, Erlick BJ, Hindman B, Academic Press, New York, 321–42.

Miller CD, Songer JR, Sullivan JF, 1987, A twenty-five year review of laboratory acquired human infections in the National Animal Disease Center, *Am Ind Hyg Assoc J*, **48:** 271–5.

Muller HE, 1988, Laboratory-acquired mycobacterial infection, *Lancet*, **2:** 331.

Pike RM, 1978, Past and present hazards of working with infectious agents, *Arch Pathol Lab Med*, **102:** 333–6.

Pike RM, 1979, Laboratory-associated infections: incidence, fatalities, causes and prevention, *Annu Rev Microbiol*, **33:** 41–66.

Richmond JY, McKinney RW, 1993, *Biosafety in Microbiological and Biomedical Laboratories*, 3rd edn, US Department of Health and Human Services, CDC, Atlanta, GA.

Segretain G, 1959, *Penicillium marnfeii*, n. sp., agent d'une mycose du système reticulo-endothelial, *Mycopathol Mycol Appl*, **11:** 327–53.

Sewell DL, 1995, Laboratory-associated infections and biosafety, *Clin Microbiol Rev*, **8:** 383–405.

Sulkin SE, Pike RM, 1949, Viral infections contracted in the laboratory, *N Engl J Med*, **241:** 205–13.

Sulkin SE, Pike RM, 1981, Survey of laboratory acquired infections, *Am J Public Health*, **41:** 769–81.

Thucydides, 1972, *The Peloponnesian War*, 2nd edn, transl. Warner R, Penguin, Harmondsworth, 154, 158.

Williams REO, 1981, In pursuit of safety, *J Clin Pathol*, **34:** 232–9.

World Health Organization, 1993, *Laboratory Biosafety Manual*, 2nd edn, WHO, Geneva.

Chapter 20

ACTINOMYCES

G H W Bowden

1 DEFINITION

Actinomyces spp. are gram-positive rods, 0.4–1.0 μm wide, which may be straight, curved, or pleomorphic and occur singly, in pairs, clusters or short chains. Filaments up to 50 μm in length are formed by members of some species. Some show true branching. They are non-acid-fast, non-motile and do not form endospores or conidia. The majority of species are facultative anaerobes; some are anaerobic. Growth is stimulated by CO_2 and sodium carbonate in broth media and members of several species grow well aerobically with added CO_2. The optimum temperature for growth of all species except *Actinomyces humiferus*, which grows at 30°C, is 35–37°C. Carbohydrates are fermented, generally with the production of formic, acetic, lactic and succinic acids. There is little action on proteins, although organic nitrogen is required for growth. Species can be α-, β- or γ-haemolytic and haemolysis may depend on culture conditions. Some species show antigenic diversity and have more than one serotype. The cell wall peptidoglycan is one of 3 types: the majority of the species have Orn-Lys-Glu, whereas *Actinomyces bovis* has Lys-Lys-D-Asp and in *Actinomyces bernardiae*, *Actinomyces suis* and *Actinomyces pyogenes* the peptidoglycan includes Lys-Ala-Lys-D-Glu. Diaminopimelic acid and mycolic acids are absent. Cell wall polysaccharides include, fucose, glucose, galactose, mannose, rhamnose, and 6-deoxytalose and amino sugars; arabinose and xylose have not been detected. The major cellular fatty acids of *Actinomyces* comprise myristic (14:0), palmitic (16:0), stearic (18:0) and oleic acids (18:1ω9). The relative amounts of these acids vary among species. Smaller amounts of other acids (10:0, 16:1) may

be found. The range of G + C content of the DNA is 55–71 mol% and the type species is *A. bovis*.

2 INTRODUCTION AND HISTORICAL PERSPECTIVE

The early history of the classification of *Actinomyces* was complicated by their histological resemblance to fungi. As pointed out by Slack and Gerencser (1975), as early as 1827 (Meyen 1827), the name *Actinomyces* (ray fungus) had been given incorrectly to a previously named fungus. Slack and Gerencser (1975) list 16 generic names proposed from 1875 to 1934 to include organisms now considered to be *Actinomyces*. Harz (1879) initially provided a detailed histological description of an organism that formed granules in lesions in the jaws of cattle, which he named *Actinomyces bovis*. Harz could not cultivate the organism and it was not possible to compare it to those described subsequently by other workers. Apparently, Mosselman and Lienaux (1890) first isolated *A. bovis* as it is known today. However, a variety of organisms, including aerobes (Bostroem 1891) were also identified as *A. bovis*, hindering further the accurate definition of the genus.

Wolff and Israel (1891) described an anaerobic pathogen (*Actinomyces israelii*) isolated from 2 cases of actinomycosis in humans and demonstrated the pathogenicity and virulence of their isolates. However, new genera, often with the species names *bovis* or *israelii* continued to be proposed to include branching pathogens of humans and other animals. It remained a problem to distinguish *Actinomyces* from other gram-positive genera with branching cells and to differentiate *A. bovis* and *A. israelii*. Wright (1905) defined *Actinomyces* as anaerobic and distinguished them from the aerobes identified by some workers as *A. bovis*, which he named *Nocardia*. Breed and Cohn (1919) recommended *Actinomyces* as a genus with the type species as *A. bovis* and this was accepted by Winslow et al. (1920).

Chemotaxonomic techniques made a dramatic impact on the classification of *Actinomyces*. Studies by Cummins and Harris (1958) and Cummins (1962) showed that *Actinomyces* spp. had cell walls typical of bacteria. Chemotaxonomy allowed better definition of the genus, resulting in reclassification of some species (Schaal 1986). More recently, 16S rRNA sequence data has been used to assign further species to the genus (Collins et al. 1993, Funke et al. 1994, 1995, Wüst et al. 1995) and to demonstrate the phylogenetic relationships between *Actinomyces* spp. and other actinomycetes (Embley and Stackebrandt 1994). Species currently placed into *Actinomyces* are shown in Table 20.1.

Many *Actinomyces* spp. are known to be indigenous bacteria, colonizing the mucous membranes of humans and other animals. In particular, the oral cavity is the natural and unique habitat of several species. These indigenous organisms may play a pathogenic role, often as components of mixed infections (Bowden 1984, Schaal and Beaman 1984, Schaal 1986) at various sites of the body.

3 HABITAT

The natural habitats (Table 20.1) of most of the species of *Actinomyces* are known to be intestinal surfaces of humans and animals. The exceptions are *A. bovis*, and the more recently described species. Although detailed examinations of oral samples from healthy cattle revealed new species of *Actinomyces* (Dent and Williams 1984a, 1984b, 1984c, 1986) strains of *A. bovis* were not isolated. This suggests that if this species is a member of the normal oral flora of cattle it is present in relatively low numbers in healthy animals. *Actinomyces* spp. form a significant proportion of the normal flora of the oral cavities of humans and animals, where they occur as components of dental plaque on teeth and biofilms on mucosal surfaces (Bowden and Hardie 1973, 1978, Slack and Gerencser 1975, Bowden, Ellwood and Hamilton 1979, Dent and Marsh 1981, Johnson et al. 1990). Generally, these organisms do not colonize other sites in the intestinal tract and, with certain exceptions, they can be described as uniquely oral organisms. However, some species can colonize tonsils (Slack and Gerencser 1975) and *A. israelii* is regularly present in the female genital tract (Persson and Holmberg 1984a). *Actinomyces hyovaginalis* colonizes the porcine urinary tract. *Actinomyces humiferus* is unique within the genus, with soil as its natural habitat.

4 MORPHOLOGY

4.1 Cellular morphology

Cells are gram-positive, although occasionally they may appear beaded on Gram's stain. When grown on blood agar the majority of species show diphtheroidal V and Y forms and may produce short coccobacilli. Several different cellular morphologies can occur together and often cells form clusters. Some species, including *A. israelii* (Fig. 20.1a) and *A. bovis* produce long filamentous forms and show true non-septate branching, which may also be seen with *Actinomyces viscosus*, *Actinomyces naeslundii* (Fig. 20.1b) and *Actinomyces odontolyticus*. In semi-defined broth (Bowden 1991) cells of *A. israelii*, *A. viscosus* and *A. naeslundii* tend to produce predominantly pleomorphic branching filaments. Cells of *Actinomyces* show a typical gram-positive wall structure when examined by electron microscopy (Slack and Gerencser 1975, Schaal 1986). Some species, in particular *A. naeslundii* and *A. viscosus*, have extensive fimbriae on their outer surfaces (see section 13, p. 458). Other species that have been examined (*A. pyogenes*, *A. israelii* and *A. odontolyticus*) have relatively smooth cell surfaces without fimbriae.

4.2 Colonial morphology and appearance in broth

Species such as *A. israelii*, which form long branching filaments, usually produce a granular deposit in broth with a completely clear supernate. The granules tend to be resistant to disruption. *A. naeslundii*, *A. viscosus* and *Actinomyces gerencseriae*, which produce fewer, shorter filaments, also form a deposit in broth but it is viscous and ropy and more easily suspended. Organisms that produce diphtheroidal or coccobacilliary cells usually grow as evenly dispersed suspensions.

On solid media, *Actinomyces* spp. produce a variety of colony forms. Photographs of the colonies of *Actinomyces* spp. are shown by Slack and Gerencser (1975) and Schaal (1986). Typically, *A. israelii* produces a white-coloured, rough, 'molar tooth' colony (Fig. 20.1c), whereas *A. naeslundii*, *A. viscosus* and *A. gerencseriae* usually produce convex, smooth, matt-surfaced cream-coloured colonies (Fig. 20.1d). Colonies of other species may be flat (*A. hyovaginalis*) or low convex (*Actinomyces neuii*) and the original references should be consulted for details. Species vary in their effect on blood (see Table 20.4, p. 456) and growth conditions can affect the nature of the haemolysis. Colonies of some strains of *A. odontolyticus* have a reflective metallic surface sheen and turn brownish red after incubation for 72–96 h on blood agar (Batty 1958, Johnson et al. 1990, Brander and Jousimies-Somer 1992). The morphology of early growth of the organisms (microcolonies) has been used in species identification (Slack and Gerencser 1975, Schaal 1986).

Table 20.1 *Actinomyces* species

Actinomyces species	Subdivisions within species	Pathogenicity	Natural habitat	References
A. bernardiae	None known	Pathogen in humans	Not known	Na'was et al. 1987, Funke et al. 1995
A. bovis	Serotypes I and II	Pathogen in animals	Not known	Schaal 1986
A. denticolens	None known	Non-pathogen	Oral cavity, cattle	Dent and Williams 1984a, 1984c
A. georgiae	None known	? Associated with periodontal disease	Oral cavity, humans	Johnson et al. 1990
A. gerencseriae	None known	Pathogen in humans and animals	Oral cavity, humans	Johnson et al. 1990
A. hordeovulneris	None known	Pathogen in dogs	? Oral cavity, dogs	Buchanan et al. 1984
A. howellii	None known	Non-pathogen	Oral cavity, cattle	Dent and Williams 1984b
A. humiferus	None known	Non-pathogen	Soil	Gledhill and Casida 1969
A. hyovaginalis	Not known	Pathogen in pigs	Porcine genital tract	Hommez et al. 1991, Collins et al. 1993
A. israelii	Some subdivisions (Schofield and Schaal 1981)	Pathogen in humans and animals	Oral cavity, humans	Schaal 1986
A. meyeri	? Serotypes	Pathogen in humans ? Associated with periodontal disease	Oral cavity, humans	Cato et al. 1984
A. naeslundii	Genospecies 1 and 2 Serotypes I–III Many ribotypes	Pathogen in humans ? Associated with root caries and periodontal disease	Oral cavity, humans	Johnson et al. 1990
A. neuii	Subsp. *neuii* Subsp. *anitrus*	Pathogen in humans	Not known	Funke et al. 1993, 1994
A. odontolyticus	Serotypes I and II	? Occasional pathogen in humans	Oral cavity, humans	Batty 1958, Schaal 1986
A. pyogenes	Several ribotypes Bacteriocin types	Pathogen in animals and humans	? Mucosal surfaces of animals	Collins and Jones 1982, Reddy, Cornell and Fraga 1982
A. radingae	None known	Pathogen in humans	Not known	Wüst et al. 1993, 1995
A. slackii	None known	Non-pathogen	Oral cavity, cattle	Dent and Williams 1986
A. suis	None known	Pathogen in pigs	Recovered from urine of healthy boars	Wegienek and Reddy 1982, Ludwig et al. 1992
A. turicensis	None known	Pathogen in humans	Not known	Wüst et al. 1993, 1995
A. viscosus	None known	Non-pathogen	Oral cavity, animals	Johnson et al. 1990

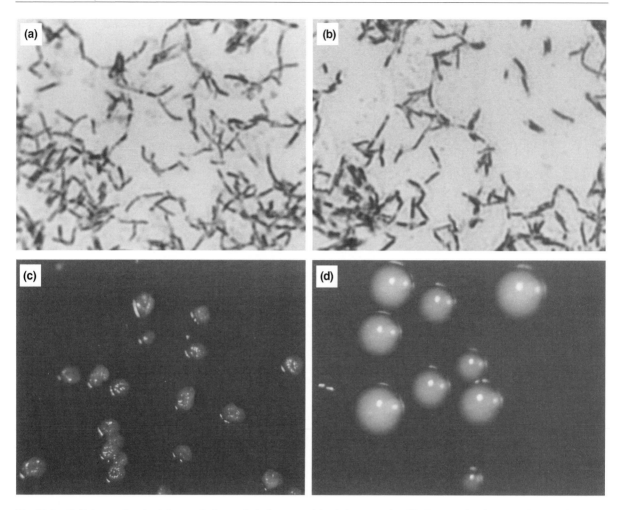

Fig. 20.1   Cellular and colonial morphology of *Actinomyces*. (a) *Actinomyces israelii*. Gram-stained smear from culture on blood agar (× 810). (b) *Actinomyces naeslundii* genospecies 2. Gram-stained smear from culture on blood agar (× 810). (c) *Actinomyces israelii* colonies on blood agar after incubation for 5 days (× 3.4). (d) *Actinomyces naeslundii* genospecies 2 colonies on blood agar after incubation for 5 days (× 3.4).

5   CULTURAL CHARACTERISTICS

The optimum temperature for growth of all species with the exception of *A. humiferus* is 35–37°C. The reported range of temperatures that support growth is 20–45°C depending on the species (Schaal 1986). *A. israelii*, *A. gerencseriae*, *A. naeslundii*, *A. bovis*, *A. odontolyticus* and *A. viscosus* grow on modern high quality nutrient agars in air with added CO_2, often without added enrichment. However, it is common practice to grow the organisms on solid media enriched with blood or, occasionally, serum. In some cases specific enrichments are recommended: *Actinomyces hordeovulneris* requires the addition of fetal calf serum (Buchanan et al. 1984); *Actinomyces meyeri* requires vitamin K1 and Tween 80 (Cato et al. 1984); and *A. pyogenes* requires haemin and bicarbonate (Reddy, Cornell and Fraga 1982). The nutrient requirements of the more recently described *Actinomyces* spp. are not known in detail.

Most species grow in high quality digest broths, often without added enrichment. The addition of serum to broth enhances growth. A feature of the growth of *Actinomyces* is their stimulation by CO_2, which can be provided in fluid media as a 1% v/v filter-sterilized solution of sodium carbonate (1% w/v) in distilled water. Reduced semi-solid and cooked meat media can also be used. A defined broth medium designed for *A. israelii* and its modification (Bowden 1991) will also support the growth of *A. gerencseriae*, *A. naeslundii*, *A. viscosus* and *A. odontolyticus*. Schaal (1986) notes that the semi-synthetic medium of Heinrich and Kurth is useful for the isolation and subsequent culture of *Actinomyces*.

The majority of the species of *Actinomyces* are facultative anaerobes, although strains of some species (*A. israelii*) may grow best under anaerobic conditions and *A. suis* is anaerobic. Growth under aerobic and anaerobic conditions is stimulated by CO_2. Some strains of *Actinomyces* may not grow under anaerobic conditions in the absence of CO_2 (Schofield and Schaal 1981). Therefore, strains of all species should be grown in 5–10% CO_2. Although it is common practice to grow *Actinomyces* under anaerobic conditions, Schaal (1984) has noted that growth of some facultative species may be inhibited in anaerobic atmospheres. Some *Acti-*

nomyces spp. have the reputation of being slow-growing and, indeed, *A. israelii*, *A. bovis* and *A. gerencseriae* may take 7–14 days to grow on initial isolation. However, once isolated and grown in pure culture, maximum growth usually occurs after incubation for 3–4 days.

6 METABOLISM

Examinations of the metabolism of glucose and CO_2 by *A. naeslundii* (*A. israelii*) were made by Buchanan and Pine (1965, 1967) and Reddy, Cornell and Fraga (1982) studied the nutritional requirements of *A. pyogenes*. Considerable interest has been shown by oral microbiologists in the biochemistry and physiology of *A. viscosus* and *A. naeslundii* (Brown, Christian and Eifert 1975, Kiel and Tanzer 1977, Miller and Somers 1978, Birkhed, Rosell and Granath 1979, de Jong et al. 1988, van der Hoeven and Gottschal 1989, van der Hoeven and van den Kieboom 1990, Takahashi and Yamada 1992, Watson et al. 1993). Nothing is known in detail of the metabolic activities of the more recently described species of *Actinomyces*.

Actinomyces spp. are fermentative, generally utilizing carbohydrates anaerobically in the presence of CO_2 or HCO_3^- to produce formic, acetic, lactic and succinic acids. Cultural conditions influence the amounts of these acids detected. The level of succinate in anaerobic cultures depends on the concentration of CO_2 or HCO_3^- available, whereas under aerobic conditions with CO_2, acetate is the major acid produced by *A. israelii* and *A. pyogenes*. Succinate is generated by *A. viscosus* via the succinate pathway (Brown and Breeding 1980). In *A. viscosus*, the stimulation of glycolysis by HCO_3^- has been related to enhanced activation of glyceraldehyde-3-phosphate dehydrogenase, resulting from the more efficient regeneration of NAD in the presence of bicarbonate (Takahashi and Yamada 1992). Different species can show variation in the pattern of acid products: *A. suis* may produce only trace amounts of succinate and strains of *A. meyeri* may not form lactic acid.

Sugar transport in *A. viscosus* is via a phosphoenolpyruvate phosphotransferase system and this organism also has an alternative system for sugar transport (Hamilton and Ellwood 1983). *Actinomyces* spp. ferment a wide range of carbohydrates, including mono-, di- and trisaccharides, sugar alcohols and some polysaccharides (see Table 20.4, p. 456). Some strains degrade starch (see Table 20.4) and human oral strains produce enzymes that degrade levans (Miller and Somers 1978) and glucans (Johnson 1990). Genes for a neuraminidase (Henningsen, Roggentin and Schauer 1991, Yeung 1993) and a sucrase–fructanase (Norman, Bunny and Giffard 1995) have been characterized from a strain of *A. viscosus*. Strains of *A. viscosus* from animals produce extracellular polysaccharides (van der Hoeven 1974, Birkhed, Rosell and Granath 1979).

Generally, *Actinomyces* spp. do not degrade proteins (see Table 20.4). They are also limited in their abilities to decarboxylate or deaminate amino acids, except for the production of ammonia from arginine. Only *A. suis* and some strains identified as *A. naeslundii* and *A. viscosus* hydrolyse urea. Schaal (1986) gives details of other enzymes associated with *Actinomyces*; often these activities are detected as characters in identification schemes.

7 GENETIC MECHANISMS

Relatively little is known of the genetics of *Actinomyces* spp., although some genes from *Actinomyces* have been cloned (Henningsen, Roggentin and Schauer 1991, Yeung and Fernandez 1991, Yeung 1993, Norman, Bunny and Giffard 1995). Almost all the information derives from studies of the molecular biology of the fimbriae of *A. viscosus* T14V (Yeung and Cisar 1990, Cisar et al. 1991, Yeung 1992). The description of a broad host range vector for *Actinomyces* (Yeung and Kozelsky 1994) will undoubtedly promote genetic studies.

8 CELL WALL COMPOSITION; ANTIGENIC STRUCTURE

8.1 Cell wall composition

Actinomyces spp. have cell walls typical of gram-positive bacteria. Species may have one of 3 types of mucopeptide based on the amino acid at position 3 of the stem peptide and the interpeptide bridge (Schleifer and Kandler 1972, Schleifer and Seidl 1985): Lys-Lys-D-Asp (*A. bovis*); Orn-Lys-D-Glu (*Actinomyces radingae*, *A. israelii*, *A. gerencseriae*, *A. viscosus*, *A. naeslundii*, *A. odontolyticus*, *A. hyovaginalis*); and Lys-Ala-Lys-D-Glu (*A. pyogenes*, *A. bernardiae*). The type strain of *A. radingae* has an unusual mucopeptide structure which has not been described previously (Wüst et al. 1995). *A. suis* has lysine as its dibasic amino acid with alanine and glutamic acid but the mucopeptide structure has not been reported (Wegienek and Reddy 1982).

Neutral carbohydrate accounts for 25–45% by weight of the cell walls of *A. israelii*, *A. gerencseriae*, *A. naeslundii*, *A. viscosus* and *A. bovis* and there is no evidence that teichoic acids are present. The wall polysaccharide component can be extracted with trichloracetic acid and yields of 5–24% by weight (Bowden, Hardie and Fillery 1976, Bowden and Fillery 1978) are obtained. These polymers can contain one or more carbohydrates, with traces of amino sugars. The composition of the wall carbohydrate reflects to some extent the species of origin (Table 20.2).

8.2 Antigenic structure

Serological analysis has been used for decades to aid the identification and serotyping of *Actinomyces* spp. (Slack and Gerencser 1975, Gerencser 1979, Schaal and Gatzer 1985, Johnson et al. 1990). In general, the technique used has been fluorescent antibody (FA) staining, with polyclonal absorbed sera. However, FA

Table 20.2 Cell wall components and fermentation products of *Actinomyces* species and other genera

Genera and species	Significant cell wall components		Acid products[c]
	Amino acids[a]	Carbohydrates[b]	
Actinomyces			
A. bovis	Ala, Lys, D-Asp	Rham, 6-Deoxyt, (Gluc)[d]	Ac, Lac, Suc
A. pyogenes	Ala, Lys, D-Glu	Gluc, Rham, (Man)	Ac, Lac, Suc
A. bernardiae	Ala, Lys, D-Glu	Not known	Suc
A. suis	Ala, Lys, D-Glu	Rham	Form, Ac
A. denticolens	Ala, Lys, Orn, D-Glu	Rham	Ac, Lac, (Suc)
A. georgiae	Not known	Not known	Ac, Lact, Suc
A. gerencseriae	Ala, Lys, Orn, D-Glu	Gal, Rham	Ac, Lac, Suc
A. hordeovulneris	Ala, Lys, Orn, D-Glu	Gluc, Gal	Ac, Lact, Suc
A. howellii	Ala, Lys, Orn, D-Glu	Gluc, Rham	Ac, Lac, (Suc)
A. humiferus	Ala, Lys, Orn, Glu, Asp	Rham, (Gluc, Fuc)	Ac, Lac, (Suc)
A. hyovaginalis	Not known	Not known	Not known
A. israelii	Ala, Lys, Orn, D-Glu	Gluc, Gal	Ac, Lac, Suc
A. meyeri	Not known	Not known	Ac, Lac, Suc
A. naeslundii	Ala, Lys, Orn, D-Glu	Rham, 6-Deoxyt,[e] (Gluc)	Ac, Lac, Suc
A. neuii	Not known	Not known	Ac, Lac, Suc
A. odontolyticus	Ala, Lys, Orn, D-Glu	Glu, Man, Rham, 6-Deoxyt	Ac, Lac, Suc
A. radingae	Ala, Lys, Orn,[f] D-Glu	Not known	Lac, Suc
A. slackii	Ala, Lys, Orn, D-Glu	Gluc, Rham, (Gal)	Ac, Lac, (Suc)
A. turicensis	Ala, Lys, Orn, D-Glu	Not known	Lac, Suc
A. viscosus	Ala, Lys, Orn, D-Glu	Glu, Rham, 6-Deoxyt, (Man, Gal)	Ac, Lac, Suc
Arcanobacterium	Ala, Lys, D-Glu	Not known	Ac, Lac, (Suc)
Propionibacterium	L-DAP, Gly (*meso*-DAP)	Glu, Gal, Man, Rham	Ac, Prop
Corynebacterium	*meso*-DAP	Gal, Arab	Ac, Prop, Lac
Rothia	Ala, Lys, D-Glu	Gal, Glu, Fruc	Ac, Lac, (Suc)

[a]Amino acids: Ala, alanine; Lys, lysine; Orn, ornithine; Glu, glutamic acid; Asp, aspartic acid; Gly, glycine; L-DAP, L-diaminopimelic acid; *meso*-DAP, *meso*-diaminopimelic acid.
[b]Carbohydrates: Gluc, glucose; Gal, galactose; Man, mannose; Rham, rhamnose; 6-Deoxyt, 6-deoxytalose; Arab, arabinose; Fuc, fucose; Fruc, fructose.
[c]Acids produced in presence of CO_2 for most species: Form, formic; Ac, acetic; Prop, propionic; Lac, lactic; Suc, succinic.
[d]( ), presence variable or present in trace amounts.
[e]6-Deoxytalose may not be present in all strains.
[f]A new peptidoglycan type, ornithine may replace lysine in position 3 of the stem peptide.

staining gives no information on the nature of the antigens that have been demonstrated and absorbed sera do not reveal the numbers of antigens common to different species. Cross-reactions between *Actinomyces* spp. demonstrated predominantly by FA are shown in Table 20.3. Serological techniques that demonstrate the nature and extent of antigenic relationships between bacteria (Bowden 1993) have also been used to examine *Actinomyces* spp. These include immunodiffusion (Bowden, Hardie and Fillery 1976, Schaal and Gatzer 1985); crossed immunoelectrophoresis (Holmberg, Nord and Wadström 1975a, Bowden and Fillery 1978); Western blotting (Putnins and Bowden 1993); and FA staining with monoclonal antibody (Firtel and Fillery 1988).

Actinomyces spp. have carbohydrate and protein antigens associated with the cell wall. In *Actinomyces denticolens*, *Actinomyces howellii*, *A. israelii*, *A. gerencseriae*, *A. naeslundii*, *A. odontolyticus* and *A. viscosus* (Cummins 1962, Bowden, Hardie and Fillery 1976, Bowden and Fillery 1978, Fillery, Bowden and Hardie 1978, Putnins and Bowden 1993), the carbohydrate antigens are responsible for both species-specific and cross-reactions. *A. israelii* and *A. gerencseriae* (*A. israelii* serotype II) share a common carbohydrate antigen but *A. gerencseriae* has a second species-specific rhamnose-containing antigen (Bowden and Fillery 1978). *Actinomyces*, as typified by *A. naeslundii* and *A. viscosus*, have a complex mixture of surface antigens and epitopes (Firtel and Fillery 1988). Many of these are proteins, which can be extracted from isolated cell walls (Fig. 20.2). In *A. naeslundii*, *A. viscosus*, *A. howellii*, *A. denticolens* and *Actinomyces slackii*, the protein antigens are responsible for species-specific and cross-reactions (Putnins and Bowden 1993). It seems that some 'genus antigens' or antigens common to *Actinomyces* could also be included among the wall proteins. Western blotting has revealed cross-reactions between *A. israelii* and other species (Fig. 20.2). Perhaps the best defined antigens of *Actinomyces* are the surface fimbriae of *A. viscosus* and *A. naeslundii* (Musada et al. 1983, Yeung and Cisar 1990, Yeung 1992). Little is known of the antigens of the more recently described *Actinomyces* spp.

Table 20.3 Serological cross-reactions among *Actinomyces* species

Antiserum	Cross-reacting species or serotype[a]
A. israelii	*A. gerencseriae, A. israelii* subtypes,[b] *A. naeslundii* genosp. 1, 2, *A. pyogenes*
A. gerencseriae	*A. israelii, A. israelii* subtypes, *A. naeslundii* genosp. 1, 2
A. naeslundii genospecies 1[c]	
A. naeslundii serotype I	*A. gerencseriae, A. israelii* subtype 1c, *A. naeslundii* genosp. 2
A. naeslundii genospecies 2[c]	
A. naeslundii serotype II	*A. naeslundii* serotypes I and III, '*A. viscosus* serotype II'
A. naeslundii serotype III	*A. naeslundii* serotypes I and II
'*A. viscosus* serotype II'	*A. gerencseriae, A. israelii, A. israelii* subtypes 1b, c, *A. naeslundii* serotypes I, II and III, *A. bovis* serotype, I, *A. meyeri, Actinomyces* serotype NV
A. viscosus	*A. naeslundii* genospecies 1, '*A. viscosus* serotype II'
A. odontolyticus serotype I	*A. israelii,* '*A. viscosus* serotype II'
A. odontolyticus serotype II	*A. israelii* subtype 1c, '*A. viscosus* serotype II', *A. bovis* serotype II, *A. pyogenes*
A. bovis serotype I	*A. viscosus,* '*A. viscosus* serotype II', *A. meyeri*
A. bovis serotype II	*A. bovis* serotype I, *A. naeslundii* serotype II
A. pyogenes	*A. odontolyticus* serotype II
A. hordeovulneris	*A. israelii, A. gerencseriae, A. viscosus,* '*A. viscosus* serotype II'

[a]It is possible that protein antigens common to most of the species and serotypes exist and could be demonstrated by Western blotting (Putnins and Bowden 1993).
[b]See Schofield and Schaal (1981) and Schaal and Gatzer (1985).
[c]The genospecies as defined by Johnson et al. (1990).
Data also taken from Gerencser (1979) and Schaal (1986).

Two types of fimbriae (types 1 and 2), which are antigenically distinct, can be detected on the cell surface of strains of *A. naeslundii* and *A. viscosus* (Cisar et al. 1991). Strains of *A. naeslundii* genospecies 2 isolates have both types 1 and 2 fimbriae, whereas those typical of *A. naeslundii* genospecies 1 only carry type 2. Testing strains using specific antibody against the fimbriae shows their wide distribution among strains of *A. viscosus* and *A. naeslundii* (Masuda et al. 1983, Cisar et al. 1991). Moreover, studies using a type 1 subunit-specific probe and specific antibody confirmed that the subunit was conserved among strains of *A. viscosus* and *A. naeslundii* from oral habitats in humans and animals and absent in *A. israelii* and *A. odontolyticus* (Yeung 1992).

9 SUSCEPTIBILITY TO ANTIMICROBIAL AGENTS

Those *Actinomyces* spp. that have been tested are susceptible to a wide range of antimicrobial agents (Schaal 1986). *Actinomyces* spp. are highly sensitive to the β-lactam antibiotics and have a high to moderate sensitivity to tetracyclines, chloramphenicol, macrolides, lincomycins, fusidic acid and vancomycin. Generally, the organisms are resistant to aminoglycosides, peptide antibiotics and metronidazole. Although, as a general rule, *Actinomyces* spp. do not develop antibiotic resistance, this phenomenon has been observed in the case of rifampicin in *A. naeslundii* (Lerner 1974). Animal isolates of *A. pyogenes* are generally highly susceptible to all the β-lactam antibiotics, although strains resistant to penicillin G or ampicillin have been described (Rhoades 1979). Strains of *A. pyogenes* are also sensitive to gentamicin, kanamycin, chloram-

phenicol, rifampicin, vancomycin and novobiocin and, unlike other *Actinomyces* spp., aminoglycosides (Guérin-Faublée et al. 1993). In contrast to other *Actinomyces* spp., 67% of the strains of *A. pyogenes* examined by Guérin-Faublée et al. (1993) were resistant to tetracycline and streptomycin. *A. pyogenes* strains from human infections (Gahrn-Hansen and Frederiksen 1992) were sensitive to penicillin, ampicillin, carbenicillin, piperacillin, cephalothin, cefuroxime, cefotaxime, tetracycline, chloramphenicol, amikacin, gentamicin, netilmicin, tobramycin and ciprofloxacin. All strains were resistant to trimethoprim and one strain was resistant to streptomycin and erythromycin. The antibiotic sensitivities of *A. meyeri* and *A. hordeovulneris* are similar, although they have not been examined in detail. Both these species are sensitive to penicillin G, tetracycline and chloramphenicol; the former has also been shown to be sensitive to erythromycin and clindamycin. *A. suis* is sensitive to penicillin G, ampicillin, erythromycin, tetracycline, chloramphenicol and clindamycin. Among the more recently described *Actinomyces* spp., *A. bernardiae* is sensitive to clindamycin, erythromycin, penicillin G, rifampicin, tetracycline and vancomycin, shows variation in sensitivity to gentamicin and is resistant to ciprofloxacin (Funke et al. 1995). *A. neuii* is similar in its antibiotic sensitivity pattern to *A. bernardiae* (Funke et al. 1993), except that one strain showed resistance to tetracycline and the strains tested did not vary in gentamicin sensitivity.

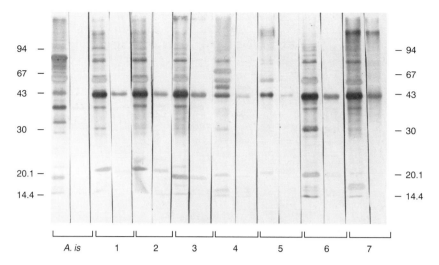

Fig. 20.2 Western blot of *Actinomyces* cell wall extracts. Cell wall protein extracts (Putnins and Bowden 1993) of *A. israelii*, *A. naeslundii* genospecies 1 and 2 and *A. viscosus*. The extracts are shown in pairs, the left lane of each pair was reacted with *A. viscosus* (ATCC 15978) antiserum and the right lane with the *A. viscosus* antiserum absorbed with *A. israelii* (NGB 17) cell walls. Lanes: *A. is.* (*A. israelii*); 1, 2, 3, 4 and 6, representatives of *A. naeslundii* genospecies 2; 5, *A. naeslundii* genospecies 1 (ATCC 12104); and 7, *A. viscosus* (ATCC 15987). The results demonstrate wide cross-reactivity among the strains and that many of the antigens are common between *A. israelii*, *A. naeslundii* and *A. viscosus*. Molecular mass standards (kDa) left and right.

10 CLASSIFICATION

The gradual expansion and development of chemotaxonomy revolutionized the classification of actinomycetes. Traditional morphological characters had proved less than satisfactory in classification and chemotaxonomy (Goodfellow and Minnikin 1985) was significant in defining these organisms at the level of the genus (Goodfellow and Cross 1984). Analysis of acid end products (Bowden and Hardie 1978, Schaal 1986), cell wall composition (Bowden and Hardie 1978) and peptidoglycan structure (Schleifer and Kandler 1972, Schleifer and Seidl 1985) of *Actinomyces* resulted in a more precise definition of the genus. Cell walls of *Actinomyces* spp. had one of 3 peptidoglycan types, a range of carbohydrates (see section 8.1, p. 449) and lacked diaminopimelic acid, arabinose and mycolic acids. Revisions to the genus were made, based on chemotaxonomic characters, e.g. *Actinomyces ericksonii* was shown to be a *Bifidobacterium* and *Actinomyces propionicus*, originally reclassified as *Arachnia propionica*, was subsequently named *Propionibacterium propionicus*. Methods to determine chemotaxonomic characters that aid the classification of *Actinomyces* are now well established (Goodfellow and Minnikin 1985, Goodfellow and O'Donnell 1993) and include cell wall composition, acid end products, protein profiles of whole cells and nucleic acid analysis.

In a numerical taxonomic study, Schofield and Schaal (1981) examined 134 strains of *Actinomyces*. *A. israelii* strains fell into a single well defined cluster, which could be subdivided into subclusters a–d, suggesting differences among the strains. Schaal and Gatzer (1985) confirmed the subdivisions among *A. israelii* and Schaal (1986) described them as 'subspecies', the first 2 being represented by *A. israelii*

serotypes I and II, the others being new groups. The majority (45 of 67) of strains of *A. naeslundii* and *A. viscosus* were recovered in 2 main clusters at 82.5% similarity. This similarity among strains of *A. naeslundii* and *A. viscosus* supported an earlier observation by Fillery, Bowden and Hardie (1978) who had demonstrated an 88% similarity between 35 human isolates of *A. viscosus* serotype II and *A. naeslundii*. In this study, a separate cluster of 3 animal strains, including the type strain of *A. viscosus* serotype I, reacted only with *A. viscosus* serotype I antisera and the authors suggested that *A. viscosus* serotype I could represent a distinct group of animal organisms. By contrast, the human strains of *A. viscosus*, i.e. serotype II, and *A. naeslundii* could be seen as serotypes, rather than separate species. However, Schaal (1986) believed that *A. naeslundii* and *A. viscosus* should be retained as separate species. *A. odontolyticus* strains were recovered by Schofield and Schaal (1981) in a single cluster, as were 3 of 4 strains of *A. bovis* and the 10 strains of *Corynebacterium pyogenes*.

Collins and Jones (1982) and Reddy, Cornell and Fraga (1982) proposed that *C. pyogenes* should be reclassified as *Actinomyces pyogenes*. Buchanan et al. (1984) studied *Actinomyces* isolates from infections in dogs and found a group of strains (*A. hordeovulneris*) that were distinct from previously described species. Strains from healthy cattle were examined by Dent and Williams (1984 a, 1984b, 1984c, 1986). Using chemotaxonomic and biochemical tests and DNA homology, they described 3 new species: *A. denticolens*, *A. howellii* and *A. slackii*. *A. meyeri* (Cato et al. 1984) was the last species included by Schaal (1986) in his detailed review and definition of the genus. However, 2 organisms '*Actinomyces suis*' and '*Actinomyces humiferus*', were considered by Schaal to be species *incertae sedis.* The former organism had been described by Franke (1973) but no type strain existed. *A. humiferus* had been validly described by Gledhill and Casida (1969) and was included in the approved list of names (Skerman, McGowan and Sneath 1980). Schaal (1986) considered that its unusual habitat in soil, low optimum growth temperature of 30°C and the relatively high G + C content of its DNA (73 mol%) made its inclusion in *Actinomyces* inappropriate.

Johnson et al. (1990) studied human oral *Actinomyces* isolates, some of which did not conform to named species or react with standard antisera. Two new species were described: *A. gerencseriae*, to include isolates previously described as serotype II of *A. israelii*, and *Actinomyces georgiae*, to include organisms from the periodontal flora, previously called '*Actinomyces* D08'. These authors made a clear distinction between the animal organism *A. viscosus* serotype I and *A. naeslundii* and human strains of *A. viscosus* (serotype II). *A. viscosus* serotype I was retained as a distinct species, which was in accord with some numerical data (Fillery, Bowden and Hardie 1978). They also showed a close relationship between *A. naeslundii* serotypes II and III, human strains of *A. viscosus* (serotype II) and serotype *Actinomyces* NV, which they considered to be examples of the same species. Because differentiation between strains in this latter group and *A. naeslundii* serotype I could be made only on the basis of serology and not on reliable phenotypic tests, they proposed 2 genospecies: *A. naeslundii* genospecies 1 to include *A. naeslundii* serotype I, and genospecies 2 to include the other group of human strains. *Actinomyces* WVA 963 was proposed as a third genospecies. The proposal by Johnson et al. (1990) for *A. viscosus* and *A. naeslundii* was supported by calculation of their antigenic similarities (Putnins and Bowden 1993).

The most recent method to be applied to *Actinomyces* classification has been determination of phylogenetic relationships, using data from sequence analysis of 16S rRNA (Embley and Stackebrandt 1994, Stackebrandt and Charfreitag 1990). This technique (Stackebrandt and Liesack 1993) has been used to determine relationships among the actinomycete clade (Stackebrandt and Charfreitag 1990, Embley and Stackebrandt 1994), although Embley and Stackebrandt (1994) point out that the phylogeny of the *Actinomyces* cannot at this time be determined with certainty, as the position of this taxon shifts in the actinomycete radiation, depending on analytical methods and the strains tested. However, *Actinomyces* seem to be most closely related to *Arthrobacter* and phylogeny confirms that *Actinomyces* is a well defined taxon. *A. hyovaginalis*, *A. suis* (previously *Eubacterium suis*) and the more recently described species, *A. neuii*, *A. bernardiae*, *A. radingae* and *Actinomyces turicensis*, have all been identified and placed in *Actinomyces* on the basis of 16S rRNA sequence data. Included in the paper by Embley and Stackebrandt is a personal communication from N Weiss stating that unpublished 16S rRNA sequencing data confirm that *Arcanobacterium haemolyticum* (see Table 20.4, p. 456) should be transferred to *Actinomyces*. Undoubtedly, phylogenetic data have already made major contributions to the classification of *Actinomyces*. Embley and Stackebrandt (1994) emphasize the need for a polyphasic approach to bacterial classification, using genotypic and phenotypic features.

11 LABORATORY ISOLATION AND IDENTIFICATION

11.1 Isolation

Schaal (1984) discusses the laboratory diagnosis of diseases caused by actinomycetes, including *Actinomyces*. Detection of *Actinomyces* in clinical specimens by FA avoids the need for culture (Gerencser 1979) and has been particularly successful in demonstrating these organisms in samples from infections involving intrauterine devices (Leslie and Garland 1991). In general, isolation of *Actinomyces* from clinical and other specimens is relatively easy if certain criteria are met. These include: appropriate sample taking and transport; use of high quality media, or in certain cases selective media; incubation in an atmosphere with CO_2 or in broth media with HCO_3^-; incubation for a sufficient period of time; adequate spreading of sample on solid media; and careful examination of colonies. Usually *Actinomyces* will survive well in clinical samples, providing that oxygen is excluded and the samples do not dry. In the past, *Actinomyces* spp. were thought of as pathogens in pyogenic mixed anaerobic infections, with some emphasis placed on actinomycosis. Whereas the newly described species are often associated with mixed anaerobic infections, recent revisions in classification mean that *Actinomyces* may be encountered in samples from other sources. *A. bernardiae* has been isolated from blood and urinary tract infections and *A. neuii* subsp. *neuii* and subsp. *anitras* from blood.

Samples of pus or exudate from mixed infections can be examined for the presence of macroscopic masses of filaments, which appear as granules (sulphur granules or druzen) and are typical of actinomycosis (Slack and Gerencser 1975, Schaal 1984). Plating of a granule will often provide an enriched culture of *Actinomyces*. In the absence of obvious granules, samples may be plated directly, or after dilution in broth or Reduced Transport Fluid (RTF) (Loesche, Hockett and Syed 1972). Isolation of individual colonies of *Actinomyces* from mixed samples is made easier if dilutions of the sample are plated. A simple spreading technique is usually effective. Samples of blood, or swabs are dealt with in the normal way, taking care that the media, cultural conditions and time of incubation are appropriate. Reliable recognition of *Actinomyces* colonies among those in mixed samples depends on experience. It is a good idea to grow known culture collection strains on the media that are being used for isolation, in order to become familiar with their colony forms.

Samples from the oral cavity can include dental plaque from different areas of the dentition, saliva, swabs of mucosal surfaces and plaque taken from the gingival margin and subgingivally. Plaque can be removed by the use of sterile dental scalers, abrasive strips (Bowden, Hardie and Slack 1975) and dental floss. Various methods have been used to remove subgingival samples (Tanner and Goodson 1986). Oral samples are usually placed into RTF, suspended by mild sonication and diluted further in RTF, before plating.

Actinomyces spp. can be isolated on most good quality digest nutrient agar media that are enriched with serum or blood (see section 5, p. 448); very often these standard media include haemin and vitamin K1 (Holdeman, Cato and Moore 1977). Schaal (1984, 1986) recommended the CC medium of Heinrich and Korth and Tarozzi broth; details of the preparation of these media are given by Schaal (1986). Currently, although selective media are available for some *Actinomyces* spp., their use is restricted to oral samples and they are not commonly used in clinical laboratories.

Selective media have been designed to isolate actinomycetes (Beighton and Colman 1976) or, more specifically, *A. naeslundii* and *A. viscosus* (Ellen and Balcerzak-Raczkowski 1975, Kornman and Loesche 1978, Zylber and Jordan 1982) from oral samples. The medium of Beighton and Colman (1976) will support the growth of strains of *A. israelii*, *A. naeslundii*, *A. viscosus*, *A. odontolyticus* and other oral pleomorphic gram-positive rods such as *Propionibacterium* (*Arachnia*), *Rothia* and *Corynebacterium* (*Bacterionema*). The media designed specifically for *A. viscosus* and *A. naeslundii* are not completely selective; they will all support some other oral organisms.

11.2 Identification

The identification of *Actinomyces* spp. has always presented a problem due to the lack of reliable, readily available tests to differentiate the species. Often isolates are identified on the basis of a few characters. Even reference laboratories find it convenient to assign these non-speciated bacteria to groups, e.g. the Centers for Disease Control (CDC) groups 1, 2 and E coryneform bacteria, which have been shown to be *Actinomyces* (Funke et al. 1994, 1995, Wüst et al. 1995) and the unknown species *Actinomyces* D08, isolated from oral samples at the Virginia Polytechnic Institute (VPI) Anaerobe Reference Laboratory (Johnson et al. 1990).

Facultative or obligatory anaerobic gram-positive pleomorphic rods can be assigned to a genus by analysis of acid end products (Holdeman, Cato and Moore 1977, Bowden and Hardie 1978, Schaal 1986, von Graevenitz et al. 1994). This well accepted, relatively simple technique is routine in most laboratories. Typically, *Actinomyces* spp. produce significant amounts of succinic acid when they are grown anaerobically in the presence of CO_2 or HCO_3^-. There are exceptions (see Table 20.2, p. 450) and gram-positive pleomorphic rods included in other genera can produce succinate (von Graevenitz et al. 1994). Despite these limitations, the analysis of acid end products remains an invaluable aid in assigning isolates to a genus. A second chemotaxonomic test that has has not gained regular acceptance in routine or reference lab-

oratories, perhaps because it is thought to be too complex, is determining cell wall composition. However, rapid methods for both preparation and analysis of *Actinomyces* walls (Boone and Pine 1968, Bousfield et al. 1985) and murein (mucopeptide) (Schleifer and Seidl 1985) have been described. Cell wall and end product analyses can be particularly valuable in differentiating *Actinomyces* from other gram-positive pleomorphic rods (see Table 20.2, p. 450).

A valuable technique in the classification of bacteria, which is becoming more routine in identification, is electrophoresis of whole cell proteins and enzymes (Vauterin, Swings and Kersters 1993). The apparatus is simple, adequate comparisons of protein profiles can be made visually without computer analysis (Dent and Williams 1985), and this technique has been used to characterize *Actinomyces* (Dent and Williams 1984a, 1984b, 1985, 1986, McCormick, Mengoli and Gerencser 1985). Although analysis of the cellular fatty acid composition is used to support identification of pleomorphic gram-positive rods (Bernard, Bellefeuille and Ewan 1991, von Graevenitz et al. 1994) and details are available on the fatty acids of *Actinomyces* spp., such analyses are not in general use.

Very often *Actinomyces* spp. have to be identified on the basis of phenotypic tests. However, species give variable results in many of the tests, which makes them of limited value. Johnson et al. (1990) noted 'that it continues to be exceedingly difficult to differentiate among the described species of *Actinomyces* by usual phenotypic tests, although a few tests are helpful'. Table 20.4 lists some selected tests that can be valuable in speciating isolates identified as *Actinomyces* on the basis of acid end product analysis. It is recommended that the original references (see Table 20.1, p. 447) are consulted whenever possible, to obtain specific details and it must be borne in mind that test results may vary, depending on the media employed.

Standardized commercial test kits could provide a valuable identification system for *Actinomyces* spp. Some use and evaluation of the efficacy of commercial identification kits for *Actinomyces* spp. have been made (Kilian 1978, Brander and Jousimies-Somer 1992, Carlson and Kontiainen 1994); also, *Actinomyces* spp. have been included in comparative studies, which emphasized other anaerobes (Marler et al. 1991). Brander and Jousimies-Somer (1992) examined 71 clinical isolates and 14 *Actinomyces* reference strains with the RapID ANA II and API ZYM systems. The accuracy of identification was assessed by comparison to identification by the standard VPI methods (Holdeman et al. 1977). The RapID ANA II gave correct identification of all the reference strains, except *A. gerencseriae* (*A. israelii* serotype II), which was identified as *A. israelii*. Among the clinical isolates this system correctly identified all *A. odontolyticus* (19 of 19) and 65% (11 of 14) of the *A. israelii* strains. A large proportion (31) of the clinical isolates were identified as *A. meyeri* by the RapID ANA II system, although only 2 were obligate anaerobes. Seven of the clinical isolates identified as *A. pyogenes* by the RapID ANA II system were classified as *Arcanobacterium haemolyticum* by the conventional tests. Relatively recently, Carlson and Kontiainen (1994) have described the differentiation of *A. pyogenes* from *A. haemolyticum*, with the Listeria-Zym kit. The conclusions of Brander and Jousimies-Somer (1992), that the RapID ANA II and API ZYM methods are useful aids in identifying *Actinomyces* but accurate identification will often require supplementary conventional tests, provides a good current assessment of the effectiveness of commercial kits for identifying *Actinomyces*.

FA staining has provided one of the most useful methods for identifying isolates of *Actinomyces* and for direct demonstration of these organisms in clinical samples (Gerencser 1979, Schaal 1984, Leslie and Garland 1991). Techniques such as gel diffusion (Bowden, Hardie and Fillery 1976, Schaal and Gatzer 1985) and crossed immunoelectrophoresis (Holmberg, Nord and Wadström 1975a, 1975b) have also been used in identification. Simple whole cell slide agglutination (Putnins and Bowden 1993) has been shown to be useful for differentiating the 2 genospecies of *A. naeslundii*.

A few studies have explored the possibility of the serodiagnosis of actinomycosis caused by *A. israelii*. Early studies by Colebrook (1920) showed that patient's serum contained antibodies to *A. israelii* and more recently Holmberg, Nord and Wadström (1975b) have used crossed immunoelectrophoresis to diagnose *A. israelii* infections. Persson and Holmberg (1984b) evaluated crossed and countercurrent electrophoresis for the detection of genital actinomycosis and showed 98% specificity with 83% sensitivity. Weil and Schaal (1990) detected significant levels of antibodies to *A. viscosus* and *A. naeslundii* in 16% and 2% of healthy subjects, respectively. No significant responses were detected against *A. israelii* antigens.

Despite the ease of use and the specificity of serological methods in identification, there are drawbacks. A major one is the availability and standardization of antisera. Sera are not generally available; also, sera can vary in their reactivity and specificity even when raised against a standard strain (Johnson et al. 1990). These authors also point out that *Actinomyces* isolates from the human gingival crevice may be phenotypically similar to some accepted species but they fail to react or cross-react only weakly with the standard sera. Thus, the range of antisera available needs to be extended constantly to include new species.

A technique with the advantages of serology without its problems is the use of nucleic acid probes (Schleifer, Ludwig and Amann 1993). To date, details of only one probe for this purpose have been published (Stackebrandt and Charfreitag 1990). The probe was prepared against *A. israelii* serotype I and did not hybridize with *A. israelii* serotype II (now *A. gerencseriae*). Although not designed for use in identification, the probe for the type 1 fimbrial subunit (Yeung 1992) could have value in placing isolates into *A. naeslundii* genospecies 2 and *A. viscosus* (see section 8.2, p. 449).

12 TYPING METHODS

Serology has been the most widely used method to type *Actinomyces* spp. and recently genetic typing methods are also being applied to *Actinomyces*. Few other typing methods have been used, although Lämmler (1990) typed *A. pyogenes* by production and sensitivity to different bacteriocins.

12.1 Serotyping

Several *Actinomyces* spp. are known to include serotypes (see Table 20.3, p. 451) (Gerencser 1979, Schaal and Gatzer 1985). Little is known of the antigens that define the serotypes (see section 8.2, p. 449). Perhaps the most complex group of *Actinomyces* with regard to serological subdivisions are those designated *A. naeslundii* genospecies 1 and 2 and phenotypically similar organisms (Johnson et al. 1990). It is apparent that *A. naeslundii* genospecies 2 (see Table 20.3, p. 451) represents an antigenically heterologous group of organisms, with 33–79% antigenic similarity among strains (Putnins and Bowden 1993). *A. naeslundii* genospecies 1 could be more antigenically homogeneous, because to date it seems to include only strains of *A. naeslundii* serotype I. Little is known of the serological diversity among the more recently described *Actinomyces*, although *A. denticolens*, *A. howellii*, *A. slackii* (Putnins and Bowden 1993) and *A. hordeovulneris* (Buchanan et al. 1984) appear to be homogeneous. Some antigenic diversity has been shown among strains of *A. pyogenes* (Tainaka et al. 1983). Little is known of any specific relationships between *Actinomyces* serotypes and pathogenicity. Details of the distribution of *Actinomyces* species, genospecies and serotypes in humans with healthy or diseased gingivae are given by Johnson et al. (1990). *A. naeslundii* serotype I (genospecies 1) appears to be more closely associated with the tooth surface than genospecies 2.

12.2 Genetic typing

It is likely that genetic typing and identification will largely replace serotyping for recognizing groups, types and specific strains within *Actinomyces* spp. *Actinomyces* spp. have been typed by restriction fragment length polymorphism (RFLP) analysis of total DNA (Barsotti et al. 1993, Guérin-Faublée et al. 1994) and ribotyping (Bowden, Johnson and Schachtele 1993, Barsotti et al. 1994). Currently, with endonucleases *Bam*H1 and *Pvu*II, over 130 ribotypes have been identified among 410 strains of *A. naeslundii* genospecies 1 and 2 (Johnson, Schachtele and Bowden, unpublished). Figure 20.3 shows the *Bam*H1 ribotype patterns of strains from a study of root surface caries (Bowden et al. 1990). Wüst et al. (1993) used ribotyping and slot hybridization to aid in differentiating between *A. pyogenes* and a group of phenotypically similar isolates (*A. radingae* and *A. turicensis*) (Wüst et al. 1995) from deep wound infections. Guérin-Faublée et al. (1994) also used RFLP and ribotyping to differentiate among strains of *A. pyogenes*. The ribotypes

Table 20.4 Characteristics of *Actinomyces* species and *Arcanobacterium haemolyticum*

Character	*A. bern*[a]	*A. bov*	*A. dent*	*A. georg*	*A. gerenc*	*A. horde*	*A. howell*	*A. humif*	*A. hyov*	*A. israel*	*A. mey*	*A. naes*	*A. neu*	*A. odont*	*A. pyog*	*A. radin*	*A. slack*	*A. suis*	*A. turic*	*A. visc*	*Ar. hae*
Growth																					
O_2	nk[b]	–	(+)	–	–	nk	nk	+	nk	–	–	(+)	–	(+)	+	nk	+	–	nk	+	+
$O_2 + CO_2$	+	(+)[b]	+	+	(+)	+	+	(+)	+	(+)	(+)	+	+	+	+	+	+	–	+	+	+
$AnO_2 + CO_2$	+	+	+	+	+	+	+	–	+	+	+	+	+	+	+	+	+	+	+	+	+
catalase	–	–	–	–	–	+	+	–	+	–	–	(+)[c]	–	–	+	–	+	nk	+	+	(–)w
haemolysis	(β)	(β)	–	(α)	–	(β)	–	nk	–	–	(α)	–	(α)/γ[d]	(α)	β	–	–	(β)	(β)w[e]	–	β
Hydrolysis of																					
aesculin	–	(+)	+	(+)	+	+	nk	+	+	+	(+)	+	–	(+)	–	–	–	–	–	+	–
gelatine	–	–	nk	(+)	–	nk	nk	(+)	+	–		–		–	+	–	nk	nk	–	–	–
casein	nk	–	nk	nk	nk	nk	nk	(+)	nk	–		–	nk	–	–	–	nk	nk	–	–	–
starch	A	AH[b]	nk	A (H)	A (H)	–	nk	AH	nk	–		–	nk	(AH)	AH	H	nk	AH	AH	–	(H)
Ammonia from																					
arginine	nk	–	nk	nk	+	nk	nk	–	–	+	(+)	(+)	nk	–	–	nk	nk	nk	nk	(+)	nk
urea	–	–	nk	nk	–	–	nk	–	–	–		(+)	–	–	–	–	nk	+	–	(+)	–
Acid from																					
adonitol	+	–	nk	nk	nk	nk	nk	–	+	(+)	(+)	–	–/+[d]	(+)	(+)	nk	nk	nk	nk	–	nk
amygdalin	–	–	–	nk	+m	–	–	nk	(+)	(+)	(+)	–	nk	–	(+)	+	–	nk	(+)	–	nk
arabinose	–	–	–	–	–	+	(+)	+	+	–	(+)	–	(+)	+	+	+	–	nk	(+)	–	+
cellobiose	–	–	–	nk	+	nk	–	(+)	(+)	–	(+)	(+)	(+)	(+)	(+)	–	–	nk	nk	+	–
erythritol	+m	+	+	+	+	+	+	(+)	(+)	+	(+)	(+)	(+)	+	(+)	–	+	+	+	+	+
glucose	+	+	+	+	+	+	+	+	+	+	(+)	(+)	(+)	+	+	+	+	+	+	+	+
glycerol	+	–	–	–	–	nk	–	(+)	nk	–	(+)	(+)	(+)	(+)	(+)	nk	–	nk	nk	(+)	–
glycogen	+m	+	nk	+w	(+)	nk	nk	nk	(+)	(+)	(+)	(+)[f]	(+)	(+)	+	+w	nk	+	–	–	–
maltose	+	(+)	+	+	+	(+)	(+)	+	+	+	+	+	+	+	+	+	nk	+	+	+	+

	1	2	3	4	5	6	7	8	9	10	11	12	13	14	15	16	17	18	19	20	21	22
mannose	−	(+)	(+)	(+)	+	+w	(+)	+	+	+	−	+m	+	−	(+)	+	nk	−	(+)	+	nk	
mannitol	−	−	(+)	(+)	+m	−	−	+	nk	+m	−	−	+	−	−	+w	−	−	(+)	−	−	
raffinose	−	−	+	(+)	+m	+w	+w	(+)	−	+	−	+	+	−	−	+	+	−	(+)	+	−	
rhamnose	−	−	−	+w	(+)	−	−	+	−	−	−	−	−	(+)	−	−	−	−	−	−	−	
ribose	+m	−	(+)	+	+m	−	−	−	nk	+m	+	(+)	+	(+)	+	+	nk	−	+	−	nk	
sucrose	−	+	+	+	+	+w	+	nk	+	+	+	+	+	(+)	(+)	+w	nk	−	+	+	(+)	
trehalose	−	−	−	+	+	+	(+)w	(+)	−	(+)	−	(+)	+	−	(+)	−	nk	−	(+)	−	nk	
xylose	−	−	−	+m	+m	+	(+)w	(+)	+	+	+m	−	+	(+)	(+)	+	−	−	−	+	−	
Enzymes[c]																						
esterase-lipase	nk	−	−	−	−	nk	nk	nk	nk	−	−	−	nk	−	−	+w	nk	nk	+	+	−	
leucine-arylamidase	+	+	+	+	+	nk	nk	nk	+	(+)	+	+	+	(+)	+	+	nk	nk	+	+	+w	
valine-arylamidase	nk	−	−	−	(+)	nk	nk	nk	nk	−	(+)	−	−	−	(+)	−	nk	nk	−	+w	−	
acid phosphatase	−	−	(+)	−	−	nk	nk	nk	nk	−	−	(+)	−	−	−	−	nk	nk	−	−	+	
β-galactosidase	nk	−	+	−	+	nk	nk	nk	+	+	−	(+)	+	(+)	+w	−	nk	nk	−	(+)	−	
α-glucosidase	+	−	+	+	+	nk	nk	nk	nk	(+)	+	(+)	−	−	+w	nk	nk	nk	−	−	−	
β-glucosidase	−	−	(+)	−	+	nk	nk	nk	nk	+	−	+w	−	(+)	−	−	nk	nk	−	+	−	
NAc β-glucosaminidase	nk	+	−	−	−	nk	nk	nk	nk	−	−	−	−	−	−	−	nk	nk	nk	nk	−	+w
α-fucosidase	−	−	−	−	−	nk	nk	nk	nk	−	−	−	−	(+)	−	−	nk	nk	+w	−	−	

[a]A. bernardiae; A. bovis; A. denticolens; A. georgiae; A. gerencseriae; A. hordeovulneris; A. howellii; A. humiferus; A. hyovaginalis; A. israelii; A. meyeri; A. naeslundii; A. neuii; A. odontolyticus; A. pyogenes; A. radingae; A. slackii; A. suis; A. turicensis; A. viscosus; Arcanobacterium haemolyticum.

[b]+, positive; −, negative; ( ), variable reaction; w, weak; m, most strains; nk, not known; A, acid; H, hydrolysis.

[c]A. naeslundii genospecies 1 is catalase −ve.

[d]A. neuii subsp. neuii/subsp. anitrus.

[e]β haemolysis O_2 + CO_2, γ-anaerobic.

[f]A. naeslundii genospecies 1 seldom ferments glycogen.

[g]APIzyme.

Data from references in Table 20.1 and Brander and Jousimies-Somer (1992).

were not related to clinical source, geographical origin or date of isolation. Barsotti et al. (1994) also ribotyped 64 strains of *Actinomyces*, in a taxonomic study. Similarities showed *A. gerencseriae*, *A. israelii*, *A. meyeri*, *A. odontolyticus* and *A. pyogenes* to be distinct species. However, *A. naeslundii* and *A. viscosus* were not clearly differentiated. To date, the use of arbitrary primed polymerase chain reaction (APPCR) to type *Actinomyces* strains has not been reported.

13 ROLE IN THE NORMAL FLORA OF HUMANS

Actinomyces spp. are common in the mouths of humans and animals (Bowden, Ellwood and Hamilton 1979, Dent and Marsh 1981). They form a significant component of dental plaque on the tooth surface and, together with the other components of the normal flora, aid in the protection of the host from colonization by exogenous pathogens. Samples from healthy sites on the gingivae harbour high proportions of several *Actinomyces* taxa, most of which can be considered to be associated with gingival health (Socransky et al. 1982, Dzink, Socransky and Haffajee 1988, Moore et al. 1991, Socransky and Haffajee 1992). *Actinomyces* play a significant role in the accumulation of dental plaque, where their early colonization of the tooth surface and specific interactions with other oral organisms contribute to the composition of the community on the tooth surface (Kolenbrander and London 1992, Kolenbrander 1993). *A. naeslundii* genospecies 1 and 2 will coaggregate with a variety of other oral bacteria (Eifuku et al. 1990, Jenkinson et al. 1993, Hsu et al. 1994), oral epithelial cells and salivary pellicles, via the type 2 fimbriae which can show subtle struc-

tural variations (Strömberg et al. 1992). The type 1 fimbriae on *A. naeslundii* genospecies 2 also promote attachment to tooth surfaces through interaction with acidic proline-rich proteins and statherin (Gibbons et al. 1988) and collagen (Liu, Gibbons and Skobe 1991). Some recent data (Li and Bowden 1995) on in vitro biofilms of *A. naeslundii* suggest that biofilms of these organisms are significantly more resistant to removal by shear forces than streptococci, suggesting a role for *Actinomyces* in maintaining the integrity of oral biofilm communities.

14 PATHOGENICITY AND VIRULENCE

Traditionally, actinomycotic infections in humans have been viewed as mixed, involving predominantly *A. israelii* and *A. gerencseriae* with *A. naeslundii*, *A. viscosus* (*A. naeslundii* genospecies 2) and *A. odontolyticus* playing minor roles (Slack and Gerencser 1975, Bowden 1984, Schaal and Beaman 1984, Schaal 1986). The lesions of actinomycosis occur most commonly in the cervicofacial region, perhaps reflecting the oral habitat of *Actinomyces*, although infections may occur at any site in the body (Schaal 1986, Leslie and Garland 1991). *A. meyeri* and some of the more recently described *Actinomyces* spp. can also be isolated from abscesses in different areas of the body.

The pathogenesis of actinomycotic infections is based on the concept of an endogenous aetiology with haematogenous spread of the organisms from the oral cavity (Bowden 1984). However, it now seems likely that *A. israelii* can persist in the genital tract of healthy females (Persson and Holmberg 1984a) and this could be the source of the organism for infections at this site. Although some of the more recently described *Actinomyces* spp. are isolated from mixed infections (*A. radingae*, *A. turicensis*), they can also occur alone in ear and eye infections (*A. neuii* subspp.), in blood (*A. neuii* subspp., *A. bernardiae*) and the urinary tract (*A. bernardiae*). As the natural habitat of these organisms is not yet known, the infections may not be of endogenous origin. *A. pyogenes*, a significant pathogen in animals (Kirkbride 1993) has also been isolated from abscesses, ulcers, otitis media, cystitis and septicaemia in humans (Gahrn-Hansen and Frederiksen 1992, Drancourt et al. 1993). The origin of the strains isolated from human infections is not known.

Actinomyces spp. have also been proposed to have a role in 2 widespread human diseases, root surface caries and periodontal disease. There is an extensive literature on the bacterial aetiology of periodontal diseases (Holt and Bramanti 1991, Moore et al. 1991, Socransky and Haffajee 1992) and although some *Actinomyces* spp. may be found in higher numbers in association with lesions, the majority are not suggested to play a direct role (Dzink, Socransky and Haffajee 1988, Moore et al. 1991). In periodontal diseases, *Actinomyces* spp. are thought to contribute to plaque development and perhaps through the increase in plaque mass, to gingivitis. Also, through coaggregation they promote colonization of the gingival crevice by gram-negative anaerobic puta-

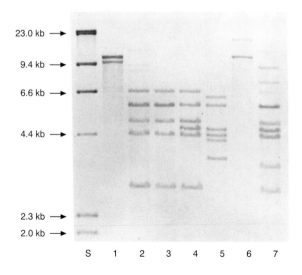

Fig. 20.3 Ribotypes of *A. naeslundii*. Ribotype patterns of strains of *A. naeslundii* genospecies 2 isolated from subjects with root surface caries. Lanes: S, *Hin*dIII fragments of lamda DNA labelled with digoxigenin; 1–7, DNA from *A. naeslundii* isolates from 7 subjects, digested with *Bam*H1 and probed with a cDNA digoxigenin-labelled probe transcribed from *E. coli* 16S and 23 S rRNA.

tive periodontal pathogens (Slots and Gibbons 1978, Ellen, Schwarz-Faulkner and Grove 1988). In root surface caries *Actinomyces* spp. are found in samples from lesions (Bowden 1990, van Houte, Lopman and Kent 1994) and one experimental model has shown that *Actinomyces* spp. can dominate the flora of lesions in root tissue (Nyvad and Kilian 1990).

Infections resembling actinomycosis occur in a variety of animals (Slack and Gerencser 1975, Schaal 1986) although the causative organisms have not always been isolated. The most well known is bovine actinomycosis or 'lumpy jaw'; the major pathogen is *A. bovis*, but *A. israelii* can cause bovine infections. *A. viscosus* has been reported to cause infections in cats and dogs, although *A. hordeovulneris* seems to be particularly associated with canine actinomycosis. Actinomycotic lesions in pigs can involve *A. israelii* and *A. viscosus*, but an organism described as '*A. suis*' (Franke 1973) has also been isolated. Although *A. suis* (Ludwig et al. 1992), previously *E. suis*, is a well known pathogen in pigs, it has phenotypic characters distinct from the original description by Franke (1973). Another porcine pathogen, *A. hyovaginalis*, has been described from purulent vaginal discharges and aborted fetuses (Collins et al. 1993).

Experimental infections have been produced in a wide range of animals (Slack and Gerencser 1975) but mice seem to be the most reliable in terms of susceptibility (Behbehani and Jordan 1982). A guinea pig groin (Grenier and Mayrand 1983) and implanted chamber models (Figdor et al. 1992) have been used to study infections with *A. israelii*. This organism will usually produce lesions typical of actinomycosis, but the mice may not die and the infection usually resolves. *A. naeslundii*, *A. viscosus* and *A. odontolyticus* may produce abscesses in mice but they are less aggressive than *A. israelii*. *A. viscosus* and *A. naeslundii* have been associated with periodontal tissue destruction and root caries in experimental infections. *A. pyogenes* is unique among the *Actinomyces* examined to date in that strains produce a soluble toxin and haemolysins, which are fatal to mice and which can be neutralized by antiserum (Lovell 1944).

Those *Actinomyces* that have been tested in experimental animals cannot be regarded as particularly virulent pathogens. With the exception of *A. pyogenes*, none has been shown to produce any toxins, although immune reactions could contribute to pathogenicity (Bowden 1984, Takada et al. 1993). There has been considerable discussion on the role that ancillary organisms may play in enhancing the virulence of *Actinomyces*. Some studies have suggested nutritional interactions (Mayrand and McBride 1980), others that the granules of *Actinomyces* play a protective role (Jordan and Kelly 1983, Figdor et al. 1992) or that gram-negative organisms enhance the survival of *Actinomyces* (Jordan, Kelly and Heeley 1984). In one study of experimental mixed infections, *A. israelii* was a component of mixtures of bacteria that produced abscesses but it was not essential for abscess formation (Grenier and Mayrand 1983).

References

Barsotti O, Morrier JJ et al., 1993, An investigation into the use of restriction endonuclease analysis for the study of transmission of *Actinomyces*, *J Clin Periodontol*, **20:** 436–42.

Barsotti O, Decoret D et al., 1994, rRNA gene restriction patterns as possible taxonomic tools for the genus *Actinomyces*, *Int J Med Microbiol Virol Parasitol Infect Dis*, **281:** 433–41.

Batty I, 1958, *Actinomyces odontolyticus*, a new species of actinomycete regularly isolated from deep carious dentine, *J Pathol Bacteriol*, **75:** 455–9.

Behbehani MJ, Jordan HV, 1982, Comparative pathogenicity of *Actinomyces* species in mice, *J Med Microbiol*, **15:** 465–73.

Beighton D, Colman G, 1976, A medium for the isolation of oral Actinomycetaceae from dental plaque, *J Dent Res*, **55:** 875–8.

Bernard KA, Bellefeuille M, Ewan EP, 1991, Cellular fatty acid composition as an adjunct to the identification of asporogenous, aerobic gram-positive rods, *J Clin Microbiol*, **29:** 83–9.

Birkhed D, Rosell K-G, Granath K, 1979, Structure of water soluble extracellular polysaccharides synthesized from sucrose by oral strains of *Streptococcus mutans*, *Streptococcus salivarius*, *Streptococcus sanguis* and *Actinomyces viscosus*, *Arch Oral Biol*, **24:** 53–61.

Boone CJ, Pine L, 1968, Rapid method for characterization of actinomycetes by cell wall composition, *Appl Microbiol*, **16:** 279–84.

Bostroem E, 1891, Untersuchungen über die aktinomykose des menschen, *Beitr Pathol Anat Allg Pathol*, **9:** 1–240.

Bousfield IJ, Keddie RM et al., 1985, Simple rapid methods of cell wall analysis as an aid in the identification of aerobic coryneform bacteria, *Chemical Methods in Bacterial Systematics*, eds Goodfellow M, Minnikin DE, Academic Press, London, 221–36.

Bowden GHW, 1984, Pathogenesis of *Actinomyces israelii*, *Biological, Biochemical and Biomedical Aspects of Actinomycetes*, eds Ortiz-Ortiz L, Bojalil LF, Yakoleff V, Academic Press, New York, 1–10.

Bowden GHW, 1990, Microbiology of root surface caries in humans, *J Dent Res*, **69:** 1205–10.

Bowden GHW, 1991, *Actinomyces* and *Arachnia*, *Anaerobes in Human Disease*, eds Duerden BI, Drasar BS, Edward Arnold, London, 131–50.

Bowden GHW, 1993, Serological identification, *Handbook of New Bacterial Systematics*, eds Goodfellow M, O'Donnell AG, Academic Press, London, 429–62.

Bowden GHW, Ellwood DE, Hamilton IR, 1979, Microbial ecology of the oral cavity, *Advances in Microbial Ecology*, vol. 3, ed. Alexander M, Plenum Press, New York, 135–217.

Bowden GHW, Fillery ED, 1978, Carbohydrate antigens of *A. israelii*, *Advances in Experimental Medicine and Biology*, vol. 107, eds McGhee JH, Mestecky J, Babb JL, Plenum Press, New York, 685–93.

Bowden GHW, Hardie JM, 1973, Commensal and pathogenic *Actinomyces* species in man, *Actinomycetes: Characteristics and Practical Importance*, eds Sykes G, Skinner FA, Academic Press, London, 277–95.

Bowden GHW, Hardie JM, 1978, Oral pleomorphic (coryneform) gram positive rods, *Coryneform Bacteria*, eds Bousfield IJ, Cally AG, Academic Press, London, 235–63.

Bowden GHW, Hardie JM, Fillery ED, 1976, Antigens from *Actinomyces* species and their value in identification, *J Dent Res*, **55, Special Issue A:** A192–204.

Bowden GHW, Hardie JM, Slack GL, 1975, Microbial variations in approximal dental plaque, *Caries Res*, **9:** 253–77.

Bowden GHW, Johnson J, Schachtele C, 1993, Characterization of *Actinomyces* with genomic DNA fingerprints and rRNA gene probes, *J Dent Res*, **72:** 1171–9.

Bowden GHW, Ekstrand J et al., 1990, The association of selected bacteria with the lesions of root surface caries, *Oral Microbiol Immunol*, **5:** 346–51.

Brander MA, Jousimies-Somer HR, 1992, Evaluation of the RapID ANA II and API ZYM systems for identification of *Acti-*

nomyces species from clinical specimens, *J Clin Microbiol*, **30:** 3112–16.

Breed RS, Cohn HJ, 1919, The nomenclature of the Actinomycetaceae, *J Bacteriol*, **4:** 585–602.

Brown AT, Breeding LC, 1980, Carbon dioxide metabolism by *Actinomyces viscosus*: pathways for succinate and aspartate production, *Infect Immun*, **28:** 82–91.

Brown AT, Christian CP, Eifert RL, 1975, Purification, characterization and regulation of a nicotinamide adenine dinucleotide-dependent lactate dehydrogenase from *Actinomyces viscosus*, *J Bacteriol*, **122:** 1126–35.

Buchanan BB, Pine L, 1965, Relationship of carbon dioxide to aspartic acid and glutamic acid in *Actinomyces naeslundii*, *J Bacteriol*, **89:** 729–33.

Buchanan BB, Pine L, 1967, Path of glucose breakdown and cell yields of a facultative anaerobe *Actinomyces naeslundii*, *J Gen Microbiol*, **46:** 225–36.

Buchanan AM, Scott JL et al., 1984, *Actinomyces hordeovulneris* sp. nov., an agent of canine actinomycosis, *Int J Syst Bacteriol*, **34:** 439–43.

Carlson P, Kontiainen S, 1994, Evaluation of a commercial kit in the identification of *Arcanobacterium haemolyticum* and *Actinomyces pyogenes*, *Eur J Clin Microbiol Infect Dis*, **13:** 507–9.

Cato EP, Moore WEC et al., 1984, *Actinomyces meyeri* sp. nov., specific epithet rev., *Int J Syst Bacteriol*, **34:** 487–9.

Cisar JO, Barsumian BL et al., 1991, Immunochemical and functional studies of *Actinomyces viscosus* T14V type 1 fimbriae with monoclonal and ployclonal antibodies directed against the fimbrial subunit, *J Gen Microbiol*, **137:** 1971–9.

Colebrook L, 1920, The mycelial and other microorganisms associated with human actinomycosis, *Br J Exp Pathol*, **1:** 197–212.

Collins MD, Jones D, 1982, Reclassification of *Corynebacterium pyogenes* (Glage) in the genus *Actinomyces* as *Actinomyces pyogenes* comb. nov., *J Gen Microbiol*, **128:** 901–3.

Collins MD, Stubbs S et al., 1993, Molecular taxonomic studies of *Actinomyces*-like bacteria from purulent lesions in pigs and description of *Actinomyces hyovaginalis* sp. nov., *Int J Syst Bacteriol*, **43:** 471–3.

Cummins CS, 1962, Chemical composition and antigenic structure of cell walls of *Corynebacterium*, *Mycobacterium*, *Nocardia*, *Actinomyces* and *Arthrobacter*, *J Gen Microbiol*, **28:** 35–50.

Cummins CS, Harris H, 1958, Studies on the cell wall composition and taxonomy of Actinomycetales and related groups, *J Gen Microbiol*, **18:** 173–89.

Dent VE, Marsh PD, 1981, Evidence for a basic plaque microbial community on the tooth surface in animals, *Arch Oral Biol*, **26:** 171–9.

Dent VE, Williams RAD, 1984a, *Actinomyces denticolens* Dent & Williams sp. nov.: a new species from the dental plaque of cattle, *J Appl Bacteriol*, **56:** 183–92.

Dent VE, Williams RAD, 1984b, *Actinomyces howellii* a new species from the dental plaque of cattle, *Int J Syst Bacteriol*, **34:** 316–20.

Dent VE, Williams RAD, 1984c, Deoxyribonucleic acid reassociation between *Actinomyces denticolens* and other *Actinomyces* species from dental plaque, *Int J Syst Bacteriol*, **34:** 501–2.

Dent VE, Williams RAD, 1985, A combined biochemical approach to the taxonomy of Gram-positive rods, *Chemical Methods in Bacterial Systematics*, ed. Goodfellow M, Academic Press, London, 341–57.

Dent VE, Williams RAD, 1986, *Actinomyces slackii* sp. nov. from dental plaque of dairy cattle, *Int J Syst Bacteriol*, **36:** 392–5.

Drancourt M, Oules O et al., 1993, Two cases of *Actinomyces pyogenes* infection in humans, *Eur J Clin Microbiol Infect Dis*, **12:** 55–7.

Dzink JL, Socransky SS, Haffajee AD, 1988, The predominant cultivable microbiota of active and inactive lesions of destructive periodontal diseases, *J Clin Periodontol*, **15:** 316–23.

Eifuku H, Yakushiji T et al., 1990, Cellular coaggregation of oral *Streptococcus milleri* with *Actinomyces*, *Infect Immun*, **58:** 161–8.

Ellen RP, Balcerzak-Raczkowski IB, 1975, Differential medium for detecting dental plaque bacteria resembling *Actinomyces viscosus* and *Actinomyces naeslundii*, *J Clin Microbiol*, **2:** 305–10.

Ellen RP, Schwarz-Faulkner S, Grove DA, 1988, Coaggregation among periodontal pathogens emphasizing *Bacteroides gingivalis–Actinomyces viscosus* cohesion on a saliva coated mineral surface, *Can J Microbiol*, **34:** 299–306.

Embley TM, Stackebrandt E, 1994, The molecular phylogeny and systematics of the actinomycetes, *Annu Rev Microbiol*, **48:** 257–89.

Figdor D, Sjögren U et al., 1992, Pathogenicity of *Actinomyces israelii* and *Arachnia propionica*: experimental infection in guinea pigs and phagocytosis and intracellular killing by human polymorphonuclear leukocytes *in vitro*, *Oral Microbiol Immunol*, **7:** 129–36.

Fillery ED, Bowden GHW, Hardie JM, 1978, A comparison of strains of bacteria designated *Actinomyces viscosus* and *Actinomyces naeslundii*, *Caries Res*, **12:** 299–312.

Firtel M, Fillery ED, 1988, Distribution of antigenic determinants between *Actinomyces viscosus* and *Actinomyces naeslundii*, *J Dent Res*, **67:** 15–20.

Franke F, 1973, Untersuchungen zur atiolgie der gesaugeaktinomycose des schweines, *Zentralbl Bakteriol Parasitenkd Infektionskr Hyg Abt 1 Orig*, **223:** 111–24.

Funke G, Lucchini GM et al., 1993, Characteristics of CDC group 1 and group 1-like coryneform bacteria isolated from clinical specimens, *J Clin Microbiol*, **31:** 2907–12.

Funke G, Stubbs S et al., 1994, Assignment of human-derived CDC group 1 coryneform bacteria and CDC group 1-like coryneform bacteria to the genus *Actinomyces* as *Actinomyces neuii* subsp. *neuii* sp. nov., subsp. nov., and *Actinomyces neuii* subsp. *anitratus* subsp. nov., *Int J Syst Bacteriol*, **44:** 167–71.

Funke G, Ramos CP et al., 1995, Description of human derived Centers for Disease Control corynebacterium group 2 bacteria as *Actinomyces bernardiae* sp. nov., *Int J Syst Bacteriol*, **45:** 57–60.

Gahrn-Hansen B, Frederiksen W, 1992, Human infections with *Actinomyces pyogenes* (*Corynebacterium pyogenes*), *Diagn Microbiol Infect Dis*, **15:** 349–54.

Gerencser MA, 1979, The application of fluorescent antibody techniques to the identification of *Actinomyces* and *Arachnia*, *Methods in Microbiology*, vol. 13, ed. Bergen T, Academic Press, London, 287–321.

Gibbons RJ, Hay DI et al., 1988, Adsorbed salivary proline-rich protein-1 and statherine: receptors for type 1 fimbriae of *Actinomyces* T14V-J1 on apatitic surfaces, *Infect Immun*, **56:** 2990–3.

Gledhill WF, Casida IE Jr, 1969, Predominant catalase negative soil bacteria II. Occurrence and characterization of *Actinomyces humiferus* sp. N., *Appl Microbiol*, **18:** 114–21.

Goodfellow M, Cross T, 1984, Classification, *The Biology of the Actinomycetes*, eds Goodfellow M, Mordarski M, Williams ST, Academic Press, London, 7–164.

Goodfellow M, Minnikin DE (eds), 1985, *Chemical Methods in Bacterial Systematics*, Academic Press, London.

Goodfellow M, O'Donnell AG (eds), 1993, *Handbook of New Bacterial Systematics*, Academic Press, London.

von Graevenitz A, Pünter V et al., 1994, Identification of coryneform and other Gram-positive rods with several methods, *APMIS*, **102:** 381–9.

Grenier D, Mayrand D, 1983, Études d'infections mixtes anaérobies comportant *Bacteroides gingivalis*, *Can J Microbiol*, **29:** 612–18.

Guérin-Faublée V, Flandrois JP et al., 1993, *Actinomyces pyogenes*: susceptibility of 103 clinical animal isolates to 22 antimicrobial agents, *Vet Res*, **24:** 251–9.

Guérin-Faublée V, Decoret D et al., 1994, Molecular typing of *Actinomyces pyogenes* isolates, *Zentralbl Bakteriol*, **281:** 174–82.

Hamilton IR, Ellwood DC, 1983, Carbohydrate metabolism by *Actinomyces viscosus* growing in continuous culture, *Infect Immun*, **42:** 19–26.

Harz CO, 1879, *Actinomyces bovis* ein neuer schimmel in dem geweben des rindes, *Jahresber Königl Centralen Thierarzneischule München*, **5:** 125–40.

Henningsen M, Roggentin P, Schauer R, 1991, Cloning, sequencing and expression of the sialidase gene from *Actinomyces viscosus* DSM 43798, *Biol Chem Hoppe Seyler*, **372:** 1065–72.

van der Hoeven JS, 1974, A slime producing organism in dental plaque of rats selected by glucose feeding: chemical composition of extracellular slime elaborated by *Actinomyces viscosus* strain NY 1, *Caries Res*, **8:** 183–210.

van der Hoeven JS, Gottschal JC, 1989, Growth of mixed cultures of *Actinomyces viscosus* and *Streptococcus mutans* under dual limitation of glucose and oxygen, *FEMS Microbiol Ecol*, **62:** 275–84.

van der Hoeven JS, van den Kieboom CWA, 1990, Oxygen-dependent lactate utilization by *Actinomyces viscosus* and *Actinomyces naeslundii*, *Oral Microbiol Immunol*, **5:** 223–5.

Holdeman LV, Cato EP, Moore WEC (eds), 1977, *Anaerobe Laboratory Manual*, 4th edn, VPI Anaerobe Laboratory, Virginia Polytechnic Institute and State University, Blacksburg, VA.

Holmberg K, Nord CE, Wadström I, 1975a, Serological studies of *A. israelii* by crossed immunoelectrophoresis: standard antigen–antibody system for *A. israelii*, *Infect Immun*, **12:** 387–97.

Holmberg K, Nord CE, Wadström I, 1975b, Serological studies of *Actinomyces israelii*: taxonomic and diagnostic applications, *Infect Immun*, **12:** 398–403.

Holt SC, Bramanti TE, 1991, Factors in virulence expression and their role in periodontal disease pathogenesis, *Crit Rev Oral Biol Med*, **2:** 177–281.

Hommez J, Devriese LA et al., 1991, Characterization of 2 groups of *Actinomyces*-like bacteria isolated from purulent lesions in pigs, *J Vet Med Ser B*, **38:** 575–80.

van Houte J, Lopman J, Kent R, 1994, The predominant flora of sound and carious human root surfaces, *J Dent Res*, **73:** 1727–34.

Hsu SD, Cisar JO et al., 1994, Adhesive properties of viridans streptococcal species, *Microbiol Ecol Health Dis*, **7:** 125–37.

Jenkinson HF, Terry SD et al., 1993, Inactivation of the gene encoding surface protein SspA in *Streptococcus gordonii* DL1 affects cell interactions with human salivary agglutinin and oral *Actinomyces*, *Infect Immun*, **61:** 3199–208.

Johnson IH, 1990, Glucanase-producing organisms in human dental plaques, *Microbios*, **61:** 89–98.

Johnson JL, Moore LVH et al., 1990, *Actinomyces georgiae* sp. nov., *Actinomyces gerencseriae* sp. nov., designation of two genospecies of *Actinomyces naeslundii*, and inclusion of *A. naeslundii* serotypes II and III and *Actinomyces viscosus* serotype II in *A. naeslundii* genospecies 2, *Int J Syst Bacteriol*, **40:** 273–86.

de Jong MH, van der Hoeven JS et al., 1988, Effects of oxygen on the growth and metabolism of *Actinomyces viscosus*, *FEMS Microbiol Ecol*, **53:** 45–52.

Jordan HV, Kelly DM, 1983, Persistence of associated gram-negative bacteria in experimental actinomycotic lesions in mice, *Infect Immun*, **40:** 847–9.

Jordan HV, Kelly DM, Heeley JD, 1984, Enhancement of experimental actinomycosis in mice by *Eikenella corrodens*, *Infect Immun*, **46:** 367–71.

Kiel RA, Tanzer JM, 1977, Regulation of invertase of *Actinomyces viscosus*, *Infect Immun*, **17:** 510–12.

Kilian M, 1978, Rapid identification of Actinomycetaceae and related bacteria, *J Clin Microbiol*, **8:** 127–33.

Kirkbride CA, 1993, Bacterial agents detected in a 10 year study of bovine abortions and stillbirths, *J Vet Diagn Invest*, **5:** 64–8.

Kolenbrander PE, 1993, Coaggregation of human oral bacteria: potential role in the accretion of dental plaque, *J Appl Bacteriol Symp Suppl*, **74:** 79S–86S.

Kolenbrander PE, London J, 1992, Ecological significance of coaggregation among oral bacteria, *Advances in Microbial Ecology*, vol. 12, ed. Marshall KC, Plenum Press, New York, 183–217.

Kornman KS, Loesche WJ, 1978, New medium for isolation of *Actinomyces viscosus* and *Actinomyces naeslundii* from dental plaque, *J Clin Microbiol*, **7:** 514–18.

Lämmler C, 1990, Typing of *Actinomyces pyogenes* by its production and susceptibility to bacteriocin-like inhibitors, *Zentralbl Bakteriol*, **273:** 173–8.

Lerner PI, 1974, Susceptibility of pathogenic actinomycetes to antimicrobial compounds, *Antimicrob Agents Chemother*, **5:** 302–9.

Leslie DE, Garland SM, 1991, Comparison of immunofluorescence and culture for the detection of *Actinomyces israelii* in wearers of intra-uterine contraceptive devices, *J Med Microbiol*, **35:** 224–8.

Li YH, Bowden GHW, 1995, Retention of biofilm cells of *A. naeslundii* and *S. mutans*, *J Dent Res*, **74, Special Issue:** 199.

Liu T, Gibbons RJ, Skobe Z, 1991, Binding of *Actinomyces viscosus* to collagen: association with the type 1 fimbrial adhesin, *Oral Microbiol Immunol*, **6:** 1–5.

Loesche WJ, Hockett RN, Syed SA, 1972, The predominant cultivable flora of tooth surface plaque removed from institutionalized subjects, *Arch Oral Biol*, **17:** 1311–25.

Lovell R, 1944, Further studies on the toxin of *Corynebacterium pyogenes*, *J Pathol Bacteriol*, **56:** 525–9.

Ludwig W, Kirchhof G et al., 1992, Phylogenetic evidence for the transfer of *Eubacterium suis* to the genus *Actinomyces* as *Actinomyces suis* comb. nov., *Int J Syst Bacteriol*, **42:** 161–5.

McCormick SS, Mengoli HF, Gerencser MA, 1985, Polyacrylamide gel electrophoresis of whole cell preparations of *Actinomyces* spp., *Int J Syst Bacteriol*, **35:** 429–33.

Marler LM, Siders JA et al., 1991, Evaluation of the new RapID-ANA II ssystem for the identification of clinical anaerobic isolates, *J Clin Microbiol*, **29:** 874–8.

Masuda N, Ellen RP et al., 1983, Chemical and immunological comparison of surface fibrils of strains representing six taxonomic groups of *Actinomyces viscosus* and *Actinomyces naeslundii*, *Infect Immun*, **39:** 1325–33.

Mayrand D, McBride BC, 1980, Ecological relationships of bacteria involved in a simple mixed anaerobic infection, *Infect Immun*, **27:** 44–50.

Meyen FJF, 1827, *Actinomyce*, Strahlenpilz Eine neue Pilz-Gattung, *Linnaea*, **2:** 433–44.

Miller CH, Somers PJB, 1978, Degradation of levan by *Actinomyces viscosus*, *Infect Immun*, **22:** 266–74.

Moore WEC, Moore LH et al., 1991, The microflora of periodontal sites showing active destructive progression, *J Clin Periodontol*, **18:** 729–39.

Mosselman G, Lienaux E, 1890, L'actinomycose et son agent infecteur, *Ann Med Vet*, **39:** 409–26.

Na'was TE, Hollis DG et al., 1987, Comparison of biochemical, morphologic, and chemical characteristics of Centers for Disease Control fermentative coryneform groups 1, 2 and A-4, *J Clin Microbiol*, **25:** 1354–8.

Norman JM, Bunny KL, Giffard PM, 1995, Characterization of *levJ*, a sucrase/fructanase-encoding gene from *Actinomyces naeslundii* T14V, and comparison of its product with other sucrose-cleaving enzymes, *Gene*, **152:** 93–8.

Nyvad B, Kilian M, 1990, Microflora associated with experimental root surface caries in humans, *Infect Immun*, **58:** 1628–33.

Persson E, Holmberg K, 1984a, A longitudinal study of *Actinomyces israelii* in the female genital tract, *Acta Obstet Gynecol Scand*, **63:** 207–16.

Persson E, Holmberg K, 1984b, Clinical evaluation of precipitin tests for genital actinomycosis, *J Clin Microbiol*, **20:** 917–22.

Putnins EE, Bowden GHW, 1993, Antigenic relationships among oral *Actinomyces* isolates, *Actinomyces naeslundii* genospecies 1 and 2, *Actinomyces howellii*, *Actinomyces denticolens*, and *Actinomyces slackii*, *J Dent Res*, **72:** 1374–85.

Reddy CA, Cornell CP, Fraga AM, 1982, Transfer of *Corynebacterium pyogenes* (Glage) Eberson to the genus *Actinomyces* as *Actinomyces pyogenes* (Glage) comb. nov., *Int J Syst Bacteriol*, **32:** 419–29.

Rhoades HE, 1979, Sensitivity of bacteria to 16 antibiotic agents, *Vet Med Small Anim Clin*, **74:** 976–9.

Schaal KP, 1984, Laboratory diagnosis of actinomycete diseases, *The Biology of the Actinomycetes*, eds Goodfellow M, Mordarski M, Williams ST, Academic Press, London, 425–56.

Schaal KP, 1986, Genus *Actinomyces* Harz 1877, *Bergey's Manual of Systematic Bacteriology*, vol. 2, ed. Sneath PHA, Williams & Wilkins, Baltimore, 1383–418.

Schaal KP, Beaman BL, 1984, Clinical significance of actinomycetes, *The Biology of the Actinomycetes*, eds Goodfellow M, Mordarski M, Williams ST, Academic Press, London, 389–424.

Schaal KP, Gatzer R, 1985, Serological and numerical phenetic classification of clinically significant fermentative actinomycetes, *Filamentous Organisms, Biomedical Aspects*, ed. Arai A, Japan Scientific Societies Press, Tokyo, 85–109.

Schleifer K, Kandler O, 1972, The peptidoglycan types of bacterial cell walls and their taxonomic implications, *Bacteriol Rev*, **36:** 407–77.

Schleifer K, Ludwig W, Amann R, 1993, Nucleic acid probes, *Handbook of New Bacterial Systematics*, eds Goodfellow M, O'Donnell AG, Academic Press, London, 463–510.

Schleifer K, Seidl PH, 1985, Chemical composition and structure of murein, *Chemical Methods in Bacterial Systematics*, eds Goodfellow M, Minnikin DE, Academic Press, London, 201–19.

Schofield GM, Schaal KP, 1981, A numerical taxonomic study of members of the Actinomycetaceae and related taxa, *J Gen Microbiol*, **127:** 237–59.

Skerman VBD, McGowan V, Sneath PHA, 1980, Approved Lists of Bacterial Names, *Int J Syst Bacteriol*, **30:** 225–420.

Slack JM, Gerencser MA, 1975, Actinomyces, *Filamentous Bacteria. Biology and Pathogenicity*, Burgess, Minneapolis, MN.

Slots J, Gibbons RJ, 1978, Attachment of *Bacteroides melaninogenicus* sub. *asaccharolyticus* to oral surfaces and its possible role in colonization of the mouth and of periodontal pockets, *Infect Immun*, **19:** 254–64.

Socransky SS, Haffajee AD, 1992, The bacterial etiology of destructive periodontal disease: current concepts, *J Periodontol*, **63:** 322–31.

Socransky SS, Tanner AC et al., 1982, Present status of studies on the microbial etiology of periodontal disease, *Host–Parasite Interactions in Periodontal Diseases*, eds Genco RJ, Mergenhagen SE, American Society for Microbiology, Washington, DC, 1–12.

Stackebrandt E, Charfreitag O, 1990, Partial 16S rRNA primary structure of five *Actinomyces* species: phylogenetic implications and development of an *Actinomyces israelii* specific oligonucleotide probe, *J Gen Microbiol*, **136:** 37–43.

Stackebrandt E, Liesack W, 1993, Nucleic acids and classification, *Handbook of New Bacterial Systematics*, eds Goodfellow M, O'Donnell AG, Academic Press, London, 151–94.

Strömberg N, Borén T et al., 1992, Salivary receptors for GalNAcβ-sensitive adherence of *Actinomyces* spp.: evidence for heterologous GalNAcβ and proline rich protein receptor properties, *Infect Immun*, **60:** 3278–86.

Tainaka MT, Kume T et al., 1983, Studies on the biological and serological properties of *Corynebacterium pyogenes*, *Kitasato Arch Exp Med*, **56:** 105–17.

Takada H, Kimura S, Hamada S, 1993, Induction of inflammatory cytokines by a soluble moiety prepared from an enzyme lysate of *Actinomyces viscosus* cell walls, *J Med Microbiol*, **38:** 395–400.

Takahashi N, Yamada T, 1992, Stimulatory effect of bicarbonate on the glycolysis of *Actinomyces viscosus* and its biochemical mechanism, *Oral Microbiol Immunol*, **7:** 165–70.

Tanner ACR, Goodson JM, 1986, Sampling of microorganisms associated with periodontal disease, *Oral Microbiol Immunol*, **1:** 15–20.

Vauterin L, Swings J, Kersters K, 1993, Protein electrophoresis and classification, *Handbook of New Bacterial Systematics*, eds Goodfellow M, O'Donnell AG, Academic Press, London, 251–80.

Watson EL, Sodhi S et al., 1993, Glucose stimulates cAMP accumulation in the oral bacterium *Actinomyces viscosus*, *Biochim Biophys Acta*, **1178:** 243–8.

Wegienek J, Reddy AC, 1982, Taxonomic study of '*Corynebacterium suis*' Soltys and Spratling: proposal of *Eubacterium suis* (nom. rev.) comb. nov., *Int J Syst Bacteriol*, **32:** 218–28.

Weil H-P, Schaal KP, 1990, Serum antibodies to pathogenic actinomycetes in the normal human population, *Zentralbl Bakteriol*, **274:** 398–405.

Winslow CE, Broadhurst AJ et al., 1920, The families and genera of bacteria, *J Bacteriol*, **5:** 191–229.

Wolff M, Israel J, 1891, Euber Reincultur des *Actinomyces* und seine Üebertragbarkeit auf Tiere, *Arch Pathol Anat Physiol Klin Med*, **126:** 11–59.

Wright JH, 1905, The biology of the organism of actinomycosis, *J Med Res*, **8:** 349–404.

Wüst J, Lucchini ML et al., 1993, Isolation of gram positive rods that resemble but are clearly distinct from *Actinomyces pyogenes* from mixed wound infections, *J Clin Microbiol*, **31:** 1127–35.

Wüst J, Stubbs S et al., 1995, Assignment of *Actinomyces pyogenes*-like (CDC coryneform group E) bacteria to the genus *Actinomyces* as *Actinomyces radingae* sp. nov. and *Actinomyces turicensis* sp. nov., *Letts Appl Microbiol*, **20:** 76–81.

Yeung MK, 1992, Conservation of an *Actinomyces viscosus* T14V Type 1 fimbrial subunit homolog among divergent groups of *Actinomyces* spp., *Infect Immun*, **60:** 1047–54.

Yeung MK, 1993, Complete nucleotide sequence of the *Actinomyces viscosus* T14V sialidase gene: presence of a conserved repeating sequence among strains of *Actinomyces* spp., *Infect Immun*, **61:** 109–16.

Yeung MK, Cisar JO, 1990, Sequence homology between the subunits of two immunologically and functionally distinct types of fimbriae of *Actinomyces* spp., *J Bacteriol*, **172:** 2462–8.

Yeung MK, Fernandez SR, 1991, Isolation of a neuraminidase gene from *Actinomyces viscosus* T14V, *Appl Environ Microbiol*, **57:** 3062–9.

Yeung MK, Kozelsky CS, 1994, Transformation of *Actinomyces* spp. by a gram-negative broad host range plasmid, *J Bacteriol*, 4173–6.

Zylber LJ, Jordan HV, 1982, Development of a selective medium for detection and enumeration of *Actinomyces viscosus* and *Actinomyces naeslundii* in dental plaque, *J Clin Microbiol*, **15:** 253–9.

Chapter 21

NOCARDIA AND RELATED GENERA

M Goodfellow

NOCARDIA

1 DEFINITION

The nocardiae have extensively branched vegetative hyphae, 0.5–1.2 μm in diameter, that grow on the surface of and penetrate agar media; these hyphae often fragment in situ or on mechanical disruption into rod-shaped to coccoid elements. Aerial hyphae, at times visible only microscopically, are almost always formed. Short-to-long chains of well-to-poorly formed conidia may occasionally be found on the aerial hyphae and, more rarely, on both aerial and vegetative hyphae. Nocardiae are aerobic, catalase-positive, non-motile, gram-variable to gram-positive and are typically acid–alcohol fast at some stage of the growth cycle. They are chemo-organotrophic, having an oxidative type of carbohydrate metabolism. The peptidoglycan, which is of the A1γ type, contains *meso*-diaminopimelic acid as the diamino acid and muramic acid in the N-glycolated form. The wall envelope contains mycolic acids with 44–64 carbon atoms and up to 3 double bonds and major proportions of straight-chain, unsaturated, and 10-methyl (tuberculostearic)-branched fatty acids. Fatty acid esters released on pyrolysis gas chromatography of mycolic esters have 12–18 carbon atoms and may be saturated or unsaturated. The polysaccharide fraction of the wall is rich in arabinose and galactose. Cells contain diphosphatidylglycerol, phosphatidylethanolamine, phosphatidyl-inositol and phosphatidylinositol mannosides as major phospholipids and a hexahydrogenated menaquinone with 8 isoprene units in which the end 2 units are cyclized (i.e. II,III-tetrahydro-ω[2,6,6-trimethylcyclohex-2-enylmethyl]menaquinone-6) as the predominant menaquinone. The range of G + C content of the DNA is 64–72 mol% (T_m). Nocardiae are widely distributed and are abundant in soil. Some strains are opportunistic pathogens for humans and animals. The type species is *Nocardia asteroides*.

2 INTRODUCTION AND HISTORICAL PERSPECTIVE

The first actinomycete, isolated from a human tear duct, was named *Streptothrix foersteri* (Cohn 1875). It is evident from Cohn's drawings that the organism showed true branching. A further species, *Streptothrix farcinica*, was isolated by Nocard (1888) from caseous lymph nodes of cattle with farcy on the island of Guadeloupe. The genus *Nocardia* was introduced by Trevisan (1889) to encompass 5 species including these 2. *Nocardia actinomyces*, the *Actinomyces bovis* of Harz (1879), was also included in the genus. The classification of what subsequently became accepted as an anaerobic species with the strictly aerobic *Nocardia farcinica* was not surprising as Harz had not succeeded in growing his actinomycete; hence its oxygen requirements were not known at the time Trevisan published. What is remarkable is that several authors (Buchanan

1918, Ørskov 1923, Jensen 1931) failed to see any contradiction in classifying *A. bovis* and *N. farcinica* in the same genus. It was left to Wright (1905) to propose that the anaerobic pathogenic actinomycetes be classified in the genus *Actinomyces*, leaving the genus *Nocardia* for aerobic actinomycetes that produced aerial mycelium and spores (*Nocardia* plus *Streptomyces*). He also introduced the term nocardiosis for infections caused by members of the genus *Nocardia*.

In 1891, Eppinger isolated an aerobic, gram-positive, acid-fast organism from a fatal case of meningitis with a brain abscess, considered it to be a fungus, and called it *Cladothrix asteroides*. The organism was renamed *Nocardia asteroides* by Blanchard (1896). An additional species, *Nocardia brasiliensis*, was proposed by Castellani and Chalmers (1913) for an organism isolated from the leg of a patient in Brazil and named *Discomyces brasiliensis* by Lindenberg (1909). *Nocardia otitidiscaviarum*, an organism isolated from the infected ear of a guinea pig, was described by Snijders (1924).

The genus *Nocardia* subsequently became a 'catch-all' for a variety of aerobic actinomycetes considered to form a mycelium that fragmented into bacillary and coccoid elements. Lechevalier (1976) has detailed the twists and turns in the early taxonomic history of the genus and spelt out the difficulties involved with retaining *N. farcinica* as the type species of the genus. Trevisan did not specify a type species. It was only with the application of modern taxonomic methods, notably chemical, molecular and numerical taxonomy, that measures were taken to revise what was a notably heterogeneous taxon (Goodfellow 1992). The redefined genus was shown to be related to the genera *Corynebacterium*, *Mycobacterium* and *Rhodococcus*, not with the genus *Actinomyces*. Furthermore, *N. asteroides* was designated the type species of the genus (Judicial Commission 1985), a course recommended by Ruth Gordon years before (Gordon and Mihm 1962).

The genus *Nocardia* is now largely defined using chemotaxonomic properties (Goodfellow and Lechevalier 1989, Goodfellow 1992). It is recommended that only actinomycetes with the following properties should be assigned to the genus:

1 a peptidoglycan composed of *N*-acetylglucosamine, L-alanine, D-alanine, D-glutamic acid with *meso*-diaminopimelic acid (*meso*-A$_2$pm) as the diamino acid and muramic acid in the N-glycolated form (Bordet et al. 1972, Uchida and Aida 1977, 1979)

2 a polysaccharide wall fraction containing arabinose and galactose (i.e. nocardiae have a wall chemotype IV and whole-organism sugar pattern A *sensu* Lechevalier HA and Lechevalier MP 1970)

3 a phospholipid pattern composed of diphosphatidylglycerol, phosphatidylethanolamine, phosphatidylinositol and phosphatidylinositol mannosides (i.e. a phospholipid pattern 2 *sensu* Lechevalier, De Biévre and Lechevalier 1977)

4 a fatty acid profile consisting of major amounts of straight-chain, saturated and unsaturated fatty acids (Kroppenstedt 1985)

5 mycolic acids with 46–60 carbon atoms (Lechevalier and Lechevalier 1980, Goodfellow 1992) and

6 an isoprenoid quinone fraction rich in a hexahydrogenated menaquinone with 8 isoprene units in which the 2 end units are cyclized (Howarth et al. 1986, Collins et al. 1987).

Species excluded from the redefined genus have been reclassified mainly using chemical, molecular systematic, morphological and numerical phenetic data (Goodfellow 1989, 1992). The genus *Actinomadura* (see section on '*Actinomadura* and other sporoactinomycetes', pp. 473–478) was proposed for organisms previously known as *Nocardia dassonvillei*, *Nocardia madurae* and *Nocardia pelletieri* (Lechevalier MP and Lechevalier HA 1970); the genera *Amycolata* and *Amycolatopsis* for *Nocardia autotrophica*, *Nocardia hydrocarbonoxydans*, *Nocardia mediterranei*, *Nocardia orientalis*, *Nocardia rugosa*, *Nocardia saturnea* and *Nocardia sulphurea* (Lechevalier et al. 1986); the genus *Oerskovia* for *Nocardia turbata* (Prauser, Lechevalier and Lechevalier 1970); the genus *Rothia* for *Nocardia dentocariosa* and *Nocardia salivae* (Georg and Brown 1967); the genus *Saccharothrix* for *Nocardia aerocolonigenes* (Labeda et al. 1984) and the genus *Skermania* for actinomycetes previously called *Nocardia pinensis* (Chun et al. 1997). Similarly, *Nocardia amarae* was transferred to the genus *Gordona* as *Gordona amarae* (Klatte, Rainey and Kroppenstedt 1994). The discovery that the genus *Actinomadura* was heterogeneous led to the description of *Actinomadura dassonvillei* as the type species of the genus *Nocardiopsis* (Meyer 1976) and to a redescription of the taxon following the transfer of several *Actinomadura* spp. to the revised genus *Microtetraspora* (Kroppenstedt, Stackebrandt and Goodfellow 1990). It has also been proposed that the genus *Amycolata* become a synonym of the genus *Pseudonocardia* (Bowen et al. 1989). The new and revised taxa can be distinguished from the redefined genus *Nocardia*, and from one another, using a combination of phenotypic properties (see Tables 21.1 and 21.2).

3 HABITAT

Nocardiae are a widely distributed group of actinomycetes which are predominantly saprophytic (Orchard 1981, Goodfellow and Williams 1983) but also include species forming parasitic associations with animals and plants (Goodfellow 1992, Beaman and Beaman 1994, McNeil and Brown 1994). They occur in a wide range of man-made and natural habitats including activated sewage sludge, soil, water and the tissues of plants and animals, including humans.

4 MORPHOLOGY AND CULTURAL APPEARANCES

The only constant morphological feature of nocardiae is their ability to form filamentous, branched cells which fragment into pleomorphic, rod-shaped and coccoid elements (Fig. 21.1). The growth and stability of both aerial and substrate hyphae often depends on the conditions of culture (Locci 1976, Williams et al. 1976, Beaman and Beaman 1994). Ecologically, fragmentation may confer advantages for both survival and dispersal (Orchard 1981). Scanning electron microscopy has been used to study the morphogenesis of *N. asteroides* fragments (Locci 1976) and shows that both lateral buds and terminal extension occur when fragments germinate in agar or in soil. Nocardiae, when growing in the animal body, generally form tangled mycelia. The well known acid-fastness of *Nocardia* spp. is often more pronounced in clinical than cultural material.

Other morphological features include well developed conidia in *Nocardia brevicatena* and less well differentiated spores in some strains of *N. asteroides* (Goodfellow and Lechevalier 1989). The spores, borne on both vegetative and aerial hyphae, develop into mycelia on fresh media. Aerial hyphae may be lacking (Fig. 21.1a), sparse (Fig. 21.1b) or abundant and visible to the naked eye (Fig. 21.1c). Most nocardiae produce carotenoid-like pigments that result in colonies with various shades of orange, pink, red or yellow. Soluble brown or yellowish pigments may be produced. Colonies may be smooth or granular and irregular, wrinkled or heaped. Mesosomes are common. L-forms of *N. asteroides* and *N. otitidiscaviarum* may be important in pathogenesis (Beaman and Beaman 1994).

Nocardiae often form a thick, dry, scaly or leathery pigmented surface pellicle in broth culture. Aerial hyphae may develop on the surface of the pellicle and may extend up the sides of the tube. Broths tend to be clear although some cultures produce a fine granular turbidity, others a ropy or membranous sediment that might be pigmented. Growth may occasionally start at the bottom of the tubes, giving rise to fluffy masses of mycelium.

5 METABOLISM

Nocardiae have an oxidative type of carbohydrate metabolism. Many of the metabolic properties generally associated with nocardiae can be attributed to *Rhodococcus* strains that were misclassified because of the emphasis once placed on the fragmentation property in nocardial systematics (Peczyńska-Coch and Mordarski 1988, Finnerty 1992). Glucose, acetate and propionate are metabolized but nocardiae can also use a diverse range of fatty acids, hydrocarbons, steroids and sugars as sole sources of carbon for energy and growth (Goodfellow 1971). Most strains grow on media containing simple nitrogen sources such as amino acids, ammonium and nitrate and on media supplemented with casein, meat extract, soy, or yeast peptones and hydrolysates. Nocardiae do not seem to have specific growth requirements.

Some nocardiae are able to grow at rather extreme

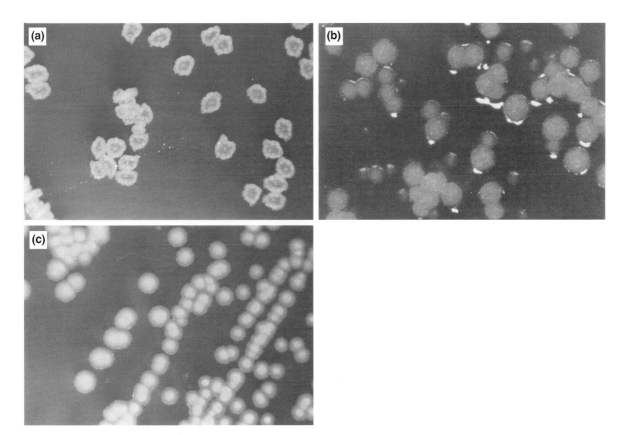

Fig. 21.1 Colonies of *Nocardia* spp. on sheep blood agar (3 days at 37°C) (× 1.4): (a) *Nocardia otitidiscaviarum*; (b) *Nocardia brasiliensis*; (c) *Nocardia asteroides*.

Table 21.1 Chemical, morphological and physiological properties separating nocardiae from other wall-chemotype IV actinomycetes containing mycolic acids[a]

Characteristics	Corynebacterium	Dietzia	Gordona	Mycobacterium	Nocardia	Rhodococcus	Skermania	Tsukamurella
Morphological characters								
Cell morphology	Straight to slightly curved rods which reproduce by snapping division; club-shaped elements may also be formed	Short rods and cocci	Rods and cocci	Slightly curved or straight rods, sometimes branching filaments that fragment into rods and coccoid elements	Substrate mycelium fragments into rods and coccoid elements	Rods to extensively branched substrate mycelium that fragments into irregular rods and cocci	Substrate mycelium resembles that of a pine-tree in early stage of growth (24h); short microscopically visible aerial hyphae formed	Straight to slightly curved rods occur singly, in pairs, or in masses
Aerial hyphae	Absent	Absent	Absent	Usually absent	Present	Absent	Present	Absent
Degree of acid-fastness	Sometimes weakly acid-fast	Not acid-fast	Often partially acid-fast	Usually strongly acid-fast	Often partially acid-fast	Often partially acid-fast	Not acid-fast	Weak to strongly acid-fast
Time for visible colonies to appear (days)	1–2	1–3	1–3	2–40	1–5	1–3	9–21	1–3
Chemical characters								
Fatty acids								
Tuberculostearic acid[b]	–[c]	+	+	+[c]	+	+	+	+
Mycolic acids:								
Overall size (number of carbon atoms)	22–38	34–38	46–66	60–90	44–64	34–52	58–64	62–78

Number of double bonds[d]	0–2	ND	1–4	1–3	0–3	0–4	2–6	1–6
Fatty acid esters released on pyrolysis (number of carbon atoms)[e]	8–18	ND	16–18	22–26	12–18	12–18	16–20	20–22
Phospholipid type[f,g]	1	2	2	2	2	2	2	2
Predominant menaquinones[h]	MK-8(H_2) or MK-9(H_2)	MK-8(H_2)	MK-9(H_2)	MK-9(H_2)	MK-8(H_4, ω-cycl)	MK-8(H_2)	MK-8(H_4, ω-cycl)	MK-9
Guanine and cytosine content of DNA (mol%)	51–67	73	63–69	61–71	64–72	63–73	67.5	68–74
Physiological characters								
Sensitivity to								
5-Fluorouracil (20 µg ml⁻¹)	ND	ND	+	ND	–	+	+	–
Lysozyme (50 µg ml⁻¹)	ND	ND	+	–	–	+	+	–
Mitomycin C (5 µg ml⁻¹)	ND	ND	+	ND	–	+	+	–

+, positive; –, negative; ND, not determined.

[a]Adapted from Goodfellow (1992), Boiron et al. (1992), Holt et al. (1994) and Chun et al. (1997).

[b]Determined by gas liquid chromatography (Embley and Wait 1994).

[c]*C. bovis* contains tuberculostearic acid (Lechevalier, De Bièvre and Lechevalier 1977, Collins, Goodfellow and Minnikin 1982a); *M. gordonae* lacks substantial amounts of tuberculostearic acid (Tisdall, Roberts and Anhalt 1979, Minnikin et al. 1985).

[d]Detected by mass spectrometry (Alshamaony, Goodfellow and Minnikin 1976, Collins, Goodfellow and Minnikin 1982b). The double bonds in mycobacterial mycolic acids may be converted to cyclopropane rings; methyl branches and oxygen functions may be present (Minnikin et al. 1984, Dobson et al. 1985).

[e]Esters of fatty acids detected by gas chromatography of mycolate esters (Lechevalier, Lechevalier and Gerber 1971, Goodfellow et al. 1978, Collins, Goodfellow and Minnikin 1982b).

[f]Phospholipid types: 1, phosphatidylglycerol (variable) and phosphatidylinositol; 2, phosphatidylethanolamine (Lechevalier, Goodfellow and Minnikin 1977, Lechevalier, Stern and Lechevalier 1981).

[g]Phospholipid patterns are determined by thin layer chromatography and chemical analysis (Embley and Wait 1984).

[h]Menaquinones detected by chromatographic or physicochemical analysis (Collins 1994). Abbreviations exemplified by MK-9(H_2), menaquinones having 2 of the 9 isoprene units hydrogenated. Hexahydrogenated menaquinones with 8 isoprene units of which the end 2 units are cyclized (Howarth et al. 1986, Collins et al. 1987).

temperatures such as 10°C and 50°C, but all grow well between 25 and 37°C. Good growth occurs in media at pH 6–9. A generation time of 5.5 h has been reported for *N. asteroides* and *N. brasiliensis* strains (Beadles et al. 1980). Some strains reach stationary phase in 3–7 days, others grow more slowly.

6 BIOCHEMISTRY AND GENETICS

Very little is known about the biochemistry or genetics of the genus *Nocardia*. Members of the genus are catalase-positive, hydrolyse aesculin and allantoin, but do not show arylsulphatase or oxidase activity. They can also metabolize a diverse range of carbon compounds for energy and growth (Tsukamura 1969, Goodfellow 1971). Most strains form acid aerobically from fructose, glucose, glycerol and trehalose but not from cellobiose, lactose, melezitose, melibiose, raffinose or xylose.

Genetic recombination and plasmids have been reported in *N. asteroides* (Kasweck and Little 1982, Kasweck, Little and Bradley 1982) and nocardiophages for *N. asteroides* (Pulverer, Schütt-Gerowitt and Schaal 1975, Prauser 1976, 1981, Andrzejewski et al. 1978), *N. brasiliensis* (Pulverer, Schütt-Gerowitt and Schaal 1975), *Nocardia carnae* (Williams, Wellington and Tipler 1980), *N. otitidiscaviarum* and *Nocardia vaccinii* (Prauser 1976).

7 CELL WALL COMPOSITION

The walls of nocardiae consist of a peptidoglycan, lipid constituents and other polysaccharide or polypeptide fractions (Michel and Bordet 1976). The composition and taxonomic significance of the peptidoglycan has already been mentioned (p. 464). Sugars were reported in the nocardial wall during early investigations on actinomycete wall composition (Cummins and Harris 1956, Romano and Sohler 1956) and a polysaccharide that contained arabinose and galactose was isolated from *N. asteroides* (Bishop and Blank 1958). The presence of arabinose and galactose in the wall was later found to be a common feature of all nocardiae. Glucose has also been detected in the nocardial wall (Michel and Bordet 1976), as have amino acids that are not part of the peptidoglycan (Sohler, Romano and Nickerson 1958).

Mycolic acids, α-branched, β-hydroxylated long-chain fatty acids, are the most characteristic component of the walls of nocardiae and related actinomycetes (Minnikin and Goodfellow 1980, Minnikin 1993, Chun et al. 1997). These compounds, which are covalently linked to arabinose units of the wall arabinogalactan, are found in strains of *Corynebacterium*, *Dietzia*, *Gordona*, *Nocardia*, *Rhodococcus*, *Skermania* and *Tsukamurella* but were discovered in *Mycobacterium*. Mycolic acids with between 44 and 64 carbon atoms have been isolated from *N. asteroides* (Bordet et al. 1965), *N. brasiliensis* (Lanéelle and Asselineau 1970), *N. farcinica* (Yano, Imaeda and Tsukamura 1990), *Nocardia nova* (Yano, Imaeda and Tsukamura

1990), *N. otitidiscaviarum* (Alshamaony, Goodfellow and Minnikin 1976) and *Nocardia seriolae* (Kudo, Hatai and Seino 1988). Some nocardiae have also been found to contain shorter chain mycolic acids (Pommier and Michel 1985).

Several methods are available for the detection and characterization of the different structural types of mycolic acids (Minnikin and Goodfellow 1980, Minnikin 1993, Embley and Wait 1994). Qualitative evaluation of mycolic acids can be achieved by thin layer chromatography (TLC, Minnikin, Alshamaony and Goodfellow 1975); mycolic acids can be positively identified on chromatograms by their characteristic immobility when plates are washed with methanol:water (5:2, v/v). Methanolysates of mycobacteria typically give a multispot pattern, tsukamurellae a characteristic 2-spot configuration and nocardiae and other mycolic acid-containing actinomycetes single spots whose mobilities reflect the chain length and structure of the constituent mycolic acids (Minnikin 1993, Yassin, Binder and Schaal 1993). *Mycobacterium brumae*, *Mycobacterium fallax* and *Mycobacterium triviale* are not typical mycobacteria in the sense that they give single spot patterns (Dobson et al. 1985, Luquin et al. 1993) and can thereby be confused with gordonae and nocardiae. However, mycobacterial mycolic acids can readily be recognized as they are precipitated when treated with a mixture of acetonitrile and toluene (3:2, v/v; Hamid, Minnikin and Goodfellow 1993). By contrast, the shorter-chain components from nocardiae and other mycolic acid-containing actinomycetes remain in solution.

Once mycolic acids have been detected, their esters can be isolated and examined by pyrolysis gas chromatography, high performance liquid chromatography (HPLC), mass spectrometry, or by gas chromatography-mass spectrometry (GC-MS). Nocardial mycolic acids give C_{12}–C_{18} esters on pyrolysis (Lechevalier, Lechevalier and Gerber 1971, Hamid, Minnikin and Goodfellow 1993); mycolic acids with unsaturation in the β-position have been observed in strains of *N. carnae* and *N. vaccinii* (Lechevalier and Lechevalier 1974). Reverse-phase HPLC of *p*-bromophenacyl esters of mycolic acids has been used to distinguish between members of mycolic acid-containing genera (Butler, Kilburn and Kubica 1987, Butler, Jost and Kilburn 1991, De Briel et al. 1993).

The overall size of mycolates, their degree of unsaturation, and the nature of the long alkyl chain can be measured by mass spectrometry (Maurice, Vacheron and Michel 1971, Alshamaony, Goodfellow and Minnikin 1976). Chemical analysis can be taken further by using GC-MS of trimethylsilyl and tertbutyldimethylsilyl derivatives of mycolic acids (Yano et al. 1978, Pommier and Michel 1985, Kudo, Hatai and Seino 1988, Yano, Imaeda and Tsukamura 1990). This procedure separates mycolic ester derivatives into their homologous components each of which can be analysed by mass spectrometry. Detailed chemical analyses of mycolic acids can be used to assign mycolic acid-containing organisms to species (Yano et al. 1986, Ruimy et al. 1996).

8 ANTIGENIC PROPERTIES

Agglutination, complement fixation, immunodiffusion, immunoelectrophoresis and skin testing have all been applied to nocardiae (Lind and Ridell 1976, Magnusson 1976, Pier 1984). It has been demonstrated that representatives of the genera *Corynebacterium*, *Mycobacterium*, *Nocardia* and *Rhodococcus* (including *Gordona*) have antigens in common

(Cummins 1962, 1965, Ridell 1974, 1977, 1981a, Ridell et al. 1979) and that ribosomes account for many of the cross-reactions observed between representatives of these taxa (Ridell 1981a). Immunodiffusion analysis, with disintegrated cells as antigens, allowed the definition of 3 groups of *N. asteroides* and one of *N. otitidiscaviarum* (Ridell 1981b).

Serological procedures and testing for cutaneous hypersensitivity have been used in the diagnosis of nocardiosis in animals and humans (Bojalil and Zamora 1963, Shainhaus, Pier and Stevens 1978). Antigenic preparations of 2 main types have been used. Culture-filtrate antigens have been employed without further absorption or chemical manipulation, as have polysaccharide antigens extracted and chemically purified from nocardial cells. These latter antigens are highly specific and have been used extensively in tests for cutaneous hypersensitivity and in immunodiffusion (Zamora, Bojalil and Bastarrachea 1963). Antigens in culture filtrates have been used to establish 4 serotypes within *N. asteroides*, to define a species-specific antigen for *N. otitidiscaviarum* (Pier and Fichtner 1971), and to determine cutaneous hypersensitivity in human patients and cattle infected with *N. asteroides*, *N. brasiliensis* and *N. otitidiscaviarum* (Pier, Thurston and Larson 1968, Salman, Bushnell and Pier 1982). These antigens have also been used successfully in epidemiological studies of group infections in both humans (Stevens et al. 1981) and cattle (Pier and Fichtner 1981).

Tests designed to demonstrate delayed cutaneous hypersensitivity and humoral antibodies have been described for the diagnosis of nocardiosis (Boiron et al. 1993). An enzyme-linked immunosorbent assay (ELISA) technique based on a 55 kDa protein specific to *Nocardia* allowed the detection of antibodies in over 90% of patients with cutaneous or pulmonary nocardiosis (Angeles and Sugar 1987). The value of the immunoblot technique has also been demonstrated in the diagnosis of nocardiosis (Boiron and Provost 1990a, Boiron and Stynen 1992). Monoclonal antibodies raised against a specific 54 kDa protein may prove to be of value in the detection of this antigen in sera of patients with nocardiosis (Boiron et al. 1992b).

9 RESISTANCE TO PHYSICAL AND CHEMICAL AGENTS

Nocardiae are quite resistant to heat and desiccation. Most strains can withstand 50°C for 8 h; a strain of *N. asteroides* (*Nocardia sebivorans*) withstood exposure to 90°C for 10 min when dispersed in phosphate solution (Erikson 1955). Lysozyme resistance is characteristic of nocardiae (Gordon and Barnett 1977, Mordarska et al. 1978), as is their ability to grow in the presence of bleomycin (25 µg ml^{-1}; Tsukamura 1982a), 5-fluorouracil (20 µg ml^{-1}; Tsukamura 1981a), mitomycin C (10 µg ml^{-1}; Tsukamura 1981b) and picric acid (0.2%, w/v; Tsukamura 1965).

Antimicrobial susceptibility testing is difficult as results may be influenced by factors such as pH,

inoculum size, composition of agar assay media and by spontaneous drug degradation due to the slow growth rate of the organism (McNeil and Brown 1994). Nevertheless, several antimicrobial susceptibility testing methods have been recommended, but none of them has been accepted as the standard method. Once a standardized method has been accepted, inter- and intralaboratory reproducibility can be evaluated and the role of antimicrobial susceptibility patterns as predictors of clinical outcome and taxonomic relationships can be established.

The most commonly used antimicrobial testing procedures are the modified disk diffusion method (Wallace et al. 1977, Boiron and Provost 1988, 1990b, Boiron et al. 1992a), the agar dilution method (Carroll, Brown and Haley 1977, Yazawa, Mikami and Uno 1989) and the broth microdiffusion method (Wallace et al. 1988, McNeil et al. 1990). The different antimicrobial susceptibility profiles of pathogenic species may be of taxonomic importance (Boiron et al. 1993). *N. otitidiscaviarum* strains are sensitive to amikacin, chloramphenicol, clindamycin, erythromycin, tetracyclines and to the association trimethoprim + sulphonamides and thereby can be distinguished from *N. asteroides* and *N. brasiliensis* (Boiron and Provost 1988). Similarly, strains of *N. nova* are sensitive to ampicillin and erythromycin, but are resistant to carbenicillin (Wallace et al. 1991). *N. farcinica* strains are resistant to cephamandole, cefotaxime and tobramycin (Wallace et al. 1990). Members of the *N. asteroides* complex can be assigned to several major antibiotypes (Wallace and Steele 1988, Wallace et al. 1988). Antibiotic sensitivity of *N. asteroides* varies with the stage of growth (Locci 1980).

10 PATHOGENICITY

Nocardiae cause a variety of suppurative infections in humans and animals (Schaal and Lee 1992, Beaman and Beaman 1994, McNeil and Brown 1994) (see also Volume 3, Chapter 39). Infection may occur by inhalation, and through contaminated wounds and traumatic implantations. Three distinct clinical symptoms may develop:

1 primary pulmonary and systemic
2 primary cutaneous and
3 primary subcutaneous nocardiosis.

Primary pulmonary nocardiosis may be subclinical or pneumonic; it may be chronic or acute with possible secondary, often fatal, involvement with other organs, notably the brain. In non-tropical countries, most infections are caused by *N. asteroides*, *N. farcinica* and *N. nova*, relatively few by *N. brasiliensis*, *N. otitidiscaviarum* and *Nocardia transvalensis*. *N. farcinica* shows a greater degree of virulence than *N. asteroides* (Schaal and Lee 1992). Localized cutaneous and subcutaneous nocardioses are encountered less frequently. Their aetiological agents include *N. asteroides* and *N. brasiliensis*, and to a lesser extent *N. farcinica*, *N. otitidiscaviarum* and *N. transvalensis*.

Nocardiosis usually develops as an opportunist infection complicating debilitating primary diseases such as leukaemia, lymphoma and other neoplasms, or in patients undergoing immunosuppression (McNeil and Brown 1994). Clinical, radiological and histopathological findings are not sufficient for the recognition of the disease. Definitive diagnosis depends on the isolation and identification of the causal organism from clinical material. These procedures are not straightforward; hence, the true incidence of the disease is masked, a problem which is compounded by poor documentation. Recent increases in the reported frequency of human nocardial infections can be attributed to the widespread use of immunosuppressive drugs, improved selective isolation procedures and increased clinical and microbiological awareness. In France, it has been estimated that up to 250 new cases of nocardiosis occur each year (Boiron et al. 1990). Current estimates indicate that considerably more than 1000 cases of the disease are diagnosed each year in the USA (Beaman 1988).

Nocardiosis is usually considered to be a late-presenting, community-acquired infection but there is growing evidence that the disease is transmissible. Clusters of patients with *N. asteroides* infections have been reported from liver (Sahathevan et al. 1991) and renal transplant units (Houang et al. 1980, Baddour et al. 1986). In another outbreak, Schaal (1991) suggested that nosocomial air-borne transmission, possibly in the operating room environment, was the cause of a cluster of *N. farcinica* postoperative wound infections in patients undergoing cardiac and other vascular surgeries at a university hospital. Nocardial infections also occur in HIV patients (Kim, Minamato and Grieco 1991, Javaly, Horowitz and Wormser 1992) though the suggestion by some clinicians that nocardiosis is a rare complication in AIDS patients is probably more apparent than real (Beaman and Beaman 1994).

Reliable and reproducible information has been obtained over the past 25 years about the mechanism of pathogenesis and host immunity to nocardial infection (Beaman and Beaman 1994). It has been shown that virulent strains of *N. asteroides* are facultative intracellular pathogens that can grow in a variety of cells from humans and experimental animals. The mechanisms of pathogenesis are multiple, complex, and not yet fully understood (Beaman et al. 1992). The virulence of *N. asteroides* appears to be associated with its stage of growth and with its capacity to inhibit phagosome–lysozyme fusion, neutralize phagosomal acidification, resist oxidative killing mechanisms of phagocytes, alter lysosomal enzymes within phagocytes, and by its ability to invade and grow within the brains of experimental animals. The mechanisms of host resistance to nocardiae are also complex and poorly understood (Beaman 1992). Although L-forms can be isolated from humans, their role in human disease is not known (Beaman 1982).

Actinomycete mycetomas are localized, chronic progressive infections of the skin and subcutaneous tissue that are endemic in many tropical and subtropical countries (see also Volume 3, Chapter 39). They are characterized by subcutaneous granulomata and abscesses and by areas of induration. Sinus tracts, often multiple, may discharge granules that have a characteristic size, shape and colour. The granules consist of small colonies of the infective agent surrounded by masses of inflammatory cells. *N. brasiliensis* is the most frequently recognized cause of *Nocardia*-induced mycetomas. However, *N. asteroides*, *N. otitidiscaviarum* and *N. transvalensis* can also induce mycetomas (Beaman and Beaman 1994). Mycetomas may occasionally be seen in patients from temperate countries. The disease process usually begins at the site of a localized injury such as a puncture wound caused by a thorn or splinter. Human mycetoma has been simulated in a mouse model (González-Ochoa 1973) which has been used to study aspects of host–parasite relationships (Ortiz-Ortiz, Melendro and Conde 1984).

Pathogenic nocardiae not only cause disease in humans but are also agents of similar diseases in a wide range of animals (Beaman and Sugar 1983, Beaman and Beaman 1994). Animals susceptible to nocardial infections include cattle, cats, dogs, chickens, ducks, fish, goats, sheep and swine. Pulmonary and systemic nocardioses, including infections of the brain, are the most frequently recognized conditions; however, cutaneous and mycetomatous lesions also occur. In dairy animals, especially cows, mastitis is a distinct clinical manifestation of major significance (Battig et al. 1990, Stark and Anderson 1992, Manninen, Smith and Kim 1993). The most frequently recognized pathogen of animals is *N. asteroides* followed by *N. brasiliensis* and *N. otitidiscaviarum*. Strains involved in the recent Canadian mastitis epizootic were presumptively identified as *N. farcinica* (Manninen, Smith and Kim 1993). In addition, *N. seriolae* has been isolated from infections in fish (Kudo, Hatai and Seino 1988).

11 ISOLATION AND CULTIVATION

In patients with a suspected nocardial infection and a compatible clinical picture, a definitive diagnosis usually depends on the demonstration of the organisms in smears or sections examined microscopically prior to the isolation and identification of the causal agent (Schaal 1984, McNeil and Brown 1992, Goodfellow 1996). Clinical material, such as bronchial washings, sinus discharge and biopsy and autopsy specimens, need to be examined as soon as possible to prevent overgrowth by contaminants. Fluid material can be examined in wet mounts under the microscope without staining. Gram-positive branched filaments (c. 1 μm in diameter) can be seen at high magnification ($\times 1000$); the filaments may show evidence of fragmentation into rod and coccoid-like elements. Acid-fastness, which is usually more pronounced in clinical than cultured material, is best seen using the modified Kinyoun acid-fast procedure (Berd 1973). Even with this technique, nocardiae may be only partially acid-fast; that is, they show both acid-fast and non-acid-fast bacilli and filaments.

Sputum is the most readily available material from pulmonary nocardial infections. However, several fresh samples may need to be examined as some specimens may not contain nocardiae. It is also necessary to culture the same organism from a number of independent samples to ensure its aetiological role. Invasive procedures, such as bronchoscopic biopsy and fine needle aspiration, may be needed when repeated sputum cultures fail to yield nocardiae. In the case of systemic nocardiosis, abscesses can be punctured or incised to obtain pus. Involvement of the central nervous system is diagnosed from brain abscess material or cerebrospinal fluid. The latter may give negative results, even in cases of serious infection, as the pathogen can be present as L-forms or restricted to an abscess. Exudate from discharging sinuses and biopsy material should be examined in cases of actinomycetoma and cutaneous infections.

Several general purpose media can be used to isolate nocardiae from clinical material. They include brain–heart infusion, Sabouraud dextrose and yeast extract–malt extract agars (Goodfellow 1992). Nevertheless, selective media are needed to isolate nocardiae from clinical specimens that harbour large numbers of contaminating bacteria. Several media have been recommended for the selective isolation of nocardiae, notably chemically defined formulations supplemented with paraffin (Shawar, Moore and LaRocco 1990), Czapek's agar amended with yeast extract (Higgins and Lechevalier 1969), Diagnostic Sensitivity Test (DST) agar supplemented with tetracyclines (Orchard and Goodfellow 1974), *Nocardia* selective agar (Schaal 1972), buffered charcoal yeast extract agar supplemented with anisomycin, polymixin and vancomycin (Garrett, Holmes and Nolte 1992) and Sabouraud dextrose agar supplemented with chloramphenicol (Ajello and Roberts 1981). The pretreatment of material with the concentration and digestion–decontamination procedures used in the isolation of mycobacteria should not be employed as they reduce the isolation rate of nocardiae (Schaal 1977).

Nocardiae usually form well sized colonies on most standard laboratory media, including modified Bennett's, brain–heart infusion, Sabouraud dextrose, modified Sauton's, yeast extract–glucose and yeast extract–malt extract agars, within 14 days at 37°C.

12 CLASSIFICATION

The marked improvements made in recent years in the classification of mycolic acid-containing actinomycetes have been extensively reviewed (Goodfellow 1992, Goodfellow and Magee 1997). The continued application of chemotaxonomic, numerical phenetic and molecular systematic methods has led to improved descriptions of established genera, the recognition of new genera and species, and the reduction of some poorly described taxa to synonyms of previously proposed species. The improved taxonomy provides an essential framework for the classification of novel mycolata strains. It is clear from numerical taxonomic and molecular systematic studies that additional mycolata strains have still to be fully characterized and named (Schuppler et al. 1995, Goodfellow et al. 1996).

12.1 Suprageneric relationships

Analyses of 16S rRNA sequence data show that mycolic acid-containing actinomycetes form a well defined clade within the evolutionary radiation occupied by actinomycetes (Embley and Stackebrandt 1994, Pascual et al. 1995, Ruimy et al. 1995). *Nocardia* forms

a distinct phyletic line within this clade (Chun and Goodfellow 1995) and has a phylogenetic depth comparable to that of the other mycolata genera (Fig. 21.2). Mycolata strains have many properties in common, notably chemical characters. They contain *meso*-A$_2$pm as the diamino acid of the wall peptidoglycan, arabinose and galactose as major wall sugars, high proportions of straight-chain saturated and monounsaturated fatty acids, and diphosphatidylglycerol, phosphatidylinositol and phosphatidylinositol mannosides as predominant phospholipids. Glycolipids have not been systematically investigated but representative corynebacteria, mycobacteria, nocardiae and rhodococci contain 6,6′-dimycolic esters of trehalose, the so-called chord factors. Mycolic acid-containing actinomycetes also have antigens in common (see p. 468).

The congruence found between the discontinuous distribution of certain chemical markers and the emerging phylogeny provides the kernal of a proposal to assign mycolata strains to 2 suprageneric taxa, namely the families Corynebacteriaceae and Mycobacteriaceae (Chun et al. 1996). The emended family Corynebacteriaceae accommodates the genera *Corynebacterium* and *Dietzia*, and the revised family Mycobacteriaceae, the genera *Gordona*, *Mycobacterium*, *Nocardia*, *Rhodococcus*, *Skermania* and *Tsukamurella*. *Corynebacterium amycolatum* (Collins, Burton and Jones 1988) and *Turicella otitidis* (Funke et al. 1994), which lack mycolic acids, fall within the evolutionary radiation of the family Corynebacteriaceae (Fig. 21.2).

12.2 Subgeneric relationships

The redefined genus *Nocardia* forms a homogeneous taxon which contains 11 validly described species. The latter can be assigned to at least 3 rRNA subgroups centred on the earliest described species, namely *N. asteroides*, *N. brasiliensis* and *N. otitidiscaviarum*. The *N. asteroides* and *N. otitidiscaviarum* subclades are supported by high bootstrap values (Fig. 21.2). *N. brasiliensis*, *N. farcinica*, *N. otitidiscaviarum* and *N. seriolae* are usually seen as homogeneous species (Goodfellow 1992) but *N. asteroides* is markedly heterogeneous. The heterogeneity of the latter has been established in antimicrobial susceptibility (Wallace et al. 1988, 1990), DNA relatedness (Bradley and Mordarski 1976, Mordarski et al. 1977), immunological (Pier and Fichtner 1971, Magnusson 1976, Ridell 1981a), mycolic acid (Yano, Imaeda and Tsukamura 1990), numerical taxonomic (Goodfellow 1971, Orchard and Goodfellow 1980, Tsukamura 1982b), phage sensitivity (Pulverer, Schütt-Gerowitt and Schaal 1975) and molecular fingerprinting (Laurent et al. 1996) studies.

Investigations such as those outlined above have shown that many strains isolated from clinical specimens and previously identified as *N. asteroides* actually belong to different species. One of these new taxa, *N. nova*, was cited as a species *incertae sedis* in the current edition of *Bergey's Manual of Determinative Bacteriology* (Goodfellow and Lechevalier 1989). However, in 1990, Yano, Imaeda and Tsukamura were able to sep-

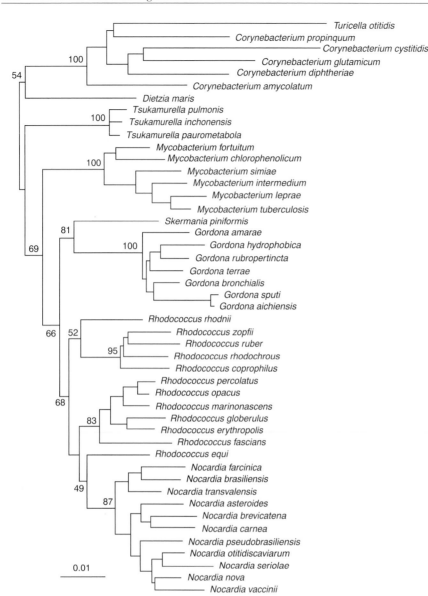

Fig. 21.2 Phylogenetic tree showing relationships between mycolic acid-containing taxa based on full 16S rRNA sequences. The tree was generated using the neighbor-joining method (Saitou and Nei 1987). The numbers at the nodes indicate the levels of bootstrap support based on data for 1000 replicates.

arate *N. nova* from *N. asteroides* and *N. farcinica* by DNA relatedness analysis, mycolic acid profiles and numerical taxonomy. The taxonomic status of this species was also supported by a distinct antimicrobial resistance pattern (Wallace et al. 1991). The most recent addition to the genus, *Nocardia pseudobrasiliensis*, was also circumscribed using a rich combination of genotypic and phenotypic data (Ruimy et al. 1996).

13 IDENTIFICATION

The improved classification of the genus *Nocardia* provides a sound base for the continued search for better diagnostic methods to distinguish between members of clinically significant taxa.

13.1 Differentiation at genus level

Nocardiae are most easily distinguished from actinomadurae, streptomycetes and other sporoactinomy-

cetes (Table 21.1) as they alone have whole-organism hydrolysates containing mycolic acids. Qualitative evaluation of mycolic acids can be easily and quickly achieved by the TLC technique of Minnikin, Alshamaony and Goodfellow (1975). By contrast, a combination of chemical, morphological and physiological tests is necessary to distinguish between the mycolata genera (Table 21.2). Simplified chemical procedures applicable in clinical laboratories are available for the detection of diagnostic amino acids and sugars (Hancock 1994), fatty acids, including mycolic acids (Embley and Wait 1994), menaquinones (Collins 1994) and polar lipids (Suzuki, Goodfellow and O'Donnell 1993). The resistance of nocardiae to bleomycin (Tsukamura 1982a), 5-fluorouracil (Tsukamura 1981a), lysozyme (Gordon and Barnett 1977, Mordarska et al. 1978) and mitomycin C (Tsukamura 1981b) may be useful in distinguishing them from most other mycolata strains.

13.2 Differentiation at species level

Nocardia spp. can be difficult to identify due to a dearth of suitable phenotypic tests. The phenotypic identification tests recommended by a number of investigators (Goodfellow and Lechevalier 1989, Boiron et al. 1993) are inadequate and only give presumptive identifications. Partial identification of the major causal agents of nocardiosis can be achieved with a few simple biochemical, degradation and growth tests (Table 21.3) though the time required from specimen submission to species identification may take several weeks. Supplementary tests based on antibiotic sensitivity and enzymatic profiles have been proposed for the separation of key nocardial species but have still to be extensively applied (Boiron and Provost 1990c, Boiron et al. 1993). The use of polymerase chain reaction (PCR) coupled with restriction endonuclease analysis of PCR products has been the focus of recent interest for the separation of *Nocardia* spp. (Lungu et al. 1994, Steingrube et al. 1995). This approach promises to provide a rapid, sensitive and effective way of identifying clinically significant nocardiae. Agents of actinomycetoma other than nocardiae lack mycolic acids (Table 21.1).

13.3 Other diagnostic methods

Serological tests for the diagnosis of nocardial infections have already been considered (see p. 469) but their practical value remains limited at present, as does the use of DNA probes (Boiron et al. 1993, Goodfellow 1996). Monoclonal antibodies developed for use in the localization, purification and characterization of *Nocardia* antigens may possibly serve as diagnostic reagents (Jimenez, Diaz and Zlotnik 1990), as may those raised against the specific 54 kDa protein mentioned earlier (see p. 469). A conventional solid-phase ELISA, based on 2 immunodominant antigens, can be used to confirm the diagnosis of *N. brasiliensis* infections in human mycetoma cases (Salinas-Carmona, Welsh and Casillas 1993). DNA probes have been prepared for the rapid identification of *N. asteroides* using genomic libraries generated for selected strains of *N. asteroides* (Brownell and Belcher 1990).

13.4 Typing methods

Several typing systems have been used in epidemiological studies of nocardial outbreaks. *N. asteroides* strains involved in human or animal infections produce 1–4 antigens which can be detected by gel diffusion (Pier and Fichtner 1971). This technique was successfully used in an investigation of an outbreak of nocardiosis in immunocompromised patients in a renal transplant unit (Stevens et al. 1981). Isolates from the patients and the environment were found to have a characteristic type III antigen pattern. There is also evidence that comparisons of plasmid (Jonsson et al. 1986) and restriction fragment length polymorphism (RFLP; Patterson et al. 1992) profiles can be used to type *N. asteroides* isolates. Patterson and his colleagues showed

that 18 out of 19 clinical isolates had an identical RFLP pattern when examined with the restriction enzyme *Pvu*III. Ribotyping has also been used to distinguish between strains assigned to the *N. asteroides* complex (Laurent et al. 1996).

ACTINOMADURA AND OTHER SPOROACTINOMYCETES

14 *ACTINOMADURA*

14.1 Definition

Actinomadurae are aerobic, gram-positive, non-acid alcohol-fast, non-motile actinomycetes that form a non-fragmenting, extensively branched substrate mycelium. When present, aerial hyphae carry chains of up to 15 spores. Spore chains may be straight, hooked (open loops) or irregular spirals (1–4 turns) and spore surfaces folded, irregular, smooth, spiny or warty. The aerial mycelium may be blue, brown, cream, grey, green, pink, red, white or yellow. In the absence of aerial mycelium, colonies have a leathery or cartilagenous appearance. The organism is chemo-organotrophic with an oxidative type of carbohydrate metabolism. The temperature range is 10–60°C.

The peptidoglycan contains *meso*-diaminopimelic acid, N-acetylated muramic acid and is of the A1γ type. Whole-organism hydrolysates contain galactose, glucose, mannose, ribose and madurose, the latter sometimes in trace amounts. Actinomadurae contain major proportions of hexahydrogenated menaquinones with 9 isoprene units saturated at sites II, III and VIII, diphosphatidylglycerol and phosphatidylinositol as major phospholipids, and complex mixtures of fatty acids with hexadecanoic, 14-methylpentadecanoic and 10-methyloctadecanoic acids predominating. Mycolic acids are not produced. The G + C composition of the DNA is 66–72 mol%. The organism is widely distributed in soil. Some strains are pathogenic for humans and animals. The type species is *Actinomadura madurae*.

14.2 Introduction and historical perspective

The genus *Actinomadura* was proposed by Lechevalier MP and Lechevalier HA (1970) for nocardiae that formed stable mycelia with walls containing *meso*-A₂pm without characteristic sugars (wall chemotype III *sensu* Lechevalier and Lechevalier 1970). The taxon was listed as a genus *incertae sedis* in the eighth edition of *Bergey's Manual of Determinative Bacteriology* (McClung 1974) but was included on the 'Approved Lists of Bacterial Names' (Skerman, McGowan and Sneath 1980). The genus was introduced for 3 species, *dasson-*

Table 21.2 Characteristics of *Nocardia* and non-mycolic acid containing taxa encompassing actinomycetes previously associated with the genus

Character	Nocardia	Actinomadura	Amycolatopsis	Microtetraspora	Nocardiopsis	Oerskovia	Pseudonocardia	Rothia	Saccharothrix
Morphological properties									
Substrate mycelium	Fragments into rods and cocci	Stable, extensively branched	Fragments into squarish elements	Stable, extensively branched	May fragment into rods and cocci	Fragments into rod-shaped motile, flagellate elements	Hyphae are segmented and may be zig-zag shaped. They carry chains of spores	When formed fragments into rods and cocci	Fragments into ovoid to bacillary elements
Aerial mycelium	Sparse to moderate, nearly always formed	Moderately developed or absent, may bear chains up to 15 spores	When formed may be sterile or differentiated into squarish or oval elements	Moderately developed or absent, may bear chains up to 30 spores	Well developed forms long spore chains	Absent	Aerial hyphae when formed are segmented and often zig-zag shaped. They bear chains of spores formed by acropetal budding or septation.	Absent	Fragments into ovoid to bacillary elements
Acid-fastness	Usually partially acid-fast	Negative	Negative	Negative	Negative	Negative	Negative	Negative	Negative

Chemical properties

Metabolism of glucose	Oxidative	Oxidative	Oxidative	Oxidative	Oxidative	Fermentative and oxidative	Oxidative	Fermentative and oxidative	Oxidative
Wall chemotype[a]	IV	III	IV	III	III	VI	IV	VI	III
Characteristic sugars	Arabinose, galactose	Madurose	Arabinose, galactose	Madurose	None	Galactose	Arabinose, galactose	None	Galactose, rhamnose
Peptidoglycan types[b]	A1γ	A1γ	A1γ	A1γ	Not determined	A4α	A1γ	A3α	Not determined
Major fatty acids[c]	S,U,T	S,U,I,A	S,U,I,A	S,U,I,A	S,U,I,A	S,I,A	S,U,I,A	S,I,A	S,U,I,A,T
Major menaquinones (MK)[d]	Present -8(H₄) or -9(H₂)	Absent -9(H₆)	Absent -9(H₂,H₄)	Absent -9(H₄)	Absent -10(H₂, H₄,H₆)	Absent -9(H₄)	Absent -8(H₄)	Absent -7	Absent -8(H₄) or -9(H₄)
Phospholipid type[e]	2	1	2	4	3	5	3	1	2
DNA G + C mol%	64–72	66–72	66–69	66–69	64–69	70–75	68–79	65–70	70–76

[a]Major constituents in cell walls of types: III, *meso*-A₂pm; IV, *meso*-A₂pm, arabinose, galactose; VI, lysine (with variable presence of aspartic acid and galactose).

[b]According to Schleifer and Kandler (1972) and Schleifer and Seidl (1985).

[c]Abbreviations: S, straight-chain saturated; U, monounsaturated; A, *anteiso*-methyl-branched; I, *iso*-methyl-branched; T, 10-methyl-branched (tuberculostearic acid).

[d]Abbreviations exemplified by MK-9(H₂), menaquinone with 2 of the 9 isoprene units hydrogenated.

[e]Characteristic phospholipids: 1, phosphatidylglycerol (variable); 2, only phosphatidylethanolamine; 3, phosphatidylcholine (with phosphatidylethanolamine, phosphatidylmethylethanolamine and phosphatidylglycerol variable, no phospholipids containing glucosamine); 4, phospholipids containing glucosamine (with phosphatidylethanolamine and phosphatidylmethylethanolamine); 5, phospholipids containing glucosamine and phosphatidylglycerol; all preparations contain phosphatidylinositol (Lechevalier, De Bièvre and Lechevalier 1977, Lechevalier, Stern and Lechevalier 1981).

Table 21.3   Characters differentiating species of the genus *Nocardia*

Character	N. asteroides	N. brasiliensis	N. brevicatena	N. carnea	N. farcinica	N. noza	N. otitidis-caviarum	N. pseudobrasiliensis	N. seriolae	N. transvalensis	N. vaccinii
Decomposition of											
Adenine	-	-	-	-	-	-	-	+	-	v	-
Casein	-	+	-	-	-	-	-	+	-	-	-
Elastin	-	+	-	-	-	-	-	v	-	-	-
Hypoxanthine	-	+	-	-	+	-	+	+	-	+	+
Testosterone	+	+	+	+	+	+	+	-	v	-	-
Tyrosine	-	+	-	-	-	+	-	+	-	-	-
Xanthine	-	-	-	-	-	-	+	-	-	v	-
Growth on sole carbon sources (1%, w/v)											
L-Arabinose	-	-	-	+	-	-	-	ND	ND	-	v
D-Mannitol	-	+	-	-	-	-	+	ND	-	-	+
L-Rhamnose	-[a]	-	+	-	+	-	-	ND	-	-	+
Production of											
Nitrate reductase	+	+	-	+	+	+	+	-	ND	+	+
Urease	+	+	-	-	+	+	+	+	-	+	+

Symbols: +, ≥90% of strains are positive; −, ≥90% of strains are negative; v, variable; ND, not determined.
For details of test procedures see Goodfellow (1971), Goodfellow and Pirouz (1982), and Boiron et al. (1993).
[a]*N. asteroides* and *N. farcinica* can also be distinguished by the ability of the latter to use *iso*-amyl alcohol, 2,3-butylene glycol and 1,2-propylene glycol as sole carbon sources (Schaal 1977). Similarly, *N. farcinica* and *N. nova* can be distinguished by the capacity of the former to grow on acetamide and 1,3-butylene glycol as a sole carbon source (Boiron et al. 1993).

villei, madurae and *pelletieri*, a number that rose to 26 (Meyer 1989). In 1976, Meyer transferred '*A. dassonvillei*' to the new genus *Nocardiopsis*, as *Nocardiopsis dassonvillei*.

The taxonomy of the genus *Actinomadura* has undergone marked revision due to the application of chemical, numerical taxonomic and molecular systematic methods (Goodfellow, Trujillo and Alderson 1995). Fischer, Kroppenstedt and Stackebrandt (1983) were amongst the first to realize that the genus was markedly heterogeneous; they assigned representative strains to 2 aggregate groups, based on *A. madurae* and *Actinomadura pusilla*. This division was formalized by Kroppenstedt, Stackebrandt and Goodfellow (1990) who proposed that the genus *Actinomadura* be retained for *A. madurae* and related species and that the *A. pusilla* group be reclassified in the genus *Microtetraspora*. This proposition was subsequently strongly supported by analyses of the ribosomal protein AT-L30 (Ochi, Miiyadoh and Tamura 1991) and 16S rRNA (Wang, Zhang and Ruan 1996). Three out of the 27 validly described species of *Actinomadura* are clinically significant. One of these species, *Actinomadura latina*, was proposed by Trujillo and Goodfellow (1996) for strains previously classified as *Actinomadura pelletieri*. Other sporoactinomycetes that cause human infections include *Nocardiopsis dassonvillei* and *Streptomyces somaliensis*.

14.3 Pathogenic species

The taxonomic integrity of *A. latina* is supported by a rich blend of genotypic and phenotypic data (Trujillo and Goodfellow 1997). The organism forms cream to pink colonies that rarely bear aerial hyphae. Little is known about the geographical distribution of the organism or its prevalence as an agent of actinomycetoma.

A. madurae was first isolated from an Algerian case of Madura foot and described by Vincent (1894) as *Streptothrix madurae*, this organism was later assigned to several genera before being classified in the genus *Actinomadura* (Lacey, Goodfellow and Alderson 1978). It forms greyish-yellow colonies that may carry sparse-to-moderate amounts of aerial hyphae, which may differentiate to give short, hooked or curled spore chains of up to 12 spores. The latter are elliptical or round with warty surfaces. Details of the biochemical, chemical and physiological properties of the organism are available (Fischer, Kroppenstedt and Stackebrandt 1983, Athalye, Goodfellow and Minnikin 1984, Athalye et al. 1985, Trujillo and Goodfellow 1997). The pigment formed is nonylprodigiosin (Gerber 1969). In *A. madurae* infections, the pus contains granules that are soft, white-to-yellow or reddish, usually 1–5 mm in diameter, and spherical or angular with lobes.

A. pelletieri was first observed by Laveran (1906) in a fistulous tumour of the knee in Senegal. It appeared to be a micrococcus arranged in zoogloeal masses and short chains, and was called *Micrococcus pelletieri*. Another strain was isolated by Thiroux and Pelletier (1912) from a large tumour of the thorax that was ulcerating and discharging pus containing red granules. Similar granules were present in the purulent sputum. The name *Nocardia pelletieri* was proposed by Pinoy (1912). *A. pelletieri* strains form characteristic red colonies on Sabouraud's glucose agar when incubated at 25–28°C for 10 days. Aerial hyphae are rarely found in old laboratory cultures. However, hooked or spiral chains of up to 6 spores have been observed on the aerial mycelium. The spores are subspherical with warty surfaces. Details of some of the biological properties of the organism have been recorded (Fischer, Kroppenstedt and Stackebrandt 1983, Athalye, Goodfellow and Minnikin 1984, Athalye et al. 1985, Trujillo and Goodfellow 1997). In infections caused by *A. pelletieri*, the pus contains granules that are soft, deep red, 0.3–0.5 mm in diameter and usually spherical-to-oval.

The first *Nocardiopsis dassonvillei* strains were isolated from mildewed grain and named '*Streptothrix dassonvillei*' by Brocq-Rousseu (1904). In 1911, Liégard and Landrieu isolated a similar organism from a patient with conjunctivitis but labelled it *Nocardia dassonvillei*. Most of the 26 strains of *Nocardiopsis dassonvillei* examined by Gordon and Horan (1968) were from human and animal infections, but their status as pathogens was uncertain. However, there have been 3 reports of cutaneous infections caused by *N. dassonvillei*: one was a case of mycetoma (Sindhuphak, MacDonald and Head 1985), the second a familial cluster of skin infections (Singh et al. 1991) and the third occurred in an elderly man, who developed a hand abscess following a soil-contaminated injury (Philip and Roberts 1984). Recognition of *N. dassonvillei* is based largely on morphology, but chemical markers can also be used to distinguish it from *Actinomadura* and other sporoactinomycetes (Table 21.1). The organism forms abundant aerial hyphae which typically differentiate into chains of smooth spores of variable length. During sporogenesis, hyphae have a zig-zag appearance due to developing spores subtending angles of varying degree to adjacent spores. The latter are enriched within a fibrillar sheath and have thickened polar walls. *Nocardiopsis* strains are common in soil, mouldy hay and grain.

Streptomyces somaliensis, first isolated by Bouffard in French Somaliland from patients affected with mycetoma, was described by Brumpt in 1906 as *Indiella somaliensis*. Infections due to this organism have been reported from the African continent, the Arabian peninsula, India, Mexico, Venezuela and the USA (Tight and Bartlett 1981, Serrano et al. 1986, Hay et al. 1992). The organism has been associated in particular with mycetomas affecting the head and neck, causing Madura skull, and involving the cranial vault. In *S. somaliensis* infections, the pus contains hard, yellow to brown, round-to-oval granules which are 1–2 mm in diameter. There are reports that other species of *Streptomyces*, notably *Streptomyces albus*, *Streptomyces anulatus* (*griseus*), *Streptomyces lavendulae*, *Streptomyces rimosus* and *Streptomyces violaceoruber*, may be of medical importance (Berd 1973, Mishra, Gordon and Barnett 1980, McNeil et al. 1990).

14.4 Diagnosis and treatment of actinomycetoma

Actinomycetoma has a world-wide distribution but is a major health problem in some tropical and subtropical regions (Serrano et al. 1986) (see also Volume 3, Chapter 39). Climatic conditions may play an important role in the distribution of the causal agents. *N. brasiliensis* is the predominant organism in many tropical areas, such as the sugar plantations in Mexico. In India, *A. madurae* is reported to be the major pathogen whereas *A. pelletieri* and *S. somaliensis* are prevalent in the African continent and on the Arabian peninsula. *A. madurae* seems to be widely distributed in soil but *A. latina* and *A. pelletieri* have only been isolated from clinical material. Non-mycetomic infections caused by *A. madurae* have been reported (Wust et al. 1990), including one involving an immunocompromised patient (McNeil et al. 1990).

The diagnosis of actinomycetoma is currently based on the isolation and identification of the causal agent. A stepwise approach from the collection of specimens through to identification has been described by Goodfellow (1996). In practice, the isolation of the causal organism is not always possible; identification to the genus level depends on the detection of key chemical markers (Table 21.1). Several simple phenotypic tests are available to distinguish the 3 pathogenic *Actinomadura* spp. both from one another and from the remaining causal agents of the disease which lack mycolic acids (Table 21.4).

Favourable in vitro susceptibilities have been reported with amikacin, impenem, minocycline, tobramycin and vancomycin against *A. madurae*, *A. pelletieri* and *S. somaliensis* (Boiron et al. 1992b). These results are in good agreement with those of an earlier study (McNeil et al. 1990) though some inconsistencies were apparent with certain cephalosporins and penicillins and with trimethoprim–sulphamethoxazole. These antimicrobial agents were either only moderately effective or ineffective. It has still to be seen whether the results of these investigations can be extrapolated to antibiotic activity in subcutaneous granulomas and abscesses formed in mycetomas.

GORDONA, RHODOCOCCUS AND TSUKAMURELLA

These genera form distinct clades in the evolutionary radiation of the mycolata (see Fig. 21.2). Members of these taxa can be separated using a battery of phenotypic properties, notably by detecting chemical markers (Table 21.2).

15 GORDONA

The genus *Gordona* (Tsukamura 1971) was proposed for some slightly acid-fast actinomycetes isolated from soil and sputa of patients with pulmonary disease. The 3 original species, *Gordona bronchialis*, *Gordona rubra* and *Gordona terrae*, were later reclassified in the revived and redescribed genus *Rhodococcus* (Tsukamura 1974, Goodfellow and Alderson 1977). Rhodococcal species were subsequently divided into 2 aggregate groups recognized mainly by chemical and serological properties (Goodfellow 1989). The species initially classified in the genus *Gordona* contained mycolic acids with between 48 and 66 carbon atoms and large amounts of dihydrogenated menaquinones with 9 isoprene units. By contrast, the remaining strains were characterized by shorter chain mycolic acids (C_{34}–C_{52}) and a dihydrogenated menaquinone with 8 isoprene units as the predominant isoprenologue (Collins et al. 1985). The 2 aggregate groups were also distinguished on the basis of their antibiotic sensitivity profiles (Goodfellow and Orchard 1974), delayed skin reaction on sensitized guinea pigs, and polyacrylamide gel electrophoresis of cell extracts (Hyman and Chaparas 1977). Gordonae were also found to contain mycobactins whereas rhodococci were unable to synthesize these compounds under iron-limited growth conditions (Hall and Ratledge 1986).

The discovery that the 2 aggregate groups were phylogenetically distinct led Stackebrandt, Smida and Collins (1988) to reintroduce the genus *Gordona* Tsukamura 1971 for organisms classified as *Rhodococcus bronchialis*, *Rhodococcus rubropertincta*, *Rhococococcus sputi* and *Rhodococcus terrae*. The genus currently accommodates 8 validly described species due to the addition of 4 new species, including *Gordona amarae*. The taxonomic status of most of these species is supported by 16S rRNA sequence (Rainey et al. 1995, Klatte et al. 1996), DNA relatedness (Mordarski et al. 1977, 1980) and numerical taxonomic data (Goodfellow et al. 1982, 1991). The key properties of the genus are given below.

Gordonae are aerobic, gram-positive to gram-variable, non-motile, catalase-positive actinomycetes that form short rods and cocci. They are usually partially acid–alcohol-fast. Rough brownish, pink, or orange to red colonies are formed on glucose yeast extract agar, Sauton's agar and egg media. The organism has an oxidative carbohydrate metabolism, produces mycobactins, is sensitive to lysozyme and is arylsulphatase-negative. The peptidoglycan is of the A1γ type, contains *meso*-A_2pm as the diamino acid and muramic acid with N-glycolyl residues. The polysaccharide fraction of the wall is rich in arabinose and galactose. The wall envelope contains mycolic acids with 46–66 carbon atoms and up to 4 double bonds and major proportions of straight-chain saturated, monounsaturated, and 10-methyl (tuberculostearic)-branched fatty acids. Fatty acid esters released on pyrolysis gas chromatography of mycolic esters have 16–18 carbon atoms. Cells contain diphosphatidylglycerol, phosphatidylethanolamine and phosphatidylinositol mannosides as major phospholipids. Dihydrogenated menaquinone with 9 isoprene units [MK-9(H_2)] is the predominant isoprenologue. The range of G + C content of the DNA is 63–69 mol%. It is isolated from activated sludge foam, biofilters, soil and from sputa of patients with bronchiectasis and cavitary pulmonary tuberculosis. The type species is *Gordona bronchialis*.

Simple and reproducible phenotypic markers are needed

Table 21.4 Characters differentiating the main causal agents of actinomycetoma

Character	Actinomadura			Nocardia			Streptomyces
	latina	madurae	pelletieri	asteroides	brasiliensis	otitidis-caviarum	somaliensis
Whole-organism hydrolysate analysis							
A₂pm-DL	+	+	+	+	+	+	−
A₂pm-LL	−	−	−	−	−	−	+
Arabinose	−	−	−	+	+	+	−
Galactose	+	+	+	+	+	+	−
Madurose	+	+	+	−	−	−	−
Mycolic acids	−	−	−	+	+	+	−
Degradation tests							
Aesculin	+	+	−	+	+	+	−
Casein	+	+	+	−	+	−	+
Elastin	v	+	+	−	+	−	+
Hypoxanthine	v	+	+	−	+	+	+
Tyrosine	+	+	+	−	+	−	+
Urea	−	−	−	+	+	+	−
Xanthine	−	−	−	−	−	+	−
Sensitivity to penicillin (10 units)	−[a]	−[a]	+[a]	−	−	−	−

Symbols for the degradation and antibiotic sensitivity tests: +, ≥90% of strains are positive; −, ≥90% of strains are negative; v, variable. For details of test procedures see Boiron et al. (1993) and Goodfellow (1996).
[a]*A. latina* and *A. pelletieri* can also be distinguished by the inability of the latter to use L-arabinose, fructose, mannose and mannitol as sole sources of carbon for energy and growth. Similarly, *A. madurae* can metabolize adonitol, L-arabinose, mannitol, rhamnose and xylose as sole carbon sources whereas *A. pelletieri* is unable to do so.

to distinguish between *Gordona* spp. However, there is evidence that rapid enzyme and nutritional tests should help to address this situation (Tsukamura 1971, Goodfellow et al. 1991). Plasmid profiling, restriction endonuclease analysis, and ribosomal fingerprinting have been found useful in typing *G. bronchialis* isolates (Richet et al. 1991). Similarly, a digoxigen-labelled rDNA gene probe has been used to identify clinically significant gordonae (Buchman et al. 1992, Lasker, Brown and McNeil 1992).

16 *RHODOCOCCUS*

Rhodococci have a long and chequered taxonomic history (Bousfield and Goodfellow 1976, Goodfellow 1989). The epithet *rhodochrous* (Zopf 1891) was reintroduced by Gordon and Mihm (1957) for actinomycetes bearing numerous generic and specific names but with many phenotypic properties in common with both mycobacteria and nocardiae. The taxon was provisionally assigned to the genus *Mycobacterium* but was later considered to merit generic status. The genus *Rhodococcus* was eventually resurrected (Tsukamura 1974, Goodfellow and Alderson 1977). Sixteen rhodococcal species are described in the current edition of *Bergey's Manual of Systematic Bacteriology* (Goodfellow 1989). Recent taxonomic revisions that have reassigned certain members of the genus to 3 new genera,

namely *Dietzia*, *Gordona* and *Tsukamurella*, have left *Rhodococcus* as a more homogeneous taxon. At present, the genus contains 12 validly described species. The key properties shared by rhodococci are given below.

Rhodococci are aerobic, gram-positive, non-motile, catalase-positive actinomycetes that form rods to extensively branched vegetative mycelium. They are usually partially acid–alcohol-fast. In all strains the morphogenetic cycle starts with the coccus or short rod stage, with different organisms showing a succession of more or less complex morphological stages by which the completion of the growth cycle is achieved: cocci may germinate only into short rods, or form filaments with side projections, or show elementary branching, or in the most differentiated forms produce extensively branched hyphae. The next generation of cocci or short rods is formed by fragmentation of the rods, filaments and hyphae. Some strains produce feeble, microscopically visible aerial hyphae, which may be branched, or aerial synnemata consisting of unbranched filaments that coalesce and project upwards. Colonies may be rough, smooth, or mucoid and pigmented buff, cream, yellow, orange or red, although colourless variants do occur. The organism has an oxidative carbohydrate metabolism, is sensitive to lysozyme, does not produce mycobactins and is arylsulphatase-negative. The peptidoglycan is of the A1γ type, contains *meso*-A₂pm as the diamino acid and muramic acid with *N*-glycolyl residues. The polysaccharide fraction of the wall is rich in arabinose and galactose. The wall envelope contains mycolic acids with 34–

52 carbon atoms and up to 3 double bonds and major proportions of straight-chain saturated, unsaturated, and 10-methyl (tuberculostearic)-branched fatty acids. Fatty acid esters released on pyrolysis gas chromatography of mycolic esters have 12–18 carbon atoms. Cells contain diphosphatidylglycerol, phosphatidylethanolamine and phosphatidylinositol dimannosides as major phospholipids. Dihydrogenated menaquinone with 8 isoprene units [MK-8(H$_2$)] is the predominant isoprenologue. The range of G + C content of the DNA is 63–73 mol%. The organism is widely distributed but is particularly abundant in soil, activated sludge foam and herbivore dung. Some strains are pathogenic for animals, including humans. The type species is *Rhodococcus rhodochrous*.

Criteria useful for differentiating *Rhodococcus* spp. are shown in Table 21.5. However, a better panel of phenotypic tests is needed to improve further the identification of rhodococcal species. Rapid enzyme tests should prove useful in this respect (Goodfellow et al. 1990, Boiron et al. 1993, Klatte, Kroppenstedt and Rainey 1994). There is also evidence that PCR primers can be used to distinguish *Rhodococcus equi* from other mycolata strains (Bell et al. 1996). Good correlation has been found between ribotype patterns and DNA relatedness data (Lasker, Brown and McNeil 1992). These investigators also found that ribotyping was a potentially useful epidemiological tool for determining interstrain relationships of *R. equi* isolates. There are grounds for believing that *R. equi* is a heterogeneous taxon (Butler, Kilburn and Kubica 1987, Gotoh et al. 1991, McNeil and Brown 1994).

17 TSUKAMURELLA

This genus was proposed by Collins et al. (1988) for actinomycetes previously known as *Corynebacterium paurometabolum*, *Gordona aurantiaca* and *Rhodococcus aurantiacus*. *Tsukamurella paurometabola* was first discovered in humans in 1971 by Tsukamura and Mizuno following its isolation from the sputum of patients with tuberculosis in Japan. Three additional species, *Tsukamurella inchonensis* (Yassin et al. 1995), *Tsukamurella pulmonis* (Yassin et al. 1996) and *Tsukamurella tyrosinosolvens* (Yassin et al. 1997), also contain organisms isolated from clinical material. A fifth species, *Tsukamurella wratislaviensis*, has properties consistent with its classification in the genus *Rhodococcus*. The salient features of the genus are given below.

Tsukamurellae are obligately aerobic, gram-positive, non-motile, catalase-positive actinomycetes that form straight to slightly curved rods. True mycelium is not formed though cells may present a pseudomycelial appearance. The organisms are weakly to strongly acid–alcohol-fast. Rough, dry, creamy to orange colonies are formed on Lowenstein–Jensen medium and brain–heart infusion agar. The organism has an oxidative carbohydrate metabolism, is resistant to lysozyme and is arylsulphatase-negative. The peptidoglycan is of the A1γ type, contains *meso*-A$_2$pm as the diamino acid and muramic acid with *N*-glycolyl residues. The polysaccharide fraction of the wall is rich in arabinose and galactose. The cell envelope contains mycolic acids with 62–78 carbon atoms and up to 6 double bonds and major proportions of straight-chain, saturated, unsaturated and 10-methyl (tuberculostearic)-branched fatty acids. Fatty acid esters on pyrolysis gas chromatography of mycolic acids have 20–22 carbon atoms. Cells contain diphosphatidylglycerol, phosphatidylethanolamine, phosphatidylinositol and phosphatidylinositol mannosides as major phospholipids. Unsaturated menaquinones with 9 isoprene units form the predominant isoprenologue. The range of G + C content of the DNA is 68–74 mol%. The organisms are isolated from activated sludge foam, soil and clinical material. The type species is *T. paurometabola*.

The 4 species forming the genus *Tsukamurella* can be distinguished on the basis of DNA relatedness data (Yassin et al. 1997). Several phenotypic properties can be weighted for the provisional separation of these taxa (Table 21.6) though additional strains need to be studied to determine whether they really are predictive.

18 CLINICAL MANIFESTATIONS

Gordonae, rhodococci and tsukamurellae have only rarely been encountered as agents of human infection (see also Volume 3, Chapter 39). However, the superficial resemblance of these actinomycetes to other more common pathogens expected in immunocompromised patients, notably mycobacteria and nocardiae, has probably resulted in inadequate diagnosis and hence an underscoring of their clinical significance. Clinicians need to be aware of the pathogenic potential of these organisms, especially when treating AIDS patients and similarly immunocompromised individuals.

G. bronchialis and *Gordona sputi* have been associated with patients with pulmonary disease (Tsukamura 1971, 1978). More recently, *G. bronchialis* was shown to be the cause of a nosocomial outbreak of sternal wound infections in patients following coronary artery bypass surgery (Richet et al. 1991). The first documented case involving *Gordona rubropertincta* was a lung infection of an immunocompetent female (Hart et al. 1988). Similarly, a primary cutaneous infection of a non-immunocompromised girl with a granulomatous forearm skin lesion and axillary lymphadenopathy was associated with a *G. terrae* strain (Martin et al. 1991, Lasker, Brown and McNeil 1992). Catheter-associated sepsis has been attributed to *Gordona* strains (Buchman et al. 1992). *G. bronchialis* strains are sensitive to amoxycillin + clavulanic acid and to cefotaxin, ceftriaxone, gentamicin and minocycline (Boiron et al. 1993).

The clinical presentation of rhodococcal infections is influenced by the immune status of the host and the virulence of the infecting organism. The first reported human infection involved a patient suffering from *R. equi* pneumonia who had been given corticosteroid therapy for chronic hepatitis (Golub, Falk and Spink 1967). Subsequent reports of human infection, while rare, have emphasized the role of rhodococci as agents of pulmonary disease in severely immunoimpaired individuals (McNeil and Brown 1994). There is also evidence that rhodococci can cause actinomycetoma (Severo, Petrillo and Coutinho 1987).

R. equi has long been recognized as a causal agent

Table 21.5 Characters differentiating species of the genus *Rhodococcus*

	R. coprophilus	*R. equi*	*R. erythropolis*	*R. fascians*	*R. globerulus*	*R. marino-nascens*	*R. opacus*	*R. percolatus*	*R. rhodnii*	*R. rhodochrous*	*R. ruber*	*R. zopfii*
Morphogenetic sequence	H-R-C	R-C	EB-R-C	H-R-C	EB-R-C	H-R-C	R-C	EB-R-C	EB-R-C	EB-R-C	H-R-C	H-R-C
Degradation of												
Adenine	–	+	+	–	+	–	ND	ND	–	+	–	ND
Tyrosine	+	–	v	+	–	–	ND	ND	+	+	+	ND
Growth on sole carbon source (1%, w/v)												
Cellobiose	–	v	–	–	–	–	+	–	–	–	–	ND
Inositol	–	+	+	–	–	+	+	+	–	–	v	+
Maltose	+	–	+	–	+	–	+	–	–	+	+	+
Mannose	+	v	–	+	–	+	+	+	–	+	+	ND
Mannitol	–	+	+	+	v	+	ND	+	+	+	+	–
Sorbitol	+	+	+	+	v	–	ND	+	+	+	+	–
Sucrose	+	+	+	+	–	+	+	+	–	+	+	–
Turanose	–	–	–	v	–	ND	+	ND	–	–	–	ND

Symbols: +, ≥90% of strains positive; –, 90% of strains negative; v, variable; ND, not determined.
Data taken from Goodfellow et al. (1991), Klatte, Kroppenstedt and Rainey (1994), Stoecker, Russell and Staley (1994) and Briglia et al. (1996).

Table 21.6 Some phenotypic properties which differentiate the type strains of *Tsukamurella* species

Characteristic[a]	T. inchonensis	T. paurometabola	T. pulmonis	T. tyrosinosolvens
Acid production from				
Cellobiose	−	+	−	−
Inositol	+	+	−	+
Maltose	−	+	−	+
Mannitol	−	+	−	−
Mannose	−	+	+	+
Melezitose	−	+	−	+
Sorbitol	−	+	+	+
Growth at 45°C				
Degradation of				
Hypoxanthine	−	+	−	+
Tyrosine	−	−	−	+
Xanthine	−	−	−	+

[a]Data taken from Yassin et al. (1997).

of bronchial pneumonia, primarily in foals, but it also infects pigs, a wide range of other animals and in recent years has been implicated as a human pathogen (Lasky et al. 1991, Prescott 1991, McNeil and Brown 1994). Since the first report of a *R. equi* infection in an AIDS patient (Samies et al. 1986) more than 100 cases have been recorded. Drancourt et al. (1992) reported 51 infections due to *R. equi*, 20 of which occurred in HIV-infected patients and 9 in immunocompetent individuals. These workers also noted that patients infected with *R. equi* frequently had a history of contact with farm animals. *Rhodococcus erythropolis*, *Rhodococcus rhodnii* and *R. rhodochrous* have also been implicated in pathogenic processes (Alture-Werber, O'Hara and Louria 1968, Haburchack et al. 1978, Boughton et al. 1981). *R. equi* strains are generally sensitive to amikacin, erythromycin, gentamicin, rifampicin, streptomycin, tobramycin and vancomycin.

Tsukamurellae can cause catheter-associated sepsis, cutaneous infections, meningitis and pulmonary disease. Respiratory tract colonization occurs in both immunocompromised and non-immunocompromised patients, especially in those with underlying chronic lung diseases. Tsukamura and Kawakami (1982) first drew attention to the pathogenic role of *Tsukamurella* strains in humans when they repeatedly isolated a pure culture of *T. paurometabola* from the sputa of a patient with a tuberculosis-like disease. Individual cases of lethal meningitis (Prinz et al. 1985), severe gangrenous tendosynovitis with multiple subcutaneous abscesses (Tsukamura et al. 1988) and catheter-related bacteraemia (Shapiro et al. 1992) have been attributed to *T. paurometabola*. *T. inchonensis*, *T. pulmonis* and *T. tyrosinosolvens* have also been reported to cause lung infections (Yassin et al. 1995, 1996, 1997). Tsukamurellae are sensitive to amikacin, gentamicin, imipenem and vancomycin.

OTHER OPPORTUNIST PATHOGENIC ACTINOMYCETES

Members of the genera *Dermatophilus*, *Oerskovia*, *Rothia*, *Saccharomonospora* and *Saccharopolyspora* are occasionally encountered as primary agents of human disease (see also Volume 3, Chapter 39). Tests are available to distinguish them from one another and from other actinomycete genera (see Tables 21.1 and 21.2, pp. 466 and 474) (Holt et al. 1994). There is also evidence that *Amycolatopsis* and *Pseudonocardia* strains may be clinically significant. *Amycolatopsis orientalis* has been isolated from cerebrospinal fluid (Gordon et al. 1978) and *Pseudonocardia* (*Amycolata*) *autotrophica* has been implicated in a case of purulent pericarditis (Causey and Brown 1974). Procedures used to selectively isolate, characterize and identify this broad assortment of actinomycetes can be found elsewhere (McNeil and Brown 1994).

Dermatophilus congolensis is an obligate parasite that causes an exudative skin disease of animals and humans (Lloyd and Sellers 1976, McNeil and Brown 1994). Susceptible domestic animals include cattle, donkeys, goats, horses and sheep. The disease can cause considerable economic damage to the hides and wool of infected animals in countries where raising livestock is an important activity. Humans contract the disease through contact with infected animals or contaminated products (Yeruham, Hadini and Elad 1991). In humans, dermatophilosis is characterized by multiple pustules, furuncles, or desquamatous eczema of the head and forearms; pitted keratolysis has also been observed. The organism produces large amounts of keratinase when grown on appropriate substrates (Hanel et al. 1991). The diagnosis of dermatophilosis depends on the detection of *D. congolensis* in clinical material and the isolation and identification of the aetiological agent in culture. The organism is susceptible to many antimicrobial drugs including erythromycin, chloramphenicol, penicillin, streptomycin, tetracycline and trimethoprim–sulphamethoxazole.

In 1975, Reller et al. published the first report of an infection caused by *Oerskovia turbata*; the patient had endocarditis complicating a homograft of an aortic valve. Similarly, LeProwse, McNeil and McCarty (1989) documented a case of a child age 3 years who had *O. turbata* bacteraemia associated with an indwelling central venous catheter. In each of these patients, removal of the indwelling foreign prosthetic device was necessary for effecting a cure. Sottnek et al. (1977) examined 35 *Oerskovia* strains isolated from clinical material: 9 of the isolates were identified as *O. turbata* and 26 as *Oerskovia xanthineolytica*. Five of the 9 strains of *O. turbata* were isolated from heart valves or heart tissue. Only one of the *O. xanthineolytica* strains was associated with the heart; the remaining strains were isolated from several sources including blood, cerebrospinal fluid, sputum and granuloma of the hand. Rihs et al. (1990) reported a case of *O. xanthineolytica* in a patient receiving peritoneal dialysis. Cruickshank, Gawler and Shalson (1979) reported a strain of *Oerskovia* suspected of causing pyonephrosis. An *Oerskovia* strain has also been implicated in catheter-related sepsis developed in a female receiving parenteral nutrition therapy (Guss and Ament 1989). It can be anticipated that such infections will be encountered more frequently in future due to the increased use of long-term indwelling central venous catheters, the widespread use of home total parenteral nutrition therapy and the difficulty in sterilizing homografts with antimicrobial agents. High doses of co-trimoxazole combined with ampicillin and amoxycillin have been recommended for the treatment of infections caused by *O. turbata* (Reller et al. 1975).

Rothia dentocariosa is a normal inhabitant of the human mouth and is frequently isolated from the throat and from sputum cultures. Brown, Georg and Waters (1969) were amongst the first to report the isolation of rothiae from clinical specimens. The first report of *R. dentocariosa* as a primary pathogen involved a female with an abdominal infection

(Scharfen 1975). Clinical findings were typical of actinomycosis, and following surgery the patient was cured with penicillin treatment. Other reported infections associated with *R. dentocariosa* include a patient with a pilonidal abscess (Lutwick and Rockhill 1978), one with an infected postoperative maxillary cyst (Minato and Abiko 1984) and several with endocarditis (Pape et al. 1979, Isaacson and Grenko 1988). Rothiae are susceptible to several antibiotics including ampicillin, chlortetracycline, erythromycin, methacillin and penicillin (Dzierzanowski et al. 1978). Abscess formation has been demonstrated experimentally in mice (Roth and Flanagan 1969).

Thermophilic actinomycetes are well known agents of allergic alveolitis. In 1932, Campbell associated farmers' lung disease with white dust released from mouldy hay, but it was only in 1963 that the active component was identified as the spores of thermophilic actinomycetes (Pepys et al. 1963). It was subsequently recognized that farmers' lung was only one of a group of clinically similar occupational diseases, known as extrinsic allergic alveolitis or hypersensitivity pneumonitis, caused by the inhalation of spores. Hypersensitivity pneumonitis is due to the sensitization of susceptible individuals by inhaled antigens. The disease usually affects the middle and upper bronchi as well as the lung parenchyma and represents an interstitial lymphocytic or granulomatous allergic reaction of the pulmonary tissue. The role of actinomycetes in the disease has been extensively reviewed (Lacey 1981, 1988). Farmers' lung, which occurs in Europe and North America, is caused by 2 sporoactinomycetes, *Saccharopolyspora* (*Faenia*) *rectivirgula* and *Saccharomonospora viridis*. These organisms have also been implicated in mushroom workers' lung and humidifier fever. It is possible that other sporoactinomycetes common in mouldy hay may act as agents of allergic alveolitis.

REFERENCES

Ajello G, Roberts GD, 1981, Mycetomas, *Diagnostic Procedures for Bacterial, Mycotic and Parasitic Infections*, ed. Hausler WJ, American Public Health Association, Washington DC, 1033–54.

Alshamaony L, Goodfellow M, Minnikin DE, 1976, Free mycolic acids as criteria in the classification of *Nocardia* and the '*rhodochrous*' complex, *J Gen Microbiol*, **92:** 188–99.

Alture-Werber E, O'Hara D, Louria DB, 1968, Infections caused by *Mycobacterium rhodochrous* and scotochromogens, *Am Rev Respir Dis*, **97:** 694–8.

Andrzejewski J, Müller G et al., 1978, Isolation characterisation and classification of *Nocardia asteroides* bacteriophage, *Zentralbl Bakteriol Suppl*, **6:** 319–26.

Angeles AM, Sugar AM, 1987, Rapid diagnosis of nocardiosis with an enzyme immunoassay, *J Infect Dis*, **155:** 292–6.

Athalye M, Goodfellow M, Minnikin DE, 1984, Menaquinone composition in the classification of *Actinomadura* and related taxa, *J Gen Microbiol*, **130:** 817–23.

Athalye M, Goodfellow M et al., 1985, Numerical classification of *Actinomadura* and *Nocardiopsis*, *Int J Syst Bacteriol*, **35:** 86–98.

Baddour LM, Baselski VS et al., 1986, Nocardiosis in recipients of renal transplants: evidence for nosocomial acquisition, *Am J Infect Control*, **14:** 214–19.

Battig U, Wegmann P et al., 1990, *Nocardia* mastitis in cattle. 1. Clinical observations and diagnosis in 7 particular cases, *Schweiz Arch Tierheilkd*, **132:** 315–22.

Beadles TA, Land GA et al., 1980, An ultrastructural comparison of the cell envelopes of selected strains of *Nocardia asteroides* and *Nocardia brasiliensis*, *Mycopathologia*, **70:** 25–32.

Beaman BL, 1982, Nocardiosis: role of the cell wall deficient state of *Nocardia*, *Cell Wall Defective Bacteria: Basic Principles and Clinical Significance*, ed. Dominque GJ, Addison-Wesley Publishing Co. Inc., Reading, MA, 231–55.

Beaman BL, 1988, Actinomycetes as opportunistic pathogens, *3rd International Symposium of the Research Center for Pathogenic Fungi and Microbial Toxicoses*, Chiba University, Japan, 3.

Beaman BL, 1992, *Nocardia* as a pathogen of the brain: mechanisms of interactions in the murein brain – a review, *Gene*, **115:** 213–17.

Beaman BL, Beaman L, 1994, *Nocardia* species: host–parasite relationships, *Clin Microbiol Rev*, **7:** 213–64.

Beaman BL, Sugar AM, 1983, *Nocardia* in naturally acquired and experimental infections in animals, *J Hyg (Lond)*, **91:** 393–419.

Beaman BL, Boiron P et al., 1992, *Nocardia* and nocardiosis, **30, Suppl. I:** 317–31.

Bell KS, Philp JC et al., 1996, Identification of *Rhodococcus equi* using the polymerase chain reaction, *Lett Appl Microbiol*, **23:** 72–4.

Berd D, 1973, Laboratory identification of clinically important aerobic actinomycetes, *Appl Microbiol*, **25:** 665–81.

Bishop CT, Blank F, 1958, The chemical composition of the Actinomycetales: isolation of a polysaccharide containing D-arabinose and D-galactose from *Nocardia asteroides*, *Can J Microbiol*, **4:** 35–42.

Blanchard R, 1896, Parasites végétaux à l'exclusion des bactéries, *Traite de Pathologie Generale*, vol. II, G Masson, Paris, 811–923.

Boiron P, Provost F, 1988, *In vitro* susceptibility testing of *Nocardia* spp. and its taxonomic implication, *J Antimicrob Chemother*, **22:** 623–9.

Boiron P, Provost F, 1990a, Use of partially purified 54-kilodalton antigen for diagnosis of nocardiosis by Western blot (immunoblot) assay, *J Clin Microbiol*, **28:** 328–31.

Boiron P, Provost F, 1990b, Characterisation of *Nocardia*, *Rhodococcus* and *Gordona* species by *in vitro* susceptibility testing, *Zentralbl Bakteriol Abt I Orig*, **274:** 203–13.

Boiron P, Provost F, 1990c, Enzymatic characterisation of *Nocardia* spp. and related bacteria by API ZYM profile, *Mycopathologia*, **110:** 51–6.

Boiron P, Stynen D, 1992, Immunodiagnosis of nocardiosis, *Gene*, **115:** 219–22.

Boiron P, Provost G et al., 1990, Review of nocardial infections in France 1987 to 1990, *Eur J Clin Microbiol Infect Dis*, **11:** 709–14.

Boiron P, Provost F et al., 1992a, *In vitro* antibiotic susceptibility testing of agents of actinomycetoma, *Med Microbiol Lett*, **1:** 38–42.

Boiron P, Stynen D et al., 1992b, Monoclonal antibodies to a specific 54-kilodalton antigen of *Nocardia* spp., *J Clin Microbiol*, **30:** 1033–5.

Boiron P, Provost F et al., 1993, *Laboratory Methods for the Diagnosis of Nocardiosis*, Institut Pasteur, Paris.

Bojalil LF, Zamora A, 1963, Precipitin and skin tests in the diagnosis of mycetoma due to *Nocardia brasiliensis*, *Proc Soc Exp Biol Med*, **113:** 40–53.

Bordet C, Etémadi AH et al., 1965, Structure des acides nocardiques de *Nocardia asteroides*, *Bull Soc Chim Fr*, 234–5.

Bordet C, Karahjoli M et al., 1972, Cell walls of nocardiae and related actinomycetes. Identification of the genus *Nocardia* by cell wall analysis, *Int J Syst Bacteriol*, **22:** 251–9.

Boughton RA, Wilson HD et al., 1981, Septic arthritis and osteomyelitis caused by an organism of the genus *Rhodococcus*, *J Clin Microbiol*, **13:** 209–13.

Bousfield IJ, Goodfellow M, 1976, The 'rhodochrous' complex and its relationships with allied taxa, *The Biology of the Nocardiae*, eds Goodfellow M, Brownell GH, Serrano JA, Academic Press, London, 39–65.

Bowen T, Stackebrandt E et al., 1989, The phylogeny of *Amycolata autotrophica*, *Kibdelosporangium aridum* and *Saccharothrix australiensis*, *J Gen Microbiol*, **135:** 2529–36.

Bradley SG, Mordarski M, 1976, Association of polydeoxyribonucleotides of deoxyribonucleic acids from nocardioform bacteria, *The Biology of the Nocardiae*, eds Goodfellow M, Brownell GH, Serrano JA, Academic Press, London, 310–36.

Briglia M, Rainey FA et al., 1996, *Rhodococcus percolatus* sp. nov., a bacterium degrading 2,4,6-trichlorophenol, *Int J Syst Bacteriol*, **46:** 23–30.

Brocq-Rousseu D, 1904, Sur un *Streptothrix* cause de l'alteration des avomes moisies, *Rev Bot*, **16:** 219–30.

Brown JM, Georg LK, Waters LC, 1969, Laboratory identification of *Rothia dentocariosa* and its occurrence in human clinical materials, *Appl Microbiol*, **17:** 150–6.

Brownell GH, Belcher KE, 1990, DNA probes for the identification of *Nocardia asteroides*, *J Clin Microbiol*, **28:** 2082–6.

Brumpt E, 1906, Les mycétomes, *Arch Parasitol*, **10:** 489–527.

Buchanan RE, 1918, Studies in the classification and nomenclature of the bacteria. VIII. The subgroups and genera of the Actinomycetales, *J Bacteriol*, **3:** 403–6.

Buchman AL, McNeil MM et al., 1992, Central venous catheter sepsis caused by unusual *Gordona* (*Rhodococcus*) species: identification with a digoxigenin-labelled rDNA probe, *Clin Infect Dis*, **15:** 694–7.

Butler WR, Jost KC, Kilburn JO, 1991, Identification of mycobacteria by high performance liquid chromatography, *J Clin Microbiol*, **29:** 2468–72.

Butler WR, Kilburn O, Kubica GP, 1987, High performance liquid chromatography analysis of mycolic acids as an aid in laboratory identification of *Rhodococcus* and *Nocardia* species, *J Clin Microbiol*, **25:** 2126–31.

Campbell JM, 1932, Acute symptoms following work with hay, *Br Med J*, **2:** 1143–4.

Carroll GF, Brown JM, Haley LD, 1977, A method for determining *in vitro* susceptibilities of some nocardiae and actinomadurae, *Am J Clin Pathol*, **68:** 279–83.

Castellani A, Chalmers AJ, 1913, *Manual of Tropical Medicine*, 2nd edn, Baillière, Tindall and Cox, London.

Causey WA, Brown JM, 1974, Characterization of isolates of *Nocardia autotrophica* (Takamiya and Tubaki) Hirsch recovered from clinical sources, *Proceedings of the 1st International Conference on the Biology of the Nocardiae*, ed. Brownell GH, McGowen Printing Co., Augusta, GA, USA, 100–1.

Chun J, Goodfellow M, 1995, A phylogenetic analysis of the genus *Nocardia* with 16S rRNA gene sequences, *Int J Syst Bacteriol*, **45:** 240–5.

Chun J, Kang SO et al., 1996, Phylogeny of mycolic acid-containing actinomycetes, *J Ind Microbiol*, **17:** 205–13.

Chun J, Blackall LL et al., 1997, A proposal to reclassify *Nocardia pinensis* Blackall et al. as *Skermania piniformis* gen. nov., comb. nov., *Int J Syst Bacteriol*, **47:** 127–31.

Cohn F, 1875, Untersuchungen über Bacterien. II, *Beitr Biol Pfl*, **I:** 141–207.

Collins DM, 1994, Isoprenoid quinones, *Chemical Methods in Prokaryotic Systematics*, eds Goodfellow M, O'Donnell AG, John Wiley & Sons, Chichester, 265–309.

Collins MD, Burton RA, Jones D, 1988, *Corynebacterium amycolatum* sp. nov. A new mycolic acid-less *Corynebacterium* species from human skin, *FEMS Microbiol Lett*, **49:** 349–52.

Collins MD, Goodfellow M, Minnikin DE, 1982a, Fatty acid composition of some mycolic acid-containing coryneform bacteria, *J Gen Microbiol*, **128:** 2503–9.

Collins MD, Goodfellow M, Minnikin DE, 1982b, A survey of the structure of mycolic acids in *Corynebacterium* and related taxa, *J Gen Microbiol*, **128:** 129–49.

Collins MD, Goodfellow M et al., 1985, The menaquinone composition of mycolic acid-containing actinomycetes and some sporoactinomycetes, *J Appl Bacteriol*, **58:** 77–86.

Collins MD, Howarth OW et al., 1987, Isolation and structural determination of new members of the vitamin K_2 series from *Nocardia brasiliensis*, *FEMS Microbiol Lett*, **41:** 35–9.

Collins MD, Smida J et al., 1988, *Tsukamurella* gen. nov. harboring *Corynebacterium paurometabolum* and *Rhodococcus aurantiacus*, *Int J Syst Bacteriol*, **38:** 385–91.

Cruickshank JG, Gawler AH, Shalson C, 1979, *Oerskovia* species: rare opportunistic pathogens, *J Med Microbiol*, **12:** 513–15.

Cummins CS, 1962, Chemical composition and antigenic structure of cell walls of *Corynebacterium*, *Mycobacterium*, *Nocardia*, *Actinomyces* and *Arthrobacter*, *J Gen Microbiol*, **28:** 35–50.

Cummins CS, 1965, Chemical and antigenic studies on cell walls of mycobacteria, corynebacteria and nocardias, *Am Rev Respir Dis*, **92:** 63–72.

Cummins CS, Harris H, 1956, The chemical composition of the cell wall in some Gram-positive bacteria and its possible value as taxonomic character, *J Gen Microbiol*, **14:** 583–600.

De Briel, Piedmont Y et al., 1993, Eight deep abscesses due to nocardioforms over a two-year period, *Abstract 93rd General Meeting of the American Society for Microbiology*, American Society for Microbiology, Washington, DC, 493.

Dobson G, Minnikin DE et al., 1985, Systematic analysis of complex mycobacterial lipids, *Chemical Methods in Bacterial Systematics*, eds Goodfellow M, Minnikin DE, Academic Press, London, 237–65.

Drancourt M, Bonnet E et al., 1992, *Rhodococcus equi* infection in patients with AIDS, *J Infect*, **24:** 123–31.

Dzierzanowska DS, Miksza-Zytkiewicz R et al., 1978, Sensitivity of *Rothia dentocariosa*, *J Antimicrob Chemother*, **4:** 469–71.

Embley TM, Stackebrandt E, 1994, The molecular phylogeny and systematics of the actinomycetes, *Annu Rev Microbiol*, **48:** 257–89.

Embley TM, Wait R, 1994, Structural lipids of eubacteria, *Chemical Methods in Prokaryotic Systematics*, eds Goodfellow M, O'Donnell AG, John Wiley & Sons, Chichester, 121–61.

Eppinger H, 1891, Über eine neue pathogene *Cladothrix* und eine durch sie hervorgerufene Pseudotuberculosis (Cladotrichia), *Beitr Pathol Anat Allg Pathol*, **9:** 287–328.

Erikson D, 1955, Thermoduric properties of *Nocardia sebivorans* and other pathogenic aerobic actinomycetes, *J Gen Microbiol*, **13:** 127–35.

Finnerty WR, 1992, The biology and genetics of the genus *Rhodococcus*, *Annu Rev Microbiol*, **46:** 193–218.

Fischer A, Kroppenstedt RM, Stackebrandt E, 1983, Molecular-genetic and chemotaxonomic studies on *Actinomadura* and *Nocardiopsis*, *J Gen Microbiol*, **129**: 3433–46.

Funke G, Stubbs S et al., 1994, *Turicella otitidis* gen. nov., sp. nov., a coryneform bacterium isolated from patients with otitis media, *Int J Syst Bacteriol*, **44**: 270–3.

Garrett MA, Holmes HT, Nolte FS, 1992, Selected buffered charcoal-yeast extract medium for isolation of nocardiae from mixed cultures, *J Clin Microbiol*, **30**: 1891–2.

Georg LK, Brown JM, 1967, *Rothia* gen. nov., an aerobic genus of the family Actinomycetaceae, *Am Rev Respir Dis*, **84**: 337–47.

Gerber NN, 1969, Prodigiosin-like pigments from *Actinomadura* (*Nocardia*) *pelletieri* and *Actinomadura madurae*, *Appl Microbiol*, **18**: 1–3.

Golub B, Falk G, Spink WW, 1967, Lung abscess due to *Corynebacterium equi*. Report of first human infection, *Ann Intern Med*, **66**: 1174–7.

González-Ochoa A, 1973, Virulence of nocardiae, *Can J Microbiol*, **19**: 901–4.

Goodfellow M, 1971, Numerical taxonomy of some nocardioform bacteria, *J Gen Microbiol*, **69**: 33–80.

Goodfellow M, 1989, Genus *Rhodococcus* Zopf 1891, 28[AL], *Bergey's Manual of Systematic Bacteriology*, vol. 4, eds Williams ST, Sharpe ME, Holt JG, Williams & Wilkins, Baltimore, 2362–71.

Goodfellow M, 1992, The Family *Nocardiaceae*, *The Prokaryotes*, vol. 2, 2nd edn, eds Balows A, Trüper HG et al., Springer-Verlag, New York, 1188–213.

Goodfellow M, 1996, Actinomycetes: *Actinomyces, Actinomadura, Nocardia, Streptomyces* and related genera, *Mackie & McCartney Practical Medical Microbiology*, 14th edn, Churchill Livingstone, Edinburgh, 343–59.

Goodfellow M, Alderson G, 1977, The actinomycete genus *Rhodococcus*. A home for the '*rhodochrous*' complex, *J Gen Microbiol*, **100**: 99–122.

Goodfellow M, Lechevalier MP, 1989, Genus *Nocardia* Trevisan 1889, 9[AL], *Bergey's Manual of Systematic Bacteriology*, vol. 4, ed. Williams ST, Williams & Wilkins, Baltimore, 2350–61.

Goodfellow M, Magee J, 1997, Taxonomy of mycobacteria, *Mycobacteria. Volume I: Basic Aspects*, eds Gangadharam P, Jenkins PA, Chapman & Hall, New York, in press.

Goodfellow M, Orchard VA, 1974, Antibiotic sensitivity of some nocardioform bacteria and its value as a criterion for taxonomy, *J Gen Microbiol*, **83**: 375–87.

Goodfellow M, Pirouz T, 1982, Numerical classification of sporoactinomycetes containing *meso*-diaminopimelic acid in the cell wall, *J Gen Microbiol*, **128**: 503–7.

Goodfellow M, Trujillo ME, Alderson G, 1995, Approaches towards the identification of sporoactinomycetes that cause actinomycetoma, *The Biology of the Actinomycetes '94*, eds Debabov VG, Dudnik YV, Danilenko VN, All Russia Scientific Research Institute for Genetics, Moscow, 271–86.

Goodfellow M, Williams ST, 1983, Ecology of actinomycetes, *Annu Rev Microbiol*, **37**: 189–216.

Goodfellow M, Orlean PAB et al., 1978, Chemical and numerical taxonomy of some strains received as *Gordona aurantiaca*, *J Gen Microbiol*, **109**: 57–68.

Goodfellow M, Weaver CR et al., 1982, Numerical classification of some rhodococci, corynebacteria and related organisms, *J Gen Microbiol*, **128**: 731–45.

Goodfellow M, Thomas EG et al., 1990, Classification and identification of rhodococci, *Zentralbl Bakteriol*, **274**: 299–315.

Goodfellow M, Zakrzewska-Czerwinska J et al., 1991, Polyphasic taxonomic study of the genera *Gordona* and *Tsukamurella* including the description of *Tsukamurella wratislaviensis*, *Zentralbl Bakteriol*, **275**: 162–78.

Goodfellow M, Davenport R et al., 1996, Actinomycete diversity associated with foaming in activated sludge plants, *J Ind Microbiol*, **17**: 268–80.

Gordon RE, Barnett JE, 1977, Resistance to rifampicin and lysozyme of strains of some species of *Mycobacterium* and *Nocardia* as a taxonomic tool, *Int J Syst Bacteriol*, **27**: 176–8.

Gordon RE, Horan AC, 1968, *Nocardia dassonvillei*, a macroscopic replica of *Streptomyces griseus*, *J Gen Microbiol*, **50**: 235–50.

Gordon RE, Mihm JM, 1957, A comparative study of some new strains received as nocardiae, *J Bacteriol*, **50**: 15–27.

Gordon RE, Mihm JM, 1962, The type species of the genus *Nocardia*, *J Gen Microbiol*, **27**: 1–10.

Gordon RE, Mihm JM et al., 1978, Some bits and pieces of the genus *Nocardia*: *N. carnae, N. vaccinii, N. transvalensis, N. orientalis* and *N. aerocolonigenes*, *J Gen Microbiol*, **109**: 69–78.

Gotoh K, Mitsuyama M et al., 1991, Mycolic acid-containing glycolipid as a possible virulence factor of *R. equi* for mice, *Microbiol Immunol*, **35**: 175–85.

Guss WJ, Ament ME, 1989, *Oerskovia* infection caused by contaminated home parenteral nutrition solution, *Arch Intern Med*, **149**: 1457–8.

Haburchack DR, Jeffrey B et al., 1978, Infections caused by *rhodochrous*, *Am J Med*, **65**: 298–302.

Hall RM, Ratledge CA, 1986, Distribution and application of mycobactins for the characterisation of species within the genus *Nocardia*, *J Gen Microbiol*, **132**: 853–6.

Hamid ME, Minnikin DE, Goodfellow M, 1993, A simple chemical test to distinguish mycobacteria from other mycolic acid-containing actinomycetes, *J Gen Microbiol*, **139**: 2203–13.

Hancock IC, 1994, Analysis of cell wall constituents of Gram-positive bacteria, *Chemical Methods in Prokaryotic Systematics*, eds Goodfellow M, O'Donnell AG, John Wiley & Sons, Chichester, 63–84.

Hanel H, Kalisch M et al., 1991, Quantification of keratolytic activity from *Dermatophilus congolensis*, *Med Microbiol Immunol*, **180**: 45–51.

Hart DHL, Peel MM et al., 1988, Lung infection caused by *Rhodococcus*, *Aust N Z J Med*, **18**: 790–1.

Harz CO, 1879, *Actinomyces bovis*, ein neuer Schimmel in den Geweben des Rindes, *Z Tiermed*, **5**: 125–40.

Hay RJ, Mahgoub ES et al., 1992, Mycetoma, *J Med Vet Mycol*, **30, Suppl. 1**: 41–9.

Higgins ML, Lechevalier MP, 1969, Poorly lytic bacteriophage from *Dactyosporangium thailandensis*, *J Virol*, **3**: 210–16.

Holt JG, Kreig NR et al. (eds), 1994, *Bergey's Manual of Determinative Bacteriology*, 9th edn, Williams & Wilkins, Baltimore.

Houang ET, Lovett IS et al., 1980, *Nocardia asteroides* infection – a transmissible disease, *J Hosp Infect*, **1**: 31–40.

Howarth OW, Grund E et al., 1986, Structural determination of a new naturally occurring cyclic vitamin K, *Biochem Biophys Res Commun*, **140**: 916–23.

Hyman IS, Chaparas SD, 1977, A comparative study of the '*rhodochrous*' complex and related taxa by delayed type skin reactions on guinea pigs and by polyacrylamide gel electrophoresis, *J Gen Microbiol*, **100**: 363–71.

Isaacson JH, Grenko RT, 1988, *Rothia dentocariosa* endocarditis complicated by brain abscess, *Am J Med*, **84**: 352–4.

Javaly K, Horowitz HW, Wormser GP, 1992, Nocardiosis in patients with human immunodeficiency virus infection. Report of 2 cases and review of the literature, *Medicine (Baltimore)*, **71**: 128–38.

Jensen JL, 1931, Contributions to our knowledge of the Actinomycetales. II. The definition and subdivision of the genus *Actinomyces*, with a preliminary account of Australian soil actinomycetes, *Proc Linnean Soc NSW*, **56**: 345–70.

Jimenez T, Diaz M, Zlotnik H, 1990, Monoclonal antibodies to *Nocardia asteroides* and *Nocardia brasiliensis* antigens, *J Clin Microbiol*, **28**: 87–91.

Jonsson S, Wallace RJ et al., 1986, Recurrent *Nocardia* pneumonia in an adult with chronic granulomatous disease, *Am Rev Respir Dis*, **133**: 932–4.

Judicial Commission, 1985, Confirmation of the types in the Approved Lists as nomenclatural types including recognition of *Nocardia asteroides* (Eppinger 1891) Blanchard 1896 and *Pasteuria multocida* (Lehmann and Neumann 1899) Rosenbusch and Merchant 1939 as the respective type species of the genera *Nocardia* and *Pasteurella* and rejection of the species name *Pasteurella gallicida* (Burrill 1883) Buchanan 1925, *Int J Syst Bacteriol*, **35:** 538.

Kasweck KL, Little ML, 1982, Genetic recombination in *Nocardia asteroides*, *J Bacteriol*, **149:** 403–6.

Kasweck KL, Little ML, Bradley SG, 1982, Plasmids in mating strains of *Nocardia asteroides*, *Dev Ind Microbiol*, **23:** 279–86.

Kim J, Minamato GY, Grieco MH, 1991, Nocardial infection as a complication of AIDS: report of six cases and review, *Rev Infect Dis*, **13:** 624–9.

Klatte S, Kroppenstedt RM, Rainey FA, 1994, *Rhodococcus opacus* sp. nov., an unusual nutritionally versatile *Rhodococcus* species, *Syst Appl Microbiol*, **17:** 355–60.

Klatte S, Rainey FA, Kroppenstedt RM, 1994, Transfer of *Rhodococcus aichiensis* Tsukamura 1982 and *Nocardia amarae* Lechevalier and Lechevalier 1974 to the genus *Gordona* as *Gordona aichiensis* comb. nov. and *Gordona amarae* comb. nov., *Int J Syst Bacteriol*, **44:** 769–73.

Klatte S, Kroppenstedt RM et al., 1996, *Gordona hirsuta* sp. nov., *Int J Syst Bacteriol*, **46:** 876–80.

Kroppenstedt RM, 1985, Fatty acid and menaquinone analysis of actinomycetes and related organisms, *Chemical Methods in Bacterial Systematics*, eds Goodfellow M, Minnikin DE, Academic Press, London, 173–99.

Kroppenstedt RM, Stackebrandt E, Goodfellow M, 1990, Taxonomic revision of the actinomycete genera *Actinomadura* and *Microtetraspora*, *Syst Appl Microbiol*, **13:** 148–60.

Kudo T, Hatai K, Seino A, 1988, *Nocardia seriolae* sp. nov. causing nocardiosis of cultured fish, *Int J Syst Bacteriol*, **38:** 173–8.

Labeda DP, Testa RT et al., 1984, *Saccharothrix*, a new genus of the Actinomycetales related to *Nocardiopsis*, *Int J Syst Bacteriol*, **38:** 287–90.

Lacey J, 1981, Airborne actinomycete spores as respiratory allergens, *Zentralbl Bakteriol Suppl*, **11:** 243–50.

Lacey J, 1988, Actinomycetes as biodeteriogens and pollutants of the environment, *Actinomycetes in Biotechnology*, eds Goodfellow M, Mordarski M, Williams ST, Academic Press, London, 359–432.

Lacey J, Goodfellow M, Alderson G, 1978, The genus *Actinomadura* Lechevalier and Lechevalier, *Zentralbl Bakteriol Suppl*, **6:** 107–17.

Lanéelle MA, Asselineau J, 1970, Caractérisation de glycolipides dans une souche de *Nocardia brasiliensis*, *Fed Eur Biochem Soc Lett*, **7:** 64–7.

Lasker BA, Brown JM, McNeil MM, 1992, Identification and epidemiological typing of clinical and environmental isolates of the genus *Rhodococcus* with use of a digoxigenin-labelled rDNA gene probe, *Clin Infect Dis*, **15:** 223–33.

Lasky JA, Pulkingham N et al., 1991, *Rhodococcus equi* causing human pulmonary infection: preview of 29 cases, *South Med J*, **84:** 1217–20.

Laurent F, Carlotti A et al., 1996, Ribotyping: a tool for taxonomy and identification of the *Nocardia asteroides* complex species, *J Clin Microbiol*, **34:** 1079–82.

Laveran M, 1906, Tumeur provoquée par un microcoque rose en zooglées, *C R Hebd Soc Biol*, **2:** 340–1.

Lechevalier HA, Lechevalier MP, 1970, Chemical composition as a criterion in the classification of aerobic actinomycetes, *Int J Syst Bacteriol*, **20:** 435–43.

Lechevalier HA, Lechevalier MP, Gerber NN, 1971, Chemical composition as a criterion in the classification of actinomycetes, *Adv Appl Microbiol*, **14:** 47–72.

Lechevalier MP, 1976, The taxonomy of the genus *Nocardia*: some light at the end of the tunnel?, *The Biology of the Nocardiae*, eds Goodfellow M, Brownell GH, Serrano JA, Academic Press, London, 1–38.

Lechevalier MP, De Biévre C, Lechevalier HA, 1977, Chemotaxonomy of aerobic actinomycetes: phospholipid composition, *Biochem Syst Ecol*, **5:** 249–60.

Lechevalier MP, Lechevalier HA, 1970, A critical evaluation of the genera of aerobic actinomycetes, *The Actinomycetales*, ed. Prauser H, Gustav Fischer Verlag, Jena, 393–405.

Lechevalier MP, Lechevalier HA, 1974, *Nocardia amarae* sp. nov., an actinomycete common in foaming activated sludge, *Int J Syst Bacteriol*, **24:** 278–88.

Lechevalier MP, Lechevalier HA, 1980, The chemotaxonomy of actinomycetes, *Actinomycete Taxonomy, Special Publication 6*, eds Dietz A, Thayer D, Society for Industrial Microbiology, Arlington, USA, 227–91.

Lechevalier MP, Stern AE, Lechevalier HA, 1981, Phospholipids in the taxonomy of actinomycetes, *Zentralbl Bakteriol Suppl*, **11:** 111–16.

Lechevalier MP, Prauser H et al., 1986, Two new genera of nocardioform actinomycetes: *Amycolata* gen. nov. and *Amycolatopsis* gen. nov., *Int J Syst Bacteriol*, **36:** 29–37.

LeProwse CR, McNeil MM, McCarty JM, 1989, Catheter-related bacteremia caused by *Oerskovia turbata*, *J Clin Microbiol*, **27:** 571–2.

Liégard H, Landrieu M, 1911, Un cas de mycose conjonctivale, *Ann Ocul*, **146:** 418–26.

Lind A, Ridell M, 1976, Serological relationships between *Nocardia*, *Mycobacterium*, *Corynebacterium* and the '*rhodochrous*' taxon, *The Biology of the Nocardiae*, eds Goodfellow M, Brownell GH, Serrano JA, Academic Press, London, 220–35.

Lindenberg A, 1909, Un nouveau mycétome, *Arch Parasitol*, **13:** 265–82.

Lloyd DH, Sellers KC (eds), 1976, Dermatophilus *Infection in Animals and Man*, Academic Press, London.

Locci R, 1976, Developmental micromorphology of actinomycetes, *Actinomycetes: The Boundary Microorganisms*, ed. Arai T, Toppan Company Limited, Tokyo, 249–97.

Locci R, 1980, Response of developing branched bacteria to adverse environments. I Membrane-transfer techniques for assessment and SEM visualisation of drug activity against *Nocardia asteroides*, *Zentralbl Bakteriol I Abt Orig A*, **246:** 98–111.

Lungu O, Latta PD et al., 1994, Differentiation of *Nocardia* from rapidly growing *Mycobacterium* species by PCR-RFLP analysis, *Diagn Microbiol Infect Dis*, **18:** 13–18.

Luquin M, Ausina V et al., 1993, *Mycobacterium brumae* sp. nov., a rapidly growing, nonphotochromogenic *Mycobacterium*, *Int J Syst Bacteriol*, **43:** 405–13.

Lutwick LI, Rockhill RC, 1978, Abscess associated with *Rothia dentocariosa*, *J Clin Microbiol*, **8:** 612–13.

McClung NM, 1974, Family VI. Nocardiaceae Castellani and Chalmers 1919, 1040, *Bergey's Manual of Determinative Bacteriology*, 8th edn, eds Buchanan RE, Gibbons NE, Williams & Wilkins, Baltimore, 726–46.

McNeil MM, Brown JM, 1992, Distribution and antimicrobial susceptibility of *Rhodococcus equi* from clinical specimens, *Eur J Epidemiol*, **8:** 437–43.

McNeil MM, Brown JM, 1994, The medically important aerobic actinomycetes: epidemiology and microbiology, *Clin Microbiol Rev*, **7:** 357–417.

McNeil MM, Brown JM et al., 1990, Comparison of species distribution and antimicrobial susceptibility of aerobic actinomycetes from clinical specimens, *Rev Infect Dis*, **12:** 778–83.

Magnusson M, 1976, Sensitin tests as an aid in the taxonomy of *Nocardia* and its pathogenicity, *The Biology of the Nocardiae*, eds Goodfellow M, Brownell GH, Serrano JA, Academic Press, London, 236–65.

Manninen KI, Smith RA, Kim LO, 1993, Highly presumptive identification of bacterial isolates associated with the recent Canada-wide mastitis epizootic as *Nocardia farcinica*, *Can J Microbiol*, **39:** 635–41.

Martin T, Hogan DJ et al., 1991, *Rhodococcus* infection of the skin with lymphadenitis in a nonimmunocompromised girl, *J Am Acad Dermatol*, **24:** 328–32.

Maurice MT, Vacheron MJ, Michel G, 1971, Isolément d'acides nocardiques de plusieurs espèces de *Nocardia*, *Chem Phys Lipids*, **7:** 9–18.

Meyer J, 1976, *Nocardiopsis*, a new genus of the order Actinomycetales, *Int J Syst Bacteriol*, **26:** 487–93.

Meyer J, 1989, Genus *Actinomadura* Lechevalier and Lechevalier

1970a, 400^AL, *Bergey's Manual of Systematic Bacteriology*, vol. 4, ed. Williams ST, Williams & Wilkins, Baltimore, 2511–26.

Michel G, Bordet C, 1976, Cell walls of nocardiae, *The Biology of the Nocardiae*, eds Goodfellow M, Brownell GH, Serrano JA, Academic Press, London, 141–59.

Minato K, Abiko Y, 1984, Beta-lactam antibiotic resistant *Rothia dentocariosa* from infected postoperative maxillary cyst: studies on R-plasmid and beta-lactamase, *Gen Pharmacol*, **15**: 287–92.

Minnikin DE, 1993, Mycolic acids, *CRC Handbook of Chromatography: Analysis of Lipids*, CRC Press, Cleveland, Ohio, 339–48.

Minnikin DE, Alshamaony L, Goodfellow M, 1975, Differentiation of *Mycobacterium*, *Nocardia* and related taxa by thin-layer chromatographic analysis of whole-organism methanolysates, *J Gen Microbiol*, **88**: 200–4.

Minnikin DE, Goodfellow M, 1980, Lipid composition in the classification and identification of acid-fast bacteria, *Microbiological Classification and Identification*, eds Goodfellow M, Board RG, Academic Press, London, 189–256.

Minnikin DE, Minnikin SM et al., 1984, Mycolic acid patterns of some species of *Mycobacterium*, *Arch Microbiol*, **139**: 225–31.

Minnikin DE, Dobson G et al., 1985, Quantitative comparison of the mycolic acid and fatty acid compositions of *Mycobacterium leprae* and *Mycobacterium gordonae*, *J Gen Microbiol*, **131**: 2013–21.

Mishra SK, Gordon RE, Barnett DA, 1980, Identification of nocardiae and streptomycetes of medical importance, *J Clin Microbiol*, **11**: 728–36.

Mordarska H, Cebrât S et al., 1978, Differentiation of nocardioform actinomycetes by lysozyme sensitivity, *J Gen Microbiol*, **109**: 381–4.

Mordarski M, Goodfellow M et al., 1977, Classification of the '*rhodochrous*' complex and allied taxa based upon deoxyribonucleic acid reassociation, *Int J Syst Bacteriol*, **27**: 31–7.

Mordarski M, Goodfellow M et al., 1980, Deoxyribonucleic acid reassociation in the classification of the genus *Rhodococcus*, *Int J Syst Bacteriol*, **30**: 521–7.

Nocard E, 1888, Note sur la maladie de boeufs de la Guadeloupe, comsue sous le nom de farcin, *Ann Inst Pasteur (Paris)*, **2**: 293–302.

Ochi K, Miyadoh S, Tamura T, 1991, Polyacrylamide gel electrophoresis analysis of ribosomal protein AT-L30 as a novel approach to actinomycete taxonomy: application to the genera *Actinomadura* and *Microtetraspora*, *Int J Syst Bacteriol*, **41**: 234–9.

Orchard VA, 1981, The ecology of *Nocardia* and related taxa, *Zentralbl Bakteriol Suppl*, **11**: 167–80.

Orchard VA, Goodfellow M, 1974, The selective isolation of *Nocardia* from soil using antibiotics, *J Gen Microbiol*, **85**: 160–2.

Orchard VA, Goodfellow M, 1980, Numerical classification of some named strains of *Nocardia asteroides* and related isolates from soil, *J Gen Microbiol*, **118**: 295–312.

Ørskov J, 1923, *Investigations into the Morphology of the Ray Fungi*, Levin and Munksgaard, Copenhagen.

Ortiz-Ortiz L, Melendro EI, Conde C, 1984, Host–parasite relationship in infections due to *Nocardia brasiliensis*, *Biological, Biochemical, and Biomedical Aspects of Actinomycetes*, eds Ortiz-Ortiz L, Bojalil LF, Yakoleff V, Academic Press, Orlando, 119–33.

Pape J, Singer T et al., 1979, Infective endocarditis caused by *Rothia dentocariosa*, *Ann Intern Med*, **91**: 746–7.

Pascual C, Lawson PA et al., 1995, Phylogenetic analysis of the genus *Corynebacterium* based on 16S rRNA gene sequences, *Int J Syst Bacteriol*, **45**: 724–8.

Patterson JE, Chapin-Robertson K et al., 1992, Pseudoepidemic of *Nocardia asteroides* associated with a mycobacterial culture system, *J Clin Microbiol*, **30**: 1357–60.

Peczyńska-Czoch W, Mordarski M, 1988, Actinomycete enzymes, *Actinomycetes in Biotechnology*, eds Goodfellow M, Mordarski M, Williams ST, Academic Press, London, 219–83.

Pepys J, Jenkins PA et al., 1963, Farmers' lung: thermophilic actinomycetes as sources of 'farmers' lung hay' antigen, *Lancet*, **1**: 607–9.

Philip A, Roberts GD, 1984, *Nocardiopsis dassonvillei* cellulitis of the arm, *Clin Microbiol Newslett*, **6**: 14–15.

Pier AC, 1984, Serological relationships among aerobic and anaerobic actinomycetes in human and animal diseases, *Biological, Biochemical and Biomedical Aspects of Actinomycetes*, eds Ortiz-Ortiz L, Bojalil LF, Yakoleff V, Academic Press, Orlando, 135–43.

Pier AC, Fichtner RE, 1971, Serological typing of *Nocardia asteroides* by immunodiffusion, *Am Rev Respir Dis*, **103**: 698–707.

Pier AC, Fichtner RE, 1981, Distribution of serotypes of *Nocardia asteroides* from animal, human and environmental sources, *J Clin Microbiol*, **13**: 548–53.

Pier AC, Thurston JR, Larson AB, 1968, A diagnostic antigen for nocardiosis: comparative tests in cattle with nocardiosis and mycobacteriosis, *Am J Vet Res*, **29**: 397–403.

Pinoy E, 1912, Isolement et culture d'une nouvelle oospora pathogene, *Bull Soc Path Exot*, **5**: 585–9.

Pommier MT, Michel G, 1985, Occurrence of corynomycolic acids in strains of *Nocardia otitidis-caviarum*, *J Gen Microbiol*, **131**: 2637–41.

Prauser H, 1976, Host–parasite relationships in nocardioform organisms, *The Biology of the Nocardiae*, eds Goodfellow M, Brownell GH, Serrano JA, Academic Press, London, 266–84.

Prauser H, 1981, Taxon specificity of lytic actinophages that do not multiply in the cells affected, *Zentralbl Bakteriol Suppl*, **11**: 87–92.

Prauser H, Lechevalier MP, Lechevalier HA, 1970, Description of *Oerskovia* gen. nov. to harbor Ørskov's motile nocardia, *Appl Microbiol*, **19**: 534.

Prescott JF, 1991, *Rhodococcus equi*: an animal and human pathogen, *Clin Microbiol Rev*, **4**: 20–34.

Prinz G, Ban E et al., 1985, Meningitis caused by *Gordona aurantiaca* (*Rhodococcus aurantiacus*), *J Clin Microbiol*, **22**: 472–4.

Pulverer G, Schütt-Gerowitt H, Schaal KP, 1975, Bacteriophages of *Nocardia asteroides*, *Med Microbiol Immunol*, **161**: 113–22.

Rainey FA, Burghardt J et al., 1995, Phylogenetic analysis of the genera *Rhodococcus* and *Nocardia* and evidence for the evolutionary origin of the genus *Nocardia* from within the radiation of *Rhodococcus* species, *Microbiology*, **141**: 523–8.

Reller LB, Maddoux GL et al., 1975, Bacterial endocarditis caused by *Oerskovia turbata*, *Ann Intern Med*, **83**: 664–6.

Richet H, Craven PC et al., 1991, A cluster of *Rhodococcus* (*Gordona*) *bronchialis* sternal-wound infections after coronary-artery bypass surgery, *N Engl J Med*, **324**: 104–9.

Ridell M, 1974, Serological study of nocardiae and mycobacteria by using '*Mycobacterium*' *pellegrino* and *Nocardia corallina* precipitation reference systems, *Int J Syst Bacteriol*, **24**: 64–72.

Ridell M, 1977, Studies on corynebacterial precipitinogens common to mycobacteria, nocardiae and rhodococci, *Int Arch Allergy Appl Immunol*, **55**: 468–75.

Ridell M, 1981a, Immunodiffusion studies of *Mycobacterium*, *Nocardia* and *Rhodococcus* for taxonomic purposes, *Zentralbl Bakteriol Suppl*, **11**: 235–41.

Ridell M, 1981b, Immunodiffusion studies of some *Nocardia* strains, *J Gen Microbiol*, **123**: 69–74.

Ridell M, Baker R et al., 1979, Immunodiffusion studies of ribosomes in classification of mycobacteria and related taxa, *Int Arch Allergy Appl Immunol*, **59**: 162–72.

Rihs JD, McNeil MM et al., 1990, *Oerskovia xanthineolytica* implicated in peritonitis associated with peritoneal dialysis, *J Clin Microbiol*, **28**: 1934–7.

Romano AH, Sohler A, 1956, Biochemistry of the Actinomycetales. II. A comparison of the cell wall composition of species of the genera *Streptomyces* and *Nocardia*, *J Bacteriol*, **72**: 865–8.

Roth GD, Flanagan V, 1969, The pathogenicity of *Rothia dentocariosa* inoculated into mice, *J Dent Res*, **49**: 957–8.

Ruimy R, Boiron P et al., 1995, Phylogeny of the genus *Corynebacterium* deduced from analyses of small-subunit ribosomal DNA sequences, *Int J Syst Bacteriol*, **45**: 740–6.

Ruimy R, Riegel P et al., 1996, *Nocardia pseudobrasiliensis* sp. nov., a new species of *Nocardia* which groups bacterial strains previously identified as *Nocardia brasiliensis* and associated with invasive diseases, *Int J Syst Bacteriol*, **46**: 259–64.

Sahathevan M, Harvey FAH et al., 1991, Epidemiology, bacteriology and control of an outbreak of *Nocardia asteroides* infection in a liver unit, *J Hosp Infect*, **18, Suppl. A:** 473–80.

Saitou N, Nei M, 1987, The neighbor-joining method: a new method for reconstructing phylogenetic trees, *Mol Biol Evol*, **4:** 406–25.

Salinas-Carmona MC, Welsh O, Casillas SM, 1993, Enzyme-linked immunosorbent assay for serological diagnosis of *Nocardia brasiliensis* and clinical correlation with mycetoma infections, *J Clin Microbiol*, **31:** 2901–6.

Salman MD, Bushnell RB, Pier AC, 1982, Determination of sensitivity and specificity of the *Nocardia asteroides* skin test for detection of bovine mammary infections caused by *Nocardia asteroides* and *Nocardia caviae*, *Am J Vet Res*, **43:** 332–5.

Samies JH, Hathaway BN et al., 1986, Lung abscess due to *Corynebacterium equi*. Report of the first case in a patient with acquired immune deficiency syndrome, *Am J Med*, **80:** 685–8.

Schaal KP, 1972, Zur mikrobiologischer Diagnostik der Nocardiose, *Zentralbl Bakteriol I Abt Orig*, **220:** 242–6.

Schaal KP, 1977, *Nocardia, Actinomadura* and *Streptomyces*, CRC Handbook Series in Clinical Laboratory Sciences, Section E, Clinical Microbiology, vol. I, ed. von Graevenitz A, CRC Press, Cleveland, Ohio, 131–58.

Schaal KP, 1985, Laboratory diagnosis of actinomycete diseases, *Chemical Methods in Bacterial Systematics*, eds Goodfellow M, Minnikin DE, Academic Press, London, 359–81.

Schaal KP, 1991, Medical and microbiological problems arising from airborne infection in hospitals, *J Hosp Infect*, **18, Suppl. A:** 451–9.

Schaal KP, Lee H-J, 1992, Actinomycete infections in humans – a review, *Gene*, **115:** 201–11.

Scharfen J, 1975, Untraditional glucose fermenting actinomycetes as human pathogens. Part II. *Rothia dentocariosa* as a cause of abdominal actinomycosis and a pathogen for mice, *Zentralbl Bakteriol Abt I Orig A*, **233:** 80–92.

Schleifer K-H, Kandler O, 1972, Peptidoglycan types of bacterial cell walls and their taxonomic implications, *Bacteriol Rev*, **36:** 407–77.

Schleifer K-H, Seidl PH, 1985, Chemical composition of structure of murein, *Chemical Methods in Bacterial Systematics*, eds Goodfellow M, Minnikin DE, Academic Press, London, 201–19.

Schuppler M, Mertens F et al., 1995, Molecular characterisation of nocardioform actinomycetes in activated sludge by 16S rRNA analysis, *Microbiology*, **141:** 513–21.

Serrano JA, Beaman BL et al., 1986, Histological and ultrastructural studies on human actinomycetoma, *Biological, Biochemical and Biomedical Aspects of Actinomycetes*, eds Szabó G, Bíró S, Goodfellow M, Akadémiai Kiadó, Budapest, 647–62.

Severo LC, Petrillo VF, Coutinho LM, 1987, Actinomycetoma caused by *Rhodococcus* spp., *Mycopathologia*, **98:** 129–31.

Shainhouse JZ, Pier AC, Stevens DA, 1978, Complement fixation antibody test for human nocardiosis, *J Clin Microbiol*, **8:** 516–19.

Shapiro CL, Haft RF et al., 1992, *Tsukamurella paurometabolum*: a novel pathogen causing catheter-related bacteremia in patients with cancer, *Clin Infect Dis*, **14:** 200–3.

Shawar RM, Moore DG, LaRocco MT, 1990, Cultivation of *Nocardia* spp. on chemically defined media for selective recovery of isolates from clinical specimens, *J Clin Microbiol*, **28:** 508–12.

Sindhuphak W, MacDonald E, Head E, 1985, Actinomycetoma caused by *Nocardiopsis dassonvillei*, *Arch Dermatol*, **121:** 1332–4.

Singh SM, Naidu J et al., 1991, Cutaneous infections due to *Nocardiopsis dassonvillei* (Brocq-Rousseu) Meyer 1976, endemic in members of a family up to fifth degree relatives, *XI Congress of the International Society for Human and Animal Mycology*, Program Abstracts, 85.

Skerman VBD, McGowan V, Sneath PHA, 1980, Approved lists of bacterial names, *Int J Syst Bacteriol*, **30:** 225–340.

Snijders EP, 1924, Cavia-scheefkopperij, een nocardiose, *Geneeskd Tijdschr Ned Ind*, **64:** 85–7.

Sohler A, Romano AH, Nickerson WJ, 1958, Biochemistry of the Actinomycetales. III. Cell wall composition and the action of lysozyme upon cells and cell walls of the Actinomycetales, *J Bacteriol*, **75:** 282–90.

Sottnek FO, Brown JM et al., 1977, Recognition of *Oerskovia* species in the clinical laboratory: characterisation of 35 isolates, *Int J Syst Bacteriol*, **27:** 263–70.

Stackebrandt E, Smida J, Collins MD, 1988, Evidence of phylogenetic heterogeneity within the genus *Rhodococcus*: revival of the genus *Gordona* (Tsukamura), *J Gen Microbiol*, **35:** 364–8.

Stark DA, Anderson NG, 1990, A case-control study of *Nocardia* mastitis in Ontario dairy herds, *Can Vet J*, **31:** 197–201.

Steingrube VA, Brown BA et al., 1995, DNA amplification and restriction endonuclease analysis for differentiation of 12 species and taxa of *Nocardia*, including recognition of four new taxa within the *Nocardia asteroides* complex, *J Clin Microbiol*, **33:** 3096–101.

Stevens DA, Pier AC et al., 1981, Laboratory evaluation of an outbreak of nocardiosis in immunocompromised hosts, *Am J Med*, **71:** 928–34.

Stoecker MA, Russell HP, Staley JT, 1994, *Rhodococcus zopfii* sp. nov., a toxicant-degrading bacterium, *Int J Syst Bacteriol*, **44:** 106–10.

Suzuki K, Goodfellow M, O'Donnell AG, 1993, Cell envelopes and classification, *Handbook of New Bacterial Systematics*, Academic Press, London, 195–250.

Thiroux A, Pelletier J, 1912, Mycetome à grains rouges de la paroi thoracique. Isolement et culture d'une nouvelle oospora à pathogène, *Bull Soc Pathol Exot*, 585–9.

Tight RR, Bartlett MS, 1981, Actinomycetoma in the United States, *Rev Infect Dis*, **3:** 1139–50.

Tisdall PA, Roberts GD, Anhalt JP, 1979, Identification of clinical isolates of mycobacteria with gas-liquid chromatography alone, *J Clin Microbiol*, **10:** 506–14.

Trevisan V, 1889, *I Generi e le Specie delle Batteriacee*, Zanaboni and Gabuzzi, Milan.

Trujillo ME, Goodfellow M, 1997, Polyphasic taxonomic study of clinically significant actinomadurae including the description of *Actinomadura latina* sp. nov., *Zentralbl Bakteriol*, **25:** 212–33.

Tsukamura M, 1965, Differentiation of mycobacteria by picric acid tolerance, *Am Rev Respir Dis*, **92:** 491–2.

Tsukamura M, 1969, Numerical taxonomy of the genus *Nocardia*, *J Gen Microbiol*, **56:** 265–87.

Tsukamura M, 1971, Proposal of a new genus, *Gordona*, for slightly acid-fast organisms occurring in sputa of patients with pulmonary disease and in soil, *J Gen Microbiol*, **68:** 15–26.

Tsukamura M, 1974, A further numerical taxonomic study of the *rhodochrous* group, *Jpn J Microbiol*, **18:** 37–44.

Tsukamura M, 1978, Numerical classification of *Rhodococcus* (formerly *Gordona*) organisms recently isolated from sputa of patients: description of *Rhodococcus sputi* Tsukamura sp. nov., *Int J Syst Bacteriol*, **28:** 169–81.

Tsukamura M, 1981a, Differentiation between the genera *Mycobacterium, Rhodococcus* and *Nocardia* by susceptibility to 5-fluorouracil, *J Gen Microbiol*, **125:** 205–8.

Tsukamura M, 1981b, Tests for susceptibility to mitomycin C as aids in differentiating the genus *Rhodococcus* from the genus *Nocardia* and for differentiating *Mycobacterium fortuitum* and *Mycobacterium chelonei* from other rapidly growing mycobacteria, *Microbiol Immunol*, **25:** 1197–9.

Tsukamura M, 1982a, Differentiation between the genera *Rhodococcus* and *Nocardia* and between species of the genus *Mycobacterium* by susceptibility to bleomycin, *J Gen Microbiol*, **128:** 2385–8.

Tsukamura M, 1982b, Numerical analysis of the taxonomy of nocardiae and rhodococci. Division of *Nocardia asteroides sensu stricto* into two species and descriptions of *Nocardia pseudotuberculosis* sp. nov. Tsukamura (formerly the Kyoto-I-group of Tsukamura), *Nocardia nova* sp. nov. Tsukamura, *Rhodococcus aichiensis* sp. nov. Tsukamura, *Rhodococcus chubiensis* sp. nov. Tsukamura, *Microbiol Immunol*, **26:** 1101–19.

Tsukamura M, Kawakami K, 1982, Lung infection caused by *Gordona aurantiaca* (*Rhodococcus aurantiacus*), *J Clin Microbiol*, **16:** 604–7.

Tsukamura M, Hikosaka K et al., 1988, Severe progressive subcutaneous abscess and necrotizing tenosynovitis caused by *Rhodococcus aurantiacus*, *J Clin Microbiol*, **26:** 201–5.

Uchida K, Aida K, 1977, Acyl type of bacteria cell wall: its simple identification by colorimetric method, *J Gen Appl Microbiol*, **23:** 249–60.

Uchida K, Aida K, 1979, Taxonomic significance of cell-wall acyl type in *Corynebacterium-Mycobacterium-Nocardia* group by a glycolate test, *J Gen Appl Microbiol*, **25:** 169–83.

Vincent H, 1894, Étude sur le parasite du pied le madura, *Ann Inst Pasteur (Paris)*, **8:** 129–51.

Wallace RJ Jr, Steele LC, 1988, Susceptibility testing of *Nocardia* species for the clinical laboratory, *Diagn Microbiol Infect Dis*, **9:** 155–66.

Wallace RJ Jr, Septimus EJ et al., 1977, Disk diffusion susceptibility testing of *Nocardia* species, *J Infect Dis*, **35:** 568–76.

Wallace RJ Jr, Steele LC et al., 1988, Antimicrobial susceptibility patterns of *Nocardia asteroides*, *Antimicrob Agents Chemother*, **32:** 1776–9.

Wallace RJ Jr, Tsukamura M et al., 1990, Cefotaxime-resistant *Nocardia asteroides* strains are isolates of the controversial species *Nocardia farcinica*, *J Clin Microbiol*, **28:** 2726–32.

Wallace RJ Jr, Brown BA et al., 1991, Clinical and laboratory features of *Nocardia nova*, *J Clin Microbiol*, **29:** 2407–11.

Wang Y, Zhang Z, Ruan J, 1996, Phylogenetic analysis reveals new relationships among members of the genera *Microtetraspora* and *Microbispora*, *Int J Syst Bacteriol*, **46:** 658–63.

Williams ST, Wellington EMH, Tipler LS, 1980, The taxonomic implications of the reactions of representative *Nocardia* strains to actinophage, *J Gen Microbiol*, **119:** 173–8.

Williams ST, Sharples GP et al., 1976, The micromorphology and fine structure of nocardioform organisms, *The Biology of the Nocardiae*, eds Goodfellow M, Brownell GH, Serrano JA, Academic Press, London, 103–40.

Wright JH, 1905, The biology of microorganisms of actinomycosis, *J Med Res*, **13:** 349–404.

Wust J, Lanzendorfer H et al., 1990, Peritonitis caused by *Actinomadura madurae* in a patient on CAPD, *Eur J Clin Microbiol Infect Dis*, **9:** 700–1.

Yano I, Imaeda T, Tsukamura M, 1990, Characterisation of *Nocardia nova*, *Int J Syst Bacteriol*, **40:** 170–4.

Yano I, Kageyama K et al., 1978, Separation and analysis of molecular species of mycolic acids in *Nocardia* and related taxa by gas chromatography, *Biomed Mass Spectrom*, **5:** 14–24.

Yano I, Tomiyasu I et al., 1986, GC/MS analysis of mycolic acids molecular species and contribution to the chemotaxonomy of new *Rhodococcus* species, *Biological, Biochemical and Biomedical Aspects of Actinomycetes*, Part B, eds Szabó G, Biró S, Goodfellow M, Akadémiai Kiadó, Budapest, 567–70.

Yassin AF, Binder C, Schaal KP, 1993, Identification of mycobacterial isolates by thin-layer and capillary gas-liquid chromatography under diagnostic routine conditions, *Zentralbl Bakteriol*, **278:** 34–48.

Yassin AF, Rainey FA et al., 1995, *Tsukamurella inchonensis* sp. nov., *Int J Syst Bacteriol*, **45:** 522–7.

Yassin AF, Rainey FA et al., 1996, *Tsukamurella pulmonis* sp. nov., *Int J Syst Bacteriol*, **46:** 429–36.

Yassin AF, Rainey FA et al., 1997, *Tsukamurella tyrosinosolvens* sp. nov., *Int J Syst Bacteriol*, in press.

Yazawa K, Mikami Y, Uno J, 1989, *In vitro* susceptibility of *Nocardia* spp. to a new fluoroquinolone, tosufloxacin T-3262, *Antimicrob Agents Chemother*, **33:** 2140–1.

Yeruham I, Hadini A, Elad D, 1991, Human dermatophilosis *Dermatophilus congolensis* in dairymen in Israel, *Isr J Vet Med*, **46:** 114–16.

Zamora A, Bojalil LF, Bastarrachea F, 1963, Immunologically active polysaccharides from *Nocardia asteroides* and *Nocardia brasiliensis*, *J Bacteriol*, **85:** 549–55.

Zopf W, 1891, Uber Ausscheidung von Fellfarbstoffen (Lysochromen) seitens geiusér Spattjulze, *Ber Dtsch Bot Ges*, **9:** 22–8.

THE ACTINOMYCETES: *MICROCOCCUS* AND RELATED GENERA

M Goodfellow

1 *MICROCOCCUS*

1.1 Definition

Micrococcus species are gram-positive, non-encapsulated, non-halophilic actinomycetes which form spherical cells (0.8–1.8 μm in diameter) arranged in tetrads or irregular clusters of tetrads that are non-motile and asporogenous. They are aerobic, chemo-organotrophic, catalase- and oxidase-positive and have a strictly respiratory metabolism. The optimal growth range is 25–37°C. The peptidoglycan contains L-lysine as the diagnostic diamino acid. The peptidoglycan variation is either A2, with the interpeptide bridge consisting of a polymerized peptide subunit, or A4α. Galactosamine or mannosamine-uronic acid may be present as an amino sugar in the cell wall polysaccharide. The major menaquinones are either MK-8 and MK-8(H_2) or MK-8(H_2); MK-7 or MK-7(H_2) and MK-9(H_2) occur in minor amounts. Micrococci contain cytochromes aa_3, b_{557}, and d_{626}; cytochromes b_{563}, b_{564}, b_{567}, c_{550} and c_{551} may be present. They are also rich in *iso-* and *anteiso*-branched fatty acids, with 12 and 13-methyltetradecanoic acids predominating. Teichuronic acids may be present but mycolic acids and teichoic acids are absent. The predominant polar lipids are phosphatidylglycerol, diphosphatidylglycerol, unknown ninhydrin-negative phospholipids and glycolipids; phosphatidylinositol may be present. The major aliphatic hydrocarbons (br-Δ-C) are C_{27} to C_{29} components. The range of G + C content of the DNA is 69–76 mol% (T_m). The primary natural habitat is the mammalian skin. The type species is *Micrococcus luteus* (Schroeter 1872) Cohn 1872.

2 AEROBIC, GRAM-POSITIVE, CATALASE-POSITIVE COCCI

Initial problems in the systematics of these organisms can be attributed to the absence of reliable features for their classification and identification. Indeed, the separate processes of classification and identification were often confused by early investigators who based much of their work on a few subjectively weighted morphological and behavioural features that were rarely examined under rigorously standardized conditions. The situation was further complicated by a tendency to lump micrococci and staphylococci together first in the genus *Micrococcus* (Hucker 1924, 1948) and later in the genus *Staphylococcus* (Shaw, Stitt and Cowan 1951).

The merger of *Micrococcus* and *Staphylococcus* in the sixth edition of *Bergey's Manual of Determinative Bacteriology* (Hucker 1948) prompted disbelievers to redouble their efforts to separate the 2 genera. Evans, Bradford and Niven (1955) proposed separating micrococci from staphylococci on the basis of oxygen requirements. The obligate aerobes were classified in the genus *Micrococcus* and the facultative cocci in the genus *Staphylococcus*. This division was recognized in the seventh edition of *Bergey's Manual of Determinative Bacteriology* (Breed, Murray and Smith 1957). Detailed accounts of the intricacies of the early taxonomic history of micrococci and staphylococci are available (Hill 1981, Kloos, Schleifer and Götz 1992).

A clear distinction between micrococci and staphylococci was eventually drawn on the basis of their DNA base composition (Silvestri and Hill 1965, Rosypal, Rosypalová and Horejš 1966, Kocur, Bergan and Mortensen 1971). These investigators found that the G + C content of the DNA of micrococci fell within the range 63–73 mol%; the corresponding range for staphylococci was 30–39 mol%. This wide divergence in DNA base composition shows that these genera are not closely related. More recent taxonomic studies have distinguished micrococci from staphylococci on the basis of the chemical composition of cell walls (Schleifer and Kandler 1972, Endl et al. 1983), comparative immunology of catalases (Schleifer 1986) and antibiotic susceptibility patterns (Schleifer and Kloos 1975a, Falk and Guering 1983). These organisms also contain different types of menaquinones (Jeffries et al. 1969, Yamada et al. 1976) and have contrasting cytochrome patterns (Faller, Götz and Schleifer 1980).

The first comprehensive comparative study on the taxonomy of aerobic, gram-positive, catalase-positive cocci was carried out by Baird-Parker (1963, 1965) who examined isolates from diverse habitats for a battery of biochemical and physiological features. He used a modification of the anaerobic glucose utilization test to separate micrococci from staphylococci and assigned the former to 8 subgroups, the first 4 of which were subsequently transferred to the genus *Staphylococcus* as *Staphylococcus saprophyticus* (Schleifer and Kloos 1975b). Baird-Parker (1974) recognized 3 species of *Micrococcus* in the eighth edition of *Bergey's Manual of Determinative Bacteriology*, namely *M. luteus*, *Micrococcus roseus* and *Micrococcus varians*. This number rose to 9 in the current edition of *Bergey's Manual* (Kocur 1986) due to the addition of *Micrococcus agilis*, *Micrococcus halobius*, *Micrococcus kristinae*, *Micrococcus lylae*, *Micrococcus nishinomiyaensis* and *Micrococcus sedentarius*.

Stomatococcus mucilaginosus was introduced by Bergan and Kocur (1982) for bacteria previously known as '*Micrococcus mucilaginosus*' or '*Staphylococcus salivarius*'; a similar organism was described by Gaffky (1883) as '*Micrococcus tetragenus*'. This monospecific genus accommodates gram-positive, non-motile, capsulate, asporogenous, facultatively anaerobic cocci (0.9–1.3 μm in diameter) that are arranged in clusters and occasionally in pairs and tetrads. Stomatococci give a weak or negative catalase reaction and have a metabolism that is respiratory and fermentative. Acid, but not gas, is produced from glucose and various sugars. Colonies are usually mucoid, transparent or whitish, and adhere to agar surfaces. Stomatococci appear to be normal inhabitants of the human oral cavity and upper respiratory tract.

The genus *Stomatococcus* was distinguished from *Micrococcus* and *Staphylococcus* on the basis of DNA base and fatty acid composition and shown to have supra-generic affinities with *Arthrobacter* and *Micrococcus* (Ludwig et al. 1981, Stackebrandt, Scheuerlein and Schleifer 1983, Koch, Rainey and Stackebrandt 1994). Several phenotypic properties, notably the presence of a thick capsule, poor growth on nutrient agar, a weak

to negative catalase reaction and lack of growth on agar supplemented with 5% NaCl served to distinguish *S. mucilaginosus* from *Micrococcus* spp. (Bergan and Kocur 1986). Isolates of *S. mucilaginosus* that are catalase-negative may be misidentified as streptococci but their adherence to agar is a simple indicator of identity.

It is now widely accepted that nomenclature should reflect genomic relationships (Goodfellow, Manfio and Chun 1997) and that all preconceived notions should be examined within this context (Murray et al. 1990). These propositions have far reaching implications for the classification of the genus *Micrococcus* and related taxa. Constituent members of the genus *Micrococcus*, as defined in the current edition of *Bergey's Manual of Determinative Bacteriology*, have been assigned to 4 new centres of taxonomic variation, namely the genera *Dermacoccus*, *Kocuria*, *Kytococcus* and *Nesterenkonia*, primarily on the basis of chemotaxonomic and 16S rRNA sequence data (Stackebrandt et al. 1995). Similarly, *M. agilis* has been transferred to the genus *Arthrobacter* as *Arthrobacter agilis* (Koch, Schumann and Stackebrandt 1995). These developments leave the amended genus *Micrococcus* as a relatively homogeneous taxon (Stackebrandt et al. 1995) the properties of which were given earlier. Members of the new genera are gram-positive, asporogenous, non-capsular, catalase-positive, non-haemolytic cocci that have an essentially respiratory metabolism. The chemical characteristics of organisms previously classified in the genus *Micrococcus* are shown in Table 22.1.

The genus *Dermacoccus* is monospecific. *Dermacoccus nishinomiyaensis* strains produce spherical cells (0.9–1.6 μm diameter) that occur in pairs, tetrads or irregular clusters of tetrads. The organism is aerobic though weak growth sometimes occurs under micro-aerophilic conditions. Colonies are circular, entire, slightly convex, smooth with glistening (rarely matt) surfaces and bright orange; they may be up to 2 mm in diameter. Colony morphology and colour become more distinct with age; cell morphology is neither culture age nor medium dependent. Some strains produce a water-soluble orange exopigment. Cysteine or methionine and niacin are required; growth is stimulated by aspartic acid, glutamic acid, lysine, proline and tryptophan. Gelatin and starch, but not aesculin, are hydrolysed. The organism is oxidase-positive but negative for free and bound coagulase and DNAase; acetoin, indole and hydrogen sulphide are not produced. Dermacocci grow well at 25–37°C and in the presence of 5%, but not 7%, sodium chloride. They are found on mammalian skin.

The genus *Kocuria* accommodates *Kocuria rosea* (the type species), *Kocuria kristinae* and *Kocuria varians*. Members of the genus produce spherical cells (0.7–1.5 μm diameter) in pairs, tetrads or clusters. Colonies are circular and convex and may be pink or red, pale cream to pale orange or yellow. Colony morphology and colour become more distinct with age; cell morphology is neither culture age nor medium dependent. Water-soluble pigments are not produced. Growth may be stimulated by cysteine, methionine, pantothenic acid or thiamine. Some strains hydrolyse aesculin, gelatin and starch and produce acetoin and oxidase. The organism, which grows well in the range 22–37°C, and in the presence of up to 7.5% sodium chloride, is found in a variety of habitats, notably mammalian skin, soil and water.

Table 22.1   Chemotaxonomic properties of organisms previously assigned to the genus *Micrococcus*[a]

Characteristics	Micrococcus	Dermacoccus	Kocuria	Kytococcus	Nesterenkonia	Stomatococcus
Amino sugar in cell wall polysaccharide	Mannosamine-uronic acid or galactosamine	ND	Galactosamine	Galactosamine	ND	ND
Cytochrome pattern	aa_3, b_{557}, (b_{563}), (b_{564}), (b_{567}), (c_{550}), (c_{551}), d_{624}	aa_3, b_{555}, b_{559}, b_{564}, c_{549}, d_{626}	aa_3, b_{557}, (b_{562}), b_{564}, (c_{548}), (c_{549}), (c_{550}), d_{626}	aa_3, b_{557}, b_{561}, b_{564}, c_{550}, d_{626}	ND	ND
Lysozyme susceptibility	Susceptible–slightly resistant	Slightly resistant–resistant	Slightly resistant–resistant	Slightly resistant–resistant	Resistant	Resistant
Major aliphatic hydrocarbons (br-Δ-C)	C_{27}–C_{29}	C_{22}–C_{23}	C_{24}–C_{29}	C_{22}–C_{27}	ND	ND
Major menaquinone (s) (MK-)[b]	8 or 8(H_2)	8(H_2)	7(H_2), 8(H_2)	8, 9, 10	8, 9	7
Peptidoglycan type[c]	L-Lys-peptide subunit or L-Lys-D-Asp	L-Lys-D-Glu$_2$	L-Lys-L-Ala$_{3-4}$	L-Lys-L-Ser$_2$-(L-Ala)-D-Glu	L-Lys-Gly-L-Glu	L-Lys-(L-Ala)-L-Ser
Peptidoglycan variation[d]	A2 or A4α	A4α	A3α	A4α	A4α	A3α
Predominant fatty acids[e]	*Anteiso*-C$_{15:0}$, *iso*-C$_{15:0}$	C$_{15:0}$, *anteiso* and *iso*-C$_{17:0}$, *iso*-C$_{17:1}$, C$_{17:0}$	*Anteiso*-C$_{15:0}$, (*iso*-C$_{16:0}$), *anteiso*-C$_{17:0}$	*Iso*-C$_{15:0}$, *iso*-C$_{17:0}$, *anteiso*-C$_{17:0}$, *iso*-C$_{17:1}$	*Anteiso*-C$_{15:0}$, *anteiso*-C$_{17:0}$	*Anteiso*-C$_{15:0}$, *anteiso*-C$_{17:0}$, *iso*-C$_{15:0}$, *iso*-C$_{16:0}$
Predominant polar lipids	DPG, PG, (PI), GL, PL	DPG, PG, PI	DPG, PG, (PI, GL, PL)	DPG, PG, PI	DPG, PG, PI, GL, PL	DPG, PG, GL
G + C content of DNA (mol%; T$_m$)	69–76	66–71	66–75	68–69	70–72	56–60

[a]Data taken from Tornabene, Morrison and Kloos (1970); Schleifer and Kandler (1972), Kloos, Tornabene and Schleifer (1974), Faller and Schleifer (1981), Amadi, Alderson and Minnikin (1988) and Stackebrandt et al. (1995). Abbreviations: ND, not determined; ( ) components showing variable occurrence.

[b]Abbreviations exemplified by MK-8, unsaturated menaquinone with 8 isoprene units.

[c]Abbreviations: L-Ala, L-alanine; D-Asp, D-aspartic acid; D-Glu, D-glutamic acid; Gly, glycine; L-lys, L-lysine and L-Ser, L-serine.

[d]Tridigital classification of peptidoglycans after Schleifer and Kandler (1972).

[e]Abbreviations exemplified by *anteiso*-C$_{15}$, 12-methyltetradecanoic acid; *iso*-C$_{15}$, 13-methyltetradecanoic acid and C$_{15:0}$, pentadecanoic acid. Abbreviations: DPG, diphosphatidylglycerol; PG, phosphatidylglycerol; PI, phosphatidylinositol; GL, glycolipid; PL, phospholipid.

The sole species of the genus *Kytococcus* is *Kytococcus sedentarius*. This organism forms spherical cells (0.8–1.1 μm diameter) which usually occur in tetrads or in tetrads in cubical packets. In smears, cells are often enveloped by a slimy gram-negative layer. Colonies are circular, entire, convex to pulvinate, usually smooth and deep white or buttercup yellow. They develop slowly and may be up to 3.5 mm in diameter. Colony morphology and colour become more distinct with age; cell morphology is neither culture age nor medium dependent. Some strains produce a brownish exopigment. The organism is acetoin-negative and metabolically inert for acid production from carbohydrates. Gelatin is hydrolysed but aesculin and starch are not; most strains are oxidase-negative. Methionine is required; many strains also need arginine, leucine, lysine, pantothenic acid, tyrosine and valine for growth. Good growth occurs in the presence of 10% sodium chloride and within the temperature range 28–36°C. The primary habitat is human skin.

The genus *Nesterenkonia* is also monospecific. *Nesterenkonia halobia* produces spheres (0.8–1.5 μm diameter) which occur singly, in pairs and sometimes in tetrads or irregular clusters. The organism is moderately halophilic and forms circular, smooth, opaque and non-pigmented colonies on nutrient agar supplemented with 5% sodium chloride. Optimal growth occurs on media containing 1–2 M sodium chloride and moderate growth is evident in the presence of 4 M sodium chloride; growth does not occur in the absence of sodium or potassium chloride. Acid is produced aerobically from a range of sugars, acetoin and oxidase activity is seen but neither hydrogen sulphide nor indole is produced. Starch, but not gelatin, is hydrolysed. The growth temperature range is 20–40°C. The organism was isolated from unrefined salt and presumably inhabits saline habitats.

It is evident that considerable care is needed to distinguish *Dermacoccus*, *Kocuria*, *Kytococcus*, *Micrococcus*, *Nesterenkonia* and *Stomatococcus* from one another, from phylogenetically related taxa (Fig. 22.1), and from other gram-positive, catalase-positive cocci, such as those classified in the genera *Deinococcus*, *Luteococcus*, *Planococcus* and *Salinicoccus*. A number of taxonomic features can be weighted for this purpose (Table 22.2). Molecular systematic data led to the reclassification of '*Micrococcus conglomeratus*' strains as *Brachybacterium conglomeratus* (Takeuchi, Fang and Yokota 1995) and to the assignment of 2 red-pigmented, moderately halophilic organisms, previously misclassified as *Micrococcus roseus*, to the genus *Salinicoccus* (Ventosa et al. 1993). Similarly, *Deinococcus erythromyxa* has been transferred to the genus *Kocuria* (Rainey et al. 1997).

The radical nomenclatural changes outlined above make it difficult to interpret the significance of much of the earlier literature on the genus *Micrococcus sensu lato* as it is not always clear which particular taxa are being considered. Consequently, in the rest of this chapter the term 'micrococci' is used to cover organisms now classified in the genera *Dermacoccus*, *Kocuria*, *Kytococcus*, *Micrococcus sensu stricto*, *Nesterenkonia* and *Stomatococcus*.

3   HABITAT

Micrococci are widely distributed in nature but their primary habitat is mammalian skin. Kloos, Tornabene and Schleifer (1974) showed that nearly all of 115 individuals living in 18 different states in the USA carried cutaneous populations of micrococci. The percentages of individuals carrying the various species were as follows: *M. luteus*, 90%; *K. varians*, 75%; *M. lylae*, 33%; *D. nishinomiyaensis*, 28%; *M. kristinae*, 25%; *K. rosea*, 15% and *K. sedentarius*, 13%. The *M. luteus* populations were usually relatively large, occupying, on average, just over half the skin sites sampled on individuals carrying this species. Certain strains of *M. luteus*, *K. varians*, *K. kristinae* and *K. sedentarius* have been shown to persist on specific individuals for up to a year, suggesting that they form part of the resident microflora (Kloos and Musselwhite 1975); *S. mucilaginosus* is also a member of the normal human oral flora. Carr and Kloos (1977) noted an increase in the occurrence of micrococci on infant skin with increasing age up to 10 weeks. However, micrococci were rarely isolated from infants less than one week old.

The skin of other mammals, such as cattle, dogs, horses, pigs, squirrels, rats and primates, is also a rich source of micrococci (Kloos, Zimmerman and Smith 1976). *M. luteus* has only rarely been isolated from non-human mammals; the predominant isolate from such sources appears to be *K. varians*. Members of other micrococcal taxa found on human skin seem to have a narrower host range, possibly due to their requirement of one or more amino acids and vitamins for growth (Farrior and Kloos 1975, 1976). A coherent picture of the distribution of micrococci on other animals, notably amphibians, birds, fish and reptiles, awaits further study. Micrococci have also been isolated from diverse environmental samples, especially animal and dairy products, but such habitats are usually considered as secondary sources of the organisms. Indeed, *M. luteus* cells die relatively quickly when added to natural soil (Casida 1980a, 1980b). In ecological surveys great care needs to be taken to ensure that environmental samples do not become contaminated with micrococci from the skin of investigators.

4   MORPHOLOGY AND CULTURAL CHARACTERISTICS

On standard complex media such as nutrient agar, micrococci usually appear as typical gram-positive spheres (0.7–1.8 μm in diameter) arranged predominantly in tetrads or diplococci. *S. mucilaginosus* grows as cocci arranged in large and irregular clusters. The cells of this organism form extensive capsules composed of polysaccharide (Silva, Polonia and Kocur 1977). The colonies of micrococci are usually circular, convex, entire and smooth. Some strains, such as *K. varians*, may form matted colonies. Colonies may have an orange, orange-red, pink-red, red or yellow pigment. The colonies of some species, notably *D. nishinomiyaensis* and *K. varians*, may be confused with those of certain coryneform bacteria (Kloos, Tornabene and Schleifer 1974). By contrast, those of *S. mucilaginosus* are distinctive as they are mucoid and adhere to agar surfaces.

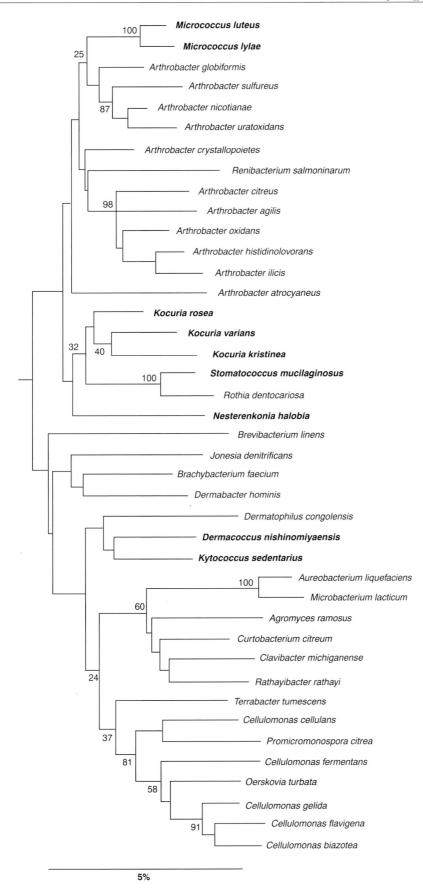

Fig. 22.1 Phylogenetic tree showing relationships between *Dermacoccus*, *Kocuria*, *Kytococcus*, *Micrococcus*, *Nesterenkonia*, *Stomatococcus* and related genera. The tree was constructed using the least squares method (De Soete 1983). The numbers at the nodes indicate the levels of bootstrap support (Felsenstein 1985) based on data for 300 replicates; only values greater than 30% are shown. The scale bar indicates 5 nucleotide substitutions per 100 nucleotides (modified from Stackebrandt et al. 1995).

Table 22.2 Morphological and chemotaxonomic features of aerobic, asporogenous, catalase-positive cocci and some related taxa[a]

	Cell morphology	Motility	Wall diamino acid	Peptidoglycan variation	Fatty acids[b]	Major menaquinones (MK-)	Polar lipids	Mol% G + C content
Micrococcus and related taxa								
Micrococcus	Coccoid	−	Lysine	A2, A4α	S,A,I	8, 8(H$_2$)	DPG, PG, PL, GL, (PI)	69–76
Arthrobacter	Rod-coccus	+, −	Lysine	A3α, A4α	S,A,I	8, 9	DPG, PG, PI, DMDG	60–66
Brachybacterium	Short rods, coccoid	−	*meso*-Diaminopimelic acid	A4γ	S,A,I	7	DPG, PG, GL	68–72
Dermacoccus	Coccoid	−	Lysine	A4α	S,A,I	8(H$_2$)	DPG, PG, PL	66–71
Dermabacter	Short rods	−	*meso*-Diaminopimelic acid	A1γ	S,A,I	7, 8, 9	DPG, PG, PL, GL	62
Kocuria	Coccoid	−	Lysine	A3α	S,A,I	7(H$_2$), 8(H$_2$)	DPG, PG, (PI, PL, GL)	66–75
Kytococcus	Coccoid	−	Lysine	A4α	(S),A,I	8, 9, 10	DPG, PG, PI	68–69
Nesterenkonia	Coccoid	−	Lysine	A4α	(S),A,I	8, 9	DPG, PG, PI, PL, GL	70–72
Renibacterium	Short rods	−	Lysine	A3α	S,A,I	9, 10	DPG, GL	52–54
Rothia	Irregular rods, coccoid	−	Lysine	A3α	S,A,I	7	DPG, PG	49–53
Stomatococcus	Coccoid	−	Lysine	A3α	S,A,I	7	DPG, PG	56–60
Other gram-positive cocci								
Deinococcus	Coccoid	−	Ornithine	A3α, A3β	S,A,I	8	Unusual pattern	62–71
Kineococcus	Coccoid	+	*meso*-Diaminopimelic acid	A1γ	Mainly *anteiso*-C$_{15:0}$	9(H$_2$)	DPG, PG, GL	74
Luteococcus	Coccoid	−	LL-*meso*-Diaminopimelic acid	A3γ	Mainly C$_{16:1}$, C$_{17:1}$, C$_{18:1}$	9(H$_4$)	DPG, PG, PI	66–68
Planococcus	Coccoid	+	Lysine, *meso*-diaminopimelic acid	A4α[c]	S,A,I	8	DPG, PG, PI	39–52
Salinicoccus	Coccoid	−	Lysine	A3α	(S),A,I	....	ND	51
Staphylococcus	Coccoid	−	Lysine	A3α	Mainly C$_{15Br}$, C$_{18:0}$, C$_{20:0}$	6, 7, 8	GL, PG, lys PG, DGD	30–38

[a]Data taken from Komura, Yamada and Komagata (1975), Kocur (1986), Ventosa et al. (1990), Tamura, Takeuchi and Yokota (1994) and Stackebrandt et al. (1995).
[b]S, straight chain saturated; A, *anteiso*-methyl branched; I, *iso*-methyl branched.
[c]Data for *Planococcus citreus*.
Abbreviations: DPG, diphosphatidylglycerol; PG, phosphatidylglycerol; GL, glycolipid; PI, phosphatidylinositol; PL, phospholipid.

5 METABOLISM

Most micrococci are strict aerobes that grow well on nutrient media at 37°C. They oxidize a wide range of carbon compounds to carbon dioxide and water. Glucose is metabolized by the fructose-1,6-biphosphate and hexose monophosphate pathways and citric acid enzymes (Dawes and Holmes 1958, Perry and Evans 1960, Blevins, Perry and Evans 1969). Like most bacteria, micrococci have a class II D-fructose-1,6-biphosphate aldolase (Götz, Nürnberger and Schleifer 1979) though some strains of *K. kristinae* and *K. varians* grow as facultative anaerobes and produce L-lactic acid from glucose. *M. luteus* produces an NAD-dependent and NAD-independent malic dehydrogenase which oxidizes malic acid to oxalacetic acid (Cohn 1956), a tyramine oxidase which catalyses the oxidation of tyramine and dopamine (Yamada et al. 1967) and a phosphoglucomutase which is responsible for the interconversion of glucose-1-phosphate and glucose-6-phosphate (Hanabusa et al. 1966). The metabolism of exogenous pyrimidine bases and nucleosides has also been studied in this organism (Auling, Prella and Diekmann 1982, Auling and Moss 1984). The flavin adenine dinucleotide-containing putrescine oxidase of a strain labelled '*Micrococcus rubens*' catalyses oxidative deamination of putrescine (Ishizuka, Horinouchi and Beppu 1993). Various sugars are fermented by *S. mucilaginosus* though information is lacking on acid end products (Bergan and Kocur 1986). Members of this species may be catalase-negative.

Micrococci contain a range of cytochromes and menaquinones (Table 22.2). In addition to these compounds, *M. luteus* also contains NADH, lactate, malate and succinate dehydrogenases as part of the electron transport system (Erikson and Parker 1969, Crow and Owen 1983a, 1983b). The proton-translocating ATP synthase of *M. luteus* is of the typical F0F1 complex (Salton and Schor 1974, Schmitt et al. 1978). The cytoplasmic membrane of *M. luteus* is also the site of enzymes involved in peptidoglycan, phospholipid and teichuronic acid biosynthesis (De Siervo and Salton 1971, Traxler, Goustin and Anderson 1982, Park and Matsuhashi 1984).

Chemically defined media have been formulated for the growth of *K. varians* and *M. luteus* (Wolin and Naylor 1957, Grula, Luk and Chu 1961, Cooney and Thierry 1966). *M. luteus* strains may grow in a chemically defined medium containing pyruvate or glutamate as carbon and energy source, biotin and mineral salts (Perry and Evans 1960). Initiation of growth of this organism in a defined medium depends upon the presence of iron-binding compounds such as catechol or ferrichrome (Salton 1964, Walsh, O'Dor and Warren 1971). Micrococci require one or more amino acids and vitamins for growth (Aaronson 1955, Wolin and Naylor 1957, Eisenberg and Evans 1963, Farrior and Kloos 1975). Some micrococci can grow with ammonium phosphate as sole nitrogen source; *M. luteus* strains grow on inorganic nitrogen agar and *K. varians* on Simmons' citrate agar (Kloos, Tornabene

and Schleifer 1974). Under aerobic conditions, stomatococci grow well within 24–30 h on complex media such as brain–heart infusion agar. Colonies of this organism are smaller and firmly adherent to the agar surface under anaerobic conditions (Gordon 1967).

6 GENETICS

Genetic exchange has been demonstrated in *M. luteus* (Mahler and Grossman 1968, Okubo and Nakayama 1968, Kloos 1969, Kloos and Schultes 1969). Transformation of an auxotrophic *M. luteus* strain occurred between 1 and 5% of homologous values with DNA isolated from *M. lylae* (Kloos, Tornabene and Schleifer 1974). These low transformation rates suggest a considerable divergence between the 2 species, but nevertheless demonstrate a significant genetic relationship. By contrast, corresponding experiments between *M. luteus*, *K. sedentarius* and the 3 *Kocuria* spp. were negative. An epigenetic relationship between *M. lylae* and *M. luteus* has been established by comparative immunological studies of catalase in both double-immunodiffusion tests and quantitative microcomplement fixation assays (Rupprecht and Schleifer 1977). In addition, DNA probes specific for *M. lylae*–*M. luteus* (pAR28) and for arthrobacters and all micrococci have been constructed (Regensburger, Ludwig and Schleifer 1988).

Kloos (1969) determined the optimal conditions for transformation, thereby paving the way for a transformation procedure for use in genetic mapping (Kloos and Rose 1970). The histidine and tryptophan biosynthesis genes of *M. luteus* were mapped in studies which showed that at least 2 histidine genes are closely linked to the tryptophan gene cluster (Kloos and Rose 1970, Kane-Falce and Kloos 1975). The purine biosynthesis genes of *M. luteus* have also been mapped (Mohapatra and Kloos 1974, 1975). A preliminary physical map has been constructed for an extreme alkaliphile, designated *Micrococcus* sp. Y-1 (Park et al. 1994). In *M. luteus* there is a strong correlation between the relative amount of isoacceptor tRNAs for an amino acid and the usage of the corresponding synonymous codons (Kano et al. 1991).

Plasmids have been detected in some micrococci (Mathis and Kloos 1984) but not in *K. sedentarius* or *M. lylae*. To date, many micrococcal plasmids remain cryptic. Most strains with plasmids show only one or 2 types, ranging in size from 1.5 to 150 kDa. Slightly more complex plasmid patterns have been detected in *N. nishinomiyaensis*. Several small plasmids identified in *K. rosea*, *M. luteus* and *N. nishinomiyaensis* have been the subject of restriction endonuclease analyses and may be suitable for use as cloning vectors following some modifications (Kocur, Kloos and Schleifer 1992). A detailed physical map has been constructed of a plasmid isolated from a cholesterol biotransforming strain of *Micrococcus* (Verma et al. 1993).

7 CELL ENVELOPE COMPOSITION

The cell envelopes of micrococci consist of layers of peptidoglycan, lipid constituents and other polysaccharide fractions. The amino acid composition of the peptidoglycan of representative micrococci has been determined (Schleifer and Kandler 1972, Kocur 1986, Stackebrandt et al. 1995). All micrococci have a group A peptidoglycan (cross-linkage from the dicarboxylic acid at position 3 of the peptide subunit, which is L-lysine). However, the amino acid composition of the interpeptide subunits show considerable variation (see Table 22.1, p. 493). *M. luteus* shows the most unusual composition as the interpeptide bridge has the same composition as the peptide subunit (variation A2). By contrast, the interpeptide bridges of *K. sedentarius* and *M. lylae* contain a single dicarboxylic amino acid (glutamic acid and aspartic acid moieties, respectively; variation A4α), those of *D. nishinomiyaensis* and *N. halobia* a monocarboxylic acid and a dicarboxylic acid (serine and glutamic acid and glycine and glutamic acid, respectively; variation A4α), and those of *K. kristinae*, *K. rosea* and *K. varians* several monocarboxylic acids (alanine; variation A3α). The peptidoglycan type of *S. mucilaginosus* strains differs as the interpeptide bridge consists of either L-alanine, D-serine, or glycine (Schleifer and Kandler 1972, Stackebrandt, Scheuerlein and Schleifer 1983). Glycine, when present in the interpeptide bridges of micrococci, is linked to the carboxyl group of glutamic acid with only one molecule of glycine per molecule of glutamic acid present.

Neither teichoic acid nor lipoteichoic acid is present in the micrococcal wall (Bowden 1969, Schleifer and Kandler 1972, Sutcliffe 1994), though *M. luteus* has been reported to contain teichuronic acid (Perkins 1963, Yamada, Hirose and Matsuhashi 1975). However, macroamphiphilic polymers, described as 'atypical lipoteichoic acids' or lipoglycans, are usually found in organisms that lack lipoteichoic acids (Sutcliffe and Shaw 1991, Sutcliffe 1994). *M. luteus* was one of the first bacteria reported to produce a lipoglycan which did not contain a polyglycerophosphate (PGP) moiety (Powell, Duckworth and Baddiley 1974); a phenol-extractable succinylated lipomannan was subsequently characterized (Owen and Salton 1975, Pless, Schmitt and Lennarz 1975, Powell, Duckworth and Baddiley 1975) and similar structures consisting of around 50 mannose units and membrane anchored by a diglyceride unit were proposed (Pless, Schmitt and Lennarz 1975, Powell, Duckworth and Baddiley 1975). This lipomannan may be a multiglycosylated form of the dimannosyldiglyceride glycolipid of *M. luteus* (Lennarz and Talamo 1966, Scher and Lennarz 1969). Like lipoteichoic acid, the lipomannan formed micelles in aqueous solution and the succinyl esters gave it an overall negative charge, allowing it to bind Mg^{2+} ions effectively (Powell, Duckworth and Baddiley 1975). Lipomannans have also been detected in representatives of the genera *Dermacoccus*, *Kocuria* and *Kytococcus* (Sutcliffe and Alderson 1995). It is also interesting that these organisms have fatty acid methyl ester patterns broadly consistent

with the variations noted below. *S. mucilaginosus* also produces a lipoglycan distinct from lipoteichoic acid (Sutcliffe 1994, Sutcliffe and Old 1995) whereas a strain labelled '*M. conglomeratus*' was found to lack detectable PGP antigen (Hamada, Mizuno and Kotani 1978).

Methyl branched fatty acids, distinctive for many gram-positive bacteria, are the dominant class of cellular fatty acids found in micrococci (Ishizuka, Ueta and Yamakawa 1966, Girard 1971, Morrison, Tornabene and Kloos 1971, Onishi and Kamekura 1972, Jantzen, Bergan and Bøvre 1974, Brooks et al. 1980, Amadi, Alderson and Minnikin 1988). Stackebrandt et al. (1995) found that *M. luteus* and *M. lylae* gave similar fatty acid patterns with 13-methyltetradecanoic acid (iso-$C_{15:0}$) and 12-methyltetradecanoic acid ($anteiso$-$C_{15:0}$) as major components. *K. kristinae*, *K. rosea* and *K. varians* contained major amounts of 12-methyltetradecanoic acid and strain-dependent amounts of other fatty acids, including 14-methylpentadecanoic acid (iso-$C_{16:0}$), hexadecanoic acid ($C_{16:0}$), 14-methylhexadecanoic acid ($anteiso$-$C_{17:0}$), 13-methyltetradecanoic acid (iso-$C_{15:0}$) and hexadecenoic acid ($C_{16:1}$). *N. halobia* showed a similar fatty acid profile albeit with much higher levels of 14-methylhexadecanoic acid than in the *Kocuria* strains. By contrast, *K. sedentarius* contained several fatty acids absent in the other species, such as pentadecanoic ($C_{15:0}$), heptadecanoic ($C_{17:0}$) and 15-methylhexadecanoic (iso-$C_{17:0}$) acids, and *D. nishinomiyaensis* major amounts of 13-methyltetradecanoic, 15-methylhexadecanoic and 14-methylhexadecanoic acids. The fatty acid profiles of *S. mucilaginosus* and *Rothia dentocariosa* were found to be similar as they included a broad range of fatty acids from $C_{12:0}$ to $C_{18:2}$.

Less variation is shown in the polar lipid patterns of micrococci (Stackebrandt et al. 1995). *K. kristinae*, *M. luteus* and *N. halobia* contain diphosphatidylglycerol, phosphatidylglycerol, phosphatidylinositol and unknown ninhydrin-negative phospholipids and glycolipids. A similar pattern but without phosphatidylinositol was found in *M. lylae* and *S. mucilaginosus*. *D. nishinomiyaensis* and *K. sedentarius* had similar patterns, as did *K. rosea* and *K. varians*. A characteristic glycolipid, G1, found in stomatococci, has the chromatographic mobility of dimannosyl diacylglycerol (Amadi, Alderson and Minnikin 1988), a component that has also been detected in *R. dentocariosa* (Pandhi and Hammond 1975, Embley et al. 1984).

Micrococci show a number of menaquinone patterns (Jeffries 1969, Jeffries et al. 1969, Amadi, Alderson and Minnikin 1988, Amadi and Alderson 1991, Stackebrandt et al. 1995). *M. luteus* contains major amounts of a fully unsaturated menaquinone with 8 isoprene units (MK-8) and substantial proportions of a dihydrogenated menaquinone with 8 isoprene units [MK-8(H_2)]. By contrast, *M. lylae* possesses dihydrogenated menaquinones with 7, 8 and 9 isoprene units, the MK-8(H_2) component predominating. Similar patterns are found in *D. nishinomiyaensis* and *Kocuria* spp. *K. sedentarius* and *N. halobia* are characterized by the presence of fully unsaturated menaquinones (see Table 22.1, p. 493).

Serological relationships have not been found amongst species of *Kocuria*, *Micrococcus*, *Staphylococcus* and *Stomatococcus* (Bergan and Kocur 1986). *K. rosea*, *K. varians* and *M. luteus* have a number of agglutinogens without any systematic pattern. No relationship has been found between their specific agglutinogens and biochemical features (Hasselgren and Oeding 1972, Oeding and Hasselgren 1972). Simple serological tests have been described for the separation of micrococci from staphylococci based on the presence or absence of cell wall teichoic acid and peptidoglycan types (Hamada, Mizuno and Kotani 1978, Seidl and Schleifer 1978).

8 SUSCEPTIBILITY TO CHEMICALS AND PHAGES

A characteristic feature of micrococci is their resistance to lysostaphin (Gordon 1967, Klesius and Schuhardt 1968, Bergan, Bøvre and Hovig 1970, Schleifer and Kloos 1975a). Micrococci also tend to be slightly resistant or resistant to lysosyme (Jeffries 1968, Kloos, Tornabene and Schleifer 1974) and susceptible to a wide range of antibiotics, including chloramphenicol, erythromycin, kanamycin, neomycin, novobiocin, penicillin, streptomycin, tetracycline and vancomycin (Kloos, Tornabene and Schleifer 1974). *K. sedentarius* is resistant to methicillin and penicillin.

Bacteriophages isolated from micrococci, notably *K. varians* and *M. luteus*, lyse only micrococci (Naylor and Burgi 1956, Peters and Pulverer 1975, Bauske, Peters and Pulverer 1978). *Stomatococcus*-specific phages have yet to be found. Micrococci are resistant to staphylococcal phages (Peters, Pulverer and Pillich 1976, Bauske, Peters and Pulverer 1978) and do not absorb polyvalent phages isolated from coagulase-negative staphylococci (Schumacher-Perdreau, Pulverer and Schleifer 1979).

9 PATHOGENICITY

Compelling evidence is still needed to determine whether micrococci can be pathogenic for humans. Early reports associating micrococci with various infections, notably those of the urinary tract (Roberts 1967, Meers, Whyte and Sandys 1975, Sellin et al. 1975, Telander and Wallmark 1975) are difficult to evaluate due to poor strain characterization or incorrect identification. Consequently, only relatively recent case histories implicating micrococci can be taken into consideration.

K. sedentarius has been associated with pitted keratolysis (Nordstrom et al. 1987) and *M. luteus* with meningitis (Fosse et al. 1986), septic shock (Albertson, Natsions and Gleckman 1978), intracranial suppuration (Selladurai et al. 1993) and cavitating pneumonia in an immunosuppressed patient (Souhami et al. 1979). Similarly, *S. mucilaginosus* has been isolated from blood cultures taken from intravenous drug abusers with endocarditis (Coudron et al. 1987, Relman, Ruoff and Ferraro 1987) and from immunocompromised patients with bacteraemia (Barlow, Vogele and Dzintars 1986, Kaufhold, Reinert and Kern 1992), aggressive endocarditis of native heart valves (Rubin, Lyons and Murcia 1978, Prag, Kjoller and Espersen 1985) and recurrent peritonitis (Ragnoud et al. 1981). Micrococci, possibly *M. lylae*, have been isolated from blood and surgical specimens of patients associated with heart diseases and septic complications following cardiac surgery (Kocur, Kloos and Schleifer 1992). The increasing number of reports implicating micrococci in clinical cases cannot be ignored. Painstaking studies are needed to demonstrate whether micrococci should be considered as opportunistic pathogens.

10 ISOLATION AND CULTIVATION

Several semiquantitative methods have been described for isolating aerobic bacteria from human skin. The procedure described by Kloos and Musselwhite (1975) has been used for the isolation of micrococci and is suitable for use with human as well as mammalian skin.

Sterile cotton swabs are moistened with detergent containing Triton X-100 (0.1%) in 0.075 M phosphate buffer at pH 9 (Williamson 1965) and rubbed vigorously, with rotation, over approximately 8 cm² sites. Swabbing needs to be done for 5 s on sites such as the axillae, cheek, chin, forehead and nares, which usually support large populations of bacteria, and for 15 s on sites on arms and legs, which usually have relatively smaller populations. Swabs taken from the arm, cheek, chin and external nares, forehead and legs can be applied directly to agar media, such as P agar (Naylor and Burgi 1956), by rubbing, with rotation, over the entire surface of 100 mm diameter plates for 2 consecutive times. Swabs taken from the axillae and anterior nares, or from other sites found to support large populations, should be rinsed immediately in 5 ml of detergent, and the rinse applied to the surface of agar media. Inoculation media should be incubated under aerobic conditions for 4 days at 34°C and colonies counted and recorded according to morphology and pigmentation.

The procedure outlined above can be modified for use with other mammalian skin (Kloos, Zimmerman and Smith 1976). In some instances it may be necessary to supplement P agar with cyclohexamide (50 µg ml^{-1}; Kloos, Tornabene and Schleifer 1974, Kloos, Zimmerman and Smith 1976) in order to inhibit fungal growth. Similarly, P agar supplemented with 7% sodium chloride can be used to inhibit spreading colonies of aerobic, endospore-forming bacilli. Another selective medium, known as FTO agar, allows the growth of micrococci but prevents that of staphylococci (Curry and Borovian 1976). This medium, which contains nitrofuran as the selective agent, is especially useful for sampling areas of the skin, such as the axillae, nares and perineum, where staphylococci occur in large numbers.

In the case of stomatococci swab samples taken

Table 22.3 Chemical and biochemical characters separating micrococci from staphylococci

Character	Micrococci	Staphylococci
Acid (aerobically) from glycerol on erythromycin medium	–	+
Anaerobic fermentation of glucose	$-^a$	+
Cytochrome pattern	aa_3, b, c, d	a, b^b
Fructose-1,6-diphosphate aldolase class	II	I^c
Susceptibility to:		
bacitracin (0.04 unit disc)	+	–
furazolidone (100 µg disc)	–	+
lysostaphin (200 mg l^{-1})	–	+
Peptidoglycan composition (>2 mol glycine: 1 mol lysine)	–	+
DNA base composition (mol% G + C)	66–76	30–39

^{a}*K. kristinae* produces acid from glucose anaerobically.
^{b}*Staphylococcus caseolyticus, Staphylococcus lentus* and *Staphylococcus sciuri* also contain cytochrome *c*.
^{c}*Staphylococcus hyicus* and *Staphylococcus intermedius* contain both class I and II enzymes; *S. caseolyticus* contains only enzyme of class II.
+, Positive; –, negative.

from the human tongue or other parts of the oral cavity are inoculated onto blood agar or trypticase soy agar plates, which need to be incubated at 30–37°C for 1–2 days. Stomatococci grow well on brain–heart infusion agar under aerobic conditions. Most micrococci show good growth on nutrient agar and P agar at 37°C. These media need to be supplemented with 5% sodium chloride to support good growth of *N. halobia*.

11 CLASSIFICATION

The application of modern taxonomic methods has revolutionized the classification of aerobic, gram-positive, catalase-positive cocci. Recent studies have led to improved descriptions of established genera, the validation of new genera and species, the reduction of poorly described taxa to synonyms of previously proposed species, and the reassortment of mis-classified strains. The resultant improved taxonomy provides an invaluable basis for determining the biological properties of these poorly studied organisms and for recognizing new centres of taxonomic variation.

11.1 Intergeneric relationships of micrococci, planococci and staphylococci

The family Micrococcaceae Prévot 1961 encompasses the genera *Micrococcus, Planococcus, Staphylococcus* and *Stomatococcus*. However, there is a wealth of taxonomic evidence, notably from chemotaxonomic (Alderson 1985, Stackebrandt et al. 1995), DNA relatedness (Schleifer et al. 1979a, 1979b) and nucleic acid sequencing studies (Stackebrandt and Woese 1979, Ludwig et al. 1981, Stackebrandt, Lewis and Woese 1980, Stackebrandt, Scheuerlein and Schleifer 1983, Stackebrandt et al. 1995), which unequivocally show that the 4 genera should not be combined into a single family. It is clear that micrococci and stomato-cocci are related to an assortment of mainly amycelial

actinomycetes whereas planococci and staphylococci belong to the bacilli–lactobacilli–streptococci phyletic line. The close relationship of morphologically diverse bacteria demonstrates that shape can be a poor indicator of suprageneric relationships. It is very likely that the genera *Micrococcus, Planococcus, Staphylococcus* and *Stomatococcus* will be classified in different families when phylogenetic studies on these and related organisms have been completed.

11.2 Suprageneric relationships of micrococci

Analyses of almost complete 16S rDNA sequences of representative micrococci show that these organisms can be assigned to several phyletic lines (Fig. 22.1; Stackebrandt et al. 1995); these results confirm and extend those of previous phylogenetic studies (Stackebrandt and Woese 1979, Stackebrandt, Lewis and Woese 1980, Ludwig et al. 1981, Stackebrandt, Scheuerlein and Schleifer 1983, Koch, Rainey and Stackebrandt 1994). It is evident from the figure that *M. luteus* and *M. lylae* are related to one another and to the type species of the genus *Arthrobacter*, *Arthrobacter globiformis*, and its relatives. This group also contains *A. agilis*, which was recently transferred from the genus *Micrococcus* (Koch, Schumann and Stackebrandt 1995), and the fish pathogen, *Renibacterium salmoninarum*. A close relationship exists between *S. mucilaginosus* and *R. dentocariosa*; the 3 *Kocuria* spp. are loosely associated with this group. *N. halobia* lies at the periphery of the resultant aggregate group. A loose association is also evident between *D. nishinomiyaensis* and *K. sedentarius*, the most distantly related micrococci.

The branching pattern of the various micrococcal sublines (Fig. 22.1) were not markedly influenced by the treeing algorithms applied by Stackebrandt et al. (1995). However, some deviations were detected in the dendrogram based on the maximum-parsimony method. These deviations were particularly pronounced in distantly related organisms, notably *Jonesia denitrificans* and *N. halobia*, and in the formation of

Table 22.4 Phenotypic properties differentiating micrococci[a]

Characteristics	Dermacoccus		Kocuria		Kytococcus	Micrococcus		Nesterenkonia	Stomatococcus
	nishinomiyaensis	*kristinae*	*rosea*	*varians*	*sedentarius*	*luteus*	*lylae*	*halobia*	*mucilaginosus*
Acid aerobically from:									
glucose	d	+	+	+	−	−	−	+	+
glycerol	−	+	−	−	−	−	−	+	+
lactose	−	−	−	−	−	−	−	+	−
mannose	−	+	−	−	+	−	−	−	+
Arginine hydrolase	−	−	−	−	−	−	−	−	−
Nitrate to nitrite	d	−	+	+	−	−	−	−	+
Oxidase	+	+	−	−	−	+	+	+	−
Hydrolysis of:									
aesculin	−	+	−	−	−	−	−	ND	+
gelatin	+	−	−	+	+	+	+	−	+
Growth on:									
inorganic nitrogen agar	−	−	−	−	−	+	−	ND	ND
nutrient agar with 7% NaCl	−	+	+	+	+	+	+	+	−
Simmons' citrate agar	−	−	−	+	−	−	−	−	−
Colour of colonies	Orange	Pale orange	Pink/orange-red	Yellow	Cream-white/buttercup yellow	Yellow	Cream-white	Non-pigmented	Whitish
DNA mol% G+C	66–71	66–67	66–75	66–72	67–68	70–75	68–69	70–72	56–60

[a]Data taken from Bergan and Kocur (1982), Holt et al. (1994) and Stackebrandt et al. (1995).
Symbols: +, 90% or more strains positive; −, 90% or more of strains negative; d, 11–89% of strains positive; ND, not determined.

distinct phyletic lines for the *R. dentocariosa–S. mucila-ginosus* group and the *Kocuria* spp. A broader rDNA database is needed to clarify the detailed phylogenetic relationships between micrococci and related organisms. Nevertheless, micrococci can be distinguished both from one another and from related taxa on the basis of chemotaxonomic and morphological properties (Tables 22.1 and 22.2).

The heterogeneity of the micrococcal assemblage is underpinned by DNA relatedness (Ogasawara-Fujita and Sakahuchi 1976, Schleifer, Heise and Meyer 1979), chemotaxonomic (Jeffries et al. 1969, Schleifer and Kandler 1972, Jantzen, Bergan and Bøvre 1974, Faller, Götz and Schleifer 1980, Amadi, Alderson and Minnikin 1988, Amadi and Alderson 1991) and numerical taxonomic data (Alderson et al. 1991). Early DNA relatedness studies on what are now the type strains of *K. rosea*, *K. varians* and *M. luteus* revealed complementary DNA relatedness values below 10% (Ogasawara-Fujita and Sakahuchi 1976). These results were confirmed by Schleifer, Heise and Meyer (1979) who also found that *M. luteus* and *M. lylae* shared a DNA relatedness value of 40% under optimal hybridization conditions. The close relationship between these 2 species is also apparent from transformation experiments (Kloos 1969, Kloos, Tornabene and Schleifer 1974) and from numerical taxonomic data (Alderson et al. 1991). Oligonucleotide probe experiments directed against the 23S rRNA of *M. luteus* provide further evidence of an affinity between this organism and *M. lylae* (Regensburger, Ludwig and Schleifer 1988). The DNA of *M. lylae* showed a positive hybridization signal whereas DNAs from other micrococci gave negative results. It is also interesting that *R. dentocariosa* and *S. mucilaginosus* have several chemotaxonomic properties in common (Table 22.2) given their evolutionary closeness.

11.3 Subgeneric classification

A more reliable and comprehensive approach to the circumscription of bacterial species is emerging based on the integrated use of genotypic and phenotypic data (Goodfellow, Manfio and Chun 1997). This approach, known as polyphasic taxonomy, was introduced by Colwell (1970) to signify successive or simultaneous taxonomic studies on groups of related organisms using an array of methods designed to provide genotypic and phenotypic data. The improved classification of micrococci and related taxa makes it possible to choose objectively sets of strains for comparative taxonomic studies. Such investigations can be expected to yield improved species definitions and thereby provide a framework for the recognition of novel species. They will also provide a stable

nomenclature and a sound basis for devising improved identification and typing procedures.

12 IDENTIFICATION

Rapid and reliable methods are needed to distinguish between the various types of micrococci and between these organisms and phylogenetically related actinomycetes. In addition, it is important to distinguish between micrococci and staphylococci because of their differing significance as potential pathogens and their occurrence together on the body surface and in the environment of humans and many animals (Kloos 1980).

12.1 Separation of micrococci and staphylococci

Several tests that can be used to differentiate between these 2 groups of organisms are shown in Table 22.3. Micrococci and staphylococci can also be separated by the analysis of aliphatic hydrocarbons (Tornabene, Morrison and Kloos 1970), fatty acids (Jantzen, Bergan and Bøvre 1974) and polar lipids (Nahaie et al. 1984), and by serological tests (Rupprecht and Schleifer 1977, 1979, Seidl and Schleifer 1978). Further, staphylococci contain teichoic acids but micrococci do not (Schleifer and Kandler 1972, Endl et al. 1983); staphylococci also differ from micrococci in causing bacteriolysis of *M. luteus* (Varaldo et al. 1979). Many of these tests allow a clear distinction to be drawn between micrococci and staphylococci but few are suitable for routine use in clinical diagnostic laboratories. According to Oeding (1983), the most useful tests in practice are the glucose fermentation test and the combined glycerol–erythromycin plate test. A numerical code system based on a selected panel of conventional biochemical tests has been established for the identification of micrococcal, staphylococcal and stomatococcal species (Rhoden, Hancock and Miller 1993).

12.2 Separation of micrococci and related taxa

Tests which can be used to distinguish between the different types of micrococci and related genera are presented in Tables 22.1 and 22.2. Additional differential phenotypic tests which can be used to separate the different kinds of micrococci are shown in Table 22.4. It is possible that lipomannans may eventually feature prominently in the separation of micrococcal and related genera given the chemical diversity and discontinuous distribution of these cell surface components (Sutcliffe 1994).

REFERENCES

Aaranson S, 1955, Biotin assay with a coccus, *Micrococcus sodonensis* nov. sp., *J Bacteriol*, **69**: 67–70.

Albertson D, Natsions GA, Gleckman R, 1978, Septic shock with *Micrococcus luteus*, *Arch Intern Med*, **138**: 487–8.

Alderson G, 1985, The current taxonomic status of the genus *Micrococcus*, *Zentralbl Bakteriol Suppl*, **14**: 117–24.

Alderson G, Amadi EN et al., 1991, Recent advances in the classification and identification of the genus *Micrococcus*, *Zentralbl Bakteriol Suppl*, **21**: 103–9.

Amadi EN, Alderson G, 1991, Menaquinone composition of some micrococci determined by high performance liquid chromatography, *J Appl Bacteriol*, **70**: 517–21.

Amadi EN, Alderson G, Minnikin DE, 1988, Lipids in the classification of the genus *Stomatococcus*, *Syst Appl Microbiol*, **10**: 111–15.

Auling G, Moss B, 1984, Metabolism of pyrimidine bases and nucleosides in the coryneform bacteria *Brevibacterium ammoniagenes* and *Micrococcus luteus*, *J Bacteriol*, **158**: 733–6.

Auling G, Prelle H, Diekmann H, 1982, Incorporation of deoxyribonucleosides into DNA of coryneform bacteria and the relevance of deoxyribonucleoside kinases, *Eur J Biochem*, **121**: 365–70.

Baird-Parker AC, 1963, A classification of micrococci and staphylococci based on physiological and biochemical tests, *J Gen Microbiol*, **30**: 409–27.

Baird-Parker AC, 1965, The classification of staphylococci and micrococci from world-wide sources, *J Gen Microbiol*, **38**: 363–87.

Baird-Parker AC, 1974, Genus I. *Micrococcus* Cohn 1872, 151, *Bergey's Manual of Determinative Bacteriology*, 8th edn, eds Buchanan RE, Gibbons NE, Williams & Wilkins, Baltimore, 478–83.

Barlow JF, Vogele KA, Dzintars PF, 1986, Septicaemia with *Stomatococcus mucilaginosus*, *Clin Microbiol Newslett*, **8**: 22.

Bauske R, Peters G, Pulverer G, 1978, Activity spectrum of micrococcal and staphylococcal phages, *Zentralbl Bakteriol Hyg Abt Orig A*, **241**: 24–9.

Bergan T, Bøvre K, Hovig B, 1970, Priority of *Micrococcus mucilaginosus* Migula 1900 over *Staphylococcus salivarius* Andrews and Gordon 1907 with proposal of a neotype strain, *Int J Syst Bacteriol*, **20**: 107–13.

Bergan T, Kocur M, 1982, *Stomatococcus mucilaginosus* gen. nov., sp. nov., ep. rev., a member of the family Micrococcaceae, *Int J Syst Bacteriol*, **32**: 374–7.

Bergan T, Kocur M, 1986, Genus II. *Stomatococcus* Bergan and Kocur, 1982, 375[VP], *Bergey's Manual of Systematic Bacteriology*, vol. 2, ed. Sneath PHA, Williams & Wilkins, Baltimore, 1008–10.

Blevins WT, Perry JJ, Evans JB, 1969, Growth and macromolecular biosynthesis by *Micrococcus sodonensis* during the utilisation of glucose and lactate, *Can J Microbiol*, **15**: 383–8.

Bowden GH, 1969, The components of cell walls and extracellular slime of four strains of *Staphylococcus salivarius* isolated from human dental plaque, *Arch Oral Biol*, **14**: 685–97.

Breed RS, Murray EGD, Smith NR (eds), 1957, *Bergey's Manual of Determinative Bacteriology*, 7th edn, Williams & Wilkins, Baltimore.

Brooks BW, Murray RG et al., 1980, Red pigmented micrococci: a basis for taxonomy, *Int J Syst Bacteriol*, **30**: 627–46.

Buchanan RE, Gibbons NE (eds), 1974, *Bergey's Manual of Determinative Bacteriology*, 8th edn, Williams & Wilkins, Baltimore.

Carr DL, Kloos WE, 1977, Temporal study of the staphylococci and micrococci of normal infant skin, *Appl Environ Microbiol*, **34**: 673–80.

Casida LE Jr, 1980a, Death of *Micrococcus luteus* in soil, *Appl Environ Microbiol*, **39**: 1031–4.

Casida LE Jr, 1980b, Bacterial predators of *Micrococcus luteus* in soil, *Appl Environ Microbiol*, **39**: 1035–41.

Cohn DV, 1956, The oxidation of malic acid by *Micrococcus lysodeikticus*, *J Biol Chem*, **221**: 413–20.

Cohn F, 1872, Untersuchungen über Bakterien, *Beitr Biol Planz*, **2**: 127–224.

Colwell RR, 1970, Polyphasic taxonomy of bacteria, *Culture Collections of Microorganisms*, eds Iizuka H, Hasegawa T, University of Tokyo Press, Tokyo, 421–36.

Cooney JJ, Thierry OC, 1966, A defined medium for growth and pigment synthesis of *Micrococcus roseus*, *Can J Microbiol*, **12**: 83–9.

Coudron PE, Markowitz SM et al., 1987, Isolation of *Stomatococcus mucilaginosus* from drug user with endocarditis, *J Clin Microbiol*, **25**: 1359–63.

Crow BA, Owen P, 1983a, Immunochemical analysis of respiratory-chain components of *Micrococcus luteus* (*lysodeikticus*), *J Bacteriol*, **153**: 498–505.

Crow BA, Owen P, 1983b, Molecular properties of succinate dehydrogenase isolated from *Micrococcus luteus* (*lysodeikticus*), *J Bacteriol*, **153**: 1493–501.

Curry JC, Borovian GE, 1976, Selective medium for distinguishing micrococci from staphylococci in the clinical laboratory, *J Clin Microbiol*, **4**: 455–7.

Dawes EA, Holmes WH, 1958, On the quantitative evaluation of routes of glucose metabolism by the use of radioactive glucose, *Biophys Acta*, **34**: 551–2.

De Siervo AJ, Salton MRJ, 1971, Biosynthesis of cardiolipin in the membranes of *Micrococcus lysodeikticus*, *Biochem Biophys Acta*, **239**: 280–92.

De Soete G, 1983, A least squares algorithm for fitting additive trees to proximity data, *Psychometrica*, **48**: 621–6.

Eisenberg RC, Evans JB, 1963, Energy and nitrogen requirements of *Micrococcus luteus*, *Can J Microbiol*, **9**: 633–42.

Embley TM, Goodfellow M et al., 1984, Lipid and wall amino acid composition in the classification of *Rothia dentocariosa*, *Zentralbl Bakteriol Mikrobiol Hyg Abt 1 A*, **257**: 285–95.

Endl J, Seidl F et al., 1983, Chemical structure of cell wall teichoic acids of staphylococci, *Arch Microbiol*, **110**: 305–14.

Erickson SK, Parker GL, 1969, The electron-transport system of *Micrococcus luteus* (*Sarcina lutea*), *Biochem Biophys Acta*, **180**: 56–62.

Evans JB, Bradford WL, Niven CF Jr, 1955, Comments concerning the taxonomy of the genera *Micrococcus* and *Staphylococcus*, *Int Bull Bacteriol Nomencl Taxon*, **5**: 61–6.

Falk D, Guering SJ, 1983, Differentiation of *Staphylococcus* and *Micrococcus* spp. with the taxa A bacitracin disk, *J Clin Microbiol*, **18**: 719–21.

Faller A, Götz F, Schleifer KH, 1980, Cytochrome patterns of staphylococci and micrococci and their taxonomic implications, *Zentralbl Bakteriol Mikrobiol Hyg Orig C*, **1**: 26–39.

Faller A, Schleifer KH, 1981, Modified oxidase and benzidine tests for separation of staphylococci from micrococci, *Zentralbl Bakteriol Mikrobiol Hyg*, **Suppl. 10**: 49.

Farrior JW, Kloos WE, 1975, Amino acid and vitamin requirements of *Micrococcus* species isolated from human skin, *Int J Syst Bacteriol*, **25**: 80–2.

Farrior JW, Kloos WE, 1976, Sulfur amino acid autotrophy in *Micrococcus* species isolated from human skin, *Can J Microbiol*, **22**: 1680–90.

Felsenstein J, 1985, Confidence limits on phylogenies: an approach using the bootstrap, *Evolution*, **39**: 783–91.

Fosse T, Peloux Y et al., 1986, Meningitis due to *Micrococcus luteus*, *Eur J Clin Study Treat Infect*, **13**: 280–1.

Gaffky G, 1883, Über antiseptische Eigenschaften des in der Esmarchschuen Klinik als Verbandmittel benutzten Torfmulls, *Arch Klin Chir*, **28**: 495–507.

Girard AE, 1971, A comparative study of the fatty acids of some micrococci, *Can J Microbiol*, **17**: 1503–8.

Goodfellow M, Manfio GP, Chun J, 1997, Towards a practical species concept for cultivable bacteria, *The Units of Biodi-*

versity – *Species in Practice*, eds Claridge MF, Dawah HA, Wilson MR, Chapman and Hall, London, 25–59.

Gordon RE, 1967, The taxonomy of soil bacteria, *The Ecology of Soil Bacteria*, eds Gray TRG, Parkinson D, University of Liverpool Press, Liverpool, 293–321.

Götz F, Nürnberger E, Schleifer KH, 1979, Distribution of class I and class II D-fructose-1,6-biphosphate aldolase in various Gram-positive bacteria, *FEMS Microbiol Lett*, **5**: 253–7.

Grula EA, Luk S-K, Chu YC, 1961, Chemically defined medium for growth of *Micrococcus lysodeikticus*, *Can J Microbiol*, **7**: 27–32.

Hamada S, Mizuno J, Kotani S, 1978, A separation of staphylococci and micrococci based on serological reactivity with antiserum specific for polyglycerolphosphate, *Microbiös*, **18**: 213–21.

Hanabusa K, Dougherty HW et al., 1966, Phosphoglucomutase. II. Preparation and properties of phosphoglucomutases from *Micrococcus lysodeikticus* and *Bacillus cereus*, *J Biol Chem*, **241**: 3930–9.

Hasselgren IL, Oeding P, 1972, Antigenic studies of genus *Micrococcus*, *Acta Pathol Microbiol Scand Sect B*, **80**: 257–64.

Hill LR, 1981, Taxonomy of the staphylococci, *The Staphylococci, Proceedings of the Alexander Ogston Centennial Conference*, eds Macdonald A, Smith G, University Press, Aberdeen, 33–62.

Holt JG, Krieg NR et al. (eds), 1994, *Bergey's Manual of Determinative Bacteriology*, 9th edn, 534.

Hucker GJ, 1924, Studies on the Coccaceae. IV. The classification of the genus *Micrococcus* Cohn, *Tech Bull NY St Agric Exp Sta Cornell University*, **102**.

Hucker GJ, 1948, Micrococcaceae, *Bergey's Manual of Systematic Bacteriology*, 6th edn, eds Breed RS, Murray EGD, Hitchens AP, Williams & Wilkins, Baltimore, 235–94.

Ishizuka H, Horinouchi S, Beppu T, 1993, Putrescine oxidase of *Micrococcus rubens*: primary structure and *Escherichia coli*, *J Gen Microbiol*, **139**: 425–32.

Ishizuka I, Ueta N, Yamakawa T, 1966, Gas chromatographic studies of microbial components. II. Carbohydrate and fatty acid constitution of the family Micrococcaceae, *Jpn J Exp Med*, **36**: 73–83.

Jantzen E, Bergan T, Bøvre K, 1974, Gas chromatography of bacterial whole cell methanolysates. VI. Fatty acid composition of strains within Micrococcaceae, *Acta Pathol Microbiol Scand Sect B*, **82**: 785–98.

Jeffries L, 1968, Sensitivity to novobiocin and lysozyme in the classification of Micrococcaceae, *J Appl Bacteriol*, **31**: 436–42.

Jeffries L, 1969, Menaquinone in the classification of Micrococcaceae with observations on the application of lysozyme and novobiocin sensitivity tests, *Int J Syst Bacteriol*, **19**: 183–7.

Jeffries L, Cawthorne A et al., 1969, Menaquinone determination in the taxonomy of Micrococcaceae, *J Gen Microbiol*, **54**: 365–80.

Jones D, Collins MD, 1988, Taxonomic studies on some human cutaneous coryneform bacteria: description of *Dermabacter hominis* gen. nov., spec. nov., *FEMS Microbiol Lett*, **51**: 51–6.

Kane-Falce CM, Kloos WE, 1975, A genetic and biochemical study of histidine biosynthesis in *Micrococcus luteus*, *Genetics*, **79**: 361–76.

Kano A, Andachi Y et al., 1991, Novel anticodon composition of transfer RNAs in *Micrococcus luteus*, a bacterium with a high genomic G + C content. Correlation with codon usage, *J Mol Biol*, **221**: 387–401.

Kaufhold A, Reinert RR, Kern W, 1992, Bacteremia caused by *Stomatococcus mucilaginosus* – a report of 7 cases, *Infection*, **20**: 213–20.

Klesius PH, Schuhardt VT, 1968, Use of lysostaphin in the isolation of highly polymerized deoxyribonucleic acid and in the taxonomy of aerobic Micrococcaceae, *J Bacteriol*, **95**: 739–43.

Kloos WE, 1969, Transformation of *Micrococcus lysodeikticus* by various members of the family Micrococcaceae, *J Gen Microbiol*, **59**: 247–55.

Kloos WE, 1980, Populations of the genus *Staphylococcus*, *Annu Rev Microbiol*, **34**: 559–92.

Kloos WE, Musselwhite MS, 1975, Distribution and persistence of *Staphylococcus* and *Micrococcus* species and other aerobic bacteria on human skin, *Appl Microbiol*, **30**: 381–95.

Kloos WE, Rose NE, 1970, Transformation mapping of tryptophan loci in *Micrococcus luteus*, *Genetics*, **66**: 595–605.

Kloos WE, Schleifer KH, Götz F, 1992, The genus *Staphylococcus*, *The Prokaryotes*, 2nd edn, eds Balows A, Trüper HG et al., Springer-Verlag, Berlin, 1369–420.

Kloos WE, Schultes LM, 1969, Transformation in *Micrococcus lysodeikticus*, *J Gen Microbiol*, **55**: 307–17.

Kloos WE, Tornabene TG, Schleifer KH, 1974, Isolation and characterization of micrococci from human skin, including two new species: *Micrococcus lylae* and *Micrococcus kristinae*, *Int J Syst Bacteriol*, **24**: 79–101.

Kloos WE, Zimmerman RJ, Smith RF, 1976, Preliminary studies on the characterization and distribution of *Staphylococcus* and *Micrococcus* species on animal skin, *Appl Environ Microbiol*, **31**: 53–9.

Koch C, Rainey FA, Stackebrandt E, 1994, 16S rDNA studies on members of *Arthrobacter* and *Micrococcus*: an aid to their future taxonomic restructuring, *FEMS Microbiol Lett*, **123**: 167–72.

Koch C, Schumann P, Stackebrandt E, 1995, Reclassification of *Micrococcus agilis* (Ali-Cohen 1889) to the genus *Arthrobacter* as *Arthrobacter agilis* comb. nov. and emendation of the genus *Arthrobacter*, *Int J Syst Bacteriol*, **45**: 837–9.

Kocur M, 1986, Genus I. *Micrococcus* Cohn 1872, 151^AL, *Bergey's Manual of Systematic Bacteriology*, vol. 2, ed. Sneath PHA, Williams & Wilkins, Baltimore, 1004–8.

Kocur M, Bergan T, Mortensen N, 1971, DNA base composition of Gram-positive cocci, *J Gen Microbiol*, **69**: 167–83.

Kocur M, Kloos WE, Schleifer KH, 1992, The genus *Micrococcus*, *The Prokaryotes*, 2nd edn, eds Balows A, Trüper HG et al., Springer-Verlag, Berlin, 1300–11.

Komura I, Yamada K, Komagata K, 1975, Taxonomic significance of phospholipid composition in aerobic Gram-positive cocci, *J Gen Appl Microbiol*, **21**: 97–107.

Lennarz WJ, Talamo B, 1966, The chemical characterization and enzymatic synthesis of mannolipids in *Micrococcus lysodeikticus*, *J Biol Chem*, **241**: 2702–19.

Ludwig W, Schleifer KH et al., 1981, A phylogenetic analysis of staphylococci, *Peptococcus saccharolyticus* and *Micrococcus mucilaginosus*, *J Gen Microbiol*, **125**: 357–66.

Mahler I, Grossman L, 1968, Transformation of radiation sensitive strains of *Micrococcus lysodeikticus*, *Biochem Biophys Res Commun*, **32**: 776–81.

Mathis JN, Kloos WE, 1984, Isolation and characterization of *Micrococcus* plasmids, *Curr Microbiol*, **10**: 163–71.

Meers PD, Whyte W, Sandys G, 1975, Coagulase-negative staphylococci and micrococci in urinary tract infections, *J Clin Pathol*, **28**: 270–3.

Mohapatra N, Kloos WE, 1974, Biochemical and genetic studies of laboratory purine auxotrophic strains of *Micrococcus luteus*, *Can J Microbiol*, **20**: 1751–4.

Mohapatra N, Kloos WE, 1975, Biochemical characterization and genetic mapping of purine genes in *Micrococcus luteus*, *Genet Res Camb*, **26**: 163–71.

Morrison SJ, Tornabene TG, Kloos WE, 1971, Neutral lipids in the study of relationships of members of the family Micrococcaceae, *J Bacteriol*, **108**: 353–8.

Murray RGE, Brenner DJ et al., 1990, Report of the *ad hoc* committee on approaches to taxonomy within the Proteobacteria, *Int J Syst Bacteriol*, **40**: 213–15.

Nahaie MR, Goodfellow M et al., 1984, Polar lipid and isoprenoid quinone composition in the classification of *Staphylococcus*, *J Gen Microbiol*, **130**: 2427–37.

Naylor HB, Burgi E, 1956, Observations on abortive infections of *Micrococcus lysodeikticus* with bacteriophage, *Virology*, **2**: 577–93.

Nordstom KM, McGinley KJ et al., 1987, Similarities between

Dermatophilus congolensis and *Micrococcus sedentarius*: identity of the etiologic agent of pitted keratolysis, *Abst Annu Meet Am Soc Microbiol*, 244.

Oeding P, 1983, Taxonomy and identification, *Staphylococci and Staphylococcal Infections*, vol. 1, eds Easmon CSF, Adlam C, Academic Press, London, 1.

Oeding P, Hasselgren IL, 1972, Antigenic studies on the genus *Micrococcus*. 2. Double diffusion in agar gel with particular emphasis on teichoic acids, *Acta Pathol Microbiol Scand Sect B*, **80:** 265–9.

Ogasawara-Fujita N, Sakahuchi K, 1976, Classification of micrococci on the basis of deoxyribonucleic acid homology, *J Gen Microbiol*, **94:** 97–106.

Okubo S, Nakayama H, 1968, Evidence of transformation in *Micrococcus lysodeikticus*, *Biochem Biophys Res Commun*, **32:** 825–30.

Onishi H, Kamekura H, 1972, *Micrococcus halobius* sp. n., *Int J Syst Bacteriol*, **22:** 233–6.

Owen P, Salton MRJ, 1975, A succinylated mannan in the membrane system of *Micrococcus lysodeikticus*, *Biochem Biophys Res Commun*, **63:** 875–80.

Pandhi PN, Hammond BF, 1975, A glycolipid from *Rothia dentocariosa*, *Arch Oral Biol*, **20:** 399–401.

Park JH, Song JC et al., 1994, Determination of genome size and a preliminary physical map of an extreme alkaliphile, *Micrococcus* sp. Y1, by pulse-field gel electrophoresis, *Microbiology*, **140:** 2247–50.

Park W, Matsuhashi M, 1984, *Staphylococcus aureus* and *Micrococcus luteus* peptidoglycan transglycosylases that are not penicillin-binding proteins, *J Bacteriol*, **157:** 538–44.

Perkins HR, 1963, A polymer containing glucose and aminohexuronic acid isolated from the cell walls of *Micrococcus lysodeikticus*, *Biochem J*, **86:** 475–83.

Perry JJ, Evans JB, 1960, Oxidative metabolism of lactate and acetate by *Micrococcus sodonensis*, *J Bacteriol*, **79:** 113–18.

Peters G, Pulverer G, 1975, Bakteriophagen aus Mikrokokken, *Zentralbl Bakteriol Abt 1 Orig A*, **232:** 221–6.

Peters G, Pulverer G, Pillich J, 1976, Bacteriophages of micrococci, *Zentralbl Bakteriol Suppl*, **5:** 159–63.

Pless DD, Schmit AS, Lennarz WJ, 1975, The characterisation of mannan of *Micrococcus lysodeikticus* as an acidic lipopolysaccharide, *J Biol Chem*, **250:** 1319–27.

Powell DA, Duckworth M, Baddiley J, 1974, An acetylated mannan in the membrane of *Micrococcus lysodeikticus*, *FEBS Lett*, **41:** 259–63.

Powell DA, Duckworth M, Baddiley J, 1975, A membrane-associated lipomannan in micrococci, *Biochem J*, **151:** 387–97.

Prag J, Kjoller E, Espersen F, 1985, *Stomatococcus mucilaginosus* endocarditis, *Eur J Clin Microbiol*, **4:** 422–4.

Prévot AR, 1961, *Traité de Systématique Bactérienne*, vol. 2, Dunod, Paris, 31.

Ragnaud JM, Marceau C et al., 1981, Péritonite a rechute à *Stomatococcus mucilaginosus* chez une malade traitée par dialyse péritoneale continue ambulatoire, *Presse Med*, **14:** 2063.

Rainey FA, Nobre M et al., 1997, Phylogenetic diversity of the deinococci as determined by 16S rDNA sequence comparison, *Int J Syst Bacteriol*, **47:** 510–4.

Regensburger A, Ludwig W, Schleifer KH, 1988, DNA probes with different specificities from a cloned 16S rRNA gene of *Micrococcus luteus*, *J Gen Microbiol*, **134:** 1197–204.

Relman DA, Ruoff K, Ferraro MJ, 1987, *Stomatococcus mucilaginosus* endocarditis in an intravenous drug abuser, *J Infect Dis*, **155:** 1080–2.

Rhoden DL, Hancock GA, Miller JM, 1993, Numerical approach to reference identification of *Staphylococcus*, *Stomatococcus* and *Micrococcus* spp., *J Clin Microbiol*, **31:** 490–3.

Roberts AP, 1967, Micrococcaceae from the urinary tract in pregnancy, *J Clin Pathol*, **20:** 631–2.

Rosypal S, Rosypalová A, Horejš J, 1966, The classification of micrococci and staphylococci based on their DNA base composition and Adansonian analysis, *J Gen Microbiol*, **44:** 281–92.

Rubin SJ, Lyons RW, Murcia AJ, 1978, Endocarditis associated with cardial catheterization due to a Gram-positive coccus designated *Micrococcus mucilaginosus incertae sedis*, *J Clin Microbiol*, **7:** 546–9.

Rupprecht M, Schleifer KH, 1977, Comparative immunological study of catalases in the genus *Micrococcus*, *Arch Microbiol*, **114:** 61–6.

Rupprecht M, Schleifer KH, 1979, A comparative immunological study of catalases from coagulase-positive staphylococci, *Arch Microbiol*, **120:** 53–6.

Salton MRJ, 1964, Requirements of dehydroxyphenols for the growth of *Micrococcus lysodeikticus* in synthetic media, *Biochem Biophys Acta*, **86:** 421–2.

Salton MRJ, Schor MT, 1974, Release and purification of *Micrococcus lysodeikticus* ATPase from membranes extracted with n-butanol, *Biochem Biophys Acta*, **345:** 74–82.

Scher M, Lennarz WJ, 1969, Studies on the biosynthesis of mannan in *Micrococcus lysodeikticus*, *J Biol Chem*, **244:** 2777–89.

Schleifer KH, 1986, Section 12. Gram-positive cocci, *Bergey's Manual of Systematic Bacteriology*, vol. 2, ed. Sneath PHA, Williams & Wilkins, Baltimore, 999–1003.

Schleifer KH, Heise W, Meyer SA, 1979, Deoxyribonucleic acid hybridisation studies among some micrococci, *FEMS Microbiol Lett*, **6:** 33–6.

Schleifer KH, Kandler O, 1972, Peptidoglycan types of bacterial cell walls and their taxonomic implications, *Bacteriol Rev*, **6:** 407–77.

Schleifer KH, Kloos WE, 1975a, A simple test system for the separation of staphylococci and micrococci, *J Clin Microbiol*, **1:** 327–38.

Schleifer KH, Kloos WE, 1975b, Isolation and characterisation of staphylococci from human skin. I. Amended descriptions of *Staphylococcus epidermidis* and *Staphylococcus saprophyticus* and descriptions of three new species: *Staphylococcus cohnii*, *Staphylococcus haemolyticus*, and *Staphylococcus xylosus*, *Int J Syst Bacteriol*, **25:** 50–61.

Schmitt M, Rittinghaus K et al., 1978, Immunological properties of membrane-bound adenosine triphosphatase: immunological identification of rutamycin-sensitive F0.F1ATPase from *Micrococcus luteus* ATCC 4698 established by crossed immunoelectrophoresis, *Biochim Biophys Acta*, **509:** 410–18.

Schroeter J, in Cohn F, 1872, Untersuchungen über Bakterien, *Beitr Biol Pflanz*, **1:** 127–224.

Schumacher-Perdreau F, Pulverer G, Schleifer KH, 1979, The phage adsorption test: a simple method for differentiation between staphylococci and micrococci, *J Infect Dis*, **138:** 392–5.

Seidl HP, Schleifer KH, 1978, A rapid test for the serological separation of staphylococci from micrococci, *Appl Environ Microbiol*, **35:** 479–82.

Selladurai BM, Sivakumaran S et al., 1993, Intracranial suppuration caused by *Micrococcus luteus*, *Br J Neurosurg*, **7:** 205–7.

Sellin MA, Cooke DI et al., 1975, Micrococcal urinary tract infections in young women, *Lancet*, **2:** 570–2.

Shaw C, Stitt JM, Cowan ST, 1951, Staphylococci and their classification, *J Gen Microbiol*, **5:** 1010–23.

Silva MT, Polonia JJ, Kocur M, 1977, The fine structure of *Micrococcus mucilaginosus*, *J Submicrosc Cytol*, **9:** 53–66.

Silvestri LG, Hill LR, 1965, Agreement between deoxyribonucleic acid base composition and taxonomic classification of Gram-positive cocci, *J Bacteriol*, **90:** 136–40.

Souhami L, Field R et al., 1979, *Micrococcus luteus* pneumonia: a case report and review of the literature, *Med Pediatr Oncol*, **7:** 309–14.

Stackebrandt E, Lewis BJ, Woese CR, 1980, The phylogenetic structure of the coryneform group of bacteria, *Zentralbl Bakteriol Mikrobiol Hyg Abt II Orig C*, **1:** 137–49.

Stackebrandt E, Scheuerlein C, Schleifer KH, 1983, Phylogenetic and biochemical studies on *Stomatococcus mucilaginosus*, *Syst Appl Microbiol*, **4:** 207–17.

Stackebrandt E, Woese CR, 1979, A phylogenetic dissection of the family Micrococcaceae, *Curr Microbiol*, **2:** 317–22.

Stackebrandt E, Koch C et al., 1995, Taxonomic dissection of the genus *Micrococcus*: *Kocuria* gen. nov., *Nesterenkonia* gen. nov., *Kytococcus* gen. nov., *Dermacoccus* gen. nov., and *Micrococcus* Cohn 1872 gen. emend., *Int J Syst Bacteriol*, **45**: 682–92.

Sutcliffe IC, 1994, The lipoteichoic acids and lipoglycans of Gram-positive bacteria: a chemotaxonomic perspective, *Syst Appl Microbiol*, **17**: 467–80.

Sutcliffe IC, Alderson G, 1995, A chemotaxonomic appraisal of the distribution of lipomannans within the genus *Micrococcus*, *FEMS Microbiol Lett*, **133**: 233–7.

Sutcliffe IC, Old LA, 1995, *Stomatococcus mucilaginosus* produces a mannose-containing lipoglycan rather than lipoteichoic acid, *Arch Microbiol*, **163**: 70–5.

Sutcliffe IC, Shaw N, 1991, Atypical lipoteichoic acids of Gram-positive bacteria, *J Bacteriol*, **173**: 7065–9.

Takeuchi M, Fang CX, Yokota A, 1995, Taxonomic study of the genus *Brachybacterium*: proposal of *Brachybacterium conglomeratum* sp. nov., nom. rev., *Brachybacterium paraconglomeratum* sp. nov., and *Brachybacterium rhamnosum* sp. nov., *Int J Syst Bacteriol*, **45**: 160–8.

Tamura T, Takeuchi M, Yokota A, 1994, *Luteococcus japonicus* gen. nov., sp. nov., a new Gram-positive coccus with LL-diaminopimelic acid in the cell walls, *Int J Syst Bacteriol*, **44**: 348–56.

Telander B, Wallmark G, 1975, *Micrococcus* subgroup 3 – a common cause of urinary tract infection in women, *Lakartidningen*, **72**: 1675–7.

Tornabene TG, Morrison SJ, Kloos WE, 1970, Aliphatic hydrocarbon contents of various members of the family Micrococcaceae, *Lipids*, **5**: 929–37.

Traxler CI, Goustin AS, Anderson JS, 1982, Elongation of teichuronic acid chains by a wall-membrane preparation from *Micrococcus luteus*, *J Bacteriol*, **150**: 649–56.

Varaldo PE, Grazi G et al., 1979, Routine separation of micrococci from staphylococci based on bacteriolytic activity production, *J Clin Microbiol*, **9**: 147–8.

Ventosa A, Marquez MC et al., 1993, Comparative study of '*Micrococcus* sp.' strains CCM 168 and CCM 1405 and members of the genus *Salinicoccus*, *Int J Syst Bacteriol*, **43**: 245–8.

Verma V, Felder M et al., 1993, Physical characterization of plasmid pMQV10 from a steroid biotransforming strain of *Micrococcus*, *Plasmid*, **30**: 281–3.

Walsh BL, O'Dor J, Warren RAJ, 1971, Chelating agents and the growth of *Micrococcus lysodeikticus*, *Can J Microbiol*, **17**: 593–7.

Williamson P, 1965, Quantitative estimation of cutaneous bacteria, *Skin Bacteria and their Role in Infection*, eds Maibach HI, Hildick-Smith G, McGraw-Hill, New York, 3–11.

Wolin HL, Naylor HB, 1957, Basic nutritional requirements of *Micrococcus lysodeikticus*, *J Bacteriol*, **74**: 163–7.

Yamada H, Uwajima T et al., 1967, Crystalline tyramine oxidase from *Sarcina lutea*, *Biochem Biophys Res Commun*, **27**: 350–5.

Yamada M, Hirose A, Matsuhashi M, 1975, Association of lack of cell wall teichuronic acid with formation of cell packets of *Micrococcus lysodeikticus* (*luteus*) mutants, *J Bacteriol*, **123**: 678–86.

Yamada Y, Inouye G et al., 1976, The menaquinone system in the classification of aerobic Gram-positive cocci in the genera *Micrococcus, Staphylococcus, Planococcus* and *Sporosarcina*, *J Gen Appl Microbiol*, **22**: 227–36.

Chapter 23

MOBILUNCUS, GARDNERELLA, VEILLONELLA AND OTHER GRAM-NEGATIVE COCCI

C A Spiegel

MOBILUNCUS

1 GENUS/SPECIES DEFINITION

Members of the genus *Mobiluncus* are curved, gram-variable, non-spore-forming, anaerobic rods. Although they may give a variable gram-stain reaction, the chemical composition of their cell wall and their antimicrobial susceptibility pattern suggest gram-positivity. They generally possess multiple flagella with a subpolar attachment or originating at a more central location on the concave side.

2 INTRODUCTION AND BRIEF HISTORICAL PERSPECTIVE

Organisms morphologically resembling *Mobiluncus* were described in vaginal fluid before the turn of the century (Krönig 1895). Strains growing in symbiosis with an anaerobic streptococcus were recovered but did not survive further passage on artificial media. The first pure culture was isolated by Curtis (1913) from vaginal and uterine material in a woman with postpartum endometritis. He also detected such organisms microscopically in women with leucorrhoea. Laughton (1948) identified curved vaginal organisms as probable corynebacteria. Moore (1954) characterized 10 strains from vaginal fluid. Two gram-stain morphotypes, each producing a specific colony type, were identified and may have represented the 2 currently recognized species. Twenty-six years later, the biochemical characteristics of 2 morphotypes, named *Vibrions succinoproducteurs* groups 1 and 2, were documented (Durieux and Dublanchet 1980). Peloux and Thomas (1981) named one strain *Vibrio mulieris*. At this same time interest in bacterial vaginosis (then called non-specific vaginitis) rose and the association of these curved organisms with that syndrome led to their independent and almost simultaneous description as *Mobiluncus curtisii* and *M. mulieris* (Spiegel and Roberts 1984) and as *Falcivibrio grandis* and *Falcivibrio vaginalis* (Hammann et al. 1984).

3   HABITAT

The prevalence of curved rods detected by wet mount or gram stain in women with signs of bacterial vaginosis ranged from 10.9 to 77% compared to none in controls (Durieux and Dublanchet 1980, Hjelm et al. 1981, Skarin and Mårdh 1982, Spiegel et al. 1983). Using culture, the prevalence has been as high as 88% in women with vaginosis (Holst 1990) and <6% in controls (Sprott et al. 1983, Hallén, Påhlson and Forsum 1987).

Mobiluncus has also been recovered from the genitourinary tract of men (Holst 1990). Of 82 male partners of women with bacterial vaginosis (BV), 3 had colonization of the urethra with *Mobiluncus* spp., 3 the coronal sulcus and 2 seminal fluid. None of the 49 male partners of women without BV were so colonized.

3.1   Extravaginal sources

Few studies have sought an extravaginal reservoir of *Mobiluncus* spp. Holst (1990) recently examined 148 women with BV, 82 male partners of 82 women with BV, 69 women without BV, 49 male partners of 49 women without BV, 4 homosexual men (2 monogamous couples), 12 virginal girls, and 12 virginal boys for rectal, oral and pharyngeal colonization by *M. mulieris*, *M. curtisii* and other BV-associated organisms. Rectal colonization with one ($n = 81$) or both ($n = 47$) *Mobiluncus* spp. occurred in 128 women with BV. Women with BV were more frequently colonized. Colonization rates for all other groups of subjects were similar to one another. Colonization by these organisms of male partners of women with BV was greater than that of partners of healthy women and homosexual males, but the numbers were too low to reach statistical significance. Forty-four male partners of women with BV were again cultured after 2 weeks, during which condoms were used during intercourse. Although rectal colonization persisted, colonization of the urethra and coronal sulcus did not and colonization rates at the 2-week follow-up were similar between the 2 groups of patients. *Mobiluncus* spp. were not recovered from any oropharyngeal cultures.

4   MORPHOLOGY, INCLUDING STAINING REACTIONS

Mobiluncus is a curved, motile, anaerobic organism that may appear gram-positive, gram-negative or gram-variable, depending on the age of the cells, the staining method and the medium on which they were grown. The smaller form, *M. curtisii*, is only slightly bent and may appear coryneform. Branching forms have been observed by electron microscopy (Taylor and Owen 1984). Cells range in length from 0.8 to 3 μm long (mean 1.5–1.7 μm), 0.4–0.6 μm wide and are more likely to retain crystal violet than are the larger form. *M. mulieris* are generally more crescentic or moon-like, some forming half circles. These cells range from 1.9 to 5 or 6 μm in length (mean 2.9–3.9 μm) and are 0.4–0.6 μm wide. The presence of a central dark-staining body has been described (Moore 1954) so that cells resemble small trypanosomes.

Mobiluncus spp. demonstrate very active motility. Flagellar attachment is either subpolar or more centrally located on the concave side. *M. curtisii* has 1–6 flagella per cell with a common origin whereas *M. mulieris* has 1–8 flagella with multiple origins (Sprott et al. 1983, Hammann et al. 1984, Taylor and Owens 1984). *M. curtisii* subsp. *curtisii* is differentiated from *M. curtisii* subsp. *holmesii* based, in part, on the ability of the former to migrate through soft agar (Spiegel and Roberts 1984), a characteristic presumed due to motility.

5   CULTURAL CHARACTERISTICS AND GROWTH REQUIREMENTS

An enriched medium, such as Columbia blood agar base (Jager), brain–heart infusion, Oxoid DST, glucose, peptone–yeast extract–glucose (PYG) or Schaedler agar, is required for growth. Growth is stimulated by addition of horse, human, sheep, guinea pig, goat or rabbit blood or by serum. Growth in broth is stimulated by horse or rabbit serum or fermentable carbohydrate such as maltose or glycogen, but not fumaric acid.

Mobiluncus spp. require an anaerobic atmosphere for primary isolation. The optimum temperature is 35–37°C with poor or no growth at 20, 43 or 45°C. A pH range of 6.0–7.2 supports growth on solid media. *Mobiluncus* spp. tolerate a pH of 12.0, which is the basis of a selective method for their recovery (Påhlson, Hallén and Forsum 1986a).

Colonies are colourless, translucent, smooth, convex and entire; they reach a maximum diameter of 2–3 mm after 5 days of incubation.

6   METABOLISM

The major metabolic products from growth of *Mobiluncus* spp. in PYG are succinic, acetic and lactic acids. Malic acid is produced from fumarate (Hammann et al. 1984, Spiegel and Roberts 1984).

7 CELL WALL COMPOSITION; ANTIGENIC STRUCTURE

Although *Mobiluncus* spp. tend to stain gram-negative to gram-variable, electron micrographs reveal a multilayered gram-positive cell wall lacking an outer membrane. The peptidoglycan layer is thin, perhaps providing an explanation for the tendency to stain gram-negative (Hammann et al. 1984, Spiegel and Roberts 1984). Biochemically the cell wall lacks lipopolysaccharide and showed minimal activity in the *Limulus* amoebocyte lysate test (Carlone et al. 1986). The cellular fatty acids include myristic (14:0), hexadecenoic (16:1), hexadecanoic (16:0), heptodecanoic (17:0), octadecadienoic (18:2), octadecenoic (18:1) and octodecanoic (18:0) acids; 16:0, 18:2 and 18:1 comprise greater than 50% of the total fatty acids. The absence of hydroxy fatty acids supports the contention that *Mobiluncus* is a gram-positive organism.

Genus-specific, species-specific and subspecies-specific antigens have been detected using monoclonal antibodies (Fohn, Lukehart and Hillier 1988). Additional antigenic subgroups have been identified among atypical strains (Påhlson, Hallén and Forsum 1986b, Schwebke et al. 1991). The heterogeneity of protein and antigenic profiles among *Mobiluncus* spp. indicates that further subdivision of the genus may be appropriate (Schwebke et al. 1991).

8 CLASSIFICATION

Although the morphology and metabolic end product pattern most closely resembled *Actinomyces* spp., the biochemical and electron microscopic characteristics of *Mobiluncus* (motile, G + C 49–52 mol%) excluded them from the families Actinomycetaceae (non-motile, G + C 60–63 mol%), Propionibacteriaceae (non-motile, G + C 59–66 mol%, propionic acid as the major metabolic product) and Bacteroidaceae (non-motile or peritrichous; gram-negative organisms). However, because it appeared most similar to Bacteroidaceae, the genus was tentatively placed in that family (Spiegel and Roberts 1984). Partial reverse transcriptase sequencing of *M. curtisii* and *M. mulieris* 16S rRNA has since indicated that *Mobiluncus* is related to *Actinomyces* (Lassnig et al. 1989).

9 LABORATORY ISOLATION AND IDENTIFICATION

9.1 Isolation

Mobiluncus is a fastidious organism requiring an enriched medium for growth. Various basal media will support growth of *Mobiluncus*, including Columbia, blood agar base (Jagar), brain–heart infusion, Oxoid DST, glucose, PYG and Schaedler agars. As noted above (see section 5, p. 508), growth is stimulated by blood or serum. Inhibitory agents to suppress coinfecting flora have included colistin plus nalidixic

acid (Durieux and Dublanchet 1980), trimethoprim–sulphamethoxazole plus polymyxin B (Holst, Hofmann and Mårdh 1984), tinidazole plus colistin or nalidixic acid (Holst, Hofmann and Mårdh 1984, Smith and Moore 1988) and colistin, nalidixic acid, tinidazole and Nile blue A (Spiegel 1991a).

9.2 Enrichment

Two pretreatment methods have been shown to increase the recovery of *Mobiluncus* spp. from clinical specimens. Using pure cultures of 10 strains of *M. curtisii* and 6 of *M. mulieris*, more than 90% of cells survived exposure to pH 12.0 buffer for 30 and 5 min, respectively. Cold enrichment has also been described (Smith and Moore 1988). Recovery of *Mobiluncus* from clinical specimens was enhanced by their immediate storage at 4–5°C for 1–21 h prior to cultivation.

9.3 Direct detection

Monoclonal antibodies described above have been used for the direct detection of *Mobiluncus* in clinical specimens. In one study indirect immunofluorescence was as sensitive as gram stain (92%). By use of 2 species-specific antibodies, speciation could be achieved. Monoclonal antibodies failed to detect 2 specimens with 'atypical' *M. curtisii* recovered by culture.

Whole cell ^{32}P-labelled or biotinylated DNA has been used to identify isolates of *Mobiluncus* using a filter blot technique. Twenty-six (47%) of 56 specimens that had *Mobiluncus* on direct gram stain were culture- and probe-positive, 17 (30%) were detected only by culture, 3 (5%) only by probe, and 10 (18%) by neither method (Roberts et al. 1985). Påhlson et al. (1992) developed a ^{32}P-labelled oligonucleotide probe complementary to a nucleotide sequence in the variable region V8 of *Mobiluncus* 16S ribosomal RNA. It was positive in 6 of 9 clinical samples from women with bacterial vaginosis in whom *Mobiluncus* was detected on wet mount, one of 10 with no *Mobiluncus* on wet mount and 8 of 37 asymptomatic women with no *Mobiluncus* on wet mount.

9.4 Identification

Members of the genus *Mobiluncus* are anaerobic, gram-variable or gram-negative, curved, non-sporing and rod-shaped with tapered ends, occurring singly or in pairs with a gull-wing appearance. They are weakly or strongly saccharolytic. Fermentation products include succinic and acetic acids with or without lactic acid. Growth is not stimulated by formate–fumarate. Oxidase, catalase, urease and H_2S are not produced.

Two species, one with 2 subspecies, have been described (Spiegel and Roberts 1984), the differentiating characteristics of which are given in Table 23.1.

Some have questioned the validity of subspeciating *M. curtisii* because nitrate reductase detection is poorly reproducible and because of the lack of subspecies-specific monoclonal antibodies in some studies. Morphological, biochemical and serological characteristics have demonstrated heterogeneity among isolates of *Mobiluncus*, more so

Table 23.1 Differential characteristics of *Mobiluncus* spp.

Characteristics	M. curtisii[a]	M. mulieris
Length of cells (μm)	1.7	2.9
Gram reaction	Variable	Negative
Stimulated by arginine	+[b]	−
NH_4^+ from arginine	+	−
Hippurate hydrolysed	+	−
CAMP reaction	Weak	Strong
β-Galactosidase (ONPG)	+	−
Leucine aminopeptidase	−	+
Acid (pH <5.5) from glycogen	−	+
Acid (pH ≤6.0) from melibiose	v	−
Acid (pH <5.5) from trehalose	−	v

[a] *M. curtisii* subsp. *curtsii* shows migration through soft agar but no reduction of nitrate whereas *M. curtisii* subsp. *holmesii* is nitrate-positive and migration-negative.
[b] +, positive; −, negative; v, variable.

among *M. curtisii* than *M. mulieris* (Christiansen et al. 1984, Påhlson, Hallén and Forsum 1986b, Vetere et al. 1987, Garlind, Påhlsson and Forsum 1989, Schwebke et al. 1991). It has been suggested that further subdivision of the genus may be appropriate.

10 SUSCEPTIBILITY TO ANTIMICROBIAL AGENTS

Most studies have reported susceptibility of *Mobiluncus* to penicillins, cephalosporins and aminoglycosides, resistance to colistin, nalidixic acid and cycloserine and resistance of *M. curtisii* but usual susceptibility of *M. mulieris* to metronidazole and tinidazole as reviewed (Spiegel 1991a). β-Lactamase activity has not been detected.

11 ROLE IN NORMAL FLORA OF HUMANS

The prevalence of *Mobiluncus* in the endogenous human flora is described above (see section 3, p. 508). The role played by these organisms is unknown.

12 PATHOGENICITY AND VIRULENCE FACTORS

The role of *Mobiluncus* spp. in bacterial vaginosis and the extravaginal abscesses has not been determined. As is true for most anaerobic infections, *Mobiluncus* has not been found in pure culture but rather mixed with other anaerobic organisms also of uncertain pathogenicity, including *Prevotella* and *Porphyromonas* (see Chapter 58) and *Peptostreptococcus* (see Chapter 33). *Gardnerella vaginalis* (see section on 'Gardnerella', p. 511) and *Mycoplasma hominis* (see Chapter 34) are also associated with bacterial vaginosis. There is no demonstrable difference in the severity of bacterial vaginosis between women with or without *Mobiluncus* spp., nor is there a difference in their response to therapy (Spiegel et al. 1983, Jones et al. 1985). This is true in spite of the fact that *M. curtisii* and some *M. mulieris* are resistant to metronidazole, the antimicro-

bial agent most commonly used to treat bacterial vaginosis. This suggests that survival of *Mobiluncus* spp. is dependent on the presence of one or more other organisms that are inhibited by metronidazole.

Signs of ascending infection or urinary tract symptoms are not more common in bacterial vaginosis with versus without *Mobiluncus* spp. (Pattman 1984). Vaginal bleeding has been reported in women with bacterial vaginosis, some of whom had *Mobiluncus* spp. (Larsson and Bergman 1986). Curved rods have been seen inside phagocytic vacuoles in vaginal polymorphonuclear leucocytes (DeBoer and Plantema 1988). Malic acid, an irritant, is produced from fumarate by *Mobiluncus*.

Women who have bacterial vaginosis in late pregnancy are at increased risk of developing chorioamnionitis, premature labour, preterm delivery and delivering low birth weight infants (Hillier et al. 1988, 1995, Martius et al. 1988). The role of *Mobiluncus* spp. in the sequelae of bacterial vaginosis is yet to be elucidated.

Pure cultures of *Mobiluncus* have been injected intravenously (Curtis 1913, Moore 1954), intraperitoneally or intramuscularly (Moore 1954) into rabbits, guinea pigs and mice (Curtis 1913, Moore 1954) with no resulting illness.

A thin watery discharge was seen in grivet monkeys challenged with *M. mulieris* morphotype plus *Gardnerella vaginalis*, but not *M. curtisii* morphotype with *G. vaginalis* or any of these species alone (Mårdh, Holst and Möller 1984). In one monkey the *M. mulieris* morphotype persisted in the vagina after 9 months.

Using untreated whole bacterial cells as the antigen, no circulating antibody was detected in 25 women with bacterial vaginosis and *Mobiluncus* spp. Vaginal immunoglobulin A (IgA) was not sought (Moi and Danielsson 1984). Immunoglobulin G (IgG) to *M. curtisii* was demonstrated in a woman with postoperative vaginal infection and *Mobiluncus* morphotype was detected microscopically (Larsson et al. 1986).

GARDNERELLA

13 GENUS/SPECIES DEFINITION

Gardnerella is a gram-variable to gram-negative pleomorphic rod with laminated cell walls. It is non-sporing, non-motile and facultatively anaerobic. It ferments various carbohydrates with the production mainly of acetic acid, and starch is hydrolysed. Catalase, oxidase, indole and urease reactions are negative. β-Haemolysis is seen on rabbit and human blood agar but not on sheep blood agar. The G + C content of the DNA is 42–44 mol%. The type species is *G. vaginalis*.

14 INTRODUCTION AND HISTORICAL PERSPECTIVE

This organism was first described by Leopold (1953). Gardner and Dukes (1955) placed it in the genus *Haemophilus* as *H. vaginalis*, but Dunkelberg and McVeigh (1969) were unable to show that it required either haemin or nicotinamide adenine dinucleotide as a growth factor. Zinneman and Turner (1963) considered it to be gram-positive and suggested it be included in the genus *Corynebacterium* as *C. vaginalis*. However, its cell wall composition and the G + C composition of its DNA differ from those of *Corynebacterium* (55–60 mol%). Greenwood and Pickett (1980) proposed its removal to a new genus, *Gardnerella*, on the evidence of its cell wall composition, electron microscopic appearance and the results of DNA hybridization tests. This proposal received support from the taxonomic study of Piot et al. (1980). To date only one species, *G. vaginalis*, has been described.

15 HABITAT

Gardnerella is a member of the endogenous vaginal flora in up to 69% of women with a normal vaginal examination (Totten et al. 1982). It has also been recovered from the rectum of 2–7% of healthy women, heterosexual but not homosexual men, and children (Holst 1990). In the same study *G. vaginalis* was not found in the oropharynx of any patient group.

16 MORPHOLOGY, INCLUDING STAINING REACTIONS

Gardnerellae are small (1.5–2.5 μm × c. 0.5 μm), pleomorphic rods. Clusters of cells may palisade, giving the appearance of Chinese letters as often seen in corynebacteria. Bifurcated cells are common due to snapping that accompanies cell division. The gram reaction varies with medium, age and atmosphere. Cells are usually gram-positive when stained directly in clinical material, blood cultures, or when grown anaerobically or in Loeffler's or Roux medium (Catlin 1992). Metaphosphate (volutin) granules are produced when the organism is grown in the presence of a fermentable compound (Edmunds 1960) or sodium phosphate (Zinneman and Turner 1963). The granules appear positive by gram stain or metachromatic with alkaline methylene blue stain.

17 CULTURAL CHARACTERISTICS AND GROWTH REQUIREMENTS

Gardnerellae are facultative organisms; growth occurs in air but is stimulated by 5–10% CO_2. A candle extinction jar provides the appropriate environment. Optimum growth is obtained at 35–37°C, but occurs between 25 and 42°C. The optimum pH range is 6.0–6.5. Round, opaque, smooth colonies are produced. Gardnerellae are nutritionally fastidious organisms, requiring biotin, folic acid, niacin, thiamine, riboflavin and 2 or more purines, pyrimidines, or both (Dunkelberg and McVeigh 1969). Growth is stimulated by fermentable carbohydrates and certain peptones. Colonies on V agar, which contains Columbia agar base (BBL, Cockeysville MD), 1% proteose peptone and 5% human blood, are 0.5 mm in diameter after 48 h. Colonies are β-haemolytic on horse or human but not sheep blood.

18 METABOLISM

G. vaginalis is chemo-organotrophic, having a fermentative type of metabolism. Acid is produced from dextrose, dextrin, maltose, ribose and starch. Acid production from L-arabinose, fructose, galactose, inulin, lactose, mannose, sucrose and xylose is variable. Acetic acid is the major metabolic end product. Indole and urease are not produced. Nitrate is not reduced to nitrite. Starch is hydrolysed. Hippurate is hydrolysed by 85% of strains (see section 22, p. 512).

19 IMPORTANT GENETIC MECHANISMS, INCLUDING PLASMID ACTIVITY

Gardnerellae possess the *tetM* determinant which codes for tetracycline resistance (Roberts et al. 1986).

20 CELL WALL COMPOSITION; ANTIGENIC STRUCTURE

Electron microscopic studies have described either a gram-positive (Reyn, Birch-Andersen and Lapage 1966, Sadhu et al. 1989), gram-negative (Criswell et al. 1971) or laminated organism (Greenwood and Pickett 1980). The cell wall contains alanine, glutamic acid, glycine and lysine (Harper and Davis 1982) and the cell membrane contains predominantly hexadecanoic (16:0), octadecenoic (18:1) and octadecanoic (18:0) acids without hydroxy fatty acids (Csango, Hagen and Jagars 1982). These profiles are typical of gram-positive organisms. Endotoxic activity was detected in cell extracts using the *Limulus* amoebocyte assay, but lipid A was not present (Greenwood and Pickett 1980).

Gardnerellae possess pili (Johnson and Davies 1984) and an exopolysaccharide layer (Sadhu et al. 1989). Seven serogroups (Edmunds 1960) and 20 serotypes (Ison et al. 1987) have been identified. A 41 kDa species-specific antigen has been identified (Boustouller, Johnson and Taylor-Robinson 1986).

21 CLASSIFICATION

DNA–DNA hybridization studies have shown that *Gardnerella* is not closely related to morphologically or physiologically similar genera (Greenwood and Pickett 1980, Piot et al. 1980). More studies are needed to delineate its relationship to other genera.

22 LABORATORY ISOLATION AND IDENTIFICATION

Isolation of *Gardnerella* can be achieved by culture on enriched media such as chocolate agar and Columbia agar with 5% sheep blood. Because *G. vaginalis* is susceptible to sodium polyanethol sulphonate (SPS), SPS-free or gelatin-supplemented blood culture media may enhance its recovery from women with postpartum sepsis (Reimer and Reller 1985).

Detection of *G. vaginalis* in specimens from the vagina where other endogenous flora are present is optimized by use of human blood bilayer Tween agar (HBT) (Totten et al. 1982). Thin, gram-negative or gram-variable short rods that are catalase-negative and produce a 1–2 mm zone of β-haemolysis with diffuse edges on HBT after 48 h of incubation in CO_2 will be *G. vaginalis* 97.5% of the time (Piot et al. 1982). The Rapid Identification Method (RIM; Austin Biological Laboratories) identified 96 (91.4%) of 105 clinical isolates of *G. vaginalis* (Lien and Hillier 1989). The API20 Strep system can be used to identify *G. vaginalis* based on starch fermentation, hippurate hydrolysis and the presence of leucine aminopeptidase (Human and Tillotson 1985).

For definitive identification of *G. vaginalis* multiple biochemical tests are needed including presence of α-glucosidase, absence of β-glucosidase, starch and hippurate hydrolysis and characteristic haemolysis. Care must be taken to differentiate *G. vaginalis* isolates from haemolytic or non-haemolytic unclassified catalase-negative coryneform (UCNC) organisms (Catlin 1992). The results of carbohydrate fermentation tests vary with age, quantity of inoculum and basal medium used.

23 SUSCEPTIBILITY TO ANTIMICROBIAL AGENTS

In a recent study (Kharsany, Hoosen and van den Ende 1993) of 93 vaginal isolates of *G. vaginalis*, 90% of the strains were susceptible to penicillin (0.5 μg ml⁻¹), ampicillin (0.5

μg ml⁻¹), second generation cephalosporins such as cefoxitin (1.0 μg ml⁻¹), third generation cephalosporins such as cefotaxime (2.0 μg ml⁻¹), imipenem (1.0 μg ml⁻¹), erythromycin (0.06 μg ml⁻¹), clindamycin (0.3 μg ml⁻¹) and vancomycin (0.5 μg ml⁻¹). Aztreonam (32.0 μg ml⁻¹), tetracycline (64 μg ml⁻¹), amikacin (128 μg ml⁻¹) and trimethoprim–sulphamethoxazole (64.0 μg ml⁻¹) had poor activity. The MIC90 of 2-hydroxymetronidazole (4 μg ml⁻¹) was more active than metronidazole (16 μg ml⁻¹). These data are in agreement with previously published studies as reviewed (Catlin 1992).

24 TYPING METHODS

Biotyping schemes based on detection of hippurate hydrolysis, β-galactosidase and lipase (Piot et al. 1984, Briselden and Hillier 1990) plus fermentation of arabinose, galactose and xylose (Benito et al. 1986) have been described.

A serotyping scheme has also been described (Ison et al. 1987). Using antibodies raised to 9 strains of *G. vaginalis*, 20 serogroups were identified. They did not coincide with the biotypes previously described (Piot et al. 1984).

25 ROLE IN NORMAL FLORA OF HUMANS

G. vaginalis is found as a member of the endogenous vaginal flora in as many as 69% of women of reproductive age (Totten et al. 1982). The reported prevalence has varied widely depending on the medium used for isolation (Catlin 1992). *G. vaginalis* was recovered more frequently from the vagina of sexually abused girls than those who had no history of abuse (Bartley, Morgan and Rimsza 1987). The colony-forming units of *Gardnerella* per ml vaginal wash are generally lower in the normal vagina ($<10^7$) than in bacterial vaginosis ($>10^6$; see section 26.1).

The biochemical role played in the vagina by *G. vaginalis* is unknown.

26 PATHOGENICITY AND VIRULENCE FACTORS

26.1 Bacterial vaginosis

G. vaginalis is well recognized for its association with bacterial vaginosis (BV) as recently reviewed (Spiegel 1991b, Catlin 1992). BV is the most common cause of vaginitis or vaginosis in women of reproductive age. It is diagnosed by the presence of 3 of the following 4 clinical signs:

1 homogeneous adherent discharge
2 'clue cells', vaginal epithelial cells coated with coccobacillary organisms such that the cell borders are obliterated
3 vaginal fluid pH >4.5 and
4 presence of a 'fishy odour' when 10% KOH is added to vaginal fluid.

Up to 69% of normal vaginae are colonized by *G. vaginalis* and this organism is present in nearly all women with BV, suggesting that either precolonization or new acquisition of *G. vaginalis* is a prerequisite for development of BV. Other organisms associated with BV include species of *Prevotella*, *Bacteroides*, *Peptostreptococcus*, *Mobiluncus* and *Mycoplasma hominis* (see Chapters 33, 34 and 58). The role played by *G. vaginalis* in the pathogenesis of BV is unclear. *G. vaginalis* is the predominant organism forming the clue cells seen in BV (Cook et al. 1989). Adherence to epithelial tissue culture cells has been associated with an outer fibrillar coat whereas adherence to red blood cells was mediated by fimbriae (Scott, Curran and Smyth 1989). Haemagglutinating activity is strongest with human 'O' cells (Deodhar and Karnad 1994).

The haemolysin of *G. vaginalis* is a 59 kDa cytolytic exotoxin that forms voltage-dependent cationic channels when incorporated into lipid membranes (Moran et al. 1992, Cauci et al. 1993). It is active on human but not animal red blood cells and is less active on human leucocytes and endothelial cells than erythrocytes (Rottini et al. 1990). BV is characterized by a paucity of inflammation in the vagina. *G. vaginalis* is a poor stimulator, and in fact an inhibitor, of chemotaxis (Sturm 1989).

26.2 Obstetric, gynaecological and fetal infections

BV late in pregnancy and *G. vaginalis* are associated with intrauterine and intra-amniotic infections, chorioamnionitis, postpartum and post-abortal pelvic inflammatory disease, and neonatal scalp wounds as recently reviewed (Catlin 1992, Spiegel 1991b). *G. vaginalis* is an agent of postpartum and neonatal sepsis. Bloodstream invasion may be facilitated by its serum resistance (Boustouller and Johnson 1986). *G. vaginalis* is one of the BV-associated organisms with phospholipase A2 activity (Bejar et al. 1981). This enzyme releases arachidonic acid which stimulates prostaglandin synthesis, resulting in labour.

26.3 Urinary tract infections

G. vaginalis is a relatively infrequent (<0.5%) urinary tract isolate and may be present with or without pyuria. Because the presence of *G. vaginalis* in midstream urine can represent vaginal contamination, its clinical significance can be difficult to ascertain. However, it has been recovered from suprapubic bladder aspirates in symptomatic women without conventional uropathogens (Lam, Birch and Fairley 1988), from pregnant women (McFadyen and Eykyn 1968) and in association with renal disease (McDowall et al. 1981) and interstitial cystitis (Wilkins et al. 1989). The majority of male sexual partners of women with BV have *G. vaginalis* recoverable from the urethra. Genitourinary tract infections in the male, including prostatitis and urosepsis, have been reported and reviewed (Catlin 1992).

VEILLONELLA AND OTHER GRAM-NEGATIVE COCCI

27 GENUS/SPECIES DEFINITION

Veillonella are anaerobic gram-negative cocci, 0.3–0.5 μm in diameter, that are found in pairs, masses or short chains (Rogosa 1984).

28 INTRODUCTION AND BRIEF HISTORY

The type species was originally described by Veillon and Zuber in 1898 as *Staphylococcus parvulus* and renamed by Prévot in 1933 as *Veillonella parvula* (Rogosa 1984).

29 HABITAT

Each species in the genus *Veillonella* is a member of the endogenous oral flora of one or more mammals. Three of the 7 species of *Veillonella* are found in humans: *V. parvula* in the mouth and intestine, *Veillonella atypica* in the mouth, and *Veillonella dispar* in the mouth and respiratory tract. The remaining species are found in the oral and intestinal tracts of rats, rabbits, hamsters and guinea pigs.

Veillonella spp. are the most numerous anaerobes in human saliva (Sutter 1984). Those found on the dorsum of the tongue are *V. atypica* and *V. dispar* (Hughes et al. 1988), those in subgingival plaque are *V. parvula* (Moore et al. 1985, 1987), and those from saliva and on the buccal mucosa are *V. atypica* and *V. dispar* (Hughes et al. 1988). Veillonellae are present on the mucosal surfaces and in the saliva of edentulous infants (Kononen, Asikainen and Jousimies-Somer 1992).

30 MORPHOLOGY

Veillonellae are gram-negative cocci that are 0.3–0.5 μm in diameter. They are found in pairs, masses or short chains. Diplococci may be flattened at their adjacent sides.

31 CULTURAL CHARACTERISTICS AND GROWTH REQUIREMENTS

Veillonellae are anaerobic, non-spore-forming, non-motile organisms. Optimum growth is obtained at 30–37°C, poor growth at 40°C and 24°C, no growth at 18°C or 45°C. They are oxidase-, catalase- and indole-negative. Veillonellae are chemo-organotrophic organisms requiring complex media for growth.

32 Metabolism

The species of *Veillonella* found in humans do not ferment carbohydrates or polyols. Lactate is used as an energy source, as are pyruvate, fumarate, malate, α-ketoglutarate and some purines. Succinic acid alone cannot serve as a sole energy source; however, succinate decarboxylation simultaneous with lactate or malate fermentation is stimulatory (Denger and Schenk 1992). L-Serine stimulates conversion of oxalacetic acid to fumarate in starved cells (Hoshino 1987). Propionic acid is the major metabolic end product along with acetic acid, carbon dioxide and hydrogen. Nitrate is reduced to nitrite. Menaquinones are produced by some veillonellae (Ramotar et al. 1984).

33 Important genetic mechanisms, including plasmid activity

The species of veillonellae are difficult to distinguish from one another based on phenotypic differences. They have been divided into 7 species based on DNA homology (Mays et al. 1982).

34 Cell wall composition; antigenic structure

Some veillonellae require putrescine or cadaverine for growth, incorporating them into peptidoglycan. Requirement for these amines varies with the species: *V. atypica* does not require them, nor do most *V. parvula*, whereas *V. dispar* do.

Veillonellae have a gram-negative cell wall containing lipopolysaccharide with endotoxic activity. Eight serogroups have been described (Mays et al. 1982). Of 44 strains of *V. parvula*, 40 belonged to serogroup II, the remaining 4 to serogroup VI; 29 of 31 *V. atypica* were serogroup VI and 2 were serogroup V; 8 of 8 *V. dispar* were in serogroup VII.

35 Classification

Veillonella is the type genus of the family Veillonellaceae which also contains the genera *Acidaminococcus* and *Megasphaera* (Rogosa 1984). The mol% G + C of *Veillonella* is 40.3–44.4, *Acidaminococcus* 56.6 and *Megasphaera* 53.1–54.1. *Acidaminococcus* (0.6–1.0 μm) and *Megasphaera* (2.4–2.6 μm) are larger on wet mount than *Veillonella*. *Acidaminococcus* is distinct in its ability to use amino acids as its main energy source, from which it produces acetate and butyrate. *Megasphaera* spp. ferments carbohydrates, lactate and pyruvate (but not succinate), from which they produce acetate, butyrate, caproate, valerate, propionate, isobutyrate and isovalerate. Only veillonellae demonstrate red fluorescence under longwave (360 nm) light when grown on enriched medium supplemented with sheep or horse blood and δ-aminolaevulinic acid. Most

recently it has been reported that *Dialister pneumosintes* (formerly *Bacteroides pneumosintes*) is related to *Veillonella* (Willems and Collins 1995).

36 Laboratory isolation and identification

Veillonella spp. will grow on enriched blood-containing media such as *Brucella*, brain–heart infusion and trypticase soy agars supplemented with sheep blood. A selective medium developed by Rogosa et al. (1958) contains per litre: 5.0 g tryptone, 3.0 g yeast extract, 0.75 g thioglycolate, 0.002 g basic fuchsin, 1.0 g Tween 80, 21.0 ml sodium lactate (60%) and 15 g agar. The pH is adjusted to 7.5 prior to autoclaving and vancomycin is added after autoclaving to achieve 7.5 μg ml^{-1}. Colonies on lactate agar are 1–3 mm, smooth, entire, opaque, greyish white and butyrous. No haemolysis is seen on blood agar. Isolates can be identified by their requirement for anaerobiosis, gram stain morphology (gram-negative cocci) and fermentation of lactate but not glucose with production of propionate. These tests will distinguish *Veillonella* spp. from other Veillonellaceae and from *Porphyromonas* spp. which can have a similar gram stain morphology and show red fluorescence under longwave UV light.

37 Susceptibility to antimicrobial agents

Clinical isolates of *Veillonella* were susceptible to meropenem, imipenem, piperacillin, chloramphenicol and cefoxitin (Murray and Niles 1990). All but one were susceptible to clindamycin. Neither aminoglycosides nor vancomycin is active. Penicillin resistance among subgingival isolates from patients with adult periodontitis was more common when the patient had received penicillin treatment within the preceding 6 months (Kinder, Holt and Korman 1986).

38 Bacteriocins and bacteriophages

Temperate (Shimizu 1968) and lytic (Totsuho 1976) phages have been isolated from human oral veillonellae.

39 Role in normal flora of humans

Veillonellae commonly colonize the oral cavity in infancy (Kolenbrander and Moore 1992, Kononen, Asikainen and Jousimies-Somer 1992); 100% of children were culture-positive by 1 year of age. Unlike certain species of oral streptococci, e.g. *Streptococcus salivarius* and *Streptococcus mutans*, veillonellae do not adhere well to buccal epithelial cells or tooth surfaces. They do, however, coaggregate with other oral organisms including *S. salivarius* (Hughes et al. 1988) and *Fusobacterium nucleatum* (Kolenbrander, Anderson and Moore 1989), the latter of which is associated with adult periodontitis.

Veillonella spp. are not thought to play a role in the development of dental caries. Their association with carious lesions is thought to be due to coaggregation with cariogenic streptococci. *Veillonella* spp. may play a protective role by conversion of streptococcal lactic acid to propionate, a milder acid not associated with caries formation.

Acidaminococcus and *Megasphaera* are frequently found in the intestinal contents of humans.

40 PATHOGENICITY AND VIRULENCE FACTORS

Although *Veillonella* spp. are not considered pathogens on the tooth surface, they have clearly been associated with sinusitis, bite wounds, intra-abdominal, pelvic and oral (apical) abscesses, sepsis, osteomyelitis and gynaecological infections (Kolenbrander and Moore 1992). Meningitis has been reported following an injury to the eyelid with a toothbrush (Nukina, Hibi and Nishida 1989). Infections associated with *Acidaminococcus* or *Megasphaera* are quite rare.

Several virulence factors of *Veillonella* have been identified. Lipopolysaccharide (LPS) and lipoteichoic acid from *Veillonella* induced human blood mononuclear cells to release collagenase, thus inducing cytokines (Heath et al. 1987). LPS induced PMN migration in a monkey model (Warfvinge, Dahlen and Bergenholtz 1985) and monocyte migration in vitro (Nagashima 1990). Whole cell sonicate induced production of IL-1 and was mitogenic for spleen cells with polyclonal activation of B cells (Nagashima 1990). Soluble antigens stimulate lymphocytes in vitro (Ivanyi, Newman and Marsh 1991).

A sonicate of *V. parvula* contained 11 antigens from 76 to 13 kDa. The 76 kDa antigen was found more frequently in serum from control patients with mild periodontitis whereas the 39 kDa antigen was associated with severe periodontitis (Watanabe, Marsh and Ivanyi 1989). A 45 kDa protein is an adhesin that mediates coaggregation (Hughes, Anderson and Kolenbrander 1992).

REFERENCES

Bartley DL, Morgan L, Rimsza ME, 1987, *Gardnerella vaginalis* in prepubertal girls, *Am J Dis Child*, **14:** 1014–17.

Bejar R, Curbelo V et al., 1981, Premature labor. ll. Bacterial sources of phospholipase, *Obstet Gynecol*, **57:** 479–82.

Benito R, Vazquez JA et al., 1986, A modified scheme for biotyping *Gardnerella vaginalis*, *J Med Microbiol*, **21:** 357–9.

Boustouller YL, Johnson AP, 1986, Resistance of *Gardnerella vaginalis* to bactericidal activity of human serum, *Genitourin Med*, **62:** 380–3.

Boustouller YL, Johnson AP, Taylor-Robinson D, 1986, Detection of a species-specific antigen of *Gardnerella vaginalis* by Western blot analysis, *J Gen Microbiol*, **132:** 1969–73.

Briselden AM, Hillier SL, 1990, Longitudinal study of the biotypes of *Gardnerella vaginalis*, *J Clin Microbiol*, **28:** 2761–4.

Carlone GM, Thomas ML et al., 1986, Cell wall characteristics of *Mobiluncus* species, *Int J Syst Bacteriol*, **36:** 288–96.

Catlin BW, 1992, *Gardnerella vaginalis*: characteristics, clinical considerations, and controversies, *Clin Microbiol Rev*, **5:** 213–37.

Cauci S, Monte R et al., 1993, Pore-forming and haemolytic properties of the *Gardnerella vaginalis* cytolysin, *Mol Microbiol*, **9:** 1143–55.

Christiansen G, Hansen E et al., 1984, Genetic relationship of short and long anaerobic curved rods isolated from the vagina, *Scand J Urol Nephrol Suppl*, **86:** 75–8.

Cook RL, Reid G et al., 1989, Clue cells in bacterial vaginosis: immunofluorescent identification of the adherent gramnegative bacteria as *Gardnerella vaginalis*, *J Infect Dis*, **160:** 490–6.

Criswell BS, Marston JH et al., 1971, *Haemophilus vaginalis* 594, a gram-negative organism? *Can J Microbiol*, **17:** 865–9.

Csango PA, Hagen N, Jagars G, 1982, Method for isolation of *Gardnerella vaginalis* (*Haemophilus vaginalis*): characterization of isolates by gas chromatography, *Acta Pathol Microbiol Scand Sect B*, **90:** 89–93.

Curtis AH, 1913, A motile curved anaerobic bacillus in uterine discharges, *J Infect Dis*, **12:** 165–9.

DeBoer JM, Plantema FHF, 1988, Ultrastructure of the in situ adherence of *Mobiluncus* to the vaginal epithelial cells, *Can J Microbiol*, **34:** 757–66.

Denger K, Schenk B, 1992, Energy conservation by succinate decarboxylation in *Veillonella parvula*, *J Gen Microbiol*, **138:** 967–71.

Deodhar L, Karnad J, 1994, In vitro adhesiveness of *Gardnerella*

vaginalis strains in relation to the occurrence of clue cells in vaginal discharge, *Indian J Med Res*, **100:** 59–61.

Dunkelberg WE Jr, McVeigh I, 1969, Growth requirements of *Haemophilus vaginalis*, *Antonie van Leeuwenhoek J Microbiol Serol*, **35:** 129–45.

Durieux R, Dublanchet A, 1980, Les 'Vibrions' anaérobies des leucorrhées. I Technique d'isolement et sensibilité aux antibiotiques, *Med Mal Infect*, **10:** 109–15.

Edmunds PN, 1960, *Haemophilus vaginalis*: morphology, cultural characteristics and viability, *J Pathol Bacteriol*, **79:** 273–83.

Fohn MJ, Lukehart SA, Hillier SL, 1988, Production and characterization of monoclonal antibodies to *Mobiluncus* species, *J Clin Microbiol*, **26:** 2598–603.

Gardner HL, Dukes CD, 1955, *Haemophilus vaginalis* vaginitis: a newly defined specific infection previously classified 'nonspecific' vaginitis, *Am J Obstet Gynecol*, **69:** 962–76.

Garlind A, Påhlsson C, Forsum U, 1989, Phenotypic complexity in *Mobiluncus*, *APMIS*, **97:** 38–42.

Greenwood JR, Pickett MJ, 1980, Transfer of *Haemophilus vaginalis* Gardner and Dukes to a new genus *Gardnerella*: *G. vaginalis* (Gardner and Dukes) comb. nov., *Int J Syst Bacteriol*, **30:** 170–81.

Greenwood JR, Pickett MJ, 1986, Genus *Gardnerella*, *Bergey's Manual of Systematic Bacteriology*, 9th edn, vol. 2, ed. Sneath PHA, Williams & Wilkins, Baltimore, 1283–6.

Hallén A, Påhlson C, Forsum U, 1987, Bacterial vaginosis in women attending STD clinic: diagnostic criteria and prevalence of *Mobiluncus* spp., *Genitourin Med*, **63:** 386–9.

Hammann R, Kronibus A et al., 1984, *Falcivibrio grandis* gen. nov. sp. nov., and *Falcivibrio vaginalis* gen. nov. sp. nov., a new genus and species to accommodate anaerobic motile curved rods formerly described as 'Vibrio mulieris' (Prévot 1940) Breed et al 1948, *Syst Appl Microbiol*, **5:** 81–96.

Harper JJ, Davis GHG, 1982, Cell wall analysis of *Gardnerella vaginalis* (*Haemophilus vaginalis*), *Int J Syst Bacteriol*, **32:** 48–50.

Heath JK, Atkinson SJ et al., 1987, Bacterial antigens induce collagenase and prostaglandin E2 synthesis in human gingival fibroblasts through a primary effect on circulating mononuclear cells, *Infect Immun*, **55:** 2148–54.

Hillier SL, Martius J et al., 1988, A case-control study of chorioamnionic infection and histologic chorioamnionitis in prematurity, *N Engl J Med*, **319:** 972–8.

Hillier SL, Nugent RP et al., 1995, Association between bacterial vaginosis and preterm delivery of a low birth weight infant, *N Engl J Med*, **333:** 1737–42.

Hjelm E, Hallén A et al., 1981, Anaerobic curved rods in vaginitis, *Lancet*, **2**: 1353–4.

Holst E, 1990, Reservoir of four organisms associated with bacterial vaginosis suggests lack of sexual transmission, *J Clin Microbiol*, **28**: 2035–9.

Holst E, Hofmann H, Mårdh PA, 1984, Anaerobic curved rods in genital samples of women, *Bacterial Vaginosis*, eds Mårdh PA, Taylor-Robinson D, Almqvist and Wiksell International, Stockholm, 117–24.

Hoshino E, 1987, L-serine enhances the anaerobic lactate metabolism of *Veillonella dispar* ATCC 17745, *J Dent Res*, **66**: 1162–5.

Hughes CV, Anderson RN, Kolenbrander PE, 1992, Characterization of *Veillonella atypica* PK 1910 adhesin-mediated coaggregation with oral *Streptococcus* spp., *Infect Immun*, **60**: 1178–86.

Hughes CV, Kolenbrander PE et al., 1988, Coaggregation properties of human oral *Veillonella* spp.: relationship to colonization site and oral ecology, *Appl Environ Microbiol*, **54**: 1957–63.

Human RP, Tillotson GC, 1985, Identification of *Gardnerella vaginalis* with the API 20 Strep strip, *J Clin Microbiol*, **21**: 985–6.

Ison CA, Harvey DG et al., 1987, Development and evaluation of scheme for serotyping *Gardnerella vaginalis*, *Genitourin Med*, **63**: 196–201.

Ivanyi L, Newman HN, Marsh PD, 1991, T cell proliferative responses to molecular fractions of periodontopathic bacteria, *Clin Exp Immunol*, **83**: 108–11.

Johnson AP, Davies HA, 1984, Demonstration by electron microscopy of pili on *Gardnerella vaginalis*, *Br J Vener Dis*, **60**: 396–7.

Jones BM, Geary I et al., 1985, In-vitro and in-vivo activity of metronidazole against *Garderella vaginalis*, *Bacteroides* spp. and *Mobiluncus* spp. in bacterial vaginosis, *J Antimicrob Chemother*, **16**: 189–97.

Kharsany ABM, Hoosen AA, van den Ende J, 1993, Antimicrobial susceptibilities of *Gardnerella vaginalis*, *Antimicrob Agents Chemother*, **37**: 2733–5.

Kinder SA, Holt SC, Korman KS, 1986, Penicillin resistance in the subgingival microbiota associated with adult periodontitis, *J Clin Microbiol*, **23**: 1127–33.

Kolenbrander PE, Anderson RN, Moore LVH, 1989, Coaggregation of *Fusobacterium nucleatum*, *Selenomonas flueggei*, *Selenomonas infelix*, *Selenomonas noxia*, and *Selenomonas sputigena* with strains from eleven genera of oral bacteria, *Infect Immun*, **57**: 3194–203.

Kolenbrander PE, Moore LVH, 1992, The genus *Veillonella*, *Prokaryotes*, 2nd edn, eds Balows A, Trüper HG et al., Springer-Verlag, New York, 2034–47.

Kononen E, Asikainen S, Jousimies-Somer H, 1992, The early colonization of gram-negative anaerobic bacteria in edentulous infants, *Oral Microbiol Immunol*, **7**: 28–31.

Krönig I, 1895, Über die Natur der Scheidenheme, speciell über das vorkommen anaërober Streptokakken in Scheidensekret Schwangerer, *Zentralbl Gynakol*, **19**: 409–12.

Lam MH, Birch DF, Fairley KF, 1988, Prevalence of *Gardnerella vaginalis* in the urinary tract, *J Clin Microbiol*, **26**: 1130–3.

Larsson P-G, Bergman BB, 1986, Is there a causal connection between motile curved rod, *Mobiluncus* species, and bleeding complications? *Am J Obstet Gynecol*, **154**: 107–8.

Larsson P-G, Bergman B et al., 1986, *Mobiluncus*-specific antibodies in a postoperative infection, *Am J Obstet Gynecol*, **154**: 1167–8.

Lassnig C, Dorsch M et al., 1989, Phylogenetic evidence for the relationship between the genera *Mobiluncus* and *Actinomyces*, *FEMS Microbiol Lett*, **65**: 17–22.

Laughton N, 1948, The bacteriological interpretation of vaginal smears, *J Hyg*, **46**: 262–4.

Leopold S, 1953, Heretofore undescribed organism isolated from genitourinary system, *US Armed Forces Med J*, **4**: 263–6.

Lien EA, Hillier SL, 1989, Evaluation of the enhanced rapid

identification method for *Gardnerella vaginalis*, *J Clin Microbiol*, **27**: 566–7.

McDowall DR, Buchanan JD et al., 1981, Anaerobic and other fastidious microorganisms in asymptomatic bacteriuria in pregnant women, *J Infect Dis*, **144**: 114–22.

McFadyen IR, Eykyn SJ, 1968, Suprapubic aspiration of urine in pregnancy, *Lancet*, **1**: 1112–14.

Mårdh P-A, Holst E, Möller BR, 1984, The grivet monkey as a model for study of vaginitis. Challenge with anaerobic curved rods and *Gardnerella vaginalis*, *Bacterial Vaginosis*, eds Mårdh P-A, Taylor-Robinson D, Almqvist and Wiksell International, Stockholm, 201–6.

Martius J, Krohn MA et al., 1988, Relationships of vaginal *Lactobacillus* species, cervical *Chlamydia trachomatis*, and bacterial vaginosis to preterm birth, *Obstet Gynecol*, **71**: 89–95.

Mays TD, Holdeman LV et al., 1982, Taxonomy of the genus *Veillonella*, *Int J Syst Bacteriol*, **32**: 28–36.

Moi H, Danielsson D, 1984, Studies on rabbit hyperimmune, patient and blood donor serum with regards to bactericidal activity and serum antibodies against anaerobic curved rods from patients with bacterial vaginosis, *Bacterial Vaginosis*, eds Mårdh P-A, Taylor-Robinson D, Almqvist and Wiksell International, Stockholm, 89–92.

Moore B, 1954, Observations on a group of anaerobic vaginal vibrios, *J Pathol Bacteriol*, **67**: 461–73.

Moore LVH, Moore WEC et al., 1987, Bacteriology of human gingivitis, *J Dent Res*, **66**: 989–95.

Moore WEC, Holdeman LV et al., 1985, Comparative bacteriology of juvenile periodontitis, *Infect Immun*, **48**: 507–19.

Moran O, Zegarra-Moran D et al., 1992, Physical characterization of the pore forming cytolysine from *Gardnerella vaginalis*, *FEMS Microbiol Immunol*, **5**: 63–9.

Murray PR, Niles AC, 1990, In vitro activity of meropenem (SM-7338), imipenem, and five other antibiotics against anaerobic clinical isolates, *Diagn Microbiol Infect Dis*, **13**: 57–61.

Nagashima Y, 1990, Immunobiological activities of *Veillonella parvula* isolated from infected root canals, *Kanagawa Shigaku*, **25**: 209–20.

Nukina S, Hibi A, Nishida K, 1989, Bacterial meningitis caused by *Veillonella parvula*, *Acta Paediatr Jpn*, **31**: 609–14.

Påhlson C, Hallén A, Forsum U, 1986a, Improved yield of *Mobiluncus* species from clinical specimens after alkaline treatment, *Acta Pathol Microbiol Immunol Scand Sect B*, **94**: 113–16.

Påhlson C, Hallén A, Forsum U, 1986b, Curved rods related to *Mobiluncus* phenotypes as defined by monoclonal antibodies, *Acta Pathol Microbiol Immunol Scand Sect B*, **94**: 117–25.

Påhlson C, Mattsson JG et al., 1992, Detection and identification of *Mobiluncus* species by direct filter hybridization with an oligonucleotide probe complementary to rRNA, *APMIS*, **100**: 655–62.

Pattman RS, 1984, The significance of finding curved rods in the vaginal secretions of patients attending a genito-urinary medical clinic, *Bacterial Vaginosis*, eds Mårdh P-A, Taylor-Robinson D, Almqvist and Wiksell International, Stockholm, 143–6.

Peloux Y, Thomas P, 1981, A propos de quelques bactéries mobiles anaerobies gram négatives, *Rev Inst Pasteur (Lyon)*, **14**: 103–11.

Piot P, van Dyck E et al., 1980, A taxonomic study of *Gardnerella vaginalis* (*Haemophilus vaginalis*) Gardner and Dukes 1955, *J Gen Microbiol*, **119**: 373–96.

Piot P, van Dyck E et al., 1982, Identification of *Gardnerella* (*Haemophilus*) *vaginalis*, *J Clin Microbiol*, **15**: 19–24.

Piot P, van Dyck E et al., 1984, Biotypes of *Gardnerella vaginalis*, *J Clin Microbiol*, **20**: 677–9.

Ramotar K, Conly JM et al., 1984, Production of menaquinones by intestinal anaerobes, *J Infect Dis*, **150**: 213–18.

Reimer LG, Reller LB, 1985, Effect of sodium polyanetholesulfonate and gelatin on the recovery of *Gardnerella vaginalis* from blood culture media, *J Clin Microbiol*, **21**: 686–8.

Reyn A, Birch-Andersen A, Lapage SP, 1966, An electron microscope study of thin sections of *Haemophilus vaginalis* (Gardner and Dukes) and some possibly related species, *Can J Microbiol*, **12:** 1125–36.

Roberts MC, Hillier SL et al., 1985, Comparison of Gram stain, DNA probe, and culture for the identification of species of *Mobiluncus* in female genital specimens, *J Infect Dis*, **152:** 74–7.

Roberts MC, Hillier SL et al., 1986, Tetracycline resistance and tetM in pathogenic urogenital bacteria, *Antimicrob Agents Chemother*, **30:** 810–12.

Rogosa M, 1984, Anaerobic gram-negative cocci, *Bergey's Manual of Systematic Bacteriology*, 9th edn, vol. 1, ed. Sneath PHA, Williams & Wilkins, Baltimore and London, 680–5.

Rogosa M, Fitzgerald RJ et al., 1958, Improved medium for selective isolation of *Veillonella*, *J Bacteriol*, **76:** 455–6.

Rottini G, Dobrina A et al., 1990, Identification and partial characterization of a cytolytic toxin produced by *Gardnerella vaginalis*, *Infect Immun*, **58:** 3751–8.

Sadhu K, Domingue PAG et al., 1989, *Gardnerella vaginalis* has a gram-positive cell-wall ultrastructure and lacks classical cell-wall lipopolysaccharide, *J Med Microbiol*, **29:** 229–35.

Schwebke JR, Lukehart SA et al., 1991, Identification of two new antigenic subgroups within the genus *Mobiluncus*, *J Clin Microbiol*, **29:** 2204–8.

Scott TG, Curran B, Smyth CJ, 1989, Electron microscopy of adhesive interactions between *Gardnerella vaginalis* and vaginal epithelial cells, McCoy cells and human red blood cells, *J Gen Microbiol*, **135:** 475–80.

Shimizu Y, 1968, Experimental studies on the bacteriophages of the *Veillonella* strains isolated from the oral cavity, *Odontology (Tokyo)*, **55:** 533–41.

Skarin A, Mårdh PA, 1982, Comma-shaped bacteria associated with vaginitis, *Lancet*, **1:** 342–3.

Smith H, Moore HB, 1988, Isolation of *Mobiluncus* species from clinical specimens using cold enrichment and selective media, *J Clin Microbiol*, **26:** 1134–7.

Spiegel CA, 1991a, The genus *Mobiluncus*, *Prokaryotes*, 2nd edn, vol. 1, eds Balows A, Trüper HG et al., Springer-Verlag, New York, 906–17.

Spiegel CA, 1991b, Bacterial vaginosis, *Clin Microbiol Rev*, **4:** 485–502.

Spiegel CA, Roberts M, 1984, *Mobiluncus* gen. nov., *Mobiluncus curtisii* subspecies *curtisii* sp. nov., *Mobiluncus curtisii* subspec-

ies *holmesii* subsp. nov., and *Mobiluncus mulieris* sp. nov., curved rods from the human vagina, *Int J Syst Bacteriol*, **34:** 177–84.

Spiegel CA, Eschenbach DA et al., 1983, Curved anaerobic bacteria in bacterial (nonspecific) vaginosis and their response to antimicrobial therapy, *J Infect Dis*, **148:** 817–22.

Sprott MS, Ingham HR et al., 1983, Characteristics of motile curved rods in vaginal secretions, *J Med Microbiol*, **16:** 175–82.

Sturm AW, 1989, Chemotaxis inhibition by *Gardnerella vaginalis* and succinate producing vaginal anaerobes: composition of vaginal discharge associated with *G. vaginalis*, *Genitourin Med*, **65:** 109–12.

Sutter VL, 1984, Anaerobes as normal oral flora, *Rev Infect Dis*, **6:** 562–6.

Taylor AJ, Owens RS, 1984, Morphological and chemical characteristics of anaerobic curved rod-shaped bacteria from the female genital tract, *Bacterial Vaginosis*, eds Mårdh P-A, Taylor-Robinson D, Almqvist and Wiksell International, Stockholm, 97–106.

Totsuka M, 1976, Studies on veillonellophages isolated from washings of human oral cavity, *Bull Tokyo Med Dent Univ*, **23:** 261–73.

Totten PA, Amsel R et al., 1982, Selective differential human blood bilayer media for isolation of *Gardnerella* (*Haemophilus*) *vaginalis*, *J Clin Microbiol*, **5:** 141–7.

Vetere A, Borriello SP et al., 1987, Characterization of anaerobic curved rods (*Mobiluncus* spp.) isolated from the urogenital tract, *J Med Microbiol*, **23:** 279–88.

Warfvinge J, Dahlen G, Bergenholtz G, 1985, Dental pulp response to bacterial cell wall material, *J Dent Res*, **64:** 1046–50.

Watanabe H, Marsh PD, Ivanyi L, 1989, Detection of immunodominant antigens of periodontopathic bacteria in human periodontal disease, *Oral Microbiol Immunol*, **4:** 159–64.

Wilkins EGL, Payne SR et al., 1989, Interstitial cystitis and the urethral syndrome: a possible answer, *Br J Urol*, **64:** 39–44.

Willems A, Collins MD, 1995, Phylogenetic placement of *Dialister pneumosintes* (formerly *Bacteroides pneumosintes*) within the *Sporomusa* subbranch of the *Clostridium* subphylum of the gram-positive bacteria, *Int J Syst Bacteriol*, **45:** 403–5.

Zinneman K, Turner GC, 1963, The taxonomic position of *Haemophilus vaginalis* (*Corynebacterium vaginale*), *J Pathol Bacteriol*, **85:** 213–19.

Chapter 24

PROPIONIBACTERIUM, BIFIDOBACTERIUM, EUBACTERIUM AND RELATED ORGANISMS

W C Noble and W G Wade

PROPIONIBACTERIUM

1 HABITAT

Some species of *Propionibacterium*, often referred to as the 'classical' propionibacteria, are found in milk and cheese and sometimes in other foodstuffs but 3 species, *Propionibacterium acnes*, *Propionibacterium avidum* and *Propionibacterium granulosum*, are normal inhabitants of human skin and also appear in pathological material. A fourth species, *Propionibacterium propionicus*, an inhabitant of the oral cavity, has been transferred into the genus from *Actinomyces* via *Arachnia*; *Propionibacterium innocuum*, also a member of the normal skin flora, has now been transferred to a new genus *Propioniferax*.

2 GENUS DEFINITION

Propionibacteria are pleomorphic, sometimes branching, gram-positive coryneform rods, non-acid fast and non-motile. They are aerotolerant and growth of the skin species may occasionally be obtained in primary culture if skin lipid is carried over (Evans and Mattern 1979) but, with the exception of *P. innocuum*, they are best treated as anaerobes. *Propioniferax innocuum* grows well as an aerobe, the remaining species will form colonies in 2–3 days at 37°C on media containing lipid such as Tween 80 in an atmosphere of N_2 and CO_2. A suitable medium contains, per litre, tryptone soya broth 30 g, yeast extract 10 g, agar 10 g, Tween 80 10 ml. They ferment sugars with the production of propionic and acetic acids. Catalase is demonstrable if cultures grown anaerobically are exposed to air for at least 30 min before testing. The cell wall peptidoglycan of *P. propionicus* contains either diaminopimelic acid (DAP) or lysine (Charfreitag, Collins and Stackebrandt 1988); that of other species contains DAP (Johnson and Cummins 1972). Most isolates of the 'skin' species possess LL-DAP but a minority of *P. acnes* and *P. avidum* have *meso*-DAP though they do not differ in G + C mol% or DNA homology from reference strains for the species (Johnson and Cummins 1972). The G + C mol% of 'classical' species of propionibacteria is 65–68; that of the skin species tends to be lower: *P. acnes* 57–60, *P. granulosum* 61–63, *P. avidum* 62–63, *P. propionicum* 63–65. The chief fatty acids are C_{15} unsaturated (Moss et al. 1967, Cummins and Moss 1990).

3 PROPIONIBACTERIUM ACNES

P. acnes is the commonest coryneform bacterium, probably the most common micro-organism on human skin; after puberty heavy colonization of lipid-rich skin areas with skin surface densities of 10^5–10^7 cm^{-2} is probably universal (Somerville and Murphy 1973, Matta 1974, McGinley, Webster and Leyden 1978). The primary site of growth is the sebaceous gland (Leeming, Holland and Cunliffe 1984) and the initiation of colonization is most probably the result of changes in skin lipid composition, especially in the balance of the C_{18} saturated and unsaturated lipids (Nordstrom and Noble 1985, Patel and Noble 1993). Although this organism is rare on animal skin, probably due to differences in skin lipid (Webster, Ruggieri and McGinley 1981), *P. acnes* indistinguishable from those found on human skin form a minor component of the skin flora of dogs (Harvey, Noble and Lloyd 1993, Goodacre et al. 1994).

Colonies on lipid-containing media are domed and whiteish, 0.5 mm in diameter after incubation anaerobically at 37°C for 3 days. Acid is formed from glucose but not sucrose or maltose. *P. acnes* is distinguished from other skin species by being DNAase-negative, gelatinase- and casein hydrolase-positive, indole-positive and nitrate-reducing (Marples and McGinley 1974). They are divisible by their susceptibility to a phage into 2 groups that tend to differ, though not absolutely, in several other respects. Phage-susceptible strains (group I) generally acidify sorbitol but phage-resistant strains (group II) do not. Group II strains belong to serogroup II but group I strains belong to serogroups I or II with serogroup I predominating (Webster and Cummins 1978). On casein yeast lactate glucose agar, group I strains forms colonies 1–2 mm in diameter after incubation anaerobically for 7 days at 37°C; the colonies are domed, opaque, cream-yellow and butyrous. Group II strains form more variable colonies that are generally larger and of a distinct reddish-brown colour. Gel electrophoresis of whole cell protein does not reveal useful differences between isolates (Nordstrom 1985) though strains may be speciated and the serogroups of *P. acnes* and *P. avidum* determined (Gross, Ferguson and Cummins 1978). Other attempts at subspecies 'typing' include extension of phage typing to 7 types (Jong, Ko and Pulverer 1975) and biotyping by 'fer-

mentation tests' to yield 5 biotypes (Kishishita et al. 1979). However, pyrolysis mass spectrometry discriminated between strains of *P. acnes* isolated from the foreheads of 6 independent normal adults; 3 adults carried more than one strain (Goodacre et al. 1996).

P. acnes is cytotoxic to cultured Vero cells and human diploid fibroblast cells, probably because of its production of propionate (Allaker, Greenman and Osborne 1987); it also produces histamine (Allaker, Greenman and Osborne 1986). Proteases and hyaluronate lyases are also produced at sharp pH and Po_2 optima in vitro (Ingham et al. 1979, 1983). The cell wall carbohydrate of *P. acnes* activates the complement cycle by the alternative pathway (Webster and McArthur 1982). All these activities may contribute to its role as a pathogen. Claims that prostaglandins are produced (Abrahamsson, Hellgren and Vincent 1978) have not been substantiated. The production of porphyrins by *P. acnes* causes sebaceous glands to fluoresce under long wave UV light; in vitro coproporphyrin III is synthesized (Lee, Shalita and Poh-Fitzpatrick 1978).

The precise role of *P. acnes* in acne vulgaris remains a matter for conjecture (Holland, Ingham and Cunliffe 1981, Winston and Shalita 1991). Although some inflamed follicles show no evidence of micro-organisms (Leeming, Holland and Cunliffe, 1988), measures directed at reducing the microbial load are effective in ameliorating the condition in some patients, though other therapies aimed at modifying the follicles themselves or altering hormone balance are also effective. A strong case can be made for the involvement of *P. acnes* in the inflammatory processes but not in the initiation of lesion formation. Antibody to *P. acnes* enzymes is higher only in those with severe acne (Ingham et al. 1987); cellular immunity to *P. acnes* is a late event (Gowland et al. 1978).

The presence of *P. acnes* in deep lesions, especially those involving the head, must always raise the question of contamination or colonization rather than primary pathogenicity. Brook and Frazier (1991) in a review of infection by *Propionibacterium* species concluded that in only 94 (12%) of 816 lesions yielding propionibacteria was the organism the cause of infection. Nevertheless, infection with *P. acnes* has been reported to follow craniotomy (van Ek et al. 1986, Estaban et al. 1995), midbrain encephalitis (Camarata et al. 1990) and lesions of the central nervous system (Richards et al. 1989), and infection of ventriculoatrial shunts have been described (Schiff and Oakes 1989, Setz et al. 1994). Other deep infections reported include osteomyelitis (Noble and Overman, 1987) and bacteraemia (Brook 1990).

Since the introduction of topical tetracycline, erythromycin and clindamycin for treatment of acne, there has been a sharp rise in resistance to these antibiotics (Leyden et al. 1983, Eady et al. 1993) such that amongst patients so treated more than 30% now carry strains resistant to erythromycin and more than 15% strains resistant to tetracycline. The fact that patients with resistant organisms suffer acne refractory to treatment with these antibiotics is further confirmation that *P. acnes* does play a role in acne vulgaris. The mechanism of antibiotic resistance has not yet been determined but does not appear to reflect the acquisition of genes from other organisms. Nevertheless, erythromycin resistance is phenotypically indistinguishable from that of the majority of bacteria where resistance is due to methylation of the 23S ribosomal RNA since most resistant *P. acnes* are inducibly or constitutively resistant to macrolide, lincosamide and streptogramin B antibiotics (Eady et al. 1989a, 1989b).

Prior to topical therapy, only a few per cent of strains were reported resistant to erythromycin or tetracycline though most were resistant to aminoglycosides and fusidic acid (Höffler, Niederau and Pulverer 1980); all were sensitive to penicillins and cephalosporins.

4 *PROPIONIBACTERIUM GRANULOSUM*

P. granulosum is also found in the sebaceous glands and on the human skin surface but generally at densities about 100-fold lower than those of *P. acnes*. Colonies on lipid-containing media are larger than those of *P. acnes* after incubation for 3 days anaerobically and are generally reddish pigmented. *P. granulosum* is not susceptible to *P. acnes* phage, is DNAase-positive, gelatinase- and casein hydrolase-negative, indole- and nitrate-negative. The DNA of *P. granulosum* has only about 12–15% homology with that of *P. acnes* or *P. avidum*.

Like *P. acnes*, *P. granulosum* may be found in some lesions of the skin and deeper tissue and is occasionally recognized as an opportunist pathogen such as in septicaemia of an immunocompromised host (Branger, Bruneau and Goullet 1987).

Studies of *P. granulosum* or *P. avidum* as immunostimulators (Hof and Pulverer 1987) are reminiscent of the use of 'Corynebacterium parvum', a commercially available product now acknowledged to be a mixture of the *Propionibacterium* spp. found on human skin (Cummins and Johnson 1974). The effects of 'C. parvum' were varied and depended on the experimental conditions (Milas and Scott, 1978, Hart 1985); this is no doubt a reflection of the effect of propionibacterium cell wall on the complement system.

5 *PROPIONIBACTERIUM AVIDUM*

P. avidum is frequently found on the moist areas of skin, such as the axillae, and is very much less common on lipid-rich areas (Nordstrom and Noble 1984) but, like the other species, is most common on post-pubertal individuals. After anaerobic incubation for 3 days, colonies are larger than those of *P. acnes* and are generally not pigmented. *P. avidum* is not susceptible to *P. acnes* phage, is DNAase-positive, gelatinase- and casein hydrolase-positive, indole- and nitrate-negative. *P. avidum* is less fastidious in amino acid requirements than the other 2 species (Ferguson and Cummins 1978), but shows about 50% homology of 16S RNA sequences with *P. acnes* (Charfreitag and Stackebrandt 1989).

As with the other skin species, *P. avidum* is occasionally reported from deep lesions such as splenic abscess (Dunne et al. 1986).

6 *PROPIONIBACTERIUM PROPIONICUS*

P. propionicus was formerly assigned to the genus *Actinomyces*, chiefly because branched bacilli may be seen. It was then transferred to the genus *Arachnia* and from there to *Propionibacterium* (Charfreitag, Collins and Stackebrandt 1988) on the basis of sequence homology of ribosomal RNA. On grammatical grounds the specific epithet should read 'propionicum'.

Anaerobic growth after 48 h on blood agar media is grey-white, dry and rough. The crumb-like colonies cause pitting of the agar. Microscopically cells may be filamentous or branching. Much propionic acid is produced. Porphyrin production is sufficient to produce red fluorescence of the colonies under UV light.

P. propionicus is a normal inhabitant of the human oral cavity but is found causing infection of the lachrymal apparatus, especially in older women (Brazier and Hall 1993, Csukas et al. 1993). Although some eye infections with *P. acnes* are reported, it may be that these are in fact *P. propionicus*. Eye infections may be difficult to treat with topical antibiotics and strains are reported resistant to gentamicin, neomycin and sulphonamides (Seal et al. 1981).

7 *PROPIONIFERAX INNOCUUM*

P. innocuum was originally described on the basis of its cell wall composition as a new coryneform from human skin (Pitcher 1976). It was formerly allocated to the genus *Propionibacterium* (Pitcher and Collins 1991) from which it differs chiefly in growing well aerobically and in possessing arabinose in its cell wall. It has now been elevated to monotypic genus status as *Propioniferax innocuum* (Yokata et al. 1994).

BIFIDOBACTERIUM

8 GENUS DEFINITION

Bifidobacterium spp. are pleomorphic gram-positive rods showing true and false branching. They are non-motile and non-sporing. Most species are strictly anaerobic; they grow between 20 and 45°C with optimum growth at 38°C. The organisms are aciduric, but killed by heat at 60°C in 5 min. They ferment various carbohydrates with production of acetic and lactic acids in the ratio 3:2. CO_2 is not produced. Glucose metabolism is characteristically and exclusively by the fructose-6-phosphate shunt. There is no proteolytic activity. They do not form oxidase, indole or H_2S and are generally non-pathogenic to man and animals. *Bifidobacterium* spp. are normal flora of the mouth and intestine. The G + C content of the DNA is c. 60 mol%. The type species is *Bifidobacterium bifidum*.

9 INTRODUCTION AND HISTORICAL PERSPECTIVE

The first member of this genus to be recognized was isolated from infants' stools by Tissier (1900), who called it *Bacillus bifidus*. The classification of the bifidobacteria has presented difficulties, but most workers consider that the bifidobacteria should be classed in a genus of their own, as suggested by Orla-Jensen (1924). This has been confirmed by phylogenetic studies that have demonstrated that the bifidobacteria are confined to a single deep cluster within the high G + C gram-positive group (Maidak et al. 1994). Furthermore, all the bifidobacteria share the property peculiar to them among the non-sporing gram-positive anerobes of degrading glucose by the fructose-6-phosphate shunt. Species definitions have been the subject to extensive revision. Several biotypes or species were described by Dehnert (1957, 1961). Gyllenberg and Carlberg (1958) and Reuter (1963, 1971) recognized and named 8 separate species from human sources. However, by means of DNA homology studies, Scardovi and his colleagues (1971) found that some of these species were homologous, and they reduced the number to 5, whilst adding 4 more. Subsequent studies have proposed a number of new species; they are currently 29, 10 of which have been isolated from humans. Bifidobacteria make up a high proportion of the bacteria in the gut flora of human infants and adults.The protective effects of bifidobacteria against enteric infection and cancer are now widely appreciated and the inclusion of bifidobacteria in probiotic products is widespread.

10 HABITAT

Bifidobacteria are found in the human mouth, the lower gut of humans and animals and in sewage; they are occasionally isolated from clinical material.

11 MORPHOLOGY

A wide variety of cell morphologies are displayed and even a single strain may appear different under different cultural conditions. The classic bifid club-shaped protusions are shown by most species under conditions of nutrient limitation. Otherwise, morphologies range from the large, curved, irregular-shaped cells of *B. bifidum* and the palisade arrangement of *Bifidobacterium angulatum* to the characteristic star-like clusters of *Bifidobacterium asteroides*. Although it has been suggested that species identification is possible by examination of cell morphology (Scardovi 1986), this is not recommended without substantial experience of the genus.

12 CULTURAL CHARACTERISTICS

Most species are strict anaerobes, but a few species, isolated from animals or bees, will tolerate O_2 in the presence of added CO_2, growing in 90% air + 10% CO_2.

13 METABOLISM

Biochemically, one of the more striking features of bifidobacteria is the formation of acetic acid in addition to lactic acid during the fermentation of glucose. This property, and the failure to form detectable gas, separate the bifidobacteria from the heterofermentative group of lactobacilli (Beerens, Gerard and Guillaume 1957). The absence of propionic acid from the products of fermentation separates *Bifidobacterium* from *Propionibacterium*. Glucose is utilized by the fructose-6-phosphate shunt, and detection of fructose-6-phosphate phosphoketolase is the most reliable test for assigning an organism to this genus (for method, see Scardovi 1986). Urease production is uncommon among human isolates, but ureolytic strains occur in all species. One of the animal species, *Bifidobacterium suis*, is most often strongly ureolytic. The catalase reaction is usually negative, but some oxygen-tolerant strains liberate O_2 from H_2O_2 when grown in air + 10% CO_2. Nitrate reduction cannot be demonstrated by the usual tests. Many of the bifidobacteria isolated from the human gut are able to hydrolyse cholic acid and conjugated bile acids such as sodium glycocholate and sodium taurocholate (Drasar and Hill 1974, Ferrari, Pacini and Canzi 1980).

14 CELL WALL COMPOSITION; ANTIGENIC STRUCTURE

Studies of cell wall murein of bifidobacteria have shown that the amino acid composition of the peptide side chains can be useful in species identification. However, closely related species may have the same cross-links, e.g. *Bifidobacterium longum* and *Bifidobacterium infantis* (Kandler and Lauer 1974). Other chemotaxonomic studies, such as the analysis of cellular fatty acids and phosphoglycerides, have not proved useful for species identification (Exterkate et al. 1971, Veerkamp 1971).

The antigenic structure is complex and most workers have found a fairly high degree of strain specificity by agglutination reactions. The antigens taking part in these reactions are heat stable; the results are the same whether living or boiled organisms are used for the preparation of antisera. Unlike the lactobacilli, bifidobacteria do not seem to contain an extractable precipitinogen.

15 SUSCEPTIBILITY TO ANTIMICROBIAL AGENTS

Bifidobacteria are uniformly susceptible to benzylpenicillin, the macrolides and lincosamines, chloramphenicol and vancomycin, but are usually resistant to the aminoglycosides, nalidixic acid and metronidazole.

16 CLASSIFICATION

Study of the DNA composition reveals a G + C content of 57.2–64.2 mol%, with a mean of 60.1. These figures differ from the much lower ones of 33.0–52.5 for the lactobacilli and the higher ones of 66.4–70.4 for the propionibacteria (Sebald, Gasser and Werner 1965, Werner, Gasser and Sebald 1965). Substantial revision of the classification has taken place in recent years, based primarily on DNA–DNA homology data. *B. bifidum* and *Bifidobacterium adolescentis* have been shown to form distinct genetic groups. *B. bifidum* biotypes a and b are closely related to each other, as are the 4 biotypes of *B. adolescentis*. The 4 species, *Bifidobacterium dentium*, *Bifidobacterium angulatum*, *Bifidobacterium catenulatum* and *Bifidobacterium pseudocatenulatum*, which are difficult to distinguish from *B. adolescentis* on the basis of fermentation patterns, are genetically distinct from each other and from *B. adolescentis*. *Bifidobacterium longum* and *Bifidobacterium infantis* are the most closely related species with about 50% homology, and *Bifidobacterium breve* shows 40–50% homology with *B. infantis* (Scardovi et al. 1971, Biavati et al. 1984).

At present, 29 species in all are recognized (Table 24.1). Of these, 10 (*B. bifidum*, *B. breve*, *B. gallicum*, *B. infantis*, *B. longum*, *B. adolescentis*, *B. catenulatum*, *B. dentium*, *B. angulatum* and *B. pseudocatenulatum*) have been isolated from the human mouth, faeces or vagina; 14 other species have been found in the intestines and faeces of other vertebrate animals, including pigs, cattle, chickens and rabbits. Three species are unique to the intestine of the honey bee and 2 species have been found only in sewage. Species have been proposed on the basis of DNA–DNA homology studies supported by phenotypic tests and immunological and chemotaxonomic investigations.

17 LABORATORY ISOLATION AND IDENTIFICATION

The nutritional requirements of bifidobacteria are still imperfectly known. Since the discovery that milk stimulated the growth of *B. bifidum*, considerable attention has been given to the study of 'bifidus factors' in human milk, but these studies have added little to our knowledge (Poupard, Hussain and Norris 1973). Bifidobacteria are very heterogeneous in their requirements for growth factors and vitamins; riboflavin and pantothenate are the most common requirements, but nicotinic acid, pyridoxine, thiamine,

Table 24.1 Current species of *Bifidobacterium*

Species	Typical sites of isolation
B. adolescentis	Human adult faeces
B. angulatum	Human adult faeces, sewage
B. catenulatum	Human adult and infant faeces
B. gallicum	Human adult faeces
B. longum	Human adult and infant faeces, vagina
B. bifidum	Human adult and infant faeces, calf faeces
B. breve	Human infant faeces, human vagina, calf faeces
B. infantis	Human infant faeces
B. pseudocatenulatum	Human adult and infant faeces, calf faeces
B. dentium	Human dental caries, faeces, vagina, miscellaneous human infections including abscesses and wound infections
B. merycicum	Bovine rumen
B. ruminantium	Bovine rumen
B. globosum	Bovine rumen, faeces of man and animals
B. boum	Bovine rumen, pig faeces
B. thermophilum	Bovine rumen, pig and calf faeces
B. pseudolongum	Bovine rumen, pig faeces
B. animalis	Chicken, rat, rabbit faeces
B. gallinarum	Chicken faeces
B. pullorum	Chicken faeces
B. asteroides	Bee intestine
B. indicum	Bee intestine
B. coryneforme	Bee intestine
B. choerinum	Pig faeces
B. suis	Pig faeces
B. cuniculi	Rabbit faeces
B. magnum	Rabbit faeces
B. saeculare	Rabbit faeces
B. minimum	Sewage
B. subtile	Sewage

folic acid and *p*-aminobenzoic acid may also be needed (Scardovi 1986). Most species are able to use ammonium salts as the sole source of nitrogen, but some species isolated from animals will not grow in the absence of organic nitrogen.

Many different media have been devised for isolating or enumerating the bifidobacteria in faeces and sewage. The media contain a carbohydrate such as glucose, lactose, fructose or maltose and complex mixtures of peptones, yeast extract, growth factors and reducing agents. Antibiotics, particularly aminoglycosides, have been used to improve selectivity, but no universally satisfactory selective medium is at present available. Non-selective media that give good growth of the strains present in the habitat being studied are to be preferred (see Scardovi 1981).

Fermentation tests have been used traditionally to distinguish individual species. However, some species such as *B. infantis*, *B. longum*, *B. dentium* and *B. adolescentis* show similar patterns of sugar fermentation and this method cannot be used reliably for identification purposes. Biavati, Scardovi and Moore (1982) showed that the generation protein profiles of soluble wholesale proteins, using SDS-PAGE, was a reliable method for the identification of species. Members of a single species have identical or nearly identical protein patterns. This method has been widely used subsequently both for identification and as a method for the preliminary characterization of new strains for classification purposes. Recently developed molecular methods have also been employed for this purpose. Ribotyping, using 23S ribosomal RNA to probe digested chromosomal DNA, has resulted in both species and strain identification (Mangin et al. 1994). Oligonucleotide probes, designed from 16S rRNA sequence data, have been shown to be specific for *B. adolescentis*, *B. breve* and *B. longum*; probes for *B. bifidum* and *B. infantis* showed specificity adequate for the identification of isolates from human material (Yamamoto, Morotomi and Tanaka 1992). Extension and refinement of these approaches should permit rapid and even automated identification in the foreseeable future.

Although fermentation tests with simple sugars do not allow discrimination of species (Gavini et al. 1991), the use of complex carbohydrates has been shown by Crociani et al. (1994) to discriminate between species commonly isolated from human specimens (Table 24.2).

Isoenzyme patterns (of transaldolases and 6-phosphogluconate dehydrogenases) have proved useful for characterizing species of *Bifidobacterium*. Antisera against purified transaldolases have been used to distinguish groups of species from different habitats (Sgorbati and London 1982). Furthermore, β-galactosidase electrophoretic patterns successfully differentiated animal and human species of bifidobacteria and were more discriminatory than numerical analysis based on 45 tests in a comparative study (Roy, Berger and Reuter 1994).

18 ROLE IN NORMAL FLORA OF HUMANS

Bifidobacteria are reported to play an important regulatory role in the large intestine, controlling pH and protecting against infection by exogenous pathogens, particularly in infants (Modler, McKellar and Yaguchi 1990, Saavedra et al. 1994). It has further been proposed that bifidobacteria may offer protection against cancer, not only of the lower gut but also at other body sites (Reddy and Rivenson 1993). These findings have led to considerable interest in the use of bifidobacteria in probiotics and a number of dairy products, which include bifidobacteria, are being developed (Fuller 1989, Puhan 1990). The need for quality control and safety of such products has stimulated taxonomic studies of the genus and the development and refinement of identification systems.

The species most often found are: in babies, *B. infantis* and *B. breve*, and in adults, *B. adolescentis*, *B. longum* and *B. pseudocatenulatum* (Dehnert 1957, 1961, Reuter 1963, Beerens, Romond and Neut 1980, Biavati et al. 1984, Mitsuoka 1984). *B. dentium* is part of the normal oral flora and can be isolated readily from dental plaque (Biavati, Scardovi and Moore 1982).

19 PATHOGENICITY AND VIRULENCE FACTORS

B. dentium and 2 unnamed taxa are associated with dental caries and periodontal disease although whether they play a pathogenic role in these diseases is unknown (Moore et al. 1983). *B. dentium* has also been isolated from clinical specimens obtained from a variety of sites. These are principally mixed infections, typically abscesses or wound infections around the head and neck area or the lungs. *B. dentium* can probably be classed as an opportunist pathogen like many other members of the oral microflora. Other bifidobacteria that have been isolated from clinical material, albeit rarely, include *B. longum*, *B. adolescentis* and *B. breve*, recovered from abscesses, urinary tract infections and septicaemia (Darbas et al. 1991).

20 *BIFIDOBACTERIUM BIFIDUM*

B. bifidum is common in the faeces of breast-fed and bottle-fed infants and in the faeces of adults and of animals. It is non-pathogenic to man and laboratory animals. The G + C content of DNA is c. 60.1 mol% and DNA–DNA homology studies show *B. bifidum* to be a distinct species related to but separate from other bifidobacteria.

In faeces it is a delicate bacillus, about 4 μm long and 0.7 μm broad, with tapering, pointed ends. Arranged in pairs end to end, with the distal ends pointed and the proximal ends swollen, they generally lie parallel to one another, rarely intertwined. Two or 3 bacilli often radiate from a single point, forming a Y-shaped structure; clubbed forms and forms ending

Table 24.2 Key for differentiation of *Bifidobacterium* species of human origin (Crociani et al. 1994)

Substrate						Suggested species
α-L-F	D-G	Ar	Ga	Gu	Am	
+	+					
						B. infantis
	−					*B. breve*
						(*B. pseudocatenulatum*)
−	−	+				
						B. longum
		−	+			
						B. bifidum
			−	+		
						B. dentium
				−	+	*B. adolescentis*
						(*B. pseudocatenulatum*)
					−	
						B. catenulatum

α-L-F, α-L-fucose; D-G, D-glucuronate; Ar, arabinogalactan; Ga, gastric mucin; Gu, gum guar; Am, amylopectin.
Species in parentheses is less likely.
B. angulatum and *B. gallicum* are not included because of the low number of strains available.

in knobs are not uncommon. They are often arranged in palisades or Chinese letters. The general appearance is not unlike a diphtheroid bacillus. In culture its morphology varies with the medium. Its characteristic appearance is that of a highly pleomorphic bacillus showing irregularly clubbed forms with branching often at both ends. Geniculate forms, forms ending in knobs, forms with lateral buds, bladder forms, and candle-flame forms may be seen. The absence of chain formation and of long filaments is noteworthy. The species is non-motile and non-sporing, stains uniformly in young cultures, but in older cultures irregular or granular staining is not uncommon. It is gram-positive in young cultures; later gram-negative forms appear. *B. bifidum* is non-acid fast. For a description of the morphology with illustrations, see Orla-Jensen (1943), Dehnert (1957, 1961) and Scardovi (1986).

Ammonium salts are utilized as sole source of nitrogen, but good growth is obtained on peptone–yeast extract–glucose agar with added cysteine and Tween 80 (Scardovi 1981). No growth occurs on nutrient agar. On glucose agar and human milk agar incubated anaerobically, colonies are usually low convex, greyish-brown, lenticular or ovoid, 0.5–2 mm in diameter, showing under the microscope a delicately granular structure, a brownish opaque centre, a finer translucent periphery and a finely crenated edge. In glucose broth growth is moderate; in 3 or 4 days the organisms fall to the bottom of the tube, forming an abundant loose flocculogranular deposit, easily disintegrated on shaking. Very slight or no growth occurs at 20°C; optimum temperature is 38–39°C; upper limit is 45°C. Optimum pH is 6.5–7.0. The organism grows only in the absence of O_2; CO_2 is beneficial. Growth is improved by extracts of liver, yeast and faeces (Orla-Jensen 1943). Some strains are stimulated by 'bifidus factor' present in human milk. The organism requires riboflavin, nicotinic acid, folic acid and *p*-aminobenzoic acid for growth; it is stimulated by Tween 80.

Glucose, lactose and galactose are fermented; in addition, most strains ferment fructose and some attack sucrose, maltose or melibiose. The addition of Tween 80 improves reliability of fermentation reactions. D-Lactic acid and acetic acid are the main end products of metabolism. Oxidase, catalase, urease, indole and H_2S are not produced, nitrate is not reduced and arginine is not hydrolysed.

In fluid cultures the organisms often die within 3 days. They are killed by heat at 55°C in 30 min and at 60°C in 5 min. They are resistant to acids; for preservation they should be subcultured weekly or freeze-dried.

The antigens are, as yet, incompletely studied. Cells are agglutinated by sera prepared against live or heat-killed organisms. The organism belongs to immunological specificity group B on the basis of its reaction with antitransaldolase sera (Sgorbati and London 1982).

EUBACTERIUM

21 GENUS DEFINITION

Eubacteria are uniform or pleomorphic gram-positive rods, motile or non-motile and non-sporing. The are strictly anaerobic and grow between 30 and 37°C. They may ferment various carbohydrates or peptone to produce mixtures of organic acids; gas is usually produced. They do not produce:

1 the large amounts of propionic acid characteristic of propionibacteria

2 more acetic than lactic acid as do the bifidobacteria

3 lactic acid as the sole major product like the lactobacilli or

4 the mixture of succinic and lactic acid formed by actinomycetes.

Some species are proteolytic; indole and H_2S may be produced. The G + C content of the DNA 25–55 mol%. The type species is *Eubacterium limosum*.

22 INTRODUCTION AND HISTORICAL PERSPECTIVE

The first members of this genus to be described were isolated from the faeces of man by Eggerth (1935), who assigned them to the genus *Bacteroides* as a temporary expedient. The genus *Eubacterium* was described by Prévot (1938). Since then, it has become a genus of convenience in that, as implied by its description above, it has become a repository for non-sporing gram-positive anaerobic bacilli that do not correspond to other, better defined, genera. *Eubacterium* currently encompasses an extraordinary variety of organisms and the necessary taxonomic revision of the group will require considerable time and effort.

23 HABITAT

Eubacterium species are found in the mouths and intestines of humans and animals, in the rumen, in abscesses and soft tissue infections, in the environment in soil and in extreme conditions.

24 MORPHOLOGY

The cell morphology is extremely variable, ranging from small coccobacilli to large filamentous bacilli. Cells often stain gram-variable. Eubacteria may be confused with peptostreptococci; indeed, a recent phylogenetic study has shown that *Peptostreptococcus heliotrinreducens*, previously classified as an anaerobic coccus, shows most similarity to *Eubacterium* spp. (unpublished data).

25 CULTURAL CHARACTERISTICS

Growth is extremely variable but in the main eubacteria tend to be fastidious and many species are extremely slow growing. *Eubacterium* spp. found in clinical specimens can be isolated on complex media suitable for anaerobes (Moore and Holdeman Moore 1986). Isolation media should usually contain haemin and menadione, but different species have different requirements. Extended incubation of at least 7 days is recommended. All eubacteria are strict anaerobes; some are extremely sensitive to oxygen and require pre-reduced and anaerobically sterilized media for growth. The growth of a number of species found in the mouth and in clinical specimens is enhanced by the inclusion of arginine or lysine, or both, in culture media (Hill, Ayers and Kohan 1987).

26 METABOLISM

As might be expected given such a diverse group, metabolism is extremely variable. Saccharolytic, non-fermentative and proteolytic species have been described. A wide variety of patterns of production of volatile and non-volatile fatty acids is seen. Some species reduce nitrate. *Eubacterium budayi* and *Eubacterium tenue* produce lecithinase (Moore and Holdeman Moore 1986). Some rumen strains such as *Eubacterium cellulosolvens*, *Eubacterium uniforme* and *Eubacterium xylanophilum* can degrade fibre (van Gylswick and van der Toorn 1985, 1986). *E. limosum* is a versatile organism that can degrade amino acids, lactate and methanol; conversely, this species can grow autotrophically on hydrogen and carbon dioxide or just carbon monoxide (Genthner, Davis and Bryant 1981, Genthner and Bryant 1982). For the majority of species, however, metabolic pathways are unknown.

27 CELL WALL COMPOSITION; ANTIGENIC STRUCTURE

The chemical composition of cell wall peptidoglycans shows wide variation between species and includes *meso*-diaminopimelic acid direct, LL-diaminopimelic acid–glycine types and a type where peptide bridges are connected to the D-glutamic acid residue (Andreeson 1992), although relatively few species have been examined.

28 SUSCEPTIBILITY TO ANTIMICROBIAL AGENTS

In general, *Eubacterium* species are susceptible to all the major classes of antimicrobial agents. A detailed description of antimicrobial susceptibility by species is given by Moore and Holdeman Moore (1986).

29 CLASSIFICATION

At present, 45 species are recognized in the genus but the classification of *Eubacterium* has long been unsatisfactory. A recent phylogenetic study has shown that *Eubacterium* spp. are intimately associated with the clostridia, itself a genus of considerable complexity (Collins et al. 1994). *Eubacterium* spp. are widely distributed among the low G + C gram-positive organisms. The only criterion for the placing of a species in *Eubacterium* or *Clostridium* is spore formation by the latter. However, individual lines of descent include both sporing and non-sporing species. The reason for this is unknown. Either spore formation is a feature that has emerged a number of times throughout evolution or, more likely, non-sporing species carry sporulation genes that are either dormant or non-functional.

Even within groups of related organisms, there is considerable heterogeneity among *Eubacterium* spp. For example, the oral asaccharolytic *Eubacterium* spp., *E. brachy*, *E. nodatum*, *E. saphenum* and *E. timidum*, although found on one line of descent by 16S rRNA analysis, show negligible DNA homology (Nakazawa and Hoshino 1994) and their rRNA similarity is such that they all appear to represent new genera (unpublished data). It is likely that a large number of new genera will be created when comprehensive systematic studies have been completed.

30 LABORATORY ISOLATION AND IDENTIFICATION

Careful specimen collection, and strict anaerobic transport, processing and culture are undoubtedly important as is the use of a good nutritious culture medium. Incubation for 7 days is recommended as many species are slow growing. Identification of isolates can be difficult because most species tend to be unreactive in conventional biochemical tests. A scheme for the identification of commonly encountered species is shown in Table 24.3.

A substantial proportion of fresh isolates do not correspond to named species; there are a large number of, as yet, unnamed taxa. Protein profile analysis is a useful but time-consuming method for definitive speciation (Wade, Slayne and Aldred 1990) of characterized species.

31 ROLE IN NORMAL FLORA OF HUMANS

Eubacterium spp. comprise a substantial part of the normal flora of the intestine (Finegold, Sutter and Mathisen 1983). *E. saburreum* is a frequently isolated member of the normal oral flora. The oral asaccharolytic species are not normally found in oral health.

32 PATHOGENICITY AND VIRULENCE FACTORS

Seventeen species of eubacteria have been isolated from infections; these include *E. aerofaciens*, *E. alactolyticum*, *E. combesii*, *E. contortum*, *E. cylindroides*, *E. lentum*, *E. limosum*, *E. saburreum*, *E. tenue* and *E. rectale*; *E. lentum* is the most frequently seen (Lewis and Sutter 1981, Sutter et al. 1986). *Eubacterium* spp. are typically recovered as part of a mixed flora from abscesses at various body sites. There have been several reports of the isolation of *Eubacterium* spp. from oral infections but because, in general, they are slow growing and have fastidious nutritional requirements, they have not been widely studied. However, Moore et al. (1982, 1983) found that *E. brachy*, *E. nodatum*, *E. timidum*, *E. alactolyticum*, *E. saburreum* and 17 unnamed taxa made up a significant proportion of the subgingival microflora in chronic and severe advanced periodontitis. Higher isolation rates were reported by Uematsu and Hoshino (1992) who found that the genus made up 54% of the anaerobic flora of periodontal pockets. In addition, *Eubacterium* spp. are regularly isolated from carious dentine and endodontic and periapical infections (Hoshino 1985, Sundqvist 1992, Wasfy et al.

1992, Sato et al. 1993). Furthermore, oral asaccharolytic *Eubacterium* spp. are found in infections at a range of non-oral sites, albeit mainly in the head and neck region (Hill et al. 1987).

33 VIRULENCE FACTORS

The numerical associations between *Eubacterium* spp. and oral infections are strong. However, whether these bacteria play a causative role or merely colonize diseased sites is unknown. Because the majority of oral *Eubacterium* spp. have been described only recently, little work has been done in investigating these organisms for possible virulence factors. Preliminary work (unpublished data) suggests that the asaccharolytic species do not produce proteases but exhibit acid phosphatases, esterases and aminopeptidases. Since these organisms are always found in mixed infections, they may act in concert with other bacteria in the degradation of host tissues.

34 *EUBACTERIUM LIMOSUM*

This organism is isolated from the intestine of humans and vertebrate animals, including rats, poultry and fish, and from sewage-sludge and mud. It may be isolated from wounds and abscesses, usually in mixed culture.

E. limosum is a gram-positive, non-motile, irregular, club-shaped rod with occasional bifurcations; it may be gram-negative in old cultures. Ammonium salts are used as the main source of nitrogen. Good growth occurs on peptone–yeast extract agar or in peptone–yeast extract broth. Growth is often improved by the presence of fermentable carbohydrate. On blood agar incubated anaerobically, colonies are usually circular, entire, convex, up to 2 mm in diameter and translucent or slightly opaque. Growth in glucose broth is good, the broth becoming turbid with a smooth or viscous deposit. Slight or no growth occurs at 25°C; optimum temperature is 37°C; upper limit is 45°C. Glucose, fructose, mannitol, erythritol and ribose are fermented; some strains attack maltose, mannose and xylose. Acid and gas are produced. Major end products of metabolism are acetic, butyric and lactic acids together with CO_2 and H_2. Gelatin, but not meat, is digested by some strains. Indole is not produced. Nitrate is not reduced. The G + C content of DNA is 47 mol%.

For further information, see Moore and Cato (1965) and Moore and Holdeman Moore (1986).

35 *EUBACTERIUM LENTUM*

E. lentum is isolated from human faeces and from blood, postoperative wounds and abscesses, commonly in mixed culture. It is a gram-positive, non-motile coccobacillus. Growth is limited by the availability of arginine. On blood agar incubated anaerobically colonies are circular, entire, 0.5–2 mm in diameter. Growth in glucose broth is moderate with a slight sediment. Carbohydrates are not fermented. Energy is obtained by the arginine dihydrolase pathway (Sperry and Wilkins 1976). Acetate is the major end product of metabolism with trace amounts of lactate and succinate. Bile acids and corticosteroids are metabolized. The ability to metabolize digoxin may be clinically significant (Dobkin et al. 1983).

For more information, see Moore, Cato and Holdeman (1971) and Moore and Holdeman Moore (1986).

Table 24.3 Differential characteristics of *Eubacterium* species encountered in human clinical materials

Species	Glucose	Indole	Maltose	Lactose	Mannose	Starch hydrolysis	Aesculin hydrolysis	Nitrate	Metabolic products in PYG[a]
E. aerofaciens	+	–	+	V	+	–	V	–	A, F, L
E. alactolyticum	+	–	–	–	–	–	–	–	A, B, C
E. contortum	+	–	+	+	V	–	+	–	A, f
E. cylindroides	+	–	–	–	+	V	+	–	a, B, L
E. limosum	+	–	V	–	–	V	+	–	A, B
E. moniliforme	+	–	V	+	+	V	–	V	a, B, L
E. multiforme	+	–	–	+	+	–	+	+	A, p, B, L
E. rectale	+	–	+	+	V	+	+	–	B, L
E. saburreum	+	+	+	–	–	–	+	–	a, b, l
E. tenue	+	+	–	–	–	V	–	–	a, f
E. brachy	–	–	–	–	–	–	–	–	a, IB, IV, IC, s
E. combesii	–	–	–	–	–	–	V	–	A, ib, B, iv
E. lentum	–	–	–	–	–	–	–	V	a
E. nodatum	–	–	–	–	–	–	–	–	a, B, s
E. saphenum	–	–	–	–	–	–	–	–	ab
E. timidum	–	–	–	–	–	–	–	–	a, s

[a]Metabolic product analysis determined on peptone–yeast extract–glucose (PYG) broth cultures.
Abbreviations: A, acetic acid; F, formic acid; P, propionic acid; IB, isobutyric acid; B, butyric acid; IV, isovaleric acid; IC, isocaproic acid; C, caproic acid; L, lactic acid; S, succinic acid. Capital letters indicate major products.
Adapted from Allen (1985).

REFERENCES

Abrahamsson S, Hellgren L, Vincent J, 1978, Prostaglandin-like substances in *Propionibacterium acnes, Experientia*, **34**: 1446–7.

Allaker RP, Greenman J, Osborne RH, 1986, Histamine production by *Propionibacterium acnes* in batch and continuous culture, *Microbios*, **48**: 165–72.

Allaker RP, Greenman J, Osborne RH, 1987, The production of inflammatory compounds by *Propionibacterium acnes* and other skin organisms, *Br J Dermatol*, **117**: 175–83.

Allen SD, 1985, Gram-positive nonsporeforming anaerobic bacilli, *Manual of Clinical Microbiology*, 4th edn, eds Lennette EH, Balows A et al., American Society for Microbiology, Washington DC, 461–72.

Andreesen JR, 1992, The genus *Eubacterium, The Prokaryotes: a Handbook on the Biology of Bacteria: Ecophysiology, Isolation, Identification, Applications*, 2nd edn, eds Balows A, Truper HG et al., Springer-Verlag, New York, 1914–24.

Beerens H, Gerard A, Guillaume J, 1957, Étude de 30 souches de *Bifidobacterium bifidum* (*Lactobacillus bifidus*). Caractérization d'une variété buccale. Comparison avec les souches d'originale fécale, *Ann Inst Pasteur (Lille)*, **9**: 77–85.

Beerens H, Romond C, Neut C, 1980, Influence of breast feeding on the bifid flora of the newborn intestine, *Am J Clin Nutr*, **33**: 2434–39.

Biavati B, Scardovi V, Moore WEC, 1982, Electrophoretic patterns of proteins in the genus *Bifidobacterium* and proposal of four new species, *Int J Syst Bacteriol*, **32**: 358–73.

Biavati B, Castagnoli P et al., 1984, Species of the genus *Bifidobacterium* in the faeces of infants, *Microbiologica*, **7**: 341–5.

Branger C, Bruneau B, Goullet P, 1987, Septicemia caused by *Propionibacterium granulosum* in a compromised host, *J Clin Microbiol*, **25**: 2405–6.

Brazier JS, Hall V, 1993, *Propionibacterium propionicum* and infections of the lachrymal apparatus, *Clin Infect Dis*, **17**: 892–3.

Brook I, 1990, Bacteremia due to anaerobic bacteria in newborns, *J Perinatol*, **10**: 351–6.

Brook I, Frazier EH, 1991, Infections caused by *Propionibacterium acnes, Rev Infect Dis*, **13**: 819–22.

Camarata PJ, McGeachie RE, Haines SJ, 1990, Dorsal midbrain encephalitis caused by *Propionibacterium acnes*. Report of two cases and comment, *J Neurosurg*, **72**: 654–9.

Charfreitag D, Collins MD, Stackebrandt E, 1988, Reclassification of *Arachnia propionica* as *Propionibacterium propionicus* comb. nov., *Int J Syst Bacteriol*, **38**: 354–7.

Charfreitag O, Stackebrandt E, 1989, Inter- and intrageneric relationships of the genus *Propionibacterium* as determined by 16S RNA sequences, *J Gen Microbiol*, **135**: 2035–70.

Collins MD, Lawson PA et al., 1994, The phylogeny of the genus *Clostridium*: proposal of five new genera and eleven new species combinations, *Int J Syst Bacteriol*, **44**: 812–26.

Crociani F, Alessandrini A et al., 1994, Degradation of complex carbohydrates by *Bifidobacterium* spp., *Int J Food Microbiol*, **24**: 199–210.

Csukas Z, Palfalvi M, Kiss R, 1993, The role of *Propionibacterium propionicus* in chronic canaliculitis, *Acta Microbiol Hung*, **40**: 107–13.

Cummins CS, Johnson JL, 1974, *Corynebacterium parvum*: a synonym for *Propionibacterium acnes*?, *J Gen Microbiol*, **80**: 433–42.

Cummins CS, Moss CW, 1990, Fatty acid composition of *Propionibacterium propionicum* (*Arachnia propionica*), *Int J Syst Bacteriol*, **40**: 307–8.

Darbas H, Jean-Pierre H et al., 1991, Septicémie à *Bifidobacterium longum, Méd Mal Infect*, **21**: 707–9.

Dehnert J, 1957, Untersuchung über die gram-positive Stuhlflora des Brustmilchkindes, *Zentralbl Bakteriol Parasitenkd Infektionskr Hyg Abt 1 Orig*, **169**: 66–83.

Dehnert J, 1961, *Uber die Bedeutung der Intestinalbesiedlung beim Menschen. Bakteriologische Untersuchungen als Beitrag zum Bifidoproblem*, Habilistationsschrift, Heidelberg.

Dobkin JF, Saha JR et al., 1983, Digoxin-inactivating bacteria: identification in human gut flora, *Science*, **220**: 325–7.

Drasar BS, Hill MJ, 1974, *Human Intestinal Flora*, Academic Press, London.

Dunne WM, Kurschenbaum HA et al., 1986, *Propionibacterium avidum* as the etiologic agent of splenic abscess, *Diagn Microbiol Infect Dis*, **4**: 87–92.

Eady EA, Cove JH et al., 1989a, Erythromycin-resistant propionibacteria in antibiotic treated acne patients, association with therapeutic failure, *Br J Dermatol*, **121**: 51–7.

Eady EA, Ross JI et al., 1989b, Macrolide-lincosamide-streptogramin B (MLS) resistance in cutaneous propionibacteria: definition of phenotypes, *J Antimicrob Chemother*, **23**: 493–502.

Eady EA, Jones CE et al., 1993, Antibiotic-resistant propionibacteria in acne: need for policies to modify antibiotic usage, *Br Med J*, **306**: 555–6.

Eggerth AH, 1935, The gram-positive non-spore-bearing anaerobic bacilli of human feces, *J Bacteriol*, **30**: 277–90.

Estaban J, Ramos JM et al., 1995, Surgical wound infections due to *Propionibacterium acnes*: a study of 10 cases, *J Hosp Infect*, **30**: 229–32.

Evans CA, Mattern KL, 1979, The aerobic growth of *Propionibacterium acnes* in primary cultures from skin, *J Invest Dermatol*, **72**: 103–6.

Exterkate FA, Otten BJ et al., 1971, Comparison of the phospholipid composition of *Bifidobacterium* and *Lactobacillus* strains, *J Bacteriol*, **106**: 824–9.

Ferguson DA, Cummins CS, 1978, Nutritional requirements of anaerobic coryneforms, *J Bacteriol*, **135**: 858–67.

Ferrari A, Pacini N, Canzi E, 1980, A note on bile acids transformation by strains of *Bifidobacterium, J Appl Bacteriol*, **49**: 193–7.

Finegold SM, Sutter VL, Mathisen GE, 1983, *Human Intestinal Microflora in Health and Disease*, ed. Hentges DJ, Academic Press, New York, 3–31.

Fuller R, 1989, Probiotics in man and animals, *J Appl Bacteriol*, **66**: 365–78.

Gavini F, Pourcher A-M et al., 1991, Phenotypic differentiation of bifidobacteria of human and animal origins, *Int J Syst Bacteriol*, **41**: 548–57.

Genthner BRS, Bryant MP, 1982, Growth of *Eubacterium limosum* with carbon monoxide as the energy source, *Appl Environ Microbiol*, **43**: 70–4.

Genthner BRS, Davis CL, Bryant MP, 1981, Features of rumen and sewage sludge strains of *Eubacterium limosum*, a methanol- and H_2-CO_2-utilizing species, *Appl Environ Microbiol*, **42**: 12–19.

Goodacre R, Neal MJ et al., 1994, Rapid identification using pyrolysis mass spectrometry and artificial neural networks of *Propionibacterium acnes* isolated from dogs, *J Appl Bacteriol*, **76**: 124–34.

Goodacre R, Howell SA et al., 1996, Subspecies discrimination, using pyrolysis mass spectrometry and self-organising neural networks, of *Propionibacterium acnes* isolated from normal skin, *Zentralbl Bakteriol, Int J Med Microbiol, Virol, Parasitol Infect Dis*, **284**: 501–15.

Gowland G, Ward RM et al., 1978, Cellular immunity to *P. acnes* in the normal population and patients with acne vulgaris, *Br J Dermatol*, **99**: 43–7.

Gross CS, Ferguson DA, Cummins CS, 1978, Electrophoretic protein patterns and enzyme mobilties in anaerobic coryneforms, *Appl Environ Microbiol*, **35**: 1102–8.

Gyllenberg H, Carlberg G, 1958, Specific contaminants in cultures of bifidobacteria (*Lactobacillus bifidus*), *Acta Pathol Microbiol Scand*, **44**: 293–8.

van Gylswyk NO, van der Toorn JJTK, 1985, *Eubacterium uniforme* sp. nov. and *Eubacterium xylanophilum* sp. nov., fiber-digesting bacteria from the rumina of sheep fed corn stover, *Int J Syst Bacteriol*, **35**: 323–6.

van Gylswyk NO, van der Toorn JJTK, 1986, Description and designation of a neotype strain of *Eubacterium cellulosolvens* (*Cillobacterium cellulosolvens* Bryant, Small, Bouma and Robinson) Holdeman and Moore, *Int J Syst Bacteriol*, **36:** 275–7.

Hart DA, 1985, Increased sensitivity of *Corynebacterium parvum*-treated mice to toxic effects of indomethacin and lipopolysaccharide, *Infect Immun*, **47:** 408–14.

Harvey RG, Noble WC, Lloyd DH, 1993, Distribution of propionibacteria on dogs: a preliminary report of the findings on 11 dogs, *J Small Anim Pract*, **34:** 80–4.

Hill GB, Ayers OM, Kohan AP, 1987, Characteristics and sites of infection of *Eubacterium nodatum*, *Eubacterium timidum*, *Eubacterium brachy*, and other asaccharolytic Eubacteria, *J Clin Microbiol*, **25:** 1540–5.

Hof H, Pulverer G, 1987, The influence of killed *Propionibacterium granulosum* on experimental infection with *Escherichia coli*, *Med Microbiol Immunol*, **176:** 75–8.

Höffler V, Niederau W, Pulverer G, 1980, Susceptibility of cutaneous propionibacteria to newer antibiotics, *Chemotherapy*, **26:** 7–11.

Holland KT, Ingham E, Cunliffe WJ, 1981, The microbiology of acne, *J Appl Bacteriol*, **51:** 195–215.

Hoshino E, 1985, Predominant obligate anaerobes in human carious dentine, *J Dent Res*, **64:** 1195–8.

Ingham E, Holland KT et al., 1979, Purification and partial characterization of hyaluronate lyase (EC 4.2.2.1) from *Propionibacterium acnes*, *J Gen Microbiol*, **115:** 411–18.

Ingham E, Holland KT et al., 1983, Studies of the extracellular proteolytic activity produced by *Propionibacterium acnes*, *J Appl Bacteriol*, **54:** 263–71.

Ingham E, Gowland G et al., 1987, Antibodies to *P. acnes* and *P. acnes* exocellular enzymes in the normal population at various ages and in patients with acne vulgaris, *Br J Dermatol*, **116:** 805–12.

Johnson JL, Cummins CS, 1972, Cell wall composition and deoxyribonucleic acid similarities among the anaerobic coryneforms, classical propionibacteria, and strains of *Arachnia propionica*, *J Bacteriol*, **109:** 1047–66.

Jong EC, Ko HL, Pulverer G, 1975, Studies on bacteriophages of *Propionibacterium acnes*, *Med Microbiol Immunol*, **161:** 263–71.

Kandler O, Lauer E, 1974, Neuere Vorstellungen zur Taxonomie der Bifidobacterien, *Zentralbl Bakteriol Orig A*, **228:** 29–45.

Kishishita M, Ushijima T et al., 1979, Biotyping of *Propionibacterium acnes* isolated from normal human facial skin, *Appl Environ Microbiol*, **38:** 589–9.

Lee W-LS, Shalita AR, Poh-Fitzpatrick MB, 1978, Comparative studies of porphyrin production in *Propionibacterium acnes* and *Propionibacterium granulosum*, *J Bacteriol*, **133:** 811–15.

Leeming JP, Holland KT, Cunliffe WJ, 1984, The microbial ecology of pilosebaceous units isolated from human skin, *J Gen Microbiol*, **130:** 803–7.

Leeming JP, Holland KT, Cunliffe WJ, 1988, The microbial colonization of inflamed acne vulgaris lesions, *Br J Dermatol*, **118:** 203–8.

Lewis RP, Sutter VL, 1981, *The Prokaryotes: a Handbook on Habitats, Isolation, and Identification of Bacteria*, vol. 2, eds Starr MP, Stolp H et al., Springer-Verlag, Berlin, 1903–11.

Leyden JJ, McGinley KJ et al., 1983, *Propionibacterium acnes* resistance to antibiotics in acne patients, *J Am Acad Dermatol*, **8:** 41–5.

McGinley KJ, Webster GF, Leyden JJ, 1978, Regional variations of cutaneous propionibacteria, *Appl Environ Microbiol*, **35:** 62–6.

Maidak BL, Larsen MJ et al., 1994, The Ribosomal Database Project, *Nucleic Acids Res*, **22:** 3485–7.

Mangin I, Bourget N et al., 1994, Identification of *Bifidobacterium* strains by rRNA gene restriction patterns, *Appl Environ Microbiol*, **60:** 1451–8.

Marples RR, McGinley KJ, 1974, *Corynebacterium acnes* and other anaerobic diphtheroids from human skin, *J Med Microbiol*, **7:** 349–57.

Matta M, 1974, Carriage of *Corynebacterium acnes* in school children in relation to age and sex, *Br J Dermatol*, **91:** 557–61.

Milas L, Scott MT, 1978, Antitumor activity of *Corynebacterium parvum*, *Adv Cancer Res*, **26:** 257–306.

Mitsuoka T, 1984, Taxonomy and ecology of bifidobacteria, *Bifid Microflor*, **3:** 11–28.

Modler HW, McKellar RC, Yaguchi M, 1990, Bifidobacteria and bifidogenic factors, *Can Inst Food Sci Technol J*, **23:** 29–41.

Moore WEC, Cato EP, 1965, *Eubacterium limosum* and *Butyribacterium rettgeri*: *Butyribacterium limosum* comb. nov., *Int Bull Bacteriol Nomencl Taxon*, **15:** 69–80.

Moore WEC, Cato EP, Holdeman LV, 1971, *Eubacterium lentum* (Eggerth) Prévot 1938: emendation of description and designation of the neotype strain, *Int J Syst Bacteriol*, **21:** 299–303.

Moore WEC, Holdeman Moore LV, 1986, Genus *Eubacterium* Prévot 1938, *Bergey's Manual of Systemic Bacteriology*, vol. 2, ed. Sneath PHA, Williams & Wilkins, Baltimore, 1353–73.

Moore WEC, Holdeman LV et al., 1982, Bacteriology of severe periodontitis in young adults, *Infect Immun*, **38:** 1137–45.

Moore WEC, Holdeman LV et al., 1983, Bacteriology of moderate (chronic) periodontitis in mature adult humans, *Infect Immun*, **52:** 510–15.

Moss CW, Dowell VR et al., 1967, Cultural characteristics and fatty acid composition of *Corynebacterium acnes*, *J Bacteriol*, **94:** 1300–5.

Nakazawa F, Hoshino E, 1994, Genetic relationships among *Eubacterium* species, *Int J Syst Bacteriol*, **44:** 787–90.

Noble RC, Overman SB, 1987, *Propionibacterium acnes* osteomyelitis: case report and review of the literature, *J Clin Microbiol*, **25:** 251–4.

Nordstrom NKM, 1985, Polyacrylamide gel electrophoresis (PAGE) of whole-cell proteins of cutaneous *Propionibacterium* species, *J Med Microbiol*, **19:** 9–14.

Nordstrom NKM, Noble WC, 1984, Colonization of the axilla by *Propionibacterium avidum* in relation to age, *Appl Environ Microbiol*, **47:** 1360–2.

Nordstrom NKM, Noble WC, 1985, Application of computer taxonomic techniques to the study of cutaneous propionibacteria and skin surface lipid, *Arch Dermatol Res*, **278:** 107–13.

Orla-Jensen S, 1924, La classification des bactéries lactiques, *Le Lait*, **4:** 468–74.

Orla-Jensen S, 1943, *Die echten Milchsaurebakterien*, Ejnar Munksgaard, Copenhagen.

Patel S, Noble WC, 1993, Analyses of skin surface lipid in patients with microbially associated skin disease, *Clin Exp Dermatol*, **18:** 405–9.

Pitcher DG, 1976, Arabinose with LL diaminopimelic acid in the cell wall of an aerobic coryneform organism isolated from human skin, *J Gen Microbiol*, **94:** 225–7.

Pitcher DG, Collins MD, 1991, Phylogenetic analysis of some LL diaminopimelic acid-containing coryneform bacteria from human skin: description of *Propionibacterium innocuum* sp. nov., *FEMS Microbiol Lett*, **84:** 295–300.

Poupard JA, Husain I, Norris RF, 1973, Biology of the bifidobacteria, *Bacteriol Rev*, **37:** 136–65.

Prévot AR, 1938, Études de systématique bactérienne. III. Invalidité du genre *Bacteroides* Castellani et Chalmers démembrement et reclassification, *Ann Inst Pasteur (Paris)*, **60:** 285–307.

Puhan Z, 1990, Developments in the technology of fermented milk products, *Cult Dairy Prod J*, **25:** 4–9.

Reddy BS, Rivenson A, 1993, Inhibitory effect of *Bifidobacterium longum* on colon, mammary, and liver carcinogenesis induced by 2-amino-3-methylimidazo[4,5-*f*]quinoline, a food mutagen, *Cancer Res*, **53:** 3914–18.

Reuter G, 1963, Vergleichende Untersuchungen über die Bifidus-Flora im Säuglings- und Erwachsenenstuhl, *Zentralbl Bakteriol Parasitenkd Infektionskr Hyg Abt 1 Orig*, **191:** 486–507.

Reuter G, 1971, Designation of typestrains for *Bifidobacterium* species, *Int J Syst Bacteriol*, **21:** 273–5.

Richards J, Ingham HR et al., 1989, Focal infections of the central nervous system due to *Propionibacterium acnes*, *J Infect*, **18**: 279–82.

Roy D, Berger J-L, Reuter G, 1994, Characterization of dairy-related *Bifidobacterium* spp. based on their β-galactosidase electrophoretic patterns, *Int J Food Microbiol*, **23**: 55–70.

Saavedra JM, Bauman NA et al., 1994, Feeding of *Bifidobacterium bifidum* and *Streptococcus thermophilus* to infants in hospital for prevention of diarrhoea and shedding of rotavirus, *Lancet*, **344**: 1046–9.

Sato T, Hoshino E et al., 1993, Predominant obligate anaerobes in necrotic pulps of human deciduous teeth, *Microbial Ecol Health Dis*, **6**: 269–75.

Scardovi V, 1981, The genus *Bifidobacterium*, *The Prokaryotes*, vol. 2, eds Starr MP, Stolp H et al., Springer-Verlag, New York, 1418–34.

Scardovi V, 1986, Genus *Bifidobacterium* Orla-Jensen 1924, *Bergey's Manual of Systemic Bacteriology*, vol. 2, ed. Sneath PHA, Williams & Wilkins, Baltimore, 1418–34.

Scardovi V, Trovatelli LD et al., 1971, Deoxyribonucleic acid homology among species of the genus *Bifidobacterium*, *Int J Syst Bacteriol*, **21**: 276–94.

Schiff SJ, Oakes WJ, 1989, Delayed cerebrospinal-fluid shunt infections in children, *Pediatr Neurosci*, **15**: 131–5.

Seal DV, McGill J et al., 1981, Lachrymal canaliculitis due to *Arachnia* (*Actinomyces*) *propionica*, *Br J Ophthalmol*, **65**: 10–13.

Sebald M, Gasser F, Werner H, 1965, Teneur GC percentage et classification. Application au groupe des bifidobactéries et à quelques genres voisirs, *Ann Inst Pasteur (Paris)*, **109**: 251–69.

Setz U, Frank V et al., 1994, Shunt nephritis associated with *Propionibacterium acnes*, *Infection*, **22**: 99–101.

Sgorbati B, London J, 1982, Demonstration of phylogenetic relatedness among members of the genus *Bifidobacterium* by means of the enzyme transaldolase as an evolutionary marker, *Int J Syst Bacteriol*, **32**: 37–42.

Somerville DA, Murphy CT, 1973, Quantitation of *Corynebacterium acnes* on healthy human skin, *J Invest Dermatol*, **60**: 231–3.

Sperry JF, Wilkins TD, 1976, Arginine, a growth-limiting factor for *Eubacterium lentum*, *J Bacteriol*, **127**: 780–4.

Sundqvist G, 1992, Associations between microbial species in dental root canal infections, *Oral Microbiol Immunol*, **7**: 257–62.

Sutter VL, Citron DM et al., 1986, *Wadsworth Anaerobic Bacteriology Manual*, 4th edn, Star, Belmont, California.

Tissier H, 1900, *Recherches sur la Flore intestinale des Nourissons (état normal et pathologique)*, Thesis, University of Paris, Paris.

Uematsu H, Hoshino E, 1992, Predominant obligate anaerobes in human periodontal pockets, *J Periodont Res*, **27**: 15–19.

Van Ek B, Bakker FP et al., 1986, Infections after craniotomy: a retrospective study, *J Infect*, **12**: 105–9.

Veerkamp JH, 1971, Fatty acid composition of *Bifidobacterium* and *Lactobacillus* strains, *J Bacteriol*, **108**: 861–7.

Wade WG, Slayne MA, Aldred MJ, 1990, Comparison of identification methods for asaccharolytic *Eubacterium* species, *J Med Microbiol*, **33**: 239–42.

Wasfy MO, McMahon KT et al., 1992, Microbiological evaluation of periapical infections in Egypt, *Oral Microbiol Immunol*, **7**: 100–105.

Webster GF, Cummins CS, 1978, Use of bacteriophage typing to distinguish *Propionibacterium acnes* types I and II, *J Clin Microbiol*, **7**: 84–90.

Webster GF, McArthur WP, 1982, Activation of components of the alternative pathway of complement by *Propionibacterium acnes* cell wall carbohydrate, *J Invest Dermatol*, **79**: 137–40.

Webster GF, Ruggieri MR, McGinley KJ, 1981, Correlation of *Propionibacterium acnes* population with the presence of triglycerides on non-human skin, *Appl Environ Microbiol*, **41**: 1269–70.

Werner H, Gasser F, Sebald M, 1965, DNS - Basenbestimmungen an 28 Bifidus - Stämmen und an Stämmen morphologisch ähnlicher Gattungen, *Zentralbl Bakteriol Parasitenkd Infektionskr Hyg Abt 1 Orig*, **198**: 504–16.

Winston MH, Shalita AR, 1991, Acne vulgaris: pathogenesis and treatment, *Pediatr Clin North Am*, **38**: 889–903.

Yamamoto T, Morotomi M, Tanaka R, 1992, Species-specific oligonucleotide probes for five *Bifidobacterium* species detected in human intestinal microflora, *Appl Environ Microbiol*, **58**: 4076–9.

Yokota A, Tamura T, 1994, Transfer of *Propionibacterium innocuum*. Pitcher and Collins 1991 to *Propioniferax* gen. nov. as *Propioniferax innocua* comb. nov., *Int J Syst Bacteriol*, **44**: 579–82.

Chapter 25

CORYNEBACTERIA AND RARE CORYNEFORMS

A W C von Graevenitz, M B Coyle and G Funke

1 COMMON FEATURES OF THE 'CORYNEFORM' GROUP

'Coryneform' bacteria do not form a taxonomic entity but rather are characterized by morphological traits, i.e. as non-spore-forming, non partially acid-fast gram-positive rods showing a 'diphtheroid' morphology (straight or slightly curved, club-like or ellipsoidal shapes with round or tapered ends). Staining may be uneven and there may be metachromatic granules consisting of polymetaphosphate that stain reddish purple with methylene blue and may retain other stains (Fig. 25.1).

In recent years, taxonomic investigations of large collections of gram-positive rods have been successful in delineating new genera and species which will be discussed here (see Tables 25.1, 25.2 and 25.3). New genera and species are probably yet to be discovered and characterized.

With the exception of the so-called lipophilic *Corynebacterium* species (see section 2.3, p. 542), these bacteria are nutritionally non-fastidious: they grow on nutrient agar at 37°C and on agar media containing blood but not on enteric agar formulations. With very few exceptions, they are catalase-positive, indole-negative and oxidase-negative. Selection of *Corynebacterium* spp. may be accomplished by inoculating media inhibitory to gram-negative bacteria such as those containing colistin sulphate and nalidixic acid.

Initially only certain members of the genus *Corynebacterium* were thought to cause human infections, but this view has changed with the thorough identification and taxonomic delineation of human strains, initiated by Hollis and Weaver (1981) and now continued by several other groups.

In the diagnostic laboratory identification to the species level is desirable at least for all pure cultures including those that appear to be 'contaminants'. Several systems are available for this purpose: traditional multimedia ones (Hollis and Weaver 1981, von Graevenitz et al. 1994), a commercial one (APICoryne, bioMérieux, La Balme-les-Grottes, France) and an automated cellular fatty acid analyser (MIDI, Microbial ID, Newark, DE, USA). These systems have been evaluated recently (von Graevenitz et al. 1994). For the separation of some taxa, chemotaxonomic analyses will have to be performed. The system API-Zym is useful for characterization of various species but is strongly inoculum-dependent and lacks specificity (von Graevenitz et al. 1994).

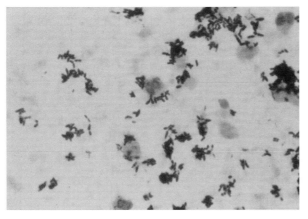

Fig. 25.1 Coryneform morphology. See also Plate 25.1.

Table 25.1 Some chemotaxonomic characteristics of coryneform genera

	Corynebacterium	*Turicella*	*Brevibacterium*	*Dermabacter*	*Oerskovia*	*Cellulomonas*	*Sanguibacter*	*Microbacterium*	*Aureobacterium*	*'C. aquaticum'*
G + C mol%[a]	46–74	65–72	60–64	62	71–75	71–76	69–70	69–75	67–70	73
Mycolic acids	v[b] (C_{22-38})	–	–	–	–	–	–	–	–	–
Cellular fatty acids rank	18:1 ωc9 16:0 18:0	18:1 ωc9 16:0 18:0	15:0 ai 17:0 ai 15:0 i	17:0 ai 15:0 ai 16:0 i	15:0 ai 15:0 i 17:0 ai	15:0 ai 16:0	16:0 15:0 ai 14:0	15:0 ai 17:0 ai 16:0 i	15:0 ai 17:0 ai 16:0 i	17:0 ai 15:0 ai 16:0 i
TBSA[c]	v	+								
Diamino acid[d]	*m*-DAP	*m*-DAP	*m*-DAP	*m*-DAP	L-Lys	L-Orn	L-Lys	L-Lys	Orn	DAB
Arabinogalactan	+	+	–	–	–	–	–	–	–	–
Main menaquinones	MK-9 (H$_2$) MK-8 (H$_2$)	MK-10 MK-11	MK-8 (H$_2$)	MK-9 MK-8 MK-7	MK-9 (H$_4$)	MK-9 (H$_4$)	MK-9 (H$_4$)	MK-12 MK-11	MK-11 MK-12	MK-10 MK-11
Microscopy	Irregular, V forms, clubbing, palisading	Irregular, V forms, long rods	Rod–coccus cycle	Short to coccoid	Coccoid to rudimentary filaments, vegetative hyphae	Short, thin, branching	Irregular, short	Short, thin	Irregular, V forms, coccoid	Short, irregular, slender

[a]G + C, guanine + cytosine.
[b]v, variable.
[c]TBSA, tuberculostearic acid (10-methyl-octadecanoic acid).
[d]*m*-DAP, *meso*-diaminopimelic acid; Lys, lysine; Orn, ornithine; DAB, diaminobutyric acid.

Table 25.2 Biochemical and morphological characteristics of coryneform genera

	Corynebacterium	*Turicella*	*Brevibacterium*	*Dermabacter*	*Oerskovia*	*Cellulomonas*	*Sanguibacter*	*Microbacterium*	*Aureobacterium*	*'C. aquaticum'*
Pigment[a]	– to w to y	w	w to sl y to t	– to w	w to y	w to y	sl y	y to o	y	y
Motility	–[b]	–	–	–	+	v	+	v	v[b]	+[b]
NO$_3 \rightarrow$ NO$_2$	v	–	v	–	+	+	v	v	v	v
Urea[c]	v	–	–	–	–	–	ND[b]	–	v	–
Aesculin[c]	v	–	+	+	+	+	+	+	+	v
Gelatin[c]	v	–	–	+	+	+	v	v	v	–
Casein[c]	v	ND	+	+	+	–	ND	v	v	v
Starch[c]	v			+	+	+	ND	v	v	ND
DNA[c]	v	–[d]	+	+	+	v	ND	+		+
Sugars[e]	F/O[e]	O	O	F	F	F	F	F	O	O
Glucose	v	–	v	+	+	+	+	+	+	+
Maltose	v	–	–	+	+	+	+	+	+	v
Sucrose	v	–	–	+	+	+	–	+	+/(+)	v
Mannitol	v	–	–	–		v	+	+	v	+
Xylose	v[c]	–	–	v	+	+		v	v	+
CAMP	v	+	–	–	–[f]		ND	–	–	–
Others (unique)			Some exhibit 'cheese-like odour'		Agar penetration. Xanthine hydrolysis separates *O. x.* from *O. t.*	Cellulose hydrolysis + (except *C. hominis*)				

[a] o, orange; sl, slight; t, tan; w, white; y, yellow.
[b] v, variable; –, negative in ≥90% of strains; +, positive in ≥90% of strains; (), rare reactions; ND, no data.
[c] Hydrolysis.
[d] Authors' experience.
[e] F, fermentative; O, oxidative or non-oxidative/non-fermentative.
[f] *O. xanthineolytica* may show a slight reverse CAMP reaction (authors' experience). For further differentiation, see text.

Table 25.3   Biochemical characteristics of *Corynebacterium* spp.

	Fermentation/ oxidation	Lipophilism	Nitrate	Urease	Aesculin	Pyrazin-amidase	Alkaline phosphatase	Glu	Mal	Suc	Man	Xyl	CAMP	Other characteristics
C. accolens	F	+	+	−	−	V	−	+	+	V	V	−	−	
C. afermentans subsp. *afermentans*	O	−	−	−	−	+	+	−	−	−	−	−	V	
C. afermentans subsp. *lipophilum*	O	+	−	−	−	+	+	−	−	−	−	−	V	
C. amycolatum	O	−	V	V	−	+	+	+	V	V	−	−	−	
C. argentoratense	F	−	−	−	−	+	V	+	−	−	−	−	−	
C. auris	O	−	−	−	−	+	+	−	−	−	−	−	+	Dry, slight adherence
C. bovis	O	+	−	+	−	V	+	+	−	−	−	−	−	β-Galactosidase+
C. cystitidis	F	−	+	+	−	+	+	+	−	−	−	−	−	
C. diphtheriae gravis	F	−	+	−	−	+	−	+	+	−	−	−	−	See text
C. diphtheriae intermedius	F	+	+/−[a]	−	−	−	−	+	+	+	−	−	−	
C. diphtheriae mitis	F	−	V	−	−	−	−	+	+	−	−	−	−	
C. glucuronolyticum	F	−	V	V	V	+	V	+	V	+	−	V	+	β-Glucuronidase+ Fructose−
C. jeikeium	O	+	−	−	−	+	+	+	V	−	−	−	−	
C. kutscheri	F	−	V	+	−	V	−	+	V	+	−	−	−	
C. macginleyi	F	+	+	−	−	−	+	+	−	+	V	−	−	
C. matruchotii	F	−	+	V	−	+	+	+	+	V	V	−	−	'Whip handle'
C. minutissimum	F	−	−	−	−	+	+	+	+	−	−	−	−	
C. pilosum	F	−	+	+	−	V	V	+	+	−	−	−	−	Yellow pigment
C. propinquum	O	−	+	−	−	+	V	−	−	−	−	−	−	
C. pseudodiphtheriticum	O	−	+	+	−	+	V	−	−	−	−	−	−	
C. pseudotuberculosis	F	−	V	+	−	V	−	+	+	V	−	−	Rev[b]	
C. renale	F	−	−	+	−	+	+	+	−	−	−	−	+	
C. striatum	F	−	+	−	−	+	+	+	+	V	−	−	V	
C. ulcerans	F	−	−	+	−	+	V	+	+	−	−	−	−	
C. urealyticum	O	+	−	+	−	+	−	−	−	−	−	−	−	
C. xerosis	F	−	+	−	−	+	+	+	+	+	−	−	−	Glycogen+
CDC group F-1	F	+	V	+	−	+	−	+	V	+	−	−	−	
CDC group G	F	+	V	−	−	+	+	+	V	V	−	−	−	

[a]var. *belfanti* is nitrate negative.
[b]Rev, reverse CAMP reaction.

2 THE GENUS *CORYNEBACTERIUM*

The microscopic characteristics of members of this genus have been described above. Moreover, coryne-bacteria are non-motile, catalase-positive and are either facultatively anaerobic (fermentative) or strictly aerobic (non-fermentative).

Chemotaxonomic features of the genus are listed in Table 25.1. The presence of mycolic acids is not considered a pertinent feature of members of the genus as at least one species, i.e. *Corynebacterium amyco-latum*, does not contain mycolic acids. The cellular fatty acids (Bernard, Bellefeuille and Ewan 1991, von Graevenitz, Osterhout and Dick 1991) are mainly pal-mitic (hexadecanoic, C16:0) and oleic (*cis*-9-octade-cenoic; C18:1ω9c) acids, and smaller amounts of ste-aric (octadecanoic, C18:0) acid. Members of the 'Corynebacterium diphtheriae group' have, in addition, large amounts of palmitoleic acid (*cis*-9-hexadecenoic acid, C16:1ω7c). Several species also show C18:2 acid (*Corynebacterium jeikeium*, *Corynebacterium urealyticum*, 'Corynebacterium genitalium', 'Corynebacterium pseudogeni-talium', the F-1 and G groups), whereas *C. urealyticum* and some G-2 and *Corynebacterium minutissimum* strains show tuberculostearic acid (10-methyl-octadecanoic acid). Glucose metabolism results mainly in acetate, lactate and sometimes propionate as well as succinate. This is important because *C. striatum* and *C. minutissi-mum* both produce succinate.

Most corynebacteria are nutritionally exacting but, with the exception of the 'lipophilic' ones (whose growth is either stimulated by, or fully dependent on lipids like Tween 80, oleic acid, egg yolk or serum), they will grow on the usual non-selective laboratory media. Selection can be accomplished by the addition of fosfomycin (Wirsing von König et al. 1988) or furoxone (Smith 1969). Thus far, all species have been susceptible to vancomycin; susceptibility to other anti-biotics has varied.

2.1 The *Corynebacterium diphtheriae* group

Members of this group are separated from other corynebacteria by their ability to form exotoxin, lack of pyrazinamidase, and presence of palmitoleic acid.

CORYNEBACTERIUM DIPHTHERIAE
Colonial morphology

Anderson et al. (1933) described 3 types of *C. diph-theriae* on the basis of cultural and biochemical differ-ences (including colonial morphology) of 48 h cul-tures on McLeod's tellurite chocolate agar that clearly distinguished the minute *intermedius* colonies (≤0.5 mm in diameter) from the *mitis* and *gravis* col-onies (2.0–4.0 mm in diameter). The ability to reduce tellurium salts to tellurium, which is precipitated in the cell to colour the colonies grey, brown or black, is characteristic not only of *C. diphtheriae* but also to a lesser extent of other members of the *Corynebacterium* genus. However, on a medium described by Tinsdale

(1947) containing L-cystine and potassium tellurite and modified by Moore and Parsons (1958), only *C. diphtheriae*, *Corynebacterium ulcerans* and *Corynebac-terium pseudotuberculosis* produce a well delineated brown halo around the greyish-black colonies. A brown halo results when H_2S is produced by the action of cystinase on L-cystine and potassium tellurite is reduced to metallic tellurium. Halo formation also depends upon the organism acidifying the medium. It is accelerated by stabbing the medium with the inoculum, which is especially useful to detect biotype *intermedius* strains within 18–24 h rather than 48 h of incubation. Hoyle's lysed blood tellurite agar, pre-pared with horse, sheep or ox blood, has proved to be an excellent medium to distinguish the 3 biotypes (Hoyle 1941).

On blood agar the tiny, transparent colonies of the *intermedius* variety are typical of lipophilic coryneforms and distinguish them from the larger, denser colonies of the non-lipophilic *gravis* and *mitis* biotypes. Most *mitis* and some *gravis* strains produce a narrow zone of weak β-haemolysis on sheep, rabbit or horse blood agar, whereas *intermedius* strains are non-haemolytic. Frobisher, Adams and Kuhns (1945) proposed a fourth biotype of *C. diphtheriae*, named *minimus*, but these strains are not clearly distinguishable from *intermedius* strains (Johnstone and McLeod 1949, Coyle et al. 1993b).

The initial report that *gravis* strains caused the most severe cases of diphtheria (McLeod 1943) and that *mitis* strains were associated with milder clinical cases was not confirmed but the ability of laboratories to recognize these different types continues to provide useful epidemiological data on diphtheria outbreaks (McLeod 1943, Saragea, Maximescu and Meitert 1979, Dixon 1984, Coyle et al. 1989, Harnisch et al. 1989, Krech 1994) (see also section on 'Bacteriophage and molecular typing', p. 539).

Cellular morphology

The cellular morphology of *C. diphtheriae* varies with medium, biotype and strain. Colonies from serum-based media (Pai or Loeffler slants) show pleo-morphic rods some of which may be club-shaped (Fig.

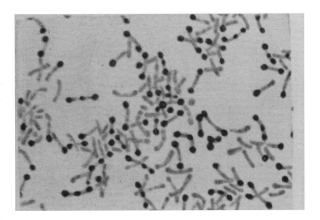

Fig. 25.2 *Corynebacterium diphtheriae* with metachromatic granules. See also Plate 25.2.

25.2). Cells may contain a few mostly terminal reddish-purple (metachromatic) polyphosphate granules which confer a beaded or barred appearance. Biotypes *mitis* and *intermedius* produce long bacilli with metachromatic granules (*mitis*) or are barred with poorly developed granules (*intermedius*). *C. diphtheriae gravis* cells are short and tend to stain uniformly but may have a few granules. Like other corynebacteria, *C. diphtheriae* cells are arranged in parallel groups or at various angles to form clusters resembling cuneiform letters. These arrangements result from incomplete separation of daughter cells which remain attached at one side of the dividing septum. *C. diphtheriae* is non-encapsulated and non-motile. Fimbriae are formed (Yanagawa and Honda 1976). For a detailed review of morphology and ultrastructure of *C. diphtheriae* see Barksdale (1970).

Biochemical reactions

C. diphtheriae usually acidifies glucose and maltose but not sucrose. Rarely strains may attack sucrose (Frobisher, Adams and Kuhns 1945, Butterworth et al. 1974, Jones et al. 1984). Fermentation of carbohydrates occurs without the production of gas; the major products are acetic, lactic, formic and propionic acids. A simple test for distinguishing the *intermedius* biotype from the others is its stimulation of growth by a lipid supplement such as 0.2% Tween 80 (Ward 1948, Coyle et al. 1993b). Biotype *gravis* is distinguished from *mitis* by its ability to produce acid from glycogen and starch. The glycogen utilization test is preferable as technical problems with the starch test, such as the need to check the suitability of the soluble starch and the choice of serum for Hiss's starch serum water, are bothersome. Rabbit serum is preferred to horse serum which contains a heat-labile diastase that may hydrolyse the starch. Andrade's indicator is the best for detecting starch hydrolysis. Other biochemical reactions are shown in Table 25.3. With the exception of a variety of biotype *mitis* known as *belfanti* (which is usually non-toxinogenic) (Chang, Laughren and Chalvardjian 1978), *C. diphtheriae* reduces nitrate to nitrite. H$_2$S production is evident on modified Tinsdale medium only.

The 3 species with the potential to produce diphtheria toxin, *C. diphtheriae*, *C. ulcerans* and *C. pseudotuberculosis*, are distinguished from almost all other *Corynebacterium* species by their inability to attack pyrazinamide and their capacity to hydrolyse cystine (Colman, Weaver and Efstratiou 1992). The pyrazinamide utilization test should not be the sole screening test for *C. diphtheriae* (Colman, Weaver and Efstratiou 1992) because *Corynebacterium macginleyi* and some strains of *Corynebacterium accolens* (Riegel et al. 1995a) do not produce pyrazine carboxylamidase.

Susceptibility to physical, chemical and antimicrobial agents

C. diphtheriae is readily killed by heating at 58°C for 10–min. It is also susceptible to the usual disinfectants, but is relatively resistant to drying. Crosbie and Wright (1941) observed that diphtheria bacilli survived for 3 months or longer in dust collected from hospital floors and stored in the dark.

Most strains of *C. diphtheriae* are susceptible to penicillin, ampicillin, erythromycin, clindamycin, rifampicin, tetracycline, ciprofloxacin, chloramphenicol, gentamicin, cephalothin and trimethoprim (Gordon et al. 1971, Maple et al. 1994). Occasional strains are resistant to erythromycin, clindamycin and lincomycin (Jellard and Lipinski 1973, Coyle, Minshew and Hsu 1979, Dixon 1984), tetracycline (Rockhill et al. 1982) and rifampicin and trimethoprim (Maple et al. 1994). Erythromycin resistance in *C. diphtheriae* is plasmid mediated and is an expression of inducible cross-resistance to macrolides, lincosamides and streptogramin B (MLS resistance) (Coyle, Minshew and Hsu 1979, Schiller, Groman and Coyle 1980).

Toxin production

Diphtheria toxin is synthesized by strains of *C. diphtheriae* that are lysogenic for one of a family of bacteriophages carrying *tox*, the structural gene for the exotoxin (see section on *tox*+ Bacteriophages, p. 539). It is a protein and the only recognized virulence factor of *C. diphtheriae*. Virulence factors for obviously pathogenic non-toxinogenic strains, e.g. those causing endocarditis (Gruner et al. 1992), have not been investigated thus far. Although the toxin inhibits protein synthesis in cell-free extracts of virtually all eukaryotic organisms, it is only toxic to the intact cells of certain mammals. Diphtheria toxin is a 535 amino acid, 58 kDa protein consisting of 2 fragments: an N-terminal catalytic fragment A (21 kDa amino acid 1–193) and fragment B (37 kDa), with 2 domains, an internal translocating one (205–378) and a C-terminal receptor-binding one (386–535). The process likely follows these steps: the proteolytic 'nicking' into fragments A (21 kDa) and B (37 kDa) occurs before or shortly after binding. Following binding to the receptor, the toxin enters the cell through receptor mediated endocytosis. An acid pH triggers the translocation of fragment A across the endosomal membrane into the cytosol. The A fragment becomes enzymatically active following reduction of the disulphide bridge which connects it to the B fragment. Then it catalyses ADP ribosylation of the GTP-binding elongation factor 2 (EF-2) on diphthamide, a post-translationally modified histidine. EF-2 normally effects the translocation of the growing polypeptide chain from the aminoacyl-tRNA to the peptidyl tRNA position on the ribosome. The energy for this reaction is provided by hydrolysis of GTP-ATP. Ribosylation of EF-2 inhibits this GTP-dependent translocation on the ribosome and thus the building of the polypeptide chain (Krueger and Barbieri 1995). When introduced into the cell cytoplasm, a single molecule of subunit A is lethal for a cell within a few hours (Collier 1975). Similarities between diphtheria toxin and other microbial toxins including *Pseudomonas* exotoxin A have been reviewed by Pappenheimer (1984).

Addition of iron to the growth medium of *C. diphtheriae* inhibits production of diphtheria toxin (Pappenheimer and Johnson 1936). The regulation of diphtheria toxin expression by varying iron concentrations in the growth medium occurs at the level of transcription of the *tox* gene (Russell, Cryz and Holmes 1984, Kaczorek et al. 1985, Leong and Murphy 1985, Tai et al. 1990). The repressor molecule that regulates the *tox* gene is an iron-dependent protein that binds DNA by a sequence-specific mechanism and also regulates iron uptake by *C. diphtheriae* (Schmitt, Twiddy and Holmes 1992, Schmitt and Holmes 1994).

Nowadays, most strains of *C. diphtheriae* that are isolated outside epidemic areas from routine throat swabs are non-toxinogenic (Wilson et al. 1992, Efstratiou et al. 1993).

Pathogenicity and toxin testing in laboratory animals

Guinea pigs and rabbits are most susceptible to experimental infection with *C. diphtheriae* whereas rats and mice are resistant (see review by Barksdale 1970). Subcutaneous inoculation with a toxigenic culture or filtrate into the flank of a guinea pig leads within 12–18 h to a local oedematous swelling that gradually spreads. Depending on the dose, death usually occurs between 18 and 96 h. Haemorrhagic oedema with a central necrotic area is present at the injection site; regional lymph nodes and abdominal viscera are congested, but the most striking lesion is the swelling and congestion of the adrenal glands, with scattered haemorrhages in the medulla or cortex, or both. The intradermal route of inoculation with either live bacilli or toxin causes a local erythematous lesion within 48 h in guinea pigs or 72 h in rabbits. The intradermal testing of toxin has the advantage of allowing several strains to be tested on one animal.

The immunodiffusion test described by Elek (1949) offers an economical alternative to animal tests. A strip of filter paper impregnated with diphtheria antitoxin (100–200 units ml⁻¹) is placed in a horse serum agar plate while the medium is still fluid. When the agar has set, organisms are streaked at right angles to the strip. If toxin is produced a precipitate appears within 24–48 h in the form of double arrow-headed lines. Precipitin lines from adjacent toxinogenic control and test organisms should merge to form a single line of identity. Because a limiting concentration of iron is essential for the expression of the *tox* gene by *C. diphtheriae*, an agar medium with a low ash content is required for the Elek test medium. A modified recipe for improving the performance of the Elek test medium was described by Colman, Weaver and Efstratiou (1992).

The use of a serum substitute in the Elek test medium as described by Hermann, Moore and Parsons (1958) can be reliable provided all the components have been performance tested in advance by the manufacturer or an experienced reference laboratory (Bickham and Jones 1972). False positive Elek tests have been reported from laboratories that rarely perform the test (Snell et al. 1984) but when done correctly by experienced workers the immunodiffusion test can be used instead of animal tests.

Pallen (1991) first used a polymerase chain reaction (PCR) to screen for toxinogenic *C. diphtheriae*. Using oligonucleotide primers based on published diphtheria toxin gene sequences, he amplified a 246 base pair fragment of the toxin gene from boiled cells. Subsequent studies with routine clinical isolates have confirmed the sensitivity of Pallen's method and showed that false positive reactions are unlikely to occur in tests of routine clinical isolates (Martinetti Lucchini, Gruner and Altwegg 1992, Pallen et al. 1994, Aravena-Román, Bowman and O'Neill 1995). However, a collection of 33 non-toxinogenic *C. diphtheriae* strains from 6 countries did include one strain that gave a false positive result (Pallen et al. 1994). False negative PCR reactions are readily recognized if an internal control template is added to every reaction tube. PCR has several advantages over the Elek test: it takes as little as 5 or 6 h from the selection of colonies to the final result, works on mixed cultures, is relatively easy to perform, and gives clear-cut results. Reagents, including the *Taq* DNA polymerase, have a long shelf life and PCR does not require the highly variable reagents used in immunoassays. The presence of an amplification product correlates with ADP-ribosylation activity (Hauser et al. 1993).

tox+ Bacteriophages

Freeman (1951) discovered that a lysogenic bacteriophage can convert non-toxigenic strains of *C. diphtheriae* to toxin producers. Murphy, Pappenheimer and de Borms (1974) demonstrated that the diphtheria toxin gene (*tox*) is located on the genome of the phage. DNA analyses showed that, with one exception, all of the *tox*-bearing phages, including those with a mutated *tox* gene, share extensive homology and similar restriction fragment patterns with the original β-converting phage (Buck et al. 1985). Phages that carry *tox* integrate into the chromosome of *C. diphtheriae* by a process analogous to λ lysogenization of *Escherichia coli* (Buck and Groman 1981). Site-specific recombination occurs between an attachment site on the phage (*attP*) and one or 2 attachment sites on the bacterial chromosome (*attB1*, *attB2*) (Rappuoli and Ratti 1984). Conversion of *C. ulcerans* and *C. pseudotuberculosis* also occurs with integration of a β-related phage by specifc recombination between the *attP* and *attB* attachment sites (Cianciotto, Rappuoli and Groman 1986). Although *attB*-related sequences also occur in a wide variety of *Corynebacterium* species, the only species that are known either to be lysogenized by β phage or to produce diphtheria toxin are *C. diphtheriae*, *C. ulcerans* and *C. pseudotuberculosis* (Cianciotto, Rappuoli and Groman 1986).

Bacteriophage and molecular typing

Following earlier efforts to develop a bacteriophage typing system to distinguish strains of *C. diphtheriae*, Saragea, Maximescu and Meitert (1979) introduced a scheme that has been widely accepted.

Molecular typing methods have replaced phage typing for epidemiological studies of diphtheria (Krech 1994). Phage typing requires maintenance of a large collection of phage preparations in high titres and fails to type many isolates, especially non-toxinogenic strains, whereas molecular methods require relatively stable reagents and are capable of reproducibly typing all strains. One of the earliest applications was the experiment characterizing 3 epidemiologically linked isolates by hybridizing 3 DNA probes to Southern blots of chromosomal DNAs digested with a variety of restriction enzymes (Pappenheimer and Murphy 1983).

Rappuoli, Perugini and Falsen (1988) used an insertion element as a DNA probe in Southern hybridizations to demonstrate that there were 16 different patterns among 35 strains of *C. diphtheriae* isolated from Sweden and Denmark between 1976 and 1986. Other authors (Gruner et al. 1992, Wilson et al. 1992, Efstratiou et al. 1993) have used an *E. coli* DNA probe for the ribosomal RNA gene in Southern hybridization experiments (ribotyping). Whole cell polypeptide profiling from sodium dodecyl sulphate polyacrylamide gel electrophoresis (SDS-PAGE) is a relatively rapid typing method that agrees with phage typing (Krech, de Chastonay and Falsen 1988) and ribotyping (Wilson et al. 1992, Efstratiou et al. 1993) but gel-to-gel variation is a disadvantage (Hallas 1988, Krech, de Chastonay and Falsen 1988). De Zoysa et al. (1995) used both ribotyping and pulse field gel electrophoresis (PFGE) to analyse DNA patterns of *C. diphtheriae* isolates recovered in 1993 from patients and carriers in Russia, Finland and Estonia. Both typing methods provided clearly distinguishable profiles of DNA fragments that could be expressed numerically and were in good agreement; the minor exception was 3 closely related ribotypes that were indistinguishable by PFGE.

CORYNEBACTERIUM ULCERANS

Although 4 h culture of *C. ulcerans* on Loeffler's slants consists of rods that are similar to *C. diphtheriae* except for staining evenly, cells from cultures of 18–24 h are predominantly short coccoid rods. The practice of screening diphtheria cultures for microscopic morphology will cause laboratories to overlook *C. ulcerans* (Hermann and Parsons 1957). Colonies resemble those of *C. diphtheriae* biotype *gravis*, including production of a narrow zone of haemolysis on blood agar and brown halos on Tinsdale's medium. The key reactions for identification of *C. ulcerans* are fermentation of glycogen (and starch), production of urease, digestion of gelatin (at 25°C but not at 37°C) and failure to reduce nitrates.

The uncertain taxonomic status of *C. ulcerans* was resolved in 1995 when Riegel et al. (1995c) demonstrated on the basis of DNA–DNA homology and sequences of the rRNA genes that it is a species distinct from *C. diphtheriae*. However, *C. ulcerans* and *C. pseudotuberculosis* are phylogenetically very closely related.

C. ulcerans may produce both diphtheria toxin and phospholipase D (PLD). A toxin believed to be PLD can be detected by intradermal injection of guinea pigs, which produces a characteristic ulcerating lesion

that is not neutralized by 1000 IU of diphtheria antitoxin.

CORYNEBACTERIUM PSEUDOTUBERCULOSIS

C. pseudotuberculosis causes caseous lymphadenitis in sheep and goats and ulcerative lymphangitis and abscesses in horses. It is a major cause of morbiditiy in sheep that acquire the infections from superficial wounds inflicted during shearing (Serikawa et al. 1993). Infections acquired as occupational disease are rarely reported in humans and usually present as caseating lymphadenitis.

After 48 h of incubation, colonies of *C. pseudotuberculosis* are 0.5–1 mm in diameter, opaque, white and dry with a barely visible zone of β-haemolysis. Cells from blood agar are small coccoidal rods. Both *C. ulcerans* and *C. pseudotuberculosis* are similar to *C. diphtheriae* in their production of haloes on Tinsdale media and failure to hydrolyse pyrazinamide. The best biochemical tests for distinguishing these 2 species are the hydrolysis of glycogen by *C. ulcerans* and the lipid-stimulated growth of *C. pseudotuberculosis*. *C. pseudotuberculosis* comprises 2 biovars, *equi* and *ovis*, that are distinguished by the ability of biovar *equi* to reduce nitrate (Songer et al. 1988). In vitro susceptibility tests show that *C. pseudotuberculosis* is susceptible to β-lactams, macrolides, tetracyclines, chloramphenicol and rifampicin (Judson and Songer 1991).

PLD is a potential virulence factor of *C. pseudotuberculosis* that hydrolyses sphingomyelin in mammalian cell membranes and releases choline (Soucek, Michalic and Souckova 1971). It does not lyse red blood cell (RBC) membranes but it enhances RBC lysis by *Rhodococcus equi* and, conversely, inhibits the β-haemolysin of *Staphylococcus aureus*. The PLD genes and gene products from *C. pseudotuberculosis* and *C. ulcerans* have 80% DNA sequence homology and 87% amino acid sequence homology as well as antigenic relationships (Cuevas and Songer 1993). These highly conserved enzymes share over 60% DNA and amino acid sequence homology with the PLD of *Arcanobacterium haemolyticum* (McNamara, Cuevas and Songer 1995), which lends support to the assumption that they act as virulence factors. Over 10% of *C. pseudotuberculosis* isolates produce the diphtheria toxin (Maximescu et al. 1974) but the authors are unaware of human diphtheria cases due to this organism.

2.2 Other non-lipophilic corynebacteria

CORYNEBACTERIUM AMYCOLATUM

C. amycolatum is one of the most under-recognized *Corynebacterium* species. In the authors' experience, it is the most frequently encountered non-lipophilic *Corynebacterium* species in clinical samples. It was first described in 1988 for some mycolic acid-free coryneform bacteria isolated from the human skin (Collins, Burton and Jones 1988). Later investigations suggested that 'Corynebacterium asperum' as well as CDC coryneform group F-2 and I-2 bacteria are synonyms of *C. amycolatum* (Barreau et al. 1993). *C. amycolatum* grows well at 37°C with colonies ranging from 1 to

1.5 mm in diameter after 24–48 h; colonies are dry and waxy, and gram stains show typical diphtheroids. *C. amycolatum* strains have been isolated from blood cultures, intravascular catheters, abscesses, urines and respiratory specimens. Usually *C. amycolatum* strains are isolated from sites anatomically closely related to the skin. Susceptibility to antimicrobial agents is unpredictable as many strains are multiresistant (Funke, Pünter and von Graevenitz 1996). *C. amycolatum* strains may have been misidentified as *Corynebacterium minutissimum*, *Corynebacterium striatum* or *Corynebacterium xerosis* in the past (Barreau et al. 1993, Funke et al. 1996, Zinkernagel, von Graevenitz and Funke 1996).

CORYNEBACTERIUM XEROSIS

C. xerosis is considered a commensal of human skin and mucous membranes. The true identity of reported *C. xerosis* isolates warrants further study because there is phenotypic and genomic diversity in the representative strains deposited by contributors to the ATCC and the NCTC (Coyle et al. 1993a). At this time the only authentic reference strains for the species are the type strain, ATCC 373, and strain ATCC 7711 (Funke et al. 1996) which are not closely related to other *C. xerosis* strains in either the ATCC or NCTC.

Identification of *C. xerosis* requires distinguishing it from *C. striatum* that differs in a single conventional test, maltose fermentation (see Table 25.2, p. 575). The Hollis and Weaver (1981) scheme for identification of pleomorphic gram-positive rods accurately describes *C. xerosis* ATCC 373.

After growth for 48 h on sheep blood agar plates, *C. xerosis* ATCC 373 produces dry colonies that are 0.5 mm in diameter with slight yellow-tan pigmentation. The 72 h colonies have irregular edges. This organism grows with a pellicle in heart infusion broth. Cellular morphology after 24 h on heart infusion broth or trypticase soy blood agar is characterized by short, straight, gram-positive rods that become coccobacillary with longer incubation.

It has been demonstrated that most *C. xerosis* strains identified in the routine clinical laboratory (e.g. Porschen, Goodman and Rafai 1977) actually represent misidentified *C. amycolatum* strains (Funke et al. 1996). The authors suggested that most strains, including those with multiple resistance against antimicrobials reported in the literature as *C. xerosis*, correspond to *C. amycolatum*. True *C. xerosis* strains are susceptible to the vibriocidal compound O/129 whereas *C. amycolatum* strains are usually resistant to this antimicrobial agent.

CORYNEBACTERIUM STRIATUM

C. striatum is a commensal of the nasopharynx and skin. Recognized infections with this organism have been limited to a few compromised patients who developed respiratory disease, native valve endocarditis, or sepsis (Markowitz and Coudron 1990). Hospital-acquired colonization was demonstrated in the sputum of 9 intensive care patients harbouring a unique strain that produced a diffusible brown pigment (Leonard et al. 1994).

After incubation on blood agar for 48 h the 1–2 mm colonies of *C. striatum* are flat and whitish-grey with a creamy consistency and can be mistaken for coagulase-negative staphylococci. The inability of *C. striatum* to attack maltose is the key to differentiation from *C. xerosis*. Some strains called *C. striatum* in the past were actually *C. amycolatum* (see section on '*C. amycolatum*', p. 540). Some CDC coryneform group I-1 strains (sucrose fermentation negative) were shown to be identical with *C. striatum* (De Briel et al. 1992). All *C. striatum* strains hydrolyse tyrosine; some strains, including 2 ATCC strains, produce a positive CAMP reaction with *S. aureus* (Martinez-Martinez et al. 1995).

C. striatum strains usually are susceptible to β-lactams but resistant ones have also been described. Resistance to clindamycin, erythromycin and tetracycline is also not uncommon (Roberts et al. 1992, Martinez-Martinez et al. 1995).

CORYNEBACTERIUM MINUTISSIMUM

This *Corynebacterium* species has frequently been isolated from clinical specimens. Since the species designation was not included in the Approved List of Bacterial Names in 1980 it was revived in 1983 (Collins and Jones 1983). *C. minutissimum* is part of the normal skin flora. Strains grow well on blood agar at 35–37°C to a colony size of 1–1.5 mm in diameter after 24–48 h; gram stain shows typical diphtheroids. *C. minutissimum* strains do not reduce nitrate which separates them from the phylogenetically closely related *C. striatum*. Recent investigations have demonstrated that some *C. minutissimum* strains ferment mannitol (Zinkernagel, von Graevenitz and Funke 1996). Some strains called *C. minutissimum* in the past were actually *C. amycolatum* (see section on '*C. amycolatum*', p. 540). Early work described *C. minutissimum* as the causative agent of erythrasma whereas there are now reports which strongly question this association (Coyle and Lipsky 1990). *C. minutissimum* was isolated from cases of endocarditis, bacteraemia, infected venous catheters, and recurrent abscesses, mostly in patients with skin disruptions. Multiresistant strains of *C. minutissimum* are rarely seen. Specific virulence factors of *C. minutissimum* are not known.

CORYNEBACTERIUM GLUCURONOLYTICUM

C. glucuronolyticum is a fermentative bacterium that has been isolated from patients with genitourinary disease (Funke et al. 1995). Characteristic is a positive β-glucuronidase test which is, however, not specific since it also occurs in *Corynebacterium renale* and *Corynebacterium pilosum*. However, *C. glucuronolyticum* can be distinguished by a positive CAMP reaction and fermentation reaction from related bacteria (see Table 25.3, p. 536).

CORYNEBACTERIUM RENALE GROUP AND CORYNEBACTERIUM KUTSCHERI

Organisms of the *C. renale* group cause cystitis and pyelonephritis in cows and bulls (Collins and Cummins 1986). *C. renale sensu stricto* differs from *C. pilosum* and *Corynebacterium cystitidis* in some parameters (nitrate reduction, hydrolysis of casein and Tween 80, xylose and starch fermentation); the degree of DNA homology is also not sufficient to establish a single species. Occasional human strains have been reported in the early 1980s but there is reason to doubt their identity as *C. renale*.

The same is true for human isolates of *C. kutscheri*. This organism is a common commensal in mice, rats and voles that will develop lesions when their immune status is altered (Collins and Cummins 1986).

CORYNEBACTERIUM MATRUCHOTII

C. matruchotii, formerly *Bacterionema matruchotii* (Gilmour 1974), is found in the human oral cavity, particularly in plaque and calculus deposits on the teeth. Young microcolonies of *C. matruchotii* are flat, filamentous, spider-like and may have a dense centre. Mature colonies have diameters of 0.5–1.5 mm. Colonies can be circular, convex, rough, with entire or filamentous margin; or irregular, molar-toothed, rough, with an entire to filamentous margin at the base; or irregular with a low convex rough centre and raised curled-up lobate margin. All mature colony types are opaque, tough and adherent (Collins 1982). Cells are pleomorphic, comprising non-septate and septate branching filaments and bacilli. Occasionally single bacilli attach in a terminal position along the side of the filaments and resemble whip handles.

Almost 90% of the *C. matruchotii* isolates submitted to the CDC for identification were recovered from the eye (Hollis and Weaver 1981) yet there is no report of this species acting as the sole cause of an infection of the eye or any other site. Wilhelmus, Robinson and Jones (1979) described 3 patients with a structurally altered eye that developed either endophthalmitis or corneal ulceration; *C. matruchotii* was recovered in mixed culture.

CORYNEBACTERIUM ARGENTORATENSE

C. argentoratense is a diphtheroid that has been isolated from human throat cultures. In contrast to *C. diphtheriae*, it is pyrazinamidase positive. No diphtheria toxin production has been observed in these strains (Riegel et al. 1995b).

CORYNEBACTERIUM PSEUDODIPHTHERITICUM

C. pseudodiphtheriticum is a commensal of the human nasopharynx that infrequently causes infections. It is characterized morphologically as short regular rods that stain evenly. Colonies are non-haemolytic, white, smooth and butyrous or dry. *C. pseudodiphtheriticum* is a non-fermentative organism that reduces nitrate and hydrolyses urea. Endocarditis due to this organism has been reported in 18 patients, half of whom had prosthetic devices (Morris and Guild 1991). Reports have documented that *C. pseudodiphtheriticum* can cause bronchitis and pneumonia in patients with underlying disease (Ahmed et al. 1995, Manzella, Kellog and Parsey 1995).

CORYNEBACTERIUM PROPINQUUM

C. propinquum was proposed for CDC coryneform absolute non-fermenting (ANF)-3 bacteria (Riegel et al. 1993a). Like the phylogenetically closely related *C. pseudodiphtheriticum*, most *C. propinquum* strains are isolated from respiratory tract specimens. *C. propinquum* colonies have a matted whitish-greyish surface and measure 1–2 mm in diameter after 24 h of incubation on sheep blood agar. They do not hydrolyse urea but reduce nitrate. Infections due to 'true' *C. propinquum* have not yet been described. *C. propinquum* strains are susceptible to nearly all agents used in the treatment of *Corynebacterium* infections.

CORYNEBACTERIUM AFERMENTANS SUBSP. AFERMENTANS

C. afermentans was formerly included in the CDC coryneform ANF-1 group of bacteria (Riegel et al. 1993b). Presently, it is the only defined *Corynebacterium* species apart from *C. diphtheriae* that includes both non-lipophilic and lipophilic strains. *C. afermentans* subsp. *afermentans* grows with a colony size of 1–2 mm in diameter after 24 h of incubation on sheep blood agar. Colonies are creamy whitish. Some strains exhibit a positive CAMP reaction. *C. afermentans* subsp. *afermentans* has frequently been isolated from blood cultures. Nearly all isolates are susceptible to β-lactams.

CORYNEBACTERIUM AURIS

C. auris resembles group ANF corynebacteria (*C. afermentans*) and *Turicella otitidis* phenotypically and by its CAMP positivity, but can be separated from these by its slightly dry colonies and by carbon source assimilation tests. It has been isolated from the ears of patients with otitis (Funke, Lawson and Collins 1995).

2.3   Lipophilic *Corynebacterium* spp.

This group of fastidious bacteria comprises at present 6 named species (except *C. diphtheriae* biotype *intermedius*) and 2 unnamed taxa (see Table 25.3, p. 536). Most of these species have been proposed and validated within the last few years only, which may be a result of their under-recognition in clinical specimens, perhaps due to nutritional requirements and prolonged incubation necessary for isolation. The authors prefer the term 'lipophilic' rather than 'lipid-requiring' because lipid dependency of growth is difficult to determine as it requires a medium completely free of lipids; moreover, the comparison of growth on a medium with or without supplement of fatty acids, e.g. Tween 80 (polyethoxysorbate oleate), or serum is easy to perform. Therefore, those *Corynebacterium* species whose growth is significantly increased by these supplements are referred to as lipophilic.

All lipophilic *Corynebacterium* spp. show very small (less than 1 mm in diameter), non-β-haemolytic colonies after 24–48 h at 37°C on sheep blood agar but colony size increases to 2–4 mm in diameter when 1% Tween 80 is supplemented to the agar. Gram stains of all lipophilic *Corynebacterium* spp. show small diphtheroids.

CORYNEBACTERIUM JEIKEIUM

Clinically, *C. jeikeium* is regarded as the most important lipophilic *Corynebacterium* species. It consists of the isolates previously designated as CDC coryneform group JK bacteria (Jackman et al. 1987). *C. jeikeium* can be isolated from the skin of healthy individuals, mainly from perineum, inguina and axilla, and has also been found as an environmental contaminant in a hospital setting (Coyle and Lipsky 1990). It is at present unclear whether nosocomial infections with *C. jeikeium* strains occur.

Quantitative DNA–DNA hybridizations have revealed 3 genomospecies within *C. jeikeium* strains (Riegel et al. 1994). The first genomospecies includes the type strain, other strains which are highly resistant to penicillin G and gentamicin, and the reference strain of '*C. genitalium*' biotype 2 (Furness and Evangelista 1978); the other 2 genomospecies of *C. jeikeium* comprise low level penicillin G-resistant and gentamicin-susceptible strains. Until further distinguishing phenotypic data are published, strains belonging to one of the latter 2 genomospecies should be identified as *C. jeikeium*. *C. jeikeium* strains will not grow under strict anaerobic conditions nor do they produce acid from fructose. The differentiation of *C. jeikeium* strains from other lipophilic *Corynebacterium* species is outlined in Table 25.3 (see p. 536).

C. jeikeium may cause endocarditis, septicaemia, meningitis, osteomyelitis, soft tissue infections, wound infections, pulmonary infiltration and other infections (Coyle and Lipsky 1990). Risk factors for acquiring or developing serious infections caused by *C. jeikeium* include immunosuppression (especially in patients with malignancies), prosthetic devices, skin lesions, prolonged hospitalization and exposure to broad spectrum antibiotics. *C. jeikeium* endocarditis is more commonly associated with prosthetic than with normal heart valves (Petit et al. 1994).

Most *C. jeikeium* strains are resistant to β-lactams, erythromycin, clindamycin and aminoglycosides; some strains are susceptible to quinolones, tetracycline and glycopeptides (Williams, Selepak and Gill 1993, Soriano, Zapardiel and Nieto 1995). Plasmids have only very rarely been found in *C. jeikeium* strains and their relation to the intrinsic resistance of *C. jeikeium* to certain antibiotics is not clear (Kerry-Williams and Noble 1988). Specific virulence factors have not been reported although *C. jeikeium* strains were shown to colonize catheters by extracellular slime production (Bayston, Compton and Richards 1994).

CORYNEBACTERIUM UREALYTICUM

Among the lipophilic *Corynebacterium* species, *C. urealyticum* is another taxon of well established clinical significance. It was previously known as CDC coryneform group D-2 but has been validly described as *C. urealyticum* (Pitcher et al. 1992). The habitat of *C. urealyticum* is the human skin and it readily colonizes the urinary tract. *C. urealyticum* is asaccharolytic and exhibits abundant urease activity. It is one of the very few *Corynebacterium* species that consistently contain tuberculostearic acid as cellular fatty acid (Bernard,

Bellefeuille and Ewan 1991, von Graevenitz, Osterhout and Dick 1991).

The predominant diseases caused by *C. urealyticum* are lower and upper urinary tract infections (Soriano et al. 1990) and an alkaline encrusted cystitis. The prevalence of urinary tract infections due to *C. urealyticum* is usually less than 1%. Bacteraemia and wound infections due to *C. urealyticum* have also been described (Soriano et al. 1993). Risk factors for *C. urealyticum* infections include genitourinary disorders, urological manipulation, age, immunosuppression and long-term hospitalization. *C. urealyticum* is often resistant to β-lactams, aminoglycosides and trimethoprim–sulphamethoxazole, but susceptible to vancomycin. The molecular factors responsible for the multiresistance of *C. urealyticum* are not known. The ability of *C. urealyticum* to produce struvite crystals has been demonstrated as a virulence factor (Soriano et al. 1986).

CDC CORYNEFORM GROUP G BACTERIA

Initially, the CDC Special Bacteriology Reference Laboratory established the taxa G-1 (nitrate reduction positive) and G-2 (nitrate reduction negative) (Hollis and Weaver 1981) but recent taxonomic investigations have shown that both taxa belong to the same genomospecies (Riegel et al. 1995a). Due to lack of phenotypic traits that differentiate these strains from related taxa, group G bacteria have not been given a species designation. Group G bacteria also include some invalidated taxa referred to as '*C. pseudogenitalium*' biotypes 2–4 (Furness and Evangelista 1978) and '*C. tuberculostearicum*' (Riegel et al. 1995a). The habitat of group G bacteria are the skin, the oropharynx and the eye. However, only a few reports on infections caused by group G bacteria are found in the literature (Quinn, Comaish and Pedler 1991). Some authors have described group G bacteria as multiresistant (Williams et al. 1993) although in the authors' experience they are usually susceptible to many antibiotics. To avoid misidentification of group G bacteria it is stressed that growth under anaerobic conditions differentiates them from *C. jeikeium* strains.

CORYNEBACTERIUM MACGINLEYI

This species was most recently sequestered from CDC coryneform G-1 strains (Riegel et al. 1995a). Only 3 strains, all of them from eye specimens, have been described in the literature; their pathogenic role is not known. *C. macginleyi* can be differentiated from group G bacteria by a negative pyrazinamidase reaction; some *C. macginleyi* strains ferment mannitol which is an unusual feature in *Corynebacterium* spp. (see Table 25.3, p. 536).

CORYNEBACTERIUM ACCOLENS

C. accolens is another newly described *Corynebacterium* (Neubauer et al. 1991). It exhibits increased growth in the vicinity of *S. aureus* colonies, which may simply indicate its lipophilism. Most strains have been isolated from human ear, eye and respiratory specimens. *C. accolens* is phylogenetically closely related to *C.*

macginleyi (Riegel et al. 1995a). Phenotypic differentiation is mainly based on a negative alkaline phosphatase reaction whereas this enzyme can be detected in *C. macginleyi*. According to the descriptions given, *C. accolens* is strictly aerobic whereas *C. macginleyi* also grows under anaerobic conditions.

CDC CORYNEFORM GROUP F-1 BACTERIA

This is another taxon that was established by the Special Bacteriology Reference Laboratory at the Centers for Disease Control and Prevention (Hollis and Weaver 1981). Since 2 genomospecies, which could not be phenotypically separated, have been described within group F-1 bacteria, these strains have not been given a species name (Riegel et al. 1995a). Apart from *C. urealyticum*, group F-1 bacteria are the only other lipophilic *Corynebacterium* species that are urea-splitting (see Table 25.2, p. 535). The majority of these strains has been isolated from the genitourinary tract and in very few instances group F-1 strains have been reported causative agents of urinary tract infections (Digenis et al. 1992).

CORYNEBACTERIUM BOVIS

C. bovis is probably one of the most controversial *Corynebacterium* species. From molecular analysis it is now evident that *C. bovis* is a true member of the genus *Corynebacterium* (Pascual et al. 1995) although it possesses mycolic acids with lower molecular weight than other *Corynebacterium* species and has a relatively high G + C content (68%) (Collins and Cummins 1986). *C. bovis* is a commensal of the bovine udder and has been described as causing infections in cattle. In the authors' experience, *C. bovis* has been reported to occur in clinical specimens; most likely, however, those strains were misidentified *C. jeikeium*. *C. bovis* can be readily distinguished from *C. jeikeium* by its positive β-galactosidase reaction.

CORYNEBACTERIUM AFERMENTANS SUBSP. *LIPOPHILUM*

Some strains of CDC coryneform group ANF-1 bacteria were defined as *C. afermentans* (Riegel et al. 1993b). This species contains the well growing subspecies *afermentans* (see section on '*Corynebacterium afermentans* subsp. *afermentans*', p. 542) and the subspecies *lipophilum*. The habitat of *C. afermentans* subsp. *lipophilum* strains probably include the human skin and mucous membranes. Strains of *C. afermentans* subsp. *lipophilum* were described as being isolated from human blood cultures and as causing prosthetic valve endocarditis (Riegel et al. 1993b, Sewell, Coyle and Funke 1995).

3   THE GENUS *TURICELLA*

This genus, named after the city of Zurich, consists of non-motile, non-spore-forming, obligately aerobic (non-fermentative and non-oxidative) gram-positive rods that show a long diphtheroid morphology with V-shaped forms (Funke et al. 1994a) (for the main chemotaxonomic and biochemical characteristics, see Tables 25.1 and 25.2, pp. 534 and 535). The genus is nutritionally non-fastidious. It is catalase-positive, grows in 6.5% NaCl and is phenotypically closely related to non-fermentative members of the genus *Corynebacterium* (*C. afermentans* subsp. *afermentans* as well as *C. auris*) but differs from them in G + C content, the absence of mycolic acids, the presence of tuberculostearic acid, and the main menaquinones. The colonies of the single species, *T. otitidis*, are circular, convex, whitish, 1–2 mm in diameter after 48 h of incubation at 37°C. *T. otitidis* has been isolated from patients with otitis media but its role in the disease is unclear.

4   THE GENUS *BREVIBACTERIUM*

This genus, established in 1953, consists of non-spore-forming, non-motile, obligately aerobic (non-fermentative) gram-positive rods that are nutritionally non-fastidious and show a rod–coccus cycle when grown on complex media; older cultures are coccoid and decolourize easily (Jones and Keddie 1986). The main chemotaxonomic and biochemical properties of the genus are shown in Tables 25.1 and 25.2, respectively (see pp. 534 and 535). Brevibacteria are catalase-positive, proteolytic, grow in NaCl concentrations of ≥6.5%, and form methanethiol from methionine (Pitcher and Malnick 1984), which, among other factors, accounts for the smell of colonies and of the habitats in which they are found in large numbers. According to earlier work, habitats include raw milk and surface-ripened cheeses (*Brevibacterium iodinum*, *Brevibacterium linens*, *Brevibacterium casei*), the human skin (*Brevibacterium epidermidis*) and animal sources (Jones and Keddie 1986). Recent studies have shown most human skin isolates belong to the species *B. casei* (Funke and Carlotti 1994); there seems to be a new species, *Brevibacterium mcbrellneri*, that occurs with *Trichosporon beigelii* in white piedra (McBride et al. 1993); the former CDC groups B-1 and B-3 belong to the genus *Brevibacterium* (Gruner et al. 1994); and brevibacteria may also cause human infections, particularly in normally sterile areas such as the bloodstream and peritoneum (continuous ambulatory peritoneal dialysis [CAPD] peritonitis) (Pitcher and Malnick 1984, Gruner, Pfyffer and von Graevenitz 1993, Funke and Carlotti 1994, Gruner et al. 1994).

Whereas *B. linens* forms an orange to red pigment and *B. iodinum* a purple one on suitable media and both have growth maxima below 37°C (Jones and Keddie 1986), separation of the other 3 species by traditional means is difficult but may be accomplished by carbohydrate utilization tests (Funke and Carlotti 1994). Clinical isolates grow within 24–48 h, producing colonies of 1–2 mm diameter that are convex and white or slightly yellow.

Brevibacteria generally are susceptible to gentamicin, rifampicin, tetracycline and vancomycin, but may exhibit minimal inhibitory concentrations of >1 mg l⁻¹ against penicillins (Gruner, Pfyffer and von

Graevenitz 1993, Funke, Pünter and von Graevenitz 1996).

5 THE GENUS *DERMABACTER*

The genus *Dermabacter* was described by Jones and Collins in 1988. It consists of non-spore-forming, non-motile, facultatively anaerobic (fermentative) gram-positive rods with a diphtheroid morphology. The main chemotaxonomic and biochemical data are listed in Tables 25.1 and 25.2 (see pp. 534 and 535). *Dermabacter* strains are seen as very short ('coccoid') rods. Particularly noteworthy is their ability to decarboxylate lysine and ornithine (Funke et al. 1994b). The only species, *Dermabacter hominis* (Jones and Collins 1988), has been isolated from human skin and various other sources, notably blood cultures (Funke et al. 1994b). There are no case reports at the time of writing. The species is identical with the CDC coryneform groups 3 and 5 (Hollis 1992, Funke et al. 1994b); the only difference between these groups is the fermentation of xylose. Colonies are non-fastidious, small, whitish, low convex and can be mistaken for coagulase-negative staphylococci. They are susceptible to vancomycin and occasionally resistant to aminoglycosides (Funke et al. 1994b).

6 YELLOW PIGMENTED GENERA: *OERSKOVIA*, *CELLULOMONAS*, *SANGUIBACTER*, *MICROBACTERIUM*, *AUREOBACTERIUM* AND '*CORYNEBACTERIUM AQUATICUM*'

In the past few years, reports of yellow pigmented diphtheroids in human samples have multiplied. They belong to the genera listed in Tables 25.1 and 25.2 (see pp. 534 and 535).

6.1 *Oerskovia* spp. (CDC groups A-1 and A-2)

These organisms are characterized by extensively branching vegetative hyphae that grow into the underlying agar and break up into coccoid to rudimentary branched, often gram-variable, motile (first monotrichous, later peritrichous) or non-motile ('NMO') filaments. There is no aerial mycelium. The normal habitats of *Oerskovia* spp. are soil and plants. Several reports of clinically significant strains exist, most strains having infected immunocompromised hosts (Sottnek et al. 1977, McDonald et al. 1994), resulting in bacteraemia, CAPD peritonitis, etc. Phenotypically, the species *Oerskovia xanthineolytica* can best be differentiated from *Oerskovia turbata* by hydrolysis of xan-

thine and hypoxanthine (Sottnek et al. 1977). The genus is susceptible only to vancomycin.

6.2 *Cellulomonas* spp.

Recently, clinical isolates (blood and spinal fluid) have been placed in the genus *Cellulomonas*; *Cellulomonas hominis* has been proposed as a species name for the CDC A-3 strains (Funke, Pascual Ramos and Collins 1995). This genus is closely related to *Oerskovia* but does not form mycelia. Characteristic is lysis of cellulose (except in *C. hominis*). These strains are susceptible to many antimicrobials.

6.3 *Sanguibacter*

Members of this recently described genus (Fernandez-Garayzabal et al. 1995) have thus far been isolated from the blood of apparently healthy cows. Phenotypically, they resemble *Oerskovia* spp. and are considered members of the family *Cellulomonadaceae* (Stackebrandt and Prauser 1991) but differ from *Oerskovia* in the composition of cell wall amino acids and cellular fatty acids.

6.4 *Microbacterium* spp.

Some clinical CDC group A-4 strains and all CDC group A-5 strains (differentiated by xylose fermentation) have been found to belong to the genus *Microbacterium* (Funke, Falsen and Barreau 1995). Species identification was possible only in a minority of them. Orange-pigmented strains are easy to recognize as *Microbacterium*, but separation of yellowish ones from *Cellulomonas* is based mainly on chemotaxonomic analyses. Most strains came from blood cultures and were susceptible to many antimicrobials (except aminoglycosides).

6.5 *Aureobacterium* and '*Corynebacterium aquaticum*'

Clinical strains reported under the latter name (in quotation marks because the group does not fit the criteria for *Corynebacterium*, see Table 25.1, p. 534) are biochemically close to *Aureobacterium* (see Table 25.1) but can be differentiated from this genus by chemotaxonomic tests (see Table 25.1) (Funke, von Graevenitz and Weiss 1994), particularly peptidoglycan analysis. Clinical strains of both *Aureobacterium* and '*C. aquaticum*' have been described (Funke, von Graevenitz and Weiss 1994), mostly from normally sterile fluids. Of note is susceptibility to vancomycin: *Aureobacterium* have so far been fully susceptible, whereas most '*C. aquaticum*' strains have moderate (intermediate) susceptibility. Otherwise, both groups were susceptible to erythromycin and tetracycline but often resistant to aminoglycosides.

REFERENCES

Ahmed K, Kewakami K et al., 1995, *Corynebacterium pseudodiphtheriticum*: a respiratory tract pathogen, *Clin Infect Dis*, **20**: 41–6.

Anderson JS, Cooper KE et al., 1933, Incidence and correlation with clinical severity of *gravis, mitis*, and *intermediate* types of diphtheria bacillus in a series of 500 cases at Leeds, *J Pathol Bacteriol*, **36**: 169–82.

Aravena-Román M, Bowman R, O'Neill G, 1995, Polymerase chain reaction for the detection of toxigenic *Corynebacterium diphtheriae*, *Pathology*, **27**: 71–3.

Barksdale L, 1970, *Corynebacterium diphtheriae* and its relatives, *Bacteriol Rev*, **4**: 378–422.

Barreau C, Bimet F et al., 1993, Comparative chemotaxonomic studies of mycolic acid-free coryneform bacteria of human origin, *J Clin Microbiol*, **31**: 2085–90.

Bayston R, Compton C, Richards K, 1994, Production of extracellular slime by coryneforms colonizing hydrocephalus shunts, *J Clin Microbiol*, **32**: 1705–9.

Bernard KA, Bellefeuille M, Ewan EP, 1991, Cellular fatty acid composition as an adjunct to the identification of aspogenous, aerobic gram-positive rods, *J Clin Microbiol*, **29**: 83–9.

Bickham ST, Jones WL, 1972, Problems in the use of the *in vitro* toxigenicity test for *Corynebacterium diphtheriae*, *Am J Clin Pathol*, **57**: 244–6.

Buck GA, Cross RE et al., 1985, DNA relationships among some *tox*-bearing corynebacteriophages, *Infect Immun*, **49**: 679–84.

Buck GA, Groman NB, 1981, Physical mapping of β-converting and γ-nonconverting corynebacteriophage genomes, *J Bacteriol*, **148**: 131–42.

Butterworth A, Abbott JD et al., 1974, Diphtheria in the Manchester area 1967–1971, *Lancet*, **2**: 1558–61.

Chang DN, Laughren GS, Chalvardjian NE, 1978, Three variants of *Corynebacterium diphtheriae* subsp. *mitis* (*belfanti*) isolated from a throat specimen, *J Clin Microbiol*, **8**: 767–8.

Cianciotto N, Rappuoli R, Groman N, 1986, Detection of homology to the beta bacteriophage integration site in a wide variety of *Corynebacterium* spp., *J Bacteriol*, **168**: 103–6.

Collier RJ, 1975, Diphtheria toxin: mode of action and structure, *Bacteriol Rev*, **39**: 54–85.

Collins MD, 1982, Reclassification of *Bacterionema matruchotii* (Mendel) in the genus *Corynebacterium* as *Corynebacterium matruchotti*, *Zentralbl Bakteriol Hyg Abt 1 Orig C*, **3**: 364–7.

Collins MD, Burton RA, Jones D, 1988, *Corynebacterium amycolatum* sp. nov. a new mycolic acid-less *Corynebacterium* species from human skin, *FEMS Microbiol Lett*, **49**: 349–52.

Collins MD, Cummins CS, 1986, Genus *Corynebacterium* Lehmann and Neumann 1896, 350[AL], *Bergey's Manual of Systematic Bacteriology*, vol. 2, eds Sneath PHA, Mair NS et al., Williams and Wilkins, Baltimore, 1266–76.

Collins MD, Jones D, 1983, *Corynebacterium minutissimum* sp. nov., nom. rev., *Int J Syst Bacteriol*, **33**: 870–1.

Colman G, Weaver E, Efstratiou A, 1992, Screening tests for pathogenic corynebacteria, *J Clin Pathol*, **45**: 46–9.

Coyle MB, Lipsky BA, 1990, Coryneform bacteria in infectious diseases: clinical and laboratory aspects, *Clin Microbiol Rev*, **3**: 227–46.

Coyle MB, Minshew BH, Hsu PC, 1979, Erythromycin and clindamycin resistance in *Corynebacterium diphtheriae* from skin lesions, *Antimicrob Agents Chemother*, **16**: 525–7.

Coyle MB, Groman NB et al., 1989, The molecular epidemiology of three biotypes of *Corynebacterium diphtheriae* in the Seattle outbreak of 1972–1982, *J Infect Dis*, **159**: 670–9.

Coyle MB, Leonard RB et al., 1993a, Evidence of multiple taxa within commercially available reference strains of *Corynebacterium xerosis*, *J Clin Microbiol*, **31**: 1788–93.

Coyle MB, Nowowiejski DJ et al., 1993b, Laboratory review of reference strains of *Corynebacterium diphtheriae* indicates mistyped *intermedius* strains, *J Clin Microbiol*, **31**: 3060–2.

Crosbie WE, Wright HD, 1941, Diphtheria bacilli in floor dust, *Lancet*, **1**: 656.

Cuevas WA, Songer JG, 1993, *Arcanobacterium haemolyticum* phospholipase D is genetically and functionally similar to *Corynebacterium pseudotuberculosis* phospholipase–D, *Infect Immun*, **61**: 4310–16.

De Briel D, Couderc F et al., 1992, High-performance liquid chromatography of corynomycolic acids as a tool in identification of *Corynebacterium* species and related organisms, *J Clin Microbiol*, **30**: 1407–17.

De Zoysa A, Efstratiou A et al., 1995, Molecular epidemiology of *Corynebacterium diphtheriae* from northwestern Russia and surrounding countries studied by using ribotyping and pulsed-field gel electrophoresis, *J Clin Microbiol*, **33**: 1080–3.

Digenis G, Dombros N et al., 1992, Struvite stone formation by *Corynebacterium* group F1: a case report, *J Urol*, **147**: 169–70.

Dixon JM, 1984, Diphtheria in North America, *J Hyg Camb*, **93**: 419–32.

Efstratiou A, Tiley SM et al., 1993, Invasive disease caused by multiple clones of *Corynebacterium diphtheriae*, *Clin Infect Dis*, **17**: 136.

Elek SD, 1949, The plate virulence test for diphtheria, *J Clin Pathol*, **2**: 250–8.

Fernandez-Garayzabal JF, Dominguez L et al., 1995, Phenotypic and phylogenetic characterization of some unknown coryneform bacteria isolated from bovine blood and milk: description of *Sanguibacter* gen. nov., *Lett Appl Microbiol*, **20**: 69–75.

Freeman VJ, 1951, Studies on the virulence of bacteriophage-infected strains of *Corynebacterium diphtheriae*, *J Bacteriol*, **61**: 675–8.

Frobisher M, Adams ML, Kuhns WJ, 1945, Characteristics of diphtheria bacilli found in Baltimore since November, 1942, *Proc Soc Exp Biol Med*, **58**: 330–4.

Funke G, Carlotti A, 1994, Differentiation of *Brevibacterium* spp. encountered in clinical specimens, *J Clin Microbiol*, **32**: 1729–32.

Funke G, Falsen E, Barreau C, 1995, Primary identification of *Microbacterium* spp. encountered in clinical specimens as CDC coryneform group A-4 and A-5 bacteria, *J Clin Microbiol*, **33**: 188–92.

Funke G, von Graevenitz A, Weiss N, 1994, Primary identification of *Aureobacterium* spp. from clinical specimens as 'Corynebacterium aquaticum', *J Clin Microbiol*, **32**: 2686–91.

Funke G, Lawson PA, Collins MD, 1995, Heterogeneity within human-derived Centers for Disease Control and Prevention (CDC) coryneform ANF-1-like bacteria and description of *Corynebacterium auris* sp. nov., *Int J Syst Bacteriol*, **45**: 735–9.

Funke G, Pascual Ramos C, Collins MD, 1995, Identification of some clinical strains of CDC coryneform group A-3 and A-4 bacteria as *Cellulomonas* species and proposal of *Cellulomonas hominis* sp. nov. for some group A-3 strains, *J Clin Microbiol*, **33**: 2091–7.

Funke G, Pünter V, von Graevenitz A, 1996, Antimicrobial susceptibility patterns of recently established coryneform bacteria, *Antimicrob Agents Chemother*, **40**: in press.

Funke G, Stubbs S et al., 1994a, *Turicella otitidis* gen. nov., sp. nov., a coryneform bacterium isolated from patients with otitis media, *Int J Syst Bacteriol*, **44**: 270–3.

Funke G, Stubbs S et al., 1994b, Characteristics of CDC group 3 and group 5 coryneform bacteria isolated from clinical specimens and assignment to the genus *Dermabacter*, *J Clin Microbiol*, **32**: 1223–8.

Funke G, Bernard KA et al., 1995, *Corynebacterium glucuronolyticum* sp. nov. isolated from male patients with genitourinary infections, *Med Microbiol Lett*, **4**: 204–15.

Funke G, Lawson PA et al., 1996, Most *Corynebacterium xerosis* strains identified in the routine clinical laboratory correspond to *Corynebacterium amycolatum*, *J Clin Microbiol*, **34**: 1124–8.

Furness G, Evangelista AT, 1978, A diagnostic key employing biological reactions for differentiating pathogenic *Corynebac-*

terium genitalium (NSU corynebacteria) from commensals of the urogenital tract, *Invest Urol*, **16**: 1–4.

Gilmour MN, 1974, Genus IV, *Bacterionema*,Gilmour, Howell and Bibby 1961, 139, *Bergey's Manual of Determinative Bacteriology*, 8th edn, eds Buchanan RE, Gibbons NE, Williams and Wilkins, Baltimore, 676–9.

Gordon RD, Yow MD et al., 1971, *In vitro* susceptibility of *Corynebacterium diphtheriae* to thirteen antibiotics, *Appl Microbiol*, **21**: 548–9.

von Graevenitz A, Osterhout G, Dick J, 1991, Grouping of some clinically relevant gram-positive rods by automated fatty acid analysis, *APMIS*, **99**: 147–54.

von Graevenitz A, Pünter V et al., 1994, Identification of coryneform and other gram-positive rods with several methods, *APMIS*, **102**: 381–9.

Gruner E, Pfyffer GE, von Graevenitz A, 1993, Characterization of *Brevibacterium* spp. from clinical specimens, *J Clin Microbiol*, **31**: 1408–12.

Gruner E, Zuber PLF et al., 1992, A cluster of non-toxigenic *Corynebacterium diphtheriae* infections among Swiss intravenous drug abusers, *Med Microbiol Lett*, **1**: 160–7.

Gruner E, Steigerwalt AG et al., 1994, Human infections caused by *Brevibacterium casei*, formerly CDC groups B-1 and B-3, *J Clin Microbiol*, **32**: 1511–18.

Hallas G, 1988, The use of SDS-polyacrylamide gel electrophoresis in epidemiological studies of *Corynebacterium diphtheriae*, *Epidemiol Infect*, **100**: 83–90.

Harnisch JP, Tronca E et al., 1989, Diphtheria among alcoholic urban adults. A decade of experience in Seattle, *Ann Intern Med*, **111**: 71–82.

Hauser D, Popoff M et al., 1993, Polymerase chain reaction assay for diagnosis of potentially toxinogenic *Corynebacterium diphtheriae* strains: correlation with ADP-ribosylation activity assay, *J Clin Microbiol*, **31**: 2720–3.

Hermann GJ, Moore MS, Parsons EJ, 1958, A substitute for serum in the diphtheriae *in vitro* toxigenicity test, *Am J Clin Pathol*, **29**: 181–3.

Hermann GJ, Parsons EJ, 1957, Recognition of *C. diphtheriae*-like corynebacteria (*Corynebacterium ulcerans*) in the laboratory, *Public Health Lab*, **15**: 34–7.

Hollis DG, 1992, *Gram-positive Organisms: Potential New CDC Coryneform Groups*, Centers for Disease Control and Prevention, Atlanta.

Hollis DG, Weaver RE, 1981, *Gram-positive Organisms: a Guide to Identification*, Centers for Disease Control, Atlanta.

Hoyle L, 1941, A tellurite blood agar medium for the rapid diagnosis of diphtheria, *Lancet*, **1**: 175–6.

Jackman PJH, Pitcher DG et al., 1987, Classification of corynebacteria associated with endocarditis (group JK) as *Corynebacterium jeikeium* sp. nov., *Syst Appl Microbiol*, **9**: 83–90.

Jellard CH, Lipinski AE, 1973, *Corynebacterium diphtheriae* resistant to erythromycin and lincomycin, *Lancet*, **1**: 156.

Johnstone KI, McLeod JW, 1949, Nomenclature of strains of *Corynebacterium diphtheriae*, *Public Health Rep*, **64**: 1181–7.

Jones D, Collins MD, 1988, Taxonomic studies on some human cutaneous coryneform bacteria: description of *Dermabacter hominis* gen. nov., sp. nov., *FEMS Microbiol Lett*, **51**: 51–6.

Jones D, Keddie RM, 1986, Genus *Brevibacterium* Breed 1953, 13^AL^ emend Collins et al.1980,6, *Bergey's Manual of Systematic Bacteriology*, vol. 2, eds Sneath PHA, Mair–NS et al., Williams and Wilkins, Baltimore, 1301–13.

Jones SA, Miller HJ et al., 1984, An experience of diphtheria in Westminster, *Public Health (London)*, **98**: 3–7.

Judson R, Songer JG, 1991, *Corynebacterium pseudotuberculosis*: in vitro susceptibility of 39 antimicrobial agents, *Vet Microbiol*, **27**: 145–50.

Kaczorek M, Zettlmeissl G et al., 1985, Diphtheria toxin promoter function in *Corynebacterium diphtheriae* and *Escherichia coli*, *Nucleic Acids Res*, **13**: 3147–59.

Kerry-Williams SM, Noble WC, 1988, Plasmids in coryneform bacteria of human origin, *J Appl Bacteriol*, **64**: 475–82.

Krech T, 1994, Epidemiological typing of *Corynebacterium diphtheriae*, *Med Microbiol Lett*, **3**: 1–8.

Krech T, de Chastonay J, Falsen E, 1988, Epidemiology of diphtheria: polypeptide and restriction enzyme analysis in comparison with conventional phage typing, *Eur J Clin Microbiol Infect Dis*, **7**: 232–7.

Krueger KM, Barbieri JT, 1995, The family of bacterial ADP-ribosylating exotoxins, *Clin Microbiol Rev*, **8**: 38–47.

Leonard RB, Nowowiejski DJ et al., 1994, Molecular evidence of person-to-person transmission of a pigmented strain of *Corynebacterium striatum* in intensive care units, *J Clin Microbiol*, **32**: 164–9.

Leong D, Murphy JR, 1985, Characterization of the diphtheria *tox* transcript in *Corynebacterium diphtheriae* and *Escherichia coli*, *J Bacteriol*, **163**: 1114–19.

McBride ME, Ellner KM et al., 1993, A new *Brevibacterium* sp. isolated from infected genital hair of patients with white piedra, *J Med Microbiol*, **39**: 255–61.

McDonald CL, Chapin-Robertson K et al., 1994, *Oerskovia xanthineolytica* bacteremia in an immunocompromised patient with pneumonia, *Diagn Microbiol Infect Dis*, **18**: 259–61.

McLeod JW, 1943, The types *mitis*, *intermedius* and *gravis* of *Corynebacterium diphtheriae*. A review of observations during the past 10 years, *Bacteriol Rev*, **7**: 1–41.

McNamara PJ, Cuevas WA, Songer JG, 1995, Toxic phospholipases D of *Corynebacterium pseudotuberculosis*, *C. ulcerans* and *Arcanobacterium haemolyticum*: cloning and sequence homology, *Gene*, **156**: 113–18.

Manzella JP, Kellogg JA, Parsey KS, 1995, *Corynebacterium pseudodiphtheriticum*: a respiratory tract pathogen in adults, *Clin Infect Dis*, **20**: 37–40.

Maple PA, Efstratiou A et al., 1994, The *in-vitro* susceptibilities of toxigenic strains of *Corynebacterium diphtheriae* isolated in northwestern Russia and surrounding areas to ten antibiotics, *J Antimicrob Chemother*, **34**: 1037–40.

Markowitz SM, Coudron PE, 1990, Native valve endocarditis caused by an organism resembling *Corynebacterium striatum*, *J Clin Microbiol*, **28**: 8–10.

Martinetti Lucchini M, Gruner E, Altwegg M, 1992, Rapid detection of diphtheria toxin by the polymerase chain reaction, *Med Microbiol Lett*, **1**: 276–83.

Martinez-Martinez L, Suarez I et al., 1995, Phenotypic characteristics of 31 strains of *Corynebacterium striatum* isolated from clinical samples, *J Clin Microbiol*, **33**: 2458–61.

Maximescu P, Oprisan A et al., 1974, Further studies on *Corynebacterium* species capable of producing diphtheria toxin (*C. diphtheriae*, *C. ulcerans*, *C. ovis*), *J Gen Microbiol*, **82**: 49–56.

Moore MS, Parsons EI, 1958, A study of modified Tinsdale's medium for the primary isolation of *Corynebacterium diphtheriae*, *J Infect Dis*, **102**: 88–93.

Morris A, Guild I, 1991, Endocarditis due to *Corynebacterium pseudodiphtheriticum*: five case reports, review, and antibiotic susceptibilities of nine strains, *Rev Infect Dis*, **13**: 887–92.

Murphy JR, Pappenheimer AM Jr, de Borms ST, 1974, Synthesis of diphtheria *tox*-gene products in *Escherichia coli* extracts, *Proc Natl Acad Sci USA*, **71**: 11–15.

Neubauer M, Sourek J et al., 1991, *Corynebacterium accolens* sp. nov., a gram-positive rod exhibiting satellitism, from clinical material, *Syst Appl Microbiol*, **14**: 46–51.

Pallen MJ, 1991, Rapid screening for toxigenic *Corynebacterium diphtheriae* by the polymerase chain reaction, *J Clin Pathol*, **44**: 1025–6.

Pallen MJ, Hay AJ et al., 1994, Polymerase chain reaction for screening clinical isolates of corynebacteria for the production of diphtheria toxin, *J Clin Pathol*, **47**: 353–6.

Pappenheimer AM Jr, 1984, The diphtheria bacillus and its toxin: a model system, *J Hyg Camb*, **93**: 397–404.

Pappenheimer AM Jr, Johnson SJ, 1936, Studies in diphtheria toxin production. I. The effect of iron and copper, *Br J Exp Pathol*, **17**: 335–41.

Pappenheimer AM Jr, Murphy JR, 1983, Studies on the molecular epidemiology of diphtheria, *Lancet*, **2**: 923–6.

Pascual C, Lawson PA et al., 1995, Phylogenetic analysis of the genus *Corynebacterium* based on 16S rRNA gene sequences, *Int J Syst Bacteriol*, **45**: 724–8.

Petit PLC, Bok JW et al., 1994, Native-valve endocarditis due to CDC coryneform group ANF-3: report of a case and review of corynebacterial endocarditis, *Clin Infect Dis*, **19**: 897–901.

Pitcher DG, Malnick H, 1984, Identification of *Brevibacterium* from clinical sources, *J Clin Pathol*, **37**: 1395–8.

Pitcher DG, Soto A et al., 1992, Classification of coryneform bacteria associated with human urinary tract infection (group D2) as *Corynebacterium urealyticum* sp. nov., *Int J Syst Bacteriol*, **42**: 178–81.

Porschen RK, Goodman Z, Rafai B, 1977, Isolation of *Corynebacterium xerosis* from clinical specimens, *Am J Clin Pathol*, **68**: 290–3.

Quinn AG, Comaish JS, Pedler SJ, 1991, Septic arthritis and endocarditis due to group G-2 coryneform organism, *Lancet*, **338**: 62–3.

Rappuoli R, Perugini M, Falsen E, 1988, Molecular epidemiology of the 1984–1986 outbreaks of diphtheria in Sweden, *N Engl J Med*, **318**: 12–14.

Rappuoli R, Ratti G, 1984, Physical map of the chromosomal region of *Corynebacterium diphtheriae* containing corynephage attachments sites *attB1* and *attB2*, *J Bacteriol*, **158**: 325–30.

Riegel P, de Briel D et al., 1993a, Proposal of *Corynebacterium afermentans* sp. nov. containing the subspecies *C. afermentans* subsp. *afermentans* subsp. nov. and *C. afermentans* subsp. *lipophilum* subsp. nov., *FEMS Microbiol Lett*, **113**: 229–34.

Riegel P, de Briel D et al., 1993b, Taxonomic study of *Corynebacterium* group ANF-1 strains: proposal of *Corynebacterium* sp. nov. containing the subspecies *C. afermentans* subsp. nov. and *C. afermentans* subsp. nov., *Int J Syst Bacteriol*, **43**: 287–92.

Riegel P, de Briel D et al., 1994, Genomic diversity among *Corynebacterium jeikeium* strains and comparison with biochemical characteristics and antimicrobial susceptibilities, *J Clin Microbiol*, **32**: 1860–5.

Riegel P, Ruimy R et al., 1995a, Genomic diversity and phylogenetic relationships among lipid-requiring diphtheroids from humans and characterization of *Corynebacterium macginleyi* sp. nov., *Int J Syst Bacteriol*, **45**: 128–33.

Riegel P, Ruimy R et al., 1995b, *Corynebacterium argentoratense* sp. nov. from the human throat, *Int J Syst Bacteriol*, **45**: 533–7.

Riegel P, Ruimy R et al., 1995c, Taxonomy of *Corynebacterium diphtheriae* and related taxa, with recognition of *Corynebacterium ulcerans* sp. nov., nom. rev., *FEMS Microbiol Lett*, **126**: 271–6.

Roberts MC, Leonard RB et al., 1992, Characterization of antibiotic-resistant *Corynebacterium striatum* strains, *J Antimicrob Chemother*, **30**: 463–74.

Rockhill RC, Sumarmo L et al., 1982, Tetracycline resistance in *Corynebacterium diphtheriae* isolated from diphtheria patients in Jakarta, Indonesia, *Antimicrob Agents Chemother*, **21**: 842–3.

Russell LM, Cryz SJ, Holmes RK, 1984, Genetic and biochemical evidence for a siderophore-dependent iron transport system in *Corynebacterium diphtheriae*, *Infect Immun*, **45**: 143–9.

Saragea A, Maximescu P, Meitert E, 1979, *Corynebacterium diphtheriae*: microbiological methods used in clinical and epidemiological investigations, *Methods in Microbiology*, eds Bergan T, Norris JR, Academic Press, New York, 61–176.

Schiller A, Groman N, Coyle M, 1980, Plasmids in *Corynebacterium diphtheriae* and diphtheroids mediating erythromycin resistance, *Antimicrob Agents Chemother*, **18**: 814–21.

Schmitt MP, Holmes RK, 1994, Cloning, sequence, and footprint analysis of two promoter/operators from *Corynebacterium diphtheriae* that are regulated by the diphtheria toxin repressor (DtxR) and iron, *J Bacteriol*, **176**: 1141–9.

Schmitt MP, Twiddy EM, Holmes RK, 1992, Purification and characterization of the diphtheria toxin repressor, *Proc Natl Acad Sci USA*, **89**: 7576–80.

Serikawa S, Ito S et al., 1993, Seroepidemiological evidence that shearing wounds are mainly responsible for *Corynebacterium pseudotuberculosis* infection in sheep, *J Vet Med Sci*, **55**: 691–2.

Sewell DL, Coyle MB, Funke G, 1995, Prosthetic valve endocarditis caused by *Corynebacterium afermentans* subsp. *lipophilum* (CDC coryneform group ANF-1), *J Clin Microbiol*, **33**: 759–61.

Smith RF, 1969, A medium for the study of the ecology of human cutaneous diphtheroids, *J Gen Microbiol*, **57**: 411–17.

Snell JJ, Demello JV et al., 1984, Detection of toxin production by *Corynebacterium diphtheriae*: results of a trial organized as part of the United Kingdom National External Microbiological Quality Assessment Scheme, *J Clin Pathol*, **37**: 796–9.

Songer JG, Beckenbach K et al., 1988, Biochemical and genetic characterization of *Corynebacterium pseudotuberculosis*, *Am J Vet Res*, **49**: 223–6.

Soriano F, Zapardiel J, Nieto E, 1995, Antimicrobial susceptibilities of *Corynebacterium* species and other non-spore-forming gram-positive bacilli to 18 antimicrobial agents, *Antimicrob Agents Chemother*, **39**: 208–14.

Soriano F, Ponte C et al., 1986, In vitro and in vivo study of stone formation by *Corynebacterium* group D2 (*Corynebacterium urealyticum*), *J Clin Microbiol*, **23**: 691–4.

Soriano F, Aguado JM et al., 1990, Urinary tract infection caused by *Corynebacterium* group D2: report of 82 cases and review, *Clin Infect Dis*, **12**: 1019–34.

Soriano F, Ponte C et al., 1993, Non-urinary tract infections caused by multiply antibiotic-resistant *Corynebacterium urealyticum*, *Clin Infect Dis*, **17**: 890–1.

Sottnek FO, Brown JM et al., 1977, Recognition of *Oerskovia* species in the clinical laboratory: characterization of 35 isolates, *Int J Syst Bacteriol*, **27**: 263–70.

Soucek A, Michalic C, Souckova A, 1971, Identification and characterization of a new enzyme of the group 'phospholipase D' isolated from *Corynebacterium ovis*, *Biochem Biophys Acta*, **227**: 116–28.

Stackebrandt E, Prauser H, 1991, Assignment of the genera *Cellulomonas*, *Oerskovia*, *Promicromonospora* and *Jonesia* to *Cellulomonadaceae* fam. nov., *Syst Appl Microbiol*, **14**: 261–5.

Tai SP, Krafft AE et al., 1980, Coordinate regulation of siderophore and diphtheria toxin production by iron in *Corynebacterium diphtheriae*, *Microb Pathog*, **9**: 267–73.

Tinsdale GFW, 1947, A new medium for the isolation and identification of *C. diphtheriae* based on the production of hydrogen sulphide, *J Pathol Bacteriol*, **59**: 461–6.

Ward KW, 1948, Effect of Tween 80 on certain strains of *C. diphtheriae*, *Proc Soc Exp Biol Med*, **67**: 527–8.

Wilhelmus KR, Robinson NM, Jones DB, 1979, *Bacterionema matruchotii* ocular infections, *Am J Ophthalmol*, **87**: 143–7.

Williams DY, Selepak ST, Gill VJ, 1993, Identification of clinical isolates of non-diphtherial *Corynebacterium* species and their antibiotic susceptibility patterns, *Diagn Microbiol Infect Dis*, **17**: 23–8.

Wilson APR, Efstratiou A et al., 1992, Unusual non-toxigenic *Corynebacterium diphtheriae* in homosexual man, *Lancet*, **339**: 998.

Wirsing von König CH, Krech T et al., 1988, Use of fosfomycin disks for isolation of diphtheroids, *Eur J Clin Microbiol Infect Dis*, **7**: 190–3.

Yanagawa R, Honda E, 1976, Presence of pili in species of human and animal parasites and pathogens of the genus *Corynebacterium*, *Infect Immun*, **13**: 1293–5.

Zinkernagel A, von Graevenitz A, Funke G, 1996, Heterogeneity within *Corynebacterium minutissimum* strains is explained by misidentified *Corynebacterium amycolatum* strains, *Am J Clin Pathol*, **106**: 378–83.

Chapter 26

MYCOBACTERIUM

R C Good and T M Shinnick

1 DEFINITION

The genus *Mycobacterium* is currently the only genus in the family Mycobacteriaceae, order Actinomycetales, although there has been a proposal to include the genera *Nocardia* and *Rhodococcus* in this family (Fox and Stackebrandt 1987). The minimal standards for including a species in this genus are:

1 acid–alcohol fastness (i.e. resist decolorization by acidified alcohol after being stained with a basic fuschin dye)
2 the presence of mycolic acids containing 60–90 carbon atoms which are cleaved to C_{22}–C_{26} fatty acid methyl esters by pyrolysis and
3 a G + C content of the DNA of 61–71 mol% (Levy-Frebault and Portaels 1992).

Mycobacteria are non-motile, non-sporing, weakly gram-positive, aerobic or micro-aerophilic, straight or slightly curved rod-shaped bacteria (Wayne and Kubica 1986). Some mycobacteria display coccobacillary, filamentous, or branched forms, and some produce yellow to orange pigment in the dark or after exposure to light. The species fall into 2 main groups based on growth rate. Slowly growing species require more than 7 days to form visible colonies on solid media whereas rapidly growing species require fewer than 7 days. Slowly growing species are often pathogenic for humans or animals. Rapidly growing species are usually considered non-pathogenic for humans, although important exceptions exist.

The type species is *Mycobacterium tuberculosis*.

Mycobacteria were among the first bacteria to be ascribed to specific diseases. In 1874, Armauer Hansen identified a rod-shaped bacillus (*Bacillus leprae*) in a tissue biopsy from a lepromatous leprosy patient and suggested that it was the aetiological agent of leprosy (Hansen 1880). Eight years later, Robert Koch identified a rod-shaped bacillus (*Bacterium tuberculosis*) as the causative agent of tuberculosis and formulated Koch's postulates for establishing a causal relationship between a suspected pathogen and a given disease (Koch 1882, Zopf 1883). These species were subsequently renamed *Mycobacterium leprae* and *Mycobacterium tuberculosis*, respectively, and placed in the genus *Mycobacterium* ('fungus bacterium', named to reflect the mould-like pellicle formed by *M. tuberculosis* on liquid media) (Lehmann and Neumann 1896).

At the beginning of this century, *M. tuberculosis* was the only species of *Mycobacterium* routinely isolated from, and associated with, human disease. As other species of *Mycobacterium* were recognized as causes of human disease, they were often simply categorized as non-tuberculosis mycobacteria without further speciation. Other names given to this group of pathogenic species of *Mycobacterium* include 'MOTT' (mycobacteria other than tubercle) bacilli, 'atypical', 'opportunistic', 'nyrocine' and 'environmental' mycobacteria (Timpe and Runyon 1954, Runyon 1959, Grange and Collins 1983, Good 1985). Although such names are routinely used in the published literature and in clinical laboratories, they have little informational value and represent inappropriate clustering of distantly related species which cause different diseases and which require different treatment regimens.

There are currently 71 recognized or proposed species of *Mycobacterium* (Table 26.1) (Wayne and Kubica 1986, Shinnick and Good 1994), that are usually grouped into 2 major divisions, 'rapidly growing' and 'slowly growing', based on the time required for visible colonies to appear on a solid medium after plating sufficiently dilute suspensions to give well separated colonies. Colonies of rapidly growing species appear in 7 days or less and colonies of slowly growing species in more than 7 days. The slowly growing species are further divided into 3 groups based on pigmentation (Timpe and Runyon 1954, Runyon 1959): photochromogens (Runyon group I), scotochromogens (Runyon group II) and non-photochromogens (Runyon group III). These divisions have no formal taxonomic standing but are useful in identification schemes.

The genus *Mycobacterium* contains several important

Table 26.1 *Mycobacterium* species

Pathogenic	Non-pathogenic
Slow growers	Slow growers
M. africanum	M. cookii
M. asiaticum	M. gastri
M. avium	M. gordonae
M. bovis	M. hiberniae
M. celatum	M. nonchromogenicum
M. farcinogenes[a]	M. terrae
M. genavense	M. triviale
M. haemophilum	
M. interjectum	Rapid growers
M. intermedium	M. agri
M. intracellulare	M. aichense
M. kansasii	M. alvei
M. leprae	M. aurum
M. lepraemurium[a]	M. austroafricanum
M. malmoense	M. brumae
M. marinum	M. chitae
M. microti[a]	M. chubuense
M. paratuberculosis[a]	M. confluentis
M. scrofulaceum	M. diernhoferi
M. shimoidei	M. duvalii
M. simiae	M. fallax
M. szulgai	M. flavescens
M. tuberculosis	M. gadium
M. ulcerans	M. gilvum
M. xenopi	M. komossense
	M. madagascariense
Rapid growers	M. methylovorum
M. abscessus	M. moriokaense
M. chelonae	M. neoaurum
M. fortuitum	M. obuense
M. peregrinum	M. parafortuitum
M. porcinum[a]	M. phlei
M. senegalense[a]	M. poriferae
	M. pulveris
	M. rhodesiae
	M. shanghaiense
	M. smegmatis
	M. sphagni
	M. thermoresistibile
	M. tokaiense
	M. vaccae
	M. yunnanense

[a]Pathogenic for animals.

pathogens of animals and humans (Table 26.1) including the causative agents of tuberculosis (see Volume 3, Chapter 21), Hansen disease or leprosy (see Volume 3, Chapter 23), Johne's disease (see Volume 3, Chapter 23) and infections in immunocompromised persons (see Volume 3, Chapter 22). In general, slowly growing species can cause disease in humans or animals, whereas the rapidly growing species cannot, although there are several significant exceptions to this correlation (Good 1992, Hartmans and De Bont 1992). However, for the immunocompromised individual, non-pathogenic species of *Mycobacterium* may not really exist (Good 1985, Horsburgh and Selik 1989).

2 SPECIES DIFFERENTIATION

Mycobacterium species have been extensively characterized in a series of co-operative studies co-ordinated by the International Working Group on Mycobacterial Taxonomy (IWGMT), and the genus is one of most thoroughly described of the bacterial genera (Wayne et al. 1981, 1983, 1989, 1991). The keys to this were differentiating species according to their patterns of reactivity in a large battery of biochemical tests rather than according to one or 2 essential properties (Gordon and Smith 1955) and the phenetic data were analysed using an Adansonian classification scheme known as numerical taxonomy (Wayne 1981). However, a limitation of numerical taxonomy is that it measures phenetic similarities which do not necessarily reflect genetic relatedness. Usually, the overall genetic relatedness of bacteria is measured using DNA–DNA hybridization techniques, and strains displaying >70% hybridization are considered to be members of the same species (Wayne et al. 1987). However, only one or a few strains of a small number of species have been analysed in this manner because the techniques for extraction of DNA from mycobacteria are technically demanding and labour intensive (Baess 1979).

Phylogenetic trees of the genus *Mycobacterium* have been constructed using sequences of 16S rRNA genes to assess genetic relatedness (Fox and Stackebrandt 1987, Rogall et al. 1990, Stahl and Urbance 1990, Pituille et al. 1992). In these trees, all recognized species of *Mycobacterium* are closely related to each other and distantly related to members of other genera. Furthermore, the major phenotypic division of *Mycobacterium* spp. (rapidly versus slowly growing species) also appears as a major branch point in the phylogenetic tree (Stahl and Urbance 1990). Clusters identified by numerical analysis of phenotypic traits generally correlate well with the results of the 16S rRNA phylogenetic analysis, although exceptions exist. For example, *Mycobacterium kansasii* and *Mycobacterium gastri* can be clearly distinguished by numerical taxonomy (Wayne et al. 1978), but these species have identical 16S rRNA sequences (Rogall et al. 1990).

Although each of the recognized species of *Mycobacterium* can be clearly differentiated from each of the other species, diagnostic laboratories often identify isolates only as a member of a group or complex of closely related species where a 'complex' is defined as 2 or more species whose distinction is of little or no medical importance. For example, pulmonary tuberculosis caused by *Mycobacterium africanum* is treated in the same manner as pulmonary tuberculosis caused by *M. tuberculosis*, so it is sufficient to identify the causative agent of pulmonary tuberculosis as a member of the *M. tuberculosis* complex (*M. africanum*, *M. bovis*, *M. tuberculosis*).

3 HABITAT

Mycobacteria can be isolated from a wide variety of environmental samples including water, soil, dust and *Sphagnum* vegetation (reviewed by Kazda 1983, Collins, Grange and Yates 1984, Hartmans and De Bont 1992). However, this does not mean that mycobacteria actually grow in these materials in nature. For example, *Mycobacterium paratuberculosis* bacilli are shed in large numbers in the faeces of infected cattle, and although these bacilli can survive for long periods of time in the soil, there is no evidence that they actually multiply outside their animal hosts (Kazda 1983).

Mycobacteria have been classified as obligate pathogens, facultative or opportunistic pathogens, or free-living saprophytes, based on their ability to multiply in various environments (Kazda 1983). Obligate pathogens are species that do not appear to multiply outside their hosts and include *M. tuberculosis*, *M. bovis*, *M. africanum*, *M. asiaticum*, *M. farcinogenes*, *M. haemophilum*, *M. leprae*, *M. malmoense*, *M. microti*, *M. paratuberculosis*, *M. shimodei*, *M. simiae* and *M. szulgai*. Some of these mycobacterial species can infect several different animal species. For example, naturally occurring tuberculosis infections have been observed in humans, other primates, cattle, deer and badgers, and there is evidence for zoonotic transmission of the tubercle bacilli (Good 1992, Thoen 1994a). Facultative pathogens can multiply outside the host as well as cause infections in animals or humans and include *M. avium*, *M. chelonae*, *M. fortuitum*, *M. kansasii*, *M. intracellulare*, *M. marinum*, *M. senegalense*, *M. scrofulaceum*, *M. ulcerans* and *M. xenopi*. Free-living saprophytes do not cause a progressive infection or disease in immunocompetent humans or animals and are often found in soil and watery habitats such as marshes and estuaries. The saprophytic species include *M. gastri*, *M. gordonae*, *M. nonchromogenicum*, *M. terrae*, *M. triviale* and all of the rapidly growing species except *M. abscessus*, *M. chelonae*, *M. fortuitum*, *M. peregrinum*, *M. porcinum* and *M. senegalense*.

Humans are exposed to environmentally derived mycobacteria in a variety of ways. Viable mycobacteria are present in municipal water supplies, and some species may be able to colonize water pipes and faucets (e.g. *M. fortuitum*, *M. kansasii* and *M. scrofulaceum*); thus providing a potential source for infection of humans. For example, the source of an outbreak of pulmonary *M. kansasii* infections among coal miners was traced to bacilli present in water used for showering (Kubin et al. 1980), and *M. chelonae* infections in patients with chronic renal failure were traced to water used in a haemodialysis centre (Bolan et al. 1985).

The presence of mycobacteria in water supplies also complicates diagnostic laboratory tests, because mycobacteria can contaminate reagents and vessels, leading to false positive results. For example, pseudoepidemics of *M. abscessus* isolation from bronchoscopic washings have been traced to contamination of the bronchoscopes, and pseudoepidemics of *M. fortuitum* isolation from sputum have been traced to contaminated water (reviewed by Wallace 1994). Also, because of their environmental distribution, saprophytic species can be isolated from a variety of pathological specimens including saliva, sputum, skin and intestine, although such bacilli are usually regarded as transitory contaminants. Hence, diagnostic laboratories must take care to identify these species as a part of the proper diagnosis of disease.

Another medically important aspect of exposure to environmental mycobacteria is their potential impact on the immune response. Exposure to environmental mycobacteria has been suggested to influence immune responsiveness to the pathogenic mycobacteria (Stanford, Shields and Rook 1981) and to sensitize individuals to skin test reagents. For example, sensitization by exposure to *M. fortuitum* in the soil is thought to be responsible for a portion of the false positive tuberculin skin test reactions found in persons from the southeastern USA (Edwards et al. 1969).

4 MORPHOLOGY

The general description of the microscopic morphology of bacilli in the genus *Mycobacterium* given in section 1 (see p. 549) is consistent with the descriptions found in most texts; however, it is based primarily on observations of bacilli that were grown in vitro on laboratory media and may not represent the morphology of bacilli as they occur in their natural habitat (Youmans 1979). Even the steps taken to decontaminate and concentrate specimens such as sputum may alter the appearance of bacilli in stained smears. Bacilli in sputum specimens stained by the Ziehl–Neelsen technique frequently are much longer, more curved and sometimes more beaded than cells found in culture. Stained preparations of mycobacteria also often show beading, i.e. darkly stained spheres within the cell. This has been associated with cell wall deficient and filterable forms. The many implications of the occurrence of L-forms, the conditions that lead to their existence and effect on disease processes are unclear and often contradictory (Imaeda 1984).

4.1 Staining reactions

Mycobacteria are described as being acid–alcohol fast, i.e. once stained with a specific dye the cells resist decolorization with acidified ethanol. This staining characteristic is shared only by species of related genera that have mycolic acids as a constituent of the cell wall, e.g. *Nocardia*, *Rhodococcus*, *Corynebacterium* (Goodfellow and Minnikin 1984). The basis of the acid-fast staining reaction is not clearly understood, but appears to be related to the presence of mycolic acids in the cell wall, to the integrity of the cell and to the viability of the cell (Kölbel 1984). Clinically, the detection of acid-fast bacilli by microscopic examination is used in many developing countries as the only test to confirm the diagnosis of tuberculosis and in developed countries to measure the relative infectiousness of a patient and to follow the effects of chemotherapy.

To confirm a physician's diagnosis of tuberculosis, a sputum specimen is collected from the patient in a clean, sterile container, and the caseous, bloody or purulent particles found in it are used to prepare smears. A volume of 0.01 ml, delivered usually with a 3 mm inoculating loop, is smeared over a 2 cm² area of the slide, which is then stained by one of 3 standard methods: Ziehl–Neelsen acid-fast stain (hot staining procedure), Kinyoun acid-fast stain (cold staining procedure), or auramine O fluorescence acid-fast stain (Collins, Grange and Yates 1985, Kent and Kubica 1985). For example, in the Ziehl–Neelsen procedure, stain is prepared by disolving 0.3 g basic fuchsin in 10 ml 90–95% ethanol or methylated spirits and mixing with 90 ml of phenol solution (5 g phenol crystals in 95 ml distilled water). The specimen is smeared on the slide, heat fixed and covered with absorbent paper. Approximately 5 drops of fuchsin–phenol solution is added and the bottom of the slide heated with a bunsen burner or electric heater until the stain begins to steam. After heating for 5 min, the paper is removed and the smears rinsed with tap water and drained. Next, the smears are flooded with an acid–alcohol solution (3 ml concentrated hydrochloric acid plus 97 ml 90–95% ethanol or methylated spirits) for at least 2 min, rinsed in tap water and drained. The smear is then counterstained with methylene blue for 1–2 min.

Fuchsin-stained smears should be examined with a light microscope by making 3 longitudinal sweeps of the stained area along the length of the slide. About 100 fields will be seen in a single sweep at a magnification of 1000-fold for a total of 300 fields. Mycobacteria appear as red rods on a blue background (Fig. 26.1, see also plate 26.1). Auramine-stained smears are examined with a fluorescence microscope at a magnification of 250 × and only 30 fields need to be examined. If fluorescent particles are seen, they must be observed with higher magnification to confirm morphology typical of a tubercle bacillus. A smear can be examined in approximately 1.5 min with fluorescence microscopy (30 fields) as opposed to about 15 min by light microscopy (300 fields). A smear is considered negative unless 3 or more bacilli are seen during the examination, and 1–2 bacilli per 300 fields indicates that another specimen should be requested (Smithwick 1976).

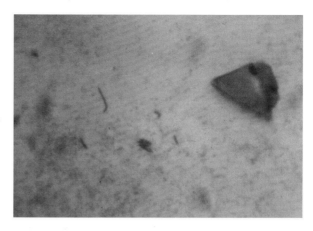

Fig. 26.1 *M. tuberculosis* in sputum stained by the Kinyoun cold staining procedure. See plate 26.1 for colour. (Photograph kindly provided by R W Smithwick, CDC).

5 CULTURAL CHARACTERISTICS

5.1 Culture media

Recovery of mycobacteria from their normal habitats is dependent on providing the conditions that are necessary for optimal growth. Most species are not very fastidious, but convincing evidence has not been presented to show growth of *M. leprae* in culture, and *M. genavense* has been grown in specific liquid medium but not on solid medium. Many media have been tried

from the time that Koch used heat-coagulated bovine or ovine serum as a solid medium and glycerinated beef broth as a liquid medium. Currently, 3 media are routinely used in most laboratories for primary isolation, drug susceptibility testing, biochemical tests and determination of colonial morphology. Löwenstein–Jensen (LJ) medium is most commonly used for growth of all mycobacteria. The medium is prepared with glycerol for the cultivation of *M. tuberculosis* or with sodium pyruvate for the cultivation of *M. bovis*, which grows poorly or not at all on the medium prepared with glycerol. Middlebrook 7H10 and 7H11 media are agar-based and used in many laboratories for general growth of mycobacteria, particularly for studies of colonial morphology. The latter 2 media were developed particularly to encourage the growth of isoniazid-resistant strains of *M. tuberculosis*, but they also encourage the growth of many species that require auxiliary growth factors. Middlebrook 7H9 liquid medium can be used to recover strains from stock culture, prepare inocula for tests of identification or drug susceptibility and make dilutions. Formulations for these media are described by Kent and Kubica (1985) and Collins, Grange and Yates (1985).

In clinical laboratories equipped to handle mycobacteria, slants of LJ medium are inoculated with a specimen that has been digested, decontaminated and concentrated (see section 5.5, p. 554). The usual inoculum is 0.1 ml of a treated clinical specimen or concentrated material from an environmental source. After spreading the inoculum over the surface of the slant, the tube is left in the slanted position for at least 7 days to permit even distribution of the inoculum over the entire surface of the medium. The tubes are then placed upright and incubation continues, at least 6 weeks for clinical specimens, but up to 12 or more weeks in rare instances when mycobacteria are suspected to be present but are not detected after 6 weeks. Incubation temperatures commonly used in the clinical laboratory are 35–37°C for growth of tubercle bacilli, 30–33°C for *M. marinum* and *M. ulcerans* and 42–43°C for *M. xenopi*.

5.2 Appearance on solid media

Colonies on solid media may appear as either smooth or rough, transparent or opaque. Colonial morphology is often suggested as a feature for identification; however, too much variation occurs in this characteristic for it to be used except as an indication of what the species might be. Characteristically, strains of *M. tuberculosis* form cords when growing on solid medium as shown in Fig. 26.2 (see also plate 26.2). When colonies are suspended in liquid or when they are grown in liquid culture, the cording characteristic can be seen clearly in stained preparations (Fig. 26.3, see also plate 26.3). Colonies of tubercle bacilli on solid medium typically appear as intertwined cords that are heaped up and dry and that may often have a smoother veil of growth surrounding the central formation (Fig. 26.2, see also plate 26.2). This eugonic colony form has often been described to have the appearance of bread crumbs and is in contrast to the dysgonic growth of *M. bovis* on a medium that contains glycerol.

Colonies of *M. avium* complex (*M. avium*, *M. intracelluare*, MAC) strains are smooth and transparent (T) in primary cultures of clinical specimens, but opaque (O) and rough (R) colonies develop in subcultures. The O forms are less virulent and less resistant to antimicrobial agents than the T colony types (Thoen, Himes and Karlson 1984). The basis of T and O variation, colonial morphology and serological types of MAC species and *M. scrofulaceum* appears to be related to the chemical structure of their surface antigens, exopolysaccharides and cell envelope (Brennan 1984,

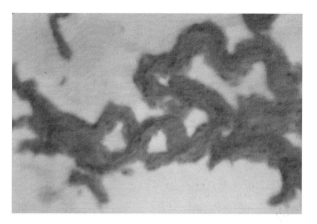

Fig. 26.3 Cording characteristic of *M. tuberculosis* grown in liquid culture (Kinyoun stain). See plate 26.3 for colour. (Photograph kindly provided by R W Smithwick, CDC).

Belisle and Brennan 1994). In addition, the virulence of *M. avium* strains may be associated with the presence of a particular surface glycopeptidolipid. These reactions are under study using newer procedures for clarification of the morphological changes and their associated host–parasite activities.

5.3 Appearance in liquid media

Mycobacteria grow as a surface pellicle in liquid medium unless a surfactant, such as the non-ionic detergent Tween 80, is added to lower the surface tension and permit diffuse growth (Youmans 1979). Pellicle growth has been used in many studies to maintain strain characteristics such as virulence. For example, growth of tubercle bacilli as a smooth pellicle on Proskauer and Beck synthetic medium helps maintain their virulence. However, growth in liquid media other than those containing Tween 80 have limited application in clinical laboratories, because mycobacteria grow most rapidly in liquid medium prepared with a surfactant.

5.4 Pigmentation

Runyon (1959, 1965) simplified the classification of *Mycobacterium* spp. by placing them into one of 4 groups with 2 easily determined cultural characteristics: speed of growth and pigmentation. Thus, species are described as rapidly growing or as slowly growing and photochromogenic, scotochromogenic, or non-photochromogenic. Scotochromogens produce yellow or orange pigment in the dark whereas photochromogens produce pigment after exposure to light.

The orange and yellow colours of the colonies result from an accumulation of carotenoid pigments, which are tetraterpenes of the general formula $C_{40}H_{56}$ (David 1984). The synthesis of the carotenoids is influenced by the composition of the medium and the growth conditions. Leprotene and β-carotene are the principal carotenes that accumulate, and whereas some species accumulate both, others will accumulate only one or the other. Distribution of carotenoid pigments in *Mycobacterium* spp. is reviewed by David (1984); how-

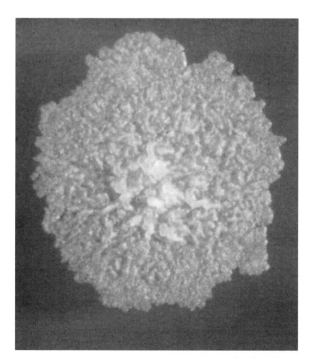

Fig. 26.2 Rough colony morphology of *M. tuberculosis* growing in Middlebrook 7H10 agar medium. See plate 26.2 for colour. (Photograph kindly provided by R W Smithwick, CDC).

ever, carotene content is not used for species identification because a standard content of pigment for each species has not been determined.

5.5 Preparation of specimens for primary culture

Patient specimens, especially sputum specimens, often contain micro-organisms other than mycobacteria and the organisms may be entrapped in mucus. Treatment with a mucolytic agent frees the mycobacteria and makes the specimen easier to process. Treatment with a toxic agent kills contaminating micro-organisms (Collin, Grange and Yates 1985, Kent and Kubica 1985), but overtreatment will also kill many of the mycobacteria. The N-acetyl-L-cysteine–sodium hydroxide (NALC–NaOH) method is the procedure used in most clinical laboratories in the USA (Kent and Kubica 1985, Heifets and Good 1994, Smithwick 1994). Other methods are available for use when contamination is heavy or when mycobacteria must be protected from harsh procedures. Specimens can also be inoculated into media containing antimicrobial agents such as penicillin which will control the growth of contaminants.

5.6 Conditions for growth

Media inoculated for primary isolation of mycobacteria should be incubated in an atmosphere of 10% CO_2 and 90% air to obtain optimal growth (Kent and Kubica 1985). Inoculated Middlebrook agar media require a CO_2 atmosphere to ensure growth, but CO_2 is not essential for growth on egg-based media, although it stimulates earlier, more luxuriant growth. To ensure penetration of the gas into containers, tubes should be incubated in the slanted position with caps loose for at least a week before caps are tightened, and plates should be placed medium side down in CO_2-permeable plastic bags until the inoculum has been absorbed. The optimal temperature for recovery of mycobacteria in the clinical laboratory is 35–37°C. However, if the specimen was obtained from skin or a superficial lesion suspected to contain M. marinum, M. ulcerans or M. haemophilum, incubation should be at 25–33°C, which is optimal for these species. Specimens suspected of containing M. avium or M. xenopi should be incubated at 40–42°C. In general, the optimal pH for growth of mycobacteria is 6.0–6.5, but this may vary from species to species.

Many Mycobacterium spp. are obligate aerobes that will grow at or near the surface of semisolid Middlebrook or Kirchner medium after inoculation with 0.2 ml of a suspension about 1 cm below the surface (Collins, Grange and Yates 1984). The inoculum must be mixed carefully with the medium to avoid air bubbles, and the bottle or tube must then be incubated without agitation for 18 days. Micro-aerophilic species grow as a narrow band 10–20 mm below the surface of the medium. Oxygen preference tested in this way is one of several tests used to identify species in the M. tuberculosis complex.

6 NUTRITIONAL REQUIREMENTS AND METABOLIC ACTIVITIES

Most Mycobacterium spp. do not require specific growth factors or vitamins, and the basic nutritional requirements of mycobacteria growing in axenic media are similar to those of other bacteria. These include carbon, nitrogen, oxygen, phosphorus, sulphur, iron, potassium, magnesium and trace elements (reviewed by Ratledge 1982, Wheeler and Ratledge 1994). Given the wide spectrum of ecological niches occupied by Mycobacterium spp., it is not surprising that the various species can use a wide range of compounds as sources of essential nutrients.

6.1 Carbon sources

As a whole, mycobacteria are metabolically very versatile, and various species of Mycobacterium can grow on a wide range of carbon sources including carbohydrates, organic acids, hydrocarbons and even CO_2. Laboratory culture medium traditionally contains glycerol as the carbon source because it is the only carbon source that can be utilized by all species of Mycobacterium, although it is not the optimal carbon source for many species. Pyruvate is a better carbon source for many species such as M. bovis. Various sugars, including glucose, fructose, sucrose, mannose, trehalose, inositol and mannitol, can also serve as preferred carbon sources. Organic acids, including short chain (pyruvic, acetic and citric) and long chain (oleic and palmitic) acids, can be utilized as carbon sources by many species. In fact, the oxidation of ^{14}C-labelled palmitic acid to release ^{14}C-labelled CO_2 forms the basis of a rapid automated system for the radiometric detection of mycobacterial growth.

Mycobacteria also express a number of hydrolytic and degradative activities, which suggests that they may be able to utilize additional sources of carbon. For example, Tween 80 can be hydrolysed to produce oleic acid which can then be used as a carbon source. Certain species can degrade polycyclic aromatic hydrocarbons. The ability to utilize or degrade certain carbon sources varies considerably between different species and is used in species identification tests.

6.2 Nitrogen sources

For laboratory media, the preferred nitrogen source is asparagine or glutamine, although mycobacteria can obtain nitrogen from many inorganic (e.g. NH_4^+ salts) and organic sources (e.g. amides, amines, amino acids, nucleosides). A few species may be able to assimilate nitrate or nitrite via nitrate and nitrite reductases to generate NH_3. Variation in nitrogen utilization and metabolism, particularly nitrate reduction and amidase activities, is used for species identification.

6.3 Acquisition of iron

Iron is essential for the growth of mycobacteria both in vivo and in vitro, and mycobacteria have evolved a sophisticated system for scavenging iron from the environment and their eukaryotic hosts (reviewed by Wheeler and Ratledge 1994). Mycobacteria secrete small, water-soluble iron-binding siderophores called exochelins. The MS-type of exochelin (e.g. produced by *M. smegmatis*) remain water-soluble at all stages, whereas the MB-type (e.g. produced by *M. tuberculosis*) become chloroform extractable when complexed with Fe(III). Each type of exochelin actually encompasses a family of small molecules whose masses range from approximately 0.7 to 0.8 kDa, which reflects varying numbers of CH_2 groups on an alkyl side chain (Gobin et al. 1995). Exochelins extract iron from various iron-containing molecules in their vicinity (e.g. ferritin) by virtue of their very high affinity for ferric ions (K_s of c. 10^{25} M). The ferriexochelin can then interact with a specific protein receptor on the mycobacterial cell surface and be transported to the interior of the cell. Alternatively, the ferric iron may be transferred to a related membrane-bound molecule called mycobactin (K_s of c. 10^{36} M). Mycobactins and exochelins share a common iron-binding core but differ in alkyl side chains which accounts for the differences in polarity. Mycobactins can also bind free ferric ion and facilitate the transport of it across the membrane to the interior of the bacterium. Release of the iron from either ferri-exochelin or ferrimycobactin is accomplished by reduction of the ferric ion to ferrous ion by a NADH-dependent reductase.

Members of all species of *Mycobacterium*, except *M. paratuberculosis* and some strains of *M. avium*, produce mycobactins and growth of these bacilli requires the addition of mycobactin to culture medium. Mycobactins isolated from various species differ in substitutions in the iron-binding core; within a species, mycobactins differ in the length of alkyl chains. Because of the efficient iron scavenging systems, most mycobacteria require only small amounts of iron (1 μg Fe per ml) in culture medium for growth. *M. haemophilum* is unusual in that it requires high iron concentrations (2% ferric ammonium citrate or 40 μg haemin per ml) for growth.

6.4 Other requirements for growth

Mycobacteria require several inorganic elements for growth including sodium, potassium, magnesium, sulphur and phosphorus as well as a variety of trace elements, primarily zinc and manganese. CO_2 is essential for optimal growth of many species (Ratledge 1982) and is usually included in media as $NaHCO_3/Na_2CO_3$ or as CO_2 in the gas phase (5–10%).

7 METABOLIC PATHWAYS IN MYCOBACTERIA

In general, metabolic activities of mycobacteria are similar to those of other bacteria, and basic pathways for assimilation of nutrients, energy production, metabolism and biosynthesis of macromolecules are like those of most bacteria. General metabolic pathways and enzyme systems have been reviewed

(Ratledge 1982, Wheeler and Ratledge 1994). Of course, mycobacteria do have several unique biochemical activities related to the synthesis of mycobacteria-specific compounds such as mycolic acids or phenolic glycolipid I of *M. leprae*. Also, individual species express characteristic sets of enzymatic activities, probably related to their ecological niches, and these characteristic activities are exploited in species identification tests (see section 15.4, p. 571).

The reasons mycobacteria grow so slowly (generation times of c. 3 h for rapid growers and 18–24 h for slow growers) are not known. Possible explanations include:

1 decreased diffusion or transport of required nutrients across the thick, hydrophobic cell wall
2 differences in key respiratory enzymes or energy production
3 decreased rates of nucleic acid biosynthesis
4 increased energy and nutrient requirements for production of large amounts of cell wall lipids, which can account for 10% of the cell dry weight and
5 fewer ribosomal RNA genes (one copy in *M. tuberculosis*, 2 copies in *M. smegmatis*, 7 in *Escherichia coli*).

Also, relatively little is known about metabolic activities in 2 environments which are important in mycobacteria-caused diseases. First, the environment encountered by an intracellular pathogen is quite different from that encountered on an agar slant. So far, few studies have analysed the metabolic activities of in vivo grown mycobacteria, although Barclay and Wheeler (1989) characterized some of the nutritional features of the intracellular environment and the corresponding mycobacterial metabolic activities. Second, both *M. tuberculosis* and *M. leprae* can persist in the human host for long periods in an apparently metabolically dormant state. An in vitro model of persisters has been developed by Wayne and Lin (1982) in which tubercle bacilli are allowed to settle to the bottom of a liquid culture. These bacilli cease to replicate, reduce their oxidative metabolism and survive in anaerobic conditions much longer than actively metabolizing cells. Analyses of these bacilli may provide clues to the nature of in vivo dormancy and persistence (Wayne 1994).

7.1 Metabolic activities used in identification tests

In the diagnostic laboratory, species of *Mycobacterium* are routinely identified based on their metabolic activities (see section 15.4, p. 571). This is possible, in part, because highly reproducible and standardized tests for various metabolic activities were developed through co-operative studies directed by the IWGMT (Wayne et al. 1974, 1976). Key identification tests include those for niacin production, arylsulphatase activity, catalase activity, nitrate reductase activity, acid phosphatase activity (Collins, Grange and Yates 1985, Kent and Kubica 1985, Nolte and Metchock 1995).

8 SUSCEPTIBILITY TO CHEMICAL AND PHYSICAL AGENTS

Mycobacteria are as susceptible as other non-spore-forming bacteria to heat and to some other physical and chemical agents, although some early work on the heat susceptibility of mycobacteria may have suggested otherwise (reviewed by Corper and Cohn 1937). For example, the conditions for pasteurization of milk were selected on the basis of the killing curves for tubercle bacilli (55°C for 1 h), because at that time they were considered the most heat-resistant organisms in milk. The discrepancies in the early studies were probably due to differences in methodology and selection of an end point. Materials containing mycobacteria can be readily sterilized by the standard conditions used (15 min at 121°C for clean materials and 30–60 min for infectious wastes) (Marsik and Denys 1995).

Heat susceptibility varies among the *Mycobacterium* spp. For example, the kill rate for a strain of *M. avium* isolated from human and porcine tissues was not significant at 60°C, whereas the decimal reduction values (D values) were 4 min or less at 65°C and 1.5 min or less at 70°C (Merkal and Crawford 1979). The temperature required to kill *M. bovis* was 6–7°C lower than that for *M. avium* in meat products (Merkal and Whipple 1980), and in a study of 9 species frequently isolated from domestic water supplies (Schulze-Robbecke and Buchholtz 1992), D values at 55°C ranged from 6 min for an isolate of *M. kansasii* to about 6 h for an isolate of *M. xenopi*. Of the other isolates tested, *M. phlei* was rather heat-resistant, *M. marinum* was rather susceptible, and the 6 other species tested (*M. avium*, *M. chelonae*, *M. fortuitum*, *M. intracellulare* and *M. scrofulaceum*) were intermediate in their susceptibility to heat. A confounding variable in these studies, however, is that growth conditions affect D values. For example, a population of cultured *M. avium* bacilli inoculated into a processed meat product had a D value of 28 min at 60°C, whereas bacilli harvested from tubercles in the liver and spleen of a naturally infected pig were found to have a D value of 1 min at 60°C (Merkal, Lyle and Whipple 1981).

Mycobacteria are generally resistant to acids and alkalis, and this feature is used to advantage in isolation procedures. As much as 2% sodium hydroxide, 2% sulphuric acid or 2.5% oxalic acid can be used to kill contaminants in specimens prior to culture. However, the killing activity of acids and alkalis increases with increasing temperature of exposure, and resistance varies greatly among different species, so care must be taken in any decontamination procedure to avoid killing the mycobacteria of interest. Tubercle bacilli are also resistant to quaternary ammonium compounds and, indeed, cetylpyridinium chloride has been used for decontamination of clinical specimens prior to culture (Kent and Kubica 1985).

With respect to chemical disinfectants, mycobacteria are susceptible to a variety of chemical agents including: alcohols (ethyl and isopropyl although the latter is not as active as the former), chlorine, glutaraldehyde, iodophores, phenolic compounds, ethylene oxide, formaldehyde and hydrogen peroxide (Marsik and Denys 1995). Derivatives of phenol, in which a functional group (e.g. chloro, benzyl, phenyl or amyl) replaces one of the hydrogen atoms on the aromatic ring, are effective and safe to use (Marsik and Denys 1995). The 3 most commonly used derivatives are *ortho*-phenylphenol, *ortho*-benzyl-*para*-chlorophenol

and *para*-tertiary amylphenol. A 10-fold dilution of household bleach (5.25% sodium hypochlorite) provides a solution with approximately 5000 ppm available chlorine, which may be used for immersion of contaminated glassware, in discard pans in biological safety cabinets and for general laboratory clean-up. However, the amount of chlorine needed to kill the various species of *Mycobacterium* ranges from 1000 to 10 000 ppm (Best et al. 1990, Marsik and Denys 1995). Vaporization of *para*-formaldehyde crystals is used for the disinfection of large areas. The conditions for this procedure are very detailed since the area must be sealed to prevent the escape of toxic gas (CDC/NIH 1993).

Endoscopes are a potential source for the spread of mycobacteria and represent a challenge for disinfection. Alkaline 2% solutions of glutaraldehyde at pH 7.4–8.5 have been used, but Marsik and Denys (1995) caution that the claims for its activity against mycobacteria must be evaluated carefully and the exposure time must be adequate to assure tuberculocidal activity. Rutala and Weber (1995) reviewed studies relating to the tuberculocidal activity of glutaraldehyde and concluded that the number of bacilli on endoscopes could be reduced by 4 logs by a standardized cleaning protocol including immersion in a glutaraldehyde solution for 20 min at 20°C. Current requirements are that endoscopes be immersed in the glutaraldehyde solution at 25°C for 45 min.

Mycobacteria are resistant to drying and can survive for long periods on inanimate objects if protected from ultraviolet (UV) light, which is highly tuberculocidal. For example, 90% of a population of 10^6–10^7 cells of *M. tuberculosis* suspended in tap water at a depth of 2 cm can be killed by exposure to 5000 μW s cm^{-2} of UV light or by 99.99% with exposure to 20 000 μW s cm^{-2} of UV light, doses that are similar to those required to kill other bacteria (Rubbo and Gardner 1965). Tubercle bacilli can remain suspended as a stable aerosol in air for many hours. The persistence of tubercle bacilli on surfaces and in air prompted development of methods for removal including treatment of the air and surfaces with UV light (Riley 1957, 1961), filtration of room air through high efficiency particulate air filters (Rutala et al. 1995) and the use of respirators by health care personnel (Nettleman et al.1994). Each procedure can clearly reduce the number of tubercle bacilli available to be inhaled, but the overall efficiency of each procedure for preventing transmission must be evaluated case by case, and the chosen method tailored to the specific conditions of control (Iseman 1992, Nardell 1993). These aspects of tuberculosis control procedures are discussed further in Volume 3 (see Volume 3, Chapter 21).

8.1 Susceptibility to antimicrobial agents

Diseases caused by *Mycobacterium* spp. are difficult to treat and the search for effective drugs has been active, the most intensive search being for drugs effective against tuberculosis, the mycobacterial disease of greatest public health significance. Doub (1979) recounts some of the early events leading to the development of antituberculosis drugs and concludes that 'of those that succeed (as antituberculosis drugs), it is a story of serendipity and of chemical intermediates for planned drugs'. Synthetic drugs developed include *p*-aminosalicylic acid (PAS), thiacetazone, pyrazinamide (PZA), isoniazid (INH), ethionamide and ethambutol. Antibiotics active against tuberculosis are streptomycin, viomycin, cycloserine, kanamycin, capreomycin and rifampicin. One of the newer active drugs is ofloxacin, a fluorinated carboxyquinolone. Other compounds effective against mycobacteria other than *M. tuberculosis* include dapsone, clofazimine, clarithromycin and tetracycline. The modes of action of the antimycobacterial drugs have been reviewed (Winder 1982, Rastogi and David 1992, Musser 1995) and current treatment recommendations are discussed in Volume 3 (see Volume 3, Chapters 21, 23 and 22).

The reliability and standardization of methods for testing the susceptibility of *M. tuberculosis* isolates to antituberculosis drugs were discussed by Canetti et al. (1969) and the methods used routinely in most mycobacteriology laboratories have been reviewed (Collins et al. 1985, Kent and Kubica 1985, Heifets and Good 1994, Inderlied and Salfinger 1995). A key to producing reliable results is the use of standardized drug concentrations to determine if a strain is resistant. As defined by Canetti et al. (1963): 'Resistance is clinically significant when at least 1% of the total bacterial population develops at the so-called critical concentrations.' The 'critical concentration' is the weakest concentration of drug that inhibits the growth of >95% of wild-type isolates of a given species using precisely defined experimental conditions. For *M. tuberculosis*, the critical concentration of isoniazid in 7H10 medium is 0.2 μg ml^{-1}, rifampin is 1.0 μg ml^{-1}, PZA is 25.0 μg ml^{-1}, and ethambutol is 5.0 μg ml^{-1} (Kent and Kubica 1985). Additional concentrations are often tested to provide information to physicians to assist them in designing a therapeutic regimen. Therefore, isoniazid is routinely tested at 0.2, 1.0 and 5.0 μg ml^{-1}, and streptomycin is tested at 2.0 and 10 μg ml^{-1}. However, the critical concentration is always included so that there is a historical basis to determine if resistance increases in specific populations over time. Recognition of the emergence of resistance and the need to insert new drugs into a treatment regimen are dependent on collection of accurate data.

ISONIAZID

INH (isonicotinic acid hydrazide) was first synthesized in the early part of the twentieth century, but its activity against tubercle bacilli was not discovered until mid-century. The drug has been the mainstay of antituberculosis therapy for more than 40 years, but neither the target site in the mycobacterial cell nor the mode of action is well understood (Zhang and Young 1993, Musser 1995). The antibacterial spectrum of INH is limited largely to inhibition of strains of *M. tuberculosis*. The MIC for susceptible strains of *M. tuberculosis* is usually less than 0.05 μg ml^{-1}, and other species in the *M. tuberculosis* complex are also highly susceptible. However, MAC strains and strains of other species are not susceptible to INH. Middle-

brook (1954) found that there was a link between INH resistance and reduced catalase activity. However, the exact relationship and molecular basis are still unknown, although one working hypothesis that INH or an INH metabolite blocks the synthesis of mycolic acids (Zhang and Young 1993, Musser 1995). In fact, INH can inhibit the activity of a particulate enzyme complex that controls the synthesis of mycolic acids (Rastogi and David 1992). The molecular basis of INH resistance may involve mutations in the *katG* gene, but INH resistance in all strains cannot be ascribed to changes in this gene (Zhang and Young 1993, Banerjee et al. 1994, Musser 1995).

RIFAMPICIN

Rifampicin was introduced in 1968 for the treatment of tuberculosis and is a first-line drug along with isoniazid, pyrazinamide and ethambutol. It is a broad spectrum antibiotic which is active against *M. leprae*, *M. kansasii*, *M. haemophilum* and *M. marinum* as well as bacteria in other genera. The mechanism of action is similar to that in *E. coli* and involves inhibition of DNA-dependent RNA polymerase (Jin and Gross 1988, Musser 1995). A derivative, rifabutin, is widely used for the treatment of *M. avium* infections (Horsburgh 1991) and in prophylactic regimens to prevent infection with *M. avium* in AIDS patients (Masur et al. 1993, Nightingale et al. 1993, Havlir 1994).

PYRAZINAMIDE

Pyrazinamide (PZA) is a synthetic derivative of nicotinamide which is rapidly bactericidal for reproducing cells of *M. tuberculosis* and the average MIC is 20 μg ml^{-1} (Inderlied and Salfinger 1995). The drug is inactive against non-replicating tubercle bacilli and against all other species of mycobacteria including *M. bovis*, MAC and rapid growers. Optimal in vitro activity of PZA is observed at pH 5.5–6.0. Neither the mechanism of action nor the molecular basis for resistance is fully known (Musser 1995) although there is evidence that the enzyme that hydrolyses PZA to pyrazinoic acid is essential to susceptibility to the drug (Butler and Kilburn 1983).

ETHAMBUTOL

Ethambutol (EMB) is a synthetic compound introduced in 1961 for the treatment of tuberculosis. Preliminary studies were carried out with the racemic mixture of the compound, but only the D isomer is effective. The D isomer is also less toxic than the racemic mixture. MICs against wild-type isolates of *M. tuberculosis* are 1–5 μg ml^{-1}, but the drug is rather inactive against other species (Inderlied and Salfinger 1995). EMB inhibits cell wall synthesis and is bacteriostatic. The mechanism of action probably involves inhibition of arabinogalactan synthesis (Takayama and Kilburn 1989) or synthesis of precursors of cell wall components (Musser 1995). The drug has a synergistic effect in combination with ciprofloxacin, amikacin and rifampicin against *M. malmoense* (Hoffner, Hjelm and Kallenius 1993).

DAPSONE

Dapsone, diaminodiphenyl sulphone, is a synthetic compound that inhibits folic acid synthesis. It is bacteriostatic or weakly bactericidal against *M. leprae* and has been the drug of choice for treatment of leprosy since the 1940s (Shepard 1981, Shinnick 1992). However, as is typical for mycobacteria-caused diseases, treatment with just one drug led to the development of drug-resistant bacilli. Hence, in more recent years, the drug has been used with great success in combination therapy with rifampicin and clofazimine. Entry of this hydrophilic drug into the cell may be by diffusion through an aqueous porin channel in the same manner as other antimycobacterial agents, such as INH, PZA, PAS and cycloserine (Connell and Nikaido 1994).

CLOFAZIMINE

Clofazimine, a synthetic bright red dye, is highly active in vitro against *M. tuberculosis* and other mycobacteria. Unfortunately, the drug is not as effective in vivo for the treatment of tuberculosis and other mycobacterial infections even though it is deposited in fatty tissues and in cells of the reticuloendothelial system where it may be present for long periods. The effectiveness of the drug for treatment of MAC infection is probably due to the rather high serum level which helps control bacteraemia. Recommendations for treating disseminated MAC disease include clofazimine in combination with other drugs (Masur et al. 1993). Clofazimine has weak bactericidal activity against *M. leprae* and is used in combination with rifampicin and dapsone for the treatment of leprosy (Inderlied and Salfinger 1995).

AZITHROMYCIN AND CLARITHROMYCIN

Azithromycin and clarithromycin are macrolide antibiotics that are active against MAC infections, disease caused by rapidly growing mycobacteria and leprosy (Inderlied and Salfinger 1995). Clarithromycin inhibits 90% of MAC isolates at MICs of 0.25–0.5 μg ml^{-1}, and a positive clinical response was obtained in HIV-infected patients treated with 500 mg of the drug twice a day. Unfortunately, clarithromycin monotherapy led to the development of drug-resistant bacilli, and the resistance to clarithromycin was associated with changes in the 23S rRNA gene as in other bacteria (Musser 1995).

STREPTOMYCIN

Streptomycin is an aminoglycoside antibiotic that has been used extensively in the treatment of tuberculosis. However, the drug must be given by injection and, over the years, it lost popularity and became difficult to obtain. Ototoxicity is the major side effect associated with the drug. It is active in vitro against *M. tuberculosis*, *M. kansasii* and *M. marinum*. About 66% of streptomycin-resistant strains of *M. tuberculosis* display changes in the *rpsL* or 16S rRNA gene, as is seen in other bacteria (Musser 1995). This observation implies that there is at least one additional mechanism conferring resistance.

9 CELL WALL STRUCTURE AND COMPONENTS

Mycobacteria have a complex outer envelope composed of several distinct layers (reviewed by Besra and Chatterjee 1994, Brennan and Draper 1994). The innermost layer is the plasma membrane which displays an asymmetric bilayer structure. Inserted into it are proteins, phosphatidylinositol mannosides and lipoarabinomannan. Next is the peptidoglycan layer, which determines the shape of the cell and which is similar to peptidoglycans of other gram-positive bacteria. It contains repeating disaccharide units of *N*-acetylglucosamine-(β1–4)-*N*-glycolylmuramic acid cross-linked via L-alanyl-D-isoglutaminyl-*meso*-diaminopimelyl-D-alanine tetrapeptides, except in *M. leprae* where the L-alanine is replaced by glycine (Draper 1986). About 10% of the *N*-glycolylmuramic acid residues are covalently attached to a branched chain polysaccharide, arabinogalactan, via phosphodiester bonds. The terminal and penultimate arabinose residues of the arabinogalactan molecules are esterified to high molecular weight mycolic acids. Finally, the outer surface of the mycobacterium is formed by the intercalation of medium chain (e.g. mycocerosates) and short chain (e.g. acylglycerols) lipids, glycolipids and peptidoglycolipids into the uneven, hydrophobic layer of mycolic acids. Proteins (e.g. porins, transport proteins) are found throughout the various layers.

Several components of the mycobacterial envelope are strongly immunologically active (Stewart-Tull 1983). For example, whole heat-killed mycobacteria are strong adjuvants and are the basis of Freund's complete adjuvant (heat-killed mycobacteria in oil). It is the peptidoglycan (murein) layer which contains this adjuvant activity, and a water-soluble fragment of the peptidoglycan called muramyl dipeptide (MDP, *N*-acetylmuramyl-L-alanyl-D-isoglutamine) also acts as an adjuvant. MDP has the advantages over heat-killed mycobacteria that it can be chemically synthesized, it is commercially available and it is not immunogenic (i.e. does not elicit an immune response to itself). Lipoarabinomannan is also highly immunoreactive (see section on 'Lipoarabinomannan').

9.1 Lipids

A prominent feature of the outer surface of mycobacteria is its high content of lipid, which accounts for up to 60% of the cell wall weight and which contributes to several biological features, including the hydrophobicity of mycobacteria, the tendency of mycobacteria to form clumps or cords, the resistance of mycobacteria to common lysis procedures, and the ability of mycobacteria to survive intracellularly (reviewed by Brennan et al. 1990, Besra and Chatterjee 1994). In general, the lipids are long chain fatty acids (e.g. $CH_3(CH_2)_nCOOH$) which are often modified by the presence of unsaturated bonds, cyclopropane rings, or side groups such as methyl, methoxy, hydroxyl and keto groups. Well characterized mycobacterial fatty acids include tuberculostearic acid and mycoserosic acid.

LIPOARABINOMANNAN

Lipoarabinomannan (LAM) is structurally and functionally related to the O-antigenic lipopolysaccharides of other bacteria (reviewed by Brennan et al. 1990, Besra and Chatterjee 1994). LAM is thought to be anchored in the plasma membrane and to extend through the cell wall to the surface of the mycobacterium. The membrane anchor is a diacylglycerol moiety, which in *M. tuberculosis* contains palmitic and tuberculostearic acids and which is attached to a phosphatidylinositol residue via a phosphodiester linkage. The polysaccharide backbone is also attached to the phosphatidylinositol and consists of α(1–6)-linked D-mannose residues to which short side chains of α(1–2)-linked D-mannose residues and α(1–5)-linked D-arabinose residues are attached. The termini of the LAM molecules may be branched hexa-arabinosides or linear tetra-arabinosides (Chatterjee et al. 1992a) and the arabinose termini may be capped with 1–3 mannose residues (Chatterjee et al. 1992b). Capped LAM molecules are called manLAM and uncapped ones are called araLAM.

Biological activities of LAM include strong seroreactivity, inhibition of interferon-γ mediated activation of macrophages, induction of cytokine production and release by macrophages, scavenging reactive oxygen intermediates and suppression of T cell proliferation (Kaplan et al. 1987, Sibley et al. 1988, Barnes et al. 1992, Chatterjee et al. 1992c). Several parts of LAM are involved in these biological activities (reviewed by Besra and Chatterjee 1994). The terminal arabinose units are targets of circulating antibodies, and the degree of mannosylation of the terminal arabinose units influences the biological activities of LAM (e.g. ability to induce TNF-α production) (Chatterjee et al. 1992c). This difference may be related to virulence. The acyl groups are also required for some biological activities, such as the induction of cytokine production, because removal of the acyl groups by mild alkali treatment abolishes the activity.

MYCOLIC ACIDS

Mycolic acids are a defining characteristic of members of the genus *Mycobacterium*, although related long chain fatty acids are found in the genera *Corynebacterium* (corynomycolic acids containing 28–40 carbon atoms) and *Nocardia* (nocardomycolic acids containing 40–60 carbon atoms). The mycobacterial mycolic acids are α-branched, β-hydroxy fatty acids with 60–90 carbon atoms in the primary chain. The alkyl branches are attached to the α-position (the CH_2 group adjacent to the terminal carboxylic acid) and typically contain 22–26 carbon atoms. Mycolic acids are categorized according to oxygen-containing modifications found in the primary chain. Mycolic acids that do not contain any oxygen functions in addition to the β-hydroxy group are called α-mycolates, those containing keto groups are ketomycolates, those with methoxy groups are methoxymycolates, and those with epoxy groups are epoxymycolates.

Each species of *Mycobacterium* appears to synthesize a unique set of mycolic acids (Minnikin and Goodfellow 1980, Butler and Kilburn 1988), and this has been exploited for speciating mycobacteria (Fig. 26.4). In this procedure, mycolic acids are extracted from saponified mycobacteria, converted to *p*-bromophenacyl esters and analysed by high performance liquid chromatography (HPLC). The resulting pattern is compared to a library of reference patterns to identify the species. This rapid assay can provide definitive species identification for essentially any of more than 50 *Mycobacterium* spp. in less than 4 h (plus the time required for producing a pure culture), in contrast to the weeks required for conventional tests for speciation.

ACEYLATED TREHALOSES

In 1950, Bloch isolated 6,6'-dimycolyl-α,α'-D-trehalose (trehalose dimycolate or TDM) and suggested it was the cell surface component responsible for the ability of virulent tubercle bacilli to form serpentine cords and to absorb the cationic phenazine dye neutral red. Subsequent studies have not borne out a role for trehalose dimycolate in either cord formation or virulence. Regardless, biological activities associated with cord factor include systemic toxicity, granulomagenic activity and cytokine induction (Goren 1982).

Other trehalose-based lipids found in *M. tuberculosis* are sulpholipids, which are thought to play a role in the intracellular survival of tubercle bacilli by inhibiting phagosome activation (Goren, Vatter and Fiscus 1987). The sulpholipids are based on trehalose

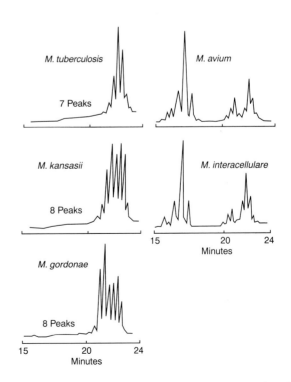

Fig. 26.4 HPLC patterns of mycolic acids from 5 species of *Mycobacterium*. (Photograph kindly provided by W R Butler, CDC).

2'-sulphate acetylated with hydroxyphthioceranic, phthioceranic and saturated straight chain fatty acids such as palmitate and stearate. Additional polar (Minnikin et al. 1985) and non-polar (Besra et al. 1992) acetylated trehaloses have been described and suggested to be virulence factors, because these compounds have been found only in virulent strains of *M. tuberculosis*.

Mycosides

The outer surface of a mycobacterium contains a heterogenous group of biologically and immunologically active medium and short chain lipids, which are analogous structurally and functionally to the O antigens of gram-negative enteric bacteria (reviewed by Minnikin 1982, Besra and Chatterjee 1994). These substances, collectively called mycosides, were discovered in 1957 by infrared microscopy of cell wall extracts and defined as type-specific glycolipids of mycobacteria (Smith et al. 1957). The mycosides fall into 2 major classes:

1 peptidoglycolipids which contain mycoserosic acid, sugars and amino acids and
2 phenol-phthiocerol glycosides.

Peptidoglycolipids often contain unusual sugar residues such as O-methyl rhamnose, fucose or deoxytalose and play roles in determining serotype, colony morphology and virulence. For example, peptidoglycolipids form the basis of an agglutination serotyping scheme for members of the *M. avium* complex. A peptidolipid also serves as the receptor for phage D4 attachment to mycobacterial cells.

Mycosides lacking amino acids are typically derivatives of phenol-phthiocerol and have been isolated and characterized from *M. kansasii*, *M. bovis*, *M. marinum* and *M. leprae*. Phenolic glycolipid I (PGL-I) is found only in *M. leprae* and is synthesized and shed in large amounts (reviewed by Shinnick 1992). The immune response to the trisaccharide component of PGL-I has been used in immunodiagnostic tests to detect persons infected with *M. leprae*. In addition, PGL-I can scavenge reactive oxygen intermediates and hence may play a role in the ability of *M. leprae* to survive within macrophages (Chan et al. 1989). PGL-I has also been implicated as playing a role in the specific immunosuppression seen in lepromatous leprosy patients (Mehra et al. 1984).

A few mycosides, including one that was isolated from an attenuated strain of *M. tuberculosis*, lack sugar residues. Because this mycoside appears to be characteristic of the attenuated strain, it has been named the 'attenuation indicator lipid' (Goren, Brokl and Schaefer 1974). The role of this mycoside in virulence is not known.

10 Antigens

Robert Koch's studies with antigens present in filtrates of cultures of *M. tuberculosis* were the beginning of a great deal of research, which still continues today, to define and characterize mycobacterial antigens. The importance of this work lies in the use of the antigens to detect infections or disease caused by mycobacteria or to classify, identify, or subtype mycobacteria.

10.1 Tuberculins

A key tool in many tuberculosis control programmes is the tuberculin skin test, which measures the cellular immune response to mycobacterial antigens. Koch developed 2 tuberculins, Old Tuberculin, which was a filtrate of several-week-old broth cultures of *M. tuberculosis* concentrated by evaporation, and New Tuberculin, which was a finely ground, vacuum-dried preparation of tubercle bacilli reconstituted in a glycerol–water mixture (Koch 1891). Many studies followed to improve the specificity of Old Tuberculin or to remove impurities by ammonium sulphate or trichloroacetic acid precipitation and culminated in the development of Purified Protein Derivative (PPD) (Seibert and Glenn 1941), which is still used throughout the world today. Subsequent attempts to improve PPD by the isolation of individual antigens have not yet produced a clinically useful reagent (reviewed by Daniel and Janicki 1978). In attempts to circumvent potential problems caused by the denaturation of proteins during the production of PPD, Stanford improved 'New Tuberculin' by harvesting bacilli from Sauton's medium, washing them, disrupting them in an ultrasonicator, separating cytoplasm from cell wall debris by centrifugation, sterilizing the supernatant by repeated membrane filtration and standardizing the protein concentration of the filtrate (Stanford 1983).

Skin test reagents have also been developed for other species of *Mycobacterium*. For example, Stanford and colleagues developed 'new tuberculins' for a variety of pathogenic and environmental mycobacteria, including Burulin which has been used in studies of *M. ulcerans* infections (Stanford et al. 1975, Stanford 1983). Lepromin, a heat-sterilized homogenate of *M. leprae*-laden tissue, is a skin test reagent used in the diagnosis of leprosy.

10.2 Soluble antigens

Mycobacterial antigens have been classified generally in terms of their chemical nature and distribution among species. Soluble antigens are the antigens found in the supernatant following high speed centrifugation of a lysate of mycobacteria, which removes cell wall fragments and other particulate matter. These antigens include most cytoplasmic and secreted proteins and soluble carbohydrates. The soluble antigens have been divided into 4 groups based on their distribution among species of *Mycobacterium* (Stanford and Grange 1974). Group I antigens are common to all species of *Mycobacterium* and some may also be found in species of *Nocardia* and *Corynebacterium*. Group II antigens are found only in slowly growing *Mycobacterium* spp. Group III antigens are found in rapidly growing species of *Mycobacterium* and may also be found in species of *Nocardia*. Group IV antigens are those unique to an individual species. Overall, these groupings suggest that mycobacteria evolved from a common ancestral form and that the rapid and slow growers diverged early in evolution, consistent with the interpretation of 16S rRNA phylogenetic trees (see section 2, p. 550). Also, the sharing of antigens by the various species probably accounts for the lack of specificity of serological tests for tuberculosis.

Various chemical and immunochemical techniques have been used to characterize soluble antigens, including immunoelectrophoresis (Daniel and Janicki 1978), double diffusion in agar gel (Stanford and Grange 1974) and crossed immunoelectrophoresis (Closs et al. 1980). Although these tests identifed up to 90 distinct lines of precipitation or antigens, until recently, only limited progress was made in characterizing a few of the precipitins because of difficulties in isolating and purifying the individual antigens. These difficulties were partially circumvented by the use of recombinant DNA technologies (see section 11). Currently, mycobacterial antigens are being systematically characterized using a variety of sophisticated techniques including 2-dimensional gel electrophoresis, mass spectroscopy and HPLC. Overall, the combination of immunological studies, sophisticated biochemistry, recombinant DNA technologies and the genome sequencing projects is producing a valuable catalogue of mycobacterial antigens (reviewed by Young et al. 1992, Anderson and Brennan 1994, Cole and Smith 1994).

One subset of soluble antigens contains proteins that are secreted during growth. The secreted proteins are the main antigenic constituents of culture filtrates of young, log-phase cultures of *M. tuberculosis*. Older cultures contain secreted proteins as well as many proteins released by autolysis of the tubercle bacilli. Secreted antigens have been suggested to be key targets of a protective immune response to *M. tuberculosis* (Horwitz et al. 1995, Roberts et al. 1995).

10.3 Insoluble antigens

Insoluble antigens are those that are in the pellet following high speed centifugation of lysates and include cell wall components, membrane-bound proteins, high molecular weight carbohydrates, lipids, mycolic acids, phenolic glycolipids, etc. Their immunoreactivity is discussed in section 9 (p. 558).

The antigenic behaviour of whole mycobacteria has been used for the subtyping of strains. That is, mycobacteria that form stable smooth suspensions can be typed using seroagglutination tests. For example, serotyping of *M. avium* complex strains has been used extensively in identification and epidemiological studies (Wolinsky and Schafer 1973, Stanford 1983). The antigens responsible for serotyping behaviour have been identified as sugar moieties on mycosides or peptidoglycolipids (see section 9, p. 558).

11 THE GENOME

The genomes of mycobacteria display a typical bacterial chromosomal structure (a single large circular DNA molecule), contain about 3×10^6 base pairs of DNA and have a G + C content of 60–70 mol% (except *M. leprae*, which is 55 mol%). Molecular and recombi-

nant DNA analyses of mycobacterial genomes revealed that:

1 the genomes of most species of *Mycobacterium* contain repetitive DNA elements
2 mycobacteria have only one or 2 copies of the genes encoding the ribosomal RNAs and these genes are arranged in the typical rRNA operon and
3 the genomic DNAs of *M. leprae* and *M. tuberculosis* display surprisingly little variation in strains isolated from around the world (reviewed by Clark-Curtiss 1990).

The ultimate definition of the structure of the mycobacterial genome will come from determination of the nucleotide sequence of the entire genome; because so much information can be gained from such a nucleotide sequence, great efforts are being expended on determining the sequences of the genomes of *M. leprae* and *M. tuberculosis* (reviewed by Bergh and Cole 1994, Cole and Smith 1994). These data will be a tremendous resource for researchers and will allow them to concentrate on addressing the biologically important questions of the regulation of gene expression and the structure and function of the gene products.

11.1 Repeated sequences

Mycobacterial repeated DNA elements range from short stretches of sequences rich in G + C to insertion elements and transposons. Individual repeated DNA elements may be found only in certain species of *Mycobacterium* (e.g. IS6110 in the *M. tuberculosis* complex or IS900 in *M. paratuberculosis*) or may be found in many species (e.g. the major polymorphic tandem repeat) (Eisenach, Crawford and Bates 1986, McFadden et al. 1987, Clark-Curtiss and Docherty 1989, Hermans, van Soolingen and van Embden 1992). Species-specific elements have been used as hybridization probes and targets of polymerase chain reaction assays to detect and identify mycobacteria in clinical specimens (reviewed by Crawford 1996). Because the location of repetitive elements in the genome can vary dramatically among isolates of a given species, certain repetitive DNA elements have also been exploited in strain identification and fingerprinting systems (see section on 'IS6110 fingerprinting', p. 563).

11.2 Genes and gene products

The vast majority of the characterized genes of mycobacteria are structurally similar to those of other bacterial genera. By contrast, the *recA* genes of *M. tuberculosis* and *M. leprae* are quite unusual (reviewed by Colston and Davis 1994). That is, the *recA* gene of *M. tuberculosis* encodes an 85 kDa protein, although the mature *M. tuberculosis* RecA protein has a molecular mass of only c. 38 kDa. The primary translation product of the *M. tuberculosis recA* gene contains an internal amino acid sequence, called an intein, which is removed by a protein splicing mechanism to produce an enzymatically active RecA protein. This is an interesting phenomenon because so few examples of protein splicing are known and because it may be a novel way to regulate protein expression and function. The *M. leprae recA* gene also contains an intein, but its structure and location are different from those of the *M. tuberculosis* intein.

11.3 Mycobacterial proteins

Much of the early work into characterizing mycobacterial proteins was aimed at producing better immunological reagents to detect tuberculosis. Unfortunately, classic biochemical approaches met with limited success because of difficulties in growing large quantities of highly pathogenic mycobacteria and in disrupting the bacilli and isolating native proteins. Recently, however, Brennan and colleagues began using state-of-the-art analytical procedures to isolate and characterize proteins of *M. tuberculosis* and *M. leprae*. Their efforts have produced:

1 reliable protocols for isolating and fractionating mycobacterial proteins
2 relatively large amounts of many purified native mycobacterial proteins
3 amino-terminal amino acid sequence information for many proteins
4 and one- and 2-dimensional electrophoretic maps of *M. tuberculosis* proteins (reviewed by Anderson and Brennan 1994).

Because of the difficulties in purifying proteins from mycobacteria, many researchers turned to recombinant DNA techniques to facilitate the isolation and characterization of immunoreactive mycobacterial proteins (Clark-Curtiss et al. 1985, Young et al. 1985a, Young et al. 1985b). In early studies, recombinant DNA libraries in the λ-gt11 expression vector were tested for reactivity with a panel of monoclonal antibodies that had been collected and characterized by the World Health Organization; genes encoding 7 mycobacterial proteins were isolated (reviewed by Young and Mehlert 1989, Young 1990). The nucleotide sequences of the genes were determined, the encoded proteins were expressed and the immunoreactivity of the proteins characterized in detail. It turns out that many of the initially identified immunoreactive mycobacterial proteins displayed homology with heat shock proteins, which led to a great deal of experimentation into their possible roles in autoimmunity and arthritis (reviewed by Young 1990, Shinnick 1991, van Eden 1991).

Other recombinant DNA studies and the genome sequence projects also generated information about potential mycobacterial gene products. Comparison of the predicted amino acid sequences with those available in the international sequence databases identified a number of similarities between the putative mycobacterial gene products and proteins with known functions (reviewed by Bergh and Cole 1994, Cole and Smith 1994). This information is helping direct studies to purify and characterize particular mycobacterial proteins.

11.4 Mutation

Mutants of mycobacteria arise spontaneously at low frequency or can be induced by treatment with a variety of mutagens including ultraviolet light, γ-irradiation and chemical mutagens (Greenberg and

Woodley 1984). In general, the spontaneous and induced mutation rates of mycobacteria are similar to those of other bacterial genera. For example, the spontaneous mutation rate to rifampicin resistance is about one mutation in 10^8 organisms in both *M. tuberculosis* and *E. coli* (Tsukamura 1972, Jin and Gross 1988). Despite the similarities in mutation rates with other bacteria, the genomes of 3 pathogenic species of *Mycobacterium* display surprisingly little sequence variation among strains isolated from around the world. For example, it is estimated that *M. leprae* isolates contain <0.26% base substitutions (Clark-Curtiss and Walsh 1989), *M. paratuberculosis* isolates contain <0.15% base substitutions (McFadden et al. 1987) and *M. tuberculosis* genes contain <1 synonymous substitution per 10 000 synonymous sites in the absence of selective pressure (Kapur, Whittam and Musser 1994). The biological implications of such unusually high sequence conservation in 3 pathogenic *Mycobacterium* spp. is unclear. One possible explanation is that these 3 pathogenic species evolved or established environmental niches recently, perhaps within the last 15 000 years (Kapur, Whittam and Musser 1994).

11.5 Genetic transfer

There have been sporadic reports of gene transfer between mycobacteria by conjugation (Mizuguchi, Suga and Tokunaga 1976), transduction by phage I3 (Sundaraj and Ramakrishnan 1971), transfection and transformation under artificial laboratory conditions. For example, Katanuma and Nakasato (1954) transformed mycobacteria from streptomycin-susceptible to resistant by the addition of chromosomal DNA from streptomycin-resistant mycobacteria. Similarly, Tokunaga and Sellers (1964) demonstrated that mycobacteriophage D29 DNA could transfect *M. smegmatis*. It is not known whether any of these processes play a biologically significant role in genetic transfer between mycobacteria in nature.

11.6 Mycobacteriophages

Mycobacteriophages can be readily isolated from soil and water samples (reviewed by Mizuguchi 1984, Hatfull and Jacobs 1994). The first mycobacteriophage was isolated from a strain of *M. smegmatis* in 1947 (Gardner and Weiser 1947), and the first phage that could infect *M. tuberculosis* was described in 1954. So far, more than 250 bacteriophages have been described that infect various species of *Mycobacterium*. Mycobacteriophages are morphologically similar to phages of other bacteria and typically have hexagonal, icosahedral or oval heads and long non-contractile tails. Phage I3 is the only mycobacteriophage with a contractile tail. The genomes of most mycobacteriophages are linear, double-stranded DNA molecules with a G + C content of 60–70 mol% and cohesive ends, although phage I3 and BxbI appear to have terminally redundant or irregular ends, and the genome of I3 contains several single-stranded gaps.

Mycobacteriophages undergo the typical phage life

cycle of adsorption, infection, replication, assembly and release. Relatively little is known about the mycobacterial surface receptors used by the phage (although mycoside C has been shown to be used by phage D4), or about the process by which phage DNA crosses the complex mycobacterial cell wall. Mycobacteriophages can produce bursts of 4–400 phage particles per infected cell or can establish a lysogenic state. A few phages establish true lysogeny (integration of a copy of the phage genome into the bacterial chromosome and immunity to superinfection) whereas many form pseudolysogens. In the psuedolysogenic state, phage DNA is maintained as an episomal plasmid instead of being integrated into the chromosome and is only transmitted to some of the daughter cells.

Mycobacteriophages have played important roles in the development of mycobacterial molecular biology. Phage D29 was used to develop procedures to introduce foreign DNA into mycobacteria (Tokunaga and Sellers 1964, Jacobs, Tuckman and Bloom 1987). Phage L1 was used to construct plasmids that could integrate into the host chromosome and show that kanamycin resistance was a useful selectable marker for studies with mycobacteria (Snapper et al. 1988).

The most thoroughly analysed mycobacteriophage is L5 (reviewed by Hatfull and Jacobs 1994). The nucleotide sequence of this phage has been determined, open reading frames and potential protein products identified, and gene products and their functions characterized (Hatfull and Sarkis 1993). For example, the genes and gene products required for integration of this temperate mycobacteriophage into the mycobacterial chromosome have been identified and the mechanism of integration elucidated. This information led to the development of recombinant DNA vectors that can integrate foreign DNA into the mycobacterial genome (Lee et al. 1991). Ongoing studies with L5 are providing important insights into gene structure, expression and function as well as novel tools for manipulating genes in mycobacteria.

PHAGE TYPING

Initial interest in mycobacteriophages centred around potential use in the speciation of mycobacteria. Unfortunately, many mycobacteriophages have broad host ranges that cross species boundaries, which makes them unsuitable as taxonomic tools. Despite this broad cross-reactivity, most phages can lyse only a few strains of a given species, which makes them useful in strain-typing studies. Indeed, mycobacteriophages have been used to subtype strains of *M. tuberculosis*, *M. avium*, *M. kansasii*, *M. fortuitum* and *M. xenopi*, although only phage typing of *M. tuberculosis* isolates has been exploited for epidemiological studies (reviewed by Crawford and Bates 1984). However, because many *M. tuberculosis* isolates cluster in a few phage types and because of difficulties in standardizing phage typing protocols and producing reagents, phage typing has been replaced by IS6110 fingerprinting as the standard method to subtype *M. tuberculosis* isolates (van Embden et al. 1993, Crawford 1996).

IS6110 FINGERPRINTING

The repetitive DNA element IS6110 is found only in members of the *M. tuberculosis* complex. Most *M. tuberculosis* strains contain 1–20 copies of IS6110 and the precise locations of the copies in the genome vary dramatically among individual isolates (reviewed by Crawford 1996). IS6110 fingerprinting or restriction fragment length polymorphism (RFLP) has been used extensively in epidemiological investigations of tuberculosis. In this procedure (van Embden et al. 1993), genomic DNA is isolated from a *M. tuberculosis* isolate, cleaved with the *Pvu*II restriction enzyme and electrophoresed through agarose gels. The separated DNA fragments are transferred to a nitrocellulose membrane and hybridized with a labelled probe corresponding to a portion of the IS6110 element. The pattern of hybridizing bands is considered characteristic (i.e. a fingerprint) of the isolate.

11.7 Plasmids

Extrachromosomal plasmids are common in strains of *M. avium*, *M. intracellulare*, *M. scrofulaceum*, *M. fortuitum* and *M. chelonae* (reviewed by Falkinham and Crawford 1994). Naturally occurring plasmids have not been found in the *M. tuberculosis* complex. In the *M. avium* complex, plasmids tend to be small (<30 kb) or very large (>150 kb) with few plasmids of intermediate size. Little is known about the functions of these plasmids, although there are hints that some plasmids may be involved in mercury resistance or in virulence.

12 MYCOBACTERIAL MOLECULAR BIOLOGY

The development of mycobacterial molecular biology was hindered by the facts that:

1 mycobacteria grow very slowly
2 mycobacteria are hydrophobic and tend to grow in clumps, which makes it difficult to purify individual cells for genetic analysis
3 there is no known efficient, naturally occurring genetic exchange between mycobacteria and
4 few genetic markers have been identified in mycobacteria which could be exploited for the development of molecular biological tools, such as cloning vehicles.

Because of these difficulties, studies of molecular genetics in mycobacteria began with the cloning of mycobacterial DNA into *E. coli*. However, the general usefulness of this molecular approach was limited because many important biological questions could only be answered by studying mycobacterial genes in mycobacteria. Critical advances in mycobacterial molecular biology were:

1 the discovery that electroporation (exposing a mixture of DNA and bacteria briefly to a strong electrical field) is an efficient method for introducing exogenously added DNA into mycobacteria
2 the identification of a reliable selectable genetic marker for use with mycobacteria and
3 the development of recombinant DNA vectors that could be stably maintained in mycobacteria.

Numerous molecular tools and techniques are currently available for use in mycobacteria (reviewed by Hatfull 1993, Jacobs and Bloom 1994) including vectors for cosmid cloning, for expressing cloned genes and for characterizing promoters. Most mycobacterial plasmid vectors use an origin of replication from the *M. fortuitum* plasmid pAL5000, which allows the vectors to be maintained in *M. bovis* BCG or *M. smegmatis* at 5–10 plasmids per cell. Other plasmid vectors use origins of replication derived from mycobacteriophage D29 or from naturally occurring plasmids of *M. scrofulaceum*, *M. avium*, *Corynebacterium* spp. or gram-negative bacteria. Another type of vector replicates as a plasmid in *E. coli* but integrates into a specific site in the mycobacterial genome. Such integrating vectors are based on the integrase and attachment sites of mycobacteriophage L5 or of *Streptomyces ambofaciens* plasmid pSAM2.

Useful selectable genetic markers include genes that confer resistance to kanamycin (the most frequently used marker), chloramphenicol, gentamicin, thiostrepton, hygromycin, streptomycin, sulphonamide or superinfection by mycobacteriophage L5 and genes that encode biosynthetic enzymes that allow growth of the recipient strains in the absence of specific nutrients such as uridine or valine (reviewed by Hatfull 1993). Useful phenotypic markers include β-galactosidase, agarase, firefly and *Vibrio* luciferases, alkaline phosphatase, chloramphenicol acetyltransferase and catechol 2,3-dioxygenase. Available molecular genetic techniques include vectors and protocols for:

1 replacing genes in *M. smegmatis* by homologous recombination
2 mutating genes in mycobacteria by the insertion of foreign DNA (e.g. transposon-mediated mutagenesis)
3 stably expressing proteins in mycobacteria
4 strongly expressing reporter enzyme activities and
5 identifying genes that are differentially expressed (reviewed by Hatfull 1993, Burlein et al. 1994, Jacobs and Bloom 1994).

13 PATHOGENICITY AND VIRULENCE FACTORS

An interesting aspect of mycobacteria-caused diseases is that only a small percentage of infected persons develop clinically overt symptoms. That is, only about 10% of immunocompetent persons infected with *M. tuberculosis* will develop active tuberculosis during their lifetimes (Comstock 1982). This may reflect differences in the virulence of the infecting bacilli, or differences in the host, or both. Differences in the immunocompetence of the host are clearly important because immunocompromised persons such as those with AIDS have a much higher rate of developing disease – perhaps as much as 8% per year (Selwyn et al. 1989).

No factors have been identified which distinguish bacilli whose infection is controlled from those that cause clinically evident disease. Indeed, identifying virulence factors of mycobacteria is experimentally difficult because of the complexity of the interactions of the bacterium and the host immune systems and the limitations of animal models. For example, although strains of *M. tuberculosis* differ in their ability to cause disease in various animal models, the differences between the strains have not been clearly defined. One complication is that different animal models and even different laboratories using the same animal model can produce quite different results in virulence testing. Nevertheless, studies in several systems suggest that production of catalase-peroxidase activity and resistance to hydrogen peroxide may be related to the virulence of *M. tuberculosis* strains in animal models of pulmonary tuberculosis.

In general, pathogenic mycobacteria are relatively non-toxic for eukaryotic cells, and much of the tissue damage in mycobacteria-caused diseases results from the host's immune response to the mycobacterium. Possible exceptions to this are the cytotoxin produced by *M. ulcerans*, which may play a role in the ulcerating skin lesions characteristic of infections with this pathogen, and various substances made by mycobacteria (e.g. sulpholipids and trehalose dimycolate), which are toxic to eukaryotic cells in vitro, but whose role in vivo is not known.

In the infected animal or human, slowly growing pathogenic species of *Mycobacterium* survive and replicate within the host's phagocytic cells, primarily within macrophages. Entry of *M. leprae* and *M. tuberculosis* into human monocytes appears to be by a phagocytic mechanism mediated by complement component C3 and complement receptor or by lipoarabinomannan and the macrophage mannose receptors when complement is absent, which may be the case in the fluids lining the alveolar spaces (Schlesinger and Horwitz 1990, Schlesinger et al. 1990, Schlesinger 1993). Once inside the macrophage, the intracellular mycobacteria employ a variety of survival strategies. Mechanisms hypothesized for how tubercle bacilli avoid being killed by macrophages include:

1 prevention of an oxidative burst in phagocytosing cells
2 inhibition of phagosome–lysosome fusion
3 resistance to lysosomal enzymes such as lysozyme
4 secretion of inhibitors or inactivators of bactericidal agents such as peroxide or oxygen radicals
5 exudation of lipids or capsules to block the access of bactericidal agents to their targets and
6 escape from the phagosome into the cytoplasm (reviewed by Horwitz 1988, Sathish and Shinnick 1994).

Several bacterial components have been implicated in these various hypotheses and, by analogy with other bacterial pathogens, are suspected to be virulence factors of mycobacteria. For example, phenolic glycolipids can act as scavengers of free radicals and the mycolic acid layer can act as a hydrophobic barrier to bactericidal agents. Similarly, a recently described cytolytic activity might be involved in the ability of mycobacteria to enter and exit host cells or perhaps escape from the phagosome (King et al. 1993).

Phagocytized tubercle bacilli appear to inhibit acidification of the phagosome and subsequent phagosome–lysosome fusion (Crowle et al. 1990). Potential fusion-inhibiting substances made by the mycobacteria include ammonia, polyglutamic acid and sulpholipids, although the key molecule has not been identified. The next step in the intracellular trafficking of tubercle bacilli is presently unclear. Some electron microscopic evidence suggests that the tubercle bacilli escape from the phagosome and replicate in the cytoplasm (Myrvick, Leake and Wright 1984, McDonough, Kress and Bloom 1993), whereas other data suggest that *M. tuberculosis* ends up in another membrane-bound vacuole which contains proteins characteristic of phagosomes and early and late endosomes (Clemens and Horwitz

1995). Similar conflicting data suggest that *M. leprae* bacilli escape from the phagosome and replicate in the cytoplasm of macrophages and Schwann cells (Mor 1983) and also inhibit phagosome–lysosome fusion and reside in membrane-bound vacuoles (Sibley, Franzblau and Krahenbuhl 1987, Steinhoff et al. 1989). Pathogenic *M. avium* complex strains appear to inhibit phagosome–lysosome fusion and reside in unacidified vacuoles; they also appear to survive and replicate in phagolysosomes. In the latter case, a thick 'electron transparent zone' (ETZ) may protect the bacilli from the bactericidal activities found in phagolysosomes (Frehel and Rastogi 1989). The ETZ is probably a hydrophobic layer of mycolic acids.

The ability of the pathogenic bacteria to survive within the host and produce clinically evident disease relies both on the ability to survive intracellularly and to avoid a protective immune response. Survival within macrophages may inhibit the ability of the macrophages to process and present mycobacterial antigens as well as the production of cytokines required for eliciting a protective cellular immune response. This subversion of the host immune response may produce an anergic state as seen in some tuberculosis patients and in lepromatous leprosy patients or to a destructive cellular immune response, which may be responsible for tissue destruction and cavity formation in tuberculosis and various reactional states and neuropathies in leprosy.

14 ANIMAL MODELS

Mycobacteria that cause human disease also cause disease in animals (reviewed by Thoen 1994a, 1994b). For example, *M. bovis* naturally infects cattle and swine, *M. avium* infects birds, cattle, swine, horses, sheep and goats, *M. paratuberculosis* causes disease in ruminants, and 9 species have been isolated from cold-blooded animals and invertebrates. The diseases of greatest public health significance are tuberculosis, leprosy and *M. avium* infections, and animal models of these human diseases are needed for detailed study of pathogenic mechanisms and therapeutic strategies.

Studies of experimental infection with *M. tuberculosis* in animals must be carried out under Animal Biosafety Level 3 (ABS 3) conditions to prevent spread of the disease to other animals and to care takers (CDC/NIH 1993). Enforcement of ABS 3 conditions is essential for studies with all animal species because monkeys expel bacilli by coughing, rodents excrete bacilli in urine and stool and the bedding of all animal species becomes contaminated. The infectious dose of *M. tuberculosis* for humans has been estimated to be 1–10 bacilli carried in 1–3 droplet nuclei (Balasubramanian et al. 1994), i.e. a particle 1–5 μm in size that is respirable and forms a stable aerosol. Routine procedures should be established that assure safety in all steps of a study, and an animal study should be considered only if it will provide answers that cannot be obtained in another way. Mycobacterial strains should also be selected to minimize biohazards.

14.1 Tuberculosis

GUINEA PIG

Guinea pigs are highly susceptible to induced disease with *M. tuberculosis* and they were used for many years for the isolation of bacilli from clinical specimens. However, more gentle decontamination procedures for specimens and improved primary isolation media led to the removal of animal inoculation from current recommendations for recovering tubercle bacilli from clinical material. Nevertheless, animal inoculation may still be valuable for isolating tubercle bacilli from sputum consistently contaminated on culture or from urine, cerebral spinal fluid and other specimens which may contain few bacilli (Kubica 1984).

The guinea pig's susceptibility to infection and its ability to develop delayed hypersensitivity have allowed many types of studies to be carried out (Youmans 1979). Experimental infection in early studies involved subcutaneous, intramuscular or intraperitoneal injection of approximagely 1 mg of bacilli (10^7–10^8 cfu) which resulted in disease in the spleen and liver with minimal lung involvement; the 'Feldman' index was used to evaluate the extent of disease and effects of intervention (Youmans 1979). For example, to show differences in the virulence of strains of tubercle bacilli, Mitchison et al. (1960) inoculated guinea pigs intramuscularly with 1 mg of cells and sacrificed them after 6 and 12 weeks. The extent of disease was then scored in the organs and the total divided by the time of survival (42 or 84 days) to give a root index of virulence. In this way, many isolates from patients in south India and many isolates that were resistant to isoniazid were found to be less virulent than classical strains of *M. tuberculosis*, but this does not imply that they were any less virulent for humans or that the disease was any less severe.

Major advances in the utility of the guinea pig model of tuberculosis were the development of a method for infecting guinea pigs via the aerosol route with small numbers of tubercle bacilli and careful standardization of the experimental protocols, e.g. strain and age of the animal and strain and amount of tubercle bacilli (reviewed by Smith 1984, McMurray 1994). The aerosol-challenge model can provide a precise evaluation of the disease process and has been used to evaluate the protective efficacy of BCG strains and experimental vaccines (Smith 1984). Studies of chemotherapeutic agents must be conducted with care in guinea pigs since drugs that alter the microbial population in the gastrointestinal tract adversely affect the health of the animal and may lead to its death. Studies with isoniazid were successfully performed in this model because of the limited spectrum of action of this drug.

RABBIT

Tuberculosis in wild rabbits is rare. Rabbits are susceptible to infection with *M. bovis*, but resistant to infection with *M. tuberculosis* (reviewed by Dannenberg 1994, Thoen 1994a). The outstanding work of Max B Lurie was crucial to the development of the rabbit model of *M. bovis* infection (Dannenberg 1994). An important feature of this model is that the inhalation of *M. bovis* bacilli by an inbred strain of rabbits resistant to tuberculosis produced cavitary disease resembling that seen in immunocompetent adults. By contrast, induced disease in an inbred strain susceptible to tuberculosis was haematogenously spread and resembled that found in immunocompromised persons and infants. The rabbit model was used for extensive studies of the pathogenesis of tuberculosis, protective immunity and evaluation of antituberculosis drugs. Unfortunately the rabbit strains were lost because the inbreeding resulted in infertility.

MICE AND RATS

The mouse model has been used extensively in the search for new chemotherapeutic drugs and for evaluating vaccine efficacy (reviewed by Youmans 1979, Orme and Collins 1994). For example, Youmans, Doub and Youmans (1953) examined the in vitro bacteriostatic effect of 3500 compounds and further tested 184 at 1–4 dosage levels for bacteriostatic effects in the mouse model. Only 11 of the compounds showed any suppressive effect on experimental tuberculosis. Disease following intravenous challenge of selected susceptible species of mice with 10^6 or 10^7 bacilli occurs primarily in the lungs. Variations in disease in animals in the same group is small because of the absence of caseation in mice and rats (Lefford 1984). Therefore, the major parameters of disease, survival time and the number of bacilli in each organ, can be measured accurately. The high level of specific acquired immunity that develops in the rat makes it suitable for studies of chronic pulmonary tuberculosis and associated immune responses such as protective immunity, tuberculin delayed-type hypersensitivity and production of tuberculin-induced migratory inhibitory factor. In more recent years the mouse model has been used extensively in studies of host responses, particularly for studying cytokines and CD4, CD8 and γ/δ subsets of T cells (Orme and Collins 1994). The T cell response is easily studied in this animal model because of the relative ease and economy of maintaining the model. As immunological techniques improve, the murine model will continue to be a valuable tool.

NON-HUMAN PRIMATES

Tuberculosis among free-living primates is probably rare because normal social behaviours such as grooming would lead to rapid spread of the disease and destruction of the colony. Mycobacterioses were reported in 15 New World and Old World primate species between 1968 and 1980 (Good 1984). M. tuberculosis is the most serious infection since it is routinely pulmonary and is spread by the aerosol route from animal to animal, probably through coughing. Because sputum is swallowed, large numbers of bacilli may be present in faeces. Contamination of traumatized skin and use of a common rectal thermometer have been described as routes of infection.

Schmidt (1972) reported that as few as 10 tubercle bacilli instilled into the trachea of a rhesus monkey led to progressive, fatal disease. The final outcome was the same despite the strain used for infection although there were differences in rate of disease development. By systematic studies, he established a disease model in which juvenile rhesus monkeys were infected by the instillation of 400–1000 cfu of M.

tuberculosis into the right or left mainstem bronchus. Following inoculation, tuberculin skin reactivity was measured and the extent of disease was followed by radiography. The model is highly reproducible because the rhesus monkey is highly susceptible to infection with M. tuberculosis and because a large inoculum was used to establish the infection. Good (1968) and Schmidt (1972) used this model to assess the activity of vaccines. Viable BCG vaccines given by the intracutaneous or subcutaneous route afforded substantial but not complete protection from challenge, whereas vaccination with 12.5×10^6 cfu of BCG given intravenously gave remarkable protection against challenge. Since the challenge dose in these studies was considered excessive, rhesus monkeys vaccinated by inhalation of 8.0×10^5 cfu were compared to intracutaneous and intravenous administration of 3.3×10^6 cfu of the vaccine for protection against challenge with 12–16 cfu of M. tuberculosis strain H37Rv (Barclay et al. 1973). When the more pathogenic Erdman strain was used for challenge, protective immunity was demonstrated (Good and McCarroll 1978), but it was not as great as when the H37Rv strain was used for challenge. In the course of this study, it was found that protection against the challenge infection was as great 72 weeks following vaccination as it was at 8 weeks. Lymphocyte transformation tests were more sensitive than tuberculin skin tests for following the immune response elicited by the inhalation of 10^5 cfu of BCG or by challenge with 47 cfu of M. tuberculosis (Chaparas, Good and Janicki 1975). Other procedures to detect the immune response were not as predictive of infection as the skin test, but increases in immunoglobulins G, A and M occurred in animals vaccinated by the intravenous route (Janicki et al. 1973).

The parameters of disease that can be studied in the non-human primate model of tuberculosis have only been approached in the studies reviewed here. Unfortunately, the work was interrupted and has not been resumed. Additional work is needed to develop a model of disease that is similar to that seen in the adult rather than the fulminant disease that is similar to that seen in infants and immunocompromised individuals. New work in the area should involve scientists in many fields so that a single experiment will yield data useful in the study of many parameters of the disease.

14.2 *M. avium* infections

M. avium infects a wide range of hosts including chickens, cattle and swine. The disease occurs most often in the lymph nodes, spleen and liver, but other tissues may be involved including lungs, kidneys, brain, intestinal mucosa, tonsils, ovaries and the skin (Thoen, Himes and Karlson 1984, Thoen 1994b). Infections in animals are often caused by M. avium serovars 1–3 and disease in humans has been found to be due to M. avium serotypes 4, 8 and 1. For example, intravenous infection of rabbits with M. avium serotypes 1, 2 and 3 can cause extensive disease which is rapidly fatal, whereas other serovars may cause slowly progressive lesions, often involving joints and tendon sheaths (Thoen and Karlson 1984). The beige mouse (C57BL/6/bgj/bgj) has been developed as a model of human disease caused by *M. avium* serotypes 1, 4 and 8 (reviewed by Gangadharam and Reddy 1994). The model can be used to discover new drugs and to develop new therapeutic regimens that include combinations of drugs. For example, of 60 compounds found active against *M. avium* in vitro, only rifabutin, clofazimine, amikacin, clarithromycin and ethambutol were active in the mouse model and are now accepted in current clinical applications (Inderlied and Salfinger 1995).

14.3 *M. leprae* infections

Leprosy is a human disease caused by *M. leprae*, although naturally acquired, leprosy-like infections have been observed in armadillos (*Dasypus novemcinctus*), chimpanzees (*Pan troglodytes*) and mangabey monkeys (*Cercocebus torquatas atys*) (reviewed by Shinnick 1992). The disease progresses slowly in chimpanzees and mangabeys, but disease in the armadillo resembles human lepromatous leprosy with bacillary loads in lesions reaching 10^{10} bacilli per gram of tissue; the total bacillary load can exceed 10^{12} bacilli per animal. Shepard (1981) reviewed the advantages and disadvantages of the normal mouse (CFW, CBA or BALB/c strains) model that he developed 20 years earlier. The primary advantages are that uniform infections occur after inoculation of 10^3–10^4 bacilli into the footpad and reach a maximum level of 10^6 150–180 days after inoculation. The model has been used for the evaluation of drug regimens and experimental vaccines by Shepard and others. New bactericidal antileprosy drugs discovered in this system are minocycline, clarithromycin and fluoroquinolones, and the opportunity exists to combine them with the bactericidal drug rifampicin (Gelber 1994).

14.4 Other mycobacterioses

M. lepraemurium is a natural pathogen of rats and mice and the disease is used as a model of human leprosy (Lefford 1984, Pattyn 1984b). The disease may remain localized in rat lymph nodes or deeper tissues may become infected as the musculocutaneous form develops. There is almost complete absence of any inflammatory reaction as though the infection represented immunological tolerance. In this respect the disease is similar to the immunosuppressive state in human lepromatous leprosy. Other species of mycobacteria will establish disease in animals if the infecting dose is high (Thoen, Francis and Haagsma 1984), but these infections have not been standardized for routine investigations. Generally, the mouse is susceptible to infection with most mycobacteria so that routine methods could be developed in this model.

15 SPECIES OF *MYCOBACTERIUM*

15.1 Slowly growing mycobacteria

M. TUBERCULOSIS COMPLEX

M. tuberculosis, *M. bovis*, *M. africanum* and *M. microti* are grouped into the *M. tuberculosis* complex on the basis of DNA homology (Baess 1979, Imaeda 1985). *M. microti*, a pathogen of the vole bacillus, is of such limited pathogenicity for humans that it has been used as a vaccine against tuberculosis. It is rarely encountered and is not considered an important pathogen for animals or humans (Thoen, Karlson and Himes 1984). The other 3 species in the *M. tuberculosis* complex can cause tuberculosis and are of public health significance. They can be distinguished by biochemical reactions (Shinnick and Good 1994), but display identical mycolic acid profiles when assayed by HPLC (Butler, Jost and Kilburn 1991) and react identically with procedures based on nucleic acid hybridization or gene amplification (reviewed by Kohne 1989, Shinnick and Jonas 1994). Most clinical laboratories use probe procedures and simply report *M. tuberculosis* complex. In most instances, this reflects infection with *M. tuberculosis* because this species causes greater than 95% of cases in the USA (Good, Silcox and Kilburn 1985, Kent and Kubica 1985). None the less, species identification is important for epidemiological studies.

M. tuberculosis

M. tuberculosis grows well (eugonic) on Löwenstein–Jensen medium and Middlebrook 7H10 agar. Well grown colonies are usually visible between 14 and 35 days at the optimal temperature of 35–37°C. The bacilli grow more rapidly in BACTEC 7H12 selective medium (Becton Dickinson Diagnostic Instrument Systems, Sparks, MD, USA) and are detectable in 14 days or less. Colonies on solid media are an off-white or cream colour and are usually heaped up and rough in appearance (Fig. 26.2, see also plate 26.2). Isolates are aerobic, reduce nitrate, produce niacin, have strong catalase activity that is resistant to heating at 68°C for 30 min, are susceptible to PZA and are resistant to thiophen-2-carboxylic acid hydrazide (TCH). Six biotypes can be distinguished (Collins, Grange and Yates 1985). Fingerprints of isolates using the *IS*6110 insertion are used extensively in epidemiological studies of tuberculosis (reviewed by Crawford 1996).

M. bovis

M. bovis is dysgonic, particularly on media containing glycerol. It is micro-aerophilic, resistant to PZA, susceptible to TCH, does not reduce nitrate, does not produce niacin and does not produce a heat-stable catalase. BCG was derived from *M. bovis*, but strains grow well on media containing glycerol, are aerobic and are resistant to cycloserine (Collins, Grange and Yates 1985). Both *M. bovis* and the BCG variant react with commercial DNA probes for *M. tuberculosis* complex; *M. bovis*, but not BCG strains, have a mycolic acid pattern identical to *M. tuberculosis* (Butler, Jost and Kilburn 1991).

M. africanum

Strains with biochemical reactions that place them as intermediate between *M. tuberculosis* and *M. bovis* are *M. africanum*. David et al. (1978) found that those strains isolated from patients in West Africa are similar to *M. tuberculosis* whereas those isolated from patients in Rwanda and Burundi appear closely related to *M. bovis*. In this study *M. africanum* did not separate by numerical taxonomy into a cluster apart from *M. tuberculosis* and *M. bovis*, and Wayne (1984) concludes that it should not be treated as a separate distinct species. Isolation of this species is from patients in certain parts of Africa or from former residents who have resettled in other areas.

SLOWLY GROWING PHOTOCHROMOGENS

Differential reactions are reviewed in Shinnick and Good (1994).

M. kansasii

M. kansasii is the third most common, potentially pathogenic species isolated by state public health laboratories. A range of clinical manifestations from colonization to fatal infection is associated with specimens received in the laboratory. Trehalose-containing lipo-oligosaccharides occur on the surface of variants with rough colony morphology but not on variants with smooth morphology. Belisle and Brennan (1994) suggest that this may be a factor in the pathogenesis of certain strains. Most infections in the USA have been reported from California, Texas, Louisiana, Florida, Illinois and Missouri, and those in Europe have been from the coal mining regions of the UK and Europe (Hoffner 1994).

M. marinum

Skin abrasions may become infected with *M. marinum*, a photochromogenic species with an optimal growth temperature of 25–35°C. This species is commonly isolated from diseased fish. Humans are infected through exposure to water in swimming pools and tropical fish aquariums. Superficial infections usually heal spontaneously, but the course is very prolonged and associated with discomfort. Most strains of *M. marinum* are susceptible to streptomycin, cycloserine, cotrimoxazole, rifampicin and ethambutol and partially susceptible to tetracyclines (Pattyn 1984a).

M. simiae and M. asiaticum

M. simiae and *M. asiaticum* are photochromogenic strains that were isolated from monkeys. The former synthesizes niacin and may be incorrectly identified unless tested for photochromogenicity. It grows well at 37°C, is nitrate negative and does not hydrolyse Tween 80 in 10 days. *M. asiaticum* is phenotypically similar to *M. gordonae* and a test for photochromogenicity is the most reliable differential character.

SLOWLY GROWING SCOTOCHROMOGENS

Differential reactions are reviewed in Shinnick and Good (1994).

M. gordonae

M. gordonae is the third most frequently isolated species in mycobacteriology laboratories in the USA. It is commonly associated with water, and isolation conditions rarely meet the criteria of the American Thoracic Society for diagnosis of a disease caused by non-tuberculous mycobacteria (Wallace et al. 1990). *M. gordonae* is scotochromogenic and key differential reactions include hydrolysis of Tween 80 in 5 days and failure to hydrolyse pyrazinamide, nicotinamide and urea. Other differential characters include a unique mycolic acid profile and reaction with a specific, commercially available hybridization probe.

M. scrofulaceum

M. scrofulaceum causes cervical adenitis in children and has been isolated from sputum specimens, gastric aspirates and the environment. It is sometimes incorrectly included in a complex with MAC, but it is not related to these species. The species is scotochromogenic, grows at both 22 and 42°C, hydrolyses urea and produces large amounts of catalase.

M. szulgai

Distinguishing characteristics of *M. szulgai* are the growth rate, 1 week Tween opacity and resistance to 5% NaCl. A comparison of 16S rRNA sequences shows a close relationship to *M. malmoense*, but phenotypic characters are differential. This species is rarely found as a cause of human disease, but it has been responsible for pulmonary disease that is indistinguishable from tuberculosis. *M. szulgai* has been isolated from 2 patients with AIDS.

SLOWLY GROWING NON-PHOTOCHROMOGENS

Differential reactions are reviewed in Shinnick and Good (1994).

M. avium complex (MAC)

M. avium and *M. intracellulare* cannot be easily differentiated on the basis of biochemical tests, and often *M. scrofulaceum* may be confused with pigmented strains of *M. avium*. MAC species are grouped with non-photochromogens, not because they are non-pigmented, but because induction of pigment is not influenced by exposure to light. Strains of *M. avium* are serotypes 1–6 and 8–11 whereas *M. intracellulare* strains are serotypes 7 and 12–20, *M. scrofulaceum* strains are serotypes 42–43, and the strains that type 21–28 may be of different species (Good 1992, Wayne et al. 1993).

M. avium infects a wide range of hosts including humans, chickens, cattle and swine (reviewed by Thoen 1994b, see also Volume 3, Chapter 22). *M. avium* complex occurs widely in the environment and has been isolated from raw and treated water sources throughout the world, including hospital hot water supplies (du Moulin et al. 1988, von Reyn et al. 1993, 1994). The temperature of hot water supplies in hospitals may run as low as 51°C (Sniadak et al. 1992), but a temperature of 70°C for 5–60 min is required to kill 99% of *M. avium* cells (du Moulin et al. 1988).

As part of an epidemiological study of MAC infections, Yajko et al. (1995) cultured water, food and soil from the home environments of 290 persons infected with HIV. Mycobacteria were isolated from many of the samples, but isolates reacting with MAC-specific DNA probe were recovered from only 4 (one *M. avium* isolate) of 528 water specimens and one (*M. avium*) of 397 food samples. From 140 soil samples, MAC was isolated from 86 and 43 of these were *M. avium*. On the basis of their data the authors concluded that soil might be a significant reservoir of *M. avium* since patients were all infected with *M. avium* serovars.

Epidemiological markers for tracking and relating MAC types include serological typing (Good and Beam 1984), multilocus enzyme electrophoresis (Yakrus, Reeves and Hunter 1992), PCR-RFLP assays based on the 65 kDa antigen gene and rRNA (Plikaytis et al. 1992), plasmid profiles, pulse field gel electrophoresis of large restriction fragments and random amplified polymorphic DNA procedures (reviewed by Crawford 1994, Falkinham 1994). These markers have been used to suggest that polyclonal infections with *M. avium* have been underdetected (15–25% of patients) because too few colonies were selected for typing (Falkinham 1994).

M. paratuberculosis

M. paratuberculosis is the aetiological agent of Johne's disease, a chronic intestinal disease in ruminants. The species fails to synthesize mycobactin and growth media must be supplemented with iron. Mycobactin-dependent organisms resembling *M. paratuberculosis* have been isolated from wood pigeons; *M. paratuberculosis*, *M. avium* and the isolates from wood pigeons are closely related by DNA–DNA homologies and may represent subspecies of a single species (Levy-Frebault et al. 1989). *M. paratuberculosis* has been suspected as a cause of Crohn's disease, a human intestinal illness with characteristic lesions resembling those of Johne's disease (reviewed by Chiodini 1989). There is evidence suggesting that the organisms may occur as spheroplasts in intestinal lesions and recovery of this cell wall free form with a requirement for mycobactin from a highly contaminated source may be the reason culture has been so unsuccessful.

M. ulcerans

M. ulcerans causes ulcerations that are usually located on the extremities and may occur also on the neck, head and trunk, particularly in young children (Pattyn 1984c). Lesions first appear as circumscribed, hard, painless areas that rupture in 2–8 weeks to leave an ulcer with a necrotic centre and undetermined edges. Ulcers heal spontaneously after many months or years and leave extensive scars which are disfiguring. The disease seems to be limited to warm climates, almost exclusively to savannah areas. The first cases were described in Australia where they were called Bairnsdale ulcer, and later cases in Africa where they were called Buruli ulcer. *M. ulcerans* is very slowly growing in vitro at the restricted temperature range of 31–34°C. It is not reactive in the routine tests used for identification.

M. haemophilum

M. haemophilum is a pathogen of immunocompromised patients, particularly those with AIDS and organ transplants (Kiehn and White 1994, Straus et al. 1994). Adults usually present with granulomatous or ulcerating skin lesions, septic arthritis or pneumonia. Children have perihilar, cervical or submandibular adenitis. For growth in vitro strains need high levels of iron which can be supplied by the addition of blood, haem or ferric ammonium citrate. The organisms grow best at 30–32°C and can be detected 2 weeks after inoculation.

M. xenopi

M. xenopi is infrequently isolated in laboratories in the USA, but is endemic in regions of Canada and Europe. It represents 39% of all MOTT bacilli identified in Belgium (Fauville-Dufaux et al. 1995). Strains of this species require 6–8 weeks to form visible colonies on primary isolation. It does not grow at 25°C and grows better at 45°C than at 37°C (Collins, Grange and Yates 1985). It gives a strong positive sulphatase reaction, does not reduce nitrate, gives a weak catalase reaction and is negative in the Tween 80 hydrolysis and nitrate reduction tests. Besides biochemical reactions, this species can be identified using hybridization probes (Fauville-Dufaux et al. 1995, Picardeau and Vincent 1995) or by its mycolic acid pattern (Butler, Thibert and Kilburn 1992). *M. xenopi* is an opportunistic pathogen in human lung disease, but is rarely significant as a cause of disease when found in other sites. It is a common contaminant of pathological material in England where it occurs in piped water supplies.

M. celatum

M. celatum is similar to *M. xenopi* biochemically and morphologically (Butler et al. 1993). Primary differential reactions for *M. celatum* include poor growth at 45°C, production of large colonies on 7H10 agar and production of detectable amounts of 2-docosanol. Most strains have been isolated from respiratory tract secretions collected throughout the USA, Finland and Somalia. The clinical significance of the isolates is not known, but in one series 32% of patients with cultures positive for *M. celatum* were infected with HIV.

M. genavense

M. genavense bacilli have unusual fastidious growth requirements and grow poorly and variably in vitro (reviewed by Böttger 1994). Isolation has been most successful using radiometric detection techniques (e.g. BACTEC), preferably with the medium adjusted to a more acidic pH. Specimens stained for acid-fast bacilli (AFB) must be observed carefully to detect small coccobacillary rods which are considered diagnostic for *M. genavense*. Growth is inhibited in the NAP (p-nitro-α-acetylamino-β-propiophenone) test. Disseminated infections with this organism have been recognized in AIDS patients in the USA, Europe and Australia. It probably occurs frequently but is not detected because of failure to inoculate the proper medium, the requirement for a long incubation period and the poor methods for identification.

M. lepraemurium

The rat leprosy bacillus, *M. lepraemurium*, causes induration and ulceration in the skin and lymph nodes of mice, rats and cats in all areas of the world (Pattyn 1984b). *M. lepraemurium* is difficult to grow on laboratory media, but it has been cultivated on Ogawa egg medium and on agar-based medium containing added cytochrome *c* and α-ketoglutarate.

M. gastri

This species was isolated from gastric washings and isolates have formed a clear and separate cluster in studies based on numerical taxonomy (Wayne 1984). The species has not been associated with disease in man or animals and is encountered only rarely, even though it has been isolated from sputum and soil. Differential reactions include lack of heat-stable catalase, Tween hydrolysis and urease activity (Kent and Kubica 1985).

M. malmoense

M. malmoense was first isolated from patients with chronic pulmonary disease in Malmo, Sweden. It has since been recognized as occurring in other parts of Europe and in the USA. Differential characteristics include positive urease activity and reaction in the semiquantitative catalase test (Wayne 1984). The strains grow very slowly and colonies may not be observed on solid media for 8–12 weeks.

M. terrae complex

In the clinical laboratory, *M. terrae*, *M. nonchromogenicum* and *M. triviale* are grouped into a complex that contains species with little or no clinical significance (Wayne 1984). The complex can be characterized by the lack of yellow pigment (some colonies may produce a pink pigment), rapid hydrolysis of Tween 80, strong catalase activity and failure to hydrolyse urea.

M. shimoidei

This species is the cause of rare cases of pulmonary disease in Japan. It grows at 45°C, but not at 25°C. In general, *M. shimoidei* bacilli are unreactive in standard biochemical identification tests.

15.2 Rapidly growing mycobacteria

Eight rapidly growing *Mycobacterium* spp. are considered pathogenic for humans (reviewed by Wallace 1994). At one time *M. chelonae* and *M. fortuitum* with their various subspecies and biovariants were grouped together into the *M. fortuitum* complex, largely because they hydrolysed phenolphthalein sulphate within 3 days (Wayne 1984). Growth on MacConkey agar without crystal violet and the lack of pigmentation provided the keys to separate the clinically significant species from saprophytic species (Silcox, Good and Floyd 1981). Growth on mannitol and inositol can be used to differentiate *M. fortuitum*, *M. peregrinum* and the third biovar of *M. fortuitum*. *M. chelonae* and *M. abscessus* can be differentiated by tolerance to NaCl at 28°C and the utilization of sodium citrate. Those classified as *M. chelonae*-like organisms (MCLO) develop a tan colour in the iron uptake test rather than the characteristic deep rust colour, and they will use both mannitol and sodium citrate as a sole carbon source for growth. *M. smegmatis* is negative for 3 day

arylsulphatase and does not use citrate as a sole source of carbon. Wallace (1994) splits the third biovar group on the basis of sorbitol utilization.

Approximately 90% of clinical disease is due to *M. fortuitum*, *M. chelonae* and *M. abscessus* (Wallace 1994). The most common disease manifestation is post-traumatic wound infection and surgical wound infection (reviewed by Good 1992). MCLO were first isolated from people undergoing automated peritoneal dialysis. About 62% of recent isolates were from the respiratory tract and were not considered a cause of disease (Wallace 1994). The majority of non-respiratory isolates were from post-traumatic wound infection and catheter-related sepsis. Susceptibility of the rapidly growing mycobacteria to drugs is variable and the selection of a chemotherapeutic regimen should be based on minimal inhibitory concentrations determined for the particular strain by the in vitro susceptibility test described by Swenson, Thornsberry and Silcox (1982).

Clinical manifestations of disease with the biovariants of *M. fortuitum* divided on the basis of sorbitol utilization include post-traumatic wound or bone infection. Infections tend to occur after metal puncture wounds or open fractures (Wallace 1994). The sorbitol-positive isolates were resistant to cefoxitin and clarithromycin whereas the sorbitol-negative isolates were susceptible. Additional studies with the developing DNA fingerprinting technology have incorporated the improved data for expansion of epidemiological investigations (Wallace 1994).

M. phlei is rarely isolated from either environmental or clinical sources, and it is not associated with disease in man or animals. It and *M. thermoresistibile* are thermophilic and will grow at 52°C. They will also withstand heating at 60°C for 4 h. *M. thermoresistibile* has been associated with human infection (Weitzman et al. 1981), a finding that suggests that any *Mycobacterium* species can invade the human host and cause progressive pathological changes. Other scotochromogenic rapid growers include *M. flavescens*, which is frequently found in water and very rarely as a cause of disease in man; *M. duvali* and *M. gilvum* are also species that have not been associated with disease. Characteristics of other rapidly growing species not associated with human disease are reviewed by Tsukamura (1984).

15.3 Non-cultivatable mycobacteria

M. leprae is the primary species in this group and is the cause of leprosy (Hansen disease), a chronic infectious granulomatous disease that primarily affects the peripheral nervous system, skin and mucous membranes, especially nasal mucosa (see Volume 3, Chapter 23). Data have accumulated over the past few years on the structure and biology of *M. leprae*, but the organism still cannot be propagated outside an animal host. Other 'non-cultivatable' mycobacteria have included *M. paratuberculosis*, *M. haemophilum* and *M. genavense*. Perhaps additional study will yet lead to a way of growing *M. leprae* in the laboratory setting.

15.4 Laboratory isolation and identification

Mycobacteriology laboratories are most active in the isolation and identification of clinically significant species infecting humans and animals and manuals for these specific purposes have been published (Collins, Grange and Yates 1985, Kent and Kubica 1985, Inderlied and Salfinger 1995, Nolte and Metchock 1995). Recent advances in this area include the radiometric BACTEC system for isolation and identification (Siddiqi 1988), HPLC analysis of mycolic acids for speciation (Butler, Thibert and Kilburn 1992), various molecular procedures for identification (Shinnick and Jonas 1994) and fingerprinting techniques and their application to epidemiological studies (Crawford 1996). Unfortunately, many diagnostic laboratories have been slow to incorporate new procedures that speed up identification and drug susceptibility testing (Huebner, Good and Tokar 1993, Woods and Witebsky 1993).

In the model diagnostic mycobacteriology laboratory described by Salfinger and Pfyffer (1994), specimen decontamination and concentration, staining with fluorochrome dye and inoculation of primary isolation media are done on the day the specimen is received. Depending on growth, identification tests can start as early as 4 days after inoculation of liquid media or 14–21 days for solid media. Species identification by HPLC and DNA probes can be completed in one day, or identification of *M. tuberculosis* by the NAP test can be completed in 4 days. Biochemical tests for identification of other species can take 7–21 days after the primary culture is fully grown. Drug susceptibility testing can be completed in 7–10 days using the BACTEC system and in 21 days using the conventional agar method. Because of the need for rapid turn around in some mycobacteriology laboratories, particularly for identification of *M. tuberculosis*, the authors emphasized procedures that streamline laboratory performance and identified subsets of activities for 'point-of-care', 'fast track' and 'specialty' laboratories. Taken together, these laboratories form a 'dynamic acid-fast network to improve mycobacteriology laboratory service'.

REFERENCES

Anderson AB, Brennan P, 1994, Proteins and antigens of *Mycobacterium tuberculosis*, Tuberculosis: Pathogenesis, Protection, and Control, ed. Bloom BR, American Society for Microbiology Press, Washington, DC, 307–32.
Baess I, 1979, Deoxyribonucleic acid relatedness among species of slowly growing mycobacteria, *Acta Pathol Microbiol Scand*, **87:** 221–6.
Balasubramanian V, Wiegeshaus EH et al., 1994, Pathogenesis of tuberculosis: pathway to apical localization, *Tuber Lung Dis*, **75:** 168–78.
Banerjee A, Dubnau E et al., 1994, inhA, a gene encoding a target for isoniazid and ethionamide in *Mycobacetrium tuberculosis*, *Science*, **263:** 227–30.
Barclay R, Wheeler PR, 1989, Metabolism of mycobacteria in tissues, The Biology of the Mycobacteria, vol. 3, eds Ratledge C, Stanford JL, Grange JM, Academic Press, London, 37–196.
Barclay WR, Busey WM et al., 1973, Protection of monkeys against airborne tuberculosis by aerosol vaccination with Bacillus Calmette–Guérin, *Am Rev Respir Dis*, **107:** 351–8.
Barnes PF, Chatterjee D et al., 1992, Cytokine production induced by *Mycobacterium tuberculosis* lipoarabinomannan: relationship to chemical structure, *J Immunol*, **149:** 541–7.
Belisle JT, Brennan PJ, 1994, Molecular basis of colony morphology in *Mycobacterium avium*, *Res Microbiol*, **145:** 237–42.
Bergh S, Cole ST, 1994, MycDB: an integrated mycobacterial database, *Mol Microbiol*, **12:** 517–34.
Besra GS, Chatterjee D, 1994, Lipids and carbohydrates of *Mycobacterium tuberculosis*, Tuberculosis: Pathogenesis, Protection, and Control, ed. Bloom BR, American Society for Microbiology Press, Washington, DC, 285–306.
Besra GS, Bolton RC et al., 1992, Structural elucidation of a novel family of acyltrehaloses from *Mycobacterium tuberculosis*, *Biochemistry*, **31:** 9832–7.
Best M, Sattar SA et al., 1990, Efficacies of selected disinfectants against *Mycobacterium tuberculosis*, *J Clin Microbiol*, **28:** 2234–9.
Bloch H, 1950, Studies on the virulence of tubercle bacilli. Isolation and biological properties of a constituent of virulent organisms, *J Exp Med*, **91:** 197–218.
Bolan G, Reingold AL et al., 1985, Infections with *Mycobacterium chelonei* in patients receiving dialysis and using processed hemodialyzer, *J Infect Dis*, **152:** 1013–19.

Böttger EC, 1994, *Mycobacterium genavense*: an emerging pathogen, *Eur J Clin Microbiol Infect Dis*, **13:** 932–6.
Brennan PJ, 1984, Antigenic peptidoglycolipids, phospholipids and glycolipids, The Mycobacteria: A Sourcebook, eds Kubica GP, Wayne LG, Marcel Dekker, New York, 467–89.
Brennan PJ, Draper P, 1994, Ultrastructure of *Mycobacterium tuberculosis*, Tuberculosis: Pathogenesis, Protection, and Control, ed. Bloom BR, American Society for Microbiology Press, Washington, DC, 271–84.
Brennan PJ, Hunter SW et al., 1990, Reappraisal of the chemistry of mycobacterial cell walls, with a view to understanding the roles of individual entities in disease processes, Microbial Determinants of Virulence and Host Response, eds Ayoub EM, Cassell GH et al., American Society for Microbiology Press, Washington, DC, 55–75.
Burlein JE, Stover CK et al., 1994, Expression of foreign genes in mycobacteria, Tuberculosis: Pathogenesis, Protection, and Control, ed. Bloom BR, American Society for Microbiology Press, Washington, DC, 239–52.
Butler WR, Jost KC, Kilburn JO, 1991, Identification of mycobacteria by high-performance liquid chromatography, *J Clin Microbiol*, **29:** 2468–72.
Butler WR, Kilburn JO, 1983, Susceptibility of *Mycobacterium tuberculosis* to pyrazinamide and its relationship to pyrazinamidase activity, *Antimicrob Agents Chemother*, **24:** 600–1.
Butler WR, Kilburn JO, 1988, Identification of major slow growing pathogenic mycobacteria and *Mycobacterium gordonae* by high-performance liquid chromatography of their mycolic acids, *J Clin Microbiol*, **26:** 50–3.
Butler WR, Thibert L, Kilburn JO, 1992, Identification of *Mycobacterium avium* complex strains and some similar species by high-performance liquid chromatography, *J Clin Microbiol*, **30:** 2698–704.
Butler WR, O'Connor SP et al., 1993, *Mycobacterium celatum* sp. nov., *Int J Syst Bacteriol*, **43:** 539–48.
Canetti G, Froman S et al., 1963, Mycobacteria: laboratory methods for testing drug sensitivity and resistance, *Bull WHO*, **29:** 565–78.
Canetti G, Fox W et al., 1969, Advances in techniques of testing mycobacterial drug sensitivity, and the use of sensitivity tests in tuberculosis control programs, *Bull W H O*, **41:** 21–43.

CDC/NIH, 1993, *Biosafety in Microbiological and Biomedical Laboratories*, 3rd edn, DHHS Publication No. (CDC) 93-8395, US Department of Health and Human Services, Public Health Service.

Chan J, Fujiwara T et al., 1989, Microbial glycolipids: possible virulence factors that scavenge oxygen radicals, *Proc Natl Acad Sci USA*, **86:** 2543–7.

Chaparas SD, Good RC, Janicki BW, 1975, Tuberculin-induced lymphocyte transformation and skin reactivity in monkeys vaccinated or not vaccinated with Bacille Calmette–Guérin, then challenged with virulent *Mycobacterium tuberculosis*, *Am Rev Respir Dis*, **112:** 43–77.

Chatterjee D, Hunter SW et al., 1992a, Lipoarabinomannan: multiglycosylated form of the mycobacterial mannosylphosphatidylinositols, *J Biol Chem*, **267:** 6228–33.

Chatterjee D, Lowell K et al., 1992b, Lipoarabinomannan of *Mycobacterium tuberculosis*: capping with mannosyl residue in some strains, *J Biol Chem*, **267:** 6234–9.

Chatterjee D, Roberts AD et al., 1992c, Structural basis of capacity of lipoarabinomannan to induce secretion of tumor necrosis factor, *Infect Immun*, **60:** 1249–53.

Chiodini RJ, 1989, Crohn's disease and the mycobacterioses: a review and comparison of two disease entities, *Clin Microbiol Rev*, **2:** 90–117.

Clark-Curtiss JE, 1990, Genome structure of mycobacteria, *Molecular Biology of the Mycobacteria*, ed. McFadden JJ, Harcourt Brace Jovanovich, London, 77–96.

Clark-Curtiss JE, Docherty MA, 1989, A species-specific repetitive sequence in *Mycobacterium leprae* DNA, *J Infect Dis*, **159:** 7–15.

Clark-Curtiss JE, Walsh GP, 1989, Conservation of genomic sequences among isolates of *Mycobacterium leprae*, *J Bacteriol*, **171:** 4844–51.

Clark-Curtiss J, Jacobs W et al., 1985, Molecular analysis of DNA and construction of genomic libraries of *Mycobacterium leprae*, *J Bacteriol*, **161:** 1093–102.

Clemens DL, Horwitz MA, 1995, Characterization of the *Mycobacterium tuberculosis* phagosome and evidence that phagosomal maturation is inhibited, *J Exp Med*, **181:** 257–70.

Closs O, Harboe M et al., 1980, The antigens of *Mycobacterium bovis*, strain BCG, studied by crossed immunoelectrophoresis: a reference system, *Scand J Immunol*, **12:** 249–63.

Cole ST, Smith DR, 1994, Toward mapping and sequencing the genome of *Mycobacterium tuberculosis*, *Tuberculosis: Pathogenesis, Protection, and Control*, ed. Bloom BR, American Society for Microbiology Press, Washington, DC, 227–38.

Collins CH, Grange JM, Yates MD, 1984, Mycobacteria in water, *J Appl Bacteriol*, **57:** 193–211.

Collins CH, Grange JM, Yates MD, 1985, Organization and practice in tuberculosis bacteriology, Butterworths, London.

Colston MJ, Davis EO, 1994, Homologous recombination, DNA repair, and mycobacterial *recA* genes, *Tuberculosis: Pathogenesis, Protection, and Control*, ed. Bloom BR, American Society for Microbiology Press, Washington, DC, 217–26.

Comstock GW, 1982, Epidemiology of tuberculosis, *Am Rev Respir Dis*, **125, Suppl.:** 8–16.

Connell ND, Nikaido H, 1994, Membrane permeability and transport in *Mycobacterium tuberculosis*, *Tuberculosis: Pathogenesis, Protection, and Control*, ed. Bloom BR, American Society for Microbiology, Washington, DC, 333–52.

Corper HJ, Cohn ML, 1937, The thermolability of the tubercle bacillus, *Am Rev Tuberc*, **35:** 663.

Crawford JT, 1994, Development of rapid techniques for identification of *M. avium* infections, *Res Microbiol*, **145:** 177–81.

Crawford JT, 1996, Molecular approaches to the detection of mycobacteria, *Mycobacteria, Volume 1: Basic Aspects*, eds Gangadharam P, Jenkins PA, Chapman and Hall, New York, in press.

Crawford JT, Bates JH, 1984, Phage typing of mycobacteria, *The Mycobacteria: A Sourcebook*, eds Kubica GP, Wayne LG, Marcel Dekker, New York, 123–32.

Crowle A, Dahl R et al., 1990, Evidence that vesicles containing living virulent *M. tuberculosis* or *M. avium* in cultured human macrophages are not acidic, *Infect Immun*, **59:** 1823–31.

Daniel TM, Janicki BW, 1978, Mycobacterial antigens: a review of their isolation, chemistry, and immunological properties, *Microbiol Rev*, **42:** 84–113.

Dannenberg AM Jr, 1994, Rabbit model of tuberculosis, *Tuberculosis: Pathogenesis, Protection, and Control*, ed. Bloom BR, American Society for Microbiology, Washington, DC, 149–56.

David HL, 1984, Carotenoid pigments of the mycobacteria, *The Mycobacteria: A Sourcebook*, eds Kubica GP, Wayne LG, Marcel Dekker, New York, 537–45.

David HL, Jahan M-T et al., 1978, Numerical taxonomy analysis of *Mycobacterium africanum*, *Int J Syst Bacteriol*, **28:** 467–72.

Doub L, 1979, The chemical structures, properties, and mechanisms of action of the antituberculosis drugs, *Tuberculosis*, ed. Youmans GP, WB Saunders, Philadelphia, 435–56.

Draper P, 1986, Structure of *Mycobacterium leprae*, *Lepr Rev*, **57, Suppl. 2:** 15–20.

van Eden W, 1991, Heat-shock proteins as immunogenic bacterial antigens with the potential to induce and regulate autoimmune arthritis, *Immunol Rev*, **121:** 5–28.

Edwards LB, Acqaviva FA et al., 1969, An atlas of sensitivity to tuberculin, PPD-B and histoplasmin in the United States, *Am Rev Respir Dis*, **99, Suppl.:** 1–131.

Eisenach KD, Crawford JT, Bates JH, 1986, Genetic relatedness among strains of the *Mycobacterium tuberculosis* complex, *Am Rev Respir Dis*, **133:** 1065–8.

Ellner JJ, Goldberger MJ, Parenti DM, 1991, *Mycobacterium avium* infection and AIDS: a therapeutic dilemma in rapid evolution, *J Infect Dis*, **163:** 1326–35.

van Embden JDA, Cave MD et al., 1993, Strain identification of *Mycobacterium tuberculosis* by DNA fingerprinting: recommendations for a standardized methodology, *J Clin Microbiol*, **31:** 406–9.

Falkinham JO III, 1994, Epidemiology of *Mycobacterium avium* infection in the pre- and post-HIV era, *Res Microbiol*, **145:** 169–72.

Falkinham JO, Crawford JT, 1994, Plasmids, *Tuberculosis: Pathogenesis, Protection, and Control*, ed. Bloom BR, American Society for Microbiology Press, Washington, DC, 185–98.

Fauville-Dufax M, Maes N et al., 1995, Rapid identification of *Mycobacterium xenopi* from bacterial colonies or 'Bactec' culture by the polymerase chain reaction and a luminescent sandwich hybridization assay, *Res Microbiol*, **146:** 349–56.

Fox GE, Stackebrandt E, 1987, The application of 16S rRNA cataloging and 5S rRNA sequencing in bacterial systematics, *Methods in Microbiology*, vol. 19, eds Colwell R, Grigorova R, Academic Press, London, 405–58.

Frehel C, Rastogi N, 1989, Phagosome–lysosome fusions in macrophages infected with *Mycobacterium avium*: role of mycosides-C and other cell surface components, *Acta Leprol*, **7, Suppl. 1:** 173–4.

Gangadharam PRJ, Reddy MV, 1994, Contributions of animal and macrophage models to the understanding of host parasite interaction of *Mycobacterium avium* complex (MAC) disease, *Res Microbiol*, **145:** 214–24.

Gardner GM, Weiser RS, 1947, A bacteriophage for *Mycobacterium smegmatis*, *Proc Soc Exp Biol Med*, **66:** 205–6.

Gelber RH, 1994, Chemotherapy of lepromatous leprosy: recent developments and prospects for the future, *Eur J Clin Microbiol Infect Dis*, **13:** 942–52.

Gobin J, Moore CH et al., 1995, Iron acquisition by *Mycobacterium tuberculosis*: isolation and characterization of a family of iron-binding exochelins, *Proc Natl Acad Sci USA*, **92:** 5189–93.

Good RC, 1968, Simian tuberculosis: immunologic aspects, *Ann NY Acad Sci*, **154:** 200–13.

Good RC, 1984, Diseases in nonhuman primates, *The Mycobacteria: A Sourcebook*, eds Kubica GP, Wayne LG, Marcel Dekker, New York, 903–24.

Good RC, 1985, Opportunistic pathogens in the genus *Mycobacterium*, *Ann Rev Microbiol*, **39:** 347–69.

Good RC, 1992, The genus *Mycobacterium* – medical, *The Prokaryotes: a Handbook on the Biology of Bacteria: Ecophysiology, Isolation, Identification, Applications*, 2nd edn, vol. 2, eds Balows A, Truper HG et al., Springer-Verlag, New York, 1238–70.

Good RC, Beam RE, 1984, Seroagglutination, *The Mycobacteria: A Sourcebook*, eds Kubica GP, Wayne LG, Marcel Dekker, New York, 105–22.

Good RC, McCarroll NE, 1978, BCG vaccination in rhesus monkeys: study of skin hypersensitivity and duration of protective immunity, *Mycobacterial Infections of Zoo Animals*, ed. Montali RJ, Smithsonian Institution Press, Washington, DC, 115–21.

Good RC, Silcox VA, Kilburn JO, 1985, Identification and drug susceptibility test results for *Mycobacterium* spp., *Clin Microbiol Newslett*, **7**: 133–6.

Goodfellow M, Minnikin DE, 1984, Circumscription of the genus, *The Mycobacteria: A Sourcebook*, eds Kubica GP, Wayne LG, Marcel Dekker, New York, 1–24.

Gordon RE, Smith MM, 1955, Rapidly growing acid fast bacteria. II. Species description of *Mycobacterium fortuitum* Cruz, *J Bacteriol*, **69**: 502–7.

Goren MB, 1982, Immunoreactive substances of mycobacteria, *Am Rev Respir Dis*, **125**: 50–69.

Goren MB, Brokl O, Schaefer WB, 1974, Lipids of putative relevance to virulence in *Mycobacterium tuberculosis*: correlation of virulence and elaboration of sulfatides and strongly acidic lipids, *Infect Immun*, **9**: 150–8.

Goren MB, Vatter AE, Fiscus J, 1987, Polyanionic agents do not inhibit phagosome–lysosome fusion in cultured macrophages, *J Leuk Biol*, **41**: 122–9.

Grange JM, Collins CH, 1983, Mycobacterial pathogenicity and nomenclature: the 'nyrocine mycobacteria' [letter], *Tubercle*, **64**: 141–2.

Greenberg J, Woodley CL, 1984, Genetics of mycobacteria, *The Mycobacteria: A Sourcebook*, eds Kubica GP, Wayne LG, Marcel Dekker, New York, 629–39.

Hansen GA, 1880, *Bacillus leprae, Virchows Archiv*, **79**: 32–42.

Hartmans S, De Bont JAM, 1992, The genus *Mycobacterium* – nonmedical, *The Prokaryotes: a Handbook on the Biology of Bacteria: Ecophysiology, Isolation, Identification, Applications*, 2nd edn, vol. 2, eds Balows A, Truper HG et al., Springer-Verlag, New York, 1214–37.

Hatfull GF, 1993, Genetic transformation of mycobacteria, *Trends Microbiol*, **1**: 310–14.

Hatfull GF, Jacobs WR, 1994, Mycobacteriophages: cornerstones of mycobacterial research, *Tuberculosis: Pathogenesis, Protection, and Control*, ed. Bloom BR, American Society for Microbiology Press, Washington, DC, 165–83.

Hatfull GF, Sarkis GJ, 1993, DNA sequence, structure, and gene expression of mycobacteriophage L5: a phage system for mycobacterial genetics, *Mol Microbiol*, **7**: 395–405.

Havlir DV, 1994, *Mycobacterium avium* complex: advances in therapy, *Eur J Clin Microbiol Infect Dis*, **13**: 915–24.

Heifets LB, Good RC, 1994, Current laboratory methods for the diagnosis of tuberculosis, *Tuberculosis: Pathogenesis, Protection, and Control*, ed. Bloom BR, American Society for Microbiology, Washington, DC, 85–110.

Hermans PWM, van Soolingen D, van Embden JDA, 1992, Characterization of a major polymorphic tandem repeat in *Mycobacterium tuberculosis* and its potential use in the epidemiology of *Mycobacterium kansasii* and *Mycobacterium gordonae*, *J Bacteriol*, **174**: 4157–65.

Hoffner SE, 1994, Pulmonary infections caused by less frequently encountered slow-growing environmental mycobacteria, *Eur J Clin Microbiol Infect Dis*, **13**: 937–41.

Hoffner SE, Hjelm U, Kallenius G, 1993, Susceptibility of *Mycobacterium malmoense* to antibacterial drugs and drug combinations, *Antimicrob Agents Chemother*, **37**: 1285–8.

Horsburgh CR Jr, 1991, *Mycobacterium avium* complex infection in the acquired immunodeficiency syndrome, *N Engl J Med*, **324**: 1332–8.

Horsburgh CR Jr, Selik RM, 1989, The epidemiology of disseminated nontuberculous mycobacterial infection in the acquired immunodeficiency syndrome (AIDS), *Am Rev Respir Dis*, **139**: 4–7.

Horwitz MA, 1988, Intracellular parasitism, *Curr Opin Immunol*, **1**: 41–6.

Horwitz MA, Lee BWE et al., 1995, Protective immunity against tuberculosis induced by vaccination with major extracellular proteins of *Mycobacterium tuberculosis*, *Proc Natl Acad Sci USA*, **92**: 1530–4.

Huebner RE, Good RC, Tokars JI, 1993, Current practices in mycobacteriology: results of a survey of state laboratories, *J Clin Microbiol*, **31**: 771–5.

Imaeda T, 1984, Cell wall deficient forms, *The Mycobacteria: A Sourcebook*, eds Kubica GP, Wayne LG, Marcel Dekker, New York, 671–80.

Imaeda T, 1985, Deoxyribonucleic acid relatedness among selected strains of *Mycobacterium tuberculosis, Mycobacterium bovis, Mycobacterium bovis* BCG, *Mycobacterium microti*, and *Mycobacterium africanum*, *Int J Syst Bacteriol*, **35**: 147–50.

Inderlied CB, Salfinger M, 1995, Antimicrobial agents and susceptibility tests: mycobacteria, *Manual of Clinical Microbiology*, 6th edn, eds Murray PR, Baron EJ et al., American Society for Microbiology, Washington, DC, 1385–404.

Iseman MD, 1992, A leap of faith. What can we do to curtail intrainstitutional transmission of tuberculosis?, *Ann Intern Med*, **117**: 251–3.

Jacobs WR, Bloom BR, 1994, Molecular genetic strategies for identifying virulence determinants of *Mycobacterium tuberculosis, Tuberculosis: Pathogenesis, Protection, and Control*, ed. Bloom BR, American Society for Microbiology Press, Washington, DC, 253–68.

Jacobs WR, Tuckman M, Bloom BR, 1987, Introduction of foreign DNA into mycobacteria using a shuttle phasmid, *Nature (London)*, **327**: 532–5.

Janicki BW, Good RC et al., 1973, Immune responses in rhesus monkeys after Bacillus Calmette–Guérin vaccination and aerosol challenge with *Mycobacterium tuberculosis*, *Am Rev Respir Dis*, **107**: 359–66.

Jin DJ, Gross CA, 1988, Mapping and sequencing of mutations in the *Escherichia coli rpoB* gene that lead to rifampin resistance, *J Mol Biol*, **202**: 45–58.

Kaplan G, Gandhi RR et al., 1987, *Mycobacterium leprae* antigen-induced suppression of T cell proliferation in vitro, *J Immunol*, **138**: 3028–34.

Kapur V, Whittam TS, Musser JM, 1994, Is *Mycobacterium tuberculosis* 15,000 years old?, *J Infect Dis*, **170**: 1348–9.

Katanuma N, Nakasato H, 1954, A study of the mechanism of the development of streptomycin resistant organisms by addition of deoxyribonucleic acid prepared from resistant bacilli, *Kekkaku*, **29**: 19–22.

Kazda JF, 1983, The principles of the ecology of mycobacteria, *The Biology of the Mycobacteria*, vol. 2, eds Ratledge C, Stanford J, Academic Press, London, 323–415.

Kent PT, Kubica GP, 1985, *Public Health Mycobacteriology: A Guide for the Level III Laboratory*, US Department of Health and Human Services, Public Health Service, Centers for Disease Control, Atlanta, 1–207.

Kiehn TE, White M, 1994, *Mycobacterium haemophilum*: an emerging pathogen, *Eur J Clin Microbiol Infect Dis*, **13**: 925–31.

King CH, Sathish M et al., 1993, Expression of contact-dependent cytolytic activity by *Mycobacterium tuberculosis* and isolation of the genomic locus that encodes the activity, *Infect Immun*, **61**: 2708–12.

Koch R, 1882, Die Aetiologie der Tuberkulose, *Berl Klin Wochenschr*, **19**: 221–30.

Koch R, 1891, Weitere Mittheilung uber das Tuberkulin, *Dtsch Med Wochenschr*, **17**: 1189–92.

Kohne DE, 1989, The use of DNA probes to detect and identify microorganisms, *Rapid Methods in Clinical Microbiology*, eds Kleger B, Jungkind D et al., Plenum Press, New York, 11–35.

Kölbel HK, 1984, Electron microscopy, *The Mycobacteria: A Source-*

book, eds Kubica GP, Wayne LG, Marcel Dekker, New York, 249–313.

Kubica GP, 1984, Clinical microbiology, *The Mycobacteria: A Sourcebook*, eds Kubica GP, Wayne LG, Marcel Dekker, New York, 133–75.

Kubin N, Svandova E et al., 1980, *Mycobacterium kansasii* infection in an endemic area of Czechoslovakia, *Tubercle*, **61:** 207–12.

Lee MH, Pascopella L et al., 1991, Site specific integration of mycobacteriophage L5: integration-proficient vectors for *Mycobacterium smegmatis*, BCG, and *M. tuberculosis*, *Proc Natl Acad Sci USA*, **88:** 3111–15.

Lefford MJ, 1984, Diseases in mice and rats, *The Mycobacteria: A Sourcebook*, eds Kubica GP, Wayne LG, Marcel Dekker, New York, 947–77.

Lehmann KB, Neumann R, 1896, *Atlas und Grundis der Bakteriologie und Lehrbuch der speciellen bakteriologischen Diagnostik*, JF Lehmann, Munchen, Germany.

Levy-Frebault V, Portaels F, 1992, Proposed minimal standards for the genus *Mycobacterium* and for description of new slowly growing *Mycobacterium* species, *Int J Syst Bacteriol*, **42:** 315–23.

Levy-Frebault VV, Thorel MF et al., 1989, DNA polymorphism in *Mycobacterium paratuberculosis*, 'wood pigeon mycobacteria', and related mycobacteria analyzed by field inversion gel electrophoresis, *J Clin Microbiol*, **27:** 2823–6.

McDonough KA, Kress Y, Bloom BR, 1993, Pathogenesis of tuberculosis: interaction of *Mycobacterium tuberculosis* with macrophages, *Infect Immun*, **61:** 2763–73.

McFadden JJ, Butcher PD et al., 1987, Crohn's disease-associated mycobacteria are identical to *Mycobacterium paratuberculosis* as determined by DNA probes that distinguish between mycobacterial species, *J Clin Microbiol*, **25:** 796–801.

McMurray DN, 1994, Guinea pig model of tuberculosis, *Tuberculosis: Pathogenesis, Protection, and Control*, ed. Bloom BR, American Society for Microbiology, Washington, DC, 135–47.

Marsik FJ, Denys GA, 1995, Sterilization, decontamination, and disinfection procedures for the microbiology laboratory, *Manual of Clinical Microbiology*, 6th edn, eds Murray PR, Baron EJ et al., American Society for Microbiology, Washington, DC, 86–98.

Masur H, Public Health Service Task Force on Prophylaxis and Therapy for *Mycobacterium avium* Complex, 1993, Recommendations on prophylaxis and therapy for disseminated *Mycobacterium avium* complex disease in patients infected with the human immunodeficiency virus, *N Engl J Med*, **329:** 898–904.

Mehra V, Brennan PJ et al., 1984, Lymphocyte suppression in leprosy induced by unique *M. leprae* glycolipid, *Nature (London)*, **308:** 194–6.

Merkal RS, Crawford JA, 1979, Heat inactivation of *Mycobacterium avium-Mycobacterium intracellulare* complex organisms in aqueous suspension, *Appl Environ Microbiol*, **38:** 827–30.

Merkal RS, Lyle PS, Whipple DL, 1981, Heat inactivation of in vivo- and in vitro-grown mycobacteria in meat products, *Appl Environ Microbiol*, **41:** 1484–5.

Merkal RS, Whipple DL, 1980, Inactivation of *Mycobacterium bovis* in meat products, *Appl Environ Microbiol*, **40:** 282–4.

Middlebrook G, 1954, Isoniazid-resistance and catalase activity of tubercle bacilli, *Am Rev Tuberc*, **69:** 471–2.

Minnikin DE, 1982, Lipids: complex lipids, their chemistry, biosynthesis and roles, *The Biology of the Mycobacteria*, eds Ratledge C, Stanford JL, Academic Press, London, 96–184.

Minnikin DE, Goodfellow M, 1980, Lipid composition in the classification and identification of acid-fast bacteria, *Microbiological Classification and Identification*, eds Goodfellow M, Board RG, Academic Press, London, 189–256.

Minnikin DE, Dobson G et al., 1985, Mycolipenates and mycolipanolates of trehalose from *Mycobacterium tuberculosis*, *J Gen Microbiol*, **131:** 1369–74.

Mitchison DA, Wallace JG et al., 1960, A comparison of the virulence in guinea pigs of South Indian and British tubercle bacilli, *Tubercle*, **41:** 1–22.

Mizuguchi Y, 1984, Mycobacteriophages, *The Mycobacteria: A Sourcebook*, eds Kubica GP, Wayne LG, Marcel Dekker, New York, 641–62.

Mizuguchi Y, Suga K, Tokunaga T, 1976, Multiple mating types of *Mycobacterium smegmatis*, *Jpn J Microbiol*, **20:** 435–43.

Mor N, 1983, Intracellular location of *Mycobacterium leprae* in macrophages of normal and immunodeficient mice and the effect of rifampin, *Infect Immun*, **42:** 802–11.

du Moulin GC, Stottmeier KD et al., 1988, Concentration of *Mycobacterium avium* in hospital hot water systems, *JAMA*, **260:** 1599–601.

Musser JM, 1995, Antimicrobial agent resistance in mycobacteria: molecular genetic insights, *Clin Microbiol Rev*, **8:** 496–514.

Myrvick QN, Leake ES, Wright MJ, 1984, Disruption of phagosomal membranes of normal alveolar macrophages by the H37Rv strain of *Mycobacterium tuberculosis*, *Am Rev Respir Dis*, **129:** 322–8.

Nardell EA, 1993, Fans, filters, or rays? Pros and cons of the current environmental tuberculosis control technologies, *Infect Control Hosp Epidemiol*, **14:** 681–5.

Nettleman MD, Fredrickson M et al., 1994, Tuberculosis control strategies: the cost of particulate respirators, *Ann Intern Med*, **121:** 37–40.

Nightingale SD, Cameron DW et al., 1993, Two controlled trials of rifabutin prophylaxis against *Mycobacterium avium* complex infection in AIDS, *N Engl J Med*, **329:** 828–33.

Nolte FS, Metchock B, 1995, *Mycobacterium*, *Manual of Clinical Microbiology*, 6th edn, eds Murray PR, Baron EJ, American Society for Microbiology, Washington, DC, 400–37.

Orme IM, Collins FM, 1994, Mouse model of tuberculosis, *Tuberculosis: Pathogenesis, Protection, and Control*, ed. Bloom BR, American Society for Microbiology, Washington, DC, 113–34.

Pattyn SR, 1984a, *Mycobacterium marinum*, *The Mycobacteria: A Sourcebook*, eds Kubica GP, Wayne LG, Marcel Dekker, New York, 1137–9.

Pattyn SR, 1984b, *Mycobacterium lepraemurium*, *The Mycobacteria: A Sourcebook*, eds Kubica GP, Wayne LG, Marcel Dekker, New York, 1277–86.

Pattyn SR, 1984c, *Mycobacterium ulcerans*, *The Mycobacteria: A Sourcebook*, eds Kubica GP, Wayne LG, Marcel Dekker, New York, 1129–33.

Picardeau M, Vincent V, 1995, Development of a species-specific probe for *Mycobacterium xenopi*, *Res Microbiol*, **146:** 237–43.

Pitulle C, Dorsch M et al., 1992, Phylogeny of rapidly growing members of the genus *Mycobacterium*, *Int J Syst Bacteriol*, **42:** 337–43.

Plikaytis BB, Plikaytis BD et al., 1992, Differentiation of slow growing *Mycobacterium* species including *Mycobacterium tuberculosis* by gene amplification and restriction fragment length polymorphism, *J Clin Microbiol*, **30:** 1815–22.

Rastogi N, David HL, 1992, Mode of action of antituberculous drugs and mechanisms of drug resistance in *Mycobacterium tuberculosis*, *Res Microbiol*, **143:** 133–43.

Ratledge C, 1982, Nutrition, growth and metabolism, *The Biology of the Mycobacteria*, vol. 1, eds Ratledge C, Stanford JL, Academic Press, London, 286–312.

von Reyn CF, Waddell RD et al., 1993, Isolation of *Mycobacterium avium* complex from water in the United States, Finland, Zaire, and Kenya, *J Clin Microbiol*, **31:** 3227–30.

von Reyn CF, Maslow JN et al., 1994, Persistent colonisation of potable water as a source of *Mycobacterium avium* infection in AIDS, *Lancet*, **343:** 1137–41.

Riley RL, 1957, Aerial dissemination of pulmonary tuberculosis, *Am Rev Tuberc Pulm Dis*, **76:** 931–41.

Riley RL, 1961, Airborne pulmonary tuberculosis, *Bacteriol Rev*, **25:** 243–8.

Roberts AD, Sonnenberg MG et al., 1995, Characteristics of protective immunity engendered by vaccination of mice with purified culture filtrate protein antigens of *Mycobacterium tuberculosis*, *Immunology*, **85:** 502–8.

Rogall T, Wolters J et al., 1990, Towards a phylogeny and definition of species at the molecular level within the genus *Mycobacterium, Int J Syst Bacteriol*, **40**: 323–30.

Rubbo SD, Gardner JF, 1965, *A Review of Sterilization and Disinfection as Applied to Medical, Industrial and Laboratory Practice*, Year Book Medical Publishers, Chicago, IL, 85.

Runyon EH, 1959, Anonymous mycobacteria in pulmonary disease, *Med Clin North Am*, **43**: 273–90.

Runyon EH, 1965, Pathogenic mycobacteria, *Adv Tuberc Res*, **14**: 235–87.

Rutala WA, Weber DJ, 1995, FDA labeling requirements for disinfection of endoscopes: a counterpoint, *Infect Control Hosp Epidemiol*, **16**: 231–5.

Rutala WA, Jones SM et al., 1995, Efficacy of portable filtration units in reducing aerosolized particles in the size range of *Mycobacterium tuberculosis*, *Infect Control Hosp Epidemiol*, **16**: 391–8.

Salfinger M, Pfyffer GE, 1994, The new diagnostic mycobacteriology laboratory, *Eur J Clin Microbiol Infect Dis*, **13**: 961–79.

Sathish M, Shinnick TM, 1994, Identification of genes involved in the resistance of mycobacteria to killing by macrophages, *Ann NY Acad Sci*, **730**: 26–36.

Schlesinger LS, 1993, Macrophage phagocytosis of virulent but not attenuated strains of *Mycobacterium tuberculosis* is mediated by mannose receptors in addition to complement receptors, *J Immunol*, **150**: 2920–30.

Schlesinger LS, Horwitz MA, 1990, Phagocytosis of leprosy bacilli is mediated by complement receptors CR1 and CR3 on human monocytes and complement component C3 in serum, *J Clin Invest*, **85**: 1304–11.

Schlesinger LS, Bellinger-Kawahara CG et al., 1990, Phagocytosis of *Mycobacterium tuberculosis* is mediated by human monocyte complement receptors and complement component C3, *J Immunol*, **144**: 2771–80.

Schmidt LH, 1972, Improving existing methods of control of tuberculosis: a prime challenge to the experimentalist, *Am Rev Respir Dis*, **105**: 183–205.

Schulze-Röbbecke R, Buchholtz K, 1992, Heat susceptibility of aquatic mycobacteria, *Appl Environ Microbiol*, **58**: 1869–73.

Seibert FB, Glenn JT, 1941, Tuberculin purified protein derivative: preparation and analysis of a large quantity for standard, *Am Rev Tuberc*, **44**: 9–25.

Selwyn PA, Hartel D et al., 1989, A prospective study of the risk of tuberculosis among intravenous drug users with human immunodeficiency virus infection, *N Engl J Med*, **320**: 545–50.

Shepard CC, 1981, *Mycobacterium leprae, The Prokaryotes*, eds Starr MP, Stolp H et al., Springer-Verlag, Berlin, 1985–90.

Shinnick TM, 1991, Heat shock proteins as antigens of bacterial and parasitic pathogens, *Curr Top Microbiol Immunol*, **167**: 145–60.

Shinnick TM, 1992, *Mycobacterium leprae, The Prokaryotes, a Handbook on the Biology of Bacteria: Ecophysiology, Isolation, Identification, Applications*, 2nd edn, eds Balows A, Trüper HG et al., Springer-Verlag, New York, 1271–82.

Shinnick TM, Good RC, 1994, Mycobacterial taxonomy, *Eur J Clin Microbiol Infect Dis*, **13**: 884–901.

Shinnick TM, Jonas V, 1994, Molecular approaches to the diagnosis of tuberculosis, *Tuberculosis: Pathogenesis, Protection, and Control*, ed. Bloom BR, American Society for Microbiology Press, Washington, DC, 517–30.

Sibley LD, Franzblau SG, Krahenbuhl JL, 1987, Intracellular fate of *Mycobacterium leprae* in normal and activated macrophages, *Infect Immun*, **55**: 680–5.

Sibley LD, Hunter SW et al., 1988, Mycobacterial lipoarabinomannan inhibits gama interferon-mediated activation of macrophages, *Infect Immun*, **56**: 1232–6.

Siddiqi SH, 1988, *BACTEC TB System: Product and Procedure Manual*, Becton Dickinson Diagnostic Instrument Systems, Inc., Towson, MD.

Silcox VA, Good RC, Floyd MM, 1981, Identification of clinically significant *Mycobacterium fortuitum* complex isolates, *J Clin Microbiol*, **14**: 686–91.

Smith DW, 1984, Diseases in guinea pigs, *The Mycobacteria: A Sourcebook*, eds Kubica GP, Wayne LG, Marcel Dekker, New York, 925–46.

Smith DW, Randall HM et al., 1957, The characterization of mycobacterial strains by composition of their lipid extracts, *Ann NY Acad Sci*, **69**: 145–57.

Smithwick RW, 1976, *Laboratory Manual for Acid-fast Microscopy*, 2nd edn, US Department of Health, Education and Welfare, Public Health Service, Center for Disease Control, Atlanta, 1–40.

Smithwick RW, 1994, The working mycobacteriology laboratory, *Tuberculosis: Current Concepts and Treatment*, ed. Friedman LN, CRC Press, Boca Raton, FL, 71–80.

Snapper SB, Lugosi L et al., 1988, Lysogeny and transformation in mycobacteria: stable expression of foreign genes, *Proc Natl Acad Sci USA*, **85**: 6987–91.

Sniadack DE, Ostroff SD et al., 1992, A nosocomial pseudo-outbreak of *Mycobacterium xenopi* due to a contaminated potable water supply: lessons in prevention, *Infect Control Hosp Epidemiol*, **14**: 636–41.

Stahl DA, Urbance JW, 1990, The division between fast- and slow-growing species corresponds to natural relationships among the mycobacteria, *J Bacteriol*, **172**: 116–24.

Stanford JL, 1983, Immunologically important constituents of mycobacteria: antigens, *The Biology of the Mycobacteria*, vol. 2, eds Ratledge C, Stanford JL, Academic Press, London, 85–127.

Stanford JL, Grange YM, 1974, The meaning and structure of species as applied to mycobacteria, *Tubercle*, **55**: 143–52.

Stanford JL, Shields MJ, Rook GAW, 1981, How mycobacteria may predetermine the protective efficiency of BCG, *Tubercle*, **62**: 55–62.

Stanford JL, Revill WDL et al., 1975, The production and preliminary investigation of Burulin, a new skin test reagent for *Mycobacterium ulcerans* infection, *J Hyg*, **74**: 7–16.

Steinhoff U, Golecki JR et al., 1989, Evidence for phagosome–lysosome fusion in *Mycobacterium leprae*-infected murine Schwann cells, *Infect Immun*, **57**: 1008–10.

Stewart-Tull DES, 1983, Immunologically important constituents of mycobacteria: adjuvants, *The Biology of the Mycobacteria*, vol. 2, eds Ratledge C, Stanford JL, Academic Press, London, 3–84.

Straus WL, Ostroff SM et al., 1994, Clinical and epidemiologic characteristics of *Mycobacterium haemophilum*, an emerging pathogen of immunocompromised patients, *Ann Intern Med*, **120**: 118–25.

Sundaraj CV, Ramakrishnan T, 1971, Transduction in *Mycobacterium smegmatis*, *Nature (London)*, **228**: 456–60.

Swenson JM, Thornsberry C, Silcox VA, 1982, Rapidly growing mycobacteria: testing of susceptibility to 34 antimicrobial agents by broth microdilution, *Antimicrob Agents Chemother*, **22**: 186–92.

Takayama K, Kilburn JO, 1989, Inhibition of synthesis of arabinogalactan by ethambutol in *Mycobacterium smegmatis*, *Antimicrob Agents Chemother*, **33**: 1493–9.

Thoen CO, 1994a, Tuberculosis in wild and domestic animals, *Tuberculosis: Pathogenesis, Protection, and Control*, ed. Bloom BR, American Society for Microbiology Press, Washington, DC, 157–62.

Thoen CO, 1994b, *Mycobacterium avium* infection in animals, *Res Microbiol*, **145**: 173–7.

Thoen CO, Francis J, Haagsma J, 1984, Experimental mycobacterial infections in some domestic animals, *The Mycobacteria: A Sourcebook*, eds Kubica GP, Wayne LG, Marcel Dekker, New York, 1287–96.

Thoen CO, Himes EM, Karlson AG, 1984, *Mycobacterium avium* complex, *The Mycobacteria: A Sourcebook*, eds Kubica GP, Wayne LG, Marcel Dekker, New York, 1251–75.

Thoen CO, Karlson AG, 1984, Experimental tuberculosis in rabbits, *The Mycobacteria: A Sourcebook*, eds Kubica GP, Wayne LG, Marcel Dekker, New York, 979–89.

Thoen CO, Karlson AG, Himes EW, 1984, *Mycobacterium tuberculosis* complex, *The Mycobacteria: A Sourcebook*, eds Kubica GP, Wayne LG, Marcel Dekker, New York, 1209–35.

Timpe A, Runyon EH, 1954, The relationship of 'atypical' acid-fast bacteria to human disease, *J Lab Clin Med*, **44**: 202–9.

Tokunaga T, Sellers MI, 1964, Infection of *Mycobacterium smegmatis* and D29 phage DNA, *J Exp Med*, **119**: 139–49.

Tsukamura M, 1972, The pattern of rifampin resistance in *Mycobacterium tuberculosis*, *Tubercle*, **53**: 111–17.

Tsukamura M, 1984, The 'non-pathogenic' species of mycobacteria: their distribution and ecology in non-living reservoirs, *The Mycobacteria: A Sourcebook*, eds Kubica GP, Wayne LG, Marcel Dekker, New York, 1339–59.

Wallace RJ Jr, 1994, Recent changes in taxonomy and disease manifestations of the rapidly growing mycobacteria, *Eur J Clin Microbiol Infect Dis*, **13**: 953–60.

Wallace RJ Jr, O'Brien R et al., 1990, Diagnosis and treatment of disease caused by nontuberculous mycobacteria, *Am Rev Respir Dis*, **142**: 940–53.

Wayne LG, 1981, Numerical taxonomy and cooperative studies: roles and limits, *Rev Infect Dis*, **3**: 822–8.

Wayne LG, 1984, Mycobacterial speciation, *The Mycobacteria: A Sourcebook*, eds Kubica GP, Wayne LG, Marcel Dekker, New York, 25–65.

Wayne LG, 1994, Dormancy of *Mycobacterium tuberculosis* and latency of disease, *Eur J Clin Microbiol Infect Dis*, **13**: 908–14.

Wayne LG, Kubica GP, 1986, The mycobacteria, *Bergey's Manual of Systematic Bacteriology*, 8th edn, eds Sneath PHA, Mair NS et al., Williams & Wilkins, Baltimore, MD, 1436–57.

Wayne LG, Lin K-Y, 1982, Glyoxylate metabolism and adaption of *Mycobacterium tuberculosis* to survival under anaerobic conditions, *Infect Immun*, **37**: 1042–9.

Wayne LG, Engbaek HC et al., 1974, Highly reproducible techniques for use in systematic bacteriology in the genus *Mycobacterium*: tests for pigment, urease, resistance to sodium chloride, hydrolysis of Tween 80, and β-galactosidase, *Int J Syst Bacteriol*, **24**: 412–19.

Wayne LG, Engel HWB et al., 1976, Highly reproducible techniques for use in systematic bacteriology in the genus *Mycobacterium*: tests for niacin and catalase and resistance to isoniazid, thiophene 2-carboxylic acid hydrazide, hydroxylamine, and p-nitrobenzoate, *Int J Syst Bacteriol*, **26**: 311–18.

Wayne LG, Andrade L et al., 1978, A cooperative numerical analysis of *Mycobacterium gastri*, *Mycobacterium kansasii* and *Mycobacterium marinum*, *J Gen Microbiol*, **109**: 319–27.

Wayne LG, Good RC et al., 1981, First report of the cooperative, open-ended study of slowly growing mycobacteria by the International Working Group on Mycobacterial Taxonomy, *Int J Syst Bacteriol*, **31**: 1–20.

Wayne LG, Good RC et al., 1983, Second report of the cooperative, open-ended study of slowly growing mycobacteria by the International Working Group on Mycobacterial Taxonomy, *Int J Syst Bacteriol*, **33**: 265–74.

Wayne LG, Brenner DJ et al., 1987, Report of the ad hoc committee on the reconciliation of approaches to bacterial systematics, *Int J Syst Bacteriol*, **437**: 463–4.

Wayne LG, Good RC et al., 1989, Third report of the cooperative, open-ended study of slowly growing mycobacteria by the

International Working Group on Mycobacterial Taxonomy, *Int J Syst Bacteriol*, **39**: 267–78.

Wayne LG, Good RC et al., 1991, Fourth report of the cooperative, open-ended study of slowly growing mycobacteria by the International Working Group on Mycobacterial Taxonomy, *Int J Syst Bacteriol*, **41**: 463–72.

Wayne LG, Good RC et al., 1993, Serovar determination and molecular taxonomic correlation in *Mycobacterium avium*, *Mycobacterium intracellulare* and *Mycobacterium scrofulaceum*: a cooperative study of the International Working Group on Mycobacterial Taxonomy, *Int J Syst Bacteriol*, **43**: 482–9.

Weitzman I, Osadcyzi D et al., 1981, *Mycobacterium thermoresistibile*: a new pathogen for humans, *J Clin Microbiol*, **14**: 593–5.

Wheeler PR, Ratledge C, 1994, Metabolism of *Mycobacterium tuberculosis*, *Tuberculosis: Pathogenesis, Protection, and Control*, ed. Bloom BR, American Society for Microbiology Press, Washington, DC, 353–85.

Winder FG, 1982, Mode of action of the antimycobacterial agents and associated aspects of the molecular biology of the mycobacteria, *The Biology of the Mycobacteria*, vol. 1, eds Ratledge C, Stanford J, Academic Press, London, 352–438.

Wolinski E, Schaefer WB, 1973, Proposed numbering scheme for mycobacterial serotypes by agglutination, *Int J Syst Bacteriol*, **23**: 182–3.

Woods GL, Witebsky FG, 1993, Current status of mycobacterial testing in clinical laboratories: results of a questionnaire completed by participants in the College of American Pathologists mycobacteriology E survey, *Arch Pathol Lab Med*, **117**: 876–84.

Yajko DM, Chin DP et al., 1995, *Mycobacterium avium* complex in water, food, and soil samples collected from the environment of HIV-infected individuals, *J Acquir Immune Defic Syndr Hum Retrovirol*, **9**: 176–82.

Yakrus MA, Reeves MW, Hunter SB, 1992, Characterization of isolates of *Mycobacterium avium* serotypes 4 and 8 from patients with AIDS by multilocus enzyme electrophoresis, *J Clin Microbiol*, **30**: 1474–8.

Youmans GP, 1979, *Tuberculosis*, WB Saunders, Philadelphia, 9–25.

Youmans GP, Doub L, Youmans AS, 1953, *The Bacteriostatic Activity of 3500 Organic Compounds for* Mycobacterium tuberculosis *var.* hominis, Chemical-Biological Coordination Center, National Research Council, Washington, DC, 1–713.

Young DB, Mehlert A, 1989, Serology of mycobacteria: characterization of antigens recognized by monoclonal antibodies, *Rev Infect Dis*, **11**: S431–5.

Young DB, Kaufmann SHE et al., 1992, Mycobacterial protein antigens: a compilation, *Mol Microbiol*, **6**: 133–45.

Young RA, 1990, Stress proteins and immunology, *Annu Rev Immunol*, **8**: 401–20.

Young RA, Bloom BR et al., 1985a, Dissection of *Mycobacterium tuberculosis* antigens using recombinant DNA, *Proc Natl Acad Sci USA*, **82**: 2583–7.

Young RA, Mehra V et al., 1985b, Genes for the major protein antigens of the leprosy parasite *Mycobacterium leprae*, *Nature (London)*, **316**: 450–2.

Zhang Y, Young DB, 1993, Molecular mechanisms of isoniazid: a drug in the front line of tuberculosis control, *Trends Microbiol*, **1**: 109–13.

Zopf W, 1883, *Die Spaltpilze*, Edward Trewendt, Breslau.

Chapter 27

STAPHYLOCOCCUS

W E Kloos

1 Historical perspective	8 Cellular components
2 Definition of the genus	9 Genetic mechanisms
3 Classification of species and subspecies	10 Resistance to antimicrobial agents
4 Habitat	11 Laboratory isolation and identification
5 Cell morphology	12 Typing methods for the identification of
6 Cultural characteristics	infrasubspecific forms
7 Metabolism	13 Pathogenicity

1 HISTORICAL PERSPECTIVE

Cohn described 4 tribes of bacteria and placed the spherical types, including the bacteria that are recognized today as staphylococci, streptococci, and micrococci, into the genus *Micrococcus* of the tribe Sphaerobacteria (Kugelbacterien). Koch noted the presence of small spherical bacteria in pus, abscesses, and the blood of people with pyaemia and referred to them as micrococci. Ogston introduced the name *Staphylococcus* (σταφυλή, a bunch of grapes) for the group-micrococci causing inflammation and suppuration. Pasteur observed the presence of small spherical bacteria in the pus of furuncles and osteomyelitis and thought that these bacteria might be pathogenic. Based on the description of these organisms, it is likely that Pasteur was observing Ogston's staphylococci.

Rosenbach provided the first formal description of the genus *Staphylococcus* and divided the genus into 2 species, *Staphylococcus aureus* and *Staphylococcus albus*. Passet added a third species, *Staphylococcus citreus*. Cell morphology and type of cell aggregation provided the criteria for genus classification. Colony colour was the criterion for species classification. Zopf placed the staphylococci and a group of saprophytic, tetrad-forming micrococci back into the genus *Micrococcus* and Flügge rearranged the cocci and separated the genus *Staphylococcus* from the genus *Micrococcus*. He differentiated the 2 genera primarily on the basis of their action on gelatin and on the symbiotic relationship to their hosts. Staphylococci liquefied gelatin and were considered to be parasitic or pathogenic, or both, whereas micrococci were variable in their action on gelatin and were thought to be saprophytic. Evans, Bradford and Niven (1955) proposed separating staphylococci from micrococci on the basis of their relation to oxygen using a standard oxidation–fermentation (OF) test for glucose fermentation. The facultative anaerobic cocci were placed in the genus *Staphylococcus* and the obligate aerobes were placed in the genus *Micrococcus*. The separation of the genera solely on the basis of

the OF test continued as a practice until it became apparent that some staphylococci formed very little acid from glucose and gave a negative reaction with the OF test, whereas some micrococci produced sufficient acid from glucose under anaerobic conditions to give a positive reaction. A clear distinction could be made between staphylococci and micrococci on the basis of DNA base composition (Silvestri and Hill 1965); however, this property could not be determined in the routine diagnostic laboratory. Surveys of gram-positive, catalase-positive cocci indicated that staphylococci have a G + C content of DNA of 30–39 mol%, whereas micrococci have a G + C content of 63–73 mol%. Although both genera were placed in the family Micrococcaceae (Prévot 1961), the very wide divergence in DNA base composition indicates that they are not significantly related. More recent systematic studies have distinguished staphylococci from micrococci and other bacteria on the basis of cell wall composition (Schleifer and Kandler 1972), cytochromes (Faller, Götz and Schleifer 1980), menaquinones (Collins and Jones 1981), cellular fatty acids, polar lipids (Nahaie et al. 1984), DNA–rRNA hybridization (Kilpper, Buhl and Schleifer 1980, Schleifer 1986), and comparative oligonucleotide cataloguing of 16S rRNA (Ludwig et al. 1981). It is now recognized that the genus *Staphylococcus* belongs to the broad *Bacillus–Lactobacillus–Streptococcus* cluster consisting of gram-positive bacteria that have a low G + C content of DNA. The closest relatives of staphylococci are the macrococci (Kloos et al. 1997a), and on the basis of partial oligonucleotide sequencing of 16S rRNA and rDNA, staphylococci are also related to salinicocci, enterococci, planococci, bacilli and listeriae (Ludwig et al. 1985, Stackebrandt et al. 1987). The closest relatives of the micrococci are the arthrobacters, renibacteria, rothias, dermatophili and stomatococci (Koch, Rainey and Stackebrandt 1994). The genus *Micrococcus* has been recently dissected into 6 genera (*Micrococcus*, *Kocuria*, *Nesterenkonia*, *Kytococcus*, *Dermacoccus* and *Arthrobacter*) on the basis of 16S rDNA sequence relationships and several chemotaxonomic characters (Koch, Schumann and Stackebrandt 1995, Stackebrandt et al. 1995).

Early medical bacteriologists placed major emphasis on distinguishing the pathogenic species *S. aureus* from the presumed commensal staphylococci, referred to as *S. albus*, *Staphylococcus epidermidis albus* (Welch 1891), or *Staphylococcus epidermidis* (Evans 1916). The distinction was of considerable importance since *S. aureus* was a major cause of morbidity and mortality and clinical specimens often carried both types of organisms. Von Darányi (1925) was the first person to draw attention to the practical value of the coagulating principle (coagulase) test to identify *S. aureus* and it remains one of the most important tests used by the clinical laboratory to identify this species. Baird-Parker (1963, 1965a) attempted to subdivide the genera *Staphylococcus* and *Micrococcus* by using many classical morphological, physiological and biochemical tests. He first divided staphylococci into 6 subgroups (I–VI) and micrococci into 8 subgroups (1–8). In subsequent schemes, Baird-Parker (1965b, 1974) recognized the species *S. aureus*, *S. epidermidis* and *Staphylococcus saprophyticus* and divided the latter 2 species into several biotypes. His schemes were widely used for more than a decade, especially by medical and food diagnostic laboratories. Meyer (1967) and Hájek and Maršálek (1971) divided the species *S. aureus* into several biotypes on the basis of physiological, biochemical and phage typing properties, and host preferences.

2 DEFINITION OF THE GENUS

Members of the genus *Staphylococcus* are gram-positive cocci (0.5–1.5 μm) that occur singly, in pairs, tetrads, short chains, and irregular 'grape-like' clusters. They are non-motile and non-spore-forming. Most species demonstrate catalase activity and are facultative anaerobes, growing better under aerobic than anaerobic conditions; the anaerobic species *Staphylococcus saccharolyticus* and subspecies *S. aureus* subsp. *anaerobius* are exceptions. Most species grow in the presence of 10% sodium chloride and at 18–40°C. Staphylococci are susceptible to furazolidone (100 μg furazolidone disc) and resistant to low levels of bacitracin (0.04 unit TAXO A bacitracin disc). They are susceptible to lysis by lysostaphin (some species more than others) and are relatively resistant to lysis by lysozyme. The cell wall contains peptidoglycan and teichoic acid. The diamino acid present in the peptidoglycan is L-lysine; the interpeptide bridge of the peptidoglycan consists of oligoglycine peptides that are susceptible to the action of lysostaphin. Depending on the particular species, some glycine residues may be substituted by L-serine or L-alanine. The teichoic acids of staphylococci are either of the poly(polyolphosphate), poly(glycerolphosphate-glycosylphosphate), or poly(glycosylphosphate) class. Glycerol or ribitol or both occur as typical components of poly(polyolphosphate) teichoic acids. Species contain either *a*- and *b*-type cytochromes or *a*-, *b*- and *c*-type cytochromes. Staphylococci contain unsaturated polyisoprenoid side chains in their menaquinones. The major isoprenologues are MK-6, MK-7 or MK-8. The principal cellular fatty acids are $C_{16:0}$, $C_{18:0}$ and $C_{20:0}$ and *iso*- and *anteiso*-methyl-branched $C_{15:0}$ and $C_{17:0}$. The G + C content of DNA is 30–40 mol%. Staphylococci have genus-, species- and subspecies-specific chromosome *Eco*RI fragments containing portions of rRNA operons (Cole et al. 1994, Webster et al. 1994).

Recent investigations on cell structure, cell wall composition, G + C content of DNA, DNA–DNA hybridization, 16S rRNA sequence similarities, and the genome sizes of *Staphylococcus caseolyticus* (Schleifer et al. 1982) and the newly introduced species *Staphylococcus bovicus*, *Staphylococcus carouselicus* and *Staphylococcus equipercicus* (Ballard et al. 1995) have indicated that this group of 4 species should be placed into a separate, but closely related genus, which has been given the name *Macrococcus* (Kloos et al. 1997a). Cells of these organisms are generally larger (1.5–2.5 μm diameter) than the cells of staphylococcal species. *S. caseolyticus* (proposed to be renamed *Macrococcus caseolyticus*) has an unusual cell wall teichoic acid and the other species of this genus fail to demonstrate teichoic acid. The G + C content of DNA is 38–45 mol%. The estimated genome size of the members of the genus *Macrococcus* is 1500–1820 kbp, which is significantly smaller than the genome size of 2000–3000 shown for *Staphylococcus* spp.

3 CLASSIFICATION OF SPECIES AND SUBSPECIES

3.1 Species

There are 32 species currently recognized in the genus *Staphylococcus* (Table 27.1). *Staphylococcus* spp. are classified first of all on the basis of DNA–DNA hybridization (DNA relatedness) as determined by the relative binding of DNAs in reassociation reactions conducted at non-restrictive (optimal), restrictive (stringent) conditions, or a combination of both (Kloos 1980, Schleifer 1986, Kloos, Schleifer and Götz 1991). Members of the same species demonstrate relative DNA-binding values of generally 70% or greater when reactions are performed at the optimal criterion. Organisms representing different species demonstrate relative DNA-binding values of less than 70% at the optimal criterion and have a much lower relative binding percentage at the stringent criterion. A dendrogram depicting the DNA relationships of species is shown in Fig. 27.1. The thermal stability ($\Delta T_{m(e)}$) of the DNA duplexes formed in reassociation reactions conducted at non-restrictive conditions supports the conclusions drawn from the relative DNA-binding studies, although not all species have been investigated by this approach. Comparative immunological studies of catalases (Rupprecht and Schleifer 1979, Schleifer, Meyer and Rupprecht 1979) and fructose-1,6-biphosphate (FBP) aldolases (Fischer et al. 1983), using microcomplement fixation techniques, have indicated essentially the same relatedness as DNA–DNA hybridization.

Chemical properties of the cell wall, especially the amino acid composition and sequence of the interpeptide bridges of the peptidoglycan (Schleifer 1983, 1986) and teichoic acid composition (Endl et al. 1984), provide useful chemotaxonomic markers for the classification of species (Table 27.2). Penta- and hexaglycine interpeptide bridges are found in the

Table 27.1 Currently recognized *Staphylococcus* species

Species	Reference
S. epidermidis	Winslow and Winslow 1908, Evans 1916, Schleifer and Kloos 1975
S. capitis	Kloos and Schleifer 1975a
S. caprae	Devriese et al. 1983
S. saccharolyticus	Foubert and Douglas 1948, Kilpper-Bälz and Schleifer 1981
S. hominis	Kloos and Schleifer 1975a
S. haemolyticus	Schleifer and Kloos 1975
S. warneri	Kloos and Schleifer 1975a
S. pasteuri	Chesneau et al. 1993
S. lugdunensis	Freney et al. 1988
S. auricularis	Kloos and Schleifer 1983
S. aureus	Rosenbach 1884
S. saprophyticus	Shaw, Stitt and Cowan 1951, Schleifer and Kloos 1975
S. cohnii	Schleifer and Kloos 1975
S. xylosus	Schleifer and Kloos 1975
S. kloosii	Schleifer, Kilpper-Bälz and Devriese 1984
S. equorum	Schleifer, Kilpper-Bälz and Devriese 1984
S. arlettae	Schleifer, Kilpper-Bälz and Devriese 1984
S. gallinarum	Devriese et al. 1983
S. simulans	Kloos and Schleifer 1975a
S. carnosus	Schleifer and Fischer 1982
S. piscifermentans	Tanasupawat et al. 1992
S. felis	Igimi et al. 1989
S. intermedius	Hájek 1976
S. schleiferi	Freney et al. 1988
S. delphini	Varaldo et al. 1988
S. hyicus	Devriese et al. 1978
S. chromogenes	Devriese et al. 1978, Hájek et al. 1986
S. muscae	Hájek et al. 1992
S. sciuri	Kloos, Schleifer and Smith 1976
S. lentus	Kloos, Schleifer and Smith 1976, Schleifer et al. 1983
S. vitulus	Webster et al. 1994
S. caseolyticus	Schleifer et al. 1982

peptidoglycan in about half the species, whereas in the other half a minor portion of the glycine residues are replaced by L-serine. In 3 species (*Staphylococcus sciuri, Staphylococcus lentus, Staphylococcus vitulus*), an L-alanine residue, in place of glycine, is bound to lysine of the peptide subunit. Most species have cell wall teichoic acids of the poly(glycerolphosphate) and/or poly(ribitolphosphate) type that are substituted with various combinations of sugars and/or N-acetylamino sugar residues. Some strains of *S. sciuri, S. vitulus* and *Staphylococcus hyicus* have the poly(glycerolphosphate-N-acetylglucosaminylphosphate) type and *Staphylococcus auricularis* and *S. caseolyticus* have the poly(N-acetylglucosaminylphosphate) type, where the N-acetylamino sugar residues form an integral part of the polymer chain.

Certain other biochemical properties of staphylococci are useful for the differentiation of species. Many species produce lactic acid from glucose when grown under anaerobic conditions, although some produce only trace amounts (Schleifer 1986). Some of the species differ with regard to the lactate isomer formed and the occurrence of NAD-dependent L- and/or D-lactate dehydrogenases. Most of the species form L-lactate or L- and D-lactate from glucose. The

closely related species *Staphylococcus hominis* and *Staphylococcus haemolyticus* form D-lactate from glucose. *Staphylococcus intermedius, Staphylococcus capitis, Staphylococcus epidermidis* and *Staphylococcus warneri* have an L-lactate dehydrogenase which is specifically activated by FBP (Götz and Schleifer 1976). Most species possess a class I FBP aldolase, which is an aldolase that functions via the formation of a Schiff base intermediate between the substrate and the amino group of a lysine residue of the enzyme (Götz, Nürnberger and Schleifer 1979). *S. intermedius, S. hyicus* and *Staphylococcus chromogenes* possess class I and class II FBP aldolases and *S. caseolyticus* possesses only a class II aldolase (Fischer, Luczak and Schleifer 1982). Class II aldolases do not form a Schiff base intermediate and require an essential divalent cation. Staphylococci contain *a*- and *b*-type cytochromes in their respiratory chains (Faller, Götz and Schleifer 1980). The species *S. sciuri, S. lentus, S. vitulus* and *S. caseolyticus* also contain *c*-type cytochromes (Faller, Götz and Schleifer 1980, Schleifer et al. 1982, Webster et al. 1994). Many of the staphylococcal species can be distinguished on the basis of their relative percentages of cellular fatty acid components, as determined by gas-liquid chromatography (Durham and Kloos 1978, Kotilainen, Houvinen and Eerola 1991). For example, *S. warneri* can be clearly distinguished from the related species *S. hominis* and *S. haemolyticus* by its high percentage of $C_{20:0}$ fatty acid and relatively low percentages of methyl-branched *iso*-

% DNA relatedness at optimal conditions

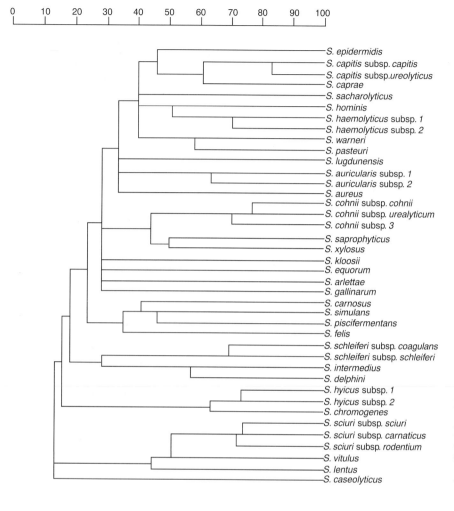

Fig. 27.1 Dendrogram of the DNA relationships of *Staphylococcus* species and subspecies based on the relative % of DNA–DNA hybridization (reassociation). Optimal DNA reassociation conditions were performed at 55°C (29–31°C below the T_m of the DNA) (Kloos and Wolfshohl 1979).

and *anteiso*-$C_{15:0}$, $C_{17:0}$ and $C_{19:0}$ fatty acids. *S. capitis* can be distinguished from the closely related species *S. epidermidis* by its high percentage of $C_{18:0}$ fatty acid and relatively low percentages of methyl-branched *iso*- and *anteiso*-$C_{15:0}$, $C_{17:0}$ and $C_{19:0}$ fatty acids. Some of the biochemical and physiological properties of staphylococci can be determined by simple conventional tests and rapid identification systems. These include various enzyme activities, haemolysins, oxygen requirements, products of glucose metabolism, utilization of substrates, production of acid from carbohydrates and intrinsic resistance to certain antibiotics (Kloos, Schleifer and Götz 1991, Kloos and Bannerman 1995). Colony morphology and pigment can serve as secondary characters for the classification of species and are valuable markers for the initial identification of staphylococci growing on primary isolation plates (Kloos and Bannerman 1994). Specific combinations of the above phenotypic characters have been quite accurate in predicting the identification of species based on DNA relatedness.

Three recent molecular approaches showing promise for the classification of species are:

1 ribotyping (De Buyser et al. 1992, Webster et al. 1994)
2 macrorestriction analysis using pulse field gel electrophoresis (PFGE) (Lina et al. 1992b, George and Kloos 1994, Bannerman et al. 1995, Goering 1995) or field-inversion gel electrophoresis (FIGE) (Goering and Winters 1992) and

3 polymerase chain reaction (PCR)-amplified ribosomal DNA spacer and tDNA intergenic spacer fingerprinting (Welsh and McClelland 1992, Jensen, Webster and Straus 1993).

The comprehensive ribotyping studies of Webster and colleagues (Cole et al. 1994, Webster et al. 1994) have identified conserved, chromosome *Eco*RI fragments containing portions of the rRNA operons that are species-specific. PFGE studies have identified conserved, chromosome *Sma*I fragments that are species-specific (George and Kloos 1994, Ballard et al. 1995, Bannerman et al. 1995, Shimizu et al. 1996). Although only a relatively small number of species have been analysed by either rDNA–PCR or tDNA–PCR fingerprinting to date, each of the species examined could be clearly distinguished on the basis of species-specific length polymorphisms.

Some of the staphylococcal species can be placed into species groups because of their close genomic relationships, as determined by DNA–DNA relatedness (Kloos, Schleifer and Götz 1991) and ribotyping (Webster et al. 1994). Members of the same staphylococcal species group generally produce resident populations on hosts that are closely related or have been in close contact with one another throughout a long history (e.g. humans and domestic animals). The following 6 species groups are informally recognized (member species are listed in parentheses):

Table 27.2 Types of cell wall peptidoglycan and teichoic acid of *Staphylococcus* species

Species	Peptidoglycan type: interpeptide bridge[a]	Teichoic acid type Poly(repeating unit)[b]	Teichoic acid main substituent[c]
S. epidermidis	L-Lys-Gly$_4$, L-Ser	GroP	Glc, GlcNAc
S. capitis	L-Lys-Gly$_4$, L-Ser	GroP	GlcNAc
S. caprae	L-Lys-Gly$_4$, L-Ser	GroP	Glc, GlcNAc
S. saccharolyticus	L-Lys-Gly$_4$, L-Ser	GroP	Glc, GlcNAc
S. hominis	L-Lys-Gly$_4$, L-Ser	GroP	GlcNAc
S. haemolyticus	L-Lys-Gly$_4$, L-Ser	GroP	GlcNAc
S. warneri	L-Lys-Gly$_4$, L-Ser	GroP	Glc, GlcNAc
S. pasteuri	L-Lys-Gly$_4$, L-Ser	GroP	Glc, (GlcNAc)
S. lugdunensis	L-Lys-Gly$_5$	GroP	Glc, GlcNAc
S. aureus	L-Lys-Gly$_5$	RitP	GlcNAc
S. saprophyticus	L-Lys-Gly$_5$, (L-Ser) or L-Lys-Gly$_4$, L-Ser	GroP + RitP	GlcNAc
S. cohnii	L-Lys-Gly$_5$	GroP or GroP + (RitP)	Glc, (GlcNAc) or (GalNAc)
S. xylosus	L-Lys-Gly$_5$	GroP + RitP	GlcNAc
S. kloosii	L-Lys-Gly$_5$ or L-Lys-Gly$_5$, (L-Ser)	GroP + RitP	Glc, GlcNAc or GalNAc
S. equorum	L-Lys-Gly$_5$	GroP + (RitP)	GlcNAc
S. arlettae	L-Lys-Gly$_5$	GroP + RitP	GlcNAc
S. gallinarum	L-Lys-Gly$_4$, L-Ser or L-Lys-Gly$_5$, (L-Ser)	GroP	Glc, (GlcNAc)
S. simulans	L-Lys-Gly$_5$	GroP	GlcNAc, GalNAc
S. carnosus	L-Lys-Gly$_5$	GroP	Glc, GalNAc, (GlcNAc)
S. piscifermentans	L-Lys-Gly$_5$	ND	ND
S. felis	L-Lys-Gly$_5$, (L-Ser)	ND	ND
S. intermedius	L-Lys-Gly$_4$, L-Ser or L-Lys-Gly$_5$, (L-Ser)	GroP	GlcNAc and/or Glc
S. schleiferi	L-Lys-Gly$_5$, (L-Ser)	GroP	Glc, GlcNAc
S. delphini	L-Lys-Gly$_5$	GroP	GlcNAc
S. muscae	L-Lys-Gly$_5$ or L-Lys-Gly$_5$, (L-Ser)	ND	ND
S. hyicus	L-Lys-Gly$_5$ or L-Lys-Gly$_5$, (L-Ser)	Grop-GlcNAcP	None
S. chromogenes	L-Lys-Gly$_5$ or L-Lys-Gly$_5$, (L-Ser)	GroP-GlcNAcP	None
S. sciuri	L-Lys-L-Ala-Gly$_4$	GroP-GlcNAcP, GroP-GlcP, or RitP-GlcNAcP	None None None
S. lentus	L-Lys-L-Ala-Gly$_4$	GroP-GlcNAcP or GroP	None or GlcNAc
S. vitulus	L-Lys-L-Ala-Gly$_4$	GroP-GlcNAcP or GroP	None, GalNAc, or (GLcNAc)
S. auricularis	L-Lys-Gly$_5$ or L-Lys-Gly$_5$, (L-Ser)	GlcNAcP	None
S. caseolyticus	L-Lys-Gly$_5$, (L-Ser) or L-Lys-Gly$_4$, L-Ser	GlcNAcP	None

[a]L-Lys, L-lysine; L-Ala, L-alanine; Gly, glycine; L-Ser, L-serine; (L-Ser), low amounts (0.2–0.6 mol mol^{-1} glutamic acid) of L-serine.
[b]GroP, glycerolphosphate; RitP, ribitolphosphate; (RitP), GroP-GlcNAcP, glycerolphosphate-*N*-acetylglucosaminylphosphate; RitP-GlcNAcP, ribitolphosphate-*N*-acetylglucosaminylphosphate; GlcNAcP, *N*-acetylglucosaminylphosphate; GroP-GlcP, glycerolphosphate-glucosephosphate; ( ), low amount of polyol; ND, not determined.
[c]Glc, glucose; GlcNAc, *N*-acetylglucosamine; GalNAc, *N*-acetylgalactosamine; ( ), low amount of substituent; ND, not determined.
From Hájek et al. (1986, 1992), Schleifer (1986), Freney et al. (1988), Varaldo et al. (1988), Igimi et al. (1989), Kloos, Schleifer and Götz (1991), Tanasupawat et al. (1992), Chesneau et al. (1993) and Webster et al. (1994).

1 *S. epidermidis* species group (*S. epidermidis*, *S. capitis*, *Staphylococcus caprae*, *S. saccharolyticus*, *S. warneri*, *Staphylococcus pasteuri*, *S. haemolyticus*, *S. hominis*), *Staphylococcus lugdunensis* is at the periphery of the group

2 *S. saprophyticus* species group (*S. saprophyticus*, *Staphylococcus cohnii*, *Staphylococcus xylosus*), *Staphylococcus equorum*, *Staphylococcus arlettae*, *Staphylococcus kloosii* and *Staphylococcus gallinarum* are at the periphery

3 *Staphylococcus simulans* species group (*S. simulans*, *Staphylococcus carnosus*, *Staphylococcus piscifermentans*), *Staphylococcus felis* is at the periphery

4 *S. intermedius* species group (*S. intermedius, Staphylococcus delphini*), *Staphylococcus schleiferi* is at the periphery
5 *S. hyicus* species group (*S. hyicus, S. chromogenes*) and
6 *S. sciuri* species group (*S. sciuri, S. lentus, S. vitulus*).

Members of the same species group also share several key phenotypic characteristics. For example, the *S. saprophyticus* species group is intrinsically resistant to novobiocin and the *S. sciuri* species group possesses *c*-type cytochromes and a peptidoglycan interpeptide bridge containing glycine and L-alanine.

3.2 Subspecies

Mayr (1963) defines a subspecies in higher organisms as an aggregate of local populations of a species, inhabiting a geographical subdivision of the range of the species and differing taxonomically from other populations of the species. In the case of the host-adapted staphylococci, host range takes the place of geographical range, though perhaps not entirely, since these organisms are not obligate parasites. Staphylococcal subspecies (Table 27.3) are being classified on the basis of phenotypic characters and DNA relatedness (Igimi, Takahashi and Mitsuoka 1990, Bannerman and Kloos 1991, Kloos et al. 1997b), ribotyping (De Buyser at al. 1992, Kloos et al. 1997b) and PFGE (George and Kloos 1994). Members of the same subspecies demonstrate relative DNA-binding values of generally 80% or greater when DNA–DNA hybridization reactions are performed at either optimal or stringent conditions. Different subspecies demonstrate relative DNA-binding values of generally 65–80% at the optimal criterion, but have significantly lower relative DNA-binding values, in the range of 30–70%, at the stringent criterion. *S. pasteuri* (Chesneau et al. 1993) is a borderline species-subspecies, as it demonstrates relative DNA-binding values of 50–67% at the optimal criterion and relative DNA-binding values of 19–36% at the stringent criterion when its DNA is hybridized to *S. warneri* DNA (Kloos and Wolfshohl 1979). The DNA relationships of subspecies are shown in Fig. 27.1. Subspecies can be distinguished from one another by one or a few phenotypic characters. Ribotyping (Fig. 27.2) and PFGE (Fig. 27.3) have proved to be accurate methods for distinguishing subspecies and they are concordant with the classification based on phenotypic characters and DNA relatedness.

4 HABITAT

4.1 Cutaneous habitats

Staphylococci are one of the major groups of bacteria inhabiting the skin, skin glands and mucous membranes of mammals (Noble and Somerville 1974, Kloos 1980, 1986a, Devriese 1986, Kloos, Schleifer and Götz 1991). Staphylococci have been isolated sporadically from the skin of birds (Devriese et al. 1978, 1983, Akatov et al. 1985). Since the residency status of avian staphylococci has not been adequately determined, one cannot be certain that birds constitute a major natural host. Price (1938) defines cutaneous residents as bacteria that produce relatively stable populations and increase in number mainly by the multiplication of cells already present in the habitat. Bacteria that are relatively rare on unexposed skin, but occur more frequently on exposed skin are considered to be transients. Noble and Somerville (1974) proposed 3 categories of skin microbes according to their host relationship:

1 transients, contaminating organisms that do not multiply
2 temporary residents, contaminants that multiply and persist for short periods of time and
3 residents, the natural inhabitants of the skin.

These ecological concepts are important to understand when identifying the natural habitats of staphylococci. An important feature of resident staphylococcal species and subspecies is that they are represented by at least several different strains on an individual host and, depending on the species, many of these strains may persist for a period of several weeks to several years (Kloos 1986a, George and Kloos 1994, Kloos and Bannerman 1994).

The largest populations of cutaneous staphylococci (c. 10^4–10^6 cfu cm^{-2}) are found in regions of the skin of mammals supplied with large numbers of pilosebaceous units and sweat glands and on the skin and mucous membranes surrounding openings to the body surface. Staphylococcal populations living on human skin have been observed in the follicular canals (usually in the more superficial areas or infundibulum), openings to sweat glands, the capacious lumen of sebaceous follicles, and on the surface and beneath desquamating epithelial scales (Noble and Somerville 1974, Noble and Pitcher 1978). They appear on the skin surface as microcolonies or aggregates ranging in size from several cells to hundreds of cells.

Human skin provides staphylococci and other micro-organisms with a wide variety of habitats and niches. The scalp provides a unique region of skin, that is richly supplied with nutrients via numerous blood vessels and sweat and sebaceous glands. A marked increase in sebaceous gland activity occurs at puberty, resulting in an increase in the quantity of lipids and fatty acids on the scalp. *S. capitis* reaches a climax population on the scalp following puberty and becomes the predominant species. In many adults, it comprises more than 90% of the staphylococci present in this habitat. In pre-adolescent children, *S. epidermidis*, *S. hominis* and *S. haemolyticus* are the major staphylococci found living on the scalp. *S. capitis* subsp. *capitis* has a strong preference and *S. capitis* subsp. *ureolyticus* has a moderate preference for the human head (scalp, forehead, eyebrows, external auditory meatus). The face provides several different habitats, most of which are exposed to the external environment. The forehead is richly supplied with sweat and sebaceous glands and is covered often with an oily film. The cheeks and chin of the face have fewer sweat glands and are usually drier than the forehead. The predominant species of the face are members of the *S. epidermidis* species group.

The external auditory meatus of the ear provides a unique habitat that is largely protected from the external environment. The outer two-thirds of the

Table 27.3 *Staphylococcus* subspecies

Subspecies	Reference[a]
S. capitis subsp. *capitis* and *S. capitis* subsp. *ureolyticus*	Bannerman and Kloos 1991[VP]
S. caprae subsp. 1 and *S. caprae* subsp. 2	Cole et al. 1994, George and Kloos 1994, Bannerman, Ayers and Kloos, unpublished
S. haemolyticus subsp. 1 and *S. haemolyticus* subsp. 2	Kloos and Wolfshohl 1979, Cole et al. 1994
S. auricularis subsp. 1 and *S. auricularis* subsp. 2	Kloos 1986a, 1986b
S. aureus subsp. *aureus* and *S. aureus* subsp. *anaerobius*	De la Fuente, Suarez and Schleifer 1985[VP]
S. cohnii subsp. *cohnii*, *S. cohnii* subsp. *urealyticum* and *S. cohnii* subsp. 3	Kloos and Wolfshohl 1983, 1991[VP]
S. schleiferi subsp. *schleiferi* and *S. schleiferi* subsp. *coagulans*	Igimi, Takahashi and Mitsuoka 1990[VP]
S. hyicus subsp. 1 and *S. hyicus* subsp. 2	Phillips and Kloos 1981, Cole et al. 1994, Shimizu et al. unpublished
S. sciuri subsp. *sciuri*, *S. sciuri* subsp. *rodentium* and *S. sciuri* subsp. *carnaticus*	Kloos et al. 1997b

[a]Superscript *VP* designates a valid publication.

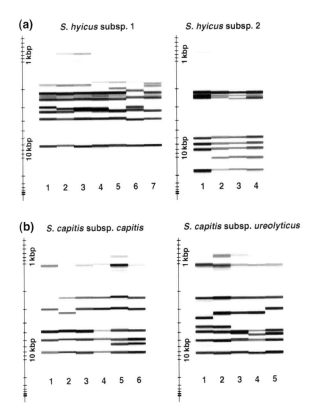

Fig. 27.2 Patterns of *Eco*RI chromosome fragments containing rRNA operon sequences derived from image data (Cole et al. 1994). The image data for each lane were processed to normalize band positions relative to standards, to reduce background, and to scale the band intensity (Webster et al. 1994). Each numbered lane represents a pattern type observed for the designated subspecies. (Courtesy of J Webster and R Hubner, EI Du Pont de Nemours & Company, Experimental Station, Wilmington, DE, USA).

canal contains sebaceous and ceruminous glands. Eccrine sweat glands are not present. Nutrients are supplied to the area by the processes of keratinization, sebaceous secretion and ceruminous secretion. Although amino acids and proteins are present, there is only a very small amount of urea. The major species and subspecies found living in the external auditory meatus of adults, *S. auricularis* and *S. capitis* subsp. *capitis*, do not exhibit urease activity. *S. auricularis* has a strong preference for this habitat and reaches a climax population in young adults, following the onset of ceruminous gland activity.

The anterior nares are a major passageway, providing a habitat for staphylococci and certain other bacteria between the outer skin surface of the nose and the mucous membranes of the pharynx. The region is ventilated but usually remains wet and warm, being supplied with water and nutrients, mainly from nasal secretions. Staphylococci produce very large populations (c. 10^3–10^6 cfu ml^{-1} of wash) on the skin of the vestibule. The anterior nares are the main headquarters for *S. aureus* in adults and provide one of the major habitats for *S. epidermidis*. Both these species demonstrate a specific adherence to nasal epithelial (mucosal) cells (Aly, Shinefield and Maibach 1981). The adherence of *S. aureus* to nasal mucosal cells is significantly greater for human carriers of this species than for non-carriers. Nasal carriage ability may be genetically determined in humans (Kinsman, McKenna and Noble 1983). In general, the carriage rate for *S. aureus* is higher in pre-adolescent children than in adults, and it is more widely dispersed on the body of children than on adults. Nasal carriage rates range from less than 10% to more than 40% in normal adult populations residing in the community (Noble and Somerville 1974). *S. aureus* is one of the major species living on non-human primates, where it occupies a variety of habitats. Different ecovars of this species can be found living on other animals. *S. epider-*

(a)

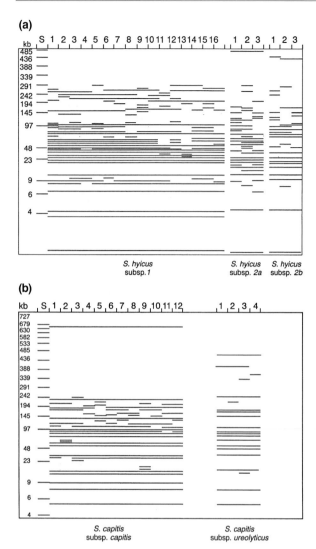

S. hyicus subsp. 1   S. hyicus subsp. 2a   S. hyicus subsp. 2b

(b)

S. capitis subsp. capitis   S. capitis subsp. ureolyticus

Fig. 27.3 Patterns of *Sma*I chromosome fragments resulting from PFGE and derived from photographic data (George and Kloos 1994, A Shimizu, unpublished data). The photographic data for each lane were converted to a line drawing and processed to normalize band positions relative to standards. The upper portion of each lane (97 kbp and above) was taken from gels run at a ramped pulse of 15–55 s at 200 V for 22 h and the lower portion (4–97 kbp) was taken from gels run at a ramped pulse of 1–12 s at 150 V for 20 h. Each numbered lane represents a pattern type observed for the designated subspecies.

midis is almost always found living in the anterior nares and often is the predominant species (Kloos and Musselwhite 1975). This species colonizes a wide variety of habitats and niches on human skin and it is the predominant residing species in most of them. Certain strains of *S. aureus* and *S. epidermidis* can be detected on individuals for a relatively long period, from several months to several years. In one survey, it was shown that strains of *S. epidermidis* capable of persisting in communities on skin for more than 2 months to several years produced a polysaccharide adhesin (PS/A) and an extensive biofilm (Kloos et al. 1992, Lambe et al. 1994).

The axilla contains a rich supply of both eccrine and apocrine glands and is characterized by high humidity (near-aqueous conditions), rich supply of nutrients, near-body temperature, and a higher pH (6.8–7.9) than is found on the general skin surface, factors that enhance the growth of staphylococci and certain other bacteria. Populations of staphylococci reach very high densities in this habitat (c. 10^4–10^6 cfu cm^{-2}). The major species of the axillae are *S. epidermidis* and *S. hominis*, though some individuals may carry also moderate-size populations of the closely related species *S. haemolyticus*. The species *S. hominis* colonizes a wide variety of habitats on human skin and is often second to *S. epidermidis* in population size. Both these species appear to tolerate higher levels of certain fatty acids found on skin than other staphylococci (Lacey and Lord 1981, Ushijima, Takahashi and Ozaki 1984). Strains of *S. hominis* and *S. haemolyticus* usually colonize human skin for relatively short periods. The inguinal and perineal area is in several ways very similar to the axilla as a habitat. The region differs from the axilla in receiving urine, faeces and genital secretions that supply additional nutrients, salts and water to the area, and in being contaminated with faecal organisms. Like the axilla, the major species of the inguinal and perineal area are *S. epidermidis* and *S. hominis*. Populations of *S. capitis* subsp. *ureolyticus* may reach a relatively large size in this habitat in some adults. All of these staphylococci demonstrate high levels of urease activity, which may of particular benefit to them, considering the high levels of substrate urea normally present. The opportunistic pathogens, *S. aureus* and *S. saprophyticus*, are found sometimes in the inguinal and perineal area, and may use this region as a staging area for colonization of the genitourinary tract. The urease activity of these species may play a role in the pathogenesis of urinary tract infections, including infection-induced stones and pyelonephritis (Mobley and Hausinger 1989).

The skin of the arms and legs provides a large region that is approximately half the total area of the human body. The arms and legs provide a rather similar habitat composed of glabrous skin. The skin surface is relatively dry to moderately moist and is bathed in an emulsion of lipids and eccrine sweat containing lactic acid–lactate, amino acids, urea and electrolytes. These habitats support small populations of staphylococci (c. 10–10^3 cfu cm^{-2}). A wide variety of staphylococcal species may be isolated from the arms and legs, though many are transients and arrive on the skin surface as a result of contamination. Bacteria of the axillary community are often dispersed to adjacent areas of the upper arm and, likewise, bacteria of the inguinal and perineal community are dispersed to adjacent areas of the thigh. The major resident species are members of the *S. epidermidis* species group. The proportion of *S. hominis* to other species is often higher here than in other body regions.

The cutaneous habitats of other mammals are different from those of humans, especially with respect to the number, distribution and anatomy of hair follicles and glands

(Montagna and Ellis 1963, Ford and Perkins 1970, Sokolov 1982) and lipid composition (Nicolaides 1974). The skin of man's closest relative, the chimpanzee (*Pan troglodytes*), has many similarities to that of humans, but also has some definite differences. There are striking differences between the cutaneous lipids of chimpanzees (including other primates) and humans. Humans are unique in having much of the cutaneous lipid originate from the sebaceous glands and its composition differs markedly from that of other mammals by the high percentage of triglycerides and their breakdown products. The major staphylococcal species found living on the skin of the chimpanzee are *S. aureus*, *S. pasteuri* and *S. haemolyticus*. A comparison of the resident, staphylococcal species of humans and chimpanzees leads one to consider that *S. pasteuri* has been replaced by the closely related species *S. epidermidis* and *S. warneri*, on humans, but perhaps not completely. Very small populations of *S. pasteuri* can occasionally be located on human skin. It appears that *S. haemolyticus* is in the process of being replaced by the closely related species *S. hominis*, on humans.

4.2 Host range

Many of the staphylococcal species and subspecies living on mammals demonstrate host preferences for the establishment of residency (Table 27.4). The host range may be narrow to wide, depending on the particular species or subspecies. With the exception of staphylococci that prefer the single host species *Homo sapiens*, preferences are either at the host subfamilial, familial, or ordinal levels. Generally, staphylococci from closely related hosts are more closely related to one another than staphylococci from distantly related hosts. A comparison of the dendrogram of resident, mammalian staphylococcal species and subspecies, based on DNA–DNA hybridization data (Kloos, Schleifer and Götz 1991, Webster et al. 1994), and proposed consensus trees of mammalian orders, based on amino acid sequence data (Goodman, Czelusniak and Beeber 1985, Prothero 1993) and nucleotide sequence data (Goodman, Czelusniak and Beeber 1985, Saccone, Pesole and Sbisá 1991, Milinkovitch 1992) indicates a close alignment between the position of most staphylococcal taxa and their corresponding mammalian hosts. The agreement seems to be too good to be accidental and supports the idea of a parallel cladogenesis or mutual descent. These observations lead one to consider the possibility that staphylococci, like the eukaryotic parasites of mammals, may have coevolved with their hosts (Kloos and Wolfshohl 1979, Kloos 1980, Brooks and Glen 1982, Kim 1985). Although staphylococci can interact with their hosts in a variety of ways ranging from commensal to parasitic relationships, effective isolation on certain kinds of hosts might have led to the formation of new subspecies and species in much the same way that free-living organisms undergo speciation during geographical isolation. Some investigations of the resident staphylococci and macrococci of cetaceans (whales, dolphins, porpoises), artiodactyls (cattle, pigs, sheep, goats), and perissodactyls (horses and ponies, donkeys) have corroborated the assertion by Milinkovitch, Orti and Meyer (1993) that ungulates, and in particular the artiodactyls, appear to be the closest relatives of cetaceans (Webster et al. 1994, Ballard et al. 1995). *S. xylosus*, the principal resident species of rodents, is an exceptional species in that populations are very widespread in nature. Its extensive distribution appears to be primarily the result of host and environmental transfer rather than by descent, and this is perhaps a consequence of the very large population size and geographical range of rodents. Survival of this species in environments frequented by rodents and other animals may be facilitated by its unusual ability to utilize inorganic nitrogen as the sole source of substrate nitrogen (Emmett and Kloos 1975). *S. aureus* and *S. caprae*, resident species of primates, are also exceptional in that distinct ecovars can be found living on various domestic animals, though individual strains generally have a relatively short residency status. The ecovars can be recognized by their phenotypic characteristics (Devriese 1984, Musser and Selander 1990) and ribotype (Cole et al. 1994) and PFGE (George and Kloos 1994) fragment patterns. Their distinction within each of the species cannot be made on the basis of DNA–DNA hybridization. One attractive hypothesis is that these species were transferred from human handlers to animals during early animal domestication. Over thousands of years, these staphylococci became somewhat adapted to their new hosts and, in the process of adaptation, they were provided with an opportunity for divergence into separate distinct populations. An alternative hypothesis is that these species were transferred from non-human primates to certain animals, e.g. ungulates, prior to their domestication by humans, as a consequence of contact by these mammals in their natural ranges.

4.3 Other habitats

Staphylococci have been detected in the pharynx, conjunctiva, mouth, blood, mammary glands, faeces, bodily discharges, excretions and intestinal, genitourinary and respiratory tracts of their hosts (Elek 1959). Infected tissues of the host may support large populations of staphylococci and, in some situations, they may persist for long periods. Staphylococci have generally a benign relationship with their host; however, if the cutaneous organ system is damaged by trauma, inoculation by needles, or direct implantation of medical devices (foreign bodies), these organisms can gain entry into the host tissues and may develop the life-style of a pathogen. The success of the new life-style will depend on the ability of the organism to adhere to host or foreign body surfaces, to breach or avoid the immune system, and to produce harmful products. The occurrence of contaminating staphylococci in various food products has been investigated extensively (Bergdoll 1989, Genigeorgis 1989, Mossel and Van Netten 1990, Lambe, Kloos and Lachica 1994). The presence of enterotoxigenic strains of *S. aureus* in foods is regarded as a public health hazard because of the ability of these strains to produce intoxication or food poisoning. Small numbers of staphylococci have been found in air, dust, soil and water, and on inanimate surfaces or fomites, molluscs, insects and plants in areas frequented by mammals and birds (Elek 1959, Kloos and Schleifer 1981, Hájek and Balusek 1985).

5 CELL MORPHOLOGY

5.1 Light microscopy and staining reactions

Gram-stained cells of staphylococci are uniformly gram-positive in young (18–24 h) cultures and appear spherical with an average diameter of 0.5–1.5 μm

Table 27.4 Host range of *Staphylococcus* species and subspecies

Species and subspecies[a]	Natural host	Temporary (recent) host
S. epidermidis	Humans	
S. capitis subsp. *capitis*	Humans	
S. capitis subsp. *ureolyticus*	Primates	
S. caprae subsp. 1	Humans	
S. caprae subsp. 2		Domestic goats
S. saccharolyticus	Humans	
S. hominis	Humans	
S. haemolyticus subsp. 1	Humans	Domestic artiodactyls and horses
S. haemolyticus subsp. 2	Primates	
S. warneri	Humans	Domestic artiodactyls and horses
S. pasteuri	Primates	Domestic artiodactyls and horses
S. lugdunensis	Humans	
S. auricularis subsp. 1	Humans	
S. auricularis subsp. 2	Primates	
S. aureus subsp. *aureus* (A)	Primates	Domestic artiodactyls, poultry
S. aureus subsp. *aureus* (B)		Domestic pigs, poultry
S. aureus subsp. *aureus* (C)		Domestic artiodactyls
S. aureus subsp. *aureus* (D)		Lagamorpha, Rodentia
S. aureus subsp. *anaerobius*		Domestic sheep
S. saprophyticus	Primates, Scandentia	Rodentia
S. cohnii subsp. *cohnii*	Humans	
S. cohnii subsp. *urealyticum*	Primates, Scandentia	
S. cohnii subsp. 3	New-world monkeys	
S. xylosus	Rodentia	Mammals and birds
S. kloosii	Rodentia	Domestic artiodactyls
S. equorum		Domestic horses and cattle
S. arlettae		Poultry
S. gallinarum		Poultry
S. simulans	Carnivora	Domestic artiodactyla, humans
S. carnosus		Domestic artiodactyla
S. felis	Carnivora	
S. intermedius	Carnivora	Domestic horses, poultry
S. schleiferi subsp. *schleiferi*	Carnivora	Humans
S. schleiferi subsp. *coagulans*	Carnivora	
S. delphini	Cetacea	
S. hyicus subsp. 1	Artiodactyla (Suidae)	
S. hyicus subsp. 2	Artiodactyla (Bovidae)	Poultry
S. chromogenes	Artiodactyla, Perissodactyla	
S. sciuri subsp. *sciuri*	Rodentia, Artiodactyla, Perissodactyla, Cetacea, Marsupialia	Poultry
S. sciuri subsp. *rodentium*	Rodentia, Cetacea	
S. sciuri subsp. *carnaticus*	Artiodactyla, Cetacea	
S. lentus	Artiodactyla, Perissodactyla, Cetacea	
S. vitulus	Artiodactyla, Perissodactyla, Cetacea	
S. caseolyticus	Artiodactyla, Cetacea	

[a]The host range of *S. muscae* and *S. piscifermentans* is unknown. *S. aureus* subsp. *aureus* biotypes are designated by the letters (A–D). From Kloos, Schleifer and Götz (1991) and Kloos and Bannerman (1994, 1995).

when being viewed under the light microscope. The cells of old cultures (>48 h) are often gram-variable to nearly gram-negative. The cells of most *S. aureus* strains are noticeably smaller than those of other species. Cells divide in more than one plane to form irregular clusters and aggregates of pairs, tetrads and short chains, depending on the species. For example, *S. aureus* mainly produces irregular clusters of cells; *S. hominis*, *S. haemolyticus* and *S. capitis* mainly produce aggregates of tetrads and pairs; and *S. saprophyticus* and *S. cohnii* produce loose aggregates of single cells and pairs.

Uncommon cell wall defective or deficient (L-form) cells are variable in size and the smallest viable forms may pass through filters with a pore size as small as 50–450 nm. They are osmotically fragile and fail to take the Gram stain. Due to the absence of most or all of the rigid cell wall, L-form cells do not appear as true coccal forms. L-forms have been recognized in *S. aureus* (Kagan 1972) and members of the *S. epidermidis* species group (Acevedo, Campbell-Acevedo and Kloos 1985). Most of the L-form strains have been isolated from chronic infections, malignant tumours and body fluids of immunodeficient patients. They may be induced by benzylpenicillin, methicillin and lysostaphin, or may develop naturally in a variety of lesions. Since L-forms are osmotically fragile and are not easily cultured on the usual isolation media, their natural populations and role in nature are not known.

Encapsulated cells (e.g. from mucoid, glistening colonies) are surrounded by a capsular layer (>200 nm thickness) outside the cell wall that has a definite external surface, demonstrable by light microscopy (Wilkinson 1983). These cells can be detected by the India ink method, which makes encapsulated organisms appear white against a dark background. Yoshida (1971) has shown that 5–18% of fresh isolates of *S. aureus* are encapsulated as detected by the India ink method. Encapsulation has been observed occasionally in species of the *S. epidermidis* species group, *S. saprophyticus* species group and *S. simulans* species group (Wilkinson et al. 1987). Another method for demonstrating capsules is the quellung test or specific capsular reaction, which depends upon the combination of capsular substance with its homologous antibody (Tomcsik 1956). In this test, a microprecipitation reaction occurs and the antigen–antibody complex outlines the surface of the capsule, giving the impression of capsular swelling. Staphylococci may also have capsules that are thinner than 200 nm (microcapsules), which are not visible by light microscopy or staining by the India ink method. The incidence of *S. aureus* strains exhibiting microcapsules is quite high and may approach 80–90% (Hochkeppel et al. 1987).

5.2 Electron microscopy

Most of what is understood about the basic fine structure of staphylococcal cells comes from transmission electron microscopic studies of the species *S. aureus* (Suganuma 1972, Suganuma, Yokoto and Morioka 1973). The cell wall shows simple structural differentiations. It has outer and inner dense layers with an intervening layer that is much less dense. The thickness of the wall varies (15–80 nm) according to the particular strain and age of the culture. The inner dense layer is a conjoint structure made up of the inner part of the cell wall and the outer part of the plasma (cell) membrane. By using a variety of special techniques, including freeze-etching and thin sectioning, Suganuma and colleagues were able to demonstrate clearly a typical triple-layered unit membrane structure for the cell membrane of *S. aureus*. Septum formation during cell division takes place as the cell wall of the septum forms centripetally along with the cell membrane. Membranous structures (mesosomes) have been observed in the cytoplasm of sections of cells of *S. aureus*. The mesosome appears to be continuous with the plasma membrane and also appears frequently in the vicinity of the nucleoid.

Capsules of *S. aureus* have been observed by treating organisms with either homologous antisera or ferritin-labelled homologous antisera (Yoshida and Minegishi 1976, Lee, Hopkins and Pier 1985). Electron micrographs demonstrate the localization of capsular-type antigen on the outer side of the capsule. Glycocalyx or slime has been observed bound to staphylococcal cells and in areas surrounding cells by both transmission electron microscopy (Lambe et al. 1994) and scanning electron microscopy (Peters, Locci and Pulverer 1981, 1982). This exocellular material is not as clearly defined or as firmly attached to the cell surface as a capsule. Although slime production is a common property of staphylococci, the amount may vary considerably depending on the species, strain and cultural conditions. Slime production is especially noteworthy in the species *S. epidermidis*.

6 CULTURAL CHARACTERISTICS

6.1 Colony morphology

Staphylococci produce distinctive colonies on a variety of commercial, selective and non-selective agar media. The commonly used selective media include mannitol–salt agar, lipase–salt–mannitol agar, phenylethyl alcohol agar, Columbia colistin–nalidixic acid (CNA) agar, and Baird-Parker agar base supplemented with egg yolk tellurite enrichment. These media inhibit the growth of gram-negative bacteria, but allow the growth of staphylococci and certain other gram-positive bacteria. Baird-Parker agar base when supplemented with egg yolk tellurite enrichment is widely recommended for the detection and enumeration of *S. aureus* in foods (Schwab, Leininger and Powers 1984). This medium and the other selective media were designed to distinguish *S. aureus* from other species on the basis of colonial and biochemical properties; however, with the discovery of additional staphylococcal species that share some properties with *S. aureus*, it is now recognized that such a distinction cannot be made accurately. Schleifer–Krämer agar (Schleifer and Krämer 1980) is used by some laboratories for the selective isolation and enumeration of staphylococci from foods and other heavily contaminated sources. Incubation of cultures on selective media should be for at least 48–72 h at 35–37°C for colony development.

Staphylococci from a variety of clinical specimens are usually isolated in primary culture on blood agar (e.g. tryptic soy agar supplemented with 5% sheep blood), following an incubation period of 18–24 h at 35–37°C. In this short time, most staphylococcal species will produce abundant growth and well isolated colonies will be 1–3 mm in diameter, circular, smooth and raised, with a butyrous consistency; however, unfortunately colonies of most of the species and subspecies cannot be distinguished from one another. Considering the necessity for the rapid identification of *S. aureus* in clinical specimens, it is most fortunate that colonies of pigmented, haemolytic strains of *S. aureus* can be tentatively identified within 24 h. Suggestions to extend the incubation period, to allow for the development of species-, subspecies-, and strain-specific colonial features, have been largely ignored, until recently. Now there is an appreciation that certain coagulase-negative staphylococcal species (CNS) are opportunistic pathogens and that individual species, subspecies and strains should be identified in multiple specimens taken from the site(s) of infection when determining the aetiological agent. The identification of staphylococci should start with the chacterization of colony morphology. The first encounter of a staphylococcal isolate is usually on the primary isolation plate, where colonies are screened and selected as inoculum for identification. Primary isolation plates will often contain more than one strain of one or more staphylococcal species; however, sometimes the specimen will contain a pure culture, especially if it is taken from a normally sterile site. The best method for identification allows for colonies to develop over a period of 72 h at 35–37°C and then 48 h longer at room temperature (Kloos and Bannerman 1994, 1995). Following these conditions, colonies will be 2–10 mm in diameter and, in most species, will develop distinctive clonal characteristics. If colonies are not allowed to develop for several days, the following errors may result:

1   selection of more than one species, subspecies, or strain if 2 or more colonies are sampled to produce an inoculum, which could lead to errors in identification
2   selection of an organism that is not the aetiological agent or the desired organism if the specimen contains 2 or more species, subspecies, or strains and
3   incorrect labelling of a mixed culture as a pure culture.

Colonies of the same strain generally exhibit similar features of size, consistency, edge, profile, luster and pigment. Some strains may produce 2 or more morphotype(s). In this situation, classical and molecular typing methods should clarify the relationship of each morphotype. Several unusual morphotypes of *S. aureus* have been described that depart significantly from the normal colony morphology, and include certain encapsulated strains (Wiley 1972), L-forms (Kagan 1972) and dwarf or small colony variants (Quie 1969, Balwit et al. 1994). They are of particular clinical interest because of their enhanced virulence and/or persistence in tissues. Different strains of *S. capitis* subsp. *capitis* and *S. cohnii* subsp. *cohnii* are often difficult to distinguish because the colonies of these subspecies are unpigmented and opaque (appear uniformly white) and demonstrate little variation in colonial features.

P agar (Kloos, Tornabene and Schleifer 1974) and tryptic soy agar have been widely used in the primary culture and subculture of staphylococci from cutaneous habitats (Kloos, Schleifer and Götz 1991). Colonies of each of the recognized species and subspecies can be distinguished from one another on these media with considerable accuracy, provided reference strains of each of the taxa are included for comparison. Detailed descriptions (and in some cases colour photographs) of colonies have been reported in the original taxonomic descriptions of the species and subspecies. Pigmentation and pigment sectoring patterns are usually more pronounced in colonies growing on these media than on blood agar. When pigment is present, colonies are usually different shades of cream-yellow, yellow, yellow-orange, or orange, depending on the particular species and strain. Some strains of *S. epidermidis*, *S. intermedius* and *S. lentus* demonstrate a subtle violet, pinkish, or brownish pigment. All staphylococcal species grow well on tryptic soy agar, but *S. vitulus*, *S. lentus*, *S. caseolyticus* and some strains of *S. sciuri* grow poorly on P agar. These species should be cultured on tryptic soy agar or tryptic soy agar supplemented with blood. The anaerobic species *S. saccharolyticus* and subspecies *S. aureus* subsp. *anaerobius* grow well on the above nonselective media under anaerobic conditions, but grow very poorly under aerobic conditions. Brain–heart infusion agar and nutrient agar support good growth of staphylococci, although not many species comparisons have been made of colonies growing on these media.

6.2   Growth in broth and semi-solid media

Staphylococci grow well in a variety of commercial broth media, including tryptic soy broth, brain–heart infusion broth, nutrient broth and tryptose phosphate broth, with or without the addition of blood. Most of the species are butyrous and easy to emulsify, but the *S. sciuri* species group, *S. caseolyticus* and the strong slime-producing strains of *S. epidermidis* are glutinous and difficult to emulsify. Many of the staphylococcal species can produce abundant anaerobic growth in a semi-solid Brewer's thioglycollate medium within 24–72 h at 35–37°C (Kloos and Schleifer 1975b, Kloos and Bannerman 1995). Species such as *S. aureus*, *S. epidermidis*, *S. lugdunensis* and *S. schleiferi*, which are among the most pathogenic species, produce abundant anaerobic growth with overnight incubation. Some species such as *S. hominis*, *S. auricularis*, *S. kloosii*, *S. equorum*, *S. arlettae*, *S. caseolyticus*, *S. vitulus* and *S. lentus* fail to grow or grow only very slowly in the anaerobic portion of this medium.

7   METABOLISM

7.1   Carbohydrate metabolism

Although glucose is a major carbohydrate supplied by the diet and utilized by the tissues of the host, it is probably not a major exogenous source of carbon for staphylococci growing in their primary habitat. In the sweat and aqueous surface film of the human cutaneous habitat, glucose and other reducing sugars are present in very small amounts. Somewhat higher levels of glucose may be found in certain host tissues (e.g. blood, liver, kidneys, muscle), and these may be made available to invading staphylococci. Lactic acid and lactate, in addition to contributing to the buffer capacity of the skin surface, are major sources of carbon for staphylococci and certain other bacteria living on skin. These compounds are derived mainly from glycolysis in host tissues and the breakdown of glycogen in the sweat glands. The lactic acid–lactate concentration in sweat may vary from 45 to 350 mg per 100 ml (Rothman 1954). Staphylococci can readily and reversibly convert these end products into pyruvic acid, thereby allowing them to enter the pathways of pyruvate metabolism and assimilation.

Staphylococci are capable of using a variety of carbohydrates as carbon and energy sources. Carbohydrate uptake can occur in either of 2 ways. The carbohydrate can be taken up and accumulated inside the cell without a change in its form or it can be covalently modified during uptake. In the latter type of carbohydrate uptake, which has been studied extensively in *S. aureus*, the carbohydrate is phosphorylated during the transport process mediated by the phosphoenolpyruvate (PEP)–carbohydrate phosphotransferase system (PTS). Glucose, mannose, glucosamine, fructose, lactose, galactose, mannitol, *N*-acetylglucosamine and β-glucosides are taken up by the PTS (Reizer et al. 1988). The lactose-specific PTS of *S. aureus* is composed of 4 enzymes, enzyme I (EI), Hpr, enzyme III (EIII)^{lac} and enzyme II (EII)^{lac}, that appear to form a membrane-bound multienzyme complex (Kalbitzer et al. 1981, Sobek et al. 1984). Comparisons of the primary structure of Hprs of *S. aureus* and 2 close relatives of staphylococci, *Bacillus subtilis* and *Enterococcus faecalis*, indicated that all these organisms had Hprs of very similar size that contain 3 highly conserved centres: the active centre around His-15, an adjacent region around Tyr-37, and a region around Ser-46 (Reizer et al. 1988). Some carbohydrates are not taken up via the PTS. Examples of these are the pentoses ribose, xylose and arabinose, and the corresponding pentitols. They are taken up unsubstituted in the species *S. saprophyticus* and *S. xylosus* (Lehmer and Schleifer 1980).

The Embden–Meyerhof–Parnas (EMP, glycolytic) pathway and the oxidative hexose monophosphate pathway (HMP) are the 2 central routes used by staphylococci for glucose metabolism (Strasters and Winkler 1963, Blumenthal 1972). *S. aureus* and *S. epidermidis* metabolize glucose mainly by glycolysis, and to a limited extent by the HMP (Sivakanesan and Dawes 1980). The major end product of anaerobic glucose metabolism in *S. aureus* is lactate (73–94%); smaller quantities of acetate (4–7%) and traces of pyruvate are also formed. Under aerobic conditions, only 5–10% of the glucose carbon appears as lactate and most of it appears as acetate and CO_2. In *S. epidermidis*, lactate is the major end product of anaerobic glucose metabolism. The other end products are acetate, formate and CO_2 and these are formed in only trace amounts. *S. saccharolyticus* appears to be an exceptional species in that it ferments glucose mainly to ethanol, acetic acid and CO_2; only small amounts of lactic and formic acid are produced (Kilpper-Bälz and Schleifer 1981). In members of the *S. saprophyticus* species group and *S. intermedius*, *S. capitis*, *S. haemolyticus* and *S. warneri*, lactose and galactose are metabolized via the Leloir pathway whereby galactose-1-phosphate is epimerized to glucose-1-phosphate (Schleifer, Hartinger and Götz 1978, Schleifer 1986). *S. aureus*, *S. epidermidis*, *S. hominis*, *S. chromogenes*, *S. sciuri* and *S. lentus* metabolize lactose and galactose via the tagatose-6-phosphate pathway, whereby galactose-6-phosphate is isomerized to tagatose-6-phosphate, which is further converted to tagatose-1,6-diphosphate and then cleaved to triosephosphates (Schleifer, Hartinger and Götz 1978, Schleifer 1986).

7.2 Respiration

Cytochromes and unsaturated menaquinones form the membrane-bound electron transport system. The major cytochromes of the respiratory chains of staphylococci are a_{602}, b_{557} and o_{555} (previously b_{555}) (Faller, Götz and Schleifer 1980). However, it has been suggested that cytochrome *a* does not play a major role in the respiration of at least some staphylococci. The minor cytochromes b_{552}, b_{560} and b_{566} are widely distributed in staphylococci. Cytochrome b_{552} is not found in *S. sciuri* and *S. lentus*. Members of the *S. sciuri* species group and *S. caseolyticus* and its related species have cytochromes of the *c* type, in addition to cytochromes *a* and *b*. The cytochrome *c*s of *S. sciuri* and *S. lentus* are c_{549} and c_{554}. Cytochrome b_{557} appears to be an intermediate electron carrier of the cytochrome *b* or b_1 type. Cytochrome o_{555} binds carbon monoxide and is probably the major terminal oxidase. The role of cytochrome a_{602} is not clear, though it may be involved with membrane-associated nitrate reductase activity. Menaquinones (MK-6 through MK-9) are the sole isoprenoid quinones of staphylococci and play important roles in electron transport and oxidative phosphorylation (Collins and Jones 1981). Most staphylococcal species contain MK-7 as the major isoprenologue. MK-8 is a major isoprenologue in *S. aureus* and *S. lugdunensis* and MK-6 is a major isoprenologue in *S. hyicus*, *S. equorum* and members of the *S. sciuri* species group (Collins 1981, Nahaie et al. 1984, Schleifer and Kroppenstedt 1990).

7.3 Amino acid biosynthesis and nitrogen requirements

Most staphylococcal species are capable of synthesizing a large proportion of the different amino acids needed for growth. The genetic control of histidine (Kloos and Pattee 1965), isoleucine and valine (Smith and Pattee 1967), lysine (Barnes, Bondi and Fuscaldo 1971), tryptophan (Proctor and Kloos 1970), leucine (Pattee et al. 1974) and alanine, threonine, tyrosine and methionine (Schroeder and Pattee 1984, Mahairas et al. 1989) biosynthesis has been studied extensively in the type species *S. aureus*. The histidine (*hisEABCDG*), isoleucine–valine (*ilvABCD*) and leucine (*leuABCD*), lysine (*lysOABFG*) and tryptophan (*trpABFCDE*) genes of *S. aureus* are each clustered in what appear to be individual operons. Many naturally occurring strains have mutations in one or more of the amino acid biosynthesis genes, resulting in certain amino acid requirements. The amino acid requirements of approximately half the recognized species of staphylococci have been determined in vitro with the use of chemically defined media (Tschäpe 1973, Emmett and Kloos 1975, 1979, Hussain, Hastings and White 1991). Members of the *S. epidermidis* species group have numerous (c. 5–13) amino acid requirements (Emmett and Kloos 1975). All require arginine, the principal amino acid of human sweat and one that is present in moderate amounts (10–18 mg per 100 ml) (Heir, Cornbleet and Bergeim 1946). Most of the strains of species in this group also require isoleucine–valine and proline, and with the exception of *S. epidermidis*, most require histidine. *S. capitis* generally requires more different amino acids than other members of the group. *S. aureus* requires arginine and has either an absolute or partial requirement for proline. Most strains of this species also require isoleucine–valine and have either an absolute or partial requirement for cysteine and leucine. Different ecovars of *S. aureus* demonstrate some differences in their amino acid requirements (Tschäpe 1973). *S. simulans* requires arginine and most strains of this species require also proline, isoleucine–valine, leucine and alanine. Members of the *S. saprophyticus* and *S. sciuri* species groups require fewer amino acids than the other species and some do not even require an amino acid or an organic nitrogen source. Some strains of *S. saprophyticus* have an absolute or partial requirement for proline and isoleucine–valine and some strains of *S. cohnii* require arginine and proline. Most strains (89–95%) of *S. xylosus*, *S. kloosii* and *S. sciuri* do not require an organic nitrogen source (Emmett and Kloos 1979). They can grow well with $(NH_4)_2SO_4$ as the nitrogen source. Relatively high levels of ammonia (3–78 mg per 100 ml) and urea (24–620 mg per 100 ml) are present in the sweat of humans (Rothman 1954) and certain animals (Montagna and Parakkal 1974), making them available to staphylococci as additional sources of substrate nitrogen. These nitrogenous compounds may also reach the skin surface of mammals by urination practices. Many of the amino acid requirements of staphylococci exhibit spontaneous reversion to an independence. *S. capitis* is an exceptional species in that it has a large number (9–13) of amino acid requirements and, of these, only requirements for alanine, glycine, proline and cysteine have been known to exhibit reversion, either spontaneously or in response to alkylating mutagens (Emmett and Kloos 1979).

Vitamin requirements have been determined for about a third of the recognized staphylococcal species. Nicotinic acid and thiamine are usually required by *S. aureus* and members of the *S. epidermidis* and *S. saprophyticus* species groups (Tschäpe 1973, Cove et al. 1983). Biotin, or pantothenic acid, or both are also required by many strains of species in the *S. epidermidis* species group (Emmett and Kloos 1975). Some strains in the *S. saprophyticus* species group may also require pantothenic acid.

8 CELLULAR COMPONENTS

8.1 Cell surface components

The principal structures of the cell envelope or surface of staphylococci are the cell membrane, cell wall and exocellular material. Many of the components of these structures have biological activities and play a vital role in the interaction of staphylococci with their habitat or environment. The cell surface is a mosaic in which the cell wall components and certain membrane components may be exposed sufficiently to interact with external factors. Some of these components may be submerged beneath the surface in staphylococci producing large amounts of exocellular material.

CELL MEMBRANE

The cell membrane appears to be a typical lipid–protein bilayer, being composed mainly of phospholipids and proteins. It represents a selective barrier and fulfils many functions, including electron transport, active transport, participation in septum formation, and segregation of DNA. The cytochromes and menaquinones bound to cell membranes are important components of the electron transport system. Phospholipids, glycolipids, menaquinones and carotenoids make up the major lipid components of the membrane. The major polar lipids are phospholipids and glycolipids (Shaw 1975, Nahaie et al. 1984). The major

phospholipids are phosphatidylglycerol, diphosphatidylglycerol (cardiolipin) and phosphatidic acid. Lysylphosphatidylglucose is also a major component of the cell membrane of *S. aureus* and *S. intermedius*. The glycolipids are monoglucosyl and β-diglucosyl diglycerides and phosphatidyl glucose. The $(1\rightarrow6)$-β-linked diglucosyl (gentiobiosyl) diacylglycerol of staphylococci is also found in the membrane of *Bacillus* species.

The pigments of staphylococci are triterpenoid carotenoids having a C_{30} chain (Marshall and Wilmoth 1981a). In *S. aureus*, carotenoids range from colourless polyisoprene compounds such as squalene, diapophytoene and diapophytofluene to the yellow, orange and red triterpenoid carotenoids. The main pigment is staphyloxanthin, a compound in which glucose is esterified with both a triterpenoid carotenoid carboxylic acid and an *anteiso*-methyl-branched C_{15} fatty acid (12-methyl tetradecanoic acid). It is accompanied by some isomers containing other hexoses and homologues containing C_{17} fatty acids. In addition, several different carotenes and xanthophylls are present, along with some of their isomers and breakdown products. Some of these compounds are probably intermediates in the pathway for biosynthesis of staphyloxanthin (Marshall and Wilmoth 1981b). The main fatty acid components of the cell membrane are *iso*- and *anteiso*-methyl-branched $C_{15:0}$ and unbranched $C_{18:0}$ and $C_{20:0}$ (Durham and Kloos 1978, Kotilainen, Houvinen and Eerola 1991).

Although the protein and fatty acid composition of mesosomal vescicles and the cell membrane are almost identical qualitatively, there are some differences quantitatively. The lipid content of mesosomal vesicles is higher than that of the cell membrane (Beining et al. 1975), and lipoteichoic acid (LTA) is localized in the mesosomal vesicles and not in the cell membrane (Huff, Cole and Theodore 1974). LTA in *S. aureus* consists of a 1,3-phosphodiester-linked glycerol phosphate polymer which is substituted by ester-linked alanine and diglucosyl (gentiobiose) residues. It is attached to the membrane by a covalent linkage between the teichoic acid and a membrane glycolipid (Knox and Wicken 1973). Staphylococcal LTA can act as an adhesin in binding *S. saprophyticus* to mammalian cells (Teti et al. 1987, Beuth et al. 1988). It can also act as an immunomodulator by stimulating the proliferation and maturation of human monocytes, murein thymocytes and peripheral blood lymphocytes, and by promoting antitumour immunity (Ohshima et al. 1991, Pulverer et al. 1994).

Various proteins have been isolated from the membranes of *S. aureus*, such as adenosine triphosphatase (Gross and Coles 1968), polyprenolphosphokinase (Sandermann and Strominger 1972), various oxidases and dehydrogenases (Theodore and Weinbach 1974), and several penicillin-binding proteins (PBPs), which catalyse terminal reactions of peptidoglycan biosynthesis (Hayes et al. 1981, Hartman and Tomasz 1984). Some PBPs are species- or species group-specific (Canepari et al. 1985, Pierre et al. 1990).

Certain iron-regulated cell membrane proteins are

expressed under iron limitation in *S. aureus* (Domingue, Lambert and Brown 1989) and members of the *S. epidermidis* species group (Smith et al. 1991, Wilcox et al. 1991). These proteins are possibly siderophore receptors and part of a siderophore mediated iron uptake system used by staphylococci to overcome a shortage of iron in their natural habitats. Two different, complexone type siderophores are known to be produced extracellularly by staphylococci: staphyloferrin A, consisting of 2 molecules of citric acid, each linked to D-ornithine by an amide bond (Meiwes et al. 1990) and staphyloferrin B, having the structural components 2,3-diaminopropionic acid, ethylenediamine, citric acid and 2-ketoglutaric acid (Haag et al. 1994). Staphyloferrin A, B, or both, are produced by a wide range of staphylococcal species. In addition to the above membrane proteins, a 42 kDa cell wall protein that binds human transferrin, the major iron-binding protein in serum, has been detected in *S. aureus* and certain members of the *S. epidermidis* species group (Modun, Kendall and Williams 1994) and a 450 kDa protein that binds human lactoferrin, an iron-binding protein found in milk, tears, saliva and some other body fluids, has been identified in *S. aureus* (Naidu, Andersson and Forsgren 1992).

CELL WALL

Peptidoglycan and teichoic acid are the major components of the staphylococcal cell wall. The peptidoglycan amounts to about 50–60% of the dry weight (Schleifer and Kandler 1972, Schleifer 1983). The cell wall teichoic acid amounts to about 30–50% of the dry weight, and it is covalently linked to peptidoglycan. The peptidoglycan is the main structural polymer in the wall and it plays an important role in maintaining the spherical shape of the cell. It is a heteropolymer consisting of glycan chains that are cross-linked by short peptides. The glycan moiety is made up of alternating β-1,4-linked units of *N*-acetylglucosamine and *N*-acetylmuramic acid. Some of the C-6 hydroxyl groups of muramic acid are phosphorylated and the resulting muramyl-6-phosphate residue represents the attachment point between peptidoglycan and teichoic acid (Kojima, Araki and Ito 1985). The carboxyl group of muramic acid is substituted by an oligopeptide (peptide subunit) containing alternating L- and D-amino acids. The peptide subunits are cross-linked by the insertion of an interpeptide bridge that extends from the COOH-terminal D-alanine in position 4 of one peptide subunit to the ε-amino group of L-lysine in position 3 of an adjacent peptide subunit (Schleifer 1973). Interpeptide bridges consist of oligoglycine peptides, though some glycine residues may be replaced by L-serine or L-alanine (see Table 27.2, p. 581). Seidl and Schleifer (1978) have developed a latex agglutination method that can distinguish staphylococci from other bacteria based on the recognition of the NH$_2$-terminal glycine of the interpeptide bridge. Peptidoglycan antibodies can be found in normal human and animal sera. The biological activities of peptidoglycans include endotoxin-like properties (pyrogenicity, complement activation, generation of chemotactic factors, aggregation and lysis of animal blood platelets), inflammatory skin reactions, inhibition of leucocyte migration, adjuvant activity, mitogenic activity and induction of immunosuppressive cells (Schleifer 1983).

The cell wall teichoic acids of staphylococci are water-soluble polymers composed of alditol (glycerol, ribitol), sugar and/or *N*-acetylamino sugar, and sometimes D-alanine (Schleifer 1983). Most staphylococcal species contain ribitol, or glycerol teichoic acids, or both (see Table 27.2, p. 581). Cell wall teichoic acids are at least partially exposed to the cell surface where they contribute to the binding of antibodies (Knox and Wicken 1973), bacteriophages (Schleifer and Steber 1974) and lectins (Reeder and Ekstedt 1971). Precipitating antibodies to teichoic acids can be found in the sera of patients with staphylococcal infections (Daugharty, Martin and White 1967, Crowder and White 1972). Hussain, Hastings and White (1991, 1992) have suggested that glycerol teichoic acid is a component of the extracellular slime produced by *S. epidermidis*. Teichoic acids, in conjunction with lipoteichoic acids, act as a cation-exchange system and reservoir of bound divalent cations, especially magnesium.

PROTEIN A

Protein A (SpA) of *S. aureus* has been detected in 90–99% of biotype A strains isolated from man (Hájek and Maršálek 1976, Forsgren et al. 1983). It is detected less frequently in *S. aureus* biotype B strains (2–5%), isolated from pigs and poultry and in biotype C strains (6–40%), isolated from cattle, pigs, sheep and goats. *S. hyicus* produces a type of SpA that is different from that of *S. aureus* (Muller, Schaeg and Blobel 1981). About 85% of *S. intermedius* strains produce an extracellular type of SpA, whereas 4% of strains produce a cell-bound form (Cox, Schmeer and Newman 1986). SpA from *S. aureus* is a 42 kDa polypeptide that has a very extended shape (Björk, Peterson and Sjöquist 1972) and it is encoded by the gene *spa* that appears to have evolved through multiple duplications (Uhlén et al. 1984). SpA is generally regarded as a cell wall protein and it was thought that the COOH terminus was anchored in the cell wall (Sjöquist et al. 1972); however, sequence data have indicated a stretch of hydrophobic amino acids at the C terminus, suggesting anchoring in the cell membrane (Uhlén et al. 1984). The C-terminal part has an 8 amino acid unit that is repeated 12 times. By electron microscopy using immunocytochemical methods, conjugated SpA can be observed on the cell wall and cross-wall of cells (Morioka and Suganuma 1985). In *S. aureus* strain A676 and many methicillin-resistant strains, SpA is an extracellular protein excreted into the culture supernatant. The NH-terminal region protrudes through the cell wall and has 5 repetitive, homologous Fc-binding domains, each of which binds to the Fc region of immunoglobulin G (IgG) from many different mammalian species (Moks et al. 1986). The main biological effects include complement activation, induction of hypersensitivity reactions, mitogenic stimulation of lymphocytes, inhibition of opsonization, cell mediated cytotoxicity, and enhancement of virulence (Forsgren et al. 1983).

CELL SURFACE ADHESINS

Staphylococci have a group of cell surface proteins that act as adhesins (known also as microbial surface components recognizing adhesive matrix molecules, MSCRAMMs) and bind to the extracellular matrix proteins, such as fibronectin, vitronectin, fibrinogen, laminin, bone sialoprotein, thrombospondin, elastin and collagen types I, II and IV, of their host (Wadström and Rozgonyi 1986, Rydén et al. 1983, 1989, 1990, Switalski, Höök and Beachey 1989, Wadström 1991). The matrix proteins play important roles in the systematic organization of host tissues (e.g. connective tissue, bone tissue) and maintenance of homoeostasis. They can also serve as ligands for pathogenic micro-organisms, especially when they are exposed to the environment following a loss of tissue integrity by trauma. These proteins bind to eukaryotic host cells via the cell surface receptor proteins (integrins) (Edelman and Buck 1992). The adhesins act as targeting factors, attaching bacteria to certain host tissues via the matrix proteins. This attachment may be considered an early step in the process of pathogenesis, leading to colonization and subsequent invasion of tissue cells (Lindberg et al. 1990).

The 2 fibronectin-binding adhesins (FnBPs) of *S. aureus* are encoded by 2 distinct, but highly homologous, genes, *fnbA* and *fnbB* (Jönsson et al. 1991, Höök et al. 1994). In the 108 kDa *fnbA* product (FnBPA), the N-terminal signal peptide sequence is followed by a long unique sequence, which is interrupted by a 31 amino acid long motif that is repeated twice. This motif is not present in the 98 kDa *fnbB* product (FnBPB). The main fibronectin-binding activity of both gene products is attributed to a 38 amino acid long motif that is repeated in an essentially intact form 3 times and in a partial form a fourth time. This fibronectin-binding domain is located near the C-terminal end of the protein and is presumably associated with the cell wall. Following this domain is the LPXTGX motif, which is located just outside a hydrophobic segment and presumably represents a membrane-spanning domain.

S. aureus produces a collagen-binding adhesin that is encoded by the gene *cna* (Patti et al. 1992). The 135 kDa *cna* gene product is composed of a unique sequence followed by a domain containing a motif of 157 amino acids repeated 2 or 3 times, depending on the particular strain of *S. aureus*. The collagen-binding domain is located in the N-terminal half of the protein in the A region that is located outside the repeating units. This protein aids in targeting staphylococci to collagen-rich tissues such as joints. *S. aureus* colonization of the articular cartilage within the joint space appears to be an important factor contributing to the development of septic arthritis. It is, therefore, not surprising that most *S. aureus* strains isolated from septic arthritis contain the gene *cna* and express a collagen-binding protein (Höök et al. 1994). Strains expressing a bone sialoprotein adhesin are often associated with osteomyelitis (Rydén et al. 1989).

The cell surface fibrinogen-binding adhesin (also known as clumping factor) of *S. aureus* is encoded by gene *clfA* (McDevitt et al. 1995). This protein has a molecular weight of 185 kDa (about twice that predicted from the nucleotide sequence) and contains an interesting 308 amino acid domain consisting mainly of the dipeptide aspartic acid and serine, which is repeated 154 times. The fibrinogen-binding domain is located in the carboxy-terminal half of a region (A) that is outside the repeating units. Staphylocoagulase (coagulase) is mainly an extracellular protein of *S. aureus* and certain other species that binds prothrombin and activates the coagulation pathway (Hemker, Bas and Muller 1975). However, a small fraction of the coagulase molecules remains bound to the cell wall and this fraction can bind fibrinogen as well as prothrombin (Bodén and Flock 1989).

Staphylococcal species other than *S. aureus* can also interact with some of the components of the extracellular matrix (Switalski et al. 1983, Paulsson and Wadström 1990, Rydén et al. 1990, Paulsson, Ljungh and Wadström 1992, Paulsson, Petersson and Ljungh 1993, Rozgonyi et al. 1994). In general, *S. lugdunensis* and *S. haemolyticus* bind fibronectin, vitronectin, laminin and collagen I and IV to a greater extent than does *S. epidermidis*. The level of fibronectin binding is generally lower for these species compared to *S. aureus*. A proteinaceous surface antigen of *S. epidermidis*, which mediates attachment to polystyrene, might play a role in the attachment of this species to foreign bodies such as catheters and other medical devices (Timmerman et al. 1991). *S. saprophyticus* has a 95 kDa surface fibrillar protein (Ssp) that appears to be involved in interactions of this species with eukaryotic host cells (Gatermann et al. 1992).

EXOCELLULAR MATERIAL

Staphylococcal capsules are located external to the cell wall and they are primarily composed of antigenic (capsular) polysaccharides (Sutherland 1977). The capsular polysaccharides of *S. aureus* are made up of different combinations of either amino uronic acids (*N*-acetyl-D-aminoglucuronic acid, *N*-acetyl-D-aminogalacturonic acid, or *N*-acetyl-D-aminomannuronic acid) or non-amidated uronic acids (glucuronic acid or galacturonic acid), and *N*-acetyl-D-fucosamine or galactose, depending upon the particular strain (Wilkinson 1983). Some *S. aureus* strains also contain taurine in their capsule and it is linked to the carboxyl group of *N*-acetyl-D-aminogalacturonic acid via an amide bond (Liau and Hash 1977, Lee et al. 1987). *S. aureus* strains can be assigned to a least 11 capsular serotypes by means of polyclonal rabbit antiserum specific for their associated capsular polysaccharides. Of these, serotypes 5 and 8 are associated with microcapsules and are the ones most frequently encountered in bacteraemia (Arbeit et al. 1984) and a variety of other infections (Hochkeppel et al. 1987, Albus et al. 1988). Highly encapsulated *S. aureus* isolates of serotypes 1 and 2 are more virulent in mouse lethality tests than isolates of serotypes 5 and 8 (Lee et al. 1987, 1993). Furthermore, they are relatively resistant to phagocytosis, are not phage typable, and have negative clumping factor reactions and diminished coagulase reactions. The capsule acts in varying degrees as a diffusion barrier, molecular sieve and adsorbant. Phagocytosis may be prevented by the inability of encapsulated staphylococci to attach to phagocytic cells.

Slime is a complex extracellular substance produced in varying amounts by many, if not most, staphylococci. The amounts of slime produced by a particular strain may vary widely according to genetic factors and growth conditions. Many strains of *S. epidermidis* and some strains of *S. capitis* subsp. *ureolyticus* produce copious amounts of this substance (Peters et al. 1987, Kloos et al. 1992). Other members of the *S. epidermidis* species group such as *S. capitis* subsp. *capitis*, *S. hominis*, *S. haemolyticus* and *S. warneri* generally produce much smaller amounts of slime, and although many strains of these species may fail to produce detectable quantities of slime by standard tests (Christensen et al. 1986), it can usually be detected by transmission electron microscopy (Lambe et al. 1994). Slime appears to be rather loosely bound to the cell and it is water-soluble. It can be observed trailing from the cell surface and also detached from the cell. Continued production of slime by a growing clone of cells attached to a polymer surface (e.g. an implanted catheter) results in encasement and formation of connective cell-slime clusters (biofilm) (Peters et al 1987). Once established, the bacterial biofilm may act as a penetration barrier to antibiotics (Gristina et al. 1987, Peters et al. 1987). Crude slime is a very heterogeneous substance, which is usually composed of a variety of monosaccharides, including mannose, galactose, glucose, glucosamine and glucuronic acid, and proteins and small peptides. It is not clear whether slime is mainly a carbohydrate polymer or a complex glycoconjugate. The chemical composition of slime may vary according to the medium used for cell propagation. Under some growth conditions, components of teichoic acids may be present in slime (Hussain, Hastings and White 1991). Some strains of *S. epidermidis* and *S. capitis* subsp. *ureolyticus*, especially those from foreign body infections or demonstrating a long-term persistence on their host, produce a slime containing PS/A that is rich in galactose (Tojo et al. 1988, Kloos et al 1992, Muller et al. 1993). PS/A appears to enhance the very early stages of colonization of these species on biomaterials and perhaps also on the surfaces of their natural habitat. It is highly immunogenic in its purified form and may play a role in protective immunity. Somewhat similar polysaccharide antigens have been described that appear to be important for the surface proliferation of cells (Christensen et al. 1990, Mack, Siemssen and Laufs 1992). Most *S. epidermidis* strains can be serotyped and belong to either polysaccharide surface antigen type 1 (14%) or type 2 (77%) (Fattom, Shepherd and Karakawa 1992). There is growing evidence that slime interferes with host defence mechanisms such as opsonization and phagocytosis (Gray, Regelmann and Peters 1987, Johnson, Carparas and Peters 1989, Stout et al. 1992).

8.2 Extracellular proteins

Staphylococci produce a variety of different extracellular proteins acting as either toxins, non-toxic enzymes, or enzyme activators (Table 27.5). The toxins can attack or regulate cellular components of the host, thus presumably facilitating the successful invasion and proliferation of staphylococci within the host. Some of the non-toxic enzymes and polypeptides provide staphylococci with an ability to survive or defend themselves in the presence of competing micro-organisms. Other enzymes are capable of degrading various macromolecules such as lipids, nucleic acids, proteins and polysaccharides, thereby providing low molecular weight nutrients for growth. Most of the extracellular proteins that have been investigated in detail have been derived from *S. aureus*, a species that produces a wide range of different kinds of these proteins.

Many of the staphylococcal species produce toxins that damage the plasma membrane of eukaryotic cells (Thelestam 1983, Wadström 1983). The haemolytic toxins (haemolysins) attack the membranes of erythrocytes, as well as some other cells, from various host species. The leucocidins restrict their action to leucocytes (granulocytes and macrophages). *S. aureus* produces at least 4 types of haemolysins known as α-, β-, γ- and δ-toxins. The α-toxin has been studied extensively, and the wide range of information obtained on its structure and function has been reviewed by Bhakdi and Tranum-Jensen (1991). A high percentage (86–95%) of human *S. aureus* strains produce α-toxin, although many produce only small amounts and most strains producing toxic shock syndrome toxin-1 (TSST-1) do not produce it (Clyne et al. 1988), due to a nonsense mutation generating a stop codon within the α-toxin gene (O'Reilly, Kreiswirth and Foster 1990). The *trans*-active, global regulator, *agr*, regulates the production of α-toxin as well as several other exoproteins and some cell surface proteins (Kornblum et al. 1990, Vandenesch, Kornblum and Novick 1991). The secreted exoproteins are up-regulated, whereas the cell surface proteins are down-regulated. A 514 nt transcript, RNA III, is believed to be the effector molecule acting primarily on the initiation of transcription and secondarily on translation (Novick et al. 1993). Another regulator, *xpr*, affects the level of *agr* mRNA and consequently the amount of *agr* regulated proteins produced (Hart, Smeltzer and Iandolo 1993). A third regulatory gene designated *sar* affects the phenotype of these same proteins differently from that of *agr*, although the mode of action appears to be similarly at the transcriptional level (Cheung and Ying 1994). It is suspected that the γ-toxin is produced by many strains of *S. aureus*, since elevated titres of antibody against this toxin can be detected in most staphylococcal osteomyelitis patients (Taylor, Fincham and Cook 1976) and in most strains producing TSST-1 (Clyne et al. 1988). δ-Toxin is produced by a high percentage (86–

Table 27.5 Staphylococcal extracellular proteins

Protein	MW (kDa)	Major biochemical and biological activities	Gene	Gene location	Species distribution	References
Membrane damaging toxins						
α-Toxin (α-haemolysin)	33 mono	Lethal to man and animals Dermonecrotic, neurotoxic Hexamers form pores in membrane of erythrocytes Cytolytic and cytotoxic	hla (hly+)	Chromosome: Sma I fragment B	S. aureus: biotype A> biotypes B and C	Bhakdi and Tranum-Jensen 1991
β-Toxin (β-haemolysin)	30	Phospholipase C activity specific for sphingomyelin and lysophosphatidylcholine Collapse of erythrocyte membrane at <10°C	hlb (plc)	Chromosome: Sma I fragment F	S. aureus: biotype C> biotype A	Doery et al. 1965, Smyth, Möllby, and Wadström 1975, Coleman et al. 1989
γ-Toxin (γ-haemolysin)	32 and 36	Both proteins act in concert Cytolytic for erythrocytes and leucocytes	hlgA and hlgB	Chromosome: Sma I fragment C	S. aureus	Fackrell and Wiseman 1976, Cooney et al. 1988
δ-Toxin (δ-haemolysin)	2.9 mono Multimers up to 210	Surfactant on various cells: erythrocytes, leucocytes, bacterial protoplasts Penetrates membranes: affinity for phospholipids Synergistic with β-toxin	hld	Chromosome: Sma I fragment F	S. aureus S. epidermidis S. haemolyticus	Turner and Pickard 1979, Fitton, Dell, and Shaw 1980, Gemmell and Thelestam 1981
Leucocidin	S: 31–35 F: 32	Cytolytic for leucocytes S component activates membrane phospholipase A_2 S and F synergistic inducing an ion channel for K+	lukS	Chromosome	S. aureus	Scheifele et al. 1987 Noda et al. 1980, Rahman et al. 1991
Pyrogenic exotoxins (superantigens)						
Enterotoxin A (SE-A)	27.8	Gastrointestinal intoxication resulting in emesis, diarrhoea, and enteritis Mitogenic activity for T cells: stimulate T lymphocytes by cross-linking T cell receptor with major histocompatibility complex class II molecules	sea (entA)	Temperate phage: preferential insert in chromosome Sma I fragment F but may occur on other fragments Phage conversion	S. aureus: major type for biotype A	Mallonee, Glatz and Pattee 1982, Betley, Miller and Makalanos 1986, Bergdoll 1989, Fleischer 1994

Toxin	(kDa)	Gene	Activity	Location	Organism	References
Enterotoxin B (SE-B)	28.3	seb (entB)	Gastrointestinal intoxication; Mitogenic activity for T cells	Defective phage or chromosomally integrated plasmid	S. aureus	Johns and Khan 1988, same references as for SE-A (1986–1994)
Enterotoxin C (SE-C1, SE-C2, SE-C3)	C1: 26; C2: 26; C3: 28.9	C1: sec (entC)	Gastrointestinal intoxication; Mitogenic activity for T cells	Chromosome or plasmid 56.2 kbp plasmid pZA10 carries both seb and sec	S. aureus major type for biotype C	Altboum, Hertman and Sarid 1985, Bohach and Schlievert 1987, same references as for SE-A (1986–1994)
Enterotoxin D (SE-D, closely related to SE-A)	27.3	sed (entD)	Gastrointestinal intoxication; Mitogenic activity for T cells	27.6 kbp plasmid of prototype pIB485	S. aureus	Iandolo 1989, same references as for SE-A (1986–1994)
Enterotoxin E (SE-E)	29.6	see (entE)	Gastrointestinal intoxication; Mitogenic activity for T cells	Chromosome: possibly on defective phage	S. aureus	Couch, Soltis and Betley 1988
Enterotoxin G (SE-G)	27.1	seg	Gastrointestinal intoxication	Chromosome	S. aureus	Betley, Borst and Regassa 1992
Enterotoxin H (SE-H)	25.1 or 27.3	seh	Gastrointestinal intoxication; Mitogenic activity for T cells	Chromosome	S. aureus	Ren et al. 1994, Su and Wong 1995
Toxic shock syndrome toxin-1 (TSST-1)	22	tst	Toxic shock syndrome; Mitogenic activity for T cells	Chromosome: Sma I fragment A on heterologous insertion element in trp operon or att φ12 site	S. aureus: mainly phage group I	Bergdoll et al. 1981, Schlievert et al. 1981, Kreiswirth et al. 1983, Chu et al. 1988
Epidermolytic toxins						
Exfoliatin A (ETA)	26.9	eta	Staphylococcal scalded skin syndrome; Binds to profilaggrin of stratum granulosum; Catalytic triad similarity with serine proteinases	Chromosome	S. aureus: phage group II> phage groups I and III	Melish and Glasgow 1970, Rogolsky 1979, Lee et al. 1987, Smith, John and Bailey 1989, Dancer et al. 1990
Exfoliatin B (ETB)	27.3	etb	Staphylococcal scalded skin syndrome; Binds to profilaggrin; Catalytic triad similarity with serine proteinases	39.4–43.9 kbp plasmid of prototype pRW001	S. aureus: phage group II> phage groups I and III	Jackson and Iandolo 1986, O'Toole and Foster 1986, Lee et al. 1987

Table 27.5 Continued

Protein	MW (kDa)	Major biochemical and biological activities	Gene	Gene location	Species distribution	References
Fibrin-forming and fibrinolytic enzymes						
Staphylocoagulase (coagulase)	40–64 Multiple forms	Clots plasma in the absence of Ca^{2+}. Coagulase reacts with coagulase-reacting factor (CRF) and the resulting complex (staphylothrombin) converts fibrinogen to fibrin	coa	Chromosome: Sma I fragment E	S. aureus S. intermedius S. hyicus S. delphini S. schleiferi subsp. coagulans	Drummond and Tager 1963, Phonimdaeng et al. 1988, 1990
Staphylokinase (SAK)	13–15	Binds to plasminogen and activates it to become the fibrinolytic enzyme plasmin. Activates plasminogen from specific mammalian species	sak	Chromosome: possibly on a converting phage	S. aureus: biotype A> biotype C	Papke and Blobel 1978, Sako and Tsuchida 1983
Bacteriolytic enzymes						
Endo-β-N-acetyl-glucosaminidases	31–80 Different species types	Bacterial cell lysis. Cleaves β 1–4 glucosaminidic bonds of Bacillus and Micrococcus cell wall peptidoglycan. Interferes with phagocytosis			S. aureus Many species of staphylococci	Wadström and Hisatsune 1970, Varaldo and Sattas 1978, Valisena, Varaldo and Satta 1982, Guardati et al. 1993
Lysostaphin endopeptidase (lysostaphin)	59 pro 26	Staphylococcal cell lysis. Cleaves glycyl–glycyl bonds of interpeptide bridge of staphylococcal cell wall peptidoglycan. Zinc metalloenzyme	end	Plasmid	S. simulans: biovar staphylolyticus	Schindler and Schuhardt 1965, Sloan, Robinson and Kloos 1982, Heath, Heath and Sloan 1987, Recsei, Gruss and Novick 1987
Hydrolytic enzymes						
Lipase	71 pre 46	Hydrolyses triglycerides, Tweens, phosphatidylcholines, lysophospholipids	geh	Chromosome Chromosome: Sma I fragment E	S. hyicus S. aureus Many other species	Götz et al. 1985, Lee and Iandolo 1986, 1988, van Oort et al. 1989

Enzyme	Molecular weight (kDa)	Function	Gene	Location	Species	References
Staphylococcal nuclease (thermonuclease)	A: 16.8	Hydrolyses RNA and DNA to 3'-phosphomono-nucleotides. Phosphodiesterase requiring Ca^{2+}	*nuc*	Chromosome	*S. aureus* *S. intermedius* *S. hyicus* *S. schleiferi*	Anfinsen, Cuatrecasas and Taniuchi 1971, Davis et al. 1977, Shortle 1983
Urease	Subunits: α: 72.4 β: 20.4 γ: 13.9 Multimer: 420	Hydrolyses urea to ammonia and carbamate. Nickel requirement. Plays role in invasiveness of *S. saprophyticus* in urinary tract	*ure*	Chromosome	*S. saprophyticus* *S. aureus* *S. xylosus* Many other species	Gatermann, John, and Marre 1989, Jose et al. 1991, Jose, Schafer, and Kaltwasser 1994, Schafer and Kaltwasser 1994
Hyaluronate lyase (hyaluronidase)	84	Hydrolyses hyaluronate at 1–4 hexosaminidic bonds. Aids in invasiveness by breakdown of hyaluronate-rich tissue barriers	*hysA*	Chromosome	*S. aureus* *S. hyicus*	Rautela and Abramson 1973, Farrell, Taylor and Holland 1995
Serine proteinase (or endopeptidase)	27	Cleaves peptide bonds at carboxy-terminal side of dicarboxylic amino acids. Increases influenza virus infectivity by cleavage activation of haemagglutinin	*sprV8 (sasP)*	Chromosome	*S. aureus* *S. epidermidis*	Drapeau 1978, Carmona and Gray 1987, Tashiro et al. 1987

97%) of *S. aureus* strains of human and animal origin. The δ-toxin or a δ-like toxin is produced by some strains of *S. epidermidis* and *S. haemolyticus* (Gemmell and Thelestam 1981, Scheifele et al. 1987). Wadström and coworkers (Wadström, Kjellgren and Ljungh 1976) partially characterized the haemolysins produced by several strains of *S. haemolyticus*, *S. capitis* and *S. simulans* and concluded that they were not identical to the known staphylococcal toxins.

The species *S. aureus* produces a group of functionally related pyrogenic toxins that cause fever and shock in their hosts. These toxins are classified as superantigens (SAgs) and include the enterotoxins (SE) and TSST-1, which have in common a potent mitogenic activity for T lymphocytes of several host species (Iandolo 1989, Fleischer 1994). *S. aureus* is clearly the major staphylococcal species capable of forming enterotoxins. About 50% of human *S. aureus* strains of biotype A produce enterotoxins, with a preponderance of SE-A (Bergdoll 1989). The percentage of enterotoxigenic *S. aureus* strains of biotype C from cattle is relatively low (0–15%), and when enterotoxin is produced it is usually SE-C. Some *S. intermedius* and *S. hyicus* strains may produce enterotoxins (SE-C, SE-D, or SE-E), but this remains to be substantiated at the genotypic level (Devriese and Hájek 1980, Hirooka et al. 1988, Valle et al. 1990). TSST-1 causes approximately 75% of all staphylococcal TSS cases (Bergdoll et al. 1981, Schlievert et al. 1981). About 90% of *S. aureus* strains isolated from the vagina of patients with TSS produce TSST-1. Most of these strains belong to the *S. aureus* typing phage group I and are lysed by bacteriophages 29, or 52, or both. The incidence of TSST-1 is much lower (15%) in *S. aureus* strains isolated from other types of patients or healthy individuals, and it has not been detected in other staphylococcal species. The *S. aureus* epidermolytic toxins (ETs) known as exfoliatin A (ETA) and B (ETB) are recognized as the agents causing the staphylococcal scalded skin syndrome (SSSS), a disease associated with severe blistering or scalding of the skin, especially in young children (Rogolsky 1979). ETs are produced by a low percentage (≤5%) of *S. aureus* strains.

Coagulase is a protein that clots plasma in the absence of Ca^{2+} but requires a plasma constituent known as coagulase-reacting factor (CRF). CRF, perhaps a derivative of prothrombin, reacts with coagulase, and the resulting coagulase–CRF complex (staphylothrombin) converts fibrinogen to fibrin (Drummond and Tager 1963). A very high percentage (98–99%) of *S. aureus* strains exhibit coagulase activity. Coagulase activity is also exhibited by the species *S. intermedius*, *S. hyicus*, *S. delphini* and *S. schleiferi* subsp. *coagulans*. Staphylokinase (SAK), a protein that exhibits fibrinolytic activity indirectly by binding to plasminogen, is produced by a relatively high percentage (60–95%) of human *S. aureus* strains of biotype A, but by only a small percentage (5–10%) of bovine *S. aureus* strains of biotype C (Hájek and Maršálek 1969).

The bacteriolytic enzymes *endo*-β-*N*-acetylglucosaminidase and *N*-acetylmuramyl-L-alanine amidase (Wadström and Hisatsune 1970) are produced by *S.* *aureus* and many other staphylococcal species. The former enzyme is especially active against the cells of *Bacillus* and *Micrococcus* spp., which compete for some of the same cutaneous habitats as staphylococci. The bacteriolytic enzyme known as lysostaphin (or lysostaphin endopeptidase) is a zinc metalloenzyme that has as its main target the polyglycyl bridge of the cell wall peptidoglycan of staphylococci (Schindler and Schuhardt 1964, Trayer and Buckley 1970) and salinicocci (Ventosa et al. 1990). Lysostaphin is produced by *S. simulans* biovar staphylolyticus (Sloan, Robinson and Kloos 1982). The plasmid containing the endopeptidase gene *end* also contains the lysostaphin endopeptidase resistance gene *epr* that specifies modification of the interpeptide bridge of the peptidoglycan, making the host *S. simulans* strain resistant to the lysostaphin endopeptidase that it produces (DeHart et al. 1995). The modification of the interpeptide bridge involves a replacement of many of the glycine residues by serine residues. Most strains of *S. sciuri* produce a staphylolytic enzyme that is immunologically related to lysostaphin, but it is determined by a gene sharing little nucleotide sequence homology with *end* (Kloos et al. 1997b).

Various lipases (and esterases) are produced by staphylococci (Saggers and Stewart 1968, Zimmerman and Kloos 1976). Staphylococcal lipases hydrolyse a wide range of substrates, including both water-soluble and water-insoluble triglycerides, as well as oxyethylene-sorbitan fatty acids (Tweens), phosphatidylcholines and lysophospholipids (Rollof, Hedström and Nilsson-Ehle 1987, van Oort et al. 1989). Both heat-stable and heat-labile nucleases are produced by staphylococci. A large percentage (95–100%) of the strains of *S. aureus*, *S. hyicus*, *S. intermedius* and *S. schleiferi* produce detectable levels of the heat-stable nuclease (or thermonuclease) (Devriese et al. 1978, Freney et al. 1988). Some staphyococcal species exhibit proteolytic activity on casein and gelatin, especially *S. aureus* (Abramson 1972), *S. sciuri* (Kloos, Schleifer and Smith 1976) and *S. hyicus* (Devriese et al. 1978). Several different proteinases (proteases) of *S. aureus* have been characterized, including the serine, metallo-, and thiol proteases (Arvidson 1983). Urease activity is exhibited by many staphylococcal species, and it apparently plays a role in the invasiveness of *S. saprophyticus* in the urinary tract (Gatermann, John and Marre 1989). Hyaluronate lyase (hyaluronidase) is a glycoprotein produced by *S. aureus* and *S. hyicus* that hydrolyses the mucopolysaccharide hyaluronate (Rautela and Abramson 1973). Pathogenic staphylococci that produce this enzyme have the capacity to break down hyaluronate-rich tissue barriers, thereby increasing their invasiveness.

8.3 Bacteriocins

Lantibiotics are low molecular weight bacteriocins produced by a wide range of gram-positive bacteria including staphylococci, lactococci, bacilli and streptomycetes (Jack, Tagg and Ray 1995). They are small polypeptides of 19–34 amino acids and have several sulphide rings consisting of 2 unusual amino acids, *meso*-lanthionine and 3-methyllanthionine (Schnell et al. 1988). Epidermin (staphylococcin 1580) and Pep5 are lantibiotics produced by *S. epidermidis* (Allgaier et al. 1986, Kellner, Jung and Sahl 1991). The 52 amino acid epidermin is encoded by the gene *epiA* contained within an operon located on a 54 kbp plasmid (Schnell et al. 1988, 1992). The epidermin operon contains a minimum of 6 genes (*epiABCD* and *epiQ*, *epiP*). The *epiP* gene product is homologous to serine proteases and may be involved in the cleavage of the 30 amino acid leader from the epidermin prepeptide molecule. *pepA* encodes the 60 amino acid Pep5 and is contained within a gene cluster (*pepI*, *pepT*, ORF X and *pepA*, *pepP*, *pepB*, *pepC*) found on a plasmid (Kaletta et al. 1989, Reis et al. 1993). The *pepI* gene product is essential for Pep5 immunity. Gallidermin is produced by *S. gallinarum* (Kellner et al. 1988). The activity of these lantibiotics is directed mainly against gram-positive bacteria, many of which interact or compete with staphylococci in their natural habitats. These lantibiotics depolarize bacterial and planar lipid membranes in a voltage-dependent manner and they can also form pores (up to 1 nm in diameter) in the membrane (Kordel, Benz and Sahl 1988). Some strains of *S. haemolyticus* produce one or more small, 44 amino acid peptides (sharing 65–75% sequence homology) that exhibit antibacterial activity, especially antigonococcal activity (Frenette et al. 1984, Watson et al. 1988). It has been suggested that these peptides are released signal sequences of secreted and/or membrane-bound proteins.

9 GENETIC MECHANISMS

9.1 Genetic exchange mechanisms

Transduction has been demonstrated in both laboratory and natural populations of *S. aureus* (Novick and Morse 1967, Richmond and Lacey 1973). Transduction methods were used for the fine structure mapping of amino acid biosynthesis genes (Kloos and Pattee 1965, Smith and Pattee 1967, Proctor and Kloos 1970, Barnes, Bondi and Fuscaldo 1971, Pattee et al. 1974). The generalized transducing phages of *S. aureus* belong to the serological group B (Pattee and Baldwin 1961). The size of the chromosomal DNA packaged into the phage head is similar to that of the phage DNA (Beryhill and Pattee 1969). Transducing DNA fragments appear to be highly uniform in size (Kloos and Pattee 1965, Pattee et al. 1968). Small plasmids of *S. aureus* (1–5 kbp) may be transduced by being packaged in a phage head as a phage genome-sized plasmid concatemer, whose formation requires plasmid-specific initiation of replication (Novick, Edelman and Löfdahl 1986). The plasmid concatemer is processed to the monomeric form in the recipient. The cotransduction of different plasmids can occur via a stable cointegrate formed between the plasmid DNAs, which is apparently not resolved in the recipient cell (Novick et al. 1981). The cointegration

involves recombination at specific sites on certain small class I plasmids (Novick et al. 1984). The larger class II plasmids may also be transduced, though plasmid replication is not required (Novick 1989). Transduction of plasmids and their maintenance are affected by the host restriction–modification system, which may limit to some extent the distribution of plasmids in staphylococcal communities. Transduction of chromosomal markers and plasmid DNA has also been demonstrated in *S. epidermidis* (Olsen et al. 1979).

Transformation of chromosomal and plasmid markers was first described in *S. aureus* strain NCTC 8325 by Lindberg and coworkers (Lindberg, Sjöström and Johansson 1972). The ability of this strain to become competent for transformation (and transfection) depends on the presence of high concentrations of Ca^{2+} and the presence of certain bacteriophages of serotype B (e.g. $\phi11$, $\phi14$, 83A, 80α) (Ruden et al. 1973, Thompson and Pattee 1981). The involvement of bacteriophage 80α in conferring competence is believed to be due to an interaction of externally supplied phage components with the surface of the cell (Birmingham and Pattee 1981). Transformation has played a major role in determining the genetic map of the chromosome of *S. aureus* strain NCTC 8325 (Pattee 1993). Transformation by plasmid DNA occurs at a low frequency (10^3–10^4 transformants μg^{-1} plasmid DNA), and it is lower for plasmids than for chromosomal markers (Lindberg, Sjöström and Johansson 1972, Lindberg and Novick 1973). The transformation frequency is greatly influenced by the restriction–modification system of the recipient cell. Heterologous plasmids (isolated from a different *S. aureus* strain or species) are associated with very low transformation frequencies (Sjöström, Löfdahl and Philipson 1979).

Relatively high transformation frequencies (10^6 transformants μg^{-1} plasmid DNA) can be obtained with protoplast transformation of *S. carnosus* by plasmid DNA (Götz and Schumacher 1987). Protoplast transformation is inefficient for *S. epidermidis* and other species that are not very susceptible to lysostaphin. Transformation of *S. aureus*, *S. epidermidis*, *S. carnosus* and *S. simulans* by plasmid DNA has been accomplished using electroporation techniques, which provide low to moderate transformation frequencies (10^3–10^5 transformants μg^{-1} plasmid DNA) (Augustin and Götz 1990).

Plasmid mediated conjugative transfer has been demonstrated both in laboratory and natural populations of *S. aureus*, *S. epidermidis*, *S. hominis* and *S. haemolyticus*, and includes both intra- and interspecies transfer (Archer and Johnston 1983, Forbes and Schaberg 1983, Goering and Ruff 1983, McDonnell, Sweeney and Cohen 1983, Naidoo and Noble 1987). Most of the conjugative plasmids are class III plasmids that encode resistance to gentamicin and certain other aminoglycosides, such as tobramycin and kanamycin. Many also encode resistance to ethidium bromide and quaternary amines, whereas some also encode resistance to penicillin and trimethoprim.

These plasmids are relatively large (30–60 kbp) and have a conjugative transfer (*tra*) region that is often flanked by directly repeated 900 bp IS*257* elements (Thomas and Archer 1989a). They are also capable of mobilizing or cotransferring certain smaller coresident plasmids which are not independently transferable. Class I plasmids that can form DNA–protein relaxation complexes can be mobilized, whereas nonrelaxable plasmids cannot be mobilized or can be mobilized only at a very low frequency (McDonnell, Sweeney and Cohen 1983, Projan and Archer 1989). Conjugative gentamicin-resistance plasmids from *S. aureus* and *S. epidermidis* strains isolated from different geographical regions in the USA are very closely related in their structure and may have had a clonal origin (Jaffe et al. 1982, Goering, Teeman and Ruff 1985). Two other types of conjugative plasmids have been detected in *S. aureus* (Townsend et al. 1986, Udo, Townsend and Grubb 1987, Udo, Love and Grubb 1992). One of these appears to be unable to mobilize other plasmids and encodes for the production of a diffusible pigment, in addition to encoding resistance to one or more antibiotics. The other type is cryptic except that it is conjugative and can mobilize non-conjugative plasmids. Transposon-labelled derivatives of these plasmids have been transferred from *S. aureus* to *S. epidermidis* and *E. faecalis* and back to *S. aureus* (Udo and Grubb 1990).

Fusion of lysostaphin–lysozyme-prepared, staphylococcal protoplasts can be accomplished by treatment of the protoplast mixture with polyethylene glycol (Götz, Ahrné and Lindberg 1981). By this method, plasmids can be transferred between strains of the same species and between strains of different species. In fusions between different species, the frequency of transfer is reduced somewhat from that of intraspecific fusions. A very low frequency of recombination of chromosomal genes by protoplast fusion has been demonstrated for strains of *S. aureus*.

9.2   Chromosome map of *S. aureus*

The genome of staphylococci consists of a chromosome to which may be added or subtracted various accessory elements, such as prophages, plasmids and transposons. The chromosome of *S. aureus* strain NCTC 8325 is about 2800 kbp, and has been mapped by genetic and physical methods by Pattee (Pattee 1993, Iandolo and Stewart 1997) (Fig. 27.4). More than 100 loci have been mapped to date, including phenotypic markers and silent transposon insertions. The average size of the *S. aureus* chromosome is 2741 ± 277 kbp.

9.3   Plasmids

Plasmids are facultative extrachromosomal genetic systems (elements) and, for the most part, they may be regarded as endosymbionts supplying the host cell with protective and various other adaptive functions. Plasmids are common in natural populations of most staphylococcal species (Lacey 1975, Kloos, Orban and

Walker 1981, Weinstein et al. 1982). They are rare (<2% of strains) in the species *S. auricularis* (Kloos 1990) and relatively uncommon (≤20% of strains) in *S. schleiferi* (Etienne et al. 1990a) and members of the *S. sciuri* species group (Kloos, Orban and Walker 1981). The characteristics of many of the plasmids from *S. aureus* have been reviewed by Lyon and Skurray (1987) and Novick (1989). *S. aureus* plasmids have been classified into 3 general classes, I through III. Class I plasmids are of small size (1–5 kbp) and have a high copy number (10–55 copies per cell), and they usually encode a single antibiotic resistance or are cryptic. These plasmids are the most widespread throughout the genus *Staphylococcus*. Novick (1989) has subdivided class I plasmids into 4 subgroups or families on the basis of their nucleotide sequence and functional organization. Plasmids in this class are largely composed of cassettes or specific segments that are not transposons. They represent at least 10 different incompatibility groups and replicate by an asymmetric rolling-circle mechanism (Ruby and Novick 1975, Iordănescu and Surdeanu 1980). The pT181 family is made up of a group of small (4–4.6 kbp) plasmids that usually encode tetracycline or chloramphenicol resistance and it is defined by homologous minimal replicons, consisting of an initiator (Rep) protein cistron containing the leading-strand replication origin (Novick 1989). All major transcription units are codirectional with replication. Tetracycline-resistance plasmids belonging to this family are highly conserved and are very common in a wide range of staphylococcal species (Kloos, Orban and Walker 1981, Cooksey and Baldwin 1985, Dodd et al. 1985, Wells and Kloos 1987). The pC194 family contains plasmids with homologous Rep protein cistrons and replication origins, though the functional organization of plasmids and their phenotype varies considerably. Some members of this family are very closely related to certain *Bacillus* plasmids (Polak and Novick 1982, Muller et al. 1986) and *E. faecalis* plasmids (Perkins and Youngman 1983). The pSN2 family plasmids have a direction of replication that appears to be opposite that of the Rep protein coding frame. Most plasmids of this family encode erythromycin resistance and contain the recombination site RS$_A$. Some, such as pSN2, are cryptic. The erythromycin-resistance plasmids belonging to this family are usually 2–2.5 kbp in size and except for variation in the control region of the *ermC* gene, are highly conserved (Iordănescu and Surdeanu 1980, Lampson and Parisi 1986, Catchpole et al. 1988, Kloos, George and Jones-Park 1992). They, like the tetracycline-resistance plasmids of the pT181 family, are very common in a wide range of staphylococcal species. A naturally occurring plasmid found in *B. subtilis* is a member of this family (Projan et al. 1987). The pE194 family is currently represented by the 3.7 kbp plasmid pE194 of *S. aureus* that contains an *ermC* gene, which is nearly identical to the *ermC* of the pSN2 family, but the plasmid functional organization is similar to certain pT181 family plasmids. Somewhat similar erythromycin-resistance plasmids have also been iso-

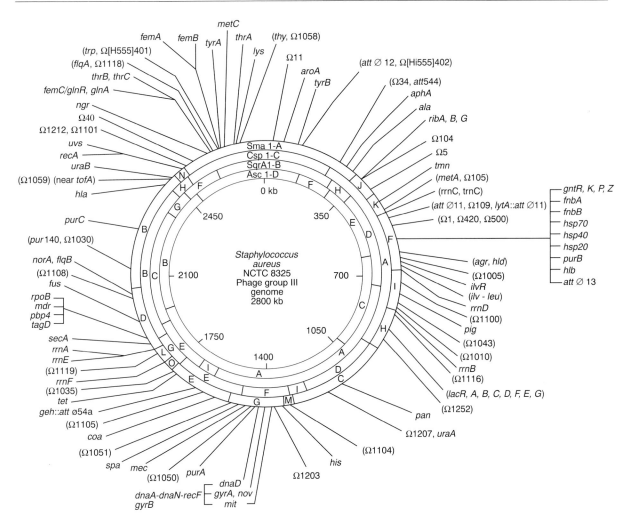

Fig. 27.4 Genetic and physical map of the chromosome of *S. aureus* NCTC 8325 (Pattee 1993, Iandolo and Stewart 1997). The order of the majority of the markers shown is based on genetic analysis and DNA hybridization analysis of *Sma*I, *Csp*I, *Sgr*AI and *Asc*I restriction fragments resolved by PFGE and hybridized with appropriate labelled probes. The markers *lys*, *thy*, Ω11, Ω402, *aphA*, *att*Φ11, Ω420, Ω500, *purB*, *bla*, *ilvR*, *leu*, *pig*, *uraA*, *his*, *mit*, *nov*, *dnaD*, *purA*, *fus*, *pur-140*, *tofA*, *ngr*, *thrC*, *cfxB*, *ofxC*, Ω401, *tyrA* and *metC* have not been physically mapped, and their map locations are based only on multifactorial transformation analysis. Each of the ribosomal RNA operons (*rrnA–F*) contains an internal *Sma*I recognition site which defines the junctions between *Sma*I L/D, H/I, K/F, I/F and L/O. The orientation of markers shown in parentheses is not known relative to the remainder of the map. The entire chromosome is about 2800 kbp, of which approximately 125–150 kbp represents the 3 known prophages Φ11, Φ12 and Φ13. The few small DNA fragments not placed on the physical map include *Sgr*AI fragments G, J and K (total of about 300 kbp), 2 *Csp*I fragments (total of about 100 kbp) and 2 *Sma*I fragments (total of about 25 kbp). (Courtesy of J Iandolo and G Stewart, Department of Diagnostic Medicine and Pathobiology, Kansas State University, Manhattan, KS, USA).

lated from members of the *S. saprophyticus* species group.

Class II plasmids of *S. aureus* have been subdivided into 2 major families on the basis of incompatibility (Novick and Richmond 1965). These plasmids, commonly referred to as penicillinase or β-lactamase plasmids, are relatively large (15–33 kbp), have a low copy number (4–6 per cell), and replicate using the θ replication mechanism (Sheehy and Novick 1975). They carry various combinations of antibiotic and heavy metal resistance genes, many of which are located on transposons (Shalita, Murphy and Novick 1980, Lyon and Skurray 1987). Class II plasmids have been identified in many other staphylococcal species but, unlike class I plasmids, they are very uncommon in the spec-

ies *S. hyicus*, *S. intermedius*, *S. simulans* and *S. lugdunensis* (Kloos, Orban and Walker 1981, Götz et al. 1983, Etienne et al. 1990a, 1990b). Class III plasmids include the large conjugative plasmids discussed above (see section 9.1, p. 599). Like class II plasmids, they appear to be assemblages of transposons and transposon remnants (Gillespie et al. 1987).

9.4 Bacteriophages

The phage typing of *S. aureus* became possible due to the readily available source of phages with a narrow spectrum of activity on strains of this species. Phage typing has been generally regarded as a means of excluding possible sources of infection rather than as a means for defining groups of epidemiologically related strains (Parker 1983). For several decades since its inception in 1952–1953, typing of *S. aureus* strains by an official International Basic Set of phages has found wide use as an established method for epidemiology (Williams and Rippon 1952). By 1970, it became apparent that the Basic Set could not type *S. aureus* strains isolated from a wide range of animal species, so it was redesigned and limited to a Basic Set of Typing Phages for Human Strains of *S. aureus*, which could identify many strains from human sources as belonging to phage groups I, II, III or V. A separate set of typing phages was established for bovine strains. Some unofficial sets of *S. epidermidis* phages have been used for the typing of *S. epidermidis* strains (Verhoef, Van Boven and Winkler 1971, Pulverer, Pillich and Haklová 1976). The use of phage typing in epidemiology is now being re-evaluated in the light of the newer molecular typing methods (Bannerman et al. 1995). In general, phage typing appears not to be as discriminatory or as reproducible as PFGE and ribotyping.

Although the future of phage typing appears to be less certain now than it did a decade ago, it can serve as a reminder that staphylococci interact with these organisms. Genetic and molecular studies of staphylococcal phages began as a consequence of the availability of typing phages and their temperate behaviour. Most strains of *S. aureus* and *S. epidermidis* (and probably many other species) are multiply lysogenic and the phages can usually be induced by UV and mitomycin C (Verhoef, Van Boven and Winkler 1971, Pulverer, Pillich and Haklová 1976). The temperate phages of *S. aureus* can be subdivided into 3 main serological groups, A, B and C. Serological group B contains most of the known transducing phages and phages that can confer competence in transformation. Members of this group exhibit considerable DNA sequence homology (Inglis, Waldron and Stewart 1987). The group B transducing phage φ11 has been studied extensively (Löfdahl, Zabielski and Philipson 1981, Chapple and Stewart 1987). It has a 45 kbp genome that is circularly permuted and terminally redundant with a blunt end. Examples of lysogenic conversion have been mentioned above (see section 8.2, p. 593) and include the prophage carriage of genes encoding SE-A and SAK. The phage φ11 genome has also been shown to acquire the transposon Tn554 from its primary chromosomal site during lytic infection. It may transfer Tn554, via transduction, directly or through a plasmid intermediate, to the chromosome of the recipient cell (Murphy et al. 1981). Phage S1 can exhibit recombination with the tetracycline-resistance gene of a class I plasmid, producing a hybrid phage–plasmid element (Inoue and Mitsuhashi 1976). Negative lysogenic conversion has been demonstrated for the *geh* (Lee and Iandolo 1986) and *hlb* (Coleman et al. 1986) genes, which contain phage attachment sites within their sequence. Several *S. epidermidis* (Verhoef, Van Boven and Winkler 1971, Verhoef et al. 1971) and *S. saprophyticus* (Fournet et al. 1985) phages have been characterized, but not to the extent of the *S. aureus* phages.

10 RESISTANCE TO ANTIMICROBIAL AGENTS

Staphylococci have a record of developing resistance quickly and successfully to antibiotics. This defensive response is a consequence of the acquisition and transfer of antibiotic-resistance plasmids and the possession of intrinsic resistance mechanisms, some of which may have evolved prior to the formation of the genus *Staphylococcus*. The acquired defence systems by staphylococci may have originated from antibiotic-producing organisms, where they may have been developed and then passed on to other genera. Presumably the genus *Staphylococcus* has been one of the recipient genera as a consequence of coming in contact with antibiotic-producing bacteria and fungi in their natural habitats. Staphylococci are sometimes exposed to heavy metal ions present in their natural habitat or in the environment, e.g. by contact with certain metal-containing cosmetics, ointments, antiseptics and soils. They may also participate in genetic exchange with related soil bacteria, acting as reservoirs of heavy metal ion resistance genes. The various major antibiotic and heavy metal resistance mechanisms described for staphylococci are outlined in Table 27.6.

Three different mechanisms of resistance to β-lactam antibiotics have been identified for staphylococci: the inactivation of penicillin (and cephalosporin) by penicillinase (β-lactamase) mediated hydrolysis of the β-lactam ring of the antibiotic; an intrinsic resistance resulting from a reduction in the affinity or the amount of the PBPs; and tolerance to the bactericidal effect of β-lactam antibiotics due to an excess of autolysin inhibitor (Lyon and Skurray 1987). Penicillin-resistant *S. aureus* strains began emerging shortly after the introduction of penicillin in medicine in the early 1940s. Today the percentage of penicillin-resistant strains has risen to 75–95%, with the highest percentages found among hospital (nosocomial) strains. Similar percentages have been observed for penicillin-resistant strains of the *S. epidermidis* species group. Most penicillin-resistant staphylococcal strains produce β-lactamase. β-Lactamase genes (*bla*) are most often found on class II plasmids that are distributed among many staphylococcal species (Baldwin, Strickland and Cox 1969, Archer and Scott 1991). Resistance to methicillin and other β-lactamase-resistant penicillins was first observed in *S. aureus* soon after the introduction of methicillin into clinical use in Britain (Jevons 1961). The methicillin-resistant strains isolated in Britain came from hospitalized patients, were multiply antibiotic-resistant, belonged to phage group III, and their resistance to methicillin was heterogeneous, affecting only a minority of the cell population (Barber 1961). After the mid-1970s, large outbreaks of infection by methicillin-resistant *S. aureus* (MRSA) were recorded in many hospitals in Australia (Pavillard et al. 1982), the USA (Schaefler et al. 1981), Britain (Shanson, Kensit and Duke 1976, Cookson and Phillips 1988) and Ireland (Cafferkey et al. 1983). Many of these outbreaks appear to have been caused by a single epidemic strain that was transferred between hospitals by the movement of patients (Duckworth, Lothian and Williams 1988). Genetic analyses and molecular typing methods have indicated that various isolates of MRSA may have had a clonal origin, and suggest that the methicillin-resistance determinant was acquired by *S. aureus* at some point in time before or around the time of the introduction of methicillin (Ichiyama et al. 1991, Kreiswirth et al. 1993). During the 1980s, attention was drawn to the high incidence (20–85% of strains) of methicillin-resistant *S. epidermidis*

Table 27.6 Major antibiotic and heavy metal resistance mechanisms for staphylococci

Resistance phenotype and responsible protein	MW (kDa)	Major activity or mechanism	Gene	Gene location	Species distribution	References
Penicillin (β-lactams)						
Penicillinase (A–D) (β-lactamase)	A: 28.8	Inactivation of penicillin and cephalosporin by hydrolysis of the β-lactam ring A, B and C require induction by penicillin or its analogues	*blaZ*	Plasmids (mainly class II and III) >chromosome *blaI-blaR1-blaZ* region is often on transposon (Tn552, Tn4002, Tn4201)	*S. aureus* *S. epidermidis* Most species of staphylococci	Dyke 1979, Murphy and Novick 1979, Weber and Goering 1988, Wang, Projan and Novick 1991
β-Lactamase repressor BlaI	14.9	Transcriptional repressor for the system	*blaI*			
β-Lactamase antirepressor BlaR1	69.2	Receptor for β-lactams and the derepression of *blaZ*	*blaR1*			
Methicillin (β-lactamase resistant penicillins)						
Penicillin-binding protein PBP 2a (PBP2′)	74–78	Low-affinity penicillin-binding protein substituting activities of essential PBPs MIC range: 1.5–1500 $mg\ ml^{-1}$ Variation not solely *mecA*, but also *fem* and other antibiotic response genes	*mecA*	Chromosome: *Sma* I fragment G *mecI-mecR1-mecA* region may be on a transposon and sometimes on plasmids	*S. aureus* *S. epidermidis* *S. haemolyticus* Several other species	Sjöström, Löfdahl, and Philipson 1975, Hartman and Tomasz 1986, Mathews, Inglis, and Stewart 1990, De Lencastre and Tomasz 1994
Methicillin-resistance repressor MecI	14.8	Transcriptional repressor for the system	*mecI*			
Methicillin-resistance MecR1 protein (or antirepressor)	68.5	Derepression of *mecA* BlaI and BlaR1 can substitute for MecI and MecR1	*mecR1*			

Table 27.6 Continued

Resistance phenotype and responsible protein	MW (kDa)	Major activity or mechanism	Gene	Gene location	Species distribution	References
Aux (auxiliary) or Fem (factors essential for expression of methicillin resistance) (A–D)	A: 50.6 B: 49.7	A and B: biosynthesis of pentaglycine interpeptide bridge of peptidoglycan	$femA$, $femB$	Chromosome: Sma I fragment A	$S.$ $aureus$	Berger-Bächi et al. 1992, De Jonge et al. 1992, 1993, Ornelas-Soares et al. 1993, De Lencastre et al. 1994, Gustafson et al. 1994
		C: amidation of α-carboxyl group of D-glutamic acid in peptide subunits of the peptidoglycan	$femC$	Chromosome: Sma I fragment A	$S.$ $aureus$	
		D: controls rate of synthesis of unsubstituted disaccharide pentapeptide precursor	$femD$	Chromosome: Sma I fragment I	$S.$ $aureus$	

Macrolide, lincosamide, and streptogramin B (MLS)

Resistance phenotype and responsible protein	MW (kDa)	Major activity or mechanism	Gene	Gene location	Species distribution	References
23S rRNA methylases (or methyltransferases) A–C	28.3–29	N^6,N^6-dimethylation of adenine-2058 residues at peptidyl transferase centre of 23S rRNA, resulting in a decreased affinity of 50S ribosomal subunit for MLS antibiotics	$ermA$	Chromosome: on transposon Tn554 which prefers a single att site	$S.$ $aureus$ $S.$ $epidermidis$ Frequently found in $mecA$ strains Several other species	Murphy 1985a, Murphy, Huwyler and Bastos 1985, Thakker-Varia et al. 1987
		Require induction by erythromycin or are made constitutively	$ermB$	Plasmids and chromosome: on transposon Tn551 which can transpose to many sites	$S.$ $aureus$ $S.$ $intermedius$ $S.$ $hyicus$ $S.$ $xylosus$ Several other genera	Novick et al. 1979, Khan and Novick 1980, Luchansky and Pattee 1984, Eady et al. 1993
		Regulation by translational attenuation	$ermC$	Plasmids (mainly class I) > chromosome	$S.$ $aureus$ $S.$ $epidermidis$ Most species of staphylococci $Bacillus$ $subtilis$	Iordănescu and Surdeanu 1980, Horinouchi and Weisblum 1982, Weisblum 1985, Lampson and Parisi 1986, Kloos, George and Jones-Park 1992

		Gene	Function	Location	Species	References
Macrolide and streptogramin B (MS) ATP-dependent efflux protein MsrA (member of ATP-binding cassette transporter superfamily)		*msrA*	Plays a role as ATP-dependent efflux pump to remove MS antibiotics and requires a transmembrane complex. Possibly inactivate macrolides	Chromosome and plasmids	*S. hominis, S. cohnii* > *S. epidermidis* Several other species	Jenssen et al. 1987, Ross et al. 1989, 1990, Eady et al. 1993, Wondrack and Sutcliffe 1995
Lincosamide 3-Lincomycin, 4-clindamycin *O*-nucleotidyltransferase	19	*linA, linA'* (*lin* gene group)	Inactivates lincosamides. Requires a nucleoside 5'-triphosphate as nucleotidyl donor and Mg^{2+} as cofactor	Plasmids (class I)	*S. haemolyticus, S. aureus, S. hominis, S. cohnii* Several other species	Leclercq et al. 1985, 1987, Brisson-Noël et al. 1988, Kloos, George and Jones-Park 1992
Tetracycline Tetracycline efflux proteins (metal–tetracycline/H+ antiporters)	32–35	*tetK*	Plays role as energy-dependent efflux pump to remove tetracycline. Uses antiport mechanism of transport exchanging a proton for a metal–tetracycline complex. Requires induction by very low amounts of tetracycline. Regulation by translational attenuation	Plasmids (class I) > chromosome	*S. aureus, S. epidermidis* Many other species of staphylococci *Bacillus subtilis*	Iordănescu et al. 1978, Kloos, Orban and Walker 1981, Cooksey and Baldwin 1985, Wells and Kloos 1987
		tetL		Plasmids	*S. hyicus, Bacillus* species	Schwarz et al. 1993
Tetracycline and minocycline Ribosomal protection protein TetM	72.6	*tetM*	Permits productive binding of aminoacyl-tRNAs to ribosomes in the presence of tetracycline and minocycline. Requires tRNA modification (miaA) activity. Homology with elongation factors G and Tu and has GTPase activity	Chromosome	*S. intermedius, S. aureus*	Schaefler, Francois, and Ruby 1976, Wells and Kloos 1987, Nesin et al. 1990, Burdett 1993, Schwarz, Werckenthin and Ellendorff 1994
				Chromosome: Tn*916* and Tn*916*-like transposons Plasmids	Other gram positive genera Gram-negative genera	

Table 27.6 Continued

Resistance phenotype and responsible protein	MW (kDa)	Major activity or mechanism	Gene	Gene location	Species distribution	References
Aminoglycosides Aminoglycoside-modifying enzymes:						
Aminoglycoside 6'-acetyltransferase-aminoglycoside 2"-phosphotransferase [AAC(6') + APH(2")]	56	Bifunctional: 2 domains AAC(6') acetylates amino groups of tobramycin, netilmicin, amikacin, and gentamicin C at 6' position APH(2") phosphorylates 2"-hydroxyl groups	aac(6')-aph(2')	Plasmids (mainly class III) and chromosome on transposons (Tn4001 and Tn4001-like, Tn4031, Tn3851)	S. aureus S. epidermidis Enterococcus and some other gram-positive genera	Le Goffic et al. 1977, Townsend, Grubb and Ashdown 1983, Townsend et al. 1984, Ubukata et al. 1984, Rouch et al. 1987, Thomas and Archer 1989b
Aminoglycoside 3'-phosphotransferase [APH(3')-III]	31	Phosphorylates 3'-hydroxyl groups of kanamycin, neomycin, paromomycin, amikacin and gentamicin B	aph(3')-IIIa (aphA)	Plasmids and chromosome: Sma I fragment A	S. aureus Enterococcus	Gray and Fitch 1983, Coleman et al. 1985, El Solh, Moreau and Ehrlich 1986
Aminoglycoside-aminocyclitol-4'-adenylyltransferase (aminoglycoside 4'-adenylyltransferase) [ANT(4',4")-I]	34	Adenylylates tobramycin, amikacin, isepamicin, paromomycin, kanamycin, neomycin and gentamicin A at 4'-hydroxyl groups and also dibekacin at the 4"-hydroxyl group	ant(4')-Ia (aadD)	Plasmids	S. aureus S. epidermidis	Schwotzer, Kayser and Schwotzer 1978, El Solh et al. 1985, Thomas and Archer 1989b
Aminoglycoside 9-adenylyltransferase [ANT(9)-I]	29	Adenylylates spectinomycin	ant(9)-Ia (spc)	Chromosome: on transposon Tn554	S. aureus S. epidermidis Frequently found in mecA strains Several other species	Murphy 1985b, Thakker-Varia et al. 1987

Trimethoprim S1 Dihydrofolate reductase (S1 DFHR)	18–19	*dfrA*	Marked reduced affinity for trimethoprim High-level resistance: (MIC > 1000 mg ml⁻¹) Phe → Tyr change at position 98 (compared with native DHFR) is major determinant of resistance	Plasmid > chromosome: on transposon-like Tn4003 in an operon with *thyE* and ORF	*S. aureus* *S. epidermidis* *S. hominis* Several other species	Lyon et al. 1986, Coughter, Johnston and Archer 1987, Tennent et al. 1988, Rouch et al. 1989, Dale et al. 1995
Chloramphenicol Chloramphenicol acetyltransferase (CAT)	22.5–23 mono Native: trimeric	*cat*	Acetylates chloramphenicol via acetyl coenzyme A to yield mono- and diacetylated derivatives unable to bind to the ribosome Requires induction by chloramphenicol Regulated by translational attenuation	Plasmids (class I) Chromosome: with *cat* plasmid integrated	*S. aureus* Several other species *S. intermedius*	Iordănescu et al. 1978, Shaw 1983, Schwarz, Cardoso and Blobel 1989, 1990, Lovett 1990, Cardoso and Schwarz 1992, Schwarz et al. 1995
Fluoroquinolones DNA gyrase subunits [DNA topoisomerase (ATP-hydrolysing)]	A: 99.2 B: 72.5	*gyrA* *gyrB* (*nov*)	Subunit A: Ser → Leu or Phe change at position 84 and Glu → Lys change at position 88 result in moderate to high fluoroquinolone resistance Subunit B: mutations may result in novobiocin resistance and a slight reduction in fluoroquinolone susceptibility	Chromosome: *Sma* I fragment G Part of operon: *redF-gyrB-gyrA*	*S. aureus* *S. epidermidis* Many other species *Bacillus subtilis*	Sreedharan, Peterson and Fisher 1991, Goswitz et al. 1992, Margerrison, Hopewell and Fisher 1992, Brockbank and Barth 1993, Ito et al. 1994

Table 27.6 Continued

Resistance phenotype and responsible protein	MW (kDa)	Major activity or mechanism	Gene	Gene location	Species distribution	References
Multidrug efflux protein (or transporter) NorA	42.2	Plays role as energy-dependent efflux pump to remove hydrophilic fluoroquinolones and some other unrelated antibiotics. Related to tetracycline and *Bacillus*-Bmr efflux proteins. Change in NorA or increased transcription rate of *norA* can result in resistance	*norA* or its regulatory region; *flqB* may affect level of expression of *norA*	Chromosome: *Sma* I fragment D; Infrequently on plasmids	*S. aureus* *S. epidermidis* *S. haemolyticus* Many other species	Ohshita, Hiramatsu and Yokota, 1990, Yoshida et al. 1990, Kaatz, Seo and Ruble 1993, Ng, Trucksis and Hooper 1994
DNA topoisomerase IV subunit A	A: 90 B: 74.4	Subunit A: Ser → Phe or Tyr change at position 80 results in either high or low fluoroquinolone resistance. Subunits A and B are closely related to subunits A and B of DNA gyrase. *grlA* mutations may be prerequisite for resistance by *gyrA* mutations	*grlA* (*cfxB*, *ofxC* of *flq* locus) *grlB*	Chromosome: *Sma* I fragment A; Part of operon: *grlB-grlA*	*S. aureus*	Trucksis, Wolfson and Hooper 1991, Ferrero et al. 1994, Ferrero, Cameron and Crozet 1995
Rifampin DNA-dependent RNA polymerase β subunit	142–151	Mutations in rifampin binding area (area 1) of β subunit may result in rifampicin, rifamycin, and streptovaricin resistance. Specific amino acid changes have not been documented	*rpoB* (*rif*)	Chromosome: *Sma* I fragment D; Part of operon: *rpL-rpoB-rpoC*	*S. aureus* *S. epidermidis*	Aboshkiwa et al. 1992, Aboshkiwa, Rowland and Coleman 1995, Deora and Misra 1995
Cadmium and zinc Cadmium-efflux ATPase (an E_1E_2 cation-translocating ATPase)	78.8	Exports Cd^{2+} and Zn^{2+} to the outside of the cell	*cadA*	Plasmids (class II); In operon: *cadC-cadA*; Infrequently on chromosome	*S. aureus*	Nucifora et al. 1989, Endo and Silver 1995

Protein	MW (kDa)	Function	Gene	Location	Organism	References
Cadmium efflux system accessory protein	13.8	Transcriptional regulatory protein for system Induction by calcium	cadC			
Cadmium-binding protein CadB		Binds Cd^{2+} and Zn^{2+}	cadB	Plasmids (class I and II) Infrequently on chromosome	S. aureus S. lugdunensis	Smith and Novick 1972, Shalita, Murphy and Novick 1980, El Solh and Ehrlich 1982, Poitevin-Later et al. 1992
Mercury and organomercurial compounds						
Mercuric reductase	58.6	Reduces Hg^{2+} to the volatile Hg^o	merA	Plasmids (class II) Occasionally on chromosome	S. aureus	Weiss, Murphy and Silver 1977, Novick et al. 1979, Laddaga et al. 1987, Lyon and Skurray 1987, Chu et al. 1992
Organomercurial lyase (alkylmercury lyase)	23.6	Cleaves the carbon–mercury bond of organomercurials The Hg^{2+} product is subsequently reduced by mercuric reductase	merB	Located in mer operon: merR-ORF3-ORF4-ORF5-merA-merB		
Mercuric resistance operon regulatory protein	15.7	Transcriptional regulatory protein for system Induction by mercury	merR	Mer region is provisionally noted as Tn4004		
Arsenic and antimony						
Arsenical pump membrane protein (arsenite efflux protein)	46.5	Exports arsenite [As(III)] and antimonite [Sb(III)] to the outside of the cell	arsB	Plasmids (class II) Located in ars operon: arsR-arsB-arsC	S. aureus S. xylosus	Novick and Roth 1968, Silver et al. 1981, Götz et al. 1983, Ji and Silver 1992, Rosenstein et al. 1992, Bröer et al. 1993, Ji et al. 1994, Rosenstein, Nikoleit and Götz 1994
Arsenate reductase	14.8	Reduces arsenate [As(V)] to arsenite [As(III)]	arsC			
Arsenical resistance operon repressor (DNA-binding negative regulatory protein)	11.9	Transcriptional repressor for the system Induction by arsenate, arsenite, antimonite and bismuth	arsR			

(MRSE) in nosocomial infections (Karchmer, Archer and Dismukes 1983, Jones et al. 1989, Schaberg, Culver and Gaines 1991). Methicillin resistance has now been detected in several other staphylococcal species, including *S. haemolyticus*, *S. hominis*, *S. capitis*, *S. warneri*, *S. caprae*, *S. simulans*, *S. saprophyticus* and *S. sciuri* (Archer and Pennell 1990, Pierre et al. 1990, Murakami et al. 1991, Suzuki, Hiramatsu and Yokota 1992). More recently, it has been shown that many strains of *S. sciuri* are either resistant or intermediate resistant to oxacillin and methicillin, and some strains are intermediate resistant to cefazolin (Kloos et al. 1997b). The frequency and level of resistance to these antibiotics are generally higher in *S. sciuri* subsp. *rodentium* compared to those of the other subspecies. Chromosomal DNA of *S. sciuri* hybridizes with *mecA*-specific DNA probes, suggesting the presence of an intrinsic gene homologue in this species that is closely related to the *mecA* gene of methicillin-resistant strains of *S. aureus*. This property raises the possibility that *S. sciuri* may serve as an important reservoir of genetic determinants of methicillin resistance.

Methicillin-resistant staphylococci still pose a serious problem for patients in health care institutions and these organisms are beginning to appear in animals in veterinary hospitals. The accurate detection of methicillin resistance has been hampered by the variability of techniques used to identify heterotypic expression of resistance, though improvement in detection can generally be made by using relatively large inocula, supplementation of Mueller–Hinton agar with 2–4% sodium chloride, and incubation times of up to 48 h (Woods et al. 1986, National Committee for Clinical Laboratory Standards 1993). Genotypic testing using PCR or DNA hybridization to identify isolates containing the *mecA* gene is more sensitive and more specific than standard broth microdilution, agar dilution, or agar screening tests based on phenotypic expression (Archer and Pennell 1990, De Lencastre et al. 1991, Suzuki, Hiramatsu and Yokota 1992, Ubukata et al. 1992). Some *mecA⁻ S. aureus* strains, which harbour β-lactamase plasmids and belong to phage group 94/96, exhibit borderline susceptibility to methicillin and other β-lactamase-resistant penicillins (McMurray, Kernodle and Barg 1990, Barg, Chambers and Kernodle 1991). The slight increase in resistance of these closely related strains (oxacillin MIC, 1–2 μg ml⁻¹) is partly due to the hyperproduction of β-lactamase type A, resulting in some inactivation of β-lactamase-resistant penicillins (McDougal and Thornsberry 1986, Chambers, Archer and Matsuhashi 1989). A low-level intrinsic mechanism has been proposed to explain the moderately increased methicillin MICs (4–8 μg ml⁻¹) of *mecA⁻*, borderline methicillin-resistant strains of *S. aureus* (Berger-Bächi, Strassle and Kayser 1986, De Lencastre et al. 1991). Although the mechanism is not fully understood, it at least partly involves the presence of modified PBPs with decreased β-lactam affinity (Tomasz et al. 1989).

Erythromycin-resistant staphylococci often have cross-resistance to macrolides (erythromycin, oleandomycin, spiramycin, clarithromycin, azithromycin), lincosamides (lincomycin, clindamycin) and streptogramin type B antibiotics (designated MLS-resistant). The different types of MLS antibiotics bind to the 50S ribosomal subunit at overlapping binding sites, and binding interferes with transpeptidation and translocation reactions needed for peptide chain elongation. These sites are protected by the N^6,N^6-dimethylation of an adenine-2058 residue at the peptidyl transferase centre of 23S rRNA, a reaction performed by an rRNA methylase (Weisblum 1985). Three distinct rRNA methylase genes have been detected in staphylococci: *ermA* (Murphy 1985a), *ermB* (Novick and Murphy 1985, Leclercq and Courvalin 1991), and *ermC* (Horinouchi and Weisblum 1982, Projan et al. 1987). Even though each of the *erm* gene classes can be distinguished by hybridization, the amino acid sequences of the encoded methylases are highly conserved, which suggests that they evolved from a common ancestor, possibly originating in the antibiotic-producing organism (Arthur, Brisson-Noël and Courvalin 1987). The chromosomal *ermA* gene is common among methicillin-resistant (*mecA*) strains of *S. aureus* and *S. epidermidis*, but it is relatively uncommon in *mecA⁻* strains and usually accounts for only 6–11% of those resistant to MLS antibiotics (Thakker-Varia et al. 1987, Kloos, George and Jones-Park 1992, Eady et al. 1993). *ermB* is usually not found in staphylococcal species indigenous to primates; however, it appears to be relatively common in MLS-resistant strains of *S. intermedius* from dogs, in which expression can be either inducible or constitutive, and in MLS-resistant strains of *S. hyicus* and *S. xylosus* from pigs, in which expression is constitutive (Eady et al. 1993). The *ermC* gene is most often located on class I plasmids of the pSN2 and pE194 families (Iordănescu and Surdeanu 1980, Dunny et al. 1981, Parisi et al. 1981, Thakker-Varia et al. 1987, Kloos, George and Jones-Park 1992). These plasmids are present in very high frequencies (85–98% of strains) in most staphylococcal populations following treatment of the host with tylosin (a member of the spiramycin group) (Dunny et al. 1981), eythromycin (Vowels et al. 1995), or clindamycin (Kloos, George and Jones-Park 1992). Constitutive *ermC* genes have been selected in laboratory populations of *S. aureus* by the growth of inducible strains in the presence of tylosin (Horinouchi and Weisblum 1981) and in natural populations of staphylococci exposed to clindamycin. On the skin of out-patients receiving topical clindamycin for acne vulgaris, the percentage of total staphylococcal strains represented by constitutive MLS-resistant strains increased from 1%, prior to treatment, to 60% after one month of treatment, and to 71% by 2 months of treatment (Kloos, George and Jones-Park 1992). Approximately 95% of these strains had the constitutive *ermC* gene. As an exceptional species, *S. capitis* responded very slowly to clindamycin pressure, with only 12–15% of its strains expressing constitutive MLS resistance. This species also responds slowly to penicillin, erythromycin, or tetracycline pressure and it is seldom multiply resistant to antibiotics (Wells and Kloos 1987). Clinical isolates of constitutive MLS-resistant staphylococci are continuing to increase in frequency and this trend may be a reflection of the increased clinical use of clindamycin (Jenssen et al. 1987). The inducible macrolide and streptogramin (MS) resistance phenotype involves erythromycin cross-resistance to other 14–16-membered ring macrolides and streptogramin type B, but not lincosamides (Jenssen et al. 1987, Ross et al. 1989, Wondrack and Sutcliffe 1995). MS resistance appears to be most prevalent in members of the *S. epidermidis* and *S. saprophyticus* species groups, especially in *S. hominis* and *S. cohnii* (Kloos, George and Jones-Park 1992, Eady et al. 1993, Vowels et al. 1995).

Tetracycline resistance is widespread among staphylococcal species and ranks along with β-lactam and MLS resistance as one of the most frequent types of antibiotic resistance found in natural populations of staphylococci (Cooksey and Baldwin 1985, Wells and Kloos 1987, Bismuth et al. 1990, Archer and Scott 1991, Schwarz et al. 1993). There are 2 mechanisms of tetracycline resistance recognized in staphylococci. The most common one involves an energy-dependent pumping (efflux) of tetracycline and doxycycline from the cell, so that levels of these antibiotics are reduced below that required to inhibit the ribosome. The efflux protein is most often encoded by the inducible gene *tetK* which is located on class I plasmids of the pT181 family. The second mechanism, one that is controlled by the gene *tetM*, involves ribosome protection such that protein synthesis is unaffected by the presence of tetracycline, doxycycline, or minocycline (Schaefler, Francois and Ruby 1976).

There are 3 major mechanisms responsible for aminoglycoside resistance in staphylococci. One mechanism involves changes in ribosomal proteins as a consequence of certain mutations in their structural genes, such that ribosomes can no longer bind streptomycin. A second mechanism involves the energization and permeability of the cell membrane. Some energy-deficient, small-colony mutants of *S. aureus* have been shown to be resistant to aminoglycosides due to a diminished uptake of the antibiotics, presumably as a consequence of cell membrane impermeability (Miller et al. 1980). The third and most common mechanism of resistance involves modification of aminoglycosides by aminoglycoside-modifying enzymes so that the antibiotics are no longer capable of binding to ribosomes. Genes encoding these enzymes are either located on plasmids (e.g. gentamicin-resistance plasmids and neomycin- and kanamycin-resistance plasmids) or on the chromosome (Jaffe et al. 1982, Lyon et al. 1984, Coleman et al. 1985, El Solh, Moreau and Ehrlich 1986, Thomas and Archer 1989b).

Trimethoprim resistance is either mediated by alterations in the expression of the intrinsic chromosomal *dfr* gene (e.g. *dfrB* of *S. aureus* or *dfrC* of *S. epidermidis*), possibly resulting in overproduction of the native dihydrofolate reductase (DHFR) or a reduced affinity of the native DHFR for trimethoprim, or by the acquisition of a second chromosomal or plasmid *dfr* gene (e.g. *dfrA* in *S. aureus*, *S. epidermidis* and *S. hominis*) that

encodes a trimethoprim-resistant DHFR capable of rescuing the reduction step leading to tetrahydrofolate in the presence of trimethoprim (Galetto, Johnston and Archer 1987, Rouch et al. 1989, Dale et al. 1995). In Australian *S. aureus* strains, the *drfA* gene is usually carried by non-conjugative plasmids, whereas in USA *S. aureus* strains, the gene is frequently carried by both conjugative and non-conjugative plasmids, and occasionally is found on the chromosome.

The glycopeptide antibiotics teicoplanin and vancomycin bind to the peptidyl-D-alanyl-D-alanine termini of peptidoglycan precursors and prevent the transglycosylation and transpeptidation steps of cell wall peptidoglycan synthesis. Since this mode of action is different from that of β-lactams, glycopeptides are being used to treat severe infections caused by methicillin- and other β-lactam-resistant staphylococci. Teicoplanin resistance (MIC >16 µg ml^{-1}) and/or moderate vancomycin susceptibility (MIC 8–16 µg ml^{-1}) have been observed in *S. haemolyticus*, especially in methicillin-resistant strains of this species (Goldstein et al. 1990, Bannerman, Wadiak and Kloos 1991a). Strains of *S. haemolyticus* and *S. epidermidis* that are moderately susceptible to teicoplanin (MIC 16 µg ml^{-1}) are relatively common. Vancomycin and teicoplanin resistance can be selected in vitro in *S. haemolyticus* (Schwalbe et al. 1990, Herwaldt, Boyken and Pfaller 1991). Even though vancomycin resistance appears not to be established in natural populations of staphylococci, the threat of it appearing is very real because the closely related enterococci can carry and transfer *van* resistance genes located on the transposon Tn1546 (Leclercq et al. 1988, Arthur et al. 1993). Furthermore, under laboratory conditions, *van* genes have been transferred from *E. faecalis* to *S. aureus* by conjugation, with the concomitant expression of vancomycin resistance (Noble, Virani and Cree 1992).

Three mechanisms for fluoroquinolone resistance have been postulated for staphylococci. One mechanism found in *S. aureus* and *S. epidermidis* involves mutations in the chromosomal gene *gyrA*, encoding the DNA gyrase subunit A, so that its function is no longer inhibited by the antibiotic (Sreedharan, Peterson and Fisher 1991, Goswitz et al. 1992). A second mechanism found in *S. aureus*, *S. epidermidis* and *S. haemolyticus* involves mutations in the chromosomal gene *norA* (or its regulatory region) that encodes a membrane efflux protein for hydrophilic fluoroquinolones and other unrelated antibiotics (Yoshida et al. 1990, Kaatz, Seo and Ruble 1993). A third mechanism found in *S. aureus* involves mutations in the chromosomal gene *grlA* that encodes the A subunit of DNA topoisomerase IV (Trucksis, Wolfson and Hooper 1991, Ferrero et al. 1994, Ferrero, Cameron and Crouzet 1995). Clinical isolates of *S. aureus* that have mutations in both *gryA* and *grlA* genes generally exhibit higher levels of ciprofloxacin resistance (MIC 16–>128 µg ml^{-1}) than isolates with only mutations in *grlA* (MIC 2–16 µg ml^{-1}). Wide use of the fluoroquinolone ciprofloxacin has resulted in a steady increase in the incidence of fluoroquinolone-resistant (MIC ≥8 µg ml^{-1}) staphylococci, especially among clinical isolates

(Kotilainen, Nikoskelainen and Huovinen 1990, Bannerman, Wadiak and Kloos 1991b, Archer and Climo 1994). The newer fluoroquinolones such as fleroxacin, levofloxacin and clinafloxacin are more active than ciprofloxacin against ciprofloxacin-susceptible staphylococci by in vitro testing; however, the problem still remains that fluoroquinolone-resistant mutants emerge following exposure to these antibiotics. Fluoroquinolone resistance has been identified in the species *S. aureus*, *S. epidermidis*, *S. haemolyticus*, *S. hominis* and *S. warneri*. The *S. saprophyticus* and *S. sciuri* species groups exhibit an intermediate susceptibility (MIC 1–4 μg ml^{-1}) to fluoroquinolones and this property may be related to their intrinsic novobiocin resistance (MIC 1.6–64 μg ml^{-1}) and nalidixic acid resistance (MIC 64–1024 μg ml^{-1}) (Schleifer 1986, Magni and Soltész 1986), presumably due to modifications of the *gyrB* gene and/or its regulation.

Some strains of *S. aureus*, *S. lugdunensis* and members of the *S. epidermidis* and *S. saprophyticus* species groups demonstrate resistance to various combinations of the heavy metal ions: cadmium, zinc, bismuth, lead, mercury, arsenate, arsenite and antimony(III) (Novick and Roth 1968, Weiss, Murphy and Silver 1977, Götz et al. 1983, Poitevin-Later et al. 1992). The genes controlling heavy metal resistance are usually carried by plasmids, but they may be integrated into the chromosome either as a result of transposon insertion or integration of the resistance plasmid (Novick and Roth 1968, Novick et al. 1979, Shalita, Murphy and Novick 1980, Silver et al. 1981, Witte et al. 1986). Cadmium ions enter the cell via a specific, energy-dependent transport system that normally takes up manganese ions (Tynecka, Gos and Zajac 1981). One of the main toxic effects of cadmium is the inhibition of respiration caused by its binding to sulfhydryl groups on essential proteins. Both cadmium and zinc resistance in *S. aureus* are determined by the same mechanisms. One mechanism involves the *cadA* gene product, which is a membrane-translocating ATPase that prevents internal accumulation of cadmium and zinc by exporting these cations to the outside of the cell (Nucifora et al. 1989, Endo and Silver 1995). Mercury and organomercurial compounds are toxic primarily because of their ability to bind to the sulphydryl groups of enzymes, resulting in their inactivation. Mercury-resistant staphylococci have been selected in the clinical setting perhaps as a consequence of the therapeutic use of mercurial diuretics and the common usage of organomercurials as hospital disinfectants (Porter et al. 1982). Resistance to inorganic mercury is determined by the gene *merA*, which encodes a mercuric reductase capable of reducing the Hg^{2+} ion to the volatile, metallic Hg^0 (Weiss, Murphy and Silver 1977). Resistance to organomercurials is determined by the gene *merB* that encodes an organomercurial lyase which cleaves carbon–mercury bonds, resulting in the liberation of Hg^{2+} ions. These ions can then be acted upon by mercuric reductase for volatilization. Arsenicals are toxic to staphylococci and other bacteria. Arsenate is an anologue of phosphate and therefore inhibits kinases and can interrupt energy transfer during glycolysis; arsenite can bind to the cysteine residues of proteins and inhibit many enzymes with essential thiol groups. The primary mechanism for arsenic resistance is plasmid mediated and involves an energy-dependent arsenic efflux pump (Silver et al. 1981, Silver and Keach 1982). The gene *arsB* encodes a membrane efflux protein specific for arsenite and antimonite(III), and *arsC* encodes a thioredoxin-dependent arsenate reductase that reduces arsenate to arsenite (Bröer et al. 1993, Ji et al. 1994).

11 LABORATORY ISOLATION AND IDENTIFICATION

11.1 Laboratory isolation

Considering the widespread distribution of staphylococci and other bacteria on their hosts, considerable care should be taken when attempting to isolate organisms from the focus of infection to prevent isolation of surrounding normal flora (Kloos and Bannerman 1994). Some reasonably good isolation procedures are available for the diagnosis of central venous catheter infections and include quantitative blood cultures taken from blood drawn from a peripheral catheter (Flynn et al. 1987) and semiquantitative counts taken from a distal segment of the catheter (Aufwerber, Ringertz and Ransjö 1991). The most convincing laboratory findings for native valve endocarditis and prosthetic valve endocarditis (prior to removal of the prosthetic valve) are the rapid isolation of the same staphylococcal strain(s) from more than one blood culture (especially sequential cultures) and a high intensity bacteraemia (Archer 1985, Karchmer and Caputo 1986). Blood for culture should be collected aseptically from more than one venepuncture site in the event that normal skin flora or a contaminant is accidently introduced into the blood at one of the sites. For infections of hip prostheses, aspiration of the joint space and washing of the prosthesis with sterile broth often yield the infecting organisms. Ultrasonic oscillation can be used to shake off adherent organisms imbedded in a biofilm matrix on various prosthetic devices (Tollefson et al. 1987, Bandyk et al. 1991). A freshly voided, midstream, clean-catch sample is usually satisfactory for determining a urinary tract infection. However, suprapubic aspiration may be necessary for neonates, young infants and patients with clinical symptoms who have a low bacterial count in clean-catch specimens. For staphylococcal species other than *S. aureus*, it has been suggested that colony counts of as low as 100 to 100 000 cfu ml^{-1} should be considered a significant bacteriuria, especially if the isolated colonies represent a single strain or only one species (Hovelius 1986, Hedman and Ringertz 1991).

Basic culture procedures should be followed as soon as the specimen is received in the laboratory to minimize changes in the microbial composition from that originally present in the specimen. Regardless of the source of the specimen, a blood agar medium (preferably tryptic soy agar supplemented with 5% sheep blood) should be inoculated to provide a number of well isolated colonies from which to choose for subsequent testing. Specimens from heavily contaminated sources, such as faeces and sputum, should also be inoculated on a selective agar medium. It is advisable to inoculate a liquid medium from which to obtain additional inocula in case of failure or overgrowth on the primary isolation plate. However, during incubation, the proportions of various taxa in mixed cultures may change considerably from those originally present in the specimen. At least one, but preferably several, colonies representing each discernible morphotype should be gram-stained, subcultured and tested for genus, species, subspecies and strain properties.

The direct microscopic examination of normally sterile fluids (e.g. cerbrospinal fluid, joint aspirates and pulmonary secretions collected by transtracheal aspiration) may be helpful in obtaining a presumptive report of gram-positive cocci·resembling staphylococci. Microscopic examination of certain non-sterile fluids may also be helpful if the microscopist carefully evaluates the specimen by noting the relative proportion of inflammatory cells to other cell types.

11.2 Identification of *Staphylococcus* species and subspecies

The most prevalent staphylococcal species and subspecies in human infections are *S. aureus*, *S. epidermidis*, *S. haemolyticus* and *S. saprophyticus*, followed by *S. hominis*, *S. warneri*, *S. lugdunensis*, *S. schleiferi* subsp. *schleiferi*, *S. capitis* subsp. *ureolyticus* and *S. simulans* (Kloos and Bannerman 1994). Those of special veterinary interest include *S. aureus*, *S. intermedius*, *S. hyicus*, *S. felis* and *S. schleiferi* subsp. *coagulans* (Devriese 1986, Igimi et al. 1989, Igimi, Takahashi and Mitsuoka 1990). The above staphylococcal species and subspecies can be distinguished on the basis of the minimal key characters shown in Table 27.7.

CONVENTIONAL METHODS FOR IDENTIFICATION

Methods used to determine colony morphology have been mentioned above (see section 6.1, p. 587). Coagulase activity can be determined by a standard tube test that is best performed by suspending a well isolated colony or mixing 0.1 ml of an overnight culture with 0.5 ml of reconstituted plasma, incubating the mixture at 37°C in a water bath or heat block for 4 h, and observing the tube for clot formation by slowly tilting the tube 90° from the vertical. Any degree of clotting should be considered a positive test. Tests which are negative at 4 h should be incubated and observed again for clotting at 24 h. *S. hyicus* and some strains of *S. aureus* and *S. intermedius* require longer than 4 h for clot formation. Clumping factor can be detected by a standard slide test performed by making a heavy suspension of cells in distilled water, stirring the mixture to a homogeneous composition, and then adding a drop of plasma. The mixture should be examined for clumping within about 10 s. Approximately 85–90% of *S. aureus* and 10–15% of *S. intermedius* strains are clumping factor-positive. *S. lugdunensis* and *S. schleiferi* subsp. *schleiferi* are usually clumping factor-positive if human plasma is used in the slide test (Freney et al. 1988). Slide tests for clumping factor based on latex agglutination (detecting both clumping

factor and protein A) are commercially available from a number of manufacturers in the USA and Europe. A new latex agglutination test is now available that detects clumping factor, protein A and serotype 5 and 8 capsular polysaccharides of *S. aureus* (Pastorex Staph-Plus, Sanofi Diagnostics Pasteur, Marnes-la-Coquette, France). Thermonuclease (TNase) activity is a common property of the coagulase-positive species and *S. schleiferi* subsp. *schleiferi*. It can be detected using a metachromatic-agar diffusion procedure and DNA–toluidine blue agar (Lachica, Hoeprich and Genigeorgis 1972). The DNA–touilidine blue agar test can be interpreted in 4–6 h. A positive reaction is indicated by a wide zone of pink colour surrounding the agar well filled with a heat-treated suspension of the organism. DNA–toluidine blue agar plates are commercially available (Remel, Lenexa KS, USA). A seroinhibition test has been developed to distinguish the TNase of *S. aureus* from those of other species (Lachica, Jang and Hoeprich 1979).

Alkaline phosphatase activity can be determined by using a modification of the method of Pennock and Huddy (1967), in which a 0.005 M solution of phenolphthalein diphosphate (sodium salt in 0.01 M citric acid–sodium citrate buffer, pH 5.8) is used as substrate. A positive test is indicated by the development of a red colour following the addition of 4-aminoantipyrine and potassium ferricyanide to the suspension. Pyrrolidonyl arylamidase activity can be determined with a kit containing pyrrolidonyl-β-naphthylamide (PYR) broth and PYR reagent (Carr-Scarborough Microbiologicals, Inc., Stone Mountain, GA, USA) (Hébert et al. 1988). A loopful of an overnight slant culture is dispersed in the PYR broth tube to the turbidity of a McFarland no. 2 and the cell suspension is incubated at 35–37°C for 2 h. After incubation, 2 drops of PYR reagent are added to each tube without mixing. A positive activity is indicated by the development of a purple-red colour within 2 min. The PYR CARD TEST of Oxoid (Basingstoke, England) is a rapid test involving the application of a loopful of cells onto a PYR CARD and then observing the inoculum for 2 min for the development of a red colour (positive reaction). Ornithine decarboxylase activity can be determined by a modification of the test described by Moeller (1955). Decarboxylase basal medium (Becton Dickinson Microbiology Systems, Cockeysville, MD, USA, Difco, Detroit, MI, USA, GIBCO Laboratories, Grand Island, NY, USA) is supplemented by 1% (w/v) L-ornithine dihydrochloride and the final medium is adjusted to pH 6 prior to sterilization. The medium is dispersed in 3–4 ml amounts into small (13 by 100 mm) tubes and sterilized. A loopful of an overnight slant culture is suspended in the test broth, and the suspension is overlaid with 4–5 mm of sterile mineral oil. Inoculated tubes should be incubated at 35–37°C for up to 24 h. A positive test is indicated by the formation of a deep violet colour. *S. lugdunensis* produces a positive reaction by 8–12 h. Urease activity can be determined by using either urea both or urea agar (Oxoid, Difco, Becton Dickinson Microbiology Systems, Carr-Scarborough), following the instructions of the manufacturer. These media contain the indicator phenol red and can detect the release of ammonia from urea by the increase in alkalinity. Urease-positive staphylococci will change the colour of the medium from yellow-orange to red or cerise by 4–12 h. Acetoin (acetylmethylcarbinol) production can be detected by the rapid paper disc method of Davis and Hoyling (1973) or the classical Voges–Proskauer (VP) test using MR-VP broth (Oxoid, Difco, Becton Dickinson Microbiology Systems). Using the paper disc method, a 1 cm disc of Whatman 3M paper freshly soaked in 10% sodium pyruvate solution is placed on a 48 h patch of culture growing on the surface of a tryptone–yeast extract–glucose agar plate; the treated cul-

Table 27.7   Identification of clinically significant *Staphylococcus* species and subspecies

Species and subspecies	Colony pigment	Anaerobic growth	Staphylocoagulase	Clumping factor	Thermonuclease	Alkaline phosphatase	Pyrrolidonyl arylamidase	Ornithine decarboxylase	Urease	β-Glucuronidase	β-Galactosidase	Acetoin production	Novobiocin resistance	D-Trehalose	D-Mannitol	D-Mannose	D-Turanose	Maltose	Sucrose	N-Acetylglucosamine
S. epidermidis	−	+	−	−	−	+[b]	−	(d)	+	−	−	+	−	−	−	(+)	(d)	+	+	−
S. capitis subsp. *capitis*	−	(+)	−	−	−	−	−	−	−	−	−	d	−	−	+	+	−	−	(+)	−
S. capitis subsp. *ureolyticus*	(d)	(+)	−	−	−	−	(d)	−	+	−	−	d	−	−	+	+	−	+	+	−
S. hominis	d	−	−	−	−	−	−	−	+	−	d	−	d	d	−[c]	−	+	+	(+)	d
S. haemolyticus	d	(+)	−	−	−	−	+	−	−	d	−	+	−	+	d	−	(d)	+	+	+
S. warneri	d	+	−	−	−	−	+	−	−	d	−	+	−	+	d	−	(d)	(+)	+	−
S. lugdunensis	d	+	−	(+)	−	−	+	+	d	−	−	+	−	+	−	+	(d)	+	+	+
S. aureus	+[d]	+	+	+	+	+	−	−	d	−	−	+	−	+	+	+	+	+	+	+
S. saprophyticus	d	(+)	−	−	−	−	−	−	+	−	+	+	+	+	d	−	+	+	+	d
S. simulans	−	+	−	−	−	(d)	+	−	+	d	+	d	−	d	+	d	−	(±)	+	+
S. felis	−	+	−	−	−	+	ND	−	+	−	+	−	−	+	+	+	ND	−	d	+
S. intermedius	−	(+)	+	d	+	+	+	−	+	−	+	−	−	+	(d)	+	d	(±)	+	+
S. schleiferi subsp. *schleiferi*	−	+	−	+	+	+	+	−	−	−	(+)	(+)	−	d	−	+	−	−	−	(+)
S. schleiferi subsp. *coagulans*	−	+	+	−	+	+	ND	−	ND	−	(+)	+	−	−	d	+	−	−	d	ND
S. hyicus	−	+	d	−	+	+	−	−	d	d	−	−	−	+	−	+	−	−	+	+

[a]Symbols: +, 90% or more strains positive; ±, 90% or more strains weakly positive; −, 90% or more strains negative; d, 11–89% of strains positive. Parentheses indicate a delayed reaction. All species listed are negative for the modified oxidase test, arginine arylamidase, aesculin hydrolysis and acid (aerobically) from D-xylose, D-cellobiose, L-arabinose and raffinose. The characteristics of *S. capitis* subsp. *ureolyticus* are shown for making a comparison with the clinically significant subspecies *S. capitis* subsp. *ureolyticus*.
[b]Alkaline phosphatase activity is negative for 6–15% of the strains of *S. epidermidis*.
[c]Acid is produced aerobically from D-mannitol in 5–12% of the strains of *S. hominis*.
[d]Approximately 6–11% of *S. aureus* strains fail to produce detectable pigment on commercial agar media.
From Kloos and Bannerman (1995).

ture is then incubated at 30°C for an additional 3 h. Acetoin is detected by spotting a drop each of 40% potassium hydroxide, 1% creatinine and 1% α-naphthol (alcoholic) solution onto the disc and observing the development of a pink-red colour within 1 h. For the classical VP test, a positive reaction is indicated by the development of an orange-red to red colour within 30 min after adding the α-naphthol and potassium hydroxide reagents to a 48 h MR-VP broth culture.

Novobiocin resistance can be determined by a disc diffusion method using a 5 μg novobiocin disc placed on Mueller–Hinton agar or on tryptic soy sheep blood agar. One-tenth ml of an inoculum suspension (McFarland no. 0.5) is spread uniformly on the surface of an agar plate, a novobiocin disc is then applied to the inoculated surface, and the test plate is incubated at 35–37°C for overnight to 24 h. Resistance is indicated by an inhibition zone diameter of ≤16 mm.

Acid production from carbohydrates can be detected by using the agar plate method of Kloos and Schleifer (1975b).

Carbohydrate agars are prepared by adding a filter-sterilized carbohydrate stock solution to an autoclaved-sterilized purple agar base medium (Difco), containing bromocresol purple indicator, to give a final carbohydrate concentration of 1%. Partitioned quadrant plates are prepared for each of the carbohydrates to be examined. Each culture is tested for acid production by lightly inoculating a 0.5–1 cm long streak of a 24 h culture on the surface of one quadrant of carbohydrate agar (4 cultures per plate) and then incubating the inoculated plates at 34–37°C for 72 h. The cultures are examined at 24, 48 and 72 h for evidence of acid production, indicated by a yellow colour.

Anaerobic growth in a semi-solid thioglycollate medium (Oxoid, Difco, Becton Dickinson Microbiology Systems), supplemented with 0.3% agar, can be determined by adding a 0.1 ml saline suspension (McFarland no. 0.5–1) of an overnight agar slant culture into a tube (150 by 16 mm) containing 8 ml of cooled (50–52°C) autoclaved medium, gently mixing the contents, and then incubating the culture without shaking for up to 3 days at 34–37°C (Kloos and Schleifer 1975b).

COMMERCIAL RAPID IDENTIFICATION KITS AND AUTOMATED SYSTEMS

To expedite the process of identifying staphylococcal species and subspecies in the clinical laboratory, several manufacturers have developed rapid identification kits and automated systems requiring only a few hours to one day for completing tests. With these products, identification of most species and subspecies can be made with an accuracy of 70–>90% (Kloos and Wolfshohl 1982, Crouch, Pearson and Parham 1987, Kloos and George 1991, Bannerman, Kleeman and Kloos 1993). Currently, *S. aureus*, *S. epidermidis*, *S. haemolyticus*, *S. capitis* subsp. *capitis*, *S. saprophyticus*, *S. cohnii* subsp. *cohnii*, *S. simulans*, *S. intermedius* and *S. sciuri* can be identified reliably by most of the commercial systems available. Some additional testing may be required to increase the accuracy of identification to above 90%. The rapid identification systems now available include the following: API-STAPH-IDENT, STAPH Trac System and ID 32 STAPH kits and the fully automated Vitek and Vitek, Jr systems, which utilize a Gram Positive Identification (GPI) Card (bioMérieux Vitek Inc., Hazelwood, MO, USA); MicroScan Pos ID panel (read manually or on MicroScan instrumentation), MicroScan Rapid Pos ID panel (read by AutoScan-W/A), and the Pos Combo and Rapid Pos Combo panels, which combine species identification and antimicrobial susceptibility tests (Dade MicroScan Inc., West Sacramento, CA, USA); Minitek Gram-Positive Set (Becton Dickinson Microbiology Systems); Sceptor *Staphylococcus* MIC/ID panel and Sceptor Gram Positive Breakpoint/ID Panel (Becton Dickinson Instrument Systems, Towson, MD, USA); GP MicroPlate test panel (read manually using Biolog computer software for interpretation or automatically with the Biolog MicroStation) (Biolog, Haywood, CA, USA); and the Microbial Identification System (MIS) that automates identification by combining cellular fatty acid analysis with computerized high-resolution gas chromatography (MIDI, Newark, DE, USA).

Rapid identification of the species *S. aureus* can be made using the AccuProbe culture identification test for *S. aureus* (Gen-Probe Inc., San Diego, CA, USA). The test is a DNA probe assay directed against rRNA and it is very accurate. This species can also be identified by a new immunoenzymatic assay based on a monoclonal antibody prepared against the *S. aureus* endo-β-*N*-acetylglucosaminidase (Guardati et al. 1993). These specific tests are especially useful in identifying coagulase-negative, protein A-negative, and/or clumping factor-negative mutants of *S. aureus*, that would otherwise be misidentified by coagulase and latex agglutination tests.

As mentioned above (see section 3, p. 578), several DNA molecular typing methods are proving to be very promising for the identification of species and subspecies. They include ribotyping, PFGE and PCR fingerprinting and are based on the rationale that each species and subspecies has conserved and recognizable DNA sequences or patterns that are taxon-specific. The accuracy of molecular typing methods is very high and the procedures can be automated and computerized. DuPont has recently developed a fully automated RiboPrinter Microbial Characterization System designed for food and industrial microbiology applications that can ribotype 32 cultures per day, and results are available in 8 h (DuPont, Wilmington, DE, USA). This system has a large database of ribotype patterns of *Staphylococcus* strains representing all the recognized species and subspecies.

12 TYPING METHODS FOR THE IDENTIFICATION OF INFRASUBSPECIFIC FORMS AND STRAINS

Most epidemiological studies of staphylococci attempt to identify aetiological agents and determine their source and distribution. An important rationale for typing staphylococci is that the repeated isolation of a particular strain is more clinically significant than only the repeated isolation of a species. The typing methods selected should be able to identify the specific strain responsible for the infection. Typing systems are based on the premise that isolates originating from a clonal population, i.e. representing a particular strain, exhibit similar characteristics and have one or more features that distinguish them from other strains. A single typing system divides a species or subspecies into a number of infrasubspecific forms and, depending on the number of polymorphisms present in a taxon, it may or may not have the discriminatory power to identify a strain. It is important to note that staphylococcal species demonstrate considerable variation with respect to the extent of their polymorphisms as revealed by typing methods. In any epidemiological study of staphylococci, strain identity should begin with a good characterization of colony morphology. As yet, it is the only practical way to select prospective strains on the primary isolation plate. The most discriminitory, interpretable and reproducible molecular typing methods for staphylococci include ribotyping, PFGE (or FIGE), multilocus enzyme electrophoresis (MLEE) and plasmid profiling (reviewed by Kloos and Bannerman 1994, Arbeit 1995). Ribotyping and PFGE are now well developed methods that are represented by large databases (see section 3, p. 578). MLEE has been used to examine *S. aureus* strains from a wide range of sources (Musser and Selander 1990, Musser and Kapur 1992) and should also have application with other species. Plasmid profiling and plasmid restriction endonuclease analysis have been applied to all the recognized species and subspecies (Kloos, Orban and Walker 1981, Archer, Vishniavsky and Stiver 1982, Parisi 1985, Wells and Kloos 1987, Etienne et al. 1990a, 1990b, Kloos, George and Jones-Park 1992). PCR techniques for random amplified polymorphic DNA (Welsh and McClelland 1991, Marquet-Van Der Mee et al. 1995) and specific gene sequences, e.g. *mecA* sequences combined with variable DNA sequence motifs (van Belkum et al. 1993) or *coa* sequences and subsequent enzyme digestion of the PCR product(s) (Goh et al. 1992), have been used to identify certain strains of *S. aureus*.

The choice of typing methods depends on the particular species being examined. For example, *S. aureus* exhibits a very high degree of polymorphism with respect to ribotype, PFGE and MLEE patterns, but often has no or only a simple plasmid profile (0–3 plasmids per strain). In this species, more than 100 infrasubspecific forms can be identified by either ribotyping, PFGE, or MLEE. However, unless a pattern is rare in the species population, it may represent more than one strain or clonal population. If the isolates being evaluated are from limited geographical range, e.g. from the same host or group of hosts living in close proximity, a particular pattern is more likely to represent an individual strain than if the isolates were taken from a wide geographical range. Discrimination can be increased if a combination of 2 or more of the current typing methods is used.

S. epidermidis exhibits a moderately high degree of polymorphism with respect to ribotype and PFGE patterns and, like other members of the *S. epidermidis* group, it usually exhibits complex plasmid profiles useful for typing. Approximately 5–15% of *S. epidermidis* strains do not carry plasmids, though about 70% carry 2–6 plasmids. *S. haemolyticus* and *S. hominis* exhibit less polymorphism than *S. epidermidis* with ribotyping and PFGE, but their plasmid profiles are as complex. *S. capitis* subsp. *capitis* and *S. capitis* subsp. *ureolyticus* can be clearly distinguished from one another by ribotyping and PFGE, but these subspecies exhibit a low degree of polymorphism with these typing methods. Their plasmid profiles are moderately complex and are useful for typing. Other species and subspecies exhibiting a low or moderately low degree of polymorphism with ribotyping and PFGE methods include *S. caprae*, *S. lugdunensis*, *S. schleiferi* subsp. *schleiferi*, *S. auricularis*, *S. saprophyticus* and *S. chromogenes*.

The ecological, genetic and molecular typing data that are now available on strains of the various staphylococcal species, can lead one to the proposition that the main source of infra-subspecific variation in ribotype and PFGE patterns is the insertion and/or deletion of extrachromosomal or accessory DNA elements, e.g. prophages, plasmids and transposons. The specific effects of staphylococcal phages on PFGE fragment patterns (Lina et al. 1993, Arbeit 1995) support this proposition. The following observations are also supportive:

1   Each recognized species and subspecies demonstrates one or more conserved chromosome fragments providing each taxon with specific markers. The basic species pattern or spacing of the enzyme restriction sites on the chromosome appears to be disrupted by the insertion or deletion of a relatively large segment of DNA. In specific clonal populations of *S. aureus* and *S. epidermidis* that have been monitored on human hosts for several years, changes in PFGE fragment patterns were associated with an increase or decrease in the size of 1–3 fragments of 15–60 kbp per fragment, which approximates the size of staphylococcal phage genomes, plasmids and large transposons. Strains producing very large and persistent populations on their respective hosts characteristically exhibit, at any point in time, 2–3 different pattern forms, each differing from one another by 1–3 fragments. In the case of *S. epidermidis* strains, a particular pattern may be associated with a subpopulation of the strain located in a specific cutaneous niche.

2   Some species and subspecies exhibit a conserved fragment pattern, whereas others exhibit a high degree of polymorphism, which is associated with a marked variation in chromosome size, but with little or no difference in the total number of fragments of the profile. The mean chromosome size is generally larger in the more polymorphic species, though they generally do not have more fragments than the conserved species. The degree of fragment polymorphism is usually directly related to fragment size, especially in the more polymorphic species. These correlations are consistent with the idea that insertion or deletion events involving relatively large segments of DNA are occurring more frequently in fragments providing a larger target, and that the number of restriction enzyme sites are not significantly increasing or decreasing.

3   Species and subspecies exhibiting the most conserved fragment patterns demonstrate a narrow host range and strong niche preference. *S. capitis* and *S. auricularis* respond very slowly to antibiotic pressure in the cutaneous habitat, perhaps because of the protection afforded by their specific niches and/or their difficulty to acquire accessory DNA elements. Their main populations are imbedded in protected lipid-rich niches where there is little exposure to most antibiotics or competition from other staphylococcal species. Several questions

seem appropriate with regard to the intrinsic mechanisms that might be operating in the different species. For example, does the chromosome of the most conserved species have a sufficient supply of phage attachment sites, insertion sequences, or other recombination sites to be able to acquire accessory DNA sequences? Are these species having problems taking up extrachromosomal DNA elements into the cell or presenting their DNA for integration? It is known that the polymorphic species *S. aureus* and *S. epidermidis* have the ability to acquire and lose accessory DNA elements and have chromosomes containing a variety of phage attachment sites and insertion sequences. These species respond rapidly to antibiotic pressure and live in a variety of habitats subject to considerable competition from other species, including each other. Were some of the conserved species formed relatively recently?

13   PATHOGENICITY

Certain of the cell surface adhesins, exocellular materials and extracellular proteins produced by *S. aureus* are believed to play important roles in the pathogenicity of this organism (see sections on 'Cell surface adhesins', p. 592, 'Exocellular material', p. 593, and section 8.2, p. 592). The species is well supported with accessory DNA elements carrying a variety of virulence and resistance factors, which act together with intrinsic mechanisms to make this organism one of the most successful opportunistic pathogens known to mankind and animals. Infections caused by this species are often acute and pyogenic and, if untreated, may spread to surrounding tissue or to metastatic sites involving other organs. Some of the more common infections of the skin include furuncles or boils, cellulitis and impetigo. *S. aureus* is a common aetiological agent of postoperative wound infections, bacteraemia, pneumonia, osteomyelitis, acute endocarditis, mastitis, toxic shock syndrome and abscesses of the muscle, urogenital tract, central nervous system and various intra-abdominal organs. Food poisoning is frequently attributed to staphylococcal enterotoxin (see section 8.2, p. 593). Comprehensive reviews on the nature of human and animal model infections can be found in the following texts: Elek (1959), Cohen (1972), Jeljaszewicz (1973, 1976, 1981, 1985), Easmon and Adlam (1983) and Wadström, Holder and Kronvall (1994). Reviews on domestic animal infections are published in the following texts: Stableforth and Galloway (1959), Heidrich and Renk (1967), Easmon and Adlam (1983) and Timoney et al. (1988). Many of the infections produced in animals are rather similar to those produced in humans. Staphylococcal mastitis in either a clinical or subclinical form may have considerable economic consequences in the dairy industry. *S. aureus* subsp. *anaerobius* is the aetiological agent of an abscess disease (caseous lymphadenitis) in sheep.

S. intermedius is a common opportunistic pathogen of dogs and may cause otitis media, pyoderma, abscesses in various organs, mastitis, reproductive tract infections and purulent wound infections (Devriese and Hájek 1980, Phillips and Kloos 1981, Raus and Love 1983, Szynkiewicz et al. 1985). This species can also produce wound infections in humans following dog bites. *S. hyicus* is the aetiological agent of infectious exudative epidermitis (greasy pig disease) (Devriese and Hájek 1980, Phillips and Kloos 1981) and can also cause septic polyarthritis in pigs (Phillips, King and Kloos 1980), skin lesions in cattle and horses (Devriese and Derycke 1979, Devriese et al. 1983), osteomyelitis in cattle and poultry (Carnaghan 1966, Wise 1971, De Kesel and Devriese 1982), and may on occasion be associated with mastitis in cattle (Devriese and De Keyser 1980). *S. delphini* has been implicated in purulent skin lesions of dolphins (Varaldo et al. 1988). *S. felis* can cause skin lesions, external otitis, cystitis and abscesses and wound infections in the cat (Igimi et al. 1989). *S. schleiferi* subsp. *coagulans* can produce external otitis in dogs (Igimi, Takahashi and Mitsuoka 1990).

Members of the *S. epidermidis* species group are a major cause of foreign body infections, e.g. infections of intravascular catheters, catheters for continuous ambulatory peritoneal dialysis (CAPD), fluid shunt systems, prosthetic heart valves, joint prostheses and pacemaker electrodes. The most noteworthy species is *S. epidermidis*. The process of foreign body infections proceeds by a series of steps starting with a race for the surface of the biomaterial implant (Gristina et al. 1994). Portions of the exposed surface of the implant will rapidly acquire a conditioning film of matrix proteins (e.g. the glycoproteins albumin, collagen, fibronectin, fibrinogen and vitronectin) and host tissue cells (e.g. macrophages and neutrophils), whereas other available portions, as well as those conditioned with matrix protein films, will rapidly be covered with adherent microbial cells. The first step in adhesion of bacteria to biomaterials is most likely a non-specific one that involves attracting van der Waals forces and hydrophobic interactions (Fleer and Verhoef 1989). In general, strains of *S. epidermidis* that exhibit high hydrophobicity adhere more strongly to polymer surfaces (Ludwicka et al. 1984). For the initial non-specific adhesion of bacterial cells to be successful toward colonization, other more specific types of adhesion are probably required. The adhesion of *S. epidermidis* and *S. capitis* subsp. *ureolyticus* to catheter surfaces is facilitated by a capsular PS/A (see section on 'Exocellular material', p. 592) (Tojo et al. 1988, Kloos et al. 1992, Muller et al. 1993). More than one type of adhesin may be involved with the adherence of *S. epidermidis* to biomaterials. Some strains of this species produce a 220 kDa proteinaceous surface antigen that mediates adhesion to polystyrene (Timmerman et al. 1991). In addition, specific receptor–ligand interactions by adhesins and their respective protein ligand components provide an effective adhesion of staphylococci to conditioned matrix protein films located on the implant surface. *S. haemolyticus*, *S. lugdunensis* and *S. epidermidis* react well with many of the matrix proteins immobilized on latex beads (Paulsson, Ljungh and Wadström 1992). Establishment of colonization and the ensuing development of biofilm is facilitated by the elaboration of slime polysaccharide, which acts like a non-specific glue adhesin binding the population of cells to the biomaterial surface as well as to each other. Under appropriate conditions, the population of cells will become progressively embedded in a deep slime layer, and in the process become protected from the host immune system and antimicrobial agents (Peters, Locci and Pulverer 1982, Peters and Pulverer 1984, Gray, Regelmann and Peters 1987, Gristina et al. 1989). Furthermore, the presence of a foreign body affects the host cellular defence response. A long-term presence can result in a constant stimulation of macrophages, leading to macrophage exhaustion and adjacent tissue damage, and a cytokine cascade is initiated (Zimmerli, Lew and Waldvogel 1984). One of the consequences of a foreign body infection is a chronic inflammatory reaction about the biomaterial implant that can lead to tissue and device failure (Gristina et al. 1994).

S. epidermidis and other members of the *S. epidermidis* species group are commonly associated with hospital-acquired bacteraemia, especially in patients in intensive therapy units (ITUs) or in neonatal intensive therapy units (NITUs) (Freeman et al. 1987, Low et al. 1992). In most cases, the focus of infection is an intravascular catheter. These species have also been implicated in native valve endocarditis (Karchmer and Caputo 1986, Caputo et al. 1987, Westblom et al. 1990, Bandres and Darouiche 1992, Kamath, Singer and Isenberg 1992, Lina et al. 1992a). *S. epidermidis* is a common cause of peritonitis during continuous ambulatory peritoneal dialysis (Kraus and Spector 1983). Nosocomial methicillin-resistant *S. epidermidis* strains have become a serious problem in patients who have prosthetic heart valves or who have undergone other forms of cardiac surgery (Archer and Tenenbaum 1980, Karchmer, Archer and Dismukes 1983). *S. lugdunensis* can cause native valve endocarditis, prosthetic valve endocarditis and other foreign body infections, bacteraemia, chronic osteoarthritis and abscesses in various organs, especially involving soft tissues (Etienne et al. 1989, Fleurette et al. 1989, Herchline and Ayers 1991, Shuttleworth and Colby 1992). *S. schleiferi* subsp. *schleiferi* has been implicated in bacteraemia, brain empyema, rachis osteitis, wound infections, and catheter and hip prosthesis infections (Fleurette et al. 1989, Jean-Pierre et al. 1989).

S. saprophyticus is an important opportunistic pathogen in human urinary tract infections such as cystitis, urethritis and pyelonephritis, especially frequent in young, sexually active females (Marrie et al. 1982, Hovelius and Mårdh 1984). It is second to *Escherichia coli* as the most common cause of urinary tract infections in both males and females. This species adheres more readily to human urothelium and periurethral cells than to human buccal and skin cells (Colleen et al. 1979). Other members of the *S. saprophyticus* species group may be infrequently associated with urinary tract infections in humans. Occasionally, members of this species group are implicated in bacteraemia and native valve endocarditis (Golledge 1988, Singh and Raad 1990). Comprehensive reviews on the nature of human and animal model infections caused by coagulase-negative staphylococcal species can be found in the following texts: Jeljaszewicz (1985), Mårdh and Schleifer (1986), Pulverer, Quie and Peters (1987) and Wadström, Holder and Kronvall (1994).

REFERENCES

Aboshkiwa M, Rowland G, Coleman G, 1995, Nucleotide sequence of the *Staphylococcus aureus* RNA polymerase *rpoB* gene and comparison of its predicted amino acid sequence with those of other bacteria, *Biochim Biophys Acta*, **1262:** 73–8.

Aboshkiwa M, al-Ani B et al., 1992, Cloning and physical mapping of the *Staphylococcus aureus rplL, rpoB* and *rpoC* genes, encoding ribosomal protein L7/L12 and RNA polymerase subunits beta and beta', *J Gen Microbiol*, **138:** 1875–80.

Abramson C, 1972, Staphylococcal enzymes, *The Staphylococci*, ed. Cohen JO, John Wiley, New York, 187–248.

Acevedo HF, Campbell-Acevedo E, Kloos WE, 1985, Expression of human choriogonadotropin-like material in coagulase-negative *Staphylococcus* species, *Infect Immun*, **50:** 860–8.

Akatov AK, Hájek V et al., 1985, Classification and drug resistance of coagulase-negative staphylococci isolated from wild birds, *The Staphylococci*, ed. Jeljaszewicz J, Gustav Fischer Verlag, Stuttgart, 125–7.

Albus A, Fournier JM et al., 1988, *Staphylococcus aureus* capsular types and antibody response to lung infection in patients with cystic fibrosis, *J Clin Microbiol*, **26:** 2505–9.

Allgaier H, Jung G et al., 1986, Epidermin: sequencing of a heterodet tetracyclic 21-peptide amide antibiotic, *Eur J Biochem*, **160:** 9–22.

Altboum Z, Hertman I, Sarid S, 1985, Penicillinase plasmid-linked genetic determinants for enterotoxins B and C$_1$ production in *Staphylococcus aureus*, *Infect Immun*, **47:** 514–21.

Aly R, Shinefield HR, Maibach HI, 1981, *Staphylococcus aureus* adherence to nasal epithelial cells: studies of some parameters, *Skin Microbiology: Relevance to Clinical Infection*, eds Maibach HI, Aly R, Springer-Verlag, New York, 177–9.

Anfinsen CB, Cuatrecasas P, Taniuchi H, 1971, Staphylococcal nuclease, chemical properties and catalysis, *The Enzymes*, vol. 4, ed. Boyer P, Academic Press, New York, 177–204.

Arbeit RD, 1995, Laboratory procedures for the epidemiologic analysis of microorganisms, *Manual of Clinical Microbiology*, 6th edn, eds Murray PR, Baron EJ et al., ASM Press, Washington, DC, 190–208.

Arbeit RD, Karakawa WW et al., 1984, Predominance of two newly described capsular polysaccharide types among clinical isolates of *Staphylococcus aureus*, *Diagn Microbiol Infect Dis*, **2:** 85–91.

Archer GL, 1985, Coagulase-negative staphylococci in blood cultures: a clinicians dilemma, *Infect Control*, **6:** 477–8.

Archer GL, Climo MW, 1994, Antimicrobial susceptibility of coagulase-negative staphylococci, *Antimicrob Agents Chemother*, **38:** 2231–7.

Archer GL, Johnston JL, 1983, Self-transmissible plasmids in staphylococci that encode resistance to aminoglycosides, *Antimicrob Agents Chemother*, **24:** 70–7.

Archer GL, Pennell E, 1990, Detection of methicillin resistance in staphylococci by using a DNA probe, *Antimicrob Agents Chemother*, **34:** 1720–4.

Archer GL, Scott J, 1991, Conjugative transfer genes in staphylococcal isolates from the United States, *Antimicrob Agents Chemother*, **35:** 2500–4.

Archer GL, Tenenbaum MJ, 1980, Antibiotic-resistant *Staphylococcus epidermidis* in patients undergoing cardiac surgery, *Antimicrob Agents Chemother*, **17:** 269–72.

Archer GL, Vishniavsky N, Stiver HG, 1982, Plasmid pattern analysis of *Staphylococcus epidermidis* isolates from patients with prosthetic valve endocarditis, *Infect Immun*, **35:** 627–32.

Arthur M, Brisson-Noël A, Courvalin P, 1987, Origin and evolution of genes specifying resistance to macrolide, lincosamide, and streptogramin antibiotics: data and hypotheses, *J Antimicrob Chemother*, **20:** 783–802.

Arthur M, Molinas C et al., 1993, Characterization of Tn*1546*, a Tn*3*-related transposon conferring glycopeptide resistance by synthesis of depsipeptide peptidoglycan precursors in *Enterococcus faecium* BM4147, *J Bacteriol*, **175:** 117–27.

Arvidson SO, 1983, Extracellular enzymes from *Staphylococcus aureus*, *Staphylococci and Staphylococcal Infections*, vol. 2, eds Easmon CSF, Adlam C, Academic Press, London, 745–808.

Aufwerber E, Ringertz S, Ransjö U, 1991, Routine semi-quantitative cultures and central venous catheter-related bacteraemia, *Acta Pathol Microbiol Immunol Scand*, **99:** 627–30.

Augustin J, Götz F, 1990, Transformation of *Staphylococcus epidermidis* and other staphylococcal species with plasmid DNA by electroporation, *FEMS Microbiol Lett*, **66:** 203–8.

Baird-Parker AC, 1963, A classification of micrococci and staphylococci based on physiological and biochemical tests, *J Gen Microbiol*, **30:** 409–27.

Baird-Parker AC, 1965a, The classification of staphylococci and micrococci from world-wide sources, *J Gen Microbiol*, **38:** 363–87.

Baird-Parker AC, 1965b, Staphylococci and their classification, *Ann NY Acad Sci*, **128:** 4–25.

Baird-Parker AC, 1974, The basis for the present classification of staphylococci and micrococci, *Ann NY Acad Sci*, **236:** 7–14.

Baldwin JN, Strickland RH, Cox MF, 1969, Some properties of the beta-lactamase genes in *Staphylococcus epidermidis*, *Appl Microbiol*, **18:** 628–30.

Ballard D, Kloos WE et al., 1995, Rediscovery of *Staphylococcus caseolyticus* and description of the related species group, new species isolated from cattle, horses, and food, *Abstr 95th Gen Meet ASM*, 480.

Balwit JM, Vann JM et al., 1994, Role of *Staphylococcus aureus* small-colony variants in persistent infections, *Molecular Pathogenesis of Surgical Infections*, eds in Wadström T, Holder IA, Kronvall G, Gustav Fischer Verlag, Stuttgart, 31–6.

Bandres JC, Darouiche RO, 1992, *Staphylococcus capitis* endocarditis: a new cause of an old disease, *Clin Infect Dis*, **14:** 366–7.

Bandyk DF, Bergamini TM et al., 1991, In situ replacement of vascular prostheses infected by bacterial biofilms, *J Vasc Surg*, **13:** 575–83.

Bannerman TL, Kleeman KT, Kloos WE, 1993, Evaluation of Vitek systems Gram-positive identification card for species identification of coagulase-negative staphylococci, *J Clin Microbiol*, **31:** 1322–5.

Bannerman TL, Kloos WE, 1991, *Staphylococcus capitis* subsp. *ureolyticus* subsp. nov. from human skin, *Int J Syst Bacteriol*, **41:** 144–7.

Bannerman TL, Wadiak DL, Kloos WE, 1991a, Susceptibility of *Staphylococcus* species and subspecies to teicoplanin, *Antimicrob Agents Chemother*, **35:** 1919–22.

Bannerman TL, Wadiak DL, Kloos WE, 1991b, Susceptibility of *Staphylococcus* species and subspecies to fleroxacin, *Antimicrob Agents Chemother*, **35:** 2135–9.

Bannerman TL, Hancock GA et al., 1995, Pulsed-field gel electrophoresis as a replacement for bacteriophage typing of *Staphylococcus aureus*, *J Clin Microbiol*, **33:** 551–5.

Barber M, 1961, Methicillin-resistant staphylococci, *J Clin Pathol*, **14:** 385–93.

Barg N, Chambers H, Kernodle D, 1991, Borderline susceptibility to antistaphylococcal penicillins is not conferred exclusively by the hyperproduction of β-lactamase, *Antimicrob Agents Chemother*, **35:** 1975–9.

Barnes IJ, Bondi A, Fuscaldo KE, 1971, Genetic analysis of lysine auxotrophs of *Staphylococcus aureus*, *J Bacteriol*, **105**: 553–5.

Beining PR, Huff E et al., 1975, Characterization of the lipids of mesosomal vesicles and plasma membranes from *Staphylococcus aureus*, *J Bacteriol*, **121**: 137–43.

van Belkum A, Bax R et al., 1993, Comparison of phage typing and DNA fingerprinting by polymerase chain reaction for discrimination of methicillin-resistant *Staphylococcus aureus* strains, *J Clin Microbiol*, **31**: 798–803.

Bergdoll MS, 1989, *Staphylococcus aureus, Foodborne Bacterial Pathogens*, ed. Dole MP, Marcel Dekker, New York, 463–523.

Bergdoll MS, Cass BA et al., 1981, A new staphylococcal enterotoxin, enterotoxin F associated with toxic-shock-syndrome *Staphylococcus aureus* isolates, *Lancet*, **1**: 1017–21.

Berger-Bächi B, Strassle A, Kayser F, 1986, Characterization of an isogenic set of methicillin-resistant and susceptible mutants of *Staphylococcus aureus*, *Eur J Clin Microbiol*, **5**: 697–701.

Berger-Bächi B, Strassle A et al., 1992, Mapping and characterization of multiple chromosomal factors involved in methicillin resistance in *Staphylococcus aureus*, *Antimicrob Agents Chemother*, **36**: 1367–73.

Beryhill DL, Pattee PA, 1969, Buoyant density analysis of staphylococcal bacteriophage 80 transducing particles, *J Virol*, **4**: 804–6.

Betley MJ, Borst DW, Regassa LB, 1992, Staphylococcal enterotoxins, toxic shock syndrome toxin and streptococcal pyrogenic exotoxins: a comparative study of their molecular biology, *Biological Significance of Superantigens*, ed. Fleischer B, Karger, Basel, 1–35.

Betley MJ, Miller VL, Mekalanos JJ, 1986, Genetics of bacterial enterotoxins, *Annu Rev Microbiol*, **40**: 577–605.

Beuth J, Ko HL et al., 1988, *The role of lectins and lipoteichoic acid in adherence of Staphylococcus saprophyticus*, Zentralbl Bakteriol Parasitenkd Infektionskr Hyg Abt 1 Orig A, **268**: 357–61.

Bhakdi S, Tranum-Jensen J, 1991, Alpha-toxin of *Staphylococcus aureus*, *Microbiol Rev*, **55**: 733–51.

Birmingham VA, Pattee PA, 1981, Genetic transformation in *Staphylococcus aureus*: isolation and characterization of a competence-conferring factor from bacteriophage 80α lysates, *J Bacteriol*, **148**: 301–7.

Bismuth R, Zilhao R et al., 1990, Gene heterogeneity for tetracycline resistance in *Staphylococcus* spp., *Antimicrob Agents Chemother*, **34**: 1611–14.

Björk I, Peterson B-Å, Sjöquist J, 1972, Some physiological properties of protein A from *Staphylococcus aureus*, *Eur J Biochem*, **29**: 579–84.

Blumenthal HJ, 1972, Glucose catabolism in staphylococci, *The Staphylococci*, ed. Cohen JO, John Wiley, New York, 111–35.

Bodén MK, Flock JI, 1989, Fibrinogen-binding protein/clumping factor from *Staphylococcus aureus*, *Infect Immun*, **57**: 2358–63.

Bohach GA, Schlievert PM, 1987, Nucleotide sequence of staphylococcal enterotoxin C_1 gene and relatedness to other pyrogenic toxins, *Mol Gen Genet*, **209**: 15–20.

Brisson-Noël A, Delrieu P et al., 1988, Inactivation of lincosamide antibiotics in *Staphylococcus*, *J Biol Chem*, **263**: 15880–7.

Brockbank SM, Barth PT, 1993, Cloning, sequencing, and expression of the DNA gyrase genes from *Staphylococcus aureus*, *J Bacteriol*, **175**: 3269–77.

Bröer S, Ji G et al., 1993, Arsenic efflux governed by arsenic resistance determinant of *Staphylococcus aureus* plasmid pI258, *J Bacteriol*, **175**: 3480–5.

Brooks DR, Glen DR, 1982, Pinworms and primates: a case study in coevolution, *Proc Helminth Soc Wash*, **49**: 76–85.

Burdett V, 1993, tRNA modification activity is necessary for Tet(M)-mediated tetracycline resistance, *J Bacteriol*, **175**: 7209–15.

Cafferkey MT, Hone R et al., 1983, Gentamicin and methicillin resistant *Staphylococcus aureus* in Dublin hospitals, *Lancet*, **2**: 705–8.

Canepari P, Varaldo PE et al., 1985, Different staphylococcal species contain various numbers of penicillin-binding proteins ranging from four (*Staphylococcus aureus*) to only one (*Staphylococcus hyicus*), *J Bacteriol*, **163**: 796–8.

Caputo GM, Archer GL et al., 1987, Native valve endocarditis due to coagulase-negative staphylococci, *Am J Med*, **83**: 619–25.

Cardoso M, Schwarz S, 1992, Nucleotide sequence and structural relationships of a chloramphenicol acetyltransferase encoded by the plasmid pSCS6 from *Staphylococcus aureus*, *J Appl Bacteriol*, **72**: 289–93.

Carmona C, Gray GL, 1987, Nucleotide sequence of the serine protease gene of *Staphylococcus aureus*, strain V8, *Nucleic Acids Res*, **15**: 6757.

Carnaghan RBA, 1966, Spinal cord compression in fowls due to spondylitis caused by *Staphylococcus pyogenes*, *J Comp Pathol*, **76**: 9–14.

Catchpole I, Thomas C et al., 1988, The nucleotide sequence of *Staphylococcus aureus* plasmid pT48 conferring inducible macrolide-lincosamide-streptogramin B resistance and comparison with similar plasmids expressing constitutive resistance, *J Gen Microbiol*, **134**: 697–709.

Chambers HF, Archer GL, Matsuhashi M, 1989, Low-level methicillin resistance in strains of *Staphylococcus aureus*, *Antimicrob Agents Chemother*, **33**: 424–8.

Chapple R, Stewart PR, 1987, Polypeptide synthesis during lytic induction of phage 11 of *Staphylococcus aureus*, *Virology*, **68**: 1401–9.

Chesneau O, Morvan A et al., 1993, *Staphylococcus pasteuri* sp. nov., isolated from human, animal, and food specimens, *Int J Syst Bacteriol*, **43**: 237–44.

Cheung AL, Ying P, 1994, Regulation of alpha- and beta-hemolysins by the *sar* locus of *Staphylococcus aureus*, *J Bacteriol*, **176**: 580–5.

Christensen GD, Simpson WA et al., 1986, Adherence of coagulase-negative staphylococci to plastic tissue culture plates: a quantitative model for the adherence of staphylococci to medical devices, *J Clin Microbiol*, **22**: 996–1006.

Christensen GD, Barker LP et al., 1990, Identification of an antigenic marker of slime production for *Staphylococcus epidermidis*, *Infect Immun*, **58**: 2906–11.

Chu L, Mukhopadhyay D et al., 1992, Regulation of the *Staphylococcus aureus* plasmid pI258 mercury resistance operon, *J Bacteriol*, **174**: 7044–7.

Chu MC, Kreiswirth BN et al., 1988, Association of toxic shock toxin-1 determinant with a heterologous insertion at multiple loci in the *Staphylococcus aureus* chromosome, *Infect Immun*, **56**: 2702–8.

Clyne M, De Azavedo J et al., 1988, Production of gamma-hemolysin and lack of production of alpha-hemolysin by *Staphylococcus aureus* strains associated with toxic shock syndrome, *J Clin Microbiol*, **26**: 535–9.

Cohen JO (ed.), 1972, *The Staphylococci*, John Wiley, New York.

Cole E, Kloos WE et al., 1994, Classification of staphylococci by patterns of conserved *Eco*RI fragments containing ribosomal RNA operon sequences, *Abstr 94th Gen Meet ASM*, 315.

Coleman DC, Pomeroy H et al., 1985, Susceptibility to antimicrobial agents and analysis of plasmids in gentamicin- and methicillin-resistant *Staphylococcus aureus* from Dublin hospitals, *J Med Microbiol*, **20**: 157–67.

Coleman DC, Arbuthnott JP et al., 1986, Cloning and expression in *Escherichia coli* and *Staphylococcus aureus* of the beta-lysin determinant from *Staphylococcus aureus*: evidence that bacteriophage conversion of beta-lysin activity is caused by insertional inactivation of the beta-lysin determinant, *Microb Pathog*, **1**: 549–64.

Coleman DC, Sullivan DJ et al., 1989, *Staphylococcus aureus* bacteriophages mediating the simultaneous lysogenic conversion of β-lysin, staphylokinase and enterotoxin A: molecular mechanisms of triple-conversion, *J Gen Microbiol*, **135**: 1679–97.

Colleen S, Hovelius B et al., 1979, Surface properties of *Staphylococcus saprophyticus* and *Staphylococcus epidermidis* as studied by adherence tests and two-polymer, aqueous phase systems, *Acta Pathol Microbiol Immunol Scand Sect B*, **87**: 321–8.

Collins MD, 1981, Distribution of menaquinones within members of the genus *Staphylococcus*, *FEMS Microbiol Lett*, **12**: 83–5.

Collins MD, Jones D, 1981, Distribution of isoprenoid quinone structural types and their taxonomic implications, *Microbiol Rev*, **45**: 316–54.

Cooksey RC, Baldwin JN, 1985, Relatedness of tetracycline resistance plasmids among species of coagulase-negative staphylococci, *Antimicrob Agents Chemother*, **27**: 234–8.

Cookson BD, Phillips I, 1988, Epidemic methicillin-resistant *Staphylococcus aureus*, *J Antimicrob Chemother*, **24, Suppl. C:** 57–65.

Cooney J, Mulvey M et al., 1988, Molecular cloning and genetic analysis of the determinant for gamma-lysin, a two-component toxin of *Staphylococcus aureus*, *J Gen Microbiol*, **134**: 2179–88.

Couch JL, Soltis MT, Betley MJ, 1988, Cloning and nucleotide sequence of the type E staphylococcal enterotoxin gene, *J Bacteriol*, **170**: 2954–60.

Coughter JP, Johnston JL, Archer GL, 1987, Characterization of a staphylococcal trimethoprim resistance gene and its product, *Antimicrob Agents Chemother*, **31**: 1027–32.

Cove JH, Keareney JN et al., 1983, The vitamin requirements of *Staphylococcus cohnii*, *J Appl Bacteriol*, **54**: 203–8.

Cox HU, Schmeer N, Newman SS, 1986, Protein A in *Staphylococcus intermedius* isolates from dogs and cats, *Am J Vet Res*, **47**: 1881–4.

Crouch SF, Pearson TA, Parham DM, 1987, Comparison of modified Minitek system with Staph-Ident system for species identification of coagulase-negative staphylococci, *J Clin Microbiol*, **25**: 1626–8.

Crowder JG, White A, 1972, Teichoic acid antibodies in staphylococcal and nonstaphylococcal infections, *Ann Intern Med*, **77**: 87–90.

Dale GE, Broger C et al., 1995, Characterization of the gene for the chromosomal dihydrofolate reductase (DHFR) of *Staphylococcus epidermidis* ATCC 14990: the origin of the trimethoprim-resistant S1 DHFR from *Staphylococcus aureus?*, *J Bacteriol*, **177**: 2965–70.

Dancer SJ, Garratt R et al., 1990, The epidermolytic toxins are serine proteases, *FEBS Lett*, **268**: 129–32.

Daugharty H, Martin RR, White A, 1967, Antibodies against staphylococcal teichoic acids and type specific antigens in man, *J Immunol*, **98**: 1123–9.

Davis A, Moore IB et al., 1977, Nuclease B, a possible precursor of nuclease A, an extracellular nuclease of *Staphylococcus aureus*, *J Biol Chem*, **252**: 6544–53.

Davis GHG, Hoyling B, 1973, Use of a rapid acetoin test in the identification of staphylococci and micrococci, *Int J Syst Bacteriol*, **23**: 281–2.

De Buyser M-L, Morvan A et al., 1992, Evaluation of a ribosomal gene probe for the identification of species and subspecies within the genus *Staphylococcus*, *J Gen Microbiol*, **138**: 889–99.

DeHart HP, Heath HE et al., 1995, The lysostaphin endopeptidase resistance gene (*epr*) specifies modification of peptidoglycan cross bridges in *Staphylococcus simulans* and *Staphylococcus aureus*, *Appl Environ Microbiol*, **61**: 1475–9.

De Jonge BLM, Chang Y-S et al., 1992, Peptidoglycan composition of a highly methicillin-resistant *Staphylococcus aureus* strain, *J Biol Chem*, **267**: 11248–54.

De Jonge BLM, Sidow T et al., 1993, Altered muropeptide composition in *Staphylococcus aureus* strains with an inactivated *femA* locus, *J Bacteriol*, **175**: 2779–82.

De Kesel A, Devriese LA, 1982, Successful treatment of a case of osteomyelitis caused by a *Staphylococcus hyicus* in a heifer, *Vlaams Diergeneesk Tijdschr*, **51**: 222–5.

De la Fuente R, Suarez G, Schleifer KH, 1985, *Staphylococcus aureus* subsp. *anaerobius* subsp. Nov., the causal agent of abscess disease of sheep, *Int J Syst Bacteriol*, **35**: 99–102.

De Lencastre H, Tomasz A, 1994, Reassessment of the number

of auxiliary genes essential for expression of high-level methicillin resistance in *Staphylococcus aureus*, *Antimicrob Agents Chemother*, **38**: 2590–8.

De Lencastre H, Sá Figueiredo AM et al., 1991, Multiple mechanisms of methicillin resistance and improved methods for detection in clinical isolates of *Staphylococcus aureus*, *Antimicrob Agents Chemother*, **35**: 632–9.

De Lencastre H, De Jonge BLM et al., 1994, Molecular aspects of methicillin resistance in *Staphylococcus aureus*, *J Antimicrob Chemother*, **33**: 7–24.

Deora R, Misra TK, 1995, Purification and characterization of DNA dependent RNA polymerase from *Staphylococcus aureus*, *Biochem Biophys Res Commun*, **208**: 610–16.

Devriese LA, 1984, A simplified system for biotyping *Staphylococcus aureus* strains isolated from different animal species, *J Appl Bacteriol*, **56**: 215–20.

Devriese LA, 1986, Coagulase-negative staphylococci in animals, *Coagulase-negative Staphylococci*, eds Mårdh P-A, Schleifer KH, Almqvist and Wiksell International, Stockholm, 51–7.

Devriese LA, De Keyser H, 1980, Prevalence of different species of coagulase-negative staphylococci on teats and in milk samples from dairy cows, *J Dairy Res*, **47**: 151–8.

Devriese LA, Derycke J, 1979, *Staphylococcus hyicus* in cattle, *Res Vet Sci*, **26**: 356–8.

Devriese LA, Hájek V, 1980, Identification of pathogenic staphylococci isolated from animals and foods derived from animals, *J Appl Bacteriol*, **49**: 1–11.

Devriese LA, Hájek V et al., 1978, *Staphylococcus hyicus* (Sompolinsky 1953) comb. nov. and *Staphylococcus hyicus* subsp. *chromogenes* subsp. nov., *Int J Syst Bacteriol*, **28**: 482–90.

Devriese LA, Poutrel B et al., 1983, *Staphylococcus gallinarum* and *Staphylococcus caprae*, two new species from animals, *Int J Syst Bacteriol*, **33**: 480–6.

Dodd CER, Nahaie MR et al., 1985, Distribution of tetracycline resistance plasmids amongst representatives of the genus *Staphylococcus*, *The Staphylococci*, ed. Jeljaszewicz J, Gustav Fischer Verlag, Suttgart, 481–2.

Doery HM, Magnusson BJ et al., 1965, The properties of phospholipase enzymes in staphylococcal toxins, *J Gen Microbiol*, **40**: 283–96.

Domingue PAG, Lambert PA, Brown MRW, 1989, Iron depletion alters surface-associated properties of *Staphylococcus aureus* and its association to human neutrophils in chemiluminescence, *FEMS Microbiol Lett*, **59**: 265–8.

Drapeau GR, 1978, The primary structure of staphylococcal protease, *Can J Biochem*, **56**: 534–44.

Drummond MC, Tager M, 1963, Fibrinogen clotting and fibrinopeptide formation by staphylocoagulase and the coagulase-reacting factor, *J Bacteriol*, **85**: 628–35.

Duckworth GJ, Lothian JL, Williams JD, 1988, Methicillin-resistant *Staphylococcus aureus*: report of an outbreak in a London teaching hospital, *J Hosp Infect*, **11**: 1–15.

Dunny GM, Christie PJ et al., 1981, Effects of antibiotics in animal feed on the antibiotic resistance of the Gram-positive bacterial flora of animals and man, *Molecular Biology, Pathogenicity, and Ecology of Bacterial Plasmids*, eds Levy SB, Clowes RC, Koenig EL, Plenum Press, New York, 557–65.

Durham DR, Kloos WE, 1978, A comparative study of the total cellular fatty acids of *Staphylococcus* species of human origin, *Int J Syst Bacteriol*, **28**: 223–8.

Dyke KGH, 1979, β-Lactamases of *Staphylococcus aureus*, *Beta-Lactamases*, eds Hamilton-Miller JMT, Smith JT, Academic Press, London, 291–310.

Eady EA, Ross JI et al., 1993, Distribution of genes encoding erythromycin ribosomal methylases and an erythromycin efflux pump in epidemiologically distinct groups of staphylococci, *J Antimicrob Chemother*, **31**: 211–17.

Easmon CSF, Adlam C (eds), 1983, *Staphylococci and Staphylococcal Infections*, vols 1 and 2, Academic Press, London.

Edelman JM, Buck CA, 1992, The integrins: a general overview,

Microbial Adhesion and Invasion, eds Höök, M, Switalski L, Springer Verlag, New York, 15–31.

Elek SD, 1959, Staphylococcus pyogenes *and its Relation to Disease*, E & S Livingstone, Edinburgh, 152–77 and 313–75.

El Solh N, Ehrlich SD, 1982, A small cadmium resistance plasmid isolated from *Staphylococcus aureus*, *Plasmid*, **7:** 77–84.

El Solh N, Moreau N, Ehrlich SD, 1986, Molecular cloning and analysis of *Staphylococcus aureus* chromosomal aminoglycoside resistance genes, *Plasmid*, **15:** 104–18.

El Solh N, Moreau N et al., 1985, Analysis of the genes specifying aminoglycoside resistance in 'methicillin-resistant' *Staphylococcus aureus* strains isolated in France, *The Staphylococci*, ed. Jeljaszewicz J, Gustav Fischer Verlag, Stuttgart, 575–6.

Emmett M, Kloos WE, 1975, Amino acid requirements of staphylococci isolated from human skin, *Can J Microbiol*, **21:** 729–33.

Emmett M, Kloos WE, 1979, The nature of arginine auxotrophy in cutaneous populations of staphylococci, *J Gen Microbiol*, **110:** 305–14.

Endl J, Seidl PH et al., 1984, Determination of cell wall teichoic acid structures of staphylococci by rapid chemical and serological screening methods, *Arch Microbiol*, **137:** 272–80.

Endo G, Silver S, 1995, CadC, the transcriptional regulatory protein of the cadmium resistance system of *Staphylococcus aureus* plasmid pI258, *J Bacteriol*, **177:** 4437–41.

Etienne J, Pangon B et al., 1989, *Staphylococcus lugdunensis* endocarditis, *Lancet*, **1:** 390.

Etienne J, Grattard F et al., 1990a, Plasmid profiles of 60 independent strains of *Staphylococcus lugdunensis* and *Staphylococcus schleiferi*, *Abstr 90th Gen Meet ASM*, 402.

Etienne J, Poitevin-Later F et al., 1990b, Plasmid profiles and genomic DNA restriction endonuclease patterns of 30 independent *Staphylococcus lugdunensis* strains, *FEMS Microbiol Lett*, **67:** 93–8.

Evans AC, 1916, The bacteria of milk freshly drawn from normal udders, *J Infect Dis*, **18:** 437–76.

Evans JB, Bradford WL Jr, Niven CF, 1955, Comments concerning the taxonomy of the genera *Micrococcus* and *Staphylococcus*, *Int Bull Bacteriol Nomencl Taxon*, **5:** 61–6.

Fackrell HB, Wiseman GM, 1976, Properties of the gamma haemolysin of *Staphylococcus aureus* 'Smith 5R', *J Gen Microbiol*, **92:** 11–24.

Faller AH, Götz F, Schleifer KH, 1980, Cytochrome patterns of staphylococci and micrococci and their taxonomic implications, *Zentralbl Bakteriol Parasitenkd Infektionskr Hyg Abt 1 Orig C*, **1:** 26–39.

Farrell AM, Taylor D, Holland KT, 1995, Cloning, sequencing and expression of the hyaluronate lyase gene of *Staphylococcus aureus*, *FEMS Microbiol Lett*, **130:** 81–5.

Fattom A, Shepherd S, Karakawa W, 1992, Capsular polysaccharide serotyping scheme for *Staphylococcus epidermidis*, *J Clin Microbiol*, **30:** 3270–3.

Ferrero L, Cameron B, Crouzet J, 1995, Analysis of *gyrA* and *grlA* mutations in stepwise-selected ciprofloxacin-resistant mutants of *Staphylococcus aureus*, *Antimicrob Agents Chemother*, **39:** 1554–8.

Ferrero L, Cameron B et al., 1994, Cloning and primary structure of *Staphylococcus aureus* DNA topoisomerase IV: a primary target of fluoroquinolones, *Mol Microbiol*, **13:** 641–53.

Fischer S, Luczak H, Schleifer KH, 1982, Improved methods for the detection of class I and class II fructose-1,6-biphosphate aldolases in bacteria, *FEMS Microbiol Lett*, **15:** 103–8.

Fischer S, Tsugita A et al., 1983, Immunochemical and proteinchemical studies of class I fructose-1,6-biphosphate aldolases from staphylococci, *Int J Syst Bacteriol*, **33:** 443–50.

Fitton JE, Dell A, Shaw WV, 1980, The amino acid sequence of the delta haemolysin of *Staphylococcus aureus*, *FEBS Lett*, **115:** 209–12.

Fleer A, Verhoef J, 1989, An evaluation of the role of surface hydrophobicity and extracellular slime in the pathogenesis of foreign-body-related infections due to coagulase-negative staphylococci, *J Invest Surg*, **2:** 391–6.

Fleischer B, 1994, Lymphocyte stimulating 'superantigens' of *Staphylococcus aureus* and *Streptococcus pyogenes*, *Molecular Pathogenesis of Surgical Infections*, eds Wadström T, Holder IA, Kronvall G, Gustav Fischer Verlag, Stuttgart, 171–81.

Fleurette J, Bès M et al., 1989, Clinical isolates of *Staphylococcus lugdunensis* and *S. schleiferi*: bacteriological characteristics and susceptibility to antimicrobial agents, *Res Microbiol*, **140:** 107–18.

Flynn PM, Shenep JL et al., 1987, *In situ* management of confirmed central venous catheter-related bacteremia, *Pediatr Infect Dis J*, **6:** 729–34.

Forbes BA, Schaberg DR, 1983, Transfer of resistance plasmids from *Staphylococcus epidermidis* to *Staphylococcus aureus*: evidence for conjugative exchange of resistance, *J Bacteriol*, **153:** 627–34.

Ford DM, Perkins EM, 1970, The skin of the chimpanzee, *The Chimpanzee*, vol. 3, ed. Bourne GH, S Karger, Basel, 82–119.

Forsgren A, Ghetie V et al., 1983, Protein A and its exploitation, *Staphylococci and Staphylococcal Infections*, vol. 2, eds Easmon CSF, Adlam C, Academic Press, London, 429–80.

Foubert EL Jr, Douglas HC, 1948, Studies on the anaerobic micrococci. I. Taxonomic considerations, *J Bacteriol*, **56:** 25–34.

Fournet F, Brun Y et al., 1985, Production and propagation of *Staphylococcus saprophyticus* phages, *The Staphylococci*, ed. Jeljaszewicz J, Gustav Fischer Verlag, Stuttgart, 499–502.

Freeman J, Platt R et al., 1987, Coagulase-negative staphylococcal bacteremia in the changing neonatal intensive care unit population, *JAMA*, **258:** 2548–52.

Frenette M, Beaudet R et al., 1984, Chemical and biological characterization of a gonococcal growth inhibitor produced by *Staphylococcus haemolyticus* isolated from urogenital flora, *Infect Immun*, **46:** 340–5.

Freney J, Brun Y et al., 1988, *Staphylococcus lugdunensis* sp. nov. and *Staphylococcus schleiferi* sp. nov., two species from human clinical specimens, *Int J Syst Bacteriol*, **38:** 168–72.

Galetto DW, Johnston JL, Archer GL, 1987, Molecular epidemiology of trimethoprim resistance among coagulase-negative staphylococci, *Antimicrob Agents Chemother*, **31:** 1683–8.

Gatermann S, John J, Marre R, 1989, *Staphylococcus saprophyticus* urease: characterization and contribution to uropathogenicity in unobstructed urinary tract infection of rats, *Infect Immun*, **57:** 110–16.

Gatermann S, Kreft B et al., 1992, Identification and characterization of a surface-associated protein (Ssp) of *Staphylococcus saprophyticus*, *Infect Immun*, **60:** 1055–60.

Gemmell CG, Thelestam M, 1981, Toxigenicity of clinical isolates of coagulase-negative staphylococci towards various animal cells, *Acta Pathol Microbiol Scand Sect B*, **89:** 417–21.

Genigeorgis C, 1989, Present state of knowledge of staphylococcal intoxication, *Int J Food Microbiol*, **9:** 327–60.

George CG, Kloos WE, 1994, Comparison of the *Sma*I-digested chromosomes of *Staphylococcus epidermidis* and the closely related species *Staphylococcus capitis* and *Staphylococcus caprae*, *Int J Syst Bacteriol*, **44:** 404–9.

Gillespie MT, Lyon BR et al., 1987, Chromosome- and plasmid-mediated gentamicin resistance in *Staphylococcus aureus* encoded by Tn*4001*, *J Med Microbiol*, **24:** 139–44.

Goering RV, 1995, The application of pulsed field gel electrophoresis to analysis of the global dissemination of methicillin-resistant *Staphylococcus aureus*, *Methicillin Resistant Staphylococci*, eds Brun-Buisson C, Casewell MW et al., Médecine-Sciences Flammarion, Paris, 75–81.

Goering RV, Ruff EA, 1983, Comparative analysis of conjugative plasmids mediating gentamicin resistance in *Staphylococcus aureus*, *Antimicrob Agents Chemother*, **24:** 450–2.

Goering RV, Teeman BA, Ruff EA, 1985, Comparative physical and genetic maps of conjugal plasmids mediating aminoglycoside resistance in *Staphylococcus aureus* strains in the United

States, *The Staphylococci*, ed. Jeljaszewicz J, Gustav Fisher Verlag, Stuttgart, 625–8.

Goering RV, Winters MA, 1992, Rapid method for epidemiological evaluation of Gram-positive cocci by field inversion gel electrophoresis, *J Clin Microbiol*, **30**: 577–80.

Goh S-H, Byrne SK et al., 1992, Molecular typing of *Staphylococcus aureus* on the basis of coagulase gene polymorphisms, *J Clin Microbiol*, **30**: 1642–5.

Goldstein FW, Coutrot A et al., 1990, Percentages and distributions of teicoplanin- and vancomycin-resistant strains among coagulase-negative staphylococci, *Antimicrob Agents Chemother*, **34**: 899–900.

Golledge CL, 1988, *Staphylococcus saprophyticus* bacteremia, *J Infect Dis*, **157**: 215.

Goodman M, Czelusniak J, Beeber JE, 1985, Phylogeny of primates and other Eutherian orders: cladistic analysis using amino acid and nucleotide sequence data, *Cladistics*, **1**: 171–85.

Goswitz JJ, Willard KE et al., 1992, Detection of *gyrA* gene mutations associated with ciprofloxacin resistance in methicillin-resistant *Staphylococcus aureus*: analysis by polymerase chain reaction and automated direct DNA sequencing, *Antimicrob Agents Chemother*, **36**: 1166–9.

Götz F, Ahrné S, Lindberg M, 1981, Plasmid transfer and genetic recombination by protoplast fusion in staphylococci, *J Bacteriol*, **145**: 74–81.

Götz F, Nürnberger E, Schleifer KH, 1979, Distribution of class I and class II fructose-1,6-biphosphate aldolase in various Gram-positive bacteria, *FEMS Microbiol Lett*, **5**: 253–7.

Götz F, Schleifer KH, 1976, Comparative biochemistry of lactate dehydrogenase from staphylococci, *Staphylococci and Staphylococcal Diseases*, ed. Jeljaszewicz J, Gustav Fischer Verlag, Stuttgart, 245–52.

Götz F, Schumacher B, 1987, Improvements of protoplast transformation in *Staphylococcus carnosus*, *FEMS Microbiol Lett*, **40**: 285–8.

Götz F, Zabielski J et al., 1983, DNA homology between the arsenate resistance plasmid pSX267 from *Staphylococcus xylosus* and the penicillinase plasmid pI258 from *Staphylococcus aureus*, *Plasmid*, **9**: 126–37.

Götz F, Popp F et al., 1985, Complete nucleotide sequence of the lipase gene from *Staphylococcus hyicus* cloned in *Staphylococcus carnosus*, *Nucleic Acids Res*, **13**: 5895–906.

Gray ED, Regelmann WE, Peters G, 1987, Staphylococcal slime and host defenses: effects on lymphocytes and immune function, *Pathogenicity and Clinical Significance of Coagulase-negative Staphylococci*, eds Pulverer G, Quie PG, Peters G, Gustav Fischer Verlag, Stuttgart, 45–54.

Gray GS, Fitch WM, 1983, Evolution of antibiotic resistance genes: the DNA sequences of a kanamycin resistance gene from *Staphylococcus aureus*, *Mol Biol Evol*, **1**: 57–66.

Gristina AG, Hobgood CD et al., 1987, Adhesive colonization of biomaterials and antibiotic resistance, *Biomaterials*, **8**: 423–6.

Gristina AG, Jennings RA et al., 1989, Comparative in vitro antibiotic resistance of surface-colonizing coagulase-negative staphylococci, *Antimicrob Agents Chemother*, **33**: 813–16.

Gristina AG, Giridhar G et al., 1994, The present status of biomaterial-associated infection, *Molecular Pathogenesis of Surgical Infections*, eds Wadström T, Holder IA, Kronvall G, Gustav Fischer Verlag, Stuttgart, 313–33.

Gross R, Coles NW, 1968, Adenosine triphosphatase in isolated membranes of *Staphylococcus aureus*, *J Bacteriol*, **95**: 1322–6.

Guardati MC, Guzmán CA et al., 1993, Rapid methods for identification of *Staphylococcus aureus* when both human and animal staphylococci are tested: comparison with a new immuno-enzymatic assay, *J Clin Microbiol*, **31**: 1606–8.

Gustafson J, Strassle A et al., 1994, The *femC* locus of *Staphylococcus aureus* required for methicillin resistance includes the glutamine synthetase operon, *J Bacteriol*, **176**: 1460–7.

Haag H, Fiedler H-P et al., 1994, Isolation and biological charac-

terization of staphyloferrin B, a compound with siderophore activity from staphylococci, *FEMS Microbiol Lett*, **115**: 125–30.

Hájek V, 1976, *Staphylococcus intermedius*, a new species isolated from animals, *Int J Syst Bacteriol*, **26**: 401–8.

Hájek V, Balusek J, 1985, Staphylococci from flies of different environments, *The Staphylococci*, ed. Jeljaszewicz J, Gustav Fischer Verlag, Stuttgart, 129–33.

Hájek V, Maršálek E, 1969, A study of staphylococci of bovine origin. *Staphylococcus aureus* var. *bovis*, *Zentralbl Bakteriol Parasitenkd Infektionskr Hyg Abt 1 Orig*, **209**: 154–60.

Hájek V, Maršálek E, 1971, The differentiation of pathogenic staphylococci and a suggestion for their taxonomic classification, *Zentralbl Bakteriol Parasitenkd Infektionskr Hyg Abt 1 Orig A*, **217**: 176–82.

Hájek V, Maršálek E, 1976, Evaluation of classificatory criteria for staphylococci, *Staphylococci and Staphylococcal Diseases*, ed. Jeljaszewicz J, Gustav Fischer Verlag, Stuttgart, 11–21.

Hájek V, Devriese LA et al., 1986, Elevation of *Staphylococcus hyicus* subsp. *chromogenes* (Devriese et al., 1978) to species status: *Staphylococcus chromogenes* (Devriese et al., 1978) comb. nov., *Syst Appl Microbiol*, **8**: 169–73.

Hájek V, Ludwig W et al., 1992, *Staphylococcus muscae*, a new species isolated from flies, *Int J Syst Bacteriol*, **42**: 97–101.

Hart ME, Smeltzer MS, Iandolo JJ, 1993, The extracellular protein regulator (*xpr*) affects exoprotein and *agr* mRNA levels in *Staphylococcus aureus*, *J Bacteriol*, **175**: 7875–9.

Hartman BJ, Tomasz A, 1984, Low-affinity penicillin-binding protein associated with beta-lactam resistance in *Staphylococcus aureus*, *J Bacteriol*, **158**: 513–16.

Hartman BJ, Tomasz A, 1986, Expression of methicillin resistance in heterogenous strains of *Staphylococcus aureus*, *Antimicrob Agents Chemother*, **29**: 85–92.

Hayes MV, Curtiss NAC et al., 1981, Decreased affinity of a penicillin-binding protein for beta-lactam antibiotics in a clinical isolate of *Staphylococcus aureus* resistant to methicillin, *FEMS Microbiol Lett*, **10**: 119–22.

Heath LS, Heath HE, Sloan GL, 1987, Plasmid-encoded lysostaphin endopeptidase gene of *Staphylococcus simulans* biovar *staphylolyticus*, *FEMS Microbiol Lett*, **44**: 129–33.

Hébert GA, Cooksey RC et al., 1988, Biotyping coagulase-negative staphylococci, *J Clin Microbiol*, **26**: 1950–6.

Hedman P, Ringertz O, 1991, Urinary tract infections caused by *Staphylococcus saprophyticus*. A matched case control study, *J Infect*, **23**: 145–53.

Heidrich HJ, Renk W, 1967, *Diseases of the Mammary Glands of Domestic Animals*, transl. Van Den Heever LW, WB Saunders, Philadelphia.

Heir SW, Cornbleet T, Bergeim O, 1946, The amino-acids of human sweat, *J Biol Chem*, **166**: 327–33.

Hemker HC, Bas BM, Muller AD, 1975, Activation of a proenzyme by a stoichiometric reaction with another protein. The reaction between prothrombin and staphylocoagulase, *Biochim Biophys Acta*, **379**: 180–8.

Herchline TE, Ayers LW, 1991, Occurrence of *Staphylococcus lugdunensis* in consecutive clinical cultures and relationship of isolation to infection, *J Clin Microbiol*, **29**: 419–21.

Herwaldt LA, Boyken L, Pfaller M, 1991, *In vitro* selection of resistance to vancomycin in bloodstream isolates of *Staphylococcus haemolyticus* and *Staphylococcus epidermidis*, *Eur J Clin Microbiol Infect Dis*, **10**: 1007–12.

Hirooka EY, Muller EE et al., 1988, Enterotoxinogenicity of *Staphylococcus intermedius* of canine origin, *Int J Food Microbiol*, **7**: 185–91.

Hochkeppel HK, Braun DG et al., 1987, Serotyping and electron microscopy studies of *Staphylococcus aureus* clinical isolates with monoclonal antibodies to capsular polysaccharide types 5 and 8, *J Clin Microbiol*, **25**: 526–30.

Höök M, Patti JM et al., 1994, MSCRAMMs – microbial recognition systems for extracellular matrix molecules, *Molecular Pathogenesis of Surgical Infections*, eds Wadström T, Holder IA, Kronvall G, Gustav Fischer Verlag, Stuttgart, 137–44.

Horinouchi S, Weisblum B, 1981, The control region for erythromycin resistance: free energy changes related to induction and mutation to constitutive expression, *Mol Gen Genet*, **182**: 341–8.

Horinouchi S, Weisblum B, 1982, Nucleotide sequence and functional map of pE194, a plasmid that specifies inducible resistance to macrolide, lincosamide, and streptogramin type B antibiotics, *J Bacteriol*, **150**: 804–14.

Hovelius B, 1986, Epidemiological and clinical aspects of urinary tract infections caused by *Staphylococcus saprophyticus*, *Coagulase-negative Staphylococci*, eds Mårdh P-A, Schleifer KH, Almqvist & Wiksell International, Stockholm, 195–202.

Hovelius B, Mårdh P-A, 1984, *Staphylococcus saprophyticus* as a common cause of urinary tract infections, *Rev Infect Dis*, **6**: 328–37.

Huff E, Cole RM, Theodore TS, 1974, Lipoteichoic acid localization in mesosomal vesicles of *Staphylococcus aureus*, *J Bacteriol*, **120**: 273–81.

Hussain M, Hastings JGM, White PJ, 1991, Isolation and composition of the extracellular slime made by coagulase-negative staphylococci in a chemically defined medium, *J Infect Dis*, **163**: 534–41.

Hussain M, Hastings JGM, White PJ, 1992, Comparison of cell-wall teichoic acid with high-molecular-weight extracellular slime material from *Staphylococcus epidermidis*, *J Med Microbiol*, **37**: 368–75.

Iandolo JJ, 1989, Genetic analysis of extracellular toxins of *Staphylococcus aureus*, *Annu Rev Microbiol*, **43**: 375–402.

Iandolo JJ, Stewart GC, 1997, The *Staphylococcus aureus* genome map, *Bacterial Genomes: Physical Structure and Analysis*, eds De Bruijn FJ, Lupski JR, Weinstock G, Chapman and Hall, New York, in press.

Ichiyama S, Ohta M et al., 1991, Genomic DNA fingerprinting by pulsed field gel electrophoresis as an epidemiological marker for study of nosocomial infections caused by methicillin-resistant *Staphylococcus aureus*, *J Clin Microbiol*, **29**: 2690–5.

Igimi S, Takahashi E, Mitsuoka T, 1990, *Staphylococcus schleiferi* subsp. *coagulans* subsp. nov., isolated from the external auditory meatus of dogs with external ear otitis, *Int J Syst Bacteriol*, **40**: 409–11.

Igimi S, Kawamura S et al., 1989, *Staphylococcus felis*, a new species from clinical specimens from cats, *Int J Syst Bacteriol*, **39**: 373–7.

Inglis B, Waldron H, Stewart PR, 1987, Molecular relatedness of *Staphylococcus aureus* typing phages measured by DNA hybridization and by high resolution thermal denaturation analysis, *Arch Virol*, **93**: 69–80.

Inoue M, Mitsuhashi S, 1976, Recombination between phage S1 and the Tc resistant gene on *Staphylococcus aureus* plasmid, *Virology*, **72**: 322–9.

Iordănescu S, Surdeanu M, 1980, New incompatibility groups for *Staphylococcus aureus* plasmids, *Plasmid*, **4**: 256–60.

Iordănescu S, Surdeanu M et al., 1978, Incompatibility and molecular relationships between small staphylococcal plasmids carrying the same resistance marker, *Plasmid*, **1**: 468–79.

Ito H, Yoshida H et al., 1994, Quinolone resistance mutations in the DNA gyrase *gyrA* and *gyrB* genes of *Staphylococcus aureus*, *Antimicrob Agents Chemother*, **38**: 2014–23.

Jack RW, Tagg JR, Ray B, 1995, Bacteriocins of Gram-positive bacteria, *Microbiol Rev*, **59**: 171–200.

Jackson MP, Iandolo JJ, 1986, Sequence of the exfoliative toxin B gene of *Staphylococcus aureus*, *J Bacteriol*, **167**: 726–8.

Jaffe HW, Sweeney HM et al., 1982, Structural and phenotypic varieties of gentamicin resistance plasmids in hospital strains of *Staphylococcus aureus* and coagulase-negative staphylococci, *Antimicrob Agents Chemother*, **21**: 773–9.

Jean-Pierre H, Darbas H et al., 1989, Pathogenicity in two cases of *Staphylococcus schleiferi*, a recently described species, *J Clin Microbiol*, **27**: 2110–11.

Jeljaszewicz J (ed.), 1973, *Staphylococci and Staphylococcal Infections*, Polish Medical Publishers, Warszawa.

Jeljaszewicz J (ed.), 1976, *Staphylococci and Staphylococcal Diseases*, Gustav Fischer Verlag, Stuttgart.

Jeljaszewicz J (ed.), 1981, *Staphylococci and Staphylococcal Infections*, Gustav Fischer Verlag, Stuttgart.

Jeljaszewicz J (ed.), 1985, *The Staphylococci*, Gustav Fischer Verlag, Stuttgart.

Jensen MA, Webster JA, Straus N, 1993, Rapid identification of bacteria on the basis of polymerase chain reaction-amplified ribosomal DNA spacer polymorphisms, *Appl Environ Microbiol*, **59**: 945–52.

Jenssen WD, Thakker-Varia S et al., 1987, Prevalence of macrolide-lincosamide-streptogramin B resistance and *erm* gene classes among clinical strains of staphylococci and streptococci, *Antimicrob Agents Chemother*, **31**: 883–8.

Jevons MP, 1961, 'Celbenin' resistant staphylococci, *Br Med J*, **1**: 124–5.

Ji G, Silver S, 1992, Regulation and expression of the arsenic resistance operon from *Staphylococcus aureus* plasmid pI258, *J Bacteriol*, **174**: 3684–94.

Ji G, Garber EA et al., 1994, Arsenate reductase of *Staphylococcus aureus* plasmid pI258, *Biochemistry*, **33**: 7294–9.

Johns MB, Khan SA, 1988, Staphylococcal enterotoxin B gene is associated with a discrete genetic element, *J Bacteriol*, **170**: 4033–9.

Johnson GM, Carparas LS, Peters G, 1989, Slime production enhances resistance of *Staphylococcus epidermidis* to phagocytic killing: interference with opsonization and oxidative burst, *Pediatr Res*, **25**: 181.

Jones RN, Barry AL et al., 1989, The prevalence of staphylococcal resistance to penicillinase-resistant penicillins. Retrospective and prospective national surveillance trial of isolates from 40 medical centers, *Diagn Microbiol Infect Dis*, **12**: 385–94.

Jönsson K, Signäs C et al., 1991, Two different genes encode fibronectin binding proteins in *Staphylococcus aureus*: the complete nucleotide sequence and characterization of the second gene, *Eur J Biochem*, **202**: 1041–8.

Jose J, Schafer UK, Kaltwasser H, 1994, Threonine is present instead of cysteine at the active site of urease from *Staphylococcus xylosus*, *Arch Microbiol*, **161**: 384–92.

Jose J, Christians S et al., 1991, Cloning and expression of various staphylococcal genes encoding urease in *Staphylococcus carnosus*, *FEMS Microbiol Lett*, **80**: 277–82.

Kaatz GW, Seo SM, Ruble CA, 1993, Efflux-mediated fluoroquinolone resistance in *Staphylococcus aureus*, *Antimicrob Agents Chemother*, **37**: 1086–94.

Kagan BM, 1972, L-forms, *The Staphylococci*, ed. Cohen JO, Wiley-Interscience, New York, 65–74.

Kalbitzer HR, Deutscher J et al., 1981, Phosphoenolpyruvate-dependent phosphotransferase system of *Staphylococcus aureus*. ^{1}H-NMR studies of phosphorylated and unphosphorylated Factor III[lac] and its interaction with the phospho-carrier protein HPr, *Biochemistry*, **21**: 6178–85.

Kaletta C, Entian K-D et al., 1989, Pep5, a new lantibiotic: structural gene isolation and prepeptide sequence, *Arch Microbiol*, **152**: 16–19.

Kamath U, Singer C, Isenberg HD, 1992, Clinical significance of *Staphylococcus warneri* bacteremia, *J Clin Microbiol*, **30**: 261–4.

Karchmer AW, Archer GL, Dismukes WE, 1983, *Staphylococcus epidermidis* causing prosthetic valve endocarditis: microbiologic and clinical observations as guides to therapy, *Ann Intern Med*, **98**: 447–55.

Karchmer AW, Caputo GM, 1986, Endocarditis due to coagulase-negative staphylococci, *Coagulase-negative Staphylococci*, eds Mårdh P-A, Schleifer KH, Almqvist & Wiksell International, Stockholm, 179–87.

Kellner R, Jung G, Sahl H-G, 1991, Structure elucidation of the tricyclic lantibiotic Pep5 containing eight positively charged amino acids, *Nisin and Novel Lantibiotics*, eds Jung G, Sahl H-G, Escom Publishers, Leiden, 141–58.

Kellner R, Jung G et al., 1988, Gallidermin: a new lanthionine-containing polypeptide antibiotic, *Eur J Biochem*, **177**: 53–9.

Khan SA, Novick RP, 1980, Terminal nucleotide sequences of Tn551, a transposon specifying erythromycin resistance in *Staphylococcus aureus*: homology with Tn3, *Plasmid*, **4**: 148–54.

Khan SA, Novick RP, 1983, Complete nucleotide sequence of pT181, a tetracycline-resistance plasmid from *Staphylococcus aureus*, *Plasmid*, **10**: 251–9.

Kilpper, R, Buhl U, Schleifer KH, 1980, Nucleic acid homology studies between *Peptococcus saccharolyticus* and various anaerobic and facultative anaerobic Gram-positive cocci, *FEMS Microbiol Lett*, **8**: 205–10.

Kilpper-Bälz R, Schleifer KH, 1981, Transfer of *Peptococcus saccharolyticus* Foubert and Douglas to the genus *Staphylococcus*: *Staphylococcus saccharolyticus* (Foubert and Douglas) comb. nov., *Zentralbl Bakteriol Mikrobiol Hyg Abt 1 Orig C*, **2**: 324–31.

Kim KC, 1985, Parasitism and coevolution. Epilogue, *Coevolution of Parasitic Arthropods and Mammals*, ed. Kim KC, Wiley-Interscience, New York, 661–82.

Kinsman OS, McKenna R, Noble WC, 1983, Association between histocompatibility antigens (HLA) and nasal carriage of *Staphylococcus aureus*, *J Med Microbiol*, **16**: 215–20.

Kloos WE, 1980, Natural populations of the genus *Staphylococcus*, *Annu Rev Microbiol*, **34**: 559–92.

Kloos WE, 1986a, Ecology of human skin, *Coagulase-negative Staphylococci*, eds Mårdh P-A, Schleifer KH, Almqvist & Wiksell International, Stockholm, 37–50.

Kloos WE, 1986b, *Staphylococcus*, *McGraw-Hill 1986 Yearbook of Science and Technology*, ed. Parker SP, McGraw-Hill, New York, 431–4.

Kloos WE, 1990, Systematics and the natural history of staphylococci.1, *Staphylococci*, eds Jones D, Board RG, Sussman M, Blackwell Scientific Publications, Oxford, 25S–37S.

Kloos WE, Bannerman TL, 1994, Update on the clinical significance of coagulase-negative staphylococci, *Clin Microbiol Rev*, **7**: 117–40.

Kloos WE, Bannerman TL, 1995, *Staphylococcus* and *Micrococcus*, *Manual of Clinical Microbiology*, 6th edn, eds Murray PR, Baron EJ et al., ASM Press, Washington, DC, 282–98.

Kloos WE, George CG, 1991, Identification of *Staphylococcus* species and subspecies with the Microscan Pos ID and Rapid Pos ID panel systems, *J Clin Microbiol*, **29**: 738–44.

Kloos WE, George CG, Jones-Park LA, 1992, Effect of topical clindamycin therapy on cutaneous *Staphylococcus* species, *Abstr 92nd Gen Meet ASM*, 11.

Kloos WE, Musselwhite MS, 1975, Distribution and persistence of *Staphylococcus* and *Micrococcus* species and other aerobic bacteria on human skin, *Appl Microbiol*, **30**: 381–95.

Kloos WE, Orban BS, Walker DD, 1981, Plasmid composition of *Staphylococcus* species, *Can J Microbiol*, **27**: 271–8.

Kloos WE, Pattee PA, 1965, Transduction analysis of the histidine region in *Staphylococcus aureus*, *J Gen Microbiol*, **39**: 195–207.

Kloos WE, Schleifer KH, 1975a, Isolation and characterization of staphylococci from human skin. II. Descriptions of four new species: *Staphylococcus warneri*, *Staphylococcus capitis*, *Staphylococcus hominis*, and *Staphylococcus simulans*, *Int J Syst Bacteriol*, **25**: 62–79.

Kloos WE, Schleifer KH, 1975b, Simplified scheme for routine identification of human *Staphylococcus* species, *J Clin Microbiol*, **1**: 82–8.

Kloos WE, Schleifer KH, 1981, The genus *Staphylococcus*, *The Prokaryotes*, eds Starr MP, Stolp H et al., Springer-Verlag, New York, 1548–69.

Kloos WE, Schleifer KH, 1983, *Staphylococcus auricularis* sp. nov.: an inhabitant of the human external ear, *Int J Syst Bacteriol*, **33**: 9–14.

Kloos WE, Schleifer KH, Götz F, 1991, The genus *Staphylococcus*, *The Prokaryotes*, eds Balows A, Trüper HG et al., Springer-Verlag, New York, 1369–420.

Kloos WE, Schleifer KH, Smith RF, 1976, Characterization of *Staphylococcus sciuri* sp. nov. and its subspecies, *Int J Syst Bacteriol*, **26**: 22–37.

Kloos WE, Tornabene TG, Schleifer KH, 1974, Isolation and characterization of micrococci from human skin, including two new species: *Micrococcus lylae* and *Micrococcus kristinae*, *Int J Syst Bacteriol*, **24**: 79–101.

Kloos WE, Wolfshohl JF, 1979, Evidence for deoxyribonucleotide sequence divergence between staphylococci living on human and other primate skin, *Curr Microbiol*, **3**: 167–72.

Kloos WE, Wolfshohl JF, 1982, Identification of *Staphylococcus* species with the API STAPH-IDENT system, *J Clin Microbiol*, **16**: 509–16.

Kloos WE, Wolfshohl JF, 1983, Deoxyribonucleotide sequence divergence between *Staphylococcus cohnii* subspecies populations living on primate skin, *Curr Microbiol*, **8**: 115–21.

Kloos WE, Wolfshohl JF, 1991, *Staphylococcus cohnii* subspecies: *Staphylococcus cohnii* subsp. *cohnii* subsp. nov. and *Staphylococcus cohnii* subsp. *urealyticum* subsp. nov., *Int J Syst Bacteriol*, **41**: 284–9.

Kloos WE, Berkhoff HA et al., 1992, Relationship between cutaneous persistence in natural populations of coagulase-negative staphylococci and their ability to produce catheter infections, biofilm, and polysaccharide adhesin, *Abstr 92nd Gen Meet ASM*, 66.

Kloos WE, Ballard DN et al., 1997a, Delimiting the genus *Staphylococcus* through description of *Macrococcus caseolyticus* gen. nov., comb. nov., *M. equipercicus* sp. nov., *M. bovicus* sp. nov., and *M. carouselicus* sp. nov., *Int J Syst Bacteriol*, **47**: in press.

Kloos WE, Ballard DN et al., 1997b, Ribotype delineation and description of *Staphylococcus sciuri* subspecies and their potential as reservoirs of methicillin resistance and staphylolytic enzyme genes, *Int J Syst Bacteriol*, **47**: 313–23.

Knox KW, Wicken AJ, 1973, Immunological properties of teichoic acids, *Bacteriol Rev*, **37**: 215–57.

Koch C, Rainey FA, Stackebrandt E, 1994, 16S rDNA studies on members of *Arthrobacter* and *Micrococcus*: an aid for their future taxonomic restructuring, *FEMS Microbiol Lett*, **123**: 167–72.

Koch C, Schumann P, Stackebrandt E, 1995, Reclassification of *Micrococcus agilis* (Ali-Cohen 1889) to *Arthrobacter* as *Arthrobacter agilis* comb. nov. and emendation of the genus *Arthrobacter*, *Int J Syst Bacteriol*, **45**: 837–9.

Kojima N, Araki Y, Ito E, 1985, Structure of the linkage units between ribitol teichoic acids and peptidoglycan, *J Bacteriol*, **161**: 299–306.

Kordel M, Benz R, Sahl H-G, 1988, Mode of action of the staphylococcin-like peptide Pep5: voltage-dependent depolarization of bacterial and artificial membranes, *J Bacteriol*, **170**: 84–8.

Kornblum J, Kreiswirth BN et al., 1990, Agr: a polycistronic locus regulating exoprotein synthesis in *Staphylococcus aureus*, *Molecular Biology of the Staphylococci*, ed. in Novick RP, VCH Publishers, New York, 373–402.

Kotilainen P, Huovinen P, Eerola E, 1991, Application of gas-liquid chromatographic analysis of cellular fatty acids for species identification and typing of coagulase-negative staphylococci, *J Clin Microbiol*, **29**: 315–22.

Kotilainen P, Nikoskelainen J, Huovinen P, 1990, Emergence of ciprofloxacin-resistant coagulase-negative staphylococcal skin flora in immunocompromised patients receiving ciprofloxacin, *J Infect Dis*, **161**: 41–4.

Kraus ES, Spector DA, 1983, Characteristics and sequelae of peritonitis in diabetics and nondiabetics receiving chronic intermittent peritoneal dialysis, *Medicine (Baltimore)*, **62**: 52–7.

Kreiswirth B, Kornblum J et al., 1993, Evidence for a clonal origin of methicillin resistance in *Staphylococcus aureus*, *Science*, **259**: 227–30.

Lacey RW, 1975, Antibiotic resistance plasmids of *Staphylococcus aureus* and their clinical importance, *J Bacteriol Rev*, **39**: 1–32.

Lacey RW, Lord VL, 1981, Sensitivity of staphylococci to fatty acids: novel inactivation of linolenic acid by serum, *J Med Microbiol*, **14**: 41–9.

Lachica RVF, Hoeprich PD, Genigeorgis C, 1972, Metachromatic agar-diffusion microslide technique for detecting staphylococcal nuclease in foods, *Appl Microbiol*, **23**: 168–9.

Lachica RVF, Jang SS, Hoeprich PD, 1979, Thermonuclease seroinhibition test for distinguishing *Staphylococcus aureus* and other coagulase-positive staphylococci, *J Clin Microbiol*, **9**: 141–3.

Laddaga RA, Chu L et al., 1987, Nucleotide sequence and expression of the mercurial-resistance operon from *Staphylococcus aureus* plasmid pI258, *Proc Natl Acad Sci USA*, **84**: 5106–10.

Lambe DW Jr, Kloos WE, Lachica V, 1994, Staphylococcal food poisoning, *Handbook of Zoonoses: Bacterial, Rickettsial, Chlamydial, and Mycotic*, 2nd edn, ed. Beran GW, CRC Press, Boca Raton, FL, 369–76.

Lambe DW Jr, Berkhoff H et al., 1994, Pathogenicity of *Staphylococcus* species: abscess formation in three mouse models, *Molecular Pathogenesis of Surgical Infections*, eds Wadström T, Holder IA, Kronvall G, Gustav Fischer Verlag, Stuttgart, 453–67.

Lampson BC, Parisi JT, 1986, Naturally occurring *Staphylococcus epidermidis* plasmid expressing constitutive macrolide-lincosamide-streptogramin B resistance contains a deleted attenuator, *J Bacteriol*, **166**: 479–83.

Leclercq R, Courvalin P, 1991, Bacterial resistance to macrolide, lincosamide, streptogramin antibiotics by target modification, *Antimicrob Agents Chemother*, **35**: 1267–72.

Leclercq R, Carlier C et al., 1985, Plasmid-mediated resistance to lincomycin by inactivation in *Staphylococcus haemolyticus*, *Antimicrob Agents Chemother*, **28**: 421–4.

Leclercq R, Brisson-Noël A et al., 1987, Phenotypic expression and genetic heterogeneity of lincosamide inactivation in *Staphylococcus* spp., *Antimicrob Agents Chemother*, **31**: 1887–91.

Leclercq R, Derlot E et al., 1988, Plasmid-mediated resistance to vancomycin and teicoplanin in *Enterococcus faecium*, *N Engl J Med*, **319**: 157–61.

Lee CY, Iandolo JJ, 1986, Lysogenic conversion of staphylococcal lipase is caused by insertion of the bacteriophage L54a genome into the lipase structural gene, *J Bacteriol*, **166**: 385–91.

Lee CY, Iandolo JJ, 1988, Structural analysis of staphylococcal bacteriophage φ11 attachment sites, *J Bacteriol*, **170**: 2409–11.

Lee CY, Schmidt JJ et al., 1987, Sequence determination and comparison of the exfoliative toxin A and toxin B genes from *Staphylococcus aureus*, *J Bacteriol*, **169**: 3904–9.

Lee JC, Hopkins CA, Pier GB, 1985, The role of the *Staphylococcus aureus* capsule in abscess formation, *The Staphylococci*, ed. Jeljaszewicz J, Gustav Fischer Verlag, Stuttgart, 219–24.

Lee JC, Michon F et al., 1987, Chemical characterization and immunogenicity of capsular polysaccharide isolated from mucoid *Staphylococcus aureus*, *Infect Immun*, **55**: 2191–7.

Lee JC, Takeda S et al., 1993, Effects of in vitro and in vivo growth conditions on expression of type 8 capsular polysaccharide by *Staphylococcus aureus*, *Infect Immun*, **61**: 1853–8.

Le Goffic F, Martel A et al., 1977, 2 -*O*-Phosphorylation of gentamicin components by a *Staphylococcus aureus* strain carrying a plasmid, *Antimicrob Agents Chemother*, **12**: 26–30.

Lehmer A, Schleifer KH, 1980, Untersuchunger zum pentose- und pentitolstoffwechsel bei *Staphylococcus xylosus* und *Staphylococcus saprophyticus*, *Zentralbl Bakteriol Mikrobiol Hyg Abt 1 Orig C*, **1**: 109–23.

Liau DF, Hash JH, 1977, Structural analysis of the surface polysaccharide of *Staphylococcus aureus* M, *J Bacteriol*, **131**: 194–200.

Lina B, Celard M et al., 1992a, Infective endocarditis due to *Staphylococcus capitis*, *Clin Infect Dis*, **15**: 173–4.

Lina B, Vandenesch F et al., 1992b, Comparison of coagulase-negative staphylococci by pulsed-field gel electrophoresis, *FEMS Microbiol Lett*, **92**: 133–8.

Lina B, Bes M et al., 1993, Role of bacteriophages in genomic variability of related coagulase-negative staphylococci, *FEMS Microbiol Lett*, **109**: 273–8.

Lindberg M, Novick RP, 1973, Plasmid-specific transformation in *Staphylococcus aureus*, *J Bacteriol*, **115**: 139–45.

Lindberg M, Sjöström JE, Johansson T, 1972, Transformation of chromosomal and plasmid characters in *Staphylococcus aureus*, *J Bacteriol*, **109**: 844–7.

Lindberg M, Jonsson K et al., 1990, Fibronectin-binding proteins in *Staphylococcus aureus*, *The Molecular Biology of the Staphylococci*, ed. Novick RP, VCH Publishers, New York, 327–56.

Löfdahl S, Zabielski J, Philipson L, 1981, Structure and restriction enzyme maps of the circularly permuted DNA of staphylococcal bacteriophage φ11, *J Virol*, **37**: 784–94.

Lovett PS, 1990, Translational attenuation as the regulator of inducible *cat* genes, *J Bacteriol*, **172**: 1–6.

Low DE, Schmidt BK et al., 1992, An endemic strain of *Staphylococcus haemolyticus* colonizing and causing bacteremia in neonatal intensive care unit patients, *Pediatrics*, **89**: 696–700.

Luchansky JB, Pattee PA, 1984, Isolation of transposon Tn*551* insertions near chromosomal markers of interest in *Staphylococcus aureus*, *J Bacteriol*, **159**: 894–9.

Ludwicka A, Jansen B et al., 1984, Attachment of staphylococci to various synthetic polymers, *Zentralbl Bakteriol Mikrobiol Hyg Abt 1 Orig*, **256**: 479–89.

Ludwig W, Schleifer KH et al., 1981, A phylogenetic analysis of staphylococci, *Peptococcus saccharolyticus* and *Micrococcus mucilaginosus*, *J Gen Microbiol*, **125**: 357–66.

Ludwig W, Seewaldt E et al., 1985, The phylogenetic position of *Streptococcus* and *Enterococcus*, *J Gen Microbiol*, **131**: 543–51.

Lyon BR, Skurray R, 1987, Antimicrobial resistance of *Staphylococcus aureus*: genetic basis, *Microbiol Rev*, **51**: 88–134.

Lyon BR, Iuorio JL et al., 1984, Molecular epidemiology of multiresistant *Staphylococcus aureus* in Australian hospitals, *J Med Microbiol*, **17**: 79–89.

Lyon BR, Tennent JM et al., 1986, Trimethoprim resistance encoded on a *Staphylococcus aureus* gentamicin resistance plasmid: cloning and transposon mutagenesis, *FEMS Microbiol Lett*, **33**: 189–92.

McDevitt D, Francois P et al., 1995, Identification of the ligand-binding domain of the surface-located fibrinogen receptor (clumping factor) of *Staphylococcus aureus*, *Mol Microbiol*, **16**: 895–907.

McDonnell RW, Sweeney HM, Cohen S, 1983, Conjugational transfer of gentamicin resistance plasmids intra- and interspecifically in *Staphylococcus aureus* and *Staphylococcus epidermidis*, *Antimicrob Agents Chemother*, **23**: 151–60.

McDougal LK, Thornsberry C, 1986, The role of β-lactamase in staphylococcal resistance to penicillinase-resistant penicillins and cephalosporins, *J Clin Microbiol*, **23**: 832–9.

McMurray LW, Kernodle DS, Barg NL, 1990, Characterization of a widespread strain of methicillin-susceptible *Staphylococcus aureus* associated with nosocomial infections, *J Infect Dis*, **162**: 759–62.

Mack D, Siemssen N, Laufs R, 1992, Parallel induction by glucose of adherence and a polysaccharide antigen specific for plastic-adherent *Staphylococcus epidermidis*: evidence for functional relation to intercellular adhesion, *Infect Immun*, **60**: 2048–57.

Magni L, Soltész LV, 1986, Antibiotic susceptibility of *Staphylococcus saprophyticus*, *Coagulase-negative Staphylococci*, eds Mårdh P-A, Schleifer KH, Almqvist & Wiksell International, Stockholm, 93–6.

Mahairas GG, Lyon BR et al., 1989, Genetic analysis of *Staphylococcus aureus* with Tn*4001*, *J Bacteriol*, **171**: 3968–72.

Mallonee DH, Glatz BA, Pattee PA, 1982, Chromosomal mapping of a gene affecting enterotoxin A production in *Staphylococcus aureus*, *Appl Environ Microbiol*, **43**: 397–402.

Mårdh P-A, Schleifer KH (eds), 1986, *Coagulase-negative Staphylococci*, Almqvist & Wiksell International, Stockholm.

Margerrison EE, Hopewell R, Fisher LM, 1992, Nucleotide sequence of the *Staphylococcus aureus gyrB-gyrA* locus encoding the DNA gyrase A and B proteins, *J Bacteriol*, **174**: 1596–603.

Marquet-Van Der Mee N, Mallet S et al., 1995, Typing of *Staphylococcus epidermidis* strains by random amplification of polymorphic DNA, *FEMS Microbiol Lett*, **128**: 39–44.

Marrie TJ, Kwan C et al., 1982, *Staphylococcus saprophyticus* as a cause of urinary tract infections, *J Clin Microbiol*, **16:** 427–31.

Marshall JH, Wilmoth GJ, 1981a, Pigments of *Staphylococcus aureus*, a series of triterpenoid carotenoids, *J Bacteriol*, **147:** 900–13.

Marshall JH, Wilmoth GJ, 1981b, Proposed pathway of triterpenoid carotenoid biosynthesis in *Staphylococcus aureus*: evidence from a study of mutants, *J Bacteriol*, **147:** 914–19.

Mathews PR, Inglis B, Stewart PR, 1990, Clustering of resistance genes in the *mec* region of the chromosome of *Staphylococcus aureus*, *Molecular Biology of the Staphylococci*, ed. Novick RP, VCH Publishers, New York, 69–83.

Mayr E, 1963, *Populations, Species, and Evolution*, Belknap Press of Harvard University Press, Cambridge, MA, 209–11.

Meiwes J, Fiedler H-P et al., 1990, Isolation and characterization of staphyloferrin A, a compound with siderophore activity from *Staphylococcus hyicus* DSM 20459, *FEMS Microbiol Lett*, **67:** 201–6.

Melish ME, Glasgow LA, 1970, The staphylococcal scalded skin syndrome: development of an experimental model, *N Engl J Med*, **282:** 1114–19.

Meyer W, 1967, A proposal for subdividing the species *Staphylococcus aureus*, *Int J Syst Bacteriol*, **17:** 387–9.

Milinkovitch MC, 1992, DNA-DNA hybridizations support ungulate ancestry of Cetacea, *J Evol Biol*, **5:** 149–60.

Milinkovitch MC, Orti G, Meyer A, 1993, Revised phylogeny of whales suggested by mitochondrial ribosomal DNA sequences, *Nature (London)*, **361:** 346–8.

Miller MH, Edberg SC et al., 1980, Gentamicin uptake in wild-type and aminoglycoside-resistant small-colony mutants of *Staphylococcus aureus*, *Antimicrob Agents Chemother*, **18:** 722–9.

Mobley HL, Hausinger RP, 1989, Microbial ureases: significance, regulation, and molecular characterization, *Microbiol Rev*, **53:** 85–108.

Modun B, Kendall D, Williams P, 1994, Staphylococci express a receptor for human transferrin: identification of a 42-kilodalton cell wall transferrin-binding protein, *Infect Immun*, **62:** 3850–8.

Moeller V, 1955, Simplified tests for some amino acid decarboxylases and for the arginine dihydrolase system, *Acta Pathol Microbiol Scand*, **36:** 158–72.

Moks T, Abrahamsen L et al., 1986, Staphylococcal protein A consists of five IgG-binding domains, *Eur J Biochem*, **156:** 637–43.

Montagna W, Ellis RA, 1963, New approaches to the study of the skin of primates, *Evolutionary and Genetic Biology of Primates*, vol. 1, ed. Buettner-Janusch J, Academic Press, New York, 179–96.

Montagna W, Parakkal PF, 1974, *The Structure and Function of Skin*, 3rd edn, Academic Press, New York, 280–411.

Morioka H, Suganuma A, 1985, Electron-microscopic observations of staphylococci by protein A gold and immunogold method, *The Staphylococci*, ed. Jeljaszewicz J, Gustav Fischer Verlag, Stuttgart, 227–8.

Mossel DAA, Van Netten P, 1990, *Staphylococcus aureus* and related staphylococci in foods: ecology, proliferation, toxinogenesis, control and monitoring, *Staphylococci*, eds Jones D, Board RG, Sussman M, Blackwell Scientific Publications, Oxford, 123S–45S.

Muller E, Hübner J et al., 1993, Isolation and characterization of transposon mutants of *Staphylococcus epidermidis* deficient in capsular polysaccharide/adhesin and slime, *Infect Immun*, **61:** 551–8.

Muller HP, Schaeg W, Blobel H, 1981, Protein A activity of *Staphylococcus hyicus* in comparison to protein A of *Staphylococcus aureus*, *Zentralbl Bakteriol Mikrobiol Hyg Orig A*, **249:** 443–51.

Muller RE, Ano T et al., 1986, Complete nucleotide sequences of *Bacillus* plasmids pUB110dB, pRBH1 and its copy mutants, *Mol Gen Genet*, **202:** 169–71.

Murakami K, Minamide W et al., 1991, Identification of methicillin-resistant strains of staphylococci by polymerase chain reaction, *J Clin Microbiol*, **29:** 2240–4.

Murphy E, 1985a, Nucleotide sequence of *ermA*, a macrolide-lincosamide-streptogramin B determinant in *Staphylococcus aureus*, *J Bacteriol*, **162:** 633–40.

Murphy E, 1985b, Nucleotide sequence of a spectinomycin adenyltransferase AAD(9) determinant from *Staphylococcus aureus* and its relationship to AAD(3)(9), *Mol Gen Genet*, **200:** 33–9.

Murphy E, Huwyler L, Bastos MCF, 1985, Transposon Tn554: complete nucleotide sequence and isolation of transposition-defective and antibiotic-sensitive mutants, *EMBO J*, **4:** 3357–65.

Murphy E, Novick RP, 1979, Physical mapping of *Staphylococcus aureus* penicillinase plasmid pI524: characterization of an invertible region, *Mol Gen Genet*, **175:** 19–30.

Murphy E, Phillips S et al., 1981, Tn554: isolation and characterization of plasmid insertions, *Plasmid*, **5:** 292–305.

Musser JM, Kapur V, 1992, Clonal analysis of methicillin-resistant *Staphylococcus aureus* strains from intercontinental sources: association of the *mec* gene with divergent phylogenetic lineages implies dissemination by horizontal transfer and recombination, *J Clin Microbiol*, **30:** 2058–63.

Musser JM, Selander RK, 1990, Genetic analysis of natural populations of *Staphylococcus aureus*, *Molecular Biology of the Staphylococci*, ed. Novick RP, VCH Publishers, New York, 59–67.

Nahaie MR, Goodfellow M et al., 1984, Polar lipid and isoprenoid quinone composition in the classification of *Staphylococcus*, *J Gen Microbiol*, **130:** 2427–37.

Naidoo J, Noble WC, 1987, Skin as a source of transmissible antibiotic resistance in coagulase-negative staphylococci, *Pathogenicity and Clinical Significance of Coagulase-negative Staphylococci*, eds Pulverer G, Quie PG, Peters G, Gustav Fischer Verlag, Stuttgart, 225–34.

Naidu AS, Andersson M, Forsgren A, 1992, Identification of a human lactoferrin-binding protein in *Staphylococcus aureus*, *J Med Microbiol*, **36:** 177–83.

National Committee for Clinical Laboratory Standards, 1993, *Performance Standards for Antimicrobial Disk Susceptibility Tests. Approved Standard M2-A5*, NCCLS, Villanova, PA.

Nesin M, Svec P et al., 1990, Cloning and nucleotide sequence of a chromosomally encoded tetracycline resistance determinant, *tetA(M)*, from a pathogenic methicillin-resistant strain of *Staphylococcus aureus*, *Antimicrob Agents Chemother*, **34:** 2273–6.

Ng EY, Trucksis M, Hooper DC, 1994, Quinolone resistance mediated by *norA*: physiological characterization and relationship to *flqB*, a quinolone resistance locus on the *Staphylococcus aureus* chromosome, *Antimicrob Agents Chemother*, **38:** 1345–55.

Nicolaides N, 1974, Skin lipids: their biochemical uniqueness, *Science*, **186:** 19–26.

Noble WC, Pitcher DG, 1978, Microbial ecology of the human skin, *Adv Microb Ecol*, **2:** 245–89.

Noble WC, Somerville DA, 1974, *Microbiology of Human Skin*, WB Saunders, London.

Noble WC, Virani Z, Cree RGA, 1992, Cotransfer of vancomycin and other resistance genes from *Enterococcus faecalis* NCTC 12201 to *Staphylococcus aureus*, *FEMS Microbiol Lett*, **93:** 195–8.

Noda M, Hirayama T et al., 1980, Crystallization and properties of staphylococcal leukocidin, *Biochim Biophys Acta*, **633:** 33–44.

Novick RP, 1989, Staphylococcal plasmids and their replication, *Annu Rev Microbiol*, **43:** 537–65.

Novick RP, Edelman I, Löfdahl S, 1986, Small *Staphylococcus aureus* plasmids are transduced as linear multimers that are formed and resolved by recombination processes, *J Mol Biol*, **192:** 209–20.

Novick RP, Morse SI, 1967, *In vivo* transmission of drug resistance factors between strains of *Staphylococcus aureus*, *J Exp Med*, **125:** 45–59.

Novick RP, Murphy E, 1985, MLS-resistance determinants in *Staphylococcus aureus* and their molecular evolution, *J Antimicrob Chemother*, **16, Suppl. A:** 101–10.

Novick RP, Richmond MH, 1965, Nature and interactions of the genetic elements governing penicillinase synthesis in *Staphylococcus aureus*, *J Bacteriol*, **90**: 467–80.

Novick RP, Roth C, 1968, Plasmid-linked resistance to inorganic salts in *Staphylococcus aureus*, *J Bacteriol*, **95**: 1335–42.

Novick RP, Murphy E et al., 1979, Penicillinase plasmids of *Staphylococcus aureus*: restriction-deletion maps, *Plasmid*, **2**: 109–29.

Novick RP, Iordănescu S et al., 1981, Transduction-related cointegrate formation between staphylococcal plasmids: a new type of site-specific recombination, *Plasmid*, **6**: 159–72.

Novick RP, Projan SJ et al., 1984, Staphylococcal plasmid cointegrates are formed by host- and phage-mediated general *rec* systems that act on short regions of homology, *Mol Gen Genet*, **195**: 374–7.

Novick RP, Ross HF et al., 1993, Synthesis of staphylococcal virulence factors is controlled by a regulatory RNA molecule, *EMBO J*, **12**: 3967–75.

Nucifora G, Chu L et al., 1989, Cadmium resistance from *Staphylococcus aureus* plasmid pI258 *cadA* gene results from a cadmium-efflux ATPase, *Proc Natl Acad Sci USA*, **86**: 3544–8.

Ohshima Y, Ko HL et al., 1991, Activation of mononuclear immune cells in response to staphylococcal lipoteichoic acid, *Zentralbl Bakteriol Hyg Abt 1 Orig A*, **275**: 374–81.

Ohshita Y, Hiramatsu K, Yokota T, 1990, A point mutation in *norA* gene is responsible for quinolone resistance in *Staphylococcus aureus*, *Biochem Biophys Res Commun*, **172**: 1028–34.

Olsen WC Jr, Parisi JT et al., 1979, Transduction of penicillinase production in *Staphylococcus epidermidis* and nature of the genetic determinant, *Can J Microbiol*, **25**: 508–11.

van Oort MG, Deveer AM et al., 1989, Purification and substrate specificity of *Staphylococcus hyicus* lipase, *Biochemistry*, **28**: 9278–85.

Ornelas-Soares O, de Lencastre H et al., 1993, The peptidoglycan composition of a *Staphylococcus aureus* mutant selected for reduced methicillin resistance, *J Biol Chem*, **269**: 26268–72.

O'Reilly M, Kreiswirth B, Foster TJ, 1990, Cryptic alpha-toxin gene in toxic shock syndrome and septicaemia strains of *Staphylococcus aureus*, *Mol Microbiol*, **4**: 1947–55.

O'Toole PW, Foster TJ, 1986, Epidermolytic toxin serotype B of *Staphylococcus aureus* is plasmid encoded, *FEMS Microbiol Lett*, **36**: 311–14.

Papke G, Blobel H, 1978, Qualitative and quantitative determinations of staphylokinase activity, *Zentralbl Bakteriol Parasitenkd Infektionskr Hyg Abt 1 Orig A*, **242**: 456–61.

Parisi JT, 1985, Coagulase-negative staphylococci and the epidemiological typing of *Staphylococcus epidermidis*, *Microbiol Rev*, **49**: 126–39.

Parisi JT, Robbins J et al., 1981, Characterization of a macrolide, lincosamide, and streptogramin resistance plasmid in *Staphylococcus epidermidis*, *J Bacteriol*, **148**: 559–64.

Parker MT, 1983, The significance of phage-typing patterns in *Staphylococcus aureus*, *Staphylococci and Staphylococcal Infections*, vol. 1, eds Easmon CSF, Adlam C, Academic Press, London, 33–62.

Pattee PA, 1993, Genetic and physical map of *Staphylococcus aureus* NCTC 8325, *Genetic Maps: Locus Maps of Complex Genomes*, 6th edn, ed. O'Brien SJ, Cold Spring Harbor Laboratory Press, Cold Spring Harbor, NY, 2.106–2.113.

Pattee PA, Baldwin JN, 1961, Transduction of resistance to chlortetracycline and novobiocin in *Staphylococcus aureus*, *J Bacteriol*, **82**: 875–81.

Pattee PA, Kloos WE et al., 1968, Homogeneity in a *Staphylococcus aureus* transducing fragment, *J Virol*, **2**: 652–4.

Pattee PA, Schutzlank T et al., 1974, Genetic analysis of the leucine biosynthetic genes and their relationship to the *ilv* gene cluster, *Ann NY Acad Sci*, **236**: 175–86.

Patti JM, Jönsson K et al., 1992, Molecular characterization and expression of a gene encoding a *Staphylococcus aureus* collagen adhesin, *J Biol Chem*, **267**: 4766–72.

Paulsson M, Ljungh Å, Wadström T, 1992, Rapid identification of fibronectin, vitronectin, laminin, and collagen cell surface

binding proteins on coagulase-negative staphylococci by particle agglutination assays, *J Clin Microbiol*, **30**: 2006–12.

Paulsson M, Petersson A-C, Ljungh Å, 1993, Serum and tissue protein binding and cell surface properties of *Staphylococcus lugdunensis*, *J Med Microbiol*, **38**: 96–102.

Paulsson M, Wadström T, 1990, Vitronectin and type-I collagen binding by *Staphylococcus aureus* and coagulase-negative staphylococci, *FEMS Microbiol Immunol*, **65**: 55–62.

Pavillard R, Harvey K et al., 1982, Epidemic of hospital-acquired infection due to methicillin-resistant *Staphylococcus aureus* in major Victorian hospitals, *Med J Aust*, **1**: 451–4.

Pennock CA, Huddy RB, 1967, Phosphatase reaction of coagulase-negative staphylococci and micrococci, *J Pathol Bacteriol*, **93**: 685–8.

Perkins JB, Youngman PJ, 1983, *Streptococcus* plasmid pAMα1 is a composite of two separable replicons, one of which is closely related to *Bacillus* plasmid pBC16, *J Bacteriol*, **155**: 607–15.

Peters G, Locci R, Pulverer G, 1981, Microbial colonization of prosthetic devices. II. Scanning electron microscopy of naturally infected intravenous catheters, *Zentralbl Bakteriol Hyg Abt 1 Orig B*, **173**: 293–9.

Peters G, Locci R, Pulverer G, 1982, Adherence and growth of coagulase-negative staphylococci on surfaces of intravenous catheters, *J Infect Dis*, **146**: 479–82.

Peters G, Pulverer G, 1984, Pathogenesis and management of *Staphylococcus epidermidis* plastic foreign body infections, *J Antimicrob Chemother*, **14, Suppl. D**: 67–71.

Peters G, Schumacher-Perdreau F et al., 1987, Biology of *S. epidermidis* extracellular slime, *Pathogenicity and Clinical Significance of Coagulase-negative Staphylococci*, eds Pulverer G, Quie PG, Peters G, Gustav Fischer Verlag, Stuttgart, 15–32.

Phillips WE Jr, King RE, Kloos WE, 1980, Isolation of *Staphylococcus hyicus* subsp. *hyicus* from a pig with septic polyarthritis, *Am J Vet Res*, **41**: 274–6.

Phillips WE Jr, Kloos WE, 1981, Identification of coagulase-positive *Staphylococcus intermedius* and *Staphylococcus hyicus* subsp. *hyicus* isolates from veterinary clinical specimens, *J Clin Microbiol*, **14**: 671–3.

Phonimdaeng P, O'Reilly M et al., 1988, Molecular cloning and expression of the coagulase gene of *Staphylococcus aureus* 8325-4, *J Gen Microbiol*, **134**: 75–83.

Phonimdaeng P, O'Reilly M et al., 1990, The coagulase of *Staphylococcus aureus* 8325-4. Sequence analysis and virulence of site-specific coagulase-deficient mutants, *Mol Microbiol*, **4**: 393–404.

Pierre J, Williamson M et al., 1990, Presence of an additional penicillin-binding protein in methicillin-resistant *Staphylococcus epidermidis*, *Staphylococcus haemolyticus*, *Staphylococcus hominis*, and *Staphylococcus simulans* with a low affinity for methicillin, cephalothin, and cefamandole, *Antimicrob Agents Chemother*, **34**: 1691–4.

Poitevin-Later F, Vandenesch F et al., 1992, Cadmium-resistance plasmid in *Staphylococcus lugdunensis*, *FEMS Microbiol Lett*, **78**: 59–63.

Polak J, Novick RP, 1982, Closely related plasmids from *Staphylococcus aureus* and soil bacilli, *Plasmid*, **7**: 152–62.

Porter FD, Silver S et al., 1982, Selection for mercurial resistance in hospital settings, *Antimicrob Agents Chemother*, **22**: 852–8.

Prévot AR, 1961, *Traité de Systématique Bactérienne*, vol. 2, Dunod, Paris.

Price PB, 1938, The bacteriology of normal skin: a new quantitative test applied to a study of the bacterial flora and the disinfectant action of mechanical cleansing, *J Infect Dis*, **63**: 301–18.

Proctor AR, Kloos WE, 1970, The tryptophan gene cluster of *Staphylococcus aureus*, *J Gen Microbiol*, **64**: 319–27.

Projan SJ, Archer GL, 1989, Mobilization of the relaxable *Staphylococcus aureus* plasmid pC221 by the conjugative plasmid pG01 involves three pC221 loci, *J Bacteriol*, **171**: 1841–5.

Projan SJ, Monod M et al., 1987, Replication properties of pIM13, a naturally occurring plasmid found in *Bacillus subtilis*, and of its close relative pE5, a plasmid native to *Staphylococcus aureus*, *J Bacteriol*, **169:** 5131–9.

Prothero D, 1993, Ungulate phylogeny: molecular vs. morphological evidence, *Mammal Phylogeny. Placentals*, vol. 2, eds Szalay FS, Novacek MJ, McKenna MC, Springer-Verlag, New York, 173–81.

Pulverer G, Pillich J, Haklová M, 1976, Phage-typing set for the species *Staphylococcus albus*, *Staphylococci and Staphylococcal Diseases*, ed. Jeljaszewicz J, Gustav Fischer Verlag, Stuttgart, 153–7.

Pulverer G, Quie PG, Peters G (eds), 1987, *Pathogenicity and Clinical Significance of Coagulase-negative Staphylococci*, Gustav Fischer Verlag, Stuttgart.

Pulverer G, Ohshima Y et al., 1994, Staphylococcal LTA – a potent immunomodulator, *Molecular Pathogenesis of Surgical Infections*, eds Wadström T, Holder IA, Kronvall G, Gustav Fischer Verlag, Stuttgart, 205–10.

Quie PG, 1969, Microcolonies (G variants) of *Staphylococcus aureus*, *Yale J Biol Med*, **41:** 394–403.

Rahman A, Izaki K et al., 1991, Nucleotide sequence of leukocidin S-component gene (*lukS*) from methicillin-resistant *Staphylococcus aureus*, *Biochem Biophys Res Commun*, **181:** 138–44.

Raus J, Love DN, 1983, Characterization of coagulase-positive *Staphylococcus intermedius* and *Staphylococcus aureus* isolated from veterinary clinical specimens, *J Clin Microbiol*, **18:** 789–92.

Rautela GS, Abramson C, 1973, Crystallization and partial characterization of *Staphylococcus aureus* hyaluronate lyase, *Arch Biochem Biophys*, **158:** 687–94.

Recsei T, Gruss A, Novick R, 1987, Cloning, sequence, and expression of the lysostaphin gene from *Staphylococcus simulans*, *Proc Natl Acad Sci USA*, **84:** 1127–31.

Reeder WJ, Ekstedt RD, 1971, Study of the interaction of concanavalin A with staphylococcal teichoic acids, *Infect Immun*, **7:** 586–8.

Reis M, Eschbach-Bludau M et al., 1993, Producer immunity towards the lantibiotic Pep5: identification of the immunity gene *pepI* and localization and functional analysis of its gene product, *Appl Environ Microbiol*, **60:** 2876–83.

Reizer J, Saier MH Jr et al., 1988, The phosphoenolpyruvate:sugar phosphotransferase system in Gram-positive bacteria: properties, mechanisms, and regulation, *Crit Rev Microbiol*, **15:** 297–338.

Ren K, Bannan JD et al., 1994, Characterization and biological properties of a new staphylococcal exotoxin, *J Exp Med*, **180:** 1675–83.

Richmond MH, Lacey RW, 1973, Gene transfer between strains of *Staphylococcus aureus*, *Contrib Microbiol Immunol*, **1:** 135–43.

Rogolsky M, 1979, Nonenteric toxins of *Staphylococcus aureus*, *Microbiol Rev*, **43:** 320–60.

Rollof J, Hedström SA, Nilsson-Ehle P, 1987, Purification and characterization of a lipase from *Staphylococcus aureus*, *Biochim Biophys Acta*, **921:** 364–9.

Rosenbach FJ, 1884, *Mikro-organismen bei den Wund Infections Krankheiten des Menschen*, JF Bergmann, Weisbaden.

Rosenstein R, Nikoleit K, Götz F, 1994, Binding of ArsR, the repressor of the *Staphylococcus xylosus* (pSX267) arsenic resistance operon, to a sequence with dyad symmetry within the *ars* promoter, *Mol Gen Genet*, **242:** 566–72.

Rosenstein R, Peschel A et al., 1992, Expression and regulation of the antimonite, arsenite, and arsenate resistance operon of *Staphylococcus xylosus* plasmid pSX267, *J Bacteriol*, **174:** 3676–83.

Ross J, Farrell AM et al., 1989, Characterization and molecular cloning of the novel macrolide-streptogramin B resistance determinant from *Staphylococcus epidermidis*, *J Antimicrob Chemother*, **24:** 851–62.

Ross JI, Eady EA et al., 1990, Inducible erythromycin resistance in staphylococci is encoded by a member of the ATP-binding transport super-gene family, *Mol Microbiol*, **4:** 1207–14.

Rothman S, 1954, *Physiology and Biochemistry of the Skin*, University of Chicago Press, Chicago, IL, 201–20.

Rouch DA, Byrne ME et al., 1987, The *aacA-aphD* gentamicin and kanamycin resistance determinant of Tn*4001* from *Staphylococcus aureus*: expression and nucleotide sequence analysis, *J Gen Microbiol*, **133:** 3039–52.

Rouch DA, Messerotti LJ et al., 1989, Trimethoprim resistance transposon Tn*4003* from *Staphylococcus aureus* encodes genes for a dihydrofolate reductase and thymidylate synthetase flanked by three copies of IS*257*, *Mol Microbiol*, **3:** 161–75.

Rozgonyi F, Bíró A et al., 1994, Comparative studies on cell surface hydrophobicity, protein binding, haemolysis, virulence, and persistence of staphylococci of different species, *Molecular Pathogenesis of Surgical Infections*, eds Wadström T, Holder IA, Kronvall G, Gustav Fischer Verlag, Stuttgart, 57–65.

Ruby C, Novick RP, 1975, Plasmid interactions in *Staphylococcus aureus*. Non-additivity of compatible plasmid DNA pools, *Proc Natl Acad Sci USA*, **72:** 5031–5.

Ruden L, Sjöström JE et al., 1973, Factors affecting competence for transformation in *Staphylococcus aureus*, *J Bacteriol*, **118:** 155–64.

Rupprecht M, Schleifer KH, 1979, A comparative immunological study of catalases from coagulase-positive staphylococci, *Arch Microbiol*, **120:** 53–6.

Rydén C, Rubin K et al., 1983, Fibronectin receptors from *Staphylococcus aureus*, *J Biol Chem*, **258:** 3396–401.

Rydén C, Yacoub AI et al., 1989, Specific binding of bone sialoprotein to *Staphylococcus aureus* isolated from patients with osteomyelitis, *Eur J Biochem*, **184:** 331–6.

Rydén C, Hirsch G et al., 1990, Binding of bone sialoprotein to coagulase-negative staphylococci isolated from patients with chronic recurrent multifocal osteomyelitis, *J Infect Dis*, **161:** 814–15.

Saccone C, Pesole G, Sbisá E, 1991, The main regulatory region of mammalian mitochondrial DNA: structure-function model and evolutionary pattern, *J Mol Evol*, **33:** 83–91.

Saggers BA, Stewart GT, 1968, Lipolytic esterases in staphylococci, *J Bacteriol*, **96:** 1006–10.

Sako T, Tsuchida N, 1983, Nucleotide sequence of the staphylokinase gene from *Staphylococcus aureus*, *Nucleic Acids Res*, **11:** 7679–93.

Sandermann H Jr, Strominger JL, 1972, Purification and properties of C_{55}-isoprenoid alcohol phosphokinase from *Staphylococcus aureus*, *J Biol Chem*, **247:** 5123–31.

Schaberg DR, Culver DH, Gaines RP, 1991, Major trends in the microbial etiology of nosocomial infection, *Am J Med*, **91, Suppl. 3B:** 725–35.

Schaefler S, Francois W, Ruby CL, 1976, Minocycline resistance in *Staphylococcus aureus*: effect on phage susceptibility, *Antimicrob Agents Chemother*, **9:** 600–13.

Schaefler S, Jones D et al., 1981, Emergence of gentamicin- and methicillin-resistant *Staphylococcus aureus* strains in New York City hospitals, *J Clin Microbiol*, **13:** 754–9.

Schafer UK, Kaltwasser H, 1994, Urease from *Staphylococcus saprophyticus*: purification, characterization, and comparison to *Staphylococcus xylosus* urease, *Arch Microbiol*, **161:** 393–9.

Scheifele DW, Bjornson GL et al., 1987, Delta-like toxin produced by coagulase-negative staphylococci is associated with neonatal necrotizing enterocolitis, *Infect Immun*, **55:** 2268–73.

Schindler CA, Schuhardt VT, 1964, Lysostaphin: a new bacteriolytic agent for the *Staphylococcus*, *Proc Natl Acad Sci USA*, **51:** 414–21.

Schleifer KH, 1973, Chemical composition of staphylococcal cell walls, *Staphylococci and Staphylococcal Infections*, ed. Jeljaszewicz J, Polish Medical Publishers, Warszawa, 13–23.

Schleifer KH, 1983, The cell envelope, *Staphylococci and Staphylococcal Infections*, vol. 2, eds Easmon CSF, Adlam C, Academic Press, London, 358–428.

Schleifer KH, 1986, Taxonomy of coagulase-negative staphylococci, *Coagulase-negative Staphylococci*, eds Mårdh P-A, Schleifer KH, Almqvist & Wiksell International, Stockholm, 11–26.

Schleifer KH, Fischer U, 1982, Description of a new species of the genus *Staphylococcus: Staphylococcus carnosus, Int J Syst Bacteriol*, **32:** 153–6.

Schleifer KH, Hartinger A, Götz F, 1978, Occurrence of D-tagatose-6-phosphate pathway of D-galactose metabolism among staphylococci, *FEMS Microbiol Lett*, **3:** 9–11.

Schleifer KH, Kandler O, 1972, Peptidoglycan types of bacterial cell walls and their taxonomic implications, *Bacteriol Rev*, **36:** 401–77.

Schleifer KH, Kilpper-Bälz R, Devriese LA, 1984, *Staphylococcus arlettae* sp. nov., *S. equorum* sp. nov., and *S. kloosii* sp. nov.: three new coagulase-negative novobiocin-resistant species from animals, *Syst Appl Microbiol*, **5:** 501–9.

Schleifer KH, Kloos WE, 1975, Isolation and characterization of staphylococci from human skin. I. Amended description of *Staphylococcus epidermidis* and *Staphylococcus saprophyticus* and descriptions of three new species: *Staphylococcus cohnii*, *Staphylococcus haemolyticus*, and *Staphylococcus xylosus, Int J Syst Bacteriol*, **25:** 50–61.

Schleifer KH, Krämer E, 1980, Selective medium for isolating staphylococci, *Zentralbl Bakteriol Hyg Abt 1 Orig C*, **12:** 70–80.

Schleifer KH, Kroppenstedt RM, 1990, Chemical and molecular classification of staphylococci, *Staphylococci*, eds Jones D, Board RG, Sussman M, Blackwell Scientific Publications, Oxford, 9S–24S.

Schleifer KH, Meyer SA, Rupprecht M, 1979, Relatedness among coagulase-negative staphylococci: deoxyribonucleic acid reassociation and comparative immunological studies, *Arch Microbiol*, **122:** 93–101.

Schleifer KH, Steber J, 1974, Chemische Untersuchungen am Phagenrezeptor von *Staphylococcus epidermidis*, *Arch Microbiol*, **98:** 251–70.

Schleifer KH, Kilpper-Bälz R et al., 1982, Identification of 'Micrococcus candidus' ATCC 14852 as a strain of *Staphylococcus epidermidis* and of '*Micrococcus caseolyticus*' ATCC 13548 and *Micrococcus varians* ATCC 29750 as members of a new species, *Staphylococcus caseolyticus, Int J Syst Bacteriol*, **32:** 15–20.

Schleifer KH, Geyer U et al., 1983, Elevation of *Staphylococcus sciuri* subsp. *lentus* (Kloos et al.) to species status: *Staphylococcus lentus* (Kloos et al.) comb. nov., *Syst Appl Microbiol*, **4:** 382–7.

Schlievert PM, Shands KN et al., 1981, Identification and characterization of an exotoxin from *Staphylococcus aureus* associated with toxic shock syndrome, *J Infect Dis*, **143:** 509–16.

Schnell N, Entian K-D et al., 1988, Prepeptide sequence of epidermin, a ribosomally synthesized antibiotic with four sulphide rings, *Nature (London)*, **333:** 276–8.

Schnell N, Engelke G et al., 1992, Analysis of the genes involved in the biosynthesis of the lantibiotic epidermin, *Eur J Biochem*, **204:** 57–68.

Schroeder CJ, Pattee PA, 1984, Transduction analysis of transposon Tn551 insertions in the *trp-thy* region of the *Staphylococcus aureus* chromosome, *J Bacteriol*, **157:** 533–7.

Schwab AH, Leininger HV, Powers EM, 1984, Media, reagents, and stains, *Compendium of Methods for the Microbiological Examination of Foods*, 2nd edn, ed. Speck ML, American Public Health Association, Washington, DC, 788–897.

Schwalbe RS, Ritz WJ et al., 1990, Selection for vancomycin resistance in clinical isolates of *Staphylococcus haemolyticus*, *J Infect Dis*, **161:** 45–51.

Schwarz S, Cardoso M, Blobel H, 1989, Plasmid-mediated chloramphenicol resistance in *Staphylococcus hyicus, J Gen Microbiol*, **135:** 3329–36.

Schwarz S, Cardoso M, Blobel H, 1990, Detection of a novel chloramphenicol resistance plasmid from equine *Staphylococcus sciuri, J Vet Med*, **37:** 674–9.

Schwarz S, Werckenthin C, Ellendorff F, 1994, Heterogeneity of tetracycline resistance genes in *Staphylococcus intermedius* and *Staphylococcus lentus* from pigeons, *Abstr 94th Gen Meet ASM*, 22.

Schwarz S, Noble WC et al., 1993, Tetracycline resistance plasmids in *Staphylococcus hyicus, Abstr 93rd Gen Meet ASM*, 20.

Schwarz S, Werckenthin C et al., 1995, Chloramphenicol resistance in *Staphylococcus intermedius* from a single veterinary centre: evidence for plasmid and chromosomal location of the resistance genes, *Vet Microbiol*, **43:** 151–9.

Schwotzer U, Kayser FH, Schwotzer W, 1978, R-plasmid mediated aminoglycoside resistance in *Staphylococcus epidermidis*: structure determination of the products of an enzyme nucleotidylating the 4 and 4 hydroxyl group of aminoglycoside antibiotics, *FEMS Microbiol Lett*, **3:** 29–33.

Seidl PH, Schleifer KH, 1978, Rapid test for the separation of staphylococci from micrococci, *Appl Environ Microbiol*, **35:** 479–82.

Shalita Z, Murphy E, Novick RP, 1980, Penicillinase plasmids of *Staphylococcus aureus*: structural and evolutionary relationships, *Plasmid*, **3:** 291–311.

Shanson DC, Kensit JG, Duke R, 1976, Outbreak of hospital infection with a strain of *Staphylococcus aureus* resistant to gentamicin and methicillin, *Lancet*, **2:** 1347–8.

Shaw C, Stitt JM, Cowan ST, 1951, Staphylococci and their classification, *J Gen Microbiol*, **5:** 1010–23.

Shaw N, 1975, Bacterial glycolipids and glycophospholipids, *Adv Microbiol Physiol*, **12:** 141–67.

Shaw WV, 1983, Chloramphenicol acetyltransferase: enzymology and molecular biology, *Crit Rev Biochem*, **14:** 1–46.

Sheehy RJ, Novick RP, 1975, Studies on plasmid replication. IV. Replicative intermediates, *J Mol Biol*, **93:** 237–58.

Shimizu A, Berkhoff HA et al., 1996, Genomic DNA fingerprinting, using pulsed-field gel electrophoresis, of *Staphylococcus intermedius* isolated from dogs, *Am J Vet Res*, **57:** 1458–62.

Shortle D, 1983, A genetic system for analysis of staphylococcal nuclease, *Gene*, **22:** 181–9.

Shuttleworth R, Colby WD, 1992, *Staphylococcus lugdunensis* endocarditis, *J Clin Microbiol*, **30:** 1948–52.

Silver S, Keach D, 1982, Energy-dependent arsenate efflux: the mechanism of plasmid-mediated resistance, *Proc Natl Acad Sci USA*, **79:** 6114–18.

Silver S, Budd K et al., 1981, Inducible plasmid-determined resistance to arsenate, arsenite and antimony (III) in *Escherichia coli* and *Staphylococcus aureus, J Bacteriol*, **146:** 983–96.

Silvestri LG, Hill LR, 1965, Agreement between deoxyribonucleic acid base composition and taxonomic classification of Gram-positive cocci, *J Bacteriol*, **90:** 136–40.

Singh VR, Raad I, 1990, Fatal *Staphylococcus saprophyticus* native valve endocarditis in an intravenous drug addict, *J Infect Dis*, **162:** 784–5.

Sivakanesan R, Dawes EA, 1980, Anaerobic glucose and serine metabolism in *Staphylococcus epidermidis, J Gen Microbiol*, **118:** 143–57.

Sjöquist J, Movitz J et al., 1972, Localization of protein A in the bacteria, *Eur J Biochem*, **30:** 190–4.

Sjöström JE, Löfdahl S, Philipson L, 1975, Transformation reveals a chromosomal locus of the gene(s) for methicillin resistance in *Staphylococcus aureus, J Bacteriol*, **123:** 905–15.

Sjöström JE, Löfdahl S, Philipson L, 1979, Transformation of *Staphylococcus aureus* by heterologous plasmids, *Plasmid*, **2:** 529–35.

Sloan GL, Robinson JM, Kloos WE, 1982, Identification of '*Staphylococcus staphylolyticus*' NRRL B-2628 as a biovar of *Staphylococcus simulans, Int J Syst Bacteriol*, **32:** 170–4.

Smith CD, Pattee PA, 1967, Biochemical and genetic analysis of isoleucine and valine biosynthesis in *Staphylococcus aureus, J Bacteriol*, **93:** 1832–8.

Smith DGE, Wilcox NH et al., 1991, Characterization of cell envelope proteins of *Staphylococcus epidermidis* cultured in human peritoneal dialysate, *Infect Immun*, **59:** 617–24.

Smith K, Novick RP, 1972, Genetic studies on plasmid-linked cadmium resistance in *Staphylococcus aureus, J Bacteriol*, **112:** 761–72.

Smith TP, John DA, Bailey CJ, 1989, Epidermolytic toxin binds to components in the epidermis of a resistant species, *Eur J Cell Biol*, **49:** 341–9.

Smyth CJ, Möllby R, Wadström T, 1975, The phenomenon of hot-cold haemolysis. Studies on chelator-induced lysis of sphingomyelinase-treated erythrocytes, *Infect Immun*, **12:** 1104–11.

Sobek HM, Stüber K et al., 1984, Staphylococcal phosphoenolpyruvate-dependent phosphotransferase system: purification and characterization of a defective lactose-specific Factor III protein, *Biochemistry*, **23:** 4460–4.

Sokolov VE, 1982, *Mammal Skin*, University of California Press, Berkeley, CA.

Sreedharan S, Peterson LM, Fisher LM, 1991, Ciprofloxacin resistance in coagulase-positive and -negative staphylococci: role of mutations at serine 84 in the DNA gyrase A protein of *Staphylococcus aureus* and *Staphylococcus epidermidis*, *Antimicrob Agents Chemother*, **35:** 2151–4.

Stableforth AW, Galloway IA (eds), 1959, *Infectious Diseases of Animals. Diseases due to Bacteria*, vol. 2, Academic Press, London.

Stackebrandt E, Ludwig W et al., 1987, Comparative 16S rRNA oligonucleotide analysis and murein types of round-spore-forming bacilli and non-spore-forming bacilli and non-spore-forming relatives, *J Gen Microbiol*, **133:** 2523–9.

Stackebrandt E, Koch C et al., 1995, Taxonomic dissection of the genus *Micrococcus*: *Kocuria* gen. nov., *Nesterenkonia* gen. nov., *Kytococcus* gen. nov., *Dermacoccus* gen. nov., and *Micrococcus* Cohn 1872 gen. emend., *Int J Syst Bacteriol*, **45:** 682–92.

Stout RD, Ferguson KP et al., 1992, Staphylococcal exopolysaccharides inhibit lymphocyte proliferative responses by activation of monocyte prostaglandin production, *Infect Immun*, **60:** 922–7.

Strasters KC, Winkler KC, 1963, Carbohydrate metabolism of *Staphylococcus aureus*, *J Gen Microbiol*, **33:** 213–29.

Su Y-C, Wong ACL, 1995, Identification and purification of a new staphylococcal enterotoxin, H, *Appl Environ Microbiol*, **61:** 1438–43.

Suganuma A, 1972, Fine structure of the staphylococci: electron microscopy, *The Staphylococci*, ed. Cohen JO, Wiley-Interscience, New York, 21–40.

Suganuma A, Yokota Y, Morioka H, 1973, Plasma membrane of staphylococci as revealed by freeze-etching and thin sectioning, *J Kyoto Pref Univ Med*, **82:** 523–7.

Sutherland IV, 1977, *Surface Carbohydrates of the Prokaryotic Cell*, Academic Press, New York.

Suzuki E, Hiramatsu K, Yokota T, 1992, Survey of methicillin-resistant clinical strains of coagulase-negative staphylococci for *mecA* gene distribution, *Antimicrob Agents Chemother*, **36:** 429–34.

Switalski LM, Höök M, Beachey EH, 1989, *Molecular Mechanisms of Microbial Adhesion*, Springer Verlag, New York.

Switalski LM, Rydén C et al., 1983, Binding of fibronectin to *Staphylococcus* strains, *Infect Immun*, **42:** 628–33.

Szynkiewicz ZM, Kryński S et al., 1985, *Staphylococcus intermedius* infection in dogs in the years 1978 to 1983 and characteristics of isolated strains, *The Staphylococci*, ed. Jeljaszewicz J, Gustav Fischer Verlag, Stuttgart, 641–5.

Tanasupawat S, Hashimoto Y et al., 1992, *Staphylococcus piscifermentans* sp. nov. from fermented fish in Thialand, *Int J Syst Bacteriol*, **42:** 577–81.

Tashiro M, Ciborowski P et al., 1987, Role of *Staphylococcus* protease in the development of influenza pneumonia, *Nature (London)*, **325:** 536–7.

Taylor AG, Fincham WJ, Cook J, 1976, Staphylococcal antibodies in osteomyelitis: the use of anti-staphylococcal nuclease levels in diagnosis, *Staphylococci and Staphylococcal Diseases*, ed. Jeljaszewicz J, Gustav Fischer Verlag, Stuttgart, 911–16.

Tennent JM, Young H et al., 1988, Timethoprim resistance determinants encoding a dihydrofolate reductase in clinical isolates of *Staphylococcus aureus* and coagulase-negative staphylococci, *J Med Microbiol*, **26:** 67–73.

Teti G, Chiofalo MS et al., 1987, Mediation of *Staphylococcus sapro-*

phyticus adherence to uroepithelial cells by lipoteichoic acid, *Infect Immun*, **55:** 839–42.

Thakker-Varia S, Jenssen W et al., 1987, Molecular epidemiology of macrolides-lincosamides-streptogramin B resistance in *Staphylococcus aureus* and coagulase-negative staphylococci, *Antimicrob Agents Chemother*, **31:** 735–43.

Thelestam M, 1983, Modes of membrane damaging action of staphylococcal toxins, *Staphylococci and Staphylococcal Infections*, vol. 2, eds Easmon CSF, Adlam C, Academic Press, London, 705–44.

Theodore TS, Weinbach EC, 1974, Respiratory activities associated with mesosomal vesicles and protoplast membranes of *Staphylococcus aureus*, *J Bacteriol*, **120:** 562–4.

Thomas WD Jr, Archer GL, 1989a, Identification and cloning of the conjugative transfer region of the *Staphylococcus aureus* plasmid pG01, *J Bacteriol*, **171:** 684–91.

Thomas WD Jr, Archer GL, 1989b, Mobility of gentamicin resistance genes from staphylococci isolated in the United States: identification of Tn*4031*, a gentamicin resistance transposon from *Staphylococcus epidermidis*, *Antimicrob Agents Chemother*, **33:** 1335–41.

Thompson NE, Pattee PA, 1981, Genetic transformation in *Staphylococcus aureus*: demonstration of a competence-confering factor of bacteriophage origin in bacteriophage 80α lysates, *J Bacteriol*, **148:** 294–300.

Timmerman CP, Fleer A et al., 1991, Characterization of a proteinaceous adhesin of *Staphylococcus epidermidis* which mediates attachment to polystyrene, *Infect Immun*, **59:** 4187–92.

Timoney JF, Gillespie JH et al. (eds), 1988, *Hagan and Brunner's Microbiology and Infectious Diseases of Domestic Animals*, 8th edn, Comstock Publishing, Ithaca, NY.

Tojo M, Yamashita N et al., 1988, Isolation and characterization of a capsular polysaccharide adhesin from *Staphylococcus epidermidis*, *J Infect Dis*, **157:** 713–22.

Tollefson DF, Bandyk DF et al., 1987, Surface biofilm disruption-enhanced recovery of microorganisms from vascular prostheses, *Arch Surg*, **122:** 38–43.

Tomasz A, Drugeon HB et al., 1989, New mechanism for methicillin resistance in *Staphylococcus aureus*: clinical isolates that lack the PBP 2a gene and contain normal penicillin-binding proteins with modified penicillin-binding capacity, *Antimicrob Agents Chemother*, **33:** 1869–74.

Tomcsik J, 1956, Bacterial capsules and their relation to the cell wall, *Bacterial Anatomy*, eds Spooner ETC, Stocker BAD, Cambridge University Press, London, 41–67.

Townsend DE, Grubb WB, Ashdown N, 1983, Gentamicin resistance in methicillin-resistant *Staphylococcus aureus*, *Pathology*, **15:** 169–74.

Townsend DE, Ashdown N et al., 1984, Transposition of gentamicin resistance to staphylococcal plasmids encoding resistance to cationic agents, *J Antimicrob Chemother*, **13:** 347–52.

Townsend DE, Bolton S et al., 1986, Conjugative, staphylococcal plasmids carrying hitch-hiking transposons similar to Tn*554*; intra- and interspecies dissemination of erythromycin resistance, *Aust J Exp Biol Sci*, **64:** 367–79.

Trayer HR, Buckley CE III, 1970, Molecular properties of lysostaphin, a bacteriolytic agent specific for *Staphylococcus aureus*, *J Biol Chem*, **245:** 4842–6.

Trucksis M, Wolfson JS, Hooper DC, 1991, A novel locus conferring fluoroquinolone resistance in *Staphylococcus aureus*, *J Bacteriol*, **173:** 5854–60.

Tschäpe H, 1973, Genetic studies on nutrient markers and their taxonomic importance, *Staphylococci and Staphylococcal Infections*, ed. Jeljaszewicz J, Polish Medical Publishers, Warszawa, 57–62.

Turner WH, Pickard DJ, 1979, Immunological relationship between delta-haemolysins of *Staphylococcus aureus* and coagulase-negative strains of staphylococci, *Infect Immun*, **23:** 910–11.

Tynecka Z, Gos Z, Zajac J, 1981, Energy-dependent efflux of cadmium coded by a plasmid resistance determinant in *Staphylococcus aureus*, *J Bacteriol*, **147**: 313–19.

Ubukata K, Yamashita N et al., 1984, Purification and characterization of aminoglycoside-modifying enzymes from *Staphylococcus aureus* and *Staphylococcus epidermidis*, *Antimicrob Agents Chemother*, **25**: 754–9.

Ubukata K, Nakagami S et al., 1992, Rapid detection of the *mecA* gene in methicillin-resistant staphylococci by enzymatic detection of polymerase chain reaction products, *J Clin Microbiol*, **30**: 1728–33.

Udo EE, Grubb WB, 1990, Conjugal transfer of plasmid pWBG637 from *Staphylococcus aureus* to *Staphylococcus epidermidis* and *Streptococcus faecalis*, *FEMS Microbiol Lett*, **60**: 183–7.

Udo EE, Love H, Grubb WB, 1992, Intra- and inter-species mobilization of non-conjugative plasmids in staphylococci, *J Med Microbiol*, **37**: 180–6.

Udo E, Townsend DE, Grubb WB, 1987, A conjugative staphylococcal plasmid with no resistance phenotype, *FEMS Microbiol Lett*, **40**: 279–83.

Uhlén M, Guss B et al., 1984, Complete sequence of the staphylococcal gene encoding protein A: a gene evolved through multiple duplications, *J Biol Chem*, **259**: 1695–702.

Ushijima T, Takahashi N, Ozaki Y, 1984, Acetic, propionic, and oleic acids as the possible factors influencing the predominant residence of some species of *Propionibacterium* and coagulase-negative *Staphylococcus* on normal human skin, *Can J Microbiol*, **30**: 647–52.

Valisena S, Varaldo PE, Satta G, 1982, Purification and characterization of three separate bacteriolytic enzymes excreted by *Staphylococcus aureus*, *Staphylococcus simulans*, and *Staphylococcus saprophyticus*, *J Bacteriol*, **151**: 636–47.

Valle J, Gomez-Lucia E et al., 1990, Enterotoxin production by staphylococci isolated from healthy goats, *Appl Environ Microbiol*, **56**: 1323–6.

Vandenesch F, Kornblum J, Novick RP, 1991, A temporal signal, independent of *agr*, is required for *hla* but not *spa* transcription in *Staphylococcus aureus*, *J Bacteriol*, **173**: 6313–20.

Varaldo PE, Satta G, 1978, Grouping of staphylococci on the basis of their bacteriolytic activity patterns: a new approach to the taxonomy of the Micrococcaceae. II. Main characters of 1,054 strains subdivided into 'lyogroups', *Int J Syst Bacteriol*, **28**: 148–53.

Varaldo PE, Kilpper-Bälz R et al., 1988, *Staphylococcus delphini* sp. nov., a coagulase-positive species isolated from dolphins, *Int J Syst Bacteriol*, **38**: 436–9.

Ventosa A, Márquez MC et al., 1990, *Salinicoccus roseus* gen. nov., sp. nov., a new moderately halophilic Gram-positive coccus, *Syst Appl Microbiol*, **13**: 29–33.

Verhoef J, Van Boven CPA, Winkler KC, 1971, Character of phages from coagulase-negative staphylococci, *J Med Microbiol*, **4**: 413–24.

Verhoef J, Hoff AJ et al., 1971, Deoxyribonucleic acid base composition of *Staphylococcus epidermidis* and its phages, *J Gen Microbiol*, **69**: 279–83.

Von Darányi J, 1925, Qualitativ Untersuchungen der Luftbakterien, *Arch Hyg (Berlin)*, **96**: 182–4.

Vowels BR, Ordoukhanian E et al., 1995, Dynamic alteration of erythromycin-resistance gene usage in coagulase-negative staphylococci by topical erythromycin treatment, *Abstr 95th Gen Meet ASM*, 158.

Wadström T, 1983, Biological effects of cell damaging toxins, *Staphylococci and Staphylococcal Infections*, vol. 2, eds Easmon CSF, Adlam C, Academic Press, London, 671–704.

Wadström T, 1991, Molecular aspects on pathogenesis of staphylococcal wound and foreign body infections: bacterial cell surface hydrophobicity, fibronectin, fibrinogen, collagen, binding surface proteins, determine ability of staphylococci to colonize in damaged tissues and on prothesis materials, *The Staphylococci*, eds Jeljaszewicz J, Ciborowski P, Gustav Fischer Verlag, Stuttgart, 37–52.

Wadström T, Hisatsune K, 1970, Bacteriolytic enzymes from *Staphylococcus aureus*. Purification of an endo-β-*N*-acetylglucosaminidase, *Biochem J*, **120**: 725–34.

Wadström T, Holder IA, Kronvall G (eds), 1994, *Molecular Pathogenesis of Surgical Infections*, Gustav Fisher Verlag, Stuttgart.

Wadström T, Kjellgren M, Ljungh Å, 1976, Extracellular proteins from different *Staphylococcus* species: a preliminary study, *Staphylococci and Staphylococcal Diseases*, ed. Jeljaszewicz J, Gustav Fischer Verlag, Stuttgart, 623–34.

Wadström T, Rozgonyi F, 1986, Virulence determinants of coagulase-negative staphylococci, *Coagulase-negative Staphylococci*, eds Mårdh P-A, Schleifer KH, Almqvist & Wiksell International, Stockholm, 123–30.

Wang P-Z, Projan SJ, Novick RP, 1991, Nucleotide sequence of β-lactamase regulatory genes from staphylococcal plasmid pI258, *Nucleic Acids Res*, **19**: 4000.

Watson DC, Yaguchi M et al., 1988, The amino acid sequence of a gonococcal growth inhibitor from *Staphylococcus haemolyticus*, *Biochem J*, **252**: 87–93.

Weber DA, Goering RV, 1988, Tn*4201*, a β-lactamase transposon in *Staphylococcus aureus*, *Antimicrob Agents Chemother*, **32**: 1164–9.

Webster JA, Bannerman TL et al., 1994, Identification of the *Staphylococcus sciuri* species group with *Eco*RI fragments containing rRNA sequences and description of *Staphylococcus vitulus* sp. nov., *Int J Syst Bacteriol*, **44**: 454–60.

Weinstein RA, Kabins SA et al., 1982, Gentamicin-resistant staphylococci as hospital flora: epidemiology and resistance plasmids, *J Infect Dis*, **145**: 374–82.

Weisblum B, 1985, Inducible resistance to macrolides, lincosamides, and streptogramin type B antibiotics: the resistance phenotype, its biological diversity, and structural elements that regulate expression – a review, *J Antimicrob Chemother*, **16, Suppl. A:** 63–90.

Weiss AA, Murphy SD, Silver S, 1977, Mercury and organomercurial resistances determined by plasmids in *Staphylococcus aureus*, *J Bacteriol*, **132**: 197–208.

Welch WH, 1891, Conditions underlying the infection of wounds, *Am J Med Sci*, **102**: 439–65.

Wells SE, Kloos WE, 1987, Conservation of tetracycline resistance plasmids in staphylococci resistant to tetracycline and minocycline, *Abstr 87th Annu Meet ASM*, 163.

Welsh J, McClelland M, 1991, Species-specific genomic fingerprints produced by PCR with consensus tRNA gene primers, *Nucleic Acids Res*, **19**: 861–6.

Welsh J, McClelland M, 1992, PCR-amplified length polymorphisms in tRNA intergenic spacers for categorizing staphylococci, *Mol Microbiol*, **6**: 1673–80.

Westblom TU, Gorse GJ et al., 1990, Anaerobic endocarditis caused by *Staphylococcus saccharolyticus*, *J Clin Microbiol*, **28**: 2818–19.

Wilcox MH, Williams P et al., 1991, Variation in the expression of cell envelope proteins of coagulase-negative staphylococci cultured under iron-restricted conditions in human peritoneal dialysates, *J Gen Microbiol*, **137**: 2561–70.

Wiley BB, 1972, Capsules and pseudocapsules of *Staphylococcus aureus*, *The Staphylococci*, ed. Cohen JO, Wiley-Interscience, New York, 41–63.

Wilkinson BJ, 1983, Staphylococcal capsules and slime, *Staphylococci and Staphylococcal Infections*, vol. 2, eds Easmon CSF, Adlam C, Academic Press, London, 481–523.

Wilkinson BJ, Reifsteck F III et al., 1987, Coagulase-negative staphylococcal cell surface. Overview and specific aspects, *Pathogenicity and Clinical Significance of Coagulase-negative Staphylococci*, eds Pulverer G, Quie PG, Peters G, Gustav Fischer Verlag, Stuttgart, 67–75.

Williams REO, Rippon JE, 1952, Bacteriophage typing of *Staphylococcus aureus*, *J Hyg (Lond)*, **50**: 320–53.

Winslow CEA, Winslow A, 1908, *The Systematic Relationships of the Coccaceae*, John Wiley & Sons, New York.

Wise DR, 1971, Staphylococcal osteomyelitis of the avian vertebral column, *Res Vet Sci*, **12**: 169–71.

Witte W, Green L et al., 1986, Resistance to mercury and to cadmium in chromosomally resistant *Staphylococcus aureus, Antimicrob Agents Chemother*, **29:** 663–9.

Wondrack L, Sutcliffe J, 1995, *Staphylococcus* strains with MS phenotype efflux and inactivate erythromycin, a 14-membered macrolide, *Abstr 95th Gen Meet ASM*, 158.

Woods GL, Hall GS et al., 1986, Detection of methicillin-resistant *Staphylococcus epidermidis, J Clin Microbiol*, **24:** 349–52.

Yoshida H, Bogaki M et al., 1990, Nucleotide sequence and characterization of the *Staphylococcus aureus norA* gene, which confers resistance to quinolones, *J Bacteriol*, **172:** 6942–9.

Yoshida K, 1971, Demonstration of serologically different capsular types among strains of *Staphylococcus aureus* by the serum-soft agar technique, *Infect Immun*, **3:** 535–9.

Yoshida K, Minegishi Y, 1976, Capsular substance production in unencapsulated strains of *Staphylococcus aureus, Staphylococci and Staphylococcal Diseases*, ed. Jeljaszewicz J, Gustav Fischer Verlag, Stuttgart, 359–75.

Zimmerli W, Lew PD, Waldvogel FA, 1984, Pathogenesis of foreign body infections: evidence for a local granulocyte defect, *J Clin Invest*, **73:** 1191–200.

Zimmerman RJ, Kloos WE, 1976, Comparative zone electrophoresis of esterases of *Staphylococcus* species isolated from mammalian skin, *Can J Microbiol*, **22:** 771–9.

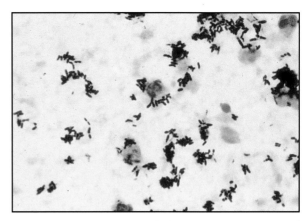

Plate 25.1 Coryneform morphology.

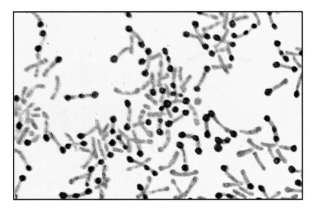

Plate 25.2 *Corynebacterium diphtheriae* with metachromatic granules.

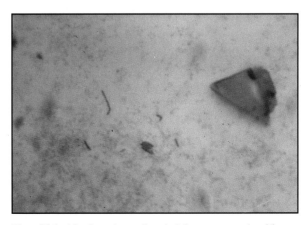

Plate 26.1 *Mycobacterium tuberculosis* in sputum stained by the Kinyoun cold staining procedure. (Photograph kindly provided by R W Smithwick, CDC).

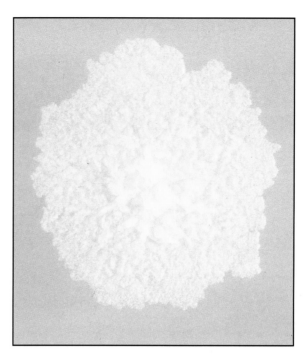

Plate 26.2 Rough colony morphology of *Mycobacterium tuberculosis* growing in Middlebrook 7H10 agar medium. (Photograph kindly provided by R W Smithwick, CDC).

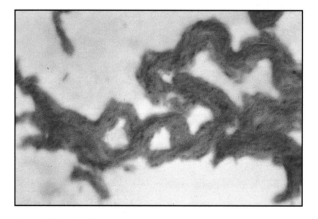

Plate 26.3 Cording characteristic of *Mycobacterium tuberculosis* grown in liquid culture (Kinyoun stain). (Photograph kindly provided by R W Smithwick, CDC).

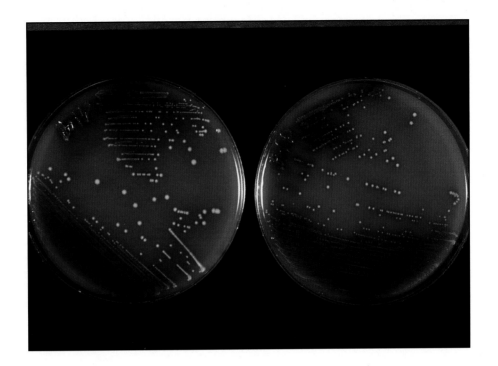

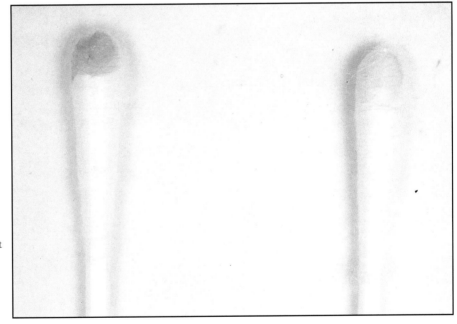

Plate 29.2 Culture and pigmentation test demonstrating yellow pigment produced by *Enterococcus* species; *E. casseliflavus* (pigmented) on left and *E. faecium* (non-pigmented) on right.

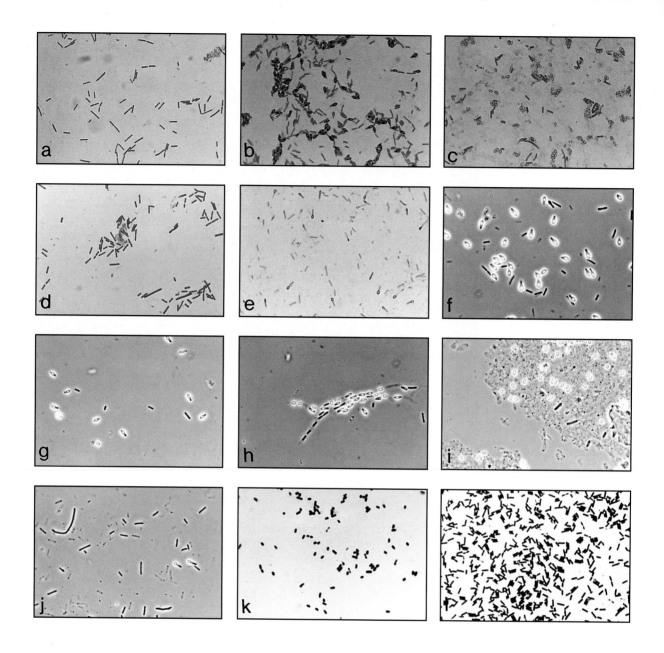

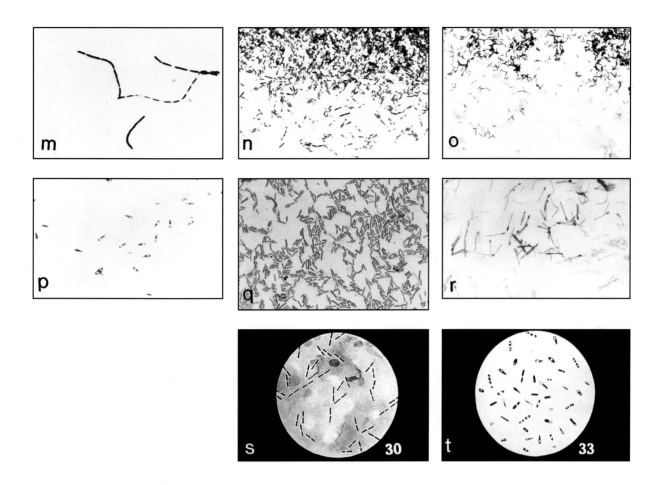

Plate 32.2 Photomicrographs (x c. 1500) of some representative species of *Clostridium*: (a) *C. botulinum* type A, 24 h CMGS, gram stain; (b) *C. botulinum* type A, 72 h EYA, gram stain; (c) *C. botulinum* type B (nonproteolytic), 72 h EYA, gram stain; (d) *C. botulinum* type E, 24h CMGS, gram stain; (e) *C. tetani*, 7 day EYA, gram stain; (f) *C. botulinum* type A, 4 day EYA; phase contrast; (g) *C. botulinum* type B, 4 day EYA, phase contrast; (h) *C. botulinum* type B, 4 day EYA, phase contrast; (i) *C. botulinum* type E, 4 day EYA, phase contrast; (j) *C. tetani*, 4 day EYA, phase contrast; (k) *C. perfringens*, 24 h CM, gram stain; (l) *C. perfringens*, 24 h Schaedler agar, gram stain; (m) *C. novyi*, 24 h CM, gram stain; (n) *C. difficile*, 72 h BAP, gram stain; (o) *C. paraputrificum*, 24 h CM, gram stain; (p) *C. subterminale*, 48 h BAP, gram stain; (q) *C. argentinense*, 72 h EYA, gram stain; (r) *C. innocuum*, 24 h thioglycollate broth, gram stain; (s) *C. septicum*, 24 h CM, methylene blue; (t) *C. chauvoei*, 24 h CM, methylene blue.

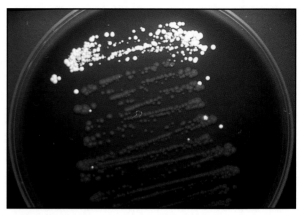

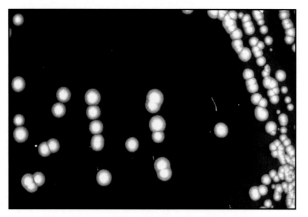

Plate 49.4 Colonies of *Legionella pneumophila* serogroup 1, strain Nottingham N7 after 4 days of incubation on BCYE agar. A bluish iridescence can be seen at the periphery of the colonies.

Plate 49.6 Colonies of *Legionella pneumophila* serogroup 1, strain Nottingham N7 and *Legionella bozemanii* serogroup 1 grown on BCYE agar and illuminated with longwave UV light at 366 nm. *L. bozemanii colonies* autofluoresce brilliant blue–white whereas those of *L. pneumophila* do not autofluoresce (see Table 49.1).

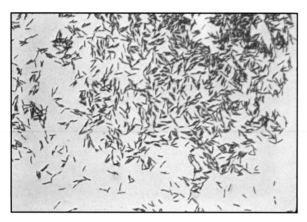

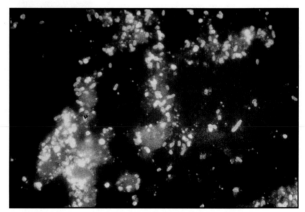

Plate 49.5 Gram stain of *Legionella pneumophila* after cultivation on bacteriological media. The preparation was counterstained with carbol fuchsin and shows slender gram negative rods with tapered ends.

Plate 49.7 Suspension smear from a postmortem lung specimen specifically stained with FITC–conjugated *Legionella* antiserum. Brightly fluorescing *Legionella* organisms are evident as are *Legionella* antigens released from lysed infected lung cells.

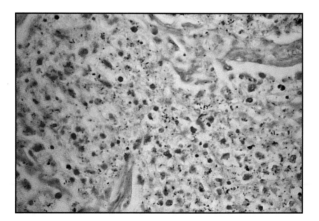

Plate 49.8 *Legionella pneumonia.* Histological section stained non–specifically by Dieterle's silver impregnation technique. Darkly staining legionellae can be seen in association with pale staining lung cells. Such a result may be suggestive of Legionnaire's disease when a tissue gram stain is negative and no other pneumonic pathogens are isolated on routine bacteriological media. Antigen detection methods and culture for *Legionella* should be attempted.

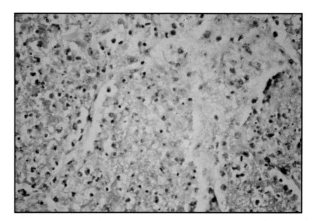

Plate 49.12 Haematoxylin and eosin stained section from a postmortem lung specimen from a fatal case of Legionnaire's disease. Note pneumonic presentation with inflammatory exudates in the alveolar sacs along with fibrin-rich debris. Organisms are not evident.

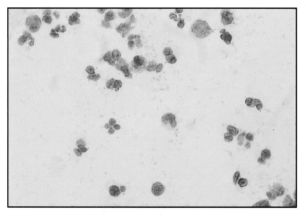

Plate 50.1 Gram–stained smear of cerebrospinal fluid from a case of *Haemophilus influenzae* type b meningitis (Bar = 5 μm).

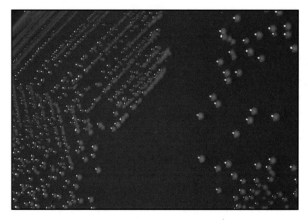

Plate 50.3 Culture of *Haemophilus influenzae* on chocolate agar.

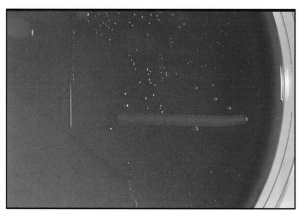

Plate 50.4 Culture of *Haemophilus influenzae* on whole horse blood agar showing satellitism of colonies adjacent to a streak of *Staphylococcus aureus*.

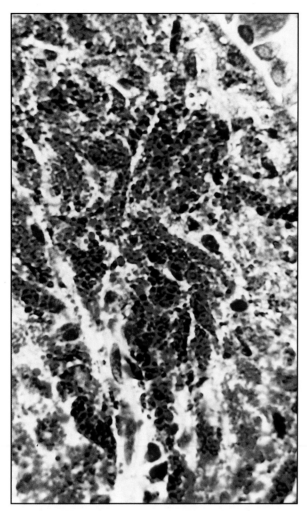

Plate 63.1 Periodic acid–Schiff positive staining macrophages in the duodenum in Whipple's disease. Transparency slide from ASCP, Anatomic Pathology II Check Sample exercise APII 8812 (APII–144), 'Gastric Xanthoma', Baddoura F, Someren A, Copyright 1988, American Society of Clinical Pathologists. Reproduced with permission.

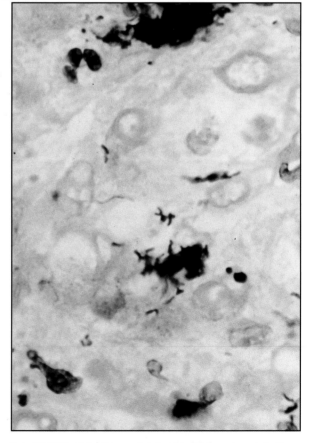

Pate 63.2 Warthin–Starry staining bacilli in cat scratch disease.

STREPTOCOCCUS AND LACTOBACILLUS

M Kilian

The genera *Streptococcus* and *Lactobacillus* belong to the lactic acid bacteria which is a taxonomically diverse group of gram-positive, non-spore-forming cocci and rods defined by the formation of lactic acid as a sole or major end-product of carbohydrate metabolism (Wood and Holzapfel 1995). Based on 16S and 23S rRNA sequence data, the gram-positive bacteria form 2 lines of descent. The typical lactic acid bacteria, which are characterized by a G + C content of less than 50 mol%, belong to the 'Clostridium branch' (Schleifer and Ludwig 1995). For many years the genera *Streptococcus* and *Lactobacillus* were both allocated to the family *Lactobacillaceae* but now belong to separate families *Streptococcaceae* and *Lactobacillaceae*.

STREPTOCOCCUS

1 GENUS DEFINITION

Streptococci are spherical or ovoid cells, arranged in chains or pairs. They are gram-positive. All species are non-motile, non-sporing, and catalase negative, with complex nutritional requirements. All are facultatively anaerobic; most will grow in air but some require the addition of carbon dioxide for growth. All species fail to reduce nitrate. They ferment glucose with the production mainly of lactic acid, never of gas. Many species are members of the commensal microflora on mucosal membranes of humans or animals, and some are highly pathogenic. The G + C content of the DNA is 36–46 mol%. The genus, named according to its typical morphology (from the Greek *streptos*, pliant; *coccos*, a grain or berry) includes 37 species which are listed in Table 28.1. The type species is *Streptococcus pyogenes*.

2 INTRODUCTION AND HISTORICAL PERSPECTIVE

The term *Streptococcus* was first applied by Billroth (1874) to a chain-forming coccus he saw in infected wounds. The first good accounts of *S. pyogenes* appear to be those of Pasteur (1879) and Rosenbach (1884) who described its morphology, cultural appearance and virulence for mice and rabbits. Since then the genus has accommodated a broad spectrum of bacteria from benign organisms used in the dairy industry to true pathogens of humans and several animal species. As a result of more recent taxonomic studies this complex situation has been resolved to some extent with the transfer of the dairy species to the new genera

Table 28.1 Species of the genus *Streptococcus*: serological and haemolytic reactions, peptidoglycan type, and main habitat

Pyogenic group	Lancefield serogroup	Serotype antigen	Haemolysis	Peptidoglycan type	Main habitat
S. pyogenes	A	M– and T–antigens (protein)	β	Lys–Ala$_{1-3}$	Humans
S. agalactiae	B	Capsular polysaccharide	β(CAMP+)	Lys–Ala$_{1-3}$(Ser)	Humans, cattle
S. equi					
subsp. *equi*	C		β	Lys–Ala$_{1-3}$	Horses, donkeys
subsp. *zooepidemicus*	C		β	Lys–Ala$_{2-3}$	Many animals
S. dysgalactiae					
subsp. *dysgalactiae*	C, L		α, β,–	Lys–Ala$_{1-3}$	Pigs, cattle
subsp. *equisimilis*	C, G		β	Lys–Ala$_{1-3}$	Humans
S. canis	G		β (CAMP+)	Lys–Thr–Gly	Many animals
S. iniae	–		β, α	Lys–Ala$_{1-3}$	Freshwater dolphins
S. porcinus	E, P, U, V		β (CAMP+)	Lys–Ala$_{2-4}$	Pigs
S. uberis	–, E		α	Lys–Ala$_{1-3}$	Cattle
S. parauberis	–, E		α	ND	Cattle
S. hyointestinalis	–		α	Lys–Ala(Ser)	Pigs
Anginosus group					
S. anginosus	–, F, A, C, G		α, β	Lys–Ala$_{1-3}$	Humans
S. constellatus	–, A, C		α, β	Lys–Ala$_{1-3}$	Humans
S. intermedius	–, F, G.		α, β	Lys–Ala$_{1-3}$	Humans
Mitis group					
S. mitis	O, K, –		α	Lys–direct	Humans
S. oralis	–		α	Lys–direct	Humans
S. pneumoniae	–	Capsular polysaccharide	α	Lys–Ala$_2$(Ser)	Humans
S. gordonii	H1, H2, –[a]		α	Lys–Ala$_{1-3}$	Humans
S. sanguis	H1, –		α	Lys–Ala$_{1-3}$	Humans
S. parasanguis	–		α	ND[b]	Humans
S. crista	–		α	ND	Humans
Salivarius group					
S. salivarius	H2, K, –		–	Lys–Ala$_{2-3}$, Lys–Thr–Gly	Humans
S. vestibularis	–		–	ND	Humans
S. thermophilus	–		–	Lys–Ala$_{2-3}$	Milk, dairy products
Bovis group					
S. bovis	D		–, α	Lys–Thr–Ala	Cattle, sheep, pigs, humans, dogs, pigeons
S. equinus	D		α	Lys–Thr–Ala	Horses, other animals
S. alactolyticus	D		α, –	ND	Pigs, chickens
Mutans group					
S. mutans	–, E	c, e, f	–, β, α	Lys–Ala$_{2-3}$	Humans
S. cricetus	–	a	–, α	Lys–Thr–Ala	Hamster, rats, humans
S. sobrinus	–	d, h, g, (or–) cell wall carbohydrate	α, –	Lys–Thr–Ala	Humans
S. downeii	–	h	–	Lys–Thr–Ala	Monkeys
S. rattus	–	b	–	Lys–Ala$_{2-3}$	Rats, humans
S. macacae	–	c	–	ND	Monkeys
S. ferus	–	c	–	Lys–Ala$_{2-3}$	Rats

Table 28.1 Continued

Pyogenic group	Lancefield serogroup	Serotype antigen	Haemolysis	Peptidoglycan type	Main habitat
Other streptococci					
S. suis	D[c]	Capsular polysaccharide	β, α, –	Lys–direct	Pigs, cattle
S. acidominimus	–		α	Lys–Ser–Gly	Cattle
S. intestinalis	–, G		β	ND	Pigs
S. caprinus				ND	Feral goats

[a]H1, Reaction detected in antiserum against strain Blackburn ('European group H'); H2, Reaction detected in antiserum against strain F90A ('American group H').
[b]ND, Not determined.
[c]Previously designated group antigens R, S and T are capsular polysaccharide types 2, 1 and 15 respectively.

Lactococcus and the motile *Vagococcus*, the enteric streptococci to the genus *Enterococcus* (Chapter 29), the anaerobic streptococci to *Peptostreptococcus* (Chapter 33), and some species to the genus *Gemella*. Recently, the so-called 'nutritionally variant streptococci', which for many years were considered variants of recognized *Streptococcus* species, were transferred to a new genus *Abiotrophia* (Kawamura et al. 1995b) which will be discussed in this chapter. For a comprehensive discussion of catalase-negative gram-positive cocci other than *Streptococcus* the reader is referred to a recent review by Facklam and Elliott (1995a).

The phylogenetic relationships between the genus *Streptococcus* and the numerous genera of catalase negative, gram-positive cocci of which several have been recently described, have been studied extensively by Collins and his coworkers and others (Aguirre et al. 1993, Collins et al. 1989, Williams, Farrow and Collins 1989, Stackebrandt and Teuber 1988, Ludwig et al. 1985). A comprehensive discussion of this topic has been recently published by Schleifer and Ludwig (1995).

3 HABITATS

All the *Streptococcus* species are obligate parasites of mucosal membranes and, for some species, tooth surfaces of humans and several animals. Many of the species are life-long and dominant members of the commensal microflora on mucosal membranes of the upper respiratory tract and some colonize the intestinal and genital tracts of humans and various animals. A few species colonize exclusively tooth surfaces and are present only after tooth eruption. Most of these members of the resident flora may cause infection when introduced into normally sterile compartments of the body or in immunocompromised patients. Other species are true pathogens which spread from patient to patient and cause infection in non-immune individuals.

4 MORPHOLOGY

Streptococci are spherical cells that may be more or less elongated and arranged in pairs or in chains of up to 50 cells or more. Chain formation is most pronounced in broth media. Individual cells are typically 0.5–1.0 μm × 1.0–2.0 μm. Growth occurs by elongation on the axis parallel to the chain. Cross-walls form at right angles to the chain and after division an appearance of pairing may remain (Fig. 28.1). Some species may develop rod-like cells depending on the growth conditions (Clarke 1924, Rosan and Eisenberg 1973). Members of the genus are non-motile in the conventional sense, although a twitching motility associated with polar fimbriae has been described for *S. sanguis* isolates (Henriksen and Henrichsen 1975).

A variety of proteinaceous surface fibrils and filaments, sometimes organized in tufts, have been described in some streptococcal species (Swanson, Hsu and Gotschlich 1969, Handley 1990). Some of these structures form a 'fuzzy coat' on the entire surface of the cells and appear to play a role in adherence and in some cases as a layer protecting against phagocytosis.

Capsulation is not a regular feature of streptococci but some form a capsule of hyaluronic acid or of other distinct polysaccharides. Several of the oral streptococci form extracellular polysaccharides when grown

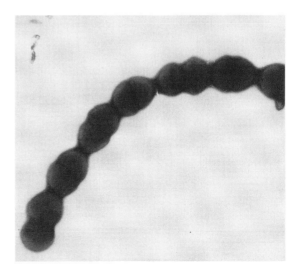

Fig. 28.1 Electron micrograph of *S. pyogenes* M-type 2 from a broth culture (× 12 500) (kindly supplied by Dr CAM Fraser and Mr AA Porter).

in the presence of sucrose, but these polysaccharides do not constitute capsules covalently linked to the cell wall (see p. 647).

Streptococci stain readily with ordinary dyes and are almost frankly gram-positive although old cultures may show variable staining.

5   CULTURAL CHARACTERISTICS

Growth on ordinary nutrient media is generally poor, in contrast to that of enterococci. On media enriched with blood, serum or a fermentable carbohydrate growth is more profuse, but colonies on blood agar seldom exceed 1 mm in diameter after 24 h at 37°C. Some species characteristically form relatively large colonies whereas others form colonies of pinpoint size (see p. 641). Growth on agar media by some strains of *S. pneumoniae*, the mutans streptococci, and *S. anginosus* requires a supplement of carbon dioxide to the incubation atmosphere. Many streptococci grow more readily under anaerobic conditions than in air plus carbon dioxide.

In general, colonies of streptococci on blood agar are non-pigmented. The exception is the majority of members of the species *S. agalactiae* which form an orange-red pigment which presumably is a β-carotenoid (Tapsall 1986).

When cultivated on sucrose-containing agar media, such as Mitis Salivarius agar, some of the viridans streptococci and *S. bovis* biotype 1 produce extracellular polysaccharides which may facilitate their recognition (Fig. 28.2). The polysaccharide will in some of the species (*S. sanguis*, *S. gordonii*, *S. oralis* and the mutans streptococci) result in coherent and adherent colonies that may be difficult to subcultivate on to agar plates or into fluid media.

The yield of cells from broth cultures is increased by the addition of a fermentable carbohydrate but the rapid fall in pH becomes inhibitory and the bacteria eventually die. In buffered media containing glucose, such as Todd–Hewitt broth, or in media with a high glucose content in which a neutral pH is maintained

by the regulated addition of alkali, a heavy yield of streptococci is obtained.

5.1   Haemolysis

The ability of certain clinically important streptococci to induce zones of complete haemolysis (**β-haemolysis**) around colonies on blood-containing agar media was one of the first characters to be recognized and used for distinguishing between isolates. Other isolates of streptococci induce a zone of greenish discoloration (**α-haemolysis**) on blood agar, and yet others cause no detectable changes to the red blood cells. β-Haemolysis is caused by well-characterized haemolysins (see below) whereas α-haemolysis is due to hydrogen peroxide released from the colonies and inducing a change of haemoglobin to methaemoglobin.

6   METABOLISM

Members of the genus *Streptococcus* are facultatively anaerobic with a preference for anaerobic conditions. They are unique amongst bacteria able to grow aerobically in that they do not synthesize porphyrins, cytochromes or catalase, and are not capable of forming ATP via an electron transport system. They generate energy, as well as some precursors for the synthesis of cellular material, through fermentation of carbohydrates.

6.1   Carbohydrate metabolism

Streptococci degrade glucose via the Embden–Meyerhof glycolytic pathway which is driven by constitutive enzymes. Most of the streptococci are able to ferment various other sugars and sugar alcohols by means of inducible enzymes that are synthesized only in the presence of each of the carbohydrates and in the absence of glucose.

Active transport of several monosaccharides, disaccharides and sugar alcohols through the cytoplasmic membrane into the cytoplasma takes place with the help of the **phosphoenolpyruvate : sugar phosphotransferase system**. This is a high-affinity 'group translocation' process which utilizes phosphoenolpyruvate as an energy source and results in the transport and phosphorylation of the sugar to the inner surface of the cell (Reizen and Peterkofsky 1987).

Many of the streptococci produce various glycosidases that enable them to take advantage of the sugar residues in glycoproteins present in the secretions in their natural habitat (Pinter, Hayashi and Bahn 1969). However, some of the streptococci, in particular oral streptococci, may encounter considerable fluctuations in the amount of carbohydrate available in their natural habitat and adjust their metabolism accordingly. When glucose is supplied in excess the vast majority is converted to L-lactate through pyruvate. However, with low sugar levels, other more energy efficient pathways of pyruvate conversion are operating. Under

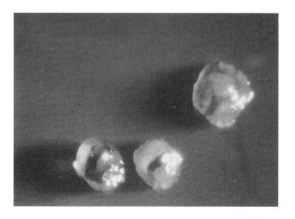

Fig. 28.2 *S. mutans* grown on sucrose-containing Mitis Salivarius agar (× 10). Incubated in N_2 (90%) + CO_2 (10%), 24 h, 37°C and then in air, 24 h, room temperature.

anaerobic conditions, streptococci use the pyruvate–formate lyase pathway and generate formic and acetic acids and ethanol as end products (Fig. 28.3). Under aerobic conditions, mutans streptococci use pyruvate dehydrogenase to convert pyruvate to acetic acid and ethanol, while some of the other oral streptococci use pyruvate oxidase with the formation of acetic acid and hydrogen peroxide as end products (Carlsson and Hamilton 1994).

In times of carbohydrate excess streptococci may synthesize intracellular polysaccharide (glycogen), which is utilized to provide maintenance energy when exogenous sources are absent. In addition, some of the species synthesize extracellular polysaccharides but only from sucrose (see Table 28.3). Some of these polysaccharides may function as storage of carbohydrate whereas others seem to perform other functions.

6.2 Other nutritional requirements

The nutritional requirements of streptococci in general are complex and include amino acids, peptides, purines, pyrimidines, vitamins and salts in addition to the energy source. However, some of the oral streptococci will grow in the presence of sugar, vitamins and salts with ammonia as the sole nitrogen source. These requirements are usually met in blood agar which combines meat extract, peptones and blood. The nutritionally variant streptococci (*Abiotrophia* spp., see p. 655) will grow only in media that contain supplements of cysteine or pyridoxal hydrochloride.

In their natural habitats the requirements for nitrogenous compounds may be satisfied by amino acids excreted by other members of the resident microflora or released from local secretions or tissues by bacterial proteinases. The utilization of peptides depends upon adequate mechanisms for transport across the cytoplasmic membrane and intracellular peptidases capable of hydrolysing the peptides to amino acids. Some of the streptococci are able to

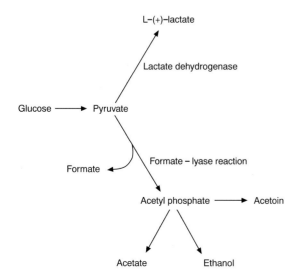

Fig. 28.3 Pathways of pyruvate metabolism in streptococci.

degrade arginine by the arginine deaminase system, which is an energy-yielding reaction. Accordingly, animal experiments have demonstrated that arginine in the diet favours the selection in the mouth of arginine-utilizing streptococci such as *S. sanguis* and *S. anginosus* (van der Hoeven, De Jong and Rogers 1985, Rogers et al. 1990).

7 GENETIC MECHANISMS

Streptococcal genetics has a long history and has been of paramount importance in the developments of genetics and biology in general. **Transformation** of a bacterial property (capsule production) was first demonstrated in pneumococci by Griffith in 1928. These studies subsequently led to the identification of DNA as the genetic material ('transforming principle') (Avery, MacLeod and McCarty 1944).

Molecular genetic studies of streptococci have provided substantial evidence that horizontal gene transfer and recombination play an important role in the evolution of *Streptococcus* species and in the generation of diversity of some genes within natural populations of streptococci (Simpson and Musser 1992, Hollingshead et al. 1994, Whatmore et al. 1994). Such processes, including the rapid spread of certain alleles of genes determining virulence factors, appear to be responsible for fluctuations observed in the prevalence of serious infections due to pyogenic streptococci (Musser et al. 1993a,b). Furthermore, horizontal transfer play a significant role in the spread of drug resistance genes between streptococci and other bacteria. However, the genetic mechanisms involved differ, as does the frequency of horizontal gene transfer in natural population of the individual species.

Transformation appears to be the principal mechanism of horizontal gene transfer in some streptococcal species such as *S. pneumoniae* and *S. gordonii*. Competence for genetic transformation, which arises in exponentially growing cultures at a critical cell density, is dependent on the release of a soluble molecule termed **competence factor** (Pakula and Walczak 1963, Tomasz and Hotchkiss 1964), which involves a heptadecapeptide pheromone (Håvarstein, Coomaraswarmi and Morrison 1995).

Many *Streptococcus* species contain conjugative as well as non-conjugative plasmids of several sizes (LeBlanc and Lee 1979, Simpson and Tagg 1984) that may encode antibiotic resistance traits. However, early reports demonstrated the en bloc transfer of resistance to several antibiotics by a mechanism unrelated to plasmids (Buu-Hoi and Horodniceanu 1980, Horodniceanu, Bougueleret and Bieth 1981, 1982). Clewell and coworkers have provided a molecular basis for plasmid-free resistance transfer with the characterization of a streptococcal tetracycline resistance conjugative transposon (Gawron-Burke and Clewell 1982).

Conjugative transposons are widespread among streptococci and play a significant role in the dissemination of drug resistance (Clewell and Gawron-Burke

1986, Horaud et al. 1991). One of the transposon families found in streptococci, Tn*916*/Tn*1545* displays a remarkable broad host range which encompasses a large number of both gram-positive and gram-negative bacteria. Tn*916* is a 18 kb element originally discovered in *Enterococcus faecalis* and Tn*1545* a 25.3 kb element first detected in *S. pneumoniae*. The transposons are transferred between bacterial cells by a conjugation-like mechanism requiring contact between donor and recipient. They become integrated in the bacterial genome by an excision/insertion process that can take place at numerous AT-rich target sites. In this way transposons are capable of disrupting the expression of particular genes, a property that provides an important method for the development of streptococcal strains deficient in defined properties and for identification of genes (transposon mutagensis).

Tn*916*-like chromosomal elements have been reported to exist in *S. pyogenes*, *S. agalactiae*, *S. equisimilis*, *S. anginosus*, *S. mitis*, *S. oralis*, *S. pneumoniae*, *S. sanguis*, and *S. bovis* and in multiple other gram-positive and gram-negative species (Clewell, Flannagan and Jaworski 1995).

As discussed below, many streptococci are lysogenic and the expression of some virulence genes is associated with prophages (Zabriskie, Read and Fischetti 1972, Malke 1972). M-type specificity, opacity factor activity (see p. 652), bacteriocin determinants and other properties can be transduced between *S. pyogenes* strains (Tagg, Skjold and Wannamaker 1976, Totolian 1979).

8 CELL WALL COMPOSITION; ANTIGENIC STRUCTURE

The cell wall of streptococci consists of the shape-forming peptidoglycan (murein), various carbohydrate structures including teichoic acids, and a number of proteins. It was previously assumed that these structures are arranged in concentric layers with the peptidoglycan as the innermost layer, followed by the so-called **group carbohydrate**, and several proteins forming the outermost layer. However, several observations discussed below do not support this view.

Reliable methods for the preparation of cells walls from streptococci have been described by Salton and Horne (1951). The bacterial cells are broken by rapid oscillation with small glass beads. Adherent intracellular debris and cell membranes are then removed by washing with buffers or detergents followed by enzymatic digestion. Extraction of the isolated walls with hot formamide removes the cell wall carbohydrate. The insoluble residue after formamide extraction is the peptidoglycan. Extraction with trichloroacetic acid is the classical method for extraction of teichoic acids from the cell wall, but the extract is not necessarily representative of the various forms present (Knox and Wicken 1973).

8.1 Cell wall peptidoglycan

As in other gram-positive cell walls the peptidoglycan consists of multiple glycan chains that are cross-linked though short peptides (Schleifer and Kandler 1972). The glycan moiety is composed of alternating β-1,4-linked units of *N*-acetylglucosamine and *N*-acetylmuramic acid. The carboxyl group of muramic acid is substituted by an oligopeptide that contains alternating L-and D-amino acids, which in streptococci always include lysine (Fig. 28.4). Adjacent oligopeptide chains from parallel glycan chains are cross-linked either directly or via an interpeptide bridge between the ε-amino group of lysine in one peptide and the D-alanine of a second chain. The type of bridge is consistent within most species and shows some characteristic differences (Table 28.1). The most common interpeptide bridge in streptococci consists of 1–4 L-alanine residues (Lys-Ala$_n$). In some species (e.g. members of the bovis and mutans groups) the alanine residues can be partly replaced by L-threonine and/or L-serine. The 2 species *S. oralis* and *S. mitis* lack an interpeptide bridge and have directly linked oligopeptide chains (Lys-direct). Detailed studies of the pneumococcal peptidoglycan have disclosed several types of cross-linking, one of which resembles that found in gram-negative bacteria (Fischer and Tomasz 1985, Garcia-Bustos, Chait and Tomasz 1987). Most of the enterococci and lactococci, which are now allocated to separate genera, have different types of interpeptide bridges (Lys-D-Asp) with the exception of *E. faecalis* (Lys-Ala$_{2-3}$) (Schleifer and Kilpper-Bälz 1987). The methods that can be employed for the determination of the composition and structure of peptidoglycans are outlined by Schleifer and Seidl (1985).

8.2 Cell wall carbohydrates

The streptococcal cell wall may contain several forms of polysaccharides, one of which, in some species, constitutes the **Lancefield group antigen** (see p. 640). Although initially believed to form a continuous layer outside the peptidoglycan, ultrastructural studies revealed that it traverses the wall and may be found both on the inner and the outer surfaces of isolated cell walls (Rýc, Beachey and Whitnack 1989, Sørensen et al. 1988, Wagner and Wagner 1985).

The qualitative composition of the cell wall polysaccharide is known for most of the *Streptococcus* species. With the exception of the 3 closely related species (*S. pneumoniae*, *S. oralis*, and *S. mitis*) all streptococcal cell walls contain rhamnose (Colman and Williams 1965). The structure of some of the wall polysaccharides, including some of those that form the basis of the Lancefield serological grouping has been determined. The polysaccharides of groups A (*S. pyogenes*) and C (*S. dysgalactiae* and *S. equi*) contain an identical backbone consisting of α-1,2- and α-1,3-glycosidically linked rhamnose molecules, but differ in their limited side branches: Group A carries *N*-acetylglucosamine residues and group C disaccharides of *N*-acetylgalactosamine, which are the immunodominant substituents (McCarty 1958, Coligan, Kindt and Krause 1978). The so-called group A-variant polysaccharide, which may be detected in strains of *S. pyogenes* after several mouse passages, is not substituted (Coligan, Kindt and Krause 1978). The group B polysaccharide of *S. agalactiae* consists of a backbone composed of rhamnose, glucitol and phosphate, and trisaccharide side chains composed of rhamnose, galactose and *N*-acetylglucosamine that are linked to the 4-position of a rhamnose in the backbone of the polysaccharide (Pritchard, Gray and Dillon 1984).

The wall polysaccharides of many oral species contain the lectin recognition determinant involved in adhesion to other microorganisms (**coaggregation**) (Glushka et al. 1992, Cisar

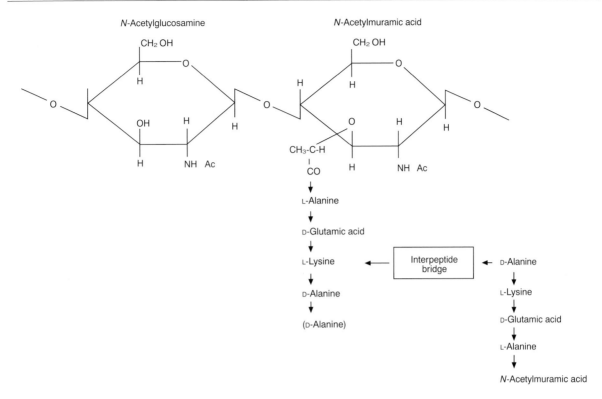

Fig. 28.4 Repeating unit of cell wall peptidoglycan of *Streptococcus* species. The major variability between species is in the structure of the interpeptide bridge (see Table 28.1).

et al. 1995, Holmes, Gopal and Jenkinson 1995). Structural studies of these polysaccharides in members of the species *S. oralis, S. mitis, S. sanguis* and *S. gordonii* revealed that each consists of a different hexa- or heptasaccharide repeating unit linked end to end by phosphodiester bonds (McIntire et al. 1988, Abeygunawardana and Bush 1989, Abeyguna-wardana et al., 1990, 1991, Reddy et al. 1993, 1994). Some of the polysaccharides contain limited branching. Most, if not all, of the cell wall polysaccharides found in *S. mitis* and *S. oralis* contain ribitol, confirming the original analyses reported by Colman and Williams (1965) (exceptions may be due to incorrect classification of the strains studied). Ribitol is also a characteristic constituent of the cell wall polysaccharide of *S. pneumoniae*.

Many of the cell wall polysaccharides may be classified as teichoic acids as they contain phosphodiester groups, polyols and/or sugar residues (Ward 1981). Thus, *S. pneumoniae, S. mitis*, and *S. oralis* contain ribitol teichoic acids (Colman and Williams 1965, Rosan 1978). Presumably all other streptococcal species contain typical glycerol teichoic acids in addition to the polysaccharides described above. The glycerol teichoic acid of *S. pyogenes* is composed of a chain of 25–30 glycerol phosphate units joined by phosphodiester linkages with ester-linked molecules of D-alanine of the peptidoglycan layers (wall teichoic acid) or fatty acid of the plasma membrane (lipoteichoic acid). For further details on the pneumococcal cell wall polysaccharides see p. 654.

Lipoteichoic acid is synthesized in the cytoplasmic membrane where it may remain anchored though the glycolipid tail. However, in the model proposed for *S. pyogenes* lipoteichoic acid is not anchored in the cytoplasmic membrane but remains associated with the cell surface by interactions with M protein (Beachey and Simpson 1982). Similar models have been proposed for oral streptococci (Shockman et al. 1986). In the case of some of the oral streptococci, lipote-

ichoic acid may become associated with extracellular polysaccharide (Rölla et al. 1980, Hogg and Lightfoot 1992) and considerable amounts are released into the environment depending on the growth conditions (Jacques et al. 1979, Wicken et al. 1982). Quantitative studies have shown that lipoteichoic acid represents only 2–4% of phenol extractable contents from *S. sanguis* (Hogg and Old 1993).

Although a definitive function for lipoteichoic acid has yet to be described, there has been considerable interest in its potential as a mediator of bacterial adhesion, particularly in the case of *S. pyogenes* (Ofek et al. 1975, Beachey and Courtney 1987), *S. agalactiae* (Nealon and Mattingly 1984) and *S. mutans* (Rölla, Iversen and Bonesvoll 1978).

8.3   Cell wall proteins

Streptococci produce an array of proteins associated with the cell wall (Kehoe 1994). They are generally exposed on the outer surface of the cell wall. Many of them protrude as filamentous structures of different length and may even protrude through the capsule as in *S. pyogenes* and *S. agalactiae* (Wagner and Wagner 1985, Fischetti 1989). The biological functions and structure of some of the surface exposed proteins in pyogenic streptococci are discussed under virulence factors.

8.4   Antigenic structure

Antigenic analysis of cell wall components and capsules has played a major, and sometimes excessive, role in the classification of members of the genus *Streptococcus* and as an epidemiological tool. Historically, the cell wall carbohydrates have received most attention as a result of the original work of Rebecca

Lancefield on pyogenic streptococci isolated from infections. The cell wall carbohydrate that can be extracted from whole streptococcal cells by a number of techniques including treatment with hot hydrochloric acid (Lancefield extraction) (Facklam and Washington 1991) will in some cases show a specific precipitate with antisera prepared by injecting whole cells into rabbits (Lancefield 1933). Such carbohydrate antigens are the Lancefield group antigens and are termed A–W (with the exception of I and J). Although serological grouping remains a valuable means of characterizing streptococci of medical importance, attempts to equate the Lancefield groups with species have generally failed. The association of group antigens with streptococcal species is shown in Table 28.1. As shown in this table the group A antigen is characteristic of *S. pyogenes* but occasional strains of other species may also react with group A antisera. The group B antigen is an exclusive characteristic of *S. agalactiae*, whereas several species may carry antigens reactive with group C, F, and G antisera. The group D and N antigens, which are teichoic acids, are associated mainly with streptococci now allocated to the genera *Enterococcus* and *Lactococcus*, respectively.

The group antigens can be demonstrated by various techniques. Thus, group-specific, precipitating, agglutinating and fluorescently labelled antibody preparations, which can be used with extracts, cell suspensions, and spent broth media, are commercially available. Most valuable are group A, B, C, F and G antisera for characterization of β-haemolytic streptococci and group B and D antisera for characterization of non-β-haemolytic isolates (Facklam and Washington 1991). There is some confusion concerning the group H antigen as 2 different strains with distinct carbohydrate antigens have been used for production of group H antisera. One is referred to as 'American group H' and the other as 'British group H' (Cole et al. 1976) (see Table 28.1).

A similar serotyping strategy has been applied to differentiate among the mutans streptococci although there has been no attempt to include this in the grouping system (Bratthall 1970, Perch, Kjems and Ravn 1974, Beighton, Russell and Hayday 1981) (see Table 28.1).

The highly diverse filamentous M and T protein antigens of *S. pyogenes* (p. 648) form the basis of serologic typing of this species and have played a significant role in epidemiological studies (Colman et al. 1993). Likewise, the diverse polysaccharide capsules produced by members of the species *S. pneumoniae, S. agalactiae*, and *S. suis* form the basis of valuable typing systems for these bacteria (see below).

9 SUSCEPTIBILITY TO ANTIMICROBIAL AGENTS

Members of the genus *Streptococcus* are naturally susceptible to a wide range of therapeutically useful antibiotics. The pyogenic streptococci and some but not all pneumococci and other viridans streptococci are inhibited by readily achievable blood levels of benzylpenicillin. Streptococci are more or less resistant to all the aminoglycoside antibiotics (Horodiceanu et al. 1982).

As mentioned above, streptococci may be resistant to multiple antibiotics such as tetracycline, streptomycin, erythromycin and chloramphenicol as a result of the acquisition of resistance genes on transposons or conjugative plasmids. Of special clinical concern is the increasing prevalence of penicillin resistance of *S. pneumoniae* strains in several parts of the world. Penicillin resistance is often associated with resistance to multiple other antibiotics (Appelbaum 1992, Doern et al. 1996).

Penicillin resistance in *S. pneumoniae* is due to alterations of **penicillin-binding proteins**, the enzymes that assemble the cell wall peptidoglycan layers (Tomasz 1987). These penicillin-binding proteins become modified as a result of recombination with homologous genes of related species such as *S. oralis* and *S. mitis*, in which penicillin resistance has evolved by the accumulation of point mutations (Dowson et al. 1993, Sibold et al. 1994). Penicillin resistance is primarily associated with pneumococci of serotypes 6B, 14 19A and 23F.

Differences in susceptibility to certain agents are useful for the presumptive identification of particular streptococci: for example, sensitivity to bacitracin and optochin (p. 645), which can be detected by means of standardized disc tests. The frequent resistance of leuconostocs to vancomycin is similarly of value in distinguishing them from streptococci.

Streptococci are destroyed by the usual strengths of disinfectants but may survive for months in dry dust in buildings. *Streptococcus* species are killed by moist heat at 55°C for 30 min, in contrast to the enterococci and some of the lactic streptococci and the exceptional *S. thermophilus*.

10 CLASSIFICATION

Since its original description the genus *Streptococcus* has undergone numerous revisions. Several subgroups of species have been transferred to new genera, new species have been added and existing species have been redefined or deleted. The major part of this development occurred at about the time of or after the publication of the second volume of *Bergey's Manual of Systematic Bacteriology* (Hardie 1986a,b,c, Rotta 1986), and is a result of the application of molecular and chemotaxonomic approaches to this group of bacteria. A comprehensive discussion of the history of streptococcal taxonomy has been provided by Jones (1978).

The slow development of a satisfactory taxonomy of streptococci is due, to a large extent, to an overriding belief in serological reactions and haemolytic activities as reliable taxonomic criteria. Although serological grouping based on cell wall carbohydrates has been a valuable tool when applied to the more pathogenic streptococci, as originally intended by Lancefield

(1933), this approach was less successful and sometimes misleading for the rest of the streptococci, in which group-specific antigens may be absent or shared by several distinct taxa. The same limitations apply to haemolysis. Although type of haemolysis is a useful marker in the initial recognition and examination of clinical isolates (Table 28.1) it is important to recognize that differences occur within species and that reactions depend on incubation procedures, and the origin of the blood incorporated in the agar.

10.1 Intrageneric structure

Comparative analyses of 16S rRNA sequences of members of the genus *Streptococcus* have revealed interesting phylogenetic relationships between species and an intrageneric structure with correlation to pathogenic properties and ecology (Whiley et al. 1990b, Williams and Collins 1990, Bentley et al. 1991, Kawamura et al. 1995a). The subdivision of the genus into 6 major clusters based on 16S rRNA sequences (Fig. 28.5) corroborates results of studies based on nucleic acid hybridization, and numerical taxonomic analyses (Carlsson 1968, Colman and Williams 1972, Coykendall and Specht 1975, Coykendall and Munzenmaier 1978, Bridge and Sneath 1983, Kilpper-Bälz and Schleifer 1984, 1987, Kilpper-Bälz, Wenzig and Schleifer 1985, Coykendall, Wesbecher and Gustavson 1987, Whiley and Hardie 1989, Whiley et al. 1990a, Whiley and Beighton 1991).

The 6 clusters are:

1. the pyogenic group consisting predominantly of β-haemolytic species that are pathogenic in humans or animal species
2. the anginosus group of streptococci found in the human oral cavity, gastrointestinal and genital tracts and sometimes isolated from infections
3. the mitis group which includes the pathogen *S. pneumoniae* and several oral streptococci
4. the salivarius group consisting of both dairy streptococci and species found in the human oral cavity
5. the bovis group of species inhabiting the intestinal canal of several animal species and sometimes humans
6. the mutans group of streptococci which exclusively colonize tooth surfaces of humans and a number of animal species.

Species not related to any particular group are *S. suis, S. acidominimus* and the only distantly related *S. pleomorphus* (Fig. 28.5). Additional species that have not yet been sufficiently examined are *S. crista, S. ferus, S. intestinalis* and *S. caprinus.*

PYOGENIC GROUP

Ten species can be distinguished within the pyogenic group of streptococci. The classic pathogens *S. pyogenes* and *S. agalactiae* are well-defined species that present no taxonomic problems. *S. canis* is a species proposed by Devriese et al. (1986) for streptococci isolated from dogs and cows and possessing the group G antigen.

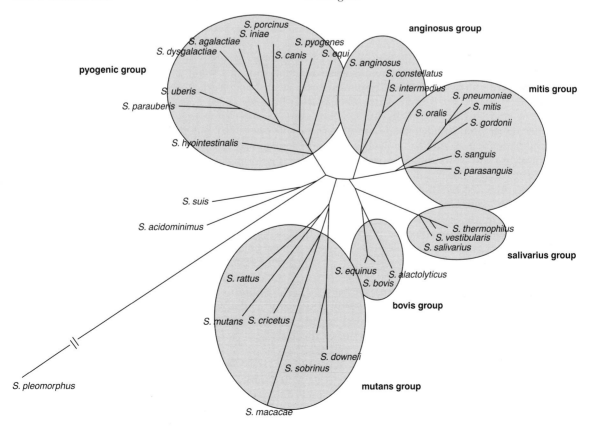

Fig. 28.5 Phylogenetic relationships of *Streptococcus* species. Distances were calculated by the neighbour-joining (NJ) method (Kawamura et al. 1995a) (reprinted with permission).

The taxonomic situation of several of the other species in this group has been confused. *S. dysgalactiae* was originally proposed for certain distinct streptococci causing bovine mastitis (Diernhofer 1932). For reasons that remain unclear the species was not included on the 'Approved lists of bacterial names' published in 1980 (Skerman, McGowan and Sneath 1980), but the name was later revived to accommodate exclusively α-haemolytic group C strains of bovine origin (Garvie, Farrow and Collins 1983). Several studies have demonstrated that the species should include also human isolates of group C streptococci previously designated '*S. equisimilis*' as well as certain streptococci that possess the group G (large colony type) or L antigens (Feltham 1979, Farrow and Collins 1984b, Kilpper-Bälz and Schleifer 1984). Historically, the name '*S. equisimilis*' was given to human isolates resembling *S. equi*, but the name has had no formal standing since 1980 (Skerman, McGowan and Sneath 1980) although it is still often used in the literature and by many clinical microbiologists. Thus, the species *S. dysgalactiae*, as currently defined, includes streptococci both from humans and from various animal species. It has been clear, however, that such strains, although genetically closely related, may differ, not only in their ecological preferences, but also in their biochemical activities (Devriese et al. 1991, Efstratiou et al. 1994). This situation has recently been resolved by the demonstration of 2 mutually distinct and genetically homogeneous clusters consisting of animal and human isolates respectively (Vandamme et al. 1996). The 2 clusters have been proposed as separate subspecies, i.e. *S. dysgalactiae* subsp. *dysgalactiae* and *S. dysgalactiae* subsp. *equisimilis*. Subspecies *dysgalactiae* accommodates strains of animal origin, with group C or L antigens, and α-, β-, or no haemolysis, whereas subspecies *equisimilis* includes human isolates with group C or G antigens and is invariably β-haemolytic. The adaptation of the latter subspecies to the human host is reflected in the fact that it shows streptokinase activity on human plasminogen and proteolytic activity on human fibrin in contrast to animal isolates belonging in subsp. *dysgalactiae*. The 2 subspecies can, furthermore, be differentiated by whole cell protein electrophoretic patterns and biochemical properties. One may argue that it would be practical and in agreement with current clinical usage to give the 2 taxa status of separate species, as originally proposed, as *S. dysgalactiae* and *S. equisimilis*, respectively.

Like '*S. equisimilis*', the species '*S. zooepidemicus*' was not included on the 'Approved lists of bacterial names' (Skerman, McGowan and Sneath 1980). This is justified on the grounds that '*S. zooepidemicus*' is genetically closely related to *S. equi*, which also carries the group C antigen, and has been proposed as a subspecies of that species (Feltham 1979, Farrow and Collins 1984b).

As described, streptococci that react with Lancefield group C antiserum may belong to *S. dysgalactiae* (both subspecies) and *S. equi* (both subspecies). These are often referred to as 'large colony-forming group C streptococci' in contrast to members of the anginosus group (see p. 641), some of which also carry the group C antigen, but form small ('minute') colonies. Likewise, streptococci with the group G antigen may belong to *S. dysgalactiae* subsp. *equisimilis*, *S. canis*, or *S. intestinalis* which form large colonies, but also to members of the anginosus group, which form small colonies. Although it is clear that streptococci belonging to these groups cause various disease in humans and animals (Jelinková and Kubin 1974, Carmeli and Ruoff 1995), the exact role of the individual species, in particular in human infections, remains obscured by the failure to differentiate between them in most clinical studies. The species *S. porcinus* was established to accommodate β-haemolytic pyogenic streptococci with a distinct phenotypic profile that are usually associated with infections in swine (Collins et al. 1984). Although it is infrequently isolated from human infections, recent findings suggest that it may become more prevalent in infections with a genitourinary source (Facklam et al. 1995b). Porcine isolates may carry Lancefield group E, P, U, V or other non-recognized antigens, whereas human isolates appear to be serologically distinct. Streptococci now included in the species *S. porcinus* have previously been referred to as '*Streptococcus infrequens*', '*Streptococcus lentus*', '*Streptococcus subacidus*', or 'Lancefield group E, P, U or V streptococci'.

S. uberis is one of the important aetiologic agents of bovine mastitis, first recognized by Diernhofer (1932). Subsequent studies demonstrated that the species included 2 distinct genetic groups ('*S. uberis* type I and II') which are now recognized as *S. uberis* and *S. parauberis*, respectively (Williams and Collins 1990). In contrast to most other streptococci in the pyogenic group *S. uberis* and *S. parauberis* are α- or non-haemolytic. Some strains have been shown to react with Lancefield group E, P, or G antisera (Garvie and Bramley 1979).

S. hyointestinalis is the name proposed by Devriese, Klipper-Bälz and Schleifer (1988) for α-haemolytic streptococci that may be isolated from the intestinal tract of pigs and are phenotypically distinct from both *S. porcinus* and *S. intestinalis* which have the same ecological niche.

The species '*S. shiloi*', which was proposed to accommodate streptococci causing septicemia in fish, has been shown to be identical to *S. iniae* and the name may be considered a junior synonym of *S. iniae* (Eldar et al. 1995). *S. iniae* is the name given to pyogenic streptococci isolated from abscesses on the thorax and abdomen of freshwater dolphins (*Inia geoffrensis*) living in the Amazon river (Pier and Madin 1976) but has been found to be pathogenic for other animals also.

ANGINOSUS GROUP

The anginosus group has been a source of considerable confusion, partly as a result of lack of international consensus on nomenclature (Facklam 1984) and partly because it has been difficult to identify reliable phenotypic differences between taxa within the group (Jones 1978, Kilian, Mikkelsen and

Henrichsen 1989, Taketoshi et al. 1993). European and Japanese microbiologists have used the term '*Streptococcus milleri*' to embrace all members of the group, whereas North American workers have used various terms such as '*Streptococcus* MG-*intermedius*' and '*Streptococcus anginosus-constellatus*' (Facklam 1984). Dependent on methods employed, DNA–DNA hybridization studies have concluded that the group includes from 1–3 distinct species (Welborn et al. 1983, Coykendall, Wesbecher and Gustafson 1987, Schleifer and Kilpper-Bälz 1987, Whiley and Hardie 1989). The currently recognized proposal, which is supported by 16S rRNA sequence data, and to some extent by phenotypic differences, is that the group includes 3 distinct species: *S. anginosus*, *S. constellatus* and *S. intermedius* (Whiley and Hardie 1989, Whiley and Beighton 1991, Bentley, Leigh and Collins 1991). DNA–DNA reassociation studies (Kilpper-Bälz et al. 1984, Whiley and Hardie 1989) and 16S rRNA gene sequence data (Bentley, Leigh and Collins 1991) reveal that *S. constellatus* and *S. intermedius* are closely related (Fig. 28.5). Curiously, *S. intermedius* is phenotypically quite distinct, whereas *S. constellatus* and *S. anginosus* may be difficult to differentiate on the basis of biochemical reactivities (Whiley et al. 1990b).

It is likely that future studies will disclose additional distinct species within this group of streptococci. Thus, Bergman et al. (1995) described a group of streptococci that belong in the anginosus group but are distinct from the 3 existing species based on 16S rRNA gene sequences. These strains form characteristic spreading colonies on agar plates. Likewise, a recent study by Whiley and coworkers (1995) of 16S–23S rRNA intergenic spacer sequences among bacteria belonging to this group show heterogeneity and suggest additional distinct taxa.

The 3 species are members of the resident microflora of the human mouth, and gastrointestinal and genital tracts (Frandsen, Pedrazzoli and Kilian 1991, Whiley et al. 1993). They show considerable phenotypic and antigenic heterogeneity and include strains that react with group A, C, F or G antisera (Table 28.1). Such strains are often referred to as 'minute (or small) colony type' strains of the respective serological groups.

The group has been referred to by various terms such as 'the milleri streptococci' or '*Streptococcus milleri* group (SMG)'. Use of the term 'anginosus group' as suggested by Kawamura et al. (1991a) is to be preferred as it may eliminate much of the confusion.

MITIS GROUP

Although *S. pneumoniae* has previously been placed among the pyogenic streptococci (Rotta 1986) 16S rRNA sequences and nucleic acid hybridization data show that it is closely related to *S. oralis* and *S. mitis* (Welborn et al. 1983, Klipper-Bälz, Wenzig and Schleifer 1985, Bentley, Leigh and Collins 1991), in agreement with the distinct cell wall composition of the 3 species among all the streptococcal species. In addition to these 3 species, the mitis group includes *S. sanguis*, *S. gordonii*, *S. parasanguis*, and presumably

S. crista (Table 28.1). All species are primarily associated with humans, but closely similar, though not necessarily identical, species may be isolated from the upper respiratory tract of various animal species (Dent, Hardie and Bowden 1978).

For many years this group of streptococci has been curiously refractory to satisfactory taxonomic solutions. The individual species have been poorly defined and several synonyms have been applied to the same species. A further source of confusion in many published studies was that the type strain of *S. mitis* did not conform with the description of the species (Welborn et al. 1983, Kilian, Mikkelsen and Henrichsen 1989). The strain was subsequently identified as an atypical *S. gordonii* and has been replaced by another type (Kilian, Mikkelsen and Henrichsen 1989). For a historical account of the nomenclature of the recognized species and a list of synonyms applied to them, the reader is referred to previous publications (Coykendall 1989, Kilian, Mikkelsen and Henrichsen 1989).

The present taxonomy of the oral members of the mitis group is the result of numerous phenotypic and genetic studies (Carlsson 1968, Colman and Williams 1972, Coykendall and Specht 1975, Coykendall and Munzenmaier 1978, Welborn et al. 1983, Klipper-Bälz, Wenzig and Schleifer 1985, Schmidhuber, Klipper-Bälz, and Schleifer 1987, Kilian, Mikkelsen and Henrichsen 1989).

Two new species genetically related to but distinct from *S. sanguis* and present in the human oral cavity have been described, *S. crista* and *S. parasanguis*. The description of *S. crista* (Handley et al. 1991) was based on the examination of 4 isolates that were characterized by laterally positioned tufted fibrils. These bacteria have previously been referred to as '*S. sanguis* I with tufted fibrils', the 'CR group', or the 'tufted-fibril group'. They show phenotypic resemblance to *S. mitis* biovar 2 (Table 28.3). *S. parasanguis* is the name proposed for some oral atypical streptococci related to *S. sanguis* (Whiley et al. 1990a).

SALIVARIUS GROUP

The 3 species in the salivarius group, *S. salivarius*, *S. thermophilus*, and *S. vestibularis*, are genetically closely related and are usually non-haemolytic. *S. salivarius* is a member of the resident microflora of mucosal membranes of the human oral cavity and pharynx (Carlsson 1967, Frandsen, Pedrazzoli and Kilian 1991). It produces characteristic large mucoid colonies (2–3 mm) on sucrose-containing media as a result of the production of extracellular fructan (levan). It usually does not colonize tooth surfaces like other oral streptococci (Nyvad and Kilian 1990), but occasional strains which produce insoluble glucan in addition to fructan may do so. These strains show characteristic large rough colonies on sucrose-containing media.

S. salivarius is genetically homogeneous but phenotypically heterogenous (Coykendall and Gustafson 1985, Beighton, Hardie and Whiley 1991). It is distinct from *S. thermophilus* which may be isolated from milk products (Bridge and Sneath 1983) although the latter species was temporarily included in the species *S. salivarius* as 'subspecies *thermophilus*' on the basis of their close genetic relationship (Farrow and Collins 1984a).

The species *S. vestibularis* (Whiley and Hardie 1988) resembles *S. salivarius* in its ecological preferences and biochemical characteristics but does not produce extracellular polysaccharide.

BOVIS GROUP

The bovis group includes 3 species, *S. bovis*, *S. equinus* and *S. alactolyticus*. The former 2 species occur in the intestinal tract of cows, horses, sheep and other ruminants. *S. bovis* sometimes also occurs in the human intestinal tract and is occasionally isolated from blood of patents with endocarditis with and underlying colonic disorder, such as malignancy or peridiverticulitis. Both phenotypic and genetic analyses of the type strains of *S. bovis* and *S. equinus* have demonstrated their close relationship, suggesting that the 2 species should be combined in a single species, *S. equinus*, which has priority (Farrow et al. 1984). This is supported by the close identity of 16S rRNA sequences (Ludwig et al. 1985, Bentley, Leigh and Collins 1991) as illustrated in Fig. 28.5. However, it is also recognized that the species *S. bovis*, as currently defined, is genetically very heterogenous (Farrow et al. 1984, Coykendall and Gustafson 1985, Knight and Shlaes 1985). This heterogeneity may cover differences between strains of human and animal origin.

The third species in the group, *S. alactolyticus*, was proposed by Farrow et al. (1984) for porcine and chicken isolates that resemble *S. bovis*.

MUTANS GROUP

The mutans group includes 7 species which exclusively colonize tooth surfaces in humans and in some animal species. The name *S. mutans* was first applied by Clarke (1924) to strongly acidogenic streptococci isolated from carious lesions in humans. These streptococci were able to induce carious lesions in extracted teeth and were considered by Clarke to be the cause of dental caries. Attempts to subdivide the species by serological means based on cell wall carbohydrates disclosed 8 serotypes (a–h) (Bratthall 1970, Perch, Kjems and Ravn 1974, Beighton, Russell and Hayday 1981). This was followed by the discovery of an unexpected degree of genetic heterogeneity (Coykendall 1971) which eventually led to the recognition of 7 separate species including species encompassing strains isolated from monkeys and rodents (Table 28.1) (Coykendall 1977 1983, Beighton, Russell and Hayday 1984, Whiley, Russell and Hardie 1988). The 7 species and their primary habitat are listed in Table 28.1. Phenotypically the mutans group of streptococci is relatively homogeneous, but several studies have shown species-associated differences in cell wall carbohydrates reflected in serotypes, cell wall peptidoglycan type (Table 28.1), and other characteristics (Hamada et al. 1986).

OTHER *STREPTOCOCCUS* SPECIES

S. suis is an important pathogen of pigs. The species was proposed by Elliott in 1966 (see Kilpper-Bälz and Schliefer 1987) and includes streptococci that carry the group D or related antigens. It is encapsulated, and more than 30 capsular serotypes have been detected. The antigens previously referred to as Lancefield group R, S and T antigens are capsular polysaccharides that characterize capsular serotypes 2, 1 and 15 respectively (Perch, Pedersen and Henrichsen 1983, Gottschalk et al. 1989). *S. suis* may cause meningitis, septicaemia, arthritis and bronchopneumonia in pig, and may also be found in the nasal cavity and tonsils of healthy pigs. It is a zoonotic cause of rare cases of meningitis in humans, most of which occur in slaughterhouse workers (Hampson et al. 1993).

DNA–rRNA hybridization and 16S rRNA sequence studies have confirmed that *S. acidominimus* is a member of the genus *Streptococcus* but it does not cluster with any of the other species in the genus (Kilpper-Bälz, Wenzig and Schleifer 1985, Bentley, Leigh and Collins 1991). The species is associated with cattle and differs from other *Streptococcus* species by being weakly acidogenic. *S. caprinus* is a recently observed species of streptococcus that inhabits the digestive tract of wild goats (Brooker et al. 1994).

11 LABORATORY ISOLATION AND IDENTIFICATION

All the *Streptococcus* species, except for *S. thermophilus*, grow well on blood agar incubated at 37°C in air plus carbon dioxide or anaerobically. Species of clinical significance will usually predominate even when members of the resident microflora are present. The pyogenic streptococci are detected initially by their haemolytic activity. Colonies of β-haemolytic streptococci on blood agar may resemble those of *Haemophilus parahaemolyticus*, but the 2 are easily distinguished upon subculture and Gram's staining. Colonies of the α-haemolytic pneumococci are smooth and may vary in size according to the amount of capsular polysaccharide produced; those of serotype 3 are usually larger than the rest and have a watery or mucoid appearance. During prolonged incubation, the centre of the colony becomes depressed as a result of autolysis.

Once it has been established that the isolates are catalase-negative, gram-positive cocci a tendency to form chains they are identified by a combination of serological and biochemical examinations. The essential discriminatory tests for the pyogenic group of streptococci and *S. suis* are summarized in Table 28.2. An additional test that is helpful in the identification of *S. pyogenes* is the bacitracin sensitivity test. *S. pyogenes* is uniformly sensitive but sensitivity can also be detected in some haemolytic strains of groups C, E, G and L and in *S. suis*. If the end-point is taken as absence of any zone of inhibition, the disc should contain 0.04 units of bacitracin. *S. pyogenes* will give a zone of diameter ≥ 11 mm around a 6 mm disc containing 0.1 unit of bacitracin. The bacitracin sensitivity test should not be performed on primary culture plates. Comprehensive lists of the characteristics of pyogenic and other streptococci have been compiled by Hardie and Whiley (1995).

Pneumococci are not readily identified by biochemical tests but can in most cases be identified on the basis of their sensitivity to optochin, bile solubility and autolysis. Pneumococci are uniformly sensitive to optochin (ethylhydrocupreine) which provides a valuable means of distinguishing pneumococci from other α-haemolytic streptococci. The test can be performed conveniently with a paper disc containing 5 µg optochin. Some of the oral streptococci may show small zones of inhibition.

All capsulate pneumococci, but not all non-capsulate variants, are lysed by bile. The bile, or other detergents, activates the autolysin *N*-acetylmuramyl-L-alanine amidase which results in the lysis of cultures of pneumococci by attacking the peptidoglycan. Presumptive identification of pneumococci may furthermore be achieved by the demonstration of a reaction in so-called 'omni-serum' which is a concentrate of pooled typing sera (Lund and Henrichsen 1978). Non-capsulate strains of *S. pneumoniae* may show atypical biochemical reactions (Pease, Douglas and Spencer 1986) and may be difficult to distinguish from *S. mitis*.

Oral streptococci are often examined on the selective medium Mitis Salivarius agar on which some species produce extracellular polysaccharide from sucrose in the medium resulting in characteristic colonies. *S. salivarius* produces large (2–3 mm) soft and glossy colonies which collapse after prolonged incubation. Mutans streptococci produce hard adherent colonies resembling frosted glass. Drops of extracellular polysaccharide often accumulate on the top or at the side of the colonies (Fig. 28.2). Colonies of the polysaccharide-producing *S. sanguis*, *S. gordonii* and *S. oralis* are regular, dome-shaped, smooth, hard and adherent, and indistinguishable. The species that do not produce extracellular polysaccharides (*S. mitis*, *S. parasanguis*, *S. crista*, *S. anginosus*, *S. intermedius*, *S. constellatus*, *S. vestibularis*) form flat or raised uncharacteristic colonies. Biochemical reactivities important for the identification of oral streptococci are summarized in Table 28.3. Characteristics that allow differentiation of biovars of *S. sanguis* and *S. gordonii* have been published by Kilian, Mikkelesen and Henrichsen (1989), and tests that allow differentiation of species within the mutans group and genotypes within *S. bovis* have been compiled by Hardie and Whiley (1995).

Commercial kits are available for the rapid identification of *Streptococcus* species. Evaluations demonstrate good agreements with traditional methods although there are problems with several new species, for which data are either incomplete or lacking in the identification data bases (Freney et al. 1992, Kikuchi et al. 1995). Identification of streptococci may also be achieved with DNA probes that hybridize exclusively with the respective species (Schmidhuber, Ludwig and Schleifer 1988, Bentley and Leigh 1995, Jacobs et al. 1996).

12 BACTERIOCINS AND BACTERIOPHAGES

12.1 Bacteriocins

Many strains of streptococci produce **bacteriocin-like inhibitory substances** (BLIS) which inhibit growth of a wide range of bacteria (Tagg 1992). One example is the intensely investigated nicin produced by some *Lactococcus lactis* strains. Nicin has a long history of application in food preservation, especially of dairy products (Jack, Tagg and Bibek 1995). BLIS activity among *Streptococcus* species associated with humans and animals are believed to play a role in their ability to interfere with growth of other bacteria in their local environment along with other released inhibitory substances such as hydrogen peroxide and lactic acid (Rogers, Van der Hoeven and Mikx 1978, Jack, Tagg and Bibek 1995).

BLIS activity has been detected in several *Streptococcus* species, with the highest prevalence among *S. salivarius* and other oral streptococci (Kelstrup and Gibbons 1969, Dempster and Tagg 1982). A survey of clinical isolates of *S. pyogenes* revealed BLIS activity in approximately 10% of strains (Tagg, Read and McGiven 1971). The activity is confined to strains of particular M types, and the overall occurrence within these M types is very high (50–100%). The BLIS of *S. pyogenes* inhibited a wide range of gram-positive bacteria and a single strain of *Prevotella intermedia* (Hynes and Tagg 1985). BLIS activity has also been demonstrated in occasional strains of *S. agalactiae*, *S. dysgalactiae* and *S. equi* (Schofield and Tagg 1983). The majority of BLIS characterized from *Streptococcus* are relatively small (<5 kDa) heat-stable proteins termed **lantibiotics** because they contain the unusual amino acids lanthionine and/or 3-methyllanthionine (Jung 1991, Hynes, Ferretti and Tagg 1993, Ross et al. 1993, Jack, Tagg and Bibek 1995). Some appear to be considerably larger (30 kDa) such as the so-called zoocin A produced by some strains of *S. equi* subspecies *zooepidemicus* (Simmonds et al. 1995), the streptococcin A-M57 of *S. pyogenes* M-type 57 (Simpson and Tagg 1983), and a bacteriocin detected in *S. mutans* (Paul and Slade 1975, Fukushima et al. 1983). Although bacteriocins in many gram-positive bacteria are encoded by plasmid-borne genes neither of the currently documented lantibiotic-producing strains of *S. pyogenes* and *S. salivarius* appears to contain plasmids (Simpson and Tagg 1984).

Bacteriocin production and sensitivity has been used as a fingerprinting method in epidemiological studies of streptococci (Kelstrup et al. 1970, Tagg 1985, Ragland and Tagg 1990).

12.2 Bacteriophages

Two kinds of phages active against streptococci are known: **virulent phages** which attack various strains; and **temperate phages** which lysogenize streptococcal strains and have a narrower host range (Maxted 1964). During the course of a virulent phage infection a

Streptococcus *and* Lactobacillus

Table 28.2 Differential characteristics of the species of the pyogenic group and *S. suis*

Species	Lancefield serogroup	Haemolysis	Hydrolysis of			Presence of				Fermentation of						
			Hip	Aes	Arg	VP	PA	βG	AP	Rib	Man	Sor	Lac	Tre	Inu	Raf
S. pyogenes	A	β	−	V[c]	+	−	+	V	+	−	V	−	+	+	−	−
S. agalactiae	B	β (CAMP+)	+	−	+	+	−	V	+	+	−	−	V	+	−	−
S. equi subsp. *equi*	C	β	−	−	+	−	−	+	+	−	−	−	−	−	−	−
S. equi subsp. *zooepidemicus*	C	β	−	V	+	−	−	+	+	V	−	+	+	−	−	−
S. dysgalactiae subsp. *dysgalactiae*	C, L	α, β, −[a]	−	−	+	−	−	+	+	+	−	+	+	+	−	−
S. dysgalactiae subsp. *equisimilis*	C, G	β	−	V	+	−	−	+	+	+	−	−	V	+	−	−
S. canis	G	β (CAMP+)[b]	−	V	+	−	−	+	+	+	−	−	V	+	−	−
S. iniae	−	β, α	−	+	NT[d]	NT	NT	NT	NT	NT	+	−	−	+	−	−
S. porcinus	E, P, U, V³, −	β (CAMP+)	−	+	+	+	+	+	+	+	+	+	V	+	−	−
S. uberis	−, E	α	+	+	+	+	+	+	V	+	+	+	+	+	+	−
S. parauberis	−, E	α	V	+	+	+	+	−	+	+	+	+	+	+	V	V
S. hyointestinals	−	α	−	+	−	+	−	−	−	−	−	−	+	+	NT	NT
S. suis	D	β, α, −	−	+	+	−	V	+	−	−	−	−	+	V	V	V

Abbreviations: Aes, aesculine; AP, alkaline phosphatase; *Arg*, arginine; βG, β-glucuronidase; Hip, hippurate; Inu, inulin; Lac, lactose; Man, mannitol; VP, production of acetoin; PA, pyrrolydonyl-amylamidase; Raf raffinose; Rib, ribose; Sor, sorbitol; Tre, trehalose.
[a]Bovine strains are never β-haemolytic.
[b]Only canine strains are CAMP positive.
[c]V, variable.
[d]NT, not tested.

Table 28.3 Differential characteristics of species of the *mitis*, *anginosus*, *salivarius*, *mutans* and *bovis* groups

Species	Production of	Hydrolysis of		Presence of									Fermentation of				
	EP[a]	Aes	Arg	VP	H$_2$O$_2$	IP	Ne	AP	βG	αF	αG	Hy	Amy	Arb	Inu	Man	Sor
S. mitis biovar 1	−	−	−	−	+	V	V	V	−	−	V	−	−	−	V	−	−
S. mitis biovar 2	−	−	+	−	+	−	−	V	−	−	+	−	−	−	−	−	V
S. oralis	G	−	−	−	+	+	+	+	+	−	+	+	−	−	−	−	−
S. pneumoniae	−	A	−	−	+	+	+	−	+	V	+	+	−	−	+	·	−
S. crista	−	V	+	−	+	−	−	−	V	+	−	−	−	−	−	−	−
S. sanguis	G	V	+	−	+	+	−	V	+	+	+	−	−	+	+	−	V
S. gordonii	G	+	+	−	+	+	−	−	+	+	−	V	−	+	+	+	−
S. parasanguis	−	A	+	−	−	−	−	A	+	A	−	−	V	A	−	−	−
S. anginosus	−	+	+	+	+	−	−	+	−	−	−	−	+	+	−	V	−
S. constellatus	−	+	+	+	V	−	−	+	−	−	−	V	V	+	−	−	−
S. intermedius	−	+	+	+	−	−	+	+	+	+	V	+	V	+	−	−	−
S. salivarius	F	+	−	V	−	−	−	+	−	−	+	−	+	V	V	−	−
S. vestibularis	−	V	−	V	−	−	−	−	−	−	V	−	V	V	−	−	−
S. thermophilus	NT	−	−	V	−	−	NT	−	−	−	V	NT	−	V	V	−	−
Mutans group	G	−	V	+	V	+	−	−	−	+	+	−	V	+	−	+	V
S. bovis	V	+	NT[2]	+	−	−	NT	NT	NT	NT	NT	NT	NT	V	−	V	NT
S. equinus	−	+	+	+	NT	−	NT	NT	NT	NT	NT	NT	NT	+	V	−	NT
S. alactolyticus	−	V	−	+	NT	−	NT	NT	−	NT	NT	NT	NT	V	V	V	NT

Abbreviations: Aes, aesculine hydrolysis; αF, α-L-fucosidase; αG, α-N-glucosidase; Amy, amygdalin; AP, alkaline phosphatase; Arb, arbutin; Arg, arginine hydrolysis; βG, β-glucosaminidase; EP, extracellular polysaccharide; Inu, inulin; IP, IgA1 protease; Ne, neuraminidase; Hy, hyaluronidase; Man, mannitol; Sor, sorbitol; VP, production of acetoin.
[a]G, glucan; F, fructan; V, variable.
[b]NT, not tested.

lysozyme-like lytic enzyme (phage-associated lysin) is produced. One such enzyme produced by phages infecting group C streptococci is able to degrade the cell wall peptidoglycan of *S. pyogenes* and has been extensively employed in procedures for isolation of wall-associated proteins in that species (Fischetti 1989).

Many *Streptococcus* species including *S. pyogenes*, *S. agalactiae* and *S. pneumoniae* are usually lysogenic may carry 2–3 prophages. Phage-associated genes encode various virulence factors (see p. 652) (Zabriskie, Read and Fischetti 1972).

13 ROLE IN NORMAL HUMAN FLORA

Soon after birth, streptococci comprise a considerable proportion of the commensal microflora of human mucosal membranes of the upper respiratory tract and female genital tract. Almost half of the bacteria that can be isolated from oral mucosae and from saliva are streptococci. These are primarily the streptococci of the mitis (except *S. pneumoniae*) and salivarius groups. Each of the species in these groups shows a characteristic predilection for specific sites. While *S. salivarius* and *S. mitis* biovar 2 predominate on the tongue surface and in the pharynx, others such as *S. sanguis*, *S. oralis* and *S. mitis* colonize tooth surfaces and the buccal and pharyngeal mucosa (Carlsson 1967, Carlsson et al. 1970, Gibbons and van Houte 1971, Hardie and Bowen 1974, Nyvad and Kilian 1990, Frandsen, Pedrazzoli and Kilian 1991, Pearce et al. 1995). The 3 species of the anginosus group are found in dental plaque and in the intestinal canal (Whiley et al. 1992). The mutans streptococci colonize exclusively tooth surfaces and are not found in the oral cavity until after tooth eruption. They may be found in high proportions in dental plaque associated with caries lesions. The extensive literature on the mutans streptococci and their aetiological implications in dental caries have been reviewed by Hamada et al. (1986).

The commensal streptococci of the respiratory tract play an important role in preventing colonization by potentially pathogenic bacteria including *S. pyogenes*, partly owing to their secretion of bacteriocins (Ross et al. 1993, Jack, Tagg and Bibek 1995). Some of these commensal streptococci (*S. sanguis*, *S. oralis* and *S. mitis*) release IgA1 protease and may theoretically interfere with the protective function of secretory IgA. Significantly increased proportions of IgA1 protease-producing *S. mitis* have been demonstrated in the pharynx of infants who develop atopic disease (Kilian et al. 1995).

S. pyogenes is almost totally restricted to humans. The carrier rate of *S. pyogenes* in the respiratory tract is only a few percent in adults and just over 10% in children attending kindergarten. It may be considerably higher before or during an epidemic (Hoffman 1985).

The intestinal tract appears to be the primary habitat of *S. agalactiae* and the main source of vaginal colonization (Ross 1970, Jelinková 1977). In a large longitudinal study, Dillon, Khare and Gray (1987) documented carriage in 18% of women by anorectal culture and in 4% by vaginal culture. During the second and third trimesters of pregnancy carriage rates were 31% and 38%, respectively. However, only 17% were carriers in both trimesters, which suggests that colonization is short-lived.

Pneumococci may be detected in the nasopharynx of 10–20% of healthy adults but constitute only a minor part of the microflora. When infants are studied prospectively, nearly all are found to be colonized with pneumococci on at least one occasion in the first 2 years of life (Gray, Converse and Dillon 1980). During episodes of disease, for example otitis media, pneumococci often predominate in the microflora of the upper respiratory tract. In developing countries rates exceeding 90% have been documented.

14 PATHOGENICITY AND VIRULENCE FACTORS

The description here of streptococcal virulence factors focuses mainly on those demonstrated in the principal human pathogens *S. pyogenes*, *S. agalactiae* and *S. pneumoniae*. Closely related factors are produced by several of the other species in the group and will only be mentioned. For a complete historical account of the virulence factors the reader is referred to the 8th edition of this book (Colman 1990).

14.1 *S. pyogenes*

S. pyogenes is among the most prevalent human pathogens, capable of causing various severe suppurative skin and mucosal infections, necrotizing fasciitis, scarlet fever and non-suppurative sequelae such as streptococcal glomerulonephritis and rheumatic fever. Since the mid-1980s, a resurgence in severe streptococcal infections and a high mortality rate due to streptococcal sepsis and toxic shock-like syndrome have been reported (Veasy et al. 1987, Colman et al. 1993). Numerous virulence factors that are potentially involved in the different types of disease have been described.

M AND M-LIKE PROTEINS
M protein

The ability of *S. pyogenes* to persist in infected tissues is due primarily to the cell surface-exposed M protein (Lancefield 1928), a molecule which confers to *S. pyogenes* the ability to resist phagocytosis by polymorphonuclear leukocytes in the absence of specific antibodies. Resistance to infections by *S. pyogenes* appears to be related to the presence of antibodies in secretions and sera to the M protein molecule (Lancefield 1959, Bessen et al. 1988). However, as there are approximately 100 different serotypes of M proteins (M1, M2, M3, etc.), though not all with antiphagocytic properties (see p. 650), individuals may suffer from recurrent *S. pyogenes* infections with strains expressing different serotypes of the M protein.

The M protein may be detected by electron microscopy on the surface of *S. pyogenes* cells as fibrils protruding up to 200 nm outwards from the cell (Swanson, Hsu and Gotschlich 1969). However, the protein is anchored in the cytoplasmic membrane and spans the entire cell wall. Each fibre consists of a dimeric M protein molecule, which, with few exceptional domains, has an α-helical coiled-coil structure with a 7-residue periodicity (Fischetti 1989). The major part of the M protein is composed of several sequence repeat regions designated by capital letters (A, B, C) (Fig. 28.6). The number of A and B tandem repeats within each region varies.

The N-terminal 25% of the M protein molecule, which is distal to the cell surface, represents a hypervariable region as a result of the above-mentioned variation in the number of repeats combined with diversity generated by intergenic recombination involving slightly different repeats (Hollingshead, Fischetti and Scott 1987) and horizontal gene transfer involving related genes (see below) (Whatmore and Kehoe 1994). The C-terminal half, which includes the wall-spanning region, is considerably more conserved and shows homology with several proteins in other gram-positive bacteria such as staphylococcal protein A (Fischetti 1989).

The short non-helical region at the exposed N-terminal end is distinct in size and sequence from one M type to another but is highly conserved within an M type (this sequence is lacking in M49). Antibodies to this part of the molecule effectively opsonize the streptococci for phagocytosis.

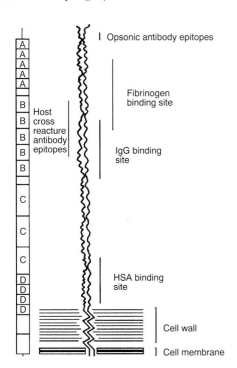

Fig. 28.6 Structure of an M protein and its gene. The diagram to the left illustrates the gene encoding the M6 protein with the characteristic A, B, C and D repeats (Fischetti 1989). The location of the functional domains in the protein are indicated on the protein shown to the right.

The majority of M proteins can be divided into 2 major classes. Those of Class I share surface-exposed antigenic epitopes with the C repeat region of M6 proteins, whereas Class II M proteins are deficient in such cross-reactive epitopes. The latter are associated with strains that produce **opacity factor**, a lipoproteinase whose activity induces increased opalescence of serum (Bessen et al. 1989). Although both classes are associated with suppurative infections and glomerulonephritis the majority of strains associated with outbreaks of rheumatic fever express M proteins of Class I (Bessen and Fischetti 1989). This association is supported by the recent observation that rheumatic fever patients display elevated levels of serum IgG antibodies to the Class I-specific epitope but lack immunoreactivity to the Class II epitope (Bessen et al. 1995).

Recent studies with M-positive and M-negative isogenic strains have demonstrated that the M protein is not an adhesin but may promote bacterial accumulation at the site of infection as a result of coaggregation between bacterial cells, presumably mediated by interactions with host proteins (Caparon et al. 1991). Some M proteins display receptors for human fibrinogen, β_2-microglobulin, factor H of the alternative complement cascade, IgG of various subclasses and serum albumin (Kronvall, Schonbeck and Myhre 1979, Rýc, Beachy and Whitnack 1989, Johansson et al. 1994, Retnoningrum and Cleary 1994).

Proteins closely related to or identical to M proteins have been demonstrated in several other pyogenic streptococci such as *S. agalactiae*, *S. equi* and *S. dysgalactiae* (Woolcock 1974, Bisno, Craven and McCabe 1987, Jones and Fischetti 1987, Fischetti 1989, Simpson et al. 1992, Schnitzler et al. 1995) and in *S. sanguis* (Demuth, Golub and Malamud 1990).

M-like surface proteins

The M protein is one of a family of proteins which share overall structure, homologous sequences, and the ability to interact with various host proteins including immunoglobulins (Kehoe 1994). Like the M protein, many of the other proteins of the family have several functions. Many bind to the Fc region of IgG (Mrp, FcRA) and IgA (Arp) (Frithz, Heden and Lindahl 1989, Heath and Cleary 1989, Lindahl and Åkerström 1989, Gomi et al. 1990, Bessen and Fischetti 1992, O'Toole et al. 1992), and some bind fibrinogen (Mrp), fibronectin, human serum albumin, α_2-macroglobulin, or factor H (ProtH) (Wagner et al. 1986, Horstmann et al. 1992, Frick et al. 1994, Natanson et al. 1995). Although it is believed that these proteins serve immune escape purposes their exact functions in the pathogenesis of *S. pyogenes* infections is not understood.

The distinction between M proteins and M-like proteins is not always clear. Kehoe (1994) has suggested restricting the designation M protein to those type-specific antigens that have been clearly demonstrated to possess antiphagocytic properties.

emm genes

The individual proteins of the M protein family are encoded by genes of the *emm* gene family, which are located in a cluster occupying 3–6 kb between the regulatory gene *mga* (previously *mry/virR*) and the coregulated *scpA* gene encoding C5a peptidase (see below) within the *vir* regulon on the chromosome of *S. pyogenes* (Caparon and Scott 1987, Simpson et al. 1990, Perez-Casal et al. 1991). Most strains contain 1–3 tandemly arranged genes which have evolved through gene duplication followed by sequence and functional divergence (Hollingshead et al. 1994, Kehoe 1994).

Cross-reactions with host tissues

M proteins share physicochemical properties and significant sequence homology with a number of mammalian fibrillar proteins. For example, the M5, M6, M12 and M24 proteins have up to 30% overall sequence homology with myosin heavy chain and type I keratins, and M5, M6 and M24 share a similar level of homology with human α-tropomyosin (Fischetti 1989). Potential common epitopes provide a theoretical basis to explain the induction of cross-reactive antibodies associated with post-streptococcal autoimmune disease in genetically predisposed hosts (Khanna et al. 1989). There is a strong association between autoimmune sequelae and particular M types of *S. pyogenes*. However, there is no clear correlation between rheumatogenic or nephritogenic potential and the pattern of tissue cross-reactivity of antibodies to a particular M type (Robinson and Kehoe 1992).

CAPSULE

Some strains of *S. pyogenes* form a capsule composed of hyaluronic acid, which results in their forming mucoid colonies on blood agar. The capsular material is not immunogenic presumably because it is indistinguishable from the hyaluronic acid of mammalian connective tissues (linear polysaccharide composed of β-1-4-linked repeating disaccharide units of glucuronic acid β-1-3 linked to *N*-acetylglucosamine). The capsule may, in this way, serve antigenic mimicry purposes. The notion that the capsule is a virulence factor is supported by the observation that the capsule is formed by 3% of isolates from patients with uncomplicated pharyngitis, 21% of isolates from severe streptococcal infections and 42% of rheumatic fever isolates (Johnson, Stevens and Kaplan 1992). Among the frequently isolated serotype M1 the prevalence of capsule production is even higher (6, 22 and 80%, respectively). Capsule-producing strains are highly virulent in animal models. Recent studies of capsule-deficient strains constructed by transposon mutagenesis have confirmed that it is an important antiphagocytic factor but that the relative significance of the M protein and the capsule differs among strains (Wessels et al. 1991b, Dale et al. 1996).

Capsule production is encoded by the *HAS* operon, which contains at least 3 genes (*has*A, hyaluronate synthase; *has*B, UDP-glucose dehydrogenase; *has*C, UDP-glucose pyrophosphorylase). The operon appears to be present in all strains of *S. pyogenes* and is also detected in strains of group C streptococci (Crater and Van de Rijn 1995) which sometimes express a hyaluronic acid capsule (*S. equi* but not '*S. equisimilis*'). The capsule is produced in vitro only during exponential growth, but the regulatory mechanisms determining expression of the operon have not been identified.

PROTEIN F

Interaction with host fibronectin has long been considered the mechanism by which *S. pyogenes* adheres to epithelial cells. This notion is supported by the observation that exogenous fibronectin inhibits adherence and that the organism preferentially adheres to fibronectin-coated epithelial cells (Simpson and Beachey 1983, Abraham, Beachey and Simpson 1983). Cloning and mutagenesis studies reveal that fibronectin binding is mediated by a surface protein (MW 120 kDa) known as protein F, which may be considered the adhesin of *S. pyogenes* (Hanski and Caparon 1992).

STREPTOCOCCAL PYROGENIC EXOTOXINS

The intradermal injection of culture filtrate of *S. pyogenes* is followed, in some individuals, by the development of an area of erythema. This reaction (the **Dick test**) is the direct and indirect effect of one or more pyrogenic exotoxins (SPE) produced by *S. pyogenes*. Three different toxins (SPE A, B and C) have been identified, and most strains of *S. pyogenes* produce one or more. The streptococcal pyrogenic exotoxins are members of a family of bacterial pyrogenic toxins, which share biological and biochemical properties. Other members include staphylococcal enterotoxin serotypes A–F, staphylococcal pyrogenic exotoxins A and B and staphylococcal toxic shock syndrome toxin 1. Properties characteristic of this family of toxins are pyrogenicity and a number of effects on the immune system.

The fact that a genetically diverse array of *S. pyogenes* clones expressing many different combinations of the pyrogenic exotoxins is recovered from contemporary invasive disease episodes suggests that no single toxin is responsible for toxic shock-like syndrome (Musser et al. 1991).

SPE A

SPE A is a polypeptide of 221 amino acids released from a somewhat larger precursor. The gene, which occurs in several allelic forms, has been cloned and sequenced and shows extensive homology to the staphylococcal enterotoxins B and C (Johnson, L'Italien and Schlievert 1986, Hynes et al. 1987). The gene was detected in 40% of isolates from cases of scarlet fever in several countries and 16% of isolates from other conditions (Ferretti et al. 1987, Musser et al. 1991). Nontoxigenic strains may be converted to toxin production with a temperate bacteriophage and toxin production appears to depend on lysogeny (Zabriskie, Read and Fischetti, 1972).

Besides being pyrogenic SPE A enhances susceptibility to lethal shock by endotoxins (Kim and Watson 1970), streptolysin O (Schwab, Watson and Cromartie 1955) and other substances. When administered to young rabbits, together with a protein to which they have been sensitized, a skin reaction resembling that seen in scarlet fever patients develops; injection of anti-exotoxin antibodies prevents this reaction (Schlievert, Bettin and Watson 1979). Like the related toxins of *Staphylococcus aureus*, SPE A is a superantigen which explains many of its biological effects (see p. 651).

SPE A is also referred to as erythrogenic exotoxin A, blastogen A, exotoxin A, or scarlet fever toxin.

SPE B

SPE B is different from the 2 other pyrogenic exotoxins in a number of ways. It is released from cells of virtually all *S. pyogenes* strains as a 398 amino acid protein (M_r c. 40 kDa). The protein is subsequently converted into a 253 amino acid protein by proteolysis or autocatalytic truncation which requires reducing conditions (Gerlach et al. 1983, Hauser and Schlievert 1990). The truncated protein is a cysteine proteinase which cleaves a number of host proteins including fibronectin and vitronectin (2 abundant extracellular matrix proteins), and human interleukin-1β precursor to generate biologically active IL-1β, suggesting an important role in inflammation and shock (Kapur et al. 1993a,b). Purified proteinase injected into experimental animals produces myocardial necrosis and death (Keller and Robertson 1954). Its critical role in the pathogenesis of *S. pyogenes* infections is supported by several observations:

1. an inhibitor of cysteine proteinases (*N*-benzyloxycarbonyl-leucyl-valyl-glycine diazomethyl ketone) can cure mice from an otherwise lethal dose of *S. pyogenes* (Björck et al. 1989)
2. immunization of mice with the cysteine proteinase generates protection of mice against intraperitoneal challenge (Kapur et al. 1994)
3. in patients with recent invasive infection there is a significant association between lack of antibody to SPE B and more severe disease course (Holm et al. 1992).

The gene encoding SPE B is highly conserved in the *S. pyogenes* population (Kapur et al. 1993b). Although SPE B is not a superantigen that may exert indirect toxic effects on the host (see below), its proteolytic activity may be directly responsible for the extensive tissue destruction (cellulitis, fasciitis and myositis) observed in many patients with severe invasive and toxic shock-like syndrome. SPE B has previously been referred to as streptococcal proteinase precursor and interleukin-1β convertase.

SPE C

SPE C resembles SPE A in several ways. It is secreted as a precursor which after cleavage attains a size somewhat larger than SPE A. In accordance with the observation that its production is associated with lysogeny the gene (*spe* C) is variably present among *S. pyogenes* strains. Its biological effects are very similar to those of SPE A.

Superantigens

The pyrogenic exotoxins SPE A and SPE C discussed above have so-called superantigen activity. Superantigens share the ability to bind to major histocompatibility complex (MHC) class II molecules to form a complex that interacts with T-cell subsets bearing Vβ regions on their T-cell receptors. This causes T-cell proliferation and the release of cytokines such as interleukins (IL-1, IL-2), tumour necrosis factor α and interferon γ, which are involved in the pathogenesis of shock. Recently, an additional 260 amino acid protein with superantigen activity, **streptococcal superantigen**, has been identified in *S. pyogenes* (Mollick et al. 1993, Reda et al. 1994). The protein shows 60%

identity to staphylococcal enterotoxin B and 49% identity to SPE A. Streptococcal superantigen is expressed only by some evolutionary lineages of *S. pyogenes*, suggesting that the gene has been acquired only relatively recently (Mollick et al. 1993, Reda et al. 1994). Previously reported superantigen activity of SPE B and of M proteins may be ascribed to contamination of the preparations used (Braun et al. 1993).

STREPTOLYSINS

S. pyogenes and many other pyogenic streptococci produce 2 distinct haemolysins, one which is haemolytic in the reduced form and the other is oxygen stable and released in serum-containing media. They have been termed streptolysin O (oxygen labile) and streptolysin S (serum soluble).

Streptolysin O is one of a family of lysins formed by various bacteria including pyogenic streptococci, *S. pneumoniae* (pneumolysin), *Clostridium tetani* (tetanolysin), *C. perfringens* (θ-toxin), *Bacillus cereus* (cereolysin) and *Listeria monocytogenes*. All are activated by sulphydryl compounds and inhibited by cholesterol and related sterols. They are antigenically related (Cowell and Bernheimer 1977) although the similarity is not evident from sequence comparison of the respective genes encoding these toxins (Kehoe and Timmis 1984). The O streptolysin is a protein of approximately 60 kDa (Kehoe et al. 1987).

There is good evidence that streptolysin O binds to cholesterol on the cell surface (Alouf 1980). Erythrocytes of all readily available animal species, except the mouse, are lysed, as are polymorphonuclear leukocytes and platelets.

The exact biological significance of streptolysin O is not known. However, intravenous injection of streptolysin O preparations into mice, rabbits and guineapigs causes death within seconds. Death is the result of an acute toxic action on the heart (Halbert, Bircher and Dahle 1961). It has been suggested that streptolysin O plays a role in the development of rheumatic fever (Gupta et al. 1986). Serum antibodies to streptolysin O can be demonstrated after streptococcal infection, with a frequency that increases with the severity of the infection. The highest titers are found in patients with rheumatic fever.

Streptolysin S is responsible for the β-haemolysis around colonies of most pyogenic streptococci on aerobically incubated blood agar. Most of these oxygen-stable haemolysins of pyogenic streptococci have similar properties, but that produced by *S. agalactiae* is distinct (Marchlewicz and Duncan 1980). The evidence available suggests that streptolysin S is composed of a polypeptide attached to an oligonucleotide (Lai et al. 1978). It has not been possible to demonstrate that streptolysin S is produced in vivo, in part because it is not antigenic.

STREPTOKINASE

Strains of *S. pyogenes* produce a streptokinase also referred to as **fibrinolysin**. It binds to human plasminogen and triggers a conformational change and self-cleavage that results in the formation of the active serine protease plasmin which is responsible for cleavage of fibrin and fibrinogen (Wulf and Mertz 1968). Streptokinase has been referred to as streptococcal spreading factor because of its ability to induce lysis of clots and fibrin deposits that limit areas of infection.

Streptokinase activity has also been detected in *S. dysgalactiae* isolates from infections in humans and various animal species and in isolates of *S. equi*, *S. uberis* and *S. porcinus* (group E). Although these enzymes all bind human plasminogen, their ability to activate is restricted to plasminogen from their own host. *S. dysgalactiae* subsp. *dysgalactiae* (group C) activates equine or porcine plasminogen depending on its origin, whereas strains of *S. dysgalactiae* subsp. *equisimilis* (group C and G) activate human plasminogen (McCoy, Broder and Lottenberg 1991, Vandamme et al. 1996). The streptokinases produced by *S. porcinus* and *S. uberis*, similarly, act only on porcine and bovine plasminogen, respectively (Ellis and Armstrong 1971, Leigh 1993).

The streptokinase from *S. pyogenes* is a 46 kDa extracellular protein encoded by the *ska* gene which has been cloned and sequenced (Ohkuni et al. 1992). There is substantial diversity of the *ska* gene, giving rise to antigenic and chemical diversity (Gerlach and Köhler 1979, Huang, Malke and Ferretti 1989, Reed, Kussie and Parhami-Seren 1993).

C5a peptidase

C5a peptidase is a surface-associated serine proteinase produced by all members of *S. pyogenes*. The enzyme specifically cleaves human C5a, one of the principal chemoattractants of polymorphonuclear leukocytes (Wexler, Chenoweth and Cleary 1985). The enzyme is produced as a precursor protein of approximately 128 kDa which includes membrane and wall-spanning domains (Chen and Cleary 1990). It cleaves a specific Lys-Asp peptide bond near the C-terminus of C5a, thereby destroying its ability to attract of polymorphonuclear leukocytes (O'Connor and Cleary 1987). Neutralizing antibodies to the C5a peptidase can be detected in sera and secretions of patients recovering from *S. pyogenes* infections (O'Connor et al. 1991).

Closely related C5a peptidases are produced by strains of *S. agalactiae* and by certain group G streptococci, presumably *S. dysgalactiae* subsp. *equisimilis* (Cleary et al. 1991, 1992).

Hyaluronidase

Hyaluronidase activity can be detected in virtually all strains of *S. pyogenes*, and antibodies can be detected in human convalescent sera. The activity in some M types of *S. pyogenes* (M12 and M49) is phage-associated (Hynes and Ferretti 1989). Hyaluronidase activity is also present in some strains of *S. agalactiae* (Hauge et al. 1996), *S. equi*, *S. dysgalactiae*, *S. uberis*, *S. suis*, *S. intermedius*, *S. constellatus*, and *S. pneumoniae*, and is often bacteriophage-associated (Schaufuss et al. 1989, Homer et al. 1993). Although the enzyme is believed to be a spreading factor favouring invasion of tissues, there is no direct evidence to support this.

Nucleases

All strains of *S. pyogenes* form at least one DNase. Of the 4 enzymes (A–D) that have been detected (Gray 1972), the B enzyme is the predominant nuclease in *S. pyogenes*. Antibodies to the B nuclease appear after most infections with *S. pyogenes*. Similar nucleases have been demonstrated in strains of group C streptococci.

Neuraminidase

Neuraminidase (sialidase) activity has been detected in *S. pyogenes*, *S. dysgalactiae*, *S. oralis*, *S. intermedius*, and in some strains of *S. mitis* (Hayano, Tanaka and Okuyama 1969, Kilian, Mikkelsen and Henrichsen 1989, Whiley et al. 1990b). In contrast to neuraminidases of *Vibrio cholerae* and clostridia, the streptococcal enzyme acts also on *O*-acetylated sialic acids (Varki and Diaz 1983). The enzyme is a candidate colonization factor for pathogens and commensals that survive on mucosal surfaces.

Serum-opacity factor

Many strains of *S. pyogenes* grown in a medium consisting of 3 parts horse serum to one of broth induce an opalescence of the serum. Top and Wannamaker (1968) demonstrated that production of the opacity factor is closely related to some M types. Subsequent studies have shown that the factor is produced exclusively by strains expressing M protein of class II (Bessen et al. 1989). The opacity factor is extractable with hot acid from M-positive strains but not from M-negative variants of them. Purification of M antigen from positive strains yields material progressively richer in opacity factor but the 2 substances can be partly separated (Hallas and Widdowson 1983). The exact mechanism or biological significance of its action is not known. The reaction is neutralized by antisera, particularly those prepared in guinea-pigs which may be employed as an adjunct to M-serotyping procedures (see below). Neutralizing antibodies can be detected in some human convalescent sera.

Typing of *S. pyogenes* based on M and T antigens

The variation in the M protein molecule between different strains is the basis of the Lancefield M serotyping scheme for *S. pyogenes* (Lancefield 1962). Typing is usually performed as a precipitation reaction with extensively absorbed antisera prepared against whole bacteria. The antigenic determinants of the M-typing procedure are resistant to heat and acid, are precipitated by ethanol and destroyed by trypsin. Recent experience based on sequence analyses of a large number of M protein genes (*emm*) suggests that it is possible to type clinical isolates by PCR sequencing or with sequence-specific oligonucleotide probes (Scott et al. 1985, Kaufhold et al. 1992, Beall, Franklin and Thompson 1996), although sequence variations within single M types occur (Fischetti 1989, Kaufhold et al. 1992, Whatmore et al. 1994, Musser et al. 1995). This method has also been applied to isolates that do not react with available antisera (Relf, Martin and

Sripakash 1992). However, for the majority of M types, a direct correlation between the M-typing reaction and a specific M protein has not been established and it remains possible that type specificity might reflect variation in more than one of the proteins (Kaufhold et al. 1994). Strains expressing the same M protein are not necessarily closely related. Thus, studies of large numbers of strains by multilocus enzyme electrophoresis and DNA-based techniques demonstrated substantial genetic diversity within single M-types (Norgren, Norrby and Holm 1992, Haase et al. 1994, Seppälä et al. 1994, Musser et al. 1995).

The second typing system developed by Lancefield is based on the T antigens, which are less resistant to heat and acid, are not precipitated by ethanol, and are trypsin resistant. It was recognized from the beginning (Lancefield 1940) that M and T antigens are not necessarily separate chemical entities. Occasionally, strains with the same M type show different T type reactivity. T typing is therefore a powerful adjunct to M typing and may provide markers for typing of strains in which no recognized M antigen can be detected (Gaworzewska and Colman 1988). It is likely that these typing methods will be replaced by typing based on genomic DNA sequences.

14.2 *S. agalactiae*

S. agalactiae or group B streptococci (GBS) are important causes of mastitis in cattle and have more recently been recognized as the leading cause of early- and late-onset septicemia and meningitis in neonates and as an important cause of invasive infections in elderly or immunocompromised adults. Its ability to survive in the host is to a high degree dependent on its ability to resist phagocytosis.

Capsule

Clinical isolates of *S. agalactiae* produce a polysaccharide capsule. A total of 9 different capsular serotypes (Ia, Ib, and II–VIII) has been demonstrated (Lancefield 1934, 1938, Perch, Kjems and Henrichsen 1979, Kogan et al. 1994, 1995, 1996). They are all polysaccharides composed of galactose and glucose, combined with 2-acetamido-2-deoxyglucose, rhamnose or *N*-acetylglucosamine and with terminally positioned sialic acid which gives them a net negative charge (Jennings et al. 1983, Schifferle et al. 1985, Wessels et al. 1987, 1991, DiFabio et al. 1989, Kogan et al. 1994, 1995, 1996). The serotype designation Ic is no longer used. The c antigen is a protein which is present in nearly all strains of type Ib, some of Ia and also in other serotypes. Strains containing the c antigen are now designated Ib/c, II/c, III/c, NT/c etc. (NT indicates that the strain is nontypable with recognized antisera) (Henrichsen et al. 1984).

The capsular polysaccharides are essential virulence factors (Rubens et al. 1987). They inhibit phagocytosis and complement activation in the absence of specific antibody. The latter effect is eliminated by the removal of sialic acid residues, and serum lacking antibodies to the complete antigen is not opsonic (Edwards et al. 1982, Wessels et al. 1989). Although invasive infection may be associated with all serotypes, strains with serotype III capsule predominate among isolates from neonatal infection (Baker and Barrett 1974, Dillon, Khare and Gray 1987, Musser et al. 1989). Most of the serotypes constitute separate evolutionary lineages which correlate with the expression of other properties such as α, β, and Rib proteins and hyaluronidase (Stålhammar-Carlemalm, Sternberg and Lindahl 1993, Hauge et al. 1996, Wästfelt et al. 1996). Two separate evolutionary lineages, which may differ in pathogenic potential, express serotype III capsular polysaccharide (Musser et al. 1989, Hauge et al. 1996).

CAMP factor and haemolysin

Most strains of *S. agalactiae* isolated from human sources give a narrow and indistinct zone of β-haemolysis. Bovine strains are more often non-haemolytic. However, practically all strains, whether haemolytic or not, give a positive CAMP reaction: they produce a diffusible substance that completes the lysis of sheep erythrocytes exposed to a sphingomyelinase C such as staphylococcal β-toxin or the α-toxin of *C. perfringens* (Sterzik and Fehrenbach 1985).

Purified CAMP factor is lethal to rabbits when injected intravenously (Skalka and Smola 1981). Furthermore, its role as a virulence factor is supported by its ability to bind immunoglobulins G and M of humans and several animal species via the Fc part (Jürgens, Sterzik and Fehrenbach 1987). It has also been referred to as protein B.

The haemolysin of *S. agalactiae*, which has been cloned and sequenced (Conrads, Podbielski and Luttiken 1991), is not related to the streptolysins of *S. pyogenes*. It has been considered a virulence factor, but isogenic strains with and without expression of the haemolysin show no significant difference in virulence in a neonatal rat model (Weiser and Rubens 1987).

Other virulence factors

Like *S. pyogenes*, strains of *S. agalactiae* produce several M-like proteins which bind various host proteins, a C5a peptidase and hyaluronidase although strains differ in their expression of the respective factors (Musser et al. 1989, Hauge et al. 1996). Earlier studies demonstrated enhanced neuraminidase production in *S. agalactiae* isolates from babies with invasive disease compared to those from colonized infants (Milligan et al. 1978, Musser et al. 1989). However, recent studies have shown that *S. agalactiae* does not have neuraminidase activity and that its detection was an artefact due to contamination of experimental substrates with hyaluronic acid (Pritchard and Lin 1993).

14.3 *S. pneumoniae*

Pneumococci are diplococci, hence the former name 'Diplococcus pneumoniae'. Although genetically closely associated with oral streptococci, *S. pneumoniae* is an important pathogen which to a high degree is ascribed to its polysaccharide capsule.

Capsule

The sizes of pneumococcal capsules vary depending on the strain, the capsular type and the growth conditions (McLeod and Krauss 1950, Sørensen et al. 1988). The capsular polysaccharides can be isolated by alcohol precipitation but most preparations, including commercial vaccine preparations, contain contaminants of cell wall polysaccharide (C polysaccharide) which cannot be eliminated owing to covalent linking through the cell wall petidoglycan (Sørensen and Henrichsen 1984, Sørensen et al. 1990).

A total of 90 distinct capsular serotypes has been demonstrated (Kauffmann, Lund and Eddy 1960, Henrichsen 1995). Although they were identified by serological techniques, the chemical structures of many have been determined (for reviews see Kenne and Lindberg 1983, van Dam, Fleer and Snippe 1990). Two different numbering systems have been used. The American system numbered all distinguishable types in order of discovery. The Danish system places antigenically closely related types together in groups (for example, Danish group 19 includes types 19F, 19A, 19B and 19C which in the American system were types 19, 57, 58 and 59, respectively) (Henrichsen 1979, 1995, van Dam et al. 1990). The Danish method of numbering has prevailed. Six of the pneumococcal capsular polysaccharides (24A, 27, 28A, 28F, 32A, 32F) cross-react with C polysaccharide (see below) (Sørensen 1986) because they contain phosphorylcholine in their structure. A few may be characterized as teichoic acids as they include phosphodiester linkages.

The capsule of *S. pneumoniae* enables the bacteria to resist phagocytosis either by resident pulmonary macrophages or by recruited polymorphonuclear leukocytes. Antibodies to the capsule confer protection.

The genes that are essential for synthesis of the type 19F capsular polysaccharide have been cloned and sequenced (Guidolin et al. 1994).

Other antigenic components

The term **C polysaccharide** (C substance) has been used for the immunochemically defined polysaccharide that can be isolated from pneumococcal cell walls (Tomasz 1981). It is composed of 2 parts: the chemically defined wall teichoic acid linked to fragments of peptidoglycan. The wall teichoic acid is a ribitol teichoic acid associated with 2 phosphorylcholine units per chain (Jennings, Lugowski and Young 1980, Behr et al. 1992, Fischer et al. 1993).

Another immunochemically defined pneumococcal antigen is the so-called **F antigen** (Forsman antigen), which is lipoteichoic acid, i.e. teichoic acid covalently linked to lipid in the plasma membrane (Briles and Tomasz 1973). It is designated F antigen because is can evoke heterophilic antibodies that cross-react with antigens of the Forsman series (e.g. on sheep erytrocytes). Antibodies against the F antigen cross-react with streptococcal group C polysaccharide (Sørensen and Henrichsen 1987).

IgA1 protease

Pneumococci of all serotypes secrete a highly specific endopeptidase which cleaves a Pro-Thr peptide bond in the hinge region of human IgA1, which is the principal mediator of specific immunity in the upper respiratory tract and the predominant IgA subclass in human serum. Cleavage of IgA1 in the hinge region abolishes the cross-binding activity and all secondary effector functions associated with the Fc portion of the antibody molecules. In addition, it has been hypothesized that the bacteria mask surface epitopes with the released monomeric Fab fragments which also inhibit complement activation (Kilian et al. 1996). The enzyme shows significant antigenic diversity within the pneumococcal population (Lomholt 1995). Genetically and functionally closely related IgA1 proteases are produced by *S. oralis*, *S. mitis* and *S. sanguis* and functionally identical IgA1 proteases are secreted by strains of *Haemophilus influenzae*, *Neisseria meningitidis* and *N. gonorrhoeae* (Kilian et al. 1996).

Other virulence factors

Pneumococci produce an intracellular haemolysin (**pneumolysin**) which is liberated by autolysis. Like streptolysin O of *S. pyogenes*, pneumolysin belongs to the family of thiol-activated toxins, which lose their activity on oxidation (Smyth and Duncan 1978). The 2 lysins are very similar in structure and contain a single cysteine residue (Walker et al. 1987); they are irreversibly inactivated by cholesterol and are immunogenic during infection (Kanclerski et al. 1988). Pneumolysin inhibits neutrophil chemotaxis, phagocytosis and the respiratory burst and, furthermore, inhibits lymphocyte proliferation and immunoglobulin synthesis (Paton and Ferrante 1983, Ferrante et al. 1984).

Many pneumococci carry a surface protein (**pneumococcal surface protein**, PspA) which shows some similarities to M proteins of *S. pyogenes* (Yother et al. 1991). Although PspA shows considerable antigenic diversity, immunization of mice with a recombinant PspA from one pneumococcal serotype conferred protection to challenge with different serotypes (McDaniel et al. 1991).

The autolysin of pneumococci which, when activated, breaks the peptide cross-linking of the cell-wall peptidoglycan, enabling the release of pneumolysin (Lee and Liu 1977). In addition, cell wall fragments released during autolysis lead to a self-perpetuating inflammatory response which is an important part of the pathogenesis of pneumococcal pneumonia and meningitis (Johnson et al. 1981, Tuomanen et al. 1985).

Like several of the pyogenic streptococci, pneumococci produce neuraminidase and a hyaluronidase which are believed to contribute to the virulence of pneumococci. Proteolytic activity resulting in degradation of complement factor C3 has been demonstrated (Angel, Ruzek and Hostetter 1994). A comprehensive review of virulence factors of *S. pneumoniae* has been published by Boulnois (1992).

ABIOTROPHIA

Members of the genus *Abiotrophia*, which contains 2 species, are the so-called **nutritionally variant streptococci** (NVS). They grow as satellite colonies around other microorganisms and in complex media only when supplemented with sulphydryl compounds such as cysteine. They have previously been referred to as satellite or symbiotic streptococci, thiol-requiring streptococci, vitamin B_6- or pyridoxal-dependent streptococci or NVS. They were previously considered nutritional variants of other streptococcal species, in particular *S. mitis*, but Bouvet and coworkers (1985, 1989) demonstrated that they form 2 distinct taxa proposed as '*Streptococcus adjacens*' and '*S. defectivus*' respectively. Subsequent comparisons of 16S rRNA sequences revealed that they are quite distinct from other species in the genus *Streptococcus*, which led to the proposal that they be placed in a new genus *Abiotrophia* as *A. adjacens* and *A. defectiva*, respectively (Kawamura et al. 1995b).

Members of the 2 species form minute α-haemolytic colonies on sheep blood agar supplemented with 10 mg l^{-1} pyridoxal hydrochloride or 100 mg l^{-1} cysteine. Their cell morphology depends upon growth conditions and phase. When cultivated in pyridoxal-or cysteine-supplemented complex media they are pleomorphic with chains that include cocci, coccobacilli, and rod-shaped cells. A tendency towards rod formation is observed in the stationary growth phase. In a semisynthetic medium (CDMT) they form small ovoid cocci (diameter 0.4–0.55 μm) which occur singly, in pairs or in chains of variable length. They do not produce extracellular polysaccharides from sucrose and may be easily distinguished from the mitis group of streptococci by their growth characteristics and the production of pyrrolidonyl-arylamidase (Bouvet, Grimont and Grimont 1989). A comprehensive study of their enzymatic activities have been presented by Beighton et al. 1995.

Abiotrophia species form part of the resident microflora of the human upper respiratory tract and may be isolated from vaginal and intestinal tracts. Like most members of the mitis group of streptococci they have been isolated from various human infections including subacute endocarditis, brain abscesses and wound infections, and from urine (Ruoff 1991).

LACTOBACILLUS

15 GENUS DEFINITION

Lactobacilli are straight or curved rods of varying length and thickness, with parallel sides, arranged singly or in chains, sometimes filamentous or pleomorphic, without branching, clubbing or bifid formation. They are gram positive and non-sporing. Colonies on agar media are usually small. They have complex nutritional requirements. Growth is favoured by anaerobic or microaerophilic conditions and by carbon dioxide. Energy is obtained by the fermentation of sugars; glucose is fermented, and either lactic acid alone or lactic acid along with other volatile acids and carbon dioxide is formed. Most strains have cell wall bound proteinases and peptidases. There is no production of catalase, oxidase or indole and no

reduction of nitrate. The organisms are readily killed by heat but unusually tolerant of acid. Lactobacilli are widely distributed in fermenting vegetable and animal products and in the alimentary tract of humans and animals. They are rarely pathogenic for humans. The G+C content of DNA is 32–53 mol%. The genus includes 56 recognized species. The type species is *Lactobacillus delbrueckii*.

16 INTRODUCTION AND HISTORICAL PERSPECTIVE

The type species of the genus *Lactobacillus*, *L. delbrueckii*, was originally isolated from milk by Leichmann (1896). A similar bacillus was observed by Döderlein in 1892 in the vaginal secretion of women, but the identity of this organism is in doubt (Sharpe 1981). In 1900 Moro cultured a slender gram-positive bacillus, *L. acidophilus*, from the faeces of breast-fed babies. Lactobacilli from cheese were named *L. casei* by Orla-Jensen (1904) and Heinemann and Hefferan (1909) isolated lactobacilli from human saliva, gastric juice, soil and various foods. An organism isolated from carious teeth and named *L. odontolyticus* (McIntosh et al. 1922, 1924) is probably the same as *L. plantarum* which was described by Pederson (1936). For other references on early work with lactobacilli see previous editions of this book.

The decision to describe *Streptococcus* and *Lactobacillus* in the same chapter follows Orla-Jensen's (1919, 1943) concept of a cluster of 'lactic-acid bacteria'. Orla Jensen's primary division was between the homofermentative thermobacteria and streptobacteria on one hand and the heterofermentative betabacteria on the other. The streptobacteria will grow at 15°C and most thermobacteria at 45°C. One organism currently classified as a streptobacterium, *L. casei* var. *rhamnosus*, will grow at either temperature.

The species of lactobacilli described here include those isolated most commonly in medical laboratories. Kandler and Weiss (1986), Sharpe (1981), Hammes, Weiss and Holzapfel (1991) and Hammes and Vogel (1995) offer more comprehensive descriptions and review their classification. The review by Hammes, Weiss and Holzapfel (1991) provides a comprehensive survey of the isolation, ecophysiology, identification and application of lactobacilli. Schillinger and Lücke (1987) give an account of the lactobacilli present in meat and meat products.

There is renewed interest in lactobacilli in human medicine because of the probiotic effects of some species (see p. 658).

17 HABITATS

Lactobacilli are found where rich carbohydrate-containing substrates are available; they live in a variety of habitats such as on mucosal membranes of humans and animal (oral cavity, intestine and vagina), in plant materials such as silage, and in foodstuffs and agricultural products, particularly milk, cheese and fermented milk products and in fermented beverages such as wine and cider. In some of these products the multiplication of lactobacilli brings about desirable changes, in others it causes spoilage. In the body flora lactobacilli are present in moderately large numbers in the mouth, gut and vagina but seldom predominate (Salminen, Deighton and Gorbach 1993). Members of several species of lactobacilli are found at each of these sites. In general those most often present in the body flora are: in the mouth, *L. casei*, *L. fermentum*, *L. breve* and *L. acidophilus* (Rogosa et al. 1953); in the small intestine, *L. acidophilus*, *L. fermentum*, *L. salivarius* and *L. reuteri* (Molin et al. 1993) and in the vagina, *L. acidophilus*, *L. fermentum*, *L. casei* and *L. cellobiosus* (Sharpe 1981).

18 MORPHOLOGY

Lactobacilli are in general fairly large non-sporing, gram-positive rods, but they vary in length and breadth and in old cultures tend to be gram negative. A few strains are motile by peritrichous flagella. Metachromatic granules are prominent in some species, notably *L. lactis*, *L. leichmannii* and *L. bulgaricus*. Some members form long chains with cells coiled or twisted. The thermobacteria are usually large, thick and often filamentous. Among the streptobacteria, *L. casei* is a short square-ended rod, forming chains of varying length. *L. plantarum* varies in length from coccoid to short filamentous forms. Two variants of streptococci previously classified as 'Streptococcus lactis' with a tendency to form elongated cells have been reclassified as *L. xylosus* and *L. hordniae* (Garvie, Farrow and Phillips 1981, Schleifer et al. 1985).

19 CULTURAL CHARACTERISTICS

All media for the isolation of lactobacilli are complex. A widely used non-selective medium, at pH 6.2–6.4, is the MRS medium of de Man, Rogosa and Sharpe (1960). For selective isolation the acetate medium (SL) of Rogosa, Mitchell and Wiseman (1951) is the medium of choice particularly when prepared in the manner described by Sharpe (1981). The presence of Tween 80 stimulates the growth of many lactobacilli and a high content of acetate at pH 5.4 is selective for them. Sharpe (1981) recommends additional media for the isolation of lactobacilli from foods and beverages because those from specialized environments may require more specific supplements.

Colonies on agar media are usually small, 1–3 mm in diameter, with entire margins. Some species form rough colonies. Rogosa and Sharpe (1959) made the general observation that colonies of streptobacteria are smooth and those of thermobacteria are rough. Some strains isolated from foodstuffs form slime.

20 METABOLISM

In the homofermentative species, the streptobacteria and the thermobacteria, glucose is broken down to lactic acid almost exclusively by the Embden–Meyerhof pathway. The heterofermentative species, the betabacteria, possess the 6-phosphogluconate pathway in which the end products are carbon dioxide, acetic acid, ethanol and lactic acid (see Kandler 1982). Because carbon dioxide is soluble in water the conventional Durham tube is inapplicable and other methods, such as a shake culture in MRS agar in a tube with a plain agar overlay as a seal, are required to demonstrate carbon dioxide production. Practically all of the streptobacteria and betabacteria, but none of the thermobacteria, ferment ribose.

The lactobacilli are acidophilic and grow best in medium at about pH 6. They are aciduric and the final pH in glucose broth with some species can be as low as 3.5. For testing the fermentation of carbohydrates, Rogosa and Sharpe (1959) recommend a medium with an initial pH of 5.5–6.0. Kits in which patterns of fermentation are determined against many different carbohydrates are often employed for identification (Hammes, Weiss and Holzapfel 1991).

Most of the lactobacilli will grow in air but grow best in an atmosphere lacking oxygen but supplemented with carbon dioxide (Rogosa and Sharpe 1959). A few are strict anaerobes. The catalase test is nearly always negative and the occasional weakly positive reaction can be attributed to a pseudocatalase action because negative benzidine tests indicate the absence of a cytochrome system (Sharpe 1981).

The temperature at which growth occurs varies with the species. Thermobacteria grow best at 37–40°C; none grows at 15°C and most will grow at 45°C. The optimum for streptobacteria is about 30°C; all grow at 15°C. Among the betabacteria *L. brevis*, *L. buchneri* and *L. viridescens* resemble streptobacteria, *L. fermentum* resembles thermobacteria, *L. cellobiosus* is variable in this characteristic.

20.1 Other nutritional requirements

The nutritional requirements of lactobacilli are complex and varied but are normally met by media which, in addition to fermentable carbohydrate, contain peptone, meat and yeast extract. Supplements that are stimulatory, or even essential, include tomato juice, manganese, acetate and oleic acid esters and Tween 80 in particular. Requirements for vitamins are scattered throughout the species and vitamin-dependent strains are used for bioassays. Thiamine is necessary for the growth of nearly all the heterofermentative organisms but not those that are homofermentative (Ledesma et al. 1977). Requirements for amino acids and peptides seem to be met by a combination of cell wall bound proteinases and peptidases and mechanisms for active transport across the cell membrane (Law and Kolstad 1983).

21 CELL WALL COMPOSITION; ANTIGENIC STRUCTURE

The chief amino acid in the peptidoglycan of most species of lactobacilli is lysine, but in some it is diaminopimelic acid and in others ornithine. All of the thermobacteria considered here have interpeptide bridges of the L-lysine–D-aspartate type. Among the streptobacteria, *L. casei* has a peptidoglycan bridge of the L-lysine–D-aspartate type and *L. plantarum* one of the *meso*-diaminopimelic type. Three types of peptidoglycan are found in the species of betabacteria described here: (1) L-lysine–D-aspartate in *L. brevis* and *L. buchneri*; (2) L-ornithine–D-aspartate in *L. fermentum* and *L. cellobiosus*; and (3) L-lysine–L-alanine–L-serine in *L. viridescens* (Schleifer and Kandler 1972).

Many lactobacilli share an antigen present in the cell membrane (Sharpe et al. 1973a). This corresponds to the 1–3 linked glycerol phosphate units of the membrane glycerol-teichoic acid. This antigen is distinct from the group antigens described by Sharpe (1955), which she identified by precipitation reactions between hot-acid extracts and antisera. The chemical composition of these antigens was reviewed by Knox and Wicken (1976) and is shown in Table 28.4. It will be noted that the *L. casei* strains, except those of subspecies *rhamnosus*, may possess one of 2 group antigens, and that the group E antigen occurs in members of 4 species, 2 of them thermobacteria and 2 betabacteria.

22 SUSCEPTIBILITY TO PHYSICAL AND CHEMICAL AGENTS

The lactobacilli have no particular resistance to heat and are destroyed by exposure to 60° or 65° for 30 min. They are, however, specially resistant to acid and are able to grow in concentrations of acid that are fatal to most other bacteria. The tolerance to bile varies and has been used to distinguish between species (Sharpe 1981).

Lactobacilli of several species can be resistant to many antibiotics including vancomycin, the peptide antibiotics, the macrolides, tetracycline and the aminoglycosides. In these strains loss of plasmids was usually accompanied by a change to sensitivity with several antibiotics (Vescovo, Morelli and Bottazzi 1982).

Lactobacilli are refractory to transformation and transduction, but the transmission of the plasmid that determines the ability of *L. casei* to ferment lactose does occur naturally.

23 CLASSIFICATION

Orla-Jensen (1919, 1943), whose monographs have influenced all subsequent workers, laid particular stress on fermentative ability and the type of lactic acid produced from glucose in his classification of lactobacilli. His 3 primary divisions of the lactobacilli into thermobacteria, streptobacteria and betabacteria were followed for many years, though not his proposal to consider them as separate genera. However, recent comparative studies of 16S rRNA sequences revealed that the 3 groups lack phylogenetic foundation. Fur-

thermore, such studies indicate that lactobacilli are phylogenetically intermixed with members of the genera *Leuconostoc* and *Pediococcus* despite differences in morphology and fermentation patterns (for review see Schleifer and Ludwig 1995). Three phylogenetic groups are evident although the first 2 may be difficult to distinguish:

1 *Obligate homofermenters.* This group includes the type species *L. delbrueckii* and other obligately homofermentative lactobacilli including *L. acidophilus.*
2 *Facultative heterofermenters.* This group comprises more than 30 *Lactobacillus* species including *L. rhamnosus*, *L. intestinalis*, and *L. sake* most of which are facultatively heterofermentative. In addition to the lactobacilli the group includes 5 *Pediococcus* species.
3 *Obligate heterofermenters* which are closely related to the leuconostocs.

These sequence studies also revealed that several taxa were erroneously placed in the genus *Lactobacillus*. As a result some were transferred to the genus *Clostridium* and 2 recently described anaerobic species '*L. uli*' and '*L. rimae*' isolated from human gingival crevices (Olsen et al. 1991) were transferred to the new genus *Atopobium* (Collins and Wallbanks 1992).

Hammes and Vogel (1995) have proposed a grouping based on a combination of phylogenetic data and biochemical and physiological characteristics of the species. They provide details about cell wall composition and identification criteria. It is remarkable that for an unequivocal identification of a *Lactobacillus* isolate it is not always sufficient to use the classical physiological and biochemical tests. A review by Pot et al. (1994) provides a discussion of methods for identification of lactobacilli including a critical evaluation of their limitations.

24 PATHOGENICITY

The relationship of lactobacilli to dental caries has been reviewed (Hardie and Bowden 1974). Lactobacilli are occasionally isolated from bacteraemic patients (Sharpe, Hill and Lapage 1973b). The selection of

Table 28.4 Group antigens of lactobacilli

Species	Group	Antigen	Location	Determinant
L. helveticus	A	Glycerol teichoic acid	Wall–membrane	α-D-Glucose
L. casei	B	Polysaccharide	Wall	α-L-Rhamnose
L. casei	C	Polysaccharide	Wall	β-D-Glucose
L. plantarum	D	Ribitol teichoic acid	Wall	α-D-Glucose
L. lactis	E	Glycerol teichoic acid	Wall	α-D-Glucose
L. bulgaricus				
L. brevis				
L. buchneri				
L. fermentum	F	Glycerol teichoic acid	Membrane	α-D-Galactose

Based on Knox and Wicken (1976).

antibiotics for the treatment of these patients has been difficult (Bayer et al. 1978).

25 ROLE IN NORMAL HUMAN FLORA

Lactobacilli are members of the commensal microflora of human mucosal membranes in the mouth, intestines and vagina, although they usually comprise a minor part of the flora (London 1976). In the oral cavity lactobacilli usually amount to less than 1% of the microflora although their proportion increases in individuals with a frequent intake of sugar. Studies of the intestinal lactobacillus flora of piglets have demonstrated a rapid turnover of clones (Tannock, Fuller and Pedersen 1990).

Due to production of bacteriocins and to their acidogenic potential, which reduces the pH in the local environments, lactobacilli play an important role in inhibiting the establishment of potential pathogens on mucosal surfaces (Roach and Tannock 1979, Hentjes 1983). Although the probiotic effect of lactobacilli is an old concept described by Metchnikoff in 1901 (see review by Bibel 1988), there is considerable renewed interest in this topic. Recent studies have demonstrated that lactobacilli administered orally to patients with viral and bacterial intestinal infections augment mucosal immune responses and promote recovery (Kaila et al. 1992, Perdigon et al. 1995). Furthermore, it has been demonstrated in a rat model that lactobacilli increase the barrier functions of the gut mucosa (Isolauri et al. 1993).

REFERENCES

Abeygunawardana C, Bush CA, 1989, The complete structure of the capsular polysaccharide from *Streptococcus sanguis* 34, *Carbohyd Res*, **191**: 279–93.

Abeygunawardana C, Bush CA, Cisar JO, 1990, Complete structure of the polysaccharide from *Streptococcus sanguis* J22, *Biochem*, **29**: 234–48.

Abeygunawardana C, Bush CA, Cisar JO, 1991, Complete structure of the cell surface polysaccharide of *Streptococcus oralis* C104: A 600-Mhz NMR study, *Biochemistry*, **30**: 8568–77.

Abraham SN, Beachey EH, Simpson WA, 1983, Adherence of *Streptococcus pyogenes*, *Escherichia coli*, and *Pseudomonas aeruginosa* to fibronectin-coated and uncoated epithelial cells, *Infect Immun*, **41**: 1261–68.

Aguirre M, Morrison D et al., 1993, Phenotypic and phylogenetic characterization of some *Gemella*-like organisms from human infections: description of *Dolosigranulum pigrum* gen. nov., sp. nov., *J Appl Bacteriol*, **75**: 608–12.

Alouf JE, 1980, Streptococcal toxins (streptolysin O, streptolysin S, erythrogenic toxin), *Pharmacol Ther*, **11**: 661–717.

Angel CS, Ruzek M, Hostetter MK, 1994, Degradation of C3 by *Streptococcus pneumoniae*, *J Infect Dis*, **170**: 600–8.

Appelbaum PC, 1992, Antimicrobial resistance in *Streptococcus pneumoniae*: an overview, *Clin Infect Dis*, **15**: 77–83.

Avery OT, MacLeod CM, McCarty M, 1944, Studies on the chemical nature of the substance inducing transformation of pneumococcal types, *J Exp Med*, **79**: 137–58.

Baker CJ, Barrett FF, 1974, Group B streptococcal infection in infants: the importance of the various serotypes, *JAMA*, **230**: 1158–60.

Bayer AS, Chow AW et al., 1978, Lactobacillemia – report of nine cases. Important clinical and therapeutic considerations, *Am J Med*, **64**: 808–13.

Beachey EH, Courtney HS, 1987, Bacterial adherence: the attachment of group A streptococci to mucosal surfaces, *Rev Infect Dis*, **9 suppl**: S475–81.

Beachey EH, Simpson WA, 1982, The adherence of group A streptococci to oropharyngeal cells: the lipoteichoic acid adhesin and fibronectin receptor, *Infection*, **10**: 107–11.

Beall B, Facklam R, Thompson T, 1996, Sequencing *emm*-specific PCR products for routine and accurate typin of group A streptococci, *J Clin Microbiol*, **34**: 953–8.

Behr T, Fischer W et al., 1992, The structure of pneumococcal lipoteichoic acid. Improved preparation, chemical and mass spectrometric studies, *Eur J Biochem*, **207**: 1063–75.

Beighton D, Hardie JM, Whiley RA, 1991, A scheme for the identification of viridans streptococci, *J Med Microbiol*, **35**: 367–72.

Beighton D, Homer KA et al., 1995, Analysis of enzymatic activities for differentiation of two species of nutritionally variant streptococci, *Streptococcus defectivus* and *Streptococcus adjacens*, *J Clin Microbiol*, **33**: 1584–7.

Beighton D, Russell RRB, Hayday H, 1981, The isolation and characterization of *Streptococcus mutans* serotype h from dental plaque of monkeys (*Macaca fascicularis*), *J Gen Microbiol*, **124**: 271–79.

Bentley RW, Leigh JA, Collins MD, 1991, Intrageneric structure of *Streptococcus* based on comparative analysis of small-subunit rRNA sequences, *Int J Syst Bacteriol*, **41**: 487–94.

Bentley RW, Leigh JA, 1995, Development of PCR-based hybridization protocol for identification of streptococcal species, *J Clin Microbiol*, **33**: 1296–301.

Bergman S, Selig M et al., 1995, *Streptococcus milleri* strains displaying a gliding type of motility, *Int J Syst Bacteriol*, **45**: 235–9.

Bessen D, Fischetti VA, 1988, Influence of intranasal immunization with synthetic peptides corresponding to conserved epitopes of M protein on mucosal colonization by group A streptococci, *Infect Immun*, **56**: 2666–72.

Bessen D, Fischetti VA, 1992, Nucleotide sequences of two adjacent M or M-like protein genes of group A streptococci: different RNA transcript levels and identification of a unique IgA-binding protein, *Infect Immun*, **60**: 124–35.

Bessen D, Jones KF et al., 1989, Evidence for two distinct classes of streptococcal M protein and their relationship to rheumatic fever, *J Exp Med*, **169**: 269–83.

Bessen DE, Veasy G et al., 1995, Serologic evidence for a class I group A streptococcal infection among rheumatic fever patients, *J Infect Dis*, **172**: 1608–11.

Bibel DJ, 1988, Elie Metchnikoff's bacillus of long life, *ASM News*, **54**: 661–5.

Billroth AW, 1874, *Untersuchungen über die Vegetationsformen von Coccobacteria Septica*, Georg Reimer, Berlin.

Bisno AL, Craven DE, McCabe WR, 1987, M proteins of group G streptococci isolated from bacteremic human infections, *Infect Immun*, **55**: 753–7.

Björck L, Åkesson P et al., 1989, Bacterial growth blocked by a synthetic peptide based on the structure of a human proteinase inhibitor, *Nature (London)*, **337**: 385–6.

Boulnois GJ, 1992, Pneumococcal proteins and the pathogenesis of disease caused by *Streptococcus pneumoniae*, *J Gen Microbiol*, **138**: 249–59.

Bouvet A, Grimont F, Grimont P, 1989, *Streptococcus defectivus* sp. nov. and *Streptococcus adjacens* sp. nov., nutritionally variant streptococci from human clinical specimens, *Int J Syst Bacteriol*, **39**: 290–4.

Bouvet A, Villeroy F et al., 1985, Characterization of nutritionally variant streptococci by biochemical tests and penicillin-binding proteins, *J Clin Microbiol*, **22**: 1030–4.

Bratthall D, 1970, Demonstration of five serological groups of streptococcal strains resembling *Streptococcus mutans*, *Odontol Rev*, **21**: 143–52.

Braun MA, Gerlach D et al., 1993, Stimulation of human T cells by streptococcal 'superantigen' erythrogenic toxins (Scarlet fever toxins), *J Immunol*, **150**: 2457–66.

Bridge PD, Sneath PH, 1983, Numerical taxonomy of *Streptococcus*, *J Gen Microbiol*, **129**: 565–97.

Briles EB, Tomasz A, 1973, Pneumococcal Forsmann antigen. A choline-containing lipoteichoic acid, *J Biol Chem*, **248**: 6394–7.

Brooker JD, O'Donovan LA et al., 1994, *Streptococcus caprinus* sp. nov. a tannin-resistant ruminal bacterium from feral goats, *Lett Appl Microbiol*, **18**: 313–16.

Buu-Hoi A, Horodniceanu T, 1980, Conjugative transfer of multiple antibiotic-resistance markers in *Streptococcus pneumoniae*, *J Bacteriol*, **143**: 313–20.

Caparon MG, Scott JR, 1987, Identification of a gene that regulates expression of M protein, the major virulence determinant of group A streptococci, *Proc Natl Acad Sci USA*, **84**: 8677–81.

Caparon MG, Stephens DS et al., 1991, Role of M protein in adherence of group A streptococci, *Infect Immun*, **59**: 1811–17.

Carlsson J, 1967, Presence of various types of nonhaemolytic streptococci in dental plaque and in other sites of the oral cavity in man, *Odontol Rev*, **18**: 55–74.

Carlsson J, 1968, A numerical taxonomic study of human oral streptococci, *Odontol Rev*, **19**: 137–60.

Carlsson J, Grahnén H et al., 1970, Early establishment of *Streptococcus salivarius* in the mouth of infants, *J Dent Res*, **49**: 415–19.

Carlsson J, Hamilton I, 1994, Metabolic activity of oral bacteria, *Textbook of Clinical Cariology*, eds Thylstrup A, Fejerskov O, Munksgaard, Copenhagen, 71–88.

Carmeli Y, Ruoff KL, 1995, Report of cases of and taxonomic considerations for large colony forming Lancefield group C streptococcal bacteremia, *J Clin Microbiol*, **33**: 2114–17.

Chen CC, Cleary PP, 1990, Complete nucleotide sequence of the streptococcal C5a peptidase gene of *Streptococcus pyogenes*, *J Biol Chem*, **265**: 3161–7.

Cisar JO, Sandberg AL et al., 1995, Lectin recognition of host-like saccharide motifs in streptococcal cell wall polysaccharides, *Glycobiology*, **5**: 655–62.

Clarke JK, 1924, On the bacterial factor in the aetiology of dental caries, *Br J Exp Pathol*, **5**: 141–7.

Cleary PP, Handley J et al., 1992, Similarity between the group B and A streptococcal C5a peptidase genes, *Infect Immun*, **60**: 4239–44.

Cleary PP, Peterson J et al., 1991, Virulent human strains of group G streptococci express a C5a peptidase enzyme similar to that produced by group A streptococci, *Infect Immun*, **59**: 2305–10.

Clewell DB, Flannagan SE, Jaworski DD, 1995, Unconstrained bacterial promiscuity: the Tn*916*-Tn*1545* family of conjugative transposons, *Trends Microbiol*, **3**: 229–36.

Clewell DB, Gawron-Burke C, 1986, Conjugative tranposons and the dissemination of antibiotic resistance in streptococci, **40**: 635–59.

Cole RM, Calandra GB et al., 1976, Attributes of potential utility in differentiating among 'Group H' streptococci or *Streptococcus sanugis*, *J Dent Res*, **55**: A142–53.

Coligan JE, Kindt TJ, Krause RM, 1978, Structure of the streptococcal groups A, A-variant and C carbohydrates, *Immunochemistry*, **15**: 755–60.

Collins MDC, Ash JAE et al., 1989, 16S Ribosomal ribonucleic acid sequences analysis of lactococci and related taxa. Description of *Vagococcus fluvialis* gen. nov., sp. nov., *J Appl Bacteriol*, **67**: 453–60.

Collins MD, Farrow JAE et al., 1984, Taxonomic studies on streptococci of serological groups E, P, U and V. Description of *Streptococcus porcinus* sp. nov., *Syst Appl Microbiol*, **5**: 402–13.

Collins MD, Wallbanks S, 1992, Comparative sequence analysis of the 16S rRNA genes of *Lactobacillis minutus*, *Lactobacillus*

rimae, and *Streptococcus parvulus*: Proposal for the creation of a new genus *Atopobium*, *FEMS Microbiol Let*, **95**: 235–40.

Colman G, 1990, *Streptococcus* and *Lactobacillus*, *Topley and Wilson's Principles of Bacteriology, Virology and Immunity*, Vol. 2, 8th edn, eds Baker MT, Collier LH, Edward Arnold, London, 119–59.

Colman G, Tanna A et al., 1993, The serotypes of *Streptococcus pyogenes* present in Britain during 1980–1990 and their association with disease, *J Med Microbiol*, **39**: 165–78.

Colman G, Williams REO, 1965, The cell walls of streptococci, *J Gen Microbiol*, **41**: 375–87.

Colman G, Williams EO, 1972, Taxonomy of some human viridans streptococci, *Streptococci and Streptococcal Disease*, eds Wannamaker LW, Matsen JM, Academic Press, New York, 282–99.

Conrads G, Podbielski A, Lutticken R, 1991, Molecular cloning and nucleotide sequence of the group B streptococcal hemolysin, *Int J Med Microbiol*, **275**: 179–84.

Cowell JL, Bernheimer AW, 1977, Antigenic relationships among thiol-activated cytolysins, *Infect Immun*, **16**: 397.

Coykendall AL, 1971, Genetic heterogeneity in *Streptococcus mutans*, *J Bacteriol*, **106**: 192–6.

Coykendall AL, 1977, Proposal to elevate the subspecies of *Streptococcus mutans* to species status, based on their molecular composition, *Int J Syst Bacteriol*, **27**: 26–30.

Coykendall AL, 1983, *Streptococcus sobrinus* nom. rev. and *Streptococcus ferus* nom. rev.: habitat of these and other mutant streptococci, *Int J Syst Bacteriol*, **33**: 883–5.

Coykendall AL, 1989, Classification and identification of the viridans streptococci, *Clin Microbiol Rev*, **2**: 315–28.

Coykendall AL, Gustafson KB, 1985, Deoxyribonucleic acid hybridizations among strains of *Streptococcus salivarius* and *Streptococcus bovis*, *Int J Syst Bacteriol*, **35**: 274–80.

Coykendall AL, Munzenmaier AJ, 1978, Deoxyribonucleic acid base sequence studies on glucan-producing and glucan-negative strains of *Streptococcus mitior*, *Int J Syst Bacteriol*, **28**: 511–15.

Coykendall AL, Specht PA, 1975, DNA base sequence homologies among strains of *Streptococcus sanguis*, *J Gen Microbiol*, **91**: 92–8.

Coykendall AL, Wesbecher PM, Gustafson KB, 1987, '*Streptococcus milleri*', *Streptococcus constellatus*, and *Streptococcus intermedius* are later synonyms of *Streptococcus anginosus*, *Int J Syst Bacteriol*, **37**: 222–8.

Crater DL, van de Rijn I, 1995, Hyaluronic acid synthesis operon (has) expression in group A streptococci, *J Biol Chem*, **270**: 18452–8.

Dale JB, Washburn RG et al., 1996, Hyaluronate capsule and surface M protein in resistance to opsonization of group A streptococci, *Infect Immun*, **64**: 1495–501.

Dempster RP, Tagg JR, 1982, The production of bacteriocin-like substances by the oral bacterium *Streptococcus salivarius*, *Arch Oral Biol*, **27**: 151–7.

Demuth DR, Golub EE, Malamud D, 1990, Streptococcal-host interactions, *J Biol Chem*, **265**: 7120–6.

Dent VE, Hardie JM, Bowden GH, 1978, Streptococci isolated from dental plaque of animals, *J Appl Bacteriol*, **44**: 249–58.

Devriese LA, 1991, Streptococcal ecovars associated with different animal species: epidemiological significance of serogroups and biotypes, *J Appl Bacteriol*, **71**: 478–83.

Devriese LA, Hommez AJ et al., 1986, *Streptococcus canis* sp. nov.: a species of group G streptococci from animals, *J Syst Bacteriol*, **36**: 422–5.

Devriese LA, Kilpper-Bälz R, Schleifer KH, 1988, *Streptococcus hyointestinalis* sp. nov. from the gut of swine, *Int J Syst Bacteriol*, **38**: 440–1.

Diernhofer K, 1932, Aesculinbouillon as Hilfsmittel für die Differenzierung von Euter- und Milchstreptokokken bei Masseuntersuchungen, *Milchwirtsch Forsch*, **13**: 368–74.

DiFabio JL, Michon F et al., 1989, Structure of the capsular polysaccharide antigen of type IV group B *Streptococcus*, *Can J Chem*, **67**: 877–82.

Dillon HC Jr, Khare S, Gray BM, 1987, Group B streptococcal carriage and disease: a 6-year prospective study, *J Pediatr*, **110**: 31–6.

Doern GV, Brueggemann A et al., 1996, Antimicrobial resistance of *Streptococcus pneumoniae* recovered from outpatients in the United States during the winter months of 1994 to 1995: Results of a 30-center national surveillance study, *Antimicrob Agents Chemother*, **40**: 1208–13.

Dowson CG, Coffey TJ et al., 1993, Evolution of penicillin resistance in *Streptococcus pneumoniae*, the role of *Streptococcus mitis* in the formation of a low affinity PBP2B in *S. pneumoniae*, *Mol Microbiol*, **9**: 635–43.

Döderlein A, 1892, *Das Scheidensekret und seine Bedeutung für das Puerperalfieber*, Leipzig, 1–86.

Edwards MS, Kasper DL et al., 1982, Capsular sialic acid prevents activation of the alternative complement pathway by type III, group B streptococci, *J Immunol*, **128**: 1278–83.

Efstratiou A, Colman G et al., 1994, Biochemical differences among human and animal streptococci of Lancefield group C or group G, *J Med Microbiol*, **41**: 145–8.

Eldar A, Frelier PF et al., 1995, *Streptococcus shiloi*, the name for an agent causing septicemic infection in fish, is a junior synonym of *Streptococcus iniae*, *Int J Syst Bacteriol*, **45**: 840–42.

Ellis RP, Armstrong CH, 1971, Production of capsules, streptokinase, and streptodornase by *Streptococcus* group E, *Am J Vet Res*, **32**: 349–56.

Facklam RR, 1984, The major differences in the American and British *Streptococcus* taxonomy schemes with special reference to *Streptococcus milleri*, *Eur J Clin Microbiol*, **3**: 91–3.

Facklam RR, Washington JA II, 1991, *Streptococcus* and related catalase-negative gram-positive cocci, *Manual of Clinical Microbiology*, 5th edn, eds Balows A, Hausler WJ Jr et al., American Society for Microbiology, Washington DC, 238–57.

Facklam R, Elliott JA, 1995a, Identification, classification, and clinical relevance of catalase-negative, gram-positive cocci, excluding the streptococci and enterococci, *Clin Microbiol Rev*, **8**: 479–95.

Facklam R, Elliott J et al., 1995b, Identification of *Streptococcus porcinus* from human sources, *J Clin Microbiol*, **33**: 385–8.

Farrow JAE, Collins MD, 1984a, DNA base composition, DNA-DNA homology and long-chain fatty acid studies on *Streptococcus thermophilus* and *Streptococcus salivarius*, *J Gen Microbiol*, **130**: 357–62.

Farrow JAE, Collins MD, 1984b, Taxonomic studies on streptococci of serological groups C, G and L and possibly related taxa, *System Appl Microbiol*, **5**: 483–93.

Farrow JAE, Kruze J et al., 1984, Taxonomic studies on *Streptococcus bovis* and *Streptococcus equinus*: Description of *Streptococcus alactolyticus* sp.nov. and *Streptococcus saccharolyticus* sp. nov., *System Appl Microbiol*, **5**: 467–82.

Feltham RKA, 1979, A taxonomic study of the genus *Streptococcus*, *Pathogenic Streptococci*, ed. Parker MT, Chertsey, Surrey, 247–8.

Ferrante A, Rowan-Kelley B et al., 1984, Inhibition of *in vitro* human lymphocyte response by the pneumococcal toxin pneumolysin, *Infect Immun*, **46**: 585–9.

Ferretti JJ, En Yu C et al., 1987, Molecular characterization of the group A streptococcal exotoxin type A (Erythrogenic toxin) gene and product, *Streptococcal Genetics*, eds Ferretti JJ, Curtiss R, American Society for Microbiology, Washington, DC, 130–7.

Fischer W, Behr T et al., 1993, Teichoic acid and lipoteichoic acid of *Streptococcus pneumoniae* possess identical chain structures. A reinvestigation of teichoic acid (C polysaccharide), *Eur J Biochem*, **215**: 815–57.

Fischer H, Tomasz A, 1985, Peptidoglycan cross-linking and teichoic acid attachment in *Streptococcus pneumoniae*, *J Bacteriol*, **163**: 46–54.

Fischetti VA, 1989, Streptococcal M protein: molecular design and biological behaviour, *Clin Microbiol Rev*, **2**: 285–314.

Frandsen EV, Pedrazzoli V, Kilian M, 1991, Ecology of viridans streptococci in the oral cavity and pharynx, *Oral Microbiol Immunol*, **6**: 129–33.

Freney J, Bland S et al., 1992, Description and evaluation of the semiautomated 4-hour rapid ID 32 strep method for identification of streptococci and members of related genera, *J Clin Microbiol*, **30**: 2657–61.

Frick I-M, Åkesson P et al., 1994, Protein H – a surface protein of *Streptococcus pyogenes* with separate binding sites for IgG and albumin, *Mol Microbiol*, **12**: 143–51.

Frithz E, Heden L-O, Lindahl G, 1989, Extensive sequence homology between IgA receptor and M proteins in *Streptococcus pyogenes*, *Mol Microbiol*, **3**: 1111–19.

Fukushima H, Kelstrup J et al., 1983, Isolation, partial purification and preliminary characterization of a bacteriocin from *Streptococcus mutans* Rm-10, *Antonie van Leeuwenhoek*, **49**: 41–50.

Garcia-Bustos JF, Chait BT, Tomasz A, 1987, Structure of the peptide network of pneumococcal peptidoglycan, *J Biol Chem*, **262**: 15400–5.

Garvie EI, Bramley AJ, 1979, *Streptococcus uberis*: an approach to its classification, *J Appl Bacteriol*, **46**: 295–304.

Garvie EI, Farrow JAE, Collins MD, 1983, *Streptococcus dysgalactiae* (Diernhofer) nom. rev., *Int J Syst Bacteriol*, **33**: 404–5.

Garvie EI, Farrow JAE, Phillips BA, 1981, A taxonomic study of some strains of streptococci which grow at 10°C but not at 45°C including *Streptococcus lactis* and *Streptococcus cremoris*, *Zentralbl Bakteriol Mikrobiol Hyg*, **1 Abt. Orig. C2**: 151.

Gaworzewska E, Colman G, 1988, Changes in the pattern of infection caused by *Streptococcus pyogenes*, *Epidemiol Infect*, **100**: 257–69.

Gawron-Burke C, Clewell DB, 1982, A transposon in *Streptococcus faecalis* with fertility properties, *Nature* (London), **300**: 281–4.

Gerlach DH, Knoll W et al., 1983, Isolation and characterization of erythrogenic toxins V. Communication: identity of erythrogenic toxin type B and streptococcal proteinase precursor, *Zentralbl Bakteriol Parasitenkd Infektionskr Hyg Abt 1*, **255**: 221–33.

Gerlach D, Köhler W, 1979, Studies of the heterogeneity of streptokinases. II. Communication: composition of amino acids and serological activity, *Zentralbl. Bakteriol Parasitenkd Infektionskr Hyg. 1 Orig. Reihe A*, **244**: 210–21.

Gibbons RJ, van Houte J, 1971, Selective bacterial adherence to oral epithelial surfaces and its role as an ecological determinant, *Infect Immun*, **3**: 567–73.

Gillespie SH, McWhinney PHM et al., 1993, Species of alpha-hemolytic streptococci possessing a C-polysaccharide phosphorylcholine-containing antigen, *Infect Immun*, **61**: 3076–7.

Glushka J, Cassels FJ et al., 1992, Complete structure of the adhesion receptor polysaccharide of *Streptococcus oralis* ATCC-55229 (*Streptococcus sanguis* H1), *Biochemistry*, **31**: 10741–6.

Gomi H, Hozumi T et al., 1990, The gene sequence and some properties of protein H: a novel IgG-binding protein, *J Immunol*, **144**: 4046–52.

Gottschalk M, Higgins R et al., 1989, Description of 14 new capsular types of *Streptococcus suis*, *J Clin Microbiol*, **27**: 2633–6.

Gray BM, Converse GM III, Dillon HC Jr, 1980, Epidemiologic studies of *Streptococcus pneumoniae* in infants: acquisition, carriage, and infection during the first 24 months of life, *J Infect Dis*, **142**: 923–33.

Gray ED, 1972, Nucleases of group A streptococci, *Streptococci and streptococcal diseases*, eds Wannamaker LW, Matsen JM, Academic Press, New York, 143–55.

Griffith F, 1928, The significance of pneumococcal types, *J Hyg*, **27**: 113–59.

Guidolin A, Morona JK et al., 1994, Nucleotide sequence analysis of genes essential for capsular polysaccharide biosynthesis in *Streptococcus pneumoniae* type 19F, *Infect Immun*, **62**: 5384–96.

Gupta RC, Badhwar AK et al., 1986, Detection of C-reactive protein, streptolysin O, and anti-streptolysin O antibodies in immune complexes isolated from the sera of patients with acute rheumatic fever, *J Immunol*, **137**: 2173–9.

Haase AM, Melder A et al., 1994, Clonal diversity of *Streptococcus pyogenes* within some M-types revealed by multilocus enzyme electrophoresis, *Epidemiol Infect*, **113**: 455–62.

Halbert SP, Bircher R, Dahle E, 1961, The analysis of streptococcal infections. V. Cardiotoxicity of streptolysin O for rabbits in vivo, *J Exp Med*, **113**: 759.

Hallas G, Widdowson JP, 1983, The relationship between opacity factor and M protein in *Streptococcus pyogenes*, *J Med Microbiol*, **16**: 13–26.

Hamada S, Michalek SM et al., 1986, *Molecular Microbiology and Immunology of* Streptococcus mutans, Elsevier, Amsterdam.

Hammes WP, Vogel RF, 1995, The genus *Lactobacillus*, *The Lactic Acid Bacteria. Vol. 2. The Genera of Lactic Acid Bacteria*, eds Wood BJB, Holzapfel WH, Blackie, Glasgow, 19–54.

Hammes WP, Weiss, N, Holzapfel WH, 1991, The genera *Lactobacillus* and *Carnobacterium*, *The Prokaryotes. Handbook on the Biology of Bacteria: Ecophysiology, Isolation, Identification, Applications*, eds Balows A, Trüper HG et al., Springer, New York, USA, 1535–94.

Hampson DJ, Trott DJ et al., 1993, Population structure of Australian isolates of *Streptococcus suis*, *J Clin Microbiol*, **31**: 2895–900.

Handley PS, 1990, Structure, composition and functions of surface structures of oral bacteria, *Biofouling*, **2**: 239–64.

Handley P, Coykendall A et al., 1991, *Streptococcus crista* sp. nov. a viridans streptococcus with tufted fibrils, isolated from the human oral cavity and throat, *Int J System Bacteriol*, **41**: 543–7.

Hanski E, Caparon M, 1992, Protein F, a fibronectin-binding protein, is an adhesin of the group A streptococcus *Streptococcus pyogenes*, *Proc Natl Acad Sci USA*, **89**: 6172–6.

Hardie JM, 1986a, Genus *Streptococcus* Rosenbach 1984, *Bergey's Manual of Systematic Bacteriology*, eds Sneath PHS, Mair NS, Sharpe ME, Williams and Wilkins, Baltimore, 1043–47.

Hardie JM, 1986b, Oral streptococci, *Bergey's Manual of Systematic Bacteriology*, eds Sneath PHS, Mair NS, Sharpe ME, Williams and Wilkins, Baltimore, 1054–63.

Hardie JM, 1986c, Other streptococci, *Bergey's Manual of Systematic Bacteriology*, eds Sneath PHS., Mair NS, Sharpe ME, Williams and Wilkins, Baltimore, 1068–71.

Hardie JM, Bowden GH, 1974, The normal microbial flora of the mouth, *The Normal Flora of Man*, Skinner FA, Carr JG, Academic Press, London, 47–83.

Hardie JM, Whiley RA, 1995, The genus *Streptococcus*, *The Lactic Acid Bacteria. Volume 2. The Genera of Lactic Acid Bacteria*, eds Wood BJB, Holzapfel WH, Blackie, Glasgow, 55–124.

Hauge M, Jespersgaard C et al., 1996, Population structure of *Streptococcus agalactiae* reveals an association between specific evolutionary lineages and putative virulence factors but not disease, *Infect Immun*, **64**: 919–25.

Hauser AR, Schlievert PM, 1990, Nucleotide sequence of the streptococcal pyrogenic exotoxin type B gene and relationship between the toxin and the streptococcal proteinase precursor, *J Bacteriol*, **172**: 4536–42.

Hayano S, Tanaka A, Okuyama Y, 1969, Distribution and serological specificity of sialidase produced by various groups of streptococci, *J Bacteriol*, **100**: 354–7.

Heath DG, Cleary PP, 1989, Fc-receptor and M-protein genes of group A streptococci and products of gene duplication, *Proc Natl Acad Sci USA*, **86**: 4741–5.

Heinemann PG, Hefferan M, 1909, A study of *Bacillus bulgaricus*, *J Infect Dis*, **6**: 304–18.

Henrichsen J, 1979, The pneumococcal typing system and pneumococcal surveillance, *J Infect Dis*, **1 (Suppl. 2)**: 31–37.

Henrichsen J, 1995, Six newly recognized types of *Streptococcus pneumoniae*, *J Clin Microbiol*, **33**: 2759–62.

Henrichsen J, Ferrieri P et al., 1984, Nomenclature of antigens of group B streptococci, *Int J Syst Bacteriol*, **34**: 500.

Henriksen SD, Henrichsen J, 1975, Twitching motility and possession of polar fimbriae in spreading *Streptococcus sanguis*

isolates from the human throat, *Acta Path Microbiol Scand B*, **83**: 133–40.

Hentges DJ, 1983, *Human Intestinal Microflora in Health and Disease*, Academic Press, New York.

Hoffmann S, 1985, The throat carrier rate of group A and other beta hemolytic streptococci among patients in general practice, *Acta Path Microbiol Immunol Scand Sect B*, **93**: 347–51.

Hogg SD, Old LA, 1993, The wall associated lipoteichoic acid of *Streptococcus sanguis*, *Antonie van Leeuwenhoek*, **63**: 29–34.

Hogg SD, Lightfoot I, 1992, Retention of lipoteichoic acid at the surface of sucrose grown *Streptococcus sanguis* and *Streptococcus mutans* strains, *New Perspectives on Streptococci and Streptococcal Infections*, ed. Orefici G, Gustav Fischer, Stuttgart, 512–14.

Hollingshead SK, Arnold J et al., 1994, Molecular evolution of a multigene family in group A streptococci, *Mol Biol Evol*, **11**: 208–19.

Hollingshead SK, Fischetti VA, Scott JR, 1987, Size variation in group A streptococcal M protein is generated by homologous recombination between intragenic repeats, *Mol Gen Genet*, **207**: 196–203.

Holm SE, Norrby A et al., 1992, Aspects of pathogenesis of serious group A streptococcal infections in Sweden, *J Infect Dis*, **166**: 31–7.

Holmes AR, Gopal PK, Jenkinson HF, 1995, Adherence of *Candida albicans* to a cell surface polysaccharide receptor on *Streptococcus gordonii*, *Infect Immun*, **63**: 1827–34.

Homer KA, Denbow L et al., 1993, Chondroitin sulfate depolymerase and hyaluronidase activities of viridans streptococci determinined by a sensitive spectrophotometric assay, *J Clin Microbiol*, **31**: 1648–51.

Horaud T, de Cespedes G et al., 1991, Variability of chromosomal genetic elements in streptococci, *Genetics and Molecular Biology of Streptococci, Lactococci and Enterococci*, eds Dunny GM, Cleary PP, McKay LL, American Society for Microbiology, Washington DC, 16–20.

Horodniceanu T, Bougueleret L, Bieth G, 1981, Conjugative transfer of multiple-antibiotic resistance markers in beta-hemolytic group A, B, F, and G streptococci in the absence of extrachromosomal deoxyribonucleic acid, *Plasmid*, **5**: 127–37.

Horodniceanu T, Buu-Hoi A et al., 1982, High-level aminoglycoside resistance in group A, B, G, D (*Streptococcus bovis*), and viridans streptococci, *Antimicrob Agents Chemother*, **21**: 176–79.

Horstmann RD, Sievertsen HJ et al., 1992, Role of fibrinogen in complement inhibition by streptococcal M protein, *Infect Immun*, **60**: 5036–41.

Huang TT, Malke H, Ferretti JJ, 1989, Heterogeneity of the streptokinase gene in group A streptococci, *Infect Immun*, **57**: 502–6.

Hynes WL, Ferretti JJ, 1989, Sequence analysis and expression in *Escherichia coli* of the hyaluronidase gene of *Streptococcus pyogenes* bacteriophage H4489A, *Infect Immun*, **57**: 533–9.

Hynes WL, Ferretti JJ, Tagg JR, 1993, Cloning of the gene encoding Streptococcin A-FF22, a novel antibiotic produced by *Streptococcus pyogenes*, and determination of its nucleotide sequence, *Appl Environ Microbiol*, **59**: 1969–71.

Hynes WL, Tagg JR, 1985, Production of broad-spectrum bacteriocin-like activity by group A streptococci of particular M-types, *Zbl Bakt Hyg A*, **259**: 155–64.

Hynes WL, Weeks CR et al., 1987, Immunologic cross-reactivity of type A streptococcal exotoxin (Erythrogenic toxin) and staphylococcal enterotoxins B and C1, *Infect Immun*, **55**: 837–8.

Håvarstein LS, Coomaraswami G, Morrison DA, 1995, An unmodified heptadecapeptide pheromone induces competence for genetic transformation in *Streptococcus pneumoniae*, *Proc Natl Acad Sci USA*, **92**: 11140–4.

Isolauri E, Majamaa H et al., 1993, *Lactobacillus casei* strain GG reverses increased intestinal permeability induced by cow milk in suckling rats, *Gastroenterol*, **105**: 1643–50.

Jack RW, Tagg JR, Bibek R, 1995, Bacteriocins of gram-positive bacteria, *Microbiol Rev*, **59**: 171–200.

Jacobs JA, Schot CS et al., 1996, Rapid species identification of 'Streptococcus milleri' strains by line blot hybridization: Identification of a distinct 16S rRNA population closely related to Streptococcus constellatus, *J Clin Microbiol*, **34**: 1717–21.

Jacques NA, Hardy L et al., 1979, Effect of growth conditions on the formation of extracellular lipoteichoic acid by Streptococcus mutans BHT, *Infect Immun*, **25**: 75–84.

Jelinková J, 1977, Group B streptococci in the human population, *Curr Topics Microbiol Immunol*, **76**: 127–65.

Jelinková J, Kubin V, 1974, Proposal of a new serological group ('V') of hemolytic streptococci isolated from serine lymph nodes, *Int J Syst Bacteriol*, **24**: 434–7.

Jennings HJ, Lugowski C, Young NM, 1980, Structure of the complex polysaccharide C-substance from Streptococcus pneumoniae type 1, *Biochemistry*, **19**: 4712–19.

Jennings HJ, Rosell K et al., 1983, Structural determination of the capsular polysaccharide antigen of type II group B Streptococcus, *J Biol Chem*, **258**: 1793–8.

Johansson PJ, Malone CC et al., 1994, Streptococcus pyogenes type M12 protein shows selective binding to some human immunoglobulin G3 myeloma proteins, *Infect Immun*, **62**: 3559–63.

Johnson DR, Stevens DL, Kaplan EL, 1992, Epidemiologic analysis of group A streptococcal serotypes associated with sever systemic infections, rheumatic fever, or uncomplicated pharyngitis, *J Infect Dis*, **166**: 374–82.

Johnson MK, Boese-Marrazzo D, Pierce WA, 1981, Effects on pneumolysin on human polymorphonuclear leukocytes and platelets, *Infect Immun*, **34**: 171–6.

Johnson LP, L'Italien JJ, Schlievert PM, 1986, Streptococcal pyrogenic exotoxin type A (scarlet fever toxin) is related to Staphylococcus aureus enterotoxin B, *Mol Gen Gent*, **203**: 354–6.

Jones D, 1978, Composition and differentiation of the genus Streptococcus, *Streptococci*, eds Skinner FA, Quesnel LB, Academic Press, London, 1–49.

Jones KF, Fischetti VA, 1987, Biological and immunochemical identity of M protein and group G streptococci with M protein on group A streptococci, *Infect Immun*, **55**: 502–6.

Jung G, 1991, Lantibiotics ribosomally synthesized biologically active polypeptides containing sulfide bridges and α,β-didehydroamino acids, *Angew Chem Int Ed Engl*, **30**: 1051–68.

Jürgens D, Sterzik B, Fehrenbach FJ, 1987, Unspecific binding of group B streptococcal cocytolysin (CAMP factor) to immunoglobulins and its possible role in pathogenicity, *J Exp Med*, **165**: 720–32.

Kaila M et Isolauri E et al., 1992, Enhancement of the circulating antibody secreting cell response in human diarrhea by human s Lactobacillus strain, *Ped Res*, **32**: 141–4.

Kanclerski K, Blomquist et al., 1988, Serum antibodies to pneumolysin in patients with pneumonia, *J Clin Microbiol*, **26**: 96–100.

Kandler O, 1982, Carbohydrate metabolism in lactic acid bacteria, *Antonie van Leeuwenhoek*, **49**: 209–24.

Kandler O, Weiss N, 1986, Regular, nonsporing gram-positive rods, *Bergey's Manual of Systematic Bacteriology*, vol. 2, eds Sneath PHA, Mair MS, Williams and Wilkins, Baltimore, 1208–34.

Kapur V, Maffei JT et al., 1994a, Vaccination with streptococcal extracellular cysteine protease (interleukin-1 beta convertase) protects mice against challenge with heterologous group A streptococci, *Microb Pathog*, **16**: 443–50.

Kapur V, Majesky MW et al., 1993b, Cleavage of interleukin 1 beta (IL-1beta) precursor to produce active IL-1 beta by a conserved extracellular cysteine protease from Streptococcus pyogenes, *Proc Natl Acad Sci USA*, **90**: 7676–80.

Kapur V, Topouzis S et al., 1993, A conserved Streptococcus pyogenes extracellular cysteine protease cleaves human fibronectin and degrades vitronectin, *Microb Pathog*, **15**: 327–46.

Kaufhold A, Podbielski A et al., 1992, M protein gene typing of Streptococcus pyogenes by nonradioactively labeled oligonucleotide probes, *J Clin Microbiol*, **30**: 2391–97.

Kaufhold A, Podbielski A et al., 1994, Rapid typing of group A streptococci by the use of DNA amplification and nonradioactive allele-specific oligonucleotide probes, *FEMS Microbiol Lett*, **119**: 19–25.

Kaufmann F, Lund E, Eddy BE, 1960, Proposal for a change in the nomenclature of Diplococcus pneumoniae and a comparison of the Danish and American type designations, *Int Bull Bacteriol Taxon*, **10**: 31–40.

Kawamura Y, Hou XG et al., 1995a, Determination of 16S rRNA sequences of Streptococcus mitis and Streptococcus gordonii and phylogenetic relationships among members of the genus Streptococcus, *Int J Syst Bacteriol*, **45**: 406–8.

Kawamura Y, Hou XG et al., 1995b, Transfer of Streptococcus adjacens and Streptococcus defectivus to Abiotrophia gen. nov. as Abiotrophia adiacens comb. nov. and Abiotrophia defectiva comb. nov., respectively, *Int J Syst Bacteriol*, **45**: 798–803.

Kehoe MA, 1994, Cell-wall-associated proteins in Gram positive bacteria, *Bacterial Cell Wall*, eds Ghuysen J-M, Hackenbeck R, Elsevier, Amsterdam, 217–61.

Kehoe MA, Miller L et al., 1987, Nucleotide sequence of the streptolysin O (SLO) gene: structural homologies between SLO and other membrane-damaging thiol-activated toxins, *Infect Immun*, **55**: 3228–32.

Kehoe M, Timmis KN, 1984, Cloning and expression in Escherichia coli of the streptolysin O determinant from Streptococcus pyogenes: characterization of the cloned streptolysin O derminant and demonstration of the absence of substantial homology with determinants of other thiol-activated toxins, *Infect Immun*, **43**: 804–10.

Kellner A, Robertson T, 1954, Myocardial necrosis produced in animals by means of crystalline streptococcal proteinase, *J Exp Med*, **99**: 495–504.

Kelstrup J, Gibbons RJ, 1969, Bacteriocins from human and rodent streptococci, *Arch Oral Biol*, **14**: 251–58.

Kelstrup J, Richmond S et al., 1970, Fingerprinting human oral streptococci by bacteriocin production and sensitivity, *Arch Oral Biol*, **15**: 1109–16.

Kenne L, Lindberg B, 1983, Bacterial polysaccharides, *The polysaccharides*, vol. 2, ed. Aspinall GO, Academic Press, New York, 287–363.

Khanna AK, Williams RC et al., 1989, The presence of a non HLA B-cell antigen in rheumatic fever patients and their famililes as defined by a monoclonal antibody, *J Clin Invest*, **83**: 1710–16.

Kikuchi K, Enari T et al., 1995, Comparison of phenotypic characteristics, DNA-DNA hybridization results, and results with a commercial rapid biochemical and enzymatic reaction system for identification of viridans group streptococci, *J Clin Microbiol*, **33**: 1215–22.

Kilian M, Husby S et al., 1995, Increased proportions of bacteria capable of cleaving IgA1 in the pharynx of infants with atopic disease, *Ped Res*, **38**: 182–6.

Kilian M, Mikkelsen L, Henrichsen J, 1989, Taxonomic study of viridans streptococci: Description of Streptococcus gordonii sp. nov. and emended descriptions of Streptococcus sanguis (White and Niven 1946), Streptococcus oralis (Bridge and Sneath 1982), and Streptococcus mitis (Andrewes and Horder 1906), *Int J Syst Bacteriol*, **39**: 471–84.

Kilian M, Reinholdt J et al., 1996, Biological significance of IgA1 proteases in bacterial colonization and pathogenesis: critical evaluation of experimental evidence, *APMIS*, **104**: 321–38.

Kilpper-Bälz R, Rischer G, Schleifer KH, 1982, Nucleic acid hybridization of group N and group D streptococci, *Curr Microbiol*, **7**: 245–50.

Kilpper-Bälz R, Schleifer KH, 1984, Nucleic acid hybridization and cell wall composition studies of pyogenic streptococci, *FEMS Microbiol Lett*, **24**: 355–64.

Kilpper-Bälz R, Schleifer KH, 1987, Description of Streptococcus suis nom. rev., *Int J Syst Bacteriol*, **37**: 160–62.

Kilpper-Bälz R, Wenzig P, Schleifer KH, 1985, Molecular relationships and classification of some viridans streptococci as *Streptococcus oralis* and emended description of *Streptococcus oralis* (Bridge and Sneath 1982), *Int J Syst Bacteriol*, **35**: 482–88.

Kilpper-Bälz R, Williams BL et al., 1984, Relatedness of '*Streptococcus milleri*' with *Streptococcus anginosus* and *Streptococcus constellatus*, *Syst Appl Microbiol*, **5**: 494–500.

Kim YB, Watson DW, 1970, A purified group A streptococcal pyrogenic exotoxin. Physicochemical and biological properties including the enhancement of suceptibility to endotoxin lethal shock, *J Exp Med*, **131**: 611–22.

Knight RG, Shlaes DM, 1985, Physiological characteristics and deoxyribonucleic acid relatedness of human isolates of *Streptococcus bovis* and *Streptococcus bovis* (var.), *Int J Syst Bacteriol*, **35**: 357–61.

Knox KW, Wicken AJ, 1973, Immunological properties of teichoic acids, *Bacteriol Rev*, **37**: 215–57.

Knox KW, Wicken AJ, 1976, Grouping and cross-reacting antigens of oral lactic acid bacteria, *J Dent Res*, **55**: A116–22.

Kogan G, Uhrín D et al., 1994, Structure of the type VI of group B *Streptococcus* capsular polysaccharide determined by high resolution NMR spectroscopy, *J Carbohydr Chem*, **13**: 1071–8.

Kogan G, Brisson JR et al., 1995, Structural elucidation of the novel type VII group B *Streptococcus* capsular polysaccharide by high resolution NMR spectroscopy, *Carbohydr Res*, **277**: 1–9.

Kogan G, Uhrin D et al., 1996, Structural and immunochemical characterization of the type VIII group B *Streptococcus* capsular polysaccharide, *J Biol Chem*, **271**: 8786–90.

Kronvall G, Schonbeck C, Myhre E, 1979, Fibrinogen binding structures in beta hemolytic streptococci group A, C and G: comparisons with receptors for IgG and aggregated beta-2 microglobulin, *Acta Pathol Microbiol Scand, Sect. B*, **87**: 303–10.

Lai CY, Wang MT et al., 1978, Streptolysin S: improved purification and characterization, *Arch Biochem Biophys*, **191**: 804–12.

Lancefield RC, 1928, The antigenic complex of *Streptococcus hemolyticus*. I. Demonstration of a type-specific substance in extracts of *Streptococcus hemolyticus*, *J Exp Med*, **47**: 91–103.

Lancefield RC, 1933, A serological differentiation of human and other groups of hemolytic streptococci, *J Exp Med*, **59**: 571–91.

Lancefield RC, 1934, A serological differentiation of specific types of bovine hemolytic streptococci (Group B), *J Exp Med*, **59**: 441–58.

Lancefield RC, 1938, Two serological types of group B haemolytic streptococci with related, but not identical, type-specific substances, *J Exp Med*, **67**: 25–39.

Lancefield RC, 1940, Type-specific antigens, M and T, of matt and glossy variants of group A hemolytic streptococci, *J Exp Med*, **71**: 521.

Lancefield RC, 1959, Persistence of type specific antibodies in man following infection with group A streptococci, *J Exp Med*, **110**: 271–92.

Lancefield RC, 1962, Current knowledge of type-specific M antigens of group A streptococci, *J Immunol*, **89**: 307–13.

Law BA, Kolstad J, 1983, Proteolytic systems in lactic acid bacteria, *Antonie van Leeuwenhoek*, **49**: 225–45.

LeBlanc DJ, Lee LN, 1979, Rapid screening procedure for detection of plasmids in streptococci, *J Bacteriol*, **140**: 1112–15.

Ledesma OV, de Ruiz Holgado AP et al., 1977, A synthetic medium for comparative nutritional studies of lactobacilli, *J Appl Bact*, **42**: 123–33.

Lee CJ, Liu TY, 1977, The autolytic enzyme activity upon pneumococcal cell wall, *J Biochem*, **8**: 573–80.

Leichmann G, 1896, Über die im Brennereiprozess bei der bereitung der Kunsthefe auftretende spontane Milchsäuregärung, *Zentralbl Bakteriol II Abt*, **2**: 281–5.

Leigh JA, 1993, Activation of bovine plasminogen by *Streptococcus uberis*, *FEMS Microbiol Lett*, **114**: 67–71.

Lindahl G, Åkerström B, 1989, Receptor for IgA in group A streptococci: cloning of the gene and characterization of the protein expressed in *Escherichia coli*, *Mol Microbiol*, **3**: 239–47.

Lomholt H, 1995, Evidence of recombination and an anti-

genically diverse immunoglobulin A1 protease among strains of *Streptococcus pneumoniae*, *Infect Immun*, **63**: 4238–43.

London J, 1976, The ecology and taxonomic status of the lactobacilli, *Annu Rev Microbiol*, **30**: 279–301.

Ludwig W, Seewaldt E et al., 1985, The phylogenetic position of *Streptococcus* and *Enterococcus*, *J Gen Microbiol*, **131**: 543–51.

Lund E, Henrichsen, J, 1978, Laboratory diagnosis, serology and epidemiology of *Streptococcus pneumoniae*, *Methods in Microbiology*, eds Bergan T, Norris JR, Academic Press, London, 241–62.

MacLeod CM, Krauss MR, 1950, Relation of virulence of pneumococcal strains for mice to the quantity of capsular polysaccharide formed in vitro, *J Exp Med*, **92**: 1–9.

McCarty M, 1959, The occurrence of polyglycerophosphates as an antigenic component of various gram-positive bacterial species, *J Exp Med*, **109**: 361–78.

McCoy HE, Broder CC, Lottenberg R, 1991, Streptokinases produced by pathogenic group C streptococci demonstrate species-specific plasminogen activation, *J Infect Dis*, **164**: 515–21.

McDaniel LS, Sheffield JS et al., 1991, PspA, a surface protein of *Streptococcus pneumoniae*, is capable of eliciting protection against pneumococci of more than one serotype, *Infect Immun*, **59**: 222–8.

McIntire FC , Crosby LK et al., 1988, A polysaccharide from *Streptococcus sanguis* 34 that inhibits coaggregation of *S. sanguis* 34 with *Actinomyces viscosus* T14V, *J Bacteriol*, **170**: 2229–35.

McIntosh J, James WW, Lazarus-Barlow P, 1922, An investigation into the aetiology of of dental caries. I. The nature of the destructive agent and the production of artificial caries, *Br J Exp Pathol*, **3**: 138–45.

McIntosh J, James WW, Lazarus-Barlow P, 1924, An investigation into the aetiology of of dental caries. II. The biological characteristics and distribution of *B. acidophilus odotolyticus*, *Br J Exp Pathol*, **5**: 175–81.

Malke H, 1972, Transduction in group A streptococci, *Streptococci and Streptococcal Diseases*, eds Wannamaker LW, Matsen JM, Academic Press, New York, 119–33.

Man JC de, Rogosa M, Sharpe EM, 1960, A medium used for the cultivation of lactobacilli, *J Appl Bacteriol*, **23**: 130–5.

Marchlewicz BA, Duncan JL, 1980, Properties of a hemolysin produced by group B streptococci, *Infect Immun*, **30**: 805–13.

Maxted WR, 1964, Streptococcal bacteriophages, *The Streptococcus, Rheumatic Fever and Glomerulonephritis*, ed. Uhr JW, Williams and Wilkins, Baltimore, 25–44.

Milligan TW, Baker CJ et al., 1978, Association of elevated levels of extracellular neuraminidase with clinical isolates of type III group B streptococci, *Infect Immun*, **21**: 738–46.

Molin G, Jeppsson B et al., 1993, Numerical taxonomy of *Lactobacillus* spp. associated with healthy and diseased mucosa of the human intestines, *J Appl Bacteriol*, **74**: 314–23.

Mollick JA, Miller GG et al., 1993, A novel superantigen isolated from pathogenic strains of *Streptococcus pyogenes* with aminoterminal homology to staphylococcal enterotoxins B and C, *J Clin Invest*, **92**: 710–19.

Moro E, 1900, Über die nach Gram farbbaren Bacillen des Säuglingsstuhles, *Wien Klin Wochenschr*, **13**: 114–15.

Musser JM, Hauser AR et al., 1991, *Streptococcus pyogenes* causing toxic-shock-like syndrome and other invasive diseases: clonal diversity and pyrogenic exotoxin expression, *Proc Natl Acad Sci USA*, **88**: 2668–72.

Musser JM, Kapur V et al., 1993a, Geographic and temporal distribution and molecular characterization of two highly pathogenic clones of *Streptococcus pyogenes* expressing allelic variants of pyrogenic exotoxin A (scarlet fever toxin), *J Infect Dis*, **167**: 337–46.

Musser JM, Kapur V et al., 1995, Genetic diversity and relationships among *Streptococcus pyogenes* strains expressing serotype M1 protein: recent intercontinental spread of a subclone causing episodes of invasive disease, *Infect Immun*, **63**: 994–1003.

Musser JM, Mattingly SJ et al., 1989, Identification of a high-virulence clone of *Streptococcus agalactiae* (group B *Streptococcus*) causing invasive neonatal disease, *Proc Natl Acad Sci USA*, **86**: 4731–5.

Musser JM, Nelson K et al., 1993b, Temporal variation in bacterial disease frequency: Molecular population genetic analysis of scarlet fever epidemics in Ottawa and in Eastern Germany, *J Infect Dis*, **167**: 759–62.

Natanson S, Sela S et al., 1995, Distribution of fibronectin-binding proteins among group A streptococci of different M types, *J Infect Dis*, **171**: 871–8.

Nealon TJ, Mattingly SJ, 1984, Role of cellular lipoteichoic acids in mediating adherence of serotype III strains of group B streptococci to human embryonic, fetal, and adult epithelial cells, *Infect Immun*, **43**: 523–30.

Norgren M, Norrby A, Holm SE, 1992, Genetic diversity in T1M1 group A streptococci in relation to clinical outcome of infection, *J Infect Dis*, **166**: 1014–20.

Nyvad B, Kilian M, 1990, Comparison of the initial streptococcal microflora on dental enamel in caries-active and in caries-inactive individuals, *Caries Res*, **24**: 267–72.

O'Connor SP, Cleary PP, 1987, In vivo *Streptococcus pyogenes* C5a peptidase activity: analysis using transposon and nitrosoguanidine induced mutants, *J Infect Dis*, **156**: 495–504.

O'Connor SP, Darip D et al., 1991, The human antibody response to streptococcal C5a peptidase, *J Infect Dis*, **163**: 109–16.

Ofek I, Beachey EH et al., 1975, Cell membrane-binding properties of group A streptococcal lipoteichoic acid, *J Exp Med*, **141**: 990–1003.

Ohkuni H, Todome Y et al., 1992, Immunochemical studies and complete amino acid sequence of the streptokinase from *Streptococcus pyogenes* (Group A) M Type 12 strain A374, **60**: 278–83.

Olsen I, Johnson JL et al., 1991, *Lactobacillus uli* sp.nov. and *Lactobacillus rimae* sp. nov. from the human gingival crevice and emended descriptions of *Lactobacillus minutus* and *Streptococcus parvulus*, *Int J Syst Bacteriol*, **41**: 261–6.

Orla-Jensen S, 1904, Studien über die fluchtigen Fettsäuren im Käse nebst Beiträgen zur Biologie der Käsefermente, *Zbl Bakteriol Parasitenk Infektionskr Hyg II Abt. Ref.*, **13**: 161–70.

Orla-Jensen S, 1919, *The Lactic Acid Bacteria*, Mémoires de l'Académie Royale des Sciences et des Lettres de Danemark, Copenhagen.

Orla-Jensen S, 1943, *The Lactic Acid Bacteria*, Einar Munksgaard, Copenhagen.

O'Toole P, Stenberg L et al., 1992, Two major classes in the M protein family in group A streptococci, *Proc Natl Acad Sci USA*, **89**: 8661–5.

Pakula R, Walczak, 1963, On the nature of competence of transformable streptococci, *J Gen Microbiol*, **31**: 125.

Paton JC, Ferrante A, 1983, Inhibition of human polymorphonuclear leukocyte respiratory burst, bactericidal activity, and migration by pneumolysin, *Infect Immun*, **41**: 1212–16.

Paul D, Slade HD, 1975, Production and properties of an extracellular bacteriocin from *Streptococcus mutans* bacteriocidal for group A and other streptococci, *Infect Immun*, **12**: 1375–85.

Pearce C, Bowden GH et al., 1995, Identification of pioneer viridans streptococci in the oral cavity of human neonates, *J Med Microbiol*, **42**: 67–72.

Pease AA, Douglas CWI, Spencer RC, 1986, Identifying non-capsulate strains of *Streptococcus pneumoniae* isolated from eyes, *J Clin Pathol*, **39**: 871–5.

Pederson CS, 1936, A study of the species *Lactobacillus plantarum* (Orla-Jensen) Bergey et al., *J Bacteriol*, **31**: 217–24.

Perch B, Kjems E, Henrichsen J, 1979, New serotypes of group B streptococci isolated from human sources, *J Clin Microbiol*, **10**: 109–10.

Perch B, Kjems E, Ravn T, 1974, Biochemical and serological properties of *Streptococcus mutans* from various human and animal sources, *Acta Pathol Microbiol Scand Ser B*, **82**: 357–70.

Perch B, Pedersen KB, Henrichsen J, 1983, Serology of capsulated stteptococci pathogenic for pigs: six new serotypes of *Streptococcus suis*, *J Clin Microbiol*, **17**: 993–6.

Perdigon G, Alvarez S et al., 1995, Probiotic bacteria for humans: Clinical systems for evaluation of effectiveness. Immune System stimulation by probiotics (Symposium), *J Dairy Sci*, **78**: 1597–606.

Perez-Casal J, Caparon MG et al., 1991, Mry, a *trans*-acting positive regulator of the M protein gene of *Streptococcus pyogenes* with similarity to the receptor proteins of two-component regulatory systems, *J Bacteriol*, **173**: 2617–24.

Pier GB, Madin SH, 1976, *Streptococcus iniae* sp. nov., a beta hemolytic *Streptococcus* isolated from an Amazon freshwater dolphin, *Inia geoffrensis*, *Int J Syst Bacteriol*, **26**: 545–53.

Pinter JK, Hayashi JA, Bahn AN, 1969, Carbohydrate hydrolases of oral streptococci, *Arch Oral Biol*, **14**: 735–44.

Pot B, Ludwig W et al., 1994, Taxonomy of lactic acid bacteria, *Bacteriocins of Lactic Acid Bacteria: Genetics and Applications*, eds De Vuyst L, Vandamme EJ, Chapman and Hall, Glasgow, 13–89.

Pritchard DG, Gray BM, Dillon HC Jr, 1984, Characterization of the group-specific polysaccharide of group B *Streptococcus*, *Arch Biochem Biophys*, **235**: 385–92.

Pritchard DG, Lin B, 1993, Group B streptococcal neuraminidase is actually a hyaluronidase, *Infect Immun*, **61**: 3234–39.

Ragland N, Tagg J, 1990, Applications of bacteriocin-like inhibitory substance (BLIS) typing in a longitudinal study of the oral carriage of β-haemolytic streptococci by a group of Dunedin schoolchildren, *Zbl Bakteriol*, **274**: 100–8.

Reda KB, Kapur V et al., 1994, Molecular characterization and phylogenetic distribution of the streptococcal superantigen gene (*ssa*) from *Streptococcus pyogenes*, *Infect Immun*, **62**: 1867–74.

Reddy GP, Abeygunawardana C et al., 1994, The cell wall polysaccharide of *Streptococcus gordonii* 38: structure and immunochemical comparison with the receptor polysaccharides of *Streptococcus oralis* 34 and *Streptococcus mitis* J22, *Glycobiology*, **4**: 183–92.

Reddy GP, Chang CC, Bush CA, 1993, Determination by heteronuclear NMR spectroscopy of the complete structure of the cell wall polysaccharide of *Streptococcus sanguis* K103, *Anal Chem*, **65**: 913–21.

Reed GL, Kussie P, Parhami-Seren B, 1993, A functional analysis of the antigenicity of streptokinase using monoclonal antibody mapping and recombinant streptokinase fragments, *J Immunol*, **150**: 4407–15.

Reizen J and Peterkofsky A (eds), 1987, *Sugar Transport and Metabolism in Gram-positive Bacteria*, Ellis Horwood, Chichester.

Relf WA, Martin DR, Sriprakash KS, 1992, Identification of sequence types among the M-nontypeable group A streptococci, *J Clin Microbiol*, **30**: 3190–4.

Retnoningrum D, Cleary PP, 1994, M12 protein from *Streptococcus pyogenes* is a receptor for immunoglobulin G3 and human albumin, *Infect Immun*, **62**: 2387–94.

Roach S, Tannock W, 1979, Indigenous bacteria influence the number of *Salmonella typhimurium* in the ileum of gnotobiotic mice, *Can J Microbiol*, **25**: 1352–8.

Robinson JH, Kehoe MA, 1992, Group A streptococcal M proteins: virulence factors and protective antigens, *Immunol Today*, **13**: 362–7.

Rogers AH, Van der Hoeven JS, Mikx JS, 1978, Inhibition of *Actinomyces viscosus* by bacteriocin-producing strains of *Streptococcus mutans* in the dental plaque of gnotobiotic rats, *Arch Oral Biol*, **23**: 477–84.

Rogers AH, Zihm PS et al., 1990, Some aspects of protease production by a strain of *Streptococcus sanguis*, *Oral Microbiol Immunol*, **5**: 72–6.

Rogosa M, Mitchell JA, Wiseman RF, 1951, A selective medium for the isolation of oral and faecal lactobacilli, *J Bacteriol*, **62**: 132–3.

Rogosa M, Wiseman RF et al., 1953, Species differentiation of oral lactobacilli from man including descriptions of *Lactobacillus salivarius* nov. spec. and *Lactobacillus cellobiosus* nov. spec., *J Bacteriol*, **65:** 681–99.

Rölla G, Iversen OJ, Bonesvoll P, 1978, Lipotichoic acid – the key to the adhesiveness of sucrose grown *Streptococcus mutans*, *Adv Exp Med Biol*, **107:** 607–17.

Rölla G, Oppermann RV et al., 1980, High amounts of lipoteichoic acid in sucrose-induced plaque *in vivo*, *Caries Res*, **14:** 235–8.

Rosan B, 1978, Absence of glycerol teichoic acids in certain oral streptococci, *Science*, **201:** 918–20.

Rosan B, Eisenberg RJ, 1973, Morphological changes in *Streptococcus sanguis* associated with growth in the presence of oxygen, *Arc Oral Biol*, **18:** 1441–4.

Rosenbach FJ, 1884, *Mikro-organismen bei den Wund-Infections-Krankheiten des Menschen*, JF Bergmann, Wiesbaden.

Ross K, Grahén E et al., 1993, Interfering alpha-streptococci as a protection against recurrent streptococcal tonsillitis in children, *Int J Pediatr Otorhinolaryngol*, **25:** 141–8.

Ross PW, 1970, Ecology of group B streptococci, *Streptococci*, Society for Applied Bacteriology Symposium Series No. 7, eds Skinner FA, Quesnel LB, Academic Press, London, 127–42.

Ross KF et al., 1993, Isolation and characterization of the lantibiotic salivaricin A and its structural gene *salA* from *Streptococcus salivarius* 20P3, *Appl Environ Microbiol*, **59:** 2014–21.

Rotta J, 1986, Pyogenic hemolytic streptococci, *Bergey's Manual of Systematic Bacteriology*, eds Sneath PHA, Mair NS, Sharpe ME, Williams and Wilkins, Baltimore, 1047–54.

Rubens CE, Wessels MR et al., 1987, Transposon mutagenesis of type III group B *Streptococcus*: Correlation of capsule expression with virulence, *Proc Natl Acad Sci USA*, **84:** 7208–12.

Ruoff KL, 1991, Nutritionally variant streptococci, *Clin Microbiol Rev*, **4:** 184–90.

Rýc M, Beachey EH, Whitnack EH, 1989, Ultrastructural localisation of the fibrinogen-binding domain of streptococcal M protein, *Infect Immunol*, **57:** 2397–404.

Salminen S, Deighton M, Gorbach S, 1993, Lactic acid bacteria in health and disease, *Lactic Acid Bacteria*, eds Salminen S, von Wright A, Marcel Dekker, New York, 237–94.

Salton MRJ, Horne RW, 1951, Studies of the bacterial cell wall. II. Methods of preparation and some properties of cell walls, *Biochim Biophys Acta*, **7:** 177–97.

Schaufuss P, Sting R et al., 1989, Isolation and characterization of hyaluronidase from *Streptococcus uberis*, *Zbl Bakteriol*, **271:** 46–53.

Schifferle RE, Jennings HJ et al., 1985, Immunochemical analysis of the types Ia and Ib group B streptococcal polysaccharides, *J Immunol*, **135:** 4164–70.

Schillinger U, Lücke F-K, 1987, Identification of lactobacilli from meat and meat products, *Food Microbiol*, **4:** 199–208.

Schleifer KH, Kandler O, 1972, Peptidoglycan types of bacterial cell walls and their taxonomic implications, *Bacteriol Rev*, **36:** 407–77.

Schleifer KH, Kilpper-Bälz R, 1987, Molecular and chemotaxonomic approaches to the classification of streptococci, enterococci and lactococci: a review, *Syst Appl Microbiol*, **10:** 1–19.

Schleifer KH, Kraus J et al., 1985, Transfer of *Streptococcus lactis* and related streptococci to the genus *Lactococcus* gen. nov., *Syst Appl Micrbiol*, **6:** 183–95.

Schleifer KH, Ludwig W, 1995, Phylogenetic relationships of lactic acid bacteria, *The Lactic Acid Bacteria. Volume 2. The Genera of Lactic Acid Bacteria*, eds Wood BJB, Holzapfel WH, Blackie, Glasgow, 7–18.

Schleifer KH, Seidl PH, 1985, Chemical composition and structue of murein, *Chemical methods in bacterial systematics*, eds Goodfellow M, Minnikin DE, Academic Press, London, 201–219.

Schlievert PM, Bettin KM, Watson DW, 1979, Reinterpretation of the Dick test: Role of group A streptococcal pyrogenic exotoxin, *Infect Immunol*, **26:** 467–72.

Schmidhuber S, Kilpper-Bälz R, Schleifer KH, 1987, A taxonomic

study of *Streptococcus mitis*, *S. oralis*, and *S., sanguis*, *System Appl Microbiol*, **10:** 74–7.

Schmidhuber S, Ludwig W, Schleiftr KH, 1988, Construction of a DNA probe for the specific identification of *Streptococcus oralis*, *J Clin Microbiol*, **26:** 1042–4.

Schnitzler N, Podbielski A et al., 1995, M or a M-like protein gene polymorphisms in human group G streptococci, *J Clin Microbiol*, **33:** 356–63.

Schofield CR, Tagg JR, 1983, Bacteriocin-like activity of group B and group C streptococci of human and of animal origin, *J Hyg Camb*, **90:** 7–18.

Schwab JH, Watson DW, Cromartie WJ, 1955, Further studies of group A streptococcal factors with lethal and cardiotoxic properties, *J Infect Dis*, **96:** 14–18.

Scott JR, Pulliam M et al., 1985, Relationship of M protein genes in group A streptococci, *Proc Natl Acad Sci USA*, **82:** 1822–6.

Seppälä H, Vuopio-Varkila J et al., 1994, Evaluation of methods for epidemiologic typing of group A streptococci, *J Infect Dis*, **169:** 519–25.

Sharpe ME, 1955, A serological classification of lactobacilli, *J Gen Microbiol*, **12:** 107–22.

Sharpe ME, 1981, The genus *Lactobacillus*, *The Prokaryocytes*, vol. II, eds Starr MP, Stolp H et al., Springer-Verlag, Berlin, 1653–74.

Sharpe ME, Brock JH et al., 1973a, Glycerol teichoic acid as a common antigenic factor in lactobacilli and some other gram-positive organisms, *J Gen Microbiol*, **74:** 119–26.

Sharpe ME, Hill LR, Lapage SR, 1973b, Pathogenic lactobacilli, *J Med Microbiol*, **6:** 281–6.

Shockman GD, Tice G et al., 1986, Biochemical aspects of the *Streptococcus mutans* cell wall, *Molecular Microbiology and Immunobiology of* Streptococcus mutans, eds Hamada S, Michalek SM et al., Elsevier, Amsterdam, 71–80.

Sibold C, Henrichsen J et al., 1994, Mosaic *pbpX* genes of major clones of penicillin-resistant *Streptococcus pneumoniae* have evolved from *pbpX* genes of a penicillin-sensitive *Streptococcus oralis*, *Mol Microbiol*, **12:** 1013–23.

Simmonds RS, Naidoo et al., 1995, The streptococcal bacteriocin-like inhibitory substance, zoocin A, reduces the proportion of *Streptococcus mutans* in an artificial plaque, *Microb Ecol Health Dis*, **8:** 281–92.

Simpson WA, Beachey EH, 1983, Adherence of group A streptococci to fibronectin on oral epithelial cells, *Infect Immun*, **39:** 275–9.

Simpson WJ, LaPenta D et al., 1990, Coregulation of type 12 M protein and streptococcal C5a peptidase genes in group A streptococci: evidence for a virulence regulon controlled by the *virR* locus, *J Bacteriol*, **172:** 696–700.

Simpson WJ, Musser JM, Cleary PP, 1992, Evidence consistent with the horizontal transfer of the gene (*emm*12) encoding serotype M12 protein between group A and group G pathogenic streptococci, *Infect Immun*, **60:** 1890–3.

Simpson WJ, Tagg JR, 1983, M-type 57 group A streptococcus bacteriocin, *Can J Microbiol*, **29:** 1445–51.

Simpson WJ, Tagg JR, 1984, Survey of the plasmid content of group A streptococci, *FEMS Microbiol Lett*, **23:** 195–9.

Skalka B, Smola J, 1981, Lethal effect of CAMP-factor and UBERIS factor – a new finding about diffusible exosubstances of *Streptococcus agalactiae* and *Streptococcus uberis*, *Zentralbl Bakteriol A*, **249:** 190–4.

Skerman VBD, McGowan V, Sneath PHA (eds), 1980, Approved lists of bacterial names, *Int J Syst Bacteriol*, **30:** 225–420.

Smyth CJ, Duncan JL, 1978, Thiol-activated (oxygen-labile) cytolysins, *Bacterial Toxins and Cell Membranes*, eds Jelijaszewicz J, Wadstrom T, Academic Press, New York, 129–83.

Stackebrandt E, Teuber M, 1988, Molecular taxonomy and phylogenetic position of lactic acid bacteria, *Biochimie*, **70:** 317–24.

Stålhammar-Carlemalm M, Stenberg L, Lindahl G, 1993, Protein Rib: A novel group B streptococcal cell surface protein that confers protective immunity and is expressed by most strains causing invasive infections, *J Exp Med*, **177:** 1593–603.

Sterzik B, Fehrenbach FJ, 1985, Reaction components influencing CAMP factor induced lysis, *J Gen Microbiol*, **131:** 817–20.

Swanson J, Hsu KC, Gotschlich EC, 1969, Electron microscopic studies on streptococci. I. M antigen, *J Exp Med*, **130:** 1063–91.

Sørensen UBS, 1986, Monoclonal phosporylcholine antibody binds to beta-lipoprotein from different animal species, *Infect Immun*, **53:** 264–6.

Sørensen UBS, Blom J et al., 1988, Ultrastructural localization of capsules, cell wall polysaccharide, cell wall proteins, and F antigen in pneumococci, *Infect Immun*, **56:** 1890–6.

Sørensen UBS, Henrichsen J, 1984, C-polysaccharide in a pneumococcal vaccine, *Acta Path Microbiol Immunol Scand C*, **92:** 351–6.

Sørensen UBS, Henrichsen J, 1987, Cross-reactions between pneumococci and other streptococci due to C polysaccharide and F antigen, *J Clin Microbiol*, **25:** 1854–9.

Sørensen UBS, Henrichsen J et al., 1990, Covalent linkage between the capsular polysaccharide and the cell wall peptidoglycan of *Streptococcus pneumoniae* revealed by immunochemical methods, *Microb Pathogen*, **8:** 325–34.

Tagg JR, 1985, An inhibitor typing scheme applicable to Lancefield group E streptococci, *Can J Microbiol*, **31:** 1056–57.

Tagg JR, 1992, BLIS production in the genus *Streptococcus*, *Bacteriocins, Microcins and Antibiotics*, eds Lazdunski RJC, Pattus F, 417–20.

Tagg JR, Read RSD, McGiven AR, 1971, Bacteriocine production by group A streptococci, *Pathology*, **3:** 277–78.

Tagg JR, Skjold S, Wannamaker LW, 1976, Transduction of bacteriocin determinants in group A streptococci, *J Exp Med*, **143:** 1540–4.

Taketoshi M, Kitada K et al., 1993, Enzymatic differentiation and biochemical and serological characteristics of the clinical isolates of *Streptococcus anginosus*, *S. intermedius* and *S. constellatus*, *Microbios*, **76:** 115–29.

Tannock GW, Fuller R, Pedersen K, 1990, Lactobacillus succession in the piglet digestive tract demonstrated by plasmid profiling, *Appl Environmental Microbiol*, **56:** 1310–16.

Tapsall JW, 1986, Pigment production by Lancefield-group-B streptococci (*Streptococcus agalactiae*), *J Med Microbiol*, **21:** 75–81.

Tomasz A, 1981, Surface components of *Streptococcus pneumoniae*, *Rev Infect Dis*, **3:** 190–211.

Tomasz A, 1987, Biochemistry and genetics of penicillin resistance in penumococci, *Streptococcal Genetics*, eds Ferretti JJ, Curtiss R, American Society for Microbiology, Washington DC, 87–92.

Tomasz A, Hotchkiss RD, 1964, Regulation of the transformability of pneumococcal cultures by macromolecular cell products, *Proc Nat Acad Sci USA*, **51:** 480–7.

Top FH Jr, Wannamaker LW, 1968, The serum opacity reaction of *Streptococcus pyogenes*: frequency of production of streptococcal lipoproteinase by strains of different serological types and the relationship of M protein production, *J Hyg Lond*, **66:** 49–58.

Totolian AA, 1979, Transduction of M-protein and serum opacity-factor in group A streptococci, *Pathogenic Streptococci*, ed Parker MT, Reed Books, Chertsey, Surrey, 38–39.

Tuomanen E, Liu H et al., 1985, The induction of meningeal inflammation by components of the pneumococcal cell wall, *J Infect Dis*, **151:** 859–68.

van Dam JEG, Fleer A, Snippe H, 1990, Immunogenicity and immunochemistry of *Streptococcus pneumoniae* capsular polysaccharides, *Antonie van Leeuwenhoek*, **58:** 1–47.

Vandamme P, Pot B et al., 1996, Taxonomic study of Lancefield streptococcal groups C, G, and L (*Streptococcus dysgalactiae*) and proposal of *S. dysgalactiae* subsp. *equisimilis* subsp. nov., *Int J Syst Bacteriol*, **46:** 774–81.

van der Hoeven JS, De Jong MH, Rogers AH, 1985, Effect of utilization of substrates on the composition of dental plaque, *FEMS Microbiol Ecol*, **31:** 129–33.

Varki A, Diaz S, 1983, A neuraminidase from *Streptococcus sanguis* that can release O-acetylated sialic acids, *J Biol Chem*, **258:** 12465–71.

Veasy LG, Wiedmeier SE et al., 1987, Resurgence of acute rheumatic fever in the intermountain area of the United States, *N Engl J Med*, **316:** 421–7.

Vescovo M, Morelli L, Bottazzi V, 1982, Drug resistance plasmids in *Lactobacillus acidophilus* and *Lactobacillus reuteri*, *Appl Environ Microbiol*, **43:** 50–6.

Wagner BK et al., 1986, Albumin bound to the surface of M protein-positive streptococci increased their phagocytosis by human polymorphonuclear leukocytes in the absence of complement and bactericidal antibodies, *Zentralbl Bakteriol Hyg A*, **261:** 432–46.

Wagner M, Wagner B, 1985, Immunoelectron microscopical demonstration of the cell wall and capsular antigens of GBS, *Antibiotics and Chemotherapy*, Vol. 35, eds Schönfeld H, Hahn FE, Karger, Basel, 119–27.

Walker JA, Allen RL et al., 1987, Molecular cloning, characterization and complete nucleotide sequence of the gene for pneumolysin, the sulfhydryl-activated toxin of *Streptococcus pneumoniae*, *Infect Immun*, **55:** 1184–9.

Ward JB, 1981, Teichoic and teichuronic acids: Biosynthesis, assembly, and location, *Microbiol Rev*, **45:** 211–43.

Wästfelt M, Stalhammer-Carlmalm M et al., 1996, Identification of a family of streptococcal surface proteins with extremely repetitive structure, *J Biol Chem*, **271:** 18892–7.

Weiser JN, Rubens CE, 1987, Transposon mutagenesis of group B streptococcus beta-hemolysin biosynthesis, *Infect Immun*, **55:** 2314–16.

Welborn PP, Hadley WK et al., 1983, Characterization of strains of viridans streptococci by deoxyribonucleic acid hybridization and physiological tests, *Int J Syst Bacteriol*, **33:** 293–9.

Wessels MR, DiFabio JL et al., 1991a, Structural determination and immunochemical characterization of the type V group B streptococcus capsular polysaccharide, *J Biol Chem*, **266:** 6714–19.

Wessels MR, Moses AE et al., 1991b, Hyaluronic acid capsule is a virulence factor for mucoid group A streptococci, *Proc Natl Acad Sci USA*, **88:** 8317–21.

Wessels MR, Pozsgay V et al., 1987, Structure and immunochemistry of an oligosaccharide repeating unit of the capsular polysaccharide of type III group B streptococcus, *J Biol Chem*, **262:** 8262–7.

Wessels MR, Rubens CE et al., 1989, Definition of a bacterial virulence factor: Sialylation of the group B streptococcal capsule, *Proc Natl Acad Sci USA*, **86:** 8983–7.

Wexler DE, Chenoweth DE, Cleary PP, 1985, Mechanism of action of the group A streptococcal C5a inactivator, *Proc Natl Acad Sci USA*, **82:** 8144–8.

Whatmore AM, Kapur V et al., 1994, Non-congruent relationships between variation in *emm* gene sequences and the population genetic structure of group A streptococci, *Mol Microbiol*, **14:** 619–31.

Whatmore AM, Kehoe MA, 1994, Horizontal gene transfer in the evolution of group A streptococcal *emm*-like genes: gene mosaics and variation in Vir regulons, *Mol Microbiol*, **11:** 363–74.

Whiley RA, Beighton D, 1991, Emended descriptions and recognition of *Streptococcus constellatus*, *Streptococcus intermedius* and *Streptococcus anginosus* as distinct species, *Int J Syst Bacteriol*, **41:** 1–5.

Whiley RA, Beighton D et al., 1992, *Streptococcus intermedius*, *Streptococcus constellatus* and *Streptococcus anginosus* (the *Streptococcus milleri* group): association with different body sites and clinical infections, *J Clin Microbiol*, **30:** 243–4.

Whiley RA, Duke B et al., 1995, Heterogeneity among 16S–23S rRNA intergenic spacers of species within the *Streptococcus milleri* group, *Microbiology*, **141:** 1461–7.

Whiley RA, Fraser HY et al., 1990a, *Streptococcus parasanguis* sp. nov. An atypical viridans streptococcus from human clinical specimens, *FEMS Microbiol Let*, **68**: 115–22.

Whiley RA, Fraser HY et al., 1990b, Phenotypic differentiation of *Streptococcus intermedius, Streptococcus constellatus,* and *Streptococcus anginosus* strains wihin the '*Streptococcus milleri* group', *J Clin Microbiol*, **28**: 1497–1501.

Whiley RA, Freemantle L et al., 1993, Isolation, identification and prevalence of *Streptococcus anginosus, S. intermedius* and *S. constellatus* from the human mouth, *Microb Ecol Hlth Dis*, **6**: 285–91.

Whiley RA, Hardie JM, 1988, *Streptococcus vestibularis* sp. nov. from the human oral cavity, *Int J Syst Bact*, **38**: 335–9.

Whiley RA, Hardie JM, 1989, DNA–DNA hybridization studies and phenotypic characteristics of strains within the '*Streptococcus milleri*' group, *J Gen Microbiol*, **28**: 1497–501.

Whiley RA, Russell RRB, Hardie JM, 1988, *Streptococcus downei* sp. nov. for strains previously described as *Streptococcus mutans* serotype h, *Int J Syst Bacteriol*, **38**: 25–29.

Wicken AJ, Broady KW et al., 1982, Production of lipoteichoic acid by lactobacilli and streptococci grown in different environments, *Infect Immun*, **36**: 864–9.

Williams AM, Collins MD, 1990, Molecular taxonomic studies on *Streptococcus uberis* types I and II. Description of *Streptococcus parauberis* sp. nov., *J Appl Bacteriol*, **68**: 485–90.

Williams AM, Farrow JAE, Collins MD, 1989, Reverse transcriptase sequencing of 16S ribosomal RNA from *Streptococcus cecorum, Lett Appl Microbiol*, **8**: 185–90.

Wood BJB, Holzapfel WH (eds), 1995, *The Lactic Acid Bacteria. Volume 2. The Genera of Lactic Acid Bacteria*, Blackie, Glasgow.

Woolcock JB, 1974, Purification and antigenicity of an M-like protein of *Streptococcus equi, Infect Immun*, **10**: 116–22.

Wulf RJ, Mertz ET, 1968, Studies on plasminogen. VIII. Species specificity of streptokinase, *Can J Biochem*, **47**: 927–31.

Yother J, McDaniel LS et al., 1991, Pneumococcal surface protein A: structural analysis and biological significance, *Genetics and Molecular Biology of* Streptococci, Lactococci*, and* Enterococci, eds Dunny GM, Cleary PP, McKay LL, American Society for Microbiology, Washington, DC, 88–91.

Zabriskie JB, Read SE, Fischetti VA, 1972, Lysogeny in streptococci, *Streptococci and Streptococcal Diseases*, eds Wannamaker LW, Matsen JM, Academic Press, New York, 99–118.

Chapter 29

ENTEROCOCCUS

R R Facklam and L M Teixeira

1   GENUS DEFINITION

Enterococci are gram-positive cocci that occur singly, in pairs or as short chains. They may be coccobacillary in gram-stained films prepared from agar cultures, but tend to be ovoid and in chains when prepared from thioglycollate broth cultures. Enterococci are facultative anaerobes with an optimum growth temperature of 35°C and a growth range from 10 to 45°C. They all grow in broth containing 6.5% NaCl and they hydrolyse aesculin in the presence of 40% bile salts (bile–aesculin medium). Some species are motile. Most enterococci, apart from *Enterococcus cecorum*, *Enterococcus columbae* and *Enterococcus saccharolyticus*, hydrolyse pyrrolidonyl-β-naphthylamide (PYR); all strains produce leucine aminopeptidase (LAP). The tests listed in Table 29.1 can be used to identify and distinguish most enterococci from other catalase-negative, gram-positive cocci (Facklam and Elliott 1995).

Enterococci do not contain cytochrome enzymes, but they occasionally produce a pseudo-catalase and appear catalase-positive with a weak effervescence. Almost all strains are homofermentative with lactic acid as the end product of glucose fermentation; gas is not produced. Most strains produce a cell wall associated glycerol teichoic acid antigen, the streptococcal group D antigen, but its detection is sometimes difficult and depends on the extraction procedure and the quality of the antiserum used (Facklam and Washington 1991, Knudtson and Hartman 1993, Truant and Satishchandran 1993). The DNA G + C content ranges from 37 to 45 mol% (Schleifer and Kilpper-Balz 1984).

The streptococcal species *Streptococcus faecalis* and *Streptococcus faecium* were split from *Streptococcus* to form the genus *Enterococcus* (Schleifer and Kilpper-Balz 1984). Since that time, 17 other species have been proposed for inclusion in the genus *Enterococcus* (Table 29.2). Genetic evidence for these proposals has been provided by DNA–DNA and DNA–rRNA hybridizations as well as by 16S rRNA sequencing.

Additional tests that aid in the identification of related gram-positive bacteria are described in another chapter (see Chapter 28).

2   HISTORICAL PERSPECTIVE

The term 'enterococcus' probably originated with the discovery of the first organism; Thiercelin (1899) used the term to describe bacteria seen in pairs and short chains in faeces. The name *Streptococcus faecalis* was used by Andrews and Horder (1906) to identify an organism of faecal origin that clotted milk and fermented mannitol and lactose but not raffinose. Orla-Jensen (1919) described a second organism, *S. faecium*, which differed from the fermentation patterns of *S. faecalis*. A third species, *Streptococcus durans*, proposed by Sherman and Wing (1935) and Sherman (1937), was similar to *S. faecium* but had less fermentation activity. The term 'enterococcal group' was used by Sherman (1938) to describe streptococci that grew at 10 and 45° C, grew in broth with pH adjusted to 9.6 and in broth containing 6.5% NaCl, and survived heating to 60°C for 30 min. Sherman's enterococcal group included all the known enterococcal species for that time. Sherman's other groups were the 'pyogenic, lactic, and viridans' groups. In 1967, Nowlan and Deibel (1967) added *Streptococcus avium* to the enterococcal group. In 1970, Kalina proposed that a genus

Table 29.1 Phenotypic characteristics of facultatively anaerobic, catalase-negative, gram-positive coccus genera[a]

	Cell arrang	VAN	GAS	PYR	LAP	BE	NaCl	Growth at: 10°C	45°C	MOT	HEM
Enterococcus	ch	S[b]	−	+	+	+	+	+	+	V	α/β/n
Vagococcus	ch	S	−	+	+	+	+[c]	+	−[d]	+	α/n
Lactococcus	ch	S	−	+	+	+	V	+	−[e]	−	α/n
Leuconostoc	ch	R	+	−	−	V	V	+	V	−	α/n
Streptococcus	ch	S	−	−[f]	+	−	−[g]	V	V	−	α/β/n
Globicatella	ch	S	−	+	−	−	+	−	−	−	α
Pediococcus	cl/te	R	−	−	+	+	V	−	+	−	α
Tetragenococcus	cl/te	S	−	−	+	+	+	−	+	−	α
Aerococcus	cl/te	S	−	+	−	V	+	−	+	−	α
Gemella	cl/te	S	−	+	V	−	−	−	−	−	α/n
Helcococcus	cl/te	S	−	+	−	+	+	−	−	−	n
Alloiococcus[h]	cl/te	S	−	+	+	−	+	−	−	−	n

[a]Abbreviations and symbols: arrang, arrangement; VAN, susceptibility to vancomycin (30 μg disc); GAS, gas produced from glucose in Mann, Rogosa, Sharpe *Lactobacillus* broth; PYR, production of pyrrolydonyl arylamidase; LAP, production of leucine aminopeptidase; BE, reaction on bile–aesculin medium; NaCl, growth in broth containing 6.5% NaCl; MOT, motility; Hem, haemolysis on blood agar containing 5% sheep blood; ch, chains; cl, clumps; te, tetrads; S, susceptible; R, resistant; −, ≤5% negative reactions; +, ≥95% positive reactions; V, variable reactions; α, α-haemolysis; β, β-haemolysis; n, no haemolysis.
[b]Some enterococcal strains are vancomycin resistant but still show a small inhibition around the disc; other strains grow right up to the disc and are vancomycin resistant under the defined screening test criteria.
[c]Strains are generally positive after long incubation (5 or more days).
[d]Some strains of vagococci grow slowly at 45°C.
[e]Some strains of lactococci grow very slowly at 45°C.
[f]Group A streptococci and nutritionally variant streptococci are PYR positive; all others are negative.
[g]*Streptococcus bovis, S. equinus* and 5–10% of the viridans streptococci are bile–aesculin positive.
[h]*Alloiococcus* strains grow anaerobically only under defined conditions.

Table 29.2 Proposals of species to be included in the genus *Enterococcus*

Species	References
E. faecalis	Schleifer and Kilpper-Balz 1984
E. faecium	Schleifer and Kilpper-Balz 1984
E. avium	Collins et al. 1984
E. casseliflavus	Collins et al. 1984
E. durans	Collins et al. 1984
E. gallinarum	Collins et al. 1984
E. malodoratus	Collins et al. 1984
E. hirae	Farrow and Collins 1985
E. mundtii	Collins, Farrow and Jones 1986
E. raffinosus	Collins et al. 1989b
E. solitarius[a]	Collins et al. 1989b
E. pseudoavium	Collins et al. 1989b
E. cecorum	Williams et al. 1989
E. columbae	Devriese et al. 1990
E. saccharolyticus	Rodrigues and Collins 1990
E. dispar	Collins et al. 1991
E. sulfureus	Martinez-Murcia and Collins 1991
E. seriolicida[a]	Kusuda et al. 1991
E. flavescens[b]	Pompei et al. 1992

[a]DNA reassociation and/or 16S rRNA sequencing studies indicated that these species do not belong to the *Enterococcus* genus.
[b]DNA reassociation studies showed that *E. flavescens* and *E. casseliflavus* are related at the species level and constitute a single species.

for the enterococcal streptococci be established and suggested that, based on cellular arrangement and phenotypic characteristics, *S. faecalis* and *S. faecium* and the subspecies of these 2 taxons be named *Entero-*

coccus. No action on this proposal was ever taken and the use of the genus name *Streptococcus* continued. Genetic evidence that *S. faecalis* and *S. faecium* were sufficiently different from the other members of the genus to merit a separate genus was provided by Schleifer and Kilpper-Balz (1984). It is generally accepted that the genus *Enterococcus* is valid.

3 HABITAT

The nature of these bacteria, which allows them to grow and survive in harsh environments, allows them to persist almost everywhere. Enterococci can be found in soil, food and water, and in animals, birds and insects (Mundt, Graham and McCarty 1967, Dutka and Kwan 1978, Kibbey, Hagedorn and McCoy 1978, Devriese et al. 1992a, 1992b). In humans and in other animals, the enterococci inhabit the gastrointestinal tract and the genitourinary tract. *Enterococcus faecalis* is one of the most common bacteria isolated from the gastrointestinal tract of humans. Because of changes in taxonomy, it is difficult to determine the distribution of other enterococcal species in humans. It is likely that *Enterococcus faecium* is also commonly found in the gastrointestinal tract of humans (Mead 1978).

4 CULTURAL CHARACTERISTICS AND MORPHOLOGY

Enterococci may be spherical, oval, or coccobacillary and are arranged in pairs and short chains. All species are gram-positive and most are non-motile, *Enterococcus gallinarum* and *Enterococcus casseliflavus* being the exceptions. The motility reaction is shown in Fig. 29.1. The culture on the left side of Fig. 29.1 is motile and the culture on the right is non-motile. Note the lack of defined line of growth in the culture on the left.

Colonies on blood agar media are usually between 1 and 2 mm in diameter, although some variants may appear smaller. Some (about one-third) cultures of *E. faecalis* may be β-haemolytic on agar containing rabbit, horse, or human blood but non-haemolytic on agar containing sheep blood. Some cultures of *Enterococcus durans* are β-haemolytic regardless of the type of blood used. All other species are usually α-haemolytic or non-haemolytic. Strains that appear α-haemolytic are actually non-haemolytic strains that produce peroxide. This 'greening' of the agar is due to peroxide action on the blood cells in the medium and not to the production of an α toxin. *Enterococcus casseliflavus*, *Enterococcus mundtii* and *Enterococcus sulfureus* produce a yellow pigment on blood agar medium (Fig. 29.2, top, see also Plate 29.2). The pigment is detected by using a white cotton swab to pick up the growth and examining the swab for a yellow colour (Fig. 29.2, bottom, see also Plate 29.2). The colonies of enterococci on selective media will depend on the chemicals used in the medium. For example, on bile–aesculin–azide medium (Sabbaj, Sutter and Finegold 1971) the colonies will appear grey-white surrounded by a black halo, whereas on agar containing tetrazolium salts the centre of the colony will appear brick red (Barnes 1956).

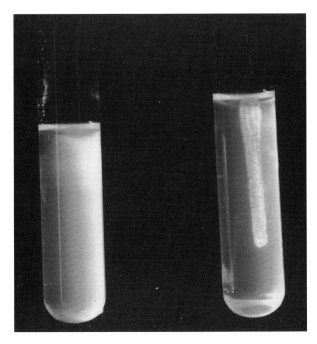

Fig. 29.1 Motility test for *Enterococcus* species; *E. gallinarum* (motile) on left and *E. faecium* (non-motile) on right.

5 METABOLISM AND GROWTH REQUIREMENTS

The nutritional requirements of the enterococci are complex (Deibel 1964). There is little in the recent literature that addresses the growth requirements of the enterococci (Murray et al. 1993). Most studies have been done with *E. faecalis* and in some cases have misidentified strains. Growth requirements include the B vitamins, nucleic acid bases and a carbon source, usually glucose. The most recent work by Murray and colleagues (1993) indicates that all 23 strains of *E. faecalis* tested had an absolute requirement for histidine, isoleucine, methionine and tryptophan; whereas some strains required arginine, glutamate, glycine, leucine and valine, others did not. This implies that there are strain-to-strain differences in growth requirements. Intensive antimicrobial pressures have created atypical growth requirements such as vancomycin-requiring strains (Fraimow et al. 1994). It is likely that the different species of enterococci have different growth requirements.

6 IMPORTANT GENETIC MECHANISMS

The enterococci are capable of transmitting genetic information by both plasmid and transposon exchange. In *E. faecalis*, the exchange of plasmids is unique and involves the production of sex pheromones (Clewell and Weaver 1989, Clewell 1993a, Tanimoto, An and Clewell 1993). Plasmid-free recipient strains produce extracellular pheromones. The pheromone-induced mating response results in the production of a proteinaceous substance on the outer surface of the donor cells called aggregation substance (Dunny 1990, Clewell 1993a). The aggregation substance then reacts with a binding substance on the surface of the recipient cell. The plasmid exchange occurs when the cells are clumped together. The pheromone-induced transfer increases the frequency of transfer of plasmids 10^5–10^6-fold (Clewell 1993b). Other species of enterococci have the capacity to acquire and exchange plasmids, but the mechanism of exchange is not pheromone induced. The genetic material included on enterococcal plasmids may be drug resistance and/or virulence genes. These factors will be discussed in the sections on antimicrobial resistance and virulence.

The enterococci are also capable of genetic exchange by conjugative transposons. The process requires cell-to-cell contact. The excised DNA can be viewed as being transferred to the recipient cell by a 'plasmid-like' process, followed by insertion into the target chromosome (Clewell and Flannagan 1993). The transposons frequently carry resistance determinants for antimicrobial agents such as tetracycline, erythromycin, gentamicin, kanamycin and other aminoglycosides (Clewell and Gawron-Burke 1986, Clewell 1990, Su and Clewell 1993). Transposons have a very broad host range and are commonly found in

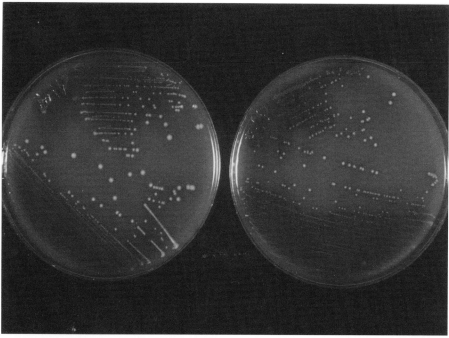

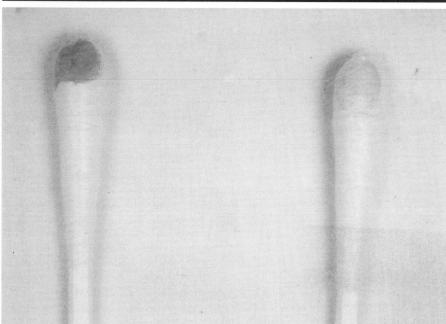

Fig. 29.2 Culture and pigmentation test demonstrating yellow pigment produced by *Enterococcus* species; *E. casseliflavus* (pigmented) on left and *E. faecium* (non-pigmented) on right. See Plate 29.2 for colour.

several *Enterococcus* species as well as species of *Streptococcus*, *Lactococcus* and other gram-positive bacteria.

7 CELL WALL COMPOSITION AND ANTIGENIC STRUCTURES

Peptidoglycan polymers are the main structural and shape-maintaining components of gram-positive bacteria. A comprehensive review of the cell wall chemistry of enterococci and related bacteria was reported by Schleifer and Kilpper-Balz (1987). The so-called 'streptococcal group D antigen' is usually associated with the *Enterococcus* species but it is not exclusive; this antigen is also found in *Streptococcus bovis* and in some *Pediococcus* and *Leuconostoc* species (Facklam, Hollis and Collins 1989). The group D antigen is a glycerol teichoic acid located intracellularly (Deibel 1964). Type antigens, carbohydrate in nature, are also present on the surface of the cells of many of the strains of *E. faecalis*, *E. faecium* and *E. durans* (Sharpe and Shattock 1952, Barnes 1964, Sharpe 1964).

8 CLASSIFICATION AND IDENTIFICATION OF SPECIES

Recent information, including unpublished data from

our laboratory, indicates that 2 of the 19 proposed species should not be included in the *Enterococcus* genus. *Enterococcus solitarius* was shown by 16S rRNA to be more closely related to *Tetragenococcus halophilus* than to any species of the genus *Enterococcus* (Williams, Rodrigues and Collins 1991). DNA reassociation studies indicate that *E. solitarius* was equally related to the reference strains of *Enterococcus* and *Tetragenococcus* (Collins, Williams and Wallbanks 1990). Therefore, the true taxonomic status of this species remains in question. The rRNA sequence of *Enterococcus seriolicida* has been shown to be identical to the rRNA sequence of *Lactococcus garvieae* (Domenech et al. 1993). Using whole-cell protein analysis (Elliott et al. 1991, Teixeira et al. 1996) and DNA reassociation studies (Teixeira et al. 1996), we have found that the protein profiles of *E. seriolicida* and *L. garvieae* are identical and the type strains of both species have a high-level relatedness (77% at optimal and stringent conditions) and are a single species. Since *L. garvieae* was named first, it should be retained as the species name. In addition to the above evidence that *E. seriolicida* and *E. solitarius* strains do not belong in the *Enterococcus*, these 2 species also fail to react positively with the AccuProbe *Enterococcus* probe manufactured by Gen-Probe, LaJolla, CA. This probe is based on a DNA oligomer having a structure complementary to a segment of enterococcal rRNA (Enns 1988, Daly, Clifton and Seskin 1991). All strains of known *Enterococcus* species, except the type strains of *E. cecorum*, *E. columbae* and *E. saccharolyticus*, react positively with this probe. We have also found that there are insufficient differences between *E. casseliflavus* and *Enterococcus flavescens* to merit a separate species for each. DNA–DNA reassociation studies show that the type strains of these 2 species are related at levels of 82%, demonstrating that they are a single species (unpublished studies). Since *E. casseliflavus* was described first it is the senior subjective synonym of *E. flavescens* and it should be retained as the species denomination.

Once it is established that an unknown catalase-negative gram-positive coccus is an enterococcus, the tests listed in Table 29.3 can be used to identify the species. The 3 species *E. cecorum*, *E. columbae* and *E. saccharolyticus* are included even though they are PYR-ase-negative and may grow very poorly in broth containing 6.5% NaCl (Devriese, Pot and Collins 1993). The capacity to grow in broth may be dependent on the base medium because we observed growth in our media formulation with the type strains. It is best to separate the species into 5 groups based on acid formation in mannitol, sorbitol and sorbose broths and hydrolysis of arginine.

All the tests listed in Table 29.3 have been previously described (Facklam and Collins 1989, Facklam, Hollis and Collins 1989, Facklam and Washington 1991, Facklam and Sahm 1995).

Group I consists of *Enterococcus avium*, *Enterococcus malodoratus*, *Enterococcus raffinosus*, *Enterococcus pseudoavium* and *Enterococcus saccharolyticus*. These 5 species form acid in all 3 of the aforementioned carbohydrate broths but do not hydrolyse arginine. The species in this group are identified by the reactions in arabinose and raffinose broth and the capacity to utilize pyruvate. *E. avium* forms acid in arabinose but not raffinose broth. *E. malodoratus* forms acid in raffinose but not arabinose broth. *E. raffinosus* forms acid in both, whereas *E. pseudoavium* forms acid in neither arabinose nor raffinose broth. *E. saccharolyticus* is differentiated from *E. malodoratus* only by its inability to utilize pyruvate.

Group II consists of *E. faecalis*, *E. faecium*, *E. casseliflavus*, *E. mundtii* and *E. gallinarum*. These 5 species form acid in mannitol broth and hydrolyse arginine, but fail to form acid in sorbose broth and give variable reactions in sorbitol broth. *Lactococcus* spp. are also listed in this group because of the similarities between the genera *Enterococcus* and *Lactococcus* (Table 29.1) and in some cases the phenotypic characteristics of *L. garvieae* will lead to the misidentification of this species as an *Enterococcus*. *E. faecalis* is the only member of group II to tolerate tellurite and utilize pyruvate. *L. garvieae* is differentiated from *E. faecalis* by negative reactions in sorbitol, tellurite and pyruvate. *L. garvieae* does not form acid in arabinose broth, differentiating it from the other group II enterococci. *E. faecium* and *E. gallinarum* have similar characteristics but can be differentiated by the motility test. *E. gallinarum* is motile but *E. faecium* is not. *E. casseliflavus* and *E. mundtii* are pigmented (yellow) and also similar to each other in other characteristics; however, *E. casseliflavus* is motile but *E. mundtii* is not.

Group III consists of *E. durans*, *Enterococcus hirae*, *Enterococcus dispar* and mannitol-negative variants of *E. faecalis* and *E. faecium*. These 5 species hydrolyse arginine but do not form acid in mannitol, sorbitol, or sorbose broths. The members of this group are easily identified by the reactions in the pyruvate, arabinose, raffinose and sucrose tests. *E. durans* is negative in these 4 tests. *E. hirae* is positive in one or both raffinose and sucrose tests and negative in the pyruvate and acid from arabinose tests. *E. dispar* is positive for acid production from raffinose and sucrose and utilizes pyruvate but does not form acid in arabinose broth. *E. faecalis* variant strain is positive in the test for pyruvate utilization but not for acid formation in arabinose, raffinose, or sucrose broth. *E. faecium* is the only member of this group to form acid in arabinose broth.

Two species are found in group IV: *E. sulfureus* and *E. cecorum*. These 2 species are negative for acid formation in mannitol and sorbose broths and do not hydrolyse arginine. *E. cecorum* forms acid in sorbitol broth and is non-pigmented, which differentiates this species from *E. sulfureus*.

Group V consists of the variant strains of *E. casseliflavus*, *E. gallinarum* and *E. faecalis* that fail to hydrolyse arginine. These species have characteristics similar to the strains that hydrolyse arginine and can be differentiated by these same phenotypic tests. *E. columbae* is also included in this group because strains of this species also do not hydrolyse arginine or form acid in sorbose broth. *E. columbae* is similar to the arginine-negative variants of *E. faecalis*; however, *E. columbae* forms acid in raffinose broth and *E. faecalis* does not.

Table 29.3 Phenotypic characteristics used for identification of *Enterococcus* species[a]

Species	MAN	SOR	ARG	ARA	SBL	RAF	TEL	MOT	PIG	SUC	PYU
Group I											
E. avium	+	+	−	+	+	−	−	−	−	+	+
E. malodoratus	+	+	−	−	+	+	−	−	−	+	+
E. raffinosus	+	+	−	+	+	+	−	−	−	+	+
E. pseudoavium	+	+	−	−	+	−	−	−	−	+	+
E. saccharolyticus[b]	+	+	−	−	+	+	−	−	−	+	−
Group II											
E. faecalis	+	−	+	−	+	−	+	−	−	+*	+
Lactococcus spp.	+	−	+	−	−	−	−	−	−	+	−
E. faecium	+	−	+	+	v	v	−	−	−	+*	−
E. casseliflavus	+	−	+	+	v	+	−*	+	+	+	v
E. mundtii	+	−	+	+	v	+	−	−	+	+	−
E. gallinarum	+	−	+	+	−	+	−	+	−	+	−
Group III											
E. durans	−	−	+	−	−	−	−	−	−	−	−
E. hirae	−	−	+	−	−	v	−	−	−	+	−
E. dispar	−	−	+	−	−	+	−	−	−	+	+
E. faecalis (var)	−	−	+	−	−	−	+	−	−	−	+
E. faecium	−	−	+	+	−	v	−	−	−	+	−
Group IV											
E. sulfureus	−	−	−	−	−	+	−	−	+	+	−
E. cecorum[b]	−	−	−	−	+	+	−	−	−	+	+
Group V											
E. casseliflavus	+	−	−	+	v	+	v	+	+	+	v
E. gallinarum	+	−	−	+	−	+	−	+	−	+	−
E. faecalis	+	−	−	−	+	−	+	−	−	+	+
E. columbae[b]	+	−	−	+	+	+	−	−	−	+	+
Vagococcus spp.	+	−	−	−	+	−	−	+	−	+	−

[a]Abbreviations and symbols: MAN, mannitol; SOR, sorbose; ARG, arginine; ARA, arabinose; SBL, sorbitol; RAF, raffinose; TEL, 0.04% tellurite; MOT, motility; PIG, pigment; SUC, sucrose; PYU, pyruvate; +, >90% positive; −, <10% positive; +* or −*, occasional exceptions (<3% of strains show aberrant reactions).
[b]Phenotypic characteristics based on data from type strains and data included in Devriese, Pot and Collins (1993).

E. faecalis variant strains also tolerate tellurite while *E. columbae* do not. *Vagococcus* spp. are listed here for the same reason for listing the lactococci in group II. The phenotypic characteristics of *Vagococcus fluvialis* are very similar to those of the genus *Enterococcus* and some strains may be identified as enterococci (Collins et al. 1989a, Facklam and Elliott 1995). In addition to the determination of physiological characteristics, analysis of electrophoretic whole-cell protein profiles has been shown to be reliable for the characterization of typical *Enterococcus* species (Fig. 29.3) (Niemi et al. 1993, Merquior et al. 1994). Atypical strains of *E. faecium* were also correctly identified by this procedure (Teixeira et al. 1995).

Species-specific ribosomal RNA probes for *E. faecalis* and *E. faecium* were used for identifying these 2 species from milk samples (Beimfohr et al. 1993). Restriction fragment length polymorphism (RFLP) was used to identify several species of streptococci as well as 4 species of enterococci (Jayarao et al. 1992). RFLPs of ribosomal DNA identified 12 different species isolated from bovine sources. Donabedian and colleagues (1995) tested contour-clamped homogeneous electric field electrophoresis (CHEF) for identification of 5

different *Enterococcus* species. It was not clear from the data presented that this procedure would clearly differentiate the species; perhaps additional work will improve the differentiation.

Still another approach to differentiating the *Enterococcus* species was suggested by Berlutti and colleagues (1993). The authors provided evidence that different enterococcal species produced different bacteriolytic enzymes with certain indicator (substrate) strains. Of these procedures, only whole-cell protein analysis has been performed in more than one laboratory and would appear to be valid for differentiating the *Enterococcus* species. Solid evidence that RFLP, CHEF, or bacteriolytic enzymes will perform as well as physiological tests or whole-cell protein analysis is lacking at this time.

9 LABORATORY ISOLATION

Trypticase–soy–5% sheep blood agar, brain–heart infusion–5% sheep blood agar, or any blood agar base containing 5% animal blood supports the growth of enterococci. Some strains of *E. faecalis* are β-haemo-

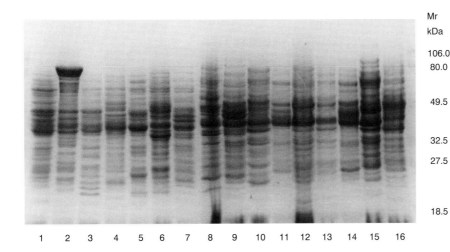

Fig. 29.3 SDS-PAGE patterns of whole-cell protein extracts of *Enterococcus* species. Lanes A, molecular weight standards; 1, SS-1314 *E. sulfureus*; 2, SS-1310 *E. columbae*; 3, SS-1297 *E. saccharolyticus*; 4, SS-1296 *E. cecorum*; 5, SS-1295 *E. dispar*; 6, SS-1278 *E. raffinosus*; 7, SS-1277 *E. pseudoavium*; 8, 1999-89 *E. malodoratus*; 9, SS-1274 *E. faecium*; 10, SS-1273 *E. faecalis*; 11, SS-1232 *E. mundtii*; 12, SS-1229 *E. casseliflavus*; 13, SS-1228 *E. gallinarum*; 14, SS-1227 *E. hirae*; 15, SS-1225 *E. durans*; 16, SS-559 *E. avium*.

lytic on agar bases containing rabbit or horse blood but non-β-haemolytic on the same base media containing sheep blood. If the sample is likely to contain gram-negative bacteria, bile–aesculin azide (Sabbaj, Sutter and Finegold 1971), Pfizer selective enterococcus (Isenberg, Goldberg and Sampson 1970), or some other commercially prepared medium containing azide, are excellent primary isolation media. The azide inhibits the gram-negative bacteria and the enterococci appear as black colonies because of hydrolysis of aesculin. Other media such as Columbia colistin–nalidixic acid agar (CNA) (Ellner et al. 1966) or phenylethyl alcohol agar (PEA) (Dayton et al. 1974) have been used successfully to isolate enterococci. The advantage CNA has over PEA is that the haemolytic reaction can be read from CNA, but not from PEA. We have previously reviewed the isolation and use of selective media for the enterococci (Facklam 1976). Willinger and Manafi (1995) have described a new medium for the isolation of enterococci from urine. The medium contains several chromogenic substrates that react selectively with certain groups of bacteria. On this medium, *E. faecalis* and *E. faecium* could not be differentiated, i.e. they appeared alike. Other enterococci or closely related strains such as lactococci and leuconostocs were not tested.

All enterococci grow at 35–37°C and do not require an atmosphere containing increased levels of carbon dioxide. However, some strains grow better in atmospheres containing increased levels of carbon dioxide.

10 SUSCEPTIBILITY TO ANTIMICROBIAL AGENTS

Resistance to the inhibitory and bactericidal activities of several commonly used antimicrobial agents is a remarkable characteristic of most of the enterococcal species. Antimicrobial resistance markers can be either intrinsic or acquired. Intrinsic (or inherent) resistance traits are present in all or most of the strains and, therefore, appear to be chromosomally coded.

Acquired resistance markers result from either mutation in existing DNA or acquisition of new DNA found in plasmid or transposons (van Asselt et al. 1992, Hodel-Christian and Murray 1992, Leclerq et al. 1992).

Enterococcal intrinsic resistance includes resistance to 2 major groups of antimicrobial therapeutic drugs: the β-lactams and the aminoglycosides (Murray 1990, Shlaes, Binczewski and Rice 1993). Intrinsic resistance of enterococci to the β-lactam antibiotics (penicillin and ampicillin among others) is due to low affinity of the penicillin-binding proteins (Fontana et al. 1992). Resistance to therapeutic achievable concentrations of aminoglycosides is also intrinsic and it is due to the low uptake of these agents. Because of this inherent antimicrobial resistance, the recommended therapy for serious infections (i.e. endocarditis, meningitis and other systemic infections, especially in immuno-compromised patients) includes a combination of a cell wall active agent, such as a β-lactam drug (usually penicillin) or vancomycin, combined with an aminoglycoside (usually gentamicin or streptomycin) (Eliopoulos and Eliopoulos 1990, Murray 1990). These combinations overcome the intrinsic resistance exhibited by enterococci and a synergistic effect is generally achieved since the intracellular penetration of the aminoglycoside is facilitated by the cell wall active agent.

However, in the last 2 decades, antimicrobial resistance among enterococci strains has been increasingly reported throughout the world. Several antimicrobial resistance traits, especially high-level resistance to aminoglycoside, β-lactam antibiotics and, more recently, vancomycin, have been acquired. Strains with such characteristics are resistant to the synergistic effects of combination therapy and constitute an even more serious problem concerning the effective therapy for enterococcal infections. A variety of antimicrobial resistance patterns involving different mechanisms in enterococcal strains is presented in Table 29.4.

Strains exhibiting high-level resistance to one or

Table 29.4 Major patterns and mechanisms of resistance to antimicrobial agents in enterococci

Pattern of resistance	Mechanism of resistance

High-level resistance to aminoglycosides[a]
  Gentamicin
  Kanamycin
  Streptomycin
	Enzymatic
	  (Production of aminoglycoside-modifying enzymes–AMES[b])
	  AAC(6′) + APH(2′)
	  AAC(6′)
	  APH(3′)
	  ANT(6′)
	  ANT(4′)
	Alteration of the target
	  (Leading to decreased ribosomal binding)

Resistance to glycopeptides[c]
  Vancomycin
  Teicoplanin
    VanA
    VanB
    VanC
    VanC-like
	Alteration of the target
	  (Production of inducible proteins related to the binding to
	  and subsequent enzymatic modification of the pentapeptide
	  precursor of the peptidoglycan, the natural target of the
	  glycopeptides, has been described)

Resistance to β-lactams[d]
  Penicillin
  Ampicillin
	Alteration of the target
	  (Altered penicillin-binding proteins–PBPs)
	Enzymatic
	  (Production of β-lactamase)

Resistance to quinolones	Alteration of the target (Subunit A of DNA gyrase)
Resistance to chloramphenicol	Enzymatic (Production of chloramphenicol acetyl transferase–CAT)

Resistance to the MLS group
  Macrolides (erythromycin)
  Lincosamides (clindamycin)
  Streptogramin B
	Enzymatic
	  (Production of methylating enzymes)

[a]Found in increasing frequencies in *E. faecalis* and *E. faecium*.
[b]AAC, acetyltransferases; APH, phosphotransferases; ANT, nucleotidyltransferases.
[c]VanA and VanB phenotypes are usually found in *E. faecalis* and *E. faecium*; VanC is usually associated with *E. gallinarum* and VanC-like with *E. casseliflavus*.
[d]Found in *E. faecalis* and *E. faecium*. Also described among *E. raffinosus* strains.

more aminoglycosides have emerged and have been described with increasing frequency among clinical and environmental enterococcal isolates (Murray 1990, van Asselt et al. 1992, Leclerq et al. 1992, Rice et al. 1995). Strains expressing acquired high-level resistance to aminoglycosides have minimal inhibitory concentrations (MICs) ≥2000 μg ml^{-1} and cannot be detected by diffusion tests with conventional discs. To circumvent this problem, special tests using high content gentamicin (120 μg) and streptomycin (300 μg) discs were developed to screen for this type of resistance (Sahm and Torres 1988). The National Committee for Clinical Laboratory Standards (NCCLS 1993) has completed the studies on methods for determining high-level aminoglycoside resistance and alternative methods for screening for aminoglycoside resistance are now available.

Strains producing β-lactamase (Murray and Mederski-Samoraj 1983, Lopardo et al. 1990, Murray 1990, 1992, Gordon et al. 1992, Tenover et al. 1993) or exhibiting high-level resistance to penicillin and ampicillin due to altered penicillin-binding proteins have also been identified (Bush et al. 1989, Sapico et al. 1989,

Oster et al. 1990, Chirurgi et al. 1991, Tenover et al. 1993). The occurrence of enterococci with plasmid-mediated β-lactamase genes is still sporadic, but it is expected to increase. This characteristic is not detected by routine diffusion or dilution susceptibility tests, but can be detected by using a chromogenic cephalosporin assay.

During the last few years, enterococcal strains with variable degrees of glycopeptide resistance (especially vancomycin resistance) have been isolated in Europe and in the USA (Kaplan, Gilligan and Facklam 1988, Leclerq et al. 1992, Tenover et al. 1993). Four phenotypes of glycopeptide resistance have been reported among enterococci: VanA phenotype, with inducible high-level resistance to vancomycin and to teicoplanin; VanB phenotype, with variable (moderate to high) levels of inducible resistance to vancomycin only, and VanC and VanC-like phenotypes, with non-inducible low-level resistance to vancomycin (Arthur and Courvallin 1993). VanA and VanB phenotypes are usually associated with *E. faecium* and *E. faecalis* strains whereas VanC and VanC-like phenotypes are seen, respectively, in *E. gallinarum* and *E. casseliflavus* strains.

The high-level resistance appears to be more readily transferable than the low and moderate levels.

The diversity and, in some cases, species specificity of emerging antimicrobial resistance markers among enterococcal isolates created an additional need for accurate identification at the species level and continuous surveillance of the resistance characteristics. Because of the diverse antimicrobial resistance mechanisms, successful treatment and control of enterococcal infections are becoming increasingly difficult. On the other hand, several of such special drug-resistance characteristics acquired by enterococcal strains are not adequately detected by the routine susceptibility tests most commonly used in the clinical microbiology laboratories, so they require modifications of the usual procedures. Thus, several resistance traits may remain undetected because clinical laboratories still neither routinely identify the different enterococcal species nor use the special methods recommended for the recognition of resistance in enterococci. Early detection of these strains would be of great value to the selection of the more appropriate therapy for the treatment of serious enterococcal infections, leading to better patient management since treatment failure, selection and spreading of resistant strains can be minimized.

11 TYPING METHODS

Because enterococci are a leading cause of nosocomial infections and frequently exhibit multiple antibiotic resistance, there has been an increasing need to type and subtype isolates as a means of assisting infection control and epidemiological studies both within and among various medical institutions. Classic typing methods have included bacteriocin typing (Pleceas, Bogdan and Vereanu 1972, Sadatsune et al. 1978), phage typing (Caprioli, Zaccour and Kasatiya 1975, Kuhnen, Rommelshein and Andries 1987), biochemical reaction profiles (Coudron and Mayhall et al. 1984, Luginbuhl et al. 1987, Smyth et al. 1987), antimicrobial resistance patterns (Murray et al. 1992) and serological characterization (Smyth et al. 1987, Maekawa, Yoshioka and Kumamoto 1992). Although these approaches have occasionally yielded useful information, they generally are time-consuming, expensive, somewhat subjective and esoteric, and they frequently fail to discriminate adequately among strains.

The advent of various molecular techniques has substantially enhanced our ability to 'type' enterococci. Plasmid profiling may be helpful in some instances (Luginbuhl et al. 1987, Boyce et al. 1992), but plasmid yield is often inconsistent and accurate interpretations of the electrophoretic patterns are frequently difficult, if not impossible. Similar interpretation problems are encountered with the use of conventional electrophoresis of endonuclease-digested genomic DNA (Hall et al. 1992, Kaufhold and Ferrieri 1993). Currently, the most useful methods include contour-clamped homogeneous electric field electrophoresis (CHEF; Murray et al. 1990, Green et al. 1995), field

inversion gel electrophoresis (FIGE; Goering and Winters 1992, Boyle et al. 1993) and ribotyping (Woodford et al. 1993). Some investigators have used more than one method, such as CHEF and plasmid analysis, for their studies (Donabedian et al. 1992, Boyle and Soumakis et al. 1993). However, among these techniques CHEF appears to be widely applied and widely useful for studying enterococcal species exhibiting a variety of antimicrobial resistance patterns (Miranda, Singh and Murray 1991, Murray et al. 1990, 1992, Patterson, Singh and Murray 1991, Donabedian et al. 1992, Chow et al. 1993a, Thal et al. 1993); in at least one direct comparison with ribotyping, CHEF showed definite advantages regarding strain discrimination (Gordillo, Singh and Murray 1993).

12 BACTERIOCINS AND BACTERIOPHAGES

Bacteriocins are proteins that prevent the growth of other bacteria, usually closely related bacteria. Among the enterococci, *E. faecalis* (Salzano et al. 1992, Villani et al. 1993), *E. faecium* (Kato et al. 1993, Laukova, Marekova and Javorsky 1993) and *E. hirae* (Siragusa 1992) are known to produce bacteriocins. These bacteriocins are inhibitory to *Listeria monocytogenes*, *Staphylococcus aureus*, *Lactococcus* spp. and other *Enterococcus* species. The detection of bacteriocin production is related to the various species of bacteria used as indicators. A high percentage of enterococci produce bacteriocins (Galvez et al. 1985). Bacteriocin production is linked to a conjugative plasmid in some cases (Tomura et al. 1973, Reichelt, Kennes and Kramer 1984, Salzano et al. 1992). The haemolytic activity of *E. faecalis* is linked to bacteriocin activity and both these activities are associated with a conjugative plasmid (Ike et al. 1990). Haemolysin activity is associated with strain virulence (see section 14, p. 678). There is additional interest in bacteriocins for their potential use as food preservatives (Kato et al. 1993). Bacteriocins have been used as a typing system for enterococci (Pleceas, Bogdan and Vereanu 1972, Sharma and Shriniwas Bhujwala 1976, Sadatsume et al. 1978).

Phage typing of enterococci has been performed in several laboratories. In some cases phage typing has been combined with bacteriocin typing to discriminate between strains (Herman and Hoch 1971, Hoch and Herman 1971, Caprioli, Zaccour and Kasatiya 1975, Kuhnen, Rommelshein and Andries 1987, Kuhnen et al. 1988).

13 ROLE IN NORMAL FLORA OF HUMANS

In all likelihood, most *Enterococcus* species are normal inhabitants of the gastrointestinal tract of humans. Since the enterococci are opportunistic pathogens, the incidence of each species found in human infections probably reflects the distribution of the different

Enterococcus species in the human gastrointestinal tract.

The majority of enterococcal clinical isolates from human sources (80–90%) are *E. faecalis*. *E. faecium* is found in 5–10% of enterococcal infections (Ruoff et al. 1990, Bryce, Zemcov and Clarke 1991, Gordon et al. 1992, Buschelman, Bale and Jones 1993, Guiney and Urwin 1993, McNamara, King and Smyth 1995). The other enterococcal species are identified less frequently. However, clusters of infections with *E. raffinosus* (Chirurgi et al. 1991) and *E. casseliflavus* (Nauschuetz et al. 1993) have been reported. Therefore, the distribution of species varies with each clinical setting. *E. avium*, *E. gallinarum*, *E. mundtii*, *E. durans*, *E. hirae* and *E. faecalis* variant strains have been isolated only rarely from human sources (Facklam and Collins 1989). *E. malodoratus*, *E. pseudoavium* and *E. sulfureus* have not been isolated from human sources. Information on the incidence of the different species of enterococci from sources other than humans is limited because of the changes in taxonomy of the genus. Recent studies using the latest taxonomic recommendations indicate that the distribution of enterococcal species in animals (Devriese et al. 1990, 1992a, 1992b, Rodrigues and Collins 1990, Stern, Carvalho and Teixeira 1994) and the environment (Niemi et al. 1993, Stern, Carvalho and Teixeira 1994) is different from that in humans.

14 PATHOGENICITY AND VIRULENCE FACTORS

The ubiquitous nature of enterococci requires caution in establishing the clinical significance of a particular isolate. Murray (1990) has thoroughly reviewed and summarized the variety of infections in which enterococci are involved. Urinary tract infections are the most common; enterococci are implicated in approximately 10% of all such infections (Felmingham et al. 1992) and in 16% of nosocomial urinary tract infections (Schaberg, Culver and Gaynes 1991). Intra-abdominal or pelvic wound infections are the next most commonly encountered infections. However, these cultures are frequently polymicrobial and the role of enterococci in this setting remains controversial (Nichols and Muzik 1992). Enterococci are being recovered from wound infections at increasing rates, probably the result of increased antibiotic usage and emerging resistance among these organisms (Murray 1990, Schaberg, Culver and Gaynes 1991, Moellering 1992). Bacteraemia is the third most common type of infection and enterococci are the third leading cause of nosocomial bacteraemia (Gullberg, Homann and Phair 1989, Schaberg, Culver and Gaynes 1991, Graninger and Ragette 1992, Moellering 1992). Although endocarditis is a serious enterococcal infection, it is less common than bacteraemia. Enterococci are estimated to cause between 5 and 20% of bacterial endocarditis cases (Megran 1992, Watanakunakorn and Burkett 1993). *E. faecalis* is the most commonly encountered species in this setting, but various other species have also been implicated as causes of endocarditis (Facklam, Hollis and Collins 1989).

Enterococcal infections of the respiratory tract or the central nervous system may occur, but are rare (Murray 1990). Although the spectrum of infections caused by enterococci has remained relatively unchanged since the review by Murray in 1990, the prevalence of these organisms as nosocomial pathogens is clearly increasing. Enterococci are second only to *Escherichia coli* as agents of nosocomial urinary tract infections and third, behind *S. aureus* and coagulase-negative staphylococci, as a cause of nosocomial bacteraemia (Schaberg, Culver and Gaynes 1991). This trend is likely to continue as the overall population ages and more people become at risk of infection due to a generalized deterioration of health (Megran 1992).

Several properties of enterococci have been suggested as potential virulence factors reviewed by Jett, Huycke and Gilmore (1994); the production of haemolysin, aggregative substance and adhesins are the most studied. The haemolysin is a cytotoxin that lyses human, horse and rabbit erythrocytes. Its production is coded by plasmid pAD1, which also confers bacteriocin production (Clewell and Weaver 1989, Weaver, Clewell and An 1993). The production of haemolysin was reported to be more common in strains of *E. faecalis* isolated from human infections than in strains isolated from faecal sources of healthy persons (Ike, Hashimoto and Clewell 1987). Haemolysin production by *E. faecalis* has also been associated with enhanced virulence in mice (Ike, Hashimoto and Clewell 1984) and was found to contribute to the severity of *E. faecalis* experimental endophthalmitis (Jett et al. 1992, Stevens et al. 1992). Haemolysin and aggregative substance contributed to enhanced virulence in experimental endocarditis (Chow et al. 1993b). However, the mechanism ·by which haemolysin and aggregation substance enhance virulence is not completely understood. It is conceivable that these substances have an effect on colonization, invasion, platelet aggregation, or fibrin generation (Chow et al. 1993b). Coque and colleagues (1995) reported that they were unable to find an increase in incidence of production of haemolysin or aggregation substance in *E. faecalis* strains isolated from patients with endocarditis and patients without endocarditis or normal flora of healthy persons.

The production of aggregation substance is induced by pheromones (small linear peptides). The immediate effect of the production of such substance is the aggregation of plasmid-free and plasmid donor cells. Exchange of plasmids carrying the haemolysin–bacteriocin genes as well as antimicrobial resistance genes occurs. Aggregation substances have been shown to enhance colonization in a tissue culture model for adherence to urinary epithelium (Hirt et al. 1993). Olmsted et al. (1994) reported that aggregation substance facilitated *E. faecalis* internalization by host epithelial cells.

Properties involved in the adherence to host tissues are considered important virulence factors for bacteria to establish infections. Guzman et al. (1989, 1991) reported that *E. faecalis* strains isolated from urinary tract infections adhered to urinary tract epithelial cells more efficiently than to human embryonic kidney cells or Girardi heart cell lines. *E. faecalis* strains isolated from endocarditis strains preferentially adhered to Girardi heart cell lines. These findings indicate that strain-specific adhesins may be necessary to establish initial colonization.

The investigation of the haemagglutination properties can be a convenient approach to detect the presence of adhesins on bacteria. Results of a recent study by Carvalho and Teixeira (1995) indicated that the surface structures related to the enterococcal adhesin are diverse. Most of the enterococcal strains analysed were shown to possess haemagglutinins, both proteins and non-proteins, that are involved in the attachment to sialic acid-containing receptors on the surface of rabbit erythrocytes. Other investigators have demonstrated that an adhesin similar to that found in oral streptococci is produced by *E. faecalis* (Lowe, Lambert and Smith 1995) and postulated that this molecule may function as an adhesin in endocarditis. Guzman et al. (1991) described a non-protein molecule that promoted the adhesin of *E. faecalis* to human Girardi heart cell line.

Enterococcal invasive properties under certain circumstances has been investigated. Evidence on the capacity of enterococci to translocate across intact intestinal mucosa in a murine model of antibiotic-induced superinfection was provided by the studies of Wells, Jechorek and Erlandsen (1990) and Wells and Erlandsen (1991). Translocation of enterococci across normal intestinal epithelium occurred in mice orally inoculated with *E. faecalis* and given broad spectrum antimicrobials that favour enterococcal overgrowth, resulting in disseminated infection.

Neutrophils (polymorphonuclear leucocytes) are one of the primary participants in host defence response to invading bacteria. Complement-dependent killing of enterococci has been demonstrated with strains of *E. faecalis* (Harvey, Baker and Edwards 1992, Arduino, Murray and Rakita 1994). Neutrophil-mediated killing of *E. faecium* was ineffective in some cases which led the investigators to postulate that resistance to neutrophil-mediated killing could be an additional virulence factor (Arduino et al. 1994).

The results of the studies mentioned, among others, indicate that we are only beginning to understand the pathogenicity and the virulence mechanisms of the enterococci.

REFERENCES

Andrews F, Horder T, 1906, A study of streptococci pathogenic for man, *Lancet*, **2:** 708–13.

Arduino RC, Murray BE, Rakita RM, 1994, Roles of antibodies and complement in phagocytic killing of enterococci, *Infect Immun*, **62:** 987–93.

Arduino RC, Jacques-Palaz K et al., 1994, Resistance of *Enterococcus faecium* to neutrophil-mediated phagocytosis, *Infect Immun*, **62:** 5587–94.

Arthur M, Courvallin P, 1993, Genetics and mechanisms of glycopeptide resistance in enterococci, *Antimicrob Agents Chemother*, **37:** 1563–71.

van Asselt GJ, Vliegenthart JS et al., 1992, High-level aminoglycoside resistance among enterococci and group A streptococci, *J Antimicrob Chemother*, **30:** 651–9.

Barnes EM, 1956, Tetrazolium reduction as a means of differentiating *S. faecalis* from *S. faecium*, *J Gen Microbiol*, **14:** 57–68.

Barnes EM, 1964, Distribution and properties of serological types of *Streptococcus faecium, Streptococcus durans* and related strains, *J Appl Bacteriol*, **27:** 461–70.

Beimfohr C, Krause A et al., 1993, In situ identification of lactococci, enterococci and streptococci, *Syst Appl Microbiol*, **16:** 450–6.

Berlutti F, Thaller MC et al., 1993, A new approach to use of bacteriolytic enzymes as a tool for species identification: selection of species-specific indicator strains with bacteriolytic activity towards *Enterococcus* strains, *Int J Syst Bacteriol*, **43:** 63–8.

Boyce JM, Opal SM et al., 1992, Emergence and nosocomial transmission of ampicillin-resistant enterococci, *Antimicrob Agents Chemother*, **36:** 1032–9.

Boyle JF, Soumakis SA et al., 1993, Epidemiologic analysis and genotypic characterization of a nosocomial outbreak of vancomycin-resistant enterococci, *J Clin Microbiol*, **31:** 1280–5.

Bryce EA, Zemcov SJV, Clarke AM, 1991, Species identification and antibiotic resistance patterns of the enterococci, *Eur J Clin Microbiol Infect Dis*, **10:** 745–7.

Buschelman BJ, Bale BJ, Jones RN, 1993, Species identification and determination of high-level aminoglycoside resistance among enterococci. Comparison study of sterile body fluid isolates, 1985–1991, *Diagn Microbiol Infect Dis*, **16:** 119–22.

Bush LM, Calmon J et al., 1989, High-level penicillin resistance among isolates of enterococci: implications for treatment of enterococcal infections, *Ann Intern Med*, **110:** 515–20.

Caprioli T, Zaccour F, Kasatiya SS, 1975, Phage typing scheme for group D streptococci isolated from human urogenital tract, *J Clin Microbiol*, **2:** 311–17.

Carvalho MGS, Teixeira LM, 1995, Hemagglutination properties of *Enterococcus*, *Curr Microbiol*, **30:** 265–8.

Chirurgi VA, Oster SE et al., 1991, Ampicillin-resistant *Enterococcus raffinosus* in an acute-care hospital: case-control study and antimicrobial susceptibilities, *J Clin Microbiol*, **29:** 2663–5.

Chow JW, Kuritza A et al., 1993a, Clonal spread of vancomycin-resistant *Enterococcus faecium* between patients in three hospitals in two states, *J Clin Microbiol*, **31:** 1609–11.

Chow JW, Thal LA et al., 1993b, Plasmid-associated hemolysin and aggregation substance production contribute to virulence in experimental enterococcal endocarditis, *Antimicrob Agents Chemother*, **37:** 2474–7.

Clewell DB, 1990, Movable genetic elements and antibiotic resistance in enterococci, *Eur J Clin Microbiol Infect Dis*, **9:** 90–102.

Clewell DB, 1993a, Sex pheromones and the plasmid-encoded mating response in *Enterococcus faecalis*, *Bacterial Conjugation*, ed. Clewell DB, Plenum Press, New York, 349–67.

Clewell DB, 1993b, Bacterial sex pheromone-induced plasmid transfer, *Cell*, **73:** 9–12.

Clewell DB, Flannagan SE, 1993, The conjugative transposons of gram-positive bacteria, *Bacterial Conjugation*, ed. Clewell DB, Plenum Press, New York, 369–93.

Clewell DB, Gawron-Burke C, 1986, Conjugative transposons and the dissemination of antibiotic resistance in streptococci, *Annu Rev Microbiol*, **40:** 635–59.

Clewell DB, Weaver KE, 1989, Sex pheromones and plasmid transfer in *Enterococcus faecalis*, *Plasmid*, **21:** 175–84.

Collins MD, Farrow JAE, Jones D, 1986, *Enterococcus mundtii* sp. nov., *Int J Syst Bacteriol*, **36:** 8–12.

Collins MD, Williams AM, Wallbanks S, 1990, The phylogeny of *Aerococcus* and *Pediococcus* as determined by 16S RNA sequence analysis, description of *Tetragenococcus*, *FEMS Microbiol Lett*, **70:** 255–62.

Collins MD, Jones D et al., 1984, *Enterococcus avium* nom. rev., comb. nov.; *E. casseliflavus* nom. rev.; *E. durans* nom. rev., comb. nov.; *E. gallinarum* comb. nov.; and E. *malodoratus* sp. nov., *Int J Syst Bacteriol*, **34:** 220–3.

Collins MD, Ash C et al., 1989a, 16S Ribosomal ribonucleic acid sequence analyses of lactococci and related taxa. Description of *Vagococcus fluvalis* gen. nov., sp. nov., *J Appl Bacteriol*, **67:** 453–60.

Collins MD, Facklam RR et al., 1989b, *Enterococcus raffinosus* sp. nov., *Enterococcus solitarius* sp. nov. and *Enterococcus pseudoavium* sp. nov., *FEMS Microbiol Lett*, **57:** 283–8.

Collins MD, Rodrigues UM et al., 1991, *Enterococcus dispar* sp. nov., a new *Enterococcus* species from human sources, *Lett Appl Microbiol*, **12:** 95–8.

Coque TM, Patterson JE et al., 1995, Incidence of hemolysin, gelatinase, and aggregation substance among enterococci isolated from patients with endocarditis and other infections and from feces of hospitalized and community-based persons, *J Infect Dis*, **171:** 1223–9.

Coudron PE, Mayhall CG et al., 1984, *Streptococcus faecium* outbreak in a neonatel intensive care unit, *J Clin Microbiol*, **20:** 1044–8.

Daly JA, Clifton NL, Seskin K, 1991, Use of rapid, nonradioactive DNA probes in culture confirmation tests to detect *Streptococcus agalactiae*, *Haemophilus influenzae*, and *Enterococcus* spp. from pediatric patients with significant infections, *J Clin Microbiol*, **29:** 80–2.

Dayton SL, Chipps DD et al., 1974, Evaluation of three media for selective isolation of gram positive bacteria from wounds, *Appl Microbiol*, **27:** 420–2.

Deibel RH, 1964, The group D streptococci, *Bacteriol Rev*, **28:** 330–66.

Devriese LA, Pot B, Collins MD, 1993, Phenotypic identification of the genus *Enterococcus* and differentiation of phylogenetically distinct enterococcal species and species groups, *J Appl Bacteriol*, **75:** 399–408.

Devriese LA, Ceyssens K et al., 1990, *Enterococcus columbae*, a species from pigeon instestines, *FEMS Microbiol Lett*, **71:** 247–52.

Devriese LA, Cruz Cloque JI et al., 1992a, Identification and composition of the tonsillar and anal enterococci and streptococcal flora of dogs and cats, *J Appl Bacteriol*, **73:** 421–5.

Devriese LA, Laurier L et al., 1992b, Enterococcal and streptococcal species isolated from faeces of calves, young cattle and dairy cows, *J Appl Bacteriol*, **72:** 29–31.

Domenech A, Prieta J et al., 1993, Phenotypic and phylogenetic evidence for a close relationship between *Lactococcus garvieae* and *Enterococcus seriolicida*, *Microbiologia Semin*, **9:** 63–8.

Donabedian SM, Chow JW et al., 1992, Molecular typing of ampicillin-resistant, non-β-lactamase-producing *Enterococcus faecium* isolates from diverse geographic areas, *J Clin Microbiol*, **30:** 2757–61.

Donabedian S, Chow JW et al., 1995, DNA hybridization and contour-clamped homogeneous electric field electrophoresis for identification of enterococci to the species level, *J Clin Microbiol*, **33:** 141–5.

Dunny GM, 1990, Genetic functions and cell–cell interactions in the pheromone-inducible plasmid transfer system of *Enterococcus faecalis*, *Mol Microbiol*, **4:** 689–96.

Dutka BJ, Kwan KK, 1978, Comparison of eight media procedures for recovering faecal streptococci from water under winter conditions, *J Appl Bacteriol*, **45:** 333–40.

Eliopoulos GM, Eliopoulos CT, 1990, Therapy of enterococcal infections, *Eur J Clin Microbiol Infect Dis*, **9:** 118–26.

Elliott JA, Collins MD et al., 1991, Differentiation of *Lactococcus lactis* and *Lactococcus garvieae* from humans by comparison of whole-cell protein patterns, *J Clin Microbiol*, **29:** 2731–4.

Ellner PD, Stoessel DJ et al., 1966, A new culture medium for medical bacteriology, *Am J Clin Pathol*, **45:** 502–3.

Enns RK, 1988, DNA probes: an overview and comparison with current methods, *Lab Med*, **19:** 295–300.

Facklam RR, 1976, A review of the microbiological techniques for the isolation and identification of streptococci, *Crit Rev Clin Lab Sci*, **6:** 287–317.

Facklam RR, Collins MD, 1989, Identification of *Enterococcus* species isolated from human infections by a conventional test scheme, *J Clin Microbiol*, **27:** 731–4.

Facklam RR, Elliott JA, 1995, Identification, classification, and clinical relevance of catalase-negative, gram-positive cocci, excluding the streptococci and enterococci, *Clin Microbiol Rev*, **8:** 479–95.

Facklam RR, Hollis D, Collins MD, 1989, Identification of gram-positive coccal and coccobacillary vancomycin-resistant bacteria, *J Clin Microbiol*, **27:** 724–30.

Facklam RR, Sahm DF, 1995, *Manual of Clinical Microbiology*, 6th edn, American Society for Microbiology, Washington, DC, 308–14.

Facklam RR, Washington II JA, 1991, *Manual of Clinical Microbiology*, 5th edn, American Society for Microbiology, Washington, DC, 238–57.

Farrow JAE, Collins MD, 1985, *Enterococcus hirae*, a new species that includes amino acid assay strain NCDO 1258 and strains causing growth depression in young chickens, *Int J Syst Bacteriol*, **35:** 73–5.

Felmingham D, Wilson APR et al., 1992, *Enterococcus* species in urinary tract infection, *Clin Infect Dis*, **15:** 295–301.

Fontana R, Amalfitano G et al., 1992, Mechanisms of resistance to growth inhibition and killing by β-lactam antibiotics in enterococci, *Clin Infect Dis*, **15:** 486–9.

Fraimow HS, Jungkind DL et al., 1994, Urinary tract infection with an *Enterococcus faecalis* isolate that requires vancomycin for growth, *Ann Intern Med*, **121:** 22–6.

Galvez A, Valdivia E et al., 1985, Production of bacteriocin-like substances by group D streptococci of human origin, *Microbios*, **43:** 223–32.

Goering RV, Winters MA, 1992, Rapid method for epidemiological evaluation of gram-positive cocci by field inversion gel electrophoresis, *J Clin Microbiol*, **30:** 577–80.

Gordillo ME, Singh KV, Murray BE, 1993, Comparison of ribotyping and pulsed-field gel electrophorsis for subspecies differentiation of strains of *Enterococcus faecalis*, *J Clin Microbiol*, **31:** 1570–4.

Gordon S, Swensen JS et al., 1992, Antimicrobial susceptibility patterns of common and unusual species of enterococci causing infections in the United States, *J Clin Microbiol*, **30:** 2373–8.

Graninger W, Ragette R, 1992, Nosocomial bacteremia due to *Enterococcus faecalis* without endocarditis, *Clin Infect Dis*, **15:** 49–57.

Green M, Barbadora K et al., 1995, Comparison of field inversion gel electrophoresis with contour-clamped homogeneous electric field electrophoresis as a typing method for *Enterococcus faecium*, *J Clin Microbiol*, **33:** 1554–7.

Guiney M, Urwin G, 1993, Frequency and antimicrobial susceptibility of clinical isolates of enterococci, *Eur J Clin Microbiol Infect Dis*, **12:** 362–6.

Gullberg RM, Homann SR, Phair JP, 1989, Enterococcal bacteremia: analysis of 75 episodes, *Rev Infect Dis*, **11:** 74–85.

Guzman CA, Pruzzo C et al., 1989, Role of adherence in pathogenesis of *Enterococcus faecalis* urinary tract infection and endocarditis, *Infect Immun*, **57:** 1834–8.

Guzman CA, Pruzzo C et al., 1991, Serum dependent expression of *Enterococcus faecalis* adhesins involved in the colonization of heart cells, *Microb Pathog*, **11:** 399–409.

Hall LMC, Duke B et al., 1992a, Typing of *Enterococcus* species by DNA restriction fragment analysis, *J Clin Microbiol*, **30:** 915–19.

Harvey BS, Baker CJ, Edwards MS, 1992, Contributions of complement and immunoglobulin to neutrophil-mediated killing of enterococci, *Infect Immun*, **60:** 3635–40.

Herman G, Hoch V, 1971, Phage typing of D group streptococci. II. Isolation of supplementary phages for classification of enterococci untypable with Roumanian phages, *Acta Microbiol Acad Sci Hung*, **18:** 101–4.

Hirt H, Wanner G et al., 1993, Biochemical, immunological and ultrastructural characterization of aggregation substances encoded by *Enterococcus faecalis* sex-pheromone plasmids, *Eur J Biochem*, **211**: 711–16.

Hoch V, Herman G, 1971, Phage typing of D group streptococci. I. Typing of enterococci with Roumanian phages, *Acta Microbiol Acad Sci Hung*, **18**: 95–9.

Hodel-Christian SL, Murray BE, 1992, Comparison of the gentamicin resistance transposon Tn*5281* with regions encoding gentamicin resistance in *Enterococcus faecalis* isolates from diverse geographic locations, *Antimicrob Agents Chemother*, **36**: 2259–64.

Ike Y, Hashimoto H, Clewell DB, 1984, Hemolysin of *Streptococcus faecalis* subspecies zymogenes contributes to virulence in mice, *Infect Immun*, **45**: 528–30.

Ike Y, Hashimoto H, Clewell DB, 1987, High incidence of hemolysin production by *Enterococcus* (*Streptococcus*) *faecalis* strains associated with human parenteral infections, *J Clin Microbiol*, **25**: 1524–8.

Ike Y, Clewell DB et al., 1990, Genetic analysis of the pAD1 hemolysin/bacteriocin determinant in *Enterococcus faecalis* Tn*917* insertional mutagenesis and cloning, *J Bacteriol*, **172**: 155–63.

Isenberg HD, Goldberg D, Sampson J, 1970, Laboratory studies with a selective *Enterococcus* medium, *Appl Microbiol*, **20**: 433–6.

Jayarao BM, Dore JJE, Oliver SP, 1992, Restriction fragment length polymorphism analysis of 16S ribosomal DNA of *Streptococcus* and *Enterococcus* species of bovine origin, *J Clin Microbiol*, **30**: 2235–40.

Jett BD, Huycke MM, Gilmore MS, 1994, Virulence of enterococci, *Clin Microbiol Rev*, **7**: 462–78.

Jett BD, Jensen HG et al., 1992, Contribution of the pAD1 encoded cytolysin to the severity of experimental *Enterococcus faecalis* endophthalmitis, *Infect Immun*, **60**: 2445–52.

Kalina AP, 1970, The taxonomy and nomenclature of enterococci, *Int J Syst Bacteriol*, **20**: 185–9.

Kaplan AH, Gilligan PH, Facklam RR, 1988, Recovery of resistant enterococci during vancomycin prophylaxis, *J Clin Microbiol*, **26**: 1216–18.

Kato T, Matsuda T et al., 1993, Isolation of *Enterococcus faecium* with antibacterial activity and characterization of its bacteriocin, *Biosci Biotechnol Biochem*, **57**: 551–6.

Kaufhold A, Ferrieri P, 1993, Molecular investigation of clinical *Enterococcus faecium* isolates highly resistant to gentamicin, *Zentralbl Bakteriol Parasitenkd Infektionskr Hyg Abt I Orig*, **278**: 83–101.

Kibbey HJ, Hagedorn C, McCoy EL, 1978, Use of fecal streptococci as indicators of pollution in soil, *Appl Environ Microbiol*, **35**: 711–17.

Knudtson LM, Hartman PA, 1993, Comparison of four latex agglutination kits to rapidly identify Lancefield group D enterococci and fecal streptococci, *J Rapid Methods Autom Microbiol*, **1**: 301–4.

Kuhnen E, Rommelshein K, Andries L, 1987, Combined use of phage typing, enterococcinotyping and specied differentiation of group D streptococci as an effective epidemiological tool, *Zentralbl Bakteriol Parasitenkd Infektionskr Hyg Abt 1 Orig*, **266**: 586–95.

Kuhnen E, Richter F et al., 1988, Establishment of a typing system for group D streptococci, *Zentralbl Bakteriol Parasitenkd Infektionskr Hyg Abt 1 Orig*, **267**: 322–30.

Kusuda R, Kawai K et al., 1991, *Enterococcus seriolicida* sp. nov., a fish pathogen, *Int J Syst Bacteriol*, **41**: 406–9.

Laukova A, Marekova M, Javorsky P, 1993, Detection and antimicrobial spectrum of a bacteriocin-like substance produced by *Enterococcus faecium* CCM4231, *Lett Appl Microbiol*, **16**: 257–60.

Leclerq R, Dutka-Malen S et al., 1992, Resistance to enterococci to aminoglycosides and glycopeptides, *Clin Infect Dis*, **15**: 495–501.

Lopardo H, Casimir L et al., 1990, Isolation of three strains of beta-lactamase-producing *Enterococcus faecalis* in Argentina, *Eur J Clin Microbiol Infect Dis*, **9**: 402–5.

Lowe AM, Lambert PA, Smith AW, 1995, Cloning of an *Enterococcus faecalis* endocarditis antigen: homology with adhesins from some oral streptococci, *Infect Immun*, **63**: 703–6.

Luginbuhl LM, Rotbart HA et al., 1987, Neonatal enterococcal sepsis: case-control study and description of an outbreak, *Pediatr Infect Dis J*, **6**: 1022–30.

McNamara EB, King EM, Smyth EG, 1995, A survey of antimicrobial susceptibility of clinical isolates of *Enterococcus* spp. from Irish hospitals, *J Antimicrob Chemother*, **35**: 185–9.

Maekawa S, Yoshioka M, Kumamoto Y, 1992, Proposal of a new scheme for the serological typing of *Enterococcus faecalis* strains, *Microbiol Immunol*, **36**: 671–81.

Martinez-Murcia AJ, Collins MD, 1991, *Enterococus sulfureus*, a new yellow-pigmented *Enterococcus* species, *FEMS Microbiol Lett*, **80**: 69–74.

Mead GC, 1978, *Streptococci*, Academic Press, London, 245–61.

Megran DW, 1992, Enterococcal endocarditis, *Clin Infect Dis*, **15**: 63–71.

Merquior VLC, Peralta JM et al., 1994, Analysis of electrophoretic whole-cell protein profiles as a tool for characterization of *Enterococcus* species, *Curr Microbiol*, **28**: 149–53.

Miranda AG, Singh KV, Murray BE, 1991, DNA fingerprinting of *Enterococcus faecium* by pulse-field gel electrophoresis may be a useful epidemiologic tool, *J Clin Microbiol*, **29**: 2752–7.

Moellering RC Jr, 1992, Emergence of *Enterococcus* as a significant pathogen, *Clin Infect Dis*, **14**: 1173–8.

Mundt JO, Graham WF, McCarty IE, 1967, Spherical lactic acid-producing bacteria of southern-grown raw and processed vegetables, *Appl Environ Microbiol*, **15**: 1303–8.

Murray BE, 1990, The life and times of the *Enterococcus*, *Clin Microbiol Rev*, **3**: 46–65.

Murray BE, 1992, β-Lactamase-producing enterococci, *Antimicrob Agents Chemother*, **36**: 2355–9.

Murray BE, Mederki-Samoraj B, 1983, A new mechanism for in vitro penicillin resistance, *J Clin Invest*, **72**: 1168–71.

Murray BE, Singh KV et al., 1990, Comparison of genomic DNAs of different enterococcal isolates using restriction endonucleases with infrequent recognition sites, *J Clin Microbiol*, **28**: 2059–63.

Murray BE, Lopardo HA et al., 1992, Intrahospital spread of a single gentamicin-resistant, β-lactamase producing strain of *Enterococcus faecalis* in Argentina, *Antimicrob Agents Chemother*, **36**: 230–2.

Murray BE, Singh KV et al., 1993, Generation of restriction map of *Enterococcus faecalis* OG1 and investigation of growth requirements and regions encoding biosynthetic function, *J Bacteriol*, **175**: 5216–23.

National Committee for Clinical Laboratory Standards (NCCLS), 1993, *Methods for Dilution Antimicrobial Susceptibility Tests for Bacteria that grow Aerobically*, M7-A, NCCLS, Villanova PA, 579–618.

Nauschuetz WF, Trevino SB et al., 1993, *Enterococcus casseliflavus* as an agent of nosocomial bloodstream infections, *Med Microbiol Lett*, **2**: 102–8.

Nichols RL, Muzik AC, 1992, Enterococcal infections in surgical patients: the mystery continues, *Clin Infect Dis*, **15**: 72–6.

Niemi RM, Niemela SI et al., 1993, Presumptive fecal streptococci in environmental samples characterized by one-dimensional sodium dodecyl sulfate-polyacrylamide gel electrophoresis, *Appl Environ Microbiol*, **59**: 2190–6.

Nowlan SS, Deibel RH, 1967, Group Q streptococci, I. Ecology, serology, physiology, and relationship to established enterococci, *J Bacteriol*, **94**: 291–6.

Olmsted SB, Dunny GM et al., 1994, A plasmid-encoded surface protein on *Enterococcus faecalis* augments its internalization by cultured intestinal epithelial cells, *J Infect Dis*, **170**: 1549–56.

Orla-Jensen S, 1919, The lactic acid bacteria, *Mem Acad Roy Sci Danemark*, *Sect Sci Ser 2*, **5**: 81–197.

Oster SE, Chirurgi VA et al., 1990, Ampicillin-resistant enterococcal species in an acute care hospital, *Antimicrob Agents Chemother*, **34**: 1821–3.

Patterson JE, Singh KV, Murray BE, 1991, Epidemiology of an endemic strain of β-lactamase-producing *Enterococcus faecalis*, *J Clin Microbiol*, **29**: 2513–16.

Pleceas P, Bogdan C, Vereanu A, 1972, Enterocine-typing of group D streptococci, *Zentralbl Bakteriol Parasitenkd Infektionskr Hyg Abt 1 Orig*, **221**: 173–81.

Pompei R, Berlutti F et al., 1992, *Enterococcus flavescens* sp. nov., a new species of enterococci of clinical origin, *Int J Syst Bacteriol*, **42**: 365–9.

Reichelt T, Kennes J, Kramer J, 1984, Co-transfer of two plasmids determining bacteriocin production and sucrose utilization in *Streptococcus faecium*, *FEMS Microbiol Lett*, **23**: 147–50.

Rice EW, Messer JW et al., 1995, Occurrence of high-level aminoglycoside resistance in environmental isolates of enterococci, *Appl Environ Microbiol*, **61**: 374–6.

Rodrigues U, Collins MD, 1990, Phylogenetic analysis of *Streptococcus saccharolyticus* based on 16S rRNA sequencing, *FEMS Microbiol Lett*, **71**: 231–4.

Ruoff KL, De La Maza L et al., 1990, Species identities of enterococci isolated from clinical specimens, *J Clin Microbiol*, **28**: 435–7.

Sabbaj J, Sutter VL, Finegold SM, 1971, Comparison of selective media for isolation of presumptive group D streptococci from human feces, *Appl Microbiol*, **22**: 1008–11.

Sadatsune T, Kuwakara M et al., 1978, Bacteriocin type of enterococci, *Hiroshima J Med Sci*, **27**: 241–6.

Sahm DF, Torres C, 1988, High-content aminoglycoside disks for determining aminoglyside-penicillin synergy against *Enterococcus faecalis*, *J Clin Microbiol*, **26**: 257–60.

Salzano G, Villani F et al., 1992, Conjugal transfer of plasmid-borne bacteriocin production in *Enterococcus faecalis* 226 NWC, *FEMS Microbiol Lett*, **99**: 1–6.

Sapico FL, Canawati HN et al., 1989, Enterococci highly resistant to penicillin and ampicillin: an emerging clinical problem?, *J Clin Microbiol*, **27**: 2091–5.

Schaberg DR, Culver DH, Gaynes RP, 1991, Major trends in the microbial etiology of nosocomial infection, *Am J Med*, **91**: 79S–82S.

Schleifer KH, Kilpper-Balz R, 1984, Transfer of *Streptococcus faecalis* and *Streptococcus faecium* to the genus *Enterococcus* nom. rev. as *Enterococcus faecalis* comb. nov. and *Enterococcus faecium* comb. nov., *Int J Syst Bacteriol*, **34**: 31–4.

Schleifer KH, Kilpper-Balz R, 1987, Molecular and chemotaxonomic approaches to the classification of streptococci, enterococci and lactococci: a review, *Syst Appl Microbiol*, **10**: 1–19.

Sharma DP, Shriniwas Bhujwala RA, 1976, Enterocin typing of group 'D' streptococci, *Jpn J Microbiol*, **20**: 559–60.

Sharpe ME, 1964, Serological types of *Streptococcus faecalis* and its varieties and their cell wall type antigen, *J Gen Microbiol*, **36**: 151–60.

Sharpe ME, Shattock PMF, 1952, The serological typing of group D streptococci associated with outbreaks of neonatal diarrhoea, *J Gen Microbiol*, **6**: 150–65.

Sherman JM, 1937, The streptococci, *Bacteriol Rev*, **1**: 3–97.

Sherman JM, 1938, The enterococci and related streptococci, *J Bacteriol*, **35**: 81–93.

Sherman JM, Wing HU, 1935, An unnoted hemolytic *Streptococcus* associated with milk products, *J Dairy Sci*, **18**: 656–60.

Sherman JM, Wing HU, 1937, *Streptococcus durans*, *J Dairy Sci*, **20**: 165–7.

Shlaes DM, Binczewski B, Rice LB, 1993, Emerging antimicrobial resistance and the immunocompromised host, *Clin Infect Dis*, **17**: S527–36.

Siragusa GR, 1992, Production of bacteriocin inhibitory to *Listeria* species by *Enterococcus hirae*, *Appl Environ Microbiol*, **58**: 3508–13.

Smyth CJ, Matthews H et al., 1987, Biotyping, serotyping and phage typing of *Streptococcus faecalis* isolated from dental plaque in the human mouth, *J Med Microbiol*, **23**: 45–54.

Stern CS, Carvalho MGS, Teixeira LM, 1994, Characterization of enterococci isolated from human and nonhuman sources in Brazil, *Diagn Microbiol Infect Dis*, **20**: 61–7.

Stevens SX, Jensen HG et al., 1992, A hemolysin-encoding plasmid contributes to bacterial virulence in experimental *Enterococcus faecalis* endophthalmitis, *Invest Ophthalmol Vis Sci*, **33**: 1650–6.

Su YA, Clewell DB, 1993, Characterization of the left 4kb conjugative transposon Tn*916*: determinants involved in excision, *Plasmid*, **30**: 234–50.

Tanimoto K, An FY, Clewell DB, 1993, Characterization of the *traC* determinant of the *Enterococcus faecalis* hemolysin-bacteriocin plasmid pAD1: binding of sex pheromone, *J Bacteriol*, **175**: 5260–4.

Teixeira LM, Facklam RR et al., 1995, Correlation between phenotypic characteristics and DNA relatedness with *Enterococcus faecium* strains, *J Clin Microbiol*, **33**: 1520–3.

Teixeira LM, Merquior VLC et al., 1996, Phenotypic and genotypic characterization of atypical *Lactococcus garvieae* strains isolated from water buffalos with subclinical mastitis and confirmation of *L. garvieae* as a senior subjective synonym of *Enterococcus seriolicida*, *Int J Syst Bacteriol*, **46**: in press.

Tenover FC, Tokars J et al., 1993, Ability of clinical laboratories to detect antimicrobial agent-resistant enterococci, *J Clin Microbiol*, **31**: 1695–9.

Thal LA, Chow JW et al., 1993, Molecular characterization of highly gentamicin-resistant *Enterococcus faecalis* isolates lacking high-level streptomycin resistance, *Antimicrob Agents Chemother*, **37**: 134–7.

Thiercelin E, 1899, Sur un diplocoque saprophyte de l'intestin susceptible de devenir pathogene, *C R Soc Biol*, **5**: 269–71.

Tomura T, Hirano T et al., 1973, Transmission of bacteriocinogenicity by conjugation in group D streptococci, *Jpn J Microbiol*, **17**: 445–52.

Truant AL, Satishchandran V, 1993, Comparison of Streptex versus PathoDx for group D typing of vancomycin-resistant *Enterococcus*, *Diagn Microbiol Infect Dis*, **16**: 89–91.

Villani F, Salzano G et al., 1993, Enterocin 226NWC, a bacteriocin produced by *Enterococcus faecalis* 226, active against *Listeria monocytogenes*, *J Appl Bacteriol*, **74**: 380–7.

Watanakunakorn C, Burkert T, 1993, Infective endocarditis at a large community teaching hospital 1980–1990, *Medicine (Baltimore)*, **72**: 90–102.

Weaver KE, Clewell DB, An F, 1993, Identification, characterization, and nucleotide sequence of a region of *Enterococcus faecalis* pheromone responsive plasmid pAD1 capable of autonomous replication, *J Bacteriol*, **175**: 1900–9.

Wells CL, Erlandsen SL, 1991, Localization of translocating *Escherichia coli*, *Proteus mirabilis*, and *Enterococcus faecalis* within cecal and colonic tissues of monoassociated mice, *Infect Immun*, **59**: 4693–7.

Wells CL, Jechorek RP, Erlandsen SL, 1990, Evidence for the translocation of *Enterococcus faecalis* across the mouse intestinal tract, *J Infect Dis*, **162**: 82–90.

Williams AM, Farrow JAE, Collins MD, 1989, Reverse transcriptase sequencing of 16S ribosomal RNA from *Streptococcus cecorum*, *Lett Appl Microbiol*, **8**: 185–9.

Williams AM, Rodrigues UM, Collins MD, 1991, Intrageneric relationships of enterococci as determined by reverse transcriptase sequencing of small-subunit rRNA, *Res Microbiol*, **142**: 67–74.

Willinger B, Manafi M, 1995, Evaluation of new chromogenic agar medium for the identification of urinary tract pathogens, *Lett Appl Microbiol*, **20**: 300–2.

Woodford N, Morrison D et al., 1993, Application of DNA probes for rRNA and *vanA* genes to investigation of a nosocomial cluster of vancomycin-resistant enterococci, *J Clin Microbiol*, **31**: 653–8.

Chapter 30

ERYSIPELOTHRIX AND LISTERIA

J McLauchlin and D Jones

1 INTRODUCTION

Erysipelothrix and *Listeria* are treated together in this chapter because of the superficial phenotypic resemblance between the species of the 2 genera. Both contain small, gram-positive, non-sporing rods with somewhat similar morphological and cultural appearances, and have similar growth requirements and G + C content of DNA. In addition, *Erysipelothrix rhusiopathiae* and *Listeria monocytogenes* are pathogenic to a wide variety of animals and cause disease in humans. In the last 20 years, however, more detailed comparative studies have shown that *Erysipelothrix* and *Listeria* are phenotypically distinct genera. Further recent comparative analysis of their 16S rRNA gene sequences indicate that the 2 genera are phylogenetically distinct. *Listeria* is more closely related to the genus *Brochothrix*, whereas *Erysipelothrix* forms a distinct subline within the clostridial group of organisms and exhibits significant, albeit loose, association with certain clostridial species, including *Clostridium innocuum* and *Clostridium ramosus*, and with some other nonsporing bacteria such as *Lactobacillus vitulinus* and *Streptococcus pleomorphus* (Collins et al. 1994).

ERYSIPELOTHRIX

2 GENUS/SPECIES DEFINITION

Erysipelothrix are slender, rod-shaped bacteria with a tendency to form long filaments. They are non-motile and non-sporing, gram-positive but decolorize easily, and may appear gram-negative. The organisms are facultatively anaerobic, not acid-fast and growth is improved in the presence of 5–10% CO_2. They grow between 5 and 42°C; optimum growth temperature is 30–37°C and organic growth factors are required. The fermentative activity of *Erysipelothrix* spp. is very weak; acid but no gas is produced from glucose and certain other carbohydrates. *Erysipelothrix* spp. are catalase- and oxidase-negative. Typical strains form H_2S on triple sugar iron agar. There are at least 26 serotypes. The genus consists of 2 species *Erysipelothrix rhusiopathiae* and *Erysipelothrix tonsillarum*. *E. rhusiopathiae* is naturally pathogenic to a wide range of mammals, including humans, and to birds. In humans, infection may manifest as septicaemia, arthritis, endocarditis and skin lesions. *E. tonsillarum*, isolated from the tonsils of apparently healthy pigs, has been implicated as a cause of endocarditis in dogs. The G + C content of DNA of both species 36–40 mol%. The type species is *E. rhusiopathiae*.

3 INTRODUCTION AND HISTORICAL PERSPECTIVE

The bacterium now known as *Erysipelothrix rhusiopathiae* was first isolated in 1876 by Koch (1878, 1880) from the blood of mice that had been inoculated subcutaneously with the blood exudate of putrefied meat. The first good description of the organism was provided by Loeffler (1886) who, in 1882, isolated a slender bacillus from the cutaneous blood vessels of a pig that had died of 'rotlauf' (swine erysipelas). Although the published descriptions are sparse, it is most probable that the same bacteria were noted at about the same time by Pasteur and Dumas (1882) and Pasteur and Thuiller (1883) in the blood of pigs dying of 'rouget'(swine erysipelas). The latter authors were able to protect pigs against spontaneous infections of 'rouget' by injecting cultures of a strain that had been passed through rabbits (Pasteur and Thuiller 1883); this was the first demonstration of artificial immunization by means of live attenuated bacteria. Trevisan (1885) proposed the name *Erysipelothrix insidiosa* and Migula (1900) used the name *Bacterium rhusiopathiae* for the pig isolates. The first human infection with *Erysipelothrix* was reported by Rosenbach (1909) who isolated the organism from a patient with localized cutaneous lesions and first used the term 'erysipeloid' to distinguish the infection from that of human erysipelas.

Rosenbach (1909) conducted a comparative study of the different isolates and suggested the names *Erysipelothrix porci*, *Erysipelothrix murisepticus* [sic] and *Erysipelothrix erysipeloides* for the pig, mouse and human isolates, respectively, on the grounds that, although very similar, they were sufficiently distinct to merit separate species status. The species name *E. porci* was antedated by the name *Bacterium rhusiopathiae* (Migula 1900); consequently, the new combination *Erysipelothrix rhusiopathiae* (Migula) was proposed by Buchanan (1918). This name became firmly established in the veterinary literature. Over the years a number of comparative studies indicated that all the then recognized species of *Erysipelothrix* belonged to a single species (see Woodbine 1950). For this reason Langford and Hansen (1953) revived the species epithet *insidiosa* (Trevisan 1885) and proposed that strains then designated *E. rhusiopathiae*, *E. muriseptica* and *E. erysipeloides* be included in one species, *E. insidiosa*. This proposal caused unnecessary confusion because the species epithet *insidiosa* had not been used in the literature for some 50 years. Shuman and Wellmann (1966) therefore requested that the Judicial Commission issue an opinion conserving the name *Erysipelothrix rhusiopathiae*. *E. rhusiopathiae* remained the type and only species in the genus until the description of a second species, *E. tonsillarum*, by Takahashi et al. (1987a).

Most of the information on the genus is derived from the results of studies on *E. rhusiopathiae* because of its long history as a pathogen of humans and animals, especially pigs. However, more information has become available on the apparently non-, or far less pathogenic species *E. tonsillarum*. More detailed accounts of *E. rhusiopathiae* and the infections caused by the organism are given by Woodbine (1950), Grieco and Sheldon (1970), Conklin and Steele (1979), Jones (1986) and Reboli and Farrar (1991).

4 HABITAT

E. rhusiopathiae is widely distributed in nature and infections caused by the organism occur world wide. It has been found as a commensal or a pathogen in a wide variety of vertebrate and invertebrate species including pigs, sheep, cattle, horses, dogs, wild rodents, crustaceans, house flies, ticks, chickens, turkeys, ducks, geese, a number of wild birds and fish. The major reservoir of *E. rhusiopathiae* is almost certainly domestic pigs but rodents and birds are frequently infected (Conklin and Steele 1979, Reboli and Farrar 1991). It is not known to cause disease in fish but it has been isolated from apparently healthy fish tissue and is known to grow and persist for long periods in the surface slime of fishes (Wood 1975).

E. rhusiopathiae is widely distributed in the soil and surface waters of farms and in the sewage effluent of abattoirs. It is now generally accepted that the organism is not indigenous to the soil and that its presence reflects contamination by infected animals. Pathogenic strains have been isolated from the faeces of apparently healthy as well as diseased pigs (Wood 1974, Reboli and Farrar 1991). Although killed by moist heat at 55°C for 15 min, *E. rhusiopathiae* can survive in the dried state for many years. In soil the organism is favoured by an alkaline pH and high organic content (Ewald 1981). Soil that may retain viable organisms serves as a medium for infection of animals by the oral route. Wood and Packer (1972) recovered *E. rhusiopathiae* from a number of soil and manure samples from pig farms where there had been no reported incidence of swine erysipelas for 5 years.

Most human infections are related to occupational exposure and probably occur via scratches or puncture wounds of the skin. Individuals at greatest risk of infection include butchers, fish handlers, abattoir workers, farmers and veterinarians (Wood 1975). Human-to-human infection has not been documented. In addition to its resistance to drying, *E. rhusiopathiae* is resistant to salting, pickling and smoking. Meat and bacon may contain the organisms after pickling for 170 days or after 30 days in a mixture of salt and potassium nitrate (Reboli and Farrar 1991). Hunter (1974) reported a case of widespread urticaria in a butcher who had eaten sausages from a pig slaughtered because of swine erysipelas. A relatively recent survey of pork, herring and cod from retail stores in southern Sweden revealed the presence of *E. rhusiopathiae* in 50% of the pork samples, 60% of the cod samples and 30% of the herring samples. Serotype

2 was the dominant serotype in all the products although other serotypes were also isolated (Stenstrom et al. 1992). The presence of virulent strains of *Erysipelothrix* on such products is probably more widespread than currently recognized.

Less is known about the habitats of the more recently described species *E. tonsillarum*. Isolated from the tonsils of apparently healthy pigs (Takahashi et al. 1987a), the organisms are almost certainly more widespread and have recently been incriminated as the cause of endocarditis in dogs (Takahashi et al. 1993).

5 MORPHOLOGY

Members of the genus exist in a rough and smooth form, each characterized by closely associated morphological and colonial appearances. In the smooth form (S-form) the cells appear as small, straight or slightly curved, non-motile, gram-positive rods 0.3–0.6 μm in diameter and 0.8–2.5 μm long with rounded ends. The cells occur singly, in pairs at an angle to give V forms, in clusters and in short chains. In the rough form (R-form) long filaments more than 60 μm long predominate (Fig. 30.1).

Both forms decolorize easily when gram-stained and both rods and filaments may appear as gram-negative

containing bands of gram-positive staining that give a beaded effect. Metachromatic granules are absent. The cell morphology varies to some extent with the conditions of culture. It has been claimed that, at pH 7.6–8.2, S-forms predominate whereas pH values of 5.2–7.0 favour the production of R-forms (Zák, Grigelová and Cernik 1965). It has also been reported that S-forms grow better at 33°C and R-forms at 37°C (Grieco and Sheldon 1970). In smears of blood and tissue taken from acute cases of infection, especially septicaemia, the organisms are usually of the S-form of morphology; in chronic infections, arthritis and endocarditis, R-forms are frequently detected together with S-forms (Ewald 1981). Capsules are considered to be absent (Ewald 1981, Jones 1986, Reboli and Farrar 1991) but Shimoji et al. (1994) noted the presence by electron microscopy of a capsule-like structure in virulent strains of *E. rhusiopathiae*.

6 CULTURAL CHARACTERS

After incubation for 24–48 h at 37°C, S-form colonies are very small, circular, low convex, with a smooth glistening surface and entire edge. Further incubation does not result in an increase in size but the centre of the colony becomes more opaque. R-form colonies are somewhat larger and flatter; the matt, uneven sur-

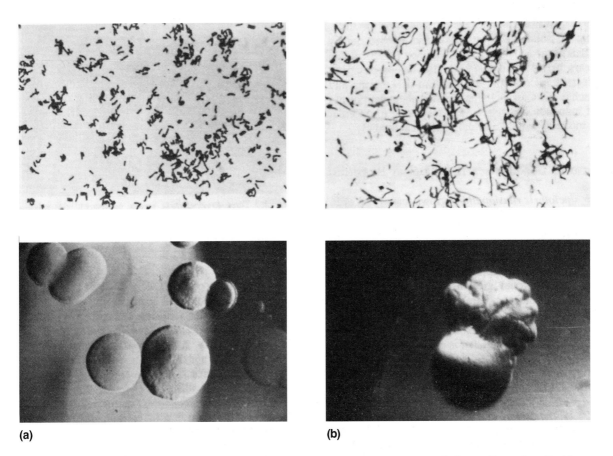

(a)　　　　　　　　　　　　　　　**(b)**

Fig. 30.1 (a) *Erysipelothrix rhusiopathiae* smooth form; (b) *Erysipelothrix rhusiopathiae* rough form. (Reproduced, with permission, from Starr MP, Stolp H et al. (eds), 1981, *The Prokaryotes: a Handbook on Habitats, Isolation and Identification of Bacteria*, Springer-Verlag, New York, p. 1691).

face, curled structure and irregular fimbriate edge are reminiscent of anthrax colonies. The colonies of both forms exhibit a light blue colour and sometimes a shimmering green colour when viewed by oblique illumination. The distinction between smooth and rough colonies is not always sharp; intermediate forms may exist (Barber 1939, Ewald 1981). In general, S-form colonies breed true but on agar plates streaked from old cultures smooth colonies frequently are seen to form rough sectors caused by dissociation to the R-form during growth; R-form colonies give rise to occasional smooth colonies.

On blood agar, α-haemolysis (greening) may be so intense that after incubation for 48 h a slight clearing may be apparent around colonies. Care must be taken because true β-haemolysis never occurs. All cultures of *E. rhusiopathiae* and those of *E. tonsillarum* examined so far produce a characteristic 'pipe cleaner' or 'test tube brush' type of growth in gelatin stab cultures incubated at 22°C for 2–3 days. The column of growth along the line of inoculation is composed of fine, lateral outgrowths that are more marked in R-forms.

7 GROWTH REQUIREMENTS AND METABOLISM

Erysipelothrix spp. are facultatively anaerobic. On first isolation, growth occurs in the form of a band just below the surface of a soft agar culture; whether this is due to a preference for CO_2 or for a reduced oxygen level is not clear. Growth is scant on the usual laboratory media. It is improved by glucose (0.2–0.5%) and to a lesser degree by blood or serum (5–10%). The optimum temperature for growth is 30–37°C; growth occurs between 5 and 42°C. The optimum pH for growth is 7.2–7.6, range 6.8–8.2 (Karlson and Merchant 1941).

The exact growth requirements of *Erysipelothrix* spp. have not been determined; several amino acids, riboflavin and small amounts of oleic acid are required (Hutner 1942). Growth is improved by tryptophan (Ewald 1981).

Glucose catabolism in *E. rhusiopathiae* is via the Embden–Meyerhof–Parnas pathway, although a small amount of glucose is dissimilated by the hexose monophosphate shunt (Robertson and McCullough 1968). Fermentation of glucose results in the production of mainly L(+) lactic acid with smaller amounts of acetic acid, formic acid, ethyl alcohol and carbon dioxide. The evidence indicates that the tricarboxylic acid cycle is relatively unimportant (Robertson and McCullough 1968). Exogenous citrate is not utilized. The organisms are catalase-negative and cytochromes and isoprenoid quinones are absent (Jones 1986).

8 GENETIC MECHANISMS

The G + C content of *Erysipelothrix* is 36–40 mol% (Flossman and Erler 1972, White and Mirikitani 1976, Takahashi et al. 1987a, 1992). DNA relatedness studies (Takahashi et al. 1992) indicate the presence of 3

genomic groups of species status within the genus (see section 11, p. 687). 16S rRNA oligonucleotide and gene sequences have been performed only with *E. rhusiopathiae* (Collins et al. 1994, Olsen, Woese and Overbeek 1994). Comparative partial 16S rRNA gene sequences have been reported for *E. tonsillarum* and *E. rhusiopathiae* (Ahrné et al. 1995).

Genetic studies with *Erysipelothrix* are relatively recent. Gene cloning of the *dnaK* gene of *E. rhusiopathiae* in *Escherichia coli* (Partridge et al. 1993) and DNA sequence analysis of chromosomal DNA from *E. rhusiopathiae* (Rockabrand et al. 1993) have identified genes that express the heat shock proteins DnaK and DnaJ, respectively. Transposon mutagenesis with the self-conjugative transposon Tn*916* has been used to obtain 3 avirulent insertional mutants of *E. rhusiopathiae* (Shimoji et al. 1994). Galán and Timoney (1990) cloned and expressed a protective antigen of *E. rhusiopathiae* in *Escherichia coli*.

Noguchi et al. (1993) detected 1–6 plasmids per strain in 7 strains out of 43 isolated from pigs with chronic swine erysipelas. The plasmids ranged in size from 1.4 to 86 kb but their functions remain unknown.

9 CELL WALL AND ENVELOPE COMPOSITION; ANTIGENIC STRUCTURE

The cell wall of *Erysipelothrix* is of the gram-positive type. The cell wall peptidoglycan diamino acid is lysine (Feist 1972) and the peptidoglycan type is the unusual B1δ (Schleifer and Kandler 1972). Mycolic acids are absent. Teichoic acids have not been detected (Feist 1972). Erler (1971) noted the presence of a large number of sugars in the cell wall of *E. rhusiopathiae*: galactose, glucose, arabinose, xylose, ribose, glucose-6-phosphate and galactose-6-phosphate. A later study (Erler 1972a) indicated the presence of the amino sugars galactosamine, glucosamine and fucosamine. From the monosaccharide and amino sugar patterns, Erler (1971, 1972a) recognized 3 chemotypes but there appears to be no correlation between these and serotypes (Erler 1972b). L-forms of *E. rhusiopathiae* have been described (Pachas and Currid 1974, Todorov 1976).

The cellular fatty acids are of the 2- and 3-hydroxy and non-hydroxylated long-chain types. The hydroxylated fatty acids are primarily of the straight-chain series; the non-hydroxylated fatty acids are predominantly of the straight-chain saturated and monounsaturated series; small amounts of *iso* and *anteiso*-methyl branched fatty acids are also present (Tadayon and Carroll 1971, Takahashi et al. 1994).

Watts (1940) and Atkinson and Collins (1940) showed that, on the basis of absorption and agglutination tests, strains of *Erysipelothrix* could be divided into 2 main types. Watts (1940) noted that each type possessed a heat-stable specific antigen and 2 heat-labile antigens present in different proportions in the 2 types and responsible for cross-agglutination when antiserum is prepared with unboiled strains. Dedié (1949) extracted the type-specific antigens by Lancefield's acid method and showed by precipitation methods that the strains fell into 2 types, A and B, and proposed that all those strains that did not react with A- or B-type specific antiserum be designated N. A number of additional serotypes labelled A, B, C, etc. were later detected among type B strains by the use of type-specific, acid-soluble antigens, or later autoclaved bacilli, in the double agar-gel precipitation test (Kucsera 1972, 1973). Kucsera (1973) proposed that the serotypes be designated by Arabic numerals instead of capital letters; small letters were retained to distinguish subtypes. Type A became type 1, etc.; the letter N was retained for the designation of strains that lacked a type specific antigen. Until the 1980s there were 22 recognized serotypes (Wood, Huabrich and Harrington 1978, Nørrung 1979) but there are now at least 26 in addition to N (Enoe and Nørrung 1992, Chooromoney et al. 1994). Chinese workers (Xu Ke-quin et al. 1984, 1986) described 2 new serotypes as numbers 23 and 24. Nørrung, Munch and Larsen (1987), unaware of this work, described a different serotype as 23; this led to 2 different serotypes with the same designation. The problem was resolved by the designation of Nørrung's serotype 23 as 25 (Nørrung and Molin 1991). Of the 26 serotypes, 1 and 2 are isolated most commonly (Nørrung 1979). The recommended method for serological investigation is the double agar-gel diffusion precipitation test with autoclaved antigens and type specific antisera.

The antigens on which serotyping and immunization depend are not the same although some components may be shared. The immunizing antigen has been described as a glycolipoprotein with a molecular weight of >200 kDa (Wood 1984). Information on the complexity of the heat-stable and heat-labile antigens is given by Gledhill (1945, 1947) and technical information on the typing of strains by Wellmann, Kucsera and Nørrung (1983a, 1983b).

Bacteriophages active on *E. rhusiopathiae* have been reported (Valerianov, Toschkoff and Cholakova 1976) and Brill and Politynska (1961) found that serotype B strains (serotype 2) were latently infected with a bacteriophage that lysed strains of serotype A (serotype 1).

10 SUSCEPTIBILITY TO ANTIMICROBIAL AGENTS

E. rhusiopathiae is resistant to a number of chemical agents. Growth occurs in the presence of 0.05% potassium tellurite, 0.02% thallous acetate, 0.001% crystal violet and at the relatively high concentration of 0.1% sodium azide (Jones 1986, Smith, McLauchlin and Taylor 1990).

Most strains of *E. rhusiopathiae* are resistant to sulphonomides, colistin, gentamicin, kanamycin, neomycin, vancomycin, novobiocin and polymyxins. Resistance to vancomycin is important because this antibiotic is frequently used in the empirical treatment of endocarditis due to gram-positive bacteria (including *E. rhusiopathiae*) in persons allergic to penicillin (Reboli and Farrar 1991). The majority of strains are very susceptible in vitro to penicillins, cephalosporins, erythromycin and clindamycin (Reboli and Farrar 1991). Minimal inhibitory concentrations for penicillins have been reported to range from 0.0025 to 0.06 μg ml^{-1} (Gorby and Peacock 1988). Penicillin G is the drug of choice for the treatment of *Erysipelothrix* infections (Poretz 1985, Azofra et al. 1991). Cephalosporins are suitable alternatives in patients allergic to penicillin because both clindamycin and erythromycin are only bacteriostatic (Reboli and Farrar 1991). MacGowan et al. (1991b) have reported the successful treatment of tricuspid value endocarditis due to *E. rhusiopathiae* with high doses of ciprofloxacin.

Susceptibility to chloramphenicol and tetracycline is variable. Takahashi et al. (1984) noted various patterns of resistance to erythromycin, oleandomycin, oxytetracycline and dihydrostreptomycin in strains from chronic swine erysipelas. There appear to be no reports of plasmid-borne antibiotic resistance.

11 CLASSIFICATION

The intra- and intergeneric classification of *Erysipelothrix* has been modified and clarified in recent years. Until 1987 the genus was monospecific with *E. rhusiopathiae* as the type and only species (Jones 1986). The genus now contains 2 species, *E. rhusiopathiae* and *E. tonsillarum* (Takahashi et al. 1987a), and there is evidence for the existence of a third, as yet unnamed, genomic species (Takahashi et al. 1992, Tamura et al. 1993, Ahrné et al. 1995). Differentiation of the species was first achieved by DNA–DNA relatedness studies (Takahashi et al. 1987a) and the results were confirmed by protein electrophoresis (Tamura et al. 1993) and by restriction fragment length polymorphism (RFLP) studies (Ahrné et al. 1995). The results of multilocus enzyme studies of 94 strains of *Erysipelothrix* detected only 2 species, *E. rhusiopathiae* and *E. tonsillarum* (Chooromoney et al. 1994), but this may well be a reflection of the strains studied. Phenotypically *E. rhusiopathiae* and *E. tonsillarum* are very similar, differing only in the ability of *E. tonsillarum* to produce acid from sucrose and its lack of virulence for pigs (Takahashi et al. 1992). There are also some differences between the serotypes most commonly found in the 2 species (Takahashi et al. 1992, Chooromoney et al. 1994) but the suggestion of Takahashi et al. (1992) that strains of serotype 7 are *E. tonsillarum* and strains of serotype 2 are *E. rhusiopathiae* has not been borne out by further studies (Chooromoney et al. 1994, Ahrné et al. 1995).

Multilocus enzyme studies indicate a greater degree of genetic variation in strains of *E. rhusiopathiae* than that detected in *E. tonsillarum* strains (Chooromoney et al. 1994). The results of RFLP studies of 16S rRNA of 39 strains of *Erysipelothrix*, representing the 26 serotypes, detected 9 ribopatterns (Ahrné et al. 1995). *E.*

rhusiopathiae strains, designated on the basis of DNA–DNA hybridization, were found in 3 ribopatterns, A, B and C; *E. tonsillarum* strains were found in 2 ribopatterns, E and I. The ribopatterns were relatively homogeneous; all had 2 fragments in common, unusual among ribopatterns of different species (Ahrné et al. 1995). Partial sequencing of a small portion of the 16S rRNA gene of 9 selected strains revealed the presence of 3 different sequences corresponding to *E. rhusiopathiae*, *E. tonsillarum* and a third sequence represented by 2 strains, one of ribopattern C, the other ribopattern I (Ahrné et al. 1995). Strains exhibiting the third sequence may represent the third genomic species detected by other workers (Takahashi et al. 1992, Tamura et al. 1993). Of interest, and indicative of the complexity of the genus, is the observation that one strain, 715, with low DNA–DNA homology to the type strain of *E. rhusiopathiae* (47%) and *E. tonsillarum* (16%), exhibited a unique ribopattern, H, distinct from those typical of *E. rhusiopathiae* and *E. tonsillarum*, but had the same partial 16S rRNA gene sequence as the type strain of *E. rhusiopathiae* (Ahrné et al. 1995). The fact that strains representing 2 apparently different species have the same 16S rRNA sequence is uncommon but has been described previously for *Lactobacillus plantarum* (Collins et al. 1991a). Another strain, L136, exhibited the same partial sequence as *E. tonsillarum* but had a ribopattern different from those of *E. rhusiopathiae* and *E. tonsillarum*; no DNA–DNA homology data are available for this strain (Ahrné et al. 1995).

Erysipelothrix is not, as indicated previously, closely related to *Listeria* (Barber 1939, Hutner 1942) or to the streptococci (Wilkinson and Jones 1977). On the basis of 16S rRNA gene sequencing studies, *E. rhusiopathiae* forms a distinct subline within the clostridial group of bacteria and exhibits a significant degree of relatedness with certain clostridial species, including *C. innocuum* and *C. ramosum*, and with some nonsporing bacteria such as *Eubacterium biforme*, *L. vitulinus* and *S. pleomorphus* (Collins et al. 1994, Olsen, Woese and Overbeek 1994). Further comparative studies are required to determine the precise position of the genus with regard to other members of the clostridial group.

12 LABORATORY ISOLATION AND IDENTIFICATION

12.1 Isolation techniques

Isolation from the blood of suspected cases of sepsis or endocarditis is relatively straightforward; routine blood culture techniques are adequate. Successful isolation of *E. rhusiopathiae* from skin requires the removal of a small piece of the dermis because the organisms are located in the deeper portions of the skin. *E. rhusiopathiae* may also be obtained from skin lesions by injecting saline into the edge of the lesion and aspirating some of the injected saline for culture (Smith 1983). After collection, biopsy specimens or tissue aspirates should be put into an infusion broth with 1% glucose and incubated in air or 5–10% CO_2 at 35°C (Weaver 1985); subcultures on blood agar should then be made at intervals of 24 h. In cases of chronic infection where the number of bacteria is small, enrichment by the addition of 5% horse serum and incubation for up to 10 days is recommended.

The use of selective media is necessary only when the specimen is heavily contaminated with other bacteria, e.g. soil, faeces or certain animal tissues (Wood 1965, Wood and Packer 1972). Many selective media have been described. Isolation from heavily contaminated skin or tissues is best achieved by placing the specimen in 10 ml of modified *Erysipelothrix* Selective Broth (ESB) (Wood 1965). After overnight incubation at 35°C, 5 ml of the broth is placed in a sterile tube and centrifuged for 20 min at approximately 1400 *g*. The supernate is then discarded, the sediment resuspended in 1–2 ml of physiological saline and a portion is plated on modified blood–azide agar (MBA) medium (Harrington and Hulse 1971). After incubation for 24–48 h at 35°C, the plate is examined for colonies.

Isolation from faeces or contaminated soil may be achieved in much the same way. The sample (c. 100 g) is placed in a sterile blender containing 220 ml of sterile 0.1 M phosphate buffer. After mixing for 10 min, the whole is transferred to a sterile centrifuge bottle and centrifuged at low speed for 10 min. The cloudy supernate is then decanted into a sterile 1 litre screw-capped flask containing 200 ml of double strength ESB broth (Wood 1965). After incubation for 24–48 h, samples are plated on to the medium of Packer with 5% horse serum (Packer 1943), incubated for 24–48 h and the plates are examined for colonies. The medium of Packer is preferred for grossly contaminated specimens such as faeces or soil because it is more selective for *E. rhusiopathiae* than MBA medium (Jones 1986).

A fluorescent antibody technique has been used to detect *E. rhusiopathiae* in tissues (Seidler, Trautwein and Bohm 1971) and enrichment broth cultures (Harrington, Wood and Hulse 1974). Makino et al. (1994) describe a polymerase chain reaction (PCR)-based method for the direct detection of *Erysipelothrix* DNA in joint and spleen samples in mice. The probe is genus specific; it does not distinguish between *E. rhusiopathiae* and *E. tonsillarum* but could be useful for pig tissue because only *E. rhusiopathiae* is pathogenic for pigs.

After isolation the organisms may be preserved for many months by stab inoculation into screw-capped tubes of nutrient agar. Longer-term preservation may be achieved by freezing in glass beads (Feltham et al. 1978). The organisms can also be preserved by freeze drying.

12.2 Identification of the genus *Erysipelothrix*

Identification of new isolates is based on examination of cell morphology, lack of haemolysis on blood agar, growth characteristics in nutrient gelatin, catalase and oxidase tests, production of acid from carbohydrates in a suitable medium and hydrogen sulphide production. In specimens from suspected infections, bacteria with which *Erysipelothrix* is likely to be confused include *Actinomyces pyogenes, Arcanobacterium haemolyticum* and *Listeria monocytogenes.* These bacteria are all β-haemolytic on blood but care is required because colonies of *A. haemolyticum* display only very weak haemolysis after 24 h; none produces hydrogen sulphide in the base of TSI slants and *L. monocytogenes* is catalase-positive and motile. The resistance of *Erysipelothrix* to neomycin can also be used to distinguish it from *L. monocytogenes. E. rhusiopathiae* has been misidentified as a viridans streptococcus (Gorby and Peacock 1988). It has also been dismissed as a coryneform contaminant.

Salient properties useful for the identification of *Erysipelothrix* spp. are listed in Table 30.1.

Acid production from carbohydrates is frequently poor and inconsistent in peptone water. Many workers have recommended the addition of sterile horse serum to the basal medium (Jones 1986). This is not always convenient; good results are achieved by testing for acid production in a nutrient broth plus the test carbohydrate (0.5%), with phenol red as indicator. The use of different basal media can result in different fermentation patterns. It is advisable to test the pattern of known strains in the medium to be used (Jones 1986). Soto, Zapardiel and Soriano (1994) reported the APl Coryne System to be suitable for the identification of *E. rhusiopathiae.* All new isolates of *Erysipelothrix* produce hydrogen sulphide but the results are dependent on the medium used. Lead acetate paper with cultures in a liquid medium does not always detect hydrogen sulphide production. Tests should be performed in triple sugar agar slants in which the hydrogen sulphide causes a blackened butt. An occasional old laboratory strain does not produce hydrogen sulphide in this medium.

In addition to the properties listed in Table 30.1, indole and acetoin (Voges–Proskauer; VP) are not produced and the methyl red test is usually negative. Urea, aesculin, sodium hippurate, starch, cellulose and casein are not hydrolysed. Xanthine and tyrosine are not degraded. There is no discernible change in

Table 30.1 Characteristics of *Erysipelothrix* species

	E. rhusiopathiae	*E. tonsillarum*
Aerobic growth	+	+
Anaerobic growth	+	+
β-Haemolysis	−	−
α-Haemolysis	+	+
Motility	−	−
'Test tube brush' growth in gelatin	+	+
H₂S production[a]	+	+
Aesculin hydrolysis	−	−
Acid from:		
Glucose	+	+
Mannose	+	±
Sucrose	−	+
Lactose	+	+
Maltose	+	+
Galactose	+	+
Rhamnose	−	−
Raffinose	−	−
Arabinose	−	−
Trehalose	−	−
Xylose	−	−
Glycerol	−	−
Inositol	−	−
Sorbitol	−	−
Mannitol	−	−
Dulcitol	−	−
Inulin	−	−
Salicin	−	±
Sensitivity in vitro to:		
Penicillin G (0.1 U ml⁻¹)	+	+
Ampicillin (0.1 μg ml⁻¹)	+	+
Kanamycin (100 μg ml⁻¹)	−	−
Pathogenic for swine	+	−

[a]In triple sugar iron agar.
±, Variable, not all strains able to perform this reaction.

litmus milk and nitrate is not reduced (Reboli and Farrar 1991).

Erysipelothrix strains may also be identified serologically by the method of Kucsera (1973).

12.3 Identification of *Erysipelothrix* species

The 2 named species, *E. rhusiopathiae* and *E. tonsillarum*, and the putative third genomic species are phenotypically very similar (Takahashi et al. 1987a, 1992). The species were originally described on the basis of DNA–DNA relatedness studies (Takahashi et al. 1987a). *E. rhusiopathiae* is pathogenic for pigs whereas *E. tonsillarum* is not; one strain of *E. tonsillarum* is reported to have induced a local urticarial lesion in a pig at the site of inoculation (Takahashi et al. 1987a). *E. tonsillarum* produces acid from sucrose, *E. rhusiopathiae* does not (Table 30.1).

Contrary to an earlier report that whole cell protein patterns are unreliable for the identification of *E. rhusiopathiae* (White and Mirikitani 1976), a more recent study, performed under standard conditions, achieved sufficient discrimination between *E. rhusiopathiae* and *E. tonsillarum* to be used for identification purposes (Tamura et al. 1993).

Serological differentiation between the species is possible to some degree (Takahashi et al. 1992, Tamura et al. 1993, Chooromoney et al. 1994). However, the serotypes characteristic of *E. rhusiopathiae*, *E. tonsillarum* and the putative third genomic species differentiated on the basis of DNA–DNA relatedness (Takahashi et al. 1992) do not correspond completely with the serotypes of the species differentiated by whole cell protein patterns (Tamura et al. 1993), multilocus enzyme studies (Chooromoney et al. 1994) or restriction fragment length polymorphisms (Ahrné et al. 1995).

Many veterinary workers think that the mouse protection test is the best method to identify new isolates of *E. rhusiopathiae* with certainty. The test is done by subcutaneous injection of 0.1 ml from a 24 h culture of the suspected organism along with 0.3 ml of commercially available antierysipelothrix serum into another site. A control group of mice is inoculated with the broth culture alone. If the organism is *E. rhusiopathiae*, the mice that did not receive the antiserum die in 5–7 days, but those receiving the antiserum survive (Weaver 1985).

13 TYPING METHODS

There is little information on typing methods for *E. rhusiopathiae*. There is no information on biotyping as a practical aid for epidemiological purposes. Bacteriophages have been isolated (Valerianov, Toschkoff and Cholakova 1976) and a phage typing system may prove to be useful (Ewald 1981, Reboli and Farrar 1991). Serological methods have limited use. As noted earlier, 26 serotypes plus the N strains have been detected. In a reference laboratory new isolates can be allocated to one of these serotypes but the value of this approach for epidemiological purposes has been questioned by Chooromoney et al. (1994) and Ahrné et al. (1995). Multilocus enzyme studies of 96 strains of *Erysipelothrix* indicated such a diversity among electrophoretic types (ETs) of the same serotype that serotyping is an unreliable technique for tracing sources of isolates of *E. rhusiopathiae* in epidemiological studies (Chooromoney et al. 1994). However, the presence of isolates of different serotypes and subtypes in the same ET suggests that serotyping could be useful if used in conjunction with multilocus enzyme studies because it further differentiates isolates of the same ET (Chooromoney et al. 1994). Nucleic acid based methods could prove to be useful in the future (Ahrné et al. 1995).

14 ROLE IN THE NORMAL FLORA OF HUMANS

There is no information on the role of *Erysipelothrix* spp. in the normal flora of humans. It is possible, especially in view of their presence in various retail meats and fish, that they could occur as transient inhabitants of the gut.

15 PATHOGENICITY AND VIRULENCE FACTORS

E. rhusiopathiae has been recognized as a pathogen of mice, pigs and humans for almost 100 years. It is now recognized as a pathogen under natural conditions for a wide range of animals and birds (Reboli and Farrar 1991). *E. tonsillarum*, considered to be non-pathogenic for pigs, has been incriminated as the cause of endocarditis in dogs in Belgium (Takahashi et al. 1993).

The basis for the virulence of *E. rhusiopathiae* is not fully understood. Most strains isolated from erysipelas in pigs belong to serotypes 1a, 1b and 2. Serotype 1a is the most common in cases of septicaemia (Reboli and Farrar 1991). The ability to adhere to mammalian cells is probably an important virulence determinant. Virulent strains of *E. rhusiopathiae* are reported to adhere more avidly to porcine kidney cell lines than do avirulent strains (Takahashi et al. 1987b). Similarly, strains of *E. rhusiopathiae* isolated from pig endocarditis or septicaemia have been shown to adhere more strongly to pig heart valve tissue in vitro than do other *E. rhusiopathiae* isolates (Bratberg 1981).

E. rhusiopathiae strains produce a hyaluronidase and a neuraminidase, which cleaves α-glycosidic linkages of sialic acid, a mucopolysaccharide on the surface of mammalian cells. Neuraminidase activity is higher in virulent than in avirulent strains (Krasemann and Müller 1975). There is some evidence that this enzyme might play a role in the pathogenesis of arthritis and thrombocytopenia in rats experimentally infected with *E. rhusiopathiae* (Shinomiya and Nakato 1985, Nakato, Shinomiya and Mikawa 1986).

The use of molecular biological techniques will undoubtedly play a major role in clarifying the basis of the pathogenicity of the organism. Studies with 3 avirulent mutant strains produced by transposon mutagenesis and the virulent parent strain of *E. rhusiopathiae* showed that in the presence of normal serum, the virulent parent strain was resistant to phagocytosis whereas the avirulent mutant strains were phagocytosed. In the presence of immune serum both virulent and avirulent strains were efficiently phagocytosed. Examination of the parent strain by electron microscopy demonstrated the presence of a capsule-like structure absent in the avirulent mutant strains (Shimoji et al. 1994). The results strongly suggest that the virulence of *E. rhusiopathiae* is associated, at least in part, with the possession of a capsule-like structure that confers resistance to phagocytosis.

Cloning experiments with *E. rhusiopathiae* have demonstrated the expression of an encoded 65 kDa *E. rhusiopathiae* protein in *E. coli*. This protein shares a 56% identity with the *E. coli* DnaK heat shock protein. Analysis of the total protein extracts from *E. rhusiopathiae* indicate that DnaK is a highly expressed protein in this organism. Its role in pathogenicity, if any, is unknown (Partridge et al. 1993). Genetic analysis of *E. rhusiopathiae* has also shown the production of a DnaJ heat shock protein (Rockabrand et al. 1993).

Tamura et al. (1993), in a comparative study of protein profiles of *E. rhusiopathiae* and *E. tonsillarum*, noted the *E. rhusiopathiae* contained 2 major protein antigens with molecular masses of 32 and 56 kDa. By contrast, the non-virulent *E. tonsillarum* contained only the 32 kDa protein. These authors speculated that the 56 kDa protein may play a role in the pathogenesis of *E. rhusiopathiae*.

15.1 Inoculation into animals

PIGS

Loeffler (1886), who first isolated *E. rhusiopathiae* from swine erysipelas, failed to reproduce the disease in pigs with pure cultures of the organism; however, Schütz (1886) succeeded in doing so. Broth cultures injected subcutaneously into pigs proved fatal in 3–4 days; the organisms were recovered in pure culture from the blood, spleen and from pleural and peritoneal exudates. Laboratory maintained cultures rapidly lose their virulence for pigs (Smith, McLauchlin and Taylor 1990). Collins and Goldie (1940) produced polyarthritis by repeated intravenous inoculation of culture; they also noted focal inflammatory polyarthritis, focal necrosis of the liver and myocardium, lymphadenopathy, a monocytosis and endocarditis, but they failed to produce skin lesions. The rhomboidal skin lesions described in pigs are the result of thrombotic vasculitus of end arterioles (Grieco and Sheldon 1970).

MICE

A 24 h broth culture (0.001–0.1 ml) of *E. rhusiopathiae* injected subcutaneously or intraperitoneally is usually fatal in 2–3 days (see discussion of the mouse protection test, section 12.3, p. 690). During life the mice develop conjuctivitis and arching of the back and

constipation frequently occur (Smith, McLauchlin and Taylor 1990). After death the vessels of the skin and subcutaneous tissue are congested, the spleen is enlarged and the lungs oedematous. The organisms are abundant in the blood, especially the phagocytic cells, in which they appear to multiply (Tenbroeck 1920). Serotype 1a isolates from acute disease in pigs have been reported to be more highly virulent for mice than those from chronic disease (Takahashi et al. 1985).

PIGEONS

An intramuscular injection of 0.001–0.1 ml of a broth culture usually proves fatal in 3 or 4 days. Death is often preceded by paralysis of the legs, dyspnoea and convulsions. After death the organisms are fairly abundant in the blood and organs, the spleen is enlarged, there is a black haemorrhagic mass in the muscle at the site of inoculation and there is almost always a clear lemon-yellow exudate in the pericardium (Smith, McLauchlin and Taylor 1990).

RABBITS

An intravenous injection of 0.5 ml of a 24 h broth culture of *E. rhusiopathiae* into the ear sometimes proves fatal in 2–3 days. An oedematous swelling or erysipelous rash develops at the site of injection and there is a rise in temperature and loss of weight. After death there is congestion of the organs, sometimes large haemorrhages in the lungs, and often a clear lemon-yellow pericardial exudate. The organisms are scarce. If the disease is not rapidly fatal a monocytosis occurs, reaching its maximum in 3–7 days. In animals that die at this time tiny areas of focal necrosis may be found in the liver and areas of mononuclear cell reaction may be seen in sections of the spleen. Inoculation into the conjunctiva gives rise to conjuctivitis that often proves fatal. Subcutaneous inoculation seldom results in death (Smith, Mclauchlin and Taylor 1990).

FISH

It has been shown that fish can be infected readily by feeding or intraperitoneal injection of *E. rhusiopathiae* (Hettche 1937). The organisms are widely distributed in the tissues and may be recovered after several weeks. The highest concentration is in the kidneys and the organism is excreted in the urine; the fish show no evidence of illness (Smith, McLauchlin and Taylor 1990).

LISTERIA

16 GENUS/SPECIES DEFINITION

Listeria are coccobacillary- to bacillus-shaped gram-positive organisms. They are non-sporing and motile by peritrichate flagella. They are aerobic and micro-aerophilic organisms that grow between <0 and 45°C.

The organisms exhibit fermentative activities on carbohydrates, producing lactate and no gas from glucose. *Listeria* spp. are catalase-positive and oxidase-negative. The genus *Listeria* consists of 6 species: *monocytogenes*, *grayi*, *innocua*, *ivanovii*, *seeligeri* and *welshimeri*. *Listeria monocytogenes* is the major pathogen for a wide variety of animals, including man, causing septic lesions in various organs. The G + C content of DNA is 36–42 mol% and the type species is *L. monocytogenes*.

17 INTRODUCTION AND HISTORICAL PERSPECTIVE

In England in 1926, Murray, Webb and Swann described a disease of rabbits and guinea pigs characterized by a marked mononuclear leucocytosis caused by a gram-positive bacillus which they termed *Bacterium monocytogenes* (Murray, Webb and Swann 1926). Pirie (1927) isolated the same bacterium from infected wild gerbils in South Africa, and proposed the generic name *Listerella* in honour of the surgeon Lord Lister; later this was changed, for reasons of accurate nomenclature, to *Listeria* (Pirie 1940).

In Denmark in 1929, Nyfeldt isolated *L. monocytogenes* from the blood cultures of patients with a mononucleosis-like infection (a rare manifestation of the disease); Burn (1936) in the USA established listeriosis as a cause of both sepsis during the perinatal period and of meningitis in adults. Prior to 1926 there were published descriptions of disease likely to have been listeriosis; indeed, a 'diphtheroid' isolated from the cerebrospinal fluid of a soldier in Paris in 1919 was later identified as *L. monocytogenes* (Cotoni 1942). Listeriosis remained a relatively obscure disease, attracting limited attention until the 1980s when a rise in the numbers of human and animal cases in several countries (including the UK) and a series of human food-borne outbreaks in North America and Europe led to much renewed interest in the disease and the causative organism (McLauchlin 1993).

Listeriosis occurs in various animals, including humans, and most often affects the pregnant uterus, the central nervous system or the bloodstream. During pregnancy, infection spreads to the fetus, which will either be born severely ill or die in utero. Listeriosis usually presents as meningitis, encephalitis, or septicaemia in non-pregnant individuals. In humans, infection occurs most often in the immunocompromised and elderly patients, pregnant women, and unborn or newly delivered babies. Infection can be treated successfully with antibiotics, but human infection has a mortality of 20–40% (McLauchlin 1990a, 1990b). In domestic animals (especially in sheep and goats), listeriosis usually presents as encephalitis, abortion or septicaemia, and is a cause of considerable economic loss (Gitter 1989). Consumption of contaminated food or feed is believed to be the principal route of infection (WHO 1988). However, in humans, infection can be transmitted by contact with infected animals (usually resulting in cutaneous lesions; McLauchlin and Low 1994) or by cross-infection during the neonatal period (Schlech 1991).

L. monocytogenes is the major pathogenic species in both animals and humans (Rocourt and Seeliger 1985, McLauchlin 1987). However, in humans, occasional infections due to *L. ivanovii* (Cummins, Fielding and McLauchlin 1994) and *L. seeligeri* (Rocourt et al. 1987a) have been reported. *L. ivanovii* infections may account for a significant proportion of cases of listeriosis in domestic animals, especially in sheep (Low et al. 1993). Rare infections due to *L. innocua* in domestic animals have occurred (Rocourt and Seeliger 1985, Walker et al. 1994). *L. welshimeri* and *L. grayi* have not been shown to cause disease.

A more exhaustive account of the genus and the disease may be found in reviews by Seeliger (1961), Gray and Killinger (1966), Seeliger and Jones (1986), WHO (1988), Gellin and Broome (1989), Jones (1990), Miller, Smith and Somkuti (1990), Farber and Peterkin (1991), Ryser and Marth (1991), Schuchat, Swaminathan and Broome (1991), McLauchin (1993) and Bortolussi and Schlech (1995).

18 HABITAT

Listeria are found ubiquitously in the environment and are distributed world wide. Species of *Listeria* have been isolated from fresh water, waste water, mud and soil, especially when decaying vegetable material is present. Pirie (1927) first suggested that listeriosis may be transmitted through food, and since this route is now generally believed to be the principal route of infections for humans (WHO 1988) and animals, the distribution of *Listeria* in the environment is of importance in the transmission of the disease.

An extremely wide range of animals (mammals, birds, fish and invertebrates) has been reported to carry *Listeria* spp. without apparent disease. In humans, carriage rates of *Listeria* in faeces vary from 0.6 to 70% (Kampelmacher and van Noorle Jansen 1969, Ralovich 1984), although figures of <3% for carriage of *Listeria* spp. and <1% for carriage of *L. monocytogenes* are most commonly reported (MacGowan et al. 1991a, 1994, Oakley et al. 1992, Jensen 1993). Carriage of *L. monocytogenes* in the genital tract in the absence of disease is very rare (Chattopadhyay, James and Hussain 1991, Oakley et al. 1992). *Listeria* spp. have been isolated from the upper respiratory tract and from seminal fluid of healthy animals (Gray and Killinger 1966, Ralovich 1984). Because of the occurrence of *Listeria* in the gut of animals and its survival in the environment, it is not surprising that *Listeria* spp. have been isolated from sites contaminated with human sewage, sewage sludge or animal slurry.

The association of consumption of contaminated food with both outbreaks and sporadic human cases (McLauchlin 1993) has resulted in much interest in food-borne listeriosis. *L. monocytogenes* has been isolated from a very wide range of foods for human consumption, including raw and processed meat, dairy products, vegetables and seafood products (Farber and Peterkin 1991), and from food production and storage environments (Cox et al. 1989). The ability to grow at refrigeration temperatures and tolerate preserving agents makes *Listeria* of particular concern if present in refrigerated foods that are consumed without further cooking. *Listeria* in end-product foods results from either incomplete eradication during processing, or from contamination from sites within the food production environment. Contamination of food directly from infected animals is probably rare; however, *L. monocytogenes* can cause mastitis in cows in which large numbers of the bacteria can then be shed in the milk (Gitter, Bradley and Blampied 1980).

The relationship between the feeding of silage to domestic animals and the development of listeriosis has long been realized (Gray 1960). This is of particular importance when the pH is >5.5 and the silage is of poor quality or has had prolonged exposure to aerobic conditions (Irvin 1968). Modern practices of producing silage in large polythene covered bales ('big bale') favours the growth of *L. monocytogenes* (Fenlon 1985) in comparison with production in the more traditional clamps, and may, in part, explain the recent apparent increase in the incidence of listeriosis in domestic animals in Britain (Gitter 1989, Anon 1994).

Although frequently found as gut commensals, *Listeria* spp. show many of the characteristics of bacteria adapted to a saprophytic existence, i.e. growth at low temperature, tolerance of sodium chloride and alkaline conditions, resistance to desiccation, motility at temperatures less than 25°C, presence in soil and decaying vegetable material, and, where pathogenic, a failure to produce host-specific clinical syndromes. However, there are specific adaptations that allow invasion of and multiplication in eukaryotic cells by *L. monocytogenes* (see section 29.2, p. 700); these may have evolved for survival in unicellular and multicellular soil organisms. The 'true' habitat for the genus *Listeria* may be that of decaying plant material with occasional transitory residence in the gastrointestinal tract of animals; additional properties may allow the utilization of the intracellular environments of free-living eukaryotic soil organisms by *L. monocytogenes*.

19 MORPHOLOGY

Young cultures consist predominantly of coccobacillary forms 1–3 μm long and 0.5 μm broad. As cultures age, short chains or 'diphtheroid-like' palisade formations may be observed. The poles of the cells are blunt. Smooth forms are almost always seen on fresh isolation. However, in older cultures (3–5 days) and with strains that have been subcultured on artificial media over many years, 'rough' forms with filamentous cells (6–20 μm long) may occur. Cultures are non-motile at 37°C, but at temperatures <30°C, cells are motile by means of peritrichous flagella, with up to 6 flagella on each individual cell (Peel, Donachie and Shaw 1988a). In hanging drop preparations, characteristic tumbling movements are seen. Motility may

also be demonstrated by the clouding of medium approximately 1–2 mm below the surface in soft agar in an 'umbrella-like' formation.

20 CULTURAL CHARACTERS

Listeria usually grows on most non-selective bacteriological culture media, especially when blood, serum or a fermentable carbohydrate is added. For non-selective maintenance media, tryptose, tryptose soy or brain–heart infusion agars are preferred. When cultured overnight on solid media containing blood, round, translucent colonies 1–2 mm in diameter with a 'ground glass' crystalline appearance in the centre are formed. The colonies are slightly raised, have an entire margin, a watery consistency, are easily emulsifiable, and are non-pigmented. The rough forms have larger, flatter colonies, with an irregular indented edge, are umbonate with a central crater, friable and difficult to emulsify. All cultures have a characteristic sweet, buttermilk-like smell.

When growing on blood containing agar, colonies of *L. monocytogenes* are surrounded by a narrow zone of β-haemolysis with an indistinct margin. *L. seeligeri* has a similar appearance to *L. monocytogenes*, but exhibits a weaker zone of haemolysis. Colonies of *L. ivanovii* are surrounded by a wider and clearer β-haemolytic zone, which takes on a double appearance after 36–48 h. In semi-solid stab cultures, growth occurs most abundantly 2–4 mm below the surface of the medium. In gelatin stab cultures, filiform growth without lateral branches occurs; the gelatin is not liquefied.

Growth in broth is usually poor, but is greatly improved by the addition of 0.5–1% glucose. In this medium the smooth forms give rise within 24 h to a fairly dense suspension; after some days the organisms settle to the bottom in floccules. The organisms multiply rapidly in milk (Pine et al. 1989).

21 METABOLISM

A source of carbohydrate is essential for the growth of *Listeria* and a number of fully chemically defined media to support growth have been described (Friedman and Roessler 1961, Ralovich, Shaahamat and Woodbine 1977, Siddiqi and Khan 1982, 1989, Premaratne, Lin and Johnson 1991, Jones et al. 1995). Growth occurs at temperatures between <0 and 45°C (Walker, Archer and Banks 1990); optimal growth occurs between 30 and 35°C. *L. monocytogenes* is one of the few pathogenic bacteria that can grow at 4°C, with a maximum doubling time of about 1–2 days. Growth does not generally occur outside the pH range 5.5–9.6.

Under anaerobic conditions the catabolism of glucose by all *Listeria* spp. is homofermentative, i.e. lactate is produced exclusively (Pine et al. 1989). Under aerobic conditions cell yields are considerably increased, and all species produce lactic, acetic, isobutyric and isovaleric acids; there are differences between strains in the relative amounts of lactic and acetic acids produced (Pine et al. 1989). Friedman and Alm (1962) and Daneshvar et al. (1989) also reported the production of acetoin and pyruvate by *L. monocytogenes* under aerobic conditions. *L. monocytogenes* possesses enzymes of the Embden–Meyerhof pathway (Miller and Silverman 1959), and a split non-cyclic citric acid pathway which has an oxidative and a reductive portion (Trivett and Meyer 1971). It has been suggested (Jones 1975) that this latter pathway is important in biosynthesis but not for the net gain of energy which is supplied by glycolysis. *Listeria* spp. are catalase-positive; however, under some conditions this activity may be weak (Jones 1975). The catalase enzyme is of the 'haem' type; it is inhibited by KCN and NaN_3 (Jones 1975) and is electrophoretically homogeneous (Robinson 1968). Cytochromes b, a_1, o and d are produced (Seeliger and Jones 1986). Menaquinones are the sole isoprenoid quinones, and all species contain menaquinone-7 with minor amounts of menaquinone-6 and menaquinone-5 (Seeliger and Jones 1986).

22 GENETIC MECHANISMS

DNA base composition studies (Rocourt et al. 1982, Hartford and Sneath 1993) and 16S rRNA sequence studies (Collins et al. 1991b) show that all species of the genus *Listeria* form a homogeneous group. The chromosome of *L. monocytogenes* has been estimated to be about 3150 kb in size and a physical and genetic map has been established on which a number of genes have now been located (Michel and Cossart 1992). The genes involved with pathogenesis are almost all clustered at a single locus (see section 29.2, p. 700).

Sequence information is available for some *L. monocytogenes* genes including: 16S and 23S rRNA genes (Collins et al. 1991b, Thompson et al. 1992), a flagellin gene (Dons, Rasmussen and Olsen 1992), and a number of genes associated with pathogenicity (Sheehan et al. 1994). For further information on this last group see section 29.2 (p. 700). Sequence information for the 16S rRNA is available for the remainder of the genus (Collins et al. 1991b).

Transposons Tn*1545*, Tn*916* and Tn*917* (and their derivatives) introduced and expressed in *L. monocytogenes* have proved to be extremely useful tools in understanding the basis of virulence in the bacterium (Sheehan et al. 1994). Transfer of Tn*1545* has been demonstrated between *Enterococcus faecalis* and *L. monocytogenes* in the digestive tract of gnotobiotic mice (Doucet-Populaire et al. 1991). Native plasmid DNA has been detected in some strains of *L. monocytogenes*, *L. innocua*, *L. ivanovii*, *L. seeligeri* and *L. grayi* (Péréz-Díaz, Vicente and Baquero 1982, Kolstad, Rørvik and Granum 1990, Slade and Collins-Thompson 1990, Peterkin et al. 1992, Dykes et al. 1994). A transposon, similar to Tn*917* (designated Tn*5422*) that encodes resistance to cadmium has been recognized in plasmids from *L. monocytogenes* (Lebrun et al. 1994b). The plasmid-borne cadmium resistance genes show a high

degree of similarity to cadmium resistance genes found in *Staphylococcus aureus* (Lebrun et al. 1994a). Plasmids encoding resistance to tetracycline alone (Poyart-Salmeron et al. 1992) and for multiresistance to chloramphenicol, erythromycin, streptomycin and tetracycline have been observed (Poyart-Salmeron et al. 1990, Quentin et al. 1990, Hadorn et al. 1993), although these are rare. Transfer of native listerial plasmids has been demonstrated in vitro between strains of *L. monocytogenes*, to other *Listeria* spp., and to other species of bacteria including *Bacillus subtilis*, *E. faecalis*, *Streptococcus agalactiae* and *S. aureus* (Péréz-Díaz, Vicente and Baquero 1982, Flamm, Hinrichs and Thomashow 1984, Vicente, Baquero and Péréz-Díaz 1988).

Lysogenic phages are commonly carried by *Listeria* spp. They are generally morphologically similar with isometric heads, long non-contractile tails and correspond to the Myoviridae or Styloviridae families (Rocourt 1986, Rocourt et al. 1986, Loessner et al. 1994). A lytic phage has been described of a further (un-named) phage species (Loessner et al. 1994). The phage genomes are linear, double-stranded DNA of 35–116 kb (Rocourt, Catimel and Schrettenbrunner 1985, Loessner et al. 1994) with G + C base compositions of 37–39 mol% (Loessner et al. 1994). Lytic properties of sets of phages have been used for subtyping *L. monocytogenes* (see section 27, p. 699).

In addition to transposon mutagenesis, plasmid complementation experiments, techniques to generate in-frame point mutations by allelic exchange, and the introduction of genetic material by electroporation have been used to study the genetics of *L. monocytogenes* (Portnoy et al. 1992). These techniques, together with the expression of *L. monocytogenes* genes in *L. innocua* and *B. subtilis* and the behaviour of *L. monocytogenes* either in mammalian tissue culture or in experimentally infected mice have led to a great increase in the understanding of the genes involved with virulence (Sheehan et al. 1994). For further information see section 29.2 (p. 700).

23 CELL WALL AND ENVELOPE COMPOSITION; ANTIGENIC STRUCTURE

The cell wall of *Listeria* has the appearance of a thick multilayered structure typical of gram-positive bacteria (Ghosh and Murray 1967). The peptidoglycan of all species of *Listeria* is of the A1γ type of Schleifer and Kandler (1972), which contains L-alanine, D-glutamine, *meso*-diaminopimelic acid (as the diamino acid) and D-alanine (Kamisango et al. 1982, Fiedler et al. 1984).

Ribitol teichoic acids and lipoteichoic acid are present in all species (Hether and Jackson 1983, Kamisango et al. 1983, Fiedler et al. 1984, Uchikawa, Sekikawa and Azuma 1986b, Fiedler and Ruhland 1987). In *L. monocytogenes* serovar 4b the teichoic acid consists of chains of ribitol, phosphate and *N*-acetylglucosamine, the *N*-acetylglucosamine substituted with glucose and galactose residues (Uchikawa, Sekikawa and Azuma 1986a). The ribitol teichoic acid is linked to the peptidoglycan through a novel linkage unit (Kaya, Araki and Ito 1985). In *L. monocytogenes* the lipoteichoic acid consists of 16–33 glycerol phosphate units substituted with a glycosyl side chain and attached to a galactose and glucose containing glycolipid (Uchikawa, Sekikawa and Azuma 1986b).

The plasma membrane of *Listeria* spp. shows the typical trilamellar appearance with mesosomes (Ghosh and Murray 1967). The major phospholipids present in *L. monocytogenes* are phosphatidylglycerol, diphosphatidylglycerol, galactosylglucosyl diacylglycerol and an unidentified phosphoglycolipid (Kosaric and Carrol 1971, Shaw 1974). In all *Listeria* spp., 14-methylhexadecanoic (17:0a) and 12-methyltetradecanoic acid (15:0a) predominate, with minor amounts of other saturated fatty acids (Seeliger and Jones 1986, Ninet et al. 1992). Mycolic acids are not present.

Paterson (1939, 1940a) used bacterial agglutination and absorption experiments with hyperimmune antisera to recognize O (somatic) and H (flagellar) antigens, and described 4 serological types. The scheme was extended further by Seeliger and Donker-Voet (Seeliger and Höhne 1979) to include additional O antigen factors. In the Seeliger–Donker-Voet scheme, *L. monocytogenes* is subdivided into 13 serovars, and the remaining 7 species are similarly subdivided (Table 30.2). Fiedler et al. (1984) suggested that teichoic acids represent the immunochemical determinants in the serotyping scheme because there is a direct correlation between the ribitol teichoic acid structure and serotypes and species of *Listeria*.

Cell wall and cell surface located antigens have been described in *L. monocytogenes* (Carlier et al. 1980, Belyi, Tartakovskii and Prosorovskii 1992, 1993, Taboret, de Rycke and Dubray 1992, Sheehan et al. 1994). The flagella protein has been partially characterized (Peel, Donachie and Shaw 1988a, 1988b), and comprises a 29 kDa moiety. Three cell surface proteins have been reported to be associated with pathogenicity (Sheehan et al. 1994): the p60 protein (60 kDa) with murein hydrolase activity that is also secreted into culture supernates; the ActA protein (90 kDa) which is preferentially produced on the older pole of the cell; the internalin protein (80 kDa), located over all the cell surface and which is reminiscent of the M protein of *Streptococcus pyogenes*. For further information on the role of these in the pathogenicity of *L. monocytogenes* see section 29.2 (p. 700).

24 SUSCEPTIBILITY TO ANTIMICROBIAL AGENTS

All strains are sensitive to ampicillin, and this, in combination with an aminoglycoside, remains the treatment of choice in vivo (MacGowan 1990). Apart from the reported plasmid-encoded resistance to chloramphenicol, erythromycin, streptomycin and tetracycline (Poyart-Salmeron et al. 1990, Quentin et al. 1990, Hadorn et al. 1993), strains are universally sensitive to amikacin, amoxycillin, ampicillin, azlocillin, ciprofloxacin, chloramphenicol, clindamycin, coumermycin, doxycycline, enoxacin, erythromycin, gentamicin, imipenem, netilmicin, penicillin, rifampicin, trimethoprim and vancomycin. Norfloxacin and ofloxacin have less activity, and *Listeria* spp. are resistant to the cephalosporins, phosphomycin and polymyxin (MacGowan et al. 1990, Riviera, Dubini and Bellotti 1993).

Tetracycline is not very active against *L. monocytogenes* and 2–5% of strains are highly resistant to this antibiotic (Poyart-Salmeron et al. 1992). Most of these highly resistant cultures contain a chromosomally encoded *tetM* (together with a transposon, *int-*Tn), which also confers resistance to minocycline (Poyart-Salmeron et al. 1992). The *tetM* gene has also been detected in *L. innocua* (Facinelli et al. 1993). The plasmid-encoded tetracycline resistance in *L. monocytogenes* is rarer than the chromosomally encoded element, which is encoded by a *tetL* (minocycline sensitive; Poyart-Salmeron et al. 1992), or the *tetS* determinant (minocycline resistant; Charpentier, Gerbaud and Courvalin 1993, Hadorn et al. 1993). The *tetS* gene was first described in *L. monocytogenes*, but has since been detected in *E. faecalis* (Charpentier, Gerbaud and Courvalin 1994).

25 CLASSIFICATION

Although originally described as a monospecific genus containing only *L. monocytogenes* (Pirie 1940), 6 species of *Listeria* are now recognized (Skerman, McGowan and Sneath 1980, Moore, Cato and Moore 1985). The group of bacteria originally named *L. monocytogenes* (*L. monocytogenes sensu lato*) was redefined on the basis of DNA–DNA hybridization studies (Rocourt et al. 1982) to comprise the species *L. innocua* (Seeliger 1981), *L. welshimeri* (Rocourt and Grimont 1983), *L. seeligeri* (Rocourt and Grimont 1983), *L. ivanovii* (Seeliger et al. 1984) and *L. monocytogenes sensu stricto*. The genus includes one other species, *L. grayi* (Errebo Larsen and Seeliger 1966). This classification was supported by the results of a second DNA–DNA homology study (Hartford and Sneath 1993) and an analysis by multilocus enzyme electrophoresis (Boerlin, Rocourt and Piffaretti 1991). The study by Hartford and Sneath (1993) suggested a very close relationship between *L. monocytogenes* and *L. innocua* and there may be some overlap between these 2 species.

On the basis of both multilocus enzyme electrophoresis (Piffaretti et al. 1989, Bibb et al. 1990) and restriction fragment and sequence analysis of specific genes (Rasmussen et al. 1991, Gutekunst, Holloway and Carlone 1992, Vines et al. 1992), 2 genetic 'sublines' of *L. monocytogenes* have been identified. These 'sublines' correspond to the serotypes with H antigens ABC (serovars 1/2b, 3b and 4b), and those with H antigens AB or BD (serovars 1/2a, 1/2c, 3a and 3c). These 2 groups may represent subspecies of *L. monocytogenes* although phenotypic characters have not been found to distinguish the 2 groups.

Table 30.2 Somatic and flagellar antigens used for serotyping *Listeria*

Serovar	Somatic (O factor) antigens	Flagellar (H factor) antigens
L. monocytogenes		
1/2a	I II III	AB
1/2b	I II III	ABC
1/2c	I II III	BD
3a	II III IV	AB
3b	II III IV (XII) (XIII)	ABC
3c	II III IV (XII) (XIII)	BD
4a	III (V) VII IX	ABC
4ab	III V VI VII IX X	ABC
4b	III V VI	ABC
4c	III V VII	ABC
4d	III (V) VI VIII	ABC
4e	III V VI (VIII) (IX)	ABC
7	III XII XIII	ABC
L. ivanovii		
5	III (V) VI (VIII) X	ABC
L. innocua[a]		
4ab	III V VI VII IX X	ABC
6a	III V (VI) (VII) (IX) XV	ABC
6b	III (V) (VI) (VII) IX X XI	ABC
L. welshimeri		
6a	III V (VI) (VII) (IX) XV	ABC
6b	III (V) (VI) (VII) IX X XI	ABC
L. seeligeri[a]		
1/2b	I II III	ABC
4c	III V VII	ABC
4d	III (V) VI VIII	ABC
6b	III (V) (VI) (VII) IX X XI	ABC
L. grayi	III XII XIV	E

[a]*L. seeligeri* and *L. innocua* also contain undesignated combination of O antigens. Factor III is heat labile.
() Denotes factors not always present.

There are 2 subspecies of *L. ivanovii*, *L. ivanovii* subsp. *ivanovii* and *L. ivanovii* subsp. *londoniensis* (Boerlin et al. 1992).

On the basis of both phenotypic and genotypic characters, *L. grayi* shows a more distant relationship to the rest of the genus (Wilkinson and Jones 1977, Rocourt et al. 1982, Feresu and Jones 1988, Boerlin, Rocourt and Piffaretti 1991, Collins et al. 1991b, Kämpfer et al. 1991, Hartford and Sneath 1993), but there is clear justification for the retention of *L. grayi* within the genus (Rocourt et al. 1987b, Collins et al. 1991b). There are 2 subspecies of *L. grayi* (Rocourt et al. 1992): *L. grayi* subsp. *grayi* and *L. grayi* subsp. *murrayi* (previously named '*L. murrayi*') (Welshimer and Meredith 1971).

The species previously known as '*Listeria denitrificans*' (Prevot 1961) is not a member of the genus *Listeria* and has been reclassified in a new genus as *Jonesia denitrificans* (Rocourt, Wehmeyer and Stackebrandt 1987).

Despite the genomic heterogeneity within the genus *Listeria* outlined above, there are surprisingly few phenotypic characters that distinguish between the different species (see section 26, p. 696).

Analysis of sequence data from the 16S rRNA confirms the close relationship within the genus *Listeria* and indicates a close phylogenetic relationship (93% sequence similarity) with the genus *Brochothrix*. This latter genus comprises 2 species (*Brochothrix thermosphacta* and *Brochothrix campestris*) which have many phenotypic properties in common with *Listeria* (Seeliger and Jones 1986, Sneath and Jones 1986, Collins et al. 1991b). Members of the genus *Brochothrix* have not been implicated in disease, but are of economic importance as food spoilage organisms, particularly of meat products (Sneath and Jones 1986). 16S rRNA sequence analysis shows relationships with other gram-positive genera of low G + C mol% content, including members of the genera *Bacillus*, *Carnobacterium*, *Vagococcus*, *Enterococcus*, *Aerococcus*, *Lactobacillus*, *Leuconostoc* and *Streptococcus* (Collins et al. 1991b).

26 LABORATORY ISOLATION AND IDENTIFICATION

Culture from blood or cerebrospinal fluid does not require special media. Tissues should be homogenized, suspended in broth and subcultured on to blood agar. The incubation of medulla homogenates at refrigeration temperatures for some weeks has been reported as necessary to obtain cultures that grow on artificial media (Gray and Killinger 1966). For specimens such as faeces, vaginal secretions, food and environmental samples, special selective media are necessary.

26.1 Selective isolation techniques

Prior to the mid-1980s, 'cold enrichment', utilizing the ability of *Listeria* to outgrow competing organisms at refrigeration temperatures in non-selective broths, was the main method used for selective isolation (Gray and Killinger 1966). When growing on transparent media illuminated by oblique transmitted light and viewed at low magnification ('Henry' illumination technique) all *Listeria* colonies have a characteristic blue colour with a central 'ground glass' appearance (Gray 1957). However, because of the degree of skill required in recognizing characteristic colonies, the lack of specificity and the slowness of these methods (some workers subcultured broths for up to 6 months), procedures have been much improved.

Media have been developed that rely on a number of selective agents, including acriflavin, lithium chloride, colistin, ceftazidime, cefotetan, fosfomycin, moxolactam, nalidixic acid, cycloheximide and polymyxin. These media have resulted in the widespread ability of microbiology laboratories to isolate *Listeria* selectively. Numerous enrichment and selective isolation media have now been developed. Those mentioned here (or modifications of them) are used most frequently for the examination of foods. For selective broths, the US Food and Drugs Administration (FDA) method (Lovett, Francis and Hunt 1987), the US Department of Agriculture (USDA) method (McClain and Lee 1988), or the Netherlands Government Food Inspection Service (NGFIS) method described by Van Netten et al. (1989) are used most often. Selective agars most frequently used are those of Curtis et al. (1989; 'Oxford' formulation) or the PALCAM agar of Van Netten et al. (1989).

The FDA method is a single enrichment broth containing acriflavin, nalidixic acid and cycloheximide. The USDA method consists of a double enrichment with first a University of Vermont primary enrichment broth 1 (UVM1; containing aesculin, nalidixic acid and acriflavin) which is subcultured into a Fraser broth (containing aesculin, nalidixic acid, lithium chloride and acriflavin). The NGFIS method uses a single L-PALCAM (or Liquid-PALCAM) broth, the name of which is an acronym of the ingredients, polymyxin B, acriflavin, lithium chloride, ceftazidime, aesculin and mannitol.

After incubation the selective broths are subcultured on to selective agars, most frequently PALCAM agar (with the same agents as the L-PALCAM broth) or Oxford agar. The latter contains aesculin, lithium chloride, cycloheximide, colistin, acriflavin, cefotetan and phosphomycin. On Oxford agar all *Listeria* spp. show a typical colonial appearance and hydrolyse aesculin, to produce black zones around the colonies. On PALCAM agar the colonies have a cherry red back-

ground. It is beyond the scope of this chapter to describe the preparation of these media; for further details see Baird et al. (1989). For comparisons of the efficiency of the different selective techniques for the isolation of *Listeria* from foods, see Warburton et al. (1991) and Hayes et al. (1992).

Techniques based upon nucleic acid hybridization, the polymerase chain reaction and immunoassays are now used increasingly for the detection of *Listeria* in foods (McLauchlin 1989, Noah, Ramos and Gipson 1991, Niederhauser et al. 1992, Okwumabua et al. 1992, Fluit et al. 1993).

26.2 Identification of the genus *Listeria*

In addition to the properties outlined in Table 30.3, *Listeria* spp. produce acid without gas from a range of sugars. The choice of basal medium and pH indicator to demonstrate the production of acid is important; peptone water with phenol red or bromocresol purple as indicator and adjusted to pH 7 is recommended (Rocourt, Schrettenbrunner and Seeliger 1983, Seeliger and Jones 1986). Almost all cultures of *Listeria* produce acid from glucose, trehalose, salicin, amygdalin, cellobiose, aesculin, fructose, mannose, maltose and glycerol. Acid is not produced from adonitol, dulcitol, erythritol, inulin, α-methyl-D-glucoside, raffinose, sorbose, arabinose, glycogen, or melibiose. Aesculin is hydrolysed. Litmus milk is acidified and slowly decolorized. The methyl red reaction and Voges–Proskauer (VP) test (O'Meara's or Barritt's method; Barrow and Feltham 1993) are positive. Catalase is produced, and the oxidase test is negative. H_2S, indole and urease are not produced and there is no growth in citrate medium. Ornithine, lysine, glutamic acid, arginine decarboxylases and arginine dihydrolase are not produced. Phosphatase is produced and methylene blue is decolorized. Tributyrinase activity is negative, and Tweens 20, 40, 60 and 80 are hydrolysed only slowly (Seeliger and Jones 1986).

26.3 Identification of *Listeria* species and subspecies

Members of the genus *Listeria* are remarkably similar in their phenotypic characters (Wilkinson and Jones 1977, Rocourt, Schrettenbrunner and Seeliger 1983, Rocourt and Catimel 1985, Feresu and Jones 1988, Kämpfer et al. 1991). Rocourt, Schrettenbrunner and Seeliger (1983) showed that the species of *Listeria* could be distinguished by the results of a small number of tests, and these, together with other tests to identify the members of this genus, are shown in Table 30.3.

Kämpfer and colleagues (Kämpfer et al. 1991, Kämpfer 1992) showed that *L. monocytogenes* could be distinguished from other members of the genus by the absence of an arylesterase active against alanine-substituted substrates. Arylesterase activity on glycine-substituted substrates may be used for the identification of *Listeria* (Monget 1992) and this reaction is used in a commercially available identification kit

Table 30.3   Differential characteristics of *Listeria* species

	β-Haemolysis on blood sugar	Nitrate reduction	Acid produced from				CAMP test with	
			D-mannitol	L-rhamnose	D-xylose	α-MM	S. aureus	R. equi
L. monocytogenes	+	–	–	+[a]	–	+	+	–
L. ivanovii	+	–	–	–	+	–	–	+
L. innocua	–	–	–	±[b]	–	+	–	–
L. welshimeri	–	–	–	±	+	+	–	–
L. seeligeri	(+)	–	–	–	+	±	(+)	–
L. grayi subsp. *grayi*	–	–	+	–	–	NS	–	–
L. grayi subsp. *murrayi*	–	+	+	±	–	NS	–	–

[a]Some strains do not ferment rhamnose but these are rare.

[b]Approximately 60% ferment rhamnose.

Strains of *L. monocytogenes* occur which are non-haemolytic and do not produce a positive CAMP reaction. These are rare, and probably non-virulent.

α-MM, α-methyl-D-mannoside (methyl α-D-mannopyranoside); ±, variable; not all strains able to perform this reaction; NS, not stated; (+), weak reaction.

(Bille et al. 1992). The detection of phosphatidylinositol-specific phospholipase C has been advocated for the discrimination of *L. monocytogenes* and *L. ivanovii* from the rest of the genus *Listeria* (Notermans et al. 1991).

27 TYPING METHODS

The considerable recent interest in *L. monocytogenes* and in the epidemiology of listeriosis has resulted in the development of discriminatory subtyping methods. These methods utilize a range of phenotypic and genotypic characters.

27.1 Serotyping

L. monocytogenes can be subdivided into 13 serovars by agglutination reactions with absorbed rabbit antisera (see section 23, p. 694 and Table 30.2). However, this offers only limited practical discrimination for epidemiological studies since the majority of strains causing disease (usually >90%) in humans and animals belong to serovars 1/2a, 1/2b and 4b (Seeliger and Höhne 1979, McLauchlin 1987, Low et al. 1993); the highest proportion of human isolates usually belongs to serovar 4b (Seeliger and Höhne 1979, McLauchlin 1990c) and those from animals to serovar 1/2a (Low et al. 1993). Almost all the large outbreaks of human listeriosis have been due to serovar 4b.

The serovars of *L. monocytogenes* do not occur in the same proportions in different clinical groups of human patients (McLauchlin 1990c) or in different categories of disease in animals (Low et al. 1993). The reason for this is not known.

27.2 Bacteriophages and phage typing

Lysogenic phages commonly occur in strains of *Listeria*. Patterns of lytic reactions with sets of phages offer systems of high discrimination which are capable of application to relatively large numbers of cultures (Rocourt et al. 1985, Loessner 1991, Gerner-Smidt, Rosdahl and Frederiksen 1993). Although a high proportion of the strains causing human infection are usually phage typable, some groups of strains (particularly those belonging to serogroups 1/2 and 3) are often not phage typable and additional typing schemes may be necessary.

27.3 Bacteriocins

Within the genus *Listeria*, bacteriocin (monocin) production is as common as the carriage of lysogenic phage (Rocourt 1986, Curtis and Mitchell 1992). However, the use of monocins for subtyping has not provided good discrimination (Curtis and Mitchell 1992).

27.4 Multilocus enzyme electrophoresis

Analysis of the electrophoretic mobilities of constitutive enzymes (multilocus enzyme electrophoresis) has provided a method of good discrimination for *L. monocytogenes* (Piffaretti et al. 1989, Bibb et al. 1990).

27.5 Nucleic acid based methods

The extraction of total chromosomal DNA and the separation of restriction endonuclease digests by electrophoresis has been used to characterize *L. monocytogenes* strains (Nocera et al. 1990, Wesley and Ashton 1991). Analysis of the large number of fragments generated and the complexity of resulting patterns present some considerable difficulty. The method can be improved by probing Southern blots of similar restriction endonuclease digests with probes for rRNA genes (Graves et al. 1991, Jacquet, Billie and Rocourt 1992) or randomly cloned chromosomal DNA fragments (Ridley 1995).

The separation by pulse field gel electrophoresis of large DNA fragments obtained with low frequency cleavage restriction endonucleases offers a method of characterizing whole listeria chromosomes (Brosh, Buchrieser and Rocourt 1991, Buchrieser, Brosch and Rocourt 1991). This nucleic acid based method offers particularly high discrimination. Analysis of DNA fragments generated by the random amplification of polymorphic DNA (Mazurier and Wernars 1992) has also been described for subtyping *L. monocytogenes*.

A combination of genetic and phenotypic methods offers typing systems of high discrimination (Bologa and Harlander 1991, Nocera et al. 1993, McLauchlin 1996). However, these systems require considerable investment in time, personnel and equipment, and are usually only practicable in laboratories such as national reference centres with a particular interest in *Listeria*.

Analysis by phage typing, multilocus enzyme electrophoresis and pulsed-field gel electrophoresis of *L. monocytogenes* isolates from the recent large human food-borne outbreaks in North America and Europe have indicated that these strains show a high degree of similarity (Piffaretti et al. 1989, Buchrieser et al. 1993).

28 ROLE IN THE NORMAL FLORA OF HUMANS

As outlined in section 18 (see p. 692), *L. monocytogenes* occurs in the gastrointestinal tract, which is presumably the initial site of invasion in most cases. Carriage in the gut is probably transitory. However, there is good evidence that some patients show long incubation periods (up to 90 days with a median of 35 days) after the consumption of contaminated food (Linnan et al. 1988). Two episodes of infection have been reported in individual immunocompromised patients, some of these >1 year apart. On the basis that the same strain was shown to be responsible for the 2 episodes, it has been suggested that this represents long-term carriage and reactivation of the original infection (McLauchlin, Audurier and Taylor 1991). The basis and site of the long-term carriage suggested here is not understood.

29 PATHOGENICITY AND VIRULENCE FACTORS

L. monocytogenes has long been used as a low-grade intracellular pathogen to study cellular immunity (Kaufmann 1993). More recent advances in molecular biological techniques have further assisted in the understanding of listeriosis at the cellular level (Sheehan et al. 1994). However, much still remains obscure as to how this disease occurs in nature.

It is characteristic of the natural disease that the attack rate in both humans and animals is usually low. Susceptibility to infection may be increased by external factors, but *L. monocytogenes* is a somewhat marginal pathogen. Hence experimental models that attempt to reflect the natural infection may work poorly, and it may be necessary to challenge relatively large numbers of animals to produce clinical symptoms of disease in a small proportion. The majority of isolates of *L. monocytogenes* are capable of causing disease (Conner et al. 1989, Taboret et al. 1991, Brosch et al. 1993) and all should be treated as potentially pathogenic. There may be differences in virulence between strains (Conner et al. 1989, Brosch et al. 1993).

29.1 Animal models and invasion of mammalian cells growing in vitro

A wide range of animals are susceptible to experimental listeric infection, but rabbits and mice are used most frequently because both die following inoculation with live bacteria by the intravenous or interperitoneal route. Only strains of *L. monocytogenes* and *L. ivanovii* are virulent as measured by LD50 determination, the kinetics of bacterial growth in host tissue, survival in the liver and spleen, or the death of the experimental animal. All the non-haemolytic species of *Listeria* (*L. innocua*, *L. welshimeri* and *L. grayi*) and the weakly haemolytic *L. seeligeri* are non-virulent in mouse pathogenicity tests (Mainou-Fowler, MacGowan and Postlethwaite 1988) or by invasion and growth in mammalian cells in tissue culture (Farber and Speirs 1987).

ANIMAL MODELS

The production of experimental keratoconjunctivitis (Anton's eye test) in guinea pigs or rabbits by instilling a live bacterial suspension into the conjunctiva (Anton 1934) has been used for 60 years to demonstrate the virulence of *L. monocytogenes*. A purulent conjunctivitis (and occasionally a keratitis) develops within 24–48 h. This usually heals spontaneously and the animal rarely dies (Seeliger 1961).

In mice, subcutaneous, intraperitoneal, intravenous, or oral inoculation with *L. monocytogenes* causes death after 1 and 7 days, the mortality rate depending upon the dose and route of inoculation. The LD50 for mice after intraperi-

toneal or intravenous inoculation ranges from 10^2 to 10^7 cfu (Audurier et al. 1980, 1981, Conner et al. 1989, Brosch et al. 1993). At postmortem examination, listeric septicaemia is characterized by multiple tiny focal necroses scattered most conspicuously throughout the liver, and also in the spleen, lungs, adrenal glands, tonsils and intestinal tract (Gray and Killinger 1966). The organisms can be recovered from the spleen and heart blood. Marked differences in susceptibility to infection between different strains of inbred mice have been reported (Skamene 1983). Intraperitoneal carrageenan may be given to mice before inoculation with listeria to increase susceptibility to infection (Conner et al. 1989).

In rabbits (as in monogastric animals) a marked monocytosis is produced following parenteral inoculation, unless overwhelming numbers of bacteria are used, which results in very rapid death. The monocytosis reaches its maximum in 3–7 days (Gray and Killinger 1966).

Ovine encephalitis with characteristic histological features has been achieved experimentally by inoculating listeria into the dental pulp. Histological encephalitis is evident after 6 days, but the onset of clinical neurological disease varied from 20 to 40 days (Barlow and McGorum 1985).

Oral inoculation of mice, rats and guinea pigs has been described (Audurier et al. 1981, Czuprynski and Balish 1981, Lammerding et al. 1992, Schlech, Chase and Badley 1993, Bracegirdle et al. 1994). Infection showed most consistency in gnotobiotic animals and interference with colonization by the natural microflora of the gastrointestinal tract has been suggested (Czuprynski and Balish 1981). An increase in the virulence of *L. monocytogenes* when grown at refrigeration temperatures has been reported in mice experimentally infected by the intravenous but not by the oral route (Czuprynski, Brown and Roll 1989, Stephens et al. 1991). Oesophageal inoculation of juvenile rats with 10^6 cfu of *L. monocytogenes* showed a c. 50% infection rate in the liver or spleen (Schlech, Chase and Badley 1993). A reduction in the acidity of the stomach by cimetidine treatment reduced the infective dose (Schlech, Chase and Badley 1993). Infection of mice with *L. monocytogenes* via an aerosol has been reported (Bracegirdle et al. 1994). LD50 values after 4 days were 10^3–10^5 cfu.

Feeding trials in cynomolgous monkeys showed that only those receiving 10^9 cfu developed fever, septicaemia, loss of appetite, irritability and occasional diarrhoea; those fed $\geq 10^7$ cfu, some of which were completely asymptomatic, shed the organism in the faeces for up to 21 days (Farber et al. 1991). In chick embryos inoculated by the intra-allantoic route, the LD50 is around 10^2 cfu. Lesions occur in the chorioallantoic membrane, liver and heart, and the bacterium can be readily cultured from these sites (Paterson 1940b, Basher, Seaman and Woodbine 1983, Basher et al. 1984, Terplan and Steinmeyer 1989). Chronic mastitis has been induced experimentally in cows by intramammary injection. Bacteraemia was not detected and typically 10^3–10^4 *L. monocytogenes* cfu ml^{-1} were shed into milk for 9–12 months of the remaining lactation period (Bryner, Wesley and van der Maaten 1989).

GROWTH IN TISSUE CULTURE

L. monocytogenes is able to infect a range of cell types growing in vitro, including enterocytes, macrophages and fibroblasts (Farber and Spiers 1987, Kathariou et al. 1990, Sheehan et al. 1994). The use of such models has contributed much to understanding of the factors involved in intracellular invasion and growth (see section 29.2).

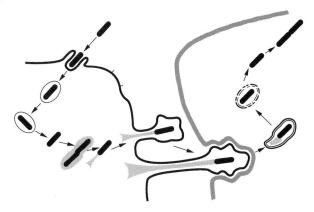

Fig. 30.2 Schematic representation for invasion of eukaryotic cells by *L. monocytogenes.*

29.2 Disease mechanisms for the invasion of mammalian cells

The stages occurring during growth and cell-to-cell spread of *L. monocytogenes* are depicted in Fig. 30.2. The organism enters both phagocytic and non-phagocytic cells. CR3 complement receptors together with other uncharacterized factors may be involved in the adhesion to phagocytes. A listerial surface protein, internalin (which is similar to the M protein of the group A streptococcus), has been shown to be involved in the initial stages of invasion of all cell types. A second cell surface protein, p60 (with murein hydrolase activity), may also be involved in the invasion of some cell types. After internalization, *L. monocytogenes* becomes encapsulated in a membrane-bound compartment. In the phagocyte, the majority of cells in the phagocytic vacuole are probably killed. However, those surviving in the vacuole and those in the membrane-bound compartment of the non-professional phagocyte mediate the dissolution of the vacuole membrane by means of a thiol-activated haemolysin (listeriolysin O), and also possibly by the action of a phospholipase C. *L. monocytogenes* then enters the host cell cytoplasm where growth occurs. In the cytoplasm, the organism becomes surrounded by polymerized host cell actin, which is preferentially polymerized at the older pole of the bacterium. The ability to polymerize actin confers intracellular

mobility to the bacterium and may be involved also with binding of host cell profilin. The resulting 'comet tail'-like structure pushes the bacterial cell into an adjacent mammalian cell, where it again becomes encapsulated in a vacuole. In this stage the vacuole is double membrane bound from the 2 host cells. A lecithinase is involved in the dissolution of these membranes, although the haemolysin may also contribute in this process. Intracellular growth and movement in the newly invaded cell is then repeated (Sheehan et al. 1994).

The genes involved in the invasion of and intracellular movement in mammalian cells are shown in Fig. 30.3. These comprise the *plcA* gene encoding a phospholipase C, the *hly* gene encoding the listeriolysin, and the *actA* gene encoding a cell surface protein involved with actin nucleation. The *plcB* gene encodes the lecithinase, which is activated by a metalloprotease (*mpl* gene). The genes *plcA*, *hly*, *mpl*, *actaA* and *plcB* are located in 3 adjacent operons. Three further open reading frames (ORF X, Y and Z) of unknown function are located adjacent to the lecithinase gene. The operon containing the internalin gene (*inlA*) is located quite closely on the bacterial chromosome (Sheehan et al. 1994).

All the above mentioned genes (or a very similar set) are present in *L. ivanovii*, which follows the same general pattern of cellular invasion and movement. Unlike *L. monocytogenes*, *L. ivanovii* does not cause plaque formation in fibroblasts growing in vitro, and it has been suggested that the lower virulence of this species may be related to lack of as yet uncharacterized cytotoxic factors. There is evidence to support the presence of these genes in *L. seeligeri*, although it is only weakly invasive to mammalian cells. It is not clear whether *L. seeligeri* also lacks additional essential virulence factors or whether the genes are poorly functional (Sheehan et al. 1994). An alternative explanation may be that *L. seeligeri* is adapted to survive in quite different eukaryotic environments.

Regulation of the genes involved with the virulence of *L. monocytogenes* is under the control of the positive regulation factor (*prfA*) gene product, and 6 promoters have been identified which interact with this protein (marked by '+' in Fig. 30.3), including a promoter for its own production. Listeriolysin is one of

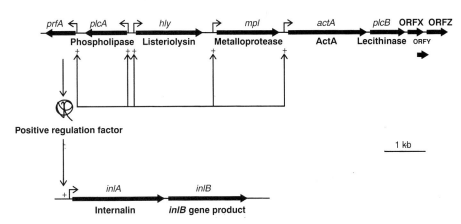

Fig. 30.3 Regulation of genes involved with the virulence of *L. monocytogenes.*

the major extracellular proteins produced by *L. mono-cytogenes* under heat shock conditions, and there is evidence to suggest that some of the above mentioned genes are also regulated by the stage of the cell cycle and temperature. Recent work has shown that the disaccharide cellobiose represses the expression of the listeriolysin and phosholipase genes by an as yet uncharacterized mechanism (Park and Kroll 1993). It is tempting to speculate that the absence of this environmentally ubiquitous plant-derived molecule allows the induction of genes as a pathogenic response to the environment of eukaryotic cells.

REFERENCES

Ahrné S, Stenstrom I-M et al., 1995, Classification of *Erysipelothrix* strains on the basis of restriction fragment length polymorphisms, *Int J Syst Bacteriol*, **45**: 382–5.

Anon, 1994, *Veterinary Investigation, Diagnosis and Analysis III*, Ministery of Agriculture, Fisheries and Food, London.

Anton W, 1934, Kritisch-experimenteller beitrag zur Biologie des *Bacterium monocytogenes*, *Zentralbl Bakteriol Parasitenkd Infektionskr*, **131**: 89–103.

Atkinson N, Collins FV, 1940, Swine erysipelas in South Australia, *Aust Vet J*, **16**: 193–9.

Audurier A, Pardon P et al., 1980, Experimental infection of mice with *Listeria monocytogenes* and *L. innocua*, *Ann Microbiol*, **131B**: 47–57.

Audurier A, Pardon P et al., 1981, Mesure de la virulence chez la souris de différentes bactéries appartenant au genre *Listeria*, *Ann Immunol*, **132D**: 191–200.

Azofra J, Torres R et al., 1991, Endocarditis por *Erysipelothrix rhusiopathiae*. Estudis de 2 casos y revision de la literature, *Enferm Infec Microbiol Clin*, **9**: 102–5.

Baird RM, Corry JEL et al., 1989, Pharmacopoeia of culture media for food microbiology, *Int J Food Microbiol*, **9**: 89–128.

Barber M, 1939, A comparative study of *Listerella* and *Erysipelothrix*, *J Pathol Bacteriol*, **48**: 11–23.

Barlow RM, McGorum B, 1985, Ovine listerial encephalitis: analysis, hypothesis and synthesis, *Vet Rec*, **116**: 233–6.

Barrow GI, Feltham RKA (eds), 1993, *Cowan and Steel's Manual for the Identification of Medical Bacteria*, 3rd edn, Cambridge University Press, Cambridge.

Basher HA, Seaman A, Woodbine M, 1983, Infection, haemorrhagia and death of chick embryos experimentally inoculated with *Listeria monocytogenes* by the intra-allantoic route, *Zentralbl Bakteriol Hyg Abt 1 Orig A*, **255**: 239–46.

Basher HA, Fowler DR et al., 1984, Pathogenesis and growth of *Listeria monocytogenes* in fertile hen's eggs, *Zentralbl Bakteriol Hyg A*, **256**: 497–509.

Belyi YF, Tartakovskii IS, Prosorovskii SV, 1992, Purification and characterization of cell wall proteins of *Listeria monocytogenes*, *Med Microbiol Immunol*, **181**: 283–91.

Belyi YF, Tartakovskii IS, Prosorovskii SV, 1993, Purification and characterization of a 58-kDa cell wall-associated protein from *Listeria monocytogenes*, *Med Microbiol Immunol*, **182**: 87–95.

Bibb WF, Gellin BG et al., 1990, Analysis of clinical and foodborne isolates of *Listeria monocytogenes* in the United States by multilocus enzyme electrophoresis and application of the method to epidemiological investigations, *Appl Environ Microbiol*, **56**: 2133–41.

Bille J, Catimel B et al., 1992, API Listeria, a new and promising one day system to identify *Listeria* isolates, *Appl Environ Microbiol*, **58**: 1857–60.

Boerlin P, Rocourt J, Piffaretti JC, 1991, Taxonomy of the genus *Listeria* using multilocus enzyme electrophoresis, *Int J Syst Bacteriol*, **41**: 59–64.

Boerlin PK, Rocourt J et al., 1992, *Listeria ivanovii* subs. *londoniensis* subs. nov., *Int J Syst Bacteriol*, **42**: 69–73.

Bologa AO, Harlander SK, 1991, Comparison of methods for discrimination between strains of *Listeria monocytogenes* from epidemiological surveys, *Appl Environ Microbiol*, **57**: 2324–31.

Bortolussi R, Schlech WF, 1995, Listeriosis, *Infectious Diseases of the Fetus and Newborn Infant*, 4th edn, eds Remington JS, Klein JO, WB Saunders, Philadelphia, 1055–73.

Bracegirdle P, West AA et al., 1994, A comparison of aerosol and intragastric routes of infection with *Listeria* spp., *Epidemiol Infect*, **112**: 69–79.

Bratberg AM, 1981, Selective adherence of *Erysipelothrix rhusiopathiae* to heart valves of swine investigated in an *in vitro* test, *Acta Vet Scand*, **22**: 39–45.

Brill J, Politynska E, 1961, Die Differenzierung von *Erysipelothrix rhusiopathiae* – Stämmen mit Bakterteriophagen, *Zentralbl Bakteriol Parasitenkd Infektionskr Hyg Abt l Orig*, **181**: 473–7.

Brosch R, Buchrieser C, Rocourt J, 1991, Subtyping of *Listeria monocytogenes* serovar 4b by use of low-frequency-cleavage restriction endonucleases and pulsed-field gel electrophoresis, *Res Microbiol*, **142**: 667–75.

Brosch R, Catimel B et al., 1993, Virulence heterogeneity of *Listeria monocytogenes* strains from various sources (food, human, animal) in immunocompetent mice and its association with typing characteristics, *J Food Prot*, **56**: 296–301.

Bryner J, Wesley I, van der Maaten M, 1989, Research on listeriosis in milk cows with intramammary inoculation of *Listeria monocytogenes*, *Acta Microbiol Hung*, **36**: 137–40.

Buchanan RE, 1918, Studies in the nomenclature and classification of the bacteria, *J Bacteriol*, **3**: 27–61.

Buchrieser C, Brosch R, Rocourt J, 1991, Use of pulsed field gel electrophoresis to compare large DNA-restriction fragments of *Listeria monocytogenes* strains belonging to serogroups 1/2 and 3, *Int J Food Microbiol*, **14**: 297–304.

Buchrieser C, Brosch R et al., 1993, Pulsed field gel electrophoresis applied for comparing *Listeria monocytogenes* strains involved in outbreaks, *Can J Microbiol*, **39**: 395–401.

Burn CG, 1936, Clinical and pathological features of an infection caused by a new pathogen of the genus *Listerella*, *Am J Pathol*, **12**: 341–8.

Carlier Y, Bout D et al., 1980, Physiochemical characteristics of *Listeria* specific antigen 2, *J Gen Microbiol*, **116**: 549–52.

Charpentier E, Gerbaud G, Courvalin P, 1993, Characterization of a new class of tetracycline-resistance gene tet(S) in *Listeria monocytogenes* BM4210, *Gene*, **131**: 27–34.

Charpentier E, Gerbaud G, Courvalin P, 1994, Presence of *Listeria* tetracycline resitance gene tet(S) in *Enterococcus faecalis*, *Antimicrob Agents Chemother*, **38**: 2330–5.

Chattopadhyay B, James E, Hussain R, 1991, Low rate of vaginal carriage of *Listeria monocytogenes*, *J Infect*, **22**: 206–8.

Chooromoney KN, Hampson DJ et al., 1994, Analysis of *Erysipelothrix rhusiopathiae* and *Erysipelothrix tonsillarum* by multilocus enzyme electrophoresis, *J Clin Microbiol*, **32**: 371–6.

Collins DH, Goldie W, 1940, Observations on polyarthriris and on experimental *Erysipelothrix* infection in swine, *J Pathol Bacteriol*, **50**: 323–53.

Collins MD, Rodrigues U et al., 1991a, Phylogenetic analysis of the genus *Lactobacillus* and related lactic acid bacteria as determined by reverse transcriptase sequencing of 16S rRNA, *FEMS Microbiol Lett*, **77**: 5–12.

Collins MD, Wallbanks S et al., 1991b, Phylogenetic analysis of the genus *Listeria* based on reverse transcriptase sequencing of 16S rRNA, *Int J Syst Bacteriol*, **41**: 240–6.

Collins MD, Lawson PA et al., 1994, The phylogeny of the genus *Clostridium*: proposal of five new genera and eleven new species combinations, *Int J Syst Bacteriol*, **44**: 812–26.

Conklin RH, Steele JH, 1979, *Erysipelothrix* infections, *CRC Handbook. Series in Zoonoses*, vol. 1, section A, CRC Press, Boca Raton, FL, 327–37.

Conner DE, Scott VN et al., 1989, Pathogenicity of foodborne, environmental and clinical isolates of *Listeria monocytogenes* in mice, *J Food Sci*, **54:** 1553–6.

Cotoni L, 1942, A propos des bactéries dénommées *Listerella* rappel d'une observation ancienne de méningite chez l'homme, *Ann Inst Pasteur (Paris)*, **68:** 92–5.

Cox LJ, Kleiss T et al., 1989, *Listeria* spp. in food processing, non-food and domestic environments, *Food Microbiol*, **6:** 49–61.

Cummins AJ, Fielding AK, McLauchlin J, 1994, *Listeria ivanovii* infection in a patient with AIDS, *J Infect*, **28:** 89–91.

Curtis GDW, Mitchell RG, 1992, Bacteriocin (monocin) interactions among *Listeria monocytogenes* strains, *Int J Food Microbiol*, **16:** 283–92.

Curtis GDW, Mitchell RG et al., 1989, A selective differential medium for the isolation of *Listeria monocytogenes*, *Lett Appl Microbiol*, **8:** 95–8.

Czuprynski CJ, Balish E, 1981, Pathogenesis of *Listeria monocytogenes* from gnotobiotic rats, *Infect Immun*, **32:** 323–31.

Czuprynski CJ, Brown JF, Roll JT, 1989, Growth at reduced temperatures increases the virulence of *Listeria monocytogenes* for intravenously but not intragastrically inoculated mice, *Microb Pathog*, **7:** 213–23.

Daneshvar MI, Brooks JB et al., 1989, Analysis of fermentation products of *Listeria* species by frequency-pulsed electron-capture gas-liquid chromatography, *Can J Microbiol*, **35:** 786–93.

Dedié K, 1949, Die saureslichen Antigene von *Erysipelothrix rhusiopathiae*, *Mh VetMed*, **4:** 7–10.

Dons L, Rasmussen OF, Olsen JE, 1992, Cloning and characterization of a gene encoding flagellin of *Listeria monocytogenes*, *Mol Microbiol*, **6:** 2919–29.

Doucet-Populaire F, Trieu-Cuot P et al., 1991, Inducible transfer of conjugative transposon Tn1545 from *Enterococcus faecalis* to *Listeria monocytogenes* in the digestive tracts of gnotobiotic mice, *Antimicrob Agents Chemother*, **35:** 185–7.

Dykes GA, Geornaras I et al., 1994, Plasmid profiles of *Listeria* species associated with poultry processing, *Food Microbiol*, **11:** 519–23.

Enoe C, Nørrung V, 1992, Experimental infection of pigs with serotypes of *Erysipelothrix rhusiopathiae*, *Proceedings of the International Pig Veterinary Society Conference*, The Hague, The Netherlands, 345.

Erler W, 1971, Serologische, chemische und immunchemische Untersuchungen an Rotlauf bakterien VIII. Mitteilung: die Neutralzucker der Zellwände, *Arch Exp Veterinarmed*, **25:** 503–12.

Erler W, 1972a, Serologische, chemische und immunchemische Untersuchungen an Rotlaufbakterien IX. Die Aminozucker der Zellwände, *Arch Exp Veterinarmed*, **26:** 797–807.

Erler W, 1972b, Serologische, chemische und immunchemische Untersuchungen an Rotlaufbakterien X. Die Differenzierung der Rotlaufbakterien nach Chemischen Merkmalen, *Arch Exp Veterinarmed*, **26:** 809–16.

Errebo Larsen H, Seeliger HPR, 1966, A mannitol fermenting *Listeria*: *Listeria grayi* sp.n., *Proceedings of the 3rd International Symposium on Listeriosis*, Bilthoven, The Netherlands, 35–9.

Ewald FW, 1981, The genus *Erysipelothrix*, *The Prokaryotes: a Handbook on Habitats, Isolation and Identification of Bacteria*, eds Starr MP, Stolp H et al., Springer, New York, 1688–700.

Facinelli B, Roberts MC et al., 1993, Genetic basis of tetracycline resistance in foodborne isolates of *Listeria innocua*, *Appl Environ Microbiol*, **59:** 614–6.

Farber JM, Peterkin PI, 1991, *Listeria monocytogenes*, a food-borne pathogen, *Microbiol Rev*, **55:** 476–511.

Farber JM, Speirs JI, 1987, Potential use of continuous cell lines to distinguish between pathogenic and nonpathogenic *Listeria* spp, *J Clin Microbiol*, **25:** 1463–6.

Farber JM, Daley E et al., 1991, Feeding trials of *Listeria monocytogenes* with a nonhuman primate model, *J Clin Microbiol*, **29:** 2606–8.

Feist H, 1972, Serologische, chemische und immunchemische

Untersuchungen an Rotlaufbakterien. XII. Das Murein der Rotlaufbakterien, *Arch Exp Veterinarmed*, **26:** 825–34.

Feltham RKA, Power AK et al., 1978, A simple method for storage of bacteria at −76°C, *J Appl Bacteriol*, **44:** 313–6.

Fenlon DR, 1985, Wild birds and silage as reservoirs of *Listeria* in the agricultural environment, *J Appl Bacteriol*, **59:** 537–43.

Feresu SB, Jones D, 1988, Taxonomic studies on *Brochothrix*, *Erysipelothrix*, *Listeria* and atypical lactobacilli, *J Gen Microbiol*, **134:** 1165–83.

Fiedler F, Ruhland GJ, 1987, Structure of *Listeria monocytogenes* cell walls, *Bull Inst Pasteur*, **85:** 287–300.

Fiedler F, Seger J et al., 1984, The biochemistry of murein and cell wall teichoic acids in the genus *Listeria*, *Syst Appl Microbiol*, **5:** 360–76.

Flamm RK, Hinrichs DJ, Thomashow MF, 1984, Introduction of pAMβ1 into *Listeria monocytogenes* by conjugation and homology between native *L. monocytogenes* plasmids, *Infect Immun*, **44:** 157–61.

Flossman K-D, Erler W, 1972, Serologische, chemische und immunchemische Untersuchungen an Rotlaufbakterien XI. Isolierung und Charakterisierung von Desoxyribonukleinsaüren aus Rotlaufbakterien, *Arch Exp Veterinarmed*, **26:** 817–24.

Fluit AC, Torensma R et al., 1993, Detection of *Listeria monocytogenes* in cheese with the magnetic immuno-polymerase chain reaction assay, *Appl Environ Microbiol*, **59:** 1289–93.

Friedman ME, Alm WL, 1962, Effect of glucose concentration in the growth medium on some metabolic activities of *Listeria monocytogenes*, *J Bacteriol*, **84:** 375–7.

Friedman ME, Roessler WG, 1961, Growth of *Listeria monocytogenes* in defined media, *J Bacteriol*, **82:** 528–37.

Galán JE, Timoney JF, 1990, Cloning and expression in *Escherichia coli* of a protective antigen of *Erysipelothrix rhusiopathiae*, *Infect Immun*, **58:** 3116–21.

Gellin BG, Broome CV, 1989, Listeriosis, *JAMA*, **261:** 1313–20.

Gerner-Smidt P, Rosdahl VT, Frederiksen W, 1993, A new Danish *Listeria monocytogenes* phage typing system, *APMIS*, **101:** 160–7.

Ghosh BK, Murray RGE, 1967, Fractionation and characterization of the plasma and mesosome membrane of *Listeria monocytogenes*, *J Bacteriol*, **97:** 426–40.

Gitter M, 1989, Veterinary aspects of listeriosis, *PHLS Microbiol Dig*, **6:** 38–42.

Gitter M, Bradley R, Blampied PH, 1980, *Listeria monocytogenes* infection in bovine mastitis, *Vet Rec*, **107:** 390–3.

Gledhill AW, 1945, The antigenic structure of *Erysipelothrix*, *J Pathol Bacteriol*, **57:** 179–89.

Gledhill AW, 1947, Some properties of a thermolabile antigen of *Erysipelothrix rhusiopathiae*, *J Gen Microbiol*, **1:** 211–20.

Gorby GL, Peacock JE, 1988, *Erysipelothrix rhusiopathiae* endocarditis: microbiologic, epidemiologic, and clinical features of an occupational disease, *Rev Infect Dis*, **10:** 317–25.

Graves LM, Swaminathan B et al., 1991, Ribosomal DNA fingerprinting of *Listeria monocytogenes* using digoxigenin-labeled DNA probe, *Eur J Epidemiol*, **7:** 77–82.

Gray ML, 1957, A rapid method for the detection of colonies of *Listeria monocytogenes*, *Zentralbl Bakteriol Mikrobiol Hyg*, **169:** 373–7.

Gray ML, 1960, Isolation of *Listeria monocytogenes* from oat silage, *Science*, **132:** 1767–8.

Gray ML, Killinger AH, 1966, *Listeria monocytogenes* and listeric infections, *Bacteriol Rev*, **30:** 309–82.

Grieco MH, Sheldon C, 1970, *Erysipelothrix rhusiopathiae*, *Ann NY Acad Sci*, **174:** 523–32.

Gutekunst KA, Holloway BP, Carlone GM, 1992, DNA sequence heterogeneity in the gene encoding a 60-kilodalton extracellular protein of *Listeria monocytogenes* and other *Listeria* species, *Can J Microbiol*, **38:** 865–70.

Hadorn K, Hächler H et al., 1993, Genetic characterization of plasmid encoded multiple antibiotic resistance in a strain of

Listeria monocytogenes causing endocarditis, *Eur J Clin Microbiol*, **12:** 928–37.

Harrington R, Hulse DC, 1971, Comparison of two plating media for the isolation of *Erysipelothrix rhusiopathiae* from enrichment culture broth, *Appl Microbiol*, **22:** 141–2.

Harrington R, Wood RL, Hulse DC, 1974, Comparison of a fluorescent antibody technique and cultural method for the detection of *Erysipelothrix rhusiopathiae* in primary broth cultures, *Am J Vet Res*, **35:** 461–2.

Hartford T, Sneath PHA, 1993, Optical DNA–DNA homology in the genus *Listeria*, *Int J Syst Bacteriol*, **43:** 26–31.

Hayes PS, Graves LM et al., 1992, Comparison of three selective enrichment methods for the isolation of *Listeria monocytogenes* from naturally contaminated foods, *J Food Prot*, **55:** 952–9.

Hether NW, Jackson LL, 1983, Lipoteichoic acid from *Listeria monocytogenes*, *J Bacteriol*, **156:** 809–17.

Hettche HO, 1937, Zur Ätiologie der Rotlautinfektion, *Arch Hyg Bakteriol*, **119:** 178–83.

Hunter D, 1974, *The Diseases of Occupations*, 5th edn, The English Universities Press Ltd, London, 709–12.

Hutner SH, 1942, Some growth requirements of *Erysipelothrix* and *Listerella*, *J Bacteriol*, **43:** 629–40.

Irvin AD, 1968, The effect of pH on the multiplication of *Listeria monocytogenes* in grass silage media, *Vet Rec*, **82:** 115–6.

Jacquet C, Bille J, Rocourt J, 1992, Typing of *Listeria monocytogenes* by restriction polymorphism of the ribosomal ribonucleic acid gene region, *Zentralbl Bakteriol*, **276:** 356–65.

Jensen A, 1993, *Listeria* in faecal and genital specimens, *Med Microbiol Lett*, **2:** 125–30.

Jones CE, Shama G et al., 1995, Comparative study of the growth of *Listeria monocytogenes* in defined media and demonstration of growth in continuous culture, *J Appl Bacteriol*, **78:** 66–70.

Jones D, 1975, The taxonomic position of *Listeria*, *Problems of Listeriosis*, ed. Woodbine M, Leicester University Press, Leicester, 4–17.

Jones D, 1986, Genus *Erysipelothrix*, *Bergey's Manual of Systematic Bacteriology*, vol. 2, eds Sneath PHA, Mair NS et al., Williams & Wilkins, Baltimore, 1245–9.

Jones D, 1990, Foodborne listeriosis, *Lancet*, **336:** 1171–4.

Kamisango K, Saiki I et al., 1982, Structures and biological activities of peptidoglycans of *Listeria monocytogenes* and *Propionibacterium acnes*, *J Biochem (Tokyo)*, **92:** 23–33.

Kamisango K, Fujii H et al., 1983, Structures and immunochemical studies of teichoic acid of *Listeria monocytogenes*, *J Biochem (Tokyo)*, **93:** 1401–09.

Kampelmacher EH, van Noorle Jansen LM, 1969, Isolation of *Listeria monocytogenes* from faeces of clinically healthy humans and animals, *Zentralbl Bakteriol Mikrobiol Hyg A*, **211:** 353–9.

Kämpfer P, 1992, Differentiation of *Corynebacterium* spp., *Listeria* spp., and related organisms by using fluorogenic substrates, *J Cin Microbiol*, **30:** 1067–71.

Kämpfer P, Böttcher S et al., 1991, Physiological characterization and identification of *Listeria* species, *Zentralbl Bakteriol*, **275:** 423–35.

Karlson AG, Merchant IA, 1941, The cultural and biochemical properties of *Erysipelothrix rhusiopathiae*, *Am J Vet Res*, **2:** 5–10.

Kathariou S, Pine L et al., 1990, Nonhemolytic *Listeria monocytogenes* mutants that are also noninvasive for mammalian cells in culture: evidence for coordinate regulation of virulence, *Infect Immun*, **58:** 3988–95.

Kaufmann SHE, 1993, Immunity to intracellular bacteria, *Annu Rev Immunol*, **11:** 129–63.

Kaya S, Araki Y, Ito E, 1985, Characterization of a novel linkage unit between ribitol teichoic acid and peptidoglycan in *Listeria monocytogenes* cell walls, *Eur J Biochem*, **146:** 517–22.

Koch R, 1878, *Untersuchungen uber die Atiologie der Wundinfektionskrankheiten*, Vogel, Leipzig.

Koch R, 1880, *Investigations into the Etiology of Traumatic Infectious Diseases*, New Sydenham Society, London.

Kolstad J, Rørvik LM, Granum PE, 1990, Characterization of plasmids from *Listeria* sp., *Int J Food Microbiol*, **12:** 123–32.

Kosaric N, Carroll KK, 1971, Phospholipids of *Listeria monocytogenes*, *Biochim Biophys Acta*, **239:** 428–42.

Krasemann C, Müller HE, 1975, Die Virulenz von *Erysipelothrix rhusiopathiae* – Stammen und Neuraminidase-produktion, *Zentralbl Bakteriol Parasitenkd Infektionskr Hyg Abt 1 Orig A*, **231:** 206–13.

Kucsera G, 1972, Comparative study on special serotypes of *Erysipelothrix rhusiopathiae* strains isolated in Hungary and abroad, *Acta Vet Acad Scient Hung*, **22:** 251–61.

Kucsera G, 1973, Proposal for standardisation of the designations used for serotypes of *Erysipelothrix rhusiopathiae* (Migula) Buchanan, *Int J Syst Bacteriol*, **23:** 184–8.

Lammerding AM, Glass KA et al., 1992, Determination of virulence of different strains of *Listeria monocytogenes* and *Listeria innocua* by oral inoculation of pregnant mice, *Appl Environ Microbiol*, **58:** 3991–4000.

Langford GC, Hansen PA, 1953, *Erysipelothrix insidiosa*, *Riass: Commun VI Congr Int Microbiol Roma*, **1:** 18.

Lebrun M, Audurier A, Cossart P, 1994a, Plasmid borne cadmium resistance genes in *Listeria monocytogenes* are similar to *cadA* and *cadC* of *Staphylococcus aureus* and are induced by cadmium, *J Bacteriol*, **176:** 3040–8.

Lebrun M, Audurier A, Cossart P, 1994b, Plasmid borne cadmium resistance genes in *Listeria monocytogenes* are present on Tn*5422*, a novel transposon closely related to Tn*917*, *J Bacteriol*, **176:** 3049–61.

Linnan MJ, Mascola L et al., 1988, Epidemic listeriosis associated with Mexican-style cheese, *N Engl J Med*, **319:** 823–8.

Loeffler F, 1886, Experimentelle Untersuchungen uber Schweinerotlauf Arbeiten aus dem Kaiserlichen, *Gesundheitsamt*, **1:** 46–55.

Loessner MJ, 1991, Improved procedure for bacteriophage typing of *Listeria* strains and evaluation of new phages, *Appl Environ Microbiol*, **57:** 882–4.

Loessner MJ, Krause IB et al., 1994, Structural proteins and DNA characteristics of 14 *Listeria* typing bacteriophages, *J Gen Virol*, **75:** 701–10.

Lovett J, Francis DW, Hunt JM, 1987, *Listeria monocytogenes* in raw milk: detection, incidence and pathogenicity, *J Food Prot*, **50:** 188–92.

Low JC, Wright F et al., 1993, Serotyping and distribution of *Listeria* isolates from cases of ovine listeriosis, *Vet Rec*, **133:** 165–6.

McClain D, Lee WH, 1988, Development of the 'USDA-FSIS' method for isolation of *Listeria monocytogenes* from raw meat and poultry, *J Assoc Off Anal Chem*, **71:** 660–4.

MacGowan AP, 1990, Listeriosis – the therapeutic options, *J Antimicrob Chemother*, **26:** 721–2.

MacGowan AP, Holt HA et al., 1990, In vitro antimicrobial susceptibility of *Listeria monocytogenes* isolated in the UK and other *Listeria* species, *Eur J Clin Microbiol Infect Dis*, **9:** 767–70.

MacGowan AP, Marshall RJ et al., 1991a, *Listeria* faecal carriage by renal transplant recipients, haemodialysis patients and patients in general practice: its relation to season, drug therapy, foriegn travel, animal exposure and diet, *Epidemiol Infect*, **106:** 157–66.

MacGowan AP, Reeves DS et al., 1991b, Tricuspid value infective endocarditis and pulmonary sepsis due to *Erysipelothrix rhusiopathiae* successfully treated with high doses of ciprofloxacin but complicated by gynaecomastia (letter), *J Infect*, **22:** 100–1.

MacGowan AP, Bowker K et al., 1994, The occurrence and seasonal changes in the isolation of *Listeria* spp. in shop bought food stuffs, human faeces, sewage and soil from urban sources, *Int J Food Microbiol*, **21:** 325–34.

McLauchlin J, 1987, *Listeria monocytogenes*, recent advances in the taxonomy and epidemiology of listeriosis in humans, *J Appl Bacteriol*, **63:** 1–11.

McLauchlin J, 1989, Rapid non-cultural methods for the detection of *Listeria* in food, *Microbiol Aliment Nutr*, **7:** 279–84.

McLauchlin J, 1990a, Human listeriosis in Britain, 1967–1985, a summary of 722 cases: 1 Listeriosis during pregnancy and in the newborn, *Epidemiol Infect*, **104**: 181–9.

McLauchlin J, 1990b, Human listeriosis in Britain, 1967–1985, a summary of 722 cases: 2 Listeriosis in non-pregnant individuals, a changing pattern of infection and seasonal incidence, *Epidemiol Infect*, **104**: 191–201.

McLauchlin J, 1990c, Distribution of serovars of *Listeria monocytogenes* isolated from different categories of patients with listeriosis, *Eur J Clin Microbiol Infect Dis*, **9**: 210–13.

McLauchlin J, 1993, Listeriosis and *Listeria monocytogenes*, *Environ Policy Pract*, **3**: 201–14.

McLauchlin J, 1995, Molecular and conventional typing methods for *Listeria monocytogenes*: the UK approach, *J Food Prot*, **59**: 1102–5.

McLauchlin J, Audurier A, Taylor AG, 1991, Treatment failure and recurrent human listeriosis, *J Antimicrob Chemother*, **27**: 851–7.

McLauchlin J, Low JC, 1994, Primary cutaneous listeriosis in adults: an occupational disease of veterinarians and farmers, *Vet Rec*, **24**: 615–7.

Mainou-Fowler T, MacGowan AP, Postlethwaite R, 1988, Virulence of *Listeria* spp.: course of infection in resistant and susceptible mice, *J Med Microbiol*, **27**: 131–40.

Makino S, Okada Y et al., 1994, Direct and rapid detection of *Erysipelothrix rhusiopathiae* DNA in animals by PCR, *J Clin Microbiol*, **32**: 1526–31.

Mazurier SI, Wernars K, 1992, Typing of *Listeria* strains by random amplification of polymorphic DNA, *Res Microbiol*, **143**: 499–505.

Michel E, Cossart P, 1992, Physical map of the *Listeria monocytogenes* chromosome, *J Bacteriol*, **174**: 7098–103.

Migula W, 1900, *System der Bakterien Handbuch der Morphologie Entwicklungsgeschichte und Systematik der Bakterie*, vol. 2, G Fischer, Jena.

Miller AL, Smith JL, Somkuti GA, 1990, *Foodborne Listeriosis*, Elsevier, Amsterdam.

Miller IL, Silverman SJ, 1959, Glucose metabolism of *Listeria monocytogenes*, *Bacteriol Proc*, 103.

Monget D, 1992, Procédé et milieu d'identification de bactéries du genre *Listeria*, *Europäisches Patentamt*, 0 496 680 A1, G01N 33/569.

Moore WEC, Cato EP, Moore LVH, 1985, Index of the bacterial and yeast nomenclatural changes published in the International Journal of Systematic Bacteriology since the 1980 Approved Lists of Bacterial Names (1 January 1980 to 1 January 1985), *Int J Syst Bacteriol*, **35**: 382–407.

Murray EGD, Webb RA, Swann MBR, 1926, A disease of rabbits characterised by a large mononuclear leucocytosis, caused by a hitherto undescribed bacillus *Bacterium monocytogenes* (n.sp.), *J Pathol Bacteriol*, **29**: 407–39.

Nakato H, Shinomiya K, Mikawa H, 1986, Possible role of neuraminidase in the pathogenesis of arteritis and thrombocytopenia induced in rats by *Erysipelothrix rhusiopathiae*, *Pathol Res Pract*, **181**: 311–9.

Niederhauser C, Candrian U et al., 1992, Use of polymerase chain reaction for the detection of *Listeria monocytogenes* in food, *Appl Environ Microbiol*, **58**: 1564–8.

Ninet B, Traitler H et al., 1992, Quantitative analysis of cellular fatty acids (CFAs) composition of the seven species of *Listeria*, *Syst Appl Microbiol*, **15**: 76–81.

Noah CW, Ramos NC, Gipson MV, 1991, Efficiency of two commercial ELISA kits compared with the BAM culture method for detecting *Listeria* in naturally contaminated foods, *J Assoc Off Anal Chem*, **74**: 819–21.

Nocera D, Bannerman E et al., 1990, Characterization by DNA restriction endonuclease analysis of *Listeria monocytogenes* strains related to the Swiss epidemic of listeriosis, *J Clin Microbiol*, **28**: 2259–63.

Nocera D, Altwegg M et al., 1993, Characterization of *Listeria* strains from a foodborne listeriosis outbreak by rDNA gene restriction patterns campared to four other typing methods, *Eur J Clin Microbiol Infect Dis*, **12**: 162–9.

Noguchi N, Sasatsu M et al., 1993, Detection of plasmid DNA in *Erysipelothrix rhusiopathiae*, *J Vet Med Sci*, **55**: 349–50.

Nørrung V, 1979, Two new serotypes of *Erysipelothrix rhusiopathiae*, *Nord Vet Med*, **34**: 462–5.

Nørrung V, Molin G, 1991, A new serotype of *Erysipelothrix rhusiopathiae* isolated from pig slurry, *Acta Vet Hung*, **39**: 137–8.

Nørrung V, Munch B, Larsen HE, 1987, Occurrence, isolation and serotyping of *Erysipelothrix rhusiopathiae* in cattle and pig slurry, *Acta Vet Scand*, **28**: 9–14.

Notermans SHW, Dufrenne J et al., 1991, Phosphatidylinositol-specific phospholipase C activity as a marker to distinguish between pathogenic and nonpathogenic *Listeria* species, *Appl Environ Microbiol*, **57**: 2666–70.

Nyfeldt A, 1929, Etiologie de la mononucleose infectieuse, *C R Soc Biol*, **101**: 590–1.

Oakley W, MacVicar J et al., 1992, Vaginal and faecal carriage of *Listeria* during pregnancy, *Health Trends*, **24**: 117–9.

Okwumabua O, Swaminathan B et al., 1992, Evaluation of a chemiluminescent DNA probe assay for the rapid confirmation of *Listeria monocytogenes*, *Res Microbiol*, **143**: 183–9.

Olsen GJ, Woese CR, Overbeek R, 1994, The winds of (evolutionary) change: breathing new life into microbiology, *J Bacteriol*, **176**: 1–6.

Pachas WN, Currid VR, 1974, L-form induction, morphology, and development in two related strains of *Erysipelothrix rhusiopathiae*, *J Bacteriol*, **119**: 576–82.

Packer RA, 1943, The use of sodium azide (NaN_3) and crystal violet in a selective medium for streptococci and *Erysipelothrix rhusiopathiae*, *J Bacteriol*, **46**: 343–9.

Park SF, Kroll RG, 1993, Expression of listeriolysin and phosphatidylinositol specific phospholipase C is repressed by the plant-derived molecule cellobiose in *Listeria monocytogenes*, *Mol Microbiol*, **8**: 653–61.

Partridge J, King J et al., 1993, Cloning, heterologous expression and characterization of the *Erysipelothrix rhusiopathiae* DnaK protein, *Infect Immun*, **61**: 411–7.

Pasteur L, Dumas M, 1882, Sur le rouget, ou mal rouge des porcs. Extrait d'une lettre, *C R Acad Sci (Paris)*, **95**: 1120–1.

Pasteur L, Thuiller L, 1883, Le vaccination du rouget des porcs à l'aide du virus mortel atténué de cette maladie, *C R Acad Sci (Paris)*, **97**: 1163–71.

Paterson JS, 1939, Flagellar antigens of organisms of the genus *Listerella*, *J Pathol Bacteriol*, **48**: 25–32.

Paterson JS, 1940a, The antigenic structure of organisms of the genus *Listerella*, *J Pathol Bacteriol*, **51**: 427–36.

Paterson JS, 1940b, Experimental infection of the chick embryo with organisms of the genus *Listerella*, *J Pathol Bacteriol*, **51**: 437–40.

Peel M, Donachie W, Shaw A, 1988a, Temperature-dependent expression of flagella of *Listeria monocytogenes* studied by electrol microscopy, SDS-PAGE and Western blotting, *J Gen Microbiol*, **134**: 2171–8.

Peel M, Donachie W, Shaw A, 1988b, Physical and antigenic heterogeneity in the flagellins of *Listeria monocytogenes* and *L. ivanovii*, *J Gen Microbiol*, **134**: 2593–8.

Péréz-Díaz JC, Vicente MF, Baquero F, 1982, Plasmids in *Listeria*, *Plasmid*, **8**: 112–8.

Peterkin PI, Gardiner MA et al., 1992, Plasmids in *Listeria monocytogenes* and other *Listeria* species, *Can J Microbiol*, **38**: 161–4.

Piffaretti JC, Kressebuch H et al., 1989, Genetic characterization of clones of the bacterium *Listeria monocytogenes* causing epidemic disease, *Proc Natl Acad Sci USA*, **86**: 3818–22.

Pine L, Malcolm GB et al., 1989, Physiological studies on the growth and utilization of sugars by *Listeria* species, *Can J Microbiol*, **35**: 245–54.

Pirie JHH, 1927, A new disease of veld rodents, 'Tiger River Disease', *Publ S Afr Inst Med Res*, **3**: 163–86.

Pirie JHH, 1940, *Listeria*: change of name for a genus of bacteria, *Nature (London)*, **145**: 264.

Poretz DM, 1985, *Erysipelothrix rhusiopathiae, Principles and Practice of Infectious Diseases*, 2nd edn, eds Mandell GL, Douglas RG, Bennett JE, Edinburgh, Churchill Livingstone, 1185–6.

Portnoy DA, Chakraborty T et al., 1992, Molecular determinants of *Listeria monocytogenes* pathogenesis, *Infect Immun*, **60:** 1263–7.

Poyart-Salmeron C, Carlier C et al., 1990, Transferable plasmid-mediated antibiotic resistance in *Listeria monocytogenes*, *Lancet*, **335:** 1422–6.

Poyart-Salmeron C, Trieu-Cuot P et al., 1992, Genetic basis of tetracycline resistance in clinical isolates of *Listeria monocytogenes*, *Antimicrob Agents Chemother*, **36:** 463–6.

Premaratne RJ, Lin WJ, Johnson EA, 1991, Development of an improved chemically defined minimal medium for *Listeria monocytogenes*, *Appl Environ Microbiol*, **57:** 3046–8.

Prévot AR, 1961, *Listeria, Traité de Systématique Bactérienne*, vol. 2, Paris, Dunod, 511–2.

Quentin C, Thibaut MC et al., 1990, Multiresistant strain of *Listeria monocytogenes* in septic abortion, *Lancet*, **336:** 375.

Ralovich B, 1984, *Listeriosis Research: Present Situation and Perspectives*, Akademiai Kiado, Budapest.

Ralovich BS, Shaahamat M, Woodbine M, 1977, Further data on characters of *Listeria* strains, *Med Microbiol Immunol*, **163:** 125–39.

Rasmussen OF, Beck T et al., 1991, *Listeria monocytogenes* isolates can be classified into two major types according to the sequence of the listeriolysin gene, *Infect Immun*, **59:** 3945–51.

Reboli AC, Farrar WE, 1991, The genus *Erysipelothrix, The Prokaryotes, a Handbook on the Biology of Bacteria: Ecophysiology, Isolation, Identification, Applications*, 2nd edn, eds Balows A, Trüper H et al., Springer, New York, 1629–42.

Ridley AM, 1995, Evaluation of a restriction fragment length polymorphism typing method for *Listeria monocytogenes*, *Res Microbiol*, **146:** 21–34.

Riviera L, Dubini F, Bellotti MG, 1993, *Listeria monocytogenes* infections: the organism, its pathogenicity and antimicrobial drugs susceptibility, *Microbiologica*, **16:** 189–204.

Robertston DC, McCullough WG, 1968, Glucose catabolism of *Erysipelothrix rhusiopathiae*, *J Bacteriol*, **95:** 2112–6.

Robinson K, 1968, The use of cell wall analysis and gel electrophoresis for the identification of coryneform bacteria, *Identification Methods for Microbiologists*, Part B, eds Gibbs BM, Shapton DA, Academic Press, London, 85–92.

Rockabrand D, Partridge J et al., 1993, Nucleotide sequence analysis and heterologous expression of the *Erysipelothrix rhusiopathiae dnaJ* gene, *FEMS Microbiol Lett*, **111:** 79–85.

Rocourt J, 1986, Bactériophages et bactériocines du genre *Listeria*, *Zentralbl Bakteriol Hyg A*, **261:** 12–28.

Rocourt J, Catimel B, 1985, Charactérisation biochemique des espèces du genre *Listeria*, *Zentralbl Bakteriol Hyg A*, **260:** 221–31.

Rocourt J, Catimel B, Schrettenbrunner A, 1985, Isolement de bactériophages de *Listeria seeligeri* et *L. welshimeri*: lysotypie de *L. monocytogenes, L. ivanovii, L. innocua, L. seeligeri* et *L. welshimeri*, *Zentralbl Bakteriol Mikrobiol Hyg A*, **359:** 341–50.

Rocourt J, Grimont PAD, 1983, *Listeria welshimeri* sp. nov. and *Listeria seeligeri* sp. nov., *Int J Syst Bacteriol*, **33:** 866–9.

Rocourt J, Schrettenbrunner A, Seeliger HPR, 1983, Différenciation biochemique des groupes génomiques de *Listeria monocytogenes* (sensu lato), *Ann Microbiol (Paris)*, **134A:** 65–71.

Rocourt J, Seeliger HPR, 1985, Distribution des espèces du genre *Listeria*, *Zentralbl Bakteriol Mikrobiol Hyg A*, **259:** 317–30.

Rocourt J, Wehmeyer U, Stackebrandt E, 1987, Transfer of *Listeria denitrificans* to a new genus *Jonesia* gen. nov. as *Jonesia denitrificans* comb. nov., *Int J Syst Bacteriol*, **37:** 266–70.

Rocourt J, Grimont F et al., 1982, DNA relatedness among serovars of *Listeria monocytogenes* sensu lato, *Curr Microbiol*, **7:** 383–8.

Rocourt J, Audurier A et al., 1985, A multi-centre study on the phage typing of *Listeria monocytogenes*, *Zentralbl Bakteriol Hyg A*, **259:** 489–97.

Rocourt J, Gilmore M et al., 1986, DNA relatedness among *Listeria monocytogenes* and *Listeria innocua* bacteriophages, *Syst Appl Microbiol*, **8:** 42–7.

Rocourt J, Schrettenbrunner A et al., 1987a, Une nouvelle espèce du genre *Listeria: Listeria seeligeri*, *Pathol Biol*, **35:** 1075–80.

Rocourt J, Wehmeyer U et al., 1987b, Proposal to retain *Listeria murrayi* and *Listeria grayi* in the genus *Listeria*, *Int J Syst Bacteriol*, **37:** 298–300.

Rocourt J, Boerlin P et al., 1992, Assignment of *Listeria grayi* and *Listeria murrayi* to a single species, *Listeria grayi*, with a revised description of *Listeria grayi*, *Int J Syst Bacteriol*, **42:** 171–4.

Rosenbach FJ, 1909, Experimentelle morphologische und klinishe Studien der Erreger des Schweinerotlaufs, Erysipeloid und Mäusenseptikamie, *Zentralbl Hyg Infektionskr*, **63:** 343–71.

Ryser ET, Marth EH, 1991, *Listeria, Listeriosis, and Food Safety*, Marcel Dekker, New York.

Schlech WF, 1991, Listeriosis: epidemiology, virulence and significance of contaminated foodstuffs, *J Hosp Infect*, **19:** 211–24.

Schlech WF, Chase DP, Badley A, 1993, A model of food-borne *Listeria monocytogenes* infection in the Sprague–Dawley rat using gastric inoculation: development and effect of gastric acidity on infective dose, *Int J Food Microbiol*, **18:** 15–24.

Schleifer KH, Kandler O, 1972, Peptidoglycan types of bacterial cell walls and their taxonomic implications, *Bacteriol Rev*, **36:** 407–77.

Schuchat A, Swaminathan B, Broome CV, 1991, Epidemiology of human listeriosis, *Clin Microbiol Rev*, **4:** 169–83.

Schütz, 1886, Ueber den Rothlauf der Schweine und die Impfung desselben, *Arb K GesundhAmt*, **1:** 56–76.

Seeliger HPR, 1961, *Listeriosis*, Karger, Basel.

Seeliger HPR, 1981, Apathogene *Listerien: L. innocua* sp. n., *Zentralbl Bakteriol Hyg Abt 1 Orig A*, **249:** 487–93.

Seeliger HPR, Höhne K, 1979, Serotyping of *Listeria monocytogenes* and related species, *Methods in Microbiology*, vol. 13, eds Bergan T, Norris JR, Academic Press, London, 31–49.

Seeliger HPR, Jones D, 1986, Genus *Listeria, Bergey's Manual of Systematic Bacteriology*, vol. 2, eds Sneath PHA, Mair NS et al., Williams & Wilkins, Baltimore, 1235–45.

Seeliger HPR, Rocourt J et al., 1984, *Listeria ivanovii* sp. nov., *Int J Syst Bacteriol*, **34:** 336–7.

Seidler D, Trautwein G, Bohm KH, 1971, Nachweis von *Erysipelothrix insidiosa* mit Fluoreszieren den Antikorpern, *Zentralbl Veterinarmed B*, **18:** 280–92.

Shaw N, 1974, Lipid composition as a guide to the classification of bacteria, *Adv Appl Microbiol*, **17:** 63–108.

Sheehan B, Kocks C et al., 1994, Molecular and genetic determinants of the *Listeria monocytogenes* infectious process, *Curr Top Microbiol Immunol*, **192:** 187–216.

Shimoji Y, Yokomizo Y et al., 1994, Presence of capsule in *Erysipelothrix rhusiopathiae* and its relationships to virulence for mice, *Infect Immun*, **62:** 2806–10.

Shinomiya K, Nakato H, 1985, An experimental model of arteritis: periarteritis induced by *Erysipelothrix rhusiopathiae* in young rats, *Int J Tissue React*, **7:** 267–71.

Shuman RD, Wellmann G, 1966, Status of the species name *Erysipelothrix rhusiopathiae* with request for an opinion, *Int J Syst Bacteriol*, **16:** 195–6.

Siddiqi R, Khan MA, 1982, Vitamin and nitrogen base requirements for *Listeria monocytogenes* and haemolysin production, *Zentralbl Bakteriol Hyg Abt 1 Orig A*, **253:** 225–35.

Siddiqi R, Khan MA, 1989, Amino acid requirements of six strains of *Listeria monocytogenes*, *Zentralbl Bakteriol*, **271:** 146–52.

Skamene E, 1983, Genetic regulation of host resistance to bacterial infection, *Rev Infect Dis*, **5:** S823–32.

Skerman VBD, McGowan V, Sneath PHA, 1980, Approved lists of bacterial names, *Int J Syst Bacteriol*, **30:** 225–420.

Slade PJ, Collins-Thompson DL, 1990, *Listeria*, plasmids, antibiotic resistance, and food, *Lancet*, **336:** 1004.

Smith GR, 1983, *Erysipelothrix* and *Listeria*, *Topley and Wilson's*

Principles of Bacteriology, Virology and Immunity, vol. 2, 7th edn, eds Wilson G, Miles A, Parker MT, Edward Arnold, London, 50–9.

Smith, GR, McLauchlin J, Taylor AG, 1990, *Erysipelothrix* and *Listeria*, *Topley and Wilson's Principles of Bacteriology, Virology and Immunity*, vol. 2, 8th edn, eds Parker MT, Collier LH, Edward Arnold, London, 59–71.

Sneath PHA, Jones D, 1986, Genus *Brochothrix*, *Bergey's Manual of Systematic Bacteriology*, vol. 2, eds Sneath PHA, Mair NS et al., Williams & Wilkins, Baltimore, 1249–53.

Soto A, Zapardiel J, Soriano F, 1994, Evaluation of API Coryne system for identifying coryneform bacteria, *J Clin Pathol*, **47:** 756–9.

Stenstrom IM, Nørrung V et al., 1992, Occurrence of different serotypes of *Erysipelothrix rhusiopathiae* in retail pork and fish, *Acta Vet Scand*, **33:** 169–73.

Stephens JC, Roberts IS et al., 1991, Effect of growth temperature on virulence of strains of *Listeria monocytogenes* in the mouse: evidence for a dose dependence, *J Appl Bacteriol*, **70:** 239–44.

Taboret M, de Rycke J, Dubray G, 1992, Analysis of surface proteins of *Listeria* in relation to species, serovar and pathogenicity, *J Gen Microbiol*, **138:** 743–53.

Taboret M, de Rycke J et al., 1991, Pathogenicity of *Listeria monocytogenes* isolates in immunocompromised mice in relation to listeriolysin production, *J Med Microbiol*, **34:** 13–18.

Tadayon RA, Carroll KK, 1971, Effect of growth conditions on the fatty acid composition of *Listeria monocytogenes* and comparison with the fatty acids of *Erysipelothrix* and *Corynebacterium*, *Lipids*, **6:** 820–5.

Takahashi T, Sawada T et al., 1984, Antibiotic resistance of *Erysipelothrix rhusiopathiae* isolated from pigs with chronic swine erysipelas, *Antimicrob Agents Chemother*, **25:** 385–6.

Takahashi T, Sawada T et al., 1985, Pathogenicity of *Erysipelothrix rhusiopathiae* strains serovars 1a, 3, 5, 6, 8, 11, 21, and type N isolated from slaughter pigs affected with chronic erysipelas, *Nippon Juigaku Zasshi*, **47:** 1–8.

Takahashi T, Fujisawa T et al., 1987a, *Erysipelothrix tonsillarum* sp. nov. isolated from tonsils of apparently healthy pigs, *Int J Syst Bacteriol*, **37:** 166–8.

Takahashi T, Hirayama N et al., 1987b, Correlation between adherence of *Erysipelothrix rhusiopathiae* strains of serovar 1a to tissue culture cells originated from porcine kidney and their pathogenicity in mice and swine, *Vet Microbiol*, **13:** 57–64.

Takahashi T, Fujisawa T et al., 1992, DNA relatedness among *Erysipelothrix rhusiopathiae* strains representing all twenty-three serovars and *Erysipelothrix tonsillarum*, *Int J Syst Bacteriol*, **42:** 469–73.

Takahashi T, Tamura Y et al., 1993, *Erysipelothrix tonsillarum* isolated from dogs with endocarditis in Belgium, *Res Vet Sci*, **54:** 264–5.

Takahashi T, Tamura Y et al., 1994, Cellular fatty acid composition of *Erysipelothrix rhusiopathiae* and *Erysipelothrix tonsillarum*, *J Vet Med Sci*, **56:** 385–7.

Tamura Y, Takahashi T et al., 1993, Differentiation of *Erysipelothrix rhusiopathiae* and *Erysipelothrix tonsillarum* by sodium dodecyl sulfate–polyacrylamide gel electrophoresis of cell proteins, *Int J Syst Bacteriol*, **43:** 111–14.

Tenbroeck C, 1920, Studies on *Bacillus murisepticus* or the rotlauf *Bacillus* isolated from swine in the United States, *J Exp Med*, **32:** 331–43.

Terplan G, Steinmeyer S, 1989, Investigations on the pathogenicity of *Listeria* spp. by experimental infection of the chick embryo, *Int J Food Microbiol*, **8:** 277–80.

Thompson DE, Balsdon JT et al., 1992, Studies on the ribosomal RNA operons of *Listeria monocytogenes*, *FEMS Microbiol Lett*, **96:** 219–24.

Todorov T, 1976, Induction of L-forms of *Erysipelothrix insidiosa* using antibiotics and lysozyme, *Acta Microbiol Virol Immunol (Sofia)*, **4:** 39–45.

Trevisan V, 1885, Caratteri di alcuni nuovi generi di Batteria-

ceae. Atti della Accadmeia Fisio-Medico-Statistica in Milano. Ser 4, 3, 92–107, *Int Bull Bacteriol Nomencl Taxon*, **2:** 11–29.

Trivett TL, Meyer EA, 1971, Citrate cycle and related metabolism of *Listeria monocytogenes*, *J Bacteriol*, **107:** 770–9.

Uchikawa K, Sekikawa I, Azuma I, 1986a, Structural studies on teichoic acids in cell walls of several serotypes of *Listeria monocytogenes*, *J Biochem*, **99:** 315–27.

Uchikawa KI, Sekikawa I, Azuma I, 1986b, Structural studies on lipoteichoic acids from four *Listeria* strains, *J Bacteriol*, **168:** 115–22.

Valerianov TS, Toschkoff A, Cholakova S, 1976, Biological properties of *Erysipelothrix* phages isolated from lysogenic cultures, *Acta Microbiol Virol Immun (Sofia)*, **3:** 32–8.

Van Netten P, Perales A et al., 1989, Liquid and solid selective differential media for the detection and enumeration of *L. monocytogenes* and other *Listeria* spp., *Int J Food Microbiol*, **8:** 299–316.

Vicente MF, Baquero F, Péréz-Díaz JC, 1988, Conjugative acquisition and expression of antibiotic resistance determinants in *Listeria* spp., *J Antimicrob Chemother*, **21:** 309–18.

Vines A, Reeves MW et al., 1992, Restriction fragment length polymorphism in four virulence-associated genes of *Listeria monocytogenes*, *Res Microbiol*, **143:** 281–94.

Walker JK, Morgan JH et al., 1994, *Listeria innocua* isolated from a case of ovine meningoencephalitis, *Vet Microbiol*, **42:** 245–53.

Walker SJ, Archer P, Banks JG, 1990, Growth of *Listeria monocytogenes* at refrigeration temperatures, *J Appl Bacteriol*, **68:** 157–62.

Warburton DW, Farber JM et al., 1991, A comparative study on the FDA and USDA methods for the detection of *Listeria monocytogenes* in foods, *Int J Food Microbiol*, **13:** 105–18.

Watts PS, 1940, Studies on *Erysipelothrix rhusiopathiae*, *J Pathol Bacteriol*, **50:** 355–69.

Weaver RE, 1985, *Erysipelothrix*, *Manual of Clinical Microbiology*, 4th edn, eds Lennette EH, Balows A et al., American Society for Microbiology, Washington, DC, 209–10.

Wellmann G, Kucsera G, Nørrung V, 1983a, Comparative studies on different methods in typing strains of *Erysipethothrix rhusiopathiae*. I Methods and influence of some factors on their results, *Zentralbl Bakteriol Parasitenkd Infektionskr Hyg Abt 1 Orig A*, **254:** 42–54.

Wellmann G, Kucsera G, Nørrung V, 1983b, Comparative studies on different methods in typing strains of *Erysipethothrix rhusiopathiae*. II. Comments on the methods and type classification tests of *E. rhusiopathiae* strains, *Zentralbl Bakteriol Parasitenkd Infektionskr Hyg Abt 1 Orig A*, **254:** 55–63.

Welshimer HJ, Meredith AL, 1971, *Listeria murrayi* sp. n.: a nitrate-reducing mannitol-fermenting *Listeria*, *Int J Syst Bacteriol*, **21:** 3–7.

Wesley IV, Ashton F, 1991, Restriction fragment analysis of *Listeria monocytogenes* strains associated with food-borne epidemics, *Appl Environ Microbiol*, **57:** 969–75.

White TG, Mirikitani FK, 1976, Some biological and physical chemical properties of *Erysipelothrix rhusiopathiae*, *Cornell Vet*, **66:** 152–63.

WHO Working Group, 1988, Foodborne listeriosis, *Bull W H O*, **66:** 421–8.

Wilkinson BJ, Jones D, 1977, A numerical taxonomic survey of *Listeria* and related bacteria, *J Gen Microbiol*, **98:** 399–421.

Wood RL, 1965, A selective liquid medium utilizing antibiotics for isolation of *Erysipelothrix insidiosa*, *Am J Vet Res*, **26:** 1303–8.

Wood RL, 1974, Isolation of pathogenic *Erysipelothrix rhusiopathiae* from feces of apparently healthy swine, *Am J Vet Res*, **35:** 41–3.

Wood RL, 1975, *Erysipelothrix* infection, *Diseases Transmitted from Animals to Man*, 6th edn, eds Hubbert WT, McCullough WF, Schnurenberger PR, Charles C Thomas, Springfield, IL, 271–81.

Wood RL, 1984, Swine erysipelas – a review of prevalence and research, *J Am Vet Med Assoc*, **184:** 944–9.

Wood RL, Huabrich DR, Harrington R, 1978, Isolation of previously unreported serotypes of *Erysipelothrix rhusiopathiae* from swine, *Am J Vet Res*, **39**: 1958–61.

Wood RL, Packer R, 1972, Isolation of *Erysipelothrix rhusiopathiae* from soil and manure of swine-raising premises, *Am J Vet Res*, **33**: 1611–20.

Woodbine M, 1950, *Erysipelothrix rhusiopathiae.* Bacteriology and chemotherapy, *Bacteriol Rev*, **14**: 161–78.

Xu Ke-quin, Gao Cheng-hua, Hu Xiu-fang, 1986, Study on a new serotype of *Erysipelothrix rhusiopathiae* isolated from marine fish, *Anim Infect Dis*, **48**: 6–7.

Xu Ke-quin, Hu Xiu-fang et al., 1984, A new serotype of *Erysipelothrix rhusiopathiae*, *Anim Infect Dis*, **46**: 11–14.

Zák O, Grigelová K, Cernik K, 1965, Variability of the microorganism *Erysipelothrix insidiosa* and its metabolic activity, *Folia Microbiol (Praha)*, **10**: 211.

Chapter 31

BACILLUS

M J Rosovitz, M I Voskuil and G H Chambliss

1 DEFINITION

Bacillus species are rod-shaped, endospore-forming aerobes or facultative anaerobes. Cells stain gram-positive; some are gram-variable, especially in older cultures. Most are motile with peritrichous flagella. Spores, one per cell, contain dipicolinic acid and are resistant to adverse environmental conditions. The genus encompasses species varying widely in physiological characteristics, including species that are psychrophiles, mesophiles and thermophiles; alkalophiles and acidophiles; halotolerant and halophilic organisms. Although most are catalase-positive, their diversity is exemplified by the fact that their G + C content varies from 33 to 69 mol%. The type species is *Bacillus subtilis*.

The genus *Bacillus* is a member of the family Bacillaceae, which encompasses gram-positive or variable bacilli capable of endospore formation. Anaerobic members of the family belong to the genus *Clostridium*, whereas the aerobes and the facultative anaerobes are classified as *Bacillus*. *Bacillus* spp. can be found in almost every environment, primarily because the spores formed by the organisms are resistant to adverse conditions and are readily dispersed to many habitats. Most are considered soil organisms, although some, such as *B. subtilis* and *Bacillus licheniformis*, are often found in marine and estuarine environments. Fastidious members of this genus, such as *Bacillus larvae* and *Bacillus popilliae*, are obligate insect pathogens and sporulate well only in insect haemolymph. Human pathogens of the genus include *Bacillus anthracis*, the causative agent of anthrax, and *Bacillus cereus*, an organism associated with food poisoning as well as several types of opportunistic infection.

2 IMPORTANCE OF THE GENUS

Members of the genus *Bacillus* have been important in several areas of basic research, such as the discovery of spores in *B. subtilis* and *B. anthracis* by Cohn and Koch and the establishment of the germ theory of disease (Gordon 1981). Pasteur developed the first vaccine against *B. anthracis* in 1881 (Keynan and Sandler 1983). The first alternative σ factors, important in directing transcription by bacterial RNA polymerase, were purified from *B. subtilis* infected with the bacteriophage, SP0-1, in the mid 1970s (Haldenwang 1995). Extensive research into the sporulation process in *B. subtilis* has made it perhaps the best understood developmental system.

In addition to being central to basic research studies, members of the genus are also of great commercial importance. Many proteins secreted by members of the genus *Bacillus* are commercially useful. The biggest share of the industrial enzymes are produced by bacilli, the laundry industry consuming the most, specifically the various subtilisins, cellulases and amylases produced by species of *Bacillus* (Jarnagin and Ferrari 1992). Subtilisins, the generic name for alkaline serine proteases produced by several *Bacillus* spp., are also used in contact lens cleaners, collagen and gelatin processing, and many other industrial processes (Zukowski 1992). Other uses of enzymes isolated from *Bacillus* strains include: modification of milk protein in dairy products by neutral proteases, starch and maltose syrup production by the different amylases and pullulanase, high fructose corn syrup (found in soft drinks and other foods) production utilizing glucose isomerase, and modification of the barley cell wall in brewing processes by β-glucanase (Zukowski 1992). Additionally, insecticides (Bella et al. 1985), nucleotides and nucleosides (Demain 1987), and amino acids (Priest 1989) are produced by *Bacillus* spp., as are several recombinant proteins such as pertussis toxin subunits, β-lactamase and human proinsulin (Arbige et al. 1993).

In the pharmaceutical industry, several peptide antibiotics of importance are the products of *Bacillus* spp. A few of the more common antibiotics are bacitracin (from *B. licheniformis*), polymyxin (*Bacillus polymyxa*), linear and cyclic gramicidin (*Bacillus brevis*), tyrocidine (*B. brevis*), subtilin (*B. subtilis*), and bacilysin (*B. subtilis*). A number of other substances with biocontrol activities have also been isolated from species of *Bacillus*. Iturins, cyclic lipoproteins isolated from *B. subtilis*, are toxic to a wide range of pathogenic fungi and yeasts (Maget-Dana and Peypoux 1994). A strain of *B. cereus* produces 2 antibiotics, zwittermicin A and antibiotic B, which suppress damping-off disease in alfalfa caused by the fungus *Phytophthora* (Silo-Suh et al. 1994).

Species of *Bacillus* are also important to the food industry, where they are frequent causes of contamination and spoilage. The proteolytic, lipolytic and saccharolytic enzymes (mentioned above) which are beneficial commercially can also cause spoilage of several food products. *Bacillus stearothermophilus*, *Bacillus coagulans*, *Bacillus licheniformis*, *Bacillus macerans* and *Bacillus subtilis* have been implicated in flat sour spoilage of evaporated milk. In flat sour spoilage, the sugars present in the milk are fermented, producing acid (and hence the sour taste) without gas production (hence the flat description). In another type of spoilage caused by *B. polymyxa* and *B. macerans*, the fermentation of sugars produces acid and gas, leading to can swells and cheese defects. *B. cereus* causes the spoilage of cream known as 'bitty' or 'broken' cream or as 'sweet curdling'. *Bacillus* spp. are also found in pasteurized milk and can cause spoilage of milk if inadequately refrigerated. *B. subtilis* causes a type of spoilage called 'rope' in homemade breads. In this spoilage, the bread proteins, carbohydrates, or both, are broken down by the organism. In strains which cause the bread to become alkaline, capsular material is formed from sugars released from the bread starch by the bacterial amylases. This leads to the appearance of a slimy string or 'rope' when the bread loaf is broken apart. Both *B. subtilis* and *B. licheniformis* have been implicated in the spoilage of hermetically sealed pasteurized sausage stored above proper temperatures (Rodel and Lucke 1990).

3 HABITAT

Due to the longevity of the spore, members of the genus *Bacillus* can be isolated from many environments. The isolation of spores from a particular environment does not necessarily signify that the environment is populated by actively growing *Bacillus*. For instance, spores of acidophiles may be found in alkaline soil, but that finding would not correlate to growth of the isolate in that environment. This type of problem can lead to confusion when trying to evaluate the ecology of species in the genus (Priest 1993).

In spite of this complication, several diverse habitats supporting the growth of the various species of *Bacillus* have been identified. The most commonly associated habitat is the soil, with different types of soil supporting different species. For example, *B. subtilis*, *B. licheniformis* and *B. cereus*, which do not have complex nutrient requirements, are commonly found in low nutrient soil and on straw and rice, whereas other species such as *B. polymyxa* and *Bacillus azotofixans* are not common in low nutrient soils, but instead associate with plant rhizospheres and rhizoplanes where nutrients are available; *B. macerans* and *Bacillus circulans* also require complex nutrients and are found in decomposing plant matter (Priest 1989).

In addition to inhabiting soil environments, many *Bacillus* spp. are found in marine waters and sediments. Non-polluted seawater contains large numbers of *B. licheniformis*, *B. subtilis* and *Bacillus pumilus*. Sediments are dominated by the latter 2 species, although other *Bacillus* species are also common (Priest 1989). Members of the genus are less common in fresh water, although they are often found in fresh water sediments.

Some of the insect pathogens such as *Bacillus popilliae* and *Bacillus lentimorbus* grow and sporulate well only in insect larvae, whereas another insect pathogen, *Bacillus thuringiensis*, is found often in soils and on plants and does not require an insect host to sporulate. Due to larval association, however, *Bacillus* insect pathogens are often found in sites favourable for larval growth, such as drainage ditches and sediments of pools and lakes. *B. thuringiensis* var. *israelensis* was first isolated as a spore from mud containing insect larvae (Margalit and Dean 1985).

Several species of *Bacillus* are capable of growth in extreme conditions. *Bacillus pasteurii* is found in environments high in urea and is a common inhabitant of urinals and urban soils (Priest 1989). *Bacillus psychrophilus* and *Bacillus insolitus* are found in frozen foods. At the other extreme, *Bacillus acidocaldarius* grows only in acid hotsprings and soil in surrounding areas (Priest 1989), growing optimally from pH 2 to 6. Other thermophilic species, *B. coagulans* and *B. stearothermophilus*, are commonly found in foods that require heat processing, such as beet sugar and canned foods. Many of the thermophilic species also populate soils and muds in temperate areas (Priest 1993).

4 PHYLOGENY AND TAXONOMY

As presently defined, the genus *Bacillus* is composed of gram-positive, rod-shaped, aerobic or facultatively anaerobic, endospore-forming bacteria (Claus and Berkeley 1986). The broad morphological and physiological definition of the genus has resulted in the inclusion of a diverse assemblage of bacteria. It has become increasingly clear that the current taxonomy of the genus is unsatisfactory and in need of revision. The genus *Bacillus* encompasses a wide range of phenotypes: strict aerobes, facultative anaerobes, acidophiles, alkalophiles, chemolithotrophs, halophiles, psychrophiles and thermophiles (Claus and Berkeley 1986). DNA base composition studies have also indicated extreme heterogeneity within the genus. According to Del Ley (1978), the base composition within a genus typically varies no more than 15%. The mol% G + C content of the genus *Bacillus* varies from 33 (*B. anthracis*) to 69 (*Bacillus thermocatenulatus*), far more than the variation of a typical genus (Priest 1993).

In addition to phenotypic diversity, there is evidence of significant phylogenetic diversity. In the most comprehensive study to date Ash et al. (1991b) compared 16S rRNA sequences from 51 *Bacillus* spp. and demonstrated at least 5 phylogenetically distinct groups within the *Bacillus* genus (Fig. 31.1). Group 1 consists of 28 species including the genus type species, *B. subtilis*, as well as most pathogenic *Bacillus* spp. The 4 other groups are organized as follows: group 2 includes *Bacillus sphaericus* and 5 other species, group 3 includes *B. polymyxa* and 9 other species, group 4 consists of 2 species, and group 5 contains 3 species. Although classical phenotypic characteristics often reflect phylogenetic relationships, the advance of molecular techniques has brought about a recognition that molecular criteria more clearly reveal evolutionary relationships and provide a more appropriate basis for the grouping of organisms.

In response to the initial rRNA analysis of the genus, attempts at reclassification have begun. One recent proposal has been to reclassify group 3 into the new genus *Paenibacillus* (Ash, Priest and Collins 1993). It seems likely with increasing molecular data that new genera will be formed out of the genus *Bacillus* and will include organisms that, by some phenotypic characteristics, may appear to belong to other genera but at the DNA level are more closely related to species of the currently defined genus *Bacillus*. One example is the rod-shaped endospore-forming bacterium *Bacillus oleronius* isolated from the hindgut of termites (Kuhnigk et al. 1995). Even though *B. oleronius* stains gram-negative, 16S rRNA analysis, as well as some phenotypic characteristics, place this bacterium within group 1 of the genus *Bacillus*, most closely related to *Bacillus lentus*.

5   IDENTIFICATION

5.1   Isolation

To isolate a particular species from a complex environment containing many species, the conditions employed should promote the growth of the desired bacterium while inhibiting the growth of others. In an environment where the desired bacterium comprises the majority of the population, simply streaking material onto solid media and further subculturing may be all that is required for isolation. The majority of *Bacillus* spp. grow well on a rich medium such as blood agar base (see Fig. 31.2). In environments where the desired organism is found in low numbers,

contaminating microflora can make isolation difficult, and specific isolation methods are necessary. Due to the general non-pathogenic nature of *Bacillus* spp., few methods for *Bacillus* isolation have been developed. Many of the selective and enrichment methods that have been developed are summarized in Norris et al. (1981) and Claus and Berkeley (1986). The emergence of *B. cereus* as an agent of food poisoning, spoilage and infections has led to the development of a variety of methods for the detection and enumeration of *B. cereus*. A summary of these methods can be found in van Netten and Kramer (1992).

Generally, the ability of *Bacillus* spp. to form heat- and chemical-resistant spores is a useful trait for the isolation of these spore-forming bacteria. Pasteurization of a sample at 80°C for 10 min will kill most bacteria while leaving many spores viable. Heat sensitivity of spores can vary considerably, especially from spores isolated directly from the environment, thus making it difficult to obtain some species using heat sterilization (Roberts, Ingram and Skulberg 1965). Isolation difficulties due to heat sensitivity can often be overcome by sterilization with 95% ethanol instead of pasteurization (Bond et al. 1970). However, in conditions when spore-forming bacteria are growing vegetatively, or conditions when spore germination and subsequent growth are not favourable, isolation by pasteurization or ethanol treatment is not possible.

5.2   Traditional identification

Identification and classification have relied heavily on spore morphology. The location of the spore within the mother cell, either central or terminal, and the spore shape are used to differentiate between species. Gordon, Hayes and Pang (1973) divided the genus into 3 groups based on spore morphology. Group 1 consists of *B. subtilis*, *B. megaterium*, *B. cereus* and others with spores that do not distend the mother cell. Group 2 consists of *B. polymyxa*, *B. stearothermophilus*, *B. alvei* and others with oval spores that distend the mother cell. Group 3 consists of species that form round spores (Fig. 31.3). Some of this classical grouping is similar to the recent classification of *Bacillus* spp. by rRNA analysis as seen in Fig. 31.1, whereas many of the species classified by spore morphology and other means are now being recategorized into groups based on rRNA similarity.

In addittion to spore morphology, a large battery of tests have been utilized for *Bacillus* identification. Gordon, Hayes and Pang (1973) published the prime authority on the morphology and biochemical characteristics of the genus *Bacillus*. These criteria have been used to differentiate 19 *Bacillus* species. Table 31.1 lists these species and the corresponding characteristics used for their identification.

5.3   API and molecular identification

The identification of *Bacillus* spp. is complicated and many laboratories often go no further than simply '*Bacillus* spp.' or 'aerobic spore-forming rod'. Classical

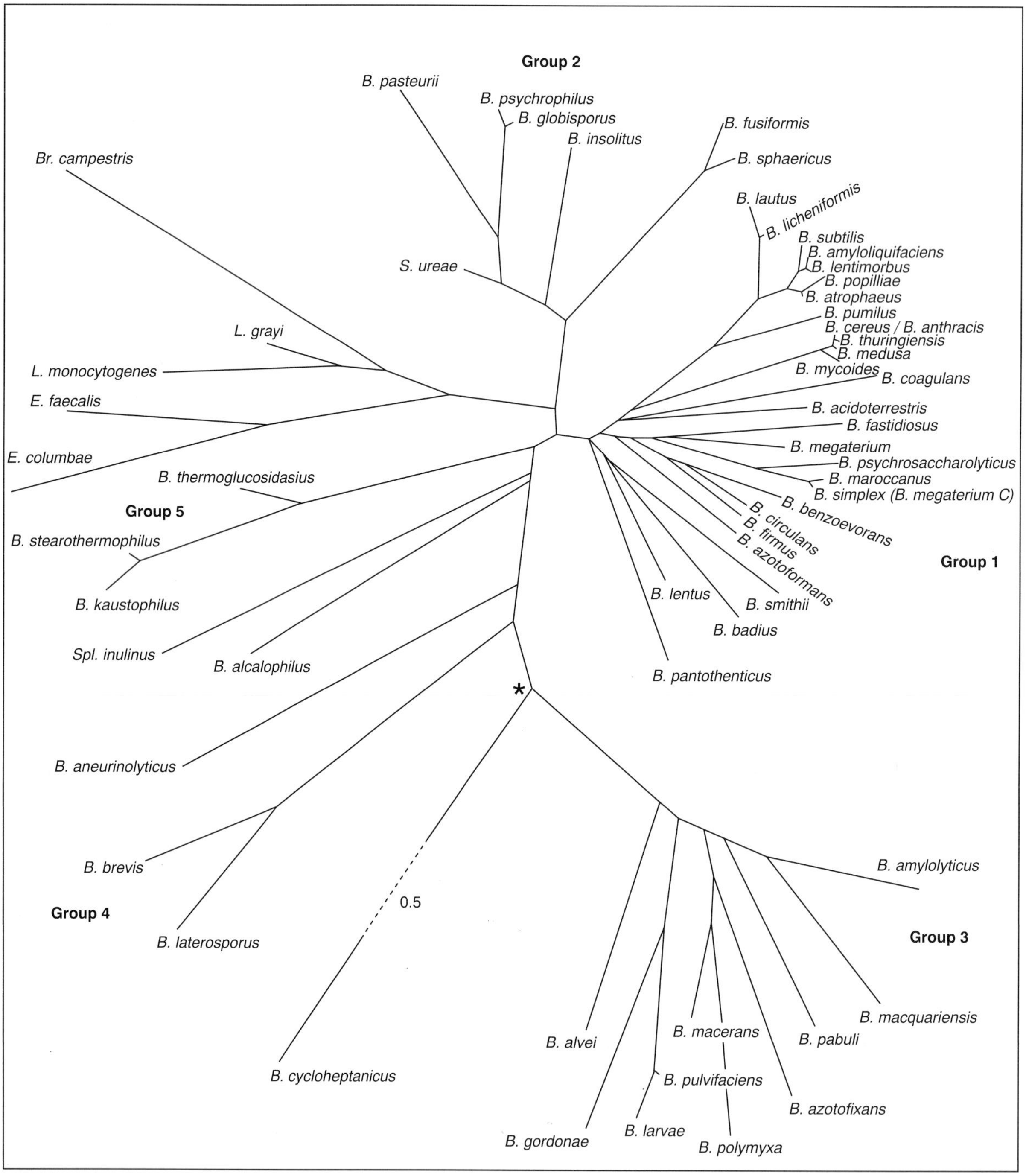

Fig. 31.1 Phylogenetic tree of 51 *Bacillus* spp. based on 16S rRNA sequence analysis. Genus abbreviations: *B.*, *Bacillus*; *Br.*, *Brochothrix*; *E.*, *Enterococcus*; *L.*, *Listeria*; *S.*, *Sporosarcina*; *Spl.*, *Sporolactobacillus*. (From Ash et al. 1991b. Reproduced with permission of Blackwell Science Ltd).

tests for identification require special media which is expensive, difficult to store, and can lead to inconsistent results. The high degree of heterogeneity within the genus can also make identification by standardized tests difficult. Logan and Berkeley (1981, 1984) reported a rapid and accurate system for the identification of *Bacillus* spp. using API strips (API Laboratory Products, Basingstoke, Hants, UK). The combination of 12 tests from the API 20E test kit, and 49 tests from the API 50 CHB test kit, and a few supplementary tests

was found to be more reproducible and less time consuming than classical tests. API tests are a significant tool for *Bacillus* identification, especially in laboratories where it is not feasible to maintain a supply of the materials needed for classical tests.

In addition to classical tests and the API system, several molecular tests can be performed to differentiate between species. Estimation of chromosomal DNA base composition [mol% (G + C)] and DNA–DNA liquid hybridization have been used for identification.

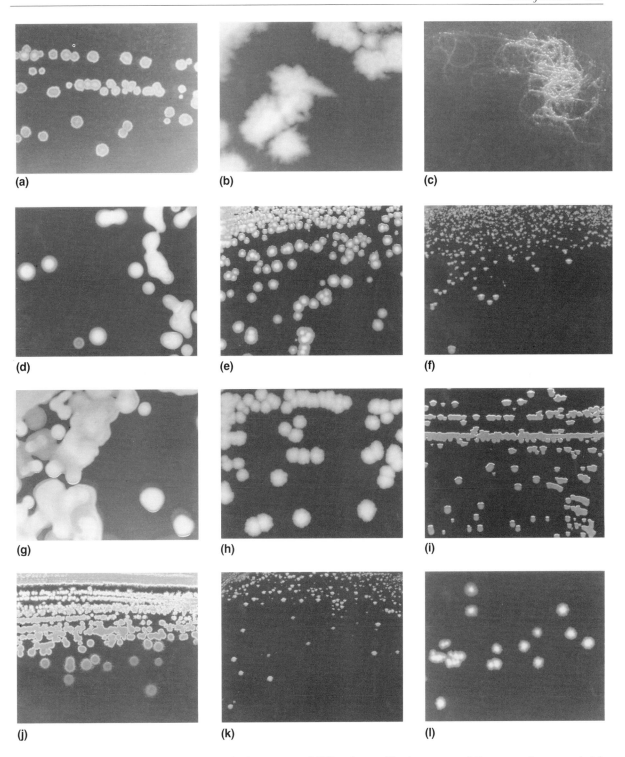

Fig. 31.2 Colonies on blood agar base. Incubations were at 30°C and magnifications were × 1.6, except where noted: (a) type species, *B. subtilis*; (b) *B. cereus* (note spreading colony morphology); (c) *B. cereus* var. *mycoides* (note rhizoid colony morphology; × 2.2); (d) *B. megaterium*; (e) *B. brevis*; (f) *B. stearothermophilus* (50°C incubation; × 2.2); (g) *B. sphaericus* (note mucoid spreading morphology); (h) *B. circulans*; (i) *B. pumilus* (× 2.7); (j) *B. licheniformis*; (k) *B. polymyxa*; and (l) *B. coagulans* (37°C).

In the future, testing methods employing specific DNA probes and polymerase chain reaction (PCR) should increase the speed and accuracy of identification.

5.4 Antigenic constitution

In general, the use of antigens has not been very successful in differentiating among different *Bacillus* spp.

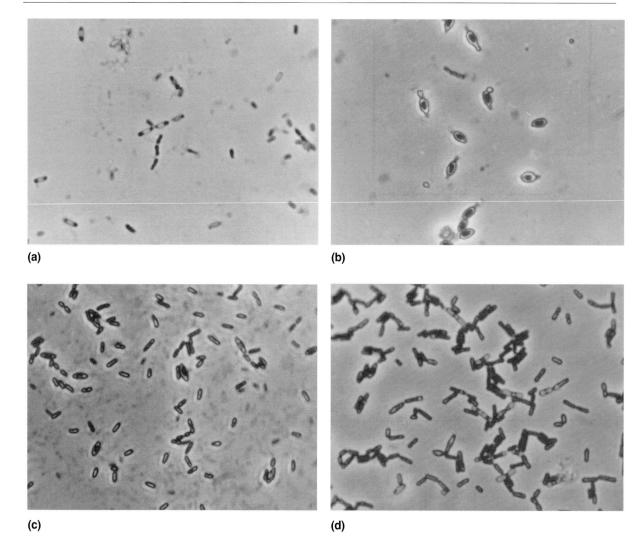

Fig. 31.3 Phase contrast microscopy of spores and sporangia, illustrating the different spore morphological groups established by Gordon, Hayes and Pang (1973): (a) group 1 (*B. licheniformis*); (b) group 2 (*B. brevis*); (c) group 2 (*B. laterosporus*); (d) group 3 (*B. sphaericus*).

Spore antigens confer the highest species specificity, but cross-agglutination is observed between *B. thuringiensis* and *B. cereus*, as well as between *B. anthracis* and *B. cereus* (Berkeley et al. 1984). Another problem with utilizing spore antigens for identification is a technical difficulty caused by the hydrophobic nature of the spore surface, which results in significant autoagglutination during the assay. Somatic antigens, or O antigens, have not been used successfully in identifying the different species either, again due to cross-reactivity between species. The flagellar antigens, or H antigens, although not overly useful in differentiating at the species level, have found application in serological studies of different strains within a species. In particular, serological studies of H antigens have been utilized to follow *B. cereus* epidemiology in food poisoning outbreaks and to help differentiate new strains of *B. thuringiensis* as they are characterized.

5.5 *B. cereus* and related species

Much effort has been directed at differentiating between *B. cereus* and closely related species (Table 31.2). The main characteristics that distinguish *B. cereus* from the closely related organisms are the 2 virulence plasmids of *B. anthracis*, the production of δ-endotoxin by *B. thuringiensis*, and the rhizoid growth of *B. cereus* var. *mycoides*, thus making differentiation between them difficult. Other characteristics are nearly identical, leading many to consider these species as variations of *B. cereus*. For example, analysis of *B. cereus* and *B. anthracis* rRNA revealed identical 16S rRNA and only 2 differences in their 23S rRNA (Ash et al. 1991a, Ash and Collins 1992). The recent discovery by Andersen, Simchock and Wilson (1996) of a region of DNA sequence variability among *B. cereus*, *B. anthracis* and *B. mycoides* suggests that molecular

Table 31.1 Summary of characters used to identify 19 *Bacillus* spp.

	Catalase production	Voges–Proskauer (VP) reaction	Anaerobic growth	Growth at 50°C	Growth in 7% NaCl	Acid + gas from AS* glucose	Nitrate reduction	Starch hydrolysis	Growth at 65°C	Cell width ≥1.0 μm	pH in VP medium <6.0	Acid from AS* glucose	Casein hydrolysis	Parasporal bodies
B. megaterium	+	−	−	−	+	−	v	+	−	+	v	+	+	−
B. cereus	+	+	+	−	+	−	+	+	−	+	+	+	+	v
B. thuringiensis	+	+	+	−	+	−	+	+	−	+	+	+	+	+
B. licheniformis	+	+	+	+	+	−	+	+	−	−	v	+	+	−
B. subtilis	+	+	−	+	+	−	+	+	−	−	v	+	+	−
B. pumilus	+	+	−	+	+	−	−	−	−	−	+	+	+	−
B. firmus	+	−	−	−	+	−	+	+	−	−	−	+	+	−
B. coagulans	+	+	+	+	−	−	v	+	−	v	+	+	v	−
B. polymyxa	+	+	+	−	−	+	+	+	−	−	v	+	+	−
B. macerans	+	−	+	+	−	+	+	+	−	−	−	+	−	−
B. circulans	+	−	v	+	v	−	v	+	−	−	v	+	v	−
B. stearothermophilus	v	−	−	+	−	−	v	+	+	v	+	+	v	−
B. alvei	+	+	+	+	−	−	−	+	−	v	+	+	+	−
B. laterosporus	+	−	+	+	−	−	+	−	−	−	−	+	+	+
B. brevis	+	−	−	+	−	−	v	−	−	−	−	+	+	−
B. larvae	−	−	+	−	−	−	v	−	−	−	−	+	−	−
B. popilliae	−	−	+	−	−	−	−	+	−	−	−	+	−	+
B. lentimorbus	−	−	+	−	−	−	−	−	−	−	−	+	−	−
B. sphaericus	+	−	−	−	v	−	−	−	−	v	−	−	v	−

*AS, ammonium-salt basal medium.
+, >85% of strains examined by Gordon, Hayes and Pang (1973) positive; −, >85% of strains negative; v, variable character.
Table modified from Norris et al. (1981).

techniques will make it easier to distinguish between these organisms in the future.

6 VEGETATIVE AND MOTHER CELLS

6.1 Morphology

Vegetative *Bacillus* cells exist as single cells or in chains. The cells are rod-shaped, rounded, or squared at the ends and range in size from 0.5 × 1.2 μm to as large as 2.5 × 10 μm (Claus and Berkeley 1986). They typically stain gram-positive, although positive staining is often difficult to obtain in older cultures. Upon limitation of necessary nutrients, growing cells enter stationary phase and, under proper conditions, endospores are formed within the mother cell. Some vegetative cells may be vacuolate, often containing protein crystals such as those found in *B. thuringiensis*, or globules of stored metabolic material such as poly-β-hydroxybutyrate.

Bacillus cells are covered by a cytoplasmic membrane, a cell wall and in some strains, other layers. Unlike gram-negative eubacteria, cells of *Bacillus* spp. do not contain outer membranes or membrane-enclosed periplasms. The cell wall enclosures are composed of several sheets of peptidoglycan and one or more anionic polymers, forming a thick barrier around the cell. Peptidoglycan murein, made of glycan strands cross-linked with short peptides, is the most common polymer found in bacterial cell walls.

The majority of *Bacillus* peptidoglycan types are members of the directly cross-linked *meso*-diaminopimelic acid (m-Dpm or mA$_2$pm) type (Schleifer and Kandler 1972). Interestingly, besides '*Bacillus aminovorans*', all exceptions to *meso*-diaminopimelic acid peptidoglycan type form round endospores (Stackebrandt et al. 1987). *Bacillus* cell surfaces contain paracrystalline cell wall surface layers (S layers) consisting of a single protein or glycoprotein and possessing a high degree of structural regularity (Sleytr and Messner 1983). Carbohydrate capsules are produced by several *Bacillus* spp. such as the poly-D-glutamic acid capsule produced by *B. anthracis* in vivo, or in vitro under conditions of virulence factor expression (Meynell and Meynell 1964) (Fig. 31.4).

Bacillus spp. are typically motile by means of peritrichous flagella (Fig. 31.5); however, *B. anthracis* is non-motile whereas its closest relatives, *B. cereus* and *B. thuringiensis*, are motile. Exceptions include one motile strain of *B. anthracis* (Brown and Cherry 1955) and several non-motile strains of *B. cereus* (Logan and Berkeley 1984). Flagellar antigens have been useful for the identification of *B. cereus*, *B. thuringiensis* and *B. sphaericus* (Turnbull, Kramer and Melling 1990).

Colony characteristics of *Bacillus* spp. vary greatly depending on environmental conditions. Quality and quantity of media, age of the colony, and number of colonies on a petri dish frequently affect the diameter of colonies as well as other features. Differences in the percentage of sporulating cells often result in a mixture of translucent and opaque colonies on the same

Table 31.2 Characters used to identify *B. cereus* and related species

Property	B. cereus	B. anthracis	B. thuringiensis	B. cereus var. mycoides
Lecithinase reaction	+	(+)	+	+
Acid from mannitol	−	−	−	−
Gram reaction	+	+	+	+
Catalase	+	+	+	+
Motility	+	−	+	−
Anaerobic glucose utilization	+	+	+	+
Haemolysis (sheep or horse erythrocytes)	+	−	+	(+)
Rhizoid growth	−	−	−	+
Crystalline parasporal inclusion	−	−	+	−
Lipid globules in protoplasm	+	+	+	+
Lysis by γ-phage	−	+	−	−
'String of pearls' effect (with penicillin G 0.5–10 units ml^{-1})	−	+	−	−
Reduction of nitrate	+	+	+	+
Acetylmethylcarbinol production (VP)	+	+	+	+
Citrate utilization	+	b	+	a
Growth in 7% NaCl	+	+	+	a
Tyrosine decomposition	+	−	+	a
Possession of plasmids pX01, pX02, and corresponding elaboration of toxin and capsule	−	+	−	−

+, 85–100% of strains positive; −, 0–14% strains positive; (+), usually weakly positive; a, 50–84% strains positive; b, 15–49% strains positive; VP, Voges–Proskauer.
Table adapted and modified from Gordon (1977).

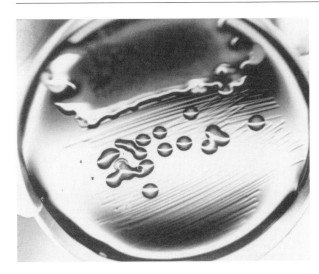

Fig. 31.4 Capsule formation of *B. anthracis* colonies incubated in a high CO_2 environment. (Courtesy of J Lindquist).

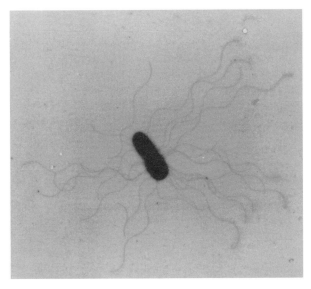

Fig. 31.5 *B. cereus* peritrichous flagella ($\times$ 4470). (From Parry et al. 1983, reproduced by permission of I Popiel and Wolfe Medical Publications Ltd.)

plate of a pure culture. Due to the great variation in colony morphology of *Bacillus* spp., it is difficult to utilize colony appearance in distinguishing species; however, under defined conditions colony morphology can be useful. Several species grown on blood agar base medium plates can be seen in Fig. 31.2. *B. mycoides* produces an unusual colony structure which exhibits rhizoid growth usually turning left, that eventually covers the entire plate (Stapp and Zycha 1931). Further descriptions of *Bacillus* colonies can be found in Smith, Gordon and Clark (1952).

6.2 Metabolism

The genus *Bacillus* is composed of a diverse assortment of gram-positive, aerobic or facultatively anaerobic, endospore-forming bacteria. As such, members of the genus have a wide variety of metabolic abilities, nutritional requirements and growth conditions. The majority of species will grow well on a rich medium such as nutrient agar. As previously mentioned (see section 5.2, p. 711), Gordon, Hayes and Pang (1973) divided the genus into 3 groups. In this classification system species in group 1 have the simplest nutritional requirements. Group 2 species have more complex requirements and group 3 species have the most fastidious requirements.

Claus and Berkeley (1986) list many of the diverse metabolic characteristics of several *Bacillus* spp. A few, including *B. polymyxa* and *B. macerans*, are capable of fixing nitrogen. *B. azotoformans* and *B. licheniformis* can reduce nitrate. *Bacillus schlegelii* can grow autotrophically in an O_2–CO_2–H_2 or O_2–CO environment, and heterotrophically, aerobically in medium supplemented with a carbon source such as acetate or succinate. *B. pumilus* can utilize and is resistant to cyanide. Several species can metabolize aromatic and hydroxyaromatic compounds and have been used in the bioremediation of gasoline spills. Several species grow at either high or low temperatures, whereas others can grow at high or low pH. A common feature of the genus *Bacillus* is the production of catalase, differentiating *Bacillus* spp. from species of *Clostridium* and *Sporolactobacillus*; however, a few species – *B. larvae*, *B. lentimorbus*, *B. popilliae* and some strains of *B. stearothermophilus* – produce little to no catalase (Turnbull, Kramer and Melling 1990).

Species of *Bacillus* are attractive micro-organisms for industrial application due to several characteristics:

1 they synthesize products of commercial interest
2 they have a large range of metabolic properties
3 they have relatively well developed gene transfer systems and
4 most are non-pathogenic.

Many have simple growth requirements and can express and secrete large amounts of proteins and metabolites. Enzymes isolated from *Bacillus* spp. account for over half the total enzyme sales annually (Arbige and Pitcher 1989). The predominant enzymes of commercial interest have been discussed (see section 2, p. 709).

7 THE SPORE

7.1 Spore formation as a developmental model system

The study of sporulation in the *Bacillus* type organism, *B. subtilis*, has provided an excellent model system in which to study development. During the process of sporulation, 2 cell compartments starting out with identical genomes differentiate into 2 distinct cells types, a forespore, which subsequently becomes the mature endospore, and the mother cell, which ultimately lyses, releasing the spore. The regulation of sporulation is controlled in part by a cascade of transcriptional regulatory proteins including σ factors, transcription activators and repressors, and by mechanisms that couple activities in each cell compartment to those in the other (for recent reviews see Errington 1993, 1996).

The entry into sporulation is controlled by signals related to starvation (reviewed in Sonenshein 1989), cell density (Grossman and Losick 1988) and the cell cycle (see, for example, Mandelstam and Higgs 1974, Clark and Mandelstam 1980). Signals from these conditions trigger the conversion of cellular physiology from active growth to sporulation. The trigger mechanism operates via the phosphorelay system (Grossman 1991, Burbulys, Trach and Hoch 1991), a complex signal transduction system pivotal in the decision to sporulate. Phosphorylation of Spo0A by the phosphorelay system results in the activation of genes essential in early sporulation and the repression of genes whose products block sporulation.

The contributions of many researchers have led to our current understanding of the development of the spore and its properties. A brief summary of some of the control mechanisms thus far elucidated will be presented here; readers are referred to Errington (1993, 1996) and Haldenwang (1995) for reviews on the many contributions to the current understanding of sporulation and σ factors and to Moir and Smith (1990) for those on spore germination.

Initiation of sporulation involves Spo0A, a response regulator activated by phosphorylation through the phosphorelay system mentioned above, and σ^H, a σ factor active early in sporulation. These factors in part control the formation of an asymmetric septum, leading to the creation of the 2 compartments of unequal size, the larger mother cell and the smaller forespore. Once sporulation has commenced, transcription in the mother cell is largely directed first by σ^E, followed by σ^K in late sporulation, along with transcription regulators SpoIIID in earlier stages and GerE in later stages. In the forespore first σ^F and then σ^G direct transcription.

The complex mechanisms controlling the cascade of gene expression in appropriate cell compartments co-ordinately with morphological stages in sporulation have been the subject of a great deal of research, and are now becoming understood. Each σ factor directs transcription of a specific set of genes, or regulon. Included in the σ^E and σ^F regulons are the genes encoding for pro-σ^K and σ^G, respectively, ensuring that σ^E and σ^F are active before the latter 2 σ factors are produced. Two of the σ factors (σ^E and σ^K) are made as inactive proteins, pro-σ^E and pro-σ^K, whose activations by processing are coupled to development of the forespore, leading to an additional level of regulation ensuring that genes in the σ^E and σ^K regulons are expressed at the appropriate developmental time. The first forespore-specific σ factor, σ^F, is held inactive by an anti-σ factor, and is released from this repression by another protein which is capable of binding the anti-σ protein when certain physiological conditions are attained in the post-septational sporulating cell. Regulation of the later prespore-specific σ factor, σ^G, is not well understood. The mechanisms for

its regulation may include interaction with the anti-σ factor mentioned above, transcription of certain genes in the mother cell, and a mechanism coupling its activation to complete forespore engulfment.

In the forespore, as sporulation progresses, the α/β small acid-soluble proteins (α/β-type SASPs) involved in UV resistance are produced, as are products necessary for germination of the spore, and dipicolinic acid (made in the mother cell) is accumulated in the spore. From the mother cell, the spore cortex and spore coats are laid down on the forespore, giving the spore some of its resistance properties.

The cascade of protein expression in the developing forespore is complex, with multiple layers of regulation ensuring that the developmental process proceeds in the proper order to produce a viable spore. A simplified version of the cascade is illustrated in Fig. 31.6. Briefly, the cell receives a variety of inputs signalling a need to shift from vegetative growth to sporulation. Spo0A is phosphorylated, and together with σ^H, controls in part, at least, the switch from vegetative growth to sporulation and the formation of the asymmetric septum. Following this septation, σ^F is released from the anti-σ factor and becomes active in the forespore. One of the proteins (SpoIIR) required to convert pro-σ^E to active σ^E in the mother cell is encoded by a gene (spoIIR) transcribed in the forespore σ^F regulon. Thus σ^E is activated in the mother cell after σ^F activation in the forespore. Shortly after σ^E activation the forespore is engulfed by the mother cell, creating a free forespore within the mother cell cytoplasm. At this stage, σ^E (with the SpoIIID protein in some cases) directs the transcription of genes required early in production of the coat (cotE) and cortical layers of the spore, the gene encoding pro-σ^K (sigK), and some scavenging enzymes. In the forespore, the transcription of the gene encoding σ^G is initially directed by σ^F (once active, σ^G can direct transcription of its own gene), but this transcription is dependent on σ^E activity in the mother cell, again connecting development of the 2 compartments. Once active, σ^G controls the transcription of genes in its regulon, leading to the production of several forespore products (such as the SASPs) necessary for spore survival and germination. Active σ^G is also required for SpoIVB production, which in turn is needed for the conversion of pro-σ^K to active σ^K in the mother cell. σ^K (with GerE in some cases) directs the activation of a number of genes in the mother cell, causing the completion of the spore cortex and coat. Fig. 31.7 is an electron micrograph of a forespore within a mother cell late in sporulation, with the forespore surrounded by the cortex and coat.

7.2 Spore susceptibility to physical and chemical agents

The bacterial spore has long been known for its resistance properties. It was discovered independently by both Cohn and Koch in 1876: Cohn in studying the sterilization of hay infusions by boiling, and Koch in studying the bacilli causing anthrax (B. anthracis)

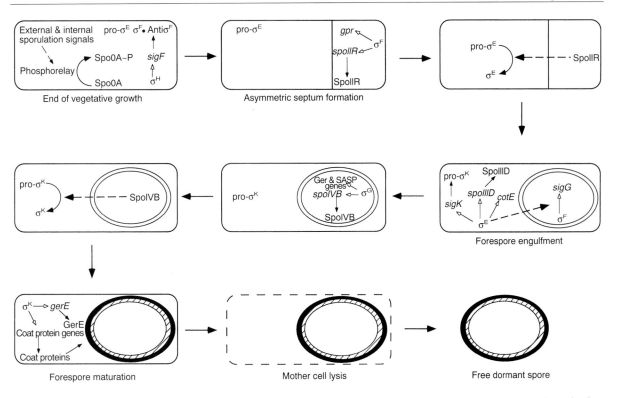

Fig. 31.6 Simplified step diagram of sporulation in *B. subtilis* from the end of vegetative growth to the formation of a free dormant spore. Arrows with unfilled heads denote transcriptional regulation; arrows with filled heads denote a direct connection; dashed arrows denote an indirect or multistep connection. See text for a detailed description of sporulation.

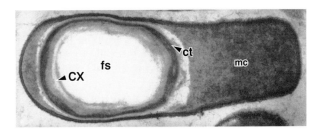

Fig. 31.7 Electron micrograph of sporulating *B. subtilis* cell with the forespore (fs) surrounded by the cortex (cx) and coat (ct) in the mother cell (mc). (From Beall et al. 1993, reproduced by permission of A Driks and the American Society for Microbiology).

(Keynan and Sandler 1983). The resistance properties of spores allow them to survive for long periods. Spores stored by Louis Pasteur were still viable 70 years later. Cano and Borucki (1995) have reported the revival of spores of an ancient *B. sphaericus* relative from the abdomen of bees preserved in amber for 25–40 million years. Modern day *B. sphaericus*, as well as other *Bacillus* spp., are commonly found in symbioses with bees. If the discovery of viable spores that have survived millions of years of dormancy is substantiated, it will be the microbial equivalent of discovering a viable dinosaur egg. The comparison of an ancient bacterium with its modern day counterparts may provide insights into the evolution of present day organisms.

Because of the extreme longevity of the spore, much effort has been expended to understand the mechanisms by which it is resistant to agents that kill most other bacteria and vegetatively growing cells of the spore-forming strains, and to finding ways of effectively killing spores during sterilization. The resistances of the spore to heat, irradiation and chemicals will be discussed below.

HEAT

In general, spores are 10^5 more resistant to heat than their vegetative cell counterparts (Slepecky 1992). There are many factors influencing the resistance of spores to heat, including: the particular species of *Bacillus*, the temperature at which the spores were formed, the type of heat (moist or dry), spore core mineralization, the production of α/β-type SASPs, and the spore core water content, which is believed to be maintained by the spore cortex (Gould 1983, Molin 1992, Slepecky 1992, Setlow 1994). In practice, spores can be killed by both dry and moist heat, and since spores are more resistant to heat than other cells, the killing of spores is often used as a biological indicator of successful sterilization. *B. stearothermophilus* is used as an indicator in moist heat sterilization, and *B. subtilis* var. *niger* as an indicator in dry heat sterilization (Greene 1992).

IRRADIATION

Spores are approximately 7–50 times more resistant to UV irradiation than are vegetatively growing cells (Setlow 1994). The forespore expressed α/β-type

SASPs mentioned above are essential for UV resistance. The SASPs are believed to bind to the DNA in the spore, changing its conformation and protecting it from the UV-induced formation of certain dimers, promoting the formation of a photoproduct repaired early in spore germination (Setlow 1994).

Spores are also more resistant to γ-irradiation than are vegetative cells (Gould 1983). The mechanism for this resistance is unknown, although it may parallel the formation of spore coat proteins rich in cystine (Setlow 1994). SASPs are not involved in the resistance of spores (Setlow 1994) to γ-irradiation. Due to their high resistances, *B. pumilus*, *B. cereus* and *B. sphaericus* are often used as biological indicators in monitoring the efficacy of ionizing radiation procedures (Greene 1992).

CHEMICALS

The increased resistance of spores to various chemical agents is believed to be due to the impermeability of the spore due to its spore coats, cortex and the membrane surrounding the spore core (Slepecky 1992, Setlow 1994). Chemical sterilization is used mainly when the materials to be sterilized are thermolabile or cannot be easily sterilized by other means; for example, glutaraldehyde is used to sterilize equipment (Bloomfield 1992). Active sporicidal agents include: glutaraldehyde and formaldehyde, chlorine, iodine, acids and alkali, and hydrogen peroxide and other peroxygen compounds. These agents require greater concentrations and times of contact to kill spores than to kill vegetative cells (Bloomfield 1992). Often the sporicidal activities can be increased by combining the sporicidal compounds. Mixes of formaldehyde and glutaraldehyde are 10 times more effective than either alone (Bloomfield 1992), and combinations of peracetic acid and hydrogen peroxide were found to be more effective than the individual compounds in sterilizing ultrafiltration membranes used in water treatment (Alasri et al. 1993).

8 PATHOGENICITY

8.1 *Bacillus anthracis*

B. anthracis is the aetiological agent of anthrax. The disease has afflicted domestic livestock and humans for millennia, and due to the survival of *B. anthracis* spores in the soil, will likely persist into the foreseeable future. Human anthrax results from a cutaneous infection in 90–95% of all cases (Hunter, Corbett and Grinden 1989). Ingestion and inhalation are alternative routes for the acquisition of human anthrax (Watson and Keir 1994). The vaccination of livestock has controlled outbreaks in industrialized countries, whereas anthrax continues to be a problem in less developed countries where vaccines are less widely used. In modern times, *B. anthracis* as a biological warfare agent has become a serious concern. It has been determined that 96 cases of human anthrax, resulting in 64 deaths in 1979, were a result of an accident at

a military facility in Sverdlovsk, in the former Soviet Union (Meselsen et al. 1994). Further information on *B. anthracis* and anthrax can be found in Volume 3 (see Volume 3, Chapter 40).

VIRULENCE FACTORS

B. anthracis possesses 2 main virulence factors: a poly-D-glutamic acid capsule and a tripartite toxin consisting of a protective antigen (PA, 82.7 kDa), an oedema factor (EF, 88.8 kDa) and the lethal factor (LF, 90.2 kDa) (Leppla 1988). The capsule and the tripartite toxin are both necessary for normal virulence of this bacterium. The capsule is thought to inhibit phagocytosis by leucocytes during infection (Green et al. 1985). Whereas the capsule protects the *B. anthracis*, the toxin components are thought to be responsible for oedema and death. Little is known about the specific mechanism(s) of toxicity in the cytosol mediated by the toxin components, although a mechanism has recently emerged for how the toxin components gain access to the cytosol.

The anthrax toxin is a unique member of the A-B family of toxins (e.g. cholera, diphtheria, tetanus, botulinum) (Gill 1978). A-B toxins contain 2 proteins. The A moiety is the actual cause of cell death, whereas the B moiety is required for the A moiety to cross the plasma membrane of the target cell. Unlike other A-B toxins, anthrax toxin contains 2 A moieties, EF and LF, each of which requires the B moiety, PA, to access the cytosol. EF and LF act in binary combination with PA to generate 2 independent toxic effects. As their names imply, PA-EF without LF results in gross local oedema, and PA-LF without EF results in death. The combination of all 3 act synergistically to cause oedema and death (Smith and Stoner 1967, Lincoln and Fish 1970).

The first step in the mechanism of anthrax toxin uptake (Fig. 31.8) is the attachment of PA to a specific cell surface receptor (Escuyer and Collier 1991), at which point PA is cleaved at the tetrabasic site (RKKR167: R, arginine; K, lysine) into 63 kDa (PA63) and 20 kDa (PA20) fragments, leaving PA63 bound to the receptor (Leppla 1991). Several proteases have been implicated in the cleavage of PA; furin, a subtilisin-like protease, has been shown to cleave PA (Molloy et al. 1992) and recently the prohormone convertases PC1 and PC2 were shown in vitro to be responsible for the majority of the PA-cleaving activity (Friedman 1995). The removal of the PA20 fragment from PA63 exposes a site on PA63 that can bind either EF or LF (Leppla 1991). The PA63 EF or LF complex is internalized by endocytosis into an endosome, where PA63 facilitates the crossing of EF or LF into the cytosol (Friedlander 1986, Gordon, Leppla and Hewlett 1988). It appears that both the proteolytic cleavage of PA and the acidic pH of the endosome are necessary for PA63 to assist EF and LF across the endosomal membrane (Blaustein et al. 1989, Milne and Collier 1993). Milne et al. (1994) have demonstrated that PA63 oligomerizes to form heptameric rings which appear to act as ion channels that EF and LF can utilize for translocation into the cytosol. Growing evidence indicates that the PA20 fragment is necessary to keep native PA in a water-soluble form and prevent it from binding effector molecules (Milne and Collier 1993). Once in the cytosol, EF and LF exert their toxic effects. EF is characterized as an adenylate cyclase which requires calmodulin as a cofactor (Leppla 1984). EF activity, resulting in increased levels of intracellular cyclic AMP in monocytes, is believed to cause accumulation of cytokines (interleukin-6 and tumour necrosis factor α) and contribute to localized oedema (Hoover et al. 1994). The lethal function of LF has recently been attributed to a zinc metallopeptidase activity (Klimpel, Arora and Leppla 1994). The protein or protein family that is the substrate of LF has yet to be identified.

ANTIBIOTIC TREATMENT

B. anthracis is generally sensitive to penicillins, therefore penicillin G is the first line of treatment against *B. anthracis* infections. Erythromycin and doxycycline are second choices of treatment. The first generation A cephalosporin and chloramphenicol are third lines of treatment (Chambers and Sande 1996).

GENETICS AND REGULATION OF VIRULENCE

Fully virulent strains of *B. anthracis* contain the 2 large plasmids pX01 and pX02 (Mikesell et al. 1983). Genes that encode all 3 toxin components are carried on pX01, and genes responsible for the poly-D-glutamic acid capsule are carried on pX02. Loss of either plasmid results in the loss of one of the 2 virulence factors, resulting in significant attenuation of virulence. The genes for PA, EF and LF, designated *pag*, *cya* and *lef*, respectively, have been cloned in *E. coli* (Vodkin and

Leppla 1983, Robertson and Leppla 1986, Mock et al. 1988) and their nucleotide sequences determined (Welkos et al. 1988, Robertson, Tippetts and Leppla 1988, Robertson and Bragg 1990). Insertion mutations have been made in each of the toxin genes, resulting in the loss of the corresponding toxin component (Pezard, Duflot and Mock 1993). Mutant strains with only one or 2 functional toxin components are making it possible to study the roles of the individual components. The region of pX02 required for capsule formation (*cap*) has also been cloned and sequenced (Makino et al. 1988, 1989). The *cap* region contains 3 putative structural genes necessary for encapsulation.

The first vaccine developed against anthrax by Pasteur in 1881 was a pX01–/pX02+ strain. The Pasteur vaccine was obtained by inadvertently heat curing the strain of pX01 by passsing the bacteria through chickens, which have an elevated body temperature in comparison to humans (Mikesell et al. 1983). However, the weak immunogenicity of the Pasteur strain most likely came from small numbers of fully virulent residual pX01+/pX02+ cells and not the cured strain (Farrar 1994). The Sterne vaccine is composed of pX01+/pX02–*B. anthracis* cells and therefore is not encapsulated but contains the 3 toxin components (Farrar 1994). The Sterne vaccine is widely used for veterinary vaccinations but remains slightly virulent, and therefore is not useful for human vaccinations. A non-encapsulated strain which produces high levels of PA is used for the primary human vaccination in the USA (Hambleton, Carman and Melling 1984).

B. anthracis cultured in vitro requires the addition of bicarbonate or serum for production of the polyglutamate capsule and for full production of the 3 toxin

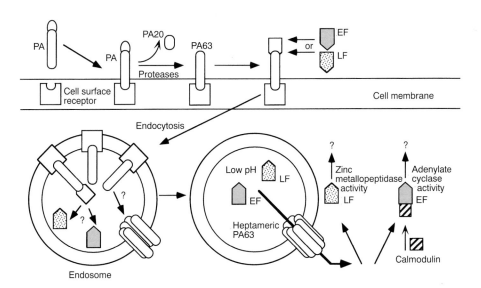

Fig. 31.8 Current model of anthrax toxin uptake and action. Protective antigen (PA) attaches to a cell surface receptor, subsequent proteolytic cleavage of PA removes a 20 kDa fragment (PA20), leaving a 63 kDA molecule (PA63) attached to the receptor. Removal of PA20 allows PA63 to interact with either oedema factor (EF) or lethal factor (LF) and eventually allows for the formation of a heptameric structure of PA63 monomers. The PA–EF and PA–LF complexes are internalized by receptor mediated endocytosis. The heptamer of PA63 molecules and low pH are thought to facilitate the crossing of EF and LF into the cytosol, but the mechanism of heptamer formation is unknown. Once EF and LF cross into the cytosol they assert their toxic effects, EF possessing adenylate cyclase activity (activated by calmodulin) and LF possessing zinc metallopeptidase activity. The specific targets of the toxins are not known. see p.717.

components. Bicarbonate regulation of the 3 anthrax toxin components appears to be accomplished by a positive *trans*-acting regulatory factor and an unknown negative regulatory factor. Strains carrying mutations obtained by insertion of the transposon Tn917 into pX01 were found to be deficient in synthesis of all 3 toxin components (Uchida et al. 1993). The strains deficient in toxin production were complimented by *atxA*, which indicated that this gene encoded a regulatory factor necessary for optimal expression of the toxin components. The *atxA* gene is located on pX01 between the *cya* and *pag* genes and encodes for AtxA, a protein with a predicted molecular weight of 55.7 kDa. An additional mutation made by Uchida et al. (1993) allowed all 3 toxin components to be produced in the absence of bicarbonate, indicating that a negative regulator is also involved in the regulation of the toxin component genes.

Sirard, Mock and Fouet (1994) have shown that the 3 toxin component genes are also regulated by temperature. Expression of these genes was found to be 4–6 times higher at 37°C than 28°C. The temperature dependence of the toxin components may help explain why cold-blooded animals are less susceptible to anthrax than warm-blooded animals.

8.2   *Bacillus cereus*

B. cereus is a causative agent of diarrhoeal and emetic food poisoning and of several clinical infections not related to gastroenteritis including endophthalmitis and other ocular infections, local wound infections, bacteraemia and septicaemia, central nervous system infections, endocarditis and pericarditis, and respiratory infections. Groups likely to be infected include imunocompromised individuals, intravenous drug users, and neonates (reviewed in Drobniewski 1993). In a 19 month study in an orthopaedic ward, *B. cereus* was isolated from 19 of 24 patients with postoperative or post-traumatic wounds (Åkesson, Hedström and Ripa 1991).

Toxins

B. cereus elaborates a number of toxins believed to play a role in its pathogenicity. The study of the toxins has focused on particular activities that the toxins possess, but it has proven difficult to assign those activities to single toxins. Instead, it has become apparent that at least some of the toxins are present in multicomponent complexes. Historically, the toxins have been broken down into 4 classes: the phospholipases C, the haemolysins, diarrhoeal enterotoxin and emetic toxin (Turnbull 1986). Recent studies have blurred the lines between the 4 classes, but for the sake of continuity, they will be presented here under the subgroups of toxins. A good review can be found in Drobniewski (1993).

Phospholipases C

The 3 enzymes in this toxin group have specificities for phosphatidylcholine, phosphatidylinositol and sphingomyelin. The phosphatidylinositol-specific phospholipase (34.5 kDa) does not require metal or divalent ions for activity and causes the release of some membrane proteins through the hydrolysis of their phosphatidylinositol-containing membrane anchor (Kuppe et al. 1989). Gilmore et al. (1989) demonstrated that the phosphatidylcholine hydrolase (23 kDa) and sphingomyelinase (29 kDa) are present in a cytolytic complex referred to as cereolysin AB. The phosphatidylcholine enzyme requires zinc for activity, whereas the sphingomyelinase requires divalent cations. The 2 enzymes act synergistically, causing haemolysis of erythrocytes.

Haemolysins

Cereolysin (not related to cereolysin AB), or haemolysin I, is a well characterized haemolysin of *B. cereus*. This thiol-activated haemolysin (49–59 kDa) belongs to the streptolysin O family of haemolysins. It is heat-labile, reversibly inactivated by oxygen, and is inactivated by preincubation with cholesterol, its membrane receptor. Another factor described as haemolysin II is said to be a thermolabile protein unaffected by cholesterol or antistreptolysin O antibody. Not much is known about this haemolysin, although Shinagawa et al. (1991) purified a mouse lethal toxin which was haemolytic to sheep erythrocytes and was unaffected by cholesterol, dithiothreitol and papain. Further study is required to determine whether the mouse lethal toxin will prove to be the elusive haemolysin II or a component of another toxin complex.

Diarrhoeal enterotoxin

The enterotoxin(s) causing diarrhoea have proven difficult to purify due to the large number of toxins produced by *B. cereus* and the various activities associated with the toxins. Toxins labelled diarrhoeagenic factor, mouse lethal factor, necrotic factor, vascular permeability factor and oedema factor have been partially or completely purified from *B. cereus* isolates causing diarrhoea and are increasingly considered to be part of an enterotoxin complex. Thompson et al. (1984) partially purified an enterotoxin complex with haemolytic activity. Granum and Nissen (1993) attempted to purify the components of the complex and found that one component was identical to sphingomyelinase (see section on 'Phospholipases C'). Beecher and Macmillan (1991) purified a haemolysin complex they termed haemolysin BL. The complex components B, L_1 and L_2 had molecular weights, isoelectric focusing points and biological activities consistent with those described earlier for the enterotoxin. The B component is required for binding to the target cell, followed by binding of the L components to give maximum haemolytic and vascular permeability activities. Subsequent sequencing of the gene encoding the B component revealed that it was the same as one of the components purified by Granum and Nissen (Heinrichs et al. 1993). Dermonecrotic activity of haemolysin BL was described by Beecher and Wong (1994). In addition, Beecher, Schoeni and Wong (1995) demonstrated enterotoxic activity by the haemolysin BL complex as shown by the accumulation of fluid in ligated rabbit ileal loops. Haemolysin BL is not inhibited by cholesterol and the activity formerly referred to as haemolysin II may be this enterotoxin complex (Beecher and Macmillan 1991).

Emetic toxin

Cereulide, a dodecadepsipeptide, was purified from a strain of *B. cereus* causing emetic food poisoning (Agata et al. 1994). Cereulide was shown to be a vacuolation factor of HEp-2 cells, an activity Hughes et al. (1988) correlated to emetic toxin activity. Cereulide is stable to trypsin, pepsin, heating to 121°C for 20 min, and low and high pH conditions (pH 2 and pH 12). Vomiting was induced in monkeys orally fed purified cereulide as well as partially pure vacuolation factor, suggesting cereulide is an emetic toxin (Shinagawa et al. 1995).

Although much is now known about the various toxins produced by *B. cereus*, not much is known about how the toxins affect non-gastrointestinal infections caused by the organism. It is presumed that the exotoxins and proteases produced by *B. cereus* are involved, but there is little evidence to support the production of a particular toxin or toxin complex with specific clinical diseases.

One toxin that has been implicated in non-gastrointestinal disease is haemolysin BL. When injected intravitreally in a rabbit model system, pure haemolysin BL caused endophthalmitis characteristic of *B. cereus* infection (Beecher et al. 1995). Toxicity was greater in crude extracts than with purified haemolysin, and inactivating haemolysin BL decreased, but did not eliminate, crude extract toxicity in vitro. The authors concluded that haemolysin BL contributes to multifactorial virulence in *B. cereus* ocular infections.

ANTIBIOTIC TREATMENT

B. cereus produces β-lactamases, making it resistant to penicillins and third generation cephalosporins such as cefotaxime. The species is usually sensitive to aminoglycosides, clindamycin, vancomycin, gentamicin, erythromycin and chloramphenicol. In reviewing cases of endocarditis caused by *B. cereus*, Steen et al. (1992) noted that some strains resistant to aminoglycosides, erythromycin and chloramphenicol were isolated, although most were still sensitive to clindamycin. Culturing the isolate and determining its susceptibilities may be useful in such cases. However, in ocular infections that are aggressive and can result in blindness within less than 24 h, immediate antimicrobial therapy is required. Combinations of clindamycin and gentamicin have been successful, as has vancomycin. Topical, systemic and intravenous antibiotic treatment may be necessary to deliver antibiotics to all parts of the eye (Drobniewski 1993). The fluoroquinolone compound, ciprofloxacin, has been successful in treating cases of recurrent pneumonia, bacteraemia, and local wound infection caused by *B. cereus* (Gascoigne et al. 1991, Kemmerly and Pankey 1993).

GENETICS AND REGULATION OF TOXIN EXPRESSION

Progress has been made in cloning some of the toxin genes from *B. cereus*. The genes encoding the components of cereolysin AB are found in tandem, with *cerA* encoding for the phosphatidylcholine phospholipase and *cerB* encoding the sphingomyelinase (Gilmore et al. 1989). The phosphatidylinositol phospholipase gene has also been cloned and found to be unlinked to the components of cereolysin AB (Kuppe et al. 1989). Heinrichs et al. (1993) cloned the *hblA* gene encoding for the B subunit of haemolysin BL. Another putative toxin gene, *bceT*, has been cloned into *E. coli* and conferred enterotoxin activities on *E. coli* lysates (Agata et al. 1995). Further work with purified protein encoded by the gene and demonstration of its presence in *B. cereus* culture supernatants is needed to confirm that *bceT* encodes an enterotoxin. Cloned toxin genes can be used to help produce large amounts of the various toxin components in order to study their biochemical properties further. As more toxin genes are cloned, it will be feasible to gain a better understanding of the regulation of toxin production and how it affects the pathogenicity of *B. cereus*.

Although it is not known whether the enterotoxin of *B. cereus* is preformed or produced in the gut upon infection, regulation studies have indicated that various growth medium properties influence diarrhoeal toxin production in laboratory cultures and dairy foods inoculated with *B. cereus* spores. Whereas starch enhances toxin production, high sugar levels and low pH levels do not support toxin production by *B. cereus* (Sutherland 1993, Sutherland and Limond 1993).

8.3 *Bacillus thuringiensis*

B. thuringiensis is noted for its use as a biocontrol agent for various insects including several disease vectors. Its toxicity to insect larvae is due to the production of insecticidal protein crystals made of δ-endotoxins (Fig. 31.9). The crystalline protein inclusions distinguish *B. thuringiensis* from its close relative, *B. cereus*, and the study of δ-endotoxin production and activity has been the centre of *B. thuringiensis* research.

TOXINS

The endotoxins have been classified into 5 groups (CryI, CryII, CryIII, CryIV and CryV) based on insecticidal and molecular properties (Höfte and Whiteley 1989, Tailor et al. 1992). Subclassifications (A, B, C etc.) were made based on sequence information.

The δ-endotoxins are made as precursor protoxins during the stationary phase while the cell is sporulating; crystal protoxin inclusions may account for 25% of the dry cell weight (Agaisse and Lereclus 1995). Upon ingestion by filter-feeding insect larvae, the crystal protoxins are solubilized in the alkaline larval midgut and converted into active toxin molecules. The toxins then bind to specific larval midgut receptors. The specificity of binding to receptors determines, in part, the larvae against which the toxins are active (reviewed in Aronson 1993). The correlation

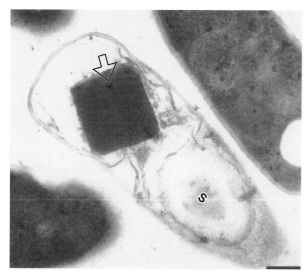

Fig. 31.9 Cell of *B. thuringiensis* containing a δ-endotoxin crystalline inclusion (arrow) and a forespore (S). (From Parry *et al.* 1983, reproduced by permission of I. Popiel and Wolfe Medical Publications Ltd.)

between larval toxicity and receptor binding is not perfect, however, and other factors such as crystal protein solubility have been implicated in determining insecticidal specificity (Aronson et al. 1991, Bradley et al. 1995). After successfully binding, the toxin molecules are believed to insert into the cell membrane and create an ion pore or channel leading to cell lysis.

A strain of *B. thuringiensis* may produce several protoxins which comprise the crystal inclusion. The production of a combination of protoxins extends the range of insects that the *B. thuringiensis* strain can affect. Chestukhina et al. (1994) have reported the identification of 8 different δ-endotoxins by a single strain of *B. thuringiensis*. Due to the insecticidal activity of the toxins, *B. thuringiensis* is attractive as a biocontrol agent to deplete populations of insect crop pests and human disease vectors such as mosquitoes. One strain, *B. thuringiensis israelensis*, has been effective against blackfly and mosquito larvae as it is toxic for vector species of *Aedes*, *Culex*, *Anopheles* and *Simulium* (Federici 1995). Although the search continues for new *B. thuringiensis* isolates with different insecticidal properties, the technology for introducing protoxin genes from one strain of *B. thuringiensis* to another (in order to broaden insect toxicity ranges) is being developed (Kalman et al. 1995). One limitation of using *B. thuringiensis* as an insecticide is that it is only effective as a larvicidal agent since it cannot penetrate the insect cuticle and is not ingested by adult insects (Federici 1995).

B. thuringiensis elaborates several other toxins, although none has been studied in as great detail as the δ-endotoxins. It produces a bacteriocin (termed thuricin) which attacks gram-positive bacteria (Favret and Yousten 1989), thuringiolysin (or haemolysin I), a second haemolysin (haemolysin II), and a β-exotoxin termed thuringiensin. Thuringiensin is a thermostable nucleotide analogue of ATP formed in some strains

of *B. thuringiensis* and causes extensive damage in the mosquito larval midgut (Weiser and Žiňka 1994).

B. thuringiensis has not been widely recognized as a human pathogen. However, it has become clear that *B. thuringiensis* has some of the same virulence factors as its close relative, *B. cereus*. One study found that among 14 strains of *B. thuringiensis* and 13 strains of *B. cereus*, haemolysin II (the haemolysin identified in *B. cereus* that is not inhibited by cholesterol) is actually more characteristic of *B. thuringiensis* than of *B. cereus* with 13 of 14 of the former and only 4 of 13 of the latter containing haemolysin II (Budarina et al. 1994). Another study, in which haemolysins were purified from both *B. cereus* and *B. thuringiensis*, demonstrated that the toxins (presumably cereolysin and thuringiolysin) behaved identically in immunological and biochemical assays (Honda et al. 1991). Because *B. thuringiensis* is not generally considered a human pathogen, it may be misidentified as *B. cereus* in cases of infection. Jackson et al. (1995) note such a case where isolates from an outbreak of gastroenteritis were presumptively identified as *B. cereus* and were later discovered to be *B. thuringiensis* when the isolates were stained for crystal proteins. These studies and others carry implications for the safety of using *B. thuringiensis* as an insecticidal agent, and more study is required in this area.

ANTIBIOTIC TREATMENT

As not much attention has been given to *B. thuringiensis* as a human pathogen, antibiotic susceptibilities have not been widely tested. As the species produces β-lactamases, the penicillins and cephalosporins are ineffective against *B. thuringiensis*. Antibiotic treatment effective for *B. cereus* should be applicable to this close relative.

GENETICS AND REGULATION OF TOXIN PRODUCTION

Most of the progress in *B. thuringiensis* genetics has been focused on the δ-endotoxins. The protoxin genes, or *cry* genes, are usually plasmid encoded. Some *B. thuringiensis* strains have several toxin encoding plasmids, some of which may be unstable (Aronson 1993). In addition, many *B. thuringiensis* transposable elements are near the protoxin genes, mostly on large conjugative plasmids (reviewed in Mahillon et al. 1994). In subspecies *B. thuringiensis israelensis* a single 112 kb plasmid encodes all 4 protoxin genes and a cytolytic factor, with at least 2 δ-endotoxins located near insertion sequences. The mobility of the transposable elements and the conjugative plasmids leads to the possibility of producing strains carrying a variety of protoxin genes.

Expression studies of the protoxin genes have revealed that some of the genes are transcribed by the *B. thuringiensis* homologues (σ^{35} and σ^{28}) of the *B. subtilis* sporulation σ factors, σ^{E} and σ^{K} (Adams, Brown and Whiteley 1991) and are expressed while the cell is sporulating. At least one protoxin gene, *cryIIIA*, is expressed at low levels prior to sporulation initiation and is activated at the end of exponential growth.

Table 31.3 *Bacillus* infections reported since 1960

Species	Clinical condition(s)	Reports or occurrence*
B. alvei	Sepsis, meningitis	+
B. anthracis	Anthrax	
	Cutaneous (eschar, malignant pustule)	++++
	Intestinal	++
	Pulmonary	+
	Meningitis (secondary to cutaneous)	+
B. brevis	Bacteraemia	+
B. cereus	Infected wounds, mild to severe, necrotic or gangrenous	++++
	Bovine mastitis	++++
	Bacteraemia or septicaemia, including drug abuse	+++
	Bovine abortion	+++
	Pneumonia, pleurisy, empyema, meningitis, endocarditis, osteomyelitis, panophthalmitis or endophthalmitis	+++
	Other (burns, ear infection, peritonitis, urinary tract infection)	+
	Food poisoning	++++
B. circulans	Wound infection, bacteraemia, septicaemia, abscesses	+++
	Meningitis	+
B. coagulans	Bacteraemia or septicaemia	+
B. licheniformis	Bacteraemia or septicaemia	+++
	Other (peritonitis, ophthalmitis, bovine toxaemia)	+
	Food poisoning	++++
B. macerans	Bacteraemia or septicaemia	+
B. pumilus	Food poisoning	++
	Rectal fistula	+
B. sphaericus	Bacteraemia, endocarditis, meningitis, pseudotumour	+
	Food poisoning	+
B. subtilis	Bacteraemia or septicaemia, endocarditis, respiratory infections	++
	Food poisoning	++++
B. thuringiensis	Wound, eye infection, bovine mastitis	+

+, One or two reports (of each clinical entity shown); ++, a few (≥2) reports; +++, several reports; ++++, many reports or frequent and regular occurrence now accepted.
Table modified from Turnbull, Kramer and Melling (1990) and updated from Turnbull and Kramer (1995).
*The majority of relevant reports can be found in Norris et al. (1981), Anonymous (1983), Parry, Turnbull and Gibson (1983), Chastel and Masure (1986), Kramer and Gilbert (1989), Drobniewski (1993), Granum, Brynstead and Kramer (1993).

When placed in *B. subtilis* to study expression, transcription of *cryIIIA* was independent of σ^E and σ^K (Agaisse and Lereclus 1994a). Sequence analysis revealed that the *cryIIIA* promoter resembles a promoter recognized by the vegetative 'housekeeping' σ factor (σ^A) of *B. subtilis* (Agaisse and Lereclus 1994b). Other factors such as mRNA stability, gene copy number and crystallization of the proteins also play a role in supporting the production of the large amounts of toxins in the inclusion crystals (see Agaisse and Lereclus 1995 for a review).

8.4 Other *Bacillus* pathogens

In general, most *Bacillus* spp. are considered to have little pathogenic potential to humans; however, several *Bacillus* spp. besides *B. anthracis* and *B. cereus* have

been implicated in human disease (Table 31.3). Many of these have been found in mixed infections or in infections of immunosuppressed patients. The *Bacillus* spp. are most often in infections as secondary invaders in association with other micro-organisms and act to exacerbate or maintain the infection (Norris et al. 1981).

The safety of the genus type strain, *B. subtilis*, and of *Bacillus amyloliquefaciens* has been reviewed by de Boer and Diderichsen (1991). They found these species to be non-invasive and safe except in a few cases of drug abusers or severely debilitated patients. *B. subtilis* has been reported in some cases of food poisoning (Kramer and Gilbert 1989), although it is readily consumed in large amounts in the Japanese food natto, which is prepared by fermenting soybeans with *B. subtilis natto* (Djien and Hesseltine 1979).

REFERENCES

Adams LF, Brown KL, Whiteley HR, 1991, Molecular cloning and characterization of two genes encoding sigma factors that direct transcription from a *Bacillus thuringiensis* crystal protein gene promoter, *J Bacteriol*, **173:** 3846–54.

Agaisse H, Lereclus D, 1994a, Expression in *Bacillus subtilis* of the *Bacillus thuringiensis cryIIIA* toxin gene is not dependent on a sporulation-specific sigma factor and is increased in a *spoOA* mutant, *J Bacteriol*, **176:** 4734–41.

Agaisse H, Lereclus D, 1994b, Structural and functional analysis of the promoter region involved in full expression of the *cryIIIA* toxin gene of *Bacillus thuringiensis*, *Mol Microbiol*, **13:** 97–107.

Agaisse H, Lereclus D, 1995, How does *Bacillus thuringiensis* produce so much insecticidal crystal protein?, *J Bacteriol*, **177:** 6027–32.

Agata N, Mori M et al., 1994, A novel dodecadepsipeptide, cereulide, isolated from *Bacillus cereus* causes vacuole formation in HEp-2 cells, *FEMS Microbiol Lett*, **121:** 31–4.

Agata N, Ohta M et al., 1995, The *bceT* gene of *Bacillus cereus* encodes an enterotoxic protein, *Microbiology*, **141:** 983–8.

Åkesson A, Hedström SÅ, Ripa T, 1991, *Bacillus cereus*: a significant pathogen in postoperative and post-traumatic wounds on orthopaedic wards, *Scand J Infect Dis*, **23:** 71.

Alasri A, Valverde M et al., 1993, Sporocidal properties of peracetic acid and hydrogen peroxide, alone and in combination, in comparison with chlorine and formaldehyde for ultrafiltration membrane disinfection, *Can J Microbiol*, **39:** 52–60.

Anderson GL, Simchock JM, Wilson KH, 1996, Identification of a region of genetic variability among *Bacillus anthracis* strains and related species, *J Bacteriol*, **178:** 377–84.

Anonymous, 1983, Bacillus cereus as a systemic pathogen, *Lancet*, **2:** 1469.

Arbige MV, Pitcher WH , 1989, Industrial enzymology: a look towards the future, *Trends Biotechnol*, **7:** 330–5.

Arbige MV, Bulthuis BA et al., 1993, Bacillus subtilis *and other gram-positive bacteria: biochemistry, physiology, and molecular genetics*, ed. Sonenshein AL , American Society for Microbiology, Washington, DC, 871–95.

Aronson AI, 1993, The two faces of *Bacillus thuringiensis*: insecticidal proteins and post-exponential survival, *Mol Microbiol*, **7:** 489–96.

Aronson AI, Han ES et al., 1991, The solubility of inclusion proteins from *Bacillus thuringiensis* is dependent upon protoxin composition and is a factor in toxicity to insects, *Appl Environ Microbiol*, **57:** 981–6.

Ash C, Collins MD, 1992, Comparative analysis of 23S ribosomal RNA gene sequences of *Bacillus anthracis* and emetic *Bacillus cereus* determined by PCR-direct sequencing, *FEMS Microbiol Lett*, **94:** 75–80.

Ash C, Priest FG, Collins MD, 1993, Molecular identification of rRNA group 3 bacilli (Ash, Farrow, Wallbanks and Collins) using a PCR probe test, *Antonie van Leeuwenhoek*, **64:** 253–60.

Ash C, Farrow JAE et al., 1991a, Comparative analysis of *Bacillus anthracis*, *Bacillus cereus*, and related species on the basis of reverse transcriptase sequencing of 16S rRNA, *Int J Syst Bacteriol*, **41:** 343–6.

Ash C, Farrow JAE et al., 1991b, Phylogenetic heterogeneity of the genus *Bacillus* revealed by comparative analysis of small-subunit ribosomal RNA sequences, *Lett Appl Microbiol*, **13:** 202–6.

Beall B, Driks A et al., 1993, Cloning and characterization of a gene required for assembly of the *Bacillus subtilis* sporecoat, *J Bacteriol*, **175:** 1705–16.

Beecher DJ, Macmillan JD, 1991, Characterization of the components of hemolysin BL from *Bacillus cereus*, *Infect Immun*, **59:** 1778–84.

Beecher DJ, Schoeni JL, Wong ACL, 1995, Enterotoxic activity of hemolysin BL from *Bacillus cereus*, *Infect Immun*, **63:** 4423–8.

Beecher DJ, Wong ACL, 1994, Improved purification and characterization of hemolysin BL, a hemolytic dermonecrotic vascular permeability factor from *Bacillus cereus*, *Infect Immun*, **62:** 980–6.

Beecher DJ, Pulido JS et al., 1995, Extracellular virulence factors in *Bacillus cereus* endophthalmitis: methods and implication of involvement of hemolysin BL, *Infect Immun*, **63:** 632–9.

Bella LA, Faust RM et al., 1985, Insecticidal bacilli, *Molecular Biology of the Bacilli*, vol. 2, ed. Dubnau, Academic Press, Orlando, FL, 186–210.

Berkeley RCW, Logan NA et al., 1984, Identification of *Bacillus* species, *Methods in Microbiology*, vol. 16, ed. Bergen T, Academic Press, London, 291–328.

Blaustein RO, Koehler TM et al., 1989, Anthrax toxins: channel-forming activity of protective antigen in planar phospholipid bilayers, *Proc Natl Acad Sci USA*, **86:** 2209–13.

Bloomfield SF, 1992, Resistance of bacterial spores to chemical agents, *Principles and Practice of Disinfection, Preservation, and Sterilization*, eds Russell AS, Hugo WB, Ayliffe GAJ, Blackwell Scientific Publications, Oxford, 230–45.

de Boer AS, Diderichsen B, 1991, On the safety of *Bacillus subtilis* and *B. amyloliquefaciens*: a review, *Appl Microbiol Biotechnol*, **36:** 1–4.

Bond WW, Favero MS et al., 1970, Dry-heat inactivation kinetics of naturally occurring spore populations, *Appl Microbiol*, **20:** 573–8.

Bradley D, Harkey MA et al., 1995, The insecticidal CryIB crystal protein of *Bacillus thuringiensis* has dual specificity to coleopteran and lepidopteran larvae, *J Invertebr Pathol*, **65:** 162–73.

Brown ER, Cherry WB, 1955, Specific identification of *Bacillus anthracis* by means of a variant bacteriophage, *J Infect Dis*, **96:** 34–9.

Budarina ZI, Sinev MA et al., 1994, Hemolysin II is more characteristic of *Bacillus thuringiensis* than *Bacillus cereus*, *Arch Microbiol*, **161:** 252–7.

Burbulys D, Trach KA, Hoch JA, 1991, Initiation of sporulation in *Bacillus subtilis* is controlled by a multicomponent phosphorelay, *Cell*, **64:** 545–52.

Cano RJ, Borucki MK, 1995, Revival and identification of bacterial spores in 25- to 40-million-year-old Dominican amber, *Science*, **268:** 1060–4.

Chambers HF, Sande MA, 1996, Antimicrobial agents: general considerations, *Goodman & Gilman's The Pharmacological Basis of Therapeutics*, eds Hardman JG, Limbird LE, McGraw-Hill, New York, 1029–56.

Chastel C, Masure O, 1986, Bactériémies, septicémies et infections diverses de *Bacillus licheniformis*, *Méd Mal Infect*, **4:** 226.

Chestukhina GG, Kostina LI et al., 1994, Production of multiple δ-endotoxins by *Bacillus thuringiensis*: δ-endotoxins produced by strains of the subspecies *galleriae* and *wuhanensis*, *Can J Microbiol*, **40:** 1026–34.

Clark S, Mandelstam J, 1980, Dissociation of an early event in sporulation from chromosome replication in *Bacillus subtilis*, *J Gen Microbiol*, **121:** 487–90.

Claus D, Berkeley RCW, 1986, Genus *Bacillus* Cohn 1872, *Bergey's Manual of Systematic Bacteriology*, vol. 2, eds Sneath PHA, Mair NS et al., Williams & Wilkins, Baltimore, 1105–39.

De Ley J, 1978, *Proceedings of the 4th International Conference on Plant Pathology and Bacteriology*, 347.

Demain AL, 1987, Production of nucleotides by microorganisms, *Economic Microbiology*, vol. 2, ed. Rose AH, Academic Press, London, 178–208.

Djien KS, Hesseltine CW, 1979, Tempe and related foods, *Economic Microbiology*, vol. 4, ed. Rose AH, Academic Press, London, 116–40.

Drobniewski FA, 1993, *Bacillus cereus* and related species, *Clin Microbiol Rev*, **6:** 324–38.

Errington J, 1993, *Bacillus subtilis* sporulation: regulation of gene expression and control of morphogenesis, *Microbiol Rev*, **57**: 1–33.

Errington J, 1996, Determination of cell fate in *Bacillus subtilis*, *Trends Genet*, **12**: 31–4.

Escuyer V, Collier RJ, 1991, Anthrax protective antigen interacts with a specific receptor on the surface of CHO-K1 cells, *Infect Immun*, **59**: 3381–6.

Farrar WE, 1994, Anthrax: virulence and vaccines, *Ann Intern Med*, **121**: 379–80.

Favret ME, Yousten AA, 1989, Thuricin: the bacteriocin produced by *Bacillus thuringiensis*, *J Invertebr Pathol*, **53**: 206–16.

Federici BA, 1995, The future of microbial insecticides as vector control agents, *J Am Mosq Control Assoc*, **11**: 260–8.

Friedlander AM, 1986, Macrophages are sensitive to anthrax lethal toxin through an acid-dependent process, *J Biol Chem*, **261**: 7123–6.

Friedman TC, Gordon VM et al., 1995, *In vitro* processing of anthrax toxin protective antigen by recombinant PC1 (SPC3) and bovine intermediate lobe secretory vesicle membranes, *Arch Biochem Biophys*, **316**: 5–13.

Gascoigne AD, Richards J et al., 1991, Successful treatment of *Bacillus cereus* infection with ciprofloxacin, *Thorax*, **46**: 220–1.

Gill DM, 1978, Seven toxin peptides that cross cell membranes, *Bacterial Toxins and Cell Membranes*, eds Jeljaszewicz J, Wadstrom T, Academic Press, New York, 291–332.

Gilmore MS, Cruz-Rodz AL et al., 1989, A *Bacillus cereus* cytolytic determinant, cereolysin AB, which comprises the phospholipase C and sphingomyelinase genes: nucleotide sequence and genetic linkage, *J Bacteriol*, **171**: 744–53.

Gordon RE, 1977, The genus *Bacillus*, *CRC Handbook of Microbiology*, 2nd edn, vol. 1, eds Laskin AI, Lechevalier HA, CRC Press, Cleveland, Ohio, 319–36.

Gordon RE, 1981, One hundred and seven years of the genus *Bacillus*, *The Aerobic Endospore-forming Bacteria: Classification and Identification*, eds Berkeley RCW, Goodfellow M, Academic Press, London, 1–16.

Gordon RE, Hayes WC, Pang CH-N, 1973, *The genus* Bacillus, United States Department of Agriculture, Agriculture Research Service, Agriculture Handbook no. 427, US Government Printing Office, Washington, DC, 2040.

Gordon VM, Leppla SH, Hewlett EL, 1988, Inhibitors of receptor-mediated endocytosis block entry of *Bacillus anthracis* adenylate cyclase toxin but not that of *Bordetella pertussis* adenylate cyclase, *Infect Immun*, **56**: 1066–9.

Gould GW, 1983, Mechanisms of resistance and dormancy, *The Bacterial Spore*, vol. 2, eds Hurst A, Gould GW, Academic Press, London, 173–209.

Granum PE, Brynstead S, Kramer JM, 1993, Analysis of enterotoxin production by *Bacillus cereus* from dairy products, food poisoning incidents and non-gastrointestinal infections, *Int J Food Microbiol*, **17**: 269–79.

Granum PE, Nissen H, 1993, Sphingomyelinase is part of the 'enterotoxin complex' produced by *Bacillus cereus*, *FEMS Microbiol Lett*, **110**: 97–100.

Green BD, Battisti L et al., 1985, Demonstration of a capsule plasmid in *Bacillus anthracis*, *Infect Immun*, **49**: 291–7.

Greene VW, 1992, Sterility assurance: concepts, methods and problems, *Principles and Practice of Disinfection, Preservation, and Sterilization*, eds Russell AD, Hugo WB, Ayliffe GAJ, Blackwell Scientific Publications, Oxford, 605–24.

Grossman AD, 1991, Integration of developmental signals and the initiation of sporulation in *Bacillus subtilis*, *Cell*, **65**: 5–8.

Grossman AD, Losick R, 1988, Extracellular control of spore formation in *Bacillus subtilis*, *Proc Natl Acad Sci USA*, **85**: 4369–73.

Haldenwang WG, 1995, The sigma factors of *Bacillus subtilis*, *Microbiol Rev*, **59**: 1–30.

Hambleton P, Carman JA, Melling J, 1984, Anthrax: the disease in relation to vaccines, *Vaccine*, **2**: 125–32.

Heinrichs JH, Beecher DJ et al., 1993, Molecular cloning and characterization of the *hblA* gene encoding the B component of hemolysin BL from *Bacillus cereus*, *J Bacteriol*, **175**: 6760–6.

Höfte H, Whiteley HR, 1989, Insecticidal crystal proteins of *Bacillus thuringiensis*, *Microbiol Rev*, **53**: 242–55.

Honda T, Shiba A et al., 1991, Identity of hemolysins produced by *Bacillus thuringiensis* and *Bacillus cereus*, *FEMS Microbiol Lett*, **79**: 205–10.

Hoover DL, Friedlander AM et al., 1994, Anthrax edema toxin differentially regulates lipopolysaccharide-induced monocyte production of tumor necrosis factor alpha and interleukin-6 by increasing intracellular cyclic AMP, *Infect Immun*, **62**: 4432–9.

Hughes S, Bartholomew B et al., 1988, Potential application of a HEp-2 cell assay in the investigation of *Bacillus cereus* emetic-syndrome food poisoning, *FEMS Microbiol Lett*, **52**: 7–12.

Hunter L, Corbett W, Grinden C, 1989, Anthrax, *J Am Vet Med Assoc*, **194**: 1028–31.

Jackson SG, Goodbrand RB et al., 1995, *Bacillus cereus* and *Bacillus thuringiensis* isolated in a gastroenteritis outbreak investigation, *Lett Appl Microbiol*, **21**: 103–5.

Jarnagin AS, Ferrari E, 1992, Extracellular enzymes: gene regulation and structure function relationship studies, *Biology of Bacilli: Applications to Industry*, eds Doi RE, McGloughlin M, Butterworth-Hoffman, Boston, 189–224.

Kalman S, Kiehne K et al., 1995, Enhanced production of insecticidal proteins in *Bacillus thuringiensis* strains carrying an additional crystal protein gene in their chromosomes, *Appl Environ Microbiol*, **61**: 3063–8.

Kemmerly SA, Pankey GA, 1993, Oral ciprofloxacin therapy for *Bacillus cereus* wound infection and bacteremia, *Clin Infect Dis*, **16**: 189.

Keynan A, Sandler N, 1983, Spore research in historical perspective, *The Bacterial Spore*, vol. 2, eds Hurst A, Gould GW, Academic Press, London, 2–49.

Klimpel KR, Arora N, Leppla SH, 1994, Anthrax toxin lethal factor contains a zinc metalloprotease consensus sequence which is required for lethal toxin activity, *Mol Microbiol*, **13**: 1093–100.

Kramer JM, Gilbert RJ, 1989, *Bacillus cereus* and other ' *Bacillus* species, *Foodborne Bacterial Pathogens*, ed. Doyle MP, Marcel Dekker, New York, 21–70.

Kuhnigk T, Borst EM et al., 1995, *Bacillus oleronius* sp. nov., a member of the hindgut flora of the termite *Reticultitermes santonensis* (Feytaud), *Can J Microbiol*, **41**: 699–706.

Kuppe A, Evans LM et al., 1989, Phosphatidylinositol-specific phospholipase C of *Bacillus cereus*: cloning, sequencing, and relationship to other phospholipases, *J Bacteriol*, **171**: 6077–83.

Leppla SH, 1984, *Bacillus anthracis* calmodulin-dependent adenylate cyclase: chemical and enzymatic properties and interactions with eucaryotic cells, *Advances in Cyclic Nucleotide and Protein Phosphorylation Research*, vol. 17, ed. Greengard P, Raven Press, New York, 189–98.

Leppla SH, 1988, Production and purification of anthrax toxin, *Methods Enzymol*, **165**: 103–16.

Leppla SH, 1991, The anthrax toxin complex, *Sourcebook of Bacterial Protein Toxins*, ed. Alouf J, Academic Press, New York, 277–302.

Lincoln RE, Fish DC, 1970, Anthrax toxin, *Microbial Toxins*, vol. 3, eds Montie TC, Kadis S, Ajl SJ, Academic Press, New York, 361–414.

Logan NA, Berkeley RCW, 1981, Classification and identification of members of the genus *Bacillus* using API tests, *The Aerobic Endospore-forming Bacteria: Classification and Identification*, eds Berkeley RCW, Goodfellow M, Academic Press, London, 104–40.

Logan NA, Berkeley RCW, 1984, Identification of *Bacillus* strains using the API system, *J Gen Microbiol*, **130**: 1871–82.

Maget-Dana R, Peypoux F, 1994, Iturins, a special class of pore-forming lipopeptides: biological and physicochemical properties, *Toxicology*, **87**: 151–74.

Mahillon J, Rezsöhazy R et al., 1994, IS*231* and other *Bacillus* *thuringiensis* transposable elements: a review, *Genetica*, **93**: 13–26.

Makino S, Sasakawa C et al., 1988, Cloning and CO$_2$-dependent expression of the genetic region for encapsulation from *Bacillus anthracis*, *Mol Microbiol*, **2**: 371–6.

Makino S, Uchida I et al., 1989, Molecular cloning and protein analysis of the *cap* region which is essential for encapsulation in *Bacillus anthracis*, *J Bacteriol*, **171**: 722–30.

Mandelstam J, Higgs SA, 1974, Induction of sporulation during synchronized chromosome replication in *Bacillus subtilis*, *J Bacteriol*, **120**: 38–42.

Margalit J, Dean D, 1985, The study of *Bacillus thuringiensis* var. *israelensis* (*B.t.i.*), *J Am Mosq Control Assoc*, **1**: 1–7.

Meselson M, Guillemin J et al., 1994, The Sverdlovsk anthrax outbreak of 1979, *Science*, **266**: 1202–8.

Meynell E, Meynell GG, 1964, The roles of serum and carbon dioxide in capsule formation by *Bacillus anthracis*, *J Gen Microbiol*, **34**: 153–64.

Mikesell P, Ivins BE et al., 1983, Evidence for plasmid-mediated toxin production in *Bacillus anthracis*, *Infect Immun*, **39**: 371–6.

Milne JC, Collier RJ, 1993, pH-dependent permeabilization of the plasma membrane of mammalian cells by anthrax protective antigen, *Mol Microbiol*, **10**: 647–53.

Milne JC, Deirdre F et al., 1994, Anthrax protective antigen forms oligomers during intoxication of mammalian cells, *J Biol Chem*, **269**: 20607–12.

Mock M, Labruyere E et al., 1988, Cloning and expression of the calmodulin-sensitive *Bacillus anthracis* adenylate cyclase in *Escherichia coli*, *Gene*, **64**: 277–84.

Moir A, Smith DA, 1990, The genetics of bacterial spore germination, *Annu Rev Microbiol*, **44**: 531–53.

Molin G, 1992, Destruction of bacterial spores by thermal methods, *Principles and Practice of Disinfection, Preservation, and Sterilization*, eds Russell AD, Hugo WB, Ayliffe GAJ, Blackwell Scientific Publications, Oxford, 499–511.

Molloy SS, Bresnahan PA et al., 1992, Human furin is a calcium-dependent serine endoprotease that recognizes the sequence Arg-X-X-Arg and efficiently cleaves anthrax toxin protective antigen, *J Biol Chem*, **267**: 16396–402.

van Netten P, Kramer JM, 1992, Media for the detection and enumeration of *Bacillus cereus* in foods: a review, *Int J Food Microbiol*, **17**: 85–99.

Norris JR, Berkeley RCW et al., 1981, The genera *Bacillus* and *Sporolactobacillus*, *The Prokaryotes: a Handbook on Habitats, Isolation and Identification of Bacteria*, vol. 2, eds Starr MP, Stolp H et al., Springer-Verlag, Berlin, 1711–42.

Parry JM, Turnbull PCB, Gibson JR, 1983, *A Color Atlas of Bacillus species*, Wolfe Medical Atlases, Series no. 19, Wolfe Medical Publishers, London.

Pezard C, Duflot E, Mock M, 1993, Construction of *Bacillus anthracis* mutant strains producing a single toxin component, *J Gen Microbiol*, **139**: 2459–63.

Priest FG, 1989, Isolation and identification of aerobic endospore-forming bacteria, Bacillus, Biotechnology Handbooks, vol. 2, ed. Harwood CR, Plenum Press, New York, 27–56.

Priest FG, 1993, Systematics and ecology of *Bacillus*, Bacillus subtilis *and other gram positive bacteria: biochemistry, physiology, and molecular genetics*, eds Sonenshein AL, Hoch JA, Losick R, American Society for Microbiology, Washington, DC, 3–16.

Roberts TA, Ingram M, Skulberg A, 1965, The resistance of spores of *Clostridium botulinum* type E to heat and radiation, *J Appl Bacteriol*, **28**: 125–41.

Robertson DL, Bragg TS, 1990, Nucleotide sequence of the lethal factor (*lef*) and edema factor (*cya*) genes from *Bacillus anthracis*: elucidation of the EF and LF functional domains, *Salisbury Med Bull*, **Special Supplement 68**: 59.

Robertson DL, Leppla SH, 1986, Molecular cloning and expression in *Escherichia coli* of the lethal factor gene of *Bacillus anthracis*, *Gene*, **44**: 71–8.

Robertson DL, Tippetts MT, Leppla SH, 1988, Nucleotide sequence of the *Bacillus anthracis* edema factor gene (*cya*): a calmodulin-dependent adenylate cyclase, *Gene*, **73**: 363–71.

Rodel W, Lucke FK, 1990, Effect of redox potential on *Bacillus subtilis* and *Bacillus licheniformis* in broth and in pasteurized sausage mixtures, *Int J Food Microbiol*, **3–4**: 291–301.

Schleifer KH, Kandler O, 1972, Peptidoglycan types of bacterial cell walls and their taxonomic implications, *Bacteriol Rev*, **36**: 407–77.

Setlow P, 1994, Mechanisms which contribute to the long-term survival of spores of *Bacillus* species, *Fundamental and Applied Aspects of Bacterial Spores*, Society for Applied Bacteriology, Symposium Series, no. 23, eds Gould GW, Russell AD, Stewart-Tull DES, Blackwell Scientific Publications, Oxford, 49S–60S.

Shinagawa K, Ichikawa K et al., 1991, Purification and some properties of a *Bacillus cereus* mouse lethal toxin, *J Vet Med Sci*, **53**: 469–74.

Shinagawa K, Konuma H et al., 1995, Emesis of rhesus monkeys induced by intragastric administration with the HEp-2 vacuolation factor (cereulide) produced by *Bacillus cereus*, *FEMS Microbiol Lett*, **130**: 87–90.

Silo-Suh LA, Lethbridge BJ et al., 1994, Biological activities of two fungistatic antibiotics produced by *Bacillus cereus* UW85, *Appl Environ Microbiol*, **60**: 2023–30.

Sirard JC, Mock M, Fouet A, 1994, The three *Bacillus anthracis* toxin genes are coordinately regulated by bicarbonate and temperature, *J Bacteriol*, **176**: 5188–92.

Slepecky RA, 1992, What is a *Bacillus*?, *Biology of Bacilli: Applications to Industry*, eds Doi RE, McGloughlin M, Butterworth-Hoffman, Boston, 1–22.

Sleytr UB, Messner P, 1983, Crystalline surface layers on bacteria, *Annu Rev Microbiol*, **37**: 311–39.

Smith H, Stoner HB, 1967, Anthrax toxin complex, *Fed Proc*, **26**: 1554–7.

Smith NR, Gordon RE, Clark FE, 1952, *Aerobic Spore-forming Bacteria*, US Department of Agriculture, Agriculture Monograph, no. 16, US Government Printing Office, Washington, DC.

Sonenshein AL, 1989, Metabolic regulation of sporulation and other stationary-phase phenomena, *Regulation of Prokaryotic Development: a Structural and Functional Analysis*, eds Smith I, Slepecky RA, Setlow P, American Society for Microbiology, Washington, DC, 109–30.

Stackebrandt E, Ludwig W et al., 1987, Comparative 16S rRNA oligonucleotide analysis and murein types of round-spore-forming bacilli and non-spore-forming relatives, *J Gen Microbiol*, **133**: 2523–9.

Stapp C, Zycha H, 1931, Morphologische Untersuchungen an *Bacillus mycoides*; ein Beitrag zur Frage des Pleomorphismus der Bakterien, *Arch Mikrobiol*, **2**: 493–536.

Steen MK, Bruno-Murtha LA et al., 1992, *Bacillus cereus* endocarditis: report of a case and review, *Clin Infect Dis*, **14**: 945–6.

Sutherland AD, 1993, Toxin production by *Bacillus cereus* in dairy products, *J Dairy Res*, **60**: 569–74.

Sutherland AD, Limond AM, 1993, Influence of pH and sugars on the growth and production of diarrhoeagenic toxin by *Bacillus cereus*, *J Dairy Res*, **60**: 575–80.

Tailor R, Tippett J et al., 1992, Identification and characterization of a novel *Bacillus thuringiensis* δ-endotoxin entomocidal to coleopteran and lepidopteran larvae, *Mol Microbiol*, **6**: 1211–17.

Thompson NE, Ketterhagen MJ et al., 1984, Isolation and some properties of an enterotoxin produced by *Bacillus cereus*, *Infect Immun*, **43**: 887–94.

Turnbull PCB, 1986, Pharmacology of bacterial protein toxins, *International Encyclopedia of Pharmacology and Therapeutics*, section 119, eds Dorner F, Drews J, Pergamon Press, Oxford, 397–448.

Turnbull PCB, Kramer JM, 1995, *Bacillus, Manual of Clinical Microbiology*, 6th edn, ed. Murray P, American Society for Microbiology, Washington, DC, 349–56.

Turnbull PCB, Kramer JM, Melling J, 1990, *Bacillus, Topley &*

Wilson's Principles of Bacteriology, Virology and Immunity, 8th edn, vol. 2, eds Parker MT, Collier LH, Edward Arnold, London/BC Decker, Philadelphia, 187–210.

Uchida I, Hornung JM et al., 1993, Cloning and characterization of a gene whose product is a *trans*-activator of anthrax toxin synthesis, *J Bacteriol*, **175:** 5329–38.

Vodkin MH, Leppla SH, 1983, Cloning of the protective antigen gene of *Bacillus anthracis*, *Cell*, **34:** 693–7.

Watson A, Keir D, 1994, Information on which to base assessments of risk from environments contaminated with anthrax spores, *Epidemiol Infect*, **113:** 479–90.

Weiser J, Žiňka Z, 1994, Effect of *Bacillus thuringiensis* beta exotoxin on ultrastructures of midgut cells of *Culex sitiens*, *Cytobios*, **77:** 19–27.

Welkos SL, Lowe JR et al., 1988, Sequence analysis of the DNA encoding protective antigen of *Bacillus anthracis*, *Gene*, **69:** 287–300.

Zukowski MM, 1992, Production of commercially valuable products, *Biology of Bacilli: Applications to Industry*, eds Doi RE, McGloughlin M, Butterworth-Hoffman, Boston, 311–37.

Chapter 32

CLOSTRIDIUM: THE SPORE-BEARING ANAEROBES

C L Hatheway and E A Johnson

1 GENUS DEFINITION

The organisms are anaerobic or aerotolerant rods, producing endospores which are usually wider than the vegetative organisms in which they arise, giving the spindle shapes, the so-called **clostridium forms**. They generally stain gram-positive, but strains failing to show positive reaction possess the gram-positive cell wall structure, devoid of an outer membrane. They often vigorously decompose proteins and often ferment carbohydrates, but do not carry out a dissimilatory sulphate reaction. Many species produce antigens with biological activity, some of which are lethal to animals, and are responsible for the pathogenicity of the organisms. The G + C content of DNA is 26–32 mol%, but some species presently included in the genus have G + C contents of 38–56 mol%. The type species is *Clostridium butyricum*.

2 HISTORICAL BACKGROUND

In 1861, Pasteur discovered **anaerobiosis** by noting that butyric fermentation occurred in the absence of oxygen, due to a rod-shaped organism which he called *Vibrion butyrique*, which possibly corresponds to *Clostridium butyricum* (Pasteur 1861a,b, 1863a,b, Willis 1969). Thus, the first known anaerobe was probably *C. butyricum*, and this is the organism that serves as the type species for the genus *Clostridium*. In 1875, Bollinger observed that the disease of livestock known as blackleg (Rauschbrand, charbon symptomatique) was distinct from anthrax and was caused by a different organism (Bollinger 1875). The causative organism, now known as *C. chauvoei*, was described by Feser (1876), and cultured in artificial liquid medium by Arloing, Cornevin and Thomas (1880). In 1877, Pasteur discovered *C. septicum* which he called *Vibrion septique* (Pasteur and Joubert 1877). The organism, originating in the intestinal tract, appeared in the blood of animals which had died of anthrax. The blood samples had been taken at post mortem intervals after which the anthrax bacillus had disappeared from the blood, and investigators were troubled by the unexpected symptoms in animals injected with the samples in an attempt to reproduce the anthrax. Pasteur explained that upon death of the animal, the aerobic anthrax bacillus died from lack of oxygen, but the anaerobic conditions favoured the anaerobic *Vibrion*.

Although tetanus had been known since ancient times, the causative agent, *C. tetani*, was not discovered until 1884 (Kobel and Marti 1985). *C. perfringens* was isolated from a patient who had died of tuberculosis in 1892 (Welch and Nuttall 1892). *C. novyi* was discovered in an extract of milk protein after it was injected into guinea-pigs and caused severe pathology and deaths (Novy 1894). The organism was recovered from the dead guinea-pigs and found to be distinct from the earlier pathogenic anaerobes. Botulism, like tetanus, had been known for a long time before its aetiology was elucidated. In 1897 van Ermengem published the findings from his thorough investigation of a large outbreak of botulism in Ellezelles, Belgium. He showed that he illness was due to a potent toxin in the food, produced by an anaerobic bacterium which he isolated, characterized and named *Bacillus botulinus* (Van Ermengem 1897).

In 1902, Tissier isolated *C. bifermentans* from putrefying meat (Tissier and Martelly 1902). The name applied at that time, *Bacillus bifermentans*, was chosen because this was the first anaerobe noted with the capacity to degrade both proteins and carbohydrates. This organism is non-pathogenic, but a similar, pathogenic organism was isolated from human gas gangrene cases 20 years later by Sordelli (1922); the organism is known as *C. sordellii*. In 1935, Hall and O'Toole reported on a new anaerobic spore-forming organism (*C. difficile*) from 4 of 10 infants during the first 10 days of life (Hall and O'Toole 1935). Although the infants showed no illness, pure cultures of the isolates were pathogenic when injected into guinea-pigs.

Clostridial wound infections have been of particular concern because of their association with **gas gangrene** (clostridial myositis), especially in those occurring on the battlefield (MacLennan 1962). The pathology is due to the action or interaction on the tissues of one or more of the soluble serologically recognizable toxins produced by the infecting organisms. Among the species involved in this malady, *C. perfringens* has been found most frequently. It was a surprise to find this same organism involved in a rather common, relatively mild enteric disturbance (food-borne illness) due to an enterotoxin which it produces in addition to its previously recognized toxins (McClung 1945).

Early on, the organisms were classified in the genus *Bacillus* because of their cylindrical shape, but in 1880 a new genus, *Clostridium*, described by Prazmowski (Cato and Stackebrandt 1989), was proposed for the anaerobic spore-forming organisms. The early discoveries were prompted by an interest in microbial diseases and problems with food spoilage. The definition of the genus subsequently was found to accommodate many organisms isolated from the environment that have no obvious role in human or animal disease. Many of these organisms are of biotechnological interest because of their ability to convert readily available substrates into commercially and industrially important organic solvents, acids and other compounds. Recent studies using newer techniques show that the genus contains a rather diverse collection of organisms.

3 CLASSIFICATION

Classification of bacteria has been carried out or proposed on the basis of morphology, disease association, pathogenicity, toxigenicity, source of isolation, physiological and metabolic characteristics, staining reactions, serologic properties, DNA relatedness and ribosomal RNA gene sequence homology.

Bergey's Manual of Systematic Bacteriology (Cato, George and Finegold 1986) lists 83 species in the genus *Clostridium*. Seventy-five species are listed by the International Committee on Systematic Bacteriology in the Approved Lists of Bacterial Names (Skerman, McGowan and Sneath 1989). An additional 46 species names have been added to the list and 3 deleted in a recent update (Moore and Moore 1992), for a total of 118 official *Clostridium* species. The diversity in the nucleotide base composition of the DNA among the species has made it obvious that the genus would have to be subdivided into at least 2 genera (Cato, George and Finegold 1986). The diversity of organisms classified as clostridia has been further emphasized by 16S rRNA gene homology studies (Collins et al. 1994).

In a study comparing mol% G+C content of DNA and 23 S rRNA homologies of 56 species of *Clostridium* (Johnson and Francis 1975), 4 groups were established. Three homology groups were seen among the low G + C strains (22–33%), and the high G + C strains (41–45%) formed another (Table 32.1). The first group included 47 strains of 33 species (most of the pathogenic clostridia; 22–29% G+C). The RNA from these organisms competed to the extent of 50% or more with labelled RNA from one or more of the reference strains *C. butyricum*, *C. perfringens*, *C. carnis*, *C. sporogenes*, *C. novyi* type A and *C. pasteurianum*. Subgroups which contained organisms with compatible characteristics were established within group I on the basis of either a very high homology with a given reference RNA or on the pattern of homologies with the 6 reference RNA preparations in the study. Group II contained 1 strain of each of 11 species (26–29% G+C) including *C. tetani* and *C. sordellii* of clinical interest. These strains had a range in homology of 69–89% with the 23S rRNA preparation of *C. lituseburense*. Group III included a total of 7 strains from 6 species (26–33% G+C), which showed little relationship with each other, or any of the reference strains in the genus on the basis of 23S rRNA homology. Group IV included 13 strains of 5 species that share high (41–45%) G+C content, but little relationship by rRNA homology.

A recent analysis of the 16S rRNA gene sequences of 129 clostridia and 69 representative species of other low G + C content gram-positive genera was undertaken in an attempt to resolve the taxonomic discrepancies (Collins et al. 1994). The resulting dendrogram was subdivided into 19 clusters. Most of the species of medical interest were contained in cluster I which is equivalent to rRNA group I of Johnson and Francis (1975) (see Fig. 32.1). In cluster I, one can see the close grouping of similar organisms such as the nonproteolytic strains of *C. botulinum*, and elsewhere, the proteolytic strains, linked with *C. sporogenes*. The close similarity between *C. argentinense* (*C. botulinum* type G) and *C. subterminale* is apparent, but *C. hastiforme* which is rather difficult to distinguish from *C. subterminale* on the basis of phenotypic characteristerics is separated by a long distance, in cluster XII. More recently, it has been established that *C. hastiforme* is identical with *Tissierella (Bacteroides) praeacuta* on the basis of 16S rRNA gene sequence analysis (Farrow et al. 1995); only one base difference was found in a sequence of 1475 nucleotides.

Table 32.1 *Clostridium* species groups of Johnson and Francis (1975) (modified)

Group	Subgroup	%G + C
Group I		
C. butyricum	I-A	28
C. pseudotetanicum		27
C. beijerinckii		25
C. botulinum type B (NP)		27–29
C. botulinum type E (NP)		27–29
C. botulinum type F (NP)		27–29
C. aurantibutyricum	I-B	27
C. paraputrificum		26
C. paraperfringens		28
C. perfringens A	I-C	24
C. perfringens B		25
C. perfringens C		26
C. perfringens D		27
C. plagarum		25
C. perenne	I-D	25
C. carnis		28
C. sartagoformum		28
C. chauvoei		27
C. septicum		21
C. scatologenes		27
C. fallax	I-E	26
C. sporogenes	I-F	26–28
C. botulinum type A (P)		26
C. botulinum type B (P)		29
C. botulinum type F (P)		26
C. putrificum		27
C. oceanicum	I-G	23
C. cadaveris		27
C. botulinum type C	I-H	26–28
C. botulinum type D		27
C. haemolyticum		26
C. novyi type A		29
C. novyi type B		26
C. novyi type C		27
C. lentoputrescens	I-J	27
C. pasteurianum		26
C. acetobutylicum		28
C. tyrobutyricum		28
C. malenominatum	I-K	28
C. subterminale		28
C. histolyticum		–
C. argentinense		28–30
C. limosum		24
Group II		
C. lituseburense		27
C. tertium		28
C. ghoni		27
C. sordellii		26
C. bifermentans		27
C. tetani		26
C. cellobioparum		28
C. rectum		26

Group	Subgroup	%G + C
C. cochlearium		28
C. glycolicum		29
C. mangenoti		–
Group III		
C. ramosum		26
C. propionicum		–
C. sticklandii		31
C. sporospheroides		27
C. aminovalericum		33
C. thermosaccharolyticum		32
Group IV		
C. innocuum		43–44
C. sphenoides		41
C. indolis		44
C. barkeri		45
C. oroticum		44

Several other important pathogens are included in other clusters: *C. histolyticum* is in cluster II, and *C. difficile* and *C. sordellii* are in cluster XI, which contains the organisms of Johnson and Francis group II (except for *C. tetani*, which is solidly within cluster I). This chapter deals with the organisms of medical and veterinary importance heretofore classified as *Clostridium* species, and these organisms are found in 16S rRNA clusters I, II and XI.

4 HABITAT

The clostridia are widely distributed in nature, but they seem to have 2 principal habitats, the soil and the intestine of animals (Smith and Williams 1984). Some of them appear to be common inhabitants of the intestinal canal of humans and animals. In a review of the literature, 38 species have been found in human faeces (George and Finegold 1985). Among the most frequently found are *C. perfringens*, *C. tetani*, *C. sporogenes*, *C. tertium*, *C. paraputrificum*, *C. putrificum*, *C. bifermentans* and *C. difficile*. *C. perfringens* has been found in almost every soil sample in which it was actively sought (Smith and Williams 1984). *C. difficile* is commonly present in the faeces of infants, but is infrequent and sparse in healthy adult faeces. *C. tetani* is found in most soils world wide that have been surveyed. It has been held by some that the intestinal canal is the main habitat of many of the clostridia and that their presence in the soil is due to faecal contamination. It is more likely that the primary habitat of most anaerobes is the soil; that they are ingested frequently with vegetable foods; and that some of them have adapted themselves temporarily or permanently to a life in the intestinal canal. They frequently appear in dust, milk and sewage. Though they usually lead a saprophytic existence, some species are causally related to well recognized diseases in humans and ani-

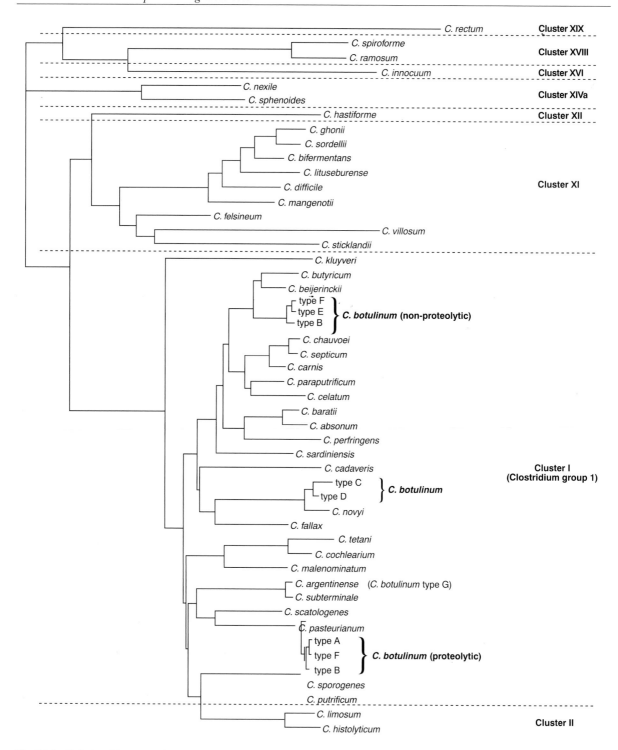

Fig. 32.1 Relationship of medically important *Clostridium* species based on 16S rRNA gene sequences. Data from Collins et al. (1994). Dendrogram for selected species provided by Paul A. Lawson, Institute for Food Research, Reading, UK.

mals. It is with the pathogenic species, and those found in close association with humans and animals, that we are most concerned with here.

5 PHYSICAL FEATURES

5.1 Morphology

Many of the clostridia are so pleomorphic that their

identification on a morphological basis is difficult. The morphology of a strain varies widely, both within and between cultures. Photomicrographs of smears and wet mounts of some representative species are seen in Fig. 32.2 and Plate 32.2.

Like the aerobic spore-bearing bacilli, they are large, rod-shaped organisms. In length they range from about 3 μm to 7–8 μm, but long filamentous forms are common. Their breadth ranges from about 0.4 to 1.2 μm. The vegetative bacilli are straight or curved, their sides parallel, and their ends rounded or somewhat truncated. Most are arranged singly, but some occur in pairs or in chains, others in bundles the members of which are arranged parallel to each other. Irregular forms include navicular, or boat-shaped, organisms; citron forms shaped like a lemon with a small knob at each end; large swollen, non-sporing rods; snake-like filaments; deeply stained bulb-shaped types: and a great variety of so-called involution forms varying both in shape and in depth of staining. Autolysis frequently sets in when sporulation begins so that shadow forms are numerous particularly in certain species. L-forms occur in clostridia, including *C. tetani* (Willis 1969).

5.2   Staining reactions

All members stain readily with the usual dyes. Great irregularity is noticeable in the depth of staining, especially in cultures more than a day or 2 old. Sometimes metachromatic granules or points of more intense colouration are seen, especially when acetone is used for decolorization. In young cultures, the bacilli are all gram-positive. Some species rapidly lose this property, and some are readily decolourized by the ethanol. In the early stages of spore formation, the position of the spore is often marked by an area of intense staining; as it matures, however, the spore presents a colourless centre surrounded by a peripherally stained ring. For initial visualization of the organisms in the diagnostic laboratory, Gram's stain is most commonly used. The clostridia are considered gram-positive organisms, although many strains show the positive (violet) staining reaction only in young cultures (less than 18 h), and sometimes identification has to be made without this observation. Often, gram-stained smears of pure cultures reveal a mixture of positive and negative organisms. Note Gram stains of *C. perfringens* and *C. difficile* (panels k and n, respectively, in Fig. 32.2 and Plate 32.2); also, the cells of *C. botulinum* containing spores in panel b are gram-positive, while those without spores are gram-negative.

5.3   Spores

Sporulation is common to all members, but there is considerable variation in the readiness with which it occurs. *C. sporogenes*, for example, spores readily on all media; *C. perfringens* only in particular media (Duncan and Strong 1968, Sacks and Thompson 1978). All the pathogenic members are able to form spores in the animal body, though *C. perfringens* does so rarely in the tissues; however, extensive sporulation of ingested vegetative organisms in the intestine, concurrently with the release of enterotoxin, appears to be involved in *C. perfringens* food-borne diarrhoea (Hauschild, Niilo and Dorward 1967). The spores of most members are wider than the vegetative bacilli; they therefore confer on the organism a distinctive appearance according to the position in which they arise. When they are formed at the equator the clostridium is spindle-shaped; when subterminally, club-shaped; with

an oval terminal spore the organism may look like a tennis racket; with a spherical terminal spore like a drumstick. Spores are easily visualized on a gram-stained smear, or by phase-contrast illumination of a wet mount (see Fig. 32.2 and Plate 32.2). Special spore stains are not necessary. Sporulation of clostridia has been reviewed by Woods and Jones (1986) and Setlow and Johnson (1997).

Spores of most pathogenic species can be produced in chopped meat broth or agar (Holdeman, Cato and Moore 1977) or in clear, complex media such as trypticase–peptone–glucose–yeast extract (TPGY) broth. Spores can be purified to over 99% purity by density gradient centrifugation from the clear media (Kihm et al. 1988). The clostridial spore released from the mother cell is structurally distinct from the vegetative cell. The outermost spore layer, the **exosporium**, varies among species, but is prominent in many pathogenic clostridia including *C. botulinum* (Setlow and Johnson 1997). Underlying the exosporium are the **spore coats**, consisting of unusual structural proteins. The central region of the spore, or the core, contains the spore's DNA, ribosomes, most of the enzymes, and deposits of divalent cations. The metal content of purified *C. botulinum* spores is different from metals in *Bacillus* (Kihm et al. 1988). Proteolytic strains of *C. botulinum* can produce spores of high heat resistance and are the most important spore-former in public health safety of thermally processed foods.

The clostridia are classifiable according to the shape of the spore and its position in the rod: those with (1) an equatorial or subterminal spore; (2) an oval terminal spore (racket form); and (3) a spherical terminal spore (drumstick form). The division is useful, but must not be used too rigidly. It is common, for instance, to find organisms that usually form subterminal spores giving rise to strictly terminal spores: and it may be hard to distinguish a spherical from an oval subterminal spore.

Spores are resistant to exposure to oxygen and chemical agents, heating and drying,. The spores of some strains of some species, e.g. *C. botulinum* and *C. sporogenes* will remain viable after boiling in aqueous media for more than 1 h. This is the reason that spoilage and food-borne illness sometimes occur with foods that have been heat processed. The heat resistance of spores is often used to advantage in isolation of clostridia from mixed cultures.

The germination of spores depends on a number of factors. For example, for germination of *C. perfringens*, the optimal pH is 6.0 at a temperature of 30°, and preliminary heat activation at 75° for 20 min is required (Willis 1990). Heat-shock of bacterial spore suspensions is widely used to initiate germination, while resistance of spores to ethanol is used for so called alcohol-shock treatment which merely destroys vegetative forms (Koransky, Allen and Dowell 1978). Cooked meat medium containing 0.2 % soluble starch (CMGS) is recommended for recovery of sporulated clostridia (Dowell et al. 1977a). The starch will bind certain lipid components of the medium and inoculum that might inhibit germination.

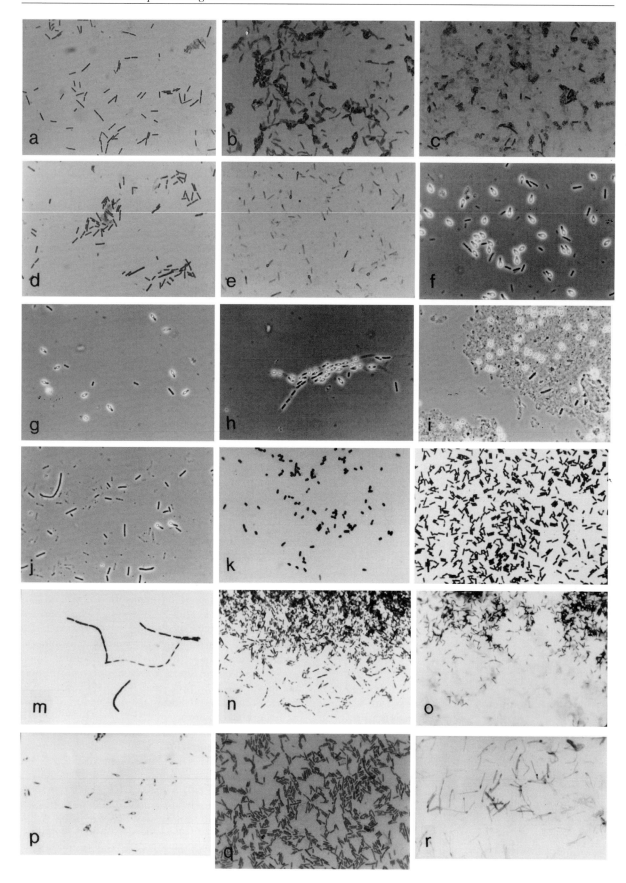

Fig. 32.2   Caption overleaf.

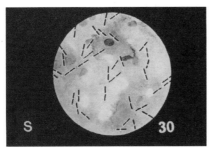 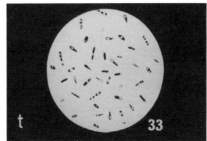

Fig. 32.2 Photomicrographs (× c. 1500) of some representative species of *Clostridium*: (a) *C. botulinum* type A, 24 h CMGS, gram stain; (b) *C. botulinum* type A, 72 h EYA, gram stain; (c) *C. botulinum* type B (non-proteolytic), 72 h EYA, gram stain; (d) *C. botulinum* type E, 24 h CMGS, gram stain; (e) *C. tetani*, 7 day EYA, gram stain; (f) *C. botulinum* type A, 4 day EYA; phase contrast; (g) *C. botulinum* type B, 4 day EYA, phase contrast; (h) *C. botulinum* type B, 4 day EYA, phase contrast; (i) *C. botulinum* type E, 4 day EYA, phase contrast; (j) *C. tetani*, 4 day EYA, phase contrast; (k) *C. perfringens*, 24 h CM, gram stain; (l) *C. perfringens*, 24 h Schaedler agar, gram stain; (m) *C. novyi*, 24 h CM, gram stain;(n) *C. difficile*, 72 h BAP, gram stain; (o) *C. paraputrificum*, 24 h CM, gram stain; (p) *C. subterminale*, 48 h BAP, gram stain; (q) *C. argentinense*, 72 h EYA, gram stain; (r) *C. innocuum*, 24 h thioglycollate broth, gram stain; (s) *C. septicum*, 24 h CM, methylene blue; (t) *C. chauvoei*, 24 h CM, methylene blue (see also Plate 32.2).

5.4 Flagella

With the exception of *C. perfringens* and a few non-pathogenic species, all the members are motile, by peritrichous flagella. Motility, however, is often difficult to demonstrate, especially in strains that have been subcultured for some time. Young cultures in fluid medium, not more than 6–24 h old, are the most suitable for examination. Motility may be observed by examining a drop of culture overlaid with a coverslip under the microscope using phase contrast or dark field illumination. Motility is not always obvious, and is often slow and stately. Alternatively, growth in a tube of motility medium (containing 0.5% agar) (Dowell et al. 1977a) will reveal diffuse growth throughout the medium with a motile organism; the growth of a non-motile organism will remain confined to the immediate area of inoculation. Flagella can be visualized with Liefson's Flagellar Stain (Dowell and Hawkins 1974, Paik 1980).

5.5 Cell walls

As noted in the definition of the genus, the clostridia are considered gram-positive organisms, although sometimes the gram reaction is equivocal, and in some cases gram-positive organisms are not seen. However, even those strains of clostridia failing to show the reaction possess a gram-positive cell wall, i.e. they lack an outer membrane. This remains an important taxonomic criterion, since members of the genus *Sporomusa*, also anaerobic spore formers, possess a gram-negative cell wall (Andreesen, Bahl and Gottschalk 1989). With gram-positive organisms, the peptidoglycan accounts for 80–90% of the cell wall components (Gottschalk 1986), while it amounts to only about 10% in gram-negative organisms. **Diaminopimelic acid** (DAP) provides the crosslink in the peptidoglycan for 53 of the 64 *Clostridium* species for which the information is available in *Bergey's Manual* (Cato, George and Finegold 1986). It is the *meso*-form for 47 species and the LL-form for 6 species (*C. carnis*,

C. fallax, C. perfringens, C. putrefaciens, C. thermoaceticum and *C. thermoautotrophicum*). Among the 11 species lacking DAP are *C. septicum, C. chauvoei*, and *C. tertium*. Lysine is usually the crosslinking component for the DAP-negative clostridia.

5.6 Capsules

C. butyricum and *C. perfringens* are the only members with a capsule; that of *C. perfringens* is noticeable in the animal body, and sometimes in cultures containing serum. The serology of the capsular polysaccharide antigens of *C. perfringens* is so diverse that it could not be used practically for species identification (Klotz 1965). This diversity has been employed for establishing a common vehicle in outbreaks of food-borne diarrhoea (Hatheway, Whaley and Dowell 1980, Stringer, Turnbull and Gilbert 1980).

5.7 Plasmids

Rood and Cole (1991) have reviewed the incidence of plasmids in *C. perfringens*. Many cryptic plasmids have been found. *C. perfringens* is the only *Clostridium* in which conjugative antibiotic resistance plasmids (R plasmids) have been identified. All of the conjugative R plasmids found in *C. perfringens* so far carry the same tetracycline resistance determinant. One non-conjugative R plasmid which confers resistance to the macrolide–lincosamide–streptogramin B antibiotics has been found. Studies have shown that the neurotoxin genes for *C. tetani* and *C. argentinense* are present on plasmids (Finn et al. 1984, Eklund et al. 1988, Zhou et al. 1995). The gene for the enterotoxin of *C. perfringens* may be present on either the chromosome or a plasmid (Cornillot et al. 1995). Plasmid profiles have been used for strain identification of *C. difficile* (Steinberg, Beckerdite and Westenfelder 1987) and *C. perfringens* (Mahony et al. 1987).

5.8 Bacteriophages

Bacteriophages have been described for many of the clostridia and their properties investigated (see Guelin, Beerens and Petiprez 1966, Prescott and Altenbern 1967, Sebald and Popovitch 1967, Mahony and Kalz 1968, Dolman and Chang 1972, Grant and Riemann 1976, Paquette and Fredette 1977, Mahony 1979, Ogata and Hongo 1979, Mahony, Bell and Easterbrook 1985). Phages are associated with neuro-toxigenicity of *C. botulinum* types C and D, as well as production of α-toxin by *C. novyi*. Betz and Anderson (Betz and Anderson 1964), besides grouping the phages of *C. sporogenes*, found that many strains of this organism produced bacteriocin-like substances acting on other strains of the same species.

5.9 Bacteriocins

Bacteriocins are produced by a number of clostridia, for example *C. perfringens* (Mahony and Butler 1971, Mahony and Swantee 1978, Mahony 1979) and *C. botulinum* (Kautter et al. 1966).The technique of bacteriocin typing of *C. perfringens* has been used as a complement to serotyping in the laboratory confirmation of *C. perfringens* food poisoning outbreaks. It was helpful when the causative strain was serologically non-typable (Scott and Mahony 1982, Watson et al. 1982). As might be expected, bacteria of unrelated species sometimes produce bacteriocins active upon the cells of others; Smith (1975) isolated from soil strains of *Bacillus cereus*, *C. sporogenes* and *C. perfringens* that produced bacteriocins active against *C. botulinum*.

6 ANTIGENIC STRUCTURE

Antigenic structure was used as the basis of early attempts at establishing a systematic identification schema for the clostridia (e.g., see Mandia 1951, 1955). With the application of nucleic acid homologies to bacteriological taxonomy (Cummins and Johnson 1971, Brenner 1973, Johnson 1973), interest in the serological approach has waned.

Three groups of clostridial antigens have been studied in detail: (1) the antigens of the flagella and the bacterial bodies, (2) capsular polysaccharides and (3) toxins or other factors found in filtrates of cultures. The capsular antigen studies have largely been restricted to *C. perfringens*. The third group, although originally examined for their pathogenic significance, have been, like the first, useful in determining the relationships among clostridia. The relationships among the clostridia based on antigenic structure are reviewed in detail in the previous edition of this text (Willis 1990).

A practical aim of the serological approach was to reliably identify organisms by species, e.g. by fluorescent antibody (FA) staining, thus allowing identification without isolation and performing the necessary battery of tests. FA reagents for a number of the pathogenic species were available commercially in the past, but are no longer available. The use of FA reagents for confirmation of infant botulism by identification of *C. botulinum* in the patients' stools was studied (Glasby and Hatheway 1983, 1984a). Since some strains of *C. sporogenes* also reacted with the reagents, toxicity tests remained necessary and largely negated the advantage of FA identification. An example of the difficulties encountered with attempted serological identification of a *Clostridium* species was the discovery that the capsular antigens involved in agglutination and FA reactions of *C. perfringens* are so diverse that a very large collection of reagents is necessary for detecting all of the strains (Klotz 1965). This diversity has been used to distinguish among strains for epidemiologic purposes in *C. perfringens* food-borne diarrhoea outbreaks (Hatheway, Whaley and Dowell 1980, Stringer, Turnbull and Gilbert 1980). However, successful pursuit of such studies required continual supplementation of reagents with new ones each time another non-agglutinable strain was encountered, and it was not possible to make a constantly changing battery of reagents available to all interested investigators. This approach to subtyping of strains, requiring specific serological reagents has lost its appeal because alternative approaches using newer molecular methodologies, e.g. pulsed field gel electrophoresis of chromosome digests and ribotyping, appear to offer more universally applicable approaches.

7 TOXINS AND BIOLOGICALLY ACTIVE ANTIGENS OF CLOSTRIDIA

One of the most interesting features of the clostridia is their production of a wide diversity of biologically active proteins, many of which have roles in diseases of humans or animals. These agents include neurotoxins, lipases, lecithinases, haemolysins, enterotoxins, cytotoxins, collagenases, permeases, necrotizing toxins, proteinases, hyaluronidases, DNAases, ADP-ribosyltransferases, neuraminidases and some that are just described as 'lethal toxins'. The clostridial toxins are listed in Table 32.2 by organism. Some of them, e.g. the botulism and tetanus neurotoxins, are notable because of their extreme lethal potency. The lethality of some of the clostridial toxins for mice is listed in Table 32.3. Greek letters have commonly been assigned as names of the toxins produced by many of the clostridia. The letter reflects the chronology of the discovery of each, rather than any indication of function or biological activity. There is no intended relationship between toxins with the same Greek letter designation produced by different species. This can be a source of confusion. A review of clostridial toxins published previously is the source of most of the information presented here (Hatheway 1990). Since the neurotoxins and oxygen-labile haemolysins are produced by a number of species, and their structures and mechanisms of action are similar regardless of which organism is the source, they will be described here. The other toxins will be presented in the sections dealing with the species that produce them.

Recently, pathogenic clostridia have been shown to produce extracellular toxins or lipoteichoid acid-like molecules that act as superantigens, greatly stimulating the immune system (Bowness et al. 1992, Campos-Neto et al. 1995). *C. perfringens* enterotoxin selectively stimulates peripheral blood lymphocytes bearing T cell receptors. *C. botulinum* types C and D also produce a high molecular weight mitogen that potently activates B lymphocytes. These superantigens probably contribute to pathogenesis by stimulating a hyperactive response of the immune system of mammalian hosts.

7.1 Genetics of toxigenesis

The clostridia produce many more toxins than any other bacterial genus (van Heyningen 1950, Hatheway 1990). More than 20 distinct toxins as well as other extracellular proteins contributing to virulence such as spreading factors, phospholipases, and proteolytic enzymes have been identified in *Clostridium* spp. The genes encoding for several clostridial toxins are located on integrative lysogenic bacteriophages, while others are believed to be located on the chromosome and have not been shown to be associated with lysogenic bacteriophages (Johnson 1997, Rood et al. 1997). Genes encoding clostridial toxins that reside on the chromosome are those of *C. difficile* and *C. perfringens* enterotoxin (human isolates). Genes encoding toxins that reside at least temporally on extrachromosomal virulence plasmids or bacteriophages are those of *C. botulinum* types C, D and G, enterotoxigenic *C. perfringens* (animal isolates), and *C. tetani*. Analysis of toxin genes by gene probes, pulsed field gel electrophoresis and other molecular approaches has demonstrated that these genes are frequently associated with unstable genetic elements such as plasmids, transposons and bacteriophages. The presence of genes for virulence factors on extrachromosomal and movable genetic elements often results in phenotypic properties such as genetic instability and the capacity of toxigenicity to be dispersed by horizontal gene transfer to other microbial species.

7.2 Neurotoxins

The clostridial neurotoxins that cause tetanus and botulism are the most lethal substances known (Table 32.3). The tetanus toxin is known as **TeTx** and the botulinum neurotoxin as **BoNT** (Niemann 1992). The botulinum type is indicated by a letter, for example BoNT/A for type A. The structures of tetanus and botulinum toxins are quite similar, despite the striking differences in the manifestations of the 2 diseases, or the serological diversity among the toxins causing botulism; 7 serological types (type A–G) have been identified. The neurotoxins are synthesized as single 150 kDa polypeptide chains (Fig. 32.3; Niemann 1992). The molecule is activated by cleavage into a light chain (L; 50 kDa) and a heavy chain (H; 100kDa)

by a protease, either endogenous in the case of a proteolytic organism, or exogenous in the case of a non-proteolytic organism. Trypsin can serve as the exogenous enzyme for a non-proteolytic organism in the laboratory. The L and H chains remain linked by an interchain sulphydryl bridge formed between 2 cysteine residues; the 2 peptides can be separated by reduction of this disulphide bond. The H chain can be cleaved into 2 fragments by papain: the N-terminal (H_N) and the C-terminal (H_C) portions. The active form of the neurotoxin is the dichain (H + L) linked through the disulphide bond. Trypsin treatment is necessary for realizing maximum potency of the type B, E and F botulinum neurotoxins produced by non-proteolytic strains. Tetanus toxin has been observed only with *C. tetani*, but neurotoxins that cause botulism are known to be produced by 3 groups (equivalent to 3 distinct species) of *C. botulinum*, *C. argentinense* (also known as *C. botulinum* type G) and rare toxigenic strains of *C. butyricum* and *C. baratii*. Both the structure and mechanism of action of the toxins causing the 2 diseases are very similar. The gene encoding tetanus neurotoxin (or tetanospasmin) is located on a plasmid (Laird et al. 1980, Finn et al. 1984, Eisel et al. 1986). The genes for BoNT/C and BoNT/D are phage associated (Eklund et al. 1987) and for BoNT/G, the gene appears to be plasmid associated (Eklund et al. 1988). Those for the other toxin types have been generally been assumed to be chromosomal, although evidence for phage transfer of BoNT/E from toxigenic *C. butyricum* has been shown (Zhou, Sugiyama and Johnson 1993).

Amino acid sequences

Early approaches to the elucidation of the chemical nature of the neurotoxins were by determination of amino acid composition of purified preparations of the toxins, then by determining amino acid sequences of selected fragments of the molecule (DasGupta 1989). Satisfactory answers came only with the technologies that made it possible to determine the nucleotide sequences of the genes encoding the neurotoxins.

The complete primary structure of tetanus toxin was reported in 1986 (Eisel et al. 1986). Since then, the sequences of each serologic variant of botulinum neurotoxin have been elucidated: type A (Binz et al. 1990a, Thompson et al. 1990); type B (Whelan et al. 1992b, Hutson et al. 1994); type C (Hauser et al. 1990, Kimura et al. 1990); type D (Binz et al. 1990b); type E (Whelan et al. 1992a); type F (East et al. 1992, Elmore et al. 1995); and type G (Campbell, Collins and East 1993). The sequences for the type E toxin produced by a toxigenic strain of *C. butyricum* (Fujii et al. 1993) and the type F toxin produced by a strain of *C. baratii* (Thompson et al. 1993) have also been determined and compared with those from strains of *C. botulinum*.

Botulinum neurotoxin in the native state exists as part of a complex with non-toxic proteins, one of which may exhibit haemagglutinating activity (Sakaguchi 1983). The neurotoxin molecule itself has a molecular mass of 150 kDa. The size of the com-

Table 32.2 Toxins and biologically active antigens of clostridia (from Hatheway 1990)

Species	Toxins	Size of molecule (kDa)	Activity/disease
C. botulinum	Neurotoxin	150	Botulism
	C₂ (binary)		Permease/
	component I	50	ADP-ribosylation
	component II	105	Binding
	C₃	25	ADP-ribosylation
C. argentinense (C. botulinum type G)	Neurotoxin	150	Botulism (experimental)
C. tetani	Neurotoxin	150	Tetanus
	Tetanolysin	48	Oxygen-labile haemolysin
C. perfringens	Major		
	α	43	Phospholipase C/myonecrosis
	β	40	Lethal, necrotic/enterotoxaemia
	ε	34	Lethal, permease/enterotoxaemia
	ι (binary)		Enterotoxaemia
	Component a	40	ADP-ribosylation
	Component b	81	Binding
	Other		
	Enterotoxin	35	Food-borne diarrhoea
	δ	42	Haemolysin
	θ	51	Oxygen-labile haemolysin
	κ	80	Collagenase
	λ		Protease
	μ		Hyaluronidase
	ν		Deoxyribonuclease
	Neuraminidase	43, 64, 105, 310	N-acetylneuraminic acid glycohydrolase
C. difficile	Toxin A	400–500	Enterotoxin/AAPMC[c]
	Toxin B	360–470	Cytotoxin/AAPMC
	CDT	43	ADP-ribosylation
C. sordelii (C. bifermentans)	α	43	Phospholipase C
	β		Lethal
	HT	525	equiv. to C. difficile toxin A
	LT	250	equiv. to C. difficile toxin B
	Haemolysin	43	Oxygen-labile haemolysin
C. novyi/C. haemolyticum	α	260–280	Lethal
	β	32	Phospholipase C
	γ	30	Phospholipase C
	δ		Oxygen-labile haemolysin
	ε		Lipase
C. chauvoei/C. septicum	α	27	Lethal, necrotizing
	β	45	Deoxyribonuclease
	γ		Hyaluronidase
	δ		Oxygen-labile haemolysin
C. histolyticum	α		Necrotizing
	β		Collagenases
	Class I	68, 115, 79, 130	
	Class II	100, 110, 125	
	γ	50	Proteinase, thiol-activated
	δ	>10, <50	Proteinase
	ε		Oxygen-labile haemolysin
C. spiroforme	ι (binary)		Diarrhoea in rabbits
	Component a	45	ADP-ribosylation
	Component b	92	Binding
C. butyricum	Neurotoxin	145	Botulism, type E
C. baratii	Neurotoxin	141	Botulism, type F

[c]AAPMC, antibiotic-associated pseudomembranous colitis.

Table 32.3 Mouse lethal doses of selected clostridial toxins (from Hatheway 1990)

Species	Type	Toxin	Mouse LD$_{50}$ (ng)[a]	Reference
C. botulinum	A	Neurotoxin	0.00625 (i.p.)	Sakaguchi (1983)
C. tetani		Neurotoxin	0.015 (i.p.)	Helting and Zwisler (1977)
C. perfringens	B, D	ε	0.32	Habeeb (1969)
C. perfringens	B, C	β	8	Sakurai and Fujii (1987)
C. difficile		Toxin A	26 (i.p.)	Banno et al. (1984)
C. botulinum	C	C2	45 (i.p.)	Ohishi et al. (1980)
C. perfringens	A	α	50	Tso and Seibel (1989)
C. perfringens	B, C	δ	60	Alouf and Jolivet-Reynaud (1981)
C. perfringens	A	θ	167	Yamakawa et al. (1977)
C. perfringens	A	Enterotoxin	1400	Stark and Duncan (1972)
C. difficile		Toxin B	1500	Banno et al. (1984)
C. perfringens	E	ι	1560	Stiles and Wilkins (1986)
C. bifermentans		Lecithinase	2500	Tso and Seibel (1989)
C. perfringens	A	κ	30000	Kameyama and Akama (1971)

[a]Dose determined by intravenous injection unless indicated otherwise; i.p., intraperitoneal. Published values expressed in terms of N were converted to protein by multiplying by 6.25; those in MLD were converted to LD50 by multiplying by 0.5; and those expressed per kg of body weight were recalculated for 25 g mice.

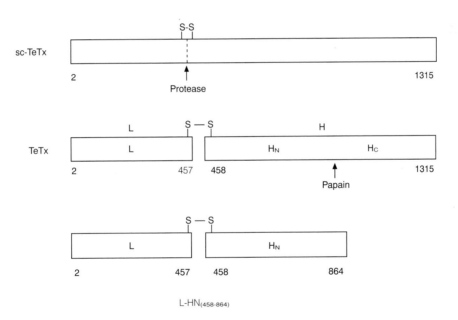

Fig. 32.3 Conventions for *Clostridium* neurotoxin nomenclature (Niemann, 1992). The designations are TeTx and BoNT for tetanus toxin and botulinum neurotoxins, respectively. The botulinum type is indicated by the letter such as BoNT/A for type A. The diagram depicts the tetanus toxin molecule: the single-chain tetanus toxin molecule (sc-TeTx) is activated by protease cleavage of a peptide bond, forming a dichain molecule (TeTx), consisting of a heavy (H) and light (L) chain held together by a disulphide bond; the heavy chain may be subdivided in the laboratory by cleavage at a papain-sensitive site, forming the N-terminal (H$_N$) and the C-terminal (H$_C$) fragments. The numbers indicate the the amino acids of the single-chain peptide sequence.

plexes range from approximately 300 to 900 kDa (generally the sizes in the literature are indicated by sedimentation values; 7S, 12S, 16S and 19S). The neurotoxin in the complex is stabilized against conditions in the environment and in the gastrointestinal tract. The complex dissociates under mildly alkaline conditions such as in the small intestine whence it is absorbed and enters the circulation.

MECHANISM OF NEUROTOXICITY

Tetanus and botulism are neuroparalytic diseases due to the inhibition of neurotransmitter release. With tetanus, the blockage of the inhibitory pathways in the central nervous system results in spasticity and convulsions due to aberrant neuron firing. The neurotransmitter for these pathways is γ-aminobutyric acid (GABA). Botulism is a flaccid paralysis due to blockage of the neurotransmitter (acetylcholine) release at the neuromuscular junction. TeTx and BoNT intoxication of nerve cells can be described as a 4-step process (Montecucco and Schiavo 1994): (1) cell binding, (2) internalization, (3) membrane translocation and (4) target modification in the cytosol. Binding results from recognition of toxin receptors on the motor neuron plasmalemma at the neuromuscular junction by the binding area on the H_C domain of the toxin molecule. The toxin is internalized into the nerve cell within a vesicle formed from the the the cell membrane. The vesicles formed with TeTx are different from those formed with BoNT because the TeTx vesicles move backward along the motor neuron axon into the soma, from where they gain entrance into the CNS by trans-synaptic movement from the motorneuron into the afferent terminals (Bizzini 1989); the BoNT vesicles remain within the neuromuscular junction. Membrane translocation is thought to be mediated by the H_N region, placing the L-chain, or at least the L-catalytic domain, into the cytosol. The final step is the cleavage of specific vesicular proteins by the peptidase activity of the L-chain in the cytosol. The catalytic component of each neurotoxin acts as a zinc-endopeptidase with a specific peptide bond target on one of 3 vesicular structural proteins known as **vesicle-associated membrane protein** (VAMP), **synaptosomal-associated protein** (SNAP) or **syntaxin** (see Montecucco and Schiavo 1994). The targets are unique, except for TeTx and BoNT/B which surprisingly cleave the same Ser-Gln-Phe-Glu site on VAMP. The modification of the vesicular proteins prevents neurotransmitter release.

The means of detection, identification and measurement of the neurotoxins is the mouse bioassay which includes specific neutralization as described for investigation of botulism (Hatheway 1988). Although many in vitro assays have been proposed, none has been sufficiently evaluated for reliable use (see review by Hatheway and Ferreira 1996). The serological diversity of BoNT complicates the problem, and at this stage of our understanding would require at least 7 sets of reagents for universal detection. The problem is simpler in the case of TeTx which exists in only one serological type (as far as is known), but there is little need for laboratory investigation of tetanus and it is rarely done, except for establishing toxigenicity of organisms.

7.3 Oxygen-labile haemolysins

Oxygen-labile haemolysins produced by clostridia are designated **tetanolysin** (*C. tetani*), **θ-toxin** (*C. perfringens*), **δ-toxin** (*C. novyi* type A, *C. septicum*, and *C. chauvoei*) and **ε-toxin** (*C. histolyticum*). They lyse a variety of cells in addition to erythrocytes. These cytolysins are serologically related to each other and to streptolysin-O, pneumolysin, cereolysin, thuringiolysin, aveolysin, laterosporolysin and listeriolysin, produced by bacteria in other genera (Bernheimer 1976). They are inactivated by mild oxidizing conditions, reactivated by thiol compounds, and inhibited by a

small amount of cholesterol. Bernheimer (1976) also includes *C. bifermentans* (and *C. sordellii*) and *C. botulinum* types C and D among the organisms that produce these haemolysins. The gene for *C. perfringens* θ-toxin has been cloned and the amino acid sequence of the protein is now known (Tweten 1988a, 1988b). Streptolysin-O and pneumolysin possess considerable homology, with a common identical 12-amino acid segment. Oxygen-labile haemolysins have been shown to have lethal and cardiotoxic effects in vivo and to cause intravascular lysis (Hardegree, Palmer and Duffin 1971, Bernheimer 1976). The role they play in diseases caused by the organisms that produce them is difficult to assess. With such a widespread occurrence of these cytolysins in bacteria, they must serve some advantageous function.

7.4 Laboratory cultures as sources of clostridial toxins

Many *Clostridium* spp. produce low quantities of toxins in laboratory culture, and decreasing quantities of toxin are produced on progressive subcultures (Schantz and Johnson 1992). For consistent toxin production, it may be necessary to isolate high producing strains by single colony isolation, and to preserve the strains at low temperatures or lyophilization. Specially formulated media have resulted in production of consistent quality and high titres of botulinum and tetanus toxins (Schantz and Johnson 1992).

8 GROWTH AND APPEARANCE ON CULTURE MEDIA

Most of the clostridia with which we are concerned grow best at about 37°C, though many of them are capable of growing at temperatures of 20°C and even lower. There is a group of thermophilic clostridia which have an optimum temperature about 50–60°C, and which sometimes do not grow at all below 30°C. The optimum hydrogen ion concentration for growth is about pH 7.0–7.4. Anaerobes will grow in liquid media from which oxygen has been excluded and which contain a reducing agent such as thioglycollate or metallic iron. For growth on solid media, an anaerobic environment such as in a chamber containing an atmosphere of 85% nitrogen, 10% hydrogen and 5% carbon dioxide must be provided.

On solid media growth is relatively slow, and sometimes takes the form of a thin, effuse, often spreading film, which may be difficult to distinguish from the underlying medium. Film formation is promoted by moisture. On first isolation *C. septicum*, and particularly *C. tetani*, tend to spread rapidly over a moist surface. *C. tetani* inoculated into the condensation water of an agar slant, or laterally on a blood agar plate, in the course of a day spreads over the whole medium; the film is so thin that were it not for its dentate spreading edge it might escape detection. Advantage may be taken of this property in the isolation of the organism (Fildes 1925). The spreading of clostridia is inhibited by certain chemicals; most of them, however, are to some extent bacteriostatic; inhibition of spreading without bacteriostasis may be effected by increasing the concentration of agar up to about 4% (Dowell et al. 1977a), or by the addition of agglutinating antibody to the medium (Williams and Willis 1970). Certain clostridia also produce on agar motile daughter colonies, which rotate and wander over the surface of the medium (Turner and Eales 1941). Concentrated agar is less effective as an inhibitor of this type of spread.

Some clostridia produce colonies that fluoresce in longwave ultraviolet light (Willis 1990). *C. putrificum* produces red fluorescent colonies in the presence of blood and a fermentable carbohydrate due to the production of protoporphyrin. Colonies of *C. difficile* show yellow-green or chartreuse fluorescence on blood agar after incubation for 48 h; it is quite distinct from the non-specific yellow fluorescence seen in cultures growing in the presence of neutral red, a property which *C. difficile* shares with a number of clostridia and is well recognized in cultures on MacConkey's agar.

For formulae of media for clostridia see Dowell et al. (1977a), Holdeman, Cato and Moore (1977), Willis (1977); for an illustrated description of the morphological and colonial appearance of the pathogenic anaerobes see Batty and Walker (1966).

8.1 Culture media

AGAR PLATES

Single colonies are rounded, generally effuse, and have crenated, fimbriate or rhizoid edges. They generally are translucent, not frankly opaque; grayish or exhibiting something of the colour of the agar medium. *C. perfringens*, which is one of the less strict anaerobes, forms low convex colonies with an entire edge; *C. sporogenes* and *C. histolyticum* may form umbonate colonies with a raised centre and a flat periphery. The colonial appearances are often characteristic, but some species give rise to variants which not only are unlike the typical colony but which strongly suggest the occurrence of contamination; and the colonies of some aerobic spore-bearing bacilli, growing anaerobically, simulate those of clostridia. Several different types of colony may be formed, for example, by *C. sporogenes*. Dezfulian and Dowell (1980) and Dowell and Dezfulian (1981) observed 2 colonial forms of type A and type B strains of *C. botulinum*, which they designated opaque (Op) and transparent (Tr). After isolation, Tr isolates gave rise only to Tr offspring, whereas Op isolates occasionally yielded some Tr colonial types. The Op organisms produced abundant spores, whereas Tr organisms produced only rare spores or none. Differences in growth rates and amounts of certain volatile fatty acids were also noted between the colony types.

DEEP CULTURES IN SOFT AGAR

Most clostridia grow in media with enough agar to prevent gross convection movements in the liquid. The medium devised by Brewer (1940) containing thiogly-

collic acid is one of this type. Separate diffuse 'colonies' may be found, but these readily become confluent, especially with motile forms. Mandia (1950) observed 'motile' colonies of the non-motile *C. perfringens* in these circumstances.

BLOOD AGAR PLATES

On blood agar plates, both the colonial form and the degree and type of haemolysis may be characteristic. Haemolysis is well developed after incubation for 24–48 h at 37°C; when the plates are stored in the dark at room temperature it often continues to increase. With a thick seeding the whole plate may be completely lysed. The nature and extent of haemolysis produced by different organisms may vary according to the species of erythrocyte used (see Willis 1969).

Many organisms give incomplete haemolysis after incubation for 24 h; after further incubation this passes into the fully developed β-variety. In some cases, it is possible to specify the haemolytic factors concerned. For instance the relatively wide zone of haemolysis produced by toxigenic strains of *C. perfringens* on routine horse-blood agar is usually due to the θ-toxin; when the action of θ-toxin is suppressed by θ-antitoxin, a narrower, ill-defined zone of partial haemolysis is revealed, due to α-toxin. On horse-blood agar containing added calcium chloride (0.5%) enhancement of α-toxin activity leads to the characteristic appearance of 'target' haemolysis (Evans 1945).

EGG YOLK AGAR MEDIA

Egg yolk agar media are very useful for the detection of the lecithinases and lipases that characterize certain pathogenic clostridia (Nagler 1939, MacFarlane and Knight 1941, McClung and Toabe 1947, Willis 1969). The intense **diffuse opacity** produced by some clostridia in egg yolk agar is due to lecithinases C which are inhibited by specific antitoxins; the lecithinase producing organisms include *C. perfringens*, *C. bifermentans*, *C. sordellii*, and *C. novyi* types A, B and D (*C. haemolyticum*). Some species produce an intense **restricted opacity** accompanied by a fine **pearly layer** overlying the colonies due to lipases; lipolytic species include *C. novyi* type A. *C. sporogenes* and *C. botulinum* types A–F. These 2 effects, which are easily distinguished from one another, are also developed on the more complex lactose–egg yolk–milk agar (Willis 1990). This medium additionally shows lactose fermentation and proteinase effects, thus permitting an early presumptive identification of a number of different species (Table 32.4).

MACCONKEY'S AGAR

Production of green fluorescent colonies by some clostridia on MacConkey's agar has been recognized for some time (Willis 1990); *C. perfringens* is particularly active in this respect. Fluorescence does not appear to be produced by facultative anaerobes. The fluorescence first becomes visible under ultraviolet light after incubation for 18–24 h, and is seen with ordinary illumination at about 24 h. It is due to some alteration in the neutral red that occurs under highly reduced

Table 32.4 Reactions of some clostridia on half-antitoxin[a] lactose egg-yolk agar milk agar (from Willis and Hobbs 1959, modified)

Species	Type	Diffuse lecithinase C opacity		Restricted opacity and pearly layer (lipase)	Lactose fermentation	Proteolysis
		Produced	**Inhibited**			
C. perfringens	A–E	+	+	–	+	–
C. bifermentans		+	+	–	–	+
C. sordellii		+	+	–	–	+
C. botulinum	A	–		+	–	+
	B	–		+	–	+ or –
	C	–		+	–	–
	D	–		+	–	–
	E	–		+	–	–
	F	–		+	–	+ or –
C. argentinense	(G)	–		–	–	+
C. sporogenes		–		+	–	+
C. novyi	A	+	+[b]	+	–	–
	B	+		–	–	–
	C	–		–	–	–
C. haemolyticum[c]		+	–	–	–	–
C. histolyticum		–		–	–	+
C. septicum		–		–	+	–
C. chauvoei		–		–	+	–
C. tetani		–		–	–	–
C. cochlearium		–		–	–	–
C. cadaveris		–		–	–	–
C. sphenoides		–		–	+	–
C. tertium		–		–	+	–
C. butyricum		–		–	+	–
C. fallax		–		–	+	–

[a]Mixture of *C. perfringens* type A and *C. novyi* type A antitoxic sera.
[b]Note that the restricted lipase opacity is obscured on the non-antitoxin half of the plate by the lecithinase opacity.
[c]*C. haemolyticum* formerly known as *C. novyi* type D.

conditions. The same effect is seen on other media containing neutral red, e.g. in cultures of *C. difficile* on CCF agar (George et al. 1979).

COOKED MEAT MEDIUM

Most clostridia grow well in cooked meat medium. All render the fluid turbid and most produce gas. The proteolytic species turn the meat black and may obviously digest it; the saccharolytic organisms do not digest the meat, and frequently turn it pink. The proteolytic organisms produce characteristic foul and pervasive odours, whereas with the saccharolytic organisms the odour is not foul, or is undetectable. This medium has the advantage of maintaining viability of many clostridia, sometimes for weeks at room temperature, and for years under refrigeration.

GELATIN

All strongly proteolytic clostridia hydrolyse gelatin, but there are many gelatinolytic species that do not attack complex proteins. Gelatin liquefaction is a key distinguishing feature in the identification of clostridial species (note sections (a) and (b) of Table 32.7). A good way of identifying gelatinase activity is by culturing the test organisms on gelatin agar; see, for example, Dowell et al. (1981). The results are developed by precipitating undegraded gelatin with acid mercuric chloride solution. Another common method is to inoculate the culture into Thiogel medium (Dowell et al. 1977a), which is liquid at incubation temperature, but solid at refrigerator temperature. After incubation up to 7 days, the inoculated tubes are placed in a refrigerator or cold water until the control tube (uninoculated medium) has solidified. If the inoculated tube remains liquid, the organism has digested the gelatin.

MILK MEDIA

Iron milk medium (as well as coagulated serum and coagulated egg) has been used for testing the proteolytic powers of clostridia. Less subjective and more rapid identification of proteinase activity can be obtained in cultures on agar plates containing skim milk or soluble casein (Willis 1977, Dowell et al. 1981).

SELECTIVE MEDIA

Selective media for the isolation of clostridia are based on the relative lack of inhibitory action of polymyxin

B, neomycin and crystal violet (see Willis 1990), phenylethyl alcohol (Dowell, Hill and Altemeier 1964), cycloserine (Hauschild and Hilsheimer 1974), and trimethoprim/sulphamethoxazol (Dezfulian et al. 1981, Mills, Midura and Arnon 1985).

9 METABOLISM

9.1 Anaerobiosis

Clostridia are anaerobic organisms that possess neither cytochrome oxidase nor oxygenases (Decker, Jungermann and Thauer 1970). They derive their energy from fermentation of organic compounds rather than from oxidative processes involving oxygen (Andreesen, Bahl and Gottschalk 1989). In the fermentation process, organic compounds serve as the primary electron donor and also as the terminal electron acceptor (Morris 1975). This leads to the accumulation of reduced organic products. ATP is formed by substrate level phosphorylation only, not by a respiratory process involving electron transport. The organisms do not carry out a dissimilatory sulphate reduction in which sulphate serves as an inorganic electron acceptor; this is referred to as **anaerobic respiration** (Decker, Jungermann and Thauer 1970).

Since anaerobic organisms cannot use molecular oxygen and can thrive in its absence, they often (or usually) are unable to cope with oxygen or the toxic products of oxygen consumption. In contrast, aerobes which are dependent on oxygen must be equipped to operate and survive under aerobic conditions. The clostridia in general lack catalase, although low levels of superoxide dismutase have been detected in some strains (Morris 1976). Oxygen may interfere with metabolism by oxidizing NADH through reactions catalysed by NADH oxidases which many clostridia possess in substantial quantities (Andreesen, Bahl and Gottschalk 1989). For many clostridia, oxygen seems to be not bactericidal, but bacteriostatic. Agar plate cultures of some species, e.g. *C. butyricum* or *C. botulinum* can be removed from the anaerobic chamber for an hour or more, and growth of colonies will recommence after they are returned to the chamber. *C. haemolyticum* or *C. novyi* type B may survive for only a few minutes of exposure (Andreesen 1994). Sometimes oxygen resistance of the organisms is attributed to the spores, noting the normal presence of clostridia in soils and the viability of their spores in the dust carried by the wind. For growth, however, most clostridia require a greatly diminished oxygen level. Some attribute the inhibitory effect of oxygen to an increased oxidation–reduction potential (E_h), because many anaerobic bacteria can be grown in the presence of air provided a sufficiently low E_h is established in the medium. This can be done by reducing substances, some of which act mainly by absorbing oxygen, others establishing a low E_h after the molecular oxygen has been nearly used up or removed by mechanical means (Willis 1990). However, Morris points out the unreliability of E_h measurements in culture media and shows evidence that the inhibitory effect is possibly more dependent on oxygen than on E_h (Morris 1975). *C. histolyticum*, *C. tertium* and *C. carnis* are exceptional in growing to a limited extent in the presence of air, though they are said to form no spores under these conditions (Willis 1990). Media for culturing the clostridia usually contain reducing compounds such as cysteine, thioglycollate, glutathione, sulphites, iron or reduced iron compounds. Cooked meat medium, in addition to providing many essential nutrients and an environment conducive to germination of spores as well as to sporulation of vegetative organisms, maintains anaerobic conditions through tying up the oxygen by unsaturated fatty acids catalysed by hematin of the muscle, and the presence of sulphydryl compounds which bring about a negative oxidation–reduction potential (Willis 1990).

9.2 Metabolism of carbohydrates, proteins and nucleotide bases

Polysaccharides may be broken down into their sugar components. Monosaccharides are utilized through the Embden–Meyerhof–Parnas pathway (Andreesen, Bahl and Gottschalk 1989). Fermentation end products formed through the central intermediate of pyruvate are acetate, butyrate lactate and ethanol. Other alcohols such as isopropanol, butanol and 1,2-propandiol may be formed by some species and under certain conditions.

Proteins are digested, obviously by the proteolytic clostridia as well as other organisms in nature and serve as the source of amino acids. The clostridia are diverse in their utilization of these as energy sources, as is evidenced by metabolic end products (Holdeman, Cato and Moore 1977, Lombard and Dowell 1982). Many amino acids may be fermented singly, and can serve as sole carbon, nitrogen and energy sources (Andreesen, Bahl and Gottschalk 1989). However, the fermentation of amino acids often takes place in pairs with one serving as electron donor (equation 1, Fig. 32.4) and the other as electron acceptor (equation 2, Fig. 32.4) in what is known as the **Stickland reaction** (Gottschalk 1986). The electron donor loses one carbon while the electron acceptor maintains its original carbon chain length. In general, alanine, leucine, isoleucine, valine, histidine, tyrosine, phenylalanine and tyrosine serve as electron donors; and glycine, proline, hydroxyproline, ornithine and arginine as electron acceptors (Ljungdahl, Hugenholtz and Wiegel 1989). However, some such as leucine, phenylalanine and tryptophan can serve as either substrate for certain organisms (Gottschalk 1986). Straight chain amino acids yield acetate, propionate, butyrate and valerate as end products; branched chain amino acids are converted to isobutyrate, isovalerate and isocaproate. Phenylalanine is converted to phenylpropionate, phenylacetate and phenol, while tyrosine and tryptophan are metabolized to their hydroxyphenyl and indole equivalents, respectively (Andreesen, Bahl and Gottschalk 1989).

$$R\text{-}CHNH_2COOH \rightarrow R\text{-}COCOOH + NH_3 + 2H$$
$$\downarrow +H_2O$$
$$R\text{-}COOH + CO_2 + 2H \qquad \text{(Equation 1)}$$

$$2R\text{-}CHNH_2COOH + 4H \rightarrow 2R\text{-}CH_2COOH + 2NH_3 \qquad \text{(Equation 2)}$$

Fig. 32.4 The Stickland reaction.

The degradation of purines and pyrimidines follows pathways through conversions to glycine and β-alanine intermediates, respectively, then generally to acetate end products.

10 SUSCEPTIBILITY TO PHYSICAL AND CHEMICAL AGENTS

Because of their ability to sporulate, all clostridia have a pronounced but variable resistance to heat, drying and disinfectants. In the vegetative state, they are about as resistant to heat and disinfectants as nonsporing aerobes, but anaerobes may have a slightly greater susceptibility to a large number of organic bactericides. The spores of *C. botulinum* may withstand boiling for 3–4 h, and even at 105°C may not be killed completely in less than 100 min. *C. novyi* is a little less resistant than *C. botulinum*. Spores of most strains of *C. perfringens* are destroyed by boiling in less than 5 min, but those of some food poisoning strains are often more heat resistant (Hobbs 1965). *C. sporogenes* can survive exposure for 8 days to a 5% phenol solution. Among hospital disinfectants the greatest sporicidal activity is shown by alcoholic hypochlorite and glutaraldehyde; iodophors, formalin and phenolics are less effective (Willis 1990). In dried earth or dust *C. tetani* may survive for years. Stock cultures of most members in cooked meat medium remain viable for months; some, such as *C. fallax* and *C. cochlearium*, are more delicate and require transferring frequently.

The results of studies on susceptibility of clostridia to antimicrobial agents have been summarized by Willis (1990). Swenson et al. (1980) and Dezfulian and Dowell (1980) established that *C. botulinum* is susceptible to most common antimicrobial agents but is resistant to nalidixic acid, trimethoprim/sulphamethoxazole, gentamicin and cycloserine. Drugs of choice for the prevention and treatment of clostridial wound infections are metronidazole and benzylpenicillin. Metronidazole is uniformly bactericidal for all anaerobic micro-organisms, but is inactive against aerobes and facultative anaerobes. The aminoglycosides, on the other hand, show broad spectrum activity against aerobes and facultative anaerobes, but are inactive against anaerobes. Under highly reduced conditions the activity of aminoglycosides is greatly diminished or abolished. Vancomycin is the drug of choice for treatment of pseudomembranous colitis due to *C. difficile*, and metronidazole has also been shown to be effective (Borriello and Larson 1985).

11 LABORATORY ISOLATION AND IDENTIFICATION

The conventional approach to diagnosis of a clostridial disease is usually to isolate the organism from or to detect the toxin in a suitable specimen. The organism is identified by performing appropriate differential tests on the isolated organism. Alternative methods such as use of FA reagents have been attempted for identification of the organism without isolation, with variable success (Klotz 1965, Hunter and Rosen 1966, Glasby and Hatheway 1984a). The polymerase chain reaction (PCR) for detection of toxin genes has been proposed as a means of detecting toxigenic organisms without culturing them (Szabo et al. 1994, Arzese et al. 1995, Baez and Juneja 1995, Buogo et al. 1995, Ferreira and Hamdy 1995, Franciosa et al. 1996). Staining of organisms with FA reagents (Batty and Walker 1963, 1966), determining electrophoretic patterns of soluble proteins (Cato et al. 1982), and cellular fatty acid analysis (Ghanem et al. 1991) have been used or proposed for use in identification of *Clostridium* species.

Attempts at isolation of clostridia will often be prompted by symptoms in a patient suggestive of a clostridial disease. Infections involving clostridia may be suggested by observing clostridial forms in gram stains of smears from wounds or wound exudates. Isolation from agar cultures of materials containing a single or predominating organism is quite straightforward. For isolation from highly contaminated materials such as faeces or soils, advantage is made of resistance of spores to heat and bactericidal agents such as ethanol. Sometimes cultures of the samples are tested for toxin (in particular, neurotoxin), and toxin-positive samples are worked further for recovery of the toxigenic organism. Selective and differential agar media are often very helpful (George et al. 1979, Mills, Midura and Arnon 1985). The lecithinase and lipase reactions detectable on egg yolk based media are useful in selecting colonies for attempted isolation of *C. perfringens*, *C. botulinum*, *C. novyi*, *C. sordellii* and *C. baratii*.

12 DIFFERENTIAL CHARACTERIZATION OF THE CLOSTRIDIA

The differential characteristics include morphological features such as spore position and shape, biochemical reactions in liquid and on solid media, metabolic products detected by gas–liquid chromatography (GLC), and the production of toxins and other biologically active antigenic agents.

12.1 Biochemical reactions

The biochemical reactions which reveal the physiological capabilities of the organisms in pure culture are determined using differential media and procedures described by others (Willis 1969, Dowell and

Hawkins 1974, Dowell et al. 1977a, Holdeman, Cato and Moore 1977). Some of the important differential characteristics are listed in Table 32.5.

12.2   Metabolic products

An important adjunct to performing the tests on the differential media is the determination of the metabolic end products by GLC (Holdeman, Cato and Moore 1977, Lombard and Dowell 1982). Pure cultures are grown in peptone–yeast extract–glucose medium for 48 h. The volatile fatty acids are extracted from a sample of acidified culture with ethyl ether and analysed by GLC. Non-volatile acid products are converted to their methyl esters by treatment with methanol under acidic conditions; the esters are extracted with chloroform and likewise analysed. Volatile and non-volatile products for 21 clostridia are listed in Table 32.6. In general, proteolytic organisms produce the 'isoacids' (IB, IV, IC), however, *C. histolyticum* is one notable exception. It is evident that the phenylacetic and phenylpropionic acids produced from phenylalanine are detectable by this procedure, but the corresponding products from tyrosine (hydroxyphenyl derivatives) and tryptophan (indole derivatives) are not. Those products of amino acid metabolism have to be detected by alternative procedures (Moss et al. 1980).

12.3   Detection of lethal toxins

Bioassays are performed to detect neurotoxins for identification of *C. botulinum* and *C. tetani*, as well as to establish pathogenicity of rare strains of other species implicated in botulism. Neutralization by type-specific *C. botulinum* antitoxins assures positive identification as well as establishing the toxin type. *C. botulinum* group I (proteolytic) cannot be distinguished from *C. sporogenes* without determining toxigenicity. Identification of *C. botulinum* requires toxigenicity, but this feature has not been required for *C. tetani*, as non-toxigenic strains of this species are allowed. Detection of lethal toxins in other clostridia is important for type determination in some of the other species (e.g. *C. perfringens*), but not necessary for species identification.

12.4   Identifying the organism

On the basis of the characteristics determined by the above tests, the identity of the organism can be established with the dichotomous key devised by Holdeman et al. (1977), shown in Table 32.7.

12.5   Subtyping of strains of *Clostridium* species

Sometimes it is of interest to establish identity or non-identity between or among strains of a species with no distinguishing phenotypic characteristics, for epidemiological purposes, or to establish the source of contaminating or infecting organisms. This has been done with modest success in the serotyping (Hatheway, Whaley and Dowell 1980, Stringer, Turnbull and Gilbert 1980), bacteriocin typing (Mahony and Swantee 1978) and plasmid analysis (Mahony et al. 1987) of *C. perfringens*, and in investigation of outbreaks of antibiotic associated pseudomembranous colitis caused by *C. difficile* (Clabots et al. 1993, Chachaty et al. 1994, Kato et al. 1994, Killgore and Kato 1994, Cartwright et al. 1995, Talon et al. 1995, Tang et al. 1995). Further development of subtyping means for other species (notably *C. botulinum*) is needed.

13   CLOSTRIDIAL DISEASES

Diseases caused by various *Clostridium* species are botulism (see Volume 3, Chapter 37), tetanus (see Volume 3, Chapter 36), gas gangrene (see Volume 3, Chapter 35), antibiotic associated diarrhoea and pseudomembranous colitis, food-borne diarrhoea (see Volume 3, Chapter 28), necrotic enteritis of humans (see Volume 3, Chapter 59) and domestic animals, and blackleg and malignant oedema in cattle and sheep. The diseases are listed in Tables 32.8 and 32.9.

Gas gangrene can be caused by at least 6 different species. Clostridia usually have low potential for infection in the normal tissues of living animals. They have been referred to as primarily saprophytic, and only facultative pathogens (MacLennan 1962). The presence of clostridia in a wound often represents clostridial contamination rather than clostridial infection. The organisms that can cause gas gangrene are *C. perfringens*, *C. novyi*, *C. septicum*, *C. bifermentans*, *C. sordellii* and *C. fallax*. Under appropriate conditions, these organisms can become infective in themselves and generate the dreaded condition commonly known as gas gangrene; clostridial myonecrosis might be a more properly descriptive term. These conditions are most notably initiated with a lowered oxidation–reduction potential such as results from a disrupted or impaired blood supply, which results in a lowering of the pH to about 6.8 and autolysis of some tissue proteins, making available amino acids such as cysteine and tryptophan which are normally not available but necessary for initiation of growth (MacLennan 1962, Smith and Williams 1984).

14   CLOSTRIDIA OF MEDICAL INTEREST

14.1   *C. butyricum*

C. butyricum is of particular interest because (1) it serves as the type strain for the genus, (2) it is associated with Pasteur's *Vibrion butyrique* which is reputed to be the first known anaerobic organism, (3) it is often isolated from clinical specimens and (4) neurotoxigenic strains have been discovered.

Microscopically, the organism is seen as gram-

Table 32.5 Reactions of some commonly encountered clostridia (after Willis 1977, modified)

Species	Type	Acid from sugars				Gelatinase	Indole	Milk digestion	Egg-yolk agar		Pathogenic for laboratory animals
		Glu	Mal	Lac	Suc				Lecithinase	Lipase	
C. butyricum		+	+	+	+	–	–	–	–	–	–
C. baratii		+	+	+	+	–	–	–	+	–	–
C. perfringens	A–E	+	+	+	+	+	–	–	+	–	v
C. tertium		+	+	+	+	–	–	–	–	–	–
C. fallax		+	+	+	+	–	–	–	–	–	v
C. carnis		+	+	+	+	+	–	–	–	–	+
C. chauvoei		+	+	+	+	+	–	–	–	–	+
C. septicum		+	+	+	–	+	–	–	–	–	+
C. paraputrificum		+	+	+	+	–	–	–	–	–	–
C. sphenoides		+	+	–	+	–	+	–	–	–	–
C. sporogenes		+	+	–	–	+	–	+	–	+	–
C. botulinum	I: (A,B,F; proteolytic) II: (B,E,F; non-proteolytic) III (C,D)	+	+	–	+	+	–	+	–	+	+
C. argentinense		+	v	–	–	+	–	v	–	+	+
C. novyi	(A) (B) (C)	–	–	–	–	+	–	+	+	–	+
C. haemolyticum		+	+	–	–	+	–	+	+	+	+
C. difficile		+	+	–	–	+	–	+	–	+	+
C. bifermentans		+	–	–	+	+	+	–	+	–	–
C. sordellii		+	–	–	–	+	+	–	+	–	+
C. cadaveris		+	+	–	–	+	v	–	+	–	+
C. cochlearium		–	+	–	–	–	–	–	+	–	–
C. tetani		–	–	–	–	+	+	–	–	–	v
C. histolyticum		–	–	–	–	+	–	+	–	–	–
C. putrificum		–	–	–	–	+	+	+	–	–	–
C. hastiforme		+	–	–	–	+	–	+	v	–	v
C. ramosum		+	+	+	+	–	–	–	–	–	+

+, Positive reaction; –, negative reaction; v, some strains give a positive reaction, others do not.

Table 32.6 Metabolic endpoint products for selected clostridia detectable by gas–liquid chromatography (from Lombard and Dowell 1982, modified)

Species	Type	Acid products[a]	
		Volatile	Non-volatile
C. argentinense		A,IB,B,IV,V	PA
C. bifermentans		A,IC(P),(IB),(IV)	PP
C. baratii		A,B	(L)
C. botulinum	A,B,E (group I)	A,IB,B,IV,(P),(V),(IC)	PP
	B,E,F (group II)	A,B	
	C,D (group III)	A,P,B	
C. butyricum		A,B	
C. difficile		A,IB,B,IV,V,IC,(P)	PP
C. histolyticum		A	(PP)
C. innocuum		A,B	(L)
C. limosum		A	
C. novyi	A	A,P,B(V)	
C. paraputrificum		A,B	(L)
C. perfringens		A,B,(P)	(L)
C. ramosum		A	L,(PY)
C. septicum		A,B	
C. sordellii		A,IC,(P),(IB),(IV)	
C. sporogenes		A,IB,B,IV,(P),(V),(IC)	PP
C. subterminale		A,IB,B,IV,(P),(V),(IC)	PA
C. tertium		A,B	(L),(PP)
C. tetani		A,P,B	(PP)

[a]A, acetic; P, propionic; B, butyric; V, valeric; C, caproic; IB, isobutyric; IV, isovaleric; IC, isocaproic; L, lactic; PA, phenylacetic; PP, phenylpropionic (hydrocinnamic).
Products which may or may not be found are shown in parentheses.

positive rods, 0.7 μm × 3–4 μm with parallel sides; spores are oval, 1.3 μm × 1.6 μm, situated subterminally, forcing the spindle shape. The cells are motile by peritrichous flagella. The organism ferments glucose, maltose, lactose and sucrose. It is entirely non-proteolytic, non-haemolytic and does not produce indole, lecithinase or lipase. It does not require amino acids or vitamins other than biotin. It will grow well in a medium containing glucose, mineral salts and biotin; this capability distinguishes *C. butyricum* from *C. beijerinckii* (Table 32.7).

C. butyricum has been considered entirely non-pathogenic (Willis 1990); however, neurotoxigenic strains have been implicated as the cause of 2 cases of type E infant botulism (Aureli et al. 1986). The nucleotide and derived amino acid sequence for the neurotoxin has been determined and compared with those of the neurotoxin of *C. botulinum* strain Beluga (Poulet et al. 1992); only 39 of 1251 amino acid were altered (97% amino acid identity). Zhou, Sugiyama and Johnson (1993) found evidence that the neurotoxin gene in a culture derived from *C. butyricum* strain ATCC 43181 could be transferred to a non-toxigenic strain, type E-like *C. botulinum*. A phage induced from the toxigenic strain in the presence of a helper phage recovered from the type strain (ATCC 19398; non-toxigenic) transduced the neurotoxin gene to the non-toxigenic type E-like *C. botulinum* strain.

14.2   *C. botulinum*

Organisms known under this species designation share the ability to produce BoNT and cause botulism in humans and animals. The neurotoxins can be distinguished serologically as types A–F (type G toxin has thus far been associated with *C. argentinense*). *C. botulinum* consists of 3 groups (see Table 32.1 and Fig. 32.1) of organisms which are genetically equivalent to 3 distinct species. The organisms in all 3 groups are motile, produce lipase as demonstrated on egg yolk agar (Table 32.4), liquefy gelatin and ferment glucose. Morphologically the organisms are generally large spores, 0.9 μm × 4–6 μm, with oval, subterminal spores. There is variation from strain to strain and there is no characteristic morphology for distinguishing between physiological groups or toxin types.

GROUPING
Group I

Organisms in group I, generally known as proteolytic *C. botulinum*, may produce either type A, type B or type F neurotoxin. They digest complex proteins such as casein, meat particles, or coagulated egg albumin; produce isoacids (isobutyric and isovaleric, as is common among proteolytic clostridia) and phenylpropionic (hydrocinnamic) acid as metabolic end products;

Table 32.7 Identification key for selected *Clostridium* spp. (Holdeman, Cato and Moore 1977)

(a) Species liquefying gelatin

Glucose	Indole produced	Lipase	Butyric produced	Lactose	Sucrose	Mannitol	Mannose	Lecithinase	Lipase	Lactic major	Lecithinase	Urease	Aesculin hydrolysed	Toxic	Starch acid	Motile	Products from PYG	Suggested species
+	+	+															BP(alsf)	*C. botulinum* type C
	−						+	+									Aic2(Fpivslibb)	*C. sordellii*
									−								AF(picibivhbsl2,4)	*C. bifermentans*
																	PBA(ls)	*C. haemolyticum*
																	Pba(vfs)	*C. novyi* type B
									−								AB4(lfp)	*C. cadaveris*
	−					+	+	+					+				BA(Lspf)	*C. sardiniensis*
													−				AB(Lfps)	*C. perfringens*
									−		+		+				ABLsp	*C. aurantibutyricum*
											−						BA4(lsf)	*C. felsineum*
											−						BAF(sl)	*C. chauvoei*
									−								AB(Fpls2)	*C. septicum*
						−	+		+								Bbivibp2(ic)	*C. lituseburense*
									−	+							BA(fsl)	*C. botulinum* types B,E,F (non-prot.)
									−								ABl(fps)	*C. perfringens*
					−	+											Abibivic(vfplcs)	*C. difficile*
							−	+		+							BP(aflsv)	*C. botulinum* types C,D
								−	+								Lab(ivsfic)	*C. oceanicum*
									−								Pba(vfs)	*C. novyi* type B
									−	+							Bpa(slf)	*C. novyi* type A
																	Abivib2,3i5,5(icspvl)	*C. sporogenes*
									−	+			+				BaiVibp4(icv5i42lfs)	*C. botulinum* types A,B,F (prot.)
											−						Abivib2,3,i4,4,i5,5(icspvl)	*C. sporogenes*
											−						Abivib(slfpic2)	*C. putrificum*
	+												+				AiCbicib2i4(p4)	*C. ghoni*
										−	+						Abp4(s)	*C. tetani*
											−						Ba(pfls)	*C. malenominatum*
																	Afivicibpsl	*C. mangenoti*
−	+												+				Abivibp4(icv5i4,2lfs)	*C. botulinum* types A,B,F (prot.)
											−						Abivib2,3i4,4i55(icspv)	*C. sporogenes*
−	+												+				Abp4(s)	*C. tetani*
																	Aivbibl	*C. argentinense*
											−						Abivibp(slicf2,3i4,4)	*C. hastiforme*
																	Aivbib2,4(lsfp)	*C. subterminale*
									−				+				A(slf)	*C. limosum*
											−						A(fls)	*C. histolyticum*
																	Aibiv(lfpiC)	*C. irregularis*

Table 32.7 Continued

(b) Species not liquefying gelatin

Glucose	Gr. on aero.BAP	Grows at 37°C	Lecithinase	Caproic produced	Indole produced	Butyric produced	Aesculin hydrolysed	Iv from glucose	Fructose	Sucrose	Maltose	Aesculin hydrolysed	Spore location	Starch (pH)	Melibiose	Mannitol	Mannose	Lactose	Ribose	Req. ferm. CHO*	Xylose	Grows in GMB	Products from PYG	Suggested Species
+	+																+		+				Alb(fs)	*C. tertium*
																			−				La(f)	*C. inulinum*
																	−						LFA2	*C. durum*
																							Bafl(s)	*C. carnis*
	−	+	+										T										BA(Lps)	*C. perenne*
													ST										BLA(sfp)	*C. baratii*
			−	+																			ABCivvib(fls)	*C. scatologenes*
				−	+												+						A2(Fsl)	*C. sphenoides*
															−		+						A(Fls2)	*C. clostridiiforme*
																	−						AF2(plb)	*C. indolis*
	−	+	+		+	+							T				+		+				BAFl(sp4)	*C. sartagoformum*
																	−						LBA(fs)	*C. innocuum*
																	−			+			BAF(lp)	*C. pseudotetanicum*
																	−						LBA(Fs)	*C. paraputrificum*
													ST	+				+					BA4(Ls)	*C. acetobutylicum*
																		−		+			BAF(ls)	*C. butyricum*
																		−					BA(4Fpls)	*C. beijerinckii*
																	−			+			BA4(lsf)	*C. felsineum*
																		−					Fab(2s)	*C. celatum*
																							Bapv	*C. rectum*
											−						+						LBA(fs)	*C. innocuum*
											−												AB(Ls2,4)	*C. fallax*
										−													BL(4sp)	*C. barkeri*
												−		+									BA(lsf4)	*C. pasteurianum*
																							AbiViblps4	*C. sticklandii*
												−											BAs(lfp)	*C. tyrobutyricum*
			−			+																	Avib(pslf2,3,4,5)	*C. glycolicum*
							−			+	+			+									FAL(sp2)	*C. ramosum*
											−							+					Fal2(s)	*C. oroticum*
											−												A(Fls2)	*C. clostridiiforme*
												−											AF2(ls)	*C. nexile*
											−												Alfs	*C. cellobioparum*
	−																						ALB(sf)	*C. thermosaccharolyticum*
−	+	+																					BA(fpls)	*C. malenominatum*
	−										+												A(2ls)	*C. leptum*
											−	+											A(2lfs)	*C. aminovalericum*

Table 32.7 Continued

(b) Species not liquefying gelatin

Glucose	Gr. on aero.BAP	Grows at 37°C	Lecithinase	Caproic produced	Indole produced	Butyric produced	Aesculin hydrolysed	Iv from glucose	Fructose	Sucrose	Maltose	Aesculin hydrolysed	Spore location	Starch (pH)	Melibiose	Mannitol	Mannose	Lactose	Ribose	Req. ferm. CHO*	Xylose	Grows in GMB	Products from PYG	Suggested Species
																		−					Afs(ivl)	*C. formicoaceticum*
																							Abp(l)	*C. sporosphaeroides*
																							Bap(fls)	*C. cochlearium*
																							Pivibbsla	*C. propionicum*
−																							a(lsf)	*C. putrefaciens*

+, positive reaction for 90–100% of strains; −, negative reaction for 90–100% of strains.
Spore location: T, terminal; ST, subterminal.
Products from peptone–yeast–glucose (PYG): **Acids:** F, formic; A, acetic; P, propionic; B, butyric; V, valeric; C, caproic; iB, isobutyric; iV, isovaleric; iC, isocaproic; L, lactic; S, succinic. **Alcohols:** 2, ethanol; 3, propanol; 4, butanol; 5, pentanol; 6, hexanol; i4, isobutanol; i5 isopentanol; (upper case), symbols denote products detected at >1 mEq per 100 ml; lower case symbols denote products detected at >1 mEq per 100 ml; symbols within parentheses are products produced by occasional strains.

Table 32.8 Diseases caused by clostridia[a] other than those caused exclusively by *Clostridium perfringens*

Disease	Organisms	Types	Remarks
Botulism	*C. botulinum*	A,B,E	Human food-borne
		A,B	Human infant, wound infection
		B	Equine, shaker foal
		C	Avian, bovine, canine
		D	Bovine
		F	Human food-borne (very rare)
	C. baratii (neurotoxigenic)	F	Human: infant, adult colonization
	C. butyricum (neurotoxigenic)	E	Human infant
	C. argentinense	G	(reports of autopsy isolates, but no clinical evidence of botulism)
Tetanus	*C. tetani*		Human, equine
Gas gangrene	*C. perfringens*, *C. novyi*, *C. septicum*, *C. histolyticum*, *C. sordellii*, *C. fallax*		Human (often mixed clostridial infection)
Pseudomembranous colitis	*C. difficile*		Human
Blackleg	*C. chauvoei*		Bovine, ovine

[a]Diseases caused exclusively by *C. perfringens* are listed in Table 32.9 by toxin type.

form highly heat-resistant spores (they may survive boiling for more than 1 h); and have an optimum growth temperature of 30–40°C. These organisms are distinguished from *C. sporogenes* genetically and phenotypically only on the basis of their ability to produce neurotoxin. They are most often implicated in human botulism, although type F botulism is most rare. Only group I organisms have been associated with wound botulism. Also, excluding the cases caused by *C. butyricum* (Aureli et al. 1986) and *C. baratii* (Hall et al. 1985), and one case reported as type C (Oguma et al. 1990), only group I strains have been implicated in infant botulism.

Group II

Group II organisms are commonly known as non-proteolytic, and sometimes referred to as saccharolytic *C. botulinum*. They produce either type B, type E or

Table 32.9 Diseases caused by *Clostridium perfringens* toxin types A, B, C, D and E

Toxin type	Diseases
A	Gas gangrene (myonecrosis), food-borne illness, and infectious diarrhoea in humans; enterotoxaemia of lambs, cattle, goats, horses, dogs, alpacas, and others; necrotic enteritis in fowl; equine intestinal clostridiosis; acute gastric dilatation in non-human primates, various animal species, and humans
B	Lamb dysentery, sheep and goat enterotoxaemia (Europe, Middle East); guinea-pig enterotoxaemia
C	Darmbrand (Germany) and pig-bel (New Guinea) in humans, 'struck' in sheep, enterotoxaemia in lambs and pigs; necrotic enteritis in fowl
D	Enterotoxaemia of sheep, pulpy kidney disease of lambs
E	Enterotoxaemia in calves, lamb dysentery; guinea-pig enterotoxaemia; rabbit 'iota' enterotoxaemia

type F neurotoxin. They generally ferment sugars such as sucrose, maltose and mannose, which are not fermented by group I strains. Their cultures do not show the isoacids on GLC. They have a lower optimum growth temperature (20–30°C) and some strains will grow at refrigerator temperatures (Eklund, Wieler and Poysky 1967). Spores formed by these organisms are not nearly so heat-resistant as those formed by group I strains; this might explain why group II organisms are not associated with botulism from heat-processed home-canned foods. Similarly, the lower growth temperature requirement makes it less likely that they will grow in the living body to cause botulism by growth in an infected wound or colonization of the intestine. Strains that produce type E toxin often cause botulism from contaminated fish or marine products (Wainwright et al. 1988, Weber et al. 1993b). Group II strains that produce type B toxin are associated with botulism from salt-cured meat (Luecke, Hechelmann and Leistner 1981). This appears to be the same organism originally described by Van Ermengem 1897). Only one incident of botulism due to non-proteolytic type F *C. botulinum* has been reported (Midura et al. 1972); the vehicle was dried deer meat (venison jerky).

Group III

Strains belonging to group III produce type C and D toxin and are responsible for botulism occurring in non-human species, especially in birds (Eklund and Dowell 1987). These organisms are genetically related to *C. novyi* (Nakamura et al. 1983a; see Table 32.1, Fig. 32.1, and below under *C. novyi*). Neurotoxigenicity of these organisms is dependent on their carrying a bacteriophage that contains the gene for either type C or type D neurotoxin (Eklund et al. 1987). Interspecies conversions between group III organisms and *C. novyi* have been demonstrated by phage manipulations (Eklund et al. 1974). There is disagreement as to whether these organisms are proteolytic or non-proteolytic, but the isoacid end products associated with proteolytic organisms are not found in their cultures (Table 32.6). The optimal growth temperature is in the range 25–37°C (Smith and Sugiyama 1988). The organisms are less aerotolerant than those in groups I and II. Detection of neurotoxin in cultures of samples from animals dying from type C botulism is rather straightforward, but isolation of toxigenic organisms in pure culture is another matter. Under certain conditions, the phage is lost from many of the cells and the isolates from the plates are predominantly, if not completely non-toxigenic. Although growing at temperatures higher than 30°C can produce highly toxic cultures, many of the organisms recovered from them are non-toxigenic. Culturing at temperatures below 30°C has been shown to maintain toxigenicity of stock cultures (Eklund et al. 1987). After death of an animal harbouring the organism, the carcass serves as a suitable milieu for intensive growth and toxin production by group III organisms.

Inoue and Iida (1971) noted a close relation between lysogenicity and toxigenicity among strains of *C. botulinum* types C and D and succeeded in converting non-toxigenic into toxigenic strains by lysogenization. Not only can phages effect conversion of one type of *C. botulinum* to another, but they can also bring about interspecific conversion from *C. botulinum* type C to *C. novyi* type A (Eklund et al. 1974). A strain of *C. botulinum* type C was cured of its phage and thus converted into a non-toxigenic variant. On infection with one or 2 phages from *C. novyi* type A it produced *C. novyi* lecithinase (α-toxin).

Type C strains have been referred to as C_α and C_β subtypes (Smith and Williams 1984). Initially it was thought that the neurotoxin had slightly different serological features. Jansen (1971) demonstrated that type C strains produced 3 toxins: C_1, C_2, and a small amount of type D toxin. Type D strains produced mostly type D toxin but also a minor amount of C_1; C_α strains produce both C_1 and C_2, while C_β strains produce mainly, if not exclusively, C_2. As noted above, C_2 is not a neurotoxin, but a binary toxin that acts as a permease, causing its own pathology but no paralysis. It is conceivable that it enhances the uptake of C_1 neurotoxin from the gut.

In addition, a third factor produced by type C and type D strains known as exoenzyme C_3 has been found (Aktories, Weller and Chhatwal 1987). It is an ADP-ribosyltransferase for which no pathogenic role has been established.

There seem to be problems unique to the culture and isolation of neurotoxigenic group III organisms.

These problems stem from the fact that toxigenicity is dependent on a pseudolysogenic relationship with the bacteriophage that encodes the toxin gene. Eklund et al. (1987) noted that incubation temperature for type C organisms is critical. The optimum growing temperature is stated by several sources as 30–37°C, and that most type C and D strains grow well at 45°C, and poorly or not at all at 25°C (Cato, George and Finegold 1986). If the cultures are incubated at 37°C, the phages multiply within the cells and induce toxin production. At this temperature the phage becomes virulent and lyses the bacterial cells. Almost all of the recoverable organisms are non-toxigenic. A maximum temperature of 30°C is recommended at which toxicity of stock cultures is seldom lost (Eklund et al. 1987). This may explain the experience of many workers who have reported success in demonstrating toxin in enrichment cultures, but consistent failure in recovering pure isolates of toxigenic organisms.

CLINICAL ASPECTS OF BOTULISM

Botulism has also been known for a long time before its bacterial aetiology and toxicological mechanism were elucidated (Van Ermengem 1897). It has been and still is recognized primarily as a food-borne disease, although 4 forms of the disease are now recognized: (1) food-borne botulism, (2) wound botulism, (3) infant botulism and (4) botulism due to intestinal colonization of non-infants. Although the means of presentation of the botulinum toxin differs, the mechanism of the paralytic disease is the same for all forms, as described in the discussion of the neurotoxins. Signs and symptoms include blurred and or double vision, ptosis, slurred speech, difficulty swallowing, dry mouth, muscular weakness (progressing to severe paralysis) and respiratory impairment sometimes resulting in respiratory arrest (Hughes et al. 1981). Treatment includes supportive intensive care and administration of therapeutic antitoxin (Morris 1981). Recovery involves regeneration of nerve endings to restore muscle function.

Food-borne botulism

Food-borne botulism remains a problem in many countries, usually due to home prepared or processed foods. The countries having the highest incidence are Poland, China, Iran, countries of the former Soviet Union, Italy, the USA, Germany and France (Hauschild 1993). The toxin types associated with food-borne botulism are almost exclusively A, B and E; rare incidents due to type F have been documented. The organisms have been *C. botulinum* of either group I or II. Confirmation is made of the basis of detecting the neurotoxin in the patient's circulation, the patient's stool or remnants of a food consumed by the patient before the onset of illness (Hatheway 1988). Recovery of *C. botulinum* from the patient's stool is also good confirmatory evidence, because the organism is rarely, if ever, found in human faeces in the absence of botulism.

Wound botulism

Wound botulism, the rarest form of the disease, is analogous to tetanus, being a systemic intoxication caused by toxin elaborated by the organisms growing in a wound. Between 1943 and 1990, 47 cases were documented in the USA (Weber et al. 1993a). All cases encountered so far have been caused by *C. botulinum* (group I) type A or type B. In the 1980s, wound botulism was found in several patients with wound infections due to illicit drug use (MacDonald et al. 1985). Most recently, within the calendar year 1995, 19 laboratory-confirmed cases of wound botulism associated with drug use infections were reported in California (CDC 1995). Wound botulism is confirmed by detection of neurotoxin in serum and recovery of the toxigenic organism from the infected site.

Infant botulism

Infant botulism has been confirmed only rarely outside the USA. It was first recognized as a form of the disease distinct from food-borne botulism in 1976 (Midura and Arnon 1976, Pickett et al. 1976). The disease occurs because the environment within the infant intestine during the first 6 months of life can at times provide satisfactory conditions for colonization by *C. botulinum*. Neurotoxin produced in the intestine is absorbed into the circulation and causes the paralytic disease similarly as in food-borne botulism. Examination of faecal specimens for confirmation of botulism was introduced in the early 1970s and became part of the routine protocol about 1974; this provided the necessary means for confirmation since there is no toxic food involved, and infant serum specimens are usually too scanty for adequate bioassay and also usually negative when tested. Stools obtained during the acute phase of the illness usually show unquestionable levels of neurotoxin and readily yield the toxigenic organism upon culture (Hatheway and McCroskey 1987).

Through 1990, 14 countries had confirmed at least one case of infant botulism (Dodds 1993). The US had confirmed 932, Argentina 23, Australia 11 and Japan 10; the remainder had confirmed 4 or less. Infant botulism has become the most frequent form of the disease in the USA. Approximately one half of the confirmed cases were found in California. Practically all of the infant cases have been caused by *C. botulinum* (group I), either type A or type B. Unusual cases are as follows: 2 type F cases in the US caused by *C. baratii* (Hall et al. 1985); 2 type E cases in Italy caused by *C. butyricum* (Aureli et al. 1986); 1 type C case in Japan (Oguma et al. 1990).

Non-infant botulism due to colonization

Botulism of non-infants due to colonization had been suspected from time to time, and after recognition of botulism in infants, the search for analogous adult forms gained impetus. Evidence suggestive of a colonization mechanism has been found in cases associated with food-borne vehicles of the organism and in patients with surgical alteration of the gastrointestinal tract (Chia et al. 1986, McCroskey and Hatheway

1988). A 67-year old man with Crohn's disease developed type A botulism and was found to yield positive stool cultures for *C. botulinum* for 19 weeks (Griffin et al. 1997). It cannot be concluded whether the organism persisted by intestinal lumen colonization or by infection of intestinal lesions. More recently, type F botulism caused by *C. baratii* probably by intestinal colonization has been documented (McCroskey et al. 1991). Since then, 4 more cases of probable adult colonization type F botulism from which toxigenic *C. baratii* has been isolated have been documented (CDC, unpublished records).

Botulism in non-human species

Botulism occurs quite frequently in nature in many non-human species. Most spectacular are extensive outbreaks of type C botulism in wild waterfowl (Eklund and Dowell 1987, Jensen and Price 1987). Type C botulism also occurs in cattle, sheep, horses, dogs and mink (Smith and Sugiyama 1988). Type D botulism has been documented only very rarely; its discovery was made with the investigation of an outbreak in cattle in South Africa (Seddon 1922). Horses seem to be very susceptible to type B toxin (Johnston and Whitlock 1987). A condition in foals known as shaker foal has been shown to be botulism, and when determination was made, the type was B (Swerczek 1980a,b).

LABORATORY INVESTIGATION OF BOTULISM

Botulism is confirmed by detecting botulinum neurotoxin (BoNT) in the patient's blood or in a sample of a food consumed within a few hours to a few days before onset of symptoms. Toxin in a patient's faeces indicates residual toxin from the ingested contaminated food, or toxin produced in the gastrointestinal tract by organisms colonizing the gut, such as occurs in infant botulism. In either case, the toxigenic organism should be recoverable from cultures of the faecal samples. In infant botulism, large numbers are usually found (Wilcke, Midura and Arnon 1980), and isolation can often be done from a directly streaked egg yolk agar plate, especially if the medium contains antibiotics for selection of *C. botulinum* (Glasby and Hatheway 1984b, Mills, Midura and Arnon 1985). Finding *C. botulinum* in the absence of toxin in the faeces of a patient showing signs and symptoms consistent with botulism is considered good confirmatory evidence, since the organism is rarely, if ever, found in humans in the absence of botulism (Easton and Meyer 1924, Dowell et al. 1977b).

Detection and identification of neurotoxin

BoNT is routinely detected and identified in clinical specimens and food samples using the mouse bioassay, employing type-specific diagnostic antisera for neutralizing the lethal activity (Hatheway 1988). Identification of the neurotoxin is also necessary for identifying the isolated organism. Close observation over the first 6–24 hours should allow the laboratorian to additionally confirm the toxin identity by noting signs of botulism in the injected mice. Although the assay is considered a 4-day test, positive results are almost always apparent in less than 24 h. Liquid samples such as serum are injected directly (intraperitoneally) into mice, usually 0.4 ml, and when antitoxin is added, 0.5 ml of the mixture (containing 0.1 ml of the reagent) is injected. For testing solid or semisolid samples, an extract is made by suspending (grinding with mortar and pestle when necessary) the material in buffered gelatin (0.2% gelatin, 0.4% Na_2HPO_4, adjusted to pH 6.2 with HCl), then centrifuging the suspension and recovering the supernatant for testing. Some faecal samples yield non-specifically toxic extracts, and cause mouse deaths that cannot be prevented by any of the antitoxins, and which are not accompanied by any signs of botulism. Sometimes this problem can be overcome by retesting the extract at a dilution at which the BoNT is still lethal but the non-specific factor is not. Such can be the case with infant botulism faecal samples for which toxin can often be demonstrated at extract dilutions of greater than 1 : 100; the non-specific lethality usually has a titre of less than 1 : 10. When the nonspecific toxicity cannot be resolved, the culture results become much more important. It is rare that toxin is ever found in faecal samples that do not yield a neurotoxigenic organism (Dowell et al. 1977b, Hatheway and McCroskey 1987). The activity of neurotoxins, especially those derived from non-proteolytic (group II) strains can be enhanced by exposure to proteolytic enzymes. Thus, in some cases it has been possible to demonstrate toxin in samples after trypsin treatment, when tests on the untreated samples were negative. One part trypsin solution (1.5% trypsin, Difco 1 : 250) is added to 4 parts of sample, the mixture is incubated at 37°C for 30 min, and 0.5 ml is injected into each mouse. If neutralization tests are performed, one part of antitoxin is added to 5 parts of trypsinized sample, and 0.6 ml of the neutralization mixture is enjected.

Culturing of samples for recovery of neurotoxigenic organisms

It is always important to culture faecal samples for neurotoxigenic organisms. Recovery of the organism from a toxin-positive sample confirms the toxin identification and provides a tangible piece of evidence that can be stored and re-examined indefinitely. With toxin-negative samples, of course, the recovered organism serves as the only confirmatory evidence. Sometimes the isolated organisms show some surprising features, such as the ability to produce more than one type of toxin, or that they even are identifiable as different species (Hatheway and McCroskey 1989). Type A and type E toxin-producing strains of *C. botulinum* belong only to group I or group II respectively, but type B and type F strains can belong to either.

The recovery of *C. botulinum* from a food in which no preformed toxin was found, however, is of questionable value in food-borne botulism, since the organism is frequently found, for example, on fresh fruits and vegetables that pose no problem for consumers of those foods (Easton and Meyer 1924). In infant botulism, however, recovery of the organism from a food item, notably honey (Arnon et al. 1979), has provided insight into the probable source of colonization.

For routine culture of investigative samples, and in environmental studies, samples are inoculated into 2 tubes of cooked meet medium containing 0.3% glucose and 0.2% starch (CMGS). One inoculated tube is placed into a waterbath at 80°C and held for 10 min to kill the vegetative organisms, thus selecting for spores; the other tube is not treated. Both tubes are incubated in an anaerobic environment for at least 4 days, at 35–37°C. The cultures are screened for toxicity in mice by injecting 0.4 ml of culture supernatant; some laboratories simultaneously inject 0.4 ml of heated (100°C, 10 min) supernatant to ascertain heat lability, and another sample to which 0.1 ml of a 1% solution of crude trypsin (Difco 1 : 250) to enhance toxicity of non-proteolytic organisms. Lethal samples are retested with the addition of relevant types of antitoxin for positive identification and determination of type.

When type E organisms are considered, a third tube of medium, TPGY (Solomon, Rhodehamel and Kautter 1995), to which trypsin is added (for inactivation of interfering bacteriocins, Kautter et al. 1966) is also inoculated. All 3 tubes are incubated at 30°C for at least 4 days, and then screened for toxicity. This approach might be followed when any of the group II organisms are sought. Since the spores of group II organisms are less heat-resistant than those of group I, the 80°C treatment is usually less successful. For these, alcohol treatment (Koransky, Allen and Dowell 1978) may be a more effective method of spore selection. An equal volume of 95% ethanol is added to the sample, and the mixture is held at room temperature for 1 h with occasional gentle mixing before inoculating into the CMGS. As noted above, cultures for recovery of type C and type D organisms must be incubated at no more than 30°C.

Isolation and identification of toxigenic organisms

Isolation of the toxigenic organism from the enrichment cultures as well as on occasion from the directly streaked plates is usually done by picking lipase-positive colonies from the egg yolk based agar medium. However, sometimes this is complicated by the presence of non-toxigenic lipase-positive organisms, and numerous colonies may have to be picked and screened for toxicity. On rare occasions, the toxigenic organisms have been lipase-negative, conforming to the species *C. baratii* (Hall et al. 1985, McCroskey et al. 1991) and *C. butyricum* (Aureli et al. 1986).

Usually, the only criteria needed for proper identification of the isolate are establishing toxigenicity and toxin type; finding that the organism is lipase-positive, gram-positive (in young cultures), spore-forming, and grows anaerobically; and establishing proteolytic status by milk digestion. For a type G toxin-producing organism, the identity should conform to *C. argentinense* which is lipase-negative and asaccharolytic. For lipase-negative organisms producing type E or type F toxin,

sufficient tests for identification of *C. butyricum* or *C. baratii* need to be done. If a new organism not conforming to the characteristics of any previously encountered neurotoxigenic organism, a complete characterization will have to be done.

14.3 *C. tetani*

C. tetani is one of the best known clostridia because it is the cause of tetanus. It was first isolated by Kitasato from a patient with tetanus in 1889 (Bytchenko 1981). It is a strict anaerobe, and will grow on the surface of agar media only in an anaerobic environment. On the basis of 16S rRNA gene homology, the organism is placed in cluster I (Fig. 32.1), and is closely related to *C. cochlearium*. The bacilli are 0.5–1.7×2.1–18.1 μm and often possess terminal endospores that give them a drumstick appearance (Fig. 32.2 and Plate 32.2). Cells in cultures older than 24 h may appear gram-negative. They are motile by means of peritrichous flagella. Optimal growth occurs at 37°C, while little or no growth takes place at 25°C or 42°C. Growth may not be apparent until after 48 h and may appear as a film rather than as discrete colonies because of swarming due to the vigourous motility. Media containing 3–4% agar are more conducive to formation of discrete colonies. On blood agar the colonies are 4–6 mm in diameter, flat, translucent, gray with a matt surface, showing a narrow zone of clear (β-type) haemolysis. Colonies have irregular and rhizoid margins (Cato, George and Finegold 1986).

Most common biochemical tests are negative. No sugars are fermented; milk and other complex proteins are not digested. Neither lecithinase nor lipase is produced and nitrate is not reduced. Gelatin is liquified slowly, requiring perhaps 7 days for complete liquefaction. Hydrogen sulphide and indole are produced. GLC of peptone–yeast extract broth cultures shows butanol, and acetic, propionic and butyric acids as metabolic end products (Holdeman, Cato and Moore 1977). Spores generally survive moderate heating (75–80°C for 10 min) but usually are destroyed after 100°C for 1 h (Adams, Lawrence and Smith 1969).

C. tetani is similar culturally and biochemically to *C. cochlearium* and organisms identified as *C. tetanomorphum* (the latter is no longer listed in *Bergey's Manual*: Cato, George and Finegold 1986), but all 3 groups could be clearly distinguished on the basis of DNA homology (Nakamura et al. 1979). Non-toxigenic strains of *C. tetani* are found that correlate well with toxigenic strains by DNA comparison. Soluble cellular proteins of *C. tetani* and *C. cochlearium* may be distinct (Cato et al. 1982), but otherwise it seems difficult to distinguish between the latter and non-toxigenic *C. tetani* without DNA studies.

C. tetani is commonly found in soil samples in all parts of the world. Surveys in Japan, Canada, Brazil and the USA have yielded 30–42% positive samples (Smith and Williams 1984). It is also commonly found in human and animal faeces. Bauer and Meyer (1926), Ten Broeck and Bauer (1922), and Tulloch (1919) found the organism in about 25–35% of human faecal specimens in the USA, China and England. However, many of the more recent studies on human faecal flora failed to find *C. tetani* (George and Finegold 1985). Intestinal carriage may be responsible for naturally acquired immunity to the toxin (Veronesi et al. 1983). Antitoxin, but no toxin, has been found in the serum of animals experimentally colonized with organisms (Wells and Balish 1983).

Since the clinical features of tetanus are so recognizable, laboratory investigation of cases is very rarely done. Few organisms actually involved in tetanus have been studied, and our knowledge of *C. tetani* is based almost entirely on environmental isolates, or those obtained from normal humans or animals. Perhaps we are missing some important and interesting bacteriological and pathological information that clinical isolates might reveal.

CULTURE AND ISOLATION

Culture and isolation of *C. tetani* from wound specimens and environmental samples can be attempted by the same methods. Pieces of dead tissues taken from deep wounds of tetanus patients should be satisfactory, although attempts may be made with wound swabs. Cooked meat medium to which starch has been added may be superior to CMGS since *C. tetani* does not utilize glucose, and this might provide an unnecessary energy source that may be used by competing organisms. Heat treatment for spore selection might be used to advantage. Adams, Lawrence and Smith (1969) recommend inoculating 3 broth cultures, heating the first at 80°C for 15 min, the second for 5 min, and not heating the third. Beland and Rossier (1973) recommend inoculating soil samples after suspending in sterile saline; one portion is inoculated without treatment, and another after heating at 60°C for 10 min. After incubating for 2 days at 37°C, the broth cultures are inoculated onto a small area on one side of a blood agar plate. The plates are incubated anaerobically at 37°C and observed at 24 h and 48 h for swarming growth. The bacteria at the leading edge of the swarming growth is picked and inoculated into chopped meat broth. After incubation of these cultures, they are observed microscopically, tested for toxin and examined for physiological characteristics.

TETANUS

Tetanus has been known since ancient times (Adams, Lawrence and Smith 1969). Its cause was first hypothesized to be an infectious agent in 1867; the drumstick-like forms of the organism were first described by Fleugge and by Rosenbach, and a pure culture of the organism was obtained by Kitasato in 1889 (Bytchenko 1981). The disease was shown to be due to a soluble product of the bacterial culture; Behring and Kitasato (1890) demonstrated that animals could be immunized with tetanus toxin inactivated with iodine trichloride.

The disease results from poisoning of the nerves by TeTx, also known as **tetanospasmin**, produced by *C. tetani* growing in a wound. The spastic and convulsive condition ensues according to the neurotoxic mechanism described above. The condition may be local or generalized (Bleck 1989). Local tetanus occurs in muscle groups near the site of infection and usually progresses to generalized tetanus. Partial immunity may be responsible for restricting the condition. Neonatal tetanus is due to infection of the umbilical stump. This form has a very poor prognosis, but tragically could have been prevented by maternal antibody, had the mother been immunized. The diagnosis of tetanus is usually, if not invariably, made on the basis of the clinical signs. Rarely is any laboratory confirmation attempted.

Tetanus toxoid has almost eliminated tetanus in the developed countries where immunization is almost universal, but the disease, especially in neonates, remains a serious problem in some areas of the world. Between 1983 and 1992, an average of 63 (range: 45–91) cases of human tetanus per year were reported in the USA (CDC 1993).

TOXINS

C. tetani produces 2 biologically active agents: the neurotoxin TeTx or tetanospasmin, and an oxygen-labile haemolysin known as **tetanolysin**. TeTx, described above, is encoded by a gene that is carried on a plasmid. Some strains identified as *C. tetani* lack the plasmid and are non-toxigenic (Laird et al. 1980). Although non-toxigenic strains are allowable in the species, complete characterization requires establishing toxigenicity. Toxicity and neutralization tests can be performed by intramuscular injection of 0.1 ml of toxic culture supernatant into the rear leg muscle of a mouse; a second mouse is injected with a mixture of 0.1 ml of supernatant and 0.1 ml of tetanus antitoxin. A positive culture will cause the development of a rigid paralysis in the injected muscle, with subsequent progression of the paralysis into the rest of the musculature of the lower body. No paralysis should be observed with the neutralized sample, unless the amount of toxin in the sample overwhelms the neutralizing capacity of the antitoxin. Beland and Rossier (1973) recommend testing cultures for toxigenicity by mixing equal volumes of broth cultures and 2% $CaCl_2$ and injecting 0.5 ml of the mixture at the base of the tail of a mouse for each test sample. Mice pretreated with 1500 IU of tetanus antitoxin 1 h before challenge serve as controls. Test animals should be killed as soon as a conclusive judgement can be made on the basis of paralytic signs.

Tetanolysin is related functionally and serologically to streptolysin-O and to the oxygen-sensitive haemolysins of a variety of other organisms, including at least 6 species of *Clostridium* (Bernheimer 1976). Purified tetanolysin has a molecular mass of 48±3 kDa and appears to have several molecular species based on ionic charge, exhibiting pI values of 5.3, 5.6, 6.1 and 6.6 (Lucain and Piffaretti 1977, Mitsui, Mitsui and Hase 1980). Some of the isoelectric point variation may be due to differences in charge between oxidized and reduced forms of the same molecule (Cowell, Grushoff and Bernheimer 1976). This group of haemolysins lyses a variety of cells such as erythrocytes, polymorphonuclear leukocytes, macrophages, fibroblasts, ascites tumour cells, HeLa cells and platelets (Bernheimer 1976). Lytic activity is reversibly inactivated by mild oxidizing conditions such as aeration or hydrogen peroxide, and reactivated by thiol reagents such as cysteine, reduced glutathione or thioglycollate. The active toxin has an affinity for cholesterol and related sterols, and its lytic and lethal activities are inhibited by these compounds. Hardegree, Palmer and Duffin (1971) showed in vivo effects of tetanolysin after intravenous injection into animals. In mice pulmonary oedema rapidly developed, followed by death. In rabbits and monkeys evidence showed intravascular haemolysis. Monkeys showed electrocardiographic changes and a decreased heart rate indicating a cardiotoxic effect of tetanolysin. It is questionable if this toxin plays any role in *C. tetani* infections. The amount of tetanolysin produced by the organism in vivo is unknown, and serum that contains cholesterol is known to inhibit its activity in vitro.

14.4 *C. perfringens*

C. perfringens is the most widely occurring pathogenic bacterium (Smith and Williams 1984). It is readily found in soil samples and intestinal contents of animals and humans. The organism, first described by Welch and Nuttall in 1892 as *Bacillus aerogenes capsulatus* (Welch and Nuttall 1892), has also been commonly known as *C. welchii*, especially in the UK. The organism belongs to cluster I of the 16S rRNA dendrogram (Fig. 32.1), and is most closely related to *C. baratii* and *C. absonum*. Spores of *C. perfringens* usually are rare or not observed in cultures grown in ordinary media, so it must be recognized by its other characteristics (Holdeman, Cato and Moore 1977). It grows vigorously at temperatures between 20 and 50°C with an optimum of 45°C for most strains (Cato, George and Finegold 1986), at which it has a generation time of about 8 min. This provides an easy means of isolation. A sample containing *C. perfringens* is inoculated into chopped meat broth (or CMGS) and is incubated for 4 h at 45°C, or until the first indication of bacterial growth is observed. If the culture is transferred after several 4 h intervals, the only organism present in the later transfers should be *C. perfringens* because of its ability to outgrow any other organisms (Smith and Williams 1984).

Colonies on blood agar usually show a characteristic double-zone haemolysis around the colony: an inner, clear zone due to θ-toxin, and an outer, hazy zone due to α-toxin. On McClung–Toabe egg yolk agar, the colonies are surrounded by a wide circular opaque zone, recognized as the lecithinase reaction due to the α-toxin (Cato, George and Finegold 1986). The organisms are gram-positive, straight rods with blunt ends, that occur singly or in pairs, 0.6–2.4 μm wide × 1.3–19.0 μm long. Stained smears often show coccobacillus or short rod forms (Fig 32.2k,l). They are nonmotile, reduce nitrate, ferment glucose, lactose, maltose, sucrose and other sugars, and liquefy gelatin.

'Stormy fermentation' in milk is seen, due to the fermentation of lactose, production of gas and clotting but not digestion of casein.

Toxin type A is readily found in the environment, and is considered a part of the normal flora of humans and many animal species (Smith and Williams 1984). The other types do not seem to survive in soils and therefore appear to be obligate parasites, being carried in the gut of immune hosts. The differences between toxin types seem to be restricted to which of the genes encoding the 4 major toxins are possessed. They cannot be differentiated on the basis of morphology, biochemical reactions, metabolic end products (Cato, George and Finegold 1986), or electrophoretic analysis of soluble proteins (Cato et al. 1982). Types A–D were identical by 23S rRNA homology studies (Johnson and Francis 1975). The type strain is in *Clostridium* cluster I by 16S rRNA gene sequence analysis (Collins et al. 1994).

C. perfringens is probably the most highly studied anaerobic bacterium. This is because of its ubiquity, the ease with which it can be grown, its low pathogenicity, the multiplicity of biological and antigenic products, and its involvement with various human and veterinary diseases. The status of our knowledge of the molecular genetics of *C. perfringens* has been reviewed by Rood and Cole (1991). The chromosome maps for strains of toxin types A, B, D and E show remarkably constant chromosome organization, and regardless of type, the strains represent a homogeneous group of closely related organisms. Type C could not be included in the comparison because the only available strain produced a very potent DNAase.

TOXINS AND TOXIN TYPES OF *C. PERFRINGENS*

The toxin types of *C. perfringens* A–D were initially established in 1931 on the basis of the studies of Wilsdon (cited by Glenny et al. 1933) and expanded to include type E after its discovery in 1943 (Bosworth 1943). The types are distinguished according to the production of the major toxins, α, β, ε, and ι, as indicated in Table 32.10. Toxin typing has generally been done by mouse lethality of culture fluids and neutralization with anti A (anti-α), anti B (anti-α + anti-β + anti-ε), anti C (anti-α + anti-β), anti D (anti-α + anti-ε), and anti E (anti-α + anti-ι) antitoxin reagents (Dowell and Hawkins 1974). In recent years, commercial sources of typing reagents have been difficult to find (types A, C, D and E reagents are currently available from TechLab, Blacksburg, VA, USA). Type B toxin type is determined by using the type C and D reagents. α-Toxin can be assumed by the lecithinase reaction on egg yolk agar (Table 32.4). Immunoassays for β-, ε-, and ι-toxins have been proposed (Nagahama et al. 1991), but reagents for these tests are not available, and must be prepared by each prospective user. Since the nucleotide sequences for the genes for α-, β-, ε- and ι-toxins have been published, gene probes or PCR could be used for determining toxin types (Songer and Meer 1996).

Table 32.10 Toxin types of *Clostridium perfringens* and major and minor toxins they produce (from Hatheway 1990)

Toxins	Biological activity	Toxin type				
		A	B	C	D	E
Major						
(lethal)						
α	Lethal, lecithinase (phospholipase C)	+	+	+	+	+
β	Lethal, necrotizing, trypsin labile	−	+	+	−	−
ε	Lethal, permease, trypsin activatable	−	+	−	+	−
ι	Lethal, dermonecrotic, binary, ADP-ribosylating, trypsin activatable	−	−	−	−	+
Minor						
γ	Not defined, existence questionable	−	±	±	−	−
δ	Haemolysin	−	±	+	−	−
η	Not defined, existence questionable	±	−	−	−	−
θ	Haemolysin (O₂-labile), cytolysin	±	+	+	+	+
κ	Collagenase, gelatinase	+	+	+	+	+
λ	Protease	−	+	−	+	+
μ	Hyaluronidase	±	+	±	±	±
ν	Deoxyribonuclease	±	+	+	±	±
Neuraminidase	*N*-acetylneuraminic acid glycohydrolase	+	+	+	+	+
Other						
Enterotoxin	Enterotoxic, cytotoxic	+	nt	+	+	nt

[a]+, produced by most strains; ±, produced by some of the strains; −, no strain of the indicated toxin type has been shown to produce the toxin; nt, insufficient studies have been done with strains of the indicated toxin type.

α-Toxin

Produced in large amounts by type A strains, α-toxin is a phospholipase C (EC 3.1.4.3) and appears to play a major role in gas gangrene. It hydrolyses phosphatidylcholine and sphingomyelin, but not other phospholipids (Jolivet-Reynaud, Moreau and Alouf 1988). It is a zinc metal protein and requires calcium ions for interaction with substrate. It is responsible for the lecithinase reaction on egg yolk agar and for the hazy zone of haemolysis on blood agar. The gene encoding α-toxin has been cloned and sequenced; the results show that the gene product is a 399-amino acid peptide with a molecular mass of 43 kDa (Okabe, Shimizu and Hayashi 1989, Titball et al. 1989, Tso and Seibel 1989). Immunization of guinea-pigs with α-toxin protects them against gas gangrene when challenged with *C. perfringens* and toxin (Kameyama, Sato and Muratoa 1972).

β-Toxin

β-Toxin is a major lethal toxin produced by type B and C toxin types. It is responsible for the lesions of necrotic enteritis of pig-bel (Murrell et al. 1966) and Darmbrand (Zeissler and Rassfeld-Sternberg 1949). The toxin purified by affinity chromatography has a molecular mass of 40 kDa and an isoelectric pH of 5.6 (Sakurai et al. 1981). Nucleotide sequencing of the gene encoding the β-toxin reveals an open reading frame of 1008 nucleotides that encodes a protein of 336 amino acids with a molecular mass of 34.9 kDa (Hunter et al. 1993).

ε-Toxin

ε-Toxin is a prototoxin that is activated by proteolytic enzymes and is produced by both type B and type D strains. It increases the permeability of the intestine, thus enhancing its own uptake, and acts systemically as a lethal toxin (Buxton 1978). In the circulation, it causes swollen, hyperaemic kidneys, oedema in the lungs and excess pericardial fluid (McDonel 1980a). The nucleotide sequence of the gene encoding ε-toxin shows that the mature prototoxin consists of 297 amino acids with a molecular mass of 33 kDa (Hunter et al. 1992). A 13 amino acid N-terminal peptide is cleaved during activation.

ι-Toxin

ι-Toxin is a binary toxin consisting of 2 subunits, ι-a and ι-b, which are immunologically and biochemically distinct (Stiles and Wilkins 1986a, 1986b). The gene sequences encoding these subunits have been determined and the deduced amino acid sequences for the functionally active proteins correspond to peptides with molecular masses of about 40 and 81 kDa, respectively (Perelle et al. 1993). A mixture of both components is needed to demonstrate biological activity by mouse lethality or dermonecrosis. The light chain (ι-a) is an enzyme that ADP-ribosylates polyarginine (Simpson et al. 1987) and skeletal muscle and nonmuscle actin (Vandekerckhove et al. 1987, Schering et al. 1988). ι-a must gain entrance into the target cell before it can have any effect, but cannot do this of itself; ι-b recognizes a binding site on the cell membrane, binds to the site, and interacts with ι-a to facilitate its entry. ι-Toxin of *C. perfringens* is similar to ι-toxin of *C. spiroforme* in serological, biological, and enzymatic activities (Popoff and Boquet 1988).

Minor toxins

Nine other factors produced by at least some strains of *C. perfringens* referred to as *minor toxins* have been identified and are listed in Table 32.10. At least some strains of all toxin types produce θ, κ, μ, ν, and neuraminidase. δ-**Toxin** is a haemolysin produced by type B and C strains, but not by type A, D, and E strains. λ-**Toxin** has not been detected in type A and C strains. It is a proteinase that digests gelatin, haemoglobin and casein to some extent, but not collagen (Smith and Williams 1984). Strains of any toxin type may be encountered which fail to produce one or more of the indicated minor toxins. The minor toxins have been of primary interest in the early attempts at classifying members of the species. κ-**Toxin** (collagenase), μ-**toxin** (hyaluronidase), and λ-**toxin** (protease) appear to play roles in pathogenesis because of their ability to break down host tissues. γ- **and** η-**Toxins** have been proposed to account for discrepancies in neutralizing results obtained with specific antisera, but specific active substances related to those supposed entities have not yet been isolated (McDonel 1980a).

δ-**Toxin** has been recovered from *C. perfringens* type C and purified (Tixier and Alouf 1976, Alouf and Jolivet-Reynaud 1981). It has a molecular mass of 42 kDa and an isoelectric pH of 9.1. It has high haemolytic activity for erythrocytes from sheep, goats and pigs, but is relatively inactive against those from humans, horses, rabbits, mice and other mammals. The activity is inhibited by gangliosides (especially G_{M2}), but not by other lipid compounds such as sphingomyelin, lecithin or cholesterol.

θ-**toxin**, also known as perfringolysin-O, is responsible for the clear zone of haemolysis produced by at least some strains of all toxin types (McDonel 1980a, Smith and Williams 1984). It is an oxygen-labile, thiol-activated cytolysin, similar to but not identical with some haemolysins produced by other species (*Streptococcus pyogenes, Streptococcus pneumoniae, C. tetani* and *C. novyi*) (Bernheimer 1976, Smith and Williams 1984). θ-Toxin has been purified by anion exchange and gel permeation chromatography (Yamakawa, Ito and Sato 1977) and has a molecular size of 51 kDa by polyacrylamide gel electrophoretic (PAGE) analysis. This estimate agrees with amino acid analysis. θ-Toxin, activated by cysteine, is lethal for mice (intravenous injection) and the lethality is reportedly due to the cardiodepressant effect of toxin-induced release of endogenous mediators such as platelet-activating factor (Stevens et al. 1988).

Tweten (1988a,b) has cloned and expressed the gene for θ-toxin in *E. coli*. The gene product was identical to the θ-toxin produced by the donor strain in amino terminal sequence and in SDS gel electrophoretic analysis. Both had an estimated molecular mass of 54 kDa and were of comparable haemolytic activity. The 1.8 kb chromosomal fragment generated a peptide of 499 amino acids that included a 27 residue

signal peptide. The secreted form of the θ-toxin has a calculated molecular weight of 52.5 kDa. The toxin has 65% homology with streptolysin-O and 42% with pneumolysin. All 3 haemolysins share an identical region of 12 amino acid residues that include the single cysteine residue of the molecule, which is involved in the thiol activation.

Neuraminidase, or sialidase, serves many micro-organisms as a pathogenicity factor in a variety of ways (Mueller 1976). Its action on erythrocytes may render them panagglutinable, resulting in increase of blood viscosity and promoting capillary thrombosis. Its modification of gangliosides on host cell surfaces may allow more direct contact of pathogens with the host, or it can provide suitable receptors for other toxins produced by the same or other micro-organisms.

Nees, Veh and Schauer (1975) recovered and purified neuraminidase from *C. perfringens* strain ATCC 10543 and found it to be a single peptide with a molecular mass of about 64 kDa and exhibiting 5 components on isoelectric focusing, each with a different isoelectric pH, ranging between 4.7 and 5.4. After denaturation with SDS or 8 M urea those differences disappeared and only a single component with an isoelectric pH of 4.3 was seen. Rood and Wilkinson (1976) recovered 3 different neuraminidases from strain CN 3870 with molecular masses of 310, 105 and 64 kDa. The 2 larger enzyme species were associated with haemagglutinin potency, but the 64 kDa species was devoid of that activity. Roggentin et al. (1988) cloned a 2.1 kb Sau3A DNA fragment from *C. perfringens* strain A99, whose product had neuraminidase activity. The active product was a peptide of 382 amino acids with a molecular mass of 42.8 kDa. Thus, different neuraminidase enzymes have been recovered from different *C. perfringens* strains.

Enterotoxin

Enterotoxin produced by *C. perfringens* is responsible for food-borne diarrhoea which occurs after consumption of foods containing large numbers of the vegetative organism. It has been found in toxin types A, C and D, but type B and E strains have not been sufficiently tested to establish whether they also produce it. Many, but not all, type A strains produce it. Enterotoxin studies have primarily involved toxin derived from type A strains. Enterotoxin is produced in the intestine during sporulation of vegetative organisms and it reacts with the surface of intestinal epithelial cells, causing tissue destruction, and accumulation of fluids in the intestinal lumen (McClane 1992).

C. perfringens enterotoxin was isolated and purified (Hauschild and Hilsheimer 1971, Stark and Duncan 1972, Sakaguchi, Uemura and Riemann 1973) and found to be a protein with a molecular mass of 35 kDa and an isoelectric pH of 4.3. The amino acid sequence has been determined (Richardson and Granum 1985, Granum 1986). The toxin consists of one peptide of 309 amino acids with a molecular weight of 34 262. The peptide has one free sulphydryl group. The activity of the enterotoxin is enhanced 3-fold by treatment with trypsin (Granum, Whitaker and Skjelkvale 1981). Trypsin cleaves at 2 sites, each involving a lysine residue, cleaving 15 or an additional 10 amino acids from the N-terminal end of the toxin (Richardson and Granum 1983). The trypsinized toxin then consists of 284 amino acids and 2 short peptides of 10 and 15 amino acids. Evidence shows that the short peptides do not separate from the main molecule in the absence of SDS or other denaturants. More recently, the nucleotide sequence of the enterotoxin gene has been determined; it encodes a 319 amino acid protein with a deduced molecular mass of 35.3 kDa (Czeczulin, Hanna and McClane 1993).

The mechanism of action of the enterotoxin seems to involve direct binding of the toxin to receptors on the surface of intestinal epithelial cells. Wnek and McClane (1983) isolated a 50 kDa protein from rabbit intestinal brush border membranes that specifically inhibits cytotoxicity for Vero cells. This molecule may be the specific receptor for the enterotoxin. Binding is followed by insertion of the entire molecule into the cell membrane, but no internalization into the cell (McClane, Hanna and Wnek 1988). A sudden change of ion fluxes occurs, affecting cellular metabolism and macromolecular synthesis. As intracellular calcium ion levels increase, morphological damage occurs, resulting in greatly altered membrane permeability and loss of cellular fluid and ions and moderate-sized molecules (up to 3.5 kDa). Under some conditions a loss of protein molecules may occur, but this may reflect cell death (McClane, Hanna and Wnek 1988). Based on rabbit studies, the enterotoxin is most active in the ileum, moderately active in the jejunum and essentially inactive in the duodenum (McDonel 1980b). It has been demonstrated that the enterotoxin acts as a superantigen, stimulating T lymphocyte activity (Bowness et al. 1992). The observations suggest that superantigenic and enterotoxigenic properties are linked.

Several assays for detecting and measuring enterotoxin, including Western immunoblotting (Kokai-Kun et al. 1994), Vero cell toxicity, reversed passive latex agglutination (RPLA), and enzyme-linked immunosorbent assay (ELISA) (Berry et al. 1988) have been used. Kits for ELISA and RPLA are currently available from TechLab (Blacksburg, VA, USA) and Oxoid USA (Columbia, MD, USA), respectively). All of the tests for enterotoxigenicity require sporulation of cultures. Detecting the gene by use of a gene probe (Kokai-Kun et al. 1994) can show the potential of a strain for producing enterotoxin without requiring in vitro sporulation, but do not allow one to conclude that the strain can sporulate and produce enterotoxin in vivo.

DISEASES CAUSED BY *C. PERFRINGENS*

The diseases caused by *C. perfringens* are listed in Table 32.9. Songer has reviewed the enteric diseases of domestic animals that are caused by this organism (Songer 1996).

Gas gangrene

C. perfringens has been implicated as the most common cause of gas gangrene and the toxin type of the organisms is assumed as type A (MacLennan 1962). It has been found in 60–80% of all cases. The most critical condition for establishing the clostridial infection and development of the gas gangrene is a lowered oxidation–reduction potential. This can result from failure of the blood supply due to trauma to the vessels, pressure of tourniquets, casts or dressings, presence of foreign bodies in the wound, presence of necrotic tissue and haemorrhage in the wound due to direct trauma, the action of necrotizing agents which may be found in soil (such as calcium chloride), or in applied medications, and the presence and multiplication of other less exacting bacteria in the wound. Injuries and conditions favouring gas gangrene are common under battlefield situations, but are rare otherwise. The pathology is certainly due to soluble toxins produced by the organisms such as α-toxin and might involve the combined action of several of these factors. The α-toxin appears to be the factor of overriding importance (MacLennan 1962).

Enterotoxaemias

Enterotoxaemias in animals caused by type A toxin strains are evidenced by the the presence of lethal toxin in the intestine and the destruction of capillary walls in the peritoneal and thoracic cavities. The presence of type A strains in the intestine in the absence of pathology is not significant; these organisms are considered by many to be normal flora. The pathology associated with the different toxin types is a reflection of the toxins produced by the organisms. Most of the diseases occur in young animals because of their lack of immunity, while the source of the organisms is immune adult carriers. Enteritis due to β-toxin may result because of lack of gastrointestinal proteolytic enzymes, or because of their inhibition by constituents in their diet of colostrum or milk. Type B and D strains produce ε-toxin which is not only trypsin resistant, but trypsin activatable, and acts as a permease; it enhances not only its own uptake into the circulation, but also other proteins responsible for cardiac, pulmonary, kidney and brain oedema (Smith and Williams 1984). Enterotoxaemias due to type E strains (ι-toxin) have been documented, but the incidents and the isolation of these strains have been rare.

Necrotic enteritis in humans

This condition is caused by the β-toxin of *C. perfringens* type C. This sporadically occurs among populations in New Guinea in a form known as pig-bel (Murrell et al. 1966). The organism is acquired from consumption of pork from animals carrying it, and the β-toxin is not inactivated by gastrointestinal proteases because of the normally low protein diet of the victims, and the simultaneous consumption of yams which contain large amounts of protease inhibitor. This same disease had been first recognized in Europe under the name 'Darmbrand' shortly after World War II, apparently because of the unusual dietary conditions in the aftermath of the war (Zeissler and Rassfeld-Sternberg 1949). At the time, the toxin type was designated type F on the basis of unusually high heat resistance of the spores, and the lack of 3 minor toxins noted in previous type C strains (δ, θ and κ); since the toxin type designations depend only on major toxins, type F was later dropped. The disease is characterized by acute abdominal pain, bloody diarrhoea, vomiting, ulceration of the small intestine and perforation of the intestinal wall and acute toxaemia (Smith and Williams 1984). The case/fatality ratio for both the European and the New Guinea outbreaks is about 40%.

Food-borne diarrhoea

Many type A strains produce an enterotoxin that causes a severe, but usually self-limiting diarrhoea. Meat dishes (usually containing beef, chicken or turkey) held at temperatures under 60°C (optimum 46°C) allow spores of *C. perfringens* that have survived the cooking temperature to germinate and multiply to high numbers of vegetative organisms. After consumption of a minimum of approximately 10^8 vegetative organisms, the victim experiences intensive diarrhoea and gas caused by the enterotoxin produced simultaneously with sporulation of the organisms in the small intestine (Hauschild 1975). Incubation is about 10 h and symptoms persist for 24–48 h. Confirmation is made on the basis of finding $>10^4$ organisms in a food epidemiologically associated with the outbreak, a median count of $>10^6$ *C. perfringens* g^{-1} of stool obtained from the victims within 48 h after onset of diarrhoea, and or detecting enterotoxin in the faeces of the victims (Harmon and Kautter 1986). Identifying an outbreak strain by serotyping and establishing strain identity among isolates from patients, and between patient isolates and the food isolates, has been recommended, but in view of the problems of maintaining an adequate set of reagents required to identify all isolates of such a serologically diverse species, interest in this approach has waned (Hatheway, Whaley and Dowell 1980).

Another form of diarrhoea caused by *C. perfringens* enterotoxin appears to be antibiotic associated (Borriello 1985). The enterotoxin and very high numbers of enterotoxigenic organisms are found in diarrheic stools. Studies on 26 mostly sporadic cases indicate an association with treatment with penicillins, and that the effective site of colonization is the small bowel. The diarrhoea is self-limiting, though in some cases it may be protracted. Treatment with metronidazole has been effective.

14.5   *C. difficile*

C. difficile was discovered in 1935 as a member of the microflora of the intestine of normal infants (Hall and O'Toole 1935). The organism is a motile, gram-positive rod, with dimensions of 0.5–1.9 × 3.0–16.9 μm, which forms oval, subterminal spores. Cells stain uniformly gram-positive in young cultures, but may become gram-negative after 24–48 h. *C. difficile* lique-

fies gelatin but is non-proteolytic with respect to milk and meat proteins. It ferments fructose, glucose, mannitol, mannose and usually xylose. It is negative for lecithinase and lipase, and is non-haemolytic on horse blood. It produces acetic, isobutyric, butyric, isovaleric, valeric, isocaproic, formic and lactic acids in PYG (Holdeman, Cato and Moore 1977, Cato, George and Finegold 1986), and converts tyrosine to *p*-cresol. The organisms produce 2 major toxins, toxin A (enterotoxic) and toxin B (cytotoxic).

The organism was isolated on rare occasions from abscesses and infected tissues but it was considered as non-pathogenic (Willis 1969). Involvement of *C. difficile* in rare cases of gas gangrene has been suspected, but not clearly documented (MacLennan 1962). Its recognition as the cause of antibiotic-associated pseudomembranous colitis (Bartlett et al. 1978, Larson et al. 1978) has generated an intense interest in *C. difficile*. Several cases of *C. difficile* infections involving bones and joints have also been reported (Pron et al. 1995). Little has been published on the bacteriology of the organism, but the literature dealing with its toxins and pathology is extensive. Several reviews are available (Lyerly, Krivan and Wilkins 1988, Knoop, Owens and Crocker 1993, Bongaerts and Lyerly 1994, Wolfhagen et al. 1994).

The organism may be isolated from faecal specimens using cycloserine–mannitol agar (CMA) or cycloserine–mannitol blood agar (CMBA) (Dowell 1981), or cycloserine–egg yolk–fructose agar (CFA), or cycloserine–cefoxitin–egg yolk–fructose agar (CCFA) (George et al. 1979). There have been many efforts using various techniques to develop typing systems, because of the importance of identifying strains involved in hospital outbreaks (Brazier 1995).

According to *Bergey's Manual* (Cato, George and Finegold 1986), *C. difficile* phenotypically resembles *C. sporogenes* most closely. However, it is related to *C. sordellii* and *C. bifermentans*, which are classified outside of the mainstream of the pathogenic clostridia. Most of the pathogenic clostridia are in Johnson and Francis group I (Table 32.1) and cluster I of the 16S rRNA dendrogram (Fig. 32.1). These 3 organisms are in Johnson and Francis group II, and in 16S rRNA gene sequence cluster XI (Collins et al. 1994).

TOXINS PRODUCED BY *C. DIFFICILE*

Toxins A and B

C. difficile was not known to be pathogenic until it was implicated as the cause of antibiotic associated pseudomembranous colitis. A toxin neutralized by *C. sordellii* antitoxin was found in the faeces of patients (Larson et al. 1977, Rifkin, Fekety and Silva 1977), but the organism that produced it was actually *C. difficile* (Bartlett et al. 1978, Larson et al. 1978). The toxin had both enterotoxic and cytotoxic activities, which were subsequently separated from each other and designated as toxin A and toxin B, respectively (Taylor, Thorne and Bartlett 1981). Purification of toxins A and B has been done by several researchers. Sullivan, Pellett and Wilkins (1982) separated the 2 toxins and purified them by DEAE ion-exchange chromatography and observed molecular masses of 440–500 kDa for toxin A and 360–470 kDa for toxin B. Banno et al. (1984) purified the corresponding toxins (designated D-1 and D-2) to homogeneity as determined by PAGE analysis using gel filtration and ion-exchange chromatography. Their molecular masses were 550–600 kDa and 450–500 kDa, respectively. Each of the 2 toxins, D-1 and D-2, was converted to an apparent single, smaller molecular form, 190–200 kDa, determined by SDS–PAGE analysis after heating at 100°C for 5 min in the presence of SDS and 2-mercaptoethanol. The toxins were found to be immunologically differentiable by cross-neutralization studies in cytotoxicity and mouse lethal assays (Libby and Wilkins 1982, Banno et al. 1984). Cross-reactivity without neutralization between the toxins and corresponding heterologous monoclonal antibodies have, however, been observed (Eichel-Striber et al. 1987, Rothman et al. 1988), thus indicating common epitopes.

Toxin A is primarily responsible for the enterotoxic activity of *C. difficile* (Triadafilopoulos et al. 1987), but toxin B is much more potent as a cytotoxin than toxin A (Rothman et al. 1984, Pothoulakis et al. 1986a, Lima et al. 1988). Both toxins are lethal for mice, with toxin A having a potency 50–400 times that of toxin B (Taylor, Thorne and Bartlett 1981, Banno et al. 1984). The physical characteristics and biological activities of the 2 toxins are compared in Table 32.11. The data for similar toxins produced by *C. sordellii* are also listed.

The enterotoxic effect of toxin A in the rabbit intestine appears to be due to tissue damage resulting from an inflammatory process induced by the toxin (Triadafilopoulos et al. 1987). Following injection of toxin A (but not toxin B) an infiltration of neutrophils into the ileum and a release of inflammatory mediators occur, causing fluid secretion, altered membrane permeability, and haemorrhagic necrosis. It has also been observed in vitro that toxin A acts as a powerful chemotactic agent for human neutrophils (Pothoulakis et al. 1986b).

The cytotoxic action of toxin B appears to involve depolymerization of filamentous actin, causing a destructuring of the cell cytoskeleton and thus, a rounding of the cell (Pothoulakis et al. 1986a, Ottinger and Lin 1988). In light of the high potency of toxin B, the effect may be due to an indirect action, perhaps an enzymatic action on proteins involved in actin polymerization (Pothoulakis et al. 1986a).

The gene for toxin A and portions of it have been cloned and expressed in *E. coli*. Muldrow et al. (1987) cloned a 300 base fragment from the *C. difficile* genome that coded for a peptide serologically related to toxin A, but not active biologically. Price et al. (1987) recovered a 4.7 kb DNA fragment that codes for a peptide with haemagglutinating activity corresponding to that of toxin A; this is believed to be related to the specific binding by which the toxin binds to target cells. The peptide was not cytotoxic or enterotoxic in hamsters. Wren et al. (1987) obtained a recombinant λ phage carrying a 14.3 kb DNA fragment from *C. difficile* encoding for a 250 kDa protein that cross-reacted antigenically with antitoxin A. The lysate caused elongation (and destruction at higher concentrations) of Chinese hamster ovary (CHO) cells, and haemagglutination of rabbit erythrocytes. Both of these activities could be neutralized with antitoxin A and *C. sordelli* antitoxin. Nucleotide sequencing of the toxin genes has provided the definitive characterization of toxins A and B (von Eichel-Streiber et al. 1992). Molecular weights of 308 and 270 kDa, and pIs of 5.3 and 4.1 are calculated for toxins A and B, respectively. Amino acid sequences are 49% identical between the toxins, and 14% show conservative substitutions. In spite of the high degree of homology, polyclonal antisera against the toxins are specific and do not react with both toxins. C-terminal repetitive structures consisting of groups of repetitive peptides with lengths of 21–50 amino acids occur in each of the toxins and each provides the immunodominant portion of the molecule. It is hypothesized that these repetitive regions serve as the ligand domain and that they recognize different toxin-binding molecules on

Table 32.11 Physical characteristics and biological activities of toxins A and B of *C. difficile*[a] and HT[b] and LT[c] of *C. sordellii*

Toxin	Molecular size (kDa)	Isoelectric pH	Dose (ng)			Vascular permeability
			Tissue culture	Enterotoxic	Lethal (mouse)	
C. difficile						
A	308[d]	5.3	10	1000[e]	50	1–10
B	270[d]	4.1	0.0002–0.001	Negative[e]	50	1–10
C. sordellii						
HT	450–525	6.1	500	2000[e]	120	
LT	240–250	4.55	16.4	Positive[f]	2.94	

[a]Lyerly et al. (1988).
[b]Martinez and Wilkins (1988).
[c]Popoff (1987).
[d]Wolfhagen et al. (1994).
[e]Rabbit loop.
[f]Guinea-pig loop.

cell surfaces, and are thus responsible for the different in vivo activities of the toxins.

ADP-ribosyltransferase (CDT)

In addition to toxins A and B, a biologically active protein with ADP-ribosyltransferase activity (CDT) has been found in a strain (CD196) of *C. difficile* (Popoff et al. 1988). It was shown to modify cell actin in a manner similar to that of *C. botulinum* C_2 and *C. perfringens* ι toxin. This protein cross-reacts antigenically with the light chains of the ι binary toxins from *C. perfringens* type E and *C. spiroforme* (Popoff and Boquet 1988). CDT has a molecular mass of 43 kDa. Although it has no complementary binding component as have the binary toxins, it acts as a binary toxin in Vero cell cytotoxicity and mouse lethality assays when complemented by the binding pepide (ι-b) of either *C. perfringens* type E or *C. spiroforme* ι toxins but not by the binding molecule of C_2 toxin (C_2II). CDT thus far has been found in only one strain of *C. difficile*.

ANTIBIOTIC ASSOCIATED INFECTION BY *C. DIFFICILE*

Antibiotic associated diarrhoea and pseudomembranous colitis due to *C. difficile* is probably the most common clostridial human disease at present. The organism is a common nosocomial pathogen that infects 15–25% of hospitalized patients (Knoop, Owens and Crocker 1993). Most of these patients are asymtomatic carriers. Numbers for determining the actual incidence of the illness are difficult to find, but a French review estimates between 1 and 30 cases per 1000 patient admissions (Barbut and Petit 1996).

The severity of the disease may range from a mild diarrhoea to a fulminant pancolitis, including megacolon and bowel perforation (Knoop, Owens and Crocker 1993). Symptoms may occur after 5–10 days of antimicrobial therapy. Most cases will have brown or clear watery diarrhoea, whereas about 5% will experience bloody diarrhoea. Patients with pseudomembranous colitis have mucoid faeces. Elevated temperature and leucocytosis are common features. Treatment with vancomycin or metronidazole have been effective (Borriello and Larson 1985).

14.6 *C. sordellii* and *C. bifermentans*

C. bifermentans was recovered from a study on the putrefaction of meat (Tissier and Martelly 1902). The name *Bacillus bifermentans sporogenes* was applied because of its ability to ferment carbohydrates as well as amino acids. *C. sordellii* was first recognized because of its involvement in gangrenous wound infections (Sordelli 1922)

Cells of *C. bifermentans* grown in PYG are described as gram-positive straight rods, 0.6–1.9 μm × 1.6–11.0 μm, motile, occurring singly, in pairs or in short chains, with oval central to subterminal spores which usually do not swell the cells (Cato, George and Finegold 1986). The description for *C. sordellii* is gram-positive straight rods, usually motile, 0.5–1.7 × 1.6–20.6 μm, occurring singly or in pairs, with oval, central

or subterminal spores. Both organisms liquefy gelatin, ferment glucose, maltose and often fructose, produce indole and lecithinase, and show a β-type haemolysis on blood agar. In PYG medium they produce acetic, formic, propionic, isobutyric, isovaleric and isocaproic acids as metabolic end products. Optimal growth temperature is 30–37°C, and most strains grow nearly as well at 25 and 45°C. *C. sordellii* is distinguished from *C. bifermentans* most readily by its ability to produce urease (Willis 1969, Holdeman, Cato and Moore 1977, Smith and Williams 1984, Cato, George and Finegold 1986). Hall (1929) reported on the potent virulence of strains of *Bacillus sordellii* and demonstrated that pathogenicity was due to a toxin that caused severe oedema and could be neutralized by a specific antiserum. For a while, *C. sordellii* was considered as a subgroup of *C. bifermentans*, distinguished by its ability to produce the potent lethal toxin responsible for the severe gelatinous oedema. These organisms are related to *C. difficile* (see above), and belong to 16S rRNA gene cluster XI (Fig. 32.1).

TOXINS PRODUCED BY *C. SORDELLII* AND *C. BIFERMENTANS*

C. sordellii produces 3 toxins in common with the non-pathogenic *C. bifermentans*: (1) a lecithinase; (2) an oxygen-labile haemolysin and (3) a fibrinolysin. The lecithinase is a phospholipase C, serologically related to the α-toxin of *C. perfringens* as evidenced by the positive Nagler reaction (Willis 1969). It is relatively non-toxic for mice. The gene for the α-toxin of *C. bifermentans* has been cloned and found to be 64% homologous in coding sequence in comparison with the *C. perfringens* gene (Tso and Seibel 1989). It codes for a mature protein consisting of about 376 amino acids. This lecithinase from *C. bifermentans* has about 1/50 the activity of *C. perfringens* α-toxin in enzymic, haemolytic, and mouse lethality assays. The calculated molecular weight, although not given for the *C. bifermentans* lecithinase would be similar to the 43 kDa calculated for the *C. perfringens* α-toxin.

Major lethal toxins

A lethal factor referred to as β-toxin (Willis 1969) responsible for the pathogenicity of *C. sordellii* distinguishes it from *C. bifermentans*. Arsecularatne, Panabokke and Wijesundra (1969) found 2 different activities associated with the major lethal toxin, which were separable from each other in different preparations. Both toxic factors were dermonecrotic and haemorrhagic when injected into the skin of rats and guinea-pigs. The first activity (oedematizing) caused massive oedema and moderate areas of bright red haemorrhage when injected intradermally, subcutaneously, or intramuscularly into guinea-pigs, with death occurring within 24–36 h. The second factor (haemorrhagic) caused minimal oedema but confluent areas of brownish haemorrhage in the skin; and in the omentum, mesentery, and contiguous viscera when injected intravenously. or intraperitoneally. The haemorrhagic factor appeared to be associated with sporulating cultures. Little lethality was noted for this toxin at doses with high haemorrhagic activity.

Nakamura et al. (1983b) examined 55 strains of *C. sordellii* for mouse lethality and cytotoxicity. They found a close correlation between the 2 activities. All 34 strains negative for mouse lethal toxin lacked cytotoxin. Lethal toxin titres paralleled cytotoxicity titres. Yamakawa et al. (1983) found that only 2 of 15 cytotoxigenic strains produced positive rabbit ileal loop responses (fluid accumulation). The lethal and cytotoxic effects, as well as the ileal loop response, were eliminated by preincubation of active culture fluid with either *C. sordellii* or *C. difficile* antitoxin. Two cytotoxins (I and II) were produced by one strain (3703), and were separated from each other by DEAE ion-exchange chromatography (Yamakawa, Nakamura and Nishida 1985). They could be distinguished from one other by specific antitoxins produced against each of them.

It appears that the lethal toxin classically designated as β-toxin (Willis 1969) actually consists of 2 components: **lethal toxin** (LT) and **haemorrhagic toxin** (HT). Popoff (1987) purified LT from a strain of *C. sordellii* and found it to be a protein with a molecular mass of 250 kDa and an isoelectric pH of 4.55. It was antigenically related to toxin B of *C. difficile*, but not to toxin A. Martinez and Wilkins (1988) purified HT and found a molecular mass of 525 kDa under nondenaturing conditions and an isoelectric pH of 6.l. HT is cytotoxic for cultured cells, lethal for mice, and causes an accumulation of haemorrhagic fluid in ligated rabbit ileal loops. It is immunologically related to toxin A of *C. difficile*. The properties and activities of HT and LT are listed and may be compared with the *C. difficile* toxins in Table 32.11. In summary: HT is equivalent to cytotoxin I (Yamakawa, Nakamura and Nishida 1985) and is related antigenically and in biological activity to toxin A of *C. difficile*; LT is equivalent to cytotoxin II and is related antigenically and in biological activity to toxin B of *C. difficile*.

Diseases caused by *C. sordellii*

The first strains of *C. sordellii* were isolated from acute oedematous wound infections in humans (Sordelli 1922). Subsequently the organism was implicated as the cause of a fatal cattle disease in Nevada (Hall 1929). MacLennan lists *C. sordellii* as one of 6 clostridia involved in histotoxic, gas gangrene-like infections (MacLennan 1962). More recently, fatal *C. sordellii* infections have been noted in association with obstetrical surgical incisions (episiotomy) (Soper 1986, McGregor et al. 1989). Fatality in these cases was due to clinical shock, presumably toxin induced. The described cases were characterized by sudden onset of shock with severe hypotension, generalized tissue oedema, accumulation of fluids in the peritoneum and other body cavities, increased haematocrit, marked neutrophilia, absence of rash or fever, limited or no myonecrosis and a rapid, lethal course. A case of spontaneous endometritis due to *C. sordellii*, having the same rapidly fatal clinical course has been described (Hogan and Ireland 1989). A fatality due to

C. sordellii infection in a deep laceration of a thigh has also been reported (Browdie et al. 1975). Intramuscular injection of sterile fluid from cultures of *C. sordellii* isolated from the thigh wound caused oedema and haemoconcentration in mice, and death within 12–48 h, the time until death depending on dose.

Pathogenicity of *C. bifermentans*

The involvement of *C. bifermentans* in infections has been indicated by its association with liver abscess (Nachman et al. 1989), endocarditis (Kolander, Cosgrove and Molavi 1989), abdominal abscess (Rechtman and Nadler 1991), panophthalmitis (Rehany et al. 1994) and metastatic osteomyelitis (Scanlan et al. 1994).

14.7 *C. novyi* and *C. haemolyticum*

C. novyi, previously known as *C. oedematiens*, was first described by Novy (1894). It was isolated from guinea-pigs who had died of 'malignant oedema' after injections of casein (Willis 1969).

C. novyi and *C. haemolyticum* are motile, gram-variable rods (positive in young cultures, often negative in older cultures). Cell dimensions are 0.5–1.6 μm × 1.6–18 μm, except for *C. novyi* type B which are larger (1.1–2.5 μm × 3.3–22.5 μm) (Cato, George and Finegold 1986). They ferment glucose and liquefy gelatin. Proteolytic activity is variable. Although *C. haemolyticum* is indole positive, a few strains (notably type A) of *C. novyi* are indole negative (Holdeman, Cato and Moore 1977, Cato, George and Finegold 1986). All *C. novyi* strains produce acetic, propionic, and butyric acids as metabolic products. These organisms are included in 16S rRNA gene cluster I, and are closely related to *C. botulinum* types C and D on this basis (Fig. 32.1).

C. novyi and *C. haemolyticum* are among the most fastidious and oxygen-sensitive bacterial pathogens known. They die rapidly on exposure to air (Willis 1969). Only freshly prepared agar plates and broth media should be used to cultivate these organisms. Cooked meat–glucose has been recommended as an enrichment medium. Cultures on agar media should be incubated at least 2–4 days before removal from the anaerobic system. Some strains grow too slowly to form recognizable colonies in shorter incubation times, and exposure to air may prevent further growth. On blood agar, zones of haemolysis may be seen, due to β, γ, or δ toxins (Table 32.12); the β and γ toxins are 'hot-cold' haemolysins and thus, the haemolytic activity is more pronounced if the plates are cooled after incubation (Willis 1969). On egg yolk agar plates, an opaque zone in the agar surrounding the colonies due to the lecithinase activity of β- or γ-toxin is apparent, and a pearly layer associated with the colony surface or its periphery is seen with strains that produce the ε-toxin. Spores of these organisms survive heating 5 min at 100°C (Willis 1969), so heat treatment of certain specimens and mixed cultures may be helpful for isolation of the organism.

Because of the difficulties encountered in growing

Table 32.12 Toxins of *C. novyi* and *C. haemolyticum*[a]

Toxin	Activity	*C. novyi* Type			*C. haemolyticum*[b]
		A	**B**	**C**	
α	Necrotizing, lethal	+	+	–	–
β	Lecithinase; necrotizing lethal; haemolytic	–	+	–	+
γ	Lecithinase; necrotizing; haemolytic	+	–	–	–
δ	Oxygen-labile haemolysin	+	–	–	–
ε	Lipase (pearly layer)	+	–	–	–
ζ	Haemolysin	–	+	–	–
η	Tropomyosinase	–	+	–	–
θ	Opalescence in egg yolk	–	tr	–	+

[a]From Hatheway (1990).
[b]Sometimes referred to as *C. novyi* type D.

the organism and isolating it from wound cultures, it was not initially recognized as an important and frequent cause of gas gangrene in humans (MacLennan 1962). It is now known that *C. novyi* is involved in more than one-third of such cases, and the fatality rate in wound infection with this organism, especially in combination with *C. sporogenes*, is very high (Smith and Williams 1984). The pathology and mortality are apparently due to the lethal α-toxin. The organism also is the cause of infections in domestic animals, most notably in infectious necrotic hepatitis in sheep. The infection follows parasitic liver infestation, usually involving the liver fluke.

C. haemolyticum is an organism so similar to *C. novyi* in physiological characteristics that it is considered by some to be a toxin variant (type D) of the latter. It is closely related to some strains of *C. novyi* (type B) by DNA relatedness criteria (Nakamura et al. 1983a). It is the causative agent of haemoglobinuria, also known as 'red water disease,' a highly fatal disease of cattle (Smith and Williams 1984). Diseases caused by pathogenic strains of *C. novyi* and *C. haemolyticum* appear to involve primarily the α-toxin of the former and the β-toxin of the latter. In gas gangrene in humans the α-toxin causes massive oedema due to its effect on capillary permeability. In bacillary haemoglobinuria, the β-toxin destroys the circulating erythrocytes resulting in excretion of the haemoglobin in the urine; simultaneously, blood is lost into the intestine because of destruction of the capillary endothelium. The grossly different pathological presentation of these 2 diseases has led to maintaining 2 separate species for the causative organisms (Smith and Williams 1984, Cato, George and Finegold 1986).

Toxins produced by *C. novyi*

Classification of 3 types of *C. novyi* is based on production of several toxic, antigenic factors. *C. novyi* types A, B and C, and *C. haemolyticum* are distinguished from each other by the toxins designated as α and β (Willis 1969, Smith and Williams 1984) (Table 32.12), based on the studies of Oakley and coworkers (Oakley, Warrack and Clarke 1947, Oakley 1955, Oakley and Warrack 1959). Type A produces α only, *C. haemolyticum* produces β only, and type B produces both.

Production of 6 other toxins by species and toxin type is also shown in Table 32.12. Type C strains produce none of the known toxins and are considered non-pathogenic. Non-pathogenic strains phenotypically similar to *C. novyi* type A, or to *C. botulinum* type C or D may be derived from pathogenic strains that have lost their infecting phages (Cato, George and Finegold 1986).

The lecithovitellin reaction has often been used to identify toxins of the *C. novyi* group. Rutter and Collee (Rutter and Collee 1969) noted that positive lecithovitellin reactions could be due to (1) lecithinase, (2) lipase or (3) both lecithinase and lipase activities. They pointed out that type A strains produce γ-toxin (a haemolytic lecithinase) and ε-toxin (a lipase); type B and *C. haemolyticum* strains produce β-toxin (a haemolytic lecithinase), and also θ-toxin, which may be a lipase, though not demonstrable by a visible reaction on egg yolk agar. The β and γ lecithinases are serologically distinct. Rutter and Collee showed by thin-layer chromatography that *C. novyi* type B and *C. haemolyticum* strains break down lecithin into diglycerides, while *C. novyi* type A strains initially convert lecithin into diglycerides but subsequently break down the diglycerides from the lecithinase reaction as well as those present in the egg yolk suspension into free fatty acids and glycerol (Rutter and Collee 1969). Thus, *C. novyi* type A, *C. novyi* type B, and *C. haemolyticum* all possess lecithinase activity, but only type A possesses a readily demonstrable lipase. Those authors also showed a correlation between the mouse lethal activity of the α-toxin of types A and B strains and cytotoxicity of the cultures.

α-Toxin

Phillips, Batty and Wood (1970) purified the α-toxin of *C. novyi* type B by gel filtration, adsorption onto alumina, and ultrafiltration, and reported it as a protein with a molecular mass of 132 kDa. Izumi, Niiro and Kondo (1983) reported a molecular mass of 260–280 kDa for the toxin purified by a combination of ion-exchange and gel filtration chromatography. The purified toxin had an isoelectric pH of 6.1. It had lethal, oedematizing, and permeability activities but was free of the haemolytic and lecithinase activities that were present in starting culture fluid concentrate. The LD50 of the purified toxin for mice was 17 ng, and the OeD50 (50% oedematizing dose) was 1.7 ng.

Eklund et al. (1976) found that α-toxin production in strains of *C. novyi* type A and type B was due to phages. Curing the organisms of their phages, NAI^tox+ and NBI^tox+, respectively, rendered them non-toxigenic (with respect to α-toxin) and susceptible to reinfection by the homologous, but not the heterologous tox+ phage. Reinfection resulted in their regaining toxigenicity. These phages affected only α-toxin production. Thus, the cured type A strain resembles nontoxigenic *C. botulinum* type C, and the cured type B strain resembles *C. haemolyticum*, since it continues to produce the β-toxin. Schallehn and Eklund (1980) infected a strain of *C. haemolyticum* with a tox+ phage from type A strains, rendering it capable of producing α-toxin; it was thus indistinguishable from *C. novyi* type B on the basis of the major toxins it produced.

β-Toxin

The β-toxin is lethal, haemolytic, necrotizing, and has lecithinase activity (Willis 1969). Darakhshan and Lauerman (1981) report a molecular weight of 32 kDa for β-toxin from *C. haemolyticum* purified by gel filtration chromatography. The toxin was labile at 60°C and rapidly inactivated by exposure to trypsin. The β-toxins of *C. novyi* type B and *C. haemolyticum* appear to be serologically identical (MacFarlane 1950). Although the enzymatic activity is that of phospholipase C, it is not related serologically to *C. perfringens* α- toxin or to the γ-toxin of *C. novyi* type A. *C. botulinum* type C produces a lecithinase that is comparable serologically to β-toxin of *C. novyi* type B and *C. haemolyticum* (Nakamura et al. 1983a). The lethality and pathogenicity of *C. haemolyticum* appear to be due to β-toxin that is produced in large amounts by this organism, more so than by *C. novyi* type B.

γ-Toxin

The γ-toxin produced by *C. novyi* type A is also a phospholipase C, but is serologically distinct from β-toxin as well as from the α-toxin of *C. perfringens* (MacFarlane 1948). γ-Toxin was purified by Taguchi and Ikezawa (1975) by gel filtration chromatography, and the estimated molecular mass was 30 kDa. In addition to hydrolysis of lecithin, γ-toxin catalyses the hydrolysis of phosphatidylinositol and phosphatidylglycerol, substrates not utilized by *C. perfringens* α-toxin. β- and γ-Toxins may be determined and differentiated by haemolytic or lipovitellin assays using specific antitoxins (Willis 1969).

δ-Toxin

The δ-toxin is an oxygen-labile haemolysin that is serologically related to similar haemolysins such as the θ-toxin of *C. perfringens* and the tetanolysin of. *C. tetani* (Willis 1969, Smith and Williams 1984). It is produced only by type A strains.

ε-Toxin

ε-Toxin is a lipase that is responsible for the 'pearly layer' associated with the bacterial colonies on egg yolk agar. This factor is seen only with type A strains, and is shared in common with *C. botulinum* types C and D. The ε-toxin decomposes triglycerides and diglycerides in the egg yolk medium as well as diglycerides formed by hydrolysis of lecithin by γ-toxin (Rutter and Collee 1969).

ζ-Toxin

ζ-Toxin is a haemolysin is produced only by type B strains. It is not related serologically to δ-toxin nor to any of the other oxygen-labile haemolysins, nor is it sensitive to oxygen (Willis 1969). There is no known role for these haemolysins in pathogenicity of the organisms that produce them.

η-Toxin

η-Toxin is a proteolytic enzyme produced by *C. novyi* type B and *C. haemolyticum*. It is active on the muscle proteins, myosin and, tropomyosin, and has been named **tropomyosinase** (MacFarlane 1955). Tropomyosin is hydrolysed more completely than is myosin; 74 and 25% of the nitrogen of those respective substrates was converted to acid-soluble form. The enzyme is activated by sulphydryl reagents such as cysteine, glutathione and thiolactate. It is not inhibited by soybean trypsin inhibitor. It is neutralized by antisera prepared against *C. novyi* type B cultures. Its pathogenic action in muscle infection may be important, but this has not been studied (Smith and Williams 1984).

θ-Toxin

θ-Toxin, produced by *C. haemolyticum* (and possibly by *C. novyi* type B on the basis of antibodies produced against those strains), causes opalescence in egg yolk emulsions, but has not been characterized. It might be a lipase, serologically distinct from ε-toxin, and non-haemolytic (Willis 1969).

GENETIC RELATEDNESS OF *C. NOVYI*, *C. HAEMOLYTICUM* AND *C. BOTULINUM*

Nakamura et al. (1983a) examined 4 strains each of *C. novyi* type A, type B, and *C. haemolyticum* and 5 strains of *C. botulinum* type C. They found 3 groups of closely related organisms as indicated in Table 32.13. *C. novyi* type A is less related than either *C. novyi* type B or *C. haemolyticum* to *C. botulinum* type C. *C. novyi* type B and *C. haemolyticum* are very closely related to each other. One strain of *C. botulinum* type C (the Stockholm strain) is more closely related to the *C. novyi* type B/ *C. haemolyticum* group than to the other 4 strains of *C. botulinum* type C.

14.8 *C. septicum* and *C. chauvoei*

C. chauvoei and *C. septicum* are difficult to distinguish from each other on the basis of their physiological and toxigenic characteristics. Both are rather oxygen toler-

Table 32.13 DNA relatedness of *C. novyi*, *C. haemolyticum* and *C. botulinum* type C[a]

Species	No. of strains	Relation to reference strain (%)[b] from:		
		Group I	Group II	Group III
Group I				
C. novyi A	4	80–100	44–45	33–36
Group II				
C. novyi B	4	28–49	93–100	50–62
C. haemolyticum	4	26–38	93–100	50–62
C. botulinum C	1	42	85	54
Group III				
C. botulinum C	4	36–48	68–70	91–100

[a]From Hatheway (1990); data condensed from Nakamura et al. (1983a).
[b]Values indicate relatedness between DNA from the test strain and that of the reference strain.

ant and easy to culture, although they may be difficult to isolate because of their vigorous motility and tendency to swarm on the surface of agar media (Willis 1969). The organisms are gram-positive rods (often gram-negative in older cultures). The cell dimensions listed for *C. chauvoei* are 0.5–1.7 μm × 1.6–9.7 μm, and are slightly greater for *C. septicum*, 0.6–1.9 μm × 1.9–35 μm, indicating that more pleomorphism of the latter has been observed. These organisms belong in 16S rRNA gene cluster I (Fig. 32.1), and are closely related to each other on this basis.

Both organisms ferment glucose, fructose, lactose, maltose and mannose. They liquefy gelatin but do not digest meat or milk proteins. Both produce acetic and butyric acids as metabolic end products. A differential characteristic that is widely accepted is sucrose fermentation which is positive for *C. chauvoei* and negative for *C. septicum* (Holdeman, Cato and Moore 1977, Cato, George and Finegold 1986), but Al-Khatib (1969) has reported that this distinction is unreliable. It has also been reported that long chains of bacilli or long filaments in the serous cavities and on the liver surface in infected animals are formed by *C. septicum* but not by *C. chauvoei* (Heller 1920, Willis 1969). This means of differentiation is also disputed by Al-Khatib (1969).

It appears the only reliable means of differentiation are serological, pathological or toxicological (Heller 1920). Moussa studied 37 strains of *C. septicum* and 38 strains of *C. chauvoei* serologically and found 8 different serologic groups (Moussa 1959). Five groups contained only *C. septicum* and 2 groups contained only *C. chauvoei*. The one mixed group contained only one strain of *C. septicum* and 2 of *C. chauvoei*. With the exception of the mixed group, the 2 species can be distinguished on the basis of their somatic antigens. *C. septicum* strains possess O-antigens 1 or 2, while *C. chauvoei* strains possess O-antigen 3. Within each O-antigen group, strains may be differentiated on the basis of their H (flagellar) antigens. A common spore antigen was found for all strains regardless of species designation (Moussa 1959). The O-antigen differences provide the basis for distinguishing the 2 organisms by using specific FA reagents (Batty and Walker 1963). Vaccines for protection of animals against infection by

C. chauvoei (Macheak, Claus and Malloy 1970) and *C. septicum* (Claus and Kolbe 1979) appear to be effective; but protection by *C. septicum* vaccines, is somewhat strain specific and may be related to the antigenic diversity of those organisms as indicated by Moussa's studies (Moussa 1959).

C. septicum and *C. chauvoei* belong in 23S rRNA homology group I-D of Johnson and Francis (1975) and cluster I on the basis of 16S rRNA gene sequence homology (Fig. 32.1).

14.9 *C. histolyticum*

C. histolyticum is of interest because of its isolation from gangrenous and non-gangrenous war wounds, its production of a lethal toxin that cross-reacts serologically with the α-toxin of *C. septicum*, and its production of a mixture of collagenases and other proteolytic enzymes that are unique in their efficiency of converting tissue proteins to amino acids and peptides. The organism was first described by Weinberg and Seguin (1916). Its isolation from wounds and implication as a cause of gas gangrene is rather infrequent (MacLennan 1962, Willis 1969, Smith and Williams 1984). However, it may play an important role as a component of a virulent mixture of organisms, for example in combination with *C. perfringens* in gas gangrene infections (Weinberg and Seguin 1916). Its infrequent isolation may be due to certain difficulties in culturing the organism. Although it is not a strict anaerobe (it may grow on agar media in the presence of air) and its nutritional requirements are not more stringent than many other clostridia, its growth may be inhibited by the presence of sugar in the medium, and contrary to some reports (Zeissler 1930, Prevot 1957), the heat resistance of spores may be rather low (Nishida and Imaizumi 1966).

C. histolyticum is a gram-positive rod, 0.5–0.9 μm × 1.3–9.3 μm appearing singly, in pairs, or as short chains. It falls into 16S rRNA cluster II, which it shares with *C. limosum*, slightly outside cluster I. It is asaccharolytic and strongly proteolytic, but not unique, as *C. subterminale*, *C. hastiforme* and *C. argentinense* are also asaccharolytic and proteolytic (Cato, George and Finegold 1986, Suen et al. 1988a). It is unusual among proteolytic clostridia in not producing isoacids (isobutyric, isocaproic) as metabolic end products. Only acetic acid is formed (Holdeman, Cato and Moore 1977). It digests casein, gelatin, haemoglobin, albumin, collagen (Smith and Williams 1984) and elastin, the latter by means of its δ-toxin (Willis 1969). Little or no gas is detected in cultures. It is negative for the lecithinase and lipase reactions. Thus, with the exception of the protein reactions, all commonly used culture tests are negative.

TOXINS OF *C. HISTOLYTICUM*

C. histolyticum produces 5 toxins, designated by the first 5 letters of the Greek alphabet, in the order of their recognition. It is pathogenic for laboratory animals (Willis 1969). Strains that produce appreciable amounts of α-(lethal) toxin cause death of a laboratory animal within 24 h of intramuscular injection of the organism. In the absence of α-toxin no toxaemia ensues, but a progressive gangrenous infection may take place, with tissue destruction due largely to actions of the organism's collagenolytic and proteolytic toxins. The skin over the area of infected muscle is completely destroyed and the underlying tissues are grossly digested as are also the soft parts of the bones (Aikat and Dible 1960). Ultimately the digestive process may terminate with autoamputation of the infected limb, but in some cases infection may spread into the trunk of the body, damaging vital organs and resulting in death (Weinberg and Seguin 1916, Willis 1969).

α-Toxin

Lethal toxicity of culture filtrates of *C. histolyticum* was reported by Weinberg and Seguin (1916). This lethal factor was designated α-toxin and noted to be necrotizing but not haemolytic (Oakley and Warrack 1950). It has been noted that the α-toxin of *C. histolyticum* can be neutralized by antisera produced against toxic filtrates of *C. septicum* cultures; similarly, the lethality of *C. septicum* cultures can be neutralized by *C. histolyticum* antisera (Sterne and Warrack 1964). Cross-neutralizations can be demonstrated both in mouse lethality and intradermal necrosis reactions.

Nishida and Imaizumi (1966) found that only 6 of 21 strains of *C. histolyticum* isolated from soil samples in Japan produced α-toxin in culture. The pharmacological and molecular properties of this toxin have not been studied in depth, probably because it is rather unstable. It is readily inactivated by proteolytic enzymes (Smith and Williams 1984). Bowen (Bowen 1952) reported 85 LD50 per mg toxin per kg of body weight for mice for α-toxin partially purified by ethanol precipitation.

β-Toxin

β-Toxin has been identified as a collagenase (EC 3.4.24.3) or more recently as a group of 7 collagenases (Bond and Van Wart 1984b, Van Wart and Steinbrink 1985). Collagenase is a zinc metalloprotease that cleaves native triple-helix collagen as well as gelatin into small fragments (Dixon and Webb 1979). Col-

lagen is the most abundant protein in the animal body, constituting one-fourth to one-third of the total protein forming the insoluble fibre of connective tissue (White et al. 1978). Yoshida and Noda (1965) first separated *C. histolyticum* collagenase into 2 fractions designated as I and II. Both degraded collagen at similar rates, but collagenase II split more peptide bonds in the collagen molecule and was more efficient in degrading lower molecular weight polypeptides. Bond and Van Wart (1984a,b) and Van Wart and Steinbrink (1985) have identified 7 distinguishable molecular forms of *C. histolyticum* collagenase, and designated each by a Greek letter; unfortunately 5 of these can be confused with the 5 toxins of this organism designated by the same Greek letters. Each collagenase is distinguished by its molecular mass, determined as 68, 115, 79, 100, 110, 125 and 130 kDa for collagenases α, β, γ, δ, ε, ζ and η, respectively. Two subspecies of the α- and β collagenases are noted on the basis of different isoelectric points. Class I collagenase activity is found with the α, β, γ and η molecular species, and class II with the δ, ε and ζ. The class I collagenases have extensive amino acid sequence homology with each other, and similar homology is found among the class II enzymes, but the 2 classes have substantially different sequences (Bond and Van Wart 1984c). Evidence shows intragenic duplication in the β molecule, which may account for its higher molecular weight. This duplication may be true also for the other higher molecular weight collagenases. The collagenases are all related serologically, but some distinctions are evident by immunodiffusion analysis in agar gels. The 2 classes of collagenases have been shown to have similar but complementary substrate amino acid sequence specificities by which they synergistically digest collagen (Mookhtiar, Steinbrink and Van Wart 1985, Van Wart and Steinbrink 1985). β-Toxin no doubt plays a major role in the pathology of *C. histolyticum* infections in view of its ability to destroy collagen fibres. The toxin induces haemorrhage when placed on the surface of the lungs of animals, and causes haemorrhage and oedema when injected into rat paws (Vargaftig, Lefort and Giroux 1976). It causes a lethal intrapulmonary haemorrhage when injected intravenously (Smith and Williams 1984).

γ-Toxin

γ-Toxin is a thiol-activated proteinase that digests hide powder, azocoll, gelatin and casein, but is inactive against collagen (Willis 1969). Its molecular weight is about 50 kDa (Smith and Williams 1984).

δ-Toxin

The δ-toxin is also a proteolytic enzyme; more specifically, it is an elastase (Willis 1969). It is reversibly inactivated by reducing agents. Takahashi, Seifter and Binder (1970) partially purified δ-toxin and found that it passed through a 50 kDa ultramembrane filter but was retained by a 10 kDa membrane. The active fraction obtained by gel filtration and ion-exchange chromatography had high specific caseinolytic as well as elastolytic activity. It was not active on collagen. The elastolytic and caseinolytic activities were not affected by chelating agents.

ε-Toxin

The ε-toxin is an oxygen-labile haemolysin similar serologically to those produced by other clostridia such as *C. tetani*, *C. septicum* and *C. novyi* (Willis 1969, Bernheimer 1976, Smith and Williams 1984).

14.10   *C. argentinense*

Organisms that produce BoNT/G were designated *C. botulinum* type G, since all other organisms producing botulism neurotoxins of the various serological types were known by the one species name. The original strain of this organism, as well as a second strain isolated from soil samples in Argentina (Giménez and Ciccarelli 1970, Ciccarelli, Giulietti and Giménez 1976), were quite different from organisms classified as *C. botulinum* groups I–III, in that they were asaccharolytic and did not produce lipase. Phenotypically they closely resembled *C. subterminale*, which some speculated to be non-toxigenic variants. Although the 2 organisms show little relationship by DNA homology (Suen et al. 1988a), they are very closely related on the basis of 16S rRNA gene sequence homology, and are found in cluster I (Fig. 32.1). Cells in PYG broth are 1.3–1.9 μm × 1.6–9.4 μm. Spores are rarely observed (Fig. 32.2q), but are reported as oval, subterminal and causing swelling of the cells (Giménez and Ciccarelli 1970). Surface colonies on blood agar are β-haemolytic. The organism digests proteins and liquefies gelatin. Products of metabolism are acetic, butyric, isobutyric, isovaleric and phenylacetic acids.

DNA relatedness studies on 9 strains known as *C. botulinum* type G, 11 strains identified as *C. subterminale* and 3 strains identified as *C. hastiforme* showed that the toxigenic organisms were distinct from the type strain of *C. subterminale*, but closely related to 2 other phenotypically similar, non-toxigenic organisms, and marginally related to a third strain (Suen et al. 1988a). The name *C. argentinense* was proposed for the closely related toxigenic and non-toxigenic organisms. This could be justified with the recognition of other clostridial species that can produce BoNT, namely *C. baratii* and *C. butyricum* (Suen et al. 1988b). Phenotypic differentiation was based on detection of an 'indole derivative' (Lombard and Dowell 1983; possibly 3-indolepropionic acid) in cultures of *C. argentinense*, but not in cultures of *C. subterminale*, *C. hastiforme* or members of the other DNA relatedness groups (Suen et al. 1988a).

The nucleotide sequence of the gene encoding the type G neurotoxin (strain 113/30, NCFB 3012) was determined and shows that the toxin consists of 1297 amino acid residues (Campbell, Collins and East 1993) with a molecular mass of 149 kDa. It has the highest sequence relatedness with type B neurotoxin (approximately 58% for both proteolytic and non-proteolytic strains).

Besides the isolates from soil in Argentina, isolation of BoNT/G-producing organisms from specimens taken at autopsy have been reported from one laboratory in Switzerland (Sonnabend et al. 1981, 1985). The same laboratory has reported the isolation of type G neurotoxigenic organisms from Swiss soil (Sonnabend, Sonnabend and Krech 1987). In view of the lack of documentation of any evidence of botulism in any of the cases, the significance of the reported autopsy isolates is questionable. There has not been any symptomatic case of human or non-human botulism in which BoNT/G has been detected nor from which organisms producing type G neurotoxin have been isolated.

14.11   *C. subterminale*

C. subterminale is a proteolytic, asaccharolytic organism with soil and the intestinal tract of humans and animals as habitat (Smith and Williams 1984). Cells in PYG are gram-positive straight rods, 0.5–1.9 μm × 1.6–11.0 μm. The organisms produce isobutyric and isovaleric acids as metabolic end products on GLC analysis as expected for proteolytic clostridia, as well as acetic, butyric and phenylacetic acids. A few strains produce a small amount of lecithinase. It is non-toxigenic and non-pathogenic for laboratory animals. Its frequent isolation from specimens is probably of little clinical significance. Although the DNA relatedness between the type strain and that of *C. argentinense* was only 20% (Suen et al. 1988a), the 2 species are placed very closely, within cluster I (Fig. 32.1) on the basis of 16S-ribosomal RNA homology. (Collins et al. 1994).

14.12   *C. hastiforme*

C. hastiforme is non-toxigenic and non-pathogenic, and has its habitat in the soil. It is often encountered in clinical specimens and is sometimes difficult to identify. This organism has been difficult to distinguish from *C. subterminale* on the basis of phenotypic characteristics, but it shows less than 10% relatedness by DNA hybridization studies (Suen et al. 1988a). The type strains of these 2 species have been distinguished on the basis of differences in the soluble protein patterns seen on polyacrylamide gel electrophoresis (Cato et al. 1982), and the formation of terminal spores and lack of hydrogen production by *C. hastiforme* (Cato, George and Finegold 1986). The 2 organisms are widely separated on the basis of 16S-rRNA gene sequence analysis (Collins et al. 1994; clusters I and XII, respectively). A recent study of available data shows virtual identity of the 16S rRNA genes of the type strains of *C. hastiforme* and *Tissierella praeacuta* (Farrow et al. 1995). The next organism most closely related to *C. hastiforme* by 16S rRNA gene homology in that study was *Tissierella creatinini*. Those observations question the continued inclusion of *C. hastiforme* in the genus *Clostridium*.

14.13 *C. sporogenes*

C. sporogenes was first described and named (*Bacillus sporogenes*) by Metchnikoff (1908). It is of particular interest because it so widely distributed in the environment and frequently found in human faeces and recovered from wound specimens. It closely resembles *C. botulinum* phenotypically and genetically so that it is sometimes considered a non-toxigenic variant. It is very closely related to proteolytic strains of *C. botulinum* as well as to *C. putrificum* by 16S rRNA gene homology (Fig. 32.1). *C. sporogenes* is a frequent contaminant in other anaerobic cultures because of its ubiquitous distribution (Willis 1969), and thus must be identified frequently. Although by itself it is not pathogenic, it is able to colonize devitalized tissue and may modify the appearance and course of infections by other histotoxic clostridia.

Cells in PYG are gram-positive, motile, straight rods, 0.3–1.4 μm × 1.3–16.0 μm. The organisms ferment glucose, liquefy gelatin, digest meat and milk proteins, and produce lipase. They produce acetic, butyric, isobutyric, isovaleric and hydrocinnamic (phenylpropionic) acids (Holdeman, Cato and Moore 1977). With regard to these phenotypic characteristics, *C. sporogenes* is not distinguishable from *C. botulinum* group I (toxin types A, B and F). *C. sporogenes* does not produce any lethal toxins and is distinguished by a negative bioassay.

Two varieties of this species have been observed by a number of workers, beginning with Metchnikoff. Nakamura et al. (1977) designate a rhizoidal-colony variant as type I and a circular- or crenate-colony variant as type II. Type I strains showed much more abundant spores, but type II strains were generally more heat resistant, even when spores were not apparent on the stained slide. Type II strains were 81–91% related to a reference strain of *C. botulinum* type A by DNA hybridization, while type I strains were only 66–73% related.

C. sporogenes is sometimes used as a surrogate organism for *C. botulinum* is studying sporocidal processing techniques because of the high heat resistance of its spores and obviating the need for working with a hazardous toxigenic organism, e.g. PA (putrefactive anaerobe) 3679 = ATCC7955. The spores of *C. sporogenes* PA 3679 have a $D_{121.1}$ = 1–5 min, compared to $D_{121.1} \leq 0.21$ min for *C. botulinum* type A.

14.14 *C. baratii*

C. baratii has been generally recognized as a non-pathogenic organism isolated from soil, normal human faeces, war wounds, various human infections and marine sediments (Cato, George and Finegold 1986). On the basis of its phenotypical characteristics it resembles *C. perfringens*, and is most closely related to it by 16S rRNA gene homology. The phospholipase C of *C. baratii* is completely inhibited by antibodies to *C. perfringens* α-toxin (Smith and Williams 1984). This species is distinguished most easily because of its inability to liquefy gelatin. *C. perenne* and *C. paraperfringens* were found to be synonyms of *C. baratii*, based on comparison of electrophoretic protein patterns (Cato, Holdeman and Moore 1982).

Cultures in PYG broth show non-motile, straight rods measuring 0.5–1.9 μm × 1.6–10.2 μm. Most strains ferment glucose, fructose, maltose, lactose, mannose and mannitol. They are non-proteolytic and do not liquefy gelatin. They produce formic, acetic, propionic and butyric acids as volatile products as well as lactic, and sometimes succinic acids.

C. baratii has been known as a non-toxigenic organism, but in recent times toxigenic strains that produce a type F-like botulinum neurotoxin have been implicated in a number of cases of human botulism. Two cases of infant botulism have been reported (Hall et al. 1985, Trethon et al. 1995), and another has been documented (CDC, unpublished data). One case of botulism due to intestinal colonization has been reported (McCroskey et al. 1991), and at least 3 other such cases have been documented (CDC, unpublished data). The nucleotide sequence of the gene encoding the neurotoxin has been determined (Thompson et al. 1993). A comparison of the gene sequences from *C. botulinum* and *C. baratii* shows 73.6% and 64.2 % homology for the heavy and light chain sequences, respectively. This is less than expected in view of the much higher homology for the type E toxin genes found in *C. botulinum* and *C. butyricum* (98.1% and 96.0% for the heavy and light chain sequences, respectively). The low sequence homology finding is, however, consistent with the low efficiency of neutralization of the *C. baratii* toxin with the type F antitoxin (McCroskey et al. 1991).

14.15 *C. spiroforme*

Since 1964 there have been several reports of helically coiled, gram-positive anaerobic organisms isolated from animal faeces and caecum contents (Bladen, Nylen and Fitzgerald 1964, Fitzgerald et al. 1965). Because spore formation was noted in some of these strains, they were recognized as clostridia (Koopman and Kennis 1977). Kaneuchi et al. (1979) compared 33 strains of coiled spore-forming organisms recovered from humans and animals. All of the organisms were non-proteolytic and non-gelatinolytic, fermented glucose, and produced terminal to subterminal round spores. Two main groups were established on the basis of physiological characteristics and DNA relatedness; 21 strains were designated as *C. cocleatum* and 8 as *C. spiroforme*. Each of these 2 species has 46–60% relatedness with reference strains of the opposite species and 74–100% relatedness in comparison of strains within each species. The phenotypic differences noted (Kaneuchi et al. 1979) were fermentation of galactose by *C. cocleatum* and a more pronounced coiling by *C. spiroforme*. Both species were related to *C. ramosum*; 35–52% for *C. cocleatum*, and 32–53% for *C. spiroforme*. *C. ramosum* has a straight rod morphology and has α-methylmannosidase activities that are not found in the 2 coiled organisms. The relationship of *C. spiroforme* to *C. ramosum* on the basis of characteristics other than morphology is indicated further by their 16S rRNA similarity, as seen in Fig. 32.1, with both organisms occupying cluster XVIII.

After *C. spiroforme* cultures are heated at 80°C for 10 min, uncoiled, straight cells are found that do not revert to the coiled structure upon subculture (Kaneuchi et al. 1979). No alterations of any other features of the organism are observed. The helical structure of the native organism consists of numerous single semicircular cells joined end to end (Borriello, Davies and Carman 1986). The individual cells are non-motile and gram-positive, with dimensions of 0.3–0.5 × 2.0–10 μm (Cato, George and Finegold 1986).

Much clinical interest in *C. spiroforme* arose when an organism with similar morphological and physiological characteristics which produced a toxin neutralizable with type E antitoxin of *C. perfringens* was consistently isolated from faeces of scouring rabbits (Carman and Borriello 1982). Borriello and Carman (1983) reported complete agreement between the characteristics of toxigenic isolates from rabbits and the type strain of *C. spiroforme*, but the validity of the identity of the toxigenic strains has been questioned (Moore, Cato and Moore 1987). ι-Toxin had been found previously in rabbit enterotoxaemia, but investigators had attempted to recover ι-toxigenic *C. perfringens* (Patton et al. 1978, Baskerville, Wood and Seamer 1980). The toxigenic organism identified as *C. spiroforme* was subsequently implicated as the cause of both spontaneous and antibiotic-induced diarrhoea and colitis in rabbits (Borriello and Carman 1983, Carman and Borriello 1984). Holmes, Sonn and Patton (1988) found that isolation of the organism from rabbit intestinal contents can be facilitated by high-speed centrifugation (20 000 × g) of caecal contents and culturing the material at the supernatant–pellet interface. The helical shape of the organism perhaps is responsible for its slower sedimentation than that of other microorganisms in the samples and thus, its accumulation on the top of the pellet.

ι-Toxin

The ι-toxin of *C. spiroforme* is a binary toxin with components ι-a and ι-b that correspond serologically and electrophoretically to the components of *C. perfringens* ι-toxin (Stiles and Wilkins 1986a). The electrophoretic mobilities of the latter are slightly faster. Although the *C. spiroforme* antiserum formed precipitates with both components of the toxin from either species, *C. perfringens* antiserum formed visible precipitates only with the b-component of the *C. spiroforme* toxin on immunoelectrophoretic plates.

Popoff and Boquet (1988) purified the a-component of *C. spiroforme* ι-toxin by immunoaffinity and reported that it consists of a heterogeneous population of molecules with molecular masses ranging from 43 to 47 kDa. This is similar to the 47.5 kDa size of the ι-a component of *C. perfringens*. This component has ADP-ribosyltransferase activity towards actin. It was inactive in both cytotoxic and mouse lethality assays by itself, but was potentiated by the component ι-b from *C. spiroforme* or *C. perfringens*. ι-b from *C. spiro-*

forme potentiated ι-a from *C. perfringens* and also an ADP-ribosyltransferase (CDT) from *C. difficile* in those same assays. The components of the binary C_2 toxin of *C. botulinum* did not synergize with any of the binary components of the other 3 species.

14.16   *C. colinum*

C. colinum is of interest because it is the aetiological agent of acute or chronic ulcerative enteritis of wild game birds, notably quail, as well as domestic fowl (Songer 1996). The nature of its pathology in birds suggests a toxigenic mechanism, but testing of culture supernatants in laboratory animals has no effect. Further studies on possible toxigenicity of pathogenic strains need to be done. The organism is typical of clostridia in the Gram reaction, being positive in young cultures, but becoming gram-negative with further incubation. Cells are motile, 1 × 3–4 μm rods, with rare spores which are oval and subterminal when observed. The organism is isolated from other pathogenic clostridia by 16S rRNA homology (Collins et al. 1994; not shown in Fig. 32.1), falling into cluster XIVb.

14.17   *C. fallax*

C. fallax is one of 6 *Clostridium* species listed by MacLennan as causes of gas gangrene (MacLennan 1962). It was first isolated in 1915 from war wounds (Weinberg and Seguin 1915), but rarely encountered thereafter, except for less than a dozen cases of gas gangrene during World War II (MacLennan 1962). The organism has been isolated from soil, marine sediments and human faeces (Cato, George and Finegold 1986). It is a motile, gram-positive bacillus, 0.6 μm × 1.2–5 μm, with rounded ends, arranged singly. It belongs in 16S rRNA gene cluster I (Fig. 32.1). Spores, which are rarely formed, are subterminal, oval and wider than the bacillus. The organism ferments glucose, maltose, lactose and sucrose. It is non-proteolytic but coagulates milk in 7 days, and usually fails to liquefy gelatin. It produces acetic, butyric and lactic acids, and is negative for lecithinase and lipase. Culture supernatants are considered non-toxic for mice, although there are reports that freshly isolated organisms produce a soluble toxin and are pathogenic for mice and guinea-pigs (Willis 1990).

15   OTHER *CLOSTRIDIUM* SPECIES

15.1   *C. cadaveris*

C. cadaveris, formerly known as *C. capitovale*, was isolated by Snyder and Hall (1935) from a number of sources, including the pleural fluid of a sheep that had died of gas gangrene, the heart blood and peritoneal fluid at necropsy of cases of septic infection in humans and the faeces of normal infants. It is a slender, motile, gram-positive rod with rounded ends, measuring 0.5–0.8 μm × 2.0–2.5 μm, and forming oval terminal spores. It is found in 16S rRNA gene cluster I. *C. cadaveris* is non-haemolytic and negative for lecithinase and lipase on egg yolk agar. It ferments glucose, but not maltose, lactose or sucrose. It liquefies gelatin, is mildly proteolytic, clots milk irregularly and sometimes digests the clot. Products of metabolism are acetic and butyric acids. It is non-pathogenic to guinea-pigs and rabbits inoculated subcutaneously and appears to be antigenically homogeneous.

15.2   *C. carnis*

C. carnis was first isolated from putrifying beef infusion and described by Klein (1904). It is a gram-positive rod, sluggishly motile by peritrichous flagella, 0.5–0.7 μm × 1.5–4.5 μm. It is found in 16S rRNA gene cluster I and is rather closely related to *C. septicum* and *C. chauvoei* by this criterion. *C. carnis* readily forms subterminal elongated spores, slightly wider than the bacillus, which later appear to be terminal. It is aerotolerant, but spores are not formed under aerobic conditions. It ferments glucose, maltose, lactose and sucrose. It is egg yolk negative and non-proteolytic; it does not produce indole or hydrogen sulphide, and does not liquefy gelatin. It produces a soluble exotoxin and is pathogenic to mice, rats and rabbits, with production of an oedematous and congested local lesion.

15.3   *C. cochlearium*

C. cochlearium was encountered in a study of organisms recovered from war wounds, and so named because of its likeness to a spoon (Douglas, Fleming and Colebrook 1920). It is a slender rod, weakly gram-positive only in young cultures, 0.5–0.6 μm × 3–5 μm, actively motile by peritrichous flagella. It belongs to 16S rRNA cluster I and is closely related to *C. tetani*. Oval subterminal spores, twice the width of the bacillus are formed late. It is non-haemolytic, non-proteolytic, asaccharolytic, and egg yolk negative. It produces hydrogen sulphide, but not ammonia or indole. Volatile products of metabolism include a major amount of butyric acid with smaller amounts of acetic and propionic acids. It is antigenically homogeneous and non-pathogenic to guinea-pigs.

15.4   *C. limosum*

The interest in *C. limosum* is mainly due to the frequency of its isolation from clinical and environmental samples. It is considered a pathogen in various animals, but it does not appear to pose a serious hazard for any species (Smith and Williams 1984). The organism is proteolytic, hydrolysing gelatin, cooked meat and casein, and produces lecithinase and collagenase, but does not ferment any of the usual substrates. *C. limosum* is unusual among the proteolytic clostridia (but like *C. histolyticum*) in not producing the isoacids as metabolic end products. Pathogenicity may be due to lecithinase and collagenase, which seem to be readily lost in laboratory cultures. The organism has sometimes been mistaken for *C. histolyticum*, which is closely related by 16S rRNA gene homology in cluster II (Fig. 32.1). The cells are motile, straight rods, 0.6–1.6 × 1.7–16 μm with oval, subterminal spores which usually swell the cells.

15.5   *C. putrificum*

C. putrificum was described by Bienstock, who isolated it from faeces (Bienstock 1906). There has been some confusion concerning the actual isolate of the original organism, but the name now applies to the isolate described by Reddish and Rettger (1922). *C. putrificum* is a slender bacillus, gram-positive only in young cultures, 0.3–1.3 μm × 1.3–11 μm, with oval or round terminal or subterminal spores. It is found in 16S rRNA gene cluster I, and closely related to proteolytic *C. botulinum* and *C. sporogenes*. It is motile by peritrichate flagella. It is proteolytic, liquefying coagulated serum and gelatin in 7–20 days, and blackens cooked meat medium slightly; haemolytic, hydrogen sulphide positive, indole and egg yolk negative. It ferments glucose only; and produces acetic, isobutyric, butyric, and isobutyric acids as metabolic products. Culture supernatants are non-toxic for mice.

15.6   *C. paraputrificum*

This organism was described by Bienstock (1906). It is found in faeces, particularly of infants, both normal and ill nourished. It is a slender, motile, gram-variable bacillus with large terminal oval spores, and belongs to 16S rRNA cluster I. It is non-proteolytic; ferments glucose, maltose, lactose and sucrose. It produces major amounts of lactic, acetic and butyric acids as metabolic products. It is non-pathogenic for guinea-pigs and rabbits.

15.7   *C. ramosum*

The name *C. ramosum* was proposed in 1971 as a new combination to include organisms previously named *Bacillus ramosus*, *Nocardia ramosa*, *Actinomyces ramosus*, *Bacteroides ramosus* and *Ramibacterium ramosum* (Holdeman, Cato and Moore 1971), since the organisms were shown to be anaerobic, spore-forming rods with a G+C ratio of 27%. This organism is frequently isolated from clinical specimens, especially in intra-abdominal sepsis (Smith and Williams 1984) and appendicitis. It is gram-positive, non-motile, and arranged in pairs or short chains. The V- and Y-forms to which the species epithet refers are common. Terminal spores are formed scantily and resist heating at 80°C for 10 min. It is found in 16S rRNA cluster XVIII which it shares with *C. spiroforme*. Cultures have a fetid odour, but form little gas. The organism ferments glucose, maltose, lactose and sucrose, but is entirely non-proteolytic and generally does not liquefy gelatin. It is non-haemolytic; and negative for hydrogen sulphide, indole, lecithinase and lipase. Main products of metabolism are acetic and formic acids with smaller amounts of lactic acid. Culture supernatants are nontoxic for mice, but strains are pathogenic for guineapigs; pathogenicity may be lost in laboratory cultures (Cato, George and Finegold 1986).

15.8   *C. sphenoides*

C. sphenoides is another species isolated by Douglas in his study of organisms recovered from war wounds (Douglas, Fleming and Colebrook 1920). It is so named because of the wedge shape of the sporing bacillus. It is small, motile, and weakly gram-positive. Vegetative bacilli are fusiform in shape and arranged in pairs end to end. Spores are large and round, appearing subterminally, but soon become strictly terminal. It is found in 16S rRNA cluster XIVa with *C. nexile*. The organism is non-proteolytic. It ferments glucose, maltose, and lactose, and produces acetic and formic acids. It is indole positive, haemolytic, hydro-

gen sulphide and egg yolk negative, and non-pathogenic.

15.9   *C. tertium*

C. tertium was isolated from war wounds and described by Henry (1916). The name *tertium* (meaning third) was applied because it was the third most frequently isolated organism in Henry's study. It is a thin, slightly curved bacillus, 3–5 μm long, sluggishly motile, grampositive, often showing granular staining. It sporulates freely, giving rise to large, oval, elongated terminal spores. It ferments glucose, maltose lactose and sucrose. It is negative on egg yolk, non-proteolytic and does not liquefy gelatin. It is indole negative, but usually nitrate positive. Main products of metabolism include acetic and lactic acids with lesser amounts of butyric and formic acids. It is aerotolerant, rather than strictly anaerobic, but forms spores only under anaerobic conditions. It is non-pathogenic for guinea-pigs.

REFERENCES

Adams EB, Lawrence DR, Smith JWG, 1969, *Tetanus*, Blackwell Scientific, Oxford.

Aikat BK, Dible JH, 1960, The local and general effects of culture and culture-filtrates of *Clostridium oedematiens, Cl. septicum, Cl. sporogenes* and *Cl. histolyticum, J Pathol Bacteriol*, **79:** 227–41.

Aktories K, Weller V, Chhatwal GS, 1987, *Clostridium botulinum* type C produces a novel ADP-ribosyltransferase distinct from C2 toxin, *FEBS Lett*, **212:** 109–13.

Al-Khatib G, 1969, Beitrage zur Clostridiendifferenzierung. IV. Zur Differenzierung von *Cl. septicum* und *Cl. chauvoei, Arch Exp Vet Med*, **23:** 963–70.

Alouf JE, Jolivet-Reynaud C, 1981, Purification and characterization of *Clostridium perfringens* delta toxin, *Infect Immun*, **31:** 536–46.

Andreesen JR, 1994, Glycine metabolism in anaerobes, *Antonie Van Leeuwenhoek*, **66:** 223–37.

Andreesen JR, Bahl H, Gottschalk G, 1989, Introduction to the physiology and biochemistry of the genus *Clostridium, Clostridia*, eds Minton NP, Clarke DJ, Plenum Press, New York, 27–62.

Arloing S, Cornevin, Thomas, 1880, De l'inoculation du charbon symptomatique par injection intra-veneuse, et de i'immunité conférée au veau, au mouton, et à la chévee par ce procédé [On the intravenous inoculation of 'black disease' and the immunity conferred on the calf, sheep and horse by this procedure], *CR Acad Sci Paris*, **91:** 734–6.

Arnon SS, Midura TF et al., 1979, Honey and other environmental risk factors for infant botulism, *J Pediatr*, **94:** 331–6.

Arsecularatne SN, Panabokke RG, Wijesundra S, 1969, The toxins responsible for the lesions of *Clostridium sordellii* gas gangrene, *J Med Microbiol*, **2:** 237–53.

Arzese A, Trani G et al., 1995, Rapid polymerase chain reaction method for specific detection of toxigenic *Clostridium difficile, Eur J Clin Microbiol Infect Dis*, **14:** 716–19.

Aureli P, Fenicia L et al., 1986, Two cases of type E infant botulism caused by neurotoxigenic *Clostridium butyricum* in Italy, *J Infect Dis*, **154:** 201–6.

Baez LA, Juneja VK, 1995, Detection of enterotoxigenic *Clostridium perfringens* in raw beef by polymerase chain reaction, *J Food Protect*, **58:** 154–9.

Banno Y, Kobayashi T et al., 1984, Biochemical characterization and biologic actions of two toxins (D-1 and D-2) from *Clostridium difficile, Rev Infect Dis*, **6:** S11–20.

Barbut F, Petit JC, 1996, Epidemiology of nosocomial infections due to *Clostridium difficile* [French], *Presse Méd*, **25:** 385–92.

Bartlett JG, Moon N et al., 1978, Role of *Clostridium difficile* in antibiotic-associated pseudomembranous colitis, *Gastroenterology*, **75:** 778–82.

Baskerville M, Wood M, SeAm JH, 1980, *Clostridium perfringens* type E enterotoxaemia in rabbits, *Vet Rec*, **107:** 18–9.

Batty I, Walker PD, 1963, The differentiation of *Clostridium septicum* and *Clostridium chauvoei* by the use of fluorescent-labelled antibodies, *J Pathol Biol*, **85:** 517–21.

Batty I, Walker PD, 1966, Colonial morphology and fluorescent-labelled antibody staining in the identification of species of the species *Clostridium, J Appl Bacteriol*, **28:** 112–18.

Bauer JH, Meyer KF, 1926, Human intestinal carriers of tetanus spores in California, *J Infect Dis*, **38:** 295–305.

Behring E, Kitasato S, 1890, Ueber das Zustandekommen der Diptherie-Immunität und der Tetanus-Immunität bei Thieren, *Dtsch Med Wochenschr*, **16:** 113–14.

Beland S, Rossier E, 1973, Isolement et identification de *Clostridium tetani* dans le sol des cantons de l'Est de la Province de Quebec, *Can J Microbiol*, **19:** 1513–18.

Bernheimer AW, 1976, Sulfhydryl activated toxins, *Mechanisms in Bacterial Toxinology*, ed. Bernheimer AW, Wiley, New York, 85–97.

Berry PR, Rodhouse JC et al., 1988, Evaluation of ELISA, RPLA, and Vero cell assays for detecting *Clostridium perfringens* enterotoxin in faecal specimens, *J Clin Pathol*, **41:** 458–61.

Betz JV, Anderson KE, 1964, Isolation and characterization of bacteriophages active in *Clostridium sporogenes, J Bacteriol*, **87:** 408–15.

Bienstock B, 1906, *Bacillus putrificus, Ann Inst Pasteur*, **20:** 407.

Binz T, Kurazono H et al., 1990a, The complete sequence of botulinum neurotoxin type A and comparison with other clostridial neurotoxins, *J Biol Chem*, **265:** 9153–8.

Binz T, Kurazono H et al., 1990b, Nucleotide sequence of the gene encoding for *Clostridium botulinum* neurotoxin type D, *Nucleic Acids Res*, **18:** 5556.

Bizzini B, 1989, Axoplasmic transport and transsynaptic movement of tetanus toxin, *Botulinum Neurotoxin and Tetanus Toxin*, ed Simpson LL, Academic Press, San Diego, 203–29.

Bladen HA, Nylen MV, Fitzgerald RJ, 1964, Internal structures of a *Eubacterium* sp. demonstrated by the negative-staining technique, *J Bacteriol*, **88:** 763–70.

Bleck TP, 1989, Clinical aspects of tetanus, *Botulinum Neurotoxin and Tetanus Toxin*, ed Simpson LL, Academic Press, San Diego, 379–98.

Bollinger O, 1875, Beitrag zur Kenntnis des sogenantes 'Gerausches', einer angeblichen Milzbrandform, *Dtsch Z Tiermed Vergl Pathol*, **1**: 297–9.

Bond MD, Van Wart HE, 1984a, Characterization of the individual collagenases from *Clostridium histolyticum*, *Biochemistry*, **23**: 3085–91.

Bond MD, Van Wart HE, 1984b, Purification of individual collagenase of *Clostridium histolyticum* using red dye ligand chromatography, *Biochemistry*, **23**: 3077–85.

Bond MD, Van Wart HE, 1984c, Relationship between the individual collagenases of *Clostridium histolyticum*: evidence for evolution by gene duplication, *Biochemistry*, **23**: 3092–9.

Bongaerts GPA, Lyerly DM, 1994, Role of toxins A and B in the pathogenesis of *Clostridium difficile* disease, *Microb Pathog*, **17**: 1–12.

Borriello SP, 1985, Newly described clostridial diseases of the gastrointestinal tract: *Clostridium perfringens* enterotoxin-associated diarrhea and neutropenic enterocolitis due to *Clostridium septicum*, *Clostridia in Gastrointestinal Disease*, ed Borriello SP, CRC Press, Boca Raton, FL, 223–9.

Borriello SP, Carman RJ, 1983, Association of iota-like toxin and *Clostridium spiroforme* with both spontaneous and antibiotic-associated diarrhea and colitis in rabbits, *J Clin Microbiol*, **17**: 414–18.

Borriello SP, Davies HA, Carman RJ, 1986, Cellular morphology of *Clostridium spiroforme*, *Vet Microbiol*, **11**: 191–5.

Borriello SP, Larson HE, 1985, Pseudomembranous and antibiotic-associated colitis, *Clostridia in Gastrointestinal Disease*, ed Borriello SP, CRC Press, Boca Raton, FL, 145–64.

Bosworth TJ, 1943, On a new type of toxin produced by *Clostridium welchii*, *J Comp Pathol*, **53**: 245–55.

Bowen HE, 1952–53, A comparison of the lethal and hemolytic toxins of *Clostridium histolyticum*, *Yale J Biol Med*, **25**: 124–38.

Bowness P, Moss PAH et al., 1992, *Clostridium perfringens* enterotoxin is a superantigen reactive wuth human T cell receptors Vβ6.9 and Vβ22, *J Exp Med*, **176**: 893–6.

Brazier JS, 1995, An international study on the unification of the nomenclature for typing of *Clostridium difficile*, *Clin Infect Dis*, **20**: S325–6.

Brenner DJ, 1973, Deoxyribonucleic acid reassociation in the taxonomy of enteric bacteria, *Int J Syst Bacteriol*, **23**: 298–307.

Brewer JH, 1940, A clear medium for the 'aerobic' cultivation of anaerobes, *J Bacteriol*, **39**: 10.

Browdie DA, Davis JH et al., 1975, *Clostridium sordellii* infection, *J Trauma*, **15**: 515–18.

Buogo C, Capaul S et al., 1995, Diagnosis of *Clostridium perfringens* type C enteritis in pigs using a DNA amplification technique (PCR), *J Vet Med B*, **42**: 51–8.

Buxton D, 1978, Further studies on the mode of action of *Clostridium welchii* type D epsilon toxin, *J Med Microbiol*, **11**: 293–8.

Bytchenko B, 1981, Microbiology of tetanus, *Tetanus, Important New Concepts*, ed Veronesi R, Excerpta Medica, Amsterdam, 28–39.

Campbell K, Collins MD, East AK, 1993, Nucleotide sequence of the gene coding for *Clostridium botulinum* (*Clostridium argentinense*) type G neurotoxin: genealogical comparison with other clostridial neurotoxins, *Biochim Biophys Acta*, **1216**: 487–91.

Campos-Neto A, Mengel JP et al., 1995, Potent stimulation of murine B cells to proliferate and to secrete immunoglobulins by a lipoteichoic acid-like molecule produced by *Clostridium botulinum* C and D, *Braz J Med Biol Res*, **28**: 575–84.

Carman RJ, Borriello SP, 1982, *Clostridium spiroforme* isolated from rabbits with diarrhea, *Vet Rec*, **111**: 461–2.

Carman RJ, Borriello SP, 1984, Infectious nature of *Clostridium spiroforme*-mediated rabbit enterotoxaemia, *Vet Microbiol*, **9**: 497–502.

Cartwright CP, Stock F et al., 1995, PCR amplification of rRNA intragenic spacer regions as a method for epidemiologic typing of *Clostridium difficile*, *J Clin Microbiol*, **33**: 184–7.

Cato EP, George WL, Finegold SM, 1986, Genus *Clostridium*,

Bergey's Manual of Systematic Bacteriology, eds Sneath PHA, Mair NS et al., Williams and Wilkins, Baltimore, 1141–200.

Cato EP, Holdeman LV, Moore WEC, 1982, *Clostridium perenne* and *Clostridium paraperfringens*: later subjective synonyms of *Clostridium barati*, *Int J Syst Bacteriol*, **32**: 77–81.

Cato EP, Stackebrandt E, 1989, Taxonomy and phylogeny, *Clostridia*, eds Minton NP, Clarke DJ, Plenum Press, New York, 1–26.

Cato EP, Dash DE et al., 1982, Electrophoretic study of *Clostridium* species, *J Clin Microbiol*, **15**: 688–702.

CDC, 1993, Summary of notifiable diseases, United States 1992, *Morbid Mortal Weekly Rep*, **41**: 1–65.

CDC, 1995, Wound botulism – California, 1995, *Morbid Mortal Weekly Rep*, **44 (no. 48)**: 890–2.

Chachaty E, Saulnier P et al., 1994, Comparison of ribotyping, pulsed-field gel electrophoresis and random amplified polymorphic DNA for typing *Clostridium difficile* strains, *FEMS Microbiol Lett*, **122**: 61–8.

Chia JK, Clark JB et al., 1986, Botulism in an adult associated with food-borne intestinal infection with *Clostridium botulinum*, *N Engl J Med*, **315**: 239–41.

Ciccarelli AS, Giulietti AM, Giménez GF, 1976, Segunda cepa de *Clostridium botulinum* tipo G, *Primer Congresso y IV Jornadas Argentinas de Microbiologia*, 21.

Clabots CR, Johnson S et al., 1993, Development of a rapid and efficient restriction endonuclease analysis typing system for *Clostridium difficile* and correlation with other typing systems, *J Clin Microbiol*, **31**: 1870–5.

Claus KD, Kolbe DR, 1979, Immunogenicity of *Clostridium septicum* in guinea pigs, *Am J Vet Res*, **40**: 1752–6.

Collins MD, Lawson PA et al., 1994, The phylogeny of the genus *Clostridium*: proposal of five new genera and eleven new species combinations, *Int J Syst Bacteriol*, **44**: 812–26.

Cornillot E, Saint-Joanis B et al., 1995, The enterotoxin gene (cpe) of *Clostridium perfringens* can be chromosomal or plasmid-borne, *Mol Biol*, **15**: 639–47.

Cowell JL, Grushoff PS, Bernheimer AW, 1976, Purification of cereolysin and the electrophoretic separation of the active (reduced) and inactive (oxidized) forms of the purified toxin, *Infect Immun*, **14**: 144–54.

Cummins CS, Johnson JL, 1971, Taxonomy of the clostridia: Wall composition and DNA homologies in *Clostridium butyricum* and other butyric acid-producing clostridia, *J Gen Microbiol*, **67**: 33–46.

Czeczulin JR, Hanna PC, McClane BA, 1993, Cloning, nucleotide sequencing, and expression of the *Clostridium perfringens* enterotoxin gene in *Escherichia coli*, *Infect Immun*, **61**: 3429–39.

Darakhshan H, Lauerman LH, 1981, Some properties of beta toxin produced by *Clostridium haemolyticum* strain iRP-135, *Comp Immunol Microbiol Infect Dis*, **4**: 307–16.

DasGupta BR, 1989, The structure of botulinum neurotoxin, *Botulinum Neurotoxin and Tetanus Toxin*, ed Simpson LL, Academic Press, San Diego, 53–67.

Decker K, Jungermann K, Thauer RK, 1970, Energy production in anaerobic organisms, *Angew Chem (Int Ed)*, **9**: 138–58.

Dezfulian M, Dowell VRJ, 1980, Cultural and physiological characteristics and antimicrobial susceptibility of *Clostridium botulinum* isolates from foodborne and infant botulism cases, *J Clin Microbiol*, **11**: 604–9.

Dezfulian M, McCroskey LM et al., 1981, Selective medium for isolation of *Clostridium botulinum* from human feces, *J Clin Microbiol*, **13**: 526–31.

Dixon M, Webb EC, 1979, *Enzymes*, Academic Press, New York.

Dodds KL, 1993, Worldwide incidence and ecology of infant botulism, *Clostridium botulinum: Ecology and Control in Foods*, eds Hauschild AHW, Dodds KL, Marcel Dekker, New York, 105–17.

Dolman CE, Chang E, 1972, Bacteriophages of *Clostridium botulinum*, *Can J Microbiol*, **18**: 67–76.

Douglas SR, Fleming A, Colebrook L, 1920, *Special Report Series of the Medical Research Council*, HMSO, London.

Dowell VRJ, Dezfulian M, 1981, Physiological characterization of *Clostridium botulinum* and development of practical isolation and identification procedures, *Biomedical Aspects of Botulism*, ed Lewis GEJ, Academic Press, New York, 205–16.

Dowell VRJ, Hill EO, Altemeier WA, 1964, Use of phenylethyl alcohol in media for isolation of anaerobic bacteria, *J Bacteriol*, **88:** 1811–13.

Dowell VRJ, Lombard GL et al., 1977a, *Media for Isolation, Characterization and Identification of Obligately Anaerobic Bacteria*, US Department of Health and Human Servicies, Public Health Service, Centers for Disease Control, Atlanta.

Dowell VRJ, McCroskey LM et al., 1977b, Copro-examination for botulinal toxin and *Clostridium botulinum*; a new procedure for laboratory diagnosis of botulism, *JAMA*, **238:** 1829–32.

Dowell VRJ, Lombard GL et al., 1981, Procedures for use of differential media in the identification of anaerobic bacteria, *CDC Laboratory Improvement through Education in Bacteriology*, US Department of Health and Human Servicies, Public Health Service, Centers for Disease Control, Atlanta.

Dowell VR Jr, 1981, Anaerobes in the clinical laboratory, *Les Anaerobies: Microbiologie-Pathologie; Symposium International*, Masson, New York, 23–35.

Dowell VR Jr, Hawkins TM, 1974, *Laboratory Methods in Anaerobic Bacteriology*, Centers for Disease Control, Atlanta.

Duncan CL, Strong DH, 1968, Improved medium for sporulation of *Clostridium perfringens*, *Appl Microbiol*, **16:** 82–9.

East AK, Richardson PT et al., 1992, Sequence of the gene encoding type F neurotoxin of *Clostridium botulinum*, *FEMS Microbiol Lett*, **96:** 225–30.

Easton EJ, Meyer KF, 1924, Occurrence of *Bacillus botulinus* in human and animal excreta, *J Infect Dis*, **35:** 207–12.

von Eichel-Streiber C, Laufenberg-Feldmann R et al., 1992, Comparative sequence analysis of the *Clostridium difficile* toxins A and B, *Mol Gen Genet*, **233:** 260–8.

Eichel-Striber CV, Harperath V et al., 1987, Purification of two high molecular weight toxins of *Clostridium difficile* which are antigenically related, *Microb Pathog*, **2:** 307–18.

Eisel U, Jarausch W et al., 1986, Tetanus toxin: primary structure, expression in *E. coli* and homology with botulinum toxins, *EMBO J*, **5:** 2495–502.

Eklund MW, Dowell VR Jr, 1987, *Avian Botulism: An International Perspective*, Charles C. Thomas, Springfield, IL.

Eklund MW, Wieler DI, Poysky FT, 1967, Outgrowth and toxin production of non-proteolytic type B *Clostridium botulinum* at 3.3 – 5.6 deg.C, *J Bacteriol*, **93:** 1461–2.

Eklund MW, Poysky FT et al., 1974, Interspecies conversion of *Clostridium botulinum* type C to *Clostridium novyi* type A by bacteriophage, *Science*, **186:** 456–8.

Eklund MW, Poysky FT et al., 1976, Relationship of bacteriophages to alpha toxin production in *Clostridium novyi* types A and B, *Infect Immun*, **14:** 793–803.

Eklund MW, Poysky F et al., 1987, Relationship of bacteriophages to toxin and hemagglutinin production and its significance in avian botulism outbreaks, *Avian Botulism*, eds Eklund MW, Dowell VR Jr, Charles C. Thomas, Springfield, IL, 191–222.

Eklund MW, Poysky FT et al., 1988, Evidence for plasmid-mediated toxin and bacteriocin production in *Clostridium botulinum* type G, *Appl Environ Microbiol*, **54:** 1405–8.

Elmore MJ, Hutson RA et al., 1995, Nucleotide sequence of the gene coding for proteolytic (Group I) *Clostridium botulinum* type F neurotoxin: genealogical comparison with other clostridial neurotoxins, *Syst Appl Microbiol*, **18:** 23–31.

Evans DG, 1945, The *in vitro* production of α-toxin, θ-haemolysin and hyaluronidase by strains of *Cl. welchii* type A, and the relationship of *in vitro* properties to virulence for guinea pigs, *J Pathol Bacteriol*, **57:** 75–87.

Farrow JAE, Lawson PA et al., 1995, Phylogenetic evidence that the gram-negative nonsporulating bacterium *Tissierella (Bacteroides) praeacuta* is a member of the *Clostridium* subphy-lum of the gram-positive bacteria and description of *Tissierella creatinini* sp.nov., *Int J Syst Bacteriol*, **45:** 436–40.

Ferreira JL, Hamdy MK, 1995, Detection of botulinal toxin genes: types A and E or B and F using the multiplex polymerase chain reaction, *J Rapid Meth Automat Microbiol*, **3:** 177–83.

Feser J, 1876, Studien über den sogenannten Rauschbrand des Rindes, *Z prakt vet Wiss*, **4:** 13–26.

Fildes P, 1925, Tetanus. I. Isolation, morphology, and cultural reactions of *B. tetani*, *Br J Exp Pathol*, **6:** 62–9.

Finn CW, Silver RP et al., 1984, The structural gene for tetanus neurotoxin is on a plasmid, *Science*, **224:** 881–4.

Fitzgerald RJ, McBride JA et al., 1965, Helically coiled microorganism from cecum contents of the rat, *Nature (London)*, **205:** 1133–4.

Franciosa G, Fenicia L et al., 1996, PCR for detection of *Clostridium botulinum* type C in avian and environmental samples, *J Clin Microbiol*, **34:** 882–5.

Fujii N, Kimura K et al., 1993, Similarity in nucleotide sequence of the gene encoding nontoxic component of botulinum toxin produced by toxigenic *Clostridium butyricum* strain 6340 and *Clostridium botulinum* type E strain Mashike, *Microbiol Immunol*, **37:** 395–8.

George WL, Finegold SM, 1985, Clostridia in the human gastrointestinal flora, *Clostridia in Gastrointestinal Disease*, ed Borriello SP, CRC Press, Boca Raton, FL, 1–37.

George WL, Sutter VL et al., 1979, Selective and differential medium for isolation of *Clostridium difficile*, *J Clin Microbiol*, **9:** 214–9.

Ghanem FM, Ridpath AC et al., 1991, Identification of *Clostridium botulinum*, *Clostridium argentinense*, and related organisms by cellular fatty acid analysis, *J Clin Microbiol*, **29:** 1114–24.

Giménez DF, Ciccarelli AS, 1970, Another type of *Clostridium botulinum*, *Zentralbl Bakteriol I, Abt Orig A*, **215:** 221–4.

Glasby C, Hatheway CL, 1983, Fluorescent-antibody reagents for the identification of *Clostridium botulinum*, *J Clin Microbiol*, **18:** 1378–83.

Glasby C, Hatheway CL, 1984a, Evaluation of fluorescent-antibody tests as a means of confirming infant botulism, *J Clin Microbiol*, **20:** 1209–12.

Glasby C, Hatheway CL, 1984b, Isolation and enumeration of *Clostridium botulinum* by direct inoculation of infant fecal specimens on egg yolk agar and *Clostridium botulinum* isolation media, *J Clin Microbiol*, **21:** 264–6.

Glenny AT, Barr M et al., 1933, Multiple toxins produced by some organisms of the *Cl. welchii* group, *J Pathol Bacteriol*, **37:** 53–74.

Gottschalk G, 1986, *Bacterial Metabolism*, 2nd edn, Springer-Verlag, New York.

Grant RB, Riemann HP, 1976, Temperate phages of *Clostridium perfringens* type C, *Can J Microbiol*, **22:** 603–10.

Granum PE, 1986, Structure and mechanism of action of the enterotoxin from *Clostridium perfringens*, *Proc. II Eur. Workshop Bact. Prot. Toxins*, eds Falmagne P, Jeljaszewicz J, Thelestam M, Gustav Fischer, Stuttgart, 327–34.

Granum PE, Whitaker JR, Skjelkvale R, 1981, Trypsin activation of enterotoxin from Clostridium perfringens type A, *Biochim Biophys Acta*, **668:** 325–32.

Griffin PM, Hatheway CL et al., 1997, Endogenous antibody production to botulinum toxin in an adult with intestinal colonization botulism and underlying Crohn's disease, *J Infect Dis*, **175:** 633–7.

Guelin A, Beerens H, Petiprez A, 1966, Un bacteriophage des anaerobies actif sur *Clostridium histolyticum*, *Ann Inst Past*, **111:** 141–8.

Habeeb AFSA, 1969, Studies on epsilon prototoxin of *Clostridium perfringens* type D. I. Purification methods: evidence for multiple forms of epsilon prototoxin, *Arch Biochem Biophys*, **130:** 430–40.

Hall IC, 1929, The occurrence of *Bacillus sordellii* in icterohemoglobinuria of cattle in Nevada, *J Infect Dis*, **45:** 156–62.

Hall IC, O'Toole E, 1935, Intestinal flora in new-born infants with a description of a new pathogenic anaerobe *Bacillus difficilis*, *Am J Dis Child*, **49**: 390–402.

Hall JD, McCroskey LM et al., 1985, Isolation of an organism resembling *Clostridium barati* which produces type F botulinal toxin from an infant with botulism, *J Clin Microbiol*, **21**: 654–5.

Hardegree MC, Palmer AE, Duffin N, 1971, Tetanolysin: in-vivo effects in animals, *J Infect Dis*, **123**: 51–60.

Harmon SM, Kautter DA, 1986, Evaluation of a reversed passive latex agglutination test kit for *Clostridium perfringens* enterotoxin, *J Food Protect*, **49**: 523–5.

Hatheway CL, 1988, Botulism, *Laboratory Diagnosis of Infectious Diseases: Principles and Practice*, eds Balows A, Hausler WH Jr et al., Springer-Verlag, New York, 111–33.

Hatheway CL, 1990, Toxigenic clostridia, *Clin Microbiol Rev*, **3**: 67–98.

Hatheway CL, Ferreira JL, 1996, Detection and identification of *Clostridium botulinum* neurotoxins, *Natural Toxins II: Proceedings of a Symposium; 209th Am. Chem. Soc. National Meeting, Anaheim, California, April 2–7, 1995*, eds Singh BR, Tu AT, Plenum, New York, 481–98.

Hatheway CL, McCroskey LM, 1987, Examination of feces and serum for diagnosis of infant botulism in 336 patients, *J Clin Microbiol*, **25**: 2334–8.

Hatheway CL, McCroskey LM, 1989, Unusual neurotoxigenic clostridia recovered from human fecal specimens in the investigation of botulism, *Recent Advances in Microbial Ecology,*, eds Hattori T, Ishida Y et al., Japan Scientific Societies Press, Tokyo, 477–81.

Hatheway CL, Whaley DN, Dowell VR Jr, 1980, Epidemiological aspects of *Clostridium perfringens* foodborne illness, *Food Technol*, **34**: 77–9.

Hauschild AHW, 1975, Criteria and procedures for implicating *Clostridium perfringens* in foodborne outbreaks, *Can J Public Health*, **66**: 388–92.

Hauschild AHW, 1993, Epidemiology of human foodborne botulism, Clostridium botulinum*: Ecology and Control in Foods*, eds Hauschild AHW, Dodds KL, Marcel Dekker, New York, 69–104.

Hauschild AHW, Hilsheimer R, 1971, Purification and characteristics of the enterotoxin of *Clostridium perfringens* type A, *Can J Microbiol*, **17**: 1425–33.

Hauschild AHW, Hilsheimer R, 1974, Evaluation and modifications of media for enumeration of *Clostridium perfringens*, *Appl Microbiol*, **27**: 78–82.

Hauschild AHW, Niilo L, Dorward WJ, 1967, Experimental enteritis with food poisoning and classical strains of *Clostridium perfringens* type A in lambs, *J Infect Dis*, **117**: 379–86.

Hauser D, Eklund MW et al., 1990, Nucleotide sequence of *Clostridium botulinum* C1 neurotoxin, *Nucleic Acids Res*, **18**: 4924.

Heller HH, 1920, Aetiology of acute gangrenous infections of animals: a discussion of blackleg, braxy, malignant oedema and whale septicemia, *J Infect Dis*, **27**: 385–451.

Helting TB, Zwisler O, 1977, Structure of tetanus toxin. I. Breakdown of the toxin molecule and discrimination between polypeptide fragments, *J Biol Chem*, **252**: 187–93.

Henry H, 1916–17, On investigation of the cultural reactions of certain anaerobes found in wounds, *J Pathol Bacteriol*, **21**: 344–51.

Hobbs BC, 1965, *Clostridium welchii* as a food poisoning organism, *J Appl Bacteriol*, **28**: 74–82.

Hogan SF, Ireland K, 1989, Fatal acute spontaneous endometritis resulting from *Clostridium sordellii*, *Am J Clin Pathol*, **91**: 104–6.

Holdeman LV, Cato EP, Moore WEC, 1971, *Clostridium ramosum* (Vuillemin comb. nov.: Emended description and proposed neotype strain, *Int J Syst Bacteriol*, **21**: 35–9.

Holdeman LV, Cato EP, Moore WEC, 1977, *Anaerobe Laboratory Manual*, 4th edn, Department of Anaerobic Microbiology, Virginia Polytechnic Institute and State University, Blacksburg.

Holmes HT, Sonn RJ, Patton NM, 1988, Isolation of *Clostridium spiroforme* from rabbits, *Lab Anim Sci*, **38**: 167–8.

Hughes JM, Blumenthal JR et al., 1981, Clinical features of types A and B food-borne botulism, *Ann Intern Med*, **95**: 442–5.

Hunter BF, Rosen MN, 1966, Detection of *Clostridium botulinum* type C cells and toxin by the fluorescent antibody technique, *Avian Dis*, **11**: 345–53.

Hunter SE, Clarke IN et al., 1992, Cloning and nucleotide sequencing of the *Clostridium perfringens* epsilon-toxin gene and its expression in *Escherichia coli*, *Infect Immun*, **60**: 102–10.

Hunter SEC, Brown JE et al., 1993, Molecular genetic analysis of beta-toxin of *Clostridium perfringens* reveals sequence homology with alpha-toxin, gamma-toxin, and leukocidin of *Staphylococcus aureus*, *Infect Immun*, **61**: 3958–65.

Hutson RA, Collins MD et al., 1994, Nucleotide sequence of the gene coding for non-proteolytic *Clostridium botulinum* type B neurotoxin: comparison with other clostridial neurotoxins, *Curr Microbiol*, **28**: 101–10.

Inoue K, Iida H, 1971, Phage-conversion of toxigenicity in *Clostridium botulinum* types C and D, *Jpn J Med Sci Biol*, **24**: 53–6.

Izumi N, Niiro M, Kondo H, 1983, *Clostridium oedematiens* type A toxin: the correlation between the lethal and edematizing activities, *Jpn J Med Sci Biol*, **36**: 67–74.

Izumi N, Kondo H et al., 1983, Purification and characterization of alpha toxin of *Clostridium oedematiens* type A, *Jpn J Med Sci Biol*, **36**: 135–46.

Jansen BC, 1971, The toxic antigenic factors produced by *Clostridium botulinum* types C and D, *Onderstepoort J Vet Res*, **38**: 93–8.

Jensen WI, Price JI, 1987, The global importance of type C botulism in wild birds, *Avian Botulism: an International Perspective*, eds Eklund MW, Dowell VR Jr, Charles C Thomas, Springfield, IL, 33–54.

Johnson EA, 1997, Extrachromosomal virulence determinants in the clostridia, *Molecular Genetics and Pathogenesis of the Clostridia*, eds Rood J, Songer JG et al., Academic Press, London.

Johnson JL, 1973, Use of nucleic-acid homologies in the taxonomy of anaerobic bacteria, *Int J Syst Bacteriol*, **23**: 308–15.

Johnson JL, Francis BS, 1975, Taxonomy of the clostridia: ribosomal ribonucleic acid homologies among the species, *J Gen Microbiol*, **88**: 229–44.

Johnston J, Whitlock RH, 1987, Botulism, *Current Therapy in Equine Medicine*, 2nd edn, ed. Robinson NE, WB Saunders, Philadelphia, 367–70.

Jolivet-Reynaud C, Moreau H, Alouf JE, 1988, Purification of alpha toxin from *Clostridium perfringens*: phospholipase C, *Methods Enzymol*, **165**: 91–4.

Kameyama S, Akama K, 1971, Purification and some properties of kappa toxin of *Clostridium perfringens*, *Jpn J Med Sci Biol*, **24**: 9–23.

Kameyama S, Sato H, Muratoa R, 1972, The role of alpha-toxin of *Clostridium perfringens* in experimental gas gangrene in guinea pigs, *Jpn J Med Sci Biol*, **25**: 200.

Kaneuchi C, Miyazato T et al., 1979, Taxonomic study of helically coiled spore-forming anaerobes isolated from the intestines of humans and other animals: *Clostridium cocleatum* sp. nov. and *Clostridium spiroforme* sp. nov, *Int J Syst Bacteriol*, **29**: 1–12.

Kato H, Kato N et al., 1994, Application of typing of pulsed-field gel electrophoresis to the study of *Clostridium difficile* in a neonatal intensive care unit, *J Clin Microbiol*, **32**: 2067–70.

Kautter DA, Harmon SM et al., 1966, Antagonistic effect on *Clostridium botulinum* type E by organisms resembling it, *Appl Microbiol*, **14**: 616–22.

Kihm DJ, Hutton MT et al., 1988, Zinc stimulates sporulation in *Clostridium botulinum* 113B, *Curr Microbiol*, **17**: 193–8.

Killgore GE, Kato H, 1994, Use of arbitrary primer PCR to type *Clostridium difficile* and comparison of results with those by immunoblot typing, *J Clin Microbiol*, **32**: 1591–3.

Kimura K, Fujii N et al., 1990, The complete nucleotide sequence of the gene coding for botulinum type C1 toxin in the C-ST phage genome, *Biochem Biophys Res Commun*, **171**: 1304–11.

Klein E, 1904, Ein neuer tierpathogener Mikrobe – *Bacillus carnis, Zentralbl Bakteriol I, Abt Orig A,* **35:** 459–61.

Klotz AW, 1965, Application of FA techniques to detection of *Clostridium perfringens, Public Health Rep,* **80:** 305–11.

Knoop FC, Owens M, Crocker IC, 1993, *Clostridium difficile:* clinical disease and diagnosis, *Clin Microbiol Rev,* **6:** 251–65.

Kobel T, Marti MC, 1985, Decouverte du bacille de tetanos (1884), *Rev Med Suisse Romande,* **105:** 547–56.

Kokai-Kun JF, Songer JG et al., 1994, Comparison of Western immunoblots and gene detection assays for identification of potentially enterotoxigenic isolates of *Clostridium perfringens, J Clin Microbiol,* **32:** 2533–9.

Kolander SA, Cosgrove EM, Molavi A, 1989, Clostridial endocarditis: Report of a case caused by *Clostridium bifermentans* and review of the literature, *Arch Intern Med,* **149:** 455–6.

Koopman JP, Kennis HM, 1977, Differentiation of bacteria isolated from mouse ceca, *Z Versuchstierk,* **19:** 174–81.

Koransky JR, Allen SD, Dowell VRJ, 1978, Use of ethanol for selective isolation of sporeforming microorganisms, *Appl Environ Microbiol,* **35:** 762–5.

Laird WJ, Aaronson W et al., 1980, Plasmid-associated toxigenicity in *Clostridium tetani, J Infect Dis,* **142:** 623.

Larson HE, Parry JV et al., 1977, Undescribed toxin in pseudomembranous colitis, *Br Med J,* **1:** 1246–8.

Larson HE, Honour P et al., 1978, *Clostridium difficile* and the etiology of pseudomembranous colitis, *Lancet,* **i:** 1063–6.

Libby JM, Wilkins TD, 1982, Production of antitoxins to two toxins of *Clostridium difficile* and immunological comparison of the toxins by cross-neutralization studies, *Infect Immun,* **35:** 374–6.

Lima AA, Lyerly DM et al., 1988, Effects of *Clostridium difficile* toxins A and B in rabbit small and large intestine *in vivo* and on cultured cells *in vitro, Infect Immun,* **56:** 582–8.

Ljungdahl LG, Hugenholtz J, Wiegel J, 1989, Acetogenic and acid-producing clostridia, *Clostridia,* eds Minton NP, Clarke DJ, Plenum Press, New York, 145–91.

Lombard GL, Dowell VRJ, 1982, *Gas-Liquid Chromatography Analysis of the Acid Products of Bacteria,* US Department of Health and Human Services, Public Health Service, Centers for Disease Control, Center for Infectious Diseases, Atlanta.

Lombard GL, Dowell VRJ, 1983, Comparison of three reagents for detecting indole production by anaerobic bacteria in microtest systems, *J Clin Microbiol,* **18:** 609–13.

Lucain C, Piffaretti JC, 1977, Characterization of the haemolysins of different serotypes of *Clostridium tetani, FEMS Microbiol Lett,* **1:** 231–4.

Luecke FK, Hechelmann H, Leistner L, 1981, The relevance to meat products of psycrotrophic strains of *Clostridium botulinum, Psychrotrophic Microorganisms in Spoilage and Pathogenicity,* eds Roberts TA, Hobbs G et al., Academic Press, London, 491–7.

Lyerly DM, Krivan HC, Wilkins TD, 1988, *Clostridium difficile:* its disease and toxins, *Clin Microbiol Rev,* **1:** 1–18.

MacDonald KL, Rutherford GW et al., 1985, Botulism and botulism-like illness in chronic drug abusers, *Ann Intern Med,* **102:** 616–18.

MacFarlane MG, 1948, The biochemistry of bacterial toxins. 3. The identification and immunological relations of lecithinases present in *Clostridium oedematiens* and *Clostridium sordellii* toxins, *Biochem J,* **42:** 590–5.

MacFarlane MG, 1950, The biochemistry of bacterial toxins. 4. The lecithinase activity of *Clostridium haemolyticum* toxin, *Biochem J,* **47:** 267–70.

MacFarlane MG, 1955, *Clostridium oedematiens* eta-antigen, an enzyme decomposing tropomyosin, *Biochem J,* **61:** 308–15.

MacFarlane MG, Knight BCJG, 1941, The biochemistry of bacterial toxins. 1. The lecithinase activity of *Cl. welchii* toxins, *Biochem J,* **34:** 884–902.

Macheak ME, Claus KD, Malloy SE, 1970, Potency testing of *Clostridium chauvoei*-containing bacterins: relationship of aggluti-nation titers and potency tests in cattle, *Am J Vet Res,* **33:** 1053–8.

MacLennan JD, 1962, The histotoxic clostridial infections of man, *Bacteriol Rev,* **26:** 177–276.

Mahony DE, 1979, Bacteriocin, bacteriophage and other epidemiological typing methods for the genus *Clostridium, Methods in Microbiology,* eds Bergan T, Norris JR, Academic Press, New York, 1–30.

Mahony DE, Bell PD, Easterbrook KB, 1985, Two bacteriophages of *Clostridium difficile, J Clin Microbiol,* **21:** 251–4.

Mahony DE, Butler ME, 1971, Bacteriocins of *Clostridium perfringens.* 1. Isolation and preliminary studies, *Can J Microbiol,* **17:** 1–6.

Mahony DE, Kalz GG, 1968, A temperate bacteriophage of *Clostridium perfringens, Can J Microbiol,* **14:** 1085–93.

Mahony DE, Swantee CA, 1978, Bacteriocin typing of *Clostridium perfringens, J Clin Microbiol,* **7:** 307–9.

Mahony DE, Stringer MF et al., 1987, Plasmid analysis as a means of strain differentiation in *Clostridium perfringens, J Clin Microbiol,* **25:** 1333–5.

Mandia JW, 1950, The migration of cultures of *Clostridium perfringens* in semisolid medium, *J Bacteriol,* **60:** 275–82.

Mandia JW, 1951, The serological indentification of cultures of *Clostridium histolyticum* as group III of the proteolytic clostridia, *J Infect Dis,* **30:** 445–504.

Mandia JW, 1955, The position of *Clostridium tetani* within the serological schema for the proteolytic clostridia, *J Infect Dis,* **97:** 66–72.

Martinez RD, Wilkins TD, 1988, Purification and characterization of *Clostridium sordellii* hemorrhagic toxin and cross-reactivity with *Clostridium difficile* toxin A (enterotoxin), *Infect Immun,* **56:** 1215–21.

McClane BA, 1992, *Clostridium perfringens* enterotoxin: structure, action and detection, *J Food Safety,* **12:** 237–52.

McClane BA, Hanna PC, Wnek AP, 1988, *Clostridium perfringens* enterotoxin, *Microbial Pathogenesis,* **4:** 317–23.

McClung LS, 1945, Human food poisoning due to growth of *Clostridium perfringens* (*C. welchii*) in freshly cooked chicken: Preliminary note, *J Bacteriol,* **50:** 229–31.

McClung LS, Toabe R, 1947, The egg yolk plate reaction for the presumptive diagnosis of *Clostridium sporogenes* and certain species of the gangrene and botulism groups, *J Bacteriol,* **53:** 139–47.

McCroskey LM, Hatheway CL, 1988, Laboratory findings in four cases of adult botulism suggest colonization of the intestinal tract, *J Clin Microbiol,* **26:** 1052–4.

McCroskey LM, Hatheway CL et al., 1991, Type F botulism due to neurotoxigenic *Clostridium baratii* from an unknown source in an adult, *J Clin Microbiol,* **29:** 2618–20.

McDonel JL, 1980a, *Clostridium perfringens* toxins (type A, B, C, D, E), *Pharmacol Ther,* **10:** 617–55.

McDonel JL, 1980b, Mechanism of action of *Clostridium perfringens* enterotoxin, *Food Technol,* **34:** 91–5.

McGregor JA, Soper DE et al., 1989, Maternal deaths associated with *Clostridium sordellii* infection, *Am J Obstet Gynecol,* **161:** 987–95.

Metchnikoff E, 1908, Études sur la flore intestinale, *Ann Inst Pasteur,* **22:** 929–55.

Midura TF, Arnon SS, 1976, Infant botulism: Identification of *Clostridium botulinum* and its toxin in faeces, *Lancet,* **ii:** 934–6.

Midura TF, Nygaard GS et al., 1972, *Clostridium botulinum* type F: isolation from venison jerky, *Appl Microbiol,* **24:** 165–7.

Mills DC, Midura TF, Arnon SS, 1985, Improved selective medium for the isolation of lipase-positive *Clostridium botulinum* from feces of human infants, *J Clin Microbiol,* **21:** 947–50.

Mitsui N, Mitsui K, Hase J, 1980, Purification and some properties of tetanolysin, *Microbiol Immunol,* **24:** 575–84.

Montecucco C, Schiavo G, 1994, Mechanism of action of tetanus and botulinum neurotoxins, *Mol Microbiol,* **13:** 1–8.

Mookhtiar KA, Steinbrink DR, Van Wart HE, 1985, Mode of hydrolysis of collagen-like peptides by class I and class II *Clos-*

tridium histolyticum collagenases: evidence for both endopeptidase and tripeptidylcarboxpeptidase activities, *Biochemistry*, **24**: 6527–33.

Moore LVH, Cato EP, Moore WEC, 1987, *Anaerobe Manual Update*, Supplement to the VPI Anaerobe Laboratory Manual, 4th edn, Department of Anaerobic Microbiology, Virginia Polytechnic Institute and State University, Blacksburg, VA.

Moore WEC, Moore LVH, 1992, *Index of the Bacterial and Yeast Nomenclatural Changes*, American Society for Microbiology, Washington, DC, 19–21.

Morris JG, 1975, The physiology of obligate anaerobiosis, *Adv Microbiol Physiol*, **12**: 169–245.

Morris JG, 1976, Fifth Stenhouse-Williams Memorial Lecture: oxygen and the obligate anaerobe, *J Appl Bacteriol*, **40**: 229–44.

Morris JG, 1981, Current trends in therapy of botulism in the United States, *Biomedical Aspects of Botulism*, ed Lewis GE Jr, Academic Press, New York, 317–26.

Moss CW, Hatheway CL et al., 1980, Production of phenylacetic and hydroxyphenylacetic acids by *Clostridium botulinum* type G, *J Clin Microbiol*, **11**: 743–5.

Moussa RS, 1959, Antigenic formulae of *Cl. septicum* and *Cl. chauvoei*, *J Pathol Bacteriol*, **77**: 341–50.

Mueller HE, 1976, Neuraminidase als Pathogenitaetsfaktor bei mikrobiellen Infektionen, *Zentralbl Bakteriol Hyg I Abt Orig A*, **235**: 106–10.

Muldrow LL, Ibeanu GC et al., 1987, Molecular cloning of *Clostridium difficile* toxin A gene fragment in lambda gt11, *FEBS Lett*, **213**: 249–53.

Murrell TCG, Egerton JR et al., 1966, The ecology and epidemiology of the pig-bel syndrome in New Guinea, *J Hyg*, **64**: 375–96.

Nachman S, Kaul A et al., 1989, Liver abcess caused by *Clostridium bifermentans* following blunt abdominal trauma, *J Clin Microbiol*, **27**: 1137–8.

Nagahama M, Kobayashi K et al., 1991, Enzyme-linked immunosorbant assay for rapid detection of toxins from *Clostridium perfringens*, *FEMS Microbiol Lett*, **84**: 41–4.

Nagler FPO, 1939, Observations on a reaction between the lethal toxin of *Cl. welchii* (type A) and human serum, *Br J Exp Pathol*, **20**: 473–85.

Nakamura S, Okado I et al., 1977, *Clostridium sporogenes* isolates and their relationship to *C. botulinum* based on deoxyribonucleic acid reassociation, *J Gen Microbiol*, **100**: 395–401.

Nakamura S, Okado I et al., 1979, Taxonomy of *Clostridium tetani* and related species, *J Gen Microbiol*, **113**: 29–35.

Nakamura S, Kimura I et al., 1983a, Taxonomic relationships among *Clostridium novyi* types A and B, *Clostridium haemolyticum* and *Clostridium botulinum* type C, *J Gen Microbiol*, **129**: 1473–9.

Nakamura S, Tanabe N et al., 1983b, Cytotoxin production by *Clostridium sordellii* strains, *Microbiol Immunol*, **27**: 495–502.

Nees S, Veh RW, Schauer R, 1975, Purification and characterization of neuraminadase from *Clostridium perfringens*, *Hoppe Seyler's Z Physiol Chem*, **356**: 1027–42.

Niemann H, 1992, Clostridial neurotoxins – proposal of a common nomenclature, *Toxicon*, **30**: 223–5.

Nishida S, Imaizumi M, 1966, Toxigenicity of *Clostridium histolyticum*, *J Bacteriol*, **91**: 477–83.

Novy FG, 1894, Ein neuer anaerober Bacillus des malignen Oedems, *Z Hyg Infektionskrankh*, **17**: 209–32.

Oakley CL, 1955, Bacterial toxins and classification, *J Gen Microbiol*, **12**: 344–7.

Oakley CL, Warrack GH, 1950, The alpha, beta, and gamma antigens of *Clostridium histolyticum* (Weinberg and Sequin, 1916), *J Gen Microbiol*, **4**: 365–73.

Oakley CL, Warrack GH, 1959, The soluble antigens of *Clostridium oedematiens* type D (*Cl. haemolyticum*), *J Pathol Bacteriol*, **78**: 543–51.

Oakley CL, Warrack GH, Clarke PH, 1947, The toxins of *Clostridium oedematiens* (*Cl. novyi*), *J Gen Microbiol*, **1**: 91–107.

Ogata S, Hongo M, 1979, Bacteriophages of the genus *Clostridium*, *Adv Appl Microbiol*, **40**: 241–73.

Oguma K, Yokota K et al., 1990, Infant botulism due to *Clostridium botulinum* type C toxin, *Lancet*, **336**: 1449–50.

Ohishi I, Iwasaki M, Sakaguchi G, 1980, Purification and characterization of two components of botulinum C2 toxin, *Infect Immun*, **30**: 668–73.

Okabe A, Shimizu T, Hayashi H, 1989, Cloning and sequencing of phospholipase C gene of *Clostridium perfringens*, *Biochem Biophys Res Commun*, **150**: 33–9.

Ottinger ME, Lin S, 1988, *Clostridium difficile* toxin B induces reorganization of actin, vinculin, and talin in cultured cells, *Exp Cell Res*, **174**: 215–29.

Paik G, 1980, Reagents, stains, and miscellaneous test procedures, *Manual of Clinical Microbiology*, 3rd edn, eds Lennette EH, Balows A et al., American Society for Microbiology, Washington, DC, 1000–24.

Paquette G, Fredette V, 1977, Properties of four temperate bacteriophages active on *Clostridium perfringens* type A, *Rev Can Bacteriol*, **36**: 205–15.

Pasteur L, 1861a, Animalcules infusores vivant sans gaz oxygene libre et determinant des fermentations, *CR Acad Sci Paris*, **52**: 344–7.

Pasteur L, 1861b, Experiences et vues nouvelles sur la nature des fermentations, *CR Acad Sci Paris*, **52**: 1260–4.

Pasteur L, 1863a, Nouvel exemple de fermentation déterminée par des animalcules infusoires pouvant vivre sans gaz oxygene libre, et en dehors de tout contact avec l'air de l'atmosphere, *CR Acad Sci Paris*, **56**: 416–21.

Pasteur L, 1863b, Recherches sur la putrefaction, *CR Acad Sci Paris*, **56**: 1189–94.

Pasteur L, Joubert J, 1877, Charbon et septicemie, *Bull Acad Med*, **6**: 781–98.

Patton NM, Holmes HT et al., 1978, Enterotoxemia in rabbits, *Lab Anim Sci*, **28**: 536–40.

Perelle S, Gibert M et al., 1993, Characterization of *Clostridium perfringens* iota-toxin genes and expression in *Escherichia coli*, *Infect Immun*, **61**: 5147–56.

Phillips AW, Batty I, Wood RD, 1970, A partial characterization of the alpha toxin of *Clostridium oedematiens* type B, *Eur J Biochem*, **14**: 367–71.

Pickett J, Berg B et al., 1976, Syndrome of botulism in infancy: clinical and electrophysiologic study, *N Engl J Med*, **295**: 770–2.

Popoff MR, 1987, Purification and characterization of *Clostridium sordellii* lethal toxin and cross-reactivity with *Clostridium difficile* cytotoxin, *Infect Immun*, **55**: 35–43.

Popoff MR, Boquet P, 1988, *Clostridium spiroforme* toxin is a binary toxin which ADP-ribosylates cellular actin, *Biochem Biophys Res Commun*, **152**: 1361–8.

Popoff MR, Rubin EJ et al., 1988, Actin-specific ADP-ribosyltransferase produced by a *Clostridium difficile* strain, *Infect Immun*, **56**: 2299–306.

Pothoulakis C, Barone LM et al., 1986a, Purification and properties of *Clostridium difficile* cytotoxin B, *J Biol Chem*, **261**: 1316–21.

Pothoulakis C, Sullivan DA et al., 1986b, *Clostridium difficile* toxins A and B stimulate intracellular calcium release in human neutrophils, *Clin Res*, **34**: 530A.

Poulet S, Hauser D et al., 1992, Sequences of the botulinal neurotoxin E derived from *Clostridium botulinum* type E (strain Beluga) and *Clostridium butyricum* (strains ATCC 43181 and ATCC 43755), *Biochem Biophys Res Commun*, **183**: 107–13.

Prescott LM, Altenbern RA, 1967, Detection of bacteriophages from two strains of *Clostridium tetani*, *J Virol*, **1**: 1085–6.

Prevot AR, 1957, *Manual de Classification et de Determination des Bacteries Anaerobies*, 3rd edn, Masson, Paris.

Price SB, Phelps CJ et al., 1987, Cloning of the carbohydrate-binding portion of the toxin A gene of *Clostridium difficile*, *Curr Microbiol*, **16**: 55–60.

Pron B, Merckx J et al., 1995, Chronic septic arthritis and osteomyelitis in a prosthetic knee joint due to *Clostridium difficile*, *Eur J Clin Microbiol Infect Dis*, **14:** 599–601.

Rechtman DJ, Nadler JP, 1991, Abdominal abcess due to *Cardiobacterium hominis* and *Clostridium bifermentans*, *Rev Infect Dis*, **13:** 418–19.

Reddish GF, Rettger LF, 1922, *J Bacteriol*, **9:** 13.

Rehany U, Dorenboim Y et al., 1994, *Clostridium bifermentans* panophthalmitis after penetrating eye injury, *Ophthalmology*, **101:** 839–42.

Richardson M, Granum PE, 1983, Sequence of the aminoterminal part of enterotoxin from *Clostridium perfringens* type A: identification of points of trypsin activation, *Infect Immun*, **40:** 943–9.

Richardson M, Granum PE, 1985, The amino acid sequence of the enterotoxin from *Clostridium perfringens* type A, *FEBS Lett*, **182:** 479–84.

Rifkin GD, Fekety FR, Silva J Jr, 1977, Antibiotic-induced colitis: implication of a toxin neutralized by *Clostridium sordellii* antitoxin, *Lancet*, **ii:** 1103–6.

Roggentin P, Rothe B et al., 1988, Cloning and sequencing of a *Clostridium perfringens* sialidase gene, *FEBS Lett*, **238:** 31–4.

Rood JI, Cole ST, 1991, Molecular genetics and pathogenesis of *Clostridium perfringens*, *Microbiol Rev*, **55:** 621–48.

Rood JI, Wilkinson RG, 1976, Relationship between hemagglutinin and sialidase from *Clostridium perfringens* CN 3870: chromatographic characterization of the biologically active proteins, *J Bacteriol*, **126:** 831–44.

Rood J, Songer G et al., 1997, *Molecular Genetics and Pathogenesis of the Clostridia*, Academic Press, London.

Rothman SW, Brown JE et al., 1984, Differential cytotoxic effects of toxins A and B isolated from *Clostridium difficile*, *Infect Immun*, **46:** 324–31.

Rothman SW, Gentry MK et al., 1988, Immunochemical and structural similarities in toxin A and toxin B of *Clostridium difficile* shown by binding to monoclonal antibodies, *Toxicon*, **26:** 583–97.

Rutter JM, Collee JG, 1969, Studies on the soluble antigens of *Clostridium oedematiens* (*Cl. novyi*), *J Med Microbiol*, **2:** 395–417.

Sacks LE, Thompson PA, 1978, Clear, defined medium for the sporulation of *Clostridium perfringens*, *Appl Environ Microbiol*, **35:** 405–10.

Sakaguchi G, 1983, *Clostridium botulinum* toxins, *Pharmacol Ther*, **19:** 165–94.

Sakaguchi G, Uemura T, Riemann H, 1973, Simplified method for purification of *Clostridium perfringens* type A enterotoxin, *Appl Microbiol*, **26:** 762–7.

Sakurai J, Fujii Y, 1987, Purification and characterization of *Clostridium perfringens* beta toxin, *Toxicon*, **25:** 1301–10.

Sakurai J, Fujii Y et al., 1981, Pharmacological effect of beta toxin of *Clostridium perfringens* type C on rats, *Microbiol Immunol*, **25:** 423–32.

Scanlan DR, Smith MA et al., 1994, *Clostridium bifermentans* bacteremia with metastatic osteomyelitis, *J Clin Microbiol*, **32:** 2867–8.

Schallehn G, Eklund MW, 1980, Conversion of *Clostridium novyi* type D (*Clostridium haemolyticum*) to alpha toxin production by phages of *Clostridium novyi* type A, *FEMS Microbiol Lett*, **7:** 83–6.

Schantz EJ, Johnson EA, 1992, Properties and use of botulinum toxin and other microbial neurotoxins in medicine, *Microbiol Rev*, **56:** 80–99.

Schering B, Baermann M et al., 1988, ADP-ribosylation of skeletal muscle and non-muscle actin by *Clostridium perfringens* iota toxin, *Eur J Biochem*, **171:** 225–9.

Scott HG, Mahony DE, 1982, Further development of a bacteriocin typing system for *Clostridium perfringens*, *J Appl Bacteriol*, **53:** 363–9.

Sebald M, Popovitch M, 1967, Etude des bacteriophages de *Clostridium histolyticum* souche P, *Ann Inst Pasteur*, **113:** 781–9.

Seddon HR, 1922, Bulbar paralysis in cattle due to the action of a toxicogenic bacillus with a discussion of the relationship of the condition to forage poisoning (botulism), *J Comp Pathol Ther*, **35:** 147–90.

Setlow P, Johnson EA, 1997, Spores and their significance, *Fundamentals of Food Microbiology*, eds Doyle MP, Beuchat LR, Montville T, American Society for Microbiology, Washington, DC.

Simpson LL, Stiles BG et al., 1987, Molecular basis for the pathological actions of *Clostridium perfringens* iota toxin, *Infect Immun*, **55:** 118–22.

Skerman VBD, McGowan V, Sneath PHA, 1989, *Approved List of Bacterial Names*, American Society for Microbiology, Washington, DC, 46–54.

Smith LDS, 1975, Inhibition of *Clostridium botulinum* by strains of *Clostridium perfringens* isolated from soil, *Appl Microbiol*, **30:** 319–23.

Smith LDS, Sugiyama H, 1988, *Botulism: the Organism, its Toxins, the Disease*, 2nd edn, Charles C. Thomas, Springfield, IL.

Smith LDS, Williams BL, 1984, *The Pathogenic Anaerobic Bacteria*, 3rd edn, Charles C. Thomas, Springfield, IL.

Snyder ML, Hall IC, 1935, *Bacillus capitovalis*, a new species of obligate anaerobe encountered in post-mortem materials, in a wound infection, and in the faeces of infants, *Zentralbl Bakteriol Parasitenkde, Infektionskr Hyg I Abt. Orig.*, **135:** 290–7.

Solomon HM, Rhodehamel EJ, Kautter DA, 1995, *Clostridium botulinum*, *FDA Bacteriological Analytical Manual*, 8th edn, US Food and Drug Administration, Washington, DC, 17.01–10.

Songer JG, 1996, Clostridial enteric diseases of domestic animals, *Clin Microbiol Rev*, **9:** 216–34.

Songer JG, Meer RR, 1996, Genotyping of *Clostridium perfringens* by polymerase chain reaction is a useful adjunct to diagnosis of clostridial enteric disease in animals, *Anaerobe*, **2:** 197–203.

Sonnabend O, Sonnabend W et al., 1981, Isolation of *Clostridium botulinum* type G and identification of type G botulinal toxin in humans: report of five sudden unexpected deaths, *J Infect Dis*, **143:** 22–7.

Sonnabend OA, Sonnabend WF et al., 1985, Continuous microbiological study of 70 sudden and unexpected infant deaths: toxigenic intestinal *Clostridium botulinum* infection in 9 cases of sudden infant death syndrome, *Lancet*, **ii:** 237–41.

Sonnabend WF, Sonnabend UP, Krech T, 1987, Isolation of *Clostridium botulinum* type G from Swiss soil specimens using sequential steps in an identification scheme, *Appl Environ Microbiol*, **53:** 1880–4.

Soper DD, 1986, Clostridial myonecrosis arising from an episiotomy, *Obstet Gynecol*, **68:** 265–85.

Sordelli A, 1922, Un germen anaerobico de las gangrenas gasosas, *Rev Assoc Med Argent*, **35:** 217–21.

Stark RL, Duncan CL, 1972, Purification and biochemical properties of *Clostridium perfringens* type A enterotoxin, *Infect Immun*, **6:** 662–73.

Steinberg JP, Beckerdite ME, Westenfelder GO, 1987, Plasmid profiles of *Clostridium difficile* isolates from patients with antibiotic-associated colitis in two community hospitals, *J Infect Dis*, **156:** 1036–8.

Sterne M, Warrack GH, 1964, The types of *Clostridium perfringens*, *J Pathol Bacteriol*, **88:** 279–83.

Stevens DL, Troyer BE et al., 1988, Lethal effects and cardiovascular effects of purified alpha and theta thoxins from *Clostridium perfringens*, *J Infect Dis*, **157:** 272–9.

Stiles BG, Wilkins TD, 1986a, *Clostridium perfringens* iota toxin: synergism between two proteins, *Toxicon*, **24:** 767–73.

Stiles BG, Wilkins TD, 1986b, Purification and characterization of *Clostridium perfringens* iota toxin: dependence on two non-linked proteins for biological activity, *Infect Immun*, **54:** 683–8.

Stringer MF, Turnbull PCB, Gilbert RJ, 1980, Application of serological typing to the investigation of outbreaks of *Clostridium perfringens* food poisoning, 1970–1978, *J Hyg Camb*, **84:** 443–56.

Suen JC, Hatheway CL et al., 1988a, *Clostridium argentinense*, sp. nov: a genetically homogenous group composed of all strains of *Clostridium botulinum* toxin type G and some nontoxigenic strains previously identified as *Clostridium subterminale* or *Clostridium hastiforme*, *Int J Syst Bacteriol*, **38:** 375–81.

Suen JC, Hatheway CL et al., 1988b, Genetic confirmation of identities of neurotoxigenic *Clostridium baratii* and *Clostridium butyricum* implicated as agents of infant botulism, *J Clin Microbiol*, **26:** 2191–2.

Sullivan NM, Pellett S, Wilkins TD, 1982, Purification and characterization of toxins A and B of *Clostridium difficile*, *Infect Immun*, **35:** 1032–40.

Swenson JM, Thornsberry C et al., 1980, Susceptibility of *Clostridium botulinum* to thirteen antimicrobial agents, *Antimicrob Agents Chemother*, **18:** 13–9.

Swerczek TW, 1980a, Experimentally induced toxicoinfectious botulism in horses and foals, *Am J Vet Res*, **41:** 348–50.

Swerczek TW, 1980b, Toxicoinfectious botulism in foals and adult horses, *J Am Vet Med Assoc*, **176:** 217.

Szabo EA, Pemberton JM et al., 1994, Polymerase chain reaction for detection of *Clostridium botulinum* types A, B, and E in food, soil and infant feces, *J Appl Bacteriol*, **76:** 539–45.

Taguchi R, Ikezawa H, 1975, Phospholipase C from *Clostridium novyi* type A, *Biochim Biophys Acta*, **409:** 75–85.

Takahashi S, Seifter S, Binder M, 1970, Elastolytic activities of *Clostridium histolyticum*, *Biochem Biophys Res Commun*, **39:** 1058–64.

Talon D, Bailly P et al., 1995, Use of pulsed-field gel electrophoresis for investigation of an outbreak of *Clostridium difficile* infection among geriatric patients, *Eur J Microbiol Infect Dis*, **14:** 987–93.

Tang YJ, Houston ST et al., 1995, Comparison of arbitrarily primed PCR with restriction endonuclease and immunoblot analysis for typing of *Clostridium difficile* isolates, *J Clin Microbiol*, **33:** 3169–73.

Taylor NS, Thorne GM, Bartlett JG, 1981, Comparison of two toxins produced by *Clostridium difficile*, *Infect Immun*, **34:** 1036–43.

Ten Broeck C, Bauer JH, 1922, The tetanus bacillus as an intestinal saprophyte in man, *J Exp Med*, **36:** 261.

Thompson DE, Brehm JK et al., 1990, The complete amino acid sequence of the *Clostridium botulinum* type A neurotoxin, deduced by nucleotide sequence analysis of the encoding gene, *Eur J Biochem*, **189:** 73–81.

Thompson DE, Hutson RA et al., 1993, Nucleotide sequence of the gene coding for *Clostridium barati* type F neurotoxin: comparison with other clostridial neurotoxins, *FEMS Microbiol Lett*, **108:** 175–82.

Tissier H, Martelly X, 1902, Recherches sur la putréfaction de la viande de boucherie, *Ann Inst Pasteur*, **16:** 865–903.

Titball RW, Hunter SEC et al., 1989, Molecular cloning and nucleotide sequence of the alpha-toxin (phospholipase C) of *Clostridium perfringens*, *Infect Immun*, **57:** 367–76.

Tixier G, Alouf JE, 1976, Essai de purification et proprieties de la toxine delta de *Clostridium perfringens* type C, *Ann Microbiol (Inst Pasteur)*, **127B:** 509–24.

Trethon A, Budai J et al., 1995, Csecsemokori botulizmus, *Orvosi Hetilap*, **28:** 1497–9.

Triadafilopoulos G, Pothoulakis C et al., 1987, Differential effects of *Clostridium difficile* toxins A and B on rabbit ileum, *Gastroenterology*, **93:** 273–9.

Tso JY, Seibel C, 1989, Cloning and expression of the phospholipase C gene from *Clostridium perfringens* and *Clostridium bifermentans*, *Infect Immun*, **57:** 468–76.

Tulloch WJ, 1919–20, Report of bacteriological investigations of tetanus on behalf of the war office, *J Hyg*, **18:** 103.

Turner TB, Eales CE, 1941, Motile daughter cells in the *Clostridium oedematiens* group and some other clostridia (*Cl. botulinum* C, *Cl. tetani*, *Cl. septicum*), *Austr J Exp Biol Med Sci*, **19:** 167–78.

Tweten RK, 1988a, Cloning and expression in *Escherichia coli* of the perfringolysin-O (theta toxin) from *Clostridium perfringens* and characterization of the gene product, *Infect Immun*, **56:** 3228–34.

Tweten RK, 1988b, Nucleotide sequence of the gene for perfringolysin-O (theta toxin) from *Clostridium perfringens*: significant homology with the genes for streptolysin-O and pneumolysin, *Infect Immun*, **56:** 3235–40.

Vandekerckhove J, Schering B et al., 1987, *Clostridium perfringens* iota toxin ADP-ribosylates skeletal muscle actin in arg-177, *FEBS Lett*, **225:** 48–52.

Van Ermengem E, 1897, Ueber einen neuen anaeroben Bacillus und seine Beziehungen zum Botulismus, *Z Hyg Infektionskh*, **26:** 1–56.

van Heyningen WE, 1950, *Bacterial Toxins*, Blackwell Scientific, Oxford.

Van Wart HE, Steinbrink DR, 1985, Complementary substrate specificities of Class I and Class II collagenases from *Clostridium histolyticum*, *Biochemistry*, **24:** 6520–6.

Vargaftig BB, Lefort J, Giroux EL, 1976, Hemorrhagic and inflammatory properties of collagenase from *C. histolyticum*, *Agents and Actions*, **6:** 627–35.

Veronesi R, Bizzini B et al., 1983, Naturally acquired antibodies to tetanus toxin in humans and animals from the Galapagos Islands, *J Infect Dis*, **147:** 308–11.

Wainwright RB, Heyward WL et al., 1988, Foodborne botulism in Alaska, 1947–1985: epidemiology and clinical findings, *J Infect Dis*, **157:** 1158–62.

Watson GN, Stringer MF et al., 1982, The potential of bacteriocin typing in the study of *Clostridium perfringens* food poisoning, *J Clin Pathol*, **35:** 1361–5.

Weber JT, Goodpasture HC et al., 1993a, Wound botulism in a patient with a tooth abscess: case report and review, *Clin Infect Dis*, **16:** 635–9.

Weber JT, Hibbs RG et al., 1993b, A massive outbreak of type E botulism associated with traditional salted fish in Cairo, Egypt, *J Infect Dis*, **167:** 451–4.

Weinberg M, Seguin P, 1915, Flore microbienne de la gangrène gazeuse: le *B. fallax*, *CR Soc Biol Paris*, **78:** 686–9.

Weinberg M, Seguin P, 1916, Contribution a l'etiologie de la gangrene gazeuse, *CR Acad Sci Paris*, **163:** 449–51.

Welch WH, Nuttall GHF, 1892, A gas producing bacillus (*Bacillus aerogenes capsulatus*, Nov. Spec.) capable of rapid development in the blood vessels after death, *Bull Johns Hopkins Hosp*, **3:** 81–91.

Wells CL, Balish E, 1983, *Clostridium tetani* growth and toxin production in the intestines of germfree rats, *Infect Immun*, **41:** 826–8.

Whelan SM, Elmore MJ et al., 1992a, The complete amino acid sequence of *Clostridium botulinum* type E neurotoxin, derived by nucleotide-sequence analysis of the encoding gene, *Eur J Biochem*, **204:** 657–67.

Whelan SM, Elmore MJ et al., 1992b, Molecular cloning of the *Clostridium botulinum* structural gene encoding the type B neurotoxin and determination of its entire sequence, *Appl Environ Microbiol*, **58:** 2345–54.

White A, Handler P et al., 1978, *Principles of Biochemistry*, 6th edn, McGraw-Hill, New York.

Wilcke BW Jr, Midura TF, Arnon SS, 1980, Quantitative evidence of intestinal colonization by *Clostridium botulinum* in four cases of infant botulism, *J Infect Dis*, **141:** 419–23.

Williams K, Willis AT, 1970, A method of performing surface viable counts with *Clostridium tetani*, *Microbiology*, **4:** 639–42.

Willis AT, 1969, *Clostridia of Wound Infection*, Butterworths, London.

Willis AT, 1977, *Anaerobic Bacteriology: Clinical and Laboratory Practice*, 3rd edn, Butterworths, London.

Willis AT, 1990, *Clostridium*: the sporebearing anaerobes, *Topley and Wilson's Principles of Bacteriology, Virology, and Immunology*, 8th edn, eds Parker MT, Collier LH, Arnold, London, 211–46.

Willis AT, Hobbs G, 1959, Some new media for the isolation and identification of clostridia, *J Pathol Bacteriol*, **77:** 511–21.

Wnek AP, McClane B, 1983, Identification of a 50,000 Mr Protein from rabbit brush border membranes that binds Clostrid-

ium perfringens enterotoxin, *Biochem Biophys Res Commun*, **112**: 1094–105.

Wolfhagen MJHM, Torensma R et al., 1994, Toxins A and B of *Clostridium difficile*, *FEMS Microbiol Rev*, **13**: 59–64.

Woods DR, Jones DT, 1986, Physiological responses of *Bacteroides* and *Clostridium* strains to environmental stress, *Adv Microbiol Physiol*, **28**: 1–64.

Wren BW, Clayton CL et al., 1987, Molecular cloning and expression of *Clostridium difficile* toxin A in *Escherichia coli* K12, *FEBS Lett*, **225**: 82–6.

Yamakawa K, Nakamura S, Nishida S, 1985, Separation of two cytotoxins of *Clostridium sordellii* strains, *Microbiol Immunol*, **29**: 553–7.

Yamakawa K, Tanabe N et al., 1983, Rabbit ileal loop responses to *Clostridium sordellii* strains, *Microbiol Immunol*, **27**: 807–89.

Yamakawa Y, Ito A, Sato H, 1977, Theta toxin of *Clostridium perfringens*. I. Purification and some properties, *Biochim Biophys Acta*, **494**: 301–13.

Yoshida E, Noda H, 1965, Isolation and characterization of collagenases I and II from *Clostridium histolyticum*, *Biochim Biophys Acta*, **105**: 562–74.

Zeissler J, 1930, Anaerobenzuchtung, *Handbuch der pathogenen Mikroorganismen*, 3rd edn, eds Kolle W, Kraus R, Ulenhuth P, Gustav Fischer, Berlin, 35–41.

Zeissler J, Rassfeld-Sternberg L, 1949, Enteritis necroticans due to *Clostridium welchii* type F, *Br Med J*, **1**: 267–9.

Zhou Y, Sugiyama H, Johnson EA, 1993, Transfer of neurotoxigenicity from *Clostridium butyricum* to a nontoxigenic *Clostridium botulinum* type E-like strain, *Appl Environ Microbiol*, **59**: 3825–31.

Zhou Y, Sugiyama H et al., 1995, The genes for the *Clostridium botulinum* type G toxin complex are on a plasmid, *Infect Immun*, **63**: 2087–91.

Chapter 33

GRAM-POSITIVE ANAEROBIC COCCI

D A Murdoch

1 INTRODUCTION

The first description of 'anaerobic streptococci' was by Veillon, who isolated an organism he named *Micrococcus foetidus* from a case of bartholinitis in 1893. Other workers soon cultured similar organisms from a variety of infections, notably puerperal fever, abscesses and gynaecological sepsis. However, the classification has never been satisfactory; previous schemes relied on inconsistent morphological characteristics and included capnophilic strains, which are now placed in other genera such as *Streptococcus* (Holdeman and Moore 1974, Cato 1983) and *Staphylococcus* (Kilpper-Baelz and Schleifer 1981). Watt and Jack (1977) defined anaerobic cocci as 'cocci that grow well under satisfactory conditions of anaerobiosis and do not grow on suitable solid media in 10% CO_2 in air even after incubation for 7 days at 37°C'. This definition is valuable for distinguishing obligate anaerobes from micro-aerophilic organisms and has been followed here.

Gram-positive anaerobic cocci (GPAC) are now recognized as a major part of the normal human flora of the mouth, gastrointestinal tract, female genital tract and skin. They are often isolated from clinical specimens but seldom in pure culture, making it difficult to determine their importance in human disease. They have received much less study than some other anaerobic groups and most aspects of their biology are poorly understood.

2 CLASSIFICATION

There have been several attempts to develop a satisfactory classification for GPAC. The genera *Peptococcus* and *Peptostreptococcus* were proposed by Kluyver and van Neil (1936), who separated them by morphological characteristics: peptococci were arranged in clumps and peptostreptococci in chains. This distinction is unreliable because it is greatly influenced by many variables, for instance composition of the medium. Prevot (1948) divided anaerobic cocci into 8 genera on the basis of their microscopic appearance; individual species were differentiated by tests such as indole production, liquefaction of gelatin and growth in litmus milk, which are now recognized to be of little validity. Hare and coworkers (1952) distinguished 10 groups of anaerobic cocci by fermentation and gas production from carbohydrates and inorganic acids; wisely, they did not add more names to a classification already confused by poorly defined species. Rogosa (1971) created the family Peptococcaceae for *Peptococcus*, *Peptostreptococcus* and *Ruminococcus*. Shortly afterwards, Holdeman and Moore (1974) proposed the genus *Coprococcus* and assigned it with *Sarcina* to the Peptococcaceae, which now contained 5 genera classified together purely on morphological grounds. Some authorities consider that the Peptococcaceae are too heterogeneous to be considered a valid taxon (Holdeman Moore, Johnson and Moore 1986, Holdeman Moore and Moore 1986) but others (Ezaki et al. 1994) still use it.

In recent years, a wide range of analytical techniques has been used, including DNA G + C content, DNA–DNA homology studies, comparison of 16S rRNA sequences, analysis of cell wall fatty acids and peptidoglycan structure, and whole cell composition by pyrolysis mass spectrometry (PMS). These studies have emphasized the heterogeneity of GPAC; major changes at the genus level are likely in the near future (Li, Hashimoto and Ezaki 1994).

2.1 Recent changes at the genus level

The results of DNA–DNA homology studies led Ezaki et al. (1983) to propose that most species in the genus *Peptococcus* should be placed in the genus *Peptostreptococcus*. However, similar studies by Huss, Festl and Schleifer (1984) suggested that these organisms were considerably more heterogeneous. The genus *Peptococcus* now includes only one species, *Peptococcus niger*, with a G + C content of 50–51 mol%, but there are 13 species in the genus *Peptostreptococcus*, with a G + C range of 27–37 mol% (Table 33.1). Recent comparisons of 16S rRNA sequences indicate that *Pc. niger*, the type species of the family Peptococcaceae, is not related to other members of the family (Ezaki et al. 1994); and *Peptostreptococcus anaerobius*, the type species of its genus, is more closely related to some members of the genus *Clostridium* than it is to other peptostreptococci (Lawson et al. 1993, Paster et al. 1993, Collins et al. 1994, Ezaki et al. 1994). It is now clear that the genus *Peptostreptococcus* is not a genetically valid taxon (Lawson et al. 1993, Ezaki et al. 1994); Li, Hashimoto and Ezaki (1994) have recommended that it be divided into at least 7 genera. A recent study of whole cell composition by PMS agreed with these conclusions (Murdoch and Magee 1995).

Ezaki et al. (1994) recently proposed moving *Peptostreptococcus productus*, a strongly saccharolytic species with a G + C content of 45 mol%, and *Streptococcus hansenii*, another obligately anaerobic coccus, to the genus *Ruminococcus*; they also suggested that members of the genera *Coprococcus* and *Ruminococcus* might be better classified in a single genus. Unfortunately, this study did not include the type species of the genus, *Ruminococcus flavefaciens*. Recent studies using 16S rRNA sequence comparisons (Collins et al. 1994, Rainey and Janssen 1995) confirm that the genus *Ruminococcus* contains at least 2 genetic clusters; it is likely that *Ruminococcus productus* will be placed in a new genus. *Streptococcus parvulus*, an obligately anaerobic coccus previously in the genus *Peptostreptococcus* (Cato 1983), has now been placed in a new genus, *Atopobium*, with species formerly in the genus *Lactobacillus* (Collins and Wallbanks 1992). *Peptostreptococcus heliotrinreducens* is only distantly related to other anaerobic cocci (Li, Hashimoto and Ezaki 1994, Murdoch and Magee 1995) and appears closer to some organisms at present in the genus *Eubacterium*. Thus the taxonomic problems that have always held back studies of GPAC are not yet resolved.

2.2 Recent changes in the genus *Peptostreptococcus*

It has become increasingly clear that *Peptostreptococcus asaccharolyticus* and *Peptostreptococcus prevotii* are genetically heterogeneous (Ezaki et al. 1983, Harpold and Wasilauskas 1987, Murdoch and Mitchelmore 1991, Ng and Dillon 1991, Murdoch and Magee 1995). Several new species have recently been described: *Peptostreptococcus barnesae* (Schiefer-Ullrich and Andreesen 1985), *Peptostreptococcus hydrogenalis* (Ezaki et al. 1990), *Peptostreptococcus vaginalis*, *Peptostreptococcus lactolyticus* and *Peptostreptococcus lacrimalis* (Li et al. 1992), but there is good evidence from DNA hybridization and PMS studies (Li et al. 1992, Murdoch and Magee

Table 33.1 Changes in classification of GPAC since Skerman, MacGowan and Sneath (1980)[a]

Current classification	Previous approved name[a]	Other designations
P. asaccharolyticus	*Pc. asaccharolyticus*	
P. anaerobius	Unchanged	
P. barnesae	New species	
P. heliotrinreducens		*Pc. heliotrinreducens*
P. hydrogenalis	New species	
P. indolicus	*Pc. indolicus*	
P. lacrimalis	New species	
P. lactolyticus	New species	
P. magnus	*Pc. magnus*	
P. micros	Unchanged	
	Pc. glycinophilus	
P. prevotii	*Pc. prevotii*	
P. tetradius		'Ga. anaerobia'
P. vaginalis	New species	
Pc. niger	Unchanged	
Staph. saccharolyticus	*Pc. saccharolyticus*	
A. parvulum	*P. parvulus*	*Str. parvulus*
R. productus	*P. productus*	
R. hansenii	*Str. hansenii*	
Str. constellatus	Unchanged	*Pc. constellatus*
Str. intermedius	Unchanged	*P. intermedius*
Ge. morbillorum	*Str. morbillorum*	*P. morbillorum*

[a]Skerman, MacGowan and Sneath (1980) approved list of bacterial names.
P., *Peptostreptococcus*; *Pc.*, *Peptococcus*; *R.*, *Ruminococcus*; *Str.*, *Streptococcus*; *Staph.*, *Staphylococcus*; *A.*, *Atopobium*; *Ga.*, *Gaffkya*; *Ge.*, *Gemella*.

1995), that further species await description. *Peptostreptococcus magnus*, *Peptostreptococcus micros* and *P. anaerobius*, the other species most often isolated from human material, appear to be valid and homogeneous taxa (Ezaki et al. 1983, Murdoch and Magee 1995). There are some data from protein electrophoretic studies (Cato et al. 1983, Taylor, Jackman and Phillips 1991) that ATCC 14955, the type strain of '*Peptococcus variabilis*', is distinct from *P. magnus*, but most workers have found no evidence that *P. magnus* is heterogeneous.

3 LABORATORY ISOLATION AND MAINTENANCE

Peptostreptococci are strict anaerobes in that they need an anaerobic atmosphere for multiplication (Watt and Jack 1977), but the limited data available suggest that most clinical strains are moderately aerotolerant. The 14 clinical strains studied by Tally et al. (1975) all survived 8 h or more of exposure to oxygen; 9 (63%) survived more than 72 h. Personal investigations of fresh clinical isolates indicate that 1% of cells of *P. magnus* and *P. micros* were still viable after exposure to air for 48 h. Most workers consider that anaerobic conditions are necessary during specimen transport, though opinions differ (Smith, Cumming and Ross 1986a, Ezaki, Oyaizi and Yabuuchi 1992). Growth is best in the temperature range 35–37°C and is enhanced by the presence of 10% CO_2 in the atmosphere (Watt and Smith 1990); a palladium catalyst should be present to remove traces of oxygen. Peptostreptococci require complex but ill-defined nutrients; commercial non-selective media vary in their ability to support the growth of fresh clinical isolates (Heginbotham et al. 1990). Sodium oleate (Tween 80, final concentration 0.02%) enhances growth of some species but is not essential; nor are vitamin K or haemin supplements (Holdeman Moore, Johnson and Moore 1986). In the author's experience, pre-reduced media are not necessary for growth, though others disagree (Ezaki, Oyaizu and Yabuuchi 1992). Viability in chopped meat broth depends on the commercial source; some preparations do not support growth at all. Solid media without blood can also be used (Ezaki, Oyaizu and Yabuuchi 1992).

Ruminococci, coprococci and sarcinae (see section 10.4, page 794) are more sensitive to oxygen and will grow only in well maintained anaerobic conditions (Ezaki, Oyaizu and Yabuuchi 1992). Carbohydrates stimulate the growth of coprococci but are essential for ruminococci and sarcinae. Few strains of these genera are likely to grow on standard commercial media; Bryant (1986) and Ezaki, Oyaizu and Yabuuchi (1992) give excellent guidelines for their isolation and culture.

The development of selective media has been neglected. This is an area that deserves active study; as clinical isolates grow slowly on standard media and are usually present in mixed culture, they are likely to be overgrown by more rapidly growing organisms, thus many clinical studies will give a falsely low estimate of their frequency. However, GPAC are so heterogeneous that any single selective medium is unlikely to be satisfactory for all. Wren (1980) found that nalidixic acid–Tween agar was superior to a non-selective enriched blood agar as an isolation medium but a combination of different media was necessary to maximize recovery rates. Peptostreptococci are very sensitive to most antibiotics but are usually resistant to bicozamycin (Watt and Brown 1983, Smith, Cumming and Ross 1986a); however, this agent may no longer be available. Ezaki, Oyaizu and Yabuuchi (1992) recommend the use of phenylethylalcohol blood agar.

GPAC retain viability well at −80°C or in liquid nitrogen. For long-term storage, Holdeman Moore, Johnson and Moore (1986) recommend lyophilization of cultures in the early stationary stage of growth in a medium containing less than 0.2% fermentable carbohydrate. For short-term storage, most strains survive well on the open bench in high quality chopped meat broth.

4 LABORATORY IDENTIFICATION

4.1 Identification to the genus level

Obligately anaerobic cocci must be distinguished from micro-aerophilic and capnophilic organisms at present classified in the genera *Streptococcus*, *Staphylococcus* and *Gemella*, which may appear only on anaerobic plates on primary isolation but will grow in 10% CO_2 on repeated subculture. Streptococci and gemellae also produce large quantities of lactic acid which can be detected by gas-liquid chromatography (GLC). *Staphylococcus saccharolyticus*, a normal part of the skin flora, will usually grow only in an anaerobic atmosphere on primary incubation; strains ferment several carbohydrates, produce urease and catalase and reduce nitrate (Evans, Mattern and Hallam 1978, Ezaki, Oyaizu and Yabuuchi 1992). The species of GPAC of major medical importance are at present classified in the genus *Peptostreptococcus*, but the definition of Watt and Jack (1977) also embraces *Peptococcus*, *Ruminococcus*, *Coprococcus*, *Sarcina* and *Atopobium* (Table 33.2); isolates of these genera have rarely been reported from human clinical specimens, perhaps because techniques for their isolation and identification are difficult.

Antibiotic disc susceptibility tests have been widely used for the presumptive identification of gram-negative anaerobic rods (Sutter and Finegold 1971) but not for GPAC. Watt and Jack (1977) and Murdoch and Mitchelmore (1991) used sensitivity to metronidazole as a simple screening method for separating GPAC from facultative organisms; GPAC gave a zone of inhibition greater than 15 mm in width around a 5 μg disc. Metronidazole-resistant GPAC have been reported but incompletely characterized (Edson et al. 1982, Sanchez, Jones and Croco 1992). Many isolates of GPAC retain Gram's stain poorly and can be confused with gram-negative organisms; sensitivity to vancomycin is a simple and reliable method of separation (Murdoch and Mitchelmore 1991).

Table 33.2   Characteristics differentiating genera of GPAC and microscopically similar genera

| Genus | G + C content (mol%) | Microscopic arrangement | Major fatty acid end products | | | Utilization of | | Metronidazole susceptibility |
			butyrate	caproate	lactate	carbohydrates	peptides	
Peptostreptococcus[a]	27–37	Variable	v	v	–	v	+	S
Peptococcus[a]	50–51	Clumps	+	+	–	–	+	S
Ruminococcus[a]	39–46	Pairs, chains	–	–	v	+[b]	–	S
Coprococcus[a]	39–44	Pairs, chains	+	–	v	+	–	S
Sarcina[a]	28–31	Tetrads	v	–	–	+[b]	–	S
Atopobium[a]	35–46	Pairs, chains	–	–	+	+	–	R
Streptococcus	30–46	Pairs, chains	–	–	+	+	+	R
Gemella	30	Chains	–	–	+	+	+	R
Staphylococcus	30–39	Clumps	–	–	–	+	+	R

Note: several of these characteristics, notably cell arrangement, are generalizations and should only be used as a guide.
[a]Denotes genera of GPAC.
[b]Carbohydrates are required for growth of ruminococci and sarcinae.

4.2 Identification to species level

Many standard manuals still base identification on microscopic appearance, detection of volatile fatty acids (VFAs) by GLC, ability to ferment carbohydrates, and standard biochemical tests such as nitrate reduction and indole production (Holdeman, Cato and Moore 1977, Sutter et al. 1985, Summanen et al. 1993, Hillier and Moncla 1995). The results of GLC correlate well with cell wall peptidoglycan structure (Ezaki et al. 1983, Li et al. 1992) and whole cell composition (Murdoch and Magee 1995) but they are of limited discrimination; they permit a useful if arbitrary division into 3 VFA groups (Murdoch and Mitchelmore 1991):

1. an 'acetate group', of species producing acetic acid alone or no VFAs at all
2. a 'butyrate group', in which the major terminal VFA formed is butyric acid and
3. a 'caproate group', in which the species produce terminal peaks of isovaleric, isocaproic or *n*-caproic acid (Table 33.3).

Production of non-volatile fatty acids (NVFAs) has been little studied, except by Ezaki et al. (1983), but appears to be of little value except to exclude streptococci. Few species of GPAC produce acid from carbohydrates or are active in standard biochemical tests (Ezaki and Yabuuchi 1985, Holdeman Moore, Johnson and Moore 1986, Summanen et al. 1993). Therefore most species have been identified on the basis of negative reactions. *P. anaerobius* can be presumptively identified by sodium polyanethol sulphonate (SPS) disc testing (Graves, Morello and Kocka 1974, Wideman et al. 1976); Murdoch and Mitchelmore (1991) found that this test had a sensitivity and specificity approaching 100%.

The products of protein decomposition are a major energy source for most species of *Peptostreptococcus* (Rogosa 1974, Holdeman Moore, Johnson and Moore 1986). Ezaki and Yabuuchi (1985) showed that tests for amidase and oligopeptidase activity clearly and reproducibly distinguished between most species of peptostreptococci and micro-aerophilic streptococci. Commercial preformed enzyme kits for the detection of proteolytic and saccharolytic enzymes (Karachewski, Busch and Wells 1985, Murdoch, Mitchelmore and Tabaqchali 1988a, Murdoch and Mitchelmore 1991) have now made rapid, reliable identification straightforward for routine diagnostic laboratories (Table 33.3). However, as the classification is still incomplete, particularly for butyrate-producing strains previously identified as *P. prevotii*, about 10% of isolates still cannot be identified to recognized species (Murdoch, Mitchelmore and Tabaqchali 1994).

DNA probes provide a sensitive and specific method for the rapid identification of single bacterial colonies. ^{32}P-labelled probes for the identification of *P. anaerobius* (Yasui et al. 1989) and *P. micros* (Yasui 1989) are limited by the short half-life of the radioisotope and problems with its disposal. The development of a 'cold' digoxigenin-labelled probe for *P. micros*

(Gunaratnam et al. 1992) could be of considerable value, particularly in oral microbiology.

5 ROLE IN NORMAL FLORA OF HUMANS

GPAC are a major part of the normal flora of skin and mucosal surfaces (Neut et al. 1985, Bartlett 1990, Summanen et al. 1993) but reports have usually not attempted identification to the species level; many commensals of low pathogenicity are poorly studied and cannot be placed in recognized species (Murdoch and Mitchelmore 1991, Summanen et al. 1993). There is considerable variation between reports, partly because of genuine differences between the populations studied, partly because of difficulties with nomenclature and identification. In particular, organisms described in earlier reports as *P. asaccharolyticus* and *P. prevotii* are likely to be heterogeneous. As the endogenous flora is believed to be the source of most anaerobic infections (Finegold and George 1989), further studies of commensal GPAC are required, with identification when possible to the species level.

GPAC constitute 1–15% of the normal oral flora (Sutter 1984), the major species being *P. micros* and, according to some reports, *P. anaerobius* (Neut et al. 1985, Holdeman Moore, Johnson and Moore 1986, Rams et al. 1992). The gastrointestinal tract hosts most species of GPAC, with many little known commensals such as coprococci, sarcinae and ruminococci (Holdeman and Moore 1974, Ezaki, Oyaizu and Yabuuchi 1992), which have rarely been isolated from infectious processes. *Ruminococcus productus*, *P. micros*, '*P. prevotii*' and *P. magnus* are reported as being particularly common; the composition varies with diet (Finegold, Attebury and Sutter 1974, Neut et al. 1985). The female genitourinary tract contains high numbers of GPAC, including *P. magnus*, '*P. prevotii*', *P. asaccharolyticus*, *P. anaerobius* and *P. micros* (Bartlett et al. 1977, Neut et al. 1985); counts vary considerably with physiological features such as the stage of the menstrual cycle. GPAC are part of the skin flora (Bartlett 1990, Summanen et al. 1993) but its composition at the species level appears to have been little studied; *P. magnus*, *P. asaccharolyticus* and *P. vaginalis* are likely to be present as they are the predominant species in superficial wound infections and abscesses (Murdoch, Mitchelmore and Tabaqchali 1994).

6 CLINICAL IMPORTANCE

GPAC are the second commonest group of anaerobes cultured from human clinical material; they consistently account for 20–35% of all anaerobic isolates (Holland, Hill and Altemeier 1977, Wren et al. 1977, Rosenblatt 1985, Brook 1988a, Murdoch, Mitchelmore and Tabaqchali 1994). They can be cultured from a wide variety of sites, particularly gynaecological, oral, cutaneous and upper respiratory tract infections (Brook 1995). They are major causes of serious obstetric infections, particularly puerperal fever

Table 33.3 Biochemical characteristics of *Peptostreptococcus* species, *Ruminococcus productus* and *Peptococcus niger*

	Species								
	P. magnus	*P. micros*	*P. heliotrin-reducens*	*R. productus*	*P. barnesae*	*P. asaccharo-lyticus*	*P. indolicus*	*P. hydrogen-alis*	*'P. trisimilis'*
No. strains examined	87	31	6	1	1	50	4	9	4
Terminal major VFA	−/A	−/A	−/A	A	A	B	B	B	B
Indole	−	−	−	−	w	v	+	+	w/+
Urease	−	−	−	−	−	−	−	v	−
ALP	v	+	−	−	−	−	+	−/w	−
Catalase	v	−	−	−	−	v	−	−	v
ADH	v	−	+	−	−	v	−	−	−
Carbohydrate fermentation tests									
Glucose	−/w	−	−	+	−	−	−	+	+
Lactose	−	−	−	+	−	−	−	+	NT
Maltose	−	−	−	+	−	−	−	+	NT
Sucrose	−	−	−	+	−	−	−	+	NT
Fructose	−/w	−	−	+	−	−	−	+	+
Mannose	−	−	−	+	−	−	−	v	+
Raffinose	−	−	−	+	−	−	−	v	v
Saccharolytic enzymes									
αGAL	−	−	−	+	−	−	−	−	−
βGAL	−	−	−	−	−	−	−	−	v
αGLU	−	−	−	+	−	−	−	v	−
βGUR	−	−	−	−	−	−	−	−	−
Proteolytic enzymes									
ArgA	+	+	v	−	−	+	+	−	−
ProA	−	+[a]	+	−	−	−	−	−	−
PheA	−	+[a]	+	−	−	−	−	−	−
LeuA	+	+	+	−	−	v	−	−	−
PyrA	+	+	−	−	−	−	−	−	+
TyrA	−/w	+	w	−	−	v	+	−	−
HisA	w	+	w	−	−	v	+	−	−
GGA	−	+[a]	−	−	−	−	−	−	−
SPS sensitivity	R	R	R	R	R	R	R	R	R

P., *Peptostreptococcus*; *Pc.*, *Peptococcus*; *R.*, *Ruminococcus*. +, positive in >90%; −, negative in >90%; w, weak; v, variable; NT, not tested; VFA, volatile fatty acid; A, acetate; B, butyrate; IV, isovalerate; IC isocaproate; C, *n*-caproate; ALP, alkaline phosphatase; ADH, arginine dihydrolase.
Saccharolytic enzymes: αGAL, α-galactosidase; βGAL, β-galactosidase; αGLU, α-glucosidase; βGUR, β-glucuronidase.
Proteolytic enzymes (all arylamidases): Arg, arginine; Pro, proline; Phe, phenylalanine; Leu, leucine; Pyr, pyroglutamyl; Tyr, tyrosine; His, histidine; GG, glutamylglutamyl.
SPS, sodium polyanethol sulphonate; S, sensitive; R, resistant; V, variable.
The results of indole, urease, ALP and ADH production, and saccharolytic and proteolytic enzyme reactions, are based on a commercial kit (ATB 32A, API-BioMérieux, Basingstoke, Hants, UK).
[a]8 of the 11 genital tract isolates of *P. micros* tested by Ng et al. (1994) did not produce ProA, PheA or GGA.

(Schwarz and Dieckman 1926, Colebrook and Hare 1933, Hare and Polunin 1960, Hillier et al. 1990). Isolation from the blood is uncommon except in obstetric cases (DiZerega et al. 1980, Topiel and Simon 1986, Brook 1989a); endocarditis is rare (Felner and Dowell 1970, Cofsky and Seligman 1985). Central nervous system infections usually present as abscesses (Brook 1981, Murdoch, Mitchelmore and Tabaqchali 1988b); meningitis has been reported after head and neck surgery (Brown et al. 1994). Careful investigations have shown that GPAC are common in superficial infections (Wheat et al. 1986, Brook 1989b, Edmiston et al. 1990, Brook, Frazier and Thompson 1992). Most infections are mixed, particularly abdominal wounds and deep organ abscesses, which may yield a characteristic flora of anaerobes and micro-aerophilic streptococci (Murdoch, Mitchelmore and Tabaqchali 1988b). However, GPAC are sometimes isolated in pure culture, particularly from soft tissue infections and cases of septic arthritis and osteomyelitis (Bourgault, Rosenblatt and Fitzgerald 1980, Fitzgerald et al. 1982, Murdoch, Mitchelmore and

Table 33.3 Continued

	Species								
	P. lacrimalis	*P. lactolyticus*	*P. vaginalis*	*P. prevotii*	*P. tetradius*	*'P. ivoricus'*	*P. anaerobius*	Hare group VIII	*Pc. niger*
No. strains examined	1	1	19	1	5	4	47	4	1
Terminal major VFA	B	B	B	B	B	IV	IC	C	C
Indole	–	–	–	–	–	–	–	–	–
Urease	–	+	–	+	+	–	–	–	–
ALP	–	–	w	–	–	–	–	–	–
Catalase	–	–	v	+	v	–	–	v	+
ADH	–	–	+	–	–	–	–	–	–
Carbohydrate fermentation tests									
Glucose	–	+	w	w	+	–	w	+	–
Lactose	–	+	–	–	–	–	–	–	–
Maltose	–	+	w	–	+	–	w	–/w	–
Sucrose	–	–	–	–	+	–	–	–/w	–
Fructose	–	+	+	+	+	–	w	+	–
Mannose	–	+	v	w	+	–	w	+	–
Raffinose	–	–	–	+	v	–	–	–	–
Saccharolytic enzymes									
αGAL	–	–	–	+	–	–	–	–	–
βGAL	–	+	–	–	–	–	–	–	–
αGLU	–	–	–	+	+	–	+	–	–
βGUR	–	–	–	+	+	–	–	–	–
Proteolytic enzymes									
ArgA	w	+	+	+	v	–	–	–	–
ProA	–	–	–	–	–	+	+	+	–
PheA	–	–	–	–	–	–	–	–	–
LeuA	+	–	+	–	–	–	–	–	–
PyrA	–	–	–	+	v	–	–	w	–
TyrA	–	–	–	–	v	–	–	–	–
HisA	–	–	+	+	+	–	–	–	–
GGA	–	–	–	–	–	–	–	–	–
SPS sensitivity	R	R	R	R	R	V	S	R	R

Tabaqchali 1994). Prosthetic joints provide potential foci for low grade infections which can easily be overlooked (Fitzgerald et al. 1982, Davies, Leak and Dave 1988).

The species of greatest clinical importance appear to be *P. anaerobius*, *P. asaccharolyticus*, *P. micros* and, in particular, *P. magnus*; these species constituted 77% of all isolates in a recent series (Murdoch, Mitchelmore and Tabaqchali 1994). The most frequently isolated in pure culture is *P. magnus* (Bourgault, Rosenblatt and Fitzgerald 1980, Murdoch, Mitchelmore and Tabaqchali 1994). Previous series reported *P. prevotii* as one of the commonest pathogens; these organisms are likely to have been heterogeneous.

7 PATHOGENICITY AND VIRULENCE FACTORS

The pathogenicity of GPAC has been little studied; clinical observations suggest that it is most often expressed via a synergic interaction with other anaerobes, facultative or obligate. However, as most infections are mixed, it is difficult to evaluate the relative importance of different organisms. Synergy of GPAC with facultative and anaerobic organisms has been demonstrated in an animal model, with increased mortality, ability to induce abscesses and enhanced growth of the bacterial components (Brook 1988b). The ability to produce capsules is an important virulence mechanism in this model (Brook 1986). Few other virulence factors have been described. Tam and Chan (1983) isolated hyaluronidase-producing pepto-streptococci (not fully identified) in higher numbers from diseased periodontium than from healthy periodontium. Murdoch, Mitchelmore and Tabaqchali (1988b) noted the strong proteolytic activity of *P. micros* and suggested that it might contribute to the formation of deep organ abscesses. Krepel et al. (1991, 1992) studied the production by *P. magnus* of proteolytic enzymes, particularly collagenase and gelatinase; strains from non-puerperal breast abscesses and diabetic foot infections had significantly greater enzymic activity than those from intra-abdominal sepsis. They proposed that these proteolytic enzymes could be important virulence factors in the causation of soft tissue infections by *P. magnus*. Protein L is a cell surface protein formed by some strains of *P. magnus* which can bind to the κ light chain variable domain of human Ig molecules (Nilson et al. 1992); its expression has been linked to clinical infection (Kastern et al. 1990).

8 TYPING METHODS

There have been several attempts to devise a serologically based classification of GPAC but they have had little success (Porschen and Spaulding 1974, Wong, Catena and Hadley 1980, Collins et al. 1989). Several antigens are shared between strains of *P. anaerobius* (Smith, Cumming and Ross 1986b, Collins et al. 1989). Bacteriophage and bacteriocin typing schemes have not been developed.

9 SUSCEPTIBILITY TO ANTIBIOTICS

GPAC are usually susceptible to the antibiotics used for anaerobic infections (Garcia-Rodriguez, Garcia-Sanchez and Munoz-Bellido 1995). This predictability has led some authorities (Finegold 1988) to suggest that routine susceptibility testing is required only in limited, well defined circumstances. Guidelines for quantitative susceptibility testing have been published (King and Phillips 1988, National Committee for Clinical Laboratory Standards 1990). Almost all strains tested have been susceptible to vancomycin, rifampicin, chloramphenicol, broad spectrum penicillins, cefotaxime and cefoxitin, imipenem and combinations of β-lactam with β-lactamase inhibitor (Watt, Young and McCurdy 1979, Edson et al. 1982, Watt and Brown 1986, Wexler and Finegold 1988). Most studies have found that strictly anaerobic cocci are very susceptible to metronidazole (Watt, Young and McCurdy 1979, Panichi et al. 1990, Wexler, Molitoris and Finegold 1993); Edson et al. (1982) and Sanchez, Jones and Croco (1992) reported resistance rates of 10–15% but did not give the species identity of their strains; some may have been micro-aerophilic streptococci. Penicillin G is usually considered to be highly effective but Panichi et al. (1990) reported a resistance rate of 10%; 24% of the strains tested by Greenwood and

Palfreyman (1987) and 10% of *P. anaerobius* (Murdoch DA, personal observation) showed MICs of greater than 1 mg l^{-1} but did not exhibit β-lactamase activity. Four strains of *P. anaerobius* studied by Reig and Baquero (1994) had a modal MIC to amoxycillin of 8 mg l^{-1}; the MIC was unaffected by the addition of β-lactamase inhibitors. These observations suggest that β-lactam resistance may be mediated via modified penicillin-binding proteins. Ciprofloxacin has borderline activity (Watt and Brown 1986) but recently developed quinolones are more active (Wexler, Molitoris and Finegold 1993). Susceptibility to tetracycline, erythromycin and clindamycin appears to be variable (Edson et al. 1982, Reig, Moreno and Baquero 1992, Sanchez, Jones and Croco 1992) and selection of clindamycin-resistant strains following clindamycin therapy has been described (Ohm-Smith, Sweet and Hadley 1986). Inducible macrolide–lincosamide resistance has been demonstrated (Reig, Moreno and Baquero 1992, Sanchez, Jones and Croco 1992), though regrettably the species identities of the relevant strains were not reported. Sanchez recommended testing erythromycin susceptibility so that inducible clindamycin resistance can be detected.

As GPAC are usually isolated from polymicrobial infections, frequently with other anaerobes and micro-aerophilic streptococci, therapy should consist of a combination of a penicillin and metronidazole; a β-lactam with a β-lactamase inhibitor is a reasonable alternative. More work would be valuable, particularly on the frequency and mechanisms of resistance to penicillin, metronidazole and clindamycin. Reports of significant antibiotic resistance in GPAC are rare and identification of most strains is now straightforward; therefore such isolates should be identified to the species level.

10 SPECIES DESCRIPTIONS

10.1 Genus *Peptostreptococcus*

DEFINITION

Peptostreptococcus spp. are gram-positive cocci (though often retaining gram stain poorly). They are obligate anaerobes, though many strains are relatively aerotolerant. They occur in pairs, tetrads, chains or irregular masses. They do not form spores. Several species produce characteristic colonies and odours on blood agar medium. They are almost always non-haemolytic. Production of catalase, indole and urease is variable as is nitrate reduction. Products of protein digestion appear to be the main energy sources for most species. Carbohydrate utilization varies: some species are asaccharolytic but others ferment a wide range of carbohydrates. *Peptostreptococcus* spp. are genetically heterogeneous. The G + C content of DNA is 27–37 mol% and the type species is *P. anaerobius*.

PEPTOSTREPTOCOCCUS ANAEROBIUS

P. anaerobius cells are 0.5–0.9 μm in diameter, often coccobacillary with a variety of pleomorphic forms;

cells usually occur in pairs or chains. *P. anaerobius* is the most rapidly growing species in the genus; colonies reach 1 mm in diameter after incubation for 24 h; after 5 days they reach 2–4 mm, are grey, flat, entire, with slightly raised whitish centres and a distinctive, sickly sweet smell. Growth is inhibited by polyanethol sulphonate (SPS). This species does not produce indole, urease, ALP (alkaline phosphatase) or catalase and is a weak fermenter of carbohydrates; it produces α-glucosidase and proline arylamidase. Various VFAs are formed, usually terminating in isocaproic acid, but 5–10% of strains produce a terminal isovaleric peak. *P. anaerobius* is a normal part of the human flora of the genitourinary and gastrointestinal tracts, commonly isolated from human clinical specimens, particularly from abdominal sites, but rarely in pure culture. The G + C content of DNA is 33–34 mol% and the type strain is NCTC 11460 (= ATCC 27337). Recent taxonomic studies suggest a closer relationship to some clostridia than to other peptostreptococci.

PEPTOSTREPTOCOCCUS ASACCHAROLYTICUS

P. asaccharolyticus is a genetically heterogeneous species (Ezaki et al. 1983, Holdeman Moore, Johnson and Moore 1986, Murdoch and Magee 1995). Typical strains form cells 0.7–0.9 μm in diameter which vary little in size, occur in clumps and retain Gram's stain poorly. Colonies after 5 days are 2–3 mm in diameter, glistening, lemon-yellow, low convex, circular, entire, often with a musty smell; 80–90% of strains form indole but urease, catalase, coagulase and ALP are not produced. The species is asaccharolytic and moderately proteolytic. The terminal VFA is butyric acid. *P. asaccharolyticus* is a normal part of the human flora of the gastrointestinal system; the species is commonly isolated from clinical specimens, sometimes in pure growth (Murdoch, Mitchelmore and Tabaqchali 1994). The G + C content of DNA is 30–34 mol% and the type strain is NCTC 11461 (= ATCC 14963). Approximately 25% of clinical isolates can be distinguished from typical strains by cell and colonial morphology, but not yet satisfactorily by biochemical tests; whole cell composition and 16S rRNA sequence are distinct. On microscopy, atypical strains show marked variation in cell size and shape (cell diameter 0.5–1.5 μm), with oval and elliptical forms; they grow more slowly, forming colonies 1 mm in diameter, translucent, matt, flat, entire after 5 days. Indole production is weak, catalase production is variable. Atypical strains can be isolated from human pathological specimens, occasionally in pure growth (Murdoch, Mitchelmore and Tabaqchali 1994).

PEPTOSTREPTOCOCCUS BARNESAE

P. barnesae cells are 0.5–0.9 μm in diameter, usually occurring in pairs. Colonies of the type strain are white, up to 1 mm in diameter after incubation for 5 days. Growth is enhanced by bile salts. *P. barnesae* forms indole feebly but not urease or ALP; catalase activity is variable; nitrate is not reduced. *P. barnesae* is asaccharolytic but utilizes purines and glycine, alone of amino acids tested (Schiefer-Ullrich and Andreesen

1985). Acetate is the terminal VFA. *P. barnesae* has been isolated from chicken faeces. The G + C content of DNA is 33–35 mol% and the type strain is DSM 3244.

PEPTOSTREPTOCOCCUS HELIOTRINREDUCENS

P. heliotrinreducens cells are 0.3–0.6 μm in diameter, and occur in pairs, chains and clumps, often with elongated pleomorphic forms. They are very slowly growing, forming translucent, glistening, low convex, entire, circular colonies, 1 mm in diameter after incubation for 5 days. *P. heliotrinreducens* strains produce arginine dihydrolase (ADH) but not ALP, thus distinguishing them from *P. micros*; they do not produce urease or catalase. Nitrate may be reduced. *P. heliotrinreducens* strains are asaccharolytic but strongly proteolytic (Murdoch and Mitchelmore 1991). Acetate is the terminal VFA. The type strain was isolated from sheep rumen (Lanigan 1976); similar isolates cultured from human polymicrobial anaerobic abscesses (Murdoch and Mitchelmore 1989) may belong to a different species, but both may be better classified with some species of eubacteria. The G + C content of DNA is 35–37 mol% and the type strain is NCTC 11029 (= ATCC 29202).

PEPTOSTREPTOCOCCUS HYDROGENALIS

P. hydrogenalis cells are 0.5–1.8 μm in diameter, and occur in clumps, diplococci and tetrads, sometimes in short chains. Colonies are usually 2–3 mm, grey-white, low convex, entire, circular after incubation for 5 days, often with an unpleasant smell. They produce indole and ALP but not coagulase; urease and catalase production are variable and they do not reduce nitrate. *P. hydrogenalis* is strongly saccharolytic but weakly or not proteolytic. Butyrate is the terminal VFA produced. *P. hydrogenalis* has been isolated from human faeces, vaginal discharge (Ezaki et al. 1990), infected superficial sites (Murdoch, Mitchelmore and Tabaqchali 1994), ulcers and urine. Pathogenicity is unknown. The G + C content of DNA is 30–31 mol% and the type strain is DSM 7454. *P. hydrogenalis* is synonymous with Hare group III (Thomas and Hare 1954, Murdoch and Magee 1995).

PEPTOSTREPTOCOCCUS INDOLICUS

P. indolicus cells are 0.7–1.6 μm in diameter and occur mainly in clumps; they often retain Gram's stain poorly. Colonies are usually 3–4 mm (though with considerable variation), raised, yellow-buff, circular, entire, smooth, after incubation for 5 days. They produce indole but not urease or catalase. Biochemical activity is similar to typical *P. asaccharolyticus* but distinguished by production of coagulase (Ezaki et al. 1983) and, possibly, ALP (Murdoch and Mitchelmore 1991) and, in some test systems, reduction of nitrate to nitrite (Ezaki et al. 1983). *P. indolicus* is asaccharolytic but strongly proteolytic. Butyrate is the terminal VFA produced. *P. indolicus* is a species of veterinary importance, causing bovine summer mastitis (Madsen, Aalbaek and Hansen 1992), but it is rarely isolated from human clinical specimens. The G + C content of DNA is 32–34 mol% and the type strain is NCTC 11088 (= ATCC 29427).

PEPTOSTREPTOCOCCUS LACRIMALIS

Cells of the type strain of *P. lacrimalis* are 0.5–0.7 μm in diameter, and occur in short chains or clumps; after 5 days, colonies are pink-white, 1–2 mm in diameter but with considerable size variation. They are asaccharolytic and inactive in classic biochemical tests, using peptones and oligopeptides as energy source (Li et al. 1992). Butyrate is the terminal VFA produced. Both strains described by Li et al. (1992) were isolated from human eyes. The G + C content of DNA is 30–31 mol% and the type strain is DSM 7455.

PEPTOSTREPTOCOCCUS LACTOLYTICUS

The type strain of *P. lactolyticus* is slow growing, forming translucent colonies 1 mm in diameter after 5 days; cells are 0.5–1.5 μm in diameter and occur in short chains or clumps. *P. lactolyticus* produces urease, ALP and β-galactosidase but not indole; it is strongly saccharolytic but weakly proteolytic (Li et al. 1992). Butyrate is the terminal VFA produced. Both strains described by Li et al. (1992) were from vaginal discharges. The G + C content of DNA is 34 mol% and the type strain is DSM 7456.

PEPTOSTREPTOCOCCUS MAGNUS

P. magnus cells are 0.8–1.6 μm in diameter, and arranged in clumps. The colonial morphology is highly variable: most commonly translucent but colour varies from white to greyish or yellowish; surface glistening or matt; entire, circular, low convex; up to 2 mm diameter after 5 days but marked size variation; occasionally β-haemolytic. *P. magnus* does not produce urease or indole or reduce nitrate; activity of ADH, ALP and catalase is variable. There is weak saccharolytic activity but marked proteolytic activity. The terminal VFA is acetate. *P. magnus* is part of the normal flora of the gastrointestinal and female reproductive tracts and probably of the skin. It is the commonest species of GPAC isolated from human pathological specimens (Bourgault, Rosenblatt and Fitzgerald 1980) and is frequently cultured from soft tissue infections (Bourgault, Rosenblatt and Fitzgerald 1980, Murdoch, Mitchelmore and Tabaqchali 1994), septic joints, particularly in the presence of prosthetic material (Fitzgerald et al. 1982), diabetic foot infections (Sanderson 1977, Wheat et al. 1986), breast abscesses (Edmiston et al. 1990) and superficial wound infections (Brook 1989b, Murdoch, Mitchelmore and Tabaqchali 1994). It is often isolated in pure culture and can be a primary pathogen (Cofsky and Seligman 1985, Phelps and Jacobs 1985, Panagou, Papandreou and Bouros 1991, Pouedras et al. 1992, Brown et al. 1994). Collagenase (Krepel et al. 1992) and protein L (Nilson et al. 1992) may be virulence factors. The G + C content of DNA is 32–34 mol% and the type strain is NCTC 11804 (= ATCC 15794). *Peptococcus variabilis* is probably a synonym.

PEPTOSTREPTOCOCCUS MICROS

P. micros cells are 0.3–0.7 μm in diameter, and arranged in chains and clumps. Colonies grow slowly and are usually distinctive: glistening, white (sometimes grey), domed, entire, circular, 1 mm in diameter after incubation for 5 days, often surrounded by a yellow-brown halo of discoloration in the medium about 2 mm wide (Murdoch and Mitchelmore 1991). A rough morphotype possessing fibrillar structures forms dry, white, haemolytic colonies (van Dalen et al. 1993). *P. micros* produces ALP but not indole, urease, ADH or catalase. It is asaccharolytic but very strongly proteolytic; it can be distinguished from *P. magnus* by production of proline, phenylalanine and glutamylglutamyl aminopeptidases, though Ng et al. (1994) reported that these tests were not reliable for vaginal strains of *P. micros*. *P. micros* produces acetic acid or no VFAs. It is a normal part of the mouth flora, associated with other anaerobes in periodontitis (Moore et al. 1982, Socransky et al. 1988, Rams et al. 1992), peritonsillar abscess (Jokipii et al. 1988, Murdoch, Mitchelmore and Tabaqchali 1988b) and endodontic abscesses (Williams, McCann and Schoenknecht 1983). It is rarely isolated from outside the mouth but it is probably under-recorded; it can be cultured from a wide range of human polymicrobial abscesses, including brain (Murdoch, Mitchelmore and Tabaqchali 1988b). The G + C content of DNA is 27–29 mol% and the type strain is NCTC 11808 (= ATCC 33270). *Peptococcus glycinophilus* is a synonym (Cato et al. 1983).

PEPTOSTREPTOCOCCUS PREVOTII

P. prevotii cells are 0.6–1.2 μm in diameter, varying markedly in size, usually occurring in clumps and tetrads. Colonies are matt grey with whiter centres, low convex, circular, entire, 2 mm in diameter after 5 days but showing marked variation in size and shape. *P. prevotii* produces urease but not indole or ALP; catalase production is variable. There is weak saccharolytic and proteolytic activity; butyrate is the terminal VFA. *P. prevotii* is a constituent of the normal flora but its pathogenic potential is unclear. The G + C content of DNA is 29–33 mol% and the type strain is NCTC 11806 (= ATCC 9321).

Taxonomic note

The original description of this species (Foubert and Douglas 1948) was based on 6 strains, some saccharolytic and some asaccharolytic. Rogosa (1974) considered that *P. prevotii* was a 'composite description of two organisms', one similar to '*Gaffkya anaerobia*' (now *P. tetradius*) and the other to indole-negative strains of *P. asaccharolyticus*; he recommended that the name should be rejected. The type strain is weakly saccharolytic and closely related to *P. tetradius* (Ezaki et al. 1983, Li, Hashimoto and Ezaki 1994). Until recently, identification manuals and clinical papers described most or all indole-negative, butyrate-producing strains of GPAC as *P. prevotii*. However, strictly defined isolates are infrequently isolated from human clinical material (Murdoch, Mitchelmore and Tabaqchali

1994); strains previously reported as *P. prevotii* probably belong to a variety of species such as *P. vaginalis*.

PEPTOSTREPTOCOCCUS TETRADIUS

P. tetradius (formerly '*Gaffkya anaerobia*') cells are 0.5–1.8 μm in diameter, occurring in clumps and tetrads. Colonies after 5 days are usually 2 mm in diameter, matt grey with whiter centres, low convex, circular and entire, often showing marked variation in size and shape. *P. tetradius* produces urease but not indole or ALP; nitrate is not reduced and catalase production is variable. The species is strongly saccharolytic but proteolytic activity is very weak. Butyrate is the terminal VFA. *P. tetradius* is probably a constituent of the normal vaginal flora; it is rarely isolated from human clinical specimens but has been little studied. The G + C content of DNA is 30–32 mol% and the type strain is ATCC 35098 (= DSM 2951).

PEPTOSTREPTOCOCCUS VAGINALIS

P. vaginalis cells are 0.5–1.5 μm in diameter and usually occur in clumps or tetrads. Colonies are 2–3 mm, grey-white, low convex and circular after incubation for 5 days, often with an unpleasant smell. *P. vaginalis* produces ADH but not urease or indole; ALP and catalase production is variable. There is moderate saccharolytic and proteolytic activity. Butyrate is the terminal VFA produced. *P. vaginalis* is part of the vaginal flora (Li et al. 1992) and a significant human pathogen, accounting for 6% of all isolates of GPAC in one survey (Murdoch, Mitchelmore and Tabaqchali 1994); it has been cultured from pleural empyema, superficial and post-surgical wound infections, sometimes in pure culture. The G + C content of DNA is 28–30 mol% and the type strain is DSM 7457.

SPECIES AWAITING DESCRIPTION

Numerous species await description, particularly in the butyrate group. The following have been well characterized.

'*Peptostreptococcus trisimilis*'

'*P. trisimilis*' is similar to *P. hydrogenalis* (Hare group III; Murdoch and Magee 1995); cells are 0.8–1.5 μm in diameter, occurring in clumps and tetrads. Colonies are grey with whiter centres, entire, circular, 1–2 mm in diameter after 5 days. '*P. trisimilis*' produces indole but not ALP or urease; there is weak catalase activity. The organism is strongly saccharolytic but weakly proteolytic. The terminal VFA is butyric acid. '*P. trisimilis*' has been isolated from blood, infected mastoid and sternotomy wounds.

'*Peptostreptococcus ivoricus*'

'*P. ivoricus*' cells are 0.4–1.5 μm in diameter, occurring in clumps. Colonies grow slowly; they are 1–2 mm in diameter, whitish, low convex, entire and circular after 5 days. The organism does not produce indole, urease, ALP or catalase. The 4 strains tested (Murdoch and Mitchelmore 1991) are asaccharolytic and weakly proteolytic. The terminal VFA produced is isovaleric acid but large quantities of butyric acid are also formed.

'*P. ivoricus*' has been isolated from superficial human flora (Murdoch, Mitchelmore and Tabaqchali 1994); its pathogenicity is unknown.

Hare group VIII

Hare group VIII cells are 0.7–0.9 μm in diameter, occurring in clumps. Colonies after 5 days are 1–2 mm in diameter, yellow-white, glistening, circular, raised and entire (Murdoch and Mitchelmore 1991). Catalase production is variable; indole, urease and ALP are not produced. Strains of Hare group VIII are strongly saccharolytic but weakly proteolytic; they produce large quantities of butyric acid and some isovaleric acid; the terminal VFA is *n*-caproic acid. Fifteen strains studied by Thomas and Hare (1954) and 2 strains studied by Murdoch, Mitchelmore and Tabaqchali (1994) came from nasal flora; their pathogenicity is unknown.

10.2 *Peptococcus*

This genus now contains only the type species, *Pc. niger*.

PEPTOCOCCUS NIGER

Pc. niger cells are 0.3–1.3 μm in diameter, occurring in singles, pairs and clumps. The type strain grows slowly to form raised, circular, entire colonies 1 mm in diameter after incubation for 5 days. Black colonies may be seen on initial isolation but become grey on exposure to air; pigment is often absent after several laboratory transfers (Wilkins et al. 1975). The type strain forms catalase but is inactive in other presently available tests (Ezaki and Yabuuchi 1985). The distinctive VFA profile includes butyric, isovaleric and terminal *n*-caproic acids. The neotype and other strains were isolated from human navel flora by Wilkins et al. (1975); very rarely the organism is isolated from pathological specimens (Ezaki, Oyaizu and Yabuuchi 1992, Murdoch, Mitchelmore and Tabaqchali 1994). The G + C content of DNA is 51 mol%. Although it is the type species of the family Peptococcaceae, *Pc. niger* is only distantly related to other members (Ezaki et al. 1994). The type strain is NCTC 11805 (= ATCC 27731).

10.3 *Ruminococcus*

DEFINITION

Ruminococcus spp. are gram-positive coccobacilli (though often retaining stain poorly) with ends that can be rounded or pointed. They occur in pairs and chains. They are obligate anaerobes and do not form spores; they require carbohydrates, which are fermented to form various proportions of acetate, formate, succinate, lactate, ethanol, CO_2 and H_2. Amino acids and peptides are not fermented; most strains require ammonia as their nitrogen source. The G + C content of DNA is 39–46 mol% and the type species is *Ruminococcus flavefaciens*.

Most strains have been isolated from the gastrointestinal tract of animals, including humans, and appear to be of very low pathogenicity (Bryant 1986); however, the culture methods used in diagnostic laboratories are unlikely to lead to their isolation (Ezaki, Oyaizu and Yabuuchi 1992). Bryant (1986) listed 8 species; Ezaki et al. (1994) have since proposed that *P. productus* and *S. hansenii* should be transferred to the genus *Ruminococcus*. Collins et al. (1994) and Rainey and Janssen (1995) disagree; Collins et al. (1994) place *P. productus* and *S. hansenii* in *Clostridium* Cluster XIVa. *R. productus* is a major part of the human gastrointestinal flora; it will grow on routine anaerobic media and can be readily identified using preformed enzyme kits (Murdoch and Mitchelmore 1991).

Ruminococcus productus

R. productus cells are elliptical, (0.6–0.9) × (0.8–2.0) μm; they occur in pairs or short chains and will grow on enriched blood agar to form circular, convex, glistening grey colonies, 1–3 mm in diameter, after 2 days. They are strongly saccharolytic enzyme activity, forming acid from many carbohydrates, but have no proteolytic activity. Nitrate reduction, catalase, urease, ALP and indole production are all negative; aesculin is weakly fermented. VFAs formed are formate and acetate. The organism has rarely been isolated from human clinical specimens. The G + C content of DNA is 43–45 mol% and the type strain is NCTC 11829 (= ATCC 27340).

10.4   Other genera

Coprococcus

This genus was proposed by Holdeman and Moore (1974) to include gram-positive, obligately anaerobic cocci for which fermentable carbohydrates are required or highly stimulatory, and which form butyric acid. They do not form spores and are differentiated from *Ruminococcus* by production of butyric acid; however, Ezaki et al. (1994) suggested that these genera

might be better classified together. Coprococci are unlikely to grow on routine media; methods for their isolation have been described (Holdeman, Cato and Moore 1977, Ezaki, Oyaizu and Yabuuchi 1992). There are 3 species, all described from the human gastrointestinal tract; they have not yet been reported from clinical specimens (Holdeman Moore and Moore 1986). The G + C content of DNA is 39–42 mol%.

Sarcina

This is a little-studied genus of gram-positive, obligately anaerobic cocci characteristically arranged in packets of 8. The organisms can form endospores and 16S rRNA sequence data indicate that *Sarcina ventriculi* is closely related to *Clostridium perfringens* and *P. anaerobius* (Collins et al. 1994, Ezaki et al. 1994). *S. ventriculi* is placed by Collins et al. (1994) in *Clostridium* cluster I. The species require fermentable carbohydrate, will grow at pH 2.0–2.5, and can be selected out using *Bifidobacterium* medium (Ezaki, Oyaizu and Yabuuchi 1992). Two species have been described, both isolated from the human gastrointestinal tract and also from soil. *S. ventriculi* has been cultured from human vomitus (Ezaki, Oyaizu and Yabuuchi 1992). The G + C content of DNA is 28–31 mol%.

Atopobium

The genus *Atopobium* was proposed by Collins and Wallbanks (1992) on the basis of 16S rRNA sequence data. The organisms are gram-positive, obligately anaerobic cocci or rods occurring in pairs or short chains; they do not form spores. Major metabolic products are acetic and lactic acids. *Atopobium parvulum*, formerly in the genus *Peptostreptococcus*, later *Streptococcus* (Cato 1983), is weakly saccharolytic and proteolytic. The type strain will grow slowly on commercial media to form tiny translucent colonies after 5 days; its growth is stimulated by Tween 80. Its principal habitat is unknown. The G + C content of DNA is 35–46 mol% and the type strain is ATCC 33793.

References

Bartlett JG, 1990, Anaerobic cocci, *The Principles and Practice of Infectious Diseases*, 3rd edn, eds Mandell GL, Douglas RG, Bennett JE, Churchill Livingstone, New York, 1867–9.

Bartlett JG, Onderdonk AB et al., 1977, Quantitative bacteriology of the vaginal flora, *J Infect Dis*, **136:** 271–7.

Bourgault A-M, Rosenblatt JE, Fitzgerald RH, 1980, *Peptococcus magnus*: a significant human pathogen, *Ann Intern Med*, **93:** 244–8.

Brook I, 1981, Bacteriology of intracranial abscess in children, *J Neurosurg*, **54:** 484–8.

Brook I, 1986, Encapsulated anaerobic bacteria in synergistic infections, *Microbiol Rev*, **50:** 452–7.

Brook I, 1988a, Recovery of anaerobic bacteria from clinical specimens in 12 years at two military hospitals, *J Clin Microbiol*, **26:** 1181–8.

Brook I, 1988b, Enhancement of growth of aerobic, anaerobic, and facultative bacteria in mixed infections with anaerobic and facultative Gram-positive cocci, *J Surg Res*, **45:** 222–7.

Brook I, 1989a, Anaerobic bacterial bacteremia: 12-year experience in two military hospitals, *J Infect Dis*, **160:** 1071–5.

Brook I, 1989b, Microbiology of post-thoracotomy sternal wound infection, *J Clin Microbiol*, **27:** 806–7.

Brook I, 1995, Anaerobic cocci, *The Principles and Practice of Infectious Diseases*, 4th edn, eds Mandell GL, Bennett JE, Dolin R, Churchill Livingstone, New York, 2204–6.

Brook I, Frazier EH, Thompson DH, 1992, Aerobic and anaerobic microbiology of external otitis, *Clin Infect Dis*, **15:** 955–8.

Brown MA, Greene JN et al., 1994, Anaerobic meningitis caused by *Peptostreptococcus magnus* after head and neck surgery, *Am J Med Sci*, **308:** 184–5.

Bryant MP, 1986, Genus *Ruminococcus*, *Bergey's Manual of Systematic Bacteriology*, vol. 2, ed. Sneath PHA, Williams & Wilkins, Baltimore, 1093–7.

Cato EP, 1983, Transfer of *Peptostreptococcus parvulus* (Weinberg, Nativelle, and Prevot 1937) Smith 1957 to the genus *Streptococcus*: *Streptococcus parvulus* (Weinberg, Nativelle, and Prevot 1937) comb. nov., nom. rev., emend., *Int J Syst Bacteriol*, **33:** 82–4.

Cato EP, Johnson JL et al., 1983, Synonymy of *Peptococcus glycinophilus* (Cardon and Barker 1946) Douglas 1957 with *Peptostreptococcus micros* (Prevot 1933) Smith 1957 and electrophoretic differentiation of *Peptostreptococcus micros* from *Peptococcus magnus* (Prevot 1933) Holdeman and Moore 1972, *Int J Syst Bacteriol*, **33:** 207–10.

Cofsky RD, Seligman SJ, 1985, *Peptococcus magnus* endocarditis, *South Med J*, **78**: 361–2.

Colebrook L, Hare R, 1933, The anaerobic streptococci associated with puerperal fever, *J Obstet Gynaecol*, **40**: 609–30.

Collins MD, Wallbanks S, 1992, Comparative sequence analyses of the 16S rRNA genes of *Lactobacillus minutus*, *Lactobacillus rimae* and *Streptococcus parvulus*: proposal for the creation of a new genus *Atopobium*, *FEMS Microbiol Lett*, **74**: 235–40.

Collins MD, Lawson PA et al., 1994, The phylogeny of the genus *Clostridium*: proposal of five new genera and eleven new species combinations, *Int J Syst Bacteriol*, **44**: 812–26.

Collins MLZ, Falkler WA et al., 1989, Serological studies of peptostreptococci using an indirect fluorescent antibody test, *J Dent Res*, **68**: 1508–12.

van Dalen PJ, van Steenbergen TJ et al., 1993, Description of two morphotypes of *Peptostreptococcus micros*, *Int J Syst Bacteriol*, **43**: 787–93.

Davies UM, Leak AM, Dave J, 1988, Infection of a prosthetic knee joint with *Peptostreptococcus magnus*, *Ann Rheum Dis*, **47**: 866–8.

DiZerega GS, Yonekura ML et al., 1980, Bacteremia in post-caesarean section endomyometritis: differential response to therapy, *Obstet Gynecol*, **55**: 587–90.

Edmiston CE, Walker AP et al., 1990, The non-puerperal breast infection: aerobic and anaerobic microbial recovery from acute and chronic disease, *J Infect Dis*, **162**: 695–9.

Edson RS, Rosenblatt JE et al., 1982, Recent experience with antimicrobial susceptibility of anaerobic bacteria; increasing resistance to penicillin, *Mayo Clin Proc*, **57**: 737–41.

Evans CA, Mattern KL, Hallam SL, 1978, Isolation and identification of *Peptococcus saccharolyticus* from human skin, *J Clin Microbiol*, **7**: 261–4.

Ezaki T, Oyaizu H, Yabuuchi E, 1992, The anaerobic gram-positive cocci, *The Prokaryotes*, 2nd edn, ed Balows A, Springer-Verlag, New York, 1879–92.

Ezaki T, Yabuuchi E, 1985, Oligopeptidase activity of Gram-positive anaerobic cocci used for rapid identification, *J Gen Appl Microbiol*, **31**: 255–65.

Ezaki T, Yamamoto N et al., 1983, Transfer of *Peptococcus indolicus*, *Peptococcus asaccharolyticus*, *Peptococcus prevotii* and *Peptococcus magnus* to the genus *Peptostreptococcus* and proposal of *Peptostreptococcus tetradius* sp. nov., *Int J Syst Bacteriol*, **33**: 683–98.

Ezaki T, Liu S-L et al., 1990, *Peptostreptococcus hydrogenalis* sp. nov. from human faecal and vaginal flora, *Int J Syst Bacteriol*, **40**: 305–6.

Ezaki T, Li N et al., 1994, 16S ribosomal DNA sequences of anaerobic cocci and proposal of *Ruminococcus hansenii* comb. nov. and *Ruminococcus productus* comb. nov., *Int J Syst Bacteriol*, **44**: 130–6.

Felner JM, Dowell VR, 1970, Anaerobic bacterial endocarditis, *N Engl J Med*, **22**: 1188–92.

Finegold SM, 1988, Susceptibility testing of anaerobic bacteria, *J Clin Microbiol*, **26**: 1253–6.

Finegold SM, Attebery HR, Sutter VL, 1974, Effect of diet on human fecal flora: comparison of Japanese and American diets, *Am J Clin Nutr*, **27**: 1456–69.

Finegold SM, George WL, 1989, *Anaerobic Infections in Humans*, Academic Press, New York.

Fitzgerald RH, Rosenblatt JE et al., 1982, Anaerobic septic arthritis, *Clin Orthop*, **164**: 141–8.

Foubert EL, Douglas HC, 1948, Studies on the anaerobic micrococci. I. Taxonomic considerations, *J Bacteriol*, **56**: 25–34.

Garcia-Rodriguez JA, Garcia-Sanchez JE, Munoz-Bellido JL, 1995, Antimicrobial resistance in anaerobic bacteria: current situation, *Anaerobe*, **1**: 69–80.

Graves MH, Morello JA, Kocka FE, 1974, Sodium polyanethol sulfonate sensitivity of anaerobic cocci, *Appl Microbiol*, **27**: 1131–3.

Greenwood D, Palfreyman J, 1987, Comparative activity of

LY146032 against anaerobic cocci, *Eur J Clin Microbiol*, **6**: 682–4.

Gunaratnam M, Smith GLF et al., 1992, Enumeration of subgingival species on primary isolation plates using colony lifts, *Oral Microbiol Immunol*, **7**: 14–18.

Hare R, Polunin I, 1960, Anaerobic cocci in the vagina of native women in British North Borneo, *J Obstet Gynaecol Br Empire*, **67**: 985–9.

Hare R, Wildy P et al., 1952, The anaerobic cocci: gas formation, fermentation reactions, sensitivity to antibiotics and sulphonamides. Classification, *J Hyg*, **50**: 295–319.

Harpold DJ, Wasilauskas BL, 1987, Rapid identification of obligately anaerobic Gram-positive cocci using high-pressure liquid chromatography, *J Clin Microbiol*, **25**: 996–1001.

Heginbothom M, Fitzgerald TC, Wade WG, 1990, Comparison of solid media for cultivation of anaerobes, *J Clin Pathol*, **43**: 253–6.

Hillier SL, Watts DH et al., 1990, Etiology and treatment of post caesarean section endometritis after cephalosporin prophylaxis, *J Reprod Med*, **35**: 322–8.

Hillier SL, Moncla BJ, 1995, *Peptostreptococcus*, *Propionibacterium*, *Eubacterium* and other nonsporeforming anaerobic Gram-positive bacteria, *Manual of Clinical Microbiology*, 6th edn, eds Murray PR, Baron EJ et al., ASM Press, Washington, DC, 587–602.

Holdeman LV, Cato EP, Moore WEC, 1977, *Anaerobe Laboratory Manual*, 4th edn, Anaerobe Laboratory, Virginia Polytechnic Institute and State University, Blacksburg.

Holdeman LV, Moore WEC, 1974, New genus, *Coprococcus*, twelve new species, and emended descriptions of four previously described species of bacteria from human faeces, *Int J Syst Bacteriol*, **24**: 260–77.

Holdeman Moore LV, Johnson JL, Moore WEC, 1986, Genus *Peptococcus*, genus *Peptostreptococcus*, *Bergey's Manual of Systematic Bacteriology*, vol. 2, ed. Sneath PHA, Williams & Wilkins, Baltimore, 1082–92.

Holdeman Moore LV, Moore WEC, 1986, Genus *Coprococcus*, *Bergey's Manual of Systematic Bacteriology*, vol. 2, ed. Sneath PHA, Williams & Wilkins, Baltimore, 1097–9.

Holland JW, Hill EO, Altemeier WA, 1977, Numbers and types of anaerobic bacteria isolated from clinical specimens since 1960, *J Clin Microbiol*, **5**: 20–5.

Huss VAR, Festl H, Schleifer KH, 1984, Nucleic acid hybridisation studies and deoxyribonucleic acid base compositions of anaerobic Gram-positive cocci, *Int J Syst Bacteriol*, **34**: 95–101.

Jokipii AMM, Jokipii L et al., 1988, Semiquantitative culture results and pathogenic significance of obligate anaerobes in peritonsillar abscesses, *J Clin Microbiol*, **26**: 957–61.

Karachewski NO, Busch EL, Wells CL, 1985, Comparison of PRAS II, RapID ANA, and API 20A systems for identification of anaerobic bacteria, *J Clin Microbiol*, **21**: 122–6.

Kastern W, Holst E et al., 1990, Protein L, a bacterial immunoglobulin-binding protein and possible virulence determinant, *Infect Immun*, **58**: 1217–22.

Kilpper-Baelz R, Schleifer KH, 1981, Transfer of *Peptococcus saccharolyticus* Foubert and Douglas to the genus, *Staphylococcus*: *Staphylococcus saccharolyticus* (Foubert and Douglas) comb. nov. *Zentralbl Bakteriol Parasitenkd Infektionskr Hyg Abt I Orig Reihe C*, **2**: 324–31.

King A, Phillips I, 1988, European collaborative study of reproducibility of quantitative sensitivity testing of anaerobes, *J Antimicrob Chemother*, **21**: 425–38.

Kluyver AJ, van Niel CB, 1936, Prospects for a natural system of classification of bacteria, *Zentralbl Bakteriol Parasitenkd Infektionskr Hyg Abt II*, **94**: 369–403.

Krepel CJ, Gohr CM et al., 1991, Anaerobic pathogenesis: collagenase production by *Peptostreptococcus magnus* and its relationship to site of infection, *J Infect Dis*, **163**: 1148–50.

Krepel CJ, Gohr CM et al., 1992, Enzymatically active *Peptostreptococcus magnus*: association with site of infection, *J Clin Microbiol*, **30**: 2330–4.

Lanigan GW, 1976, *Peptococcus heliotrinreducens* sp. nov., a cytochrome-reducing anaerobe which, metabolises pyrrolizidine alkaloids, *J Gen Microbiol*, **94**: 1–10.

Lawson PA, Llop-Perez P et al., 1993, Towards a phylogeny of the clostridia based on 16S rRNA sequences, *FEMS Microbiol Lett*, **113**: 87–92.

Li N, Hashimoto Y, Ezaki T, 1994, Determination of 16S ribosomal RNA sequences of all members of the genus *Peptostreptococcus* and their phylogenetic position, *FEMS Microbiol Lett*, **116**: 1–6.

Li N, Hashimoto Y et al., 1992, Three new species of the genus *Peptostreptococcus* isolated from humans: *Peptostreptococcus vaginalis* sp. nov., *Peptostreptococcus lacrimalis* sp. nov. and *Peptostreptococcus lactolyticus* sp. nov., *Int J Syst Bacteriol*, **42**: 602–5.

Madsen M, Aalbaek B, Hansen JW, 1992, Comparative bacteriological studies on summer mastitis in grazing cattle and pyogenes mastitis in stabled cattle in Denmark, *Vet Microbiol*, **32**: 81–8.

Moore WEC, Holdeman LVH et al., 1982, Bacteriology of severe periodontitis in young adult humans, *Infect Immun*, **38**: 1137–1148.

Murdoch DA, Magee JT, 1995, A numerical taxonomic study of the gram-positive anaerobic cocci, *J Med Microbiol*, **43**: 148–55.

Murdoch DA, Mitchelmore IJ, 1989, Isolation of *Peptostreptococcus heliotrinreducens* from human polymicrobial abscesses, *Lett Appl Microbiol*, **9**: 223–5.

Murdoch DA, Mitchelmore IJ, 1991, The laboratory identification of Gram-positive anaerobic cocci, *J Med Microbiol*, **34**: 295–308.

Murdoch DA, Mitchelmore IJ, Tabaqchali S, 1988a, Identification of Gram-positive anaerobic cocci by use of systems for detecting preformed enzymes, *J Med Microbiol*, **25**: 289–93.

Murdoch DA, Mitchelmore IJ, Tabaqchali S, 1988b, *Peptostreptococcus micros* in polymicrobial abscesses, *Lancet*, **1**: 594.

Murdoch DA, Mitchelmore IJ, Tabaqchali S, 1994, The clinical importance of gram-positive anaerobic cocci isolated at St Bartholomew's Hospital, London, in 1987, *J Med Microbiol*, **41**: 36–44.

National Committee for Clinical Laboratory Standards, 1990, *Methods for Antimicrobial Susceptibility Testing of Anaerobic Bacteria*, 2nd edn, NCCLS, Villanova, PA, 218.

Neut C, Lesieur V et al., 1985, Analysis of Gram-positive anaerobic cocci in oral, faecal and vaginal flora, *Eur J Clin Microbiol*, **4**: 435–7.

Ng J, Ng L-K et al., 1994, Identification of five *Peptostreptococcus* species isolated predominantly from the female genital tract by using the rapid ID32A system, *J Clin Microbiol*, **32**: 1302–7.

Ng L-K, Dillon J-A R, 1991, Molecular fingerprinting of isolates of the genus *Peptostreptococcus* using rRNA genes from *Escherichia coli* and *P. anaerobius*, *J Gen Microbiol*, **137**: 1323–31.

Nilson BH, Solomon A et al., 1992, Protein L from *Peptostreptococcus magnus* binds to the kappa light chain variable domain, *J Biol Chem*, **267**: 2234–9.

Ohm-Smith MJ, Sweet RL, Hadley WK, 1986, Occurrence of clindamycin-resistant anaerobic bacteria isolated from cultures taken following clindamycin therapy, *Antimicrob Agents Chemother*, **30**: 11–14.

Panagou P, Papandreou L, Bouros D, 1991, Severe anaerobic necrotizing pneumonia complicated by pyopneumothorax and anaerobic monoarthritis due to *Peptostreptococcus magnus*, *Respiration*, **58**: 223–5.

Panichi G, Di Rosa R et al., 1990, Anaerobic bacteria and bacterial infections: perspectives on treatment and resistance in Italy, *Rev Infect Dis*, **12**: S1252–6.

Paster BJ, Russell JB et al., 1993, Phylogeny of the ammonia-producing ruminal bacteria *Peptostreptococcus anaerobius*, *Clostridium sticklandii* and *Clostridium aminophilum* sp. nov., *Int J Syst Bacteriol*, **43**: 107–10.

Phelps R, Jacobs RA, 1985, Purulent pericarditis and mediastinitis due to *Peptococcus magnus*, *JAMA*, **254**: 947–8.

Porschen RK, Spaulding EH, 1974, Fluorescent antibody study of the Gram-positive anaerobic cocci, *Appl Microbiol*, **28**: 851–5.

Pouedras P, Donnio PY et al., 1992, Prosthetic valve endocarditis and paravalvular abscess caused by *Peptostreptococcus magnus*, *Clin Infect Dis*, **15**: 185.

Prevot AR, 1948, *Manuel de Classification et de Determination des Bacteries Anaerobies*, 2nd edn, Masson, Paris.

Rainey FA, Janssen PH, 1995, Phylogenetic analysis by 16S ribosomal DNA sequence comparison reveals two unrelated groups of species within the genus *Ruminococcus*, *FEMS Microbiol Lett*, **129**: 69–74.

Rams TE, Feik D et al., 1992, *Peptostreptococcus micros* in human periodontitis, *Oral Microbiol Immunol*, **7**: 1–6.

Reig M, Baquero F, 1994, Antibacterial activity of clavulanate and tazobactam on *Peptostreptococcus* spp., *J Antimicrob Chemother*, **33**: 358–9.

Reig M, Moreno A, Baquero F, 1992, Resistance of *Peptostreptococcus* spp. to macrolides and lincosamides: inducible and constitutive phenotypes, *Antimicrob Agents Chemother*, **36**: 662–4.

Rogosa M, 1971, Peptococcaceae, a new family to include the Gram-positive, anaerobic cocci of the genera *Peptococcus*, *Peptostreptococcus*, and *Ruminococcus*, *Int J Syst Bacteriol*, **21**: 234–7.

Rogosa M, 1974, Family III. Peptococcaceae, *Bergey's Manual of Determinative Bacteriology*, 8th edn, eds Buchanan RE, Gibbons NE, Williams & Wilkins, Baltimore, 517–27.

Rosenblatt JE, 1985, Anaerobic cocci, *Manual of Clinical Microbiology*, 4th edn, eds Lennette EH, Balows A et al., American Society for Microbiology, Washington, DC, 445–9.

Sanchez ML, Jones RN, Croco JL, 1992, Use of the E-Test to assess macrolide-lincosamide resistance patterns among *Peptostreptococcus* species, *Antimicrobic Newslett*, **8**: 45–52.

Sanderson PJ, 1977, Infection of the foot with *Peptococcus magnus*, *J Clin Pathol*, **30**: 266–8.

Schiefer-Ullrich H, Andreesen JR, 1985, *Peptostreptococcus barnesae* sp. nov., a Gram-positive, anaerobic, obligately purine-utilising coccus from chicken faeces, *Arch Microbiol*, **143**: 26–31.

Schwarz O, Dieckman WJ, 1926, Anaerobic streptococci: their role in puerperal infection, *South Med J*, **19**: 470–9.

Skerman VBD, MacGowan V, Sneath PHA, 1980, Approved lists of bacterial names, *Int J Syst Bacteriol*, **30**: 225–40.

Smith GLF, Cumming CG, Ross PW, 1986a, Survival of Gram-positive anaerobic cocci on swabs and their isolation from the mouth and vagina, *J Clin Pathol*, **39**: 93–8.

Smith GLF, Cumming CG, Ross PW, 1986b, Analysis of EDTA-soluble cell surface components of Gram-positive anaerobic cocci, *J Gen Microbiol*, **132**: 1591–7.

Socransky SS, Haffajee AD et al., 1988, Associations between microbial species in subgingival plaque samples, *Oral Microbiol Immunol*, **3**: 1–7.

Summanen P, Baron EJ et al., 1993, *Wadsworth Anaerobic Bacteriology Manual*, 5th edn, Star, Los Angeles.

Sutter VL, 1984, Anaerobes as normal oral flora, *Rev Infect Dis*, **6, Suppl. 1**: S62–3.

Sutter VL, Finegold SM, 1971, Antibiotic disc susceptibility tests for rapid presumptive identification of Gram-negative anaerobic bacilli, *Appl Microbiol*, **21**: 13–20.

Sutter VL, Citron DM et al., 1985, *Wadsworth Anaerobic Bacteriology Manual*, 4th edn, Star, Los Angeles.

Tally FP, Stewart PR et al., 1975, Oxygen tolerance of fresh clinical anaerobic bacteria, *J Clin Microbiol*, **1**: 161–4.

Tam Y-C, Chan ECS, 1983, Phase variation of hyaluronidase-producing peptostreptococci associated with periodontal disease, *J Dent Res*, **62**: 1009–12.

Taylor EA, Jackman PJH, Phillips I, 1991, The differentiation of asaccharolytic anaerobic Gram-positive cocci by protein electrophoresis, *J Med Microbiol*, **34**: 339–48.

Thomas CGA, Hare R, 1954, The classification of anaerobic cocci and their isolation in normal human beings and pathological processes, *J Clin Pathol*, **7**: 300–4.

Topiel MS, Simon GL, 1986, Peptococcaceae bacteremia, *Diagn Microbiol Infect Dis*, **4**: 109–17.

Watt B, Brown FV, 1983, A selective agent for anaerobic cocci, *J Clin Pathol*, **36**: 605–6.

Watt B, Brown FV, 1986, Is ciprofloxacin active against clinically important anaerobes? *J Antimicrob Chemother*, **17**: 605–13.

Watt B, Jack EP, 1977, What are anaerobic cocci? *J Med Microbiol*, **10**: 461–8.

Watt B, Smith GLF, 1990, Anaerobic cocci, *Topley & Wilson's Principles of Bacteriology, Virology and Immunology*, 8th edn, eds Parker MT, Collier LH, Edward Arnold, London, 247–53.

Watt B, Young O, McCurdy G, 1979, The susceptibility of anaerobic cocci from clinical samples to six antimicrobial agents, *J Infect Dis*, **1**: 143–9.

Wexler HM, Finegold SM, 1988, In vitro activity of cefoperazone plus sulbactam compared with that of other antimicrobial agents against anaerobic bacteria, *Antimicrob Agents Chemother*, **32**: 403–6.

Wexler HM, Molitoris E, Finegold SM, 1993, In vitro activity of Bay Y3118 against anaerobic bacteria, *Antimicrob Agents Chemother*, **37**: 2509–13.

Wheat LJ, Allen SD et al., 1986, Diabetic foot infections, *Arch Intern Med*, **146**: 1935–40.

Wideman PA, Vargo VL et al., 1976, Evaluation of the sodium polyanethol sulfonate disk test for the identification of *Peptostreptococcus anaerobius*, *J Clin Microbiol*, **4**: 330–3.

Wilkins DT, Moore WEC et al., 1975, *Peptococcus niger* (Hall) Kluyver and van Niel 1936: emendation of description and designation of neotype strain, *Int J Syst Bacteriol*, **25**: 47–9.

Williams BL, McCann GF, Schoenknecht FD, 1983, Bacteriology of dental abscesses of endodontic origin, *J Clin Microbiol*, **18**: 770–4.

Wong M, Catena A, Hadley WK, 1980, Antigenic relationships and rapid identification of *Peptostreptococcus* species, *J Clin Microbiol*, **11**: 515–21.

Wren MWD, 1980, Multiple selective media for the isolation of anaerobic bacteria from clinical specimens, *J Clin Pathol*, **33**: 61–5.

Wren MWD, Baldwin AWF et al., 1977, The anaerobic culture of clinical specimens: a 14-month study, *J Med Microbiol*, **10**: 49–61.

Yasui S, 1989, Development and clinical application of DNA probe specific for *Peptostreptococcus micros*, *Bull Tokyo Med Dent Univ*, **36**: 49–62.

Yasui S, Reynolds HS et al., 1989, Development of specific DNA probe for the identification of *Peptostreptococcus anaerobius*, *J Dent Res*, **68**: 256.

Chapter 34

Mycoplasmas, Ureaplasmas, Spiroplasmas and Related Organisms

D Taylor-Robinson and J G Tully

1 Class, genus and species definition	10 Metabolism and biochemical and biological reactions
2 Introduction and historical perspective	11 Susceptibility to physical and chemical agents
3 Classification, nomenclature and phylogeny	12 Antigenic composition and serological behaviour
4 Habitat	13 Mycoplasma viruses and plasmids
5 Cellular morphology	14 Mollicutes in cell cultures
6 Mode of reproduction	15 Pathogenicity
7 Growth requirements and media formulations	
8 Colonial morphology	
9 Chemical and structural composition	

1 CLASS, GENUS AND SPECIES DEFINITION

Organisms in the class Mollicutes are microscopically visible and extremely pleomorphic. Most cells vary in shape from coccoid to branched or unbranched filamentous forms, whereas others have a definite helical structure. They possess a triple-layered limiting membrane but no rigid cell wall. The smallest viable forms can pass through membrane filters of average pore diameter between 450 and 200 nm. Although most viable spherical cells are around 300 nm, some helical filaments can be as small as 200 nm in diameter. They possess no flagella or pili but many are motile and exhibit translational movement, especially helical mollicutes. They are gram-negative, stain poorly with other bacterial stains but stain well with Giemsa. Growth occurs in nutrient media in the absence of living tissue cells but most species require animal protein; organisms of the genera *Mycoplasma*, *Ureaplasma*, *Entomoplasma*, *Anaeroplasma* and most *Spiroplasma* species require sterol for growth. Species in the genera *Acholeplasma*, *Asteroleplasma*, *Mesoplasma* and a few *Spiroplasma* species have no sterol requirement. Apart from the strictly anaerobic mollicutes (anaeroplasmas and asteroleplasmas), most other mollicutes are facultatively anaerobic, growth often being optimal anaerobically or in an atmosphere containing added CO_2. Most species on solid media form characteristic small 'fried-egg' colonies showing central growth in the medium; the smallest colonies are produced by organisms of the genus *Ureaplasma*. Many species ferment carbohydrates, others hydrolyse arginine, and organisms of the genus *Ureaplasma* hydrolyse urea. All are readily destroyed by heat. Antigenic specificity is usual, and growth is inhibited by specific antiserum and by broad spectrum antibiotics, such as the tetracyclines, but not by the penicillins. The organisms exhibit a considerable degree of host specificity. Some species are pathogenic, causing mainly respiratory tract and genital tract disease in vertebrates, or plant and insect diseases. A large cluster of the plant pathogenic mollicutes (now termed phytoplasmas), which are transmitted by insect vectors or grafting, has not been cultured successfully on artificial medium. Many species of mollicutes occur as part of the normal vertebrate or plant/insect flora. The G + C content of DNA is mostly in the range 24–36 mol%.

The type species are: *Mycoplasma mycoides* subsp. *mycoides*; *Acholeplasma laidlawii*; *Ureaplasma urealyticum*; *Spiroplasma citri*; *Mesoplasma florum*; *Entomoplasma ellychniae*; *Anaeroplasma abactoclasticum*; and *Asteroleplasma anaerobium*.

2 INTRODUCTION AND HISTORICAL PERSPECTIVE

The organism causing bovine pleuropneumonia, later

designated *Mycoplasma mycoides* subsp. *mycoides* (Borrel et al. 1910), was grown in cell-free medium 100 years ago (Nocard et al. 1896) and organisms of a similar nature isolated subsequently from other sources were called pleuropneumonia-like organisms (PPLO). Only much later were they termed mycoplasmas and then mollicutes (see section 3). Interest in them was stimulated in the late 1930s and early 1940s by their isolation from laboratory animals and fowl and the finding that, in some instances, they were the cause of disease. In particular, the work of Klieneberger (later Klieneberger-Nobel) in the UK, and Sabin and Nelson in the USA, during this period did much to illuminate the nature and pathogenicity of mycoplasmas, especially for rats and mice (Tully 1980). Furthermore, the first account of the isolation of a mycoplasma of human origin also appeared at this time (Dienes and Edsall 1937), coming from a Bartholin's abscess. Twenty-five years later, the realization that the organism that caused some cases of primary atypical pneumonia of humans, first termed the Eaton agent, was not a virus but a mycoplasma (Chanock, Hayflick and Barile 1962) had a stimulating effect on research in the whole field. Indeed, there are now few mammalian or avian species from which a mycoplasma has not been isolated. Some of these organisms are responsible primarily for the disease with which they are associated, others are looked upon as opportunist pathogens or secondary invaders and some appear to be simply part of the commensal flora of various hosts. Since their first recognition in eukaryotic cell cultures (Robinson, Wichelhausen and Roizman 1956), mycoplasmas have been found frequently as cell contaminants, particularly in continuous cell lines and in hybridomas, and they continue to have a major deleterious impact on the quality and reliability of research undertaken with such cells. However, the use of cell cultures has enabled the relationship between mycoplasmas and tissues to be studied in greater detail (Barile 1979), including the more recent finding that some mollicutes clearly become intracellular (Lo et al. 1989, Baseman et al. 1995, Taylor-Robinson 1996a). Furthermore, growth of some of the more fastidious mycoplasmas has been accomplished only through use of cell culture systems (Montagnier et al. 1990, Hackett and Lynn 1995). Finally, the last 3 decades have seen an unfolding of an enormous number and diversity of new mollicutes discovered in plants and insects. These developments have contributed to a better understanding of the host relationships of mollicutes and of the ability of these wall-less prokaryotes to incite disease in a variety of hosts, including both plants and insects (Whitcomb and Tully 1989, Tully and Whitcomb 1991). Studies on the occurrence and biology of these new mollicutes have also advanced knowledge on mollicutes of man and animals, since the use of new culture medium formulations developed for plant and insect mollicutes (such as that designated SP-4) (see section 7, p. 806) has resulted in primary isolation of previously unknown species of *Mycoplasma* from both man and animals (Tully et al. 1981, McGarrity et al. 1983, Lo et al. 1992).

3 CLASSIFICATION, NOMENCLATURE AND PHYLOGENY

The term 'mycoplasma' was introduced in 1929 by Nowak and was the first acceptable generic name for what appeared to be related wall-less organisms. This designation, which joined 'myco' (Greek *mykes*, meaning fungus) with 'plasma' (Latin or Greek, meaning something formed or moulded), referred to the mycelial-like, filamentous or pleomorphic forms of the organisms and to the plasticity of their outer membrane. The latter is attributable to the absence of a cell wall and to the inability of mycoplasmas to synthesize the peptidoglycan polymer or its precursors. The major features that distinguish the mollicutes from other bacteria and viruses are summarized in Table 34.1.

The order Mycoplasmatales, first proposed by Freundt (1955) for about 12 distinct species, was later incorporated into the joint proposal of Edward and Freundt (1967) for elevation of wall-less bacteria to the taxonomic level of class Mollicutes. These developments were based upon the isolation and description of an expanding and diverse group of organisms within the 'mycoplasmas', including wall-less organisms that differed in some biochemical activities (ureaplasmas) or sterol requirements (acholeplasmas) from classical mycoplasmas. Within the next decade, new helical mollicutes (genus *Spiroplasma*) and a group of strictly anaerobic mollicutes (genera *Anaeroplasma* and *Asteroleplasma*) were discovered. By 1989 the class Mollicutes had come to represent over 100 distinct species within 6 genera and 3 orders (Mycoplasmatales, Acholeplasmatales and Anaeroplasmatales) (Tully 1989).

Although attempts to classify mollicutes on the bases of immunological, nutritional and some limited molecular features (such as DNA base composition and genome size) offered obvious advantages, these approaches lacked the value of a classification scheme based upon phylogenetic relationships. The initial characterization of mollicute 16S rRNA oligonucleotide cataloguing by Woese, Maniloff and Zablen (1980) indicated that the organisms were phylogenetically related to the gram-positive bacteria with low G + C DNA compositions, the bacillus-lactobacillus cluster, and more specifically to a small subgroup represented by *Clostridium innocuum* and *Clostridium ramosum*. These evolutionary relationships were confirmed by the use of 5S rRNA sequence analysis (Hori et al. 1981, Rogers et al. 1985) and it was proposed that the divergence of mollicutes from the clostridial branch involved a major genome reduction to form the *Acholeplasma* branch of the mollicutes, with further divergence to form the *Spiroplasma/Mycoplasma* stem (Rogers et al. 1985). These findings were further confirmed and considerably extended in the phylogenetic analysis by Weisburg et al. (1989), which compared 16S rRNA sequences of more than 40 species of mollicutes and 6 of their walled bacterial relatives. This

Table 34.1 Characteristics of mycoplasmas compared to those of bacteria, chlamydiae and viruses

Character	Mycoplasmas	Bacteria	Chlamydiae	Viruses
Size (diameter)	0.3 μm[a]	1–2 μm	0.3 μm	<0.5 μm
Cell wall	–	+	+	–
Contain both DNA and RNA	+	+	+	–
Multiply in cell-free medium	+	+	–	–
Multiplication dependent on host-cell nucleic acid	–	–	–	+
Usually require sterol and native protein for propagation	+	–	–	–
Intrinsic energy metabolism	+	+	+	–
Range of host specificity usually narrow	+	–	–	+
Growth inhibited by specific antibody alone	+	–	+	+
Resist cell-wall active antibiotics (e.g. penicillins)	+	–	–	+
Resist antibiotics which inhibit metabolism (e.g. tetracyclines)	–	–	–	+

[a]Smallest organism capable of propagation.

work resulted in the proposal of 5 specific phylogenetic groups: pneumoniae (including the ureaplasmas), hominis, spiroplasma (including some mycoplasmas), acholeplasma/anaeroplasma and the asteroleplasmas.

Although these results provided a firm assurance that most of the current classification of the mollicutes followed phylogenetic relationships, several sterol-non-requiring plant and insect mollicutes assigned to the genus *Acholeplasma* were shown to be more closely related to the spiroplasma branch (Weisburg et al. 1989). These organisms were also found to differ significantly from other *Acholeplasma* spp. in their genome size, sugar transport enzyme systems and codon usage (Carle et al. 1992, Navas-Castillo et al. 1992a, 1992b). Accordingly, a proposed revision of the taxonomy of the Mollicutes provided for several new taxa to accommodate and differentiate plant and insect mollicutes with sterol needs (genus *Entomoplasma*) from such mollicutes lacking sterol for growth (genus *Mesoplasma*) (Tully et al. 1993).

More than 158 species within 4 orders and 7 genera have been described within the class Mollicutes (Table 34.2). The potential number of mollicute species now seems almost unlimited, especially in view of the increasing number of mollicutes isolated recently from insect hosts and the potential that each insect species, of the more than 30 million estimated insect species in nature, might have its own unique mollicute flora (Tully 1989, Williamson, Tully and Whitcomb 1989).

The major features that separate members of the class Mollicutes are host origin and temperature or atmospheric growth requirements (Table 34.2). Genome size and sterol requirements, which were earlier used to distinguish major taxa, have become less valuable as taxonomic markers (see sections 9 and 10, pp. 812–814). In attempts to improve the description of new species in the class Mollicutes, a revision of the minimum standards for such descriptions has been published (Subcommittee on the Taxonomy of Mollicutes 1995).

It should be noted that the terms 'mycoplasma' and 'mycoplasmas' are often used in a trivial fashion to refer to any member of the class Mollicutes, irrespective of whether they belong to the genus *Mycoplasma*. Although this usage is common, it is more accurate and less confusing to refer to the class with the trivial 'mollicute(s)', and to individual organisms with the trivial term for the genus (that is 'acholeplasmas', 'mesoplasmas', etc.). The established species in the 8 genera, including their base composition values and major biochemical activities, are given in Tables 34.3–34.7.

4 HABITAT

Mollicutes occur widely in nature, as parasites or commensals in humans, other primates and mammals, in reptiles and fish, in numerous arthropods (including insects), and in many plants (Tables 34.3–34.7). Acquisition of mollicutes is generally through direct host-to-host contact, or through a number of secondary transmissions, including aerosols or fomites, food or water, insect vectors or carriers, and nosocomial acquisition (organ or tissue transplants) (Tully 1996). Many mollicutes are inhabitants of the host genitourinary or respiratory tract and are transferred through direct oral-to-oral, genital-to-genital, or oral-to-genital contacts. Direct transmission of *U. urealyticum* from mother to neonate through in utero infection has also been documented (Waites et al. 1988). Secondary transmission through aerosols and fomites accounts for transfer of mollicutes involved in respiratory diseases of humans and animals, as well as the transfer of mollicutes considered to be part of the normal oral commensal flora. Food, such as nectar or sap, and intestinal secretions deposited on plant or other surfaces, play an important role in acquisition of mollicutes by arthropods, as does the direct ingestion of infected or colonized insects by other predatory species. Milk also accounts for some transmission of both non-pathogenic and pathogenic mollicutes to animal offspring. Insect vectors play a predominant

Table 34.2 Taxonomy and characteristics of members of the class Mollicutes

Classification	Number of recognized species	Guanine + cytosine content (mol%)	Genome size (kbp)[a]	Cholesterol requirement	Habitat	Other distinctive features
Order I: **Mycoplasmatales**						
Family I: Mycoplasmataceae						
Genus I: *Mycoplasma*	100	23–40	600–1350	Yes	Humans, animals	Optimum growth usually at 37°C
Genus II: *Ureaplasma*	6	27–30	760–1170	Yes	Humans, animals	Urea hydrolysis
Order II: **Entomoplasmatales**						
Family I: Entomoplasmataceae						
Genus I: *Entomoplasma*	5	27–29	790–1140	Yes	Insects, plants	Optimum growth 30°C
Genus II: *Mesoplasma*	12	27–30	870–1100	No	Insects, plants	Optimum growth 30°C; sustained growth in serum-free medium only with 0.04% Tween 80
Family II: Spiroplasmataceae						
Genus I: *Spiroplasma*	17	25–30	940–2400	Yes	Insects, plants	Helical filaments; optimum growth at 30–37°C
Order III: **Acholeplasmatales**						
Family I: Acholeplasmataceae						
Genus I: *Acholeplasma*	13	26–36	1500–1650	No	Animals, some plants/insects	Optimum growth at 30–37°C
Order IV: **Anaeroplasmatales**						
Family I: Anaeroplasmataceae						
Genus I: *Anaeroplasma*	4	29–34	1500–1600	Yes	Bovine/ovine rumen	Oxygen-sensitive anaerobes
Genus II: *Asteroleplasma*	1	40	1500	No	Bovine/ovine rumen	Oxygen-sensitive anaerobes

[a]Range of genome sizes, in kilobase pairs, as reported in literature.

Table 34.3 Genus mycoplasma and major characteristics

Species and type strain	DNA base composition (G + C mol%)	Metabolism of glucose/arginine[a]	Principal host
M. adleri G-145	29.6	−/+	Caprine
M. agalactiae PG2	30.5–34.2	−/−	Caprine/ovine
M. alkalescens D12	25.9	−/+	Bovine
M. alvi Ilsley	26.4	+/+	Bovine
M. anatis 1340	26.6	+/−	Avian
M. anseris 1219	24.7–26.0	−/+	Avian
M. arginini G230	27.6–28.6	−/+	Caprine/ovine
M. arthritidis PG6	30.0–32.6	−/+	Murine
M. auris U1AT	26.9	−/+	Caprine
M. bovigenitalium PG11	28.1–30.4	−/−	Bovine
M. bovirhinis PG43	24.5–27.3	+/−	Bovine
M. bovis Donetta	27.8–32.9	−/−	Bovine
M. bovoculi M165/69	29.0	+/−	Bovine
M. buccale CH20247	25.0–26.4	−/+	Human/primate
M. buteonis BbT2g	27.0	+/−	Avian
M. californicum ST-6	31.9	−/−	Bovine
M. canadense 275C	29.0	−/+	Bovine
M. canis PG14	28.4–29.1	+/−	Canine/bovine
M. capricolum			
subsp. *capricolum* Calif.Kid	24.1–25.5	+/+	Caprine
subsp. *capripneumoniae* F38	24.4	+/−	Caprine
M. caviae G122	nd[b]	+/−	Rodent/g.pig
M. cavipharyngis 117C	30.0	+/−	Rodent/g.pig
M. citelli RG-2C	27.4	+/−	Rodent/squirrel
M. cloacale 383	26.0	−/+	Avian
M. collis 58B	28.0	+/−	Canine
M. columbinasale 694	32.0	−/+	Avian
M. columbinum MMP-1	27.3	−/+	Avian
M. columborale MMP-4	29.2	+/−	Avian
M. conjunctivae HRC581	nd	+/−	Ovine/bovine
M. corogypsi BV1	28.0	+/−	Avian
M. cottewii VIS	27.0	+/−	Caprine
M. cricetuli CH	nd	+/−	Rodent/hamster
M. cynos H831	25.8	+/−	Canine
M. dispar 462/2	28.5–29.3	+/−	Bovine
M. edwardii PG24	29.2	+/−	Canine
M. equigenitalium T37	31.5	+/−	Equine
M. equirhinis M432/72	nd	−/+	Equine
M. falconis H/T1	27.5	−/+	Avian
M. fastidiosum 4822	32.3	+/−	Equine
M. faucium DC333	nd	−/+	Human/primate
M. felifaucium PU	31.0	−/+	Feline
M. feliminutum Ben	29.1	+/−	Feline
M. felis CO	25.2	+/−	Feline/equine
M. fermentans PG18	27.5–28.7	+/+	Human/primate
M. flocculare Ms42	33.0	−/−	Porcine
M. gallinaceum DD	28.0	+/−	Avian
M. gallinarum PG16	26.5–28.0	−/+	Avian
M. gallisepticum PG31	31.8–35.7	+/−	Avian
M. gallopavonis WR1	27.0	+/−	Avian
M. gateae CS	28.5	−/+	Feline
M. genitalium G37	32.4	+/−	Human
M. glycophilum 486	27.5	+/−	Avian
M. gypis B1/T1	27.1	−/+	Avian
M. hominis PG21	27.3–33.7	−/+	Human
M. hyopharyngis H3-6BF	24.0	−/+	Porcine

Table 34.3 Continued

Species and type strain	DNA base composition (G + C mol%)	Metabolism of glucose/arginine[a]	Principal host
M. hyopneumoniae J	27.5–33.0	−/−	Porcine
M. hyorhinis BTS7	27.3–27.8	+/−	Porcine
M. hyosynoviae S16	28.0	−/+	Porcine
M. imitans 4229	31.9	+/−	Avian
M. indiense 3	32.0	−/+	Primate
M. iners PG30	29.1–29.6	−/+	Avian
M. iowae 695	25.0	+/+	Avian
M. leocaptivus 3L2	27.0	+/−	Feline
M. leopharyngis LL2	28.0	−/−	Feline
M. lipofaciens R171	24.5	+/+	Avian
M. lipophilum MaBy	29.7	−/+	Human/primate
M. maculosum PG15	26.7–29.6	−/+	Canine
M. meleagridis 17529	27.0–28.6	−/+	Avian
M. moatsii MK405	25.7	+/+	Primate
M. mobile 163K	23.5	+/−	Piscine
M. molare H542	26.0	+/−	Canine
M. muris RIII4	24.9	−/+	Rodent/mice
M. mustelae MX9	28.2	+/−	Rodent/mink
M. mycoides			
subsp. *mycoides* PG1	26.1–27.1	+/−	Bovine/caprine
subsp. *capri* PG3	24.0–26.0	+/−	Caprine
M. neurolyticum Type A	22.8–26.2	+/−	Murine
M. opalescens MH5408	29.2	−/+	Canine
M. orale CH19299	24.0–28.2	−/+	Human/primate
M. ovipneumoniae Y98	25.7	+/−	Ovine
M. oxoniensis 128	29.0	+/−	Rodent/hamster
M. penetrans GTU54	30.5	+/−	Human
M. phocacerebrale 1049	25.9	−/+	Aquatic/seal
M. phocarhinis 852	26.5	−/+	Aquatic/seal
M. phocidae 105	27.8	−/+	Aquatic/seal
M. pirum 70-159	25.5	+/+	Human
M. pneumoniae FH	38.6–40.8	+/−	Human
M. primatum HRC292	28.6	−/+	Primate/human
M. pullorum CKK	29.0	+/−	Avian
M. pulmonis PG34	27.5–29.2	+/−	Murine
M. putrefaciens KS-1	28.9	+/−	Caprine
M. salivarium PG20	27.3–31.4	−/+	Human
M. simbae LX	37.0	−/+	Primate
M. spermatophilum AH159	32.0	−/+	Human
M. spumans PG13	28.4–29.1	−/+	Canine
M. sualvi Mayfield B	23.7	+/+	Porcine
M. subdolum TB	28.8	−/+	Equine
M. synoviae WVU 1853	34.2	+/−	Avian
M. testudinis 01008	35.0	+/−	Reptile/turtle
M. yeatsii GIH	26.6	+/+	Caprine
M. verecundum 107	27.0–29.2	−/−	Bovine

[a]Positive or negative responses in glucose fermentation/arginine hydrolysis tests.
[b]nd, not done.

role in transmission of spiroplasmas that cause plant diseases (citrus stubborn, corn stunt, etc.) and of phytoplasmas that cause so-called plant 'yellows' diseases. This transfer involves a clearly defined biological cycle within the insect of acquisition of organisms, multiplication in the host, and reintroduction into susceptible plants. The transmission of mollicutes through infected plant grafts to healthy rootstock and through transplantation of infected organs or tissues to healthy hosts has been demonstrated. The presence of mollicutes in semen plays some role in their sexual transmission in humans and animals, and may complicate artificial insemination programmes in such hosts.

Table 34.4   Genera *Ureaplasma* and *Acholeplasma*

Species and type strain	DNA base composition (G + C mol%)	Principal host
U. canigenitalium D6P-C	28.7	Canine
U. cati F2	28.1	Feline
U. diversum A417	26.9–27.8	Bovine
U. felinum FT2-B	27.1	Feline
U. gallorale D6-1	27.6	Avian
U. urealyticum T960	26.9–27.8	Human/primate
A. axanthum S-743	31.0	Bovine/porcine/plants
A. brassicae 0502	35.5	Plants
A. cavigenitalium GP3	36.0	Rodent/guinea pig
A. equifetale C112	30.5	Equine
A. granularum BTS39	30.0–32.0	Porcine/caprine/ovine
A. hippikon C1	33.1	Equine
A. laidlawii PG8	31.0–36.0	Many animals/plants
A. modicum PG49	29.0	Bovine/equine
A. morum 72-043	34.0	Bovine
A. multilocale PN525	31.0	Equine
A. oculi 19L	26.0–27.0	Caprine/equine
A. palmae J-233	30.0	Plants
A. parvum H23M	29.1	Equine

All *U.* species hydrolyse urea and do not ferment glucose or hydrolyse arginine. All *A.* species, except *A. parvum*, ferment glucose and do not hydrolyse arginine or urea.

Table 34.5   Genera *Anaeroplasma* and *Asteroleplasma*

Species and type strain[a]	Base composition (G + C mol%)
An. abactoclasticum 6-1	29.3–30.1
An. bactoclasticum JR	32.8–33.7
An. intermedium 7LA	32.5
An. varium A-2	33.4
Ast. anaerobium 161	39.2–40.5

[a]All species ferment glucose and do not hydrolyse arginine.

5   CELLULAR MORPHOLOGY

5.1   Light microscopy

The morphology of individual mollicutes is best seen by darkfield or phase contrast microscopy at a magnification near × 1250. The cell shape varies according to the species, the environmental conditions, and the stage of the growth cycle. Many cells are pleomorphic, ranging from spherical (300–960 nm in diameter) through coccoid, coccobacillary, ring and dumb-bell forms, to short and long branching, beaded, or segmented filaments, 300–400 nm in diameter to ≥1000 nm long (Boatman 1979). Genome replication precedes but is not necessarily synchronized with cell division, which is thought to account for the various morphological forms observed in mollicutes. The helical shape of spiroplasmas is usually characteristic, with individual cells around 200 nm in diameter, but length (from 3 to 15 μm) will vary with species (Tully and Whitcomb 1991). Some spiroplasmas may lose helicity in the stationary phase of growth, when exposed to certain fixatives, or when present in insect tissues, but cell viability is usually maintained.

5.2   Electron microscopy

The morphology of mycoplasma organisms seen by electron microscopy after negative staining reflects that seen by light microscopy. However, several mycoplasmas, including *Mycoplasma genitalium* (human) (Fig. 34.1), *Mycoplasma pneumoniae* (human) (Fig. 34.2), *Mycoplasma penetrans* (human) (Fig. 34.3), *Mycoplasma pirum* (human), *Mycoplasma alvi* (bovine), *Mycoplasma sualvi* (porcine), *Mycoplasma pulmonis* (murine), *Mycoplasma gallisepticum* (avian) and *Mycoplasma mobile* (piscine) are characterized by having specialized structures at one or both ends (Collier 1972, Tully et al. 1981, Kirchhoff et al. 1984, Tully 1986). These structures were noted first with *M. gallisepticum* ('pear-shaped blebs') (Maniloff, Morowitz and Barnett 1965) and later with *M. pneumoniae* (Biberfeld and Biberfeld 1970), and it was later established that adhesin proteins, in the form of projections (Figs 34.1 and 34.4) located at the tip structure, are involved in the attachment of the organisms to the respiratory or genital tract mucosal surface (Baseman et al. 1982, Razin and Jacobs 1992, Baseman 1993) (Fig. 34.2). Specialized terminal structures also may be involved in motion; several mycoplasmas with such structures exhibit a gliding motility in which they move tip first (Bredt 1979, Taylor-Robinson and Bredt 1983, Kirchhoff 1992). Spiroplasmas with a helical structure show rotatory and flexional movement, frequently with translational motility, and exhibit morphological polarity (namely, a blunt and a tapered

Table 34.6 Genera *Entomoplasma* and *Mesoplasma*

Species and type strain[a]	Base composition (G + C mol%)	Principal host
E. ellychniae ELCN-1	27.5	Firefly
E. lucivorax PIPN-2	27.4	Firefly
E. luminosum PIMN-1	28.8	Firefly
E. melaleucae M1	27.0	Plant/bee
E. somnilux PYAN-1	27.4	Firefly larva
Me. chauliocola CHPA-2	28.3	Beetles
Me. coleopterae BARC-779	27.8	Beetles/plants
Me. corruscae ELCA-2	26.5	Firefly
Me. entomophilum TAC	30.0	Beetles, horseflies, bees, moths, butterflies, plants
Me. florum L1	27.3	Plants/beetles
Me. grammopteriae GRUA-1	29.1	Beetles/bee
Me. lactucae 831-C4	30.0	Plant
Me. photuris PUPA-2	29.8	Fireflies
Me. pleciae PS-1	31.6	Fly maggot
Me. seiffertii F7	30.0	Plants/deerfly/mosquitoes
Me. syrphidae YJS	27.6	Flies/bee/butterfly
Me. tabanidae BARC-857	28.1	Horse fly

[a]All species ferment glucose, and with exception of *M. photuris*, do not hydrolyse arginine.

end) (Cole et al. 1973, Bové et al. 1989, Williamson, Tully and Whitcomb 1989).

Transmission electron microscopy of sections of the organisms shows various ultrastructural features. Characteristically, in all members of the mollicutes, there is an outer triple-layered membrane, 7.5–10 nm wide, the middle layer of which is less electron dense than the other 2 (Boatman 1979) (Figs 34.5 and 34.6). No cell wall of the type seen in conventional bacteria can be distinguished and its absence clearly accounts for the plasticity of the organisms. Capsular material external to the cell membrane can be observed in some mycoplasmas, the most notable being the layer of galactan seen in freshly isolated strains of *M. mycoides* subsp. *mycoides* (Buttery and Plackett 1960) and an undefined capsule in *Mycoplasma dispar* (Howard and Gourlay 1974). The capsules and other undefined surface material (Fig. 34.6), especially that observed in *M. pulmonis* (Taylor-Robinson et al. 1981), are thought to have some role in pathogenicity of the organisms.

Apart from a few species with specialized internal structures, the ultrastructure of the cytoplasm of the various members of the class Mollicutes is fairly uniform. However, the terminal structure of several mycoplasmas (for example, *M. genitalium* and *M. pneumoniae*) may exhibit a dense, central rod-like core (Figs 34.2 and 34.7) (Collier 1972, Cole et al. 1973) and some bovine or caprine mycoplasmas show a striated banding at periodic intervals along filamentous cells (Rodwell et al. 1975). Strains of *M. penetrans*, a newly isolated organism from the urine of HIV-positive patients, exhibit an elongated, flask-shape morphology and tip structure similar to *M. genitalium* (Fig. 34.3). The internal structure, however, is divided into 2 distinct compartments, containing densely packed fine granules at the narrow end of the cell and loosely packed coarse granules at the broad end of the cell (Lo et al. 1992, 1993a, Giron, Lange and Baseman 1996). The function of such internal organization is as yet unknown.

6 MODE OF REPRODUCTION

Although the mode of reproduction in mollicutes was a matter of considerable dispute in the early history of these organisms, classic binary fission is now regarded as the principal means of replication. As noted above, the numerous morphological shapes and forms observed relate to the fact that cytoplasmic division is not always synchronous with genome replication. Many of the smaller and aberrant shaped cells probably have received insufficient genetic material and are unable to replicate. In spiroplasmas, binary fission is also the mode of reproduction but cell division appears more synchronized with genome replication (Bové et al. 1989).

7 GROWTH REQUIREMENTS AND MEDIA FORMULATIONS

Mollicutes have limited biosynthetic abilities, reflecting their small genome and parasitic mode of life. Consequently, they need a rich medium containing natural animal protein and, with the exception of the acholeplasmas, asteroleplasmas and mesoplasmas, require a sterol component. Of the natural animal proteins, a combination of bovine heart infusion and an animal serum (horse, or fetal bovine), at a concentration of 10–20%, is most commonly used. Serum supplies not only cholesterol but also saturated and unsaturated fatty acids for membrane synthesis, components which the organisms are unable to synthesize (McElhaney 1992). The medium used most

Table 34.7 Group classification of the genus *Spiroplasma*

Binomial and/or common name	Group[a]	Strains[b]	G + C content (mol%)	Metabolism of glucose/arginine	Principal host	Disease incited
S. citri	I-1	Maroc-R8A2[T] (27556) C189 (27665) Israel	26	+/+	Dicots, leaf-hoppers	Citrus stubborn
S. melliferum	I-2	BC-3[T] (33219) AS 576 (29416)	26	+/+	Bees	Honeybee spiroplasmosis
S. kunkelii	I-3	E275[T] (29320) I-747 (29051) B655 (33289)	26	+/+	Maize, leaf-hoppers	Corn stunt
277F spiroplasma	I-4	277F (29761)	26	+/+	Rabbit tick	None known
Green leaf bug	I-5	LB-12 (33649)	26	+/+	Green leaf bug	None known
S. insolitum	I-6	M55[T] (33502)	28	+/+	Flowers, *Eristalis* fly	None known
Cocos spiroplasma	I-7	N525 (33287) N628	26	+/+	Coconut palm	None known
S. phoeniceum	I-8	P40[T] (43115)	26	+/+	*Catharanthus roseus*	Periwinkle disease
Sex-ratio spiroplasmas	II	DW-1 (43153)	26	nd	*Drosophila*	Sex ratio trait
S. floricola	III	23-6[T] (29989) BNR1 (33220) OBMG (33221)	26	+/−	Insects, flowers	None known
S. apis	IV	B31[T] (33834) SR3 (33095) PPS1 (33450)	30	+/+	Bees, flowers	'May disease'
S. mirum	V	SMCA[T] (29335) GT-48 (29334) TP-2 (33503)	30	+/+	Rabbit ticks	Suckling mouse cataract disease
S. ixodetis	VI	Y32[T] (33835)	25	+/−	*Ixodes pacificus* ticks	None known
S. monobiae	VII	MQ-1[T] (33825)	28	+/−	*Monobia* wasp	None known
Syrphid spiroplasma	VIII-1	EA-1 (33826)	30	+/+	*Eristalis arbustorum* fly	None known
	VIII-2	DF-1 (43209)	29	+/+	*Chrysops* deerfly	None known
	VIII-3	TAAS-1 (51123)	30	+/+	*Tabanus atratus* horsefly	None known
S. clarkii	IX	CN-5[T] (33827)	29	+/+	*Cotinus* beetle	None known
S. culicicola	X	AES-1[T] (35112)	26	+/−	*Aedes* mosquito	None known
S. velocicresens	XI	MQ-4[T] (35262)	26	+/+	*Monobia* wasp	None known

Table 34.7 Continued

Binomial and/or common name	Group[a]	Strains[b]	G + C content (mol%)	Metabolism of glucose/arginine	Principal host	Disease incited
Cucumber beetle	XII	DU-1 (43210)	25	+/−	*Diabrotica undecimpunctata* beetle	None known
S. sabaudiense	XIII	Ar-1343[T] (43303)	30	+/+	*Aedes* mosquito	None known
Ellychnia	XIV	EC-1 (43212)	26	+/−	*Ellychnia cornusca* beetle	None known
Leafhopper	XV	I-25 (43262)	26	+/−	*Cicadulina* leafhopper	None known
S. cantharicola	XVI-1	CC-1[T] (43207)	26	+/−	*Cantharis* beetle	None known
	XVI-2	CB-1 (43208)	26	+/−	beetle	None known
	XVI-3	Ar-1357 (51126)	26	+/−	mosquito	None known
VACANT[c]	XVII					
Tabanid spiroplasma	XVIII	TN-1 (43211)	25	+/−	*Tabanus nigrovittatus* horsefly	None known
Firefly spiroplasma	XIX	PUP-1 (43206)	26	+/−	*Photuris pennsylvanicus* beetle	None known
Colorado potato beetle spiroplasma	XX	LD-1 (43213)	25	+/nd	*Leptinotarsa decemlineata* beetle	None known
Flower spiroplasma	XXI	W115 (43260)	24	+/nd	*Prunus* sp. flower	None known
S. taiwanense	XXII	CT-1[T] (43302)	25	+/−	*Culex tritaeniorhynchus* mosquito	None known
Tabanid spiroplasma	XXIII	TG-1 (43525)	26	+/−	*Tabanus gladiator* horsefly	None known
S. chinense	XXIV	CCH[T] (43960)	29	+/−	*Calystegia hederaceae* flowers	None known
S. diminutum	XXV	CUAS-1[T] (49235)	26	+/+	*Culex annulus* mosquito	None known
Tentative group designations[c]	(XXVI)	PLHS-1 (51752)	31	+/+	Scorpionfly	
	(XXVII)	TALS-2 (51749)	25	+/−	Horsefly	
	(XXVIII)	PALS-1 (51748)	29	+/−	Dragonfly	
	(XXIX)	TIUS-1 (51751)	28	+/−	Tiphiid wasp	
	(XXX)	BIUS-1 (51750)	28	+/−	Flower	
	(XXXI)	HYOS-1 (51745)	28	+/+	Horsefly	
	(XXXII)	TABS-2 (51746)	28	+/−	Horsefly	
	(XXXIII)	TAUS-1 (51747)	26	+/−	Horsefly	

[a]Groups assigned on the basis of failure to cross-react in growth inhibition, metabolism inhibition and deformation serological tests.
[b]Superscript T denotes type strains. Accession numbers (in parentheses) from ATCC.
[c]Strain DF-1 previously assigned this group designation has been reclassified to group VIII-2.
nd, not done.

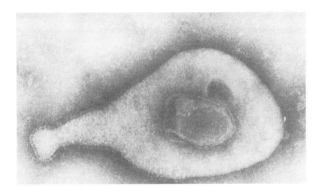

Fig. 34.1 Electron micrograph of negatively stained preparation of *Mycoplasma genitalium*; note terminal structure with surface projections (×114 000).

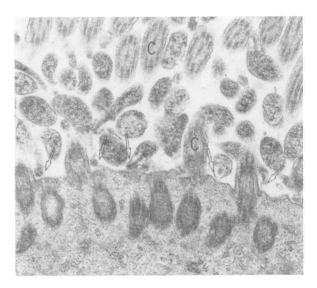

Fig. 34.2 Electron micrograph of *Mycoplasma pneumoniae* organisms (arrowed) associated with a ciliated (c) hamster tracheal cell in organ culture (×30 800).

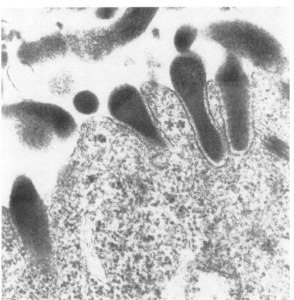

Fig. 34.3 Electron micrograph of *Mycoplasma penetrans* showing invasion of a human umbilical vein endothelial cell (×44 000).

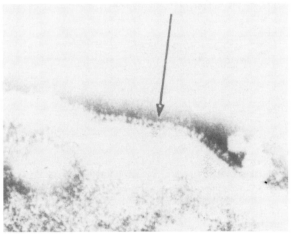

Fig. 34.4 Electron micrograph of negatively stained preparation of *Mycoplasma gallisepticum*; note coarse surface projections (arrowed) (×228 000).

widely for the isolation and growth of mycoplasmas is based on a formulation developed originally by Edward (1947). This contains a basal component of bovine heart infusion and peptone, to which are added 10% v/v of a 25% w/v extract of fresh bakers' yeast and 20% v/v of horse serum. This basic formulation, or other subsequent minor modifications reported in the literature, still provides the most useful medium for the isolation of the majority of non-fastidious mollicutes (Freundt 1983). However, in the early 1950s, it became apparent that a number of special supplements to this basic medium were essential for primary isolation, or greatly increased the isolation rate, of a number of animal mycoplasmas. Adenine dinucleotide (NAD) was found to be required for the growth of the avian species *Mycoplasma synoviae* (Chalquest 1962), and was incorporated in the formulation developed by Frey (Freundt 1983). The growth of fastidious strains of *Mycoplasma hyopneumoniae* or *Mycoplasma flocculare* from swine was enhanced by special additives (lactalbumin hydrolysate) and swine

serum supplements (Goodwin and Whittlestone 1964, Friis 1971, Freundt 1983).

The first sustained culture of *S. citri* was accomplished on a basic Edward-type medium (BSR) to which sorbitol was added to elevate the osmolarity (Saglio et al. 1971, Whitcomb 1983). However, cultivation of other spiroplasmas proved more difficult and required media modifications. A medium, designated SP-4, was developed to cultivate *Spiroplasma mirum* strains (Tully et al. 1977) and is essentially an Edward formulation containing tryptone, a mammalian cell culture supplement (CMRL 1066), Yeastolate, and fetal bovine serum in place of horse serum (Whitcomb 1983). This medium also enhanced the primary isolation of *M. pneumoniae* from respiratory tract specimens and was responsible for the primary isolation of

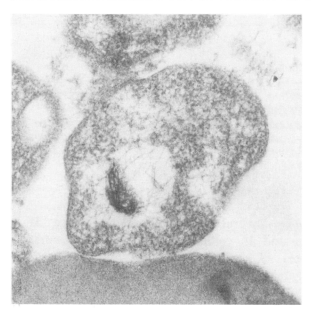

Fig. 34.5 Electron micrograph of thin section of *Mycoplasma pulmonis*. The organism is associated with the surface of a human erythrocyte and has a triple layered membrane (×55 700).

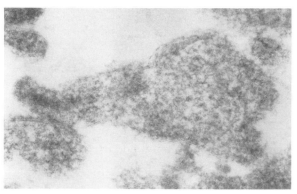

Fig. 34.7 Electron micrograph of thin section of *Mycoplasma genitalium*; note the electron-dense rod-like core within the terminal structure (×85 500).

enhanced growth occurs on SP-4 or Edward media when supplemented with 3–5% horse serum. The mesoplasmas, which have no sterol requirements for growth, do require a fatty acid supplement (0.04% polyoxyethylene sorbitan [Tween 80]) for adequate growth (Rose et al. 1993).

7.1 Toxic components in media or tissues

Certain strains of *Mycoplasma hyorhinis* (cultivar α) isolated from contaminated cell cultures grow with ease in cell cultures but usually not at all in cell-free media (Hopps et al. 1973). Such strains of *M. hyorhinis*, frequently incorrectly designated as unculturable, are especially sensitive to toxic factors found mostly in yeast extract or peptone supplements (Del Giudice, Gardella and Hopps 1980). These strains have now been grown on a minimal chemically defined medium containing a tissue culture supplement (CMRL 1066), L-glutamine and fetal bovine serum (Gardella and Del Giudice 1995).

The addition of bacterial inhibitors to culture medium is crucial in the isolation of most mollicutes, since the rich medium required actively promotes the growth of almost all bacteria present in the specimen (Tully 1983a). However, caution should be exercised because some of these substances may be toxic for some mollicutes. Penicillin G at a final concentration of 500–1000 U ml^{-1} is the recommended additive to inhibit most gram-positive bacteria. For mollicutes apparently sensitive to penicillin G (that is, *M. hyopneumoniae*, *M. flocculare* and *M. dispar*), ampicillin at a final concentration of 0.5–1.0 mg ml^{-1} might be considered as a substitute. Thallium acetate has often been used to inhibit gram-negative bacteria but the potential for human toxicity has persuaded the staff of many laboratories to replace this compound with polymyxin B (final concentration of 500 U ml^{-1}) (Tully 1983a, 1985). Thallium is also inhibitory to the growth of ureaplasmas, *M. hominis* and *M. genitalium*. Excess amounts of arginine in the culture medium (≥0.5%) can also inhibit growth of some mycoplasmas (Leach 1976). Unwashed agars that contain sulphonated polysaccharides and other impurities inhibit col-

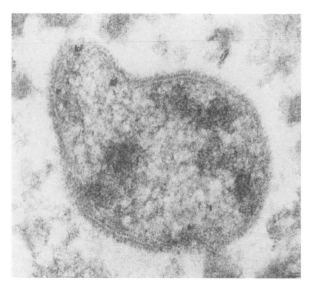

Fig. 34.6 Electron micrograph of thin section of *Ureaplasma urealyticum* (serotype 8). A 'fuzzy' layer is seen external to the membrane (×165 000).

such important or potentially important human mycoplasmas as *M. genitalium* (Tully et al. 1981) and *M. penetrans* (Lo et al. 1991). This medium supports the primary isolation and maintenance of a wide variety of animal or plant and insect mollicutes (Tully 1995a). For ureaplasmas, the medium described by Shepard (1983) is probably the preferred formulation for both primary isolation and maintenance of the organisms, although the Edward and SP-4 formulations with added urea and an initial medium pH of 6.0 are also suitable. The sterol-independent acholeplasmas will grow on medium devoid of animal serum, but ony growth of many mollicutes. Solid media should be formulated with approximately 0.6–0.8% of one of the washed agar preparations (namely Columbia agar, Noble agar, Oxoid Ion agar, etc.), or with more highly purified agarose (Tully 1985). Inhibitory substances in host tissues, fluids, or both can also have a critical influence on the successful isolation of mollicutes. Mechanical tissue maceration frequently releases lyso-lecithins and other tissue components that inhibit mollicute growth. Recommended techniques to circumvent these problems involve mild maceration of tissues, specimen collection in a transport medium using swabs containing inert materials, or dilution of toxic substances by serial dilution of tissues, fluids, or transport specimens in culture medium (Clyde and McCormack 1983, Taylor-Robinson and Chen 1983).

7.2 Conditions of pH, atmosphere and temperature

The initial pH value of the growth medium should be adjusted to 7.3–7.8 for fermentative organisms, to c. 7.0 for arginine-metabolizing organisms and to 6.0–6.5 for the ureaplasmas. Most mollicutes are facultatively anaerobic, but since organisms from primary tissue specimens frequently grow only under anaerobic conditions, an atmosphere of N_2 95% + CO_2 5% is preferred for primary isolation. The 'Gaspak' anaerobic jar (BBL Microbiology Systems) with addition of envelopes for either anaerobic or CO_2 environments is a convenient method for such incubation. A number of *Mycoplasma* spp., such as *M. muris* and *M. spermatophilum*, and several unclassified strains have been shown to require more reduced environments for both primary isolation and maintenance (McGarrity et al. 1983), apart from the strictly anaerobic species in the genus *Anaeroplasma*. The temperature range for growth varies according to species, and to fatty acid and cholesterol composition of the growth medium, but the optimum temperature for most mycoplasmas and ureaplasmas of human or animal origin is 36–38°C. Although acholeplasmas replicate at temperatures as low as 22°C, optimal growth takes place near 37°C. Mesoplasmas and entomoplasmas usually have an optimum at 30°C, and most species in these genera cannot replicate at 37°C. The spiroplasmas multiply over an unsually wide temperature range, from 5° to 41°C (Konai, Clarke and Whitcomb 1996), with most growing optimally at 30°C. However, some *Spiroplasma* spp. can grow well at 37°C, particularly those isolated from ticks (*S. mirum*) or other haematophagous, arthropod (insect) hosts (i.e. mosquitos, horseflies, deerflies, etc.). Mollicutes isolated from fish (*M. mobile*) or other poikilotherms (such as tortoises) usually have a optimum growth temperature near 25°C.

8 COLONIAL MORPHOLOGY

Under low power magnification (×25–×100), colonies of most members of the Mollicutes are umbonate by reflected light (Fig. 34.8). By transmitted light, the col-

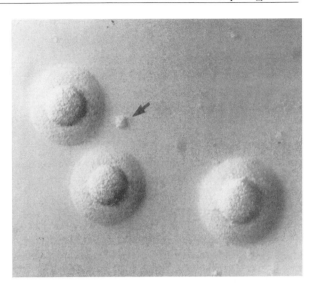

Fig. 34.8 Colonial morphology by reflected light; three umbonate colonies (90–110 μm diameter) of *Mycoplasma hominis* and one colony (15 μm diameter, arrowed) of *Ureaplasma urealyticum* (×300).

onies have a characteristic fried-egg appearance (Figs 34.9 and 34.10) representing an opaque central zone of growth deep in the agar and a translucent peripheral zone on the surface. The small colonies of ureaplasmas usually lack the peripheral zone (Fig. 34.8); they form darker colonies when manganous or calcium chloride is added to the medium, so aiding identification (Shepard and Lunceford 1976) (Fig. 34.11).

The spectrum of colony size is wide, some bovine mycoplasmas, and most acholeplasmas, mesoplasmas and entomoplasmas producing colonies as large as 2 mm in diameter, and easily visible to the naked eye, whereas those of the ureaplasmas characteristically

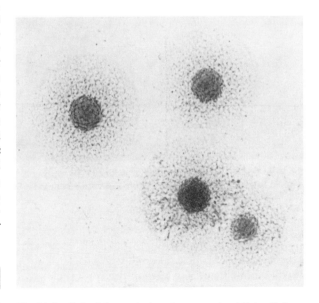

Fig. 34.9 Colonial morphology by transmitted light. Colonies of *Mycoplasma agalactiae* (150 μm diameter) exhibiting a characteristic 'fried-egg' appearance (×192).

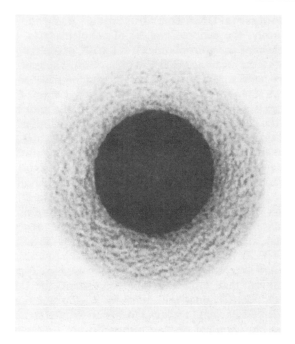

Fig. 34.10 Colonial morphology by transmitted light. Colony of *Acholeplasma laidlawii* (250 μm diameter) with an opaque centre and translucent periphery ('fried-egg' appearance) (×144).

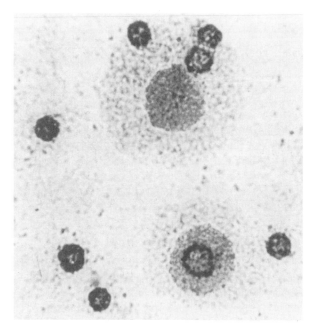

Fig. 34.11 Colonial morphology by transmitted light. Two colonies of *Mycoplasma hominis* with a 'fried-egg' appearance and 7 smaller dark colonies of *Ureaplasma urealyticum* on agar medium containing manganous chloride (×192).

produce very small colonies (15–60 μm in diameter). However, size and appearance depend not only on the species of mollicute, but also on the constituents and degree of hydration of the medium, the agar concentration, the atmospheric conditions and the age of the culture. Thus, on medium buffered to maintain a pH of <6.5, ureaplasma colonies may be up to 300 μm

and have a fried-egg appearance (Manchee and Taylor-Robinson 1969a) (Fig. 34.12). Colony size is always reduced by crowding; under suboptimal conditions the initial central growth within the agar may occur without formation of the peripheral surface growth (Razin and Oliver 1961). However, on primary isolation under the best conditions, *M. pneumoniae* and other species in the genus usually produce colonies without a translucent peripheral zone (Fig. 34.13) that are mulberry-like in appearance, although larger colonies with a periphery sometimes develop after subculture. By contrast, others, such as *M. hyopneumoniae*, show little central growth. Motile spiroplasmas usually do not exhibit typical fried-egg colony formation, especially on conventional 'soft' (0.6–0.8%) agar, but frequently produce a small area of central growth into the agar, with numerous small satellite colonies around the central core. Spiroplasmas plated onto 'hard' (2.25–2.5%) agar may show fried-egg colonies or only central growth into the agar, and without satellite colonies.

PSEUDOCOLONIES

Agar plates containing high concentrations of serum and subjected to extended periods of incubation may exhibit pseudocolonies. These surface forms may easily confuse the inexperienced observer to mistake them for genuine mycoplasmal colonies. A central point with a 'whorled' periphery mimics a genuine colony but these formations do not stain with vital dyes, such as methylene blue, since they consist of calcium and magnesium soaps. They can give rise to fresh centres of crystallization when transferred to uninoculated serum agar plates by push-block transfer, thereby producing the further erroneous impression that they are caused by reproducible viable organisms.

9 CHEMICAL AND STRUCTURAL COMPOSITION

9.1 Lipids, proteins and carbohydrates

Unlike other bacterial membranes, the cell membrane of mollicutes contains cholesterol but lacks α,ε-diaminopimelic acid (McElhaney 1992, Smith 1992, Wieslander, Boyer and Wroblewski 1992, Rottem and Kahane 1993). It is a typical prokaryotic plasma membrane built of about one-third lipid and two-thirds protein. The lipids are neutral, mostly cholesterol, and polar phospholipids, and in some mycoplasmas are composed also of glycolipids and phosphoglycolipids. Membrane proteins are important; apart from their structural and catalytic roles, they make a major contribution to the immunological activities of the cell. Deposition onto the membrane of proteins from the medium must be taken into account in assessing those in the membrane. Spiralin is a dominant membrane protein first identified and characterized (MW 26 kDa) in both helical and non-helical strains of *S. citri*. The amino acid sequence of the protein has been determined and the gene encoding spiralin has been

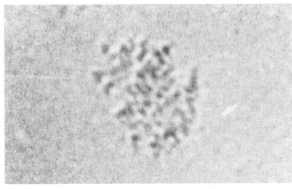

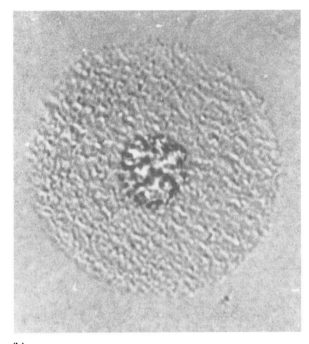

(a)

(b)

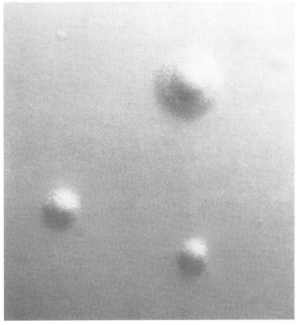

Fig. 34.13 Colonies of *Mycoplasma pneumoniae* after few subcultures. Two colonies, lacking a peripheral zone, are characteristic of the appearance on primary isolation.

Fig. 34.12 (a) Colony of *Ureaplasma urealyticum* 30–40 μm diameter. (b) Colony of same strain of *U. urealyticum*, 120 μm diameter, on agar medium containing 0.05 m HEPES buffer and 0.01% w/v urea (×480).

fully sequenced (Bové et al. 1989). Spiralin-like membrane proteins with somewhat similar molecular weights, but serologically dissimilar, have also been identified in 2 *Spiroplasma melliferum* strains. Ribosomal proteins (and DNA) are the only structures observed in the cytoplasm of mollicutes (Glaser, Hyman and Razin 1992). It has been estimated that approximately 500 proteins are required for the minimal biosynthetic mechanisms in *Mycoplasma capricolum* (Muto, Yamao and Osawa 1987). About one-half of this number of proteins (287) has been detected in the organism from detailed sequence analysis of only 214 kb of the expected 1070 kb total gene size of the organism (Bové 1993, Bork et al. 1995). As noted earlier, some mollicutes possess carbohydrates in the form of an extracellular capsule. Information on their chemical composition and biology and their possible role in

pathogenesis has been summarized by Rosenbusch and Minion (1992).

9.2 Mycoplasma genome size and DNA base composition

Earlier estimates of the genome size of mollicutes obtained by renaturation kinetics divided the mollicutes into genera with a genome of 750 kb (500 000 kDa) (*Mycoplasma, Ureaplasma*) from those with a genome of 1500 kb (1 000 000 kDa) (*Acholeplasma, Spiroplasma, Anaeroplasma, Asteroleplasma*) and the assumed validity of the differences resulted in their use as part of earlier taxonomic criteria (Subcommittee on the Taxonomy of Mollicutes 1995). The advent of pulsed field gel electrophoresis as a method for measuring large DNA molecules with minimum degradation, and for genome sizing of both cultured and uncultured mollicutes (Neimark and Carle 1995), provided much new data on the genome size of prokaryotes. Genome size among mollicutes is now viewed as a continuum from around 580 kb (*M. genitalium*) to 2220 kb (*Spiroplasma ixodetis*) (Su and Baseman 1990, Carle et al. 1995) with overlapping values between mollicute genera (Table 34.2). Although genome size cannot now be used as a definitive taxonomic marker, those mollicutes with phylogenetic relationships suggesting that they are early ancestors of the group (acholeplasma/anaeroplasma and spiroplasma branches) have genomes larger than those recorded for mycoplasmas and ureaplasmas. The smallest genome recorded for a mollicute (*M. genitalium* at 580 kb) is also the smallest genome currently known for any self-replicating prokaryote, an observation that conforms with an earlier estimate of the theoretical minimum amount of genetic machinery necessary for a microbial cell to be fully functional and capable of sustained replication (Morowitz 1984).

The G + C content of the DNA of mollicutes is low, most species falling in the range 24–33 mol% (Tables 34.3–34.7), the exception being *M. pneumoniae* (38.6–40.8 mol%). Among other prokaryotes, such low values are found in certain clostridia, a property used to support the notion that mollicutes are descendants of these bacteria. G + C values that differ by 1.5–2.0 mol% are considered sufficient to exclude inclusion within the same species, but identical or close values do not necessarily indicate genetic relatedness.

9.3 Genome mapping

Availability of restriction endonucleases and pulsed field gel electrophoresis has considerably enhanced the available restriction maps for various mollicutes, beginning with that produced for *M. pneumoniae* (Wenzel and Herrmann 1988). In addition, the use of cloned conserved prokaryotic genes as hybridization probes has materially assisted in locating assigned genes in physical mapping of the mollicute genome (Proft and Herrmann 1995). A fairly large number of genetic maps are available for the mollicutes and they have been important in comparing strains of a single species or species among different genera. Since the mollicute genome represents only about 20% of the total genomic content of conventional prokaryotes, many have argued for the obvious advantages in knowing the full DNA sequence of a mollicute. This position has received some acceptance in the recent report of the complete DNA sequencing of *M. genitalium* (Fraser et al. 1995), only the second prokaryote to have been fully sequenced. The complete genomic map will have a long-term major impact on understanding the genetics and metabolic activity of mollicutes. Efforts are also underway for full genomic sequencing of both *M. pneumoniae* (Hilbert et al. 1994) and *M. capricolum* (Bork et al. 1995).

9.4 Ribosomal RNA genes, operons and codon usage

As noted earlier, mycoplasmal ribosomal genes function in protein synthesis in a similar manner to those of other prokaryotes and their organization generally resembles the typical eubacterial order of 16S-23S-5S, functioning as an operon. These genes are highly conserved and serve as important phylogenetic markers. Mollicute genomes usually carry only one or 2 rRNA gene sets, with the exception that *Mesoplasma lactucae* (strain 831-C4) has 3 operons. This compares to 4 or 5 rRNA sets in the 2 clostridial species phylogenetically close to the mollicutes, and to as many as 7–10 rRNA gene sets in other prokaryotes (Bové 1993). The uncultured plant-pathogenic phytoplasmas have been shown to have 2 sets of operons, consistent with their putative evolutionary relationship to the acholeplasmas (Schneider and Seemuller 1994). In *M. capricolum*, there are 29 tRNA species encoded by 30

tRNA genes, with only one anticodon duplicated (Muto et al. 1990). Certain eubacteria (*Bacillus* and *Escherichia*) have 50–78 tRNA genes, which suggests that a significant deletion of tRNA genes occurred during the regressive evolution of the mollicutes. Codon usage among mollicutes generally follows that recorded for other eubacteria, but with a few notable exceptions (Bové 1993). The CGG (arginine) codon has evolved from an assigned codon (in *S. citri*) to an unassigned codon (in *M. capricolum* and other mycoplasmas) during the evolution from the spiroplasma precursor branch to the mycoplasma subbranch. The UGA codon in the universal genetic code is one of 3 stop codons, in addition to UAA and UAG. However, in members of the orders Mycoplasmatales and Entomoplasmatales UGA is used as a tryptophan codon, whereas UGG encodes tryptophan and UGA functions as a stop codon in the Acholeplasmatales and Anaeroplasmatales. Again, codon usage has been significantly modified during the evolutionary changes from the acholeplasma/anaeroplasma branch to the spiroplasma/mycoplasma branch. The use of UGA as a tryptophan codon in spiroplasmas and mycoplasmas and not as a termination codon has created major problems in the full expression of such genes in normal, non-suppressive bacterial clones. A possible solution to this dilemma is the use of a spiroplasmal viral vector (see p. 819) for both mycoplasma and spiroplasma gene cloning and expression in *S. citri* (Renaudin et al. 1995).

10 METABOLISM AND BIOCHEMICAL AND BIOLOGICAL REACTIONS

Members of the Mollicutes differ widely in the metabolic pathways they use and in their biochemical activity. They multiply generally at a slower rate than conventional bacteria. The mean generation time for many mycoplasmas, including ureaplasmas, is 1–3 h; for some species it is 6–9 h. Spiroplasmas have been shown to have a much wider growth rate, varying from 0.6 h for *Spiroplasma monobiae* (MQ-4) to c. 37 h for a strain (B655) of *Spiroplasma kunkelii* (Konai, Clarke and Whitcomb 1996).

10.1 Energy sources

Mycoplasmas utilize either glucose (and other carbohydrates, for example, mannose, maltose, starch and glycogen) or arginine as a major source of energy. Of the 100 *Mycoplasma* spp. listed in Table 34.3, 45 ferment glucose, 38 hydrolyse arginine, 9 use both substrates, and 8 appear to lack pathways for either glucose or arginine. Six species of *Ureaplasma* have been described and all hydrolyse urea, but lack evidence of glucose fermentation or arginine hydrolysis (Table 34.4). Of 13 recognized *Acholeplasma* species (Table 34.4), all except *Acholeplasma parvum* ferment glucose, and usually some other carbohydrates, but none degrades arginine. The anaerobic mollicutes (Table

34.5) are all glycolytic, with no evidence of arginine hydrolysis. All non-helical mollicutes from plants and insects (mesoplasmas and entomoplasmas) are glycolytic and currently only a single species has been shown to hydrolyse arginine (Table 34.6). All established species or groups, subgroups, or putative groups within the spiroplasmas (Table 34.7) ferment glucose and about half the species apparently also have pathways for arginine metabolism. The carbohydrate-fermenting species catabolize glucose or other carbohydrates by glycolytic pathways mainly to lactic acid and, to a lesser extent, to pyruvic acid, acetic acid and acetylmethylcarbinol (Pollack 1992). Hexokinase activity in glycolysis has been reported in only a few mollicutes (acholeplasmas and anaeroplasmas) and not in other groups of mollicutes. However, a functional phosphotransferase system (PEP) seems to be absent in acholeplasmas and some non-fermentative mycoplasmas but is present in spiroplasmas, mesoplasmas and some fermentative mycoplasmas (Cirillo 1979, Tarshis 1991, Navas-Castillo et al. 1992a, 1992b). In most but not all mycoplasmas, the respiratory pathways are flavin-terminated so that cytochrome, cytochrome pigments and catalase are absent. Some mycoplasmas cleave glutamine to yield glutamic acid, ammonia and ATP but arginine is the main energy source for the non-fermentative mycoplasmas (Pollack 1992). They metabolize arginine through a 3-enzyme system. The first step is mediated by arginine deiminase which converts arginine to citrulline and ammonia. The subsequent reaction sequence involves the phosphorolysis of citrulline to ornithine and carbamoyl phosphate. The latter with ADP and Mg^{2+} is cleaved by carbamoyl phosphate synthetase to ammonia, CO_2 and ATP. These energy-yielding pathways may not, however, be the sole ones in non-fermentative mycoplasmas, since ATP can be derived also from acetylcoenzyme A through reactions catalysed by phosphate acetyltransferase and acetate kinase. As noted, *Mycoplasma* species (Table 34.3) that do not metabolize sugars or arginine are capable of oxidation of organic acids, such as lactate and pyruvate, to acetate and carbon dioxide (Miles et al. 1994). Ureaplasmas exhibit various enzyme activities (Pollack 1992), but their distinctive feature is the conversion of urea to ammonia by means of a urease (Purcell et al. 1966, Shepard 1966). The source of energy in ureaplasmas has been much debated but the possibility that ATP is generated through the formation of an ion gradient coupled to urea hydrolysis has received support (Romano, Lolicata and Alesi 1986).

As a means of detecting mollicutes in specimens from man, animals, plants and insects, as well as a first step in identification and classification, testing for the fermentation of glucose and for the hydrolysis of arginine or urea is invaluable. Fermentative organisms cause a fall in the pH of the medium whereas the non-fermentative ones cause a rise due to the production of ammonia. The change in pH is detected by a change in colour of media incorporating a pH indicator, often phenol red. Details of various isolation and identification procedures and methodology for biochemical and biological tests applicable to mollicutes from humans, animals, plants and insects have been extensively reviewed (Tully and Razin 1996).

10.2 Other biochemical and biological features

Most mollicutes have an absolute sterol requirement for growth, although this characteristic now has less value as a classification marker. All *Mycoplasma*, *Ureaplasma*, *Entomoplasma* and *Anaeroplasma* species fail to grow in media devoid of cholesterol or serum, but the amount of sterol required will vary considerably within genera and species. The usual serum supplement in a culture medium is 15–20%, although some species can grow well in 5% serum. The genus *Spiroplasma* consists of both sterol-requiring and sterol-non-requiring species (Rose et al. 1993), with a majority of members belonging to the former group. Acholeplasmas and asteroleplasmas are capable of growing in the absence of serum or sterol supplements, although growth is considerably enhanced in the presence of 5–20% serum. The mesoplasmas are incapable of growing in a serum-free medium, but growth occurs in such a medium containing a small supplement (0.04%) of polyoxyethylene sorbitan (Tween 80) (Rose et al. 1993). Several standard tests for measuring cholesterol or serum requirements have been reviewed recently (Tully 1995b). Other biochemical or biological tests useful in characterizing mollicutes, in addition to the genetic markers (genome size, base composition, etc.) and serological characteristics (see section 12, p. 818), include filterability, haemadsorptive and β-D-glucosidase activity. Most mollicutes will pass through 450 and 300 nm porosity membranes with little reduction in the number of viable organisms, and organisms of many species will also pass to some extent through 220 nm pore membranes (Tully 1983b). Most *Mycoplasma* spp., and also ureaplasmas, cause some degree of lysis of guinea pig or other erythrocytes suspended in agar (Fig. 34.14) and *M. pneumoniae* causes complete lysis (β-haemolysis). Haemolysis is due to hydrogen peroxide production (Somerson, Walls and Chanock 1965). Erythrocytes may be used also to test the haemadsorptive capacity of colonies. This is measured by covering the colonies with an erythrocyte suspension (usually of guinea pig, sheep or human origin) and observing adherence of the erythrocytes to them after removing excess, unattached cells by washing (Fig. 34.15) (Manchee and Taylor-Robinson 1968). Adhesion of spermatozoa (Taylor-Robinson and Manchee 1967) and tissue-culture cells (Manchee and Taylor-Robinson 1969b) (Fig. 34.16) may be demonstrated in a similar manner. Testing for β-D-glucosidase from hydrolysis of arbutin or aesculin is useful in the detection of some acholeplasmas (Rose and Tully 1983). More extensive details of the tests useful for characterization and taxonomy and recommended methodology have been presented elsewhere (Subcommittee on the Taxonomy of Mollicutes 1995).

11 SUSCEPTIBILITY TO PHYSICAL AND CHEMICAL AGENTS

Although a high concentration of serum in the suspending fluid tends to be protective, most if not all mollicutes are killed if held at 56°C for 30 min; for some species a much shorter time is sufficient. Broth or agar cultures held at room temperature or even at

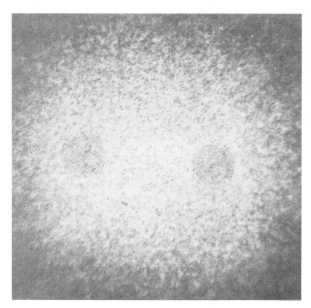

Fig. 34.14 Lysis of guinea pig erythrocytes suspended in agar around 2 colonies of a bovine ureaplasma (×66).

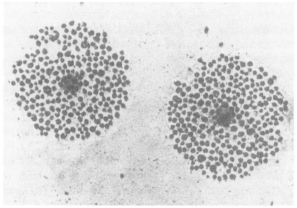

Fig. 34.16 HeLa cells adherent to the surface of 2 colonies of *Mycoplasma gallisepticum* (×120).

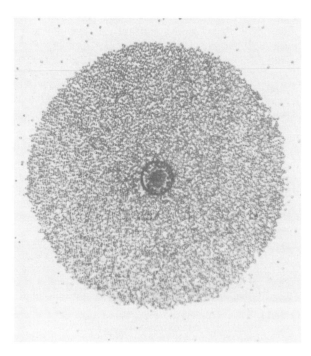

Fig. 34.15 Guinea pig erythrocytes covering completely the surface of a colony of *Mycoplasma agalactiae* (phenomenon of haemadsorption). A few erythrocytes remain on the agar surface after washing.

4°C will often retain viability for only a few days and usually for not more than one to 2 weeks, depending on species, growth rate and medium composition. Ureaplasmas die within a few hours of maximal growth, being susceptible to ammonium ions and particularly to high pH values, but can survive a little longer if the medium is well buffered at a low pH value (≤6.5). Broth cultures of both acholeplasmas and spiroplasmas held at room temperature can fre-

quently remain viable for as long as a month, especially, in the case of acholeplasmas, if the medium lacks serum. Most mollicutes frozen at −20°C will usually not remain viable for more than 1–2 months. For long-term preservation, lyophilization or freezing broth cultures at −70°C (or in liquid nitrogen) are the preferred storage methods (Leach 1983). Freeze drying of a broth culture at the logarithmic phase of growth, sealing under vacuum, with storage at 4°C, retains viability for many years. Swabs, tissues or fluid specimens taken to test for mollicutes should not be subjected to drying or held at incubator or refrigerator temperatures. Optimum collection techniques include either direct inoculation of broth medium and proper incubation, or inoculation of a suitable transport medium with eventual inoculation of culture media (Clyde and McCormack 1983, Taylor-Robinson and Chen 1983).

The absence of a cell wall in mollicutes makes the organisms highly susceptible to most disinfectants and antiseptics (Brunner and Laber 1985). However, the effect of such agents again depends upon the specific organism and the suspending medium. Spiroplasmas isolated from a variety of insect hosts displayed an increased resistance to glutaraldehyde, formaldehyde, ethanol and phenol when compared to bacteria with cell walls or to spiroplasmas isolated from plants or ticks (Stanek, Hirschl and Laber 1981). The use of antiseptics, analgesics and lubricants in reduction of patient discomfort in a variety of urological, obstetrical and gynaecological manipulations can have serious inhibitory effects on the isolation and growth of *U. urealyticum* and *M. hominis*, and possibly other mollicutes (Furr and Taylor-Robinson 1981).

11.1 Susceptibility to antibiotics

It has long been recognized that members of the mollicutes are normally sensitive to antibiotics that inhibit protein synthesis (for example, tetracyclines) and are resistant to antibiotics that act on the cell wall (for example, penicillins). The susceptibility of *M. pneumoniae*, *M. genitalium*, *M. hominis*, *M. fermentans* and *U. urealyticum* to various antimicrobial agents in vitro is shown in Table 34.8. Sensitivity has been measured usually by a metabolism-inhibition technique (Taylor-Robinson 1983, Bébéar and Robertson 1996) in which different investigators have used different strains or numbers of organisms, and different periods of incubation. Thus, a compilation of a list of inhibitory concentrations of antibiotics to any one mollicute is open to some variation, although the general pattern shown in Table 34.8 is unlikely to be misleading (Roberts 1992, Bébéar and Robertson 1996).

It has been customary to use tetracyclines for the treatment of many mollicute infections and for *M. pneumoniae* infections, erythromycin too. However, the newer macrolides (such as clarithromycin and azithromycin), the ketolides and the newer quinolones have equal or sometimes greater activity, at least in vitro (Taylor-Robinson and Bébéar 1997). Rifampicin, trimethoprim, the sulphonamides and the penicillins have no activity, and erythromycin is inactive against *M. hominis*. Many of these statements are applicable also to *U. urealyticum* (Table 34.8), but this organism, unlike *M. hominis*, is sensitive to erythromycin and resistant to lincomycin. Indeed, lincomycin has been used as a selective agent in media for the isolation of ureaplasmas from animal sources (Koshimizu et al. 1983).

It is important to emphasize that most antibiotics that are used successfully in treating mollicute infections have a mycoplasmastatic effect rather that a lethal one on the organisms. The newer quinolones, for example sparfloxacin, and the ketolides are the most likely to have some cidal effect (Taylor-Robinson and Bébéar 1997), but there are few well documented instances of an antibiotic, at drug levels consistent with clinical application, inducing a permanent lethal effect against a variety of strains of the mollicute, if laboratory procedures to distinguish between a static

and cidal effect (Taylor-Robinson 1996b) have been applied. Support for this contention comes from the almost consistent failure of antibiotics to eradicate mollicutes from contaminated cell cultures (see section 14, p. 819), or from plants that lack a functioning immune system (McCoy et al. 1989) and from the reported difficulties of controlling mollicute infections in patients with immune deficiencies (Furr, Taylor-Robinson and Webster 1994). Thus, successful chemotherapeutic intervention in a mollicute infection depends not only on the type of antibiotic but also on the ability of the host to mount an adequate immune response, including a humoral antibody response (Gelfand 1993).

11.2 Antibiotic resistance

Mycoplasmas may be innately resistant to antibiotics, as mentioned before, or develop resistance to antibiotics to which they are considered usually sensitive. Streptomycin resistance may develop as a one-step process (Blyth 1958). Resistance of *M. hominis* to tetracyclines has been observed (Bygdeman and Mårdh 1983, Taylor-Robinson et al. 1983) and in some areas 30% of strains have been resistant (Koutsky et al. 1983). The reason for this is the acquisition of a streptococcal *tetM* gene (Roberts et al. 1985). *U. urealyticum* strains also may be resistant to tetracyclines (Taylor-Robinson and Furr 1986) for the same reason (Roberts and Kenny 1986), and in London 10% of strains have been recorded as resistant (Taylor-Robinson and Furr 1986). Erythromycin resistance has been noted in about 10% of ureaplasma strains in the same area (Taylor-Robinson and Furr 1986), but multiresistant strains appear to be very infrequent. Tetracycline-resistant strains of *M. hominis* are sensitive to the glycylcyclines (new tetracycline derivatives), as

Table 34.8 Susceptibilities of *M. pneumoniae, M. genitalium, M. hominis, M. fermentans* and *U. urealyticum* to various antibiotics[a]

Antibiotic(s)	*M. pneumoniae*	*M. genitalium*	*M. hominis*	*M. fermentans*	*U. urealyticum*
Tetracyclines	++	++	++	++	++
Erythromycin	++	++	–	+	++
Clarithromycin	++	++	–	–	++
Azithromycin	++	++	–	++	+
Pristinamycin	++	++	++	?	++
Streptomycin	++	++	–	–	+
Spectinomycin	++	?	+	+	+
Sparfloxacin	++	++	++	++	++
Gentamicin	+	?	+	+	+
Chloramphenicol	+	+	+	+	+
Clindamycin	+	+	++	++	–
Lincomycin	+	+	++	++	–
Ciprofloxacin	+	+	++	++	+
Difloxacin	+	?	++	?	+
Nalidixic acid	–	–	–	–	–
Cephalosporins	–	–	–	–	–
Penicillins	–	–	–	–	–
Rifampicin	–	–	–	–	–

[a]++, susceptible (MICs <1 mg ml⁻¹); +, partially susceptible (MICs 1–10 mg ml⁻¹); –, resistant (MICs >10 mg ml⁻¹). Results presented in order of diminishing activity for *M. pneumoniae*.

are some tetracycline-resistant ureaplasma strains. However, all resistant ureaplasmas seem to be sensitive to the ketolides (Taylor-Robinson and Bébéar 1997). The difficulties in eradicating erythromycin-sensitive ureaplasmas from the vagina and erythromycin-sensitive *M. pneumoniae* strains from the respiratory tract (Smith, Friedewald and Chanock 1967) by erythromycin therapy indicate that the promise of in vitro tests does not always correlate with clinical outcome.

12 ANTIGENIC COMPOSITION AND SEROLOGICAL BEHAVIOUR

12.1 Membrane antigens

Mollicute antigens that are recognized by the host assume particular importance in host–parasite relationships. Although cytoplasmic mollicute antigens can be immunogenic, the major antigenic determinants are membrane proteins, lipoproteins and glycolipids (Howard and Taylor 1985, Wise, Yogev and Rosengarten 1992). The glucose- and galactose-containing glycolipids of *M. pneumoniae* are haptens, which are antigenic only when bound to membrane protein. They induce antibodies that react in tests of complement fixation, metabolism inhibition and growth inhibition. Glycolipids of similar structure and serological activity have been found in some other mollicutes, for example *A. laidlawii*, *M. neurolyticum* and *M. fermentans*, in most plants, and in the human brain. The cross-reactivity of human brain tissue antigens with antibodies to *M. pneumoniae* could account for the neurological manifestations of *M. pneumoniae* infection (see section 15, p. 820). In contrast, a glycoprotein fraction of *M. pneumoniae*, rather than the glycolipid moiety, is involved in the development of a cell mediated immune response to this mycoplasma. Furthermore, major surface proteins involved in attachment, the P1 and P30 adhesins of *M. pneumoniae* and the P140 adhesin of *M. genitalium*, are recognized regularly by the host. Thus, antibody to these adhesins has been detected in convalescent sera and in respiratory secretions (Leith et al. 1983, Vu et al. 1987, Tully et al. 1995, Jacobs et al. 1996).

12.2 Variable membrane proteins

Major membrane lipoproteins have been identified in *M. bovis*, *M. fermentans*, *M. gallisepticum*, *M. genitalium*, *M. hominis*, *M. hyopneumoniae*, *M. hyorhinis*, *M. penetrans*, *M. pulmonis* and *U. urealyticum*. The nature and function of these components and the methods used for their isolation and characterization have been reviewed (Wise, Yogev and Rosengarten 1992, Razin 1995, Wang and Lo 1995, Wise, Kim and Watson-McGown 1995). These acylated membrane proteins are bound to fatty acids, particularly to palmitic and myristic acids, and appear to be major components of a mycoplasmal antigenic variation system. Since the mollicute plasma membrane is the one cell component that comes in direct contact with the host

immune system, the ability of an organism to develop a complicated mechanism for reversible switching of both expression and modification of membrane proteins provides an active means of escaping from the host immune response. Many of the genes that encode for these lipoproteins have been cloned and sequenced. Although these variable lipoproteins were thought to account for serological heterogeneity observed in some mollicutes, the variations are restricted to a small number of protein antigens and do not appear to alter total cell protein profiles of the organisms. However, the lipoproteins of both *M. penetrans* and *M. genitalium* have been used in enzyme-linked immunosorbent assays (ELISA) to test a variety of human sera, with evidence that these lipoproteins are the major components of the humoral response to the 2 mycoplasmas (Wang et al. 1993, Ferris et al. 1995, Grau et al. 1995, Wang and Lo 1995).

12.3 Serological techniques

The ability of mollicutes to stimulate antibody production has long been recognized; serology still plays an important role in the diagnosis of mollicute infections and detection and identification of the organisms. Many of the earlier tests developed for species identification of the organisms, such as growth inhibition (Clyde 1983), metabolism inhibition (Taylor-Robinson 1983) and immunofluorescence (Gardella, Del Giudice and Tully 1983), continue to be valuable laboratory procedures. The growth-inhibition and immunofluorescence tests are performed on agar colonies and both are fairly specific and rapid techniques for identification of most species in the class. The immunofluorescence test can also be adapted to specifically identify some mycoplasmas (*M. genitalium*, *M. pneumoniae*) that occur in mixed cultures and have close serological relationships (Tully et al. 1995). The metabolism-inhibition test carried out with broth suspensions of viable organisms is most useful in the speciation of ureaplasmas and spiroplasmas, although this technique can also be applied to measure specific antibody to these and other mollicutes (Taylor-Robinson 1983, 1996c, Williamson 1983). Rapid serological identification of spiroplasmas can be accomplished with the microscopic deformation test, in which specific antibody alters the helical structure of the organisms (Williamson 1983, Whitcomb and Hackett 1996). The use of monoclonal antibodies in ELISA procedures has also improved the detection of mollicute antigens in biological materials and in cultures, particularly in some plant and animal infections when the aetiological agent is more difficult to cultivate (Thomas, Garnier and Boothby 1996). More sensitive and specific tests are required, along with reproducibility and ease of performance, for seroepidemiological studies and serological diagnosis of mycoplasmal infections. The diagnosis of *M. pneumoniae* infections in humans is still based primarily on serological responses, but more sensitive and specific antigen–enzyme immunoassay or indirect haemagglutination procedures are replacing the conventional complement fixation test (Harris et al. 1996). Enzyme immunoassays also have the advantage of measuring immune responses to all 3 antibody classes; such procedures are also being applied more frequently to detect antibody to urogenital mycoplasmas, in which the above mentioned lipoprotein antigens are used (Taylor-Robinson 1996c). Other newly described enzyme immunoassays for detecting antibody following mollicute infections of a variety of animals (bovine, caprine, ovine, porcine, rodents, birds, etc.) have been published (Tully and Razin 1996).

13 MYCOPLASMA VIRUSES AND PLASMIDS

As with other bacteria, some members of the mollicutes are susceptible to infection by viruses; the first virus was identified in a strain of *A. laidlawii* by Gourlay (1970). The occurrence, molecular biology and host distribution of mollicute viruses have been reviewed (Maniloff 1992, Renaudin and Bové 1994). Fourteen viruses have been identified so far, 6 in *Acholeplasma*, 4 in *Spiroplasma* and 4 in *Mycoplasma* spp., the most recent isolation being made from strains of *Mycoplasma arthritidis* (Voelker et al. 1995). Morphologically, the viruses consist of filamentous rods or enveloped spheres that bud from the mollicute cell membrane or are polyhedron viruses with short to medium tails. Although not all viruses have been well characterized, those propagated and examined to date have all been identified as DNA viruses with single- or double-stranded DNA in either a circular or linear form. Whether morphologically similar viruses infecting different mollicute genera are genetically related is still not established. However, evidence is available that whole viral genomes are integrated into the mollicute chromosome, especially in spiroplasmas (Renaudin and Bové 1994). These observations provide a mechanism for natural chromosomal rearrangement and gene transfer within mollicutes and promotion of genetic diversity within the group. A successful experimental gene transfer system between mollicutes has recently been developed with the SPV-1 virus of *S. citri*. The occurrence of DNA viruses in *M. arthritidis* is the first report of an association between viral infections in mollicutes and host pathogenicity (Voelker et al. 1995). The occurrence of such viral agents and their host responses have contributed much new information to the molecular biology of mollicutes. In addition to viral DNA, plasmids have also been found as extrachromosomal DNA, mostly in *Spiroplasma* spp. and in strains of *M. mycoides* (Bové and Saillard 1979, Ranhand et al. 1980, 1987, Bergmann and Finch 1988, Dybvig and Khaled 1990, Gasparich et al. 1993, Gasparich and Hackett 1994). The separation of spiroplasmal plasmid DNA from the replicative form of viral DNA can sometimes be difficult considering the frequent occurrence of viral infections in these organisms. As with viral DNA, some spiroplasma plasmids have apparently been integrated into the spiroplasma chromosome. However, there is

no evidence presently available that integrated plasmid DNA has any relationship to pathogenicity, drug resistance, or other phenotypic modifications, and so these extrachromosomal elements are currently considered to be cryptic. It is interesting that the mollicutes with clearly identified plasmids have all come from a single evolutionary clade (spiroplasma/mycoides branch) of the group (Weisburg et al. 1989).

14 MOLLICUTES IN CELL CULTURES

Although the first report of mollicutes in uninoculated HeLa cell cultures occurred 4 decades ago (Robinson, Wichelhausen and Roizman 1956), such contamination in cultivated cells remains a serious and formidable problem. Contamination is now observed frequently in many continuous cell lines of human or animal origin, in primary human, animal, or insect cell lines and in such other cultured cells as hybridomas. The occurrence, detection and control of such infections have been reviewed extensively by McGarrity, Kotani and Butler (1992) and in a recent methodology series (Tully and Razin 1996). The extent of the contamination is variable, depending upon geographical location and quality control endeavours, but is estimated to occur in about 10–25% of all cell lines examined. Six mollicutes currently are responsible for almost all the reported infections, 3 species of animal origin (*Mycoplasma arginini*, *M. hyorhinis* and *A. laidlawii*) and 3 species found in humans (*Mycoplasma orale*, *Mycoplasma salivarium* and *M. fermentans*). Cell infections with animal mycoplasmas or acholeplasmas can usually be traced to contaminated serum (usually fetal bovine) employed in cell culture media. Contamination with mycoplasmas of human origin usually comes from breaks in sterility within the cell culture laboratory that allow normal human respiratory tract organisms (*M. orale* and *M. salivarium*) into cell lines, or to an infection of human primary lymphocyte or macrophage cells with *M. fermentans*. The observed effects of mollicute infection extend to essentially every parameter of cell structure, growth, metabolism and viability, including the induction of chromosomal aberrations, alterations in nucleic acid metabolism of cells, inhibition of lymphocyte stimulation, altering cytokine production and promoting or suppressing virus production.

14.1 Detection, elimination and control procedures

The most consistently effective detection system is based upon an adequate microbiological culture scheme (Del Giudice and Tully 1996) and the use of a clean, mollicute-free, indicator cell system for detection of contamination with a 2-step staining procedure (for identification of DNA and type-specific α strains of *M. hyorhinis*) (Del Giudice and Hopps 1978, Masover and Becker 1996). The presence of antibiotics in cell cultures used for testing is detrimental to most detection schemes and testing should only be performed after cells receive at least 3 passages in antibiotic-free medium. Proper culture methods and serological techniques will identify most mollicute contaminants of these cells, but these procedures may not identify α strains of *M. hyorhinis* unless the medium is modified (Gardella and Del Giudice 1995). Sterile cover-slips containing cell sheets of the indicator cells inoculated with test material are incubated for 2–3 days. Some fixed cells are then stained with the Hoechst 33258 DNA dye and examined microscopically for the presence of a fluorescent stippling effect over the cell surfaces from mollicute DNA. Other fixed cells are stained with a fluorescein-conjugated antiserum specific to *M. hyorhinis*, and are also examined microscopically for fluorescence on cell surfaces. Numerous DNA probes and polymerase chain reaction (PCR)-based detection schemes for mollicutes in cell infections have been described over the past 5 years, and have been reviewed (Razin 1994, Rawadi and Dussurget 1995, Veilleux, Razin and May 1996). Although the results of many of the PCR detection methods have not been correlated with those of culture or indicator cell methodology, the newer techniques when standardized and properly evaluated may supersede procedures currently recommended.

As with detection systems, numerous procedures have been described to eliminate mycoplasmas from cell cultures. Since no procedure is successful consistently, the number of techniques described being testimony to their inadequacy, it is easier to discard contaminated cell cultures, replace them with mycoplasma-free cells and adhere to simple guidelines to prevent contamination (see below). However, in a few instances when a cell line is valuable, an eradication procedure based upon antibiotic treatment of the cells can be labour-intensive, but worthwhile (Del Giudice and Gardella 1996). The technique requires identification and isolation of the contaminant, extensive pretesting to determine the most effective antibiotic against the organism, adequate treatment time, and an intensive follow-up period with proper detection methods to establish that eradication has been achieved. Preparation and use of a specific antiserum may also be helpful.

Primary prevention and control of cell culture contamination involves an awareness of the origin and status of cells introduced into the laboratory, quarantine of such lines until their status has been defined, and cell banking of documented clean lines for possible later needs (McGarrity, Kotani and Butler 1992, Smith and Mowles 1996). Probably the single most useful approach in the control of cell culture infections is the discontinuance of the use of antibiotics in cell cultivation. This would lead to the easier recognition of a break in sterility and would initiate efforts to eliminate the progressive and persistent development of mollicute contamination that will spread within the laboratory.

15 PATHOGENICITY

Although the molecular basis of mollicute pathogenicity is still not well understood, considerable advances have been made recently in defining the interactions that occur between mollicutes and host cells or systems that relate to induction or enhancement of disease patterns. Thus, there is new information on the mechanisms and genetic control of host cell adherence by mollicutes, evidence of their ability to induce intracellular infections, and further information on the ability of the organisms to activate and alter widespread aspects of the host immune system. These factors and other potential host interactions play an important role in well established mollicute infections

of man, such as *M. pneumoniae* respiratory disease, and in mycoplasmal and ureaplasmal infections in hosts immunocompromised by genetic immune deficiencies, AIDS, or following organ or tissue transplantation. Similar factors must also play a role in the numerous animal mycoplasmal infections on record, and possibly even in mollicute-induced diseases of plants and insects.

15.1 Attachment and intracellular infections

Adherence of organisms to host tissues is a major prerequisite for pathogenicity, but some non-pathogenic and pathogenic mollicutes possess the ability to adhere to mucosal or epithelial surfaces lining the oral cavity and the respiratory and urogenital tracts of vertebrates. Likewise, both pathogenic helical mollicutes and those that are part of the commensal flora of insects and other arthropods attach to selected cells of the gut epithelium and salivary gland. In fact, most mollicutes, regardless of their pathogenic potential, have the ability to adhere to cells, but the avidity of attachment by different mycoplasmas is unknown and may be very weak for some. Such differences are reflected, perhaps, in haemadsorption, another expression of adherence, where there is a greater tendency for pathogenic mycoplasmas to haemadsorb than for those that are non-pathogenic. The erythrocyte receptors for haemadsorption are sialylated glycoproteins and it is thought that other membrane glycoproteins may play some role in the generalized cytadherence of non-pathogenic mollicutes (Razin and Jacobs 1992). Of special interest is the possession by several *Mycoplasma* spp. pathogenic for humans and some other species of an organized tip structure containing unique adhesin proteins that promote eukaryotic cell attachment. Techniques to localize adhesins or other antigens on the mycoplasma cell surface or on tip structures have been described (Krause and Stevens 1995). The adhesins of *M. pneumoniae* (P1 and P30) and the 140 kDa adhesin of *M. genitalium* are the most extensively characterized (Razin and Jacobs 1992, Tryon and Baseman 1992, Baseman 1993). The genes and full nucleotide sequence of each of the encoded proteins have been detailed and some structural similarities and differences noted. Variation in the P1 protein of *M. pneumoniae* (Su et al. 1990) has led to strains being placed in 2 groups which may differ in epidemiology and pathogenicity (Jacobs et al. 1996). Other putative adhesin proteins (or lipoproteins) have been described in *M. hominis* (Henrich, Feldmann and Hadding 1993), *M. bovis* (Sachse 1994), *M. hyopneumoniae* (Zhang, Young and Ross 1994) and *M. pirum* (Tham et al. 1994). A cloned and sequenced gene of the *M. pirum* protein was found to encode a 127 kDa polypeptide that had a 46% amino acid homology with both the P1 and 140 kDa adhesins of *M. pneumoniae* and *M. genitalium*, respectively.

The early event of adherence allows intimate contact between mollicute and host cell and provides the opportunity for various metabolites of the organism to cause cell injury or otherwise alter or interfere with host metabolism. Such putative pathogenic determinants as surface capsules (see section 5, p. 805), toxins (as produced by *M. neurolyticum* and *M. gallisepticum*), oxidation (from hydrogen peroxide), and nucleases, arginine deiminase and phospholipases (Shibata, Sasaki and Watanabe 1995) causing damage, have been reviewed (Tryon and Baseman 1992).

Whether mollicutes actively enter eukaryotic cells has long been a matter of some dispute, beginning with early experimental studies (Zucker-Franklin, Davidson and Thomas 1966) in which several mollicutes were found to be taken up by leucocytes and macrophages. More recently, techniques employing electron microscopic examination of sectioned cells (Taylor-Robinson 1996a) and immunohistochemistry, in situ hybridization, or both, for mycoplasma-specific DNA (Wear and Lo 1995) have yielded more convincing evidence that some *Mycoplasma* spp. are to be found in intracellular locations (Lo et al. 1992, 1993a, Mernaugh et al. 1993, Stadtländer et al. 1993, Taylor-Robinson, Sarathchandra and Furr 1993, Jensen, Blom and Lind 1994). The use of confocal microscopy to examine the internal structure of the cell and the ability to separate cell nuclei and identify mollicutes attached to nuclear material by specific staining techniques has offered additional evidence for the ability of *M. genitalium*, *M. pneumoniae* and *M. penetrans* to reach intracellular sites (Baseman et al. 1995). In addition, recent scanning electron microscopy of HEp-2 cell cultures infected with *M. penetrans* has revealed numerous mycoplasmas actively penetrating the cell surface (Giron, Lange and Baseman 1996) (see Fig. 34.3).

15.2 Evasion and modulation of the host immune response

Recent observations on the occurrence and extent of antigenic variation in lipid-modified proteins in mollicute membranes and the basic gene rearrangements responsible have cast new light on the ability of mollicutes to evade host immune responses. Modulation or activation of host immune reactions now appears to play a critical role in the pathogenesis of mollicute infections in vertebrates, although regulation and interaction between the various cellular components of the response are complex and variable. Potent B cell mitogens have been demonstrated in many mollicutes (mycoplasmas, acholeplasmas and spiroplasmas) where the organisms act as polyclonal B cell activators (Naot 1995); both *M. fermentans* and *M. penetrans* lipoprotein membrane components have been shown to be B cell mitogens (Feng and Lo 1994). A cytoplasmic component of *M. arthritidis* (MAM) has been found to be a potent mycoplasma activator or superantigen, a class of T cell mitogens dependent upon major histocompatibility complex accessory molecules (Cole and Adkin 1995). The interest in superantigens relates to their ability to modulate the immune system in a manner that promotes the devel-

opment or enhancement of human autoimmune disease (see below). Various mollicutes, their membranes or extracts, have also been shown to activate macrophages and monocytes, leading to the expression and secretion of the major proinflammatory cytokines – specifically, tumour necrosis factor α, interleukin (IL-1, IL-1β, IL-6, IL-8, IL-12) and interferon-γ (Faulkner et al. 1995, Gallily et al. 1995, Kostyal, Butler and Beezhold 1995). In addition to modulation of the immune response by mollicutes, it has long been suggested that mollicutes pathogenic for man and animals could provoke an immune response that is effectively anti-self (Biberfeld 1971, 1985), or based upon molecular mimicry (Tryon and Baseman 1992). Thus, cross-reactions between the galactan of *M. mycoides* and bovine lung, or between *M. pneumoniae* glycolipids and human brain and lung, are responsible for the production of autoantibodies that could be responsible for the damaging immunopathological consequences of infection. These concepts have been revived and further supported by observations on both *M. pneumoniae* and *M. genitalium* (Baseman and Tryon 1990, Baseman 1993). The family of adhesin-related molecules shared by these 2 mycoplasmas (and possibly other species) exhibits high levels of sequence homology with mammalian cytoskeletal components (keratin, myosin, fibrinogen, etc.). In addition, elevated levels of antibodies to keratin were observed in the serum of a patient convalescing from a mixed *M. pneumoniae–M. genitalium* infection, and immunoblotting of the antikeratin antibodies revealed immunoreactivities to the 2 dominant adhesin proteins of the 2 mollicutes involved (Tully et al. 1995). Although it remains uncertain whether mollicutes elicit immunopathological processes through molecular mimicry, or through modulation of the immune response by immune cell activation or cytokine production, or by a combination of these factors, the biological properties of the organisms appear to be consistent with the changes observed in mollicute-associated diseases.

15.3 Pathogenicity for vertebrates

Mollicutes currently known to be pathogenic for vertebrates are confined to the genera *Mycoplasma* and *Ureaplasma*. About half the 100 *Mycoplasma* spp. listed in Table 34.3 are considered to cause disease at one or more anatomical sites in vertebrates. However, the pathogenicity of other species is much less easy to determine. Part of the difficulty lies in their frequent occurrence in the absence of disease, which tends to cast doubt on the significance of finding them in the diseased state. Even for those that are considered to be important pathogens for humans or other vertebrate hosts, the strength of evidence varies (Krause and Taylor-Robinson 1992, Taylor-Robinson 1995) (see also Volume 3, Chapter 54). In humans, *M. pneumoniae*, *M. genitalium*, *M. fermentans*, *M. hominis* and possibly *M. penetrans* are considered the principal pathogens (Krause and Taylor-Robinson 1992, Lo et al. 1992, Tully 1993). *M. hominis* occurs infrequently in the normal male urogenital tract, more frequently in the normal female genital tract, and most often in the genital tract of women attending sexually transmitted disease clinics (Tully et al. 1983) and those with bacterial vaginosis. However, the organism is clearly associated with extragenital infections, often in septicaemias occurring postpartum or from various traumas, and in transplant or joint infections in immunosuppressed patients (Krause and Taylor-Robinson 1992, Tully 1993). Likewise, *M. salivarium*, a normal oral commensal in humans, has been associated with septic arthritis in patients with hypogammaglobulinaemia (Furr, Taylor-Robinson and Webster 1994). The majority of mycoplasmas isolated from cattle, rats, mice, sheep, goats and swine are pathogenic. Their specific association with animal disease and the techniques available for laboratory diagnosis have been reviewed (Simecka et al. 1992, Whitford, Rosenbuch and Lauerman 1994, Taylor-Robinson 1995, Tully and Razin 1996) (see also Volume 3, Chapter 54).

The principal pathogenic *Ureaplasma* spp. (Table 34.4) include *U. urealyticum* in humans and *Ureaplasma diversum* in cattle. Although *U. urealyticum* organisms occur frequently in the urogenital tract of normal males and females, they have been shown to have a role in non-gonococcal urethritis in males and in septic arthritis in hypogammaglobulinaemic individuals (Furr, Taylor-Robinson and Webster 1994). These organisms have also been associated with neonatal respiratory disease, particularly in infants with very low birth weight, in whom acquisition apparently occurs sometimes in utero (Krause and Taylor-Robinson 1992, Cassell et al. 1993). *U. diversum* plays an important role in bovine reproductive failure (ter Laak and Ruhnke 1996). A few *Acholeplasma* spp. have been isolated from humans and many more species identified in animal hosts, but little evidence exists for a primary role in disease of vertebrates (Tully 1993, 1996).

15.4 Pathogenicity for insects and arthropods

Although several mollicute species (mesoplasmas, entomoplasmas, spiroplasmas) have been isolated from a wide range of insects and other arthropods, including a number of haematophagous species (mosquitos, horseflies, deerflies, etc.), the only overt pathogens for such hosts are currently confined to the genus *Spiroplasma* (Table 34.7). These include *S. melliferum* and *Spiroplasma apis*, both agents of a lethal infection in honey bees (*Apis mellifera*). The sex ratio spiroplasma isolated from several neotropical *Drosophila* (fruitfly) species is a transovarially transmitted organism that induces selective male death in the offspring of infected females (Williamson, Tully and Whitcomb 1989, Tully and Whitcomb 1991). *Spiroplasma floricola*, an organism found mainly on floral surfaces, has been associated with a natural disease in certain beetles (Tully and Whitcomb 1991).

15.5 Pathogenicity for plants

The first mollicutes to be associated with plant disease were a group of uncultivable, non-helical, wall-less prokaryotes

termed mycoplasma-like organisms (MLOs). Now termed phytoplasmas, this group has expanded into more than 300 different, insect vector-transmitted organisms causing plant diseases, which to date still remain uncultivable (McCoy et al. 1989). The results of attempts at molecular and genetic characterization indicate that the organisms are phylogenetically related to acholeplasmas and that the available representatives might be subdivided into at least 11–12 genetically distinct organisms (Schneider et al. 1995). Several spiroplasmas are pathogenic for plants and represent economically important diseases in many geographical locations. *S. citri* is the aetiological agent of citrus stubborn disease and brittle root disease in horseradish (Calavan and Bové 1989). Under natural conditions, these diseases are transmitted by leafhoppers, although transfer can occur also during plant grafting. Other natural *S. citri* infections occur in more than 35 different species of annual weeds and cultivated plants or flowers, which act as important reservoirs for insect transmission of *S. citri* to citrus or horseradish. *S. kunkelii* infections are the cause of at least one form of corn stunt disease, with viruses and phytoplasmas also able to induce a similar disease in corn (Whitcomb 1989). These organisms are also naturally transmitted by various leafhopper species. *Spiroplasma phoeniceum* infections have so far only been found in Syria in naturally infected periwinkle plants (Saillard et al. 1987).

15.6 Experimental infections

Inoculation of animals, plants or insects with mollicutes in an attempt to fulfil Koch's postulates is an important aspect of determining pathogenicity. However, mollicutes, like other microbial agents, often quickly lose virulence when passaged in artificial media, so that the use of low-passage strains, following preservation by freezing or lyophilization, is advisable. Then, characteristic disease, for example pneumonia, may sometimes be reproduced experimentally in the larger domestic animals (bovine, ovine, porcine, etc.) (Cassell, Clyde and Davis 1985, Bradbury and Levisohn 1996, Kobisch and Ross 1996, Rosenbusch and Ruhnke 1996). Furthermore, non-human primates have been used extensively to examine the pathogenicity of mycoplasmas of human origin, for example *M. pneumoniae* (Barile et al. 1987), *M. fermentans* (Lo et al. 1993b), *M. genitalium* (Tully et al. 1986, Taylor-Robinson et al. 1987) and *M. penetrans* (Grau et al. 1995). Laboratory rodents have been employed to study both respiratory and urogenital tract infections (Cassell and Yancy 1996, Furr and Taylor-Robinson 1996) and as models for joint infections (Washburn 1996). Some small laboratory animals may become susceptible, or more susceptible to genital tract infection by mollicutes after receiving sex hormones (Furr and Taylor-Robinson 1996). Unnatural laboratory-animal hosts, that is those receiving mycoplasmas from quite dissimilar animal species, tend to be more refractory to infection. Such host specificity provokes questions about the mechanisms of pathogenicity, including the role of specific cell receptors for mycoplasmas. Experimental spiroplasma infections with *S. citri*, *S. kunkelii* and *S. phoeniceum* have been useful in establishing the host range of these organisms and the role of various insect species in transmission (Foissac et al. 1996). *S. mirum*, an organism isolated naturally from rabbit ticks (*Haemaphysalis leporispalustris*), has been shown to induce central nervous system disease and ocular cataracts in experimentally infected mice and rats (Tully and Whitcomb 1991). Experimental phytoplasma infections in plants have been an important factor in maintaining the agents in the laboratory and in understanding the capacity of various insects as transmission vectors (Purcell 1996).

REFERENCES

Barile MF, 1979, Mycoplasma–tissue cell interactions, *The Mycoplasmas*, vol. 2, eds Tully JG, Whitcomb RF, Academic Press, New York, 425–74.

Barile MF, Grabowski MW et al., 1987, Superiority of the chimpanzee animal model to study pathogenicity of known *Mycoplasma pneumoniae* and reputed mycoplasma pathogens, *Isr J Med Sci*, **23:** 556–60.

Baseman JB, 1993, The cytadhesins of *Mycoplasma pneumoniae* and *M. genitalium*, *Subcellular Biochemistry, Mycoplasma Membranes*, vol. 20, eds Rottem S, Kahane I, Plenum, New York, 243–59.

Baseman JG, Tryon VV, 1990, Microbial adhesion and arthritides: other pathogens, *Musculoskeletal Pathogens*, eds Esterhai JE, Gristina AG, Poss R, American Academy Orthopedic Surgeons, 89–115.

Baseman JB, Cole RM et al., 1982, Molecular basis for cytadsorption of *Mycoplasma pneumoniae*, *J Bacteriol*, **151:** 1514–22.

Baseman JB, Lange M et al., 1995, Interplay between mycoplasmas and host target cells, *Microb Pathog* **19:** 105–16.

Bébéar C, Robertson J, 1996, Determination of minimal inhibitory concentration, *Molecular and Diagnostic Procedures in Mycoplasmology*, vol. 2, eds Tully JG, Razin S, Academic Press, San Diego, 189–97.

Bergmann AD, Finch LR, 1988, Isolation and restriction endonuclease analysis of a mycoplasma plasmid, *Plasmid*, **16:** 68–70.

Biberfeld G, 1971, Antibodies to brain and other tissues in cases of *M. pneumoniae* infection, *Clin Exp Immunol*, **8:** 319–33.

Biberfeld G, 1985, Infection sequelae and autoimmune reactions in *Mycoplasma pneumoniae* infection, *The Mycoplasmas*, vol. 4, eds Razin S, Barile MF, Academic Press, San Diego, 293–311.

Biberfeld G, Biberfeld P, 1970, Ultrastructural features of *Mycoplasma pneumoniae*, *J Bacteriol*, **102:** 855–61.

Blyth WA, 1958, PhD thesis, London University.

Boatman E, 1979, Morphology and ultrastructure of the Mycoplasmatales, *The Mycoplasmas*, vol. 1, eds Barile MF, Razin S, Academic Press, San Diego, 63–102.

Bork P, Ouzounis C et al., 1995, Exploring the *Mycoplasma capricolum* genome: a minimal cell reveals its physiology, *Mol Microbiol*, **16:** 955–67.

Borrel A, Dujardin-Beaumetz E et al., 1910, Le microbe de la peripneumonie, *Ann Inst Pasteur (Paris)*, **24:** 168–79.

Bové JM, 1993, Molecular features of mollicutes, *Clin Infect Dis*, **17, Suppl. 1:** S10–31.

Bové JM, Saillard C, 1979, Cell biology of spiroplasmas, *The Mycoplasmas*, vol. 3, eds Whitcomb RF, Tully JG, Academic Press, San Diego, 83–153.

Bové JM, Carle P et al., 1989, Molecular and cellular biology of spiroplasmas, *The Mycoplasmas*, vol. 5, eds Whitcomb RF, Tully JG, Academic Press, San Diego, 243–364.

Bradbury JM, Levisohn S, 1996, Experimental infections in poultry, *Molecular and Diagnostic Procedures in Mycoplasmology*, vol. 2, eds Tully JG, Razin S, Academic Press, San Diego, 361–79.

Bredt W, 1979, Motility, *The Mycoplasmas*, vol. 1, eds Barile MF, Razin S, Academic Press, San Diego, 141–55.

Brunner H, Laber G, 1985, Chemotherapy of mycoplasma infections, *The Mycoplasmas*, vol. 4, eds Razin S, Barile MF, Academic Press, San Diego, 403–50.

Buttery SH, Plackett P, 1960, A specific polysaccharide from *Mycoplasma mycoides*, *J Gen Microbiol*, **23:** 357–68.

Bygdeman SM, Mårdh P-A, 1983, Antimicrobial susceptibility and susceptibility testing of *Mycoplasma hominis*: a review, *Sex Transm Dis*, **10, Suppl.:** 366–70.

Calavan EC, Bové JM, 1989, Ecology of *Spiroplasma citri*, *The Mycoplasmas*, vol. 5, eds Whitcomb RF, Tully JG, Academic Press, San Diego, 425–85.

Carle P, Rose DL et al., 1992, The genome size of spiroplasmas and other mollicutes, *IOM Lett*, **2:** 263.

Carle P, Laigret F et al., 1995, Heterogeneity of genome sizes within the genus *Spiroplasma*, *Int J Syst Bacteriol*, **45:** 178–81.

Cassell GH, Clyde WA Jr, Davis JK, 1985, Mycoplasmal respiratory infections, *The Mycoplasmas*, vol. 4, eds Razin S, Barile MF, Academic Press, San Diego, 65–106.

Cassell GH, Yancy A, 1996, Experimental mycoplasmal respiratory infections in rodents, *Molecular and Diagnostic Procedures in Mycoplasmology*, vol. 2, eds Tully JG, Razin S, Academic Press, San Diego, 327–36.

Cassell GH, Waites KB et al., 1993, *Ureaplasma urealyticum*: role in prematurity and disease in newborns, *Clin Microbiol Rev*, **6:** 69–87.

Chalquest RR, 1962, Cultivation of the infectious-synovitis-type pleuropneumonia-like organisms, *Avian Dis*, **6:** 36–43.

Chanock RM, Hayflick L, Barile M, 1962, Growth on artificial medium of an agent associated with atypical pneumonia and its identification as a PPLO, *Proc Natl Acad Sci USA*, **48:** 41–9.

Cirillo VP, 1979, Transport systems, *The Mycoplasmas*, vol. 1, eds Barile MF, Razin S, Academic Press, San Diego, 323–49.

Clyde WA Jr, 1983, Growth inhibition tests, *Methods in Mycoplasmology*, vol. 1, eds Razin S, Tully JG, Academic Press, San Diego, 405–10.

Clyde WA Jr, McCormack WM, 1983, Collection and transport of specimens, *Methods in Mycoplasmology*, vol. 1, eds Razin S, Tully JG, Academic Press, San Diego, 103–7.

Cole BC, Adkin CL, 1995, Identification, characterization, and purification of mycoplasmal superantigens, *Molecular and Diagnostic Procedures in Mycoplasmology*, vol. 1, eds Razin S, Tully JG, Academic Press, San Diego, 439–49.

Cole RM, Tully JG et al., 1973, Morphology, ultrastructure, and bacteriophage infection of the helical mycoplasma-like organisms (*Spiroplasma citri* gen. nov., sp. nov.) cultured from 'stubborn' disease of citrus, *J Bacteriol*, **115:** 367–86.

Collier AM, 1972, Pathogenesis of *Mycoplasma pneumoniae* infection as studied in the human foetal trachea in organ culture, *Pathogenic Mycoplasmas*, Ciba Symposium, Elsevier, New York, 307–27.

Del Giudice RA, Gardella RS, 1996, Antibiotic treatment of mycoplasma-infected cell cultures, *Molecular and Diagnostic Procedures in Mycoplasmology*, vol. 2, eds Tully JG, Razin S, Academic Press, San Diego, 439–43.

Del Giudice RA, Gardella RB, Hopps HE, 1980, Cultivation of formerly noncultivable strains of *Mycoplasma hyorhinis*, *Curr Microbiol*, **4:** 75–80.

Del Giudice RA, Hopps H, 1978, Microbiological methods and fluorescent microscopy for the direct demonstration of mycoplasma infection on cell cultures, *Mycoplasma Infection of Cell Cultures*, eds McGarrity GJ, Murphy DG, Nichols WW, Plenum Press, New York, 57–69.

Del Giudice RA, Tully JG, 1996, Isolation of mycoplasmas from cell cultures by axenic cultivation techniques, *Molecular and Diagnostic Procedures in Mycoplasmology*, vol. 2, eds Tully JG, Razin S, Academic Press, San Diego, 411–18.

Dienes L, Edsall G, 1937, Observations on the L-organism of Klieneberger, *Proc Soc Exp Biol Med*, **36:** 740–4.

Dybvig K, Khaled M, 1990, Isolation of a second cryptic plasmid from *Mycoplasma mycoides* subsp. *mycoides*, *Plasmid*, **24:** 153–5.

Edward DGff, 1947, A selective medium for pleuropneumonia-like organisms, *J Gen Microbiol*, **1**: 238–43.

Edward DGff, Freundt EA, 1967, Proposal for Mollicutes as name of the class established for the order *Mycoplasmatales*, *Int J Syst Bacteriol*, **17**: 267–8.

Faulkner CB, Simecka JW et al., 1995, Gene expression and production of tumor necrosis factor alpha, interleukin 1, interleukin 6, and gamma interferon in C3H/HeN and C57BL/6N mice in acute *Mycoplasma pulmonis* disease, *Infect Immun*, **63**: 4084–90.

Feng S-H, Lo S-C, 1994, Induced mouse spleen B-cell proliferation and secretion of immunoglobulins by lipid-associated membrane proteins of *Mycoplasma fermentans* incognitus and *Mycoplasma penetrans*, *Infect Immun*, **62**: 3916–21.

Ferris S, Watson HL et al., 1995, Characterization of a major *Mycoplasma penetrans* lipoprotein and of its gene, *FEMS Microbiol Lett*, **130**: 313–20.

Foissac X, Danet JL et al., 1996, Experimental infections of plants by spiroplasmas, *Molecular and Diagnostic Procedures in Mycoplasmology*, vol. 2, eds Tully JG, Razin S, Academic Press, San Diego, 385–9.

Fraser CM, Gocayne JD et al., 1995, The minimal gene complement of *Mycoplasma genitalium*, *Science*, **270**: 397–403.

Freundt EA, 1955, The classification of the pleuropneumonia group of organisms (Borrelomycetales), *Int Bull Bacteriol Nomencl Taxon*, **5**: 67–78.

Freundt EA, 1983, Culture medium for classic mycoplasmas, *Methods in Mycoplasmology*, vol. 1, eds Razin S, Tully JG, Academic Press, San Diego, 127–35.

Friis NF, 1971, Mycoplasma cultivated from the respiratory tract of Danish pigs, *Acta Vet Scand*, **12**: 69–79.

Furr PM, Taylor-Robinson D, 1981, The inhibitory effect of various antiseptics, analgesics and lubricants on mycoplasmas, *J Antimicrob Chemother*, **8**: 115–19.

Furr PM, Taylor-Robinson D, 1996, Urogenital infections in rodents, *Molecular and Diagnostic Procedures in Mycoplasmology*, vol. 2, eds Tully JG, Razin S, Academic Press, San Diego, 337–47.

Furr PM, Taylor-Robinson D, Webster ADB, 1994, Mycoplasmas and ureaplasmas in patients with hypogammaglobulinaemia and their role in arthritis: microbiological observations over twenty years, *Ann Rheum Dis*, **53**: 183–7.

Gallily R, Avron A et al., 1995, Activation of macrophages and monocytes by mycoplasmas, *Molecular and Diagnostic Procedures in Mycoplasmology*, vol. 1, eds Razin S, Tully JG, Academic Press, San Diego, 421–38.

Gardella RB, Del Giudice RA, 1995, Growth of *Mycoplasma hyorhinis* cultivar α on semisynthetic medium, *Appl Environ Microbiol*, **61**: 1976–9.

Gardella RB, Del Giudice RA, Tully JG, 1983, Immunofluorescence, *Methods in Mycoplasmology*, vol. 1, eds Razin S, Tully JG, Academic Press, San Diego, 431–9.

Gasparich G, Hackett KJ, 1994, Characterization of a cryptic extrachromosomal element isolated from the mollicute *Spiroplasma taiwanense*, *Plasmid*, **32**: 342–3.

Gasparich G, Hackett KJ et al., 1993, Occurrence of extra-chromosomal deoxyribonucleic acids in spiroplasmas associated with plants, insects, and ticks, *Plasmid*, **29**: 81–93.

Gelfand EW, 1993, Unique susceptibility of patients with antibody deficiency to mycoplasma infections, *Clin Infect Dis*, **17, Suppl. 1**: S250–3.

Giron JA, Lange M, Baseman JB, 1996, Adherence, fibronectin binding and induction of cytoskeleton reorganization in cultured human cells by *Mycoplasma penetrans*, *Infect Immun*, **64**: 197–208.

Glaser G, Hyman HC, Razin S, 1992, Ribosomes, *Mycoplasmas: Molecular Biology and Pathogenicity*, lst edn, eds Maniloff J, McElhaney RN et al., American Society for Microbiology, Washington, DC, 169–77.

Goodwin RFW, Whittlestone P, 1964, Production of enzootic pneumonia of pigs with a microorganism grown in a medium free of living cells, *Vet Rec*, **76**: 611.

Gourlay RN, 1970, Isolation of a virus infecting a strain of *Mycoplasma laidlawii*, *Nature (London)*, **225**: 1165.

Grau O, Slizewicz B et al., 1995, Association of *Mycoplasma penetrans* with human immunodeficiency virus, *J Infect Dis*, **172**: 672–81.

Hackett KJ, Lynn DE, 1995, Insect cell culture approaches in cultivating spiroplasmas, *Molecular and Diagnostic Procedures in Mycoplasmology*, vol. 1, eds Razin S, Tully JG, Academic Press, San Diego, 55–64.

Harris, R, Williamson J et al., 1996, Laboratory diagnosis of *Mycoplasma pneumoniae* infection, *Molecular and Diagnostic Procedures in Mycoplasmology*, vol. 2, eds Tully JG, Razin S, Academic Press, San Diego, 211–23.

Henrich B, Feldmann R-C, Hadding U, 1993, Cytoadhesins of *Mycoplasma hominis*, *Infect Immun*, **61**: 2945–51.

Hilbert H, Himmelreich R et al., 1994, DNA sequence analysis of the complete *Mycoplasma pneumoniae* genome and identification of genes and gene products, *IOM Lett*, **3**: 338.

Hopps H, Meyer BC et al., 1973, Problems concerning 'non-cultivable' mycoplasma contaminants in tissue culture, *Ann N Y Acad Sci*, **225**: 265–76.

Hori H, Sawada M et al., 1981, The nucleotide sequence of 5S rRNA from *Mycoplasma capricolum*, *Nucleic Acids Res*, **9**: 5407–10.

Howard CJ, Gourlay RN, 1974, An electron-microscopic examination of certain bovine mycoplasmas stained with ruthenium red and the demonstration of a capsule on *Mycoplasma dispar*, *J Gen Microbiol*, **83**: 393–8.

Howard CJ, Taylor G, 1985, Humoral and cell-mediated immunity, *The Mycoplasmas*, vol. 4, eds Razin S, Barile MF, Academic Press, New York, 259–92.

Jacobs E, Vonski M et al., 1996, Are outbreaks and sporadic respiratory infections by *Mycoplasma pneumoniae* due to two distinct subtypes?, *Eur J Clin Microbiol Infect Dis*, **15**: 38–44.

Jensen JS, Blom J, Lind K, 1994, Intracellular location of *Mycoplasma genitalium* in cultured Vero cells as demonstrated by electron microscopy, *Int J Exp Pathol*, **75**: 91–8.

Kirchhoff H, 1992, Motility, *Mycoplasmas: Molecular Biology and Pathogenicity*, eds Maniloff J, McElhaney RN et al., American Society for Microbiology, Washington, DC, 289–306.

Kirchhoff H, Rosengarten R et al., 1984, Flask-shaped mycoplasmas: properties and pathogenicity for man and animals, *Isr J Med Sci*, **20**: 848–53.

Kobisch M, Ross RF, 1996, Experimental infections of swine, *Molecular and Diagnostic Procedures in Mycoplasmology*, vol. 2, eds Tully JG, Razin S, Academic Press, San Diego, 371–6.

Konai M, Clark EA, Whitcomb RF, 1996, Temperature ranges and growth optima of *Spiroplasma* species (*Spiroplasmataceae; class Mollicutes*), *Microb Ecol*, **32**: 1–7.

Koshimizu K, Ito M et al., 1983, Selective medium for isolation of ureaplasmas from animals, *Jpn J Vet Sci*, **45**: 263–8.

Kostyal DA, Butler GH, Beezhold DH, 1995, *Mycoplasma hyorhinis* molecules that induce tumor necrosis factor alpha secretion by human monocytes, *Infect Immun*, **63**: 3858–63.

Koutsky LA, Stamm WE et al., 1983, Persistence of *Mycoplasma hominis* after therapy: importance of tetracycline resistance and of coexisting vaginal flora, *Sex Transm Dis*, **10, Suppl.**: 374–81.

Krause DC, Stevens MK, 1995, Localization of antigens on mycoplasma cell surface and tip structures, *Molecular and Diagnostic Procedures in Mycoplasmology*, vol. 1, eds Razin S, Tully JG, Academic Press, San Diego, 89–98.

Krause DC, Taylor-Robinson D, 1992, Mycoplasmas which infect humans, *Mycoplasmas: Molecular Biology and Pathogenesis*, eds Maniloff J, McElhaney RN et al., American Society for Microbiology, Washington, DC, 417–44.

ter Laak EA, Ruhnke HL, 1996, Mycoplasma infections of cattle, *Molecular and Diagnostic Procedures in Mycoplasmology*, vol. 2, eds Tully JG, Razin S, Academic Press, San Diego, 255–64.

Leach RH, 1976, The inhibitory effect of arginine on growth of some mycoplasmas, *J Appl Bacteriol*, **41**: 259–64.

Leach RH, 1983, Preservation of mycoplasma cultures and culture collections, *Methods in Mycoplasmology*, vol. 1, eds Razin S, Tully JG, Academic Press, San Diego, 197–204.

Leith DK, Trevino LB et al., 1983, Host discrimination of *Mycoplasma pneumoniae* proteinaceous immunogens, *J Exp Med*, **157:** 502–14.

Lo S-C, Dawson MS et al., 1989, Association of the virus-like infectious agent originally reported in patients with AIDS with acute fatal disease in previously healthy non-AIDS patients, *Am J Trop Med Hyg*, **41:** 364–76.

Lo S-C, Hayes MM et al., 1991, Newly discovered mycoplasma isolated from patients infected with HIV, *Lancet*, **338:** 1415–18.

Lo S-C, Hayes MM et al., 1992, *Mycoplasma penetrans* sp. nov., from the urogenital tract of patients with AIDS, *Int J Syst Bacteriol*, **42:** 357–64.

Lo S-C, Hayes MM et al., 1993a, Adhesion onto and invasion of mammalian cells by *Mycoplasma penetrans* – a newly isolated mycoplasma from patients with AIDS, *Mod Pathol*, **6:** 276–80.

Lo S-C, Wear DJ et al., 1993b, Fatal systemic infections of nonhuman primates by *Mycoplasma fermentans* (incognitus strain), *Clin Infect Dis*, **17, Suppl.:** S283–8.

McCoy, RE, Caudwell A et al., 1989, Plant diseases associated with mycoplasma-like organisms, *The Mycoplasmas*, vol. 5, eds Whitcomb RF, Tully JG, Academic Press, San Diego, 545–640.

McElhaney RN, 1992, Membrane structure, *Mycoplasmas: Molecular Biology and Pathogenesis*, eds Maniloff J, McElhaney RN et al., American Society for Microbiology, Washington, DC, 113–55.

McGarrity GJ, Kotani H, Butler GH, 1992, Mycoplasmas and tissue culture cells, *Mycoplasmas: Molecular Biology and Pathogenesis*, eds Maniloff J, McElhaney RN et al., American Society for Microbiology, Washington, DC, 445–54.

McGarrity GJ, Rose DL et al., 1983, *Mycoplasma muris*, a new species from mice, *Int J Syst Bacteriol*, **33:** 350–5.

Manchee RJ, Taylor-Robinson D, 1968, Haemadsorption and haemagglutination by mycoplasmas, *J Gen Microbiol*, **50:** 465–78.

Manchee RJ, Taylor-Robinson D, 1969a, Enhanced growth of T-strain mycoplasmas with N-2-hydroxy-ethylpiperazine-N′-2-ethanesulfonic acid buffer, *J Bacteriol*, **100:** 78–85.

Manchee RJ, Taylor-Robinson D, 1969b, Studies on the nature of receptors involved in attachment of tissue culture cells to mycoplasmas, *Br J Exp Pathol*, **50:** 66–75.

Maniloff J, 1992, Mycoplasma viruses, *Mycoplasmas: Molecular Biology and Pathogenesis*, eds Maniloff J, McElhaney RN et al., American Society for Microbiology, Washington, DC, 41–59.

Maniloff J, Morowitz H, Barnett RJ, 1965, Ultrastructure and ribosomes of *Mycoplasma gallisepticum*, *J Bacteriol*, **90:** 193–204.

Masover GK, Becker F, 1996, Detection of mycoplasmas by DNA staining and fluorescent antibody methodology, *Molecular and Diagnostic Procedures in Mycoplasmology*, vol. 2, eds Tully JG, Razin S, Academic Press, San Diego, 419–29.

Mernaugh GR, Dallo SF et al., 1993, Properties of adhering and nonadhering populations of *Mycoplasma genitalium*, *Clin Infect Dis*, **17, Suppl.:** S69–78.

Miles RJ, Taylor RR et al., 1994, Diversity of energy-yielding metabolism in *Mycoplasma* spp., *IOM Lett*, **3:** 165–6.

Montagnier L, Blanchard A et al., 1990, A possible role of mycoplasmas as co-factor in AIDS, *Retroviruses of human AIDS and related animal diseases*, eds Girard M, Valette L, Fondation Merieux, Lyon, France, 9–17.

Morowitz HJ, 1984, The completeness of molecular biology, *Isr J Med Sci*, **20:** 750–3.

Muto A, Yamao F, Osawa S, 1987, The genome of *Mycoplasma capricolum*, *Prog Nucleic Acid Res*, **34:** 28–58.

Muto A, Andachi Y et al., 1990, The organization and evolution of transfer RNA genes in *Mycoplasma capricolum*, *Nucleic Acids Res*, **18:** 5037–43.

Naot Y, 1995, Mycoplasmal B-cell mitogens, *Molecular and Diagnostic Procedures in Mycoplasmology*, vol. 1, eds Razin S, Tully JG, Academic Press, San Diego, 451–60.

Navas-Castillo J, Laigret F et al., 1992a, Le mollicute *Acholeplasma florum* possède un gène du système phosphoenolpyruvate sucre-phosphotransferase et il utilise UGA comme codon tryptophane, *C R Acad Sci (Paris)*, **315:** 43–8.

Navas-Castillo J, Laigret F et al., 1992b, Evidence for a phosphoenolpyruvate-dependent sugar-phosphotransferase system in the mollicute *Acholeplasma florum*, *Biochimie*, **75:** 675–9.

Neimark HC, Carle P, 1995, Molecular chromosome size determination and characterization of chromosomes from uncultured mollicutes, *Molecular and Diagnostic Procedures in Mycoplasmology*, vol. 1, eds Razin S, Tully JG, Academic Press, New York, 119–31.

Nocard E, Roux ER et al., 1896, Le microbe de la peripneumonia, *Ann Inst Pasteur (Paris)*, **12:** 240–62.

Nowak J, 1929, Morphologie, nature et cycle évolutif du microbe de la péripneumonie des bovidés, *Ann Inst Pasteur (Paris)*, **43:** 1330.

Pollack JD, 1992, Carbohydrate metabolism and energy conservation, *Mycoplasmas: Molecular Biology and Pathogenesis*, eds Maniloff J, McElhaney RN et al., American Society for Microbiology, Washington, DC, 181–200.

Proft T, Herrmann R, 1995, Physical and genetic mapping, *Molecular and Diagnostic Procedures in Mycoplasmology*, vol. 1, eds Razin S, Tully JG, Academic Press, San Diego, 133–57.

Purcell AH, 1996, Experimental phytoplasma infections in plants and insects, *Molecular and Diagnostic Procedures in Mycoplasmology*, vol. 2, eds Tully JG, Razin S, Academic Press, San Diego, 391–8.

Purcell RH, Taylor-Robinson D et al., 1966, Color test for the measurement of antibody to T-strain mycoplasmas, *J Bacteriol*, **92:** 6–12.

Ranhand JM, Mitchell WO et al., 1980, Covalently closed circular deoxyribonucleic acids in spiroplasmas, *J Bacteriol*, **143:** 1194–9.

Ranhand JM, Nur I et al., 1987, *Spiroplasma* species share common DNA sequences among their viruses, plasmids and genomes, *Ann Microbiol (Inst Pasteur)*, **138:** 509–22.

Rawadi G, Dussurget O, 1995, Advances in PRC-based detection of mycoplasmas contaminating cell cultures, *PCR Methods Appl*, **4:** 199–208.

Razin S, 1994, DNA probes and PCR in diagnosis of mycoplasma infections, *Mol Cell Probes*, **8:** 497–511.

Razin S, 1995, Molecular properties of mollicutes: a synopsis, *Molecular and Diagnostic Procedures in Mycoplasmology*, vol. 1, eds Razin S, Tully JG, Academic Press, New York, 1–25.

Razin S, Jacobs E, 1992, Mycoplasma adhesion, *J Gen Microbiol*, **138:** 407–22.

Razin S, Oliver O, 1961, Morphogenesis of mycoplasma and bacterial L-form colonies, *J Gen Microbiol*, **24:** 225–37.

Renaudin J, Bové JM, 1994, SpV1 and SpV4 spiroplasma viruses with circular, single-stranded DNA genomes, and their contribution to the molecular biology of spiroplasmas, *Adv Virus Res*, **44:** 429–63.

Renaudin J, Marais A et al., 1995, Integrative and free *Spiroplasma citri* oriC plasmids: expression of the *Spiroplasma phoeniceum* spiralin in *Spiroplasma citri*, *J Bacteriol*, **177:** 2870–7.

Roberts MC, 1992, Antibiotic resistance, *Mycoplasmas: Molecular Biology and Pathogenesis*, eds Maniloff J, McElhaney RN et al., American Society for Microbiology, Washington, DC, 513–23.

Roberts MC, Kenny GE, 1986, Dissemination of the *tet*M tetracycline resistant determinant to *Ureaplasma urealyticum*, *Antimicrob Agents Chemother*, **29:** 350–2.

Roberts MC, Koutsky LA et al., 1985, Tetracycline resistant *Mycoplasma hominis* strains containing streptococcal *tet*M sequences, *Antimicrob Agents Chemother*, **28:** 141–3.

Robinson LB, Wichelhausen RH, Roizman B, 1956, Contamination of human cell cultures by pleuropneumonia-like organisms, *Science*, **124:** 1147–8.

Rodwell A, Peterson JE et al., 1975, Striated fibers of the rho form of mycoplasma: in vitro assembly, composition, and structure, *J Bacteriol*, **122:** 1216–29.

Rogers MJ, Simmons J et al., 1985, Construction of the mycoplasma evolutionary tree from 5S rRNA sequence data, *Proc Natl Acad Sci USA*, **82:** 1160–4.

Romano N, LaLicata R, Alesi DR, 1986, Energy production in *Ureaplasma urealyticum*, *Pediatr Infect Dis*, **5, Suppl.:** S308–12.

Rose DL, Tully JG, 1983, Detection of β-D-glucosidase: hydrolysis of esculin and arbutin, *Methods in Mycoplasmology*, vol. 1, eds Razin S, Tully JG, Academic Press, San Diego, 385–9.

Rose DL, Tully JG et al., 1993, A test for measuring growth responses of mollicutes to serum and polyoxyethylene sorbitan, *Int J Syst Bacteriol*, **43:** 527–32.

Rosenbusch RF, Minion FC, 1992, Cell envelope: morphology and biochemistry, *Mycoplasmas: Molecular Biology and Pathogenesis*, eds Maniloff J, McElhaney RN et al., American Society for Microbiology, Washington, DC, 73–7.

Rosenbusch RF, Ruhnke HL, 1996, Experimental infections in cattle, *Molecular and Diagnostic Procedures in Mycoplasmology*, vol. 2, eds Tully JG, Razin S, Academic Press, San Diego, 377–84.

Rottem S, Kahane I (eds), 1993, *Mycoplasma Cell Membranes, Subcellular Biochemistry*, Plenum, New York.

Sachse K, 1994, Characteristics of *Mycoplasma bovis* cytadherence, *IOM Lett*, **3:** 431–2.

Saglio P, Lefléche D et al., 1971, Isolement, culture et observation au microscope électronique des structures de type mycoplasme associées à la maladie du stubborn des agrumes et leur comparaison avec les structures observées dans le cas de la maladie du greening des agrumes, *Physiol Veg*, **9:** 569–82.

Saillard C, Vignault JC et al., 1987, *Spiroplasma phoeniceum* sp. nov., a new plant pathogenic species from Syria, *Int J Syst Bacteriol*, **37:** 106–15.

Schneider B, Seemuller E, 1994, Presence of two sets of ribosomal genes in phytopathogenic mollicutes, *Appl Environ Microbiol*, **60:** 3409–12.

Schneider B, Seemuller E et al., 1995, Phylogenetic classification of plant pathogenic mycoplasma-like organisms or phytoplasmas, *Molecular and Diagnostic Procedures in Mycoplasmology*, vol. 1, eds Razin S, Tully JG, Academic Press, San Diego, 369–80.

Shepard MC, 1966, Human mycoplasma infections, *Health Lab Sci*, **3:** 163–9.

Shepard MC, 1983, Culture media for ureaplasmas, *Methods in Mycoplasmology*, vol. 1, eds Razin S, Tully JG, Academic Press, San Diego, 137–46.

Shepard MC, Lunceford CD, 1976, Differential agar medium (A7) for identification of *Ureaplasma urealyticum* (human T mycoplasmas) in primary cultures of clinical material, *J Clin Microbiol*, **3:** 613–25.

Shibata K-I, Sasaki T, Watanabe T, 1995, AIDS-associated mycoplasmas possess phospholipases C in the membrane, *Infect Immun*, **63:** 4174–7.

Simecka JW, Davis JK et al., 1992, Mycoplasma diseases of animals, *Mycoplasmas: Molecular Biology and Pathogenesis*, eds Maniloff J, McElhaney RN et al., American Society for Microbiology, Washington, DC, 391–444.

Smith A, Mowles J, 1996, Prevention and control of infections of cell cultures, *Molecular and Diagnostic Procedures in Mycoplasmology*, vol. 2, eds Tully JG, Razin S, Academic Press, San Diego, 445–51.

Smith CB, Friedewald WT, Chanock RM, 1967, Shedding of *Mycoplasma pneumoniae* after tetracycline and erythromycin therapy, *N Engl J Med*, **276:** 1172–5.

Smith PF, 1992, Membrane lipid and lipopolysaccharide structures, *Mycoplasmas: Molecular Biology and Pathogenesis*, eds Maniloff J, McElhaney RN et al., American Society for Microbiology, Washington, DC, 79–91.

Somerson NL, Walls BE, Chanock RM, 1965, Hemolysin of *Mycoplasma pneumoniae*: tentative identification as a peroxide, *Science*, **150:** 226–8.

Stanek G, Hirschl A, Laber G, 1981, Sensitivity of various spiroplasma strains against ethanol, formalin, glutaraldehyde and phenol, *Zentralbl Bakteriol Parasitenkd Infektionskr Hyg*, **174:** 348–54.

Stadtländer CTK-H, Watson HL et al., 1993, Cytopathogenicity of *Mycoplasma fermentans* (including strain incognitus), *Clin Infect Dis*, **17, Suppl.:** S289–301.

Su CJ, Baseman JB, 1990, Genome size of *Mycoplasma genitalium*, *J Bacteriol*, **172:** 4705–7.

Su CJ, Charoya A et al., 1990, Sequence divergency of the cytadhesin gene of *Mycoplasma pneumoniae*, *Infect Immun*, **58:** 2669–74.

Subcommittee on the Taxonomy of Mollicutes, 1995, Revised minimum standards for description of new species of the class *Mollicutes*, *Int J Syst Bacteriol*, **45:** 605–12.

Tarshis M, 1991, Spiroplasma cells utilize carbohydrates via the phospho-enolpyruvate-dependent sugar phosphotransferase system, *Can J Microbiol*, **37:** 477–9.

Taylor-Robinson D, 1983, Metabolism inhibition tests, *Methods in Mycoplasmology*, vol. 1, eds Razin S, Tully JG, Academic Press, San Diego, 411–17.

Taylor-Robinson D, 1995, *Mycoplasma* and *Ureaplasma*, *Manual of Clinical Microbiology*, 6th edn, eds Murray PR, Baron EJ et al., American Society for Microbiology Press, Washington, DC, 652–62.

Taylor-Robinson D, 1996a, Intracellular location of mycoplasmas, *Molecular and Diagnostic Procedures in Mycoplasmology*, vol. 2, eds Tully JG, Razin S, Academic Press, San Diego, 73–80.

Taylor-Robinson D, 1996b, Cidal activity testing, *Molecular and Diagnostic Procedures in Mycoplasmology*, vol. 2, eds Tully JG, Razin S, Academic Press, San Diego, 199–204.

Taylor-Robinson D, 1996c, Diagnosis of sexually transmitted diseases, *Molecular and Diagnostic Procedures in Mycoplasmology*, vol. 2, eds Tully JG, Razin S, Academic Press, San Diego, 225–36.

Taylor-Robinson D, Bébéar C, 1997, Antibiotic susceptibilities of mycoplasmas and treatment of mycoplasmal infections, *J Antimicrob Chemother*, in press.

Taylor-Robinson D, Bredt W, 1983, Motility of *Mycoplasma* strain G37, *Yale J Biol Med*, **56:** 910.

Taylor-Robinson D, Chen TA, 1983, Growth inhibitory factors in animal and plant tissues, *Methods in Mycoplasmology*, vol. 1, eds Razin S, Tully JG, Academic Press, San Diego, 109–14.

Taylor-Robinson D, Furr PM, 1986, Clinical antibiotic resistance of *Ureaplasma urealyticum*, *Pediatr Infect Dis*, **5, Suppl.:** 335–7.

Taylor-Robinson D, Manchee RJ, 1967, Spermadsorption and spermagglutination by mycoplasmas, *Nature (London)*, **215:** 484–7.

Taylor-Robinson D, Sarathchandra P, Furr PM, 1993, *Mycoplasma fermentans*–HeLa cell interactions, *Clin Infect Dis*, **17, Suppl.:** S302–4.

Taylor-Robinson D, Furr PM et al., 1981, Mycoplasma adherence with particular reference to the pathogenicity of *Mycoplasma pulmonis*, *Isr J Med Sci*, **17:** 599–603.

Taylor-Robinson D, Thomas BJ et al., 1983, The association of *Mycoplasma hominis* with arthritis, *Sex Transm Dis*, **10, Suppl.:** 191–8.

Taylor-Robinson D, Furr PM et al., 1987, Animal models of *Mycoplasma genitalium* urogenital infection, *Isr J Med Sci*, **23:** 561–4.

Tham NT, Ferris S et al., 1994, Identification of a P1-like adhesin gene from *Mycoplasma pirum*, *IOM Lett*, **3:** 419–20.

Thomas CB, Garnier M, Boothby JT, 1996, Monoclonal antibodies as diagnostic tools, *Molecular and Diagnostic Procedures in Mycoplasmology*, vol. 2, eds Tully JG, Razin S, Academic Press, San Diego, 137–46.

Tryon VV, Baseman JB, 1992, Pathogenic determinants and mechanisms, *Mycoplasmas: Molecular Biology and Pathogenesis*, eds Maniloff J, McElhaney RN et al., American Society for Microbiology, Washington, DC, 457–71.

Tully JG, 1980, Foreword, *Memoirs of E Klieneberger-Nobel*, Academic Press, London, i–ii.

Tully JG, 1983a, Bacterial and fungal inhibitors in mycoplasma culture media, *Methods in Mycoplasmology*, vol. 1, eds Razin S, Tully JG, Academic Press, San Diego, 205–9.

Tully JG, 1983b, Cloning and filtration techniques for mycoplasmas, *Methods in Mycoplasmology*, vol. 1, eds Razin S, Tully JG, Academic Press, San Diego, 173–7.

Tully JG, 1985, Newly discovered mollicutes, *The Mycoplasmas*, vol. 4, eds Razin S, Barile MF, Academic Press, San Diego, 1–26.

Tully JG, 1986, Biology of rodent mycoplasmas, *Viral and Mycoplasma Infections in Laboratory Rodents: Effects on Biomedical Research*, eds Bhatt PN, Jacoby RO et al., Academic Press, San Diego, 63–85.

Tully JG, 1989, Class Mollicutes: new perspectives from plant and arthropod studies, *The Mycoplasmas*, vol. 5, eds Whitcomb RF, Tully JG, Academic Press, San Diego, 1–31.

Tully JG, 1993, Current status of the mollicute flora of humans, *Clin Infect Dis*, **17, Suppl.**: S2–9.

Tully JG, 1995a, Culture medium formulation for primary isolation and maintenance of mollicutes, *Molecular and Diagnostic Procedures in Mycoplasmology*, vol. 1, eds Razin S, Tully JG, Academic Press, San Diego, 33–9.

Tully JG, 1995b, Determination of cholesterol and polyoxyethylene sorbitan growth requirements of mollicutes, *Molecular and Diagnostic Procedures in Mycoplasmology*, vol. 1, eds Razin S, Tully JG, Academic Press, New York, 381–9.

Tully JG, 1996, Mollicute–host interrelationships – current concepts and diagnostic implications, *Molecular and Diagnostic Procedures in Mycoplasmology*, vol. 2, eds Tully JG, Razin S, Academic Press, San Diego, 1–21.

Tully JG, Razin S (eds), 1996, *Molecular and Diagnostic Procedures in Mycoplasmology*, vol. 2, Academic Press, San Diego.

Tully JG, Whitcomb RF, 1991, The genus *Spiroplasma*, *The Prokaryotes*, vol. 2, 2nd edn, eds Balows A, Trüper HG et al., Springer-Verlag, New York, 1960–80.

Tully JG, Whitcomb RF et al., 1977, Pathogenic mycoplasmas: cultivation and vertebrate pathogenicity of a new spiroplasma, *Science*, **195**: 892–4.

Tully JG, Taylor-Robinson D et al., 1981, A newly discovered mycoplasma in the human urogenital tract, *Lancet*, **337**: 1288–91.

Tully JG, Taylor-Robinson D et al., 1983, Evaluation of culture media for the recovery of *Mycoplasma hominis* from the human urogenital tract, *Sex Transm Dis*, **10, Suppl.**: 256–60.

Tully JG, Taylor-Robinson D et al., 1986, Urogenital challenge of primate species with *Mycoplasma genitalium* and characteristics of infection induced in chimpanzees, *J Infect Dis*, **153**: 1046–54.

Tully JG, Bove JM et al., 1993, Revised taxonomy of the class *Mollicutes*: proposed elevation of a monophyletic cluster of arthropod-associated mollicutes to ordinal rank (*Entomoplasmatales* ord. nov.), with provision for familial rank to separate species with nonhelical morphology (*Entomoplasmataceae* fam. nov.) from helical species (*Spiroplasmataceae*), and emended descriptions of the order *Mycoplasmatales*, family *Mycoplasmataceae*, *Int J Syst Bacteriol*, **43**: 378–85.

Tully JG, Rose DL et al., 1995, *Mycoplasma pneumoniae* and *Mycoplasma genitalium* mixture in synovial fluid isolate, *J Clin Microbiol*, **33**: 1851–5.

Veilleux C, Razin S, May LH, 1996, Detection of mycoplasma infection by PCR, *Molecular and Diagnostic Procedures in Mycoplasmology*, vol. 2, eds Tully JG, Razin S, Academic Press, San Diego, 431–8.

Voelker LL, Weaver KE et al., 1995, Association of lysogenic bacteriophage MAV1 with virulence of *Mycoplasma arthritidis*, *Infect Immun*, **63**: 4016–23.

Vu AC, Foy HM et al., 1987, The principal protein antigens of isolates of *Mycoplasma pneumoniae* as measured by levels of immunoglobulin G in human serum are stable in strains collected over a 10 year period, *Infect Immun*, **55**: 1830–6.

Waites KB, Rudd PT et al., 1988, Chronic *Ureaplasma urealyticum* and *Mycoplasma hominis* central nervous system infections in preterm infants, *Lancet*, **2**: 17–21.

Wang R-HY, Lo S-C, 1995, ELISA in human urogenital infections and AIDS, *Molecular and Diagnostic Procedures in Mycoplasmology*, vol. 2, Academic Press, San Diego, 115–21.

Wang R-HY, Grandinetti T et al., 1993, Antibodies to *M. genitalium* in patients with AIDS and patients attending sexual transmitted diseases clinics, *Bacteriology Proceedings*, vol. G-17, American Society for Microbiology, Washington, DC, 165.

Washburn LR, 1996, Experimental models of arthritis, *Molecular and Diagnostic Procedures in Mycoplasmology*, vol. 2, eds Tully JG, Razin S, Academic Press, San Diego, 349–59.

Wear DJ, Lo S-C, 1995, Localization of mycoplasmas in tissues, *Molecular and Diagnostic Procedures in Mycoplasmology*, vol. 1, eds Razin S, Tully JG, Academic Press, San Diego, 81–7.

Weisburg WG, Tully JG et al., 1989, A phylogenetic analysis of the mycoplasmas: basis for their classification, *J Bacteriol*, **171**: 6455–67.

Wenzel R, Herrmann R, 1988, Repetitive DNA sequences in *Mycoplasma pneumoniae*, *Nucleic Acids Res*, **16**: 8337–50.

Whitcomb RF, 1983, Culture media for spiroplasmas, *Methods in Mycoplasmology*, vol. 1, eds Razin S, Tully JG, Academic Press, San Diego, 147–58.

Whitcomb RF, 1989, *Spiroplasma kunkelii*: biology and ecology, *The Mycoplasmas*, vol. 5, eds Whitcomb RF, Tully JG, Academic Press, San Diego, 487–544.

Whitcomb RF, Hackett KJ, 1996, Identification of mollicutes from insects, *Molecular and Diagnostic Procedures in Mycoplasmology*, vol. 2, eds Tully JG, Razin S, Academic Press, San Diego, 313–22.

Whitcomb RF, Tully JG (eds), 1989, *The Mycoplasmas*, vol. 5, Academic Press, San Diego.

Whitford HW, Rosenbusch RF, Lauerman LH (eds), 1994, *Mycoplasmosis in Animals: Laboratory Diagnosis*, Iowa State University Press, Ames, Iowa.

Wieslander A, Boyer MJ, Wroblewski H, 1992, Membrane protein structure, *Mycoplasmas: Molecular Biology and Pathogenesis*, eds Maniloff J, McElhaney RN et al., American Society for Microbiology, Washington, DC, 93–112.

Williamson DL, 1983, The combined deformation-metabolism inhibition test, *Methods in Mycoplasmology*, vol. 1, eds Razin S, Tully JG, Academic Press, San Diego, 477–83.

Williamson DL, Tully JG, Whitcomb RF, 1989, The genus *Spiroplasma*, *The Mycoplasmas*, vol. 5, eds Whitcomb RF, Tully JG, Academic Press, San Diego, 71–111.

Wise K, Kim KF, Watson-McGown R, 1995, Variant membrane proteins, *Molecular and Diagnostic Procedures in Mycoplasmology*, vol. 1, eds Razin S, Tully JG, Academic Press, San Diego, 227–41.

Wise K, Yogev D, Rosengarten R, 1992, Antigenic variation, *Mycoplasmas: Molecular Biology and Pathogenesis*, eds Maniloff J, McElhaney RN et al., American Society for Microbiology, Washington, DC, 473–89.

Woese C, Maniloff J, Zablen LB, 1980, Phylogenetic analysis of the mycoplasmas, *Proc Natl Acad Sci USA*, **77**: 494–8.

Zhang Q, Young TF, Ross RF, 1994, Identification and characterization of *Mycoplasma hyopneumoniae* adhesins, *IOM Lett*, **3**: 433–4.

Zucker-Franklin D, Davidson M, Thomas L, 1966, The interaction of mycoplasmas with mammalian cells, *J Exp Med*, **124**: 521–42.

BRUCELLA

M J Corbel

1   DEFINITION

Brucellae are small non-motile, non-sporing, gram-negative coccobacilli or short rods. They grow rather slowly on ordinary nutrient media; growth is improved by serum or blood. Metabolism is aerobic; there is no growth under strictly anaerobic conditions. Growth is often improved by carbon dioxide, which is essential for some strains. The organisms have little or no fermentative action on carbohydrates in conventional media. They oxidize certain amino acids, urea cycle intermediates and carbohydrates; oxidative patterns are useful for speciation. They are catalase positive and usually oxidase positive, reduce nitrates and hydrolyse urea to a variable extent. They are susceptible to genus-specific phages, with the lytic pattern dependent on species and colonial phase. The smooth phase expresses a distinctive outer-membrane lipopolysaccharide; the O chain is a homopolymer of 4-formamido-4,6-dideoxymannose. The genus is a member of the α_2 subdivision of the Proteobacteria. The species are intracellular parasites of humans and animals producing characteristic infections, particularly of the reticuloendothelial and reproductive systems. They contain 2 chromosomes, and the G + C content of the DNA is 58–59 mol%. Sequence homogeneity is so high that the existence of separate species is doubtful. The type species is *B. melitensis*.

2   INTRODUCTION

The genus *Brucella* comprises a group of very closely related bacteria. Molecular genetic studies have indicated that the genus contains only a single species differentiated into a number of biovars, with certain host preferences (Verger et al. 1985). The taxonomic validity of this viewpoint has been accepted but the proposed new nomenclature, which would identify all members of the genus as biovars of *B. melitensis*, has met with opposition on practical grounds (see section 12, pp. 844–5). For this reason, the traditional nomenclature is retained in the present work.

The first member of the group, *B. melitensis*, was isolated by Bruce in 1887 from the spleen tissue of patients who had died of Malta fever. Because of its coccoid morphology in vivo and on primary culture in vitro, the organism was described as a micrococcus. The name *Micrococcus melitensis* appeared in the earlier literature. Sheep and goats are the preferred natural hosts of *B. melitensis*, but other animals may also be infected. As with the other members of the genus, *B. melitensis* tends to localize in the reticuloendothelial system and the genital tract; genital infection of the pregnant female typically results in abortion. Humans are susceptible to infection, often manifest initially as an acute febrile illness which has been described by various names including **Malta fever**, **Mediterranean fever** and **undulant fever**. Chronic complications may succeed the acute phase and the term **brucellosis** is used as a convenient description for all phases of the disease. *B. melitensis* is fairly widely distributed throughout the world but is particularly common in countries around the Mediterranean littoral, the Arabian peninsula, central Asia and parts of Latin America. It probably accounts for the majority of cases of brucellosis in humans. This species is not found in North America, northern Europe, Australia or New Zealand.

The second member of the group, *B. abortus*, was

discovered by Bang in 1897, who isolated the organism from cows with contagious abortion, and by a series of experiments demonstrated its specific role in this disease. Cattle are the preferred natural hosts of this organism but it can also infect other animals. Although usually less virulent than *B. melitensis*, it can also cause brucellosis in humans. *B. abortus* is even more widespread than *B. melitensis* and has, at one time or another, been isolated in virtually all cattle-raising countries of the world. Over the past few decades, control campaigns have dramatically reduced the prevalence of *B. abortus* infection in most developed countries and eliminated it altogether from some. Countries which have reported the eradication of bovine brucellosis include Australia, Canada, the Czech Republic, Germany, Holland, Japan, the Scandinavian countries and New Zealand. It is now uncommon in the USA and most countries of western Europe. There are indications of a resurgence in some parts of eastern Europe which formerly reported a low incidence, including Russia and Ukraine.

The relationship between *B. abortus* and *B. melitensis* was not appreciated until attention was drawn to their similarities by Evans (1918). This led Meyer and Shaw (1920) to propose the genus *Brucella* to include both organisms.

The third member, *B. suis*, was first recorded in 1914 by Traum, who reported its isolation from the fetus of a sow. It is a natural parasite of pigs, frequently producing a generalized infection but with a tendency to localize in the genital tract. Infection can also be transmitted to other animals, although the host range tends to be narrower than that of *B. abortus* and *B. melitensis*, possibly for geographical rather than biological reasons. Infection is now rare in the USA but is prevalent in parts of Latin America, southern China and South East Asia. In Australia, it occurs in feral swine. In contrast with the *B. suis* strains typified by those described by Traum, other types have been found which show a different host range and pathogenicity. Thus, Thomsen (1934) isolated from pigs in Denmark, strains which differed in certain cultural properties from those found in the USA and were less pathogenic for humans. These Danish or European porcine strains have hares and swine as their natural hosts, and have been classified as *B. suis* biogroup ('biovar') 2; the American strains have been assigned to *B. suis* biogroups 1 and 3. Two additional *B. suis* biogroups have also been defined, neither of which causes natural infections in swine. *B. suis* biogroup 4 was originally described as a separate species, *B. rangiferi tarandi* (Davydov 1961), and infects reindeer in Alaska, Canada and northern Russia, causing reproductive failure. It is transmissible to humans and causes an undulant-fever syndrome. *B. suis* biogroup 5 has only been found in mouse-like rodents in the Caucasus (Vershilova et al. 1983). However, it is known to be pathogenic for humans and causes a disease similar to that produced by the other *B. suis* biogroups. Generally, *B. suis* strains are less widely distributed geographically than *B. abortus* or *B. melitensis*.

The fourth member of the *Brucella* group, *B. ovis*, was first observed at about the same time in Australia and New Zealand (Buddle and Boyes 1953, Simmons and Hall 1953) and identified as the cause of sexually transmitted epididymitis in rams. It has since been found in most other sheep-raising countries including Argentina, Chile, France, Germany, South Africa, USA, Spain and countries of the former Soviet Union. Although serological evidence suggests that humans can be infected by this organism, it has not been confirmed to be a cause of overt disease.

The fifth member, *B. neotomae*, was isolated by Stoenner and Lackman (1957) from desert wood rats in a remote area of Utah, USA. It has not been associated with disease in humans or other species and further isolates have not been recorded.

The sixth member of the genus, *B. canis*, was reported by Carmichael and Bruner (1968) as the cause of abortion among beagle dogs in the USA. It has since been found in dogs of various breeds in many countries including Argentina, Brazil, China, the Czech Republic, Germany, Japan, Madagascar, Mexico, Papua New Guinea, Peru and the Philippines. Occasional cases of infection have also been reported in humans, usually presenting as a mild pyrexial illness (Weber 1982).

Unlike *B. abortus*, *B. melitensis* and *B. suis*, in which virulence is associated with the smooth colonial form, *B. canis* and *B. ovis* have been found only in the non-smooth phase. This has implications for the serological diagnosis of infections caused by these organisms because, as will be shown, smooth and non-smooth *Brucella* strains are antigenically distinct.

Recently, *Brucella* strains have been isolated from marine mammals (Ross et al. 1994). The isolates comprise at least 2 distinct biogroups corresponding to strains of cetacean and phocine origin. Within these groups there is some variation in metabolic and antigenic properties. However, it is apparent that these isolates differ from the *Brucella* strains infecting terrestrial mammals. They appear to have low pathogenicity for ruminants but circumstantial evidence suggests that they are pathogenic for humans.

3 MORPHOLOGY

Typically *Brucella* spp. occur as small gram-negative coccobacilli, but coccal and bacillary forms also occur. The cells are short and slender; the axis is straight; the ends are rounded; the sides may be parallel or convex outwards. In length they vary from about 0.6 to 1.5 μm, and in breadth from 0.5 to 0.7 μm. The short forms may appear as oval cocci, or, if they are arranged singly, in pairs end to end, or in small groups; sometimes short chains of 4–6 members may be seen, especially in liquid media. Because of their frequently coccoid appearance, their bacillary nature may be in doubt, but it may be noted that they are smaller than any of the gram-negative cocci. Moreover, when arranged in pairs, their long diameter is in the same axis as that in which they are lying, as distinct from the gram-negative diplococci, whose long axis is generally at right angles to that in which they are lying (Fig. 35.1).

B. melitensis tends to be more coccal in form than *B. abortus* but this is not consistent enough to be of value for identification. The bacillary forms of *B. abortus* and *B. suis* are most readily apparent when grown on a rich medium, when individual cells may reach 2–3 μm in length. *B. melitensis* usually remains coccoid and rarely exceeds 1 μm in length. The organisms stain fairly well with the ordinary dyes. They are gram-negative, non-acid-fast, non-motile and non-sporing. Bipolar staining can occur and irregularity in the depth of colour may be seen especially in old cultures in which irregular forms appear. ʟ-forms have been isolated from natural sources (Nelson and Pickett 1951, Corbel, Scott and Ross 1980) and from cultures treated with penicillin, glycine or hormones (Hines, Freeman and Pearson 1964, Roux and Sassine 1971, Meyer 1976). They have the morphology and structure typical of bacteria that are cell wall defective. Although sometimes isolated from infected individuals, it has not been shown that these organisms retain their pathogenicity.

Brucella cells resist decolorization by dilute solutions of acids and alkalis and advantage has been taken of this in differential staining procedures for the examination of infected tissues. Modified Ziehl–Neelsen, Macchiavello, or Hansen and Köster's methods may be used (Christoffersen and Ottosen 1941, Stamp et al. 1950). These procedures are not absolutely specific for *Brucella* and false positive reactions may be given by chlamydiae, *Coxiella burnetii* and several species of gram-negative bacilli. Immunospecific staining with labelled immunoglobulins will differentiate *Brucella* from most other organisms but not from *Yersinia enterocolitica* O9. False positive staining reactions may also be given by gram-positive cocci containing protein A or protein G (Corbel 1973a, Brewer and Corbel 1980).

3.1 Ultrastructure

Brucella strains have many structural features in common with other gram-negative bacteria. Nevertheless, they show a number of important differences from the gram-negative bacilli typified by *Escherichia coli*. In electron micrographs from negatively stained preparations, the cell surface appears rugose, probably because of the presence of structures formed from the lipopolysaccharide (LPS)–protein complex which comprises the outer membrane. This layer, which is about 9 nm thick, encloses a muramic acid-containing peptidoglycan layer 3–5 nm thick which is much more prominent in *Brucella* cells than in *E. coli* (Dubray and Plommet 1976). Internal to this layer is a zone of low electron density, the **periplasmic** region. Closely associated with the inner cell membrane are polyribosome complexes. The cytoplasm contains small vacuoles and polysaccharide-containing granules (Dubray 1972). The chromosomal material has been located as an osmiophobic mass interspersed with delicate osmiophilic filaments (De Petris, Karlsbad and Kessel 1964, Peschkov and Feodorov 1978) (Fig. 35.2).

4 CULTURAL ASPECTS

4.1 Biohazard aspects

Brucella strains have frequently been implicated in laboratory-acquired infections and are appropriately classified as dangerous pathogens. In Britain they are assigned as Class 3 pathogens in the hazard classification of the Advisory Committee on Dangerous Pathogens (1994). Cultures and other materials potentially containing *Brucella* should only be handled under adequate containment conditions. Clinical specimens and isolates from patients with febrile disease should always be regarded with suspicion until positively identified. Accidental infections have occurred among unsuspecting laboratory staff.

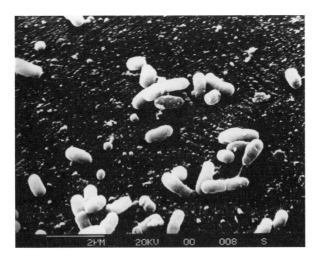

Fig. 35.1 Scanning electron micrograph of *B. abortus* strain 19 (bar = 2 μm).

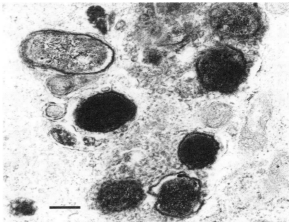

Fig. 35.2 Negatively stained thin section of bovine macrophage infected with *B. abortus* biogroup 1. The bacteria are enclosed in vacuoles and their outer membranes and internal structure are visible (bar = 0.25 μm).

Misidentification of cultures through the use of inadequate methods can present a particular hazard. The incorrect identification of *B. melitensis* as *Moraxella phenylpyruvica* through the use of API20NE rapid identification tests has resulted in several cases of laboratory-acquired brucellosis (Batchelor et al. 1992, Luzzi et al. 1993).

4.2   Cultural properties

Apart from different carbon dioxide requirements, all members of the genus resemble each other closely in cultural properties. Although most strains will grow on nutrient agar, growth tends to be slow and colony size small. Growth is much improved by the addition of blood, serum and tissue extracts. Liver-infusion agar was formerly recommended for the culture of *Brucella* spp. but has been superseded by more consistent media based on high quality peptone preparations, usually tryptic digests of soybean protein. These will support the growth of all but the most fastidious strains. *B. ovis*, *B. abortus* biogroup 2 and some strains of biogroups 3 and 4 grow very poorly in the absence of blood or serum, and media enriched with these are essential for their isolation.

On serum dextrose agar or similar medium, most *Brucella* strains produce raised, convex, circular, translucent colonies, 0.5–1 mm in diameter, after incubation for 48 h at 37°C. In direct light the colonies of smooth strains appear a clear honey colour, but in reflected light they have a distinctive bluish-grey translucency. Non-smooth strains produce colonies of similar size but of much more variable colour and consistency. They are usually more opaque than smooth colonies, with a granular dull surface and range in colour from off-white or yellowish to buff or even brown. Unlike smooth colonies, which are soft and easily emulsifiable, non-smooth colonies can be friable, tacky or obviously slimy.

Strains of the less fastidious types, especially *B. melitensis* and *B. suis*, will grow on bile-salt media producing small lactose-negative colonies. Growth in gelatin is poor and liquefaction is not produced. On blood agar, the colonial appearance is not distinctive; true haemolysis is not produced but a greenish brown discoloration develops around the colonies. In static liquid culture, maximum turbidity is produced after 7 days or longer. Most strains produce a uniform turbidity with a variable deposit. A surface pellicle may also be produced, especially by carbon dioxide-independent strains. Dissociation from smooth to non-smooth colonial forms occurs readily in static liquid media and may be marked by a change in the deposit from light and powdery to extremely viscous.

Dissociation is best detected by examination of 4 day old cultures on glycerol dextrose agar under a stereoscopic plate-microscope with obliquely reflected light (Henry 1933, FAO/WHO 1958). Smooth colonies appear small, circular, convex, translucent and greyish-blue with a smooth glistening surface. The undivided cells are uniformly short rods or coccobacilli arranged singly. Colonies of rough strains are of much the same size, but are less convex, more opaque and have a dull dry yellowish-white granular appearance. The individual cells are rather larger than those of the smooth form, and occasional long slender rods are present. Mucoid colonies are transparent, greyish or slightly orange, and slimy. The distinction between smooth and rough colonies can be increased by flooding plates with a 0.05% aqueous solution of crystal violet and pouring off the excess dye 15 s later. Smooth colonies then appear a light bluish-green, rough colonies are red or purple (White and Wilson 1951). (Fig. 35.3.)

Smooth colonies form uniform suspensions in saline or aqueous acriflavine. Non-smooth colonies are autoagglutinable in unbuffered saline solutions and in the presence of acriflavine. They can also be agglutinated by heating and by antiserum to the R antigenic determinant, or by the lectin concanavalin A (for further details see Corbel et al. 1979).

When inoculated on to the chorioallantoic membrane of the developing chick embryo, *B. abortus*, *B. melitensis*, *B. suis* and *B. canis* are able to multiply and to cause death of the embryo in a few days with lesions in the spleen and liver. All these organisms grow intracellularly – *B. melitensis* in the ectodermal epithelium, *B. abortus* and *B. suis* in cells of mesodermal origin and in the vascular endothelium. Rough strains of *B. abortus* and *B. melitensis* are usually non-invasive (Goodpasture and Anderson 1937). *B. canis*, in contrast, grows well in the chick embryo (Weber 1976). This procedure is no longer recommended for primary isolation of *Brucella*.

4.3   Growth requirements

Although laboratory-adapted strains can often be induced to grow in simple minimal media containing ammonium ion as sole nitrogen source (Gerhardt 1958), most *Brucella* strains have much more exacting nutritional requirements, especially on primary isolation. In general, several amino acids, thiamin, biotin, nicotinamide, magnesium, iron and manganese are

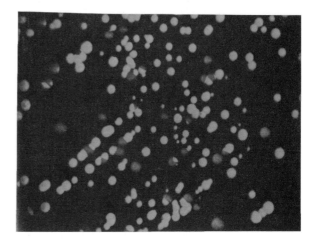

Fig. 35.3 Colonies of *B. melitensis* biogroup 1 grown on glycerol-dextose agar. Addition of 1% crystal violet solution to the plate has produced dark staining of the non-smooth (R) colonies but left the smooth (S) colonies unstained.

required for growth. The growth of many strains is improved by pantothenate and isoerythritol. Indeed, the latter substance is used by *B. abortus*, *B. melitensis* and *B. suis* as an energy source in preference to glucose.

All *Brucella* strains are aerobic but many are carboxyphilic and grow best in a carbon dioxide-enriched atmosphere. No growth occurs in strictly anaerobic conditions although it is reported that nitrate can substitute for molecular oxygen in some circumstances. The optimum temperature for growth is about 37°C but this occurs in the range 20–40°C. The thermal cutoff point for growth is difficult to identify precisely but the viability of cultures declines rapidly at temperatures above 45°C. The optimum pH is near neutrality and cultures are rapidly killed by extremes of acidity or alkalinity. Many strains produce alkali during metabolism and will turn litmus milk blue. It is essential to use media well buffered between pH 6.6 and 6.8 to prevent growth inhibition by alkali production. The optimum osmolarity is equivalent to between 0.05 M and 0.15 M sodium chloride.

4.4 Carbon dioxide requirement

Many strains of *B. abortus* and nearly all of *B. ovis* require for growth a partial pressure of carbon dioxide substantially in excess of that normally present in the atmosphere (0.03–0.04%). This is best supplied by a carbon dioxide incubator set to produce an atmosphere containing 5–10% carbon dioxide. The carbon dioxide serves as a metabolite and not simply to lower the pH or the oxygen tension. Radioactive-isotope studies have shown that *B. abortus* incorporates labelled carbon dioxide into alanine, glycine and pyrimidines (Newton et al. 1954). For further details of early studies on the carbon dioxide requirement of *B. abortus*, see Wilson (1983).

4.5 Selective media

For the isolation of *Brucella* from contaminated material, the use of selective media is generally required. Various formulations have been developed but the most generally useful are based on that of Farrell (1974). This contains bacitracin, cycloheximide, nalidixic acid, nystatin, polymyxin B and vancomycin in a serum dextrose agar base. A liquid medium containing a similar formulation with the addition of amphotericin B and D-cycloserine was devised by Brodie and Sinton (1975) for enrichment of *Brucella* and suppression of contaminants in milk samples. An improved version of this has been recommended by the joint FAO/WHO Expert Committee on Brucellosis (FAO/WHO 1986). It is suitable for the enrichment of milk or tissue homogenates from contaminated sources. A biphasic combination of these 2 selective media has also been described (Corbel and Hendry 1985).

These formulations are, however, too inhibitory for the isolation of some *Brucella* strains, particularly *B. ovis*. For this, a medium containing vancomycin, colistimethate, nystatin and nitrofurantoin has been recommended (Brown, Ranger and Kelly 1971). For the isolation of *Brucella* from human blood or bone marrow samples, a 2-phase culture system of the type devised by Castañeda (1947) is recommended. The sensitivity of isolation can be improved by using the lysis-concentration method for processing samples (Kolman et al. 1991). The time taken to detect positive cultures can also be reduced by using rapid, automated detection methods. Caution should be observed before discarding cultures as small inocula may take a considerable time to produce a positive result (Solomon and Jackson 1992). These methods have received most attention for the isolation of *B. melitensis*; *B. abortus* and other carboxyphilic strains may give significantly slower and possibly false negative results with systems which depend on radiometric measurement of carbon dioxide. (For further information see Corbel 1993.) Cultures should always be incubated in an atmosphere containing 5–10% carbon dioxide and retained for up to 6 weeks as growth may be slow, particularly if the patient has received previous antibiotic treatment. For further details of media, see Corbel and Morgan (1984).

4.6 Cultivation in the presence of dyes

Huddleson (1929) devised a method for distinguishing between *B. abortus*, *B. melitensis* and *B. suis* based on their differing susceptibility to inhibition by certain synthetic dyes. The method is still valid but does not produce absolute definition of these species because the sensitivity varies between biogroups, particularly in the case of *B. abortus* (see Table 35.1). The most useful dyes are basic fuchsin and thionin. When incorporated in a suitable basal medium, such as serum dextrose agar, basic fuchsin at a final concentration of c. 20 mg l^{-1} will permit the growth of all *B. abortus* biogroups except for 2 and some strains of 4, all *B. melitensis* biogroups but only biogroup 3 of *B. suis*. *B. neotomae* is inhibited as are most strains of *B. canis* and *B. ovis*.

Thionine at the same concentration inhibits the growth of *B. abortus* biogroups 1, 2 and 4 and *B. neotomae*, but permits the growth of all other types. Occasional variations in these patterns are encountered, e.g. *B. suis* biogroup 1 strains from South America are frequently resistant to basic fuchsin (Corbel, Thomas and Garcia-Carillo 1984) and atypical strains of *B. melitensis* are encountered (Corbel 1991). Two other dyes useful for certain purposes are thionine blue (not to be confused with thionin) and safranin O. Thionine blue in a concentration of 2 mg l^{-1} allows the growth of all 3 main species, but inhibits the attenuated vaccine strain *B. abortus* S19 and *B. abortus* biogroup 2. Safranin O in a concentration of 100–200 mg l^{-1} inhibits *B. suis* but, with a few exceptions, not other strains of *Brucella* (Moreira-Jacob 1963, Jones 1964).

The molecular basis of dye sensitivity has been explained by Douglas et al. (1984) in relation to the expression of specific porins (36 kDa outer-membrane proteins). The genes for these have been cloned

Table 35.1 Characters of the species and biogroups ('biovars') of *Brucella*[a]

Species	Biogroup	CO₂ requirement	H₂S production	Growth in presence of 1 in 50 000 (20 μg ml⁻¹)		Agglutination by monospecific serum[b]			Preferred natural host	Remarks
				Thionin	Basic fuchsin	A	M	R		
B. melitensis	1	–	–	+	+	–	+	–	Sheep, goat	Typical melitensis
	2	–	–	+	+	+	–	–	Sheep, goat	
	3	–	–	+	+	+	+	–	Sheep, goat	
B. abortus	1	(+)	+	–	+	+	–	–	Cattle	Typical abortus
	2	(+)	+	–	(+)	+	–	–	Cattle	Wilson II type
	3	(+)	+	+[c]	+	+	–	–	Cattle	Rhodesian type
	4	(+)	+	–	+	–	+	–	Cattle	British 'melitensis'
	5	–	–	+	+	–	+	–	Cattle	
	6	–	+	+[c]	+	+	–	–	Cattle	
	9	–	+	+	+	+	+	–	Cattle	
B. suis	1	–	+	+	(–)	+	–	–	Pig	American suis
	2	–	–	+	–	+	–	–	Pig, hare	Danish suis
	3	–	–	+	+	+	–	–	Pig	American 'melitensis'
	4	–	–	+	(–)	+	+	–	Reindeer	'*B. rangiferi tarandi*'
	5	–	–	+	–	–	+	–	Rodents	Caucasus only
B. neotomae		–	+	–	–	+	–	–	Desert wood rat	USA only
B. canis		–	–	+	(–)	–	–	+	Dog	Canine abortion organism
B. ovis		+	–	+	(–)	–	–	+	Sheep	Ram epididymitis organism
B. 'maris'		+ or –	–	+	+	+	+ or –	–	Marine mammals	Pathogenicity unknown

+, positive; –, negative; (+), usually positive; (–), usually negative.
[a] For oxidative metabolism, see Table 35.2; for phage susceptibility see Table 35.4.
[b] A, abortus; M, melitensis; R, rough.
[c] *B. abortus*, biogroup 3 grows in the presence of 1 in 25 000 thionin; biogroup 6 does not.
Former *B. abortus* biogroups 7 and 8 are no longer regarded as valid.

(Ficht et al. 1989) and shown to be polymorphic. In *B. abortus* at least, 2 variants of the porin gene exist, *omp2a* and *omp2b*. Only the latter is expressed under normal cultural conditions.

B. abortus S19 may also be differentiated from virulent strains of *B. abortus* biogroup 1 by its sensitivity to penicillin 3 mg l⁻¹ (Jones, Montgomery and Wilson 1965) and mitomycin C 1 mg l⁻¹ (Myers and Dobosch 1969). Most current vaccine seed cultures are also inhibited by isoerythritol 1–2 mg l⁻¹ but it is not clear if this was a property of the original strain (Thomas, Bracewell and Corbel 1981). PCR with primers specific for the *Hin*dIII region of the erythritol catabolism gene *eri* also differentiates strain S19 (Sangari et al. 1994).

The vaccine strain Rev 1 of *B. melitensis* grows more slowly, is more sensitive to penicillin and more resistant to streptomycin, and displays weaker urease activity than field strains. No different characters have been reported for distinguishing the vaccine strain 2 of *B. suis* from field strains of biogroup 1.

Further information on the use of dye tests is given in Wilson and Miles (1964).

5 METABOLISM AND BIOCHEMICAL PROPERTIES

All *Brucella* strains are aerobic and require oxygen for growth. No growth occurs under strictly anaerobic conditions. The requirement of some strains for supplementary carbon dioxide has been mentioned. Although acid production from sugars has been demonstrated under special conditions (Pickett and Nelson 1955), metabolism is essentially oxidative. *Brucella* strains are catalase positive and most are oxidase positive. They also have superoxide dismutase activity mediated by 2 distinct enzymes, a manganese superoxide dismutase of typical prokaryote type (Sriranganathan et al. 1991) and a copper-zinc enzyme (Beck, Tabatabai and Mayfield 1990). In the case of *B. abortus*, the respiratory system has been shown to make use of cytochromes *a* and *a₃*, cytochrome *b*, cytochrome *c*, cytochrome *o*, flavoproteins and ubiquinone (Rest and Robertson 1975). Energy-yielding processes involve the monophosphate pathway and the tricarboxylic acid cycle (Robertson and McCullough 1968). Glucose is metabolized by most strains but isoerythritol is used preferentially by *B. abortus*, *B. melitensis* and *B. suis*. *B. ovis* shows little activity towards either substrate; its preferred energy source is unknown, but it has been shown to oxidize water-soluble components of various ovine tissues very actively (Redwood and Corbel 1983).

Most *Brucella* strains produce nitrate reductase and will reduce nitrate to nitrite and may also reduce nitrite, especially *B. suis* biogroup 1. *B. ovis* and, occasionally, strains of other species, do not reduce nitrate. Hydrogen sulphide is produced from sulphur-containing amino acids. Strains of *B. abortus*, *B. neotomae* and *B. suis* biogroup 1 produce it in sufficient quantity to assist in their identification; the other species produce it in small quantities or not at all. *Brucella*

strains do not produce indole from tryptophan. They have the capacity to synthesize most if not all amino acids essential to growth. The genes for biosynthesis of proline and leucine have been cloned (Essenberg and Sharma 1993).

Brucellae do not form acetylmethylcarbinol from glucose and hence give negative results in the Voges–Proskauer test. They also give negative reactions in the methyl red test although acid production from glucose can be demonstrated by sensitive techniques (Pickett 1994). The reaction for *o*-nitro-phenol β-D-galactosidase is usually also negative. Urease is produced by most strains but the activity varies considerably between species and even between strains within species. *B. canis* and *B. suis* consistently give strong urease reactions, producing a magenta colour on Christensen's medium with 5 min. At the other extreme, *B. ovis* is a weak producer of urease and some strains may give negative reactions even after incubation for 7 days. Strains of *B. abortus*, *B. melitensis* and *B. neotomae* fall between these extremes and usually give positive urease reactions after 1 h or more. Nevertheless, variation occurs between strains and the test is of limited value for species identification (Corbel and Hendry 1985).

The oxidative activity of *Brucella* strains towards selected amino acid and carbohydrate substrates varies in a manner which correlates closely with other properties used to define the species. Originally, manometric methods were used to detect oxidation (McCullough and Beal 1951, Meyer and Cameron 1957, 1961a,b) and although hazardous and time-consuming to perform, they are still useful when quantitative studies are to be performed. Nevertheless, quantitative variations in activity between strains within a species can cause confusion. To overcome this problem, Verger and Grayon (1977) established 3 levels of oxidative activity, corresponding to low, medium and high oxygen uptake, which they used to produce a metabolic profile for each of the main species. The metabolic activity towards selected substrates can also be determined qualitatively by thin layer chromatography (Balke, Weber and Fronk 1977, Corbel and Morgan 1984). The patterns of oxidative activity characteristic of the species are shown in Table 35.2.

There is some variation in oxidative pattern between the biogroups of *B. suis*, but in our experience this is not sufficiently reliable for identification. With an extended range of substrates, further differentiation of *B. melitensis* strains beyond the 3 currently recognized biogroups has been reported (Arnaud-Bosq et al. 1987). Caution should be exercised, however, in attributing significance to minor differences in oxidative activity as this can be influenced by many factors including method of preservation of the strain and cultural conditions.

6 SUSCEPTIBILITY TO PHYSICAL AND CHEMICAL AGENTS

The members of this group exhibit the usual suscepti-

Table 35.2   Oxidative metabolism of species of *Brucella*

	Species					
	B. melitensis	*B. abortus*	*B. suis*	*B. neotomae*	*B. canis*	*B. ovis*
Amino acids						
L-Alanine	+	+	v*	v	v	v
L-Asparagine	+	+	v*	+	−	+
L-Glutamate	+	+	v*	+	+	+
L-Arginine	−	−	+	−	+	−
DL-Citrulline	−	−	+	−	+	−
L-Lysine	−	−	v*	−	+	−
DL-Ornithine	−	−	+	−	+	−
Carbohydrates						
L-Arabinose	−	+	v*	+	v	−
D-Galactose	−	+	v*	+	v	−
D-Ribose	−	+	+	v	+	−
D-Xylose	−	v	−	−	−	−
D-Glucose	+	+	+	+	+	−
Isoerythritol	+	+	+	+	v	−

+, positive; −, negative; v, variation between strains; v*, variation between biogroups of some assistance in classification.

bility of vegetative bacteria to heat and disinfectants. In aqueous suspensions of moderate density they are destroyed by heating for about 10 min at 60°C but in very dense suspensions they may survive much higher temperatures (Swann et al. 1981). In agar cultures kept sealed at 4°C they generally survive for at least 1 month, and often longer. If lyophilized, especially in the presence of a protecting agent, they will survive for decades.

Considerable attention has been paid to their resistance under natural conditions and this subject is discussed in the report of the Mediterranean Fever Commission (1905–7). So many factors determine the exact outcome of any given observation under natural conditions that it is dangerous to draw general conclusions. In favourable circumstances, however, *B. melitensis* may remain viable for 6 days in urine, 6 weeks in dust and 10 weeks in water or soil. In pickled hams from naturally infected pigs, *B. suis* can live for as long as 3 weeks, but it is apparently destroyed by smoking (Hutchings et al. 1951). *B. suis* may live on sacking for 4 weeks and in sterile faeces for 100 days in the dark. *B. abortus* may survive for 7 months in infected uterine exudate kept at about freezing point (Bang 1897). It can also survive in bovine urine for 4 days, faeces for 120 days, aborted fetuses for 75 days and liquid manure for up to 2.5 years. In raw milk at room temperature it seems to die out fairly rapidly with the production of acid. Acid production also seems to be the cause of its rapid death in butter, cheese and yoghurt although variable reports exist on its survival in these materials. In general, survival in soft, non-acid cheeses is much longer than in hard, lactic- or propionic-acid-fermented cheeses. Pasteurization, whether by holder or high-temperature short-time cycles, kills *Brucella* in milk. Ultraviolet and γ-radiation at normal sterilizing dosage are rapidly lethal to *Brucella* provided that the organisms are not protected by the suspending medium. Ethanol, isopropanol, iodophors, phenols, hypochlorite, ethylene oxide and formaldehyde (either gaseous or as aqueous formalin) are effective disinfectants for *Brucella* under appropriate conditions; they are killed by 1.0% phenol in 15 min. Xylene and calcium cyanamide have been

recommended for killing *Brucella* in manure but prolonged contact times are required (FAO/WHO 1986).

7   SUSCEPTIBILITY TO ANTIMICROBIAL AGENTS

Good intracellular penetration is essential for in vivo activity against *Brucella* and thus there is limited correlation between in vitro performance and therapeutic efficacy. β-Lactam antibiotics show limited activity against *Brucella* (Hall and Manion 1970). Some strains are inhibited by benzylpenicillin, ampicillin and amoxycillin. Most strains are resistant to methicillin, nafcillin, ticarcillin and piperacillin. Similarly, first and second generation cephalosporins show limited activity against *Brucella* but some third generation cephalosporins such as cefotaxime, ceftizoxime and ceftriaxone have MICs in the range 0.25–2 mg l^{-1}(Palenque, Otero and Noriga 1986). Latamoxef is also active and has been used therapeutically, alone or in combination with rifampicin (Tosi and Nelson 1982). The MIC for chloramphenicol is in the range 2–3 mg l^{-1} for most strains. Sensitivity to macrolides is variable. With the exception of *B. abortus* biogroup 2 and *B. ovis*, most strains are resistant to erythromycin, with $MIC_{90} \geq 16$ mg l^{-1}. Sensitivity to dirithromycin and roxithromycin is similar but clarithromycin and azithromycin show 2–8 fold greater activity (Garcia Rodriguez et al. 1993).

Most *Brucella* strains are inhibited by streptomycin, gentamicin, kanamycin, tobramycin and amikacin at concentrations of 1–4 mg l^{-1}(Mortensen et al. 1986). Streptomycin augments the activity of tetracycline in infected cell cultures and this is borne out by therapeutic experience (Richardson and Holt 1962, Colmenero et al. 1989). Sensitivity to tetracyclines is universal, with MICs in the region of 0.1 mg l^{-1}(Hall and Manion 1970). *Brucella* strains are also highly sensitive to rifamycins; the MICs for rifampicin are in the range 0.1–2 mg l⁻¹ with MBCs at approximately 4 times this concentration (Hall and Manion 1970, Corbel 1976a). Single step resistance develops rapidly in vitro (Corbel 1976a) and has also been observed during the course of therapy (de Rautlin de la Roy et al. 1986). Rifapentine has similar activity to rifampicin but has superior pharmacokinetic properties (Garcia Rodriguez et al. 1993).

Brucella strains are generally resistant to nalidixic acid but show in vitro sensitivity to the fluoroquinolones. The MICs for ciprofloxacin are in the range 0.5–1 mg l⁻¹ but therapeutic results have been disappointing (Bosch et al. 1986). Sensitivity to co-trimoxazole is borderline with the MIC₉₀ being just within the breakpoint (García Rodriguez et al. 1993). This is consistent with the high relapse rate observed with this drug.

For further information on the antibiotic treatment of brucellosis, see Volume 3, Chapter 41.

8 CELLULAR COMPOSITION

The gross cellular composition is similar to that of other gram-negative bacteria. Thus the dry weight of the cell comprises an average 40–50% protein, 20–25% carbohydrate, c. 7% total lipid (2.5% bound lipid, 2% phospholipid and 2.5% neutral lipids), 10–15% RNA and 1.5–3% DNA. The precise proportions of these constituents are very dependent on conditions of growth.

In relation to detailed chemical composition, brucellae strains show some distinctive features. *Brucella* cells are more resistant to the action of lysozyme, even in the presence of chelating agents and non-ionic detergents, than are enterobacterial cells which suggests some unusual features in peptidoglycan structure. The latter comprises a glycan skeleton of D-glucosamine and muramic acid linked by short chains of alanine, glutamic acid and α,ε-diaminopimelic acid. However, it also contains covalently linked proteins and lipids. (Cherwonogrodzky et al. 1990).

In *B. abortus* the outer-membrane proteins include the 88–94 kDa high molecular weight group 1, the 43 kDa and 36–38 kDa porin proteins of group 2 (Douglas et al. 1984) and the 25–27 kDa proteins of group 3, as well as minor proteins of 15–31 kDa. A lipoprotein of 8 kDa is also covalently linked to the peptidoglycan skeleton. These components are also present in the other nomen species but with quantitative differences (Santos et al. 1984, Verstreate and Winter 1984). In addition to the above, *B. melitensis* contains a 31 kDa outer-membrane protein and another of 39–40 kDa.

In all *Brucella* strains, the group 2 proteins are by far the most abundant. The genes for the 36 kDa porins (*omp2a* and *omp2b*) have been cloned and the peptide sequences determined (Ficht et al. 1989). The group 3 proteins were assumed to be analogues of OMP A but sequence data have not confirmed this.

The 8 kDa lipoprotein resembles the Braun lipoprotein of *E. coli* in molecular weight, isoelectric point and amino acid composition but differs from it in being surface exposed (Gomez Miguel et al. 1987). *Brucella* is also distinguished by being particularly rich in myristic, palmitic and stearic acids, in containing moderate quantities of *cis*-vaccenic and arachidonic acids, low quantities of C17 and C19 cyclopropane fatty acids and no hydroxy fatty acids. It is believed that this unusual fatty acid composition contributes to hydrophobic interactions in the *Brucella* outer membrane and enhances its stability (Cherwonogrodzky et al. 1990).

The unusual glycose composition of the LPS is discussed elsewhere (see section 9, Antigenic structure). Another distinctive polysaccharide component is the material identified as polysaccharide B, also known as component 1 or second component. This was thought to be an antigen related to the O polysaccharide (Diaz et al. 1979). However, it was subsequently shown to be a cyclic polymer of 17–24 β-1,2 linked D-glucose residues (Bundle, Gerken and Peters 1988). It is apparently non-antigenic and similar to the cyclic β-D-glucans synthesized by many other bacteria. It readily forms non-covalently linked complexes with *Brucella* LPS and O chain.

The lipid composition of *Brucella* cells has a number of distinctive features which reinforce the taxonomic affiliation of the genus to the α₂ subdivision of the Proteobacteria.

The free lipid fraction comprises mainly phospholipids and neutral lipids. Phosphatidylcholine is the principal phospholipid, in contrast to most bacterial species (Thiele and Schwinn 1973), although it is also present in *Agrobacterium tumefaciens*. Its presence confers distinctive properties on the outer membrane and may account for its reduced susceptibility to phospholipases and lysozyme. Phosphatidylglycerol and diphosphatidylglycerol are also present as major lipids. Phosphatidyl ethanolamine, phosphatidyl serine and candiolipin are represented as minor components. The fatty acids associated with the phospholipid fraction are unusual in that lactobacillic (C19: cyclic) acid, typical of gram-positive but not gram-negative species, is usually the major cyclopropane fatty acid, together with its metabolic precursor *cis*-vaccenic (C18:1 cyclic) acid. It should be noted that *B. canis* is an exception to this and has *cis*-vaccenic acid as the major fatty acid with lactobacillic acid in only trace amounts. This largely accounts for the distinct position of *B. canis* vis-à-vis the other nomen species when fatty acid composition is used for taxonomic analysis (Tanaka et al. 1977).

The neutral lipids include unusual wax-like esters containing large quantities of palmitic (C16:0) acid and moderate amounts of myristic (C14:0), palmitoleic (C16:1), stearic (C18:0) and *cis*-vaccenic (C18:1) acids. Lactobacillic acid is absent from these compounds.

Other distinctive free lipid components of *Brucella* include ubiquinone Q10 and ornithine-containing lipids (Thiele and Schwinn 1973). The latter make up 32% of the total neutral lipid. They contain lactobacillic, *cis*-vaccenic and palmitoleic acids in ester linkage and palmitic and stearic acids in amide linkage but no hydroxy fatty acid. The function of the ornithine lipids is unknown but they are structural components of the outer membrane and it has been suggested that they are implicated in the attachment of *Brucella* cells to the surface of macrophages and lymphocytes (Cherwonogrodzky et al. 1990). Minor free lipid components include 1,3 and 1,2 diesters of glycerol and monoesters of ethylene glycol.

The bound lipids are mainly associated with the LPS, lipoprotein and glycolipid fractions of the outer membrane. The composition of the LPS is unusual in that the lipid A backbone is formed of 2,3-diamino-2,3-dideoxy-D-glucose as well as D-glucosamine. This feature is present in some other members of the Proteobacteria (Weckesser and Mayer 1988). Both amide- and ester-linked fatty acids are attached to the aminoglycose skeleton. The amide-linked acids include 3-O-(C16:0) 12:0 (25%), 3-O-(C16:0) 13:0 (4%), 3-O-(C16:0) 14:(64%) and 3-O-(C18:0) 14:(7%) as diesters with 3-OH(C16:0) as the unsubstituted fatty acid. The ester-linked acids comprise C:16:0, 3-OH-C16:0, 3– -C18:0 and C18:0 acids which account for 37%, 12.5%, 3.5% and 4.5% respectively of the total fatty acids. Lactobacillic and unsaturated fatty acids are absent from the lipid A of *Brucella* although represented in many other lipid components (Cherwonogrodzky et al. 1990).

9 ANTIGENIC STRUCTURE

9.1 Surface antigens

LPS ANTIGENS

The antigenic composition of the *Brucella* cell surface varies with the colonial phase of the organism. All smooth *Brucella* strains cross-react extensively in agglutination tests with antisera prepared against smooth cultures. Similarly, all rough strains show extensive cross-reactions in tests with antisera to non-smooth cultures. However, there is little or no cross-reactivity between the major surface antigens of smooth and completely non-smooth cultures, with varying degrees between strains in transition from smooth to rough phases. Failure to appreciate these differences led to much confusion in earlier studies on the antigenic structure of *Brucella* (for details, see Wilson and Miles 1964). The studies of Wilson and Miles (1932) represented a major advance in the understanding of the antigenic structure of the *Brucella* cell surface. By careful cross-adsorption of antiserum to typical *B. abortus* strains with cells of *B. melitensis* and vice versa, they produced antisera that were monospecific for the A determinant of *B. abortus* or the M determinant of *B. melitensis*. They attributed the cross-reactivity of smooth strains to the presence of a small proportion of the heterospecific antigen in the homologous strain. Subsequently, Miles and Pirie (1939a,b) identified the serological activity with a formylated phospholipid-aminopoly-hydroxy compound isolated from culture supernates. Later studies showed that the A and M epitopes were associated with the LPS complexes that partitioned into the phenol phase on extraction by the Westphal method (Diaz et al. 1968).

Initial attempts at chemical characterization of the structures responsible for the cross-reactivity of smooth strains and the A and M specificity were unsuccessful. Subsequently Perry and colleagues concluded that the O chain of smooth LPS was degraded by conventional hydrolysis procedures. By carbon-13 and proton nuclear magnetic resonance spectroscopy in combination with polarimetry and methylation analysis, they demonstrated that the O chains from smooth *B. abortus* and smooth *B. melitensis* were both homo-

polymers of 4,6 dideoxy-4-formamido-D-mannose (N-formyl-D-perosamine) (Caroff, Bundle and Perry 1984, Caroff et al. 1984, Bundle et al. 1987). In the case of *B. abortus* LPS, the O chain consists of about 100 glycose residues nearly all linked α-1,2 but with a very small proportion linked α-1,3.

In the case of *B. melitensis* LPS, the O chains consist of unbranched linear polymers of pentasaccharide units comprising 4 residues linked α-1,2 and one residue linked α-1,3. The difference in linkage produces penta- or hexasaccharide units with different preferred conformations (Figure 35.4). This hypothesis has been confirmed by crystallographic studies with monoclonal antibodies which differentiate the rod-like A epitope from the kinked M structure (Rose et al. 1993). The common presence of non-terminal tetrasaccharide units of α-1,2 linked N-formyl-D-perosamine explains the cross-reactivity observed between the LPS of all smooth *Brucella* strains. The A- and M-specific epitopes are actually present as minority structures in both types of LPS. In the case of strains typified by *B. abortus* biogroup 1, the O chains contain predominantly A epitopes with a very small proportion of M epitope attributable to the few α-1,3 linked residues. In strains typified by *B. melitensis* biogroup 1, the reverse situation applies. This confirms the hypothesis of Wilson and Miles (1932) that A and M epitopes resided on a single molecule, the observed specificity being determined by the relative proportions of each.

By means of slide agglutination, agglutinin absorption or enzyme immunoassays with polyclonal antisera or monoclonal antibodies specific for the A and M epitopes, the A or M antigen predominance of *Brucella* strains can be determined (Wilson and Miles 1932, Olin 1935, Meikle et al. 1989, Bundle et al. 1989). This information is useful in classifying the smooth *Brucella* nomen species into biogroups. It should be noted that strains of *B. abortus*, *B. melitensis* or *B. suis* can be A, M or A and M antigen positive (see Table 35.1 and Dubray and Limet 1987). Strains that are both A and M antigen positive synthesize LPS with O chains that contain both A and M structural features in relatively high proportion (Perry and Bundle 1990).

N-Acylated-D-perosamine also occurs in the O chains of the LPS complexes of *E. coli* 0157, *Salmonella* Kauffmann–White group N (Bundle et al. 1987), *Stenotrophomonas maltophilia* strain 555, *Vibrio cholerae* (Redmond 1979, Kenne et al. 1982) and *Yersinia enterocolitica* 09 (Caroff, Bundle and Perry 1984), all of which cross-react serologically with smooth *Brucella* (for references, see Corbel 1985). Cross-reactions also occur between *Brucella* and *Francisella tularensis* (Francis and Evans 1926, Ohara, Sato and Homma 1974), but it is not known if the latter organism contains D-perosamine.

The structure of the LPS of rough *Brucella* strains is basically similar to that of smooth strains. Both contain the same lipid A in which both 2,3-diamino-2,3-dideoxyglucose and 2-amino-2-dioxyglucose occur in the glycose backbone. This is linked through 2-keto-3-deoxyoctulosonic acid (KDO) to the core polysaccharide composed of glucose, mannose and 6-amino-6-deoxglucose (quinovosamine). Heptose is notably absent from *Brucella* LPS. A short homopolymer of N-formyl perosamine has been reported in the LPS of some rough *B. abortus* strains and *B. canis* (Perry and Bundle 1990). How-

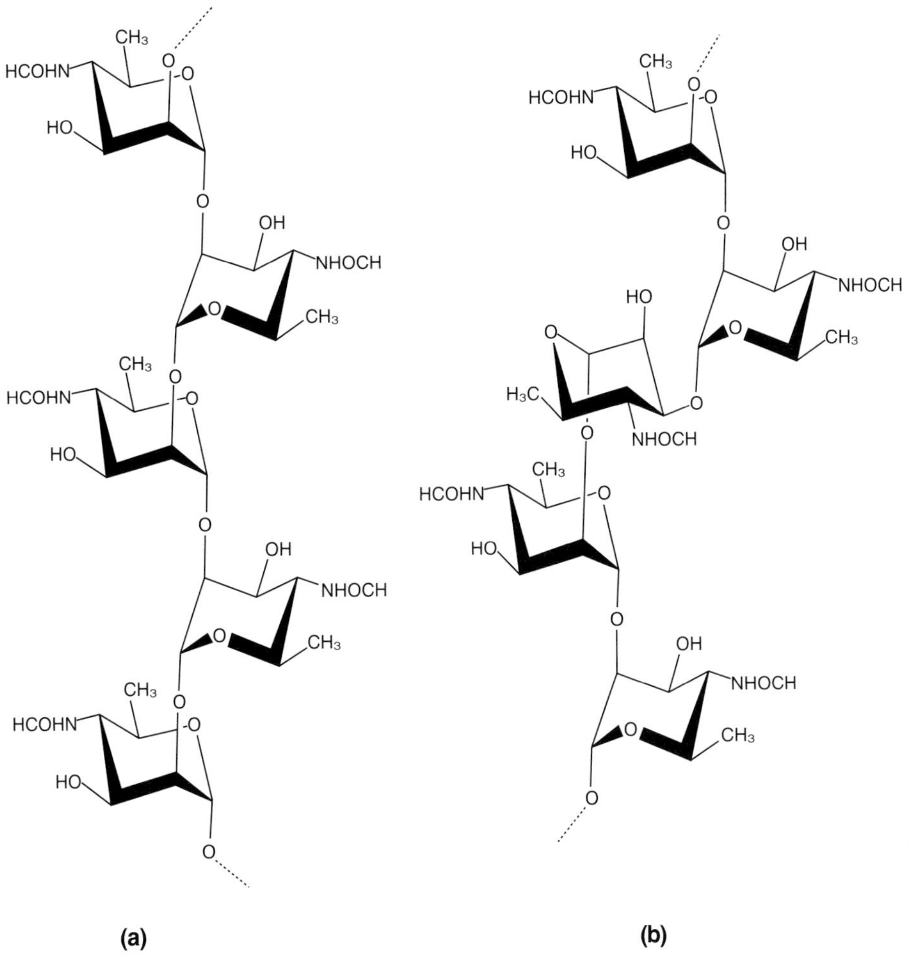

Fig. 35.4 Structures of (a) A type LPS of *B. abortus* biogroup 1 and (b) M type LPS of *B. melitensis* biogroup 1 (after Bundle et al. 1989).

ever, some rough LPS preparations do not contain quinovosamine suggesting that this is the terminal glycose of the core oligosaccharide and that the glucose, mannose residues are the main determinants of R specificity (Moreno, Jones and Berman 1984). If non-smooth *Brucella* strains are to be examined in agglutination procedures, the suspensions need to be stabilized by special buffers (Corbel et al. 1979). Serological cross-reactions have been reported between rough *Brucella* strains and *Actinobacillus equuli*, *Pasteurella multocida* and mucoid strains of *Pseudomonas aeruginosa* (Weber 1976, Carmichael, Flores Castro and Zoha 1980).

The smooth LPS is the immunodominant antigen of the *Brucella* cell surface and a major virulence factor. It has endotoxic activity but shows some major differences in activity from enteric endotoxins typified by *E. coli* LPS. For example, it is much less toxic for rabbits, chick embryos and endotoxin-sensitive mouse strains. It is much more toxic than *E. coli* endotoxin for endotoxin-resistant mouse strains and is effective in stimulating interleukin-1 and tumour necrosis factor-α production in these. It is also toxic for macrophages and is antigenic for spleen cells and B- but not T-lymphocytes. Its lipid A does not bind polymyxin B and this does not inhibit its mitogenic or toxic activity. *Brucella* LPS has an unusual adjuvant activity in that it stimulates high levels of IgM and IgG$_3$ antibodies in mice. It is a major protective antigen in mice and other species, including cattle.

OTHER POLYSACCHARIDE ANTIGENS

Various polysaccharides structurally related to *Brucella* LPS O chain have been described. These include 'native antigen' or 'native hapten'. This can be extracted from LPS or whole cells by mild methods (Moreno, Borowiak and Mayer 1987, Moreno et al. 1979). Its association with lipid and protein is controversial. It is believed to be O chain which has not been incorporated into LPS. The rough strain *B. melitensis* B115 has been shown to synthesize smooth O chain which accumulates in the cytoplasm but is not assembled into complete LPS nor exported to the cell surface (Cloeckaert, Zygmunt et al. 1992).

The component identified as polysaccharide B and formerly advocated as a diagnostic reagent (Diaz et al. 1979) is now known to be a non-antigenic cyclic D-glucose which forms complexes with smooth LPS or O chain (Perry and Bundle 1990).

OUTER-MEMBRANE PROTEINS

The outer-membrane proteins have been described earlier (see section 8, Cellular composition). They include the outer-membrane proteins of groups 1, 2 and 3, the most quantitatively important of which are the group 2 porins. These and other proteins associated with the peptidoglycan fraction of the outer membrane have been investigated as candidate protective antigens. In general, attempts to demonstrate protection with monoclonal or polyclonal antibodies to these have indicated low activity in the absence of antibody to smooth LPS (Jacques et al. 1992). However, this does not disprove their role in protective immunity as they could still be implicated in relevant cell-mediated responses.

The role of outer-membrane proteins in the response of cattle to *Brucella* infection has been investigated. Proteins with molecular masses of 10, 16.5, 19, 25–27 and 36–38 kDa elicited antibody responses in cattle infected with *B. abortus* although the pattern of response to each varied between individual animals. Antibodies to the 89 kDa protein were not specific for *Brucella* (Cloeckaert, Kerkhofs and Limet 1992, Cloeckaert et al. 1992). The 8 kDa lipoprotein covalently linked to peptidoglycan is antigenically related to the Braun lipoprotein of *E. coli* and is thus a potential source of cross-reaction (Gomez Miguel et al. 1987).

9.2 Intracellular antigens

The internal antigens released on breakage of *Brucella* cells are for the most part proteins, glycoproteins and peptides common to all strains irrespective of colonial phase and biogroup. With polyclonal antisera raised against homogenates of disrupted cells, 30–40 individual precipitating components have been detected by western blotting or 2-dimensional immunoelectrophoresis procedures. Most of these are still detected by antisera adsorbed with washed whole cells indicating that they are not exposed on the cell surface. Few have been identified with structural components of the cell but attempts have been made to characterize those most relevant to serological responses in infected animals or humans (Stemshorn and Nielsen 1977, 1981, Schurig et al. 1978, Stemshorn, Nielsen and Samach 1981).

Some internal antigens are associated with the ribosomal fraction. They may be involved in both antibody and cell-mediated responses to infection (Corbel 1976b). The L7/L12 ribosomal protein has been identified as an important component of brucellin INRA and shown to elicit delayed hypersensitivity reactions in sensitized animals (Bachrach et al. 1994).

The antigens designated A1, A2, A3, A4, B1, B2 and C by Schurig et al. (1978) have been examined for their role as indicators of infection status. The A2 antigen is identical with the heat-stable glycoprotein described by Stemshorn and Nielsen (1981) and Stemshorn, Nielsen and Samach (1981) and the 20 kDa protein described by Zygmunt, Gilbert and Dubray (1992). An 18 kDa cytoplasmic protein has been described as an indicator of active infection in cattle and humans (Goldbaum et al. 1993). Hitherto, experience of protein antigens has indicated a high specificity but relatively low sensitivity for detection of infected individuals. In brucellosis, the antibody response is dominated by the LPS antigen.

9.3 In vivo antigens

Evidence that *Brucella* cells grown in vivo exhibited differences from cells grown in culture media has been presented (Smith and Fitzgeorge 1964, Fitzgeorge and Smith 1966). They reported that virulent *B. abortus* extracted from infected bovine placenta was more resistant to intracellular killing by bovine buffy coat phagocytes than the same strain grown in vitro. Furthermore, the effect was neutralized by antiserum from infected animals. The protective factor was associated with the cell envelope, preparations of which from in vivo grown organisms promoted the intracellular survival of attenuated strains. Similar effects were observed if the virulent strain was grown in culture medium supplemented with bovine allantoic fluid. These important observations have not been followed up and the composition of the protective factor produced in vivo has not been determined.

It is now well established for other bacteria that growth under conditions analogous to those found in vivo induces environmentally-regulated antigens. The most extensively studied have been the iron-regulated proteins and it has been clearly demonstrated for a number of bacteria, including the pathogenic *Neisseria*, *Pasteurella* and *Yersinia* species, that novel proteins associated with iron acquisition are produced under such 'in vivo' conditions. These proteins are essential for growth of the organisms and for the establishment of infection (for further information see Griffiths 1993). Little information is available on the effect of iron restriction on the growth of *Brucella* in vivo. It is known however, that *Brucella* responds to adverse environmental conditions by synthesis of chaperonins or **heat shock proteins** analogous to the GroEL and Htr proteins of *Escherichia coli* (Tatum, Cheville and Morfitt 1994).

Brucella also responds to an acidic environment by synthesis of stress-related proteins. These are produced in at least 2 phases; between pH 6.5 and 4.5 the proteins synthesized are probably involved in pre-acid shock inducible pH homeostasis, whereas those induced at pH 3.8 are probably involved in acid tolerance (Lin and Ficht, 1995). During intracellular growth in a macrophage cell line, production of novel proteins of 62, 28, 24 and 17 kDa was observed. The 62 kDa protein was identified as Hsp 62, a GroEL homologue. The 24 kDa protein was probably equivalent to the Asp 24 acid-induced protein whereas the 17 and 28 kDa proteins were apparently specific to macrophage-induced stress. These observations are clearly relevant to understanding the mechanisms of intracellular survival of *Brucella* and are discussed further below (see section 11, Virulence and pathogenicity).

10 GENETICS

In recent years there have been considerable advances in knowledge of the molecular genetics of *Brucella*. These have provided an indication of the phylogenetic relationships of the genus and its possible origins and have pointed the way towards a system of classification based on genetic rather than phenotypic characteristics.

10.1 Genome composition

The average genome complexity for *Brucella* and the closely related *Ochrobactrum* and *Phyllobacterium* genera falls within the range 2.37–2.82×10^6 kDa (de Ley et al. 1987, Allardet-Servent et al. 1988). The DNA of all members of the genus contains approximately 58–59 mole% G + C. This is quite different from the values for *Bordetella bronchiseptica* and *Francisella tularensis* which were formerly classified as *Brucella* species on the basis of superficial phenotypic similarity. It is identical with the value for *Ochrobactrum anthropi* (formerly CDC group Vd, see Cieslak et al. (1992)) and very close to those for *Agrobacterium*, *Rhizobium* and *Phyllobacterium* (Table 35.3).

A partial physical map of the *Brucella* genome was produced by Allardet Servent et al. (1991). Extension of this study led to the conclusion that the genome comprised 2 chromosomes of 2.1 and 1.5 mbp respectively. This has been confirmed by insertion of unique restriction sites (Jumas-Bilak et al. 1995). Two rRNA operons and the gene for the DnaK heat shock protein are located on the larger replicon and another rRNA operon and the gene for the GroEL chaperonin are located on the smaller one. This indicates that both replicons encode functions essential for survival and replication and hence are chromosomes and not plasmids (Michaux et al. 1993). The presence of multiple replicons is also typical of the *Agrobacterium* and *Rhizobium* genera, now known to have genetic affinity with *Brucella*.

DNA–DNA hybridization studies have indicated a high degree of homogeneity within the genus (Hoyer and McCullough 1968a,b; Verger et al. 1985, de Ley et al. 1987). The DNA relatedness of all the nomen species is $96 \pm 4\%$ in the most recent studies. The apparent deletion of 6% of sequences in *B. ovis* relative to the other species reported by Hoyer and McCullough (1968b) has not been confirmed but is close to the limits of error of the methodology used. It is notable that *B. ovis* has been reported to show slight differences from the others in restriction endonuclease digestion pattern (O'Hara, Sato and Homma 1985).

In general restriction endonuclease analysis of whole DNA with frequently cutting enzymes has been of limited value in differentiating the members of the group. The use of infrequently cutting enzymes combined with pulsed field gel electrophoresis has differentiated *B. abortus*, *B. melitensis*, *B. suis*, *B. ovis* and *B. canis* along conventional lines although it has not distinguished the biogroups (Allardet-Servent et al. 1988).

Restriction endonuclease analysis combined with probes for specific genes has demonstrated a number of polymorphisms. Of most taxonomic significance are polymorphisms in the *omp2* porin gene encoding the 36 kDa outer-membrane protein responsible for determining sensitivity to dyes (Ficht et al. 1988). Polymorphism has also been demonstrated in the gene encoding the BCSP 31 surface protein. This is associated with a 0.9 kb insertion sequence which is present at higher frequency in *B. ovis* than in the other nomen species (Halling and Zehr 1990).

10.2 RNA analysis

Both the 5S and 16S rRNA have been sequenced and have disclosed previously unexpected relationships to other genera. The 16S rRNA sequence is typical of the α-2 subdivision of the Proteobacteria. A high degree of sequence homology (over 95%) has been reported with the rRNA of *Agrobacterium*, *Ochrobactrum* and the *Bartonella/Rochalimaea* group (Dorsch et al. 1989, Relman et al. 1992). Comparison of 16S rRNA/DNA

Table 35.3 Comparison of DNA and rRNA composition of *Brucella* and other bacteria

Species	DNA G + C (mol%)	DNA homology (%)	16S rRNA/DNA binding	$T_m(e)$ (°C)	5S rRNA homology (%)
B. melitensis	57.9–59.2	96 ± 4	0.19	80.2	100
B. abortus	58.2–58.9	96 ± 4	0.18	80.0	100
B. suis	57.9–58.2	96 ± 4	0.18	80.1	100
B. neotomae	57.9	96 ± 4	0.18	80.3	100
B. ovis	58.1	96 ± 4	0.18	80.5	100
B. canis	57.9	96 ± 4	0.18	80.3	100
Agrobacterium tumefaciens	60.2–60.6	≥6	0.10	72.6	95.1
Bartonella bacilliformis	39	<5	–	–	95.4
Bartonella quintana	38.3–39	<5	–	–	95.8
Bordetella bronchiseptica	68.9	<5	0.06	57.4	–
Francisella tularensis	32.8	<5	0.08	56.7	–
Mycoplana dimorpha	63.8	~6	0.14	74.2	–
Ochrobactrum anthropi	57.6–59	23 ± 7	0.15	77.7	~98
Rhizobium meliloti	62.3	~6	0.07	72.0	–

–, not available.

binding patterns and sequence homology has confirmed the relationship of *Brucella* to *O. anthropi* and, less closely, to *Agrobacterium*, *Mycoplana*, *Phyllobacterium* and *Rhizobium*. It has also indicated an affiliation to other intracellular pathogens including *Bartonella bacilliformis*, *B. (Rochalimaea) henselae* and *B. (Rochalimaea) quintana*. Observations on the 5S rRNA sequences have indicated that *Brucella* is distinct from the *Bartonella* group, with a sequence homology of 86.6% compared with 92%. However, it shows 95% sequence homology with the 5S rRNA of an inadequately characterized bacterium identified as '*Vibrio cyclosites*' (Minnick and Stiegler 1993).

DNA–DNA hybridization studies have confirmed the close relationship between *Brucella* and *Ochrobactrum*. The similarity to *Agrobacterium* and *Rhizobium* is less evident and no relatedness to *Bartonella* has been found by this method (Table 35.3).

10.3 Plasmids and genetic exchange

Unequivocal evidence of naturally occuring plasmids in *Brucella* has not been presented. Similarly, spontaneous conjugation or transformation by chromosomal DNA has not been reported. However, conjugative transfer of the broad host-range plasmid R751 from *E. coli* to *Brucella* and thence between *Brucella* species has been demonstrated (Verger et al. 1993). This was associated with transfer of trimethoprim resistance. Transfer of tetracycline resistance to *Brucella* by an *E. coli* plasmid had been reported previously by Rigby and Fraser (1989). These observations suggest that *Brucella* strains could acquire multiple antibiotic resistance by plasmid transfer.

The transduction of antibiotic resistance by phages isolated from atypical *Brucella* strains has also been described (Rigby 1990).

10.4 Molecular cloning

Numerous *Brucella* genes have now been cloned and expressed in heterologous systems. These have included the genes for the 36 kDa porin protein (Ficht et al. 1988), the copper–zinc superoxide dismutase (Bricker et al. 1993), the BCSP 31 protein (Mayfield et al. 1988), various outer-envelope proteins (Wergifosse et al. 1995), heat shock proteins (Cellier et al. 1992) and many others. The regulatory proteins for some of these genes have also been identified and resemble those of *E. coli* (Mayfield et al. 1988).

Deletion mutants of *Brucella* have also been produced by genetic modification, mainly with the objective of determining the role of specific genes such as *htrA*, *recA* and the copper–zinc superoxide dismutase (*sodC*) gene in pathogenesis (Tatum et al. 1993).

10.5 Phages

Although the occurrence of bacteriocins specific for *Brucella* has not been confirmed, numerous phages lytic for *Brucella* have been isolated. These phages are all closely related DNA phages of the same morpho-logical group (Pedoviridae), with a base composition of 45–47 mol% G + C and a genome size of 25×10^3 kDa. They are stable to anionic and non-ionic detergents and to common organic solvents with the exception of chloroform, but are inactivated by heat, cationic detergents and oxidizing agents. Their stability to proteolytic enzymes varies between strains. Restriction endonuclease and serological studies have indicated that all are very similar and can be regarded as host-range variants of a single type of phage. For convenience, they have been classified into 6 groups on the basis of host range (Corbel and Thomas 1983).

The phages of group 1, typified by the Tbilisi (Tb) strains, replicate only in smooth *B. abortus* and to a much lesser extent in *B. neotomae* cultures. They can produce 'lysis-from-without' on smooth *B. suis* cultures when applied at high concentration. Tb phage alone can be used for identification of smooth *Brucella* species if preparations standardized at routine test dilution (RTD) and 10 000 RTD are used. It is of no value for the identification of non-smooth cultures and in practice identification is facilitated by using a battery of phages selected from groups 1, 3, 5 and 6.

The phages of group 2, typified by the Firenze (Fi75/13) strain, replicate in smooth *B. abortus* and *B. neotomae* and to a much smaller extent in *B. suis* cultures. Those of group 3, typified by the Weybridge (Wb) strain, replicate with similar efficiency in smooth cultures of *B. abortus*, *B. neotomae* and *B. suis* but not usually in *B. melitensis* cultures although this varies with strains from different geographical locations (Corbel 1987). Phages of group 4, typified by the Berkeley (BK₂) strain, replicate in smooth cultures of all *Brucella* species although *B. melitensis* strains from some localities may be lysed with low efficiency' (Corbel 1987). The group 5 phages R (rough), R/O and R/C are lytic for rough strains of *B. abortus*, *B. ovis* or *B. canis* but not for smooth cultures (Corbel and Thomas 1985). The group 6 phages, represented by the Izatnagar (Iz₁) strain, are lytic for smooth cultures of all *Brucella* species and for rough cultures of *B. melitensis* and *B. suis* and to a much smaller extent, *B. ovis* and *B. canis* (Corbel, Tolari and Yadava 1988). Another set of phages, the Nepean (Np) strains, resemble those of Group 1 in host range but do not lyse *B. suis* strains at 10^4 RTD. They have been proposed as a seventh group (Rigby 1990). The lytic patterns produced by representatives of these groups are shown in Table 35.4. For further information on *Brucella* phages and phage typing see Corbel and Thomas (1983), Corbel (1984a, 1987) and Young and Corbel (1989). The earlier studies on *Brucella* phages were summarized by Droževkina (1963).

11 VIRULENCE AND PATHOGENICITY

Although epidemiological evidence suggests that *B. abortus*, *B. melitensis* and *B. suis* show distinct host preferences, this only marks a general trend and the organisms are capable of establishing infection in a

Table 35.4 Lytic activity of phages for smooth (S) and rough (R) *Brucella* species

Phage group	Phage strain	Titre	B. abortus S	B. abortus R	B. suis S	B. suis R	B. melitensis S	B. melitensis R	B. neotomae S	B. neotomae R	B. canis R	B. ovis R
1	Tb	RTD	L	NL	NL	NL	NL	NL	NL or PL	NL	NL	NL
		RTD × 10⁴	L	NL	L	NL	NL	NL	L	NL	NL	NL
2	Fi 75/13	RTD	L	NL	PL	NL	NL	NL	L	NL	NL	NL
3	Wb	RTD	L	NL	L	NL	V	NL	L	NL	NL	NL
4	BK₂	RTD	L	NL	L	NL	L or PL	NL	L	NL	NL	NL
5	R	RTD	V	L	NL	NL	NL	NL	NL	NL	NL	L
	R/O	RTD	V	L	V	NL	NL	NL	V	NL	L	L
	R/C	RTD	NL	L	NL	NL	NL	NL	NL	NL	L	L
6	Iz₁	RTD	L	NL	Lᵃ PLᵇ	Vᵃ NLᵇ	L or PL	V	L	PL	NL	NL
7	Np	RTD	L	NL	NL	NL	NL	NL	L	NL	NL	NL
		RTD × 10⁴	L	NL	NL	NL	NL	NL	L	NL	NL	NL

L, confluent lysis; PL, partial lysis; single plaques or growth inhibition; NL, no lysis; V, variable, some strains lysed; RTD, routine test dilution.
ᵃBiogroups 1 and 4.
ᵇBiogroups 2, 3 and 5.

wide range of host species, including humans. *B. neotomae*, *B. canis* and *B. ovis*, in contrast, show much greater host specificity, and with the exception of occasional *B. canis* infections in other carnivores and in humans seem to have little capacity to spread beyond their usual hosts.

Typically, in all host species *Brucella* grows intracellularly, producing a variable bacteraemic phase followed by localization in the reticuloendothelial system. In the preferred host, localization also occurs in the tissues of the genital tract and in the mammary glands. In the case of *B. abortus*, *B. melitensis* and *B. suis* this has been attributed to the presence of isoerythritol in the target tissues of cattle, sheep, goats and pigs (Smith et al. 1961, 1962). Abortion is a frequent consequence of infection in the pregnant female, and orchitis and epididymitis can result in the male. Sexually immature animals are often less susceptible to the disease.

All species of *Brucella* can establish infection in guinea pigs and mice but the severity and duration varies considerably. In general, *B. melitensis* and *B. suis* strains produce the most severe effect, *B. abortus* produces less severe but more obviously granulomatous lesions, and the remaining species produce a more transient infection accompanied by few, if any, gross lesions (Braude 1951, Isayama et al. 1977). There is some evidence that *B. melitensis* and *B. abortus* induce different cellular responses (Young et al. 1979).

The basis of the virulence of *Brucella* strains is incompletely understood. Non-smooth variants of the normally smooth species are usually of greatly reduced virulence. This suggests a role for the O chain of the smooth LPS in determining virulence; supportive evidence for this is provided by the protective effect of monoclonal antibodies directed towards A or M determinants (Montaraz et al. 1986).

LPS and possibly another cell-envelope component have also been implicated in the blocking of the bactericidal action of normal serum and of phagocytes, permitting the survival of *Brucella* in polymorphonuclear and mononuclear phagocytes (Smith and Fitzgeorge 1964, Kreutzer and Robertson 1979). However, other factors are also involved in this process. The organisms are able to suppress the oxidative burst at least in polymorphonuclear phagocytes. *B. abortus* releases a low molecular weight nucleotide fraction containing guanine monophosphate and adenine which inhibits the intracellular bactericidal mechanisms of bovine phagocytes (Canning, Roth and Deyoe 1986). The organisms also release low molecular weight RNA which may block the action of cationic proteins including lysozyme and defensins (Corbel and Brewer 1980).

The copper–zinc superoxide dismutase also plays a part in facilitating intracellular survival of *Brucella* by blocking the formation of activated oxygen and probably also hypohalogen acids. Mutants unable to synthesize the enzyme produce tenfold lower infection levels in mice than wild type strains (Tatum et al. 1992).

Survival within macrophages is associated with the synthesis of proteins of molecular weight 17, 24, 28, 60 and 62 kDa. The 62 kDa protein corresponds to the Gro EL homologue Hsp 62 and the 60 kDa protein is an acid-induced variant of this. The 24 kDa protein is also acid-induced and its production correlates with bacterial survival under acidic conditions (pH <4). The 17 and 28 kDa proteins are apparently specifically induced by macrophages and correlated with intracellular survival (Lin and Ficht 1995).

Another stress-induced protein, HtrA, was shown to be involved in the induction of an early granulomatous response to *B. abortus* in mice. This was associated with a reduction in the levels of infection during the early phase. However, it did not prevent a subsequent increase in bacterial numbers and *htrA*-deficient mutants ultimately produced levels of splenic infection similar to those given by wild-type *B. abortus* (Tatum, Cherville and Morfitt 1994). Similarly, *recA*-deleted mutants produced a lower initial spleen viable count than *recA*-positive strains but still established persistent infection (Tatum, Morfitt and Halling 1993). Clearly a number of still unknown factors are involved in promoting protective immune responses to *Brucella*.

Antibodies to LPS provide some protection against infection but this is incomplete. Even opsonized bacteria are not effectively killed by macrophages (Caron et al. 1994). Antibodies to cell-surface proteins are even less effective than LPS in eliminating *Brucella* (Dubray 1987). However, protein antigens may play a significant role in triggering cell-mediated responses. The clearance of infection is dependent upon Th1-type responses; the stimulation of γ-interferon producing CD4+ cells is crucial. These are most effectively induced by live *Brucella* cells (Zhan, Kelso and Cheers 1995). Tumour necrosis factor (TNF)-α is also important for intracellular killing of *Brucella* and its production is suppressed by live but not by killed cells (Caron et al. 1994). Interestingly, purines or nucleosides appear to be involved in the suppression (Caron et al. 1994). The mechanisms whereby infection with *Brucella* results in tissue damage and disease are still unknown. No exotoxins have been detected and not all of the effects observed can be explained by the presence of endotoxin. Indeed, although *Brucella* LPS shares many of the properties of the endotoxins of other gram-negative bacteria, it is intrinsically less toxic than enterobacterial LPS, possibly because of a lower efficiency in releasing inflammatory cytokines and particularly TNF-α (Berman and Kurtz 1987, Caron et al. 1994).

12   CLASSIFICATION AND IDENTIFICATION

Criteria for the classification of an organism as a member of the *Brucella* genus have been defined by the *Brucella* Sub-Committee of the International Committee on Systematic Bacteriology (Corbel and Morgan 1975). With some modifications these still apply. Thus the minimum requirements for establishing a hitherto unidentified organism as a *Brucella* are as follows.

Gram-negative coccobacillary morphology; non-motile; DNA G+C content of 58–59 mol%; a minimum of 90% homology with the DNA of reference strains; complete homology of 5S and 16S rRNA sequences with presence of signature sequences; coincidence of the majority of protein bands with those of reference strains on sodium dodecyl sulphate–polyacrylamide gel electrophoresis; characteristic fatty acid composition; synthesis of LPS devoid of heptose and with O chain homopolymer composed of 4-formamido-4,6-dideoxymannose; extensive serological cross-reactions of intracellular antigens with those of reference strains.

Subdivision into nomen species depends on principal natural host, oxidative metabolic pattern and phage sensitivity; restriction fragment polymorphism with selected enzymes may also be useful. The PCR reaction with appropriate primers is effective for identification at genus and possibly sub-genus level (Fekete et al. 1992). Classification into 'biovars' (biogroups) is based on carbon dioxide requirement, hydrogen sulphide production, dye sensitivity and agglutination by monospecific sera to A, M and R antigens. In practice, presumptive identification of isolates is made on the basis of cultural characteristics, cellular morphology and serological reactivity. Association with particular disease patterns may give an indication of identity (see Robertson et al. 1980, Corbel 1993).

On the basis of DNA–DNA homology the genus has been defined as monospecific and a system of nomenclature proposed which identifies each type as a biogroup of *B. melitensis* (Verger et al. 1985). Although this is in accordance with taxonomic practice, this nomenclature has not been widely accepted because of the confusion that could be caused to non-specialists. It is recommended that the current terminology should be retained for practical purposes until a system based on detailed molecular genetic data has evolved.

Some aspects of the current nomenclature may also be confusing and should be rationalized. Thus *B. abortus* is currently divided into 7 biogroups (1–6 and 9). Biogroups 7 and 8 have been discarded as invalid. *B. melitensis* is divided into 3 biogroups but as these are differentiated solely on the basis of reactions with antisera specific for A and M antigenic determinants, they should more properly be termed serogroups. *B. suis* is divided into 5 biogroups, of these only the first 3 have swine as their natural hosts. *B. suis* biogroup 4 was formerly classified as *B. rangiferi tarandi* (Davydov 1961). *B. suis* biogroup 5 includes M antigen-dominant strains isolated from rodents in the Caucasus (Vershilova et al. 1983) and should not be confused with strains previously described under this designation (Renoux and Philippon 1969) but subsequently shown not to be *Brucella* (Corbel 1973b). No biogroups have been defined for other species but there is evidence of heterogeneity within the *B. ovis* and *B. canis* groups (Corbel and Thomas 1985).

12.1 Epidemiological aspects

The distribution of biogroups may vary between localities or even within a locality and can provide useful epidemiological information. However, in many instances a single biogroup predominates and this makes the tracing of sources of infection difficult. This situation arose in the UK during the latter stages of the eradication campaign. Before initiation of eradication, about 78% of isolates were *B. abortus* biogroup 1, 6% biogroup 2, 1% biogroup 3, 2% biogroup 4, 10% biogroup 5, 0.5% biogroup 6 and 2.5% biogroup 9. Towards the end of the campaign only strains of *B. abortus* biogroup 1 were isolated. To facilitate epidemi-

ological tracing of the sources of these infections, additional methods had to be devised, of which antibiotic resistogram patterns were of the most value. Most of the isolates could be assigned to one of 5 groups on the basis of resistance pattern. Examination of old stock cultures suggested that these resistance patterns had been conserved for at least 40 years and predated the use of antibiotics (Corbel 1993).

Worldwide, *B. abortus* biogroup 1 is usually the most common cause of brucellosis in cattle in developed countries and in others in which intensive systems of management are used. *B. abortus* biogroup 3 tends to predominate in indigenous cattle populations in Africa and Asia but is now the most common type in western Europe. *B. melitensis* biogroup 1 is probably the most common type worldwide but biogroup 2 predominates in Italy and is at least as common as biogroup 1 in countries surrounding the Arabian Gulf. *B. suis* biogroup 2 is now uncommon but occurs sporadically in hare populations throughout Europe from the Baltic to the Adriatic Sea. *B. suis* biogroups 1 and 3 are now uncommon in the USA but frequent in Mexico, Colombia and Argentina, southern China and Indonesia. *B. suis* biogroup 4 is confined to reindeer populations in the Arctic regions of Alaska, Canada and Russia. *B. suis* biogroup 5 is found only in rodents in the Caucasus.

For further information on *Brucella* see Regamey et al. 1970, Elberg 1973, Regamey et al. 1976, Corbel and Gargani 1977, Crawford and Hidalgo 1977, Corbel et al. 1979, Corbel, Gill and Redwood 1979, Blobel and Schliesser 1982, Wundt 1982, Corbel, Gill and Thomas 1983, Corbel and Morgan 1984, Valette and Hennessen 1984, Verger and Plommet 1985, Plommet 1987, Alton et al. 1988, Corbel 1988a,b, Madkour 1989, Young and Corbel 1989, Adams 1990, Nielsen and Duncan 1990, Tümbay, Hilmi and Ang 1991, and also reports (FAO/WHO 1951, 1953, 1958, 1964, 1971, 1986) from the FAO/WHO Expert Committee on Brucellosis and Reports of the ICSB Sub-Committee on Taxonomy of *Brucella* (Stableforth and Jones 1963, Jones 1967, Jones and Wundt 1971, Wundt and Morgan 1975, Corbel 1982, 1984b).

13 SUMMARIZED DESCRIPTIONS OF SPECIES

13.1 *Brucella abortus*

The organisms are gram-negative coccobacilli or short rods, 0.8–1.5 μm long by 0.6–0.8 μm wide. The species is catalase and oxidase positive and usually requires supplementary carbon dioxide for growth, especially on primary isolation. It usually produces hydrogen sulphide from sulphur-containing amino acids or proteins. Most isolates hydrolyse urea but some may not. They generally grow in the presence of basic fuchsin, methyl violet, pyronin and safranin O but not thionin, at standard concentrations. They reduce nitrate to nitrite and may also reduce nitrite. Isolates are normally smooth on primary isolation. Smooth strains may have A or M surface antigens reactive in tests with monospecific antisera, depending upon biogroup. They oxidize L-alanine, D-alanine, L-asparagine, L-glutamic acid, D-galactose, D-glucose, D-ribose and isoerythritol but do not oxidize D-xylose, L-arginine, DL-citrulline, DL-ornithine or L-lysine. Cultures in the smooth or smooth-intermediate phase are lysed by *Brucella* phages of groups 1, 2, 3, 4 and 6, non-smooth strains are lysed by phages of group 5 at routine test dilution (RTD) and

10^4 RTD. Non-smooth cultures are lysed by *Brucella*-phage R at RTD. The species is usually pathogenic for cattle, causing abortion, but may also infect other species including sheep, goats, dogs, horses and humans. Guinea-pigs, rabbits and mice are susceptible to experimental infection. Seven biogroups are recognized: former biogroups 7 and 8 are no longer considered valid. See Table 35.5 for reference strains.

13.2 *Brucella melitensis*

The organisms are gram-negative cocci or coccobacilli, rarely rods; 0.6–1.2 μm long by 0.5–0.7 μm wide. They are catalase and oxidase positive, and do not require supplementary carbon dioxide for growth. They do not produce hydrogen sulphide, or no more than a trace, when grown on recommended media. They usually hydrolyse urea but some strains may not. They usually grow in the presence of basic fuchsin, thionin, methyl violet, pyronin and thionine blue at the standard concentrations. They reduce nitrate to nitrite and may also reduce nitrite. Smooth cultures may have the A, M or both A and M surface antigens reactive in tests with monospecific sera. They oxidize D-glucose, isoerythritol, L-alanine, D-alanine, L-asparagine and L-glutamic acid, but do not oxidize L-arabinose, D-galactose, D-ribose, D-xylose, L-arginine, DL-citrulline, DL-ornithine or L-lysine. Cultures in the smooth phase are usually susceptible to lysis by phages of groups 4 and 6 at RTD and 10^4 RTD. The species is usually pathogenic for sheep and goats but may also infect other species, including humans. Guinea-pigs, rabbits and mice are susceptible to experimental infection. See Table 35.5 for reference strains.

13.3 *Brucella suis*

The organisms are gram-negative coccobacilli or rods, 0.8–1.5 μm long by 0.6–0.8 μm wide. They are catalase and oxidase positive, and supplementary carbon dioxide is not required for growth. They produces large amounts of hydrogen sulphide (biogroup 1) or none at all (other biogroups) and hydrolyse urea rapidly. They usually grow in the presence of thionin but most strains are inhibited by basic fuchsin, methyl violet, pyronin and safranin O at standard concentrations. Isolates are normally in the smooth phase on primary isolation. In smooth cultures the A surface antigen is predominant except for cultures of biogroup 4 which react equally with antisera monospecific for the A and M surface antigens, and biogroup 5 which reacts only with M monospecific serum. They usually oxidize D-ribose, D-glucose, isoerythritol, D-xylose, L-arginine, DL-citrulline, DL-ornithine and L-lysine. Oxidation of L-asparagine, L-glutamic acid, L-arabinose and D-galactose varies with the biogroups, and they do not oxidize L-alanine or D-alanine. Smooth or smooth-intermediate cultures are lysed by *Brucella* phage of groups 3, 4 and 6 at RTD and 10^4 RTD. Phages of group 2 produce partial lysis at RTD; those of group 1 do not produce lysis at RTD but are lytic at 10^4 RTD. The species is usually pathogenic for pigs, except biogroups 4 and 5 which are usually pathogenic for reindeer and rodents respectively. Biogroup 2 also naturally infects hares. Many other species are susceptible to the other biogroups, including humans. Guinea pigs, rabbits and mice are susceptible to infection but the severity varies with the biogroup. See Table 35.5 for reference strains.

13.4 *Brucella neotomae*

The organisms are gram-negative coccobacilli 0.6–1.4 μg long by 0.6 μm wide. They are catalase positive and oxidase negative and do not require supplementary carbon dioxide for growth. They usually produce hydrgen sulphide profusely and hydrolyse urea rapidly. They do not grow in the presence of basic fuchsin even at 7.5 mg l⁻¹, nor in the presence of safranin O at 100 mg l⁻¹ or thionine blue at 2 mg l⁻¹ but will grow in the presence of thionin at 7.5 mg l⁻¹. They reduce nitrate to nitrite. Cultures are usually smooth on primarily isolation. In smooth cultures the A surface antigen is predominant. They oxidize L-asparagine, L-glutamic acid, L-arabinose, D-galactose, D-glucose, isoerythritol, D-xylose, but do not oxidize L-alanine, D-alanine, L-arginine, DL-citrulline, DL-ornithine or L-lysine. Oxidation of D-ribose may be variable. Smooth or smooth-intermediate cultures are lysed

Table 35.5 *Brucella* reference strains

Species	Biogroup	Strain	NCTC no.	ATCC no.
B. abortus	1	544	10093	23448
	2	86/8/59	10501	23449
	3	Tulya	10502	23450
	4	292	10503	23451
	5	B3196	10504	23452
	6	870	10505	23453
	9	C68	10507	23455
B. melitensis	1	16M	10094	23456
	2	63/9	10508	23457
	3	Ether	10509	23458
B. suis	1	1330	10316	23444
	2	Thomsen	10510	23445
	3	686	10511	23446
	4	40	11364	23447
	5	513	11996	
B. neotomae		5K33	10084	23459
B. ovis		63/290	10512	25840
B. canis		RM6/66	10854	23365

by *Brucella* phages of groups 2, 3, 4 and 6 at RTD. Phages of group 1 produce partial lysis with few very small plaques at RTD, complete lysis at 10^4 RTD. Rough or mucoid cultures are not lysed by these phages at RTD or 10^4 RTD. The species is pathogenic for the desert wood rat (*Neotoma lepida* Thomas). Authenticated natural infections of other species have not been reported. Mice are more susceptible than guinea pigs to experimental infection. No biogroups are recognized. For reference strain see Table 35.5.

13.5 *Brucella ovis*

The organisms are gram-negative cocci, coccobacilli or short rods, 0.7–1.2 μm long by 0.5–0.7 μm wide. They are catalase positive and oxidase negative. They require supplementary carbon dioxide for growth, do not produce hydrogen sulphide and hydrolyse urea weakly or not at all. They usually grow in the presence of basic fuchsin and thionin at standard concentrations. Production of nitrite from nitrate is variable. A true smooth phase on primary isolation has not been described. Rough (R)-specific surface antigens cross-reacting with other non-smooth *Brucella* are predominant. They oxidize L-alanine, D-alanine, L-asparagine, D-asparagine, L-glutamic acid, DL-serine and adonitol but do not oxidize L-arabinose, D-galactose, D-glucose, D-ribose, isoerythritol, D-xylose, L-arginine, DL-citrulline, DL-ornithine or L-lysine. The cultures are not lysed by *Brucella* phages of groups 1, 2, 3, 4 and 6 at RTD or 10^4 RTD but are lysed by pages R/O and R/C of group 5 at RTD. The species is pathogenic for sheep, causing epididymitis in rams and sometimes abortion in ewes; it produces low-grade splenic infection in guinea pigs and mice. No biogroups are recognized. See Table 35.5 for reference strain.

13.6 *Brucella canis*

The organisms are gram-negative coccobacilli or rods, 0.5–2 μm long by 0.5–0.6 μm wide. They are catalase positive and oxidase positive. They do not require supplementary carbon dioxide for growth, do not produce hydrogen sulphide and hydrolyse urea very rapidly. Most strains reduce nitrate to nitrite. Growth is usually inhibited by basic fuchsin but not by thionin at the standard concentrations. A smooth phase is not known; cultures are always in the rough or mucoid phase on primary isolation. Cultures form a mucoid sediment in liquid media. Rough-specific surface antigens cross-react with other non-smooth strains of *Brucella*. They oxidize D-ribose, D-glucose, L-arginine, DL-citrulline, DL-ornithine and L-lysine. Oxidation of isoerythritol is variable, and they do not oxidize L-alanine, D-alanine, L-asparagine, L-glutamic acid, L-arabinose and D-galactose. They are not lysed by *Brucella* phages of groups 1, 2, 3, 4 or 6 but are lysed by phages of group 5 at RTD and 10^4 RTD. The species is pathogenic for dogs, causing abortion in pregnant females and epididymo-orchitis in males. It is occasionally transmitted to humans. It produces splenic infection, sometimes accompanied by 'tapioca-grain' nodules, in guinea pigs; also produce low-grade infection in mice. No biogroups are recognized. See Table 35.5 for reference strain.

13.7 *'Brucella maris'*

The organisms are gram-negative cocci or coccobacilli, 0.5–1.5 μm long by 0.5–0.6 μm wide. They are catalase positive and oxidase positive. Supplementary carbon dioxide is required by strains of seal origin but not by those isolated from cetaceans. Hydrogen sulphide is not produced; urea is hydrolysed. They grow in the presence of basic fuchsin, thionin and safranin O at standard concentration. Smooth cultures may have the A, the M, or both A and M surface antigens reactive in tests with monospecific sera. They oxidize L-glutamic acid, D-ribose, D-xylose and isoerythritol. Oxidation of L-alanine and L-asparagine is slow or absent. Strains of cetacean origin also oxidize D-galactose. They are usually lysed by phages of groups 2, 3, 4 and 6 at RTD and 10^4 RTD but are not lysed by phages of group 1 or show only partial lysis at RTD or 10^4 RTD. They are not lysed by phages of group 5 at RTD or 10^4 RTD.

This species causes natural infections in marine mammals (seals, sea otters, dolphins, porpoises). Experimental infections in mice and guinea pigs are mild. There are probably several biogroups: strains are distinguishable by preferred natural host, carbon dioxide requirement, antigenic specificity and oxidation of D-galactose.

REFERENCES

Adams LG (ed), 1990, *Advances in Brucellosis Research*, Texas A& M University Press, Austin.

Advisory Committee on Dangerous Pathogens, 1994, *Categorization of Pathogens According to Hazard and Categories of Containment*, 3rd edn, interim issue 1994, HMSO, London.

Allardet-Servent A, Bourg G et al., 1988, DNA polymorphism in strains of the genus *Brucella*, *J Bacteriol*, **170**: 4603–7.

Allardet-Servent A, Carles-Nurit M-J et al., 1991, Physical map of the *Brucella melitensis* 16M chromosome, *J Bacteriol*, **173**: 2219–4.

Alton GG, Jones LM et al., 1988, *Techniques for the Brucellosis Laboratory*, Institut National de la Recherche Agronomique, Paris.

Arnaud-Bosq CJ, Brousson-Jalaguier J et al., 1987, Détermination des biovars de *Brucella melitensis* par les caractères manométriques: interet épidemiologique et relation avec les sérovars, *Ann Inst Pasteur Microbiol (Paris)*, **138**: 189–200.

Bachrach G, Banai M et al., 1994, Brucella ribosomal protein L7/L12 is a major component in the antigenicity of Brucellin INRA for delayed type hypersensitivity in *Brucella*-sensitized guinea-pigs, *Infect Immun*, **62**: 5361–6.

Balke E, Weber A, Fronk B, 1977, Untersuchungen des Amino säurestoffwechsels mit der Dünnschichtchromatographie zur Differenzierung von Brucellen, *Zentralbl Bakteriol Parasitenkd Infektionskr Hyg*, **A237**: 523–9.

Bang B, 1897, The aetiology of contagious abortion, *Z Tiermed*, **1**: 241–78.

Batchelor BI, Brindle RJ et al., 1992, Biochemical misidentification of *Brucella melitensis* and subsequent laboratory-acquired infections, *J Hosp Infect*, **22**: 159–62.

Beck BL, Tabatabai LB, Mayfield JE, 1990, A protein isolated from *Brucella abortus* is a Cu-Zn superoxide dismutase, *Biochemistry*, **29**: 372–5.

Berman DT, Kurtz RS, 1987, Relationship of biological activities to structures of *Brucella abortus* endotoxin and LPS, *Ann Inst Pasteur Microbiol (Paris)*, **138**: 98–101.

Blobel H, Schliesser T (eds), 1982, *Handbuch der bakteriellen Infektionen bei Tieren*, Vol IV, VEB Gustav Fischer Verlag, Jena, 17, 53, 214, 261, 293, 309, 329, 370, 408.

Bosch J, Linares J et al., 1986, *In vitro* activity of ciprofloxacin, ceftriaxone and five other antimicrobial agents against 95 strains of *Brucella melitensis*, *J Antimicrob Chemother*, **17**: 459–61.

Braude AI, 1951, Studies in the pathology and pathogenesis of experimental brucellosis. I. A comparison of the pathogenicity of *Brucella abortus*, *Brucella melitensis* and *Brucella suis* for guinea pigs, *J Infect Dis*, **89**: 76–86.

Brewer RA, Corbel MJ, 1980, An immunospecific double staining procedure for rapid quantitative assessment of dissociation by *Brucella* cultures, *Br Vet J*, **136**: 484–7.

Bricker BJ, Tabatabai LB et al., 1990, Cloning, expression and occurrence of the *Brucella* Cu-Zn superoxide dismutase, *Infect Immun*, **58**: 2935–9.

Brodie J, Sinton GP, 1975, Fluid and solid media for isolation of *Brucella abortus*, *J Hyg Camb*, **74**: 359–67.

Brown GM, Ranger CR, Kelley DT, 1971, Selective media for the isolation of *Brucella ovis*, *Cornell Vet*, **61**: 265–80.

Bruce D, 1887, Note on the recovery of a micro-organism in Malta Fever, *Practitioner*, **39**: 161.

Buddle MB, Boyes BW, 1953, A *Brucella* mutant causing genital disease in sheep in New Zealand, *Aust Vet J*, **29**: 145–53.

Bundle DR, Cherwonogrodzky JW et al., 1987, The lipopolysaccharides of *Brucella abortus* and *B. melitensis*, *Ann Inst Pasteur Microbiol (Paris)*, **138**: 92–8.

Bundle DR, Cherwonogrodzky JC et al., 1989, Definition of *Brucella* A and M epitopes by monoclonal typing reagents and synthetic oligosaccharides, *Infect Immun*, **57**: 2829–36.

Bundle DR, Gerken M, Peters T, 1988, Synthesis of antigenic determinants of the *Brucella* A antigen, utilizing methyl 4-azido-4,6-dideoxy-I-D-mannopyranoside efficiently derived from D-mannose, *Carbohydr Res*, **174**: 239–51.

Canning PC, Roth JA, Deyoe BL, 1986, Release of 5′-guanosine monophosphate and adenine by *Brucella abortus* and their role in the intracellular survival of the bacteria, *J Infect Dis*, **154**: 464–70.

Carmichael LE, Bruner DW, 1968, Characteristics of a newly-recognized species of *Brucella* responsible for infectious canine abortion, *Cornell Vet*, **58**: 579–92.

Carmichael LE, Flores Castro R, Zoha S, 1980, Brucellosis caused by *Brucella canis* (*B. canis*): An update of infection in animals and man, *World Health Organization Brucellosis Document*, WHO/BRUC/80361.

Caroff M, Bundle DR et al., 1984a, Antigenic S-type lipopolysaccharide of *Brucella abortus* 1119–3, *Infect Immun*, 384–8.

Caroff M, Bundle DR, Perry MB, 1984b, Structure of the O-chain of the phenol-phase soluble lipopolysaccharide of *Yersinia enterocolitica* serotype 0:9, *Eur J Biochem*, 195–200.

Caron E, Peyrard T et al., 1994, Live *Brucella* spp fail to induce tumor necrosis factor alpha excretion upon infection of U937-derived phagocytes, *Infect Immun*, **62**: 5267–74.

Castañeda MR, 1947, A practical method for routine blood cultures in brucellosis, *Proc Soc Exp Biol Med NY*, **64**: 114–15.

Cellier MFM, Teyssier J et al., 1992, Cloning and characterisation of the *Brucella ovis* heat shock protein DnaK functionally expressed in *Escherichia coli*, *J Bacteriol*, **174**: 8036–42.

Cherwonogrodzky JW, Dubray G et al., 1990, Antigens of *Brucella*, *Animal Brucellosis*, eds Nielsen K, Duncan JR, CRC Press, Boca Raton, FL, 19–64.

Christofferson PA, Ottosen HE, 1941, Recent staining methods, *Skand Vet Tidskr*, **31**: 599–607.

Cieslak TJ, Robb ML et al., 1992, Catheter-associated sepsis caused by *Ochrobactrum anthropi*: report of a case and review of related nonfermentative bacteria, *Clin Infect Dis*, **14**: 902–7.

Cloeckaert A, Kerkhofs P, Limet JN, 1992, Antibody response to *Brucella* outer membrane proteins in bovine brucellosis: immunoblot analysis and competitive enzyme-linked immunosorbent assay using monoclonal antibodies, *J Clin Microbiol*, **30**: 3168–74.

Cloeckaert A, Zygmunt MS et al., 1992, O chain expression in the rough *Brucella melitensis* strain B115: induction of O-polysaccharide-specific monoclonal antibodies and intracellular localization by immunoelectron microscopy, *J Gen Microbiol*, **138**: 1211–19.

Colmenero JD, Hernandez S et al., 1989, Comparative trial of doxycycline plus streptomycin versus doxycycline plus rifampin for the therapy of human brucellosis, *Chemotherapy (Basel)*, **35**: 146–52.

Commission on Mediterranean fever, 1905–1907, *Report, Parts I, III and IV*, Harrison and Sons, London.

Corbel MJ, 1973a, The direct fluorescent antibody test for detection of *Brucella abortus* in bovine abortion material, *J Hyg Camb*, **71**: 123–9.

Corbel MJ, 1973b, Examination of two bacterial strains designated 'Brucella suis biotype 5', *J Hyg Camb*, **71**: 271–85.

Corbel MJ, 1976a, Determination of the *in vitro* sensitivity of *Brucella* strains to rifampicin, *Br Vet J*, **132**: 266–75.

Corbel MJ, 1976b, The immunogenic activity of ribosomal fractions derived from *Brucella abortus*, *J Hyg Camb*, **76**: 65–74.

Corbel MJ, 1982, International Committee on Systematic Bacteriology. Sub Committee on Taxonomy of *Brucella*. Minutes of the Meeting, 4 and 5 September 1978, Munich, FRG, *Int J Syst Bacteriol*, **32**: 260–61.

Corbel MJ, 1984a, Recent advances in brucella-phage research, *Vet Bull*, **54**: 65–74.

Corbel MJ, 1984b, International Committee on Systematic Bacteriology. Sub Committee on Taxonomy of *Brucella*. Minutes of the Meeting, 10 August 1982, Boston, Massachusetts, *Int J Syst Bacteriol*, **34**: 366–7.

Corbel MJ, 1985, Recent advances in the study of *Brucella* antigens and their serological cross-reactions, *Vet Bull*, **55**: 927–42.

Corbel MJ, 1987, Brucella phages: advances in the development of a reliable phage typing system for growth and non-smooth *Brucella* isolates, *Ann Inst Pasteur Microbiol (Paris)*, **138**: 70–5.

Corbel MJ, 1988a, International Committee on Systematic Bacteriology. Sub-Committee on the Taxonomy of *Brucella*. Report of the Meeting, 5 September 1986, Manchester, England, *Int J Syst Bacteriol*, **38**: 450–452.

Corbel MJ, 1988b, Brucellosis, *Fertility and Infertility in Veterinary Practice*, 4th edn, eds Laing JA, Brinley Morgan WJ, Wagner WC, 189–221.

Corbel MJ, Identification of dye-sensitive strains of *Brucella melitensis*, *J Clin Microbiol*, **29**: 1066–8.

Corbel MJ, 1993, Microbiological aspects of brucellosis, *Saudi Med J*, **14**: 489–502.

Corbel MJ, Brewer RA, 1980, Isolation and properties of an RNA fraction present in *Brucella* culture supernatants, *J Hyg Camb*, **84**: 223–36.

Corbel MJ, Gargani G (eds), 1977, Articoli sul genera 'Brucella' in memoria di Alice Evans, *Annali Sclavo*, **19(1)**.

Corbel MJ, Gill KPW, Redwood DW, 1979, Diagnostic Procedures for Non-smooth *Brucella* Strains, Ministry of Agriculture, Fisheries and Food, Pinner, Middlesex.

Corbel MJ, Hendry DMFD, 1985, Urease activity of *Brucella* species, *Res Vet Sci*, **38**: 252–3.

Corbel MJ, Morgan WJB, 1975, Proposals for minimal standards for descriptions of new species and biotypes of the genus *Brucella*, *Int J Syst Bacteriol*, **25**: 83–9.

Corbel MJ, Morgan WJB, 1984, Genus *Brucella* Meyer and Shaw 1920, 173[AL], *Bergey's Manual of Systematic Bacteriology*, Vol 1, Williams and Wilkins, Baltimore, 377–88.

Corbel MJ, Thomas EL, 1983, *The Brucella-phages, Their Properties, Characterisation and Applications*, 2nd edn, Ministry of Agriculture, Fisheries and Food, Alnwick, Northumberland: HMSO.

Corbel MJ, Thomas EL, 1985, Use of phage for the identification of *Brucella canis* and *Brucella ovis* cultures, *Res Vet Sci*, **38**: 35–40.

Corbel MJ, Bracewell CD et al., 1979, *Identification Methods for Microbiologists*, 2nd edn, eds Skinner FA, Lovelock DW, Technical Series No 14, Society for Applied Bacteriology, Academic Press, London, 71–122.

Corbel MJ, Scott AC, Ross HM, 1980, Properties of a cell-wall-defective variant of *Brucella abortus* of bovine origin, *J Hyg Camb*, **85**: 103–13.

Corbel MJ, Gill KPW, Thomas EL, 1983, *Methods for the Identification of* Brucella, 2nd end, Ministry of Agriculture, Fisheries and Food: HMSO, London.

Corbel MJ, Thomas EL, Garcia-Carillo C, 1984, Taxonomic studies on some atypical strains of *Brucella suis*, *Br Vet J*, **140**: 34–43.

Corbel MJ, Tolari F, Yadava VK, 1988, Characterisation of a new phage lytic for both smooth and non-smooth *Brucella* species, *Res Vet Sci*, **44:** 45–9.

Crawford RP, Hidalgo RJ (eds), 1977, *Brucellosis, an International Symposium*, Texas A&M University Press, Austin.

Davydov NN, 1961, Properties of *Brucella* isolated from reindeer (in Russian), *Trudy Vsyesoyuz Inst Eksp Vet*, **27:** 24–31.

de Ley J, Mannheim W et al., 1987, Ribosomal ribonucleic acid cistron similarities and taxonomic neighbourhood of *Brucella* and CDC group Vd, *Int J Syst Bacteriol*, **37:** 35–42.

Diaz R, Jones LM et al., 1968, Surface antigens of smooth brucella, *J Bacteriol*, **96:** 893–901.

Diaz R, Garatea P et al., 1979, Radial immunodiffusion test with a *Brucella* polysaccharide antigen for differentiating infected from vaccinated cattle, *J Clin Microbiol*, **10:** 37–41.

Dorsch M, Moreno E, Stackebrandt E, 1989, Nucleotide sequence of the 16S rRNA from *Brucella abortus*, *Nucleic Acids Res*, **17:** 1765.

Douglas JT, Rosenberg EY et al., 1984, Porins of *Brucella* species, *Infect Immun*, **44:** 16–21.

Droževkina MS, 1963, The present position in *Brucella* phage research A review of the literature, *Bull WHO*, **29:** 43–57.

Dubray G, 1972, Etude ultrastructurale des bactéries de colonies lisses (S) et rugueuses (R) du genre *Brucella*, *Ann Inst Pasteur (Paris)*, **123:** 171–93.

Dubray G, 1987, Protective antigens in brucellosis, *Ann Inst Pasteur Microbiol (Paris)*, **138:** 84–7.

Dubray G, Limet J, 1987, Evidence of heterogeneity of lipopolysaccharides among *Brucella* biovars in relation to A and M specificities, *Ann Inst Pasteur Microbiol (Paris)*, **138:** 27–37.

Dubray G, Plommet M, 1976, Structure et constituants de *Brucella*. Characterisation des fractions et propriétés biologiques, *Dev Biol Stand*, **31:** 68–91.

Elberg SS, 1973, Immunity to brucella infection, *Medicine*, **52:** 339–56.

Essenberg RC, Sharma YK, 1993, Cloning of genes for proline and leucine biosynthesis from *Brucella abortus* by functional complementation in *Escherichia coli*, *J Gen Microbiol*, **139:** 87–93.

Evans AC, 1918, Further studies on *Bacterium abortus* and related bacteria. II. A comparison of *Bacterium abortus* with *Bacterium bronchisepticus* and with the organism which causes Malta fever, *J Infect Dis*, **22:** 580–93.

FAO/WHO, 1951, *Report, Joint FAO/WHO Expert Committee on Brucellosis*, Technical Report Series No. 37, WHO, Geneva.

FAO/WHO, 1953, *Report, Joint FAO/WHO Expert Committee on Brucellosis*, Techical Report Series No. 67, WHO, Geneva.

FAO/WHO, 1958, *Report, Joint FAO/WHO Expert Committee on Brucellosis*, Techical Report Series No. 148, WHO, Geneva.

FAO/WHO, 1964, *Report, Joint FAO/WHO Expert Committee on Brucellosis*, Technical Report Series No. 289, WHO, Geneva.

FAO/WHO, 1971, *Report, Joint FAO/WHO Expert Committee on Brucellosis*, Technical Report Series No. 464, WHO, Geneva.

FAO/WHO, 1986, *Report, Joint FAO/WHO Expert Committee on Brucellosis*, Techical Report Series No. 740, WHO, Geneva.

Farrell ID, 1974, The development of a new selective medium for the isolation of *Brucella abortus* from contaminated sources, *Res Vet Sci*, **16:** 280–286.

Fekete A, Bantle JA et al, 1992, Amplification fragment length polymorphism in *Brucella* strains by use of polymerase chain reaction with arbitrary primers, *J Bacteriol*, **174:** 7778–83.

Ficht TA, Bearden SW et al., 1988, A 36 kilodalton *Brucella abortus* cell envelope protein is encoded by repeated sequences closely linked in the genomic DNA, *Infect Immun*, **56:** 2036–46.

Ficht TA, Bearden SW et al., 1989, DNA sequence and expression of the 36-kilodalton outer membrane protein gene of *Brucella abortus*, *Infect Immun*, **57:** 3281–91.

Fitzgeorge RB, Smith H, 1966, The chemical basis of the virulence of *Brucella abortus* VII The production *in vitro* of organisms with an enhanced capacity to survive intracellularly, *Br J Exp Pathol*, **47:** 558–62.

Francis E, Evans AC, 1926, Agglutination, cross-agglutination and agglutinin absorption in tularaemia, *Publ Hlth Reps, Washington DC*, **41:** 1273–1295.

Garcia-Rodriguez JA, Munoz Bellido JL et al., 1993, In vitro activities of new macrolides and rifapentine against *Brucella* spp., *Antimicrob Agent Chemother*, **37:** 911–13.

Gerhardt P, 1958, The nutrition of Brucellae, *Bacteriol Revs*, **22:** 81–98.

Goldbaum FA, Leoni J et al., 1993, Characterisation of an 18-kilodalton *Brucella* cytoplasmic protein which appears to be a serological marker of active infection of both human and bovine brucellosis, *J Clin Microbiol*, **31:** 2141–5.

Gomez Miguel MJ, Moriyon I, Lopez J, 1987, *Brucella* outer membrane lipoprotein shares antigenic determinants with *Escherichia col* Braun lipoprotein and is exposed on the cell surface, *Infect Immun*, **55:** 258–62.

Goodpasture EW, Anderson K, 1937, The problem of infection as presented by bacterial invasion of the chorioallantoic membrane of chick embryos, *Am J Pathol*, **13:** 149–74.

Griffiths E, 1993, Iron and infection: better understanding at the molecular level but little progress on the clinical front (editorial), *J Med Microbiol*, **38:** 389–90.

Hall WH, Manion RE, 1970, *In vitro* susceptibility of *Brucella* to various antibiotics, *Appl Microbiol*, **20:** 600–4.

Halling SM, Zehr ES, 1990, Polymorphism in *Brucella* due to highly repeated DNA, *J Bacteriol*, **172:** 6637–40.

Henry BS, 1933, Dissociation in the genus *Brucella*, *J Infect Dis*, **52:** 374–402.

Hines WD, Freeman BA, Pearson GA, 1964, Production and characterisation of *Brucella* spheroplasts, *J Bacteriol*, **87:** 438–45.

Hoyer BH, McCullough NB, 1968a, Polynucleotide homologies of *Brucella* nucleic acids, *J Bacteriol*, **95:** 444–8.

Hoyer B, McCullough NB, 1968b, Homologies of deoxyribonucleic acids from *Brucella ovis*, canine abortion organisms, and other *Brucella* species, *J Bacteriol*, **96:** 1783–90.

Huddleson IF, 1929, The differentiation of the species of the genus *Brucella*, *Bull Mich Agric Exp Sta*, **100:** 1–6.

Hutchings LM, Bunnel DE et al., 1951, The viability of *Br melitensis* in naturally infected cured hams, *Publ Hlth Rep, Washington DC*, **66:** 1402–8.

Isayama Y, Azuma R et al., 1977, Chemo-taxonomical studies on fatty acids of *Brucella* species, *Ann Sclavo*, **19:** 67–82.

Jacques I, Cloeckaert A et al., 1992, Protection conferred on mice by combinations of monoclonal antibodies directed against outer membrane proteins or smooth lipopolysaccharide of *Brucella*, *J Med Microbiol*, **37:** 100–3.

Jones LM, 1964, Use of safranin O for characterization of *Brucella* species, *J Bacteriol*, **88:** 1527.

Jones LM, 1967, Report to the International Committee on Nomenclature of Bacteria by the Subcommittee on Taxonomy of Brucellae. Minutes of Meeting, 22– 23 July 1966, Moscow, USSR, *Int J Syst Bacteriol*, **17:** 371–5.

Jones LM, Montgomery V, Wilson JB, 1965, Characteristics of carbon dioxide-independent cultures of *Brucella abortus* isolated from cattle vaccinated with strain 19, *J Infect Dis*, **115:** 312–20.

Jones LM, Wundt W, 1971, International Committee on Nomenclature of Bacteria. Subcommittee on the Taxonomy of *Brucella*. Minutes of Meeting, 7 August 1970, Mexico City, *Int J Syst Bacteriol*, **21:** 126–8.

Jumas-Bitlak E, Maugard C et al., 1995, Study of the organization of the genomes of *Escherichia coli*, *Brucella melitensis* and *Agrobacterium tumefaciens* by insertion of a unique restriction site, *Microbiology*, **141:** 2425–32.

Kenne L, Lindberg B et al., 1982, Structural studies of the *Vibrio cholerae* antigen, *Carbohydr Res*, **100:** 341–9.

Kolman S, Maayan MC et al., 1991, Comparison of the Bactec and lysis concentration method for recovery of *Brucella* species from clinical specimens, *Eur J Clin Microbial Infect Dis*, **10:** 647–8.

Kreutzer DL, Robertson DC, 1979, Surface macromolecules and virulence in intracellular parasitism: Comparison of cell envelope components of smooth and rough strains of *Brucella abortus*, *Infect Immun*, **23**: 819–28.

Lin J, Ficht TA, 1995, Protein synthesis in *Brucella abortus* induced during macrophage infection, *Infect Immun*, **63**: 1409–14.

Luzzi GA, Brindle R et al., 1993, Brucellosis: imported and laboratory-acquired cases, and an overview of treatment trials, *Trans R Soc Trop Med Hyg*, **87**: 138–41.

Madkour MM (ed), 1989, *Brucellosis*, Butterworths, London.

Mayfield JE, Bricker BJ et al., 1988, The cloning, expression and nucleotide sequence of a gene coding for an immunogenic *Brucella abortus* protein, *Gene*, **63**: 1–9.

McCullough NB, Beal GA, 1951, Growth and manometric studies on carbohydrate utilization of *Brucella*, *J Infect Dis*, **89**: 266–71.

Meikle PJ, Perry MB et al., 1989, The fine structure of A and M antigens from *Brucella* biovars, *Infect Immun*, **57**: 2870–8.

Meyer KF, Shaw EB, 1920, A comparison of the morphological, cultural and biochemical characteristics of *B. abortus* and *B. melitensis* Studies on genus *Brucella* nov. gen., *J Infect Dis*, **27**: 173–84.

Meyer ME, 1976, Evolution and taxonomy in the genus *Brucella*: steroid hormone induction of filterable forms with altered characteristics after reversion, *Ann J Vet Res*, **37**: 207–10.

Meyer ME, Cameron HS, 1957, Species metabolic patterns in morphologically similar Gram negative pathogens, *J Bacteriol*, **73**: 158–61.

Meyer ME, Cameron HS, 1961a, Metabolic characterisation of the genus *Brucella*. I. Statistical evaluation of the oxidative rates by which type I of each species can be identified, *J Bacteriol*, **82**: 387–95.

Meyer ME, Cameron HS, 1961b, Metabolic characterisation of the genus *Brucella*. II. Oxidative metabolic patterns of the described species, *J Bacteriol*, **82**: 396–400.

Michaux S, Paillisson J et al., 1993, Presence of two independent chromosomes in the *Brucella melitensis* 16M genome, *J Bacteriol*, **175**: 701–5.

Miles AA, Pirie NW, 1939a, The properties of antigenic preparations from *Brucella melitensis*. IV. The hydrolysis of the formamide linkage, *Biochem J*, **33**: 1709–15.

Miles AA, Pirie NW, 1939b, The properties of antigenic preparations from *Brucella melitensis*. V. Hydrolysis and acetylation of the amino-poly-hydroxy compound derived from the antigen, *Biochem J*, **33**: 1716–24.

Minnick MF, Stiegler GL, 1993, Nucleotide sequence and comparison of the 5S ribosomal RNA genes of *Rochalimaea henselae*, *R. quintana* and *Brucella abortus*, *Nucleic Acids Res*, **21**: 2518.

Montaraz JA, Winter AJ et al., 1986, Protection against *Brucella abortus* in mice with O-polysaccharide-specific monoclonal antibodies, *Infect Immun*, **51**: 961–3.

Moreira-Jacob M, 1963, Safranine O: reliable selective dye for characterization of *Brucella suis*, *J Bacteriol*, **86**: 599–600.

Moreno E, Pitt MW et al., 1979, Purification and characterisation of smooth and rough lipopolysaccharide from *Brucella abortus*, *J Bacteriol*, **138**: 361–9.

Moreno E, Jones LM, Berman DT, 1984, Immunochemical characterisation of rough *Brucella* lipopolysaccharides, *Infect Immun*, **43**: 779–82.

Moreno E, Borowiak D, Mayer H, 1987, *Brucella* lipopolysaccharides and polysaccharides, *Ann Inst Pasteur Microbiol (Paris)*, **138**: 102–5.

Moriyon I, Berman DT, 1982, Effects of non-ionic, ionic and dipolar ionic detergents and EDTA on the *Brucella* cell envelope, *J Bacteriol*, **152**: 822–8.

Mortenson JE, Moore DG et al., 1986, Antimicrobial susceptibility of clinical isolates of *Brucella*, *Diagn Microbiol Infect Dis*, **5**: 163–9.

Myers DM, Dobosch D, 1969, Use of mitomycin C to distinguish *Brucella abortus* field strains from the vaccinal *Brucella abortus* strain 19, *Appl Microbiol*, **18**: 511–12.

Nelson EL, Pickett MJ, 1951, The recovery of L-forms of *Brucella* and their relation to *Brucella* phage, *J Infect Dis*, **89**: 226–32.

Newton JW, Marr AG, Wilson JB, 1954, Fixation of $C^{14}O_2$ with nucleic acid constituents by *Brucella abortus*, *J Bacteriol*, **67**: 233–6.

Nielsen K, Duncan JR, 1990, *Animal Brucellosis*, CRC Press, Boca Raton, FL.

O'Hara MJ, Collins DM, Lisle GW, 1985, Restriction endonuclease analysis of *Brucella ovis* and other *Brucella* species, *Vet Microbiol*, **10**: 425–9.

Ohara S, Sato T, Homma M, 1974, Serological studies on *Francisella tularensis*, *Francisella novicida*, *Yersinia philomeragia* and *Brucella abortus*, *Int J Syst Bacteriol*, **24**: 191–6.

Olin G, 1935, *Studien uber das Undulantfieber in Schweden*, Isaac Marcus Boktryckin–Aktiebolag, Stockholm.

Palenque E, Otero JR, Noriga AR, 1986, In vitro susceptibility of *Brucella melitensis* to new cephalosporins crossing the blood-brain barrier, *Antimicrob Agents Chemother*, **29**: 182–3.

Perry MB, Bundle DR, 1990, Lipopolysaccharide antigens and carbohydrates of *Brucella*, *Advances in Brucellosis Research*, Chapter 5, ed Adams LG, Texas A&M University, Austin, 76–88.

Peschkov JJ, Feodorov V, 1978, Comparative study on the ultrastructure of L-forms obtained from S and R variants of *Brucella suis* 1330, *Zentralbl Bakteriol Parasitenkd Infektionskr Hyg*, **240, Abt 1 Orig A**: 94–105.

de Petris S, Karlsbad G, Kessel RWI, 1964, Ultrastructure of S and R variants of *Brucella abortus* grown on a lifeless medium, *J Gen Microbiol*, **35**: 373–82.

Pickett MJ, 1994, Identification of *Brucella* species with a procedure for detecting acidification of glucose, *Clin Infect Dis*, **19**: 976–7.

Pickett MJ, Nelson EL, 1955, Speciation within the genus *Brucella*. IV. Fermentation of carbohydrates, *J Bacteriol*, **69**: 333–6.

Plommet M (ed), 1987, Brucella and brucellosis: an update, *Ann Inst Pasteur Microbiol (Paris)*, **138**: 69–144.

Rautlin de la Roy YM, Grignon B et al., 1986, Rifampicin resistance in a strain of *Brucella melitensis* after treatment with doxycycline and rifampin, *J Antimicrob Chemother*, **18**: 648–9.

Redmond JW, 1979, The structure of the O-antigenic side chain of the lipopolysaccharide of *Vibrio cholerae* 569B (Inaba), *Biochim Biophys Acta*, **584**: 346–52.

Redwood DW, Corbel MJ, 1983, Interaction of *Brucella ovis* with ovine tissue extracts, *Vet Rec*, **113**: 220.

Regamey RH, de Barbieri A et al. (eds), 1970, International Symposium on Brucellosis, Tunis 1968, *Symp Ser Immunobiol Stand*, **12**.

Regamey RH, Hulse EC, Valette L (eds), 1976, International Symposium on Brucellosis (II) Rabat 1975, *Dev Biol Standard*, **31**.

Relman Da, Lepp PW et al., 1992, Phylogenetic relationships among the agent of bacillary angiomatosis, *Bartonella bacilliformis* and other alpha-proteobacteria, *Mol Microbiol*, **6**: 1801–7.

Renoux G, Philippon A, 1969, Position taxonomique dans le genre *Brucella* de bactéries isolées de brebis et de vaches, *Ann Inst Pasteur (Paris)*, **117**: 524–8.

Rest RF, Robertson DC, 1975, Characterisation of the electron transport system in *Brucella abortus*, *J Bacteriol*, **122**: 139–44.

Richardson M, Holt JN, 1962, Synergistic action of streptomycin with other antibiotics on intracellular *Brucella abortus in vitro*, *J Bacteriol*, **84**: 638–46.

Rigby CE, 1990, The brucella phages, *Animal Brucellosis*, Chapter 6, eds Nielsen K, Duncan JR, CRC Press, Boca Raton, FL, 121–30.

Rigby CE, Fraser ADE, 1989, Plasmid transfer and plasmid-mediated genetic exchange in *Brucella abortus*, *Can J Vet Res*, **53**: 326–30.

Robertson DC, McCullough WG, 1968, The carbohydrate catabolism of the genus *Brucella* I Evaluation of pathwways, *Archs Biochim Biophys*, **127**: 263–73.

Robertson L, Farrell ID et al., 1980, *Benchbook on Brucella*, PHLS Monograph Series No. 14, HMSO, London.

Rose DR, Przybylska M et al., 1993, Crystal structure to 245Å resolution of a monoclonal Fab specific for the *Brucella* A cell wall polysaccharide antigen, *Protein Sci*, **2**: 1106–13.

Ross HM, Foster G et al., 1994, *Brucella* species infection in sea-mammals, *Vet Rec*, **132**: 359.

Roux J, Sassine J, 1971, Etude d'une souche fixée de sphero-plastes (formes L) de *Brucella melitensis*, *Ann Inst Pasteur (Paris)*, **120**: 174–85.

Sangari FJ, Garcia-Lobo JM, Agüero J, 1994, The *Brucella abortus* vaccine strain B19 carries a deletion in the erythritol catabolic genes, *FEMS Microbiol Lett*, **121**: 337–42.

Santos JM, Verstreate DK et al., 1984, Outer membrane proteins from rough strains of four *Brucella* species, *Infect Immun*, **46**: 188–94.

Schurig GG, Jones LM et al., 1978, Antibody response to antigens distinct from smooth lipopolysaccharide complex in *Brucella* infection, *Infect Immun*, **21**: 994–1002.

Simmons GC, Hall WTK, 1953, Epididymitis in rams. Preliminary studies on the occurrence and pathogenicity of a *Brucella*-like organism, *Aust Vet J*, **29**: 33–40.

Smith H, Fitzgeorge RB, 1964, The chemical basis of the viru-lence of *Brucella abortus*. V. The basis of intracellular survival and growth in bovine phagocytes, *Br J Exp Pathol*, **45**: 174–86.

Smith H, Keppie J et al., 1961, The chemical basis of the viru-lence of *Brucella abortus*. I. Isolation of *B. abortus* from bovine foetal tissue, *Br J Exp Pathol*, **42**: 631–7.

Smith H, Keppie J et al., 1962, The chemical basis of the viru-lence of *Brucella abortus*. IV. Immunogenic products from *Brucella abortus* grown *in vivo* and *in vitro*, *Br J Exp Pathol*, **43**: 538–48.

Solomon HM, Jackson D, 1992, Rapid diagnosis of *Brucella melitensis* in blood: some operational characteristics of the BACT/ALERT, *J Clin Microbiol*, **28**: 2139–41.

Sriranganathan N, Boyle SM et al., 1991, Superoxide dismutases of virulent and avirulent strains of *Brucella abortus*, *Vet Microbiol*, **26**: 359–366.

Stableforth AW, Jones LM, 1963, Report of the Subcommittee on Taxonomy of the genus *Brucella*. Speciation in the genus *Brucella*, *Inst Bull Bacteriol Nomencl Taxon*, **13**: 145–58.

Stamp JT, McEwen AD et al., 1950, Enzootic abortion of ewes. I. Transmission of the disease, *Vet Rec*, **62**: 251–4.

Stemshorn B, Nielsen K, 1977, The bovine immune response to *Brucella abortus*. I. A water soluble antigen precipitated by sera of some naturally infected cattle, *Can J Comp Med*, **41**: 152–9.

Stemshorn B, Nielsen K, 1981, The bovine immune response to *Brucella abortus*. IV. Studies with a double immunodiffusion test for antibody against antigen A2, *Can J Comp Med*, **45**: 147–53.

Stemshorn B, Nielsen K, Samagh B, 1981, The bovine immune response to *Brucella abortus* III Preparation to antisera against a *Brucella* component precipitated by sera of some infected cattle, *Can J Comp Med*, **45**: 77–81.

Stoenner HG, Lackman DB, 1957, A new species of *Brucella* isol-ated from the desert wood rat, *Neotoma lepida* Thomas, *Ann J Vet Res*, **18**: 947–51.

Swann AI, Garby CL et al., 1981, Safety aspects in preparing sus-pensions of field strains of *Brucella abortus* for serological identification, *Vet Rec*, **109**: 254–5.

Tanaka S, Suto T et al., 1977, Chemotaxonomical studies on fatty acids of *Brucella* species, *Ann Sclavo*, **19**: 67–82.

Tatum FM, Cheville NF, Morfitt D, 1994, Cloning, characteris-ation and construction of *htr* A and htr A – like mutants of *Brucella abortus* and their survival in BALB/C mice, *Microb Pathog*, **17**: 23–36.

Tatum FM, Detilleux PG et al., 1992, Construction of Cu-Zn superoxide dismutase deletion mutants of *Brucella abortus*: analysis of survival *in vitro* in epithelial and phagocytic cells and *in vivo* in mice, *Infect Immun*, **60**: 2863–9.

Tatum FM, Morfitt DC, Halling SM, 1993, Construction of a *Bru-cella abortus* Rec A mutant and its survival in mice, *Microb Pathog*, **14**: 177–85.

Thiele OW, Schwinn G, 1973, The free lipids of *Brucella melitensis* and *Bordetella pertussis*, *Eur J Biochem*, **34**: 337–44.

Thomas EL, Bracewell CD, Corbel MJ, 1981, Characterisation of *Brucella abortus* strain 19 cultures isolated from vaccinated cattle, *Vet Rec*, **108**: 90–3.

Thomsen A, 1934, *Brucella infection in swine*, Thesis, Copenhagen.

Tosi MF, Nelson TJ, 1982, *Brucella canis* infection in a 17 month old child successfully treated with moxalactam, *J Pediatr*, **101**: 725–7.

Traum JE, 1914, Immature and hairless pigs. Report of the Department of Agriculture for the year ended June 30, 1914, Report of the Chief of the Bureau of Animal Industry, Washington DC, 30.

Tümbay E, Hilmi S, Anğ O, 1991, Brucella *and Brucellosis in Man and Animals*, Turkish Microbiological Society No 16, Ege Uni-versity Press, Izmir.

Valette L, Hennessen W (eds), 1984, IIIrd International Sym-posium on Brucellosis, Algiers, *Dev Biol Stand*, **56**.

Verger JM, Grayon M, 1977, Oxidative metabolic profiles of *Bru-cella* species, *Ann Sclavo*, **19**: 45–60.

Verger JM, Grayon M et al., 1993, Conjugative transfer and *in vitro/in vivo* stability of the broad host range Inc P R751 plas-mid in *Brucella* spp., *Plasmid*, **29**: 142–6.

Verger JM, Grimont F et al., 1985, *Brucella*, a monospecific genus as shown by dioxyribonucleic acid hybridization, *Int J Syst Bac-teriol*, **35**: 292–5.

Verger JM, Plommet M (eds), 1985, *Brucella melitensis*, Martinus Nojhoff Publishers, Dordrecht.

Vershilova PA, Liamkin GI et al., 1983, *Brucella* strains isolated from mouse-like rodents in South Western USSR, *Int J Syst Bacteriol*, **33**: 399–400.

Verstreate DR, Winter AJ, 1984, Comparison of sodium dodecyl sulphate-polyacrylamide gel electrophoresis profiles and anti-genic relatedness among outer membrane proteins of 49 *Bru-cella abortus* strains, *Infect Immun*, **46**: 182–7.

Weber A, 1976, *Untersuchungen zur mikrobiologischen Diagnose und Epidemiologie der Brucella canis – Infektion des Hundes*, Thesis, Giessen.

Weber A, 1982, *Brucella canis, Handbuch der bakteriellen Infektionen bei Tieren*, Vol. IV, eds Blobel H, Schliesser, VEB Gustav Fischer Verlag, Jena, 329–69.

Weckesser J, Mayer H, 1988, Different lipid A types in lipopoly-saccharides of phototrophic and related non-phototrophic bacteria, *FEMS Microbiol Rev*, **54**: 143–54.

De Wergifosse P, Lintermans P et al., 1995, Cloning and nucleot-ide sequence of the gene coding for the major 25-kilodalton outer membrane protein of *Brucella abortus*, *J Bacteriol*, **172**: 1911–14.

White PG, Wilson JB, 1951, Differentiation of smooth and non-smooth colonies of *Brucellae*, *J Bacteriol*, **61**: 239–40.

Wilson GS, Miles AA, 1932, The serological differentiation of smooth strains of the *Brucella* group, *Br J Exp Pathol*, **13**: 1–13.

Wilson GS, 1983, *Brucella, Topley and Wilson's Principles of Bacteri-ology, Virology and Immunology*, 7th edn, Vol. 2, Chapter 40, Wilson GS, Miles AA, Parker MT, eds, Edward Arnold, London, 409–10.

Wilson GS, Miles AA (eds), 1964, *Brucella, Topley and Wilson's Principles of Bacteriology and Immunology*, 5th edn, Vol. 1, Chap-ter 35, 998–1003.

Winter AJ, 1987, Outer membrane proteins of *Brucella*, *Ann Inst Pasteur Microbiol (Paris)*, **138**: 87–9.

Wundt W, 1982, Brucellose des Menschen, *Handbuch der Bakteri-ellen Infektionen bei Tieren*, Vol. IV, eds Blobel H, Schliesser T, VEB Gustav Fischer Verlag, Jena, 408–465.

Wundt W, Morgan WJ, 1975, *International Committee on Systematic Bacteriology. Subcommittee on Taxonomy of* Brucella. *Minutes of Meeting, 3 September 1974, Tokyo, Japan*, **25**: 235–36.

Young EJ, Corbel MJ (eds), 1989, *Brucellosis: Clinical and Labora-tory Aspects*, CRC Press, Boca Raton, FL.

Young EJ, Gomez CI et al., 1979, Comparison of *Brucella abortus* and *Brucella melitensis* infection of mice and their effect on acquired cellular resistance, *Infect Immun*, 680–5.

Zhan Y, Kelso A, Cheers C, 1995, Differential activation of *Brucella*-reactive CD4+ T cells by *Brucella* infection or immunization with antigenic extracts, *Infect Immun*, 63: 969–75.

Zygmunt MS, Gilbert FB, Dubray G, 1992, Purification, characterization, and seroactivity of a 20-kilodalton *Brucella* protein antigen, *J Clin Microbiol*, 30: 2662–7.

Chapter 36

THE RICKETTSIAE

G A Dasch and E Weiss

1 INTRODUCTION

In the past, the taxonomy of the rickettsiae was based principally on comparisons of phenotypic characteristics. More so than in other bacteria, historical and environmental considerations also played important roles in classification. In the eighth edition of Topley and Wilson, the principal genera discussed were *Rickettsia*, *Rochalimaea* and *Coxiella*. Other genera were discussed briefly. More recently, classification of rickettsiae and other bacteria have been based increasingly on DNA sequences, particularly on 16S and 23S rDNA sequence comparisons. The genera *Rickettsia* and *Ehrlichia* belong in distinct branches of the α subdivision of Proteobacteria (Roux and Raoult 1995, Stothard and Fuerst 1995), whereas *Rochalimaea* belong in the α_2 subdivision and are most closely related to the agrobacteria and rhizobacteria. *Bartonella* and *Rochalimaea* have similar 16S rDNA sequences and DNA homology by DNA–DNA hybridization and both can be cultivated on cell-free media. Consequently, the genera *Bartonella* and *Rochalimaea* were combined in *Bartonella* and the family Bartonellaceae was removed from the order Rickettsiales (Brenner et al. 1993). Thus, the genus *Bartonella* is discussed in Chapter 63 of this edition. Recently, species of the genus *Grahamella* were also renamed *Bartonella* (Birtles et al. 1995). *Rickettsia tsutsugamushi* is sufficiently different from the typhus and spotted fever groups (SFG) of rickettsiae to be placed in a separate genus, *Orientia* (Ohashi et al. 1995, Tamura et al. 1995). Considerable information has also been accumulated on the genus *Ehrlichia* and related genera, *Cowdria*, *Neorickettsia* and *Anaplasma*. Some

reclassification may be expected in the 3 major divisions of the ehrlichiae (Walker and Dasch 1995, Wen et al. 1996).

Wolbachia persica and *Coxiella burnetii* are the only rickettsiae in the γ Proteobacteria (Weisburg et al. 1989). *Wolbachia* is polyphyletic as *W. persica* is cultivable and will be renamed as a species of *Francisella* (it is discussed in Chapter 60) whereas the *Wolbachia pipientis* complex contains α Proteobacteria with affinities to the ehrlichiae (Werren, Zhang and Guo 1995). It is discussed briefly in this chapter. Since close relatives of *C. burnetii* have not yet been defined, this micro-organism is still retained in this chapter. This is justified by similarities in the technology used for this micro-organism and typical rickettsiae and, in some cases, by similarities in ecology.

2 HISTORICAL PERSPECTIVES

Some of the rickettsiae are very important pathogens of man and animals. Outbreaks of typhus fever, for example, on many occasions have changed the course of human history. This topic is discussed in Volume 3. The designation 'Rickettsia' honours Howard Taylor Ricketts who, in a series of brilliant experiments conducted between 1906 and 1909, isolated the aetiological agent of Rocky Mountain spotted fever and established the role of the tick in its transmission (Harden 1990). Ricketts recognized that the bacteria causing Rocky Mountain spotted fever and epidemic typhus were similar, but distinct. In 1909, Charles Nicolle had shown that typhus is transmitted by the body louse, which led to the establishment of delousing procedures as a means of controlling epidemics. *Rickettsia prowazekii* was named after Von Prowazek who also contributed greatly to our understanding of the epidemiology of typhus. The diagnosis of rickettsial diseases was greatly aided by the discovery in 1916 by Weil and Felix that patient sera agglutinated certain *Proteus* antigens. The Weil–Felix reaction is still widely used but has been gradually replaced by more accurate and sensitive procedures (Weiss 1992).

Early research workers experienced great difficulty in cultivating rickettsiae. Guinea pigs or mice were used most frequently. In 1938 Harold Cox found that embryonated chicken eggs supported growth of most rickettsiae. Derrick isolated the agent of Q fever in guinea pigs from ill workers in a meat-packing plant in Brisbane, Australia. Burnet and Freeman characterized it as a rickettsia. At about the same time, an agent was isolated in Montana and named *Rickettsia diaporica* because, unlike other rickettsial agents, it was filterable. Because of its differences from other rickettsiae, the agent was renamed *Coxiella burnetii* in honour of Cox and Burnet (Weiss 1992).

The discovery of animal pathogens had similar histories of arthropod associations and difficulty in cultivation. Perhaps the most important is *Cowdria ruminantium*, which is responsible for heartwater, a widespread disease of sheep, goats and cattle in sub-Saharan Africa. The disease was probably encountered as early as 1838. In 1925, EV Cowdry recognized the rickettsial aetiology of the disease, as well as the mode of transmission by the bont tick, *Amblyomma hebraeum* (Weiss 1992). Our knowledge of the ehrlichiae has greatly expanded recently. Once believed to include primarily agents of veterinary importance including *Ehrlichia canis* and *Ehrlichia risticii*, the genus now includes 2 monocytic agents, *Ehrlichia chaffeensis* and *Ehrlichia sennetsu*, and a granulocytic *Ehrlichia equi*-like agent, as agents of human disease (Dumler and Bakken 1995).

3 HABITAT

A common feature of the habitat of the pathogenic rickettsiae is an association with arthropods, vertebrate animals and humans. There are, however, considerable differences in the details of such associations and each species (or groups of closely related species) needs to be discussed separately (Tables 36.1 and 36.2).

Epidemic typhus, caused by *R. prowazekii*, is essentially a disease of humans, transmitted by its vector, the human body louse (Dasch and Weiss 1992, Weiss 1992). The main reason for its historical importance is that, in many societies, the louse has been a constant companion of humans. This has been particularly true in times of war and other catastrophes and where, in cold climates, one or 2 layers of clothing were constantly worn and infrequently changed. The louse becomes infected by ingesting infected blood. The rickettsiae multiply rapidly in the gut cells of the lice and are discharged in louse faeces. The lice are killed

by the infection, but survive long enough (about 2 weeks) to carry the infection to other individuals. Migration of lice from one person to another is stimulated by the patient's fever or by death. Infection is usually acquired by the scarification of the skin bites, rather than by the skin bites themselves. The rickettsiae are quite stable in louse faeces and may also cause infection by aerosol. Knowledge of the interepidemic survival of *R. prowazekii* stems from the observation that patients who recover from typhus occasionally suffer a relatively mild disease, called Brill–Zinsser disease, which has some of the features of typhus. In 1933, Zinsser and Castaneda isolated *R. prowazekii* from such patients. Thus, former patients are the main habitat of *R. prowazekii* during interepidemic periods. Although *R. prowazekii* infection is almost exclusively a human disease, a sylvatic cycle has been described, involving the American flying squirrel *Glaucomys volans*. The infection is transmitted from squirrel to squirrel by the squirrel's louse and to humans probably by its fleas. A few human cases occur during the winter months, when the squirrels seek refuge from cold weather in the attics of houses.

Rickettsia typhi induces a milder disease in humans than *R. prowazekii* and it is not always recognized (Dasch and Weiss 1992, Weiss 1992). It has a worldwide distribution like that of its chief reservoir, the rats *Rattus norvegicus* and *Rattus rattus*, but other vertebrate hosts may be involved. Increase in incidence is often associated with destruction of buildings and other factors which lead to the increase of rat populations near human habitations. Rat lice play an important role in transmission from rat to rat, but the oriental rat flea, *Xenopsylla cheopis*, is the chief transmitter of the disease to humans. The rickettsiae grow profusely in the midgut epithelial cells of the flea and are excreted in the faeces, but the longevity of the flea is not curtailed by the infection. Infection, as in the case of epidemic typhus, is often due to scarification of flea bite sites, but aerosol infection may also occur. A new typhus-like rickettsia, ELB, has been isolated from the cat flea, *Ctenocephalides felis*, which can maintain it by efficient transovarial passage (Radulovic et al. 1995). It has been identified in opossum tissues and from one patient originally thought to have had murine typhus (Schriefer et al. 1994). *Rickettsia canada*, another typhus-like rickettsia, was isolated from *Haemaphysalis* ticks from Richmond, Canada and Mendocino County, California, but its epidemiology is not understood (Weiss 1992). Human infection has been suspected, but not confirmed.

Ricketts elucidated the main features of the habitat of *Rickettsia rickettsii* in the Rocky Mountains (Weiss 1992, Walker 1995). Ticks that acquire the infection by feeding on infected animals remain infected throughout their lifetime and females transmit the agent transovarially to their offspring. Some ticks are not infectious after a cold winter, but the infection is reactivated by a blood meal or incubation at elevated temperature. *R. rickettsii* is found throughout the western hemisphere, not just in the Rocky Mountains where it is transmitted by the wood tick, *Dermacentor*

Table 36.1 Diseases and habitats of species of the genera *Rickettsia*, *Orientia* and *Coxiella*

Species[a]	Human disease[b]	Arthropod association[c]	Vertebrate reservoirs[d]	Geographical distribution
Typhus group				
R. prowazekii	Epidemic typhus	Human body louse	**Human**	World wide
	Sylvatic typhus	Flea, louse	**Flying squirrels**	Eastern USA
	Brill–Zinsser	None	**Human**	World wide
R. typhi	Endemic (murine) typhus	Rat flea, louse	**Rats, other rodents**	World wide
R. felis (ELB)	Murine typhus-like	Cat flea	**Opossum**, rats	Texas, California
R. canada	?	*Haemaphysalis* ticks	Rabbits, hares, birds	Ontario, California
Spotted fever group				
R. akari	Rickettsialpox	Mouse mite	**Rodents**	World wide
R. rickettsii	Rocky Mountain SF	*Dermacentor* ticks, *Amblyomma cajennense* tick	**Rodents, lagomorph, canines**, birds	North America / South America
R. rickettsii HLP	?	*Haemaphysalis* ticks		North America
R. amblyommii	? Suspected mild SF	*Amblyomma americanum* tick	Rabbits, birds	Southern USA
R. parkeri	?	*Amblyomma maculatum* tick	Rodents, birds, ruminants	North America
R. montana	?	*Dermacentor* ticks	Rodents, birds, ruminants	North America
R. rhipicephali	?	*Rhipicephalus sanguineus* tick	**Rodents**, dogs	North America
R. conorii	Boutonneuse fever, Mediterranean SF	*Rhipicephalus*, *Haemaphysalis* ticks	Dogs / **Rodents, dogs**, lagomorphs	Africa, southern Europe to India
R. helvetica	?	*Ixodes ricinus* ticks	Rodents, deer, cattle	Europe
R. slovaca	?	*Dermacentor* ticks	**Rodents, lagomorphs**, ruminants	Europe, Asia
R. massiliae	?	*Rhipicephalus* ticks	Rodents, dogs, ruminants	Europe, Africa
R. sibirica	North Asian tick typhus	*Dermacentor*, *Haemaphysalis* ticks	**Rodents**, canines, ruminants	Eurasia, Asia
R. africae	African tick bite fever	*Amblyomma* ticks	**Ruminants**, rodents	Sub-Saharan Africa
R. australis	Queensland tick typhus	*Ixodes holocyclus* ticks	Rodents, marsupials	Australia
R. honei	Flinders Island SF	*Ixodes cornuatus* tick	Rodents, dogs	Australia
R. japonica	Oriental SF	*Haemaphysalis*, *Dermacentor* ticks	Rodents, dogs	Japan
R. heilongjiangi	?	*Dermacentor*, *Haemophysalis* ticks	Rodents	China
R. sharonii	Israeli tick typhus	*Rhipicephalus* ticks	Rodents	Israel
R. sp.	Astrakhan SF	*Rhipicephalus pumilio* tick	Dogs, rodents, hedgehog	Europe
Other species				
R. bellii	?	Ixodid and argasid ticks	Rodents	USA
R. sp. AB agent	?	*Adalia bipunctata* ladybird beetle	None	Europe, Japan?
O. tsutsugamushi	Scrub typhus, tsutsugamushi fever	Trombiculid mites	**Rodents, marsupials**	Southern Asia, Australia
C. burnetii	Q fever (acute and chronic)	Ticks and other arthropods	**Domestic and wild animals**	World wide

[a]For other unclassified isolates of the spotted fever group see Dasch and Weiss (1992), Eremeeva et al. (1994, 1995b) and Roux and Raoult (1995).

[b]Spotted fever (SF).

[c]Primary vectors are indicated. Many vectors, but not all, serve as the primary rickettsial reservoir.

[d]Vertebrate hosts that have been shown to be rickettsial reservoirs are in bold print. The other vertebrates listed serve as hosts for the vectors and frequently have antibodies to rickettsiae but rickettsiae have not yet been isolated from their tissues or blood.

andersoni. The dog tick, *Dermacentor variabilis*, is the chief vector in the eastern USA, where human infection is now much more frequent. *Rhipicephalus sanguineus* and *Amblyomma cajennense* ticks have been implicated as vectors of human infection in Mexico and South America. Other named SFG rickettsiae, including *Rickettsia bellii*, *Rickettsia montana*, *Rickettsia amblyommii* and *Rickettsia parkeri* as well as other unnamed agents, are found in North America (Dasch and Weiss 1992). They are generally believed to be non-pathogenic for man but may cause seroconversion.

Numerous other spotted fever rickettsiae cause disease in man (Dasch and Weiss 1992). *Rickettsia conorii* causes the diseases known as boutonneuse fever, Marseilles fever or Mediterranean spotted fever; *Rickettsia sibirica* causes North Asian tick typhus. The precise geographical range of *R. conorii* is not known but the brown dog tick, *Rhipicephalus sanguineus*, is the principal vector in the Mediterranean and North African countries. Other rickettsiae, including *Rickettsia massiliae*, *Rickettsia slovaca* and *Rickettsia helvetica*, believed to be non-pathogenic, also occur in Europe. Spotted fever agents causing diseases known as Israeli tick typhus, Astrakhan fever and *Amblyomma*-transmitted tick typhus in sub-Saharan Africa are closely related to the highly variable species *R. conorii* (Walker et al. 1995), but only the latter rickettsia has been elevated to specific status as *Rickettsia africae* (PJ Kelly et al. 1994). *Rickettsia australis*, *Rickettsia honei* and *Rickettsia japonica* are agents of human disease in Australia, Flinders Island, and Japan, respectively. Other tickborne spotted fever agents whose pathogenicity has not been established are known from Asia.

Rickettsia akari differs from the other rickettsiae, since its main vector is not a tick, but a mite, *Liponysoides sanguineus*, that feeds on the house mouse, *Mus musculus* (Kass et al. 1994). The mite appears to be the chief reservoir of the disease, as it can pass the rickettsiae transtadially and transovarially to its progeny. The distribution of this rickettsia is probably world wide, because human infection has been recorded in North America, Asia and Europe.

Various micro-organisms living in intracellular symbioses with arthropods cause sex ratio distortion and alteration of sex determination of their hosts, such as parthenogenesis, female-biased sex ratios and sterility of offspring of crosses between infected males and uninfected females. Most such micro-organisms are relatives of the species *W. pipientis* (Werren, Zhang and Guo 1995). This species was first described in 1936 by Hertig, as occurring in the gonads and gut epithelium of the mosquito *Culex pipiens*. Another bacterium found in the ladybird beetle, *Adalia bipunctata*, has been shown to cause sex ratio distortion in its host. Surprisingly, this bacterium (AB bacterium) is closely related to typhus and spotted fever rickettsiae (Werren et al. 1994, Balayeva et al. 1995).

Scrub typhus was first recognized in Japan as early as 1810 and attributed to the bite of a mite, usually the red mite or 'akamushi' (Dasch and Weiss 1992, Tamura et al. 1995). 'Tsutsugamushi' means mite disease. *Orientia tsutsugamushi* is often found in 'ecological islands', which have the proper vegetation for supporting the mites and their wild rodent hosts. The habitats are often characterized by the presence of changing ecological conditions, wrought by humans or nature, and expressed by transitional types of vegetation. Trombiculid mites, particularly of the genus *Leptotrombidium*, are important vectors for the rickettsiae. Only the larval stage (chigger) is parasitic on a vertebrate host. Shortly after its emergence from the egg, the larva travels to the grass or dead vegetation and remains there until it can burrow into the skin of an animal it happens to contact, usually a rodent. Following a meal of tissue juices, it returns to the soil to resume a free-living existence. The chigger is not host-specific and humans are also infected by their bites. Scrub typhus occurs in an area of the Orient that extends from Afghanistan and Tadzhikistan to Korea and Japan, from the maritime provinces of Russia to the northern part of Australia and to the intervening islands of the Pacific Ocean in the east.

C. burnetii is widespread in the natural environment due in part to its high degree of stability under conditions unfavourable for growth and to its transmission from animal to animal and to humans primarily by aerosol (Raoult and Marrie 1995). It has been reported from virtually every part of the world. Ticks undoubtedly play an important role in natural infection, but many vertebrate animals are also heavily infected and play a role in transmission. *C. burnetii* is often an occupational disease in individuals working in slaughterhouses. The bacterium is particularly abundant in the placenta of a parturient animal. Parturient cats in a household can also cause infection.

E. canis, a world-wide pathogen of dogs, is transmitted by the brown dog tick, *R. sanguineus*. Similarly, *Amblyomma* ticks transmit *Cowdria ruminantium* and *Anaplasma marginale* to ruminants. *E. chaffeensis*, first isolated from military recruits in Fort Chaffee, Arkansas, has been shown to occur in the tick vector, *Amblyomma americanum*. It occurs most frequently in southeastern and south-central USA and has been reported from other parts of the USA. Serological evidence of infection has been reported in a few cases in Europe and Africa (Dumler and Bakken 1995). The white-tailed deer and the tick, *A. americanum*, are the most likely reservoir and vector (Lockhart et al. 1996). An ehrlichia very similar to *E. equi* and *Ehrlichia phagocytophila* is responsible for human granulocytic ehrlichiosis in the northern USA and Europe, and is probably transmitted by *Ixodes* ticks (Richter et al. 1996). However, the habitat of a number of ehrlichiae is not well understood. Fluke transmission has been suspected in the case of *E. sennetsu* and *E. risticii* and has been demonstrated for the related ehrlichiae, *Neorickettsia helminthoeca* and the *Stellantchasmus falcatus* (SF) agent (Wen et al. 1996).

Table 36.2 Diseases and habitats of species of the ehrlichias

Genetic group species	Animals affected	Disease	Invertebrate host	Geographical distribution
Group I ehrlichias				
Ehrlichia sennetsu	Human	Sennetsu ehrlichiosis	Fluke?	Japan, Malaysia USA, Europe
Ehrlichia risticii	Horse	Potomac horse fever, equine monocytic ehrlichiosis	Fluke?	
Neorickettsia helminthoeca	Canidae	Salmon poisoning, Elokomin fluke fever	Fluke (*Nanophyetus salmincola*)	West coast of USA
SF agent	Human, Canidae	Hyuganetsu disease	Fluke (*Stallantchasmus falcatus*)	Japan
Group II ehrlichias				
Ehrlichia canis	Canidae	Tropical canine pantocytopenia	Tick (*Rhipicephalus sanguineus*)	Tropical and subtropical areas, world wide
Ehrlichia chaffeensis	Human	Human ehrlichiosis	Tick (*Amblyomma americanum*)	USA, Portugal? Spain?
Ehrlichia ewingii	Canidae	Canine granulocytic ehrlichiosis	Tick (*Amblyomma americanum?*)	USA
Ehrlichia muris	Mouse	Unnamed	?	Japan
Cowdria ruminantium	Ruminants	Heartwater	Tick (*Amblyomma hebraeum*)	Sub-Saharan Africa, Carribean Islands
Group III ehrlichias				
Ehrlichia phagocytophila	Ruminants	Tick-borne fever	Tick (*Ixodes ricinus*)	Europe, Asia, Africa
Ehrlichia equi	Horse	Equine ehrlichiosis	Tick (*Ixodes pacificus*)	USA, Europe
HGE	Human, horse, dog	Human granulocytic ehrlichiosis	Tick (*Ixodes scapularis*)	Northern USA, Europe
Ehrlichia platys	Canidae	Canine cyclic thrombocytopenia	Tick?	USA
Ehrlichia bovis	Cattle	Bovine ehrlichiosis	Tick (*Hyalomma*)	Africa, Middle East
Anaplasma marginale	Cattle	Anaplasmosis	Ticks (*Dermacentor, Boophilus*), tabanid flies	World wide
Group IV ehrlichia-like agents				
Wolbachia pipientis-like symbionts	Arthropods, isopod	Cytoplasmic incompatibility, sex ratio distortion	Seven orders of insects, *Armadillium*	Europe, USA

4 MICROENVIRONMENT AND MORPHOLOGY

The rickettsiae are intracellular parasites of eukaryotic cells. The great majority of species induce their own phagocytosis into the phagosome. They survive by 3 different mechanisms. Species of the genera *Rickettsia* and *Orientia* rapidly escape from the phagosome into the cytoplasm and sometimes invade the nucleus. Species of the genus *Ehrlichia* and related genera prevent phagosome fusion with the lysosomes and thus remain in a favourable environment for growth. *C. burnetii* is adapted to survival and growth in the hostile environment of the phagolysosomes. A few species, such as *E. phagocytophila*, invade granulocytes, which, in addition to lysosomes, produce other antimicrobial proteins, such as myeloperoxidases and defensins. The difference in appearance of primary cultures of chick embryo endodermal cells infected, respectively, with *R. prowazekii* and *C. burnetii* is illustrated in Fig. 36.1. *R. prowazekii*, growing in the cytoplasm, does not change the vacuolar nature of its host cell, while *C. burnetii*, growing in the phagolysosome, forms a single large multilobed vacuole. This was confirmed by 3-dimensional high voltage electron microscopy (Hechemy et al. 1993).

The escape from the lysosome is probably due to the prompt activation of a phospholipase, which acts on the phagosomal membrane (Ojcius et al. 1995). *R. prowazekii* achieves high bacterial density in the cytoplasm and escapes from the cell by cell rupture, due to the heavy burden. *R. typhi* and SFG rickettsiae, on the other hand, escape earlier from the cells in the course of multiplication and invade other cells. Occasionally, SFG rickettsiae and *R. canada* invade the cell nucleus, where they achieve high density. Figure 36.2 illustrates *R. rickettsii* strain Sheila Smith, stained by the method of Giménez, with preferential growth in the cytoplasm and nucleus, respectively. *R. typhi* and SFG rickettsiae have been shown to catalyse the polymerization of actin tails which gives them active movement in the cell and facilitates their exit and invasion of other cells (Teysseire, Chiche-Portiche and Raoult 1992, Heinzen et al. 1993). *O. tsutsugamushi* also achieves a high population density in the cytoplasm of invaded cells and on rare occasions invades the nucleus.

The morphology of members of the genus *Rickettsia* is typical of small gram-negative bacterial rods. Their size is about 0.3–0.5 μm in diameter by 0.8–2.0 μm in length. They do not have flagella, pili, or attachment proteins that can be recognized morphologically. They are gram-negative, but they do not stain well by the gram stain. The morphology of *O. tsutsugamushi* is similar, except that they have a much thicker outer layer, by which they adhere tenaciously to host cell components. Figure 36.3 illustrates in detail the electron microscopic morphology of typical rickettsiae grown in chicken embryo fibroblasts, released from their host cells, fixed and sectioned.

The inhibition of phagosome–lysosome fusion by

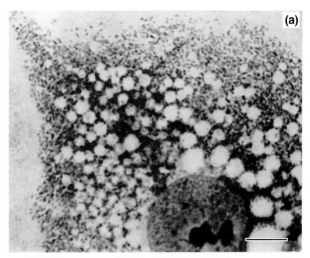

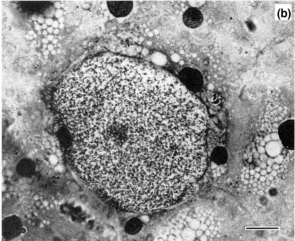

Fig. 36.1 Rickettsiae cultivated in primary cultures of chicken embryo endodermal cells stained with May–Grunwald–Giemsa. (a) *Rickettsia prowazekii* strain E. Bar = 5 μm. (b) *Coxiella burnetii*, California strain. Bar = 30 μm. Note difference in appearance of cell infected with a rickettsia growing in the cytoplasm and one growing in the phagolysosome. This illustration, as well as subsequent ones, were previously reprinted in the *Encyclopedia of Microbiology* (Weiss 1992) and reproduced here with permission from Academic Press, Inc. The original references for the figures are cited in Weiss (1992).

Ehrlichia has been demonstrated only in cells infected with *E. risticii* (Rikihisa 1991a), but there is good morphological evidence that it occurs in other species of *Ehrlichia* and related genera. Infection of canine monocytes with *E. canis* is effected by small round particles 0.5 μm in diameter. They increase in size and divide to form large particles, usually referred to as morulae. The individual particles have typical gram-negative trilaminar outer and inner membranes. The various species of *Ehrlichia* and related genera vary in the size of the morulae and time of release of the individual particles (Chaichanasiriwithaya et al. 1994, Popov et al. 1995). The morphology of ehrlichial morulae and individual particles is illustrated in Fig. 36.4. The apparent developmental cycle of the ehrlichiae is quite distinct from that of the phyloge-

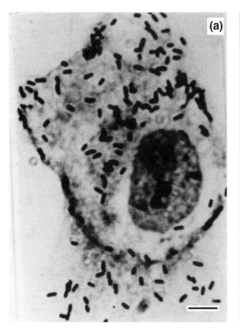

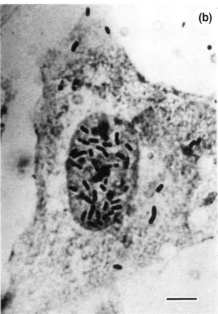

Fig. 36.2 *Rickettsia rickettsii,* strain Sheila Smith, cultivated in umbilical vein endothelial cells, stained by the method of Giménez. (a) Preferential growth in the cytoplasm; (b) in the nucleus. Bar = 5 μm.

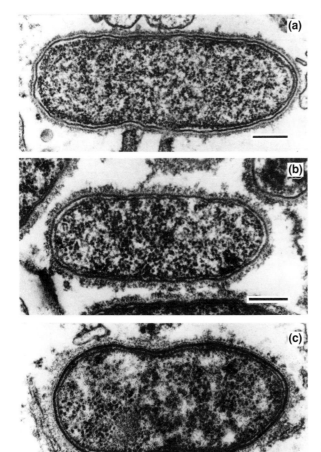

Fig. 36.3 Electron microscopy of typical rickettsias carefully separated from their host cells. Bar = 0.25 μm. (a) *R. prowazekii,* strain Breinl; (b) *R. rickettsii,* strain Sheila Smith; (c) *O. tsutsugamushi,* strain Gilliam.

netically unrelated chlamydiae. *Cowdria* grows preferentially in endothelial cells while *Anaplasma* grows in erythrocytes.

C. burnetii is a unique bacterium that combines adaptation to the acid environment of the phagolysosome with a developmental cycle that includes transverse binary fission and sporogenesis. The developmental cycle as described in detail by McCaul and Williams (1981) is shown in Fig. 36.5. In addition to the schematic representation of the cycle, the great variety of forms in a purified preparation and a cell undergoing cell division and containing a spore is shown. The usual smears of *C. burnetii* infected cells display a great variety of forms; the cells which have not yet divided are usually small rods (approximately 0.3 by 1.0 μm) which double in size or develop a spore at one end or do both. The smears also contain spores in various stages of development. In contrast to other rickettsiae, coxiellae have some gram-positive surface components and, on repeated cultivation in the laboratory, they may display lipopolysaccharide (LPS) phase variation. Phase I cells are infectious for animals, while phase II cells usually appear upon repeated cultivation in the yolk sac of chicken embryos. Phase II cells do not have the full complement of properties required for survival in professional macrophages. The adaptation to an acid environment is in part demonstrated by the fact that many metabolic activities are detectable only when the pH is 5 or lower (Redd and Thompson 1995).

5 STAINING PROCEDURES

The staining procedure developed by Giménez is used frequently for most rickettsiae. This procedure is based on the selective retention of carbol fuchsin by rickettsiae, which are seen as bright red, slender coccobacillary forms against a pale greenish-blue background. Smears are air dried and

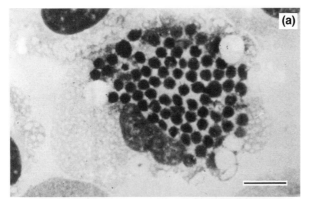

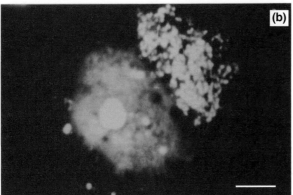

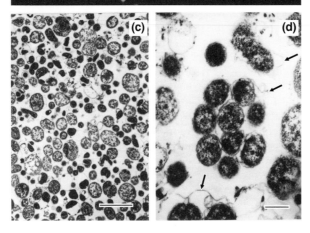

Fig. 36.4 The morphology of ehrlichiae. (a) *E. canis* in primary canine monocyte cultures, stained by Wright–Giemsa. Bar = 10 μm.; (b–d) *E. risticii* in mouse macrophage. (b) Stained by acridine orange. Note clump of organisms within the cytoplasm. Bar = 10 μm. (c) Note variety of morphological forms. Bar = 3 μm. (d) Note retention of morula structure and some host membranes (arrows), even in purified preparation. Bar = 0.5 μm.

gently heat-fixed or fixed in 1% formalin in 0.1 M sodium phosphate buffer, pH 6.8. The stock solution of carbol fuchsin is prepared by mixing 100 ml of 10% basic fuchsin in 95% ethanol with 250 ml of 4% (v/v) aqueous phenol and 650 ml of distilled water. The working solution is prepared by filtering 4 ml of carbol fuchsin stock mixed with 10 ml of 0.1 M sodium phosphate, pH 7.45. The slide is stained for 5 min, washed with tap water and counterstained briefly once or twice with 0.8% malachite green–oxalate in distilled water. The Giemsa stain is used frequently for *O. tsutsugamushi*, the ehrlichiae, *Wolbachia* and also for *Coxiella*. By this method and by the Wright–Giemsa procedure, the micro-organisms

are easily recognized in tissue cells or blood smears. Acridine orange staining of the rickettsiae combines visualization with an assessment of their physiological activity. Physiologically active, but not dead micro-organisms, fluoresce an intense bright orange to red colour against a yellow-green background. An ultraviolet microscope is required for this procedure (see Fig. 36.4b). Fluorescent antibody tests have the unique benefit of permitting simultaneous detection and identification of the rickettsiae. Since the rickettsiae vary greatly in antigenic specificity, the antibodies must be carefully selected, depending on the problem under investigation. The procedure is particularly useful when rapid identification is required or in studies involving wide surveys. More details of these procedures may be found in Dasch and Weiss (1992).

6   LABORATORY ISOLATION, CULTURAL CHARACTERISTICS AND GROWTH REQUIREMENTS

Rickettsiae cannot be cultivated in chicken embryos or tissue cultures until freed from adventitious bacteria. Guinea pigs and mice are most frequently used for such a purpose. This is in part due to the fact that infection with *R. typhi* and some of the pathogenic spotted fever rickettsiae can be suspected because they elicit scrotal oedema and erythema in male guinea pigs. This reaction does not occur in infections with *R. prowazekii* or *C. burnetii*. Fever provides evidence of infection in most cases. After a few days of fever, blood or tissue homogenates can be used for passage in yolk sacs of chicken embryos or tissue cultures for further propagation. *O. tsutsugamushi*, some of the SFG rickettsiae and *C. ruminantium* are usually isolated in voles or mice. Kidneys, spleens and peritoneal exudate are processed for passage. It must be emphasized that such procedures must be carried out in laboratories equipped to provide safety to its workers. This is particularly true when *C. burnetii* infection is suspected.

The yolk sacs of embryonated chicken embryos are a good medium for the isolation of non-pathogenic spotted fever rickettsiae and for the preparation of large pools of typhus, scrub typhus and Q fever rickettsiae. Eggs are inoculated when the embryos are 5–7 days old. The top of the egg above the air sac is surface-sterilized and a hole is punched aseptically. A 0.2–0.4 ml inoculum is delivered with a 22-gauge needle long enough (2–3 cm) to penetrate into the yolk sac. The inoculum is adjusted to kill 30% of the embryos in 5–8 days in the case of *Rickettsia* or *Coxiella* or 10–12 days in the case of *Orientia*. If yolk sac smears from the dead embryos display infection, the typhus and scrub typhus rickettsiae are rapidly harvested in the yolk sacs of the surviving eggs. Spotted fever rickettsiae continue to grow after death of the embryos and *C. burnetii* rickettsiae are quite stable so harvesting of the yolk sacs can be delayed. Suspending fluids for such harvests are brain–heart infusion (BHI) broth or sucrose phosphate glutamate (SPG) solution, consisting of 0.22 M sucrose, 0.1 M potassium phosphate, 5 mM potassium glutamate, pH 7.0. The pools of yolk sacs and their suspending medium are homogenized in bottles containing 5 mM glass beads, dispensed in vials and used as inocula or the rickettsiae are purified for use in physiological or antigenic studies. For further details of these procedures see Dasch and Weiss (1992).

Cell cultures offer many opportunities for rapid isolation and identification of the rickettsiae from infected animals or patients, isolation of rickettsiae by the plaque assay method to obtain the equivalent of pure cultures, or for the production of rickettsial stocks that can be purified from host

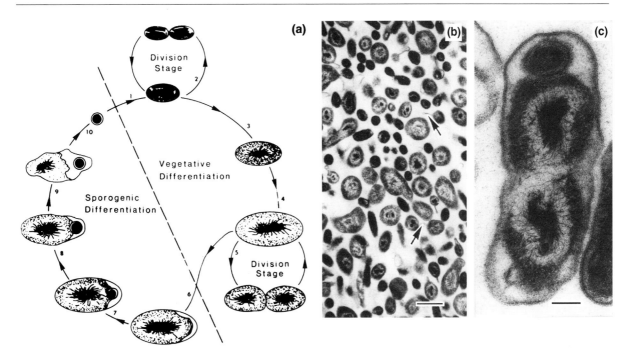

Fig. 36.5 (a) Schematic representation of the cycle of development of *Coxiella burnetii*. (b) Renografin purified coxiellae cultivated in the yolk sac of chicken embryos, illustrating the great variety of forms seen in such preparations. The outer membranes of some cells appear to form blebs (arrows). Bar = 0.6 μm. (c) Formation of an endospore in a cell undergoing cell division. Bar = 0.1 μm.

cell materials for the detailed study of their antigenic and physiological properties. The shell vial culture technique has the advantage that it concentrates a moderate volume of inoculum over a small monolayer of highly susceptible cells on a coverslip. It enhances the infection by centrifugation (usually at 700 x *g* for 1 h) prior to incubation. After centrifugation, the supernatant is removed and replaced by an appropriate medium, such as Eagle's minimal essential medium (MEM) containing 10% fetal bovine serum. If several vials are treated with the same inoculum, a duplicate coverslip can be examined a few days after inoculation and the rickettsiae identified by the indirect fluorescent antibody method. After a satisfactory level of infection is reached, the remaining vials can be used for passage of the rickettsiae into tissue culture flasks for the production of larger volumes. This method is used, for example, to isolate rickettsiae from the haemolymph, withdrawn aseptically from ticks suspected of harbouring rickettsiae. It has also been used to identify *C. burnetii* from human blood in cases of acute disease and suspected chronic endocarditis (Musso and Raoult 1995).

Isolation of rickettsiae by plaque formation is usually performed on monolayers of chicken embryo fibroblasts but can also be done on L929 or Vero cells. The tissues are obtained from decapitated 10 day old chicken embryos, thoroughly minced in Earle's balanced salt solution (EBSS), and the cells are further separated from each other by digestion with 0.25% trypsin for 20 min at 37°C. Trypsinization is terminated by the addition of fetal bovine serum. Clumps are removed by filtration over sterile cheesecloth and the isolated cells are sedimented by centrifugation and resuspended in MEM containing 10% fetal bovine serum. The suspension is dispensed into 25 cm² tissue culture flasks, 5 ml per flask, and confluent monolayers are allowed to form by incubation overnight at 37°C. The samples to be plaqued are diluted serially in BHI and, after the supernatant fluid has been removed, 0.1 ml volumes are added to the mono-

layers. Plaquing efficiency is increased by gentle rocking of the flasks for 60 min or by moderate centrifugation of the inoculum over the cells. Finally, the cultures are overlaid with an appropriate medium (such as RPMI 1640 or Medium 199 containing glutamine and 0.8% agarose). SFG rickettsial plaques are recognized 4–7 days post-inoculation and are 2–3 mm in diameter. Typhus group rickettsiae require a second feeder layer and form 1–2 mm plaques 10–14 days after inoculation. *O. tsutsugamushi* requires refeeding twice and forms 0.5–1.0 mm plaques by 16–18 days. Plaques are recognized by inspection of the monolayers by oblique light or by staining by neutral red. Plaque isolation is particularly valuable for the isolation of phase I and phase II variant forms of *C. burnetii*.

For the mass cultivation of rickettsiae and coxiellae, irradiated mouse L929 or Vero cells are often used in large flasks. When growth is sufficiently abundant, the cells are harvested with glass beads. The suspension is then centrifuged and the pellet resuspended in SPG for freezing or in BHI for further propagation. For additional information see Dasch and Weiss (1992) and Williams, Weiss and Dasch (1992). Different ehrlichiae have been grown in a variety of cells including L929, BGM, mouse embryo, Vero, P388D1, DH82, bovine endothelial, tick embryo IDE8, and HL60 human promyelocytic leukaemia cells (Rikihisa 1991a, Chen et al. 1995, Goodman et al. 1996, Wen et al. 1996).

7 METABOLISM

Although most studies of rickettsiae have focused on their importance as agents of disease, many metabolic and enzymatic activities have been detected (Austin and Winkler 1988, Winkler 1990, Thompson 1991). Because relatively large amounts can be obtained, the typhus rickettsiae have been studied most extensively.

Although the results with typhus rickettsiae are probably applicable to spotted fever rickettsiae, they may not all be applicable to *Orientia*. Typhus rickettsiae are non-glycolytic and utilize citric acid cycle intermediates, particularly glutamate or glutamine, to drive oxidative phosphorylation and ATP synthesis. They are also efficient in transporting activated sugar compounds, amino acids and phosphorylated nucleotides but not purine or pyrimidine bases or nucleosides. Purified rickettsiae can synthesize RNA and proteins, but not DNA, from nucleotide and amino acid precursors. Peak metabolic activities occur at pH 7.3–7.6. Early metabolic experiments with *C. burnetii* were disappointing because it was not realized that anabolic activities of cells of this species can only be demonstrated in an acid environment, consistent with its growth in the phagolysosomal environment. *Coxiella* is a glycolytic organism and during acid activation in medium with low concentrations of glucose, glutamate and amino acids, it synthesizes DNA, RNA and at least 30 polypeptides. Limited information is available on the metabolism of *E. sennetsu* and *E. risticii* (Weiss et al. 1989). Isolated ehrlichiae resemble rickettsiae in being non-glycolytic and in carrying out oxidative phosphorylation and ATP synthesis in the presence of citric acid cycle intermediates, particularly glutamine, when incubated at neutral pH.

8 CLASSIFICATION

As indicated in section 1 (p. 853) numerous changes in rickettsial classification have occurred since the publication of the last edition of *Bergey's Manual of Systematic Bacteriology* (Krieg and Holt 1984). Species related to the genus *Ehrlichia* particularly deserve further taxonomic examination, especially since new species, vectors, hosts and reservoirs have recently been described. Furthermore, some species, such as *Wolbachia melophagi*, because of greatly reduced environmental importance have not been examined in decades, and are only of historical interest. Tables 36.1 and 36.2, describing the habitats of the most important species, can be used as a guide to present classification.

9 GENOME AND PLASMIDS

9.1 *Rickettsia* and *Orientia*

The genome sizes of *R. typhi* and *R. prowazekii* are about 1.1 mb while those of 14 species of spotted fever rickettsiae are somewhat larger, about 1.2–1.3 mb (Eremeeva, Roux and Raoult 1993, Roux and Raoult 1993). *R. massiliae* and *R. helvetica* genomes are somewhat larger, 1.3–1.4 mb, than for the other SFG species while the genome of *R. bellii* is about 1.66 mb. Pulsed field gel electrophoresis patterns of rickettsial DNA cut with infrequently cutting restriction enzymes generally exhibit minimal variation among isolates of a species but have been very useful in confirming the identity of individual isolates (Eremeeva et al. 1995a, 1995b). The mol% G + C of typhus rickettsiae and *R. bellii* DNA is 29–30% while the DNA of 6 species of spotted fever rickettsiae is 31–33%. The 16S

rDNA sequence of most species has been characterized and used to determine relationships among the rickettsial species (Ohashi et al. 1995, Roux and Raoult 1995, Stothard and Fuerst 1995). 23S rDNA sequences have supported the view that *R. bellii*, a species with properties intermediate to the typhus and spotted fever groups, was a product of a divergence predating the origins of typhus and SFG group rickettsiae (Stothard, Clark and Fuerst 1994). However, 16S rDNA relationships of the typhus-like agents *R. canada*, ELB and AB bacterium vary depending on the analysis employed, suggesting the present typhus/spotted fever group dichotomy does not adequately reflect their evolutionary history. Similarly, other relationships are deduced when information from 17 kDa protein antigen, *rompB* and citrate synthase genes are included (Werren et al. 1994, Balayeva et al. 1995, Radulovic et al. 1995). Spotted fever group rickettsiae are closely related but *R. akari* and *R. australis* usually group as a distinct lineage and are somewhat more typhus-like biologically. Because only 0.5–2% 16S rDNA sequence divergence exists among many of the tick-transmitted SFG rickettsiae, both the validity of the species named and their interrelationships are still uncertain. The *R. prowazekii* 16S and 23S-5S rRNA operons exist as unusual separate units without associated encoded tRNA genes (Andersson et al. 1995). The 23S-5S rDNA unit was preceded by a methionyl-tRNA$_f^{Met}$ formyltransferase gene. Each rDNA gene is present in one copy.

The few characterized rickettsial antigen genes have been subject to a great deal of comparison by PCR-RFLP and sequencing. The genus-specific 17 kDa protein is a lipoprotein with a signal peptide and is found in all species including *R. bellii* (Regnery, Spruill and Plikaytis 1991). The conserved rOmpB protein is processed from a 168 kDa precursor by cleavage at a conserved carboxypeptide domain generating an amino terminal encoded surface layer protein and a 32 kDa β protein which contains a membrane anchor domain (Ching et al. 1990, Hackstadt et al. 1992). The β-protein sequence is very conserved among the sequenced *R. typhi*, *R. prowazekii* and *R. rickettsii rompB* genes (Hahn et al. 1993) and is also similar to a homologous sequence in the 190 kDa *R. rickettsii* rOmpA protein which has not been shown to undergo processing (Anderson et al. 1990). β-Protein processing of rOmpB does not occur in the avirulent Iowa strain of *R. rickettsii*. rOmpB contains a signal peptide sequence and the amino terminus in some species is blocked. PCR-RFLP using 3 segments of the *rompB* gene can be used to identify many rickettsial species except *R. bellii* which does not have an *rompB* gene and *R. helvetica* whose gene was not amplified (Eremeeva et al. 1993, Eremeeva, Yu and Raoult 1994). The rOmpA protein has a signal peptide-like sequence and tandem related 72 and 75 amino acid repeats which vary in number and order among different SFG isolates (Crocquet-Valdes, Weiss and Walker 1994). PCR-RFLP analysis of *rompA* has been used extensively to identify new isolates (Eremeeva et al. 1994, 1995b). *rompA* genes of *R. australis* and *R. canada* do not hybridize to a repeat region probe and *R. helvetica* and AB rickettsiae are not amplified with the *rompA* PCR primers tested. *R. bellii*, *R. typhi*, *R. felis* and *R. prowazekii* lack the *rompA* gene. Another 120 kDa antigen gene from *R. conorii* lacked a signal sequence and was found in the rickettsial cytoplasm. Homologues were detected in 8 spotted fever rickettsiae (Schuenke and Walker 1994). Emelyanov (1993) described the cloning of the *groE* operon and 2 outer-membrane protein genes from *R. prowazekii*.

The genome size of *O. tsutsugamushi* is unknown. The mol% G + C of DNA of 6 isolates of scrub typhus rickettsiae varied between 28 and 30.5% (Kumura et al. 1991). Eight antigen genes have been cloned from *O. tsutsugamushi* (Oaks et al. 1989). The sequences of the 16S rRNA gene, *groE* operon (encoding a 10 kDa protein and 58 kDa antigen), 47 kDa, 56 kDa variable outer-membrane protein (VOMP) and 22 kDa protein antigen genes have been obtained (Stover et al. 1990a, 1990b, Hickman et al. 1991, Ohashi et al. 1992, 1995). With monospecific sera prepared against the recombinant antigens, VOMP and 110 kDa antigens exhibited size variation among serotypes while the 22, 47, 49, 58, 72 and 150 kDa antigens were conserved. 16S rDNA and VOMP gene sequencing have confirmed that *O. tsutsugamushi* contains a diverse group of isolates that are not closely related to the typhus and spotted fever rickettsiae. The 56 kDa protein has been overexpressed as a maltose binding fusion protein and used in immunodiagnostic procedures (Kim et al. 1993a, 1993b). PCR-RFLP polymorphisms and serotype-specific PCR primers have been described for the 22, 47, 56 and 110 kDa protein antigen and *groE* genes (Furuya et al. 1993, Kawamori et al. 1993, DJ Kelly et al. 1994).

Many genes have been identified in rickettsiae, especially typhus rickettsiae, initially by detection of their encoded enzymatic activities (Austin and Winkler 1988). Although rickettsial genes have been cloned and identified by their sequence similarity to those of other bacteria, differences in their genetic organization and functional interactions with other proteins can preclude their functional expression in other hosts. The citrate synthase gene is controlled by 2 promoters. The rickettsial flavoprotein subunit gene *sdh* of succinate dehydrogenase was unable to complement an *Escherichia coli* mutant and it was not found in a *sdhCDAB*-type operon. An unusual functional rickettsial ATP/ADP translocase gene which permits the acquisition of host cell ATP has been cloned. The *recA* gene (an inducer of the SOS DNA repair process) of *R. prowazekii* complements *E. coli recA* mutants but may be regulated differently. The *R. prowazekii* A subunit of DNA gyrase, which can supercoil DNA and is a target of quinolone antibiotics, is unable to complement *E. coli* gyrase B subunit. Rickettsial homologues of the regulator of RNA polymerase sigma factor *rpoB*, *greA*, as well as 2 genes in the macromolecular synthesis operon, sigma factor *rpoD* and DNA primase *dnaG*, have also been obtained. The rickettsial *pepA* gene encoding leucine aminopeptidase, which has a role in recombination and in cell protein turnover, can be detected in *E. coli* but does not complement the recombination system. Two genes from *R. rickettsii*, *firA* and *lpxA*, involved in the lipid A biosynthetic pathway of LPS and found together with an open reading frame (ORF) encoding a 16 kDa protein, have been identified. A 34 kDa protein gene of unknown function has been identified upstream of the *R. rickettsii* 17 kDa lipoprotein gene.

9.2 Ehrlichiae

Except for *Anaplasma marginale* which has a 1.25 mb genome and 56% G + C composition (Alleman et al. 1993), the genome sizes and % G + C of the ehrlichiae are unknown. The molecular differentiation of genetic groups and species of the other ehrlichiae has depended primarily on comparison of 16S rDNA sequences (Pretzman et al. 1995). Whereas new ehrlichial isolates have also been differentiated primarily by their 16S rDNA sequences, their antigenic and biological properties have generally been consistent with this approach (Dumler et al. 1995b, Wen et al. 1995a, 1995b, 1996). By 16S rDNA sequence comparisons the ehrlichiae consist of 4 diverse genetic groups as shown in Table 36.2. DNA hybridization with a few cloned genetic fragments or total genomic DNA confirm that *E. sennetsu* and *E. risticii* are closely related but distinct from *E. canis* (Thaker et al. 1990, Shankarappa, Dutta and Mattingly-Napier 1992a). *E. risticii* isolates dif-

fering in pathogenicity have been distinguished by RFLP analysis of genomic DNA probed with specific antigen gene probes or a partial 16S rDNA PCR product (Chaichanasiriwithaya et al. 1994, Vemulapalli, Biswas and Dutta 1995). Sequences of the 16S and 23S rRNA genes and the bacterial cell division gene *ftsZ* have been very useful in characterizing 2 distinct populations of *W. pipientis*-like symbionts which diverged 60 million years ago as well as for detecting *W. pipientis*-like agents in numerous invertebrate species (Werren, Zhang and Guo 1995). The rRNA operons of *W. pipientis* are unusual in that the 16S rRNA operon is unlinked to the 23S-5S rRNA operon, neither is linked to tRNA-encoding sequence, each is present in a single genomic copy, and the antitermination boxes usually present in eubacteria are absent (Bensaadi-Merchermek et al. 1995). *Wolbachia* isolates from *Culex* and *Ephestia* differed in sequences flanking the rRNA operons although their rRNA operon sequences and organization were very conserved.

Only a few *Ehrlichia* genes have been cloned. These include the 44, 51, 55, 70 and 85 kDa antigen genes of *E. risticii* (Dutta, Shankarappa and Mattingly-Napier 1991, Vemulapalli, Biswas and Dutta 1995) and the *groE* operon and 120 kDa antigen gene of *E. chaffeensis* (Sumner et al. 1993, Yu and Walker 1995). The antigens encoded by the genes were identified by preparation of monospecific sera using the expressed full size or partial fusion protein products. The 85 kDa antigen differed among *E. risticii* isolates while some protection for mice was observed with the 55 and 44 kDa recombinant proteins (Shankarappa, Dutta and Mattingly-Napier 1992b). The *groE* genes are cotranscribed from a single promoter and a single transcription terminator and consist of open reading frames encoding 10 and 58 kDa GroES and GroEL heat shock proteins with 50% amino acid homology to other GroESL proteins. More than half of the 120 kDa antigen was comprised of multiple tandem repeat units of 80 amino acids, much as occurs in the *Anaplasma* MSP1a protein.

Two random genomic fragments and 3 genes encoding protein antigens of *C. ruminantium* have been cloned and sequenced (Mahan 1995). Both pCS20 and pCR9, which had 1306 and 754 bp inserts, respectively, were used as DNA probes but the pCS20 probe had greater specificity for *Cowdria* DNA. The *Cowdria groE* operon proteins exhibited 83% and 94% amino acid sequence identities to *E. chaffeensis* GroES and GroEL proteins, respectively (Lally et al. 1995). However, the expressed recombinant protein GroEL was recognized by antisera against 4 isolates of *Cowdria* but not by antisera to *Ehrlichia ovina*, *Ehrlichia ondiri*, *Ehrlichia bovis* or *Ehrlichia phagocytophila*. A conserved 21 kDa *Cowdria* antigen with a putative N-terminal signal peptide and homology to the conserved *A. marginale* outer-membrane protein MSP5 was obtained in pUC13. Antisera against a pFLAG expressed 21 kDa fusion protein reacted against the 21 kDa protein of 7 *Cowdria* isolates and the protein was recognized by all sera from animals with heartwater. Its cross-reactivity with antigens of other ehrlichial species is unknown. The conserved *Cowdria* 32 kDa major antigenic protein (MAP1) has sequence homology with *A. marginale* surface protein MSP4. MAP1 has a putative N-terminal signal sequence and varies somewhat in size in different isolates. A MAP1–glutathione-*S*-transferase fusion product expressed in pGEX-2T was recognized by sera prepared against 7 *Cowdria* isolates and immune sera from 4 animal species. Two immunogenic regions on the MAP1 protein were expressed in *E. coli*. MAP1A fragment reacted with *Cowdria* and *E. ovina* antisera while MAP1B fragment reacted to antisera against 9 isolates of *Cowdria*, antisera to *E. canis* and *E. chaffeensis*, but not to species infecting ruminants, *E. bovis*, *E. ovina* and *E. phagocyto*-

phila (van Vliet et al. 1995). Recombinant MAP1B fragment also did not react with 159 of 169 antisera considered to be falsely positive for heartwater. Consequently, MAP1B fragment is more suitable for specific diagnosis than intact MAP1 protein.

Nine major surface protein antigens have been identified in *A. marginale* initial bodies and the genes encoding 5 of these proteins have been cloned and sequenced (Barbet 1995). MSP1 contains 2 polypeptides: 70–105 kDa MSP1a is expressed from a single genomic copy and is exceedingly polymorphic among isolates due to differences in the number of 28–29 amino acid tandem repeats present; 97–100 kDa polypeptide MSP1b, which varies little between isolates but is encoded by multiple genes whose expression has not been studied. MSP1a was expressed in a variety of recombinant vaccinia virus constructs in which the protein localized diffusely or in the Golgi apparatus of infected cells and which were able to elicit variable amounts of antibody in mice. Functional roles as adhesins for bovine erythrocytes were demonstrated for each recombinant MSP1 polypeptide in *E. coli* and particularly when coexpressed (McGarey et al. 1994). Although MSP1a and MSP1b had no typical N-terminal signal sequences, both polypeptides were expressed on the surface of *E. coli* recombinants. MSP2 is a variable 33–36 kDa protein which is encoded by a polymorphic gene present in multiple copies dispersed through the genomes of different isolates (Palmer et al. 1994a). Different MSP2 genes may be expressed in different cells or simultaneously in the same cell. MSP2 shares extensive sequence homology with the conserved 31 kDa MSP4 protein which is encoded by a single gene; both proteins have putative N-terminal signal sequences. MSP4 is highly conserved among isolates of *A. marginale* and *Anaplasma centrale* and although of limited value for diagnosis, it may be a suitable vaccine candidate. MSP3 is a 86 kDa protein also encoded by multicopy genes but its variability in *Anaplasma* and cross-reactivity with other ehrlichiae preclude its use as a diagnostic antigen (Alleman and Barbet 1996). The 19 kDa MSP5 protein, which is present in all species of *Anaplasma,* is encoded by a single genomic copy and has a putative signal sequence. It has some amino acid homology to the 17 kDa common antigen of typhus and SFG rickettsiae. The MSP5 recombinant antigen has been used with a monoclonal antibody recognizing a highly conserved MSP5 domain in a competitive ELISA to detect antibodies to *A. marginale* and *Anaplasma ovis* (Ndung'u et al. 1995). To date *Anaplasma* genes for only 2 enzymes, glutathione synthetase II and D-alanine-D-alanine ligase, which is involved in peptidoglycan synthesis, have been cloned.

9.3   *Coxiella burnetii*

C. burnetii was thought for many years to be relatively homogeneous except for antigenic phase variation and the same organism was believed to cause both acute and chronic disease. Recent genetic studies have shown that *Coxiella* is not homogeneous but it appears the same genotype can cause both types of disease. *Coxiella* isolates exhibited 14 distinct RFLP patterns of genomic DNA by pulsed field gel electrophoresis, giving a genomic size of 1.4–1.9 mb, in good agreement with the 1.7 mb estimated by reassociation kinetics (Thiele et al. 1993, Thiele and Willems 1994). The DNA base composition of *Coxiella* is 42% G + C. Among rickettsial species, plasmids have only been discovered in *C. burnetii*. Initially, 6 different genomic

groups were distinguished among American isolates by the type of plasmid and RFLP pattern obtained using *Eco*RI or *Bam*HI digested total DNA separated on SDS-PAGE and silver stained. A 36 kb plasmid QpH1 was present in 3 genomic groups with isolates from ticks or animals or causing acute illness in humans, the 39 kb plasmid QpRS was present in an isolate causing chronic disease, and the 51 kb plasmid QpDG was present in feral rodent isolates of unknown pathogenicity. Another chronic disease isolate group contained both QpRS and QpH1 related plasmid sequences integrated into the chromosome. No unique sequences common to the plasmidless isolates and QpRS have been found that might cause 'chronic' disease. About 30 kb of core plasmid sequence is conserved in all genomic groups whereas the remainder is plasmid specific. Isolates varying only in phase state or passage history exhibit minimal differences. These plasmid sequences are not known to encode virulence factors but their conservation in all genetic groups suggests they are essential to the survival of *C. burnetii*. European isolates were also found to contain QpH1 sequences whereas a Namibian isolate contained QpRS sequences. More recently the association of specific plasmid type with pathogenicity has been questioned as only 9 of 30 European isolates, including both acute and chronic isolates, had sequences specific to QpH1 (Stein and Raoult 1993, Thiele and Willems 1994). Similarly, a new 33.5 kb plasmid QpDV, found in isolates from both acute and chronic disease, has been described (Valkova and Kazar 1995). Both the 90–95% DNA–DNA homologies exhibited between different genomic groups and the greater than 99% 16S rDNA sequence similarity in different isolates of *C. burnetii* argue for their retention as a single species (Hendrix, Samuel and Mallavia 1991, Stein et al. 1993).

Thirty-seven open reading frames have been identified in QpH1 (Thiele et al. 1994). ORF cbhE' encoded a 39.4 kDa hydrophilic protein unique to QpH1. ORFs related to *Pseudomonas* proteins ferripyochelin-binding protein (FBP), 32.4 kDa protein and replication proteins, to *Escherichia* DNA helicase I and SopA protein, to *Agrobacterium* replication protein RepB and to bacteriophage λ tail assembly protein K were recognized. FBP plays a role in iron acquisition and may be virulence determinant in *Pseudomonas*. QpH1 proteins with homology to the F plasmid partition proteins SopA and SopB were found to be also conserved in the plasmids QpRS, QpDV and QpDG but absent in plasmidless isolates (Lin and Mallavia, 1995). The QpRS-specific gene *cbbE'* was not found in plasmidless isolates and encoded a 55 kDa protein which was a surface-exposed outer-membrane protein of unknown function.

The rRNA operon of *C. burnetii* is organized in the order 16S-23S-5S rDNA (Afseth, Mo and Mallavia 1995). The 16S-23S rDNA spacer is *Coxiella* specific and encodes tRNA genes for isoleucine and alanine. The 23S rDNA contains an unusual 444 bp intervening sequence which has a stem-loop structure due to flanking 28 bp inverted repeats. The absence of intact mature 23S rRNA suggests the loop is excised. Approximately 19 copies of a 1450 bp repetitive element were found in *C. burnetii* including one associated with the *groESL* heat shock protein operon (Hoover, Vodkin and Williams 1992). The element had terminal 7 and internal 12 bp inverted repeats at each end and encoded an ORF for a 367 amino acid basic polypeptide with a DNA binding helix-turn-helix and a leucine zipper motif, suggesting it may be a transposase. Ten French isolates with 8 different PFGE patterns each contained this repetitive element (Thiele and Willems 1994). Three independent copies of this element each had additional non-homologous internal 85–93 bp inserts with strong dyad symmetry demarked by identical 7 bp inverted repeats (Hoover, Vodkin and Williams 1992). Remarkably, the *gltA-sdh* intergenic region was found to contain 3 similar nearly perfect inverted repeats (Heinzen et al. 1995). A probe to the terminal 7 bp inverted repeat sequence hybridized to multiple sequences in 4 different genomic groups. Whether the inverted repeat sequences have important regulatory functions is unknown.

Although *C. burnetii* is rather unique in its life-style, it retains many genetic functions that are organized similarly to those of other γ Proteobacteria like *E. coli*; this permits their cloning and identification by functional complementation of mutants and by sequence homology. Characterized genomic regions include a TCA cycle gene cluster similar in arrangement to that of *E. coli* (Heinzen et al. 1995) and the aspartate carbamylase catalytic subunit. The *sdhCDAB* gene cluster encodes succinate dehydrogenase enzyme complex and is adjoined by the 2-oxoglutarate dehydrogenase and citrate synthase genes. Other characterized genes express iron containing superoxide dismutase, homologues of *E. coli* heat shock GroES and GroEL proteins, the heat shock protein DnaJ and the *mucZ* gene product which has some homology to *dnaJ* and activates capsule synthesis in *E. coli*. An autonomous replication sequence was characterized that contains ORFs with homology to genes often found near bacterial chromosomal origins, including *rpmH*, *rnpA*, 9 kDa and 60 kDa membrane proteins. Some information has been obtained for genes encoding a protein similar to the *Legionella* macrophage infectivity potentiator (Mip) protein (Mo, Cianciotto and Mallavia 1995), a protein with homology to bacterial sensor proteins found in two-component regulatory systems (Mo and Mallavia 1994) and a 27 kDa surface-exposed loosely associated outer-membrane protein Com1 (Hendrix, Mallavia and Samuel 1993). The *rnc* locus of *C. burnetii* contained genes with protein homology to RNAase III, RecO and Era of *E. coli*; *rnc* suppressed capsule synthesis in *E. coli* even though *C. burnetii* does not contain a capsule. Era is a 35 kDa GTP binding protein that is essential for cell viability. RNAase III is a double stranded RNA-dependent endoribonuclease. RecO function is involved in DNA recombination and repair.

10 CELL WALL COMPOSITION AND ANTIGENIC PROPERTIES

10.1 *Rickettsia* and *Orientia*

In many respects the cell walls of typhus and SFG rickettsiae are typical of other gram-negative bacteria (Winkler 1990). They contain peptidoglycan (Pang and Winkler 1994), a smooth type LPS, a cytoplasmic membrane which has numerous proteins and an outer membrane in which a few proteins are present in large amounts. However, the rickettsiae also contain a microcapsular protein layer, often called a crystalline protein surface layer, which is comprised of one or 2 multimeric proteins arrayed in a regular periodic manner (Ching et al. 1990). The S layer is comprised of the >120 kDa rOmpB and rOmpA (species-specific surface protein antigen, SPA) surface layer proteins but the precise 3-dimensional interactions of the proteins in the arrays comprised of either one or both of these proteins is unknown. The rOmpB protein multimer of *R. prowazekii* is probably formed of at least 4 antiparallel monomers since they can be isolated as disulphide-linked forms including tetramers. Monomers are released by trypsin or chymotrypsin digestion of the carboxy-terminal region of the isolated multimers from *R. typhi* and *R. prowazekii*. The rOmpA and rOmpB proteins are very rich in β-sheet structure and are heat labile antigens. Monoclonal antibodies responsible for neutralization of rickettsial toxicity for mice recognize conformation-dependent epitopes on these proteins. One conformation-dependent epitope has been localized to the tandem repeat region of the rOmpA proteins. However, not all heat-sensitive epitopes are neutralizing and antibodies to denatured antigen or linear epitopes are not neutralizing. Numerous electron microscopic studies have detected an electron lucent zone around rickettsiae in fixed cells that was thought to be a polysaccharide layer. However, it is likely that it is a fixation artefact since a rickettsial capsule has never been isolated. Double labelling studies with monoclonal antibodies have indicated that LPS, rOmpA and rOmpB are present simultaneously in the cell envelope location (cell wall and microcapsule but not lucent zone) (Uchiyama et al. 1994). Mice immunized with typhus and SFG rickettsiae respond primarily to the rOmpA and rOmpB heat labile domains while LPS antibodies are dominant only when the SPA microcapsule is removed before immunization. Since anti-LPS antibodies bind to intact purified rickettsiae in the presence of the microcapsule, some LPS with longer O side chains intercalates between the open S-layer microcapsule as has been demonstrated in *Aeromonas salmonicida* S layer. Much of the rickettsial LPS is of low chain length and probably does not extend beyond the S-layer microcapsule but can be detected by immunocytochemistry. The rOmpA and rOmpB contain strain, species, group-specific and group-cross-reactive epitopes. Some monoclonal antibodies recognize domains that contain methylated residues on rOmpB of typhus rickettsiae (Ching, Carl and Dasch 1992,

Turco and Winkler 1994). The rOmpA and rOmpB S-layer proteins have been demonstrated to be protective subunit vaccines for both typhus and SFG rickettsiae (Carl and Dasch 1989, Sumner et al. 1995).

Rickettsial LPS is the group antigen that distinguishes typhus and SFG rickettsiae although *R. bellii* contains epitopes common to both and some antigenic heterogeneity exists in the LPS of each group. Human IgM and IgG responses to both typhus and SFG rickettsiae are primarily to the rOmpA and rOmpB proteins and to LPS (Eremeeva, Balayeva and Raoult 1994, Eremeeva et al. 1995c). The LPS of both groups share epitopes with both *Proteus* OX19 (typhus primarily) and *Proteus* OX2 (SFG stronger) Weil–Felix antigens and to *Legionella bozemanii* and *Legionella micdadei* that are detected by human IgM early after infection (Raoult and Dasch 1995). These cross-reactive antibodies can lead to misdiagnosis while IgG anti-LPS antibodies are generally rickettsia-specific (Jones et al. 1993). The 60 kDa common bacterial heat shock proteins of typhus and spotted fever rickettsiae are very similar antigenically and share epitopes with other bacteria, including *Proteus*, that may be misleading in diagnostic procedures (Dasch et al. 1990).

The cell wall structure and antigens of *O. tsutsugamushi* are distinctly different from those of typhus and spotted fever rickettsiae (Tamura, Urakami and Ohashi 1991). No electron lucent slime layer, microcapsule, peptidoglycan or LPS has been detected. The only antigenic protein shared between *Rickettsia* and *Orientia* is the highly conserved 60 kDa heat shock protein but the *Orientia* protein is poorly cross-reactive (Stover et al. 1990b). Although scrub typhus infections occasionally elicit IgM anti-*Proteus* OXK LPS Weil–Felix reactions, the rickettsial antigen responsible for this cross-reaction has not been identified (Amano et al. 1993). The serotype-specific 56 kDa VOMPs are recognized by both IgM and IgG very early in infection and these antibodies persist. Cross-reactive antibodies against the 72, 60, 47 and 22–35 kDa proteins arise commonly in early convalescence. γ-Irradiated whole cell vaccines have been effective vaccines in animal models. Although recombinant VOMPs are good candidates for use as a subunit vaccine (Kim et al. 1993a), only preliminary studies demonstrating their efficacy have been completed.

10.2   Ehrlichiae

Three factors have contributed to our relatively meagre information about the cell wall composition and antigenic properties of ehrlichiae (Rikihisa 1991a). First, although an increasing number of agents can now be cultivated in continuous cell lines, *E. equi*, some agents of bovine and ovine ehrlichioses and *W. pipientis* have not been routinely cultivated. No laboratories have expertise in cultivating all of the ehrlichial agents and restrictions on international exchange of veterinary agents has further slowed their comparison. The other major obstacles are the substantive difficulties experienced in freeing these agents from host cell components (Weiss et al. 1989) and the complex

variation in morphology and morula structures that could be considered a developmental cycle or pathological change (Popov et al. 1995). Ultrastructurally, the cell wall is gram-negative but no obvious peptidoglycan layer is visible. No convincing chemical evidence for a LPS has been reported. Western blotting with diverse polyclonal sera from natural infections and immunizations of laboratory animals has been used to identify antigens present in semipurified cells. However, this approach may fail to detect some antigens exported by ehrlichiae into the phagosome or host cell surface (Messick and Rikihisa 1992, Popov et al. 1995). *E. risticii* has also been studied by radioimmunoprecipitation of iodinated surface proteins. Eighteen protein antigens, 9 of which were prominent, have been identified in *E. risticii* with a variety of homologous polyclonal sera. Antisera from different species, as well as individual animals, exhibited differences in reactivity to *E. risticii* antigens. *E. risticii* and *E. sennetsu* share many antigens of the same size, including 110, 70, 58 and 44 kDa, but not 55 and 28 kDa, antigens as shown with monospecific sera prepared against cloned *E. risticii* genes or with monoclonal antibodies (Dasch, Weiss and Williams 1990, Shankarappa, Dutta and Mattingly-Napier 1992a). Other antigens of somewhat different size also share epitopes recognized by monoclonal antibodies. Only a few of these antigens are shared with *E. canis* but *N. helminthoeca* was more cross-reactive, a result consistent with 16S rDNA groupings (Rikihisa 1991b, Shankarappa, Dutta and Mattingly-Napier 1992a). *E. sennetsu* protected ponies against challenge with *E. risticii* and elicited strong reactivity to a shared 44 kDa protein. However, mice that were protected against *E. risticii* challenge by a killed homologous vaccine reacted primarily to 33, 57 and 100 kDa antigens (Rikihisa 1991c).

The human monocytic ehrlichia, *E. chaffeensis*, has 20 protein antigens detectable with homologous antisera. They cross-reacted most strongly with antisera to *E. canis*, *E. ewingii*, *C. ruminantium* and *E. muris* and less strongly with antisera against *E. sennetsu* and *E. risticii*, a result consistent with 16S rDNA groupings (Chen et al. 1994b, Rikihisa, Ewing and Fox 1994, Wen et al. 1995a). The 66, 64, 55, 47 and 27 kDa bands were cross-reactive with antisera from most species. *E. chaffeensis* antigens resembled *E. canis* and *E. muris* most in reactivity but each had species-specific antigens. Yu et al. (1993) described a monoclonal antibody which recognized the 27 and 29 kDa antigen bands of *E. chaffeensis* but no *E. canis* antigens. The immunoreactivity of some antigens was heat labile.

Little is known about the antigens of granulocytic ehrlichiae although IFA reactions are consistent with their close relationship and antigenic distance from the other ehrlichiae (Dumler et al. 1995a, Magnarelli et al. 1995). *E. ewingii*-specific antigens include 25, 42, 44 and 100 kDa antigens whereas 25, 56 and 75 kDa antigens appear to be shared with other ehrlichiae. A horse infected with the human granulocytic agent developed an *E. equi*-like disease and was protected against challenge by *E. equi*, suggesting they may be similar agents (Barlough et al. 1995).

Other than the cloned 32 and 21 kDa antigens and the 60 kDa GroEL proteins discussed in section 9.2 (p. 863), little is known about other *Cowdria* antigens. Western blotting of serum from infected animals or animals immunized with inactivated *Cowdria* purified from bovine endothelial cells suggests that additional conserved antigenic proteins of 25, 27, 33, 43, 70 and 80 kDa are also present in different isolates (Mahan et al. 1995). *Cowdria* antigens exhibit cross-reactivity with antisera to *E.˙ canis*, *E. equi*, *E. phagocytophila*, *E. bovis* and *E. ovina* by indirect fluorescence, probably due in part to shared epitopes on the 25 and 32 kDa protein antigens. Homologous protective responses were obtained with the killed vaccine but it is unknown whether heterologous protection will be comparable to that afforded by the infect and treat method.

Purified *A. marginale* initial bodies have 9 surface iodinatable proteins and 5 of these can be precipitated by a rabbit neutralizing antiserum. These include MSP1–5 whose cloning and properties have been described in section 9.2 (p. 863) and a 61 kDa protein. Stage-specific antigens have not been recognized. Although cytoplasmic and outer-membrane fractions obtained from initial bodies had different densities, morphology and peptide composition (except MSP4 which was present in both fractions), both fractions were protective. Vaccination with the outer membrane delayed and reduced rickettsaemia but did not eliminate anaemia after heterologous challenge (Palmer et al. 1994b). Antibodies in immunized animals were primarily against MSP2 and MSP5 of the homologous and heterologous strain. Under non-reducing conditions MSP2 and MSP5 form disulphide-linked multimers (Vidotto et al. 1994). MSP1 complex consists of both disulphide and non-covalently associated MSP1a and b polypeptides. MSP1–5 proteins could all be identified in a cross-linked aggregate. MSP2 is the major protein antigen present in purified initial bodies and possibly contains a carbohydrate epitope recognized by a monoclonal antibody. MSP2 migrated as multiple spots on 2-dimensional gels (Zakimi, Tsuji and Fujisaki 1994). Five protein spots of *A. marginale* and *A. centrale* had similar positions but another 20–30 proteins were different.

10.3 *Coxiella burnetii*

Consistent with the phylogenetic distance of *Coxiella* from the other rickettsiae, it is antigenically distinct from them. Although the gram-negative cell wall structure and composition of *C. burnetii* have been studied intensively (Williams and Waag 1991), an accurate inventory of the cell wall components and their function is difficult because of the distinct morphological forms present in its complex developmental cycle, the virulence-associated LPS phase variation unique among rickettsiae, the difficult physical solubility properties of individual components in the cell envelope, and the plethora of chemical methods used in cell fractionation. The structure of LPS is not completely known but phase I and II differences in chemical composition and size are compatible with a smooth to rough transition where the O side polysaccharide undergoes significant truncation while the core region which contains KDO and lipid A is retained. The neutral sugars virenose and dihydrohydroxystreptose are the major antigenic sugars in the O side chain but they are not unique to *Coxiella*. The branched chain fatty acid composition of the LPS is unique to *Coxiella* although other pathogenic bacteria share some components. Phase I LPS is relatively non-toxic compared with *Salmonella* LPS.

Formalin-treated phase I whole cell vaccines have been widely used in animals and are effective in man while phase II whole cells are considerably less effective (Ackland, Worswick and Marmion 1994). Unfortunately the phase I whole cell vaccines occasionally induce erythema, induration, granulomas and sterile abscesses in some individuals and such severe local and systemic reactions in immune individuals that they must be prescreened by skin test. Consequently, a chloroform–methanol residue (CMR) vaccine was developed which retained good efficacy for animals and man and fewer adverse reactions (Williams et al. 1992, Fries, Waag and Williams 1993). This vaccine retains the LPS and the majority of cellular proteins but is greatly reduced in phospholipids. Trichloroacetic acid extracts containing phase I LPS and purified phase I LPS were protective in mice but not phase II LPS or polysaccharide or lipid A fractions of phase I or II LPS (Gajdosova et al. 1994). Phase I cells contain both immunosuppressive and immunostimulatory molecules that are in part disassociated by chloroform–methanol extraction (Williams and Waag 1991, Tokarevich et al. 1993). Both tumour regression and antiviral activity of phase I and CMR fraction have been observed (Zvilich et al. 1995).

Various protein antigens have been identified by radioimmunoprecipitation of surface radioiodinated proteins and immunoblotting (Williams and Waag 1991). The best characterized is a 29 kDa protein P1 present in phase I and II cells but not in the small dense cell type or endogenous spore (McCaul, Banerjee-Bhatnagar and Williams, 1991). It is both immunogenic and protective for animals (Gadjosova et al. 1994, Lukacova et al. 1994). The 29 kDa protein P1 may be identical to the cloned 27 kDa Com1 protein or several antigenic proteins of similar size are present since another 29 kDa lipoprotein, P2, has also been described. Zhang et al. 1994 also found a 67 kDa outer-membrane protein which was protective in guinea pigs and mice. The conserved 62 kDa protein of *Coxiella* is homologous to the widely conserved chaperonin 60 heat shock protein GroEL. Its expression is regulated by heat in *E. coli* and by heat or 10% ethanol in acid-activated *Coxiella*. It is present on the surface of phase II but not phase I cells. The 62 kDa protein is immunogenic since it is recognized by sera from acute and chronic Q fever patients but it is probably not protective. Whether combinations of purified LPS and antigenic protein or peptide components will offer advantages over CMR or whole cell vaccines is unresolved.

11 IDENTIFICATION AND TYPING METHODS

11.1 *Rickettsia* and *Orientia*

PCR-RFLP analysis of the *rompA*, *rompB*, 17 kDa and citrate synthase genes and RFLP of chromosomal DNAs have become the primary means for rapid characterization of new isolates of typhus and spotted fever rickettsiae (Regnery, Spruill and Plikaytis 1991, Eremeeva, Yu and Raoult 1994). 16S rDNA sequences are also useful (Roux and Raoult 1995, Stothard and Fuerst 1995) but because of the limited amount of variability found, particularly among spotted fever rickettsiae, they are best analysed after other markers indicate that the isolates are unique. Random DNA probes as well as probes derived from specific genes like citrate synthase and the *rompA* tandem repeat region have also been employed in Southern hybridization with genomic DNA (Ralph et al. 1990, Gilmore and Hackstadt 1991, Demkin et al. 1994). PCR with specific primers coupled with specific oligonucleotide probes have been designed for *R. rickettsii*, *R. prowazekii* and for distinguishing ELB and *R. typhi* (Higgins and Azad 1995). Western blotting and SDS-PAGE analysis have also been very useful in distinguishing closely related isolates, particularly when specific mouse typing sera are utilized (Eremeeva et al. 1993, 1994, Walker et al. 1995). Specific monoclonal antibodies have been described for 7 species of typhus and spotted fever rickettsiae and these have been employed in blocking assays, capture assays, IFA and Western blotting procedures to identify rickettsiae (Raoult and Dasch 1989, Uchiyama, Ichida and Walker 1990, Radulovic et al. 1993, 1994). Polyclonal sera are often used for serotyping since no complete set of species-specific monoclonal antibodies is available.

Scrub typhus isolates are best typed by PCR-RFLP methods employing the conserved *groE* operon and the more variable 47 and 56 kDa antigen genes (DJ Kelly et al. 1994). Specific nested PCR procedures have also been described but these are not available for most genetic types (Furuya et al. 1993, Kawamori et al. 1993). The accuracy and specificity of a widely used direct fluorescent antibody serotyping procedure has been questioned (DJ Kelly et al. 1994). However, monoclonal antibody panels have proved very suitable in distinguishing isolates, particularly when employed to analyse antigens by Western blotting (Tange, Kanemitsu and Kobayashi 1991, Moree and Hanson 1992, Park et al. 1993). Protein fingerprinting by cleavage of the VOMP with *N*-chlorosuccinimide has also been used to characterize a new antigenic type (Ohashi et al. 1990).

11.2 Ehrlichiae

Originally identification of ehrlichiae in clinical or tick samples was based primarily on indirect fluorescent antibody reactivity with specific sera but it has been supplanted in part by 16S rDNA sequencing methods (Chaichanasiriwithaya et al. 1994, Wen et al. 1995b). DNA probe and PCR primers specific for *E. risticii*, *E. chaffeensis* and granulocytic agent group have been described (Thaker et al. 1990, Chen et al. 1994a, Pancholi et al. 1995). A segment of the *groEL* gene has also been used for characterizing *E. chaffeensis* but the variability of this region among ehrlichiae is unknown (Dumler et al. 1995b). Western blotting has been particularly useful in demonstrating antigen variation of *E. risticii* and a panel of monoclonal antibodies for this purpose has also been obtained (Chaichanasiriwithaya et al. 1994, Vemulapalli, Biswas and Dutta 1995). Reactivity of human ehrlichial sera with *E. chaffeensis* 22 and 30 kDa antigens or 44 kDa antigen of *E. equi* has been suggested as a specific means to distinguish monocytic or granulocytic disease (Dumler and Bakken 1995).

Serological methods for identifying *Cowdria* still suffer from potential cross-reactivity with other *Ehrlichia* species although an ELISA based on a fragment of MAP1 appears to have eliminated some of these problems (van Vliet et al. 1995). Presently 16S rDNA sequencing, hybridization with pCS20 probe or PCR primers derived from pCS20 or MAP1 protein gene are the only other specific methods available for identifying *Cowdria* (Kock et al. 1995, Peter et al. 1995). Although *Cowdria* isolates differ in virulence and serological properties, no standard typing methods exist.

Anaplasma species may be differentiated by morphology, animal host, cross-protection tests, serological assays, dot hybridization procedures with specific probes, RFLP patterns of genomic DNA with or without specific probes (described in section 9.2, p. 863) and SDS-PAGE protein profiles immunodetected with polyclonal and monoclonal antisera (Nakamura, Kawazu and Minami 1993, Eriks et al. 1994). A PCR method based on *msp1b* gene specifically detects *A. marginale* but not *A. ovis* in ticks (Stich et al. 1993). No PCR-RFLP-based methods for distinguishing *Anaplasma* isolates have been described.

11.3 *Coxiella burnetii*

Most diagnoses of Q fever infection are based on a variety of retrospective serological procedures employing phase I and phase II antigens (Uhaa et al. 1994, Waag et al. 1995). The direct identification of *C. burnetii* is most easily accomplished by direct immunofluorescent antibody staining of organisms in biopsies or after isolation (Musso and Raoult 1995). A monoclonal antibody suitable for this purpose has been described. Alternatively, PCR using primers specific for superoxide dismutase, conserved plasmid sequence, or a large conserved repetitive element (Thiele and Willems 1994) may be done. Chromosomal DNA and plasmid-based typing has been used extensively to differentiate isolates (see section 9.3, p. 864). Protein profiles and Western blotting of proteins have not been very useful for typing strains although distinct LPS profiles may be obtained, particularly among phase variants (Kovacova et al. 1994). Monoclonal and polyclonal sera can be used for distinguishing LPS variants (Yu and Raoult 1994).

12 SUSCEPTIBILITY TO ANTIMICROBIAL AGENTS

12.1 Physical stability and chemical inactivation

Rickettsiae and ehrlichiae are notorious for the difficulties they pose to investigators in their physical maintenance outside host cells under even physiological conditions (Weiss et al. 1989, Winkler 1990). High ionic strength buffers or sucrose substituted to provide osmolarity are essential for long-term maintenance of isolated organisms. Even with media designed to mimic the internal host cell environment (activated energy compounds, amino acid and cofactors, nucleotides, neutral pH), it is difficult to preserve metabolic activity or infectivity for more than several days. Consequently, chemical disinfectants and 60°C treatment are highly effective in inactivation. Scrub typhus rickettsiae are more labile than typhus group rickettsiae while *R. rickettsii* and *R. conorii* can continue to divide after host cell death. The stability of ehrlichiae after host cell death is probably comparable to SFG rickettsiae although even the preparation and maintenance of frozen blood stabilates for use as live vaccines was difficult for *Anaplasma* and *Cowdria* until cryopreservation in 10% DMSO was introduced.

Relative to all the other rickettsiae and to vegetative bacteria, *Coxiella burnetii* is notorious for its resistance to elevated temperatures, desiccation, osmotic shock, ultraviolet light and chemical disinfectants (Scott and Williams 1990). Coupled with its infectivity for humans of 1–10 organisms, contamination of food, buildings and pastures has frequently led to human and animal infections. Highly effective disinfectants of suspended organisms were 70% ethanol, 5% chloroform and 5% EnviroChem, whereas Alcide, sodium hypochlorite, benzalkonium chloride, Lysol and 5% formalin were not. Paraformaldehyde gas and ethylene oxide sterilization of surface-applied organisms was inefficient under low humidity conditions. It is probable that metabolic dormancy at pH 6 and the developmental cycle which generates spores and small dense forms both contribute to the physical and chemical resistance of *C. burnetii* to inactivation.

12.2 Sensitivity to antibiotics

Plaque reduction techniques have been used extensively for assessing antibiotic susceptibility in typhus and, particularly, SFG rickettsiae (Raoult and Drancourt 1991). Direct microscopic examination of growth inhibition in infected cells has been most useful for typhus and scrub typhus rickettsiae. Dye uptake assays have also been useful for cytotoxic rickettsial isolates (Maurin and Raoult 1993). Earlier studies more commonly employed embryonated chicken eggs or animals. Tetracyclines, chloramphenicol, rifampicin, fluoroquinolones (except for scrub typhus) and some macrolides are all effective in vitro against rickettsiae whereas penicillins, cephalosporins, aminoglycosides, sulphonamides and trimethoprim–sulphamethoxazole are not. Therapy with one of the tetracyclines is the method of choice for rickettsiae (Walker 1995). Oral or intravenous tetracycline is generally efficacious whereas doxycycline has been used as a single dose treatment for epidemic typhus and scrub typhus (Song et al. 1995). Relapses may occur with typhus and scrub typhus. Although weekly doxycycline chemoprophylaxis for scrub typhus appears effective, doxycycline resistance and treatment failures have been reported (Strickman et al. 1995). Chloramphenicol is commonly used as an alternative drug to tetracyclines but treatment failures have been reported. Delay in treatment is a major risk factor for fatal Rocky Mountain spotted fever (Dalton et al. 1995). Rifampicin resistance has been induced in *R. prowazekii* by mutagenesis. The fluoroquinolone ciprofloxacin has been used to treat Mediterranean spotted fever and murine typhus but patients responded less promptly than to doxycycline. Although the macrolide erythromycin has some activity in vitro against rickettsiae, *R. prowazekii* can acquire resistance. Newer macrolides such as josamycin have been used to treat children and pregnant women with boutonneuse fever. In vitro azithromycin was effective against doxycycline-resistant *O. tsutsugamushi* (Strickman et al. 1995) whereas clarithromycin was effective against SFG rickettsiae (Maurin and Raoult 1993).

The in vitro antibiotic susceptibility of ehrlichiae has been determined only for the type strains of *E. sennetsu*, *E. ristici*, *E. canis* and *E. chaffeensis* (Rikihisa 1991a, Brouqui and Raoult 1992). Doxycycline and rifampicin exerted bactericidal effects whereas chloramphenicol, erythromycin, co-trimoxazole, penicillin and gentamicin were not inhibitory. Ciprofloxacin was bacteriostatic for *E. chaffeensis* and *E. canis* only at high concentrations but very effective against *E. sennetsu*. Practical in vivo experience with antibiotics gained during the treatment of a wider range of human and veterinary diseases caused by the ehrlichiae is in agreement with the in vitro data (Dumler and Bakken 1995). Oxytetracycline and doxycycline are generally effective when given in an early stage of infection. Tetracyclines have been used to treat *E. canis* infections in dogs and in the infect and treat methods used to vaccinate against heartwater and anaplasmosis, but they appear ineffective in completely eliminating ehrlichial carriage (Iqbal and Rikihisa 1994). Relapses of ehrlichioses can occur after ineffective treatment. Tetracycline has also been used to eliminate *W. pipientis* from arthropods to demonstrate their role in various manifestations of cytoplasmic incompatibility (Holden, Jones and Brookfield 1993). In vivo resistance of ehrlichiae to chloramphenicol, coupled with anecdotal evidence of chloramphenicol failure in patient care, suggests it is prudent to use doxycycline rather than chloramphenicol since human ehrlichiosis can be severe or fatal. Sulphadimidine, dithiosemicarbazone, and imidocarb dipropionate treatments have also been used successfully in veterinary practice.

Since *C. burnetii* does not multiply in axenic media, animals, embryonated chicken eggs and cell culture methods have been used for testing antibiotic susceptibility. All of these methods suggest *C. burnetii* is more resistant to antibiotics like chloramphenicol, erythromycin and streptomycin than other rickettsiae. Egg survival and suppression of illness in animals are less useful than growth in tissue culture for gauging whether antibiotics are bactericidal rather than bacteriostatic. In eggs clindamycin, erythromycin, viomycin, cycloserine and cephalothin were ineffective while rifampicin, trimethoprim, doxycycline and oxytetracycline were bacteriostatic. Chlorotetracycline-resistant isolates of *C. burnetii* have been isolated by serial passage in eggs in the presence of low concentrations of antibiotic; one Cyprus isolate with enhanced natural resistance to tetracyclines was found. Since acute Q fever is often self-limiting, bacteriostatic antibiotics suffice to help the patient recover. Chronic Q fever can be managed with bacteriostatic antibiotics but the patient may not be cured unless a bactericidal regimen is employed. Although differential resistance of isolates from chronic disease patients has been noted, this may be due to changes in host cell (tetracyclines) or isolate-specific permeabilities (fluoroquinolones) (Yeaman and Baca 1991).

Suppression of primary shell vial growth in HEL cells of 13 *C. burnetii* isolates was used to evaluate bacteriostatic properties of antibiotics (Raoult 1993). Amikacin and amoxycillin were never effective. Cotrimoxazole, rifampicin, doxycycline, tetracycline, minocycline, sparfloxacin and quinolones PD127,391 and PD131,628 were always effective. Variable resistance was noted with ofloxacin, pefloxacin, chloramphenicol, ceftriaxone, fusidic acid and erythromycin. The fluoroquinolones ciprofloxacin, pefloxacin and fleroxacin were bacteriostatic in eggs and Vero cells (Keren et al. 1994). Assays employing persistently infected dividing L929 cells initially suggested that rifampicin and the quinolones pefloxacin, ofloxacin and ciprofloxacin were bactericidal but that doxycycline was not. However, this could not be confirmed for any of these antibiotics when cell growth was inhibited by cycloheximide. Using this assay or direct enumeration of viable *Coxiella* exposed to antibiotic for 24 h after infection in P388D1 macrophage cells, the lysosomotropic agents amantadine, chloroquine or ammonium chloride were used to alkalinize the pH 4.8 *C. burnetii*-containing phagolysosome to pH 5.3, 5.7 or 6.8 (Maurin et al. 1992). Pefloxacin and doxycycline were bactericidal at the more alkaline pH whereas rifampicin was not. Clarithromycin, a macrolide erythromycin derivative that can be tolerated during childhood and pregnancy, exhibited good bac-

teriostatic activity against 4 genomic types but it was not tested in the presence of lysosomotropic agents for bactericidal activity (Maurin and Raoult 1993).

13 PATHOGENICITY AND VIRULENCE FACTORS

A number of molecular factors have been associated with the virulence of rickettsiae, particularly for *R. prowazekii*, *R. rickettsii* and *O. tsutsugamushi*, but the continued lack of simple genetic systems for manipulating the genes encoding these factors or for selecting mutants has impeded their analysis. Rickettsiae are not believed to elaborate extracellular toxins causing disease and although typhus and SFG contain LPS with low endotoxin activities, LPS could not be detected in *O. tsutsugamushi*. Changes in host immune, inflammatory and coagulation mechanism responses also occur during rickettsial infection but there does not appear to be an important immunopathological component to these responses that causes disease (Walker 1989). Indeed, rickettsial direct damage to target endothelial cells and underlying vascular smooth muscle cells as a consequence of invasion and replication in the cells appears to be the primary mechanism of injury, although lysis of rickettsia-infected cells by interferon-γ and cytotoxic T cells may be a contributing factor. Endothelial cells are not even particularly efficiently infected by rickettsiae relative to the variety of cells that can be infected in cell culture; rather they are an accidental target cell exposed by the haematogenous route of arthropod dissemination of rickettsiae. However, infected endothelial cells exhibit increased platelet and neutrophil adhesion, release of von Willebrand factor multimers and increased secretion of plasminogen activator inhibitor and tissue factor expression that may participate in focal thrombotic events responsible for some of the pathological changes occurring in fulminant fatal disease (Sporn et al. 1994). Thromboxane mediated platelet activation, in vivo thrombin generation and increased plasma endothelin-1 (indicating endothelial dysfunction) occur in Mediterranean spotted fever (Davi et al. 1995). An essential protective role for macrophages in rickettsial clearance has also been demonstrated, most elegantly with the attenuated live vaccine strain E of *R. prowazekii* which does not replicate in macrophages (Winkler and Turco 1993). Two changes in the crystalline surface layer protein antigens have been correlated with alterations in rickettsial virulence: hypomethylation of the protein in the attenuated Madrid E strain of *R. prowazekii* and deficient carboxy-protein processing in the avirulent Iowa vaccine strain of *R. rickettsii* (Hackstadt et al. 1992, Turco and Winkler 1994). Mice, depleted of either interferon-γ and tumour necrosis factor α or both cytokines, experienced increased rickettsial growth after challenge and fatal disseminated rickettsial disease (Feng, Popov and Walker 1994). *R. prowazekii* and scrub typhus rickettsiae resistant to interferon or unable to induce interferon production have been described (Hanson 1991, Turco and Winkler 1994).

The adhesins involved in rickettsial attachment to host cells are uncharacterized except that antibody neutralization of plaque formation and invasion of host cells by *O. tsutsugamushi* depend on the protease sensitive VOMP. Specific antibody does not inhibit attachment and invasion of non-professional phagocytic cells by the typhus and spotted fever rickettsiae, indicating different adhesion mechanisms are employed. The host cell ligand recognized by spotted fever rickettsia is probably a protein (Li and Walker 1992) although cholesterol binding is important in adhesion of *R. prowazekii* to erythrocytes. Host cell uptake occurs by induced phagocytosis of metabolically active rickettsiae and can be blocked by cytochalasins B and D. Phospholipase A2 activity, likely of rickettsial origin, and lysophospholipase and phospholipase C activity occur during rickettsial escape from the phagosome and growth in infected cells that probably facilitates rickettsial exit (Winkler, Day and Daugherty 1994, Ojcius et al. 1995). Trypsin-like proteases have also been implicated in host cell damage. After invasion, *R. rickettsii* induce increased levels of intracellular peroxide, superoxide dismutase and reduced intracellular glutathione levels in endothelial cells. The rickettsiae probably cause these changes by reducing the activity of catalase, glucose-6-phosphate dehydrogenase (G-6-PD) and glutathione peroxidase, key enzymes involved in protection against oxidative cell damage (Devamanoharan et al. 1994). G-6-PD deficiency has been implicated as a human risk factor for severe rickettsial disease.

Antibody has been found to neutralize the infectivity of *E. risticii* for mice and P388D1 cells and to mediate antibody-dependent cellular toxicity of infected cells (Messick and Rikihisa 1992, Rikihisa et al. 1993). Intact antibody does not block adhesion or internalization but inhibits ehrlichial growth, possibly by inhibiting ehrlichial metabolism (Messick and Rikihisa 1994). *E. risticii* adhesins and receptors appear to be proteins. Interferon-γ but not tumour necrosis factor inhibited infection of treated macrophages with *E. risticii* and induced the ability to eradicate erhlichiae from infected cells, possibly by nitric oxide mediated killing. *E. risticii* does not stimulate a respiratory burst after infection of resident macrophages but activated or immune macrophages destroy the ehrlichiae (Williams and Timoney 1993, Williams, Cross and Timoney 1994). The inflammatory mediators IL-1α but not TNF-α or PGE₂ may be primary factors in the pathogenesis of disease caused by *E. risticii* (van Heeckeren et al. 1993). Strains of mice with defects in macrophage function were highly susceptible to illness due to infection with *E. risticii* whereas other strains were quite resistant (Williams and Timoney 1994). *E. chaffeensis* infection in human monocytes is also inhibited by interferon-γ but killing is mediated by limitation of cytoplasmic iron rather than due to reactive oxygen intermediates or nitric oxide (Barnewell and Rikihisa 1994). *E. chaffeensis* causes distinctive cytopathic effects in Vero, HEL, L929 and mouse embryo cells, possible systems for investigating the pathogenic mechanism of cell injury (Chen et al. 1995).

Cowdria isolates differ substantially in mouse virulence, cross-protection tests in goats, and IFA cross-reactivity with immune sera, but no specific molecular markers correlating with these differences have been described. Similarly, cell culture passaged *Cowdria* became attenuated for virulence in goats (Jongejan 1991) but the generality of this procedure for other isolates and its molecular basis is unknown. A specific role for antibody in protection appears unlikely as it does not block infectivity of *Cowdria* for bovine endothelial cells (Martinez et al. 1994). Immune CD8+ but not CD4+ T cells conferred resistance to *Cowdria* challenge on recipient mice. Interferon-α and particularly interferon-γ reduce the growth of *Cowdria* in endothelial cells, suggesting they may be important mediators of immunity in heartwater (Totte et al. 1994).

A. marginale has been shown to vary greatly in blood titres in persistently infected cattle (Kieser, Eriks and Palmer 1990). Isolates are known to vary in MSP2 protein reactivity with monoclonal antibodies and individual cells of a single isolate expressed different or coexpressed several MSP2 gene products (Palmer et al. 1994a). Consequently, emergent antigenic variation has been suggested as a mechanism of rickettsial persistence. Pathological cytokine responses have been proposed to account for anaemia in vaccinated animals otherwise protected from *Anaplasma* challenge (Palmer et al. 1994b). Antibodies to MSP1a, MSP1b, MSP2 and 61 kDa antigen, but not MSP4 or a neutralization-sensitive epitope in MSP1a, were able to block haemagglutination of bovine erythrocytes by *A. marginale* initial bodies. This suggested that the former proteins act as erythrocyte adhesins and are essential for *Anaplasma* infection (McGarey and Allred 1994). Antibody to MSP1 has been correlated with protection; it neutralizes *A. marginale* infectivity for splenectomized cattle and it opsonizes *Anaplasma* for phagocytosis by bovine macrophages (Cantor, Pontzer and Palmer 1993).

C. burnetii parasitizes the acidified phagolysosomal compartment of its host cells (Baca, Li and Kumar 1994). Both catabolic and anabolic activity, including the synthesis of DNA and protein, can be measured in defined medium at acidic pH (Thompson 1991, Redd and Thompson 1995). Following acid activation 34, 24 and 12 kDa proteins are exported by *Coxiella* but their function is unknown. The *Coxiella* 24 kDa Mip protein possesses peptidyl-prolyl-*cis-trans*-isomerase activity and is an exported protein, suggesting it has a role in protein folding and trafficking (Mo, Cianciotto and Mallavia 1995). Whether Mip is one of the exported acid activation proteins is unknown. In *Legionella* and *Chlamydia* Mip proteins have been found to have roles in establishing infection of host cells. Phase II cells more readily attach to L cells than phase I organisms and while purified phase I LPS did not inhibit attachment of *Coxiella* to host cells, protease treatment of host cells abolished attachment (Baca, Klassen and Aragon 1993). Heat- or formaldehyde-inactivated *Coxiella* could attach and enter cells whereas inhibitors of host cell phagocytosis (such as NaF and cytochalasins B and D) abolished rickettsial uptake. This suggests *Coxiella* is passively phagocytosed. *C. burnetii* also binds C-reactive protein, complement components and normal immunoglobulin which may facilitate cell infection in vivo (Williams et al. 1989). *Coxiella* adhesins or proteins essential for survival in the phagolysosome have not been identified conclusively although roles for superoxide dismutase, catalase and acid phosphatase have been suggested (Baca, Li and Kumar 1994). The acid phosphatase activity blocks superoxide anion production by stimulated human neutrophils. In *Salmonella*, acid phosphatase encoding genes are regulated by *phoQ* and *phoP* genes which enhance survival in macrophages. A similar sensor-like protein has been described in *Coxiella* (Mo and Mallavia 1994). Phase II cells are sensitive to complement mediated killing while phase I cells are not, suggesting that phase I LPS mediates resistance. Phase I LPS may mask underlying antigens from exposure to the immune system since ^{125}I-labelled antiphase II antibodies bound 10- and 44-fold more to trichloroacetic acid-extracted phase I cells and to phase II cells, respectively, than to native phase I cells (Hackstadt 1988), thus explaining, in part, the slow phase I serological response in *Coxiella* infection. LPS is an important virulence factor since intrastrain LPS phase I, intermediate and phase II variants differ significantly in virulence in guinea pig and mouse models (Kazar et al. 1993).

ACKNOWLEDGEMENTS

This investigation was supported by the Naval Medical Research and Development Command, Research Task 61102A.001.01.BJX.1293. The opinions and statements contained herein are the private ones of the authors and are not to be construed as official or reflecting the views of the Navy Department or the Naval Service at large.

We are indebted to Yuan Hsu Kang of the Naval Medical Research Institute who prepared the figures in this chapter.

REFERENCES

Ackland JR, Worswick DA, Marmion BP, 1994, Vaccine prophylaxis of Q fever. A follow-up of the efficacy of Q-Vax (CSL) 1985–1990, *Med J Aust*, **160:** 704–8.

Afseth G, Mo YY, Mallavia LP, 1995, Characterization of the 23S and 5S rRNA genes of *Coxiella burnetii* and identification of an intervening sequence within the 23S RNA gene, *J Bacteriol*, **177:** 2946–9.

Alleman AR, Barbet AF, 1996, Evalution of *Anaplasma marginale* major surface protein 3 (MSP3) as a diagnostic test antigen, *J Clin Microbiol*, **34:** 270–6.

Alleman AR, Kamper SM et al., 1993, Analysis of the *Anaplasma marginale* genome by pulsed-field electrophoresis, *J Gen Microbiol*, **139:** 2439–44.

Amano KI, Suzuki N et al., 1993, Serological reactivity of sera from scrub typhus patients against Weil–Felix test antigens, *Microbiol Immunol*, **37:** 927–33.

Anderson BE, McDonald GA et al., 1990, A protective protein antigen of *Rickettsia rickettsii* has tandemly repeated, near-identical sequences, *Infect Immun*, **58:** 2760–9.

Andersson SGE, Zomorodipour A et al., 1995, Unusual organization of the rRNA genes in *Rickettsia prowazekii*, *J Bacteriol*, **177:** 4171–5.

Austin FE, Winkler HH, 1988, *Biology of Rickettsial Diseases*, vol. 2, 1st edn, CRC Press, Boca Raton, FL, 29–50.

Baca OG, Klassen DA, Aragon AS, 1993, Entry of *Coxiella burnetii* into host cells, *Acta Virol*, **37:** 143–55.

Baca OG, Li YP, Kumar H, 1994, Survival of the Q fever agent *Coxiella burnetii* in the phagolysosome, *Trends Microbiol*, **2:** 476–80.

Balayeva NM, Eremeeva ME et al., 1995, Genotypic characterizatiion of the bacterium expressing the male-killing trait in the ladybird beetle *Adalia bipunctata* with specific rickettsial tools, *Appl Environ Microbiol*, **61:** 1431–7.

Barbet AF, 1995, Recent developments in the molecular biology of anaplasmosis, *Vet Parasitol*, **57:** 43–9.

Barlough JE, Madigan JE et al., 1995, Protection against *Ehrlichia equi* is conferred by prior infection with the human granulocytotropic ehrlichia (HGE agent), *J Clin Microbiol*, **33:** 3333–4.

Barnewall RE, Rikihisa Y, 1994, Abrogation of gamma interferon-induced inhibition of *Ehrlichia risticii* infection in human monocytes with iron transferrin, *Infect Immun*, **61:** 4804–10.

Bensaadi-Merchermek N, Salvado JC et al., 1995, Characterization of the unlinked 16S rDNA and 23S-5S rRNA operon of *Wolbachia pipientis*, a prokaryotic parasite of insect gonads, *Gene*, **165:** 81–6.

Birtles RJ, Harrison TC et al., 1995, Proposal to unify the genera *Grahamella* and *Bartonella* with descriptions of *Bartonella grahami*, sp. nov., *Bartonella taylorii*, sp. nov., and *Bartonella doshiae*, sp nov., *Int J Syst Bacteriol*, **45:** 1–8.

Brenner DJ, O'Connor SP et al., 1993, Proposal to unify the genera *Bartonella* and *Rochalimaea*, with description of *Bartonella quintana*, comb. nov., *Bartonella vinsonii*, comb. nov., *Bartonella henselae*, comb. nov., and *Bartonella elizabethae*, comb. nov., and to remove the family Bartonellaceae from the order Rickettsiales, *Int J Syst Bacteriol*, **43:** 777–86.

Brouqui P, Raoult D, 1992, In vitro antibiotic susceptibility of the newly recognized agent of ehrlichiosis in humans, *Ehrlichia chaffeensis*, *Antimicrob Agents Chemother*, **36:** 2799–803.

Carl M, Dasch GA, 1989, The importance of the crystalline surface layer protein antigens of rickettsiae in T-cell immunity, *J Autoimmun*, **2, Suppl.:** 81–91.

Cantor GH, Pontzer CH, Palmer GH, 1993, Opsonization of *Anaplasma marginale* mediated by bovine antibody against surface protein MSP-1, *Vet Immunol Immunopathol*, **37:** 343–50.

Chaichanasiriwithaya W, Rikihisa Y et al., 1994, Antigenic, morphologic, and molecular characterization of new *Ehrlichia risticii* isolates, *J Clin Microbiol*, **38:** 3026–33.

Chen SM, Dumler JS et al., 1994a, Identification of a granulocytic *Ehrlichia* species as the etiologic agent of human disease, *J Clin Microbiol*, **32:** 589–95.

Chen SM, Dumler JS et al., 1994b, Identification of the antigenic constituents of *Ehrlichia chaffeensis*, *Am J Trop Med Hyg*, **50:** 52–8.

Chen SM, Popov VL et al., 1995, Cultivation of *Ehrlichia chaffeensis* in mouse embryo, Vero, BGM, and L929 cells and study of *Ehrlichia*-induced cytopathic effect and plaque formation, *Infect Immun*, **63:** 647–55.

Ching WM, Carl M, Dasch GA, 1992, Mapping of monoclonal antibody binding sites on CNBr fragments of the S-layer protein antigens of *Rickettsia typhi* and *Rickettsia prowazekii*, *Mol Immunol*, **29:** 95–105.

Ching WM, Dasch GA et al., 1990, Structural analyses of the 120-kDa serotype protein antigens of typhus group rickettsiae. Comparison with other S-layer proteins, *Ann N Y Acad Sci*, **590:** 334–41.

Crocquet-Valdes PA, Weiss K, Walker DH, 1994, Sequence analysis of the 190-kDa antigen-encoding gene of *Rickettsia conorii* (Malish 7 strain), *Gene*, **140**: 115–9.

Dalton MJ, Clarke MJ et al., 1995, National surveillance for Rocky Mountain spotted fever, 1981–1982: epidemiologic summary and evaluation of risk factors for fatal outcome, *Am J Trop Med Hyg*, **52**: 405–13.

Dasch GA, Weiss E, 1992, *The Prokaryotes. A Handbook on the Biology of Bacteria: Ecophysiology, Isolation, Identification, Applications*, 2nd edn, Springer Verlag, New York, 2407–70.

Dasch GA, Weiss E, Williams JC, 1990, Antigenic properties of the ehrlichiae and other Rickettsiaceae, *Curr Top Vet Med Anim Sci*, **54**: 32–58.

Dasch GA, Ching WM et al., 1990, A structural and immunological comparison of rickettsial HSP60 antigens with those of other species, *Ann N Y Acad Sci*, **590**: 352–69.

Davi G, Giammarresi C et al., 1995, Demonstration of *Rickettsia conorii*-induced coagulative and platelet activation in vivo in patients with Mediterranean spotted fever, *Thromb Haemost*, **74**: 631–4.

Demkin VV, Rydkina EB et al., 1994, Genotypic characterization of rickettsiae by DNA probes generated from *Rickettsia prowazekii* DNA, *Acta Virol*, **38**: 65–70.

Devamanoharan PS, Santucci LA et al., 1994, Infection of human endothelial cells by *Rickettsia rickettsii* causes a significant reduction in the levels of key enzymes involved in protection against oxidative injury, *Infect Immun*, **62**: 2619–21.

Dumler JS, Bakken JS, 1995, Ehrlichial diseases of humans: emerging tick-borne infections, *Clin Infect Dis*, **20**: 1102–10.

Dumler JS, Asanovich KM et al., 1995a, Serologic cross-reactions among *Ehrlichia equi*, *Ehrlichia phagocytophila*, and human granulocytic ehrlichia, *J Clin Microbiol*, **33**: 1098–103.

Dumler JS, Chen SM et al., 1995b, Isolation and characterization of a new strain of *Ehrlichia chaffeensis* from a patient with nearly fatal monocytic ehrlichiosis, *J Clin Microbiol*, **33**: 1704–11.

Dutta SK, Shankarappa B, Mattingly-Napier BL, 1991, Molecular cloning and analysis of recombinant major antigens of *Ehrlichia risticii*, *Infect Immun*, **59**: 1162–9.

Emelyanov VV, 1993, Molecular cloning and expression of *Rickettsia prowazekii* genes for three outer membrane proteins in *Escherichia coli*, *Microb Pathog*, **15**: 7–16.

Eremeeva ME, Balayeva NM, Raoult D, 1994, Serological response of patients suffering from primary and recrudescent typhus: comparison of complement fixation reaction, Weil-Felix test, microimmunofluorescence, and immunoblotting, *Clin Diagn Immunol*, **1**: 318–24.

Eremeeva ME, Roux V, Raoult D, 1993, Determination of genome size and restriction pattern polymorphism of *Rickettsia prowazekii* and *Rickettsia typhi* by pulsed field gel electrophoresis, *FEMS Microbiol Lett*, **112**: 105–12.

Eremeeva M, Yu Z, Raoult D, 1994, Differentiation among spotted fever group rickettsiae species by analysis of restriction fragment length polymorphism of PCR–amplified DNA, *J Clin Microbiol*, **32**: 803–10.

Eremeeva ME, Balayeva NM et al., 1993, Proteinic and genomic identification of spotted fever group rickettsiae isolated in the former USSR, *J Clin Microbiol*, **31**: 2625–33.

Eremeeva ME, Beati L et al., 1994, Astrakhan fever rickettsiae: antigenic and genotypic analysis of isolates obtained from humans and *Rhipicephalus pumilio* ticks, *Am J Trop Med Hyg*, **51**: 697–706.

Eremeeva M, Balayeva N et al., 1995a, Genomic study of *Rickettsia akari* by pulsed-field gel electrophoresis, *J Clin Microbiol*, **33**: 3022–4.

Eremeeva M, Balayeva N et al., 1995b, Genomic and proteinic characterization of strain S, a rickettsia isolated from *Rhipicephalus sanguineus* ticks in Armenia, *J Clin Microbiol*, **33**: 2738–44.

Eremeeva ME, Balayeva NM et al., 1995c, Serologic response to rickettsial antigens in patients with Astrakhan fever, *Eur J Epidemiol*, **11**: 383–7.

Eriks IS, Stiller D et al., 1994, Molecular and biological characterization of a newly isolated *Anaplasma marginale* strain, *J Vet Diagn Invest*, **6**: 435–41.

Feng HM, Popov VL, Walker DH, 1994, Depletion of gamma interferon and tumor necrosis factor alpha in mice with *Rickettsia conorii*-infected endothelium: impairment of rickettsicidal nitric oxide production resulting in fatal overwhelming rickettsial disease, *Infect Immun*, **62**: 1952–60.

Fries LF, Waag DM, Williams JC, 1993, Safety and immunogenicity in human volunteers of a chloroform-methanol residue vaccine for Q fever, *Infect Immun*, **61**: 1251–8.

Furuya Y, Yoshida Y et al., 1993, Serotype-specific amplification of *Rickettsia tsutsugamushi* DNA by nested polymerase chain reaction, *J Clin Microbiol*, **31**: 1637–40.

Gajdosova E, Kovacova E et al., 1994, Immunogenicity of *Coxiella burnetii* whole cells and their outer membrane components, *Acta Virol*, **38**: 339–44.

Gilmore Jr RD, Hackstadt T, 1991, DNA polymorphism in the conserved 190 kDa antigen gene repeat region among spotted fever group rickettsiae, *Biochim Biophys Acta*, **1097**: 77–80.

Goodman JL, Nelson C et al., 1996, Direct cultivation of the causative agent of human granulocytic ehrlichiosis, *N Engl J Med*, **334**: 209–15.

Hackstadt T, 1988, Steric hindrance of antibody binding to surface proteins of *Coxiella burnetii* by phase I polysaccharide, *Infect Immun*, **56**: 802–7.

Hackstadt T, Messer R et al., 1992, Evidence for proteolytic cleavage of the 120-kilodalton outer membrane protein of rickettsiae: identification of an avirulent mutant deficient in processing, *Infect Immun*, **60**: 159–65.

Hahn MJ, Kim KK et al., 1993, Cloning and sequence analysis of the gene encoding the crystalline surface layer protein of *Rickettsia typhi*, *Gene*, **133**: 129–33.

Hanson B, 1991, Comparative susceptibility to mouse interferons of *Rickettsia tsutsugamushi* strains with different virulence in mice and of *Rickettsia rickettsii*, *Infect Immun*, **59**: 4134–41.

Harden VA, 1990, *Rocky Mountain Spotted Fever: History of a Twentieth-Century Disease*, 1st edn, Johns Hopkins University Press, Baltimore, 1–375.

Hechemy KE, McKee M et al., 1993, Three-dimensional reconstruction of *Coxiella burnetii*-infected L929 cells by high-voltage electron microscopy, *Infect Immun*, **61**: 4485–8.

van Heeckeren AM, Rikihisa Y et al., 1993, Tumor necrosis factor alpha, interleukin-1 α, interleukin-6, and prostaglandin E2 production in murine peritoneal macrophages infected with *Ehrlichia risticii*, *Infect Immun*, **61**: 4333–7.

Heinzen RA, Hayes SF et al., 1993, Directional actin polymerization associated with spotted fever group rickettsia infection of Vero cells, *Infect Immun*, **61**: 1926–35.

Heinzen RA, Mo YY et al., 1995, Characterization of the succinate dehydrogenase-encoding gene cluster (*sdh*) from the rickettsia *Coxiella burnetii*, *Gene*, **155**: 27–34.

Hendrix LR, Mallavia LP, Samuel JE, 1993, Cloning and sequencing of *Coxiella burnetii* outer membrane gene *com1*, *Infect Immun*, **61**: 470–7.

Hendrix LR, Samuel JE, Mallavia LP, 1991, Differentiation of *Coxiella burnetii* isolates by analysis of restriction-endonuclease-digested DNA separated by SDS-PAGE, *J Gen Microbiol*, **137**: 269–76.

Hickman CJ, Stover CK et al., 1991, Molecular cloning and sequence analysis of a *Rickettsia tsutsugamushi* 22 kDa antigen containing B- and T-cell epitopes, *Microb Pathog*, **11**: 19–31.

Higgins JA, Azad AF, 1995, Use of polymerase chain reaction to detect bacteria in arthropods: a review, *J Med Entomol*, **32**: 213–22.

Holden PR, Jones P, Brookfield JF, 1993, Evidence for a *Wolbachia* symbiont in *Drosophila melanogaster*, *Genet Res*, **62**: 23–9.

Hoover TA, Vodkin MH, Williams JC, 1992, A *Coxiella burnetii* repeated DNA element resembling a bacterial insertion sequence, *J Bacteriol*, **174**: 5540–8.

Iqbal Z, Rikihisa Y, 1994, Reisolation of *Ehrlichia canis* from blood and tissues of dogs after doxycycline treatment, *J Clin Microbiol*, **32:** 1644–9.

Jones D, Anderson B et al., 1993, Enzyme-linked immunosorbent assay for detection of human immunoglobulin G to lipopolysaccharide of spotted fever group rickettsiae, *J Clin Microbiol*, **31:** 138–41.

Jongejan F, 1991, Protective immunity to heartwater (*Cowdria ruminantium* infection) is acquired after vaccination with in vitro-attenuated rickettsiae, *Infect Immun*, **59:** 729–31.

Kass EM, Szaniawski WK et al., 1994, Rickettsialpox in a New York city hospital, 1980–1989, *N Engl J Med*, **331:** 1612–17.

Kawamori F, Akiyama M et al., 1993, Two-step polymerase chain reaction for diagnosis of scrub typhus and identification of antigenic variants of *Rickettsia tsutsugamushi*, *J Vet Med Sci*, **55:** 749–55.

Kazar J, Lesny M et al., 1993, Comparison of virulence for guinea pigs and mice of different *Coxiella burnetii* phase I strains, *Acta Virol*, **37:** 437–48.

Kelly DJ, Dasch GA et al., 1994, Detection and characterization of *Rickettsia tsutsugamushi* (Rickettsiales: Rickettsiaceae) in infected *Leptotrombidium* (*Leptotrombidium*) *fletcheri* chiggers (Acari: Trombiculidae) with the polymerase chain reaction, *J Med Entomol*, **31:** 691–9.

Kelly PJ, Beati L et al., 1994, A new pathogenic spotted fever group rickettsia from Africa, *J Trop Med Hyg*, **97:** 129–37.

Keren G, Keysary A et al., 1994, The inhibitory effect of fluoroquinolones on *Coxiella burnetii* growth in in-vitro systems, *J Antimicrob Chemother*, **33:** 1253–5.

Kieser ST, Eriks IS, Palmer GH, 1990, Cyclic rickettsemia during persistent *Anaplasma marginale* infection of cattle, *Infect Immun*, **58:** 1117–9.

Kim IS, Seong SY et al., 1993a, High-level expression of a 56-kilodalton protein gene (*bor56*) of *Rickettsia tsutsugamushi* Boryong and its application to enzyme-linked immunosorbent assays, *J Clin Microbiol*, **31:** 598–605.

Kim IS, Seong SY et al., 1993b, Rapid diagnosis of scrub typhus by a passive hemagglutination assay using recombinant 56-kilodalton polypeptides, *J Clin Microbiol*, **31:** 2057–60.

Kock ND, Van Vliet AHM et al., 1995, Detection of *Cowdria ruminantium* in blood and bone marrow samples from clinically normal, free-ranging Zimbabwean wild ungulates, *J Clin Microbiol*, **33:** 2501–4.

Kovacova E, Vavrekova J et al., 1994, Immunochemical and antigenic characterization of *Coxiella burnetii* strains isolated in Europe and Mongolia, *Eur J Epidemiol*, **10:** 9–16.

Krieg NR, Holt JB, 1984, *Bergey's Manual of Systematic Bacteriology*, 1st edn, Williams & Wilkins, Baltimore and London, 687–729.

Kumura K, Minamishima Y et al., 1991, DNA base composition of *Rickettsia tsutsugamushi* determined by reversed-phase high-performance liquid chromatography, *Int J Syst Bacteriol*, **41:** 247–8.

Lally NC, Nicoll S et al., 1995, The *Cowdria ruminantium groE* operon, *Microbiology*, **141:** 2091–100.

Li H, Walker DH, 1992, Characterization of rickettsial attachment to host cells by flow cytometry, *Infect Immun*, **60:** 2030–5.

Lin Z, Mallavia LP, 1995, The partition region of plasmid QpH1 is a member of a family of two transacting factors as implied by sequence analysis, *Gene*, **160:** 69–74.

Lockhart JM, Davidson WR et al., 1996, Site-specific geographic association between *Amblyomma americanum* (Acari: Ixodidae) infestations and *Ehrlichia chaffeensis*-reactive (Rickettsiales: Ehrlichieae) antibodies in white-tailed deer, *J Med Entomol*, **33:** 153–8.

Lukacova M, Gajdosova E et al., 1994, Characterization and protective effect of a 29 kDa protein isolated from *Coxiella burnetii* by detergent Empigen BB, *Eur J Epidemiol*, **10:** 227–30.

McCaul TF, Banerjee-Bhatnagar N, Williams JC, 1991, Antigenic differences between *Coxiella burnetii* cells revealed by postembedding immunoelectron microscopy and immunoblotting, *Infect Immun*, **59:** 3243–53.

McCaul TF, Williams JC, 1981, Developmental cycle of *Coxiella burnetii*: structure and morphogenesis of vegetative and sporogenic differentiations, *J Bacteriol*, **147:** 1063–76.

McGarey DJ, Allred DR, 1994, Characterization of hemagglutinating components on the *Anaplasma marginale* initial body surface and identification of possible adhesins, *Infect Immun*, **62:** 4587–93.

McGarey DJ, Barbet AF et al., 1994, Putative adhesins of *Anaplasma marginale*: major surface polypeptides 1a and 1b, *Infect Immun*, **62:** 4594–601.

Magnarelli LA, Stafford III KC et al., 1995, Hemocytic rickettsia-like organisms in ticks: serologic reactivity with antisera to ehrlichiae and detection of DNA of agent of human granulocytic ehrlichiosis by PCR, *J Clin Microbiol*, **33:** 2710–4.

Mahan SM, 1995, Review of the molecular biology of *Cowdria ruminantium*, *Vet Parasitol*, **57:** 51–6.

Mahan SM, Andrew HR et al., 1995, Immunisation of sheep against heartwater with inactivated *Cowdria ruminantium*, *Res Vet Sci*, **58:** 46–9.

Martinez D, Maillard JC et al., 1994, Protection of goats against heartwater acquired by immunisation with inactivated elementary bodies of *Cowdria ruminantium*, *Vet Immunol Immunopathol*, **41:** 153–63.

Maurin M, Raoult D, 1993, In vitro susceptibilities of spotted fever group rickettsiae and *Coxiella burnetii* to clarithromycin, *Antimicrob Agents Chemother*, **37:** 2633–7.

Maurin M, Benoliel AM et al., 1992, Phagolysosomal alkalinization and the bactericidal effect of antibiotics: the *Coxiella burnetii* paradigm, *J Infect Dis*, **166:** 1092–102.

Messick JB, Rikihisa Y, 1992, Presence of parasite antigen on the surface of P388D$_1$ cells infected with *Ehrlichia risticii*, *Infect Immun*, **60:** 3079–86.

Messick JB, Rikihisa Y, 1994, Inhibition of binding, entry, or intracellular proliferation of *Ehrlichia risticii* in P388D$_1$ cells by anti-*E. risticii* serum, immunoglobulin G, or Fab fragment, *Infect Immun*, **62:** 3156–61.

Mo YY, Cianciotto NP, Mallavia LP, 1995, Molecular cloning of a *Coxiella burnetii* gene encoding a macrophage infectivity potentiator (Mip) analogue, *Microbiology*, **141:** 2861–71.

Mo YY, Mallavia LP, 1994, A *Coxiella burnetii* gene encodes a sensor-like protein, *Gene*, **151:** 185–90.

Moree MF, Hanson B, 1992, Growth characteristics and proteins of plaque-purified strains of *Rickettsia tsutsugamushi*, *Infect Immun*, **60:** 3405–15.

Musso D, Raoult D, 1995, *Coxiella burnetii* blood cultures from acute and chronic Q-fever patients, *J Clin Microbiol*, **33:** 3129–32.

Nakamura Y, Kawazu SI, Minami T, 1993, Antigen profiles of *Anaplasma ovis* and *A. mesaeterum* and cross-infection trials with them and *A. marginale*, *Vet Microbiol*, **37:** 19–30.

Ndung'u LW, Aguirre C et al., 1995, Detection of *Anaplasma ovis* infection in goats by major surface protein 5 competitive inhibition enzyme-linked immunosorbent assay, *J Clin Microbiol*, **33:** 675–9.

Oaks EV, Rice RM et al., 1989, Antigenic and genetic relatedness of eight *Rickettsia tsutsugamushi* antigens, *Infect Immun*, **57:** 3116–22.

Ohashi N, Tamura A et al., 1990, Characterization of a new antigenic type, Kuroki, of *Rickettsia tsutsugamushi* isolated from a patient in Japan, *J Clin Microbiol*, **28:** 2111–13.

Ohashi N, Nashimoto H et al., 1992, Diversity of immunodominant 56-kDa type-specific antigen (TSA) of *Rickettsia tsutsugamushi*. Sequence and comparative analyses of the genes encoding TSA homologues from four antigenic variants, *J Biol Chem*, **267:** 12728–35.

Ohashi N, Fukuhara M et al., 1995, Phylogenetic position of *Rickettsia tsutsugamushi* and the relationship among its antigenic variants by analyses of 16S rRNA gene sequences, *FEMS Microbiol Lett*, **125:** 299–304.

Ojcius DM, Thibon N et al., 1995, pH and calcium dependence of hemolysis due to *Rickettsia prowazekii*: comparison with phospholipase activity, *Infect Immun*, **63:** 3069–73.

Palmer GH, Eid G et al., 1994a, The immunoprotective *Anaplasma marginale* major surface protein 2 is encoded by a polymorphic multigene family, *Infect Immun*, **62**: 3808–16.

Palmer GH, Munodzana D et al., 1994b, Heterologous strain challenge of cattle immunized with *Anaplasma marginale* outer membranes, *Vet Immunol Immunopathol*, **42**: 265–73.

Pancholi P, Kolbert CP et al., 1995, *Ixodes dammini* as a potential vector of human granulocytic ehrlichiosis, *J Infect Dis*, **172**: 1007–12.

Pang H, Winkler HH, 1994, Analysis of the peptidoglycan of *Rickettsia prowazekii*, *J Bacteriol*, **176**: 923–6.

Park CS, Kim IC et al., 1993, Analysis of antigenic characteristics of *Rickettsia tsutsugamushi* Boryong strain and antigenic heterogeneity of *Rickettsia tsutsugamushi* using monoclonal antibodies, *J Korean Med Sci*, **8**: 319–24.

Peter TF, Deem SL et al., 1995, Development and evaluation of PCR assay for detection of low levels of *Cowdria ruminantium* infection in *Amblyomma* ticks not detected by DNA probe, *J Clin Microbiol*, **33**: 166–72.

Popov VL, Chen SM et al., 1995, Ultrastructural variation of cultured *Ehrlichia chaffeensis*, *J Med Microbiol*, **43**: 411–21.

Pretzman C, Ralph D et al., 1995, 16S rRNA gene sequence of *Neorickettsia helminthoeca* and its phylogenetic alignment with members of the genus *Ehrlichia*, *Int J Syst Bacteriol*, **45**: 207–11.

Radulovic S, Speed R et al., 1993, EIA with species-specific monoclonal antibodies: a novel seroepidemiologic tool for determination of the etiologic agent of spotted fever rickettsiosis, *J Infect Dis*, **168**: 1292–5.

Radulovic S, Feng HM et al., 1994, Antigen-capture enzyme immunoassay: a comparison with other methods for the detection of spotted fever group rickettsiae in ticks, *Am J Trop Med Hyg*, **50**: 359–64.

Radulovic S, Higgins JA et al., 1995, Isolation, cultivation, and partial characterization of the ELB agent associated with cat fleas, *Infect Immun*, **63**: 4826–9.

Ralph D, Pretzman C et al., 1990, Genetic relationships among the members of the family Rickettsiaceae as shown by DNA restriction fragment polymorphism analysis, *Ann N Y Acad Sci*, **590**: 541–52.

Raoult D, 1993, Treatment of Q fever, *Antimicrob Agents Chemother*, **37**: 1733–6.

Raoult D, Dasch GA, 1989, The line blot: an immunoassay for monoclonal and other antibodies; its application to the serotyping of gram-negative bacteria, *J Immunol Methods*, **125**: 57–65.

Raoult D, Dasch GA, 1995, Immunoblot cross-reactions among *Rickettsia*, *Proteus* spp. and *Legionella* spp. in patients with Mediterranean spotted fever, *FEMS Immunol Med Microbiol*, **11**: 13–18.

Raoult D, Drancourt M, 1991, Antimicrobial therapy of rickettsial diseases, *Antimicrob Agents Chemother*, **35**: 2457–62.

Raoult D, Marrie T, 1995, Q fever, *Clin Infect Dis*, **20**: 489–96.

Redd T, Thompson HA, 1995, Secretion of proteins by *Coxiella burnetii*, *Microbiology*, **141**: 363–9.

Regnery RL, Spruill CL, Plikaytis BD, 1991, Genotypic identification of rickettsiae and estimation of intraspecies sequence divergence for portions of two rickettsial genes, *J Bacteriol*, **173**: 1576–89.

Richter Jr PJ, Kimsey RB et al., 1996, *Ixodes pacificus* (Acari: Ixodidae) as a vector of *Ehrlichia equi* (Rickettsiales: Ehrlichieae), *J Med Entomol*, **33**: 1–5.

Rikihisa Y, 1991a, The tribe Ehrlichieae and ehrlichial diseases, *Clin Microbiol Rev*, **4**: 286–308.

Rikihisa Y, 1991b, Cross-reacting antigens between *Neorickettsia helminthoeca* and *Ehrlichia* species, shown by immunofluorescence and Western immunoblotting, *J Clin Microbiol*, **29**: 2024–9.

Rikihisa Y, 1991c, Protection against murine Potomac horse fever by an inactivated *Ehrlichia risticii* vaccine, *Vet Microbiol*, **27**: 339–50.

Rikihisa Y, Ewing SA, Fox JC, 1994, Western immunoblot analysis of *Ehlichia chaffeensis*, *E. canis*, or *E. ewingii* infections in dogs and humans, *J Clin Microbiol*, **32**: 2107–12.

Rikihisa Y, Wada R et al., 1993, Development of neutralizing antibody in horses infected with *Ehrlichia risticii*, *Vet Microbiol*, **36**: 139–47.

Roux V, Raoult D, 1993, Genotypic identification and phylogenetic analysis of the spotted fever group rickettsiae by pulsed-field gel electrophoresis, *J Bacteriol*, **175**: 4895–904.

Roux V, Raoult D, 1995, Phylogenetic analysis of the genus *Rickettsia* by 16S rDNA sequencing, *Res Microbiol*, **146**: 385–94.

Schriefer ME, Sacci Jr JB et al., 1994, Murine typhus: updated roles of multiple urban components and a second typhuslike rickettsia, *J Med Entomol*, **31**: 681–5.

Schuenke K, Walker DH, 1994, Cloning, sequencing, and expression of the gene coding for an antigenic 120-kilodalton protein of *Rickettsia conorii*, *Infect Immun*, **62**: 904–9.

Scott GH, Williams JC, 1990, Susceptibility of *Coxiella burnetii* to chemical disinfectants, *Ann NY Acad Sci*, **590**: 291–6.

Shankarappa B, Dutta SK, Mattingly-Napier BL, 1992a, Antigenic and genomic relatedness among *Ehrlichia risticii*, *Ehrlichia sennetsu*, and *Ehrlichia canis*, *Int J Syst Bacteriol*, **42**: 127–32.

Shankarappa B, Dutta SK, Mattingly-Napier BL, 1992b, Identification of the protective 44-kilodalton recombinant antigen of *Ehrlichia risticii*, *Infect Immun*, **60**: 612–7.

Song JH, Lee C et al., 1995, Short-course doxycycline treatment versus conventional tetracycline therapy for scrub typhus: a multicenter randomized trial, *Clin Infect Dis*, **21**: 506–10.

Sporn LA, Haidaris PJ et al., 1994, *Rickettsia rickettsii* infection of cultured human endothelial cells induces tissue factor expression, *Blood*, **83**: 1527–34.

Stein A, Raoult D, 1993, Lack of phenotype specific gene in human *Coxiella burnetii* isolates, *Microb Pathog*, **15**: 177–85.

Stein A, Saunders NA et al., 1993, Phylogenetic homogeneity of *Coxiella burnetii* strains as determined by 16S ribosomal RNA sequencing, *FEMS Microbiol Lett*, **113**: 339–44.

Stich RW, Bantle JA et al., 1993, Detection of *Anaplasma marginale* (Rickettsiales: Anaplasmataceae) in hemolymph of *Dermacentor andersoni* (Acari: Ixodidae) with the polymerase chain reaction, *J Med Entomol*, **30**: 781–8.

Stothard DR, Clark JB, Fuerst PA, 1994, Ancestral divergence of *Rickettsia bellii* from the spotted fever and typhus groups of *Rickettsia* and antiquity of the genus *Rickettsia*, *Int J Syst Bacteriol*, **44**: 798–804.

Stothard DR, Fuerst PA, 1995, Evolutionary analysis of spotted fever and typhus groups of *Rickettsia* using rRNA gene sequences, *Syst Appl Microbiol*, **18**: 52–61.

Stover CK, Marana DP et al., 1990a, The 56-kilodalton major protein antigen of *Rickettsia tsutsugamushi*: molecular cloning and sequence analysis of the *sta56* gene and precise identification of a strain-specific epitope, *Infect Immun*, **58**: 2076–84.

Stover CK, Marana DP et al., 1990b, Molecular cloning and sequence analysis of the Sta58 major antigen gene of *Rickettsia tsutsugamushi*: sequence homology and antigenic comparison to the 60-kilodalton family of stress proteins, *Infect Immun*, **58**: 1360–8.

Strickman D, Sheer T et al., 1995, In vitro effectiveness of azithromycin against doxycycline-resistant and -susceptible strains of *Rickettsia tsutsugamushi*, etiologic agent of scrub typhus, *Antimicrob Agents Chemother*, **39**: 2406–10.

Sumner JW, Sims KG et al., 1993, *Ehrlichia chaffeensis* expresses an immunoreactive protein homologous to the *Escherichia coli* GroEL protein, *Infect Immun*, **61**: 3536–9.

Sumner JW, Sims KG et al., 1995, Protection of guinea pigs from experimental Rocky Mountain spotted fever by immunization with baculovirus-expressed *Rickettsia rickettsii* rOmpA protein, *Vaccine*, **13**: 29–35.

Tamura A, Ohashi N et al., 1995, Classification of *Rickettsia tsutsugamushi* in a new genus, *Orientia* gen. nov. as *Orientia tsutsugamushi* comb. nov., *Int J Syst Bacteriol*, **45**: 589–91.

Tamura A, Urakami H, Ohashi N, 1991, A comparative view of

Rickettsia tsutsugamushi and the other groups of rickettsiae, *Eur J Epidemiol*, **7:** 259–69.

Tange Y, Kanemitsu N, Kobayashi Y, 1991, Analysis of immunological characteristics of newly isolated strains of *Rickettsia tsutsugamushi* using monoclonal antibodies, *Am J Trop Med Hyg*, **44:** 371–81.

Teysseire N, Chiche-Portiche C, Raoult D, 1992, Intracellular movements of *Rickettsia conorii* and *R. typhi* based on actin polymerization, *Res Microbiol*, **143:** 821–9.

Thaker SR, Dutta SR et al., 1990, Molecular cloning of *Ehrlichia risticii* and development of a gene probe for the diagnosis of Potomac horse fever, *J Clin Microbiol*, **28:** 1963–7.

Thiele D, Willems H, 1994, Is plasmid based differentiation of *Coxiella burnetii* in 'acute' and 'chronic' isolates still valid?, *Eur J Epidemiol*, **20:** 427–34.

Thiele D, Willems H et al., 1993, Polymorphism in DNA restriction patterns of *Coxiella burnetii* isolates investigated by pulsed field gel electrophoresis and image analysis, *Eur J Epidemiol*, **9:** 419–25.

Thiele D, Willems H et al., 1994, Analysis of the entire nucleotide sequence of the cryptic plasmid QpH1 from *Coxiella burnetii*, *Eur J Epidemiol*, **10:** 413–20.

Thompson HA, 1991, *Q fever: The Biology of* Coxiella burnetii, 1st edn, CRC Press, Boca Raton, FL, 131–56.

Tokarevich NK, Daiter AB et al., 1993, Biological properties of chloroform/methanol extracts of *Coxiella burnetii*, *Acta Virol*, **37:** 29–40.

Totte P, Jongejan F et al., 1994, Production of alpha interferon in *Cowdria ruminantium*-infected cattle and its effect on infected endothelial cell cultures, *Infect Immun*, **62:** 2600–4.

Turco J, Winkler HH, 1994, Cytokine sensitivity and methylation of lysine in *Rickettsia prowazekii* EVir and interferon-resistant *R. prowazekii* strains, *Infect Immun*, **62:** 3172–7.

Uchiyama T, Ichida T, Walker DH, 1990, Species-specific monoclonal antibodies to *Rickettsia japonica*, a newly identified spotted fever group rickettsia, *J Clin Microbiol*, **28:** 1177–80.

Uchiyama T, Uchida T et al., 1994, Demonstration of heat-labile and heat-stable epitopes of *Rickettsia japonica* on ultrathin sections, *Lab Invest*, **71:** 432–7.

Uhaa IJ, Fishbein DB et al., 1994, Evaluation of specificity of indirect enzyme-linked immunosorbent assay for diagnosis of human Q fever, *J Clin Microbiol*, **32:** 1560–5.

Valkova D, Kazar J, 1995, A new plasmid (QpDV) common to *Coxiella burnetii* isolates associated with acute and chronic Q fever, *FEMS Microbiol Lett*, **125:** 275–80.

Vemulapalli R, Biswas B, Dutta SK, 1995, Pathogenic, immunologic, and molecular differences between two *Ehrlichia risticii* strains, *J Clin Microbiol*, **33:** 2987–93.

Vidotto MC, McGuire TC et al., 1994, Intermolecular relationships of major surface proteins of *Anaplasma marginale*, *Infect Immun*, **62:** 2940–6.

van Vliet AHM, van der Zeijst BAM et al., 1995, Use of a specific immunogenic region on the *Cowdria ruminantium* MAP1 protein in a serological assay, *J Clin Microbiol*, **33:** 2405–10.

Waag D, Chulay J et al., 1995, Validation of an enzyme immunoassay for serodiagnosis of acute Q fever, *Eur J Clin Microbiol Infect Dis*, **14:** 421–7.

Walker DH, 1989, Rocky Mountain spotted fever: a disease in need of microbiological concern, *Clin Microbiol Rev*, **2:** 227–40.

Walker DH, 1995, Rocky Mountain spotted fever: a seasonal alert, *Clin Infect Dis*, **20:** 1111–7.

Walker DH, Dasch GA, 1995, *Manual of Clinical Microbiology*, 6th edn, American Society for Microbiology, Washington DC, 665–8.

Walker DH, Feng HM et al., 1995, Comparative antigenic analysis of spotted fever group rickettsiae from Israel and other closely related organisms, *Am J Trop Med Hyg*, **52:** 569–76.

Weisburg WG, Dobson ME et al., 1989, Phylogenetic diversity of the rickettsiae, *J Bacteriol*, **17:** 4202–6.

Weiss E, 1992, *Encyclopedia of Microbiology*, vol. 3, 1st edn, Academic Press, San Diego, CA, 585–610.

Weiss E, Williams JC et al., 1989, Energy metabolism of monocytic *Ehrlichia*, *Proc Natl Acad Sci USA*, **86:** 1674–8.

Wen B, Rikihisa Y et al., 1995a, *Ehrlichia muris* sp. nov., identified on the basis of 16S rRNA base sequences and serological, morphological, and biological characteristics, *Int J Syst Bacteriol*, **45:** 250–4.

Wen B, Rikihisa Y et al., 1995b, Diversity of 16S rRNA genes of new *Ehrlichia* strains isolated from horses with clinical signs of Potomac horse fever, *Int J Syst Bacteriol*, **45:** 315–8.

Wen B, Rikihisa Y et al., 1996, Characterization of the SF agent, an *Ehrlichia* sp. isolated from the fluke *Stellantchasmus falcatus*, by 16S rRNA base sequence, serological, and morphological analyses, *Int J Syst Bacteriol*, **46:** 149–54.

Werren JH, Zhang W, Guo LR, 1995, Evolution and phylogeny of *Wolbachia*: reproductive parasites of arthropods, *Proc R Soc Lond B*, **261:** 55–63.

Werren JH, Hurst GDD et al., 1994, Rickettsial relative associated with male killing in the ladybird beetle (*Adalia bipunctata*), *J Bacteriol*, **176:** 388–94.

Williams JC, Waag DM, 1991, *Q fever: The Biology of* Coxiella burnetii, 1st edn, CRC Press, Boca Raton, FL, 175–222.

Williams JC, Weiss E, Dasch GA, 1992, *The Prokaryotes. A Handbook on the Biology of Bacteria: Ecophysiology, Isolation, Identification, Applications*, 2nd edn, Springer-Verlag, NY, 2471–84.

Williams JC, McCaul TF et al., 1989, *Intracellular Parasitism*, CRC Press, Boca Raton, FL, 127–39.

Williams JC, Peacock MG et al., 1992, Vaccines against coxiellosis and Q fever. Development of a chloroform:methanol residue subunit of phase I *Coxiella burnetii* for the immunization of animals, *Ann NY Acad Sci*, **653:** 88–111.

Williams NM, Cross RJ, Timoney PJ, 1994, Respiratory burst activity associated with phagocytosis of *Ehrlichia risticii* by mouse peritoneal macrophages, *Res Vet Sci*, **57:** 194–9.

Williams NM, Timoney PJ, 1993, In vitro killing of *Ehrlichia risticii* by activated and immune mouse peritoneal macrophages, *Infect Immun*, **61:** 861–7.

Williams NM, Timoney PJ, 1994, Variation in susceptibility of ten mouse strains to infection with a strain of *Ehrlichia risticii*, *J Comp Pathol*, **110:** 137–43.

Winkler HH, 1990, *Rickettsia* species (as organisms), *Annu Rev Microbiol*, **44:** 131–53.

Winkler HH, Day L, Daugherty R, 1994, Analysis of hydrolytic products from choline-labeled host cell phospholipids during growth of *Rickettsia prowazekii*, *Infect Immun*, **62:** 1457–9.

Winkler HH, Turco J, 1993, *Macrophage–Pathogen Interactions*, 1st edn, Marcel Dekker, New York, 401–14.

Yeaman MR, Baca OG, 1991, Mechanism that may account for differential antibiotic susceptibilities among *Coxiella burnetii* isolates, *Antimicrob Agents Chemother*, **35:** 948–54.

Yu X, Raoult D, 1994, Serotyping *Coxiella burnetii* isolates from acute and chronic Q fever patients by using monoclonal antibodies, *FEMS Microbiol Lett*, **117:** 15–20.

Yu XJ, Walker DH, 1995, Molecular cloning and sequencing of a 120 kDa immunodominant protein gene of *Ehrlichia chaffeensis*, *Am J Trop Med Hyg*, **53, Suppl.:** 166–7.

Yu X, Brouqi P et al., 1993, Detection of *Ehrlichia chaffeensis* in human tissue by using a species-specific monoclonal antibody, *J Clin Microbiol*, **31:** 3284–8.

Zakimi S, Tsuji N, Fujisaki K, 1994, Protein analysis of *Anaplasma marginale* and *Anaplasma centrale* by two-dimensional polyacrylamide gel electrophoresis, *J Vet Med Sci*, **56:** 1025–7.

Zhang YX, Zhi N et al., 1994, Protective immunity induced by 67 K outer membrane protein of phase I *Coxiella burnetii* in mice and guinea pigs, *Acta Virol*, **38:** 327–32.

Zvilich M, Williams JC et al., 1995, Efficacy of *Coxiella burnetii* and its chloroform-methanol residue (CMR) fraction against Rift Valley fever infection in mice, *Antiviral Res*, **27:** 137–49.

Chapter 37

NEISSERIA

S A Morse and C A Genco

1 INTRODUCTION

Members of the genus *Neisseria* are gram-negative diplococci that inhabit the human body. Two members of this genus are important human pathogens: *Neisseria gonorrhoeae* and *Neisseria meningitidis*. Owing to their serious disease-causing capabilities, the pathogenic properties of both organisms have been extensively studied.

2 GENERAL FEATURES

2.1 Definition

Neisseria are cocci 0.6–1.0 μm in diameter, occurring singly but more often in pairs with adjacent sides flattened; one species (*Neisseria oblongata*) is an exception and consists of short rods 0.5 μm wide, often arranged as diplobacilli or in short chains. Division of the coccal species is in 2 planes at right angles to each other, sometimes resulting in tetrads. Capsules and fimbriae (pili) may be present; endospores are not present. The cocci are gram-negative aerobes but there is a tendency to resist gram decolorization. Swimming motility does not occur and flagella are absent. Some species produce a greenish yellow carotenoid pigment and some are nutritionally fastidious and haemolytic. The optimum growth temperature is 35–37°C. Cultures are oxidase-positive and catalase-positive except *N. oblongata*. Carbonic anhydrase is produced by all species except the 'false neisseriae' *Neisseria caviae*, *Neisseria ovis* and *Neisseria cuniculi*. All species reduce nitrite except *N. gonorrhoeae*, *N. canis* and the 'false neisseriae' *N. cuniculi* and *N. ovis*. Neisseriae are chemo-organotrophic and some species are saccharolytic. The neisseriae are normal inhabitants of the mucous membranes of mammals and reptiles and some species are primary pathogens of man. The mol% G + C of the DNA is 46.5–53.5% (Vedros 1984).

The type species is *Neisseria gonorrhoeae*.

2.2 Historical

The first species of *Neisseria* to be described was *N. gonorrhoeae* (the gonococcus), which was initially observed by Albert Neisser in 1879 within polymorphonuclear leucocytes (PMNs) in smears of pus from patients with gonorrhea (Fig. 37.1). The organism was successfully cultivated by Bumm (1885a, 1885b) and by Lestikow and Loeffler (Lestikow 1882) in 1882. The meningococcus (*N. meningitidis*) was first isolated by Weichselbaum in 1887 from the cerebrospinal fluid of patients with acute meningitis. In 1906, von Lingelsheim described a number of gram-negative cocci from the nasopharynx of both healthy and diseased persons; these included *Micrococcus pharyngis siccus* (*Neisseria sicca*), *Micrococcus cinereus* (*Neisseria cinerea*) and *Micrococcus pharyngis flavus* groups I, II and III (*Neisseria subflava* and its biovars). *Neisseria flavescens* was described in 1930 by Sarah Branham (1930) and *Neisseria lactamica* was described in 1969 by Hollis, Wiggins and Weaver. Both these species were originally isolated from cerebrospinal fluid and thought to be responsible for occasional cases of meningitis. *N. gonorrhoeae* subsp. *kochii* was isolated from conjunctival cultures from patients in rural Egypt and was first described in 1986 (Mazloum et al. 1986).

2.3 Classification

The genus *Neisseria* is the type genus of the family Neisseriaceae, which currently contains the genera *Actinetobacter*, *Kingella* and *Moraxella* (Bovre 1984). However, the results of studies comparing 16S rRNA sequences and DNA hybridizations (Dewhirst, Paster and Bright 1989, Rossau et al. 1989) have suggested that the genera *Eikenella*, *Simonsiella*, *Alysiella* and the CDC groups EF-4, M-5 and M-6 should also be included in this family. Strains belonging to CDC group M-5 have been classified as *Neisseria weaverii* sp.

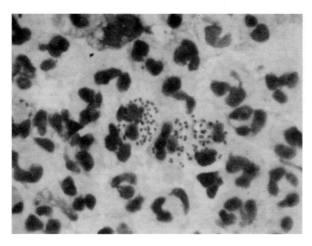

Fig. 37.1 Gram smear of pus sample obtained from a patient with gonorrhoea.

2.4 Habitat

Most human *Neisseria* spp. are non-pathogenic and are normal inhabitants only of the upper respiratory tract (oro- and nasopharyngeal mucous membranes) (Knapp and Hook 1988). Commensal species may infrequently be isolated from other mucosal sites. They have also been isolated from a variety of clinical specimens and have been associated with several infectious processes, including meningitis, osteomyelitis, endocarditis, cellulitis, arthritis and pneumonia (Herbert and Ruskin 1981, Doern et al. 1982, Davis et al. 1983, Johnson 1983, Boyce et al. 1985, Gilrane et al. 1985, Gini 1987, Wong and Janda 1992). Patients with various underlying diseases such as leukaemia and acquired immunodeficiency syndrome are at increased risk for serious infections with these organisms (Schifman and Ryan 1983, Boyce et al. 1985). *Neisseria* species that inhabit the upper respiratory tract of non-human hosts may occasionally infect humans through bites (Andersen et al. 1993). However, only *N. gonorrhoeae* and *N. meningitidis* are considered pathogens. Strains of *N. gonorrhoeae* are always considered pathogenic and infect mucosal surfaces lined with columnar epithelial cells (e.g. endocervix, urethra, rectum, oro- and nasopharynx, conjunctiva), causing symptomatic or asymptomatic infections. Strains of *N. meningitidis* may also be pathogenic; however, they frequently colonize the oro- or nasopharynx without causing disease (carrier state) as well as exposed anogenital mucosal membranes, particularly in homosexual men (Janda et al. 1983). Less frequently, *N. meningitidis* may be a cause of acute bacterial meningitis.

The normal patterns of oro- and nasopharyngeal colonization by *Neisseria* spp. were studied extensively in the early 1900s, but these data are unreliable owing to misidentification and the use of suboptimal media for isolation (Knapp 1988). More recent studies (Knapp and Hook 1988) have demonstrated that both children and adults may be colonized simultaneously by several *Neisseria* spp. or biovars. Colonization by non-pathogenic *Neisseria* species as well as by *N. meningitidis* may persist for several months (Knapp and Hook 1988). *N. lactamica* has been isolated more frequently from children than adults (Gold et al. 1978, Blakebrough et al. 1982) whereas colonization of the oropharynx by *N. polysaccharea* appears to occur infrequently and varies geographically (Riou, Guibourdenche and Popoff 1983, Boquete, Marcos and Saez-Nieto 1986). *N. mucosa*, a species commonly present in the nasopharynx of healthy adult humans (Berger 1971), has also been found to colonize mucosal surfaces of dolphins (*Lagenorhynchus obliguidens* and *Delphinus bairdi*) (Vedros, Johnson and Warren 1973).

The oropharynx of mammals is the primary habitat of non-human *Neisseria* spp. *Neisseria animalis* has been isolated from guinea pigs (Berger 1960). *N. canis* and *N. weaverii* have been isolated from the oropharynx of dogs (Berger 1962, Andersen et al. 1993) and *Neisseria macacae* from the oropharynx of rhesus monkeys

nov. (Holmes et al. 1993) whereas strains belonging to CDC group M-6 have been classified as *Neisseria elongata* subsp. *nitroreducens* (Grant et al. 1990). The results of 16S rRNA sequencing and DNA hybridization (Dewhirst, Paster and Bright 1989, Rossau et al. 1989) have also led to the recommendation that the genera *Actinetobacter*, *Moraxella* and *Branhamella*, as well as the 'false neisseriae' and *Kingella indologenes*, be removed from the family Neisseriaceae. Proposals have been made to assign *Branhamella catarrhalis* (formerly *Neisseria catarrhalis*) to the genus *Moraxella* (*Moraxella catarrhalis*) in the family Moraxellaceae or to its own genus, *Branhamella*, in the family Branhamaceae (Catlin 1991, Rossau et al. 1991).

The genus *Neisseria* is currently comprised of 15 species, subspecies and biovars that may be isolated from humans and 6 species that may be isolated from animals (Vedros 1984, Knapp 1988, Barrett et al. 1994, Holmes et al. 1993) (Table 37.1). The taxonomy of the species of human origin has undergone many changes; these and the names by which individual species have been known were summarized by Knapp (1988). Strains belonging to the genus *Neisseria* may be identified by phenotypic characteristics including pigment production, production of acid from various carbohydrates, production of polysaccharide from sucrose, and the reduction of nitrate and nitrite (Table 37.1).

Most human *Neisseria* spp. can be placed into one of 2 major groups. Strains belonging to the first group (*N. gonorrhoeae*, *N. meningitidis*, *N. lactamica*, *N. cinerea*, *N. polysaccharea*, *N. gonorrhoeae* subsp. *kochii*) grow as non-pigmented, translucent colonies on solid medium; strains belonging to the second group (*N. mucosa*, *N. sicca*, *N. subflava* [including the biovars *subflava*, *flava* and *perflava*]) are referred to as the saccharolytic species and usually grow as opaque, yellow-pigmented colonies on solid medium.

Table 37.1 Differential characteristics of *Neisseria* species of human and animal origin[a]

Species	Growth on:			Acid from:					Reduction of:		Polysaccharide from sucrose	Catalase	DnAase	Pigment
	MTM, ML and NYC media	chocolate or blood agar (22°C)	nutrient agar (35°C)	Glucose	Maltose	Lactose	Sucrose	Fructose	NO$_3^-$	NO$_2^-$				
Human species														
N. gonorrhoeae	+	−	−	+	−	−	−	−	−	−	−	+	−	−
N. meningitidis	+	−	V	+	+	−	−	−	−	V	−	+	−	−
N. gonorrhoeae subsp. kochii	−	+	+	+	−	−	−	−	−	−	−	+	−	−
N. lactamica	+	V	+	+	+	+	−	−	−	V	−	+	−	−
N. cinerea[b]	V	−	+	−	−	−	−	−	−	+	−	+	−	−
N. polysaccharea	V	−	+	+	+	−	−	−	−	V	+	+	−	+
N. subflava[c]	V	+	+	+	+	−	V	V	−	+	V	+	−	V
N. sicca	−	+	+	+	+	−	+	+	−	+	+	+	−	+
N. mucosa	−	+	+	+	+	−	+	+	+	+	+	+	−	+
N. flavescens	−	+	+	−	−	−	−	−	−	+	+	+	−	+
N. elongata subsp. elongata	−	?	−	−	−	−	−	−	−	−	−	−	−	+
N. elongata subsp. glycolytica	−	?	+	W+	−	−	−	−	−	+	−	+	−	+
N. elongata subsp. nitroreducens (formerly CDC group M-6)	−	?	+	−	−	−	−	−	+	−	−	−	−	+
Animal species														
N. animalis	?	?	?	+	−	−	+	W+	−	+	+	+	−	−
N. canis	?	?	?	−	−	−	−	−	+	−	−	+	W+	+
N. dentrificans	?	?	?	+	−	−	+	+	−	+	+	+	+	V
N. macacae	?	?	?	+	+	−	+	+	−	+	+	+	+	+
N. weaverii (formerly CD group M-5)	?	+	?	−	−	−	−	−	+	−	?	+	?	+
N. iguanae	?	?	?	W+	−	−	W+	−	+	+	+	+	−	−

[a] Symbols and abbreviations: +, strains typically positive but genetic mutants may be negative; −, most strains negative; v, strain dependent; W+, weakly positive; ?, not known; MTM, modified Thayer–Martin medium; ML, Martin–Lewis medium; NYC, New York City medium. All species contain cytochrome oxidase.

[b] Some strains grow on selective media even though they are colistin susceptible.

[c] Includes biovars *subflava*, *flava*, and *perflava*. N. *subflava* bv. *perflava* strains produce acid from sucrose and fructose and produce polysaccharide from sucrose; N. *subflava* bv. *flava* strains produce acid from fructose; N. *subflava* bv. *flava* and N. *subflava* bv. *subflava* do not produce polysaccharide from sucrose.

(Vedros, Hoke and Chun 1983). *Neisseria* spp. have also been isolated from dental plaque specimens from a variety of animals including primates (5 species), yaks, deer, kangaroos, llamas, black bears, panda bears, sheep, dairy cattle, domestic cats and iguanid lizards (Dent 1982, Barrett et al. 1994).

2.5 Morphology, structure and cell division

The *Neisseria* spp. are gram-negative cocci with the exception of *N. elongata*, which is a short rod. *Neisseria* spp. vary in the ease with which they are decolorized by alcohol. Cell morphology and arrangement are also affected by environmental conditions and may vary between cells grown in vitro and those directly observed in specimens from an infected host. Thin sections prepared from *N. gonorrhoeae* grown in vitro exhibit cell structures in electron micrographs, which are similar to those of other gram-negative bacteria (Fig. 37.2). An undulating outer membrane, approximately 7.5–8.5 nm in thickness, appears as a bilayered structure (Fitz-James 1964, Swanson, Kraus and Gotschlich 1971, Wegner, Hebeler and Morse 1977) and contains lipopolysaccharide (LPS), proteins and phospholipids (Morse 1978). The periplasmic space, the space between the cytoplasmic membrane and the outer membrane, comprises approximately 25% of the cell volume (Morse and Lysko 1980) and contains proteins which are released upon osmotic shock (Morse and Lysko 1980, Chen et al. 1993) or by treatment with chloroform (Judd and Porcella 1993). Among the periplasmic proteins that have been identified are an iron-binding protein (Chen et al. 1993), a *c*-type cytochrome (Judd and Porcella 1993) and a homologue of elongation factor Tu (Judd and Porcella 1993). An electron-dense layer, approximately 6.0 nm in thickness, corresponding to the peptidoglycan layer of the bacterial cell envelope, is located within the periplasmic space (Swanson, Kraus and Gotschlich 1971). Peptidoglycan isolated from *N. gonorrhoeae* grown at neutral pH comprises 1–2% of the cellular dry weight and has a composition similar to that of *Escherichia coli* (Hebeler and Young 1976). The peptidoglycan layer and outer membrane appear to adhere to each other at regular intervals around the periphery of the cell (Fitz-James 1964, Wolf-Watz et al. 1975). Electron microscopy has also revealed the presence of membrane-bound vesicles in the cytoplasm of some cells located proximal to the site of septum formation, which resemble mesosomes (Morse 1976, Fitz-James 1964, Murray, Reyn and Birch-Anderson 1963).

Cell-wall blebs produced by budding of the outer membrane have been observed both in log phase broth- or agar-grown cultures of *N. gonorrhoeae* and *N. meningitidis*. These blebs consist of outer-membrane components including LPS and proteins; they are produced by rapidly growing cells (Andersen and Solberg 1978, Andersen, Skjorten and Solberg 1979, Dorward, Garon and Judd 1989, Pettit and Judd 1992). Blebs produced by *N. gonorrhoeae* contain both circular and

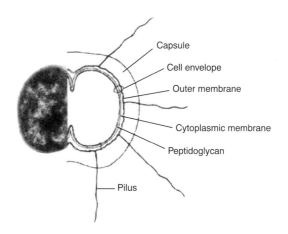

Fig. 37.2 Diagrammatic and electron micrographic representation of *N. gonorrhoeae*. To the left is a thin-section transmission electron micrograph showing the morphology of the cell membrane. The right half drawing is developed from the electron micrograph and other data.

linear DNA and may function by facilitating the intercellular transfer of plasmid or chromosomal DNA (Dorward, Garon and Judd 1989).

Most of our knowledge of cell division in *Neisseria* spp. comes from studies with *N. gonorrhoeae* and *N. meningitidis*; however, it is likely that cell division is similar in all of the diplococcal species of *Neisseria*. Cell division occurs by septation rather than by constriction (Westling-Haggstrom et al. 1977) and is initiated by an ingrowth of the cytoplasmic membrane enclosing a fold of peptidoglycan (Fig. 37.3). Division planes are formed consecutively at right angles to each other, resulting in a transient tetrad formation (Murray, Reyn and Birch-Anderson 1963, Catlin 1975, Westling-Haggstrom et al. 1977). Individual cells expand in only one dimension throughout most of the cell cycle (Westling-Haggstrom et al. 1977). Towards the end of the division period, initiation of growth in the second dimension, i.e. the former width, often

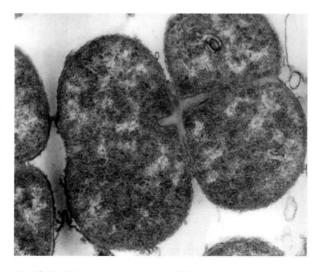

Fig. 37.3 Electron micrograph of *N. gonorrhoeae* undergoing cell division. (× 50 000).

begins before completion of the first septum. It has been suggested that this change in growth direction enables these organisms to avoid a rod–sphere–rod transition and the large fluctuations in internal pressure that would occur if growth were unidirectional (Westling-Haggstrom et al. 1977). Subinhibitory concentrations of penicillin G, which is known to induce filament formation in gram-negative rods and has been used to differentiate coccobacilli from cocci, does not induce filament formation in *N. gonorrhoeae* (Catlin 1975); however, subinhibitory concentrations of penicillin will induce filament formation in *N. elongata*, suggesting that cells of this species grow in one direction.

2.6 Growth requirements

The natural habitat of the *Neisseria* spp. suggests that some species may have complex growth requirements. Many of these requirements are fulfilled by standard laboratory media. For example, *Neisseria* spp. other than *N. gonorrhoeae* and *N. meningitidis* will grow on nutrient agar at 35–37°C (Table 37.1). Many of these non-pathogenic species will also grow in a chemically defined medium containing as few as 5 amino acids and 2 vitamins, although some require the addition of glucose, lactate or both glucose and lactose for good growth (McDonald and Johnson 1975). Some species produce large amounts of ammonia during growth in these media, which will interfere with the detection of acid production from sugars such as glucose. Consequently, the utilization of a monosaccharide such as glucose by some *Neisseria* spp. may not correlate with results of tests that measure acid production (Table 37.1) (McDonald and Johnson 1975). As a group, strains of *N. meningitidis* are relatively homogeneous and biosynthetically competent (Catlin 1973); most strains can grow on a relatively simple agar medium containing mineral salts, lactate and 5 amino acids. Cystine is required by <10% of strains (Catlin 1973). *N. gonorrhoeae* is more fastidious and will not grow in the absence of an energy source such as glucose, pyruvate or lactate (Morse 1978). All strains require cystine for growth; glutamine and cocarboxylase are required by a significant number of strains during primary isolation. For these reasons a growth factor supplement containing these nutrients is added to media used for the primary isolation of *N. gonorrhoeae*. Many strains of *N. gonorrhoeae* have additional genetic defects in the pathways used for the biosynthesis of amino acids, purines, pyrimidines and vitamins. This results in specific growth requirements and reinforces the need to use complex media for primary isolation of this micro-organism. The use of growth factor requirements to differentiate between gonococcal strains, i.e. auxotyping, is a useful tool for epidemiological studies (Catlin 1973). The development of defined media for growth of *N. gonorrhoeae* (Catlin 1973, La Scolea and Young 1974, Morse and Bartenstein 1980) has facilitated studies on gonococcal genetics and has helped to elucidate biosynthetic pathways.

2.7 Metabolism

N. gonorrhoeae and *N. meningitidis* dissimilate glucose via the Entner–Doudoroff (ED) pathway with acetate and CO_2 as the primary end products (Morse, Stein and Hines 1974, Holten 1975). With the exceptions of *N. cinerea* and *N. elongata* subsp. *elongata*, which lack 6-phosphogluconate dehydrase (Holten 1974), other *Neisseria* spp. also dissimilate glucose via the ED pathway (Holten 1975). Fermentative pathways such as the Embden–Meyerhoff pathway do not appear to function in the dissimilation of glucose by these microorganisms (Morse, Stein and Hines 1974). The lack of fermentative capability may explain why *Neisseria* spp. are aerobic and little or no growth occurs under strictly anaerobic conditions in the absence of an alternative terminal electron acceptor. Nevertheless, gonococci will remain viable for extended periods under anaerobic conditions (Short et al. 1982) and growth will occur when subtoxic concentrations of the alternative electron acceptor potassium nitrite (0.01–0.001%) are present (Knapp 1984, Knapp and Clark 1984). Nitrite, which is reduced by the constitutive enzyme, nitrite reductase, may enable gonococci to survive within aerobic or anaerobic environments in the host.

Amino acids are utilized as an energy source via the tricarboxylic acid cycle by those *Neisseria* spp. capable of growth in a chemically defined medium without glucose, pyruvate, or lactate. *N. gonorrhoeae*, which also has a functional tricarboxylic acid cycle (Hebeler and Morse 1976), is unable to grow in medium containing amino acids as the carbon and energy source.

A high relative humidity (c. 50%) is beneficial to the growth of all *Neisseria* spp. (Vedros 1984). Whereas all *Neisseria* spp. contain carbonic anhydrase, increased concentrations of carbon dioxide (5–10%) are required for the growth of *N. gonorrhoeae* and will enhance the growth of *N. meningitidis* on solid medium (Vedros 1984). Bicarbonate can replace the requirement for carbon dioxide (Talley and Baugh 1975). The carbon dioxide (Platt 1976) and bicarbonate ions (Talley and Baugh 1975, Earl et al. 1976) stimulate gonococcal growth by reducing the lag phase. Incorporation studies using ^{14}C-labelled bicarbonate revealed that the majority of the bicarbonate was used for nucleic acid and protein biosynthesis during the lag phase (Morse 1976). This would be expected since the requirement for carbon dioxide can be met in part by the addition of uracil (Griffin and Racker 1956) and oxaloacetate (Griffin and Rieder 1957) to the medium. The former is a direct precursor of RNA, whereas the latter can be used as a precursor of pyrimidines or proteins. Phosphoenolpyruvate carboxylase activity has been described in *N. gonorrhoeae* (Cox and Baugh 1977).

The optimum growth temperature of *Neisseria* spp. is 36–38.5°C (Morse 1976, Vedros 1984) with a range of 22–40°C. It has been reported that *N. gonorrhoeae* and *N. meningitidis* grow poorly or not at all below 30°C (Vedros 1984); however, several reports have suggested that some strains of *N. gonorrhoeae* may grow on solid or in liquid medium at temperatures as low as 25–28°C (Morse 1976, Annear 1981, Annear and Grubb 1982). pH has a marked effect upon the metabolism and cell composition of *N. gonorrhoeae* (Morse and Hebeler 1978, Hebeler et al. 1979, Pettit et al. 1995). *N. gonorrhoeae* will grow in a glucose-containing medium over a pH range of 6.0–8.0 (Morse and Hebeler 1978), with the shortest generation time between pH 7.0 and 7.5. When gonococci were grown in continuous culture at constant pH values ranging from 6.3 to 7.2, the highest cell yields at all dilution rates were obtained at pH 6.75 (Brookes and Sikyta 1967).

2.8 Bacteriocins

Bacteriocin production is not a widespread characteristic of the pathogenic *Neisseria* spp. Protease-sensitive bacteriocins have been isolated from only 4 of 215 strains of *N. meningitidis* (Jyssum and Allunans 1982) and have been induced by Mitomycin C in some strains of *N. meningitidis* (Kingsbury 1966). Protease-sensitive bacteriocins have been isolated from 17 of 2123 isolates of *N. gonorrhoeae* (Lawton et al. 1976). Bacteriocins from *N. gonorrhoeae* and *N. meningitidis* do not inhibit the producer strains; however, meningococcal bacteriocins have been shown to inhibit strains of *N. gonorrhoeae*, *N. lactamica*, *N. cinerea*, and *N. flavescens* (Jyssum and Allunans 1984).

Many strains of *N. gonorrhoeae* have been reported to produce bacteriocin-like substances that inhibit the growth of other gonococcal strains (Flynn and McEntegart 1972). Further investigation suggested that this bacteriocin-like activity was due to free fatty acids that are released during growth (Walstad, Reitz and Sparling 1974, Knapp, Falkow and Holmes 1975). Fatty acids may play a role in the ability of gonococcal strains to colonize the rectal mucosa (McFarland et al. 1983); rectal isolates, which are relatively resistant to faecal lipids, have a derepressed efflux system, that mediates resistance to hydrophobic agents including drugs, dyes and detergents (Shafer et al. 1995).

Some R-type bacteriocins (pyocins) from *Pseudomonas aeruginosa* exhibit bactericidal activity against *N. gonorrhoeae* (Morse et al. 1976, Sidberry and Sadoff 1977). Differential sensitivity to these pyocins suggested the feasibility of a typing system based upon pyocin sensitivity (Sidberry and Sadoff 1977, Blackwell, Young and Anderson 1979). However, pyocin susceptibility of a gonococcal strain is influenced by growth conditions (Stein, Hebeler and Young 1980). The pyocin receptor is located on the LPS of *N. gonorrhoeae* (Morse and Apicella 1982) and the selection of pyocin-resistant mutants with altered LPS structure has proved useful in elucidating the structure of the gonococcal LPS (Guymon, Esser and Shafer 1982, Morse and Apicella 1982, Dudas and Apicella 1988). Pyocin-resistant mutants have also been used to investigate the genetics of LPS biosynthesis (Sandlin, Apicella and Stein 1993) and to study the mechanisms of serum resistance in *N. gonorrhoeae* (Shafer et al. 1984).

2.9 Laboratory isolation and identification

N. GONORRHOEAE

The laboratory diagnosis of gonorrhoea is made presumptively and then confirmed: this process involves identifying characteristics that distinguish *N. gonorrhoeae* from other *Neisseria* sp. that may be present in the specimen (see Table 37.1, p. 879). Non-pathogenic *Neisseria* are normal inhabitants of the orpharynx and nasopharynx and are occasionally isolated from sites that are infected by *N. gonorrhoeae*. The presence of multiple pairs of bean-shaped, gram-negative diplococci within a neutrophil is highly characteristic of gonorrhoea when the smear is from a genital site. A gram-stained smear is about 95% sensitive in symptomatic men; however, the direct smear is only 50–70% sensitive in women and its specificity is complicated by the presence of other bacteria in the female genital tract flora that may have a similar morphology. The sensitivity and specificity of the gram stain for rectal specimens are lower than with cervical specimens.

N. gonorrhoeae can be cultured on selective media; however, attention to detail is necessary for isolation of the gonococcus in that it is a fragile organism. In men, the best specimen is urethral exudate or urethral scrapings. In women, cervical swabs are preferred over urethral or vaginal specimens. Swabs may be transported to the laboratory in a suitable transport medium although, ideally, specimens should be inoculated onto appropriate media and incubated immediately after collection. Urethral, cervical and pharyngeal specimens are inoculated onto selective media such as Thayer–Martin or Martin–Lewis. These are complex media that contain antimicrobial and antifungal agents to inhibit the growth of normal flora. Specimens collected from normally sterile sites such as blood, synovial fluid and conjunctiva may be inoculated onto a non-selective medium such as chocolate agar. Direct detection methods for *N. gonorrhoeae*, such as DNA–rRNA hybridization assays, are also available. DNA–rRNA hybridization assay has an advantage where culture is impractical, because specimen viability is not required.

N. gonorrhoeae can be distinguished from other *Neisseria* spp. by its reaction in tests that measure acid production from carbohydrates; the gonococcus is only capable of producing acid from glucose (see Table 37.1, p. 879). Gonococcal strains can be characterized according to their nutritional requirements (auxotyping) (Table 37.2). A panel of monoclonal antibodies specific for epitopes on the outer-membrane protein I have also been used to subtype strains. Strains exhibiting specific reaction patterns are termed serovars. A combined serovar–auxotype classification provides resolution among gonococcal isolates and is useful in epidemiological investigations. By combining serotyping and auxotyping it has been shown that over 80 distinct strains of gonococci are circulating in nature (Sparling, Tsai and Cornelissen 1990). Pulsed-field gel electrophoresis has recently been utilized for the genomic analysis of *N. gonorrhoeae* and may prove to be a useful tool for gonococcal epidemiological studies (Xia et al. 1995).

For further information on gonorrhoea the reader is referred to Volume 3, Chapter 33.

Table 37.2 Phenotypic classification systems of *N. gonorrhoeae* and *N. meningitidis*

Organism	System	Basis	No. of groups or types	Names
N. gonorrhoeae	Serovars	Protein I	24 PIA, 31 PIB	PIA,...PIA-24 PIB-1,...PIB-31
	Auxotypes	Nutritional requirement	35[a]	ARG⁻,PRO⁻, etc.
N. meningitidis[b]	Serogroups	Capsular polysaccharide	12	A,B,C,X,Y,Z,29E W-135,H,I,K,L[c]
	Serotypes	Class 2/3 proteins	20	1,2a,2b,2c,..21[d]
	Subserotypes	Class 1 protein	10	P1.1,P1.2,...P1.16[d]
	Immunotypes	LOS	12	L1-L12

[a]Auxotypes determined by growth response patterns on a standard set of defined media (Catlin 1978).
[b]A strain can express more than 1 serosubtype or immunotype-specific epitope, e.g. L3,7,9.
[c]See Table 37.3 for structure of the capsular polysaccharides.
[d]Not all the numbers between 1 and 21 and P1.1 and P1.16 are used.

N. MENINGITIDIS

In cases of suspected meningococcal disease, specimens of blood, cerebrospinal fluid and nasopharyngeal secretions are typically collected and examined for the presence of *N. meningitidis*. Cerebrospinal fluid should be concentrated by centrifugation and a portion cultured on chocolate agar or blood agar. Nasopharyngeal specimens are typically plated on a selective medium such as Thayer–Martin. Blood cultures are typically plated on chocolate or blood agar. The plates are then incubated in an aerobic atmosphere containing 5% CO_2. The presence of oxidase-positive, gram-negative diplococci provides a presumptive identification of *N. meningitidis*. For confirmation, production of acid from glucose and maltose but not sucrose, lactose, or fructose may be used (see Table 37.1, p. 879). Gram-stained smears of cerebrospinal fluid may also be diagnostic.

The only distinguishing structural feature between *N. meningitidis* and *N. gonorrhoeae* is the presence of a polysaccharide capsule in *N. meningitidis*. It is believed to play a role in the resistance to PMN-mediated phagocytosis; it is also used to provide the basis for grouping of these organisms. To date, 12 different serogroups have been identified based on the chemical composition of the polysaccharide (Table 37.3). The serological group is determined by a slide agglutination test, using polyvalent and monovalent antisera. In addition to classification based on the capsular polysaccharide, *N. meningitidis* strains can be grouped into specific serotypes and subserotypes based on antigenic determinants on specific outer-membrane proteins and immunotypes based on antigenic determinants on the lipopolysaccharide (see Table 37.2). A typing scheme based on isoenzyme electrophoresis has also been used to study the epidemiology and geographical distribution of *N. meningitidis* strains (Olyhoek, Crowe and Achtman 1985).

3 GENETIC MECHANISMS

To date, only transformation and conjugation have

been described in *N. gonorrhoeae* and *N. meningitidis*. Transformation and conjugation have been used as molecular tools to conduct genetic studies on the pathogenic *Neisseria* spp. and have aided in the elucidation of the role of putative virulence factors. Although conjugative plasmids exist, conjugative (high-frequency resolution [Hfr]-like) mobilization of chromosomal determinants is not known to occur under natural conditions. There have been no substantiated reports that document the presence of bacteriophage in *N. gonorrhoeae* and *N. meningitidis*. However, bacteriophages active against non-pathogenic *Neisseria* spp. have been isolated (Stone, Culbertson and Powell 1956, Phelps 1967, Steinberg et al. 1976). These bacteriophages exhibit a very narrow host range as measured by plaque formation. Lysogenic strains of *N. perflava*, *N. sicca* and *N. flavescens* have also been reported (Stone, Culbertson and Powell 1956, Phelps 1967).

3.1 Transformation

In transformation, naked DNA is taken up by a recipient cell and ultimately integrated into the chromosome. Transformation in *Neisseria* was described over 30 years ago (Catlin and Cunningham 1961), when it was demonstrated that nearly all *Neisseria* species are transformable by homologous and heterologous chromosomal DNA. *Neisseria* spp. are atypical in that they are competent for genetic transformation throughout their entire growth cycle (Sparling, Biswas and Sox 1977). Transforming DNA taken up as a linear molecule requires the RecA function and homologous sequences in the recipient DNA in order for recirculazation of a plasmid or incorporation of the DNA into the chromosome to occur (Biswas and Sparling 1986, Koomey et al. 1987). Competence for transformation is much greater in piliated (Pil⁺) colonial forms of the gonococcus than in their isogenic non-piliated (Pil⁻) colonial variants (Sparling 1966). Pilin (PilE), the major pilus subunit, and PilC, the minor pilus-associated protein, are required for DNA uptake (Meyer, Pohlner and van Putten 1994). A competence

Table 37.3 Chemical composition of capsular polysaccharides and exopolysaccharides of *Neisseria* spp[a]

Species	Structural repeating unit[b]
N. meningitidis Serogroup A[c] (homopolymer)	ManNac-(1-P$\overset{\alpha}{\rightarrow}$6)- 3 | OAc
Serogroup B (homopolymer)	NeuNAc-(2$\overset{\alpha}{\rightarrow}$8)-
Serogroup C[d] (homopolymer)	NeuNAc-(2$\overset{\alpha}{\rightarrow}$9)- 7 8 | | OAc OAc
Serogroup H (monosaccharide-glycerol repeating unit)	→4)α-D-Gal-(1→2)-Gro-(3-P→
Serogroup I (disaccharide repeating unit)	→4)α-L-GulNAcA(1→3)β-D-ManNAcA(1→ | 4OAc
Serogroup K (disaccharide repeating unit)	→3)-β-D-ManNAcA-(1→4)-β-D-ManNAcA-(1→ | 4-OAc
Serogroup L (trisaccharide repeating unit)	→3)-β-D-GlcNAc-(1→3)β-D-GlcNAc-(1→3)α- D-GlcNAc-(1-P-

factor that is involved in a transformation step subsequent to the initial DNA uptake has also recently been identified (Facius and Meyer 1993). Gonococci can be transformed by either chromosomal or plasmid DNA, although the efficiency of transformation with plasmid DNA is approximately 1000-fold lower than with chromosomal DNA (Sox, Mohammed and Sparling 1979). Electroporation of both chromosomal and plasmid DNA has also been used to introduce DNA into the gonococcus (Kapczynski and Genco 1991). DNA-containing membrane blebs produced by the gonococcus may facilitate the transfer of plasmid or chromosomal DNA (Dorward, Garon and Judd 1989).

Neisseria spp. may exchange DNA in vivo by transformation (Cannon and Sparling 1984); this mechanism may be how gonococci and other *Neisseria* spp. exchange genetic information in vivo. The evolution of the transformation process requires that free DNA be present in the environment. Neisseriae, like many other naturally competent bacteria, are highly autolytic, which results in the release of biologically active transforming DNA into their environment. Although an enzymatic activity has been implicated in the process of autolysis, the mechanistic details are not known.

3.2 Conjugation

Conjugation in *N. gonorrhoeae* is different from that of *E. coli* F, in that a plasmid-encoded pilus has not been identified and transfer only occurs when cells are on a solid surface. Two gonococcal conjugal plasmids of 24 500 and 25 200 kDa mediate the transfer of R plasmids to strains of *N. gonorrhoeae* and *N. meningitidis*, as well as to commensal *Neisseria* strains, *E. coli* and to *Haemophilus influenzae* (Biswas, Blackman and Sparling 1980, Flett, Humphreys and Saunders 1980, Genco, Knapp and Clark 1984). Although these conjugal plasmids have been found to function transiently in *E. coli*, they are not stably maintained in any species other than *N. gonorrhoeae*, *N. meningitidis* or *N. cinerea* (Genco, Knapp and Clark 1984, Sarafian et al. 1990). Chromosomal genes are not mobilized by conjugation and the phenomenon of surface exclusion does not appear to be expressed. The mobilization of R plasmids is often accompanied by transfer of the conjugal plasmids; however, no evidence of stable cointegrate formation has been found (Sox et al. 1978). Several R plasmids can be mobilized by *E. coli* conjugal plasmids and transferred to other *E. coli* strains, *Salmonella minnesota* and *H. influenzae* (Guiney and Ito 1982), sug-

Table 37.3 Continued

Species	Structural repeating unit[b]
Serogroup W-135 (disaccharide repeating unit)	6-D-Gal(1$\xrightarrow{\alpha}$4)-NeuNAc(2$\xrightarrow{\alpha}$6)
Serogroup X (homopolymer)	GlcNAc(1-P→4)-
Serogroup Y (BO)[c] (disaccharide repeating unit)	6-D-Glc(1$\xrightarrow{\alpha}$4)-NeuNAc(2$\xrightarrow{\alpha}$6) ‖ OAc
Serogroup Z (monosaccharide glycerol repeating unit)	D-GalNAc(1$\xrightarrow{\alpha}$1)-Gro-(3'-P$\xrightarrow{\alpha}$4)
Serogroup 29E (disaccharide repeating unit)	D-GalNAc(1$\xrightarrow{\beta}$7)-KDO(2$\xrightarrow{\alpha}$3)- 4 5 ‖ OAc
N. lactamica	Antigenically similar to capsular polysaccharide of *N. meningitidis* serogroup B
N. polysaccharea	Glycogen-like structure containing mainly 1,4-linked α-D-glucopyranosyl residues; ca. 6% 4,6-di-*O*-substituted α-D-glucopyranosyl branch points[f]
N. sicca	Polymer of GalNAc
N. subflava biovar *perflava*	Similar to *N. polysaccharea*[f]

[a]From Morse and Knapp, 1991.
[b]Gal, galactose; Glc, glucose; ManNAc, *N*-acetylmannosamine (2-acetamido-2-deoxy-D-mannose); NeuNAc, *N*-acetylneuraminic acid (sialic acid); OAc, *O*-acetylated; Gro, glycerol; P, phosphate; GulNAcA, 2-acetamido-2-deoxy-L-guluronic acid; ManNAcA, 2-acetamido-2-deoxy-mannuronic acid; GlcNAc, *N*-acetylglucosamine (2-acetamido-2-deoxy-D-glucose); GalNAc, *N*-acetylgalactosamine (2-acetamido-2-deoxy-D-galactose).
[c]Group A is substituted with *O*-acetyl at C3 on about 70% of the ManNAc-P residues.
[d]Group C is substituted on C7 or C8 with 1 mol of *O*-acetyl per mole of sialic acid. One quarter of the sialyl residues are not acetylated. Some di-*O*-acetylated (C7 and C8) may exist.
[e]The Y polysaccharide contains 1.3 mol of *O*-acetyl per NeuNAc residue. The most probable site for acetylation is C3, C4, or C7. ^{13}C nuclear magnetic resonance studies have shown that the serogroup BO polysaccharide is identical to serogroup Y, although BO contains 1.8 mol of *O*-acetyl per mole of NeuNAc.
[f]Produced in medium containing 1 to 5% sucrose.

gesting that *E. coli* could have played a role in the dissemination of the R plasmids to *N. gonorrhoeae*.

3.3 Transposons

Transposable elements have become valuable tools for molecular genetic analysis and manipulation of genes in many different organisms. However, no such naturally occurring transposons have been described in *Neisseria*. Investigators have exploited several exogenous transposons for use in the pathogenic *Neisseria*, including Tn*916* and derivatives of Tn*1545* (Kathariou et al. 1990, Nassif, Puaoi and So 1991). However, direct transposon mutagenesis with Tn*916* is not highly efficient in *N. meningitidis*, nor has it been developed for use in *N. gonorrhoeae* (Kathariou et al. 1990, Nassif, Puaoi and So 1991). Although several interesting *N. meningitidis* mutants have been isolated, including strains altered in capsular polysaccharide and LPS and auxotrophic mutants (Stephens et al. 1991, 1994), mutagenesis with Tn*916* has been diffi-

cult. Several shuttle mutagenesis systems have also been described for targeting and modification of distinct chromosomal genes (Seifert and So 1991, Haas et al. 1993). A mini-Tn system based on Tn*1721* transposition functions appears to be particularly useful for genetic studies in the pathogenic *Neisseria*. A member of this mini-transposon family, Tn*Max4*, includes features of Tn*phoA* that are useful for targeting secretory determinants. Tn*Max4* has been used in *N. gonorrhoeae* for the isolation of epithelial cell invasion-defective mutants (Kahrs et al. 1994). The use of Tn*Max*-mediated mutagenesis should prove useful in the identification of additional virulence-associated genes in the pathogenic *Neisseria* spp.

3.4 Plasmids and plasmid-mediated antibiotic resistance

The increase in the proportion of antibiotic-resistant strains of bacteria is of growing importance in the treatment of infectious diseases. The inappropriate use of broad spectrum antibiotics, combined with the self-adminstration of antibiotics, has provided powerful selection for antibiotic-resistant bacteria. This has facilitated the appearance and spread of antibiotic resistance encoding plasmids in many bacterial pathogens. The discovery of penicillinase-producing *N. gonorrhoeae* (PPNG) in 1976 (Ashford, Golash and Hemming 1976, Phillips 1976) foreshadowed the demise of penicillin as effective therapy for gonorrhoea and ensured that future control of this infection would require the use of more costly treatment regimens.

Two β-lactamase plasmids with molecular weights of 3200 (African) and 4400 kDa (Asian) were first described in 1976 (Ashford, Golash and Hemming 1976, Perine et al. 1977). Initially, PPNG isolates possessing the 4400 kDa Asia β-lactamase plasmid were isolated primarily in Asia and on the west coast of the USA whereas strains possessing the 3200 kDa Africa β-lactamase plasmid were found primarily in Africa, Europe and on the east coast of the USA. Since 1985, β-lactamase plasmids with molecular masses of 2900 (Rio), 3090 (Toronto) and 4000 kDa (Nimes) have also been described in *N. gonorrhoeae* isolates (Seifert and So 1991). The origin of these β-lactamase plasmids is uncertain, but the β-lactamase gene itself and some of its surrounding DNA are homologous with the ampicillin transposon Tn*A* (Roberts, Elewell and Falkow 1977). The β-lactamase encoded by Tn*A* is a TEM1 type enzyme. The left 60% of the transposon, including the structural gene for the transposase, has been lost. It is thought that the right 40% of Tn*A* found in *N. gonorrhoeae* may have originated in the Enterobacteriaceae. The non-Tn*A* sequences of the gonococcal β-lactamase plasmids appear to be deletion derivatives of *Haemophilus* plasmids with which they share an identical origin of transfer (OriT) (Roberts, Elewell and Falkow 1977). β-Lactamase plasmids in *N. gonorrhoeae* are not autotransmissible, but may be mobilized between strains by either the 24 500 kDa conjugative plasmid or the 25 200 kDa TetM-containing conjugative plasmid (Genco, Knapp and Clark 1984, Sarafian et al. 1990). In addition to the presence of various R plasmids, a majority of *N. gonorrhoeae* isolates also contain a 2600 kDa cryptic plasmid. Although *N. meningitidis* isolates have also been reported to harbour cryptic plasmids, they are extremely rare.

Although the prevalence of PPNG is still relatively low in the USA and Europe, it is much higher in other parts of the world, including the Philippines (30–70%), eastern Asia (10–30%) and parts of Africa (10–34%) (Handsfield et al. 1982). Recently, *N. gonorrhoeae* strains have been isolated in the USA with plasmid-mediated, high-level resistance to tetracycline (MIC 16–64 µg ml^{-1}) (Knapp et al. 1986, Morse et al. 1986). Tetracycline resistance in these strains is associated with the presence of the 25 200 kDa conjugative *tetM* cointegrate plasmid. The *tetM* gene is a determinant which was described originally as part of the streptococcal conjugative transposons Tn*916* and Tn*1545* (Burdett, Inamine and Rajagopalan 1982). How the *tetM* gene became associated with the gonococcal conjugal plasmid is unknown. Tetracycline-resistant *N. gonorrhoeae* isolates can transfer the 25 200 kDa plasmid to *N. meningitidis*, commensal *Neisseria* and *Haemophilus* species (Sarafian et al. 1990). Studies have also indicated that in the presence of the 25 200 kDa and β-lactamase plasmids, *N. meningitidis* and commensal *Neisseria* have the potential to act as donors to further disseminate both plasmids (Sarafian et al. 1990). This may increase the possibilities for acquisition and spread of the β-lactamase plasmids in *N. meningitidis* which could have serious consequences, since penicillins are often used to treat these infections. Because of the prevalence of tetracycline-resistant *N. gonorrhoeae*, tetracyclines are no longer recommended as sole therapy for uncomplicated urethral, endocervical, or rectal gonorrhoea infections in the USA. However, because of possible coinfections with *Chlamydia trachomatis*, dual therapy of doxycyline plus either a cephalosporin such as ceftriaxone, or a fluoroquinolone are currently recommended as standard treatment by the Centers for Disease Control (Centers for Disease Control 1983).

4 ANTIGENIC STRUCTURE

The antigenic composition of the gonococcal and meningococcal cell envelopes has been the subject of extensive investigation because this structure interfaces with the defence mechanisms of the host; knowledge of this structure may ultimately yield a suitable vaccine component.

4.1 Pili

Pili are hair-like filamentous proteins composed of repeating peptide subunits (pilin), that extend several micrometres from the bacterial cell surface. Pili have been observed on *N. gonorrhoeae* (Jephcott, Reyn and Birch-Anderson 1971, Swanson, Kraus and Gotschlich 1971), *N. meningitidis* (Devoe and Gilchrist 1974, McGee et al. 1977) and the non-pathogenic *Neisseria* spp. (Weistreich and Baker 1971, McGee et al. 1977). The length of the pili varies; short pili (175–210 nm in length) have only been observed on non-pathogenic *Neisseria* spp. (Weistreich and Baker 1971) whereas long pili (up to 4300 nm in length) have been observed on both pathogenic and non-pathogenic *Neisseria* spp. (McGee et al. 1977). Piliation is associated with a characteristic colonial morphology in *N. gonorrhoeae* (Jephcott, Reyn and Birch-Anderson 1971); pili are only observed on cells from small, domed, highlighted colonies (types 1 and 2) and not on cells from large, flat colonies (types 3 and 4) (Kellogg et al. 1963). However, there does not appear to be an association between colonial morphology and piliation with *N. meningitidis* or the non-pathogenic *Neisseria* spp. (McGee et al. 1977).

Gonococcal and meningococcal pili have been purified by repeated cycles of disaggregation and recrystallization (Olafson et al. 1985, Stephens et al. 1985,

Parge et al. 1990). Sodium dodecyl sulphate polyacrylamide gel electrophoresis (SDS-PAGE) analysis of such preparations revealed the presence of a predominant protein (pilin), with a molecular mass that varied between strains from 17 000 to 22 000 (Robertson, Vincent and Ward 1977). Pili from *N. gonorrhoeae* and *N. meningitidis* are antigenically and structurally similar (Hermodsen, Chen and Buchanan 1978, Olafson et al. 1985, Stephens et al. 1985) and exhibit extensive similarity in their amino- and carboxyl-terminal amino acid sequences to pilins from diverse bacterial species such as *Bacteroides nodosus* (McKern et al. 1985), *Moraxella bovis* (Marrs et al. 1985) and *P. aeruginosa* (Sastry et al. 1983). The first 32 amino acid residues of these pilins are nearly identical with the modified amino acid *N*-methylphenylalanine as the amino-terminal residue. Pilins belonging to this group are termed mePhe pilins (Elleman 1988). Gonococcal pilin also has been crystallized and x-ray diffraction data suggest that the pilin subunit has structural similarity to the 4-α-helix bundle fold in proteins such as the coat protein subunit of tobacco mosaic virus (Getzoff et al. 1988, Parge et al. 1990). Using an alternative procedure for pilin purification, Muir, Strungall and Davies (1988) identified a number of minor proteins that copurified with pilin. It is thought that some of these proteins are involved with pilus assembly or with adherence.

Meningococci express one of 2 quite distinct classes of pili which have been termed class 1 and class 2 pili (see Table 37.4) (Heckels 1989). Class 1 pili closely resemble gonococcal pili, whereas class 2 pili are composed of smaller pilin subunits that share conformational determinants with class 1 and gonococcal pili (Heckels 1989). The genes encoding expression of the gonococcal pilin and the meningococcal class 1 pilin have been cloned and sequenced (Meyer et al. 1984, Potts and Saunders 1987).

N. gonorrhoeae and *N. meningitidis* are highly efficient in their ability to turn on or off the expression of cell surface components such as pili (phase variation) and to vary these components (antigenic variation). Antigenic variation of surface proteins may be a means of

escape from host specific antibody directed against the initial antigen that is expressed when an infection starts. Gonococcal and meningococcal pili from different strains are antigenically diverse and a single gonococcal strain is capable of expressing multiple antigenically distinct types of pili. The control of phase variation is complex and appears to involve several mechanisms. Bergstrom et al. (1986) showed that deletions and frameshift mutations resulted in the production of truncated pilin molecules and a stable non-piliated phenotype. Reversible phase variation can result from changes in the signal peptide-coding region of *pilC*, a gene encoding a protein involved in pilus assembly (Jonsson, Nyberg and Normark 1991). Most strains of *N. gonorrhoeae* contain one copy of the expressed major pilus subunit gene, *pilE*, and multiple copies of *pilS*, which are transcriptionally silent, incomplete pilin loci carrying variant sequences (Meyer et al. 1984, Haas and Meyer 1986). Antigenic variation results from recombination events between silent and expressed loci, which result in the formation of diverse pilins either by a transformation-mediated recombination with DNA released from lysed gonococci or by recombination between a silent locus and an expressed locus on the same chromosome (Seifert, Ajioka and So 1988, Gibbs et al. 1989).

Pili facilitate the attachment of *Neisseria* spp. to host cells. They are thought to participate in the initial stage of a 2-stage attachment process whereby they overcome the electrostatic barrier which exists between the negatively charged surfaces of the bacterial and host cell (Heckels et al. 1976). Pili have been shown to facilitate the attachment of gonococci or meningococci to tissue culture cells (Swanson 1973), vaginal epithelial cells (Mardh and Westrom 1976), fallopian tube epithelium (Ward, Watt and Robertson 1974), buccal epithelial cells (Punsalang and Sawyer 1973), endothelial cells (Virji et al. 1991), nasopharyngeal cells (Stephens and McGee 1981) and erythrocytes (Lamben, Robertson and Watt 1981). Several early studies conducted before knowledge of Opa variation was available (see section 4.4, p. 889) suggested that piliated gonococci were more resistant to

Table 37.4 Outer-membrane proteins produced by *Neisseria gonorrhoeae* and *Neisseria meningitidis*

N. gonorrhoeae	*N. meningitidis*	Function
Pilin	Class I pilin Class II pilin	Adherence to epithelial cells and erythrocytes
Protein I	Class 2 and 3	Function as porins; anion-selective
	Class 1	Function as porin; cation-selective
Protein III	Class 4	Bind blocking bactericidal Ab homology to OmpA
Protein II (Opa)	Class 5	Adherence to epithelial and phagocytic cells
PilC	PilC	Epithelial cell-specific pilus-associated adherence
Pan 1	Pan 1	Anaerobically induced lipoprotein; may function in nitrate reductase system
Oxi A	–	Oxygen induced protein; function unknown
Lip (H.8)	–	Lipoprotein; function unknown
Laz	–	Lipid associated azurin
36 kDa adhesin	–	Glycolipid-binding adhesin

phagocytosis than non-piliated variants (Dilworth, Hendley and Mandell 1975, Densen and Mandell 1978). More recent studies controlling for Opa expression have suggested that pili may have little effect in resistance to phagocytosis by polymorpho-nuclear leucocytes (Virji and Heckels 1986).

4.2 Porins

The gonococcal and meningococcal outer membranes contain trimeric proteins that form pores (porins) through this structure (Leith and Morse 1980, Newhall, Sawyer and Haak 1980, Douglas, Lee and Nikaido 1981). The gonococcal porin has been termed protein I or PI. Gonococci express one of 2 structurally related forms of this protein (PIA and PIB) (Sandstrom, Chen and Buchanan 1982). A single copy of the structural gene exists in the chromosome (Gotschlich et al. 1987), suggesting that the PIA and PIB genes are alleles of the same gene. In membranes, the porin exists in 2 states, open or closed (Lynch et al. 1984). The diameter of the pore has been esti-mated to be 2.5 nm (Douglas, Lee and Nikaido 1981), with an anion-selective channel ranging in Cl^-/K^+ se-lectivity from 6:1 (for PIBs) to 3:1 (for PIAs) (Young et al. 1983, Blake and Gotschlich 1987). Porin function is necessary for the survival of these micro-organisms, allowing nutrients to pass through the outer mem-brane and waste products to exit. Antigenic hetero-geneity in PIA and PIB provides the basis for gono-coccal serotyping (see Table 37.2, p. 883).

N. meningitidis simultaneously expresses 2 porin genes. Expression of a given porin is a stable trait for a given strain; however, differences that occur between strains are responsible for antigenic diversity. One porin is the class 1 protein (PorA), produced by almost all meningococcal isolates, although there is considerable variation in the amount produced (Poolman, DeMarie and Zanen 1980). In addition, all meningococcal isolates posses a gene that encodes for either the class 2 or class 3 porin (PorB). The class 2 and 3 porins are equivalents of the gonococcal PIA and PIB proteins (see Table 37.4, p. 887) (Blake and Gotschlich 1987, Judd 1989) and also form anion-selective pores. In contrast, the class 1 protein pores are cation-selective (Tommassen et al. 1990). Anti-genic differences in class 2/3 proteins are used to serotype strains of *N. meningitidis* whereas antigenic differences in the class 1 protein are used for subsero-typing (Verheul, Snippe and Poolman 1993) (see Table 37.2, p. 883).

Although the role of neisserial porins in pathogen-esis is unclear, several studies have suggested that it may be important. With *N. gonorrhoeae*, the PI subclass has been epidemiologically associated with strains causing disseminated (PIA) and localized gonococcal (PIB) infections (Cannon, Buchanan and Sparling 1983, Sandstrom et al. 1984, Brunham et al. 1985). Studies with lipid bilayers and erythrocytes have dem-onstrated that gonococci and meningococci spon-taneously transfer their porin molecules in an inverted manner into these membranes (Lynch et al. 1984,

Blake and Gotschlich 1987). Meningococci and PIA-expressing strains of *N. gonorrhoeae* are apparently more efficient at porin transfer than PIB-expressing strains of *N. gonorrhoeae*; the non-pathogenic species *N. sicca* does not transfer its porin molecules to a lipid bilayer. Insertion of neisserial porins into cells such as human neutrophils may be important in pathogenesis as their ability to exocytose granules and other cellular functions was affected (Haines et al. 1988).

There are data suggesting that PI may be a suitable candidate for a gonorrhoea vaccine. In vitro assays have demonstrated that antibodies against PI are both bactericidal and opsonic (Virji, Zak and Heckles 1986, Virji et al. 1987). Data from a longitudinal study of a small group of prostitutes in Nairobi who experienced frequent gonococcal infections suggested that there was a 2- to 10-fold reduced risk of reinfection with most serovars (Plummer et al. 1989). Another study has suggested that bactericidal antibodies directed against PI provide serovar-specific protection against recurrent gonococcal salpingitis (Buchanan et al. 1980). The results of other studies have suggested that antibodies directed against PI may not be effective in vivo. Immunoelectron microscopy revealed that PI was variably exposed on the cell surface (Robinson et al. 1987). Furthermore, sialylation of gonococcal LPS inhibited the binding and subsequent complement-mediated killing by rabbit antisera directed against surface-exposed regions of protein I (Elkins et al. 1992).

4.3 Reduction-modifiable proteins

The outer membrane of *N. gonorrhoeae* and *N. meningit-idis* contains a protein whose apparent molecular weight in SDS-PAGE is increased upon treatment with a reducing agent (McDade and Johnson 1980). The gonococcal reduction-modifiable protein was termed protein III, while the meningococcal homologue was designated the class 4 protein (see Table 37.4, p. 887). The function of these proteins in pathogenesis or in the physiology of these organisms is unknown; how-ever, antibodies to protein III appears to increase sus-ceptibility to gonococcal infection (Plummer et al. 1993). A similar protein appears to be missing among non-pathogenic *Neisseria* spp. (Wolff and Stern 1995). Cross-linking studies with bifunctional reagents have provided data indicating that protein III is closely asso-ciated with protein I in the gonococcal outer mem-brane in an apparent ratio of 1:3 (Leith and Morse 1980, Newhall, Sawyer and Haak 1980). Protein III and the class 4 protein are both structurally and immunologically conserved among the pathogenic *Neisseria* spp. Surface-labelling studies, susceptibility to cleavage by cathepsin G and immunoprecipitation with a monoclonal antibody have provided evidence that these proteins have surface-exposed domains (Swanson, Mayer and Tam 1982, Shafer and Morse 1987). The structural genes for protein III and the class 4 protein have been cloned and sequenced (Gotschlich et al. 1986, Klugman, Gotschlich and Blake 1989). Gonococci and meningococci contain a single copy of this gene. Mutants lacking protein III and the class 4 protein have been obtained by insertional inactivation, suggesting that these proteins are not essential for cell growth (Klugman, Gotschlich and Blake 1989, Wetzler et al. 1989).

The carboxy-terminal half of protein III and that of the class 4 protein share significant sequence homology with the carboxy-terminal portion of the enterobacterial OmpA protein (Blake et al. 1989). Portions of the Omp-like region also appear to be surface-exposed (Blake et al. 1989). Human complement-fixing IgG binds to surface-exposed regions of protein III and interferes with the bactericidal activity of antibodies directed to other surface antigens such as protein I and LPS (Joiner et al. 1985, Rice et al. 1986, Rice 1989). These antibodies are termed blocking antibodies. The observation that human IgG directed at OmpA also binds to surface-exposed regions of protein III and promotes blocking activity (Rice et al. 1994) suggests that blocking antibodies may arise naturally from exposure to members of the family Enterobacteriaceae or to *N. meningitidis*. Immunization of human volunteers with protein I preparations containing trace amounts of protein III have resulted in the formation of blocking antibodies, further demonstrating that protein III is very immunogenic. Thus, any gonorrhoea vaccine will have to be free of protein III.

4.4 Opacity-associated proteins

Both *N. gonorrhoeae* and *N. meningitidis* possess a set of variably expressed heat-modifiable surface-exposed outer-membrane proteins. The gonococcal proteins have been termed protein IIs, whereas those from meningococci are referred to as class 5 proteins (see Table 37.4). Most, but not all gonococcal opacity-associated (Opa) proteins are associated with colony opacity, hence their name. However, there appears to be no relationship between colony opacity and expression of these proteins in *N. meningitidis* (Hagman and Danielsson 1989). A gene which encodes a similar protein has been identified in *N. lactamica* and other non-pathogenic *Neisseria* spp. (Aho, Murphy and Cannon 1987, Wolff and Stern 1995). The potential repertoire of Opa proteins is greater in *N. gonorrhoeae* than in *N. meningitidis*, as 12 genes in the former and 3 or 4 genes in the latter have been identified that encode Opa proteins (Meyer and van Putten 1989). However, there are no more than 2 loci present in the chromosomal DNA of *N. lactamica* and *N. flava* and only one copy in the genome of *N. mucosa*, *N. subflava* and *N. sicca* (Wolff and Stern 1995). Each of the Opa genes is complete with a functional promoter (Stern et al. 1986, Stern and Meyer 1987). All of the Opa protein genes are apparently transcribed, although not all are translated.

The Opa genes contain variable numbers of DNA base repeat units which appear to be responsible for the variable lengths of the various Opa genes. The addition or removal of these repeat units forces a given reading frame into an out of frame position. Only the correct frame can allow the individual opac-

ity transcripts to be translated into a functional protein. This is due to changes in the reading frame resulting from the presence of from 7 to 28 repeats of the pentameric sequence CTCTT in the leader peptide region of the Opa protein genes. The changes in the reading frame of these genes are RecA independent and are thought to be due to replicative slippage (Meyer and van Putten 1989). Consequently, the expression of each gene can be independently switched on and off depending on the number of pentameric sequences. These phase transitions occur frequently and may reach several per cent per cell per generation. Antigenic variation among the Opa proteins of a single strain can also occur by recombination among Opa protein genes (Connell et al. 1988).

Opa proteins have an important role in bacterial adherence. The variable expression of these proteins by *N. gonorrhoeae* and *N. meningitidis* represents important cell tropism determinants. Different Opa proteins mediate the attachment of gonococci and meningococci to epithelial cells and to neutrophils (Meyer and van Putten 1989). Recent data indicate that specific Opa proteins facilitate the invasion of epithelial cells by *N. gonorrhoeae* (Simon and Rest 1992, Kupsch et al. 1993).

The Opa proteins of *N. gonorrhoeae* and *N. meningitidis* can undergo antigenic variation during natural infections which may allow these organisms to evade the host's immune response or colonize various sites within the host. Gonococcal Opa proteins have been shown to vary during the menstrual cycle (James and Swanson 1978, Draper et al. 1980) and during infection (Zak et al. 1984). Opa protein variation has also been demonstrated in a human challenge model of infection (Jerse et al. 1994). Meningococci isolated from different anatomical sites may also differ in the expression of Opa proteins (Poolman, DeMarie and Zanen 1980, Tinsley and Heckels 1986).

4.5 Other outer-membrane proteins

Gonococci and meningococci also possess a protein called PilC, that appears to function in epithelial-cell-specific pilus-associated adherence (Rudel, Scheuerpflug and Meyer 1995). In addition, a number of other outer-membrane proteins have been described in *N. gonorrhoeae* and *N. meningitidis*. These include the H.8 antigen (a lipoprotein of unknown function), Laz (a lipid-associated azurin) and a 36 kDa glycolipid-binding adhesin (Cannon 1989, Paruchuri et al. 1990). A number of environmentally regulated outer-membrane proteins have also been identified in *N. gonorrhoeae* and *N. meningitidis* (see Table 37.4, p. 887 and Table 37.5).

4.6 Polysaccharides

Several *Neisseria* spp. synthesize polysaccharide capsules and exopolysaccharides (see Table 37.3). Antigenic differences in the capsular polysaccharides is the basis for serogrouping *N. meningitidis*. Presently A, B,

Table 37.5   Iron-regulated proteins produced by *Neisseria gonorrhoeae* and *Neisseria meningitidis*

Proteins[a]	MW	Function
Outer-membrane receptors		
Tbp1 *(tbpA)*	102 kDa	Involved in human transferrin binding
Tbp2 *(tbpB)*	85 kDa	Involved in human transferrin binding
Lbp *(lbpA)*	103 kDa	Receptor for human lactoferrin
HmBP 1	97 kDa	Proposed to be involved in haemin binding
HmBP 2	50 (44) kDa[c]	but exact functions are not known
Hpu[b]	85 kDa	Receptor for haemoglobin–haptoglobin
HmbR[b]	89.5 kDa	Receptor for haemoglobin
FrpB *(frpB)*	76.6 kDa	Unknown
Periplasmic-binding proteins		
Fbp *(fbp)*	33.5 kDa	Binds Fe from transferrin, ferric citrate and haemin
Regulatory proteins		
Fur *(fur)*	16.4 kDa	Serves as a negative transcriptional regulator
Other proteins		
FrpA[b] *(frpA)*	122 kDa	Share homology to RTX toxin family but
FrpC[b] *(frpC)*	198 kDa	functions are not known

[a]Each protein indicated is present in both *N. gonorrhoeae* and *N. meningitidis* with the exception of proteins marked by [b] which are present only in *N. meningitidis*. For genes which have been cloned, the molecular weight of the mature protein has been determined based on the predicted amino acid sequence. Gene designation is listed in ( ).
[c]50 kDa protein is present in *N. meningitidis*.
44 kDa protein is present in *N. gonorrhoeae*.

C, H, I, K, L, W-135, X, Y, Z and 29E are recognized serogroups (Frasch 1989) (see Table 37.2, p. 883). Structural and chemical characterization of meningococcal capsular polysaccharides indicates that they are either homopolymers (serogroups A, B, C and X), or heteropolymers comprised of a monosaccharide-glycerol (serogroups H and Z), disaccharide (serogroups I, K, W-135, Y and 29E), or trisaccharide (serogroup L) repeating unit. Meningococcal capsular polysaccharides also contain the hydrophobic moiety, 1,2-diacylglycerol, which is thought to help anchor one end of the polysaccharide chain in the outer membrane (Gotschlich et al. 1981) (see Table 37.3, p. 884 and 885).

By virtue of its antiphagocytic properties, the capsule of *N. meningitidis* functions as a virulence factor (Masson, Holbein and Ashton 1982). In general, meningococcal capsular polysaccharides are immunogenic in humans. Vaccine formulations based on serogroups A, C, W-135 and Y capsular polysaccharides are available for use in humans and elicit bactericidal antibodies directed against the capsule. However, the group B capsular polysaccharide is poorly immunogenic because of its similarity to sialic acid moieties found in human tissues. Both the biochemistry and genetics of group B capsular polysaccharide synthesis have been elucidated (Masson and Holbein 1983, Frosh, Weisberger and Meyer 1989).

Morphological evidence provided by several earlier studies suggested that gonococci also possess a capsule (Hendley et al. 1977, 1981, James and Swanson 1977, Richardson and Sadoff 1977, Demarco de Hormaeche, Thornley and Glavert 1978, Melly et al. 1979, Reimann, Heise and Blom 1988); however, a capsular polysaccharide has never been isolated or characterized. *N. gonorrhoeae* (and other *Neisseria* spp.) produce a high molecular weight extracellular polyphosphate that may serve the function of a capsule in this species (Noegel and Gotschlich 1983).

Under certain growth conditions, some non-pathogenic *Neisseria* spp. synthesize extracellular polysaccharides. *N. perflava* possesses the enzyme amylosucrase which transfers the glucosyl moiety of sucrose to a 1–4-α-D-glucan to form a glycogen-like polysaccharide (Okada and Hehre 1974). Other *Neisseria* spp. (i.e. *N. polysaccharea*, *N. denitrificans*, *N. canis*, *N. cinerea* and *N. subflava*) produce a similar polysaccharide during growth on a medium containing 1–5% sucrose (MacKenzie, McDonald and Johnson 1977, 1978a, 1978b, MacKenzie et al. 1978, Riou et al. 1986). The structure of these d-glucans in shown in Table 37.3 (p. 884 and 885). *N. sicca* synthesizes a galactosamine polymer, the function of which is presently unknown (Adams and Chaudhari 1972, Wagner, Cooper and Bishop 1973).

4.7   Lipopolysaccharide

Lipopolysaccharide (LPS) is the major glycolipid component of the outer membrane of gram-negative bacteria. High molecular weight LPS from enteric bacteria such as *E. coli* is comprised of a lipid A moiety, a core oligosaccharide and a repeating O-antigen polysaccharide. Gonococcal and meningococcal LPS are smaller glycolipid molecules that lack the repeating O-antigen polysaccharides (Mintz, Apicella and Morse 1984). They are similar in size to the LPS from rough mutants of *Salmonella*, but with considerable antigenic diversity. The oligosaccharide component of meningococcal and gonococcal LPS consists of relatively short, multiantennary glycans (Phillips et al. 1990). In the case of the meningococcus, a serological typing system has been developed that separates strains into 12 immunotypes (see Table 37.2, p. 883); antigenic variability of gonococcal LPS within a single strain is so marked that the development of a similar classification system has proved elusive. The size and structural differences of these molecules have led to their designation as lipo-oligosaccharides (LOS) rather than LPS. Similar glycolipids have been identified in other bacteria (e.g. *H. influenzae, Haemophilus ducreyi* and *Bordetella pertussis*) that colonize or infect the mucosal surfaces of the respiratory and genital tracts.

LOS has a number of biological activities and probably plays an important role in pathogenesis. LOS possesses potent endotoxic activity and is believed to be the toxin responsible for adrenal cortical necrosis seen in severe meningococcal disease. LOS also serves as the target antigen for much of the bactericidal antibody present in normal or convalescent sera (Rice and Kasper 1977).

The LOS may help gonococci and meningococci avoid the host's immune response. The oligosaccharide structures of these molecules mimic host antigens. The tetrasaccharide Gal-β1→4GlcNAc-β1→3Gal-β1→4Glc-β1→4 is a perfect mimic of lacto-*N*-neotetraose of the sphingolipid paragloboside (Mandrell, Griffiss and Macher 1988, Tsai and Civin 1991); the addition of a terminal *N*-acetylgalactosamine residue results in a structure that mimics gangliosides. Some gonococcal strains synthesize LOS molecules with the alternative glycan side chain Gal-α1→4Gal-β1→4Glc-β1→, which mimics the saccharide portion of globoglycolipids (Pk-like antigen) (John et al. 1991). The terminal lacto-*N*-neotetraose tetrasaccharide on gonococcal and meningococcal LOS is the target for sialylation by an endogenous sialyltransferase. Gonococci utilize exogenously supplied cytidine-5'-monophospho-*N*-acetylneuraminic acid (CMP-NANA) and add NANA to the LOS on the surface of the organism; meningococci synthesize the CMP-NANA. Gonococcal strains appear to be sialylated in vivo (Apicella et al. 1990); sialylated LOS is lost after growth in vitro. Sialylation of gonococcal LOS is associated with increased resistance to killing by normal human serum (Parsons et al. 1992). The addition of this terminal sialic acid residue may downregulate the alternative complement pathway or mask protective epitopes.

The LOS of *N. gonorrhoeae* exhibits antigenic variation at a frequency of 10^{-2}–10^{-3} (Apicella et al. 1987). This variation in LOS structure may be another mechanism for evading host defences. Experimental gonococcal infection in volunteers indicates that bacteria isolated early in the infection have a short LOS, whereas after the development of an inflammatory response a different bacterial phenotype with a long LOS species predominates (Griffiss et al. 1988). Recently, a locus involved in the biosynthesis of gonococcal LOS encoding glycosyl transferases has been cloned and sequenced (Gotschlich 1994). Several of the genes contained poly-G tracts. Slippage in such poly-G tracts may provide an explanation for the high-frequency variation of expression of these genes.

4.8 Regulatory responses

The ability of a pathogen to colonize and proliferate within a particular environmental niche in the host is essential for the initiation of an infection. Each of the diverse sites within the human host in which *N. gonorrhoeae* and *N. meningitidis* infect represents a unique niche with respect to nutrients, environmental factors and competing micro-organisms. The growth environment has a marked effect on the metabolism and cellular composition; altered cellular composition is often reflected by changes in the cell surface that can ultimately affect the interaction of these micro-organisms with the human host (Chen et al. 1989).

After entry into the human host the pathogenic *Neisseria* must multiply to colonize mucosal surfaces and to establish an infection. Growth depends in part upon the ability of these organisms to scavenge essential nutrients; of these nutrients, iron plays a crucial role in the establishment and progression of an infection (Wooldridge and Williams 1993). In response to the iron-limited environment of the host, most micro-organisms synthesize a unique class of iron-regulated proteins. These iron-regulated proteins are thought to function either in the acquisition of growth essential iron or as mediators of microbial virulence.

N. gonorrhoeae expresses a number of iron-regulated proteins when grown in vitro under iron-limited conditions (Chen et al. 1989, Genco and Desai 1996) and they possess several mechanisms for obtaining essential iron from their environment. These mechanisms differ from the typical siderophore-mediated mechanism described for many other pathogens. For example, gonococci and meningococci express both transferrin (TF) and lactoferrin (LF) receptors; these receptors are involved in the acquisition of iron from these host binding proteins. The TF receptor appears to consist of a complex of 2 TF-binding proteins (Tbps), a relatively conserved Tbp1 and an antigenically and size variable Tbp2. Although Tbp2 is required for TF-mediated iron uptake, its TF-binding activity appears to depend on the presence of Tbp1 (Cornelissen et al. 1992, Anderson, Sparling and Cornelissen 1994, Cornelissen and Sparling 1994). A LF-binding protein (Lbp1) has been shown to bind LF in vitro; studies using a *N. gonorrhoeae* insertional mutant in the Lbp1 gene (*lbpA*) have confirmed the role of Lbp1 in LF binding and utilization (Biswas and Sparling 1995). In addition to the utilization of TF and LF bound iron, *N. gonorrhoeae* and *N. meningitidis* can utilize free haemoglobin, haemoglobin bound to haptoglobin and free haem as iron sources (Dyer, West and Sparling 1987). Using haemin-agarose in batch affinity chromatography, putative haemin-binding proteins of 97 and 50 kDa and 97 and 44 kDa have been isolated from *N. meningitidis* and *N. gonorrhoeae*, respectively (Lee 1992, 1994). Biotinylated human haemoglobin has also been used as an affinity ligand to identify putative haemoglobin-binding proteins from *N. meningitidis* (Lee and Hill 1992). FrpB, an iron-regulated protein, is thought to play a role in haemin utilization; however, a function in iron uptake has not been documented (Beucher and Sparling 1995). A putative haptoglobin–haemoglobin binding protein (Hpu) has also been identified in *N. meningitidis* and thought to be involved in haemoglobin utilization (Lewis and Dyer 1995). Stojiljkovic et al. (1995) have also cloned and characterized the *N. meningitidis* haemoglobin receptor, HmbR.

In addition to the distinct nutrient-regulated expression of antigens, the pathogenic *Neisseria* spp. display a uniform stress response irrespective of the nature of the environment. A number of stress (or heat shock) proteins have been identified. The most abundant neisserial stress protein is genetically conserved among the *Neisseria* spp. and has considerable homology to the Hsp60 heat shock protein family (Pannekoek, van Putten and Dankert 1992). Analysis of patient sera indicates that this antigen is expressed and immunogenic in vivo.

Another environmental factor influencing the expression of gonococcal genes is oxygen. The growth of *N. gonorrhoeae* in the absence of oxygen with nitrite as a terminal electron acceptor results in the expression of several additional proteins and the repression of others (Keevil et al. 1986, Clark et al. 1987). The major anaerobically induced protein is a surface-exposed 54 kDa lipoprotein, designated Pan1 (Hoehn and Clark 1992). Coisolation of gonococci and obligate anaerobic micro-organisms from the site of infection and the presence of antibodies against the anaerobically induced proteins in the sera of patients with neisserial disease (Clark et al. 1988) suggest that anaerobic growth of *Neisseria* spp. occurs in vivo. Although *N. meningitidis* contains a gene for the Pan1 protein (*aniA*), the gene is expressed at significantly lower levels (Clark and Silver 1994). Transcription of *aniA* occurs from 2 promoters: the gearbox promoter and a minor σ 70 promoter.

4.9 Pathogenicity and virulence factors

Several factors have been proposed to play a crucial role in the pathogenesis of neisserial infections. These include surface components such as pili, outer-membrane proteins, capsule, LPS and the secretion of an IgA1 protease. Attachment of gonococci to mucosal cells is mediated in part by pili, although non-specific factors such as surface charge and hydrophobicity may be important. Pili formation and pilus-mediated binding of *N. gonorrhoeae* to epithelial cells is an important prerequisite for gonococcal infection in vivo. Results of in vitro studies, using transformed epithelial cell lines, suggests that gonococcal invasion is enhanced in the absence of pili. Specific Opa proteins appear to facilitate invasion under these conditions (Kupsch et al. 1993). However, additional invasion factors, some of which may be tightly regulated and induced upon Opa-mediated contact with epithelial cells, may also play a role in invasion (Kahrs et al. 1994). The production of PilC proteins, which are necessary for pilus assembly, pilus-mediated adherence and natural transformation competence, also plays a role in the invasion of human epithelial cells by *N. gonorrhoeae*

(Rudel, Scheuerpflug and Meyer 1995). Gonococci attach only to microvilli of non-ciliated columnar epithelial cells; attachment to ciliated cells is not observed. Gonococcal invasion of epithelial cells has been demonstrated in vitro but it is not clear if this represents a normal part of uncomplicated mucosal infection. There is evidence that suggests that in complicated infections, such as salpingitis and disseminated gonococcal infection, cellular invasion is an important factor in the pathogenesis of the disease. Invasion may serve as a means for *N. gonorrhoeae* to bypass transiently through polarized epithelial cells as opposed to a long-term intracellular habitat.

To cause disease the meningococcus must first breach the mucosal barrier. Adherence of *N. meningitidis* to human cells is an important virulence attribute. Meningococci attach to the non-ciliated columnar epithelial cells of the nasopharynx via pili and the class 5 outer-membrane protein. Pili are the major components that determine the attachment of meningococci to non-ciliated cells; piliated encapsulated meningococci are more capable of damaging ciliated cells than are non-piliated meningococci (Stephens, Hoffman and McGee 1983). Meningococci exert a toxic effect on ciliated cells from a distance, suggesting the release of soluble toxins by the bacteria or the induction of cytotoxic host factors by these components.

Meningococci are also capable of invasion and this process appears to be similar to that observed with the gonococcus; however, once internalized, meningococci remain in an apical location within epithelial cells. Meningococci and gonococci enter epithelial cells by parasite-directed endocytosis (Stephens et al. 1986, Stephens and Farley 1991) and large numbers of organisms can be typically found in the phagocytic vacuoles of these cells. Meningococci can also produce a cytotoxic effect, resulting in breakdown of tight junctions of epithelial cells, sloughing of ciliated cells, loss of ciliary activity and alteration of microvilli of non-ciliated cells (Stephens and Farley 1991).

Colonization of the human mucosa by *N. gonorrhoeae* and *N. meningitidis* may typically give rise to an inflammatory response with recruitment and activation of professional phagocytes. Morphological data suggest that in natural infection, the pathogenic *Neisseria* may reside inside phagocytes but prolonged survival has been difficult to establish in vitro (Devoe, Gilchrist and Storm 1973, Swanson and Zelias 1974). Gonococci associated with neutrophils in urethral exudates from males with gonorrhoea are sialylated, indicating that sialylation occurs in vivo within phagocytic cells (Schneider et al. 1991).

N. gonorrhoeae and *N. meningitidis* can also evade the host immune response through the production of molecules that precisely mimic the normal host; thus they are not recognized as foreign. The capsule of group B meningococci is immunochemically identical to a neuraminic acid of the central nervous system and therefore group B capsular polysaccharide is non-immunogenic in humans (Sparling, Tsai and Cornelissen 1990). The terminal structure on the LPS core of gonococcus closely mimics glycosphingolipids on human epithelial cells (Griffiss et al. 1988). Another mechanism utilized by the pathogenic *Neisseria* to escape the host immune response relates to the shedding of pieces of outer membrane or blebs. It is not known if this occurs in vivo, but shedding of blebs containing endotoxin has been suggested as a mechanism by which gonococci damage ciliated cells. Gonococci are highly autolytic and release peptidoglycan fragments during growth. These fragments, released by bacterial and/or host peptidoglycan hydrolases, are toxic for fallopian tube mucosa and contribute to the intense inflammatory reactions characteristic of gonococcal disease.

Infections of the bloodstream (meningococcaemia) or the meninges (meningitis) are characterized by vascular and tissue damage. Although this damage is not completely understood, it is thought to be due mainly to the effects of meningococcal LPS. Meningococcal LPS is highly toxic and has been shown to suppress leukotriene B4 synthesis in human PMNs (Verheul, Snippe and Poolman 1993). Meningococcal LPS can also stimulate release of tumour necrosis factor (TNF), resulting in damage to host cells. The events after bloodstream invasion are unclear and little is known about how the meningococcus enters the central nervous system. Although RTX toxin genes have been cloned from the meningococcus, their functions remain unknown and haemolytic or cytotoxic activity has not been observed in vitro (Verheul, Snippe and Poolman 1993). Another virulence factor of *N. meningitidis* is the antiphagocytic polysaccharide capsule. The capsule, which can mask outer-membrane protein antigens, is essential in defence against the host's immune mechanisms.

Specific antibodies and the complement system play a key role in host defence against *N. meningitidis*. They cause lysis of the bacteria, enhance phagocytosis by monocytes or PMNs, or neutralize the effects mediated by endotoxin. The presence of bactericidal antibody is extremely important; anti-polysaccharide and anti-outer-membrane protein antibodies are bactericidal and facilitate phagocytosis. The role of anti-LPS antibodies remains unclear. The serogroups differ in their susceptibility to serum bactericidal activity or phagocytosis. Group B meningococci are relatively resistant to serum bactericidal activity and are more susceptible to killing by PMNs. In contrast, group Y meningococci are relatively susceptible to the bactericidal activity of serum and resistant to killing by PMNs.

Certain strains of *N. gonorrhoeae* are very susceptible to killing by normal human serum (NHS) whereas others are quite resistant. The bactericidal antibodies are frequently directed at LPS core sugars or at PI. The blocking antibodies frequently are directed at an invariant PIII that exists in an apparent complex with PI and LPS. As mentioned above, PIII shares considerable homology to the *E. coli* OmpA membrane protein. Presumably blocking antibodies in NHS result from colonization by *E. coli* or other bacteria that express antigens such as OmpA and the resultant antibodies help to protect gonococci against killing by anti-LPS or anti-PI antibodies.

N. gonorrhoeae and *N. meningitidis* produce a type 2 IgA1 protease which cleaves this immunoglobulin within the hinge region. IgA1 protease is believed to play an important role in the ability of these organism to evade the host immune response (Mulks and Plaut 1978). The significance of the IgA1 cleavage by the protease is considered to rely on the binding of Fab fragments to the bacterial surface, thereby masking the antigenic epitopes. Genital IgA antibodies may be able to block adherence and since IgA antibodies are capable of complement-dependent lysis of meningococci, they presumably are able to kill gonococci by the same mechanism. All gonococci and meningococci, but not non-pathogenic *Neisseria* spp., produce an IgA1 protease.

For further information on pathogenicity, see Chapter 12.

5 SUSCEPTIBILITY TO ANTIMICROBIAL AGENTS

Penicillin is no longer the antimicrobial of choice for the primary treatment of gonorrhoea due to the development of resistance involving multiple mechanisms (Table 37.6). Resistance to β-lactam antibiotics results from the destruction of the antibiotics by β-lactamases or the presence of penicillin-binding proteins (PBPs) (Dowson, Coffey and Spratt 1994). The increase in the prevalence of β-lactamase producing strains of *N. gonorrhoeae* in the 1970s and 1980s has resulted in a shift to treatment with third generation cephalosporins, such as ceftriaxone, because of their high activity and resistance to β-lactamases. Resistance to penicillin in non-β-lactamase producing *N. gonorrhoeae* is chromosomally mediated and due to the production of low-affinity forms of PBPs combined with reductions in the permeability of the cell envelope to penicillin. Alterations in PBPs have also occurred in *N. meningitidis* to produce isolates with increased resistance to penicillin. In both pathogenic *Neisseria* spp. chromosomal resistance to penicillin results from low-affinity mosaic forms of PBP-2, a bifunctional enzyme with transpeptidase and transglycosylase activities. These have arisen by the replacement of parts of the PBP-2 gene (*penA*) with the corresponding regions from those of the closely related commensal species *N. flavescens* and *N. cinerea* (Dowson, Coffey and Spratt 1994). Other agents for which chromosomal resistance exists in *N. gonorrhoeae* and *N. meningitidis* include tetracycline, sulphonamides and erythromycin (see Table 37.6). In addition, strains with multiple chromosomal resistance to penicillin, tetracycline, erythromycin, and cefoxitin have been identified in the USA and most other parts of the world. Plasmid and chromosomally mediated antibiotic resistance has also been described in a number of commensal *Neisseria* spp. Of interest is the reported plasmid-mediated transferable multiple drug resistance to sulphonamides, streptomycin and penicillin (see Table 37.6) which could potentially spread to *N. meningitidis*.

Penicillin is the drug of choice to treat meningo-

Table 37.6 Antibiotic resistance in *Neisseria*[a]

	N. gonorrhoeae		N.meningitidis		Commensal Neisseria	
	Plasmid	**Chromosomal**	**Plasmid**	**Chromosomal**	**Plasmid**	**Chromosomal**
Penicillin	+	+	+	+	+	+
Tetracycline	+	+	+	+	+	+
Sulphonamides	–	+	–	+	+	+
Trimethoprim	–	+	–	?	–	+
Spectinomycin	–	+	–	?	?	?
Streptomycin	–	+	–	+	+	+
Quinolones (Ciprofloxacin)	–	+	–	?	?	?
Erythromycin	–	+	–	+	?	?
Rifampicin	–	+	–	+	?	?
Pen, Su, Sm[b]	–	–	–	–	+	–

[a]+, antibiotic resistance gene has been reported on either a plasmid or the chromosome; –, antibiotic resistance has not been reported; ?, indicates not known.
[b]Multiple antibiotic resistance to penicillin, sulphonamides, and streptomycin is encoded on a single plasmid.

coccal meningitis and meningococcaemia. Penicillin does not readily penetrate the blood–brain barrier; however, when the meninges are acutely inflamed it can readily penetrate. Recently, penicillin-resistant *N. meningitidis* strains have been described (Brett 1989), indicating that continued use of this drug may be in jeopardy. The *penA* gene from penicillin-resistant *N. meningitidis* is very diverse and 30 mosaic genes have been found in 70 different isolates. In contrast, in *N. gonorrhoeae*, only 3 different mosaic *penA* genes have been identified. It would appear that the opportunity for acquiring DNA from commensal *Neisseria* spp. is greater for *N. meningitidis* which inhabits the naso-

pharynx normally. Tetracycline resistance in *N. meningitidis* due to the acquisition of the 25 200 kDa TetM plasmid has also been described (Roberts and Knapp 1988). Sulphonamide resistance in *N. meningitidis* is due to chromosomally mediated determinants (Fermer and Kristiansen 1995). Recent evidence indicates that the origin of the sulphonamide resistance determinants genes may have been from other *Neisseria* species (Fermer and Kristiansen 1995). This observation supports the idea of interspecies transfer of genetic material in *Neisseria* species as a major mechanism for the development of chromosomally mediated resistance.

REFERENCES

Adams GA, Chaudhari AS, 1972, Galactosamine polymer isolated from the cell wall of *Neisseria sicca*, *Can J Biochem*, **50:** 345–51.

Aho EL, Murphy GL, Cannon JG, 1987, Distribution of specific DNA sequences among pathogeneic and commensal *Neisseria* species, *Infect Immun*, **55:** 1009–13.

Andersen BM, Skjorten F, Solberg O, 1979, Electron microscopical study of *Neisseria meningitidis* releasing various amounts of free endotoxin, *Acta Pathol Microbiol Scand Sect B*, **87:** 109–15.

Andersen BM, Solberg O, 1978, Liberation of endotoxin during growth of *Neisseria meningitidis* in a chemically-defined medium, *Acta Pathol Microbiol Scand Sect B*, **86:** 275–81.

Andersen BM, Steigerwalt AG et al., 1993, *Neisseria weaveri* sp. nov., formerly CDC group M-5, a gram-negative bacterium associated with dog bite wounds, *J Clin Microbiol*, **31:** 2456–66.

Anderson JE, Sparling PF, Cornelissen CN, 1994, Gonococcal transferrin-binding protein 2 facilitates but is not essential for transferrin utilization, *J Bacteriol*, **176:** 3162–70.

Annear DI, 1981, Growth of *Neisseria gonorrhoeae* in a simple medium at 28°C, *J Clin Pathol*, **34:** 688.

Annear DI, Grubb WB, 1982, Growth of *Neisseria gonorrhoeae* at 25°C, *J Clin Pathol*, **35:** 118–19.

Apicella MA, Shero M et al., 1987, Phenotypic variation in epitope expression of the *Neisseria gonorrhoeae* lipooligosaccharide, *Infect Immun*, **55:** 1755–61.

Apicella MA, Mandrell RE et al., 1990, Modification by sialic acid of *Neisseria gonorrhoeae* lipooligosaccharide expression in human urethral exudates: an immunoelectron microscopic analysis, *J Infect Dis*, **162:** 506–12.

Ashford WA, Golash RG, Hemming UG, 1976, Penicillinase producing *Neisseria gonorrhoeae*, *Lancet*, **2:** 657–8.

Barrett SJ, Schlater LK et al., 1994, A new species of *Neisseria* from iguanid lizards, *Neisseria iguanae* sp. nov., *Lett Appl Microbiol*, **18:** 200–2.

Berger U, 1960, *Neisseria animalis* n. sp., *Zentralbl Infektionskr Hyg*, **147:** 158–61.

Berger U, 1962, Uber das Vorkommen von *Neisserien* bei einigen Tieren, *Z Hyg*, **148:** 445–57.

Berger U, 1971, *Neisseria mucosa* var. *heidelbergensis*, *Z Med Mikrobiol Immunol*, **156:** 154–8.

Bergstrom S, Robbins K, et al., 1986, Piliation control mechanisms in Neisseria *gonorrhoeae*, *Proc Natl Acad Sci USA*, **83:** 3890–4.

Beucher M, Sparling PF, 1995, Cloning, sequencing, and characterization of the gene encoding FrpB, a major iron-regulated, outer membrane protein of *Neisseria gonorrhoeae*, *J Bacteriol*, **177:** 2041–9.

Biswas GD, Blackman EY, Sparling PF, 1980, High frequency conjugal transfer of a gonococcal penicillinase plasmid, *J Bacteriol*, **143:** 1318–24.

Biswas GD, Sparling PF, 1986, Linearization of donor plasmid during transformation in the gonococcus, *Abstracts 1986 American Society for Microbiology Meeting*.

Biswas GD, Sparling PF, 1995, Characterization of *lbpA*, the structural gene for a LF receptor in *Neisseria gonorrhoeae*, *Infect Immun*, **63:** 2958–67.

Blackwell CC, Young H, Anderson I, 1979, Sensitivity of *Neisseria gonorrhoeae* to partially purified R-type pyocines and a possible approach to epidemiological typing, *J Med Microbiol*, **12:** 321–35.

Blake MS, Gotschlich EC, 1987, Functional and immunogenic properties of pathogenic *Neisseria* surface proteins, *Bacterial Membranes as Model Systems*, ed. Inouye M, John Wiley & Sons, New York, 379.

Blake MS, Wetzler LM et al., 1989, Protein III: structure, function, and genetics, *Clin Microbiol Rev*, **2, Suppl.:** S60–3.

Blakebrough IS, Greenwood VM et al., 1982, The epidemiology of infections due to *Neisseria meningitidis* and *Neisseria lactamica* in a Northern Nigerian community, *J Infect Dis*, **146:** 626–37.

Boquete MT, Marcos C, Saez-Nieto JA, 1986, Characterization of *Neisseria polysacchareae* sp. nov. (Riou, 1983) in previously identified noncapsular strains of *Neisseria meningitidis*, *J Clin Microbiol*, **23:** 973–5.

Bovre K, 1984, Family VIII, Neisseriaceae Prevot 1933, *Bergey's Manual of Systematic Bacteriology*, vol. 1, eds Krieg NR, Holt JG, The William & Wilkins Co, Baltimore, 288–90.

Boyce JM, Taylor MR et al., 1985, Nosocomial pneumonia caused by a glucose-metabolizing strain of *Neisseria cinerea*, *J Clin Microbiol*, **21:** 1–3.

Branham SA, 1930, A new meningococcus-like organism (*Neisseria flavescens* sp.) from epidemic meningitis, *Public Health Rep*, **45:** 845.

Brett MSY, 1989, Conjugal transfer of gonococcal beta-lactamase and conjugative plasmids to *Neisseria meningitidis*, *J Antimicrobiol Chemother*, **24:** 875–9.

Brookes R, Sikyta B, 1967, Influence of pH on the growth characteristics of *Neisseria gonorrhoeae* in continuous culture, *Appl Microbiol*, **15:** 224–7.

Brunham RC, Plummer F et al., 1985, Correlation of auxotype and protein I type with expression of disease due to *Neisseria gonorrhoeae*, *J Infect Dis*, **152:** 339–43.

Buchanan TM, Eschenbach DA et al., 1980, Gonococcal salpingitis is less likely to recur with *Neisseria gonorrhoeae* of the same principal outer membrane protein antigenic type, *Am J Obstet Gynecol*, **138:** 978–80.

Bumm E, 1885a, *Dtsch Med Wochenschr*, **11:** 508.

Bumm E, 1885b, *Dtsch Med Wochenschr*, **11:** 910.

Burdett V, Inamine J, Rajagopalan S, 1982, Heterogeneity of tetracycline resistance determinants in *Streptococcus*, *J Bacteriol*, **149:** 995–1004.

Cannon JG, 1989, Conserved lipoproteins of pathogenic *Neisseria* spp bearing the H.8 epitope, lipid-modified azurin, and H.8 outer membrane protein, *Clin Microbiol Rev*, **2, Suppl.:** S1–4.

Cannon JG, BuchananTM, Sparling PF, 1983, Confirmation of association of protein I serotype of *Neisseria gonorrhoeae* with ability to cause disseminated infection, *Infect Immun*, **40:** 816–19.

Cannon JG, Sparling PF, 1984, The genetics of the gonococcus, *Annu Rev Microbiol*, **38:** 111–33.

Catlin BW, 1973, Nutritional profiles of *Neisseria gonorrhoeae*, *Neisseria meningitidis*, and *Neisseria lactamica* in chemically defined media and the use of growth requirements for gonococcal typing, *J Infect Dis*, **128:** 178–94.

Catlin BW, 1975, Cellular elongation under the influence of antibacterial agents: way to differentiate coccobacilli from cocci, *J Clin Microbiol*, **1:** 102–5.

Catlin BW, 1978, Characteristics and auxotyping of *Neisseria gonorrhoeae*, *Methods in Microbiology*, vol. 10, eds Bergan T, Norris JR, Academic Press, London, 345–80.

Catlin BW, 1991, Branhamaceae fam. nov., a proposed family to accommodate the genera *Branhamella* and *Moraxella*, *Int J Syst Bacteriol*, **41:** 320–3.

Catlin BW, Cunningham LS, 1961, Transforming activities and base contents of deoxyribonucleate preparations from various Neisseriae, *J Gen Microbiol*, **26:** 303–12.

Centers for Disease Control, 1993, Sexually transmitted diseases treatment guidelines, *Morbid Mortal Weekly Rep*, **42 RR-14:** 4–5.

Chen CY, Genco CA et al., 1989, Physiology and metabolism of *Neisseria gonorrhoeae* and *Neisseria meningitidis*, *Clin Microbiol Rev*, **2, Suppl.:** S35–40.

Chen CY, Berish SA et al., 1993, The ferric iron-binding protein of pathogenic *Neisseria* sp. functions as a periplasmic transport protein in iron acquisition from human transferrin, *Mol Microbiol*, **10:** 311–18.

Clark VL, Silver LE, 1994, Regulation of *aniA* expression by oxygen availability in *Neisseria gonorrhoeae* and *N. meningitidis*, *Proceedings of the Pathogeneic* Neisseria *Meeting*, eds Evans JS, Yost SE et al., 148–9.

Clark VL, Campbell LA et al., 1987, Induction and repression of outer membrane proteins by anaerobic growth of *Neisseria gonorrhoeae*, *Infect Immun*, **55:** 1359–64.

Clark VL, Knapp JS et al., 1988, Presence of antibodies to the major anaerobically induced outer membrane protein in sera from patients with gonococcal infection, *Microb Pathog*, **5:** 381–90.

Connell TD, Black WJ et al., 1988, Recombination among protein II genes of *Neisseria gonorrhoeae* generates new coding sequences and increases structural variability in the protein II family, *Mol Microbiol*, **2:** 227–36.

Cornelissen CN, Biswas GD et al., 1992, Gonococcal transferrin-binding protein 1 is required for transferrin utilization and is homologous to TonB-dependent outer membrane receptors, *J Bacteriol*, **174:** 5788–97.

Cornelissen CN, Sparling PF, 1994, Iron piracy: acquisition of transferrin-bound iron by bacterial pathogens, *Mol Microbiol*, **14:** 843–50.

Cox DL, Baugh CL, 1977, Carboxylation of phosphoenolpyruvate by extracts of *Neisseria gonorrhoeae*, *J Bacteriol*, **129:** 202–6.

Davis CL, Towns M et al., 1983, *Neisseria mucosa* endocarditis following drug abuse. Case report and review of the literature, *Arch Intern Med*, **143:** 583–5.

Demarco de Hormaeche R, Thornley MJ, Glauert AM, 1978, Demonstration by light and electron microscopy of capsules on gonococci recently grown in vivo, *J Gen Microbiol*, **106:** 81–91.

Densen P, Mandell GI, 1978, Gonococcal interactions with polymorphonuclear neutrophils: importance of the phagosome for bactericidal activity, *J Clin Invest*, **62:** 1161–71.

Dent VE, 1982, Identification of oral *Neisseria* species of animals, *J Appl Microbiol*, **52:** 21–30.

Devoe IW, Gilchrist JE, 1974, Ultrastructure of pili and annular structures on the cell wall surface of *Neisseria meningitidis*, *Infect Immun*, **10:** 872–6.

Devoe IW, Gilchrist JE, Storm DW, 1973, Ultrastructural studies on the fate of group B meningococci in human peripheral blood leucocytes, *Can J Microbiol*, **19:** 1355–9.

Dewhirst FE, Paster BJ, Bright PL, 1989, *Chromobacterium*, *Eikenella*, *Kingella*, *Neisseria*, *Simonsiella*, and *Vitreoscilla* species comprise a major branch of the beta group Protebacteria by 16S ribosomal ribonucleic acid sequence comparison: transfer of *Eikenella* and *Simonsiella* to the family Neisseriaceae (emend.), *Int J Syst Bacteriol*, **39:** 258–66.

Dilworth JA, Hendley JO, Mandell GL, 1975, Attachment and ingestion of gonococci by human neutrophils, *Infect Immun*, **11:** 512–16.

Doern GV, Blacklow NR et al., 1982, *Neisseria sicca* osteomyelitis, *J Clin Microbiol*, **16:** 595–7.

Dorward DW, Garon CF, Judd RC, 1989, Export and intercellular transfer of DNA via membrane blebs of *Neisseria gonorrhoeae*, *J Bacteriol*, **171:** 2499–505.

Douglas JT, Lee MD, Nikaido H, 1981, Protein I of *Neisseria gonorrhoeae* is a porin, *FEMS Microbiol Lett*, **12:** 305–9.

Dowson CG, Coffey TJ, Spratt BG, 1994, Origin and molecular epidemiology of penicillin-binding-protein-mediated resistance to beta-lactam antibiotics, *Trends Microbiol*, **2:** 361–6.

Draper DL, James JF et al., 1980, Comparison of virulence markers of peritoneal and fallopian tube isolates with endocervical *Neisseria gonorrhoeae* isolates from women with salpingitis, *Infect Immun*, **27:** 882–8.

Dudas KC, Apicella MA, 1988, Selection and immunochemical analysis of lipooligosaccharide mutants of *Neisseria gonorrhoeae*, *Infect Immun*, **56:** 499–504.

Dyer DW, West EP, Sparling PF, 1987, Effects of serum carrier proteins the growth of pathogenic neisseriae with heme-bound iron, *Infect Immun*, **55:** 2171–5.

Earl RG, Dennison D et al., 1976, Preliminary studies in the clinical use of a bicarbonate containing growth medium for *Neisseria gonorrhoeae*, *J Am Vener Dis Assoc*, **3:** 40–2.

Elkins C, Carbonetti NH et al., 1992, Antibodies to N-terminal peptides of gonococcal porin are bactericidal when gonococcal lipopolysaccharide is not sialylated, *Mol Microbiol*, **6:** 2617–28.

Elleman TC, 1988, Pilins of *Bacteroides nodosus*: molecular basis of serotypic variation and relationships to other bacterial pilins, *Microbiol Rev*, **52:** 233–47.

Facius D, Meyer TF, 1993, A novel determinant (comA) essential for natural transformation competence in *Neisseria gonorrhoeae* and the effect of a comA defect on pilin variation, *Mol Microbiol*, **10:** 699–712.

Fermer C, Kristiansen B-E, 1995, Sulfonamide resitance in *Neisseria meningitidis* as defined by site-directed mutagenesis could have its orgin in other species, *J Bacteriol*, **177:** 4669–75.

Fitz-James P, 1964, Thin sections of dividing *Neisseria gonorrhoeae*, *J Bacteriol*, **87:** 1477–82.

Flett F, Humphreys GO, Saunders JR, 1980, Mobilization of non-conjugative R plasmids by the 24.5 megadalton plasmid of *Neisseria gonorrhoeae*, *Genetics and Immunobiology of Pathogenic Neisseria*, eds Danielson D, Normark S, University of Umea, Umea, Sweden, 153–6.

Flynn J, McEntegart MG, 1972, Bacteriocins from *Neisseria gonorrhoeae* and their possible role in epidemiological studies, *J Clin Pathol*, **25:** 60–1.

Frasch CE, 1989, Vaccines for prevention of meningococcal disease, *Clin Microbiol Rev*, **2, Suppl.:** S134–8.

Frosch M, Weisberger C, Meyer TF, 1989, Molecular characterization and expression in *Escherichia coli* of the gene complex encoding the polysaccharide capsule of *Neisseria meningitidis* group B, *Proc Natl Acad Sci USA*, **86:** 1669–73.

Genco CA, Desai P, 1996, Iron acquisition in the pathogenic *Neisseria*: implications for pathogenesis, *Trends Microbiol*, **4:** 179–84.

Genco CA, Knapp JS, Clark VL, 1984, Conjugation of plasmids of *Neisseria gonorrhoeae* to other *Neisseria* species: potential reservoirs for the beta-lactamase plasmid, *J Infect Dis*, **150:** 397–401.

Genco CA, Chen CY et al., 1991, Isolation and characterization of a mutant of *Neisseria gonorrhoeae* that is defective in the uptake of iron from transferrin and hemoglobin and is avirulent in mouse subcutaneous chambers, *J Gen Microbiol*, **137:** 1313–21.

Getzoff ED, Parge HE et al., 1988, Understanding the structure and antigenicity of gonococcal pili, *Rev Infect Dis*, **10, Suppl. 2:** S296–9.

Gibbs CP, Reimann B-Y et al., 1989, Reassortment of pilin genes in *Neisseria gonorrhoeae* occurs by two distinct mechanisms, *Nature (London)*, **338:** 651–2.

Gilrane T, Tracy JD et al., 1985, *Neisseria sicca* pneumonia. Report of two cases and review of the literature, *Am J Med*, **78:** 1038–40.

Gini GA, 1987, Ocular infection in a newborn caused by *Neisseria mucosa*, *J Clin Microbiol*, **25:** 1574–5.

Gold R, Goldschneider I et al., 1978, Carriage of *Neisseria meningitidis* and *Neisseria lactamica* in infants and children, *J Infect Dis*, **137:** 112–21.

Gotschlich EC, 1994, Genetic locus for the biosynthesis of the variable portion of *Neisseria gonorrhoeae* lipooligosaccharide, *J Exp Med*, **180:** 2181–90.

Gotschlich EC, Fraser BA et al., 1981, Lipid on capsular polysaccharide of Gram-negative bacteria, *J Biol Chem*, **256:** 8915–21.

Gotschlich EC, Blake MS et al., 1986, Cloning of the structural genes of three H.8 antigens and of protein III of *Neisseria gonorrhoeae*, *J Exp Med*, **164:** 868–81.

Gotschlich EC, Seiff ME et al., 1987, Porin protein of *Neisseria gonorrhoeae*: cloning and gene structure, *Proc Natl Acad Sci USA*, **84:** 8135–9.

Grant PE, Brenner DJ et al., 1990, *Neisseria elongata* subsp. *nitroreducens* subsp. nov., formerly CDC group M-6, a gram-negative bacterium associated with endocarditis, *J Clin Microbiol*, **28:** 2591–6.

Griffin PJ, Racker E, 1956, The carbon dioxide requirement of *Neisseria gonorrhoeae*, *J Bacteriol*, **71:** 717–21.

Griffin PJ, Reider SV, 1957, A study of the growth requirements of *Neisseria gonorrhoeae* and its clinical application, *Yale J Biol Med*, **29:** 613–21.

Griffiss JM, Schneider H et al., 1988, Lipopolysaccharides: the principal glycolipids of the neisserial outer membrane, *Rev Infect Dis*, **10, Suppl. 2:** S287–95.

Guiney DG, Ito JI, 1982, Transfer of the gonococcal penicillinase plasmid: mobilization in *Escherchia coli* by IncP plasmids and isolation as a DNA-protein relaxation complex, *J Bacteriol*, **150:** 298–302.

Guymon LF, Esser M, Shafer WM, 1982, Pyocin resistant lipopolysaccharide mutants of *Neisseria gonorrhoeae*: alterations in sensitivity to normal human serum and polymyxin B, *Infect Immun*, **36:** 541–7.

Haas R, Meyer TF, 1986, The repertoire of silent pilus genes in *Neisseria gonorrhoeae*: evidence for gene conversion, *Cell*, **44:** 107–15.

Haas R, Kahrs AF et al., 1993, TnMax – a versatile mini-transposon for the analysis of cloned genes and shuttle mutagenesis, *Gene*, **130:** 23–31.

Hagman M, Danielsson D, 1989, Increased adherence to vaginal epithelial cells and phagocytic killing of gonococci and urethral meningococci associated with heat modifiable proteins, *APMIS*, **97:** 839–44.

Haines KA, Yeh L et al., 1988, Protein I, a translocatable ion channel from *Neisseria gonorrhoeae*, selectively inhibits exocytosis from human neutrophils without inhibiting superoxide generation, *J Biol Chem*, **263:** 945–51.

Handsfield HH, Sandstrom JS et al., 1982, Epidemiology of penicillinase-producing *Neisseria gonorrhoeae* infections: analysis by auxotyping and serotyping, *N Engl J Med*, **306:** 950–4.

Hebeler BH, Morse SA, 1976, Physiology and metabolism of pathogenic *Neisseria*: tricarboxylic acid cycle activity in *Neisseria gonorrhoeae*, *J Bacteriol*, **128:** 192–201.

Hebeler BH, Young FE, 1976, Chemical composition and turnover of peptidoglycan in *Neisseria gonorrhoeae*, *J Bacteriol*, **126:** 1180–5.

Hebeler BH, Wong W et al., 1979, Cell envelope of *Neisseria gonorrhoeae* CS-7: peptidoglycan-protein complex, *Infect Immun*, **23:** 353–9.

Heckels JE, 1989, Structure and function of pili of pathogenic *Neisseria* species, *Clin Microbiol Rev*, **2, Suppl.:** S66–73.

Heckels JE, Blackett B et al., 1976, The influence of surface charge on the adhesion of *Neisseria gonorrhoeae* to human cells, *J Gen Microbiol*, **96:** 359–64.

Hendley JO, Powell KR et al., 1977, Demonstration of a capsule on *Neisseria gonorrhoeae*, *N Engl J Med*, **296:** 608–11.

Hendley JO, Powell KR et al., 1981, Electron microscopy of the gonococcal capsule, *J Infect Dis*, **143:** 796–802.

Herbert DA, Ruskin J, 1981, Are the 'nonpathogenic' neisseriae pathogenic?, *Am J Clin Pathol*, **75:** 739–43.

Hermodsen MA, Chen KCS, Buchanan TM, 1978, *Neisseria* pili proteins: amino terminal sequences and identification of an unusual amino acid, *Biochemistry*, **17:** 442–5.

Hoehn GT, Clark VL, 1992, The major anaerobically induced outer membrane protein of *Neisseria gonorrhoeae*, Pan 1, is a lipoprotein, *Infect Immun*, **60:** 4704–8.

Hollis DG, Wiggins GL, Weaver RE, 1969, *Neisseria lactamicus* sp. n., a lactose-fermenting species resembling *Neisseria meningitidis*, *Appl Microbiol*, **17:** 71–7.

Holmes B, Costas M et al., 1993, *Neisseria weaverii* sp. nov. (formerly CDC group M5) from dog bite wounds of humans, *Int J Syst Bacteriol*, **43**: 687–93.

Holten E, 1974, 6-Phosphogluconate dehydrogenase and enzymes of the Entner–Doudoroff pathway in *Neisseria*, *Acta Pathol Microbiol Scand Sect B*, **82**: 207–13.

Holten E, 1975, Radiorespirometric studies in genus *Neisseria*. I. The catabolism of glucose, *Acta Pathol Microbiol Scand Sect B*, **84**: 353–66.

James JF, Swanson J, 1977, The capsule of the gonococcus, *J Exp Med*, **145**: 1082–6.

James JF, Swanson J, 1978, Studies on gonococcus infection. XIII. Occurrence of color/opacity colonial variants in clinical cultures, *Infect Immun*, **19**: 332–40.

Janda WM, Morello JA et al., 1983, Characteristics of pathogenic *Neisseria* spp. isolated from homosexual men, *J Clin Microbiol*, **17**: 85–91.

Jephcott AE, Reyn A, Birch-Anderson A, 1971, *Neisseria gonorrhoeae*. III. Demonstration of presumed appendages to cells from different colony types, *Acta Pathol Microbiol Scand Sect B*, **79**: 437–9.

Jerse AE, Cohen MS et al., 1994, Multiple gonococcal opacity proteins are expressed during experimental urethral infection in the male, *J Exp Med*, **179**: 911–20.

John CM, Griffiss JM et al., 1991, The structural basis for pyocin resistance in *Neisseria gonorrhoeae* lipooligosaccharides, *J Biol Chem*, **266**: 19303–11.

Johnson AP, 1983, The pathogenic potential of commensal species of *Neisseria*, *J Clin Pathol*, **36**: 213–23.

Joiner KA, Scales R et al., 1985, Mechanism of action of blocking immunoglobulin G for *Neisseria gonorrhoeae*, *J Clin Invest*, **76**: 1765–72.

Jonsson AB, Nyberg G, Normark S, 1991, Phase variation of gonococcal pili by frameshift mutation in pilC, a novel gene for pilus assembly, *EMBO J*, **10**: 477–88.

Judd RC, 1989, Protein I: structure, function, and genetics, *Clin Microbiol Rev*, **2, Suppl.**: S41–8.

Judd RC, Porcella SF, 1993, Isolation of the periplasm of *Neisseria gonorrhoeae*, *Mol Microbiol*, **10**: 567–74.

Judd RC, Shafer WM, 1989, Topographical alterations in proteins I of *Neisseria gonorrhoeae* correlated with lipooligosaccharide variation, *Mol Microbiol*, **3**: 637–43.

Jyssum K, Allunans J, 1982, Three types of inhibition among strains of *Neisseria meningitidis* isolated from patients in Norway, *Acta Pathol Microbiol Immunol Scand Sect B*, **90**: 335–40.

Jyssum K, Allunans J, 1984, Inhibitory spectrum of bacteriocin-like agents from *Neisseria meningitidis*, *Acta Pathol Microbiol Immunol Scand Sect B*, **92**: 159–63.

Kahr AF, Bihlmaier A et al., 1994, Generalized transposon shuttle mutagenesis in *Neisseria gonorrhoeae*: a method for isolating epithelia cell invasion-defective mutants, *Mol Microbiol*, **12**: 819–31.

Kapczynski DR, Genco CA, 1991, Genetic transformation of *Neisseria gonorrhoeae* using electroporation, *Neisseriae 1990*, eds Achtman M, Kohl P et al., Walter de Gruyter & Co., Berlin, Germany, 527–32.

Kathariou S, Stephens DS et al., 1990, Transposition of Tn916 to different sites in the chromosome of *Neisseria meningitidis*: a genetic tool for meningococcal mutagenesis, *Mol Microbiol*, **4**: 729–35.

Keevil CW, Major NC et al., 1986, Physiology and virulence determinants of *Neisseria gonorrhoeae* grown in glucose, oxygen or cystine-limited continuous culture, *J Gen Microbiol*, **132**: 3289–302.

Kellogg Jr DS, Peacock Jr WL et al., 1963, *Neisseria gonorrhoeae*. I. Virulence genetically linked to clonal variation, *J Bacteriol*, **85**: 1274–9.

Kingsbury DT, 1966, Bacteriocin production by strains of *Neisseria meningitidis*, *J Bacteriol*, **91**: 1696–9.

Klugman KP, Gotschlich EC, Blake MS, 1989, Sequence of the structural gene (*rmpM*) for the class 4 outer membrane protein of *Neisseria meningitidis*, homology of the protein to gonococcal protein III and *Escherichia coli* OmpA, and construction of meningococcal strains that lack class 4 protein, *Infect Immun*, **57**: 2066–71.

Knapp JS, 1984, Reduction of nitrite by *Neisseria gonorrhoeae*, *Int J Syst Bacteriol*, **34**: 376–7.

Knapp JS, 1988, Historical perspectives and identification of *Neisseria* and related species, *Clin Microbiol Rev*, **1**: 415–31.

Knapp JS, Clark VL, 1984, Anaerobic growth of *Neisseria gonorrhoeae* coupled to nitrite reduction, *Infect Immun*, **46**: 176–81.

Knapp JS, Falkow S, Holmes KK, 1975, Reevaluation of bacteriocinogeny in *Neisseria gonorrhoeae*, *J Clin Pathol*, **28**: 274–8.

Knapp JS, Hook III EW, 1988, Prevalence and persistence of *Neisseria cinerea* and other *Neisseria* spp. in adults, *J Clin Microbiol*, **26**: 896–900.

Knapp JS, Zenilman JM et al., 1986, Distribution and frequency of strains of *Neisseria gonorrhoeae* with plasmid mediated high-level resistance to tetracycline (TRNG) in the United States, *Abstracts, The Fifth Pathogenic* Neisseria *Meeting, Amsterdam, The Netherlands*.

Koomey JM, Gotschlich EC et al., 1987, Effects of RecA mutations on pilus antigenic variation and phase transitions in *Neisseria gonorrhoeae*, *Genetics*, **117**: 391–8.

Kupsch E-M, Knepper B et al., 1993, Variable opacity (Opa) outer membrane proteins account for the cell tropisms displayed by *Neisseria gonorrhoeae* for human leukocytes and epithelial cells, *EMBO J*, **12**: 641–50.

Lambden PR, Robertson JN, Watt PJ, 1981, The preparation and properties of alpha and beta pili from variants of *Neisseria gonorrhoeae* P9, *J Gen Microbiol*, **124**: 109–17.

La Scolea LJ, Young FE, 1974, Development of a defined minimal medium for the growth of *Neisseria gonorrhoeae*, *Appl Microbiol*, **28**: 70–6.

Lawton WD, Bellinger MA et al., 1976, Bacteriocin production by *Neisseria gonorrhoeae*, *Antimicrob Agents Chemother*, **10**: 417–20.

Lee BC, 1992, Isolation of haemin-binding proteins of *Neisseria gonorrhoeae*, *J Med Microbiol*, **36**: 121–7.

Lee BC, 1994, Isolation and characterization of the haemin-binding proteins from *Neisseria meningitidis*, *J Gen Microbiol*, **140**: 1473–80.

Lee BC, Hill P, 1992, Identification of an outer-membrane hemoglobin-binding protein in *Neisseria meningitidis*, *J Gen Microbiol*, **138**: 2647–56.

Leith DK, Morse SA, 1980, Cross-linking of outer membrain proteins of *Neisseria gonorrhoeae*, *J Bacteriol*, **143**: 182–7.

Lestikow, 1882, Uber Bacterien bei den venerischen Krankheiten, *Charite Ann*, **7**: 750–72.

Lewis LA, Dyer DW, 1995, Identification of an iron-regulated outer membrane protein of *Neisseria meningitidis* involved in the utilization of hemoglobin complexed to haptoglobin, *J Bacteriol*, **177**: 1299–306.

Lynch EC, Blake MS et al., 1984, Studies on porins: spontaneously transferred from whole cells and from proteins of *Neisseria gonorrhoeae* and *Neisseria meningitidis*, *Biophys J*, **45**: 104–7.

McDade Jr RL, Johnston KH, 1980, Characterization of serologically dominant outer membrane proteins of *Neisseria gonorrhoeae*, *J Bacteriol*, **41**: 1183–91.

McDonald IJ, Johnson KG, 1975, Nutritional requirements of some non-pathogenic *Neisseria* grown in simple synthetic media, *Can J Microbiol*, **21**: 1198–204.

McFarland L, Meitzner T et al., 1983, Factors affecting the sensitivity of gonococci to fecal lipids, *J Clin Microbiol*, **18**: 121–7.

McGee ZA, Dourmashkin RR et al., 1977, Relationship of pili to colonial morphology among pathogenic and nonpathogenic species of *Neisseria*, *Infect Immun*, **15**: 594–600.

MacKenzie CR, Johnston KG, McDonald IJ, 1977, Glycogen synthesis by amylosucrase from *Neisseria perflava*, *Can J Microbiol*, **23**: 1303–7.

MacKenzie CR, McDonald IJ, Johnson KG, 1978a, Glycogen

metabolism in the genus *Neisseria*: synthesis from sucrose by amylosucrase, *Can J Microbiol*, **24**: 357–62.

MacKenzie CR, McDonald IJ, Johnson KG, 1978b, Sucrose uptake by *Neisseria denitrificans*, *Can J Microbiol*, **24**: 569–73.

MacKenzie CR, Perry MB et al., 1978, Structure of the D-glucans produced by *Neisseria perflava*, *Can J Microbiol*, **24**: 1419–22.

McKern NM, O'Donnell IJ et al., 1985, Primary structure of pilin protein from *Bacteroides nodosus* strain 216: comparison with the corresponding protein from strain 198, *J Gen Microbiol*, **131**: 1–6.

Mandrell RE, Griffiss JM, Macher BA, 1988, Lipooligosaccharides (LOS) of *Neisseria gonorrhoeae* and *Neisseria meningitidis* have components that are immunochemically similar to precursors of human blood group antigens, *J Exp Med*, **168**: 107–26.

Mardh PA, Westrom L, 1976, Adherence of bacteria to vaginal epithelial cells, *Infect Immun*, **13**: 661–6.

Marrs CF, Schoolnik G et al., 1985, Cloning and sequencing of a *Moraxella bovis* pili gene, *J Bacteriol*, **163**: 132–9.

Masson L, Holbein BE, 1983, Physiology of sialic acid capsular polysaccharide synthesis in serogroup B *Neisseria meningitidis*, *J Bacteriol*, **154**: 728–36.

Masson L, Holbein BE, Ashton FE, 1982, Virulence linked to polysaccharide production in serogroup B *Neisseria meningitidis*, *FEMS Lett*, **13**: 187–90.

Mazloum H, Totten PA et al., 1986, An unusual *Neisseria* isolated from conjunctival cultures in rural Egypt, *J Infect Dis*, **154**: 212–24.

Melly MA, McGee ZA et al., 1979, An electron microscopic India ink technique for demonstrating capsules on microorganisms: studies with *Streptococcus pneumoniae*, *Staphylococcus aureus*, and *Neisseria gonorrhoeae*, *J Infect Dis*, **140**: 605–9.

Meyer TF, Pohlner J, van Putten JPM, 1994, Biology of the pathogenic Neisseriae, *Curr Top Microbiol Immunol*, **192**: 283–317.

Meyer TF, van Putten JPM, 1989, Genetic mechanisms and biological implications of phase variation in pathogenic neisseriae, *Clin Microbiol Rev*, **2, Suppl.**: S139–45.

Meyer TF, Billyard R et al., 1984, Pilus genes of *Neisseria gonorrhoeae*: chromosomal organization and DNA sequence, *Proc Natl Acad Sci USA*, **81**: 6110–14.

Mintz CS, Apicella MA, Morse SA, 1984, Electrophoretic and serological characterization of the lipopolysaccharide produced by *Neisseria gonorrhoeae*, *J Infect Dis*, **149**: 544–52.

Morse SA, 1976, Physiology and metabolism of *Neisseria gonorrhoeae*, *Microbiology 1976*, ed. Schlessinger D, American Society for Microbiology, Washington, DC, 467–90.

Morse SA, 1978, The biology of the gonococcus, *CRC Rev Microbiol*, **7**: 92–189.

Morse SA, Apicella MA, 1982, Isolation of a lipopolysaccharide mutant of *Neisseria gonorrhoeae*: an analysis of the antigenic and biologic differences, *J Infect Dis*, **145**: 206–16.

Morse SA, Bartenstein L, 1980, Purine metabolism in *Neisseria gonorrhoeae*: the requirement for hypoxanthine, *Can J Microbiol*, **26**: 13–20.

Morse SA, Hebeler BH, 1978, Effect of pH on the growth and glucose metabolism of *Neisseria gonorrhoeae*, *Infect Immun*, **21**: 87–95.

Morse SA, Knapp JS, 1991, The genus *Neisseria*, *The Prokaryotes*, 2nd edn, eds Balows A, Truper HG et al., Springer-Verlag, New York, 495–529.

Morse SA, Lysko PG, 1980, The cell envelope of *Neisseria gonorrhoeae*, *Genetics and Immunobiology of Pathogenic Neisseria*, eds Normark S, Danielsson D, EMBO Workshop, Hemavan, Sweden, 1–6.

Morse SA, Stein S, Hines J, 1974, Glucose metabolism in *Neisseria gonorrhoeae*, *J Bacteriol*, **120**: 702–14.

Morse SA, Vaughan P et al., 1976, Inhibition of *Neisseria gonorrhoeae* by a bacteriocin from *Pseudomonas aeruginosa*, *Antimicrob Agents Chemother*, **10**: 354–62.

Morse SA, Johnson SR et al., 1986, High-level tetracycline resistance in *Neisseria gonorrhoeae* is due to the acquisition of the streptococcal tetM determinant, *Abstracts, The Fifth Pathogenic* Neisseria *Meeting, Amsterdam, The Netherlands*.

Muir LL, Strugnell A, Davies JK, 1988, Proteins that appear to be associated with pili in *Neisseria gonorrhoeae*, *Infect Immun*, **56**: 1743–7.

Mulks MH, Plaut AG, 1978, IgA protease production as a characteristic distinguishing pathogeneic from harmless Neisseriacea, *N Engl J Med*, **299**: 973–6.

Murray RGE, Reyn A, Birch-Anderson A, 1963, The fine structure of *Neisseria* and possible implications in classification, *Can J Public Health*, **54**: 46–7.

Nassif X, Puaoi D, So M, 1991, Transposition of TN 1545-3 in the pathogenic neisseriae: a genetic tool for mutagenesis, *J Bacteriol*, **173**: 2147–54.

Newhall WJ, Sawyer WD, Haak RA, 1980, Cross-linking analysis of the outer membrane proteins of *Neisseria gonorrhoeae*, *Infect Immun*, **28**: 785–91.

Noegel A, Gotschlich EC, 1983, Isolation of a high molecular weight polyphosphate from *Neisseria gonorrhoeae*, *J Exp Med*, **157**: 2049–60.

Okada G, Hehre EJ, 1974, New studies on amylosucrase, a bacterial alpha-D-glucosylase that directly converts sucrose to glycogen-like-glucan, *J Biol Chem*, **249**: 126–35.

Olafson RW, McCarthy PJ et al., 1985, Structural and antigenic analysis of meningococcal piliation, *Infect Immun*, **48**: 336–42.

Olyhoek T, Crowe B, Achtman M, 1985, Epidemiological analysis and geographical distribution of *Neisseria meningitidis* Group A, *The Pathogenic Neisseriae*, ed. Schoolnik GK, American Society for Microbiology, Washington, DC, 530–5.

Pannekoek Y, van Putten JPM, Dankert J, 1992, Identification and molecular analysis of a 63-kDa gonococcal stress protein from *Neisseria gonorrhoeae*, *J Bacteriol*, **174**: 6928–37.

Parge HE, Bernstein SL et al., 1990, Biochemical purification and crystallographic characterization of the fiber-forming protein pilin from *Neisseria gonorrhoeae*, *J Biol Chem*, **265**: 2278–85.

Parsons NJ, Curry A et al., 1992, The serum resistance of gonococci in the majority of urethral exudates is due to sialylated lipooligosaccharide seen as a surface coat, *FEMS Microbiol Lett*, **90**: 295–300.

Paruchuri DK, Seifert HS et al., 1990, Identification and characterization of a *Neissera gonorrhoeae* encoding a glycolipid-binding in adhesin, *Proc Natl Acad Sci USA*, **87**: 333–7.

Perine PL, Schalla W et al., 1977, Evidence for two distinct types of penicillinase-producing *Neisseria gonorrhoeae*, *Lancet*, **2**: 993.

Pettit RK, Judd RC, 1992, Characterization of naturally elaborated blebs from serum-susceptible and serum-resistant strains of *Neisseria gonorrhoeae*, *Mol Microbiol*, **6**: 723–8.

Pettit RK, Martin ES et al., 1995, Phenotypic modulation of gonococcal lipooligosaccharide in acidic and alkaline culture, *Infect Immun*, **63**: 2773–5.

Phelps LN, 1967, Isolation and characterization of bacteriophages for *Neisseria*, *J Gen Virol*, **1**: 529–36.

Phillips I, 1976, Beta-lactamase producing penicillin-resistant gonococci, *Lancet*, **2**: 656–7.

Phillips NJ, John CM et al., 1990, Structural models for the cell surface lipooligosaccharides of *Neisseria gonorrhoeae* and *Haemophilus influenzae*, *Biomed Environ Mass Spectrom*, **19**: 731–45.

Platt DJ, 1976, Carbon dioxide requirement of *Neisseria gonorrhoeae* growing on a solid medium, *J Clin Microbiol*, **4**: 129–32.

Plummer FA, Simonsen JN et al., 1989, Epidemiologic evidence for the development of serovar-specific immunity after gonococcal infection, *J Clin Invest*, **83**: 1472–6.

Plummer FA, Chubb H et al., 1993, Antibody to Rmp (outer membrane protein 3) increases susceptibility to gonococcal infection, *J Clin Invest*, **91**: 339–43.

Poolman JT, DeMarie S, Zanen HC, 1980, Variability of low-molecular-weight, heat-modifiable outer membrane proteins of *Neisseria meningitidis*, *Infect Immun*, **30**: 642–8.

Potts W, Saunders JR, 1987, Nucleotide sequence of the structural gene for class 1 pilin from *Neisseria meningitidis*: homologies with the pilE locus of *Neisseria gonorrhoeae*, *Mol Microbiol*, **2**: 647–53.

Punsalang AP, Sawyer WD, 1973, Role of pili in the virulence of *Neisseria gonorrhoeae*, *Infect Immun*, **8**: 255–63.

Reimann K, Heise H, Blom J, 1988, Attempts to demonstrate a polysaccharide capsule in *Neisseria gonorrhoeae*, *APMIS*, **96**: 735–40.

Rice PA, 1989, Molecular basis for serum resistance in *Neisseria gonorrhoeae*, *Clin Microbiol Rev*, **2, Suppl.**: S112–17.

Rice PA, Kasper DL, 1977, Characterization of gonococcal antigens responsible for induction of bactericidal antibody in disseminated infection, *J Clin Invest*, **60**: 1149–58.

Rice PA, Vayo HE et al., 1986, Immunoglobulin G antibodies directed against protein III block killing of serum-resistant *Neisseria gonorrhoeae* by immune serum, *J Exp Med*, **164**: 1735–48.

Rice PA, McQuillen DP et al., 1994, Serum resistance of *Neisseria gonorrhoeae*. Does it thwart the inflammatory response and facilitate the transmission of infection?, *Ann NY Acad Sci*, **730**: 7–14.

Richardson WP, Sadoff JC, 1977, Production of a capsule by *Neisseria gonorrhoeae*, *Infect Immun*, **15**: 663–4.

Riou J-Y, Guibourdenche M, Popoff MY, 1983, A new taxon in the genus *Neisseria*, *Ann Microbiol (Paris)*, **134**: 257–67.

Riou J-Y, Guibourdenche M, et al., 1986, Structure of the exocellular D-glucan produced by *Neisseria polysaccharea*, *Can J Microbiol*, **32**: 909–11.

Roberts M, Elewell LP, Falkow S, 1977, Molecular characterization of two beta-lactamase-specifying plasmids isolated from *Neisseria gonorrhoeae*, *J Bacteriol*, **131**: 557–63.

Roberts MC, Knapp JS, 1988, Host range of the conjugative 25.2 Mdal tetracycline resistance plasmid from *Neisseria gonorrhoeae*, *Antimicrob Agents Chemother*, **32**: 488–91.

Robertson JN, Vincent P, Ward ME, 1977, The preparation and properties of gonococcal pili, *J Gen Microbiol*, **102**: 169–77.

Robinson Jr EN, McGee ZA et al., 1987, Probing the surface of *Neisseria gonorrhoeae*: simultaneous localization of protein I and H.8 antigens, *Infect Immun*, **55**: 1190–7.

Rossau R, Vandenbussche F et al., 1989, Ribosomal ribonucleic acid cistron similarities and deoxyribonucleic acid homologies of *Neisseria, Kingella, Simonsiella, Alysiella*, and Centers for Disease Control groups EF-4 and M5 in the emended family *Neisseriaceae*, *Int J Syst Bacteriol*, **39**: 185–98.

Rossau RG, van Landschoot A et al., 1991, Taxonomy of Moraxellaceae fam. nov., a new bacterial family to accomodate the genera *Moraxella, Acinetobacter*, and *Psychrobacter* and related organisms, *Int J Syst Bacteriol*, **41**: 310–19.

Rudel T, Scheuerpflug I, Meyer TF, 1995, *Neisseria* PilC protein identified as type-4 pilus tip-located adhesin, *Nature (London)*, **373**: 357–9.

Sandlin RC, Apicella MA, Stein DC, 1993, Cloning of a gonococcal DNA sequence that complements the lipooligosaccharide defects of *Neisseria gonorrhoeae* 1291d and 1291e, *Infect Immun*, **61**: 3360–8.

Sandstrom EG, Chen KCS, Buchanan TM, 1982, Serology of *Neisseria gonorrhoeae*: coagglutination serogroups WI and WII/III correspond to different outer membrane proteins, *Infect Immun*, **38**: 462–70.

Sandstrom EG, Knapp JS et al., 1984, Serogrouping of *Neisseria gonorrhoeae*: correlation of serogroup with disseminated gonococcal infection, *Sex Transm Dis*, **11**: 77–80.

Sarafian SK, Genco CA et al., 1990, Acquisition of beta-lactamase and TetM-containing conjugative plasmids by phenotypically different strains of *Neisseria gonorrhoeae*, *Sex Transm Dis*, **17**: 67–71.

Sastry PA, Pearlstone JR et al., 1983, Amino acid sequence of pilin isolated from *Pseudomonas aeruginosa* PAK, *FEBS Lett*, **151**: 253–6.

Schifman RB, Ryan KJ, 1983, *Neisseria lactamica* septicemia in an immunocompromised patient, *J Clin Microbiol*, **17**: 934–5.

Schneider H, Griffiss JM et al., 1991, Expression of paragloboside-like lipooligosaccharides may be a necessary component of gonococcal pathogenesis, *J Exp Med*, **174**: 1601–5.

Seifert HS, Ajioka R, So M, 1988, Alternative model for *Neisseria gonorrhoeae* pilin variation, *Vaccine*, **6**: 107–9.

Seifert HS, So M, 1991, Genetic systems in pathogenic neisseriae, *Methods Enzymol*, **204**: 342–57.

Shafer WM, Morse SA, 1987, Cleavage of the protein III and major iron-regulated protein of *Neisseria gonorrhoeae* by lysosomal cathepsin G, *J Gen Microbiol*, **133**: 155–62.

Shafer WM, Joiner KA et al., 1984, Serum sensitivity of *Neisseria gonorrhoeae*: the role of lipopolysaccharide, *J Infect Dis*, **149**: 175–83.

Shafer WM, Balthazar JT et al., 1995, Missense mutations that alter the DNA-binding domain of the MtrR protein occurs frequently in rectal isolates of *Neisseria gonorrhoeae*, *Microbiology*, **141**: 907–11.

Short HB, Clark VL et al., 1982, Anaerobic survival of clinical isolates and laboratory strains of *Neisseria gonorrhoeae*: use in stransfer and storage, *J Clin Microbiol*, **15**: 915–19.

Sidberry HD, Sadoff JC, 1977, Pyocin sensitivity of *Neisseria gonorrhoeae* and its feasibility as an epidemiological tool, *Infect Immun*, **15**: 628–37.

Simon D, Rest RF, 1992, *Escherichia coli* expressing a *Neisseria gonorrhoeae* opacity-associated outer membrane protein invade human cervical and endometrial epithelial cell lines, *Proc Natl Acad Sci USA*, **89**: 5512–16.

Sox TE, Mohammed W, Sparling PF, 1979, Transformation-derived *Neisseria gonorrhoeae* plasmids with altered structure and function, *J Bacteriol*, **138**: 510–18.

Sox TE, Mohammed W et al., 1978, Conjugative plasmids in *Neisseria gonorrhoeae*, *J Bacteriol*, **134**: 278–86.

Sparling PF, 1966, Genetic transformation of *Neisseria gonorrhoeae* to streptomycin resistance, *J Bacteriol*, **92**: 1364–71.

Sparling PF, Biswas GD, Sox TE, 1977, Transformation of the gonococcus, *The Gonococcus*, ed. Roberts RB, John Wiley & Sons, New York, 155–76.

Sparling PF, Tsai J, Cornelissen CN, 1990, Gonococci are survivors, *Scand J Infect Dis Suppl*, **69**: 125–36.

Stein DC, Hebeler BH, Young FE, 1980, Effect of environment on sensitivity of *Neisseria gonorrhoeae* to *Pseudomonas aeruginosa* bacteriocins, *Infect Immun*, **29**: 507–11.

Steinberg VI, Hart EJ et al., 1976, Isolation and characterization of a bacteriophage specific for *Neisseria perflava*, *J Clin Microbiol*, **4**: 87–91.

Stephens DS, Farley MM, 1991, Pathogenic effects during infection of the human nasopharynx with *Neisseria meningitidis* and *Haemophilus influenzae*, *Rev Infect Dis*, **13**: 22–33.

Stephens DS, Hoffman LH, McGee Z, 1983, Interaction of *Neisseria meningitidis* with nasopharyngeal mucosa: attachment and entry into columnar epithelial cells, *J Infect Dis*, **148**: 369–76.

Stephens DS, McGee Z, 1981, Attachment of *Neisseria meningitidis* to human mucosal surfaces: influence of pili and type of receptor cell, *J Infect Dis*, **143**: 525–32.

Stephens DS, Whitney AM et al., 1985, Pili of *Neisseria meningitidis*. Analysis of structure and investigation of structural and antigenic relationships to gonococcal pili, *J Exp Med*, **161**: 1539–53.

Stephens DS, Whitney AM et al., 1986, Analysis of damage to human ciliated nasopharyngeal epithelium by *Neisseria meningitidis*, *Infect Immun*, **51**: 579–85.

Stephens DS, Swartley JS et al., 1991, Insertion of Tn9916 in *Neisseria meningitidis* resulting in loss of group B capsular polysaccharide, *Infect Immun*, **59**: 4097–102.

Stephens DS, McAllister CF et al., 1994, Tn916-generated, lipooligosaccharide mutants of *Neisseria meningitidis* and *N. gonorrhoeae*, *Infect Immun*, **62**: 2947–52.

Stern A, Brown M et al., 1986, Opacity genes in *Neisseria*

gonorrhoeae: control of phase and antigenic variation, *Cell*, **47**: 61–71.

Stern A, Meyer TF, 1987, Common mechanism controlling phase and antigenic variation in pathogenic neisseriae, *Mol Microbiol*, **1**: 5–12.

Stojiljkovic I, Hwa V et al., 1995, The *Neisseria meningitidis* haemoglobin receptor: its role in iron utilization and virulence, *Mol Microbiol*, **15**: 531–41.

Stone RL, Culbertson CG, Powell HM, 1956, Studies of a bacteriophage active against a chromogenic *Neisseria*, *J Bacteriol*, **71**: 516–20.

Swanson J, 1973, Studies on gonococcal infection. IV. Pili: their role in attachment of gonococci to tissue culture cells, *J Exp Med*, **137**: 571–89.

Swanson J, Kraus SJ, Gotschlich EC, 1971, Studies on gonococcus infection. I. Pili and zones of adhesion: their relation to gonococcal growth patterns, *J Exp Med*, **134**: 886–906.

Swanson J, Mayer LW, Tam MR, 1982, Antigenicity of *Neisseria gonorrhoeae* outer membrane protein(s) III detected by immunoprecipitation and Western blot transfer with monoclonal antibodies, *Infect Immun*, **36**: 1042–53.

Swanson J, Zeligs B, 1974, Studies on the gonocuccus infection. VI. Electron microscopic study on in vitro phagocytosis by human leukocytes, *Infect Immun*, **10**: 645–56.

Talley RS, Baugh CL, 1975, Effects of bicarbonate on growth of *Neisseria gonorrhoeae*: replacement of gaseous CO_2 atmosphere, *Appl Microbiol*, **29**: 469–71.

Tinsley CR, Heckels JE, 1986, Variation in the expression of pili and outer membrane protein by *Neisseria meningitidis* during the course of meningococcal infection, *J Gen Microbiol*, **132**: 2483–90.

Tommassen J, Vermeij P et al., 1990, Isolation of *Neisseria meningitidis* mutants deficient in class 1 (PorA) and class 3(PorB) outer membrane proteins, *Infect Immun*, **58**: 1355–9.

Tsai C-M, Civin CI, 1991, Eight lipooligosaccharides of *Neisseria meningitidis* react with a monoclonal antibody which binds lacto-N-neotetraose (Gal beta1-4GlcNAc beta1-3Gal beta1-4Glc), *Infect Immun*, **59**: 3604–9.

Vedros NA, 1984, Genus I *Neisseria* Trevisan 1885, *Bergey's Manual of Systematic Bacteriology*, vol. 1, eds Krieg NR, Holt JG, Williams and Wilkins, Baltimore, 90–296.

Vedros NA, Hoke C, Chun P, 1983, *Neisseria macacae* sp. nov., a new *Neisseria* species isolated from the oropharynges of rhesus monkeys (*Macaca mulatta*), *Int J Syst Bacteriol*, **33**: 515–20.

Vedros NA, Johnston DG, Warren PI, 1973, *Neisseria* species isolated from dolphins, *J Wildl Dis*, **9**: 241–4.

Verheul AFM, Snippe H, Poolman JT, 1993, Meningococcal lipopolysaccharides: virulence factor and potential vaccine component, *Microbiol Rev*, **57**: 34–49.

Virji M, Heckels JE, 1986, The effect of protein II and pili on the interaction of *Neisseria gonorrhoeae* with human polymorphonuclear leukocytes, *J Gen Microbiol*, **132**: 503–12.

Virji M, Zak K, Heckels JE, 1986, Monoclonal antibodies to gonococcal outer membrane protein IB: use in the investigation of the potential protective effect of antibodies directed against conserved and type-specific epitopes, *J Gen Microbiol*, **132**: 1621–9.

Virji M, Fletcher JN et al., 1987, The potential protective effect of monoclonal antibodies to gonococcal outer membrane protein IA, *J Gen Microbiol*, **133**: 2639–46.

Virji M, Kayhty H et al., 1991, The role of pili in the interactions of pathogenic *Neisseria* with cultured human endothelial cells, *Mol Microbiol*, **5**: 1831–41.

Von Lingelsheim W, 1906, Die bakteriologisch Arbieten der Kgl hygienischen Station zu Beuthen O -Sch wahrend der Genickstarreepidemie in Oberschlesien im Winter 1904/05, *Klin Jahrb*, **15**: 373–489.

Wagner GH, Cooper FP, Bishop CT, 1973, Extracellular carbohydrate antigens from some non-pathogenic *Neisseria* species, *Can J Microbiol*, **19**: 703–8.

Walstad DL, Reitz RC, Sparling PF, 1974, Growth inhibition among strains of *Neisseria gonorrhoeae* due to production of inhibitory free fatty acids and lysophosphatidylethanolamine: absence of bacteriocins, *Infect Immun*, **10**: 481–8.

Ward ME, Watt PJ, Robertson JN, 1974, The human fallopian tube: a model for gonococcal infection, *J Infect Dis*, **129**: 650–9.

Wegner WS, Hebeler BH, Morse SA, 1977, Cell envelope of *Neisseria gonorrhoeae*: relationship between autolysis in buffer and the hydrolysis of peptidoglycan, *Infect Immun*, **18**: 210–19.

Weichselbaum A, 1887, *Fortschr Med*, **5**: 573.

Weistreich GA, Baker RF, 1971, The presence of fimbriae (pili) in three species of *Neisseria*, *J Gen Microbiol*, **65**: 167–73.

Westling-Haggstrom B, Elmros T et al., 1977, Growth pattern and cell division in *Neisseria gonorrhoeae*, *J Bacteriol*, **129**: 333–42.

Wetzler LM, Gotschlich EC et al., 1989, The construction and characterization of *Neisseria gonorrhoeae* lacking protein III in its outer membrane, *J Exp Med*, **169**: 2199–209.

Wolf-Watz H, Elmros T et al., 1975, Cell envelope of *Neisseria gonorrhoeae*: outer membrane and peptidoglycan composition of penicillin-sensitive and resistant strains, *Infect Immun*, **11**: 1332–41.

Wolff K, Stern A, 1995, Identification and characterization of specific sequences encoding pathogenicity associated proteins in the genome of commensal *Neisseria* species, *FEMS Microbiol Lett*, **125**: 255–64.

Wong JD, Janda JM, 1992, Association of an important *Neisseria* species, *Neisseria elongata* subsp. *nitroreducens*, with bacteremia, endocarditis, and osteomyelitis, *J Clin Microbiol*, **30**: 719–20.

Wooldridge KG, Williams PH, 1993, Iron uptake mechanisms of pathogenic bacteria, *FEMS Microbiol Rev*, **12**: 325–48.

Xia M, Whittington WL et al., 1995, Pulsed-field gel electrophoresis for genomic analysis of *Neisseria gonorrhoeae*, *J Infect Dis*, **171**: 455–8.

Young JDE, Blake M et al., 1983, Properties of the major outer membrane protein from *Neisseria gonorrhoeae* incorporated into model lipid membranes, *Proc Natl Acad Sci USA*, **80**: 3831–5.

Zak K, Diaz JL et al., 1984, Antigenic variation during infection with *Neisseria gonorrhoeae*: detection of antibodies to surface proteins in sera of patients with gonorrhea, *J Infect Dis*, **149**: 166–74.

Chapter 38

BORDETELLA

R Parton

1   DEFINITION

Bordetella spp. are minute, gram-negative, aerobic, non-acid-fast, non-sporing coccobacilli. They do not ferment carbohydrates. Their optimum temperature is 35–37°C. There are 6 named species, 3 motile and 3 non-motile. The organisms are obligatory parasites, mostly inhabiting the surface of the respiratory tract of man and other warm-blooded animals, including birds. Some species appear to be capable of intracellular survival and one species is associated with bacteraemia. Four species are known to produce a tracheal cytotoxin, a heat-labile, dermonecrotizing toxin and fimbriae (pili). Three species produce adenylate cyclase toxin and the surface protein adhesins filamentous haemagglutinin and pertactin. Only *Bordetella pertussis* produces pertussis toxin and tracheal colonization factor. The expression of virulence-associated properties and motility in some species is modulated by environmental signals. The G + C content of the DNA is 60.2–69.5% and the type species is *B. pertussis*.

2   INTRODUCTION

Until recently, there were 4 recognized species in the genus. *B. pertussis* was described by Bordet and Gengou (1906) as the cause of whooping cough. *Bordetella bronchiseptica* was first obtained by Ferry (1910) from the respiratory tract of dogs and is now known to be an important respiratory pathogen in wild and domesticated animals, and occasionally affects man. *Bordetella parapertussis* was isolated by Bradford and Slavin (1937) from cases of mild whooping cough and recog-

nized as being different from *B. pertussis*. *Bordetella avium* was first proposed as a species by Kersters et al. (1984) to include agents of respiratory disease of turkey poults originally isolated by Filion et al. (1967). Two more species have been added to the genus. The species *Bordetella holmesii* was proposed for a group of strains, isolated from 1983 onwards, from blood cultures of patients, some of whom were immunocompromised (Weyant et al. 1995). *Bordetella hinzii* was the name proposed by Vandamme et al. (1995) for a *B. avium*-like group of organisms found mainly in the respiratory tracts of chickens and turkeys and thought to be non-pathogenic. Possibly the first such isolate, however, was from human sputum in 1957 (Cookson et al. 1994).

All of the bordetellae have been known by other names. The first 3 recognized species were included in the genus *Haemophilus* before the introduction of the genus *Bordetella* by Moreno-Lopez (1952) and named in honour of the pioneering work of Jules Bordet. *B. bronchiseptica* had also been included in the genera *Alcaligenes* and *Brucella*. The original specific name *bronchicanis* was changed to *bronchiseptica* after isolation of similar organisms from animal species other than dogs. *B. avium* was originally identified as *Alcaligenes faecalis*. The *B. hinzii* group has been referred to previously as *A. faecalis* type II, TC (turkey coryza) bacterium type II, *Alcaligenes* sp. strain C_2T_2 as well as *B. avium*-like. Their present name was proposed to honour K-H Hinz, in recognition of his work on avian isolates of *Bordetella*. *B. holmesii* was formerly known as CDC non-oxidizer group 2 (NO_2) and was named in honour of B Holmes for his contribution to the study of unusual and opportunist bacteria.

The main aim of this chapter is to summarize the vast amount of recent information on the genus

Bordetella. For a more detailed, historical perspective, and access to the earlier literature, the chapter by Wardlaw (1990), in the previous edition of this volume, is recommended.

3 CLASSIFICATION

3.1 The genus *Bordetella*

On the basis of a numerical taxonomic study covering a wide range of tests and properties, Johnson and Sneath (1973) suggested that the genus *Bordetella* should be grouped in the family Brucellaceae. The 3 species then known, *B. pertussis*, *B. parapertussis* and *B. bronchiseptica*, were grouped with *A. faecalis* and *Brucella*. This group had affinities with *Acinetobacter*, *Moraxella* and *Neisseria* strains but was distinct from the *Haemophilus*, *Actinobacillus*, *Pasteurella* group. In the 8th edition of *Bergey's Manual of Determinative Bacteriology*, this family was no longer recognized and the taxonomic position of the genus *Bordetella* was undecided. In the 1984 edition, *Bordetella* was listed as a genus without a family in Section 4 (gram-negative aerobic rods and cocci) (Pittman 1984b).

After extensive DNA–rRNA hybridization and phenotypic analyses, De Ley et al. (1986) proposed that *Bordetella* should be included in a new family, Alcaligenaceae. The 4 species known at the time, now including *B. avium*, were found to belong to the third rRNA superfamily but their only close neighbour was the genus *Alcaligenes* and these 2 genera had a common separate position within the gram-negative bacteria. On the basis of the T_m parameter (melting temperature of the DNA–rRNA hybrids), the nearest neighbours to the bordetellae (T_m 79.0–81.9°C) were *Alcaligenes xylosoxidans* (T_m 79°C) followed by *Alcaligenes faecalis* (T_m 75.5°C). *Brucella* strains were quite unrelated (T_m 58°C).

Recent evidence from 16S rRNA sequence analysis on representatives of 5 *Bordetella* spp. (including *B. holmesii*) has confirmed a common phylogeny with *Alcaligenes* and has allowed assignment of the genus to the β2 subdivision of Proteobacteria (Weyant et al. 1995). The 2 genera also have similar cellular fatty acid profiles, with $C_{16:0}$ and $C_{17:0cyc}$ (except in *B. pertussis*) as their main constituents, and contain ubiquinone 8 as the major respiratory quinone. *Bordetella* and *Alcaligenes* are clearly closely related and may be difficult to differentiate on the basis of phenotypic criteria. Differential characteristics of these and other phenotypically similar genera are described elsewhere (Johnson and Sneath 1973, Kersters et al. 1984, Pittman 1984b, Vandamme et al. 1995).

3.2 Species designation

Various studies have suggested that *B. pertussis*, *B. parapertussis* and *B. bronchiseptica* are very closely related: DNA–DNA hybridization analyses; T_m values of their rRNA–DNA hybrids; mean G + C contents of their genomic DNA; similarity in their 23S rRNA gene sequences. Another estimate of genetic relatedness was obtained by Musser et al. (1986) in a survey by multilocus enzyme electrophoresis of 15 metabolic enzymes in 60 strains of mammalian bordetellae obtained from world-wide sources at different times. They found such limited genetic diversity, compared with most other pathogenic bacteria, to suggest that continued recognition of separate species was only justified on clinical and historical grounds. This and other evidence has led to the conclusion that *B. pertussis*, *B. parapertussis* and *B. bronchiseptica* are subtypes of a single genomic species (strains whose DNAs are 70% or more related, and with 5°C or less divergence in T_m values). By the same criteria, *B. avium*, *B. holmesii* and *B. hinzii* each form true (genomic) species (Vandamme et al. 1995, Weyant et al. 1995). No alternative nomenclature has been suggested and in discussing the distinctive phenotypic and pathogenic properties of the bordetellae, the traditional specific names are appropriate. Some of the differential features of these species are shown in Table 38.1 (p. 904).

3.3 Evolutionary considerations

A number of lines of evidence have been used to write a possible evolutionary history of the first 4 *Bordetella* spp. to be described (Rappuoli 1994). Their close phylogenetic relationship with *Alcaligenes* and other bacteria widespread in the environment suggests that the ancestral bordetellae were free-living and evolved to infect warm-blooded animals. Some properties still reflect this environmental origin: temperature sensing, and regulation of virulence factor expression accordingly (see section 12, p. 911); the presence of flagella in some species and greater expression of motility at low temperature; the ability of *B. bronchiseptica* and *B. avium* to grow and survive for long periods in low nutrient conditions such as natural waters. Another finding with evolutionary implications is that, on the basis of 16S rRNA analysis, some bacterial endosymbionts in insect trypanosomatid protozoa have *B. bronchiseptica* as their nearest relative.

A phylogenetic tree has been proposed based on the nucleotide sequence of the pertussis toxin (PT) gene and the presence or absence in the chromosome of 2 insertion sequences (Gross, Arico and Rappuoli 1989). During evolution, the first to diverge, to infect birds, was *B. avium*. Its distinctiveness is shown by its lower G + C content and lack of genes for PT. Later came a branch leading to *B. pertussis* and *B. parapertussis* and specialized to infect humans, leaving the line to *B. bronchiseptica* with its broad host range. The former 2 species are still very homogeneous, clonal populations, suggesting a recent adaptation to humans, whereas *B. bronchiseptica* and *B. avium* are polyclonal.

4 MORPHOLOGY AND ULTRASTRUCTURE

The bordetellae are minute rods or coccobacilli (0.2–0.5) × (0.5–2) μm, arranged singly or in pairs. Occasionally, filamentous forms several μm in length may be seen. *B. avium, B. bronchiseptica* and *B. hinzii* are motile by peritrichous flagella; the other 3 species are non-flagellate. In *B. avium*, the proportion of motile rods is greater at room temperature than at 35°C and in *B. bronchiseptica* motility is expressed only at low temperature. *B. avium* is described as capsulate. When freshly isolated, *B. pertussis* may possess a poorly defined capsule but whether this is identical with one or more of the better-characterized surface or extracellular products of this organism is not clear.

Early ultrastructural studies showed fine filamentous appendages on the surface of the bordetellae and, with *B. pertussis*, similar filaments and membranous blebs were found in the culture supernate. More recently, appendages identified as fimbriae, 3–5 nm in width and 100–250 nm in length, have been demonstrated on the surface of 4 species (see Table 38.2, p. 908). The cellular location of the various surface-related components of *B. pertussis* has been determined by immunoelectron microscopy with gold-labelled monoclonal antibodies (Blom, Heron and Hendley 1994). Antibodies to agglutinogens (AGGs) 2 and 3 labelled, respectively, long and short fimbriae protruding from the cell surface. The presence of pertactin (PRN) was revealed by intense and evenly distributed labelling of the surface of the cell. Antibody to filamentous haemagglutinin (FHA) stained aggregates of material between or adherent to the cells, which suggests that this component is readily shed. Previous work had shown that purified FHA consists of fine filaments 2 × (40–100) nm and is distinct from the fimbriae. Antibodies to pertussis toxin (PT) and adenylate cyclase toxin (ACT) labelled amorphous material adherent to or between cells, again indicating that these products are readily dispersed after export. Based on the above information and that given in section 11 (see p. 907), a diagrammatic representation of the disposition of the important cellular components of the bordetellae is shown in Fig. 38.1. Not all components are found in all species.

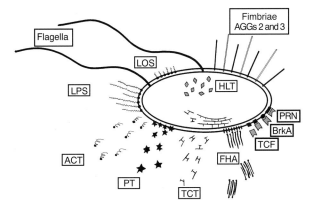

Fig. 38.1 Diagrammatic representation of the disposition of the important cellular components of the bordetellae. See sections 4 (p. 902) and 11 (p. 907) for details. Not all components are produced by all species.

5 CULTURAL CHARACTERISTICS

Growth of *B. pertussis* was first achieved by Bordet and Gengou (1906) with a glycerol–potato–extract medium, without peptone but containing 50% blood. This medium, with minor modifications, is still in general use. Sheep or horse blood is routinely used and the amount is usually reduced to 15–20%, thereby making haemolysis around the colonies easier to see. Various selective media have been developed for clinical specimens (see section 7, p. 905) and solid and liquid media without blood are available, for example, for vaccine production. *B. pertussis* is the most fastidious of the bordetellae and media suitable for *B. pertussis* is also suitable for the other species, although the latter can also be grown on peptone-containing media such as trypticase soy agar and MacConkey agar. Some of the cultural characteristics of the bordetellae are shown in Table 38.1. The time of development and size of the colonies differ between the species.

On Bordet–Gengou (BG) medium, *B. pertussis* forms tiny (0.5 mm diameter), smooth, convex, pearl-like, glistening colonies with entire edges and surrounded by a narrow zone of haemolysis. After 5–6 days, the diameter of the colonies has increased to 2–3 mm. Colonies of *B. parapertussis* develop more quickly and become slightly larger whereas those of *B. bronchiseptica* are larger still and appear within 24 h. On peptone- or tyrosine-containing agar, *B. parapertussis* and *B. holmesii* produce a brown discoloration of the medium. *B. avium* on Columbia agar containing 7% ox blood or veal infusion agar show 2 colony types. Some strains produce small, pearl-like colonies with entire edges and glistening surfaces 1 mm in diameter after 24 h. Others are larger with smooth surfaces. A few strains show dissociation into the 2 colony types whereas the majority have a stable morphology. *B. holmesii* colonies on heart infusion agar with rabbit blood are described as punctate, semiopaque, convex and round with complete edges. *B. hinzii* isolates have one of 2 distinct colony types. When grown on trypticase soy agar, some strains produce round, raised, glistening, greyish colonies about 2 mm in diameter after 48 h at 37°C in air containing 5% CO_2. Under the same conditions, other strains produce flat, dry, crinkled colonies up to 5 mm in diameter.

VARIATION DURING GROWTH

Variation during growth is a notable feature of the bordetellae, both in vitro and in vivo. Cultures frequently exhibit different colony types on the same agar surface, or after a few transfers. Changes in colony morphology on repeated subculture, with concomitant loss of antigenic and virulence attributes and alterations in growth requirements, have long been known for *B. pertussis*. Peppler and Schrumpf (1984) described phenotypic variants of *B. pertussis* that had flat, non-haemolytic colonies on BG agar, unlike the domed, haemolytic wild-type colonies; some of the variants could be selected for growth on nutrient agar. Colonial variation in *B. pertussis* is probably caused by the combined processes of serotype variation, phase variation and antigenic modulation (see section 12.1, p. 911) and similar phenomena occur in other bordetellae.

Table 38.1 Differential characteristics of *Bordetella* species

Characteristic	*B. pertussis*	*B. parapertussis*	*B. bronchiseptica*	*B. avium*	*B. hinzii*	*B. holmesii*
Growth: colonies visible in (days)	3	1–2	1	1	2	2–3
Peptone agar:						
growth	–	+	+	+	+	+
browning	–	+	–	–	–	+
Growth on MacConkey agar	–	+	+	+	+	+
Motile, peritrichous flagella	–	–	+	+	+	–
β-like haemolysis	+	+	v	v	?	–
Citrate utilization	–	v	+	v	+	–
Nitrate reduction	–	–	+	–	–	–
Oxidase	+	–	+	+	+	–
Urease	+	+	+	–	v	–
Major cellular fatty acids[a]	$C_{16:1w7c}$ $C_{16:0}$	$C_{16:0}$ $C_{17:0cyc}$	$C_{16:0}$ $C_{16:1w7c}$ $C_{17:0cyc}$	$C_{16:0}$ $C_{17:0cyc}$	$C_{16:0}$ $C_{17:0cyc}$	$C_{16:0}$ $C_{17:0cyc}$
G + C content of DNA (mol%)	67.7–68.9	68.1–69.0	68.2–69.5	61.6–62.6	65–67	61.5–62.3

+, positive; –, negative; v, some strains positive, others negative; ?, unknown.
[a]The number before the colon is the number of carbon atoms and the number after the colon is the number of double bonds; w, double bond position; c, *cis* isomer; cyc, cyclopropane ring.

6 GROWTH REQUIREMENTS

Although complex media containing blood are often used for their initial isolation, *Bordetella* spp. have relatively simple nutritional requirements (Rowatt 1957). These include amino acids as carbon and nitrogen sources, nicotinamide or nicotinic acid, and an organic source of sulphur. *B. bronchiseptica* and *B. avium* can also grow on carbon sources such as lactate or citrate plus ammonium ions in place of amino acids. Despite these simple nutritional requirements, *B. pertussis* is a fastidious organism and growth may be inhibited by various components, such as unsaturated fatty acids, present in normal media, or by contaminating detergents from the glassware. *B. parapertussis*, *B. bronchiseptica* and *B. avium* are less susceptible to these inhibitors.

Early liquid media developed for bulk growth of *B. pertussis* for vaccine production and free from blood or tissue extracts, contained salts, amino acid mixtures, growth factors and soluble starch. Despite the inclusion of starch, which helps to reduce the effects of the inhibitors, these media do not allow growth from small inocula and, when solidified with agar, do not permit single cells to form separated colonies. In place of starch, albumin, charcoal or ion-exchange resins have been used. Ammonia is formed during growth of the bordetellae and consequently media must be adequately buffered. A simple chemically defined medium for *B. pertussis* was developed by Stainer and Scholte (1971). This medium (SS) contains glutamic acid, proline and cystine, together with ascorbic acid, nicotinic acid, glutathione, salts and Tris buffer; again, it supports the growth of *B. pertussis* only from a heavy inoculum. This difficulty was overcome by Imaizumi et al. (1983) who supplemented SS medium with heptakis (2,6-*O*-dimethyl)β-cyclodextrin. Cyclodextrins form water-soluble complexes with hydrophobic molecules such as fatty acids. The resulting medium, solidified with agarose, was the first defined medium for *B. pertussis* to allow reliable growth from dilute inocula, a property only previously associated with blood-containing media such as BG agar. Supplementation of the medium with casamino acids further improved growth. Cyclodextrin not only improves the growth of *B. pertussis* but also greatly enhances the yield of PT, FHA and ACT in the culture supernate.

7 LABORATORY ISOLATION AND IDENTIFICATION

Successful isolation of *B. pertussis* from patients depends on various factors (Onorato and Wassilak 1987, Friedman 1988, Hoppe 1988, Gilchrist 1991). Cultivation of the organism is more likely to be successful early in the disease and less so during the paroxysmal stage. Age and immunization status of the patient and any preceding antimicrobial therapy are also important. Factors that can be controlled by the bacteriologist include the methods of specimen collection, transport and culture.

Nasopharyngeal swabs or nasopharyngeal aspirates give better isolation rates than cough plates, throat swabs or nasal swabs. Calcium alginate swabs have been found to be superior to those made from other materials. Although direct plating of specimens is the method of choice, transport media can be used. For swabs, Hoppe (1988) recommended the transport medium of Regan and Lowe (1977), which contains half-strength charcoal agar, horse blood and cephalexin, the latter to suppress the normal nasopharyngeal flora. For transporting nasopharyngeal secretions, casamino acids broth held at 4°C is suitable and, for longer-term preservation, there is no significant loss of viability on storage at −20°C in casamino acids or in serum inositol suspending medium (Cassiday et al. 1994). For primary isolation of *B. pertussis*, the medium developed by Regan and Lowe (1977) containing charcoal agar, with defibrinated horse blood 10% and cephalexin (40 mg l^{-1}) is recommended. Amphotericin B may be added if problems with fungal contaminants occur. A synthetic cyclodextrin-containing medium with cephalexin has a much longer shelf-life than BG agar. With simulated nasopharyngeal swab specimens, however, recovery on BG agar was 80%, and on cyclodextrin medium was <60%, of the numbers obtained on Regan and Lowe medium (Morrill et al. 1988). Plates should be incubated aerobically in a humid atmosphere at 35°C rather than 37°C and for up to 7 days. The characteristic tiny, smooth, convex, pearl-like colonies of *B. pertussis* usually become visible after 3–4 days whereas those of *B. parapertussis* appear after 2–3 days. Identity can be confirmed by gram staining, oxidase reaction and by typing with fluorescent antibody or by slide agglutination with specific antisera.

Various serological tests such as agglutination, complement fixation and ELISA have been used to confirm the diagnosis of pertussis and are valuable in epidemiological and vaccine efficacy studies. They are less suitable for rapid diagnosis and generally require seroconversion to distinguish active disease from high titres due to vaccination or maternal antibodies. ELISA tests, for example, detecting pertussis-specific IgA in a single serum sample, would suggest recent infection but results of such tests may be difficult to interpret.

The direct detection of *B. pertussis* or its components in clinical specimens is also possible. Such methods have the advantages of speed and ability to detect organisms that are no longer viable. The direct fluorescent antibody test uses fluorescein-labelled antibodies to *B. pertussis* and *B. parapertussis* to detect the bacteria in nasopharyngeal secretions. The test is technically demanding, of low sensitivity and may give false negative results if the number of organisms in the specimen is low, or false positive results, due to lack of technical expertise, poor quality slides or antigenic cross-reactions with other organisms. It is recommended as an adjunct to, rather than a replacement of, culture. Tests for the detection of *B. pertussis* components such as adenylate cyclase, by its enzymic activity, and pertussis toxin, by immunoassay or by cytotoxicity assay, either directly in respiratory secretions or after enrichment, appear to be sensitive and specific but have not found routine use.

The tests with greatest promise for rapid and sensitive detection of *B. pertussis* and other bordetellae are those involving nucleic acid probes and the polymerase chain reaction (PCR). Such techniques have attracted much interest for the diagnosis of infectious disease, especially with the advent of non-radioactive detection methods, and they are particularly suitable for fastidious, slow growing pathogens like *B. pertussis*. A PCR assay targeting multicopy species-specific insertion sequences allows the simultaneous detection and discrimination of *B. pertussis* and *B. parapertussis* and is sensitive enough to detect a single cell of either pathogen. With primers directed to the PT gene promoter, discrimination between *B. pertussis*, *B. parapertussis* and *B. bronchiseptica* is possible. PCR assays allow a much greater detection rate for *B. pertussis* infection than culture, particularly in vaccinated individuals and in patients given antibiotics. As with culture, the methods of sample collection and processing are crucial as is the choice of primers, PCR conditions and detection system (Meade and Bollen 1994).

B. bronchiseptica is readily isolated by nasal or tracheal swabbing of animals with bordetellosis. Blood agar or MacConkey agar, with or without selective agents such as penicillin, streptomycin and nystatin may be used and other selective media have been described (Goodnow 1980, Rutter 1985). Tracheal specimens from infected dogs and cats often contain high numbers of bordetellae and in pure culture (Bemis 1992). MacConkey agar is also suitable for *B. avium*.

8   TYPING METHODS

Serotyping is most commonly used for epidemiological investigations of *B. pertussis* isolates and depends on the presence or absence of specific agglutinogens (AGGs) on the bacterial cell surface. These are detected by slide agglutination tests with antisera raised in rabbits and made monospecific by absorption with heterologous strains. In an early definitive study, Eldering, Hornbeck and Baker (1957) described 14 heat-labile AGGs amongst *B. pertussis*, *B. parapertussis* and *B. bronchiseptica*. AGGs 1–6 were specific for *B. pertussis*. AGG 1 was common to all strains and AGGs 2–6 were found in various combinations on different isolates. Nowadays, only AGGs 1, 2 and 3 are widely recognized. Thus, the 4 serotypes of *B. pertussis* are 1,2,3; 1,2; 1,3; and 1. The antigenic determinants of AGGs 2 and 3 are located on fimbriae (see section 11.4, p. 909) but the nature of AGG 1 is unknown. Robinson, Ashworth and Irons (1989) suggested that monoclonal antibodies to the fimbrial subunits should be used to serotype *B. pertussis* isolates either by agglutination assays or ELISA. Such reagents would overcome problems of cross-reactions with absorbed sera and ELISA would avoid the problem of auto-agglutination seen with some strains.

9   BIOCHEMICAL ACTIVITIES AND METABOLISM

Studies on the metabolic activities of the bordetellae have been concerned mainly with defining nutritional requirements or with biochemical tests for identification and for taxonomic and phylogenetic purposes. Biochemical activity, as usually determined in the laboratory, is weak. None ferments sugars but there are species-associated differences in other biochemical tests (see Table 38.1). *B. hinzii* can be distinguished

from *B. avium* by its ability to cause alkalinization of a wider range of substrates, to assimilate caprate and to decarboxylate histidine (Vandamme et al. 1995).

Other metabolic studies have been concerned with vaccine development and virulence mechanisms. As a step towards constructing attenuated bordetellae, the *aroA* gene of *B. pertussis* has been cloned and sequenced and found to be homologous with *aroA* genes from other bacteria (Roberts et al. 1990). This gene encodes an enzyme essential for the biosynthesis of aromatic amino acids and other aromatic compounds. The enzymes catalase, superoxide dismutase and peroxidase, which are important in oxygen metabolism and for survival of some bacteria within phagocytes, are present in *B. pertussis*, *B. parapertussis* and *B. bronchiseptica* and the other 3 species are known to produce catalase. A catalase-deficient construct of *B. pertussis* was more sensitive to killing by hydrogen peroxide than the wild-type strain but its ability to survive within human polymorphs was unchanged (DeShazer, Wood and Friedman 1994). *B. bronchiseptica* has potent urease activity and, with some pathogens, this enzyme is thought to be important in host colonization and disease production. Surprisingly, Monack and Falkow (1993) found that a urease deletion mutant of *B. bronchiseptica* was better able to colonize the respiratory and digestive tracts of guinea pigs than the parent strain. They suggested that urease may be more important to *B. bronchiseptica* in a possible environmental niche rather than in pathogenicity.

Iron is an essential nutrient for bacteria and successful pathogens must be able to cope with the iron-restricted environment found in host tissues. Here, the level of free iron is kept low by the iron-binding proteins lactoferrin and transferrin. Some pathogens produce high-affinity iron chelators (siderophores) to remove iron from these proteins and others have surface receptors that bind the host proteins directly to facilitate iron transport into the cell. In the bordetellae, both mechanisms appear to operate (Redhead et al. 1987, Gorringe, Woods and Robinson 1990). Hydroxamate siderophores have been purified from *B. pertussis* and *B. bronchiseptica* and shown to be identical to alcaligin, the iron chelator of *Alcaligenes denitrificans*. Iron-regulated gene expression in *B. pertussis* appears to be controlled, as in other organisms, by the repressor protein, Fur.

10   SUSCEPTIBILITY TO ANTIMICROBIAL AGENTS

The effectiveness of antibacterial agents against bordetellae in vitro does not necessarily reflect their usefulness against the bacteria localized on the ciliated epithelium of the respiratory tract due to the difficulty in maintaining suitable concentrations of the drugs at this site. Erythromycin is recommended for the treatment of pertussis patients and for post-exposure prophylaxis of contacts; erythromycin estolate is reported to reach higher concentrations than other formulations. There is only one recorded instance of erythromycin resistance in a *B. pertussis* isolate and antibiotic susceptibility testing is usually not necessary. Antibiotic treatment in the early (catarrhal or early paroxysmal) stages can ameliorate the symptoms of pertussis and eliminate the infection but later treatment may have no clinical benefit.

In the treatment of animal bordetellosis, delivery of standard amounts of antimicrobial agents by the oral or parenteral route may be insufficient to reduce bacterial numbers in the respiratory tract and to alleviate symptoms (Bemis 1992). Increased dosage or local administration of the agent by aerosol or intratracheal injection may be beneficial. Another difficulty is the frequent development of resistant strains of *B. bronchiseptica*. In surveys on the in vitro susceptibility of *B. bronchiseptica* (Woolfrey and Moody 1991, Bemis 1992) isolates were generally susceptible to aminoglycosides, anti-pseudomonal penicillins, chloramphenicol, tetracyclines, imipenem, quinolones and polymyxins. Those that were generally ineffective were erythromycin, some cephalosporins, streptomycin, clindamycin and nitrofurans. In some cases, treatment failure has been shown to be due to R factors. Plasmids encoding multiple drug resistance have been described and some are capable of conjugal transfer to other organisms. Antibiotic resistance plasmids are also commonly encountered in *B. avium*. In a recent survey of Australian isolates, all were resistant to erythromycin and most were resistant to sulphonamides and streptomycin (Blackall, Eaves and Fegan 1995).

11 VIRULENCE FACTORS

Bordetella spp. produce an array of toxins, aggressins and adhesins that are presumed to be important in colonization of their respective hosts and ensuring their survival and propagation. The best characterized species is the human pathogen *B. pertussis* and many of its products have been rigorously purified and characterized and assessed for their protective activity in experimental animals. Following the pioneering work of Weiss, Falkow and coworkers (Weiss et al. 1983, 1984, Weiss and Falkow 1984), genes encoding the putative virulence factors have been identified by transposon mutagenesis and many have been cloned and sequenced and expressed in other bacteria to investigate their properties. Strains engineered with precise mutations have been used to determine the effect of the loss of individual factors on virulence-related properties. In some cases, however, the role of these factors in pathogenesis has been difficult to define since reliance has to be placed on in vitro assays or animal models of the human infections, particularly in the mouse, in which different conditions may prevail. With this in mind, the putative virulence factors of the bordetellae will now be described, in order of their prevalence within the genus. A summary of the species distribution of these factors is shown in Table 38.2. Further information may be found elsewhere (Wardlaw and Parton 1988b, Brennan et al. 1992, Weiss 1992, Rappuoli 1994). No information is available on the presence or absence of virulence factors in the 2 recently described species, *B. hinzii* and *B. holmesii*.

11.1 Tracheal cytotoxin (TCT)

TCT is produced by at least 4 species of bordetellae. It was discovered by Goldman and colleagues from its ability to cause ciliostasis and ciliated cell extrusion in hamster tracheal organ cultures and inhibition of DNA synthesis in hamster trachea epithelial (HTE) cell cultures. The selective destruction of ciliated cells is similar to that seen in necropsy material from human pertussis and in turkey coryza (Goldman 1988). Such effects could well account for some of the pathological events of *Bordetella* respiratory infections such as accumulation of mucus, coughing and predisposition to secondary infections. TCT is an unusual toxin, with a low MW (921 Da). It is a disaccharide tetrapeptide derived from the peptidoglycan component of the cell envelope and released into the culture supernate during the logarithmic phase of growth (Cookson et al. 1989). An identical substance is produced by *Neisseria gonorrhoeae*. These toxins belong to a family of muramyl peptides with diverse biological activities such as pyrogenicity, adjuvanticity, arthritogenicity, induction of slow-wave sleep and stimulation of IL-1 production. Nitric oxide, synthesized in response to IL-1, may be the actual cytotoxic factor (Heiss et al. 1994). There is no information on the potential immunogenicity of TCT.

11.2 Heat-labile toxin (HLT)

HLT, also known as dermonecrotizing toxin, was the first bordetella toxin to be described and yet its role in disease has not been defined. It has potent vasoconstrictive activity and in experimental animals causes death or loss of normal weight gain, spleen atrophy and ischaemic lesions or necrosis of skin. HLT activity is found in all 4 species listed in Table 38.2. Recent genetic studies (Walker and Weiss 1994) have supported earlier findings that *B. pertussis*, *B. parapertussis* and *B. bronchiseptica* produce HLTs which are indistinguishable in their physicochemical, serological and biological properties whereas that of *B. avium* is similar. HLT, a protein of 140 kDa, is a cytoplasmic component of the bacteria and is largely responsible for the mouse-lethal toxicity of freshly harvested *B. pertussis* cells. The mouse toxicity test for pertussis vaccine was introduced primarily to ensure that HLT is destroyed during vaccine manufacture. The dermonecrotizing effect of HLT appears to be due to a specific constrictive effect on vascular smooth muscle. Such an effect on the highly vascularized tissues in the respiratory tract could induce a local inflammatory reaction and thus account for some of the pathology of pertussis (Nakase and Endoh 1988). Despite its potency in various bioassays, *B. pertussis* mutants deficient in HLT production were unaltered in their ability to cause a lethal infection in mice. HLT in *B. bronchiseptica* seems to have a role in producing the turbinate atrophy associated with atrophic rhinitis in pigs (see section 13.3, p. 916) by causing degenerative changes in osteoblasts and impairing bone formation (Horiguchi, Sugimoto and Matsuda 1994).

Table 38.2 Virulence factors of *Bordetella* species

Virulence factor	B. pertussis	B. parapertussis	B. bronchiseptica	B. avium	Probable role in pathogenicity
Tracheal cytotoxin	+	+	+	+	Ciliostasis, epithelial cell cytotoxicity
Heat-labile toxin	+	+	+	+	Local inflammatory effects
Endotoxin[a]	+ LOS	+ LPS	+ LPS	+ ?	Pyrogenicity
Fimbriae	+	+	+	+	Adhesins/invasins
Filamentous haemagglutinin	+	+	+	−	Adhesin/invasin
Adenylate cyclase toxin	+	+	+	−	Interference with immune effector cells
Pertactin	+	+	+	−	Adhesin/invasin
BrkA	+	?	+	−	Adhesin/invasin, serum resistance
Tracheal colonization factor	+	−	−	−	Adhesin
Pertussis toxin	+	−	−	−	Adhesin/invasin, interference with immune effector cells

[a]LOS, lipo-oligosaccharide; LPS, lipopolysaccharide; ?, unknown.

11.3 Endotoxin

The endotoxin of *B. pertussis*, like that of some other bacterial pathogens, is generally referred to as a lipo-oligosaccharide (LOS). It contains lipid A and an oligosaccharide core with 2-keto-3-deoxyoctulosonic acid (KDO) but it does not have a long-chain polysaccharide O antigen as found in the lipopolysaccharide (LPS) of enterobacteria (Brodeur et al. 1993). By contrast, *B. parapertussis* and *B. bronchiseptica* endotoxins consist of smooth-type LPS with high molecular weight O-polysaccharide components. These are chemically and immunologically identical in the 2 species but their core oligosaccharides are different. At present, there is no clear understanding of the role of LOS in pertussis. It has the usual properties of endotoxins such as general toxicity, pyrogenicity and adjuvanticity as well as some unusual properties such as the ability to induce antiviral activity, B cell mitogenicity and polyclonal B cell activation (Chaby and Caroff 1988). LOS may be responsible for the mild fever in early pertussis. In addition, it probably causes much of the reactogenicity of whole cell vaccine and a main aim in pertussis vaccine development has been to eliminate this toxin. Nevertheless, LOS may have a role in immunity to pertussis infection. Pertussis vaccine that has been boiled to destroy all but the heat-stable LOS antigens still protects mice against lethal intranasal challenge with *B. pertussis* and some anti-LOS monoclonal antibodies are passively protective.

11.4 Fimbriae

B. pertussis produces 2 types of fimbriae (pili) which carry the antigenic determinants of the serotype 2 and 3 agglutinogens and individual strains may express one, both or neither (see section 12.1, p. 911). Serotype 2 and 3 fimbriae are composed predominantly of protein subunits of 22.5 and 22 kDa respectively. Serologically cross-reactive fimbrial subunits of different molecular weights are found in other bordetellae. Both types of *B. pertussis* fimbriae also contain FimD, a protein of 40 kDa, as a minor component. This protein enables the bacterium to bind to human monocytes via their cell-surface integrin VLA-5 and it may be located at the tip of the fimbrial structure (Mooi 1994).

Bacterial fimbriae are usually involved in adhesion but the exact role of bordetella fimbriae has not been defined. They do not appear to play a role in attachment of *B. pertussis* in its usual location, on human respiratory ciliated cells (Tuomanen 1988), but they do enable the organism to bind to other mammalian cells, including monocytes, and may serve to facilitate phagocytosis. Other evidence suggests that they are important in both pathogenesis and immunity. Of the 4 recognized serotypes (1,2,3; 1,2; 1,3; and 1) only the first 3 (possessing fimbriae) infect man. Purified fimbriae have been shown to protect mice against respiratory infection with *B. pertussis* and protection against challenge strains of different serotypes was serospecific (Robinson et al. 1989). These findings are consistent with suggestions that protection of children with whole cell pertussis vaccine is to some extent serospecific (Preston 1988). For these reasons, fimbriae (agglutinogens) are candidate antigens in acellular pertussis vaccines (see section 13.1, p. 914).

11.5 Filamentous haemagglutinin (FHA)

FHA is one of the 2 haemagglutinins of *B. pertussis*, the other being PT, and its primary role appears to be in colonization of the respiratory epithelium. Similar, but not identical, proteins are present in *B. parapertussis* and *B. bronchiseptica*. *B. avium* also has a haemagglutinin but it is unrelated to those in *B. pertussis*. FHA is synthesized as a large precursor protein of 367 kDa which is encoded by the largest prokaryotic gene known. The precursor protein is exported to the bacterial surface where it is thought to be anchored by its C-terminal moiety. Eventually, this portion is cleaved proteolytically and the N-terminal 220 kDa 'mature' FHA is released. As an adhesin, FHA is unusual in having multiple binding activities that allow *B. pertussis* to adhere to, and in some cases invade, different cell types such as ciliated cells and macrophage, possibly at different stages of infection and in conjunction with other adhesins (Locht et al. 1993, Mooi 1994). One of its binding activities is due to an Arg-Gly-Asp (RGD) domain that promotes adhesion to the macrophage integrin CR3. Such FHA-mediated binding of *B. pertussis* to macrophages leads to phagocytosis without triggering an oxidative burst and may be critical in the intracellular survival of this organism.

Infection experiments have shown that *B. pertussis* FHA mutants have a reduced ability to colonize and persist in the upper respiratory tract of mice. Immunization with FHA alone will protect mice against aerosol challenge with *B. pertussis* and FHA enhances the protective activity of pertussis toxoid (PTd) in mice against a lethal intracerebral (i.c.) challenge. This i.c. challenge test is a standard test of pertussis vaccine potency. In view of its adhesive and mouse-protective activities, FHA is one of the prime candidate antigens in acellular pertussis vaccines (see section 13.1, p. 914).

11.6 Adenylate cyclase toxin (ACT) and haemolysin (HLY)

The adenylate cyclase (AC) of *B. pertussis* was first shown to be associated with toxic activity by its ability to attenuate neutrophil superoxide production and bactericidal capabilities. Subsequently, ACT was shown to penetrate and intoxicate a wide range of cell types (Hewlett and Gordon 1988). Immune effector cells such as neutrophils, monocytes, macrophages and natural killer cells are thought to be the primary targets, when those functions necessary for combating infection are inhibited. ACT is a bifunctional protein of 177 kDa with both AC and (weak) HLY activities. DNA homology studies have revealed that ACT is a member of the RTX (repeats in toxin) family of proteins, of which the prototype is *Escherichia coli* haemolysin (Coote 1992). Most RTX proteins are pore-forming, cytolytic toxins and the C-terminal portion of ACT, with homology to the other RTX cytolysins, provides a means of entry into the target cell for the N-terminal AC moiety. Once inside the cell, the AC moiety is activated by the eukaryotic protein calmodulin and causes unregulated synthesis of cyclic AMP. *B. parapertussis* and *B. bronchiseptica* have ACT activity similar to that of *B. pertussis* but the toxins are antigenically distinct.

Studies with *B. pertussis* mutants deficient in ACT activity have confirmed its importance as a virulence factor, at least in a mouse model. ACT has been shown to be a protective antigen for mice by Guiso and colleagues (Betsou, Sebo and Guiso 1993). *B. pertussis* was cleared more rapidly from the respiratory tract of animals immunized with ACT than from controls. However, doubts have been expressed about its use as a vaccine antigen because of a cross-reaction with mammalian brain adenylate cyclase.

11.7   Pertactin (PRN)

Pertactins are a family of *bvg*-regulated (see section 12.1, p. 911), surface-associated proteins produced by the 3 closely related *Bordetella* spp. (see Table 38.2). Pertactin P.69 from *B. pertussis* has an apparent MW of 69 kDa as determined by SDS-PAGE. Homologous proteins, of slightly different size, are found in *B. parapertussis* (P.70) and *B. bronchiseptica* (P.68). Sequencing of their respective genes has shown that they are encoded as large precursor proteins. The precursor of *B. pertussis* PRN is 93.5 kDa, from which a 3 kDa N-terminal signal sequence and a 30 kDa C-terminal portion are cleaved proteolytically to yield mature PRN of 60 kDa. This molecule migrates anomalously in SDS-PAGE, hence its descriptor P.69. The cleaved C-terminal portion, designated P.30, remains in the outer membrane (Charles et al. 1994).

P.69 has been shown to mediate attachment of *B. pertussis* to, and invasion of, tissue culture cell lines and, as with FHA, this attachment involves an RGD, integrin-binding domain. In fact, P.69 and FHA may act in concert for efficient cell binding. A role in attachment to human ciliated cells, however, has not been demonstrated. P.69 is protective in mice against aerosol challenge with *B. pertussis* and a mixture of P.69 and FHA also protects mice against i.c. challenge, although neither alone is effective. The related molecule P.68 is reported to protect pigs from *B. bronchiseptica* infection. There is therefore much interest in P.69 as a vaccine component. It was shown to be present in a significant amount in one of the early Japanese acellular vaccines and it is now included as a main constituent in some of the newer acellular formulations.

11.8   Other virulence-associated, outer-membrane proteins (OMPs)

These are of particular interest because of their striking structural homology with PRN. One such protein, BrkA, has homology with P.69, 2 RGD motifs and a similar proteolytic processing site (Fernandez and Weiss 1994). Like P.69, it is synthesized as a large precursor, of 103 kDa, and processed into the N-terminal 73 kDa BrkA and a 30 kDa C-terminal fragment containing an outer-membrane localization signal. This latter fragment has homology with the C-terminal P.30 fragment of PRN. Sequences homologous to the *brk* gene are present in *B. parapertussis* and *B. bronchiseptica* and the protein has been detected in some strains of *B. bronchiseptica* by immunoblotting with a monoclonal antibody to BrkA. A *B. pertussis* mutant deficient in BrkA was less virulent for mice than the parent strain, less adherent to HeLa cells, less invasive for these cells and at least 10-fold more susceptible to killing by normal human serum.

A related protein, tracheal colonization factor (TCF), has also been described (Finn and Stevens 1995). A mutant of *B. pertussis* lacking TCF had reduced ability to colonize mouse trachea compared with the parent strain. Like PRN, this protein, of 68 kDa, migrates anomalously in gel electrophoresis (at 90 kDa), it contains an RGD sequence and has the conserved proteolytic cleavage site which releases a 30 kDa C-terminal fragment. This fragment has homology with P.30 and remains in the outer membrane. Unlike PRN and BrkA, which appear to be cell-associated, TCF is both cell-associated and released into the culture supernate. TCF production appears to be unique to *B. pertussis*.

11.9   Pertussis toxin (PT)

This toxin is the most extensively studied component of *B. pertussis* (Wardlaw and Parton 1988b, Kaslow and Burns 1992, Krueger and Barbieri 1995). PT has attracted wide interest not only because of an assumed central role in the pathogenesis of whooping cough and as a proven vaccine antigen but also because of its remarkable range of biological activities and its frequent use as a probe of eukaryotic cell signalling processes. Some of the in vitro and in vivo activities of PT are listed in Table 38.3. PT is produced only by *B. pertussis* although transcriptionally silent genes are present in *B. parapertussis* and *B. bronchiseptica*.

PT is a complex protein of 105 kDa with an enzymic moiety, the A subunit, and a heteropentameric B subunit responsible for binding to target cells and inserting the A subunit into the cytoplasm. Binding involves a lectin-like interaction in which regions of the B subunit mimic eukaryotic selectins involved in leucocyte trafficking (Sandros and Tuomanen 1993). This interaction also binds *B. pertussis* to eukaryotic cells such as human ciliated cells and macrophages and makes PT unique as both a toxin and adhesin. The haemagglutinating and T cell mitogenic activities of PT are due solely to the B subunit binding to cell

Table 38.3 Some activities of pertussis toxin

Demonstrated at cellular level in vitro
ADP-ribosylation of G proteins
Haemagglutination
Adhesion/invasion
Inhibition of neutrophil oxidative burst
Inhibition of monocyte migration
Inhibition of histamine release from mast cells
T cell mitogenicity

Demonstrated in experimental animals and *in humans
Protective antigen (in toxoided form)*
Induction of leucocytosis*
Enhancement of insulin secretion*
Inhibition of adrenaline hyperglycaemia*
Sensitization to histamine
Sensitization to anaphylaxis, anoxia, endotoxin, etc.
Adjuvanticity
Enhancement of vascular permeability
Acute toxicity/lethality

surfaces. The toxicity of PT is due to the enzymatic activity of the A subunit which is an ADP-ribosyl-transferase targeting various G proteins. The modified G proteins are unable to function in the normal signal transduction across the membrane and because different cell types and signalling systems are involved, the ensuing biological effects are numerous.

PT has been proposed as having some central role in the pathogenesis of whooping cough (Pittman 1984a) but its actual role remains obscure. Both PT and FHA are required for efficient binding to human ciliated cells and they also act co-operatively in the uptake of *B. pertussis* by macrophages. Moreover, PT and FHA released from *B. pertussis* allow other bacteria such as *Haemophilus influenzae* to bind to human ciliated cells. This phenomenon, termed 'piracy of adhesins', may contribute to the secondary infections often associated with pertussis (Tuomanen 1988). PT is essential for virulence in a mouse model of infection. One probable target is the circulating cells of the immune system and interference with their normal functioning. In view of the many common features of bordetella diseases, however, and the fact that PT is unique to *B. pertussis*, it is difficult to assign a pre-eminent role to PT in either pathogenesis (see section 13.2, p. 915) or host specificity. Nevertheless, PT, in toxoided form (PTd), has become the prime candidate antigen in acellular pertussis vaccines. Immunization with PTd protects mice against both i.c. and aerosol challenges with *B. pertussis*. A formalin-detoxified PTd has been a major component of acellular pertussis vaccines in use in Japan since 1981. Such chemical toxoiding is known to reduce immunogenicity and more promising vaccines, containing fully immunogenic recombinant PTd, are now available (Rappuoli et al. 1992).

12 GENETIC MECHANISMS

12.1 Regulation of virulence in *B. pertussis*

SEROTYPE VARIATION

The major serotype antigens (AGGs) 1, 2 and 3 occur in various combinations on different strains of *B. pertussis* and thereby differentiate the 4 widely recognized serotypes 1,2,3; 1,2; 1,3; 1. The AGGs are all lost during phase variation (see section on 'Phase variation and antigenic modulation') but AGGs 2 and 3 can also be lost or regained independently in vitro and in vivo. Such changes occur at about 1 in every 10^3–10^4 cell divisions. AGGs 2 and 3 are located on fimbriae and serotype variation, at least with AGG 3, appears to be due to spontaneous frameshift mutations in the promoter region of the fimbrial subunit gene.

PHASE VARIATION AND ANTIGENIC MODULATION

Phase variation was first described by Leslie and Gardner (1931) as a stepwise degradative process from phase I, with the characteristics of fresh isolates, to phase IV, with the different phases being distinguished by colony morphology, haemolysis and serology. Phases I and II were toxic for guinea pigs whereas phases III and IV were not. It is now clear that degradation of *B. pertussis* strains is even more complicated than the above 4 stages but the spontaneous occurrence of phase IV or 'avirulent-phase' mutants is well known. Such strains no longer express the virulence factors PT, AC, HLY, FHA, HLT, AGGs and certain OMPs associated with fresh isolates (Wardlaw and Parton 1988b, Stibitz and Miller 1994). Phase variation occurs at a frequency of 1 per 10^3–10^6 organisms and is occasionally reversible.

Expression of virulence factors is also regulated in response to growth conditions in vitro. The term 'antigenic modulation' was introduced by Lacey (1960) to describe the freely reversible phenotypic changes that occur when *B. pertussis* is grown with high levels of certain salts, organic acids or at low temperatures. The so-called C (cyanic) mode or avirulent phenotype was originally distinguished from the X (xanthic) mode or virulent phenotype by serology and cultural characteristics. Subsequent work has shown that virulence factors PT, AC, HLY, FHA, HLT and AGGs are lost during the X to C transition, as are certain OMPs, adhesiveness and hydrophobicity (Wardlaw and Parton 1988a).

The similar loss of virulence factors during antigenic modulation and phase variation suggested that a common regulatory mechanism is involved and that phase variation is the genotypic equivalent of antigenic modulation. Thus, phase I and X mode are essentially the same, as are phase IV and C mode. The difference is that the X to C change is environmentally regulated, affects all cells in the population and is freely reversible whereas the phase I to IV change is an infrequent, mutational event that requires subsequent clonal selection for recognition, and reversion is equally infrequent.

Mechanisms of phase variation and antigenic modulation

Weiss and colleagues (Weiss et al. 1983, Weiss and Falkow 1984) first demonstrated that a single Tn5 insertion in the *B. pertussis* chromosome abolished the expression of the virulence factors PT, HLY, AC, FHA and HLT. They had thus identified a virulence regulatory locus which they designated *vir*, and which was later renamed *bvg*. Subsequently, several virulence-repressed genes (*vrg*) have been identified which are regulated in a reciprocal fashion to the virulence-activated genes (*vag*) encoding the virulence factors listed above. The following description of the regulation of virulence expression in *B. pertussis* via the *bvg* locus has been distilled from recent reviews (Mooi 1994, Rappuoli 1994, Stibitz and Miller 1994) and is summarized in Fig. 38.2. The actual signal(s) for the organism to adopt the virulent (Bvg+) or avirulent (Bvg−) phase under the 'usual' growth conditions are unknown. Phase variation is caused by spontaneous mutations in the *bvg* locus and both reversible, frameshift mutations and irreversible deletions have been found in avirulent phase strains.

12.2 Significance of virulence regulation

The chameleon-like potential for change in *B. pertussis* is thus apparent (Fig. 38.3) but its significance in the life-style of the organism is less clear. There is evidence that serotype variation occurs in animal models of infection and in human infections. The fimbriae are presumed to have an important role in colonization of the host and vaccine-induced immunity appears to have a serotype-specific component. This type of variation would therefore be useful in evading the host immune response. With regard to antigenic modulation, it seems highly probable that the ability of a *B. pertussis* population to respond rapidly to environmental influences is more than just a laboratory artefact. Phase variation and serotype variation affect only a few cells in the population but the potential of these cells to adapt to changing circumstances may be advantageous. The preferred site for colonization by *B. pertussis* is the ciliated surface of the human respiratory tract where it expresses the virulent phenotype. There has been speculation, however, that it may have to undergo variation not only to evade the host immune response but to aid transmission, to prolong survival between hosts or to colonize some other site. Such a site could be within the same host, for example intracellularly, in an alternative host or in some environmental niche (Coote 1991, Parton 1991, Stibitz and Miller 1994). The idea of a significant role for the co-ordinate regulation of virulence is further strengthened by the knowledge that this process also occurs in *B. bronchiseptica* and *B. avium*, and sequences homologous to *bvg* have been shown in all 3 species. Rappuoli (1994) has suggested that the *bvg* system evolved to enable the bordetellae to distinguish between the external environment, at a low temperature, from the host environment at a higher temperature.

12.3 Genome organization

The technique of pulse field gel electrophoresis was used by Stibitz and Garletts (1992) to construct a physical map of the *B. pertussis* chromosome and to locate the positions of the virulence genes and some 'housekeeping' genes. The apparent size of the genome was 3750 kb, about 80% of the size of the *E. coli* genome. Apart from the close proximity of *fha*, *bvg* and of some genes involved in fimbrial assembly, there was no significant linkage of the virulence genes. Insertion sequence (IS) elements and associated repeated DNA sequences have been found in the bordetella genome. One such element, IS481, is unique to *B. pertussis*. Approximately 80 copies are scattered around the genome and it thus comprises about 2% of the DNA. Other such elements appear to be common to *B. pertussis*, *B. parapertussis* and *B. bronchiseptica*. In other bacteria, IS and repeated DNA sequences have been implicated in genome rearrangements and virulence factor expression but no such effects have been reported in the bordetellae. Weiss (1992), however, has speculated that mutations caused by the insertion of such elements into the genome of *B. pertussis* may be responsible for its growth deficiencies and fastidious nature.

13 HABITAT AND PATHOGENICITY

Until recently, the bordetellae were considered to be obligate, non-invasive parasites of the respiratory tracts of warm-blooded animals, including birds, with a predilection for the respiratory ciliated epithelium

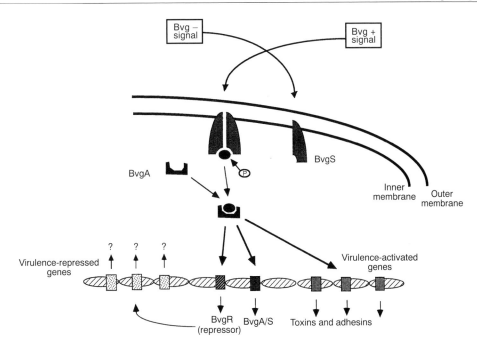

Fig. 38.2 Virulence regulation in *B. pertussis*. The *bvg* locus encodes 2 proteins BvgS and BvgA with homology to '2-component' signal-transducing proteins in other bacteria and eukaryotes. BvgS is a sensor protein spanning the inner membrane and BvgA is a cytoplasmic receiver protein able to bind to the DNA. These proteins are expressed only at a low level, from a weak promoter, under modulating conditions. Incoming (Bvg+, non-modulating, X mode) signals are transmitted to the cytoplasmic portion of BvgS which becomes active as a kinase, and possibly involves dimerization of the molecule. This in turn activates BvgA, by phosphorylation. Bvg A binds to a stronger *bvg* promoter to enhance *bvgAS* expression and causes transcription of the virulence-activated genes and repression of other genes.

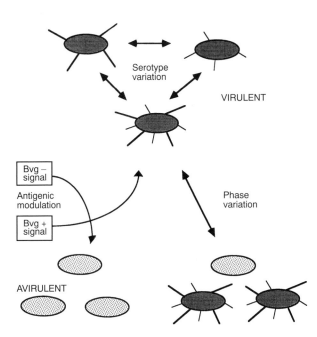

Fig. 38.3 Variation in *B. pertussis*. The combined processes of serotype variation, antigenic modulation and phase variation make *B. pertussis* a highly variable and, potentially, highly adaptable organism. These processes may be involved in evasion of host immune responses, transmission or survival at different sites in vivo or ex vivo. Antigenic modulation affects all cells in the population and is freely reversible whereas serotype and phase variation are infrequent, mutational events.

(Wardlaw 1990). This definition has been confounded by several recent observations. First, all members of the newly described species *B. holmesii* were isolated from human blood and were not associated with respiratory infection. There are single reports of the isolation of *B. pertussis* and *B. hinzii* from human blood and isolation of *B. bronchiseptica* from this site is rare. These isolations appear to have been mainly from immunocompromised patients and so an increasing number of such findings is perhaps inevitable. Second, it has become apparent that *B. pertussis*, *B. parapertussis* and *B. bronchiseptica* have mechanisms for attachment to, invasion of, and survival in, both epithelial cells and phagocytes. The significance of this habitat is not yet clear but it may be important in the protracted course of bordetella infections or in establishment of a quiescent or chronic stage. The importance of cell mediated immunity to *B. pertussis* infection, demonstrated in animal models, may be due in part to destruction of such infected cells (Redhead et al. 1993). Third, although the bordetellae are generally regarded as having little capability for growth and survival outside their hosts, this possibility must now be considered because of the ability of *B. bronchiseptica* and *B. avium* to survive and grow in low nutrient conditions such as natural waters (Porter and Wardlaw 1993). Antigenic modulation may be required for this survival. Finally, the ability of at least 4 *Bordetella* spp. to regulate virulence factor expression in response to external signals strongly suggests that they do have alternative habitats, either in vivo or ex vivo, where such regulation would be an advantage.

There is no completely satisfactory explanation for the different host specificities of the bordetellae, although adhesion mechanisms to host ciliated cells seem to be influential. *B. pertussis* has been shown to adhere best to human cilia, *B. bronchiseptica* and *B. parapertussis* adhered best to non-human mammalian, but not avian, cilia and *B. avium* adhered specifically to avian ciliated cells (Tuomanen 1988). To determine whether host specificity of the bordetellae might be related to different nutrient conditions in their respective hosts, Porter and Wardlaw (1994) collected tracheobronchial washings (TBW) from 7 vertebrate species. *B. bronchiseptica* and *B. avium* grew well in most of the TBW samples, *B. parapertussis* grew in TBW from man, sheep and certain other species but, surprisingly, *B. pertussis* did not grow in any sample, including that from man.

In considering the pathogenicity of members of the genus, the range of virulence factors produced by each species should be examined (see Table 38.2). This may provide clues as to which factors are responsible for the unique or common features of the diseases. Such evidence has been used by Goldman (1988) to propose that TCT, produced by the first 4 described species, has a central role in the pathogenesis of bordetella infections. The common features of the diseases caused by these species include age-related susceptibility to infection, adherence of organisms to ciliated epithelium and loss of ciliated cells from the respiratory tract, reduced weight gain of the host, excessive mucus production and some form of cough. Secondary infections also appear to be common and increase the mortality rate in untreated cases (Wardlaw and Parton 1988a).

13.1 *Bordetella pertussis*

The causative agent of pertussis or whooping cough is responsible for severe morbidity and mortality world wide, mainly in unvaccinated communities, with 60 million cases and more than half a million deaths estimated in 1986. Fortunately, increasing global immunization coverage by schemes such as the WHO Expanded Programme on Immunization is steadily reducing these figures. In some vaccinated communities, the problems have been rather different. In the mid-1970s, widespread concern about the possible harmful effects of whole cell vaccines, and the associated decline in vaccine uptake, resulted in recurrences of pertussis epidemics. As vaccine uptake has recovered, control has once again been established. In many countries, whether immunization is practised or not, epidemics occur every 3–4 years, presumably due to the number of susceptible individuals in the population. A lack of effect on this frequency by introduction of vaccination or changes in vaccine uptake rates seems to indicate that whole cell vaccines provide better protection against disease than against infection and that vaccination has little effect on the prevalence of *B. pertussis* in the population.

The current development of acellular pertussis vaccines,

reviewed recently (Brennan et al. 1992, Rappuoli et al. 1992, Cherry 1993), is aimed at overcoming the problems of reactogenicity, improving public acceptance of vaccination and protecting against both infection and disease. Two such vaccines, a monocomponent PTd vaccine and a 2-component PTd + FHA vaccine, were used in a large-scale, double-blind, placebo-controlled field trial in 1986–87 in Sweden where pertussis was prevalent (Ad Hoc Group 1988). Their reactogenicity was low, as expected, but efficacy results were disappointing. They were less protective against culture- or serologically confirmed pertussis than would have been expected for a whole cell vaccine. Both vaccines, however, gave good protection against severe disease and provided evidence that PTd alone or with other antigens could make effective vaccines. Further trials are now in progress to compare other vaccine formulations containing combinations of PTd or recombinant PTd, FHA, PRN and AGGs. Preliminary results suggest that the multicomponent vaccines are highly efficacious. Further pertussis vaccine developments may involve the creation of stable, genetically defined, attenuated bacterial strains suitable for use as live vaccines, or intranasal delivery of suitable antigen formulations to avoid the need for injection and to stimulate effective mucosal immunity.

Pertussis is primarily a disease of young children in that most typical cases occur in this age group, with most deaths in infants younger than 1 year. All ages are susceptible, however, and adults with waning immunity may be an important reservoir of infection. Passive protection is only poorly passed on from the mother to the newborn. Pertussis is highly communicable, especially in home exposures, and transmission can mostly be attributed to droplet infection from active cases. There is no evidence of true (i.e. long-term, asymptomatic) carriers and no natural, non-human host, vector or environmental reservoir is known. The clinical features of pertussis tend to vary with age, general health and immune status and adults and older children often show mild or atypical symptoms. Typical pertussis can be divided into the catarrhal, paroxysmal and convalescent stages. After an incubation period of 7–14 days, the catarrhal stage resembles a non-distinctive, upper respiratory tract infection with a mild cough, excessive mucus production and sometimes mild fever. The cough becomes increasingly severe and, after 7–10 days, the patient enters the paroxysmal stage. This is characterized by bouts of uncontrollable coughing, up to 20 or more in 24 h, when the patient is attempting to clear the tenacious mucus from the airways. The paroxysms are often followed by the distinctive, inspiratory whoop. Vomiting and hypoxia may also ensue. Respiratory complications and central nervous system disturbances are relatively frequent and due mainly to pressure effects and anoxia, both resulting from the severe coughing. The paroxysmal stage may last for 1–4 weeks, then the cough gradually subsides over a prolonged convalescent period. Further information on pertussis may be found elsewhere (Cherry et al. 1988, Hodder and Mortimer 1992) (see also Volume 3, Chapter 18).

The pathogenicity of *B. pertussis* has been studied in vitro, in cell and organ cultures and in vivo. The latter studies have been, of necessity, in various unnatural animal models of infection and the relative merits of each of these models have been reviewed (Sato and Sato 1988, Shahin and Cowell 1994). Mouse models are used most often but a recently decribed coughing rat model appears to have much potential for investigation of the mechanisms of cough production and immunity in pertussis (Parton, Hall and Wardlaw 1994). The results of such studies, particularly with *B. pertussis* mutants deficient in individual virulence factors, have shown clearly that pertussis pathogenesis is complex and multifactorial. Loss of any one of a number of toxins and adhesins has been shown to affect the organism's ability to colonize the host or cause pathological changes. Based on the information in the preceding sections, a possible sequence of events in pertussis is shown in Fig. 38.4.

13.2 *Bordetella parapertussis*

B. parapertussis is generally considered to cause a milder form of disease than *B. pertussis*. Although it may be true that it is isolated less frequently than *B. pertussis* and that many parapertussis infections are asymptomatic, this organism is capable of causing typical whooping cough. In 2 studies of coughing illness in Germany, paroxysmal coughing, whooping and vomiting were all features of parapertussis infections, with frequencies approaching those in pertussis cases (Heininger et al. 1994, Wirsing von Konig and Finger 1994). The main difference was that lymphocytosis, due to PT which is produced only by *B. pertussis*, was not a feature of parapertussis. These findings suggest that PT plays a minor role, if any, in causing the typical

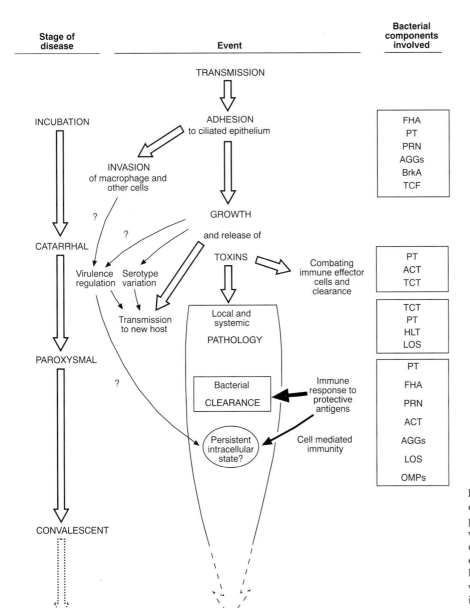

Fig. 38.4 The sequence of events in pertussis. The postulated roles for the various bacterial components at the different clinical stages of disease are based on evidence from in vitro and in vivo models of infection (see section 11, p. 907).

symptoms of whooping cough and that other toxins are responsible. In both studies, the percentage of patients who had received pertussis vaccine was greater in the parapertussis group than in the pertussis group. This observation supports previous evidence that there is little cross-immunity between the 2 infections. For example, Lautrop (1971) showed that over a 20 year period in Denmark, the epidemics of pertussis and parapertussis both occurred in 3–4 year cycles but were out of phase with each other. In view of the close relationship between *B. pertussis* and *B. parapertussis*, and their similar range of virulence factors, the lack of cross-immunity is remarkable. However, Khelef et al. (1993) showed that FHA, PRN and ACT from *B. pertussis* were protective antigens for mice against intranasal challenge with *B. pertussis* but not against *B. parapertussis*. Thus, although their virulence factors are structurally and functionally similar, they have important antigenic differences.

Until recently, *B. parapertussis* was considered to be a purely human parasite, like *B. pertussis*. Its isolation from healthy and pneumonic lambs in New Zealand and Scotland (Porter, Connor and Donachie 1994) has changed this view and may have identified a reservoir of infection for man. Such isolates have been shown to cause pneumonia in experimentally infected lambs and, when administered with *Pasteurella haemolytica*, to cause more severe disease than either agent alone. This situation parallels that with *B. bronchiseptica* and *Pasteurella multocida* in atrophic rhinitis in pigs.

13.3 *Bordetella bronchiseptica*

This organism is an important pathogen of domestic and laboratory animals and it is often carried asymptomatically. Its broad host range includes dogs, cats, pigs, guinea pigs, rats, mice, rabbits, horses, turkeys, monkeys, humans and numerous wild animals. *B. bronchiseptica* is one of the causes of atrophic rhinitis, an economically important disease of swine, characterized by inflammation of the nasal turbinates, turbinate atrophy, snout deformation and retarded growth (Rutter 1985, Woolfrey and Moody 1991). Although *B. bronchiseptica* alone is capable of causing mild to moderate turbinate atrophy, the severe, progressive disease appears to be caused by a subsequent colonization by toxigenic *P. multocida* and an interaction between the 2 species. Both produce a heat-labile, dermonecrotizing toxin that, on repeated local or parenteral administration, causes progressive turbinate atrophy. It is thought that TCT released by *B. bronchiseptica* enhances colonization by *P. multocida* by inducing ciliostasis and mucus accumulation. Another, less common, disease of pigs due to *B. bronchiseptica* is bronchopneumonia in piglets. Clinical signs include coughing, sometimes with whooping and dyspnoea. *B. bronchiseptica* also causes infectious tracheobronchitis, or kennel cough, in dogs (Goodnow 1980, Bemis 1992). This is a highly contagious disease

characterized by various degrees of coughing, sometimes paroxysmal, and purulent nasal discharge. Some pneumonia-related deaths occur but infection is generally limited to the tracheobronchial tree and the resulting pathological changes are similar to those described for whooping cough. The role of *B. bronchiseptica* in humans has been reviewed by Woolfrey and Moody (1991). They concluded that, despite the considerable exposure to animal sources of the organism, it is isolated only rarely from humans. It may be found as a respiratory tract commensal and as an opportunist in severely compromised patients.

13.4 *Bordetella avium*

This is the causative agent of turkey coryza, or turkey rhinotracheitis, although other birds are affected (Kersters et al. 1984). Turkey coryza is a highly contagious disease of turkey poults and symptoms include oculonasal discharge, tracheal mucus production, coughing, loss of appetite and decreased weight gain. It is sometimes a mild disease but conditions of stress and secondary infections, for example by *P. multocida*, can result in a high mortality rate. Histopathological examination shows attachment of the bacteria to the ciliated epithelium resulting in inflammation, loss of ciliated cells and distortion of the mucosa and tracheal rings. The clinical features similar to those of other bordetella diseases suggest that the virulence factors, such as TCT and HLT, common to these species, have a central role in bordetellosis. Alternatively, *B. avium* may possess other virulence factors to make up for those it lacks. A significant finding is that *B. avium* produces a protein, osteotoxin, that is cytotoxic for mammalian cells, including osteogenic and tracheal cells. The toxin is distinct from HLT and has β-cystathionase activity (Gentry-Weeks, Keith and Thompson 1993).

13.5 *Bordetella hinzii* and *Bordetella holmesii*

There is little information on the pathogenic potential of these 2, newly described species. All of the 15 known strains of *B. holmesii* were isolated from human blood cultures and several of these patients were known to have had an underlying condition that may have enhanced their susceptibility to infection (Weyant et al. 1995). Of the 14 characterized strains of *B. hinzii*, 12 were isolated from the respiratory tracts of turkeys and chickens but attempts to produce disease experimentally have failed (Vandamme et al. 1995). Two strains have been obtained from humans, one from sputum and one from the blood of an AIDS patient (Cookson et al. 1994). According to Vandamme (personal communication 1995), other such 'atypical' bordetellae will be described in the near future.

REFERENCES

Ad Hoc group, 1988, Placebo controlled trial of two acellular pertussis vaccines in Sweden, *Lancet*, **1:** 955–66.

Bemis DA, 1992, Bordetella and mycoplasma respiratory-infections in dogs and cats, *Vet Clin North Am Small Anim Pract*, **22:** 1173–86.

Betsou F, Sebo P, Guiso N, 1993, CyaC-mediated activation is important not only for toxic but also for protective activities of *Bordetella pertussis* adenylate cyclase-haemolysin, *Infect Immun*, **61:** 3583–9.

Blackall PJ, Eaves LE, Fegan M, 1995, Antimicrobial sensitivity testing of Australian isolates of *Bordetella avium* and the *Bordetella avium*-like organism, *Aust Vet J*, **72:** 97–100.

Blom J, Heron I, Hendley JO, 1994, Immunoelectron microscopy of antigens of *Bordetella pertussis* using monoclonal antibodies to agglutinogens 2 and 3, filamentous haemagglutinin, pertussis toxin, pertactin and adenylate cyclase toxin, *APMIS*, **102:** 681–9.

Bordet J, Gengou O, 1906, Le microbe de la coqueluche, *Ann Inst Pasteur*, **23:** 415–19.

Bradford WL, Slavin B, 1937, An organism resembling *Hemophilus pertussis*, *Am J Public Health*, **27:** 1277–82.

Brennan MJ, Burns DL et al., 1992, Recent advances in the development of pertussis vaccines, *Vaccines: New Approaches to Immunological Problems*, ed. Ellis RW, Butterworth–Heineman, Boston, 23–52.

Brodeur BR, Martin D et al., 1993, Antigenic analysis of the saccharide moiety of the lipooligosaccharide of *Bordetella pertussis*, *Springer Semin Immunopathol*, **15:** 205–15.

Cassiday PK, Sanden GN et al., 1994, Viability of *Bordetella pertussis* in four suspending solutions at three temperatures, *J Clin Microbiol*, **32:** 1550–3.

Chaby R, Caroff M, 1988, Lipopolysaccharides of *Bordetella pertussis* endotoxin, *Pathogenesis and Immunity in Pertussis*, eds Wardlaw AC, Parton R, John Wiley & Sons, Chichester, 247–71.

Charles I, Fairweather N et al., 1994, Expression of the *Bordetella pertussis* P.69 pertactin adhesin in *Escherichia coli*: fate of the carboxy-terminal domain, *Microbiology*, **140:** 3301–8.

Cherry JD, 1993, Acellular pertussis vaccines – a solution to the pertussis problem, *J Infect Dis*, **168:** 21–4.

Cherry JD, Brunell PA et al., 1988, Report of the task force on pertussis and pertussis immunization, *Pediatrics*, **81, Suppl.:** 939–84.

Cookson BT, Cho HL et al., 1989, Biological activities and chemical composition of purified tracheal cytotoxin of *Bordetella pertussis*, *Infect Immun*, **57:** 2223–9.

Cookson BT, Vandamme P et al., 1994, Bacteremia caused by a novel *Bordetella* species, 'B. hinzii', *J Clin Microbiol*, **32:** 2569–71.

Coote JG, 1991, Antigenic switching and pathogenicity: environmental effects on virulence gene expression in *Bordetella pertussis*, *J Gen Microbiol*, **137:** 2493–503.

Coote JG, 1992, Structural and functional relationships among the RTX toxin determinants of Gram-negative bacteria, *FEMS Microbiol Rev*, **88:** 137–62.

De Ley J, Segers P et al., 1986, Intra- and intergeneric similarities of the *Bordetella* ribosomal ribonucleic acid cistrons: proposal for a new family, Alcaligenaceae, *Int J Syst Bacteriol*, **36:** 405–14.

DeShazer D, Wood GE, Friedman RL, 1994, Molecular characterization of catalase from *Bordetella pertussis*: identification of the katA promoter in an upstream insertion sequence, *Mol Microbiol*, **14:** 123–30.

Eldering G, Hornbeck C, Baker J, 1957, Serological study of *Bordetella pertussis* and related species, *J Bacteriol*, **74:** 133–6.

Fernandez RC, Weiss AA, 1994, Cloning and sequencing of a *Bordetella pertussis* serum resistance locus, *Infect Immun*, **62:** 4727–38.

Ferry NS, 1910, A preliminary report of the bacterial findings in canine distemper, *Am Vet Rev*, **37:** 499–504.

Filion R, Cloutier S et al., 1967, Respiration infection in the turkey caused by a bacterium related to *Bordetella bronchiseptica*, *Can J Comp Med*, **31:** 129–34.

Finn TM, Stevens LA, 1995, Tracheal colonisation factor: a *Bordetella pertussis* secreted determinant, *Mol Microbiol*, **16:** 625–43.

Friedman RL, 1988, Pertussis: the disease and new diagnostic methods, *Clin Microbiol Rev*, **1:** 365–76.

Gentry-Weeks CR, Keith JM, Thompson J, 1993, Toxicity of *Bordetella avium* beta-cystathionase toward MC3T3-E1 osteogenic cells, *J Biol Chem*, **268:** 7298–314.

Gilchrist MJR, 1991, *Bordetella*, *Manual of Clinical Microbiology*, 5th edn, eds Balows A, Hausler WJ et al., American Society for Microbiology, Washington, DC, 471–7.

Goldman WE, 1988, Tracheal cytotoxin of *Bordetella pertussis*, *Pathogenesis and Immunity in Pertussis*, eds Wardlaw AC, Parton R, John Wiley & Sons, Chichester, 231–46.

Goodnow RA, 1980, Biology of *Bordetella bronchiseptica*, *Microbiol Rev*, **44:** 722–38.

Gorringe AR, Woods G, Robinson A, 1990, Growth and siderophore production by *Bordetella pertussis* under iron-restricted conditions, *FEMS Microbiol Lett*, **66:** 101–6.

Gross R, Arico B, Rappuoli R, 1989, Genetics of pertussis toxin, *Mol Microbiol*, **3:** 119–24.

Heininger U, Stehr K et al., 1994, Clinical characteristics of illness caused by *Bordetella parapertussis* compared with illness caused by *Bordetella pertussis*, *Pediatr Infect Dis J*, **13:** 306–9.

Heiss LN, Lancaster JRJ et al., 1994, Epithelial autotoxicity of nitric oxide: role in the respiratory cytopathology of pertussis, *Proc Natl Acad Sci USA*, **91:** 267–70.

Hewlett EL, Gordon VM, 1988, Adenylate cyclase toxin of *Bordetella pertussis*, *Pathogenesis and Immunity in Pertussis*, eds Wardlaw AC, Parton R, John Wiley & Sons, Chichester, 193–209.

Hodder SL, Mortimer EA, 1992, Epidemiology of pertussis and reactions to pertussis vaccine, *Epidemiol Rev*, **14:** 243–68.

Hoppe JE, 1988, Methods for isolation of *Bordetella pertussis* from patients with whooping cough, *Eur J Clin Microbiol Infect Dis*, **7:** 616–20.

Horiguchi Y, Sugimoto N, Matsuda M, 1994, *Bordetella bronchiseptica* dermonecrotizing toxin stimulates protein synthesis in an osteoblastic clone, MC3T3-E1 cells, *FEMS Microbiol Lett*, **120:** 19–22.

Imaizumi A, Suzuki Y et al., 1983, Heptakis(2,6-O-dimethyl)beta-cyclodextrin: a novel growth stimulant for *Bordetella pertussis* phase I, *J Clin Microbiol*, **17:** 781–6.

Johnson R, Sneath PHA, 1973, Taxonomy of *Bordetella* and related organisms of the Families Achromobacteraceae, Brucellaceae, and Neisseraceae, *Int J Syst Bacteriol*, **23:** 381–404.

Kaslow HR, Burns DL, 1992, Pertussis toxin and target eukaryotic cells: binding, entry, and activation, *FASEB J*, **6:** 2684–90.

Kersters K, Hinz KH et al., 1984, *Bordetella avium* sp. nov., isolated from the respiratory tracts of turkeys and other birds, *Int J Syst Bacteriol*, **34:** 56–70.

Khelef N, Danve B et al., 1993, *Bordetella pertussis* and *Bordetella parapertussis*: two immunologically distinct species, *Infect Immun*, **61:** 486–90.

Krueger KM, Barbieri JT, 1995, The family of bacterial ADP-ribosylating exotoxins, *Clin Microbiol Rev*, **8:** 34–47.

Lacey BW, 1960, Antigenic modulation in *Bordetella pertussis*, *J Hyg Camb*, **58:** 57–93.

Lautrop H, 1971, Epidemics of parapertussis. 20 years' observations in Denmark, *Lancet*, **1:** 1195–8.

Leslie PH, Gardner AD, 1931, The phases of *Haemophilus pertussis*, *J Hyg Camb*, **31:** 423–34.

Locht C, Bertin P et al., 1993, The filamentous haemagglutinin, a multifaceted adhesin produced by virulent *Bordetella* spp., *Mol Microbiol*, **9:** 653–60.

Meade BD, Bollen A, 1994, Recommendations for use of the polymerase chain reaction in the diagnosis of *Bordetella pertussis* infections, *J Med Microbiol*, **41:** 51–5.

Monack DM, Falkow S, 1993, Cloning of *Bordetella bronchiseptica* urease genes and analysis of colonization by a urease-negative mutant strain in a guinea-pig model, *Mol Microbiol*, **10:** 545–53.

Mooi FR, 1994, Genes for the filamentous haemagglutinin and fimbriae of *Bordetella pertussis*: colocation, coregulation and cooperation?, *Molecular Genetics of Bacterial Pathogenesis*, eds Miller VL, Kaper JB et al., American Society for Microbiology, Washington, DC, 145–55.

Moreno-Lopez M, 1952, El genero *Bordetella*, *Microbiol Esp*, **5:** 117–81.

Morrill WE, Barbaree JM et al., 1988, Effects of transport temperature and medium on recovery of *Bordetella pertussis* from nasopharyngeal swabs, *J Clin Microbiol*, **26:** 1814–17.

Musser JM, Hewlett EL et al., 1986, Genetic diversity and relationships in populations of *Bordetella* spp., *J Bacteriol*, **166:** 230–7.

Nakase Y, Endoh M, 1988, Heat-labile toxin of *Bordetella pertussis*, *Pathogenesis and Immunity in Pertussis*, eds Wardlaw AC, Parton R, John Wiley & Sons, Chichester, 211–29.

Onorato IM, Wassilak SGF, 1987, Laboratory diagnosis of pertussis: the state of the art, *Pediatr Infect Dis J*, **6:** 145–51.

Parton R, 1991, Changing perspectives on pertussis and pertussis vaccination, *Rev Med Microbiol*, **2:** 121–8.

Parton R, Hall E, Wardlaw AC, 1994, Responses to *Bordetella pertussis* mutant strains and to vaccination in the coughing rat model of pertussis, *J Med Microbiol*, **40:** 307–12.

Peppler MS, Schrumpf ME, 1984, Isolation and characterization of *Bordetella pertussis* phenotype variants capable of growing on nutrient agar: comparison with phases III and IV, *Infect Immun*, **43:** 217–23.

Pittman M, 1984a, The concept of pertussis as a toxin-mediated disease, *Pediatr Infect Dis*, **3:** 467–86.

Pittman M, 1984b, Genus *Bordetella* Moreno-Lopez 1952, 178**AL**, *Bergey's Manual of Systematic Bacteriology*, eds Krieg NR, Holt JG, Williams & Wilkins, Baltimore, 388–93.

Porter JF, Connor K, Donachie W, 1994, Isolation and characterization of *Bordetella parapertussis*-like bacteria from ovine lungs, *Microbiology*, **140:** 255–61.

Porter JF, Wardlaw AC, 1993, Long-term survival of *Bordetella bronchiseptica* in lakewater and in buffered saline without added nutrients, *FEMS Microbiol Lett*, **110:** 33–6.

Porter JF, Wardlaw AC, 1994, Tracheobronchial washings from 7 vertebrate species as growth media for the 4 species of *Bordetella*, *FEMS Immunol Med Microbiol*, **8:** 259–70.

Preston NW, 1988, Pertussis today, *Pathogenesis and Immunity in Pertussis*, eds Wardlaw AC, Parton R, John Wiley & Sons, Chichester, 1–18.

Rappuoli R, 1994, Pathogenicity mechanisms of *Bordetella*, *Bacterial Pathogenesis of Plants and Animals: Molecular and Cellular Mechanisms*, ed. Dangl JL, Springer-Verlag, Berlin, 319–36.

Rappuoli R, Podda A et al., 1992, Progress towards the development of new vaccines against whooping cough, *Vaccine*, **10:** 1027–32.

Redhead K, Hill T, Chart H, 1987, Interaction of lactoferrin and transferrins with the outer membrane of *Bordetella pertussis*, *J Gen Microbiol*, **133:** 891–8.

Redhead K, Watkins J et al., 1993, Effective immunization against *Bordetella pertussis* respiratory infection in mice is dependent on induction of cell-mediated immunity, *Infect Immun*, **61:** 3190–8.

Regan J, Lowe F, 1977, Enrichment medium for the isolation of *Bordetella*, *J Clin Microbiol*, **6:** 303–9.

Roberts M, Maskell D et al., 1990, Construction and characterization in vivo of *Bordetella pertussis* aroA mutants, *Infect Immun*, **58:** 732–9.

Robinson A, Ashworth L, Irons LI, 1989, Serotyping *Bordetella pertussis* strains, *Vaccine*, **7:** 491–4.

Robinson A, Gorringe AR et al., 1989, Serospecific protection of mice against intranasal infection with *Bordetella pertussis*, *Vaccine*, **7:** 321–4.

Rowatt E, 1957, The growth of *Bordetella pertussis*: a review, *J Gen Microbiol*, **17:** 297–326.

Rutter JM, 1985, Atrophic rhinitis in swine, *Adv Vet Sci Comp Med*, **29:** 239–79.

Sandros J, Tuomanen E, 1993, Attachment factors of *Bordetella pertussis*: mimicry of eukaryotic cell recognition molecules, *Trends Microbiol*, **1:** 192–6.

Sato Y, Sato H, 1988, Animal models of pertussis, *Pathogensis and Immunity in Pertussis*, eds Wardlaw AC, Parton R, John Wiley & Sons, Chichester, 309–25.

Shahin RD, Cowell JL, 1994, Mouse respiratory infection models for pertussis, *Methods Enzymol*, **235:** 47–58.

Stainer DW, Scholte MJ, 1971, A simple chemically defined medium for the production of phase I *Bordetella pertussis*, *J Gen Microbiol*, **63:** 211–20.

Stibitz S, Garletts TL, 1992, Derivation of a physical map of the chromosome of *Bordetella pertussis* tohama I, *J Bacteriol*, **174:** 7770–7.

Stibitz S, Miller JF, 1994, Co-ordinate regulation of virulence in *Bordetella pertussis* mediated by the *vir* (*bvg*) locus, *Molecular Genetics of Bacterial Pathogenesis*, eds Miller VL, Kaper JB et al., American Society for Microbiology, Washington, DC, 407–22.

Tuomanen E, 1988, *Bordetella pertussis* adhesins, *Pathogenesis and Immunity in Pertussis*, eds Wardlaw AC, Parton R, John Wiley & Sons, Chichester, 75–94.

Vandamme P, Hommez J et al., 1995, *Bordetella hinzii* sp. nov., isolated from poultry and humans, *Int J Syst Bacteriol*, **45:** 37–45.

Walker KE, Weiss AA, 1994, Characterization of the dermonecrotic toxin in members of the genus *Bordetella*, *Infect Immun*, **62:** 3817–28.

Wardlaw AC, 1990, *Bordetella*, *Topley and Wilson's Principles of Bacteriology, Virology and Immunity*, 8th edn, vol. 2, eds Parker MT, Duerden BI, Edward Arnold, London, 321–38.

Wardlaw AC, Parton R, 1988a, The host–parasite relationship in pertussis, *Pathogenesis and Immunity in Pertussis*, eds Wardlaw AC, Parton R, John Wiley & Sons, Chichester, 327–52.

Wardlaw AC, Parton R (eds), 1988b, *Pathogenesis and Immunity in Pertussis*, John Wiley & Sons, Chichester.

Weiss AA, 1992, The genus *Bordetella*, *The Prokaryotes*, 2nd edn, eds Balows A, Truper HG et al., Springer-Verlag, Berlin, 2530–43.

Weiss AA Falkow S, 1984, Genetic analysis of phase change in *Bordetella pertussis*, *Infect Immun*, **43:** 263–9.

Weiss AA, Hewlett EL et al., 1983, Tn5-induced mutations affecting virulence factors of *Bordetella pertussis*, *Infect Immun*, **42:** 33–41.

Weiss AA, Hewlett EL et al., 1984, Pertussis toxin and extracytoplasmic adenylate cyclase as virulence factors of *Bordetella pertussis*, *J Infect Dis*, **150:** 219–22.

Weyant RS, Hollis DG et al., 1995, *Bordetella holmesii* sp. nov., a new gram-negative species associated with septicemia, *J Clin Microbiol*, **33:** 1–7.

Wirsing von Konig CH, Finger H, 1994, Role of pertussis toxin in causing symptoms of *Bordetella parapertussis* infection, *Eur J Clin Microbiol Infect Dis*, **13:** 455–8.

Woolfrey BF, Moody JA, 1991, Human infections associated with *Bordetella bronchiseptica*, *Clin Microbiol Rev*, **4:** 243–55.

Chapter 39

THE ENTEROBACTERIACEAE: GENERAL CHARACTERS

B Holmes

1 Introduction	5 Susceptibility to physical and chemical agents
2 Morphology	6 Biochemical differentiation
3 Conditions for growth	7 Antigenic structure
4 Type of growth	

1 INTRODUCTION

1.1 Definition

The Enterobacteriaceae are gram-negative, non-sporing rods that are often motile, usually by means of peritrichate flagella. They can be capsulate or non-capsulate and are easily cultivable on ordinary laboratory media. They are aerobic and facultatively anaerobic. All species ferment glucose with the formation of acid or of acid and gas. With the exception of some strains of *Erwinia* and *Yersinia*, the Enterobacteriaceae reduce nitrate to nitrite; they are oxidase-negative and, except for *Shigella dysenteriae* 1, catalase-positive. They are typically intestinal parasites of humans and animals, though some species may occur in other parts of the body, on plants and in the soil. Many species are pathogenic. The G + C content of the DNA in most of the Enterobacteriaceae is in the range 49–59 mol%, but in *Proteus* and *Providencia* it is 37–42 mol% and in *Yersinia* 46–47 mol%.

1.2 General considerations

In the past the term '*Bacterium*' was applied to a broad group of gram-negative, non-sporing rods occurring in the intestinal tract of humans and animals, on plants and in the soil, and leading a saprophytic, commensal or pathogenic existence. These organisms have been studied for many years by groups of workers with widely differing objectives. The medical and veterinary bacteriologists concentrated their attention on those organisms that caused illness in humans and animals. The plant pathologists were most interested in those that possessed enzymes capable of digesting vegetable tissues. Industrial bacteriologists studied in detail a few strains that carried out useful fermentations or interfered with manufacturing processes. Sanitary bacteriologists were concerned in distinguishing the organisms found in the intestine from those living saprophytically outside the human or animal body. This diversity of approach led to much confusion, and the same organism was often studied independently, and under different names, by several groups of workers who used methods that were not comparable. Largely under the stimulus of the Enterobacteriaceae Sub-Committee of the International Committee on Systematic Bacteriology, attempts were made to co-ordinate the experiences of workers in the different fields, and there is now general agreement on the definition of the family Enterobacteriaceae and the main lines on which it should be subdivided.

As long ago as the early 1890s it was pointed out by Theobald Smith that certain important groups of organisms pathogenic to humans and animals differed from most of the non-pathogenic forms in failing to ferment lactose, and the genera *Salmonella* and *Shigella* were created for these non-lactose fermenters. The lactose fermenters were, for the most part, thought to be normal inhabitants of the intestinal tract of humans and the higher animals, or to exist on plants or in the soil. However, it is now known that some genera contain members that acidify lactose promptly, others that do so late and irregularly, and yet others that are lactose non-fermenting. Furthermore, it is now known that *Escherichia coli*, usually a prompt lactose fermenter, is an important cause of acute enteritis in persons of all age groups, and in animals (see Volume 3, Chapter 27). For convenience, the term 'coliform bacteria' is used in this chapter to refer to those members of the Enterobacteriaceae that generally, though by no means invariably, ferment lactose.

Although not originally classified in the Enterobacteriaceae, the inclusion of *Yersinia* in the family was proposed by Thal (1954) and supported by Sneath and Cowan (1958) and Talbot and Sneath (1960), a classification now generally accepted.

For some years there was general agreement that the genera and species of the Enterobacteriaceae should be distinguished by their biochemical characters (Report 1954a, 1954b, 1958, 1963) and that within these genera and species serological methods could be used for further subdivision. Today there are additional genomic means for defining species. The most commonly, although by no means universally, accepted definition is that members of a species show 70%, or higher, relatedness in DNA–DNA homology (at the optimum reassociation temperature) and less than 5% divergence of unpaired bases within related sequences. Strains with less than 3% divergence in related sequences are regarded as forming DNA homology subgroups. The application of these criteria has had 2 principal effects. First, a number of organisms regarded as separate species on the basis of differences in biochemical reactions have been shown to be single genomic species. Examples include: *E. coli* and *Shigella* spp.; '*Klebsiella aerogenes*', *Klebsiella ozaenae*, *Klebsiella pneumoniae* and *Klebsiella rhinoscleromatis*; all *Salmonella* 'species'; *Yersinia pestis* and *Yersinia pseudotuberculosis*. Generally the nomenclature has not been changed so as to avoid confusion amongst clinical microbiologists, epidemiologists and infectious disease clinicians. The second effect is the recognition of numerous new species, some previously regarded as aberrant biotypes within existing species. Where biochemical tests are found to differentiate them these species are named. For example, strains unable to ferment adonitol but able to ferment D-galactose and previously included in *Providencia alcalifaciens* are now known to represent the separate species *Providencia rustigianii*. Where biochemical tests for differentiation are not found, the species remain unnamed. It should be appreciated that whilst the definition of a genomic species given above works well in the Enterobacteriaceae, it has proved less readily applicable to other bacterial groups and has been criticised for arbitrarily imposing divisions upon a continuum. With the wider applicability of polyphasic taxonomy to various bacterial groups the bacterial species is now more extensively regarded as an assemblage of isolates that originated from a common ancestor population in which a steady generation of genetic diversity resulted in clones with different degrees of recombination (according to the species), characterized by a certain degree of phenotypic consistency and by a significant degree of DNA–DNA hybridization and over 97% of 16S rDNA sequence homology (Vandamme et al. 1996).

After the early separation of *Salmonella* and *Shigella* from the rest of the Enterobacteriaceae on the grounds of their pathogenicity for animals, their antigenic structure was studied intensively. Serological methods proved of great value for subdividing these genera, but yielded little information about their relation to other genera. In fact, before it was realized how often cross-reactions occurred between otherwise dissimilar organisms, undue reliance on serological methods led to the inclusion of a number of coliform bacteria in the genus *Salmonella*.

Early attempts to subdivide the coliform bacteria according to their ability to ferment a large number of carbohydrates also failed to produce a rational system of classification (Winslow et al. 1919). However, the water bacteriologists, who were mainly interested in lactose-fermenting organisms, arrived at a broad classification into 3 groups, based on a few arbitrarily selected tests, of which the Voges–Proskauer (VP) test, the methyl red (MR) test and Koser's citrate test were the most important (see Chapter 4), and recognized a coli group (MR+, VP–, citrate–), an aerogenes group (MR–, VP+, citrate+) and an intermediate group (MR+, VP–, citrate+). Attempts were later made to subdivide the late-lactose-fermenting and lactose non-fermenting 'paracolons' in the same way (Borman et al. 1944). Although nobody would now accept their suggestion of a genus '*Paracolobactrum*', divided into a coli–, an aerogenes–, and an intermediate-like species, there is no doubt that most enterobacteria do fall into one of these 3 divisions, whether or not they ferment lactose. The MR+, VP–, citrate– division includes the faecal coliform and dysentery bacteria; the MR+, VP–, citrate+ division contains the intermediate coliform bacteria and the salmonellae; and the MR–, VP+, citrate+ division includes all the aerogenes-like organisms. It must be emphasized, however, that some species, subspecies and biochemical varieties within these broad divisions may be aberrant in their MR, VP and citrate reactions. *Morganella*, *Proteus* and *Providencia* were generally believed to fall outside this classification, and form a fourth division. Ewing and Edwards (1960) advocated a similar classification into 4 groups: *Escherichia–Shigella*, *Arizona–Citrobacter–Salmonella*, '*Cloaca*'–*Klebsiella–Serratia*, and *Proteus–Providencia*, although the biochemical criteria they used were different.

The Enterobacteriaceae could thus be divided into a number of biochemical groups, each of which could be further subdivided by serological, biochemical and other methods. In the past there has been disagreement on the taxonomic rank to be given to these subdivisions but generic status is now given to the main biochemical groups. Cowan (1956, 1957) recognized 6 genera: *Citrobacter*, *Escherichia*, *Klebsiella*, *Proteus*, *Salmonella* and *Shigella*. Kauffmann (1959) divided the Enterobacteriaceae into 3 tribes and 14 genera, including, in addition to those given by Cowan, *Arizona*, '*Cloaca*', *Erwinia*, *Hafnia*, *Morganella*, *Providencia*, '*Rettgerella*' and *Serratia*. Ewing (1966) revised the earlier classification of Ewing and Edwards (1960) to comprise 4 tribes and 10 genera:

1 Escherichieae (*Escherichia*, *Shigella*)
2 Salmonelleae (*Arizona*, *Citrobacter*, *Salmonella*)
3 Klebsielleae (*Enterobacter*, *Klebsiella*, *Serratia*)

4 Proteeae (*Proteus, Providencia*),

and envisaged the addition in future of a fifth tribe Edwardsielleae for the eleventh genus, *Edwardsiella*.

By 1985 Farmer and his colleagues were able to state that there were 22 genera and 69 species in the family in addition to a further 29 unnamed biogroups. Whilst some of these biogroups have since been proposed as new species within existing genera, new species have been placed in additional genera, for example *Koserella* (Hickman-Brenner et al. 1985a). The genus *Yokenella*, with a single species *Yokenella regensburgei*, was also proposed (Kosako et al. 1984). However, the species is a subjective synonym of *Koserella trabulsii* (Kosako et al. 1987); although *Koserella* technically has priority as the name was the first to be validated, the genus *Yokenella* was the first of the 2 names to be published. The scientific community has nevertheless largely accepted *Yokenella* over *Koserella* (Holt et al. 1994) so this chapter will also use the former name. In addition, the genus *Leclercia* has been proposed to include the species previously designated *Escherichia adecarboxylata* (Tamura et al. 1986) and the genus *Pantoea* has been proposed to include the species previously designated *Enterobacter agglomerans* (Gavini et al. 1989) and referred to before that as *Erwinia herbicola*. The genera *Budvicia* (Bouvet et al. 1985), *Buttiauxella* (Ferragut et al. 1981), *Obesumbacterium* (Shimwell 1963), *Pragia* (Aldová et al. 1988), *Trabulsiella* (McWhorter et al. 1991) and *Xenorhabdus* (Thomas and Poinar 1979) have rarely, if at all, been reported from clinical specimens, so will not be considered further. This chapter will use the generic names *Citrobacter, Edwardsiella, Enterobacter, Escherichia, Hafnia, Klebsiella, Kluyvera, Morganella, Proteus, Providencia, Salmonella, Serratia, Shigella* and *Yersinia*. In addition, the more recently proposed genera *Cedecea* (Grimont et al. 1981), *Ewingella* (Grimont et al. 1983), *Leclercia* (Tamura et al. 1986), *Leminorella* (Hickman-Brenner et al. 1985b), *Moellerella* (Hickman-Brenner et al. 1984), *Pantoea* (Gavini et al. 1989), *Rahnella* (Izard et al. 1979), *Tatumella* (Hollis et al. 1981) and *Yokenella* (Kosako et al. 1984) are mentioned briefly. Although of apparently rare clinical occurrence, the species in these genera are described fully so that they may be more easily recognized and their true distribution in clinical specimens determined. The Arizona group is included in the genus *Salmonella*.

The definition of species within these genera is not consistent. For example, in the genus *Salmonella* (in reality a single genomic species) it has been customary to give a specific epithet to each of the hundreds of serotypes or 'serovars'. However, the DNA homology subgroups are separable biochemically and have been formally named as subspecies (Le Minor, Véron and Popoff 1982). By contrast, *E. coli* is still retained as a single species although divisible into a large number of serotypes, each designated by a numerical formula. Several proposals have been made to introduce some uniformity (Kauffmann 1959, Ewing 1966, Le Minor, Rohde and Taylor 1970, Le Minor, Véron and Popoff 1982, Le Minor et al. 1986, Le Minor and Popoff

1987). Further details of the classification of the genus *Salmonella* are summarized in Chapter 41.

The generic and specific names of organisms of clinical interest that are used in this book are listed alphabetically in Table 39.1, along with a few of their common synonyms. In this chapter the general characters of the Enterobacteriaceae are considered; Chapter 42 entails a more detailed account of the individual genera other than the following, which have separate chapters or parts of chapters devoted to them: *Escherichia* and *Shigella* (Chapter 40), *Salmonella* (Chapter 41), *Morganella*, *Proteus* and *Providencia* (Chapter 43), and *Yersinia* (Chapter 44).

2 MORPHOLOGY

The modal form of the individual cell is that of a rod, 2–3 μm in length and 0.6 μm in breadth, with parallel sides and rounded ends. By the usual methods of examination the cell appears to be almost devoid of internal structure. It stains evenly, forms no spores, and shows no granules. It is gram-negative and non-acid-fast. This modal form is, however, widely departed from. Some strains are almost coccal in form, others show long, sometimes filamentous rods. There is a tendency for the coccobacillary, or the elongated, form to predominate in any single strain, but some cultures show a wide diversity in this respect.

Motile strains are found in all genera of the Enterobacteriaceae except *Klebsiella* (although some authorities have proposed that *Enterobacter aerogenes* should be reclassified as *Klebsiella mobilis*; Bascomb et al. 1971, Izard et al. 1980), *Leminorella*, *Moellerella* and *Shigella*. *Y. pestis* is non-motile. Some 80% of strains of *E. coli* are motile. In the genus *Salmonella* the only constantly non-motile serotypes are Gallinarum and Pullorum. In the other genera, absence of motility is uncommon. Flagella are always peritrichate – except in *Tatumella*, in which the flagella observed tend to be polar, subpolar or lateral.

Leifson (1960), who made measurements on stained films, found the normal flagellar wavelengths to vary between 2.13 and 3.02 μm. He also described several variations in the shape of the flagella, of which the 'curly' was the most frequent. 'Curly' flagella have about half the normal wavelength, and function inefficiently. They occur as genetically stable mutants, and can also be induced phenotypically, in *Proteus* but not in other members of the Enterobacteriaceae, by growth at pH 5.5 (Hoeniger 1965). Non-motile variants may be either non-flagellate or flagellate but 'paralysed'. In the salmonellae there is an unusual type of variation – phase variation (Chapter 41) – in which the production of flagella of different antigenic constitution is rapidly alternated. A similar phenomenon may occur occasionally in *E. coli* (Ratiner 1985). For reviews of the genetic control of flagellation see Joys (1968) and Iino (1969). A study of the ultrastructure of the flagella surface in *E. coli* of different H serotypes showed that they could be grouped into a number of 'morphotypes', each containing up to 15 different H serotypes (Lawn, Ørskov and Ørskov 1977).

The upper limit of temperature for motility is often considerably lower than that for growth. Raising the temperature

Table 39.1 An alphabetical key to the genera and species of Enterobacteriaceae of clinical interest

Genera/Species and other subgeneric groups	Synonyms	Genera/Species and other subgeneric groups	Synonyms
Cedecea		*Moellerella*	
C. davisae		*M. wisconsensis*	
C. lapagei		*Morganella*	
C. neteri		*M. morganii*	
Citrobacter		*Pantoea*	
C. amalonaticus	*Levinea amalonatica*	*P. agglomerans*	*Erwinia herbicola,*
C. braakii			*Enterobacter*
C. farmeri			*agglomerans*
C. freundii		*Proteus*	
C. koseri	*Citrobacter diversus,*	*P. mirabilis*	
	Levinea malonatica	*P. penneri*	
C. sedlakii		*P. vulgaris*	
C. werkmanii		*Providencia*	
C. youngae		*P. alcalifaciens*	
Edwardsiella		*P. rettgeri*	
E. tarda	*Edwardsiella*	*P. rustigianii*	
	anguillimortifera	*P. stuartii*	
Enterobacter		*Rahnella*	
E. aerogenes	*Klebsiella mobilis*	*R. aquatilis*	
E. amnigenus		*Salmonella*	
E. asburiae		*S. choleraesuis*	*Salmonella enterica*[a]
E. cloacae		subsp. *choleraesuis*	Subgenus I, 'subsp.
E. gergoviae			*enterica*'
E. hormaechei		subsp. *salamae*	Subgenus II
E. intermedius		subsp. *arizonae*	Subgenus III a
E. sakazakii			(monophasic
E. taylorae	*Enterobacter*		strains)
	cancerogenus	subsp. *diarizonae*	Subgenus III b
Escherichia			(diphasic strains)
E. coli		subsp. *houtenae*	Subgenus IV
E. fergusonii		subsp. *bongori*	'Subgenus V'
E. hermanii			'bongor group',
E. vulneris			subsp. 6
Ewingella		subsp. *indica*	'Subgenus VI',
E. americana			subsp. 7
Hafnia		*Serratia*	
H. alvei		*S. ficaria*	
Klebsiella		*S. fonticola*	
K. ornithinolytica		*S. liquefaciens*	'Enterobacter
K. oxytoca			liquefaciens'
K. ozaenae		*S. marcescens*	
K. planticola	*Klebsiella trevisanii*	*S. odorifera*	
K. pneumoniae	includes 'Klebsiella	*S. plymuthica*	
	aerogenes'	*S. rubidaea*	*Serratia marinorubra*
K. rhinoscleromatis		*Shigella*	
K. terrigena		*S. boydii*	
Kluyvera		*S. dysenteriae*	
K. ascorbata		*S. flexneri*	
K. cryocrescens		*S. sonnei*	
K. georgiana		*Tatumella*	
Leclercia		*T. ptyseos*	
L. adecarboxylata		*Yersinia*	
Leminorella		*Y. enterocolitica*	
L. grimontii		*Y. frederiksenii*	
L. richardii		*Y. intermedia*	
		Y. kristensenii	

Table 39.1 Continued

Genera/Species and other subgeneric groups	Synonyms
Y. pestis	
Y. pseudotuberculosis	
Yokenella	
Y. regensburgei	*Koserella trabulsii*

[a] All the numerous bioserotypes ('bioserovars') of *Salmonella* belong to a single genomic species that can be divided into 7 subspecies that largely correspond to the old subgenera. The type species of *Salmonella* is *Salmonella choleraesuis* but many workers prefer the use of *Salmonella enterica* on the grounds that this name has not previously been used for any 'bioserovar' of *Salmonella* and its use for the type species is less likely to cause confusion. However, although a proposal to change the type species of the genus to *Salmonella enterica* was published, the request was denied by the Judicial Commission. For practical purposes clinical laboratories will probably continue to use 'bioserovar' names such as *Salmonella* Typhimurium as a shorthand form of the more cumbersome *Salmonella choleraesuis* subsp. *choleraesuis* bioserovar Typhimurium (the author of Chapter 41 uses the name *Salmonella enterica*). Names in quotes ('') are not in the Approved Lists of Bacterial Names and are without standing in nomenclature (see Chapter 3).

from 37 to 44°C inhibits the motility of salmonellae, and the production of flagella, while having no effect on the growth rate (Quadling and Stocker 1962). Most of the Enterobacteriaceae are motile at 37°C but some, notably *Enterobacter*, *Hafnia*, *Tatumella* and *Yersinia*, should be tested at a lower temperature. 'Swarming' over the surface of solid media is a character only of certain strains of *Proteus* (see Chapter 43).

Many of the Enterobacteriaceae are fimbriate (Duguid et al. 1955, Constable 1956, Duguid and Gillies 1957, 1958, Duguid 1959). Duguid distinguished between **common fimbriae**, which are usually present in large numbers (50–100) per cell, often influence the physicochemical characters of the organism, are chromosomally determined, and do not have an essential role in bacterial conjugation, and **sex pili**, which are present in smaller numbers, are determined by conjugative plasmids, and appear to be organs of conjugation (Duguid, Anderson and Campbell 1966, Duguid 1968). Strains may carry both **common fimbriae** and **sex pili**, and more than one type of common fimbriae. Within the strain, there are individual cells with many common fimbriae and others with none, and there is reversible variation between the fimbriate and the non-fimbriate phase.

By means of electron microscopy common fimbriae may be classified according to their number and their dimensions. In this way Duguid, Anderson and Campbell (1966) found 6 types of common fimbriae, of which 5 were found among the Enterobacteriaceae, and all are peritrichate. Type 1 fimbriae are strongly hydrophobic and render the organism adhesive to plant, fungus and animal cells, cause agglutination of untreated erythrocytes, and lead to the formation of a pellicle on the surface of liquid media. Adhesiveness and the ability to cause haemagglutination are reversed by D-mannose; fimbriae of this type are described as mannose-sensitive (MS). Type 2 fimbriae do not confer adhesiveness. Type 3 fimbriae cause adhesiveness to plant and fungal cells and to glass surfaces, but not to animal tissue cells or erythrocytes unless these are first treated with tannic acid or heated to 70°C; these properties are uninfluenced by mannose and

are termed mannose-resistant (MR). Type 4 fimbriae also cause MR adhesiveness, but this is active against untreated red cells. Type 5 fimbriae were not found in the Enterobacteriaceae. Type 6 fimbriae are rather scanty in number (4–40 per cell), longer than fimbriae of other types and do not cause adhesiveness. Fimbriae of type 1 are found in *Enterobacter*, *Escherichia*, *Klebsiella*, most salmonellae, *Shigella flexneri* and *Serratia*; of type 2 in a few of the salmonellae that do not form type 1 fimbriae; of type 3 in *Klebsiella* and *Serratia* strains together with fimbriae of type 1; of type 4 only in *Proteus* strains; and of type 6 only in otherwise non-fimbriate strains of *K. ozaenae*.

Little is known about the function of the common fimbriae. Type 1 fimbriae are able to mediate adhesion to a wide range of human and animal cells that contain mannose residues. Such adhesion might favour pathogenicity and there are some examples of this (Duguid 1968, Duguid and Old 1980). However, the possible role of type 1 fimbriae in urinary tract infection remains controversial (see the reviews of Harber 1985 and Reid and Sobel 1987 for further details). On the other hand, the ability of bacteria with type 1 fimbriae to form a pellicle on the surface of static fluids increases their access to oxygen and leads to additional multiplication of the organism (Old et al. 1968, Old and Duguid 1970). This might be an advantage to saprophytic enterobacteria in their natural environment. Adhesiveness of type 3 fimbriae to plant root hairs and fungal mycelia might serve a similar function (Duguid 1968).

More recently, a number of filamentous protein structures resembling fimbriae have been described in *E. coli*. These cause MR haemagglutination, and there is good evidence that they play an important part in the pathogenesis of diarrhoeal disease and in urinary tract infection. They include the K88 antigen found in strains causing enteritis of pigs, the K99 antigen found in strains causing enteritis of calves and lambs, and the colonization factor antigens (CFAs) found in enterotoxigenic *E. coli* of human origin. These are described in more detail in Volume 3 (see Volume 3, Chapter 27). Fimbriae that are important in urinary tract infection and cause MR haemagglutination are distinguished according to their receptor specificities. These include the P fimbriae that bind specifically to receptors present on the P blood group antigens of human erythrocytes and uroepithelial cells (see Volume 3, Chapter 32).

The sex pili or conjugative pili also vary morphologically (Bradley 1980a, 1980b). Conjugative plasmids have been classified according to their inability to coexist in the same bacterial strain (incompatibility typing) and electron microscopy reveals that 3 morphologically distinct groups of pili are determined by plasmids of different incompatibility groups. Thin flexible pili are determined by plasmids of incompatibility groups I, B and K; thick flexible pili are determined by plasmids of groups C, D, the F complex, H1, H2, J, T, V and X; and rigid pili are determined by plasmids of groups M, N, P and W.

Some species are normally **capsulate** and form mucoid colonies when first isolated, though the ability to form capsules may be lost on prolonged subculture on artificial media. The amount of capsular material varies enormously from strain to strain. Sometimes it forms a well circumscribed capsule around the organisms, but at others it becomes free in the surrounding medium as 'loose slime' (Duguid 1951). Capsulation is the rule in *Klebsiella*, and also occurs in a minority of *Enterobacter* and *E. coli* strains. *Klebsiella* capsules are composed mainly of acid polysaccharides and many antigenically distinct capsular polysaccharides have been recognized. The capsules of *E. coli* appear to contain one of 2 substances: type-specific polysaccharides (K antigens); and a more widely distributed mucoid (M) substance formed by many different strains (Kauffmann 1944). Rare strains that produce extracellular slime of the latter type occur in *Salmonella*, *Shigella* and most other genera. Slime production is the rule among forms of *Salmonella* Paratyphi B negative to D-tartrate, and is favoured by continued incubation at low temperature. When grown on medium with high osmolarity, most *Salmonella* and *E. coli* strains produce extracellular slime (Anderson 1961, Anderson and Rogers 1963). This is a colanic acid (Goebel 1963, Grant, Sutherland and Wilkinson 1969) which appears to be identical with Kauffmann's M substance (see Chapters 40 and 41).

3 CONDITIONS FOR GROWTH

Members of the Enterobacteriaceae grow readily on nutrient media without the addition of any accessory substances. They are aerobic and facultatively anaerobic, though the growth is usually far less copious under the latter conditions. The optimum temperature is, for most species isolated by medical bacteriologists, in the neighbourhood of 37°C, and the range over which growth occurs is fairly wide, extending from about 42°C to 18°C or lower. Many *Enterobacter* and *Serratia* strains grow poorly, or not at all, at 44°C, and differ in this respect from *E. coli*. Moreover, many coliform bacteria have a temperature optimum lower than 37°C, and others, which appear to grow as well at 37°C as at 30°C, are unable to carry out some of their biochemical activities at the higher temperature. These organisms frequently grow slowly at temperatures as low as −1.5°C. They form an important part of the coliform flora of water and soil, and are commonly found in chilled meat (Eddy and Kitchell 1959). Many of the coliform bacteria of water that can grow at refrigerator temperatures are *Hafnia alvei* or *Serratia* strains. *Yersinia enterocolitica* is able to multiply rapidly at 4°C (Hurvell 1981).

4 TYPE OF GROWTH

The type of growth given by the various members of the Enterobacteriaceae is very similar. When normal smooth strains are grown in broth, a uniform turbidity develops, increasing rapidly during the first 12–18 h, and then more slowly up to 48–72 h. Pellicle formation is rare except when the fimbriate phase has been selected by serial subculture in liquid medium. A slight deposit forms as growth increases, and this is easily dispersed on shaking the tube. *Y. pestis* and *Y.*

pseudotuberculosis are exceptions in that they produce little turbidity in broth but a deposit is formed on the sides and bottom of the tube.

On agar, the colonies are relatively large, with an average diameter of 2–3 mm, but vary considerably in size. They may be circular, raised and low convex, with an entire edge and smooth surface; they may be flatter with a more irregular surface, and a more effuse and irregular edge; or they may assume the well known vine-leaf form that is commonly described as characteristic of *Salmonella* Typhi. Even with freshly isolated strains the range of variation is wide and the most varied colonial forms may be seen when old laboratory strains are examined. Apart from the possible appearance of rough variants, a single strain may show several different types of colony if successive subcultures in broth are interspersed with platings and subculture of individual colonies. A few strains produce dwarf colonies on nutrient agar but form colonies of normal size when provided with a source of reduced sulphur, such as sulphide or cysteine (Gillespie 1952).

Many members of the genus *Klebsiella*, when freshly isolated, form typically mucoid colonies. The differential value of this characteristic is diminished by the fact that certain other organisms, including some strains of *E. coli*, may similarly give rise to this type of growth.

All members of the Enterobacteriaceae, with the exception of a few *Klebsiella* strains from the respiratory tract, grow in the presence of bile salts and give rise to colonies on MacConkey agar nearly as large as those on nutrient agar. Occasional strains that produce yellow or orange pigments were described previously (Parr 1937, Thomas and Elson 1957); and strains of the following more recently described species also produce yellow pigment: *Enterobacter sakazakii*, *Leclercia adecarboxylata* and *Pantoea agglomerans* (synonym: *Erwinia herbicola*). In addition, many *Serratia* strains form a red pigment called **prodigiosin**.

5 SUSCEPTIBILITY TO PHYSICAL AND CHEMICAL AGENTS

Most members of Enterobacteriaceae are killed by exposure to a temperature of 55°C for about 1 h, or to 60°C for 15–20 min. On the whole, *E. coli* strains tend to be slightly more resistant to heat than most other coliform bacteria. A small proportion of them are not completely destroyed by exposure to 60°C for 30 min in broth, or to pasteurization at 62.8°C for the same time in milk (Wilson et al. 1935). The aerogenes type tends to be slightly more resistant to chlorine in water than the coli or intermediate types (Bardsley 1938). In raw water stored under atmospheric conditions, coliform bacteria may remain alive for weeks or months. '*Klebsiella aerogenes*' (*K. pneumoniae*) tends to survive rather longer than *E. coli*, but the results are influenced by, among other things, the temperature (Platt 1935, Raghavachari and Iyer 1939b). In faeces stored at 0°C, coliform organisms may be demonstrated for a year or more, the coli types often being gradually supplanted by the intermediate and aerogenes types (Parr 1938).

Most members of the Enterobacteriaceae are susceptible to all classes of chemical disinfectants (see Chapter 7) and, like other gram-negative rods, to sodium azide (Snyder and Lichstein 1940). Differences in susceptibility to dyes and other chemicals that are of use in enrichment and selective media for the isolation of pathogenic members of the family are mentioned in Chapter 41 and Volume 3, Chapters 24 and 28. The susceptibility of individual organisms to antibiotics and other antimicrobial agents varies greatly and is described at appropriate points in Chapters 40, 43, 44, 41 and 42.

6 BIOCHEMICAL DIFFERENTIATION

It was early recognized that the fermentation of sugars provided a useful means of distinguishing certain pathogenic enterobacteria from the coliform bacteria. Theobald Smith, for instance, observed that *E. coli* fermented lactose, whereas *Salmonella* Typhi did not (Smith 1890); and the production of acid and gas from glucose by *E. coli*, but of acid only by *Salmonella* Typhi, was pointed out by Chantemesse and Widal in 1891. Shigellae were also distinguished from the coliform bacteria and divided into a few broad groups by similar methods (see Chapter 40). For many years afterwards, interest was concentrated on the serological identification of salmonellae and shigellae, and the biochemical classification of the remaining enterobacteria was left mainly in the hands of the water bacteriologists, who had a profound influence on it between 1900 and 1950.

In his original description of the coliform bacteria, Escherich (1885) noted the occurrence of 2 types: one, 'Bacterium coli', formed fairly large rods, was motile and clotted milk slowly; the other, '*Bacterium lactis aerogenes*', formed shorter, plumper rods, was non-motile and clotted milk more actively. In the next few years, the introduction of suitable indicators of acidity (Wurtz 1892) and of means of detecting gas production (Smith 1890, Durham 1898) added to the ease with which fermentation tests could be carried out. Various elaborate classifications of the coliform bacteria were made according to the range of their ability to attack sugars, but none of these proved satisfactory (Bergey and Deehan 1908, MacConkey 1905, 1909, Jackson 1911).

An important correlation between biochemical activity and natural habitat was observed at about this time; it was found that '*B. lactis aerogenes*' (later called '*Bacterium aerogenes*') was an infrequent inhabitant of the intestine, but was often found on vegetation and in the soil, whereas '*B. coli*' was a constant intestinal parasite (Winslow and Walker 1907). This was of practical as well as theoretical importance, and the presence or absence of '*B. coli*' in water supplies came to be regarded as a valuable indication of faecal pollution. The ability to distinguish between those that were of intestinal origin and those that might occur in unpolluted waters was aided by the discovery that there were differences between the results of fermentation of one and the same sugar by different coliform bacteria. Thus there were differences in the amount of gas produced from glucose and the ratio of CO_2 to H_2 in the gas (Smith 1895, Harden and Walpole 1906), in whether or not acetylmethylcarbinol was

produced, and in the final pH (see Chapter 168). Levine (1916a, 1916b) established that there was a high negative correlation between the results of the VP test for acetylmethylcarbinol and the MR test for final acidity in glucose-containing media. In a series of intensive studies he placed on a firm foundation the conclusion that the lactose-fermenting coliform bacteria could be divided into 2 primary divisions; the first comprised strains that produced a moderate amount of gas with a CO_2:H_2 ratio of about 1:1, were VP-negative and MR-positive, included most of the strains isolated from the faeces of humans and animals, and corresponded to '*B. coli*'; the second comprised strains that produced a greater amount of gas with a CO_2:H_2 ratio of about 2:1, were VP-positive and MR-negative and were found often on plants and in unpolluted water. These could be further subdivided into '*B. aerogenes*' which did not liquefy gelatin and '*Bacterium cloacae*' which did.

Later, Brown (1921) drew attention to the usefulness of a medium containing citrate for distinguishing '*B. aerogenes*' from '*B. coli*', and Koser (1923, 1924, 1926) devised a synthetic medium in which citrate was the sole source of carbon. He was able to subdivide coliform bacteria into an MR+, VP−, citrate− coli type, an MR−, VP+, citrate+ aerogenes type, and an MR+, VP−, citrate+ intermediate type; only the first of these was commonly of faecal origin.

Considerable help was also afforded by the test introduced in 1904 by Eijkman who found that 'coli' but not 'aerogenes' strains were able to form gas in a glucose broth medium incubated at 46°C. After a chequered career, this test was improved and standardized (Levine, Epstein and Vaughn 1934, Wilson et al. 1935) by the institution of accurate temperature control at 44°C and the replacement of glucose broth by MacConkey's lactose bile salt broth. It was then shown to be a highly specific test for faecal coliform bacteria in the natural waters of many countries. However, as shown by Raghavachari and Iyer (1939a) and by Boizot (1941), organisms that were MR−, VP+, citrate+ but produced gas from lactose at 44°C were common in the surface waters in some tropical countries. These organisms – referred to by British water bacteriologists as 'Irregular VI' – can be distinguished from faecal coliform bacteria by their inability to form indole at 44°C (Mackenzie, Taylor and Gilbert 1948). These tests, with the addition of indole production and gelatin liquefaction, for many years formed the basis of the classification of coliform bacteria used by British water bacteriologists. In addition to their usefulness in practice, they had the advantage of conforming in broad outline with the biochemical classification of the Enterobacteriaceae as a whole that gained general acceptance in the 1950s (Report 1954a, 1954b, Kauffmann 1956c, 1959, Kauffmann, Edwards and Ewing 1956).

For the detailed biochemical classification of the Enterobacteriaceae, however, several additional tests are required. The fermentation of sugars is of little value for the establishment of broad groupings, but action on individual substrates is often useful to distinguish between closely related groups. For example, the production of acid, with or without gas, from adonitol, cellobiose, glycerol, inositol and starch is useful in making subdivisions within *Klebsiella* and *Enterobacter* (Kauffmann 1956a, 1956b). In several genera, lactose fermentation is late or irregular. The introduction of the *o*-nitrophenyl-β-D-galactopyranoside (ONPG) test for β-galactosidase (Chapter 4), which quickly reveals potential ability to attack this sugar, has added uniformity to the characters of *Citro-*

bacter and some biochemical varieties of *Enterobacter*, *Klebsiella* and *Shigella* (Bülow 1964, Lapage and Jayaraman 1964). Other useful tests also described in Chapter 4 include those for the utilization of various organic acids as sole carbon sources or their fermentation in peptone media, for the oxidation of gluconate, the decarboxylation or deamination of amino acids and for the hydrolysis of hippurate. It must be pointed out that virtually all members of the Enterobacteriaceae produce some hydrogen sulphide under optimal conditions, and that the term 'H₂S production' is used in this group to indicate the ability to produce blackening in triple sugar iron agar, in Kligler's medium or in ferrous chloride gelatin. The test for urea hydrolysis was originally introduced for the recognition of *Proteus*, but many other members of the Enterobacteriaceae give positive reactions that are of value in classification when a suitable medium is used (see Chapter 4). Tetrathionate reductase is produced by nearly all strains of *Citrobacter*, *Proteus*, *Salmonella* and *Serratia* and by a few strains of *Enterobacter*, *E. coli* and *Klebsiella*, but is not produced by strains of *Edwardsiella* and *Shigella* (Le Minor 1967).

In general, the Enterobacteriaceae produce few exoenzymes. Rapid liquefaction of gelatin (in 1–2 days) occurs only in some *Proteus* spp. and in *Serratia*, slower liquefaction (in 3–7 days) in salmonellae of subspecies II, IIIa, IIIb and IV, and very slow liquefaction (in 15–30 days or more) in *Enterobacter* spp. and *Klebsiella oxytoca*. Deoxyribonuclease production and lipolysis are confined to *Serratia* and some *Proteus* strains (Davis and Ewing 1964, Martin and Ewing 1967) whereas strains of *Cedecea* are also lipolytic. According to Mulczyk and Szewczuk (1970), nearly all *Citrobacter*, *Enterobacter*, *Klebsiella* and *Serratia* strains, but no other enterobacteria, produce pyrrolidonyl peptidase. For further information about the biochemical characters of enterobacteria see Kauffmann (1969), Lapage et al. (1979), Farmer et al. (1985) and Ewing (1986).

Table 39.2 summarizes the usual behaviour, in some commonly used biochemical tests, of those genera of the Enterobacteriaceae that are of clinical interest. Details of the biochemical characters that differentiate between the species within these genera are given in Chapters 43, 40, 44, 41 and 42. In some genera, exceptions occur so frequently that it is difficult to describe adequately the biochemical reactions in a single table. In other genera there are distinct differences between different species, subspecies or biochemical varieties (biotypes or 'biovars'). For simplicity, the reaction of the majority of strains of each genus is indicated by using + and − signs. Reactions that vary too much to show a majority reaction are indicated by a V, regardless of whether the variation is between species, subspecies, 'biovars' or strains. For example, the reaction of *Salmonella* in the test for β-galactosidase is given a V, since strains of *Salmonella* subspecies IIIa and IIIb ('Arizona') are usually positive. Nevertheless, the great majority of *Salmonella* strains encountered belong to subspecies I or II and are usually β-galactosidase negative. Similarly, the production of gas from glucose by

Salmonella is shown as V (for 'variable', meaning that different strains give different results), since although most strains produce gas, the clinically important *Salmonella* Typhi strains are anaerogenic. On the other hand, *Salmonella* is shown as motile although strains of serotypes Gallinarum and Pullorum are non-motile, and non-motile strains occasionally occur in other serogroups. It is therefore important to consider the biochemical characters shown in Table 39.2 together with those in Chapters 43, 40, 44, 41 and 42.

7 ANTIGENIC STRUCTURE

The main structural components of the cell envelope are:

1 a thin inner layer of mucopeptide
2 a thicker outer layer composed of a polymolecular complex of lipopolysaccharide with protein and lipid and
3 probably also a lipoprotein element linked to the mucopeptide (Freer and Salton 1971).

The lipopolysaccharide (LPS) complex (see Chapter 12) is a characteristic and integral component of the outer membrane of all gram-negative bacteria. It is now recognized that LPS consists of 2 parts with contrasting properties:

1 the hydrophilic polysaccharide component consisting of the O-specific polysaccharide together with the core oligosaccharide and
2 the hydrophobic lipid A component that is responsible for the numerous pathophysiological effects of 'endotoxin' in humans and animals.

In the Enterobacteriaceae the link between the polysaccharide and lipid A components is provided by 2-keto-3-deoxyoctonic acid (KDO). Because of the acid lability of the ketosidic bond, lipid A can be obtained as a precipitate by mild acid treatment of LPS.

Lipid A is a complex phosphoglycolipid and its complete structure was established only in the comparatively recent past (Rietschel 1984). A general structure found in a number of taxonomically distinct families is characterized by a central biphosphorylated β(1→6)-linked D-glucosamine disaccharide which is substituted by up to 4 mol of ester- and amidebound (R)-3-acyloxyacyl or (R)-3-hydroxyacyl residues. Lipid A from different bacteria may vary in the chain length of its 3-hydroxy fatty acids, the substitution pattern of its 3-hydroxyl group, and that of its backbone phosphoryl groups. In *E. coli*, *Proteus* and *Salmonella* the disaccharide backbone carries 4 (R)-3-hydroxytetradecanoyl groups in positions 2, 3, 2′ and 3′ and 2 phosphoryl residues in positions 1 and 4′. The 3-hydroxyl groups of up to 3 of these hydroxy fatty acids (positions 2, 2′ and 3′) are acylated by non-hydroxylated acyl residues whereas non-acylated, nitrogen-containing residues such as 4-amino-4-deoxy-L-arabinopyranose and phosphorylethanolamine may be bound to phosphoryl groups. The hydroxyl group in position 4 of the glucosamine disaccharide is free and that in position 6′ serves as the attachment site for KDO and hence for the polysaccharide components of LPS.

Table 39.2 Differential reactions of the genera of Enterobacteriaceae

Property	*Cedecea*	*Citrobacter*	*Edwardsiella tarda*	*Enterobacter*	*Escherichia coli*	*Ewingella americana*	*Hafnia alvei*	*Klebsiella*	*Kluyvera*	*Leclercia adecarboxylata*	*Leminorella*	*Moellerella wisconsensis*	*Morganella morganii*	*Pantoea agglomerans*	*Proteus*	*Providencia*	*Rahnella aquatilis*	*Salmonella*	*Serratia*	*Shigella*	*Tatumella ptyseos*	*Yersinia*	*Yokenella regensburgei*
β-Galactosidase	+	+	−	+	+	+	+[a]	+	+	+	−	+	−	+	−	−	+	V	+	V	+[b]	+	+
Growth on Simmons's citrate medium	+	+	−	+	−	+	+[a]	+	+	−	V	−	−	V	V	V	−	V	+	−	−	−	+
Decarboxylase:																							
arginine	+	+	−	V	V	−	−	−	−	−	−	−	−	−	−	−	−	+	−	−	−	−	+
lysine	−	−	+	V	+	−	+	+	+	−	−	−	+	−	+	−	V	+	+	−	−	−	+
ornithine	V	V	+	+	V	−	+	−	+	V	−	−	+	−	+	V	V	+	V	V	−	V	+
Gelatin liquefaction	−	−	−	+	−	+	−	−	−	−	−	−	−	V	+	−	−	−	+	−	−	V	−
Gluconate oxidation	V	V	−	+	−	−	+	V	+	V	−	+	−	V	V	+	+	−	V	−	−	−	−
H₂S production[c]	−	V	+	−	−	−	−	−	−	−	+	−	−	−	+	−	−	+	−	−	−	−	−
Indole production	−	V	+	−	+	−	−	V	−	−	−	−	+	V	V	+	−	−	−	+	−	V	+
Growth in KCN medium	+	+	−	+	−	+	+	V	+	+	−	−	+	V	+	+	+	−	+	−	+	−	−
Malonate fermentation	+	V	−	+	−	+	+	V	+	+	−	+	−	+	−	−	+	+	+	−	+	−	+
Motility	+	+	+	+	V	+	+[a]	−	+	+	+	−	+	V	+	+	+	+	+	−	V[b]	V	+
Methyl red test	V	+	+	−	+	+	−	V	+	+	V	+	+	V	+	+	V	+	V	+	+	+	+
PPA reaction[d]	−	−	−	−	−	+	−	−	−	−	−	−	+	−	+	+	−	−	−	−	−	−	−
Urease production	−	V	−	V	−	−	−	V	−	−	−	−	+	V	+	+	+	−	V	−	+	+	+
Voges–Proskauer test	V	−	−	+	−	+	+[a]	V	+	+	V	+	−	V	−	−	+	−	+	−	−	−	−
Gas in glucose	V	+	+	+	V	−	+	V	+	+	−	+	−	V	+	V	+	V	V	−	−	−	+
Acid in:																							
adonitol	−	V	−	V	−	−	−	+	−	+	−	+	−	V	−	V	−	V	V	−	−	−	−
dulcitol	−	V	−	V	V	−	−	V	−	+	V	−	−	V	−	−	+	V	−	V	−	V	−
inositol	V	−	−	V	−	V	−	+	−	−	−	+	−	+	−	V	+	−	V	−	+	V	+
lactose	+	+	−	+	+	+	−	+	+	+	−	+	−	V	−	−	+	−	V	−	+	V	+
mannitol	+	+	−	+	+	+	+	+	+	+	−	−	−	+	−	V	+	+	+	V	+	+	+
salicin	V	V	−	+	V	−	V	+	+	+	−	+	−	+	V	V	+	−	+	−	+	V	+
sucrose	V	V	−	+	V	−	−	+	+	V	−	−	−	+	V	V	+	−	+	−	+	V	+
xylose	V	+	−	+	+	−	+	+	+	+	+	−	−	+	+	V	+	+	V	−	V	V	+

The following species are excluded from this table, their reactions will be found in the appropriate tables of Chapter 42: *Enterobacter asburiae, Enterobacter taylorae, Klebsiella ornithinolytica* and *Klebsiella rhinoscleromatis*; the reactions of *Escherichia* spp. other than *E. coli* will be found in Chapter 40.

+, Most strains positive; −, most strains negative. V, some strains positive, others negative.

[a] Results are those at 30°C; some strains may give positive MR test and negative VP test results and fail to grow on Simmons's citrate medium when incubated at 37°C.

[b] At 25°C, strains usually give negative results in these tests when incubated at 36°C.

[c] In triple sugar iron agar.

[d] Phenylpyruvic acid from phenylalanine.

All lipopolysaccharides of gram-negative bacteria, whether from smooth strains or rough mutants and from pathogenic and non-pathogenic strains, are potent endotoxins and the endotoxic principle is lipid A. The effects of endotoxin on the animal body are numerous; when administered parenterally to a suitable animal it gives rise to fever, leucopenia followed by leucocytosis, hyperglycaemia with a subsequent fall in the blood sugar far below the normal level, and lethal shock after a latent period; it provokes the localized and the generalized Shwartzman reaction and causes haemorrhagic necrosis in tumours and at the site of an intradermal injection of adrenaline; it gives rise to non-specific resistance to the intraperitoneal injection of a variety of gram-negative bacteria and to damage by irradiation; and it has a powerful adjuvant effect on the antibody response to unrelated protein antigens but not to polysaccharide antigens. No other biological material gives rise to such a wide variety of reactions, though some other bacterial products, for example, staphylococcal enterotoxin and the pyrogenic exotoxin of *Streptococcus pyogenes*, cause a number of similar effects. The mode of action of endotoxin is not fully understood. There is reason to believe that its action may be responsible for many of the consequences of established infections with gram-negative rods. For a review of the pathophysiology of endotoxin see Hinshaw 1985; for a review of its chemistry see Rietschel (1984).

Synthetic analogues of lipid A have been prepared and in a number of test systems, including lethal toxicity, B lymphocyte mitogenicity, macrophage activation, induction of crossed tolerance, and expression of lipid-A antigenicity, these synthetic part-structures were of activity comparable to that of free bacterial lipid A. However, in 2 test systems, pyrogenicity and local Shwartzman reaction, the synthetic analogues exhibited weak or no endotoxic activity. It is likely that distinct determinants are necessary for the expression of different biological activities of lipid A; the studies with synthetic analogues suggest that the presence of (R)-3-acyloxyacyl groups may be necessary for the full expression of pyrogenicity and the local Shwartzman reaction (Rietschel et al. 1985).

7.1   O antigens

Each of the main enterobacterial genera can be subdivided by means of agglutination tests into a number of O-antigenic groups, some characterized by a single antigen and others by a combination of antigenic 'factors', which may appear in different combinations in other members of the genus. There is also extensive sharing of O antigens between otherwise quite unrelated organisms. Nearly all the *Shigella* serotypes are antigenically related to one or more O groups of *E. coli*; the relation is sometimes unilateral, sometimes reciprocal, and sometimes one of complete identity. For example, the O antigen of *S. dysenteriae* 3 is identical with that of *E. coli* O124. Such a relation between *Salmonella* and *E. coli* serotypes is less common, but by no means infrequent. There is also considerable shar-

ing between the O antigens of *E. coli* and *Providencia*; and relationships, including some of identity, occur between *Y. enterocolitica* and certain serotypes of *E. coli* and *Salmonella* (Thomas et al. 1983).

Chemical characterizations and structural analyses have demonstrated that all salmonellae have a core oligosaccharide with the same structure (Lüderitz et al. 1971). A further 5, closely related structures have been found in *E. coli* (Jansson et al. 1981). By contrast, a great number of O-specific polysaccharides exist and differ in their composition or structure or in both. They are all made up of repeating oligosaccharide units so that each can be defined according to the structure of one of its repeating oligosaccharides and its joining linkage. Over 100 enterobacterial O antigens have been defined in this way and the details are summarized in the review of Jann and Jann (1984). For example, O-specific polysaccharides with a repeating sequence of mannose–rhamnose–galactose are found in *Salmonella* of groups A, B, D and E of the Kauffmann–White scheme (see Chapter 41). The chemical characterization of the epitopes ('immunodominant sugars') within these polysaccharides has also been described. Such polysaccharides also represent the receptors for bacteriophages that are responsible for antigenic conversions that depend on the effect of bacteriophage-induced endoglycosidases or a deacetylase. For example, groups E1 and E2 of *Salmonella* are inter-related by conversion with bacteriophage ϵ_{15}. The O-specific polysaccharides of some *E. coli* strains (but not *Klebsiella* or *Salmonella*) contain acidic components such as hexuronic acids, *N*-acetylneuraminic acid or phosphate. Thus LPS with neutral and with acidic O-specific polysaccharides exist and can be distinguished by immunoelectrophoresis (Ørskov et al. 1977). The LPS prepared from any bacterial strain is always heterogeneous with respect to chain length of the O-specific polysaccharide and this can be demonstrated by sodium dodecylsulphate polyacrylamide gel electrophoresis (SDS-PAGE) of the complete LPS (Jann, Reske and Jann 1975). This phenomenon is generally interpreted as indicating the presence of individual LPS molecules with O-specific polysaccharide chains differing in size by multiple increments of oligosaccharide repeating units.

Rough variants of the Enterobacteriaceae form lipopolysaccharide, but this does not contain any of the repeating O-specific oligosaccharides of the corresponding smooth form (Lüderitz et al. 1960). Rough variants are of 2 major classes or serogroups: RII (chemotype Ra), which contains all the core sugars, and RI (chemotype Rb), which together with a further series of mutants (chemotypes Rc to Re) have various defects in core structure (Lüderitz, Staub and Westphal 1966). A class of 'semi-rough' mutants (Naide et al. 1965), intermediate in characters between smooth and RII organisms, has core sugars but may form only part of the O-specific polysaccharide. The so-called T forms of salmonellae (see Chapter 41) have serological characters resembling those of rough mutants and have a normal core structure, but form O-specific polysaccharide composed of ribose and additional galactose in place of the sugars of the corresponding smooth form (Wheat et al. 1967).

There is uncertainty about the part played by the O antigen in the virulence of the Enterobacteriaceae. If by virulence is meant the ability to multiply in the tissues of experimental animals after intravenous or intraperitoneal injection, and to cause a fatal infection, there is little doubt that most smooth enterobacteria are more virulent than their rough variants. Semi-rough variants are usually of intermediate virulence. In studies with a strain of *E. coli* O18ac:K1:H7 that had caused meningitis in an infant, Smith and Huggins (1980) showed that mutants lacking either the O18ac or the K1 antigens were much less virulent for mice (by intraperitoneal injection) and chickens (by a variety of routes). Mäkelä, Valtonen and Valtonen (1973) have shown that even quite subtle changes in the O antigens of otherwise isogenic *Salmonella* serotype Typhimurium derivatives can affect their virulence for mice when injected intraperitoneally. Heat-killed vaccines made from smooth organisms, or lipopolysaccharide extracted from them, give protection against injections of the homologous organisms, and also sometimes against related organisms sharing the same O antigen; for example, vaccines of smooth *Salmonella* serotype Paratyphi B will protect against infection with serotype Typhimurium (Schütze 1930). Vaccines made from rough variants, or 'rough' polysaccharide, usually do not have this effect. On the other hand, protection by living vaccines, whether of smooth or rough strains, is often superior to that obtained with killed vaccines of smooth strains, and may be effective against organisms with unrelated O antigens. Very little is known about the significance of the polysaccharide portion of the O antigen in infections in the natural host. For further information about the virulence of enterobacteria and the part played in it by O antigens see Chapters 44 and 41, Roantree (1967) and Hinshaw (1985).

THE ENTEROBACTERIAL COMMON ANTIGEN

The enterobacterial common antigen (Kunin, Beard and Halmagyi 1962, Whang and Neter 1962, Böttger et al. 1987) was first observed in indirect haemagglutination tests between antisera against *E. coli* of O-group 14 and erythrocytes coated with supernatants or extracts of cultures of other enterobacteria. The antigen–antibody reaction can also be detected by haemolysis in the presence of complement and by immunofluorescence (Aoki, Merkel and McCabe 1966). The common antigen has been detected in strains of all the genera of Enterobacteriaceae tested: *Budvicia, Buttiauxella, Cedecea, Citrobacter, Edwardsiella, Enterobacter, Erwinia* (except *Erwinia chrysanthemi*), *Escherichia, Ewingella, Hafnia, Klebsiella, Kluyvera, Leminorella, Moellerella, Morganella, Obesumbacterium, Pantoea, Pragia, Proteus, Providencia, Rahnella, Salmonella, Serratia, Shigella, Tatumella, Xenorhabdus, Yersinia, Yokenella* and several unnamed groups, also in *Actinobacillus* and *Plesiomonas* (Mäkelä and Mayer 1976, Böttger et al. 1987). The latter finding might once have been surprising but several studies confirm that *Plesiomonas* and the genera *Aeromonas, Photobacterium* and *Vibrio* are phylogenetically linked with the Enterobacteriaceae and Pasteurellaceae to form a monophyletic unit within the γ3 subgroup of the Proteobacteria; in par-

ticular, *Plesiomonas shigelloides* is closely related to *Proteus* to the extent that suggestions have been made to place this oxidase-positive organism in the Enterobacteriaceae (see Ruimy et al. 1994). When vaccines of intact cells were injected into animals, only *E. coli* O14 and O56 gave rise to antibody against common antigen, but ethanol-soluble fractions of lipopolysaccharides from other members of the Enterobacteriaceae also did so (Suzuki, Gorzynski and Neter 1964). Hammarström and his colleagues (1971) were unable to separate the common antigen of *E. coli* O14 from the O polysaccharide and found only core constituents in their preparations. They concluded that *E. coli* O14 and O56 were lacking in O-specific polysaccharides; some rough strains formed much antibody to common antigen, and members of O groups with complicated O-specific polysaccharides formed little. Antigenicity was thus related to the accessibility of core constituents. Chemical analysis has shown that the common antigen is an amino sugar polymer consisting of N-acetyl-D-glucosamine and N-acetyl-D-mannoseaminuronic acid, partly esterified by acetic and palmitic acids (Mayer and Schmidt 1979). The common antigen usually occurs as a free glycolipid in the outer membrane but in certain strains, including those that are immunogenic for the common antigen, it is linked to the LPS core.

For further information about the chemistry of the O polysaccharides see Lüderitz, Staub and Westphal (1966), Stocker, Wilkinson and Mäkelä (1966), Lüderitz et al. (1971), Ørskov et al. (1977) and Rietschel (1984); for general reviews of the structure and function of O antigens see the monograph by Weinbaum, Kadis and Ajl (1971), Jann and Jann (1987) and Chapter 41.

7.2 Surface antigens

Many of the Enterobacteriaceae possess somatic antigens that are thought to be superficial to the O antigens on the ground that they are responsible for 'O inagglutinability', that is to say, absence of agglutination of living bacteria by antiserum raised by injecting heated suspensions of the homologous organism into animals. Many of these antigens have been described as heat-labile on the evidence of agglutination tests, but the main effect of heating appears to be to cause separation of the antigen from the bacterial cell. The best known representative of this group is the Vi antigen of *Salmonella* Typhi (see Chapter 41). Kauffmann (1947) recognized several classes of surface antigens in *E. coli* that caused O inagglutinability, and classified them according to the effect of heat on the agglutinability, antigenicity and antibody-binding power of bacteria that possessed them. He proposed the term K antigen to include all such surface antigens, whether present at or near the surface of non-capsulate organisms or forming part of a capsule, and it has since been widely used in this sense. Increasing knowledge of these antigens obtained by methods other than agglutination (Ørskov et al. 1971), and growing doubt about the assumption that O inagglutinability always indicates the presence of a surface antigen distinct from the lipopolysaccharide, make it necessary for the term K antigen to be more closely defined. A number of the surface antigens appear to be acid polysaccharides; these include the Vi antigen, some of the K antigens of *E. coli* and the capsular polysaccharides of *Klebsiella*. The K antigen polysaccharides enhance the virulence of invasive bacteria since they counteract the bactericidal action of complement and phagocytes (for a review of the K antigens of *E. coli* see Jann and Jann 1983). Two K antigens of *E. coli*, K88 and K99, are filamentous protein structures. These have been placed in a separate class of antigens (the F antigens) together with type 1 fimbriae, the colonization factor antigens (CFAs) of enterotoxigenic *E. coli* (see Volume 3, Chapter 27) and a number of other fimbrial antigens that cause MR haemagglutination (Ørskov and Ørskov 1983). Also referred to above (p. 924) is the mucoid substance that appears to be a colanic acid.

7.3   H antigens

The strains included in each genus of the Enterobacteriaceae possess many different H antigens. In *Salmonella* there is a close mosaic-like inter-relation between the flagellar antigens of the different serotypes. In other groups, however, the flagellar antigens are usually distinct; and H antigens common to different enterobacterial groups are rare. The genus *Salmonella* is almost unique in showing diphasic variation of the H antigen, although 2 examples of such variation have been described in *E. coli* (Ratiner 1985). The H antigens are almost certainly the fibrous proteins – flagellins – that make up the bulk of the flagella. Antigenically distinct flagella sometimes differ in amino acid composition, but specificity appears to be determined by the amino acid sequence in the flagellin molecule, and possibly also by the organization of the flagellins within the flagellum (Joys 1968, Iino 1969).

7.4   Fimbrial antigens

Antibodies to fimbriae cause the agglutination of homologous organisms that are in the fimbrial phase; loose bulky floccules closely resembling H agglutination appear rapidly at 37°C (Gillies and Duguid 1958). Heating at 100°C detaches the fimbriae and renders the organism inagglutinable by fimbrial antiserum, but the fimbrial antigen is not destroyed, and detached fimbriae retain their antibody-binding power. Organisms heated at 60°C for 30 min and treated with formalin remain fimbriate. The properties of the fimbrial antigen are thus similar to those of the X antigen described by Topley and Ayrton (1924) in *Salmonella* suspensions that had been grown in broth for several days. They may cause confusion in serum agglutination tests if the suspension is fimbriate (Cruickshank 1939), because many human sera contain fimbrial antibody (Gillies and Duguid 1958). To obtain a suitable H suspension for use in agglutination tests, a small inoculum should be taken from an agar plate or from a swarm through semi-solid agar and should be grown for not more than 6 h in broth; for O suspensions, the organism should be grown for 24 h

on a well dried agar plate. Confusion may also result if diagnostic antisera contain fimbrial antibody. The best way to avoid this is to use non-fimbrial variants for immunization.

Several antigens have been recognized among the type 1 fimbriae. All fimbriate strains of *S. flexneri* share a common antigen, and this is distinct from the 3 main fimbrial antigens found in different strains of *E. coli* (Gillies and Duguid 1958); but all fimbriate strains of *E. coli* and *S. flexneri*, and all *Klebsiella* strains that have type 1 fimbriae, share a common component that is absent from the fimbriae of *Salmonella*. On the other hand, all salmonellae with type 1 fimbriae share a major common fimbrial antigen, which is also found in *Citrobacter* strains (Duguid and Campbell 1969). Some minor *Salmonella* fimbrial antigens are less widely distributed. As noted above (see p. 923), several other *E. coli* surface antigens, including the CFAs of enterotoxigenic *E. coli*, are filamentous proteins that resemble fimbriae. Ørskov and Ørskov (1983) proposed a further series of antigens (F antigens) in which F1 represents the MS haemagglutinating type 1 'common' fimbriae, F2 and F3 are equivalent to the human colonization factor antigens CFA/I and CFA/II, F4 and F5 are the K88 and K99 antigens, F6 is the 987P antigen and F7–F12 represent antigens corresponding to additional MR haemagglutinating fimbriae. Additional fimbriae resembling type 1 fimbriae are designated 1A, 1B and 1C in this scheme.

The conjugative or sex pili that are determined by plasmids have also been studied antigenically (Bradley 1980a). Antigenic relationships exist between pili within each of the 3 morphological groups but there are no cross-reactions between the groups.

Many coliform bacteria and *Providencia* strains contain a common antigen referred to by Stamp and Stone (1944) as the α-antigen. It is more thermostable than the H antigen, withstanding a temperature of 75°C for 1 h, but is inactivated at 100°C in 15 min and by exposure for 1 h to ethanol at 65°C. It is most common in recently isolated strains and tends to be lost on subculture. Agglutinins to the α-antigen are sometimes present in rabbit sera and may lead to confusion in the identification of suspected pathogenic organisms. It appears that the α-antigen is not a single substance; Emslie-Smith (1948) distinguished between 7 separate agglutinins in rabbit sera to antigens of this description. A thermolabile β-antigen was reported by Mushin (1949) in strains of coliform bacteria, *Proteus* and *S. flexneri*. It is inactivated by boiling, gives floccular agglutination, and has an optimal agglutinating temperature of 52°C. According to Gillies and Duguid (1958), the general properties of the α- and β-antigens distinguish them from fimbrial antigens.

REFERENCES

Aldová E, Hausner O et al., 1988, *Pragia fontium* gen. nov., sp. nov. of the family *Enterobacteriaceae*, isolated from water, *Int J Syst Bacteriol*, **38**: 183–9.

Anderson ES, 1961, Slime-wall formation in the salmonellae, *Nature (London)*, **190**: 284–5.

Anderson ES, Rogers AH, 1963, Slime polysaccharides of the Enterobacteriaceae, *Nature (London)*, **198**: 714–15.

Aoki S, Merkel M, McCabe WR, 1966, Immunofluorescent demonstration of the common enterobacterial antigen, *Proc Soc Exp Biol Med*, **121**: 230–4.

Bardsley DA, 1938, A comparative study of coliform organisms found in chlorinated and in non-chlorinated swimming bath water, *J Hyg*, **38**: 721–31.

Bascomb S, Lapage SP et al., 1971, Numerical classification of the tribe Klebsielleae, *J Gen Microbiol*, **66**: 279–95.

Bergey DH, Deehan SJ, 1908, The colon:aerogenes group of bacteria, *J Med Res (Boston)*, **19**: 175–200.

Boizot GE, 1941, An examination of the modified Eijkman method applied to pure coliform cultures obtained from waters in Singapore, *J Hyg*, **41**: 566–9.

Borman EK, Stuart CA, Wheeler KM, 1944, Taxonomy of the Family Enterobacteriaceae, *J Bacteriol*, **48**: 351–67.

Böttger EC, Jürs M et al., 1987, Qualitative and quantitative determination of enterobacterial common antigen (ECA) with monoclonal antibodies: expression of ECA by two *Actinobacillus* species, *J Clin Microbiol*, **25**: 377–82.

Bouvet OMM, Grimont PAD et al., 1985, *Budvicia aquatica* gen. nov., sp. nov.: a hydrogen sulfide-producing member of the *Enterobacteriaceae*, *Int J Syst Bacteriol*, **35**: 60–4.

Bradley DE, 1980a, Morphological and serological relationships of conjugative pili, *Plasmid*, **4**: 155–69.

Bradley DE, 1980b, Determination of pili by conjugative bacterial drug resistance plasmids of incompatibility groups B, C, H, J, K, M, V, and X, *J Bacteriol*, **141**: 828–37.

Brown HC, 1921, Observations on the use of citrated media, *Lancet*, **1**: 22–3.

Bülow P, 1964, The ONPG test in diagnostic bacteriology 1. Methodological investigations, *Acta Pathol Microbiol Scand*, **60**: 376–86.

Chantemesse A, Widal F, 1891, Différenciation du bacille typhique et du bacterium coli commune; de la prétendue spontanéité de la fièvre typhoïde, *Bull Méd (Paris)*, **5**: 935.

Constable FL, 1956, Fimbriae and haemagglutinating activity in strains of *Bacterium cloacae*, *J Pathol Bacteriol*, **72**: 133–6.

Cowan ST, 1956, Taxonomic rank of Enterobacteriaceae 'groups', *J Gen Microbiol*, **15**: 345–58.

Cowan ST, 1957, Nomenclature for Enterobacteriaceae, *Bull Hyg*, **32**: 101–3.

Cruickshank JC, 1939, Somatic and 'X' agglutinins to the *Salmonella* group, *J Hyg*, **39**: 224–37.

Davis BR, Ewing WH, 1964, Lipolytic, pectolytic, and alginolytic activities of Enterobacteriaceae, *J Bacteriol*, **88**: 16–19.

Duguid JP, 1951, The demonstration of bacterial capsules and slime, *J Pathol Bacteriol*, **63**: 673–85.

Duguid JP, 1959, Fimbriae and adhesive properties in *Klebsiella* strains, *J Gen Microbiol*, **21**: 271–86.

Duguid JP, 1968, The function of bacterial fimbriae, *Arch Immunol Ther Exp*, **16**: 173–88.

Duguid JP, Anderson ES, Campbell I, 1966, Fimbriae and adhesive properties in salmonellae, *J Pathol Bacteriol*, **92**: 107–38.

Duguid JP, Campbell I, 1969, Antigens of the type-1 fimbriae of salmonellae and other enterobacteria, *J Med Microbiol*, **2**: 535–53.

Duguid JP, Gillies RR, 1957, Fimbriae and adhesive properties in dysentery bacilli, *J Pathol Bacteriol*, **74**: 397–411.

Duguid JP, Gillies RR, 1958, Fimbriae and haemagglutinating activity in *Salmonella*, *Klebsiella*, *Proteus* and *Chromobacterium*, *J Pathol Bacteriol*, **75**: 519–20.

Duguid JP, Old DC, 1980, Adhesive properties of Enterobacteriaceae, *Bacterial Adherence*, ed. Beachey EH, Chapman and Hall, London, 185–217.

Duguid JP, Smith IW et al., 1955, Non-flagellar filamentous appendages ('fimbriae') and haemagglutinating activity in *Bacterium coli*, *J Pathol Bacteriol*, **70**: 335–48.

Durham HE, 1898, A simple method for demonstrating the production of gas by bacteria, *Br Med J*, **1**: 1387.

Eddy BP, Kitchell AG, 1959, Cold-tolerant fermentative Gram-negative organisms from meat and other sources, *J Appl Bacteriol*, **22**: 57–63.

Eijkman C, 1904, Die gärungsprobe bei 46° als hilfsmittel bei der Trinkwasseruntersuchung, *Centralbl Bakteriol Parasitenkd Infektionskr*, **37**: 742–52.

Emslie-Smith AH, 1948, Agglutination of coliform bacilli by normal rabbit serum, *J Pathol Bacteriol*, **60**: 307–13.

Escherich T, 1885, Die Darmbacterien des Neugeborenen und Säuglings, *Fortschr Med*, **3**: 515–22.

Ewing WH, 1966, *Enterobacteriaceae Taxonomy and Nomenclature*, US Department of Health, Education and Welfare, Atlanta, GA.

Ewing WH, 1986, *Edwards and Ewing's Identification of Enterobacteriaceae*, 4th edn, Elsevier Science Publishing Co., New York.

Ewing WH, Edwards PR, 1960, The principal divisions and groups of Enterobacteriaceae and their differentiation, *Int Bull Bacteriol Nomencl Taxon*, **10**: 1–12.

Farmer JJ III, Davis BR et al., 1985, Biochemical identification of new species and biogroups of *Enterobacteriaceae* isolated from clinical specimens, *J Clin Microbiol*, **21**: 46–76.

Ferragut C, Izard D et al., 1981, *Buttiauxella*, a new genus of the family Enterobacteriaceae, *Zentralbl Bakteriol Mikrobiol Hyg Abt 1 Orig C*, **2**: 33–44.

Freer JH, Salton MRJ, 1971, The anatomy and chemistry of Gram-negative cell envelopes, *Microbial Toxins*, vol. 4, eds Weinbaum G, Kadis S, Ajl SJ, Academic Press, New York, 67–126.

Gavini F, Mergaert J et al., 1989, Transfer of *Enterobacter agglomerans* (Beijerinck 1888) Ewing and Fife 1972 to *Pantoea* gen. nov. as *Pantoea agglomerans* comb. nov. and description of *Pantoea dispersa* sp. nov., *Int J Syst Bacteriol*, **39**: 337–45.

Gillespie WA, 1952, Biochemical mutants of coliform bacilli in infections of the urinary tract, *J Pathol Bacteriol*, **64**: 551–7.

Gillies RR, Duguid JP, 1958, The fimbrial antigens of *Shigella flexneri*, *J Hyg*, **56**: 303–18.

Goebel WF, 1963, Colanic acid, *Proc Natl Acad Sci USA*, **49**: 464–71.

Grant WD, Sutherland IW, Wilkinson JF, 1969, Exopolysaccharide colanic acid and its occurrence in the *Enterobacteriaceae*, *J Bacteriol*, **100**: 1187–93.

Grimont PAD, Grimont F et al., 1981, *Cedecea davisae* gen. nov., sp. nov. and *Cedecea lapagei* sp. nov., new *Enterobacteriaceae* from clinical specimens, *Int J Syst Bacteriol*, **31**: 317–26.

Grimont PAD, Farmer JJ III et al., 1983, *Ewingella americana* gen. nov., sp. nov., a new *Enterobacteriaceae* isolated from clinical specimens, *Ann Microbiol (Paris)*, **134A**: 39–52.

Hammarström S, Carlsson HE et al., 1971, Immunochemistry of the common antigen of Enterobacteriaceae (Kunin), *J Exp Med*, **134**: 565–76.

Harber MJ, 1985, Bacterial adherence, *Eur J Clin Microbiol*, **4**: 257–61.

Harden A, Walpole GS, 1906, Chemical action of bacillus lactis aerogenes (Escherich) on glucose and mannitol: production of 2 3,butyleneglycol and acetylmethylcarbinol, *Proc R Soc*, **B77**: 399–405.

Hickman-Brenner FW, Huntley-Carter GP et al., 1984, *Moellerella wisconsensis*, a new genus and species of *Enterobacteriaceae* found in human stool specimens, *J Clin Microbiol*, **19**: 460–3.

Hickman-Brenner FW, Huntley-Carter GP et al., 1985a, *Koserella trabulsii*, a new genus and species of *Enterobacteriaceae* formerly known as Enteric Group 45, *J Clin Microbiol*, **21:** 39–42.

Hickman-Brenner FW, Vohra MP et al., 1985b, *Leminorella*, a new genus of *Enterobacteriaceae*: identification of *Leminorella grimontii* sp. nov. and *Leminorella richardii* sp. nov. found in clinical specimens, *J Clin Microbiol*, **21:** 234–9.

Hinshaw LB (ed.), 1985, *Handbook of Endotoxin, vol. 2: Pathophysiology of Endotoxin*, Elsevier, Amsterdam.

Hoeniger JFM, 1965, Influence of pH on *Proteus* flagella, *J Bacteriol*, **90:** 275–7.

Hollis DG, Hickman FW et al., 1981, *Tatumella ptyseos* gen. nov., sp. nov., a member of the family *Enterobacteriaceae* found in clinical specimens, *J Clin Micriobiol*, **14:** 79–88.

Holt JG, Krieg NR et al. (eds), 1994, Genus *Yokenella*, *Bergey's Manual of Determinative Bacteriology*, 9th edn, Williams & Wilkins, Baltimore, MD, 189–90.

Hurvell B, 1981, Zoonotic *Yersinia enterocolitica* infection: host range, clinical manifestations, and transmission between animals and man, Yersinia enterocolitica, ed. Bottone EJ, CRC Press, Boca Raton, FL, 145–59.

Iino T, 1969, Genetics and chemistry of bacterial flagella, *Bacteriol Rev*, **33:** 454–75.

Izard D, Gavini F et al., 1979, *Rahnella aquatilis*, nouveau membre de la famille des *Enterobacteriaceae*, *Ann Microbiol (Paris)*, **130A:** 163–77.

Izard D, Gavini F et al., 1980, Contribution of DNA–DNA hybridization to the transfer of *Enterobacter aerogenes* to the genus *Klebsiella* as *K. mobilis*, *Zentralbl Bakteriol Abt 1 Orig C*, **1:** 257–63.

Jackson DD, 1911, Classification of the *B. coli* group, *J Infect Dis*, **8:** 241–9.

Jann B, Reske K, Jann K, 1975, Heterogeneity of lipopolysaccharides. Analysis of polysaccharide chain lengths by sodium dodecylsulfate-polyacrylamide gel electrophoresis, *Eur J Biochem*, **60:** 239–46.

Jann K, Jann B, 1983, The K antigens of *Escherichia coli*, *Prog Allergy*, **33:** 53–79.

Jann K, Jann B, 1984, Structure and biosynthesis of O-antigens, *Handbook of Endotoxin, vol. 1: Chemistry of Endotoxin*, ed. Rietschel ET, Elsevier, Amsterdam, 138–86.

Jann K, Jann B, 1987, Polysaccharide antigens of *Escherichia coli*, *Rev Infect Dis*, **9:** S517–26.

Jansson PE, Lindberg AA et al., 1981, Structural studies on the hexose region of the core in lipopolysaccharides from Enterobacteriaceae, *Eur J Biochem*, **115:** 571–7.

Joys TM, 1968, The structure of flagella and the genetic control of flagellation in Eubacteriales. A review, *Antonie van Leeuwenhoek J Microbiol Serol*, **34:** 205–25.

Kauffmann F, 1944, Zur Serologie der Coli-gruppe, *Acta Pathol Microbiol Scand*, **21:** 20–45.

Kauffmann F, 1947, The serology of the coli group, *J Immunol*, **57:** 71–100.

Kauffmann F, 1956a, On biochemical investigations of Enterobacteriaceae, *Acta Pathol Microbiol Scand*, **39:** 85–93.

Kauffmann F, 1956b, A simplified biochemical table of Enterobacteriaceae, *Acta Pathol Microbiol Scand*, **39:** 103–6.

Kauffmann F, 1956c, Zur biochemischen und serologischen Gruppen- und Typen-einteilung der *Enterobacteriaceae*, *Zentralbl Bakteriol Parasitenkd Infektionshyg Abt 1 Orig*, **165:** 344–54.

Kauffmann F, 1959, On the principles of classification and nomenclature of Enterobacteriaceae, *Int Bull Bacteriol Nomencl Taxon*, **9:** 1–6.

Kauffmann F, 1969, *The Bacteriology of the Enterobacteriaceae*, 2nd edn, Munksgaard, Copenhagen.

Kauffmann F, Edwards PR, Ewing WH, 1956, The principles of group differentiation within the Enterobacteriaceae by biochemical methods, *Int Bull Bacteriol Nomencl Taxon*, **6:** 29–33.

Kosako Y, Sakazaki R, Yoshizaki E, 1984, *Yokenella regensburgei* gen. nov., sp. nov.: a new genus and species in the Family *Enterobacteriaceae*, *Jpn J Med Sci Biol*, **37:** 117–24.

Kosako Y, Sakazaki R et al., 1987, *Yokenella regensburgei* and *Koserella trabulsii* are subjective synonyms, *Int J Syst Bacteriol*, **37:** 127–9.

Koser SA, 1923, Utilization of the salts of organic acids by the colon-aerogenes group, *J Bacteriol*, **8:** 493–520.

Koser SA, 1924, Correlation of citrate utilization by members of the colon-aerogenes group with other differential characteristics and with habitat, *J Bacteriol*, **9:** 59–77.

Koser SA, 1926, Further observations on utilization of the salts of organic acids by the colon-aerogenes group, *J Bacteriol*, **11:** 409–16.

Kunin CM, Beard MV, Halmagyi NE, 1962, Evidence for a common hapten associated with endotoxin fractions of *E. coli* and other *Enterobacteriaceae*, *Proc Soc Exp Biol Med*, **111:** 160–6.

Lapage SP, Jayaraman MS, 1964, Beta-galactosidase and lactose fermentation in the identification of enterobacteria including salmonellae, *J Clin Pathol*, **17:** 117–21.

Lapage SP, Rowe B et al., 1979, Biochemical identification of Enterobacteriaceae, *Identification Methods for Microbiologists*, 2nd edn, eds Skinner FA, Lovelock DW, Academic Press, London, 123–41.

Lawn AM, Ørskov I, Ørskov F, 1977, Morphological distinction between different H serotypes of *Escherichia coli*, *J Gen Microbiol*, **101:** 111–19.

Leifson E, 1960, *Atlas of Bacterial Flagellation*, Academic Press, New York.

Le Minor L, 1967, Distribution de la tétrathionate-réductase chez divers sérotypes de *Salmonella*, *Ann Inst Pasteur (Paris)*, **113:** 117–23.

Le Minor L, Popoff MY, 1987, Request for an Opinion: designation of *Salmonella enterica* sp. nov., nom. rev., as the type and only species of the genus *Salmonella*, *Int J Syst Bacteriol*, **37:** 465–8.

Le Minor L, Rohde R, Taylor J, 1970, Nomenclature des *Salmonella*, *Ann Inst Pasteur (Paris)*, **119:** 206–10.

Le Minor L, Véron M, Popoff M, 1982, Proposition pour une nomenclature des *Salmonella*, *Ann Microbiol (Paris)*, **133B:** 245–54.

Le Minor L, Popoff MY et al., 1986, Individualisation d'une septième sous espèce de *Salmonella*: *S. choleraesuis* subsp. *indica* subsp. nov., *Ann Inst Pasteur Microbiol*, **137B:** 211–17.

Levine M, 1916a, On the correlation of the Voges–Proskauer and the methyl red reaction, *J Bacteriol*, **1:** 87.

Levine M, 1916b, On the significance of the Voges–Proskauer reaction, *J Bacteriol*, **1:** 153–64.

Levine M, Epstein SS, Vaughn RH, 1934, Differential reactions in the colon group of bacteria, *Am J Public Health*, **24:** 505–10.

Lüderitz O, Staub AM, Westphal O, 1966, Immunochemistry of O and R antigens of *Salmonella* and related *Enterobacteriaceae*, *Bacteriol Rev*, **30:** 192–255.

Lüderitz O, Kauffmann F et al., 1960, Zur Immunchemie der O-antigene von Enterobacteriaceae, *Zentralbl Bakteriol Parasitenkd Infektionskr Hyg Abt 1 Orig*, **179:** 180–6.

Lüderitz O, Westphal O et al., 1971, Isolation and chemical and immunological characterization of bacterial lipopolysaccharides, *Microbial Toxins*, vol. 4, eds Weinbaum G, Kadis S, Ajl SJ, Academic Press, New York, 145–233.

MacConkey A, 1905, Lactose-fermenting bacteria in faeces, *J Hyg*, **5:** 333–79.

MacConkey A, 1909, Further observations on the differentiation of lactose-fermenting bacilli, with special reference to those of intestinal origin, *J Hyg*, **9:** 86–103.

Mackenzie EFW, Taylor EW, Gilbert WE, 1948, Recent experiences in the rapid identification of *Bacterium coli* type 1, *J Gen Microbiol*, **2:** 197–204.

McWhorter AC, Haddock RL et al., 1991, *Trabulsiella guamensis*, a new genus and species of the family *Enterobacteriaceae* that resembles *Salmonella* subgroups 4 and 5, *J Clin Microbiol*, **29:** 1480–5.

Mäkelä PH, Mayer H, 1976, Enterobacterial common antigen, *Bacteriol Rev*, **40:** 591–632.

Mäkelä PH, Valtonen VV, Valtonen M, 1973, Role of O-antigen (lipopolysaccharide) factors in the virulence of *Salmonella*, *J Infect Dis*, **128**, Suppl.: S81–5.

Martin WJ, Ewing WH, 1967, The deoxyribonuclease test as applied to certain Gram-negative bacteria, *Can J Microbiol*, **13**: 616–18.

Mayer H, Schmidt G, 1979, Chemistry and biology of the enterobacterial common antigen (ECA), *Curr Top Microbiol Immunol*, **85**: 99–153.

Mulczyk M, Szewczuk A, 1970, Pyrrolidonyl peptidase in bacteria: a new colorimetric test for differentiation of Enterobacteriaceae, *J Gen Microbiol*, **61**: 9–13.

Mushin R, 1949, A new antigenic relationship among faecal bacilli due to a common β antigen, *J Hyg*, **47**: 227–35.

Naide Y, Nikaido H et al., 1965, Semirough strains of *Salmonella*, *Proc Natl Acad Sci USA*, **53**: 147–53.

Old DC, Duguid JP, 1970, Selective outgrowth of fimbriate bacteria in static liquid medium, *J Bacteriol*, **103**: 447–56.

Old DC, Corneil I et al., 1968, Fimbriation, pellicle formation and the amount of growth of salmonellas in broth, *J Gen Microbiol*, **51**: 1–16.

Ørskov F, Ørskov I et al., 1971, Immunoelectrophoretic patterns of extracts from all *Escherichia coli* O and K antigen test strains correlation with pathogenicity, *Acta Pathol Microbiol Scand Sect B*, **79**: 142–52.

Ørskov I, Ørskov F, 1983; Serology of *Escherichia coli* fimbriae, *Prog Allergy*, **33**: 80–105.

Ørskov I, Ørskov F et al., 1977, Serology, chemistry, and genetics of O and K antigens of *Escherichia coli*, *Bacteriol Rev*, **41**: 667–710.

Parr LW, 1937, Unrecorded form of *Bacterium aurescens*, sole colon-group representative in a fecal specimen, *Proc Soc Exp Biol Med*, **35**: 563–5.

Parr LW, 1938, Organisms involved in the pollution of water from long stored feces, *Am J Public Health*, **28**: 445–50.

Platt AE, 1935, The viability of *Bact. coli* and *Bact. aerogenes* in water. A method for the rapid enumeration of these organisms, *J Hyg*, **35**: 437–48.

Quadling C, Stocker BAD, 1962, An environmentally-induced transition from the flagellated to the non-flagellated state in *Salmonella typhimurium*: the fate of parental flagella at cell division, *J Gen Microbiol*, **28**: 257–70.

Raghavachari TNS, Iyer PVS, 1939a, The *coli aerogenes* index of pollution used in the bacteriological analysis of water, *Indian J Med Res*, **26**: 867–75.

Raghavachari TNS, Iyer PVS, 1939b, Longevity of *coliform* organisms in water stored under natural conditions, *Indian J Med Res*, **26**: 877–83.

Ratiner YA, 1985, Two genetic arrangements determining flagellar antigen specificities in two diphasic *Escherichia coli* strains, *FEMS Microbiol Lett*, **29**: 317–23.

Reid G, Sobel JD, 1987, Bacterial adherence in the pathogenesis of urinary tract infection: a review, *Rev Infect Dis*, **9**: 470–87.

Report, 1954a, *Int Bull Bacteriol Nomencl Taxon*, **4**: 1–45.

Report, 1954b, *Int Bull Bacteriol Nomencl Taxon*, **4**: 47–94.

Report, 1958, *Int Bull Bacteriol Nomencl Taxon*, **8**: 25–70.

Report, 1963, *Int Bull Bacteriol Nomencl Taxon*, **13**: 69–93.

Rietschel ET (ed.), 1984, *Handbook of Endotoxin, vol. 1: Chemistry of Endotoxin*, Elsevier, Amsterdam.

Rietschel ET, Brade H et al., 1985, Newer aspects of the chemical structure and biological activity of bacterial endotoxins, *Bacterial Endotoxins, Progress in Clinical and Biological Research*, vol. 189, eds ten Cate JW, Büller HR et al., Alan R Liss, New York, 31–50.

Roantree RJ, 1967, Salmonella O antigens and virulence, *Annu Rev Microbiol*, **21**: 443–66.

Ruimy R, Breittmayer V et al., 1994, Phylogenetic analysis and assessment of the genera *Vibrio*, *Photobacterium*, *Aeromonas*, and *Plesiomonas* deduced from small-subunit rRNA sequences, *Int J Syst Bacteriol*, **44**: 416–26.

Schütze H, 1930, The importance of somatic antigen in the production of Aertrycke and Gärtner immunity in mice, *Br J Exp Pathol*, **11**: 34–42.

Shimwell JL, 1963, *Obesumbacterium* gen. nov., *Brewers' J*, **99**: 759–60.

Smith HW, Huggins MB, 1980, The association of the O18, K1 and H7 antigens and the ColV plasmid of a strain of *Escherichia coli* with its virulence and immunogenicity, *J Gen Microbiol*, **121**: 387–400.

Smith T, 1890, Das Gährungskölbchen in der Bakteriologie, *Centralbl Bakteriol Parasitenkd*, **7**: 502–6.

Smith T, 1895, Notes on bacillus coli communis and related forms, together with some suggestions concerning the bacteriological examination of drinking-water, *Am J Med Sci*, **110**: 283–302.

Sneath PHA, Cowan ST, 1958, An electro-taxonomic survey of bacteria, *J Gen Microbiol*, **19**: 551–65.

Snyder ML, Lichstein HC, 1940, Sodium azide as an inhibiting substance for Gram-negative bacteria, *J Infect Dis*, **67**: 113–15.

Stamp (Lord), Stone DM, 1944, An agglutinogen common to certain strains of lactose and non-lactose-fermenting coliform bacilli, *J Hyg*, **43**: 266–72.

Stocker BA, Wilkinson RG, Mäkelä PH, 1966, Genetic aspects of biosynthesis and structure of *Salmonella* somatic polysaccharide, *Ann NY Acad Sci*, **133**: 334–48.

Suzuki T, Gorzynski EA, Neter E, 1964, Separation by ethanol of common and somatic antigens of Enterobacteriaceae, *J Bacteriol*, **88**: 1240–3.

Talbot JM, Sneath PHA, 1960, A taxonomic study of *Pasteurella septica*, especially of strains isolated from human sources, *J Gen Microbiol*, **22**: 303–11.

Tamura K, Sakazaki R et al., 1986, *Leclercia adecarboxylata* gen. nov., comb. nov., formerly known as *Escherichia adecarboxylata*, *Curr Microbiol*, **13**: 179–84.

Thal E, 1954, *Untersuchungen über* Pasteurella pseudotuberculosis, Berlingska Boktryckeriet, Lund.

Thomas GM, Poinar GO Jr, 1979, *Xenorhabdus* gen. nov., a genus of entomopathogenic, nematophilic bacteria of the family Enterobacteriaceae, *Int J Syst Bacteriol*, **29**: 352–60.

Thomas LV, Gross RJ et al., 1983, Antigenic relationships among type strains of *Yersinia enterocolitica* and those of *Escherichia coli*, *Salmonella* spp., and *Shigella* spp., *J Clin Microbiol*, **17**: 109–11.

Thomas SB, Elson K, 1957, Pigmented strains of coli-aerogenes bacteria, *J Appl Bacteriol*, **20**: 50–2.

Topley WWC, Ayrton J, 1924, Further investigations into the biological characteristics of *B. enteritidis* (*aertrycke*), *J Hyg*, **23**: 198–222.

Vandamme P, Pot B et al., 1996, Polyphasic taxonomy, a concensus approach to bacterial systematics, *Microbiol Rev*, **60**: 407–38.

Weinbaum G, Kadis S, Ajl SJ (eds), 1971, *Microbial Toxins*, vol. 4, Academic Press, New York.

Whang HY, Neter E, 1962, Immunological studies of a heterogenetic enterobacterial antigen (Kunin), *J Bacteriol*, **84**: 1245–50.

Wheat RW, Berst M et al., 1967, Lipopolysaccharides of *Salmonella* T mutants, *J Bacteriol*, **94**: 1366–80.

Wilson GS, Twigg RS et al., 1935, *Special Report Series, No. 206*, Medical Research Council, London.

Winslow C-EA, Kligler IJ, Rothberg W, 1919, Studies on the classification of the colon-typhoid group of bacteria with special reference to their fermentative reactions, *J Bacteriol*, **4**: 429–503.

Winslow C-EA, Walker LT, 1907, Note on the fermentative reactions of the *B. coli* group, *Science*, **26**: 797–9.

Wurtz R, 1892, Note sur deux caractères différentiels entre le bacille d'Eberth et le bacterium coli commune, *Arch Méd Exp Anat Pathol*, **4**: 85–91.

Chapter 40

ESCHERICHIA AND SHIGELLA

M Altwegg and J Bockemühl

1 Genus and species definition	8 Classification
2 Introduction and brief historical perspective	9 Laboratory isolation and identification
3 Habitat	10 Susceptibility to antimicrobial agents
4 Morphology	11 Typing methods
5 Metabolism, cultural characteristics and growth requirements	12 Role in normal flora of humans
	13 Pathogenicity and virulence factors
6 Important genetic mechanisms	
7 Cell wall composition and antigenic structure	

1 GENUS AND SPECIES DEFINITION

Based on DNA–DNA hybridization studies the genera *Escherichia* and *Shigella* are very closely related and may be combined into one genus. For practical and historical reasons both groups are still treated separately. This is especially true for the species *Escherichia coli* which includes metabolically inactive strains difficult to distinguish from 'real' *Shigella* (Holt et al. 1994). The G + C content of the DNA is 48–53 mol%.

1.1 *Escherichia*

These organisms are non-spore-forming, gram-negative bacteria, usually motile by peritrichous flagella. They are facultatively anaerobic; gas is usually produced from fermentable carbohydrates. The methyl red reaction is positive but the Voges–Proskauer reaction is negative. Many strains produce polysaccharide capsules or microcapsules.

The type species is *E. coli*. Most strains of this species promptly ferment lactose or give a positive *o*-nitrophenyl-β-D-galactopyranoside (ONPG) reaction. They produce indole, fail to hydrolyse urea and to grow in Møller's KCN broth. H_2S production is not detectable on triple sugar iron (TSI) agar or Kligler's iron agar (KIA), phenylalanine is not deaminated, and gelatin is not liquefied. Most strains decarboxylate lysine and utilize sodium acetate, but they do not grow on Simmons' citrate agar. Other species included in the genus *Escherichia* are *Escherichia fergusonii* (Farmer et al. 1985), *Escherichia hermannii* (Brenner et al. 1982a),

Escherichia vulneris (Brenner et al. 1982b) and *Escherichia blattae* (Burgess, McDermott and Whiting 1973).

Useful biochemical tests to differentiate the species of the genus *Escherichia* and to distinguish them from *Shigella* are listed in Table 40.1.

1.2 *Shigella*

In contrast to the characters described for *Escherichia*, *Shigella* is non-motile, does not produce gas from carbohydrates and does not decarboxylate lysine or hydrolyse arginine. Sodium acetate is used only occasionally, and indole is produced only by certain serovars (Table 40.2).

Shigella is classified into 4 species, *Shigella dysenteriae*, *Shigella flexneri*, *Shigella boydii* and *Shigella sonnei*, which are often referred to as subgroups A, B, C and D, respectively. They are differentiated by a combination of biochemical and serological characters.

The type species is *S. dysenteriae* 1.

2 INTRODUCTION AND BRIEF HISTORICAL PERSPECTIVE

E. coli is an organism that has been intensively studied under various aspects. In general bacteriology, it has been used as a model organism for studies of cell structure, growth and metabolism. Later, it became an important vehicle for the cloning of genes from prokaryotic and eukaryotic cells, and for the expression of gene products. *E. coli* is used as a test organism for the testing of the efficacy of antimicrobial agents and disinfectants, and is considered an indicator organism

Table 40.1 Differentiation of species of *Escherichia* (including *'E.' blattae*) and *Shigella*

Test or property	*E. coli* normal	*E. coli* inactive	*E. fergusonii*	*E. hermannii*	*E. vulneris*	*'E.' blattae*	*Shigella* subgroups A, B and C	*Shigella sonnei*
Indole production	+	v	+	+	−	−	v	−
Lysine decarboxylase	+	v	+	−	v	+	−	−
Ornithine decarboxylase	v	v	+	+	−	+	−	+
Motility	+	−	+	+	+	−	−	−
Gas produced during fermentation	+	−	+	+	+	+	−	−
Acetate utilization	+	v	+	v	v	−	−	−
Growth in KCN	−	−	−	+	v	−	−	−
Yellow pigment	−	+	−	+	v	−	−	−
Fermentation of:								
lactose	+	v	−	v	v	−	−	−
sucrose	v	v	−	v	−	−	−	−
mucate	+	v	−	+	v	v	−	−
D-mannitol	+	+	+	+	+	−	+[a]	+
adonitol	−	−	+	−	−	−	−	−
D-sorbitol	+	v	−	−	−	−	v	−
cellobiose	−	−	+	+	+	−	−	−
D-arabitol	−	−	+	−	−	−	−	−

[a] *S. dysenteriae* (subgroup A) always negative.
Incubation 48 h at 37°C.
+, ≥90% positive; −, ≤10% positive; v, variable, 11–89% positive.
Modified from Farmer (1995).

Table 40.2 Biochemical reactions of *Shigella* serovars

S. dysenteriae	All serovars mannitol −, dulcitol −, xylose −, rhamnose −, raffinose −, indole −, sodium acetate −, ornithine decarboxylase −
Serovar	Exceptions:
2	rhamnose +, indole +
5	dulcitol +
7	rhamnose +, indole +
8	xylose +, indole +
10	xylose +
S. flexneri	All serovars mannitol +, dulcitol −, xylose −, rhamnose −, raffinose v, indole v, sodium acetate −, ornithine decarboxylase −
Serovar	Exceptions:
3	rhamnose v
4	rhamnose v; some strains of subtype 4a sodium acetate +
5	indole +
6	ducitol v; some strains gas + and mannitol −
S. boydii	All serovars mannitol +, dulcitol −, xylose +, rhamnose −, raffinose −, indole −, sodium acetate −, ornithine decarboxylase −
Serovar	Exceptions
2	xylose −
3	dulcitol v, xylose v
4	dulcitol v, xylose −
5	indole +
6	ducitol +
7	indole +
9	xylose −, rhamnose v, indole +
10	ducitol +, xylose v
11	dulcitol v, indole +
12	dulcitol v, xylose −
13	xylose −, indole +, ornithine decarboxylase +, some strains gas +
14	mannitol v, some strains gas +
15	xylose −, indole +
16	indole +
17	indole +
S. sonnei	Mannitol +, dulcitol −, xylose −, rhamnose +, raffinose v, indole −, sodium acetate −, ornithine decarboxylase +, lactose (+), sucrose (+), some strains mucate (+)

Incubation 48 h at 37°C.
+, ≥90% positive; −, ≤10% positive; v, variable, 11–89% positive; (+), delayed positive reaction (3–8 days).
Modified from Ewing (1986), Rowe (1990), Wathen-Grady et al. (1990).

of faecal contamination in food, water and the environment. It is part of the intestinal microbial ecosystems in humans and warm-blooded animals. Last but not least, some strains are important pathogens for these hosts.

E. coli was first identified by the German paediatrician Theodor Escherich during his studies of the intestinal flora of infants. He described the organism in 1885 as *Bacterium coli commune* (Escherich 1885) and established its pathogenic properties in extraintestinal infections (Escherich 1894). The name *Bacterium coli* was widely used until 1919, when Castellani and Chalmers defined the genus *Escherichia* and established the type species *E. coli* (Castellani and Chalmers 1919).

The discovery of shigellae was probably impeded by the cultural problems associated with these organisms. Although Ogata (1892) in Japan and Chantemesse and Widal (1888) in France may have previously isolated the causative agents of bacterial dysentery, the discovery and first identification of these bacteria is attributed to the Japanese bacteriologist Kiyoshi Shiga (Shiga 1898). This discovery, however, was followed by numerous conflicting publications and only by 1954 was the current concept of 4 species (or subgroups) established (Enterobacteriaceae Subcommittee 1954). The historical development has been described in detail by Rowe and Gross (1981) and the interested reader is referred to this review. The genus name *Shigella* was published in 1919 by Castellani and Chalmers in honour of the discoverer.

3 HABITAT

E. coli is part of the normal intestinal flora of both humans and warm-blooded animals (mammals and birds). The organism is excreted with the faeces and may survive in the environment; however, it appears that there is no independent existence outside the body. Thus, *E. coli* is considered an indicator organism for faecal contamination and is an important parameter in food and water hygiene. In organs outside the intestinal tract, *E. coli* may cause a variety of diseases but the responsible strains as well as strains causing enteritis in humans and mammals are characterized by the presence of specific virulence factors. Infections with such strains develop either by the endogenous route (e.g. urinary tract or gall bladder infections, septicaemia), or they are spread in the hospital via contaminated equipment and by the hands of the nursing staff (urinary and respiratory tract infections, wound infections, septicaemia, meningitis). The natural reservoirs of enteropathogenic strains are the intestines of humans (EPEC, ETEC, EIEC, EAgg EC, see section 13.2, p. 953) or domestic animals (ETEC, EHEC). The organisms are transmitted by direct contact or via contaminated food and water.

E. fergusonii, *E. hermannii* and *E. vulneris* have been isolated from clinical specimens and from the intestinal contents of humans and warm-blooded animals. They are opportunistic pathogens and have occasionally been associated with wound infections in humans. The atypical *Escherichia* species '*E.*' *blattae* (see section 8, p. 943) is part of the intestinal flora of cockroaches.

Humans are the only important reservoir of *Shigella*; reports of occasional isolations of *S. flexneri* from wild monkeys in South Africa are not of epidemiological importance (Ruch 1959). Excretion of the organisms in stool is highest during the acute phase of dysenteric illness. During this phase the environment is contaminated and the organisms can survive for weeks in cool and humid locations (Rowe and Gross 1981). They survive for 5–46 days when dried on linen and kept in the dark, and for 9–12 days in soil at room temperature (Roelcke 1938). Although shigellae tolerate a low pH (<3) for short periods, they will soon perish in stools acidified by growth of coliform or other bacteria, but will remain alive for days if such specimens are kept alkaline and are prevented from drying (Rowe 1990). *S. sonnei* appears to be more resistant to detrimental conditions than *S. dysenteriae* and *S. flexneri*, although few differences in the survival in various foods have been observed between *S. sonnei* and *S. flexneri* (Rowe 1990).

Shigella of all 4 subgroups have been reported from tropical and subtropical countries around the world. During the past 30 years, *S. dysenteriae* 1 has caused major epidemics in Central America (1969–70), Bangladesh (1972) and East Africa (since 1991), whereas *S. boydii* is mainly prevalent in South Asia and the Middle East. In Europe and North America *S. sonnei* is by far predominant, followed by *S. flexneri* (Aleksic, Bockemühl and Aleksic 1987, Lee et al. 1991, CDC 1994a) and infections due to *S. boydii* and *S. dysenteriae* are almost exclusively imported by travellers or foreign-born citizens returning from visits to their home countries (Aleksic, Bockemühl and Aleksic 1987).

4 MORPHOLOGY

Escherichia and *Shigella*, as typical members of the family Enterobacteriaceae (see Chapter 39), form rod-shaped cells of 2.0–6.0 μm in length and 1.1–1.5 μm in width with rounded ends (Ørskov 1984). The shape may vary from coccal to long filamentous rods; in some strains one of these forms may prevail but others may show a wide diversity (Gross and Holmes 1990). By the usual staining methods the cells appear homogeneous without granules; spores are not formed.

Escherichia strains, with exception of the 'inactive' biovar of *E. coli*, are usually motile by a set of peritrichous flagella. These proteinaceous structures form long, slender appendages of 19–24 nm diameter which extend about 15–20 μm from the cell surface (Lawn, Ørskov and Ørskov 1977, Silverman and Simon 1977). As shown by Lawn, Ørskov and Ørskov (1977), all H antigens of *E. coli* have a morphologically distinct surface pattern that is identical within each strain and among H antigens associated with different O groups. The different morphological types could be grouped into 6 structurally related morphotypes. Shigellae by definition never possess flagella and therefore are non-motile.

Capsules or microcapsules made of acidic polysaccharides are common in *E. coli* but rare in *Shigella*. They may vary in their size and thus may be detected by light microscopy or, as microcapsules, only by serological or chemical techniques (Ørskov and Ørskov 1984). Mucoid strains sometimes produce extracellular slime which is either a polysaccharide of certain K antigen specificities, or a common acid polysaccharide formed in many *E. coli* strains as well as other Enterobacteriaceae; the latter is described as M antigen and composed of colanic acid (Ørskov and Ørskov 1984).

E. coli and, rarely, *Shigella* (some strains of *S. flexneri* serovars 1–5; Duguid and Gillies 1956, Ewing 1986) produce different kinds of fimbriae (or pili) that vary in structure and antigenic specificity. These are filamentous, proteinaceous, hair-like appendages surrounding the cell in varying numbers. If present in large numbers they may influence the physico-chemical properties of the organisms and render the strains O-inagglutinable. Fimbriae are either chromosomally or plasmid-encoded, and more than one type of fimbriae may be carried by one individual cell (Ørskov and Ørskov 1984). Within a fimbriate strain there are individual cells with many fimbriae and others with none and there is reversible variation between the fimbriate and non-fimbriate phase (Gross and Holmes 1990). Fimbriae are hydrophobic and exert host- or organ-specific adhesion properties. Thus they are important virulence factors which will be discussed later (see section 13, p. 951).

5 METABOLISM, CULTURAL CHARACTERISTICS AND GROWTH REQUIREMENTS

Escherichia and *Shigella* are facultatively anaerobic

organisms. They are chemo-organotrophic, having both a respiratory and a fermentative type of metabolism, but growth is less copious under anaerobic conditions. The optimal temperature is 37°C at which they grow well on ordinary media containing 1% peptone as carbon and nitrogen source (Holt et al. 1994). According to the state of the lipopolysaccharide of the outer membrane, the growth on solid media is characterized by glistening, smooth (S), or dry, wrinkled, rough (R) colonies, respectively. In liquid media, S forms show homogeneous turbid growth within 12–18 h whereas R forms agglutinate spontaneously, forming a sediment on the bottom of the test tubes (Ørskov 1984). Pellicle formation on the surface of liquid media can be seen in heavily fimbriated strains after prolonged incubation (>72 h) at 37°C, or can be induced by serial subcultures under these conditions.

E. coli exerts pronounced metabolic activity between 15 and 45°C (Holmes and Gross 1990); under optimal conditions the generation time is 20 min. Exotoxins such as enterotoxins and haemolysins are best produced at about 37°C, are translocated into the periplasmatic space and therefore may be liberated in higher amounts by exposition to 2000 IU ml^{-1} of polymyxin B for 30 min (Bockemühl 1992). In contrast to most other coliform bacteria, *E. coli* ferments lactose and produces indole at 44°C which is used for identification in food and water bacteriology. After 18–24 h of incubation *E. coli* forms large (2–3 mm), circular, convex and non-pigmented colonies on nutrient and blood agar; haemolysin is produced by a number of strains. *E. coli* strains are resistant to low concentrations of bile salts (e.g. 0.05 % sodium deoxycholate) and grow as large red colonies on MacConkey agar. *E. coli* is more heat resistant than most other species of Enterobacteriaceae and survives at 60°C for 15 min or at 55°C for 60 min (Holmes and Gross 1990). On the other hand, it is rather sensitive to certain dyes such as brilliant green, and to higher concentrations of deoxycholate (0.25 %) which therefore are used in selective media for the isolation of salmonellae and shigellae.

Shigellae have similar growth requirements but their growth is slower and in contaminated specimens they tend to be suppressed by the concomitant gram-negative bacterial flora. In pure cultures they form circular, glistening, translucent or slightly opaque colonies on nutrient agar and no haemolysis on blood agar. The colony size varies within the 4 subgroups with smaller colonies in *S. dysenteriae*, but most *Shigella* serovars produce colonies of 1–2 mm after 18–24 h of incubation at 37°C. *S. sonnei* may dissociate in smooth ('phase 1') and larger, flatter colonies showing an irregular edge. The latter colonial type ('phase 2') is associated with the loss of the 120 000–140 000 kDa virulence plasmid and a change of the antigenic specificity. Upon subculture, phase 1 colonies further dissociate but the change of phase 1 to phase 2 is irreversible. Phase 2 strains still grow homogeneously in broth culture but they may partially sediment after boiling at 100°C or autoagglutinate in 3.5% NaCl solution (Rowe 1990, Bockemühl 1992). Thus, phase 2 may be considered as intermediate between the smooth and the rough state of the organisms.

Due to the close relationship to *E. coli*, which is less fastidious, there are only few cultural properties which can be used for the selective isolation of *Shigella*. Most important for practical purposes is the higher tolerance of shigellae to sodium deoxycholate that is incorporated into the usual isolation media such as Leifson's deoxycholate citrate agar, *Salmonella–Shigella* agar, or xylose–lysine–deoxycholate agar, respectively. On these media and on MacConkey agar shigellae grow with colourless, translucent, smooth colonies of 1–2 mm after 18–24 h of incubation at 37°C. After prolonged incubation (>48 h) growth of *S. sonnei* becomes pinkish due to delayed fermentation of lactose and sucrose.

In common with most strains of the enterohaemorrhagic pathovars of *E. coli* (EHEC), shigellae tolerate extremely acid conditions (pH 2.5) for short periods (see section 6). However, they will soon perish if kept in an acidified environment for longer periods and therefore have to be grown at neutral or slightly alakaline pH (pH 7.0–7.4). Shigellae are not especially resistant to heat and are killed at a temperature of 55°C within 1 h (Rowe 1990).

Shigella and *Escherichia* strains can be maintained for years in tightly closed nutrient agar stabs or, better, on Dorset egg medium kept in the dark at room temperature. However, even without further subcultures such strains tend to mutate to the R form and to lose virulence plasmids. Important cultures should be preserved in tryptic soy broth containing ≥10% glycerol at −70°C or in liquid nitrogen (Ørskov 1984, Rowe and Gross 1984).

6 IMPORTANT GENETIC MECHANISMS

For decades *E. coli* has been used as a model organism to study bacterial genetics for various reasons:

1 no special nutritional requirements
2 rapid proliferation with doubling times as short as 20 min
3 non-pathogenicity
4 easy availability.

Consequently, a variety of very basic genetic mechanisms have been discovered or have at least been extensively studied in this organism. These include our basic understanding of DNA replication, transcription and translation processes; DNA restriction and modification systems where modification by methylases protects the cell's own genome from being restricted; F factor as conjugational donors of chromosomal markers at high frequency (Hfr strains); recombination; DNA repair mechanisms; organization and expression of sets of genes that determine the metabolism of various compounds, e.g. the lactose operon. It is, therefore, not astonishing that the genome of *E. coli* K12 is the one that was best analysed and was superseded only recently when the sequence of the entire genome of *Haemophilus influenzae* was published. In addition, *E. coli* has been widely used as a cloning vehicle. It is beyond the scope of this chapter to go into great detail regarding genetic mechanisms; the reader is referred to an excellent collection of reviews which cover most aspects of the cellular and molecular biology of this organism (Neidhart et al. 1996).

One genetic aspect is especially important in the context of the pathogenicity of the organisms covered in this chapter. Although results of in vitro studies of acid resistance are controversial, possibly due to different experimental methods used (Small 1994), it is clear that *Shigella* spp. (as well as some *E. coli* isolates but not necessarily the enteroinvasive variety) are more acid-resistant than other enteric pathogens such as *Salmonella* (Garrod 1937, Gorden and Small 1993). This increases the ability to survive in an environment as acidic as the contents of the normal stomach (pH below 3.0) and probably results in a lower infective dose required to induce gastrointestinal disease. Acid resistance in *S. flexneri* and *E. coli* is restricted to stationary-phase organisms and requires an alternative σ factor, *rpoS* (Small et al. 1994). Fang et al. (1993) have shown that a functional homologue of *rpoS* is also present in *Salmonella typhimurium*, yet this organism is not acid-resistant. Although the protein(s) conferring acid resistance have not been identified, they seem to be among the more than 30 proteins that are regulated by *rpoS* in stationary-phase *E. coli* (McCann, Kidwell and Matin 1991).

7   CELL WALL COMPOSITION AND ANTIGENIC STRUCTURE

7.1   Cell wall structure

First attempts to characterize the nature of the *E. coli* cell surface structures were made by Kauffmann in the 1940s using serological methods (Kauffmann 1943, 1944). During his investigations the author observed that antisera prepared from boiled cultures (O antisera) did not agglutinate many freshly isolated strains, but these cultures became agglutinable after heating at different temperatures. Kauffmann distinguished several surface antigens with different physical and serological properties and named them A, L and B antigens (Kauffmann 1965).

The elucidation of the chemical structure of the gram-negative cell wall and its outer layers (Lüderitz, Staub and Westphal 1966, Lüderitz et al. 1973, Jann and Westphal 1975, Ørskov et al. 1977, Jann and Jann 1987, Rietschel et al. 1987) not only explained the serological differences and cross-reactions between antigens but also recognized the pathophysiological importance of certain compounds now known as endotoxins.

As shown in Fig. 40.1, the outer layers of *E. coli* consist of the outer membrane with phospholipids, lipid A and proteins, from which protrude the polysaccharide (LPS) chains, overlayed by capsular polysaccharides

(CP) (Jann and Jann 1987). Both LPS and CP are the chemical basis of O and K antigens, respectively, and contribute to the pathogenicity of the organisms.

As reviewed by Jann and Jann (1987, 1992), LPS and CP are synthesized at the cytoplasmatic site of the cytoplasmic membrane of the bacteria from where they are transported to the outer membrane. Whereas CP are further secreted to form the bacterial capsule, LPS reside and are integrated into the cell wall through hydrophobic interaction. They consist of lipid A as the hydrophobic moiety linked to the O-specific polysaccharides through an oligosaccharide linkage region, called core region (Fig. 40.1).

Lipid A, of which only one chemical structure is known in *E. coli* (Jann and Jann 1987), mediates as endotoxin many different in vivo activities including pyrogenicity, local Shwartzman reactivity, lethal toxicity in mice, adjuvant activity, induction of interferon and tumour necrosis factor. In humans, these biological properties contribute to a variety of pathophysiological effects such as fever, hypotension, disseminated intravascular coagulation and septic shock (Rietschel et al. 1987).

Five different core structures have been identified in *E. coli* (Jann and Jann 1987) and 166 serological specificities of the polysaccharide chains have been defined. Loss of the O-specific polysaccharide moiety results in a mutation from smooth (S) to the rough (R) form of the bacteria; R mutants express R-LPS which consists only of lipid A and the core oligosaccharide. The polysaccharide chains consist of oligosaccharide repeating units that generally are neutral but may also have acidic components in *E. coli* (Jann and Jann 1987).

The capsular (K) antigens of *E. coli* are acidic polysaccharides that, in view of their chemical, physical and microbiological characteristics, have been divided in 2 groups. Group I CPs are of a high molecular weight (>100 000), are related to the *Klebsiella* capsular antigens and are coexpressed with O groups 8, 9, 20 and 101 of *E. coli*. They are stable at pH 6 and when heated to 100°C, and correspond to the capsular

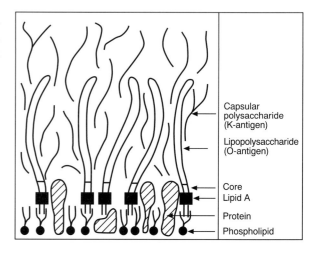

Fig. 40.1   Cell wall structure of *Escherichia coli*. (Modified from Jann and Jann 1987).

antigen type A of Kauffmann (1965). Group II capsular antigens are of lower molecular weight (<50 000), are related to the K antigens in *Neisseria meningitidis* and *H. influenzae*, and are coexpressed with many *E. coli* O groups; they are heat-labile (B- and L-type capsular antigens, Kauffmann 1965) and do not resist pH 6. The chemical identity or relatedness between certain K antigens is associated with similar pathogenic traits. Thus, *E. coli* K1 antigen is identical with the K antigen of *N. meningitidis* type b, and both are related to the capsules of *H. influenzae* types a and b, all of which are characterized by an invasive capacity of the respective strains. In these organisms the capsules are responsible for both evasion of the unspecific host defence through interruption of the complement cascade and evasion of immune recognition due to molecular mimicry of substances found in the host's tissues. For more details on this fascinating topic, the reader is referred to the reviews of Jann and Jann (1987, 1992).

With regard to their O antigens, shigellae have the same basic structure with rather distinct type-specific chemical repeating units of the polysaccharide chains in *S. dysenteriae* and the monotypic *S. sonnei* (Ewing and Lindberg 1984). Within subgroup C, *S. boydii*, several complex antigenic relationships exist with other shigellae and *E. coli*, suggesting a chemical relatedness of the respective polysaccharides.

S. flexneri is characterized by an extensive intraspecific O-antigenic relationship of its serovars. As shown by structural studies, the polysaccharides of serovars 1–5 are polymers of tetrasaccharide repeating units consisting of D-glucose, *N*-acetylglucosamine and L-rhamnose (Ewing and Lindberg 1984). The type specificity of the antigens is caused by different sequences of these sugars in the side chain (Rowe 1990). The structure of serovar 6-specific antigen is different and its tetrasaccharide repeating unit is composed of D-galactosamine, *N*-acetylgalactosamine and L-rhamnose (Ewing and Lindberg 1984). The serovars 1–5 possess group antigens designated 3, 4, 6, 7 and 8 (Table 40.3) of which the latter 3 have been chemically determined and found to form part of the same macromolecule also carrying the type antigen (Ewing and Lindberg 1984, Rowe 1990). The type-specific antigens I–V and group antigens 7 and 8 arise from the 3, 4 antigens by phage conversion (Rowe 1990); no O group antigen has been identified in *S. flexneri* serovar 6 which, however, is antigenically related to the 3, 4 group antigen (Ewing and Lindberg 1984).

Capsular material rendering *Shigella* isolates inagglutinable has been described in strains of *S. dysenteriae* and *S. boydii* (Ewing 1986, Rowe 1990).

7.2 Antigenic structure of *E. coli*

Complete serotyping of *E. coli* includes the determination of the O, K and H antigens, i.e. O:K:H, and if an additional fimbrial virulence factor is present, it is O:K:H:F. Examples given by Ørskov and Ørskov (1984) are O6:K2:H1:F7 for a typical strain from a patient with pyelonephritis, O18ac:K1:H7 for a meningitis isolate, or O111:H2 (no K antigen) for a strain from a case of infantile enteritis. Since a large number of single antigens have been described in *E. coli* and since most of these can be found in various combinations, a complete typing scheme comparable to the Kauffmann–White scheme for *Salmonella* would be too extensive and of no practical applicability. Furthermore, as shown below, K-typing is restricted to a few specialists and, therefore, complete typing has been performed only on a rather small number of strains. Certain O groups can be associated with a number of different K and H antigens and, furthermore, a number of O groups are antigenically complex and would require further subdivisions. Therefore, only standard strains for the established O, K and H antigens have been defined and listed (Ørskov et al. 1977, 1991, Ørskov and Ørskov 1984, Ewing 1986).

O ANTIGENS

Of the numbered O groups 1–173, 7 have been excluded for different reasons. Two of them (O31 and O93) proved to be identical with previously defined antigens (O1 and O8, respectively), 4 grouped strains were later identified as *Citrobacter* (O67, O72, O94, O122) and one reference strain was lost (O47) (Ørskov and Ørskov 1984, Ewing 1986). *E. coli* O antigens are not type- or species-specific but numerous cross-reactions are known between individual *E. coli* O antigens and between these and the O antigens of *Shigella*, *Citrobacter*, *Salmonella*, *Providencia* and *Yersinia* (Ørskov and Ørskov 1984, Ewing 1986, Holmes and Gross 1990). Therefore, determination of the O antigen must always be associated with a proper biochemical identification of the isolate. This is especially important for shigellae that share partial or identical O antigens with *E. coli* (Table 40.4).

O antigens are heat-stable and are not inactivated by heating at 100°C for 2.5 h (Kauffmann 1965). Such preparations are used for antiserum production in rabbits, but cultures carrying A-type capsular antigens need to be heated to 120°C for 2 h. Likewise, determi-

Table 40.3 Abbreviated antigenic scheme of *Shigella flexneri*

Serovar	Subserovar	Abbreviated antigenic formula
1	1a	I: 4 …
	1b	I: 6 …
2	2a	II: 3, 4 …
	2b	II: 7, 8
3	3a	III: 6, 7, 8 …
	3b	III: 3, 4, 6 …
4	4a	IV: 3, 4 …
	4b	IV: 6 …
5	5a	V: 3, 4 …
	5b	V: 7, 8 …
6		VI: …
X Variant		: 7, 8
Y Variant		: 3, 4

From Rowe (1990).

Table 40.4 Examples of identical O antigens in *Shigella* and *E. coli*

Shigella	Serovar	Corresponding *E. coli* O group	*Shigella*	Serovar	Corresponding *E. coli* O group
S. dysenteriae	2	112ac	*S. boydii*	1	149
	3	124		2	87
	5	58		4	53
	12	152		5	79
				8	143
S. flexneri	2b	147		11	105
	4b	135		14	32
	5	129		15	112ab

Modified from Ewing (1986).

nation of the O antigens of *E. coli* requires, as a rule, heat treatment of the strain suspensions for 1 h at 100°C. Whereas typing of all defined O antigens is very laborious, requires extensive experience and is, therefore, restricted to reference laboratories, typing of a narrow scope of O groups may be helpful for the screening of certain pathotypes such as EPEC, EIEC, or EHEC. Serogroups frequently associated with these enteropathogenic *E. coli* types are listed in Table 40.5. However, most of the virulence factors are encoded by mobile genetic elements such as plasmids or phages and therefore may be absent in such isolates, or may be present in other O groups. The problems encountered with the determination of *E. coli* O groups are discussed in the laboratory methods section (see section 9, p. 945).

Table 40.5 Serogroups and serotypes of *E. coli* frequently associated with intestinal infections in humans

Pathotype	O or OH group
EPEC	O20, O26, O44, O55, O86, O111,
Infantile diarrhoea	O114, O119, O125ac, O126, O127, O128, O142, O158
EIEC	O28ac, O112ac, O124, O136,
Enteroinvasive, dysenteric disease in all age groups	O143, O144, O152, O164, O167
EHEC	O26: H11, O111: H −, O111: H^{multiple},
Enterohaemorrhagic diarrhoea in all age groups, in young children leading to haemolytic-uraemic syndrome (HUS)	O157: H −, O157: H7

Adapted from Ørskov and Ørskov (1984), Ewing (1986), Bockemühl (1992).

K ANTIGENS

Based on different sensitivities to heat treatment, Kauffmann (1965) differentiated 3 serological groups of *E. coli* envelope antigens. Strains with type A capsular antigens mostly grew with more or less mucoid colonies, were thermostable (100°C) and became O-agglutinable only after heating at 120°C for 2 h. These antigens are now known to belong to the group of class I capsular polysaccharides according to Jann and Jann (1987). The heat-labile antigens L and B were defined by their different agglutinin-binding power following inactivation at 100°C. However, results obtained for L- and K-type antigens were often inconsistent upon repeated examination of the same culture. Finally, Ørskov et al. (Ørskov et al. 1977, Ørskov and Ørskov 1984) showed that these K antigens included a variety of surface structures such as fimbriae, flagellae, outer-membrane proteins and capsular polysaccharides that vary quantitatively according to the culture conditions. These authors also showed that the 'heat-labile' polysaccharide K antigens in principle are thermostable and eluted from the bacterial surface during boiling, thus making K agglutination of boiled suspensions of bacteria impossible. Using immunoelectrophoresis with cellular extracts, these authors demonstrated the presence of capsular antigens in all the former A- and L-containing strains but only in a few strains in which B antigens had been described. This method distinguished 5 reaction patterns to which all described K antigens could be allocated. Therefore, the term K antigen was suggested as the common name for all types of capsular polysaccharide antigens.

For the reasons described, K typing of *E. coli* is too complicated for routine purposes and is restricted to a few specialists.

F ANTIGENS

Certain fimbrial antigens are involved in the adhesion process and, therefore, are important virulence factors. They develop at 37°C but not at 18°C; chemically they are heat-labile proteins. Fimbrial antigens agglutinate a variety of erythrocytes that can be used for their characterization. Most *E. coli* strains produce a type of fimbriae whose haemagglutinating capacity is suspended in the presence of mannose (type 1 fimbriae). In addition, strains associated with diarrhoeal or extraintestinal disease may produce fimbriae that still haemagglutinate in the presence of mannose; their formation is usually genetically encoded on plasmids. Ørskov and Ørskov (1984) have developed a scheme for the serological typing of fimbrial antigens associated with different disease conditions (Table 40.6).

H ANTIGENS

Flagellar antigens are heat-labile proteins. The described 53 H antigens are numbered H1 to H56. Of these, H50 has been withdrawn and H13 and H22 were deleted after identification of the type strains as *Citrobacter freundii* (Ørskov and Ørskov 1984). Although usually one antigenic type of flagellae is produced by motile strains of *E. coli*, phase variation, as known from motile *Salmonella* strains, has been described between flagellar antigens H3 and H16, and H4 and H16 (Ratiner 1982).

H antigens are determined by slide or tube agglutination using broth cultures or growth on semisolid media from actively motile strains. As most *E. coli* strains are poorly motile when they are first isolated, one or several passages through semisolid media (e.g. in U-shaped tubes) is usually necessary to obtain well flagellated bacteria. Sometimes motility is better at 30°C than at 37°C. Most H antigens are type-specific and there are only a few antigenic relationships of practical importance (Ewing 1986). The methods applied for the determination of *E. coli* H antigens have been described by Ørskov and Ørskov (1984) and Ewing (1986). Although H typing is of importance for a precise phenotypic characterization of *E. coli* strains, its performance is usually limited to reference laboratories.

Table 40.6 Ørskov and Ørksov typing scheme for fimbrial antigens of *E. coli*

Fimbrial antigens	Previous designation	Disease association
F: 1	Type 1	Common fimbrial antigen
F: 2	CFA 1	ETEC, human
F: 3	CFA 2	ETEC, human
F: 4	K 88	ETEC, pig
F: 5	K 99	ETEC, bovine
F: 6	987	ETEC, pig
F: 7	C 1212	UTI[a], human
F: 8	C 1254–79	UTI, human
F: 9	3669	UTI, human
F: 10	C 1960–79	UTI, human
F: 11	C 1976–79	UTI, human
F: 12	C 1979–79	UTI, human

[a]UTI, urinary tract infection.
Modified from Ørksov and Ørskov (1984).

7.3 Antigenic structure of *Shigella*

Since shigellae by definition are non-motile, they never produce H (flagellar) antigens and serological typing is confined to the determination of O antigens and O-antigenic subfactors which are summarized in Tables 40.3 and 40.7. Occasional occurrence of capsules or fimbriae may render the organisms O inagglutinable and necessitate heating of the cultures at 100°C for 1 h to inactivate these structures. In addition to the intraspecific antigenic relationships discussed earlier, there exist various identical or highly related O antigens common in both *Shigella* and *E. coli* (see examples are listed in Table 40.4, p. 942). Therefore, adequate biochemical testing (see Table 40.1, p. 936) is essential to identify *Shigella* strains correctly.

8 CLASSIFICATION

The classification of the family Enterobacteriaceae has always been confusing. This is especially true for *Escherichia* and *Shigella* because DNA–DNA reassociation studies show that *E. coli* and *Shigella* belong to a single genomic species. It is, therefore, not astonishing that, biochemically, intermediate strains that are difficult to assign to one of the 2 genera do occur. In addition, it is well known that certain *E. coli* (EIEC) strains have the same pathogenic potential as *Shigella* spp., i.e. they can cause dysentery-like disease and are invasive in the Serény test. However, these strains are not necessarily the biochemically intermediate strains. Although it has been proposed that the ability to cause invasive disease might also be considered, the utilization of virulence traits for classification of these strains would create as many new problems as it would solve. The proposal of the Enterobacteriaceae Subcommittee of the International Committee on Bacteriological Nomenclature that pathogenicity should not be considered in the classification of Enterobacteriaceae and that strains with biochemical reactions that do not conform strictly with those of *Shigella* should be classified as atypical *E. coli* has, therefore, been widely accepted (Holmes and Gross 1990). For clinical laboratories, however, determining the presence of virulence factors or the ability for invasion (in cell cultures) may be more meaningful than to report *E. coli* and *Shigella* spp., respectively.

Having accepted the view that aberrant strains should be classified as *E. coli*, the main difficulty is to distinguish them from members of the genus *Shigella*. In practice, reliance is usually placed on the criteria listed in Table 40.1 (see p. 936).

Of the other species in the genus *Escherichia*, all except *E. blattae* (isolated from the hind-gut of cockroaches (Burgess, McDermott and Whiting 1973)) have been found in clinical specimens. *E. blattae* differs from 'typical' *Escherichia* spp. by its metabolic inactivity and it has, therefore, been proposed that it would be better placed in another genus in the family Enterobacteriaceae (Holmes and Gross 1990) (see Chapter

Table 40.7 Classification of *Shigella*

Subgroup	Species and serovar		Synonyms
A Mannitol not fermented Serovars antigenically distinct*	*S. dysenteriae** Serovar 1		*S. shigae*, Shiga–Kruse bacillus
	2		*S. schmitzii*; possibly some strains of *Bacillus ambiguus* (Andrewes)
	3		Q771 ⎱ *S. arabinotarda* A
	4		Q1167
	5		Q1030 ⎰ Large-Sachs group (possibly
	6		Q454 includes some strains of
	7		Q902 ⎰ *B. ambiguus*)
	8		559–52
	9		58
	10		2050
	11		3873–50
	12		3341–55
	13		I9809–73
B Mannitol usually fermented Serovars antigenically interrelated	*S. flexneri* Serovar 1	 Subtype 1a	*S. paradysenteriae; Bacillus paradysenteriae* V
		Subtype 1b	VZ
	2	Subtype 2a	W ⎱ (Andrewes and Inman)
		Subtype 2b	WX
	3	Subtype 3a	Z
		Subtype 3b	
	4	Subtype 4a	103 (Boyd)
		Subtype 4b	103Z (Rewell and Bridges)
	5	Subtype 5a	
		Subtype 5b	
	6		Boyd 88, Newcastle and Manchester biochemical subtypes
	X variant		X ⎱ (Andrews and Inman)
	Y variant		Y
C Mannitol usually fermented Serovars antigenically distinct*	*S. boydii** Serovar 1		*S. paradysenteriae* 170
	2		P288
	3		D1
	4		P274 ⎱ Boyd
	5		P143
	6		D19
	7		Lavington type T; *S. etousae*
	8		112
	9		1296/7 (1320)
	10		430 (D15)
	11		34 (732)
	12		123
	13		425
	14		2770–51
	15		703
	16		2710–54
	17		3615–53
	18		E10163

D
Mannitol usually fermented and
  lactose at 3–8 days
	S. sonnei
	Two antigenic forms
	  (phase 1, phase 2)
			Duval's bacillus; *Bacillus ceylonensis* A;
			  Kruse's *Bacillus pseudodysenteriae*
			  type E

*Three additional serovars of *S. dysenteriae* and 2 *S. boydii* serovars have been proposed by Gross et al. (1982a, 1989) and Ansaruzzaman et al. (1995).
Modified from Rowe (1990) and Wathen-Grady et al. (1990).

39) as has been done with *Escherichia adecarboxylata* which is now classified as *Leclercia adecarboxylata* (Tamura et al. 1986).

9 LABORATORY ISOLATION AND IDENTIFICATION

9.1 Isolation

Escherichia spp. may be recovered from various sites of the body either as normal flora (gastrointestinal tract) or as causative agents of a variety of infections (urinary tract and wound infections, meningitis, septicaemia, etc.), whereas shigellae are usually restricted to the human intestine, causing diarrhoea or bacillary dysentery. Transport and culture of extraintestinal specimens follow general practices as escherichiae are less fastidious than many of the other species that may be present in such materials. Specimens from normally sterile body sites are plated on the usual non-selective media such as blood, chocolate or nutrient agar. If materials are likely to be contaminated or to contain different organisms (e.g. specimens from the respiratory or the urinary tract, or from wound infections), media of low selectivity such as MacConkey or eosin–methylene blue (EMB) agar should be included in the set of plating media.

Direct culture on MacConkey or EMB agar of freshly passed stool specimens is the usual method for isolation of enterovirulent *E. coli* from patients with enteric infections. Rectal swabs are less desirable but may be taken from acutely ill patients, e.g. in hospitals.

The chance of detecting a pathogen can be increased if specimens are collected in the acute stage of the disease. Repeat examinations are of value, especially in convalescents or patients with previous antibiotic treatment. As *E. coli* is part of the normal intestinal flora, at least 10, but preferably more, colonies should be picked from the isolation media and tested for the presence of virulence markers (see section 13.2, p. 953). In the authors' laboratories cases of ETEC and EHEC infection have been identified in which one colony of pathogenic *E. coli* was detected among 200–300 'apathogenic' isolates. Alternatively, polymerase chain reaction (PCR) targeting virulence-associated gene sequences can be performed on colony sweeps from MacConkey or other moderately selective agar plates; ideally such a procedure should be followed by subculture and identification of the responsible pathogenic strain.

For the isolation of shigellae, a freshly passed stool specimen during the acute stage of illness is the material of choice. If present, mucus or blood-stained portions should be selected for culture and, if desired, for microscopic examination for the presence of faecal leucocytes (e.g. by a native or methylene blue-stained wet slide preparation). Swabs, except when taken during proctoscopy, are less suitable. If the specimens cannot be cultured within 2–4 h, they should be preserved in either a transport medium (e.g. buffered glycerol solution or Cary–Blair medium

with or without 0.2–0.5% agar) or in a combined transport–enrichment fluid (e.g. specimen preservative medium according to Hajna 1955).

Compared to *E. coli*, shigellae are more sensitive, propagate more slowly and are easily overgrown by the concomitant aerobic intestinal flora. An effective enrichment medium would, therefore, be desirable but is not available. Enrichment of stool specimens in gram-negative broth (Hajna) or selenite broth for about 6 h at 37°C can be tried. Ewing (1986) recommended ordinary infusion broth; alternatively, peptone broth supplemented by 10 mg l^{-1} novobiocin may be used (Bockemühl 1992). During acute illness, a direct culture is usually successful in isolating the organisms. A combination of non-selective (e.g. blood agar, bromthymol blue–lactose agar), moderately selective (MacConkey agar, EMB) and more selective media [xylose–lysine–deoxycholate agar (XLD), deoxycholate citrate agar (Leifson)] should be used for the isolation of *Shigella*. The cultures are incubated overnight at 37°C. For more details see Gilligan et al. (1992).

9.2 Identification

Escherichia and *Shigella* spp. are identified by biochemical reactions, combined with agglutination in group- or serovar-specific antisera for shigellae. Useful tests to differentiate the species are summarized in Table 40.1 (see p. 936). Problems may arise in separating certain metabolically inactive *E. coli* strains from *Shigella* as intermediate forms may occur. Shigellae, by definition, are non-motile and do not decarboxylate lysine or hydrolyse arginine. Except for *S. sonnei*, certain serovars within the other species, and certain strains within these serovars, they do not produce gas from glucose or decarboxylate ornithine, nor do they use sodium acetate or produce indole from tryptophan. *Shigella* serovars which are positive in the latter tests are listed in Table 40.2 (see p. 937).

Serotyping of *Shigella* strains with polyvalent, O group-, or serovar-specific diagnostic sera has to consider that identical or related O antigens do exist in *E. coli*. Therefore, proper biochemical testing is essential for the correct identification of shigellae.

Various biological, immunological and molecular methods are available to identify the different types of enterovirulent strains of *E. coli*. Unfortunately, many of these methods are not established in routine diagnostic laboratories, or simple screening methods, which only identify such strains with a certain probability, are used. Thus, collaboration with specialized or reference laboratories is usually necessary to prove infections with enterovirulent *E. coli*.

EPEC

Although this pathotype is rather heterogeneous and different virulence factors have been identified, such strains are frequently associated with certain *E. coli* O groups that can be tested by use of agglutinating antisera. Screening for '*E. coli* serogroups related to infantile diarrhoea' may be applied in outbreaks but is con-

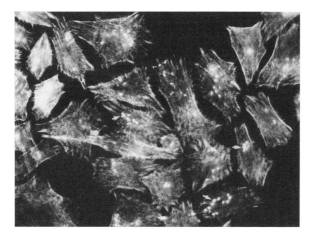

Fig. 40.2 Fluorescent actin staining (FAS) test of enterohaemorrhagic and enteropathogenic *E. coli*. Intimate adherence is characterized by actin polymerization (arrows).

troversial for sporadic diarrhoeal cases of infants below 1 year of age. Ten or more lactose-positive colonies are subcultured on blood or nutrient agar and agglutinated with a set of polyvalent and monovalent OK antisera (see Table 40.5, p. 942). A subculture yielding a clear agglutination with a monovalent OK antiserum is heated at 100°C for 30–60 min and titrated in parallel with a reference culture of the same O group. The agglutination is read after overnight incubation at 50°C. The presence of the particular O group is confirmed only if both the test and the reference O antigens are agglutinated to nearly the same titre.

Definite identification of EPEC strains includes either the fluorescence actin staining method (Knutton et al. 1989) (Fig. 40.2) and cell culture tests with HEp-2 or HeLa cells to demonstrate localized or diffuse adherence (Scaletsky, Silva and Trabulsi 1984, Cravioto et al. 1991), or molecular diagnosis by PCR (Fig. 40.3) or colony hybridization of genes encoding

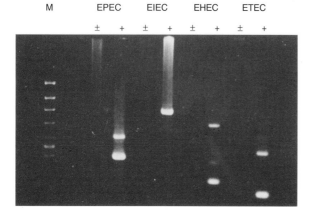

Fig. 40.3 Amplification of virulence genes of different *E. coli* pathotypes by the polymerase chain reactions: M, molecular weight marker, EPEC, *eaf* (top band), *eaeA* (lower band); EIEC, *ipaH*; EHEC, *sltIB* (top band), EHEC-specific *eaeA* (middle band), *sltIIB* (lower band); ETEC, *ltI* (top band), *stI* (lower band).

for intimin (*eaeA*), bundle-forming pili (*bfpA*) or the EPEC adherence factor (EAF) plasmid (Schmidt, Russman and Karch 1993, Franke et al. 1994, Gunzburg, Tornieporth and Riley 1995). It is likely that EPEC do not represent a homogenous group but rather consist of pathogenic strains with different virulence mechanisms (see section 13.2, p. 953). Testing for the above virulence markers may, therefore, give contradictory results.

EAggEC

These organisms are characterized by a unique, 'stacked brick-like' adherence which can be demonstrated in HEp-2 cells (Nataro et al. 1987). Some strains show the ability of bacterial clump formation at the surface of liquid cultures (Albert et al. 1993). These properties, together with production of a particular heat-stable enterotoxin, are associated with the presence of large plasmids from which a DNA probe (Baudry et al. 1990) and PCR primer pairs have been derived (Schmidt et al. 1995).

ETEC

Following earlier methods of enterotoxin detection by cell culture techniques (heat-labile enterotoxin, LT) (Fig. 40.4) or in animal models (the suckling mouse assay for the heat-stable enterotoxin, ST , and the rabbit ileal loop for LT and ST) (Figs 40.5 and 40.6), immunological tests are now commercially available

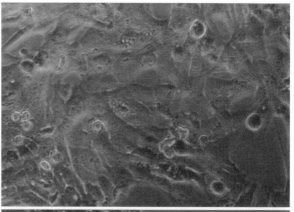

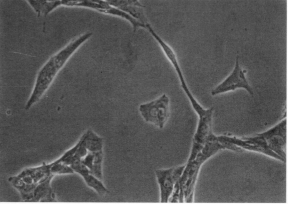

Fig. 40.4 Action of leat-labile (LT) of *E. coli* on cultured cells in vitro. (Courtesy of Virion, Switzerland).

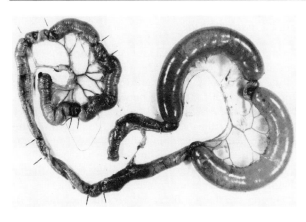

Fig. 40.5 Assay of *E. coli enterotoxin* (LT or ST) in the rabbit ileal loop test showing several negative and 2 positive loops with significant fluid accumulation.

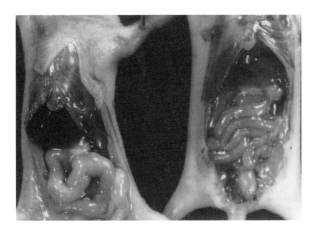

Fig. 40.6 Fluid accumulation due to *E. coli* heat-stable enterotoxin in the suckling mouse test: left, positive reaction; right, negative reaction.·

for their demonstration (enzyme immunoassays: Unipath/Oxoid, UK; latex agglutination test: Denka Seiken, Japan; immuno-diffusion/BIKEN test, see Fig. 40.7: Virion, Switzerland). Furthermore, the genes encoding for LT and ST production can be detected by PCR or DNA probes (Abe et al. 1992, Lüscher and

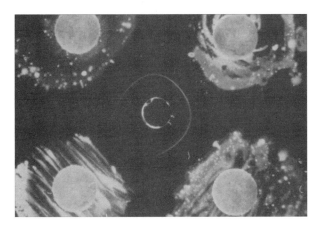

Fig. 40.7 Immunodiffusion (BIKEN) test for the demonstration of heat-labile toxin of *E. coli*.

Altwegg 1994, Schultsz et al. 1994, Stacy-Phipps, Mecca and Weiss 1995).

EIEC

EIEC do not decarboxylate lysine and are mostly non-motile. They are usually non- or late lactose fermenters and frequently belong to a set of *E. coli* serogroups that are identical with, or related to, certain *Shigella* antigens (see Tables 40.4 and 40.5, p. 942). EIEC strains are confirmed by proof of invasivenes (Serény or cell culture tests) or by demonstration of the *ipaH* gene present on the chromosome and on the virulence plasmid, which is also present in *Shigella* strains (Sethabutr et al. 1993, Lüscher and Altwegg 1994). Thus, if the invasive capacity has been established, subsequent species confirmation by biochemical tests is essential.

VTEC

Until 1994, about 160 serovars associated with the production of Shiga-like toxin (SLT or verotoxin, VT) have been identified in *E. coli* strains of human origin (World Health Organization 1994). Of these, serovars O157:H7 and O157:H-, plus a few others (see Table 40.5, p. 942), are the most important ones. VT-producing strains of O group 157 usually do not ferment sorbitol and do not produce β-glucuronidase. For their detection sorbitol MacConkey (SMAC) agar is of great value; this medium is commercially available. However, caution is needed as some strains of *E. coli* O157:H-isolated in Europe are able to ferment sorbitol rapidly (Gunzer et al. 1992); these and >90 % of the other VT-producing serovars of *E. coli* will be missed if SMAC alone is used for their detection. By supplementing SMAC with cefixime or cefixime–tellurite the selectivity for sorbitol-negative EHEC O157 can be improved (Chapman et al. 1991).

Agglutinating sera and a latex coagglutination test for O group 157 are commercially available. Due to antigenic relationship with a number of O antigens of *E. coli* and other enterobacteria (Aleksic, Karch and Bockemühl 1992), a positive slide agglutination should be confirmed by titration of heated antigens, as described for EPEC.

Most strains of *E. coli* O157:H7 and many EHEC strains of other serovars produce a plasmid-encoded haemolysin that can be detected by subculture on a special blood agar plate (Schmidt, Karch and Beutin 1994) or by PCR (Schmidt, Beutin and Karch 1995).

Detection of cytotoxin production in the Vero cell culture test, confirmed by a neutralization assay, is the standard method for identification of VT-producing *E. coli*. This test is laborious and requires extensive experience and special laboratory facilities. A commercially available enzyme immunoassay (Meridian Diagnostics, Cincinnati, USA and Milan, Italy) can be used for cytotoxin detection in both stool specimens and *E. coli* isolates. Alternatively, a latex agglutination test (Unipath/Oxoid) can be used to demonstrate separately VT1 and VT2 production in culture filtrates.

It has recently been shown by Karch et al. (1996)

that the sensitivity of EHEC O157 detection varies considerably with the diagnostic methods applied. Stool culture on SMAC as well as direct PCR from stool specimens can detect about 10^5 *E.* · *coli* O157 per gram of faeces in a background flora of 10^7 coliform bacteria. The sensitivity can be increased to 10^2–10^3 g^{-1} faeces by pre-enrichment with, and subsequent separation of, paramagnetic particles coated with O157 antibodies (immunomagnetic separation, IMS).

In view of the high proportion of concomitant *E. coli* and the comparatively low number of excreted VTEC in stool specimens, especially in patients with the haemolytic–uraemic syndrome (HUS), testing of 20–100 isolated colonies of *E. coli* is necessary to achieve a sufficient level of diagnostic sensitivity. Therefore, screening of a large number of isolates for VT genes using molecular methods such as PCR or colony hybridization (Newland and Neill 1988, Rüssmann et al. 1995) has become the method of choice in adequately equipped laboratories. Alternatively, PCR can be performed on colony sweeps from MacConkey plates (Lüscher, Graf Settah and Altwegg 1992), giving an excellent sensitivity as illustrated by the fact that up to 200 colonies would have to be screened from positive plates to allow the isolation of the VTEC strain. After identification of a VT-producing colony biochemical determination of the species must ensue (World Health Organization 1994). Identified cultures should immediately be suspended in Luria–Bertani or tryptic soy broth supplemented with 20–50% glycerol and stored at –70°C to prevent loss of the encoding genes. The same procedure is recommended for the preservation of ETEC cultures.

For a detailed description of all the media and the established test procedures the reader is referred to one of the manuals of microbiological laboratory methods (Ewing 1986, Balows et al. 1991, Burkhardt 1992, Gilligan et al. 1992, Murray et al. 1995).

Patients with *E. coli* O157 infection develop antibodies against O157 LPS which can be determined by ELISA or immunoblot, differentiating IgM and IgG antibody classes (Bitzan et al. 1991, 1993).

10 SUSCEPTIBILITY TO ANTIMICROBIAL AGENTS

Before the era of antibiotics, there was only slight resistance to antimicrobials among the species of Enterobacteriaceae. Intrinsic resistance, i.e. resistance of most strains of a given group against a particular antibiotic, is rare in the genera *Escherichia* and *Shigella* and essentially includes ampicillin and carbenicillin resistance in *E. hermannii* (Farmer 1995). Nowadays, the susceptibility of individual isolates varies greatly and, therefore, antibiograms are often used as epidemiological markers that can easily be determined. This non-intrinsic resistance is usually plasmid mediated.

10.1 *Escherichia*

E. coli strains with transferable resistance to one or multiple drugs can easily be isolated from the faeces of the general population and from animals (Holmes and Gross 1990). In fact, between 1971 and 1982, resistance of *E. coli* isolated from urinary tract infections to ampicillin, sulphonamides, tetracyclines and trimethoprim increased considerably in general practice and in hospitals. This indicates that proper antibiotic susceptibility testing technology is essential for diagnostic laboratories.

During 1980–81, 58% of strains belonging to 'enteropathogenic' serogroups of *E. coli* were resistant to one or more drugs and 37% were resistant to 3 or more (Gross et al. 1982b). Little information is available on the antibiotic susceptibility of the now recognized pathovars of enterovirulent *E. coli*. However, it seems that at least ETEC, EPEC, VTEC and EIEC do not differ significantly from other *E. coli* (Gossens et al. 1989, authors' unpublished observations); quinolones are active against almost all strains.

10.2 *Shigella*

Although mild cases of shigellosis have often responded to symptomatic therapy, specific antibiotics are usually indicated because they shorten the duration of illness and decrease the relapse rate (Hruska 1991). In addition, antibiotics result in a rapid microbiological cure. This helps prevent further spread (Hornick 1994) which is facilitated by the low infectious dose of these organisms (see Table 40.9, p. 953).

An increase in resistance against many different drugs has been observed in the last 2 decades. For example, betwen 1979 and 1982 the percentage of resistant *S. sonnei* strains isolated in a hospital in Madrid increased from 39.6 to 97.9% for ampicillin, from 34.4 to 96.9% for co-trimoxazole (SXT), from 6.3 to 18.0% for tetracycline and from 1.6 to 15.1% for chloramphenicol (Lopez-Brea et al. 1983). The first SXT-resistant strain of *S. dysenteriae* type 1 in Bangladesh was isolated in 1982. By mid-1984 most strains were resistant to this drug while still susceptible to ampicillin (Shahid et al. 1985). SXT resistance of shigellae isolated from Finnish travellers was 3% in the period 1975–82 but over 40% in 1987–88 (Heikkilä et al. 1990). Multiple drug resistance was first reported in Japan in 1956 (Elwell and Falkow 1986). In Hong Kong, 96% of 129 *Shigella* isolates were resistant to 2 or more antibiotics tested; 57% were resistant to ampicillin, 95% to tetracycline, 77% to chloramphenicol and 23% to SXT. However, all strains were susceptible to nalidixic acid and the quinolones (Ling et al. 1988). In Israel, about 13% of *Shigella* strains isolated from hospitalized children were resistant to 3 or more drugs and 1.9% were resistant to nalidixic acid (Admoni et al. 1995); there was a significant decrease in susceptibility against ampicillin and co-trimoxazole from 1988–89 to 1991–92 (Dan 1993). Reports from the USA and Germany indicated that strains isolated from imported cases of shigellosis (usually travellers to developing countries) were significantly more often multiresistant than those from domestic cases (Tauxe et al. 1990, Aleksic et al. 1993).

It is well known that antibiotic susceptibility patterns in *Shigella* may differ between geographical areas. For example, resistance of *Shigella* to ampicillin was 7% in Dacca in 1980 whereas 87% of the isolates from Bangkok between 1982 and 1983 were resistant (Murray 1986). Similar differences were found for chloramphenicol and SXT. However, these differences are not very stable, may change rapidly (especially in places where antibiotics are used excessively), and may differ between 2 adjacent countries (Murray 1986, Dan 1993). Antibiotic therapy of shigellosis should always be based on proper antibiotic susceptibility testing. If this is not possible for whatever reason, blind therapy should include a quinolone to which most strains are reportedly susceptible (Table 40.8).

Most resistance genes (e.g. those for ampicillin, tetracycline, chloramphenicol, aminoglycosides, co-trimoxazole) are carried by plasmids that are usually transferable by conjugation (Ling et al. 1993). By contrast, quinolone resistance is chromosome mediated and seems to be due to mutations of the DNA gyrase subunit A gene in *S. sonnei* (Horiuchi et al. 1993) and in *S. dysenteriae* (Rahman et al. 1994). There is one single report on plasmid mediated resistance to nalidixic acid in *S. dysenteriae* type 1 (Munshi et al. 1987) that needs confirmation before its significance can be assessed. The same is true for the recent description of a mutator plasmid, also in *S. dysenteriae* type 1, which conferred trimethoprim resistance, but not resistance to nalidixic acid, and which increased the frequency of mutation to nalidixic acid resistance in recipient strains (Ambler et al. 1993).

11 TYPING METHODS

There are numerous methods available for subtyping *Escherichia* and *Shigella* spp.; each method has advantages and disadvantages when applied to a specific situation. 'Conventional' typing methods such as biotyping, phage and colicin typing, resistotyping and serotyping have been succeeded in recent years by molecular techniques that are applicable to a wide variety of organisms with only minimal adaptation in the procedures. These newer methods are often more discriminatory but are also technically more demanding and require some specialized equipment.

11.1 Conventional typing methods

Biotyping, the most widely used typing method, includes a wide range of biochemical identification tests and characterizes an organism with regard to the presence or absence of these phenotypic markers. Such procedures have not proved very useful for subtyping *Shigella* because *Shigella* spp. are usually metabolically inactive. Nevertheless, ornithine decarboxylase allows rapid separation of *S. sonnei* from other shigellae. In some situations, biotyping has proved adequate for strain discrimination in *E. coli* (Crichton and Old 1985); recently a commercial identification panel for gram-negative enteric bacilli was shown to generate 2 unique profile numbers of *E. coli* O157:H7 strains that were not detected in other D-sorbitol-negative strains of this species (Abbott et al. 1994). Thus, this commercial identification panel might be used in preliminary screening for the most important EHEC serovar.

Typing based on variable susceptibilities to antimicrobial substances (resistotyping) is sometimes useful in distinguishing between strains. However, resistance is most often plasmid mediated and, therefore, tends to be an unstable character as resistance plasmids are easily lost or newly acquired. Because antibiograms are usually done on a routine basis for clinically significant isolates, they may provide a first hint for a common origin of 2 or more strains. Nevertheless, it should be remembered that under selective ecological pressure by antibiotics, resistance patterns may change rapidly.

Bacteriophages have been used since 1945 to subdivide shigellae. A close correspondence with recognized serovars was found (Rowe 1990). For *E. coli* serogroups O111, O55 and O26, a phage typing system

Table 40.8 Susceptibility of *Shigella* spp. to nalidixic acid and the newer quinolones

Period	Location	N	Antibiotic	% Susceptible	Reference
1977–79	Sweden[a]	43	Nalidixic acid	100	Hansson et al. 1981
1984–87	Hong Kong	129	Nalidixic acid	100	Ling et al. 1988
			New quinolones[b]	100	
1984–89	The Netherlands[a]	3313	Nalidixic acid	99.8	Voogd et al. 1992
1985–86	Switzerland[a]	107	Nalidixic acid	98	Altwegg 1986
1985–86	USA	252	Nalidixic acid	99.6	Tauxe et al. 1990
1985	Bangladesh	91	Nalidixic acid	100	Munshi et al. 1987
1986	Bangladesh	515	Nalidixic acid	68.7	Munshi et al. 1987
1987	Bangladesh	58	Nalidixic acid	40.0	Munshi et al. 1987
1987–92	Israel	262	Nalixidic acid	98.1	Admoni et al. 1995
1989–90	Germany[a]	255	Nalidixic acid	100	Aleksic et al. 1993

[a]Majority of infections imported from developing countries.
[b]Ciprofloxacin, enoxacin, pefloxacin, ofloxacin, norfloxacin.

was established in the early 1950s and was subsequently shown to provide a great deal of information about the distribution of such strains throughout the world. For further information on the phage typing of *E. coli* see the review by Milch (1978). The problem with phage typing lies in the fact that suitable phage suspensions are not readily available and are usually restricted to reference laboratories. Still, phages continue to be used, although rarely, for subtyping *Shigella* (He and Pan 1992) and *E. coli* of various origins. For example, Gershman, Markowsky and Hunter (1984) used a reduced set of 32 phages and found 178 different phage types among 866 *E. coli* isolates from cases of bovine mastitis; only 37 strains were not typable. A few years later, a phage typing scheme was introduced for isolates of *E. coli* O157:H7 that are of paramount importance in food-associated diarrhoeal disease and the haemolytic–uraemic syndrome (see below) (Ahmed et al. 1987). From the United Kingdom it was reported that the predominant phage types of *E. coli* O157 have remained unchanged between 1982 and 1991 although the proportion of strains belonging to types 2 and 49 has increased (Frost et al. 1993). In the same period the number of isolates of O157 strains has increased each year from 1 in 1982 to 532 in 1991. The superiority of phage typing (and plasmid analysis) over biotyping was confirmed during an epidemic with *S. sonnei* in Sicily (Marranzano et al. 1985).

The subdivision of O groups, or of phage types within an O group, by colicin typing has proved to be practicable (Holmes and Gross 1990). An extended scheme for colicin typing of *S. sonnei* was pubished (Horák 1994) but the method is no longer widely used because easier and more sensitive (molecular) methods with better reproducibility are now available (Gericke and Reissbrodt 1995).

Typing antisera are not readily available with the possible exception of those used for identifying O serogroups of *E. coli* that are associated with certain virulence properties and of those that allow determination of the major serogroups in *Shigella*. Full serotyping is usually restricted to reference centres but may be extremely helpful in identifying new pathogenic strains; this was demonstrated with the emergence of O157:H7 strains associated with outbreaks originating from undercooked hamburgers and other sources.

11.2 Molecular typing methods

Multilocus enzyme electrophoresis, which allows quantitative analysis of strain relationships, has revealed that the *E. coli* O157:H7 clone is most closely related to a clone of O55:H7 strains that has been associated with world-wide outbreaks of infantile diarrhoea (Whittam et al. 1993). Based on these results, the authors hypothesized that the 'new' pathogen emerged when a O55:H7-like progenitor which was already adherent to intestinal cells acquired secondary virulence factors (toxins, additional adhesins) via horizontal gene transfer and recombination. Enzyme

electrophoresis has also been used to analyse clonal relationships among bloodstream isolates of *E. coli* (Maslow et al. 1995). One cluster contained the majority of isolates and was indistinguishable from the largest cluster of each of 2 other collections of *E. coli* that caused pyelonephritis and neonatal meningitis, respectively, and thus defined a group with increased virulence.

Plasmid profiles (R plasmids and small cryptic plasmids) have been widely used to understand the epidemiology of diseases associated with escherichiae and shigellae and have proved to be more discriminative than conventional typing methods on several occasions. For example, multidrug-resistant *S. sonnei* strains were better separated into distinct clones by plasmid pattern analysis than by either phage typing, biotyping or colicinogenotyping (Tietze et al. 1984). In isolates with similar plasmid profiles further discrimination can be achieved by digestion with restriction endonucleases. It is generally agreed that plasmid profiles can be determined without great effort. In addition, results are obtained within one or 2 days, instead of several days for the more sophisticated typing methods. However, plasmid profiles are usually less sensitive when investigating disease outbreaks than methods that include digestion of high molecular weight chromosomal DNA with restriction enzymes followed by analysis of the resulting fragments by pulsed-field gel electrophoresis (PFGE) or by a combination of agarose gel electrophoresis, Southern blotting and hybridization with different kinds of probes (e.g. ribotyping). When analysing 61 isolates of *E. coli* O157:H7 isolated from patients, food samples and calf faecal samples, 21 distinct genomic profiles were generated by PFGE after digestion with endonuclease *Xba*I; only 5 different plasmid profiles were generated (Meng et al. 1995). PFGE and Southern analysis using probes derived from insertion sequences (IS) have also been useful for separating strains within *S. sonnei*, *S. dysenteriae* and *S. flexneri*, respectively (Soldati and Piffaretti 1991). In this study, IS probes showed a slightly better discrimination than PFGE.

Ribotyping has also been used extensively and with excellent results for subtyping *E. coli* and the various *Shigella* spp. The sensitivity very much depended on the selection of restriction endonucleases used (Faruque et al. 1992). Studies have focused on *S. sonnei*, the most frequent cause of shigellosis in developed countries, and suggested that ribotyping is a useful tool for epidemiological investigations (Hinojosa-Ahumada et al. 1991). In a study including 432 endemic and epidemic strains isolated over a period of 16 years in Europe, 13 ribotypes but only 5 biotypes were detected (Nastasi et al. 1993). A laboratory-acquired case of *S. sonnei* infection was studied by the authors (Altwegg and Lüthy-Hottenstein 1992); although antibiotic susceptibility testing did not allow separation of the incriminated strains the technician had been working with prior to her illness, ribotyping showed that one of the strains was identical to the strain recovered from her faeces.

Another very promising approach uses randomly

amplified polymorphic DNA (RAPD) for strain separation. This method is not necessarily dependent on purified genomic DNA and thus is both simple and rapid. Reproducibility seems to be the main obstacle, especially when comparing results obtained in different laboratories, because pattern variations may depend on the brand of *Taq* polymerase or the type of thermocyler used (Meunier and Grimont 1993). RAPD seems to be more discriminatory than other molecular methods in some situations but may be less suitable in others. In common with all typing methods, combinations are likely to give the best separation of unrelated isolates. For example, 60 *E. coli* strains previously delineated in 36 ribotypes by *Eco*RI and *Hind*III digests exhibited 28 different RAPD fingerprints (Cave et al. 1994). However, some strains of identical ribotype had clearly different RAPD patterns.

12 ROLE IN NORMAL FLORA OF HUMANS

The only site of the human body where *E. coli* is regularly found as a colonizer is the intestinal tract where it represents the most prevalent (cultivable) facultatively aerobic bacterial species (Williams Smith 1965). However, about 99% of the normal bacterial intestinal flora are strict anaerobes. Because of the extraordinary complexity of the intestinal microflora, it is very difficult to identify specific functions for individual species.

E. coli and other Enterobacteriaceae are able to synthesize a wide range of vitamins in vitro. Using gnotobiotic rats, it has been found that these animals can rely completely on their intestinal microflora for their requirement of vitamin K, folic acid, the vitamin B complex, biotin and vitamin E (Drasar and Barrow 1985). There is no doubt that intestinal bacteria contribute to the vitamin requirements of many animals but no evidence has yet been presented that this is also true for man. By contrast, the fact that gastrointestinal disturbances are relatively rare in patients who receive drugs that have no or only minimal activity against anaerobes but good activity against facultative anaerobes (e.g. quinolones), but are quite common in patients treated with substances (e.g. ampicillin) that eliminate anaerobic as well as facultatively anaerobic bacteria (Wollschlager et al. 1987), suggests that facultative anaerobes are not a very important component for maintaining the gastrointestinal equilibrium. On the other hand, colicinogenic *E. coli* have been suggested as one of the significant factors of gastrointestinal tract protection in the course of shigellosis (Bures, Horak and Duben 1979). The period of *Shigella* excretion was significantly reduced if an appropriate colicinogenic *E. coli* strain was present in the intestinal flora of patients.

Shigella spp. have no natural host other than humans and primates. Long-term carriers (usually after symptomatic infection) are considered rare but seem to be one of the reservoirs for the maintenance and spread of the disease in the community

(Benenson 1985). In a recent study of endemic shigellosis in Bangladesh, 2.1% of children under 5 years of age were found to be asymptomatic carriers (Hossain, Hasan and Albert 1994). Similar results were reported from Mexico where 55% of infants under 2 years of age infected with *Shigella* were asymptomatic (Guerrero et al. 1994). *Shigella* isolates from asymptomatic children usually carry the 120 000–140 000 kDa virulence plasmid and seem to be fully virulent (Haider et al. 1985, Guerrero et al. 1994).

13 PATHOGENICITY AND VIRULENCE FACTORS

E. coli strains can cause an impressive variety of different types of disease, including septicaemia, pneumonia, meningitis, bladder and kidney infections, HUS, diarrhoea and dysentery. However, different strains that have acquired different sets of virulence genes (see Chapter 12) cause different clinical syndromes. Despite this extremely broad spectrum of pathogenicity, the majority of *E. coli* strains have to be considered avirulent in the intestine. In contrast, *Shigella* spp. are associated with one particular disease, dysentery.

13.1 *Shigella*

HUMAN INFECTIONS

Apart from chimpanzees and monkeys that may become infected both in their natural habitat and in captivity (Ruch 1959), bacillary dysentery is a specifically human disease. It is characterized by a type of diarrhoea in which the stools contain blood and mucus and which is associated with heavy inflammation of the colonic mucosa. Although it is an invasive disease, the organisms usually do not reach tissue beyond the lamina propria and, therefore, they very rarely cause bacteraemia or systemic infections except under very special circumstances (e.g. protein-energy malnutrition in the first years of life or immunosuppression), as observed in a Bangladeshi hospital (Struelens et al. 1985). Extraintestinal complications include neurological disorders or kidney failure (HUS) and most probably result from damage to blood vessels caused by circulating Shiga toxin. HUS, first described by Gasser et al. (1955), is now better known as a complication of infection with enterohaemorrhagic *E. coli*. Very little is known about the pathogenic mechanisms leading to reactive arthritis following gastrointestinal *Shigella* infections (Hughes and Keat 1994).

Shigellosis is usually considered a self-limiting disease in otherwise healthy adults but it may be fatal in malnourished infants. Even in well nourished infants and young children a more severe course of the disease and a higher attack rate than in adults can be observed, probably due to a combination of partial immunity and better hygiene in the latter (Salyers and Whitt 1994). Apart from host factors, the severity of disease depends on the virulence of the infecting strain. In general, the disease caused by *S. sonnei* tends to be mild and of short duration whereas that caused by *S. flexneri* tends to be more severe. *S. boydii* and *S. dysenteriae* produce disease of varying severity but *S. dysenteriae* has often caused epidemics of severe infections.

Infections with *Shigella* spp. are often acquired by drinking water contaminated with human faeces or by eating food washed with contaminated water. Food-borne outbreaks of shigellosis occur, especially in the tropics and less frequently in the developed countries (Coultrip, Beaumont and Siletchnik 1977). In addition to contamination from faeces by food-handlers who have poor hygiene, flies may sometimes act as vectors in tropical countries (Khalil et al. 1994). Water-borne shigellosis presupposes sewage contamination of drinking water either by use of untreated ground and surface water or by a technical defect in the distribution system (Centers for Disease Control 1990, Swaddiwudhipong, Karintraratana and Kavinum 1995). There is also evidence for *Shigella* infection acquired by swimming in sewage-contaminated recreational waters (Rosenberg et al. 1976, Makintubee, Mallonee and Istre 1987, Sorvillo et al. 1988). In developed countries infections are usually associated with recent travel (Parsonnet et al. 1989, Lüscher and Altwegg 1994) to countries with insufficient sanitary facilities. However, outbreaks have occurred in day care centres associated with direct person-to-person transmission by the faecal–oral route, which is facilitated by the low infectious dose (10–200 organisms) necessary to induce infection (Table 40.9). Probably for the same reason shigellae are among those organisms that most often cause laboratory-acquired infections (Aleksic, Bockemühl and Degner 1981, Grist and Emslie 1989). Natural disasters and wars are frequently associated with shigellosis outbreaks and mass

encampments become breeding places, causing a high incidence of illness and fatalities. During a civil war in Burundi in 1993 dysentery accounted for 14% of all medical treatment in refugee camps situated in Rwanda. The disease was associated with an overall case fatality rate of 3.2%, which increased to 5.8% in children under 5 years of age (Centers for Disease Control 1994b). Among US troops participating in an operation in Somalia in 1992–93 diarrhoeal illness accounted for 16% of 381 hospital admissions; shigellae were obtained from 33% of the stool specimens from which enteropathogenic organisms were isolated (Sharp et al. 1995).

ANIMAL MODELS

Because *Shigella* infections are essentially restricted to primates, attempts to introduce dysenteric lesions in cats, dogs and rodents have failed, but the feeding of monkeys with large doses (c. 10^{10} organisms) of *S. flexneri* gives rise to severe dysentery (Dack and Petran 1934), with acute mucosal inflammation occurring in the stomach and colon (Kent et al. 1967). With *S. sonnei* the disease is less severe (Takasaka et al. 1969).

Large doses of dysentery bacilli given intravenously or intraperitoneally may cause death of rabbits, mice and guinea pigs but no specific lesions can be seen in the intestine. There is no increase in the LD50 for mice after intraperitoneal application of strains that have lost invasiveness as compared to fully enterovirulent strains. Under very artificial conditions (starvation plus drugs; subcutaneous carbon tetrachloride) acute infection can be induced by the oral route. There is no diarrhoea but lesions in the small intestine are similar to those in man (Formal et al. 1963).

Two aspects of *Shigella* pathogenicity can be demonstrated in animals other than monkeys: inflammation and diarrhoea. The capability of *Shigella* strains to pen-

Table 40.9 Infective doses of enterovirulent *E. coli* and *Shigella* spp.

Pathogen	Infective dose (cfu)	Reference	Type of study
Shigella spp.	Low (10–200)	DuPont et al. 1972	v
		DuPont et al. 1989	v
		Mosley, Adams and Lyman 1962	e
		Wharton et al. 1990	e
EPEC	High (10^8–10^{10})	Donnenberg et al. 1993	v
		DuPont et al. 1971	v
		Savarino 1993	v
		Ferguson and June 1952	v
ETEC	High (10^6)	Levine et al. 1979	v
EIEC	High (10^6–10^{10})	DuPont et al. 1971	v
EHEC/VTEC	Low (<100)	Griffin and Tauxe 1991	e
		Wachsmuth 1994	e
		Burnens et al. 1993	e
EAggEC	High (?)	Previously classified as EPEC	
DAEC	High (?)	Previously classified as EPEC	

Abbreviations: v, volunteer studies; e, epidemiological studies.

Table 40.10 Some known virulence factors of *Shigella* spp. and enterovirulent *E. coli*

Virulence factor	Location[a]	Putative role of gene product in disease
Shigella spp.		
ipaD	p	Attachment to host cell, induces rearrangement of cytoskeleton and phagocytosis
ipaB, ipaC	p	Induction of phagocytosis, lysis of phagosome after which cells reach the cytoplasm
mxi	p	At least 10 different loci; involved in export of Ipa proteins
icsA, icsB	p	Intercellular spread between adjacent cells
stxA, stxB	c	A1B5 toxin (Shiga toxin). A subunit specifically removes one base from eukaryotic 28S rRNA and results in inhibition of protein synthesis. B subunit is responsible for binding to receptor on host cell
virF	p	Transcriptional activator of *virB*
virB	p	Transcriptional activator of *ipa* gene family (*ipaA, ipaB, ipaC, ipaD*)
virR	c	Negative regulator of *virF*; probably mediates temperature control of virulence expression
vacC, vacB, kspA	c	Regulate *ipa* gene family and/or *icsA*
ompR, envZ	c	Osmoregulation of virulence genes located on plasmid
fur	c	Regulates *stxA* and *stxB* through regulation of iron concentration
Enteropathogenic *E. coli* (EPEC)		
bfpA	p	Bundle-forming pilus (BFP) mediates non-intimate localized adherence
dsbA	c	Disulphide isomerase which catalyses disulphide bond formation in the periplasmic space; essential for active BFP
eaeA	c	Intimin; mediates intimate adherence to epithelial cells
eaeB	c	Induction of tyrosine phosphorylation and release of inositol phosphate from cells
per	p	'plasmid encoded regulator': transcriptional activator of *eaeA*
sepA/sepB	c	Secretion of (virulence) proteins
Verotoxigenic *E. coli* (VTEC)		
eaeA	c	Mediates intimate adherence to epithelial cells; high similarity to *eaeA* of EPEC
VT (SLT) gene family	ph[b]	A1B5 toxin (similar to Shiga toxin). A subunit specifically removes one base from eukaryotic 28S rRNA and results in inhibition of protein synthesis. B subunit is responsible for binding to receptor on host cell
EHEC-hlyA	p	Enterohaemolysin, ±60% homology to α-haemolysin genes (*hlyA, hlyC*) of *E. coli*
EHEC-hlyC		
Enterotoxigenic *E. coli* (ETEC)		
LT	p	Heat-labile A1B5 toxin (similar to cholera toxin). A subunit induces an increase in intracellular cAMP via ADP-ribosylation of a G protein. B subunit mediates binding to the ganglioside GM1 receptor
ST	p	Small, heat-stable and non-immunogenic peptide toxin that induces an increase in intracellular cGMP via activation of guanylate cyclase
CFAs	(p)	Various types of colonization factor antigens that mediate adherence to the small bowel epithelium

[a]p, plasmid; (p), usually but not always located on plasmids; c, chromosome; ph, lysogenic phage.
[b]With the exception of the chromosomally encoded VT2e.

etrate into epithelial cells and to spread from cell to cell, thereby invoking intense inflammation, can be tested by placing a drop of culture in the eye of guinea pigs or mice (Serény 1957, Murayama et al. 1986) which results in mucopurulent conjunctivitis within 1–3 days and is later followed by severe keratitis. Many old cultures fail to cause keratoconjunctivitis in the Serény test, probably due to rapid loss of the virulence plasmid upon subculture (Lüscher and Altwegg 1994). Such strains fail to cause disease in the starved guinea pig, in the monkey or in humans, nor do they cause keratoconjunctivitis in guinea pigs or penetrate HeLa cells. The ability of shigellae to cause diarrhoea can be reproduced in the rabbit ileal loop assay when distention of ileal segments indicates release of fluid into the lumen.

IN VITRO MODELS

Virulent shigellae invade various tissue culture cell lines, multiply and produce a cytopathic effect. These cell lines include HeLa cells derived from a cervical carcinoma, guinea pig corneal cells, Henle intestinal epithelial cells, HEp-2 cells derived from a human larynx, or cultured macrophages. Most studies on the pathogenic mechanisms of *Shigella* have used HeLa cells because they are one of the easiest cell lines to grow in vitro and have led to the identification of a variety of virulence factors (Table 40.10).

VIRULENCE FACTORS

Invasive and toxigenic properties seem to be the main virulence factors in *Shigella* strains but the exact role of the toxin has yet to be defined. Non-invasive, toxigenic variants failed to produce disease in monkeys whereas invasive, non-toxigenic strains caused disease but of a milder nature than that produced by the fully virulent invasive and toxigenic strain. Similar results were obtained in volunteers (Levine et al. 1973).

Invasion and killing of cells

The first step in the invasion of HeLa cells by shigellae is the attachment to the host cell. This induces rearrangements in the cytoskeleton in these cells and eventually leads to phagocytosis of the bacteria. This process does not seem to be mediated through interaction with a specific receptor (Clerc and Sansonetti 1987). Although the adhesin has not yet been identified with certainty, there is some evidence that the invasion plasmid antigen (Ipa) D might be involved. Other proteins, IpaB and IpaC, which are also encoded by genes located on the virulence plasmid, can be found at the bacterial surface and in extracellular fluid. Their excretion requires the presence of membrane expression of invasion (*mxi*) genes (Menard, Sansonetti and Parsot 1994). IpaB and IpaC seem to be essential for phagocytosis and for rupture of the phagocytic vesicle which precede rapid multiplication in the cytoplasm. Intercellular spread (ICS), which again involves continuous reorganization of the host cell actin filaments, is mediated by 2 proteins, IcsA (also called VirG; Bernardini et al. 1989) and IcsB, and ultimately leads to cell death and inflammatory

response. Cell death is induced by inhibition of protein synthesis by an as yet unknown mechanism. However, this process is independent of the production of Shiga toxin (Salyers and Whitt 1994).

The invasion process as observed in cultured cell lines does not fully reflect the events occurring in vivo in that shigellae most probably are not capable of directly invading absorptive cells that make up the vast majority of the colonic mucosa (Fig. 40.8). Investigations using segments of the colons of monkeys infected with *Shigella* spp. have indicated that primary lesions occur mainly on Peyer's patches. This has led to the assumption that in vivo shigellae enter through (phagocytic) M cells and are then taken up by macrophages. However, they escape killing by these macrophages, are released and enter adjacent cells by binding to host proteins called integrins located at the basolateral surface, thereby invoking phagocytic uptake by these cells (Salyers and Whitt 1994).

Shiga toxin

S. dysenteriae produces a toxin called Shiga toxin which belongs to the family of A1/B5 toxins and which is encoded on the chromosome (Hewlett 1990). However, the activity of the A subunit is different from cholera toxin (CT), which has an ADP-ribosylating activity, in that it cleaves the 28S rRNA at one specific position (an adenine), resulting in the inhibition of protein synthesis. The B subunit is responsible for binding of the toxin to the receptor (Gb3) on the host cell surface (Table 40.11). Shiga toxin is not actively secreted from the cell but only released during cell lysis (Rowe 1990). It is not essential for invasion; however, it may add to mucosal damage as does LPS. Maximal toxin production occurs in media that are free of iron (Dubos and Geiger 1946). The toxin's main action is on small blood vessels. In addition, Louise and Obrig (1992) have described a synergistic cytotoxic effect of Shiga toxin and LPS on human vascular endothelial cells in vitro. These results are consistent with a role of Shiga toxin and LPS in the development of complications of shigellosis such as HUS.

13.2 Enterovirulent *E. coli*

E. coli strains capable of causing any type of enteric disease have often be referred to as 'enteropathogenic *E. coli* (EPEC)'. This term is now used very specifically for one of the 6 different classes of enterovirulent (or diarrhoeagenic) *E. coli* that have been associated with gastrointestinal disease by case-control studies (Kaper 1994) (see also Volume 3, Chapter 27).

For many years some of these strains were identified by serotyping based on the fact that there is an association of serogroup and virulence type (see Table 40.5, p. 942). However, the reliability of serotyping is limited because not all isolates of serogroups associated with EPEC are enteropathogenic and pathogenicity is not entirely restricted to serogroups or serovars (Valentini, Gomes and Falcao 1992, Law 1994). With the molecular characterization of the various virulence genes involved in the pathogenesis of enterovi-

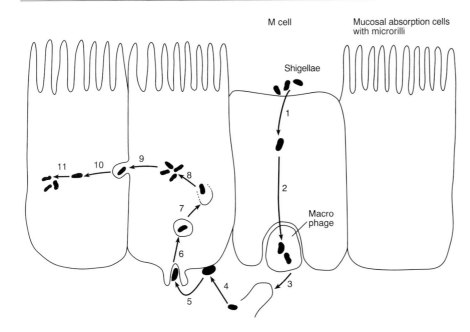

Fig. 40.8 Model proposed for invasion of the colonic mucosa by *Shigella* spp. (Modified from Salyers and Witt 1994, with permission). 1 Entering colonic mucosa through M-cells. 2 Uptake by macrophage. 3 Escape killing by macrophage. 4 Attachment to basolateral surface of host cell. 5/6 Induction of phagocytosis. 7 Rupture of phagocytic vesicle. 8 Rapid intracellular multiplication. 9/10 Intercellular spread. 11 Rapid intracellular multiplication.

rulent *E. coli*, diagnostic tests evolved that detected these genes by hybridization, PCR or a combination of both; these tests provided a much more coherent identification of these groups of diarrhoeal pathogens.

Adherence is one of the important virulence mechanisms of enterovirulent *E. coli*. Three main patterns of adherence have been described in the literature (Nataro et al. 1987): localized, diffuse and enteroaggregative (Fig. 40.9). Classification and identification of adherence patterns is confusing for several reasons (Law 1994):

1 different adhesion assay methods may give different adhesion patterns
2 some authors do not separate EPEC and diffusely adhering *E. coli* (DAEC) but rather consider them as class I EPEC (strains with localized adherence belonging to serogroups that are most commonly associated with outbreaks of infantile diarrhoea) and class II EPEC (diffusely adherent strains belonging to serogroups less often incriminated in outbreaks of diarrhoea), respectively
3 very little is as yet known about some of the mechanisms involved in adhesion of DAEC and EAggEC and, therefore, strains cannot yet be easily identified using molecular markers instead of cell culture assays.

ENTEROPATHOGENIC *E. COLI* (EPEC)

Epidemiology and disease

In 1945, a distinct *E. coli* strain (serogroup O111) was found to be associated with an outbreak of infantile diarrhoea. In the following years additional O serogroups were identified that belonged to the so-called enteropathogenic *E. coli* (EPEC) (see Table 40.5, p. 942). Such strains can cause profuse watery diarrhoea of varying severity and persistence. There is little inflammation of the intestinal mucosa but diarrhoea is often accompanied by fever and vomiting (Law 1994).

EPEC adhere to the human intestine and produce typical attaching and effacing (AE) lesions which are characterized by dissolution of the brush border membrane and destruction of microvilli (Knutton, Lloyd and McNeish 1987) and which correlate with a positive fluorescent actin-staining (FAS) test (Knutton et al. 1989).

Although the pathogenicity of EPEC strains involved in outbreaks was confirmed by volunteer studies (Ferguson and June 1952, June, Ferguson and Worfel 1953), for a long time there was no suitable animal model or reliable in vitro test available to demonstrate the pathogenicity of putative EPEC isolates. Therefore, serogrouping with all its limitations (see section 13.2, paragraph 2, p. 953) remained the only means of identifying such isolates. When enterotoxin production (ETEC, see section on 'Enterotoxigenic *E. coli* (ETEC)', p. 958) or invasive properties (EIEC, see section on 'Enteroinvasive *E. coli* (EIEC)', p. 959) were detected in some *E. coli* isolates belonging to typical EPEC serogroups, it was questioned whether EPEC should still be considered pathogenic because no specific virulence factors were known at that time. However, Levine et al. (1978) confirmed that EPEC strains are pathogenic by mechanisms other than those of ETEC and EIEC.

In developed countries, EPEC have in the past caused outbreaks as well as sporadic cases of infantile diarrhoea but infections in adults and infants have now become very rare (Levine and Edelman 1984). Their incidence has decreased in the last 2 decades for unknown reasons and, consequently, screening of infants no longer seems necessary or cost-effective (Morris and Gopal Rao 1992). In underdeveloped countries, EPEC still are a major cause of endemic infantile diarrhoea and seasonal outbreaks (Thoren 1983) and in some studies they were the most common bacterial enteropathogens of infants (Anathan et al. 1989, Katouli et al. 1990, Mubashir et al. 1990,

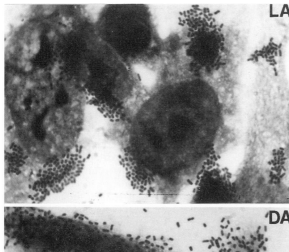

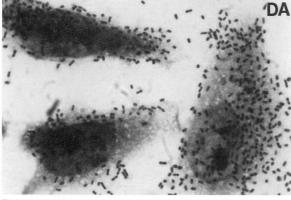

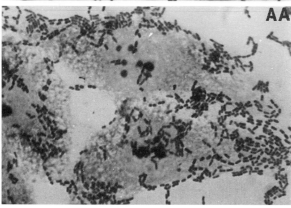

Fig. 40.9 Light microscopy of Giemsa-stained HeLa cells showing 3 types of adherence in enterovirulent *E. coli*: localized (LA, top), diffuse (DA, middle) and aggregative (AA, bottom). (Photographs courtesy of Dr S Knutton).

Gomes et al. 1991). Peak incidence is in children about 6 months old and disease rarely occurs in children over 1 year of age (Levine and Edelman 1984).

Virulence factors

EPEC pathogenesis is not yet understood in all details and several steps seem to be multifactorial. In 1992, Donnenberg and Kaper proposed a 3-stage model consisting of:

1 localized adherence
2 signal transduction and
3 intimate adherence.

In the first stage, non-intimate adherence between the bacterium and the epithelial cell is mediated by the bundle-forming pilus (BFP, Girón, Ho and Schoolnick 1991). Formation of an active BFP is dependent on 2 genes, *bfpA* and *dsbA*, located on the 55 000–70 000 kDa EPEC adherence factor (EAF) plasmid and on the chromosome, respectively. The adherence pattern is called 'localized' because organisms attach to one or 2 small areas of the cell surface in microcolonies and it is clearly different from the diffuse or aggregative adherence patterns seen in other classes of enterovirulent *E. coli* (Scaletsky, Silva and Trabulsi 1984, Nataro et al. 1987). Antibodies against BFP reduce localized adherence of EPEC significantly but not completely, which indicates that there are other fimbrial proteins involved in mediating adherence. These additional proteins share some homology with the fimbriae of uropathogenic *E. coli* and of DAEC, respectively (Girón, Ho and Schoolnick 1993).

In the second stage, tyrosine phosphorylation of a 90 kDa eukaryotic protein, an increase in intracellular levels of calcium, and the release of inositol phosphate from epithelial cells are probably mediated by the product of the *eaeB* gene and other proteins through a signal transduction event (Foubister et al. 1994). At the same time, the *eaeA* gene (named for *E. coli* attaching and effacing) is transcriptionally activated by the product of the *per* locus.

In the third stage (which probably occurs concurrently with the second stage), intimate adherence is mediated by intimin, the product of the chromosomal *eaeA* locus, and possibly other products of the *eae* gene cluster. This results in an amplification of the effects on epithelial cells. The role of the *eaeA* locus was originally identified in FAS-test negative strains after Tn*phoA* mutagenesis and sequence analysis revealed some homology with the invasin protein of *Yersinia pseudotuberculosis*. However, intimin and invasin bind to 2 different receptors (Frankel et al. 1994). EPEC isolates also have the capacity to invade epithelial cells but this does not seem to be of clinical importance as shown by the absence of faecal leucocytes in EPEC-associated disease (Kaper 1994).

DIFFUSELY ADHERENT *E. COLI* (DAEC)

Epidemiology and disease

DAEC belonging to classical EPEC serogroups were named class II EPEC because they did not hybridize with the EAF probe (Nataro et al. 1985). Their significance as a diarrhoeagenic agent is controversial. In some reports the isolation rates of strains that show diffuse adherence in the HeLa cell assay and/or that hybridize with the F1845 DNA probe (see section on 'Virulence factors', below) were similar in infants with diarrhoea and in controls (Chatkaeomorakot et al. 1987, Gomes, Blake and Traabulsi 1989, Cravioto et al. 1991). Two other studies, however, reported a strong association between DAEC and diarrhoea in Mayan and Bangladeshi children (Girón et al. 1991, Baqui et al. 1992). In this context the question arises whether only a subgroup of DAEC possessing additional virulence factors is capable of causing disease (Law 1994).

Table 40.11 Characteristics of toxins produced by enterovirulent *E. coli* and *Shigella* spp.

	Shiga toxin	VT1	VT2	VT2c	VT2e	LT	ST
Subunit structure	A1B5	A1B5	A1B5	A1B5	A1B5	A1B5	Single molecule
Eukaryotic cell surface receptor	Gb3[a]				Gb4[b]	Ganglioside GM1	
Location of genes	Chromosome	Lysogenic phage			Chromosome	Plasmid	Plasmid
Function	Subunit B: binding to host cell receptor						
	Subunit A: specific removal of one base in the of 28S rRNA of eukaryotic cells; inactivates the ribosome					Subunit A: ADP-ribosylation of host cell proteins	Induction of guanylate cyclase
Associated disease	Human HUS, haemorrhagic colitis, diarrhoea				Pig oedema disease	Diarrhoea	Diarrhoea

[a]Globotriosylceramide.
[b]Globotetraosylceramide.

Virulence factors

DAEC are clearly different from EPEC in that they are always negative in the FAS test, which correlates with attaching and effacing lesions (Knutton et al. 1989) and with hybridization with the EAF probe (Gomes, Blake and Trabulsi 1989). Their mode of adherence is different from EPEC strains and 2 adhesins have been identified: a 100 kDa, plasmid-encoded protein from an O126:H27 isolate (Benz and Schmidt 1992) and a chromosomal fimbrial adhesin from a serogroup O75 isolate (Bilge et al. 1989). A DNA probe (F1845) derived from the chromosomal adhesin gene has been used in epidemiological studies but no perfect correlation with HEp-2 assays was observed (Levine et al. 1988, Girón et al. 1991), suggesting that a number of different genetic determinants may encode diffuse adherence. In addition, Smith et al. (1994) showed that the F1845 probe cross-hybridized with 80 of 86 *E. coli* strains that exhibited aggregative adherence and that were positive to EAggEC probe. A study from France found that children carrying F1845 DNA probe-positive DAEC had significantly longer hospital stays than those with probe-negative DAEC (Poitrineau et al. 1995).

ENTEROAGGREGATIVE *E. COLI* (EAggEC)

Epidemiology and disease

Although initially isolated from adults with travellers' diarrhoea (Mathewson et al. 1985), EAggEC are now mainly considered a cause of bloody or protracted infantile diarrhoea as shown by studies in various non-industrialized countries (Law 1994). Their role in adult as well as in travellers' diarrhoea is controversial and still needs a thorough evaluation (Scotland et al. 1991, Cohen et al. 1993).

Many *E. coli* strains belonging to some of the classical EPEC serogroups (e.g. O44, O111, O86, O126) are in fact enteroaggregative (Scotland et al. 1991, Knutton et al. 1992). This is another indication that serotyping is of limited value for the identification of the various *E. coli* virulence types.

Virulence factors

EAggEC bind to small intestinal cells without any obvious histological changes and are not invasive, but knowledge of their virulence factors is very limited. Probably both toxin production and adhesion play an important role. EAggEC produce a toxin (called EAST for 'enteroaggregative heat-stable toxin') that induces fluid secretion and is antigenically related to the heat-stable toxin of ETEC (Savarino et al. 1991); they also produce a toxin similar to the α-haemolysin of *E. coli* that causes urinary tract infection (Baldwin et al. 1992). Four morphologically distinct types of fimbriae have been identified by Knutton et al. (1992), including so-called aggregative adherence fimbriae I (AAF/I; Nataro et al. 1992) that are very similar to the bundle forming pili of EPEC. AAF/I were present in 43 of 44 isolates (Knutton et al. 1992) and their presence correlated nicely with a positive hybridization signal using a DNA probe that had been derived from the 60 000 kDa plasmid of EAggEC which confers aggregative adherence when introduced into a non-adherent *E. coli* strain and which also encodes the EAST toxin (Baudry et al. 1990, Savarino et al. 1991, Nataro et al. 1992). Based on the sequence of a fragment of the EAggEC probe a PCR assay was developed that correlated nicely though not perfectly with aggregative adherence to HEp-2 cells (Schmidt et al. 1995).

ENTEROTOXIGENIC *E. COLI* (ETEC)

Epidemiology and disease

ETEC, first recognized in the late 1960s as a cause of cholera-like diarrhoea in India, resemble *Vibrio cholerae* in that they induce profuse, watery diarrhoea by elaboration of toxins that act on the mucosal cells. They adhere to the small intestinal mucosa but do not invade. There are no apparent histological changes and little inflammation.

ETEC are a common cause of dehydrating diarrhoea in children in developing countries. The disease is usually less severe than cholera (Eisenstein 1990) but can be fatal, especially in infants, and results in some kind of immunity which is directed against the colonization factor antigens. ETEC may also affect adults from industrialized countries (where these pathogens are not endemic) who visit developing nations. They are considered to be the leading cause of travellers' diarrhoea, accounting for up to 75% of these cases (Guerrant 1990b).

Virulence factors

There are 2 groups of virulence factors in ETEC, both of which are essential for their pathogenicity: enterotoxins (LT, STa, STb) and various colonization factor antigens (CFAs).

Enterotoxins can be classified according to their heat stability. Whereas heat-labile toxin (LT) is inactivated by incubation at 100°C for 30 min, heat-stable toxin (ST) retains toxin activity after such treatment (Smith and Halls 1967). LT is very similar to cholera toxin in structure (about 75% identity at the amino acid level). The mechanism of action of the 2 toxins seems to be identical: binding to the GM1 ganglioside receptor located at the apical surface of mucosal cells mediated by the B subunits, entry of subunit A into the cell followed by ADP-ribosylation of a G protein (second messenger) and activation of adenylate cyclase. The concomitant increase in intracellular cAMP concentration leads to the massive secretory diarrhoea seen with ETEC and *V. cholerae*. There is a second type of heat-labile toxin (LT II) which has the same basic structure and mechanism of action as LT I (Holmes, Twiddy and Neill 1985). However, the 2 toxins do not cross-react immunologically. In addition, LT II has a different receptor (Hewlett 1990), has been found primarily in strains of animal origin, and has not been associated with disease either in animals or humans. STs are a family of small (17–19 amino acids) and, therefore, heat-stable and non-immunogenic toxins that are either soluble (STa or ST I) or insoluble (STb or ST II) in methanol (Burgess et al. 1978, Lee et al. 1983). STa produced by human and animal strains are remarkably homogeneous, yet

2 types have been described that are referred to as STh (produced by human strains only) and STp (produced by human and animal strains), respectively. They cause an increase in cGMP levels (in contrast to cAMP by LT) in the host cells which leads to fluid loss similar to that induced by LT (Guerrant et al. 1980). STb acts by a different mechanism from that of STa and produces diarrhoea in piglets. There is no evidence that STb-positive ETEC strains are diarrhoeagenic in humans. The frequency with which LT and ST are found in ETEC isolated from persons with travellers' diarrhoea varies between studies with usually less than 50% of the strains producing both toxins (Guerrant 1990b, Wolf et al. 1993). This is important when selecting laboratory tests for the detection of ETEC because at least 25% of the cases would be missed if only tests for LT (such as the immunodiffusion test) were used.

In order to cause disease, ETEC must not only produce an enterotoxin but they must also be able to colonize the small bowel of animals and humans. There are several types of pili (fimbriae) that mediate adhesive properties: type 1 pili are usually found in *E. coli* strains from the resident microflora and do not seem to contribute to the pathogenic potential of ETEC strains (Salyers and Whitt 1994). Pili which are significant for ETEC include K88, 987P, F41, F107 and 2134P (strains infecting pigs), K99 (strains infecting pigs, lambs and calves) and various colonization factor antigens (CFAs) specific for humans. CFA/I and CFA/II are most commonly found in human ETEC but some strains do not produce either of these antigens, indicating that there are additional ETEC adhesins. At least 5 different CFAs among human ETEC are now known: CFA/I, CFA/II, E8775, 260-1 and O159:H4 (Guerrant 1990a). A new pilus has been detected and termed 'longus' because it can extend for over 20 μm from the cell surface (Girón, Levine and Kaper 1994). Its structural gene (*lngA*) is encoded on a large plasmid. In contrast to other ETEC pili, *lngA* is widely distributed among ETEC strains independent of their geographical origin, serovar, toxin production, or other pili antigens expressed. Its suitability as a vaccine component remains to be shown.

ENTEROINVASIVE *E. COLI* (EIEC)

EIEC are very similar to *Shigella* spp. in every way except for their lower acid resistance which results in a higher infectious inoculum (DuPont et al. 1971) and their inability to produce Shiga toxin which may be related to the fact that so far no complications such as HUS have been observed in EIEC infections. Although little work has been done to characterize EIEC virulence factors by molecular means, it is assumed that they are virtually identical to those of *Shigella* spp. (Fig. 40.10 (Salyers and Whitt 1994).

VEROTOXIGENIC *E. COLI* (VTEC)

Epidemiology and disease

In 1982, one particular serovar of *E. coli* (O157:H7) was identified as the causative agent involved in 2 outbreaks of a distinctive bloody diarrhoeal syndrome

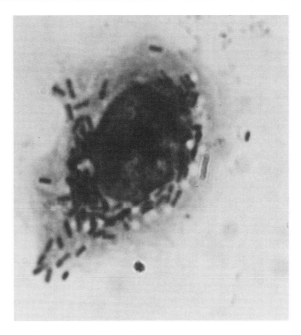

Fig. 40.10 Intracellular location of enteroinvasive *E. coli* (EIEC) in HeLa cells.

(Riley et al. 1983). Since then, these organisms have received much attention not only in the USA but also in other developed countries as a cause of epidemic or sporadic bloody and non-bloody diarrhoea, HUS and thrombotic thrombocytopenic purpura (TTP). These sometimes fatal complications occur roughly at a rate of 5–10% of all cases (Griffin and Tauxe 1991, Wachsmuth 1994).

Soon after the discovery of the special significance of *E. coli* O157:H7 it was recognized that some strains of other *E. coli* serovars may exhibit a similar virulence potential. In relation to their clinical manifestations, the entire group was named enterohaemorrhagic *E. coli* (EHEC). Because one of their major virulence factors (see section on 'Virulence factors', below) is the production of toxins that are closely related to Shiga toxin and that have a cytotoxic effect on Vero cells, these organisms have also been called Shiga-like toxin producing *E. coli* or verotoxigenic *E. coli* (VTEC). Not all VTEC cause a clinical illness similar to that of *E. coli* O157:H7 and, therefore, EHEC represent a subset of VTEC (Griffin and Tauxe 1991). Analogous to other virulence types of diarrhoeagenic *E. coli*, there seems to be a limited number of serovars that are of major importance (see Table 40.5, p. 942). However, at least 160 different VTEC serovars have so far been isolated from humans, animals and foodstuff (World Health Organization 1994). It is very likely that even this already long list is incomplete and that new EHEC-related serovars will be discovered. In addition to O157 and O26, O serogroup 111 strains may be of special epidemiological importance: the first outbreak of non-O157 associated HUS in Italy was due to serovar O111:H11 (Caprioli et al. 1994) and the same or a very closely related clone (as determined by PFGE) is the most frequently found non-O157 serovar in Germany (Karch 1994). Furthermore, a community outbreak of HUS associated with *E. coli* O111:H- was reported from Australia (Centers for Disease Control 1995). At least in Europe, the majority of sporadic cases of VTEC-associated diarrhoea are caused by *E. coli* serovars other than O157:H7 (Lüscher, Graf Settah and Altwegg 1992, Huppertz et al. 1996).

An unusual outbreak of severe disease (including cases of HUS) caused by verotoxin-producing *C. freundii* occurred in Germany (Tschäpe et al. 1995). The overall epidemiological significance of this finding is not clear but it confirms the earlier finding (Schmidt et al. 1993) that the genes coding for verotoxins, which are encoded by temperate phages, can be found in other species of the Enterobacteriaceae and might be horizontally transferred from one species to another.

The main reservoirs for VTEC strains seem to be the gastrointestinal tract of cattle, other farm animals and humans (Griffin and Tauxe 1991). Consequently, the majority of outbreaks have been the result of transmission via foods of bovine origin, such as beef and raw milk, but apple cider, potatoes and other vehicles for transmission have also been identified. In addition, direct person-to-person transmission is important, especially in families and child care facilities (Belongia et al. 1993, Reida et al. 1994, Ludwig, personal communication 1996), and is facilitated by the low infectious dose of these organisms (see Table 40.9, p. 953). Long-term shedding of *E. coli* O157 despite clinical cure has been found in 13% of patients (Karch et al. 1995).

Virulence factors

VTEC are characterized by the production of cytotoxins that are immunologically similar to Shiga toxin. These toxins have, therefore, been named Shiga-like toxins (SLTs) (O'Brien et al. 1982). Based on the work of Konowalchuk, Speirs and Stavric (1977), who demonstrated that identical toxins are cytotoxic to Vero cells, the term verotoxin (VT) was coined. It is now generally agreed that both terms may be used and that they are interchangeable. VT1 and VT2 are most often found and both can occur in a single strain. Two variants of VT2 exist and are associated with the same types of human disease (VT2c) and pig oedema disease (VT2e), respectively (see Table 40.11, p. 957). VTs are A1/B5-type toxins and are located on a lysogenic phage (Williams Smith, Green and Parsell 1983) with the exception of the chromosomally encoded VT2e. Subunit A is the actual toxic component which specifically removes the adenine base at position 4324 of eukaryotic 28S rRNA, resulting in ribosome inactivation (Endo et al. 1988), whereas subunit B mediates binding to the eukaryotic host cell receptors Gb3 and Gb4, respectively.

In newborn piglets, EHEC produce attaching and effacing lesions (Figs 40.11 and 40.12) that are very similar, if not identical, to those produced by EPEC isolates (Tzipori, Gibson and Montanaro 1989). The corresponding gene mediating this intimate adher-

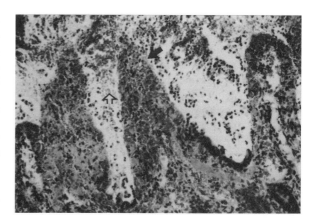

Fig. 40.11 Enteritis due to EHEC O139 in a piglet. Characteristic necrosis of villi (arrow) and presence of blood (open arrow). (Reproduced, with permission, from Dedié K, Bockemühl J et al. 1993, p. 73).

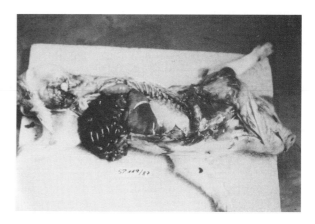

Fig. 40.12 Lethal haemorrhagic enterocolitis due to EHEC infection in a piglet. (Reproduced, with permission, from Dedié K, Bockemühl J et al. 1993, p. 72).

ence to epithelial cells shares 86% homology at the nucleotide level and 83% homology at the amino acid level with the *eaeA* gene of EPEC strains (Yu and Kaper 1992). This extremely high homology is not evenly distributed over the entire gene: 94% in the N-terminal 75% of the gene but only 49% in the C-terminal 25% of the gene which represents the putative receptor-binding site. The variability in the C-terminal region may reflect the fact that EPEC are primarily found in the small intestine whereas the major site for EHEC is the distal ileum and the colon (Kaper 1994).

A plasmid-encoded haemolysin of *E. coli* O157:H7 has been described (Schmidt, Beutin and Karch 1995). The 2 open reading frames found on a 5.4 kb *Sal*I restriction fragment share approximately 60% homology with the *hlyC* and *hlyA* genes of the *E. coli* α-haemolysin operon. This EHEC haemolysin ('enterohaemolysin') appears to be of clinical importance because it was found in all O157 strains tested (but only in 12 of 25 non-O157 VTEC) and was reactive with 19 of 20 sera of patients with HUS (but with only one of 20 control serum samples).

13.3 Uropathogenic *E. coli*

E. coli is by far the most common organism found in community-acquired urinary tract infection (UTI), being responsible for more than 80% of the cases (see also Volume 3, Chapter 32). These strains are primarily derived from the faecal flora (Plos et al. 1995) but haematogenic infections do occur (Ward and Jones 1991). In addition to host factors (sex, age, sexual activity, use of spermicides, and also genetic factors like the presence of receptors for Pap fimbriated bacteria), which probably make a particular subject more or less susceptible to UTIs, there are various possible virulence traits such as adhesion, toxins, LPS, iron acquisition, presence of capsules or serum resistance, that determine the uropathogenicity of *E. coli* strains (Salyers and Whitt 1994).

Adhesion to epithelial cells of the urogenital tract is generally accepted as being essential for uropathogenic bacteria because otherwise the bacteria would be washed out rapidly. This view has been questioned by Gordon and Riley (1992) who calculated that with a doubling time of about 50 min bacteria could maintain themselves without adhering in the bladder. However, in 100% of *E. coli* isolates from urine of patients with pyelonephritis but only in 17% of *E. coli* isolates from patients with asymptomatic bacteriuria, P or Pap

(pili associated with pyelonephritis) were found (O'Hanley et al. 1985). This suggests that these structures really are significant virulence factors. There are many different antigenic variants of Pap fimbriae. They all recognize the same type of receptors which are glycolipids containing the disaccharide α-D-galactopyranosyl-(1,4)-β-D-galactopyranose (gal-gal) (Leffler and Svanborg-Eden 1980). Gal-gal is sufficient for inhibiting haemagglutination (O'Hanley et al. 1983) and for blocking attachment (Svanborg-Eden et al. 1982) of Pap fimbriated bacteria to uroepithelial cells. Biosynthesis, assembly and regulation are encoded by a single operon located on the *E. coli* chromosome (Hultgren and Normark 1991), resulting in a single polycistronic mRNA transcript and, consequently, co-ordinated expression of all genes essential for fimbriae production. In addition, uropathogenic *E. coli* can also express afimbrial adhesins like AFA I, AFA III, or Dr adhesins which are also encoded by gene clusters (Garcia, Labigne and LeBougenec 1994). These adhesins recognize the Dr blood group antigen as receptor and mediate mannose-resistant haemagglutination (Swanson et al. 1991). When women with chronic UTI were inoculated with a mixture of an *E. coli* strain isolated from a patient with stable bacteriuria and with a strain transformed with adhesin gene sequences, the wild-type strain persisted and caused stable bacteriuria whereas the transformant strain was eliminated within 48 h (Andersson et al. 1991). These results suggest that acquisition of adherence factors may be a prerequisite but is not sufficient for survival in the urinary tract of humans.

REFERENCES

Abbott SL, Hanson DF et al., 1994, *Escherichia coli* O157:H7 generates a unique biochemical profile on Micro-Scan gram-negative identification panels, *J Clin Microbiol*, **32**: 823–4.

Abe A, Obata H et al., 1992, A sensitive method for the detection of enterotoxigenic *Escherichia coli* by the polymerase chain reaction using multiplex primer pairs, *Zentralbl Bakt*, **277**: 170–8.

Admoni O, Yagupsky P et al., 1995, Epidemiological, clinical and microbiological features of shigellosis among hospitalized children in northern Israel, *Scand J Infect Dis*, **27**: 139–44.

Ahmed R, Bopp C et al., 1987, Phage-typing scheme for *Escherichia coli* O157:H7, *J Infect Dis*, **155**: 806–9.

Albert MJ, Qadri F et al., 1993, Bacterial clump formation at the surface of liquid culture as a rapid test for identification of enteroaggregative *E. coli*, *J Clin Microbiol*, **31**: 1397–9.

Aleksic S, Bockemühl J, Aleksic V, 1987, Serologisch-epidemiologische Untersuchungen an 908 Shigella-Stämmen von Patienten in der Bundesrepublik Deutschland, 1978–1985, *Bundesgesundheitsblatt*, **30**: 207–10.

Aleksic S, Bockemühl J, Degner I, 1981, Imported shigellosis: aerogenic *Shigella boydii* 14 (Sachs A 12) in a traveller followed by two cases of laboratory-associated infections, *Tropenmed Parasitol*, **32**: 61–4.

Aleksic S, Karch H, Bockemühl J, 1992, A biotyping scheme for Shiga-like (Vero) toxin-producing *Escherichia coli* O157 and a list of serolgical cross-reactions between O157 and other gram-negative bacteria, *Zentralbl Bakteriol*, **276**: 221–30.

Aleksic S, Katz A et al., 1993, Antibiotic resistance of *Shigella* strains isolated in the Federal Republic of Germany 1989–1990, *Zentralbl Bakt – Int J Med Microbiol Virol Parasitol Infect Dis*, **279**: 484–93.

Altwegg M, 1986, Zur Resistenzlage bei Shigellen, *Schweiz Med Wochenschr*, **116**: 1848–51.

Altwegg M, Lüthy-Hottenstein J, 1992, Laboratory-acquired versus food-associated shigellosis: value of ribotyping and susceptibility testing for determining the putative source of infection, *Med Microbiol Lett*, **1**: 24–9.

Ambler JE, Drabu YJ et al., 1993, Mutator plasmid in a nalidixic acid-resistant strain of *Shigella dysenteriae* type 1, *J Antimicrob Chemother*, **31**: 831–9.

Anathan S, Subramanian S et al., 1989, Studies on the pathogenicity of classical enteropathogenic *Escherichia coli* strains isolated from acute diarrhoea among children 0–5 years of age, *Indian J Pathol Microbiol*, **32**: 92–100.

Andersson P, Engberg I et al., 1991, Persistence of *Escherichia coli* bacteriuria is not determined by bacterial adherence, *Infect Immun*, **59**: 2915–21.

Ansaruzzaman M, Kibriya AKMG et al., 1995, Detection of provisional serovars of *Shigella dysenteriae* and designation as S. *dysenteriae* serotypes 14 and 15, *J Clin Microbiol*, **33**: 1423–5.

Baldwin TJ, Knutton S et al., 1992, Enteroaggregative *Escherichia coli* strains secrete a heat-labile toxin antigenetically related to *E. coli* hemolysin, *Infect Immun*, **60**: 2092–5.

Balows A, Hausler WJ et al. (eds), 1991, *Manual of Clinical Micro-*

biology, 5th edn, American Society for Microbiology, Washington, DC.

Baqui AH, Sack RB et al., 1992, Enteropathogens associated with pathogens associated with acute and persistent diarrhea in Bangladeshi children <5 years of age, *J Infect Dis*, **166**: 792–6.

Baudry B, Savarino SJ et al., 1990, A sensitive and specific DNA probe to identify enteroaggregative *Escherichia coli*, a recently discovered diarrheal pathogen, *J Infect Dis*, **161**: 1249–51.

Belongia EA, Osterholm MT, 1993, Transmission of *Escherichia coli* O157:H7 infection in Minnesota child day-care facilities, *JAMA*, **269**: 883–8.

Benenson AS, 1985, *Control of Communicable Diseases in Man*, American Public Health Association, Washington, DC.

Benz L, Schmidt MA, 1992, Isolation and serologic characterization of AIDA-I, the adhesin mediating the diffuse adherence phenotype of the diarrhea-associated *Escherichia coli* strain 2787 (O126:H27), *Infect Immun*, **60**: 13–18.

Bernardini ML, Mounier J et al., 1989, Identification of *icsA*, a plasmid locus of *Shigella flexneri* that governs intra- and intercellular spread through interaction with F-actin, *Proc Natl Acad Sci USA*, **86**: 3867–71.

Bilge SS, Clausen CR et al., 1989, Molecular charcterization of a fimbrial adhesin, F1845, mediating diffuse adherence of diarrhea-associated *Escherichia coli* to HEP-2 cells, *J Bacteriol*, **171**: 4281–9.

Bitzan M, Moebius E et al., 1991, High incidence of serum antibodies to *Escherichia coli* O157 lipopolysaccharide in children with hemolytic uremic syndrome, *J Pediatr*, **119**: 380–5.

Bitzan M, Ludwig K et al., 1993, The role of *Escherichia coli* O157 infections in the classical (enteropathic) haemolytic uraemic syndrome: results of a central European, multicentre study, *Epidemiol Infect*, **110**: 183–96.

Bockemühl J, 1992, Enterobacteriaceae, *Mikrobiologische Diagnostik*, ed. Burkhardt F, Thieme Verlag, Stuttgart, 119–53.

Brenner DJ, Davis BR et al., 1982a, Atypical biogroups of *Escherichia coli* found in clinical specimens and description of *Escherichia hermannii* sp. nov., *J Clin Microbiol*, **15**: 703–13.

Brenner DJ, McWhorter AC et al., 1982b, *Escherichia vulneris*: a new species of Enterobacteriaceae associated with human wounds, *J Clin Microbiol*, **15**: 1133–40.

Bures J, Horak V, Duben J, 1979, Importance of colicinogeny for the course of acute bacillary dysentery, *Zentralbl Bakteriol Orig A*, **245**: 469–75.

Burgess MN, Bywater RJ et al., 1978, Biological evaluation of a methanol-soluble, heat-stable *Escherichia coli* enterotoxin in infant mice, pigs, rabbits, and calves, *Infect Immun*, **21**: 526–31.

Burgess NR, McDermott SN, Whiting J, 1973, Aerobic bacteria occurring in the hind-gut of the cockroach, *Blatta orientalis*, *J Hyg*, **71**: 1–7.

Burkhardt F (ed.), 1992, *Mikrobiologische Diagnostik*, Thieme Verlag, Stuttgart and New York.

Burnens AP, Zbinden R et al., 1993, A case of laboratory acquired infection with *Escherichia coli* O157:H7, *Zentralbl Bakteriol*, **279**: 512–17.

Caprioli A, Luzzi I et al., 1994, Community-wide outbreak of hemolytic-uremic syndrome assciated with non-O157 verocytotoxin-producing *Escherichia coli*, *J Infect Dis*, **169**: 208–11.

Castellani A, Chalmers AJ, 1919, *Manual of Tropical Medicine*, 3rd edn, Williams Wood & Co, New York.

Cave H, Bingen E et al., 1994, Differentiation of *Escherichia coli* strains using randomly amplified polymorphic DNA analysis, *Res Microbiol*, **145**: 141–50.

Centers for Disease Control, 1990, Waterborne disease outbreaks, 1986–1988, *Morbid Mortal Weekly Rep*, **39, No. SS1**: S1–13.

Centers for Disease Control, 1994a, Summary of notifiable diseases, United States 1994, *Morbid Mortal Weekly Rep*, **43**: 54.

Centers for Disease Control, 1994b, Health status of displaced persons following civil war – Burundi, December 1993–January 1994, *Morbid Mortal Weekly Rep*, **43**: 701–3.

Centers for Disease Control, 1995, Community outbreak of

hemolytic uremic syndrome attributable to *Escherichia coli* O111:NM – South Australia 1995, *Morbid Mortal Weekly Rep*, **44**: 550–8.

Chantemesse A, Widal F, 1888, Sur les microbes de la dysentérie épidémique, *Bull Acad Méd Sér 3*, **19**: 522–9.

Chapman PA, Siddons CA et al., 1991, An improved selective medium for the isolation of *Escherichia coli* O157, *J Med Microbiol*, **35**: 107–10.

Chatkaeomorakot A, Echeverria P et al., 1987, HeLa cell-adherent *Escherichia coli* in children with diarrhea in Thailand, *J Infect Dis*, **156**: 669–72.

Clerc P, Sansonetti PJ, 1987, Entry of *Shigella flexneri* into HeLa cells: evidence for directed phagocytosis involving actin polymerization and myosin accumulation, *Infect Immun*, **55**: 2681–8.

Cohen MB, Hawkins JA et al., 1993, Colonization by enteroaggregative *Escherichia coli* in travelers with and without diarrhea, *J Clin Microbiol*, **31**: 351–3.

Coultrip RL, Beaumont W, Siletchnik MD, 1977, Outbreak of shigellosis – Fort Bliss, Texas, *Morbid Mortal Weekly Rep*, **26**: 107–8.

Cravioto A, Telo A et al., 1991, Association of *Escherichia coli* HEp-2 adherence patterns with type and duration of diarrhoea, *Lancet*, **337**: 262–4.

Crichton PB, Old DC, 1985, Biotyping of *Escherichia coli*: methods and applications, *The Virulence of* Escherichia coli, ed. Sussman M, Academic Press, London, 315–32.

Dack GM, Petran E, 1934, Experimental dysentery produced by introducing *Bacterium dysenteriae* (Flexner) into isolated segments of the colon of monkeys, *J Infect Dis*, **55**: 1–6.

Dan M, 1993, Marked decrease in susceptibility of *Shigella* to ampicillin and cotrimoxazole in Israel, *Eur J Clin Microbiol Infect Dis*, **12**: 143–4.

Dedié K, Bockemühl J et al., 1993, *Bakterielle Zoonosen bei Tier und Mensch*, Ferdinand Enke Verlag, Stuttgart, 72–3.

Donnenberg MS, Kaper JB, 1992, Enteropathogenic *Escherichia coli*, *Infect Immun*, **60**: 3953–61.

Donnenberg MS, Tacker CO et al., 1993, Role of the *eaeA* gene in experimental enteropathogenic *Escherichia coli*, *J Clin Invest*, **92**: 1214–17.

Drasar BS, Barrow PA, 1985, *Intestinal Microbiology*, American Society for Microbiology, Washington, DC.

Dubos RJ, Geiger JW, 1946, Preparation and properties of Shiga toxin and toxoid, *J Exp Med*, **84**: 143–56.

Duguid JP, Gillies RR, 1956, Non-flagellar filamentous appendages ('fimbriae') and haemagglutinating activity in dysentery bacilli, *J Gen Microbiol*, **15**: vi.

DuPont HL, Formal SB et al., 1971, Pathogenesis of *Escherichia coli* diarrhea, *N Engl J Med*, **285**: 1–9.

DuPont HL, Hornick RB et al., 1972, Immunity in shigellosis. II. Protection induced by live oral vaccine or primary infection, *J Infect Dis*, **125**: 12–16.

DuPont HL, Levine MM et al., 1989, Inoculum size in shigellosis and implications for expected mode of transmission, *J Infect Dis*, **159**: 1126–8.

Eisenstein BI, 1990, Enterobacteriaceae, *Principles and Practice of Infectious Diseases*, 3rd edn, eds Mandell GL, Douglas GL, Bennett JE, Churchill Livingstone, New York, 1658–73.

Elwell LP, Falkow S, 1986, The characterization of R plasmids and the detection of plasmid-specified genes, *Antibiotics in Laboratory Medicine*, 2nd edn, ed. Lorian V, Williams & Wilkins, Baltimore, 683–721.

Endo Y, Tsurugi K et al., 1988, Site of action of verotoxin 2 (VT2) from *Escherichia coli* O157:H7 on eukaryotic ribosomes, *Eur J Biochem*, **171**: 45–50.

Enterobacteriaceae Subcommittee Reports, 1954, *Int Bull Bacteriol Nomencl Taxon*, **4**: 1–94.

Escherich T, 1885, Die Darmbakterien des Neugeborenen und Säuglings, *Fortschr Med*, **3**: 515–22, 547–54.

Escherich T, 1894, Über Cystitis bei Kindern, hervorgerufen durch das *Bacterium coli commune*, cited in Mochmann H,

Köhler W (eds), 1984, *Meilensteine der Bakteriologie*, VEB Fischer, Jena, 330–7.

Ewing WH, 1986, The genus *Escherichia*; the genus *Shigella*, *Edwards and Ewing's Identification of Enterobacteriaceae*, 4th edn, Elsevier, New York, Amsterdam, Oxford, 93–134, 135–72.

Ewing WH, Lindberg AA, 1984, Serology of *Shigella*, *Methods in Microbiology*, vol. 14, ed. Bergan T, Academic Press, London, 113–42.

Fang FC, Libby J et al., 1993, The alternative sigma factor KatF (rpos) regulates *Salmonella* virulence, *Proc Natl Acad Sci USA*, **90:** 3511–15.

Farmer III JJ, 1995, Enterobacteriaceae: introduction and identification, *Manual of Clinical Microbiology*, 6th edn, eds Murray PR, Baron EJ et al., American Society for Microbiology, Washington, DC, 438–49.

Farmer JJ, Fanning GR et al., 1985, *Escherichia fergusonii* and *Enterobacter taylorae*, two new species of Enterobacteriaceae isolated from clinical specimens, *J Clin Microbiol*, **21:** 77–81.

Faruque SM, Haider K et al., 1992, Differentiation of *Shigella flexneri* strains by rRNA gene restriction patterns, *J Clin Microbiol*, **30:** 2996–9.

Ferguson WW, June RC, 1952, Experiments on feeding adult volunteers with *Escherichia coli* 111, B4, an organism associated with infant diarrhea, *Am J Hyg*, **55:** 155–69.

Formal SB, Abrams GD et al., 1963, Experimental *Shigella* infections. VI. Role of the small intestine in an experimental infection in guinea pigs, *J Bacteriol*, **85:** 119–25.

Foubister V, Rosenshine I et al., 1994, The *eaeB* gene of enteropathogenic *Escherichia coli* is necessary for signal transduction in epithelial cells, *Infect Immun*, **62:** 3038–40.

Franke J, Franke S et al., 1994, Nucleotide sequence analysis of enteropathogenic *Escherichia coli* (EPEC) adherence factor probe and development of PCR for rapid detection of EPEC harboring virulence plasmids, *J Clin Microbiol*, **32:** 2460–3.

Frankel G, Candy DCA et al., 1994, Characterization of the C-terminal domains of intimin-like proteins of enteropathogenic and enterohemorrhagic *Escherichia coli*, *Citrobacter freundii*, and *Hafnia alvei*, *Infect Immun*, **62:** 1835–42.

Frost JA, Cheasty T et al., 1993, Phage typing of Vero cytotoxin-producing *Escherichia coli* O157 isolated in the United Kingdom: 1989–91, *Epidemiol Infect*, **110:** 469–75.

Garcia MI, Labigne A, LeBougenec C, 1994, Nucleotide sequence of the afimbrial-adhesin-encoding afa-3 gene cluster and its translocation via flanking IS1 insertion sequences, *J Bacteriol*, **176:** 7601–13.

Garrod LP, 1937, The susceptibility of different bacteria to destruction in the stomach, *J Pathol Bacteriol*, **45:** 473–4.

Gasser C, Gautier E et al., 1955, Hämolytisch-urämische Syndrome: bilaterale Nierenrindennekrosen bei akuten erworbenen hämolytischen Anämien, *Schweiz Med Wochenschr*, **85:** 905–9.

Gericke B, Reissbrodt R, 1995, Diagnostics and epidemiology of *Shigella* infections, *Biotest Bull*, **5:** 171–6.

Gershman M, Markowsky G, Hunter J, 1984, Reduced set of phages for typing *Escherichia coli*, *J Dairy Sci*, **67:** 1306–15.

Gilligan PH, Janda JM et al., 1992, *Laboratory Diagnosis of Bacterial Diarrhea. Cumitech 12A*, American Society for Microbiology, Washington, DC.

Girón JA, Ho ASY, Schoolnick GK, 1991, An inducible bundle-forming pilus of enteropathogenic *Escherichia coli*, *Science*, **254:** 710.

Girón JA, Ho ASY, Schoolnick GK, 1993, Characterization of fimbriae produced by enteropathogenic *Escherichia coli*, *J Bacteriol*, **175:** 7391–403.

Girón JA, Levine MM, Kaper JB, 1994, Longus: a long pilus ultrastructure produced by human enterotoxigenic *Escherichia coli*, *Mol Microbiol*, **12:** 71–82.

Girón JA, Jones T et al., 1991, Diffuse-adhering *Escherichia coli* (DAEC) as putative cause of diarrhea in Mayan children in Mexico, *J Infect Dis*, **163:** 507–13.

Gomes TAT, Blake PA, Trabulsi LR, 1989, Prevalence of *Escherichia coli* strains with localized, diffuse, and aggregative adherence to HeLa cells in infants with diarrhea and matched controls, *J Clin Microbiol*, **27:** 266–9.

Gomes TAT, Rassi V et al., 1991, Enteropathogens associated with acute diarrheal disease in urban infants in Sao Paulo, *J Infect Dis*, **164:** 331–7.

Goossens H, DeMol P et al., 1989, Comparative in vitro activity of lomefloxacin against enteropathogens, *Rev Infect Dis*, **11, Suppl. 5:** S1151–2.

Gorden J, Small PLC, 1993, Acid resistance in enteric bacteria, *Infect Immun*, **61:** 364–7.

Gordon DM, Riley MA, 1992, A theoretical and experimental analysis of bacterial growth in the bladder, *Mol Microbiol*, **6:** 555–62.

Griffin PM, Tauxe RV, 1991, The epidemiology of infections caused by *Escherichia coli* O157:H7, other enterohemorrhagic *E. coli*, and the associated hemolytic uremic syndrome, *Epidemiol Rev*, **13:** 60–98.

Grist NR, Emslie JAN, 1989, Infections in British clinical laboratories, 1986–7, *J Clin Pathol*, **42:** 677–81.

Gross RJ, Holmes B, 1990, The Enterobacteriaceae, *Topley & Wilson's Principles of Bacteriology, Virology and Immunity*, 8th edn, vol. 2, eds Parker MT, Collier LH, Edward Arnold, London, 401–14.

Gross RJ, Thomas LV et al., 1982a, New provisional serovar of *Shigella boydii*, *J Clin Microbiol*, **16:** 1000–2.

Gross RJ, Ward LR et al., 1982b, Drug resistance among infantile enteropathogenic *Escherichia coli* strains isolated in the United Kingdom, *Br Med J*, **285:** 472–3.

Gross RJ, Thomas LV et al., 1989, Four new provisional serovars of *Shigella*, *J Clin Microbiol*, **27:** 829–31.

Guerrant RL, 1990a, Principles and syndromes of enteric infection, *Principles and Practice of Infectious Diseases*, 3rd edn, eds Mandell GL, Douglas GL, Bennett JE, Churchill Livingstone, New York, 837–51.

Guerrant RL, 1990b, Nausea, vomiting, and noninflammatory diarrhea, *Principles and Practice of Infectious Diseases*, 3rd edn, eds Mandell GL, Douglas GL, Bennett JE, Churchill Livingstone, New York, 851–63.

Guerrant RL, Hughes JM et al., 1980, Activation of intestinal guanylate cyclase by heat-stable enterotoxin of *Escherichia coli*: studies of tissue specificity, potential receptor and intermediates, *J Infect Dis*, **142:** 220–8.

Guerrero L, Calva JJ et al., 1994, Asymptomatic *Shigella* infections in a cohort of Mexican children younger than two years of age, *Pediatr Infect Dis J*, **13:** 597–602.

Gunzburg ST, Tornieporth NG, Riley LW, 1995, Identification of enteropathogenic *Escherichia coli* by PCR-based detection of bundle-forming pilus gene, *J Clin Microbiol*, **33:** 1375–7.

Gunzer F, Böhm H et al., 1992, Molecular detection of sorbitol-fermenting *Escherichia coli* O157 in patients with hemolytic-uremic syndrome, *J Clin Microbiol*, **30:** 1807–10.

Haider K, Huq MI et al., 1985, Plasmid characterization of *Shigella* spp. isolated from children with shigellosis and asymptomatic carriers, *J Antimicrob Chemother*, **16:** 691–8.

Hajna AA, 1955, A new specimen preservative for gram-negative organisms of the intestinal group, *Public Health Lab*, **13:** 59–62.

Hale TL, Morris RE, Bonventre PF, 1979, *Shigella* infection of Henle intestinal epithelial cells: role of the host cell, *Infect Immun*, **24:** 887–94.

Hansson HB, Barkenius G et al., 1981, Controlled comparison of nalidixic acid or lactulose with placebo in shigellosis, *Scand J Infect Dis*, **13:** 191–3.

He XQ, Pan RN, 1992, Bacteriophage lytic patterns for identification of salmonellae, shigellae, *Escherichia coli*, *Citrobacter freundii*, and *Enterobacter cloacae*, *J Clin Microbiol*, **30:** 590–4.

Heikkilä E, Siitonen A et al., 1990, Increase of trimethoprim resistance among *Shigella* species, *J Infect Dis*, **161:** 1242–8.

Hewlett EL, 1990, Toxins and other virulence factors, *Principles and Practice of Infectious Diseases*, 3rd edn, eds Mandell GL,

Douglas RJ, Bennett JE, Churchill Livingstone, New York, 2–9.

Hinojosa-Ahumada M, Swaminathan B et al., 1991, Restriction fragment length polymorphisms in rRNA operons for subtyping *Shigella sonnei, J Clin Microbiol,* **29:** 2380–4.

Holmes B, Gross RJ, 1990, Coliform bacteria; various other members of the Enterobacteriaceae, *Topley & Wilson's Principles of Bacteriology, Virology and Immunity,* 8th edn, eds Parker MT, Collier LH, Edward Arnold, London, 415–41.

Holmes RK, Twiddy EM, Neill RJ, 1985, Recent advances in the study of heat-labile enterotoxins of *Escherichia coli, Bacterial Diarrheal Diseases,* 3rd edn, eds Takeda Y, Minatoni N, Martinus Nijhoff, Boston, 125–45.

Holt JG, Krieg NR et al., 1994, *Bergey's Manual of Determinative Bacteriology,* 9th edn, Williams & Wilkins, Baltimore, 179–80, 187–8.

Horák V, 1994, Seventy colicin types of *Shigella sonnei* and an indicator system for their determination, *Zentralbl Bakteriol,* **281:** 24–9.

Horiuchi S, Inagaki Y et al., 1993, Reduced susceptibilities of *Shigella sonnei* strains isolated from patients with dysentery to fluoroquinolones, *Antimicrob Agents Chemother,* **37:** 2486–9.

Hornick RB, 1994, Shigellosis, *Infectious Diseases,* 5th edn, eds Hoeprich PD, Jordan MC, Ronald AR, JB Lippincott, Philadelphia, 736–41.

Hossain MA, Hasan KZ, Albert MJ, 1994, *Shigella* carriers among non-diarrhoeal children in an endemic area of shigellosis in Bangladesh, *Trop Geogr Med,* **46:** 40–2.

Hruska JF, 1991, Gastrointestinal and intraabdominal infections, *A Practical Approach to Infectious Diseases,* 3rd edn, eds Reese RE, Betts RF, Little, Brown, Boston, 305–56.

Hughes RA, Keat AC, 1994, Reiter's syndrome andd reactive arthritis: a current view, *Semin Arthritis Rheum,* **24:** 190–210.

Hultgren SJ, Normark S, 1991, Chaperone-assisted assembly and molecular architecture of adhesive pili, *Annu Rev Microbiol,* **45:** 383–415.

Huppertz H-I, Busch D et al., 1996, Diarrhea in young children associated with *Escherichia coli* non-O157 organisms that produce Shiga-like toxin, *J Pediatr,* **128:** 341–6.

Jann K, Jann B, 1987, Polysaccharide antigens of *Escherichia coli, Rev Infect Dis,* **9, Suppl. 5:** S517–26.

Jann K, Jann B, 1992, Capsules of *Escherichia coli,* expression and biological significance, *Can J Microbiol,* **38:** 705–10.

Jann K, Westphal O, 1975, Microbial polysaccharides, *The Antigens,* vol. III, ed. Sela M, Academic Press, London, 1–125.

June RC, Ferguson WW, Worfel MT, 1953, Experiments in feeding adult volunteers with *Escherichia coli* 55, B5, a coliform organism associated with infant diarrhea, *Am J Hyg,* **57:** 222–36.

Kaper JB, 1994, Molecular pathogenesis of enteropathogenic *Escherichia coli, Molecular Genetics of Bacterial Pathogenesis,* 1st edn, eds Miller VL, Kaper JB et al., American Society for Microbiology, Washington, DC, 173–95.

Karch H, 1994, Verocytotoxin-producing *Escherichia coli* infection in Europe: diagnostics and public health perspectives, *Recent Advances in Verocytotoxin-producing* Escherichia coli *Infections,* eds Karmali MA, Goglio AG, Elsevier Science BV, Amsterdam, 13–16.

Karch H, Rüssmann H et al., 1995, Long-term shedding and clonal turnover of enterohemorrhagic *Escherichia coli* O157 in diarrheal diseases, *J Clin Microbiol,* **33:** 1602–5.

Karch H, Janetzki-Mittmann C et al., 1996, Isolation of enterohemorrhagic *Escherichia coli* O157 strains from patients with hemolytic-uremic syndrome by using immunomagnetic separation, DNA-based methods, and direct culture, *J Clin Microbiol,* **34:** 516–19.

Katouli M, Jaafari A et al., 1990, Aetiological studies of diarrhoeal diseases in infants and young children in Iran, *Iran J Trop Med Hyg,* **93:** 22–7.

Kauffmann F, 1943, Über neue thermolabile Körperantigene der Colibakterien, *Acta Pathol Microbiol Scand,* **20:** 21–44.

Kauffmann F, 1944, Zur Serologie der Coli-Gruppe, *Acta Pathol Microbiol Scand,* **21:** 20–45.

Kauffmann F, 1965, *Enterobacteriaceae,* 2nd edn, Munksgaard, Copenhagen.

Kent TH, Formal SB et al., 1967, Gastric shigellosis in rhesus monkeys, *Am J Pathol,* **51:** 259–67.

Khalil K, Lindblom GB et al., 1994, Flies and water as reservoirs for bacterial enteropathogens in urban and rural areas around Lahore, Pakistan, *Epidemiol Infect,* **113:** 435–44.

Knutton S, Lloyd DR, McNeish AS, 1987, Adhesion of enteropathogenic *Escherichia coli* to human intestinal enterocytes and cultured human intestinal mucosa, *Infect Immun,* **55:** 69–77.

Knutton S, Baldwin T et al., 1989, Actin accumulation at sites of bacterial adhesion to tissue culture cells: basis of a new diagnostic test for enteropathogenic and enterohemorrhagic *Escherichia coli, Infect Immun,* **57:** 1290–8.

Knutton S, Shaw RK et al., 1992, Ability of enteroaggregative *Escherichia coli* strains to adhere in vitro to human intestinal mucosa, *Infect Immun,* **60:** 2083–91.

Konowalchuk J, Speirs J, Stavric S, 1977, Vero response to a cytotoxin of *Escherichia coli, Infect Immun,* **18:** 775–9.

Law D, 1994, Adhesion and its role in the virulence of enteropathogenic *Escherichia coli, Clin Microbiol Rev,* **7:** 152–73.

Lawn AM, Ørskov I, Ørskov F, 1977, Morphological distinction between different H serotypes of *Escherichia coli, J Gen Microbiol,* **101:** 111–19.

Lee CH, Moseley SL et al., 1983, Characterization of the gene encoding heat-stable toxin II and preliminary molecular epidemiological studies of enterotoxigenic *Escherichia coli* heat-stable toxin II, *Infect Immun,* **42:** 264–8.

Lee LA, Shapiro CN et al., 1991, Hyperendemic shigellosis in the United States: a review of surveillance data for 1967–1988, *J Infect Dis,* **164:** 894–900.

Leffler H, Svanborg-Eden C, 1980, Chemical identification of glycosphingolipid receptor for *Escherichia coli* attaching to human urinary tract epithelial cells and agglutinating human erythrocytes, *FEMS Microbiol Lett,* **8:** 127–34.

Levine MM, Edelman R, 1984, Enteropathogenic *Escherichia coli* of classic serotypes associated with infant diarrhea: epidemiology and pathogenesis, *Epidemiol Rev,* **6:** 31–51.

Levine MM, DuPont HL et al., 1973, Pathogenesis of *Shigella dysenteriae* 1 (Shiga) dysentery, *J Infect Dis,* **127:** 261–70.

Levine MM, Bergquist EJ et al., 1978, *Escherichia coli* strains that cause diarrhoea but do not produce heat-labile or heat-stable enterotoxins and are non-invasive, *Lancet,* **1:** 1119–22.

Levine MM, Nalin DR et al., 1979, Immunity to enterotoxigenic *Escherichia coli, Infect Immun,* **23:** 729–36.

Levine MM, Prado V et al., 1988, Use of DNA probes and Hep-2 cell adherence assay to detect diarrheagenic *Escherichia coli, J Infect Dis,* **158:** 224–8.

Ling J, Kam KM et al., 1988, Susceptibilities of Hong Kong isolates of multiply resistant *Shigella* spp. to 25 antimicrobial agents, including ampicillin plus sulbactam and new 4-quinolones, *Antimicrob Agents Chemother,* **32:** 20–3.

Ling JM, Shaw PC et al., 1993, Molecular studies of plasmids of multiply-resistant *Shigella* spp. in Hong Kong, *Epidemiol Infect,* **110:** 437–46.

Lopez-Brea M, Collado L et al., 1983, Increasing antimicrobial resistance of *Shigella sonnei, J Antimicrob Chemother,* **11:** 598.

Louise CB, Obrig TG, 1992, Shiga toxin-associated hemolytic uremic syndrome: combined cytotoxic effects of Shiga toxin and lipopolysaccharide (endotoxin) on human vascular endothelial cells in vitro, *Infect Immun,* **60:** 1536–43.

Lüderitz O, Staub AM, Westphal O, 1966, Immunochemistry of O and R antigens of *Salmonella* and related Enterobacteriaceae, *Bacteriol Rev,* **30:** 193–255.

Lüderitz O, Galanos C et al., 1973, Lipid A, chemical structure and biological activity, *J Infect Dis,* **128, Suppl.:** 9–21.

Lüscher D, Altwegg M, 1994, Detection of shigellae, enteroinvasive and enterotoxigenic *Escherichia coli* using the polymerase chain reaction (PCR) in patients returning from tropical countries, *Mol Cell Probes*, **8:** 285–90.

Lüscher D, Graf Settah S, Altwegg M, 1992, Bakterielle Durchfallerreger: Nachweis von Verotoxin-produzierenden *Escherichia coli* mittels Polymerase-Kettenreaktion, *Schweiz Med Wochenschr*, **122:** 1911–18.

McCann MP, Kidwell JP, Matin A, 1991, The putative sigma factor katF has a central role in development of starvation-mediated general resistance in *Escherichia coli*, *J Bacteriol*, **173:** 4188–94.

Makintubee S, Mallonee J, Istre GR, 1987, Shigellosis outbreak associated with swimming, *JAMA*, **236:** 1849–52.

Marranzano M, Giammanco G et al., 1985, Epidemiological markers of *Shigella sonnei* infections: R-plasmid fingerprinting, phage-typing and biotyping, *Ann Inst Pasteur Microbiol*, **136A:** 339–45.

Maslow JN, Whittam TS et al., 1995, Clonal relationships among bloodstream isolates of *Escherichia coli*, *Infect Immun*, **63:** 2409–17.

Mathewson JJ, Johnson PC et al., 1985, A newly recognized cause of travelers' diarrhea: enteroadherent *Escherichia coli*, *J Infect Dis*, **151:** 471–5.

Menard R, Sansonetti P, Parsot C, 1994, The secretion of the *Shigella flexneri* Ipa invasins is activated by epithelial cells and controlled by IpaB and IpaD, *EMBO J*, **13:** 5293–302.

Meng J, Zhao S et al., 1995, Molecular characterization of *Escherichia coli* O157:H7 isolates by pulsed-field gel electrophoresis and plasmid DNA analysis, *J Med Microbiol*, **42:** 258–63.

Meunier JR, Grimont PAD, 1993, Factors affecting reproducibility of random amplified polymorphic DNA fingerprinting, *Res Microbiol*, **144:** 373–9.

Milch H, 1978, Phage typing of *Escherichia coli*, *Methods in Microbiology*, vol. 11, ed. Bergan T, Academic Press, London, 87–155.

Morris KJ, Gopal Rao G, 1992, Conventional screening for enteropathogenic *Escherichia coli* in the UK. Is it appropriate or necessary?, *J Hosp Infect*, **21:** 163–7.

Mosley WH, Adams B, Lyman ED, 1962, Epidemiologic and sociologic features of a large urban outbreak of shigellosis, *JAMA*, **182:** 1307–11.

Mubashir M, Khan A et al., 1990, Causative agents of acute diarrhoea in the first 3 years of life: hospital-based study, *J Gastroenterol Hepatol*, **5:** 264–70.

Munshi MH, Haider K et al., 1987, Plasmid-mediated resistance to nalidixic acid in *Shigella dysenteriae* type 1, *Lancet*, **2:** 419–21.

Murayama SY, Sakai T et al., 1986, The use of mice in the Sereny test as a virulence assay of shigellae and enteroinvasive *Escherichia coli*, *Infect Immun*, **51:** 696–8.

Murray BE, 1986, Resistance of *Shigella*, *Salmonella*, and other selected pathogens to antimicrobial agents, *Rev Infect Dis*, **8, Suppl. 2:** 172–81.

Murray PR, Baron EJ et al. (eds), 1995, *Manual of Clinical Microbiology*, 6th edn, ASM Press, Washington, DC.

Nastasi A, Pignato S et al., 1993, rRNA gene restriction patterns and biotypes of *Shigella sonnei*, *Epidemiol Infect*, **110:** 23–30.

Nataro JP, Scaletsky ICA et al., 1985, Plasmid-mediated factors conferring diffused and localized adherence of enteropathogenic *Escherichia coli*, *Infect Immun*, **48:** 378–83.

Nataro JP, Kaper JB et al., 1987, Patterns of adherence of diarrheagenic *Escherichia coli* to Hep-2 cells, *Pediatr Infect Dis J*, **6:** 829–31.

Nataro JP, Deng Y et al., 1992, Aggregative adherence fimbriae I of enteroaggregative *Escherichia coli* mediate adherence to Hep-2 cells and hemagglutination of human erythrocytes, *Infect Immun*, **60:** 2297–304.

Neidhart FC, Curtiss III R, et al., 1996, *Escherichia coli* and *Salmonella. Cellular and Molecular Biology*, 2nd edn, American Society for Microbiology, Washington, DC.

Newland JW, Neill RJ, 1988, DNA probes for Shiga-like toxins I and II and for toxin-converting bacteriophages, *J Clin Microbiol*, **26:** 1292–7.

O'Brien AD, LaVeck GD et al., 1982, Production of *Shigella dysenteriae* type 1-like cytotoxin by *Escherichia coli*, *J Infect Dis*, **146:** 763–9.

Ogata M, 1892, Zur Ätiologie der Dysenterie, *Zentralbl Bakteriol Parasitenkd Infektionskr Hyg*, **11:** 264–72.

O'Hanley P, Lark D et al., 1983, Mannose-sensitive and gal-gal binding pili of *Escherichia coli* from recombinant strains, *J Exp Med*, **158:** 1713–19.

O'Hanley P, Low D et al., 1985, Gal-gal binding and hemolysin phenotypes and genotypes associated with uropathogenic *Escherichia coli*, *N Engl J Med*, **313:** 414–20.

Ørskov F, 1984, Genus I. *Escherichia* Castellani and Chalmers 1919, *Bergey's Manual of Systematic Bacteriology*, vol. 1, eds Krieg N, Holt JG, Williams & Wilkins, Baltimore and London, 420–3.

Ørskov F, Ørskov I, 1984, Serotyping of *Escherichia coli*, *Methods in Microbiology*, vol. 14, ed. Bergan T, Academic Press, London, 43–112.

Ørskov I, Ørskov F et al., 1977, Serology, chemistry, and genetics of O and K antigens of *Escherichia coli*, *Bacteriol Rev*, **41:** 667–710.

Ørskov I, Wachsmuth IK et al., 1991, Two new *Escherichia coli* O groups: O172 from 'Shiga-like' toxin II-producing strains (EHEC) and O173 from enteroinvasive *E. coli* (EIEC), *APMIS*, **99:** 30–2.

Parsonnet J, Greene KD et al., 1989, *Shigella dysenteriae* type 1 infections in US travellers to Mexico, *Lancet*, **2:** 543–5.

Plos K, Connell H et al., 1995, Intestinal carriage of P fimbriated *Escherichia coli* and the susceptibility to urinary tract infection in young children, *J Infect Dis*, **171:** 625–31.

Poitrineau P, Forestier C et al., 1995, Retrospective case-control study of diffusely adhering *Escherichia coli* and clinical features in children with diarrhea, *J Clin Microbiol*, **33:** 1961–2.

Rahman M, Mauff G et al., 1994, Detection of 4-quinolone resistance mutation in *gyrA* gene of *Shigella dysenteriae* type 1 by PCR, *Antimicrob Agents Chemother*, **38:** 2488–91.

Ratiner YA, 1982, Phase variation of the H antigen in *Escherichia coli* strain Bi7327-41, the standard strain for *Escherichia coli* flagellar antigen H3, *FEMS Microbiol Lett*, **15:** 33–6.

Reida P, Wolff M et al., 1994, An outbreak due to enterohaemorrhagic *Escherichia coli* O157:H7 in a children day care centre characterized by person-to-person transmission and environmental contamination, *Zentralbl Bakteriol*, **281:** 534–43.

Rietschel ET, Brade L et al., 1987, Chemical structure and biologic activity of bacterial and synthetic lipid A, *Rev Infect Dis*, **9, Suppl. 5:** S527–36.

Riley LW, Remis RS et al., 1983, Hemorrhagic colitis associated with a rare *Escherichia coli* serotype, *N Engl J Med*, **308:** 681–5.

Roelcke K, 1938, Über die Resistenz verschiedener Ruhrkeime, *Z Hyg Infektionskr*, **120:** 307–14.

Rosenberg ML, Hazlet KK et al., 1976, Shigellosis from swimming, *JAMA*, **16:** 1849–52.

Rowe B, 1990, *Shigella, Topley & Wilson's Principles of Bacteriology, Virology and Immunity*, 8th edn, vol. 2, eds Parker MT, Collier LH, Edward Arnold, London, 455–68.

Rowe B, Gross RJ, 1981, The genus *Shigella, The Prokaryotes*, vol. II, eds Starr MP, Stolp H et al., Springer-Verlag, Berlin, Heidelberg and New York, 1248–59.

Rowe B, Gross RJ, 1984, Genus II. *Shigella* Castellani and Chalmers 1919, *Bergey's Manual of Systematic Bacteriology*, vol. 1, eds Krieg N, Holt JG, Williams & Wilkins, Baltimore and London, 423–7.

Ruch TC, 1959, *Diseases of Laboratory Primates*, Saunders, Philadelphia.

Rüssmann H, Kothe E et al., 1995, Genotyping of Shiga-like toxin genes in non-O157 *Escherichia coli* strains associated with haemolytic uraemic syndrome, *J Med Microbiol*, **42:** 404–10.

Salyers AA, Whitt DD, 1994, *Bacterial Pathogenesis: a Molecular Approach*, 1st edn, ASM Press, Washington, DC.

Savarino SJ, 1993, Diarrhoeal disease: current concepts and future challenges, *Trans R Soc Trop Med Hyg*, **87:** 49–53.

Savarino SJ, Fasano A et al., 1991, Enteroaggregative *Escherichia coli* elaborate a heat-stable enterotoxin demonstrable in an 'in vitro' rabbit intestinal model, *J Clin Invest*, **87**: 1450–5.

Savarino SJ, Fasano A et al., 1993, Enteroaggregative *Escherichia coli* heat-stable enterotoxin 1 represents another subfamily of *E. coli* heat-stable toxin, *Proc Natl Acad Sci USA*, **90**: 3093–7.

Scaletsky ICA, Silva MLM, Trabulsi LR, 1984, Distinctive patterns of adherence of enteropathogenic *Escherichia coli* to HeLa cells, *Infect Immun*, **45**: 534–6.

Schmidt H, Beutin L, Karch H, 1995, Molecular analysis of the plasmid-encoded hemolysin of *Escherichia coli* O157:H7 strain EDL 933, *Infect Immun*, **63**: 1055–61.

Schmidt H, Karch H, Beutin L, 1994, The large-sized plasmids of enterohemorrhagic *Escherichia coli* O157 strains encode hemolysins which are presumably members of the *E. coli* α-hemolysin family, *FEMS Microbiol Lett*, **117**: 189–96.

Schmidt H, Rüssmann H, Karch H, 1993, Virulence determinants in nontoxigenic *Escherichia coli* O157 strains that cause infantile diarrhea, *Infect Immun*, **61**: 4894–8.

Schmidt H, Montag M et al., 1993, Shiga-like toxin II-related cytotoxins in *Citrobacter freundii* strains from humans and beef samples, *Infect Immun*, **61**: 534–43.

Schmidt H, Knop C et al., 1995, Development of PCR for screening of enteroaggregative *Escherichia coli*, *J Clin Microbiol*, **33**: 701–5.

Schultsz C, Pool GJ et al., 1994, Detection of enterotoxigenic *Escherichia coli* in stool samples by using nonradioactively labeled oligonucleotide DNA probes and PCR, *J Clin Microbiol*, **32**: 2393–7.

Scotland SM, Smith HR et al., 1991, Identification of enteropathogenic *Escherichia coli* isolated in Britain as enteroaggregative or as members of a subclass of attaching-and-effacing *E. coli* not hybridising with the EPEC adherence-factor probe, *J Med Microbiol*, **35**: 278–83.

Serény B, 1957, Experimental keratoconjunctivitis shigellosa, *Acta Microbiol Hung*, **4**: 367–76.

Sethabutr O, Venkatesan M et al., 1993, Detection of shigellae and enteroinvasive *Escherichia coli* by amplification of the invasion plasmid antigen H DNA sequence in patients with dysentery, *J Infect Dis*, **167**: 458–61.

Shahid NS, Rahaman NM et al., 1985, Changing pattern of resistant Shiga bacillus (*Shigella dysenteriae* type 1) and *Shigella flexneri* in Bangladesh, *J Infect Dis*, **152**: 1114–19.

Sharp TW, Thornton SA et al., 1995, Diarrheal disease among military personnel during Operation Restore Hope, Somalia, 1992–1993, *Am J Trop Med Hyg*, **52**: 188–93.

Shiga K, 1898, Über den Dysenteriebacillus (*Bacillus dysentericus*), *Zentralbl Bakteriol Parasitenkd Infektionskr Hyg*, **24**: 817–28, 870–4, 913–18.

Silverman M, Simon MI, 1977, Bacterial flagella, *Annu Rev Microbiol*, **31**: 397–419.

Small P, Blankenhorn D et al., 1994, Acid and base resistance in *Escherichia coli* and *Shigella flexneri*: role of *rpoS* and growth pH, *J Bacteriol*, **176**: 1729–37.

Small PLC, 1994, How many bacteria does it take to cause diarrhea and why?, *Molecular Genetics of Bacterial Pathogenesis*, 1st edn, eds Miller VL, Kaper JB et al., American Society for Microbiology, Washington, DC, 479–89.

Smith HR, Scotland SM et al., 1994, Isolates of *Escherichia coli* O44:H18 of diverse origin are enteroaggregative, *J Infect Dis*, **170**: 1610–13.

Smith HW, Halls S, 1967, Studies on *Escherichia coli* enterotoxins, *J Pathol Bacteriol*, **93**: 531–43.

Soldati L, Piffaretti JC, 1991, Molecular typing of *Shigella* strains using pulsed field gel electrophoresis and genome hybridization with insertion sequences, *Res Microbiol*, **142**: 489–98.

Sorvillo FJ, Waterman SH et al., 1988, Shigellosis associated with recreational water contact, *Am J Trop Med Hyg*, **38**: 613–17.

Stacy-Phipps S, Mecca JJ, Weiss JB, 1995, Multiplex PCR assay and simple preparation method for stool specimens detect enterotoxigenic *Escherichia coli* DNA during course of infection, *J Clin Microbiol*, **33**: 1054–9.

Struelens MJ, Patte D et al., 1985, *Shigella* septicemia: prevalence, presentation, risk factors, and outcome, *J Infect Dis*, **152**: 784–90.

Svanborg-Eden C, Freter R et al., 1982, Inhibition of experimental ascending urinary tract infection by an epithelial cell-surface receptor analogue, *Nature (London)*, **298**: 560–2.

Swaddiwudhipong W, Karintraratana S, Kavinum S, 1995, A common-source outbreak of shigellosis involving a piped public water supply in northern Thai communities, *J Trop Med Hyg*, **98**: 145–50.

Swanson TN, Bilge SS et al., 1991, Molecular structure of the Dr adhesin: nucleotide sequence and mapping of receptor-binding domain by use of fusion constructs, *Infect Immun*, **59**: 261–8.

Takasaka M, Honjo S et al., 1969, Experimental infection with *Shigella sonnei* in cynomolgus monkeys (*Macaca irus*), *Jpn J Med Sci Biol*, **22**: 389.

Tamura K, Sakazaki R et al., 1986, *Leclercia adecarboxylata* gen. nov., comb. nov., formerly known as *Escherichia adecarboxylata*, *Curr Microbiol*, **13**: 179–84.

Tauxe RV, Puhr ND et al., 1990, Antimicrobial resistance of *Shigella* isolates in the USA: the importance of international travelers, *J Infect Dis*, **162**: 1107–11.

Thoren A, 1983, The role of enteropathogenic *Escherichia coli* in infantile diarrhoea: aspects on bacteriology, epidemiology and therapy, *Scand J Infect Dis Suppl*, **37**: 1–51.

Tietze E, Tschäpe H et al., 1984, Clonal distribution of multiple-drug-resistant *Shigella sonnei* strains: identification by means of plasmid pattern analysis, *Ann Microbiol (Paris)*, **135B**: 155–64.

Tschäpe H, Prager R et al., 1995, Verotoxigenic *Citrobacter freundii* associated with severe gastroenteritis and cases of haemolytic uraemic syndrome in a nursery school: green butter as the infection source, *Epidemiol Infect*, **114**: 441–50.

Tzipori S, Gibson R, Montanaro J, 1989, Nature and distribution of mucosal lesions associated with enteropathogenic and enterohemorrhagic *Escherichia coli* in piglets and the role of plasmid-mediated factors, *Infect Immun*, **57**: 1142–50.

Valentini SR, Gomes TAT, Falcao DF, 1992, Lack of virulence factors in *Escherichia coli* strains of enteropathogenic serogroups isolated from water, *Appl Environ Microbiol*, **58**: 412–14.

Voogd CE, Schot CS et al., 1992, Monitoring of antibiotic resistance in shigellae isolated in the Netherlands 1984–1989, *Eur J Clin Microbiol Infect Dis*, **11**: 164–7.

Wachsmuth IK, 1994, Summary: public health; epidemiology; food safety; laboratory diagnosis, *Recent Advances in Verocytotoxin-producing* Escherichia coli *Infections*, eds Karmali MA, Goglio AG, Elsevier Science BV, Amsterdam, 3–5.

Ward TT, Jones SR, 1991, Genitourinary tract infections, *A Practical Approach to Infectious Diseases*, 3rd edn, eds Reese RE, Betts RF, Little, Brown, Boston, 357–89.

Wathen-Grady HG, Britt LE et al., 1990, Characterization of *Shigella dysenteriae* serotypes 11, 12, and 13, *J Clin Microbiol*, **28**: 2580–4.

Wharton M, Spiegel RA et al., 1990, A large outbreak of antibiotic-resistant shigellosis at a mass gathering, *J Infect Dis*, **162**: 1324–8.

Whittam TS, Wolfe ML et al., 1993, Clonal relationships among *Escherichia coli* strains that cause hemorrhagic colitis and infantile diarrhea, *Infect Immun*, **61**: 1619–29.

Williams Smith H, 1965, Observations on the flora of the alimentary tract of animals and factors affecting its composition, *J Pathol Bacteriol*, **89**: 95–122.

Williams Smith H, Green P, Parsell Z, 1983, Verocell toxins in *Escherichia coli* and related bacteria: transfer by phage and conjugation and toxic action in laboratory animals, chickens and pigs, *J Gen Microbiol*, **129**: 3121–37.

Wolf MK, Taylor DN et al., 1993, Characterization of enterotoxigenic *Escherichia coli* isolated from US troops deployed to the middle east, *J Clin Microbiol*, **31**: 851–6.

Wollschlager CM, Raoof S et al., 1987, Controlled, comparative study of ciprofloxacin versus ampicillin in treatment of bacterial respiratory tract infections, *Am J Med*, **82, Suppl. 4A:** 164–8.

World Health Organization, 1994, *Report of WHO Working Group Meeting on Shiga-like Toxin producing* Escherichia coli *(SLTEC),* *with Emphasis on Zoonotic Aspects, Bergamo, Italy, 1 July 1994,* WHO, Geneva. WHO/CDS/VPH/94.136.

Yu J, Kaper JB, 1992, Cloning and characterization of the *eae* gene of enterohemorrhagic *Escherichia coli* O157:H7, *Mol Microbiol*, **6:** 411–17.

Chapter 41

SALMONELLA

D C Old and E J Threlfall

1 DEFINITION

Salmonellae are organisms that conform to the definition of the Enterobacteriaceae. Most strains are motile. Apart from a few exceptions that form acid only, they produce acid and gas from glucose and mannitol, and usually also from sorbitol; they ferment sucrose or adonitol rarely, and rarely form indole. Acetylmethylcarbinol is not formed. They do not hydrolyse urea or deaminate phenylalanine, usually form H_2S on triple sugar iron agar and use citrate as sole carbon source. They form lysine and ornithine decarboxylases. The many serotypes in the group are closely related to each other by somatic and flagellar antigens and most strains show diphasic variation of the flagellar antigens. Salmonellae are primarily intestinal parasites of vertebrates; they are pathogenic for many species of animals, giving rise to enteritis and to typhoid-like diseases. The G + C content of their DNA is 50–53 mol% and the type species is *Salmonella enterica*.

2 BACKGROUND

The genus *Salmonella* was originally created by medical bacteriologists to include organisms that gave rise to a certain type of illness in humans and animals and were related to one another antigenically. Later it became clear that salmonellae had many common biochemical characters. Now more emphasis is placed on biochemical activity than antigenic structure in their definition. Individual strains atypical in one or more biochemical tests usually have so many other biochemical characters in common with other salmonellae that there is little difficulty in classifying them. An organism which, on biochemical grounds, appears to be a salmonella will usually possess one or more antigens in common with other salmonella types but the possession of salmonella antigens is itself insufficient for an organism's inclusion in the group.

The genus *Salmonella* includes not only the familiar serotypes that are pathogens of mammals but also other serotypes formerly considered to be biochemically aberrant types. It is now considered to comprise 2 species: *S. enterica* and *Salmonella bongori*. There are 6 subspecies of *S. enterica*, the most important of which is *S. enterica* subsp. *enterica* (subspecies I) which includes the typhoid and paratyphoid bacilli and most of the other serotypes responsible for widespread disease in mammals. Members of the other 5 subspecies (II–VI) are in the main parasites of cold-blooded animals or are found in the natural environment.

3 NOMENCLATURE

The terminology introduced by early workers accorded specific rank to each antigenically distinguishable salmonella type. The species names given were generally descriptive of the disease or the host with which the serotype was associated, and were sometimes incorrect. Thereafter, the convention was established that each new type should be named after the place in which it was first isolated. Whereas the first published table contained some 20 serotypes, each considered to be a species, the current number is 2399 (Popoff, Bockemühl and Hickman-Brenner 1995).

However, they are no longer accorded specific status because more modern taxonomic techniques (Le Minor, Veron and Popoff 1982a, 1982b) suggested that all serotypes of *Salmonella* probably belonged to one DNA-hybridization group within which 7 subgroups were identified; and, following the strict rules of the Bacteriological Code (see Chapter 3), Le Minor et al. (1986) correctly proposed the name *Salmonella choleraesuis* for the only genospecies of *Salmonella*. That same name, however, had long been used to designate a salmonella serotype and its use was likely to lead to errors of interpretation by clinicians and others unfamiliar with the complexities of bacterial nomenclature. To avoid such confusion, Le Minor and Popoff (1987) requested that the name of this species be changed from *S. choleraesuis* to *S. enterica*, an epithet never before used to designate a salmonella serotype, and that proposal has been generally adopted (Ewing 1986, Old 1992, Popoff and Le Minor 1992). The 7 DNA-hybridization subgroups were designated as subspecies: *S. enterica* subspp. *enterica*, *salamae*, *arizonae*, *diarizonae*, *houtenae*, *bongori* and *indica* (Le Minor and Popoff 1987). However, the DNA–DNA hybridization studies of Le Minor and colleagues (Le Minor, Veron and Popoff 1982a, Le Minor et al. 1986) suggested that DNA subgroup V (*S. enterica* subsp. *bongori*) had evolved significantly from the other 6 subspecies. Results from multilocus enzyme electrophoresis (MLEE) studies supported that observation and the elevation of *S. enterica* subsp. *bongori* to the level of species as *S. bongori* was proposed (Reeves et al. 1989).

Because names of serotypes escape the strictures of the Bacteriological Code, they have no more nomenclatural ranking than phage type or biotype designations and are no longer given specific status (Popoff and Le Minor 1992). Serotype names should be given in Roman (**not** italic) type as, for example, serotype (ser.) Typhimurium. Furthermore, only serotypes of subsp. *enterica* are still named; serotypes of other subspecies of *S. enterica* and of *S. bongori* are no longer named but designated by their antigenic formulae. Designations such as *Salmonella* ser. Typhimurium, *Salmonella* Typhimurium or even simply Typhimurium are convenient for use in clinical situations and indicate, furthermore, that the named serotype is a member of subsp. *enterica*. This practice will be followed in this chapter.

Subtypes of serotypes recognized by phage typing or biotyping should not be named as if they were serotypes. Thus, the names of salmonellae (e.g. 'S. java') distinguishable from established serotypes by biotype characters only should not be perpetuated and most have been deleted from the Kauffmann–White scheme of serotypes (Popoff and Le Minor 1992).

4 HABITAT

Salmonellae are primarily intestinal parasites of humans and many animals, including wild birds, domestic pets and rodents; they may also be isolated from their blood and internal organs. They are found frequently in sewage, river and other waters and soil in which they do not multiply significantly. Under suitable environmental conditions, they may survive for weeks in waters and for years in soil. They have been isolated from many of the foods, including vegetables and fruit, used by humans (Rampling 1990, Report 1993) and are important contaminants of animal protein-feed supplements.

Some serotypes are adapted to specific hosts, e.g. Abortusovis, Gallinarum, Typhi and Typhisuis are confined respectively to sheep, fowl, humans and swine (or closely related species). The majority, however, are ubiquitous serotypes inhabiting a wide range of hosts. Members of subsp. *enterica* predominate among mammals; those from other subspecies are isolated infrequently from, and are rarely pathogenic for, humans and other mammals. Serotypes from subspp. *salamae*, *arizonae*, *diarizonae* and *houtenae* are found commonly in the intestinal tract of cold-blooded animals.

5 MORPHOLOGY

The morphology of salmonellae is similar to that of other enterobacteria. With the exception of Gallinarum-Pullorum, they are motile by peritrichous flagella. Non-motile strains may be isolated from clinical cases.

Most salmonellae form common fimbriae (see Chapter 39) and most fimbriate strains (80%) possess type-1 fimbriae associated with mannose-sensitive adhesive properties (Duguid, Anderson and Campbell 1966, Duguid and Old 1980). These fimbriae are composed of fimbrillin subunits (MW c. 21 kDa) containing a high proportion (40%) of hydrophobic amino acids. Failure to form type-1 fimbriae is the rule in some serotypes, e.g. Paratyphi A, Gallinarum-Pullorum and is unusual in others, e.g. Paratyphi B, Typhi and Typhimurium (Duguid et al. 1975, Duguid and Old 1980, 1994). Strains of Gallinarum-Pullorum form type-2 fimbriae which are morphologically and antigenically like type-1 fimbriae but non-adhesive (Duguid, Anderson and Campbell 1966, Crichton et al. 1989, Duguid and Old 1994).

Some strains of serotypes such as Enteritidis and Typhimurium that are usually type-1 fimbriate produce thin fimbriae (<3 nm diameter) the presence of which renders them O-inagglutinable (Rohde et al. 1975). Originally described as non-adhesive, they agglutinate tannic acid-treated red blood cells (Adegbola, Old and Aleksic 1983) and behave like type-3 fimbriae commonly present in Klebsielleae and Proteeae (Old and Adegbola 1985). Other kinds of thin fimbriae produced by strains of Enteritidis include 'SEF 14KDα' fimbriae which, unlike type-3 fimbriae, are non-haemagglutinating; thin aggregative fimbriae may also be produced by Enteritidis strains (see Clegg and Swenson 1994). About one-third of strains of subspp. *arizonae* and *diarizonae* and a few strains of subsp. *salamae* also produce thin fimbriae which, though they agglutinate tanned red blood cells, are probably not type-3 fimbriae (see Adegbola, Old and Aleksic 1983).

Strains of serotypes Salinatis and Sendai produce mannose-resistant and eluting haemagglutinins (MREHAs) which, though common in *Escherichia coli* (Duguid et al. 1955), are rare in salmonellae. MREHA production by Salinatis and Sendai is associated with thin (3.6 nm diameter) and thick (13.6 nm diameter) fimbriae, respectively (Old, Yakubu and Senior 1989, Yakubu, Senior and Old 1989).

6 CULTURAL CHARACTERS AND GROWTH REQUIREMENTS

Salmonellae grow over a wide temperature range from 7 to 48°C, at pH 4–8 and at water activities above 0.93 (Baird-Parker 1991). Under special conditions, they may proliferate at <4°C (d'Aoust 1991) and withstand extremes of pH <4 (Foster 1992). In aerobic and anaerobic conditions, salmonellae grow readily on ordinary media, producing colonies indistinguishable from those of other Enterobacteriaceae. Simple carbon compounds can be used as a source of carbon and energy and a wide range of nitrogenous compounds as nitrogen source on first isolation or after adaptation. Most salmonellae are prototrophic and grow in minimal salts medium with a suitable carbon source. Auxotrophic serotypes adapted to a single host species (see above) will grow on a minimal medium supplemented with appropriate growth factor(s). Auxotrophic strains of prototrophic serotypes are not uncommon, e.g. c. 7% of Typhimurium strains (Duguid et al. 1975).

Some serotypes of salmonellae, particularly Paratyphi B, produce mucoid colonies best developed at low temperature, low humidity and high osmolarity (Anderson and Rogers 1963). The presence of a mucoid surface layer, the M antigen of Kauffmann, inhibits O and H agglutinability. Because the M antigen is identical in all salmonella serotypes and is like the colanic acid materials of other Enterobacteriaceae, it is unimportant diagnostically. The 'mucoid-wall test' is positive with most strains of Paratyphi B that cause enteric fever (Kauffmann 1966).

7 SUSCEPTIBILITY TO CHEMICAL AGENTS

Many observations on the resistance of salmonellae to different chemical substances have been derived from attempts to devise enrichment and selective media for the isolation of salmonellae from samples containing other coliform bacilli. The use of dyes, particularly those of the triphenylmethane group, as inhibitors has been well defined since the early 1900s when malachite green and later brilliant green were used. Brilliant green-containing media are useful for the isolation of most serotypes other than Typhi. RV medium, a modification by Vassiliadis et al. (1981) of the original Rappaport medium, in which the concentration of malachite green was reduced to 0.004% w/v, is considered superior to other enrichment media. Tetrathionate broth, especially the modification of Kauffmann–Müller containing brilliant green and 0.018 M tetrathionate, is useful for a wide range of serotypes including Dublin, but not for Typhi which is best recovered through selenite broth.

Many salmonellae multiply at 43°C and incubation of enrichment media such as selenite or RV broths at that temperature is recommended for the isolation of salmonellae. Solid media containing bile salts or pure sodium deoxycholate, often in the presence of other inhibitory substances, are generally used as selective plating media. Bismuth sulphite agar, often recommended for Typhi, is perhaps even more useful for the detection of lactose-fermenting salmonellae. Many other media based on the action of yet other inhibitory substances have been devised though few are in use today. For a discussion of the use and choice of these media and modifications of those described above, the authoritative review of Fricker (1987) is invaluable (see also Volume 3, Chapters 24 and 28).

8 SUSCEPTIBILITY TO ANTIMICROBIAL AGENTS

Until about 1960 nearly all salmonellae were sensitive to a wide range of antimicrobial agents but since 1962 resistance, frequently plasmid mediated, has appeared in salmonellae world wide. The relative importance of antibiotic resistance, and the serotypes in which it occurs, differs from country to country. For example, in developed countries in western Europe such as the UK, resistance is common in serotypes associated with bovine animals, e.g. Typhimurium, but is relatively uncommon in serotypes associated with poultry, e.g. Enteritidis. It must also be realized that within Typhimurium, resistance may be concentrated in a relatively few phage types, often associated with bovine animals, e.g. definitive phage types (DTs) 29, 204c and 104, whilst remaining uncommon in phage types associated with poultry, e.g. DTs 9, 10 and 12 (Palmer and Rowe 1986, Frost, Threlfall and Rowe 1995). By contrast, in many developing countries resistance is found in several serotypes that are almost invariably linked to severe outbreaks of salmonellosis in humans without obvious animal involvement.

8.1 Developed countries

The question of whether antibiotic resistance in non-typhoidal salmonellas associated with food animals is a human public health problem in developed countries has been a contentious issue since the late 1960s. In the UK, following concern about the increasing incidence of multiresistance (to 4 or more antimicrobial agents) in strains of salmonellae, particularly Typhimurium DT 29 in humans and bovine animals (Anderson 1968), the Joint Committee on the Use of Antibiotics in Animal Husbandry and Veterinary Medicine (the Swann Committee) recommended in 1969 that certain therapeutic antibiotics, at that time widely used in food animals without prescription, should be available only on prescription (Anonymous 1969). A further recommendation of the Swann Committee was that certain antibiotics should be reserved specifically for prophylaxis and therapy and should not be used for growth promotion. By 1970, DT 29 had disappeared from bovine animals in Britain and for the next 6 years <8% of isolations of Typhimurium from cattle and 3% of isolations from humans were multiresistant (Rowe and Threlfall 1984). However, from 1975 to the mid-1980s there was a substantial upsurge in the occurrence of multiresistant Typhimurium strains in humans and food animals, particularly calves. The phage types involved were different from those that caused outbreaks in the 1960s, with the related DTs 204, 193 and 204c predominating (Threlfall, Ward and Rowe 1978, Threlfall et al. 1980, 1985). A feature of this outbreak was the sequential acquisition of plasmids and transposons coding for a wide range of antimicrobial agents, e.g. ampicillin (A), chloramphenicol (C), gentamicin (G), kanamycin (K), streptomycin (S), sulphonamides (Su), tetracyclines (T) and trimethoprim (Tm). The acquisition of resistance by strains of these phage types seemed to coincide with the introduction and use of at least some of the antimicrobial agents in attempts to combat infections in calves by Typhimurium strains resistant to an increasing range of antibiotics (reviewed by Rowe and Threlfall 1984). This epidemic also provided the first conclusive evidence of the introduction and use, in calf husbandry, of a veterinary aminoglycoside antibiotic (apramycin) giving rise to resistance to gentamicin, a related antibiotic which is used for treating severe systemic infections in humans (Threlfall et al. 1985, 1986). Over the next 5 years the incidence of drug resistance in both human and bovine isolates of Typhimurium continued to rise (Ward, Threlfall and Rowe 1990, Threlfall, Rowe and Ward 1993), and the Expert Group on Animal Feedingstuffs (The Lamming Committee) recommended not only that antibiotics giving cross-resistance to those used in human medicine should not be used as growth promoters, but also that their prophylactic use in animals should be reconsidered (Anonymous 1992a).

Since 1991 there has been a further substantial increase in the incidence of both resistance and multiple resistance in Typhimurium strains in England and Wales. In 1994, 78% of isolations from humans were resistant to at least one antimicrobial agent and 62% were multiresistant (Frost, Threlfall and Rowe 1995). Of particular importance in this increase in the incidence of multiresistance in Typhimurium since 1991 has been an epidemic in cattle and humans in England and Wales of multiresistant strains of DT 104 of R-type ACSSuT. In contrast to DTs 29 and 204c, all resistance genes in DT 104 are inserted in the chromo-some (Threlfall et al. 1994a). Furthermore, since 1992 there has been an increasing number of isolates of DT 104 which, as well as possessing chromosomally encoded resistance to ACSSuT, have also acquired plasmid mediated resistance to sulphonamides and trimethoprim (R-type ACSSuTTm) (Threlfall et al. 1996a). A further development in 1995 was the substantial increase in multiresistant DT 104 with additional chromosomally encoded resistance to ciprofloxacin (MIC 0.250 mg l^{-1}), which is now the drug of choice for the treatment of invasive salmonellosis in humans.

In other developed countries multiple antibiotic resistance has been reported in a number of serotypes from food animals. For example, in the USA, multiple resistance has been reported in Saintpaul, Heidelberg, Newport and Typhimurium (Neu et al. 1975) and such resistance has been attributed to the use of antibiotics in animal feeds. In general, however, such resistance is relatively uncommon in the majority of developed countries. As antibiotics are not recommended for the treatment of mild to moderate salmonella-induced enteritis in humans, it may be argued that in developed countries drug resistance in non-typhoidal salmonellas is of little consequence to human public health. However, antibiotics are used for the treatment of salmonellosis in immunocompromised patients and sometimes for treating particularly vulnerable patients; in such cases treatment with an appropriate antibiotic is often essential and may be life-saving. Thus, it would appear that in developed countries, and particularly in the UK, the injudicious use of antibiotics in food animals has encouraged the spread and persistence of multiresistant salmonellas in these animals. This has undoubtedly contributed to the overall occurrence of such strains in humans and has also resulted in the appearance and spread of strains resistant to antibiotics used for the treatment of invasive disease in humans.

8.2 Developing countries

In developed countries the most common presentation in patients with salmonellosis is mild to moderate gastroenteritis. The disease is normally self-limiting with <2% of infections being extraintestinal (Threlfall, Hall and Rowe 1992a) and mortality is <0.5%. Nosocomial outbreaks are uncommon and the majority of infections are related to the consumption of infected food. The majority of strains have food-animal reservoirs and the most common serotypes involved are Enteritidis, Typhimurium and Virchow. By contrast, in developing countries, particularly in South America, Africa, the Indian subcontinent and South East Asia, the most common presentation is that of severe gastroenteritis often accompanied by septicaemia (up to 40% in some outbreaks) and with up to 30% mortality. Nosocomial outbreaks are common and the main method of transmission is by person-to-person spread either in hospitals or in the community. The strains involved are invariably multiresistant, often with resistance to up to

9 antimicrobial agents. With the exception of resistance to furazolidone and, since 1990, to nalidixic acid, resistances are invariably plasmid encoded. Examples of outbreaks caused by such multiresistant strains are shown in Table 41.1.

A particular property of the majority of these multiresistant strains is the possession of a plasmid of the F_1me incompatibility group coding not only for multiple resistance but also for production of the hydroxamate siderophore aerobactin, which is a known virulence factor for some enteric and urinary tract pathogens. These plasmids, first identified in Typhimurium DT 208 which caused numerous epidemics in many Middle Eastern countries in the 1970s (Anderson et al. 1977a), were subsequently identified in a strain of Wien responsible for a massive epidemic that began in Algiers in 1969 but spread rapidly thereafter through paediatric and nursery populations in many countries throughout North Africa, Western Europe, the Middle East and eventually the Indian subcontinent over the next 10 years (Le Minor 1972, McConnell et al. 1979, Casalino et al. 1984). F_1me plasmids have also been identified in several unrelated phage types of Typhimurium that have caused substantial outbreaks in Africa (Kenya, Liberia), India and Turkey (Frost et al. 1982) (Table 41.1). Although not clinically proven, the epidemiological evidence strongly suggests that possession of the F_1me plasmid has contributed to the exceptional virulence of these epidemic clones.

SALMONELLA TYPHI

An appropriate antibiotic is essential for the treatment of patients with typhoid fever; until the mid-1970s, chloramphenicol was the undisputed drug of choice. Although a few sporadic isolations of chloramphenicol-resistant Typhi had been reported before 1970 (see Anderson and Smith 1972), the first epidemic caused by a chloramphenicol-resistant strain occurred in Mexico in 1972 (Anonymous 1972, Olarte and Galindo 1973). At about that same time, a second substantial outbreak occurred in India (Paniker and Vilma 1972) and in the succeeding 5 years outbreaks were reported in several other countries, notably Vietnam, Indonesia, Korea, Chile and Bangladesh (Anderson 1975). A feature of all chloramphenicol-resistant strains from outbreaks in Mexico, the Indian subcontinent and South East Asia was that, although the strains belonged to different Vi phage types, resistance to chloramphenicol was encoded by a plasmid of the H_1 incompatibility group, and was often found in combination with resistance to streptomycin, sulphonamides and tetracyclines (R-type CSSuT) (Anderson 1975, Threlfall, Rowe and Ward 1991). Since 1989 outbreaks caused by Typhi strains resistant to chloramphenicol, ampicillin and trimethoprim, and with additional resistances to streptomycin, sulphonamides and tetracyclines (R-type ACSSuTTm), have been reported in many developing countries, especially Pakistan and India (Threlfall et al. 1992; reviewed by Rowe, Ward and Threlfall 1997). Multiresistant strains have also caused outbreaks in Bangladesh (Albert et al. 1991), several countries in South East Asia (Tinya-Superable et al. 1995) and in both north and south Africa (Coovadia et al. 1992, Mourad et al. 1993). The recent emergence in developing countries of Typhi strains with resistance to trimethoprim and ampicillin has caused many problems because, since 1980, these antibiotics had been used extensively for the treatment of patients infected with chloramphenicol-resistant Typhi strains (Mandal 1991). Without exception, in all outbreaks involving multiresistant Typhi so far studied, the complete spectrum of multiple resistance has been encoded by plasmids of the H_1 incompatibility group (Rowe, Threlfall and Ward 1991, Threlfall et al. 1992).

Table 41.1 Multiresistant salmonellae in developing countries

Serotype and phage type	Years	Country/area	Resistance patterns[a]
Wien[b]	1970–84	Northern Africa	ACSSuT
		Southern Europe, India	ACSSuTTm
Typhimurium PT 208[b]	1974–84	Middle East	ACSSuT, ACGKSSuT
Johannesburg[b]	1974–78	South Africa	ACKSSuT
Oranienburg[c]	1974–86	Indonesia	ACKSSuT
Typhimurium PT Nc[b]	1976–80	Kenya	ACSSuT
Typhimurium PT Un[b]	1976–80	Liberia	ACKSSuT
Typhimurium PT 66/122[b]	1978–84	India	ACKSSuT, ACGKSSuT, ACGKSSuTTmNx
Bareilly[b,c]	1986–92	India	ACKSSuT
Typhimurium PT Un[b]	1978–94	India	ACKSSuT, ACKSSuTFu, ACGKSSuT, ACGKSSuTTmNx
Typhimurium PT Un	1986–94	Turkey	ACKSSuT, ACGKSSuTTm, ACGKSSuTTmNx

[a]Resistance to: A, ampicillin; C, chloramphenicol; G, gentamicin; K, kanamycin; S, streptomycin; Su, sulphonamides; T, tetracycline; Tm, trimethoprim; Fu, furazolidone; Nx, nalidixic acid.
[b]Outbreak.
[c]Sporadic.
Un, untypable; Nc, not-conforming.

In the UK, resistance to chloramphenicol was rarely encountered until 1990 (Rowe, Threlfall and Ward 1987, Rowe, Ward and Threlfall 1990), but since then Typhi strains resistant not only to chloramphenicol but also to trimethoprim and ampicillin have been isolated with increasing frequency. The majority of these strains have been isolated from travellers with a history of recent return from countries where multi-resistant strains have either caused outbreaks or have become endemic. In all multiresistant Typhi strains isolated in the UK since 1990, resistance to chloramphenicol, ampicillin and trimethoprim, together with resistance to streptomycin and sulphonamides (ACSSuTTm) has been encoded by a plasmid of the H_1 incompatibility group.

Because multiresistant Typhi is now endemic in many developing countries and is also common in travellers returning to developed countries, ciprofloxacin is generally used for the treatment of typhoid in both developing and developed countries (Anand et al. 1990, Mandal 1991). It is therefore a concern that multiresistant Typhi strains with plasmid-encoded resistance to chloramphenicol, ampicillin and trimethoprim and additional chromosomal resistance to ciprofloxacin have been reported (Rowe, Ward and Threlfall 1995).

9 BIOCHEMICAL ACTIVITIES

The common biochemical characters of the salmonellae are shown in Table 41.2 (see p. 975). Although most strains conform closely to this pattern, there are several exceptions; no organism should, therefore, be excluded on the result of a single test. The usual reactions include:

1 fermentation of glucose, maltose, mannitol and sorbitol with the production of acid and gas
2 absence of fermentation of sucrose, salicin and adonitol
3 failure to produce indole, to hydrolyse urea or to deaminate phenylalanine and
4 a positive methyl red reaction and a negative Voges–Proskauer reaction.

It should be noted, however, that members of subsp. *houtenae* acidify salicin and that strains of subsp. *indica* do not acidify sorbitol (Table 41.2). Gas is not formed by Typhi, biotype Gallinarum or by occasional strains of other serotypes; maltose is usually not fermented by biotype Pullorum strains; and Typhisuis does not ferment mannitol. Occasional strains that form acid from lactose, sucrose or raffinose, produce indole, hydrolyse malonate or split urea have been recorded. Some of these atypical properties are plasmid mediated (Le Minor et al. 1974, Buissière, Coynault and Le Minor 1977). The positive reaction to the methyl red test, and the negative reactions to the phenylalanine and Voges–Proskauer tests appear to be constant. Other biochemical characters are variable, and some of them are the means by which *S. enterica* is subdivided into subspecies (Table 41.2). Within subsp.

enterica there are several types that depart from the usual pattern; Table 41.3 shows the reactions of 5 of them, and other examples will be found in the description of individual types at the end of this chapter (pp. 985–990).

Most salmonellae grow with citrate as the sole carbon source though important exceptions include Typhi, Paratyphi A, Typhisuis and Sendai and biotype Pullorum strains of serotype Gallinarum. Most salmonellae also give a positive reaction for H_2S in triple sugar iron agar, but exceptions include strains of Paratyphi A, Choleraesuis (*sensu stricto*), Typhisuis, Sendai, Abortusequi and Berta, as well as a few strains of Typhi. Liquefaction of gelatin, which may be slow or rapid, is characteristic of members from all subspecies other than *enterica* and *S. bongori* (Table 41.2). Nearly all salmonellae produce arginine dihydrolase and lysine and ornithine decarboxylases but not glutamic acid decarboxylase. Notable exceptions are Typhi and biotype Gallinarum strains which fail to decarboxylate ornithine, and Paratyphi A, which does not attack lysine. Fermentation of organic acids is common; most salmonellae of subsp. *enterica* rapidly attack *d*-tartrate, citrate and mucate though there are exceptions. Several types, notably Paratyphi A, Sendai and most enteric fever-causing strains of Paratyphi B are *d*-tartrate negative (see p. 989). Other biochemical reactions that are variable within the *Salmonella* group, and are at times useful for the identification of individual serotypes, or for subdividing them further, have been described in earlier editions of this book.

Screening media for the simultaneous detection of several biochemical reactions are widely used in the routine identification of salmonellae. On triple sugar iron agar they show H_2S production and absence of fermentation of lactose, sucrose and salicin; on lysine iron agar they show the production of H_2S and lysine decarboxylase. The use of screening media is time-saving when appropriately controlled. For further information about the biochemical reactions of salmonellae, see Ewing (1986).

10 ANTIGENIC STRUCTURE

The antigens used to define the serological types of salmonellae include:

1 the O antigens, heat-stable polysaccharides that form part of the cell wall lipopolysaccharide (LPS)
2 the H antigens, heat-labile proteins of the flagella that in salmonellae have the almost unique character of diphasic variation and
3 surface polysaccharides that inhibit the agglutinability of the organisms by homologous O antisera, of which the Vi antigen of Typhi is the most important example (see Volume 3, Chapter 24).

The O polysaccharides have a core structure that is common to all enterobacteria and side chains of sugars attached to the core determine O specificity. Salmonellae may be classified into 'chemotypes' each of which contains organisms with the same sugars in

Table 41.2 Biochemical differentiation of species and subspecies of *Salmonella*

Reaction	Subspecies of *S. enterica*						*S. bongori*
	enterica	*salamae*	*arizonae*	*diarizonae*	*houtenae*	*indica*	
ONPG	−	−	+	+	−	d	+
Gelatinase	−	+	+	+	+	+	−
Galacturonate	−	+	−	+	+	+	+
Growth in KCN	−	−	−	−	+	−	+
Malonate	−	+	+	+	−	−	−
Dulcitol	+	+	−	−	−	d	+
Mucate	+	+	+	d	−	+	+
d-Tartrate	+	−	−	−	−	−	−
γ-Glutamyltransferase	+	+	−	+	+	+	+
β-Glucuronidase	d	d	−	+	−	d	−
Salicin	−	−	−	−	+	−	−
Sorbitol	+	+	+	+	+	−	+

+, >90% of strains positive; −, >90% of strains negative; d, some strains positive, others negative.

Table 41.3 Biochemical reactions of some *Salmonella* serotypes of subsp. *enterica* (subsp. I)

Reaction[a]	Most serotypes	Typhi	Paratyphi A	Choleraesuis	Gallinarum[b]	Pullorum[b]
Gas from sugars	+	−	+	+	−	+
Utilization of citrate	+	−	−	d	+	−
H_2S	+	w	−	−	−	−
Lysine decarboxylase	+	+	−	+	+	+
Ornithine decarboxylase	+	−	+	+	−	+
Motility	+	+	+	+	−	−

[a]For aberrant reactions of other serotypes, see text.
[b]Gallinarum and Pullorum are biotypes of serotype Gallinarum.
−, Negative reaction; +, positive reaction; d, delayed positive reaction; w, weakly positive in triple sugar iron medium.

their side chains. Chemotypes may include salmonellae with different O antigens and in many cases also *E. coli* strains of several O groups and other enterobacteria, but the organisms are serologically distinct because of differences in the sequence of sugars in the side chains, particularly at the distal end. Minor cross-reactions between salmonella O serogroups, and between the O antigens of salmonellae and other members of the Enterobacteriaceae, are quite common. The traditional method of detecting salmonella O antigens is by the agglutination of heated suspensions of organisms by rabbit antisera raised against boiled organisms; known cross-reactions are removed by suitable absorption of the sera.

Some of the H antigens of *Salmonella* are also found in *Citrobacter*; they comprise a large number of factors arranged in different combinations in the different serotypes. In most salmonellae the flagellar antigens exist in 2 alternative phases; to identify a serotype completely it is necessary to determine the antigenic factors present in both phases. For information about the practical identification of serotypes, the reader should consult reference publications (Kauffmann 1966, Ewing 1986, Popoff and Le Minor 1992). An up-to-date list of salmonella serotypes can be obtained from most national salmonella centres. Kelterborn (1967, 1987) gives a comprehensive account of the

first isolation and geographical distribution of nearly 2000 serotypes. Additions to the list of officially recognized serotypes are published annually (see Popoff, Bockemühl and Hickman-Brenner 1995).

10.1 Antigenic notation

The antigenic formula consists of 3 parts, describing the somatic O antigen, the phase-1 H antigen and the phase-2 H antigen, in this order. The 3 parts are separated by colons, and the components of each part by commas. The somatic O antigens are given arabic numerals. The phase-1 H antigens are designated a to z, a series that is complete except for j. H1 antigens described after z are designated as z with subscripts, e.g. z_1 to z_{83}. The phase-2 H antigens are designated by arabic numerals (1–12) but phase 2 may also contain antigenic components of the e series or one of the z series. Some H antigens are phase-specific, others appear in both phases.

Certain somatic factors are present in some members only of a particular serotype. For example, the O factor 5 is absent from many strains of Paratyphi B; this is indicated by placing the factor within a square bracket in the antigenic formula (see Table 41.4). Some somatic factors are underlined; this is because they are determined by the presence of a phage (see below), e.g. O factor 1 in Typhimurium and the factors 15 and 15,34 in Anatum (Table 41.4).

THE KAUFFMANN–WHITE DIAGNOSTIC SCHEME

Primary subdivision is into O serogroups, each of which shares a common somatic antigen. Where more than one O antigen is present, one of them is the major O antigen and is regarded as determining the group to which the strain shall be allocated. O serogroups were formerly designated by letters of the alphabet and some groups were subdivided into subgroups. In this chapter, however, each O serogroup is designated by its characteristic O factor(s) with the letters formerly used to designate the O serogroups shown in parentheses (see Table 41.4). The series of O antigens numbered O1–67 is not continuous because some O antigens were originally assigned to bacteria that proved subsequently not to be salmonellae. Again, some of the 67 O antigens are minor antigens (e.g. O12), which have no discriminatory value; others (e.g. O5) arise by chemical modification of a known major O antigen or are determined by phage conversion. Thus, only 46 O serogroups are defined by the 67 O antigens described (see Lindberg and Le Minor 1984, Popoff and Le Minor 1992).

The serotypes classified in the scheme include members of all subspecies and of *S. bongori*. An antigenic scheme was developed independently from the Kauffmann–White scheme for the characterization of salmonellae of subspp. *arizonae* and *diarizonae* when they were considered to belong to a separate genus ('*Arizona*') distinct from *Salmonella*. It is convenient and sensible to designate the serotypes of all subspecies of *Salmonella* by one set of symbols. Hence, the '*Arizona*' formulae have been deleted from the scheme (Popoff and Le Minor 1992). In the Kauffmann–White scheme, only antigens of diagnostic value are cited. For most purposes a simplified version of the scheme, based on only 12 O, 18 H sera and the Vi serum, gives sufficient information for routine diagnostic identifications (see Ewing 1986).

The distribution of 2399 known salmonella serotypes among the different subspecies is: *enterica* (1416), *salamae* (477), *arizonae* (94), *diarizonae* (317), *houtenae* (66), *indica* (10) and *S. bongori* (19) (Popoff, Bockemühl and Hickman-Brenner 1995). The majority (96.5%) of the serotypes of subsp. *enterica* belong to 6 O serogroups (O4–O1,3,19) and the rest are scattered throughout the remaining serogroups. Most of the serotypes from subspecies other than *enterica* belong to higher O serogroups O11–67, some of which also contain serotypes of *enterica*. Serotypes in subspp. *arizonae* and *houtenae* and *S. bongori* are monophasic.

10.2 Variation in the O antigens

The chemical basis of the smooth-to-rough variation is discussed in Chapter 39. Rough mutant strains can be classified in a series from Ra, which lacks the O-specific side chains only, through Rb to Re which show a progressive loss of sugar constituents from the core. Agglutinability in the presence of 0.3% w/v auramine and heat-stability tests are considered particularly suitable for the differentiation of smooth from rough forms. Although the different rough forms behave similarly in these tests, rough strains of chemotypes Ra–e show steady gradation in their sensitivity to antibiotics, detergents and dyes. Rough variation occurs rarely in nature but is common in strains maintained through many generations on ordinary laboratory media.

LYSOGENIC CONVERSION

The specificities of O antigens may be modified in the process of lysogenic conversion by phages which genetically determine subtle changes in the chemistry of the repeating unit of the polysaccharide (see Lindberg and Le Minor 1984). The new specificities appear in salmonellae within minutes of their infection with phage. The presence of factor O1 in serotypes of groups O2, 4 and 9 is associated with lysogenization by phages such as P22 whereas other phages determine O1 in higher serogroups such as O13, 40, 42 and 51; not all O1 factors, however, e.g. that in group O1,3,19 (Table 41.4), are phage determined.

The sequential conversions by phages ε15 and ε34 of serotypes of serogroup O3,10 (formerly E₁) resulted in the appearance of new specificities designated, respectively, 3,15 and 3,15,34. On the basis of what were minor changes in the structure of the repeating unit of the antigen O3,10, special serogroups (formerly E₂ and E₃) were established and the sequentially lysogenized variants of serotypes of serogroup E₁ were given new serotype names. Thus, when Anatum (3,10:e,h:1.6) was lysogenized with phage ε15 it became Newington (3,15:e,h:1,6) which in turn, when lysogenized by ε34 became Minneapolis (3,15,34:e,h:1,6). The serotype Anatum is now designated as 3,10[15],[15,34]:e,h:1,6 and its variants are not named. Although serotype names for the lysogenized variants of extant serotypes have been deleted from the current list of *Salmonella* serotypes (Popoff and Le Minor 1992), not all *Salmonella* reference laboratories have adopted that protocol. Phage conversions responsible for many other O antigen modifications are of little, or no, diagnostic significance and have been discussed in earlier editions.

PLASMID CONVERSION

The first observation of changes in the specificities of O antigens of *Salmonella* resulting from plasmid conversion was made with regard to O54. The serotype Tonev (21,54:b:e,n,x) contains a small plasmid, loss of which results in failure to express factor O54; thus, the plasmidless variant becomes (21:b:e,n,x), i.e. Minnesota of group O21 (Popoff and Le Minor 1985). Although strains of the other 12 serotypes of serogroup O54 contain plasmids similar to that of Tonev, plasmidless variants not expressing O54 could be derived from only 8 of them; the latter O54⁻ variants were indistinguishable from serotypes already classified in other O serogroups. Some serotypes of serogroup O54, therefore, should be deleted from the scheme; thus, if Minnesota could be redefined as 21,54:b:e,n,x in a style analogous to that used for lysogenized variants, the serotype Tonev could be suppressed. But some problems remain. With the loss of expression of O54 by Winnipeg (54:e,h:1,5), a new factor (O8) not normally expressed by that serotype appears and it is thereby converted to Ferruch (8:e,h:1,5). Neither of these serotypes, however, produces the other's O-determining antigen, i.e. strains of serotype (8,54:e,h:1,5) have not been

Table 41.4 Illustration of the Kauffmann White scheme of serological classification

O serogroup[a]	Serotype[b]	O antigens[c]	H antigens Phase 1	H antigens Phase 2
2 (A)	Paratyphi A	1,2,12	a	[1,5]
4 (B)	Paratyphi B	1,4,[5],12	b	1,2
	Stanley	1,4,[5],12,27	d	1,2
	Schwarzengrund	1,4,12,27	d	1,7
	Saintpaul	1,4,[5],12	e,h	1,2
	Derby	1,4,[5],12	f,g	[1,2]
	Agona	1,4,12	f,g,s	[1,2]
	Typhimurium	1,4,[5],12	i	1,2
	Bredeney	1,4,12,27	l,v	1,7
	Brandenburg	1,4,[5],12,27	l,v	e,n,z$_{15}$
	Heidelberg	1,4,[5],12	r	1,2
7 (C$_1$)	Choleraesuis	6,7	c	1,5
	Paratyphi C	6,7[Vi]	c	1,5
	Livingstone	6,7,14	d	l,w
	Montevideo	6,7,14	g,m,[p],s	[1,2,7]
	Thompson	6,7,14	k	1,5
	Virchow	6,7	r	1,2
	Infantis	6,7,14	r	1,5
	Mbandaka	6,7,14	z$_{10}$	e,n,z$_{15}$
8 (C$_2$–C$_3$)	Muenchen	6,8	d	1,2
	Newport	6,8,20	e,h	1,2
	Hadar	6,8	z$_{10}$	e,n,x
9 (D$_1$)	Typhi	9,12[Vi]	d	–
	Enteritidis	1,9,12	g,m	[1,7]
	Dublin	1,9,12[Vi]	g,p	–
	Panama	1,9,12	l,v	1,5
	Gallinarum	1,9,12	–	–
3, 10 (E$_1$)	Anatum	3,10,[15],[15,34]	e,h	1,6
1, 3, 19 (E$_4$)	Senftenberg	1,3,19	g,[s],t	–
11 (F)	Rubislaw	11	r	e,n,x
13 (G)	Kedougou	1,13,23	i	l,w
6, 14 (H)	VI	1,6,14,25	a	e,n,x
16 (I)	II	16	g,[m],[s],t	[e,n,x]
18 (K)	IIIa	18	z$_4$,z$_{32}$	–
21 (L)	IIIb	21	i	1,5,7
43 (U)	IV	43	z$_4$,z$_{23}$	–
48 (Y)	V	48	z$_{35}$	–
60	IIIb	60	r	e,n,x,z$_{15}$
61	IIIb	61	k	1,5,[7]

[a]Some serogroups were formerly designated by letters indicated in parentheses.
[b]Serotypes of *S. enterica* subsp. *enterica* are named; others are designated by antigenic formula only in other subspecies of *S. enterica* (II, *salamae*; IIIa, *arizonae*; IIIb, *diarizonae*; IV, *houtenae*; and VI, *indica*) and in *S. bongori* (V).
[c]Somatic factors associated with phage conversion are underlined, e.g. 14.
['x'] Antigen 'x' not present in all strains of serotype.

described in nature. Thus, Winnipeg should be retained as well as the names of 4 other serotypes from which O54⁻ variants have not yet been derived. The heterogeneous group O54 has been retained provisionally in the current scheme (Popoff and Le Minor 1992).

Form variants may show complete or partial loss of O antigen, e.g. somatic antigen O5 is not present in all cultures of Paratyphi B or Typhimurium and, hence, is designated as [5] (Table 41.4). Form and other variants, e.g. T (transient) forms, have been discussed in earlier editions of this book.

10.3 Variation in the H antigens

Most serotypes of *Salmonella* (of subspecies other than *arizonae* and *houtenae* and *S. bongori*) show the phenomenon of diphasic variation, i.e. they express alternately 2 kinds of flagella with different antigenic specificities. Typhimurium, for example, produces flagella of antigenic specificity i in phase 1 and of specificity 1,2 in phase 2. Salmonellae switch phases at characteristic frequencies and the transition can be induced in the laboratory by their cultivation in semi-solid agar containing antiserum against phase-1 or phase-2 flagellar antigens. Thus, growth of phase-2$^+$ Typhimurium in the presence of H-antiserum 1,2 induces transition to phase 1 and selects bacteria expressing flagella of i specificity.

The major components of the flagellar filaments are highly antigenic proteins called flagellins which are encoded by 2 independent, chromosomally located genes (*fliC*) (phase 1) and *fljB* (phase 2). Salmonellae in phase 1 express flagellin of the *fliC* gene and in phase 2 express flagellin of the *fljB* gene along with an associated repressor of the phase-1 gene (coded by the *fljA* gene). The regulation of the phase switching is complex but depends on a recombinational event involving a specific invertible sequence of DNA (970 bp long) that contains the promoter region of the phase-2 operon. With this invertible sequence in one orientation, the promoter is correctly positioned to allow reading of the *fljB* gene along with the repressor (from *fljA*) that switches off the phase-1 gene. In its other orientation, the phase-2 gene cannot be read, the repressor of phase-1 gene is not formed and so flagella with phase-1 antigenicity are formed. The invertible region also determines the frequency of inversion and, hence, of phase variation and functions essentially as a 'flip-flop' switch; it is related, therefore, to similar sequences involved in other phase-variable systems (see Silverman and Simon 1980).

Some serotypes of *Salmonella* are usually monophasic, expressing in nature flagella of only one phase, e.g. Paratyphi A (1,2,12:a: -). The growth of Paratyphi A in the presence of H antiserum a induces flagella with antigens 1,5 characteristic of phase 2. Thus, in the Kauffmann–White scheme Paratyphi A is written 1,2,12:a:[1,5] (Table 41.4). On the other hand, when Abortusequi (4,12: - :e,n,x), a natural serotype monophasic in phase 2, is cultivated in the presence of H antiserum, e,n,x, variants with phase-1 flagella of specificity a are selected that are monophasic in phase 1, and as stable as the naturally occurring phase-2 monophasic strain; it requires culture in H antiserum a to induce reversion to the common phase-2 only type. Natural serotypes fixed in one H phase are known to be associated with mutations linked to regulatory genes.

Other serotypes, such as Typhi (9,12:d: -), appear to be monophasic and most populations encode flagellin of phase 1 with d antigenic specificity. Culture of Typhi in the presence of H antiserum d selects variants with a different phase-1 specificity of the j type. These uncommon phase-1 (R-phase) variants occasionally arise in nature, e.g. some Typhi populations from Indonesia form a variant phase-1 j allele which arises as a result of a deletion of a portion of 261 bp from the central region of the phase-1 flagellin gene (Frankel et al. 1989). An interesting example of R-phase H antigens arising in nature (Guinée et al. 1981) comes from a series of isolates in Indonesia in 1979–80 from patients who had authentic typhoid fever, were biochemically typical of Typhi but were unreactive in the H antisera d and j (R) previously associated with Typhi. These isolates possessed a new flagellar antigen z$_{66}$, thought to be encoded by a phase-2 locus (Selander et al. 1990b), and when they were grown in the presence of H antiserum z$_{66}$, gave rise to variants with the d or j specificities usually associated with the phase-1

flagella of Typhi. This is important diagnostically because that strain of Typhi, which is restricted to Indonesia, was Vi unreactive and gave negative reactions in the Widal test with standard d suspensions.

NEW FLAGELLAR ANTIGENS

Comparison of the nucleotide sequences of the phase-1 flagellin locus (*fliC*) of strains of 5 serotypes – Paratyphi A (specificity a), Choleraesuis (c), Muenchen (d), Typhimurium (i) and Rubislaw (r) – showed that the terminal parts of the genes are highly conserved (Wei and Joys 1985, 1986) probably because of their importance in polymerization and secretion of the flagellin proteins. The central region of the gene is highly variable with marked differences in length and sequence and yet without impairment of flagellar motility; the central region of the gene, which determines the major antigenic epitopes of the flagellin exposed in the flagellar surface, is subject to little or no functional constraint. Do new flagellar antigens arise, therefore, by random mutational drift in these flagellin genes? If so, then variations in their nucleotide sequences might be expected even among strains within a serotype.

When the central regions of the genes coding for phase-1 flagellin of i specificity were sequenced for 6 strains of Typhimurium of different genetic backgrounds (i.e. of different electrophoretic types (ETs) as judged by MLEE), they were invariant (Smith and Selander 1990). Similarly, the sequences of the central parts of the phase-1 flagellin of strains of serotype Heidelberg with antigenic specificity of the r type were also invariant (Smith, Beltran and Selander 1990). Thus, the *fliC* genes are not evolving by sequence drift at unusually high rates.

The serotypes Heidelberg (1,4,[5]12:r:1,2) and Typhimurium (1,4,[5]12:i:1,2), which are indistinguishable other than by their phase-1 flagellins, are genetically close (genetic distance 0.2, as determined by MLEE), yet the *fliC* alleles (r and i) show considerable divergence with a 19% nucleotide sequence difference (Selander and Smith 1990). Likewise, strains of Typhimurium and Muenchen (which have a genetic distance of only 0.22 despite belonging to different O serogroups) showed a 50% difference in the nucleotide sequence in the *fliC* genes coding for phase-1 flagellins of antigenic types i and d.

By contrast, the sequences of the *fliC* genes coding for phase-1 flagella of antigenic specificity i in serotypes from different subspecies (Typhimurium in *enterica* and an O48$^+$ serotype in *arizonae*) that are distantly related (genetic distance of 0.72) showed at the chromosomal level a small difference of 2.2% in their phase-1 (i) alleles; likewise strains of serotypes Muenchen and Typhi (with a genetic distance of 0.47) had phase-1 (d) alleles that differed in nucleotide sequence by only 1.3% (Smith, Beltran and Selander 1990). The existence of flagellin genes that are almost identical in serotypes that are genetically unrelated is best explained by the horizontal transfer of these genes; their recombination after transfer provides an explanation of new flagellar antigen combinations. Phage mediated transfer of genetic material, demonstrated for salmonellae by Zinder and Lederberg (1952), seems the most likely method.

TRIPHASIC STRAINS

Occasional strains of *Salmonella* are found in nature that express 3 or more antigenically distinct kinds of flagella (Ewing 1986). It has long been known that when triphasic serotypes, such as Montgomery or Salinatis (now deleted from the Kauffmann–White scheme), were grown in H antiserum d, normal diphasic variants (11:a:e,n,z$_{15}$, and 1,4,12,27:e,h:e,n,z$_{15}$, respectively) were obtained from which the third flagellar antigen type d was irreversibly lost (Edwards, Kauffmann and Huey 1957). Recent genetic analysis has shown that a triphasic variant of serotype Rubislaw has, in addition to the phase-1 (*fliC*) and phase-2 (*fljB*) genes (r and e,n,x, respectively) of Rubislaw, a third flagellin gene (*flpA*) carried on a large plasmid (Smith and Selander 1991). The gene *flpA* contained a central region coding for a phase-1 antigen (d) coupled with a phase-2 promoter. In phase 2, the triphasic variant expressed its real phase-2 flagellin (e,n,x) and one (d) normally associated with phase-1 flagella. Growth of the triphasic isolate in the presence of H antiserum d gave a diphasic variant indistinguishable from Rubislaw expressing the normal phase-1 and 2 flagellar antigens (r:e,n,x) of that serotype; the *flpA* gene had been completely deleted from the plasmid (Smith and Selander 1991). When the deletion of the *flpA* gene from the plasmid was incomplete, an antigenic variant (j) of the d allele was formed in variants that were still triphasic. The existence of similar large plasmids carrying phase-1 flagellin (d) genes in distantly related triphasic serotypes (including Salinatis) in different *Salmonella* subspecies is strong evidence that horizontal transfer of flagellar genes has occurred. With their subsequent recombination new flagellar antigens are formed (Selander and Smith 1990, Smith and Selander 1991).

Non-motile strains of salmonellae may occasionally be found with flagella that are antigenically and morphologically like those of the motile parent strains. The failure of Mot⁻ strains to rotate the flagella is thought to be associated with defects in the mechanism of energy transduction (MacNab 1987). Flagellate salmonellae may give rise to non-flagellate H⁻ strains to which it is difficult to assign serotype names.

Strains of Gallinarum-Pullorum (1,9,12: - : -) are permanently non-flagellate salmonellae from which spontaneous reversions to motility have not been reported. However, in transduction experiments they have been shown to carry factors determining phase-1 flagellar antigens of the g,m type, like serotype Enteritidis (1,9,12:g,m: -). Sequencing studies have shown that the phase-1 (*fliC*) flagellin gene in most strains of Gallinarum is complete and identical to that of Enteritidis (g,m), and that in strains from 3 other Gallinarum ETs (Gal,2,2a) there was a stop codon (position 495) towards the distal part of the gene (Li et al. 1993). On the other hand, the sequence of the *fliC* gene of strains of Pullorum from different ETs differed from that of Enteritidis by having 2–3 non-synonymous substitutions in the central part of the gene and a synonymous substitution at its end; thus, if ever expressed, the flagellar specificities of Pullorum might well be other than g,m (Li et al. 1993). Similarly, the few strains of Gallinarum-Pullorum analysed seem to have complete genes encoding the flagellar-hook protein (*flgK*) that are similar to that of Enteritidis. Thus, the genetic basis of the non-motility of these strains is as yet unclear but it has been speculated that it is due to a mutation in a gene (e.g. *fliA*) of the flagellar regulon (Li et al. 1993).

10.4 Vi antigen

Vi is a capsular polysaccharide of α-(1→4)-linked *N*-acetyl-D-galactosaminouronic acid, variably acetylated at C2/C3 positions (Daniels et al. 1989); it prevents immune serum mediated killing, is antiphagocytic (by inhibiting binding of C3b and antibodies to LPS) and increases resistance to peroxide. The rate of synthesis and cell-association properties of Vi are determined by structural (*viaB*) and functional (*viaA*) elements at

distinct chromosomal sites (Makela and Stocker 1969).

Felix and Pitt (1934) demonstrated that Typhi strains cultured from the blood of patients with typhoid fever were inagglutinable in O9 serum, showed that the virulence of O-inagglutinable strains of Typhi was greater for mice than O-agglutinable strains and proposed the name Vi (virulence) antigen for the implicated surface structure. The virulence and protective roles of Vi were established by the following observations:

1 Vi⁺ strains of Typhi (and Paratyphi C) have a lower LD50 for mice than Vi⁻ strains

2 active immunization with Vi from Typhi, or other serotypes, protects mice against subsequent challenge with Typhi (but not Paratyphi C)

3 a higher incidence of disease, including bacteraemia and fever, is seen in volunteers challenged with Vi⁺ Typhi strains than with Vi⁻ strains

4 isolates of Typhi and Paratyphi C from the blood of patients with typhoid or enteric fever are invariably Vi⁺ and

5 Vi vaccine prepared under non-degrading conditions gives excellent protection in controlled trials in areas with high attack rates of typhoid fever (see Felix and Pitt 1934, Robbins and Robbins 1984, Tacket et al. 1986, Klugman et al. 1987, Daniels et al. 1989).

Vi is produced by strains of 3 salmonella serotypes – Typhi, Paratyphi C and Dublin – that are genetically distant. The presence of *via* genes in all but a few (c. 1%) strains of Typhi and Paratyphi C suggests that Vi is a property long established in these serotypes; by contrast, production of Vi by Dublin strains is restricted to Du1, a clone of limited geographical distribution, that may have acquired it recently by horizontal transfer of *via* genes (Selander et al. 1990b). Strains rich in Vi form opaque colonies but the amount of Vi present in different strains and serotypes varies considerably; thus, continued laboratory culture of Vi⁺ strains may lead to loss of Vi production. Again, isolates of Paratyphi C, 50% of which are phenotypically Vi⁻, produce less Vi per cell than Typhi, release it more rapidly into the medium and show a higher frequency of reversion from Vi⁺ to Vi⁻ than Typhi (Daniels et al. 1989). Rare strains of *Citrobacter freundii* produce large amounts of cell-associated Vi identical to that of Typhi and Paratyphi C (Daniels et al. 1989) and so are ideal sources of Vi antigen and useful for the preparation of Vi antiserum (Ewing 1986). An invertible insertion sequence located within *viaB* is responsible for variable expression of Vi by *C. freundii* strains (Snellings et al. 1981).

In the absence of positive cultures from patients with typhoid fever, other methods are needed to confirm the diagnosis. The detection of serum antibodies to LPS, flagella and Vi antigens forms the basis of the long-established Widal test. A rapid immunoblotting procedure with Enteritidis LPS and Muenchen flagella has been developed that provides same-day diagnostic results (Chart, Ward and Rowe 1995). The performance of this and other established tests for Vi has been reviewed (Chart 1995).

10.5 Fimbrial antigens

Only one of the 5 type-1 fimbrial antigens described in *Salmonella* is common to the type-1 fimbriae of all *Salmonella* serotypes (Duguid and Campbell 1969, Duguid 1985); that common antigen is also present on the type-1 fimbriae of *C. freundii* but not on those of other Enterobacteriaceae (Duguid 1985, Adegbola and Old 1987). Type-1 fimbrial antibodies, which may be produced by a majority of typhoid patients and vaccinees (Brodie 1977), are responsible for many of the false positive reactions obtained in Widal tests (Duguid 1985).

Type-3 fimbriae are commonly formed by many Enterobacteriaceae but not by *E. coli* and by only a few serotypes of *Salmonella* (Adegbola and Old 1983, Old and Adegbola 1985, Clegg and Swenson 1994); the type-3 fimbriae of *Salmonella*, *Enterobacter*, *Klebsiella* and *Yersinia* belong to a single antigenic group, distinct from those of other Enterobacteriaceae (Old and Adegbola 1985). Type-3 fimbriae, when present, render salmonellae O-inagglutinable but may be removed by heating at 100°C for 2.5 h (Rohde et al. 1975).

The ability of many of the novel types of fimbriae described in *Salmonella* (see Clegg and Swenson 1994) to mask other antigens and to give false positive results in serotyping tests is unknown. Nevertheless, consideration of the fimbriation status of salmonellae is important and much of the early work in this area needs reassessment.

11 BACTERIOPHAGE TYPING METHODS

The underlying principle of phage typing is the host specificity of bacteriophages and on this basis several phage typing schemes have been developed for serotypes of clinical or epidemiological importance.

11.1 Typhi

The first phage typing scheme based on the principle of phage adaptation was that developed for the differentiation of Typhi (Craigie and Yen 1938); in this scheme progressive adaptations were made of Vi phage II, which is specific for Vi (capsular) antigen of Typhi (Felix and Pitt 1934), is highly adaptable and shows a high degree of specificity for the last strain on which it has been propagated. The extraordinary adaptation of Vi phage II is due in part to the selection of spontaneously occurring host-range phage mutants by the bacterium and in part to a non-mutational phenotypic modification of phage by the host strain. The mechanisms underlying the Vi type specificity of Typhi have been discussed fully elsewhere (Anderson and Williams 1956).

The method of Vi phage typing was standardized in 1947

(Craigie and Felix 1947) and with further adaptations of Vi phage II, a further 95 types were defined and internationally recognized bringing the total number of Vi phage types to 106 (Edelman and Levine 1986). Vi phage typing is now the internationally accepted method for differentiation of Typhi and the scheme is used in specialized WHO-approved reference centres world wide. The types most widespread and abundant throughout the world are E1 and A, followed by B2, C1, D1 and F1; other less common types are found that are prevalent temporarily or permanently in some countries only, or even within certain geographical areas within a country (Jegathesan 1983). The value of the Vi phage typing method was demonstrated, for example, by investigations of the sudden appearance in the UK in 1990 of multiresistant strains belonging to Vi phage type M1 and associated with patients recently returned from Pakistan (Rowe, Ward and Threlfall 1990). Subsequently, multiresistant strains of Vi phage type E1 have been associated with patients returning from India (Rowe, Ward and Threlfall 1995), where strains of type E1 have caused numerous outbreaks since 1990 (Prakash and Pillai 1992). Again Vi phage typing has linked outbreaks in several countries in the Arabian Gulf to immigrant workers from the Indian subcontinent (Wallace et al. 1993, Mirza, Beeching and Hart 1996).

A serious limitation of the usefulness of Vi phage typing is that one type, usually A or E1, may be so common in a country as to limit the usefulness of epidemiological information. Several attempts have been made to overcome this problem; members of common phage types have been further discriminated by biochemical tests, by the use of a battery of unadapted O phages (Nicolle, Pavlatou and Diverneau 1954) and, more recently, by various molecular methods, e.g. insertion sequence (IS) *200* for Vi phage types E1 and M1 (Threlfall et al. 1993b) and pulsed field gel electrophoresis (PFGE) (Thong et al. 1994).

11.2 Other serotypes

In contrast to the phage typing scheme for Typhi, which is based primarily on adaptations of bacteriophage Vi II, phage typing schemes for other serotypes depend to a limited extent on phage adaptability and, for the most part, are based on patterns of lysis produced by serologically distinct phages isolated from a variety of sources. In addition to Typhi, other serotypes for which published phage typing schemes are in routine use in the UK include: Paratyphi B (Felix and Callow 1943, 1951), Typhimurium (Callow 1959, Anderson 1964), Hadar (de Sa, Ward and Rowe 1980), Enteritidis (Ward, de Sa and Rowe 1987) and Virchow (Chambers et al. 1987). More than 50 phage types are now recognized in the Enteritidis scheme, the value of which was realized on an international scale following the global pandemic of Enteritidis from the late 1980s to the early 1990s. For the Typhimurium scheme, 232 phage types were designated (Anderson et al. 1977b) and a further 40 types have been recognized subsequently. Supplementary schemes have been developed in several countries to discriminate Typhimurium strains untypable by conventional typing schemes. Again, phage typing schemes have been developed, as required, for several other serotypes which became predominant in particular areas, e.g. a phage typing scheme for Agona was developed in the UK in the 1980s when isolations of Agona were at a high level (LR Ward, unpublished), but the scheme was not put into effect until 1995 following an international outbreak associated with a contaminated kosher snack imported into the UK and the USA from Israel (Anonymous 1995). Several phage typing schemes in use in different countries of the EU are now being rationalized as part of an international collaborative venture for salmonella surveillance (Fisher et al. 1994).

It is important to realize that phage types cannot always be regarded as indicative of clonality because phage type conversions may result from the acquisition of both plasmids (Anderson and Lewis 1965, Anderson et al. 1973, Threlfall, Ward and Rowe 1978, Barker 1986, Frost, Ward and Rowe 1989) and bacteriophages (Threlfall et al. 1980, Rankin and Platt 1995).

12 BIOTYPING

Subdividing common salmonella serotypes according to their biochemical characters is sometimes of value in epidemiological investigations. In many serotypes there are few biochemical tests in which significant numbers of strains behave differently and so the number of identifiable biotypes is small. But, when available, biotyping is a useful adjunct to phage typing for it can subdivide a large group of untypable strains or members of common phage types (as in Typhi).

Its usefulness has been greatest in studying the epidemiology of infections with Typhimurium for which Duguid et al. (1975) developed a biotyping scheme based on the use of 15 biochemical characters. Thirty-two potential primary biotypes were defined by the possible combinations of positive and negative reactions in the 5 tests most discriminating for this serotype: D-xylose, m-inositol, L-rhamnose, d- and m-tartrates; primary biotypes were designated by numbers (1–32) and full biotypes by appending to these numbers letters which indicated results in 10 secondary tests. To date representatives of 24 primary and 184 full biotypes have been identified. In different studies the system has afforded a high degree of discrimination and the biotype characters have proved remarkably stable (Duguid et al. 1975, Anderson et al. 1978, Barker and Old 1979, 1980, 1989, Barker, Old and Sharp 1980, Old and Barker 1989).

When biotyping was used in conjunction with phage typing, each system complemented the other and combined data allowed characterization of 574 different 'phage biotypes' among >2000 strains of Typhimurium (Anderson et al. 1978). Strains of several phage types could be subdivided by biotype; thus, strains of phage type 141 included representatives of 3 distinct, yet stable, biotypes 1f, 9f and 31bd (Barker and Old 1979), probably reflecting the acquisition of the same phage type-determining character by different biotype lines of the serotype. Furthermore, strains of several biotypes were found that had diversified in phage type by acquisition of different phage type-determining characters. Combined phage type–biotype studies help:

1 to determine with greater confidence the fine relationships among strains

2 to characterize variants that arise from a strain in the course of its epidemic spread and

3 to indicate likely phage type interconversions (Anderson et al. 1978, Barker, Old and Sharp 1980, Barker 1986).

Modified versions of the Typhimurium biotyping scheme have been successfully applied to the epidemiology of other salmonella serotypes: Agona (Barker, Old and Tyc 1982), Livingstone (Old, Porter-Boveri and Munro 1994, Crichton, Old et al. 1996), Montevideo (Reilly et al. 1985) and Paratyphi B (Barker et al. 1988).

13 MOLECULAR TYPING METHODS

A range of molecular typing methods based on characterization of the genotype of the organism by analysis of plasmid and chromosomal DNA has now been developed either to supplement the more traditional phenotypic methods of typing (serotyping, phage typing, biotyping) or, in some cases, as methods of discrimination in their own right. Molecular typing methods based on the characterization of plasmid DNA and which have been used for the differentiation of *Salmonella* include plasmid profile typing, plasmid fingerprinting and the identification of plasmid mediated virulence genes. By contrast, more recent methods have sought to identify small regions of heterogeneity within the bacterial chromosome. Five chromosomally based methods have been used for *Salmonella*: ribotyping; random cloned chromosomal sequence (RCCS) typing; insertion sequence (IS) *200* typing; pulsed field gel electrophoresis (PFGE); and polymerase chain reaction (PCR)-based methods such as random amplified polymorphic DNA typing (RAPD), enterobacterial repetitive intergenic consensus typing (ERIC-PCR) and repetitive extragenic palindromic element typing (REP-PCR). The first 3 methods use DNA–DNA hybridization to identify restriction fragment length polymorphisms (RFLPs) following detection of single or multicopy gene sequences across the bacterial genome; the fourth method (PFGE) is a modification of conventional agarose gel electrophoresis (AGE) that permits analysis of the whole bacterial genome on a single gel (see section 13.2, p. 982). The PCR-based methods are based on amplification of specific DNA sequences by PCR to produce characteristic groups of fragments dependent upon the origin of the template DNA. A detailed review describing these methods and their applicability for salmonella epidemiology is available (Threlfall, Powell and Rowe 1994).

The methods used most extensively in support of epidemiological investigations of *Salmonella* are plasmid typing, ribotyping, RCCS typing, IS*200* fingerprinting and, more recently, PFGE.

13.1 Plasmid typing

Many wild-type strains of salmonellae carry plasmids differing in both molecular mass and number. Plasmid typing, based on the numbers and molecular weight of plasmids after extraction of partially purified plasmid DNA and AGE, has been used for differentiation within serotypes, e.g. Muenchen (Taylor et al. 1982b), Goldcoast (Threlfall, Hall and Rowe 1986) and Berta (Threlfall, Hall and Rowe 1992b), and phage types (Wray et al. 1987, Hampton et al. 1995) but is restricted to strains of serotypes possessing plasmids and is of limited use in serotypes in which the majority of isolates contain only one plasmid. Thus, plasmid profile typing has been of only limited value in Enteritidis (Erdem et al. 1994), in which the majority of isolates carry a single plasmid of 38 000 kDa (Helmuth et al. 1985). The sensitivity of the technique may be increased by cleaving plasmid DNA with a limited number of restriction endonucleases and the resultant plasmid 'fingerprint' may be used to discriminate between plasmids of similar MWs (Platt et al. 1986). As with plasmid profile typing, the use of plasmid fingerprinting is restricted to plasmid-carrying strains; furthermore, carriage of multiple plasmids may make the interpretation of results extremely difficult.

13.2 Chromosomally based methods

For salmonellae that do not carry plasmids or possess only serotype-specific plasmids (SSPs), it may be necessary to use chromosomally based methods such as ribotyping which has been used for differentiation within serotypes, e.g. Dublin (Chowdry et al. 1993) and Typhi (Altwegg, Hickman-Brenner and Farmer 1989), and within phage types, e.g. Typhi (Grimont and Grimont 1986). However, ribotyping alone is not highly discriminatory and, in general, it is used in combination with other genotypic methods such as IS200 fingerprinting (see below).

Observations of heterogeneity in chromosomal restriction enzyme-generated fragment patterns may be enhanced by the use of randomly cloned sequences of chromosomal DNA as single-stranded gene probes and this method of typing, originally developed in the USA by Tompkins and colleagues (1986), provided a method for the differentiation of strains of Typhimurium but was of limited use for Dublin and Enteritidis.

A third RFLP-based method is that of insertion sequence typing. Insertion sequences belong to a class of mobile genetic elements which contain only those genes necessary for their own transposition. In particular, the Salmonella-specific 708 bp insertion sequence IS200 (Lam and Roth 1983) has been shown to be distributed on conserved loci on the chromosome of many Salmonella serotypes with copy numbers ranging from one to 25 (Gibert, Barbe and Casadesus 1990). In some serotypes, identification of the number and distribution of IS200 elements in the genome has provided a method of discrimination suitable for epidemiological investigations. In particular, IS200 fingerprinting has been used for discrimination within serotypes such as Brandenburg (Baqúar, Burnens and Stanley 1994), Infantis (Pelkonen et al. 1994) and Heidelberg (Stanley et al. 1992) for which phage typing schemes are not available and which do not contain extrachromosomal plasmid DNA. However,

when applied to serotypes that can be subdivided by phage typing, IS200 fingerprinting appears to be of more limited value; thus, in Enteritidis the method defined only 3 clonal lineages among 27 phage types and did not differentiate within phage types (Stanley, Jones and Threlfall 1991). For both Typhimurium and Paratyphi B biotype Java, preliminary studies have suggested that IS200 fingerprinting may be as discriminatory as phage typing for some investigations (Ezquerra et al. 1993, Stanley, Chowdry-Baqúar and Threlfall 1993), a finding recently exploited in the typing of Paratyphi B strains of biotype Java from a large outbreak of human infection in France, caused by contaminated goats' milk cheese (Desenclos et al. 1996).

Although the RFLP-based methods described above provide fingerprints that are easy to interpret and reproduce, ribotyping, RCCS typing and IS200 fingerprinting may be non-discriminatory. Furthermore, in the case of IS200 fingerprinting, not all serotypes possess these elements. By contrast, PFGE, a variation of conventional AGE that uses alternation between 2 field orientations to separate linear DNA fragments of a magnitude ranging from >6000 kb to <10 kb, can provide a fingerprint of the whole genome. This method is being used increasingly for the fingerprinting of Salmonella, and has provided subdivision within both serotype, e.g. Typhi (Thong et al. 1994), and phage type, e.g. Enteritidis PT 4 (Powell et al. 1994, 1995). PFGE has recently been used for characterization of a strain of Agona PT 15 responsible for an international outbreak of salmonellosis in at least 4 countries (Threlfall et al. 1996b) and, when combined with ribotyping and IS200 fingerprinting, has also provided a genotypic method for the subdivision of strains of Panama isolated in several countries over an extended period of time (Stanley, Baqúar and Burnens 1995).

Each of the PCR-based methods – RAPD, ERIC-PCR and REP-PCR – has been used experimentally for differentiation within both serotypes and phage types. However, results are not yet sufficiently reproducible for widespread use in large-scale outbreak investigations.

14 OUTER-MEMBRANE PROTEIN (OMP) AND LIPOPOLYSACCHARIDE (LPS) PROFILES

Analysis of OMP patterns has demonstrated considerable homogeneity among strains within each of the serotypes Choleraesuis, Heidelberg, Infantis, Panama and Typhimurium; by contrast, a limited degree of heterogeneity was observed within Dublin and Enteritidis, with a few strains lacking one major OMP (Helmuth et al. 1985). Because of the limited heterogeneity observed, it is unlikely that OMP typing can be used in epidemiological investigations. However, it has demonstrated that some strains of Typhimurium are deficient in OMP F and, because of this deficiency, show low-level resistance to a range of antibiotics, including ciprofloxacin, resulting from decreased uptake of the respective antibiotics through cell wall porins.

Analysis of LPS content, though not a useful tool for subdivision within a serotype, has proved useful in investigating changes of phage type within certain serotypes; thus, irreversible loss of the ability to synthesize LPS accounts for the conversion of PT 4 to PT 7 in Enteritidis strains (Chart et al. 1989).

15 POPULATION STRUCTURE

Phenotypic methods such as serotyping, phage typing and biotyping are convenient for the primary discrimination of *Salmonella* strains and have yielded useful markers for highlighting epidemic strains in epidemiological studies. They do not, however, provide a ready means for the genetic analysis of population structure in *Salmonella*.

The work of Selander and colleagues, who pioneered the study of clonal relationships and evolutionary structure of many species of medically important bacteria, used MLEE analysis to estimate the genetic distances among *Salmonella* serotypes (Selander et al. 1986, Selander and Musser 1990). Their studies confirmed that the population structure of *Salmonella* is clonal and that many common serotypes, e.g. Typhimurium, are monophyletic, i.e. represented by one, or a few, genetically similar clones probably derived from a common ancestor, that are distributed world wide and are resident on the same branch of the salmonella phylogenetic tree. That finding explains why serotyping is so useful in the epidemiological analysis of monophyletic serotypes. Other (c. 25%) serotypes are polyphyletic and comprise clones that are genetically distant and found on different branches of the phylogenetic tree; clones of these polyphyletic serotypes, e.g. Derby, often show distinct geographical distributions and/or host associations.

Other aspects of population structure of *Salmonella* that emerged from these genetic-based MLEE studies include the following:

1 strains of the same serotype, e.g. Paratyphi B, may belong to genetically distant groups
2 strains of different serotypes, e.g. Heidelberg and Typhimurium, may be genetically indistinguishable
3 salmonellae causing typhoid and enteric fevers in humans are phylogenetically distant, implying that convergent evolution of the properties of host adaptation and invasiveness occurred recently in these human-adapted serotypes and
4 the lineages of serotypes adapted to avians and other animals may be close.

Furthermore, used in conjunction with comparative nucleotide sequencing, particularly of the *fliC* gene, MLEE has shown that the H1 flagellins of genetically similar serotypes may be extensively divergent, whereas serotypes from diverse chromosomal backgrounds, even of different subspecies, may have closely similar nucleotide sequences for the highly polymorphic central region of the H1 gene. These observations suggest that recombinational events and horizontal gene exchange of both O and H genes among different lineages of *Salmonella* are likely to have been important mechanisms for the generation of new serotypes. Further details and references can be found in the section dealing with selected serotypes of salmonellae (see section 17, p. 985).

16 PATHOGENICITY

16.1 Natural infections

Salmonellae cause disease in a wide range of species of vertebrates; most of the serotypes pathogenic in mammals and birds belong to subsp. I (but see p. 991). Broadly speaking, the disease may present in 3 ways. First, a few host-adapted serotypes (see p. 970) habitually cause systemic disease in their hosts. When the manifestations of systemic disease are mainly septicaemic, as is usually the case with typhoid and paratyphoid bacilli in humans, the clinical picture is one of enteric fever with an incubation period of 10–20 days, but with outside limits of 3 and 56 days depending on the infecting dose (Mandal 1979). Diarrhoea, starting 3–4 days after onset of fever and lasting, on average, 6 days, may occur in 50% of cases of typhoid fever and is more common in younger, than in older, children or adults (Roy et al. 1985); intestinal symptoms, however, may be absent or insignificant. Second, certain other serotypes – Blegdam, Bredeney, Choleraesuis, Dublin, Enteritidis, Panama and Virchow in humans and Gallinarum in adult fowl – are also invasive but tend to cause pyaemic infections and to localize in the viscera, meninges, bones, joints and serous cavities. Third, most other salmonellae, the ubiquitous serotypes found in a number of animal species, tend to cause an acute, but mild, enteritis with a short incubation period of 12–48 h, occasionally as long as 4 days.

Nevertheless, these distinctions are not clear cut. Local abscesses and even pyaemia may develop occasionally as a late complication of a diarrhoeal disease. Serotypes that usually cause enteritis in healthy adults may cause septicaemia or pyaemic infections in young or elderly patients. The incidence of laboratory-confirmed salmonellosis in AIDS patients is 20–100 times that in the general population (Angulo and Swerdlow 1995). In American states with a high incidence of AIDS, the proportion of salmonella isolations from blood among men 25–49 years of age increased from 2.8% before the HIV epidemic (1978–82) to 14.2% in 1983–87, with Enteritidis, Typhimurium and Dublin being more opportunistically invasive than other serotypes (Levine et al. 1991). Recurrent non-typhoidal salmonella septicaemia (RSS) has been included as an AIDS-defining illness since 1987. Typhimurium, generally associated with enteritis in humans, may give rise to more severe disease in other hosts. Again, the typhoid bacillus, often considered to cause mild and atypical infections in children, will give rise to severe infections with high mortality in children whose previous health and nutrition have been poor (Scragg, Rubidge and Wallace 1969).

Convalescent patients may continue to excrete salmonellae, usually in the faeces or urine but from other sites after pyaemic infections, long after clinical cure. Asymptomatic persons may also harbour salmonellae unknowingly. Both remain potentially infectious for weeks or months and some become life-long excreters (see Volume 3, Chapter 24).

16.2 Experimental studies and virulence determinants

Extremely large doses of typhoid bacilli given orally or intravenously to chimpanzees produce an illness closely resembling typhoid fever in humans (Gaines et al. 1968) though the incubation period is shorter and ulceration of the lymphoid tissue of the small intestine does not occur (for experimental infection in humans, see Volume 3, Chapter 24). In mice and other small laboratory animals, oral administration of Typhi does not give rise to typhoid fever; when injected in small doses, there is no evidence that Typhi multiplies freely in their tissues. With some virulent strains of Typhi, it is necessary to inject $>10^7$ bacilli into the mouse peritoneum to cause death; but similar doses of killed bacilli will cause a purely toxaemic death. Fatal infections may, however, be produced in mice when smaller doses (10^2–10^7 bacteria) are given intraperitoneally with agents such as gastric mucin that depress host resistance. Typhi, therefore, is not an invasive pathogen for small laboratory animals; its failure to cause disease in these species may result from its inability to compete successfully for iron essential for its growth (O'Brien 1982).

Typhimurium infection in the mouse is, however, a useful model for typhoid fever in humans. Orally administered organisms pass rapidly through the mouse intestine with only a small proportion found in the large intestine after the first few hours. Bacteria infect the ileal mucosa and Peyer's patches and spread thereafter to the draining lymph nodes. Typhimurium is resistant to killing by phagocytic cells and spreads through the lymphatics to form infective foci in the spleen and liver (Carter and Collins 1974).

INVASIVE INFECTION

The factors responsible for the virulence of salmonellae are still ill-defined. The following sections summarize our understanding of the complex interactions between different salmonella serotypes, their hosts and host cells. Molecular techniques have helped to elucidate some of the critical steps in these host–pathogen interactions and to identify genes involved but progress remains slow.

The ability of salmonellae to invade, survive and replicate within eukaryotic cells is essential for successful infection. Salmonellae possess several factors which contribute to the disease process; these virulence-promoting factors are generally conserved among species, as are the mechanisms by which bacteria interact with the host cell. Such factors facilitate entry into (invasion of) non-phagocytic cells, survival in the intracellular environment and replication within host cells (for reviews, see Finlay et al. 1992, Guiney et al. 1995).

After oral ingestion of organisms in sufficient numbers to promote onset of disease, the next stage in the disease process is penetration of the intestinal epithelium. Transmission electron microscopy has revealed that invasive salmonellae interact with the well defined apical microvilli of epithelial cells, thereby disrupting the brush border. Once these cells have been penetrated, the bacteria are enclosed in membrane-bound vacuoles within the host cytoplasm. Virulent salmonellae survive and multiply within these vacuoles, eventually lysing their host cells and disseminating to other parts of the body. Salmonellae also depolarize epithelial barriers by affecting the integrity of tight junctions between cells, which has the result of promoting significant cytotoxic damage to epithelial cells.

The induction of protein synthesis de novo is necessary for invasion and is regulated by the microenvironment (low oxygen), growth phase or the epithelial cell surface. Only viable, metabolically active salmonellae can adhere to host cell surfaces. Adherence is followed almost immediately by internalization into host cells. The bacterial genes necessary for salmonellae to enter eukaryotic cells have yet to be fully characterized but at least 6 different genetic loci appear to be involved and an additional hyperinvading locus has recently been identified (Finlay et al. 1992, Guiney et al. 1995).

Internalization of salmonellae through the apical surface of epithelial cells is associated with disruption of the eukaryotic brush border. After a lag period of about 4 h, invading organisms begin to multiply within the vacuoles of host epithelial cells. For Typhimurium, it has been demonstrated that this intracellular replication is essential for pathogenicity. Salmonellae remain within membrane-bound inclusions and their survival appears to involve blockage of phagosome–lysosome fusion events.

SEROTYPE-SPECIFIC PLASMIDS

Analysis of the plasmid content of salmonella strains belonging to a range of serotypes of epidemiological importance in humans and food animals has demonstrated that some (but not all) serotypes possess plasmids of high MW that may be regarded as serotype-specific plasmids (SSPs). Serotypes harbouring such plasmids include Enteritidis, Typhimurium, Dublin, Choleraesuis, Pullorum and Gallinarum. In contrast, SSPs have not been identified in serotypes such as Virchow and Hadar, both of which cause disease in humans, nor in Typhi. These plasmids, which range in MW from about 30 000 kDa (Choleraesuis) and 38 000 kDa (Enteritidis) to 62 000 kDa (Typhimurium) (Helmuth et al. 1985), are generally non-conjugative and do not carry easily identifiable phenotypic markers such as drug resistance.

The results of animal challenge experiments have indicated that SSPs are involved in the virulence in their host strains for certain strains of inbred mice, e.g. BALB/c. Studies by Pardon et al. (1986) and Gulig and Curtis (1987) have demonstrated that the 62 000 kDa SSP of Typhimurium genetically determined its spread beyond the small intestine to deeper tissues such as the mesenteric lymph nodes or the spleen. They also observed the attenuation of virulence of plasmid-cured strains in parenterally inoculated mice.

Although SSPs from different serotypes possess substantial regions of non-homologous DNA, all possess a highly conserved common region which carries salmonella plasmid virulence (*spv*) genes (Gulig et al. 1993) responsible for their virulence in mice (Williamson, Baird and Manning 1988). In Dublin *spv* genes have been shown to be clustered within an 8 kb *Sal*I–*Xho*I restriction endonuclease fragment (Williamson, Pullinger and Lax 1988) and a homologous region has been identified in the SSPs of Typhimurium, Enteritidis, Choleraesuis and several other serotypes (Williamson, Baird and Manning 1988). Within this region, a highly conserved 3.5 kb *Hind*III fragment has been shown to have homology with the virulence regions of the SSPs of Dublin and Enteritidis (Woodward, McLaren and Wray 1989).

Six *spv* genes within the common 8 kb *Sal*I–*Xho*I fragment have been sequenced, namely *spvR*, *spvA*, *spvB*, *spvC*, *spvD* and *spvE*. The *spvE* gene encodes a 13 kDa protein, the *spvD* gene a 25 kDa protein and the *spvC* gene a 28 kDa protein, which is located both in the outer membrane and the cytoplasm. The latter protein has a demonstrable role in virulence, as it has been shown that transposon insertion mutants in the *spvC* gene of SSP result in a significant drop in the number of Typhimurium isolated from the spleen of orally infected mice. Moreover, only one-fifth of these mice died after infection with an SSP transposon-attenuated strain as compared to those infected with wild-type bacteria (Norel et al. 1989). The *spvB* gene encodes a 65 kDa protein of unknown function which is located both in the outer membrane and the cytoplasm, and the *spvA* gene a 28 kDa protein also of unknown function.

Although essential for the virulence of most strains for certain strains of mice, the role of SSP virulence plasmids in the pathogenesis of disease in humans and other animal species is not clear. Results with cattle have suggested that these plasmids are required for bacteraemia (Pardon et al. 1986) but not necessarily for gastroenteritis. SSP-like plasmids have been shown to be necessary for the intracellular survival of their host organisms in mouse phagocytes (Buchmeier and Heffron 1991) and it has been suggested that they may enhance survival of bacteria in extraintestinal infections in humans (Fierer et al. 1992). However, studies have demonstrated that for Enteritidis, the possession of an SSP is not necessary for the induction of enteritis in humans (Threlfall et al. 1994c). Likewise, similar SSPs have not been identified in certain phage types of Typhimurium isolated from cases of diarrhoea in humans (Brown, Munro and Platt 1986).

Toxins

Early evidence suggesting that food-poisoning salmonellae of diverse serotypes produced 'enterotoxins' with biological and antigenic properties of cholera-like (CT) toxins (Sandefur and Peterson 1977, Jiwa 1981, Finkelstein et al. 1983) could not be confirmed by other workers (Wallis et al. 1986a, Clarke et al. 1988).

Other possible explanations for salmonella-induced diarrhoea in gastroenteritis invoke mechanisms involving some kind of immune response in the intestine or salmonella entry into enterocytes. Support for these latter hypotheses comes from the following observations:

1 interaction between salmonellae and inflammatory cells leads to release of prostaglandins mediating fluid secretion, which is reversible in monkeys by inhibitors of prostaglandin synthesis (Gianella, Rout and Formal 1977, Gianella 1979)
2 microscopy studies of experimental Typhimurium infection show that fluid secretion is preceded by extensive infiltration of inflammatory cells and that cell damage, when it occurs, is limited to the tips of the villi and shortened villi may lead to enhanced secretion (Wallis et al. 1986b)
3 salmonellae induce epithelial cells to secrete IL-8, a potent chemoattractant of neutrophils which might contribute to inflammation, cell damage and fluid secretion and
4 salmonella entry into epithelial cells in monolayers brings about many biochemical changes including the phosphorylation of epidermal growth factor (EGF) receptor and activation via phospholipase A2 of leukotriene synthesis which may result in actin rearrangements and disruption of the integrity of the tight junctions on epithelial cells, with resultant cytotoxic damage and fluid loss (Finlay et al. 1992, Pace, Haymar and Galan 1993).

There is, therefore, a range of mechanisms whereby salmonellae might cause gastroenteritis and diarrhoea production may be multifactorial.

In both experimental and natural conditions, salmonella infections may occur via the conjunctivae, by inhalation and by insect bites as well as by the oral route. No attempt will be made here to describe in detail the infections in humans and other animals by other serotypes but some information will be found in the descriptions of individual serotypes and also in earlier editions of this book. Enteric fever and certain other generalized salmonella infections are discussed in Volume 3, Chapter 24, salmonella enteritis in Volume 3, Chapter 28 and hospital-acquired salmonella infections in Volume 3, Chapter 13.

17 Notes on Selected Serotypes of Salmonellae

17.1 Subspecies I

Agona (1,4,12:f,g,s:[1,2]) Rarely isolated before 1969, this serotype was imported into the USA and many European countries in contaminated Peruvian fishmeal which was used in animal feed stuffs. Agona soon became entrenched in pigs and poultry (Lee 1974, Turnbull 1979) and by 1971 an animal-food cycle independent of imported products was established, e.g. in the UK (Palmer and Rowe 1986). Thereafter, Agona was soon present in the top 10 serotypes isolated from humans in the UK and elsewhere; its subsequent decline remains unexplained (Le Minor, Le Minor and Grimont 1985, Palmer and Rowe 1986). The combined use of phage typing and biotyping revealed little type divergence (Barker, Old and Tyc 1982). A different phage typing scheme recognizing 38 phage types (LR Ward, unpublished) was used to investigate an outbreak of Agona that occurred in the UK from late 1994 to early 1995, associated with a kosher, savoury peanut-based snack imported from Israel. All isolates from cases in the UK and from others in Israel, Canada and the USA and from the snacks belonged to PT 15 (Anonymous 1995). The clonal identity of the outbreak strain was confirmed by PFGE (Threlfall et al. 1996b).

MLEE has shown that the serotype is monophyletic; all isolates of Agona examined belonged to one clone (Reeves et al. 1989, Boyd et al. 1993). Of the 3 distinct lineages of serotype Derby ($\underline{1}$,4,[5],12:f,g:[1,2]) (Beltran et al. 1988), one (De31) is more closely related in ET to that of Agona (Ag1) (from which it differs in only 4 of 26 enzyme loci) than to those of the other Derby clones (De1, De13) (Boyd et al. 1993).

Choleraesuis (6,7:c:1,5) This swine-adapted serotype commonly causes enteritis in pigs but may be isolated occasionally from other animals including humans, e.g. in the UK from 1981 to 1990 there were only 27 isolations from humans, 74% of which were invasive (Threlfall, Hall and Rowe 1992a). About 50% of recorded human infections are associated with prolonged pyrexia, over one-third result in localized pus formation and 20% are fatal (Saphra and Winter 1957). Common pyaemic manifestations include pneumonia, septic arthritis and osteomyelitis, meningitis and endocarditis. Choleraesuis grows better in brilliant green-containing media than in selenite broth or on MacConkey or deoxycholate agars. Traditionally 3 biotypes (Choleraesuis, Decatur and Kunzendorf) have been recognized (see Table 41.5), each containing different components of the H1 antigen factors c_{1-3}. Two other salmonella serotypes with the same antigenic formula as Choleraesuis are still retained in the Kauffmann–White scheme (Popoff and Le Minor 1992): Typhisuis and Paratyphi C. Typhisuis too is swine adapted but may occasionally be isolated from other animals including humans in whom the clinical presentation is like that of Choleraesuis (Saphra and Wassermann 1954). Typhisuis grows poorly on ordinary media, produces gas sparsely and is distinguishable biochemically (Table 41.5); among salmonellae it is unusual in being mannitol non-fermenting and lysine decarboxylase-negative. Most strains of the human-adapted Paratyphi C are difficult to distinguish from Choleraesuis and Typhisuis but produce Vi antigen which, however, is rapidly lost on laboratory culture; Paratyphi C strains (Vi$^+$ or Vi$^-$) give a positive result with a *viaB*-specific probe (Selander et al. 1990b).

Analysis by MLEE indicates a very close genetic relationship among most clones of Choleraesuis, Typhisuis and Paratyphi C. Most (82%) strains of Choleraesuis belong to one dominant clone (Cs1) and all but 2 clones of Choleraesuis form a tight genetic cluster to which Typhisuis clones (Ts1, Ts2) also belong (Beltran et al. 1988, Selander et al. 1990b). About 90% of Paratyphi C strains belong to clones Pc1 and Pc2 which, with most other Pc clones, also cluster in this same lineage; it has been suggested that the major clones of Choleraesuis, Typhisuis and Paratyphi C shared a common, invasive ancestor from which they evolved with a shift to human hosts by Paratyphi C (Selander and Smith 1990). However, some clones of Choleraesuis (Cs6,13), Typhisuis (Ts3) and Paratyphi C (Pc4) are distantly related to the above major genetic group (Selander et al. 1990b). Furthermore, the 3 clones representative of biotype Decatur (Dt1–3) are distantly related to those of serotype Choleraesuis (Selander et al. 1990b); yet Decatur has been subsumed into Choleraesuis (Popoff and Le Minor 1992).

Dublin ($\underline{1}$,9,12 [Vi]:g,p: -) Dublin is highly host-adapted to cattle but other animals including humans are sporadically infected. In Britain, it is the second most common serotype in cattle (Anonymous 1994a). In infected calves, it causes severe diarrhoea whereas in adult cattle it is responsible for septic abortion associated with a 70% mortality and prolonged carriage by surviving animals. Human infections are relatively uncommon in the UK, e.g. only 430 human isolations in England and Wales between 1981 and 1990 (Threlfall, Hall and Rowe 1992a), but are more common in other parts of Western Europe such as France (Le Minor, Le Minor and Grimont 1985). Numbers of human infections, particularly in western states of the USA, increased steadily after 1964, especially among elderly, debilitated male patients in whom mortality (35%) was high (Taylor et al. 1982a). Human infection often follows the consumption of raw milk and large milk-borne outbreaks have been described (Small and Sharp 1979). There is a high incidence of bloodstream invasion; thus, 25% of isolates from humans in the UK were from blood (Threlfall, Hall and Rowe 1992a); abscess formation in bones and joints has also been noted.

Of 3 closely related clones (Du1, Du3, Du4) recognized by MLEE, 82% of strains belong to Du1 which is globally distributed (Beltran et al. 1988, Selander et al. 1992). Gene probing reveals that *viaB* genes are confined to clone Du3, restricted in its distribution to France and the UK; whether clones Du1 and Du3 differ in type or severity of infection in humans or animals is unknown (Selander et al. 1992). Both MLEE and sequencing of *fliC* genes show that Dublin is closely related to Enteritidis, ($\underline{1}$,9,12:g,m:[1,7]), particularly to clonal lineage SECLIII, and that Rostock ($\underline{1}$,9,12:g,p,u: -) is identical by MLEE to Du1 (Selander et al. 1992, Li et al. 1993, Chowdry et al. 1993). Most wild-type strains carry a large (52 000 kDa) SSP implicated in virulence for BALB/c mice, not required for blood invasion in humans and of uncertain status in bovine infections (Manning, Baird and Jones 1986, Heffernan et al. 1987). Most strains (96%) require nicotinic acid for growth. Some biotype diversification is present (Walton 1972, Fierer and Fleming 1983), but molecular techniques have been necessary for the typing of Dublin strains (see Liebisch and Schwarz 1996). Among human isolations in the UK, 2 clones (*Sd*RI, *Sd*RII) of identical IS*200* profile were identified on the basis of ribotyping; it has been suggested that strains of ribotype I may be associated with invasive disease in humans whereas those of ribotype II are associated only with non-invasive disease (Chowdry et al. 1993). Strains formerly assigned to clone Du2 belong to a new serotype ($\underline{1}$,9,12:g,m,p: -) distantly related to Dublin (Selander et al. 1992). Non-motile strains of Dublin ($\underline{1}$,9,12: -

Table 41.5 Biochemical reactions of salmonellae of antigenic formula 6,7:c:1,5

Serotype	Biotype	Fermentation of				Production of
		arabinose	trehalose	dulcitol	mucate	H$_2$S
Choleraesuis	Choleraesuis	–	–	–	–	–
Choleraesuis	Kunzendorf	–	–	–	–	+
Choleraesuis	Decatur	+	+	+	+	+
Paratyphi C[a]		+/–	+/–	+	–	+
Typhisuis		+	+	–	–	–

[a]Most strains are Vi[+] but production of Vi is rapidly lost on subculture.
–, Negative reaction (in 5 days); +, positive reaction (in 2 days); +/–, some strains are positive, others negative.

: -), indistinguishable by MLEE from Du1, carry a plasmid (52 000 kDa) the restriction pattern of which is the same as that of wild-type Dublin strains (Selander et al. 1992).

Enteritidis (1,9,12:g,m:[1,7]) This serotype usually causes food poisoning in humans but known complications include severe septicaemia and pyaemic conditions such as spinal meningitis and subcutaneous abscesses, as described, for example, among Liberian infants among whom very high mortality rates (45%) were noted in children <1 year old (Hadfield, Monson and Wachsmuth 1985). Enteritidis is commonly among the top 3 serotypes from humans in many countries world wide (Rodrigue, Tauxe and Rowe 1990, Schroeter et al. 1994); in the UK, for example, reported isolations have increased 16-fold in the period 1981–94 (Threlfall et al. 1994b, Frost, Threlfall and Rowe 1995), Enteritidis accounting for 54% of all salmonellae isolated from humans in 1995 (Anonymous 1996). Its main reservoir is in poultry flocks, poultry meat and contaminated eggs being important vehicles of human infection (Coyle et al. 1988, Cowden et al. 1989a, 1989b, de Louvois 1993, 1994). Primary differentiation of strains is best achieved by phage typing; the scheme of Ward, de Sa and Rowe (1987) with 11 phages originally recognized 32 types and has now been extended to include 15 phages recognizing >50 distinct types (LR Ward, unpublished). The unprecedented epidemic of Enteritidis in the UK and several other western European countries in the late 1980s and early 1990s was caused by a strain of PT 4 which spread in poultry flocks, selected by environmental pressures associated with poultry husbandry. An unusual feature of the epidemic was the transovarian spread of the strain in the avian host (Humphrey et al. 1989, Timoney et al. 1989). In other countries epidemics were caused by strains of other phage types: PTs 8 and 13 in the USA (Rodrigue, Tauxe and Rowe 1990), PT 6a in Greece (Vatopoulos et al. 1994) and PT 1 in several eastern European countries; other PTs associated with poultry and poultry products are 7, 7a, 23, 24 and 30 (Threlfall et al. 1993a). Although isolations of Enteritidis from humans are declining in the UK, e.g. from 63 to 54% in 1991–95, it remains the most common serotype from humans and food animals in the UK. Despite its predominance, the overall level of antimicrobial resistance in Enteritidis in the UK has remained low (15–19% in 1981–94), and multiple-

drug resistance in isolates from food animals or humans is rare (Threlfall, Rowe and Ward 1993). Further discrimination within major PTs has been obtained by use of molecular techniques (see pp. 981–982).

Enteritidis is polyphyletic and clone En2 is distantly related to other ETs of this serotype, except in its *fliC* gene sequence (Beltran et al. 1988, Li et al. 1993). The dominant clone En1 is closely related to clones of the cattle-adapted serotype Dublin (Du1,3) and to the avian-adapted types Gallinarum and Pullorum (Boyd et al. 1993, Li et al. 1993).

Gallinarum (1,9,12: - : -) Two distinct entities, distinguished by biotyping and by causing different pathologies in their avian hosts (Blaxland et al. 1956), are recognized within this non-motile serotype. Bioserotype Gallinarum is the agent of fowl typhoid, a septicaemic disease of young and adult birds, usually spread by contaminated food or water. In natural infections, mortality is high. Bioserotype Pullorum causes an acute diarrhoeal illness in chicks; adult birds may be chronically infected but remain healthy. Spread occurs by transovarian transmission to eggs in carrier hens. Now uncommon in the UK and USA, these bioserotypes have been prevalent since the 1970s in Africa, Asia and South America (da Silva 1985). Sporadic cases occur in humans and other animals. The virulence plasmids of both types are similar in size and structure (Barrow and Lovell 1989) but the mechanisms responsible for different diseases in avian hosts are unknown. Whereas Gallinarum strains grow well on ordinary enteric media, brilliant green-containing media are recommended for Pullorum strains, some of which, however, are very sensitive to brilliant green and bile salts. Pullorum, but not Gallinarum, strains exhibit phase-variable expression of antigen O12$_2$ subfactor. Most Gallinarum strains belong to PT 2 of Lilleengen (1952); the phage typing scheme of Anderson (1964) recognizes 13 phage types of Pullorum. Gallinarum strains are remarkably homogeneous in biotype: they are anaerogenic, ferment dulcitol and maltose promptly and are ornithine decarboxylase-negative (Crichton and Old 1990). At least 5 biotypes of Pullorum are recognized (Crichton and Old 1990).

MLEE analysis has shown that both Gallinarum and Pullorum are monophyletic and closely related to Enteritidis (Li et al. 1993). Only 5 ETs were identified for Gallinarum strains, most (93%) of which belonged to the globally distributed clone Ga2. By contrast, Pullorum strains showed greater evolutionary divergence with 7 ETs identified. The dominant, global Pullorum clone (Pu3 and its variants) contained 61% of strains; clones Pu2 (26% strains) and Pu4 (13%) were apparently restricted to the UK and Germany, respectively (Li et al. 1993). These groupings are in agreement with findings from ribotyping, IS200 profiles and PFGE (Olsen et al. 1996). The existence of a hybrid type, dulcitol-positive and rhamnose-negative like Gallinarum but gas-producing and ornithine decarboxylase-positive like Pullorum (Crichton and Old 1990), was confirmed by the presence of a unique ET (Ga/Pu1) closer in overall genetic structure to Gallinarum than to Pullorum (Li et al. 1993). The kind of disease produced by strains of Ga/Pu1 is not known. All 3 lineages are thought to have been derived by loss of motility and independent host adaptations to birds, from a motile Enteritidis-like ancestor of broad host range.

Hadar (6,8:z₁₀:e,n,x) Rarely isolated before 1971, Hadar became one of the prevalent serotypes isolated from humans in many countries in the 1970s–80s (Le Minor, Le Minor and Grimont 1985, Palmer and Rowe 1986, Reilly et al. 1988, Farmer 1995), its sudden epidemic spread being attributed to its introduction via contaminated feed supplements to turkey flocks; its major reservoir, in the UK, for example, is turkeys (Anonymous 1992b) with ducks and geese increasingly affected (Anonymous 1994a). Hadar remains a common serotype in the UK, accounting for c. 2% of salmonella isolations from humans in 1994–95 (Frost, Threlfall and Rowe 1995). The phage typing scheme of de Sa, Ward and Rowe (1980) has been expanded and currently 62 PTs are recognized; PTs from humans and turkeys are similar (Palmer and Rowe 1986). Resistance to antimicrobial agents has increased dramatically in Hadar isolates in the UK from 2 to 90% in the period 1981–94 and 13% of strains are multidrug-resistant (pattern, ACST); since 1991, resistance to ciprofloxacin has increased from 0 to 40% (Frost, Threlfall and Rowe 1995). The use of enrofloxacin in veterinary use has also increased in that period. MLEE indicates that Hadar is a monophyletic serotype (Reeves et al. 1989).

Heidelberg (1,4,[5],12:r:1,5) Consistently ranked among the top 10 serotypes isolated from humans in different countries in Europe and in the USA (Le Minor, Le Minor and Grimont 1985, Reilly et al. 1988, Threlfall, Hall and Rowe 1992a, Farmer 1995), Heidelberg usually causes gastroenteritis but is occasionally associated (3.3% of cases) with bloodstream invasion. It is well entrenched in poultry, particularly turkeys, in the UK (Anonymous 1992b).

Epidemiological and phylogenetic groups of Heidelberg have been distinguished by IS200 profiling; the copy number of IS200 varied from 4 to 6 with at least one insertion site being serotype-specific (Stanley et al. 1992). Seven unique, stable IS200 fingerprints identified clones: one was associated with human infections, a second comprised strains from chicken sources and a third was derived from that chicken clone; in addition, there were 4 minor clones. Clones could be further subdivided by plasmid analysis showing, for example, that all chicken isolates carried a unique (23 000

kDa) plasmid of the IncX group (Stanley et al. 1992). Populations of Heidelberg have been shown by MLEE to comprise 8 ETs which form a single cluster of closely related genotypes; most (87%) strains belong to the globally dominant clone He1 (Beltran et al. 1988). This monophyletic serotype is a member of a large phylogenetic complex to which Typhimurium, Saintpaul, (some clones of) ParatyphiB/Java and Muenchen also belong (Beltran et al. 1988, 1991).

Infantis (6,7,14:r:1,5) The primary reservoir of this serotype is poultry but it has spilled over to cattle in some countries (Anonymous 1992b, Pelkonen et al. 1994). Infantis features regularly in the top 10 prevalent serotypes isolated from humans in many developed countries (Le Minor, Le Minor and Grimont 1985, Reilly et al. 1988, Pelkonen et al. 1994), and there is some evidence of an enhanced propensity to cause invasive disease with 4.3% of strains isolated from extraintestinal sites (Wilkins and Roberts 1988). A phage typing scheme for Infantis (Kasatiya, Caprioli and Champoux 1979) has not been widely applied. Again, resistance to antimicrobial agents is rare and few (18%) strains have plasmids (Pelkonen et al. 1994).

Thus, primary strain discrimination of Infantis has been molecular based. A study in Finland, where Infantis is the most common serotype identified from cases of food poisoning in humans, showed that most Infantis isolates had 3 (97% of strains) or >4 (71%) copies of IS200. Used together with ribotyping, IS200 profiling identified 15 different genotypes and clearly differentiated between isolates from humans and other animal sources of infection; all strains from domestic, and most (96%) imported, cases of Infantis infection in humans belonged to genotypes distinct from those strains entrenched in domestic broiler chickens and cattle (Pelkonen et al. 1994). MLEE analysis has identified 4 clones and showed that 96% of isolates belong to a predominant, globally distributed clone (In1). The serotype may be polyphyletic; only one isolate of an aberrant clone (In3) of uncertain status did not cluster with the other (99%) strains (Beltran et al. 1988, Boyd et al. 1993).

Montevideo (6,7,14:g,m [p],s:[1,2,7]) Serotype Montevideo is recognized as a cause of serious illness in sheep (Sharp et al. 1983) in which it is the second most commonly isolated serotype in the UK; it is also common in poultry but less so in cattle (Anonymous 1994a). Montevideo is less commonly isolated from human cases in Scotland than in England and Wales; it is also regularly among the top 10 serotypes from humans in the USA (Farmer 1995).

Biotyping recognized 2 major biogroups, the distribution of which was different in parts of the UK. Biogroup 10di was predominant in all animal species in Scotland but only in sheep in England and Wales; biogroup 2d, on the other hand, was responsible for almost all infections in humans, poultry and cattle in England and Wales but for only one-quarter of human infections in Scotland (Reilly et al. 1985). MLEE recognized 2 genotypically distinct ETs in this monophyletic serotype (Boyd et al. 1993).

Panama (1,9,12:l,v:1,5) This serotype was rarely isolated in the UK before 1938. Imported dried-egg products were responsible for its establishment in pigs which, with pig-meat products, remain a major source of human infection; nevertheless, Panama is now isolated from a wide variety of animals in the UK (Anonymous 1992b). For many years it has ranked in the top 10 serotypes isolated from humans in the UK (Lee 1974, Turnbull 1979, Threlfall, Hall and Rowe 1992a) and elsewhere (Le Minor, Le Minor and Grimont 1985, Stanley, Baqúar and Burnens 1995). In humans, there is evidence of an above-average ability to cause infections in blood and other extraintestinal sites (Wilkins and Roberts 1988, Threlfall, Hall and Rowe 1992a).

The phage typing scheme of Guinée (1969) differentiates only 8 PTs and is of limited value epidemiologically. IS*200* profiling, which shows that 4 (of 7–9) loci are conserved among all strains, is considered to be the most appropriate genotyping method (Stanley, Baqúar and Burnens 1995). Although a high degree of discrimination has been achieved and many individual genotypes identified when IS*200* profiling is used with plasmid analysis, these techniques have not yet been applied to epidemiological investigations. MLEE analysis recognized 13 clones, the predominant one of which (Pn1) contained 75% of strains (Selander et al. 1990b). Clones of the monophyletic Panama are closely related to those of the polyphyletic serotype Miami (1̲,9,12:a:1,5) (Selander and Smith 1990, Selander et al. 1990b).

Paratyphi A (1,2,12:a:[1,5]) This serotype, host-adapted to humans, is an important cause of enteric fever in Asia, the Middle East, Africa and South America (Report 1982); it is infrequently isolated from animals and occurs naturally in the H1 phase. Among salmonellae of subsp. I, it is unusual in being H_2S-negative, xylose non-fermenting and often anaerogenic (Ewing 1986). It is auxotrophic and, hence, unable to utilize citrate as sole carbon source in Simmons's medium, and is unreactive with other organic acids (see Table 41.3).

Of 4 clones recognized by MLEE, 2 (Pa1, Pa3) are widely distributed (Selander and Smith 1990, Selander et al. 1990b). Serotype Sendai (1̲,9,12:a:1,5), a rare cause of enteric fever, resembles Paratyphi A in its biochemical properties, auxotrophy and in its host adaptation to humans; it is, however, aerogenic, ferments xylose and possesses O factor 9 rather than O2. The immunodominant sugars of factors O2 and 9, the O antigens of which are otherwise identical, are paratose and tyvelose, respectively; gene *rfbJ*, encoding cytidine 5′-diphosphate (CDP)-tyvelose epimerase which converts CDP-paratose to CDP-tyvelose, is active in strains of serogroup O9 but is present in a mutant form in strains of serogroup O2 (Verma and Reeves 1989). Four clones of Sendai (Se1–4) identified by MLEE are closely related to those of Paratyphi A (Selander et al. 1990b). Serotype Miami (1̲,9,12:a:1,5), though antigenically like Sendai, differs from it in being prototrophic, in not forming a fimbrial MREHA (see p. 971) and in causing gastroenteritis rather than enteric fever. Strains of Miami are genetically diverse and are more closely related to serotype Panama (1̲,9,12:1,v:1,5) which also causes gastroenteritis, than to Paratyphi A or Sendai. Two clones of Miami (Mi1 and Mi2) are adapted to, but not invasive for, humans. Serotype Miami is **not** a biotype variant of Sendai and is correctly distinguished from Sendai in the Kauffmann–White scheme (Popoff and Le Minor 1992). The possible derivation of Para-

typhi and Sendai from a Panama-like ancestor would have involved both a restriction in host range to humans and acquisition of invasiveness potential (Selander and Smith 1990).

Paratyphi B (1̲,4 [5],12:b:1,2) Paratyphi B is also known as Schottmuelleri, but this synonym is rarely used now. The phage typing method of Anderson (1964) differentiates 55 phage types and the biotyping scheme of Duguid et al. (1975) 56 full biotypes (Barker et al. 1988); used together, they provide excellent strain discrimination for epidemiological studies (Old and Barker 1989). Two groups of strains exist:

1 some cause enteric fever in humans, are rarely isolated from animals, usually form a mucoid (slime) wall at room temperature and 90% are *d*-tartrate non-fermenting (dT^-)

2 others cause gastroenteritis in humans, are also isolated from animals and food, do not form a slime wall and are usually *d*-tartrate fermenting (dT^+), i.e. are of biotype Java.

Cases of gastroenteritis occur sporadically but a few large, food-borne outbreaks have been reported, e.g. in the UK in 1988 (Anonymous 1994b) and in France in 1993 (Desenclos et al. 1996). In this latter outbreak, which was associated with contaminated goats' milk cheese, the symptoms were those of gastroenteritis and the implicated strain was of PT var. 3, which in the UK is normally associated with Java. Thus, it seems likely that the French outbreak was caused by strains of biotype Java, and not of Paratyphi B which is associated with paratyphoid illness in humans. This reflects clearly the present confusion in nomenclature, which is important to resolve for international comparison of salmonella-associated disease.

Of 23 ETs recognized by MLEE (Selander et al. 1990a, 1990b), only 3 are significantly represented in natural populations: 89% of dT^- strains belong to clone Pb1, and 84% of dT^+ strains (Java) belong to clones Pb3 and Pb4. The traits of adaptation to humans and ability to cause enteric fever have evolved, probably recently, in only one clone (Pb1) which is globally distributed but otherwise phenotypically similar to the clones that cause gastroenteritis and are of broad host range (Selander et al. 1990a, 1990b). The serotype is polyphyletic. Thus, clones Pb1, 2 and 3 are genetically close; but the 4 variant ETs of clone Pb5 (comprising monophasic strains) and clones Pb4, 6 and 7 are genetically closer to strains of Heidelberg, Saintpaul and Typhimurium, from which they differ antigenically in H1 only, than to clones Pb1, 2 and 3 (Selander and Smith 1990).

Typhi (9,12 [Vi̲]:d: -) This human-adapted serotype is estimated to cause annually 12–21 million cases of typhoid fever in humans and up to 700 000 deaths (Thong et al. 1994, Mirza, Beeching and Hart 1996). With appropriate antimicrobial therapy, mortality is reduced from 30% to <1%. Multidrug resistance in Typhi strains has become a problem in many countries (see p. 973) but is less so in Africa and South and Central America (Mirza, Beeching and Hart 1996). Ciprofloxacin is now the antibiotic of choice for multidrug-resistant strains. Children infected with drug-resistant strains are more ill for longer periods and have higher mortality than those infected with drug-sensitive strains (Bhutta et al. 1991). Strains are homogeneous in biotype. Primary discrimination of Vi$^+$ strains is best achieved by phage typing (Craigie and Yen 1938, Anderson and Williams 1956) which recognizes 106 PTs; Vi$^-$ strains may be discriminated by PFGE. The number of IS*200* loci varies from 10 to 25 (Gibert, Barbe and Casadesus 1990); whilst IS*200* profiling may distinguish between drug-resistant and sensitive strains within common PTs, such as E1 or M1, it is less discriminating than phage typing, e.g. the type strains of the commonest PTs (E1, M1 and A) have identical IS*200* profiles (Threlfall et al. 1993b, 1994d). Among Typhi strains from Indonesia, some (16%) express an H1 flagellar antigen of type j resulting from a deletion in the central antigen-determining part of the H1-d gene; others express a z_{66} flagellar antigen, thought to be an H2 locus (Guinée et al. 1981, Frankel et al. 1989, Selander et al. 1990b). Typhi strains of type 9,12,[Vi]:j: - are associated with milder clinical illness in older patients and are less motile and less invasive for HEp-2 cells in vitro than Typhi strains of type 9,12,[Vi]:d: - (Grossman et al. 1995).

Two clones were identified by MLEE: Tp1 (83%) was dominant world wide and Tp2 (16%) was found in Africa, particularly in Senegal; dual infections with Tp1, Tp2 were observed in some patients in Senegal (Selander et al. 1990b). Indonesian strains, whether of H type d, j or z_{66}, belonged to Tp1. A very few (<1%) Typhi strains that do not have Vi antigen genes are otherwise of similar MLEE profiles to Vi$^+$ strains of Tp1, Tp2. As measured by MLEE, Typhi strains are genetically distant from other salmonellae, including other serotypes that are host-adapted and/or invasive (Selander et al. 1990b).

Typhimurium (1,4,[5],12:i:1,2) Typhimurium is one of the top 3 serotypes isolated world wide over many decades from humans, domestic and wild animals, foodstuffs and the environment, with cattle and poultry important sources of infection for humans (Palmer and Rowe 1986). In the UK, multiple-drug resistance (MDR) to >4 antimicrobial agents has increased 12-fold in isolates from humans in the period 1981–94 (Frost, Threlfall and Rowe 1995); since 1980 the majority of isolates from bovine hosts showed MDR which also increased in pigs and, to a lesser extent, in poultry (Threlfall, Rowe and Ward 1993). In strains of types prevalent from 1981 to 1990, e.g. DTs 204, 204c and 193, MDR was plasmid mediated (Threlfall et al. 1986, 1994a). Since 1992, a particular cause for concern in the UK has been Typhimurium of DT 104 which is currently epidemic in cattle and has caused many human infections (see p. 972). Broad spectrum MDR in strains of DT 104 is chromosomally located (Threlfall et al. 1994a, 1996a), and additional chromosomal resistance to quinolones has been found in poultry isolates (Frost, Threlfall and Rowe 1995). Additional discrimination within phage types can be achieved by biotyping (Duguid et al. 1975, Anderson et al. 1978, Barker and Old 1979, 1980); their combined use is highly discriminatory and provides excel-

lent strain characterization for epidemiological purposes (Old and Barker 1989).

Detailed genetic studies of the main biotype markers identified major clones, e.g. the FIRN (fimbriation-, inositol- and rhamnose-negative) group (Old and Duguid 1979, Barker and Old 1989). Additional strain discrimination within the serotype or phage types can be achieved, where needed, by molecular methods (see Threlfall and Frost 1990, Threlfall, Powell and Rowe 1994). MLEE analysis of natural populations has identified 17 closely related clones in this monophyletic serotype that cluster with clones of Heidelberg, Saintpaul and Paratyphi B/Java (Beltran et al. 1988, 1991, Selander and Smith 1990, Selander et al. 1990a, 1990b).

Virchow (6,7:r:1,2) Before 1975, this serotype accounted for <1% of isolations from humans in the UK but during 1981–94 it became the third commonest serotype, accounting for 9% of human isolations (Frost, Threlfall and Rowe 1995). A phage typing scheme (Chambers et al. 1987), based on 13 phages and distinguishing 57 phage types (Torre et al. 1993), is the method of choice for primary strain discrimination; however, 6 phage types (PTs 8, 31, 26, 21, 19 and 2, in ranking order) account for 62% of all isolates (Threlfall, Rowe and Ward 1993). For further discrimination within major phage types, plasmid profiling is better than IS*200* sequence distribution (Torre et al. 1993). Poultry, particularly chicken, is a major source of infection for humans (Reilly et al. 1988, Threlfall, Rowe and Ward 1993).

There has been a significant increase (16–71%) in drug resistance in Virchow between 1981 and 1994 with many (9%) strains showing multiple resistance to >4 antimicrobial agents (Threlfall, Rowe and Ward 1993, Frost, Threlfall and Rowe 1995). Phage types in which resistance was common included PT 19 associated with poultry imported from France; in contrast, multiple-drug resistance was less common in home-produced poultry (Torre et al. 1993). Quinolone resistance has emerged in different phage types, possibly associated with the use of enrofloxacin. Diverse studies have shown that among non-typhoidal salmonellae, Virchow has a high potential for invasion in humans with high incidences of isolations from blood (Mani, Brennand and Mandal 1974, Todd and Murdoch 1983, Wilkins and Roberts 1988, Threlfall, Hall and Rowe 1992a). Hence, the emergence of resistance to the likely therapeutic drug of choice in invasive Virchow infection causes much concern.

Although the vast majority of salmonellae recovered from humans in developed countries are serotypes from subsp. I, e.g. 99.73% of 67 767 isolates in France in a period of 4 years (Le Minor, Le Minor and Grimont 1985), evidence increasingly suggests that some serotypes from other subspecies may be pathogens of humans and animals and these will now be considered.

17.2 Subspecies II

The biochemical characters for identification of *S. enterica* subsp. *salamae* are given in Table 41.2. The O and phase-1 H antigens of most of the 477 serotypes described are similar to those of serotypes from subsp. *enterica* (Rohde 1965, Popoff and Le Minor 1992). Most retrospective studies have confirmed their rare occurrence in humans; thus, only 27 isolates of serotypes of subsp. II were found among 81 936 isolates, mostly from humans, reported in different surveys, e.g. Central Africa before 1960 (see Schrire et al. 1987), Malaysia 1973–82 (Jegathesan 1984) and France 1980–83 (Le Minor, Le Minor and Grimont 1985). The main reservoirs of this subspecies are healthy or diseased reptiles and diverse cold-blooded animals (Rohde 1965).

The first indication that strains of subsp. II might be found more often in human populations closely associated with the indigenous fauna of remote areas in some countries came from Iveson, MacKay-Scollay and Bamford (1969) in Western Australia. More recently, a relatively high frequency (6.4%) of isolation of subsp. II strains from humans was evident in southern Africa in the period 1979–84 (Schrire et al. 1987). Many isolates were from patients with symptoms of gastroenteritis or dysentery and, whilst most of them occurred sporadically, some clustering of cases was noted, e.g. of the former serotype Mobeni from children in an institutional outbreak. Isolates belonged to 203 serotypes, 45 of them newly described types present in both Namibia and South Africa. Schrire et al. (1987) speculated that a combination of poor conditions of hygiene and contamination of food and water supplies by wild animals contributed to the greater frequency of human infections with strains of subsp. II and also to the widespread presence of so many exotic serotypes in humans in that region.

17.3 Subspecies IIIa and IIIb

The members of these 2 subspecies (previously designated as *Salmonella* subgenus III or '*Arizona hinshawii*') are now named *S. enterica* subsp. *arizonae* (monophasic strains) and *S. enterica* subsp. *diarizonae* (diphasic strains); 94 and 317 serotypes, respectively, have been identified (Popoff, Bockemühl and Hickman-Brenner 1995). The biochemical properties helpful in their identification are presented in Table 41.2. Soon after their first isolation from reptiles in western states of the USA, it became clear that they were an important cause of diarrhoeal illness in turkey poults, with spread traced from farm to farm and infection transmitted by hatchery eggs (see Edwards, Fife and Ramsey 1959). As avian pathogens, particularly of chickens and turkeys, they are still of world-wide economic importance. The major serotype of subsp. *arizonae* in turkeys for 30 years has been $18:z_4,z_{32}:\_$; but other serotypes ($18:z_4,z_{23}:$ - and $53:z_4,z_{23}:$ -), formerly important in turkeys, are now rarely isolated from them (Edwards, McWhorter and Fife 1956, Weiss et al. 1986). The serotypes present in other avian species are not necessarily those prevalent in turkeys. For example, in earlier surveys serotype $40:z_4,z_{23}:$ - of subsp. IIIa was responsible for 50% of chicken infections but was rare in turkeys (Edwards, McWhorter and Fife 1956).

Epidemiological surveys in Australia have indicated that the distribution of serotypes of these 2 subspecies in reptiles, both captive and wild, is similar and not influenced by their proximity to humans (Iveson, MacKay-Scollay and Bamford 1969). Again, there are subtle differences in the serotypes carried by different reptilian species (Weiss et al. 1986) and

wild snakes are known to yield more commonly strains of serotypes from *arizonae* than *diarizonae* (Edwards, McWhorter and Fife 1956, Weiss et al. 1986). Reptiles remain an important reservoir of these subspecies (Weiss et al. 1986). Consumption of rattlesnake meat or powder is an unusual source of extraintestinal infections in patients with chronic medical conditions including AIDS (Noskin and Clarke 1990).

Members of these subspecies are often considered uncommon human pathogens, but reports of their involvement in serious human illness are not new (Edwards, Fife and Ramsey 1959). In a survey in the USA over 30 years (Weiss et al. 1986), 374 isolates of human origin included representatives of 71 serotypes; the 4 most common were one from subsp. *arizonae* ($18:z_4,z_{32}:$-) and 3 from *diarizonae* ($61:l,v:1,5,7$; $61:k:1.5,7$; and $60:r:e,n,x,z_{15}$); together they accounted for 55% of all human isolates. Serotypes $18:z_4,z_{23}:$ - and $21:g,z_{51}:$ - from *arizonae* and $61:k:1,5,7$ from *diarizonae* were isolated more commonly from extraintestinal than intestinal sites and accounted for 50% of all extraintestinal isolates. Weiss et al. (1986) suggested that strains of these 3 serotypes are more invasive than other serotypes of these 2 subspecies and that they are associated with higher mortality in, and have enhanced virulence for, humans. The proportion of these isolates giving rise to serious septicaemic and pyaemic illnesses is greater than for most other salmonella types (see Johnson et al. 1976). In a survey in the UK over 25 years (Hall and Rowe 1992), 66 isolates of human origin included representatives of 29 serotypes; the most common was $61:l,v:1,5,7$ which was also the commonest from terrapins. Many (35%) patients had a history of foreign travel. However, 41% of UK patients were children of <4 years of age, many of whom had not been abroad and for whom contact with terrapins or other reptiles, especially pet snakes, was a potential source of infection (Hall and Rowe 1992). In the UK series, only 2 patients had extraintestinal infections.

Differences in the frequency with which individual serotypes occurred in humans over the years probably reflect corresponding adaptations of individual serotypes in different animal hosts. Thus, serotype $18:z_4,z_{32}:$ - , the prevalent one in turkeys for several decades, is now the most common type found in humans (Weiss et al. 1986) from whom it was absent 30 years ago (Edwards, McWhorter and Fife 1956). Outbreaks of human infection are predominantly food-borne (Edwards, Fife and Ramsey 1959), and important serotypes prevalent in domestic animals like cattle ($61:l,v:1,5,7$) and sheep ($18:z_4,z_{32}:$ - ; $61:l,v,:1,5,7$; $61:k:1,5,7$) are also frequently isolated from humans.

17.4 Subspecies IV–VI

Most of the 66 serotypes of *S. enterica* subsp. *houtenae* (subsp. IV) belong to high O serogroups and are usually isolated from cold-blooded animals, particularly in the tropics, and from the inanimate environment. Available evidence suggests that they are isolated infrequently from humans in developed countries (Le Minor, Le Minor and Grimont 1985). Ten serotypes of *S. enterica* subsp. *indica* (subsp. VI) and 19 serotypes of *S. bongori* (Reeves et al. 1989), formerly designated as *S. enterica* subsp. *bongori* (subsp. V), have been defined (Popoff, Bockemühl and Hickman-Brenner 1995). The biochemical properties of these 3 groups are detailed (see Table 41.2); however, information about their epidemiology is sparse.

REFERENCES

Adegbola RA, Old DC, 1983, Fimbrial haemagglutinins in *Enterobacter* species, *J Gen Microbiol*, **129:** 2175–80.

Adegbola RA, Old DC, 1987, Antigenic relationships among type-1 fimbriae of Enterobacteriaceae revealed by immuno-electronmicroscopy, *J Med Microbiol*, **24:** 21–8.

Adegbola RA, Old DC, Aleksic S, 1983, Rare MR/K-like haemagglutinins (and type 3-like fimbriae) of *Salmonella* strains, *FEMS Microbiol Lett*, **19:** 233–8.

Albert MJ, Haider K et al., 1991, Multiresistant *Salmonella typhi* in Bangladesh, *J Antimicrob Chemother*, **27:** 554–5.

Altwegg M, Hickman-Brenner FW, Farmer JJ, 1989, Ribosomal RNA gene restriction patterns provide increased sensitivity for typing *Salmonella typhi* strains, *J Infect Dis*, **160:** 145–9.

Anand AC, Kataria VK et al., 1990, Epidemic multiresistant enteric fever in eastern India, *Lancet*, **335:** 352.

Anderson ES, 1964, The phage typing of salmonellae other than *S. typhi*, *The World Problem of Salmonellosis*, ed. van Oye E, Dr W Junk, The Hague, 89–110.

Anderson ES, 1968, Drug resistance in *Salmonella typhimurium* and its implications, *Br Med J*, **3:** 333–9.

Anderson ES, 1975, The problem and implications of chloramphenicol resistance in the typhoid bacillus, *J Hyg Camb*, **74:** 289–99.

Anderson ES, Lewis MJ, 1965, Drug resistance and its transfer in *Salmonella typhimurium*, *Nature (London)*, **206:** 579–83.

Anderson ES, Rogers AH, 1963, Slime polysaccharides of the Enterobacteriaceae, *Nature (London)*, **198:** 714–15.

Anderson ES, Smith HR, 1972, Chloramphenicol resistance in the typhoid bacillus, *Br Med J*, **3:** 329–31.

Anderson ES, Williams REO, 1956, Bacteriophage typing of enteric pathogens and staphylococci and its use in epidemiology, *J Clin Pathol*, **9:** 94–127.

Anderson ES, Threlfall EJ et al., 1973, Bacteriophage restriction in *Salmonella typhimurium* by R factors and transfer factors, *J Hyg Camb*, **71:** 619–31.

Anderson ES, Threlfall EJ et al., 1977a, Clonal distribution of resistance plasmid-carrying *Salmonella typhimurium*, mainly in the Middle East, *J Hyg Camb*, **79:** 425–48.

Anderson ES, Ward LR et al., 1977b, Bacteriophage-typing designations of *Salmonella typhimurium*, *J Hyg Camb*, **78:** 297–300.

Anderson ES, Ward LR et al., 1978, Correlation of phage type, biotype and source in strains of *Salmonella typhimurium*, *J Hyg Camb*, **81:** 203–17.

Angulo FJ, Swerdlow DL, 1995, Bacterial enteric infections in persons infected with human immunodeficiency virus, *Clin Infect Dis*, **21 (Suppl. 1):** S84–93.

Anonymous, 1969, *Report of the Joint Committee on the Use of Antibiotics in Animal Husbandry and Veterinary Medicine*, HMSO, London.

Anonymous, 1972, Typhoid fever – Mexico, *Morbid Mortal Weekly Rep*, **21:** 177–8.

Anonymous, 1992a, *Report of the Expert Group on Animal Feeding Stuffs*, HMSO, London.

Anonymous, 1992b, *Salmonella in Animal and Poultry Production 1992*, Central Veterinary Laboratory, New Haw, 1–40.

Anonymous, 1994a, *Salmonella in Animal and Poultry Production 1994*, Central Veterinary Laboratory, New Haw, 1–82.

Anonymous, 1994b, An outbreak of *Salmonella paratyphi* B infection in France, *Commun Dis Rep Weekly*, **4:** 165.

Anonymous, 1995, An outbreak of *Salmonella agona* due to contaminated snacks, *Commun Dis Rep Weekly*, **5:** 29–32.

Anonymous, 1996, Salmonella infections, England and Wales: reports to the PHLS (salmonella data set), *Commun Dis Rep Weekly*, **6:** 47.

d'Aoust J-Y, 1991, Psychrotrophy and foodborne *Salmonella*, *Int J Food Microbiol*, **13:** 207–16.

Baird-Parker AC, 1991, Foodborne salmonellosis, *Lancet Review of Foodborne Illness*, Edward Arnold, London, 53–61.

Baqúar N, Burnens A, Stanley J, 1994, Comparative evaluation

of molecular typing of strains from a national epidemic due to *Salmonella brandenburg* by rRNA gene and IS*200* probes and pulsed-field gel electrophoresis, *J Clin Microbiol*, **32:** 1876–80.

Barker RM, 1986, Tracing *Salmonella typhimurium* infection, *J Hyg Camb*, **96:** 1–4.

Barker RM, Old DC, 1979, Biotyping and colicine typing of *Salmonella typhimurium* strains of phage type 141 isolated in Scotland, *J Med Microbiol*, **12:** 265–76.

Barker RM, Old DC, 1980, Biotypes of strains of *Salmonella typhimurium* of phage types 49, 204 and 193, *J Med Microbiol*, **13:** 369–71.

Barker RM, Old DC, 1989, The usefulness of biotyping in studying the epidemiology and phylogeny of salmonellae, *J Med Microbiol*, **29:** 81–8.

Barker RM, Old DC, Sharp JCM, 1980, Phage type/biotype groups of *Salmonella typhimurium* in Scotland 1974–6: variation during spread of epidemic clones, *J Hyg Camb*, **84:** 115–25.

Barker R, Old DC, Tyc Z, 1982, Differential typing of *Salmonella agona*: type divergence in a new serotype, *J Hyg Camb*, **88:** 413–23.

Barker RM, Kearney GM et al., 1988, Types of *Salmonella paratyphi* B and their phylogenetic significance, *J Med Microbiol*, **26:** 285–93.

Barrow PA, Lovell MA, 1989, Functional homology of virulence plasmids in *Salmonella gallinarum*, *S. pullorum* and *S. typhimurium*, *Infect Immun*, **57:** 3136–41.

Beltran P, Musser JM et al., 1988, Towards a population genetic analysis of *Salmonella*: genetic diversity and relationships among strains of serotypes *S. choleraesuis*, *S. derby*, *S. dublin*, *S. enteritidis*, *S. heidelberg*, *S. infantis*, *S. newport*, and *S. typhimurium*, *Proc Natl Acad Sci USA*, **85:** 7753–7.

Beltran P, Plock SA et al., 1991, Reference collection of strains of the *Salmonella typhimurium* complex from natural populations, *J Gen Microbiol*, **137:** 601–6.

Bhutta ZA, Naqui SH et al., 1991, Multidrug-resistant typhoid in children: presentation and clinical features, *Rev Infect Dis*, **13:** 832–6.

Blaxland JD, Sojka WJ et al., 1956, A study of *Salm. pullorum* and *Salm. gallinarum* strains isolated from field outbreaks of disease, *J Comp Pathol*, **66:** 270–7.

Boyd EF, Wang F-S et al., 1993, *Salmonella* reference collection B (SARB): strains of 37 serovars of subspecies I, *J Gen Microbiol*, **139:** 1125–32.

Brodie J, 1977, Antibodies and the Aberdeen typhoid outbreak of 1964 II. Coombs, complement fixation and fimbrial agglutination tests, *J Hyg Camb*, **79:** 181–92.

Brown DJ, Munro DS, Platt DJ, 1986, Recognition of the cryptic plasmid, pSLT, by restriction fingerprinting and a study of its incidence in Scottish *Salmonella* isolates, *J Hyg Camb*, **97:** 193–7.

Buchmeier NA, Heffron F, 1991, Inhibition of macrophage phagosome–lysosome fusion by *Salmonella typhimurium*, *Infect Immun*, **59:** 2232–8.

Buissière J, Coynault C, Le Minor L, 1977, Etude des conditions d'expréssion du caractère raffinose chez les *Escherichia coli* et *Salmonella*, *Ann Microbiol (Paris)*, **128A:** 167–83.

Callow BR, 1959, A new phage typing scheme for *Salmonella typhimurium*, *J Hyg Camb*, **57:** 346–59.

Carter PB, Collins FM, 1974, The route of enteric infection in normal mice, *J Exp Med*, **139:** 1189–203.

Casalino M, Comanducci A et al., 1984, Stability of plasmid content in *Salmonella wien* in late phases of the epidemic history, *Antimicrob Agents Chemother*, **25:** 499–501.

Chambers RM, McAdam P et al., 1987, A phage-typing scheme for *Salmonella virchow*, *FEMS Microbiol Lett*, **40:** 155–7.

Chart H, 1995, Detection of antibody responses to infection with *Salmonella*, *Serodiagn Immunother Infect Dis*, **7:** 34–9.

Chart H, Ward LR, Rowe B, 1995, Serological response of

patients with clinical typhoid, *Serodiagn Immunother Infect Dis*, **7**: 30–3.

Chart H, Rowe B et al., 1989, Conversion of *Salmonella enteritidis* phage type 4 to phage type 7 involves loss of lipopolysaccharide with a concomitant loss of virulence, *FEMS Microbiol Lett*, **60**: 37–40.

Chowdry N, Threlfall EJ et al., 1993, Genotype analysis of faecal and blood isolates of *Salmonella dublin* from humans, *Epidemiol Infect*, **110**: 217–25.

Clarke GJ, Qi G-M et al., 1988, Expression of an antigen in strains of *Salmonella typhimurium* which reacts with antibodies to cholera toxin, *J Med Microbiol*, **25**: 139–46.

Clegg S, Swenson DL, 1994, Salmonella fimbriae, *Fimbriæ – Adhesion, Genetics, Biogenesis and Vaccines*, ed. Klemm P, CRC Press, Boca Raton, FL, 105–13.

Coovadia YM, Gathiram V et al., 1992, An outbreak of multiresistant *Salmonella typhi* in South Africa, *Q J Med*, **82**: 91–100.

Cowden JM, Chisholm D et al., 1989a, Two outbreaks of *Salmonella enteritidis* phage type 4 infection associated with the consumption of fresh shell-egg products, *Epidemiol Infect*, **103**: 47–52.

Cowden JM, Lynch D et al., 1989b, Case-control study of infections with *Salmonella enteritidis* phage type 4 in England, *Br Med J*, **299**: 771–3.

Coyle EF, Palmer SR et al., 1988, *Salmonella enteritidis* phage type 4 infection: association with hens' eggs, *Lancet*, **2**: 1295–7.

Craigie J, Felix A, 1947, Typing of typhoid bacilli with Vi bacteriophages: suggestions for its standardisation, *Lancet*, **1**: 823–7.

Craigie J, Yen CH, 1938, Demonstration of types of *B. typhosus* by means of preparations of type II Vi phage: principles and techniques, *Can Public Health J*, **29**: 448–63.

Crichton PB, Old DC, 1990, Salmonellae of serotypes Gallinarum and Pullorum grouped by biotyping and fimbrial-gene probing, *J Med Microbiol*, **32**: 145–52.

Crichton PB, Yakubu DE et al., 1989, Immunological and genetical relatedness of type-1 and type-2 fimbriae in salmonellas of serotypes Gallinarum, Pullorum and Typhimurium, *J Appl Bacteriol*, **67**: 283–91.

Crichton PB, Old DC et al., 1996, Characterisation of strains of *Salmonella* serotype Livingstone by multiple typing, *J Med Microbiol*, **44**: 325–31.

Daniels EM, Schneerson R et al., 1989, Characterization of the *Salmonella paratyphi* C Vi polysaccharide, *Infect Immun*, **57**: 3159–64.

Desenclos J-C, Bouvet P et al., 1996, Large outbreak of *Salmonella enterica* serotype *paratyphi* B infection caused by a goats' milk cheese, France, 1993: a case finding and epidemiological study, *Br Med J*, **312**: 91–3.

Duguid JP, 1985, Antigens of type-1 fimbriae, *Immunology of the Bacterial Cell Envelope*, eds Stewart-Tull DES, Davies M, John Wiley & Sons, Chichester, 301–18.

Duguid JP, Anderson ES, Campbell I, 1966, Fimbriae and adhesive properties in salmonellae, *J Pathol Bacteriol*, **92**: 107–38.

Duguid JP, Campbell I, 1969, Antigens of the type-1 fimbriae of salmonellae and other enterobacteria, *J Med Microbiol*, **2**: 535–53.

Duguid JP, Old DC, 1980, Adhesive properties of Enterobacteriaceae, *Bacterial Adherence*, Receptors and Recognition, Series B, vol. 6, ed. Beachey EH, Chapman and Hall, London, 187–217.

Duguid JP, Old DC, 1994, Introduction: a historical perspective, *Fimbriae – Adhesion, Genetics, Biogenesis and Vaccines*, ed. Klemm P, CRC Press, Boca Raton, FL, 1–7.

Duguid JP, Smith IW et al., 1955, Non-flagellar filamentous appendages ('fimbriae') and haemagglutinating activity in *Bacterium coli*, *J Pathol Bacteriol*, **70**: 335–48.

Duguid JP, Anderson ES et al., 1975, A new biotyping scheme for *Salmonella typhimurium* and its phylogenetic significance, *J Med Microbiol*, **8**: 149–66.

Edelman R, Levine MM, 1986, Summary of an international workshop on typhoid fever, *Rev Infect Dis*, **8**: 329–49.

Edwards PR, Fife M, Ramsey CH, 1959, Studies on the Arizona group of Enterobacteriaceae, *Bacteriol Rev*, **23**: 155–74.

Edwards PR, Kauffmann F, Huey CR, 1957, An unusual salmonella type (*Salmonella montgomery*) 11:d,a:d,e,n,z_{15}, *Acta Pathol Microbiol Scand*, **41**: 517–20.

Edwards PR, McWhorter AC, Fife MA, 1956, The Arizona group of Enterobacteriaceae in animals and man. Occurrence and distribution, *Bull W H O*, **14**: 511–28.

Erdem B, Threlfall EJ et al., 1994, Plasmid profile typing provides a method for the differentiation of strains of *Salmonella enteritidis* phage type 4 isolated in Turkey, *Appl Microbiol Lett*, **19**: 265–7.

Ewing WH, 1986, *Edwards and Ewing's Identification of Enterobacteriaceae*, 4th edn, Elsevier, New York.

Ezquerra E, Burnens A et al., 1993, Genotypic typing and phylogenetic analysis of *Salmonella paratyphi* B and *S. java* with IS*200*, *J Gen Microbiol*, **139**: 2409–14.

Farmer JJ, 1995, Enterobacteriaceae: introduction and identification, *Manual of Clinical Microbiology*, 6th edn, eds Murray PR, Baron EJ et al., ASM Press, Washington, DC, 438–49.

Felix A, Callow BR, 1943, Typing of paratyphoid B bacilli by means of Vi bacteriophage, *Br Med J*, **2**: 127–30.

Felix A, Callow BR, 1951, Paratyphoid-B Vi-phage typing, *Lancet*, **2**: 10–14.

Felix A, Pitt RM, 1934, A new antigen of *B. typhosus*. Its relation to virulence and to active and passive immunization, *Lancet*, **2**: 186–91.

Fierer J, Fleming W, 1983, Distinctive biochemical features of *Salmonella dublin* isolated in California, *J Clin Microbiol*, **17**: 552–4.

Fierer J, Krause M et al., 1992, *Salmonella typhimurium* bacteremia: association with the virulence plasmid, *J Infect Dis*, **166**: 639–42.

Finkelstein RA, Marchlewicz BA et al., 1983, Isolation and characterization of a cholera-related enterotoxin from *Salmonella typhimurium*, *FEMS Microbiol Lett*, **17**: 239–41.

Finlay BB, Leung KY et al., 1992, *Salmonella* interactions with the epithelial cell, *ASM News*, **58**: 486–9.

Fisher IST, Rowe B et al., 1994, 'Salm-Net' – laboratory-based surveillance of human salmonella infections in Europe, *PHLS Microbiol Dig*, **11**: 181–2.

Foster JW, 1992, Beyond pH homeostasis: the acid tolerance response of salmonellae, *ASM News*, **58**: 266–70.

Frankel G, Newton SMC et al., 1989, Intragenic recombination in a flagellin gene: characterization of the *H1:j* gene of *Salmonella typhi*, *EMBO J*, **8**: 3149–52.

Fricker CR, 1987, The isolation of salmonellas and campylobacters, *J Appl Bacteriol*, **63**: 99–116.

Frost JA, Threlfall EJ, Rowe B, 1995, Antibiotic resistance in salmonellas from humans in England and Wales: the situation in 1994, *PHLS Microbiol Dig*, **12**: 131–3.

Frost JA, Ward LR, Rowe B, 1989, Acquisition of a drug resistance plasmid converts *Salmonella enteritidis* phage type 4 to phage type 24, *Epidemiol Infect*, **103**: 243–8.

Frost JA, Rowe B et al., 1982, Characterization of resistance plasmids and carried phages in an epidemic clone of multiresistant *Salmonella typhimurium* in India, *J Hyg Camb*, **88**: 193–204.

Gaines S, Sprinz H et al., 1968, Studies on infection and immunity in experimental typhoid fever, *J Infect Dis*, **118**: 293–306.

Gianella RA, 1979, Importance of the intestinal inflammatory reaction in salmonella-mediated intestinal secretion, *Infect Immun*, **23**: 140–5.

Gianella RA, Rout WR, Formal SB, 1977, Effect of indomethacin on intestinal water transport in salmonella-infected rhesus monkeys, *Infect Immun*, **17**: 136–9.

Gibert I, Barbe J, Casadesus J, 1990, Distribution of insertion sequence IS*200* in *Salmonella* and *Shigella*, *J Gen Microbiol*, **136**: 2555–60.

Grimont F, Grimont PAD, 1986, Ribosomal ribonucleic acid gene restriction patterns as potential taxonomic tools, *Ann Inst Pasteur (Paris)*, **137B**: 165–75.

Grossman DA, Witham ND et al., 1995, Flagellar serotypes of *Salmonella typhi* in Indonesia: relationships among motility, invasiveness and clinical illness, *J Infect Dis*, **171**: 212–16.

Guinée PAM, 1969, Phage types and resistance factors in *S. panama* strains from various countries, *Zentralbl Bakteriol Parasitenkd Infketionskr Hyg Abt I Orig*, **209**: 331–6.

Guinée PAM, Jansen WH et al., 1981, An unusual H antigen (z_{66}) in strains of *Salmonella typhi*, *Ann Microbiol (Paris)*, **132A**: 331–4.

Guiney DG, Fang FC et al., 1995, Biology and clinical significance of virulence plasmids in *Salmonella* serovars, *Clin Infect Dis*, **21 (Suppl. 2)**: S146–51.

Gulig PA, Curtis R, 1987, Plasmid-associated virulence of *Salmonella typhimurium*, *Infect Immun*, **55**: 2891–901.

Gulig PA, Danbara H et al., 1993, Molecular analysis of *spv* virulence genes of the salmonella virulence plasmids, *Mol Microbiol*, **7**: 825–30.

Hadfield TL, Monson MH, Wachsmuth IK, 1985, An outbreak of an antibiotic-resistant *Salmonella enteritidis* in Liberia, West Africa, *J Infect Dis*, **151**: 790–5.

Hall MLM, Rowe B, 1992, *Salmonella arizonae* in the United Kingdom from 1966 to 1990, *Epidemiol Infect*, **108**: 59–65.

Hampton MD, Threlfall EJ et al., 1995, *Salmonella typhimurium* DT 193: differentiation of an epidemic phage type by antibiogram, plasmid profile, plasmid fingerprint and salmonella plasmid virulence (*spv*) gene probe, *J Appl Bacteriol*, **78**: 402–8.

Heffernan EJ, Fierer J et al., 1987, Natural history of oral *Salmonella dublin* infection in BALB/c mice: effect of an 80-kilobase pair plasmid on virulence, *J Infect Dis*, **155**: 1254–9.

Helmuth R, Stephan R et al., 1985, Epidemiology of virulence-associated plasmids and outer membrane protein patterns with seven common *Salmonella* serovars, *Infect Immun*, **48**: 175–82.

Humphrey TJ, Baskerville A et al., 1989, *Salmonella enteritidis* phage type 4 from the contents of intact eggs: a study involving naturally infected hens, *Epidemiol Infect*, **103**: 415–23.

Iveson JB, Mackay-Scollay EM, Bamford V, 1969, *Salmonella* and Arizona in reptiles and man in Western Australia, *J Hyg Camb*, **67**: 135–45.

Jegathesan M, 1983, Phage types of *Salmonella typhi* isolated in Malaysia over the 10-year period 1970–1979, *J Hyg Camb*, **90**: 91–7.

Jegathesan M, 1984, Salmonella serotypes isolated from man in Malaysia over the ten-year period 1973–1982, *J Hyg Camb*, **92**: 395–9.

Jiwa SFH, 1981, Probing for enterotoxigenicity among the salmonellae: an evaluation of biological assays, *J Clin Microbiol*, **14**: 463–72.

Johnson RH, Lutwick LI et al., 1976, *Arizona hinshawii* infections. New cases, antimicrobial sensitivities and literature review, *Ann Intern Med*, **85**: 587–92.

Kasatiya S, Caprioli T, Champoux S, 1979, Bacteriophage typing scheme for *Salmonella infantis*, *J Clin Microbiol*, **10**: 637–40.

Kauffmann F, 1966, *The Bacteriology of Enterobacteriaceae*, Munksgaard, Copenhagen.

Kelterborn E, 1967, *Salmonella Species. First Isolation, Names and Occurrence*, Dr W Junk, The Hague.

Kelterborn E, 1987, *Catalogue of Salmonella First Isolations, 1965–1984*, Fisher, Jena.

Klugman KP, Gilbertson IT et al., 1987, Protective activity of Vi capsular polysaccharide vaccine against typhoid fever, *Lancet*, **2**: 1165–9.

Lam S, Roth JR, 1983, IS*200*: a *Salmonella*-specific insertion sequence, *Cell*, **34**: 951–60.

Lee JA, 1974, Recent trends in human salmonellosis in England and Wales: the epidemiology of prevalent serotypes other than *Salmonella typhimurium*, *J Hyg Camb*, **72**: 185–95.

Le Minor L, Coynault C, Pessoa G, 1974, Determinisme plasmi-

dique du caractère atypique de *S. typhimurium* et de *S. oranienburg* isolées au Bresil lors d'épidémies de 1971 a 1973, *Ann Microbiol (Paris)*, **125A**: 261–85.

Le Minor L, Le Minor S, Grimont PAD, 1985, Rapport quadriennal du Centre national des *Salmonella* sur l'origine et la répartition en sérotypes des souches isolées en France continentale au cours des années 1980 à 1983, *Rev Epidemiol Sante Publique*, **33**: 13–21.

Le Minor L, Popoff MY, 1987, Designation of *Salmonella enterica* sp. nov., nom. rev., as the type and only species of the genus *Salmonella*, *Int J Syst Bacteriol*, **37**: 465–8.

Le Minor L, Veron M, Popoff M, 1982a, Taxonomie des *Salmonella*, *Ann Microbiol (Paris)*, **133B**: 223–43.

Le Minor L, Veron M, Popoff M, 1982b, Proposition pour une nomenclature des *Salmonella*, *Ann Microbiol (Paris)*, **133B**: 245–54.

Le Minor L, Popoff MY et al., 1986, Individualisation d'une septième sous-espèce de *Salmonella*, *Ann Microbiol (Paris)*, **137B**: 211–17.

Le Minor S, 1972, Apparition en France d'une epidemie à *Salmonella wien*, *Med Mal Infect*, **2**: 441–8.

Levine WC, Buehler JW et al., 1991, Epidemiology of nontyphoidal *Salmonella* bacteremia during the human immunodeficiency virus epidemic, *J Infect Dis*, **164**: 81–7.

Li J, Smith NH et al., 1993, Evolutionary origin and radiation of the avian-adapted non-motile salmonellae, *J Med Microbiol*, **38**: 129–39.

Liebisch B, Schwarz S, 1996, Evaluation and comparison of molecular techniques for epidemiological typing of *Salmonella enterica* subsp. *enterica* serovar *dublin*, *J Clin Microbiol*, **34**: 641–6.

Lilleengen K, 1952, Typing of *Salmonella gallinarum* and *Salmonella pullorum* by means of bacteriophage, *Acta Pathol Microbiol Scand*, **30**: 194–202.

Lindberg AA, Le Minor L, 1984, Serology of *Salmonella*, *Methods in Microbiology*, vol. 15, ed. Bergan T, Academic Press, London, 1–141.

de Louvois J, 1993, Salmonella contamination of eggs: a potential source of human salmonellosis. A report of the PHLS surveys of imported and home-produced eggs, *PHLS Microbiol Dig*, **10**: 158–62.

de Louvois J, 1994, Salmonella contamination of stored hens' eggs. A PHLS Food Surveillance Group study, *PHLS Microbiol Dig*, **11**: 203–5.

McConnell MM, Smith HR et al., 1979, The value of plasmid studies in the epidemiology of infections due to drug-resistant *Salmonella wien*, *J Infect Dis*, **139**: 178–90.

MacNab RM, 1987, Flagella, *Escherichia coli and Salmonella typhimurium*, *Cellular and Molecular Biology*, vol. 1, ed. Neidhart FC, American Society for Microbiology, Washington, DC, 70–83.

Makela PH, Stocker BAD, 1969, Genetics of polysaccharide biosynthesis, *Annu Rev Genet*, **3**: 291–322.

Mandal BK, 1979, Typhoid and paratyphoid fever, *Clin Gastroenterol*, **8**: 715–35.

Mandal BK, 1991, Modern treatment of typhoid fever, *J Infect*, **22**: 1–4.

Mani V, Brennand J, Mandal BK, 1974, Invasive illness with *Salmonella virchow* infection, *Br Med J*, **2**: 143–4.

Manning EJ, Baird GD, Jones PW, 1986, The role of plasmid genes in the pathogenicity of *Salmonella dublin*, *J Med Microbiol*, **21**: 239–43.

Mirza SH, Beeching NJ, Hart CA, 1996, Multi-drug resistant typhoid: a global problem, *J Med Microbiol*, **44**: 317–19.

Mourad AS, Metwally M et al., 1993, Multiple-drug-resistant *Salmonella typhi*, *Clin Infect Dis*, **17**: 135–6.

Neu HC, Cherubin CE et al., 1975, Antimicrobial resistance and R-factor transfer among isolates of *Salmonella* in the Northeastern United States: a comparison of human and animal isolates, *J Infect Dis*, **132**: 617–22.

Nicolle P, Pavlatou M, Diverneau G, 1954, Les lysotypies auxiliaires de *Salmonella typhi*, *Ann Inst Pasteur (Paris)*, **87**: 493–509.

Norel F, Coynault C et al., 1989, Cloning and expression of plasmid DNA sequences involved in *Salmonella* serotype *typhimurium* virulence, *Mol Microbiol*, **3**: 733–43.

Noskin GA, Clarke JT, 1990, *Salmonella arizonae* bacteremia as the presenting manifestation of human immunodeficiency virus infection following rattlesnake meat ingestion, *Rev Infect Dis*, **12**: 514–17.

O'Brien AD, 1982, Innate resistance of mice to *Salmonella typhi* infection, *Infect Immun*, **38**: 948–52.

Olarte J, Galindo E, 1973, *Salmonella typhi* resistant to chloramphenicol, ampicillin and other antimicrobial agents: strains isolated during an extensive typhoid fever epidemic in Mexico, *Antimicrob Agents Chemother*, **4**: 597–601.

Old DC, 1992, Nomenclature of *Salmonella*, *J Med Microbiol*, **37**: 361–3.

Old DC, Adegbola RA, 1985, Antigenic relationships among type-3 fimbriae of Enterobacteriaceae revealed by immunoelectronmicroscopy, *J Med Microbiol*, **20**: 113–23.

Old DC, Barker RM, 1989, Numerical index of the discriminatory ability of biotyping for strains of *Salmonella typhimurium* and *Salmonella paratyphi B*, *Epidemiol Infect*, **103**: 435–43.

Old DC, Duguid JP, 1979, Transduction of fimbriation demonstrating common ancestry in FIRN strains of *Salmonella typhimurium*, *J Gen Microbiol*, **112**: 251–9.

Old DC, Porter-Boveri M, Munro DS, 1994, Human infection in Tayside, Scotland due to *Salmonella* serotype Livingstone, *J Med Microbiol*, **40**: 134–40.

Old DC, Yakubu DE, Senior BW, 1989, Characterisation of a fimbrial, mannose-resistant and eluting haemagglutinin (MREHA) produced by strains of *Salmonella* of serotype Sendai, *J Med Microbiol*, **30**: 59–68.

Olsen JE, Skov MN et al., 1996, Genomic lineage of *Salmonella enterica* serotype Gallinarum, *J Med Microbiol*, **45**: 413–18.

Pace J, Haymar J, Galan JE, 1993, Signal transduction and invasion of epithelial cells by *Salmonella typhimurium*, *Cell*, **72**: 505–14.

Palmer SR, Rowe B, 1986, Trends in salmonella infections, *PHLS Microbiol Dig*, **3**: 18–21.

Paniker CKJ, Vilma KN, 1972, Transferable chloramphenicol resistance in *Salmonella typhi*, *Nature (London)*, **239**: 109–10.

Pardon P, Popoff MY et al., 1986, Virulence-associated plasmids of *Salmonella* serotype Typhimurium in experimental murine infection, *Ann Inst Pasteur Microbiol*, **137B**: 47–60.

Pelkonen S, Rompanen E-L et al., 1994, Differentiation of *Salmonella* serovar infantis from human and animal sources by fingerprinting, IS*200* and 16S *rrn* loci, *J Clin Microbiol*, **32**: 2128–33.

Platt DJ, Chesham JS et al., 1986, Restriction enzyme fingerprinting of enterobacterial plasmids: a simple strategy with wide application, *J Hyg Camb*, **97**: 205–10.

Popoff MY, Bockemühl J, Hickman-Brenner FW, 1995, Supplement 1994 (no. 38) to the Kauffmann–White scheme, *Res Microbiol*, **146**: 799–803.

Popoff MY, Le Minor L, 1985, Expression of antigenic factor O:54 is associated with the presence of a plasmid in *Salmonella*, *Ann Inst Pasteur Microbiol*, **136B**: 169–79.

Popoff MY, Le Minor L, 1992, *Antigenic Formulas of the Salmonella Serovars*, 6th rvn, WHO Collaborating Centre for Reference and Research on Salmonella, Institut Pasteur, Paris.

Powell NG, Threlfall EJ et al., 1994, Subdivision of *Salmonella enteritidis* PT 4 by pulsed-field gel electrophoresis: potential for epidemiological surveillance, *FEMS Microbiol Lett*, **119**: 193–8.

Powell NG, Threlfall EJ et al., 1995, Correlation of change in phage type with pulsed field profile and 16S *rrn* profile in *Salmonella enteritidis* phage types 4, 7 and 9a, *Epidemiol Infect*, **114**: 403–11.

Prakash K, Pillai PK, 1992, Multidrug-resistant *Salmonella typhi* in India, *APUA Newslett*, **10**: 1–3.

Rampling A, 1990, Microbiological consequences of healthy eating, *Rev Med Microbiol*, **1**: 125–32.

Rankin S, Platt DJ, 1995, Phage conversion in *Salmonella enterica* serotype Enteritidis: implications for epidemiology, *Epidemiol Infect*, **114**: 227–36.

Reeves MW, Evins GM et al., 1989, Clonal nature of *Salmonella typhi* and its genetic relatedness to other salmonellae as shown by multilocus enzyme electrophoresis, and proposal of *Salmonella bongori* comb. nov., *J Clin Microbiol*, **27**: 313–20.

Reilly WJ, Forbes GI et al., 1988, Poultry-borne salmonellosis in Scotland, *Epidemiol Infect*, **101**: 115–22.

Reilly WJ, Old DC et al., 1985, An epidemiological study of *Salmonella montevideo* by biotyping, *J Hyg Camb*, **95**: 23–8.

Report, 1982, The geographical distribution of *Salmonella typhi* and *Salmonella paratyphi A* and *B* phage types during the period 1 January 1970 to 31 December 1973. The International Federation for Enteric Phage-Typing (IFEPT), *J Hyg Camb*, **88**: 231–54.

Report, 1993, *Advisory Committee for the Microbiological Safety of Food Report on Salmonella in Eggs*, HMSO, London, 1–58.

Robbins JD, Robbins JB, 1984, Re-examination of the protective role of the capsular polysaccharide (Vi antigen) of *Salmonella typhi*, *J Infect Dis*, **150**: 436–49.

Rodrigue DC, Tauxe RV, Rowe B, 1990, International increase in *Salmonella enteritidis*: a new pandemic? *Epidemiol Infect*, **105**: 21–7.

Rohde R, 1965, The identification, epidemiology and pathogenicity of the salmonellae of subgenus II, *J Appl Bacteriol*, **28**: 368–72.

Rohde R, Aleksic S et al., 1975, Profuse fimbriae conferring O-inagglutinability to several strains of *S. typhimurium* and *S. enteritidis* isolated from pasta products – cultural, morphological and serological experiments, *Zentralbl Bakteriol Parasitenkd Infektionskr Hyg Abt I Orig*, **230**: 38–50.

Rowe B, Threlfall EJ, 1984, Drug resistance in gram negative aerobic bacilli, *Br Med Bull*, **40**: 68–76.

Rowe B, Threlfall EJ, Ward LR, 1987, Does chloramphenicol remain the drug of choice for typhoid?, *Epidemiol Infect*, **98**: 379–83.

Rowe B, Threlfall EJ, Ward LR, 1991, Treatment of multiresistant typhoid fever, *Lancet*, **337**: 1422.

Rowe B, Ward LR, Threlfall EJ, 1990, Spread of multiresistant *Salmonella typhi*, *Lancet*, **336**: 1065.

Rowe B, Ward LR, Threlfall EJ, 1995, Ciprofloxacin-resistant *Salmonella typhi* in the UK, *Lancet*, **346**: 1302.

Rowe B, Ward LR, Threlfall EJ, 1997, Multiresistant *Salmonella typhi* – a world-wide epidemic, *Clin Infect Dis*, **24, Suppl. 1**: S106–9.

Roy SK, Speelman P et al., 1985, Diarrhea associated with typhoid fever, *J Infect Dis*, **151**: 1138–43.

de Sa JDH, Ward LR, Rowe B, 1980, A scheme for the phage typing of *Salmonella hadar*, *FEMS Microbiol Lett*, **9**: 175–7.

Sandefur PD, Peterson JW, 1977, Neutralization of *Salmonella* toxin-induced elongation of Chinese hamster ovary cells by cholera antitoxin, *Infect Immun*, **15**: 988–92.

Saphra I, Wassermann M, 1954, *Salmonella cholerae suis*. A clinical and epidemiological evaluation of 329 infections identified between 1940 and 1954 in the New York Salmonella Center, *Am J Med Sci*, **228**: 525–33.

Saphra I, Winter JW, 1957, Clinical manifestations of salmonellosis in man, *N Engl J Med*, **256**: 1128–34.

Schrire L, Crisp S et al., 1987, The prevalence of human isolates of *Salmonella* subspecies II in southern Africa, *Epidemiol Infect*, **98**: 25–31.

Schroeter A, Ward LR et al., 1994, *Salmonella enteritidis* phage types in Germany, *Eur J Epidemiol*, **10**: 645–8.

Scragg J, Rubidge C, Wallace HL, 1969, Typhoid fever in African and Indian children in Durban, *Arch Dis Child*, **44**: 18–28.

Selander RK, Musser JM, 1990, Population genetics of bacterial pathogenesis, *Molecular Basis of Bacterial Pathogenesis*, vol. 11, eds Iglewski BH, Clark VL, Academic Press, London, 11–36.

Selander RK, Smith NH, 1990, Molecular population genetics of *Salmonella, Rev Med Microbiol,* **1:** 219–28.

Selander RK, Caugant DA et al., 1986, Methods of multilocus enzyme electrophoresis for bacterial population genetics and systematics, *Appl Environ Microbiol,* **51:** 873–84.

Selander RK, Beltran P et al., 1990a, Genetic population structure, clonal phylogeny, and pathogenicity of *Salmonella paratyphi* B, *Infect Immun,* **58:** 1891–901.

Selander RK, Beltran P et al., 1990b, Evolutionary genetic relationships of clones of *Salmonella* serovars that cause human typhoid and other enteric fevers, *Infect Immun,* **58:** 2262–75.

Selander RK, Smith NH et al., 1992, Molecular evolutionary genetics of the cattle-adapted serovar *Salmonella dublin, J Bacteriol,* **174:** 3587–92.

Sharp JCM, Reilly WJ et al., 1983, *Salmonella montevideo* infection in sheep and cattle in Scotland 1970–81, *J Hyg Camb,* **90:** 225–32.

da Silva EN, 1985, The *Salmonella gallinarum* problem in central and South America, *Proceedings of the International Symposium on Salmonella,* ed. Shoeynbos GH, Am Assoc Avian Pathol, Philadelphia, PA, 150–6.

Silverman M, Simon M, 1980, Phase variation: genetic analysis of switching mutants, *Cell,* **19:** 845–54.

Small RG, Sharp JCM, 1979, A milk-borne outbreak due to *Salmonella dublin, J Hyg Camb,* **82:** 95–100.

Smith NH, Selander RK, 1990, Sequence invariance of the antigen-coding central region of the phase 1 flagellar filament gene (*fliC*) among strains of *Salmonella typhimurium, J Bacteriol,* **172:** 603–9.

Smith NH, Selander RK, 1991, Molecular genetic basis for complex flagellar antigen expression in a triphasic serovar of *Salmonella, Proc Natl Acad Sci USA,* **88:** 956–60.

Smith NH, Beltran P, Selander RK, 1990, Recombination of *Salmonella* phase 1 flagellin genes generates new serovars, *J Bacteriol,* **172:** 2209–16.

Snellings NJ, Johnson EM et al., 1981, Genetic regulation of variable Vi antigen expression in a strain of *Citrobacter freundii, J Bacteriol,* **145:** 1010–17.

Stanley J, Baqúar N, Burnens A, 1995, Molecular subtyping for *Salmonella panama, J Clin Microbiol,* **33:** 1206–11.

Stanley J, Chowdry-Baqúar N, Threlfall EJ, 1993, Genotypes and phylogenetic relationships of *Salmonella typhimurium* are defined by molecular fingerprinting of IS*200* and 16S *rrn* loci, *J Gen Microbiol,* **139:** 1133–40.

Stanley J, Jones CS, Threlfall EJ, 1991, Evolutionary lines among *Salmonella enteritidis* phage types are identified by insertion sequence IS*200* distribution, *FEMS Microbiol Lett,* **82:** 83–90.

Stanley J, Burnens N et al., 1992, The insertion sequence IS*200* fingerprints chromosomal genotypes and epidemiological relationships in *Salmonella heidelberg, J Gen Microbiol,* **138:** 2329–36.

Tacket CO, Ferreccio C et al., 1986, Safety and immunogenicity of two *Salmonella typhi* Vi capsular polysaccharide vaccines, *J Infect Dis,* **154:** 342–5.

Taylor DN, Bied JM et al., 1982a, *Salmonella dublin* infections in the United States, 1979–1980, *J Infect Dis,* **146:** 322–7.

Taylor DN, Wachsmuth IK et al., 1982b, Salmonellosis associated with marijuana. A multistate outbreak traced by plasmid fingerprinting, *N Engl J Med,* **306:** 1249–53.

Thong K-L, Cheong Y-M et al., 1994, Epidemiologic analysis of sporadic *Salmonella typhi* isolates and those from outbreaks by pulsed-field gel electrophoresis, *J Clin Microbiol,* **32:** 1135–41.

Threlfall EJ, Frost JA, 1990, The identification, typing and fingerprinting of *Salmonella:* laboratory aspects and epidemiological applications, *J Appl Bacteriol,* **68:** 5–16.

Threlfall EJ, Hall MLM, Rowe B, 1986, *Salmonella gold-coast* from outbreaks of food-poisoning in the British Isles can be differentiated by plasmid profiles, *J Hyg Camb,* **97:** 115–22.

Threlfall EJ, Hall MLM, Rowe B, 1992a, Salmonella bacteraemia in England and Wales, 1981–1990, *J Clin Pathol,* **45:** 34–6.

Threlfall EJ, Hall MLM, Rowe B, 1992b, Increase in *Salmonella berta* infections in humans in England and Wales from 1986 to 1990: association with imported poultry, *Eur J Epidemiol,* **8:** 27–33.

Threlfall EJ, Powell NG, Rowe B, 1994, Differentiation of salmonellas by molecular methods, *PHLS Microbiol Dig,* **11:** 199–202.

Threlfall EJ, Rowe B, Ward LR, 1991, Occurrence and treatment of multi-resistant *Salmonella typhi, PHLS Microbiol Dig,* **8:** 56–9.

Threlfall EJ, Rowe B, Ward LR, 1993, A comparison of multiple drug resistance in salmonellas from humans and food animals in England and Wales, 1981 and 1990, *Epidemiol Infect,* **111:** 189–97.

Threlfall EJ, Ward LR, Rowe B, 1978, Spread of multiresistant strains of *Salmonella typhimurium* phage types 204 and 193 in Britain, *Br Med J,* **2:** 997.

Threlfall EJ, Ward LR et al., 1980, Plasmid-encoded trimethoprim resistance in multiresistant epidemic *Salmonella typhimurium* phage types 204 and 193 in Britain, *Br Med J,* **280:** 1210–11.

Threlfall EJ, Rowe B et al., 1985, Increasing evidence of resistance to gentamicin and related aminoglycosides in *Salmonella typhimurium* phage type 204c in England, Wales and Scotland, *Vet Rec,* **117:** 355–7.

Threlfall EJ, Rowe B et al., 1986, Characterization of plasmids conferring resistance to gentamicin and apramycin in strains of *Salmonella typhimurium* phage type 204c isolated in Britain, *J Hyg Camb,* **97:** 419–26.

Threlfall EJ, Ward LR et al., 1992, Widespread occurrence of multiple drug-resistant *Salmonella typhi* in India, *Eur J Clin Microbiol Infect Dis,* **11:** 990–3.

Threlfall EJ, Chart H et al., 1993a, Interrelationships between strains of *Salmonella enteritidis* belonging to phage types 4, 7, 7a, 8, 13, 13a, 23, 24 and 30, *J Appl Bacteriol,* **75:** 43–8.

Threlfall E J, Torre E et al., 1993b, Insertion sequence IS*200* can differentiate drug-resistant and drug-sensitive *Salmonella typhi* of Vi-phage types E1 and M1, *J Med Microbiol,* **39:** 454–8.

Threlfall EJ, Frost JA et al., 1994a, Epidemic in cattle of *S. typhimurium* DT 104 with chromosomally-integrated multiple drug resistance, *Vet Rec,* **134:** 577.

Threlfall EJ, Hampton MD et al., 1994b, Use of plasmid profile typing for surveillance of *Salmonella enteritidis* phage type 4 from humans, poultry and eggs, *Epidemiol Infect,* **112:** 25–31.

Threlfall EJ, Hampton MD et al., 1994c, Identification of a conjugative plasmid carrying antibiotic resistance and salmonella plasmid virulence (*spv*), *Appl Microbiol Lett,* **18:** 82–5.

Threlfall EJ, Torre E et al., 1994d, Insertion sequence IS*200* fingerprinting of *Salmonella typhi:* an assessment of epidemiological applicability, *Epidemiol Infect,* **112:** 253–61.

Threlfall EJ, Frost JA et al., 1996a, Increasing spectrum of resistance in multiresistant *Salmonella typhimurium, Lancet,* **347:** 1053–4.

Threlfall EJ, Hampton MD et al., 1996b, Application of pulsed-field gel electrophoresis to an international outbreak of *Salmonella agona, Emerging Infect Dis,* **2:** 59–61.

Timoney JF, Shivaprasad HL et al., 1989, Egg transmission following experimental infection of laying hens with *Salmonella enteritidis* phage type 4, *Vet Rec,* **125:** 600–1.

Tinya-Superable JF, Castillo MTG et al., 1995, Multidrug resistant *Salmonella typhi* outbreak in Metro Manila, Philippines, *Southeast Asian J Trop Med Public Health,* **26 (Suppl. 2):** S37–8.

Todd WTA, Murdoch J McC, 1983, *Salmonella virchow:* a cause of significant bloodstream invasion, *Scott Med J,* **28:** 176–8.

Tompkins LS, Troup N et al., 1986, Cloned, random chromosomal sequences as probes to identify *Salmonella* species, *J Infect Dis,* **152:** 156–62.

Torre E, Threlfall EJ et al., 1993, Characterization of *Salmonella virchow* phage types by plasmid profile and IS*200* distribution, *J Appl Bacteriol,* **75:** 435–40.

Turnbull PCB, 1979, Food poisoning with special reference to *Salmonella* – its epidemiology, pathogenesis and control, *Clin Gastroenterol,* **8:** 663–714.

Vassiliadis P, Trichopoulos D et al., 1981, Salmonella isolation with Rappaport's enrichment medium of different compositions, *Zentralbl Bakteriol Parasitenkd Infektionskr Hyg Abt I Orig*, **173**: 382–9.

Vatopoulos AC, Mainas E et al., 1994, Molecular epidemiology of ampicillin-resistant clinical isolates of *Salmonella enteritidis*, *J Clin Microbiol*, **32**: 1322–5.

Verma N, Reeves P, 1989, Identification and sequence of *rfb*S and *rfb*E which determine antigenic specificity of group A and group D salmonellae, *J Bacteriol*, **171**: 5694–701.

Wallace MR, Yousif AA et al., 1993, Ciprofloxacin versus ceftriaxone in the treatment of multiresistant typhoid fever, *Eur J Clin Microbiol Infect Dis*, **12**: 907–10.

Wallis TS, Starkey WG et al., 1986a, Enterotoxin production by *Salmonella typhimurium* strains of different virulence, *J Med Microbiol*, **21**: 19–23.

Wallis TS, Starkey WG et al., 1986b, The nature and role of mucosal damage in relation to *Salmonella typhimurium*-induced fluid secretion in the rabbit ileum, *J Med Microbiol*, **22**: 39–49.

Walton JR, 1972, Bacteriological, biochemical and virulence studies on *Salmonella dublin* from abortion and enteric disease in cattle and sheep, *Vet Rec*, **90**: 236–40.

Ward LR, de Sa JDH, Rowe B, 1987, A phage-typing scheme for *Salmonella enteritidis*, *Epidemiol Infect*, **99**: 291–304.

Ward LR, Threlfall EJ, Rowe B, 1990, Multiple drug resistance in salmonellas isolated from humans in England and Wales: a comparison of 1981 with 1988, *J Clin Pathol*, **43**: 563–6.

Wei L-N, Joys TM, 1985, Covalent structure of three phase 1 flagellar filament proteins of *Salmonella*, *J Mol Biol*, **186**: 791–803.

Wei L-N, Joys TM, 1986, The nucleotide sequence of the H-1r gene of *Salmonella rubislaw*, *Nucleic Acids Res*, **14**: 8227.

Weiss SH, Blaser MJ et al., 1986, Occurrence and distribution of serotypes of the Arizona subgroup of *Salmonella* strains in the United States from 1967 to 1976, *J Clin Microbiol*, **23**: 1056–64.

Wilkins EGL, Roberts C, 1988, Extraintestinal salmonellosis, *Epidemiol Infect*, **100**: 361–8.

Williamson CM, Baird D, Manning EJ, 1988, A common virulence region on plasmids from eleven serotypes of *Salmonella*, *J Gen Microbiol*, **134**: 975–82.

Williamson CM, Pullinger GD, Lax AJ, 1988, Identification of an essential virulence region on *Salmonella* plasmids, *Microb Pathog*, **5**: 469–73.

Woodward MJ, Mclaren I, Wray C, 1989, Distribution of virulence plasmids within salmonellae, *J Gen Microbiol*, **135**: 503–11.

Wray C, McLaren I et al., 1987, Differentiation of *Salmonella typhimurium* DT204c by plasmid profile and biotyping, *Vet Rec*, **121**: 514–16.

Yakubu DE, Senior BW, Old DC, 1989, A novel fimbrial haemagglutinin produced by a strain of *Salmonella* of serotype Salinatis, *FEMS Microbiol Lett*, **57**: 29–34.

Zinder ND, Lederberg J, 1952, Genetic exchange in *Salmonella*, *J Bacteriol*, **64**: 679–99.

CITROBACTER, ENTEROBACTER, KLEBSIELLA, SERRATIA AND OTHER MEMBERS OF THE ENTEROBACTERIACEAE

B Holmes and H M Aucken

1 INTRODUCTION

This chapter describes important members of the Enterobacteriaceae that are (together with *Escherichia*) commonly referred to as 'coliform bacteria' (Chapter 39), i.e. members of genera in which lactose fermentation is usual, such as *Enterobacter* and *Klebsiella*. Considering these organisms together does not imply that lactose fermentation is of any great taxonomic significance. Later in the chapter shorter descriptions of other genera, in which lactose fermentation differs between strains or is absent, are given. Separate chapters or parts of chapters are devoted to *Escherichia* and *Shigella* (Chapter 40), *Proteus*, *Morganella* and *Providencia* (Chapter 43), *Salmonella* (Chapter 41), and *Yersinia* (Chapter 44).

Ahmad, Weisburg and Jensen (1990) presented a comprehensive phylogenetic tree for virtually the entire assemblage of enteric bacteria. Character states of aromatic amino acid biosynthesis were used as criteria and the results were compared with partial trees based upon sequencing of 16S rRNA, 5S rRNA, and tryptophan leader peptide. Three major clusters were apparent: enterocluster 1 possesses a gene fusion (*trpG–trpD*) encoding anthranilate synthase of tryptophan biosynthesis and includes the genera *Citrobacter*, *Enterobacter*, *Escherichia*, *Klebsiella*, *Salmonella* and *Shigella*. The remaining 2 clusters lack the *trpG–trpD* gene

fusion, but differ in the presence (enterocluster 2) or absence (enterocluster 3) of the 3-step overflow pathway to L-phenylalanine. Enterocluster 2 comprises the genera *Erwinia* and *Serratia*. Enterocluster 3 includes the genera *Cedecea*, *Edwardsiella*, *Hafnia*, *Kluyvera*, *Morganella*, *Proteus*, *Providencia* and *Yersinia*.

With a few exceptions, the genera described in this chapter conform to the general definition of the Enterobacteriaceae given in Chapter 39: they are aerobic and facultatively anaerobic organisms that ferment glucose and give a positive catalase and a negative oxidase reaction; all of them reduce nitrate to nitrite; and only in *Tatumella* are there motile strains that do not exhibit peritrichous flagella.

2 CITROBACTER

2.1 Definition

Citrobacter species are motile organisms that ferment mannitol, usually with gas production. They may or may not ferment lactose but nearly always produce β-galactosidase. They give a positive methyl red (MR) test and a negative Voges–Proskauer (VP) test. They grow in Simmons' citrate medium and may or may not hydrolyse urea; they do not decarboxylate lysine. Many strains produce a dihydrolase for arginine and most strains decarboxylate ornithine. These organisms are found in human clinical specimens, soil and water, and in the intestinal tract of animals. The G + C content of the DNA is 52–54 mol% and the type species is *Citrobacter freundii*.

2.2 Classification

Werkman and Gillen (1932) proposed the establishment of the genus *Citrobacter* to include certain 'intermediate' coliform bacteria (Chapter 39) that produced trimethylene glycol from glycerol. The name did not find immediate acceptance and these organisms were described as '*Escherichia freundii*' by Yale (1939). A number of lactose-negative or late lactose-fermenting organisms described some years later shared certain somatic antigens with salmonellae and many possessed the Vi antigen of *Salmonella* serotype Typhi. These organisms were known as the Ballerup-Bethesda group until West and Edwards (1954) showed their similarity to strains of '*E. freundii*'. Kauffmann (1956) subsequently revived the name *Citrobacter* for them and the species became known as *Citrobacter freundii*.

An outstanding feature of *C. freundii* is its ability to blacken triple sugar iron agar through the production of H_2S. In 1971, Young and her colleagues described a group of organisms that were H_2S-negative in this medium and placed them in a new genus *Levinea*, in which there were 2 species, *Levinea amalonatica* and *Levinea malonatica*. Ewing and Davis (1972) suggested that *L. malonatica* was a later synonym of *Citrobacter diversum* (see Werkman and Gillen 1932) and proposed the revival of the name *Citrobacter diversus*, with the change of spelling for grammatical reasons. However, in 1970, Frederiksen had also described a group of organisms for which he proposed the name *Citrobacter koseri*. Subsequent studies (Crosa et al. 1974, Sakazaki et al. 1976) showed that *C. diversus* and *C. koseri* are synonyms. The authors of this chapter preferred the name *C. koseri* because the description of *C. diversus* given by Ewing and Davis (1972) differs in several respects from the original description of the species (Holmes et al. 1974). The Judicial Commission of the International Committee on Systematic Bacteriology no longer recognizes *C. diversus* and has, instead, validated the name *C. koseri* in its place. Brenner and coworkers (1977) re-examined strains of *L. amalonatica* and suggested that these might also be included in the genus *Citrobacter* as a third species, *Citrobacter amalonaticus*.

In the previous edition of this book the authors accepted that the genus comprised the 3 species *C. amalonaticus*, *C. freundii* and *C. koseri* (*C. diversus*). Subsequently, the genus was determined to contain 11 genomospecies separable by their biochemical characters (Brenner et al. 1993). *C. amalonaticus* and *C. koseri* proved to be homogeneous species, as previously described. *C. amalonaticus* biogroup 1 as described by Farmer et al. (1985a), was shown to be a separate homogeneous species, which was named *Citrobacter farmeri*. The *C. freundii* complex was quite heterogeneous;

C. freundii sensu stricto, as represented by the type strain, contained only 9 of 66 strains in this complex, whereas the remaining 57 strains were members of 7 genomospecies. Genomospecies 5, containing 21 strains, was named *Citrobacter youngae*; genomospecies 6, containing 15 strains, was named *Citrobacter braakii*; genomospecies 7 and 8, each containing 6 strains, were named *Citrobacter werkmanii* and *Citrobacter sedlakii*, respectively. Genomospecies 9, 10 and 11, each containing 3 strains, were not named. The 8 named species in the genus are thus: *C. amalonaticus*, *C. braakii*, *C. farmeri*, *C. freundii*, *C. koseri*, *C. sedlakii*, *C. werkmanii* and *C. youngae* (Table 42.1).

2.3 Morphological and cultural characters

In these respects strains of *Citrobacter* resemble most other members of the Enterobacteriaceae. They grow well on ordinary media producing smooth, convex colonies 2–4 mm in diameter on nutrient agar. They are not pigmented. Rough or mucoid forms sometimes occur.

2.4 Biochemical activities

The chief biochemical reactions of the genus are shown in Chapter 39 (see Table 39.2, p. 927) and the distinguishing characters of the 8 named species are set out in Table 42.1. The expansion in number of species necessitates a wider range of, and more specialized, tests than previously if full identification is to be attempted (Table 42.1). Janda et al. (1994) attempted identification of 235 *Citrobacter* strains to the species level on the basis of the 15 conventional tests of Table 42.1; 100% of the *C. amalonaticus* group strains and 81% of the *C. freundii* complex strains could be definitively assigned to one of the previously established or more recently designated species or hybridization groups of the genus *Citrobacter*. Within the *C. freundii* complex, *C. freundii* predominated (37%), followed by *C. youngae* (24%), *C. braakii* (13%), and *C. werkmanii* (6%). The ability of commercial identification systems to identify the more recently recognized species of *Citrobacter* has been evaluated by O'Hara, Roman and Miller (1995). Strains of *C. freundii* able to produce ornithine decarboxylase but unable to produce β-galactosidase have been shown by various techniques (including DNA–DNA hybridization) to represent only a separate biotype and not a separate species (Popoff and Stoleru 1980).

2.5 Susceptibility to antimicrobial agents

C. freundii is usually susceptible to aminoglycosides and chloramphenicol and susceptibility to ampicillin, cephalosporins and tetracycline varies. Holmes and his colleagues (1974) showed that 79% of *C. freundii* strains were resistant to cephaloridine and susceptible to carbenicillin, whereas 96% of *C. koseri* strains were susceptible to cephaloridine and resistant to carbenicillin. Lund, Matsen and Blazevic (1974) found that both *C. amalonaticus* and *C. koseri* were generally resist-

Table 42.1 Differentiation of species of *Citrobacter*

Property	C. amalo-naticus	C. braakii	C. farmeri	C. freundii	C. koseri	C. sedlakii	C. werkmanii	C. youngae
Acid from								
acetate	+	+	+	V	+	+	+	V
adonitol	-	-	-	-	+	-	-	-
arabitol	-	-	-	-	+	-	-	-
dulcitol	-	V	-	-	V	+	-	+
aesculin	V	-	V	-	V	V	-	-
melibiose	-	+	+	+	-	+	-	-
raffinose	-	-	+	+	-	-	-	-
salicin	+	-	+	-	+	V	-	-
sucrose	-	-	+	+	V	-	-	V
α-CH₃-D-glucoside	V	V	+	V	+	-	-	-
Growth in KCN medium	+	+	+	+	-	+	+	+
Indole production	+	V	+	V	+	+	-	-
Malonate fermentation	-	-	-	-	+	+	+	-
Ornithine decarboxylase	+	+	+	-	+	+	-	-
Urease production	V	V	V	V	V	+	+	V
Utilization of								
benzoate	V	-	+	-	-	+	-	-
m-coumarate	-	+	-	+	-	V	+	+
dulcitol	-	V	-	-	V	+	-	+
gentisate	+	+	+	+	+	+	+	-
3-hydroxy-benzoate	+	+	+	+	+	+	+	-
4-hydroxy-benzoate	+	-	+	-	-	+	-	-
myo-inositol	-	-	-	+	+	+	-	-
5-ketogluconate	+	+	+	+	+	-	V	+
lactulose	-	V	-	+	-	+	-	-
D-lyxose	-	V	-	+	+	V	+	V
maltitol	-	V	+	V	+	-	-	-
D-melibiose	-	+	+	+	-	+	-	-
palatinose	-	V	+	V	+	-	-	-
3-phenyl-propionate	-	+	-	V	-	-	+	+
protocatechuate	+	-	+	-	-	+	-	-
D-raffinose	-	-	+	+	-	-	-	-
L-sorbose	+	-	+	+	-	-	+	+
sucrose	-	-	+	+	V	-	-	-
D-tartrate	-	-	-	-	-	-	+	-
tricarballylate	+	+	+	+	-	+	+	-
L-tyrosine	-	+	-	+	+	-	+	+
1-O-CH₃-α-galactoside	-	+	+	+	-	+	-	V
3-O-CH₃-D-glucose	+	+	+	V	-	+	+	-

+, Most strains positive: −, most strains negative: V, some strains positive, others negative.

ant to ampicillin and carbenicillin. Gross and Rowe (1983) reported that resistance to cephaloridine, gentamicin, neomycin, streptomycin and sulphonamides also occurred frequently among *C. koseri* strains.

2.6   Typing methods

Serotyping schemes have been proposed for *C. amalonaticus* (Sourek and Aldová 1976), *C. freundii* (West and Edwards 1954, Sedlák and Slajsová 1966) and *C. koseri* (Gross and Rowe 1975, Gross et al. 1981). Determination of outer-membrane protein profiles has been found potentially useful in epidemiological investigations of disease caused by *C. koseri* (Kline, Mason and Kaplan 1988, 1989). Harvey et al. (1995) evaluated the epidemiological usefulness of an automated procedure for analysis of polymerase chain reaction (PCR)-generated DNA fingerprints to confirm the vertical transmission of *C. koseri* from a mother to her infant. A monoclonal antibody has been developed against *C. freundii* O36 (Shearman et al. 1984).

2.7   Habitat and pathogenicity

Members of the genus *Citrobacter* are often found in the faeces of humans and may be isolated from a variety of clinical specimens. They do not often give rise to serious infections, except *C. koseri*, which has been responsible for several outbreaks of neonatal meningitis (Gross, Rowe and Easton 1973, Gwynn and George 1973, Duhamel et al. 1975, Parry et al. 1980, Graham and Band 1981, Lin et al. 1987). Neonatal meningitis is usually accompanied by the development of brain abscesses and tends to have high rates of morbidity and mortality. Morgan et al. (1992) described brain abscesses occurring in 2 infants; both survived, albeit with some minor degree of brain damage. Eppes et al. (1993) reported a case of a neonate with *C. koseri* meningitis and brain abscesses who relapsed after initial antibiotic therapy and from whom the same organism (but a genetically different strain) was recovered from cerebrospinal fluid 4 years later during a neurosurgical procedure. A case of brain abscesses following urinary infection in an adult was described by Booth et al. (1993). The patient was treated with surgical drainage, cefotaxime and netilmicin. Strains from cerebrospinal fluid possess a minor outer-membrane protein of 32 kDa, which may serve as a marker for strains that are likely to cause meningitis or brain abscess in human neonates.

Clonally identical isolates of verotoxinogenic *C. freundii* proved responsible for a summer outbreak of severe gastroenteritis followed by haemolytic–uraemic syndrome (HUS) and thrombotic thrombocytopenic purpura in a nursery school and kindergarten (Tschape et al. 1995). Infant food has been identified as a vehicle in a nosocomial outbreak of *C. freundii* in a neonatal intensive care unit of a large hospital where colonization and clinical diseases due to the agent had been observed (Thurm and Gericke 1994). Occasion-

ally, like *C. koseri*, this organism can also cause neonatal meningitis (Joaquin et al. 1991–2).

The next 3 sections describe 3 genera of particular clinical importance: *Enterobacter*, *Klebsiella* and *Serratia*; they occur in such material in ratios of about 2:3.4:1. In the past, they were often referred to collectively as the 'KES' group and approximately 60% of all strains may be expected from urinary specimens, 10% from respiratory secretions and 10% from wounds and abscesses. Within these genera, non-enzyme-dependent multiple-drug resistance occurs preferentially.

3   ENTEROBACTER

3.1   Definition

Enterobacter organisms are motile and less often and less heavily capsulate than *Klebsiella*. They ferment mannitol and form gas from some sugars, including cellobiose but not starch. They are generally negative to MR, positive to VP, and grow on Simmons' citrate and in Møller's KCN medium, if tested at 30°C. There is no H_2S production in triple sugar iron agar and they do not deaminate phenylalanine. Gluconate is generally oxidized and ornithine decarboxylase is produced. The organisms are non-pigmented or yellow-pigmented; many liquefy gelatin. Their habitat is soil and water, but they are occasionally found in the human bowel flora. They occasionally cause septic infection in humans. The G + C content of the DNA is 52–60 mol% and the type species is *Enterobacter cloacae*.

3.2   Classification

The organism that Escherich (1885) described as '*Bacterium lactis aerogenes*' was non-motile; it was subsequently renamed '*Bacterium aerogenes*', and in 1900 was transferred to a separate genus '*Aerobacter*' by Beijerinck. The terms '*Bacterium*', '*Aerobacter*' or '*Klebsiella aerogenes*' have been applied by successive generations of water bacteriologists to all VP-positive coliform bacteria, whether motile or non-motile, except for those that liquefy gelatin rapidly. Later, some bacteriologists defined '*Aerobacter aerogenes*' as a motile organism and so distinguished it from *Klebsiella*. Motile, gelatin-liquefying '*Aerobacter aerogenes*'-like organisms were usually described by water bacteriologists as '*Bacterium cloacae*'. When it was discovered that many of the motile organisms from water and faeces liquefied gelatin slowly they were transferred to '*Cloaca*', taking the specific epithet *aerogenes* with them. Hormaeche and Munilla (1957) and Hormaeche and Edwards (1958) recognized as 'Cloaca A' and 'Cloaca B' the organisms now called *E. cloacae* and *Enterobacter aerogenes*, respectively (Report 1963). The genus has been renamed successively '*Aerobacter*' (Hormaeche and Edwards 1958) and *Enterobacter* (Hormaeche and Edwards 1960). The latter name gained general acceptance (Report 1963), and the genus *Enterobacter* is considered to include all the motile 'Aerobacter aerogenes'-like organisms, except those that form a red pigment and strains related to them, which are placed in the genus Serratia. E. cloacae is heterogeneous and comprises at least 6 genomic groups; however, the groups could not be differentiated phenotypically so there seemed to be no reason for an attempt to split E. cloacae into 2 or more species (Lindh and Ursing 1991). Nevertheless, Kosako et al. (1996) have proposed a new species, Enterobacter kobei, which differs phenotypically little from E. cloacae except in giving a negative reaction in the VP test.

In addition to E. aerogenes and E. cloacae, other species have been subsequently recognized in the genus. In 1976 Richard and colleagues described a new group of organisms that was most similar to E. aerogenes. Subsequently the name Enterobacter gergoviae was proposed for this group, strains of which are found in various clinical specimens and in the natural environment (Brenner et al. 1980). Strains previously regarded as yellow-pigmented, non-sorbitol-fermenting variants of E. cloacae have been shown by DNA–DNA hybridization to warrant recognition as a separate species for which the name Enterobacter sakazakii has been proposed (Farmer et al. 1980). Also described from clinical isolates are Enterobacter asburiae (Brenner et al. 1986), Enterobacter hormaechei (O'Hara et al. 1989) and Enterobacter taylorae (Farmer et al. 1985b). The latter was subsequently shown to be a later synonym of Enterobacter cancerogenus (see Schonheyder, Jensen and Frederiksen 1994) so the latter has priority. However, the name E. taylorae will be used here until the name E. cancerogenus comes into more common use. Although E. hormaechei was described from clinical isolates (22 of 23), it will not be described in detail here, pending the recognition of further isolates; the organism is included in Table 42.2 to facilitate such recognition. Two further species will not be considered further because they have so far been isolated only from water: Enterobacter amnigenus (Izard et al. 1981b) and Enterobacter intermedius (Izard, Gavini and Leclerc 1980). However, the isolation of E. amnigenus has been reported from an intravenous catheter, along with Pseudomonas aeruginosa, from the blood of a heart transplant patient (Bollet et al. 1991a). Also included in Table 42.2 are 2 more species, Enterobacter dissolvens and Enterobacter nimipressuralis, purely for completeness; neither has so far been encountered in human clinical specimens.

An anaerogenic, yellow-pigmented organism, which was described as 'Bacterium typhiflavum' by Dresel and Strickl (1928), and as 'Chromobacterium typhiflavum' in some of the earlier editions of this book, deserves description here. This organism is not uncommon in the human upper respiratory tract and in swabs from superficial lesions (see Slotnick and Tulman 1967, Gilardi, Bottone and Birnbaum 1970, Bottone and Schneierson 1972, Meyers et al. 1972); it has also been isolated from various animals (Muraschi, Friend and Bolles 1965, Lev, Alexander and Sobel 1969). The 'typhiflavum' strains are indistinguishable from Erwinia herbicola, which is anaerogenic and does not liquefy pectin (Graham and Hodgkiss 1967). Although E. her-

bicola is the name accepted by many microbiologists, the name Enterobacter agglomerans has been commonly used in the American literature. The authors are reluctant to accept the name E. agglomerans proposed by Ewing and Fife (1972) because the description of this organism differs from the original description of 'Bacillus agglomerans' in several important respects; in particular, the latter was described as having polar flagella. Ewing and Fife (1972) recognized 7 anaerogenic and 4 aerogenic biochemical varieties within the species. However, this classification showed little correlation with the results of DNA–DNA hybridization, by which 10 or more DNA-relatedness groups can be identified within the species. Studies of the group by numerical taxonomic analysis of phenotypic characters obtained with a variety of commercial systems (Mergaert et al. 1984, Verdonck et al. 1987), or by correlation of phenotypic characters with DNA–DNA hybridization results (Brenner et al. 1984) have further illustrated the heterogeneity of this taxon. Further study is still necessary before more definite proposals can be made about the classification and nomenclature of these organisms. However, in the previous edition of this book the authors regarded this heterogeneous group as a single species named Erwinia herbicola. More recently, the organism has been transferred to a new genus as Pantoea agglomerans (Gavini et al. 1989). In the interests of uniformity the organism is described under that name in this chapter, in the section on Enterobacter in view of the evident similarities between these 2 genera.

3.3 Morphological and cultural characters

Although motility is the main distinguishing character between Enterobacter and Klebsiella, a few strains that in all other respects resemble E. cloacae are non-motile. In fluid media, sausage-shaped aggregations or symplasmata may occur in P. agglomerans; these appear to be chains of spherical bodies, 7–13 μm in diameter, consisting of organisms within a matrix (Lev, Alexander and Sobel 1969). The colonies of Enterobacter strains may be somewhat mucoid, but the amount of extracellular material formed is usually not great. In P. agglomerans there is pigment of an ochre or rusty yellow colour; on further incubation, granular structures corresponding to the symplasmata appear, as well as biconvex bodies with a clear-cut margin. The latter probably represent downgrowths into the medium (Cruickshank 1935, Graham and Hodgkiss 1967).

P. agglomerans grows poorly on MacConkey agar and is not haemolytic on blood agar. In a gelatin stab, liquefaction usually begins in 6–10 days. Growth occurs between 20 and 37°C, but the optimum is near 37°C.

3.4 Biochemical activities

In general, the fermentative activity of Enterobacter strains is more limited than that of typical strains of Klebsiella; the most significant restriction is that of the

Table 42.2   Differentiation of species of *Enterobacter* and *Pantoea agglomerans*

Property	*E. aerogenes*	*E. amnigenus 1*	*E. amnigenus 2*	*E. asburiae*	*E. cloacae*	*E. dissolvens*	*E. gergoviae*	*E. hormaechei*	*E. intermedius*	*E. nimipressuralis*	*E. sakazakii*	*E. taylorae*	*P. agglomerans*
Acid from													
adonitol	+	−	−	−	V	−	−	−	−	−	−	−	−
aesculin	+	+	+	+	V	+	+	−	+	+	+	+	V
arabitol	+	−	−	−	−	NK	+	−	−	NK	−	−	V
glycerol	+	−	−	−	V	NK	+	−	+	+	−	−	V
i-inositol	+	−	−	−	−	V	−	−	−	V	V	−	−
melibiose	+	+	+	−	+	+	+	−	+	+	+	−	V
mucate	+	V	+	V	V	+	−	+	+	+	−	V	V
raffinose	+	+	−	V	+	+	+	−	+	V	+	−	V
L-rhamnose	+	+	+	−	+	+	+	+	+	+	+	+	+
sorbitol	+	V	+	+	+	+	−	−	+	+	−	−	V
sucrose	+	V	−	+	+	+	+	+	V	−	+	−	+
α-methyl-D-glucoside	+	V	+	+	+	+	−	−	+	+	+	V	−
Arginine dihydrolase	−	+[a]	V	−	+	V	−	V	−	+	+	+	
Growth in KCN medium	+	+	+	+	+	+	+	−	+	V	+	+	V
Lysine decarboxylase	+	−	−	−	−	−	V	−	−	−	−	−	−
Malonate fermentation	+	+	+	−	+	+	+	+	+	+	−	+	V
Methyl red test	−	−	V	+	−	−	−	V	−[b]	−	−	−	V
Motility	+	+	+	−	+	+	+	V	+	+	+	+	+
Urease formation	−	−	−	V	V	+	+	+	−	−	−	−	−
Yellow pigmentation	−	−	−	−	−	−	−	−	−	−	+	−	V

+, Most strains positive; −, most strains negative; V, some strains positive, others negative; NK, not known.
[a]Negative according to Holt et al. (1994).
[b]Positive according to Holt et al. (1994).

ability to form gas from starch, and often also from inositol and glycerol; but most *Enterobacter* strains do form gas from cellobiose and ferment rhamnose, characters which distinguish them from most species of *Serratia*. Some *Enterobacter* strains give a weak urease reaction in Christensen's medium. In the modified medium advocated by Kauffmann (1954), however, *Klebsiella* strains are urease-positive and *Enterobacter* strains usually negative (but *E. gergoviae* and *E. hormaechei* are exceptions to this rule). Although growth at 37°C is usually good, many *Enterobacter* strains give atypical biochemical reactions unless tested at a lower temperature. When strains of *P. agglomerans* are tested at 37°C, the MR reaction is positive and the VP reaction negative, though the latter is often positive at 30°C. The main cultural and biochemical characters of the genera *Enterobacter* and *Pantoea* are given in Chapter 39 (see Table 39.2, p. 927) and the characters

of 11 *Enterobacter* species (and of *P. agglomerans*) are given in Table 42.2.

E. aerogenes resembles *Klebsiella* in its wide range of fermentative activity and in its ability to form gas from cellobiose, glycerol and inositol, but it does not form gas from starch. It also differs from *Klebsiella* in being motile and in forming lysine and ornithine decarboxylase. Liquefaction of gelatin in 7–60 days distinguishes it from all the subspecies of *Klebsiella pneumoniae* but not from *Klebsiella oxytoca*. Nevertheless, Bascomb and her colleagues (1971) believed that it should be transferred to a reconstituted *Klebsiella* genus as *Klebsiella mobilis* and this is supported by DNA–DNA hybridization data. The proposal has, however, not gained wide acceptance. *E. cloacae* differs from *E. aerogenes* in attacking arginine but not lysine and in its inability to form gas from glycerol and inositol. It sometimes fails to liquefy gelatin. *E. gergoviae* differs from *E. aerogenes* in producing urease, and in giving negative results in the following tests: KCN tolerance, and fermentation of adonitol, *i*-inositol, D-sorbitol and mucate. *E. sakazakii* differs from *E. cloacae* in being yellow-pigmented, producing extracellular deoxyribonuclease, and failing to ferment D-sorbitol. Only strains of *E. asburiae* fail to ferment malonate, give a positive result in the MR test and fail to ferment L-rhamnose; only strains of this species and of *E. hormaechei* and *E. taylorae* fail to ferment melibiose.

Clinical, animal and plant isolates of *P. agglomerans*, representing different geographical areas, have been characterized phenotypically (Lindh et al. 1991). No strain decarboxylated ornithine and 22 strains, mainly plant isolates, showed delayed acid production from α-methyl-glycoside. In these 2 characters the results differed from the description of *P. agglomerans* given by Gavini et al. (1989).

3.5 Susceptibility to antimicrobial agents

Strains of *Enterobacter* are nearly always highly resistant to first-generation cephalosporins (Benner et al. 1965) by virtue of producing a β-lactamase with predominantly cephalosporinase activity (Jack and Richmond 1970). Many are also resistant to chloramphenicol, streptomycin and tetracycline. At one time most were susceptible to kanamycin and nearly all to gentamicin (Toala et al. 1970). Most British strains of *E. cloacae* remain susceptible to the third-generation cephalosporins, amikacin, gentamicin and nalidixic acid but more than 10% show resistance to ampicillin, carbenicillin, cefuroxime and sulphamethoxazole. Following treatment with ampicillin, isolates can develop markedly elevated MICs to several agents including cefotaxime, ceftazidime, cefuroxime and piperacillin. Administration of amdinocillin in combination with ceftazidime is said to confer a protective effect against emergence of resistance to ceftazidime. In Canada, many isolates of *Enterobacter* spp. (>16%) are resistant to the third-generation cephalosporins with marked cross-resistance to aztreonam (76.6%), piperacillin (63.1%) and piperacillin–tazobactam (44.9%; Toye, Scriver and Lowe 1993). Ciprofloxacin, cefepime, cefpirome, gentamicin, imipenem and tobramycin were consistently active against most isolates of *Enterobacter* spp. including those resistant to the third-generation cephalosporins. Elsewhere, resistance to imipenem has been observed, the proportion being 1.3% of isolates in the USA; the resistance appears to be related to mutants deficient in the production of non-specific porins.

Ehrhardt and Sanders (1993) reviewed the effects of the introduction of extended-spectrum cephalosporins into clinical use, which caused the prevalence of *Enterobacter* spp. to increase because of their natural resistance to earlier cephalosporins and their ability to develop resistance rapidly to the newer drugs. β-Lactam resistance in this genus is due, for the most part, to the presence of a Bush group 1 chromosomal cephalosporinase. This enzyme is normally inducible and resistance to older cephalosporins, aminopenicil-

lins and cephamycins results from either the extreme lability of the drugs to the enzyme or from their inducer activities. Resistance to newer cephalosporins, monobactams and penicillins is attributable to the selection of mutants which express large amounts of the enzyme. Such mutants arise as the result of a spontaneous mutation in one of the regulatory genes responsible for suppressing enzyme expression. Since the enzyme has very high affinity for the newer cephalosporins, this, coupled with the slow penetration of the drugs into the cell, provides a very efficient mechanism of resistance. Recent surveys in the USA and elsewhere have shown that the increased prevalence of multi-β-lactam-resistant *Enterobacter* strains is due to the increased use of the newer cephalosporins. Attempts to prevent these problems include the more judicious use of newer β-lactam antibiotics and the development of enhanced-potency cephalosporins, which are able to evade the resistance mechanism because they have lower enzyme affinity and permeate more rapidly into the cell. Monotherapy with an extended-spectrum cephalosporin should be avoided unless the presence of resistant mutants and inducibility of β-lactamase can be excluded. Plasmids also play a role in resistance, with up to 5 aminoglycoside-modifying enzymes being detected on the same R plasmid; *E. cloacae* is thus also important as a gene pool for the spread of resistance to other bacteria of clinical relevance.

Fussle et al. (1994) traced the development of resistance by *E. cloacae* during the treatment of pulmonary infections in intensive care patients. During therapy with cefotaxime and tobramycin, the strains from 47% of the patients became resistant to cefotaxime within 6 days. In all cases, resistance encompassed all other broad spectrum penicillins and cephalosporins tested, as well as aztreonam. Development of resistance regularly led to persistence of bacteria. Resistance to ciprofloxacin, imipenem or tobramycin was not observed. Treatment of 25 patients with persisting infections was successful in 6 of 7 patients receiving ciprofloxacin and in 17 of 18 patients treated with imipenem.

Huber and Thomas (1994) described how strains of *E. aerogenes* and *E. cloacae* with inducible β-lactamase developed resistance when cefoxitin was added to cefuroxime discs; this approach can be used in routine clinical laboratories to detect latent resistance due to chromosomally mediated inducible β-lactamase in enterobacters. Yu, Chow and Yu (1996) proposed use of the spiral plater in identifying those antimicrobial agents that induce few or no spontaneous mutants and, therefore, may be more likely to be successful in treating infections due to *Enterobacter* spp. Higashitani et al. (1995) found that when *E. cloacae* strains were treated with piperacillin in combination with tazobactam, the in vitro frequency of emergence of resistant strains (mutants producing β-lactamase) was lower than with bacteria treated with piperacillin or ceftazidime. *Enterobacter* strains differ from *Serratia* strains in being susceptible to the polymyxins (Greenup and Blazevic 1971).

Outbreaks of infection may need to be controlled

by interrupting the transmission of the epidemic strain(s), by measures such as cohort nursing, diligent hand-washing before and after procedures (*E. cloacae* has been found still present on the fingertips after 15 repeated courses of hand-washing and applications of disinfectants) and thorough environmental cleaning including decontamination of any equipment believed to have acted as a persistent reservoir. Pharmacy intervention may also be necessary; increasing resistance to ceftazidime and some other β-lactam antibiotics developed among *Enterobacter* spp. after increased use of ceftazidime at a 500-bed community teaching hospital (Schentag 1993). Severe restrictions on the use of ceftazidime were imposed by pharmacy intervention. For empiric therapy of severe infections, a combination of piperacillin plus tobramycin was most frequently substituted for ceftazidime. Susceptibility patterns of *Enterobacter* returned to baseline within 3 months after active intervention reduced the use of ceftazidime by 98% of its peak. There was no development of enhanced resistance to piperacillin or tobramycin or to other antibiotics on the formulary. It was concluded that active pharmacy intervention resulted in reversion of susceptibility of *Enterobacter* spp. to baseline for ceftazidime and the other β-lactam antibiotics (i.e. aztreonam, cefotaxime, ceftriaxone, mezlocillin and piperacillin) for which covariance (i.e. parallel decline of organisms' sensitivities) or cross-resistance had developed.

3.6 Antigenic structure

According to Sakazaki and Namioka (1960), there is no significant relation between the capsular antigens of *Klebsiella* and strains with the characteristics of *E. cloacae*. In their opinion, the capsules of *E. cloacae* strains contain only M or slime antigen. Nevertheless, the capsular antigens of *E. aerogenes* are similar to those of *Klebsiella* and isolates can frequently be typed with *Klebsiella* capsular antisera (Gaston et al. 1989). An O-antigen typing scheme has been described for *E. cloacae* and currently comprises 30 O types (Gaston 1988).

3.7 Other typing methods

Schemes for biotyping and bacteriocin typing of *E. aerogenes* have been described; for biotyping there is available the PhenePlate-*Klebsiella/Enterobacter* (KE) system automated biochemical fingerprinting system, which is performed in microtitration plates (Kuhn, Tullus and Burman 1991). Georghiou et al. (1995) applied several molecular techniques to study the epidemiology of infections due to *E. aerogenes*: restriction endonuclease analysis of chromosomal DNA and repetitive-element polymerase chain reaction (rep-PCR) with primers based on repetitive extragenic palindromic (REP) and enterobacterial repetitive intergenic consensus (ERIC) bacterial DNA sequences; genomic fingerprinting with rep-PCR appeared most advantageous, especially when REP primers (rather than ERIC primers) were used.

Most interest lies in typing *E. cloacae* and the most successful approach appears to be O serology as the primary method of strain discrimination with strains of the same O

serotype then being subdivided by phage typing (Gaston 1988). Costas et al. (1989) used high-resolution SDS-PAGE of whole cell proteins and found discrimination similar to that achieved with conventional typing methods; all strain groups recognized by combined sero–phage typing were also found by SDS-PAGE. Ribotyping and arbitrarily primed PCR (Grattard et al. 1995) and random amplification of polymorphic DNA (RAPD; Davin-Regli et al. 1996) appeared to be reliable methods for typing *E. aerogenes* strains implicated in nosocomial infection. Restriction fragment length polymorphism analysis (RFLP) of total DNA and rDNA regions (Bingen et al. 1992), ribotyping (Garaizar, Kaufmann and Pitt 1991, Poilane et al. 1993), small-fragment restriction endonuclease analysis of *Eco*RI DNA digests and pulse field gel electrophoresis (PFGE) of genomic restriction fragments (Haertl and Bandlow 1993) and RAPD (Riain et al. 1994) have all similarly proved useful in the investigation of outbreaks due to *E. cloacae*.

3.8 Habitat and pathogenicity

The normal habitat of *Enterobacter* is believed to be soil and water, but the organism is occasionally found in the faeces and the respiratory tract of humans. In recent years, infection of hospital patients with *E. aerogenes* and *E. cloacae* has been reported more often than formerly, but *Enterobacter* is a much less important cause of hospital infection than is *Klebsiella*. Most infections are of the urinary tract (Eickhoff, Steinhauer and Finland 1966), although members of the genus are an important cause of bacteraemia in some hospitals (Gaston 1988). Shlaes (1993) described a prospective study of *Enterobacter* bacteraemia conducted in several patients. The results indicated that:

1 emergence of resistance was more frequent during treatment with third-generation cephalosporins than with other antibiotics

2 the addition of an aminoglycoside to the cephalosporin did not prevent emergence of resistance

3 previous treatment with cephalosporins was associated with bacteraemia caused by multiresistant *Enterobacter* spp. and

4 infection with multiresistant *Enterobacter* spp. was associated with a higher mortality than infection with susceptible strains.

The author concluded that avoidance of third-generation cephalosporins for surgical prophylaxis and therapy in patients in whom *Enterobacter* infections are suspected or proven should lower the prevalence of *Enterobacter* bacteraemias and mortality and prevent the emergence of multiresistance. The organism has been shown to have serious implications following eye surgery; in the episode described by Mirza et al. (1994) the use of contaminated swabs led to infections resulting in useful vision being retained in only one of 10 eyes. Colonization with *Enterobacter* spp. has been found to increase in cardiac surgery patients given cefazolin prophylaxis (Flynn et al. 1987).

The clinical significance of the more recently described *Enterobacter* spp. remains to be determined but *E. sakazakii* is known to have caused neonatal meningitis and sepsis (Muytjens et al. 1983, Gallagher and Ball 1991). Two unrelated hospital outbreaks, involving bacteraemia, meningitis and colonization of neonates, were investigated by a combination of typing methods: antibiograms, chromosomal restriction endonuclease analysis, multilocus enzyme electrophoresis (MEE), plasmid analysis and ribotyping. All but the antibiograms proved effective as epidemiological typing methods, especially when used in combination (Clark et al. 1990). *E. taylorae* is known to have caused osteomyelitis (Westblom and Coggins 1987). The latter organism was also reported as the cause of severe nosocomial infections in 4 patients; the isolates were not susceptible to cephalosporins or penicillins (unlike most members of the genus; Rubinstien et al. 1993). As well as being an occasional pathogen in predisposed human patients, *P. agglomerans* has caused bacteraemia when administered in contaminated intravenous fluids (Lapage, Johnson and Holmes 1973).

In mice, lipopolysaccharide from *P. agglomerans* has demonstrated relief of morphine dependence (Okutomi et al. 1992) and a protective effect on gastric ulcers (Inagawa et al. 1992). When administered intradermally, LPS was less toxic and elicited a tumour response in combination with cyclophosphamide; Goto et al. (1996) therefore foresaw an application to cancer treatment even in humans.

4 KLEBSIELLA

4.1 Definition

Klebsiella organisms are non-motile and usually capsulate. They ferment adonitol, inositol, mannitol, salicin and sorbitol, and often also lactose and sucrose. Most strains form gas from sugars; gas production from starch is an important diagnostic feature. Characteristically they give a negative MR and a positive VP reaction, but strains from the respiratory tract often give the opposite reactions and may have other atypical biochemical reactions. Nearly all grow on Simmons' citrate medium and in Møller's KCN medium. They are non-pigmented, do not deaminate phenylalanine and, with a few exceptions, fail to liquefy gelatin. They are found in the bowel and respiratory tract of humans and animals and in soil and water and cause a variety of septic infections in humans and animals. The G + C content of the DNA is 52–58 mol% and the type species is *Klebsiella pneumoniae*.

4.2 Classification

In earlier editions of this book, the name '*Klebsiella aerogenes*' was used for the non-motile, capsulate, gas-producing, acetylmethylcarbinol-forming strains commonly found in human faeces and in water. They were thought to correspond to the non-motile, gas-producing organism from faeces described by Escherich (1885) as '*Bakterium lactis aerogenes*', referred to by later workers as '*Bacterium aerogenes*', and subsequently transferred to a reconstituted genus *Klebsiella* (Report 1954). Unfortunately, the term '*Bacterium*' (later '*Aerobacter*') *aerogenes* was also used by water bacteri-

ologists to refer to organisms that were later shown to be motile and are now placed in the genus *Enterobacter*. In an attempt to resolve the resultant confusion, some taxonomists adopted *pneumoniae* as the specific epithet for the non-motile *aerogenes*-like organisms, although it had earlier been used to designate certain biochemically atypical strains of *Klebsiella* from the respiratory tract (see below). The view of these workers prevailed, and the name *K. pneumoniae* appeared in the Approved Lists of Bacterial Names (Skerman, McGowan and Sneath 1980) whereas '*K. aerogenes*' was omitted. Because of the widespread use by British clinicians of '*K. aerogenes*', in the previous edition of this book the organism was retained as an unofficial subspecies, *K. pneumoniae* subsp. '*aerogenes*'. The time has now come, however, to follow international opinion so hereinafter the name *K. pneumoniae* is used to include both the respiratory strains, to which this name was originally applied, and the biochemically typical strains formerly described in this book as either '*K. aerogenes*' or *K. pneumoniae* subsp. '*aerogenes*'.

A number of other non-motile and capsulate organisms occur in the respiratory tract of humans and other animals. In 1882, von Frisch cultivated a capsulate organism from patients with rhinoscleroma; in 1883, Friedländer isolated a similar organism – generally known as Friedländer's bacillus – from the lungs of patients who had died of pneumonia; and Abel (1896) described the ozaena bacillus. These 3 organisms, and others from the respiratory tract, form a biochemically heterogeneous group but are antigenically related to some of the more biochemically typical strains now included in *K. pneumoniae*. Various specific names, including '*Klebsiella atlantae*', '*Klebsiella edwardsii*', *Klebsiella ozaenae*, *Klebsiella pneumoniae* (as the name was initially used) and *Klebsiella rhinoscleromatis*, have been attached to biochemical varieties in this group. Both American and British authors, in the past, used the name *K. pneumoniae* to apply only to respiratory strains believed to correspond to Friedländer's bacillus. Studies of DNA–DNA hybridization (Brenner, Steigerwalt and Fanning 1972) indicated, however, that these respiratory strains are so closely related genetically to the more biochemically typical strains now included in *K. pneumoniae* that they should all form part of the single species *K. pneumoniae*. The epithets *ozaenae* and *rhinoscleromatis* have been proposed as subspecies of *K. pneumoniae* (this is reflected in Table 42.3) but for medical purposes both *K. ozaenae* and *K. rhinoscleromatis* were retained on the Approved Lists of Bacterial Names (Skerman, McGowan and Sneath 1980) as species in their own right; they will hereinafter be referred to as such.

Four other members of the genus *Klebsiella*, though biochemically similar to *K. pneumoniae*, are accorded separate specific status. An organism that formed indole and liquefied gelatin slowly was described by Flügge (1886) as '*Bacterium oxytocum*' (see Lautrop 1956). The decision to consider it a separate species – *K. oxytoca* – is supported by evidence from DNA–DNA hybridization tests, which suggest that assignment to a separate genus may even be appropriate (Jain, Radsak

Table 42.3 Differentiation of species and subspecies of *Klebsiella*

| Property | K. ornithino-lytica | K. oxytoca | K. planticola | K. pneumoniae subspecies | | | K. terrigena |
				ozaenae	pneumoniae	rhino-scleromatis	
Acid in							
D-arabinose	−	+	−	−	−	−	−
L-arabitol	−	+	−	−	−	−	−
gentibiose	NK	+	+	+	+	−	+
lactose	+	+	+	V	+	−	+
lyxose	NK	−	+	−	−	−	−
melezitose	−	V	−	−	V	−	+
sorbose	+	+	+	−	−	−	V
β-Galactosidase	+	+	+	+	+	−[a]	+
Decarboxylases							
lysine	+	+	+	V	+	−	+
ornithine	+	−	−	−	−	−	−
Gas from lactose at 44°C	NK	−	−	+	+	+	−[b]
Gluconate oxidation	+	+	+	−	V	−	+
Growth at 4°C	+		+	−	−	−	+
Growth at 10°C	NK	+	+	−	−	−	+
Growth at 42°C	+	+	NK	V	+	NK	−
Indole formation	+	+	V	−	−	−	−
Malonate	+	+	+	−	+	+	+
Pectinase	−	+	−	−	−	−	−
Urease formation	+	+	+	−	+	−	V
Voges–Proskauer	V	V	+	−	V	−	+[c]

+, Most strains positive; −, most strains negative; V, some strains positive, others negative; NK, not known.
[a]Positive according to Ewing (1986).
[b]Positive according to Podschun (1991).
[c]Negative according to Holmes, Dawson and Pinning (1986).

and Mannheim 1974). From *K. oxytoca* must be differentiated another indole-producing species, formerly known as enteric group 47, but now designated as *Klebsiella ornithinolytica* (Sakazaki et al. 1989). This species occurs only rarely in clinical specimens and is the only *Klebsiella* species to decarboxylate ornithine. Although production of indole is often relied upon to differentiate *K. oxytoca* from *K. pneumoniae*, Maslow et al. (1993) established a clonal relationship, by ribotyping and PFGE, between 2 isolates from the same urine specimen that otherwise differed only in their ability to produce indole. *Klebsiella planticola* (Bagley, Seidler and Brenner 1981) and *Klebsiella trevisanii* (Ferragut et al. 1983) have been shown to be synonyms (Gavini et al. 1986), the former name taking priority. Strains of the species also occur rarely in clinical material (Freney et al. 1986) and some produce indole but the species is not easily differentiated from some of the other *Klebsielleae* (Table 42.3). Another organism, named *Klebsiella terrigena*, also shows genetic differences from *K. pneumoniae* but is largely indistinguishable from it in routinely used tests (Izard et al. 1981a). It has been found mainly in soil and water.

4.3 Morphological and cultural characters

Members of the genus *Klebsiella* tend to be somewhat shorter and thicker than the other enterobacteria and are straight rods about 1–2 μm long and 0.5–0.8 μm wide, with parallel or bulging sides and rounded or slightly pointed ends (Fig. 42.1). The cells are either in pairs end to end or are arranged singly. In the body diplobacilli, very like pneumococci, are commonly seen. They are non-motile. When the capsule is pronounced, it can be demonstrated even by Gram's stain. The India ink method is to be preferred to the ordinary capsule stains, since distortions due to drying are avoided and the capsular material present as 'loose slime' can be seen as well as that around individual cells (Duguid 1951).

Capsular material is produced in greater amount in media containing a relative excess of carbohydrate (Duguid and Wilkinson 1953) and is a nitrogen-free polysaccharide (Toeniessen 1921, Heidelberger, Goebel and Avery 1925). Wilkinson, Dudman and Aspinall (1954) purified the capsular polysaccharides of a number of strains belonging to capsular type 54, and showed that they contained about 50% D-

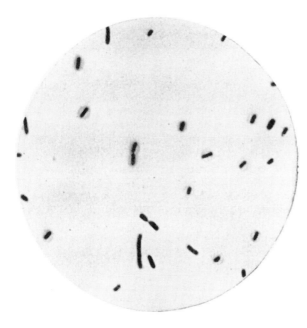

Fig. 42.1 *Klebsiella pneumoniae.* From a nutrient agar culture, 24 h, 37°C (× 1500).

glucose, 10% L-fucose and 29% of a uronic acid subsequently shown to be glucuronic acid. Mucoid strains produced the largest amount of polysaccharide, and most of it was present as capsule or slime; smooth strains produced less and nearly all of it was intracellular. Rough strains produced least (Wilkinson, Duguid and Edmunds 1954). Wherever the polysaccharide material was situated, its chemical composition was the same (Dudman and Wilkinson 1956). There were, however, differences in physical properties and in molecular weight between capsular material and loose slime (see Wilkinson 1958). The polysaccharides of the different capsular types are all complex acid polysaccharides (Dudman and Wilkinson 1956), which contain a uronic acid – usually glucuronic acid but occasionally galacturonic acid – as well as a considerable amount of pyruvic acid (Wheat, Dorsch and Godoy 1965). They resemble the group I K antigens of *Escherichia coli* (see Chapter 40 and Jann and Jann 1983).

Most strains of *Klebsiella* are fimbriate but some of the respiratory strains form an exception (Duguid 1959, 1968). Biochemically typical strains of any capsular type usually form fimbriae of both type 1 and type 3. The respiratory strains, which originally were the sole constituents of *K. pneumoniae*, form only type 1 fimbriae. *K. ozaenae* and *K. rhinoscleromatis* are invariably non-fimbriate, as are certain biochemically aberrant respiratory strains belonging to capsular types 1 and 2. The type 1 fimbriae of different species of *Klebsiella* are antigenically similar and related to those of *E. aerogenes* (Adegbola and Old 1987). In vitro, the *Klebsiella* type 3 fimbrial adhesin appears to mediate adherence to human respiratory tissue.

When much capsular material is produced, the growth on agar is luxuriant, greyish-white, mucoid and almost diffluent. This is due, no doubt, to the high proportion of water, 92% (Toenniessen 1921), in the capsular material. The condensation water on an agar slope is converted into a greyish-white mucoid mass. In broth the organism grows freely, giving rise after a few days to a pronounced viscosity, so that the medium takes on the consistency of melted gelatin.

Great stress used to be laid on the nail-headed growth in stab gelatin cultures; a circular, convex growth may occur on the surface, with a filiform growth in the stab, but this appearance is given only by some strains. Usually there is no liquefaction of the gelatin, but often a large napiform bubble of gas accumulates just beneath the surface, giving on first sight the appearance of liquefaction.

The cultural appearances of capsulate strains are subject to considerable variation. Non-mucoid variants appear on serial subculture on solid medium, particularly when the plates are incubated for several days (Toenniessen 1913), either as translucent peripheral outgrowths or as secondary colonies in the substance or on the surface of the original colonies. Sometimes the whole colony may dry up and wither away, leaving an effuse translucent layer looking like ground glass – aptly called by Collins (1924) 'suicide colonies'. Non-mucoid variants form colonies closely resembling those of *E. coli*. Reversion to the mucoid form may occur, often suddenly. For further information about colonial variation see Toenniessen (1914), Hadley (1927), Goslings (1935), Read, Keller and Cabelli (1957). Some of the respiratory strains grow poorly or not at all on MacConkey agar.

The organisms are killed by moist heat at 55°C in 30 min. They may survive drying for months (Loewenberg 1894). When kept at room temperature, cultures remain viable as a rule for weeks or months. They are facultatively anaerobic, but growth under strictly anaerobic conditions is poor. There is no haemolysis of horse or sheep red cells. The optimum temperature for growth is 37°C, the limits are 4 and 43°C, depending on the species. Some strains form a slightly brownish pigment.

Cysteine-requiring strains that are auxotrophic for this amino acid because of defects in the sulphur assimilatory pathway account for about 1.5% of urinary tract isolates of *Klebsiella* spp. (and *E. coli*); such strains may be seen as small (c. 1 mm) colonies on MacConkey agar. Problems with the isolation, identification and sensitivity testing of cysteine-requiring *Klebsiella* strains have been studied by McIver and Tapsall (1988) who suggested methods by which these may be minimized. McIver and Tapsall (1990) examined cysteine-requiring strains of *Klebsiella* to test the ease with which various test systems identified clinical isolates of cysteine auxotrophs. A significant proportion of the cysteine-requiring strains were not adequately identified by growth-dependent tests, which used various peptones as a nutrient source. Problems were encountered with all test systems examined: conventional methods and the commercial API 20E, Microbact and Vitek systems. The performance of the test systems was only partly improved when inocula were derived from appropriately supplemented media. However, the problems of the growth-dependent tests were resolved when a cysteine-supplemented suspension was used to inoculate each test system.

4.4 Biochemical activities

Members of the genus ferment a wide range of sugars, but their behaviour in this and other respects is far from uniform (Table 42.3). *K. pneumoniae* is the most active fermenter of the genus, producing acid and gas from all or nearly all the sugars usually employed, with the possible exception of dulcitol in the case of the respiratory strains. Attention should be drawn to their ability to form gas from starch. Hormaeche and Munilla (1957) advocated a medium containing non-soluble starch on which practically all strains of *K. pneumoniae*, and practically no other members of the Enterobacteriaceae, are able to form gas within 4 days. The other biochemical reactions of *K. pneumoniae* are fairly uniform. They are indole-negative, do not liquefy gelatin, and grow on Simmons' citrate medium. They are urease-positive, utilize malonate and have a lysine decarboxylase. Non-respiratory strains usually give a positive VP reaction, grow in Møller's KCN medium and oxidize gluconate, whereas respiratory strains give the opposite results. The respiratory strains that originally comprised *K. pneumoniae* were found by Cowan et al. (1960) to belong always to capsular type 3 and to be fimbriate. *K. oxytoca* resembles closely the biochemically typical *K. pneumoniae* strains, except that it liquefies gelatin slowly, forms indole and nearly always acidifies dulcitol (Malcolm 1938, Ørskov 1955c, Lautrop 1956). *K. planticola* also closely resembles the biochemically typical members of *K. pneumoniae* and indole-producing strains may easily be confused with *K. oxytoca*. More specialized tests to distinguish these taxa are given by Bagley, Seidler and Brenner (1981); of special note is growth at 10°C, positive in *K. oxytoca*, *K. planticola* and *K. terrigena* but negative in *K. pneumoniae*. Conventional methods usually fail to identify *K. planticola* and *K. terrigena*, which represent up to 19% of clinical *Klebsiella* isolates. Monnet and Freney (1994) combined 4 carbon substrate assimilation tests and 2 conventional tests; their scheme identified these species with a specificity and a sensitivity of 100%, although based on only few strains.

The respiratory klebsiellas (other than those now included in *K. pneumoniae*) are somewhat less active biochemically. Among them *K. rhinoscleromatis* is fairly well defined. It is anaerogenic, does not acidify lactose, gives a positive MR reaction and a negative VP reaction, does not grow on Simmons' citrate medium, does not form lysine decarboxylase, and is urease- and gluconate-negative. Some strains fail to grow in Møller's KCN medium. *K. ozaenae* forms a less clear-cut taxon, including strains that are late lactose and sucrose fermenters, are sometimes anaerogenic, and also give a positive MR and a negative VP reaction. They are malonate- and gluconate-negative. Few strains form lysine decarboxylase, but some attack arginine slowly.

Cowan and his colleagues (1960) described a further species, '*K. edwardsii*', of dulcitol-negative, late-lactose-fermenting, non-fimbriate members of capsular types 1 and 2 with 2 varieties: subsp. '*edwardsii*', which is anaerogenic, sometimes fails to grow on Simmons' medium but is always VP-positive; and subsp. '*atlantae*' which forms gas in sugars but is malonate-negative and sometimes VP-negative. Cowan (1974) elevated these 2 varieties to specific status but Bascomb and her colleagues (1971) were unable to confirm the existence of '*K. edwardsii*' by numerical taxonomic analysis (see also Brooke 1953, Report 1954, Henriksen 1954, Edwards and Fife 1955, Ørskov 1955c, Hormaeche and Munilla 1957, Epstein 1959, Fife, Ewing and Davis 1965, Ślopek and Durlakowa 1967, Dubay 1968).

4.5 Susceptibility to antimicrobial agents

Biochemically typical strains of *K. pneumoniae* are resistant to a wider range of antibiotics than are most *E. coli* strains. They are nearly always naturally resistant to ampicillin; they were at one time usually susceptible to cephalosporins, thus differing from strains of *Enterobacter*, which are almost invariably cephalosporin-resistant (Benner et al. 1965). Their resistance to chloramphenicol, streptomycin and tetracycline varied from strain to strain but they were usually susceptible to gentamicin and the polymyxins. Since that time, resistance to a number of antibiotics, notably various cephalosporins and gentamicin, have become common in strains found in hospitals. Transferable enzymatic resistance to third-generation cephalosporins during a nosocomial outbreak of infection with multiresistant strains has been described by Brun-Buisson et al. (1987). Other authors have also noted such transferable resistance, for example to cefotaxime and ceftazidime, in nosocomial strains due to their production of plasmid-borne extended-spectrum β-lactamases; in such circumstances, active agents are likely to include carbapenems (imipenem, meropenem), cefotetan and the monobactam carumonam as well as β-lactam–β-lactamase inhibitor combinations such as amoxycillin–clavulanic acid, ampicillin–sulbactam, cefoperazone–sulbactam, ceftazidime–clavulanic acid and piperacillin–tazobactam. Cefoxitin is said to be more active than ampicillin–sulbactam. French, Shannon and Simmons (1996), however, reported a hospital outbreak caused by a strain of *K. pneumoniae* K2 producing the extended-spectrum β-lactamase SHV-5. Some of the isolates produced up to 5 times as much enzyme as the other isolates and were resistant to β-lactam–β-lactamase inhibitor combinations. The outbreak was controlled by patient isolation and attention to hand-washing. Cefotaxime plus co-amoxiclav might usefully be considered as an alternative to imipenem for the treatment of infections with *K. pneumoniae* strains carrying an extended-spectrum β-lactamase.

Subminimal inhibitory concentrations of β-lactam drugs such as cephems, monobactams and penicillins (also cefodizime) may cause thinning of the capsule of *K. pneumoniae* with increases in the hydrophobicity and decreases in the negative charge of the cell surface. This renders *K. pneumoniae* more susceptible to phagocytic activity by reducing the physical repulsion between the bacteria and phagocytes, thereby enhancing the susceptibility of the bacteria to phagocytic killing activity (Nomura, Murata and Nagayama 1995).

Many of the respiratory strains, on the other hand, are more susceptible to antibiotics. A few of them are susceptible to as little as benzylpenicillin 2 μg ml^{-1}, and most of them are susceptible to ampicillin, chloramphenicol, streptomycin and tetracycline. Some *K. oxytoca* strains have been found resistant to aztreonam and cefuroxime, but susceptible to cefotaxime, ceftazidime and imipenem. *K. rhinoscleromatis* isolates are inhibited by clinically achievable concentrations of amoxycillin–clavulanate, cefpodoxime, cefuroxime, cephalexin, chloramphenicol, ciprofloxacin and trimethoprim–sulphamethoxazole (Perkins et al. 1992). In Canada, *Klebsiella* spp. remain highly susceptible to most antimicrobial agents with only 1 of 656 isolates tested showing resistance to third-generation cephalosporins (Toye, Scriver and Low 1993). Similarly, in Finland, resistance to cefuroxime has remained rare and cefuroxime remains an alternative to third-generation cephalosporins in the treatment of *Klebsiella* septicaemia. In neonates, ampicillin-based regimens are more likely than cefuroxime to produce drug-resistant strains (Tullus and Burman 1989).

For hand-washing, chlorhexidine 0.5% in isopropyl alcohol yielded sterile post-disinfection finger washings more often than chlorhexidine digluconate 4%; both preparations were more effective than soap and water, and with each residual action was demonstrable.

4.6 Antigenic structure

In studies of the antigenic structure of this group, most attention has been paid to the capsular (K) antigens. A great advance was made when American workers showed the presence in the group of capsular polysaccharides (Avery, Heidelberger and Goebel 1925, Heidelberger, Goebel and Avery 1925, Julianelle 1926a, 1926b, 1926c). Julianelle (1926a) recognized 3 serological types (A, B and C) among the respiratory klebsiellas, distinguishable by agglutination, absorption, precipitation and protection tests, and an undifferentiated group. The type specificity depended on a polysaccharide in the capsule. Goslings and Snijders (1936) described 3 further capsular antigens (D, E and F) among *K. ozaenae* strains, and Kauffmann (1949) described 8 more. Kauffmann proposed that the capsular types should be referred to by arabic numerals in place of the capital letters used previously. The former types A, B, C and D became types 1, 2, 3 and 4, and the new types were numbered consecutively. Since then, many further types have been recognized (Brooke 1951, Edwards and Fife 1952, Edmunds 1954, Ørskov 1955a, Durlakowa, Lachowicz and Ślopek 1967) and the present total is about 80. Unfortunately, the prevalence of non-typable strains, which can be up to 25%, limits the usefulness of capsular serology as an epidemiological tool.

In addition to the capsular antigens, there are smooth somatic antigens that occur in various combinations with the capsular antigens (Goslings 1933, Goslings and Snijders 1936). Kauffmann (1949) studied spontaneous non-capsulate variants of capsulate strains and recognized 3 of these O antigens among members of the first 14 capsular types. Ørskov (1954) examined a much larger selection of strains and was able to add only 2 more O antigens. Of these 5 *Klebsiella* O antigens, 4 were identical with or related to *E. coli* O antigens. So far 12 O antigens have been identified but 2 of these, O1 and O6, are identical (Ørskov and Ørskov 1984). It is thus possible to divide *Klebsiella* strains into a small number of O groups, which may be further subdivided into capsular types. Organisms with the same capsular antigen may, however, occur in several O groups. It is unlikely, therefore, that the identification of the O antigen, which in any case presents considerable technical difficulties, will be of much practical value in the classification of the capsulate members of the genus *Klebsiella*. In addition to the type-specific acid polysaccharide, a neutral polysaccharide, which is serologically active but not type-specific, has also been described (Gormus and Wheat 1971).

There is some association between antigenic structure, biochemical activities and habitat. Thus, members of the first 6 capsular types occur most frequently in the human respiratory tract, though occasionally they may be found in other parts of the body or even in other animals (Edwards and Fife 1955). They are not, however, by any means the only types found in the respiratory tract. Ørskov (1955b), for example, found that only 16% of strains from sputum belonged to capsular types 1–6. Nearly all the biochemically aberrant respiratory klebsiellas are to be found in capsular types 1–6, though a number of strains in types 1–3 are biochemically typical strains of *K. pneumoniae*. Capsular type 3 contains nearly all the *K. rhinoscleromatis* strains, as well as most of the respiratory strains now included in *K. pneumoniae*. The strains described by Cowan and his colleagues (1960) as '*K. edwardsii*' belong to types 1 and 2. Members of *K. ozaenae* belong to capsular types 4–6, and make up all, or nearly all, of these types. Capsule type 66 proved common in *K. oxytoca*, but not in *K. pneumoniae*, whereas K types 2, 7 and 33 were frequently found in *K. pneumoniae*, but not in *K. oxytoca* (Podschun 1990). Seventy of 81 *K. planticola* isolates (86.4%) were typable and were allocated to 35 K types. The proportion of typable strains among clinical isolates of *K. planticola* was very similar to those in *K. oxytoca* (86.0%) and *K. pneumoniae* (87.5%; Mori et al. 1989).

There is considerable overlapping between the antigens of the genus *Klebsiella* and certain quite unrelated organisms. Capsular type 2, for example, is similar immunologically to the type 2 pneumococcus (Avery, Heidelberger and Goebel 1925). Capsular antigens are usually detected by means of the capsular 'swelling' reaction, but agglutination, complement fixation, indirect immunofluorescence (Riser, Noone and Poulton 1976) and countercurrent immunoelectrophoresis (Palfreyman 1978) have also been employed.

4.7 Other typing methods

Many *Klebsiella* strains produce bacteriocins (klebocins), which appear to be distinct from colicins because they have no action on *E. coli* (Stouthamer and Tieze 1966). Many of the so-called pneumocins from *K. pneumoniae* have a narrow range of activity on other *Klebsiella* strains, often mainly on members of the same biochemical variety. Bacteriocin typing can be carried out by a traditional cross-streak method (Hall 1971) or by means of liquid preparations of bacteriocins after induction with mitomycin C (Edmondson and Cooke 1979). Epidemiological analysis may be improved by the use of bacteriocins as an adjunct to capsular serotyping (Bauernfeind, Petermuller and Schneider 1981). Phage typing by means of a set of temperate phages derived from other *Klebsiella* strains has also been advocated (Ślopek et al. 1967). Bacteriophage typing can be an effective adjunct to serotyping in distinguishing serologically cross-reactive isolates (Gaston, Ayling-Smith and Pitt 1987). Humphries (1948) described an enzyme, present in lysates of phage-infected organisms, capable of dissolving the capsule of type 1 organism. It did not inhibit growth itself nor was it toxic to the cells. Sikka, Sabherwal and Arora (1989) advocated a combination of bacteriocin and resistogram typing. Biotyping has been advocated in place of serotyping in less well equipped laboratories (Simoons-Smit et al. 1985).

The advent of molecular typing methods has seen the successful application of various approaches to the typing of isolates of *Klebsiella*. These include β-lactamase typing, MEE (Nouvellon et al. 1994) and one-dimensional sodium dodecyl sulphate polyacrylamide gel electrophoresis (SDS-PAGE) of whole cell proteins (Costas, Holmes and Sloss 1990). Twelve protein types were recognized; comparison with established typing methods indicated that the level of discrimination of SDS-PAGE was similar to that achieved with conventional typing methods but the strains were grouped differently. RAPD analysis (Wong et al. 1994, Eisen et al. 1995) of *K. pneumoniae* has been considered as discriminatory as RFLP analysis using PFGE, yet quicker and less costly. Restriction enzyme analysis by PFGE was found useful by Poh, Yap and Yeo (1993) as was ribotyping by Thompson et al. (1993).

4.8 Pathogenicity

In humans, strains of *Klebsiella* occasionally give rise in members of the general population to cases of severe bronchopneumonia, and also to more chronic destructive lesions with multiple abscess formation in the lungs (Limson, Romansky and Shea 1956). Such lesions are usually but not always associated with members of capsular types 1–5, which are frequently biochemically atypical. However, the main importance of *Klebsiella* as a pathogen for humans is in causing infections in hospital patients; the strains responsible are nearly always biochemically typical members of *K. pneumoniae*, most of which belong to higher-numbered capsular types. These strains cause widespread colonization of hospital patients. Clinical sepsis develops in surgical wounds and in the urinary tract; a number of patients have bacteraemic infections and some of them die. Colonization of the respiratory tract is very common, but its clinical significance is often difficult to assess in patients with serious underlying diseases. Some of them develop bronchopneumonia in which the klebsiella appears to be the primary infecting agent. Biochemically typical strains of *K. pneumoniae*

are also responsible for various septic diseases in animals.

Experimentally, the virulence of *K. pneumoniae* is subject to considerable variation. Apart from the fact that smooth variants tend to be pathogenic for laboratory animals and rough variants non-pathogenic, there is a great difference in the virulence of individual smooth strains. Some strains will kill mice in a dose of 0.2 ml of a 24 h broth culture diluted 10^6 times; others fail to kill even with 0.2 ml of the undiluted culture. Capsular types 1 and 2 are usually very virulent to mice when injected intraperitoneally; other types are generally non-virulent or of only low virulence to mice. Virulence does not appear to depend on capsule formation. The types just quoted as being of low virulence possess capsules in the same way as the highly virulent types 1 and 2. Moreover, non-capsulate, highly virulent variants have been described (Toenniessen 1914).

After subcutaneous injection of a very small dose – about 10 μl of a 24 h broth culture of a virulent strain – into mice, the animals die in 12–72 h. At postmortem examination, there is a local exudate, the associated lymph glands are swollen, and the spleen is enlarged. Capsulate rods are found in the blood and viscera. Guinea pigs are refractory to subcutaneous, but succumb to intraperitoneal injection, death occurring in 12–72 h. The fatal dose is about 0.01 ml of a 24 h broth culture. At postmortem examination, there is a viscous exudate in the peritoneum; the spleen may be enlarged, and the adrenals haemorrhagic. The rods are found in large numbers in the blood and viscera. Rabbits appear to be more resistant, but they succumb after intravenous or intraperitoneal injection with a dose of about 0.1 ml of a broth culture. Intraperitoneal inoculation is likewise fatal to pigeons.

Bacterial pathogens must multiply in order to establish an infection and in order to multiply they must acquire iron. *Klebsiella* strains make use of 2 high affinity iron uptake systems, one employing aerobactin, the other enterochelin (Williams, Brown and Lambert 1984). Production of aerobactin can be correlated with virulence and the genes encoding aerobactin have been found located on a plasmid (Nassif and Sansonetti 1986). In addition to aerobactin production, another phenotype can be correlated with the presence of this virulence plasmid: the mucoid phenotype of the bacterial colonies. This mucoid phenotype is considered an important virulence factor of *K. pneumoniae*; it is due to the plasmid-encoded production of a substance that is different from colanic acid and the capsular polysaccharide. *Klebsiella* strains show resistance to complement mediated serum killing and phagocytosis if both K and O antigens are present; resistance to the former seems related to the O antigens and the latter to the K antigens (Williams et al. 1983, Tomás et al. 1986). Immunization directed against the capsular polysaccharides has been successful in rats (Cryz, Furer and Germanier 1986) and humans (Cryz et al. 1986). It has been postulated that production of a capsule-like extracellular material may mediate aggregative adhesion of *K. pneumoniae*, which might explain the persistence of this organism inside the host gastrointestinal tract. Agents known to reduce capsule expression in *K. pneumoniae*, such as bismuth compounds or salicylate, also enhance phagocytic uptake of bacteria. Effecting a decrease in the production of capsular polysaccharide, the primary *K. pneumoniae* virulence factor, with salicylate may therefore have therapeutic potential (however, sodium salicylate can affect both antibiotic susceptibility and synergy). Salicylate accentuates phagocytosis of *K. pneumoniae* by making subcapsular antigens and components accessible to immune and non-immune host defences, and vaccination with subcapsular antigens may exhibit optimal protection against lethal infection when combined with salicylate therapy.

Among a survey of 439 clinical isolates of *Klebsiella*, the proportion of those identified as *K. planticola* was 81 (18.5%); of these, 52 (64%) were isolated from sputum, 17 (21%) from urine and the remaining 12 (15%) from other sources (Mori et al. 1989). Podschun (1991) investigated 5377 stool specimens from healthy persons (food handlers) and found 50 isolates of *K. terrigena*. Capsule typing revealed 30 different serotypes with K14 and K70 the most frequent. Six strains expressed capsule types K2 and K5, which are associated with virulence in *K. pneumoniae*. Podschun and Ullmann (1992) identified 10 strains of *K. terrigena* (0.4%) among 2355 indole-negative clinical *Klebsiella* isolates over a period of 3 years. Most of the isolates were from the respiratory tract. Serotyping revealed capsule types K2, K5 and K18 in 2 strains each. In antibiotic susceptibility tests the strains were similar in susceptibility to *K. pneumoniae*.

5 *SERRATIA*

5.1 **Definition**

Serratia organisms are small, motile, gram-negative rods that ferment mannitol, salicin and sucrose with the production of acid and sometimes of a small bubble of gas. They are indole-negative, generally give a negative MR and a positive VP reaction, and grow on Simmons' citrate medium. They do not deaminate phenylalanine but they do all liquefy gelatin rapidly, usually within 2–3 days and all produce lecithinase, lipase and deoxyribonuclease. Some strains produce a red non-diffusible pigment. *Serratia* species are typically found in soil and water, but some strains occur in the animal body. They may cause septic infection in humans. The G + C content of the DNA is 53–59 mol% and the type species is *Serratia marcescens*.

5.2 **Classification**

S. marcescens was first described by Bartolomeo Bizio in 1823 as a cause of 'bleeding polenta' (see Breed and Breed 1924). Similar organisms have been isolated at various times from water, soil and sewage, from contaminated foodstuffs and, less frequently, from the animal body. It has in recent times become obvious

that the pigmented strains form only a small part of a group of mainly non-pigmented organisms (Davis, Ewing and Reaven 1957), to which this name is now applied.

Numerous other species of *Serratia* have been described, but until 10 years ago only *S. marcescens* was generally recognized. Since then, several others have been added:

1 *Serratia liquefaciens* was formerly known as '*Enterobacter liquefaciens*', and was transferred to *Serratia* as a result of a numerical taxonomy study (Bascomb et al. 1971).

2 *Serratia odorifera* (see Grimont et al. 1978) comprises 2 distinct biochemical varieties, but DNA–DNA hybridization tests indicate that it forms a single species.

3 *Serratia plymuthica* (see Grimont et al. 1977) somewhat resembles *S. liquefaciens* in biochemical characters.

4 *Serratia rubidaea*: this name was used by Ewing and his colleagues (Ewing, Davis and Fife 1972, Ewing et al. 1973), but their description of this organism differs in several respects from that given originally for '*Bacterium rubidaeum*'. The authors have always accepted the reasons given by Grimont and coworkers (1977) for preferring the name *Serratia marinorubra* for this organism and it was described under this name in previous editions of this book. However, unlike the almost identical situation with *C. diversus* versus *C. koseri* described above, no-one has yet formulated a request that the Judicial Commission express an opinion as to which of these 2 names is the correct one to use. As the name *S. rubidaea* has seen most frequent use, particularly in the American literature, this name will be used here solely in the interests of uniformity.

The differential characters of these species are given in Table 42.4. There are several other proposed species that are not described in detail. *Serratia ficaria* is associated with figs and a species of fig wasp (Grimont, Grimont and Starr 1979) but it has also been isolated from human sources (Gill et al. 1981, Pien and Farmer 1983, Brouillard, Hansen and Compere 1984). *Serratia proteamaculans*, another plant-associated species, was originally thought to be the same as *S. liquefaciens* (Grimont, Grimont and Starr 1978) but more recent work suggests that it is a distinct species. Also similar to *S. liquefaciens* and *S. proteamaculans* is *Serratia grimesii*, some strains of which come from clinical specimens. The distinction of these 3 species is not easy without assimilation tests and it has been suggested that all such strains be referred to as '*S. liquefaciens*-like' (Grimont. Grimont and Irino 1982). *Serratia fonticola* (Gavini et al. 1979), a new species from water, is possibly misplaced in *Serratia*.

5.3 **Morphological and cultural characters**

S. marcescens is described in detail because it is the species most commonly encountered in clinical specimens. It is on the whole smaller than the average coli-

Table 42.4   Differentiation of species of *Serratia*

Property	*S. ficaria*	*S. fonticola*	*S. lique-faciens*[a]	*S. marcescens*	*S. odorifera* biotype 1	*S. odorifera* biotype 2	*S. plymuthica*	*S. rubidaea*
Acid from								
adonitol	V	+	–	V	V	V	–	+
arabinose	+	+	+	–	+	+	+	+
arabitol	+	NK	–	–	–	–	–	+
dulcitol	–	+	–	–	–	–	–	–
lactose	V	+	–	–	V	+	V	+
raffinose	V	+	V	–	+	–	V	+
sorbitol	+	+	+	+	+	+	V	–
sucrose	+	V	+	+	+	–	+	+
xylose	+	V	+	–	+	+	+	+
Decarboxylases								
lysine	–	+	+	+	+	+	–	V
ornithine	–	+	+	+	+	–	–	–
DNAase	+	–	+	+	+	+[b]	+	+
Gas from glucose	–	+	V	V	–	–	V	–
Gelatinase	+	–	+	+	+	+	V	+
Lipase	+	+[c]	+	+	–	–	+	+
Potato-like odour	+	NK	–	–	+	+	–	V
Red pigmentation	–	–	–	V	–	–	V	+

+, Most strains positive: –, most strains negative; V, some strains positive, others negative; NK, not known.
[a]Includes not only *S. liquefaciens sensu strictu* but also *S. grimesii* and *S. proteamaculans*.
[b]Negative according to Holmes, Dawson and Pinning (1986).
[c]Type strain negative according to Bollet et al. (1991b).

form bacterium. However, its size is subject to considerable variation; even on the same type of medium a single strain may at one time give rise to coccobacilli and at another to rods indistinguishable from other coliform bacteria (Figs 42.2 and 42.3). Capsules are not visible around cells grown on nutrient agar, but Bunting, Robinow and Bunting (1949) found that capsular material was formed on a well aerated medium poor in nitrogen and phosphate. Aucken, Wilkinson and Pitt (1997) showed that capsules could be demonstrated around cells of most of the O-serotype reference strains when grown on suitable agar media. Most *Serratia* strains are motile with peritrichous flagella. The flagella are usually best seen in cultures grown at temperatures below 37°C (Fulton, Forney and Leifson 1959).

Colonies of *S. marcescens* on agar are usually undifferentiated for the first day or 2, and then may develop a convex, pigmented and relatively opaque centre and an effuse, colourless, almost transparent periphery with an irregular crenated edge. However, the colonial characters of a strain are liable to considerable variation; colonies may vary in size, shape, opacity, surface and consistency. Similarly, there is great variation in their ability to produce the red pigment, which is formed only in the presence of oxygen and at a suitable temperature. The optimum temperature for pigment formation is not necessarily the same as that for

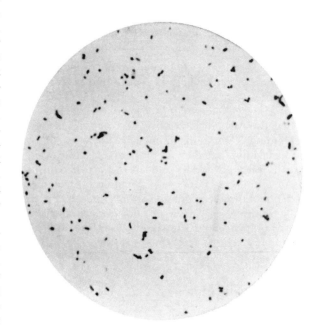

Fig. 42.2   *Serratia marcescens*, coccobacillary form, from a nutrient agar culture, 24 h, 37°C (× 1500).

growth. Thus many strains grow best at 30–37°C but form little or no pigment, whereas at lower temperatures growth is poorer and pigment formation is abundant. The ability to form pigment is commonly diminished and often irreversibly lost after repeated subculture. *S. liquefaciens* and *S. odorifera* are non-pigmented but red pigment is formed by many strains of *S. plymuthica* and *S. rubidaea*.

The red pigment, prodigiosin, is soluble in absolute alcohol, acetone, benzol, carbon disulphide, chloroform and ether, but is insoluble in water. Wrede and Rothhaas (1934) purified it and assigned to it a tripyrrylmethene structure. This was confirmed by Hubbard and Rimington (1949, 1950). Williams, Green and Rappoport (1956a, 1956b; see also Green, Rappoport and Williams 1956) consider that prodigiosin is not a single substance. They separated it into 3 red fractions and one blue fraction with different absorption spectra. Prodigiosin is also formed by some organisms unrelated to *Serratia*, including an actinomycete (Perry 1961) and certain gram-negative rods from seawater that attack sugars oxidatively, are oxidase-positive and have polar flagella (Lewis and Corpe 1964).

Except for the possibly misplaced species *S. fonticola*, all *Serratia* strains are actively proteolytic. Liquefaction of gelatin is usually obvious within 2–3 days. On blood agar, many produce a narrow zone of haemolysis in 24 or 48 h. Most strains produce opacity in egg-yolk media, due to the formation of a lecithinase C (Monsour and Colmer 1952, Klinge 1957); except for *S. fonticola*, they also produce deoxyribonuclease (Schreier 1969).

The optimum temperature for growth varies; some strains grow as well at 37°C as at 30°C, many have an optimum between 30 and 37°C, and a few fail to grow at all at 37°C. Many grow at 1–5°C.

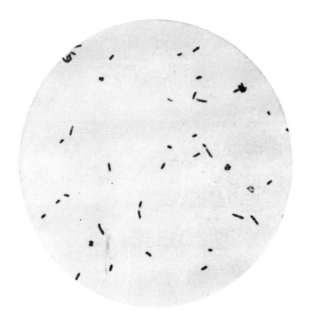

Fig. 42.3 *Serratia marcescens*, rod form, from a nutrient agar culture, 24 h, 37°C (× 1500).

5.4 Biochemical activities

The biochemical reactions of the genus are given in Chapter 39 (see Table 39.2, p. 927) and those of the various species of *Serratia* are shown in Table 42.4. Acid is usually formed promptly in glucose, glycerol, maltose, mannitol, sorbitol, sucrose and trehalose. Cellobiose and inositol may be acidified in a few days. Lactose is not acidified, except by strains of *S. fonticola* and *S. rubidaea*, or is acidified late, but β-galactosidase is always formed. Dulcitol is fermented only by *S. fonticola* and rhamnose only by strains of *S. ficaria*, *S. fonticola* and *S. odorifera*. The strains are either completely anaerogenic, or form small bubbles of gas filling no more than 5% of a Durham's tube. Gas is not formed in cellobiose, glycerol, inositol or starch.

MacConkey agar with sorbitol (1%) and colistin (200 iu ml^{-1}) has been proposed for better isolation of *S. marcescens* from clinical samples.

5.5 Susceptibility to antimicrobial agents

Serratia strains, like *Enterobacter* strains, are nearly always highly resistant to cephalosporins. Such resistance is frequently plasmid mediated and readily transferable to other members of the Enterobacteriaceae. As with other organisms described in this chapter, prior antimicrobial therapy with an extended-spectrum cephalosporin is an important risk factor for subsequent acquisition of an organism resistant to third-generation cephalosporins. Resistance to ampicillin and gentamicin varies from strain to strain, but many strains destroy these antibiotics enzymatically. *Serratia* strains, unlike *Enterobacter* strains, are resistant in vitro to polymyxins (Ramirez 1968). In an experimental model of rabbit endocarditis, Potel et al. (1992) found that intermittent amikacin dosing gave excellent bactericidal activity within the first 24 h in severe *S. marcescens* infections. Aztreonam is also effective. *S. liquefaciens* is said to be more resistant than *S. marcescens* to amikacin, aztreonam and ceftazidime.

Some strains of *S. marcescens* may grow in chlorhexidine-based disinfecting solutions; such solutions may therefore be a potential source of infection, for example, where used for contact lenses. Cells adapted to chlorhexidine may persist or grow in solutions with different antimicrobial agents, including benzalkonium chloride. The organism has also persisted in a dialyser in spite of the implementation of recommended sterilization procedures.

5.6 Antigenic structure

Davis and Woodward (1957) studied the O antigens of 16 cultures of *S. marcescens* and identified 6 O groups. There was no apparent relation between serological group and pigment production. Ewing, Davis and Reavis (1959) examined 115 *Serratia* cultures and established an antigenic typing scheme with 9 O groups, 13 separate H antigens and 46 serotypes. This scheme was then extended to 15 O groups (Ewing, Davis and Johnson 1962) and the present total is 28

(Pitt and Erdman 1984, Traub 1985, 1991c, Aucken, Wilkinson and Pitt 1996). Serogroup O14 predominates in clinical specimens. Another 7 H antigens have also been described by Traub and Kleber (1977) and Le Minor and Pigache (1977); these may conveniently be detected by motility-inhibition tests (Traub and Kleber 1977). Between 16 and 50% of all strains may belong to the combined serotype O14:H12. Gaston and Pitt (1989) developed a dot immunoassay that appeared to offer greater accuracy than agglutination tests for serotype identification in *S. marcescens*. Subsequently, 14 chemically and serologically distinct K types have been identified among the 28 O-serotype strains (Aucken, Wilkinson and Pitt 1997).

Traub (1991a) has compared bacteriocin typing, biotyping and serogrouping (O antigens) of *S. liquefaciens*. Biotyping afforded least discrimination, because 85.5% of the isolates comprised 2 biotypes; bacteriocin typing differentiated 84.3% of the isolates into 20 types; polyclonal rabbit anti-O immune sera identified 16 O antigens, and all 83 isolates could be serogrouped. Traub (1991b) differentiated 12 flagellar (H) antigens among 79 motile isolates with polyclonal anti-H rabbit immune sera.

5.7 Other typing methods

Serratia strains produce 2 different groups of bacteriocins or 'marcescins' (Prinsloo 1966, Eichenlaub and Winkler 1974). Group A bacteriocins are resistant to chloroform, heat and proteolytic enzymes; they are active against other *Serratia* strains and sometimes also against less closely related enterobacteria. Group B bacteriocins are susceptible to these agents; they are active against other enterobacteria but not against *Serratia* strains. Bacteriocin-susceptibility tests (Traub and Raymond 1971) have been used as a means of typing *S. marcescens*. According to Traub (1980), 73 patterns of susceptibility can be detected; unfortunately, however, small differences in pattern may occur on replicate typing. Nevertheless, the method may be useful to subdivide strains of the same O serogroup from an outbreak of infection. Several phage typing systems have been reviewed by Traub (1980). Biotyping has also been described and the scheme of Grimont and Grimont (1978) has been improved by Sifuentes-Osornio and Groschel (1987). Alonso et al. (1993) compared bacteriocin type, biotype and serotype with rDNA RFLP patterns (ribotypes) for the type identification of *S. marcescens*. They concluded that, due to the accessibility of biotyping and the lack of commercially available antisera for *S. marcescens*, the biotype and ribotype together provide reliable markers of strain identity. Bale et al. (1993) reached similar conclusions from a combination of biotyping and DNA restriction fragment analysis. One-dimensional SDS-PAGE of whole cell proteins has also been used (Holmes, Costas and Sloss 1990). Comparison with O serotyping indicated that the level of discrimination by SDS-PAGE was similar; however, as with O serotyping, a secondary scheme, such as phage typing, was necessary to differentiate strains of the same protein type. PCR amplification of enterobacterial repetitive intergenic consensus sequences has also been shown to provide a rapid and simple means of typing isolates for epidemiological studies (Liu et al. 1994).

Although most interest lies in typing isolates of *S. marcescens*, typing has been performed on strains of other species. Sader et al. (1994) found macrorestriction analysis of chromosomal DNA by PFGE useful for typing isolates of *S. odorifera* (biogroup 2).

5.8 Habitat and pathogenicity

S. marcescens is widely distributed in nature. Pigmented strains have at times caused alarm by giving rise to red colours in various foods (e.g. Klein 1894), by simulating the appearance of blood in the sputum (Woodward and Clarke 1913), or by producing stains on babies' napkins (Waisman and Stone 1958). Pigmented and non-pigmented strains are found from time to time in the human respiratory tract and in faeces. Accounts of human disease due to *S. marcescens* have become increasingly frequent in recent years. Most infections occur in hospital patients; they include sepsis of the meninges, of the respiratory and urinary tracts, and of wounds. Septicaemia is common, and endotoxic shock and endocarditis have been reported; some strains become established endemically in hospitals (see, for example, Wilfert et al. 1970). Outbreaks of infection are frequently reported, such as epidemic septic arthritis associated with an antiseptic (Nakashima et al. 1987), one involving a special care baby unit (Gransden et al. 1986) and one in a cardiac surgery unit (Wilhelmi et al. 1987). Only a small proportion, usually <10%, of the strains responsible for infection are pigmented. Some strains produce a cell-bound haemolysin and have a higher pathogenic potential than strains failing to produce the haemolysin. For a review of infections caused by *S. marcescens* see Acar (1986).

On **experimental inoculation** into laboratory animals, organisms of this group are harmless except in very large doses. Culture filtrates of *S. marcescens* have been used at times in the treatment of cancer, but there is no reason to believe that the substance producing haemorrhage and necrosis in the tumour is other than the endotoxin (see Wharton and Creech 1949). The inhalation of aerosols of *S. marcescens* is said to cause an acute, short-lived illness with respiratory and general constitutional symptoms (Paine 1946).

The other *Serratia* spp. also occur commonly in the natural environment, especially in water. *S. liquefaciens* and *S. odorifera* occur with some frequency in human clinical specimens whereas only occasional strains of *S. rubidaea* (Parment, Ursing and Palmer 1984) and *S. plymuthica* (Clark and Janda 1985, Horowitz et al. 1987) are seen. Chmel (1988) isolated a strain of *S. odorifera* (biotype 1) from the blood and urine of an alcoholic man with cirrhosis and signs of septic shock. Mermel and Spiegel (1992) described a case of nosocomial sepsis due to *S. odorifera* (biotype 1). *S. rubidaea* was isolated from the bile and blood of a patient with a biliary tract carcinoma obstructing the common bile duct and who underwent invasive procedures (Ursua et al. 1996). *S. plymuthica* has been documented from a case of chronic osteomyelitis and 2 cases of sepsis secondary to central venous catheter infection. Reina, Borrell and Llompart (1992) presented a case of a woman aged 50 years who was admitted to hospital as a result of a process affecting the lower respiratory tract, which was associated with a community-acquired bacteraemia due to this organism; the patient was treated with erythromycin and gentamicin and was discharged home 7 days after admission with complete clinical cure. Carrero et al. (1995) reported the isolation of *S. plymuthica* from 6 patients: 3 from blood cultures (in which the patients had lymphoblastic leukaemia, lymphoma, or stroke), 2 from exudates (following knee and abdominal surgery) and one from the peritoneal fluid of a patient with cholecystitis. The infection was considered nosocomial in 5 cases and community acquired in the other. The pathogenicity of *S. ficaria* is questionable but it has been reported as a cause of septicaemia in an elderly cancer patient (Darbas, Jean-Pierre and Paillisson 1994). *S. fonticola* has been reported from a very large leg abscess in a patient following an accident (Bollet et al. 1991b) and from pus from a severe infection of the hand following a road traffic accident (Pfyffer 1992). Bollet et al. (1993) isolated *S. proteamaculans* subsp. *quinovora* from blood cultures, pleural effusion and tracheal aspirates of a patient with pneumonia, which proved fatal.

6 CEDECEA

6.1 Definition

Cedecea organisms are usually motile and usually produce gas from glucose. Acid is produced from cellobiose, maltose, D-mannitol, salicin and trehalose. Indole is not produced. Most strains utilize citrate. They do not hydrolyse urea or produce H$_2$S detectable in triple sugar iron agar. Phenylalanine is not deaminated and gelatin is not liquefied. Most strains grow in Møller's KCN medium. Lysine is not decarboxylated. The organisms are isolated from the human respiratory tract but their clinical significance is uncertain. The G + C content of the DNA is 48–52 mol% and the type species is *Cedecea davisae*.

Cedecea and its 3 named species have been described only comparatively recently and 2 more species may eventually be recognized (Grimont et al. 1981, Farmer et al. 1982).

6.2 Cultural characters and biochemical activities

Members of the genus grow well on ordinary media, producing convex colonies about 1.5 mm in diameter on nutrient agar at 37°C.

The usual biochemical characters of *Cedecea* are summarized in Chapter 39 (see Table 39.2, p. 927). Properties not mentioned in the definition of the genus (see section 6.1) include failure to form acid from adonitol, L-arabinose, dulcitol, *i*-inositol or L-rhamnose; most strains ferment malonate and form arginine dihydrolase. The differential characters of *C. davisae*, *Cedecea lapagei* and *Cedecea neteri* are shown in Table 42.5.

6.3 Susceptibility to antimicrobial agents

Cedecea strains are susceptible to amikacin, carbenicillin, chloramphenicol, gentamicin, kanamycin, minocycline, nalidixic acid, nitrofurantoin, streptomycin, sulphonamides, tetracycline, tobramycin and tri-

Table 42.5 Differentiation of species of *Cedecea*

Property	*C. davisae*	*C. lapagei*	*C. neteri*
Acid from			
lactose	–	+	+
D-sorbitol	–	–	+
sucrose	+	–	+
D-xylose	+	–	+
Methyl red test	+	V	+
Ornithine decarboxylase	+	–	–
Voges–Proskauer test	–	+	–

+, Most strains positive; –, most strains negative; V, some strains positive, others negative.

methoprim. Strains are resistant to ampicillin, cephalothin, colistin and polymyxin B. Resistance to third-generation cephalosporins has also been reported (Berkowitz and Metchock 1995).

6.4 Habitat and pathogenicity

All *Cedecea* strains so far described have been isolated from human clinical specimens, predominantly from the respiratory tract. There is as yet little clear evidence that they play a pathogenic role although *C. davisae* and *C. neteri* have been reported to cause bacteraemia (Farmer et al. 1982, Perkins, Beckett and Bump 1986) and a *Cedecea* strain has been reported from a cutaneous ulcer (Hansen and Glupczynski 1984).

7 EDWARDSIELLA

7.1 Definition

Edwardsiella species are motile organisms that ferment glucose, often with the production of some gas. Maltose and D-mannose are also fermented, but fewer other sugars than by members of many other taxa of Enterobacteriaceae. Lysine and ornithine are decarboxylated but arginine dihydrolase is not produced. The genus is pathogenic for catfish, eels and other animals; occasional human infections have been reported. The G + C content of the DNA is 55–59 mol% and the type species is *Edwardsiella tarda*.

7.2 Classification

In 1962, Sakazaki and Murata described under the name 'Asakusa' a group of enterobacteria that appeared to be quite distinct from all others (see Sakazaki 1965). The main habitat of this organism appears to be the gastrointestinal tract of lower animals but a number of isolations have been made from human faeces, and a few cases of febrile diarrhoea and systemic infection in humans have been reported

(Okubadejo and Alausa 1968, Sonnenwirth and Kallus 1968, Jordan and Hadley 1969, Bockemühl, Pan-Urai and Burkhardt 1971). According to Gilman and his colleagues (1971) the presence of this organism in the faeces of jungle-dwelling Malaysians is closely associated with *Entamoeba histolytica* infection; however, the organism does not necessarily play a role in the pathogenesis of amoebic dysentery and may have multiplied in the gut as a result of a change in the local microenvironment.

The organism has been named *Edwardsiella tarda* (Ewing et al. 1965). Sakazaki and Tamura (1975) proposed the new combination *Edwardsiella anguillimortifera* for the organism previously known as 'Paracolobactrum anguillimortiferum' and considered this an earlier synonym of *E. tarda*. This issue remains to be settled, and the authors prefer to use the name *E. tarda* because it has been in common use for so long and because the characters of the type strain of *E. anguillimortifera* differ from those described for 'P. anguillimortiferum'. Grimont and coworkers (1980) described a distinct biochemical variety of *E. tarda* differing from typical members of the species in fermenting L-arabinose, mannitol and sucrose, but these atypical strains are closely related to *E. tarda* by DNA–DNA homology and are generally referred to as 'E. tarda biogroup 1'. However, Walton, Abbott and Janda (1993) encountered an unusual strain (H₂S-negative, fermenting sucrose) which mimicked a biogroup 1 isolate (it was isolated from a mixed infection from a woman suffering from cholelithiasis). Two other species have been described:

1 *Edwardsiella hoshinae* (Grimont et al. 1980) has been isolated only from animals and will not be described in detail and
2 *Edwardsiella ictaluri* (Hawke et al. 1981) has caused several outbreaks of enteric septicaemia in catfish and was earlier called *Edwardsiella* group GA7752 (Hawke 1979).

7.3 Cultural characters and biochemical activities

E. tarda grows well on ordinary media but produces only small colonies of 0.5–1 mm diameter after 24 h.

Biochemical activities are described in Chapter 39 (see Table 39.2, p. 927); see also Sakazaki (1967), Ewing et al. (1969) and Bascomb et al. (1971).

7.4 Susceptibility to antimicrobial agents

Studies indicate that all 3 *Edwardsiella* spp. are susceptible to most commonly prescribed antibiotics (including penicillin, which is unusual in the Enterobacteriaceae, and to β-lactam antibiotics). All strains were susceptible to 2 quinolones tested and to doxycycline and gentamicin (Reger, Mockler and Miller 1993). Nevertheless, fatal gastrointestinal and extraintestinal infections have been described. They are usually resistant to colistin and occasional strains are resistant to sulphonamides. Reger, Mockler and Miller

(1993) found *E. hoshinae* and *E. tarda* resistant to clindamycin, whereas *E. ictaluri* was moderately susceptible; β-lactamase was produced by all strains of *E. tarda*, but not by *E. hoshinae* or *E. ictaluri*.

7.5 Antigenic structure

The H and O antigens of *E. tarda* appear to be unrelated to those of other enterobacteria (Sakazaki 1965). Two different serotyping schemes were originally described:

1 Sakazaki (1967) recognized 17 O antigens, 11 H antigens and 18 O–H combinations;
2 Ewing (1986) recognized 49 O antigens, 37 H antigens and 148 O–H combinations.

The 2 systems have now been combined to form a single scheme comprising 61 O groups and 45 H antigens (Tamura et al. 1988).

7.6 Other typing methods

Some *E. tarda* strains produce bacteriocins, which are active against other *E. tarda* strains and against *Yersinia*, but not against *Proteus* (Hamon et al. 1969). *E. tarda* strains are not sensitive to colicins.

7.7 Habitat and pathogenicity

Edwardsiella strains are frequently isolated from faeces or other specimens from healthy cold-blooded animals and their environment, particularly fresh water. The natural reservoir appears to be the gastrointestinal tract of cold-blooded animals. *Edwardsiella* strains are pathogenic for catfish, eels and other animals, sometimes causing economic losses. Of the 3 recognized species, only *E. tarda* has been demonstrated to be pathogenic for humans. Principal infections associated with this species include gastroenteritis, wound infections (Jordan and Hadley 1969) such as cellulitis or gas gangrene associated with trauma to mucosal surfaces, and systemic disease such as cholecystitis, meningitis, osteomyelitis and septicaemia. Zighelboim et al. (1992) noted only 3 previous cases of patients who had documented hepatic abscess due to *E. tarda*; 2 patients died, and the third required a laparotomy and drainage. They reported a fourth case that was successfully managed with antibiotic therapy alone. Risk factors associated with *E. tarda* infections include exposure to aquatic environments or exotic animals (e.g. amphibia or reptiles), pre-existing liver disease, conditions leading to iron overload, and dietary habits (e.g. raw fish ingestion). *E. tarda* is rarely found in the faeces of healthy people. Although a higher isolation rate has been found in patients with diarrhoea (Ewing et al. 1965), the role of the species in the aetiology of diarrhoea requires further study.

The organism does have invasive capabilities. Janda et al. (1991) investigated the pathogenic characteristics of 35 *Edwardsiella* strains from clinical and environmental sources. Most *E. tarda* strains were invasive in HEp-2 cell monolayers, produced a cell-associated haemolysin and siderophores, and bound Congo red; many strains also expressed mannose-resistant haemagglutination against guinea pig erythrocytes. *E. hoshinae* strains bound Congo red and differed in their invasive and haemolytic capabilities whereas *E. ictaluri* strains did not produce either factor; neither *E. hoshinae* nor *E. ictaluri* expressed mannose-resistant haemagglutination nor elaborated siderophores. Selected strains of each species tested for mouse lethality indicated strain variability in pathogenic potential, with *E. tarda* strains the most virulent. Their findings indicate some potentially important differences in pathogenic properties that may help explain the environmental distribution of the 3 species and their differing abilities to cause disease in humans. Janda and Abbott (1993) found that *E. tarda* produces a haemolysin that is at least partially regulated by the relative availability of iron and may play a role in human disease.

8 EWINGELLA

8.1 Definition

Ewingella organisms are usually motile and do not produce gas from glucose. Acid is produced from cellobiose, glycerol, mannitol, salicin and trehalose. Indole is not produced. All strains grow on Simmons' citrate medium. They do not hydrolyse urea or produce H_2S detectable in triple sugar iron agar. Phenylalanine is not deaminated and there is no liquefaction in nutrient gelatin stab culture within 5 days but weak gelatinase production detectable by the plate test. Growth does not occur in Møller's KCN medium. Lysine and ornithine are not decarboxylated and arginine dihydrolase is not produced. The organisms are isolated predominantly from the human respiratory tract but their clinical significance is uncertain. The G + C content of the DNA is 53–55 mol% and the type species is *Ewingella americana*.

This organism was described by Grimont et al. (1983) from strains resembling *Cedecea*.

8.2 Cultural characters and biochemical activities

E. americana grows well on nutrient agar, producing convex colonies about 1.5 mm in diameter.

Biochemical activities are given in Chapter 39 (see Table 39.2, p. 927). In addition to the properties mentioned in the definition (see section 8.1), strains produce β-galactosidase and give a positive result in the VP test; they do not ferment adonitol, arabinose, dulcitol, inositol, raffinose, sorbitol or sucrose. Although thought to resemble *Cedecea*, several characters distinguish *E. americana* from this genus. More difficult, and not discussed by Grimont et al. (1983), is the differentiation of *E. americana* from *P. agglomerans*. Typically *E. americana* does not ferment malonate, sucrose or xylose (see Chapter 39, Table 39.2) but strains

atypical in these characters may not be easily assigned to one or other species. Two biotypes may be recognized among *E. americana* strains; strains of one ferment rhamnose and xylose and strains of the other fail to do so.

8.3 Susceptibility to antimicrobial agents

E. americana strains are susceptible to carbenicillin, chloramphenicol, colistin, gentamicin, kanamycin, nalidixic acid, streptomycin, sulphadiazine, tetracycline and tobramycin; they show resistance to cephalothin and penicillin G.

8.4 Habitat and pathogenicity

Although rare in occurrence, the organism is most commonly associated with the human respiratory tract (but it has also been found in molluscs). Whereas the pathogenicity of the species remains to be determined, *E. americana* has been reported from polymicrobial bacteraemia (Pien, Farmer and Weaver 1983), from 2 blood cultures from a 75-year-old man after cholecystectomy (Devreese, Claeys and Verschraegen 1992) and from wound colonization (Bear et al. 1986). The organism was isolated separately from both eyes of a woman aged 30 years (Heizmann and Michel 1991). Her clinical signs and symptoms included adhesive eyelids, itching and oedematous upper and lower lids. Relief of symptoms was effected with amoxycillin–clavulanate therapy. Plasmid profiling was used to investigate an episode of pseudobacteraemia due to the contamination of blood coagulation tubes with *E. americana* (McNeil et al. 1987a, 1987b).

9 HAFNIA

9.1 Definition

Hafnia organisms are usually motile and usually produce gas from glucose. Acid is formed from arabinose, glycerol, maltose, mannitol, rhamnose, trehalose and xylose. Indole is not produced. Most strains utilize citrate (if tested at 30°C) but do not hydrolyse urea or produce H_2S detectable in triple sugar iron agar. Phenylalanine is not deaminated and gelatin is not liquefied. Most strains grow in Møller's KCN medium. Arginine dihydrolase is not produced but both lysine and ornithine are decarboxylated. The organisms occur in the faeces of humans and other animals and are also widespread in the natural environment. The G + C content of the DNA is 52–57 mol% and the type species is *Hafnia alvei*.

9.2 Classification

This organism has at times been placed in the genus *Enterobacter* under the names 'Enterobacter alvei' and 'Enterobacter hafniae'. However, DNA–DNA hybridization studies reveal that the organism deserves separate generic status (Brenner 1978). Three DNA-relatedness groups have been recognized in *H. alvei* and these may be elevated to separate species at some future date. The organism known as *Obesumbacterium proteus* (syn. '*Hafnia protea*' biogroup I) is a brewery-adapted biochemical variety of *H. alvei*.

9.3 Morphological and cultural characters

Strains grow well on ordinary media, producing greyish convex colonies 1.0–2.0 mm in diameter on nutrient agar at 37°C after incubation for 24 h.

9.4 Biochemical activities

H. alvei ferments a much narrower range of sugars than do members of the genus *Enterobacter*: it acidifies salicin and sucrose late or not at all and lactose and sorbitol only rarely, and does not attack adonitol, dulcitol or inositol. It is not capsulate and does not liquefy gelatin. Møller (1954) greatly advanced the knowledge of this species when he showed that, although strains were able to grow at 37°C, many of their biochemical activities at this temperature were irregular. The effect of temperature on motility was also critical: many were non-motile at 37°C, but nearly all were motile at 30°C. At 22°C they all gave a positive VP reaction, grew on Simmons' citrate medium, and formed gas in sugars, though any one or all of these reactions might be inhibited at 37°C. According to Guinée and Valkenburg (1968), all *H. alvei* strains are lysed by a single phage, which is without action on any other members of the Enterobacteriaceae.

9.5 Antigenic structure

Forty-nine serotypes were recognized by Sakazaki (1961) and the total was extended to 197 by Matsumoto (1963, 1964).

9.6 Susceptibility to antimicrobial agents

Isolates that display resistance to conventional antibiotics, including cephalosporins and penicillins, have been reported (Klapholz et al. 1994).

9.7 Habitat and pathogenicity

Hafnia organisms are isolated from the faeces of humans and other animals; they are also found in sewage, soil, water and dairy products. They were rarely considered pathogenic in the past but Albert et al. (1992) described 7 strains from diarrhoeal stools of children that resembled enteropathogenic *E. coli* (EPEC) in that they produced attaching and effacing (AE) lesions in rabbit ileal loops and fluorescent actin staining in infected HEp-2 cells. In addition, a DNA probe, from a chromosomal gene required by EPEC to produce AE lesions, hybridized to chromosomal DNA from all 7 *H. alvei* strains. These findings indicated a sharing of virulence-associated properties at the phenotypic and genetic levels by *H. alvei* and EPEC.

H. alvei strains with these properties were considered diarrhoeagenic. Ridell et al. (1994) found an epidemiological association of *H. alvei* with diarrhoea, because the organism was isolated from 12 (16%) of 77 adult Finnish tourists to Morocco who developed diarrhoea and from none of 321 tourists without diarrhoea ($p < 0.001$). The strains were negative for the AE lesion by an in vitro fluorescent actin staining test and also did not show homology to the *E. coli* AE gene (*eaeA*) by PCR. The results suggested that a mechanism or mechanisms other than the AE lesion may also be involved in the association of *H. alvei* with diarrhoea. It has also been noted that *eaeA*-positive strains have characteristic biochemical properties, including the ability to assimilate 3-hydroxybenzoate and the inability to assimilate histidine and 2-ketogluconate (Ridell et al. 1995). Ginsberg and Goldsmith (1988) reported a neonate with necrotizing enterocolitis and subsequent ileal perforation from whom the organism was isolated from both blood and stool. *H. alvei* may also be a potential pathogen in patients with chronic underlying illness (Klapholz et al. 1994).

10 KLUYVERA

10.1 Definition

Kluyvera organisms are motile and usually form gas from glucose. Acid is produced from arabinose, cellobiose, glycerol, lactose, maltose, mannitol, raffinose, rhamnose, salicin, sucrose, trehalose and xylose. Indole is produced by most strains. Most strains grow on Simmons' citrate medium. They do not hydrolyse urea or form H_2S detectable in triple sugar iron agar. Phenylalanine is not deaminated and gelatin is not liquefied. Most strains grow in Møller's KCN medium. Arginine dihydrolase is not produced; most strains decarboxylate lysine and all decarboxylate ornithine. They occur in human clinical specimens and the natural environment. The G + C content of the DNA is 55–57 mol% and the type species is *Kluyvera ascorbata*.

10.2 Classification

The name *Kluyvera* was originally proposed in 1956 by Japanese workers; they recognized 2 species: '*Kluyvera citrophila*', in which citrate was utilized, and '*Kluyvera noncitrophila*', in which it was not. These names were little used in succeeding years and do not appear in the Approved Lists of Bacterial Names (Skerman, McGowan and Sneath 1980). In 1981, Farmer and coworkers re-proposed the name *Kluyvera*; their studies of DNA–DNA hybridization led them to recognize 3 genomic groups, 2 of which they named *K. ascorbata* and *Kluyvera cryocrescens*. Two new species have subsequently been proposed: *Kluyvera cochleae* from slugs and snails and *Kluyvera georgiana* from human clinical specimens (Müller et al. 1996). The latter organism is included in Table 42.6 but it will be seen that full identification in this group now requires the performance of a wide range of specialized tests.

Table 42.6   Differentiation of species of *Kluyvera*

Property	*K. ascorbata*	*K. cryocrescens*	*K. georgiana*
Acid from			
D-glucose[a]	−	+	NK
dulcitol	V	−	NK
D-sorbitol	V	V	−
Ascorbate test[b]	+	−	NK
Gas from glucose	+	V	NK
Lysine decarboxylase	+	· V	+
Utilization of			
N-acetyl-D-galactosamine	V	+	V
N-acetyl-L-glutamine	V	−	−
L-arginine	V	−	−
gentisate	+	−	V
3-hydroxybenzoate	+	−	+
3-hydroxyphenylacetate	+	+	V
malonate	+	+	V
phenylacetate	+	+	V
3-phenylpropionate	V	V	+

+, Most strains positive; −, most strains negative; V, some strains positive, others negative; NK, not known.
[a]Incubated at 5°C for 21 days.
[b]For method see Farmer et al. (1981).

10.3   Cultural characters and biochemical activities

Strains grow well on ordinary media and form colonies 1–2 mm in diameter on nutrient agar after 24 h at 37°C.

The characteristic biochemical reactions of the genus are given in Chapter 39 (see Table 39.2, p. 927). The tests used to distinguish *K. ascorbata* from *K. cryocrescens* are shown in Table 42.6 (for test methods see Farmer et al. 1981), but most workers will attempt to identify strains only to the generic level. Key biochemical characters of the genus were given in section 10.1. Neither adonitol nor *i-*(*myo*)inositol is acidified. The MR test is positive and the VP test negative. Most strains ferment malonate.

10.4   Susceptibility to antimicrobial agents

Kluyvera strains are generally susceptible to antimicrobial agents (see Farmer et al. 1981). Strains of *K. cryocrescens* often display large zones of inhibition around discs containing carbenicillin and cephalothin whereas strains of *K. ascorbata* do not.

10.5   Habitat and pathogenicity

Strains of *Kluyvera* have been isolated from milk, sewage, soil and water, but most of those so far identified have come from human sources, especially sputum and, less commonly, urine; a number were from faeces (some from patients with severe diarrhoea, Fainstein et al. 1982, Aevaliotis et al. 1985) and a few from blood cultures (one associated with a catheter-related infection, Wong 1987). Thaller, Berlutti and Thaller (1988) recorded the isolation of a *K. cryocrescens* strain in pure culture from a gall-bladder pus specimen from a 76-

year-old woman with acute cholecystitis. Yogev and Kozlowski (1990) treated a child who developed peritonitis due to *K. ascorbata*; the repeated isolation of the organism in pure culture from the peritoneal fluid and its isolation from postmortem subdiaphragmatic microabscesses suggested it was clinically significant. There is, however, as yet little definite evidence that the organisms are of clinical significance in humans. Luttrell et al. (1988) described a soft tissue infection caused by *Kluyvera* spp. in a previously healthy woman. Successful treatment required incision and drainage of the wound in addition to the administration of antibiotics. Sierra-Madero et al. (1990) described a case of bacteraemia and mediastinitis in a man following open-heart surgery. Dollberg, Gandacu and Klar (1990) described a *Kluyvera* sp. recovered from the urine of a previously healthy 5-year-old child with clinical and laboratory evidence of acute pyelonephritis; their findings suggest that this organism can cause severe disease even in previously healthy, immunocompetent children.

11   LECLERCIA

11.1   Definition

Leclercia organisms are usually motile and usually produce gas from glucose. They often form a yellow pigment. Acid is produced from adonitol, arabinose, cellobiose, dulcitol, lactose, maltose, mannitol, rhamnose, salicin, trehalose and xylose. Indole is formed. They do not grow on Simmons' citrate medium, seldom hydrolyse urea and do not produce H_2S detectable in triple sugar iron agar. Phenylalanine is not deaminated and there is no liquefaction in nutrient gelatin stab culture within 5 days but weak gelatinase production is detectable by the plate test. Strains grow in Møller's KCN medium but show no decarboxylase activity. They are isolated from various human clinical specimens, food, water and the environment; their clinical significance remains uncertain. The G + C content of the DNA is 52–55 mol% and the type species is *Leclercia adecarboxylata*.

11.2 Classification

This organism was originally described as *Escherichia adecarboxylata* by Leclerc (1962) from a collection of strains isolated from water. Strains of the species are, however, easily distinguished from *E. coli* as they acidify adonitol, ferment malonate and are KCN tolerant, as well as failing to form lysine decarboxylase or produce alkali when grown on Christensen's citrate medium. Ewing and Fife (1972) included *E. adecarboxylata* in *Enterobacter* (now *Pantoea*) *agglomerans* (syn. *Erwinia herbicola*), but the former yields gas from glucose, produces indole and acidifies dulcitol and inositol, all characters that distinguish it from typical strains of *P. agglomerans*. More recent DNA–DNA hybridization studies show that *E. adecarboxylata* should be placed in a separate genus for which the name *Leclercia* was proposed (Tamura et al. 1986).

11.3 Cultural characters and biochemical activities

Strains grow well on ordinary media.

The biochemical characteristics of the organism are given in Chapter 39 (see Table 39.2, p. 927). In addition to the characters mentioned in section 11.1, strains fail to produce acid from glycerol, inositol and sorbitol. The MR reaction is positive and VP reaction negative. Malonate is fermented and β-galactosidase produced.

11.4 Susceptibility to antimicrobial agents

All strains are susceptible to ampicillin, carbenicillin, cephaloridine, colistin, gentamicin, kanamycin and nalidixic acid but resistant to penicillin. Most strains are also susceptible to chloramphenicol, streptomycin, sulphadiazine and tetracycline.

11.5 Habitat and pathogenicity

Isolations have been made from various human clinical specimens including blood, faeces, sputum, urine and wounds. There are no definite indications of pathogenicity. Strains also occur in the environment, food and water.

12 *LEMINORELLA*

12.1 Definition

Leminorella organisms are non-motile; they may or may not produce gas from glucose. Acid is produced from arabinose and xylose and generally also from glycerol.

Indole is not formed. Strains may or may not grow on Simmons' citrate medium. They do not hydrolyse urea but produce H_2S detectable in triple sugar iron agar. Phenylalanine is not deaminated and gelatin is not liquefied. Growth does not occur in Møller's KCN medium. They do not show any decarboxylase activity. They are isolated predominantly from human faecal specimens but their clinical significance remains to be determined. The G + C content of the DNA has not been determined and the type species is *Leminorella grimontii*.

12.2 Classification

This genus, with its 2 species *L. grimontii* and *Leminorella richardii*, was described by Hickman-Brenner et al. (1985b). DNA–DNA hybridization studies indicated the existence of a third species but it was represented by only a single strain so no name was proposed for it.

12.3 Cultural characters and biochemical activities

In general, colonies are not as large as those of other species of Enterobacteriaceae, but growth occurs on MacConkey agar.

Leminorella strains are unique amongst the Enterobacteriaceae in that although they produce H_2S and ferment arabinose and xylose, they are otherwise relatively inactive. The biochemical characteristics of the genus are given in Chapter 39 (see Table 39.2, p. 927) and tests useful in differentiating the 2 named species are shown in Table 42.7. If strains grow only weakly then they may fail to give appropriate results in these tests, making species assignment difficult or incorrect; strains of *L. richardii* may fail to produce acid from glucose even though they acidify arabinose, glycerol and xylose. In the authors' experience, some strains of *L. grimontii* are anaerogenic. In addition to the characteristics given in section 12.1, strains fail to produce acid from adonitol, cellobiose, inositol, lactose, maltose, mannitol, raffinose, rhamnose, salicin, sorbitol, sucrose and trehalose. The MR reaction is positive in most strains of *L. grimontii* and negative in strains of *L. richardii*; the VP reaction is negative in both species. Malonate is not fermented and β-galactosidase is not produced.

Table 42.7 Differentiation of species of *Leminorella*

Property	L. grimontii	L. richardii
Gas from glucose	+	−
Growth on Simmons's citrate	+	−
Dulcitol: acid	V	−
Methyl red test	+	−

+, Most strains positive; −, most strains negative; V, some strains positive, others negative.

12.4 Susceptibility to antimicrobial agents

Leminorella strains are susceptible to colistin but resistant to ampicillin, carbenicillin, cephalothin and penicillin.

12.5 Habitat and pathogenicity

Two strains of *L. grimontii* were isolated from urine and all other *Leminorella* strains have come from faecal specimens. Their clinical significance remains to be determined.

13 MOELLERELLA

13.1 Definition

Moellerella organisms are non-motile and do not produce gas from glucose. Acid is produced from adonitol, glycerol, lactose, mannitol, raffinose and sucrose. Indole is not formed. Strains may or may not grow on Simmons' citrate medium. They do not hydrolyse urea or produce H_2S detectable in triple sugar iron agar. Phenylalanine is not deaminated and gelatin is not liquefied. Strains may or may not grow in Møller's KCN medium and they show no activity in decarboxylase media. They are isolated predominantly from human faeces but their clinical significance remains to be determined. The G + C content of the DNA has not been determined and the type species is *Moellerella wisconsensis*.

This genus and its single species were described by Hickman-Brenner et al. (1984).

13.2 Cultural characters and biochemical activities

Strains grow well on ordinary media. On MacConkey agar, colonies are bright red with precipitated bile around them, thus resembling *E. coli* colonies.

The characteristic biochemical reactions of *M. wisconsensis* are given in Chapter 39 (see Table 39.2, p. 927). In the original description of the species, strains were reported to grow on Simmons' citrate medium and not to ferment arabinose; strains of *M. wisconsensis* examined in the authors' laboratory, however, all failed to grow on Simmons' citrate medium (as shown in Table 39.2) and some fermented arabinose. The latter discrepancy may result from contamination of the arabinose with another sugar. In addition to the properties mentioned in section 13.1, strains do not form acid from dulcitol, inositol, maltose, rhamnose, salicin, sorbitol, trehalose or xylose. The MR reaction is positive and the VP reaction negative. Malonate is not fermented and β-galactosidase is produced.

13.3 Susceptibility to antimicrobial agents

Strains are resistant to colistin but susceptible to cephalothin, chloramphenicol, gentamicin and nalidixic acid.

13.4 Habitat and pathogenicity

The species is predominantly isolated from human faeces and although in some cases the patient was reported to have had diarrhoea there is no evidence at present that *M. wisconsensis* can cause diarrhoea. The organism has also been reported from a bronchial aspirate.

14 RAHNELLA

14.1 Definition

Rahnella organisms are motile and produce gas from glucose. Acid is produced from arabinose, dulcitol, lactose, raffinose, rhamnose and sorbitol. Indole is not formed. Strains grow on Simmons' citrate medium. They do not hydrolyse urea or produce H_2S detectable in triple sugar iron agar. Phenylalanine is not deaminated but gelatin is slowly liquefied. Strains do not grow in Møller's KCN medium and show no activity in lysine or ornithine decarboxylase media, but some strains produce a dihydrolase for arginine. The organisms are isolated predominantly from water and non-polluted soil, but their clinical significance remains to be determined. The G + C content of the DNA is 53 mol% and the type species is *Rahnella aquatilis*.

This genus and its single species were described by Izard et al. (1979).

14.2 Cultural characters and biochemical activities

Strains grow well on ordinary media at 30 and 37°C; they also grow at 4, but not at 41°C.

The biochemical characteristics of the organism are given in Chapter 39 (see Table 39.2, p. 927). In addition to the characters mentioned in section 14.1, strains acidify glycerol, maltose, mannitol, salicin, sucrose, trehalose and xylose but fail to produce acid from adonitol and inositol. The MR reaction is negative and the VP reaction is positive. Malonate is fermented and β-galactosidase is produced.

14.3 Susceptibility to antimicrobial agents

Funke and Rosner (1995), who isolated the organism from blood cultures of an HIV-infected intravenous drug abuser obtained a favourable outcome after a 14 day course of ciprofloxacin.

14.4 Habitat and pathogenicity

In the previous edition of this book this genus was mentioned only briefly because it inhabits fresh water and at that time had not been isolated from clinical specimens. Since that time, some reports have appeared of the isolation of this organism from clinical samples. Goubau et al. (1988) described a case of septicaemia in a patient with acute lymphoblastic leukaemia. Harrell, Cameron and O'Hara (1989) reported the isolation of *R. aquatilis* from the bronchial washing of a patient with acquired immunodeficiency syndrome. Alballaa et al. (1992) reported a case of urinary tract infection in a renal transplant patient and Hoppe et al. (1993) described repeated isolation of the organism from the blood of a paediatric bone marrow transplant recipient, probably related to inappropriate handling of a Hickman catheter. A case of a surgical wound infection in a patient who underwent a prosthetic surgical intervention was reported by Maraki et al. (1994); the presence of inducible β-lactamase was suggested. Oh and Tay (1995) reported isolation of *R. aquatilis* from the blood of a diabetic patient and a patient with laryngeal carcinoma; both patients recovered from the infection after treatment with parenteral antibiotics including gentamicin.

15 TATUMELLA

15.1 Definition

Tatumella organisms differ from other members of the Enterobacteriaceae in that, when grown at 25°C, over 50% of strains are motile by means of polar, subpolar or lateral flagella. Gas is not formed from glucose; acid is produced from glycerol, salicin, sucrose and trehalose. Indole is not formed. Most strains grow on Simmons' citrate medium at 25°C. The organisms do not hydrolyse urea or produce H$_2$S detectable in triple sugar iron agar. Phenylalanine is deaminated and gelatin is not liquefied. Growth does not occur in Møller's KCN medium. Lysine and ornithine are not decarboxylated, but some strains produce a dihydrolase for arginine. The organisms are isolated predominantly from the human respiratory tract but their clinical significance is as yet uncertain. The G + C content of the DNA is 53–54 mol% and the type species is *Tatumella ptyseos*.

15.2 Classification

This genus and its single species were described by Hollis and coworkers (1981). Studies of DNA–DNA hybridization show that, despite the absence of peritrichous flagellation, the species is correctly placed in the Enterobacteriaceae. Its members also differ from others in this family in growing less well and in surviving less readily on laboratory media.

15.3 Cultural characters and biochemical activities

Colonies are 0.5–1.0 mm in diameter, low convex with entire edges, semitranslucent, smooth and glossy after incubation for 24 h on blood agar. In general, colonies are not as large as those of other species of Enterobacteriaceae, but growth occurs on MacConkey agar.

The characteristic biochemical reactions of the species are given in Chapter 39 (see Table 39.2, p. 927). In addition to the properties mentioned in section 15.1, strains fail to form acid from adonitol, L-

arabinose, dulcitol, *i*-inositol, lactose, maltose, D-mannitol, raffinose, L-rhamnose, D-sorbitol and starch; the MR and VP reactions are negative, and malonate is not fermented. A few strains form arginine dihydrolase, particularly at 25°C. Strains of *Tatumella*, unlike members of all the other genera described in this chapter, deaminate phenylalanine.

15.4 Susceptibility to antimicrobial agents

Unlike most of the other members of the Enterobacteriaceae, strains of *Tatumella* are susceptible to cephalosporins and penicillins, and to aminoglycosides, chloramphenicol and tetracycline.

15.5 Habitat and pathogenicity

The organism is commonly associated with the human respiratory tract; most isolations of it have been from sputum, but it has also been found in faeces and urine and in blood cultures. Its pathogenicity is at present uncertain.

16 YOKENELLA

16.1 Definition

Yokenella organisms are usually motile and usually produce gas from glucose. Acid is formed from arabinose, cellobiose, maltose, mannitol, rhamnose, trehalose and xylose. Indole is not produced. Most strains utilize citrate but do not hydrolyse urea or produce H$_2$S detectable in triple sugar iron agar. Phenylalanine is not deaminated and gelatin is not liquefied. Generally, they grow in Møller's KCN medium. Lysine and ornithine are decarboxylated and most strains produce a dihydrolase for arginine. They are isolated predominantly from human wounds but their clinical significance is as yet uncertain. The G + C content of the DNA is 58–60 mol% and the type species is *Yokenella regensburgei*.

Y. regensburgei was described by Kosako, Sakazaki and Yoshizaki (1984); the authors referred their proposal, as required, for validation in the *International Journal of Systematic Bacteriology*. Also appearing on the same validation list was a proposal of *Koserella trabulsii* by Hickman-Brenner et al. (1985a) from a group of strains formerly considered as atypical *H. alvei*. *Y. regensburgei* was subsequently found to be a synonym of *K. trabulsii* (Kosako et al. 1987). *Y. regensburgei* was the earlier proposal and a retroactive amendment of the rules of nomenclature in 1986 indicates that this name has priority (Kosako and Sakazaki 1991). This organism was described under the name *K. trabulsii* in the previous edition of this book but given the apparent priority of the name *Y. regensburgei*, and its more frequent use, the organism is described here under the latter name.

16.2 Cultural characters and biochemical activities

Strains of *Y. regensburgei* grow well on ordinary media.

The biochemical characteristics of *Y. regensburgei* are given in Chapter 39 (see Table 39.2, p. 927). Additional characters not given in the definition of the genus include failure to form acid from adonitol, dulcitol, lactose, sorbitol and sucrose; β-galactosidase is produced. In addition to reactions given in Table 39.2, *Y. regensburgei* differs from *H. alvei* in failure to ferment glycerol, ability to produce acid from melibiose, resistance to both colistin and the *Hafnia*-specific bacteriophage, and having a very weak catalase reaction.

16.3 Susceptibility to antimicrobial agents

Strains of *Y. regensburgei* are resistant to colistin and penicillin and susceptible to chloramphenicol, gentamicin, kanamycin, nalidixic acid and sulphadiazine.

16.4 Habitat and pathogenicity

Y. regensburgei is infrequently encountered but a number of isolations have been made from human wounds. The organism has been isolated from a 74-year-old man with a septic knee and from a 35-year-old immunocompromised woman who had a transient bacteraemia without overt signs of sepsis (Abbott and Janda 1994).

17 OTHER GENERA

The following genera have been proposed, but will not be discussed in detail: *Erwinia* from plants; *Budvicia* (Bouvet et al. 1985) and *Pragia* (Aldová et al. 1988, Schindler, Potuznikova and Aldová 1992) from water; *Buttiauxella* (Ferragut et al. 1981, Müller et al. 1996) from slugs, snails and water; *Obesumbacterium* (see Shimwell 1963, Priest et al. 1973) from breweries; and *Xenorhabdus* (see Thomas and Poinar 1979) associated with certain nematodes and with insect larvae parasitized by them. The former *Xenorhabdus luminescens* now resides in a separate genus *Photorhabdus*; it has been reported in clinical material (Farmer et al. 1989), but it is rare. The authors also do not propose to discuss the organism once known by the vernacular name Enteric Group 90 and comprising strains originally considered as probable *Salmonella*, but which did not agglutinate with *Salmonella* typing antisera. McWhorter et al. (1991) proposed for this group the name *Trabulsiella guamensis*; however, only 8 strains were known.

REFERENCES

Abel R, 1896, Die aetiologie der ozaena, *Z Hyg Infektionskr*, **21**: 89–155.

Abbott SL, Janda JM, 1994, Isolation of *Yokenella regensburgei* ('*Koserella trabulsii*') from a patient with transient bacteremia and from a patient with a septic knee, *J Clin Microbiol*, **32**: 2854–5.

Acar JF, 1986, *Serratia marcescens* infections, *Infect Control*, **7**: 273–8.

Adegbola RA, Old DC, 1987, Antigenic relationships among type-1 fimbriae of Enterobacteriaceae revealed by immuno-electronmicroscopy, *J Med Microbiol*, **24**: 21–8.

Aevaliotis A, Belle AM et al., 1985, *Kluyvera ascorbata* isolated from a baby with diarrhea, *Clin Microbiol Newslett*, **7**: 51.

Ahmad S, Weisburg WG, Jensen RA, 1990, Evolution of aromatic amino acid biosynthesis and application to the fine-tuned phylogenetic positioning of enteric bacteria, *J Bacteriol*, **172**: 1051–61.

Alballaa SR, Qadri SM et al., 1992, Urinary tract infection due to *Rahnella aquatilis* in a renal transplant patient, *J Clin Microbiol*, **30**: 2948–50.

Albert MJ, Faruque SM et al., 1992, Sharing of virulence-associated properties at the phenotypic and genetic levels between enteropathogenic *Escherichia coli* and *Hafnia alvei*, *J Med Microbiol*, **37**: 310–14.

Aldová E, Hausner O et al., 1988, *Pragia fontium* gen. nov., sp. nov. of the family Enterobacteriaceae, isolated from water, *Int J Syst Bacteriol*, **38**: 183–9.

Alonso R, Aucken HM et al., 1993, Comparison of serotype, biotype and bacteriocin type with rDNA RFLP patterns for the type identification of *Serratia marcescens*, *Epidemiol Infect*, **111**: 99–107.

Aucken HM, Wilkinson SG, Pitt TL, 1996, Immunochemical characterization of two new O serotypes of *Serratia marcescens* (O27 and O28), *FEMS Microbiol Lett*, **138**: 77–82.

Aucken HM, Wilkinson SG, Pitt TL, 1997, Identification of capsular antigens in *Serratia marcescens*, *J Clin Microbiol*, **35**: 59–63.

Avery OT, Heidelberger M, Goebel WF, 1925, The soluble specific substance of Friedländer's bacillus. Paper II. Chemical and immunological relationships of pneumococcus type II and of a strain of Friedländer's bacillus, *J Exp Med*, **42**: 709–25.

Bagley ST, Seidler RJ, Brenner DJ, 1981, *Klebsiella planticola* sp. nov.: a new species of Enterobacteriaceae found primarily in nonclinical environments, *Curr Microbiol*, **6**: 105–9.

Bale M, Sanford M et al., 1993, Application of a biotyping system and DNA restriction fragment analysis to the study of *Serratia marcescens* from hospitalized patients, *Diagn Microbiol Infect Dis*, **16**: 1–7.

Bascomb S, Lapage SP et al., 1971, Numerical classification of the tribe Klebsielleae, *J Gen Microbiol*, **66**: 279–95.

Bauernfeind A, Petermuller C, Schneider R, 1981, Bacteriocins as tools in analysis of nosocomial *Klebsiella pneumoniae* infections, *J Clin Microbiol*, **14**: 15–19.

Bear N, Klugman KP et al., 1986, Wound colonization by *Ewingella americana*, *J Clin Microbiol*, **23**: 650–1.

Beijerinck MW, 1900, Schwefelwasserstoffbildung in den stadtgräben und aufstellung der gattung *Aërobacter*, *Zentralbl Bakteriol Parasitenkd Infektionskr Abt 2*, **6**: 193–206.

Benner EJ, Micklewait JS et al., 1965, Natural and acquired resistance of *Klebsiella-Aerobacter* to cephalothin and cephaloridine, *Proc Soc Exp Biol Med*, **119**: 536–41.

Berkowitz FE, Metchock B, 1995, Third generation cephalosporin-resistant gram-negative bacilli in the feces of hospitalized children, *Pediatr Infect Dis J*, **14**: 97–100.

Bingen E, Denamur E et al., 1992, Rapid genotyping shows the absence of cross-contamination in *Enterobacter cloacae* nosocomial infections, *J Hosp Infect*, **21**: 95–101.

Bockemühl J, Pan-Urai R, Burkhardt F, 1971, *Edwardsiella tarda* associated with human disease, *Pathol Microbiol*, **37**: 393–401.

Bollet C, Elkouby A et al., 1991a, Isolation of *Enterobacter amnigenus* from a heart transplant recipient, *Eur J Clin Microbiol Infect Dis*, **10**: 1071–3.

Bollet C, Gainnier M et al., 1991b, *Serratia fonticola* isolated from a leg abscess, *J Clin Microbiol*, **29:** 834–5.

Bollet C, Grimont P et al., 1993, Fatal pneumonia due to *Serratia proteamaculans* subsp. *quinovora*, *J Clin Microbiol*, **31:** 444–5.

Booth LV, Palmer JD et al., 1993, *Citrobacter diversus* ventriculitis and brain abscesses in an adult, *J Infect*, **26:** 207–9.

Bottone E, Schneierson SS, 1972, *Erwinia* species: an emerging human pathogen, *Am J Clin Pathol*, **57:** 400–5.

Bouvet OMM, Grimont PAD et al., 1985, *Budvicia aquatica* gen. nov., sp. nov.: a hydrogen sulfide-producing member of the Enterobacteriaceae, *Int J Syst Bacteriol*, **35:** 60–4.

Breed RS, Breed ME, 1924, The type species of the genus *Serratia*, commonly known as *Bacillus prodigiosus*, *J Bacteriol*, **9:** 545–57.

Brenner DJ, 1978, Characterization and clinical identification of Enterobacteriaceae by DNA hybridization, *Progr Clin Pathol*, **7:** 71–117.

Brenner DJ, Steigerwalt AG, Fanning GR, 1972, Differentiation of *Enterobacter aerogenes* from Klebsiellae by deoxyribonucleic acid reassociation, *Int J Syst Bacteriol*, **22:** 193–200.

Brenner DJ, Fanning GR et al., 1984, Attempts to classify *Herbicola* group-*Enterobacter agglomerans* strains by deoxyribonucleic acid hybridization and phenotypic tests, *Int J Syst Bacteriol*, **34:** 45–55.

Brenner DJ, Farmer JJ et al., 1977, *Taxonomic and Nomenclature Changes in Enterobacteriaceae*, Publication No. 79-8356, Centers for Disease Control, Atlanta, GA.

Brenner DJ, Richard C et al., 1980, *Enterobacter gergoviae* sp. nov.: a new species of Enterobacteriaceae found in clinical specimens and the environment, *Int J Syst Bacteriol*, **30:** 1–6.

Brenner DJ, McWhorter AC et al., 1986, *Erwinia asburiae* sp. nov., a new species found in clinical specimens and reassignment of *Erwinia dissolvens* and *Erwinia nimipressuralis* to the genus *Enterobacter* as *Erwinia dissolvens* comb. nov. and *Enterobacter nimipressuralis* comb. nov., *J Clin Microbiol*, **23:** 1114–20.

Brenner DJ, Grimont PA et al., 1993, Classification of citrobacteria by DNA hybridization: designation of *Citrobacter farmeri* sp. nov., *Citrobacter youngae* sp. nov., *Citrobacter braakii* sp. nov., *Citrobacter werkmanii* sp. nov., *Citrobacter sedlakii* sp. nov., and three unnamed *Citrobacter* genomospecies, *Int J Syst Bacteriol*, **43:** 645–58.

Brooke MS, 1951, Further capsular antigens of *Klebsiella* strains, *Acta Pathol Microbiol Scand*, **28:** 313–27.

Brooke MS, 1953, The differentiation of *Aerobacter aerogenes* and *Aerobacter cloacae*, *J Bacteriol*, **66:** 721–6.

Brouillard JA, Hansen W, Compere A, 1984, Isolation of *Serratia ficaria* from human clinical specimens, *J Clin Microbiol*, **19:** 902–4.

Brun-Buisson C, Legrand P et al., 1987, Transferable enzymatic resistance to third-generation cephalosporins during nosocomial outbreak of multiresistant *Klebsiella pneumoniae*, *Lancet*, **2:** 302–6.

Bunting MI, Robinow CF, Bunting H, 1949, Factors affecting the elaboration of pigment and polysaccharide by *Serratia marcescens*, *J Bacteriol*, **58:** 114–15.

Carrero P, Garrote JA et al., 1995, Report of six cases of human infection by *Serratia plymuthica*, *J Clin Microbiol*, **33:** 275–6.

Chmel H, 1988, *Serratia odorifera* biogroup 1 causing an invasive human infection, *J Clin Microbiol*, **26:** 1244–5.

Clark NC, Hill BC et al., 1990, Epidemiologic typing of *Enterobacter sakazakii* in two neonatal nosocomial outbreaks, *Diagn Microbiol Infect Dis*, **13:** 467–72.

Clark RB, Janda JM, 1985, Isolation of *Serratia plymuthica* from a human burn site, *J Clin Microbiol*, **21:** 656–7.

Collins G, 1924, *Studies on the Source of the Bacteriophage and on the Origin of Transmissible Bacterial Autolysis*, Thesis, University of Michigan.

Costas M, Holmes B, Sloss LL, 1990, Comparison of SDS-PAGE protein patterns with other typing methods for investigating the epidemiology of '*Klebsiella aerogenes*', *Epidemiol Infect*, **104:** 455–65.

Costas M, Sloss LL et al., 1989, Evaluation of numerical analysis of SDS-PAGE of protein patterns for typing *Enterobacter cloacae*, *Epidemiol Infect*, **103:** 265–74.

Cowan ST, 1974, *Cowan and Steel's Manual for the Identification of Medical Bacteria*, 2nd edn, Cambridge University Press, London.

Cowan ST, Steel KJ et al., 1960, A classification of the *Klebsiella* group, *J Gen Microbiol*, **23:** 601–12.

Crosa JH, Steigerwalt AG et al., 1974, Polynucleotide sequence divergence in the genus *Citrobacter*, *J Gen Microbiol*, **83:** 271–82.

Cruickshank JC, 1935, A study of the so-called *Bacterium typhi flavum*, *J Hyg (Lond)*, **35:** 354–71.

Cryz SJ, Furer E, Germanier R, 1986, Immunisation against fatal experimental *Klebsiella pneumoniae* pneumonia, *Infect Immun*, **54:** 403–7.

Cryz SJ, Mortimer PR et al., 1986, Safety and immunogenicity of a polyvalent *Klebsiella* capsular polysaccharide vaccine in humans, *Vaccine*, **4:** 15–20.

Darbas H, Jean-Pierre H, Paillisson J, 1994, Case report and review of septicemia due to *Serratia ficaria*, *J Clin Microbiol*, **32:** 2285–8.

Davin-Regli A, Saux P et al., 1996, Investigation of outbreaks of *Enterobacter aerogenes* colonisation and infection in intensive care units by random amplification of polymorphic DNA, *J Med Microbiol*, **44:** 89–98.

Davis BR, Ewing WH, Reavis RW, 1957, The biochemical reactions given by members of the *Serratia* group, *Int Bull Bacteriol Nomencl Taxon*, **7:** 151–60.

Davis BR, Woodward JM, 1957, Some relationships of the somatic antigens of a group of *Serratia marcescens* cultures, *Can J Microbiol*, **3:** 591–7.

Devreese K, Claeys G, Verschraegen G, 1992, Septicemia with *Ewingella americana*, *J Clin Microbiol*, **30:** 2746–7.

Dollberg S, Gandacu A, Klar A, 1990, Acute pyelonephritis due to a *Kluyvera* species in a child, *Eur J Clin Microbiol Infect Dis*, **9:** 281–3.

Dresel EG, Strickl O, 1928, Über reversible Mutation-formen der Typusbazillen bein Menschen, *Dtsch Med Wochenschr*, **54:** 517–19.

Dubay L, 1968, Biochemical subtypes of *Klebsiella* type 4 and their occurrence in patients, *Arch Immunol Ther Exp*, **16:** 486–90.

Dudman WF, Wilkinson JF, 1956, The composition of the extracellular polysaccharides of *Aerobacter–Klebsiella* strains, *Biochem J*, **62:** 289–95.

Duguid JP, 1951, The demonstration of bacterial capsules and slime, *J Pathol Bacteriol*, **63:** 673–85.

Duguid JP, 1959, Fimbriae and adhesive properties in *Klebsiella* strains, *J Gen Microbiol*, **21:** 271–86.

Duguid JP, 1968, The function of bacterial fimbriae, *Arch Immunol Ther Exp*, **16:** 173–98.

Duguid JP, Wilkinson JF, 1953, The influence of cultural conditions on polysaccharide production by *Aerobacter aerogenes*, *J Gen Microbiol*, **9:** 174–89.

Duhamel M, Cuvelier A et al., 1975, Septicémie et méningite néo-natales à *Levinea malonatica*, *Nouv Presse Med*, **4:** 428.

Durlakowa I, Lachowicz A, Ślopek S, 1967, Serologic characterisation of *Klebsiella* bacilli on the basis of properties of the capsular antigens, *Arch Immunol Ther Exp*, **15:** 497–504.

Edmondson AS, Cooke EM, 1979, The development and assessment of a bacteriocin typing method for *Klebsiella*, *J Hyg (Lond)*, **82:** 207–23.

Edmunds PN, 1954, Further *Klebsiella* capsule types, *J Infect Dis*, **94:** 65–71.

Edwards PR, Fife MA, 1952, Capsule types of *Klebsiella*, *J Infect Dis*, **91:** 92–104.

Edwards PR, Fife MA, 1955, Studies on the *Klebsiella–Aerobacter* group of bacteria, *J Bacteriol*, **70:** 382–90.

Ehrhardt AF, Sanders CC, 1993, β-Lactam resistance amongst *Enterobacter* species, *J Antimicrob Chemother*, **32, Suppl. B:** 1–11.

Eichenlaub R, Winkler U, 1974, Purification and mode of action of two bacteriocins produced by *Serratia marcescens* HY, *J Gen Microbiol*, **83:** 83–94.

Eickhoff TC, Steinhauer BW, Finland M, 1966, The *Klebsiella–Enterobacter–Serratia* division. Biochemical and serologic characteristics and susceptibility to antibiotics, *Ann Intern Med*, **65:** 1163–79.

Eisen D, Russell EG et al., 1995, Random amplified polymorphic DNA and plasmid analyses used in investigation of an outbreak of multiresistant *Klebsiella pneumoniae*, *J Clin Microbiol*, **33:** 713–17.

Eppes SC, Woods CR et al., 1993, Recurring ventriculitis due to *Citrobacter diversus*: clinical and bacteriologic analysis, *Clin Infect Dis*, **17:** 437–40.

Epstein SS, 1959, The biochemistry and antibiotic sensitivity of the Klebsiellae, *J Clin Pathol*, **12:** 52–8.

Escherich T, 1885, Die Darmbakterien des Neugeborenen und Säuglings, *Fortschr Med*, **3:** 515–22, 547–54.

Ewing WH, 1986, *Edwards and Ewing's Identification of Enterobacteriaceae*, 4th edn, Elsevier Science Publishing, New York.

Ewing WH, Davis BR, 1972, Biochemical characterization of *Citrobacter diversus* (Burkey) Werkman and Gillen and designation of the neotype strain, *Int J Syst Bacteriol*, **22:** 12–18.

Ewing WH, Davis BR, Fife MA, 1972, *Biochemical Characterization of* Serratia liquefaciens *and* Serratia rubidaea, US Dept of Health, Education and Welfare, Atlanta, GA.

Ewing WH, Davis BR, Johnson JG, 1962, The genus *Serratia*: its taxonomy and nomenclature, *Int Bull Bacteriol Nomencl Taxon*, **12:** 47–52.

Ewing WH, Davis BR, Reavis RW, 1959, *Studies on the* Serratia *Group*, US Dept of Health, Education and Welfare, Atlanta, GA.

Ewing WH, Fife MA, 1972, *Enterobacter agglomerans* (Beijerinck) comb. nov. (the Herbicola–Lathyri bacteria), *Int J Syst Bacteriol*, **22:** 4–11.

Ewing WH, McWhorter AC et al., 1965, *Edwardsiella*, a new genus of Enterobacteriaceae based on a new species, *E. tarda*, *Int Bull Bacteriol Nomencl Taxon*, **15:** 33–8.

Ewing WH, McWhorter AC et al., 1969, *Edwardsiella tarda*: biochemical reactions, *Public Health Lab*, **27:** 129–41.

Ewing WH, Davis BR et al., 1973, Biochemical characterization of *Serratia liquefaciens* (Grimes and Hennerty) Bascomb et al. (formerly *Enterobacter liquefaciens*) and *Serratia rubidaea* (Stapp) comb. nov. and designation of type and neotype strains, *Int J Syst Bacteriol*, **23:** 217–25.

Fainstein V, Hopfer RL et al., 1982, Colonization by or diarrhea due to *Kluyvera* species, *J Infect Dis*, **145:** 127.

Farmer JJ III, Asbury MA et al., 1980, *Enterobacter sakazakii*: a new species of 'Enterobacteriaceae' isolated from clinical specimens, *Int J Syst Bacteriol*, **30:** 569–84.

Farmer JJ III, Fanning GR et al., 1981, *Kluyvera*, a new (redefined) genus in the family Enterobacteriaceae: identification of *Kluyvera ascorbata* sp. nov. and *Kluyvera cryocrescens* sp nov. in clinical specimens, *J Clin Microbiol*, **13:** 919–33.

Farmer JJ III, Sheth NK et al., 1982, Bacteremia due to *Cedecea neteri* sp. nov., *J Clin Microbiol*, **16:** 775–8.

Farmer JJ III, Davis BR et al., 1985a, Biochemical identification of new species and biogroups of Enterobacteriaceae isolated from clinical specimens, *J Clin Microbiol*, **21:** 46–76.

Farmer JJ III, Fanning GR et al., 1985b, *Escherichia fergusonii* and *Enterobacter taylorae*, two new species of Enterobacteriaceae isolated from clinical specimens, *J Clin Microbiol*, **21:** 77–81.

Farmer JJ III, Jorgensen JH et al., 1989, *Xenorhabdus luminescens* (DNA hybridization group 5) from human clinical specimens, *J Clin Microbiol*, **27:** 1594–602.

Ferragut C, Izard D et al., 1981, *Buttiauxella*, a new genus of the family Enterobacteriaceae, *Zentralbl Bakteriol Mikrobiol Hyg Abt 1 Orig C*, **2:** 33–44.

Ferragut C, Izard D et al., 1983, *Klebsiella trevisanii*: a new species from water and soil, *Int J Syst Bacteriol*, **33:** 133–42.

Fife MA, Ewing WH, Davis BR, 1965, *The Biochemical Reactions of the Tribe Klebsielleae*, US Dept of Health, Education and Welfare, Atlanta, GA.

Flügge C, 1886, *Die Mikroorganismen*, 1st edn, Leipzig.

Flynn DM, Weinstein RA et al., 1987, Patients' endogenous flora as the source of 'nosocomial' *Enterobacter* in cardiac surgery, *J Infect Dis*, **156:** 363–8.

Frederiksen W, 1970, *Citrobacter koseri* (n. sp.) a new species within the genus *Citrobacter*, with a comment on the taxonomic position of *Citrobacter intermedium* (Werkman and Gillen), *Publ Fac Sci Univ J E Purkinye, Brno*, **47, Ser. K:** 89–94.

French GL, Shannon KP, Simmons N, 1996, Hospital outbreak of *Klebsiella pneumoniae* resistant to broad-spectrum cephalosporins and β-lactam-β-lactamase inhibitor combinations by hyperproduction of SHV-5 β-lactamase, *J Clin Microbiol*, **34:** 358–63.

Freney J, Gavini F et al., 1986, Nosocomial infection and colonization by *Klebsiella trevisanii*, *J Clin Microbiol*, **23:** 948–50.

Friedländer C, 1883, Die Mikrokokken der Pneumonie, *Fortschr Med*, **1:** 715–33.

von Frisch A, 1882, Zur Aetiologie des Rhinoskleroms, *Wiener Med Wochenschr*, **32:** 969–72.

Fulton M, Forney CE, Leifson E, 1959, Identification of *Serratia* occuring in man and animals, *Can J Microbiol*, **5:** 269–75.

Funke G, Rosner H, 1995, *Rahnella aquatilis* bacteremia in an HIV-infected intravenous drug abuser, *Diagn Microbiol Infect Dis*, **22:** 293–6.

Fussle R, Biscoping J et al., 1994, Development of resistance by *Enterobacter cloacae* during therapy of pulmonary infections in intensive care patients, *Clin Investig*, **72:** 1015–19.

Gallagher PG, Ball WS, 1991, Cerebral infarctions due to CNS infection with *Enterobacter sakazakii*, *Pediatr Radiol*, **21:** 135–6.

Garaizar J, Kaufmann ME, Pitt TL, 1991, Comparison of ribotyping with conventional methods for the type identification of *Enterobacter cloacae*, *J Clin Microbiol*, **29:** 1303–7.

Gaston M, 1988, *Enterobacter*: an emerging nosocomial pathogen, *J Hosp Infect*, **11:** 197–208.

Gaston MA, Pitt TL, 1989, Improved O-serotyping method for *Serratia marcescens*, *J Clin Microbiol*, **27:** 2702–5.

Gaston M, Ayling-Smith BA, Pitt TL, 1987, New bacteriophage typing scheme for subdivision of the frequent capsular serotypes of *Klebsiella* spp., *J Clin Microbiol*, **25:** 1228–32.

Gaston MA, Strickland MA et al., 1989, Epidemiological typing of *Enterobacter aerogenes*, *J Clin Microbiol*, **27:** 564–5.

Gavini F, Ferragut C et al., 1979, *Serratia fonticola*, a new species from water, *Int J Syst Bacteriol*, **29:** 92–101.

Gavini F, Izard D et al., 1986, Priority of *Klebsiella planticola* Bagley, Seidler, and Brenner 1982 over *Klebsiella trevisanii* Ferragut, Izard, Gavini, Kersters, De Ley, and Leclerc 1983, *Int J Syst Bacteriol*, **36:** 486–8.

Gavini F, Mergaert J et al., 1989, Transfer of *Enterobacter agglomerans* (Beijerinck 1888) Ewing and Fife 1972 to *Pantoea* gen. nov. as *Pantoea agglomerans* comb. nov. and description of *Pantoea dispersa*, *Int J Syst Bacteriol*, **39:** 337–45.

Georghiou PR, Hamill RJ et al., 1995, Molecular epidemiology of infections due to *Enterobacter aerogenes*: identification of hospital outbreak-associated strains by molecular techniques, *Clin Infect Dis*, **20:** 84–94.

Gilardi GL, Bottone E, Birnbaum M, 1970, Unusual fermentative, gram-negative bacilli isolated from clinical specimens. 1. Characterization of *Erwinia* strains of the 'lathyri-herbicola group', *Appl Microbiol*, **20:** 151–5.

Gill VJ, Farmer JJ III et al., 1981, *Serratia ficaria* isolated from a human clinical specimen, *J Clin Microbiol*, **14:** 234–6.

Gilman RH, Madasmy M et al., 1971, *Edwardsiella tarda* in jungle diarrhoea and a possible association with *Entamoeba histolytica*, *Southeast Asian J Trop Med Public Health*, **2:** 186–9.

Ginsberg HG, Goldsmith JP, 1988, *Hafnia alvei* septicemia in an infant with necrotizing enterocolitis, *J Perinatol*, **8:** 122–3.

Gormus BJ, Wheat RW, 1971, Polysaccharides of type 6 *Klebsiella*, *J Bacteriol*, **108:** 1304–9.

Goslings WRO, 1933, *Onderzoekingen over de Bacteriologie en de*

Epidemiologie van het Scleroma Respiratorium, A van Straelen, Amsterdam.

Goslings WRO, 1935, Untersuchungen über das Scleroma respiratorium. III. Mitteilung: die Variabilität bei Kapselbakterien, besonders bei Sklerombakterien, *Zentralbl Bakteriol Parasitenkd Infektionskr*, **134**: 195–209.

Goslings WRO, Snijders EP, 1936, Untersuchungen über das Scleroma respiratorium (Sklerom). IV. Mitteilung: die antigene Struktur der Skleromstämme im vergleich mit den anderen Kapselbakterien, *Zentralbl Bakteriol Parasitenkd Infektionskr*, **136**: 1–24.

Goto S, Sakai S et al., 1996, Intradermal administration of lipopolysaccharide in treatment of human cancer, *Cancer Immunol Immunother*, **42**: 255–61.

Goubau P, Van Aelst F et al., 1988, Septicaemia caused by *Rahnella aquatilis* in an immunocompromised patient, *Eur J Clin Microbiol Infect Dis*, **7**: 697–9.

Graham DC, Hodgkiss W, 1967, Identity of gram negative, yellow pigmented, fermentative bacteria isolated from plants and animals, *J Appl Bacteriol*, **30**: 175–89.

Graham DR, Band JD, 1981, *Citrobacter diversus* brain abscess and meningitis in neonates, *JAMA*, **245**: 1923–5.

Gransden WR, Webster M et al., 1986, An outbreak of *Serratia marcescens* transmitted by contaminated breast pumps in a special care baby unit, *J Hosp Infect*, **7**: 149–54.

Grattard F, Pozzetto B et al., 1995, Characterization of nosocomial strains of *Enterobacter aerogenes* by arbitrarily primed-PCR analysis and ribotyping, *Infect Control Hosp Epidemiol*, **16**: 224–30.

Green JA, Rappoport DA, Williams RP, 1956, Studies on pigmentation of *Serratia marcescens* II. Characterization of the blue and the combined red pigments of prodigiosin, *J Bacteriol*, **72**: 483–7.

Greenup P, Blazevic DJ, 1971, Antibiotic susceptibilities of *Serratia marcescens* and *Enterobacter liquefaciens*, *Appl Microbiol*, **22**: 309–14.

Grimont PAD, Grimont F, 1978, Biotyping of *Serratia marcescens* and its use in epidemiological studies, *J Clin Microbiol*, **8**: 73–83.

Grimont PAD, Grimont F, Irino K, 1982, Biochemical characterization of *Serratia liquefaciens sensu stricto*, *Serratia proteamaculans*, and *Serratia grimesii* sp. nov., *Curr Microbiol*, **7**: 69–74.

Grimont PAD, Grimont F, Starr MP, 1978, *Serratia proteamaculans* (Paine and Stansfield) comb. nov., a senior subjective synonym of *Serratia liquefaciens* (Grimes and Hennerty) Bascomb et al., *Int J Syst Bacteriol*, **28**: 503–10.

Grimont PAD, Grimont F, Starr MP, 1979, *Serratia ficaria* sp. nov., a bacterial species associated with smyrna figs and the fig wasp *Blastophaga psenes*, *Curr Microbiol*, **2**: 277–82.

Grimont PAD, Grimont F et al., 1977, Taxonomy of the genus *Serratia*, *J Gen Microbiol*, **98**: 39–66.

Grimont PAD, Grimont F et al., 1978, Deoxyribonucleic acid relatedness between *Serratia plymuthica* and other *Serratia* species, with a description of *Serratia odorifera* sp. nov. (type strain: ICPB 3995), *Int J Syst Bacteriol*, **28**: 453–63.

Grimont PAD, Grimont F et al., 1980, *Edwardsiella hoshinae*, a new species of Enterobacteriaceae, *Curr Microbiol*, **4**: 347–51.

Grimont PAD, Grimont F et al., 1981, *Cedecea davisae* gen. nov., sp. nov. and *Cedecea lapagei* sp. nov., new Enterobacteriaceae from clinical specimens, *Int J Syst Bacteriol*, **31**: 317–26.

Grimont PAD, Farmer JJ III et al., 1983, *Ewingella americana* gen nov., sp. nov., a new Enterobacteriaceae isolated from clinical specimens, *Ann Microbiol (Paris)*, **134A**: 39–52.

Gross RJ, Rowe B, 1975, *Citrobacter koseri*. I: An extended antigenic scheme for *Citrobacter koseri* (syn. *C. diversus*, *Levinea malonatica*), *J Hyg (Lond)*, **75**: 121–7.

Gross RJ, Rowe B, 1983, *Citrobacter koseri* (syn. *C. diversus*): biotype, serogroup and drug resistance patterns of 517 strains, *J Hyg (Lond)*, **90**: 233–9.

Gross RJ, Rowe B, Easton JA, 1973, Neonatal meningitis caused by *Citrobacter koseri*, *J Clin Pathol*, **26**: 138–9.

Gross RJ, Rowe B et al., 1981, Antigenic scheme for *Citrobacter koseri* (syn *C. diversus*, *Levinea malonatica*); three new antigens recognised in strains from Israel, *J Hyg (Lond)*, **86**: 111–15.

Guinée PAM, Valkenburg JJ, 1968, Diagnostic value of a *Hafnia*-specific bacteriophage, *J Bacteriol*, **96**: 564.

Gwynn CM, George RH, 1973, Neonatal *Citrobacter* meningitis, *Arch Dis Childh*, **48**: 455–8.

Hadley P, 1927, Microbic dissociation. The instability of bacterial species with special reference to active dissociation and transmissible autolysis, *J Infect Dis*, **40**: 1–312.

Haertl R, Bandlow G, 1993, Epidemiological fingerprinting of *Enterobacter cloacae* by small-fragment restriction endonuclease analysis and pulsed-field gel electrophoresis of genomic restriction fragments, *J Clin Microbiol*, **31**: 128–33.

Hall FA, 1971, Bacteriocine typing of *Klebsiella* spp., *J Clin Pathol*, **24**: 712–16.

Hamon Y, Kayser A et al., 1969, Les bactériocines d'*Edwardsiella tarda*. Intérêt taxonomique de l'étude de ces antibiotiques, *C R Acad Sci*, **268**: 2517–20.

Hansen MW, Glupczynski GY, 1984, Isolation of an unusual *Cedecea* species from a cutaneous ulcer, *Eur J Clin Microbiol*, **3**: 152–3.

Harrell LJ, Cameron ML, O'Hara CM, 1989, *Rahnella aquatilis*, an unusual gram-negative rod isolated from the bronchial washing of a patient with acquired immunodeficiency syndrome, *J Clin Microbiol*, **27**: 1671–2.

Harvey BS, Koeuth T et al., 1995, Vertical transmission of *Citrobacter diversus* documented by DNA fingerprinting, *Infect Control Hosp Epidemiol*, **16**: 564–9.

Hawke JP, 1979, A bacterium associated with disease of pond cultured channel catfish, *Ictalurus punctatus*, *J Fish Res Bd Canada*, **36**: 1508–12.

Hawke JP, McWhorter AC et al., 1981, *Edwardsiella ictaluri* sp. nov., the causative agent of enteric septicemia of catfish, *Int J Syst Bacteriol*, **31**: 396–400.

Heidelberger M, Goebel WF, Avery OT, 1925, The soluble specific substance of a strain of Friedländer's bacillus. Paper I, *J Exp Med*, **42**: 701–7.

Heizmann WR, Michel R, 1991, Isolation of *Ewingella americana* from a patient with conjunctivitis, *Eur J Clin Microbiol Infect Dis*, **10**: 957–9.

Henriksen SD, 1954, Studies on the *Klebsiella* group (Kauffmann) II. Biochemical reactions, *Acta Pathol Microbiol Scand*, **34**: 259–65.

Hickman-Brenner FW, Huntley-Carter GP et al., 1984, *Moellerella wisconsenis*, a new genus and species of Enterobacteriaceae found in human stool specimens, *J Clin Microbiol*, **19**: 460–3.

Hickman-Brenner FW, Huntley-Carter GP et al., 1985a, *Koserella trabulsii*, a new genus and species of Enterobacteriaceae formerly known as Enteric Group 45, *J Clin Microbiol*, **21**: 39–42.

Hickman-Brenner FW, Vohra MP et al., 1985b, *Leminorella*, a new genus of Enterobacteriaceae: identification of *Leminorella grimontii* sp. nov. and *Leminorella richardii* sp. nov. found in clinical specimens, *J Clin Microbiol*, **21**: 234–9.

Higashitani F, Nishida K et al., 1995, Effects of tazobactam on the frequency of the emergence of resistant strains from *Enterobacter cloacae*, *Citrobacter freundii*, and *Proteus vulgaris* (β-lactamase derepressed mutants), *J Antibiot*, **48**: 1027–33.

Hollis DG, Hickman FW et al., 1981, *Tatumella ptyseos* gen. nov., sp. nov., a new member of the family Enterobacteriaceae found in clinical specimens, *J Clin Microbiol*, **14**: 79–88.

Holmes B, Costas M, Sloss LL, 1990, Numerical analysis of SDS-PAGE protein patterns of *Serratia marcescens*: a comparison with other typing methods, *Epidemiol Infect*, **105**: 107–17.

Holmes B, Dawson CA, Pinning CA, 1986, A revised probability matrix for the identification of Gram-negative, aerobic, rod-shaped, fermentative bacteria, *J Gen Microbiol*, **132**: 3113–35.

Holmes B, King A et al., 1974, Sensitivity of *Citrobacter freundii* and *Citrobacter koseri* to cephalosporins and penicillins, *J Clin Pathol*, **27**: 729–33.

Holt JG, Krieg NR et al. (eds), 1994, *Bergey's Manual of Determinative Bacteriology*, 9th edn, Williams & Wilkins, Baltimore.

Hoppe JE, Herter M et al., 1993, Catheter-related *Rahnella aquatilis* bacteremia in a pediatric bone marrow transplant recipient, *J Clin Microbiol*, **31**: 1911–12.

Hormaeche E, Edwards PR, 1958, Observations on the genus *Aerobacter* with a description of two species, *Int Bull Bacteriol Nomencl Taxon*, **8**: 111–15.

Hormaeche E, Edwards PR, 1960, A proposed genus *Enterobacter*, *Int Bull Bacteriol Nomencl Taxon*, **10**: 71–4.

Hormaeche E, Munilla M, 1957, Biochemical tests for the differentiation of *Klebsiella* and *Cloaca*, *Int Bull Bacteriol Nomencl Taxon*, **7**: 1–20.

Horowitz HW, Nadelman RB et al., 1987, *Serratia plymuthica* sepsis associated with infection of a central venous catheter, *J Clin Microbiol*, **25**: 1562–3.

Hubbard R, Rimington C, 1949, Some properties of prodigiosin and preliminary results concerning its biosynthesis, *Biochem J*, **44**: l–li.

Hubbard R, Rimington C, 1950, The biosynthesis of prodigiosin, the tripyrrylmethene pigment from *Bacillus prodigiosus* (*Serratia marcescens*), *Biochem J*, **46**: 220–5.

Huber TW, Thomas JS, 1994, Detection of resistance due to inducible beta-lactamase in *Enterobacter aerogenes* and *Enterobacter cloacae*, *J Clin Microbiol*, **32**: 2481–6.

Humphries JC, 1948, Enzymic activity of bacteriophage-culture lysates I. A capsule lysin active against *Klebsiella pneumoniae* type A, *J Bacteriol*, **56**: 683–93.

Inagawa H, Saitoh F et al., 1992, Homeostasis as regulated by activated macrophage. III. Protective effect of LPSw (lipopolysaccharide (LPS) of wheat flour) on gastric ulcer in mice as compared with those of other LPS from various sources, *Chem Pharm Bull*, **40**: 998–1000.

Izard D, Gavini F, Leclerc H, 1980, Polynucleotide sequence relatedness and genome size among *Enterobacter intermedium* sp. nov. and the species *Enterobacter cloacae* and *Klebsiella pneumoniae*, *Zentralbl Bakteriol Abt 1 Orig C*, **1**: 51–60.

Izard D, Gavini F et al., 1979, *Rahnella aquatilis*, nouveau membre de la famille des Enterobacteriaceae, *Ann Microbiol (Paris)*, **130A**: 163–77.

Izard D, Ferragut C et al., 1981a, *Klebsiella terrigena*, a new species from soil and water, *Int J Syst Bacteriol*, **31**: 116–27.

Izard D, Gavini F et al., 1981b, Deoxyribonucleic acid relatedness between *Enterobacter cloacae* and *Enterobacter amnigenus* sp. nov., *Int J Syst Bacteriol*, **31**: 35–42.

Jack GW, Richmond MH, 1970, A comparative study of eight distinct beta-lactamases synthesised by gram-negative bacteria, *J Gen Microbiol*, **61**: 43–61.

Jain K, Radsak K, Mannheim W, 1974, Differentiation of the *Oxytocum* group from *Klebsiella* by deoxyribonucleic acid–deoxyribonucleic acid hybridization, *Int J Syst Bacteriol*, **24**: 402–7.

Janda JM, Abbott SL, 1993, Expression of an iron-regulated hemolysin by *Edwardsiella tarda*, *FEMS Microbiol Lett*, **111**: 275–80.

Janda JM, Abbott SL et al., 1991, Pathogenic properties of *Edwardsiella* species, *J Clin Microbiol*, **29**: 1997–2001.

Janda JM, Abbott SL et al., 1994, Biochemical identification of citrobacteria in the clinical laboratory, *J Clin Microbiol*, **32**: 1850–4.

Jann K, Jann B, 1983, The K antigens of *Escherichia coli*, *Prog Allergy*, **33**: 53–79.

Joaquin A, Khan S et al., 1991–2, Neonatal meningitis and bilateral cerebellar abscesses due to *Citrobacter freundii*, *Pediatr Neurosurg*, **17**: 23–4.

Jordan GW, Hadley WK, 1969, Human infection with *Edwardsiella tarda*, *Ann Intern Med*, **70**: 283–8.

Julianelle LA, 1926a, A biological classification of encapsulatus pneumoniae (Friedländer's bacillus), *J Exp Med*, **44**: 113–28.

Julianelle LA, 1926b, Immunological relationships of encapsulated and capsule-free strains of encapsulatus pneumoniae (Friedländer's bacillus), *J Exp Med*, **44**: 683–96.

Julianelle LA, 1926c, Immunological relationships of cell constituents of encapsulatus pneumoniae (Friedländer's bacillus), *J Exp Med*, **44**: 735–51.

Kauffmann F, 1949, On the serology of the *Klebsiella* group, *Acta Pathol Microbiol Scand*, **26**: 381–406.

Kauffmann F, 1954, *Enterobacteriaceae*, 2nd edn, Einar Munksgaard, Copenhagen.

Kauffmann F, 1956, Zur biochemischen und serologischen Gruppen- und Typen-einteilung der Enterobacteriaceae, *Zentralbl Bakteriol Parasitenkd Infektionskr Hyg Abt 1 Orig*, **165**: 344–54.

Klapholz A, Lessnau KD et al., 1994, *Hafnia alvei*. Respiratory tract isolates in a community hospital over a three-year period and a literature review, *Chest*, **105**: 1098–100.

Klein E, 1894, On an infection of food-stuffs by *Bacillus prodigiosus*, *J Pathol Bacteriol*, **2**: 217–18.

Kline MW, Mason EO Jr, Kaplan SL, 1988, Characterization of *Citrobacter diversus* strains causing neonatal meningitis, *J Infect Dis*, **157**: 101–5.

Kline MW, Mason EO Jr, Kaplan SL, 1989, Epidemiologic marker system for *Citrobacter diversus* using outer membrane protein profiles, *J Clin Microbiol*, **27**: 1793–6.

Klinge K, 1957, Die Eigelbreaktion und die Wirkung von Mikroorganismen auf den Eigelb-komplex, *Arch Hyg Bakteriol*, **141**: 334–47.

Kosako Y, Sakazaki R, 1991, Priority of *Yokenella regensburgei* Kosako, Sakazaki, and Yoshizaki 1985 over *Koserella trabulsii* Hickman-Brenner, Huntley-Carter, Brenner, and Farmer 1985, *Int J Syst Bacteriol*, **41**: 171.

Kosako Y, Sakazaki R, Yoshizaki E, 1984, *Yokenella regensburgei* gen. nov., sp. nov.: a new genus and species in the family Enterobacteriaceae, *Jpn J Med Sci Biol*, **37**: 117–24.

Kosako Y, Sakazaki R et al., 1987, *Yokenella regensburgei* and *Koserella trabulsii* are subjective synonyms, *Int J Syst Bacteriol*, **37**: 127–9.

Kosako Y, Tamura K et al., 1996, *Enterobacter kobei* sp. nov., a new species of the family Enterobacteriaceae resembling *Enterobacter cloacae*, *Curr Microbiol*, **33**: 261–5.

Kuhn I, Tullus K, Burman LG, 1991, The use of the PhP-KE biochemical fingerprinting system in epidemiological studies of faecal *Enterobacter cloacae* strains from infants in Swedish neonatal wards, *Epidemiol Infect*, **107**: 311–19.

Lapage SP, Johnson R, Holmes B, 1973, Bacteria from intravenous fluids, *Lancet*, **2**: 284–5.

Lautrop H, 1956, Gelatin-liquefying *Klebsiella* strains (*Bacterium oxytocum* Flügge), *Acta Pathol Microbiol Scand*, **39**: 375–84.

Leclerc H, 1962, Étude biochimique d'Enterobacteriaceae pigmentées, *Ann Inst Pasteur (Paris)*, **102**: 726–41.

Le Minor S, Pigache F, 1977, Étude antigènique de souches de *Serratia marcescens* isolées en France. I. Antigènes H: individualisation de six nouveau facteurs H, *Ann Microbiol (Paris)*, **128B**: 207–14.

Lev M, Alexander RH, Sobel HJ, 1969, A study of *Chromobacterium typhiflavum* from the rat, *J Appl Bacteriol*, **32**: 429–33.

Lewis SM, Corpe WA, 1964, Prodigiosin-producing bacteria from marine sources, *Appl Microbiol*, **12**: 13–17.

Limson BM, Romansky MJ, Shea JG, 1956, An evaluation of twenty-two patients with acute and chronic pulmonary infection with Friedländer's bacillus, *Ann Intern Med*, **44**: 1070–81.

Lin F-YC, Devoe WF et al., 1987, Outbreak of neonatal *Citrobacter diversus* meningitis in a suburban hospital, *Pediatr Infect Dis*, **6**: 50–5.

Lindh E, Kjaeldgaard P et al., 1991, Phenotypical properties of *Enterobacter agglomerans* (*Pantoea agglomerans*) from human, animal and plant sources, *APMIS*, **99**: 347–52.

Lindh E, Ursing J, 1991, Genomic groups and biochemical profiles of clinical isolates of *Enterobacter cloacae*, *APMIS*, **99**: 507–14.

Liu PY, Lau YJ et al., 1994, Use of PCR to study epidemiology of *Serratia marcescens* isolates in nosocomial infection, *J Clin Microbiol*, **32**: 1935–8.

Loewenberg B, 1894, Le microbe de l'ozène, *Ann Inst Pasteur (Paris)*, **8**: 292–317.

Lund ME, Matsen JM, Blazevic DJ, 1974, Biochemical and antibiotic susceptibility studies of H$_2$S-negative *Citrobacter*, *Appl Microbiol*, **28**: 22–5.

Luttrell RE, Rannick GA et al., 1988, *Kluyvera* species soft tissue infection: case report and review, *J Clin Microbiol*, **26**: 2650–1.

McIver CJ, Tapsall JW, 1988, Characteristics of cysteine-requiring strains of *Klebsiella* isolated from urinary tract infections, *J Med Microbiol*, **26**: 211–15.

McIver CJ, Tapsall JW, 1990, Assessment of conventional and commercial methods for identification of clinical isolates of cysteine-requiring strains of *Escherichia coli* and *Klebsiella* species, *J Clin Microbiol*, **28**: 1947–51 [Published erratum appears in *J Clin Microbiol*, 1991; **29**: 226].

McNeil MM, Davis BJ et al., 1987a, *Ewingella americana*: recurrent pseudobacteremia from a persistent environmental reservoir, *J Clin Microbiol*, **25**: 498–500.

McNeil MM, Davis BJ et al., 1987b, Plasmids of *Ewingella americana*: supplementary epidemiologic markers in an outbreak of pseudobacteraemia, *J Clin Microbiol*, **25**: 501–3 [Note: authors later amended to Clark N, McNeil MM et al., see *J Clin Microbiol*, 1987; **25**: 966].

McWhorter AC, Haddock RL et al., 1991, *Trabulsiella guamensis*, a new genus and species of the family Enterobacteriaceae that resembles *Salmonella* subgroups 4 and 5, *J Clin Microbiol*, **29**: 1480–5.

Malcolm JF, 1938, The classification of coliform bacteria, *J Hyg (Lond)*, **38**: 395–423.

Maraki S, Samonis G et al., 1994, Surgical wound infection caused by *Rahnella aquatilis*, *J Clin Microbiol*, **32**: 2706–8.

Maslow JN, Brecher SM et al., 1993, Relationship between indole production and differentiation of *Klebsiella* species: indole-positive and -negative isolates of *Klebsiella* determined to be clonal, *J Clin Microbiol*, **31**: 2000–3.

Matsumoto H, 1963, Studies on the *Hafnia* isolated from normal human, *Jpn J Microbiol*, **7**: 105–14.

Matsumoto H, 1964, Additional new antigens of *Hafnia* group, *Jpn J Microbiol*, **8**: 139–41.

Mergaert J, Verdonck L et al., 1984, Numerical taxonomy of *Erwinia* species using API systems, *J Gen Microbiol*, **130**: 1893–910.

Mermel LA, Spiegel CA, 1992, Nosocomial sepsis due to *Serratia odorifera* biovar 1, *Clin Infect Dis*, **14**: 208–10.

Meyers BR, Bottone E et al., 1972, Infections caused by organisms of the genus *Erwinia*, *Ann Intern Med*, **76**: 9–14.

Mirza GE, Karakucuk S et al., 1994, Postoperative endophthalmitis caused by an *Enterobacter* species, *J Hosp Infect*, **26**: 167–72.

Møller V, 1954, Distribution of amino acid decarboxylases in Enterobacteriaceae, *Acta Pathol Microbiol Scand*, **35**: 259–77.

Monnet D, Freney J, 1994, Method for differentiating *Klebsiella planticola* and *Klebsiella terrigena* from other *Klebsiella* species, *J Clin Microbiol*, **32**: 1121–2.

Monsour V, Colmer AR, 1952, The action of some members of the genus *Serratia* on egg yolk complex, *J Bacteriol*, **63**: 597–603.

Morgan MG, Stuart C et al., 1992, *Citrobacter diversus* brain abscess: case reports and molecular epidemiology, *J Med Microbiol*, **36**: 273–8.

Mori M, Ohta M et al., 1989, Identification of species and capsular types of *Klebsiella* clinical isolates, with special reference to *Klebsiella planticola*, *Microbiol Immunol*, **33**: 887–95.

Müller HE, Brenner DJ et al., 1996, Emended description of *Buttiauxella agrestis* with recognition of six new species of *Buttiauxella* and two new species of *Kluyvera*: *Buttiauxella ferragutiae* sp. nov., *Buttiauxella gaviniae* sp. nov., *Buttiauxella brennerae* sp. nov., *Buttiauxella izardii* sp. nov., *Buttiauxella noackiae* sp. nov., *Buttiauxella warmboldiae* sp. nov., *Kluyvera cochleae* sp. nov., and *Kluyvera georgiana* sp. nov., *Int J Syst Bacteriol*, **46**: 50–63.

Muraschi TF, Friend M, Bolles D, 1965, *Erwinia*-like microorganisms isolated from animal and human hosts, *Appl Microbiol*, **13**: 128–31.

Muytjens HL, Zanen HC et al., 1983, Analysis of eight cases of neonatal meningitis and sepsis due to *Enterobacter sakazakii*, *J Clin Microbiol*, **18**: 115–20.

Nakashima AK, McCarthy MA et al., 1987, Epidemic septic arthritis caused by *Serratia marcescens* and associated with a benzalkonium chloride antiseptic, *J Clin Microbiol*, **25**: 1014–18.

Nassif X, Sansonetti PJ, 1986, Correlation of the virulence of *Klebsiella pneumoniae* K1 and K2 with the presence of a plasmid encoding aerobactin, *Infect Immun*, **54**: 603–8.

Nomura S, Murata K, Nagayama A, 1995, Effects of sub-minimal inhibitory concentrations of antimicrobial agents on the cell surface of *Klebsiella pneumoniae* and phagocytic killing activity, *J Chemother*, **7**: 406–13.

Nouvellon M, Pons JL et al., 1994, Clonal outbreaks of extended-spectrum beta-lactamase-producing strains of *Klebsiella pneumoniae* demonstrated by antibiotic susceptibility testing, beta-lactamase typing, and multilocus enzyme electrophoresis, *J Clin Microbiol*, **32**: 2625–7.

Oh HM, Tay L, 1995, Bacteraemia caused by *Rahnella aquatilis*: report of two cases and review, *Scand J Infect Dis*, **27**: 79–80.

O'Hara CM, Roman SB, Miller JM, 1995, Ability of commercial identification systems to identify newly recognized species of *Citrobacter*, *J Clin Microbiol*, **33**: 242–5.

O'Hara CM, Steigerwalt AG et al., 1989, *Enterobacter hormaechei*, a new species of the family Enterobacteriaceae formerly known as enteric group 75, *J Clin Microbiol*, **27**: 2046–9.

Okubadejo OA, Alausa KO, 1968, Neonatal meningitis caused by *Edwardsiella tarda*, *Br Med J*, **3**: 357–8.

Okutomi T, Nishizawa T et al., 1992, Inhibition of morphine dependence by a lipopolysaccharide from *Pantoea agglomerans*, *Eur Cytokine Netw*, **3**: 417–20.

Ørskov I, 1954, O antigens in the *Klebsiella* group, *Acta Pathol Microbiol Scand*, **34**: 145–56.

Ørskov I, 1955a, Serological investigations in the *Klebsiella* group 1. New capsule types, *Acta Pathol Microbiol Scand*, **36**: 449–53.

Ørskov I, 1955b, Serological investigations in the *Klebsiella* group 2. Occurrence of *Klebsiella* in sputa, *Acta Pathol Microbiol Scand*, **36**: 454–60.

Ørskov I, 1955c, The biochemical properties of *Klebsiella* (*Klebsiella aerogenes*) strains, *Acta Pathol Microbiol Scand*, **37**: 353–68.

Ørskov I, Ørskov F, 1984, Serotyping of *Klebsiella*, *Methods Microbiol*, **14**: 143–64.

Paine TF, 1946, Illness in man following inhalation of *Serratia marcescens*, *J Infect Dis*, **79**: 226–32.

Palfreyman JM, 1978, *Klebsiella* serotyping by counter-current immunoelectrophoresis, *J Hyg (Lond)*, **81**: 219–25.

Parment PA, Ursing J, Palmer B, 1984, *Serratia rubidaea* isolated from a silastic foam dressing, *Infection*, **12**: 268–9.

Parry MF, Hutchinson JH et al., 1980, Gram-negative sepsis in neonates: a nursery outbreak due to hand carriage of *Citrobacter diversus*, *Pediatrics*, **65**: 1105–9.

Perkins BA, Hamill RJ et al., 1992, *In vitro* activities of streptomycin and 11 oral antimicrobial agents against clinical isolates of *Klebsiella rhinoscleromatis*, *Antimicrob Agents Chemother*, **36**: 1785–7.

Perkins SR, Beckett TA, Bump CM, 1986, *Cedecea davisae* bacteremia, *J Clin Microbiol*, **24**: 675–6.

Perry JJ, 1961, Prodigiosin in an actinomycete, *Nature* (London), **191**: 77–8.

Pfyffer GE, 1992, *Serratia fonticola* as an infectious agent, *Eur J Clin Microbiol Infect Dis*, **11**: 199–200.

Pien FD, Farmer JJ III, 1983, *Serratia ficaria* isolated from a leg ulcer, *South Med J*, **76**: 1591–2.

Pien FD, Farmer JJ III, Weaver RE, 1983, Polymicrobial bacteremia caused by *Ewingella americana* (family Enterobacteriaceae) and an unusual *Pseudomonas* species, *J Clin Microbiol*, **18**: 727–9.

Pitt TL, Erdman YJ, 1984, Serological typing of *Serratia marcescens*, *Methods in Microbiology*, vol. 15, ed. Bergan T, Academic Press, London, 173–211.

Podschun R, 1990, Phenotypic properties of *Klebsiella pneumoniae* and *K. oxytoca* isolated from different sources, *Zentralbl Hyg Umweltmed*, **189**: 527–35.

Podschun R, 1991, Isolation of *Klebsiella terrigena* from human feces: biochemical reactions, capsule types, and antibiotic sensitivity, *Int J Med Microbiol*, **275**: 73–8.

Podschun R, Ullmann U, 1992, Isolation of *Klebsiella terrigena* from clinical specimens, *Eur J Clin Microbiol Infect Dis*, **11**: 349–52.

Poh CL, Yap SC, Yeo M, 1993, Pulsed-field gel electrophoresis for differentiation of hospital isolates of *Klebsiella pneumoniae*, *J Hosp Infect*, **24**: 123–8.

Poilane I, Cruaud P et al., 1993, *Enterobacter cloacae* cross-colonization in neonates demonstrated by ribotyping, *Eur J Clin Microbiol Infect Dis*, **12**: 820–6.

Popoff M, Stoleru GH, 1980, Position taxonomique de variants biochimiques de *Citrobacter freundii*, *Ann Microbiol (Paris)*, **131A**: 189–96.

Potel G, Caillon J et al., 1992, Identification of factors affecting in vivo aminoglycoside activity in an experimental model of gram-negative endocarditis, *Antimicrob Agents Chemother*, **36**: 744–50.

Priest FG, Somerville HJ et al., 1973, The taxonomic position of *Obesumbacterium proteus*, a common brewery contaminant, *J Gen Microbiol*, **75**: 295–307.

Prinsloo HE, 1966, Bacteriocins and phages produced by *Serratia marcescens*, *J Gen Microbiol*, **45**: 205–12.

Ramirez MJ, 1968, Differentiation of *Klebsiella–Enterobacter* (*Aerobacter*)–*Serratia* by biochemical tests and antibiotic susceptibility, *Appl Microbiol*, **16**: 1548–50.

Read BE, Keller R, Cabelli VJ, 1957, The decapsulation phenomenon of *Klebsiella pneumoniae*, *J Bacteriol*, **73**: 765–9.

Reger PJ, Mockler DF, Miller MA, 1993, Comparison of antimicrobial susceptibility, beta-lactamase production, plasmid analysis and serum bactericidal activity in *Edwardsiella tarda*, *E. ictaluri* and *E. hoshinae*, *J Med Microbiol*, **39**: 273–81.

Reina J, Borrell N, Llompart I, 1992, Community-acquired bacteremia caused by *Serratia plymuthica*. Case report and review of the literature, *Diagn Microbiol Infect Dis*, **15**: 449–52.

Report, 1954, The Enterobacteriaceae Subcommittee of the Nomenclature Committee of the International Association of Microbiologists. Reports on the groups: *Salmonella, Shigella, Arizona, Bethesda, Escherichia, Klebsiella* (*Aerogenes, Aerobacter*) *Providence* (29911 of Stuart *et al.*), *Int Bull Bacteriol Nomencl Taxon*, **4**: 47–94.

Report, 1963, Report of the Subcommittee on Taxonomy of the Enterobacteriaceae, *Int Bull Bacteriol Nomencl Taxon*, **13**: 69–93.

Riain UN, Cormican MG et al., 1994, PCR based fingerprinting of *Enterobacter cloacae*, *J Hosp Infect*, **27**: 237–40.

Richard C, Joly B et al., 1976, Étude de souches de *Enterobacter* appartenant à un groupe particulier proche de *E. aerogenes*, *Ann Microbiol (Paris)*, **127A**: 545–8.

Ridell J, Siitonen A et al., 1994, *Hafnia alvei* in stool specimens from patients with diarrhea and healthy controls, *J Clin Microbiol*, **32**: 2335–7.

Ridell J, Siitonen A et al., 1995, Characterization of *Hafnia alvei* by biochemical tests, random amplified polymorphic DNA PCR, and partial sequencing of 16S rRNA gene, *J Clin Microbiol*, **33**: 2372–6.

Riser E, Noone P, Poulton TA, 1976, A new serotyping method for *Klebsiella* species: development of the technique, *J Clin Pathol*, **29**: 296–304.

Rubinstien EM, Klevjer-Anderson P et al., 1993, *Enterobacter taylorae*, a new opportunistic pathogen: report of four cases, *J Clin Microbiol*, **31**: 249–54.

Sader HS, Perl TM et al., 1994, Nosocomial transmission of *Serratia odorifera* biogroup 2: case report demonstration by macro-restriction analysis of chromosomal DNA using pulsed-field gel electrophoresis, *Infect Control Hosp Epidemiol*, **15**: 390–3.

Sakazaki R, 1961, Studies on the *Hafnia* group of Enterobacteriaceae, *Jpn J Med Sci Biol*, **14**: 223–41.

Sakazaki R, 1965, A proposed group of the family Enterobacteriaceae, the Asakusa group, *Int Bull Bacteriol Nomencl Taxon*, **15**: 45–7.

Sakazaki R, 1967, Studies on the Asakusa group of Enterobacteriaceae (*Edwardsiella tarda*), *Jpn J Med Sci Biol*, **20**: 205–12.

Sakazaki R, Namioka S, 1960, Serological studies on the *Cloaca* (*Aerobacter*) group of enteric bacteria, *Jpn J Med Sci Biol*, **13**: 1–12.

Sakazaki R, Tamura K, 1975, Priority of the specific epithet *anguillimortiferum* over the specific epithet *tarda* in the name of the organism presently known as *Edwardsiella tarda*, *Int J Syst Bacteriol*, **25**: 219–20.

Sakazaki R, Tamura K et al., 1976, Taxonomy of some recently described species in the family Enterobacteriaceae, *Int J Syst Bacteriol*, **26**: 158–79.

Sakazaki R, Tamura K et al., 1989, *Klebsiella ornithinolytica* sp. nov., formerly known as ornithine-positive *Klebsiella oxytoca*, *Curr Microbiol*, **18**: 201–6.

Schentag JJ, 1993, The results of a targeted pharmacy intervention program, *Clin Ther*, **15, Suppl. A**: 29–36.

Schindler J, Potuznikova B, Aldová E, 1992, Classification of strains of *Pragia fontium*, *Budvicia aquatica* and of *Leminorella* by whole-cell protein pattern, *J Hyg Epidemiol Microbiol Immunol*, **36**: 207–16.

Schonheyder HC, Jensen KT, Frederiksen W, 1994, Taxonomic notes: synonymy of *Enterobacter cancerogenus* (Urosevic 1966) Dickey and Zumoff 1988 and *Enterobacter taylorae* Farmer et al. 1985 and resolution of an ambiguity in the biochemical profile, *Int J Syst Bacteriol*, **44**: 586–7.

Schreier JB, 1969, Modification of deoxyribonuclease test medium for rapid identification of *Serratia marcescens*, *Am J Clin Pathol*, **51**: 711–16.

Sedlák J, Slajsová M, 1966, Antigenstruktur und Antigenbeziehungen der Gattung *Citrobacter*, *Zentralbl Bakteriol Parasitenkd Infektionskr Hyg*, **200**: 369–74.

Shearman PJ, Bundle DR et al., 1984, Characterization of anti-*Citrobacter* O36 specific polysaccharide monoclonal antibodies, *Can J Microbiol*, **30**: 91–7.

Shimwell JL, 1963, *Obesumbacterium* gen. nov., *Brewers' J*, **99**: 759–60.

Shlaes DM, 1993, The clinical relevance of *Enterobacter* infections, *Clin Ther*, **15, Suppl. A**: 21–8.

Sierra-Madero J, Pratt K et al., 1990, *Kluyvera* mediastinitis following open-heart surgery: a case report, *J Clin Microbiol*, **28**: 2848–9.

Sifuentes-Osornio J, Groschel DHM, 1987, Modification of Grimont biotyping system for epidemiolgic studies with nosocomial *Serratia marcescens* isolates, *J Clin Microbiol*, **25**: 567–8.

Sikka R, Sabherwal U, Arora DR, 1989, Resistotyping as a new epidemiological marker for *Klebsiella pneumoniae*, *Indian J Med Res*, **89**: 95–9.

Simoons-Smit AM, Verweij-Van Vught AMJJ et al., 1985, Biochemical and serological investigations on clinical isolates of *Klebsiella*, *J Hyg (Lond)*, **95**: 265–76.

Skerman VBD, McGowan V, Sneath PHA, 1980, Approved lists of bacterial names, *Int J Syst Bacteriol*, **30**: 225–420.

Ślopek S, Durlakowa I, 1967, Studies on the taxonomy of *Klebsiella* bacilli, *Arch Immunol Ther Exp*, **15**: 481–7.

Ślopek S, Przondo-Hessek A et al., 1967, A working scheme for bacteriophage typing of *Klebsiella* bacilli, *Arch Immunol Ther Exp*, **15**: 589–99.

Slotnick IJ, Tulman L, 1967, A human infection caused by *Erwinia* species, *Am J Med*, **43**: 147–50.

Sonnenwirth AC, Kallus BA, 1968, Meningitis due to *Edwardsiella tarda*. First report of meningitis caused by *E. tarda*, *Am J Clin Pathol*, **49**: 92–5.

Sourek J, Aldová E, 1976, Serotyping of strains belonging to the *Citrobacter–Levinea* group isolated from diagnostic material, *Zentralbl Bakteriol Parasitenkd Infektionskr Abt 1 Orig*, **234**: 480–90.

Stouthamer AH, Tieze GA, 1966, Bacteriocin production by members of the genus *Klebsiella*, *Antonie van Leeuwenhoek J Microbiol Serol*, **32**: 171–82.

Tamura K, Sakazaki R et al., 1986, *Leclercia adecarboxylata* gen. nov., comb. nov., formerly known as *Escherichia adecarboxylata*, *Curr Microbiol*, **13**: 179–84.

Tamura K, Sakazaki R et al., 1988, *Edwardsiella tarda* serotyping scheme for international use, *J Clin Microbiol*, **26**: 2343–6.

Thaller R, Berlutti F, Thaller MC, 1988, A *Kluyvera cryocrescens* strain from a gall-bladder infection, *Eur J Epidemiol*, **4**: 124–6.

Thomas GM, Poinar GO Jr, 1979, *Xenorhabdus* gen. nov., a genus of entomopathogenic, nematophilic bacteria of the family Enterobacteriaceae, *Int J Syst Bacteriol*, **29**: 352–60.

Thompson W, Romance L et al., 1993, *Klebsiella pneumoniae* infection on a rehabilitation unit: comparison of epidemiologic typing methods, *Infect Control Hosp Epidemiol*, **14**: 203–10.

Thurm V, Gericke B, 1994, Identification of infant food as a vehicle in a nosocomial outbreak of *Citrobacter freundii*: epidemiological subtyping by allozyme, whole-cell protein and antibiotic resistance, *J Appl Bacteriol*, **76**: 553–8.

Toala P, Lee YH et al., 1970, Susceptibility of *Enterobacter aerogenes* and *Enterobacter cloacae* to 19 antimicrobial agents *in vitro*, *Am J Med Sci*, **260**: 41–55.

Toenniessen E, 1913, Ueber Wesen und Ursache der Mutation bei Bakterien. Untersuchungen über die Morphologie und Variabilität des Friedländerschen Pneumoniebacillus, *Zentralbl Bakteriol Parasitenkd Infektionskr*, **69**: 391–412.

Toenniessen E, 1914, Ueber Vererbung und Variabilität bei Bakterien mit besonderer Berücksichtigung der Virulenz, *Zentralbl Bakteriol Parasitenkd Infektionskr*, **73**: 241–77.

Toenniessen E, 1921, Untersuchungen über die Kapsel (Gummihülle) der pathogenen Bakterien. II. Die chemische Beschaffenheit der Kapsel und ihr dadurch bedingtes verhalten gegenüber der Fixierung und Färbung, *Zentralbl Bakteriol Parasitenkd Infektionskr*, **85**: 225–37.

Tomás JM, Benedi VJ et al., 1986, Role of capsule and O antigen in resistance of *Klebsiella pneumoniae* to serum bactericidal activity, *Infect Immun*, **54**: 85–9.

Toye BW, Scriver SR, Low DE, 1993, Canadian survey of antimicrobial resistance in *Klebsiella* spp. and *Enterobacter* spp. The Canadian Antimicrobial Resistance Study Group, *J Antimicrob Chemother*, **32, Suppl. B**: 81–6.

Traub WH, 1980, Bacteriocin and phage typing of *Serratia*, *The Genus* Serratia, CRC Press, Boca Raton, FL, 79–100.

Traub WH, 1985, Serotyping of *Serratia marcescens*: identification of a new O-antigen (O24), *Zentralbl Bakteriol Mikrobiol Hyg A*, **259**: 485–8.

Traub WH, 1991a, Comparative biotyping, bacteriocin typing, and serogrouping (O-antigens) of *Serratia liquefaciens*, *Int J Med Microbiol*, **275**: 200–10.

Traub WH, 1991b, Serotyping of *Serratia liquefaciens*: H-antigens, *Int J Med Microbiol*, **275**: 211–15.

Traub WH, 1991c, Serotyping of *Serratia marcescens*: detection of two new O-antigens (O25 and O26), *Int J Med Microbiol*, **275**: 495–9.

Traub WH, Kleber I, 1977, Serotyping of *Serratia marcescens*: evaluation of Le Minor's H-immobilization test and description of three new flagella H antigens, *J Clin Microbiol*, **5**: 115–21.

Traub WH, Raymond EA, 1971, Epidemiological surveillance of *Serratia marcescens* infections by bacteriocin typing, *Appl Microbiol*, **22**: 1058–63.

Tschape H, Prager R et al., 1995, Verotoxinogenic *Citrobacter freundii* associated with severe gastroenteritis and cases of hae-

molytic uraemic syndrome in a nursery school: green butter as the infection source, *Epidemiol Infect*, **114**: 441–50.

Tullus K, Burman LG, 1989, Ecological impact of ampicillin and cefuroxime in neonatal units, *Lancet*, **1**: 1405–7.

Ursua PR, Unzaga MJ et al., 1996, *Serratia rubidaea* as an invasive pathogen, *J Clin Microbiol*, **34**: 216–17.

Verdonck L, Mergaert J et al., 1987, Genus *Erwinia*: numerical analysis of phenotypic features, *Int J Syst Bacteriol*, **37**: 4–18.

Waisman HA, Stone WH, 1958, The presence of *Serratia marcescens* as the predominating organism in the intestinal tract of the newborn. The occurrence of the 'red diaper syndrome', *Pediatrics*, **21**: 8–12.

Walton DT, Abbott SL, Janda JM, 1993, Sucrose-positive *Edwardsiella tarda* mimicking a biogroup 1 strain isolated from a patient with cholelithiasis, *J Clin Microbiol*, **31**: 155–6.

Werkman CH, Gillen GF, 1932, Bacteria producing trimethylene glycol, *J Bacteriol*, **23**: 167–82.

West MG, Edwards PR, 1954, *The Bethesda-Ballerup Group of Paracolon Bacteria*, US Dept of Health, Education and Welfare, Atlanta, GA.

Westblom TU, Coggins ME, 1987, Osteomyelitis caused by *Enterobacter taylorae*, formerly enteric group 19, *J Clin Microbiol*, **25**: 2432–3.

Wharton DRA, Creech HJ, 1949, Further studies of the immunological properties of polysaccharides from *Serratia marcescens* (*Bacillus prodigiosus*). II. Nature of the antigenic action and the antibody response in mice, *J Immunol*, **62**: 135–53.

Wheat RW, Dorsch C, Godoy G, 1965, Occurrence of pyruvic acid in the capsular polysaccharide of *Klebsiella rhinoscleromatis*, *J Bacteriol*, **89**: 539.

Wilfert JN, Barrett FF et al., 1970, *Serratia marcescens*: biochemical, serological and epidemiological characteristics and antibiotic susceptibility of strains isolated at Boston City Hospital, *Appl Microbiol*, **19**: 345–52.

Wilhelmi I, Bernaldo de Quiros JCL et al., 1987, Epidemic outbreak of *Serratia marcescens* infection in a cardiac surgery unit, *J Clin Microbiol*, **25**: 1298–300.

Wilkinson JF, 1958, The extracellular polysaccharides of bacteria, *Bacteriol Rev*, **22**: 46–73.

Wilkinson JF, Dudman WF, Aspinall GO, 1954, The extracellular polysaccharide of *Aerobacter aerogenes* A3 (S1) (*Klebsiella* type 54), *Biochem J*, **59**: 446–51.

Wilkinson JF, Duguid JP, Edmunds PN, 1954, The distribution of polysaccharide production in *Aerobacter* and *Escherichia* strains and its relation to antigenic structure, *J Gen Microbiol*, **11**: 59–72.

Williams P, Brown MRW, Lambert PA, 1984, Effect of iron deprivation on the production of siderophores and outer membrane proteins in *Klebsiella aerogenes*, *J Gen Microbiol*, **130**: 2357–65.

Williams P, Lambert PA et al., 1983, The role of O and K antigens in determining the resistance of *Klebsiella aerogenes* to serum killing, *J Gen Microbiol*, **129**: 2181–91.

Williams RP, Green JA, Rappoport DA, 1956a, Studies on pigmentation of *Serratia marcescens* I. Spectral and paper chromatographic properties of prodigiosin, *J Bacteriol*, **71**: 115–20.

Williams RP, Green JA, Rappoport DA, 1956b, Evidence for the incorporation of iron and calcium into the pigments of *Serratia marcescens*, *Science*, **123**: 1176–7.

Wong NA, Linton CJ et al., 1994, Randomly amplified polymorphic DNA typing: a useful tool for rapid epidemiological typing of *Klebsiella pneumoniae*, *Epidemiol Infect*, **113**: 445–54.

Wong VK, 1987, Broviac catheter infection with *Kluyvera cryocrescens*: a case report, *J Clin Microbiol*, **25**: 1115–16.

Woodward HMM, Clarke KB, 1913, A case of infection in man by the *Bacterium prodigiosum*, *Lancet*, **1**: 314–15.

Wrede F, Rothhaas A, 1934, Über das Prodigiosin, den rotem Farbstoff des *Bacillus prodigiosus*, *Z Physiol Chem*, **226**: 95–107.

Yale MW, 1939, Genus I. *Escherichia* Castellani and Chalmers, *Bergey's Manual of Determinative Bacteriology*, 5th edn, eds

Bergey DH, Breed RS et al., Williams & Wilkins, Baltimore, 389–96.

Yogev R, Kozlowski S, 1990, Peritonitis due to *Kluyvera ascorbata*: case report and review, *Rev Infect Dis*, **12**: 399–402.

Young VM, Kenton DM et al., 1971, *Levinea*, a new genus of the family Enterobacteriaceae, *Int J Syst Bacteriol*, **21**: 58–63.

Yu CM, Chow JW, Yu VL, 1996, Quantitative comparison in vitro of mutational antibiotic resistance of *Enterobacter* spp. using a spiral plater, *J Antimicrob Chemother*, **37**: 233–42.

Zighelboim J, Williams TW Jr et al., 1992, Successful medical management of a patient with multiple hepatic abscesses due to *Edwardsiella tarda*, *Clin Infect Dis*, **14**: 117–20.

Chapter 43

PROTEUS, MORGANELLA AND PROVIDENCIA

B W Senior

The bacteria of the genera *Proteus*, *Morganella* and *Providencia* belong to the tribe Proteeae in the family Enterobacteriaceae and conform to the definition of the family given in Chapter 39. They have one biochemical character that distinguishes them from all other members of the Enterobacteriaceae, with the exception of the recently defined rare genera *Tatumella* and *Rahnella*: the ability to deaminate oxidatively certain amino acids to the corresponding keto acid and ammonia. Tests for phenylalanine or tryptophan deaminase are the ones commonly made and a rapid method for this reaction has been devised (Giammanco, Pignato and Agodi 1985). Members of the tribe are also readily recognized by the red-brown, melanin-like pigment they form when cultured under aerobic conditions on media containing iron and an aromatic L-amino acid such as phenylalanine, tryptophan, tyrosine or histidine (Polster and Svobodova 1964, Müller 1985).

In general, most strains of *Proteus*, *Morganella* and *Providencia* also share the following common but not unique characteristics: motility, resistance to KCN, the ability to degrade tyrosine (Sheth and Kurup 1975) and inability to acidify lactose, dulcitol and malonate or form arginine or lysine decarboxylase, or β-galactosidase. With a few exceptions in *Proteus*, all are methylred positive and Voges–Proskauer negative.

PROTEUS

1 DEFINITION

Proteus spp. give a characteristic spreading growth ('swarming') on appropriate solid media, oxidatively deaminate amino acids, hydrolyse urea but fail to acidify mannose. G + C content of the DNA is 38–40 mol%.

The genus, named after the Greek deity Proteus who had the ability to assume different shapes, has 4 species: *Proteus mirabilis* and *Proteus vulgaris* (formerly known together as *Proteus hauseri*), *Proteus myxofaciens* described by Cosenza and Podgwaite (1966) and *Proteus penneri* by Hickman et al. (1982).

2 MORPHOLOGY

After growth for 24–48 h on solid media, most cells are rods, 1–3 μm long by 0.4–0.6 μm wide, though short, fat, coccobacillary forms are not uncommon. In young cultures that are swarming (see section 3.1, p. 1036) on solid media, many of the cells are long, curved and filamentous, reaching 10, 20 and even up to 80 μm in length. In older cultures, the organisms have no characteristic arrangement: they may be distributed singly, in pairs or in short chains. However, in young swarming cultures, the filamentous cells tend to be arranged concentrically like the isobars in a diagram of a cyclone.

Except for non-flagellate variants and those with paralysed flagella, all strains in young cultures are actively motile by peritrichate flagella. The flagella are more variable in shape than those of most other enterobacteria, normal and 'curly' forms sometimes being found together on the same organism and even in the same flagellum. The form of the flagellum is also influenced by the pH of the medium. *P. mirabilis* has several genes coding for flagella but normally only one type of flagellin, FlaA, a protein of 40 kDa is formed. However, it may undergo antigenic variation as a result of spontaneous mutation and this may be an important survival mechanism in vivo (Belas 1994).

Under appropriate cultural conditions, strains of *Proteus* species form a number of different types of peritrichous fimbriae. Some are associated with virulence and many have been purified and their genes cloned. A cell may bear more than one type of fimbria. Some of the fimbriae can be distinguished morphologically and by their haemagglutinating characteristics. Among these, mannose-resistant *Proteus*-like (MR/P), channelled, thick (7–8 nm in diameter) fimbriae and mannose-resistant *Klebsiella*-like (MR/K), non-channelled, thin (4–5 nm in diameter) fimbriae are frequently found in *Proteus* whereas mannose-sensitive (MS), channelled, thick (8–9 nm in diameter) fimbriae are found only infrequently (Old and Adegbola 1982, Adegbola, Old and Senior 1983, Yakubu, Old and Senior 1989). Other fimbriae such as ATF (ambient temperature fimbriae) (Massad, Bahrani and Mobley 1994), PMF (*Proteus mirabilis* fimbriae) (Massad et al. 1994) and UCA (uroepithelial cell adhesin) (Wray et al. 1986) are unable to agglutinate erythrocytes.

3 CULTURAL CHARACTERS

Proteus strains grow well on ordinary media, but most strains, particularly if grown at 22–30°C, do not form discrete colonies on nutrient agar. Instead they exhibit spreading growth (swarming, see section 3.1) even on the surface of appropriate well-dried media. In nutrient broth, *Proteus* gives rise to a uniform turbidity with a slight to moderate powdery deposit and a faint ammoniacal odour. A thin, fragile pellicle may develop in old cultures. In minimal salts media, *Proteus* shows a requirement for nicotinic acid.

A number of selective and indicator media have been designed for *Proteus* and the other genera of the Proteeae. That of Malinowski (1966) incorporates alanine, potassium nitrate and dyes so that the alanine decarboxylating strains of the tribe give rise to blue-grey colonies distinct in colour from both other lactose non-fermenters including *Salmonella* and *Shigella* spp. (white-grey) and also *Escherichia coli* (red) which cannot decarboxylate this amino acid. An infusion agar containing bile salts, lithium chloride, sodium thiosulphate and sodium citrate inhibits the growth of almost all enterobacteria except Proteeae (Xilinas, Papavassiliou and Legakis 1975). The medium of Hawkey, McCormick and Simpson (1986) contains clinda-

mycin to inhibit gram-positive bacteria, tryptophan and tyrosine. Through oxidative deamination of tryptophan, and tyrosine degradation, strains of the Proteeae form dark brown colonies surrounded by a clear area of degraded tyrosine crystals.

3.1 Swarming

This is a characteristic feature of *Proteus* in which a group of cells at the edge of a developing microcolony migrate to an uninoculated area of the medium. However, it is not unique to *Proteus* and similar behaviour can be found in some other bacteria outwith the tribe, such as *Serratia marcescens* and *Vibrio parahaemolyticus*. The process is exceedingly complex. After some 2–4 h, through receipt of an environmental signal such as that given by glutamine or an increasingly viscous (PVP) environment or a solid (agar) surface (Allison et al. 1993) or by inhibition of flagella rotation, the co-ordinate transcription of about 50 genes is triggered in the normally sparsely flagellate, short (2–4 μm) bacilli (referred to here as vegetative cells) and they differentiate into swarm cells. In this process, which involves genes associated with the synthesis and movement of flagella, lipopolysaccharide and peptidoglycan synthesis, cell division and proteolysis of peptides (Belas, Goldman and Ashliman 1995), the cell continues to grow in length, but not in width, because septum formation and cell division are inhibited. It synthesizes several hundreds of flagella, an acidic polysaccharide 'slime' which is thought to assist the movement of swarm cells across the agar surface, and virulence factors such as urease, haemolysin and protease (Allison, Lai and Hughes 1992). Eventually a multinucleate, densely flagellate, non-septate, elongated cell 20–80 μm in length, known as a swarm cell, is formed whose enzymic activity, antibiotic sensitivity, cell wall permeability, lipopolysaccharide composition and response to amino acid attractants differ from those of the vegetative cell. The swarm cell is also different from the vegetative cell in that it now has the ability, though not on its own, to migrate or swarm with a mass of other swarm cells over a solid surface. (The formation of swarm cells can also occur in liquid media and also in vivo.) The process is not haphazard but, by multicellular interaction and signalling, there is the simultaneous and co-ordinated migration in unison of swarm cells. They emerge from the edge of the colony in small groups and swarm a short distance – possibly mediated by the slime – and then return to the colony. As the swarming period proceeds, the cells move out in larger groups and travel further before returning. The duration and extent of this swarming period is highly variable according to the strain and the cultural conditions. The swarming growth on a plate may eventually appear as a uniform film of growth extending over the whole plate (**continuous swarming**) or as a series of concentric circles of growth around the point of inoculation (**discontinuous swarming**; Fig. 43.1). In discontinuous swarming, migration usually ceases after about 2 h and the cells enter a period of consolidation during which the swarm cells differentiate back to the vegetative short bacillary form by division at several positions along the length of the swarm cell. The vegetative cells then grow and multiply until such time as swarm cell formation is initiated again and the process is repeated. This cyclical swarming and consolidation, which may occur every 4 h or so, gives rise to the series of alternating concentric circles of thick and thin growth over a plate (Fig. 43.1).

The cause of swarming has given rise to much speculation. Lominski and Lendrum (1942, 1947) proposed that swarming was the outcome of a negative chemotactic response to metabolic products that accumulated in agar in areas of high population density. They implied that swarm cell formation was stimulated by the toxic products. This theory may not be correct, for although *Proteus* cells are believed to form toxic products (indeed the anti-swarming effect of charcoal has been attributed to the adsorption of such compounds), that may lead to the formation of filamentous cells, there is no evidence that such filaments are true swarm cells capable of swarming. Williams and Schwarzhoff (1978), on the other hand, believed that swarm cell formation was not the result of the effect of toxic compounds and that the movement of swarm cells was a non-chemotactic event (Williams et al. 1976). Others disagree with both these points of view and believe swarming to be a positive chemotactic response to deteriorating nutritional conditions. Swarm cells have been found to be chemotactic and they respond to fewer attractants than vegetative cells.

Some attractants are mutually exclusive and attract either swarm cells (glutamine) or vegetative cells (glutamate). This may indicate the presence of separate sensory components in swarm and vegetative cells that are coupled to different forms of motility (Allison et al. 1993).

Irrespective of the reasons for swarming, the ability of *Proteus* to differentiate into a population of cells capable of rapid migration over surfaces is believed to be important in enabling *Proteus* to infect the kidney by the ascension of migrating swarm cells up the ureter against a flow of urine and mucus. Recent evidence confirms that swarm formation is important for the uropathogenicity of *P. mirabilis* for mice in vivo (Allison et al. 1994).

ANTI-SWARMING AGENTS

The swarming of *Proteus* may make it difficult to isolate in pure culture other bacterial pathogens with which it is present in clinical specimens. Many ways of inhibiting swarming have been described. These include:

1   physically restricting the movement of *Proteus* cells by means of agar overlays or poured plates, or by increasing the agar concentration to 3–4% w/v
2   preventing the formation of or interfering with the structure or activity of flagella through the incorporation into media of polyvalent H antisera, ethanol 5.5%, boric acid 0.1%, detergents, bile salts or other surface-active agents (Lominski and Lend-

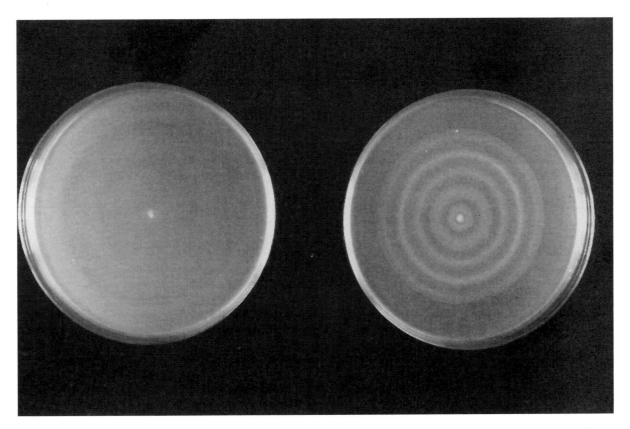

Fig. 43.1   Swarming growth given by *Proteus* strains: left, continuous swarming; right, discontinuous swarming (× 0.75).

rum 1942), or β-phenethyl alcohol (Kopp, Müller and Lemme 1966)

3 retarding the cell growth rate by incorporating into media growth inhibitors such as sulphonamide, neomycin, chloral hydrate, barbiturates, sodium azide or purine bases.

Some anti-swarming methods act by mechanisms which are as yet unexplained. Activated charcoal has been found by Smith and Alwen (1966) to inhibit swarming without affecting motility, but some components of media, notably blood, make the charcoal ineffective. Swarming is inhibited in MacConkey agar by the bile salts and in Wilson and Blair's medium by the bismuth sulphite. It rarely occurs in the absence of electrolytes. Useful alternative anti-swarming media are Lab-Lemco without added salt, and cysteine lactose electrolyte-deficient (CLED) agar (Mackey and Sandys 1966). Regrettably, many of these anti-swarming agents are unsuitable for use when isolating certain pathogenic bacteria. Some agents are toxic and prevent the growth of delicate pathogens. Others make their recognition difficult by altering the colonial morphology of the organism or by lysing red blood cells and so prevent the recognition and detection of haemolytic organisms. One exceptional anti-swarming agent is *p*-nitrophenylglycerol, which at low concentrations inhibits the formation of swarm cells without affecting the formation or motility of flagella (Kopp, Müller and Lemme 1966). It is also without effect on red blood cells, the colonial morphology of other organisms and their antibiotic sensitivity; it is non-toxic for a wide range of delicate bacterial pathogens such as *Neisseria gonorrhoeae* (Senior 1978).

3.2 Colonial appearances

Proteus strains form several sorts of discrete colony on MacConkey agar; Belyavin (1951) described 3 of these, which he designated phases. Phase A colonies are smooth, 3–4 mm in diameter, with a beaten-copper surface; morphologically they consist of regular bacillary forms 5–6 μm × 0.5 μm which on other media give rise to discontinuous swarming. Phase B colonies are smaller, smoother and more conical; they consist of highly pleomorphic cells (coccobacilli, filaments and giant cells) that do not swarm on other media. Phase C colonies are flat, rough and larger than phase A colonies. They consist of long filaments that give rise to continuous swarming on other media. The dominant type-specific O antigen is not found in phase B cells. Phase variations A → B and A → C are reversible. Coetzee and Sacks (1960) described 5 colonial variants, 3 of which, Y, W and Z, correspond to Belyavin's phases A, B and C, respectively. Cultures arising from a single cell of one particular variant eventually gave rise to all the others.

4 METABOLIC ACTIVITIES

The characteristic metabolic activity of Proteeae of the oxidative deamination of certain amino acids results in the formation of α keto acids. These have strong iron-binding properties and function as siderophores in the tribe because the Proteeae, unlike others in the family Enterobacteriaceae, are unable to form hydroxamate and catecholate siderophores (Drechsel et al. 1993). All species within the tribe also have the ability on prolonged incubation to degrade indole. It is important therefore when indole formation is to be used as an identifying character to use a standard medium such as tryptone and to read the reaction after incubation for only one day (Müller 1986).

Early reports on the haemolytic activity of *Proteus* are discrepant, probably because of variation in the culture media, conditions of assay and type of red blood cells used. Sheep red blood cells are more sensitive than human red blood cells, and mouse red blood cells are relatively resistant, to haemolysins from *P. mirabilis* (Peerbooms, Verweij and MacLaren 1983). Two distinct haemolysins, HpmA (Welch 1987) and HlyA (Koronakis et al. 1987) are found in *Proteus*. HpmA is a 166 kDa calcium-independent haemolysin and is produced by virtually all strains of *P. mirabilis*, most strains of *P. vulgaris* and some strains of *P. penneri* (Senior and Hughes 1988, Swihart and Welch 1990). HlyA, a 110 kDa calcium-dependent haemolysin, is less common in *Proteus*. It is found in some isolates of *P. vulgaris* and *P. penneri* (Koronakis et al. 1987, Senior and Hughes 1988, Senior 1993) and is very similar to the HlyA haemolysin of *Escherichia coli* and *Morganella morganii*. Some strains of *P. vulgaris* and *P. penneri* form both haemolysins. Both HpmA and HlyA cause the lysis of a wide variety of cell types in addition to erythrocytes by forming cation-selective pores in cell membranes. In *P. mirabilis*, HpmA usually remains cell-associated. As a result, strains of this species do not appear to be haemolytic on blood agar when swarming is prevented. The calcium-dependent haemolysin HlyA forms more obvious haemolytic zones on blood agar (Senior and Hughes 1988).

5 EXTRACELLULAR PRODUCTS

Most strains of *P. mirabilis*, *P. vulgaris* and *P. penneri* produce a unique EDTA-sensitive metalloproteinase which can cleave at unique sites the heavy chain of IgA1, IgA2, IgG and both free and IgA-bound secretory component (Senior, Albrechtsen and Kerr 1987, 1988, Loomes, Senior and Kerr 1990, 1992). It is thought to be an important virulence factor. Strains of *P. mirabilis* associated with urinary tract infections also form hyaluronidase.

All strains of *Proteus* spp., with rare exceptions, form potent urease enzymes whose genes have been cloned. The nickel-containing cytoplasmic enzyme is chromosomally determined and is inducible in *Proteus*. The enzyme comprises a number of subunits (α, β and γ) and in *P. mirabilis* is of the form $\alpha_2\beta_4\gamma_4$ with a mass of 212–250 kDa. The enzyme is determined by 3 structural genes, *ureA*, *ureB* and *ureC* and accessory genes *ureD*, *ureE*, *ureF* and *ureG*. Transcription is controlled by a repressor protein UreR which is specific for urea.

The urease of *P. mirabilis* hydrolyses urea 6–30 times faster than that of *Morganella* or *Providencia* spp. and this feature undoubtedly contributes to the greater virulence of this organism for the urinary tract.

6 HABITAT

P. myxofaciens has been isolated only from gypsy-moth larvae (*Porthetria dispar*), but the other *Proteus* spp. are widely distributed in nature and constitute an important part of the flora of decomposing matter of animal origin. They are constantly present in rotten meat and sewage and very frequently in the faeces of man and animals. They are commonly found in garden soil and on vegetables. In addition to their wide saprophytic existence, strains of *Proteus* cause septic infections in man and animals.

7 LABORATORY ISOLATION AND IDENTIFICATION

Proteus strains grow readily on a wide variety of media in air over a wide temperature range below 42°C but optimally at 34–37°C. For the isolation and identification of *Proteus*, the specimen should be plated directly for single colonies on either a medium that does not permit swarming, such as MacConkey or CLED agar, or one of the indicator and selective media referred to above. Enrichment culture in tetrathionate broth before subculture to solid media may be helpful. After overnight incubation at 37°C, a single colony of gram-negative pleomorphic bacilli that is oxidase-negative and unable to ferment lactose should be suspended in a small amount of nutrient broth to provide an inoculum for mannose peptone water and for either a nutrient agar medium enriched with L-tryptophan 1% and an anti-swarming agent (e.g bile salts), such as that described by Müller (1985) or Senior and Leslie (1986), or a similar medium enriched with L-phenylalanine 1% instead of tryptophan. After overnight incubation at 37°C, isolates belonging to the Proteeae form colonies surrounded by a red-brown colour on the medium containing tryptophan and form a transient green colour after the addition of aqueous ferric chloride 10% to the phenylalanine medium. Those that also acidify mannose belong to the genera *Morganella* or *Providencia* and can be identified further by biochemical tests according to Table 43.1 and the scheme in Fig. 43.2. Those that do not acidify mannose are strains of *Proteus*. Most of them swarm on nutrient agar or blood agar at 30°C and rapidly degrade urea. They are identified further according to the scheme in Fig. 43.2 by determining their ability to form indole, ornithine decarboxylase and H$_2$S, acidify maltose and xylose, and degrade aesculin. Most isolates from human clinical specimens are *P. mirabilis*. They are more readily identified from swarming growth by being indole negative and forming ornithine decarboxylase and H$_2$S. Media to examine these reactions in combinations have been devised (Senior and Leslie 1986).

7.1 Biochemical reactions

All *Proteus* strains form acid from glucose and most also form small amounts of gas. Unlike strains of *Morganella* and *Providencia*, no strain of *Proteus* forms acid from mannose, mannitol, adonitol or inositol. Lactose fermentation is rare and when present is encoded by a plasmid acquired from outside the genus. All species except *P. myxofaciens* form acid from xylose and all except *P. mirabilis* form acid from maltose. Indole is formed only by *P. vulgaris* and ornithine decarboxylase only by *P. mirabilis*. Sucrose is acidified by most strains of all species except *P. mirabilis* in which only about 15–20% strains are sucrose-positive. *P. myxofaciens* characteristically forms copious amounts of slime in broth at 25°C but does not degrade tyrosine. All species produce an inducible urease; this enzyme is distinct from the urease of *M. morganii* (Senior, Bradford and Simpson 1980, Rosenstein, Hamilton-Miller and Brumfitt 1981). All strains are catalase-positive and oxidase-negative. There are 2 biogroups in *P. vulgaris*: biogroup 2 strains acidify salicin and degrade aesculin but biogroup 3 strains do not. Growth on Simmons's citrate medium is variable but does not occur with *P. penneri* strains. Most strains of *Proteus* are methyl-red positive but only *P. myxofaciens* and a small proportion (16%) of *P. mirabilis* strains give a positive Voges–Proskauer reaction when tested at 37°C.

8 SUSCEPTIBILITY TO PHYSICAL AND CHEMICAL AGENTS

Proteus cells are readily destroyed by moist heat at 55°C for 1 h and by common disinfectants such as phenolics or halogens. However, some strains isolated in hospitals, particularly of *P. mirabilis*, have a significant resistance to chlorhexidine, of which as much as 800 mg l^{-1} may be required to prevent multiplication.

9 SUSCEPTIBILITY TO ANTIMICROBIAL AGENTS

The susceptibility of members of the Proteeae to concentrations of antibiotic attainable in the body is highly variable; some strains have resistance patterns as wide as any encountered in the clinical laboratory but others are sensitive to a number of effective agents. Individual species differ widely in antibiotic susceptibility, so the correct speciation of isolates is of great importance.

No information is available about the antibiotic susceptibility of *P. myxofaciens*. In the other species of *Proteus*, almost all strains are resistant to polymyxin B and colistin but sensitive to nalidixic acid and other quinolones (Hawkey and Hawkey 1984). The pattern of resistance of *Proteus* to penicillins and cephalosporins is complicated (see Garrod, Lambert and O'Grady 1981) and is determined partly by mechanisms of intrinsic resistance and partly by the production of β-lactamases. In general, *P. mirabilis* strains that do not

Table 43.1 Usual biochemical reactions of species of *Proteus, Morganella* and *Providencia*

Property	Proteus *mirabilis*	*vulgaris*	*penneri*	*myxofaciens*	Morganella *morganii*	Providencia *rettgeri*	*alcalifaciens*	*rustigianii*	*stuartii* biogroup 4	5	6	*heimbachae*
Gas from glucose	+	+	V	+	+	(−)	(+)	V	−	−	−	−
Acid from												
mannose	−	−	−	−	+	+	+	+	+	+	+	−
maltose	−	+	+	+	−	−	−	−	−	−	−	+
xylose	+	+	+	−	−	+	−	−	−	−	−	V
mannitol	−	−	−	−	−	+	+	−	−	−	−	−
adonitol	−	−	−	−	−	+	+	−	−	+	+	−
inositol	−	−	−	+	−	−	−	−	+	+	+	+
trehalose	+	V	V	+	V	V	−	−	−	+	+	V
rhamnose	−	−	−	−	−	+	−	−	−	−	−	−
Urease	+	+	+	+	+	+	+	−	+	+	+	+
Indole	−	+	−	−	+	+	+	+	+	+	+	−
Ornithine decarboxylase	+	−	(−)	−	(+)	−	−	−	−	−	−	−
H₂S (TSI medium)	+	+	V	+*	−	−	−	−	−	−	−	−
Gelatin liquefaction	+	+	V	+	−	−	−	−	−	−	−	−
Lipase production	+	+	+	+	+	−	−	−	−	−	−	−
Methyl red	+	+	+	+	+	+	+	V	+	+	+	+
Voges–Proskauer	V	−	−	+	−	−	−	−	−	−	−	−

The following properties are common to all: motile; acid in glucose; no acid in dulcitol, lactose, sorbitol, raffinose and arabinose; nitrate reduced to nitrite; phenylalanine deaminated; lysine and arginine decarboxylase −; malonate −; mucate−.
+, Positive reaction within 48 h; −, negative reaction; ( ), reaction of most strains; V, some strains positive, others negative; *reaction after 3–4 days.

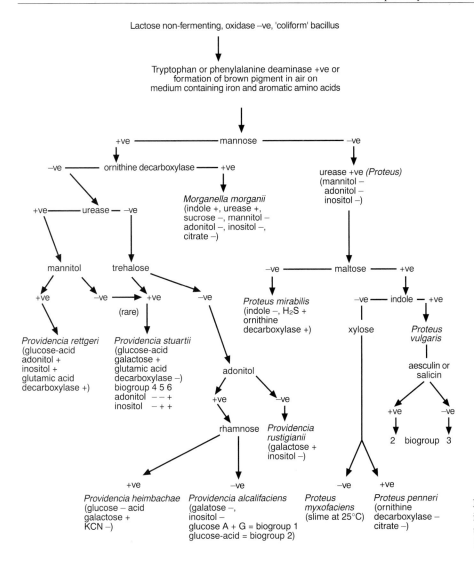

Lactose non-fermenting, oxidase −ve, 'coliform' bacillus

Tryptophan or phenylalanine deaminase +ve or
formation of brown pigment in air on
medium containing iron and aromatic amino acids

+ve ——— mannose ——— −ve

ornithine decarboxylase ——— +ve

urease +ve *(Proteus)*
(mannitol −
adonitol −
inositol −)

−ve ——— urease — −ve

Morganella morganii
(indole +, urease +,
sucrose −, mannitol −
adonitol −, inositol −,
citrate −)

+ve ——— urease — −ve

mannitol   trehalose

−ve ——— maltose ——— +ve

+ve   −ve ——— +ve ——— −ve

Proteus mirabilis
(indole −, H₂S +
ornithine
decarboxylase +)

(rare)

−ve   indole — +ve

xylose   *Proteus vulgaris*

Providencia rettgeri
(glucose-acid
adonitol +
inositol +
glutamic acid
decarboxylase +)

Providencia stuartii
(glucose-acid
galactose +
glutamic acid
decarboxylase −)
biogroup 4 5 6
adonitol − − +
inositol − + +

adonitol

aesculin or
salicin

+ve   −ve

+ve   −ve

2   biogroup   3

rhamnose   *Providencia rustigianii*
(galactose +
inositol −)

+ve   −ve   −ve   +ve

Providencia heimbachae
(glucose − acid
galactose +
KCN −)

Providencia alcalifaciens
(galatose −,
inositol −
glucose A + G = biogroup 1
glucose-acid = biogroup 2)

Proteus myxofaciens
(slime at 25°C)

Proteus penneri
(ornithine
decarboxylase −
citrate −)

Fig. 43.2 Scheme for
identification of species in
the tribe Proteeae:
( ), confirmatory reactions.

form this enzyme are unique among the Proteeae in being sensitive to amounts of benzylpenicillin that are attainable in urine; they are also fully sensitive to ampicillin, carbenicillin and the cephalosporins. However, strains that form β-lactamase are resistant to benzylpenicillin, ampicillin and carbenicillin but often remain sensitive to the cephalosporins. By contrast, *P. vulgaris* and *P. penneri* strains are resistant to benzylpenicillin, ampicillin and many cephalosporins such as cephalothin, cephaloridine, cefazolin and cefsulodin but are often sensitive to other cephalosporins such as cefuroxime, cefotaxime, cefoxitin and latamoxef (Penner et al. 1982, Fuksa, Krajden and Lee 1984). *P. vulgaris* strains are characteristically more resistant to cefamandole than other species in the Proteeae. They are also exceptional among the Enterobacteriaceae in having an inducible β-lactamase (cefuroximase) that has high activity against β-lactamase-stable cephalosporins such as cefuroxime and cefotaxime. Most strains of *P. mirabilis* and *P. vulgaris* are very susceptible to the semisynthetic penicillins such as mezlocillin, azlocillin, piperacillin, carbenicillin and ticarcillin whereas *P. penneri* strains may be somewhat more resistant to them (Hawkey, Pedler

and Turner 1983). The susceptibility of strains of *Proteus* to nitrofurantoin and tetracyclines is variable but that to chloramphenicol is mainly species-dependent: most strains of *P. mirabilis* and *P. vulgaris* biogroup 2 are sensitive but *P. penneri* strains are resistant (Hickman et al. 1982, Fuksa, Krajden and Lee 1984). Most strains of *Proteus* are susceptible to the aminoglycosides gentamicin, tobramycin, netilmicin and amikacin but from time to time strains may acquire plasmids encoding for resistance to them, to trimethoprim and to other antibiotics to which they are normally sensitive. These resistance characters may be transferred to other *Proteus* strains, to enterobacteria and to *Pseudomonas aeruginosa*.

10 CELL ENVELOPE COMPOSITION AND ANTIGENIC STRUCTURE

The peptidoglycan of *Proteus* species, and indeed all members of the Proteeae, is unusual among the enterobacteria in that the C6 hydroxyl group of many (29–57%) of the *N*-acetylmuramyl residues is O-acetylated. This modification renders the cell wall resistant to lysozyme and possibly to many muramidases and autolysins (Clarke 1993). External to the peptidoglycan is lipopolysaccharide (LPS). In *P. mirabilis* it exists in 2 forms: approximately two-thirds of it is in the form LPS I which has a relatively short O polysaccharide chain, whereas the remainder is in the form LPS II which has very long O polysaccharide chains (Gmeiner 1975). Some of these may be so long that they have been considered as capsules (Beynon et al. 1992). Analysis of the oligosaccharides in the core of the LPS shows that it can be of 6 different types.

The LPS of some strains of *Proteus* has epitopes shared with some *Rickettsia* spp. (Amano, Fujita and Suto 1993). During particular (but not all) rickettsial infections, antibody, usually of the IgM class, is formed, causing the agglutination of one or more *Proteus* strains designated X19, X2 and XK. The LPS of each of these strains has been purified and characterized (Mizushiri et al. 1990). These are, respectively, strains of *P. vulgaris* serotype O1 and serotype O2 and *P. mirabilis* serotype O3. Thus patients with epidemic louseborne typhus infected with *Rickettsia prowazekii*, or Rocky Mountain spotted fever (*Rickettsia rickettsii*) develop serum antibodies that agglutinate *Proteus* OX19 cells but not OXK cells, whereas those with scrub typhus (*Rickettsia tsutsugamushi*) develop serum antibodies that agglutinate only OXK cells. The detection of antibodies to these bacteria has been used in the past to indicate rickettsial infection (**the Weil–Felix reaction**). The test is being replaced by more specific serological and PCR methods. *P. mirabilis* strains have an outer-membrane protein of 39–40 kDa which functions as a porin. Its presence is important for the penetration of hydrophilic cephalosporins and it acts as a mitogen for B lymphocytes.

There is much antigenic heterogeneity among strains of *P. mirabilis* and *P. vulgaris* and many different O and H antigens have been described. The simplified scheme devised by Kauffmann and Perch (Kauffmann 1966) for serotyping *P. mirabilis* and *P. vulgaris* distinguished 49 O antigens and 19 H antigens. Generally, most O antigens are species specific. However, a small number of them are not species specific and may be found in both *P. mirabilis* and *P. vulgaris* (Penner and Hennessy 1980).

The O antigens of *Proteus* are resistant to heating at 100°C, to ethanol and to dilute HCl whereas the H antigens are destroyed by these treatments. Agglutination tests for the determination of O antigens should be made with cultures that have been boiled for 1 h because some living and some formalized cultures are O-inagglutinable. O agglutination tests are best read after incubation for 20 h and H agglutination tests after 4 h in a water bath at 50°C. Cross-reactions between H antigens are numerous and complex. The most frequently encountered strain in clinical infections is *P. mirabilis* serotype O3. Other frequently encountered serotypes are O6, O10, O26 and O30. The commonest flagellar antigens are H1, H2 and H3. Most workers have failed to detect K antigens in *Proteus* but Namioka and Sakazaki (1959) reported

the presence of a new type of K antigen (C antigen) in 2 non-motile strains of *Proteus*. The antigenic constitutions of *P. penneri* and *P. myxofaciens* have yet to be defined.

11 TYPING METHODS

11.1 Phage typing

Phages have been isolated from lysogenic strains and from sewage and several groups of workers have developed phage typing schemes. Lysis is generally restricted to members of the species of origin of the phage, but occasionally it is seen in members of other species in the tribe and, rarely, in other enterobacteria. The schemes of Pavlatou, Hassikou-Kaklamani and Zantioti (1965) and Schmidt and Jeffries (1974) are useful for typing strains of *Proteus* and other members of the Proteeae. Those of Vieu and Capponi (1965) and France and Markham (1968) are applicable only to typing strains of *Proteus* and allocate over 80% of strains to a type. The systems devised by Izdebska-Szymona, Monczak and Lemczak (1971) and Hickman and Farmer (1976) permit the typing only of *P. mirabilis* strains. The last of these is highly discriminatory and reproducible, permitting 94% of 200 strains to be differentiated into 113 types.

11.2 Bacteriocin typing

Cradock-Watson (1965) distinguished strains of *Proteus* by determining the range of activity of their bacteriocins on a set of indicator strains. Most strains of *P. mirabilis* have the genetic potential to produce one of 13 different bacteriocins (proticins) and to be sensitive to a different one or more of them. The scheme devised by Senior (1977a) in which *Proteus* strains were examined for both proticin production and proticin sensitivity (P/S typing) has given the greatest discrimination: 250 strains were differentiated into 90 P/S types. The proticins resemble contractile phage tails (Senior 1983a). The production of proticin 3 is associated with strains that are virulent for the urinary tract (Senior 1979). The P/S type of an isolate is independent of its O serotype (Senior and Larsson 1983).

11.3 Other typing methods

The **Dienes phenomenon** forms the basis of another typing method (Dienes 1946). When different strains of *Proteus* spp. are allowed to swarm towards each other, a line of complete or partial growth inhibition forms where the spreading growths of incompatible strains meet. Such a line does not form between identical strains (Fig. 43.3). The determinant of Dienes compatibility was thought to be the H antigen until others found serologically identical strains to be incompatible and sometimes strains with the same O antigens and different H antigens were compatible. Senior (1977b) showed that 204 swarming strains of *Proteus* could be differentiated into 98 compatibility groups and that the determinants of compatibility were the proticin production and sensitivity characters of the swarming strains. Strains of the same P/S type, irrespective of their species or O and H antigenic structure, were compatible whereas strains of different P/S types were incompatible (Senior and Larsson 1983). Kashbur, George and Ayliffe (1974) devised a scheme for resistotyping *P. mirabilis* strains. They found it discriminated between strains that appeared to be identical by other typing methods.

If only a few strains are to be compared, the rapid and simple Dienes typing method is usually adequate. When larger numbers of strains are to be examined, P/S typing or serotyping should be used. Since these latter methods are independent of each other, the best discrimination is given by a combination of P/S typing and O serotyping.

Some workers have compared the electrophoretic profiles of outer-membrane or total cell proteins of strains and used this as a typing method (Kappos et al. 1992, Costas et al. 1993). The method is relatively simple and reproducible but not very discriminatory. It can be useful in typing strains of *P. vulgaris* of biogroups 2 and 3; the latter appears to be of more than one genomic group. The discriminating power of the method is greatly increased when combined with multilocus enzyme electrophoresis (Kappos et al. 1992) but this method is labour intensive and time consuming.

Latterly, polymerase chain reaction (PCR) methods have been developed for the rapid typing of *P. mirabilis* in studies of cross-infection. That based on the use of a single arbitrary primer (Bingen et al. 1993) has been found to be as reproducible and as discrimi-

nating as ribotyping but much simpler and quicker to perform.

12 PATHOGENICITY AND VIRULENCE FACTORS

Nothing is known about the pathogenicity of *P. myxofaciens*, but members of all the other species of *Proteus* are pathogenic for man. *P. mirabilis* is the most frequently encountered species of the tribe in human infections and is responsible for 70–90% of all proteus infections in man. *P. vulgaris* and *P. penneri* cause similar types of infection to *P. mirabilis* because their habitat and virulence factors are similar. However, they are isolated less frequently and they may be less virulent.

The commonest site of proteus infection is the urinary tract and *P. mirabilis*, the species most frequently implicated, is the organism after *E. coli* most frequently associated with urinary tract infections. Proteus urinary tract infections are common in young boys and elderly patients (Senior 1979). In the latter, they are often associated in domiciliary patients with diabetes or structural abnormalities of the urinary tract and in hospital patients with various forms of urological instrumentation or manipulation. Proteus urinary tract infections tend to be more serious than those caused by *E. coli* and other coliforms for these are usually confined to the bladder whereas *Proteus* spp. have a predilection for the upper urinary tract (Fairley et al. 1971, Svanborg Eden, Larsson and Lomberg 1980).

The virulence of *P. mirabilis* for the urinary tract arises through the interplay of several virulence factors of which the most important is urease. This nickel-containing cytoplasmic enzyme is inducible solely by urea. The concentration of urea in urine is sufficiently high for the ureases of strains of all *Proteus* spp. to be able to work at the maximum rate, that of *P. mirabilis* in particular giving the greatest rate of urea hydrolysis. The enzyme hydrolyses the urea in urine to ammonia and carbon dioxide. This reaction may be important to the bacteria by providing them with a source of usable nitrogen for growth in urine. However, the formation of ammonia also leads to alkalinization of the urine and at pH values above 8, calcium and magnesium ions are precipitated in the form of struvite $(MgNH_4PO_4.6H_2O)$ and carbonate-apatite $(Ca_{10}(PO_4)CO_3)$ crystals. These are bound by the polysaccharide slime or glycocalyx formed by the cell and form bladder and kidney stones. Experiments in mice infected transurethrally with uropathogenic or isogenic urease-negative strains of *P. mirabilis* have confirmed that urease is a critical virulence determinant for colonization of the urinary tract, stone formation and the development of acute pyelonephritis (Johnson et al. 1993). Urease activity together with haemolysin (see below) also cause the death of human renal proximal tubular epithelial cells (Mobley et al. 1991). Furthermore, urease-induced formation of ammonia protects the bacterial cell from the effects of complement by inactivating it.

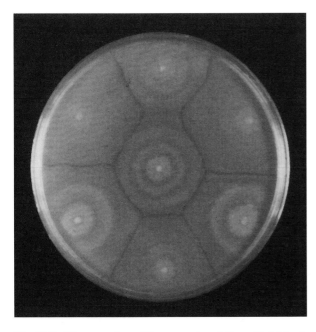

Fig. 43.3 Dienes typing of *Proteus* strains. A line of inhibited growth is formed only where the swarming growths of different strains meet. The strain at the top of the plate is the same as the one in the centre. Each one of the remaining strains is different from its immediate neighbour (× 0.85).

Fimbriae of *Proteus* spp. also play a significant but more subtle role in virulence for the urinary tract as shown by in vivo experiments with genetically designed strains. MR/P fimbriae are expressed in vivo, and though not essential for infection, appear to play a significant role in the colonization of both the bladder and the kidney and their presence correlates with the development of acute pyelonephritis (Bahrani et al. 1994). PMF appear to be important for colonization of the bladder but mutants lacking them can still invade the kidney (Massad et al. 1994). Both UCA and MR/K fimbriae bind to uroepithelial cells and the latter also bind to Bowman's capsule of the glomeruli and tubular basement membranes of the kidney (Sareneva, Holthöfer and Korhonen 1990).

Haemolysins are also known to be important virulence factors of *Proteus* spp. Haemolytic strains are much more lethal for mice than non-haemolytic ones (Peerbooms, Verweij and MacLaren 1983, 1985). Both HpmA and HlyA are cytotoxic for a wide variety of cell types and together with urease they play an important role in cell invasion and internalization (which appears to take place by a mechanism not dependent on actin polymerization) and ultimately cell death (Peerbooms, Verweij and MacLaren 1984, Allison et al. 1992, Chippendale et al. 1994). Despite having similar urease and haemolysin genes, haemolysin and urease are expressed at higher levels in *P. mirabilis* than in *P. vulgaris*. This may be the explanation for the greater virulence of *P. mirabilis*.

Motility and swarming are additional properties of *Proteus* spp. which are important, though possibly not absolutely essential, in virulence. Pazin and Braude (1974) showed that antibodies to flagella prevented *P. mirabilis* infecting the kidney. Motility is also critical for the successful infection of burns by *P. mirabilis* (Harmon et al. 1989). The development of flagella is important in swarm cell formation in which other virulence determinants, urease, haemolysin and protease, are co-ordinately expressed (Allison, Lai and Hughes 1992). *P. mirabilis* mutants lacking flagella are non-invasive to uroepithelial cells and motile but non-swarming cells are 25 times less invasive than wild-type motile, swarming cells (Allison et al. 1992).

Proteus proteinase is thought to be another important virulence factor. Active enzyme and immunoglobulin fragments can be detected in the urine of patients with a proteus urinary tract infection (Senior, Loomes and Kerr 1991), indicating it is synthesized and active in vivo. The cleaved antibody fragments have defective immune effector functions and thereby the effectiveness of the immune response to the organism is limited (Loomes, Kerr and Senior 1993). The proteinase may also play a role in generating products like glutamine to induce invasive swarm cell formation. In vivo experiments in mice have shown that proteinase-negative mutants can infect the bladder but have severely reduced ability to infect the kidney and form abscesses.

Infection of the urinary tract with *Proteus* spp. may also give rise to hyperammonaemic encephalopathy and coma. Urinary tract infection often also leads to bacteraemia. Proteus bacteraemias can be difficult to treat and have a mortality rate of 15–88% according to the severity of the underlying disease (Lewis and Feckety 1969).

Proteus spp. have also been isolated in pure culture and with other organisms from various superficial septic lesions. Their presence in mixed culture favours the multiplication of pathogenic anaerobes. Occasionally, they are isolated in pure culture from abscesses, from the meninges and from blood. Both *P. mirabilis* and *P. vulgaris* may cause osteomyelitis. In neonates, infection of the umbilical stump often leads to a highly fatal proteus bacteraemia and meningitis. Patients with active rheumatoid arthritis often have raised antibody levels specific for *Proteus* (Ebringer et al. 1985). This may be because of epitopes shared between antigens of certain HLA types associated with the disease and particular *Proteus* antigens (Ebringer et al. 1992, Senior et al. 1995) but the relationship of *Proteus* to rheumatoid arthritis remains unclear.

The pathogenicity of *Proteus* spp. for laboratory animals is variable. Virulent strains on introduction into tissue are able to proliferate and invade the bloodstream. Strains of lower virulence cause chronic inflammation, either of the suppurative or of the infective granuloma type.

The inoculation intraperitoneally of 0.5–1.0 ml of a 24 h broth culture of a virulent strain generally proves fatal to rats and mice in 18–48 h and to guinea pigs and rabbits in 1–7 days. The LD50 for mice of 21 strains ranges from 2 million to 600 million living organisms (Miles 1951). Large doses given intravenously to mice result in a fatal septicaemic illness; smaller doses of some strains produce necrotic lesions in the kidneys of survivors. Studies on the virulence of *P. mirabilis* and *P. vulgaris* for mice by determinations of the LD50 and KID50 (50% kidney infecting dose) have shown that although there can be wide variation in virulence between different strains of *P. mirabilis* (Peerbooms, Verweij and MacLaren 1982), on the basis of LD50:KID50 ratios, *P. mirabilis* strains are generally more virulent than *P. vulgaris* strains.

MORGANELLA

13 DEFINITION

Morganella spp. do not show true swarming on solid nutrient media. They acidify glucose, usually with gas formation, and mannose but not lactose, sucrose, salicin, mannitol, xylose, adonitol, or inositol. They oxidatively deaminate amino acids and produce urease but do not utilize citrate. Most strains form ornithine decarboxylase and indole but do not produce H_2S nor liquefy gelatin nor form lipase. G + C content of the DNA is 50 mol%.

Type species is *M. morganii*.

The organism is named after Morgan (1906) who isolated it from the faeces of infants with diarrhoea. Rauss (1936) suggested it was closely related to *Proteus* because, although it failed to liquefy gelatin, it formed indole, degraded urea and exhibited spreading growth on media with reduced agar concentrations at 20–28°C. The observation by Henriksen and Closs (1938) that both *Proteus* and Morgan's bacillus degraded phenylalanine to phenylpyruvic acid gave additional support to the suggestion and for many years the organism was known as *Proteus morganii*. The proposal of Kauffmann (1956) that it should be placed in a separate genus, *Morganella*, did not at first receive general acceptance, but the evidence in its favour is now overwhelming: the G + C content of the DNA of *Morganella* is considerably higher than that of *Proteus*; DNA–DNA hybridization studies show less than 20% genetic homology between the 2 genera and other members of the Proteeae (Brenner et al. 1978); there are differences in the properties of enzymes common to *Morganella* and other members of the tribe. The genus has only one species, *M. morganii*, but it has been proposed that, on the basis of DNA relatedness, it be divided into 2 subspecies, *morganii* and *sibonii* (Jensen et al. 1992).

14 GENERAL PROPERTIES

Most isolates of *M. morganii* are motile because of peritrichous flagella. These may differ in wavelength and are not formed in some strains, particularly if cultured above 30°C. Strains also form thin and thick peritrichous fimbriae (Old and Adegbola 1982). On prolonged incubation on soft (1%) agar at 22°C, growth may spread to form a film (Rauss 1936) but true swarming, which is associated with migration and consolidation on 1.5% agar and characteristic changes in cellular morphology, is not seen.

Morganella strains, unlike *Proteus* strains, require both niacin and pantothenic acid for growth. They grow readily on most culture media and nutrient broth cultures have an unpleasant smell. Approximately 30% of strains are haemolytic on blood agar through the production of a calcium-dependent haemolysin (Senior and Hughes 1988) that is serologically and functionally identical to *E. coli* haemolysin HlyA and is associated with the high virulence of strains for mice (Emódy, Vörös and Pál 1982). *M. morganii* strains form extremely high levels of phosphate irrepressible acid phosphatase, a feature rare among enterobacteria but shared with *Providencia stuartii*. Modified MacConkey media have been devised that readily and specifically reveal the presence of these organisms (Thaller et al. 1992). The biochemical characters of *M. morganii* are fairly uniform (see Table 43.1). Mannose fermentation readily distinguishes it from isolates of *Proteus*. Urease production and the ability to decarboxylate ornithine, together with an inability to utilize citrate, readily distinguish it from strains of *Providencia* spp.

M. morganii strains do not ferment many sugars, glucose and mannose being the ones characteristically acidified. Trehalose and glycerol are fermented by a few strains. Trehalose fermenters are members of the subspecies *sibonii* (named after the Danish bacteriologist Knud Siboni who first recognized them) whereas trehalose non-fermenters are members of the subspecies *morganii*. Some strains are unusual in that they are unable to decarboxylate ornithine but decarboxylate lysine. Others decarboxylate both amino acids and some decarboxylate neither. On the basis of trehalose fermentation and decarboxylation of ornithine and lysine, 7 biogroups (A–G) have been defined (Jensen et al. 1992). Other useful differentiating features include motility, glycerol fermentation and tetracycline sensitivity (Siboni 1976, Senior and Vörös 1990, Jensen et al. 1992). *Morganella* strains, unlike those of *Proteus*, produce urease constitutively. The enzyme is structurally and antigenically different from that of *Proteus* and *Providencia* and at 590 kDa is one of the largest enzymes known (Guo and Liu 1965, Smit and Coetzee 1967, Senior, Bradford and Simpson 1980, Rosenstein, Hamilton-Miller and Brumfitt 1981, Hu et al. 1990).

M. morganii strains can be typed by various methods. They can be separated into a small number of types by biotyping (Rauss and Vörös 1959, Jensen et al. 1992). Phages that lyse *M. morganii* generally do not attack strains of *Proteus* and *Providencia*. They have been used for phage typing (Schmidt and Jeffries 1974) which defines more types. Greater discrimination is given by protein profile typing (Senior and Vörös 1990). Serological typing is most useful as *M. morganii* is antigenically heterogeneous, 55 O, 4 K and 38 H antigens having been identified (Rauss et al. 1975, Vörös and Senior 1990). Typing by bacteriocin production and sensitivity (Senior 1987) is also highly discriminating. However, because the last 3 typing methods are independent of each other, the greatest discrimination is given by a combination of serotyping, protein profile and bacteriocin typing methods (Senior and Vörös 1989).

M. morganii is frequently found in human faeces and it has also been isolated from the faeces of other animals and reptiles. It is often found in diarrhoetic stools in the absence of other known bacterial enteropathogens but firm evidence for its aetiological role in enteritis has not yet been presented. Only rarely is *M. morganii* associated with urinary tract infection. This may be because of its inability to grow rapidly in urine and make it very alkaline (Senior 1983b), although the urease has high affinity for urea. Occasionally it is isolated from blood, sputum and infected wounds and can be a cause of septic arthritis. Outbreaks of hospital-acquired infections – some of them serious and even fatal – have been reported (Tucci and Isenberg 1981, Williams et al. 1983). Because it has potent histidine decarboxylase activity, *M. morganii* has the potential to cause histamine fish poisoning through the ingestion of contaminated scombroid fish such as tuna, sardines, pilchards and anchovies.

M. morganii strains are usually sensitive to carbenicillin, nalidixic acid, chloramphenicol, the aminoglycosides, cefotaxime and latamoxef, but resistant to ampicillin and cephaloridine, through formation of inducible chromosomal β-lactamases, and colistin. The enzymes are without effect on imipenem and cefoxitin. Strains show variation in their susceptibility to tetracyclines and sulphonamide.

PROVIDENCIA

15 DEFINITION

Providencia spp. do not swarm on solid nutrient media. All strains form acid from glucose and mannose, but gas formation from glucose is variable. They do not form acid from maltose or lactose; they oxidatively deaminate amino acids. Most strains of species other than *Providencia rustigianii* form acid from one or more of the sugar alcohols adonitol, arabitol, erythritol, inositol or mannitol. They do not produce ornithine decarboxylase or H_2S or form lipase or liquefy gelatin. Only some strains form urease. G + C content of the DNA is 39–42 mol%.

According to DNA hybridization studies and extensive phenotypic analyses, the genus has 5 species: *Providencia alcalifaciens*, *Providencia stuartii*, *Providencia rettgeri*, *Providencia rustigianii* and *Providencia heimbachae*.

Stuart and his colleagues (1943) described organisms they considered to be intermediate in character between *Proteus* and *Shigella*. Kauffman (1951) placed them in a new genus, *Providencia*. Ewing, Tanner and Dennard (1954) found that *Providencia* strains could be separated into 2 biochemical groups: one formed gas from glucose and fermented adonitol but not inositol, the other formed no gas from glucose and fermented inositol but not adonitol. The organisms of these groups were given the specific names *P. alcalifaciens* and *P. stuartii*, respectively (Ewing 1962).

Providencia rettgeri is the name now given to the organism isolated by Rettger (1909) from a cholera-like epidemic in chickens and found by others to be anaerogenic and capable of fermenting mannitol. Rustigian and Stuart (1943) later assigned it to the genus *Proteus* as *Proteus rettgeri* when they found it hydrolysed urea. However, Kauffmann (1953) believed the organism should be separated from the genus *Proteus* and proposed the name *Rettgerella*. The results of other workers, which indicated *Proteus rettgeri* had biochemical properties more similar to *Providencia* than to *Proteus* or *Morganella*, supported the view that the organism was classified in the wrong genus. Smit and Coetzee (1967) also showed that *Proteus rettgeri* and *Providencia* strains had similar phenylalanine deaminases. Penner and his colleagues (Penner, Hinton and Hennessy 1975, Penner et al. 1976) described a number of biotypes of *Proteus rettgeri*, one of which, apart from forming urease, resembled *P. stuartii* and had *Providencia* O antigens. Subsequent DNA hybridization studies by Brenner and his colleagues (1978) showed that the latter were in fact urease-forming strains of *P. stuartii* and that all *Proteus rettgeri* strains were more related to *Providencia* than to *Proteus*. They

proposed that the organism be known as *Providencia rettgeri*.

The name *P. rustigianii* was proposed by Hickman-Brenner et al. (1983) for strains previously called *P. alcalifaciens* biogroup 3 (Ewing, Davis and Sykes 1972). Earlier DNA hybridization studies (Brenner et al. 1978) had shown this biogroup was not closely related to any of the other biogroups of *Providencia* or to the species of other genera in the tribe. The organism isolated by Müller (1983) from penguin faeces and called *P. friedericiana* is the same as *P. rustigianii* (Hickman-Brenner et al. 1986). *P. heimbachae* is the name given to organisms originally thought to be a biogroup of *P. friedericiana* but which have since been shown by DNA pairing to form a distinct species (Müller et al. 1986).

16 GENERAL PROPERTIES

In general, strains of *Providencia* are motile at 20–25°C by means of peritrichate flagella but may be less active at 37°C. Fimbriae of 5 different morphological types have been found in members of the genus (Old and Adegbola 1982). *Providencia* strains do not swarm. They can often be recognized by their 'fruity' smell and on deoxycholate citrate agar as yellow or orange-centred colonies because the ferric hydroxide in the medium is precipitated at the alkaline pH which forms during growth. *Providencia* strains, unlike those of *Proteus* and *Morganella*, require neither niacin nor pantothenic acid for growth. The important biochemical reactions characteristic of the different species and biogroups of the genus are presented in Table 43.1.

Providencia strains differ from others of the Proteeae through their ability to form acid from mannose and utilize citrate and their inability to decarboxylate ornithine or lysine. Excepting strains of *P. rustigianii*, those of other *Providencia* spp. form acid from one or more of the polyhydric alcohols adonitol, arabitol, erythritol, inositol or mannitol.

P. rettgeri strains are readily distinguished in the genus by their ability to ferment mannitol and degrade urea. Biogroups of *P. rettgeri* can be distinguished by their reactions in rhamnose, salicin and erythritol (Penner, Hinton and Hennessy 1975).

P. stuartii is an organism of great clinical importance because of its tendency to be resistant to many antibiotics and to cause nosocomial infections. However, it is often misidentified, particularly with commercial kits, because strains frequently carry plasmids that may bear genes for the fermentation of sucrose or lactose or the hydrolysis of urea; thus the organism may show a variable phenotype. It forms, along with *M. morganii*, large amounts of phosphatase and media have been devised to simplify its recognition (Thaller et al. 1992). Strains are readily distinguished in the genus by their ability to form acid from trehalose. Unusual isolates, with some properties shared with *P. rettgeri*, can also be distinguished in that *P. stuartii* strains do not decarboxylate L-glutamic acid (Fischer et al. 1989). Some isolates (up to 30%) degrade urea through plasmid-borne genes probably derived from *P. mirabilis.*

P. rustigianii is distinguished from other species in the genus by its inability to form acid from any of the polyhydric alcohols inositol, mannitol, adonitol, arabitol or erythritol. It forms acid from galactose but not trehalose.

Strains that have the properties of the genus but do not degrade urea or form acid from trehalose but do form acid from adonitol are either *P. alcalifaciens* or *P. heimbachae. P. alcalifaciens* strains form indole but do not form acid from either rhamnose or galactose. Ribotyping information suggests there may be more than one species among strains presently bearing this name. *P. heimbachae* strains form acid from both rhamnose and galactose. They differ from other members of the Proteeae in not growing in the presence of KCN and are unusual among *Providencia* in being citrate-negative and indole-negative in certain media (but indole-positive in others). Indole reactions need to be carefully controlled with regard to medium and time of incubation, especially when identifying *Providencia* spp., for they may degrade the indole that they form (Müller 1986).

The genus *Providencia* is antigenically heterogeneous. Strains have thermostable O antigens, thermolabile H antigens and some also have capsular (K) antigens. In general, each species has its own distinctive O antigens, 46 O-antigenic groups having been defined in *P. alcalifaciens* (Penner et al. 1979a), 17 in *P. stuartii* (Penner et al. 1979b) and 93 in *P. rettgeri* (Penner and Hennessy 1979). In addition to serotyping, strains of *Providencia* can be differentiated by phage typing (Chouteau, Vieu and Brault 1974), bacteriocin typing (Stickler and Thomas 1976, McHale, Keane and Dougan 1981) and protein profile typing on SDS polyacrylamide gels (Costas, Holmes and Sloss 1987, Holmes, Costas and Sloss 1988, Costas, Holmes and Wood 1989, 1990). *P. stuartii* has also been typed on the basis of restriction fragment length polymorphisms of rRNA cistrons (Owen et al. 1988).

P. alcalifaciens is occasionally found in normal human faeces but more often in the stools of patients with diarrhoea and gastroenteritis. For many years it has been thought to cause diarrhoea. This belief has been reinforced by the demonstration in rabbits that strains can invade intestinal mucosal cells and cause diarrhoea. They can also invade HEp-2 cells and multiply a little within them before causing condensation of actin filaments in a manner similar to that caused by *Shigella flexneri* but different from that caused by enteropathogenic *E. coli* (Albert et al. 1992, 1995).

P. stuartii strains, though only occasionally isolated

from infected wounds and burns, are amongst the commonest isolates from urine of long-term catheterized elderly patients, particularly women (Rahav et al. 1994), in old people's homes and geriatric wards in hospitals. In these situations, strains can persist in patients for several months and serve as the reservoir of infection for others. Strains are particularly difficult to eradicate because of their formation of MR/K fimbriae which bind to uroepithelial cells and the catheter, and also because they are frequently resistant to many antibiotics. Such strains may give rise to a fatal bacteraemia. In animal models, isolates vary in their uropathogenicity, which is associated with motility and the ability to form urease and fimbriae.

P. rettgeri is part of the normal faecal flora of a number of reptiles and amphibians and may be found in contaminated water. It is not commonly found in human faeces but has been associated with nosocomial infections of the urinary tract, wounds, burns and of blood.

Most isolates of *P. rustigianii* have come from human faeces and those of penguins and pigs, but the organism is rare among clinical isolates of *Providencia. P. heimbachae* strains have been isolated from penguin faeces and an aborted bovine fetus but have yet to be isolated from human sources.

Providencia strains, like other Proteeae, are resistant to polymyxin B and colistin. In general, *P. alcalifaciens* strains are very sensitive to a wide range of antibiotics and antibiotic resistance is not a common problem. The opposite is true for *P. stuartii. P. rettgeri* strains have a position in between these extremes. *P. stuartii* is the most antibiotic-resistant species of the Proteeae and one of the most resistant organisms known (Hawkey 1984); most strains are resistant to tetracyclines, chloramphenicol, sulphonamides, nitrofurantoin and many penicillins, cephalosporins and aminoglycosides. *P. stuartii* is much more resistant than *P. rettgeri* and *P. alcalifaciens* to the substituted penicillins mezlocillin, azlocillin, piperacillin, carbenicillin and ticarcillin (Penner et al. 1982, Hawkey, Pedler and Turner 1983). Among the antibiotics often found useful for treating *P. stuartii* infections are the β-lactams latamoxef and cefotaxime and the monobactam aztreonam. The aminoglycoside amikacin is often useful for treating gentamicin-resistant strains. Among the quinolone antibiotics, ciprofloxacin is one of those most active against *P. stuartii* (Hawkey and Hawkey 1984). Clinical isolates of *P. stuartii* are often resistant to disinfectants such as chlorhexidine and cationic detergents such as cetrimide and benzalkonium chloride but are sensitive to phenols and glutaraldehyde.

REFERENCES

Adegbola RA, Old DC, Senior BW, 1983, The adhesins and fimbriae of *Proteus mirabilis* strains associated with high and low affinity for the urinary tract, *J Med Microbiol*, **16:** 427–31.

Albert MJ, Alam K et al., 1992, Pathogenesis of *Providencia alcalifaciens*-induced diarrhoea, *Infect Immun*, **60:** 5017–24.

Albert MJ, Ansaruzzaman M et al., 1995, Characteristics of invasion of HEp-2 cells by *Providencia alcalifaciens*, *J Med Microbiol*, **42:** 186–90.

Allison C, Lai HC, Hughes C, 1992, Co-ordinate expression of virulence genes during swarm-cell differentiation and population migration of *Proteus mirabilis*, *Mol Microbiol*, **6:** 1583–91.

Allison C, Coleman N et al., 1992, Ability of *Proteus mirabilis* to invade human urothelial cells is coupled to motility and swarming differentiation, *Infect Immun*, **60:** 4740–6.

Allison C, Lai HC et al., 1993, Cell differentiation of *Proteus mirabilis* is initiated by glutamine, a specific chemoattractant for swarming cells, *Mol Microbiol*, **8:** 53–60.

Allison C, Emödy L et al., 1994, The role of swarm cell differentiation and multicellular migration in the uropathogenicity of *Proteus mirabilis*, *J Infect Dis*, **169**: 1155–8.

Amano K, Fujita M, Suto T, 1993, Chemical properties of lipopolysaccharides from spotted fever group Rickettsiae and their common antigenicity with lipopolysaccharides from *Proteus* species, *Infect Immun*, **61**: 4350–5.

Bahrani FK, Massad G et al., 1994, Construction of a MR/P fimbrial mutant of *Proteus mirabilis*: role in virulence in a mouse model of ascending urinary tract infection, *Infect Immun*, **62**: 3363–71.

Belas R, 1994, Expression of multiple flagellin-encoding genes of *Proteus mirabilis*, *J Bacteriol*, **176**: 7169–81.

Belas R, Goldman M, Ashliman K, 1995, Genetic analysis of *Proteus mirabilis* mutants defective in swarmer cell elongation, *J Bacteriol*, **177**: 823–8.

Belyavin G, 1951, Cultural and serological phases of *Proteus vulgaris*, *J Gen Microbiol*, **5**: 197–207.

Beynon LM, Dumanski AJ et al., 1992, Capsule structure of *Proteus mirabilis* (ACTC 49565), *J Bacteriol*, **174**: 2172–7.

Bingen E, Boissinot C et al., 1993, Arbitrarily primed polymerase chain reaction provides rapid differentiation of *Proteus mirabilis* isolates from a pediatric hospital, *J Clin Microbiol*, **31**: 1055–9.

Brenner DJ, Farmer JJ et al., 1978, Deoxyribonucleic acid relatedness of *Proteus* and *Providencia* species, *Int J Syst Bacteriol*, **28**: 269–82.

Chippendale GR, Warren JW et al., 1994, Internalization of *Proteus mirabilis* by human renal epithelial cells, *Infect Immun*, **62**: 3115–21.

Chouteau J, Vieu JF, Brault G, 1974, Épidémiologie de l'infection hospitalière à *Providencia* dans un hôpital général, *Med Mal Infect*, **4**: 575–8.

Clarke AJ, 1993, Extent of peptidoglycan O acetylation in the tribe Proteeae, *J Bacteriol*, **175**: 4550–3.

Coetzee JN, Sacks TG, 1960, Morphological variants of *Proteus hauseri*, *J Gen Microbiol*, **23**: 209–16.

Cosenza BJ, Podgwaite JD, 1966, A new species of *Proteus* isolated from larvae of the gypsy moth *Porthetria dispar* (L), *Antonie van Leeuwenhoek J Microbiol Serol*, **32**: 187–91.

Costas M, Holmes B, Sloss LL, 1987, Numerical analysis of electrophoretic protein patterns of *Providencia rustigianii* strains from human diarrhoea and other sources, *J Appl Bacteriol*, **63**: 319–28.

Costas M, Holmes B, Wood AC, 1989, Numerical analysis of electrophoretic protein patterns of *Providencia rettgeri* strains from human faeces, urine and other specimens, *J Appl Bacteriol*, **67**: 441–52.

Costas M, Holmes B, Wood AC, 1990, Numerical analysis of electrophoretic protein patterns of *Providencia stuartii* strains from urine, wound and other sources, *J Appl Bacteriol*, **68**: 505–18.

Costas M, Holmes B et al., 1993, Identification and typing of *Proteus penneri* and *Proteus vulgaris* biogroups 2 and 3, from clinical sources, by computerized analysis of electrophoretic patterns, *J Appl Bacteriol*, **75**: 489–98.

Cradock-Watson JE, 1965, The production of bacteriocines by *Proteus* species, *Zentralbl Bakteriol Parasitenkd Infektionskr Hyg Abt 1 Orig*, **196**: 385–8.

Dienes L, 1946, Reproductive processes in *Proteus* cultures, *Proc Soc Exp Biol Med*, **63**: 265–70.

Drechsel H, Thieken A et al., 1993, Alpha-keto acids are novel siderophores in the genera *Proteus*, *Providencia*, and *Morganella* and are produced by amino acid deaminases, *J Bacteriol*, **175**: 2727–33.

Ebringer A, Ptaszynska T et al., 1985, Antibodies to *Proteus* in rheumatoid arthritis, *Lancet*, **2**: 305–7.

Ebringer A, Cunningham P et al., 1992, Sequence similarity between HLA-DR1 and DR4 subtypes associated with rheumatoid arthritis and proteus/serratia membrane haemolysin, *Ann Rheum Dis*, **51**: 1245–6.

Emödy L, Vörös S, Pál T, 1982, Alpha-haemolysin, a possible virulence factor in *Proteus morganii*, *FEMS Microbiol Lett*, **13**: 329–31.

Ewing WH, 1962, The tribe Proteeae: its nomenclature and taxonomy, *Int Bull Bacteriol Nomencl Taxon*, **12**: 93–102.

Ewing WH, Davis BR, Sykes JV, 1972, Biochemical characterization of *Providencia*, *Public Health Lab*, **30**: 25–38.

Ewing WH, Tanner KE, Dennard DA, 1954, The Providence group: an intermediate group of enteric bacteria, *J Infect Dis*, **94**: 134–40.

Fairley KF, Carson NE et al., 1971, Site of infection in acute urinary tract infection in general practice, *Lancet*, **2**: 615–18.

Fischer R, Penner JL et al., 1989, Usefulness of trehalose fermentation and L-glutamic acid decarboxylation for identification of biochemically aberrant *Providencia stuartii* strains, *J Clin Microbiol*, **27**: 1969–72.

France DR, Markham NP, 1968, Epidemiological aspects of *Proteus* infections with particular reference to phage typing, *J Clin Pathol*, **21**: 97–102.

Fuksa M, Krajden S, Lee A, 1984, Susceptibilities of 45 clinical isolates of *Proteus penneri*, *Antimicrob Agents Chemother*, **26**: 419–20.

Garrod LP, Lambert HP, O'Grady F, 1981, *Antibiotic and Chemotherapy*, 5th edn, Churchill Livingstone, Edinburgh.

Giammanco G, Pignato S, Agodi A, 1985, A simple chromogenic test for rapid screening of *Proteus* and *Providencia* bacteria, *Microbiologica*, **8**: 395–7.

Gmeiner J, 1975, The isolation of two different lipopolysaccharides from various *Proteus mirabilis* strains, *Eur J Biochem*, **58**: 621–6.

Guo MMS, Liu PV, 1965, Serological specificities of ureases of *Proteus* species, *J Gen Microbiol*, **38**: 417–22.

Harmon RC, Rutherford RL et al., 1989, Monoclonal antibody-mediated protection and neutralization of motility in experimental *Proteus mirabilis* infection, *Infect Immun*, **57**: 1936–41.

Hawkey PM, 1984, *Providencia stuartii*: a review of a multiply antibiotic-resistant bacterium, *J Antimicrob Chemother*, **13**: 209–26.

Hawkey PM, Hawkey CA, 1984, Comparative in-vitro activity of quinolone carboxylic acids against Proteeae, *J Antimicrob Chemother*, **14**: 485–9.

Hawkey PM, McCormick A, Simpson RA, 1986, Selective and differential medium for the primary isolation of members of the Proteeae, *J Clin Microbiol*, **23**: 600–3.

Hawkey PM, Pedler SJ, Turner A, 1983, Comparative in vitro activity of semi synthetic penicillins against Proteeae, *Antimicrob Agents Chemother*, **23**: 619–21.

Henriksen SD, Closs K, 1938, The production of phenylpyruvic acid by bacteria, *Acta Pathol Microbiol Scand*, **15**: 101–13.

Hickman FW, Farmer JJ, 1976, Differentiation of *Proteus mirabilis* by bacteriophage typing and the Dienes reaction, *J Clin Microbiol*, **3**: 350–8.

Hickman FW, Steigerwalt AG et al., 1982, Identification of *Proteus penneri* sp. nov. formerly known as *Proteus vulgaris* indole negative or as *Proteus vulgaris* biogroup 1, *J Clin Microbiol*, **15**: 1097–1102.

Hickman-Brenner FW, Farmer JJ et al., 1983, *Providencia rustigianii*: a new species in the family Enterobacteriaceae formerly known as *Providencia alcalifaciens* biogroup 3, *J Clin Microbiol*, **17**: 1057–60.

Hickman-Brenner FW, Fanning GR et al., 1986, Priority of *Providencia rustigianii* Hickman-Brenner, Farmer, Steigerwalt, and Brenner 1983 over *Providencia friedericiana* Muller 1983, *Int J Syst Bacteriol*, **36**: 565.

Holmes B, Costas M, Sloss LL, 1988, Numerical analysis of electrophoretic protein patterns of *Providencia alcalifaciens* strains from human faeces and veterinary specimens, *J Appl Bacteriol*, **64**: 27–35.

Hu L-T, Nicholson EB et al., 1990, *Morganella morganii* urease: purification, characterization, and isolation of gene sequences, *J Bacteriol*, **172**: 3073–80.

Izdebska-Szymona K, Monczak E, Lemczak B, 1971, Preliminary

scheme of phage typing *Proteus mirabilis* strains, *Exp Med Microbiol*, **23**: 18–22.

Jensen KT, Frederiksen W et al., 1992, Recognition of *Morganella* subspecies, with proposal of *Morganella morganii* subsp. *morganii* subsp. nov. and *Morganella morganii* subsp. *sibonii* subsp. nov., *Int J Syst Bacteriol*, **42**: 613–20.

Johnson DE, Russell RG et al., 1993, Contribution of *Proteus mirabilis* urease to persistence, urolithiasis, and acute pyelonephritis in a mouse model of ascending urinary tract infection, *Infect Immun*, **61**: 2748–54.

Kappos T, John MA et al., 1992, Outer membrane protein profiles and multilocus enzyme electrophoresis analysis for differentiation of clinical isolates of *Proteus mirabilis* and *Proteus vulgaris*, *J Clin Microbiol*, **30**: 2632–7.

Kashbur IM, George RH, Ayliffe GAJ, 1974, Resistotyping of *Proteus mirabilis* and a comparison with other methods of typing, *J Clin Microbiol*, **27**: 572–7.

Kauffmann F, 1951, *Enterobacteriaceae*, 1st edn, Munksgaard, Copenhagen.

Kauffmann F, 1953, On the classification and nomenclature of Enterobacteriaceae, *Riv Ist Sieroter Ital*, **28**: 485–91.

Kauffmann F, 1956, Zur biochemischen und serologischen Gruppen- und Typen- Einteilung der Enterobacteriaceae, *Zentralbl Bakteriol Parasitenkd Infektionskr Hyg Abt 1 Orig*, **165**: 344–54.

Kauffmann F, 1966, *The bacteriology of Enterobacteriaceae*, 3rd edn, Williams and Wilkins, Baltimore, 333–60.

Kopp R, Müller J, Lemme E, 1966, Inhibition of swarming of *Proteus* by sodium tetradecylsulfate, β-phenethyl alcohol, and *p*-nitrophenylglycerol, *Appl Microbiol*, **14**: 873–8.

Koronakis V, Cross M et al., 1987, The secreted hemolysins of *Proteus mirabilis*, *Proteus vulgaris*, and *Morganella morganii* are genetically related to each other and to the alpha-hemolysin of *Escherichia coli*, *J Bacteriol*, **169**: 1509–15.

Lewis J, Feckety FR, 1969, Proteus bacteremia, *Johns Hopkins Med J*, **124**: 151–6.

Lominski I, Lendrum AC, 1942, The effect of surface-active agents on *B. proteus*, *J Pathol Bacteriol*, **54**: 421–33.

Lominski I, Lendrum AC, 1947, The mechanism of swarming of *Proteus*, *J Pathol Bacteriol*, **59**: 688–91.

Loomes LM, Kerr MA, Senior BW, 1993, The cleavage of immunoglobulin G *in vitro* and *in vivo* by a proteinase secreted by the urinary tract pathogen *Proteus mirabilis*, *J Med Microbiol*, **39**: 225–32.

Loomes LM, Senior BW, Kerr MA, 1990, A proteolytic enzyme secreted by *Proteus mirabilis* degrades immunoglobulins of the immunoglobulin A1 (IgA1), IgA2, and IgG isotypes, *Infect Immun*, **58**: 1979–85.

Loomes LM, Senior BW, Kerr MA, 1992, Proteinases of *Proteus* spp.: purification, properties, and detection in urine of infected patients, *Infect Immun*, **60**: 2267–73.

McHale PJ, Keane CT, Dougan G, 1981, Antibiotic resistance in *Providencia stuartii* isolates in hospitals, *J Clin Microbiol*, **13**: 1099–104.

Mackey JP, Sandys GH, 1966, Diagnosis of urinary infections, *Br Med J*, **1**: 1173.

Malinowski F, 1966, A primary isolation medium for the differentiation of genus *Proteus* from other nonlactose and lactose fermenters, *Can J Med Technol*, **28**: 118–21.

Massad G, Bahrani FK, Mobley HLT, 1994, *Proteus mirabilis* fimbriae: identification, isolation, and characterization of a new ambient-temperature fimbria, *Infect Immun*, **62**: 1989–94.

Massad G, Lockatell CV et al., 1994, *Proteus mirabilis* fimbriae: construction of an isogenic *pmfA* mutant and analysis of virulence in a CBA mouse model of ascending urinary tract infection, *Infect Immun*, **62**: 536–42.

Miles AA, 1951, The mouse pathogenicity and toxicity of *Proteus vulgaris*, *J Gen Microbiol*, **5**: 307–16.

Mizushiri S, Amano K et al., 1990, Chemical characterization of lipopolysaccharides from *Proteus* strains used in Weil-Felix test, *Microbiol Immunol*, **34**: 121–33.

Mobley HLT, Chippendale GR et al., 1991, Cytotoxicity of the HpmA hemolysin and urease of *Proteus mirabilis* and *Proteus vulgaris* against cultured renal proximal tubular epithelial cells, *Infect Immun*, **59**: 2036–42.

Morgan H de R, 1906, Upon the bacteriology of the summer diarrhoea of infants, *Br Med J*, **1**: 908–12.

Müller HE, 1983, *Providencia friedericiana*, a new species isolated from penguins, *Int J Syst Bacteriol*, **33**: 709–15.

Müller HE, 1985, Production of brownish pigment by bacteria of the *Morganella–Proteus–Providencia* group, *Zentralbl Bakteriol Parasitkde Infektionskr Hyg Abt 1 Orig*, **260**: 428–35.

Müller HE, 1986, Production and degradation of indole by Gram-negative bacteria, *Zentralbl Bakteriol Parasitkde Infektionskr Hyg Abt 1 Orig*, **261**: 1–11.

Müller HE, O'Hara CM et al., 1986, *Providencia heimbachae*, a new species of Enterobacteriaceae isolated from animals, *Int J Syst Bacteriol*, **36**: 252–6.

Namioka S, Sakazaki R, 1959, New K antigen (C antigen) possessed by *Proteus* and *Rettgerella* cultures, *J Bacteriol*, **78**: 301–6.

Old DC, Adegbola RA, 1982, Haemagglutinins and fimbriae of *Morganella*, *Proteus*, and *Providencia*, *J Med Microbiol*, **15**: 551–64.

Owen RJ, Beck A et al., 1988, Detection of genomic variation in *Providencia stuartii* clinical isolates by analysis of DNA restriction fragment length polymorphisms containing rRNA cistrons, *J Clin Microbiol*, **26**: 2161–6.

Pavlatou M, Hassikou-Kaklamani E, Zantioti M, 1965, Lysotypie du genre *Proteus*, *Ann Inst Pasteur (Paris)*, **108**: 402–7.

Pazin GJ, Braude AI, 1974, Immobilizing antibodies in urine. II. Prevention of ascending spread of *Proteus mirabilis*, *Invest Urol*, **12**: 129–33.

Peerbooms PGH, Verweij AMJJ, MacLaren DM, 1982, Urinary virulence of *Proteus mirabilis* in two experimental mouse models, *Infect Immun*, **36**: 1246–8.

Peerbooms PGH, Verweij AMJJ, MacLaren DM, 1983, Investigation of the haemolytic activity of *Proteus mirabilis* strains, *Antonie van Leeuwenhoek J Microbiol Serol*, **49**: 1–11.

Peerbooms PGH, Verweij AMJJ, MacLaren DM, 1984, Vero cell invasiveness of *Proteus mirabilis*, *Infect Immun*, **43**: 1068–71.

Peerbooms PGH, Verweij AMJJ, MacLaren DM, 1985, Uropathogenic properties of *Proteus mirabilis* and *Proteus vulgaris*, *J Med Microbiol*, **19**: 55–60.

Penner JL, Hennessy JN, 1979, Application of O serotyping in a study of *Providencia rettgeri* (*Proteus rettgeri*) isolated from human and non-human sources, *J Clin Microbiol*, **10**: 834–40.

Penner JL, Hennessy JN, 1980, Separate O-grouping schemes for serotyping clinical isolates of *Proteus vulgaris* and *Proteus mirabilis*, *J Clin Microbiol*, **12**: 304–9.

Penner JL, Hinton NA, Hennessy J, 1975, Biotypes of *Proteus rettgeri*, *J Clin Microbiol*, **1**: 136–42.

Penner JL, Hinton NA et al., 1976, Variation in urease activity of endemic hospital strains of *Proteus rettgeri* and *Providencia rettgeri*, *J Infect Dis*, **134**: 370–6.

Penner JL, Fleming PC et al., 1979a, O serotyping *Providencia alcalifaciens*, *J Clin Microbiol*, **10**: 761–5.

Penner JL, Hinton NA et al., 1979b, O serotyping of *Providencia stuartii* isolates collected from twelve hospitals, *J Clin Microbiol*, **9**: 11–14.

Penner JL, Preston MA et al., 1982, Species differences in susceptibilities of Proteeae spp. to six cephalosporins and three aminoglycosides, *Antimicrob Agents Chemother*, **22**: 218–21.

Polster M, Svobodova M, 1964, Production of reddish-brown pigment from DL-tryptophan by enterobacteria of the *Proteus–Providencia* group, *Experientia*, **20**: 637–8.

Rahav G, Pinco E et al., 1994, Molecular epidemiology of catheter-associated bacteriuria in nursing home patients, *J Clin Microbiol*, **32**: 1031–4.

Rauss KF, 1936, The systematic position of Morgan's bacillus, *J Pathol Bacteriol*, **42**: 183–92.

Rauss K, Vörös S, 1959, The biochemical and serological properties of *Proteus morganii*, *Acta Microbiol Acad Sci Hung*, **6**: 233–48.

Rauss K, Puzova H et al., 1975, New serotypes of *Morganella morganii*, *Acta Microbiol Acad Sci Hung*, **22**: 315–21.

Rettger LF, 1909, Further studies of fatal septicaemia in young chickens, or 'white diarrhoea', *J Med Res (Boston)*, **21**: 115–23.

Rosenstein IJ, Hamilton-Miller JM, Brumfitt W, 1981, Role of urease in the formation of infection stones: comparison of ureases from different sources, *Infect Immun*, **32**: 32–7.

Rustigian R, Stuart CA, 1943, Taxonomic relationships in the genus *Proteus*, *Proc Soc Exp Biol Med*, **53**: 241–3.

Sareneva T, Holthöfer H, Korhonen TK, 1990, Tissue-binding affinity of *Proteus mirabilis* fimbriae in the human urinary tract, *Infect Immun*, **58**: 3330–6.

Schmidt WC, Jeffries CD, 1974, Bacteriophage typing of *Proteus mirabilis*, *Proteus vulgaris* and *Proteus morganii*, *Appl Microbiol*, **27**: 47–53.

Senior BW, 1977a, Typing of *Proteus* strains by proticine production and sensitivity, *J Med Microbiol*, **10**: 7–17.

Senior BW, 1977b, The Dienes phenomenon: identification of the determinants of compatibility, *J Gen Microbiol*, **102**: 235–44.

Senior BW, 1978, *p*-Nitrophenylglycerol – a superior antiswarming agent for isolating and identifying pathogens from clinical material, *J Med Microbiol*, **11**: 59–61.

Senior BW, 1979, The special affinity of particular types of *Proteus mirabilis* for the urinary tract, *J Med Microbiol*, **12**: 1–8.

Senior BW, 1983a, The purification, structure and synthesis of proticine 3, *J Med Microbiol*, **16**: 323–31.

Senior BW, 1983b, *Proteus morgani* is less frequently associated with urinary tract infections than *Proteus mirabilis* – an explanation, *J Med Microbiol*, **16**: 317–22.

Senior BW, 1987, The typing of *Morganella morgani* by bacteriocin production and sensitivity, *J Med Microbiol*, **23**: 33–9.

Senior BW, 1993, The production of HlyA toxin by *Proteus penneri* strains, *J Med Microbiol*, **39**: 282–9.

Senior BW, Albrechtsen M, Kerr MA, 1987, *Proteus mirabilis* strains of diverse type have IgA protease activity, *J Med Microbiol*, **24**: 175–80.

Senior BW, Albrechtsen M, Kerr MA, 1988, A survey of IgA protease production among clinical isolates of Proteeae, *J Med Microbiol*, **25**: 27–31.

Senior BW, Bradford NC, Simpson DS, 1980, The ureases of *Proteus* strains in relation to virulence for the urinary tract, *J Med Microbiol*, **13**: 507–12.

Senior BW, Hughes C, 1988, Production and properties of haemolysins from clinical isolates of the Proteeae, *J Med Microbiol*, **25**: 17–25.

Senior BW, Larsson P, 1983, A highly discriminatory multi-typing scheme for *Proteus mirabilis* and *Proteus vulgaris*, *J Med Microbiol*, **16**: 193–202.

Senior BW, Leslie DL, 1986, Rare occurrence of *Proteus vulgaris* in faeces: a reason for its rare association with urinary tract infections, *J Med Microbiol*, **21**: 139–44.

Senior BW, Loomes LM, Kerr MA, 1991, The production and activity *in vivo* of *Proteus mirabilis* IgA protease in infections of the urinary tract, *J Med Microbiol*, **35**: 203–7.

Senior BW, Vörös S, 1989, Discovery of new morganocin types of *Morganella morganii* strains of diverse serotype and the apparent independence of bacteriocin type from serotype of strains, *J Med Microbiol*, **29**: 89–93.

Senior BW, Vörös S, 1990, Protein profile typing – a new method of typing *Morganella morganii* strains, *J Med Microbiol*, **33**: 259–64.

Senior BW, McBride PDP et al., 1995, The detection of raised levels of IgM to *Proteus mirabilis* in sera from patients with rheumatoid arthritis, *J Med Microbiol*, **43**: 176–84.

Sheth NK, Kurup VP, 1975, Evaluation of tyrosine medium for the identification of Enterobacteriaceae, *J Clin Microbiol*, **1**: 483–5.

Siboni K, 1976, Correlation of the characters fermentation of trehalose, non-transmissible resistance to tetracycline, and relatively long flagellar wavelength in *Proteus morganii*, *Acta Pathol Microbiol Scand Sect B*, **84**: 421–7.

Smit JA, Coetzee JN, 1967, Serological specificities of phenylalanine deaminases of the Proteus–Providence group, *Nature (London)*, **214**: 1238–9.

Smith DG, Alwen J, 1966, Effect of activated charcoal on the swarming of *Proteus*, *Nature (London)*, **212**: 941–2.

Stickler DJ, Thomas B, 1976, Sensitivity of Providence to antiseptics and disinfectants, *J Clin Pathol*, **29**: 815–53.

Stuart CA, Wheeler KM et al., 1943, Biochemical and antigenic relationships of the paracolon bacteria, *J Bacteriol*, **45**: 101–9.

Svanborg Eden C, Larsson P, Lomberg H, 1980, Attachment of *Proteus mirabilis* to human urinary sediment epithelial cells in vitro is different from that of *Escherichia coli*, *Infect Immun*, **27**: 804–7.

Swihart KG, Welch RA, 1990, The HpmA hemolysin is more common than HlyA among *Proteus* isolates, *Infect Immun*, **58**: 1853–60.

Thaller MC, Berlutti F et al., 1992, Modified MacConkey medium which allows simple and reliable identification of *Providencia stuartii*, *J Clin Microbiol*, **30**: 2054–7.

Tucci V, Isenberg HD, 1981, Hospital cluster epidemic with *Morganella morganii*, *J Clin Microbiol*, **14**: 563–6.

Vieu JF, Capponi M, 1965, Lysotypie des *Proteus* OX19, OXK, OX2 et OXL, *Ann Inst Pasteur (Paris)*, **108**: 103–6.

Vörös S, Senior BW, 1990, New O antigens of *Morganella morganii* and the relationships between haemolysin production, O antigens and morganocin types of strains, *Acta Microbiol Hung*, **37**: 341–9.

Welch RA, 1987, Identification of two different hemolysin determinants in uropathogenic *Proteus* isolates, *Infect Immun*, **55**: 2183–90.

Williams EW, Hawkey PM et al., 1983, Serious nosocomial infection caused by *Morganella morganii* and *Proteus mirabilis* in a cardiac surgery unit, *J Clin Microbiol*, **18**: 5–9.

Williams FD, Schwarzhoff RH, 1978, Nature of the swarming phenomenon in *Proteus*, *Annu Rev Microbiol*, **32**: 101–22.

Williams FD, Anderson DM et al., 1976, Evidence against the involvement of chemotaxis in swarming of *Proteus mirabilis*, *J Bacteriol*, **127**: 237–48.

Wray SK, Hull SI et al., 1986, Identification and characterization of a uroepithelial cell adhesin from a uropathogenic isolate of *Proteus mirabilis*, *Infect Immun*, **54**: 43–9.

Xilinas ME, Papavassiliou JT, Legakis NJ, 1975, Selective medium for growth of *Proteus*, *J Clin Microbiol*, **2**: 459–60.

Yakubu DE, Old DC, Senior BW, 1989, The haemagglutinins and fimbriae of *Proteus penneri*, *J Med Microbiol*, **30**: 279–84.

YERSINIA

A Wanger

1 GENUS/SPECIES DEFINITION

The genus *Yersinia* belongs to the family Enterobacteriaceae. They are gram-negative rods (coccobacilli) with rounded ends. *Yersinia* are facultative anaerobes that ferment glucose in addition to other sugars without the production of gas, are oxidase-negative, catalase-positive, reduce nitrate and grow on nutrient agar. *Yersinia* are motile at 22–30°C, but not at 37°C. Their cell wall and antigenic composition also resemble other members of the family Enterobacteriaceae and some are identical. Many of the members of the genus *Yersinia* possess the ability to grow under extreme ranges in temperature and are well adapted to survival in the environment. As a genus these organisms are distinct from most other members of the family Enterobacteriaceae in that they are smaller in size and stain in a bipolar fashion, often resembling a 'safety pin'. *Yersinia pestis, Yersinia enterocolitica* and *Yersinia pseudotuberculosis* are human pathogens and *Yersinia ruckeri* is a fish pathogen whereas the other species are commensals. The G + C content of the DNA of the genus is 46–50 mol%. Eighty per cent homology exists between *Y. pestis* and *Y. pseudotuberculosis*, while only 20–55% homology exists between *Y. enterocolitica* and *Y. pseudotuberculosis* and *Y. ruckeri. Y. pestis* is the type species for the genus.

2 INTRODUCTION AND BRIEF HISTORICAL PERSPECTIVE

Members of the genus *Yersinia* were formerly included in the genus *Pasteurella* and finally removed in the 1970s, although this transfer was suggested by Thal in 1954 (Bercovier and Mollaret 1984) due to their dissimilarity with other members of this genus. The name *Yersinia* was derived from the French bacteriologist Alexander Yersin who first isolated the plague bacillus in Hong Kong in 1894 (Gyles and Thoen 1993, Solomon 1995). Included in this new genus, in addition to *Y. pestis*, was *Y. pseudotuberculosis*, first isolated by Malassez and Vignal in 1883 after inoculation of guinea pigs with material isolated from a skin lesion of a child who died of meningitis. Also moved from the genus *Pasteurella* to the newly formed genus *Yersinia* was the species *Y. enterocolitica*, described by Schleifstein and Coleman in 1939 who first called it *Bacterium entercoliticum* (Cover and Aber 1989) and later *Pasteurella pseudotuberculosis rodentium* and *Pasteurella* X. It was given its current designation of *Y. enterocolitica* in 1964 by Frederiksen (Bottone 1977).

Y. ruckeri, the causative agent of enteric redmouth disease of fish, was first described in 1955 and added to the genus *Yersinia* in 1978 on the basis of DNA analysis (Furones, Gilpin and Munn 1993). Three additional species, *Yersinia frederiksenii, Yersinia intermedia* and *Yersinia kristensenii*, were designated in 1980 and *Yersinia aldovae* in 1984 (Bercovier and Mollaret 1984). *Y. aldovae, Y. frederiksenii, Y. intermedia* and *Y. kristensenii* are often referred to as *Y. enterocolitica*-like group as a matter of convenience. Strains of *Yersinia*, isolated in the USA and Germany, that agglutinated with *Y. enterocolitica* H antisera but were untypable with O antisera and differed biochemically from other *Yersinia* by being negative for indole, Voges–Proskauer and citrate, were classified as a new species, *Yersinia rohdei* (Aleksic et al. 1987). *Y. enterocolitica* biogroup 3 was divided into 3A, which fermented L-sorbose and either *i*- or *myo*-inositol, and 3B, which did not ferment either; these were proposed as a new biogroup, number 6 (Wauters, Kandolo and Janssens 1987). However, DNA studies revealed that they were distinct enough for each to be a separate species and they were subsequently named *Yersinia mollaretii* and *Yersinia bercovieri*, respectively (Wauters et al. 1988).

The Philomiragia bacterium, isolated from a muskrat in 1959, was included in the genus *Yersinia* as proposed by Jensen in 1969 due to similar morphology and its DNA relatedness to *Y. pestis* (Hollis et al. 1989). In 1980 this categorization was reconsidered and the organism was renamed *Francisella philomiragia* and will not be discussed further in this chapter.

3 HABITAT

Y. pestis survives in nature in the stomach and proventriculus of the flea and in the soil of animal burrows. Animals that are resistant to infection with the organism act as a reservoir and enhance transmission by fleas as can be assessed by polymerase chain reaction (PCR) on tissue from fleas (Hinnebusch and Schwan 1993). *Y. pestis* is transmitted to humans either through the bite of the flea or by regurgitation during attempts at taking a blood meal; the organism causes sylvatic plague, the most common form of plague found in the USA (Gutman 1992). *Y. pestis* is also known to infect more than 200 species of rodents and small animals (Gutman 1992) which can also be a source of human infection. Once in a human host, the organism has a predilection for lymphoid tissue although *Y. pestis* can infect the lungs and can spread via respiratory secretions to other humans. Humans infected with *Y. pestis* develop lesions in the blood vessels; these lesions discolour the skin, giving the disease the name 'black plague'. Endemic areas for plague include areas of South East Asia, Africa and North and South America (see Volume 3, Chapter 44 for more clinical information regarding plague).

Y. pseudotuberculosis can also be transmitted by rodents or other infected animal species, including wild birds (Fantasia et al. 1993) although, like *Y. enterocolitica*, the most common mode of transmission is by food or water contaminated with infected faecal material (Gyles and Thoen 1993). *Y. pseudotuberculosis* causes a mesenteric lymphadenitis in infected humans, which mimics appendicitis (Fukushima 1987). Severe septicaemia can occur in immunocompromised patients (Salyers and Whitt 1994). Both *Y. enterocolitica* and *Y. pseudotuberculosis* can survive for long periods in the environment due to their ability to grow with minimal nutritional requirements and their ability to remain metabolically active at extremes of temperature (Brubaker 1991, Tashiro et al. 1991). Although *Yersinia* as a group are sensitive to inactivation by heat (56°C) or chemical disinfectants (phenol reagents), *Y.*

pestis can remain viable in dried blood for at least 3 weeks and for months in the soil. *Y. enterocolitica* is also found in the intestine of a variety of animal species; although in most cases the serotypes identified in animals are not pathogenic for humans, pathogenic serotypes have been isolated from healthy pigs (Doyle 1990). In parts of Europe and Japan the most common animal reservoir of *Y. enterocolitica* is pigs. Contamination of food such as chocolate milk and tofu has also been implicated as an outbreak source for *Y. enterocolitica*. Children infected with *Y. enterocolitica* most often present with enterocolitis; however, older children can develop severe disease, often mistaken for appendicitis (Cover and Aber 1989). Adults more often present with reactive arthritis (Reiter's syndrome) or erythema nodosum (Viitanen et al. 1991). Adults may also develop enteric disease followed in some cases by immune mediated arthritis. The HLA type B27 is associated with increased risk of arthritis. The only reported cases of human-to-human transmission of this organism were due to transfusion of contaminated blood (Cover and Aber 1989). Again, the ability of *Y. enterocolitica* to survive for extended periods at refrigeration temperatures mitigates the contamination of stored blood products (Feng, Keasler and Hill 1992). See reference Baert, Peetermans and Knockaert (1994) for a review of diseases associated with *Yersinia* species.

Y. frederiksenii is found in water and soil and is considered a human commensal of the gastrointestinal tract. Colonization of the gastrointestinal tract has been demonstrated in hospital staff as well as infection in medical residents who drank unpasteurized milk (Cafferkey et al. 1993). Both *Y. mollaretii* and *Y. bercovieri* are found in the environment and thought to be saprophytes (Wauters et al. 1988). *Y. rhodei* has been isolated from surface water, stools from 2 patients with diarrhoea and several healthy dogs (Aleksic et al. 1987). Its significance as a human or animal pathogen is unknown at this time. *Y. ruckeri* is a fish pathogen that causes an inflammation of the head region affecting trout as well as salmon (Furones et al. 1993). It is common throughout Europe, North America, South Africa and Australia.

4 MORPHOLOGY

Members of the genus *Yersinia* are gram-negative coccobacilli that exhibit bipolar staining, particularly when stained from clinical material. Wayson's dye mixture (methylene blue with carbolfuchsin) or Giemsa's is recommended for staining *Y. pestis* (Gutman 1992). *Yersinia*, especially *Y. pestis*, can also appear quite pleomorphic, particularly when colonies growing on nutrient agar medium are stained. *Yersinia* spp. produce no endospores and have no envelope except for *Y. pestis*, which has been shown to have an envelope in vivo and in vitro when grown at 37°C on a rich medium such as serum agar (Burrows 1963). The envelope is thought to represent the F1 glycoprotein antigen complex (Chen and Elberg 1975). The organisms are smaller in size then other members of the family Enterobacteriaceae (0.5–0.8 μm in diameter and 1–3 μm in length). *Y. pestis* is non-motile, whereas both *Y. enterocolitica* and *Y. pseudotuberculosis* are motile, with peritrichous or paripolar flagella, when grown at 22°C, but not at 37°C (Gutman 1992). When cultivated below 30°C all species of *Yersinia* except *Y. pestis* produce flagella and are motile. Pease (1979) demonstrated biochemically and electron microscopically that at room temperature strains of *Y. enterocolitica* could go through a transition to a spheroplast type L-form which then could revert back to an irregular shaped structure with an intact cell wall. It has also been hypothesized by Zykin (1994) that conversion of *Y. pestis* into L-forms allows them to persist in fleas or ticks for prolonged periods before conversion back to a bacillary form and transmission to a susceptible host.

5 CULTURAL CHARACTERISTICS AND GROWTH REQUIREMENTS

Yersinia are able to grow at temperatures ranging from 4 to 43°C and over a pH range of 4–10 (*Y. pestis* and *Y. pseudotuberculosis*, pH 5.0–9.6), although the optimum is pH 7.2–7.4 (Bercovier and Mollaret 1984). A combination of low pH and low temperature is used to prevent *Y. enterocolitica* from growing in foods at refrigeration temperature (Brocklehurst and Lund 1990). *Yersinia* are also salt tolerant. *Y. ruckeri* will grow in salt at a concentration of 3%, whereas *Y. pestis, Y. pseudotuberculosis* and *Y. enterocolitica* will grow in up to 5% salt. All species can grow on nutrient agar, although colony size is smaller and growth is slower for *Y. pseudotuberculosis* and *Y. pestis* (Bercovier and Mollaret 1984). Colonies of *Y. pestis* can be as small as 0.1–0.2 mm after 24 h of growth on nutrient agar at 37°C. With increased incubation the colonies reach a size of 1–1.5 mm in diameter. All other species of *Yersinia* will reach a size of 1–1.5 mm after 24 h and 2–3 mm after 48 h of incubation at 37°C, although often small colony variants remain. The colony morphology also changes to become opaque with a grey to yellow colour in the centre; they remain transparent and grey to white in colour on the periphery ('Chinese hat' shape). Growth and size of the colonies may be slightly improved by the addition of blood to the medium. Haemolysis is not observed when grown on blood agar. Most *Yersinia* will grow on MacConkey medium although growth of *Y. pseudotuberculosis* and *Y. pestis* is variable. *Y. pseudotuberculosis* is the only species of the genus that will grow as small grey to black colonies on tellurite medium (Brzin 1963).

Growth of *Yersinia* is moderate in liquid media. After 48 h of incubation some turbidity is evident whereas other Enterobacteriaceae will become turbid in less than 18 h of growth in liquid media. *Y. pestis* and *Y. pseudotuberculosis* do not show uniform turbidity, but settle to the bottom of the tube while the supernatant remains clear. A pellicle forms which disintegrates to form flocculent masses and larger deposits at the bottom of the tube (more evident in peptone water than in nutrient broth).

When grown at 25°C on minimal medium, *Y. pestis* requires L-methionine, L-phenylalanine whereas other species do not. At 37°C all species require supplements to grow on minimal medium (thiamine, biotin and other amino acids) (Burrows 1963). *Y. pestis* has the particular requirements of isoleucine, glycine, threonine, valine, a reducing agent and supplementary CO_2 when grown under these conditions (Brubaker 1991).

All species of *Yersinia* have a requirement of iron for growth. Virulent strains of *Y. pestis, Y. enterocolitica* and *Y. pseudotuberculosis* also have a requirement for a low concentration of calcium in order to express some of the antigens involved in the virulence of these species. The concentration of calcium in the medium is critical for the expression of virulence factors of *Y. pestis, Y. pseudotuberculosis* and *Y. enterocolitica*. The mechanism by which calcium affects virulence is discussed further in section 15 (p. 1059).

6 METABOLISM

Yersinia are aerobes and facultative anaerobes and therefore are both oxidative and fermentative. As with other members of the family Enterobacteriaceae, *Yersinia* ferment glucose with the production of acid and little or no gas. Fructose, galactose, maltose, mannitol, mannose, *N*-acetylglucosamine and trehalose are fermented. *Y. enterocolitica, Y. frederiksenii* and *Y. intermedia* produce acetoin when incubated at 28°C but not at 37°C. All species produce catalase, but not oxidase.

7 GENETIC MECHANISMS

Genetic mechanisms of *Yersinia* are thought to be similar to *Escherichia coli*, although no known intrinsic factors of conjugation or transduction have been specifically described. Sex factors or bacteriophages of *E. coli* have been shown to allow transfer of DNA between *E. coli* and *Yersinia* (Brubaker 1991). Although rare in clinical isolates, plasmids have been described in *Yersinia*, particularly in *Y. enterocolitica*. Plasmids involved in fermentation of both lactose and raffinose have been described. Plasmids that code for various virulence factors and antibiotic resistance genes have also been described (Ferber and Brubaker 1981). All pathogenic species of *Yersinia* possess a 70 kb plasmid, a low calcium response plasmid that contains the gene necessary for virulence of these organisms. *Y. pestis* has 2 additional plasmids, a 10 kb (pPst) encodes pesticin I and pFra that encodes the envelope antigen fraction 1 and murine toxin (Filippov et al. 1990).

In vitro transfer of DNA in *Yersinia* species has rarely been successful. Conchas and Carniel (1990) described the parameters for high efficiency transformation of *Yersinia* by electroporation, a method used extensively for *E. coli*. They were successful at transferring *E. coli* plasmid DNA into *Yersinia* at a frequency of up to 10^5–10^7 transformants per μg DNA. Cutrin et al. (1994) also used electroporation on a strain of *Y.*

ruckeri and achieved a transformation efficiency of 6×10^5 (Cutrin et al. 1994).

8 CELL WALL AND ENVELOPE COMPOSITION; ANTIGENIC STRUCTURE

The cell wall and antigenic structure of the genus *Yersinia* is in general very similar to that of other members of the family Enterobacteriaceae. The cell walls of these organisms are made up of lipopolysaccharide (LPS) consisting of a lipid A, core region and an O-specific side chain, as seen with other Enterobacteriaceae, with minor genus and species differences. The nature of the LPS of *Y. enterocolitica* does vary for certain serogroups. The pathogenic serogroups 3, 8 and 9 are composed of galactosamine, glucosamine, 3-deoxy-D-mannoctulosonic acid (KDO), 2 heptoses, glucose and galactose (Cornelis et al. 1987). *Y. pestis* lacks the extended O-group structure present in the other species. When *Y. pseudotuberculosis* is grown at 26°C instead of 37°C, short O-group side chains are formed.

Y. pestis has more than 20 antigens, many of which are shared with *Y. pseudotuberculosis* and *Y. enterocolitica* and some of which are essential for virulence of the organisms. The fraction 1 envelope antigen (F1) is a heat-labile, water-soluble antigen that stimulates immunity in both mice and humans and is only produced when the organism is grown at 37°C on protein rich media (see section 15, p. 1059 for further discussion of the role of this protein in virulence). Other antigens associated with *Yersinia* species are the V and W antigens. This complex is composed of 2 proteins both with a molecular weight of 90 kDa. The V protein is cell bound and the W protein is an excreted protein. The VW antigens as well as outer-membrane proteins, Yops, are associated with virulence of the organisms and are described in detail in section 15 (p. 1059). Two of these Yops in *Y. enterocolitica*, YopC and YopF, function as porins based on permeability studies performed with nitrocefin and cephaloridine (Brzostek and Nichols 1990). Other antigens produced by *Y. pestis* include an intracellular toxin called murine toxin, composed of 2 high molecular weight proteins (toxin A and toxin B) and a lipopolysaccharide endotoxin (Gyles and Thoen 1993).

Y. enterocolitica has more than 50 serotypes based on O and H antigens. O:3 and O:9 are the most common serotypes associated with human disease in Europe, Japan and Canada and serotype O:8 and O:5,25 in the USA. Since 1981 there has been a trend in California and New York in the increase in the prevalence of serotype O:3 as the predominant type in cases of gastroenteritis (Bissett et al. 1990). Serotypes O:1, O:2, O:3, O:5, O:6, O:7 and O:8 are responsible for most cases of severe disease in animals. There is little antigenic relationship between *Y. enterocolitica* and other *Yersinia* species; however, cross-reaction has been noted between *Y. enterocolitica* serotype O:9 and *Brucella*. There is some similarity between *Y. enterocolitica*

and *Vibrio cholerae* (Isshiki et al. 1992). Flagellar or H antigens are present but are complex, highly species specific and are not useful for serotyping (Cornelis et al. 1987). Although no true capsule has been described, some strains do have a K antigen (Cornelis et al. 1987). Pathogenic strains also produce an enterotoxin similar in nature to *E. coli* ST. A detailed discussion of the antigens of *Y. enterocolitica* can be found in Wauters (1981).

There are 6 serotypes of *Y. pseudotuberculosis* and 8 subtypes based on the presence of 15 O antigens. Serotype O:1 is associated with 90% of all cases of human disease. Some cross-reactivity has been noted between the O antigens of *Y. pseudotuberculosis* and some serotypes of *Salmonella* (Gutman 1992). At least 5 distinct flagellar (H) antigens are produced at temperatures less than 30°C in *Y. pseudotuberculosis*. O and H serotypes of *Y. pseudotuberculosis* cross-react to some extent with other members of the family Enterobacteriaceae and have some distinct geographical distributions. For a description of the LPS O antigens of *Y. ruckeri* serotype 01 and *Y. kristenseii* see Beynon et al. (1994) and L'vov et al. (1992), respectively.

9 CLASSIFICATION

Members of the genus *Yersinia* are classified into 11 species, based on biochemical analysis. The species of most concern to humans is *Y. pestis*, the agent of plague. *Y. enterocolitica* and *Y. pseudotuberculosis* are also human pathogens, whereas the other species, with the exception of *Y. ruckeri* which is a fish pathogen, are environmental, non-pathogenic organisms (Romalde 1993). *Y. pestis* and *Y. pseudotuberculosis* are biochemically homogeneous. *Y. enterocolitica* as a species is very heterogeneous and was initially divided into 5 biogroups based on the following biochemical reactions: indole production, hydrolysis of aesculin and salicin, lactose oxidation, acid from xylose, trehalose, sucrose, sorbose and sorbitol, *o*-nitrophenyl-β-D-galactopyranoside (ONPG), ornithine decarboxylase, Voges–Proskauer reaction and nitrate reduction (Wauters 1981). The scheme was later modified by Wauters to include 6 biotypes. Biogroup 1 was divided into 2 groups. Group 1A includes environmental strains that lack virulence plasmids and are pyrazinamidase, aesculin and β-D-glucosidase positive. The strains that compose biogroup 1B are aesculin, pyrazinamidase and β-D-glucosidase negative and belong to one of the following serogroups: O:4, O:8, O:13, O:18, O:20 or O:21. Biogroup 1B strains are reportedly pathogenic to humans in North America (Cornelis et al. 1987).

Y. pestis can also be divided into 3 biogroups (antigua, medievalis and orientalis), based on their ability to reduce nitrate and to ferment glycerol and melibiose. These biogroups were also found to correlate with the geographical distribution and strain-specific rodent species.

10 LABORATORY ISOLATION AND IDENTIFICATION

Because of the potential hazards to laboratory personnel, the microbiological isolation of *Y. pestis* usually is not performed in routine clinical laboratories without biosafety isolation hoods and equipment. Specimens, such as aspirates from lymph nodes or other body fluids collected from a patient suspected of having plague, should be sent to a laboratory with the proper facilities to culture the organism. Care in transport is essential.

Y. pestis is inactive in the majority of biochemical tests and is therefore difficult to identify; many commercially available identification systems do not include this species in their database. Suspected isolates should be sent to a national reference laboratory for identification and epidemiological investigation. Serological diagnosis using either microhaemagglutination, complement fixation or enzyme immunoassay can be used to detect antibodies to *Y. pestis* in the patient's serum. *Y. pestis* antigens can also be detected directly in patient samples. Amplification of 2 plasmid encoded genes, plasminogen activator and antigen fraction 1, previously sequenced by Sodeinde and Goguen in 1989 (Sodeinde et al. 1992) successfully identified *Y. pestis* in as little as 4 μl of blood from infected mice in experiments simulating the quantity of organisms found in the blood of infected humans (Norkina et al. 1994). Although some homology exists between portions of these genes of *Salmonella typhimurium* and *E. coli*, primers used were selected to avoid homologous regions. Bardarov et al. (1990) cloned and characterized a chromosomal fragment of DNA that was specific for *Y. pestis* and has the potential as a diagnostic tool for the direct identification of *Y. pestis* in clinical samples.

Culture of *Yersinia* other than *Y. pestis* can be readily performed in established clinical micriobiology laboratories. *Yersinia* will grow on non-selective media and can be isolated from specimens obtained from usually sterile sites by inoculating blood agar medium. *Yersinia* grow well at 35°C; however, a lower isolation temperature is recommended for specimens that may be contaminated with other bacteria, e.g. incubation at 25°C allows a selective advantage for the isolation of *Yersinia* from stool specimens. Cold enrichment of the stool (incubation of the sample in saline at 4°C for 1–3 weeks) has been shown to increase the frequency of isolation of the organism (Davis et al. 1980). Isolation of *Yersinia* from contaminated specimens is further enhanced by the use of a selective medium, such as cefsulodin–Irgasan–novobiocin (CIN) medium. This medium inhibits the majority of other enteric bacteria. On CIN medium *Y. enterocolitica* may be identified by its characteristic colony morphology (red pigmented colonies surrounded by a clear zone). In a review of various antimicrobials as a supplement to a broth medium for selective recovery of *Y. enterocol, itica*, Toora et al. (1994) found Irgasan to be the most effective. Addition of other antimicrobials either did not inhibit all enteric bacteria or inhibited some *Yersinia* strains as well (Toora et al. 1994). Selective enrichment for *Y. enterocolitica* from food was best achieved using Irgasan ticarcillin broth (de Boer 1992).

Specific identification of *Yersinia* requires the use of individual biochemical utilization tests. Sharma et al. (1990) successfully used the API 20E (a commercially available system containing more than 20 biochemical reactions in microtubes inoculated simultaneously) for species level identification of *Y. enterocolitica*, *Y. frederiksenii* and *Y. kristensenii* using 175 stool isolates collected in Canada. De Ryck, Struelens and Serruys (1994) proposed a screen method for the rapid identification of enteric pathogens, including *Y. enterocolitica*, from stools. Colonies resembling *Y. enterocolitica* on CIN medium were transferred to rhamnose broth. Strains which were rhamnose-negative and motility-negative as determined by a wet mount from rhamnose broth were identified presumptively as *Yersinia* species (De Ryck, Struelens and Serruys 1994). Kitch, Jacobs and Appelbaum (1994) evaluated the RapID onE (Innovative Diagnostics, Inc.), for the identification of 379 enteric organisms including *Yersinia* species. The system correctly identified 8 out of 8 isolates of *Yersinia* species. The Vitek enteric pathogens card also correctly identified 5 isolates of *Y. enterocolitica* (Imperatrice and Nachamkin 1993). Identification of *Yersinia* species can be misinterpreted due to the slow growth of the organism at 35°C. *Y. enterocolitica* and *Y. frederiksenii* differ by only one biochemical, fermentation of rhamnose, which occurs slowly at 35°C (Cafferkey et al. 1993). Therefore, biochemical analysis of *Y. enterocolitica* and the related species should be performed at temperatures of less than 30°C (see Table 44.1 for biochemical tests helpful in the identification of *Yersinia* spp.).

PCR assays have also been shown to be useful in the identification of *Y. enterocolitica* and *Y. pseudotuberculosis* directly from either food or clinical specimens, alleviating the need for the cumbersome and time-consuming biochemical identification of these isolates. Since plasmids of *Y. enterocolitica* are shared with other species of *Yersinia*, PCR assays for detection of virulence, lack species specificity (Ibrahim, Liesack and Stackebrandt 1992). Nakajima et al. (1992) described a PCR assay based on the amplification of a region of the *inv* gene of *Y. pseudotuberculosis* and the *ail* gene from pathogenic *Y. enterocolitica*. They found that the limit of detection of their assay was 10^3–10^4 cfu of bacteria in a suspension of river water. Rasmussen et al. (1994) used primers synthesized from the *inv* region of *Y. enterocolitica* and demonstrated specific detection of pathogenic *Y. enterocolitica*. Feng, Keasler and Hill (1992) developed a PCR assay for the direct detection of *Y. enterocolitica* in blood, based on the detection of a portion of the *virF* gene on the pYV plasmid and a portion of the *ail* gene located on the chromosome. The assay was able to detect 500 cfu in 100 μl of blood.

In addition to speciation, analysis of the serotype is warranted since there is an association between serotype and pathogenicity (Farmer et al. 1992); however,

Table 44.1 Biochemical reactivity of *Yersinia* sp.

	Y. pestis	Y. pseudo.	Y. ent.	Y. fred.	Y. kristen.	Y. ruckeri	Y. moll.	Y. bercovieri	Y. rohdei	Y. aldovae	Y. intermedia
Motility (25°C)	–	+	+	+	+	v	+	+	+	+	+
Ornithine decarboxylase	–	–	+	+	+	+	+	+	v	+	+
Urease	–	+	+	+	+	–	+	+	v	+	+
VP (25°C)	–	–	+	+	+	v	–	+	–	+	+
Citrate (25°C)	–	–	–	v	–	+	–	–	+	+	+
Indole	–	–	v	+	v	–	–	–	–	–	+
Rhamnose	–	+	–	+	–	–	–	–	–	+	+
Sucrose	–	–	+	+	+	–	+	+	+	–	+
Cellobiose	–	–	+	+	+	–	+	+	+	–	+
Sorbose	–	–	+	+	+	–	+	–	ND	ND	ND
Sorbitol	–	–	+	+	+	–	+	+	+	+	+
Melibiose	v	+	–	–	–	–	–	–	v	–	+
Raffinose	–	v	–	–	–	–	–	–	v	–	+
Fucose	ND	–	v	v	v	ND	+	+	ND	v	v

Y. pseudo, *Y. pseudotuberculosis*; *Y. ent.*, *Y. enterocolitica*; *Y. fred.*, *Y. frederiksenii*; *Y. kristen*, *Y. kristensenii*; *Y. moll*, *Y. mollaretii*; v, variable; ND, not done; –, negative; +, positive.
References: Bercovier and Mollaret 1984, Aleksic et al. 1987, Wauters et al. 1988, Gutman 1992, Holt et al. 1994.

O antisera for serotyping is not readily available to routine laboratories. Other methods have been described to differentiate virulent from avirulent strains of *Y. enterocolitica*, such as: presence of a 40–48 kDa plasmid, autoagglutination, tissue culture cell assay, serum resistance, hydrophobicity and virulence in animals. The majority of these methods are impractical for most laboratories although autoagglutination has been shown to be the best in vitro predictor of virulence in *Y. enterocolitica* (Kapperud et al. 1987). Other more practical methods include the use of biochemicals such as aesculin, salicin and pyrazinamide. Cimolai, Trombley and Blair (1994) defined a pathogenic biotype as strains which were negative for all 3 assays and a non-pathogenic biotype as positive for all 3. Strains belonging to the so-called pathogenic biotypes were more likely than the non-pathogenic biotypes to be isolated from young children with bloody diarrhoea. Selective media such as Congo red or Congo red magnesium oxalate (CRMOX) agar will identify strains that possess 2 factors associated with the presence of a virulence plasmid, Congo red dye uptake and calcium-dependent growth at 35°C, have also been used (Farmer et al. 1992). Other authors have proposed the use of a medium containing crystal violet in which only the virulent, plasmid-containing colonies will retain the dye. Farmer et al. (1992) described the use of reactivity in several assay systems together to increase the sensitivity and specificity: pyrazinamidase, CRMOX agar, salicin fermentation–aesculin hydrolysis and D-xylose fermentation (see Table 44.2).

PCR assays that specifically target regions of the genome responsible for virulence have also been developed, due in part to the inconsistent nature of the above-described assays (Kwaga, Iversen and Missra 1992). Wren and Tabaqchali (1990) used a PCR assay based on detection of a portion of a plasmid essential for virulence. However, plasmids can be lost on subculture, causing a false negative result (Ibrahim, Liesack and Stackebrandt 1992). Fenwick and Murray (1991) amplified a portion of the attachment invasion locus on the chromosome of pathogenic *Y. enterocolitica*. Robins-Browne et al. (1989) confirmed the use of a probe directed at all regions specific to pathogenic strains. Other more specific targets for amplification included the chromosomally encoded *yst* gene (enterotoxin) (Ibrahim, Liesack and Stackebrandt 1992).

11 SUSCEPTIBILITY TO ANTIMICROBIAL AGENTS

Alzugaray et al. (1995) studied the antimicrobial profile of clinical isolates of *Y. enterocolitica* serotype O:3. All were susceptible to amoxycillin–clavulanic acid, cefoxitin, fosfomycin, gentamicin, kanamycin, neomycin, tetracycline, naladixic acid, norfloxacin, ciprofloxacin and trimethoprim. All were resistant to ampicillin (Alzugaray et al. 1995). In a study of 375 strains of *Yersinia* species isolated from food in France, only 4 were resistant to non-β-lactam antibiotics (Ahmedy et al. 1985). According to a study by Pham, Bell and Lanzarone (1991) of 100 clinical isolates of *Y. enterocolitica* in Australia, all isolates were susceptible to chloramphenicol, ciprofloxacin, gentamicin, tetracycline, trimethoprim, sulpha drugs, ticarcillin–clavulanate and imipenem. All isolates were resistant to ampicillin (Pham, Bell and Lanzarone 1991). Biotype-related differences were observed to other β-lactam antibiotics. Biotypes 1A and 3 were resistant to cefoxitin and amoxycillin–clavulanate and biotype 3 was susceptible to ticarcillin. Biotype 4 strains were susceptible to cefoxitin and amoxycillin–clavulanate and resistant to ticarcillin. These differences are thought to be attributed to differences in types of β-lactamases produced (Pham, Bell and Lanzarone 1991). Two chromosomally mediated β-lactamases have been described in *Y. enterocolitica* (Ahmedy et al. 1985). Enzyme A is constitutive and is a broad spectrum enzyme, enzyme B is inducible and is a cephalosporinase (Pham and Bell 1993). Inducible β-lactamase was found in all isolates of *Y. enterocolitica* biotypes 1A and 3 but in none of the isolates of biotype 4 (Pham and Bell 1992). Induction of β-lactamase production can be detected using a modified disc diffusion technique, using an imipenem disc as the inducer and a cefotaxime disc as the substrate (Pham and Bell 1993).

No β-lactamases have been detected in strains of *Y. pseudotuberculosis* or *Y. pestis*; however, regardless of in vitro susceptibility to β-lactam antibiotics, in a mouse model using a pathogenic strain of *Y. pseudotuberculosis* the only antibiotic found to be effective was ofloxacin (Lemaitre, Mazigh and Scavizzi 1991). Bonacorsi et al. (1994) found that 18 strains of *Y. pestis* tested were susceptible to amoxicillin, cefotaxime, ceftriaxone, streptomycin, gentamicin, ofloxacin and doxycycline.

In a recent study of antimicrobial susceptibility of

Table 44.2 Association of biochemical reactivity with pathogenicity and the presence of the virulence plasmid

Biochemical reactivity	Pathogenicity	Presence plasmid
Red colonies CR-MOX	+	+
Pyrazinamidase production	−	−
Salicin fermentation	−	−
Aesculin hydrolysis	−	−
Retains crystal violet dye	+	+

78 strains of *Y. pestis* (57 from patients in Vietnam with plague between 1985 and 1993), the most active antimicrobials were ciprofloxacin, ofloxacin and ceftriaxone; streptomycin, tetracycline and chloramphenicol (agents most commonly used to treat patients with plague) were less active (Smith et al. 1995).

Based on serotype, *Y. ruckeri*, the fish pathogen, was found to vary in susceptibility to antimicrobial agents. Of 50 isolates tested by De Grandis and Stevenson (1985), 2 were resistant to tetracycline and sulphonamide, 2 antimicrobials commonly used for therapy of disease caused by this organism. Resistance was associated with the presence of a 3.6×10^4 kDa plasmid that was transferable to both another strain of *Y. ruckeri* and a strain of *E. coli*.

12 TYPING METHODS

As with other organisms, many methods exist for epidemiological comparison of strains of *Yersinia*, including phenotypic markers such as biotyping, serotyping, bacteriophage typing and antibiotic susceptibility patterns; genotypic differences such as restriction endonuclease digestion of either plasmid (REAP) or chromosomal (REAC) DNA; digestion of genomic DNA and separation by pulsed field gel electrophoresis (PFGE); ribotyping and analysis of PCR generated fragments. Results from multilocus enzyme electrophoresis (MLEE) studies found *Y. enterocolitica* species to be clonal, but distinct groups, correlating with virulence of the strains, were identified (Caugant et al. 1989). Fukushima et al. (1993) compared biotyping, serotyping, phage typing, REAP, REAC and antibiotic susceptibility patterns for 138 strains of *Y. enterocolitica* serotype O:5,27, isolated from both humans and animals in the USA, Japan, Canada, Australia, The Netherlands and Germany. For the epidemiological investigation of relatedness of other genera, the best method for the analysis of *Yersinia* strains was a combination of several techniques used in conjunction with the epidemiological information about the sources of the isolates. Fukushima et al. concluded that the combination of REAP, biotyping and H-antigen typing would yield the most information about the relatedness of strains of this group of organisms. Kapperud et al. (1990) also determined that multiple methods would be useful; however, in general, genotypic rather than phenotypic methods were more discriminatory. Since most isolates of *Y. enterocolitica* contain only a single virulence plasmid, typing using plasmid DNA analysis is not useful in strain differentiation (Blumberg, Kiehlbauch and Wachsmuth 1991). Although REAP or REAC seem to be useful techniques, inter- and even intra-laboratory comparisons can be difficult due to the multitude of bands on the gel. The use of gel electrophoresis of restriction digests in combination with a specific probe can facilitate the use of this method by many laboratories. Picard-Pasquier et al. (1990) compared ribotyping to MLEE and found the methods to be equivalent for

the differentiation of strains of *Y. enterocolitica*, *Y. pseudotuberculosis*, *Y. intermedia*, *Y. aldovae*, *Y. frederiksenii* and *Y. kristensenii*. Anderson and Saunders (1990) confirmed the usefulness of ribotyping to subtype serogroups of *Y. enterocolitica*. Saken et al. (1994) found PFGE following *Not*I digestion of genomic DNA of *Y. enterocolitica* strains to be more discriminatory than other genotypic methods. PFGE was also found to be a useful epidemiological tool for typing of *Y. pestis* (Lucier and Brubaker 1992).

Different typing methods have been applied to the analysis of the clonal relationship of isolates of *Y. pseudotuberculosis*. Although most isolates of *Y. pseudotuberculosis* have a single plasmid associated with virulence, analysis by REAP differentiated isolates into their serotype as well as their geographical origin (Fukushima et al. 1994). The relatedness of strains of *Y. pseudotuberculosis* has been evaluated using an advanced PCR-based genotypic technique, random amplified polymorphic DNA (RAPD) (Makino et al. 1994). This technique was found to be useful in the study of outbreak strains in Japan.

Filippov et al. (1990) analysed 242 isolates of *Y. pestis* from various areas of the former USSR, Mongolia, China, Vietnam, India, Indonesia, Brazil and Africa for the presence of plasmid DNA. The majority of the isolates possessed the same 3 plasmids; however, 20 strains from different areas contained an additional cryptic plasmid of approximately 6000 kDa. They also found changes in the size of pCad and pFra (plasmids found in all isolates of *Y. pestis*) in strains from particular regions.

13 BACTERIOCINS AND BACTERIOPHAGES

Y. pestis produces 2 bacteriocins, pesticin I and pesticin II. Pesticin I is plasmid mediated and active against *Y. pseudotuberculosis* and some strains of *E. coli* and *Y. enterocolitica* (Staggs and Perry 1992). The compound is a polypeptide with a molecular weight of 63 kDa. Its mode of action is to degrade the cell wall peptidoglycan of sensitive strains (Brubaker and Surgalla 1962, Ferber and Brubaker 1979). Pesticin II, produced by both *Y. pestis* and *Y. pseudotuberculosis*, is only active against select strains of *Y. pestis* (Fetherston, Lillard and Perry 1995). Csiszar and Toth (1992) demonstrated production of bacteriocins by clinical isolates of *Y. enterocolitica* belonging to various serogroups except O:3. The majority of the O:3 strains were sensitive to the bacteriocins produced by strains of other serogroups and are not well characterized (Rakin et al. 1994). Sensitivity of *Y. enterocolitica* strains to pesticin is associated with the production of a 65 kDa outer-membrane protein (FyuA), also thought to act as a receptor for yersiniabactin (see section 15, p. 1059) (Haag et al. 1993). Bacteriocins have also been described in *Y. intermedia* that are produced at 25°C but not at 37°C and are active against strains of *Y. enterocolitica*, *Y. intermedia*, *Y. frederiksenii* and *Y. kristensenii* (Bercovier and Mollaret 1984). Toora (1995) has described a bacteriocin in *Y. kristensenii*. The bacteriocin was found to be extracellular with activity specific for strains of *Y. enterocolitica*.

Bacteriophages active against *Yersinia* species have been described (Nilehn and Ericson 1969, Nicolle, Mollaret and Brault 1973). Typing schemes based on bacteriophage activity have been described for *Y. enterocolitica*; however, other epidemiological methods have been found to be more useful (see section 12, p. 1058).

14 ROLE IN NORMAL FLORA OF HUMANS

Although *Yersinia* species are not considered part of the normal flora in humans, *Y. enterocolitica* can occasionally be found in the intestinal tract without any associated disease (Jawetz, Melnich and Adelberg 1978).

15 PATHOGENICITY AND VIRULENCE FACTORS

Pathogenicity of *Yersinia* species is mediated by a 70–75 kb plasmid (pYV) and 2 additional plasmids in *Y. pestis* (Straley, Skrzypek and Plano 1993). These plasmids control the 4 major virulence factors in this genus: adhesin/invasin proteins, excreted antiphagocytic proteins (Yops), proteins involved in processing and excretion of the Yops (Ysc) and regulatory proteins (Lcr). The role of each of these factors in the pathogenicity of *Yersinia* species will be discussed separately. Chromosomal factors, including the production of an enterotoxin, are also thought to play a role in virulence, since strains lacking the plasmid have been found to survive within macrophages (Charnetzky and Shuford 1985) and cause disease in an animal model as well as in humans (Fukushima 1987).

Invasion of *Y. enterocolitica* and *Y. pseudotuberculosis* through mucosal surfaces and colonization of these surfaces is based, at least in part, on the production of a toxin (Yst), similar to the heat stable toxin produced by *E. coli* (Iriarte and Cornelis 1995). The role of the toxin in the production of diarrhoea has not been determined; however, it is only produced at temperatures less than 30°C, which lends evidence against it having a role in vivo. It has also been found in both pathogenic and non-pathogenic strains of *Y. enterocolitica*. The *yst* gene has been cloned and sequenced in an attempt to learn more about its role in vivo. Hybridization studies using a portion of the cloned sequence found the *yst* gene to be present in pathogenic but not in non-pathogenic serotypes of *Yersinia*. Homologous DNA was also found in some strains of *Y. kristensenii* (Delor et al. 1990). An exotoxin has also been identified, cloned and sequenced from *Y. pseudotuberculosis* (Ito et al. 1995). This toxin, *Y. pseudotuberculosis*-derived mitogen (YPM) acts as a superantigen by activation of specific human T cells in the presence

of immune cells bearing MHC class II molecules. Little homology was demonstrated with superantigens from other bacterial species (Miyoshi-Akiyama et al. 1995). It has been suggested that YPM is involved in mediating systemic symptoms associated with human disease due to *Y. pseudotuberculosis* (Abe et al. 1993).

Other invasion factors include invasin and Ail, 2 proteins under the control of chromosomal genes, and the plasmid encoded protein YadA. Invasin is produced maximally at room temperature and only at body temperature in the presence of low pH, whereas YadA and Ail are produced in higher concentrations at 37°C. Ail, the product of the *ail* gene, plays a role in adherence, invasion and serum resistance in virulent isolates of *Y. enterocolitica* (Wachtel and Miller 1995). Both invasin and YadA have been demonstrated to penetrate tissue culture cells and to bind to integrins in intestinal tissue (Pepe and Miller 1993, Skurnik et al. 1994). YadA has also been shown to bind to fibronectin (Tertti et al. 1992). YadA and *ail* are also responsible for the ability of *Yersinia* species to resist the activity of serum, a trait only expressed at 37°C in *Y. enterocolitica* and *Y. pseudotuberculosis*. The *inv* gene, encoding invasin, has been described in all strains and various species of *Yersinia* whereas *ail* has only been found in pathogenic strains of *Yersinia* spp. (Pierson and Falkow 1993).

Following colonization of mucosal surfaces, avoidance of phagocytosis is the next step in the pathogenicity of *Yersinia*. The antiphagocytic ability of this genus is under the control of at least 11 Yops at least 3 of which have been directly associated with virulence: YopE, YopH and YopM (Straley, Skrzypek and Plano 1993). Yops function in 2 ways, interfering directly with the signal transduction of the phagocytes or directly attacking the host cells, thereby inhibiting phagocytosis by macrophages (Straley, Skrzypek and Plano 1993, Visser, Annema and van Furth 1995). YopM is an example of an excreted protein which interferes with signal transduction by inhibiting platelet aggregation. YopH possesses protein tyrosine phosphatase activity, acting on host proteins specifically, inhibiting respiratory burst in macrophages (Galyov et al. 1993, Green et al. 1995). YopE acts directly on the host cell by destroying actin filaments (Rosqvist, Forsberg and Wolf-Watz 1991).

LcrV, previously designated V antigen in *Y. pestis*, is found in all species of *Yersinia* and has a role in regulation and expression of Yops as well as an unknown role in the virulence of *Yersinia* species (Salyers and Whitt 1994). Genes *yopB* and *yopD* also have a regulatory role in the control of expression of Yops. Proteins YopB and YopD are excreted under conditions of low concentrations of calcium (Hakansson et al. 1993). YopB has been demonstrated to suppress the production of tumour necrosis factor α by phagocytes (Beuscher et al. 1995). Virulence genes on *Yersinia* are controlled by 2 independent regulatory systems, temperature and cellular concentration of calcium. Secretion of Yops occurs only at 37°C and in the absence of calcium (Cornelis 1994). A chromosomal gene, *ymoA*, functions as the temperature controller

(Cornelis et al. 1991), turning on the *virF* gene which allows expression of *yop* and *ysc* genes (Michiels et al. 1991, Salyers and Whitt 1994). Calcium concentrations are regulated by *lcr* genes (LcrE [YopN] and LcrH) (Forsberg et al. 1991).

Other virulence factors of *Yersinia* species include their ability to obtain and store iron. In fact, severe disease in humans due to *Y. enterocolitica* is associated with an underlying disease, particularly disorders involving iron metabolism (Chambers and Sokol 1994). *Yersinia* produce both a siderophore, which is active at low temperature, and an iron storage system induced at 37°C. Two high molecular weight iron-regulated proteins (HMWP1 and 2) were found to be encoded on the chromosome of virulent strains of *Yersinia* (Gyles and Thoen 1993, Guilvout, Carniel and Pugsley 1995). The gene *irp2* encodes HMWP2, which is only found in virulent strains of *Y. enterocolitica* (Haag et al. 1993, Rakin et al. 1994). Haag et al. identified a siderophore from the supernatant of actively growing *Y. enterocolitica*, yersiniabactin (yersinio- phore), and by creating mutants associated the protein with virulence. The iron transport genes are thought to be regulated by Fur protein as found in other species of Enterobacteriaceae (Staggs and Perry 1992).

Yersinia species also possess a chromosomal gene which encodes a fibrillar protein in pathogenic serotypes of *Y. enterocolitica* known as Myf (Cornelis 1994). Myf is composed of MyfA (a 21 kDa protein), MyfB (a chaperone) and MyfC (an outer-membrane protein) (Iriarte and Cornelis 1995). As with other virulence factors, the fibrillar protein has homology to proteins with similar function in enterotoxigenic *E. coli*. These proteins are hypothesized to work in conjunction with Yst to aid in the colonization of mucous membranes. *Y. pseudotuberculosis* and *Y. pestis* have a protein with similar function, called pH6 antigen or pilus adhesin (PsaA), not found in *Y. enterocolitica*, which may be involved in defence once the organisms are within the phagocyte (Cornelis 1992, Salyers and Whitt 1994).

Stress proteins found in many bacterial genera are also produced by *Yersinia* species. These proteins may aid the bacteria in survival within phagocytes by neutralizing toxic products of these host cells (Yamamoto et al. 1994).

Y. pestis has 2 additional plasmids, not present in other species of *Yersinia*: the 110 kb plasmid contains the genes responsible for antiphagocytic protein capsule (Fra) and a toxin which is lethal in mice and acts by preventing the action of adrenaline (epinephrine) (Gyles and Thoen 1993); and a 9.5 kb plasmid which contains the gene(s) responsible for plasminogen activator protease (Pla), which has a role in vivo in the ability of the organism to resist the host's ability to contain the infection locally, possibly by resistance to killing by complement (Sodeinde et al. 1992, Straley, Skrzypek and Plano 1993, Friedlander et al. 1995). Pla is also capable of regulating the presence of Yops, which would allow the organisms to be ingested by monocytes when, unlike other *Yersinia* species, they would be protected from killing. Podladchikova et al. (1994) sequenced an insertion sequence (IS 100) found on the 9.5 kb plasmid of *Y. pestis*, the function of which is currently unknown. *Y. pestis* also has the ability to store haemin which occurs maximally at 26°C. Storage of iron is manifested as pigment production in virulent strains of *Y. pestis* and is regulated by the chromosomal locus *pgm* (Gyles and Thoen 1993). The F1 antigen or protein capsule is antiphagocytic and is also immunogenic (Friedlander et al. 1995).

Furones et al. (1990) compared the cell extracts of serotype I strains of *Y. ruckeri* with those of other non-pathogenic serotypes. They found the presence of a heat-sensitive lipid only in the serotype I strains. In vivo studies confirmed this substance to be a virulence factor. The addition of SDS to culture medium enhances selective growth of pathogenic strains of *Y. ruckeri*.

A 7.0×10^4 kDa plasmid thought to be involved in the virulence of *Y. ruckeri* has been described. This plasmid has been demonstrated to be unique from similar size plasmids in other species of *Yersinia* (Guilvout et al. 1988). Virulent isolates of *Y. ruckeri* have also been found to possess a heat-sensitive factor (Furones et al. 1990). This factor, designated extracellular products (ECP) by Romalde and Toranzo, was found to be involved in the pathogenesis of ERM disease in fish. Romalde, Conchas and Toranzo (1991) also hypothesized that *Y. ruckeri* produce a siderophore when grown under conditions of low iron concentrations which may have a role in the virulence of the organism.

REFERENCES

Abe JT, Takeda T et al., 1993, Evidence for superantigen production by *Yersinia pseudotuberculosis*, *J Immunol*, **151**: 4183–8.

Ahmedy A, Vido DM et al., 1985, Antimicrobial susceptibilities of food-isolated strains of *Yersinia enterocolitica*, *Y. intermedia*, *Y. frederiksenii* and *Y. kristensenii*, *Antimicrob Agents Chemother*, **28**: 351–3.

Aleksic S, Steigerwalt AG et al., 1987, *Yersinia rohdei* sp. nov. isolated from human and dog feces and surface water, *Int J Syst Bacteriol*, **37**: 327–32.

Alzugaray R, Gonzalez Hevia MA et al., 1995, *Yersinia enterocolitica* O:3 antimicrobial resistance patterns, virulence profiles and plasmids, *New Microbiol*, **18**: 215–22.

Andersen JK, Saunders NA, 1990, Epidemiological typing of *Yersinia enterocolitica* by analysis of restriction fragment length polymorphisms with a cloned ribosomal RNA gene, *J Med Microbiol*, **32**: 179–87.

Baert F, Peetermans W, Knockaert D, 1994, Yersiniosis: the clinical spectrum [Review], *Acta Clin Belg*, **42**: 76–85.

Bardarov SS, Sirakova TD et al., 1990, A cloned chromosomal DNA fragment which differentiates *Yersinia pestis* from *Yersinia pseudotuberculosis* and *Yersinia enterocolitica*, *FEMS Microbiol Lett*, **71**: 277–80.

Bercovier H, Mollaret HH, 1984, *Bergey's Manual of Systematic Bacteriology*, vol. 1, eds Krieg NR, Holt JG, Williams & Wilkins, Baltimore, MD, 498.

Beuscher HU, Rodel F et al., 1995, Bacterial evasion of host immune defense: *Yersinia enterocolitica* encodes a suppressor for tumor necrosis factor alpha expression, *Infect Immun*, **63**: 1270–7.

Beynon LM, Richards JC, Perry MB, 1994, The structure of the lipopolysaccharide O antigen from *Yersinia ruckeri* serotype O:1, *Carbohydr Res*, **256**: 303–17.

Bissett ML, Powers C et al., 1990, Epidemiologic investigations of *Yersinia enterocolitica* and related species: sources, frequency and serogroup distribution, *J Clin Microbiol*, **28**: 910–12.

Blumberg HM, Kiehlbauch JA, Wachsmuth IK, 1991, Molecular epidemiology of *Yersinia enterocolitica* O:3 infections: use of chromosomal DNA restriction fragment length polymorphisms of rRNA genes, *J Clin Microbiol*, **29**: 2368–74.

de Boer E, 1992, Isolation of *Yersinia enterocolitica* from foods [Review], *Int J Food Microbiol*, **17**: 75–84.

Bonacorsi SP, Scavizzi MR et al., 1994, Assessment of a fluoroquinolone, three β-lactams, two aminoglycosides and a tetracycline in treatment of murine *Yersinia pestis* infection, *Antimicrob Agents Chemother*, **38**: 481–6.

Bottone EJ, 1977, *Yersinia enterocolitica*: a panoramic view of a charismatic microorganism, *Crit Rev Mirobiol*, **5**: 211–41.

Brocklehurst TG, Lund BM, 1990, The influence of pH, temperature and organic acids on the initiation of growth of *Yersinia enterocolitica*, *J Appl Bacteriol*, **69**: 390–7.

Brubaker RR, 1991, Factors promoting acute and chronic diseases caused by yersiniae, *Clin Microbiol Rev*, **4**: 309–24.

Brubaker RR, Surgalla MJ, 1962, Pesticins II. Production of pesticin I and II, *J Bacteriol*, **84**: 539.

Brzin B, 1963, *Zentralbl Bakteriol Parasitenkd Infektionskr Hyg Abt 1 Orig*, **189**: 543.

Brzostek K, Nichols WW, 1990, Outer membrane permeability and porin proteins of *Yersinia enterocolitica*, *FEMS Microbiol Lett*, **70**: 275–8.

Burrows TW, 1963, Virulence of *Pasteurella pestis* and immunity to plague, *Curr Top Microbiol Immunol*, **37**: 59.

Cafferkey MT, Sloane A et al., 1993, *Yersinia frederiksenii* infection and colonization in hospital staff, *J Hosp Infect*, **24**: 109–15.

Caugant DA, Aleksic S et al., 1989, Clonal diversity and relationships among strains of *Yersinia enterocolitica*, *J Clin Microbiol*, **27**: 2678–83.

Chambers CE, Sokol PA, 1994, Comparison of siderophore production and utilization in pathogenic and environmental isolates of *Yersinia enterocolitica*, *J Clin Microbiol*, **32**: 32–9.

Charnetzky WT, Shuford WW, 1985, Survival and growth of *Yersinia pestis* within macrophages and an effect of the loss of the 47-megadalton plasmid on growth in macrophages, *Infect Immun*, **47**: 234–41.

Chen TH, Elberg SS, 1975, *Yersinia pestis*: correlation of ultra structures and immunological status, *Infect Immun*, **11**: 1382.

Cimolai NC, Trombley C, Blair GK, 1994, Implications of *Yersinia enterocolitica* biotyping, *Arch Dis Child*, **70**: 19–21.

Conchas RF, Carniel E, 1990, A highly efficient electroporation system for transformation of *Yersinia*, *Gene*, **87**: 133–7.

Cornelis GR, 1992, Yersiniae, finely tuned pathogens, *Molecular Biology of Bacterial Infection: Current Status and Future Perspectives*, eds Hormacche EE, Penn CW, Smyth CJ, Cambridge University Press, Cambridge, MA, 232–65.

Cornelis GR, 1994, *Yersinia* pathogenicity factors, *Curr Topics Microbiol Immunol*, **192**: 243–63.

Cornelis G, Laroche Y et al., 1987, *Yersinia enterocolitica* a primary model for bacterial invasiveness, *Rev Infect Dis*, **91**: 64–87.

Cornelis GR, Sluiters C et al., 1991, *ymoA* a *Yersinia enterocolitica* chromosomal gene modulating the expression of virulence functions, *Mol Microbiol*, **5**: 1023–34.

Cover TL, Aber RC, 1989, *Yersinia enterocolitica*, *N Engl J Med*, **321**: 16–24.

Csiszar K, Toth I, 1992, Bacteriocin-like antagonism in *Yersinia enterocolitica*, *Acta Microbiol Hung*, **39**: 193–201.

Cutrin JM, Conchas RF et al., 1994, Electrotransformation of *Yersinia ruckeri* by plasmid DNA, *Microbiologia*, **10**: 69–82.

Davis BP, Dulbecco R et al., 1980, *Microbiology*, 3rd edn, Harper & Row, New York, 680–4.

De Grandis SA, Stevenson RMW, 1985, Antimicrobial susceptibility patterns and R plasmid-mediated resistance of the fish pathogen *Yersinia ruckeri*, *Antimicrob Agents Chemother*, **27**: 938–42.

De Ryck R, Struelens MJ, Serruys E, 1994, Rapid biochemical screening for *Salmonella*, *Shigella*, *Yersinia* and *Aeromonas* isolates from stool specimens, *J Clin Microbiol*, **32**: 1583–5.

Delor I, Kaeckenbeeck A et al., 1990, Nucleotide sequence of *yst*, the *Yersinia enterocolitica* gene encoding the heat-stable enterotoxin and prevalence of the gene among pathogenic and nonpathogenic yersiniae, *Infect Immun*, **58**: 2983–8.

Doyle MP, 1990, Pathogenic *Escherichia coli*, *Yersinia enterocolitica* and *Vibrio parahaemolyticus*, *Lancet*, **336**: 1111–15.

Fantasia M, Mingrone MG et al., 1993, Characterisation of *Yersinia* species isolated from a kennel and from cattle and pig farms, *Vet Rec*, **132**: 532–4.

Farmer JJ III, Carter GP et al., 1992, Pyrazinamidase, CR-MOX agar, salicin fermentation-esculin hydrolysis, and D-xylose fermentation for identifying pathogenic serotypes of *Yersinia enterocolitica*, *J Clin Microbiol*, **30**: 2589–94.

Feng P, Keasler SP, Hill WE, 1992, Direct identification of *Yersinia enterocolitica* in blood by polymerase chain reaction amplification, *Transfusion*, **32**: 850–4.

Fenwick SG, Murray A, 1991, Detection of pathogenic *Yersinia enterocolitica* by polymerase chain reaction, *Lancet*, **337**: 496–7.

Ferber DM, Brubaker RR, 1979, Mode of action of pesticin: *N*-acetyl glucosaminidase, *J Bacteriol*, **139**: 495–501.

Ferber DM, Brubaker RR, 1981, Plasmids in *Yersinia pestis*, *Infect Immun*, **31**: 839.

Fetherston JD, Lillard Jr JW, Perry RD, 1995, Analysis of the pesticin receptor from *Yersinia pestis*: role in iron-deficient growth and possible regulation by its siderophore, *J Bacteriol*, **177**: 1824–33.

Filippov A, Solodovnikov NS et al., 1990, Plasmid content in *Yersinia pestis* strains of different origin, *FEMS Microbiol Lett*, **67**: 45–8.

Forsberg A, Viitanen AM et al., 1991, The surface-located YopN protein is involved in calcium signal transduction in *Yersinia pseudotuberculosis*, *Mol Microbiol*, **5**: 977–86.

Friedlander AM, Welkos SL et al., 1995, Relationship between virulence and immunity as revealed in recent studies of the F1 capsule of *Yersinia pestis*, *Clin Infect Dis*, **21**: S178–81.

Fukushima H, 1987, New selective agar medium for isolate of virulent *Yersinia enterocolitica*, *J Clin Microbiol*, **25**: 1068–73.

Fukushima H, Gomyoda M et al., 1993, Differentiation of *Yersinia enterocolitica* serotype O:527 strains by phenotypic and molecular techniques, *J Clin Microbiol*, **31**: 1672–4.

Fukushima H, Gomyoda M et al., 1994, Restriction endonuclease analysis of virulence plasmids for molecular epidemiology of *Yersinia*, *J Clin Microbiol*, **32**: 1410–14.

Furones MD, Gilpin MJ, Munn CB, 1993, Culture media for the differentiation of isolates of *Yersinia ruckeri* based on detection of a virulence factor, *J Appl Bacteriol*, **74**: 360–6.

Furones MD, Gilpin ML et al., 1990, Virulence of *Yersinia ruckeri* serotype I strains is associated with a heat sensitive factor HSF in cell extracts, *FEMS Microbiol Lett*, **66**: 339–44.

Galyov EE, Hakansson S et al., 1993, A secreted protein kinase of *Yersinia pseudotuberculosis* is an indispensable virulence determinant, *Nature (London)*, **361**: 730–2.

Green SP, Hartland EL et al., 1995, Role of YopH in the suppression of tyrosine phosphorylation and respiratory burst activity in murine macrophages infected with *Yersinia enterocolitica*, *J Leukocyte Biol*, **57**: 972–7.

Guilvout I, Carniel E, Pugsley AP, 1995, *Yersinia* spp. HMWP2, a cytosolic protein with a cryptic internal signal sequence which can promote alkaline phosphatase export, *J Bacteriol*, **177**: 1780-7.

Guilvout I, Quilici ML et al., 1988, Bam H1 restriction endonucleose analysis of *Yersinia ruckeri*, plasmids and their relatedness to the genus *Yersinia* 42 to 47 megadalton plasmid, *Appl Environ Microbiol*, **54**: 2594–7.

Gutman LT, 1992, *Zinsser Microbiology*, 20th edn, Appleton and Lange, Norwalk, CT, 584–94.

Gyles CL, Thoen CO, 1993, *Pathogenesis of bacterial infections in animals*, 2nd edn, Iowa State University Press, Ames, Iowa, 226–35.

Haag H, Hantke K et al., 1993, Purification of yersiniabactin: a siderophore and possible virulence factor of *Yersinia enterocolitica*, *J Gen Microbiol*, **139**: 2159–65.

Hakansson S, Bergman S et al., 1993, YopB and YopD constitute a novel class of *Yersinia* Yop proteins, *Infect Immun*, **61**: 71–80.

Hinnebusch J, Schwan TG, 1993, New method of plague surveillance using polymerase chain reaction to detect *Yersinia pestis* in fleas, *J Clin Microbiol*, **31**: 1511–14.

Hollis DG, Weaver RE et al., 1989, *Francisella philomiragia* comb. nov. formerly *Yersinia philomiragia* and *Francisella tularensis* biogroup novicida formerly *Francisella novicida* associated with human disease, *J Clin Microbiol*, **27**: 1601–8.

Holt JG, Krieg NR et al., eds, 1994, *Bergey's Manual of Determinative Bacteriology*, 9th edn, Williams and Wilkins, Baltimore.

Ibrahim A, Liesack W, Stackebrandt E, 1992, Polymerase chain reaction-gene probe detection system specific for pathogenic strains of *Yersinia enterocolitica*, *J Clin Microbiol*, **30**: 1942–7.

Imperatrice CA, Nachamkin I, 1993, Evaluation of the Vitek EPS enteric pathogen screen card for detecting *Salmonella*, *Shigella* and *Yersinia* spp., *J Clin Microbiol*, **31**: 433–5.

Iriarte M, Cornelis GR, 1995, MyfF, an element of the network regulating the synthesis of fibrillae in *Yersinia enterocolitica*, *J Bacteriol*, **177**: 738–44.

Isshiki Y, Haishima Y et al., 1992, Serological cross-reaction between *Yersinia enterocolitica* O9 and non-O1 *Vibrio cholerae* bio-serogroup Hakata and antigenic analysis of their relationship by their lipopolysaccharides, *Microbiol Immunol*, **36**: 575–81.

Ito Y, Abe J et al., 1995, Sequence analysis of the gene for a novel superantigen produced by *Yersinia pseudotuberculosis* and expression of the recombinant protein, *J Immunol*, **154**: 5896–906.

Jawetz E, Melnick J, Adelberg EA, 1978, *Review of Medical Microbiology*, 13th edn, Appleton and Lange, Norwalk, CT, 223–33.

Kapperud G, Namork E et al., 1987, Plasmid mediated surface fibrillae of *Yersinia pseudotuberculosis* and *Yersinia enterocolitica*: relationship to the outer membrane protein YOP1 and possible importance for virulence, *Infect Immun*, **55**: 2247–54.

Kapperud G, Nesbakken T et al., 1990, Comparison of restriction endonuclease analysis and phenotypic typing methods for differentiation of *Yersinia enterocolitica* isolates, *J Clin Microbiol*, **28**: 1125–31.

Kitch TT, Jacobs MR, Appelbaum PC, 1994, Evaluation of RapID onE system for identification of 379 strains in the family Enterobacteriaceae and oxidase-negative gram-negative nonfermenters, *J Clin Microbiol*, **32**: 931–4.

Kwaga J, Iversen JO, Misra V, 1992, Detection of pathogenic *Yersinia enterocolitica* by polymerase chain reaction and digoxigenin-labeled polynucleotide probes, *J Clin Microbiol*, **30**: 2668–73.

Lemaitre BC, Mazigh DA, Scavizzi MR, 1991, Failure of β-lactam antibiotics and marked efficacy of fluoroquinolones in treatment of murine *Yersinia pseudotuberculosis* infection, *Antimicrob Agents Chemother*, **35**: 1785–90.

Lucier TS, Brubaker RR, 1992, Determination of genome size macrorestriction pattern polymorphism and nonpigmentation-specific deletion in *Yersinia pestis* by pulsed-field gel electrophoresis, *J Bacteriol*, **174**: 2078–86.

L'vov VL, Gur 'yanova SV et al., 1992, Structure of the repeating unit of the O-specific polysaccharide of the lipopolysaccharide of *Yersinia kristensenii* strain 490 (O:12,25), *Carbohydr Res*, **228**: 415–22.

Makino S, Okada Y et al., 1994, PCR-based random amplified polymorphic DNA fingerprinting of *Yersinia pseudotuberculosis* and its practical applications, *J Clin Microbiol*, **32**: 65–9.

Malassez LC, Vignal W, 1883, Tuberculose zoogloeique, *Arch Physiol Norm Pathol*, **2**: 369.

Michiels T, Vanooteghem JC et al., 1991, Analysis of *virC*, an operon involved in the secretion of Yop proteins by *Yersinia enterocolitica*, *J Bacteriol*, **173**: 4994–5009.

Miyoshi-Akiyama T, Abe A et al., 1995, DNA sequencing of the gene encoding a bacterial superantigen *Yersinia pseudotuberculosis*-derived mitogen YPM and characterization of the gene product cloned YPM, *J Immunol*, **154**: 5228–34.

Nakajima H, Inoue M et al., 1992, Detection and identification of *Yersinia pseudotuberculosis* and pathogenic *Yersinia enterocolitica* by an improved polymerase chain reaction method, *J Clin Microbiol*, **30**: 2484–6.

Nicolle P, Mollaret H, Brault J, 1973, Recherches sur la lysogénie, la lysosensibilité, la lysotypie et al serologie de *Yersinia enterocolitica*, *Contrib Microbiol Immunol*, **2**: 54.

Nilehn B, Ericson C, 1969, Studies on *Yersinia enterocolitica*. Bacteriophages liberated from chloroform treated cultures, *Acta Pathol Microbiol Scand*, **75**: 177–87.

Norkina OV, Kulichenko AN et al., 1994, Development of a diagnostic test for *Yersinia pestis* by the polymerase chain reaction, *J Appl Bacteriol*, **76**: 240–5.

Pease P, 1979, Observations on L-forms of *Yersinia enterocolitica*, *J Med Microbiol*, **12**: 337.

Pepe JC, Miller VL, 1993, *Yersinia enterocolitica* invasin: a primary role in the initiation of infection, *Proc Natl Acad Sci USA*, **90**: 6473–7.

Pham JN, Bell SM, 1992, Beta-lactamase induction by imipenem in *Yersinia enterocolitica*, *Pathology*, **24**: 201–4.

Pham JN, Bell SM, 1993, The prevalence of inducible β-lactamase in clinical isolates of *Yersinia enterocolitica*, *Pathology*, **25**: 385–7.

Pham JN, Bell SM, Lanzarone JYM, 1991, Biotype and antibiotic sensitivity of 100 clinical isolates of *Yersinia enterocolitica*, *J Antimicrob Chemother*, **28**: 13–18.

Picard-Pasquier N, Picard B et al., 1990, Correlation between ribosomal DNA polymorphism and electrophoretic enzyme polymorphism in *Yersinia*, *J Gen Microbiol*, **136**: 1655–66.

Pierson DE, Falkow S, 1993, The *ail* gene of *Yersinia enterocolitica* has a role in the ability of the organism to survive serum killing, *Infect Immun*, **61**: 1846–52.

Podladchikova ON, Dikhanov GG et al., 1994, Nucleotide sequence and structural organization of *Yersinia pestis* insertion sequence IS100, *FEMS Microbiol Lett*, **121**: 269–74.

Rakin A, Saken E et al., 1994, The pesticin receptor of *Yersinia enterocolitica*: a novel virulence factor with dual function, *Mol Microbiol*, **13**: 253–63.

Rasmussen HN, Rasmussin OF et al., 1994, Specific detection of pathogenic *Yersinia enterocolitica* by two-step PCR using hot-start and DMSO, *Mol Cell Probes*, **8**: 99–108.

Robins-Browne RM, Miliotis MD et al., 1989, Evaluation of DNA colony hybridization and other techniques for detection of virulence in *Yersinia* species, *J Clin Microbiol*, **27**: 644–50.

Romalde JL, 1993, Pathological activities of *Yersinia ruckeri* the enteric redmouth ERM bacterium, *FEMS Microbiol Lett*, **112**: 291–300.

Romalde JL, Conchas RF, Toranzo AE, 1991, Evidence that *Yersinia ruckeri* possesses a high affinity iron uptake system, *FEMS Microbiol Lett*, **64**: 121–5.

Rosquist R, Forsberg A, Wolf-Watz H, 1991, Intracellular targeting of the *Yersinia* YopE cytotoxin in mammalian cells induces actin microfilament disruption, *Infect Immun*, **59**: 4562–9.

Saken E, Roggenkamp A et al., 1994, Characterisation of pathogenic *Yersinia enterocolitica* serogroups by pulsed-field gel electrophoresis of genomic *Not* I restriction fragments, *J Med Microbiol*, **41**: 329–38.

Salyers AA, Whitt DD, 1994, *Bacterial Pathogenesis A Molecular Approach*, ASM Press, Washington DC, 213–28.

Sharma NK, Doyle PW et al., 1990, Identification of *Yersinia* species by the API 20E, *J Clin Microbiol*, **28**: 1443–4.

Skurnik M, el Tahir Y et al., 1994, YadA mediates specific binding of enteropathogenic *Yersinia enterocolitica* to human intestinal submucosa, *Infect Immun*, **62**: 1252–61.

Smith MD, Vinh DX et al., 1995, In vitro antimicrobial susceptibilities of strains of *Yersinia pestis*, *Antimicrob Agents Chemother*, **39:** 2153–4.

Sodeinde OA, Subrahmanyam YVBK et al., 1992, A surface protease and the invasive character of plague, *Science*, **258:** 1004–7.

Solomon T, 1995, Alexandre Yersin and the plague bacillus, *J Trop Med Hyg*, **98:** 209–12.

Staggs TM, Perry RD, 1992, Fur regulation in *Yersinia* species, *Mol Microbiol*, **61:** 2507–16.

Straley SC, Skrzypek E, Plano GVE, 1993, Yops of *Yersinia* spp. pathogenic for humans, *Infect Immun*, **61:** 3105–10.

Tashiro K, Kubokura Y et al., 1991, Survival of *Yersinia enterocolitica* in soil and water, *J Vet Med Sci*, **53:** 23–7.

Tertti R, Skurnik M et al., 1992, Adhesion protein YadA of *Yersinia* species mediates binding of bacteria to fibronectin, *Infect Immun*, **60:** 3021–4.

Toora S, 1995, Partial purification and characterization of bacteriocin from *Yersinia kristensenii*, *J Appl Bacteriol*, **78:** 224–8.

Toora S, Budu-Amoako E et al., 1994, Evaluation of different antimicrobial agents used as selective supplements for isolation and recovery of *Yersinia enterocolitica*, *J Appl Bacteriol*, **77:** 67–72.

Viitanen AM, Arstila TP et al., 1991, Application of the polymerase chain reaction and immunofluorescence techniques to the detection of bacteria in *Yersinia*-triggered reactive arthritis, *Arthritis Rheum*, **34:** 89–96.

Visser LG, Annema A, van Furth R, 1995, Role of Yops in inhibition of phagocytosis and killing of opsonized *Yersinia enterocolitica* by human granulocytes, *Infect Immun*, **63:** 2570–5.

Wachtel MR, Miller VL, 1995, In vitro and in vivo characterization of an *ail* mutant of *Yersinia enterocolitica*, *Infect Immun*, **63:** 2541–8.

Wauters G, 1981, Antigens of *Yersinia enterocolitica*, *Yersinia enterocolitica*, CRC Press, Boca Raton, FL, 41–53.

Wauters G, Kandolo K, Janssens M, 1987, Revised biogrouping scheme of *Yersinia enterocolitica*, *Contrib Microbiol Immunol*, **9:** 14–21.

Wauters G, Janssens M et al., 1988, *Yersinia mollaretii* sp. nov. and *Yersinia bercovieri* sp. nov. formerly called *Yersinia enterocolitica* biogroups 3A and 3B, *Int J Syst Bacteriol*, **38:** 424–9.

Wren BW, Tabaqchali S, 1990, Detection of pathogenic *Yersinia enterocolitica* by the polymerase chain reaction, *Lancet*, **336:** 693.

Yamamoto T, Hanawa T, Ogata S, 1994, Induction of *Yersinia enterocolitica* stress proteins by phagocytosis with macrophage, *Microbiol Immunol*, **38:** 295–300.

Zykin LF, 1994, The results of a 15-year study of the persistence of *Yersinia pestis* L-forms, *Zh Mikrobiol Epidemiol Immunobiol*, **Suppl. 1:** 68–71.

Chapter 45

VIBRIO, AEROMONAS AND PLESIOMONAS

J M Janda

1 INTRODUCTION

The family Vibrionaceae was first proposed by Véron (1965) to include 3 genera (*Vibrio, Aeromonas, Plesiomonas*) that were potentially pathogenic for humans. Recent molecular and chemotaxonomic studies indicate that both *Aeromonas* and *Plesiomonas* are not closely related to true members of this family (*Vibrio, Photobacterium*). Colwell, MacDonell and De Ley (1986) have proposed that there is sufficient phylogenetic depth within the aeromonad group to warrant creation of their own family, the Aeromonadaceae. For *Plesiomonas*, most molecular studies indicate that this genus is closest to the family Enterobacteriaceae, and in particular to the genus *Proteus*. To include plesiomonads in this family, however, would require redefining the essential characteristics of this group. Despite these taxonomic uncertainties, all 3

genera share a number of features, including similar biochemical and cultural properties, ecological habitats, and disease spectrum in humans, and this chapter therefore will take a traditional approach in discussing these bacteria.

The pre-eminent pathogen of this family is *Vibrio cholerae*. Probably no disease in modern times has engendered such fear and panic in the general population as cholera (see Volume 3, Chapter 26). The causative agent, *V. cholerae*, was first described by Pacini in 1854 and later isolated in pure culture by Koch in 1886 while working in Egypt. Cholera is insidious in onset and has a high morbidity and significant mortality rate. At least 7 cholera pandemics have been reported, the last having begun in 1961 in the Celebes in Indonesia. From there it spread over the intervening 4 decades to many geographic regions of the world including Asia, the Middle East, Africa, and Eastern

Table 45.1 Key features of members of the family Vibrionaceae

Character	Vibrio	Photobacterium	Aeromonas	Plesiomonas
Oxidase	+	+	+	+
Fermentative metabolism	+	+	+	+
Flagella				
polar	+	+	+	+
sheathed	+	–	–	–
Na⁺ required	+	+	–	–
Luminescence	dᵃ	d	–	–
D-Glucose as sole carbon source	+	+	+	+
Cellular fatty acids				
3-hydroxylauric (3-OH-12:0, ≥2%)	+	+	–	+
pentadecenoic (i-15:1)	–	–	+	–
cis-9,10-methylene hexadecanoic (17-cyc, ≥3%)	–	d	–	–
Major polyamines				
norspermidine	+ᵇ	+	–	–
putrescine	–	–	+	+
cadaverine	–	–	–	+
Mol% G + C	38–51	40–44	57–63	51
Major habitat				
marine	+	+	–	–
freshwater	–	–	+	+
Pathogenicity				
humans	+	–	+	+
animals	+	–	+	+

ᵃFor some species.
ᵇExcept for *V. fischeri.*
Data from Lambert et al. 1983, Baumann and Schubert 1984, Urdaci et al. 1990, Yamamoto et al. 1991, Farmer III and Hickman-Brenner 1991.

Europe. The highest incidence of infection has been found in developing (third world) countries where poor hygiene and lack of sanitation systems exist (see Volume 3, Chapter 26).

In addition to *V. cholerae*, many other species of vibrios play important roles in the human disease process. Of increasing medical concern is *Vibrio vulnificus*, a highly invasive vibrio species affecting immunocompromised persons who have consumed raw oysters. Fatality rates in cases of *V. vulnificus* septicaemia can approach 70%. *Vibrio parahaemolyticus*, recognized for more than 40 years, is a major cause of foodborne illnesses in South East Asia, particularly Japan. Both *Aeromonas* and *Plesiomonas* can cause a wide range of serious localized and disseminated infections in humans. *Aeromonas* is the most frequently isolated genus of the family Vibrionaceae associated with human illnesses in industrialized countries. The overall clinical importance of both genera, however, will depend on whether their isolation from cases of gastroenteritis, the most frequent illness each genus is associated with, is as a bona fide aetiological agent of disease or simply as a transient colonizer.

VIBRIO

2 DEFINITION

2.1 Genus

Gram-negative, catalase-positive, and facultatively anaerobic rods. Motile by means of a single polar flagellum. Most species are oxidase-positive and reduce nitrates. Anaerogenic fermentation of many common monosaccharides, disaccharides and some alcoholic sugars (D-mannitol, glycerol). Acid not usually produced from methyl pentoses, hexoses (except L-arabinose), trisaccharides, glycosides, and non-carbohydrate compounds such as *m*-inositol. Most species are susceptible to 10 and/or 150 µg of the vibriostatic agent O/129 (2,4-diamino-6,7-di-isopropylpteridine). Nutritional requirements for most vibrios are simple. NaCl supplementation of basal medium is stimulatory and in some cases obligatory for growth. Many extracellular enzymes are produced, including cytolytic and cytotonic toxins, proteases, nucleases, lipases, sulphatases, lecithinase, chitinase and amylase. The genus is commonly found in aquatic environments and in vertebrate and invertebrate animals that inhabit these ecosystems. Some species are pathogenic for humans (Table 45.1). The G + C content of DNA is 38–51 mol%. Type species is *V. cholerae.*

2.2   Species

There are presently 36 nomenspecies in the genus *Vibrio*, the latest addition being *V. penaeicida* (Ishimaru, Akagawa-Matsushita and Muroga 1995). At least 12 species are thought to be potentially pathogenic for humans. Most recently described *Vibrio* species have been defined by DNA–DNA reassociation kinetics but some (*V. cincinnatiensis*) have been proposed using only 5S rRNA sequences (Brayton et al. 1986). Strains of *Vibrio* of a given species usually exhibit >85% similarity in phenotypic characteristics (unweighted), ≥97% homology in their 5S rRNA sequences and between 80 and 100% homology at the DNA level; ≥92% sequence homology in 5S rRNA is shared between strains from distinct *Vibrio* species (MacDonell et al. 1986).

3   HABITAT

Vibrios are normal inhabitants of the marine environment including areas contiguous with seas and oceans such as inlets, estuaries and coastal shores. As part of the normal microbial burden of the aquatic biosphere they are also intimately associated with a number of vertebrate and invertebrate species (e.g. fish, shellfish, zooplankton and in some instances plants) that inhabit these ecosystems. For non-halophilic species such as *V. cholerae* and *V. mimicus*, their environmental distribution is significantly extended as they can be isolated from freshwater rivers, streams and lakes in regions of the world far removed from the marine environment. Humans, an incidental and transient host, can promote dissemination into uncontaminated freshwater sources and foods during epidemic or pandemic conditions where sanitation and socioeconomic conditions are poor. However, such transmission probably has little impact on their long-term persistence and survival in the natural environment.

Vibrios, as typified by *V. cholerae*, can probably exist in the marine environment in several forms. First, they can be recovered as part of the water column in a free-living state, particularly during times when water temperatures and nutrient concentrations are elevated. A second phase, termed epibiotic, refers to the association of vibrios with specific substrates such as the chitinous matrix of shellfish. Under these conditions vibrios develop an intimate association with shellfish or copepods via the production of substrate-specific enzymes (chitinase) or amino sugar-binding proteins. This cycle is thought to be favoured under nutrient-poor conditions. Vibrios appear to survive longer in the epibiotic than the free-living form. Thus, the epibiotic form may not only be a mechanism for environmental persistence but also for dissemination,

as chitin-bound vibrios may be better equipped than unattached vibrios to escape the normally lethal consequences of gastric acidity upon ingestion by humans.

A third form is characterized by vibrios being recovered in a 'quiescent' state. This transformation can occur in several ways, ranging from the formation of a microvibrio (Hood et al. 1984) to a 'viable but non-culturable' vibrio (Colwell and Huq 1994). Microvibrios have altered morphologies with a decrease in size and metabolic activities. Microvibrios appear to form in response to nutrient scarcity and a limitation in particulate surfaces to which to attach (epibiotic). Viable but non-culturable *V. cholerae* cells can be detected by fluorescent staining techniques, yet they fail to grow upon plating onto routine non-selective media. Such microbial adaptation appears related to the lack of availability of sufficient nutrients in the environment. Starved vibrios can be converted to a non-culturable state in laboratory-developed microcosms where cells persist in a dormant but viable form for months. The contributory nature of each of these processes to the persistence of vibrios in the environment is a subject of conjecture.

4   MORPHOLOGY

V. cholerae bacilli are (0.5–0.8) mm × (1.5–2.5) mm in size. In young cultures vibrios may appear curved or comma-shaped and S forms may occur. However, vibrios are often indistinguishable morphologically from other enteric organisms appearing as typical straight gram-negative rods. Vibrios can also exhibit morphological pleomorphism when grown or plated onto broth or media containing suboptimal concentrations of required electrolytes (NaCl). Under these conditions, and occasionally when stained directly from body fluids, halophilic vibrios may range in appearance from thin elongated rods (with minimal curvature) to coccal-bacillary forms. In liquid media all vibrios show vigorous darting motility. Flagella are 24–30 nm thick with a central core (14–16 nm) surrounded by the sheath, which is continuous with the outer membrane of the cell envelope.

Ultrastructural studies have revealed the presence of pili (fimbriae) in select strains of *V. cholerae* O1 and non-O1 (Hall et al. 1988, Honda et al. 1988a) and *V. parahaemolyticus* (Honda et al. 1988b, Nakasone and Iwanaga 1990). Pilus-like structures have also been observed in *V. vulnificus* (Gander and LaRocco 1989). A capsule has been detected in *V. cholerae* O139 cells stained with uranyl acetate (Yamamoto, Albert and Sack 1994). Thin sections (polycationic ferritin-stained) of *V. cholerae* O139 indicate the presence of a thin electron-dense capsule (Johnson et al. 1994). Polysaccharide capsules have also been detected in strains of *V. cholerae* non-O1 (Johnson, Panigrahi and Morris 1992). In *V. vulnificus*, thin sections of ruthenium red-stained cells depict the presence of a 60 nm thick capsule with a relatively low electron density (Amako, Okada and Miake 1984). Such capsules are present on both clinical and environmental strains of *V. vulnificus* (Hayat et al. 1993).

5 CULTURAL CHARACTERISTICS AND GROWTH REQUIREMENTS

5.1 Culture

On most non-selective media containing 0.5–1.0% NaCl, vibrios appear as smooth, convex colonies 2–5 mm in diameter after overnight incubation at 35–37°C. Nutrient agar (Difco), lacking the required concentration of salt, will not support the growth of most halophilic *Vibrio* species without NaCl supplementation. Colonies are usually buff in appearance but translucent and opaque varieties are known to exist. Rough variants, termed rugose, are wrinkled in appearance and difficult to emulsify. They are occasionally recovered from both environmental and clinical specimens. Some strains of *V. alginolyticus* and *V. parahaemolyticus* can swarm on solid media, with progressive spreading across the agar surface. For *V. parahaemolyticus*, this adaptation from broth to solid media requires the formation of lateral flagella (Laf) in addition to a single polar flagellum (Fla) (McCarter and Silverman 1990). Swarming and Laf formation are dependent upon 2 environmental triggers: limited flagellar rotation and iron deprivation.

Selective media designed for the isolation of members of this genus have revolved around their resistance to toxic levels of certain organic and inorganic compounds (potassium iodide), antimicrobial agents (polymyxin B) and tolerance to highly alkaline conditions (pH 8.6). The most widely used selective medium for the isolation of vibrios is thiosulphate–citrate–bile salts–sucrose (TCBS). This medium was originally designed by Kobayashi et al. (1963) for the isolation of *V. cholerae* and *V. parahaemolyticus* and predates the discovery of most current species in the genus *Vibrio*. Although TCBS is used to isolate most *Vibrio* species, its specificity and sensitivity for detecting these non-cholera species has never been satisfactorily evaluated. The plating efficiencies of certain vibrios, notably *V. damsela*, *V. hollisae* and *V. cincinnatiensis*, are notoriously poor on TCBS. Variability in both the specificity and sensitivity of different lots of TCBS from various commercial suppliers to recover vibrios has been noted. Such variability requires rigorous quality control of each lot of TCBS before its introduction into routine use. After overnight incubation on TCBS, vibrios can be separated into 2 major groups based upon their ability to utilize sucrose. Yellow colonies, indicating sucrose fermentation, are indicative of the possible presence of *V. cholerae*, *V. alginolyticus*, or *V. fluvialis* and green (sucrose-negative) colonies are observed when *V. parahaemolyticus*, *V. vulnificus* or *V. mimicus* is present. Other media recently designed for the selective isolation or differentiation of *Vibrio* species or groups include polymyxin–mannose–tellurite agar (Shimada et al. 1990) and thiosulphate–chloride–iodide agar (Beazley and Palmer 1992). Vibrios can also be recovered on enteric media such as MacConkey, although they may be missed due to their smaller numbers or fermentation of lactose (*V. vulnificus*). One species, *V. hollisae*, fails to grow on most common media used in the bacteriology laboratory (TCBS, MacConkey). When isolated, it has almost invariably been recovered on blood agar.

BLOOD AGAR

One of the most useful media in the isolation, recognition and identification of members of the family Vibrionaceae is blood agar. Many *Vibrio* species produce zones of β-haemolysis on blood agar plates after overnight incubation at 35–37°C. This haemolytic reaction is useful in both biotype and species identification. Most strains of *V. cholerae*, *V. mimicus*, *V. fluvialis*, *V. damsela* and *V. hollisae* produce classic β-haemolysis after 24 h of incubation on blood agar containing either sheep, rabbit or horse erythrocytes. For *V. cholerae*, haemolysis of sheep red blood cells has been traditionally used as one of several tests to distinguish the 2 biotypes of *V. cholerae* O1. The classic biotype is non-haemolytic while the El Tor biotype is haemolytic; non-O1 *V. cholerae* strains are usually haemolytic. *V. parahaemolyticus*, *V. alginolyticus* and *V. vulnificus* are typically non-haemolytic or produce only α-haemolysis (greening) after similar incubation periods. Haemolysis of erythrocytes by *Vibrio* species is due to several types of enzymatic activities including cytolytic toxins (*V. fluvialis*, *V. metschnikovii*) or phospholipases (*V. damsela*). In addition to its non-selective properties (*V. hollisae* grows on blood agar), key biochemical reactions (cytochrome oxidase, tryptophanase deamination) can be tested for directly on isolated colonies using spot tests.

Although certain species do not produce overt haemolysis on standard blood agar plates, they do exhibit haemolytic activity under defined conditions. Clinical isolates of *V. parahaemolyticus* produce β-haemolysis on Wagatsuma agar, a high salt (7%) blood agar (human O, rabbit) medium containing D-mannitol as the carbohydrate source (Miyamoto et al. 1969). This reaction, termed the Kanagawa phenomenon, has diagnostic as well as pathogenic significance. *V. vulnificus* produces at least 2 different proteins which can produce a delayed haemolysis (lag period) of red blood cells in broth.

5.2 Growth requirements

The cardinal feature of all vibrios is their exacting growth requirement for salt (Baumann, Furniss and Lee 1984). All *Vibrio* species require salt supplementation for optimal growth and most will not grow in media without its addition (see Table 45.1). *Vibrio* species exhibit a broad spectrum in their salt requirements for optimal growth ranging from a low of >20 mM NaCl requirement (*V. cholerae*) to an upper end of a >600 mM NaCl required by the marine species *V. costicola*. This difference in salt requirement has diagnostic implications and has led to the classic separation of pathogenic vibrios into 2 major groups. The non-halophilic species, consisting of *V. cholerae* and *V. mimicus*, will grow on routine media such as nutrient agar (Difco) without added salt. An occasional strain of *V. fluvialis* or *V. furnissii* will produce delayed growth on unsupplemented nutrient agar after 3–4 days of incubation. The halophilic species require salt supplementation. All species (halophilic and non-halophilic) will grow in the presence of higher (6%) salt concentrations. This unique growth characteristic is of some help in separating halophilic species from non-halophilic members although the range of salt (0–12%) permitting growth of individual species is less useful since there is significant overlap between many individual groups. Because many common laboratory media contain only 0.5% NaCl, halophilic vibrios will often fail to grow in decarboxylase or nitrate broths or in the Voges–Proskauer medium. When vibrios are suspected in an unknown culture, all laboratory identification media should be additionally supplemented with 0.5–1.0% salt.

Vibrios grow over a wide temperature range (20–>40°C) with most clinically significant species exhibiting optimal growth at 35–37°C. The lower limit for most strains is 10–15°C although a few, including *V. metschnikovii* and *V. anguillarum*, will grow at 4°C. Vibrios favour alkaline over acidic conditions for optimal growth although most species grow between a pH range of 6.5 and 9.0.

6 METABOLISM

D-Glucose is anaerobically catabolized by vibrios via a constitutive Embden–Meyerhof pathway, producing formic, acetic, lactic, pyruvic and succinic acids and ethanol as end products of a mixed acid fermentation (Baumann, Furniss and Lee 1984). D-Glucose and many other sugars are transported internally via the phosphoenolpyruvate:carbohydrate phosphotransferase system whereby the sugar is transported and subsequently phosphorylated to glucose-6-phosphate (Sarker et al. 1994). In some halophilic species such as *V. alginolyticus* and *V. parahaemolyticus* amino acid and sugar transport is Na^+ dependent and an electrochemical potential across the membrane can be created by the extrusion of Na^+ which in turn drives nutrient transport into the cell (Sarker et al. 1994). Fermentation of D-glucose does not result in gas production except in the case of *V. furnissii* and rare strains of *V. damsela* (see Table 45.1).

7 GENETIC MECHANISMS

Plasmid carriage is an infrequent occurrence in pathogenic vibrios (Guidolin and Manning 1987, Nandy et al. 1995). It has been estimated that 2% of *V. cholerae* O1 strains, 38% of *V. cholerae* O139 and 25% of other *V. cholerae* non-O1 strains from both clinical and environmental sources harbour such extrachromosomal elements (Newland, Voll and McNicol 1984, Nandy et al. 1995). Most strains possess a single plasmid. Most cryptic plasmids detected in non-O1 *V. cho-*

lerae strains are of low molecular weight [$(2–4) \times 10^3$ kDa]. Twedt, Brown and Zink (1981) analysed 31 *V. parahaemolyticus* of varying phenotypes and found >10% to contain plasmids, although all 3 contained a 6×10^3 kDa plasmid. In *V. cholerae*, several types of plasmids are known to exist, including a conjugal system mediated by a plasmid sex factor designated P^+ which is similar to the F fertility factor of *Escherichia coli* (Guidolin and Manning 1987). Plasmids of the IncC incompatibility group have also been reported and have been linked to increased antimicrobial resistance among *V. cholerae* strains. In addition to drug resistance, plasmids have been implicated in decreased cholera toxin production and resistance to the vibriostatic agent O/129 in *V. cholerae* (Matsushita, Kudoh and Ohashi 1984).

V. cholerae do not undergo transformation or transfection under reproducible conditions which may be due to their copious production of extracellular deoxyribonuclease and restriction and modification systems (Guidolin and Manning 1987, Marcus et al. 1990). However, generalized vibriophage transduction and lysogenation has been reported to occur. One bacteriophage, named CP-T1, has been implicated in serotype and biotype modification via lysogenic conversion. Insertion sequences, common in many gram-negative bacteria, have been reported only once. This transposable sequence (RS1) is a 2.7 kb repeated sequence that flanks the cholera toxin in *V. cholerae* (Mekalanos 1983).

8 CELLULAR ORGANIZATION

8.1 Cell wall

The cell wall architecture of the genus *Vibrio* is typical of most gram-negative fermentative bacilli. The outer membrane consists of a lipopolysaccharide (LPS) region which contains the traditional lipid A–core–O. polysaccharide side chain regions. The LPS of *V. cholerae* has been extensively characterized. The lipid A portion consists of a $\beta(1'\rightarrow6)$-linked D-glucosamine disaccharide with 2 phosphoryl groups (Rietschel et al. 1984). Phosphorylethanolamine is linked to one of these glycosidic phosphoryl groups (Rietschel et al. 1984). The principal ester- and amide-bound acyl groups consist of a saturated O-acylated-3-hydroxy fatty acid (12:0) and an amide-bound 3-O-acylated fatty acid (14:0). The core region contains the unusual 8 carbon sugar 2-keto-3-deoxyoctonate (KDO). This sugar, which is a normal constituent of enteric LPS, was originally thought to be absent in *Vibrio* species. However, when conventional thiobarbituric acid assays were replaced by strong acid hydrolysates, KDO was detected (Brade 1985). Unlike *Salmonella* and *Escherichia coli*, the KDO moiety of *V. cholerae* possesses some unique features. First, only a single molecule of KDO exists in the core region (Kondo, Haishima and Hisatsune 1990). The C4 position of KDO in *V. cholerae* binds a phosphate molecule instead of a second KDO residue like many other enteric organisms; the C5 position of KDO binds to a distal portion of the core region (heptose) similar to the KDO–C5 binding of L-glycero-D-mannoheptose by enteric organisms. Although other vibrios have not been extensively investigated, *V. parahaemolyticus* has recently been shown to contain KDO phosphate by gas chromatography-mass spectrometry analysis (Han and Chai 1991). The outer O polysaccharide side chain region in *V. cholerae* contains a number of unusual sugars including 2-amino-2,6-dideoxy-D-glucose(quinovosamine), 4-amino-4-deoxy-L-arabinose, and 4-amino-4,6-dideoxy-D-mannose (Guidolin and Manning 1987).

8.2 Cellular fatty acids

Fatty acid methyl ester analysis of both pathogenic and non-pathogenic *Vibrio* species by capillary gas liquid chromatography have yielded similar results (Lambert et al. 1983, Urdaci, Marchand and Grimont 1990). The major fatty acids detected in all vibrios were hexadecenoic (16:1), octadecenoic (18:1) and *n*-hexadecanoic (16:0). Many other fatty acids were present in small to moderate amounts (see Table 45.1). Some species or groups could be distinguished or separated by their cellular fatty acid composition although significant overlap existed between several groups. Clusters that could not be resolved to the species level included *V. alginolyticus–V. parahaemolyticus–V. natriegens*, *V. metschnikovii–V. cincinnatiensis*, and *V. cholerae–V. mimicus* (Lambert et al. 1983, Urdaci, Marchand and Grimont 1990).

8.3 Antigenic structure

V. CHOLERAE

The antigenic characteristics of *Vibrio* species are primarily defined by 2 structural features, namely the LPS (O or somatic antigens) and the flagellum (H or flagellar antigens). There are currently 155 recognized serogroups within *V. cholerae* (Shimada et al. 1994a). Each serogroup is defined by the uniqueness of specific antisera raised in rabbits to heat-killed suspensions of smooth cultures of the reference strain (Sakazaki and Donovan 1984). Antisera for each serogroup must be absorbed with an R strain of *V. cholerae* (strain CA385) before its first use since all somatic antisera contain some R antibodies. For the flagellum, actively motile strains are obtained by multiple passages in semi-solid medium. The growth is harvested in

0.6% formalinized saline and flagella are separated from other bacterial components by mechanical shearing and differential centrifugation prior to rabbit immunization. All strains of *V. cholerae* express the same flagellar antigen as determined by immunodiffusion. H antigens of *V. cholerae* may be difficult to detect by slide or tube agglutination because the sheath may prevent access to the antigenic sites on the flagellum. This may be overcome by pretreatment with formalin or phenol or by ageing cultures to remove the sheath (Sakazaki and Donovan 1984). *V. cholerae* H antisera share partial or complete identity with the flagellum of many other *Vibrio* species including *V. mimicus*, *V. fluvialis*, *V. alginolyticus*, *V. metschnikovii*, *V. parahaemolyticus* and *V. anguillarum*.

The O1 serogroup of *V. cholerae* has held a pre-eminent position within this group for its singular association with strains responsible for epidemic and pandemic cholera. *V. cholerae* O1 strains can be detected in the laboratory using polyclonal O1 antisera in slide agglutination assays (see Table 45.2). Commercially developed monoclonal based coagglutination and colorimetric immunodiagnostic assays have been developed to detect specifically the O1 antigen of *V. cholerae* (Colwell et al. 1992, Hasan et al. 1994). These tests allow for colony confirmation (coagglutination) or direct detection (colorimetric immunoassay) of *V. cholerae* O1 with a high degree of specificity and sensitivity. Within the O1 group there are 3 distinct serotypes, Ogawa, Inaba and Hikojima, that produce 3 antigenic factors designated a, b and c. They are present in the LPS in a complex ab, ac fashion. The Hikojima serotype is not universally recognized by all investigators. For the Ogawa and Inaba serotypes, the O polysaccharide chain consists of a repeating homopolymer of perosaminyl (1→2-linked 4-amino-4,6-dideoxy-α-D-mannopyranosyl) residues (Gotoh, Barnes and Kovác 1994). Although the exact molecular changes responsible for the antigenic differences observed between these 2 serogroups are not completely understood, the presence of a novel sugar, 4-amino-4,6-dideoxy-2-*O*-methylmannose, in the LPS of Ogawa (not Inaba) and the 2-O-methylation of D-perosamine at the non-reducing terminus of Ogawa may partly explain these antigenic differences (Hisatsune et al. 1993b, Ito et al. 1994). The *rfb* locus (rough B) is apparently responsible for serotype conversion in *V. cholerae* O1 from Ogawa to Inaba. One gene product, rfbT, encodes for a 32 kDa protein involved in O-anti-

Table 45.2 Serotypes of *V. cholerae* O1

Serotype	Agglutination in polyclonal O1 antisera	Agglutination with mAb against factor			Frequency	Epidemic spread
		a	b	c		
Ogawa	+	+	+	−	Common	Yes
Inaba	+	+	−	+	Common	Yes
Hikojima	+	+	+	+	Very rare	Unknown

mAb, monoclonal antibodies to each O1 factor.

gen biosynthesis (Stroeher et al. 1992). Mutations in rfbT, causing premature termination of the gene product, invariably result in the Inaba serotype specificity (Stroeher et al. 1992, Ito et al. 1993). Some non-O1 groups of *V. cholerae* have been found to react in O1 antisera. These include *V. cholerae* O140 (Hakata serogroup) which shares the c factor in common with Inaba but does not possess either the a or b factors (Shimada et al. 1994b).

The emergence of a non-O1 serogroup ('Bengal strain') as a major cause of epidemic cholera in the Indian subcontinent and in South East Asia has broken a hard and fast cardinal rule regarding the exclusive association of epidemic cholera with the O1 serogroup of *V. cholerae*. This serogroup has been designated O139 by Shimada et al. (1994a). It shares some antigenic cross-reactivity with several other non-O1 *V. cholerae* serogroups including O22 and O155.

OTHER *VIBRIO* SPECIES

A number of serotyping schemes have been developed for non-cholera vibrios. *V. parahaemolyticus* is composed of 13 thermostable serogroups (9 chemotypes) and >60 thermolabile capsular (K) antigens (Joseph, Colwell and Kaper 1982, Hisatsune et al. 1993a). These factors are epidemiologically useful but do not have pathogenic significance as is the case with *V. cholerae*. *V. vulnificus* contains 7 serovars of which O1 and O3 appear to be the most common (Shimada and Sakazaki 1984). Serotyping of *V. vulnificus* strains requires the use of heat-killed antigens since most live strains are non-agglutinable due to a heat-labile masking antigen. A single flagellar antigen is known to exist. *V.*

fluvialis and *V. furnissii* share a combined serotyping system composed of 35 O-antigen groups (Shimada et al. 1991). Some serogroups share partial or complete serological identity with some non-O1 *V. cholerae* groups (O6, O39, O41); the O19 serogroup of *V. fluvialis*–*V. furnissii* also crosses with *V. cholerae* O1 Inaba (c factor). The flagellar antigen of *V. mimicus* is identical to that of *V. cholerae* and the LPS of most *V. mimicus* strains type with *V. cholerae* somatic antisera (Sakazaki and Donovan 1984).

9 CLASSIFICATION

Single linkage analysis of the results of rRNA–DNA hybridization investigations indicate a high degree of relatedness (≥80%) between the genera *Vibrio* and *Photobacterium* and a much lower level of relatedness (≤60%) with the genera *Aeromonas* and *Plesiomonas* (Baumann and Schubert 1984). Subsequent studies of members of the family Vibrionaceae, based upon sequence analysis of small unit, 5S and 16S rRNA, have generated similar findings (MacDonell et al. 1986, Dorsch, Lane and Stackebrandt 1992, Ruimy et al. 1994). These collective results support the removal of *Aeromonas* from this group and creation of its own family, the Aeromonadaceae (Colwell, MacDonell and De Ley 1986). *Plesiomonas* appears most closely related to the family Enterobacteriaceae and the genus *Proteus*. Even within the genus *Vibrio*, many species are not closely related on a phylogenetic basis, exhibiting <30% homology based upon DNA–DNA reassociation kinetics (Farmer III and Hickman-Brenner 1991). Sev-

Table 45.3 Key tests in the separation of the genera *Vibrio*, *Aeromonas* and *Pleisomonas*

Character	Vibrio		Aeromonas	Plesiomonas
	Non-halophilic	**Halophilic**		
Oxidase	+	+[a]	+	+
Growth on nutrient agar (Difco) with				
0% NaCl	+	−	+	+
6% NaCl	+	+	−	−
Glucose				
fermentation	+	+	+	+
gas production	−	−[b]	d	−
String test	+	+[c]	−	−
O/129 resistance				
10 µg	−[d]	d	+	−
150 µg	−[d]	d	+	−
Ampicillin (10 µg)	S	d	R[e]	R
Growth on TCBS	+	+[f]	−[g]	−

+, positive reaction; −, negative reaction; d, different for different species; S, susceptible; R, resistant; TCBS, thiosulphate–citrate–bile salts–sucrose agar.
[a]Except for *V. metschnikovii*.
[b]Except for *V. furnissii* and rare strains of *V. damsela*.
[c]Except for some strains of *V. parahaemolyticus*.
[d]Most strains (>90%) of *V. cholerae* O1 in India are resistant to both concentrations.
[e]Except for *A. trota*.
[f]Except for *V. hollisae*.
[g]Lot-to-lot variability exists.
Table adapted from Janda, Abbott and Morris Jr (1995).

eral distinct lineages exist including the *V. cholerae–V. mimicus* group, the *V. fluvialis–V. furnissii* complex, and the *V. parahaemolyticus–V. alginolyticus* line. Some species (*V. anguillarum, V. damsela*) have been proposed for transfer to other genera (*Listonella, Photobacterium*) whereas other species appear to be objective synonyms (*V. harveyi = V. carchariae*).

10 LABORATORY ISOLATION AND IDENTIFICATION

10.1 Genus identification

The most difficult aspect of the laboratory identification of members of the family Vibrionaceae is the initial assignment of unidentified isolates to the correct genus. This process is further complicated by alarming trends where major changes in the phenotype frequency of key differential tests has recently been reported. The vibriostatic agent O/129 (2,4-diamino-6,7-di-isopropylpteridine) is a pteridine compound that inhibits the synthesis of tetrahydrofolic acid from *p*-aminobenzoic acid by blocking the enzyme dihydrofolate reductase (Nath and Sanyal 1992). Resistance in *V. cholerae* O1 to the vibriostatic agent O/129, an unheard of phenotype 2 decades ago, is now the predominant pattern being reported from India (Ramamurthy et al. 1992). Such strains, though still an infrequent occurrence in most regions of the globe, have been reported from other areas of the world including the US (Abbott et al. 1992a). Most strains of *V. cholerae* O139 are also resistant to O/129 although some susceptible isolates have been identified (Yam, Yuen and Wong 1994). TCBS, once a valuable screening tool for the separation of vibrios (growth) from aeromonads and plesiomonads (no growth), is becoming less useful since significant

batch variability in the selective nature of this medium has been noted. One of the few remaining classic diagnostic tests that accurately separates the genus *Vibrio* from the genera *Aeromonas* and *Plesiomonas* is the growth of vibrios in media containing high concentrations of salt. Virtually all vibrios grow in the presence of 6–6.5% NaCl (w/v) while aeromonads and plesiomonads do not. Another useful test that aids in the separation of these genera is the 'string test', so called because organisms emulsified in 0.5% sodium deoxycholate produce a viscous DNA suspension that strings when the loop is slowly raised away from the emulsification (Farmer III and Hickman-Brenner 1991). Regardless of test reliability, no single phenotypic marker should be used to identify strains exclusively to the genus level; rather, a battery of differential tests should be utilized in determining correct generic assignments.

10.2 Species identification

Based upon salt requirements determined in screening tests (see Table 45.3), presumptive vibrios can then be identified to species using selected biochemical characteristics (Table 45.4). Of particular importance is the previously noted requirement to supplement several biochemical tests with sufficient salt in order to achieve a final concentration of ≥1% NaCl. Gram-negative bacilli misidentified in screening reactions and failing to grow in supplemental biochemical tests should be retested under salt-supplemented conditions. In identifying vibrios to species, the decarboxylase and dihydrolase reactions (lysine, LDC; ornithine, ODC; arginine, ADH) can be particularly useful as they can separate the more common halophilic species into several clusters including the LDC+/ODC+ group (*V. parahaemolyticus, V. vulnificus, V. alginolyticus*) group, the ADH+/ODC – family (*V. fluvialis, V. furnissii, V. damsela*) and *V. hollisae* which is LDC – , ODC – and ADH – (Farmer III and Hickman-

Table 45.4 Biochemical properties of pathogenic *Vibrio* species

Character	*V. cholerae*	*V. mimicus*	*V. parahaemolyticus*	*V. vulnificus*	*V. alginolyticus*	*V. fluvialis*	*V. furnissii*	*V. hollisae*	*V. damsela*	*V. metschnikovii*	*V. cincinnatiensis*
Indole	+	+	+	+	+	V	V	+	–	V	–
Moeller's decarboxylase											
lysine	+	+	+	+	+	–	–	–	V	V	V
ornithine	+	+	+	+	V	–	–	–	–	–	–
arginine	–	–	–	–	–	+	+	–	+	V	–
ONPG	+	+	–	V	–	V	V	–	–	V	V
Voges–Proskauer	+	–	–	–	+	–	–	–	+	+	+
Acid from											
L-arabinose	–	–	V	–	–	+	+	+	–	–	+
m-inositol	–	–	–	–	–	–	–	–	–	V	+
salicin	–	–	–	+	–	–	–	–	–	–	+
lactose	–	V	–	V	–	–	–	–	–	V	–
sucrose	+	–	–	V	+	+	+	–	–	+	+
Urea hydrolysis	–	–	V	–	–	–	–	–	–	–	–

ONPG, *o*-nitrophenyl-β-D-galactopyranoside; +, >90% positive; –, >90% negative; V, variable (10–90% positive).
Data from Janda et al. 1988, Farmer III and Hickman-Brenner 1991.

Brenner 1991). Both *V. metschnikovii* and *V. cincinnatiensis* are rarely isolated from clinical specimens. Strains falling into each group can be further identified using additional tests. Some individual biochemical tests are uniquely associated with individual *Vibrio* species and are a red flag with regard to their possible presence. These include *V. metschnikovii* (oxidase- and nitrate-negative), *V. cincinnatiensis* (indole-negative and acid from *m*-inositol), *V. furnissii* (gas production from D-glucose) and *V. hollisae* (triple decarboxylase- and dihydrolase-negative). Commercial identification systems are notoriously poor at identifying vibrios to the correct species. Some organisms, such as *V. fluvialis*, cannot be phenotypically separated from *Aeromonas* species (*Aeromonas caviae*) using such systems.

10.3 Biotypes

V. cholerae O1 strains can be broken down into 2 biotypes based upon several phenotypic differences. These differences, as shown in Table 45.5, involve biochemical and enzymatic properties and susceptibility to bacteriophage and antimicrobial agents. Both the classic and El Tor biotypes can be associated with each O1 serotype (Ogawa, Inaba) so that 4 common combinations exist. These combinations are of epidemiological importance as they help to monitor shifts in pandemic strains as witnessed in 1961 when the sixth pandemic of cholera due to the classic biotype of *V. cholerae* O1 was replaced by the seventh pandemic caused by El Tor. An α-^{32}P-labelled 19 bp oligonucleotide probe specifically to detect the El Tor biotype of *V. cholerae* has been constructed from a specific portion of the structural gene to the β-haemolysin gene, *hlyA* (Alm and Manning 1990). All El Tor isolates were positive with this probe whereas no classical strains reacted; non-O1 *V. cholerae* isolates that produce an immunologically and genetically related haemolysin to that of El Tor also react with this probe. *V. cholerae* O139 strains are phenotypically identical to O1 strains except that they are resistant to 150 µg of O/129 and are unreactive against El Tor phage 5 and polyclonal O1 antisera (Nair et al. 1994). However, a report of sucrose non-fermenting and late-fermenting strains of O139 raises the concern of new phenotypic differences and whether TCBS (sucrose fermentation) is adequate for detecting *V. cholerae* in outbreak situations (Ansaruzzaman et al. 1995).

Several other *Vibrio* species contain biotypes, including *V. vulnificus*, *V. pelagius* and *V. splendidus* (Tison et al. 1982,

Farmer III and Hickman Brenner 1991). The biogroups of *V. vulnificus* are distinguished from one another by several phenotypic characteristics. Biogroup 2 strains are indole- and ODC-negative, fail to grow at 42°C and do not produce acid from D-mannitol or D-sorbitol; biogroup 2 is principally recovered from eels (Tison et al. 1982). On rare occasions biogroup 2-like strains have been isolated from humans (Veenstra et al. 1992).

PHENOTYPE SWITCHING

Two biochemical properties of pathogenic vibrios are undergoing significant changes in phenotype frequency. For *V. cholerae*, both O1 and non-O1 strains are gradually becoming resistant to the vibriostatic agent O/129 at both the 10 and 150 µg concentrations. Originally reported in India, this resistotype has also been reported from Bangladesh (Huq et al. 1992), South East Asia (Mahalingam et al. 1993) and the USA (Abbott et al. 1992a). From 1970 to 1979, >80% of all *V. cholerae* strains in India were susceptible to one or both O/129 concentrations (Nath and Sanyal 1992). Now <1% are susceptible. Continued dissemination of this resistotype throughout the world will eliminate an important screening test (see Table 45.3) from the limited number presently available and may lessen accurate laboratory diagnosis. The second major phenotypic switch involves urea-hydrolysing strains of *V. parahaemolyticus*. Originally described as a negative characteristic in this species or as a rare oddity, it has over the past decade become the predominant phenotype of *V. parahaemolyticus* in the USA (Farmer III and Hickman-Brenner 1991). Some studies have linked this phenotype to a possible clonal outbreak involving a single serotype (Abbott et al. 1989). S Honda et al. (1992) has recently reported that 11.8% of persons in Japan with *V. parahaemolyticus* travellers' diarrhoea harboured urea-positive strains. Such an increase could have a significant impact on the accurate identification of this species for laboratories using triple sugar iron agar and urea slants for the screening of potentially pathogenic bacteria from faecal samples.

11 ANTIMICROBIAL SUSCEPTIBILITY

Pathogenic *Vibrio* species have traditionally been susceptible to most therapeutically active antimicrobial agents with the exception of penicillin, ampicillin, carbenicillin, trimetho-

Table 45.5 Major features of *V. cholerae* O1 biotypes

Character	V. cholerae O1 biotypes	
	Classical	**El Tor**
Genome size (kb)	3000	2500
Red blood cell		
lysis (sheep)	–	+
haemagglutination (chicken)	–	+
CAMP reaction (modified)	–	+
Polymyxin B susceptibility (50 IU)	+	–
Lysis by bacteriophage		
classical IV	+	–
FK	+	–
El Tor 5	–	+

Adapted from Janda et al. 1985, Farmer III and Hickman-Brenner 1991.
Data from Janda et al. 1985, Farmer III and Hickman-Brenner 1991, Choundhury, Bhadra and Das 1994, Lesmana et al. 1994.

prim and older first-generation cephalosporins such as cephalothin (Morris Jr, Tenney and Drusano 1985, French et al. 1989). Excellent activity against pathogenic vibrios has been noted with the newer quinolones and carbapenems (Morris Jr, Tenney and Drusano 1985, Clark 1992). β-Lactamase activity, as detected by the nitrocefin test, has been detected frequently in the halophilic vibrios, ranging from a low of 9% in *V. fluvialis* to a high of 97% in *V. alginolyticus* (French et al. 1989).

Until 1977, most strains of *V. cholerae* were universally susceptible to commonly prescribed antimicrobial agents. In that year, multiresistant *V. cholerae* El Tor, that carried R factors to ampicillin, chloramphenicol, tetracycline and others, was detected in Tanzania. Since this report, other, similar outbreaks caused by multiple drug-resistant *V. cholerae* have been described. Drug resistance in these strains has been linked to possession of an IncC group plasmid. During the outbreak of cholera in the western hemisphere, studies from Ecuador have reported high percentages (>30%) of clinical *V. cholerae* O1 isolates resistant to multiple antibiotics, including chloramphenicol, doxycycline, tetracycline and trimethoprim–sulphamethoxazole (Weber et al. 1994). Similar results were reported by Threlfall, Said and Rowe (1993). In both studies, resistant *V. cholerae* strains contained a conjugative $(100–110) \times 10^3$ kDa plasmid of the IncC group (Threlfall, Said and Rowe 1993). Exconjugants carrying various resistance markers could be detected in *Escherichia coli* K12 after matings. During this outbreak, an unusual strain of *V. cholerae* O1 El Tor that is resistant to the third generation cephalosporin cefotaxime was isolated in Argentina (Rossi et al. 1993). Cefotaxime resistance could be transferrred to a strain of *E. coli* by conjugation. In India, trimethoprim resistance has been linked to the rise in the frequency of O/129-resistant *V. cholerae* O1 (Nath and Sanyal 1992). Resistance to trimethoprim in human isolates of *V. cholerae* O1 has risen from 27% during the 1970–1979 period to 100% by 1991; high frequencies of trimethoprim-resistant *V. cholerae* O1 (68%) were also detected in environmental strains during the same interval.

12 TYPING

Outbreaks of gastrointestinal disease in the genus *Vibrio* are primarily restricted to *V. cholerae* O1 (very rarely non-O1 strains) and *V. parahaemolyticus*. For *V. cholerae* O1, initial typing methods should consist of determining the serotype (Ogawa, Inaba) and the biotype (classical, El Tor). During pandemics when a single predominant biotype exists (e.g. seventh, El Tor) the relatedness of groups of strains can be further analysed by phage typing (see section 13). In addition, powerful molecular methods have been developed to identify strain relatedness and clonal relationships within *V. cholerae* O1 El Tor. Wachsmuth and collaborators (1993) analysed 197 isolates of *V. cholerae* O1 El Tor using restriction fragment length polymorphism (RFLP), DNA sequences and multilocus enzyme electrophoresis (MEE). RFLP analysis (*Hin*dIII) of the cholera toxin A gene (*ctxA*) and DNA sequence analysis of the cholera toxin B subunit gene (*ctxB*) identified 4 clones and 3 distinct genotypes, respectively, within *V. cholerae* O1. The 4 clones identified represent the seventh pandemic, and US Gulf Coast, Australian and Latin American strains. Further diversity within these groups could be recognized by RFLP analysis (*Bg*lI) using 16S and 23S probes (14 types) and MEE (6 types). Similar strategies have been used by Faruque et al. (1993) to ribotype (*Hin*dIII, *Bg*lI) 43 classic strains of *V. cholerae* O1 isolated between 1961 and 1992 in Bangladesh. Five different ribotype patterns

could be distinguished and isolates that were genetically similar (clones) were also temporally, geographically or both temporally and geographically related. Koblavi, Grimont and Grimont (1990) ribotyped 89 *V. cholerae* O1 strains and found 4 different patterns in the classical biotype and 13 others in biotype El Tor. This suggests significant clonal diversity within each biotype.

13 BACTERIOPHAGE

Basu and Mukerjee (1968) established an international phage typing system for *V. cholerae* El Tor. This system contained 5 lytic phages (I–V) that recognized 6 different phage types. Over the past 25 years several phage types decreased in frequency whereas phage types 2 and 4 predominated. Chattopadhyay et al. (1993) have recently extended this system by incorporating 5 new phages into the typing system and redefining the routine test dilution (from confluent lysis to almost confluent lysis). Using this modified system, more than 99% of 1000 strains tested were typable into one of 146 different phage types with phage type 115 (12%) predominating.

14 NORMAL FLORA

Vibrios are not part of the normal gastrointestinal flora of humans. When recovered, they are almost invariably associated with a disease under non-epidemic conditions. However, during *V. cholerae* O1 epidemics, up to 75% of infected individuals may be asymptomatic or have only very mild gastroenteritis not requiring medical intervention. Such individuals are important vehicles in the continued propagation and dissemination of *V. cholerae* O1 into the environment during such outbreaks (Puglielli et al. 1992).

15 PATHOGENICITY

For over a century the pre-eminent pathogen of this genus has been *V. cholerae* O1 and its defining trait has been the elaboration of a potent and sometimes lethal cytotonic enterotoxin, known as cholera toxin (CT). This toxin has been studied in detail at the genetic, molecular, cellular, physiological and pathogenic levels and its role in pandemic and epidemic cholera have been unequivocally established through epidemiological investigations, volunteer studies and by use of animal model systems. However, recent discoveries have required the development of an evolving concept regarding *V. cholerae* O1 pathogenesis and CT production. CT-positive strains of *V. cholerae* O139 have emerged as the predominant cause of epidemic (and possibly the eighth pandemic) cholera in India, Bangladesh and South East Asia (Albert 1994). This solitary fact has destroyed a previously rigid dogma regarding the singular association of the O1 serogroup of *V. cholerae* with epidemic and pandemic cholera. That cholera toxin is not the exclusive extracellular product responsible for diarrhoeal disease (epidemic or otherwise) stems from 2 lines of evidence. Genetically reconstructed strains of *V. cholerae* O1 lacking the structural gene (*ctxA*) for cholera toxin can still produce diarrhoeal disease, albeit in a milder form

(Levine et al. 1988). Second, rare strains of *V. cholerae* non-O1 and *V. mimicus* possess *ctxA* and produce cholera toxin in vitro, yet they do not appear to have the inherent capacity to cause widespread disease. These facts indicate that the association of *V. cholerae* O1 and O139 with epidemic disease requires more than CT production and indicates that, as in so many other instances, bacterial pathogenicity is polygenic. These conclusions have led to the discovery of a number of co-ordinately expressed or novel virulence factors in *V. cholerae* associated with gastrointestinal symptomatology.

Despite increasing knowledge regarding the regulation and expression of virulence factors in the disease process caused by *V. cholerae*, there is very little information available regarding other pathogenic *Vibrio* species. *V. vulnificus*, a highly invasive bacterium responsible for fulminant cases of septicaemia, has been under intense scrutiny for more than 10 years. Although many potential virulence factors have been identified, no single factor or group of determinants has unambiguously been shown to correlate with pathogenicity. A major virulence factor of *V. parahaemolyticus*, the thermostable direct haemolysin (*tdh*) has been linked to foodborne gastroenteritis. Its molecular role in disease pathogenesis is, however, unknown. For many of the other pathogenic vibrios (*V. fluvialis, V. damsela, V. hollisae*) potential virulence factors have been identified but evidence linking them directly to the disease process is lacking.

16 VIRULENCE FACTORS

16.1 *V. cholerae* O1

The major virulence factor of *V. cholerae* O1 is CT, a heat-labile, multimeric protein consisting of one A subunit (holotoxin, MW 27.2 kDa) and 5 identical B subunits, each with a MW of 11.7 kDa*(Mekalanos 1985). CT is structurally and functionally related to the heat-labile enterotoxin of *E. coli* (Spangler 1992). The structural genes encoding both subunits (*ctxA, ctxB*) have been identified. The *ctxAB* operon is located on a portion of the bacterial chromosome termed the core region and is flanked by the repeat segments RS1 (Ottemann and Mekalanos 1994). In classical *V. cholerae* strains 2 copies of the CTX element are widely separated on the chromosome; for El Tor strains multiple copies are tandemly arranged (Mekalanos 1983). The B subunit serves to bind the holotoxin to the cell receptor and the A subunit provides the toxigenic activity intracellularly after proteolytic cleavage into 2 peptides, A_1 and A_2 (Kaper, Morris Jr and Levine 1995). The A_1 peptide is the active portion of the molecule acting as an ADP-ribosyltransferase from NAD to a G protein, named G_s. Activation of G_s results in increased intracellular levels of cAMP, which ultimately leads to protein kinase activation, protein dephosphorylation, altered ion transport and diarrhoeal disease (Kaper, Morris Jr and Levine 1995). The secretory effect of CT can be reproduced with live cultures, bacterial filtrates, or purified toxin in appropriate animal models such as the infant mouse assay, rabbit ligated loop or the rabbit intestinal tie-adult rabbit model (Richardson 1994). In vitro, CT acts as a cytotonic (non-lethal) enterotoxin causing rounding of Y1 adrenal cells or CHO cell elongation. Removal of CT from culture supernatant or preincubation of CT with antitoxin to CT causes Y1 and CHO cells to retain their original cell morphology. Both assays can be used in the laboratory to detect CT production. CT production in culture supernatants can also be detected using latex agglutination and ELISA methodologies or, alternatively, can be detected by colony hybridization assays (Janda et al. 1988). Genetic probes, however, have the disadvantage of detecting the structural genes rather than the active biological product.

Expression of CT is regulated by a 32 kDa integral membrane protein called ToxR (Ottemann and Mekalanos 1994). Environmental stimuli such as osmolarity, the presence of certain amino acids and temperature (heat shock response) help to regulate ToxR (gene *toxR*) expression (Parsot and Mekalanos 1990, Ottemann and Mekalanos 1994). In addition to CT, several other factors are also regulated by ToxR. One of these is the toxin co-regulated pilus, TcpA (gene *tcpA*), a 20.5 kDa protein that makes up the major subunit of the *V. cholerae* pilus (Taylor et al. 1987). TcpA fimbriae are 5–6 nm in diameter and form bundles of filaments (Hall et al. 1988). TcpA is required for virulence as TcpA mutants of O1 *V. cholerae* Ogawa (strain 395) fail to colonize mice (Taylor et al. 1987) or volunteers (Herrington et al. 1988) and elicit diarrhoea. Pre-immunization of infant mice with purified antibodies to TcpA prevented death upon challenge with fully virulent *V. cholerae* O395 (Sun, Mekalanos and Taylor 1990). ToxR forms part of the ToxR regulon which directly controls expression of a cassette of virulence-associated factors located in the core region of *V. cholerae* O1 including the zonula occludens toxin (*zot*), the accessory cholera enterotoxin (*ace*), and a core encoded pilin (*cep*). These genes are located upstream from the *ctx* operon. Zot is a heat-labile protein whose gene has the capacity to encode for a polypeptide of c. 45 kDa, which may subsequently be processed into 2 smaller peptides. Zot apparently increases the permeability of the rabbit ileal mucosa by affecting tight junctions (Fasano et al. 1991, Baudry et al. 1992). It has been hypothesized that Zot may be responsible for a milder form of diarrhoea observed in volunteers fed genetically altered strains of *V. cholerae* defective in CT production. A third toxin, Ace, with a predicted M_r of 11.3 kDa, causes differences in tissue conductivity and produces fluid accumulation in rabbit ligated ileal loops (Truckiss et al. 1993, Kaper, Morris Jr and Levine 1995). A final element of the *ctx* core region is the core encoded pilin, Cep (Pearson et al. 1993). Cep appears to code for a colonization factor for mice. Present evidence, however, does not suggest a pathogenic role in humans (Kaper, Morris Jr and Levine 1995). All of these factors are controlled at the transcription level by ToxT, a 32 kDa protein activated by ToxR (Ottemann and Mekalanos 1994).

Other potential virulence-associated factors not regulated by the ToxR regulon have been investigated. A β-haemolysin is expressed by most *V. cholerae* O1 El Tor strains. The gene (*hlyA*) encodes for a mature 84 kDa protein with haemolytic and cytolytic activity (Rader and Murphy 1988). The same identical nucleotide sequence is present in classical O1 strains (569B) except for an 11 bp deletion resulting in a truncated protein with altered haemolytic capabilities. *V. cholerae* O1 strains also produce a haemagglutinin/protease whose structural gene, *hap*, has recently been cloned and sequenced (Häse and Finkelstein 1991). Results of mutational and complementational analysis of HAP$^+$ and HAP$^-$ *V. cholerae* O1 strains suggest that the haemagglutin/protease is not a major virulence factor either in the infant rabbit model or in human disease pathogenesis (Finkelstein et al. 1992).

16.2 *V. cholerae* O139

The first non-O1 serogroup of *V. cholerae* capable of causing widespread outbreaks of cholera has been identified (Albert 1994). This serogroup, *V. cholerae* O139, is genetically similar to *V. cholerae* O1 El Tor based upon ribotypes (Faruque et al. 1994), MEE (Cravioto et al. 1994), pulsed flield gel electrophoresis of restriction digest patterns, outer-membrane protein profiles (Calia et al. 1994) and the presence of *ctxA*, *tcpA* and genes involved in iron regulation (Calia et al. 1994, Hall et al. 1994). Panji et al. (1995) have recently identified several possible precursor El Tor strains to *V. cholerae* O139. These El Tor strains share some unusual features in common with O139, that are not found in other El Tor isolates, including polymyxin B resistance, resistance to El Tor bacteriophage e4 and e5 and a high copy number and genetic polymorphism of the *ctxA* gene.

Despite these similarities, a number of differences exist between *V. cholerae* O139 and O1. At least 2 different genotypes of *ctxA* exist in O139 strains and their chromosomal location is different from that of most O1 El Tor strains based upon Southern hybridization analysis (Faruque et al. 1994). *V. cholerae* O139 also possesses a high copy number of *ctxA* genes (≥3). Calia et al. (1994) have also noted that a maltose inducible outer-membrane protein, OmpS, is constitutively expressed in O139 as opposed to O1 strains. By far the most striking differences noted in O139 are the presence of a polysaccharide capsule and distinct LPS virulence determinants (Waldor, Colwell and Mekalanos 1994). Both the capsule and LPS determinants are located in an 11 kb region of *V. cholerae* O139 not present in O1 (Comstock et al. 1995). The preliminary structure of the O139 capsule has been determined and is composed of one residue each of *N*-acetylglucosamine, *N*-acetylquinovosamine, galacturonic acid and galactose and 2 molecules of 3,6-dideoxyxylohexose (Preston et al. 1995). The capsule is thought to function potentially in serum resistance and colonization of the small intestine of newborn mice (Waldor, Colwell and Mekalanos 1994); Tn*phoA* mutants of *V. cholerae* O139 which are unable to express their LPS determinants and capsule are serum susceptible (Comstock et al. 1995). The sugar composition of the LPS of O139 contains colitose, glucose, L-glycero-D-manno-heptose, fructose, glucosamine and quinovosamine in its polysaccharide (Hisatsune et al. 1993c). Perosamine, a common sugar of O1 LPS, is absent in O139 strains. This chemical configuration most strikingly resembles the semi-R type LPS of *V. cholerae* (Hisatsune et al. 1993c).

Like O1 strains, *V. cholerae* O139 isolates contain ToxR, *ctxA*, and 3 other *ctx* core-associated genes (*cep*, *ace*, *zot*) as well as genetic factors associated with site-specific and homologous recombination (Waldor and Mekalanos 1994a, 1994b). Thus it is not surprising that O139 strains have the inherent capacity to produce epidemic cholera. Whether the presence of a capsule and distinct LPS chemotype confers additional pathogenic properties on these strains (invasiveness) awaits further clarification.

16.3 *V. cholerae* non-O1

Although *V. cholerae* non-O1 strains lack the capability to cause epidemic and pandemic cholera, some strains have been shown to produce mild to moderate gastroenteritis in adult volunteers (Morris Jr et al. 1990). Rare non-O1 strains (<4%) possess CT and Zot by colony hybridization assays; however, most clinical and environmental isolates lack these genes (Johnson, Morris Jr and Kaper 1993, Ramamurthy et al. 1993). A common phenotypic feature to almost all non-O1 isolates is the production of a β-haemolysin. Ichinose and colleagues (1987) showed that the El Tor-like haemolysin produced by one non-O1 *V. cholerae* strain was enterotoxigenic in adult rabbit ligated intestinal loops and by oral inoculation into suckling mice. Transposon inactivation of haemolytic activity in one *V. cholerae* non-O1 strain that produced fluid accumulation in adult mice caused significant reduction in this activity (Moyenuddin et al. 1993). Since this is the common phenotype found in non-O1 strains associated with gastroenteritis, it seems likely to be the major virulence determinant in this group (Ramamurthy et al. 1993, Zitzer et al. 1993).

16.4 **Other *Vibrio* species**

The best characterized virulence factor of non-cholera vibrios is the thermostable direct haemolysin (TDH) of *V. parahaemolyticus*. TDH is responsible for the Kanagawa phenomenon (KP), a reaction observed on high salt mannitol-containing blood agar that has been epidemiologically linked to the ability of pathogenic strains to produce diarrhoea in humans. The molecular weight of the holotoxin and subunits are 46 and 23 kDa respectively (Honda, Ni and Miwatani 1988). Polynucleotide (415 bp) probes constructed to TDH react with all strong KP$^+$ isolates but with <10% of non-clinical KP$^-$ strains (Nishibuchi et al. 1985). Two copies of the TDH gene (*tdh1*, *tdh2*) are present in all KP⁺ strains with the *tdh2* locus being responsible for the haemolytic phenotype observed (Nishibuchi and Kaper 1990). Both genes show greater than 97% sequence homology. The *tdh* genes are flanked by 18 bp terminal inverted repeats, or insertion sequence-like elements, suggesting possible evolutionary spread of this gene (Terai et al. 1991). TDH is a pore-forming toxin that causes cation influx (K⁺) into membrane-damaged cells (T Honda et al. 1992, Huntley et al. 1993). TDH causes fluid accumulation in the rabbit ileal loop, vascular skin permeability in rabbits and is cardiotoxic to myocardial cells in vitro. A second related toxin is the thermostable related toxin (TRH). TRH is a 48 kDa holotoxin with similar biological properties (Honda, Ni and Miwatani 1988, Honda et al. 1990). The gene *trh* shares 68% sequence homology to *tdh* (Nishibuchi et al. 1989) and can be found in some KP⁻ or weak KP⁺ isolates of *V. parahaemolyticus*. The similarity in sequences and biological activity between *tdh* and *trh* suggest a pathogenic role for the latter in the disease process. Recent genetic investigations indicate that a family of *tdh* genes exists and that most strains of *V. hollisae* and some strains of *V. mimicus* and *V. cholerae* non-O1 contain *tdh*-related genes with 93–97% homology (Terai et al. 1990, 1991). The widespread dissemination of this gene in pathogenic *Vibrio* species suggests a causal role for this toxin in the disease process.

Possession of a polysaccharide capsule appears to be an important virulence determinant in *V. vulnificus*. Encapsulated strains of *V. vulnificus* correlate with an opaque colonial morphology (heart infusion agar), utilization of transferrin-bound iron, serum resistance, antiphagocytic activity and virulence for mice (Yoshida, Ogawa and Mizuguchi 1985, Simpson et al. 1987). Acapsular Tn*phoA* mutants of *V. vulnificus* that were genetically stable demonstrated decreased serum resistance and mouse pathogenicity (Wright et al. 1990). However, studies by Hayat and collaborators (1993) indicated that many different capsular types exist among clinical isolates and suggested that serological specificity is not important in virulence. Another attractive virulence factor in *V. vulnificus* is iron regulation. Because *V. vulnificus* septicaemia arises primarily in individuals with iron overload conditions or pre-existing liver disease, iron is thought to play an important role in pathogenesis. Litwin and Calderwood (1993) have recently identified ferric uptake regulation (*fur*) sequences in *V. vulnificus*. This gene may be important in cytolysin or outer-membrane protein expression in this species.

Among the other pathogenic *Vibrio* species only the extracellular cytolysin of *V. damsela* has been characterized to any extent. This cytolysin, or damselysin, is a 69 kDa protein with phospholipase D activity (Kothary and Kreger 1985, Kreger et al. 1987). The gene has been cloned and is present in haemolytic strains of *V. damsela* but not in other pathogenic *Vibrio* species (Cutter and Kreger 1990).

AEROMONAS

17 DEFINITION

17.1 Genus

Gram-negative, oxidase- and catalase-positive, facultatively anaerobic rods. Most species and subspecies motile by means of a single polar flagellum. Nitrates reduced. Anaerogenic fermentation of many common monosaccharides, disaccharides, glycosides and some alcoholic sugars (D-mannitol, glycerol). Acid rarely produced from pentoses (except L-arabinose), methyl pentose, trisaccharides and non-carbohydrate compounds (*m*-inositol). Resistant to both 10 and 150 µg of the vibriostatic agent O/129. Nutritional requirements are simple. Salt supplementation not required for growth; high salt concentrations (6–7%) are inhibitory. Many extracellular enzymes produced including cytolytic toxins, proteases, nucleases, lipases, sulphatases, lecithinase, chitinase, amylase and stapholysin. Commonly found in freshwater reservoirs, soil and agricultural produce and in the gastrointestinal contents of fish, reptiles, amphibia and higher vertebrates. Occasionally found in the marine environment. Some species are pathogenic for humans and fish. The G + C content of DNA is 57–63 mol%. Type species is *A. hydrophila*.

17.2 Species

There are presently 14 nomenspecies in the genus *Aeromonas*, the latest addition being *A. allosaccharophila* (Martinez-Murcia et al. 1992). At least 9 of these species have been implicated in human disease (Janda 1991, Martinez-Murcia et al. 1992). Several species (e.g. *A. hydrophila*) were named prior to the advent of molecular systematics and therefore actually represent phenospecies at present. Most recently described species (genomospecies) have been defined using DNA–DNA hybridization analysis although some (*A. allosaccharophila*) have been proposed using 16S rRNA sequence data. Additional *Aeromonas* hybridization groups (HGs) which represent unnamed taxa (HG 2, HG 11) are known to exist. Most strains of a single genomospecies exhibit between 70 and 100% relatedness at the DNA level under optimal reassociation conditions and display ≥80% phenotypic similarity using the Jaccard coefficient (Kämpfer and Altwegg 1992). Comparative analysis of 16S rRNA sequences between *Aeromonas* species show ≥98% identity (Martinez-Murcia, Benlloch and Collins 1992).

18 HABITAT

Aeromonads are common inhabitants of the microbial biosphere. They can be isolated from virtually any freshwater source excluding hot springs (Hazen et al. 1978). During colder seasons they are often recovered from poikilothermic animals and freshwater environments although usually in low numbers. However, during the warmer months of the year their relative numbers increase due to elevated water temperatures. During these periods aeromonads can be isolated from potable water sources (wells, reservoirs, drinking fountains) and numerous foods including dairy products, meats and fresh produce (Millership and Chattopadhyay 1985, Nishikawa and Kishi 1988, Krovacek et al. 1992). Recovery from such diverse sources hinders epidemiological investigations attempting to link cases of *Aeromonas*-associated gastroenteritis with particular food vehicles. *Aeromonas* species can also be recovered from the marine environment, particularly from estuaries, bays and inlets where salinity values are lower. They are occasionally recovered from shellfish, although less frequently than vibrios. Aeromonads have been isolated from many other species and higher vertebrates including birds, dolphins, opossums, dogs, pigs, cattle, sheep, horses, water buffaloes, tamarins and monkeys.

19 MORPHOLOGY

Aeromonas bacilli are (0.3–1.0) mm × (1.0–3.5) mm in size. They are morphologically indistinguishable from other enteric organisms such as *E. coli*. Curved forms are not present. Cellular morphology is independent of culture conditions. The outermost surface of some strains of *A. salmonicida*, *A. hydrophila* and *A. veronii* contain a paracrystalline surface layer (S layer) which can be detected by electron microscopic analysis (thin section) of uranyl acetate stained cells (Kay and Trust 1991, Kokka et al. 1991). A single 49–53 kDa protein termed surface array protein (Sap) forms the S layer through an entropy-driven self-assembly process. Capsules have been detected microscopically in several *Aeromonas* species using India ink preparations (Kuijper et al. 1989). Although most of these capsules are poorly characterized, the capsule of *A. salmonicida* has been shown to be composed of glucose, mannose, rhamnose, *N*-acetylmannosamine and mannuronic acid (Garrote et al. 1992). Ultrastructural studies also indicate the presence of morphologically distinct fimbriae. Two major types have been described by negative-staining techniques, namely rigid (straight) and flexible (curvilinear, wavy) pili. Rigid pili have diameter of 9 nm and are composed of protein subunits with a molecular mass ranging between 17 and 21 kDa (Ho et al. 1990, Hokama, Honma and Nakasone 1990). Flexible pili are similar in size with a diameter of 7 nm and a molecular mass of 19–23 kDa. A very small mini pilin of 4 kDa has also been identified (Ho et al. 1990). The gene for this flexible mini pilin (*fxp*) has been cloned and sequenced (Ho, Sohel and Schoolnik 1992). It shares a high degree of sequence similarity with the *cep* gene of *V. cholerae* O1 (Pearson et al. 1993).

20 CULTURAL CHARACTERISTICS AND GROWTH REQUIREMENTS

On non-selective agar media *Aeromonas* isolates typically appear as buff-coloured, smooth, convex colonies 3–5 mm in diameter after overnight incubation at 35–37°C. Most *A. salmonicida* strains involved in fish infections produce a brown water-soluble pigment on tyrosine-containing agar (Donlon et al. 1983) and rare strains belonging to other groups, in particular some biotypes of *A. media* and HG 2, elaborate a similar pigment on media such as heart infusion agar (Janda, Abbott and Morris Jr 1995). Most aeromonads can grow in media containing up to 4% NaCl and over a pH range of 5–9 (Austin, McIntosh and Austin 1989). Alkaline peptone water (pH 8.6), commonly used for the isolation of vibrios, can also be used to enrich for the presence of *Aeromonas* species.

Because growth requirements are simple, aeromonads can be routinely cultured on many non-selective, differential and selective agars. Since most strains ferment sucrose, lactose or both sucrose and lactose, they can be easily missed on media like MacConkey, Hektoen enteric and xylose–lysine–desoxycholate (XLD) agars where they resemble non-pathogenic coliforms. The best differential/selective media for the isolation of pathogenic aeromonads is blood agar and cefsulodin–Irgasan–novobiocin (CIN) agar plates. Blood agar can be used as a screening medium for *Aeromonas* as spot tests for cytochrome oxidase and tryptophanase deamination (both positive for most aeromonads) can be directly performed on isolated colonies (Kelly, Stroh and Jessop 1988). Many *Aeromonas* strains also produce β-haemolysis on sheep blood agar, a phenotypic characteristic useful in separating aeromonads from other enteric bacilli. Some strains produce a double zone haemolysis, with an outer incomplete zone of clearing and an inner zone of complete β-haemolysis. CIN agar, a medium originally designed for the isolation of *Yersinia enterocolitica*, is also useful to isolate *Aeromonas* (Altorfer et al. 1985).

Classically, aeromonads have been divided into 2 large groups based upon differential temperature optima for growth. Psychrophilic strains, most commonly exemplified by the fish pathogens *A. salmonicida* ssp. *salmonicida*, *A. salmonicida* ssp. *masoucida* and *A. salmonicida* ssp. *smithia*, grow best at temperatures ranging between 22 and 28°C (Austin, McIntosh and Austin 1989). Mesophilic strains, primarily associated with human infections, grow optimally between 35 and 37°C. However, many mesophilic strains can grow at temperatures ranging between 4 and 42°C.

21 METABOLISM

Aeromonads are chemo-organotrophs using a wide variety of sugars and carbon sources for energy (Popoff 1984). Glucose is metabolized both aerobically and fermentatively with or without the production of gas (CO_2, H_2).

22 GENETIC MECHANISMS

Extrachromosomal elements are infrequently carried by aeromonads with the singular exception of *A. salmonicida*. In this latter species, close to 100% of the strains analysed carry plasmids (Toranzo et al. 1983, Belland and Trust 1989). *A. salmonicida* plasmids can be placed into 2 major groups consisting of typical strains harbouring 4–7 plasmids with molecular masses ranging from 2.3×10^3 to 9.6×10^4 kDa and atypical isolates containing 2–4 plasmids each with molecular masses ranging from 2.6×10^3 to 9.9×10^4 kDa (Belland and Trust 1989). Each group of plasmids carried by typical *A. salmonicida* strains appear highly related by restriction endonuclease digest whereas plasmids from atypical strains bear no such relationship. For other *Aeromonas* species the frequency of plasmid carriage is much lower. Chang and Bolton (1987) screened 75 wild-type isolates and found only 20 (27%) to carry plasmids. Of these 20 strains, only one (pSOB1) was found to be a conjugative plasmid upon mating experiments with *E. coli*. Most plasmids detected in *A. hydrophila* appear to belong to the IncC or IncU incompatibility groups that carry resistance (class D) to tetracycline (Hedges, Smith and Brazil 1985, Aoki and Takahashi 1987). Plasmid-mediated antibiotic resistance in select *Aeromonas* strains includes tetracycline (Toranzo et al. 1983), novobiocin and carbenicillin (Hanes and Chandler 1993), streptomycin and sulphonamides (Hedges, Smith and Brazil 1985) and kanamycin, streptomycin, tobramycin and ticarcillin (Chang and Bolton 1987). In addition to antibiotic-resistance markers, several other gene products have been found to be mobilized on individual *Aeromonas* strains including a mini pilin (Ho et al. 1990), precipitation after boiling (Toranzo et al. 1983) and attachment and haemolytic activities (Hanes and Chandler 1993).

23 CELLULAR ORGANIZATION

The outermost layer of some *Aeromonas* strains is the S layer, or paracrystalline surface layer. This layer is composed of a single 49–55 kDa acidic protein (pI 4.6–5.7) termed the surface array protein (Sap) (Dooley et al. 1988, Kokka, Vedros and Janda 1992). Sap proteins are relatively hydrophobic (41–46%) and share some sequence homology at the amino terminus. S layers can be preferentially removed by glycine hydrochloride extraction under low acid conditions and they exhibit a p4 symmetry. The gene for the S layer of *A. salmonicida* has been cloned (*vapA*) and sequenced (Belland and Trust 1987, Chu et al. 1991).

The LPS of aeromonads consist of typical lipid A–core oligosaccharide–O polysaccharide components. Early investigations by Shaw and Hodder (1978) identified 3 major core oligosaccharide chemotypes based upon the presence or absence of D-glucose, D-galactose, D-glycero-D-mannoheptose and L-glycero-D-mannoheptose in each form. Further studies have revealed the presence of some additional sugars as part of the core component, including 3-acetamido-3,6-dideoxy-L-glucose in chemotype III (Banoub and Shaw 1981) and D-glucosamine in chemotype I (Michon, Shaw and Banoub 1984). The basic structure for each of these 3 chemotypes has been published (Banoub and Shaw 1981, Banoub et al. 1983, Michon, Shaw and Banoub 1984). The O antigen structure has been determined for select strains of *A. salmonicida* and *A. hydrophila*. Chemical analysis of each species reveals a very similar backbone structure with →4)-L-Rha linked (1→3) to either N-acetylmannosamine (*A. salmonicida*) or N-acetylglucosamine for *A. hydrophila* (Shaw et al. 1983, Shaw and Squires 1984). Both backbones show partial O-acetylation of either N-acetylmannosamine at position 4 or L-rhamnose at position 2.

Analysis of the fatty acid composition of *Aeromonas* species indicates that *cis*-9-hexadecenoic acid (Δ^9-16:1), *cis*-11-octadecenoic acid (Δ^{11}-18:1) and hexadecanoic acid (16:0) are the major products produced (Lambert et al. 1983, Hansen et al. 1991, Huys et al. 1994, Kämpfer, Blasczyk and Auling 1994). Aeromonads can be distinguished from *Vibrio* species by their lack of 3-hydroxylauric acid (3-OH-12:0) and from members of the Enterobacteriaceae by their failure to produce significant amounts of cyclopropane fatty acids (Lambert et al. 1983, Hansen et al. 1991). *Aeromonas* genomospecies, however, could not be separated unambiguously from one another by cellular fatty acid analysis (Huys et al. 1994, Kämpfer, Blasczyk and Auling 1994). Quinone analysis of *Aeromonas* isolates indicates all species to contain a ubiqinone with 8 isoprenoid (Q-8) units. The major polyamines detected are putrescine and diaminopropane; members of the genus *Aeromonas* can be separated from *Vibrio* species by the absence of norspermidine in aeromonads (Kämpfer, Blasczyk and Auling 1994).

23.1 Antigenic structure

Unlike *V. cholerae* O1, the biochemical and molecular components responsible for O antigen specificity in *Aeromonas* species are poorly understood. Individual serogroups have been established based upon the uniqueness of immune antisera raised against heat-killed formalinized saline suspensions of individual strains. No international serotyping system for aeromonads presently exists although several different serogrouping schemes have been developed in Japan, England and The Netherlands (Sakazaki and Shimada 1984, Thomas et al. 1990, Shimada and Kosako 1991). The most extensive serogrouping system, that of the Japanese, recognizes 44 established and 49 provisional serogroups (Sakazaki and Shimada 1984). Individual antisera must first be absorbed with a rough strain of *Aeromonas* since all polyclonal antibodies made against O antigens contain some R antibodies. Some *Aeromonas* serogroups show complete or partial serological identity with serogroups of *V. cholerae*, *V. fluvialis* and *Plesiomonas shigelloides*. Studies on the flagellar antigen(s) of mesophilic aeromonads have not been reported.

24   CLASSIFICATION

Nowhere has there been greater confusion regarding aeromonads than their appropriate classification and taxonomic position. Members of the genus *Aeromonas* were initially classified into 2 major groups based upon optimal temperatures for growth, disease spectrum and biochemical characteristics. The psychrophilic aeromonads are a homogeneous group that inhabits freshwater environments; they are primary pathogens of fish, particularly salmon. This group is represented by a single species, *A. salmonicida*, which is non-motile, indole-negative and produces a brown diffusible pigment on tyrosine agar. The second group is composed of mesophilic strains that infect humans and fish; members of this group are motile, indole-positive and fail to produce a brown pigment. These latter strains were commonly referred to as *A. hydrophila*. Pioneering taxonomic investigations by Popoff and Véron (1976) and Popoff and colleagues (1981), using numerical taxonomy methods and DNA–DNA hybridization assays, were able to separate mesophilic aeromonads further into 3 genetically and phenotypically distinct clusters which were designated *A. hydrophila*, *A. sobria* and *A. caviae*. Within each of these species, however, multiple HGs existed, indicating that these nomenspecies were actually phenospecies, i.e. genetically dissimilar groups of organisms that could not be separated on a phenotypic basis. Later studies conducted by the Centers for Disease Control, Altanta indicated that the genus *Aeromonas* was far more diverse genetically at the species level than was first thought. Based upon the previous work of Popoff and others (1981) and the Centers for Disease Control, 12 HGs were established. The type strains of named species were then assigned to specific HGs, as in the case of *A. hydrophila* (HG 1), *A. salmonicida* (HG 3), *A. caviae* (HG 4), *A. media* (HG 5) and *A. sobria* (HG 7). Subsequent investigations using DNA–DNA reassociation kinetics identified a number of new species corresponding to recognized HGs. These included *A. eucrenophila* and HG 6 (Schubert and Hegazi 1988), *A. jandaei* and HG 9 (Carnahan, Fanning and Joseph 1991), *A. veronii* and HG 10 (Hickman-Brenner et al. 1987) and *A. schubertii* and HG 12 (Hickman-Brenner et al. 1988). HGs 2 and 11 are currently unnamed and HG 8 is actually a biotype of *A. veronii*. Two new *Aeromonas* species, which do not correspond to any of the original 12 HGs, have been proposed. These are *A. trota* (Carnahan et al. 1991) and *A. allosaccharophila* (Martinez-Murcia et al. 1992).

A final point concerns the genetic divergence that exists within the genus *Aeromonas* (Farmer III, Arduino and Hickman-Brenner 1991). Recent systematic investigations of *Aeromonas* 16S rDNA sequences indicate that this genus forms a distinct line within the γ-subclass of the Proteobacteria (Martinez-Murcia, Benlloch and Collins 1992). These studies are further supported by small-subunit rRNA sequence analysis which indicates that *Aeromonas* species deserve family rank (Ruimy et al. 1994).

25   LABORATORY ISOLATION AND IDENTIFICATION

Aeromonads can be recovered on virtually any isolation medium commonly employed in the laboratory. However, their ability to ferment sucrose, lactose or both sucrose and lactose may mask their presence on many selective media. Recovery from non-sterile specimens is therefore dependent upon the use of differential/selective media designed to highlight their appearance (blood agar, CIN) or the use of screening reactions (triple sugar iron agar, urea slants, motility, oxidase, indole, ornithine). As listed in Table 45.3, aeromonads can be easily separated from vibrios and plesiomonads by their growth on nutrient agar (Difco) containing no added salt, their resistance to O/129 (both concentrations) and by negative stringing reaction. For species identification, a battery of biochemical tests is required in order to ensure accurate identification. Table 45.6 lists a number of useful phenotypic properties helpful in separating these species.

Two major problems are still encountered in identifying aeromonads to correct species. First, it is still difficult to separate members of the *A. hydrophila*–HG 2–*A. salmonicida* group that cause infections in humans. In addition to the tests listed in Table 45.6, utilization of DL-lactate (Altwegg et al. 1990), fermentation of D-rhamnose (Abbott et al. 1992b) and utilization of urocanic acid (Hänninen 1994) are useful adjuncts to conventional tests. Second, it is not easy to separate clinical isolates of *A. caviae* from *A. media* (HG 5A). The best differential tests include DL-lactate utilization (Altwegg et al. 1990), fermentation of mannose, β-haemolysis and pyrazinamidase activity (Abbott et al. 1992b). Some species, such as *A. allosaccharophila*, do not have defined unique biochemical properties that presently allow for their separation from phenotypically related organisms. In addition to DNA–DNA hybridization, several other molecular techniques have been found to help separate aeromonads into correct genomospecies. These include ribotyping (Martinetti Lucchini and Altwegg 1992) and multilocus enzyme electrophoresis (Tonolla, Demarta and Peduzzi 1991).

26   ANTIMICROBIAL SUSCEPTIBILITY

Aeromonads are generally ampicillin resistant and susceptible to the third generation cephalosporins, aminoglycosides, tetracycline, trimethoprim–sulphamethoxazole, chloramphenicol and newer groups or classes of agents including the quinolones, carbapenems and monobactams (Burgos et al. 1990, Koehler and Ashdown 1993). In vitro susceptibility to first generation cephalosporins such as cephalothin is species associated as most strains of *A. veronii* biotype sobria are susceptible to this agent and almost all *A. hydrophila* and *A. caviae* are resistant (Motyl, McKinley and Janda 1985, Koehler and Ashdown 1993). Resistance to β-lactam antibiotics in *Aeromonas* species is often caused by inducible β-lactamases. Such resistance can be induced by a wide range of antibiotics including penicillin, cephalosporins (including cefoperazone) and carbapenems (Bakken et al. 1988). These cefoxitin and imipenem-inducible β-lactamases produced by *A. hydrophila* and *A. veronii* appear to be distinct enzymes

Table 45.6 Separation of *Aeromonas* species and *P. shigelloides*

Character	A. hydrophila	HG 2	A. salmonicida[a]	A. caviae	A. media[a]	A. veronii biotype sobria	A. veronii biotype veronii	A. jandaei	A. schubertii	A. trota	P. shigelloides
Hybridization group	1	2	3	4	5	8	10	9	12	na	na
Indole	+	+	+	+	+	+	+	+	−	+	+
Moeller's decarboxylases											
lysine	+	V	V	−	−	+	+	+	V	+	+
ornithine	−	−	−	−	−	−	+	−	−	−	+
arginine	+	+	V	+	+	+	−	+	+	+	+
Voges–Proskauer	+	V	V	−	−	+	+	+	V	−	−
Glucose (gas)	+	V	V	−	−	+	V	+	−	V	−
Acid from											
L-arabinose	+	+	+	+	+	V	−	−	−	−	−
lactose	V	V	+	+	+	V	+	V	V	−	−
D-sorbitol	−	−	V	−	−	−	−	−	−	−	−
sucrose	+	+	+	+	+	+	+	−	−	V	−
m-inositol	−	−	−	−	−	−	−	−	−	−	+
D-mannitol	+	+	+	+	+	+	+	+	−	V	−
salicin	+	−	+	+	V	−	+	−	−	−	−
Aesculin hydrolysis	+	+	+	+	+	−	+	−	−	−	−
Enzymes											
elastase	V	−	V								
β-haemolysin	+	+	V	−	V	+	+	+	V	V	−
stapholysin	+	V	V	−	−	−	−	−	−	−	−
Ampicillin (10 µg) resistance	+	V	V	+	V	+	+	+	+	−	+

[a]Human isolates only.
na, Not applicable; +, >90% positive; −, >90% negative; V, variable (10–90% positive).
Data from Janda (1991) and Abbot et al. (1992b).

based upon isoelectric focusing and molecular weight estimations (Iaconis and Sanders 1990). The gene (*cphA*) for a carbapenem-hydrolysing metallo-β-lactamase from *A. hydrophila* has been cloned in *E. coli* (Massidda, Rossolini and Satta 1991). The deduced amino acid sequence of *cphA* shows partial homology with β-lactamases of *Bacillus cereus* and *Bacteroides fragilis*.

27 TYPING

The easiest and most useful methods available to most laboratories for determining strain relatedness are biotyping and serogrouping. Most *Aeromonas* strains are 'phenotypically loose', that is they show great variability in phenotype frequency (percentage positive) to a large number of carbohydrate and enzyme-based tests. Such biochemical differences between strains can be used as a preliminary screening tool to determine identity or non-identity between 2 isolates. For a more definitive approach, serogrouping by a reference laboratory can be extremely helpful since serogroups for the most part are not genomospecies specific. Only a few serogroups of the Sakazaki and Shimada system (1984) are common (O:11, O:16, O:18, O:34) and therefore when strains type to groups exclusive of these, strain relatedness can be assumed. For molecular approaches, ribotyping has been used to establish that a single strain has chronically affected

an individual (Rautelin et al. 1995) or can link a particular food isolate to gastrointestinal infection (Altwegg et al. 1991).

28 BACTERIOPHAGE

Many *Aeromonas* bacteriophages have been identified and partially characterized (Ackermann et al. 1985). These bacteriophages exhibit different specificities for components located on the cell surface. The receptor for some phages (low MW LPS, flagellum) has been identified (Merino, Camprubi and Tomás 1990a, 1990b). No recognized phage typing system for aeromonads has been established.

29 NORMAL FLORA

Collective results from industrialized countries throughout the world suggest that aeromonads are infrequently carried as normal flora (<1%). During the warmer months of the year, the carriage rate may be slightly elevated due to increasing exposure to consumable products harbouring these bacteria.

30 PATHOGENICITY

Aeromonads are involved in both intestinal and extra-intestinal human infections (Janda and Duffey 1988). Their pathogenicity and virulence characteristics can be assessed with respect to disease presentation. In gastroenteritis, the chief *Aeromonas* virulence factor in the disease process is the enterotoxin (Janda 1991). At least 2 distinctly different molecules produced by aeromonads have been shown to contain enterotoxigenic activity. The more common enterotoxin is a cytolytic β-haemolysin, or aerolysin, produced by several different *Aeromonas* species including *A. hydrophila* and *A. veronii*. These activated aerolysins have molecular weights ranging from 51 to 54 kDa and cause fluid accumulation in infant mice and rabbit ligated ileal loops (Asao et al. 1984, Kozaki et al. 1989). The cytolytic enterotoxins (aerolysins) of both *A. hydrophila* and *A. veronii* exhibit some immunological cross-reactivity (Kozaki et al. 1989) and appear to be part of a larger family of *Aeromonas* aerolysins that have similar structural properties but distinct immunological, biological and genetic characteristics (Chopra, Houston and Kurosky 1991). The proaerolysin has been crystallized (Tucker et al. 1990) and has been shown to be a hole-forming toxin that produces a transmembrane channel that destroys the cell integrity (Parker et al. 1994). The membrane activity of aerolysins is dependent upon a prior oligomerization step which functionally hinges on key histidine and tryptophane residues (Wilmsen, Buckley and Pattus 1991, van der Goot et al. 1993). A model has been proposed for the insertion of this proteinaceous toxin into lipid bilayers based upon x-ray crystallography and computer modelling (Parker et al. 1994). A number of these aerolysin genes have been cloned and sequenced (Hirono and Aoki 1991, Hirono et al. 1992). These genes show >90% amino acid sequence homology intraspecies and 58–68% homology interspecies (Hirono et al. 1992).

A second, less common enterotoxin has also been described. This toxin differs from the aerolysin in that it is non-haemolytic and produces a cytotonic response in Y1 adrenal cells (Ljungh, Wretlind and Möllby 1981). The cytotonic enterotoxin has a reported molecular weight of 15 kDa. It causes fluid accumulation in rabbit ileal loops and in suckling mice and causes CHO cell elongation with an increase in cAMP levels (Chakraborty et al. 1984, Gosling et al. 1993). In addition to these 2 enterotoxins a number of other virulence-associated properties of *Aeromonas* may be operative in gastrointestinal disease and these include adhesins, mucinases and the ability to penetrate eukaryotic cells (Janda 1991). The inability to establish an animal model that faithfully reproduces the gastrointestinal syndrome associated with *Aeromonas* infection has hindered such investigations. One study using the removable intestinal tie adult rabbit diarrhoea model has been able partially to link histological and pathological changes in the intestine with the probable site (ileum) of infection and invasion (Pazzaglia et al. 1990).

For systemic disease, results of cumulative LD50 studies in mice support clinical data indicating that strains belonging to the phenospecies *A. hydrophila* and *A. sobria* are inherently more pathogenic than *A. caviae* (Janda and Kokka 1991, Janda et al. 1994). Virulence factors thought to play a role in invasive disease include S layers (Kokka, Vedros and Janda 1992), β-haemolysin activity (Chakraborty et al. 1987), resistance to complement-mediated lysis (Janda, Kokka and Guthertz 1994) and LPS (Merino, Camprubi and Tomás 1991). These general properties are present in many *A. hydrophila* and *A. veronii* strains and absent in most *A. caviae* isolates.

PLESIOMONAS

31 DEFINITION

Gram-negative, oxidase- and catalase-positive, facultatively anaerobic rods. Motile by means of a single polar flagellum. Nitrates reduced. Anaerogenic fermentation of only a few carbohydrates. Acid produced from *m*-inositol. Most strains susceptible to 10 and 150 μg of O/129. Nutritional requirements are simple. Salt supplementation not required for growth. Few extracellular enzymes produced. Commonly found in freshwater habitats, fish, reptiles, amphibia and snakes and occasionally shellfish. The G + C content is 51 mol%. The genus is represented by a single species, *P. shigelloides*.

32 HABITAT

Plesiomonads are commonly recovered from freshwater environments throughout the world. Medema and Schets (1993) found over 70% of all freshwater samples taken to be positive for *P. shigelloides* with densities ranging between 140 and 340 dl^{-1}. Higher *P. shigelloides* counts were associated with the trophic state (turbidity) and faecal pollution whereas lower numbers of plesiomonads were isolated during the winter. During seasonal studies Miller and Koburger (1986a) found a high rate of plesiomonads (59%) in the environment surrounding a river estuary. Samples included water sediment, eels, crabs, bream, catfish, crappies, clams and oysters. Other environmental studies have found high rates in freshwater fish, river water and sludge and the intestinal contents of many mammals including swine, cats, dogs and poultry (Arai et al. 1980, Van Damme and Vandepitte 1980). For a review of other sources of plesiomonads the reader should consult Miller and Koburger (1985).

33 MORPHOLOGY

P. shigelloides bacilli are (0.8–1.0) × 3.0 mm and typically appear as straight rods indistinguishable from other enteric organisms. Curved forms have not been noted. On solid media, c. 70% of *P. shigelloides* strains analysed produce unsheathed peritrichous flagella (Inoue et al. 1991). Cytoplasmic granules and vacuoles have also been detected in *P. shigelloides* (Pastian and Bromel 1984, Brenden, Miller and Janda 1988). Internal granules can be observed in plesiomonads using the Laybourn but not the Sudan black stains. These inclusions give cells a safety pin appearance (Pastian and Bromel 1984) and appear to be poly-phosphate granules based upon electron microscopic x-ray probe analysis (Ogawa and Amano 1987). Methods using ruthenium red staining and ultra-structural analysis have revealed a string-like material on the cell surface of *P. shigelloides* (Brenden, Miller and Janda 1988). This glycocalyx appears to be composed of acidic mucopolysaccharide material.

34 CULTURE CHARACTERISTICS AND GROWTH REQUIREMENTS

P. shigelloides strains grow over wide temperature (8–45°C) and pH (4.5–8.5) ranges, although only some strains can survive at the extremes of each of these gradients (Miller and Koburger 1986b). Plesiomonads do not require salt supplementation for growth. A majority of strains (65%) tolerate 5% NaCl whereas 6% NaCl is completely inhibitory (Miller and Koburger 1986b).

The nutritional requirements of *Plesiomonas* are simple and most strains are grown on common non-selective and differential media. On blood agar *P. shigelloides* appears as small, greyish, convex, non-haemolytic colonies (1–2 mm in diameter) after incubation of 24 h. Colonies test positive for cytochrome oxidase and tryptophanase deamination activity. Because *P. shigelloides* is sucrose-negative and lactose-negative (or delayed-positive), it should not be missed on most common selective and differential agars used in enteric workups. Several media have been designed for the isolation of plesiomonads from clinical or environmental sources and these include inositol–brilliant green–bile salts and *Plesiomonas* differential agar (von Graevenitz and Bucher 1983, Huq et al. 1991). Alkaline peptone water (pH 8.6) is a suitable enrichment broth for the recovery of *Plesiomonas*.

35 METABOLISM

Plesiomonads are chemo-organotrophs that have both a respiratory and fermentative metabolism. Most strains grow on mineral media containing ammonium salts and glucose as sole nitrogen and carbon sources (Schubert 1984).

36 CELLULAR ORGANIZATION

Very little information is available on the cellular organization of *P. shigelloides*. Basu et al. (1985) have analysed the lipid A component of the LPS. It consists of a β-(1→6)-linked glucosamine disaccharide back-bone with phosphate groups at the C-1 reducing and C-4′ non-reducing positions of glucosamine. The amino groups of the backbone are N-acylated by 3-O-(14:0)14:0 (reducing) and 3-O-(12:0)14:0 (non-reducing) by 3-hydroxyacyl residues (Basu et al. 1985). KDO is present in the core region and is linked to the C-6′ of the non-reducing glucosamine. The principal cellular fatty acids detected include *cis*-9-hexadecenoic (Δ^9-16:1) acid, hexadecanoic acid (16:0) and *cis*-11-octadecenoic (Δ^{11}-18:1) acid (Lambert et al. 1983, Chou, Aldova and Kasatiya 1991). Plesiomonads are differentiated from aeromonads by the presence of 3-hydroxylauric acid (Lambert et al. 1983). The major polyamines present in plesiomonads are putrescine, cadaverine and spermidine which clearly separate this group from aeromonads and vibrios (Yamamoto et al. 1991).

36.1 Antigenic structure

Two major serotyping schemes for *P. shigelloides* have been devised based upon somatic and flagellar antigens. The system of Shimada and Sakazaki (1985) recognized 50 O serogroups and 17 H antigens in its original form. Aldova's scheme (1994) recognizes 44 O groups and 23 H antigens. The Japanese typing scheme has since been expanded to include a number of previously unrecognized serogroups present in the Czechoslovak collection. A potential international serotyping system for *P. shigelloides* has been proposed which includes 76 O antigens and 41 H antigens (Shimada et al. 1994c). Some serogroups of *P. shigelloides* (O11, O17, O22 and O23) are known to cross with *Shigella sonnei* (form I), *Shigella boydii* 13 and *Shigella dysenteriae* 8 (Shimada and Sakazaki 1978).

37 CLASSIFICATION

The main issue regarding the genus *Plesiomonas* centres on its correct taxonomic position in the γ-subclass of the Proteobacteria. A large body of compelling evidence suggests that plesiomonads are most closely related to members of the family Enterobacteriaceae rather than the Vibrionaceae. Structurally, *P. shigelloides* contains the enterobacterial common antigen (Whang, Heller and Neter 1972) and shares the same amide-linked acyl-oxyacyl groups in the lipid A component of LPS with *S. sonnei* (Basu et al. 1985). The poly-amine composition of plesiomonads (predominant putrescine and spermidine) is more closely related to *E. coli* than to either *Vibrio* or *Aeromonas* (Yamamoto et al. 1991). Furthermore, recent phylogenetic investigations of members of the family Vibrionaceae support previous studies on 5S rRNA sequence analysis, indicating that plesiomonads are closer on an evolutionary basis to the family Enterobacteriaceae than to either vibrios or aeromonads.

38 LABORATORY ISOLATION AND IDENTIFICATION

Because of the unique biochemical characteristics of *P. shigelloides* (ADH-, ODC- and LDC-positive; sucrose- and lactose-negative) isolation and identification of this organism is not difficult (see Table 45.6). The ability of plesiomonads to produce acid from *m*-inositol, a carbohydrate-like compound, further distinguishes this bacterium from most aeromonads and vibrios (see Table 45.6). Most plesiomonads produce a variety of arylamidases, esterases, phosphatases and phosphoamidase, detected by rapid chromogenic assays (Manafi and Rotter 1992).

39 ANTIMICROBIAL SUSCEPTIBILITY

Plesiomonads are resistant to most penicillins, including ampicillin, ticarcillin and carbenicillin. All strains produce a β-lactamase as determined by the nitrocefin test (Reinhardt and George 1985) and are susceptible to antibiotic-β-lactamase inhibitor combinations (Clark et al. 1990). Other antimicrobial agents active in vitro against plesiomonads include trimethoprim–sulphamethoxazole, tetracycline, chloramphenicol, cephalosporins (all classes), carbapenems, monobactams and quinolones (Reinhardt and George 1985, Kain and Kelly 1989, Clark et al. 1990). Discrepancies in the susceptibility of plesiomonads to aminoglycosides has been noted although reasons for these observed differences have not been determined (Kain and Kelly 1989, Clark et al. 1990).

40 PATHOGENICITY

The relative pathogenicity of *P. shigelloides* is low. The mean LD50 in mice for 16 strains of *P. shigelloides* is 3.5×10^8 cfu (Abbott, Kokka and Janda 1991). Plesiomonads lack overt cytoxic activity in cell-free supernatants and are non-invasive in both animal and cell culture assay systems (Olsvik et al. 1990, Abbott, Kokka and Janda 1991). Two types of enterotoxins have been described including an iron-regulated cholera-like toxin (Gardner, Fowlston and George 1987) and a heat-stable enterotoxin (Matthews, Douglas and Guiney 1988). Neither has been characterized to any extent. Most strains harbour a large plasmid with a molecular mass $>200 \times 10^3$ kDa (Olsvik et al. 1990). One strain (but not its plasmid-cured derivative) has been shown to produce diarrhoea and inflammation in the colonic mucosa of gnotobiotic piglets; however, no strain has been shown to produce diarrhoeal illness in adult volunteers (Herrington et al. 1987). An iron-regulated haemolysin produced by most *P. shigelloides* strains has been described (Daskaleros, Stroebner and Payne 1991). Its potential role in pathogenesis is unknown.

REFERENCES

Abbott SL, Kokka RP, Janda JM, 1991, Laboratory investigations on the low pathogenic potential of *Plesiomonas shigelloides*, *J Clin Microbiol*, **29:** 148–53.

Abbott SL, Powers C et al., 1989, Emergence of a restricted bioserovar of *Vibrio parahaemolyticus* as the predominant cause of vibrio-associated gastroenteritis on the West Coast of the United States and Mexico, *J Clin Microbiol*, **27:** 2891–3.

Abbott SL, Cheung WKW et al., 1992a, Isolation of vibriostatic agent O/129-resistant *Vibrio cholerae* non-O1 from a patient with gastroenteritis, *J Clin Microbiol*, **30:** 1598–9.

Abbott SL, Cheung WKW et al., 1992b, Identification of *Aeromonas* strains to the genospecies level in the clinical laboratory, *J Clin Microbiol*, **30:** 1262–6.

Ackermann H-W, Dauguet C et al., 1985, *Aeromonas* bacteriophages: reexamination and classification, *Ann Inst Pasteur*, **136:** 175–99.

Albert MJ, 1994, *Vibrio cholerae* O139, *J Clin Microbiol*, **32:** 2345–9.

Aldova E, 1994, Serovars of *Plesiomonas shigelloides*, *Zbl Bakt*, **281:** 38–44.

Alm RA, Manning PA, 1990, Biotype-specific probe for *Vibrio cholerae* serogroup O1, *J Clin Microbiol*, **28:** 823–4.

Altorfer R, Altwegg M et al., 1985, Growth of *Aeromonas* spp. on cefsulodin-irgasan-novobiocin agar selective for *Yersinia enterocolitica*, *J Clin Microbiol*, **22:** 478–80.

Altwegg M, Steigerwalt AG et al., 1990, Biochemical identification of *Aeromonas* genospecies isolated from humans, *J Clin Microbiol*, **28:** 258–64.

Altwegg M, Martinetti Luchini G et al., 1991, *Aeromonas*-associated gastroenteritis after consumption of contaminated shrimp, *Eur J Clin Microbiol Infect Dis*, **10:** 44–5.

Amako K, Okada K, Miake S, 1984, Evidence for the presence of a capsule in *Vibrio vulnificus*, *J Gen Microbiol*, **130:** 2741–3.

Ansaruzzaman M, Rahman M et al., 1995, Isolation of sucrose late-fermenting and nonfermenting variants of *Vibrio cholerae* O139 Bengal: implications for diagnosis of cholera, *J Clin Microbiol*, **33:** 1339–40.

Aoki T, Takahashi A, 1987, Class D tetracycline resistance determinants of R plasmids from the fish pathogen *Aeromonas hydrophila*, *Edwardsiella tarda*, and *Pasteurella piscicida*, *Antimicrob Agents Chemother*, **31:** 1278–80.

Arai T, Ikejima N et al., 1980, A survey of *Plesiomonas shigelloides* from aquatic environments, domestic animals, pets and humans, *J Hyg Camb*, **84:** 203–11.

Asao T, Kinoshita Y et al., 1984, Purification and some properties of *Aeromonas hydrophila* hemolysin, *Infect Immun*, **46:** 122–7.

Austin DA, McIntosh D, Austin B, 1989, Taxonomy of fish associated *Aeromonas* spp., with the description of *Aeromonas salmonicida* subsp. *smithia* subsp. *nov.*, *Syst Appl Microbiol*, 277–90.

Bakken JS, Sanders CC et al., 1988, β-Lactam resistance in *Aeromonas* spp. caused by inducible β-lactamases active against penicillins, cephalosporins, and carbapenems, *Antimicrob Agents Chemother*, **32:** 1314–19.

Banoub JH, Shaw DH, 1981, Structural investigations on the core oligosaccharide of *Aeromonas hydrophila* (chemotype III) lipopolysaccharide, *Carbohydr Res*, **98:** 93–103.

Banoub JH, Choy Y-M et al., 1983, Structural investigations on the core oligosaccharide of *Aeromonas hydrophila* (chemotype II) lipopolysaccharide, *Carbohydr Res*, **114:** 267–76.

Basu S, Mukerjee S, 1968, Bacteriophage typing of *Vibrio* El Tor, *Experientia*, **24:** 299–300.

Basu S, Tharanathan RN et al., 1985, Chemical structure of the lipid A component of *Plesiomonas shigelloides* and its taxonomical significance, *FEMS Microbiol Lett*, **28:** 7–10.

Baudry B, Fasano A et al., 1992, Cloning of a gene (*zot*) encoding a new toxin produced by *Vibrio cholerae*, *Infect Immun*, **60:** 428–34.

Baumann P, Furniss AL, Lee JV, 1984, *Bergey's Manual of Systematic Bacteriology*, vol. 1, eds Krieg NR, Holt JG, Williams & Wilkins, Baltimore, 518–38.

Baumann P, Schubert RHW, 1984, *Bergey's Manual of Systematic Bacteriology*, vol. 1, eds Krieg NR, Holt JG, Williams & Wilkins, Baltimore, 516.

Beazley WA, Palmer GG, 1992, TCI – a new bile free medium for the isolation of *Vibrio* species, *Austr J Med Sci*, 25–7.

Belland RJ, Trust TJ, 1987, Cloning of the gene for the surface array protein of *Aeromonas salmonicida* and evidence linking loss of expression with genetic deletion, *J Bacteriol*, **169:** 4086–91.

Belland RJ, Trust TJ, 1989, *Aeromonas salmonicida* plasmids: plasmid-directed synthesis of proteins *in vitro* and in *Escherichia coli* minicells, *J Gen Microbiol*, **135:** 513–24.

Brade H, 1985, Occurrence of 2-keto-deoxyoctonic acid 5-phosphate in lipopolysaccharides of *Vibrio cholerae* Ogawa and Inaba, *J Bacteriol*, **161:** 795–8.

Brayton PR, Bode RB et al., 1986, *Vibrio cincinnatiensis* sp. nov., a new human pathogen, *J Clin Microbiol*, **23:** 104–8.

Brenden RA, Miller MA, Janda JM, 1988, Clinical disease spectrum and pathogenic factors associated with *Plesiomonas shigelloides* infections in humans, *Rev Infect Dis*, **10:** 303–16.

Burgos A, Quindós G et al., 1990, In vitro susceptibility of *Aeromonas caviae*, *Aeromonas hydrophila* and *Aeromonas sobria* to fifteen antibacterial agents, *Eur J Clin Microbiol Infect Dis*, **9:** 413–17.

Calia KE, Murtagh M et al., 1994, Comparison of *Vibrio cholerae* O139 with *V. cholerae* O1 Classical and El Tor biotypes, *Infect Immun*, **62:** 1504–6.

Carnahan A, Fanning GR, Joseph SW, 1991, *Aeromonas jandaei* (formerly genospecies DNA group 9 *A. sobria*), a new sucrose-negative species isolated from clinical specimens, *J Clin Microbiol*, **29:** 560–4.

Carrnahan AM, Chakraborty T et al., 1991, *Aeromonas trota* sp. nov., an ampicillin-susceptible species isolated from clinical specimens, *J Clin Microbiol*, **29:** 1206–10.

Chakraborty T, Montenegro MA et al., 1984, Cloning of enterotoxin gene from *Aeromonas hydrophila* provides conclusive evidence of production of a cytotonic enterotoxin, *Infect Immun*, **46:** 435–41.

Chakraborty T, Huhle B et al., 1987, Marker exchange mutagenesis of the aerolysin determinant in *Aeromonas hydrophila*, *Infect Immun*, **55:** 2274–80.

Chang BJ, Bolton SM, 1987, Plasmids and resistance to antimicrobial agents in *Aeromonas sobria* and *Aeromonas hydrophila* clinical isolates, *Antimicrob Agents Chemother*, **31:** 1281–2.

Chattopadhyay DJ, Sarkar BL et al., 1993, New phage typing scheme for *Vibrio cholerae* O1 biotype El Tor strains, *J Clin Microbiol*, **31:** 1579–85.

Chopra AK, Houston CW, Kurosky A, 1991, Genetic variation in related cytolytic toxins produced by different species of *Aeromonas*, *FEMS Microbiol Lett*, **78:** 231–8.

Chou S, Aldova E, Kasatiya S, 1991, Cellular fatty acid composition of *Plesiomonas shigelloides*, *J Clin Microbiol*, **29:** 1072–4.

Choudhury SR, Bhadra RK, Das J, 1994, Genome size and restriction fragment analysis polymorphism of *Vibrio cholerae* strains belonging to different serovars and biotypes, *FEMS Microbiol Lett*, **115:** 329–34.

Chu S, Cavaignac S et al., 1991, Structure of the tetragonal surface virulence array protein and gene of *Aeromonas salmonicida*, *J Biol Chem*, **266:** 15258–65.

Clark RB, 1992, Antibiotic susceptibilities of the Vibrionaceae to meropenem and other antimicrobial agents, *Diagn Microbiol Infect Dis*, **15:** 453–5.

Clark RB, Lister PD et al., 1990, In vitro susceptibilities of *Plesiomonas shigelloides* to 24 antibiotics and antibiotic-β-lactamase-inhibitor combinations, *Antimicrob Agents Chemother*, **34:** 159–60.

Colwell RR, Huq A, 1994, Vibrio cholerae *and Cholera: Molecular to Global Perspectives*, ASM Press, Washington DC, 117–35.

Colwell RR, MacDonell MT, De Ley J, 1986, Proposal to recognize the family Aeromonadaceae fam. nov., *Int J Syst Bacteriol*, **36:** 473–7.

Colwell RR, Hasan JAK et al., 1992, Development and evaluation of a rapid, simple, sensitive, monoclonal antibody-based co-agglutination test for direct detection of *Vibrio cholerae* O1, *FEMS Microbiol Lett*, **97:** 215–20.

Comstock LE, Maneval Jr D et al., 1995, The capsule and O antigen in *Vibrio cholerae* O139 Bengal are associated with a genetic region not present in *Vibrio cholerae* O1, *Infect Immun*, **63:** 317–23.

Cravioto A, Beltrán P et al., 1994, Non-O1 *Vibrio cholerae* O139 Bengal is genetically related to *V. cholerae* O1 El Tor Ogawa isolated in Mexico, *J Infect Dis*, **169:** 1412–13.

Cutter DL, Kreger AS, 1990, Cloning and expression of the damselysin gene from *Vibrio damsela*, *Infect Immun*, **58:** 266–8.

Daskaleros PA, Stoebner JA, Payne SM, 1991, Iron uptake in *Plesiomonas shigelloides:* cloning of the genes for the heme-iron uptake system, *Infect Immun*, **59:** 2706–11.

Donlon J, McGettigan S et al., 1983, Re-appraisal of the nature of the pigment produced by *Aeromonas salmonicida*, *FEMS Microbiol Lett*, **19:** 285–90.

Dooley JGS, McCubbin WD et al., 1988, Isolation and biochemical characterization of the S-layer protein from a pathogenic *Aeromonas hydrophila* strain, *J Bacteriol*, **170:** 2631–8.

Dorsch M, Lane D, Stackebrandt E, 1992, Towards a phylogeny of the genus *Vibrio* based on 16S rRNA sequences, *Int J Syst Bacteriol*, **42:** 58–63.

Farmer III JJ, Arduino MJ, Hickman-Brenner FW, 1991, *The Prokaryotes A Handbook on the Biology of Bacteria: Ecophysiology, Isolation, Identification, Applications*, 2nd edn, Springer-Verlag, Berlin, 3012–45.

Farmer III JJ, Hickman-Brenner FW, 1991, *The Prokaryotes A Handbook on the Biology of Bacteria: Ecophysiology, Isolation, Identification, Applications*, 2nd edn, Springer-Verlag, Berlin, 2952–3011.

Faruque SM, Abdul ARM et al., 1993, Clonal relationships among classical *Vibrio cholerae* O1 strains isolated between 1961 and 1992 in Bangladesh, *J Clin Microbiol*, **31:** 2513–16.

Faruque SM, Abdul ARM et al., 1994, Molecular analysis of rRNA and cholera toxin genes carried by the new epidemic strain of toxigenic *Vibrio cholerae* O139 synonym Bengal, *J Clin Microbiol*, **32:** 1050–3.

Fasano A, Baudry B et al., 1991, *Vibrio cholerae* produces a second enterotoxin, which affects intestinal tight junctions, *Proc Natl Acad Sci USA*, **88:** 5242–6.

Finkelstein RA, Boesman-Finkelstein M et al., 1992, *Vibrio cholerae* hemagglutinin/protease, colonial variation, virulence, and detachment, *Infect Immun*, **60:** 472–8.

French GL, Woo ML et al., 1989, Antimicrobial susceptibilities of halophilic vibrios, *J Antimicrob Chemother*, **24:** 183–94.

Gander RM, LaRocco MT, 1989, Detection of piluslike structures on clinical and environmental isolates of *Vibrio vulnificus*, *J Clin Microbiol*, **27:** 1015–21.

Gardner SE, Fowlston SE, George WL, 1987, In vitro production of cholera toxin-like activity by *Plesiomonas shigelloides*, *J Infect Dis*, **156:** 720–2.

Garrote A, Bonet R et al., 1992, Occurrence of a capsule in *Aeromonas salmonicida*, *FEMS Microbiol Lett*, **95:** 127–32.

van der Goot FG, Pattus F et al., 1993, Oligomerization of the channel-forming toxin aerolysin precedes insertion into lipid bilayers, *Biochemistry*, **32:** 2636–42.

Gosling PJ, Turnbull PCB et al., 1993, Isolation and purification of *Aeromonas sobria* cytotonic enterotoxin and β-haemolysin, *J Med Microbiol*, **38:** 227–34.

Gotoh M, Barnes CN, Kovác, 1994, Improved synthesis and the crystal structure of methyl 4,6-dideoxy-4-(3-deoxy-L-*glycero*-tetronamido)-α-D-mannopyranoside, the methyl α-glycoside of the intracatenary repeating unit of the O-polysaccharide of *Vibrio cholerae* O:1, *Carbohydr Res*, **260:** 203–18.

von Graevenitz A, Bucher C, 1983, Evaluation of differential and selective media for isolation of *Aeromonas* and *Plesiomonas* spp. from human feces, *J Clin Microbiol*, **17:** 16–21.

Guidolin A, Manning PA, 1987, Genetics of *Vibrio cholerae* and its bacteriophages, *Microbiol Rev*, **51:** 285–98.

Hall RH, Vial PA et al., 1988, Morphological studies on fimbriae expressed by *Vibrio cholerae* O1, *Microb Pathog*, **4**: 257–65.

Hall RH, Khambaty FM et al., 1994, *Infect Immun*, **62**: 3859–63.

Han T-J, Chai T-J, 1991, Occurence of 2-keto-3-deoxy-D-*manno*-octonic acid in lipopolysaccharides isolated from *Vibrio parahaemolyticus*, *J Bacteriol*, **173**: 5303–6.

Hanes DE, Chandler DKF, 1993, The role of a 40-megadalton plasmid in the adherence and hemolytic properties of *Aeromonas hydrophila*, *Microb Pathog*, **15**: 313–17.

Hänninen M-L, 1994, Phenotypic characteristics of the three hybridization groups of *Aeromonas hydrophila* complex isolated from different sources, *J Appl Bacteriol*, **76**: 455–62.

Hansen W, Freney J et al., 1991, Gas-liquid chromatographic analysis of cellular fatty acid methyl esters in *Aeromonas* species, *Zbl Bakt*, **275**: 1–10.

Hasan JAK, Huq A et al., 1994, A novel kit for rapid detection of *Vibrio cholerae* O1, *J Clin Microbiol*, **32**: 249–52.

Häse CC, Finkelstein RA, 1991, Cloning and nucleotide sequence of the *Vibrio cholerae* hemagglutinin/protease (HA/protease) gene and construction of an HA/protease-negative strain, *J Bacteriol*, **173**: 3311–17.

Hayat U, Reddy GP et al., 1993, Capsular types of *Vibrio vulnificus*: an analysis of strains from clinical and environmental sources, *J Infect Dis*, **168**: 758–62.

Hazen TC, Fliermans CB et al., 1978, Prevalence and distribution of *Aeromonas hydrophila* in the United States, *Appl Environ Microbiol*, 731–8.

Hedges RW, Smith P, Brazil G, 1985, Resistance plasmids of aeromonads, *J Gen Microbiol*, **131**: 2091–5.

Herrington DA, Tzipori S et al., 1987, In vitro and in vivo pathogenicity of *Plesiomonas shigelloides*, *Infect Immun*, **55**: 979–85.

Herrington DA, Hall RH et al., 1988, Toxin, toxin-coregulated pili, and the *toxR* regulon are essential for *Vibrio cholerae* pathogenesis in humans, *J Exp Med*, **168**: 1487–92.

Hickman-Brenner FW, MacDonald KL et al., 1987, *Aeromonas veronii*, a new ornithine decarboxylase-positive species that may cause diarrhea, *J Clin Microbiol*, **25**: 900–6.

Hickman-Brenner FW, Fanning GR et al., 1988, *Aeromonas schubertii*, a new mannitol-negative species found in human clinical specimens, *J Clin Microbiol*, **26**: 1561–4.

Hirono I, Aoki T, 1991, Nucleotide sequence and expression of an extracellular hemolysin gene of *Aeromonas hydrophila*, *Microb Pathog*, **11**: 189–97.

Hirono I, Aoki T et al., 1992, Nucleotide sequences and characterization of haemolysin genes from *Aeromonas hydrophila* and *Aeromonas sobria*, *Microb Pathog*, **13**: 433–46.

Hirschhorn N, Greenough III WB, 1971, Cholera, *Sci Amer*, **225**: 15–21.

Hisatsune K, Iguchi T et al., 1993a, Lipopolysaccharide isolated from a new O-antigenic form (O13) of *Vibrio parahaemolyticus*, *Microbiol Immunol*, **37**: 143–7.

Hisatsune K, Kondo S et al., 1993b, Occurence of 2-*O*-methyl-*N*-(3-deoxy-*L*-*glycero*-tetronyl)-*D*-perosamine (4-amino-4,6-dideoxy-*D*-*manno*-pyranose) in lipopolysaccharide from Ogawa but not from Inaba O forms of O1 *Vibrio cholerae*, *Biochem Biophys Res Commun*, **190**: 302–7.

Hisatsune K, Kondo S et al., 1993c, O-antigenic lipopolysaccharide of *Vibrio cholerae* O139 Bengal, a new epidemic strain for recent cholera in the Indian subcontinent, *Biochem Biophys Res Commun*, **196**: 1309–15.

Ho ASY, Sohel I, Schoolnik GK, 1992, Cloning and characterization of *fxp*, the flexible pilin gene of *Aeromonas hydrophila*, *Mol Microbiol*, **6**: 2725–32.

Ho ASY, Mietzner TA et al., 1990, The pili of *Aeromonas hydrophila*: identification of an environmentally regulated 'mini pilin', *J Exp Med*, **172**: 795–806.

Hokama A, Honma Y, Nakasone N, 1990, Pili of an *Aeromonas hydrophila* strain as a possible colonization factor, *Microbiol Immunol*, **34**: 901–15.

Honda S, Matsumoto S et al., 1992, A survey of urease-positive *Vibrio parahaemolyticus* strains isolated from traveller's diarrhea, sea water and imported frozen sea foods, *Eur J Epidemiol*, **8**: 861–4.

Honda T, Ni Y, Miwatani T, 1988, Purification and characterization of a hemolysin produced by a clinical isolate of Kanagawa phenomenon-negative *Vibrio parahaemolyticus* and related to the thermostable direct hemolysin, *Infect Immun*, **56**: 961–5.

Honda T, Arita M et al., 1988a, Production of pili on *Vibrio parahaemolyticus*, *Can J Microbiol*, **34**: 1279–81.

Honda T, Kasemsuksakul K et al., 1988b, Production and partial characterization of pili on non-O1 *Vibrio cholerae*, *J Infect Dis*, **157**: 217–18.

Honda T, Ni Y et al., 1990, Properties of a hemolysin related to the thermostable direct hemolysin produced by a Kanagawa phenomenon negative, clinical isolate of *Vibrio parahaemolyticus*, *Can J Microbiol*, **36**: 395–9.

Honda T, Ni Y et al., 1992, The thermostable direct hemolysin of *Vibrio parahaemolyticus* is a pore-forming toxin, *Can J Microbiol*, **38**: 1175–80.

Hood MA, Ness GE et al., 1984, *Vibrios in the Environment*, John Wiley, New York, 399–409.

Huntley JS, Hall AC et al., 1993, Cation flux studies of the lesion induced in human erythrocyte membranes by the thermostable direct hemolysin of *Vibrio parahaemolyticus*, *Infect Immun*, **61**: 4326–32.

Huq A, Akhtar A et al., 1991, Optimal growth temperature for the isolation of *Plesiomonas shigelloides*, using various selective and differential agars, *Can J Microbiol*, **37**: 800–2.

Huq A, Alam M et al., 1992, Occurrence of resistance to vibriostatic compound O/129 in *Vibrio cholerae* O1 isolated from clinical and environmental samples in Bangladesh, *J Clin Microbiol*, **30**: 219–21.

Huys G, Vancanneyt M et al., 1994, Cellular fatty acid composition as a chemotaxonomic marker for the differentiation of phenospecies and hybridization groups in the genus *Aeromonas*, *Int J Syst Bacteriol*, **44**: 651–8.

Iaconis JP, Sanders CC, 1990, Purification and characterization of inducible β-lactamases in *Aeromonas* spp., *Antimicrob Agents Chemother*, **34**: 44–51.

Ichinose Y, Yamamoto K et al., 1987, Enterotoxicity of El Tor-like hemolysis of non-O1 *Vibrio cholerae*, *Infect Immun*, **55**: 1090–3.

Inoue K, Kosako Y et al., 1991, Peritrichous flagellation in *Plesiomonas shigelloides* strains, *Japan J Med Sci Biol*, **44**: 141–6.

Ishimaru K, Akagawa-Matsushita M, Muroga K, 1995, *Int J Syst Bacteriol*, **45**: 134–8.

Ito T, Hiramatsu K et al., 1993, Mutations in the *rfbT* gene are responsible for the Ogawa to Inaba serotype conversion in *Vibrio cholerae*, *Microbiol Immunol*, **37**: 281–8.

Ito T, Higuchi T et al., 1994, Identification of a novel sugar, 4-amino-4,6-dideoxy-2-*O*-methylmannose in the lipopolysaccharide of *Vibrio cholerae* O1 serotype Ogawa, *Carbohydr Res*, **256**: 113–28.

Janda JM, 1991, Recent advances in the study of the taxonomy, pathogenicity, and infectious syndromes associated with the genus *Aeromonas*, *Clin Microbiol Rev*, **4**: 397–410.

Janda JM, Abbott SL, Morris Jr JG, 1995, *Infections of the Gastrointestinal Tract*, Raven Press, New York, 905–17.

Janda JM, Duffey PS, 1988, Mesophilic aeromonads in human disease: current taxonomy, laboratory identification, and infectious disease spectrum, *Rev Infect Dis*, **10**: 980–97.

Janda JM, Kokka RP, 1991, The pathogenicity of *Aeromonas* strains relative to genospecies and phenospecies identification, *FEMS Microbiol Lett*, **90**: 29–34.

Janda JM, Kokka RP, Guthertz LS, 1994, The susceptibility of S-layer-positive and S-layer-negative *Aeromonas* strains to complement-mediated lysis, *Microbiology*, **140**: 2899–905.

Janda JM, Powers C et al., 1988, Current perspectives on the epidemiology and pathogenesis of clinically significant *Vibrio* spp., *Clin Microbiol Rev*, **1**: 245–67.

Janda JM, Guthertz LS et al., 1994, *Aeromonas* species in septicemia: laboratory characteristics and clinical observations, *Clin Infect Dis*, **19**: 77–83.

Johnson JA, Morris Jr JG, Kaper JB, 1993, Gene encoding zonula occludens toxin (*zot*) does not occur independently from cholera enterotoxin genes (*ctx*) in *Vibrio cholerae*, *J Clin Microbiol*, **31**: 732–3.

Johnson JA, Panigrahi P, Morris Jr JG , 1992, Non-O1 *Vibrio cholerae* NRT36S produces a polysaccharide capsule that determines colony morphology, serum resistance, and virulence in mice, *Infect Immun*, **60**: 864–9.

Johnson JA, Salles CA et al., 1994, *Vibrio cholerae* O139 synonym Bengal is closely related to *Vibrio cholerae* El Tor but has important differences, *Infect Immun*, **62**: 2108–10.

Joseph SW, Colwell RR, Kaper JB, 1982, *Vibrio parahaemolyticus* and related halophilic vibrios, *Crit Rev Microbiol*, **10**: 77–124.

Kain KC, Kelly MT, 1989, Antimicrobial susceptibility of *Plesiomonas shigelloides* from patients with diarrhea, *Antimicrob Agents Chemother*, **33**: 1609–10.

Kämpfer P, Altwegg M, 1992, Numerical classification and identification of *Aeromonas* genospecies, *J Appl Bacteriol*, **72**: 341–51.

Kämpfer P, Blaszyk K, Auling G, 1994, Characterization of *Aeromonas* genomic species by using quinone, polyamine, and fatty acid patterns, *Can J Microbiol*, **40**: 844–50.

Kaper JB, Morris Jr JG, Levine MM, 1995, Cholera, *Clin Microbiol Rev*, **8**: 48–86.

Kay WW, Trust TJ, 1991, Form and functions of the regular surface array (S-layer) of *Aeromonas salmonicida*, *Experientia*, **47**: 412–14.

Kelly MT, Stroh EMD, Jessop J, 1988, Comparison of blood agar, ampicillin blood agar, MacConkey-ampicillin-tween agar, and modified cefsulodin-irgasan-novobiocin agar for isolation of *Aeromonas* spp. from stool specimens, *J Clin Microbiol*, **26**: 1738–40.

Koblavi S, Grimont F, Grimont PA, 1990, Clonal diversity of *Vibrio cholerae* O1 evidenced by rRNA gene restriction patterns, *Res Microbiol*, **141**: 645–57.

Koehler JM, Ashdown LR, 1993, In vitro susceptibilites of tropical strains of *Aeromonas* species from Queensland, Australia, to 22 antimicrobial agents, *Antimicrob Agents Chemother*, **37**: 905–7.

Kokka RP, Vedros NA, Janda JM, 1992, Immunochemical analysis and possible biological role of an *Aeromonas hydrophila* surface array protein in septicaemia, *J Gen Microbiol*, **138**: 1229–36.

Kokka RP, Janda JM et al., 1991, Biochemical and genetic characterization of autoagglutinating phenotypes of *Aeromonas* species associated with invasive and noninvasive disease, *J Infect Dis*, **163**: 890–4.

Kondo S, Haishima Y, Hisatsune K, 1990, Analysis of the 2-keto-3-deoxyoctonate (KDO) region of lipopolysaccharides isolated from non-O1 *Vibrio cholerae* 05R, *FEMS Microbiol Lett*, **68**: 155–8.

Kothary MH, Kreger AS, 1985, Purification and characterization of an extracellular cytolysin produced by *Vibrio damsela*, *Infect Immun*, **49**: 25–31.

Kozaki S, Asao T et al., 1989, Characterization of *Aeromonas sobria* hemolysin by use of monoclonal antibodies against *Aeromonas hydrophila* hemolysins, *J Clin Microbiol*, **27**: 1782–6.

Kreger AS, Bernheimer AW et al., 1987, Phospholipase D activity of *Vibrio damsela* cytolysin and its interaction with sheep erythrocytes, *Infect Immun*, **55**: 3209–12.

Krovacek K, Faris A et al., 1992, Prevalence and characterization of *Aeromonas* spp. isolated from foods in Uppsala, Sweden, *Food Microbiol*, **9**: 29–36.

Kuijper EJ, Steigerwalt AG et al., 1989, Phenotypic characterization and DNA relatedness in human fecal isolates of *Aeromonas* spp., *J Clin Microbiol*, **27**: 132–8.

Lambert MA, Hickman-Brenner FW et al., 1983, Differentiation of Vibrionaceae species by their cellular fatty acid composition, *Int J Syst Bacteriol*, **33**: 777–92.

Lee JV, 1990, *Topley and Wilson's Principles of Bacteriology, Virology*

and Immunity, vol. 2, 8th edn, eds Parker MT, Duerden BL, Edward Arnold, London, 514–30.

Lesmana M, Subekti D et al., 1994, Modified CAMP test for biogrouping *Vibrio cholerae* O1 strains and distinguishing them from strains of *V. cholerae* non-O1, *J Clin Microbiol*, **32**: 235–7.

Levine MM, Kaper JB et al., 1988, Volunteer studies of deletion mutants of *Vibrio cholerae* O1 prepared by recombinant techniques, *Infect Immun*, **56**: 161–7.

Litwin CM, Calderwood SB, 1993, Cloning and genetic analysis of the *Vibrio vulnificus fur* gene and construction of a *fur* mutant by in vivo marker exchange, *J Bacteriol*, **175**: 706–15.

Ljungh A, Wretlind B, Möllby R, 1981, Separation and characterization of enterotoxin and two haemolysins from *Aeromonas hydrophila*, *Acta Pathol Micrbiol Scand*, **89**: 387–97.

McCarter L, Silverman M, 1990, Surface-induced swarmer cell differentiation of *Vibrio parahaemolyticus*, *Mol Microbiol*, **4**: 1057–62.

MacDonell MT, Swartz DG et al., 1986, Ribosomal RNA phylogenies for the vibrio-enteric group of eubacteria, *Microbiol Sci*, **3**: 172–8.

Mahalingam S, Cheong YM et al., 1993, Occurrence of *Vibrio cholerae* O1 strains in Southeast Asia resistant to vibriostatic compound O/129, *Southeast Asian J Trop Med Publ Health*, **24**: 779–80.

Manafi M, Rotter M-L, 1992, Enzymatic profile of *Plesiomonas shigelloides*, *J Microbiol Methods*, **16**: 175–80.

Marcus H, Ketley JM et al., 1990, Effects of DNase production, plasmid size, and restriction barriers on transformation of *Vibrio cholerae* by electroporation and osmotic shock, *FEMS Microbiol Lett*, **68**: 149–54.

Martinetti Lucchini G, Altwegg M, 1992, rRNA gene restriction patterns as taxonomic tools for the genus *Aeromonas*, *Int J Syst Bacteriol*, **42**: 384–9.

Martinez-Murcia AJ, Benlloch S, Collins MD, 1992, Phylogenetic interrelationships of members of the genera *Aeromonas* and *Plesiomonas* as determined by 16S ribosomal DNA sequencing: lack of congruence with results of DNA-DNA hybridizations, *Int J Syst Bacteriol*, **42**: 412–21.

Martinez-Murcia AJ, Esteve C et al., 1992, *Aeromonas allosaccharophila* sp. nov., a new mesophilic member of the genus *Aeromonas*, *FEMS Microbiol Lett*, **91**: 199–206.

Massidda O, Rossolini GM, Satta G, 1991, The *Aeromonas hydrophila cphA* gene: molecular heterogeneity among class B metallo-β-lactamases, *J Bacteriol*, **173**: 4611–17.

Matsushita S, Kudoh Y, Ohashi M, 1984, Transferable resistance to the vibriostatic agent 2,4-diamino-6,7-diisopropyl-pteridine (O/129) in *Vibrio cholerae*, *Microbiol Immunol*, **28**: 1159–62.

Matthews BG, Douglas H, Guiney DG, 1988, Production of a heat stable enterotoxin by *Plesiomonas shigelloides*, *Microb Pathog*, **5**: 207–13.

Medema G, Schets C, 1993, Occurrence of *Plesiomonas shigelloides* in surface water: relationship with faecal pollution and trophic state, *Zbl Hyg*, **194**: 398–404.

Mekalanos JJ, 1983, Duplication and amplification of toxin genes in *Vibrio cholerae*, *Cell*, **35**: 253–63.

Mekalanos JJ, 1985, Cholera toxin: genetic analysis, regulation, and role in pathogenesis, *Curr Top Microbiol Immunol*, **118**: 97–118.

Merino S, Camprubi S, Tomás JM, 1990a, Identification of the cell receptor for bacteriophage 18 from *Aeromonas hydrophila*, *Res Microbiol*, **141**: 173–80.

Merino S, Camprubi S, Tomás JM, 1990b, Isolation and characterization of bacteriophage PM3 from *Aeromonas hydrophila* the bacterial receptor for which is the monopolar flagellum, *FEMS Microbiol Lett*, 277–82.

Merino S, Camprubi S, Tomás JM, 1991, The role of lipopolysaccharide in complement-killing of *Aeromonas hydrophila* strains of serotype O:34, *J Gen Microbiol*, **137**: 1583–90.

Michon F, Shaw DH, Banoub JH, 1984, Structure of the lipopolysaccharide core isolated from a human strain of *Aeromonas hydrophila*, *Eur J Biochem*, **145**: 107–14.

Miller ML, Koburger JA, 1985, *Plesiomonas shigelloides:* an opportunistic food and waterborne pathogen, *J Food Prot,* **48:** 449–57.

Miller ML, Koburger JA, 1986a, Evaluation of inositol brilliant green bile salts and *Plesiomonas* agars for recovery of *Plesiomonas shigelloides* from aquatic samples in a seasonal survey of the Suwannee river estuary, *J Food Prot,* **49:** 274–7.

Miller ML, Koburger JA, 1986b, Tolerance of *Plesiomonas shigelloides* to pH, sodium chloride and temperature, *J Food Prot,* **49:** 877–9.

Millership SE, Chattopadhyay B, 1985, *Aeromonas hydrophila* in chlorinated water supplies, *J Hosp Infect,* **6:** 75–80.

Miyamoto Y, Kato T et al., 1969, In vitro hemolytic characteristic of *Vibrio parahaemolyticus:* its close correlation with human pathogenicity, *J Bacteriol,* **100:** 1147–9.

Morris Jr JG, Tenney JH, Drusano GL, 1985, In vitro susceptibility of pathogenic *Vibrio* species to norfloxacin and six other antimicrobial agents, *Antimicrob Agents Chemother,* **28:** 442–5.

Morris Jr JG, Takeda T et al., 1990, Experimental non-O1 group 1 *Vibrio cholerae* gastroenteritis in humans, *J Clin Invest,* **85:** 697–705.

Motyl MR, McKinley G, Janda JM, 1985, In vitro susceptibility of *Aeromonas hydrophila, Aeromonas sobria,* and *Aeromonas caviae* to 22 antimicrobial agents, *Antimicrob Agents Chemother,* **28:** 151–3.

Moyenuddin M, Wachsmuth K et al., 1993, Potential pathogenic factors produced by a clinical nontoxigenic *Vibrio cholerae* O1, *Curr Microbiol,* **27:** 329–33.

Nair GB, Shimada T et al., 1994, Characterization of phenotypic, serological, and toxigenic traits of *Vibrio cholerae* O139 Bengal, *J Clin Microbiol,* **32:** 2775–9.

Nakasone N, Iwanaga M, 1990, Pili of a *Vibrio parahaemolyticus* strain as a possible colonization factor, *Infect Immun,* **58:** 61–9.

Nandy RK, Sengupta TK et al., 1995, A comparative study of the properties of *Vibrio cholerae* O139, O1 and other non-O1 strains, *J Med Microbiol,* **42:** 251–7.

Nath G, Sanyal SC, 1992, Emergence of *Vibrio cholerae* O1 resistant to vibriostatic agent O/129, *Lancet,* **340:** 366–7.

Newland JW, Voll MJ, McNicol LA, 1984, Serology and plasmid carriage in *Vibrio cholerae, Can J Microbiol,* **30:** 1149–56.

Nishibuchi M, Kaper JB, 1990, Duplication and variation of the thermostable direct haemolysin (*tdh*) gene in *Vibrio parahaemolyticus, Mol Microbiol,* **4:** 87–99.

Nishibuchi M, Ishibashi M et al., 1985, Detection of the thermostable direct hemolysin gene and related DNA sequences in *Vibrio parahaemolyticus* and other *Vibrio* species by the DNA colony hybridization test, *Infect Immun,* **49:** 481–6.

Nishibuchi M, Taniguchi T et al., 1989, Cloning and nucleotide sequence of the gene (*trh*) encoding the hemolysin related to the thermostable direct hemolysin of *Vibrio parahaemolyticus, Infect Immun,* **57:** 2691–7.

Nishikawa Y, Kishi T, 1988, Isolation and characterization of motile *Aeromonas* from humans, food and environmental specimens, *Epidemiol Infect,* **101:** 213–23.

Ogawa J, Amano Y, 1987, Electron microprobe X-ray analysis of polyphosphate granules in *Plesiomonas shigelloides, Microbiol Immunol,* **31:** 1121–5.

Olsvik O, Wachsmuth K et al., 1990, Laboratory observations on *Plesiomonas shigelloides* strains isolated from children with diarrhea in Peru, *J Clin Microbiol,* **28:** 886–9.

Ottemann KM, Mekalanos JJ, 1994, Vibrio cholerae *and Cholera: Molecular to Global perspectives,* ASM Press, Washington DC, 177–87.

Pacini F, 1854, Osservazione microscopiche e deduzioni pathologiche sul Cholera Asiatico, *Gaz Med Ital Toscana Firenza,* **6:** 405–12.

Pajini S, Sharma C et al., 1995, Studies on the genesis of *Vibrio cholerae* O139: identification of probable progenitor strains, *J Med Microbiol,* **42:** 20–5.

Parker MW, Buckley JT et al., 1994, Structure of the *Aeromonas*

toxin proaerolysin in its water-soluble and membrane-channel states, *Nature,* **367:** 292–5.

Parsot C, Mekalanos JJ, 1990, Expression of ToxR, the transcriptional activator of the virulence factors in *Vibrio cholerae,* is modulated by the heat shock response, *Proc Natl Acad Sci USA,* 9898–902.

Pastian MR, Bromel MC, 1984, Inclusion bodies in *Plesiomonas shigelloides, Appl Environ Microbiol,* **47:** 216–18.

Pazzaglia G, Sack RB et al., 1990, Diarrhea and intestinal invasiveness of *Aeromonas* strains in the removable intestinal tie rabbit model, *Infect Immun,* **58:** 1924–31.

Pearson GDN, Woods A et al., 1993, CTX genetic element encodes a site-specific recombination system and an essential colonization factor, *Proc Natl Acad Sci USA,* **90:** 3750–4.

Popoff M, 1984, *Bergey's Manual of Systematic Bacteriology,* vol. 1, eds Krieg NR, Holt JG, Williams & Wilkins, Baltimore, 545–6.

Popoff M, Véron M, 1976, A taxonomic study of the *Aeromonas hydrophila-Aeromonas punctata* group, *J Gen Microbiol,* **94:** 11–22.

Popoff MY, Coynault C et al., 1981, Polynucleotide sequence relatedness among motile *Aeromonas* species, *Curr Microbiol,* **5:** 109–14.

Preston LM, Xu Q et al., 1995, Preliminary structure determination of the capsular polysaccharide of *Vibrio cholerae* O139 Bengal A11837, *J Bacteriol,* **177:** 835–8.

Puglielli L, Cattrini C et al., 1992, Symptomless carriage of *Vibrio cholerae* in Peru, *Lancet,* **339:** 1056–7.

Rader AE, Murphy JR, 1988, Nucleotide sequences and comparison of the hemolysin determinants of *Vibrio cholerae* El Tor RV79(Hly⁺) and RV79(Hly⁻) and Classical 569B(Hly⁻), *Infect Immun,* **56:** 1414–19.

Ramamurthy T, Pal A et al., 1992, Taxonomical implications of the emergence of high frequency of occurrence of 2,4-diamino-6,7-diisopropylpteridine-resistant strains of *Vibrio cholerae* from clinical cases of cholera in Calcutta, India, *J Clin Microbiol,* **30:** 742–3.

Ramamurthy T, Bag PK et al., 1993, Virulence patterns of *Vibrio cholerae* non-O1 strains isolated from hospitalised patients with acute diarrhoea in Calcutta, India, *J Med Microbiol,* **39:** 310–17.

Rautelin H, Hänninen ML et al., 1995, Chronic diarrhea due to a single strain of *Aeromonas caviae, Eur J Clin Microbiol Infect Dis,* **14:** 51–3.

Reinhardt JF, George WL, 1985, Comparative in vitro activities of selected antimicrobial agents against *Aeromonas* species and *Plesiomonas shigelloides, Antimicrob Agents Chemother,* **27:** 643–5.

Richardson SH, 1994, Vibrio cholerae *and Cholera: Molecular to Global Perspectives,* ASM Press, Washington DC, 203–29.

Rietschel ET, Wollenweber H-W et al., 1984, Concepts of the chemical structure of lipid A, *Rev Infect Dis,* **6:** 432–8.

Rossi A, Galas M et al., 1993, Unusual multiresistant *Vibrio cholerae* O1 El Tor in Argentina, *Lancet,* **342:** 1172.

Ruimy R, Breittmayer V et al., 1994, Phylogenetic analysis and assessment of the genera *Vibrio, Photobacterium, Aeromonas,* and *Plesiomonas* deduced from small-subunit rRNA sequences, *Int J Syst Bacteriol,* **44:** 416–26.

Sakazaki R, Donovan TJ, 1984, *Methods in Microbiology,* vol. 16, Academic Press, London, 271–91.

Sakazaki R, Shimada T, 1984, O-serogrouping scheme for mesophilic *Aeromonas* strains, *Jpn J Med Sci Biol,* **37:** 247–55.

Sarker RI, Ogawa W et al., 1994, Characterization of a glucose transport system in *Vibrio parahaemolyticus, J Bacteriol,* **176:** 7378–82.

Schubert RHW, 1984, *Bergey's Manual of Systematic Bacteriology,* vol. 1, eds Krieg Nr, Holt JG, Williams & Wilkins, Baltimore, 548–9.

Shaw DH, Hodder HJ, 1978, Lipopolysaccharides of the motile aeromonads; core oligosaccharide analysis as an aid to taxonomic classification, *Can J Microbiol,* **24:** 864–8.

Shaw DH, Squires MJ, 1984, O-antigen structure in a virulent strain of *Aeromonas hydrophila, FEMS Microbiol Lett,* **24:** 277–80.

Shaw DH, Lee Y-Z et al., 1983, Structural studies on the O-antigen of *Aeromonas salmonicida*, *Eur J Biochem*, **131**: 633–8.

Shimada T, Kosako Y, 1991, Comparison of two O-serogrouping systems for mesophilic *Aeromonas* spp., *J Clin Microbiol*, **29**: 197–9.

Shimada T, Sakazaki R, 1978, On the serology of *Plesiomonas shigelloides*, *Jpn J Med Sci Biol*, **31**: 135–42.

Shimada T, Sakazaki R, 1984, On the serology of *Vibrio vulnificus*, *Jpn J Med Sci Biol*, **37**: 241–6.

Shimada T, Sakazaki R, 1985, New O and H antigens and additional serovars of *Plesiomonas shigelloides*, *Jpn J Med Sci Biol*, **38**: 73–6.

Shimada T, Sakazaki R et al., 1990, A new selective, differential agar medium for isolation of *Vibrio cholerae* O1: PMT (polymyxin-mannose-tellurite) agar, *Jpn J Med Sci Biol*, **43**: 37–41.

Shimada T, Kosako Y et al., 1991, *Vibrio fluvialis* and *Vibrio furnissii* serotyping scheme for international use, *Curr Microbiol*, **22**: 335–7.

Shimada T, Arakawa E et al., 1994a, Two strains of *Vibrio cholerae* non-O1 possessing somatic (O) antigen factors in common with *V. cholerae* serogroup O139 synonym 'Bengal', *Curr Microbiol*, **29**: 331–3.

Shimada T, Arakawa E et al., 1994b, Extended serotyping scheme for *Vibrio cholerae*, *Curr Microbiol*, **28**: 175–8.

Shimada T, Arakawa E et al., 1994c, New O and H antigens of *Plesiomonas shigelloides* and their O antigenic relationships to *Shigella boydii*, *Curr Microbiol*, **28**: 351–4.

Simpson LM, White VK et al., 1987, Correlation between virulence and colony morphology in *Vibrio vulnificus*, *Infect Immun*, **55**: 269–72.

Spangler BD, 1992, Structure and function of cholera toxin and the related *Escherichia coli* heat-labile enterotoxin, *Microbiol Rev*, **56**: 622–47.

Stroeher UH, Karageorgos LE et al., 1992, Serotype conversion in *Vibrio cholerae* O1, *Proc Natl Acad Sci USA*, **89**: 2566–70.

Sun D, Mekalanos JJ, Taylor RK, 1990, Antibodies directed against the toxin-coregulated pilus isolated from *Vibrio cholerae* provide protection in the infant mouse experimental cholera model, *J Infect Dis*, **161**: 1231–6.

Taylor RK, Miller VL et al., 1987, Use of *phoA* gene fusions to identify a pilus colonization factor coordinately regulated with cholera toxin, *Proc Natl Acad Sci USA*, **84**: 2833–7.

Terai A, Shirai H et al., 1990, Nucleotide sequence of the thermostable direct hemolysin gene (*tdh* gene) of *Vibrio mimicus* and its evolutionary relationship with the *tdh* genes of *Vibrio parahaemolyticus*, *FEMS Microbiol Lett*, **71**: 319–24.

Terai A, Baba K et al., 1991, Evidence for insertion sequence-mediated spread of the thermostable direct hemolysin gene among *Vibrio* species, *J Bacteriol*, **173**: 5036–46.

Thomas LV, Gross RJ et al., 1990, Extended serogrouping scheme for motile, mesophilic *Aeromonas* species, *J Clin Microbiol*, **28**: 980–4.

Threlfall EJ, Said B, Rowe B, 1993, Emergence of multiple drug resistance in *Vibrio cholerae* O1 El Tor from Ecuador, *Lancet*, **342**: 1173.

Tison DL, Nishibuchi M et al., 1982, *Appl Environ Microbiol*, **44**: 640–6.

Tonolla M, Demarta A, Peduzzi R, 1991, Multilocus genetic relationships between clinical and environmental *Aeromonas* strains, *FEMS Microbiol Lett*, **81**: 193–200.

Toranzo AE, Barja JL et al., 1983, Characterization of plasmids in bacterial fish pathogens, *Infect Immun*, **39**: 184–92.

Trucksis M, Galen JE et al., 1993, Accessory cholera enterotoxin (Ace), the third toxin of a *Vibrio cholerae* virulence cassette, *Proc Natl Acad Sci USA*, **90**: 5267–71.

Tucker AD, Parker MW et al., 1990, Crystallization of a proform of aerolysin, a hole-forming toxin from *Aeromonas hydrophila*, *J Mol Biol*, **212**: 561–2.

Twedt RM, Brown DF, Zink DL, 1981, Comparison of plasmid deoxyribonucleic acid contents, culture characteristics, and indices of pathogenicity among selected strains of *Vibrio parahaemolyticus*, *Infect Immun*, **33**: 322–5.

Urdaci MC, Marchand M, Grimont PAD, 1990, Characterization of 22 *Vibrio* species by gas chromatography analysis of their cellular fatty acids, *Res Microbiol*, **141**: 437–52.

Van Damme LR, Vandepitte J, 1980, Frequent isolation of *Edwardsiella tarda* and *Plesiomonas shigelloides* from healthy Zairese freshwater fish: a possible source of sporadic diarrhea in the tropics, *Appl Environ Microbiol*, **39**: 475–9.

Veenstra J, Rietra PJG et al., 1992, Infection caused by an indole-negative variant of *Vibrio vulnificus* transmitted by eels, *J Infect Dis*, **166**: 209–10.

Véron MM, 1965, La position taxonomique des *Vibrio* et de certaines bacteries comparables, *C R Acad Sci*, **261**: 5243–6.

Wachsmuth IK, Evins GM et al., 1993, The molecular epidemiology of cholera in Latin America, *J Infect Dis*, **167**: 621–6.

Waldor MK, Colwell RR, Mekalanos JJ, 1994, The *Vibrio cholerae* O139 serogroup antigen includes an O-antigen capsule and lipopolysaccharide virulence determinants, *Proc Natl Acad Sci USA*, **91**: 11388–92.

Waldor MK, Mekalanos JJ, 1994a, ToxR regulates virulence gene expression in non-O1 strains of *Vibrio cholerae* that cause epidemic cholera, *Infect Immun*, **62**: 72–8.

Waldor MK, Mekalanos JJ, 1994b, Emergence of a new cholera pandemic: molecular analysis of virulence determinants in *Vibrio cholerae* O139 and development of a live vaccine prototype, *J Infect Dis*, **170**: 278–83.

Weber JT, Mintz ED et al., 1994, Epidemic cholera in Ecuador: multidrug-resistance and transmission by water and seafood, *Epidemiol Infect*, **112**: 1–11.

Whang HY, Heller ME, Neter E, 1972, Production by *Aeromonas* of common enterobacterial antigen and its possible taxonomic significance, *J Bacteriol*, **110**: 161–4.

Wilmsen HU, Buckley JT, Pattus F, 1991, Site-directed mutagenesis at histidines of aerolysin from *Aeromonas hydrophila*: a lipid bilayer study, *Mol Microbiol*, **5**: 2745–51.

Wright AC, Simpson LM et al., 1990, Phenotypic evaluation of acapsular transposon mutants of *Vibrio vulnificus*, *Infect Immun*, **58**: 1769–73.

Yam W-C, Yuen K-Y, Wong S-S-Y, 1994, *Vibrio cholerae* O139 susceptible to vibriostatic agent O/129 and co-trimoxazole *Lancet*, **344**: 404–5.

Yamamoto S, Chowdhury MAR et al., 1991, Further study on polyamine compositions in Vibrionaceae, *Can J Microbiol*, **37**: 148–53.

Yamamoto T, Albert MJ, Sack RB, 1994, Adherence to human small intestines of capsulated *Vibrio cholerae* O139, *FEMS Microbiol Lett*, **119**: 229–36.

Yoshida S-I, Ogawa M, Mizuguchi Y, 1985, Relation of capsular materials and colony opacity to virulence of *Vibrio vulnificus*, *Infect Immun*, **47**: 446–51.

Zitzer AO, Nakisbekov NO et al., 1993, Entero-cytolysin (EC) from *Vibrio cholerae* non-O1 (some properties and pore-forming activity), *Zbl Bakt*, **279**: 494–50.

INTRODUCTION TO THE AEROBIC PSEUDOMONADS

N J Palleroni

1   INTRODUCTION

The name 'pseudomonads' is applied to gram-negative, aerobic non-sporulated, rod-shaped bacteria that are motile by means of polar flagella. The organisms with these characteristics are phylogenetically very diverse and cannot be allocated in a single bacterial family. Many species have a remarkable nutritional versatility, some are animal and human pathogens, and as such, they are usually considered as opportunistic. They combine a pathogenic propensity towards immunologically compromised hosts with an intrinsic capacity for tolerance to many deleterious agents, including antibiotics.

In *Bergey's Manual of Systematic Bacteriology* (Palleroni 1984) and *The Prokaryotes* (Palleroni 1992), some genera of distantly related aerobic pseudomonads were assigned to the family Pseudomonadaceae, because of their marked phenotypic resemblance to species of the genus *Pseudomonas*. This resemblance and their medical importance are why some phylogenetically unrelated organisms originally described as species of *Pseudomonas* but now assigned to newly defined genera, are included in this chapter.

The criterion of avoiding family designation for the prokaryotes described here has also been adopted in the ninth edition of *Bergey's Manual of Determinative Bacteriology* (Holt et al. 1994). The *Manual* highlights the diversity of the aerobic pseudomonads by describing an enormously complex array of gram-negative, aerobic or microaerophilic bacteria assigned to 82 genera. Approximately half these genera are characterized, in addition to the basic properties, by their polar flagella (occasionally, peritrichous ones in a mixed-type of flagellation), but the heterogeneity of a group thus defined clearly shows the inconvenience of relying on one or a few characteristics as diagnostic of a whole natural group. Essentially the same conclusion was formulated many years ago by a distinguished microbiologist: 'The recognition of ... polarly flagellated bacteria as a special group, rational and convenient as it is for determinative purposes, should not be interpreted as signifying acceptance of a natural relationship' (van Niel 1946). If we introduce further qualifications, such as an aerobic metabolism, the lack of photosynthesis and, in most cases, of dinitrogen fixation and the absence of sheaths or of cell appendages (prosthecae), a more precise circumscription is obtained; with all these limitations a great deal of phylogenetic heterogeneity still persists.

Towards the middle of this century, many international workers manifested a desire to achieve a satisfactory classification of *Pseudomonas* species. Of the various attempts, the one that was eventually more successful took place in the Department of Bacteriology of the University of California at Berkeley, where the phylogenetic diversity of the aerobic pseudomonads, even within the confines of a single genus, were precisely defined. Mentioned later in this chapter, this work has clearly demonstrated that the most important genus of the group, *Pseudomonas*, could be subdivided by various criteria into groups deserving independent generic and family designations.

The characteristics of the organisms included in this chapter are essentially those of the genus *Pseudomonas* as classically defined: straight or slightly curved gram-negative rods that do not have prosthecae or sheaths, do not produce endospores and are motile by means of polar flagella. They are strictly aerobic, with a typically respiratory metabolism, never fermentative, and they are incapable of photosynthesis and of nitrogen fixation (although some reports in the literature refer to the capacity for nitrogen fixation by some of the species). They are chemo-organotrophic, able to use other than one-carbon organic compounds as sole carbon and energy sources. The catalase reaction is positive, but, according to the species, the oxidase can be either positive or negative. The mol% of G + C in the DNA ranges from 58 to 71. Some of the species are capable of autotrophic growth at the expense of hydrogen oxidation.

2 BRIEF HISTORICAL PERSPECTIVE

The widespread occurrence of pseudomonads in nature is reflected in the vast number of species described as members of the genus *Pseudomonas* since its definition by Migula over a century ago (Migula 1894). The genus eventually became converted into a dumping ground of phylogenetically diverse organisms sharing a small set of phenotypic properties that for many years had been considered by taxonomists as valuable in bacterial classification. The *Pseudomonas* species catalogued in *Index Bergeyana* (Buchanan, Holt and Lessel 1966) and its supplement (Gibbons, Pattee and Holt 1981), and those subsequently described in journal publications, amount to more than 800 names. Many of these have been applied to plant pathogenic species. Unfortunately, the lack of proper criteria for species description added considerably to the confusion created by this nomenclatural hypertrophy and, with few exceptions, the identification of species isolated from nature became an almost hopeless task. Skerman (1949) described the state of affairs very eloquently:

Many of the descriptions of bacteria in *Bergey's Manual of Determinative Bacteriology* are decidedly poor when viewed from present-day standards. Some will be difficult to improve since a number of the original cultures have probably been lost. The original descriptions which still remain on record present us with an awkward problem in establishing priorities. Some of these descriptions are so inadequate that one description could be equally well applied to many new isolates.

An interesting approach to the characterization of the aerobic pseudomonads was introduced by den Dooren de Jong (1926). The results clearly suggested that an extensive nutritional screening of strains could provide bases for species classification. The formidable biochemical versatility of *Pseudomonas* species shown by den Dooren de Jong could not fail to attract the attention of bacterial biochemists (Stephenson 1930), but no efforts were made by bacteriologists to examine its taxonomic implications until 4 decades later.

Work performed on many strains of *Pseudomonas* at the University of California at Berkeley, mainly along the lines suggested by den Dooren de Jong (1926), resulted in the proposal of a system of classification of *Pseudomonas* species based on phenotypic characteristics with emphasis on the utilization of various organic compounds as sole carbon and energy sources. Later, this was followed by DNA–DNA hybridization studies, which confirmed the proposed system of phenotypic classification, but a clearer demonstration of the phylogenetic heterogeneity of the genus, suggested by the above studies, was eventually achieved by extension of the nucleic acid hybridization studies to an estimation of the ribosomal RNA (rRNA) similarities among the groups (Palleroni et al. 1973). Aside from providing further confirmation of the internal subdivision of the genus previously achieved by application of other approaches, the rRNA studies suggested bases for comparative studies of other bacterial genera, an approach that has been very fruitful in modern phylogenetic studies of bacteria. The development of a taxonomic system for *Pseudonomas*, therefore, has had a more general significance than simply providing bases for species classification of a single bacterial genus.

At present the genus *Pseudomonas* is reduced to one of the five rRNA homology groups (group I) into which the genus, as classically defined, was subdivided (Palleroni et al. 1973). Species of the other rRNA groups received different generic designations. A summary of the present taxonomic situation of this group of aerobic pseudomonads is presented in Table 46.1.

3 HABITATS

The capacity for growth in simple media at the expense of a wide variety of organic compounds as sole sources of carbon and energy accounts for the widespread occurrence of aerobic pseudomonads. They will grow in media in the neutral pH range, at temperatures from a few degrees above freezing to about 45°C, at the expense of many substrates in low concentrations. They are not found in habitats where either temperature or acidity are beyond these limits; in fact, there are no thermophilic or acidophilic members in the group. With the exception of the members of the genus *Brevundimonas*, the strains of species considered in this chapter grow only at pH values higher than 4.5.

Pseudomonads have been found in many different materials used in clinical laboratories and medical practice. The following references are selected among those of particular epidemiological interest. The list of materials includes water (even samples labelled 'sterile') (Lantos et al. 1969, Favero et al. 1971, Carson et al. 1973, Roberts et al. 1990), saline solution (Phillips, Curtis and Snell 1971), staining solutions (Walsh and Eberiel 1986), irrigating fluid (Mitchell and Hayward 1966), solutions purported to have antiseptic activity (Plotkin and Austrian 1958, Mitchell and Hayward 1966, Cragg and Andrews 1969, Bassett, Strokes and Thomas 1970, Phillips, Curtis and Snell 1971, Speller, Stephens and Viant 1971, Craven et al. 1981), pharmaceuticals, cosmetics and plant material preparations (Robinson 1971, Kedzia 1977, Burzynska 1977), medicaments (Shooter et al. 1969), utensils and medical instruments (Jessen 1965, Moffett, Allan and Williams 1967, Moffett and Williams 1967, Bruch 1971). Pseudomonads are found in natural or processed foods (Farmer 1976, Burzynska 1977, Wildführ and Wildführ 1977) and occasionally these materials

Table 46.1 Present generic allocation of species of different ribosomal RNA homology groups of aerobic pseudomonads[a]

Genus *Pseudomonas* (rRNA homology group I)	Other genera
Fluorescent species: *P. aeruginosa*, *P. putida*, *P. fluorescens*, *P. chlororaphis*, *P. cichorii*, *P. syringae*, *P. viridiflava*, *P. flavescens*	rRNA group II: *Burkholderia*[b]
	rRNA group III: *Comamonas*[c], *Hydrogenophaga*[d], *Acidovorax*[e]
Non-fluorescent species: *P. alcaligenes*, *P. pseudoalcaligenes*, *P. stutzeri*, *P. mendocina*	rRNA group IV: *Brevundimonas*[f]
	rRNA group V: *Stenotrophomonas*[g], *Xanthomonas*
	Not assigned to any rRNA homology group: *Sphingomonas*[h]

[a]The information in this table can be supplemented with the results of a survey by De Vos et al. 1989.
[b]Yabuuchi et al. 1992.
[c]Tamaoka, Ha and Komagata 1987.
[d]Willems et al. 1989.
[e]Willems et al. 1990.
[f]Segers et al. 1994.
[g]Palleroni and Bradbury 1993.
[h]Yabuuchi et al. 1990.

are sources of infections of patients in hospitals (Shooter et al. 1969, 1971, Kominos et al. 1972). External sources of infection can be various materials brought by visitors or health personnel, including plants and flowers (Green et al. 1974, Bergan 1975, Cho et al. 1975), which is to be expected, since pseudomonads can be isolated from healthy and diseased plants (Palleroni and Doudoroff 1972, Trust and Bartlett 1976, Schroth et al. 1977). Since pseudomonads can also occur in various parts of the animal and human body, they can spread among individuals (Matthews and Fitzsimmons 1964, Shooter et al. 1966, Hoadley and McCoy 1968).

It is evident that prevention of contamination with pseudomonads is practically impossible, and the medical concern with infection of immunologically compromised patients (in burns and neonatal units, and AIDS and cancer wards) is well justified.

4 MORPHOLOGY AND CELLULAR STRUCTURE

A discussion of the morphology of aerobic pseudomonads and details of their intracellular fine structure may be found elsewhere (Palleroni 1984). Although the definition of the strains refers to the shape of rods, in some species the cells tend to be more oval than cylindrical. A property that is fairly common in all instances is the arrangement of relatively short cells in pairs, but since the width/length ratio can vary within wide limits, strains of some species (*P. putida* and fluorescent plant pathogens) can have long cells that resemble filaments. As in other bacterial groups, the cells are shorter in the stationary phase of growth. Under certain growth conditions and oxygen limitation, filamentation can be induced in strains of *P. putida* and *P. fluorescens*, but not in *P. aeruginosa* (Jensen and Woolfolk 1985).

Poly-β-hydroxybutyrate (PHB) is accumulated in the form of refractile granules by cells of the species of genera other than those of rRNA groups I and V. However, some accumulation was observed in one of the members of group I, *P. pseudoalcaligenes* (Stanier, Palleroni and Doudoroff 1966). Synthesis may occur in other species of this genus, but is never sufficiently active to result in the formation of granules visible under the light microscope. Synthesis of other poly-β-hydroxyalkanoates has been reported for the fluorescent pseudomonads (Huijberts et al. 1992, Hori, Soga and Doi 1994), and a gene responsible for this synthesis has been cloned from *P. aeruginosa* (Timm and Steinbüchel 1992).

Membranous structures such as mesosomes (Carric and Berk 1971, Hoffman et al. 1973) and rhapidosomes (Yamamoto 1967, Baechler and Berk 1972) can be identified by electron microscopy in some of the species.

Motility is a characteristic property of the genus and is due to the presence of one or several polar flagella per cell (Fig. 46.1). One species, *Burkholderia mallei*, the agent of glanders, is permanently non-motile; occasionally non-motile strains of various other species can be isolated from nature. Lateral flagella of shorter wavelength may be observed (Palleroni et al. 1970) that may be involved in swarming over the surface of solid media (Shinoda and Okamoto 1977). In *Comamonas testosteroni* flagella are induced by growth at low temperature (personal communication from the late Professor Hans Lautrop).

Fimbriae or pili are present in most species (Fuerst and Hayward 1969), and participate in aggregation, attachment to inert or living surfaces, or may have receptors for the attachment of bacteriophages (Bradley 1972, 1974). They can even participate in causing twitching motility on the surface of solid media (Bradley 1980). The genetic determinants of

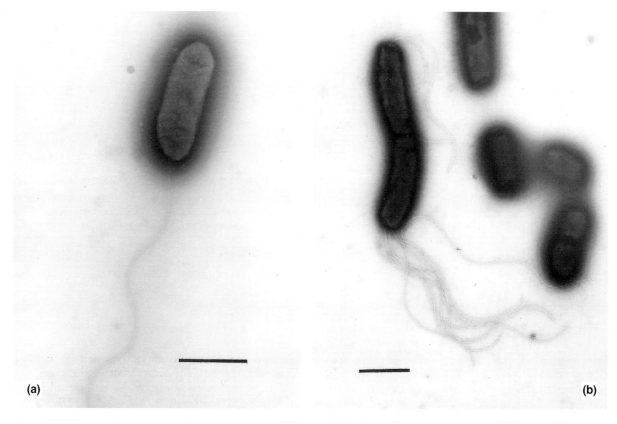

Fig. 46.1 Polar flagellation in aerobic pseudomonads: (a) *P. aeruginosa*; (b) *B. cepacia*. Bars = 1 μm. (Courtesy of Dr Kwang Shin Kim).

pili in *P. aeruginosa* may have originated by horizontal transmission from organisms of lower G + C content in their DNA, suggested by the sequence homology with pilins of unrelated organisms such as *Neisseria* and *Moraxella* (Buchanan and Pearce 1979), and by differences in codon usage, as compared with other genes of the species that have been found (West and Iglewski 1988). For these reasons, the taxonomic implications of our knowledge on the pilin markers at present are rather limited.

The composition of the cell envelopes of aerobic pseudomonads have been the subject of much research, which initially was performed mainly on well known species, such as *P. aeruginosa*, but was later extended to other species in search of correlations with their taxonomic allocations. An adequate summary of the research up to the 1980s was presented in *Bergey's Manual of Systematic Bacteriology* (Palleroni 1984), and only some supplementary information will be given here.

The cell envelopes constitute a complex system that can be resolved into 9 components by freeze-etching (Lickfield et al. 1972, Gilleland et al. 1973). Some of these compounds have structures that are removed by EDTA treatment and are reconstituted by addition of magnesium ions. Different species vary in their sensitivity to EDTA, that correlates with a high phosphorous content of the cell walls (Wilkinson 1970). Descriptions of *P. aeruginosa* outer-membrane properties and of protein components involved in per-

meability, are in excellent review articles (Nikaido and Hancock 1986, Bellido et al. 1992, Nikaido 1992).

Monoclonal antibodies for outer-membrane proteins have been isolated and characterized by Hancock et al. (1982). One of the antibodies specific for an antigenic epitope on an outer-membrane protein of *P. aeruginosa*, H2, was recommended by Mutharia and Hancock (1985) as an identification tool for use in clinical laboratories. This epitope was detected in all 17 serotype strains of the species and, in addition, in other *Pseudomonas* species (rRNA homology group I) that were tested, but not in any member of other RNA groups.

5 PIGMENTATION

Many strains of *Pseudomonas* produce pigments, some of which are water soluble and diffuse into the culture media, while others remain associated with the cell mass. Pigments are very useful for determinative purposes. In fact, their visual impact is so convincing that additional tests usually become subordinate tools when it comes to the identification of some species. However, pigments are the most striking and least reliable of taxonomic characters. Pigment formation may be erratic, often it depends on precisely defined culture conditions; it may be lost by mutation, or several pigments may be produced and it may be difficult to decide whether the diagnostically important component is present in the mixture. The following pigments are of taxonomic interest.

5.1 Fluorescent pigments

Fluorescent pigments characteristic of the fluorescent pseudomonads (*P. aeruginosa, P. putida, P. fluorescens, P. chlororaphis, P. syringae, P. cichorii, P. flavescens*), are produced abundantly in media of low iron content. These pigments are siderophores and are produced abundantly in media of low iron content; little progress was made on their chemical nature until recently. (Wendenbaum et al. 1983, Demange et al. 1986, Meyer et al. 1990).

A medium used to stimulate fluorescent pigment production has been described by King, Ward and Raney (1954) and is referred to as the 'King B' medium. The fluorescent pigments diffuse freely into the medium, with a fluorescent peak at 400 nm, and 270 nm. This is not the case with fluorescent pigments produced by some strains of genera other than *Pseudomonas* (for instance, *Burkholderia cepacia*). Fluorescent pigments different from the common ones have been described; among these are pteridine derivatives (Suzuki and Goto 1971) and the antibiotics fluopsin C and fluopsin F (Shirarata et al. 1970).

5.2 Phenazine pigments

Pyocyanin, a blue phenazine derivative characteristic of *P. aeruginosa*, is diffusible and its production can be enhanced by growth in the 'King A' medium (King, Ward and Raney 1954).

Other phenazine pigments are characteristic of *P. chlororaphis* (chlororaphin, green, which frequently crystallizes in the medium), and of *P. chlororaphis* (*P. aureofaciens*) (phenazine-α-carboxylate, orange, soluble). Some strains of *P. aeruginosa* produce phenazine-α-carboxylate (Chang and Blackwood 1969), and others produce a variety of phenazine pigments of the chlororaphin family, aside from phenazine-α-carboxylate (for references, see Palleroni and Doudoroff 1972). Several phenazine pigments of *B. cepacia* have not been chemically characterized.

5.3 Lemonnierin

Lemonnierin, an intracellular, insoluble blue pigment characteristic of *P. fluorescens* biotype IV ('*P. lemonnieri*'), is a derivative of 3,3-bipyridyl (Kuhn et al. 1965), whose structure has been determined (Ferguson et al. 1980, Jain and Whalley 1980).

5.4 Carotenoid pigments

Carotenoid pigments, usually yellow or orange, insoluble and associated with the cells, are present in *P. mendocina*, in the species of the genus *Brevundimonas* (rRNA homology group IV), and in *Sphingomonas paucimobilis* where there is a carotenoid named nostoxanthin (Fuller et al. 1971). Precise chemical characteriz-

ation is lacking for some pigments loosely classified as carotenoids.

5.5 Miscellaneous pigments

These include pigments produced by some strains of *P. aeruginosa* in addition to the pigments already mentioned. Among them there is pyorubin, which is a mixture of 2 pigments, aeruginosin A (Holliman 1957) and B (Herbert and Holliman 1964). Occasional strains of the species produce a black colour due to pyomelanin (Yabuuchi and Ohyama 1972). The yellow pigment of the recently described *P. flavescens* is different from the xanthomonadins characteristic of *Xanthomonas* (Hildebrand et al. 1994), but it has not been further characterized.

6 FATTY ACID COMPOSITION

All of 50 strains of *Pseudomonas* species analysed by Ikemoto et al. (1978) have the straight-chain saturated fatty acid $C_{16:0}$ and the straight-chain unsaturated acid of $C_{18:1}$ and are of no value as chemotaxonomic characters within the group. In contrast, the distribution of hydroxy acids, cyclopropane acids, and branched-chain acids follows the currently accepted classification (Table 46.2), and can be used as identification tools.

7 GROWTH REQUIREMENTS AND PHYSIOLOGICAL PROPERTIES

Most species of the group grow in media of simple composition without addition of organic growth factors. *Stenotrophomonas maltophilia* requires methionine or cystine and *Brevundimonas diminuta* and *B. vesicularis* require pantothenate, biotin and cyanocobalamin. None of the species considered here is thermophilic; some may reach the upper limit of the mesophilic range, e.g. *P. aeruginosa* can grow at 44°C. Strains of this species give restrictionless cells by growth at 43°C, a phenomenon that facilitates genetic manipulations (Holloway 1986).

The organisms described in this chapter are strict aerobes. There are, however, some anaerobic activities of interest; these are the ability to use nitrate as an electron acceptor under anaerobic conditions (denitrification), or to convert arginine to ornithine with production of ATP (arginine dihydrolase system), and even a weak ability to grow anaerobically at the expense of arginine in a medium containing yeast extract (Vander Wauven et al. 1984). Aerobic growth of various species on arginine and the distribution of the arginine deiminase (dihydrolase) system are summarized in Table 46.3.

Cells in suspension give the typical aerotactic response of aerobic bacteria that can be demonstrated by a method first described by Beijerinck (Schlegel 1986). Motility is linked to the provision of energy by the aerobic metabolism (Sherris, Preston and Shoe-

Table 46.2 Occurrence of hydroxy-fatty acids and ubiquinones in the aerobic pseudomonads[a]

Hydroxy-fatty acids		*Pseudomonas* (rRNA group I)	*Burkholderia* (rRNA group II)	*Comamonas* [*Hydrogenophaga*] [*Acidovorax*] (rRNA group III)	*Brevundimonas* (rRNA group IV)	*Stenotrophomonas* [*Xanthomonas*] (rRNA group V)	*Sphingomonas paucimobilis*
2-OH	12:0	(+)					
	14:0						+
	16:0		(+)				
	16:1		(+)				
	18:0		+				
3-OH	8:0						
	10:0	+		+b		+	
	11:0					+	
	i-11:0					+	
	12:0	+		+	+	+	
	i-12:0					+	
	i-13:0					+	
	14:0				+		
	16:0						
Ubiquinones		Q-9	Q-8	Q-8	Q-10	Q-8	Q-10

Symbols: (+), most strains are positive; [ ], unknown medical importance.
[a]Data from Oyaizu and Komagata (1983), and Stead (1992).
[b]Only *Hydrogenophaga palleronii* is positive.

Table 46.3 Growth on arginine and arginine deiminase system among the aerobic pseudomonads[a]

Taxa	Growth on arginine	Arginine deiminase
Pseudomonas aeruginosa	+	+
P. putida	+	+
P. fluorescens	+	+
[*P. chlororaphis*]	+	+
[*P. cichorii*]	+	+
P. mendocina	+	+
P. alcaligenes	+	+
P. pseudoalcaligenes[b]	v	v
[*P. syringae*]	v	v
[*P. viridiflava*]	v	v
P. stutzeri	−	−
[*P. flavescens*]	−	−
Burkholderia mallei	+	+
B. pseudomallei	+	+
[*B. caryophylli*]	+	+
B. cepacia	+	−
[*B. gladioli*]	+	−
B. pickettii	−	−
[*B. solanacearum*]	−	−
Comamonas spp.	−	−
[*Hydrogenophaga*]	−	−
[*Acidovorax*]	−	−
Brevundimonas spp.	−	−
Stenotrophomonas maltophilia	−	−
[*Xanthomonas* spp.][c]	−	−

[a]Data from Stanier, Palleroni and Doudoroff (1966) and from Stalon and Mercenier (1984). Symbols: +, positive; −, negative; v, not universal; [ ] unknown medical importance.
[b]Stalon and Mercenier (1984) have shown that the type strain of *P. pseudoalcaligenes* only used arginine as a nitrogen and not as a carbon source.
[c]No information is available for all species and pathovars of this genus.

smith 1957). As mentioned above, some species retain motility even in the anaerobic zones of a wet mount when the suspending liquid contains arginine, by virtue of their capacity of producing ATP in the initial steps of anaerobic degradation of arginine. The denitrifying species (for instance, *P. aeruginosa*, *P. stutzeri*, *P. mendocina*, and some biotypes of *P. fluorescens*) also retain motility anaerobically in nitrate-containing media.

8 METABOLISM

The well deserved reputation of the aerobic pseudomonads for their important role in the degradation of low molecular weight organic compounds, has its roots in the work of den Dooren de Jong (1926). The remarkable catabolic activities of the aerobic pseudomonads have made them choice subjects of research in novel catabolic pathways and their regulatory mechanisms. Our knowledge of this ability has been expanded by the discovery of the participation of these organisms in the degradation, under aerobic conditions, of xenobiotic compounds that are found in many environments as a consequence of uncontrolled human activities. Indeed, the aerobic pseudomonads are among the most active microbial agents capable of degrading, under aerobic or denitrifying conditions, many organic compounds and their

derivatives that are toxic for other bacterial groups and higher forms of life.

Some members of the genera *Pseudomonas*, *Burkholderia* and *Comamonas* that participate in these degradative activities can be a threat to human and animal health as opportunistic pathogens. *Burkholderia cepacia* is cited frequently in studies on the catabolism of organic compounds. The animal and human pathogen, *B. pseudomallei* lives freely in tropical soils and it has a nutritional versatility comparable to that of *P. cepacia*. Therefore, as a saprophyte, it may actively contribute in the mineralization of organic matter in tropical soils (Redfearn, Palleroni, and Stanier 1966).

A vast amount of literature describes the biochemical transformations of many organic compounds by pseudomonads, many of which are used as sole carbon and energy sources for growth. The book *Genetics and Biochemistry of Pseudomonas* (Clarke and Richmond 1975) is a good source of references up to the mid-1970s. More recent highly recommended sources are Sokatch (1986) and Galli, Silver and Witholt (1992). Many descriptions of biochemical activities have been included in books on bacterial metabolism and in recent years in publications dealing with the degradation of environmental contaminants and biotechnological applications. At present, studies on the degradation of natural and synthetic compounds by aerobic pseudomonads occupy a prominent position in approaches to the solution of environmental problems.

To the ever-growing literature on the aerobic degradation of aromatic compounds, the present interest in the catabolism of halogenated derivatives has acquired a particular importance, because of their toxicity for higher forms of life. Various references deal with the decomposition of these compounds by *P. aeruginosa* (Hickey and Focht 1990), *P. putida* (Hernández et al. 1991), *P. pseudoalcaligenes* (Taira et al. 1992, Gibson et al. 1993), *B. cepacia* (Fetzner, Müller and Lingens 1989, Zaitsev et al. 1991, Arensdorf and Focht 1995), *B. pickettii* (Kiyohara et al. 1992), *C. acidovorans* (Loidl et al. 1990, Hinteregger, Loidl and Streichsbier 1992, 1994). Useful general reviews are available (Neilson 1990, Chaudhry and Chapalamadugu 1991, Häggblom 1992, Fetzner and Lingens 1994). This is a sample of the published information on this subject, which has grown out of the concern created by environmental pollution and the need to develop bioremediation schemes.

9 GENETIC MECHANISMS

P. aeruginosa is the best known of all aerobic pseudomonads from the genetic standpoint. The most intensive research was performed on strain PAO of this species at Monash University in Australia, by BW Holloway, and we now have a well populated genetic map (Holloway and Carey 1993).

In *P. aeruginosa* the transfer of genetic markers can occur by conjugation, transduction and transformation. Conjugation is the most effective tool for the construction of a chromosomal map, but in *P. aeruginosa* this process differs from the more familiar *E. coli* system. Formation of high-frequency recombination (Hfr) strains is rare, and the mechanism of conjugation is still largely unknown. For years conjugation experiments relied on the chromosomal mobilization ability of fertility plasmids which have fixed points of insertion in the chromosome, a limitation that prevented the demonstration of genome circularity. Later this disadvantage was circumvented by the use of transposons and temperature-sensitive mutants of plasmids. Transposons were inserted in the chromosome by means of 'suicide' plasmids and appropriate selective techniques. The transposons created homology regions for fertility plasmids carrying the same transposons, and thus insertion at many different points of the genome could be obtained. Many of the experimental details, the plasmids used and the pertinent references have been reviewed (Holloway 1986).

As remarked by Holloway (1986), no simple system works with all species, and a different one has been developed for *P. putida*. Even so, it worked in one strain of this species (PPN) and not in others. A chromosomal map of *P. putida* has been published (Strom and Morgan 1990). A comparison of the chromosomal organization of the related species *P. aeruginosa* and *P. putida* suggests possible mechanisms of divergence from a common ancestor (Holloway et al. 1990).

A system of transfer of genetic markers in some plant pathogenic pseudomonads has been described (Errington and Vivian 1981). A chromosomal map of one of the species is also available (Nordeen and Holloway 1990).

Carlson and collaborators described a natural transformation system in *P. stutzeri* that does not require the induction of a competence state in the cells (Carlson et al. 1983, Carlson, Steenbergen and Ingraham 1984). Natural transformation seems to occur also in other non-fluorescent species of *Pseudomonas* (rRNA homology group I). Cell-to-cell contact stimulates the release of DNA by the donor cells, and the process is inhibited by DNAase, indicating that conjugation is not involved (Stewart, Carlson and Ingraham 1983). In spite of its limitations as a technique for chromosomal mapping, which is best done by conjugation, the high resolving power of transformation is advantageous for a precise estimation of marker linkage.

9.1 Genome size and structure

The genome size has been estimated for some of the species of aerobic pseudomonads. Discrepant values have been reported for *P. aeruginosa* (Palleroni 1993b) but further refinements in the technique (essentially based in the addition of sizes of restriction fragments) have resulted in determining a value around 5.9 megabase pairs (Mbp) for strain PAO (Römling et al. 1989, Romling and Tümmler 1992). This value corresponds to 3.65×10^6 kDa.

The values reported for *P. fluorescens* vary from 3.5×10^6 to 4.8×10^6 kDa and for a single strain of *P. stutzeri*, the estimation was 4.2×10^6 kDa. These and other measurements for aerobic pseudomonads have been reviewed (Herdman 1985).

A particularly interesting case is that of *B. cepacia* (strain 17616), in which the genome is constituted by 3 large circular replicons of 3.4, 2.5 and 0.9 Mbp (Cheng and Lessie 1994) which, in addition to a megaplasmid previously identified, gives a total of 7 Mbp (4.3×10^6 kDa), a large size in accordance with the nutritional and metabolic versatility of this species. The disadvantages inherent to the preservation of single genomes of large size against selective pressures, have been discussed by Stouthamer and Kooijman (1993).

Pulsed-field electrophoresis used for the separation of large fragments from the bacterial chromosome after digestion with endonucleases that cut infrequently, is the basis of the most useful methods for restriction mapping (McClelland et al. 1987). Usually, unsheared chromosomal DNA, extracted by lytic agents from cells included into low melting point agarose blocks, is subjected to digestion by endonucleases. In the method developed by Grothues and Tümmler (1991) for the analysis of 235 strains representing 32 species of *Pseudomonas*, the most appropriate enzymes were found to be *Asn*I, *Dra*I, *Spe*I, *Xba*I and *Pac*I, all of which are specific for AT-rich regions, or for sites containing the rare tetranucleotide CTAG.

The restriction patterns thus obtained are compared either by visual inspection or by the application of special algorithms. The relationships between the restriction fingerprints and taxonomic groupings defined by conventional methods, can be calculated using appropriate equations.

The results obtained on *Pseudomonas* by Grothues and Tümmler could be evaluated against the frame of reference of the extensive work performed on the taxonomy of this genus, and they were found to be generally in good agreement. The points where there is no concordance cannot be easily explained, but one possible cause may reside in differences in fragment size distribution due to mutations or chromosomal rearrangements. The fragments can be probed with cloned genes (Römling et al. 1989, Römling and Tümmler 1991) for the construction of a physical map of the chromosome. The wealth of genetic information on the *P. aeruginosa* chromosome (Holloway and Carey 1993), has been usefully combined with the above described technique to produce a physical map for strain PAO of the species. The results have been reviewed (Holloway, Römling and Tümmler 1994).

The methodology of Grothues and Tümmler was applied to the study of restriction patterns obtained from strains of *P. stutzeri* (Rainey, Thompson and Palleroni 1994), a species which is notorious for its phenotypic heterogeneity (Stanier, Palleroni and Doudoroff 1966, Palleroni et al. 1970). The results of the analysis correlate satisfactorily with those of DNA–DNA hybridization experiments and with fatty acid composition.

10 PLASMIDS

The pseudomonads are a rich source of plasmids carrying genes that code for a wide variety of functions: resistance to antibiotics and to other antibacterial agents (including simple chemicals like metals and inorganic anions), resistance to bacteriophages, to bacteriocins, or to physical agents, and induction of fertility or of particular metabolic properties. In this last category are plasmids with genes coding for enzymes of degradative pathways of aromatic compounds and their halogenated derivatives. Since many of these compounds are toxic to higher organisms and constitute a serious threat to human health, much work on environmental microbiology is now directed to a rational use of the properties that these plasmids confer to the bacterial cells, either in their natural state or after modification by recombinant DNA techniques. The best known of the catabolic plasmids of this type is TOL, found in some *P. putida* strains, which confers the ability of growth on toluene, xylenes and related aromatic compounds (Assinder and Williams 1990). The toxic compounds are often assimilated by the host cells, but plasmids can even facilitate the assimilation of simple organic compounds, like malonate (Kim and Kim 1994). It is obvious that the catabolic plasmids contribute to the nutritional diversity of the aerobic pseudomonads.

As in the case of the plasmids of the enteric bacteria, plasmids of the pseudomonads can be classified in incompatibility groups. Thirteen groups have been identified (Jacoby 1986) and in addition there are some plasmids not yet allocated to any of these groups.

Boronin (1992a, 1992b) has addressed the important questions concerning the plasmids genetic composition, ecology and diversity in the widespread species of fluorescent pseudomonads, as well as the practical consideration of determining the most appropriate combination of plasmids and hosts to take maximum advantage of their catabolic properties towards chemical contaminants in the environment. Of the 13 *Pseudomonas* incompatibility groups, most of the isolates in the survey performed by Boronin's group carried plasmids belonging to groups P1 through P5 (Boronin 1992a).

The literature on catabolic plasmids of environmental importance has been reviewed (Sayler et al. 1990). The results of this survey show that of the total of strains carrying these plasmids, about three-quarters are *Pseudomonas* (one-half of them *P. putida*). Unfortunately, the precise identification of many of the strains labelled *Pseudomonas* sp. has not been achieved, which suggests the necessity of following precisely formulated procedures now available for taxonomic analysis (Palleroni 1993a).

11 RESISTANCE TO ANTIMICROBIAL AGENTS

Plasmids conferring resistance to antibiotics are medically important, not only because they interfere with the treatment of infections caused by pathogenic pseudomonads, but also for the possibility of transfer of the plasmid genes to bacteria of other pathogenic groups. In unrelated hosts, the expression of the resistance genes may be poor (Kato et al. 1982), but since these are often located in transposons, the expression may improve after translocation to regions of other replicons (plasmids or chromosomes) where expression is enhanced.

In general, pseudomonads can be opportunistic human or animal pathogens rather than 'professional pathogens' (Nikaido 1994). The opportunistic condition is linked mainly to the intrinsic resistance to antimicrobial agents, aside from the resistance conferred by plasmids. Since some of the resistance markers are carried by promiscuous plasmids, the threat to human health is compounded by the possibility of transmission of the markers to other gram-negative pathogens. Excellent reviews on *Pseudomonas* plasmids, with particular reference to those carrying genes coding for resistance markers, are available (Jacoby 1977, 1979, 1986, Jacoby and Sutton 1989).

Part of the intrinsic antibiotic resistance of *P. aeruginosa* has to do with low outer-membrane permeability to the drugs. In addition to the low influx, there is a multidrug efflux system conferring resistance to a number of antibiotics (Li, Livermore and Nikaido

1994, Li et al. 1994, Nikaido 1994, Poole 1994). Poole et al. (1993) have identified a gene conferring resistance to several antibiotics, as part of an operon involved in pyoverdin excretion, thus showing the relationship between resistance and the efflux system. The intrinsic resistance of *P. aeruginosa* to antibiotics has been discussed by Quinn (1992).

In contrast to the high-permeability porins of other gram-negative species, *P. aeruginosa* has porins of low efficiency, and special channels are present to facilitate the entrance of nutrients. In some cases, antibacterial compounds can use these channels, but resistance can be acquired by mutation. Such is the case of the sensitivity to the β-lactam imipenem, which uses the basic amino acid channel for penetration, and many mutants have an impaired permeability to those amino acids (Quinn et al. 1986).

12 MUTUALISTIC AND ANTAGONISTIC RELATIONSHIPS

Although the pseudomonads do not excel in the production of antibiotics when compared with other groups of prokaryotes, some produce antimicrobial compounds that have attracted attention because of possible applications. Compounds such as the pseudomonic acids produced by *P. fluorescens* (Fuller et al. 1971) or pyrrolnitrin, discovered in cultures of *P. pyrrocinia* (probably a synonym of *B. cepacia* (Imanaka et al. 1965), have been known for many years. Ecological studies have indicated antagonistic activity of some of the pseudomonads within bacterial populations in the soil or in the rhizosphere region of plants, and some interesting compounds have been isolated and characterized. The beneficial effect of pseudomonads in the plant rhizosphere is not limited to their capacity to produce antimicrobial compounds active against plant pathogenic organisms, because some species have a favourable effect in stimulating plant growth (Lugtenberg and De Weger 1992).

Some references pertaining to antibiotic identification in pseudomonads follow, but the list is far from complete. Antifungal compounds are produced by *P. fluorescens* (Gurusiddaiah et al. 1986, Bin, Knudsen and Eschen 1991, Bull, Weller and Thomashow 1991, Hill et al. 1994), by *P. syringae* (Harrison et al. 1991), by *P. aureofaciens* (now renamed *P. chlororaphis*) (Pierson, Keppenne and Wood 1994), and by *B. cepacia* (Upadhyay, Visintin and Jayaswal 1991, Upadhyay and Jayaswal 1992, Abe and Nakazawa 1994, Burkhead, Schisler and Slininger 1994, Lee et al. 1994, Lim et al. 1994). Antibacterial compounds are produced by *P. aeruginosa* (Machan et al. 1992, Allison and Nolan 1994), or by *B. cepacia* (Aoki et al. 1991), and antialgal compounds are produced by *P. stutzeri* (Hayashida et al. 1991).

13 ISOLATION

Methods of isolation of pseudomonads, either directly or after an enrichment step, frequently are based on 2 oustanding properties of these organisms. One is the tolerance to antibacterial agents that can be added to the isolation medium to inhibit the growth of other bacteria. The second is the nutritional versatility of the pseudomonads, which permits the choice of substrates that are not used by most other organisms.

A good example of application of the first strategy is the use of cetrimide medium for the isolation of *P. aeruginosa*. The use of cetrimide for the isolation of this species was introduced by Lowbury (1951). The recommended concentration is 0.3% (Lowbury and Collins 1995). The fluorescent pseudomonads tolerate cetrimide, but the non-fluorescent species (e.g. *P. stutzeri*) do not. A second example is the use of specific antibiotics for the isolation of fluorescent pseudomonads, since these organisms have a high level of natural resistance to these compounds (Sands and Rovira 1970).

Application of the principle of use of particular carbon sources for growth is found in media with acetamide for the isolation of *P. aeruginosa*. Occasionally, this strategy is combined with the use of special growth conditions, to increase the specificity of the isolation or enrichment medium. For instance, an enrichment under denitrifying conditions at 37–40°C, using a variety of carbon sources, will favour the growth of some of the most common species, such as *P. aeruginosa*, *P. stutzeri*, *P. mendocina*, *Burkholderia pickettii*, and also *B. pseudomallei* when the sample is taken from tropical soil. The enriched microflora will be more heterogeneous when the denitrification is carried out at 30°C. The growth of *Bacillus* species is discouraged by the use of minimal media and the choice of carbon sources. A number of examples of special methods for isolation of pseudomonads based on the use of selected carbon sources and antibacterial compounds may be found in Palleroni (1984, 1992).

14 IDENTIFICATION

This section summarizes practical criteria for assignment of new strains of pseudomonads to genera and species, but excludes the discussion of typing methods, which are of fundamental importance for an evaluation of the intraspecific variability and for epidemiological studies. These methods will be considered in Chapter 47.

14.1 Generic assignment

There are many basic properties that are common to a large number of unrelated pseudomonads and assignment to a given genus can only be achieved by the application of special procedures, some of which will be discussed.

The method by which a satisfactory subdivision of the pseudomonads was reached was based on a ribosomal RNA–DNA hybridization procedure (Palleroni et al. 1973). Identical results were later obtained by more detailed studies of the rRNA genes, consisting of defining oligonucleotide catalogues, or in sequencing procedures. A general review of the results which led to an evolutionary scheme for prokaryotes is available (Woese 1987). The allocation of the rRNA homology groups and some of the genera of pseudomonads in a simplified phylogenetic scheme of the Proteobacteria, are shown in Fig. 46.2.

Taxonomic methods based on nucleic acid analysis have been reviewed (Stackebrandt and Liesack 1993). Ribosomal RNA components (16S or 23S) can be subjected to amplification by use of the polymerase chain reaction (PCR) (Mullis and Faloona 1987), followed by sequence determination and comparison with sequences available in databases. When the fragment amplified is only a fraction of the gene, different similarity values may be obtained according to the length of the fragment (Stackebrandt and Goebel 1994). A taxon can be characterized by a 'signature', which refers to the presence of a given nucleotide sequence found in the group and absent in others. The methodology briefly outlined is now extensively used in the characterization and identification of taxa. Probes can be prepared from the ribosomal RNA genes of organisms available in culture collection for the identification of members of the same group in natural materials (Festl, Ludwig and Schleifer 1986).

Additional approaches have different scopes, depending on how comprehensive have been the collections of organisms that have been included in the original descriptions of the respective methods. A brief description of alternative methods of group or genus assignment will follow.

FATTY ACID AND UBIQUINONE COMPOSITION

This approach has proven to be particularly useful to reach assignment at the genus and even species level, and it is now used by many laboratories as a means of quick identification. Table 46.2 summarizes the distribution of these components of the cell membranes among various groups of aerobic pseudomonads.

BIOSYNTHESIS OF AROMATIC AMINO ACIDS

The work performed by Jessen (1965) has particular interest. This group examined the enzymatic synthesis of the aromatic amino acids tyrosine and phenylalanine and defined bases for the application of the results to practical determinative procedures. Summaries of the results are presented in Tables 46.4 and 46.5. It can be seen that the results obtained by examination of the phenylalanine pathways (Table 46.5) reach a fine resolving power permitting the differentiation of subgroups which correlate with some basic phenotypic properties.

GENE ANALYSIS

The lipoprotein *oprI* gene of *P. aeruginosa* was found to be conserved among the species of the genus (rRNA homology group I). The gene was cloned and its potential usefulness as a tool for the rapid identification of members of the genus has been demonstrated (Saint-Onge et al. 1992).

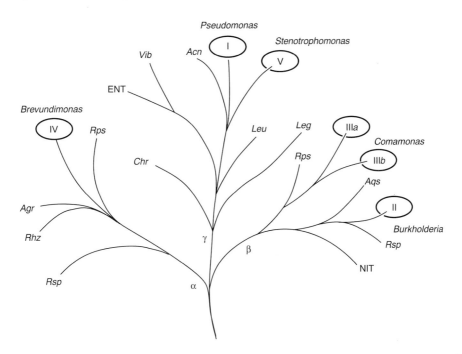

Fig. 46.2 Simplified scheme of the Proteobacteria, with the distribution of the rRNA homology groups of pseudomonads in the α, β and γ branches. Points of insertion and lengths of branches have no quantitative meaning. Only the genera of aerobic pseudomonads of medical interest are specifically indicated. Symbols: *Acn, Acinetobacter; Agr, Agrobacterium; Aqs, Acquaspirillum; Chr, Chromatium; Leg, Legionella; Leu, Leucothrix; Rhz, Rhizobium; Rps, Rhodopseudomonas; Rsp, Rhodospirillum; Vib, Vibrio;* ENT, enteric bacteria; NIT, nitrifiers. (Modified from Palleroni 1992).

Table 46.4 Tyrosine biosynthetic pathways in aerobic pseudomonads[a]

Pathway	Enzyme	Cofactor	Inhibition by tyrosine	Genus
4-Hydroxy/phenylpyruvate	Prephenate dehydrogenase	NADP	?	*Brevundimonas*
4-Hydroxy/phenylpyruvate	Prephenate dehydrogenase	NAD	–	*Pseudomonas*
4-Hydroxy/phenylpyruvate	Prephenate dehydrogenase	NAD	+	*Stenotrophomonas [Xanthomonas]*
Arogenate	Arogenate dehydrogenase	NDAP	+	*Burkholderia*
Arogenate	Arogenate dehydrogenase	NADP	–	*Comamonas [Hydrogenophaga] [Acidovorax]*
Arogenate	Arogenate dehydrogenase	NAD	+	*Pseudomonas*
Arogenate	Arogenate dehydrogenase	NAD	–	*Comamonas [Hydrogenophaga] [Acidovorax]*

[a]Data from Byng et al. (1980).
[ ] Medical importance unknown.

Table 46.5 Phenylalanine biosynthetic pathways in aerobic pseudomonads[a]

Taxon	Prephenate dehydratase activity	Arogenate dehydratase activity	Tyrosine activating factor[b]
Pseudomonas (non-fluorescent)	+	–	1
Pseudomonas (fluorescent)	+	+	1
Burkholderia cepacia	+	+	2–3
B. mallei	+	+	2–3
B. pseudomallei	+	+	2–3
[B. gladioli]	+	+	2–3
[B. caryophylli]	+	+	2–3
Burkholderia pickettii	+	+	1
[B. solanacearum]	+	+	1
Comamonas	+	–	6–12
[Acidovorax]	+	+	3–4
Brevundimonas	–	+	
Stenotrophomonas maltophilia [Xanthomonas]	+	+	1

[ ] Medical importance unknown.
[a]Data from Whitaker et al. (1981).
[b]Ratio of activity of prephenate dehydratase activity in the presence and absence of tyrosine.

Monoclonal antibody specificity

Since the determinative methods for *Pseudomonas* species may be either unsatisfactory, complicated, or expensive for use in a clinical laboratory, Mutharia and Hancock (1985) have proposed the use of a monoclonal antibody which is specific for a single antigenic epitope on the outer-membrane protein antigens of members of the rRNA group I. The specificity of the tool is not absolute, since there is also a positive reaction with *Azotobacter vinelandii*.

Polyamine analysis

It has been suggested that an analysis of polyamines and quinones composition can serve as the basis for a rapid identification of the genus *Pseudomonas* (Busse, El-Banna and Auling 1989). The most abundant of the polyamines in species of this genus were putrescine and spermidine.

14.2 Species identification

The identification of species of pseudomonads assigned to a given genus can be facilitated by the availability of the tables collected in *Bergey's Manual of Systematic Bacteriology* (Palleroni 1984), also summarized in the ninth edition of *Bergey's Manual of Determinative Bacteriology* (Holt et al. 1994). Tables are more useful than the traditional dichotomous keys because they include multiple characters, thus circumventing the problems found in the identification of aberrant strains that lack some important properties of their respective species (Palleroni and Doudoroff 1972, Palleroni 1984). Compilations of characters useful in the identification of strains isolated from clinical materials are available (Gilardi 1971, Hugh and Gilardi 1980).

Among the methods that have been proposed as practical routes to species identification is the analysis of infrared (IR) spectra. Organic materials give IR spectra often composed of a number of bands that have their origin in the vibrational and rotational motions of molecules. Conventional IR analysis can be substantially improved by the technique of Fourier transform (FT-IR) analysis, which has been applied to bacterial identification. The contribution of various cellular components can be identified in a characteristic 'spectral fingerprinting' (Giesbrecht et al. 1985, Naumann 1985). Certain regions of the spectra carry useful information on fatty acids, proteins, peptides, phosphate-containing compounds, and polysaccharides. Application of the FT-IR analysis to pseudomonads has reached a resolving power sufficiently high to allow differentiation at the species, biovar, or even strain levels (Helm et al. 1991, Naumann, Helm and Labischinski 1991).

In some cases the phenotypic exploration results in a definitive identification. In others, the identification may be only tentative, and this is confirmed by some special tests, such as DNA–DNA hybridization experiments using DNA of strains of known species as refer-ences. Doubtful or negative results of these tests may be grounds for the description of a new species; this decision should be made only after a precise allocation of the unknown strain(s) in a given rRNA homology group. Further studies may indicate a genus assignment and the relationship to known species of the genus.

No matter how sophisticated the determinative scheme may be, it is best to follow the order indicated in this section on identification without omitting the determination of basic properties of the culture under investigation. This should be as comprehensive as possible, and the 'centre of gravity' of one's attention should be the whole organism under study and not a limited number of its components, no matter how attractive or fashionable their study may appear at the moment. Bacteria are descendants of the oldest organisms that populated our planet. During evolution, aside from the characteristics that they inherited vertically from the oldest ancestors, they have incorporated genetic material received from other, unrelated, prokaryotes. A reconstruction of their phylogeny and, consequently, a solid basis for their classification, should be based on a balanced evaluation of structure and function of the various cellular components.

Below the species level, strains can be classified and identified by following typing methods based on various principles (biochemical and immunological properties, sensitivity to antibiotics, phages or bacteriocins). The classical typing methods are now facilitated by the application of modern approaches, such as the genomic analysis of the pathogenic organisms (Bingen et al. 1991, Kostman et al. 1992, Blanc et al. 1993, Sexton et al. 1993, Elaichouni et al. 1994, Römling et al. 1994a, 1994b).

ACKNOWLEDGEMENT

I am deeply grateful to Professor Kwang Shin Kim for the electron micrographs of *P. aeruginosa* and *B. cepacia*.

REFERENCES

Abe M, Nakazawa T, 1994, Characterization of hemolytic and antifungal substance, cepalycin, from *Pseudomonas cepacia*, *Microbiol Immunol*, **38:** 1–9.

Allison DG, Nolan RD, 1994, Influence of growth rate and nutrient limitation on monobactam production and peptidoglycan synthesis in *Pseudomonas aeruginosa*, *J Basic Microbiol*, **34:** 217–24.

Aoki M, Uehara K et al., 1991, An antimicrobial substance produced by *Pseudomonas cepacia* B5 against the bacterial wilt disease pathogen, *Pseudomonas solanacearum*, *Agric Biol Chem*, **55:** 715–22.

Arensdorf JJ, Focht DD, 1995, A *meta* cleavage pathway for 4–chlorobenzoate, an intermediate in the metabolism of 4–chlorobiphenyl by *Pseudomonas cepacia* P166, *Appl Environ Microbiol*, **61:** 443–7.

Assinder SJ, Williams PA, 1990, The TOL plasmids: determinants of the catabolism of toluene and the xylenes, *Adv Microb Physiol*, **31:** 1–69.

Baechler CA, Berk RS, 1972, Ultrastructural observations of *Pseudomonas aeruginosa*, *Microstructures*, **3:** 24–8.

Bassett DCJ, Stokes KJ, Thomas WRG, 1970, Wound infection with *Pseudomonas multivorans*. A water-born contaminant of disinfectant solutions, *Lancet*, **1:** 1188–91.

Bellido F, Finnen RL et al., 1992, Function and structure of *Pseudomonas aeruginosa* outer membrane protein OprF, *Pseudomonas. Molecular Biology and Biotechnology*, eds Galli E, Silver S, Witholt B, American Society for Microbiology, Washington, DC, pp 170–6.

Bergan T, 1975, Epidemiological typing of *Pseudomonas aeruginosa*, *Resistance of Pseudomonas aeruginosa*, ed. Brown MRW, Wiley & Sons, London, pp 189–235.

Bin L, Knudsen GR, Eschen DJ, 1991, Influence of an antagonistic strain of *Pseudomonas fluorescens* on growth and ability of *Trichoderma harzianum* to colonize sclerotia of *Sclerotinia sclerotiorum* in soil, *Phytopathology*, **81:** 994–1000.

Bingen EH, Denamur E et al., 1991, DNA restriction fragment length polymorphism differentiates crossed from independent infections in nosocomial *Xanthomonas maltophilia* bacteremia, *J Clin Microbiol*, **29:** 1348–50.

Blanc DS, Siegrist HH et al., 1993, Ribotyping of *Pseudomonas aeruginosa*: discriminatory power and usefulness as a tool for epidemiological studies, *J Clin Microbiol*, **31:** 71–7.

Boronin AM, 1992a, Diversity and relationships of *Pseudomonas* plasmids, *Pseudomonas. Molecular Biology and Biotechnology*, eds Galli E, Silver S, Witholt B, American Society for Microbiology, Washington, DC, pp 329–40.

Boronin AM, 1992b, Diversity of *Pseudomonas* plasmids: to what extent, *FEMS Microbiol Lett*, **100**: 461–8.

Bradley DE, 1972, Stimulation of pilus formation in *Pseudomonas aeruginosa* by RNA bacteriophage adsorption, *Biochem Biophys Res Commun*, **47**: 1080–7.

Bradley DE, 1974, The adsorption of *Pseudomonas aeruginosa* pilus-dependent bacteriophages to a host mutant with non-rectractile pili, *Virology*, **58**: 149–63.

Bradley DE, 1980, A function of *Pseudomonas aeruginosa* polar pili: twitching motility, *Can J Microbial*, **26**: 146–54.

Bruch CW, 1971, Cosmetics: sterility *vs.* microbial control, *Am Perf Cosmet*, **86**: 46–51.

Buchanan RE, Holt JG, Lessel EF Jr (eds), 1966, *Index Bergeyana*, Williams & Wilkins, Baltimore.

Buchanan TM, Pearce WA, 1979, Pathogenic aspects of outer membrane components of Gram negative bacteria, *Bacterial Outer Membranes. Biogenesis and Function*, ed. Inouye M, John Wiley & Sons, New York, pp 475–514.

Bull CT, Weller DM, Thomashow LS, 1991, Relationship between root colonization and suppression of *Gaeumannomyces graminis* var. *tritici* by *Pseudomonas fluorescens* strain 2–79, *Phytopathology*, **81**: 954–9.

Burkhead KD, Schisler DA, Slininger PJ, 1994, Pyrrolnitrin production by biological control agent *Pseudomonas cepacia* B37w in culture and in colonized wounds of potatoes, *Appl Environ Microbiol*, **60**: 2031–9.

Burzynska H, 1977, Occurrence and significance of *Pseudomonas aeruginosa* in food and cosmetics, *Pseudomonas Species*, ed. Kedzia WB, Polish Academy of Sciences, Warsaw, pp 29–34.

Busse H-J, El-Banna T, Auling G, 1989, Evaluation of different approaches for identification of xenobiotic-degrading pseudomonads, *Appl Environ Microbiol*, **55**: 1578–83.

Byng GS, Whitaker RJ et al., 1980, Variable enzymological patterning in tyrosine biosynthesis as a new means of determining natural relatedness among Pseudomonadaceae, *J Bacteriol*, **144**: 247–57.

Carlson CA, Steenbergen SM, Ingraham JL, 1984, Natural transformation of *Pseudomonas stutzeri* by plasmids that contain cloned fragments of chromosomal deoxyribonucleic acid, *Arch Microbiol*, **140**: 134–8.

Carlson CA, Pierson LS et al., 1983, *Pseudomonas stutzeri* and related species undergo natural transformation, *J Bacteriol*, **153**: 93–9.

Carric L, Berk RS, 1971, Membranous inclusions of *Pseudomonas aeruginosa*, *J Bacteriol*, **106**: 250–6.

Carson LA, Favero MS et al., 1973, Morphological, biochemical and growth characteristics of *Pseudomonas cepacia* from distilled water, *Appl Microbiol*, **25**: 476–83.

Chang PC, Blackwood AC, 1969, Simultaneous production of three phenazine pigments by *Pseudomonas aeruginosa* Mac 436, *Can J Microbiol*, **15**: 439–44.

Chaudhry GR, Chapalamadugu S, 1991, Biodegradation of halogenated organic compounds, *Microbiol Rev*, **55**: 59–79.

Cheng H-P, Lessie TG, 1994, Multiple replicons constituting the genome of *Pseudomonas cepacia* 17616, *J Bacteriol*, **176**: 4034–42.

Cho JJ, Schroth MN et al., 1975, Ornamental plants as carriers of *Pseudomonas aeruginosa*, *Phytopathology*, **65**: 425–31.

Clarke PH, Richmond MH (eds), 1975, *Genetics and Biochemistry of Pseudomonas*, John Wiley & Sons, London.

Cragg J, Andrews AV, 1969, Bacterial contamination of disinfectants, *Br Med J*, **3**: 57.

Craven DE, Moody B et al., 1981, Pseudo-bacteremia caused by providone–iodine solution contaminated with *Pseudomonas cepacia*, *N Engl J Med*, **305**: 621–3.

De Vos P, van Landschoot A et al., 1989, Genotypic relationships and taxonomic localization of unclassified *Pseudomonas* and *Pseudomonas*-like strains by deoxyribonucleic acid: ribosomal ribonucleic acid hybridizations, *Int J Syst Bacteriol*, **39**: 35–49.

Demange P, Wendenbaum S et al., 1986, Bacterial siderophores: structure of pyoverdins and related compounds, *Iron, Sider-*

ophores, and Plant Diseases, ed. Swinburne TR, Plenum Press, New York, pp 131–47.

den Dooren de Jong LE, 1926, *Bijdrage tot de kennis van het mineralisatieproces*, Nijgh & Van Ditmar, Rotterdam.

Elaichouni A, Verschraegen G et al., 1994, *Pseudomonas aeruginosa* serotype O12 outbreak studied by arbitrary primer PCR, *J Clin Microbiol*, **32**: 666–71.

Errington J, Vivian A, 1981, An indigenous system of gene transfer in the plant pathogen *Pseudomonas morsprunorum*, *J Gen Microbiol*, **124**: 439–42.

Farmer JJ, 1976, *Pseudomonas* in the hospital, *Hosp Pract*, **11**: 63–70.

Favero MS, Carson LA et al., 1971, *Pseudomonas aeruginosa*: growth in distilled water in hospitals, *Science*, **173**: 836–8.

Ferguson G, Pollard DR et al., 1980, The bacterial pigment from *Pseudomonas lemonnieri*. Part I. Structure of a degradation product, 3-n-octamido pyridine-2,5,6-trione, by X-ray crystallography, *J Chem Soc Perkin Trans I*, **8**: 1782–7.

Festl H, Ludwig W, Schleifer K-H, 1986, DNA hybridization probe for the *Pseudomonas fluorescens* group, *Appl Environ Microbiol*, **52**: 1190–4.

Fetzner S, Lingens F, 1994, Bacterial dehalogenases: biochemistry, genetics, and biotechnological applications, *Microbiol Rev*, **58**: 641–85.

Fetzner S, Müller R, Lingens F, 1989, Degradation of 2-chlorobenzoate by *Pseudomonas cepacia* 2CBS, *Biol Chem Hoppe Seyler*, **370**: 1173–82.

Fuerst JA, Hayward AC, 1969, Surface appendages similar to fimbriae (pili) on *Pseudomonas* species, *J Gen Microbiol*, **58**: 227–37.

Fuller AT, Mellows G et al., 1971, Pseudomonic acid: an antibiotic produced by *Pseudomonas fluorescens*, *Nature (London)*, **234**: 416–17.

Galli E, Silver S, Witholt B (eds), 1992, *Pseudomonas. Molecular Biology and Biotechnology*, American Society for Microbiology, Washington, DC.

Gibbons NE, Pattee KB, Holt JG (eds), 1981, *Supplement to Index Bergeyana*, Williams & Wilkins, Baltimore.

Gibson DT, Cruden DL et al., 1993, Oxidation of polychlorinated biphenyls by *Pseudomonas* sp. strain LB400 and *Pseudomonas pseudoalcaligenes* KF707, *J Bacteriol*, **175**: 4561–4.

Giesbrecht P, Naumann D et al., 1985, A new method for the rapid identification and differentiation of pathogenic microorganisms using Fourier transform infrared spectroscopy, *Rapid Methods and Automation in Microbiology and Immunology*, ed. Habermehl K-O, Springer-Verlag, Berlin, pp 198–206.

Gilardi GL, 1971, Characterization of *Pseudomonas* species isolated from clinical specimens, *Appl Microbiol*, **21**: 414–19.

Gilleland HE, Stinnett JD et al., 1973, Freeze-etch study of *Pseudomonas aeruginosa*: localization within the cell wall of an ethylenediaminetetraacetate–extractable component, *J Bacteriol*, **113**: 417–32.

Green SK, Schroth MN et al., 1974, Agricultural plants and soil as a possible reservoir for *Pseudomonas aeruginosa*, *Appl Microbiol*, **28**: 987–91.

Grothues D, Tümmler B, 1991, New approaches in genome analysis by pulsed-field gel electrophoresis: application to the analysis of *Pseudomonas* species, *Mol Microbiol*, **5**: 2763–76.

Gurusiddaiah S, Weller DM et al., 1986, Characterization of an antibiotic produced by a strain of *Pseudomonas fluorescens* inhibitory to *Gaeumannomyces graminis* var *tritici* and *Pythium* sp., *Antimicrob Agents Chemother*, **29**: 488.

Häggblom MM, 1992, Microbial breakdown of halogenated aromatic pesticides and related compounds, *FEMS Microbiol Rev*, **103**: 29–72.

Hancock REW, Wieczorek AA et al., 1982, Monoclonal antibodies against *Pseudomonas aeruginosa* outer membrane antigens: isolation and characterization, *Infect Immun*, **37**: 166–71.

Harrison L, Teplow DB et al., 1991, Pseudomycins, a family of novel peptides from *Pseudomonas syringae* possessing broad-spectrum antifungal activity, *J Gen Microbiol*, **137**: 2857–65.

Hayashida S, Tanaka S et al., 1991, Isolation of anti-algal *Pseudomonas stutzeri* strains and their lethal activity for *Chattonella antiqua*, *Agric Biol Chem*, **55:** 787–90.

Helm D, Labischinski H et al., 1991, Classification and identification of bacteria by Fourier-transform infrared spectroscopy, *J Gen Microbiol*, **137:** 69–79.

Herbert RB, Holliman FG, 1964, Aeruginosin B. A naturally occurring phenazinesulfonic acid, *Proc Chem Soc*, 19.

Herdman M, 1985, The evolution of bacterial genomes, *The Evolution of Genome Size*, ed. Cavalier-Smith T, John Wiley & Sons, Chichester, pp 37–68.

Hernández BS, Higson FK et al., 1991, Metabolism of and inhibition by chlorobenzoates in *Pseudomonas putida* P111, *Appl Environ Microbiol*, **57:** 3361–6.

Hickey WJ, Focht DD, 1990, Degradation of mono-, di-, and trihalogenated benzoic acids by *Pseudomonas aeruginosa* JB2, *Appl Environ Microbiol*, **56:** 3842–50.

Hildebrand DC, Palleroni NJ et al., 1994, *Pseudomonas flavescens* sp. nov., isolated from walnut blight cankers, *Int J Syst Bacteriol*, **44:** 410–15.

Hill DS, Stein JI et al., 1994, Cloning of genes involved in the synthesis of pyrrolnitrin from *Pseudomonas fluorescens* and role of pyrrolnitrin synthesis in biological control of plant disease, *Appl Environ Microbiol*, **60:** 78–85.

Hinteregger C, Loidl M, Streichsbier F, 1992, Characterization of isofunctional ring-cleaving enzymes in aniline and 3-chloroaniline degradation by *Pseudomonas acidovorans* CA28, *FEMS Microbiol Lett*, **97:** 261–6.

Hinteregger C, Loidl M, Streichsbier F, 1994, *Pseudomonas acidovorans*: a bacterium capable of mineralizing 2-chloroaniline, *J Basic Microbiol*, **34:** 77–85.

Hoadley AW, McCoy E, 1968, Some observations on the ecology of *Pseudomonas aeruginosa* and its occurrence in the intestinal tracts of animals, *Cornell Vet*, **58:** 354–63.

Hoffman HP, Geftic SC et al., 1973, Mesosomes in *Pseudomonas aeruginosa*, *J Bacteriol*, **114:** 434–8.

Holliman FG, 1957, Pigments from a red strain of *Pseudomonas aeruginosa*, *Chem Ind*, **28:** 1668.

Holloway BW, 1986, Chromosome mobilization and genome organization in *Pseudomonas*, *The Bacteria, Vol. X. The Biology of Pseudomonas*, ed. Sokatch JR, Academic Press, Orlando, pp 217–49.

Holloway BW, Carey E, 1993, *Pseudomonas aeruginosa* PAO, *Genetic Maps. Locus Maps of Complex Genomes*, 6th edn, ed. O'Brien SJ, Cold Spring Harbor Laboratory Press, Cold Spring Harbor, NY, pp 2.98–2.105.

Holloway BW, Römling U, Tümmler B, 1994, Genomic mapping of *Pseudomonas aeruginosa* PAO, *J Gen Microbiol*, **140:** 2907–29.

Holloway BW, Dharmsthiti S et al., 1990, Chromosome organization in *Pseudomonas aeruginosa* and *Pseudomonas putida*, *Pseudomonas: Biotransformations, Pathogenesis and Evolving Biotechnology*, eds Silver S, Chakrabarty AM et al., American Society for Microbiology, Washington, DC, pp 269–78.

Holt JG, Krieg NR et al., 1994, *Bergey's Manual of Determinative Bacteriology*, 9th edn, Williams & Wilkins, Baltimore.

Hori K, Soga K, Doi Y, 1994, Effects of culture conditions on molecular weights of poly(3-hydroxyalkanoates) produced by *Pseudomonas putida* from octanoate, *Biotechnol Lett*, **16:** 709–14.

Hugh R, Gilardi GL, 1980, *Pseudomonas, Manual of Clinical Microbiology*, 3rd edn, eds Lennette EH, Balows A, Hausler WJ Jr, Truant JP, American Society for Microbiology, Washington, DC, pp 288–317.

Huijberts GNM, Eggink G et al., 1992, *Pseudomonas putida* KT2442 cultivated on glucose accumulates poly(3-hydroxyalkanoates) consisting of saturated and unsaturated monomers, *Appl Environ Microbiol*, **58:** 536–44.

Ikemoto S, Kuraishi H et al., 1978, Cellular fatty acid composition in *Pseudomonas* species, *J Gen Appl Microbiol*, **24:** 199–213.

Imanaka H, Kousaka M et al., 1965, Studies on pyrrolnitrin, a new antibiotic. II. Taxonomic studies on pyrrolnitrin-producing strain, *J Antibiot*, **18:** 205–6.

Jacoby GA, 1977, Classification of plasmids in *Pseudomonas aeruginosa*, *Microbiology 1977*, ed. Schlessinger D, American Society for Microbiology, Washington, DC, pp 119–26.

Jacoby GA, 1979, Plasmids in *Pseudomonas aeruginosa*, *Pseudomonas aeruginosa. Clinical Manifestations of Infection and Current Therapy*, ed. Doggett RG, Academic Press, New York, pp 271–309.

Jacoby GA, 1986, Resistance plasmids of *Pseudomonas*, *The Biology of Pseudomonas*, ed. Sokatch JR, Academic Press, Orlando, pp 265–93.

Jacoby GA, Sutton L, 1989, *Pseudomonas cepacia* susceptibility to sulbactam, *Antimicrob Agents Chemother*, **33:** 583–4.

Jain KC, Whalley WB, 1980, The bacterial pigment from *Pseudomonas lemonnieri*. Part 2. The synthesis of 3 n-octanamidopyridine-2,5,6-trione: the structure and synthesis of lemonnierin, *J Chem Soc Perkin Trans I*, **8:** 1788–94.

Jensen RH, Woolfolk CA, 1985, Formation of filaments by *Pseudomonas putida*, *Appl Environ Microbiol*, **50:** 364–72.

Jessen O, 1965, *Pseudomonas aeruginosa and Other Green Fluorescent Pseudomonads. A Taxonomic Study*, Munksgaard, Copenhagen.

Kato T, Sata Y et al., 1982, Plasmid-mediated gentamicin resistance of *Pseudomonas aeruginosa* and its lack of expression in *Escherichia coli*, *Antimicrob Agents Chemother*, **22:** 358–63.

Kedzia WB, 1977, Isolation and differentiation of clinically important *Pseudomonas* species from plant drugs, *Pseudomonas Species*, ed. Kedzia WB, Polish Academy of Sciences, Warsaw, pp 63–7.

Kim YS, Kim EJ, 1994, A plasmid responsible for malonate assimilation in *Pseudomonas fluorescens*, *Plasmid*, **32:** 219–21.

King EO, Ward MK, Raney DE, 1954, Two simple media for the demonstration of pyocyanin and fluorescein, *J Lab Clin Med*, **44:** 301–7.

Kiyohara H, Hatta T et al., 1992, Isolation of *Pseudomonas pickettii* strains that degrade 2,4,6-trichlorophenol and their dechlorination of chlorophenols, *Appl Environ Microbiol*, **58:** 1276–83.

Kominos SD, Copeland CE et al., 1972, Introduction of *Pseudomonas aeruginosa* into a hospital via vegetables, *Appl Microbiol*, **24:** 567–70.

Kostman JR, Edlind TD et al., 1992, Molecular epidemiology of *Pseudomonas cepacia* determined by polymerase chain reaction ribotyping, *J Clin Microbiol*, **30:** 2084–7.

Kuhn R, Starr MP et al., 1965, Indoiodine and other pigments related to 3,3'-bypyridyl, *Arch Microbiol*, **51:** 71–84.

Lantos J, Kiss M et al., 1969, Serological and phage typing of *Pseudomonas aeruginosa* invading a municipal water supply, *Acta Microbiol Acad Sci Hung*, **16:** 333–6.

Lee C, Kim S et al., 1994, Cepacidine A, a novel antifungal antibiotic produced by *Pseudomonas cepacia*. I Taxonomy, production, isolation and biological activity, *J Antibiot*, **47:** 1402–5.

Li X-Z, Livermore DM, Nikaido H, 1994, Role of efflux pump(s) in intrinsic resistance of *Pseudomonas aeruginosa*: resistance to tetracycline, chloramphenicol, and norfloxacin, *Antimicrob Agents Chemother*, **38:** 1732–41.

Li X-Z, Ma D et al., 1994, Role of efflux pump(s) in intrinsic resistance of *Pseudomonas aeruginosa*: active efflux as a contributing factor to β-lactam resistance, *Antimicrob Agents Chemother*, **38:** 1742–52.

Lickfield KG, Achterrath H et al., 1972, Die Feinstrukturen von *Pseudomonas aeruginosa* in ihrer Deutung durch die Gefrierätztechnik, Ultramikrotomie un Kryo-Ultramikrotomie, *J Ultrastruct Res*, **38:** 27–45.

Lim Y, Suh J et al., 1994, Cepacidine A, a novel antifungal antibiotic produced by *Pseudomonas cepacia*. II. Physico-chemical properties and structure elucidation, *J Antibiot*, **47:** 1406–16.

Loidl M, Hinteregger C et al., 1990, Degradation of aniline and monochlorinated anilines by soil-born *Pseudomonas acidovorans* strains, *Arch Microbiol*, **155:** 56–61.

Lowbury EJL, 1951, Improved culture methods for the detection of *Pseudomonas pyocyanea*, *J Clin Pathol*, **4:** 66–72.

Lowbury EJL, Collins AG, 1955, The use of a new cetrimide product in a selective medium for *Pseudomonas pyocyanea*, *J Clin Pathol*, **8:** 47–8.

Lugtenberg JJ, De Weger LA, 1992, Plant root colonization by *Pseudomonas* spp., *Pseudomonas. Molecular Biology and Biotechnology*, eds Galli E, Silver S, Witholt B, American Society for Microbiology, Washington, DC, pp 13–19.

McClelland M, Jones R et al., 1987, Restriction endonucleases for pulsed field mapping of bacterial genomes, *Nucleic Acids Res*, **15:** 5985–6005.

Machan ZA, Taylor GW et al., 1992, 2-Heptyl-4-hydroxyquinoline *N*-oxide, an antistaphylococcal agent produced by *Pseudomonas aeruginosa*, *J Antimicrob Chemother*, **30:** 615–23.

Matthews PRJ, Fitzsimmons WM, 1964, The incidence and distribution of *Pseudomonas aeruginosa* in the intestinal tracts of calves, *Res Vet Sci*, **5:** 171–4.

Meyer JM, Hohnadel D et al., 1990, Pyoverdin-facilitated iron uptake in *Pseudomonas aeruginosa*: immunological characterization of the ferripyoverdin receptor, *Mol Microbiol*, **4:** 1401–5.

Migula W, 1894, Ueber ein neues System der Bakterien, *Arbeiten aus dem bakteriologischen Institut der technischen Hochschule zu Karlsruhe*, **1:** 235–8.

Mitchell RG, Hayward AC, 1966, Postoperative urinary tract infections caused by contaminated irrigating fluid, *Lancet*, **1:** 793–5.

Moffett HL, Allan D, Williams T, 1967, Survival and dissemination of bacteria in nebulizers and incubators, *Am J Dis Child*, **114:** 13–20.

Moffett HL, Williams T, 1967, Bacteria recovered from distilled water and inhalation therapy equipment, *Am J Dis Child*, **114:** 7–12.

Mullis KB, Faloona FA, 1987, Specific synthesis of DNA *in vitro* via a polymerase-catalyzed chain reaction, *Methods Enzymol*, **155:** 335–50.

Mutharia LM, Hancock REW, 1985, Monoclonal antibody specific for an outer membrane lipoprotein of the *Pseudomonas fluorescens* branch of the family Pseudomonadaceae, *Int J Syst Bacteriol*, **35:** 530–2.

Naumann D, 1985, The ultra rapid differentiation and identification of pathogenic bacteria using FT-IR techniques, *SPIE, Fourier and Computerized Infrared Spectroscopy*, eds Graselli JG, Cameron DG, International Society for Optical Engineering, Bellingham, WA, pp 268–9.

Naumann D, Helm D, Labischinski H, 1991, Microbiological characterizations by FT-IR spectroscopy, *Nature (London)*, **351:** 81–2.

Neilson AH, 1990, The biodegradation of halogenated organic compounds, *J Appl Bacteriol*, **69:** 445–70.

van Niel CB, 1946, *The Classification and Natural Relations of Bacteria*, Cold Spring Harbour Laboratory, Cold Spring Harbor, New York, pp 285–301.

Nikaido H, 1992, Nonspecific and specific permeation channels of the *Pseudomonas aeruginosa* outer membrane, *Pseudomonas. Molecular Biology and Biotechnology*, eds Galli E, Silver S, Witholt B, American Society for Microbiology, Washington DC, pp 146–53.

Nikaido H, 1994, Prevention of drug access to bacterial targets: permeability barriers and active efflux, *Science*, **264:** 382–8.

Nikaido H, Hancock REW, 1986, Outer membrane permeability of *Pseudomonas aeruginosa*, *The Bacteria: a Treatise on Structure and Function*, eds Gunsalus IC, Stanier RY, Academic Press, New York, pp 145–93.

Nordeen RO, Holloway BW, 1990, Chromosome mapping in *Pseudomonas syringae* pv. *syringae* strain PS224, *J Gen Microbiol*, **136:** 1231–9.

Oyaizu H, Komagata K, 1983, Groupings of *Pseudomonas* species on the basis of cellular fatty acid compositions and the quinone system with special reference to the existence of 3-hydroxy fatty acids, *J Gen Appl Microbiol*, **29:** 17–40.

Palleroni NJ, 1984, Genus I. *Pseudomonas* Migula 1894, *Bergey's Manual of Systematic Bacteriology*, eds Krieg NR, Holt JG, Williams & Wilkins, Baltimore, pp 141–99.

Palleroni NJ, 1992, Introduction to the family Pseudomonadaceae, *The Prokaryotes. A Handbook on the Biology of Bactreia: Ecophysiology, Isolation, Identification, Applications*, 2nd edn, eds Balows A, Trüper HG, et al., Springer-Verlag, New York, pp 3071–85.

Palleroni NJ, 1993a, *Pseudomonas* classification. A new case history in the taxonomy of Gram-negative bacteria, *Antonie Van Leeuwenhoek, J Microbiol*, **64:** 231–51.

Palleroni NJ, 1993b, Structure of the bacterial genome, *Handbook of New Bacterial Systematics*, eds Goodfellow M, O'Donnell AG, Academic Press, London, pp 57–113.

Palleroni NJ, Bradbury JF, 1993, *Stenotrophomonas*, a new bacterial genus for *Xanthomonas maltophilia* (Hugh 1980) Swings et al. 1983, *Int J Syst Bacteriol*, **43:** 606–9.

Palleroni NJ, Doudoroff M, 1972, Some properties and subdivisions of the genus *Pseudomonas*, *Annu Rev Phytopathol*, **10:** 73–100.

Palleroni NJ, Doudoroff M et al., 1970, Taxonomy of the aerobic pseudomonads: the properties of the *Pseudomonas stutzeri* group, *J Gen Microbiol*, **60:** 215–31.

Palleroni NJ, Kunisawa R et al., 1973, Nucleic acid homologies in the genus *Pseudomonas*, *Int J Syst Bacteriol*, **23:** 333–9.

Phillips I, Curtis MA, Snell JJS, 1971, *Pseudomonas cepacia (multivorans)* septicemia in an intensive-care unit, *Lancet*, **1:** 375–7.

Pierson LSI, Keppenne VD, Wood DW, 1994, Phenazine antibiotic biosynthesis in *Pseudomonas aureofaciens* 30-84 is regulated by PhzR in response to cell density, *J Bacteriol*, **176:** 3966–74.

Plotkin SA, Austrian R, 1958, Bacteremia caused by *Pseudomonas* following the use of materials stored in solutions of a cationic surface-active agent, *Am J Med Sci*, **235:** 621–7.

Poole K, 1994, Bacterial multidrug resistance – emphasis on efflux mechanisms and *Pseudomonas aeruginosa*, *J Antimicrob Chemother*, **34:** 453–6.

Poole K, Krebes K et al., 1993, Multiple antibiotic resistance in *Pseudomonas aeruginosa*: evidence for involvement in an efflux operon, *J Bacteriol*, **175:** 7363–72.

Quinn JP, 1992, Intrinsic antibiotic resistance in *Pseudomonas aeruginosa*, *Pseudomonas. Molecular Biology and Biotechnology*, eds Galli E, Silver S, Witholt B, American Society for Microbiology, Washington, DC, pp 154–60.

Quinn JP, Dudek EJ et al., 1986, Emergence of resistance to imipenem during therapy for *Pseudomonas aeruginosa* infections, *J Infect Dis*, **154:** 289–94.

Rainey PB, Thompson IP, Palleroni NJ, 1994, Genome and fatty acid analysis of *Pseudomonas stutzeri*, *Int J Syst Bacteriol*, **44:** 54–61.

Redfearn MS, Palleroni NJ, Stanier RY, 1966, A comparative study of *Pseudomonas pseudomallei* and *Bacillus mallei*, *J Gen Microbiol*, **43:** 293–313.

Roberts LA, Collignon PJ et al., 1990, An Australia-wide epidemic of *Pseudomonas pickettii* bacteraemia due to contaminated 'sterile' water for injection, *Med J Aust*, **152:** 652–5.

Robinson EP, 1971, *Pseudomonas aeruginosa* contamination of liquid antiacids: a survey, *J Pharmac Sci*, **60:** 604–5.

Römling U, Tümmler B, 1991, The impact of two-dimensional pulsed-field gel electrophoresis techniques for the consistent and complete mapping of bacterial genomes: refined physical map of *Pseudomonas aeruginosa* PAO, *Nucleic Acids Res*, **19:** 3199–206.

Römling U, Tümmler B, 1992, A *Pad/Swa*I map of the *Pseudomonas aeruginosa* PAO chromosome, *Electrophoresis*, **13:** 649–51.

Römling U, Grothues D et al., 1989, A physical genome map of *Pseudomonas aeruginosa* PAO, *EMBO J*, **8:** 4081–9.

Römling U, Fiedler B et al., 1994a, Epidemiology of chronic

Pseudomonas aeruginosa infections in cystic fibrosis, *J Infect Dis*, **170:** 1616–21.

Römling U, Wingender J et al., 1994b, A major *Pseudomonas aeruginosa* clone common to patients and aquatic habitats, *Appl Environ Microbiol*, **60:** 1734–8.

Saint-Onge A, Romeyer F et al., 1992, Specificity of the *Pseudomonas aeruginosa* PAO1 lipoprotein I gene as a DNA probe and PCR target region within the Pseudomonadaceae, *J Gen Microbiol*, **138:** 733–41.

Sands DC, Rovira AD, 1970, Isolation of fluorescent pseudomonads with a selective medium, *Appl Environ Microbiol*, **20:** 513–14.

Sayler GS, Hooper SW et al., 1990, Catabolic plasmids of environmental and ecological significance [mini review], *Microb Ecol*, **19:** 1–20.

Schlegel HG, 1986, *General Microbiology*, 6th edn, Cambridge University Press, Cambridge.

Schroth MN, Cho JJ et al., 1977, Epidemiology of *Pseudomonas aeruginosa* in agricultural areas, *Pseudomonas aeruginosa: Ecological Aspects and Patient Colonization*, ed. Young VM, Raven Press, New York, pp 1–20.

Segers P, Vancanneyt M et al., 1994, Classification of *Pseudomonas diminuta* Leifson and Hugh 1954 and *Pseudomonas vesicularis* Büsing, Döll, and Freytag 1953 in *Brevundimonas* gen. nov. as *Brevundimonas diminuta* comb. nov. and *Brevundimonas vesicularis* comb. nov., respectively, *Int J Syst Bacteriol*, **44:** 499–510.

Sexton MM, Goebel LA et al., 1993, Ribotype analysis of *Pseudomonas pseudomallei* isolates, *J Clin Microbiol*, **31:** 238–43.

Sherris JC, Preston NW, Shoesmith JG, 1957, The influence of oxygen on the motility of a strain of *Pseudomonas* sp., *J Gen Microbiol*, **16:** 86–96.

Shinoda S, Okamoto K, 1977, Formation and function of *Vibrio parahaemolyticus* lateral flagella, *J Bacteriol*, **129:** 1266–71.

Shirarata K, Deguchi T et al., 1970, The structures of fluopsins C and F, *J Antibiot*, **23:** 546–50.

Shooter RA, Walker KA et al., 1966, Fecal carriage of *Pseudomonas aeruginosa* in hospital patients. Possible spread from patient to patient, *Lancet*, **2:** 1331–4.

Shooter RA, Gaya H et al., 1969, Food and medicaments as possible sources of hospital strains of *Pseudomonas aeruginosa*, *Lancet*, **1:** 1227–9.

Shooter RA, Cooke EM et al., 1971, Isolation of *Escherichia coli*, *Pseudomonas aeruginosa*, and *Klebsiella* from food in hospitals, canteen, and schools, *Lancet*, **2:** 390–2.

Skerman VBD, 1949, A mechanical key for the generic identification of bacteria, *Bacteriol Rev*, **13:** 175–88.

Sokatch JR (ed.), 1986, *The Bacteria. Volume X: The Biology of Pseudomonas*, Academic Press, Orlando.

Speller DCE, Stephens ME, Viant AC, 1971, Hospital infection with *Pseudomonas cepacia*, *Lancet*, **1:** 798–9.

Stackebrandt E, Goebel BM, 1994, Taxonomic note: a place for DNA–DNA reassociation and 16S rRNA sequence analysis in the present species definition in bacteriology, *Int J Syst Bacteriol*, **44:** 846–9.

Stackebrandt E, Liesack W, 1993, Nucleic acids and classification, *Handbook of New Bacterial Systematics*, eds Goodfellow M, O'Donnell AG, Academic Press, London, pp 151–94.

Stalon V, Mercenier A, 1984, L-Arginine utilization by *Pseudomonas* species, *J Gen Microbiol*, **130:** 69–76.

Stanier RY, Palleroni NJ, Doudoroff M, 1966, The aerobic pseudomonads: a taxonomic study, *J Gen Microbiol*, **43:** 159–271.

Stead DE, 1992, Grouping of plant-pathogenic and some other *Pseudomonas* spp. by using cellular fatty acid profiles, *Int J Syst Bacteriol*, **42:** 281–95.

Stephenson M, 1930, *Bacterial Metabolism*, 1st edn, Longmans, Green and Co., London.

Stewart GJ, Carlson CS, Ingraham JL, 1983, Evidence for an active role of donor cells in natural transformation of *Pseudomonas stutzeri*, *J Bacteriol*, **156:** 30–5.

Southamer AH, Kooijman SALM, 1993, Why it pays for bacteria to delete disused DNA and to maintain megaplasmids, *Antonie Van Leeuwenhoek, J Microbiol*, **63:** 39–43.

Strom D, Morgan AF, 1990, *Pseudomonas putida* PPN, *Genetic Maps. Locus Maps of Complex Genomes*, 5th edn, ed. O'Brien SJ, Cold Spring Harbor Laboratory, Cold Spring Harbor, New York, pp 2.78–81.

Suzuki A, Goto M, 1971, Isolation and characterization of pteridines from *Pseudomonas ovalis*, *Bull Chem Soc (Japan)*, **44:** 1869–72.

Taira K, Hirose J et al., 1992, Analysis of *bph* operon from the polychlorinated biphenyl-degrading strain of *Pseudomonas pseudoalcaligenes* KF707, *J Biol Chem*, **267:** 4844–53.

Tamaoka J, Ha D, Komagata K, 1987, Reclassification of *Pseudomonas acidovorans* den Dooren de Jong 1926 and *Pseudomonas testosteroni* Marcus and Talalay 1946 as *Comamonas acidovorans* comb. nov. and *Comamonas testosteroni* comb. nov., with an emended description of the genus *Comamonas*, *Int J Syst Bacteriol*, **37:** 52–9.

Timm A, Steinbüchel A, 1992, Cloning and molecular analysis of the poly(3-hydroxyalkanoic acid) gene locus of *Pseudomonas aeruginosa* PAO1, *Eur J Biochem*, **209:** 15–30.

Trust T, Bartlett KH, 1976, Isolation of *Pseudomonas aeruginosa* and other bacterial species from ornamental aquarium plants, *Appl Environ Microbiol*, **31:** 992–4.

Upadhyay RS, Jayaswal RK, 1992, *Pseudomonas cepacia* causes mycelial deformities and inhibition of conidiation in phytopathogenic fungi, *Curr Microbiol*, **24:** 181–7.

Upadhyay RS, Visintin L, Jayaswal RK, 1991, Environmental factors affecting the antagonism of *Pseudomonas cepacia* against *Trichoderma viride*, *Can J Microbiol*, **37:** 880–4.

Vander Wauven C, Piérard A et al., 1984, *Pseudomonas aeruginosa* mutants affected in anaerobic growth on arginine: evidence for a four-gene cluster encoding the arginine deiminase pathway, *J Bacteriol*, **160:** 928–34.

Walsh DM, Eberiel DT, 1986, *Pseudomonas cepacia* isolated from crystal violet solution in a hospital laboratory, *J Clin Microbiol*, **23:** 962.

Wendenbaum S, Demange P et al., 1983, The structure of pyoverdine *Pa*, the siderophore of *Pseudomonas aeruginosa*, *Tetrahedron Lett*, **24:** 4877–80.

West SEH, Iglewski BH, 1988, Codon usage in *Pseudomonas aeruginosa*, *Nucleic Acids Res*, **16:** 9323–35.

Whitaker RJ, Byng GS et al., 1981, Diverse enzymological patterns of phenylalanine biosynthesis in pseudomonad bacteria are conserved in parallel with DNA/DNA homology groups, *J Bacteriol*, **147:** 526–66.

Wildführ G, Wildfür W, 1977, *Medizinische Mikrobiologie, Immunologie und Epidemiologie*, Vol. 2, VEB Georg Thieme, Leipzig.

Wilkinson SG, 1970, Cell walls of *Pseudomonas* species sensitive to ethylenediaminetetraacetic acid, *J Bacteriol*, **104:** 1035–44.

Willems A, Busse J et al., 1989, *Hydrogenophaga*, a new genus of hydrogen-oxidizing bacteria that includes *Hydrogenophaga flava* comb. nov. (formerly *Pseudomonas flava*), *Hydrogenophaga palleronii* (formerly *Pseudomonas palleronii*), *Hydrogenophaga pseudoflava* (formerly *Pseudomonas pseudoflava* and '*Pseudomonas carboxydoflava*'), and *Hydrogenophaga taeniospiralis* (formerly *Pseudomonas taeniospiralis*), *Int J Syst Bacteriol*, **39:** 319–33.

Willems A, Falsen E et al., 1990, *Acidovorax*, a new genus for *Pseudomonas facilis*, *Pseudomonas delafieldii*, E. Falsen (EF) group 13, EF group 16, and several clinical isolates, with the species *Acidovorax facilis* comb. nov., *Acidovorax delafieldii* comb. nov., and *Acidovorax temperans* sp. nov., *Int J Syst Bacteriol*, **40:** 384–98.

Woese CR, 1987, Bacteriol evolution, *Microbiol Rev*, **51:** 221–71.

Yabuuchi E, Ohyama A, 1972, Characterization of 'pyomelanin'-producing strains of *Pseudomonas aeruginosa*, Int J Syst Bacteriol, **22:** 53–64.

Yabuuchi E, Yanok I et al., 1990, Proposals of *Sphingomonas paucimobilis* gen. nov. and comb. nov., *Sphingomonas parapaucimobilis* sp. nov., *Sphingomonas yanoikuyae* sp. nov., *Sphingomonas adhaesiva* sp. nov., *Sphingomonas capsulata* comb. nov., and two genospecies of the genus *Sphingomonas, Microbiol Immunol,* **34:** 99–119.

Yabuuchi E, Kosako Y et al., 1992, Proposal of *Burkholderia* gen. nov. and transfer of seven species of the genus *Pseudomonas* homology group II to the new genus, with the type species *Burkholderia cepacia* (Palleroni and Holmes 1981) comb. nov, *Microbiol Immunol,* **36:** 1251–75.

Yamamoto T, 1967, Presence of rhapidosomes in various species of bacteria and their morphological characteristics, *J Bacteriol,* **94:** 1746–56.

Zaitsev GM, Tsoi TV et al., 1991, Genetic control of degradation of chlorinated benzoic acids in *Arthrobacter globiformis, Corynebacterium sepedonicum* and *Pseudomonas cepacia* strains, *FEMS Microbiol Lett,* **81:** 171–6.

Chapter 47

PSEUDOMONAS, BURKHOLDERIA AND RELATED GENERA

T L Pitt

1 GENUS DEFINITION

Pseudomonads are gram-negative straight or slightly curved rods. They are motile by means of one or more polar flagella, though some strains also have lateral flagella of different wavelength. They are non-sporing and not acid-fast, strict aerobes, but some grow anaerobically in the presence of nitrate. Catalase-positive, they attack sugars oxidatively; none is fermentative or photosynthetic. They are nutritionally unexacting; nearly all grow with ammonium salts and a single carbon source. Some strains are pathogenic for humans and animals. The $G + C$ content of their DNA is 57–70 mol% and the type species is *Pseudomonas aeruginosa*.

Of the pseudomonads most familiar to medical microbiologists, only the fluorescent group (*P. aeruginosa*, *Pseudomonas putida* and *Pseudomonas fluorescens*) remains within the genus *Pseudomonas*, as does the non-fluorescent *Pseudomonas stutzeri*. The other clinically significant species in human medicine have been allocated to different genera. '*Pseudomonas cepacia*', '*Pseudomonas pseudomallei*', '*Pseudomonas mallei*' and '*Pseudomonas pickettii*' are now in the genus *Burkholderia* (Yabuuchi et al. 1992). '*Pseudomonas diminuta*' and '*Pseudomonas vesicularis*' are in the genus *Brevundimonas*, and '*Pseudomonas* (subsequently *Xanthomonas*) *maltophilia*' is the sole member of the genus *Stenotrophomonas*. A comprehensive review of the present classification of aerobic pseudomonads is given in Chapter 46.

This chapter concentrates primarily on the biology of *P. aeruginosa*, and the other species of medical interest. With the exception of *Burkholderia pseudomallei* and *Burkholderia mallei*, the pseudomonads are secondary opportunist pathogens for humans. Because of their low intrinsic virulence they generally cause disease only when introduced in relatively large numbers into the bloodstream or onto mucosal membranes of the host.

PSEUDOMONAS

2 PSEUDOMONAS AERUGINOSA

2.1 Introduction and historical perspective

The organism known today as *P. aeruginosa* was earlier called *Bacillus pyocyaneus* (Gk. 'blue pus') and later *Pseudomonas pyocyanea* because of the characteristic blue-green coloration formed by cultures. Indeed, it was observed by Sédillot (1850) that the blue discoloration of surgical wound dressings was due to a transferable agent. The pigment was extracted by Fordos in 1860 and a crystalline substance, 'pyocyanine', was isolated. Lücke (1862) was the first to associate rod-shaped organisms with the pigment but these organisms were not isolated in pure culture until the classical studies of Gessard (1882). The pathogenicity of *P. aeruginosa* (Lat. 'full of copper-green rust') was established independently by Ledderhose (1888), and Charrin (1889) (cited by Bulloch 1929). The epithet *aeruginosa* has temporal priority over *pyocyanea* and is the accepted name for the organism.

2.2 Habitat

Costerton and Anwar (1994) called *P. aeruginosa* the most abundant life form on earth. It has been isolated from environments as diverse as water, jet plane fuel and disinfectant solutions, due to its ability to utilize many different organic compounds and survive in the apparent absence of nutrients. It is rarely isolated from seawater except around sewage outfalls and is not associated with disease in fish. The major sources of *P. aeruginosa* in surface waters are sewage, storm drainage and farmyard slurry, and numbers as high as $10^5 \, l^{-1}$ may be found downstream from sewage outfalls (Hoadley 1977). The species is ubiquitous in soil and the rhizosphere and consequently is often recovered from salad foods (Rhame 1980); 1 g of soil may contain 100–1000 cfu ml^{-1} (Cho et al. 1975). *P. aeruginosa* does not have a strict plant host but it can cause pathogenic processes in several plant species including bean, lettuce and potato, and is frequently recovered from chrysanthemums (Schroth et al. 1977). However, it is not a typical plant pathogen as it does not produce pectinolytic enzymes. Elrod and Braun (1942) showed that the species *Pseudomonas polycolor* isolated from plants was identical to *P. aeruginosa*. Human clinical isolates of *P. aeruginosa* are taxonomically indistinguishable by chemical and molecular techniques from environmental gasoline-utilizing strains (Foght et al. 1996).

Natural carriage of *P. aeruginosa* by humans is infrequent. In healthy subjects in the community faecal recovery rates may range from 1 to 15%; this variation may be influenced by diet. Faecal colonization appears to be short-lived in health and there is a rapid turnover of strain types. Buck and Cooke (1969) found that volunteers had to ingest at least a million *P. aeruginosa* cells before the organism could be detected in the faeces but this number was insufficient to establish colonization. This intrinsic resistance to colonization could be breached by the simultaneous administration of an antibiotic. This explains, in part, the fact that faecal isolation frequencies of *P. aeruginosa* increase dramatically in patients in hospital (rates of up to 60% have been recorded; Levison 1977) and are closely correlated with the length of stay (Shooter et al. 1969).

2.3 Morphology and cell structures

The cells of *P. aeruginosa* are rod-shaped and have parallel sides and rounded ends. They are arranged singly, in small bundles or short chains and are motile by means of a single polar flagellum (3% or fewer cells exhibit more than one flagellum per pole) (Lautrop and Jessen 1964). Molecular oxygen is necessary for motility (Shoesmith and Sherris

1960) and therefore migration through semi-solid agar is not a suitable method for tests of motility.

OUTER-MEMBRANE PROTEINS

The cell walls and membranes are structurally similar to those of other gram-negative bacteria but *P. aeruginosa* lacks the trimeric porins present in enteric bacteria. It forms a monomeric protein OprF which is structurally related to OmpA protein in *Escherichia coli*, which functions as a non-specific channel for the passage of solutes. This protein confers relatively low permeability into the cell and therefore many solutes pass through the *P. aeruginosa* membrane by specific channels (Nikaido 1992). Various workers have identified 5–8 major proteins in the outer membrane of *P. aeruginosa* and have proposed numbers or letters by which these proteins can be classified (Booth and Curtis 1977, Matsushita et al. 1978, Mizuno and Kageyama 1978); the nomenclature was unified by Hancock and Carey (1979). All strains have OprE (44 kDa), F (39 kDa), H1 (21 kDa), H2 (20.5 kDa), and I (lipoprotein, 9–12 kDa) but some strains lack G (25 kDa) and D2 (45 kDa) (Mutharia, Nicas and Hancock 1982). OprD1 (46 kDa) and D2, H2, G and F are heat-modifiable. Another protein, OprC (73 kDa), identified by Yoshihara and Nakae (1989), functions as a porin to allow the diffusion of solutes below 350–400 Da in a similar way to OprD2 and OprE1; however, OprC appears to be involved in copper utilization (Yoneyama and Nakae 1996). OprF is highly antigenic and can function as an effective vaccine to protect against subsequent challenge with *P. aeruginosa* in various infection models (Matthews-Greer et al. 1990).

FIMBRIAE

Most strains form fimbriae (pili); these are usually polar but occasionally peritrichate, and differ from those of the enterobacteria in that they do not cause haemagglutination of red cell suspensions. *P. aeruginosa* fimbriae are located at one or both poles and number 5–20 per pole. They are flexible, retractile filaments about 2500 nm in length with a mean diameter of 5.2 nm, composed of a protein, pilin, of 17.8 kDa (Paranchych and Frost 1988). Fimbriae serve as receptors for some phages (Bradley and Pitt 1974) and mediate attachment to mammalian cell membranes (see Irvin 1993). Some fimbrial elements of *P. aeruginosa* bind to different glycopeptides but the specific receptor in mammalian cell membranes is unclear. Fimbriae are strongly associated with the adherence of the micro-organism to epithelial cell surfaces but their presence is not an absolute requirement for virulence as non-fimbriate strains may be as virulent as their fimbriate counterpart (Tang, Kays and Prince 1995). Some strains have thicker non-polar fimbriae associated with the presence of certain plasmids (Bradley 1977).

FLAGELLA

Non-motile cells of *P. aeruginosa* are very rare in nature and motility is virtually always by a single polar flagellum. By electron microscopy, the width of the flagellum ranges from 16.9 ± 0.3 nm to 17.4 ± 0.3 nm (Winstanley et al. 1996). There are 2 antigenic types of flagellin, a and b; type a is heterogeneous with MWs ranging from 45 to 52 kDa whereas type b is homogeneous and of 53 kDa (Allison et al. 1985). The flagellar genes are controlled by 2 regions clustered in cistrons governing motility (*mot*), flagellate state (*fla*) and chemotaxis (*che*). The *fla* gene was cloned and expressed in *E. coli* by Kelly-Wintenberg and Montie (1989). This gene shares considerable homology with *P. putida* flagellins at the N-terminal and C-terminal ends and variation between species is most apparent in the central region of the flagellin protein (Totten and Lory 1990). The flagella of *P. aeruginosa* have been associated with virulence as non-motile mutants do not readily establish infection in an animal model and a flagellin vaccine does offer some protection to experimentally challenged animals (Drake and Montie 1987).

2.4 Cultural characteristics

P. aeruginosa grows readily on ordinary bacteriological media and is often readily identified by colonial appearances on nutrient agar. Typically it forms irregularly round, effuse colonies, 2–3 mm in diameter with a matt surface, a floccular internal structure and a butyrous consistency: colonial type 1 (Phillips 1969). Others, however, produce colonies that are smaller, raised and coliform-like (type 2). Rough forms (type 3) may be raised and umbonate or frankly rugose. Colonial types 1 and 2 form even suspensions in saline but type 3 forms a granular suspension. Any combination of these colonial forms may appear in the same culture. Mucoid colonies may have a wet or rubbery consistency, the wet forms being almost transparent. Both mucoid varieties arise from initially convex colonies that tend to coalesce on prolonged incubation.

Many mucoid isolates do not produce pyocyanin and are non-flagellate (Mahenthiralingam, Campbell and Speert 1994). Dwarf forms do not produce visible colonies unless incubated for 48–72 h and are found most often in sputum specimens from cystic fibrosis (CF) patients. Changes in colonial form may be observed on subculture from liquid to solid medium, and colonial dissociation is greatly increased in shaken cultures. No detectable differences in the heat-stable somatic antigens, phage, bacteriocin, or antibiotic susceptibility have been recognized between colonial variants from the same culture. Unlike the enteric bacteria, colonially rough strains express smooth lipopolysaccharide (LPS) antigens and can be serotyped if the soluble O antigen is extracted and tested by precipitation techniques (van den Ende 1952).

The production of a blue-green pigment that diffuses into the surrounding medium confirms the identity of *P. aeruginosa*, but many cultures do not form pyocyanin except on special media and some do not form it at all. The ability to form pyocyanin may be lost irreversibly in culture. Most but not all *P. aeruginosa* cultures have a characteristic fruity odour due to the production of *o*-aminoacetophenone from tryptophan (Habs and Mann 1967).

On nutrient agar, many cultures of *P. aeruginosa*, particularly of colonial types 1 and 3, exhibit iridescent patches with a metallic sheen. Beneath these patches crystals are visible in the medium and within the patches the organisms are lysed. These plaque-like erosions in the growth on agar were termed autoplaques by Berk (1963); he suggested that

a transferable lytic agent was responsible, but others have ruled out bacteriophage as the cause. According to Sierra and Zagt (1960), the autolysis is caused by proteolytic enzymes that digest dead cells, and the crystals are salts of fatty acids liberated by autolysis.

P. aeruginosa grows well on most formulations of MacConkey agar. On blood agar some strains cause a diffuse haemolysis which later develops into a brown discoloration of the medium. Growth in broth is abundant after 24 h but some strains from CF patients grow slowly. Broth cultures often have a thick whitish ring of slimy material adhering to the glass and most form a pellicle at the top of the broth; green pigmentation is also most evident near the surface.

SELECTIVE MEDIA

P. aeruginosa is resistant to quaternary ammonium compounds, e.g. cetyltrimethyl ammonium bromide (cetrimide). This feature has been exploited by many formulators of selective media for the isolation of the organism from heavily contaminated material (Lilly and Lowbury 1972). Cetrimide agar with nalidixic acid, and Irgasan-containing medium are commercially available. It should be noted, however, that some isolates from CF patients are hypersusceptible to these compounds and thus fail to grow on these media (Fonseca, MacDougall, and Pitt 1986). Enrichment in acetamide broth has been recommended for the isolation of *P. aeruginosa* from faeces (Kelly, Falkiner and Keane 1983).

MUCOID STRAINS

Mucoid strains of *P. aeruginosa* produce copious amounts of an extracellular polysaccharide on agar culture. The polysaccharide is chemically similar to alginic acid; it is a negatively charged copolymer of β-1,4-linked β-D-mannuronic acid and α-L-guluronic acid (Linker and Jones 1966) and is generally referred to as 'alginate'. Costerton, Brown and Sturgess (1979) proposed that alginate forms a 'glycocalyx' or loose capsule in which microcolonies are entrapped. This consortium of alginate and bacterial cells is the basis of the biofilm mode of growth and confers to the cell protection from the external environment such as complement and antibiotics. Alginate is antigenic (Pier, Matthews and Eardley 1983) in animals and humans and antibody may be demonstrated by ELISA and opsonophagocytic assays; the polymer is antigenically conserved throughout the species.

Mucoid strains are very common in the sputum of CF patients and less so in the sputum of patients with bronchiectasis. A minority ($<3\%$) of strains from other clinical sources may grow as mucoid colonies on primary culture but they are rare in the environment. However, 'mucoid' *P. aeruginosa* were isolated from 12% of 81 water samples in a recent survey (Grobe, Wingender and Truper 1995). Mucoid strains are frequently unstable on subculture and readily dissociate to the non-mucoid form, but they can be stabilized by surface-active agents such as sodium deoxycholate and lecithin (Govan 1975). The mannuronate–guluronate ratio determines the rheological properties of the polysaccharide and this is influenced by the chemical composition of the medium (Marty et al. 1992). The mucoid form generally grows less well than the non-mucoid in static broth cultures but the situation is reversed in shaken cultures. Krieg, Bass and Mattingly (1986) showed that aeration of continuous broth cultures containing both mucoid and non-mucoid varieties resulted in the preferential selection of the mucoid form. Alginate is also produced by phenotypically non-mucoid strains but this is energetically expensive (Anastassiou et al. 1987). A cluster of genes in at least 3 chromosomal loci (Govan, Martin and Deretic 1992) control the regulation and synthesis of alginate and these are influenced by environmental factors, osmotic stress, ethanol dehydration, oxygen tension and nitrogen starvation (Deretic et al. 1989, 1990, 1993, Maharaj, Zielinski and Chakrabarty 1992). The increase in ionic strength of the CF exocrine secretions caused by the elevation of sodium, chloride and calcium ions, and limitation of iron, phosphate and carbon may also influence the emergence of the mucoid form (Terry, Pina and Mattingly 1991). Speert et al. (1990) grew non-mucoid parent strains over several subcultures in near starvation conditions and obtained phenotypically mucoid colonies. They suggested that *P. aeruginosa* growing in vivo in bronchopulmonary plugs would be starved of nutrients and this environment favours the selection of alginate production.

Mucoid variants can be selected in vitro from almost any strain of *P. aeruginosa* by the action of bacteriophages (Martin 1973) and by antibiotics in sublethal concentrations (Govan and Fyfe 1978). There is little doubt that mucoid cultures arise from parent non-mucoid forms in CF patients, but the mechanism of selection is unknown. Bacteriophages that lyse *P. aeruginosa* have been found in the sputum of colonized patients (Tejedor, Foulds and Zasloff 1982) and phages isolated from mucoid strains were better able than phages from non-mucoid isolates to convert non-mucoid strains to mucoid (Miller and Rubero 1984). Ojeniyi (1988) also found bacteriophages in the sputum of CF patients and suggested that they were responsible for the selection of serologically non-typable variants frequently isolated from these patients.

The conversion of non-mucoid *P. aeruginosa* strain PAO1 to the mucoid phenotype was achieved in a chronic pulmonary infection model 6 months after inoculation. Significant decreases occurred in the expression of exotoxins A and S, phospholipase C and the siderophore pyochelin by the mucoid variants; there was also loss of LPS compared with the parent form. Conversion to the mucoid phenotype was associated with rearrangement of chromosomal DNA upstream of the exotoxin A gene due to insertion elements (Woods et al. 1991, Sokol et al. 1994).

PIGMENTS

At least 4 distinct pigments have been described in *P. aeruginosa*: pyocyanin, fluorescin, pyorubin and pyomelanin. Burton, Campbell and Eagles (1948) concluded that Mg^{2+}, SO_4^{2-}, K^+, PO_4^{3-} and Fe^{3+} were essential for the formation of pyocyanin. King, Ward and Raney (1954) devised 2 media,

A and B, for the optimal production, respectively, of pyocyanin and fluorescin; these are widely used.

Pyocyanin (*N*-methyl-1-hydroxyphenazine) is a blue phenazine pigment of 210 Da. On acidification its colour changes to yellow and then to red; at alkaline pH it is colourless. It can be extracted from fluid cultures by shaking with an equal volume of chloroform, and can be purified further by crystallization from chloroform and ether. On King's A medium, after incubation for 5 days at 37°C, c. 80% of *P. aeruginosa* strains form pyocyanin. The intensity of pigmentation often increases after agar cultures have been removed from the incubator to room temperature (18–22°C) for 3–4 h.

Fluorescin is insoluble in chloroform but soluble in water. It imparts a yellowish tinge to cultures but this is sometimes not easy to detect unless examined under ultraviolet light. Some 70% of clinical isolates form this pigment on King's B agar. A fluorescent siderophore (pyoverdin) has been characterized in a reference strain of *P. aeruginosa* (PAO1) as a 2,3-diamino-6,7-dihydroxyquinolone-derived chromophore bound to a complex octapeptide (Visca et al. 1992), which is produced optimally in iron-limited conditions. It is not clear whether this compound is the sole mediator of fluorescence by strains.

Some strains of *P. aeruginosa* elaborate a bright red water-soluble pigment designated pyorubin; it is irreversibly reduced to a colourless form in reduced oxygen concentration. Pyorubin is a chloroform-insoluble phenazine pigment that is produced by c. 2% of clinical isolates, the majority of which are from urine, and sputum of CF patients. Ogunnariwo and Hamilton-Miller (1975) showed that the addition of DL-glutamate 1% stabilized the production of pyorubin but suppressed pyomelanin formation; the reverse was shown for media supplemented with L-tyrosine1%. The production of pyomelanin, a brown-to-black pigment, is uncommon (Yabuuchi and Ohyama 1972), less than 1% of strains forming it. Pyomelanin is chemically unrelated to animal melanin.

2.5 Metabolism

P. aeruginosa is considered to be a strict aerobe but it can grow anaerobically in the presence of nitrate which it utilizes as an alternative electron acceptor. A cyanide-sensitive cytochrome *c* oxidase normally serves as a terminal enzyme but a cyanide-resistant oxidase with a lower affinity for oxygen than the former is also involved in the respiratory process (Matsushita et al. 1983, Zannoni 1989). *P. aeruginosa* converts glucose and other sugars by the Entner–Doudoroff pathway, but alternative pathways of glucose oxidation may also operate (Eisenberg et al. 1974). The oxidation of sugars yields small amounts of acid and peptone–water sugars are unsuitable for detecting this, because the acid is often neutralized by alkali produced from attack on the peptone. Hugh and Leifson's oxidation–fermentation medium is recommended for the test of glucose breakdown but acidification is more easily detected in an ammonium-salts medium in which the sugar is the only carbon source.

P. aeruginosa is unable to grow at 4°C but will grow over 3 successive subcultures at 42°C. At 37°C, a number of biochemical characters serve to distinguish it from other fluorescent pseudomonads; it oxidizes gluconate and forms slime in this medium, reduces tetrazolium salts to form red colonies, reduces selenite, and deaminates acetamide (see Cowan and Steel 1993). Most amino acids can be used as a source of carbon, nitrogen and energy, but methionine is used only as a nitrogen source. However, some strains of *P. aeruginosa* from chronic respiratory infection in CF and bronchiectatic patients are auxotrophic and require exogenous amino acids, in particular methionine, for growth; strains from other clinical sources are invariably prototrophs (Taylor, Hodson and Pitt 1992, Barth and Pitt 1995).

2.6 Virulence-associated factors and pathogenicity

PROTEASES

Most isolates of *P. aeruginosa* produce proteolytic enzymes that degrade a wide range of substrates including casein, elastin, gelatin, collagen and fibrin. At least 3 distinct proteases have been characterized: a general protease, an alkaline protease (AP) and an elastase (PE) (Morihara 1964), distinguished by their pH optima, substrate specificity and physical properties. AP has a MW of 48 kDa, an isoelectric point (pI) of 4.1, and optimum activity at pH 8–9; it is a metalloprotease but its metal cofactor is unknown. By contrast, PE is manufactured in the cell as a 54 kDa protein that is modified during passage across the inner membrane and periplasm to be secreted as a 39.5 kDa zinc metalloprotease (pI 5.9) during the late exponential or stationary phase of growth. The optimum pH for PE activity is 7–8 (Morihara and Homma 1985). AP requires calcium or cobalt for maximum activity and is inhibited by chelators; PE is also inhibited by chelators, heavy metals and reducing agents. The latter is functionally similar to several other bacterial metalloproteases such as that in *Legionella pneumophila* (Black, Quinn and Tompkins 1990). In general, AP has activity on a wider range of substrates than PE but both degrade structural proteins of the extracellular matrix such as collagen, laminin and elastin. They also have activity against a number of host-defence polypeptide components of coagulation, fibrinolysis, complement and the cytokine system (Parmely 1993). The structural gene for PE, *lasR*, controls the expression of 2 proteins LasA and LasB (Gambello and Iglewski 1991); allomorphic variants of *lasR* probably exist.

Of the proteases, PE is believed to cause destructive vascular lesions, often accompanied by haemorrhage. Keratitis has been attributed to the action of proteases, but isogenic mutants lacking proteases can cause corneal lesions in experimental animals (Ohman, Burns and Iglewski 1980). However, PE will cause liquefactive necrosis and descemetocele formation in the cornea of guinea pigs infected experimentally; AP is probably more relevant to descemetocele formation than PE (Twining, Davis and Hyndiuk 1986). Proteases also contribute to the pathogenic process in respiratory disease. PE augments the permeability of the respiratory epithelium by proteolytic attack on tight junctions (Azghani, Gray and Johnson 1993), and causes disruption of ciliary beat and detachment of epithelial cells from neighbouring cells and basement membrane (Amitani et al. 1991). In burn sepsis, much evidence suggests that *P. aeruginosa* proteases play a very important role:

1. protease-deficient strains are generally less virulent than protease producers in burned mouse models (Holder and Haidaris 1979)
2. specific antibody and chemical inhibition of protease activity increase survival of animals challenged with protease-producing strains (Holder and Neely 1989a) and
3. proteases release amino acids and peptide nutrients from burned tissue (Cicmanec and Holder 1979).

It has also been shown by Holder and Neely (1989b) that *P. aeruginosa* proteases activate host Hageman factor (a serum proenzyme), which, combined with thermal injury, results in loss of control of complement and clotting cascade pathways and leads to the accumulation of prostaglandins and subsequently tissue inflammation. Proteases may also contribute to ecthyma gangrenosum – the focal skin lesion seen in *P. aeruginosa* septicaemia – but this has not been confirmed.

The proteolytic activity of clincal isolates is best demonstrated qualitatively on casein (10% skimmed milk) agar, and quantitatively by the hydrolysis of a dye–protein complex such as azocol or a radioimmunoassay (Elsheikh et al. 1986). Isolates can also be screened specifically for elastase production on elastin–orcein agar.

HAEMOLYSINS

P. aeruginosa produces 2 distinct haemolysins: a heat-labile enzyme, phospholipase C (PLC) (Esselmann and Liu 1961), and a heat-stable rhamnolipid (Sierra 1960). PLC is a 78 kDa protein that hydrolyses phosphatidylcholine (lecithin) in erythrocyte membranes and human lung surfactant to phosphorylcholine and diacylglycerol; it is also active on sphingomyelin. An operon of 3 genes controls PLC production; *plcS* encodes for the structural gene and *plcR1* and *plcR2* encode proteins that modify PLC after translation and increase haemolytic activity (Shen et al. 1987). A second PLC enzyme of 73 kDa also has activity on phosphotidylcholine but is not haemolytic (Ostroff and Vasil 1987). This enzyme was called PLC-N to distinguish it from the haemolytic variety, termed PLC-H. The location of the PLC-N gene on the chromosome is quite distinct from that of PLC-H (Vasil, Prince and Shortridge 1993). PLC-N is produced at higher levels in phosphate limited conditions but PLC-H is not phosphate-repressed to the same degree. Both PLCs give rise to opacity around the growth on egg yolk agar after incubation at 37°C for 48 h; the enzymes can be quantitated by hydrolysis of *p*-nitrophenylphosphorylcholine (NPPC) (Berka, Gray and Vasil 1981).

There is some evidence that oxygen is involved in

PLC production and optimal enzyme production correlates well with the degree of aeration of the culture. PLC is produced by *P. aeruginosa* in the lung of CF patients and all chronically colonized patients studied by Hollsing et al. (1987) had raised antibody titres to the enzyme. PLC activity releases diacylglycerol, which, when cleaved by host or bacterial lipases, results in the release of arachidonic acid, which is a precursor of many inflammatory mediators. Purified PLC, when injected intraperitoneally into mice, induces the accumulation of inflammatory cells and the release of mediators (Meyers and Berk 1990); furthermore, in a rat chronic infection model, PLC-defective mutants did not spread throughout the lung and decreased amounts of eicosanoids were detected (Graham et al. 1990).

The rhamnolipid haemolysin alters the chemotactic responses of leucocytes at subtoxic levels and changes the electrochemical characteristics of bronchial epithelium (Shryock et al. 1984, Stutts et al. 1986); it also impairs the function of respiratory ciliated cells and has been demonstrated in the lungs of CF patients infected with *P. aeruginosa* (Hingley et al. 1986). A gene cluster encodes a regulatory protein RhlR and a rhamnosyltransferase (RhlAB), both of which are required for rhamnolipid synthesis (Ochsner and Reiser 1995).

LIPASE

Most strains of *P. aeruginosa* are lipolytic and will degrade a variety of fats and Tweens 20 and 80. Extracellular lipase is excreted during the late logarithmic growth phase and appears to be tightly bound to LPS (Stuer, Jaeger and Winkler 1986). The structural gene for the extracellular lipase of *P. aeruginosa* strain PAO1, *lipA*, codes for a proenzyme of 311 amino acids, which has a predicted MW of 30.1 kDa and an isoelectric point of 5.6. The *lipA* gene is specific for *P. aeruginosa* and *P. alcaligenes*, and an open reading frame, *lipH*, which encodes a lipophilic protein, is necessary for the expression of active lipase enzyme in strain PAO1 (Wohlfarth et al. 1992). Jaeger, Kharazmi and Hoiby (1991) suggested that lipase is released by *P. aeruginosa* as biochemically heterogeneous lipase-LPS micelles in a molecular mass of approximately 100–1000 kDa of 5–20 nm diameter; they purified a monomeric lipase of 29 kDa, which inhibited monocyte chemotaxis.

EXTRACELLULAR TOXINS

The lethal toxin of *P. aeruginosa*, exotoxin A (ETA), transfers an adenosine 5′-diphosphate-ribosyl (ADP-ribose) fragment from NAD+ to elongation factor 2 (EF-2). This reaction inactivates EF-2, terminates peptide chain elongation, and leads to inhibition of protein synthesis and death (Vasil, Kabat and Iglewski 1977). ETA consists of 2 fragments, A and B, (21 and 37 kDa respectively); overall it is a single-chain polypeptide of 613 amino acids of 66.5 kDa with a 3-dimensional structure incorporating 3 separate domains (Allured et al. 1986).

Although identical in action to diphtheria toxin, the

2 are otherwise unrelated. ETA is optimally produced by c.90% of clinical isolates of *P. aeruginosa* in iron-limited growth conditions and is encoded by a single copy of a structural gene, *toxA*, and regulated by genes *regA* and *regB* (Wick et al. 1990). Both the structural gene and the regulator genes are expressed in the lungs of CF patients infected with *P. aeruginosa* and hyperproducing-toxin strains have also been identified in this condition (Raivio et al. 1994). It is the most toxic protein elaborated by the species with an LD50 for mice of 0.3 μg kg^{-1}, and is apparently specific for *P. aeruginosa* (Vasil, Chamberlain and Grant 1986). In the native form the proenzyme is inactive but it may be converted to the active form in vitro by denaturation and reduction; the mechanism of conversion in vivo is unclear. The purified protein is highly toxic to various animals, causing hypotension and shock, hepatic necrosis and leucopenia. Histologically, it causes disruption of collagen, loss of proteoglycan ground substance and death of epithelial and endothelial cells. The toxin enters the cell via a receptor mediated endocytic pathway and the level of this receptor protein regulates susceptibility to the toxin (Mucci et al. 1995). ETA also has activity as a T cell mitogen and an inducer of interleukin-1 (Staugas et al. 1992).

Toxin expression is not absolutely required for a strain to be pathogenic as some clinical isolates lack the structural gene, but toxin-negative mutants produce less severe infections in experimental animals (Woods et al. 1982). These mutants often have a pleiotropic defect in the excretion of several other extracellular products such as elastase, alkaline phosphatase and phospholipase C, but not alkaline protease or exoenzyme S (Hamood et al. 1992). However, Miyazaki et al. (1995) found in a mouse model that an ETA-producing strain was 20 times more virulent than an isogenic mutant lacking the toxin. Antibody to ETA is protective for animals challenged with toxigenic strains (Pavlovskis et al. 1981), and patients with high levels of antitoxin at the onset of septicaemia survive more often than those with low antibody titres (Pollack and Young 1979).

Vaccines of ETA alone are poorly protective. Pavlovskis et al. (1981) showed that active immunization with a formalin toxoid, but not a glutaraldehyde toxoid, conferred a modest level of protection on burned mice even though both toxoids elicited similar levels of antitoxin. Cryz, Fürer and Germanier (1983a, 1983b) could not demonstrate appreciable passive protection by antitoxin against lethal infection by virulent strains of *P. aeruginosa*, but vaccination of humans with a toxin A–O polysaccharide conjugate gives rise to functional long-lasting elevated antitoxin antibodies (Cryz et al. 1987).

Exotoxin S (ETS) is also an ADP-ribosyl transferase but it does not modify EF-2; it mono-ADP-ribosylates the filament protein vimentin as well as GTP-binding proteins of an oncogene product (Coburn et al. 1989a, 1989b). ETS is produced as 2 forms, 49 and 53 kDa; the latter is not active enzymatically. It is immunologically distinct from ETA and is much less toxic for mice (LD50 8 μg) (Woods and Que 1987).

Only c. 40% of clinical isolates form ETS in vitro but some 90% produce it in the human body, as shown by immunoblots with sera of patients recovering from *P. aeruginosa* bacteraemia (Woods et al. 1986). Intrathecal administration of purified ETS elicits gross alterations in the pulmonary structure of rats within 2 h, and monolayers of bronchial fibroblasts become vacuolated on contact with the toxin (Woods et al. 1988).

An acidic cytotoxin of 25 kDa was described by Lutz (1979). It attacks the plasma membranes of many mammalian cells by altering the phospholipid composition of the membrane. This induces an influx of calcium, which leads to cell leakage and an increase in permeability to ions and the production of prostacyclin (Hirayama and Kato 1984). The toxin is localized in the bacterial periplasmic space as an inactive or weakly toxic form, but is converted to the active toxin by the action of proteases. The cytotoxin is probably the same protein, leucocidin, previously identified by Scharmann (1976). It is produced by c. 95% of strains and cytotoxin-deficient mutants have significantly lower toxicity in a leucopenic mouse model (Baltch et al. 1987, Woods and Vasil 1994).

SIDEROPHORES

In order to multiply in the iron-limited conditions of host tissues, *P. aeruginosa* has evolved at least 3 different siderophore compounds: pyochelin, pyoverdin and ferribactin. Pyoverdin synthesis is more important for the growth of the organism in human serum (Ankenbauer, Sriyosachati and Cox 1985), whereas the other compounds both stimulate growth under conditions of iron limitation (Cox and Graham 1979, Cox and Adams 1985). Pyoverdin has been shown to be essential for the virulence of *P. aeruginosa*; it competes directly with transferrin for iron and is necessary for iron gathering in vivo and virulence expression in a burned mouse model (Meyer et al. 1996). Siderophore activity of salicylate – a precursor of pyochelin – has also been demonstrated in *P. aeruginosa* (Visca et al. 1993).

PYOCYANIN

The pigment pyocyanin and its derivative 1-hydroxyphenazine act as inhibitors of mitochondrial enzymes in mammalian tissue (Armstrong, Stewart-Tull and Roberts 1971) and cause disruption and cessation of ciliary beat on ciliated nasal epithelium (Wilson et al. 1987). This may be significant for the ability of the organism to avoid clearance from the respiratory mucosa by primary host defences. Pyocyanin-induced ciliary slowing is associated with a fall in intracellular cyclic adenosine 5′-monophosphate (AMP) and adenosine 5′-triphosphate (ATP) and the effect can be reversed by exposure of the cells to salmeterol (Kanthakumar et al. 1994). Other activities of pyocyanin include the production of reactive nitrogen intermediates, and promotion of elastase–antielastase imbalance by increasing the release of neutrophil elastase and enhancing the oxidative inactivation of α-1-protease inhibitor (Ras et al. 1992, Shellito, Nelson and Sorensen 1992).

ENDOTOXIN

LPS from *P. aeruginosa* displays many of the biological properties of enterobacterial LPS, including mouse lethality, pyrogenic activity, the Shwartzman reaction, etc. The O side chain confers immunological specificity and lipid A is the toxic moiety. Compared with enterobacterial lipid A, that of *P. aeruginosa* contains an unusually high amount of phosphorus, probably due to the high proportion of core LPS molecules that lack O side chains (i.e. are uncapped) (Wilkinson and Galbraith 1975). The extent to which the endotoxin of *P. aeruginosa* contributes to the toxaemia of systemic sepsis is unclear; injection of *P. aeruginosa* LPS into the mouse causes endotoxic shock and death, but reports of the amount of LPS required to cause death vary from LD50 values of 450 μg to 20 μg (Dyke and Berk 1973, Barasanin et al. 1978), which is perhaps due to differences in the strains used, cultural conditions and the strain of challenge animal. However, the evidence suggests that LPS plays a major role in the virulence of the organism:

1 it confers resistance to the bactericidal action of complement in normal human serum (Young 1972)
2 it protects the bacterial cell against opsonization and phagocytosis (Engels et al. 1985)
3 antibody towards it is highly protective in experimental models (Cryz et al. 1983b) and
4 mutants deficient in O side chains are avirulent compared with their parent strain (Cryz et al. 1984).

The latter workers showed a direct correlation between virulence in a burned mouse model and the partitioning of extracted *P. aeruginosa* LPS into either the phenol or aqueous phase. LPS with a high ratio of hydrophilic O polysaccharide partitioned into the aqueous phase whereas hydrophobic short O side chains and core components were recovered from the phenol phase. Highly virulent strains (LD50 cfu $<10^2$) contained hydrophilic LPS, intermediate virulent strains (LD50 cfu 10^3–10^4) segregated into both phases, and LPS from low or avirulent strains partitioned into the phenol phase alone.

Most *P. aeruginosa* isolates from the lung of chronically colonized CF patients express LPS deficient in O side chains. These 'rough' LPS forms are avirulent in animal models and are invariably serum-sensitive. CF patients develop antibodies to both O chains and core components (Fomsgaard et al. 1988) but the contribution of these antibodies to promoting bacterial killing is not known. Pier et al. (1996) suggested that human airway cells expressing the mutant protein cystic fibrosis transmembrane conductance regulator were defective in uptake of *P. aeruginosa*. They identified LPS core oligosaccharide as the ligand for epithelial cell ingestion and postulated that the binding and internalization of *P. aeruginosa* by epithelial cells followed by desquamation was an important mechanism for the clearance of these bacteria from the lung.

Many strains of *P. aeruginosa* express a LPS antigenically and chemically distinct from type-specific LPS; this has been named A-band LPS to distinguish it from the O-specific 'B-band' polysaccharide. A-band LPS is a short-chain polymer composed of a repeating trisaccharide of D-rhamnose (Arsenault et al. 1991). The loss of B-band LPS by isolates during chronic infection does not interfere with expression of the A-band variety. The gene clusters responsible for the synthesis of A- and B-LPS are widely separated on the *P. aeruginosa* genome (Lightfoot and Lam 1993) and may involve the *algC* gene required for alginate synthesis (Coyne et al. 1994). An open reading frame region of a *rfb* gene has been identified as being involved with B-band LPS synthesis (Dasgupta and Lam 1995). Cells expressing only A-LPS demonstrate the highest surface hydrophobicity and the presence of the B-LPS results in a more hydrophilic surface. It has been suggested by Makin and Beveridge (1996) that phenotypic variation in the relative expression of A- and B-band LPS may be a mechanism by which *P. aeruginosa* can alter its overall surface characteristics to influence adhesion and favour survival.

2.7 Experimental infection

P. aeruginosa is generally only pathogenic for humans if introduced into sterile body sites in relatively large numbers. This is reflected by the range of LD50 values from 10^5 to $10^{7.5}$ required for mouse lethality by the intravenous route, and may be as high as 10^8 intraperitoneally. Many workers favour the use of experimental models in which systemic infection follows a low dose of organisms, such as mice in which an area of skin has been subjected to thermal injury before infection. Most strains of *P. aeruginosa* are lethal for burned mice with LD50s of 10–1000 cfu if the injection is made subcutaneously to the burned area; much larger doses are required if the injection is distant from the burn (Stieritz and Holder 1975). The LD50 for other micro-organisms remained unaltered in this model. It was also shown that a critical level of *P. aeruginosa* in burned skin tissue (>10^5 cfu g^{-1}) is needed before the organism can be cultured from the blood and internal organs. Therefore, this mouse model mimics human burn sepsis and is clinically relevant (Holder 1993).

A guinea pig model of acute lung infection was described by Pennington (1979) who instilled *P. aeruginosa* into the surgically exposed trachea of an anaesthetized animal to produce a bilateral haemorrhagic pneumonia. The introduction of solidified agar beads containing 10^4 cfu of *P. aeruginosa* into the exposed trachea of rats leads to the establishment of a chronic lung infection (Cash et al. 1979) with numbers of bacteria of lung tissue rising to 10^6 cfu g^{-1} and remaining stable for many weeks. The histological changes in the lung resemble those seen in human infections. This model has been used extensively to investigate the interaction between bacterial virulence factors and host defence mechanisms and to assess the efficacy of an experimental vaccine (Pennington et al. 1981). The neonatal mouse appears to be a reasonable model to study the acquisition and host response to *P. aeruginosa*; BALB/cByJ mice aged 7 days are inoculated intranasally with bacteria and the animals are killed after 24 h (Tang, Kays and Prince 1995). The *P. aeruginosa* products involved in initiating respiratory tract infection were investigated by the same group (Tang et al. 1996) in isogenic mutants lacking elastase, LPS constituents, flagella and pili.

The expression of several virulence factors was found necessary for the establishment of pneumonia in the neonatal mouse.

Neutropenia also greatly increases the susceptibility of experimental animals to infection with *P. aeruginosa* and this state can be introduced by the use of cyclophosphamide (Cryz et al. 1983a). Other animal models have been used to study *P. aeruginosa* infections in various body sites (see Baltch 1994).

2.8 Susceptibility to agents

PHYSICAL AND CHEMICAL AGENTS

P. aeruginosa is not particularly resistant to heat; it is killed by a temperature of 55°C in 1 h. It survives for many months in water at ambient temperature and has the ability to multiply in water containing minimal nutrients. When a drop of fluid containing *P. aeruginosa* dries in the air, the organism undergoes a heavy initial mortality of the order of 99% in the first 30 min but the survivors die much more slowly thereafter. Its survival time is strongly dependent on relative humidity and light (Döring et al. 1991).

The species is partially resistant to quaternary ammonium compounds, in particular to cetrimide and benzalkonium chloride, which readily become inactivated during storage in dilute solution. Indeed, it has a remarkable ability to persist and multiply in badly chosen, incorrectly compounded and improperly stored preparations of many disinfectants. It has been isolated from contaminated hexachlorophane-containing soaps and creams and from povidone-iodine and chlorhexidine solutions (Russell, Hammond and Morgan 1986).

The organism is sensitive to acid (Phillips et al. 1968) and to silver salts (Ricketts et al. 1970). Silver sensitivity has been exploited in the treatment of infections in burns but silver-resistant strains have been reported. Most strains are sensitive to *p*-aminomethylbenzene sulphonamide (mafenide) and silver sulphadiazine, both of which have been incorporated in topical creams commonly used to treat infections in burned patients. The addition of cerium to silver sulphadiazine increases its antibacterial properties as well as its penetration in the burn eschar (Munster, Helvig and Rowland 1980, Monafo and Freedman 1987).

SUSCEPTIBILITY TO ANTIMICROBIAL AGENTS

Many antibiotics inhibit the growth of *P. aeruginosa* to some extent in vitro, but only a minority of these show useful activity at therapeutically attainable concentrations. Some of the β-lactam antibiotics are active: the penicillins carbenicillin, ticarcillin, azlocillin and piperacillin; the cephalosporins cefoperazone, cefsulodin, ceftazidime, cefpirome and cefepime; the monobactam aztreonam; and the carbapenems, imipenem and meropenem. The aminoglycosides gentamicin, tobramycin and amikacin are active against most strains, and so is the fluoroquinolone ciprofloxacin. In clinical practice, an aminoglycoside is often combined with a β-lactam agent – a third generation cephalosporin, monobactam or carbapenem. There is great variation in the proportion of isolates reported to be resistant to these agents, with some countries reporting resistance rates in excess of 50%. However, a British national survey of nearly 2000 isolates (Chen et al. 1995) found the frequency of resistance to low breakpoint minimum inhibitory concentrations to be highest for gentamicin, >2 mg l^{-1}, 11.7%, and carbenicillin, >128 mg l^{-1}, 11.7%; followed by azlocillin, >16 mg l^{-1}, 10.9%; amikacin, >4 mg l^{-1}, 10.5%; ceftazidime, >4 mg l^{-1}, 9.6%; and ciprofloxacin, >1 mg l^{-1}, 8.1%. Resistance was more common among intensive care unit isolates.

The mechanisms of resistance to antibiotics include reduced cell wall permeability, production of extracellular chromosomal and plasmid mediated β-lactamases (Livermore 1989), aminoglycoside-modifying enzymes and cephalosporinases (Prince 1986), and an active multidrug efflux mechanism (Li, Livermore and Nikaido 1994, Li et al. 1994). The impermeability of the *P. aeruginosa* cell to antibiotics may have been overestimated in the past relative to the role of efflux.

There are 2 main paths by which antibiotics cross the outer membrane of *P. aeruginosa*: aminoglycosides destroy the cross-bridging of LPS through displacement of Mg^{2+} ions, whereas β-lactams and quinolones enter through non-specific porins (Bellido and Hancock 1993). The F porin is probably the key determinant of outer-membrane permeability; it forms water-filled channels in membranes and acts as a molecular sieve to exclude molecules greater than c. 9 kDa. However, it is anomalous that this protein is so populous and forms such large pores, which is inconsistent with the perceived impermeability of the species. It may be that only a minority of F-porin molecules form these channels and the small total area of channels available for the passage of antibiotics results in low outer-membrane permeability. Some workers have questioned whether other outer-membrane proteins such as the small pore-forming proteins OprC, OprD and OprE play a more pivotal role than OprF in the resistance of *P. aeruginosa* to β-lactams (Yoshihara and Nakae 1989).

All strains of *P. aeruginosa* produce a chromosomally mediated AmpC-type β-lactamase but relatively few elaborate plasmid mediated β-lactamases. The chromosomal AmpC enzyme normally is repressed but is induced strongly by first-generation cephalosporins, cefoxitin and ampicillin. As these compounds are labile to the enzyme as well as being strong inducers, they lack anti-*P. aeruginosa* activity. Third-generation cephalosporins and ureidopenicillins also are labile to the AmpC enzyme but do not induce its synthesis; therefore they remain active so long as the enzyme remains uninduced. However, stably derepressed mutants, i.e. those that elaborate AmpC copiously, arise spontaneously at moderate frequency (10^{-8}) and can be selected in vivo during cephalosporin or ureidopenicillin therapy (Livermore 1987). These mutants are resistant to all β-lactams except imipenem and sometimes carbenicillin and temocillin. Selection of derepressed mutants is rare with *P. aeruginosa*

except in chronic states such as respiratory infection in CF patients.

A large number of plasmid or transposon mediated β-lactamases have been reported in *P. aeruginosa* but their incidence is much less than in the enterobacteria. The survey by Chen, Yuan and Livermore (1995) of nearly 2000 UK isolates revealed only 13 that produced β-lactamases secondary to the chromosomal enzyme: 6 were producers of PSE-1 or PSE-4 enzymes and 7 had novel OXA types. Classical TEM and SHV β-lactamases are rare in *P. aeruginosa* and their extended spectrum mutants have scarcely been recorded. However, extended spectrum mutants of the class D β-lactamases OXA-2 and OXA-10 have been found for ceftazidime-resistant *P. aeruginosa* from Turkey (Hall et al. 1993). Furthermore, transferable imipenem resistance due to a carbapenemase has been described in the species (Watanabe et al. 1991). The gene encoding the enzyme Imp-1 is increasingly scattered in Japan though unrecorded elsewhere (Senda et al. 1996).

The efflux mechanism, in which antibiotic is actively pumped from the bacterial cell, has been widely implicated in the resistance of *P. aeruginosa* to a range of agents including tetracycline, chloramphenicol, quinolones and β-lactams (Poole 1994). Two cytoplasmic membrane proteins, one hydrophobic and spanning the membrane, the other hydrophilic and presumed to be anchored to the cytoplasmic membrane, play a pivotal role in the efflux mechanism as well as the outer-membrane protein OprM. The latter functions as a porin to allow the egress of drug molecules across the outer membrane. All *P. aeruginosa* appear to have this mechanism though its efficiency varies amongst isolates (Li, Nikaido and Poole 1995).

Resistance to imipenem appears not to be linked to resistance to other β-lactams but substantive meropenem resistance is associated with enhanced multidrug efflux as above (Chen, Yuan and Livermore 1995). Imipenem and meropenem resistance is strongly correlated with loss of D2 porin which is a specific channel for carbapenems and basic amino acids (Trias and Nikaido 1990).

Almost all strains of *P. aeruginosa* express aminoglycoside-modifying enzymes but the plasmid mediated variety are relatively infrequent. The enzymes modify aminoglycosides by acetylation, phosphorylation or adenylation. Virtually all strains possess a 6-phosphotransferase, and a 3-phosphotransferase that modifies neomycin and kanamycin (Shannon and Phillips 1982). Both 3-acetyltransferase and 2'-adenyltransferase modify gentamicin and tobramycin; and production of 6'-acetyltransferase confers resistance to amikacin. The frequency of these enzymes in resistant clinical isolates is low (Williams et al. 1984) and most aminoglycoside resistance is probably non-enzymic. β-Lactam and aminoglycoside cross-resistance is rare.

It has been suggested that the outer-membrane affinity for gentamicin is higher in strains of *P. aeruginosa* possessing the B-band LPS than in those with A-band LPS; B-band LPS strains are more susceptible to antibiotic-induced killing (Kadurugamuwa, Lam and

Beveridge 1993). Strains with both LPS forms bind more gentamicin than strains lacking one or other form and binding results in almost 50% loss of viability. These results indicate that ionic binding of aminoglycosides to the outer membrane of *P. aeruginosa* cell surfaces not only weakens the surface but also is important in cell death.

The fluorinated quinolones, in particular ciprofloxacin, are highly active against *P. aeruginosa*. Resistance may, nevertheless, emerge during long-term treatment of chronic infections (Hodson et al. 1987) but strains frequently revert to sensitivity when the drug is withdrawn. As for other bacteria, high level resistance is mostly due to mutations in DNA gyrase. However, low level resistance may be the result of impermeability or upregulation of the multidrug efflux system. Quinolones may traverse the outer membrane by porins or by a self-promoted uptake pathway similar to the aminoglycosides (Bedard et al. 1989, Young and Hancock 1992). Alterations in major outer-membrane proteins (MOMP) and LPS have both been implicated in reduced penetration of ciprofloxacin into *P. aeruginosa* (Legakis et al. 1989, Michea-Hamzehpour, Furet and Pechère 1991).

2.9   Epidemiological typing

Bacteriocin (pyocin) typing

Three varieties of bacteriocins (pyocins) are produced by *P. aeruginosa*. The R pyocins resemble the tails of contractile phages and are morphologically distinguishable from the rod-shaped flexuous F pyocins (Govan 1974a, 1974b). Pyocins R or F are produced by over 90% of strains. Some 70% also synthesize S pyocins, which are of low MW and diffuse through agar; they have no discernible structure on electron microscopy. Pyocins are active against other members of this species and occasionally against other fluorescent pseudomonads but not against non-fluorescent pseudomonads (Jones et al. 1974). They give various patterns of inhibition of gonococci (Morse et al. 1976) and serologically ungroupable meningococci (Blackwell and Law 1981).

The most widely used scheme for pyocin typing for epidemiological tracing of strains is that described by Gillies and Govan (1966) and later modified by Govan and Gillies (1969). In the original method, 8 indicator strains were streaked across an area of an agar plate that had previously supported the growth of the strain being typed. The pattern of inhibition of the indicators determined the type of the strain. Further discrimination between members of the more frequent types (1, 3, 5, 10 and untypable) was obtained by subtyping with 5 additional indicators (A–E). Govan (1978) listed 105 types and 25 subtypes; strains of different primary types could give the same subtype reactions. Since then, many new type patterns have been reported mostly in local contexts. There are some associations between pyocin type and O serotype: notably of pyocin types 2, 3 and 17 with serotype O6, of pyocin type 5 and O3, and pyocin type 11 and O1 (see Govan 1978).

Fyfe, Harris and Govan (1984) described a revised typing method in which discrimination was improved by incorporating the indicator strain in a soft agar layer over spots of growth of the producer strains. The technique was more rapid than the original and allowed the differentiation of R and F pyocins from S pyocins to be made according to the sizes of the zones of inhibition. Mucoid strains, usually untypable by the cross-streaking method, were often typable by the revised method.

Bacteriophage typing

Phages active against *P. aeruginosa* can be isolated readily from sewage and from lysogenic strains. It is often stated that 90–100% of strains are lysogenic, but phages are generally mixed with pyocins and the actual frequency of temperate phages may be somewhat lower; several antigenically different phages may be isolated from a single strain (Shionoya et al. 1967). Both DNA- and RNA-containing phages active against *P. aeruginosa* have been reported. Most of the DNA phages resemble T even phages and many morphotypes, all with tails, can be identified (Ackermann et al. 1988). They are generally resistant to heating at 60°C and exposure to chloroform; they have a latent time of 35–60 min and a burst size of 10–200 phages per host cell. The phages of the Lindberg set (see Bergan 1978) can be classified into 10 serogroups.

Both virulent and temperate phages have been used for typing *P. aeruginosa* and several phage-typing sets have been described but none has been adopted internationally (Bergan 1978). Phage typing is poorly reproducible, which is in some measure due to the diversity of cell receptors to which they attach. Most phages in the Colindale set (largely that of Lindberg) bind to LPS (Temple, Ayling and Wilkinson 1986) but others use pili (Bradley and Pitt 1974), outer-membrane proteins (Mutharia, Nicas and Hancock 1982), and slime polysaccharide as receptors (Bartell, Orr and Lam 1966). The phage patterns are random and groups are poorly defined. There is considerable overlap of patterns and a '3 major reaction-difference rule' is required before strains from the same incident of infection can be considered distinct; this results in a considerable loss of discrimination. In practice, phage typing has been used as a means of further subdividing strains of the same O serotype (Pitt 1981a). Isolates with defective LPS from CF patients are often less susceptible than isolates from other sources.

Serological typing

O antigens

The LPS of *P. aeruginosa* contain O-specific polysaccharide side chains that confer serotype specificity on the strain. O side chains usually contain fucosamine and quinovosamine (Wilkinson 1983, Knirel 1990); in some serotypes they contain D-bacillosamine. In contrast to the branched side chains of *Salmonella* spp., the side chains of *P. aeruginosa* contain unbranched tri- or tetrasaccharides rich in N-acetylated amino sugars (see Wilkinson 1983).

The O antigens are heat-stable and can be extracted with acid or formamide. They can be detected by precipitation reactions in agar gel or by tube or slide agglutination with boiled or live bacterial suspensions with antisera raised against boiled or autoclaved organisms. Purified LPS or saline extracts of strains coat sheep red cells efficiently and indirect haemagglutination or ELISA techniques are suitable for the detection of soluble O antigen. Titres of O-specific agglutinating antibody in hyperimmune rabbit antisera are generally not as high as those obtained with salmonellae; they are usually of the order of 40–160 in slide agglutination and 10-fold higher in tube agglutination tests. A short immunization course is recommended with doses of boiled cell suspension (c. 10^9 cfu ml^{-1}) consisting of 6 injections increasing from 0.25 to 2.0 ml over 15–17 days; if the course is prolonged beyond 21 days O titres tend to fall.

P. aeruginosa is serologically heterogeneous and this has been demonstrated by various workers over the past 70 years (see Liu et al. 1983). Habs (1957) described a scheme of 12 O groups that forms the basis of the most widely used International Antigenic Typing Scheme (IATS). The IATS identifies 17 serotypes; a further 3 O serotypes have been proposed (Liu and Wang 1990) but these have not been validated internationally. The scheme has been accepted almost universally but Japanese workers continue to favour that of Homma et al. (1970), although this corresponds fairly closely to the IATS. Monoclonal antibodies to the IATS serotypes have been described (Lam et al. 1987) and monoclonal reagents to the Japanese scheme are available commercially (Strickland, Gaston and Pitt 1988). Cross-reactions occur between a number of O serotypes in tests with polyclonal antisera and despite repeated serum absorptions with cells or LPS of the heterologous strain, it is often difficult to obtain a specific serum to cross-reactive O types without a dramatic decrease in homologous titre. Closely related serotypes include O2, O5, and O16; O7 and O8; and O13 and O14. Much of these cross-reactions can be attributed to similarities in the chemical structure of the LPS of the type strains. Lam et al. (1992) showed by the use of monoclonal antibodies as probes that O-specific LPS epitopes of the strains of O2, O5 and O16 involved unique chemical structures, glycosidic linkages, and some order of folding of the O side chains.

Some 5% of clinical strains of *P. aeruginosa* are agglutinated by antisera to several unrelated O groups. These polyagglutinating strains are particularly prevalent in sputum from CF patients and, to a lesser extent, in sputum from bronchiectatic patients and the urine of patients with chronic urinary tract infections. Independent studies by Hancock et al. (1983), Meadow, Rowe and Wells (1984) and Pitt et al. (1986) confirmed that these strains, and in addition non-typable isolates from chronic infections, often lack O-specific side chains in their LPS. Defects in *P. aeruginosa* LPS are not associated with changes in colonial morphology as is sometimes the case for members of the Enterobacteriaceae. Antibody to core components of LPS is probably responsible for poly-

agglutination (Pitt and Erdman 1978, Meadow, Rose and Wells 1984).

Serotypes O6 and O11 predominate in clinical material and account, respectively, for c. 20% and 15% of British isolates (Pitt 1988). Serotype O6 can be divided into 3 or 4 subgroups by the use of absorbed polyclonal, or monoclonal antibodies (Vale, Gaston and Pitt 1988). Serotype O11 is frequently associated with outbreaks of infection in hospitals, and strains of this serotype appear to be common in whirlpool-associated folliculitis (Zierdt 1986); O11 has also been reported to be a frequent cause of endocarditis in drug addicts (Levin et al. 1984). The higher-numbered serotypes of the IATS, O12–O17, with the exception of O16, are rare and together account for less than 1% of isolates from clinical material in Britain and the USA. Antibiotic multiresistant isolates of serotype O12 have been repeatedly documented throughout Europe (Legakis et al. 1982) and there is persuasive molecular genetic evidence that most of these isolates have a common evolutionary lineage (Pitt et al. 1989, Talarmin et al. 1996).

A combination of O serotyping with bacteriophage or pyocin typing is recommended for finer differentiation between strains. O serotyping is best used as a primary method to define groups; bacteriophage susceptibility or pyocin production patterns may then serve as secondary methods to subdivide strains within the same O serotype. Edmonds et al. (1972) favoured the use of the 3 methods simultaneously to differentiate isolates as each of the methods had specific disadvantages that were reduced by their combination.

O serotyping of *P. aeruginosa* is reproducible for most clinical isolates but is less so for those from CF sputum for the reasons given above. A multicentre comparison of typing methods for the organism found that when strains other than those from CF were evaluated, serotyping had a higher discriminatory power than pyocin or phage typing, and some molecular genetic approaches (Anon 1994). There are reports of phage conversion of O serotype of strains (Kuzio and Kropinski 1983) but most 'convertants' prove on further analysis to have defective LPS rather than a different polysaccharide O side chain. Indeed, LPS defective mutants may be generated by transposon mutagenesis, phage selection, or growth in gentamicin (Galbraith et al. 1984).

H antigens

Two flagellar antigens have been distinguished in motile strains of *P. aeruginosa*; type a is complex and composed of 5–7 factors and type b is uniform and serologically indivisible (Lanyi 1970, Ansorg 1978, Pitt 1981b). Antisera to formalin-killed whole bacterial cells often contain agglutinating antibody to other heat-labile constituents such as outer-membrane proteins and pili. It is therefore necessary to use purified flagella as a vaccine to ensure the specificity of the antisera (Pitt 1981b). Alternatively, H antisera raised against whole cells can be absorbed with isogenic non-flagellate variants of the vaccine strain (Pitt and Bradley 1975). Flagellar antibody titres are usually 10- to 100-fold higher than O-antibody titres and they do not decrease as rapidly as the latter.

Hence late bleedings of the immunized rabbit will contain a high ratio of H to O antibody.

The flagellar antigen can be conveniently demonstrated by inhibition of the movement of the organism through semi-solid nitrate-containing soft agar in the presence of specific antibody. This method is to be recommended particularly with unabsorbed antisera to formalin-killed cells. Ansorg (1978) preferred an indirect fluorescent antibody method for the H typing of strains but this can be time-consuming if large numbers of strains are to be examined. Pitt (1981a) detected 6 H factors that were present in strains in various combinations. Flagellar-antigen typing was useful for the differentiation of strains of the same O serotype in outbreaks, in particular among the more common serotypes O6 and O11. However, diphasic variation in some flagellar antigens may result in a degree of instability of H types in individual strains (Ansorg, Friedrichsen and Spies 1978, Pitt 1980).

Other antigens

The common fimbrial antigens of *P. aeruginosa* are serologically heterogeneous; Bradley and Pitt (1975) defined 4 different fimbrial antigens, but the apparent ease with which common fimbriae were lost, either when a plasmid encoding other fimbriae was acquired or by mutation, suggested that a fimbrial typing system might be unreliable.

Pier, Pollack and Cohen (1984) described high MW polysaccharides in *P. aeruginosa* that had the same serological specificity as the O polysaccharides but differed from the latter in their immunogenicity in animals, monosaccharide constituents and molecular size, and lacked the toxicity of intact LPS. In the standard phenol–water extraction procedure, the polysaccharide antigens of one strain partitioned in the phenol layer whereas that of another strain was recovered from the aqueous layer. The high MW polysaccharides are structurally identical to their corresponding O side chains.

Chromosomal DNA fingerprinting

Restriction endonuclease analysis

Both 'frequent' and 'rare' cutting restriction endonucleases have been effectively used for the comparison of strain types in epidemiological studies. The DNA of *P. aeruginosa* is G + C rich and thus enzymes whose recognition sites are A + T rich will cut less frequently than those with G + C rich recognition sites. Loutit and Tompkins (1991) used conventional agarose electrophoresis to separate DNA fragments generated by frequent cutting enzymes *Sal*I and *Sma*I. This was sufficiently discriminatory to differentiate strains from CF patients but the large number of bands made analysis difficult.

Enzymes such as *Dra*I, *Xba*I and *Spe*I are rare cutters for *P. aeruginosa* and have been widely used for epidemiological studies. These large DNA fragments can only be resolved by pulsed-field gel electrophoresis (PFGE) systems, in particular, field-inversion gel electrophoresis (FIGE) and contour-clamped homogeneous electric field (CHEF). Both these methods give comparable resolution of strain differences but larger fragments (up to 2000 kb) may be separated by CHEF. On the basis of macrorestriction genome mapping of *P. aeruginosa*, Grothues et al. (1988) defined 6 band differences for *Dra*I and *Xba*I digests as discriminative between clonally related and unrelated

isolates. Other investigators (Pradella et al. 1994) likewise reported up to 7 band differences with *Spe*I for genetically associated isolates but found fewer than 3 band differences in the majority of outbreak-related isolates. During outbreak situations in which the temporal and spatial distribution of isolates does not allow for the acquisition of multiple genetic alterations, fewer than 4 band differences in the *Spe*I and *Xba*I profile of different isolates are suggestive of relatedness and hence transmission. Variation of 4–7 bands seems to exclude direct transmission, but infection with a clonal variant of the same lineage is possible; with more than 7 band differences, genetic relatedness becomes increasingly unlikely (Grundmann et al. 1995). PFGE offers the highest discrimination of all the DNA-based techniques for fingerprinting *P. aeruginosa* isolates but gel-to-gel variation requires that all isolates from an outbreak or incident of infection be compared together on the same gel to ensure optimal reproducibility between isolates of the same strain.

DNA probes

Gene probes that have been used for epidemiological studies of *P. aeruginosa* include those for rDNA, exotoxin A, pilin (fimbrial) protein, alginate, and elastase. Ribotyping indexes variation in the restriction fragment length polymorphisms of the rRNA operon and its discrimination for *P. aeruginosa* is dependent on the restriction enzymes used. The enzyme *Pvu*II offers the highest discrimination between strains if used alone (Grattard et al. 1994, Grundmann et al. 1995) but a combination of *Bam*HI with *Eco*RI, *Cla*I, or *Pst*I provides almost as good strain differentiation (Blanc et al. 1993). Most strains of *P. aeruginosa* possess the ETA structural gene. This gene and its variable upstream region, a 741 bp *Pst*I–*Nru*I fragment, can be used as a probe for species identification and as a strain marker. By the use of the hypervariable region alone, Ogle et al. (1987) were able to distinguish between isolates of *P. aeruginosa* that were indistinguishable by biotype, serotype and antibiogram, from 2 unrelated CF patients. This technique was taken further by Wolz et al. (1989) who used the ETA gene and hypervariable region inserted in a plasmid, pCMtox, which gave the advantage of higher yield and sensitivity of the probe. Discrimination of *tox* typing is higher than ribotyping (Anon 1994) but less than PFGE (Grundmann et al. 1995). However, approximately 5% of clinical strains of *P. aeruginosa* are not typable with this probe.

An alternative is the pilin gene probe which is a 1.2 kbp *Hin*dIII fragment containing the *P. aeruginosa* PAK pilin gene (Speert et al. 1989). This probe defines rather broad groups and is poorly discriminatory but it gives reproducible results (Anon 1994). The alginate and elastase genes were utilized by Loutit and Tompkins (1991) for strain fingerprinting but are too highly conserved to be useful for epidemiological studies.

Polymerase chain reaction (PCR) techniques

PCR amplification of specific nucleic acid sequences has been applied for the comparative typing of *P. aeruginosa*. Two approaches have been used: random primed [random amplified polymorphic DNA fingerprinting (RAPD) or arbitrarily primed PCR (AP-PCR)], and repetitive element PCR such as the enterobacterial repetitive intergenic consensus sequence (ERIC-PCR). Both methods appear to be sufficiently discriminatory and reproducible for outbreak investigation (Grundmann et al. 1994, Lau et al. 1995). A flagellin gene-specific PCR with subsequent RFLP analysis with 7 restriction enzymes was found by Winstanley et al. (1996) to be more discriminatory than O serotyping.

Other methods

Several other methods have been used to type or fingerprint isolates of *P. aeruginosa*. They include multilocus enzyme electrophoresis (MLEE), a method in which the electrophoretic mobilities of enzymes from isolates are compared. Changes in the molecular form of the same enzyme, either in net charge or amino acid sequence, are reflected in its mobility through a gel. Many gene loci need to be screened to gain a comprehensive measure of genetic structure and this approach is laborious and consequently restricted to specialist laboratories. However, the diversity of the esterase enzymes provides reasonable discrimination between strains of *P. aeruginosa* (Pattyn and Mertens 1988, Goullet and Picard 1991). Esterase profiles can be combined with other methods such as ribotyping to improve strain discrimination (Denamur et al. 1991). Pyrolysis mass spectrometry has been reported for rapid interstrain comparison of *P. aeruginosa* (Sisson et al. 1991). The results correlated closely with O serotyping but the technique has not been evaluated sufficiently widely to be recommended for the fingerprinting of clinical isolates.

3 PSEUDOMONAS FLUORESCENS AND PSEUDOMONAS PUTIDA

These species are easily distinguishable from *P. aeruginosa* by their inability to form pyocyanin or grow at 42°C. They are motile and form more than one polar flagellum, but unlike *P. aeruginosa*, *P. putida* and many strains of *P. fluorescens* will not grow in the depths of a nitrate agar stab. *P. putida* also differs from *P. fluorescens* and *P. aeruginosa* in failing to liquefy gelatin (see Table 47.1). *P. fluorescens* does not reduce selenite or form acid from mannitol in ammonium sugars (King and Phillips 1978). Many strains form laevan from sucrose, a character not shared by other fluorescent pseudomonads; the principal distinguishing feature from *P. putida* is production of gelatinase. The LPS of both species has a low phosphorus content and this confers increased resistance to ethylenediaminetetraacetic acid (EDTA) (Wilkinson, Galbraith and Lightfoot 1973). Five biotypes of *P. fluorescens* and 2 of *P. putida* have been identified (Palleroni 1984) but these are of little value epidemiologically.

Both *P. fluorescens* and *P. putida* are usually resistant to gentamicin but *P. putida* is sensitive to sulphonamides; both are resistant to carbenicillin but vary in their susceptibility to third-generation cephalosporins. Imipenem is highly active against them, and so are the newer quinolones sparfloxacin and temafloxacin (Rolston, Messer and Ho 1990).

Both species are psychrophilic and survive storage at refrigerator temperatures. They may therefore multiply in stored blood and associated products and may give rise to fatal reactions when these are injected intravenously (Gottlieb 1993). The rate of growth of *P. fluorescens* in human blood is considerably higher at 20°C than at 4°C and contamination is due almost certainly to exogenous contamination at the time of transfusion; a survey by Puckett et al. (1992) found *P. fluorescens* on the arms of 0.3% of 782 blood donors. *P. fluorescens* and *P. putida* have a very limited ability to cause invasive infections in humans although they may be isolated from the urine and faeces and occasionally from pus and blood of cancer patients and other immunodeficient patients (see von Graevenitz 1985). The organisms are often isolated from environmental sources in hospitals such as floors and sinks but seldom from patient specimens. Recently a hypersensitivity pneumonitis associated with occupational exposure to metalworking fluid aerosols has been described in which *P. fluorescens* was implicated (Bernstein et al. 1995). Each of 6 metalworkers with the disease had serum precipitins against *P. fluorescens* and the organism was recovered from the metalworking fluid.

Several therapeutically active compounds are produced by *P. fluorescens* and *P. putida*. The latter produces an enzyme of 43 kDa that depletes plasma methionine levels and inhibits the growth of methionine-dependent tumours (Hori et al. 1996). Perhaps the best known compound produced by *P. fluorescens* is the antistaphylococcal agent mupirocin (Fuller et al. 1971); a highly active antitrypanosomal factor has also been identified in the species (Mercado, Butany and Ferrans 1986).

4 PSEUDOMONAS STUTZERI

This is a very actively denitrifying soil organism. It is an evenly staining rod frequently with monotrichous flagella. Most nutrient agar cultures exhibit 'rough', 'smooth' and intermediate forms and thus appear mixed. The rough colonies may be confused with those of *B. pseudomallei* (Dance et al. 1995), and growth may appear light brown in older cultures, but no diffusible pigment is formed. *P. stutzeri* produces large volumes of gas in nitrate broth, it is non-proteolytic and does not oxidize lactose, unlike *B. pseudomallei*. Further distinguishing features between the 2 species include the lack of KCN resistance and starch hydrolysis, by *P. stutzeri*, and the resistance of *B. pseudomallei* to colistin. The closely related soil organism *Pseudomonas mendocina* does not form wrinkled colonies, does not hydrolyse starch, and forms ammonia from arginine. *P. stutzeri* has been isolated from a number of clinical sources including blood, cerebrospinal fluid, sputum and urine. It has a wider suscepti-

Table 47.1   Characters of species of pseudomonads of medical interest

Character	Fluorescent group					Pseudomallei group							
	aer	put	flu	stu	alc	pse	mal	cep	pic	aci	dim	mal	pau
Flagella per pole	1	>1	>1	1	1	>1	0	>1	1	>1	1	>1	1
Accumulation of poly-β-hydroxybutyrate	−	−	−	−	V[a]	+	+	+	+	+	+	−	+
Pigment fluorescent	+[b]	+	+	+	−	−	−	−	−	−	−	−	−
Denitrification[c]	+	V	V	+	+	+	V	V	V	+	−	−	−
Growth at 4°C	−	V	+	−	−	+	−	+	+	−	−	−	−
Growth at 41°C	+[b]	−	−[d]	V	+	+	+	+	+	+	−	−	+
Oxidase	+	+	+	+	+	+	V	+	+	+	+[e]	−	+
NH₃ from arginine	+	+	+	V	V	+	+	+	−	+	−	−	−
Gelatinase	+	−	+	−	V[a]	+	+	+	−	−	−	+	−
Amylase	−	−	−	+	−	+	V	−	−	−	−	−	−
G + C (mol%)	67	60–63	59–61	61–66	62–68	69	69	67–68	64	65–66	66–67	67	64–67
rRNA group	I	I	I	I	I	II	II	II	II	III	IV	V	−

[a] *P. alcaligenes* does not accumulate poly-β-hydroxybutyrate, liquefies gelatin and has 66 mol% of G + C; *P. pseudoalcaligenes* accumulates poly-β-hydroxybutyrate, does not liquefy gelatin and has 62–63 mol% G + C.

[b] Only *P. aeruginosa* forms pyocyanin and grows at 42°C through 3 successive subcultures.

[c] Growth in the depths of a nitrate-agar stab.

[d] A few strains of *P. fluorescens* grow at 41°C.

[e] *B. vesicularis* gives a very weak oxidase reaction.

Abbreviations: *aer, aeruginosa; put, putida; flu, fluorescens; stu, stutzeri; alc, alcaligenes* and *pseudoalcaligenes; pse, pseudomallei; mal, mallei; cep, cepacia; pic, picketti; aci, C. acidovorans; dim, B. diminuta* and *B. vesicularis; mal, S. maltophilia; pau, S. paucimobilis;* V, some positive, others negative; + positive; − negative.

bility to antibiotics than other pseudomonads and is usually sensitive to ampicillin, carbenicillin and gentamicin but is generally resistant to first-generation cephalosporins (von Graevenitz 1985). It is much more sensitive than *P. aeruginosa* to quaternary ammonium compounds.

5   PSEUDOMONAS ALCALIGENES AND PSEUDOMONAS PSEUDOALCALIGENES

These monotrichate, non-pigmented organisms actively denitrify and rarely attack arginine; they produce little or no acid from any sugars in ammonium-salts sugars. *P. pseudoalcaligenes* is occasionally isolated from patients; it is sensitive to carbenicillin and sulphonamides (see Holmes and Howard 1994).

BURKHOLDERIA

6   BURKHOLDERIA MALLEI AND BURKHOLDERIA PSEUDOMALLEI

6.1   History

The glanders bacillus was isolated by Loeffler and Schutz in 1882 from a horse dying of glanders and was named 'Bacillus mallei' by Zopf in 1885 (see Buchanan, Holt and Lessel 1966). An organism in many respects resembling it was isolated by Whitmore and Krishnaswami (1912) from a glanders-like disease of humans in Rangoon; it was designated 'Bacillus pseudomallei' by Whitmore (1913). Subsequently, Stanton and Fletcher (1921, 1925) gave the name melioidosis to the disease and 'Bacillus whitmori' to the causative organism. Because the 2 organisms cause similar diseases they were classified together but confusion over their taxonomic position led to them being placed in a variety of bacterial genera (for early history, see the seventh edition of this book). Palleroni (1984) classified the species as members of the genus *Pseudomonas* of rRNA homology group II. However, Yabuuchi et al. (1992) proposed that all members of that rRNA group be reclassified within the genus *Burkholderia* and the new names have been validly published. Nitrogen-fixing strains of *Burkholderia vietnamiensis* may be isolated from rhizosphere macerates of rice in Vietnam but these are taxonomically distinct from *B. pseudomallei* (Gillis et al. 1995).

6.2   Habitat

B. pseudomallei occurs in soil and water in a limited geographical area – South East Asia, the Philippines and Northern Australia, parts of Africa and South and Central America – but may also be isolated in temperate climates (Dance 1991, Yabuuchi and Arakawa 1993). A damp climate and a terrain of flooded low-lying plains appear to favour the organism. Counts of *B. pseudomallei* in soil vary with region in countries such as Thailand and this may be a significant determinant of the frequency of melioidosis in the population (Smith et al. 1995). *B. mallei* is an obligate animal parasite (particularly of equine species) that was at one time widespread in the world. Isolation of the organism is exceedingly rare today and restricted to a few foci in Asia, Africa and the Middle East.

6.3   Morphology

Both species are slender rods, 0.3–0.5 μm in width; *B. mallei* is 1–3 μm in length, but *B. pseudomallei* is usually shorter (<2 μm). *B. mallei* is straight or slightly curved, with rounded ends and irregularly parallel or wavy sides; the cells are arranged singly, in pairs end to end, in parallel bundles or in Chinese-letter form. The smooth form of *B. pseudomallei* often appears as long parallel bundles of 'filaments' – really chains of closely associated rods (Miller et al. 1948) embedded in interstitial substance. In the rugose form, the shorter, oval cells are more irregularly arranged and there is no interstitial substance. Staining is irregular and bipolar staining is seen, particularly of *B. pseudomallei* in films of pus. When stained with Sudan black, both organisms show dark granules of poly-β-hydroxybutyrate.

6.4   Cultural characters

B. pseudomallei grows well on simple media, including nutrient, blood and MacConkey agar, but it does not grow on deoxycholate citrate or salmonella–shigella (SS) agars. After overnight incubation on nutrient agar at 37°C, the colonies are 1–2 mm in diameter. The growth may be smooth and mucoid or rough, with a dull wrinkled, corrugated or honeycombed surface. In the smooth form, colonies are round, low convex, amorphous, translucent and greyish-yellow, with a smooth, glistening surface and an entire edge; although mucoid in consistency, they are easily emulsified. After several days they become opaque, yellowish-brown, uneven and often umbonate. Chambon and Fournier (1956) described numerous different colonial forms, and Stanton, Fletcher and Symonds (1927) illustrated an ultra-rugose form, with an extremely corrugated surface and a tenacious consistency. Frankly mucoid forms are uncommon. The smooth colonial form of *B. pseudomallei* tends not only to die out rapidly in culture but also to kill other pseudomonads, including rough variants, in its vicinity; Rogul and Carr (1972) attribute this to the production of ammonia. The growth has a characteristic earthy or musty odour and α-haemolysis is observed on sheep blood agar; older cultures produce β-haemolysis.

B. mallei grows less well on nutrient agar and forms smooth, grey translucent colonies 0.5–1 mm in diameter in 18 h at 37°C (see Nigg et al. 1956). Neither organism forms diffusible pigment.

6.5   Metabolic and biochemical characters

Both organisms grow at 41°C, but many strains grow poorly below 25°C. The nutritional requirements of *B. mallei* are simple and, like *B. pseudomallei*, it can grow on ammonium-salt medium with a single carbon source. Both species form acid from various sugars in Hugh and Leifson's or ammonium-salts media, but *B. mallei* does this rather slowly. Both species produce ammonia from arginine and have extracellular hydrolytic enzymes that attack poly-β-hydroxy-butyrate and starch. They hydrolyse gelatin and Tween 80, and are usually KCN resistant and do not attack malonate. The following characters of *B. pseudomallei* help to distinguish it from *Burkholderia cepacia*: production of ammonia from arginine, hydrolysis of starch, formation of heat-stable phosphatase and negative lysine decarboxylase reaction. The patterns of acidification of sugars are rather similar. *B. cepacia* generally attacks salicin and adonitol but *B. pseudomallei* and *B. mallei* do not. Atypical strains occur in both species and animal pathogenicity tests may occasionally be necessary (Bremmelgaard 1975).

Dance et al. (1989a) recommend a simple screening procedure for the confirmation of identity of *B. pseudomallei*. This includes the demonstration of a bipolar or irregular staining gram-negative rod which is oxidase-positive. Organisms are tested for resistance to discs containing colistin 10 μg and gentamicin 10 μg and subcultured on a modification of the medium of Ashdown (1979) on which characteristic opaque, purple, rugose colonies appear after incubation for 48–72 h. The API 2ONE kit proved to be highly efficient for the confirmation of the identity of *B. pseudomallei* (Dance et al. 1989a) but false identification of some other pseudomonads as *B. pseudomallei* sometimes occurs. A specific latex agglutination test with a rabbit polyclonal antibody has been described for the rapid identification of the species (MD Smith et al. 1993). Wuthiekanun et al. (1990) evaluated Ashdown's medium with and without pre-enrichment in selective broth (containing colistin and crystal violet) for the isolation of *B. pseudomallei* from clinical specimens. They concluded that enrichment improved the chances of recovery of the organism from sites with an extensive normal flora. The inclusion of colistin (50 mg l⁻¹) to broth enrichments markedly improves the yield of *B. pseudomallei* from clinical specimens (Walsh et al. 1995); the antibiotic should also be added to the basal salt medium containing L-threonine (Gallimand's medium) to optimize the recovery of the organism from soil (Wuthiekanun et al. 1995).

6.6 Susceptibility to physical and chemical agents

Unlike *P. aeruginosa*, neither *B. mallei* nor *B. pseudomallei* will grow on cetrimide agar 0.1%. Both are resistant to various dyes, and 1 in 200 000 crystal violet is a useful selective agent, especially in glycerol agar (Miller et al. 1948). Neutral red and crystal violet are incorporated in the selective medium of Ashdown (1979), which also contains glycerol and gentamicin. *B. pseudomallei* survives for up to 30 months in moist clay soil (Thomas and Forbes-Faulkner 1981), but for a much shorter time in dry sandy soil. In experimental conditions, a water content in soil of <10% rendered the bacteria non-viable within 70 days, but at >40% they survived for 726 days (Tong et al. 1996). These studies also showed that the organism is killed within 18 days on nutrient medium at 0°C, at pH values below 5 and above 8, and is more susceptible to ultraviolet rays

than permanent soil bacteria. It also has a remarkable capacity to survive in nutrient-free medium and can be recoverd from triple-distilled water without any additional nutrient after more than 3 years (Wuthiekanun, Smith and White 1995). *B. mallei* survives for 4 weeks in water and then rapidly disappears (Miller et al. 1948).

Most strains of *B. pseudomallei* are sensitive to imipenem, piperacillin, doxycycline, amoxycillin–clavulanic acid, azlocillin, ceftazidime, ticarcillin–clavulanic acid, ceftriaxone and aztreonam with MICs of ≤2 mg l⁻¹; about 10% of strains exhibit resistance to chloramphenicol (Dance et al. 1989b). Of 4 carbapenems tested by Smith et al. (1996), biapenem was the most active but all carbapenems had bactericidal activity against strains resistant to ceftazidime, co-amoxiclav or both. Resistance to aminoglycosides, the polymyxins and the penicillins is uniform. *B. pseudomallei* is unusual among 'pseudomonads' in that ampicillin resistance is mediated by a clavulanate-sensitive β-lactamase (Livermore et al. 1987); 3 different mechanisms of β-lactam resistance have been described (Godfrey et al. 1991). Synergy has been observed between ampicillin and dicloxacillin, and tetracycline and novobiocin against *B. pseudomallei*. Further information about the treatment of melioidosis can be found in Volume 3 (see Volume 3, Chapter 46).

Information about the antibiotic susceptibility of *B. mallei* is scanty. The few strains reported appear to be sensitive to sulphonamides and usually also to streptomycin, tetracycline and novobiocin; some were sensitive to chloramphenicol (see Miller et al. 1948, Al Izzi and Al Bassam 1989).

6.7 Antigenic relationships

B. pseudomallei is antigenically homogeneous due to conservation of the O-antigenic LPS (Pitt, Aucken and Dance 1992). Thus polyclonal or monoclonal antibodies raised against whole cells or purified LPS of a strain will react with all strains, with rare exceptions. This common LPS antigen is largely specific to *B. pseudomallei* but some cross-reactions occur with *B. mallei* and, less so, with *B. cepacia*; nevertheless, the wide distribution of the LPS antigen makes this an ideal candidate for a vaccine and studies have demonstrated significant passive protection with anti-LPS antibodies (Bryan et al. 1994). Independent studies have shown that a single strain of *B. pseudomallei* produces 2 distinct partially O-acetylated S-type LPS molecules (Knirel et al. 1992, Perry et al. 1995); their contribution to immunogenicity and relative importance for diagnostic serology and vaccines awaits investigation. Hyperimmune antisera against the organism cross-agglutinate with *B. mallei*, and at low dilutions, with *Yersinia pestis* (Dodin and Fournier 1970), presumably due to structural similarities of LPS constituents (Knirel et al. 1992).

Steinmetz, Rohde and Brenneke (1995) described the characterization of a species-specific exopolysaccharide of *B. pseudomallei*. They isolated a monoclonal antibody, following immunization of a mouse with a mucoid strain, which showed specificity in immunoblots for a carbohydrate antigen (MW >150 kDa) poorly resolved by sodium dodecyl sulphate polyacrylamide gel electrophoresis (SDS-PAGE). The antigen had a capsule-like appearance by electron microscopy and all mucoid and non-mucoid strains tested reacted with the antibody in ELISA. Cross-reactivity was found only with *B. mallei* but no LPS was detected in the purified exopolysaccharide.

The flagellar antigens of *B. pseudomallei* are serologically homogeneous; a polyclonal serum prepared against purified flagella of a reference strain reacted with all but one of 65 strains tested by Brett, Mah and Woods (1994). Purified monomer flagellin proteins were of MW 43 kDa. Flagellin-specifc antiserum also conferred protection to infection with live organisms in an experimental model. Other miscellaneous antigens described in the species include outer-membrane proteins and a glycolipid (Anuntagool, Rugdech and Sirisinha 1993, Phung et al. 1995).

B. mallei strains are antigenically heterogeneous and form 2 or 3 groups, only one of which is related to *B. pseudomallei* (Stanton, Fletcher and Symonds 1927, Dodin and Fournier 1970).

6.8 Phages

Thirty bacteriophages active on *B. pseudomallei* were isolated from water samples around Hanoi by Leclerc and Sureau (1956) and their lytic reactions indicated the presence of 2 different strains in the area. Several temperate phages from *B. pseudomallei* will lyse *B. mallei* but not other pseudomonads (Smith and Cherry 1957, Manzenyuk, Volozhantsev and Svetoch 1994).

6.9 PCR detection and strain genotyping

An 18-base oligonucleotide probe targeting 23S rRNA sequences was used by Lew and Desmarchelier (1994) for the identification of *B. pseudomallei* either by direct PCR or by hybridization. Optimal detection was obtained by hybridization of the probe with PCR-amplified rDNA rather than total genomic DNA or colony blots. The probe also reacted with *B. mallei* but not with other pseudomonads. Approximately 100 bacterial cells could be detected in blood, and 1000 in sputum. A seminested PCR with quantitation by enzyme immunoassay was claimed to detect 75–300 *B. pseudomallei* cells in blood (Kunakorn and Markham 1995). The PCR target was intergenic spacers between the 16S and 23S rRNA genes. The 16S rRNA gene was also targeted by Dharakul et al. (1996) in a nested PCR and was reportedly able to detect as few as 2 organisms in a specimen; they did not include *B. mallei* as a control. A DNA probe which could be used to detect and type *B. pseudomallei* was advocated by Sermswan et al. (1994). This consisted of a 1.5 kb cloned chromosomal DNA fragment, a radioactively labelled insert of which could detect 40 000 *B. pseudomallei* cells. Southern blots following *Hind*III restric-

tion revealed at least 8 groups among 60 clinical isolates.

Ribotyping was first used by Lew and Desmarchelier (1993) to group strains of *B. pseudomallei*. Using the restriction enzyme *Bam*HI, they classified 22 different groups among 100 isolates from various animal, human and environmental sources. Twenty-nine isolates from different sources had the same ribotype pattern and thus the system defined groups rather than distinct strains. This was confirmed by the finding of Currie et al. (1994) who found strains of the same ribotype isolated over a period of 25 years in temperate south-western Australia. Ribotyping with *Eco*RI was proposed by Sexton et al. (1993) to distinguish a single group of strains of *B. pseudomallei*. The latter could be further divided by hybridization patterns following *Sal*I, *Hin*dIII and *Pst*I restriction endonuclease digestion. Ribotype groups of *B. pseudomallei* are further divisible by PFGE of *Xba*I digests of chromosomal DNA (Trakulsomboon, Pitt and Dance 1994).

6.10 Toxins

The role of toxic products in the pathogenesis of melioidosis is unclear. Liu (1957) showed that *B. pseudomallei* produced a lethal and dermonecrotic toxin and Heckly and Nigg (1958) separated 2 heat-labile toxic constituents, both of which were lethal for mice when injected intraperitoneally but only one of which was dermonecrotic. Proteolytic and lecithinase activity has been demonstrated in toxic fractions. Ismail et al. (1987) developed an ELISA for the detection of antibody to *B. pseudomallei* exotoxin in mice. They isolated a protein of c. 31 kDa from a broth culture that had been incubated for 7 days and raised a specific monoclonal antibody to it in mice. The protein was a potent inhibitor of DNA and protein synthesis in cultured macrophages (Mohamed et al. 1989). A non-toxic polypeptide was identified by Levine, Lein and Maurer (1959) which enhanced mortality in experimental melioidosis and plague.

An extracellular protease of c. 36 kDa was shown to be a metalloenzyme, requiring iron for maximal activity, which was inhibited by EDTA. The protease was active against various substrates, including immunoglobulins, but was weakly elastolytic. Antibodies to *P. aeruginosa* alkaline protease cross-reacted with the *B. pseudomallei* protease (Sexton et al. 1994). *B. pseudomallei* also produces an acid phosphatase enzyme that may play a role in intracellular survival (Dejsirilert et al. 1989). A survey of 100 clinical isolates of *B. pseudomallei* showed that 91% produced lecithinase, lipase and protease, but none was positive for elastase; 93% formed a haemolysin (Ashdown and Koehler 1990). *B. pseudomallei* obtains iron in serum and cells through a hydroxamate siderophore, malleobactin, which is optimally produced under iron-deficient conditions (Yang, Chaowagul and Sokol 1991). The siderophore is capable of sequestering iron from transferrin and lactoferrin at neutral and acid pH and appears to acquire iron more effectively from these sources than from the host cell (Yang, Kooi and Sokol 1993).

Intracellular growth was demonstrated in human phagocytes by Pruksachartvuthi, Aswapokee and Thankerngpol (1990) who reported up to a $\log_{10} 3$ increase in cell numbers over a period of 21 h; the phagocytes remained viable and retained their capacity to produce an oxidative burst for the first hour of incubation.

6.11   Pathogenicity

Glanders is a natural disease that spreads among equine animals, and humans are occasionally infected from them. Melioidosis occurs sporadically in a wide range of mammalian species, including humans, horses, pigs, sheep, goats, cats, dogs, several rodents, monkeys and dolphins. These diseases are considered in greater detail in Volume 3 (see Volume 3, Chapter 46), and further information on experimental infection in laboratory animals is given in earlier editions of this work. However, the diabetic rat model used by Woods, Jones and Hill (1993) warrants mention. Melioidosis is significantly associated with pre-existing diabetes mellitus (Chaowagul et al. 1989) and so these workers attempted to mimic this state experimentally by inducing diabetes in rats by the injection of streptozocin. They found that these rats were significantly more susceptible to *B. pseudomallei* septicaemia than control rats. *B. pseudomallei* grew at an increased rate in diabetic rat serum and insulin inhibited growth both in vitro and in vivo. *B. pseudomallei* has been demonstrated in clinical specimens and in soil and water submitted to the laboratory. Depending upon the nature of the laboratory work, biosafety level 2 or 3 should be employed and appropriate containment equipment and protective clothing used (see Chapter 19).

7   BURKHOLDERIA CEPACIA

7.1   Classification

This species owes its present epithet to the description by Burkholder (1950) of a bacterium responsible for rot in onion bulbs. The organism was later referred to as 'Pseudomonas multivorans' by Stanier, Palleroni and Doudoroff (1966) and as 'Pseudomonas kingii' by Jonsson (1970) but 'P. cepacia' was shown to be the correct name by Ballard et al. (1970). Following the proposal of Yabuuchi et al. (1992), the 7 species constituting rRNA group II of the genus Pseudomonas were transferred to the new genus Burkholderia with B. cepacia as the type species (type strain ATCC 25416).

7.2   Cultural characteristics

The organism is a slender rod with multitrichous flagella that accumulates poly-β-hydroxybutyrate and so stains irregularly. It is aerobic and grows well on nutrient agar but often prefers temperatures of 25–35°C for 48 h for optimal growth. Most strains grow at 41°C but not at 42°C, and none grows at 4°C. Cultures on blood agar often become non-viable after 3–4 days and survival on refrigerated slopes is poor; some workers favour maintaining cultures as suspensions in sterile tap water. Colonies on nutrient agar are opaque; those of some strains are greyish-white, but others are at first yellowish and later take on an intense reddish-purple colour due to the formation of a non-diffusible phenazine. The yellow pigment is best demonstrated on iron-containing media. The organism resembles *B. pseudomallei* in not forming ammonia from arginine and in being lysine- and ornithine decarboxylase-positive; it also forms acid from dulcitol but not from ethanol in ammonium-salts medium (see Holmes and Howard 1994). The oxidase reaction varies in strength and the nitrate reductase reaction is negative. A biotype scheme (Richard et al. 1981) has been proposed but it is relatively insensitive; the production of a melanin-like pigment on tyrosine agar may also be a reliable strain marker.

Selective media are necessary to optimize isolation of the species from specimens with mixed flora and several media, some of them also differential, have been described that exploit its biochemical diversity and intrinsic resistance to antibacterial agents. They include: an oxidation–fermentation agar base supplemented with lactose, polymyxin B and bacitracin (Welch et al. 1987); a commercially available agar containing crystal violet, bile salts, ticarcillin and polymyxin B (Gilligan et al. 1985); a medium containing the selective agents 9-chloro-9-(4-diethylaminophenyl)-10-phenylacridan and polymyxin B (Wu and Thompson 1984). For the optimal isolation of *B. cepacia* from CF patients, sputum should be liquefied, diluted and selective agar plates incubated at 37°C for 48 h and then at room temperature for up to 5 days; a liquid enrichment medium (Malka broth) supplemented with polymyxin B is recommended for the isolation of the organism from environmental swabs and soils (Butler et al. 1995). A number of pseudomonads and other gram-negative species are able to grow on *B. cepacia* selective media and care should be taken to ensure the identity of isolates by extended tests. Multiresistant isolates of bacteria, which share characteristics of both *B. cepacia* and *B. gladioli*, have also been described from CF patients.

B. cepacia is exceptionally versatile nutritionally and is able to use many simple organic compounds as sole source of carbon and energy for growth (Palleroni 1984); strains can multiply in distilled water, dilute disinfectants, and can utilize penicillin G. It also has the ability to catabolize aromatic and polyhalogeno compounds, and to produce a range of antifungal compounds (Jayaswal et al. 1993).

7.3   Habitat

It is probably inaccurate to state that *B. cepacia* is ubiquitous in nature although it can be isolated from surface waters and soil, but with varying frequency; Butler et al. (1995) isolated the species from 12 of 55 samples in a botanical complex. It is almost exclusively phytopathogenic through the production of pectolytic enzymes. It is relatively infrequent in salads and fresh foods but it was recovered from 18% of domestic environments by Mortensen, Fisher and LiPuma (1995).

7.4 Susceptibility to disinfectants and antibiotics

B. cepacia can contaminate various pharmaceutical products, especially disinfectant solutions such as chlorhexidine and cetrimide, and a number of outbreaks have arisen in hospitals as a direct consequence of the proliferation of the organism in such sources (see Martone, Tablan and Jarvis 1987). The species is resistant to most antibiotics. Nearly all strains are resistant to the aminoglycosides, polymyxin, ticarcillin, azlocillin and imipenem, whereas variable susceptibility is shown to temocillin, aztreonam, ciprofloxacin and tetracycline. A proportion of strains remain relatively susceptible to trimethoprim–sulphamethoxazole and chloramphenicol. A study of *B. cepacia* from CF patients in Britain found that about three-quarters of isolates were susceptible to ceftazidime, piperacillin (+ tazobactam) and meropenem but usually at only 'high' breakpoint levels (Pitt et al. 1996). Various combinations of 2, 3 or even 4 antibiotics exhibit synergy in vitro against *B. cepacia* (Kerr 1993). Resistance to β-lactams is a consequence of a combination of low permeability of the outer membrane and inducible β-lactamases. Decreased expression of the major porins leads to elevated resistance to β-lactams (Parr et al. 1987) and the insensitivity to cationic antibiotics results from the sparse degree of phosphorylation of its LPS coupled with the presence of protonated 4-amino-4-deoxy-L-arabinose in lipid A or core oligosaccharide (Cox and Wilkinson 1991). Resistance plasmids have been described in *B. cepacia* but their contribution to overall resistance is unknown (Sabaté, Villanueva and Prieto 1994); however, antibiotic resistance is mostly associated with large plasmids (146–222 kb). Conjugative transfer from *P. aeruginosa* to *B. cepacia*, and from *B. cepacia* transconjugants to other strains of the same species, has been demonstrated (Lennon and DeCicco 1991).

7.5 Epidemiology

A common feature of published reports of outbreaks of *B. cepacia* infections in hospitals is contamination of water supplies, often in pharmacies, disinfectant solutions, tubing for irrigation and monitoring lines (Martone, Tablan and Jarvis 1987). Today, outbreaks are less common owing to the increase in the use of prepackaged proprietary preparations, which decreases the risk of common source contamination. Nevertheless, extrinsic contamination of nebulized medications such as albuterol have been implicated in large outbreaks in intensive care units despite the presence of the preservative benzalkonium chloride in the preparation (Pegues et al. 1996). Patients tend to be colonized rather than infected and patient-to-patient spread is rare; prolonged carriage by non-CF patients has not been documented. There are conflicting reports concerning an association between *B. cepacia* and chronic granulomatous disease. Respiratory infection in these patients appears to be independent of the degree of lung damage (O'Neil et al.

1986), and the organism is found in only a minority of cases (Nakhleh, Glock and Snover 1992). Phagocytic cells from these patients do not produce peroxides necessary for the intracellular killing of bacteria. Supportive evidence of an intracellular pathogenic role for *B. cepacia* has been reported (Burns et al. 1996).

CYSTIC FIBROSIS

The major impact of *B. cepacia* infection has undoubtedly been in CF patients in whom it was first recognized in the mid-1970s. However, it did not become a clinically significant problem until 10 years later when the prevalence of the organism rose to nearly 40% of patients attending a major treatment centre in Toronto, Canada (Isles et al. 1984) and elsewhere in the USA (Thomassen et al. 1985). The clinical outcome of *B. cepacia* infection in CF patients may vary from asymptomatic carriage through a gradual but accelerated decline to a rapidly fatal fulminant septicaemia in a minority of cases. In CF patients serum antibodies are demonstrable to surface antigens (Aronoff, Quinn and Stern 1991) but the contribution of *B. cepacia* to clinical deterioration and lung damage is unclear. There is therefore a need for sensitive and specific methods of detecting and confirming the identity of *B. cepacia* and PCR assays have been reported for this purpose (Callaghan, Tanner and Boulnois 1994, Campbell et al. 1995). It has been repeatedly demonstrated that *B. cepacia* can be transmitted between CF patients both in and out of hospitals (Govan et al. 1993, DL Smith et al. 1993). Various routes of initial colonization have been implicated, but respiratory equipment, particularly nebulizers, rank among the most important (Hutchinson et al. 1996). Guidelines for patients and their carers have been put forward by various CF associations in Europe and North America in an attempt to reduce cross-infection. They stress the need to avoid intimate contact between and sharing of rooms for physiotherapy, sleeping, etc.; *B. cepacia* has been detected in air samples taken after physiotherapy (Ensor et al. 1996) and can persist in the air after the room is vacated (Humphreys et al. 1994). *B. cepacia* can survive for long periods in respiratory droplets on environmental surfaces but this property varies with the strain (Drabick et al. 1996; see also, Pankhurst and Philpott-Howard 1996).

7.6 Epidemiological typing

SEROLOGY

At least 3 serological typing systems have been described independently for the grouping of *B. cepacia* isolates (see Wilkinson and Pitt 1995a), but the scheme of Werneburg and Monteil (1989) has probably been the most widely used. This differentiates the species into 9 O and 5 H types with typability of 98% and 43%, respectively, for isolates from the environment and nosocomial infection; typability rates fall significantly with CF isolates.

BACTERIOCINS

A scheme utilizing production and sensitivity to bacteriocins was developed by Govan and Harris (1985) and identified 14 producer and 23 susceptibility types in 44 combinations among 95% of *B. cepacia* isolates. It is a simple agar overlay technique and results can be obtained within 24 h but there may be substantial variation among outbreak-related strains (Rabkin et al. 1989).

CHROMOSOMAL DNA ANALYSIS

Ribotyping has been widely applied to epidemiological studies of *B. cepacia*. LiPuma et al. (1988) found 14 different rRNA patterns based on the positions of 4–8 hybridization bands in *Eco*RI digests of DNA from CF strains and at least 50 patterns were found by Pitt et al. (1996) among strains from British CF patients. PCR can be used to detect polymorphisms in the intergenic spacer regions of rRNA (Kostman et al. 1992), and arbitrarily primed PCR reveals strain lineages similar to that obtained by PFGE of *Xba*I digests, or ribotyping (Bingen et al. 1993). Insertion sequence primers originally intended for the identification of *Bordetella pertussis* were found to differentiate between strains of *B. cepacia* from unrelated sources and show homology among epidemiologically related isolates (Cimolai and Trombley 1995).

OTHER TYPING METHODS

McKevitt and Woods (1984) found plasmids in only 23% of CF isolates and 7 had the same plasmid. However, enzyme digest lysates and salt–ethanol precipitated DNA revealed plasmids in all but one of 16 isolates (Gonzalez and Vidaver 1979), whereas 31 of 37 diverse strains proved positive for plasmids when a rapid alkaline lysis method was used (Lennon and DeCicco 1991). MLEE has proved of value for outbreak investigation and studies of the genetic structure of different strain populations (Carson et al. 1991, Yohalem and Lorbeer 1994). In particular, Wise, Shimkets and McArthur (1995) showed that there was only limited association between enzyme alleles and this was suggestive of frequent recombination within the species. MLEE in combination with ribotyping allowed the definition of various strain lineages and determination of linkage between strains from different geographical locations, which confirmed that the Toronto clone was genetically indistinguishable from the epidemic strain in the UK (Johnson, Tyler and Rozee 1994). Quantitative differences in fatty acid profiles can also be epidemiologically significant (Mukwaya and Welch 1989), and pyrolysis mass spectrometry has been reported to be more discriminating for strain identification than SDS-PAGE (Corkill et al. 1994).

7.7 Pathogenicity

B. cepacia in the rhizosphere plays an important role in the control of phytopathogenic fungi and growth promotion in plants, and as a result has attracted interest as a biological control agent (Burkhead, Schisler and Slininger 1994). Rhizospere isolates grow over a wider range of temperatures and differ in a number of other properties from CF isolates (Bevivino et al. 1994). Strains of *B. cepacia* from animal or plant sources are relatively avirulent (LD50 1×10^8 cfu) for normal mice but they persist in high numbers in a burned mouse model (Stover, Drake and Montie 1983). Adhesion to mammalian cells and respiratory mucin is mediated by fimbriae and some outer-membrane proteins, including the 37 kDa porin (Saiman, Cacalano and Prince 1990, Kuehn et al. 1992; see also Nelson et al. 1994). *B. cepacia* also produces a number of other virulence factors including exopolysaccharide (Cérantola, Marty and Montrozier 1996), lipopolysaccharide, ornithine amine lipids, proteases, lipases, haemolysin, siderophores and antibiotic resistance (see Wilkinson and Pitt 1995b). Expression of peritrichous bundles of fimbriae (pili), called cable pili (fimbriae), is the only genetically characterized virulence factor so far described. Cable pili bind specifically to CF respiratory mucin and airway epithelial cells. The presence of the *cblA* pilin subunit gene in strains is associated almost uniquely with transmissibility (Sun et al. 1995); a novel insertion sequence IS*1356* is also found in the majority of *cbl+* strains (Tyler, Rozee and Johnson 1996).

8 BURKHOLDERIA GLADIOLI

This plant pathogen is rarely encountered in clinical specimens. It was previously known as '*Pseudomonas marginata*' but is closely related in DNA hybridization to *B. cepacia* (Ballard et al. 1970). Strains grow readily on polymyxin-containing selective media but they can be differentiated from *B. cepacia* by their negative reactions for oxidase enzyme and utilization of maltose and lactose. It has been isolated sporadically from the sputum of CF patients in which it has been considered to be non-pathogenic (Christenson et al. 1989). Multiresistant isolates with shared phenotypic properties of *B. cepacia* and *B. gladioli* have been reported from CF patients by Simpson et al. (1994) who found the 'Edinburgh epidemic strain' of *B. cepacia* to give equivocal reactions in biochemical tests and fatty acid analysis. *B. gladioli* may also be confused with *Oligella ureolytica* due to its variable urea-hydrolysing properties (Trotter et al. 1990).

9 BURKHOLDERIA PICKETTII

This organism, first described by Ralston, Palleroni and Doudoroff (1973), is a non-pigmented pseudomonad that accumulates poly-β-hydroxybutyrate, is oxidase-positive and may grow at 41°C but it does not attack arginine. According to King and colleagues (1979) it is the same species as the organism earlier described as '*Pseudomonas thomasii*'. It was transferred along with other rRNA homology group II species to the genus *Burkholderia* by Yabuuchi et al. (1992). *B. pickettii* is an opportunist pathogen, especially among the immunosuppressed, and has been implicated in a number of outbreaks of infection due to contaminated water sources (Maki et al. 1991). Strains may be typed by a number of methods including PFGE of *Dra*I digests of chromosomal DNA (Dimech et al. 1993). Isolates are usually resistant to aminoglycosides, ampicillin and colistin but sensitivity to carbenicillin is variable. They are generally susceptible to chloramphenicol and second- and third-generation cephalosporins.

OTHER PSEUDOMONADS

10 *COMAMONAS ACIDOVORANS*

Although normally found in the soil, this organism has been isolated on a number of occasions from hospital patients and their environment. In addition to the characters shown in Table 47.1, it acidifies mannitol but not ethanol, glucose or maltose in ammonium-salts media. Some strains will grow on colistin-containing media but are resistant to gentamicin. It is variable in its susceptibility to carbenicillin but most are sensitive to the ureidopenicillins, tetracycline, the quinolones, and trimethoprim–sulphamethoxazole (see von Graevenitz 1985).

11 *STENOTROPHOMONAS MALTOPHILIA*

This organism was originally classified as '*P. maltophilia*' but was transferred to the genus *Xanthomonas* in 1983 and subsequently as the sole member to the genus *Stenotrophomonas* (Palleroni and Bradbury 1993). It stains evenly and on nutrient agar at 37°C forms opaque greyish colonies with a yellowish tinge; on blood agar the growth can have a faint lavender hue. Because of its requirement for methionine it will not grow in Koser's citrate medium. The oxidase reaction is negative or equivocal and it usually acidifies maltose and may acidify glucose, but it does not attack other sugars in ammonium-salts media. It decarboxylates lysine but not ornithine, and splits aesculin (see Holmes and Howard 1994).

It is ubiquitous in nature and in hospitals is occasionally associated with outbreaks of infection, particularly in intensive care units, being recovered from bypass equipment, defrost water baths in operating theatres, and ice-making machines. *S. maltophilia* has been isolated from patient specimens as the causative organism of a wide variety of infections but sepsis is unusual unless certain risk factors are prevalent in the patient population, i.e. prior surgery, shock, mechanical ventilation, and broad spectrum antimicrobial prophylaxis, particularly imipenem, to which it is intrinsically resistant (Elting et al. 1990, Laing et al. 1995). *S. maltophilia* is increasingly isolated from the sputum of CF patients and misidentification as *B. cepacia* may occur as the former grows reasonably well on selective media containing polymyxin B

(Burdge et al. 1995). Strains of *S. maltophilia* can be divided into a number of types by heat-stable antigens (Schable et al. 1989), and further subdivided by ribotyping with *Eco*RI (Bingen et al. 1991), PFGE with *Xba*I (Laing et al. 1995), and AP-PCR (Chatelut et al. 1995). Typing seldom reveals sharing of strains by different patients on a unit and often a number of unique strains selected by shared antibiotic resistances are recovered in outbreaks.

Co-trimoxazole, the tetracyclines doxycycline and minocycline, and the third-generation cephalosporins have the highest activity against the organism whereas the antipseudomonal penicillins are only moderately active. Almost all strains are resistant to aminoglycosides (Schoch and Cunha 1987, Khardori et al. 1990).

12 *BREVUNDIMONAS DIMINUTA* AND *BREVUNDIMONAS VESICULARIS*

These are closely related species of monotrichate organisms with flagella of very short wavelength. They were previously classified as rRNA homology group IV within the genus *Pseudomonas* but Segers et al. (1994) proposed the name *Brevundimonas* following a comprehensive study of phenotypic and genotypic characters. They require pantothenate, biotin and cyanocobalamin for growth; *B. diminuta* also requires cysteine or methionine. They grow rather slowly on ordinary nutrient media. Features other than growth requirements that distinguish *B. vesicularis* from *B. diminuta* are that *B. vesicularis* gives only a weak oxidase reaction, forms a carotenoid pigment and thus has yellow or orange colonies, and acidifies glucose and maltose in ammonium-salts media. Both species are extremely rare in pathological specimens and of doubtful clinical significance.

13 *SPHINGOMONAS PAUCIMOBILIS*

This is a yellow-pigmented, non-fermentative rod that is likely to be confused with flavobacteria because its motility is difficult to demonstrate (Holmes et al. 1977); in a hanging-drop preparation only a small proportion of the cells move actively. It was moved from the genus *Pseudomonas* by Yabuuchi et al. (1990). In addition to the characters shown in Table 47.1, it forms acid in ammonium-salts media from ethanol, glucose, maltose and a number of other sugars, and hydrolyses aesculin. It has been isolated often from the environment and from water or saline intended for the irrigation of wounds. Most strains are sensitive to erythromycin, tetracycline, chloramphenicol and aminoglycosides but resistant to ureidopenicillins and 'earlier' cephalosporins. Outbreaks of infection in hospitals are rare (Reina et al. 1991) but isolates can be fingerprinted by AP-PCR (Lemaitre et al. 1996).

REFERENCES

Ackermann H-W, Cartier C et al., 1988, Morphology of *Pseudomonas aeruginosa* typing phages of the Lindberg set, *Ann Inst Pasteur Virol*, **139**: 389–404.

Al Izzi SA, Al Bassam LS, 1989, *In vitro* susceptibility of *Pseudomonas mallei* to antimicrobial agents, *Comp Immunol Microbiol Infect Dis*, **12**: 5–8.

Allison JS, Dawson et al., 1985, Electrophoretic separation and molecular weight characterization of *Pseudomonas aeruginosa* H-antigen flagellins, *Infect Immun*, **49**: 770–4.

Allured VS, Collier RJ et al., 1986, Structure of exotoxin A of *Pseudomonas aeruginosa* at 3.0 Å resolution, *Proc Natl Acad Sci USA*, **83**: 1320–4.

Amitani R, Wilson R et al., 1991, Effects of human neutrophil elastase and *Pseudomonas aeruginosa* proteases on human respiratory epithelium, *Am Rev Respir Cell Mol Biol*, **4**: 26–32.

Anastassiou ED, Mintzas AC et al., 1987, Alginate production by clinical nonmucoid *Pseudomonas aeruginosa* strains, *J Clin Microbiol*, **25**: 656–9.

Ankenbauer R, Sriyosachati S, Cox CD, 1985, Effect of siderophores on the growth of *Pseudomonas aeruginosa* in human serum and transferrin, *Infect Immun*, **49**: 132–40.

Anon, 1994, A multicenter comparison of methods for typing strains of *Pseudomonas aeruginosa* predominantly from patients with cystic fibrosis, *J Infect Dis*, **169**: 134–42.

Ansorg R, 1978, Flagellaspezifisches H Antigenschema von *Pseudomonas aeruginosa*, *Zentralbl Bakteriol Parasitenkd Abt 1 Orig*, **242**: 228–38.

Ansorg R, Friedrichsen C, Spies A, 1978, Antikörper-induzierte phasenvariation von *Pseudomonas aeruginosa*, *Zentralbl Bakteriol Parasitenkd Abt 1 Orig*, **242**: 339–46.

Anuntagool N, Rugdech P, Sirisinha S, 1993, Identification of specific antigens of *Pseudomonas pseudomallei* and evaluation of their efficacies for diagnosis of melioidosis, *J Clin Microbiol*, **31**: 1232–6.

Armstrong AV, Stewart-Tull DES, Roberts JS, 1971, Characterization of the *Pseudomonas aeruginosa* factor that inhibits mouse liver mitochrondrial respiration, *J Med Microbiol*, **14**: 249–62.

Aronoff SC, Quinn FJ, Stern RC, 1991, Longitudinal serum IgG response to *Pseudomonas cepacia* surface antigens in cystic fibrosis, *Pediatr Pulmonol*, **11**: 289–93.

Arsenault TL, Hughes DW et al., 1991, Structural studies of the polysaccharide portion of 'A-band' lipopolysaccharide from a mutant (AK1401) of *Pseudomonas aeruginosa* strain PA01, *Can J Chem*, **69**: 1273–80.

Ashdown LR, 1979, An improved screening technique for isolation of *Pseudomonas pseudomallei* from clinical specimens, *Pathology*, **11**: 293–7.

Ashdown LR, Koehler JM, 1990, Production of hemolysin and other extracellular enzymes by clinical isolates of *Pseudomonas pseudomallei*, *J Clin Microbiol*, **28**: 2331–4.

Azghani AO, Gray LD, Johnson AR, 1993, A bacterial protease perturbs the paracellular barrier function of transporting epithelial monolayers in culture, *Infect Immun*, **61**: 2681–6.

Ballard RW, Palleroni NJ et al., 1970, Taxonomy of the aerobic pseudomonads: *Pseudomonas cepacia*, *P. marginata*, *P. allicola*, *P. carophylli*, *J Gen Microbiol*, **60**: 199–214.

Baltch AL, 1994, *Pseudomonas aeruginosa* bacteremia, Pseudomonas aeruginosa*: Infections and Treatment*, eds Baltch AL, Smith RP, Marcel Dekker, New York, 73–128.

Baltch AL, Obrig TG et al., 1987, Production of cytotoxin by clinical strains of *Pseudomonas aeruginosa*, *Can J Microbiol*, **33**: 104–11.

Barasanin I, Alonso ML et al., 1978, Comparative study of immunological activities of *Pseudomonas aeruginosa* and *Brucella melitensis* lipopolysaccharides, *Curr Microbiol*, **1**: 263–7.

Bartell PF, Orr TE, Lam GKH, 1966, Polysaccharide depolymerase associated with bacteriophage infection, *J Bacteriol*, **92**: 56–62.

Barth AL, Pitt TL, 1995, Auxotrophic variants of *Pseudomonas aeruginosa* are selected from prototrophic wild-type strains in respiratory infections in cystic fibrosis patients, *J Clin Microbiol*, **33**: 37–40.

Bedard J, Chamberland S et al., 1989, Contribution of permeability and sensitivity to inhibition of DNA synthesis in determining susceptibilities of *Escherichia coli*, *Pseudomonas aeruginosa* and *Alcaligenes faecalis* to ciprofloxacin, *Antimicrob Agents Chemother*, **33**: 1457–64.

Bellido F, Hancock REW, 1993, Susceptibility and resistance of *Pseudomonas aeruginosa* to antimicrobial agents, Pseudomonas aeruginosa *as an Opportunistic Pathogen*, eds Campa M, Bendinelli M, Friedman H, Plenum Press, New York, 321–48.

Bergan T, 1978, Phage typing of *Pseudomonas aeruginosa*, *Methods in Microbiology*, vol. 10, eds Bergan T, Norris J, Academic Press, London, 169–99.

Berk RS, 1963, Nutritional studies on the 'auto-plaque' phenomenon in *Pseudomonas aeruginosa*, *J Bacteriol*, **86**: 728–34.

Berka RM, Gray GL, Vasil ML, 1981, Studies of phospholipase C (heat-labile haemolysin) in *Pseudomonas aeruginosa*, *Infect Immun*, **3**: 1071–4.

Bernstein DI, Lummus ZL et al., 1995, Machine operator's lung. A hypersensitivity pneumonitis disorder associated with exposure to metalworking fluid aerosols, *Chest*, **108**: 636–41.

Bevivino A, Tabacchioni S et al., 1994, Phenotypic comparison between rhizosphere and clinical isolates of *Burkholderia cepacia*, *Microbiology*, **140**: 1069–77.

Bingen EH, Denamur E et al., 1991, DNA restriction fragment length polymorphism differentiates crossed from independent infections in nosocomial *Xanthomonas maltophilia* bacteremia, *J Clin Microbiol*, **29**: 1348–50.

Bingen EH, Weber et al., 1993, Arbitrarily primed polymerase chain reaction as a rapid method to differentiate crossed from independent *Pseudomonas cepacia* infections in cystic fibrosis patients, *J Clin Microbiol*, **31**: 2589–93.

Black WJ, Quinn FD, Tompkins LS, 1990, *Legionella pneumophila* zinc metalloprotease is structurally and functionally homologous to *Pseudomonas aeruginosa* elastase, *J Bacteriol*, **172**: 2608–13.

Blackwell CC, Law JA, 1981, Typing of non-serogroupable *Neisseria meningitidis* by means of sensitivity to R-type pyocines of *Pseudomonas aeruginosa*, *J Infect*, **3**: 370–8.

Blanc DS, Siegrist H et al., 1993, Ribotyping of *Pseudomonas aeruginosa*: discriminatory power and usefulness as a tool for epidemiological studies, *J Clin Microbiol*, **31**: 71–7.

Booth BR, Curtis NAC, 1977, Separation of the cytoplasmic and outer membrane of *Pseudomonas aeruginosa* PAO1, *Biochem Biophys Res Commun*, **74**: 1168–76.

Bradley DE, 1977, Characterisation of pili determined by drug resistance plasmids R711b and R778b, *J Gen Microbiol*, **102**: 349–63.

Bradley DE, Pitt TL, 1974, Pilus-dependence of four *Pseudomonas aeruginosa* bacteriophages with non-contractile tails, *J Gen Virol*, **23**: 1–15.

Bradley DE, Pitt TL, 1975, An immunological study of the pili of *Pseudomonas aeruginosa*, *J Hyg Camb*, **74**: 419–30.

Bremmelgaard A, 1975, Differentiation between *Pseudomonas cepacia* and *Pseudomonas pseudomallei* in clinical bacteriology, *Acta Pathol Microbiol Scand Sect B*, **83**: 65–70.

Brett PJ, Mah DCW, Woods DE, 1994, Isolation and characterization of *Pseudomonas pseudomallei* flagellin proteins, *Infect Immun*, **62**: 1914–19.

Bryan LE, Wong S et al., 1994, Passive protection of diabetic rats with antisera specific for the polysaccharide portion of the lipopolysaccharide isolated from *Pseudomonas pseudomallei*, *Can J Infect Dis*, **5**: 170–8.

Buchanan RE, Holt JG, Lessel EF, 1966, An annotated alphabetic listing of names of the taxa of the bacteria, *Index Bergeyana*, Williams & Wilkins, Baltimore.

Buck AC, Cooke EM, 1969, The fate of ingested *Pseudomonas aeruginosa* in normal persons, *J Med Microbiol*, **2**: 521–5.

Bulloch WH, 1929, *Bacillus pyocyaneus, A System of Bacteriology in Relation to Medicine*, Medical Research Council, London, 326–7.

Burdge DR, Noble MA et al., 1995, *Xanthomonas maltophilia* misidentified as *Pseudomonas cepacia* in cultures of sputum from patients with cystic fibrosis: a diagnostic pitfall with major clinical implications, *Clin Infect Dis*, **20**: 445–8.

Burkhead KD, Schisler DA, Slininger PJ, 1994, Pyrrolnitrin production by biological control agent *Pseudomonas cepacia* B37W in culture and in colonized wounds of potatoes, *Appl Environ Microbiol*, **60**: 2031–9.

Burkholder WH, 1950, Sour skin: a bacterial rot of onion bulbs, *Phytopathology*, **40–117**: 15–23.

Burns JL, Jonas M et al., 1996, Invasion of respiratory epithelial cells by *Burkholderia* (*Pseudomonas*) *cepacia*, *Infect Immun*, **64:** 4054–9.

Burton MO, Campbell JJR, Eagles BA, 1948, The mineral requirements for pyocyanin production, *Can J Res*, **26:** C15.

Butler SL, Doherty CJ et al., 1995, *Burkholderia cepacia* and cystic fibrosis: do natural environments present a potential hazard?, *J Clin Microbiol*, **33:** 1001–4.

Callaghan EM, Tanner MS, Boulnois GJ, 1994, Development of a PCR probe test for identifying *Pseudomonas aeruginosa* and *Pseudomonas* (*Burkholderia*) *cepacia*, *J Clin Pathol*, **47:** 222–6.

Campbell PW, Phillips JA et al., 1995, Detection of *Pseudomonas* (*Burkholderia*) *cepacia* using PCR, *Pediatr Pulmonol*, **20:** 44–9.

Carson LA, Anderson RL et al., 1991, Isoenzyme analysis of *Pseudomonas cepacia* as an epidemiologic tool, *Am J Med*, **91:** 252S–5S.

Cash HA, Woods DE et al., 1979, A rat model of chronic respiratory infection with *Pseudomonas aeruginosa*, *Am Rev Respir Dis*, **119:** 453–9.

Cérantola S, Marty N, Montrozier H, 1996, Structural studies of the acidic exopolysaccharide produced by a mucoid strain of *Burkholderia cepacia* isolated from cystic fibrosis, *Carbohydr Res*, **285:** 59–67.

Chambon L, Fournier J, 1956, Constitution antigénique de *Malleomyces pseudomallei*. I. Caractères morphologiques, culturaux, biochemiques et variations de type immunologique, *Ann Inst Pasteur (Paris)*, **91:** 355–62.

Chaowagul W, White NJ et al., 1989, Melioidosis: a major cause of community-acquired septicemia in north eastern Thailand, *J Infect Dis*, **159:** 890–9.

Chatelut M, Dournes JL et al., 1995, Epidemiological typing of *Stenotrophomonas* (*Xanthomonas*) *maltophilia* by PCR, *J Clin Microbiol*, **33:** 912–14.

Chen HY, Yuan M, Livermore DM, 1995, Mechanisms of resistance to β-lactam antibiotics amongst *Pseudomonas aeruginosa* isolates collected in the UK in 1993, *J Med Microbiol*, **43:** 300–9.

Chen HY, Yuan M et al., 1995, National survey of susceptibility to antimicrobials amongst clinical isolates of *Pseudomonas aeruginosa*, *J Antimicrob Chemother*, **35:** 521–34.

Cho JJ, Schroth MN et al., 1975, Ornamental plants as carriers of *Pseudomonas aeruginosa*, *Phytopathology*, **65:** 425–31.

Christenson JC, Welch DF et al., 1989, Recovery of *Pseudomonas gladioli* from respiratory tract specimens of patients with cystic fibrosis, *J Clin Microbiol*, **27:** 270–3.

Cicmanec JF, Holder IA, 1979, Growth of *Pseudomonas aeruginosa* in normal and burned skin extract: role of extracellular proteases, *Infect Immun*, **25:** 477–83.

Cimolai N, Trombley C, 1995, Insertional sequence primers for *Bordetella pertussis* diagnostic polymerase chain reaction differentiate strains of *Pseudomonas cepacia*, *J Infect Dis*, **172:** 293–5.

Coburn J, Dillon ST et al., 1989a, Exoenzyme S of *Pseudomonas aeruginosa* ADP-ribosylates the intermediate filament protein vimentin, *Infect Immun*, **57:** 996–8.

Coburn J, Wyatt RT et al., 1989b, Several GTP-binding proteins, including P21 c-H-ras, are preferred substrates of *Pseudomonas aeruginosa* exoenzyme S, *J Biol Chem*, **264:** 9004–8.

Corkill JE, Sisson PR et al., 1994, Application of pyrolysis mass spectroscopy and SDS-PAGE in the study of the epidemiology of *Pseudomonas cepacia* in cystic fibrosis, *J Med Microbiol*, **41:** 106–11.

Costerton JW, Anwar H, 1994, *Pseudomonas aeruginosa*: the microbe and pathogen, Pseudomonas aeruginosa: *Infections and Treatment*, eds Baltch AL, Smith RP, Marcel Dekker, New York, 1–20.

Costerton JW, Brown MRW, Sturgess JM, 1979, The cell envelope: its role in infection, Pseudomonas aeruginosa: *Clinical Manifestations of Infection and Current Therapy*, ed. Doggett RG, Academic Press, New York, 41–62.

Cowan ST, Steel KJ, 1993, *Cowan and Steel's Manual for the Identification of Medical Bacteria*, 3rd edn, eds Barrow GI, Feltham RKA, Cambridge University Press, Cambridge, 94–164.

Cox AD, Wilkinson SG, 1991, Ionizing groups in lipopolysaccharides of *Pseudomonas cepacia* in relation to antibiotic resistance, *Mol Microbiol*, **5:** 641–6.

Cox CD, Adams P, 1985, Siderophore activity of pyoverdin for *Pseudomonas aeruginosa*, *Infect Immun*, **48:** 130–8.

Cox CD, Graham R, 1979, Isolation of an iron-binding compound from *Pseudomonas aeruginosa*, *J Bacteriol*, **137:** 357–64.

Coyne MJ, Russell KS et al., 1994, The *Pseudomonas aeruginosa algC* gene encodes phosphoglucomutase, required for the synthesis of a complete lipopolysaccharide core, *J Bacteriol*, **176:** 3500–7.

Cryz SJ, Fürer E, Germanier R, 1983a, Passive protection against *Pseudomonas aeruginosa* infection in an experimental leukopenic mouse model, *Infect Immun*, **40:** 659–64.

Cryz SJ, Fürer E, Germanier R, 1983b, Protection against *Pseudomonas aeruginosa* infection in a murine burn wound sepsis model by passive transfer of antitoxin A, antielastase and anti-lipopolysaccharide, *Infect Immun*, **39:** 1072–9.

Cryz SJ, Pitt TL et al., 1984, Role of lipopolysaccharide in virulence of *Pseudomonas aeruginosa*, *Infect Immun*, **44:** 508–13.

Cryz SJ, Fürer E et al., 1987, Safety and immunogenicity of a *Pseudomonas aeruginosa* O-polysaccharide–toxin A conjugate vaccine in humans, *J Clin Invest*, **80:** 51–6.

Currie B, Smith-Vaughan H et al., 1994, *Pseudomonas pseudomallei* isolates collected over 25 years from a non-tropical endemic focus show clonality on the basis of ribotyping, *Epidemiol Infect*, **113:** 307–12.

Dance DAB, 1991, Melioidosis: the tip of the iceberg?, *Clin Microbiol Rev*, **4:** 52–60.

Dance DAB, Wuthiekanun V et al., 1989a, Identification of *Pseudomonas pseudomallei* in clinical practice: use of simple screening tests and API 20NE, *J Clin Pathol*, **42:** 645–8.

Dance DAB, Wuthiekanun V et al., 1989b, The antimicrobial susceptibility of *Pseudomonas pseudomallei*. Emergence of resistance *in vitro* and during treatment, *J Antimicrob Chemother*, **24:** 295–309.

Dance DAB, Sanders D et al., 1995, *Burkholderia pseudomallei* and Indian plague-like illness, *Lancet*, **346:** 904–5.

Dasgupta T, Lam JS, 1995, Identification of *rfbA*, involved in B-band lipopolysaccharide biosynthesis in *Pseudomonas aeruginosa* serotype O5, *Infect Immun*, **63:** 1674–80.

Dejsirilert S, Butraporn R et al., 1989, High activity of acid phosphatase of *Pseudomonas pseudomallei* as a possible attribute relating to its pathogenicity, *Jpn J Med Sci Biol*, **42:** 39–49.

Denamur EB, Picard B et al., 1991, Complexity of *Pseudomonas aeruginosa* infection in cystic fibrosis: combined results from esterase electrophoresis and rDNA restriction fragment length polymorphism analysis, *Epidemiol Infect*, **106:** 531–9.

Deretic V, Dikshit E et al., 1989, The *algR* gene which regulates mucoidy in *Pseudomonas aeruginosa*, belongs to a class of environmentally responsive genes, *J Bacteriol*, **171:** 1278–83.

Deretic V, Govan JRW et al., 1990, Mucoid *Pseudomonas aeruginosa* in cystic fibrosis: mutations in the *muc* loci affect transcription of the *algR* and *algD* genes in response to environmental stimuli, *Mol Microbiol*, **4:** 189–96.

Deretic V, Martin DW et al., 1993, Conversion to mucoidy in *Pseudomonas aeruginosa*, *Biotechnology*, **11:** 1133–6.

Dharakul T, Songsivilai S et al., 1996, Detection of *Burkholderia pseudomallei* DNA in patients with septicemic melioidosis, *J Clin Microbiol*, **34:** 609–14.

Dimech WJ, Hellyar AG et al., 1993, Typing of strains from a single-source outbreak of *Pseudomonas pickettii*, *J Clin Microbiol*, **31:** 3001–6.

Dodin A, Fournier J, 1970, Antigènes précipitants et agglutinants de *Pseudomonas pseudomallei* (B. de Whitmore) II. Mise en évidence d'antigènes précipitants communs à *Yersinia pestis* et *Pseudomonas pseudomallei*, *Ann Inst Pasteur (Paris)*, **119:** 738–44.

Döring G, Ulrich M et al., 1991, Generation of *Pseudomonas aeruginosa* aerosols during handwashing from contaminated sink drains, transmission to hands of hospital personnel, and its prevention by use of a new heating device, *Zentralbl Hyg Umweltmed*, **191:** 494–505.

Drabick JA, Gracely EJ et al., 1996, Survival of *Burkholderia cepacia* on environmental surfaces, *J Hosp Infect*, **32:** 267–76.

Drake D, Montie TC, 1987, Protection against *Pseudomonas aeruginosa* infection by passive transfer of antiflagellar serum, *Can J Microbiol*, **33:** 755–63.

Dyke JW, Berk RS, 1973, Comparative studies on *Pseudomonas aeruginosa* endotoxin, *Z Allg Mikrobiol*, **13:** 307–13.

Edmonds P, Suskind RR et al., 1972, Epidemiology of *Pseudomonas aeruginosa* in a burns hospital: evaluation of serological, bacteriophage, and pyocin typing methods, *Appl Microbiol*, **24:** 213–18.

Eisenberg RC, Butters SJ et al., 1974, Glucose uptake and phosphorylation in *Pseudomonas fluorescens*, *J Bacteriol*, **120:** 147–53.

Elrod RP, Braun AC, 1942, *Pseudomonas aeruginosa*: its role as a plant pathogen, *J Bacteriol*, **44:** 633–44.

Elsheikh LE, Bergman R et al., 1986, A comparison of different methods for determining elastase activity of *Pseudomonas aeruginosa* strains from mink, *Acta Pathol Microbiol Immunol Scand Sect B*, **94:** 135–8.

Elting LS, Khardori N et al., 1990, Nosocomial infection caused by *Xanthomonas maltophilia*: a case-control study of predisposing factors, *Infect Control Hosp Epidemiol*, **11:** 134–8.

van den Ende M, 1952, Observations on the antigenic structure of *Pseudomonas aeruginosa*, *J Hyg Camb*, **50:** 405–14.

Engels W, Endert J et al., 1985, Role of lipopolysaccharide in opsonization and phagocytosis of *Pseudomonas aeruginosa*, *Infect Immun*, **49:** 182–9.

Ensor E, Humphreys H et al., 1996, Is *Burkholderia (Pseudomonas) cepacia* disseminated from cystic fibrosis patients during physiotherapy, *J Hosp Infect*, **32:** 9–15.

Esselman MT, Liu PV, 1961, Lecithinase production by gram-negative bacteria, *J Bacteriol*, **81:** 939–45.

Foght JM, Westlake DWS et al., 1996, Environmental gasoline-utilizing isolates and clinical isolates of *Pseudomonas aeruginosa* are taxonomically indistinguishable by chemotaxonomic and molecular techniques, *Microbiology*, **142:** 2333–40.

Fomsgaard A, Hoiby N et al., 1988, Longitudinal study of antibody responses to lipopolysaccharides during chronic *Pseudomonas aeruginosa* lung infection in cystic fibrosis, *Infect Immun*, **56:** 2270–8.

Fonseca K, MacDougall J, Pitt TL, 1986, Inhibition of *Pseudomonas aeruginosa* from patients with cystic fibrosis, *J Clin Pathol*, **39:** 220–2.

Fordos M, 1860, Recherches sur la matiere colorante des suppurations bleues: pyocyanine, *C R Acad Sci*, **51:** 215.

Fuller AT, Mellows G et al., 1971, Pseudomonic acid: an antibiotic produced by *Pseudomonas fluorescens*, *Nature (London)*, **234:** 416–17.

Fyfe JAM, Harris G, Govan JRW, 1984, Revised pyocin typing method for *Pseudomonas aeruginosa*, *J Clin Microbiol*, **20:** 47–50.

Galbraith LS, Wilkinson SG et al., 1984, Structural alterations in the envelope of a gentamicin-resistant rough mutant of *Pseudomonas aeruginosa*, *Ann Microbiol Inst Pasteur*, **135B:** 121–36.

Gambello MJ, Iglewski BH, 1991, Cloning and characterization of the *Pseudomonas aeruginosa* lasR gene, a transcriptional activator of elastase production, *J Bacteriol*, **173:** 3000–9.

Gessard C, 1882, Sur les colorations bleues et vertes des linges à pansements, *C R Acad Sci*, **94:** 536–8.

Gillies RR, Govan JRW, 1966, Typing of *Pseudomonas aeruginosa* by pyocin production, *J Pathol Bacteriol*, **91:** 339–45.

Gilligan PH, Gage PA et al., 1985, Isolation medium for the recovery of *Pseudomonas cepacia* from respiratory specimens of patients with cystic fibrosis, *J Clin Microbiol*, **22:** 5–8.

Gillis M, Van TV et al., 1995, Polyphasic taxonomy in the genus *Burkholderia* leading to an emended description of the genus and *Burkholderia vietnamiensis* sp. nov. for N₂ fixing isolates from rice in Vietnam, *Int J Syst Bacteriol*, **45:** 274–89.

Godfrey AJ, Wong S et al., 1991, *Pseudomonas pseudomallei* resistance to β-lactamase antibiotics due to alterations in the

chromosomally encoded β-lactamase, *Antimicrob Agents Chemother*, **35:** 1635–40.

Gonzalez CF, Vidaver AK, 1979, Bacteriocin, plasmid and pectolytic diversity in *Pseudomonas cepacia* of clinical and plant origin, *J Gen Microbiol*, **110:** 161–70.

Gottlieb T, 1993, Hazards of bacterial contamination of blood products, *Anaesth Intensive Care*, **21:** 20–3.

Goullet PL, Picard B, 1991, *Pseudomonas aeruginosa* isolate typing by esterase electrophoresis, *FEMS Microbiol Lett*, **78:** 195–200.

Govan JRW, 1974a, Studies on the pyocins of *Pseudomonas aeruginosa*: morphology and mode of action of contractile pyocins, *J Gen Microbiol*, **80:** 1–15.

Govan JRW, 1974b, Studies on the pyocins of *Pseudomonas aeruginosa*: production of contractile and flexuous pyocins in *Pseudomonas aeruginosa*, *J Gen Microbiol*, **80:** 17–30.

Govan JRW, 1975, Mucoid strains of *Pseudomonas aeruginosa*: the influence of culture medium on the stability of mucus production, *J Med Microbiol*, **8:** 513–22.

Govan JRW, 1978, Pyocin typing of *Pseudomonas aeruginosa*, *Methods in Microbiology*, vol. 10, eds Bergan T, Norris J, Academic Press, London, 61–91.

Govan JRW, Fyfe JAM, 1978, Mucoid *Pseudomonas aeruginosa* and cystic fibrosis: resistance of the mucoid form to carbenicillin, flucloxacillin and tobramycin and the isolation of mucoid variants *in vitro*, *J Antmicrob Chemother*, **4:** 233–40.

Govan JRW, Gillies RR, 1969, Further studies in the pyocin typing of *Pseudomonas aeruginosa*, *J Med Microbiol*, **2:** 17–25.

Govan JRW, Harris G, 1985, Typing of *Pseudomonas cepacia* by bacteriocin susceptibility and production, *J Clin Microbiol*, **22:** 490–4.

Govan JRW, Martin DW, Deretic V, 1992, Mucoid *Pseudomonas aeruginosa* and cystic fibrosis: the role of mutations in *muc* loci, *FEMS Microbiol Lett*, **100:** 323–30.

Govan JRW, Brown PH et al., 1993, Evidence for transmission of *Pseudomonas cepacia* by social contact in cystic fibrosis, *Lancet*, **342:** 15–19.

von Graevenitz A, 1985, Ecology, clinical significance, and antimicrobial susceptibility of infrequently encountered glucose-nonfermenting gram-negative rods, *Nonfermentative Gram-negative Rods. Laboratory Identification and Clinical Aspects*, ed. Gilardi GL, Marcel Dekker, New York, 181–232.

Graham LM, Vasil ML et al., 1990, Decreased pulmonary vasoreactivity in an animal model of chronic *Pseudomonas* pneumonia, *Am Rev Respir Dis*, **142:** 221–9.

Grattard F, Pozzetto B et al., 1994, Differentiation of *Pseudomonas aeruginosa* strains by ribotyping: high discriminatory power by using a single restriction endonuclease, *J Med Microbiol*, **40:** 275–81.

Grobe S, Wingender J, Truper HG, 1995, Characterization of mucoid *Pseudomonas aeruginosa* strains isolated from technical water systems, *J Appl Bacteriol*, **79:** 94–102.

Grothues D, Koopmann U et al., 1988, Genome fingerprinting of *Pseudomonas aeruginosa* indicates colonization of cystic fibrosis siblings with closely related strains, *J Clin Microbiol*, **26:** 1973–7.

Grundmann HJ, Gräser Y et al., 1994, Randomly primed polymerase chain reaction yields comparable results to restriction fragment analysis in typing of *Pseudomonas aeruginosa*, *Med Microbiol Lett*, **3:** 42–8.

Grundmann H, Schneider C et al., 1995, Discriminatory power of three DNA-based typing techniques for *Pseudomonas aeruginosa*, *J Clin Microbiol*, **33:** 528–34.

Habs I, 1957, Untersuchungen über die O-antigene von *Pseudomonas aeruginosa*, *Z Hyg*, **144:** 218–28.

Habs H, Mann S, 1967, Die Bildung von ortho-Aminoacetophenon durch Apyocyaninogene stämme von *P. aeruginosa*, *Zentralbl Bakteriol Parasitenkd Abt 1 Orig*, **203:** 473–7.

Hall LM, Livermore DM et al., 1993, OXA-11, an extended-spectrum variant of OXA-10 (PSE-2) β-lactamase from *Pseudomonas aeruginosa*, *Antimicrob Agents Chemother*, **37:** 1637–44.

Hamood AN, Ohman DE et al., 1992, Isolation and characterization of toxin A excretion-deficient mutants of *Pseudomonas aeruginosa* PAO 1, *Infect Immun*, **60**: 510–17.

Hancock REW, Carey AM, 1979, Outer membrane of *Pseudomonas aeruginosa*: Heat- and 2-mercaptoethanol-modifiable proteins, *J Bacteriol*, **140**: 902–10.

Hancock REW, Mutharia LM et al., 1983, *Pseudomonas aeruginosa* isolates from patients with cystic fibrosis: a class of serum-sensitive nontypable strains deficient in lipopolysaccharide O side chains, *Infect Immun*, **42**: 170–7.

Heckly RJ, Nigg C, 1958, Toxins of *Pseudomonas pseudomallei* II. Characterization, *J Bacteriol*, **76**: 427–36.

Hingley ST, Hastie AT et al., 1986, Effect of ciliostatic factors from *Pseudomonas aeruginosa* on rabbit respiratory cilia, *Infect Immun*, **51**: 254–62.

Hirayama T, Kato I, 1984, Mode of cytotoxic action of pseudomonal leucocidin on phosphatidylinositol metabolism and activation of lysosomal enzyme in rabbit leukocytes, *Infect Immun*, **43**: 21–7.

Hoadley AW, 1977, *Pseudomonas aeruginosa* in surface waters, Pseudomonas aeruginosa: *Ecological Aspects and Patient Colonization*, ed. Young VM, Raven Press, New York, 31–57.

Hodson ME, Roberts CM et al., 1987, Oral ciprofloxacin compared with conventional intravenous treatment for *Pseudomonas aeruginosa* infection in adults with cystic fibrosis, *Lancet*, **1**: 235–7.

Holder IA, 1993, *Pseudomonas aeruginosa* virulence-associated factors and their role in burn wound infections, Pseudomonas aeruginosa: *the Opportunist – Pathogenesis and Disease*, ed. Fick RB, CRC Press, Boca Raton, FL, 235–45.

Holder IA, Haidaris CG, 1979, Experimental studies of the pathogenesis of infections due to *Pseudomonas aeruginosa*: extracellular protease and elastase as *in vivo* virulence factors, *Can J Microbiol*, **45**: 593–9.

Holder IA, Neely AN, 1989a, Combined host and specific antipseudomonas directed therapy for *Pseudomonas aeruginosa* infections in burned mice, *J Burn Care Rehabil*, **10**: 131–7.

Holder IA, Neely AN, 1989b, *Pseudomonas* elastase acts as a virulence factor in burned hosts by Hageman factor-dependent activation of the host kinin cascade, *J Infect Immun*, **57**: 3345–8.

Hollsing AE, Granström M et al., 1987, Prospective study of serum antibodies to *Pseudomonas aeruginosa* exoproteins in cystic fibrosis, *J Clin Microbiol*, **25**: 1868–74.

Holmes B, Howard BJ, 1994, Nonfermentative Gram-negative bacteria, *Clinical and Pathogenic Microbiology*, 2nd edn, eds Howard BJ, Keiser JF et al., Mosby, St Louis, 337–68.

Holmes B, Owen RJ et al., 1977, *Pseudomonas paucimobilis*, a new species isolated from human clinical specimens, the hospital environment, and other sources, *Int J Syst Bacteriol*, **27**: 133–46.

Homma JY, Kim KS et al., 1970, Serological typing of *Pseudomonas aeruginosa* and its cross infection, *Jpn J Exp Med*, **40**: 347–59.

Hori H, Takabayashi K et al., 1996, Gene cloning and characterization of *Pseudomonas putida* L-methionine-alpha-deamino-gamma-mercaptomethane-lyase, *Cancer Res*, **56**: 2116–22.

Humphreys H, Peckham D et al., 1994, Airborne dissemination of *Burkholderia* (*Pseudomonas*) *cepacia* from adult patients with cystic fibrosis, *Thorax*, **49**: 1157–9.

Hutchinson GR, Parker S et al., 1996, Home-use nebulizers: a potential primary source of *Burkholderia cepacia* and other colistin-resistant, Gram-negative bacteria in patients with cystic fibrosis, *J Clin Microbiol*, **34**: 584–7.

Irvin RT, 1993, Attachment and colonization of *Pseudomonas aeruginosa*, Pseudomonas aeruginosa *as an Opportunistic Pathogen*, eds Campa M, Bendinelli M, Friedman H, Plenum Press, New York, 19–42.

Isles A, Maclusky I et al., 1984, *Pseudomonas cepacia* infection in cystic fibrosis: an emerging problem, *J Pediatr*, **104**: 206–10.

Ismail G, Embi MN et al., 1987, A competitive immunosorbent assay for detection of *Pseudomonas pseudomallei* exotoxin, *J Med Microbiol*, **23**: 353–7.

Jaeger K-E, Kharazmi A, Hoiby N, 1991, Extracellular lipase of *Pseudomonas aeruginosa*: biochemical characterization and monocyte function *in vitro*, *Microb Pathog*, **10**: 173–82.

Jayaswal RK, Fernandez M et al., 1993, Antagonism of *Pseudomonas cepacia* against phytopathogenic fungi, *Curr Microbiol*, **26**: 17–22.

Johnson WM, Tyler SD, Rozee KR, 1994, Linkage analysis of geographic and clinical clusters in *Pseudomonas cepacia* infections by multilocus enzyme electrophoresis and ribotyping, *J Clin Microbiol*, **32**: 924–30.

Jones LF, Zakanycz CP et al., 1974, Pyocin typing of *Pseudomonas aeruginosa*: a simplified method, *Appl Microbiol*, **27**: 400–6.

Jonsson V, 1970, Proposal for a new species *Pseudomonas kingii*, *Int J Syst Bacteriol*, **20**: 255–7.

Kadurugamuwa JL, Lam JS, Beveridge TJ, 1993, Interaction of gentamicin with the A band and B band lipopolysaccharides of *Pseudomonas aeruginosa* and its possible lethal effect, *Antimicrob Agents Chemother*, **37**: 715–21.

Kanthakumar K, Cundell DZ et al., 1994, Effect of salmeterol on human nasal epithelial cell ciliary beating: inhibition of the ciliotoxin, pyocyanin, *Br J Pharmacol*, **112**: 493–8.

Kelly NH, Falkiner FR, Keane CT, 1983, Acetamide broth for isolation of *Pseudomonas aeruginosa* from patients with cystic fibrosis, *J Clin Microbiol*, **17**: 159.

Kelly-Wintenberg K, Montie TC, 1989, Cloning and expression of *Pseudomonas aeruginosa* flagellin in *Escherichia coli*, *J Bacteriol*, **171**: 6357–62.

Kerr JR, 1993, *In vitro* activities of two drug combinations of ceftazidime, cefotaxime, cefuroxime, chloramphenicol, imipenem and temocillin against clinical isolates of *Pseudomonas cepacia* from patients with cystic fibrosis, *Int J Antimicrob Agents*, **3**: 205–9.

Khardori N, Reuben A et al., 1990, *In vitro* susceptibility of *Xanthomonas* (*Pseudomonas*) *maltophilia* to newer antimicrobial agents, *Antimicrob Agents Chemother*, **34**: 1609–10.

King A, Phillips I, 1978, The identification of pseudomonads and related bacteria in a clinical laboratory, *J Med Microbiol*, **11**: 165–76.

King A, Holmes B et al., 1979, A taxonomic study of clinical isolates of *Pseudomonas pickettii*, '*P. thomasii*' and 'group Ivd' bacteria, *J Gen Microbiol*, **114**: 137–47.

King EO, Ward MK, Raney DE, 1954, Two simple media for the demonstration of pyocyanin and fluorescin, *J Lab Clin Med*, **44**: 301–7.

Knirel YA, 1990, Polysaccharide antigens of *Pseudomonas aeruginosa*, *Crit Rev Microbiol*, **17**: 273–304.

Knirel YA, Paramonov NA et al., 1992, Structure of the polysaccharide chains of *Pseudomonas pseudomallei* lipopolysaccharides, *Carbohydr Res*, **233**: 185–93.

Kostman JR, Edlind TD et al., 1992, Molecular epidemiology of *Pseudomonas cepacia* determined by polymerase chain reaction ribotyping, *J Clin Microbiol*, **30**: 2084–7.

Krieg D, Bass JA, Mattingly SJ, 1986, Aeration selects for mucoid phenotype of *Pseudomonas aeruginosa*, *J Clin Microbiol*, **24**: 986–90.

Kuehn M, Lent K et al., 1992, Fimbriation of *Pseudomonas cepacia*, *Infect Immun*, **60**: 2002–7.

Kunakorn M, Markham RB, 1995, Clinically practical seminested PCR for *Burkholderia pseudomallei* quantitated by enzyme immunoassay with and without solution hybridization, *J Clin Microbiol*, **33**: 2131–5.

Kuzio J, Kropinski, 1983, O-antigen conversion in *Pseudomonas aeruginosa* PAO 1 by bacteriophage D3, *J Bacteriol*, **155**: 203–12.

Laing FPY, Ramotar K et al., 1995, Molecular epidemiology of *Xanthomonas maltophilia* colonization and infection in the hospital environment, *J Clin Microbiol*, **33**: 513–18.

Lam JS, MacDonald LA et al., 1987, Production and characterization of monoclonal antibodies against serotype strains of *Pseudomonas aeruginosa*, *Infect Immun*, **55:** 1051–7.

Lam JS, Handelsman MYC et al., 1992, Monoclonal antibodies as probes to examine serotype-specific and cross-reactive epitopes of lipopolysaccharides from serotypes O2, O5, and O16 of *Pseudomonas aeruginosa*, *J Bacteriol*, **174:** 2178–84.

Lányi B, 1970, Serological properties of *Pseudomonas aeruginosa*. II. Type-specific thermolabile (flagellar) antigens, *Acta Microbiol Acad Sci Hung*, **17:** 35–48.

Lau YJ, Liu PYF et al., 1995, DNA fingerprinting of *Pseudomonas aeruginosa* serotype O11 by enterobacterial repetitive intergenic consensus-polymerase chain reaction and pulsed-field gel electrophoresis, *J Hosp Infect*, **31:** 61–6.

Lautrop H, Jessen O, 1964, On the dictinction between polar monotrichous and lophotrichous flagellation in green fluorescent pseudomonads, *Acta Pathol Microbiol Scand*, **60:** 588–98.

Leclerc H, Sureau P, 1956, Recherche des bactériophages antibacille de Whitmore dans les eaux stagnantes à Hanoi, *Bull Soc Pathol Exot*, **49:** 874–82.

Legakis NJ, Aliferopoulou M et al., 1982, Serotypes of *Pseudomonas aeruginosa* in clinical specimens in relation to antibiotic susceptibility, *J Clin Microbiol*, **16:** 458–63.

Legakis NJ, Tsouvelekis LS et al., 1989, Outer membrane alterations in multiresistant mutant of *Pseudomonas aeruginosa* selected by ciprofloxacin, *Antimicrob Agents Chemother*, **33:** 124–7.

Lemaitre D, Elaichouni A et al., 1996, Tracheal colonization with *Sphingomonas paucimobilis* in mechanically ventilated neonates due to contaminated ventilator temperature probes, *J Hosp Infect*, **32:** 199–206.

Lennon E, DeCicco BT, 1991, Plasmids of *Pseudomonas cepacia* strains of diverse origins, *Appl Environ Microbiol*, **57:** 2345–50.

Levin MH, Weinstein RA et al., 1984, Association of infection caused by *Pseudomonas aeruginosa* serotype O11 with intravenous abuse of pentazocine mixed with tripelennamine, *J Clin Microbiol*, **20:** 758–62.

Levine HB, Lein OG, Maurer RL, 1959, Mortality enhancing polypeptide constituents from *Pseudomonas pseudomallei*, *J Immunol*, **83:** 468–77.

Levison ME, 1977, Factors influencing colonization of the gastrointestinal tract with *Pseudomonas aeruginosa*, Pseudomonas aeruginosa: *Ecological Aspects and Patient Colonization*, ed. Young VM, Raven Press, New York, 97–109.

Lew A, Desmarchelier P, 1993, Molecular typing of *Pseudomonas pseudomallei*: restriction fragment length polymorphisms of rRNA genes, *J Clin Microbiol*, **31:** 533–9.

Lew AE, Desmarchelier PM, 1994, Detection of *Pseudomonas pseudomallei* by PCR and hybridization, *J Clin Microbiol*, **32:** 1326–32.

Li X-Z, Livermore DM, Nikaido H, 1994, Role of efflux pump(s) in intrinsic resistance of *Pseudomonas aeruginosa*: resistance to tetracycline, chloramphenicol, and norfloxacin, *Antimicrob Agents Chemother*, **38:** 1732–41.

Li X-Z, Nikaido H, Poole K, 1995, Role of MexA-MexB-OprM in antibiotic efflux in *Pseudomonas aeruginosa*, *Antimicrob Agents Chemother*, **39:** 1948–53.

Li X-Z, Ma D et al., 1994, Role of efflux pump(s) in intrinsic resistance of *Pseudomonas aeruginosa*: active efflux as a contributing factor to β-lactam resistance, *Antimicrob Agents Chemother*, **38:** 1742–52.

Lightfoot J, Lam JS, 1993, Chromosomal mapping, expression and synthesis of lipopolysaccharide in *Pseudomonas aeruginosa*; a role for guanosine diphospho (GDP)-D-mannose, *Mol Microbiol*, **8:** 771–82.

Lilly HA, Lowbury EJL, 1972, Cetrimide–nalidixic acid agar as a selective medium for *Pseudomonas aeruginosa*, *J Med Microbiol*, **5:** 151–3.

Linker A, Jones RS, 1966, A new polysaccharide resembling alginic acid isolated from pseudomonads, *J Biol Chem*, **241:** 3845–51.

LiPuma JJ, Mortensen JE et al., 1988, Ribotype analysis of *Pseudomonas cepacia* from cystic fibrosis treatment centres, *J Pediatr*, **113:** 859–62.

Liu PV, 1957, Survey of haemolysin production among species of pseudomonads, *J Bacteriol*, **74:** 718–27.

Liu PV, Wang S, 1990, Three new major somatic antigens of *Pseudomonas aeruginosa*, *J Clin Microbiol*, **28:** 922–5.

Liu PV, Matsumoto H et al., 1983, Survey of heat-stable major somatic antigens of *Pseudomonas aeruginosa*, *Int J Syst Bacteriol*, **33:** 256–64.

Livermore DM, 1987, Clinical significance of β-lactamase induction and stable derepression in Gram-negative rods, *Eur J Clin Microbiol*, **4:** 439–45.

Livermore DM, Chan PY et al., 1987, β-Lactamase of *Pseudomonas pseudomallei* and its contribution to antibiotic resistance, *J Antimicrob Chemother*, **20:** 313–21.

Livermore DM, 1989, Role of β-lactamase and impermeability in the resistance of *Pseudomonas aeruginosa*, *Antibiot Chemother*, **42:** 257–63.

Loutit JS, Tompkins LS, 1991, Restriction enzyme and Southern hybridization analyses of *Pseudomonas aeruginosa* strains from patients with cystic fibrosis, *J Clin Microbiol*, **29:** 2897–900.

Lücke A, 1862, Die sogenannte blaue Eiterung und ihre Ursachen, *Arch Klin Chir*, **3:** 135.

Lutz F, 1979, Purification of a cytotoxin protein from *Pseudomonas aeruginosa*, *Toxicon*, **17:** 467–75.

McKevitt A, Woods DE, 1984, Characterization of *Pseudomonas cepacia* isolates from patients with cystic fibrosis, *J Clin Microbiol*, **19:** 291–3.

Maharaj R, Zielinski NA, Chakrabarty AM, 1992, Environmental regulation of alginate gene expression by *Pseudomonas aeruginosa*, Pseudomonas: *Molecular Biology and Biotechnology*, eds Galli E, Silver S, Witholt B, American Society for Microbiology, Washington, DC, 65–74.

Mahenthiralingam E, Campbell ME, Speert DP, 1994, Nonmotility and phagocytic resistance of *Pseudomonas aeruginosa* isolates from chronically colonized patients with cystic fibrosis, *Infect Immun*, **62:** 596–605.

Maki DG, Klein BS et al., 1991, Nosocomial *Pseudomonas pickettii* bacteraemias traced to narcotic tampering, *JAMA*, **265:** 981–6.

Makin SA, Beveridge TJ, 1996, The influence of A-band and B-band lipopolysaccharide on the surface characteristics and adhesion of *Pseudomonas aeruginosa* to surfaces, *Microbiology*, **142:** 299–307.

Manzenyuk OY, Volozhantsev NV, Svetoch EA, 1994, Identification of *Pseudomonas mallei* bacteria with the help of *Pseudomonas pseudomallei* bacteriophages, *Microbiology (Moscow)*, **63:** 303–7.

Martin DR, 1973, Mucoid variation in *Pseudomonas aeruginosa* induced by the action of phage, *J Med Microbiol*, **6:** 111–18.

Martone WJ, Tablan OC, Jarvis WR, 1987, The epidemiology of nosocomial epidemic *Pseudomonas cepacia* infections, *Eur J Epidemiol*, **3:** 222–32.

Marty N, Dournes J-L et al., 1992, Influence of nutrient media on the chemical composition of the exopolysaccharide from mucoid and non-mucoid *Pseudomonas aeruginosa*, *FEMS Microbiol Lett*, **98:** 35–44.

Matsushita K, Adachi O et al., 1978, Isolation and characterization of outer and inner membranes from *Pseudomonas aeruginosa* and effect of ETDA on the membranes, *J Biochem*, **83:** 171–81.

Matsushita K, Yamada M et al., 1983, Membrane-bound respiratory chain of *Pseudomonas aeruginosa* grown aerobically. A KCN-insensitive oxidase chain and its energetics, *J Biochem*, **93:** 1137–44.

Matthews-Greer JM, Robertson DE et al., 1990, *Pseudomonas aeruginosa* outer membrane protein F produced in *Escherichia coli* retains vaccine efficiency, *Curr Microbiol*, **20:** 171–5.

Meadow PM, Rowe PSN, Wells PL, 1984, Characterization of polyagglutinating and surface antigens in *Pseudomonas aeruginosa*, *J Gen Microbiol*, **130:** 631–44.

Mercado TI, Butany JW, Ferrans VJ, 1986, *Trypanosoma cruzi*:

ultrastructural changes produced by an anti-trypanosomal factor from *Pseudomonas fluorescens*, *Exp Parasitol*, **61**: 65–75.

Meyer JM, Neely A et al., 1996, Pyoverdin is essential for virulence of *Pseudomonas aeruginosa*, *Infect Immun*, **64**: 518–23.

Meyers DJ, Berk RS, 1990, Characterization of phospholipase C from *Pseudomonas aeruginosa* as a potent inflammatory agent, *Infect Immun*, **58**: 659–66.

Michea-Hamzehpour M, Furet YV, Pechère J-C, 1991, Role of protein D2 and lipopolysaccharide in diffusion of quinolones through the outer membrane of *Pseudomonas aeruginosa*, *Antimicrob Agents Chemother*, **35**: 2091–7.

Miller WR, Pennel L et al., 1948, Studies on certain biological characteristics of *Malleomyces mallei* and *Malleomyces pseudomallei*. I. Morphology, cultivation, viability, and isolation from contaminated specimens, *J Bacteriol*, **55**: 115–26.

Miller RV, Rubero VJR, 1984, Mucoid conversion by phages of *Pseudomonas aeruginosa* strains from patients with cystic fibrosis, *J Clin Microbiol*, **19**: 717–19.

Miyazaki S, Matsumoto T et al., 1995, Role of exotoxin A in inducing severe *Pseudomonas aeruginosa* infections in mice, *J Med Microbiol*, **43**: 169–75.

Mizuno T, Kageyama M, 1978, Separation and characterization of the outer membrane of *Pseudomonas aeruginosa*, *J Biochem*, **84**: 179–81.

Mohamed R, Nathan S et al., 1989, Inhibition of macromolecular synthesis in cultured macrophages by *Pseudomonas pseudomallei* exotoxin, *Microbiol Immunol*, **33**: 811–20.

Monafo WW, Freeman B, 1987, Topical therapy for burns, *Surg Clin North Am*, **67**: 133–45.

Morihara K, 1964, Production of elastase and proteinase by *Pseudomonas aeruginosa*, *J Bacteriol*, **88**: 745–57.

Morihara K, Homma JY, 1985, *Pseudomonas* proteases, *Bacterial Enzymes and Virulence*, ed. Holder I, CRC Press, Boca Raton, FL, 41–75.

Morse SA, Vaughn P et al., 1976, Inhibition of *Neisseria gonorrhoeae* by a bacteriocin from *Pseudomonas aeruginosa*, *Antimicrob Agents Chemother*, **10**: 354–62.

Mortensen JE, Fisher MC, LiPuma JJ, 1995, Recovery of *Pseudomonas cepacia* and other *Pseudomonas* species from the environment, *Infect Control Hosp Epidemiol*, **16**: 30–2.

Mucci D, Forristal J et al., 1995, Level of receptor associated protein moderates susceptibility to *Pseudomonas aeruginosa*, *Infect Immun*, **63**: 2912–18.

Mukwaya GM, Welch DF, 1989, Subgrouping of *Pseudomonas cepacia* by cellular fatty acid composition, *J Clin Microbiol*, **27**: 2640–6.

Munster AM, Helvig E, Rowland S, 1980, Cerium nitrate–silver sulfadiazine cream in the treatment of burns, *Surgery*, **88**: 658–60.

Mutharia LM, Nicas TI, Hancock REW, 1982, Outer membrane proteins of *Pseudomonas aeruginosa* serotype strains, *J Infect Dis*, **146**: 770–9.

Nakhleh RH, Glock M, Snover DC, 1992, Hepatic pathology of chronic granulomatous disease of childhood, *Arch Pathol Lab Med*, **116**: 71–5.

Nelson JW, Butler SL et al., 1994, Virulence factors of *Burkholderia cepacia*, *FEMS Immunol Med Microbiol*, **8**: 89–98.

Nigg C, Ruch J et al., 1956, Enhancement of virulence of *Malleomyces pseudomallei*, *J Bacteriol*, **71**: 530–41.

Nikaido H, 1992, Non-specific and specific permeation channels of the *Pseudomonas aeruginosa* outer membrane, *Pseudomonas: Molecular Biology and Biotechnology*, eds Galli E, Silver S, Witholt B, American Society for Microbiology, Washington, DC, 146–53.

Ochsner UA, Reiser J, 1995, Autoinducer-mediated regulation of rhamnolipid biosurfactant synthesis in *Pseudomonas aeruginosa*, *Proc Natl Acad Sci USA*, **92**: 6424–8.

Ogle JW, Janda JM et al., 1987, Characterization and use of a probe as an epidemiological marker for *Pseudomonas aeruginosa*, *J Infect Dis*, **155**: 119–26.

Ogunnariwo J, Hamilton-Miller JMT, 1975, Brown- and red-

pigmented *Pseudomonas aeruginosa*: differentiation between melanin and pyorubrin, *J Med Microbiol*, **8**: 199–203.

Ohman DE, Burns RP, Iglewski BH, 1980, Corneal infections in mice with toxin A and elastase mutants of *Pseudomonas aeruginosa*, *J Infect Dis*, **142**: 547–55.

Ojeniyi B, 1988, Bacteriophages in sputum of cystic fibrosis patients as a possible cause of *in vivo* changes in serotypes of *Pseudomonas aeruginosa*, *APMIS*, **96**: 294–8.

O'Neil K, Herman JH et al., 1986, *Pseudomonas cepacia*: an emerging pathogen in chronic granulomatous disease, *J Pediatr*, **108**: 940–2.

Ostroff RM, Vasil ML, 1987, Identification of a new phospholipase C activity by analysis of an insertional mutation in the hemolytic phospholipase C structural gene of *Pseudomonas aeruginosa*, *J Bacteriol*, **169**: 4597–601.

Palleroni NJ, 1984, Genus I. *Pseudomonas* M. gula 1894, *Bergey's Manual of Systematic Bacteriology*, vol. 1, eds Krieg NR, Holt JG, Williams & Wilkins, Baltimore, 141–99.

Palleroni NJ, Bradbury JF, 1993, *Stenotrophomonas*, a new bacterial genus for *Xanthomonas maltophilia*, *Int J Syst Bacteriol*, **43**: 606–9.

Pankhurst CL, Philpott-Howard J, 1996, The environmental risk factors associated with medical and dental equipment in the transmission of *Burkholderia* (*Pseudomonas*) *cepacia* in cystic fibrosis patients, *J Hosp Infect*, **32**: 249–55.

Paranchych W, Frost LS, 1988, The physiology and biochemistry of pili, *Adv Microbiol Physiol*, **29**: 53–114.

Parmely MJ, 1993, *Pseudomonas* metalloproteases and the host–microbe relationship, Pseudomonas aeruginosa: *the Opportunist – Pathogenesis and Disease*, ed. Fick RB, CRC Press, Boca Raton, FL, 79–94.

Parr TR, Moore RA et al., 1987, Role of porins in intrinsic resistance of *Pseudomonas cepacia*, *Antimicrob Agents Chemother*, **31**: 121–3.

Pattyn S, Mertens G, 1988, Esterase iso-enzyme electrophoresis for epidemiological surveillance of *Pseudomonas aeruginosa* hospital infections, *Eur J Clin Microbiol Infect Dis*, **7**: 821–2.

Pavlovskis DR, Edman DC et al., 1981, Protection against experimental *Pseudomonas aeruginosa* infection in mice by active immunization with exotoxin A toxoids, *Infect Immun*, **32**: 681–9.

Pegues CF, Pegues DA et al., 1996, *Burkholderia cepacia* respiratory tract acquisition: epidemiology and molecular characterization of a large nosocomial outbreak, *Epidemiol Infect*, **116**: 309–17.

Pennington JE, 1979, Lipopolysaccharide *Pseudomonas* vaccine: efficacy against pulmonary infection with *Pseudomonas aeruginosa*, *J Infect Dis*, **140**: 73–80.

Pennington JE, Hickey W et al., 1981, Active immunization with lipopolysaccharide pseudomonas antigen for chronic pseudomonas bronchopneumonia in guinea pigs, *J Clin Invest*, **68**: 1140–8.

Perry MB, MacLean LL et al., 1995, Structural characterization of the lipopolysaccharide O antigens of *Burkholderia pseudomallei*, *Infect Immun*, **63**: 3348–52.

Phillips I, 1969, Identification of *Pseudomonas aeruginosa* in the clinical laboratory, *J Med Microbiol*, **2**: 9–16.

Phillips I, Lobo AZ et al., 1968, Acetic acid in the treatment of superficial wounds infected by *Pseudomonas aeruginosa*, *Lancet*, **1**: 11–14.

Phung LV, Han Y et al., 1995, Enzyme-linked immunosorbent assay (ELISA) using a glycolipid antigen for the serodiagnosis of melioidosis, *FEMS Immunol Med Microbiol*, **12**: 259–64.

Pier GB, Matthews WJ, Eardley DD, 1983, Immunochemical characterization of the mucoid exopolysaccharide of *Pseudomonas aeruginosa*, *J Infect Dis*, **147**: 494–503.

Pier GB, Pollack M, Cohen M, 1984, Immunochemical characterization of high-molecular-weight polysaccharide from Fisher immunotype 3 *Pseudomonas aeruginosa*, *Infect Immun*, **45**: 309–13.

Pier GB, Grout M et al., 1996, Role of mutant CFTR in hypersusceptibility of cystic fibrosis patients to lung infections, *Science*, **271:** 64–7.

Pitt TL, 1980, Diphasic variation in the flagellar antigens of *Pseudomonas aeruginosa*, *FEMS Microbiol Lett*, **9:** 301–6.

Pitt TL, 1981a, A comparison of flagellar typing and phage typing as means of subdividing the O groups of *Pseudomonas aeruginosa*, *J Med Microbiol*, **14:** 261–70.

Pitt TL, 1981b, Preparation of agglutinating antisera specific for the flagellar antigens of *Pseudomonas aeruginosa*, *J Med Microbiol*, **14:** 251–60.

Pitt TL, 1988, Epidemiological typing of *Pseudomonas aeruginosa*, *Eur J Clin Microbiol Infect Dis*, **7:** 238–47.

Pitt TL, Aucken H, Dance DAB, 1992, Homogeniety of lipopolysaccharide antigens in *Pseudomonas pseudomallei*, *J Infect*, **25:** 139–46.

Pitt TL, Bradley DE, 1975, The antibody response to the flagella of *Pseudomonas aeruginosa*, *J Med Microbiol*, **8:** 97–106.

Pitt TL, Erdman YJ, 1978, The specificity of agglutination reactions of *Pseudomonas aeruginosa* with O antisera, *J Med Microbiol*, **11:** 15–23.

Pitt TL, McDougall J et al., 1986, Polyagglutinating and nontypable strains of *Pseudomonas aeruginosa* in cystic fibrosis, *J Med Microbiol*, **21:** 179–86.

Pitt TL, Livermore DM et al., 1989, Multiresistant serotype O12 *Pseudomonas aeruginosa*: evidence for a common strain in Europe, *Epidemiol Infect*, **103:** 565–76.

Pitt TL, Kaufmann ME et al., 1996, Type characterisation and antibiotic susceptibility of *Burkholderia* (*Pseudomonas*) *cepacia* isolates from patients with cystic fibrosis in the United Kingdom and the Republic of Ireland, *J Med Microbiol*, **44:** 203–10.

Pollack M, Young LS, 1979, Protective activity of antibodies to exotoxin A and lipopolysaccharide at the onset of *Pseudomonas aeruginosa* septicemia in man, *J Clin Invest*, **63:** 276–86.

Poole K, 1994, Bacterial multidrug resistance – emphasis on efflux mechanisms and *Pseudomonas aeruginosa*, *J Antimicrob Chemother*, **34:** 453–6.

Pradella SM, Petschette F et al., 1994, Macrorestriction analysis of *Pseudomonas aeruginosa* in colonized burn patients, *Eur J Clin Microbiol Infect Dis*, **13:** 122–8.

Prince A, 1986, Antibiotic resistance of *Pseudomonas* species, *J Pediatr*, **108:** 830–4.

Pruksachartvuthi S, Aswapokee N, Thankerngpol K, 1990, Survival of *Pseudomonas pseudomallei* in human phagocytes, *J Med Microbiol*, **31:** 109–14.

Puckett A, Davison G et al., 1992, Post transfusion septicaemia 1980–1989: importance of donor arm cleansing, *J Clin Pathol*, **45:** 155–7.

Rabkin CS, Jarvis WR et al., 1989, *Pseudomonas cepacia* typing systems: collaborative study to assess their potential in epidemiologic investigations, *Rev Infect Dis*, **11:** 600–7.

Raivio TL, Vjack EE et al., 1994, Association between transcript levels of the *Pseudomonas aeruginosa* regA, regB, toxA genes in sputa of cystic fibrosis patients, *Infect Immun*, **62:** 3506–14.

Ralston E, Palleroni NJ, Doudoroff M, 1973, *Pseudomonas pickettii*, a new species of clinical origin related to *Pseudomonas solanacearum*, *Int J Syst Bacteriol*, **23:** 15–19.

Ras GJ, Theron AJ et al., 1992, Enhanced release of elastase and oxidative inactivation of α-1-protease inhibitor by stimulated human neutrophils exposed to *Pseudomonas aeruginosa* pigment 1-hydroxyphenazine, *J Infect Dis*, **166:** 568–73.

Reina J, Bassa A et al., 1991, Infections with *Pseudomonas paucimobilis*, report of four cases and review, *Rev Infect Dis*, **13:** 1072–6.

Rhame FS, 1980, The ecology and epidemiology of *Pseudomonas aeruginosa*, Pseudomonas aeruginosa: *the Organism, Diseases it Causes, and their Treatment*, ed. Sabath LD, Hans Huber, Bern, 31–51.

Richard C, Monteil H et al., 1981, Caractères phénotypiques de 100 souches de *Pseudomonas cepacia*; proposition d'un schema de biovars, *Ann Biol Clin (Paris)*, **39:** 9–15.

Ricketts CR, Lowbury EJL et al., 1970, Mechanism of prophylaxis by silver compounds against infection of burns, *Br Med J*, **1:** 444–6.

Rogul M, Carr SR, 1972, Variable ammonia production among smooth and rough strains of *Pseudomonas pseudomallei*: resemblance to bacteriocin production, *J Bacteriol*, **112:** 372–80.

Rolston KV, Messer M, Ho DH, 1990, Comparative *in vitro* activities of newer quinolones against *Pseudomonas* species and *Xanthomonas maltophilia* isolated from patients with cancer, *Antimicrob Agents Chemother*, **34:** 1812–13.

Russell AD, Hammond SA, Morgan JR, 1986, Bacterial resistance to antiseptics and disinfectants, *J Hosp Infect*, **7:** 213–25.

Sabaté J, Villanueva A, Prieto MJ, 1994, Isolation and characterization of a mercury-resistant broad-host-range plasmid from *Pseudomonas cepacia*, *FEMS Microbiol Lett*, **119:** 345–50.

Saiman L, Cacalano G, Prince A, 1990, *Pseudomonas cepacia* adherence to respiratory epithelial cells is enhanced by *Pseudomonas aeruginosa*, *Infect Immun*, **58:** 2578–84.

Schable B, Rhoden DL et al., 1989, Serological classification of *Xanthomonas maltophilia* (*Pseudomonas maltophilia*) based on heat-stable O antigens, *J Clin Microbiol*, **27:** 1011–14.

Scharmann W, 1976, Formation and isolation of leucocidin from *Pseudomonas aeruginosa*, *J Gen Microbiol*, **93:** 283–91.

Schoch PE, Cunha BA, 1987, *Pseudomonas maltophilia*, *Infect Control*, **8:** 169–72.

Schroth MN, Cho JJ et al., 1977, Epidemiology of *Pseudomonas aeruginosa* in agricultural areas, Pseudomonas aeruginosa: *Ecological Aspects and Patient Colonization*, ed. Young VM, Raven Press, New York, 1–29.

Sédillot C, 1850, Sur la nature et les causes des suppurations bleues, *Gaz Méd Paris*, **5:** 656.

Segers P, Vancanneyt M et al., 1994, Classification of *Pseudomonas diminuta* Leifson and Hugh 1954 and *Pseudomonas vesicularis* Busing, Doll and Freytag 1953 in *Brevundimonas* gen. nov. as *Brevundimonas diminuta* comb. nov., respectively, *Int J Syst Bacteriol*, **44:** 499–510.

Senda K, Arakawa Y et al., 1996, Multifocal outbreaks of metallo-β-lactamase-producing *Pseudomonas aeruginosa* resistant to broad-spectrum β-lactams, including carbapenems, *Antimicrob Agents Chemother*, **40:** 349–53.

Sermswan RW, Wongratanacheewin S et al., 1994, Construction of a specific DNA probe for diagnosis of melioidosis and use as an epidemiological marker of *Pseudomonas pseudomallei*, *Mol Cell Probes*, **8:** 1–9.

Sexton MM, Goebel LA et al., 1993, Ribotype analysis of *Pseudomonas pseudomallei* isolates, *J Clin Microbiol*, **31:** 238–43.

Sexton MM, Jones AL et al., 1994, Purification and characterization of a protease from *Pseudomonas pseudomallei*, *Can J Microbiol*, **40:** 903–10.

Shannon K, Phillips I, 1982, Mechanisms of resistance to aminoglycosides in clinical isolates, *J Antimicrob Chemother*, **9:** 91–102.

Shellito J, Nelson S, Sorensen RU, 1992, Effect of pyocyanin, a pigment of *Pseudomonas aeruginosa*, on production of reactive nitrogen intermediates by murine alveolar macrophages, *Infect Immun*, **60:** 3913–15.

Shen BF, Tai PC et al., 1987, Nucleotide sequences and expression in *Escherichia coli* of the in-phase overlapping *Pseudomonas aeruginosa plc*R genes, *J Bacteriol*, **169:** 4602–7.

Shionoya H, Goto S et al., 1967, Relationship between pyocin and temperate phage of *Pseudomonas aeruginosa*. I. Isolation of temperate phages from strain P I-III and their characteristics, *Jpn J Exp Med*, **37:** 359–72.

Shoesmith JG, Sherris JC, 1960, Studies on the mechanism of arginine-activated motility in a pseudomonas strain, *J Gen Microbiol*, **22:** 10–24.

Shooter RA, Cooke EM et al., 1969, Food and medicament as possible sources of hospital strains of *Pseudomonas aeruginosa*, *Lancet*, **1:** 1227–9.

Shryock TR, Silver SA et al., 1984, Effect of *Pseudomonas aeruginosa* rhamnolipid on human neutrophil migration, *Curr Microbiol*, **10:** 323–8.

Sierra G, 1960, Hemolytic effect of a glycolipid produced by

Pseudomonas aeruginosa, Antonie van Leeuwenhoek J Microbiol Serol, **26:** 189–92.

Sierra G, Zagt R, 1960, Some remarks on autolysis of *Pseudomonas aeruginosa*, Antonie van Leeuwenhoek J Microbiol Serol, **26:** 193–208.

Simpson IN, Finlay J et al., 1994, Multi-resistance isolates possessing characteristics of both *Burkholderia* (*Pseudomonas*) *cepacia* and *Burkholderia gladioli* from patients with cystic fibrosis, J Antimicrob Chemother, **34:** 353–61.

Sisson PR, Freeman R et al., 1991, Strain differentiation of nosocomial isolates of *Pseudomonas aeruginosa* by pyrolysis mass spectrometry, J Hosp Infect, **19:** 137–40.

Smith DL, Gumery LB et al., 1993, Epidemic of *Pseudomonas cepacia* in an adult cystic fibrosis unit: evidence of person-to-person transmission, J Clin Microbiol, **31:** 3017–22.

Smith MD, Wuthiekanun V et al., 1993, A latex agglutination test for the identification of *Pseudomonas pseudomallei*, J Clin Pathol, **46:** 374–5.

Smith MD, Wuthiekanun V et al., 1995, Quantitative recovery of *Burkholderia pseudomallei* from soil in Thailand, Trans R Soc Trop Med Hyg, **89:** 488–90.

Smith MD, Wuthiekanun V et al., 1996, *In-vitro* activity of carbapenem antibiotics against β-lactam susceptible and resistant strains of *Burkholderia pseudomallei*, J Antimicrob Chemother, **37:** 611–15.

Smith PB, Cherry WB, 1957, Identification of *Malleomyces* by specific bacteriophages, J Bacteriol, **74:** 668–72.

Sokol PA, Luan MZ et al., 1994, Genetic rearrangement associated with *in vivo* mucoid conversion of *Pseudomonas aeruginosa* PAO is due to insertion elements, J Bacteriol, **176:** 553–62.

Speert DP, Campbell M et al., 1989, Use of a pilin probe to study molecular epidemiology of *Pseudomonas aeruginosa*, J Clin Microbiol, **27:** 2589–93.

Speert DP, Farmer SW et al., 1990, Conversion of *Pseudomonas aeruginosa* to the phenotype characteristic of strains from patients with cystic fibrosis, J Clin Microbiol, **28:** 188–94.

Stanier RY, Palleroni NJ, Doudoroff M, 1966, The aerobic pseudomonads: a taxonomic study, J Gen Microbiol, **43:** 159–271.

Stanton AT, Fletcher W, 1921, Melioidosis, a new disease of the tropics, Trans Health Congr Far East Assoc Trop Med, **2:** 196–8.

Stanton AT, Fletcher W, 1925, Melioidosis, a disease of rodents communicable to man, Lancet, **1:** 10–13.

Stanton AT, Fletcher W, Symonds SL, 1927, Melioidosis in a horse, J Hyg Camb, **26:** 33–5.

Staugas RE, Harvey DP et al., 1992, Induction of tumor necrosis factor (TNF) and interleukin-1 (IL-1) by *Pseudomonas aeruginosa* and exotoxin A-induced suppression of lymphoproliferation and TNF, lymphotoxin, gamma interferon, and IL-1 production in human leukocytes, Infect Immun, **60:** 3162–8.

Steinmetz I, Rohde M, Brenneke B, 1995, Purification and characterization of an exopolysaccharide of *Burkholderia* (*Pseudomonas*) *pseudomallei*, Infect Immun, **63:** 3959–65.

Stieritz DD, Holder IA, 1975, Experimental studies of the pathogenesis of infections due to *Pseudomonas aeruginosa*: description of a burned mouse model, J Infect Dis, **131:** 688–91.

Stover GB, Drake DR, Montie TC, 1983, Virulence of different *Pseudomonas* species in a burned mouse model: tissue colonization by *Pseudomonas cepacia*, Infect Immun, **41:** 1099–104.

Strickland MA, Gaston MA, Pitt TL, 1988, Comparison of polyclonal rabbit antisera with monoclonal antibodies for serological typing of *Pseudomonas aeruginosa*, J Clin Microbiol, **26:** 768–9.

Stuer W, Jaegar KE, Winkler UK, 1986, Purification of extracellular lipase from *Pseudomonas aeruginosa*, J Bacteriol, **168:** 1070–4.

Stutts MJ, Schwab JH et al., 1986, Effects of *Pseudomonas aeruginosa* on bronchial epithelial ion transport, Am Rev Respir Dis, **134:** 17–24.

Sun L, Jiang R-Z et al., 1995, The emergence of a highly transmissible lineage of cbl⁺ *Pseudomonas* (*Burkholderia*) *cepacia* causing CF centre epidemics in North America and Britain, Nature Med, **1:** 661–6.

Talarmin A, Dubrous P et al., 1996, Study of *Pseudomonas aeruginosa* serotype O12 isolates with a common antibiotic susceptibility pattern, Eur J Clin Microbiol Infect Dis, **15:** 459–64.

Tang H, Kays M, Prince A, 1995, Role of *Pseudomonas aeruginosa* pili in acute pulmonary infection, Infect Immun, **63:** 1278–85.

Tang H, Di Mango E et al., 1996, Contribution of specific *Pseudomonas aeruginosa* virulence factors to pathogenesis of pneumonia in a neonatal mouse model of infection, Infect Immun, **64:** 37–43.

Taylor RFH, Hodson ME, Pitt TL, 1992, Auxotrophy of *Pseudomonas aeruginosa* in cystic fibrosis, FEMS Microbiol Lett, **92:** 243–6.

Tejedor C, Foulds J, Zasloff M, 1982, Bacteriophages in sputum of patients with bronchopulmonary *Pseudomonas* infection, Infect Immun, **36:** 440–1.

Temple GS, Ayling PD, Wilkinson SG, 1986, The role of lipopolysaccharide as a receptor for some bacteriophages of *Pseudomonas aeruginosa*, Microbios, **45:** 93–104.

Terry JM, Pina SE, Mattingly SJ, 1991, Environmental conditions which influence mucoid conversion in *Pseudomonas aeruginosa* PAO 1, Infect Immun, **59:** 471–7.

Thomas AD, Forbes-Faulkner JC, 1981, Persistence of *Pseudomonas pseudomallei* in soil, Aust Vet J, **57:** 535–6.

Thomassen MJ, Demko CA et al., 1985, *Pseudomonas cepacia* colonization among patients with cystic fibrosis, Am Rev Respir Dis, **131:** 791–6.

Tong S, Yang S et al., 1996, Laboratory investigation of ecological factors influencing the environmental presence of *Burkholderia pseudomallei*, Microbiol Immunol, **40:** 451–3.

Totten PA, Lory S, 1990, Characterization of a type of flagellin gene from *Pseudomonas aeruginosa*, J Bacteriol, **172:** 7188–99.

Trakulsomboon S, Pitt TL, Dance DAB, 1994, Molecular typing of *Pseudomonas pseudomallei* from imported primates in Britain, Vet Rec, **65:** 65–6.

Trias J, Nikaido H, 1990, Diffusion of antibiotics via specific pathways across the outer membrane of *P. aeruginosa*, Pseudomonas, ed. Silver S, American Society for Microbiology, Washington, DC, 319–27.

Trotter JA, Kuhls TL et al., 1990, Pneumonia caused by a newly recognized pseudomonad in a child with chronic granulomatous disease, J Clin Microbiol, **28:** 1120–4.

Twining SS, Davis SD, Hyndiuk RA, 1986, Relationship between protease and descemetocele formation in experimental *Pseudomonas* keratitis, Curr Eye Res, **5:** 503–10.

Tyler SD, Rozee KR, Johnson WM, 1996, Identification of IS*1356*, a new insertion sequence, and its association with IS*402* in epidemic strains of *Burkholderia cepacia* infecting cystic fibrosis patients, J Clin Microbiol, **34:** 1610–16.

Vale TA, Gaston MA, Pitt TL, 1988, Subdivision of O serotypes of *Pseudomonas aeruginosa* with monoclonal antibodies, J Clin Microbiol, **26:** 1779–82.

Vasil ML, Chamberlain C, Grant CCR, 1986, Molecular studies of *Pseudomonas aeruginosa* exotoxin A gene, Infect Immun, **52:** 538–48.

Vasil ML, Kabat D, Iglewski BH, 1977, Structure–activity relationships of an exotoxin of *Pseudomonas aeruginosa*, Infect Immun, **16:** 353–61.

Vasil M, Prince RW, Shortridge VD, 1993, Exoproducts: *Pseudomonas* exotoxin A and phospholipase C, Pseudomonas aeruginosa: the Opportunist – Pathogenesis and Disease, ed. Fick RB, CRC Press, Boca Raton, FL, 59–77.

Visca P, Serino L et al., 1992, Biochemical characterization of pyoverdin-defective *Pseudomonas aeruginosa* mutants and mapping of chromosomal mutations, Pseudomonas: Molecular Biology and Biotechnology, eds Galli E, Silver S, Witholt B, American Society for Microbiology, Washington, DC, 94–103.

Visca P, Ciervo A et al., 1993, Iron-regulated salicylate synthesis by *Pseudomonas* spp., J Gen Microbiol, **139:** 1995–2001.

Walsh AL, Wuthiekanun V et al., 1995, Selective broths for the isolation of *Pseudomonas pseudomallei* from clinical samples, *Trans R Soc Trop Med Hyg*, **89**: 124.

Watanabe M, Iyobe S et al., 1991, Transferable imipenem resistance in *Pseudomonas aeruginosa*, *Antimicrob Agents Chemother*, **35**: 147–51.

Welch DF, Muszynski MJ et al., 1987, Selective and differential medium for the recovery of *Pseudomonas cepacia* from the respiratory tracts of patients with cystic fibrosis, *J Clin Microbiol*, **25**: 1730–4.

Werneburg B, Monteil H, 1989, New serotypes of *Pseudomonas cepacia*, *Res Microbiol*, **140**: 17–20.

Whitmore A, 1913, An account of a glanders-like disease occurring in Rangoon, *J Hyg Camb*, **13**: 1–34.

Whitmore A, Krishnaswami CS, 1912, An account of the discovery of a hitherto undescribed infective disease occurring among the population of Rangoon, *Indian Med Gaz*, **47**: 262–7.

Wick MJ, Frank DW et al., 1990, Identification of *regB*, a gene required for optimal exotoxin A yields in *Pseudomonas aeruginosa*, *Mol Microbiol*, **4**: 489–97.

Wilkinson SG, 1983, Composition and structure of lipopolysaccharides from *Pseudomonas aeruginosa*, *Rev Infect Dis*, **5, Suppl. 5**: S941–9.

Wilkinson SG, Galbraith L, 1975, Studies of lipopolysaccharides from *Pseudomonas aeruginosa*, *Eur J Biochem*, **52**: 331–43.

Wilkinson SG, Galbraith L, Lightfoot GA, 1973, Cell walls, lipids, and lipopolysaccharides of *Pseudomonas* species, *Eur J Biochem*, **33**: 158–74.

Wilkinson SG, Pitt TL, 1995a, *Burkholderia* (*Pseudomonas*) *cepacia*: surface chemistry and typing methods, *Rev Med Microbiol*, **6**: 1–9.

Wilkinson SG, Pitt TL, 1995b, *Burkholderia* (*Pseudomonas*) *cepacia*: pathogenicity and resistance, *Rev Med Microbiol*, **6**: 10–17.

Williams RJ, Lindridge MA et al., 1984, National survey of antibiotic resistance in *Pseudomonas aeruginosa*, *J Antimicrob Chemother*, **14**: 9–16.

Wilson R, Pitt TL et al., 1987, Pyocyanin and 1-hydroxyphenazine produced by *Pseudomonas aeruginosa* inhibit the beating of human respiratory cilia *in vivo*, *J Clin Invest*, **79**: 221–9.

Winstanley C, Coulson MA et al., 1996, Flagellin gene and protein variation amongst clinical isolates of *Pseudomonas aeruginosa*, *Microbiology*, **142**: 2145–51.

Wise MG, Shimkets LJ, McArthur J, 1995, Genetic structure of a lotic population of *Burkholderia* (*Pseudomonas*) *cepacia*, *Appl Environ Microbiol*, **61**: 1791–8.

Wohlfarth S, Hoesche C et al., 1992, Molecular genetics of the extracellular lipase of *Pseudomonas aeruginosa* PAO1, *J Gen Microbiol*, **138**: 1325–35.

Wolz C, Kiosz G et al., 1989, *Pseudomonas aeruginosa* cross-colonisation and persistence in patients with cystic fibrosis. Use of a DNA probe, *Epidemiol Infect*, **102**: 205–14.

Woods DE, Jones AL, Hill PJ, 1993, Interaction of insulin with *Pseudomonas pseudomallei*, *Infect Immun*, **61**: 4045–50.

Woods DE, Que JU, 1987, Purification of *Pseudomonas aeruginosa* exoenzyme S, *Infect Immun*, **55**: 579–86.

Woods DE, Vasil ML, 1994, Pathogenesis of *Pseudomonas aeruginosa* infections, Pseudomonas aeruginosa*: Infections and Treatment*, eds Baltch AL, Smith RP, Marcel Dekker, New York, 21–50.

Woods DE, Cryz SJ et al., 1982, Contribution of toxin A and elastase to virulence of *Pseudomonas aeruginosa* in chronic lung infection of rats, *Infect Immun*, **36**: 1223–8.

Woods DE, Schaffer MS et al., 1986, Phenotypic comparison of *Pseudomonas aeruginosa* strains isolated from a variety of clinical isolates, *J Clin Microbiol*, **24**: 260–4.

Woods DE, Hwang WS et al., 1988, Alteration of pulmonary structure by *Pseudomonas aeruginosa* exoenzymes, *J Med Microbiol*, **26**: 133–41.

Woods DE, Sokol PA et al., 1991, *In vivo* regulation of virulence in *Pseudomonas aeruginosa* associated with genetic rearrangement, *J Infect Dis*, **163**: 143–9.

Wu BJ, Thompson ST, 1984, Selective medium for *Pseudomonas cepacia* containing 9-chloro-9-(4-diethylaminophenyl)-10-phenylacridan and polymyxin B sulphate, *Appl Environ Microbiol*, **48**: 743–6.

Wuthiekanun V, Smith MD, White NJ, 1995, Survival of *Burkholderia pseudomallei* in the absence of nutrients, *Trans R Soc Trop Med Hyg*, **89**: 491.

Wuthiekanun V, Dance DAB et al., 1990, The use of selective media for the isolation of *Pseudomonas pseudomallei* in clinical practice, *J Med Microbiol*, **33**: 121–6.

Wuthiekanun V, Smith MD et al., 1995, Isolation of *Pseudomonas pseudomallei* from soil in north-eastern Thailand, *Trans R Soc Trop Med Hyg*, **89**: 41–3.

Yabuuchi E, Arakawa M, 1993, *Burkholderia pseudomallei* and melioidosis be aware in temperate area, *Microbiol Immunol*, **37**: 823–36.

Yabuuchi E, Ohyama A, 1972, Characterization of 'pyomelanin'-producing strains of *Pseudomonas aeruginosa*, *Int J Syst Bacteriol*, **22**: 53–64.

Yabuuchi E, Yanok I et al., 1990, Proposals of *Sphingomonas paucimobilis* gen. nov. and comb. nov., *Sphingomonas paucimobilis* sp. nov., *Sphingomonas yanoikuyae* sp. nov., *Sphingomonas adhaesiva* sp. nov., *Sphingomonas capsulata* comb. nov., and two genospecies of the genus *Sphingomonas*, *Microbiol Immunol*, **34**: 99–119.

Yabuuchi E, Kosako Y et al., 1992, Proposal of *Burkholderia* gen nov. and transfer of seven species of the genus *Pseudomonas* homology group II to the new genus with the type species *Burkholderia cepacia* (Palleroni and Holmes 1981) comb. nov., *Microbiol Immunol*, **36**: 1251–75.

Yang H, Chaowagul W, Sokol PA, 1991, Siderophore production by *Pseudomonas pseudomallei*, *Infect Immun*, **59**: 776–80.

Yang H, Kooi CD, Sokol PA, 1993, Ability of *Pseudomonas pseudomallei* malleobactin to acquire transferrin-bound, lactoferrin-bound, and cell-derived iron, *Infect Immun*, **61**: 656–62.

Yohalem DS, Lorbeer JW, 1994, Multi-locus isoenzyme diversity among strains of *Pseudomonas cepacia* isolated from decayed onions, soils and clinical sources, *Syst Appl Microbiol*, **17**: 116–24.

Yoneyama H, Nakae T, 1996, Protein (OprC) of the outer membrane of *Pseudomonas aeruginosa* is a copper-regulated channel protein, *Microbiology*, **142**: 2137–44.

Yoshihara E, Nakae T, 1989, Identification of porins in the outer membrane of *Pseudomonas aeruginosa* that form small diffusion pores, *J Biol Chem*, **264**: 6297–301.

Young LS, 1972, Human immunity to *Pseudomonas aeruginosa*. II Relationship between heat-stabile opsonins and type-specific lipopolysaccharides, *J Infect Dis*, **126**: 277–87.

Young M, Hancock REW, 1992, Fluoroquinolone supersusceptibility mediated by outer membrane protein OprH overexpression in *Pseudomonas aeruginosa*: evidence for involvement of a nonporin pathway, *Antimicrob Agents Chemother*, **36**: 2365–9.

Zannoni D, 1989, The respiratory chains of pathogenic pseudomonads, *Biochim Biophys Acta*, **975**: 299–316.

Zierdt CH, 1986, *Pseudomonas aeruginosa*: serology, phage, and pyocin, *Non-fermentative Gram-negative Rods*, ed. Gilardi GL, Marcel Dekker, New York, 283–340.

Chapter 48

MORAXELLA, BRANHAMELLA, KINGELLA AND EIKENELLA

B K Buchanan

MORAXELLA

1 CLASSIFICATION

The exact taxonomic delineation of the genus *Moraxella* is currently the subject of debate. In the 1984 edition of *Bergey's Manual of Systematic Bacteriology*, Bovre described *Moraxella* as consisting of 2 subgenera, *Moraxella* and *Branhamella*, in the family Neisseriaceae. More recent work by Rossau et al. (1986) and Dewhirst, Paster and Bright (1989) indicates that *Moraxella* does not belong in the family Neisseriaceae based on DNA–rRNA hybridization studies and 16S rRNA anaylsis. There is agreement that *Moraxella*, *Branhamella* and the 'false *Neisseria*' (*Neisseria caviae*, *Neisseria ovis* and *Neisseria cuniculi*) all belong in the same family. Rossau et al. (1991) proposed Moraxellaceae as the family name; proposed only one genus *Moraxella* with no subgenera; and proposed inclusion of *Acinetobacter* and *Psychrobacter* in this family. In the same edition of the *International Journal of Systematic Bacteriology*, Catlin (1991) proposed the family name Branhamaceae which he felt should include *Branhamella* and *Moraxella* but not *Acinetobacter*. Later work by Veron et al. (1993) and Enright et al. (1994) both agree that *Moraxella* and *Branhamella* do not belong in the family Neisseriaceae. Veron et al. (1993) noted that more complete nucleic acid sequence data and more precise information concerning phylogenetic relationships are needed to resolve completely the issues of nomenclature. The data in support of *Moraxella* and *Branhamella* belonging to the same genus are

very strong. Catlin's (1990, 1991) arguments to the contrary are based on practicality. *Branhamella* spp. are coccoid whereas *Moraxella* spp. are rod-shaped; it is confusing for the medical community because of the differences in pathogencity between the 2 groups of organisms; it is confusing taxonomically because *Branhamella catarrhalis* was previously known as *Micrococcus* and then would be *Moraxella*; finally, it ignores the work of Dr Sarah Branham. The best solution based on current data is to accept the nomenclature approved in the latest edition of *Bergey's Manual of Systematic Bacteriology* which recognizes one genus with 2 subgenera.

2 MORAXELLA (MORAXELLA)

2.1 Definition

Moraxella (*Moraxella*) organisms are short, plump, gram-negative coccobacilli that appear predominantly in pairs, although they may be in short chains (one plane of division). They are non-flagellate, but under specialized conditions, may show sluggish motility. They are oxidase-positive, catalase-positive, strict aerobes. The asaccharolytic organisms are negative for DNAase, indole and H_2S production and have variable reactions for nitrate reduction and gelatin liquefaction. Optimal growth temperature is 33–35°C. G + C content of DNA is 40–45 mol%.

Moraxella lacunata was first isolated from cases of conjunctivitis by Morax and Axenfeld and the name '*Bacillus lacunatus*' was proposed by Eyre (Jones and Jephcott 1990). These organisms, like other members of this genus, are parasitic on the mucous membranes of humans and animals. The members of this subgenera are plump, rod-shaped, gram-negative organisms measuring 1.0–1.5 μm wide by 1.5–3 μm long. They occur in pairs or short chains, dividing in one plane. Flagella and swimming motility are not observed. Piechaud, however, observed sluggish movement on nutrient agar in a special oil chamber (Jones and Jephcott 1990). These organism are fimbriate and, with the exception of *Moraxella bovis*, do not form capsules. Pleomorphism is enhanced as the culture ages and by growth at increased temperature. Eyre described variation in size and shape ranging from short diplococci to filamentous threads.

Nutritional requirements vary from simple nutrient agar to agar supplemented with serum or blood. *Moraxella osloensis* can use citrate or ethanol as a sole carbon source. On serum agar at 37°C, *Moraxella* forms circular, raised, greyish, translucent colonies measuring 1 mm at 24 h. Continued incubation results in colonies 2–5 mm in diameter. Some species are weakly haemolytic, producing a narrow zone of haemolysis on sheep, human, ox or horse blood agar. Most strains will not grow on MacConkey agar; however, *Moraxella canis*, *M. bovis* and *Moraxella atlantae* are exceptions. Sugars are not fermented, but some species are capable of digesting gelatin, serum and casein. These oxidase-positive organisms are negative for indole and urease production and generally produce catalase. Nitrate reduction varies from species to species. In a review of 933 *Moraxella*-like species submitted to the Centers for Disease Control, Graham et al. (1990) reported that *Moraxella nonliquefaciens* was the most common isolate from nose, throat, mouth or eye.

2.2 *Moraxella (Moraxella) lacunata*

This is the type species for the genus. It is classically associated with chronic angular blepharoconjunctivitis, although it is actually the cause of only a small percentage of all eye infections. It is occasionally associated with epidemics, especially among adolescent girls who share makeup (Groschel 1995). *M. lacunata* can be isolated from polymorphonuclear leucocytes and from desquamated epithelial cells in addition to being found free in secretions. This fastidious organism prefers serum enriched growth medium such as Loeffler's. Growth on chocolate or blood agar is poor. *Moraxella liquefaciens*, a variant of *M. lacunata*, posseses the ability to liquefy gelatin rapidly, to grow at room temperature and to grow without the addition of natural animal protein. Henriksen and Bovre (1968a) considered the differences so minimal that they included it in the species *M. lacunata*. This variant has, however, been implicated in serious invasive disease.

2.3 *Moraxella (Moraxella) nonliquefaciens*

In 1955 Kaffka described an organism that was unable to liquefy gelatin or digest serum. It was isolated from a case of bronchopneumonia and also from the throat of 2 normal individuals (Jones and Jephcott 1990). It

is most frequently isolated from the human upper respiratory tract. Henriksen (1958) found it in 11.3% of 875 cultures of the nares of patients seen at an otolaryngology clinic. Later, studies by Bovre (1967) and Bovre and Henriksen (1967) noted that strains labelled *M. nonliquefaciens* actually showed great variations. Based on nutritive requirements, DNA composition and failure of genetic transformation, *M. osloensis* and *[Moraxella] phenylpyruvica* were split off. Subsequent work by Rossau et al.(1991) and Enright et al. (1994) indicates that *[M.] phenylpyruvica* probably does not belong in the genus *Moraxella* as it appears more closely related to *Psychrobacter immobilis*.

2.4 *Moraxella (Moraxella) osloensis*

Bovre and Henriksen (1967) differentiated this organsim from *M. nonliquefaciens* based on its less fastidious nutritive requirments. *M. osloensis* can grow on plain media, on Hugh and Leifson's medium and in Audureau's medium with ethanol as the sole carbon source. It also shows greater resistance to heat and a higher G + C content of 43–43.5 mol%. *M. osloensis* is a common resident of the human genital tract and can mimic gonococci although, unlike *N. gonorrhoeae*, it grows well on blood agar. There have been conflicting reports as to whether this organism belongs in the genus *Moraxella* (Rossau et al. 1991, Vandamme et al. 1993). Pathogenically *M. osloensis* has been implicated in cases of septic arthritis, osteomyeolytis and septicaemia.

2.5 *Moraxella (Moraxella) bovis*

M. bovis is the aetiological agent of infectious bovine keratoconjunctivitis (IBK). It was first isolated by Jones and Little (1923). IBK occurs primarily in summer when cattle are exposed to eye irritations from dust, flies and intense sunlight. These conditions combine to predispose the animals to infection with *M. bovis*. The syndrome may include photophobia, blepharospasm, conjunctivitis and corneal ulceration. Watt (1951) reported that *M. bovis* is capable of growing, albeit poorly, on nutrient agar and in broth. It fails to reduce nitrate but does liquefy gelatin. On blood agar it forms grey, translucent colonies 4–5 mm in diameter with a smooth convex surface. Virulence factors associated with this organism include pili for corneal adherence and a heat labile haemolysin that produces cytotoxic activity against neutrophils and corneal epithelial cells (Clinkenbeard and Theiessen 1991). The haemolysin, which needs Ca^{2+} as a cofactor, is most active against sheep RBC and least active against human RBC.

2.6 **Other** *Moraxella (Moraxella)* **species**

M. atlantae and the newly recognized *Moraxella lincolnii* are also members of the *Moraxella* subgenera. *M. atlantae* is a fastidious organism that forms colonies <0.5 mm on blood agar after 48 h of incubation. It is rarely isolated as a human pathogen. *M. lincolnii* was recently characterized by Vandamme et al. (1993). It has been isolated primarily from the human respiratory tract and forms smooth, whitish, convex colonies with a diameter of 1–3 mm at 48 h. It can grow on nutrient agar or blood agar and does not produce a zone of haemolysis. Optimal growth is at 28–33°C, but can also grow at 36–37°C. Most strains reduce nitrite but not nitrate. It is oxidase- and catalase-positive, but negative for gelatin liquefaction, urease and DNAase. G + C content is 44 mol%. *M. lincolnii* is of unknown clinical significance.

3 MORAXELLA (BRANHAMELLA)

3.1 Definition

Members of this subgenera are gram-negative diplococci measuring 0.6–1.0 μm in diameter; cell division occurs in 2 planes at right angles to each other and sometimes produces tetrads; cells may be capsulate as well as fimbriate. They are oxidase- and catalase-positive asaccharolytic organisms that are negative for indole and H_2S production but produce DNAase. Nitrate and nitrite reduction are variable. G + C content is 40–45 mol%.

3.2 *Moraxella (Branhamella) catarrhalis*

Seifert (1882) first described a purulent tracheobronchitis caused by *Micrococcus catarrhalis*. This publication served as a reference for a seminal paper by Ghon and Pfeiffer (1902) that recognized this organism as a pathogen along with pneumococci and the reputed influenza bacilli. For the next decade authors both in Europe and the USA continued to recognize the pathogenic potential of *M. catarrhalis* (Benzancon 1905, Jordan 1908, Hiss and Zinsser 1910). Gordon (1921) published results of a study designed to explore the relationship between *M. catarrhalis* and the common cold. Failing to find a link between the two, the article went on to show that individuals could be colonized with *M. catarrhalis*. Berk (1990) chronicled this historical evolution of *M. cattarhalis* from pathogen to commensal to pathogen. Part of the reason that it became known as a commensal was the misidentification of *Neisseria cinerea* which is a respiratory commensal with *M. catarrhalis*. This issue was first recognized by Berger (1963) and later by Knapp et al.(1984). The historical evolution of the organism is complicated by the fact that it has witnessed genus changes from *Micrococcus* to *Neisseria* to *Branhamella* to *Moraxella*.

Morphologically, *M. catarrhalis* are gram-negative diplococci that show a tendency to resist decolorization. On gram-stained smears from clinical samples, it resembles urethral smears of gonococci. Based on sources, such as middle ear fluid or sinus aspirate, a gram stain containing numerous neutrophils and gram-negative diplococci is almost pathognomonic for *M. catarrhalis* since *Neisseria* rarely causes infections in these locations (Doern and Morse 1980). Culturally the organism grows well on both blood and chocolate agars, producing colonies that are whitish-grey and

measure 1–3 mm after 18 h of incubation. A colony usually remains intact when dislodged from the agar with a bacteriological loop. Reports on the ability to grow on nutrient agar vary, as do media components and production lots of nutrient agar (Catlin 1974). Various investigators report the ability of some strains of *M. catarrhalis* to grow on Thayer–Martin agar and other colistin-containing agars (Blackwell, Young and Bain 1978, Doern, Miller and Winn 1981, Durussel and Siegrist 1988). Biochemically the organism fails to ferment carbohydrates, but does reduce both nitrates and nitrites. The oxidase- and catalase-positive organism can be differentiated from *Neisseria* species by its production of DNAase and butyric acid esterase. The latter test usually employs tributyrin as its substrate. Detailed reviews of this organism have been published by Catlin (1990) and Verghese and Berk (1991).

Studies by Murphy independently and with other investigators (Murphy 1989, 1990, Murphy and Bartos 1989, Murphy and Loeb 1989) have revealed interesting information about the *M. catarrhalis* cell wall. It is similar to *N. gonorrhoeae* in that no long repeating units are seen in the lipopolysaccharide (LPS) and blebs or vesicles are released from the outer membrane. Both the LPS and the outer-membrane proteins (OMP) are extremely homogeneous from strain to strain. There are 8 OMP ranging from 21 to 98 kDa (Bartos and Murphy 1988). *M. catarrhalis* also possesses a capsule that is polysaccharide in composition (Hellio et al. 1988). Fimbriation, haemagglutination and serum resistance vary among strains. Wistrich and Baker (1971) examined several ATCC strains and failed to find fimbriae but Murphy (1989), examining clinical isolates, did report fimbriae. The strains of Wistrich and Baker (1971) did not agglutinate human erythrocytes whereas Soto-Hernandez et al. (1989) reported positive findings. Jordan, Berk and Berk (1990) found that 43% of disease-producing isolates were serum resistant while only 13% of colonizing strains were serum resistant.

The ability of *M. catarrhalis* to produce β-lactamase is one that appears to have developed very rapidly and simultaneously around the world. Strains isolated before 1970 were β-lactamase negative and susceptible to penicillin (Barber and Waterworth 1962, Catlin and Cunningham 1964, Baumann, Doudoroff and Stanier 1968, Ahmad et al. 1987). The first report of strains producing β-lactamase was in 1977 in Sweden, followed by France and England (Malmvall, Brorsson and Johnsson 1977, Percival et al. 1977, Philippon et al. 1986). Wallace, Nash and Steingrube (1990) reviewed strains stored at the Centers for Disease Control and reported that by the late 1970s approximately 40% of the strains were β-lactamase positive and by 1980 the incidence was as high as 75%. The β-lactamase is of 2 types: BRO-1 and BRO-2. Approximately 90% of the *M. catarrhalis* strains producing β-lactamase possess the BRO-1 enzyme (Wallace et al. 1989, Wallace, Nash and Steingrube 1990). This organism appears to be uniformly resistant to vancomycin and clindamycin and is highly susceptible to erythromycin and rifampin.

M. catarrhalis is a frequent cause of lower respiratory tract infection, sinusitis and otitis media. Cases of pneumonia and tracheobronchitis most often occur in patients with underlying pulmonary disease. Respiratory infections typically occur in winter months regardless of location as proved by world-wide reports (Digiovanni et al. 1987, Mbaki et al. 1987, Davies and Maesen 1988). *M. catarrhalis* has also been reported to cause bacteraemia, meningitis, endocarditis, keratitis and suppurative arthritis.

3.3 *Moraxella (Branhamella) caviae*

Pelczar, Hajek and Faber (1949) described gram-negative cocci isolated from the throat of guinea pigs and named it *Neisseria caviae* (Pelczar 1953). Later studies by Veron et al. (1993) revealed that *N. caviae*, *N. ovis* and *N. cuniculi* are more closely related to *Moraxella/Branhamella* and proposed that their names be removed from *Neisseria*. *M. caviae* forms a light caramel to dirty brown colony that does not ferment carbohydrates but does reduce nitrate and nitrite and will hydrolyse both DNA and tributyrin. G + C content is 43.9 mol%.

3.4 *Moraxella (Branhamella) ovis*

M. ovis was isolated by Lindqvist (1960) from keratoconjunctivitis in sheep. On bovine blood agar it forms glossy, translucent, non-pigmented colonies. Like the other species in the *Branhamella* subgenera, it does not ferment carbohydrates, will reduce nitrate to nitrite, is both oxidase- and catalase-positive and hydrolyses tributyrin. It does not hydrolyse DNA. Its G + C content is 43.9 mol%.

3.5 *Moraxella (Branhamella) canis*

M. canis was described by Jannes et al. (1993) as oxidase-positive, catalase-positive gram-negative diplococci that had previously been confused with *M. catarrhalis*. This organism reduces nitrate and hydrolyses both DNA and tributyrin. Most of the isolates were associated with dogs, thus the name *M. canis*. It can be differentiated from the other species by its production of γ-glutamyl aminopeptidase and a brown pigment produced on Mueller–Hinton agar.

KINGELLA

4 DEFINITION

Kingella are coccoid to medium sized gram-negative bacilli appearing in pairs and short chains. They measure 1–3 μm in length and have a tendency to resist decolorization when gram stained. They are non-motile but can exhibit twitching motility. This facultative anaerobe is oxidase-positive using tetramethyl-*p*-phenylenediamine and is catalase-negative. Optimal growth occurs at 35–37°C. The organisms ferment

glucose, producing acid but no gas. Nitrate reduction is variable with species. DNA G + C content is 44.5 mol%.

Type species is *Kingella kingae*.

5 GENERAL PROPERTIES

In 1960, King described 2 β-haemolytic and saccharolytic strains of *Moraxella*; these were designated *Moraxella* new species 1 by Davis and Peel (1982) or Group M-1 by Powell and Bass (1983). Henriksen and Bovre (1968b) studied 8 strains of this organism from the King's collection and called it *Moraxella kingii*. In 1974, the spelling was amended to *kingae* to reflect King's gender (Bovre, Henriksen and Jonson 1974); in 1976, *M. kingae* was transferred by Henriksen and Bovre to the genus *Kingella*, based on lack of genetic similarity with *Moraxella* and its unique biochemical profile. Snell and Lapage (1976) added 2 new species, *Kingella indologenes* and *Kingella denitrificans*, in 1976. Bovre included this genus as a member of the family Neisseriaceae along with *Moraxella*, *Neisseria* and *Acinetobacter*. Later studies using 16S rRNA sequence and hybridization studies have confirmed a close association between the genera *Neisseria*, *Kingella*, *Eikenella*, *Simonsiella* and *Alysiella* (Rossau R et al. 1989). *K. indologenes* has been reclassified as *Suttonella indologenes* and a new species, *Kingella oralis* has been added (Dewhirst et al. 1990, 1993).

K. kingae displays 2 colony types: a convex, β-haemolytic colony with a circular edge and shiny surface and a second colony type, also β-haemolytic, forming a small depression in the agar plate with a granular surface and raised central papilla. After 2 days of incubation, the second colony type exhibits peripheral spread and when removed from the agar, corrosion in the agar may be noted. This colony type is not stable and upon subculture may be lost. The smooth colonial variant generally has no fimbriae whereas the corrosive morphotype produces numerous long, thin fimbriae that can be visualized by electron microscopy. For a more detailed description of *K. kingae*, see Odum and Frederiksen (1981).

K. kingae is the most pathogenic species of this genus and is frequently associated with septic arthritis, osteomyelitis, endocarditis and septicaemia (Vincent et al. 1981, Raymond et al. 1986). It has also been reported as the causative agent in meningitis, ophthalmic infections, pneumonia and abscesses of the head, neck and presternum (Mollee, Kelly and Tilse 1992). Morrison and Wagner (1989) provide an in-depth review of *K. kingae* infections. Henriksen and Bovre (1976) determined that the organism may be part of the normal buccal flora; many of the infections are subsequent to oropharyngeal inflammation. Bone and joint infections occur most frequently in children younger than 6 years, whereas endocarditis occurs most often in adults older than 16 years, many of whom have pre-existing heart defects (Yagupsky P and Merires M 1995). *K. denitrificans* (once known as TM-1) has been isolated from endocarditis (see review by Hassan and Hayek 1993). Case reports of *Kingella* infections have recently increased, most probably due to correct identification of the organism. There is a potential for misidentification as a β-haemolytic streptococcus because of its resistance to gram-stain decolorization, to meningococcus because of its gram-stain and oxidase reaction and the clinical manifestation of a rash that can be seen with bacteraemia; it has also been reported to cross-react with *Neisseria meningitidis* Gr. B antisera. Finally, its corrosive colony type can be misidentified as *Eikenella corrodens*, also an aetiological agent of endocarditis and septic arthritis (Goutzmanis, Gonis and Gilbert 1991). Ampicillin and penicillin are usually the drugs of choice for the treatment of *K. kingae*; however, Sordillo et al. (1993) report isolation of a strain producing β-lactamase.

EIKENELLA

6 DEFINITION

Eikenella are straight gram-negative rods measuring 1.5–4 μm in length. They do not possess flagella and are non-motile but can exhibit twitching motility on an agar surface. This facultative anaerobe is oxidase-positive and catalase-negative. Optimal growth occurs at 35–37°C. Acid is not formed from glucose nor other carbohydrates. Lysine and ornithine are decarboxylated and nitrate is reduced to nitrite. Haemin is usually required for aerobic growth. DNA G + C content is 56–58 mol%. *Eikenella corrodens* is the only recognized species, although Dewhirst et al. (1993) described a single isolate, UB-204, which represents a new species that may belong to the genus *Eikenella*.

A 'corroding bacillus' that pitted the agar was described by both Henriksen (1948) and Holm (1950). Twenty-one strains fitting that description, isolated from the oral cavity of humans, were later characterized in detail by Eiken (1958). He described these organisms as fastidious anaerobic gram-negative bacilli and proposed the name 'Bacteroides corrodens', thinking them to be obligate anaerobes. Further work by Henriksen (1969) and Jackson et al. (1971) proved that the organisms previously designated *Bacteroides corrodens* were, in fact, a phenotypically and genetically diverse group of organisms made up of both obligate and facultative anaerobes. Jackson and Goodman (1972) proposed that the facultative anaerobe be named *Eikenella corrodens* in recognition of Eiken's earlier work. The obligate anaerobes which also pitted the media were retained in the genus *Bacteroides*. Originally, *Eikenella* was tentatively placed in the family Brucellaceae by Henriksen (1969), but work by Dewhirst, Paster and Bright (1989) placed the genus in the family Neisseriaceae, based on close ribosomal RNA sequence homology with *Kingella* species and *N. gonorrhoeae*.

7 GENERAL PROPERTIES

The natural habitat of *Eikenella* appears to be the human oral cavity. Numerous investigators have reported isolating this commensal organism from supragingiva and subgingival plaque in patients with healthy periodontium. Isolation of *E. corrodens* as a normal inhabitant of the genitourinary and gastrointestinal tracts has also been reported.

A review by Casey-Chen and Wilson (1992) discusses *E. corrodens* infections and its pathogenicity. *E. corrodens* appears as a pinpoint depression found in blood or chocolate agars after 24 h of incubation. Further incubation reveals a colony with an entire or slightly irregular margin and a raised, umbonate centre that appears to pit the medium. This 'R' form is the dominant morphotype, but occasionally a non-pitting, smooth colony with a matte surface is produced. While the pitting is distinctive, further biochemical characterization is necessary for a definitive identification since other genera isolated from the oral cavity also produce pitting colonies. *Eikenella* is known for a faint bleach-like odour associated with its colonies.

Progulske and Holt (1980) used antibody studies and a staining procedure to demonstrate the presence of a loosely organized slime layer for *E. corrodens*. They also noted fibrillar structures on the surface of the organism, but concluded that these might represent a dehydration artefact. Henriksen and Blom (1975) had previously noted polar fibrils and concluded that the organism possessed pili. They further correlated the presence of the pili with the corroding colony morphology. Whether the pili are an artefact or a genetic characteristic regulated by growth conditions or strain variation is unproven at this time. Other interesting physical characteristics of the organism is the lack of 2-keto-3-deoxyoctulosonic acid (KDO), heptose and β-hydroxymyristic acid, all commonly found constituents of the lipopolysaccharide (LPS) of enteric gram-negative species. The LPS exhibits the usual biological properties of enteric LPS. In vitro, it is mitogenic for mouse spleen cells, exhibits a positive *Limulus* lysate reaction and stimulates human monocytes to release tumour necrosis factor and interleukin-1 (Progulske et al. 1984, Okuda and Kato 1987). In vivo, both fever and a Shwartzman reaction are induced in rabbits (Sasaki 1979, Mashimoto et al. 1985). The LPS of *Eikenella* also exhibits haemagglutinating activity which may play a role in pathogenesis and attachment to epithelial cells. Various investigators have examined the ability of *Eikenella* to attach to human cells. Results of these studies indicate that adherence is the result of a lectin-like bacterial protein and galactose-like host cell receptor (Slots and Gibbons 1978, Yamazaki, Ebisu and Okada 1981, 1983).

8 PATHOGENICITY

E. corrodens has been isolated in pure culture and as part of a mixed bacterial flora from a variety of infections. The true extent of its pathogenicity may be under-reported due to its fastidious nature and its proclivity for presenting as part of a mixed infection. It generally exhibits opportunistic behaviour and rarely causes life-threatening infections except for CNS infections which have a mortality rate as high as 33% (Cheng, South and French 1988). As a resident of the oral cavity, it is frequently implicated in head and neck infections, especially in association with trauma. Both human bite wounds and closed fist injuries can result in infection with *Eikenella* and in some cases lead to osteomyelitis (Goldstein 1995). The range of infections reported from *Eikenella* include bacteraemia, endocarditis, pelvic infection, sinusitis, pancreatitis, pleuropulmonary infection and parotitis (McGowan and Steinberg 1995). Infections have also been associated with haematogenous spread subsequent to dental manipulations. Bacteraemia and endocarditis are reported among intravenous drug abusers who use their saliva to 'clean' their injection site (Scheld and Sande 1995). In mixed infections, it is most commonly isolated with streptococci. The organism's role in periodontitis is controversial. It has been isolated in association with periodontitis and some patients have exhibited antibodies to *E. corrodens*. However, based on longitudinal studies and ones examining the relative numbers of organisms present, the role of *Eikenella* in periodontitis appears to be limited. For a complete discussion of this issue, see the review by Casey-Chen and Wilson (1992).

The primary treatment for *Eikenella* infections has been ampicillin or penicillin; however, there are reports of resistance to penicillin. Trallero et al. (1986) reported a β-lactamase-producing strain, whereas Goldstein and Citron (1984) reported 2 isolates with minimum inhibitory concentration (MIC) for penicillin of 8 μg ml^{-1} and negative for β-lactamase production. In vitro data have been substantiated in at least one report when a patient continued to deteriorate while on penicillin G therapy. Antibiotics to which the organism is susceptible include cefoxitin, ceftriaxone, cefuroxime, cefotetan, ciprofloxacin, norfloxacin, chloramphenicol, carbenicillin and tetracycline. *Eikenella* is resistant to clindamycin, metronidazole, methicillin, aminoglycosides and erythromycin. Susceptibility to cephalothin is variable. The presentation of infection with *Eikenella* often mimics anaerobic infection and may lead to empirical use of ineffective antibiotics such as clindamycin and metronidazole.

REFERENCES

Ahmad F, Young H et al., 1987, Characterization of *Branhamella catarrhalis* and differentiation from *Neisseria* species in a diagnostic laboratory, *J Clin Pathol*, **40**: 1369–73.

Barber M, Waterworth PM, 1962, Antibacterial activity of the penicillins, *Br Med J*, **1**: 1159–64.

Bartos LC, Murphy TF, 1988, Comparison of the outer membrane proteins of 50 strains of *Branhamella catarrhalis*, *J Infect Dis*, **158**: 761–5.

Baumann P, Doudoroff M, Stanier RY, 1968, Study of the *Moraxella* group. I. Genus *Moraxella* and the *Neisseria catarrhalis* group, *J Bacteriol*, **95**: 58–73.

Benzancon J, 1905, Caractères bacteriologiques des crachats au cours d l'epidémie actuelle dite de grippe, *Bull Mem Soc Med Hosp Paris*, **11**: 649.

Berger U, 1963, Die anspruchslosen Neisserien, *Ergeb Mikrobiol Immunitatsforsch Exp Ther*, **36**: 97–167.

Berk SL, 1990, From *Micrococcus* to *Moraxella*, *Arch Intern Med*, **150**: 2254–7.

Blackwell C, Young H, Bain SSR, 1978, Isolation of *Neisseria meningitidis* and *Neisseria catarrhalis* from the genito-urinary tract and anal canal, *Br J Vener Dis*, **54**: 41–4.

Bovre K, 1967, Transformation and DNA base composition in taxonomy, with special reference to recent studies in *Moraxella* and *Neisseria*, *Acta Pathol Microbiol Scand*, **69**: 123–44.

Bovre K, 1984, *Bergey's Manual of Systematic Bacteriology*, 8th edn, eds Krieg NR, Holt JG, Williams & Wilkins, Baltimore, 288–90.

Bovre K, Henriksen SD, 1967, A new *Moraxella* species, *Moraxella osloensis*, and a revised description of *Moraxella nonliquefaciens*, *Int J Syst Bacteriol*, **17**: 127–35.

Bovre K, Henriksen SD, Jonson V, 1974, Correction of the specific epithet *kingii* in the combinations *Moraxella kingii* and *Pseudomonas kingii* to *kingae*, *Int J Syst Bacteriol*, **24**: 307.

Casey-Chen CK, Wilson ME, 1992, *Eikenella corrodens* in human oral and non-oral infections: a review, *J Periodontol*, **63**: 941–53.

Catlin BW, 1974, *Manual of Clinical Microbiology*, 2nd edn, ASM, Washington DC, 116–23.

Catlin BW, 1990, *Branhamella catarrhalis*: an organism gaining respect as a pathogen, *Clin Microbiol Rev*, **3**: 293–320.

Catlin BW, 1991, *Branhamaceae* fam. nov., a proposed family to accommodate the genera *Branhamella* and *Moraxella*, *Int J Syst Bacteriol*, **41**: 320–3.

Catlin BW, Cunningham LS, 1964, Genetic transformation of *Neisseria catarrhalis* by deoxyribonucleate preparations having different average base compositions, *J Gen Microbiol*, **37**: 341–52.

Cheng AF, South JR, French GL, 1988, *Eikenella corrodens* as a cause of brain abscess, *Scand J Infect Dis*, **20**: 667–71.

Clinenbeard KD, Thiessen AE, 1991, Mechanism of action of *Moraxella bovis* hemolysin, *Infect Immun*, **59**: 1148–52.

Davies BI, Maesen FPV, 1988, The epidemiology of respiratory tract pathogens in southern Netherlands, *Eur Respir J*, **1**: 415–20.

Davis JM, Peel MM, 1982, Osteomyelitis and septic arthritis caused by *Kingella kingae*, *J Clin Pathol*, **35**: 219–22.

Dewhirst FE, Paster BJ, Bright PL, 1989, *Chromobacterium, Eikenella, Kingella, Neisseria, Simonsiella,* and *Vitreoscilla* species comprise a major branch of the beta group Proteobacteria by 16S ribosomal ribonucleic acid sequence comparison: transfer of *Eikenella* and *Simonsiella* to the family Neisseriaceae (emend), *Int J Syst Bacteriol*, **39**: 258–66.

Dewhirst FE, Paster BJ et al., 1990, Transfer of *K. indologenes* to the genus *Suttonella* gen. nov. as *Suttonella indologenes* comb. nov.; transfer of *Bacteroides nodosus* to the genus *Dichelobacter* gen. nov. as *Dichelobacter nodosus* comb. nov.; and assignment of the genera *Cardiobacterium, Dichelobacter,* and *Suttonella* to Cardiobacteriaceae fam. nov. in the gamma division of Proteobacteria on the basis of 16S rRNA sequence comparisons, *Int J Syst Bacteriol*, **40**: 426–33.

Dewhirst FE, Chen C-KC et al., 1993, Phylogeny of species in the family Neisseriaceae isolated from human dental plaque and description of *Kingella oralis* sp. nov., *Int J Syst Bacteriol*, **43**: 490–9.

DiGiovanni C, Riley TV et al., 1987, Respiratory tract infections due to *Branhamella catarrhalis*: epidemiological data from western Australia, *Epidemiol Infect*, **99**: 445–53.

Doern GV, Miller MJ, Winn RE, 1981, *Branhamella (Neisseria) catarrhalis* systemic disease in humans. Case reports and review of the literature, *Arch Intern Med*, **141**: 1690–2.

Doern GV, Morse SA, 1980, *Branhamella (Neisseria) catarrhalis*: criterion for laboratory identification, *J Clin Microbiol*, **11**: 193–5.

Durussel C, Siegrist HH, 1988, Evaluation of three commercial systems for the identification of pathogenic *Neisseria* and *Branhamella* species against the conventional method, *Zentrabl Bakteriol Mikrobiol Hyg Reihe*, **268**: 318–24.

Eiken M, 1958, Studies on an anaerobic, rod-shaped, gram negative microorganism: *Bacteroides corrodens* n. sp., *Acta Pathol Microbiol Scand*, **43**: 404–16.

Enright MC, Carter PE et al., 1994, Phylogenetic relationships between some members of the genera *Neisseria, Acinetobacter, Moraxella*, and *Kingella* based on partial 16S ribosomal DNA sequence analysis, *Int J Syst Bacteriol*, **44**: 387–91.

Ghon A, Pfeiffer H, 1902, Der *Mikrococcus catarrhalis* als Krankheitserreger, *Z Klin Med*, **44**: 263–81.

Goldstein EJC, 1995, *Principles and Practice of Infectious Diseases*, 4th edn, eds Mandell GL, Bennett JE, Dolin R, Churchill Livingstone, New York, 2112.

Goldstein EJC, Citron DM, 1984, Susceptibility of *Eikenella corrodens* to penicillin, apalcillin and twelve new cephalosporins, *Antimicrob Agents Chemother*, **26**: 947–8.

Gordon JE, 1921, The gram negative cocci in colds and influenza, *J Infect Dis*, **29**: 463–94.

Goutzmanis JJ, Gonis G, Gilbert GL, 1991, *Kingella kingae* infection in children: ten cases and a review of the literature, *Pediatr Infect Dis J*, **10**: 677–83.

Graham DR, Band JD et al., 1990, Infections caused by *Moraxella, M. urethralis, Moraxella*-like groups M-5 and M-6 and *Kingella kingae* in the United States 1953–1980, *Rev Infect Dis*, **12**: 423–30.

Groschel DHM, 1995, *Principles and Practice of Infectious Diseases*, 4th edn, eds Mandell GL, Bennett JE, Dolin R, Churchill Livingstone, New York, 1926–34.

Hassan IJ, Hayek L, 1993, Endocarditis caused by *Kingella denitrificans*, *J Infect*, **27**: 291–5.

Hellio RM, Guibourdenche M et al., 1988, The envelope structure of *Branhamella catarrhalis* as studied by transmission electron microscopy, *Ann Inst Pasteur*, **139**: 515–25.

Henriksen SD, 1948, Studies in gram-negative anaerobes. II. Gram negative anaerobic rods with spreading colonies, *Acta Pathol Microbiol Scand*, **25**: 368–75.

Henriksen SD, 1958, *Moraxella* duplex var *nonliquefaciens*, habitat and antibiotic sensitivity, *Acta Pathol Microbiol Scand*, **43**: 157.

Henriksen SD, 1969, Corroding bacteria from the respiratory tract. 2. *Bacteroides corrodens*, *Acta Pathol Microbiol Scand*, **75**: 91–6.

Henriksen J, Blom J, 1975, Examination of fimbriation of some gram negative rods with and without twitching and gliding motility, *Acta Pathol Microbiol Scand*, **83**: 161–70.

Henriksen SD, Bovre K, 1968a, The taxonomy of the genera *Moraxella* and *Neisseria*, *J Gen Microbiol*, **51**: 387–92.

Henriksen SD, Bovre K, 1968b, *Moraxella kingii* sp. nov., a hemolytic saccharolytic species of the genus *Moraxella*, *J Gen Microbiol*, **51**: 377–85.

Henriksen SD, Bovre K, 1976, Transfer of *Moraxella kingae* to the genus *Kingella* gen. nov. in the family Neisseriaceae, *Int J Syst Bacteriol*, **26**: 447–50.

Hiss P, Zinsser H, 1910, *A Textbook of Bacteriology*, D Appleton & Co, New York, 25.

Holm P, 1950, Studies on the aetiology of human actinomycosis. I. The 'other microbes' of actinomycosis and their importance, *Acta Pathol Microbiol Scand*, **27**: 736–51.

Jackson FL, Goodman YE, 1972, Transfer of the facultatively anaerobic organism *Bacteroides corroden* Eiken to a new genus, *Eikenella*, *Int J Syst Bacteriol*, **22**: 73–7.

Jackson FL, Goodman YE et al., 1971, Taxonomic status of facultative and strictly anaerobic 'corroding bacilli' that have been classified as *Bacteroides corrodens*, *J Med Microbiol*, **4**: 171–84.

Jannes G, Vaneechoutte M et al., 1993, Polyphasic taxonomy leading to the proposal of *Moraxella canis* sp. nov. for *Moraxella catarrhalis*-like strains, *Int J Syst Bacteriol*, **43**: 438–49.

Jones DM, Jephcott AE, 1990, *Topley and Wilson's Principles of Bacteriology, Virology and Immunity*, vol. 2, 8th edn, eds Parker MT, Duerden BI, Edward Arnold, London, 315.

Jones FS, Little RB, 1923, Infectious ophthalmia of cattle, *J Exp Med*, **38**: 139–48.

Jordan EO, 1908, *A Textbook of General Bacteriology*, WB Saunders, Philadelphia, 206.

Jordan KL, Berk SH, Berk SL, 1990, A comparison of serum bactericidal activity and phenotypic characteristics of bacteremic, pneumonia-causing strains and colonizing strains of *Branhamella catarrhalis*, *Am J Med*, **88 (5A)**: 28S–32S.

Knapp JS, Totten PA et al., 1984, Characterization of *Neisseria cinerea*, a nonpathogenic species isolated on Martin-Lewis medium selective for pathogenic *Neisseria* spp., *J Clin Microbiol*, **19**: 63–7.

Lindqvist K, 1960, A *Neisseria* species associated with infectious keratoconjunctivitis of sheep, *Neisseria ovis*, *J Infect Dis*, **106**: 162.

McGowan JE Jr, Steinberg JP, 1995, *Principles and Practice of Infectious Diseases*, 4th edn, eds Mandell GL, Bennett JE, Dolin R, Churchill Livingstone, New York, 2112.

Malmvall BE, Brorsson JE, Johnsson J, 1977, In vitro sensitivity to penicillin V and beta lactamase production of *Branhamella catarrhalis*, *J Antimicrob Chemother*, **3**: 374–5.

Mashimo J, Yoshida M et al., 1985, Fatty acid composition and Shwartzman activity of lipopolysaccharides from oral bacteria, *Microbiol Immunol*, **29**: 395–403.

Mbaki N, Rikitomi N et al., 1987, Correlation between *Branhamella catarrhalis* adherence to oropharyngeal cells and seasonal incidence of lower respiratory tract infections, *Tohoku J Exp Med*, **153**: 111–21.

Mollee T, Kelly P, Tilse M, 1992, Isolation of *Kingella kingae* from a corneal ulcer, *J Clin Microbiol*, **30**: 2516–17.

Morrison VA, Wagner KF, 1989, Clinical manifestations of *Kingella kingae* infections: case report and review, *Rev Infect Dis*, **11**: 776–82.

Murphy TF, 1989, The surface of *Branhamella catarrhalis*: a systematic approach to the surface antigens of an emerging pathogen, *Pediatr Infect Dis J*, **8, Suppl**: S75–7.

Murphy TF, 1990, Studies of the outer membrane proteins of *Branhamella catarrhalis*, *Am J Med*, **88 (5A)**: 41S–45S.

Murphy TF, Bartos LC, 1989, Surface-exposed and antigenically conserved determinants of outer membrane proteins of *Branhamella catarrhalis*, *Infect Immun*, **57**: 2938–41.

Murphy TF, Loeb MR, 1989, Isolation of the outer membrane of *Branhamella catarrhalis*, *Microb Pathog*, **6**: 159–74.

Odum L, Frederiksen W, 1981, Identification and characterization of *Kingella kingae*, *Acta Pathol Microbiol Scand*, **89**: 311–15.

Okuda K, Kato T, 1987, Hemagglutinating activity of lipopolysaccharides from subgingival plaque bacteria, *Infect Immun*, **55**: 3192–6.

Pelczar MJ, 1953, *Neisseria caviae* nov. spec., *J Bacteriol*, **65**: 744.

Pelczar MJ, Hajek JR, Faber JE, 1949, Characterization of *Neisseria* isolated from pharyngeal region of guinea pigs, *J Infect Dis*, **85**: 239.

Percival A, Corkill JE et al., 1977, Pathogenicity of and beta-lactamase production by *Branhamella (Neisseria) catarrhalis*, *Lancet*, **2**: 1175.

Philippon A, Riou JY et al., 1986, Detection, distribution and inhibition of *Branhamella catarrhalis*, *Drugs*, **31, Suppl. 3**: 64–9.

Powell JM, Bass JW, 1983, Septic arthritis caused by *Kingella kingae*, *Am J Dis Child*, **137**: 974–6.

Progulske A, Holt SC, 1980, Transmission scanning electron microscopic observations of selected *Eikenella corrodens* strains, *J Bacteriol*, **143**: 1003–18.

Progulske A, Mishell R et al., 1984, Biological activities of *Eikenella corrodens* outer membrane and lipopolysaccharide, *Infect Immun*, **43**: 178–82.

Raymond J, Bergeret M et al., 1986, Isolation of two strains of *Kingella kingae* associated with septic arthritis, *J Clin Microbiol*, **24**: 1100–1.

Rossau R, Van Landschool A et al., 1986, Inter- and intrageneric similarities of ribosomal ribonucleic acid cistrons of the Neisseriaceae, *Int J Syst Bacteriol*, **36:** 323–32.

Rossau R, Vandenbusshe G et al., 1989, Ribosomal ribonucleic acid cistron similarities and deoxyribonucleic acid homologies of *Neisseria, Kingella, Eikenella, Simonsiella, Alysiella,* and CDC groups ef-4 and M-5 in the emended family Neisseriaceae, *Int J Syst Bacteriol*, **39:** 185–98.

Rossau R, Van Lanschool A et al., 1991, Taxonomy of Moraxellaceae fam. nov., a new bacterial family to accommodate the genera *Moraxella, Acinetobacter,* and *Psychrobacter* and related organisms, *Int J Syst Bacteriol*, **41:** 310–19.

Sasaki S, 1979, Biological activity of lipopolysaccharides isolated from bacteria in human periodontal lesions, *Bull Tokyo Dent Coll*, **20:** 159–74.

Scheld WM, Sande MA, 1995, *Principles and Practice of Infectious Diseases*, 4th edn, eds Mandell GL, Bennett JE, Dolin R, Churchill Livingstone, New York, 756.

Seifert O, 1882, *Sammlungs Klinischer Vortrage, Leipzig*, **240:** 21.

Slots J, Gibbons R, 1978, Attachment of *Bacteroides melaninogenicus* subsp *asaccharolyticus* to oral surfaces and its possible role in colonization of the mouth and of periodontal pockets, *Infect Immun*, **19:** 254–64.

Snell JJS, Lapage SP, 1976, Transfer of some saccharolytic *Moraxella* species to *Kingella*, with descriptions of *Kingella indologenes* sp. nov. and *Kingella denitrificans* sp. nov., *Int J Syst Bacteriol*, **26:** 451–8.

Sordillo EM, Rendel M et al., 1993, Septicemia due to β-lactamase positive *Kingella kingae*, *Clin Infect Dis*, **17:** 818–19.

Soto-Hernandez JL, Holtsclaw-Berk S et al., 1989, Phenotypic characteristics of *Branhamella catarrhalis* strains, *J Clin Microbiol*, **27:** 903–8.

Trallero EP, Arenzan JMG et al., 1986, β-Lactamase producing *Eikenella corrodens* in an intra-abdominal abscess, *J Infect Dis*, **153:** 379–80.

Vandamme P, Gillis M et al., 1993, *Moraxella lincolnii* sp. nov., isolated from the human respiratory tract, and reevaluation of the taxonomic position of *Moraxella osloensis*, *Int J Syst Bacteriol*, **43:** 474–81.

Verghese A, Berk SL, 1991, *Moraxella (Branhamella) catarrhalis*, *Infect Dis Clin North Am*, **5:** 523–38.

Veron M, Lenvoise-Furet A et al., 1993, Relatedness of three species of 'False *Neisseriae*', *Neisseria caviae, Neisseria cuniculi,* and *Neisseria ovis*, by DNA-DNA hybridizations and fatty acid analysis, *Int J Syst Bacteriol*, **43:** 210–20.

Vincent J, Podewell C et al., 1981, Septic arthritis due to *Kingella kingae*: case report and review of the literature, *J Rheumatol*, **8:** 501–3.

Wallace RJ Jr, Nash DR, Steingrube VA, 1990, Antibiotic susceptibilities and drug resistance in *Moraxella (Branhamella) catarrhalis*, *Am J Med*, **88 (5A):** 46S–50S.

Wallace RJ Jr, Steingrube VA et al, 1989, BRO β-lactamases of *Branhamella catarrhalis* and *Moraxella* subgenus *Moraxella* including evidence for chromosomal β-lactamase transfer by conjugation in *B. catarrhalis, M. nonliquefaciens,* and *M. lacunata, Antimicrob Agents Chemother*, **33:** 1845–54.

Watt JA, 1951, *Vet Rec*, **63:** 98.

Wistreich GA, Baker RF, 1971, The presence of fimbriae (pili) in three species of *Neisseria*, *J Gen Microbiol*, **65:** 167–73.

Yagupsky P, Merires M, 1995, Evaluation of novel vancomycin-containing medium for primary isolation of *Kingella kingae* from upper respiratory tract specimens, *J Clin Microbiol*, **33:** 1426–7.

Yamazaki Y, Ebisu S, Okada H, 1983, Inhibitory effect of galactose on the establishment of *Eikenella corrodens* in the mouth of rats, *J Osaka Dent Sch*, **23:** 113–18.

Yamazaki Y, Ebisu S, Okada H, 1981, *Eikenella corrodens* adherence to human buccal epithelial cells, *Infect Immun*, **31:** 21–7.

Chapter 49

LEGIONELLA

F G Rodgers

1 DEFINITION

Legionellae are nutritionally fastidious, non-spore-forming, strictly aerobic, structurally gram-negative prokaryotes that grow as slender short rods but may form filaments following prolonged cultivation on bacteriological media. The cell wall is rich in branched-chain fatty acids and ubiquinones. They do not grow on traditional bacteriological media but require enriched agar supplemented with L-cysteine and ferric salts. Legionellae are usually motile by means of one or more polar or subpolar flagella. They do not utilize carbohydrates by oxidation or fermentation, are catalase-positive, and do not reduce nitrate. The G + C content of the DNA is 38–52 mol%. Legionellae are normal inhabitants of the fresh water environment and are pathogenic for humans.

The genus *Legionella* is the sole genus of the family Legionellaceae. There are numerous species and serogroups (Table 49.1) and they are members of the γ subgroup of the class Proteobacteria. The type species is *Legionella pneumophila* subsp. *pneumophila*.

2 HISTORICAL PERSPECTIVE

In the late summer of 1976, Legionnaires' disease entered the world stage and in doing so became the media event of the year. A series of unexplained cases of pneumonia was reported among attendees at a United States bicentennial celebration convention held by the Pennsylvania branch of the American Legion in Philadelphia in July 1976. Of the 184 legionnaires who developed disease, 29 died from the complications of pneumonia as did a further 5 individuals who, although not legionnaires, were none the less associated with the hotel where the convention was held (Fraser et al. 1977). This event ushered in not only a new species of human pathogen, but an entirely new family of hitherto unrecognized bacteria known collectively as the legionellae. The aetiological agent of the disease was isolated and identified (McDade et al. 1977) and named *Legionella pneumophila* for this outbreak and for the association of the organism with lung disease (Brenner, Steigerwalt and McDade 1979).

The agent gained enhanced notoriety as a result of a number of spectacular outbreaks which followed the initial descriptions. Retrospective serological studies revealed that epidemics of the disease had occurred more than 30 years earlier although at the time they were believed to be due to rickettsia-like organisms (McDade, Brenner and Bozeman 1979). Other investigations of a similar nature revealed that the organism was also the cause of a relatively mild, self-limiting, influenza-like illness called Pontiac fever (Glick et al. 1978). These 2 disparate conditions, collectively referred to as legionellosis, are apparently caused by phenotypically and genotypically identical strains of legionellae. Pontiac fever presents in otherwise healthy individuals as pleuritic pain in the absence of pneumonic or multisystem manifestations. The condition carries a short incubation period, a high attack rate but a very low mortality ratio (Table 49.2). Unlike Pontiac fever, Legionnaires' disease afflicts those with severe underlying disease such as lymphoma, leukaemia, pulmonary distress, congestive heart failure and acquired immune deficiency syndrome (AIDS); cigarette smoking and excessive use of alcohol are contributing factors. In the wake of the initial discovery came a plethora of problems associated with

Table 49.1 Phenotypic properties of the legionellae[a]

Species	Sero-groups	Isolated from		β-Lac-tamase	Oxi-dase	Hippu-rate	Gelatin	Brown pigment	Auto-fluor-escence	Motil-ity
		Humans	Environ-ment							
L. pneumophila[b]	14	+	+	+	V	+	+	+	–	+
L. adelaidensis	1	–	+	–	–	–	+	–	–	+
L. anisa	1	+	+	+	+	–	+	+	BW(V)	+
L. birminghamensis	1	+	–	+	V	–	+	–	YG	+
L. bozemanii[c]	2	+	+	V	V	–	+	+	BW	+
L. brunensis	1	–	+	+	–	–	+	+[e]	–	+
L. cincinnatiensis	1	+	–	–	+	–	+	+	–	+
L. cherrii	1	–	+	+	+	–	+	+	BW	+
L. dumoffii[c]	1	+	+	+	–	–	+	V	BW	+
L. erythra	2	–	+	+	+	–	+	+	R	+
L. fairfieldensis	1	–	+	–	+[e]	–	–	–	–	–
L. feeleii	2	+	+	–	–	V	–	+[e]	–	+
L. geestiae	1	–	+	–	–	+[e]	+	+[e]	–	+
L. gormanii[c]	1	+	+	+	–	–	+	+	BW	+
L. gratiana	1	–	+	+	+	–	+	–	–	+
L. hackeliae	2	+	–	+	+	–	+	+	–	+
L. israelensis	1	+	+	+	–	–	+[e]	+	–	+
L. jamestowniensis	1	–	+	+	–	–	+	+	–	+
L. jordanis	1	+	+	+	+	–	+	+	–	+
L. lansingensis	1	+	–	–	+	–	–	–	–	+
L. londoniensis	1	–	+	+	–	–/+[e]	+	+	–	–
L. longbeachae	2	+	–	V	+	–	+	+	–	+
L. maceachernii	1	+	+	–	+	–	+	+	–	+
L. micdadei[d]	1	+	+	–	+	–	–	–	–	+
L. moravica	1	–	+	+	+[e]	–	+	+[e]	–	+
L. nautarum	1	–	+	+	+	–	–	–	–	–
L. oakridgensis	1	+	+	+[e]	–	–	+	+	–	+
L. parisiensis	1	+	+	+	+	–	+	+	BW	+
L. quarteriensis	1	–	+	+	–	–	+	+	–	+
L. quinlivanii	2	–	+	–	–	–	+	+	–	+
L. rubrilucens	1	–	+	+	–	–	+	+	R	+
L. sainthelensi	2	+	+	+	+	–	+	+	–	+
L. santicrusis	1	–	+	+	+	+	+	+	–	+
L. shakespearei	1	–	+	–	+[e]	–	+	–	–	+
L. spiritensis	2	–	+	+	+	+[e]	+	+	–	+
L. steigerwaltii	1	–	+	+	–	–	+	+	BW	+
L. tucsonensis	1	+	–	+	–	–	+	–	BW	+
L. wadsworthii	1	+	–	+	–	–	+	–	–	+
L. worsliensis	1	–	+	+	–	–	+	+	–	+

[a]All strains are catalase-positive (*L. hackliae*, *L. londoniensis* and *L. worsliensis* are weakly positive), all fail to reduce nitrate, do not grow on unsupplemented blood agar and, with the exception of laboratory adapted strains of *L. oakridgensis*, none grows on BCYE agar without L-cysteine. *L. pneumophila*, *L. micdadei*, *L. feeleii* and *L. anisa* have been associated with Pontiac fever.
[b]*L. pneumophila* contains 3 subspecies: *L. pneumophila* subspecies *pneumophila* (the type species of the group); subspecies *pascullei*; and subspecies *fraseri*.
[c]*Fluoribacter* has been proposed as an alternative genus name for these species.
[d]*Tatlockia* has been proposed as an alternative genus name for this species.
[e]Some strains are weakly positive only.
V, variable; BW, blue/white fluorescence; YG, yellow/green fluorescence; R, red fluorescence.
Table adapted from Rodgers and Pasculle (1991).

developing effective means for the clinical management of the disease and for the detection of the organism, as well as for the need to generate effective therapeutic regimens and evolve preventive strategies to combat infection. The ensuing years have seen much progress in these various areas but much remains to be determined, particularly concerning the interaction of the microbe with the host's immune system and in the area of vaccine development. In addition, our understanding of the pathogenesis, molecular biology and natural history of these fascinating microorganisms is far from complete.

Table 49.2 Clinical differentiation of legionellosis

	Legionnaires' disease	Pontiac fever
Incubation period (days)	2–10	1–2
Attack rate (%)	1–5	95
Case-fatality ratio (%)	0–20	0
Named for	Philadelphia outbreak, 1976	Pontiac outbreak, 1968
Clinical syndrome	Pneumonia[a]	Non-pneumonic
Symptoms common to both	Fever, cough, headache, confusion, chest pains, nausea, malaise, diarrhoea and vomiting	
Symptoms unique to each	Dyspnoea, haemoptysis, upper respiratory tract infection, sputum production, abdominal pain	Pleuritic pain
Other organs affected	Central nervous system, gastrointestinal tract, kidneys	None

[a]Incidence rates vary but range from 1 to 30% of all pneumonias.
Table adapted from Rodgers and Pasculle (1991).

3 CLINICAL AND EPIDEMIOLOGICAL FINDINGS

3.1 The disease

Following an incubation period of 2–10 days, Legionnaires' disease manifests as an acute lobar pneumonia eventually progressing to extrapulmonary symptoms and multisystem failure (Bailey, Murray and Finegold 1985, Fang et al. 1990). Early symptoms include headache, generalized weakness, fever, myalgia, rigors and a non-productive cough. Bloody or purulent sputum may be produced late in the disease along with advancing respiratory complications. Dyspnoea, fatigue, râles, bradycardia, haemoptysis, bacteraemia and extrapulmonary abnormalities are common. Central nervous system dysfunction, involvement of the heart, spleen, bone marrow, brain, lymph nodes and renal system (Monforte et al. 1989, Armengol, Domingo and Mesalles 1992) as well as cellulitis (Waldor, Wilson and Swartz 1993) have been documented, and symptoms of disorientation, confusion, nausea, vomiting, renal insufficiency and diarrhoea are common. Laboratory investigation shows elevations in the erythrocyte sedimentation rates, creatine levels and liver function profiles in the absence of jaundice, as well as hyponatraemia, haematuria, azotaemia, proteinuria and pancytopenia (Table 49.3). Acute renal failure, disseminated intravascular coagulation, shock, respiratory insufficiency, coma and circulatory collapse are the major factors precipitating death. Pulmonary x-rays show pleural effusions, patchy infiltrates and dense consolidation that develop rapidly after the onset of symptoms. Radiological changes may be extensive, bilateral and slow to resolve. If the disease is severe, diffuse multilobar involvement of the lungs is common with focal or lobar consolidation presenting as either red or grey hepatization.

Table 49.3 Clinical abnormalities and symptoms

Symptoms and signs
Pyrexia (>39°C)
Viral prodrome
Headache
Malaise
Confusion
Cough (usually non-productive)
Pleuritic pain
Tachypnoea
Chills
Bradycardia
Dyspnoea
Anorexia
Râles
Tachycardia
Dehydration
Diarrhoea

Laboratory abnormalities
Hyponatraemia (<130 mм l^{-1})
Albuminaemia (<25 g l^{-1})
Raised ESR (>60 mm h^{-1})
Lymphocytes (<1000 mm^{-3})
Elevated urea (>10 mм l^{-1})
Haematuria
Abnormal liver function tests (typically twice normal values)
  Alkaline phosphatase (up to 300 IU l^{-1})
  Lactate dehydrogenase (up to 600 IU l^{-1})
  SGOT (up to 150 IU l^{-1})

x-Ray abnormalities
x-Ray deterioration
Patchy infiltrate
Consolidation of the lungs

3.2 Epidemiology

For Legionnaires' disease the attack rate is low and the case-to-fatality ratio varies considerably but is lowest among those for whom antibiotic therapy and aggressive management are initiated early in infection (Macfarlane et al. 1982, Woodhead et al. 1985). Males are more likely to acquire disease than are females, and infections in children are rare. Although predisposing factors include increased age, heavy smoking, underlying disease and recent major surgery, the status of the immune system at the time of infection is critical to the severity and outcome of disease (O'Mahony et al. 1990). Indeed, the prognosis is poor for those who are immunocompromised or have T cell system dysfunctions. The progression of disease is a complex multifactorial phenomenon with organism- and host-related factors playing critical roles. Although repeat infections have been recorded, and the possibility of persistent low grade infections in lung cells cannot be ruled out, a carrier state for this organism has not been reported.

Legionnaires' disease shows a world-wide incidence and accounts for 1–4% of all cases of diagnosed pneumonia, although rates as high as 30% have been reported (Macfarlane et al. 1982, Fang et al. 1990). The incidence of Pontiac fever is poorly understood. Although 1000–1300 cases of Legionnaires' disease are reported in the USA each year to the Centers for Disease Control and Prevention, this may reflect a major underestimate in the incidence of this condition. Aggressive laboratory-based investigations have resulted in increased detection; however, whether this is due to a greater awareness of the condition or to a *de facto* rise in the incidence of the disease is not clear. Asymptomatic seroconversions are not common and result from rare subclinical infections and low grade cases of Pontiac fever. Person-to-person spread does not occur. Disease not only occurs in spectacular outbreaks associated with hospitals, hotels and large building complexes, but may also be sporadic, nosocomial and community-acquired. The infectious dose is unknown. Acquisition of the disease is due to the inhalation of aerosolized water contaminated with *Legionella* organisms, major sources of which include air-conditioning evaporative condensers, cooling tower effluent, humidifiers, nebulizers, potable and hot water supplies, domestic and hospital showerheads, whirlpool spas, decorative fountains and vegetable misting machines (Arnow et al. 1982, Bartlett, Macrae and Macfarlane 1986, Mahoney et al. 1992). The disease shows a higher summer incidence due presumably to increased contact with the natural habitat of the organism.

4 HABITAT

Numerous species of *Legionella* have been isolated from a wide range of fresh water habitats including ground water, rivers, lakes and natural thermal pools (Fliermans 1985, Bartlett, Macrae and Macfarlane 1986). Isolates have also been obtained from moist potting soils, mud, river banks and rain water run-off. Despite this, organisms do not normally occur in high numbers in the aquatic environment; however, it is by entry from these sources into man-made water supplies that the hot water systems in hospitals, hotels, cooling towers and other large buildings are colonized. Long-term survival of the organism in tap water has been reported (Yee and Wadowski 1982). Although humans are readily infected, they are inopportune hosts affording no ecological advantage to the organism. Delivery of the agent to the respiratory tract in the form of water droplets 5–15 μm in diameter serve as the primary vehicle for disease induction, whereas the presence of cyanobacteria, flavobacteria, algae and other micro-organisms may serve either to stabilize the organisms in aerosols or to stimulate their growth (Tison et al. 1980, Wadowski and Yee 1985, States et al. 1987).

As with many other bacterial pathogens, the survival of legionellae in water supplies depends heavily on the efficacy of chlorination protocols (Fisher-Hoch et al. 1981, Bartlett, Macrae and Macfarlane 1986) and on the maintenance of sufficiently high water temperatures (Dennis, Green and Jones 1984, Alary and Joly 1992). Care is required in designing the plumbing systems of new buildings and those undergoing modification in order to reduce dead space volumes and sediment buildup and prevent stagnation, conditions favourable to the growth of legionellae. In addition, the nature of the materials used in the construction of plumbing systems may enhance the colonization, growth or survival of legionellae in these water supplies. The organism is not considered a thermophile *per se*; however, it has been isolated from waters at temperatures as high as 60°C. Although the agent has been removed from water systems by raising the temperature of hot water in holding tanks, this elimination has usually proved temporary. The occurrence of *Legionella* organisms in water supplies does not necessarily lead to outbreaks of disease nor to an increased incidence of sporadic infections (Dennis et al. 1982); however, aerosols containing the organism do constitute a major risk factor for nosocomial infections and for those who are immunocompromised. The seriousness of the disease and the aerosol nature of its dissemination have resulted in an increased awareness of the need to detect and eradicate the organism from colonized water supplies, especially in hospitals. Culture of multiple decontaminated water samples on semiselective media and on buffered charcoal yeast extract (BCYE) agar should be made at regular intervals when cases of legionellosis occur, or if the presence of *Legionella* in water supplies is suspected. The use of commercially available nucleic acid probes and other detection methods may prove useful on concentrated water samples; however, the presence of other cross-reacting aquatic organisms renders direct immunofluorescence antibody (DFA) assay of little value. Since the organism is ubiquitous in water, it is essential for all isolates to be typed to species and epidemiological subgroup levels if an association is to be made between the organism in the water supply and that involved in cases of disease (Barbaree 1993).

The association of *L. pneumophila* with fresh water amoebae in the aquatic environment is well documented (Rowbotham 1980). The organism multiplies intracellularly in amoebae and ciliates belonging to the genera *Hartmanella, Acanthamoeba, Naegleria, Echinamoeba, Tetrahymena* and *Cyclidium* (Barbaree et al. 1986, Breiman et al. 1990), especially when water temperatures are elevated (Anand et al. 1983). Intracellular replication within protozoa may serve this otherwise nutritionally fastidious organism well by facilitating survival in the impoverished aquatic environment (Wadowski et al. 1988). As an incidental consequence of intraprotozoal survival, virulence for humans may be augmented in that protection is afforded to the organisms within protozoal cysts which show enhanced resistance to drying and to water treatment processes such as chlorination and heating. In addition, microbial numbers may be boosted in aerosols containing these protozoa. In this fashion, delivery of the pathogen in an amplified, protected and prepackaged aerosolized form to the lungs of susceptible individuals facilitates disease induction. Those processes that allow for the survival and replication of the organism within amoebae may be reflected in human alveolar macrophages (Rowbotham 1980, Barbaree et al. 1986). Indeed, it is possible that those mechanisms involved in the molecular recognition between legionellae and protozoa or macrophages are similar; in either case, uptake, intracellular replication and dissemination follow. A precise role in the infection of either protozoa or macrophages for toxins and other products expressed by *Legionella* or of host cell-generated surface receptor molecules remains to be elucidated.

5 MORPHOLOGY

By electron microscopy, *Legionella* organisms appear as short rods approximately 0.3–0.9 μm wide and 1–3 μm long (Rodgers, Macrae and Lewis 1978, Chandler et al. 1979, Rodgers, 1979). From human or experimentally infected tissues, the pathogen appears coccobacillary in shape but filamentous forms up to 50 μm in length occur after extended cultivation on bacteriological media. In general, the bacteria have non-parallel sides with tapering ends and, like many other gram-negative bacteria, they possess wrinkled or rugose surfaces and poly-β-hydroxybutyrate (PHB) granules;

they divide by a pinching, septate binary fission (Fig. 49.1). The organisms possess polar or subpolar flagella (Chandler et al. 1980, Rodgers et al. 1980). Flagella are unsheathed, 14–20 nm wide and up to 8 μm long (Fig. 49.2) and their expression is nutrient- and temperature-dependent (Rodgers et al. 1980, Ott et al. 1991b). Motile organisms have been observed in wet mounts as well as within phagosomes of infected cells. Under conditions of exponential growth in enriched media, the legionellae also possess fimbriae or pili (Fig. 49.3), each of which is 5–6 nm in width and 1–2 μm in length (Rodgers et al. 1980); however, the role in virulence of these extruded proteins is unknown.

Negative-staining, thin-sectioning, scanning, and freeze-fracture electron microscopy of *Legionella* organisms show a cellular architecture typical for other gram-negative prokaryotes and have been reviewed by Rodgers (1985). The presence of globular PHB granules in the organism was confirmed by

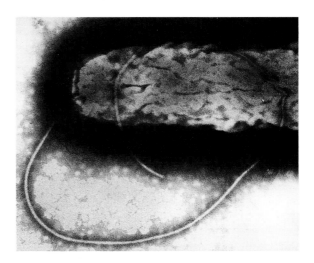

Fig. 49.2 Electron micrograph of *Legionella pneumophila* serogroup 5 stained with 1% phosphotungstic acid and showing the rugose surface of the organism and the polar attachment of a flagellum. Magnification × 66 000. (Reproduced with permission from Rodgers et al., 1980, *J Clin Pathol*, **33**: 1184–8).

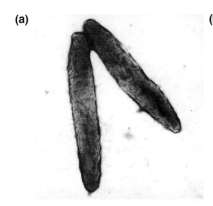
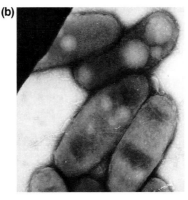

Fig. 49.1 *Legionella pneumophila* organisms negatively stained with 1% phosphotungstic acid. (a) Bloomington 2 organisms showing tapered ends and rugose surfaces. Magnification × 12 600. (b) Nottingham N7 organisms showing poly-β-hydroxybutyrate granules; fine fimbriae are also evident. Magnification × 21 000. (Reproduced with permission from Rodgers and Davey, 1982, *J Gen Microbiol*, **128**: 1547–57).

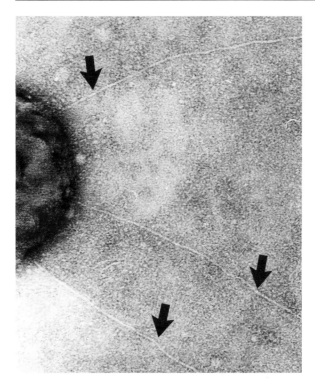

Fig. 49.3 Part of a *Legionella pneumophila* organism showing fimbriae (arrows). Stained with 1% phosphotungstic acid. Magnification × 126 000. (Reproduced with permission from Rodgers et al., 1979, *Lancet*, **2**: 753–4).

Sudan black B staining and by freeze-fracture electron microscopy. During active growth, the cytoplasm of the bacterium is rich in dispersed ribosomes each 25 nm in diameter and intermixed with a fine skein of nuclear elements. The limiting cell envelope of the organism is approximately 25 nm in thickness and comprises the periplasm located between the outer and cytoplasmic membranes, each measuring 7–10 nm. Like many of the aquatic pseudomonads, the legionellae possess a peptidoglycan cell wall that is best visualized after partial plasmolysis. A well defined capsule or glycocalyx has not been consistently reported. It should be noted, however, that individual bacteria located within the cytoplasm of infected cells are frequently surrounded by an electron-lucent zone of variable thickness suggestive of a microcapsule or slime layer. The presence of such a layer may have implications for virulence.

6 CULTURAL CHARACTERISTICS AND GROWTH REQUIREMENTS

BCYE agar with added L-cysteine, ferric pyrophosphate, α-ketoglutarate and N-2-acetamido-2-amino-ethanesulphonic acid (ACES) buffer is the medium most widely used for organism isolation (Feeley et al. 1979, Nash and Krenz 1991). A broth medium that is formulated from the same components as BCYE, but without the agar and charcoal and which is filter sterilized, also supports the growth of legionellae. After inoculation onto BCYE agar, small *Legionella* colonies

can be visualized after 2 days of incubation at 35°C using a dissecting microscope and by 3–5 days with the unaided eye. On rare occasions, colonies appear after 24 h from specimens found to contain very large numbers of organisms. The colonies show a speckled opalescence resembling ground or cut glass and have a stringy consistency that makes them difficult to pick and subculture from agar. They are round with an entire edge, glistening, convex and measure 1–4 mm in diameter (Fig. 49.4; see also plate 49.4). During early growth, colonies show a pink or blue-green iridescence which disappears with prolonged incubation, by which time large and small colony variants develop; these are grey-white in colour and appear more opaque as the ground glass and iridescent aspects diminish. At this stage, *Legionella* colonies lose their characteristic appearance and resemble those of other bacteria, but these can usually be differentiated by gram stain (Fig. 49.5; see also plate 49.5). Many species express a brown melanin-like pigment from D-phenylalanine or tyrosine (see Table 49.1). When exposed to long-wave UV light at 366 nm, the colonies of some *Legionella* spp. autofluoresce brilliant blue-white whereas *L. pneumophila* is not autofluorescent (Fig. 49.6; see also plate 49.6) and yet other species appear red or yellow-green (see Table 49.1).

For culture, the organism shows a remarkable requirement for iron and L-cysteine whereas α-ketoglutarate augments growth, and charcoal absorbs and detoxifies free fatty acids and depletes inhibitory oxygen radicals otherwise toxic to the organism (Hoffman, Pine and Bell 1983). The presence of amino acids, trace metals and a humid atmosphere containing CO_2 stimulates growth. The organism has been isolated from thermal lagoons and cooling tower plumes at temperatures in excess of 60°C and generally grows well over a relatively wide temperature range. However, for cultivation on bacteriological media, a rather narrow pH range is optimal, and media should be buffered to pH 6.85–6.95. In addition, bright lights should be avoided during media preparation to discourage the buildup of

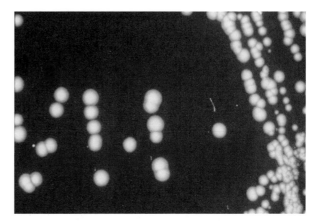

Fig. 49.4 Colonies of *Legionella pneumophila* serogroup 1, strain Nottingham N7 after 4 days of incubation on BCYE agar. A pink and blue iridescence can be seen at the periphery of colonies. See plate 49.4 for colour.

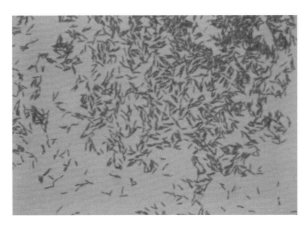

Fig. 49.5 Gram stain of *Legionella pneumophila* after cultivation on bacteriological media. The preparation was counterstained with carbol fuchsin and shows slender gramnegative rods with tapered ends. See plate 49.5 for colour.

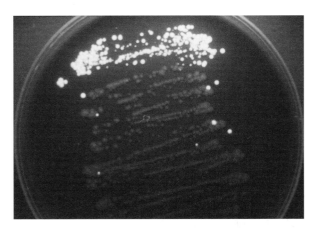

Fig. 49.6 Colonies of *Legionella pneumophila* serogroup 1, strain Nottingham N7 and *Legionella bozemanii* serogroup 1 grown on BCYE agar and illuminated with long-wave UV light at 366 nm. *L. bozemanii* colonies autofluoresce brilliant blue-white whereas those of *L. pneumophila* do not autofluoresce (see Table 49.1). See plate 49.6 for colour.

inhibitory peroxides (Hoffman, Pine and Bell 1983). Incorporation of 1% albumin into isolation and growth media enhances the isolation rate for some *Legionella* spp. including *Legionella micdadei* (Morrill et al. 1990), whereas glycine is useful for the cultivation of environmental isolates (Wadowski and Yee 1981), and bromocresol purple and bromothymol blue may assist in differentiating species (Vickers, Brown and Garrity 1981).

7 METABOLISM

Legionellae are oligotrophs and utilize amino acids rather than carbohydrates as energy sources (Tesh, Morse and Miller 1983) with sugars neither oxidized nor fermented. Glucose catabolism is achieved through the Entner–Doudoroff and pentose phosphate pathways, whereas the Krebs cycle facilitates carbon assimilation, and the gluconeogenic anabolic

enzymes of the Embden–Meyerhof pathway are responsible for sugar synthesis (Hoffman and Pine 1982). Although there are some differences in amino acid requirements between species, subspecies and strains, the amino acids arginine, cysteine, methionine, serine, threonine and valine are required as essential nutrients by all isolates, whereas other strains also need isoleucine, leucine, phenylalanine and tyrosine for growth (George et al. 1980, Tesh and Miller 1981). Proline, glutamate and glutathione have also been found to stimulate the growth of some *Legionella* strains. In keeping with the use of the Krebs cycle as the major energy-producing pathway through amino acid catabolism, the activity of NADH in the organism is high (Hoffman 1984). The presence of calcium, cobalt, copper, magnesium, manganese, molybdenum, nickel, vanadium and zinc in trace amounts all enhance bacterial growth (Reeves et al. 1981), but sodium chloride is inhibitory.

Legionellae do not possess siderophores (Reeves et al. 1983, Hoffman 1984), but they do show an absolute requirement for iron. Although the organism will grow well at iron concentrations of 0.5 μM, excess amounts are usually needed in order to achieve optimal growth of the organism and for the efficient operation of bacterial enzymes, ferredoxins and cytochromes. Iron is also involved in the bacterial processes of electron transport, regulation of gene expression and oxygen metabolism. Intracellular replication of the organism occurs during disease, and iron is essential for this process; hence iron chelators such as apolactoferrin inhibit intracellular growth of the organism. Ferritin, lactoferrin and transferrin serve as the major sources of iron for host cells. However, unbound iron is not readily available in the tissues, the plasma or the intracellular milieu of alveolar target cells and, as a consequence, it has been suggested that the organism obtains the iron it needs from the intermediate labile iron pool in free form through the action of the microbial enzyme iron reductase (Johnson, Varner and Poch 1991). One possible role for L-cysteine is that during auto-oxidation in the presence of ferric iron, soluble iron may be made more readily available to the bacterium. It has been suggested that ferritin may serve to recycle iron to the iron pool available to the organism within macrophages by undergoing degradation and releasing iron in the lysosomes (Mengaud and Horwitz 1993); however, the precise mechanism by which the element is taken up by the organism is not clear. The 85–90 kDa major iron-containing protein (MICP) in the organism is analogous with aconitase from *Escherichia coli* (Horwitz 1993). L-Cysteine is needed for incorporation into proteins by the organism, but the lack of 2 key biosynthetic enzymes, serine transacetylase and *o*-acetylserine sulphydrylase, responsible for the conversion of serine to cysteine, results in the need for added amounts of this amino acid (Hoffman 1984). These enzymes are present in *Legionella oakridgensis*, which does not require added cysteine after initial isolation.

The organisms are obligate aerobes and are catalase- and superoxide dismutase-positive, weakly peroxidase-positive, oxidase-variable and possess the cytochromes *a–d*. Nitrates are not reduced and urea is not hydrolysed. With few exceptions, the various species of *Legionella* liquefy gelatin. The positive hippurate hydrolysis of *L. pneumophila* forms a useful means to differentiate this species from many of the other members of the genus (see Table 49.1).

8 GENETIC ANALYSIS

8.1 DNA homology

The genome of the various species of *Legionella* is approximately 2.5×10^6 kDa (3900 kb) and possesses a G + C range of 38–52 mol% with the vast majority of species lying between 38 and 46 mol%. Based on DNA homology techniques, the legionellae are distinguishable from and unrelated to other bacterial genera. Indeed, following the initial isolation of *L. pneumophila*, DNA homology studies were used to determine that the organism constituted not only a new genus, but also a new bacterial family (Brenner, Steigerwalt and McDade 1979). With few exceptions, DNA relatedness is high (up to 99%) between strains and serogroups for individual species, but ranges from 1 to 67% between different species within the genus (Brenner et al. 1985). *L. pneumophila* was cleaved into 3 subspecies (see Table 49.1) based on a much reduced DNA homology of 2 of the new subspecies to the type strain Philadelphia 1 (Selander et al. 1985, Brenner et al. 1988). This divergence in DNA homology was further confirmed by reported differences in enzyme profiles and amino acid requirements for these subspecies. Some degree of genotypic and phenotypic heterogeneity has been reported between groups of legionellae, and although such variations may have future epidemiological significance, currently these do not correlate with either disease expression or species characterization. Indeed, given the relative similarity in phenotypic characteristics, definitive identification of new species of *Legionella* continues to depend on DNA homology studies.

8.2 Plasmids and genetic transfer

Plasmids ranging in size from 21 000 to 85 000 kDa have been reported from both clinical and environmental strains and serogroups (Brown et al. 1982, Nolte et al. 1984, Daaka et al. 1994) and, although the presence of such plasmids may be useful for the molecular differentiation of isolates for epidemiological purposes, there would seem to be little conclusive evidence that plasmids are associated with either enhanced or reduced virulence. The introduction of DNA into *L. pneumophila* has been achieved by transformation using electroporation, by conjugation and by transduction (Chen, Lema and Brown 1984, Dreyfus and Iglewski 1985, High and Rodgers 1991, Marra and Shuman 1992, Engleberg 1993), but cloning of *L. pneumophila* genes into *E. coli* has proved more fruitful in characterizing genes, especially those

involved in virulence. Perhaps the most intensively studied is the highly conserved *mip* gene that encodes the 29 kDa macrophage infectivity potentiator (MIP) protein that is essential for *Legionella* virulence (Engleberg 1993). The *proA* and *lly* genes are each responsible for the expression of the bacterial 38 kDa protease and 39 kDa haemolysin. Although toxic for the host, neither of these proteins plays a crucial role in intracellular replication in macrophages. Other genes, some of which have been DNA sequenced, are responsible for the expression of a variety of organism-associated and secreted proteins of the pathogen, and many have been cloned into *E. coli* and their role in virulence suggested (Table 49.4).

9 ANTIGENIC STRUCTURE

Legionellae express a variety of antigens including somatic, flagellar and outer-membrane protein antigens; however, the 2 major antigens recognized in serological assays are the lipopolysaccharide (LPS) and the cytoplasmic membrane-associated heat shock protein (Gabay and Horwitz 1985, Gabay et al. 1985). LPS from the organism is of the smooth type and functions as a weak endotoxin. The heterogeneity found in this complex molecule accounts for the diversity of the serogroups across the legionellae (see Table 49.1). LPS comprises a membrane-associated lipid portion that is rich in branched-chain fatty acids and tightly associated with the major outer-membrane protein (MOMP), a polysaccharide complex consisting of glucose, rhamnose, mannose, quinovosamine, 2-keto-3-deoxyoctonate (KDO) and glucosamine and the O-antigenic side chain which is responsible for the characteristic ladder-like banding appearance in SDS-PAGE gels as well as for the serogroup specificity detected in sera (Sonesson et al. 1989, Knirel et al. 1994, Helbig et al. 1995). It is heat-stable, pronase-resistant and stimulates interferon-γ and other cytokines. In addition, *L. pneumophila* has been shown to produce a number of potent cytotoxic exoproteases and these exacerbate the pneumonic illness by interrupting host cell oxidative metabolism, suppressing phagocytosis and inducing cytolysis.

Many legionellae share common flagella antigens. Indeed, antiserum prepared against *L. pneumophila* serogroup 1 flagella agglutinates flagellated strains of serogroups 1, 2 and 3 (Elliot and Johnson 1981). Rodgers and Laverick (1984) showed that antibodies against various *Legionella* spp. reacted in a passive haemagglutination assay against flagellar antigen prepared from *L. pneumophila* serogroup 1, suggesting that many *Legionella* spp. share common flagellar antigens. The use of flagella-specific antisera may be useful in detecting new or uncommon species or serogroups of *Legionella*. The sharing of heat-stable antigens among different serogroups of *L. pneumophila* has proved problematic in serological assays, but these have to some extent been obviated by the development of newer, molecular approaches used to redefine the interrelationship between these organisms.

Table 49.4 Virulence potentiating factors from *Legionella pneumophila*[a]

Virulence factor	Molecular mass (kDa)	Gene	Function
Macrophage infectivity potentiator protein (MIP)	24	*mip*	Macrophage internalization protein Inhibits protein kinase C Highly conserved
Heat shock protein (HSP)	58	*htpAB*	Genus common; porin molecule Major cytoplasmic membrane protein
Major outer-membrane protein (MOMP)	24–29	*ompM*	Involved in phagocytosis Binds complement C3 Closely associated with LPS
Zinc metalloprotease (MSP)	38	*proA*	Major tissue and cell damaging protein Major secretory protein Cytotoxic for cells and tissues May be 1.3 kDa subcomponent of protease
Flagella (flagellin)	47	*flaA*	Motility; common to many serogroups and species
Haemolysin/legiolysin	39	*lly*	Haemolysis
Peptidoglycan-associated lipoprotein (PAL)	19	*pal (plpAB)*	Immunogenic
Phospholipase C	50–54	●●●	Hydrolyses phosphotidylcholine

[a]Lipopolysaccharide serves as a weak endotoxin and is responsible for the serogroup reactions in detection assays. Fimbriae (pili) may play a role in adherence in vivo and/or in the environment.

10 TAXONOMY AND CLASSIFICATION

The legionellae comprise a single taxonomic group of related organisms. Following the 1976 outbreak of Legionnaires' disease, the causal agent, isolated by McDade and colleagues (1977), was shown to be a hitherto unrecognized human pathogen. The result was the establishment of a novel taxonomic group comprising a new family, the *Legionellaceae*, containing a single genus, *Legionella*, and one species, *pneumophila*. In the succeeding years the group has expanded at a staggering rate with approximately 2 new species added to the genus each year, resulting in a group containing 39 species, 3 subspecies and 60 serogroups (see Table 49.1). Following the initial isolation of the pathogen, it became clear that these agents occurred in the aquatic environment and in association with human disease and to date, 13 of the known species have been isolated from human origin and the environment, 7 from human disease only and, reflecting the aquatic nature of the organisms, 20 from the environment only (see Table 49.1).

Early in the course of investigations on these organisms and their relationship to other bacteria, the critical role of DNA homology as a tool to differentiate and classify these species became evident (Brenner, Steigerwalt and McDade 1979). Based on autofluorescence of colonies exposed to long-wave ultraviolet radiation, Garrity, Brown and Vickers (1980) suggested taxonomically subdividing the group into 3 genera: *Legionella*, *Tatlockia* and *Fluoribacter*. However, this has not been broadly accepted, nor is it supported by 16S rRNA analysis (Fry et al. 1991).

11 LABORATORY DETECTION AND IDENTIFICATION

Despite the large number of species and serogroups within the *Legionellaceae*, the vast majority of disease is of a single aetiology and is caused by *L. pneumophila* serogroup 1 (50%), serogroup 6 (10%), other serogroups of *L. pneumophila* (20%), or *L. micdadei* (5%). Detection by culture of the organisms on bacteriological media shows about a 60–75% sensitivity but is 100% specific. Antigen detection methods and serological procedures to identify antibodies in sera have been developed and these show varying degrees of specificity, sensitivity, ease of performance and cost-effectiveness (Harrison and Taylor 1988, Edelstein 1993). The use of monoclonal or polyclonal antibodies adds specificity to antigen detection systems in the DFA, enzyme-linked immunosorbent assay (ELISA), radioimmunoassay (RIA) and latex agglutination tests. In addition, the use of monoclonal antibodies has proved effective for subgrouping the legionellae, especially for epidemiological purposes, but newer molecular techniques are gaining favour. Nucleic acid probe technology has also proved useful for detection. The sensitivity of these diagnostic tests ranges between 60 and 90%, whereas the specificity approaches 99% (Table 49.5). Despite the plethora of tests available, cultivation of *Legionella* on agar-based media is the mainstay of laboratory diagnosis.

11.1 Culture

Although the organism is frequently found in the aquatic environment in the absence of infection, it does not occur in humans in the absence of disease. Hence, culture of legionellae from clinical specimens equates with infection and constitutes the 'gold standard' for diagnosis. Sensitivity of culture varies widely depending upon the laboratory attempting isolation, but a survey of clinical microbiology laboratories in the USA in 1989 indicated that only 32% were able to isolate a pure culture of *L. pneumophila* present in the sample in large numbers (Edelstein 1993). Growth on BCYE but not on 'routine' bacteriological media is a presumptive characteristic of *Legionella*. Safety precautions as well as the collection and handling of specimens used for isolation from clinical and environmental sources have been reviewed by Harrison and Taylor (1988) and by Rodgers and Pasculle (1991).

Selective media have been developed for the cultivation of *Legionella* organisms from clinical and environmental specimens that are likely to contain other microbes. The 2 most widely used are based on BCYE agar and contain cephamandole, polymyxin B and anisomycin (Edelstein 1981, Nash and Krenz 1991) or glycine, vancomycin, polymyxin B and anisomycin (Wadowski and Yee 1981, Nash and Krenz 1991). As these antibiotics are somewhat inhibitory to legionellae, growth is slower following inoculation onto these media. Putative *Legionella* isolates, especially from outbreaks, should be subcultured and identified to species and serogroup levels. Media should be quality controlled and routinely challenged on a regular basis with isolates from clinical or experimentally infected tissues.

Sputum and lung tissue should be diluted to reduce the impact of inhibitors, but pleural and lavage fluids should be concentrated by centrifugation. Environmental samples likewise should be concentrated by centrifugation or filtration methods. Should the presence of contaminating organisms be suspected or prove problematic, specimens can be treated with HCl (pH 2) for 5–20 min depending upon the levels of contamination or to a temperature of 50°C for 30 min or 60°C for 1–3 min (Buesching, Brust and Ayers 1983, Harrison and Taylor 1988, Rodgers and Pasculle 1991). Blood cultures should be taken from hospitalized patients with pneumonia, as the presence of the organism in the blood equates with infection. Smears of clinical specimens should be prepared for DFA, but for environmental samples these are of little use.

11.2 Molecular approaches

Various 'in-house' nucleic acid probes, developed for the detection of *L. pneumophila* in clinical and environmental samples, have been used to identify and type strains for which clear results are not available by other methods (Harrison and Taylor 1988). A commercial *Legionella*-specific DNA probe is available and offers an acceptable alternative to DFA but not to culture. The assay is relatively easy to perform, is cost-effective when sufficient specimen numbers merit its use, detects a wide range of *Legionella* spp. and detects approximately 10^3 cfu with a specificity of 99% and a sensitivity of 50–60% (Harrison and Taylor 1988, Edelstein 1993). A short half-life ^{125}I-labelled cDNA probe is used to hybridize with the highly conserved 16S rRNA from *Legionella* and the resultant labelled RNA–DNA duplexes are assessed by γ-counter. Polymerase chain reaction (PCR) technology using the *mip* gene and the gene encoding 5S rRNA has been applied to *Legionella* DNA probes to improve their sensitivity (Mahbubani et al. 1990, Nowicki et al. 1993) but needs to be adapted for routine clinical and environmental use.

Nucleic acid probes and serological assays have been used to identify isolated colonies and various subtyping assays have been developed, including plasmid analysis with or without peptide assay (Nolte et al. 1984, Brown et al. 1985), multilocus enzyme electrophoresis (MEE) using cytoplasmic enzymes (Selander et al. 1985), ribotyping based on 16S and

Table 49.5 Assays used in the diagnosis of *Legionella* infections[a]

Test	Commercially available reagents or kits	Specificity (%)	Sensitivity (%)
Culture and isolation	Yes	100	60–75
Nucleic acid probes	Yes	>99	50–60
Immunoassays[b]			
ELISA	No	>99	70–90
Radioimmunoassay	Yes	>99	80–90
Latex agglutination	Yes	85–99	55–90
Serological diagnosis			
IFA	Yes	>99	70–80
Rapid microagglutination test	Yes	>99	80
Direct detection[c]			
DFA	Yes	>99	25–75

[a]Many assays can be used for both clinical and environmental purposes.
[b]Haemagglutination procedures have also been developed, but these are not in regular use.
[c]Direct gram, Gimenez, silver staining and electron microscopy may be used, but these have no specificity for *Legionella*.
Table adapted from Rodgers and Pasculle (1991).

23S rRNA probes (Grimont et al. 1989), restriction fragment length polymorphism (RFLP) using the restriction endonuclease *Nci*I followed by Southern blot and biotinylated probes (Harrison and Taylor 1988, Saunders et al. 1990) and pulse field gel electrophoresis (PFGE) (Ott et al. 1991a). Such procedures serve molecular epidemiology well by subtyping isolates from outbreaks and identifying the spread of strains from the aquatic environment to humans (Barbaree 1993).

11.3 Immunoassays

All immunoassays use a specific monoclonal or polyclonal antibody to probe for the presence of bacterial soluble antigens in specimens and have the potential advantage of generating rapid results (Harrison and Taylor 1988, Edelstein 1993). *Legionella* soluble antigens present in respiratory tract secretions, sputum, serum and especially in urine have been detected by ELISA, RIA, latex agglutination and rapid microagglutination tests with varying degrees of specificity and sensitivity (see Table 49.5). The basic difference between each assay lies in the method used to detect the antibody probe binding the antigens.

Antigens in specimens are either immobilized using an antibody capture technique or are passively bound to an inert substrate such as the wells of plastic microtitre plates or latex particles. In the ELISA test the probing antibody is coupled to an enzyme that is detected using a chromogenic substrate to produce a colour change, the presence of which indicates the enzyme-linked antibody and hence the *Legionella* antigens. RIA functions similarly but the probing antibody is linked to a radioactive label which is detected in a γ-counter. Latex agglutination is a somewhat less sensitive assay but is rapid and easy to perform. This test uses latex particles coated with *Legionella* antibody to capture antigens and agglutinate or clump the latex particles. Immunoassays depend heavily upon the specificity of the reagents and on the quality of specimens and time of collection during infection.

11.4 DFA

Detection and identification of organisms in clinical specimens have been made using the specific DFA test (Cherry et al. 1978). The specificity of this assay is close to 100%, but the sensitivity is 25–75%, and this, together with a high degree of cross-reactions to microbial species commonly found in clinical and environmental specimens, render it of limited value for clinical purposes and unsuitable for environmental work.

Specimens are heat dried to slides, formalin fixed, stained with *Legionella*-specific antibody conjugated to fluorescein-isothiocyanate (FITC) and examined by fluorescence microscopy. DFA-positive clinical specimens show bright green, peripherally fluorescent coccobacilli or rod-shaped bacteria (Fig. 49.7; see also plate 49.7) often associated with fluorescent debris derived from lysed infected macrophages and bacterial products (Rodgers and Pasculle 1991). If well controlled and carefully performed, the procedure is rapid

but is plagued by problems of sensitivity and applicability due to the numerous serotypes and species of *Legionella*. Specimens must be screened with polyvalent followed by monovalent antisera to identify the causal organism, further limiting the usefulness of the test. The use of monoclonal antibodies that react with group common antigens of *Legionella* has reduced these problems somewhat (Gosting et al. 1984). Despite this, DFA should always, whenever possible, be coupled with culture procedures.

11.5 Non-specific staining

Direct staining procedures are non-specific and have little value for detecting *Legionella* organisms in those clinical or environmental specimens contaminated with other microbes. Legionellae have been visualized in clinical specimens and tissue sections using various silver impregnation stains (Fig. 49.8; see also plate 49.8), gram (counter-stained with carbol fuchsin), Gram–Weigert, Gimenez, Giemsa and electron microscopy. By this latter technique, organisms have been detected within lytic foci, alveolar macrophages and polymorphonuclear leucocytes. It is interesting to note that *L. micdadei* stains weakly acid fast, whereas other species test negative.

11.6 Serological diagnosis

Serological diagnosis is achieved by detecting antibodies in sera from infected patients by the indirect immunofluorescent antibody test (IFAT) (Wilkinson, Cruce and Broome 1981) and by the rapid microagglutination test (RMAT) (Harrison and Taylor 1988). Furthermore, the data derived from the application of these tests have served as a useful epidemiological predictor for the incidence of legionellosis in the community. Complicating this, however, is the common occurrence of cross-reacting antibodies that may lead to false positive results, as has been reported for sera from individuals infected with species of *Pseudomonas*, *Proteus*, *Bacteroides*, *Flavobacterium*, *Haemophilus*, *Rickettsia* and other microbial pathogens as well as for sera

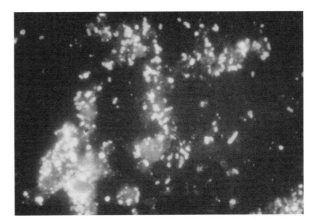

Fig. 49.7 Suspension smear from a postmortem lung specimen specifically stained with FITC-conjugated *Legionella* antiserum. Brightly fluorescing *Legionella* organisms are evident as are *Legionella* antigens released from lysed infected lung cells. See plate 49.7 for colour.

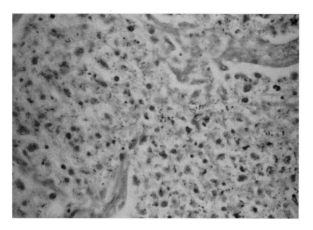

Fig. 49.8 *Legionella* pneumonia. Histological section stained non-specifically by Dieterle's silver impregnation technique. Darkly staining legionellae can be seen in association with pale staining lung cells. Such a result may be suggestive of Legionnaires' disease when a tissue gram stain is negative and no other pneumonic pathogens are isolated on routine bacteriological media. Antigen detection methods and culture for *Legionella* should be attempted. See plate 49.8 for colour.

from intravenous drug abusers. Such problems should be considered when evaluating the incidence of disease based on serological data.

To perform the test, dilutions of sera from individuals suspected of having Legionnaires' disease are allowed to react at 37°C on slides containing heat-inactivated agar-grown bacteria suspended in normal yolk sac or with formalin-fixed yolk sac-derived organisms. After washing, anti-human globulin conjugated to FITC is added, and the preparations are examined by fluorescence microscopy. As this serological diagnosis depends on determining the levels of *Legionella*-specific IgG, IgM or IgA in sera, the anti-human globulin used should be capable of detecting all classes of antibody that may be present in the serum. A positive result is indicated by the presence of brightly fluorescent bacteria, and the antibody titre is given as the highest serum dilution that shows discernible fluorescence. A drawback of the test is that infected individuals require a period of time for the immune system to mediate the development of antibodies and, as a consequence, the results are retrospective. A further disadvantage of IFAT is that the technique is labour-intensive and less suited to examining large numbers of specimens than are more automated procedures. In order to speed processing and reduce the burden of specimen screening, it is advocated that sera be examined at an initial dilution of 1:32 or 1:64 with positives selected for titration thereafter. For diagnosis, single serum samples are of less value than paired sera collected during the acute and convalescent phases of infection. However, as organisms are not carried in the absence of disease and as multiple infections are rare, antibody levels in the general population are low. As a consequence, a single serum titre of 1:128 or higher from a patient with a relevant clinical history may be suggestive of disease. Acute phase serum samples should be obtained within 1 week of onset of disease with convalescent phase sera collected 3–6 weeks later. A 4-fold increase in titre to 1:128 is considered significant (Wilkinson et al. 1983). To complicate the interpretation of results further, some patients do not seroconvert, whereas others maintain high antibody levels

for many years after the initial infection. Under ideal performance conditions, the specificity of this assay is close to 100%, the sensitivity is approximately 70–80%, and the predictive value is high (Wilkinson, Cruce and Broome 1981).

The RMAT functions in similar fashion to IFAT except that in this assay, dilutions of serum from each patient are allowed to react with heat-killed suspensions of the organism in V-bottomed microtitre plates; appropriate microagglutination patterns indicate the presence of antibody. This assay carries approximately the same specificity and sensitivity as IFAT (see Table 49.5), but it is somewhat less labour-intensive (Harrison and Taylor 1988). Immunodiffusion, counterimmunoelectrophoresis, indirect ELISA, immune adherence and haemagglutination procedures have all been applied to the serological diagnosis of legionellosis with varying degrees of success.

The use of serological assays for the diagnosis of Legionnaires' disease has proved most helpful in outbreak situations, but their effectiveness in detecting sporadic cases is less clear. In either case, serology should be used to augment diagnosis and should not be considered as a replacement for bacterial culture.

11.7 Identification

Once the organism has been isolated on bacteriological media, identification follows. From a clinical perspective, the various serogroups of *L. pneumophila* together with *L. micdadei* are the cause of most infections; therefore, a definitive identification of groups other than these is of epidemiological significance, as the therapy for legionellosis is similar irrespective of causal species.

Members of the *Legionellaceae* are asaccharolytic, and the various biochemical tests commonly used to identify non-*Legionella* bacteria in microbiology laboratories either give weak or variable results or are absent altogether. As a consequence, insufficient diversity of phenotypic characteristics occurs between the numerous species of the genus, so these are of little use for identification purposes. Incorporation of L-cysteine into isolation media is required for growth of the organism, and this phenomenon has proved useful for identification purposes. An isolate that is gram-negative, catalase-positive and grows on L-cysteine-enriched BCYE but not on blood agar or BCYE agar without L-cysteine can be tentatively identified as a member of the genus *Legionella*. However, this distinction remains presumptive, as a number of human pathogens other than legionellae may give similar results, and some may also cross-react with the *Legionella*-specific antisera in DFA assays (Benson et al. 1987, Roy, Fleming and Anderson 1989). In addition, some heterotrophic non-*Legionella* bacteria of environmental origin and thermophilic spore-forming bacilli (Thacker et al. 1981) show L-cysteine dependence. Clinical isolates provisionally identified in this fashion and which are hippurate hydrolysis positive are probably *L. pneumophila*, whereas those which are hippurate, brown pigment and gelatin negative, as well as bromocresol purple spot test positive, are probably *L. micdadei*. Colonies of some *Legionella* spp. autofluoresce when illuminated with long-wave UV light, whereas others do not (see Table 49.1). This property may prove useful in distinguishing some species of *Legionella*.

Genetic analysis using DNA hybridization is the definitive method for species identification and for the establishment of new *Legionella* spp. (Brenner, Steigerwalt and McDade 1979, Brenner et al. 1988). This procedure relies on assessing the degree of homology of the DNA from an unknown isolate with the radiolabelled DNA from well characterized species. The use of DFA, slide agglutination and other serological procedures using monoclonal and polyclonal antibodies enhances the identification process. Furthermore, selected restriction endonuclease digest profiles of the plasmids and DNA of *Legionella*, together with 16S rRNA analysis and the activity of bacterial cytoplasmic enzymes by MEE, have proved useful in characterizing isolates, especially for epidemiological purposes.

The cell wall of the legionellae, unlike most gram-negative bacteria, contains unusually high levels (>80%) of branched-chain fatty acids as shown by gas-liquid chromatography (GLC). Although there is some variation in profiles across the species, the fatty acids commonly abundant in *Legionella* strains are a-15:0-methyl-12-methyltetradecanoic acid, i-16:0-methyl-14-methylpentadecanoic acid and 16:1 methylhexadecanoic acid. In addition, using high performance liquid chromatography (HPLC), *Legionella* spp. were shown to possess a characteristic profile of isoprenoid quinones of the ubiquinone group located in the cytoplasmic membrane and involved in respiratory electron transport. The relative predominance of the ubiquinones Q9 through Q14 in each of the species, together with their fatty acid profiles, has been used effectively to identify and characterize *Legionella* isolates and to subdivide the genus into broad taxonomic groupings (Harrison and Taylor 1988, Lambert and Moss 1989).

To date, more species of *Legionella* have been isolated from environmental sources than from humans, but less is known concerning the ecological niche occupied by these bacteria and their relationship with other aquatic life. Furthermore, given the consistency with which the genus has grown over the years, our understanding concerning the diversity of organism populations within the *Legionella* group is far from complete.

12 SUSCEPTIBILITY TO PHYSICAL AND CHEMICAL AGENTS

12.1 Antibiotics

Legionella isolates are susceptible to many antimicrobial agents in vitro (Thornsberry, Baker and Kirven 1978, Edelstein and Myer 1980, Bailey, Murray and Finegold 1985); however, those antibiotics that prove clinically most effective possess high lipid solubility and hence a capacity to penetrate host cell membranes and attack the pathogen in the cytoplasm of infected target cells. Indeed, erythromycin, the drug of choice for the treatment of Legionnaires' disease, is taken up by macrophages and high concentrations are achieved intracellularly compared with the extracellular milieu (Johnson et al. 1980). Other antibiotics that have proved clinically effective include rifampicin, doxycycline, co-trimoxazole and members of the 5-fluoroquinolones. On the other hand, many antimicrobial agents, including the β-lactams and aminoglycosides, have no value in therapy despite effective minimum inhibitory concentration (MIC) values (Bailey, Murray and Finegold 1985). Many of these antibiotics have been shown to induce structural or lytic damage to the organism, but such effects are generally not sustained by the pathogen located within host cells. In addition, the various species of *Legionella* with a few exceptions produce a β-lactamase (see Table 49.1). Data from infected cell cultures and animal studies have suggested that some antibiotic combinations may act synergistically on intracellular bacteria, assisting in a more rapid clearance of the organism.

In the absence of effective therapy, prognosis is poor. Successful therapy is frequently defined by early diagnosis and an aggressive approach to patient management including the use of appropriate antibiotics, ventilation, renal dialysis, rehydration strategies and the correction of electrolyte imbalance (Macfarlane et al. 1982). However, relapse and treatment failures have been reported. Antibiotic regimens should include erythromycin with other drugs such as rifampicin added for severe cases of disease (Fraser et al. 1977, Macfarlane et al. 1982, Woodhead et al. 1985). In immunocompromised individuals the death rate is relatively high despite appropriate therapy. A lack of correlation between the effectiveness of antibiotics in clinical use and in laboratory assessments and difficulties in standardizing MIC tests for this organism have made drug susceptibility testing in the laboratory problematic. As a consequence, the use of cell cultures infected with clinical isolates of *L. pneumophila* has been advocated for evaluating the effectiveness of potentially useful antibiotics (Vilde, Dournon and Rajagopalan 1986, Havlichek, Saravolatz and Pohold 1987). However, such procedures are normally beyond the scope of the routine clinical microbiology laboratory.

12.2 Other agents and control measures

Under laboratory conditions, the legionellae are quite susceptible to a wide variety of inactivation protocols. The organism is inactivated readily by drying, and optimal survival in aerosols occurs in atmospheres of relatively high humidity (Berendt 1980). The thermal killing of legionellae varies widely depending upon the conditions and the strains used, but it was reported in one study that a population of *L. pneumophila* organisms received a $\log_{10}$ reduction in numbers in 6 min at 58°C (Dennis, Green and Jones 1984). In addition, *L. pneumophila* organisms were readily inactivated by exposure to 1.25 ppm of chlorine in 15 min and by 5 ppm in 1 min (Wang et al. 1979), and at these concentrations the electron transport of the organism was impaired and cell lysis induced. Organism killing within 1 min was also noted following treatment with 10 ppm iodophor, hydrochloric acid at pH 1.7, 70% ethanol, 0.05% phenolic and 2% formalin or glutaraldehyde (Wang et al. 1979). A 99% reduction in *L. pneumophila* bacterial cell numbers was effected in 5 min using 0.1 μg ml^{-1} ozone and in 30 min with 1 mg ml^{-1} H$_2$O$_2$ (Dominique et al. 1988), whereas a 50% inactivation rate was noted in 17 min with UV radiation used at 1 μW cm^{-2} (Gilpin 1984). Resistance to UV light at 260 nm but not to solar radiation was shown to be carried on a 36 000 kDa conjugative plasmid (Tully 1993). However, as is the case with the in vivo and in vitro evaluation of antibiotics, the disinfecting regimens described are not necessarily reflected in field trials.

Control measures depend upon eradication of the organism from contaminated water supplies especially those from which aerosols are generated. This is particularly important in the hospital environment where the number of individuals with appropriate predisposing factors may be very high. Thankfully, the organism is resistant to neither heat nor chlorine. Intermittent temperature increases in the water supply of up to 60°C as well as the use of chlorination procedures to give a continuous 1–2 mg l^{-1} (1–2 ppm) chlorine are effective (Helms et al. 1983, Shands et al. 1985). In hospital hot water systems, residual free chlorine concentrations of between 1 and 5% have proved quite effective in removing legionellae (Massanari et al. 1984, Witherell et al. 1984). Similar results have been obtained for cooling tower systems using chlorine and quaternary ammonium compounds (Kurtz et al. 1984, Fliermans 1985); however, it must be noted that the biological load in these systems profoundly influences inactivation rates. In addition to disinfection, remedial cleaning and flushing of water systems as well as the removal of sediment from hot water tanks, coupled with water treatment and constant water monitoring, are crucial to prevent the explosive outbreaks recorded to date.

13 PATHOGENICITY AND VIRULENCE FACTORS

Infection with *L. pneumophila* is a multifactorial phenomenon in which a complex of ill-defined bacterial virulence factors, the dose of infecting organisms and the status of the host's immune system play key roles in the establishment of disease. Disease in humans is initiated when *Legionella* organisms enter and replicate within unactivated alveolar macrophages (Horwitz 1993). That some serotypes and species are the major agents of disease suggests the presence of virulence traits in these organisms but not in others. Despite extensive investigations using virulent and avirulent strains, the precise nature of *Legionella* virulence remains elusive. The 24 kDa MIP protein

potentiates the infectious process for cells and is required for full expression of virulence; however, the role of other bacterial products in virulence is less clear. A 15 kDa surface expressed protein of the organism is found only during infection of amoebae (Barker, Lambert and Brown 1993), whereas in macrophages many *Legionella* proteins are repressed and yet others are induced, including a 19 kDa global stress protein (Kwaik, Eisenstein and Engleberg 1993, Kwaik and Engleberg 1994). However, the role in virulence of these products expressed in the intracellular milieu is obscure.

Binding of the pathogen to macrophage membranes followed by phagocytic uptake and intracellular replication are crucial to disease development. To this effect, the MOMP of *Legionella* binds to the complement receptors CR1 and CR3 through the mediation of complement components C3b and C3bi, respectively (Bellinger-Kawahara and Horwitz 1990). A role in pathogenesis for the bacterial fimbriae or pili has not been established but these may be important in the environment where opsonins are absent. Opsonin-independent binding to macrophages has been documented (Gibson, Tzianabos and Rodgers 1994). Uptake is often mediated by coiling phagocytosis (Fig. 49.9), by which process the organism is brought into a phagosome in the infected cell (Horwitz 1983a). Microfilament inhibitors such as cytochalasin block bacterial entry into cells and this suggests a central role for the cytoskeleton in host cell colonization. Following uptake, acidification of the phagosome does not occur. Furthermore, fusion of the phagosome with lysosomes is blocked by mechanisms as yet unknown (Horwitz 1983b). As a consequence, the organism replicates profusely within ribosome-lined vacuoles, often in association with mitochondria (Fig. 49.10) and this eventually leads to cellular destruction and organism dissemination (Oldham and Rodgers 1985). Although the organism replicates in the cytoplasm of many cell types, including fibroblasts, epithelial cells, various

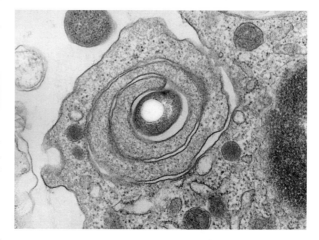

Fig. 49.9 Human monocyte ingesting *Legionella pneumophila* by coiling phagocytosis. A long monocyte pseudopod coils around the bacterium (centre) which contains a large phaselucent fat vacuole. Magnification × 28 400. (Reproduced with permission from Horwitz, 1984, *Cell*, **36**: 27–33).

transformed cells, peripheral blood monocytes, primary explants of macrophages from various animals and fresh water amoebae, alveolar macrophages serve as the major target cells for intracellular replication of the organism in human lung (Fig. 49.11). Histopathological examination of biopsy and postmortem lung tissues shows inflammatory exudates in the bronchioles and alveoli; these consist of polymorphonuclear leucocytes, macrophages, oedema fluid, fibrin-rich debris, and *Legionella* organisms (Fig. 49.12; see also plate 49.12). Leucocytoclasis or lysis of the inflammatory exudate is typical. Tissue damage in the lungs is exacerbated by the production of numerous potent exotoxins and enzymes and these facilitate coagulative necrosis, congestion, haemorrhage and abscess formation, and also act to suppress phagocytosis and interfere with host cell oxidative metabolism (Dowling, Saha and Glew 1992). In addition, these bacterial exoproducts may be responsible for the extensive non-pneumonic symptoms, such as vasculitis, frequently associated with this condition.

LPS functions as a weak endotoxin but is the major serogroup antigen of the legionellae (Ciesielski, Blaser and Wong 1986). This, together with the major cytoplasmic membrane protein (MCMP), a heat shock protein and an immunogen that is protective for guinea pigs, are the major antigens recognized by human sera. The major secretory protein, a metalloprotease, exacerbates disease in humans and guinea pigs but is not essential for infection. The protease shows structural and functional similarity to an elastase from *Pseudomonas aeruginosa* (Black, Quinn and Tompkins 1990). It is proteolytic, haemolytic and cytotoxic (Quinn and Tompkins 1989) but is not required for intracellular growth of the organism or for host cell killing (Szeto and Shuman 1990) and may inhibit the oxidative burst in macrophages and polymorpho-

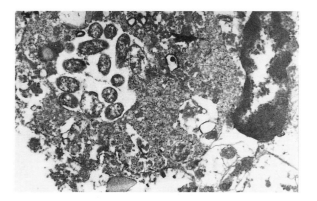

Fig. 49.11 A number of *Legionella* organisms is located within a well circumscribed phagosome within a degenerating human lung cell. From a postmortem lung specimen from a fatal case of Legionnaires' disease. Magnification × 10500. (Reproduced with permission from Rodgers et al., 1978, *Nature (London)*, **272**: 825–6).

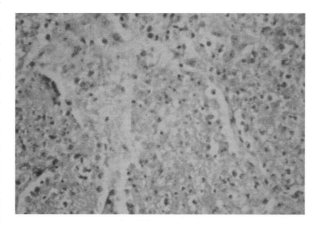

Fig. 49.12 Haematoxylin and eosin stained section from a postmortem lung specimen from a fatal case of Legionnaires' disease. Note pneumonic presentation with inflammatory exudates in the alveolar sacs along with fibrin-rich debris. Organisms are not evident. See plate 49.12 for colour.

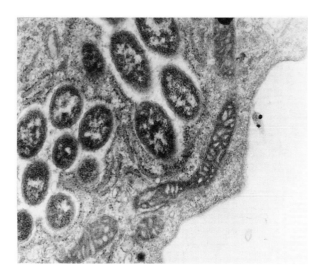

Fig. 49.10 Legionellae replicating in a U-937 cell within tight-fitting phagosomes lined with ribosomes and in close association with mitochondria. Bacteria are surrounded by an electron-diffuse zone. Magnification × 22500. (Reproduced with permission from Rodgers and Gibson, 1993, *Can J Microbiol*, **39**: 718–22).

nuclear leucocyte chemotaxis. Furthermore, the protease induces tissue damage and distal lung lesions and may also serve to inhibit the function of natural killer cells and degrade cytokines, thus enhancing organism survival. Haemolysin along with iron reductases may function by providing essential iron for the organism.

Following infection with *Legionella*, a number of cytokines is induced. Notable among these are the T lymphokine, interferon-γ (IFN-γ) and the monokine, tumour necrosis factor α (TNF-α), both of which inhibit intracellular replication but have no influence on phagocytosis (Klein et al. 1991). However, in recent studies from this and other laboratories it was shown that the cytokine interleukin-10 (IL-10) acted in an antagonistic manner to IFN-γ in *L. pneumophila*-infected cells. As a consequence, in experimental cellular infections with *L. pneumophila*, IL-10 blocked the protective effects of IFN-γ, and the resultant cellular infection proved more severe and progressed more rapidly than it did in the absence of IL-10. Whether this is also the case in human or experimental animal infections is not known. TNF-α activates mononuclear phagocytes and potentiates IFNs, and these influence the expression of a number of interleukins that may facilitate cellular killing of legionellae (Horwitz 1993, Skerrit and Martin 1993). In addition, IFN-γ reduces the iron availability for the organism by reducing the levels of intracellular ferritin and by downregulating transferrin receptors on the host cell surfaces, so dramatically lowering iron uptake. However, the impact of IFN-γ on this inhibitory process is reversible when excess iron is available. The precise role of cytokines in the development and progression of infection as well as in the recovery process is unclear. Indeed, much remains to be defined concerning the part those immune modulating molecules play in the outcome of the Legionnaire's disease.

A vaccine is not currently available. To be effective, such a vaccine would need to mobilize the bacterial killing processes of the immune system rather than elicit a humoral response only. Indeed, such a vaccine must stimulate sensitized T cells to elaborate cytokines and activate neutrophils, monocytes and macrophages for a successful outcome. Passively administered antibody does not protect in animal challenge studies, and the presence of circulating anti-*Legionella* antibody may result in a more active uptake of the organism by alveolar macrophages and may prove counterproductive. To complicate the issue further, the population at greatest risk from infection and therefore in most need of vaccination is the immunocompromised whose cell mediated responses may be diminished. For such a group, a molecular vaccine rather than a complex or whole organism product would probably prove less toxic. A lack of understanding of the mechanisms involved in pre-existing and long-term immunity currently hinders vaccine development strategies. As more information becomes available on the basic biology of this agent, the nature of its virulence factors, and how it interacts with the immune system of the host to survive and replicate within macrophages, so improved methods for prevention and control will be forthcoming for *Legionella* infections.

REFERENCES

Alary M, Joly JR, 1992, Factors contributing to the contamination of hospital water distribution systems by legionellae, *J Infect Dis*, **165:** 565–9.

Anand CM, Skinner AR et al., 1983, Interaction of *Legionella pneumophila* and free-living amoeba (*Acanthamoeba palestinensis*), *J Hyg Camb*, **91:** 167–78.

Armengol S, Domingo C, Mesalles E, 1992, Myocarditis: a rare complication during *Legionella* infection, *Int J Cardiol*, **37:** 418–20.

Arnow PM, Chow T et al., 1982, Nosocomial Legionnaires' disease caused by aerosolized tap water from respiratory devices, *J Infect Dis*, **146:** 460–7.

Bailey CC, Murray PR, Finegold SM, 1985, Clinical features of Legionnaires' disease, *Legionellosis*, ed. Katz SM, CRC Press, Boca Raton, FL, 111–50.

Barbaree JM, 1993, Selecting a subtyping technique for use in investigations of legionellosis epidemics, *Legionella: Current Status and Emerging Perspectives*, eds Barbaree JM, Breiman RF, Dufor AP, ASM, Washington, DC, 169–72.

Barbaree JM, Fields BS et al., 1986, Isolation of protozoa from water associated with a legionellosis outbreak and demonstration of intracellular replication of *Legionella pneumophila*, *Appl Environ Microbiol*, **51:** 422–4.

Barker J, Lambert PA, Brown MRW, 1993, Influence of the intra-amoebic and other growth conditions on the surface properties of *Legionella pneumophila*, *Infect Immun*, **61:** 3503–10.

Bartlett CLR, Macrae AD, Macfarlane JT, 1986, Legionella *Infections*, Edward Arnold, Baltimore, MD, 1–163.

Bellinger-Kawahara C, Horwitz MA, 1990, Complement component C3 fixes selectively to the major outer membrane protein (MOMP) of *Legionella pneumophila* and mediates phagocytosis of liposome–MOMP complexes by human monocytes, *J Exp Med*, **172:** 1201–10.

Benson RF, Thacker WL et al., 1987, Cross-reactions in *Legionella* antisera with *Bordetella pertussis* strains, *J Clin Microbiol*, **25:** 594–6.

Berendt RF, 1980, Survival of *Legionella pneumophila* in aerosols: effect of relative humidity, *J Infect Dis*, **141:** 689.

Black WJ, Quinn FD, Tompkins LS, 1990, *Legionella pneumophila* zinc metalloprotease is structurally and functionally homologous to *Pseudomonas aeruginosa* elastase, *J Bacteriol*, **172:** 2608–13.

Breiman RF, Fields BS et al., 1990, Association of shower use with Legionnaires' disease. Possible role of amoeba, *JAMA*, **263:** 2924–6.

Brenner DJ, Steigerwalt AG, McDade JE, 1979, Classification of the Legionnaires' disease bacterium: *Legionella pneumophila*, genus novum, species nova, of the family Legionellaceae, familia nova, *Ann Intern Med*, **90:** 656–8.

Brenner DJ, Steigerwalt AG et al., 1985, Ten new species of *Legionella*, *Int J Syst Bacteriol*, **35:** 50–9.

Brenner DJ, Steigerwalt AG et al., 1988, *Legionella pneumophila* serogroup Lansing 3 isolated from a patient with fatal pneumonia, and descriptions of *L. pneumophila* subsp. *pneumophila* subsp. nov., *L. pneumophila* subsp. *fraseri* subsp. nov., *L. pneumophila* subsp. *pascullei* subsp. nov., *J Clin Microbiol*, **26:** 1695–703.

Brown A, Vickers RM et al., 1982, Plasmids and surface antigen markers of endemic and epidemic *Legionella pneumophila* strains, *J Clin Microbiol*, **16:** 230–5.

Brown A, Lema M et al., 1985, Combined plasmid and peptide analysis of clinical and environmental *Legionella pneumophila* strains associated with a small cluster of Legionnaires' disease cases, *Infection*, **13:** 163–6.

Buesching WJ, Brust RA, Ayers LW, 1983, Enhanced primary isolation of *Legionella pneumophila* from clinical specimens by low-pH treatment, *J Clin Microbiol*, **17:** 1153–5.

Chandler FW, Cole RM et al., 1979, Ultrastructure of the Legionnaires' disease bacterium. A study using electron microscopy, *Ann Intern Med*, **90:** 642–7.

Chandler FW, Roth K et al., 1980, Flagella on Legionnaires' disease bacteria: ultrastructural observations, *Ann Intern Med*, **93:** 711–14.

Chen GC, Lema M, Brown A, 1984, Plasmid transfer into members of the family Legionellaceae, *J Infect Dis*, **150:** 513–16.

Cherry WB, Pittman B et al., 1978, Detection of Legionnaires' disease bacteria by direct immunofluorescent staining, *J Clin Microbiol*, **8:** 329–38.

Ciesielski CA, Blaser MJ, Wong WLL, 1986, Serogroup specificity of *Legionella pneumophila* is related to lipopolysaccharide characteristics, *Infect Immun*, **51:** 397–404.

Daaka Y, Yamamoto Y et al., 1994, Correlation of *Legionella pneumophila* virulence with the presence of a plasmid, *Curr Microbiol*, **28:** 217–23.

Dennis PJ, Green D, Jones BPC, 1984, A note on the temperature tolerance of *Legionella*, *J Appl Bacteriol*, **56**: 349–50.

Dennis PJ, Taylor JA et al., 1982, *Legionella pneumophila* in water plumbing systems, *Lancet*, **1**: 949–51.

Dominique EL, Tyndall RL et al., 1988, Effects of three oxidizing biocides on *Legionella pneumophila* serogroup 1, *Appl Environ Microbiol*, **54**: 741–7.

Dowling JN, Saha AK, Glew RH, 1992, Virulence factors of the family Legionellaceae, *Microbiol Rev*, **56**: 32–60.

Dreyfus LA, Iglewski BH, 1985, Conjugation-mediated genetic exchange in *Legionella pneumophila*, *J Bacteriol*, **161**: 80–4.

Edelstein PH, 1981, Improved semiselective medium for isolation of *Legionella pneumophila* from contaminated clinical and environmental specimens, *J Clin Microbiol*, **14**: 298–303.

Edelstein PH, 1993, Laboratory diagnosis of Legionnaires' disease: an update from 1984, *Legionella: Current Status and Emerging Perspectives*, eds Barbaree JM, Breiman RF, Dufour AP, ASM, Washington, DC, 7–11.

Edelstein PH, Myer RD, 1980, Susceptibility of *Legionella pneumophila* to twenty antimicrobial agents, *Antimicrob Agents Chemother*, **18**: 403–8.

Elliot JA, Johnson W, 1981, Immunological and biochemical relationships among flagella isolated from *Legionella pneumophila* serogroups 1, 2 and 3, *Infect Immun*, **33**: 602–10.

Engleberg NC, 1993, Genetic studies of *Legionella* pathogenesis, *Legionella: Current Status and Emerging Perspectives*, eds Barbaree JM, Breiman RF, Dufour AP, ASM, Washington, DC, 63–8.

Fang GD, Fine M et al., 1990, New and emerging etiologies for community acquired pneumonia with implications for therapy. A prospective multicenter study of 359 cases, *Medicine (Baltimore)*, **69**: 307–16.

Feeley JC, Gibson RJ et al., 1979, Charcoal yeast extract agar: primary isolation medium for *Legionella pneumophila*, *J Clin Microbiol*, **10**: 437–41.

Fisher-Hoch SP, Bartlett CLR et al., 1981, Investigation and control of an outbreak of Legionnaires' disease in a district general hospital, *Lancet*, **1**: 932–6.

Fliermans CB, 1985, Ecological niche of *Legionella pneumophila*, *Legionellosis*, vol. 2, ed. Katz SM, CRC Press, Boca Raton, FL, 75–116.

Fraser DW, Tsai TR et al., 1977, Legionnaires' disease: description of an epidemic of pneumonia, *N Engl J Med*, **297**: 1189–97.

Fry N, Warwick KS et al., 1991, The use of 16S ribosomal RNA analyses to investigate the phylogeny of the family Legionellaceae, *J Gen Microbiol*, **137**: 1215–22.

Gabay JE, Horwitz MA, 1985, Isolation and characterization of the cytoplasmic and outer membranes of the Legionnaires' disease bacterium (*Legionella pneumophila*), *J Exp Med*, **161**: 409–22.

Gabay JE, Blake MS et al., 1985, Purification of the major outer membrane protein of *Legionella pneumophila* and demonstration that it is a porin, *J Bacteriol*, **162**: 86–91.

Garrity GM, Brown A, Vickers RM, 1980, *Tatlockia* and *Fluoribacter*: two new genera of organisms resembling *Legionella pneumophila*, *Int J Syst Bacteriol*, **30**: 609–14.

George JR, Pine L et al., 1980, Amino acid requirements of *Legionella pneumophila*, *J Clin Microbiol*, **11**: 286–91.

Gibson FC, Tzianabos AO, Rodgers FG, 1994, Adherence of *Legionella pneumophila* to U-937 cells, guinea pig alveolar macrophages and MRC-5 cells by novel opsonin-independent binding mechanism, *Can J Microbiol*, **40**: 865–72.

Gilpin RW, 1984, Laboratory and field applications of UV light disinfection on six species of *Legionella* and other bacteria in water, Legionella. *Proceedings of the Second International Symposium*, eds Thornsberry C, Balows A et al., ASM, Washington, DC, 337–9.

Glick TH, Gregg MB et al., 1978, Pontiac fever. An epidemic of unknown etiology in a health department. Clinical and epidemiological aspects, *Am J Epidemiol*, **107**: 149–60.

Gosting LH, Cabrian K et al., 1984, Identification of a species-specific antigen in *Legionella pneumophila* by a monoclonal antibody, *J Clin Microbiol*, **20**: 1031–5.

Grimont F, Lefevre M et al., 1989, rRNA gene restriction patterns of *Legionella* species: molecular identification system, *Res Microbiol*, **140**: 615–26.

Harrison TG, Taylor AG (eds), 1988, *A Laboratory Manual for Legionella*, John Wiley and Sons, New York.

Havlichek D, Saravolatz L, Pohold D, 1987, Effect of quinolones and other antimicrobial agents on cell associated *Legionella pneumophila*, *Antimicrob Agents Chemother*, **31**: 1529–34.

Helbig JH, Luck PC et al., 1995, Molecular characterization of a virulence-associated epitope on the lipopolysaccharide of *Legionella pneumophila* serogroup 1, *Epidemiol Infect*, **115**: 71–8.

Helms CM, Massanari RM et al., 1983, Legionnaires' disease associated with a hospital water system: a cluster of 24 nosocomial cases, *Ann Intern Med*, **99**: 172–8.

High A, Rodgers FG, 1991, Electroporation of the major outer membrane protein-encoding genes from virulent to avirulent *Legionella pneumophila*, *Abstracts of the 91st General Meeting of the American Society for Microbiology, Dallas, Texas*, 156.

Hoffman PS, 1984, Bacterial physiology, Legionella. *Proceedings of the Second International Symposium*, eds Thornsberry C, Balows A et al., ASM, Washington, DC, 61–7.

Hoffman PS, Pine L, 1982, Respiratory physiology and cytochrome content of *Legionella pneumophila*, *Curr Microbiol*, **7**: 351–6.

Hoffman PS, Pine L, Bell S, 1983, Production of superoxide and hydrogen peroxide in medium used to culture *Legionella pneumophila*: catalytic decomposition by charcoal, *Appl Environ Microbiol*, **45**: 784–91.

Horwitz MA, 1983a, Formation of a novel phagosome by the Legionnaires' disease bacterium (*Legionella pneumophila*) in human monocytes, *J Exp Med*, **158**: 1319–31.

Horwitz MA, 1983b, The Legionnaires' disease bacterium (*Legionella pneumophila*) inhibits phagosome–lysosome fusion in human monocytes, *J Exp Med*, **158**: 2108–26.

Horwitz MA, 1984, Phagocytosis of the Legionnaires' disease bacterium (*Legionella pneumophila*) occurs by a novel mechanism: engulfment within a pseudopod coil, *Cell*, **36**: 27–33.

Horwitz MA, 1993, Toward an understanding of host and bacterial molecules mediating *Legionella pneumophila* pathogenesis, Legionella: *Current Status and Emerging Perspectives*, eds Barbaree JM, Breiman RF, Dufor AP, ASM, Washington, DC, 55–62.

Johnson JD, Hand WL et al., 1980, Antibiotic uptake by alveolar macrophages, *J Lab Clin Med*, **95**: 429–39.

Johnson W, Varner L, Poch M, 1991, Acquisition of iron by *Legionella pneumophila*: a role of iron reductase, *Infect Immun*, **59**: 2376–81.

Klein TW, Yamamoto Y et al., 1991, Interferon γ induced resistance to *Legionella pneumophila* in susceptible A/J mouse macrophages, *J Leukocyte Biol*, **49**: 98–103.

Knirel YA, Rietschel ET et al., 1994, The structure of the O-specific side chain of *Legionella* serogroup 1 lipopolysaccharide, *J Biochem*, **221**: 239–45.

Kurtz JB, Bartlett CLR et al., 1984, Field trial of biocides in control of *Legionella pneumophila* in cooling water systems, Legionella. *Proceedings of the Second International Symposium*, eds Thornsberry C, Balows A et al., ASM, Washington, DC, 340–2.

Kwaik YA, Eisenstein BI, Engleberg NC, 1993, Phenotypic modulation by *Legionella pneumophila* gene induced by intracellular infection and by various in vitro stress conditions, *Mol Microbiol*, **13**: 243–51.

Kwaik YA, Engleberg NC, 1994, Cloning and molecular characterization of *Legionella pneumophila* upon infection of macrophages, *Infect Immun*, **61**: 1320–9.

Lambert MA, Moss CW, 1989, Cellular fatty acid composition and isoprenoid quinone contents of 23 *Legionella* species, *J Clin Microbiol*, **27**: 465–73.

McDade JE, Shepard CC et al., 1977, Legionnaires' disease: isolation of bacterium and demonstration of its role in other respiratory disease, *N Engl J Med*, **297:** 1197–203.

McDade JE, Brenner DJ, Bozeman FM, 1979, Legionnaires' disease bacterium isolated in 1947, *Ann Intern Med*, **90:** 659–61.

Macfarlane JT, Finch RG et al., 1982, Hospital study of adult community acquired pneumonia, *Lancet*, **2:** 255–8.

Mahbubani MH, Bej AK et al., 1990, Detection of *Legionella* with polymerase chain reaction and gene probe methods, *Mol Cell Probes*, **4:** 175–87.

Mahoney FJ, Hoge CW et al., 1992, Community outbreak of Legionnaires' disease associated with a grocery store misting machine, *J Infect Dis*, 165, 736–9.

Marra A, Shuman HA, 1992, Genetics of *Legionella pneumophila* virulence, *Annu Rev Genet*, **26:** 51–69.

Massanari RM, Helms C et al., 1984, Continuous hyperchlorination of a potable water system for control of nosocomial *Legionella pneumophila* infections, Legionella. *Proceedings of the Second International Symposium*, eds Thornsberry C, Balows A et al., ASM, Washington, DC, 334–6.

Mengaud JM, Horwitz MA, 1993, The major iron-containing protein of *Legionella pneumophila* is an aconitase homologous with the human iron-responsive element-binding protein, *J Bacteriol*, **175:** 5666–76.

Morrill WE, Barbaree JM et al., 1990, Increased recovery of *Legionella micdadei* and *Legionella bozmanii* on buffered charcoal yeast extract agar supplemented with albumin, *J Clin Microbiol*, **28:** 616–18.

Monforte R, Marco F et al., 1989, Multiple organ involvement by *Legionella pneumophila* in a fatal case of Legionnaires' disease, *J Infect Dis*, **159:** 809.

Nash P, Krenz MM, 1991, Culture media, *Manual of Clinical Microbiology*, 5th edn, eds Balows A, Hausler WJ et al., ASM, Washington, DC, 1226–8.

Nolte FS, Conlin CA et al., 1984, Plasmids as epidemiological markers in nosocomial Legionnaires' disease, *J Infect Dis*, **149:** 251–6.

Nowicki M, Bornetein N et al., 1993, Rapid detection of legionellae in clinical and environmental samples by polymerase chain reaction, Legionella: *Current Status and Emerging Perspectives*, eds Barbaree JM, Breiman RF, Dufour AP, ASM, Washington, DC, 178–81.

Oldham LJ, Rodgers FG, 1985, Adhesion, penetration and intracellular replication of *Legionella pneumophila*: an in vitro model of pathogenesis, *J Gen Microbiol*, **131:** 697–706.

O'Mahony MC, Stanswell-Smith RE et al., 1990, The Stafford outbreak of Legionnaires' disease, *Epidemiol Infect*, **104:** 361–80.

Ott M, Bender L et al., 1991a, Pulsed field electrophoresis of genomic restriction fragments for the detection of nosocomial *Legionella pneumophila* in hospital water supplies, *J Clin Microbiol*, **29:** 813–15.

Ott M, Messner P et al., 1991b, Temperature-dependent expression of flagella in *Legionella*, *J Gen Microbiol*, **137:** 1955–61.

Quinn FD, Tompkins LS, 1989, Analysis of a cloned sequence of *Legionella pneumophila* encoding a 38 kD metalloprotease possessing haemolytic and cytotoxic activities, *Mol Microbiol*, **3:** 797–805.

Reeves MW, Pine L et al., 1981, Metal requirements of *Legionella pneumophila*, *J Clin Microbiol*, **13:** 688–95.

Reeves MW, Pine L et al., 1983, Absence of siderophore activity in *Legionella* species grown in iron deficient media, *J Bacteriol*, **154:** 324–9.

Rodgers FG, 1979, Ultrastructure of *Legionella pneumophila*, *J Clin Pathol*, **32:** 1195–202.

Rodgers FG, 1985, Morphology of *Legionella*, *Legionellosis*, ed. Katz SM, CRC Press, Boca Raton, FL, 39–82.

Rodgers FG, Davey MR, 1982, Ultrastructure of the cell envelope layers and surface details of *Legionella pneumophila*, *J Gen Microbiol*, **128:** 1547–57.

Rodgers FG, Gibson FC, 1993, Opsonin-independent adherence

and intracellular development of *Legionella pneumophila* within U-937 cells, *Can J Microbiol*, **39:** 718–22.

Rodgers FG, Laverick T, 1984, *Legionella pneumophila* serogroup 1 flagellar antigen in a passive hemagglutination test to detect antibodies to other *Legionella* species, Legionella. *Proceedings of the Second International Symposium*, eds Thornsberry C, Balows A et al., ASM, Washington, DC, 42–4.

Rodgers FG, Macrae AD, Lewis MJ, 1978, Electron microscopy of the organism of Legionnaires' disease, *Nature (London)*, **272:** 825–6.

Rodgers FG, Pasculle AW, 1991, *Legionella, Manual of Clinical Microbiology*, 5th edn, eds Balows A, Hausler WJ et al., ASM, Washington, DC, 442–53.

Rodgers FG, Greaves PW et al., 1980, Electron microscopic evidence of flagella and pili on *Legionella pneumophila*, *J Clin Pathol*, **33:** 1184–8.

Rowbotham TJ, 1980, Preliminary report on the pathogenicity of *Legionella pneumophila* for freshwater and soil amoeba, *J Clin Pathol*, **33:** 1179–83.

Roy TM, Fleming D, Anderson WH, 1989, Tularemic pneumonia mimicking Legionnaires' disease with false-positive fluorescent antibody stains for *Legionella*, *South Med J*, **82:** 1429–31.

Saunders NA, Harrison TG et al., 1990, A method for typing strains of *Legionella pneumophila* serogroup 1 by analysis of restriction fragment length polymorphisms, *J Med Microbiol*, **31:** 45–55.

Selander RK, McKinney RM et al., 1985, Genetic structure of genetic populations of *Legionella pneumophila*, *J Bacteriol*, **163:** 1021–7.

Shands KN, Ho JL et al., 1985, Potable water assource of Legionnaires' disease, *JAMA*, **253:** 1412–16.

Skerrett SJ, Martin TR, 1993, Tumor necrosis factor and lipopolysaccharide potentiate gamma interferon-induced resistance of alveolar macrophages to *Legionella pneumophila*, Legionella: *Current Status and Emerging Perspectives*, ASM, Washington, DC, 105–6.

Sonesson A, Jantzen E et al., 1989, Chemical composition of a lipopolysaccharide from *Legionella pneumophila*, *Arch Microbiol*, 153, 72–8.

States SJ, Conley LF et al., 1987, Survival and multiplication of *Legionella pneumophila* in municipal drinking water systems, *Appl Environ Microbiol*, **53:** 979–86.

Szeto L, Shuman HA, 1990, The *Legionella pneumophila* major secretor protein, a protease, is not required for intracellular growth or cell killing, *Infect Immun*, **58:** 2585–92.

Tesh MT, Miller RD, 1981, Amino acid requirements for *Legionella pneumophila* growth, *J Clin Microbiol*, **13:** 865–9.

Tesh MJ, Morse SA, Miller RD, 1983, Intermediary metabolism in *Legionella pneumophila*: utilization of amino acids and other compounds as energy sources, *J Bacteriol*, **154:** 1104–9.

Thacker L, McKinney RM et al., 1981, Thermophillic sporeforming bacilli that mimic fastidious growth characteristics and colonial morphology of *Legionella*, *J Clin Microbiol*, **13:** 794–7.

Thornsberry C, Baker CN, Kirven LA, 1978, In vitro activity of antimicrobial agents on Legionnaires' disease bacterium, *Antimicrob Agents Chemother*, **13:** 78–80.

Tison DL, Pope DH et al., 1980, Growth of *Legionella pneumophila* in association with blue-green algae (cyanobacteria), *Appl Environ Microbiol*, **39:** 456–9.

Tully M, 1993, A *Legionella* plasmid mediates resistance to UV light but not to solar radiation, Legionella: *Current Status and Emerging Perspectives*, eds Barbaree JM, Breiman RF, Dufour AP, ASM, Washington, DC, 120–4.

Vickers RM, Brown A, Garrity GM, 1981, Dye-containing buffered charcoal yeast extract medium for the differentiation of members of the Legionellaceae, *J Clin Microbiol*, **13:** 380–2.

Vilde JL, Dournon E, Rajagopalan P, 1986, Inhibition of *Legionella pneumophila* multiplication within human macrophages by antimicrobial agents, *Antimicrob Agents Chemother*, **30:** 743–8.

Wadowski RM, Yee RB, 1981, Glycine-containing selective

medium for isolation of Legionellaceae from environmental specimens, *Appl Environ Microbiol*, **42:** 768–72.

Wadowski RM, Yee RB, 1985, Effect of non-Legionellaceae bacteria on the multiplication of *Legionella pneumophila* in potable water, *Appl Environ Microbiol*, **49:** 1206–10.

Wadowski RM, Butler LJ et al., 1988, Growth supporting activity for *Legionella pneumophila* in tap water cultures and implications of hartmannellid amoebae as growth factors, *Appl Environ Microbiol*, **54:** 2677–82.

Waldor MK, Wilson B, Swartz M, 1993, Cellulitis caused by *Legionella pneumophila*, *Clin Infect Dis*, **16:** 51–3.

Wang WLL, Blaser MJ et al., 1979, Growth, survival and resistance of the Legionnaires' disease bacterium, *Ann Intern Med*, **90:** 614–18.

Wilkinson HW, Cruce DD, Broome CV, 1981, Validation of *Legionella pneumophila* indirect immunofluorescence assay with epidemic sera, *J Clin Microbiol*, **13:** 139–46.

Wilkinson HW, Reingold AL et al., 1983, Reactivity of serum from patients with suspected legionellosis against 29 antigens of Legionellaceae and *Legionella*-like organisms by indirect immunofluorescence assay, *J Infect Dis*, **147:** 23–31.

Witherell LE, Orciari LA et al., 1984, Disinfection of hospital hot water systems containing *Legionella pneumophila*, Legionella. *Proceedings of the Second International Symposium*, eds Thornsberry C, Balows A et al., ASM, Washington, DC, 336–7.

Woodhead MA, Macfarlane JT et al., 1985, Aetiology and outcome of severe community-acquired pneumonia, *J Infect*, **10:** 204–10.

Yee RB, Wadowski RM, 1982, Multiplication of *Legionella pneumophila* in unsterilized tap water, *Appl Environ Microbiol*, **43:** 1330–4.

HAEMOPHILUS

M P E Slack and J Z Jordens

1 DEFINITION

Members of this genus are small to medium-sized coccobacilli or rods, often markedly pleomorphic, sometimes filamentous. The organisms are gram-negative, non-motile, non-spore forming, non-acid-fast. They are aerobic and facultatively anaerobic, and require one or both of 2 accessory growth factors – **factor X** (haemin or other porphyrins) and **factor V** (coenzyme I; nicotinamide adenine dinucleotide, NAD^+ or NAD-phosphate, $NADP^+$) They are chemoorganotrophic with both a respiratory and a fermentative type of metabolism. Sugars are attacked fermentatively. Oxidase and catalase reactions vary between species and strains; many are positive. Nitrate is reduced to nitrite. The species are obligate parasites of humans and animals, inhabiting particularly mucous membranes. The G + C content of DNA is 37–44 mol%. The type species is *H. influenzae.*

2 INTRODUCTION AND HISTORICAL PERSPECTIVE

In 1892, Pfeiffer claimed that the small gram-negative haemophilic coccobacillus that he had isolated in large numbers from the sputum of patients suffering from epidemic influenza was the causative agent of that disease. The specific name *Haemophilus influenzae* (Winslow et al. 1917) which was given to the organism is a permanent reminder of this erroneous association. In fact, although *H. influenzae* was named as the type species it was not the first member of the genus to have been described. In 1883, Koch described a bacillus causing conjunctivitis in Egypt, now named *H. influenzae* biogroup aegyptius.

Several other small gram-negative bacteria that share many of the characteristics of *H. influenzae* have since been described. All of these organisms require one or both of 2 accessory growth factors – X factor (haemin or other porphyrins), and V factor, (nicotinamide adenine dinucleotide, NAD^+, or NAD phosphate, $NADP^+$). The use of growth-factor requirement as the major criterion for defining the genus *Haemophilus* can be questioned in the light of DNA–DNA homology studies. Occasional strains in other unrelated genera exhibit growth-factor requirements similar to those of *Haemophilus* spp. However, the majority of workers still accept that a requirement for X factor or V factor or both is a prerequisite for inclusion of a small gram-negative bacterium in the genus *Haemophilus* (Sneath and Johnston 1973, Kilian 1976, Kilian and Biberstein 1984).

3 SPECIES IN THE GENUS

The organisms we have included in the genus are listed in Table 50.1. Opinions differ on the validity of some of the species and it may be difficult to make clear cut distinctions between others. We have adopted the term *H. influenzae* biogroup aegyptius (Brenner et al. 1988) for strains formerly called *H. aegyptius*. *H. influenzae* biogroup aegyptius and *H.*

influenzae share over 90% genomic nucleotide sequence homology (Brenner et al. 1988) and are indistinguishable in routine laboratory tests.

H. aphrophilus is considered to belong to the genus because of its apparent requirement for X factor on primary isolation and is so named because it needs carbon dioxide for growth (*aphrophilus* = foam loving). The X-factor requirement is readily lost on subculture. DNA–DNA hybridization studies indicate that *H. aphrophilus* and *H. paraphrophilus* are closely related organisms (Potts et al. 1986) and possibly do not constitute separate species. Potts and Berry (1983) have suggested it may be more appropriate to designate one of these 2 organisms as a subspecies, a view endorsed by Sedlacek et al. (1993). Since *H. aphrophilus* is X-factor-dependent and *H. paraphrophilus* is V-factor-dependent we have regarded them as 2 species. DNA–DNA hybridization analyses of *Actinobacillus actinomycetemcomitans*, *H. segnis*, *H. aphrophilus* and *H. paraphrophilus* have shown these 4 species to be at least 28% related (Potts, Zambon and Genco 1985, Potts et al. 1986) consistent with their placement in a single genus. Accordingly it has been proposed that '*A*'. *actinomycetemcomitans* should be reassigned to the genus *Haemophilus* as *H. actinomycetemcomitans* despite being X- and V-factor-independent. Since we have decided to include only X- and/or V- factor requiring organisms in our consideration of the genus *Haemophilus* readers should refer to Chapter 51 for further details on this organism. Casin et al. (1985) found the level of DNA hybridization between *H. ducreyi* and other *Haemophilus* spp. was very low (0.6% relatedness) and they suggested that *H. ducreyi*, which is also phenotypically distinct from all other *Haemophilus* spp., is misplaced in this genus.

Haemophili isolated from swine and fowl have posed considerable problems of nomenclature and taxonomy (see Biberstein and White 1969, Blackall 1989). Biberstein and White (1969) proposed the name *H. parasuis* for those V-factor-dependent strains which are frequently isolated from the respiratory tract of pigs. An X- and V-factor dependent analogue, *H. suis*, described by Lewis and Shope (1931) is of uncertain validity. The organism formerly classified as *H. pleuropneumoniae* has recently been transferred to the genus *Actinobacillus* (Pohl et al. 1983) on the basis of its phenotypic and DNA relatedness to *A. lignieresii*. The emended species *A. pleuropneumoniae* is composed of V-factor requiring and V-factor-independent biovars. Two V-factor requiring *Haemophilus* spp., *H. paragallinarum* and *H. avium* have been described in poultry. The existence of a third X- and V factor-requiring organism, '*H. gallinarum*' (Schalm and Beach 1936) has been questioned (Page 1962, Roberts, Hanson and Timms 1964) and it appears likely that these strains were erroneously described as being dependent on X and V factor owing to technical limitations. Unfortunately these strains are no longer available. *H. paragallinarum* appears to be more closely related to the genus *Actinobacillus* than to *Haemophilus* on the basis of DNA hybridization studies (Mutters, Piechulla and Mannheim 1984, Piechulla, Hinz and Mannheim 1985) and its complement of respiratory quinones (Höllander and Mannheim 1975). The species *H. avium* is composed of 3 DNA homology groups, all of which are genetically closer to *Pasteurella multocida* than to *H. influenzae* (Mutters et al. 1985). The strains also fall into 3 phenotypic groups and it has been proposed to transfer *H. avium* to the genus *Pasteurella* and split it into 3 species; *P. avium sensu stricto*, *P. volantium* sp. nov. and a third un-named species *P.* species A (Mutters et al. 1985). However, Blackall (1988) found that only 64% strains of '*H. avium*' from chickens could be assigned to the 3 species (*P. avium*, *P. volantium* and *P.* species A). The taxonomy of these avian species has not been fully resolved and they may require redefinition or the inclusion of further new

Table 50.1 Species of *Haemophilus*: growth requirements, haemolytic activity and host origin

Species	Requirement for			Haemolysis on horse blood sugar	Host
	X	**V**	**CO₂**		
H. influenzae	+	+	−	−	Human
H. haemolyticus	+	+	−	+	Human
H. haemoglobinophilus	+	−	−	−	Dog
H. ducreyi	+	−	v	v	Human
H. aphrophilus	+[a]	−	+	−	Human
H. parainfluenzae	−	+	−	−	Human, monkey
H. parahaemolyticus	−	+	−	+	Human
H. paraphrohaemolyticus	−	+	+	+[b]	Human
H. paraphrophilus	−	+	+	−	Human
H. segnis	−	+	−	−	Human
H. parasuis	−	+	−	−	Pig
H. paragallinarum	−	+	+	−	Poultry
H. paracuniculus	−	+	+	−	Rabbit

+, positive; −, negative; v, variable.
[a]Requires haemin-containing media on primary isolation.
[b]May lose haemolytic activity on subculture.

species to accommodate all strains (see review by Blackall 1989).

An organism requiring V factor isolated from the small intestine of rabbits has been named *H. paracuniculus* (Targowski and Targowski 1979) but its taxonomic position has not been confirmed. Other species of *Haemophilus* have been described, but have not been validated. These include 'Haemophilus somnus' (Baillie, Coles and Weide 1973) 'Haemophilus agni' (Kennedy et al. 1958) and 'Haemophilus felis' (Inzana et al. 1992).

4 HABITAT

Haemophilus spp. are obligate parasites of the mucous membranes of humans and a wide variety of animal species (Table 50.1). They demonstrate a marked degree of host specificity; each species, with the possible exception of *H. parainfluenzae*, being associated exclusively with one host species. *Haemophilus* spp. commonly inhabit the human upper respiratory tract (Kilian, Heine-Jensen and Bulow 1972) and mouth (Kilian and Schiøtt 1975) and may also be isolated from the intestinal tract (Palmer 1981) and vagina (Kilian 1976). A similar habitat is seen in pigs (Harris, Ross and Switzer 1969), monkeys (Rayan, Flournoy and Cahill 1987), poultry (Hinz and Kunjara 1977) and other birds (Grebe and Hinz 1975). Some species are regular members of the normal flora of their host while others seem only to be associated with disease (see review by Kilian and Frederiksen 1981).

5 CELL MORPHOLOGY

H. influenzae is a slender, short, poorly staining gram-negative rod or coccobacillus, 0.3–0.5 μm × 0.5–1.0 μm with rounded ends. The organisms are relatively difficult to stain by Gram's method. Prolonged counter-staining for 5–15 min with very dilute carbol fuchsin often gives satisfactory results. Some cultures are uniformly coccobacillary. At other times they are markedly pleomorphic, with many long filamentous forms. Either form may be observed in gram-stained smears of the cerebrospinal fluid in cases of haemophilus meningitis (Fig. 50.1; see also Plate 50.1).

Capsules are found in some species, notably *H. influenzae*, *H. parasuis* and *H. paragallinarum*. Occasional capsulate strains of *H. parainfluenzae* have been described (Sims 1970). The capsules of *H. influenzae* and *H. paragallinarum* are important in pathogenicity.

6 CULTURAL CHARACTERISTICS

6.1 Growth factor requirements

Specific growth factor requirements are major criteria by which the genus *Haemophilus* is defined. These species will not grow in the absence of certain factors that are present in blood, hence the generic name *Haemo-*

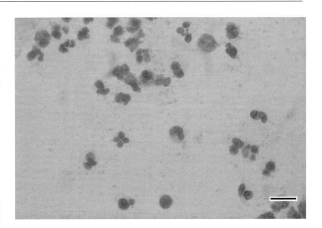

Fig. 50.1 Gram-stained smear of cerebrospinal fluid from a case of *H. influenzae* type b meningitis (Bar = 5 μm). See Plate 50.1 for colour.

philus or 'blood-loving'. *H. influenzae* requires 2 accessory growth factors, a heat-stable growth promoting substance present in red blood cells (**X factor**), and a heat-labile vitamin-like substance (**V factor**). Neither of these factors is a single substance.

X FACTOR

Fildes (1924) named haemin as X factor and suggested it plays a role as an enzyme in respiration. Various iron-containing compounds such as haems or protoporphyrin IX can satisfy a requirement for X factor. It was thought that *H. influenzae* had an absolute requirement for haem to supply both the iron requirement of the bacterium and essential porphyrin (White and Granick 1963, Coulton and Pang 1983). It now appears that, in most instances, only protoporphyrin IX is required (Pidcock et al. 1988) provided iron can be obtained from another source, because *H. influenzae* has a ferrochelatase that catalyses the insertion of iron into the protoporphyrin ring (White and Granick 1963). *H. influenzae* does not produce a haemolysin (Kilian 1976) and therefore cannot acquire its iron from the haemolysis of red blood cells. Herrington and Sparling (1985) have shown that *H. influenzae*, but not *H. parainfluenzae*, can use human transferrin as a sole source of iron. *H. influenzae* can acquire haemin from various sources, including haemoglobin–haptoglobin complexes, haem–haemopexin and haem–albumin (Pidcock et al. 1988). The requirement for X factor is substantially reduced, but not eliminated, during anaerobic growth (Gilder and Granick 1947) and strains might thus be erroneously regarded as X independent. When grown in complex media, *H. influenzae* requires NAD 0.2–1.0 mg l^{-1} and haemin up to 10 mg l^{-1} (Evans, Smith and Wicken 1974).

Haemin-dependent strains of *Haemophilus* spp. are unable to convert δ-aminolaevulinic acid (ALA) to protoporphyrin (White and Granick 1963, Biberstein, Mini and Gills 1963), a process involving 5 enzyme-mediated steps (Fig. 50.2). X-dependent strains lack some or all of these enzymes. The ability to synthesize porphobilinogen and porphyrins from ALA is the basis of the porphyrin test which was first described by Biberstein, Mini and Gills (1963) and subsequently developed by Kilian (1974) (see section 11). This test is convenient and, if properly performed, is a reliable method for demonstrating a haemin requirement. However, it does not exclude the possibility of a requirement for haemin because of a lack of enzymes later in the biosynthetic pathway. Some *Haemophilus* strains apparently require haemin itself since they lack the ferrochelatase responsible for incorporating iron into the haemin molecule (White and Granick 1963).

V FACTOR

This second factor is present in the tissues of plants and animals and is synthesized by most bacterial species other than *H. influenzae*. It was originally thought that this thermolabile substance was a vitamin, hence the name V factor (Thjøtta and Avery 1921). Pittman (1935) showed that V factor is involved in oxidation-reduction processes in the growing bacterial cell. V-factor requirement can be satisfied by nicotinamide-adenine dinucleotide (NAD⁺) and NAD phosphate (NADP⁺) or by precursors of these coenzymes. (See reviews of aspects of V-factor dependency by Cyanomon, Sorg and Patapow 1988 and Niven and O'Reilly 1990.) Although V factor is present in blood it is not available to haemophili because it is largely intracellular. Additionally the blood of many animal species contains NADase activity (Krumwiede and Kuttner 1938). Heating blood agar to about 75°C, until it acquires a chocolate colour, releases V factor from red cells and also inactivates NADase activity.

Staphylococcus aureus and some other organisms release V factor during growth. This diffuses into the surrounding medium, enhancing the growth of any organisms requiring V factor. Any V-factor-requiring species of *Haemophilus* will show satellitism, as will occasional strains of other bacterial species of unrelated genera, e.g. strains of streptococci, neisseria and diphtheroids.

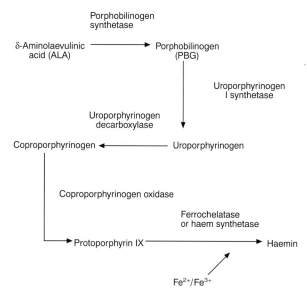

Fig. 50.2   Main steps in porphyrin and haemin biosynthesis.

Haemophilus spp. are fastidious not only in their requirements for X and V factor but also in their need for other nutritional factors, which vary among the species. *H. influenzae* requires pantothenic acid, thiamine and uracil and some strains also need a purine and cysteine (Holt 1962). *H. parasuis* requires serum. *H. paragallinarum* requires serum and sodium chloride (Rimler et al. 1977) though it is not halophilic in the usual sense.

6.2   Physical requirements for growth

The optimum temperature for growth is 35–37°C. The minimum temperature for growth is 20–25°C. Most *Haemophilus* spp. are killed by heating at 55°C for 30 min. *H. influenzae* grows better in aerobic than in anaerobic conditions. Raised carbon dioxide tension improves the growth and may be required for a number of species, including *H. aphrophilus*, *H. paraphrophilus*, *H. paraphrohaemolyticus* and *H. paragallinarum*. Under the usual conditions found in a bench incubator or incubator room some recently isolated strains of *Haemophilus* spp. may grow only feebly or not at all. Therefore, carbon dioxide should be added to the atmosphere for the primary isolation and may be beneficial for subsequent cultures of *Haemophilus* spp. Many strains that have an apparent carbon dioxide requirement on primary isolation rapidly become adapted to growing in air.

6.3   Type of growth

COLONIAL MORPHOLOGY

The colonies produced by *Haemophilus* spp. on solid media vary considerably with the individual strains and with the medium used. On blood agar, *H. influenzae* forms translucent low convex or flat pinpoint colonies. On a more favourable medium, such as chocolate agar, Levinthal's agar or Fildes' agar, colonies of non-capsulate strains are typically greyish, transparent, smooth and low convex or flat with a slightly splayed-out entire edge (Fig. 50.3; see also Plate 50.3). They attain a size of 0.5–0.8 mm after incubation for 24 h at 37°C, enlarging to 1–1.5 mm by 48 h. Morphologically atypical strains produce more granular colonies. Capsulate strains of *H. influenzae* form larger, more opaque, smooth, mucoid colonies 3–4 mm in diameter, which may appear to coalesce. Colonies of capsulate strains grown on clear media, such as Levinthal's agar, are iridescent when examined by obliquely transmitted light. The iridescence is due to dispersion of light by the arrangement of organisms in a grid-like pattern like a diffraction grating (Engbaek 1950).

Colonies of *H. influenzae* grow to a larger size in the vicinity of certain other bacterial colonies, e.g. staphylococci, that secrete V factor (satellitism) (Fig. 50.4; see also Plate 50.4). Strains from cases of meningitis and epiglottitis usually produce indole, which gives the cultures a characteristic pungent smell.

The various colonial forms of the other *Haemophilus* spp. tend to resemble non-capsulate *H. influenzae* with a few exceptions. *H. haemoglobinophilus* colonies at first

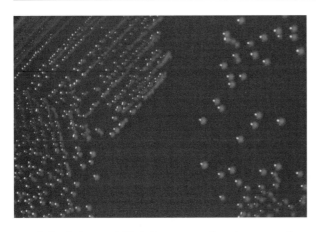

Fig. 50.3 Culture of *H. influenzae* on chocolate agar. See Plate 50.3 for colour.

Fig. 50.4 Culture of *H. influenzae* on whole horse blood agar showing satellitism of colonies adjacent to a streak of *Staphylococcus aureus*. See Plate 50.4 for colour.

resemble *H. influenzae* but become more opaque and larger, reaching 1–2 mm diameter at 24 h. They grow well on blood agar and growth is not enhanced around staphylococci. *H. aphrophilus* and *H. paraphrophilus* form small, highly convex, granular colonies. Colonies of *H. parainfluenzae* can be flat and smooth or rough and wrinkled, reaching a size of 1–2 mm at 24 h. *H. segnis* is slow growing, the colonies being smooth or granular, odour-free and about 0.5 mm after incubation for 48 h. *H. parasuis* is also slow growing, the colonies reaching a diameter of 0.5 mm after 48–72 h. *H. paragallinarum* is usually capsulate, producing iridescent colonies on transparent media.

In liquid media, such as Levinthal's broth or Filde's broth, most strains of *H. influenzae* produce a uniform turbidity. Occasional strains that produce a flocculent deposit with a slight turbidity of the supernatant suspension are found to be filamentous on microscopic examination.

HAEMOLYSIS

Pritchett and Stillman (1919) observed that gram-negative rods requiring X and V factors could be haemolytic. Pittman (1953) distinguished *H. haemolyticus* and *H. parahaemolyticus* from the non-haemolytic spe-

cies *H. influenzae* and *H. parainfluenzae*. Zinnemann et al. (1971) described the haemolytic species *H. paraphrohaemolyticus* which requires V factor and carbon dioxide. Kilian (1976) noted that in a proportion of strains of *H. parahaemolyticus* and *H. paraphrohaemolyticus* haemolysis is an unstable property.

7 METABOLISM

Holländer (1976) characterized the energy metabolism of representative strains of *H. influenzae, H. parainfluenzae* and *H. aegyptius*. All of the strains possessed functional enzymes of the Embden–Meyerhof–Parnas and Entner–Doudoroff pathways, the hexose monophosphate shunt, tricarboxylic acid cycle and gluconeogenesis, with a high activity of malate dehydrogenase.

8 GENETIC MECHANISMS

8.1 Transformation and transduction

The genome of *H. influenzae* has been shown to be a 1.9 Mb circle with a G + C content of c. 37% and genetic maps for *H. influenzae* strains Rd (capsule type d) and Eagan (capsule type b) have been constructed by use of pulsed field gel electrophoresis (Barcak et al. 1991, Butler and Moxon 1990). *H. influenzae* strain Rd is the first bacterium for which the entire DNA sequence has been determined (Fleischmann et al. 1995). Several restriction-modification systems have been identified and characterized from haemophili. *H. influenzae* is naturally transformable; under growth-limiting conditions it will become competent to bind and take up double-stranded DNA and recombine these fragments into any homologous sites on the chromosome. Temperate bacteriophages, but no virulent or transducing phage, have been identified in *H. influenzae* (Barcak et al. 1991).

8.2 Plasmids and transposons

Plasmids have been identified in *H. influenzae*. Large (c. 60 kb), conjugative plasmids are associated with multiple antibiotic resistance and are generally integrated into the chromosome (Stuy 1980, Levy et al. 1993). TnA or Tn*10*-like transposons carrying ampicillin or tetracycline resistance genes, respectively, are often carried on these plasmids and are thought to have been acquired from Enterobacteriaceae by a cryptic plasmid in *H. parainfluenzae* (Brunton, Clare and Meier 1986). Chloramphenicol resistance genes have been shown to be inserted into one of the inverted repeat sequences flanking the tetracycline resistance transposon (Brunton, Clare and Meier 1986). Indistinguishable plasmids have been identified from epidemiologically unrelated *H. influenzae*, suggesting conjugative spread in nature (Dimopoulou et al. 1992). Small (<10 kb) cytoplasmic, non-conjugative plasmids encoding TEM-1 mediated ampicillin resistance have been identified in various *Haemophilus* species; these share homology with similar plasmids from *Neisseria* (Brunton, Clare and Meier 1986). A 4.4 kb cytoplasmic plasmid has been associated with the production of ROB-1 β-lactamase in *H. influenzae* (Daum et al. 1988). These plasmids are similar to those found in *H. pleuropneumoniae* (now classified as *Actinobacillus*) (Daum et al. 1988) and Medeiros, Levesque and Jacoby (1986) have postulated an animal source for this resistance. A c. 36 kb plasmid p1031 has been associated with the majority of *H. influenzae* biogroup aegyptius strains from Brazilian purpuric fever (BPF) although not all strains possess the plasmid (Tondella, Quinn and Perkins 1995).

Insertion sequences are associated with *H. influenzae* type b (Hib) and have been detected in some non-capsulate *H. influenzae* (NCHI) (St. Geme et al. 1994). Many virulence-associated genes have been investigated; in particular, the genetics of encapsulation has been investigated in detail (Kroll 1992) and in vitro capsule loss has been shown to be due to recombination-mediated disruption of a gene involved in export (*bexB*).

8.3 Population genetics

The population genetics structure of *H. influenzae* has been reviewed by Pennington (1993). A multilocus enzyme electrophoresis (MLEE) study of 2209 capsulate strains from 30 countries showed the population structure to be clonal with 9 clones responsible for most invasive Hib disease (Musser et al. 1990). In contrast, studies of NCHI showed a panmictic structure with innumerable clones (Porras et al. 1986, Musser et al. 1986). Non-capsulate strains are thought to have arisen by convergent evolutionary loss of the ability to synthesize or express a polysaccharide capsule from a capsulate ancestor (Musser et al. 1986).

9 CELL ENVELOPE COMPOSITION: ANTIGENIC STRUCTURE

9.1 Capsule

There are 6 antigenic types of capsule in *H. influenzae*, designated a–f (Pittman 1931), each one composed of a linear polymer of disaccharide units. The capsules are negatively charged, acidic and hydrophobic. The capsules of types a, b, c and f contain phosphodiester linkages and are, therefore, teichoic acids, whereas types d and e contain glycosidic linkages with no phosphate, and unusual sugars, and are true polysaccharides (Moxon and Kroll 1990). Types a and b differ from the others in containing the 5-carbon component ribitol, and type b is unique as both sugars are pentoses. The type b capsule has been the most extensively characterized and consists of a phosphodiester-linked polymer of polyribosyl ribitol phosphate (PRP). The type b capsule antigen (PRP) cross-reacts with a wide variety of bacteria including *Streptococcus pneumoniae*, *Streptococcus pyogenes*, *Staphylococcus aureus*,

Staphylococcus epidermidis, Enterococcus faecium and E. coli K100 (reviewed by Slack 1990).

Hib disease is associated with a lack of antibodies to PRP. Infants less than about 2 years old have little or no anticapsular antibodies once maternal antibodies decline and are especially susceptible to infection with Hib. Immunization of infants with PRP fails to elicit protective levels of antibody in this age group (Peltola et al. 1977). This is due to the T-cell independent nature of the immune response to polysaccharide antigens. The conjugation of PRP to a protein carrier stimulates anti-PRP antibodies in young infants and is the basis of current Hib vaccines (Jones 1993). The PRP capsule also stimulates complement-mediated bacteriolysis (Moxon and Kroll 1990, Tunkel and Scheld 1993).

9.2 Fimbriae

Fimbriae (pili) have been demonstrated on *H. influenzae* (reviewed by van Alphen and van Ham 1994). Hib from the nasopharynx usually express fimbriae whereas isolates from blood and cerebrospinal fluid do not; this has been shown to be due to reversible phase variation. Four families of fimbriae have been described in *H. influenzae*: LKP, SNN, LNN and VNN. At least 14 serotypes of long thick haemagglutinating (LKP) fimbriae have been recognized amongst Hib and NCHI. Thin non-haemagglutinating fimbriae (SNN) have been demonstrated on Hib and all NCHI tested, including *H. influenzae* biogroup aegyptius (St. Geme, Gilsdorf and Falkow 1991). Amino acid homology between fimbrin from thin, non-haemagglutinating fimbriae and ompA proteins from other gram-negative bacteria has been demonstrated (Sirakova et al. 1994). In a chinchilla model of otitis media, antibodies to LKP fimbriae were shown to confer protection only against strains with homologous fimbriae. Antibodies specific for non-haemagglutinating fimbriae reacted with strains with homologous or heterologous fimbriae, although few strains were tested and the fimbriae preparation was impure. Recent studies suggest that antibodies to non-haemagglutinating fimbriae are partially protective in this model (Sirakova et al. 1994).

9.3 Lipopolysaccharide

The major constituent of the outer membrane is lipopolysaccharide (LPS) or lipo-oligosaccharide (LOS). In *H. influenzae*, this comprises lipid A linked to outer core oligosaccharides, via a single phosphorylated ketodeoxyoctulosonic acid moiety and 3 heptoses, but lacks a high molecular weight side chain; hence it is strictly a lipo-oligosaccharide (LOS). The lipid A backbone is a glucosamine disaccharide substituted by 2 phosphate groups, as in enterobacterial lipid A, but with a simpler fatty acid composition of only tetradecanoic and its 3-hydroxylated derivative (reviewed by Moxon and Maskell 1992). At least 2 species-specific antigenically distinct components of lipid A have been detected among capsulate and non-capsulate strains.

The outer core oligosaccharides contain mainly glucose and galactose, with the molar ratios and linkages varying between the capsular types a–f, and a sialylated terminal lactosamine (reviewed by Roche and Moxon 1995). Several LOS epitopes are similar to those in pathogenic *Neisseria* species and are cross-reactive with human glycosphingolipid epitopes. Extensive antigenic variation in LOS, between strains and within strains, has been documented for capsulate strains and NCHI. Variation in colonial morphology is also associated with variation in LPS (Roche and Moxon 1995). Antibodies to LOS have been demonstrated after infection but are not protective.

9.4 Outer-membrane proteins

The outer membrane of *H. influenzae* contains 25–35 different proteins with a few major polypeptides accounting for 80% of the total outer-membrane protein (OMP) (Loeb and Smith 1982). A numerical and an alphabetical classification system for OMPs, which are sarkosyl insoluble, are in use (reviewed by van Alphen 1993). The major OMPs are P1 (or a, M_r 43–50 kDa), P2 (or b/c, a doublet, M_r 43–50 kDa with porin activity), P4 (or e, a lipoprotein, M_r 30 kDa), P5 (or d/f; 2 conformers of the same protein) and P6 (or g, a lipoprotein, M_r 16.6 kDa). Protein c is probably a minor protein, and the OMP originally designated P3 consists of both the non-heat-modified form of P1 and the heat-modified form of P5. OMPs P1, P2 and P5 are heterogeneous in molecular weight and form the basis for typing systems (see section 13). Conserved epitopes which elicit protective antibody responses against all *H. influenzae* have been sought as candidates for inclusion in component vaccines. Antibodies to OMP P1 were shown to be partially protective against Hib in an infant rat bacteraemic model (Granoff and Munson 1986, Gonzales et al. 1987, Loeb 1987) and antibodies to P2 and P6 were shown to be protective in this model (Granoff and Munson 1986, Green, Quinn-Dey and Zlotnick 1987). OMP P4 is reported to be a conserved non-immunogenic protein and anti-P4 serum was not protective against Hib meningitis in infant rats (Granoff and Munson 1986, van Alphen 1993). In contrast, antibodies raised against P4 were shown to be bactericidal for Hib strain Eagan and 6 NCHI (Green et al. 1991). Rabbit antibodies to OMP P5 did not protect infant rats from infection with Hib in the infant rat bacteraemic model (Granoff and Munson 1986). Monoclonal antibody studies have shown OMP P1 epitopes to be non-conserved between Hib or NCHI strains (Panezutti et al. 1993). OMP P2 is conserved in type b strains but extremely diverse and shows antigenic drift in NCHI; antibodies are strain specific (Duim et al. 1994, Murphy 1994). OMP P6 has been shown to be conserved in Hib and NCHI and bactericidal antibodies demonstrated in human sera (Nelson et al. 1988, Barenkamp 1992). Human cellular immunity to the P6 OMP of NCHI has been demonstrated (Kodama and Faden 1995). Antisera against a purified outer-membrane lipoprotein PCP (M_r 15 kDa, which co-migrates

with OMP P6) was shown to be bactericidal for 9 of 11 NCHI but not Hib strain Eagan (Deich et al. 1990). A conserved epitope was detected in all 30 *H. influenzae* tested, including 27 NCHI, and *H. parainfluenzae* (Deich et al. 1990). Synergistic killing of NCHI by anti-e and anti-PCP (Green et al. 1991) and anti-PCP and anti-P6 sera (Deich et al. 1990) has been reported. Antibodies against surface exposed proteins of M_r 98 kDa and c. 103 kDa (antigen D15) have been detected in convalescent serum from the majority of infants with invasive Hib disease and shown to reduce the level of bacteraemia in infant rats (Kimura et al. 1985, Thomas et al. 1990).

10 CLASSIFICATION

Tables 50.1 and 50.2 show that members of this genus can be classified on their requirement for X and V factors, their haemolytic activity and their biochemical activities; requirement for an increased partial pressure of carbon dioxide in the atmosphere for primary isolation is also of some help. Tests of carbohydrate utilization and acid production can be of considerable value in the classification of *Haemophilus* spp. The results of these tests are, to some extent, affected by the media used, the period of observation and other conditions of the test, and thus they should be interpreted with caution. The degree of acidity may be slight and haemophili can produce acid in media devoid of sugar (Tunevall 1951). All haemophili, with the exception of *H. ducreyi*, 'ferment' glucose anaerobically (Sneath and Johnson 1973). The exact mode of carbohydrate breakdown in these tests is not known and the term 'fermentation' is being applied in a somewhat loose sense to refer to metabolism with acid production. Most strains of *H. parainfluenzae*, *H. haemolyticus*, *H. aphrophilus* and *H. paraphrophilus* produce small amounts of hydrogen and carbon dioxide from glucose (Kilian 1976). The remaining species do not produce any gas, indicating differences in the pathways of carbohydrate metabolism within the genus.

Almost all strains of *Haemophilus* reduce nitrate to nitrite (Kilian 1976). Catalase and oxidase reactions can be used to differentiate species of *Haemophilus*. Biberstein and Gills (1961) noted the catalase activity of haemophili can vary with the conditions of the test; some catalase-negative strains become catalase-positive when provided with sufficient haemin. *H. influenzae* is invariably oxidase positive, *H. aphrophilus* and *H. ducreyi* are oxidase negative, the oxidase reaction of other species is variable. Urease activity is found in many strains of *H. influenzae*, *H. parainfluenzae*, *H. parahaemolyticus* and *H. paraphrohaemolyticus* (Kilian 1976).

11 LABORATORY ISOLATION AND IDENTIFICATION

11.1 Isolation

The isolation of *Haemophilus* spp. from clinical

Table 50.2 Biochemical characteristics of *Haemophilus* spp.

Species	Production of				Acid from							
	Cat	Ox	Ind	Ure	Glu	Fru	Gal	Lac	Man	Suc	Tre	Xyl
H. influenzae	+	+	D	D	+	−	+	−	−	−	−	+
H. haemolyticus	+	+	±	+	+	W	+	−	−	−	−	V
H. haemoglobinophilus	+	+	+	−	+	−	−	−	+	+	−	+
H. ducreyi	−	+	−	−	−	−	−	−	−	−	−	−
H. aphrophilus	−	−	−	−	+	+	+	+	−	+	+	−
H. parainfluenzae	±	+	D	D	+	+	+	−	−	+	−	−
H. parahaemolyticus	±	+	−	+	+	+	±	−	−	+	−	−
H. paraphrohaemolyticus	+	+	−	+	+	+	V	−	−	+	−	−
H. paraphrophilus	−	+	−	−	+	+	−	+	−	+	+	−
H. segnis	V^w	−	−	−	W	W	±^{w}	−	−	W	−	−
H. parasuis	+	−	−	−	+	+	+	V	−	+	−	−
H. paragallinarum	−	−	−	−	+	+	−	−	+	+	−	V
H. paracuniculus	+	+	+	+	+	+	−	−	−	+	−	−

Cat, catalase; Ox, oxidase; Ind, indole; Ure, urease; Glu, glucose; Fru, fructose; Gal, galactose; Lac, lactose; Man, mannitol; Suc, sucrose; Tre, trehalose; Xyl, xylose.
+, positive; −, negative; ± = variable, most strains negative; V, variable; W, weak reaction; D, different reaction given by biotypes.
Data compiled from the work of Kristensen (1922), Lewis and Shope (1931), Tunevall (1951), Biberstein and White (1969); Sneath and Johnson (1973), Kilian (1976), Hinz and Kunjara (1977), Kilian and Theilade (1978), Targowski and Targowski (1979), Zinnemann (1980), Broom and Sneath (1981), Sturm and Zanen (1984), Kilian and Biberstein (1984).

material requires the use of media that fulfil the fastidious growth requirements of these micro-organisms. Ordinary blood agar is not suitable because growth of strains requiring V factor is limited by the V-factor deficiency of this medium. Most species grow well on chocolate agar. Rennie et al. (1992) found that GC agar base supplemented with 1% yeast autolysate and 5% sheep blood (chocolated) was superior to other medium bases and growth supplements for the primary isolation of *Haemophilus* spp. (except *H. ducreyi*). Levinthal (1918) devised a transparent and nearly colourless medium which is capable of supporting the growth of *H. influenzae*. The use of such a medium is essential for observing the iridescence of capsulate strains of *H. influenzae*. A transparent medium may also be prepared from Fildes' peptic digest of blood (Fildes 1920). Completely synthetic media have been devised by many workers but Tebbutt (1984) found none of these defined media was adequate for growth of a wide range of strains of *H. influenzae*.

For primary isolation of haemophili from specimens from the respiratory tract, a medium that supports good growth of haemophili can be made somewhat selective by the addition of substances that inhibit other members of the normal respiratory tract flora, e.g. media containing bacitracin (Barber 1969) and vancomycin, bacitracin and clindamycin (Chapin and Doern 1983) have been described. Möller et al. (1993) described NAG medium, (blood agar base supplemented with *N*-acetyl glucosamine, haemin and NAD) which improves the isolation of *H. influenzae* from the sputum of cystic fibrosis patients. Vastine et al. (1974) found IsoVitalex supplemented chocolate agar was the most useful medium for the isolation of *Haemophilus* spp. from the conjunctiva. Sturm (1986) described a selective culture medium containing van-

comycin, bacitracin, clindamycin and amphotericin B to facilitate the isolation of *H. influenzae* and *H. parainfluenzae* from genital tract specimens. Michaels, Stonebraker and Robbins (1975) described a Levinthal agar supplemented with high titre *H. influenzae* type b antiserum. Barbour, Crook and Mayon-White (1993) devised an improved antiserum agar consisting of Columbia agar supplemented with yeast extract, haemin, NAD, bacitracin and type b antiserum. On this medium colonies of *H. influenzae* type b can be readily discerned in mixed cultures from respiratory material since they have an obvious halo of antigen–antibody precipitate (Fig. 50.5).

Cultures should be incubated at 37°C in an aerobic atmosphere enhanced with 5–10% carbon dioxide.

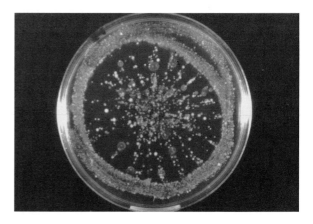

Fig. 50.5 Culture of a throat swab on antiserum agar showing halos around colonies of Hib. (By courtesy of Dr M Barbour.)

11.2 Identification

A presumptive *Haemophilus* spp. isolate should first be tested for its X- and V-factor requirements. These requirements are usually demonstrated by the absence of growth on media deficient in X and V factor but otherwise nutritionally adequate, except near paper disks or strips impregnated with X, V or X plus V factors (Fig. 50.6). Consistent results in these tests for growth factor requirements will be obtained only if a small inoculum is used, to avoid carry over of the factors. V-factor requirement of strains can be inferred by demonstrating satellitism near a streak of *Staph. aureus*. As V factor is heat-labile, media in which all the constituents have been autoclaved will reliably be free of it. Most of the basic fluid and solid media contain traces of X factor, as do some brands and batches of peptone. Doern and Chapin (1984) found trypticase soy agar to be more reliable than either brain heart infusion agar or Mueller–Hinton agar for testing the X requirement of *Haemophilus* spp. We find Columbia agar to be generally satisfactory for this purpose. Inzana, Claridge and Williams (1987) devised a broth system for the rapid determination of the X- and V-factor requirements of *Haemophilus* spp. which gives results in 4–5 hours. Kilian (1974) suggested that probably no complex medium which otherwise satisfies the growth requirements of *Haemophilus* spp. is completely free of X factor. He found that 18% of *H. influenzae* strains were misidentified as *H. parainfluenzae*, and claimed more reliable results by testing the ability of strains of *Haemophilus* spp. to synthesize porphyrins from δ-aminolaevulinic acid (ALA).

The porphyrin test (Kilian 1974) provides an accurate and reliable method for determining X-factor requirement (Fig. 50.2). A substrate of 2 mM ALA and 0.08 mM $MgSO_4$ in 0.1 M phosphate buffer pH 6.9 is used. A loopful of growth from a 24 h chocolate agar culture is added to 0.5 ml of substrate and the mixture is incubated for 4 h at 37°C. Porphyrin production is demonstrated by the development of a red fluorescence when the mixture is exposed to a Wood's lamp (maximum emission 360 nm). Alternatively the presence of porphobilinogen can be demonstrated after incubation for 24 h by adding 0.5 ml of Kovac's reagent. A red colour in the aqueous phase indicates the presence of porphobilinogen. *H. parainfluenzae* can be used as a positive control. A disc method for the porphyrin test (Lund and Blazevic 1977) and a porphyrin test agar (Gadberry and Amos 1986) have also been described.

Biochemical tests

Haemolysis of horse blood agar is of value in differentiating *H. influenzae* from *H. haemolyticus*, *H. parainfluenzae* and *H. parahaemolyticus*. Carbohydrate utilization can be studied in phenol red broth base supplemented with 1% of the carbohydrate and 10 mg l^{-1} each of NAD^+ and haemin (Kilian 1976). The results can be read after incubation for 24 h. Some species, notably *H. segnis*, show weak reactions and *H. ducreyi* does not ferment any carbohydrate in conventional tests. (See Table 50.2.)

Three biochemical tests – for indole, urease and ornithine decarboxylase – can be used to biotype *H. influenzae* and *H. parainfluenzae* (Kilian 1976) (see section 13). Biotyping can be conveniently performed in media that do not support growth since the tests detect the presence of preformed enzymes or enzyme systems (Kilian 1976). Several commercial micromethod kits have been used successfully to identify *Haemophilus* spp. and biotype *H. influenzae* and *H. parainfluenzae*. These include API 10E, API 20E and HNID (Quentin et al. 1992), API NH (Barbé et al. 1994), Rapid NH and RIM-Haemophilus (Murphy et al. 1990).

Molecular techniques are now being applied to the detection and identification of *Haemophilus* spp. in clinical specimens and for confirmatory tests on isolates. A PCR technique has also been employed to identify *H. parainfluenzae* (Hamed et al. 1994). Species-specific DNA probes and PCR-based techniques have been used to detect *H. influenzae* in clinical material (Malouin et al. 1988, Daly et al. 1991, Rådström et al. 1994, Ueyama et al. 1995) and to determine the capsular genotype of isolates (Falla et al. 1994) (see section 13).

12 SUSCEPTIBILITY TO ANTIMICROBIAL AGENTS

H. influenzae is commonly susceptible in vitro to therapeutically achievable concentrations of ampicillin, chloramphenicol, tetracycline, aminoglycosides, rifampicin, ciprofloxacin, sulphonamides, trimethoprim and co-trimoxazole. Representative minimum inhibitory concentrations (MICs) of a range of antimicrobial agents for *H. influenzae* are shown in Table 50.3.

For many years ampicillin was the treatment of choice for *H. influenzae* infections, but the increasing prevalence of resistance to ampicillin and several other antibiotics has prompted changes in the way these infections are treated.

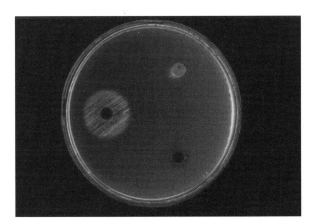

Fig. 50.6 Growth factor requirement of *H. influenzae*. Putative *Haemophilus* strain sown on Columbia agar plate. Discs containing X factor, V factor and X + V factor placed on surface of inoculated plate. Colonies of *H. influenzae* grow in vicinity of disc containing X + V factor but not near the discs containing either factor alone.

Table 50.3 Susceptibility of *Haemophilus influenzae* to antimicrobial agents

Agent	MIC[a] (mg l^{-1})
Benzyl penicillin	1–2
Ampicillin/amoxycillin[b]	0.5
Amoxycillin: clavulanic acid (2:1)[b]	0.5/0.25
Cefuroxime	0.5
Cefotaxime (desacetyl cefotaxime)	0.06 (0.25)
Ceftriaxone	0.03
Cefpodoxime	0.06
Cefixime	0.12
Cefaclor	4
Imipenem	1
Meropenem	0.5
Aztreonam	0.25
Chloramphenicol	0.5
Tetracycline	0.5
Rifampicin	1
Erythromycin	0.5–8
Clarithromycin	1–4
Azithromycin	0.5–2
Ciprofloxacin	0.015
Ofloxacin	<0.06
Trimethoprim	0.5
Sulphamethoxazole	4
Gentamicin	1

MIC determined by an agar-dilution technique; inoculum c. 10^4 colony forming units (cfu) (10^2 cfu for sulphonamide). Data compiled from Slack and Anderson (unpublished).
[a]90% of strains inhibited by concentration less than value stated.
[b]β-Lactamase negative strains.

The first reports of clinical resistance to ampicillin in cases of *H. influenzae* meningitis appeared in 1974 (Gunn et al.). The ampicillin resistance in these strains was mediated by a TEM-1 β-lactamase (Williams, Kattan and Cavanagh 1974). Ampicillin-resistant strains of *H. influenzae* are now distributed throughout the world and have become increasingly prevalent. Markedly differing rates of resistance to ampicillin have been reported in various parts of the world (Table 50.4). A second β-lactamase, designated ROB-1, has been described in *H. influenzae* (Rubin et al. 1981) and has been associated with failure of ampicillin therapy. A third, designated VAT-1, has been described recently in *H. influenzae* (Vali, Thomson and Amyes 1994, Shanahan, Thomson and Amyes 1996). Production of a β-lactamase is the most common mechanism of ampicillin resistance in *H. influenzae*, but a small number of strains exhibit reduced susceptibility to a range of β-lactam agents without β-lactamase activity being detectable (Bell and Plowman 1980, Markowitz 1980). The major mechanism of ampicillin resistance in these strains is thought to be decreased binding to penicillin binding proteins (PBP) 3A and 3B (Mendelman et al. 1984, Mendelman, Chaffin and Kalaitzoglu 1990, Clairoux et al. 1992). It has been suggested that strains with altered PBPs may be less virulent (Clairoux et al. 1992). Tolerance to β-lactam antibiotics (MBC/MIC ratio >32) has also been described in *H. influenzae* (Bergeron and Lavoie 1985) but its clinical significance is unclear.

Chloramphenicol resistance in *H. influenzae* was first noted in 1976 (Manten, van Klingeren and Dessens-Kroon 1976). The resistance is usually of a high level and is almost always due to the production of a plasmid-mediated chloramphenicol acetyl transferase (CAT) type II (Roberts et al. 1980). Non-CAT-mediated resistance has been observed. This form of resistance is chromosomally encoded, and is due to a permeability barrier to the uptake of chloramphenicol by the cell, associated with the loss of an outer-membrane protein (Burns et al. 1985). Almost all CAT-mediated chloramphenicol resistant strains are also resistant to tetracycline (Roberts et al. 1980). Resistance to both ampicillin and chloramphenicol in *H. influenzae* type b was first reported in 1980 from Bangkok (Simasthien, Dnangmani and Echeverria 1980) and has since been recognized in many parts of the world, including the USA and the UK. Strains resistant to chloramphenicol or chloramphenicol and ampicillin are still relatively uncommon, accounting for 1–2% of all isolates in most parts of the world. An explosive increase in antibiotic resistance in *H. influenzae* type b was observed in Barcelona (Campos, Garcia-Tornel and Sanfelin 1984) where resistance to ampicillin was detected in 20 (60%) of 35 strains causing meningitis; 65.7% were resistant to chloramphenicol and 57% were resistant to both agents. Most of these strains were also resistant to tetracycline and to co-trimoxazole (Campos et al. 1986).

Trimethoprim resistance was detected in 6.8% of strains monitored in the 1991 UK survey (Powell et al. 1992). The emergence of rifampicin-resistant *H. influenzae* following chemoprophylaxis with oral rifampicin has been reported (Murphy et al. 1981, Nicolle et al. 1982). The combination of rifampicin and trimethoprim (1:1) is synergic and bactericidal and might prevent the selection of rifampicin resistant mutants (Yogev, Melick and Glogowski 1982) (see Jorgensen 1992, Powell 1988, de Groot et al. 1991 for reviews of antimicrobial resistance in *H. influenzae*).

Antimicrobial resistance has been reported in a number of other *Haemophilus* spp. β-lactamase-mediated ampicillin resistance has been found more frequently in *H. parainfluenzae* than in *H. influenzae* (Green et al. 1979, Scheifele and Fussell 1981). β-Lactamase activity has been seen also in *H. parahaemolyticus, H. paraphrophilus* (Green et al. 1979, Jones, Slepack and Bigelow 1976) and *H. ducreyi* (Brunton et al. 1979). Non-β-lactamase-mediated ampicillin resistance has been noted in *H. parainfluenzae* (Walker and Smith 1980). Plasmid-mediated chloramphenicol resistance (Cavanagh, Morris and Mitchell 1975) and aminoglycoside resistance (le Goffic et al. 1977) have also been described in this species.

Table 50.4 Prevalence of antimicrobial resistance among clinical isolates of *Haemophilus influenzae* from different parts of the world

Agent (resistance criterion, MIC)	Percentage (%) of strains resistant in						
	UK	USA	Spain	Belgium	Finland	Gambia	Hong Kong
Ampicillin (β-lactamase + ve)	19.9	16.5	31.1	12.0	8.2	0	20
Ampicillin (β-lactamase − ve, MIC >2 μg l⁻¹)	4.2	0.7	<1	<1	<1	<1	<1
Chloramphenicol (ᵃCAT + ve)	<1	<1	16.7	5.3	<1	1.5	14
Tetracycline (MIC >2 mg l⁻¹)	<1	2.1	17.2	12.8	1	6.3	25

ᵃCAT, choramphenicol acetyl transferase.
Data compiled from Jorgensen et al. (1990), Powell et al. (1992), Kayser, Morenzoni and Santanam (1990), Nissinen et al. (1995), Ling et al. (1989), Bijlmer et al. (1994) and Slack and Anderson (unpublished observations).

12.1 Antimicrobial susceptibility testing

Antimicrobial susceptibility testing of *H. influenzae* by disk-diffusion procedures is significantly influenced by technical variations in inoculum size, culture medium and antimicrobial content of the discs. Jorgensen et al. (1987) have described a simple transparent susceptibility testing media for *H. influenzae*. Mueller-Hinton medium supplemented with haematin 15 mg l⁻¹, NAD 15 mg⁻¹ and yeast extract 5 g⁻¹. This medium is now commercially available as Haemophilus Test Medium. NAD agar (DST agar, Oxoid, supplemented with NAD 10 mg l⁻¹ and 5% lysed defibrinated horse blood) is a satisfactory medium for antimicrobial susceptibility testing of *H. influenzae*. *Haemophilus* spp. that produce β-lactamase may appear susceptible to ampicillin in conventional disc susceptibility tests. Disc tests can also fail to detect non-β-lactamase-mediated ampicillin resistance if the content of the ampicillin disc is too high (Philpott-Howard, Seymour and Williams 1983, Mendelman et al. 1986). More accurate results can be obtained if a low content (2 μg) ampicillin disc is used and a test for β-lactamase is employed routinely, e.g. chromogenic cephalosporin test (O'Callaghan, Morris and Kirby 1972), or acidimetric paper strip test (Slack, Wheldon and Turk 1977a). Tests for β-lactamase are especially important since there have been cases of invasive *H. influenzae* type-b infection from which mixed populations of β-lactamase-positive and β-lactamase-negative strains have been isolated (Jubelrier and Yeager 1979, Stewardson-Krieger and Naidu 1981). The chromogenic cephalosporin, Nitrocefin, is only weakly labile to the ROB-1 enzyme (Rubin et al. 1981) which therefore may not be detected with this method.

To infer the mechanism of β-lactam resistance from disc tests the zone sizes around ampicillin (2 μg), amoxycillin–clavulanate (2 μg : 1 μg) and cefaclor can be measured. Strains producing β-lactamase will appear resistant to ampicillin and cefaclor but susceptible to amoxycillin–clavulanate. Strains that are β-lactam resistant and non-β-lactamase pro-

ducing will appear resistant to all 3 compounds (Powell and Williams 1988).

For chloramphenicol susceptibility tests a low content disc (2.5, 5 or 10 μg) should be used. A test for chloramphenicol inactivation (e.g. Slack, Wheldon and Turk 1977b, Azemun et al. 1981, Howard, Williams and Proole 1986, Park, Hixon and Berger 1990) can also be applied. Doern, Daum and Tubert (1987) found that a 1 h tube assay for CAT activity (Azemun et al. 1981) was significantly more accurate than a 30 min commercially available impregnated disc test. Tests for trimethoprim and erythromycin susceptibility are prone to considerable laboratory errors and the results should be interpreted with caution. The E-test is an antimicrobial agent gradient-coated plastic test strip which allows MIC determinations on solid media, which can be conveniently used for antimicrobial susceptibility tests of *Haemophilus* spp. (Jorgensen, Howell and Maher 1991) (See review on in vitro susceptibility testing of *H. influenzae* by Doern 1992.)

The detection of antimicrobial resistance genes by the use of DNA probes or PCR is now possible for several antimicrobial agents. (See reviews by Courvalin 1991, Tenover, Popovic and Olsvik 1993.)

13 TYPING METHODS

The limited diversity of Hib from disease has been demonstrated by many techniques, including OMP subtyping, ribotyping and MLEE (Musser et al. 1990), and has been explained by clonal theory (Pennington 1993). Subtyping techniques therefore only prove useful in epidemiological studies if a strain with an infrequent subtype is involved. Defined subtyping schemes enable global comparisons. In contrast, NCHI exhibit a much wider variety of phenotypes and genotypes and can be readily characterized in local epidemiological studies by many techniques but the consequential difficulty in defining subtypes makes inter-laboratory comparisons of large numbers of strains impossible. For phylogenetic studies, MLEE remains the standard; cluster analysis based on ribotyping has been shown to be discordant with protein profiling and MLEE (Bruce and Jordens 1991, Leaves and Jordens 1994).

13.1 Capsule typing

H. influenzae strains are differentiated on the basis of capsule expression into capsulate and non-capsulate strains. Six antigenically distinct types of capsule were detected by agglutination (Pittman 1931) and designated a–f. Type e strains have been shown to possess 2 capsular antigenic components, e1 and e2: a minority have only the e2 component (Williamson and Zinneman 1951). Capsule type has long been determined by agglutination-based methods (serotyping) but autoagglutination by some strains and cross-reactions between antisera have been noted (Falla et al. 1993). DNA-based methods of determining capsular type are now available. DNA hybridization patterns obtained with a probe (pUO38) containing *cap* genes have been shown to be capsule-type specific and give a characteristic pattern for capsule-deficient mutants of type b (Hib⁻) strains (Kroll, Ely and Moxon 1991). Fourteen capsular genotypes were detected among 222 isolates of capsulate *H. influenzae* from all over the world (Musser et al. 1990) with 4 types (b[S], b[G], b[V] and b[O]) detected among 85 type b strains. A study of 425 Hib from England and Wales identified 3 rare variants (Leaves, Falla and Crook 1995). Fragments of capsule-associated DNA, specifically IS*1016* sequences, have been detected in non-capsulate strains (St. Geme et al. 1994). Primers designed to amplify products of different sizes from each of the 6 capsular types in PCR enable the unequivocal determination of capsular genotype (Falla et al. 1994) (Fig. 50.7). The detection of Hib⁻ and other unusual genetic arrangements of capsule-associated genes is also possible with PCR (Leaves, Falla and Crook 1995).

13.2 Biotyping

H. influenzae and *H. parainfluenzae* can each be subtyped on the basis of 3 biochemical tests (for indole, urease and ornithine decarboxylase) into 8 biotypes (Table 50.5) (Kilian 1976, Oberhofer and Back 1979, Gratten 1983, Sottnek and Albritton 1984).

Most clinical isolates of *H. influenzae* are distributed between 4 biotypes (I, II, III and IV); Hib isolates from invasive disease are mainly biotype I and the majority of NCHI are biotype II or III. *H. influenzae* biogroup aegyptius is contained within biotype III and a subset of NCHI biotype IV strains have been implicated as an obstetric pathogen, causing neonatal infections (reviewed by van Alphen 1993).

13.3 Outer-membrane protein (OMP) subtyping

Polyacrylamide gel electrophoresis (SDS–PAGE) of

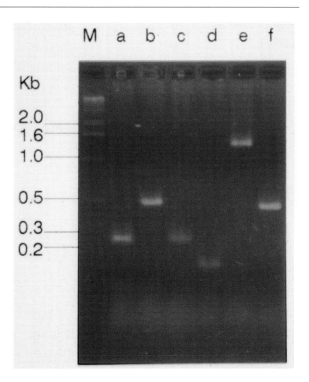

Fig. 50.7 PCR amplification products from *H. influenzae* capsule types a–f. M is a size marker. (By courtesy of Dr T Falla.)

outer-membrane proteins (OMPs) has formed the basis for subtyping Hib. Two OMP subtyping schemes, with different nomenclatures, have been advocated. With a normal SDS–PAGE system, 9 OMP subtypes have been defined in Hib (van Alphen 1994). Gradient SDS–PAGE gels classified 587 Hib isolates from all over the world into 33 subtypes (Musser et al. 1990). Five of the OMP subtypes are common to both schemes (van Alphen 1994). A few subtypes account for the majority of infections worldwide but the predominant subtypes vary geographically, in different host populations and at different times. Three OMP subtypes accounted for c. 75% of Hib in the USA (Granoff, Barenkamp and Munson 1982) whereas OMP subtype 1 (3L in the scheme of Granoff, Barenkamp and Munson 1982) accounted for 93% of Hib in the Netherlands and western Europe (van Alphen et al. 1987). OMP-enriched preparations have been used to distinguish between strains of NCHI. The enormous heterogeneity of NCHI precludes the definition of useful subtypes but OMP profiles have been used successfully to characterize strains in local outbreaks (Fig. 50.8) (Jordens et al. 1993). OMP subtyping has been shown to distinguish *H. influenzae* biogroup aegyptius from other biotype III *H. influenzae* (Carlone, Sottnek and Plikaytis 1985). Traditional methods for subtyping *H. influenzae* have been reviewed by van Alphen (1993). OMP electrophoretic patterns of *H. parainfluenzae* have been shown to be extremely heterogeneous (Quentin et al. 1989).

Table 50.5 Biotypes of *H. influenzae* and *H. parainfluenzae*

Species	Biotype	Production of		
		Indole	Urease	Ornithine decarboxylase
H. influenzae	I	+	+	+
	II	+	+	−
	III[a]	−	+	−
	IV	−	+	+
	V	+	−	+
	VI	−	−	+
	VII	+	−	−
	VIII	−	−	−
H. parainfluenzae	I	−	−	+
	II	−	+	+
	III	−	+	−
	IV	+	+	+
	V[b]	−	−	−
	VI	+	−	+
	VII	+	+	−
	VIII	+	−	−

[a]*H. influenzae* biotype III and *H. influenzae* biogroup aegyptius are indistinguishable biochemically but may be differentiated on the basis of OMP profiles.
[b]V-factor dependent strains negative in all three tests have been designated '*H. parainfluenzae* biotype V'. Similar negative reactions are given by *H. paraphrophilus* (but this is lactose positive) and *H. segnis* (poor growth and ferments slowly). (Kilian personal communication).

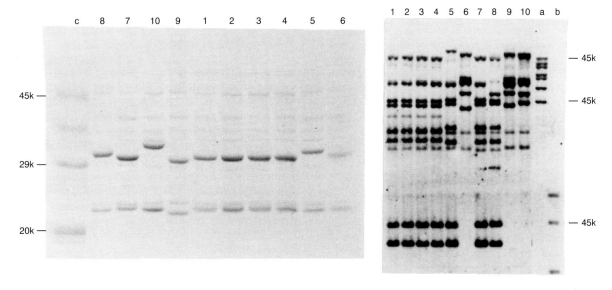

Fig. 50.8 SDS–PAGE of OMP-enriched preparations (left) and ribotyping patterns (right) of NCHI from a putative outbreak of hospital-acquired respiratory infection (tracks 1–6) and epidemiologically unrelated biotype II ampicillin resistant NCHI (tracks 7–10). a, b, c are size markers. Note: epidemiologically unrelated strains are distinct whereas isolates 1–4 are indistinguishable and probably represent spread of a single strain.

13.4 DNA-based typing and characterization

DNA-based methods for subtyping or characterizing strains of *H. influenzae* include restriction endonuclease analysis (REA) of chromosomal DNA, hybridization with probes for ribosomal RNA encoding genes (rDNA) and PCR-based methods. A subtyping scheme for Hib based on the pattern of *Eco*RI fragments of chromosomal DNA hybridizing with a probe for 16S and 23S rDNA (ribotyping) has defined 22 ribotypes (Leaves and Jordens 1994). 283 consecutive, unrelated clinical isolates from England and Wales were classified into 14 ribotypes and 4 OMP subtypes. Ribotype 1 accounted for 82% of isolates and there was good correlation between OMP subtype and ribotype. REA with *Bam*HI and ribotyping have been shown to concur with OMP analysis for characterizing NCHI (Bruce and Jordens 1991). Ribotyping has been used to discriminate NCHI strains (Fig. 50.8) (Stull, LiPuma and Edlind 1988, Bruce and Jordens 1991, Jordens et al. 1993, Smith-Vaughan et al. 1995) and *H. influenzae* biogroup aegyptius strains (Irino et al. 1988). REA with *Bam*HI has been used to characterize *H. parainfluenzae* (Kerr et al. 1993) and ribotyping to characterize *H. aphrophilus* and *H. paraphrophilus* (Sedlácek et al. 1993).

PCR-based amplification of randomly amplified polymorphic DNA (RAPD) (Fig. 50.9), inter-enterobacterial repetitive intergenic consensus (ERIC) sequences, *omp*P2 and rDNA have been used to characterize NCHI. In outbreak investigations, the results from RAPD, inter-ERIC amplification and OMP profiling were shown to correlate well (Jordens et al. 1993, van Belkum et al. 1994). Restriction analysis of the *omp*P2 amplification product was used to monitor the spread of *H. influenzae* (probably NCHI) between individuals in a closed community in Antarctica (Hobson et al. 1995). Amplification of c.6kb of rDNA, followed by restriction analysis with *Hae* III, was shown to correlate well with probe-based ribotyping (of *Xba*1 digests) for NCHI from Aboriginal children in Australia (Smith-Vaughan et al. 1995).

13.5   Typing methods for animal strains

A serotyping scheme (not based on capsules) has been reported for *H. paragallinarum* and a biotyping scheme based on the combination of serotyping, carbohydrate fermentation patterns and antimicrobial drug resistance patterns, together with REA, has been applied successfully to epidemiological studies of this species (Blackall et al. 1990). REA and ribotyping have shown that NAD-independent *H. paragallinarum* from chickens suffering from infectious coryza are indistinguish-

able and hence clonal (Miflin et al. 1995). A serotyping system has been described for *H. parasuis* (Kielstein, Rosner and Muller 1991).

14   BACTERIOCINS

Most *H. influenzae* type b produce a bacteriocin 'haemocin' (LiPuma et al. 1992), which is active against capsulate *H. influenzae* strains of other types, non-capsulate *H. influenzae*, other *Haemophilus* spp. and certain enterobacteria, but not against gram-positive bacteria. *Haemophilus* spp. vary in their susceptibility; non-typable *H. influenzae*, *H. haemolyticus* and *H. parainfluenzae* have been shown to be the most susceptible and *H. parahaemolyticus* the least susceptible (Venezia, Matusiak and Robertson 1977). A large proportion of strains of *E. coli* and related genera was susceptible to haemocin. Less closely related genera, including *Klebsiella*, *Proteus* and *Enterobacter* were uniformly resistant. This bacteriocin appears to act by inhibiting DNA synthesis (Streker, Venezia and Robertson 1978).

15   ROLE IN NORMAL HUMAN FLORA

Humans are the hosts of *H. influenzae*, *H. haemolyticus*, *H. aphrophilus*, *H. parainfluenzae*, *H. parahaemolyticus* and *H. segnis*. Haemophili can be found almost universally in the human pharynx by use of selective culture media. Kilian, Heine-Jensen and Bulow (1972) found haemophili in the nasopharynx of c. 80% of infants less than 1 year old; the carriage rate rose to nearly 100% during early childhood. In the mouth, haemophili are found on the tongue, palate, cheeks and teeth, in dental plaque and in saliva (Sims 1970).

H. influenzae can be isolated from the pharyngeal mucosa of 60–80% of young children. The colonization rate is considerably lower in older children and adults (see Turk and May 1967). *H. influenzae* constitutes only about 10% of the haemophili found in the pharynx and is virtually absent from the extensive haemophilus flora of the oral cavity (Kilian and Frederiksen 1981).

Several studies have measured the nasopharyngeal and oropharyngeal carriage rates of *H. influenzae* type b (Hib) prior to the introduction of routine Hib immunization of infants. Oropharyngeal carriage of Hib is uncommon during the first 6 months of life, rises to an average 3–5% among children aged 3–5 years and then gradually declines with increasing age. Many factors influence reported colonization rates, including age (Sell, Turner and Federspiel 1973), ethnic origin (Turk 1963) day-care attendance (Ginsburg et al. 1977) close family contact with a case of invasive Hib disease (Turk 1975, Michaels and Norden 1977), season of the year (Henderson et al. 1982), recent antibiotic therapy (Howard, Dunkin and Miller 1988) and sampling (Michaels et al. 1976) and cultural techniques (Chapin and Doern 1983). The use of standardized swabbing techniques and Hib antiserum agar

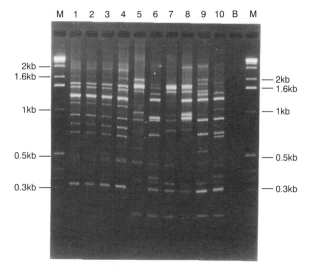

Fig. 50.9   Randomly amplified polymorphic DNA (RAPD) generated fingerprints of NCHI. Track numbers correspond to isolates shown in Fig. 50.8. B, reagent blank; M, size marker. Note: epidemiologically unrelated strains distinct whereas isolates 1–4 are indistinguishable and probably represent spread of a single strain.

(Barbour, Crook and Mayon-White 1993, Barbour et al. 1993) is recommended for these studies. *H. influenzae* types e and f are also carried in the pharynx at similar rates to Hib (Barbour et al. 1995). The carriage of *H. influenzae* including Hib is a dynamic process with intermittent colonization but tends to persist for weeks or months (Michaels and Nordern 1977, Glode et al. 1985) (See review of Hib carriage by Moxon 1986.) Hib immunization of infants results in reduced pharyngeal carriage of Hib (Takala, Eskola and Leinonen 1991, Takala et al. 1993, Mohle-Boetani et al. 1993). This appears to be the result of reduced or delayed acquisition of Hib in the first year of life (Barbour et al. 1995). Giving Hib vaccine to a child does not rapidly terminate carriage (Barbour et al. 1995). To date, carriage rates of *H. influenzae* type e and f appear to be unaffected by Hib immunization.

The haemolytic species *H. parahaemolyticus* and *H. paraphrohaemolyticus* have been isolated from the pharynx (Kilian, Heine-Jensen and Bulow 1972, Kawakami, Okimura and Kanai 1982) and oral cavity (Sims 1970). *H. haemolyticus* is found in the nasopharyngeal flora of c. 1% of the population (Kilian, Heine-Jensen and Bulow 1972). *H. parainfluenzae* is a regular member of the flora of the nasopharynx and mouth, accounting for c. 75% of the haemophili isolated from these sites (Kilian and Schiøtt 1975). It may also be found in the normal vaginal flora (Kilian 1976) and has been reported in 26% of faecal specimens (Palmer 1981). *H. segnis* forms a significant proportion of the flora of dental plaque (Liljemark et al. 1984) and is also found to a lesser extent in the oropharynx. *H. paraphrophilus* and *H. aphrophilus* show a predilection for teeth (Kilian and Schiøtt 1975, Kraut et al. 1972). *H. aphrophilus* has been found in dental plaque in about one quarter of the adult population (Kraut et al. 1972).

16 PATHOGENICITY AND VIRULENCE FACTORS

16.1 Pathogenicity

CAPSULATE *H. INFLUENZAE*

Within the genus *Haemophilus*, *H. influenzae* is the most important species causing human disease. *H. influenzae* is strictly a parasite of humans and is associated with the normal commensal flora of the respiratory tract (see section 15). Infections caused by *H. influenzae* generally result from invasion of the bloodstream or contiguous spread from the respiratory tract. Hib causes serious invasive disease in children under 5 years of age. This is predominantly meningitis, but also includes epiglottitis, pneumonia, cellulitis, osteomyelitis and septic arthritis (reviewed by Jordens and Slack 1995). Up to 20% of survivors of Hib meningitis have long term neurological sequelae. Risk factors for Hib disease are mainly socioeconomic and include overcrowding, attendance at day-care centres, chronic illness and lack of access to good health care facilities. Other capsular types may also cause invasive disease, notably type a, especially in non-industrialized countries. The introduction of vaccines effective against Hib in infants has dramatically reduced the incidence of Hib disease in children (Morbid Mortal Weekly Rep 1995) and consequently the epidemiology of Hib disease is changing (Hargreaves et al. 1995).

NON-CAPSULATE *H. INFLUENZAE* (NCHI)

NCHI are often associated with infection of previously damaged tissues, causing respiratory infections in patients with chronic bronchitis, bronchiectasis or cystic fibrosis. They can also cause pneumonia, sinusitis, otitis media and conjunctivitis, often in older children or adults. Recent reports show that NCHI are also an important cause of invasive disease in both adults and children (reviewed by Jordens and Slack 1995). In most cases there are predisposing factors such as head injury, with or without a cerebrospinal fluid leak, otitis media or sinusitis, and the infection is presumed to result from direct extension (Bol et al. 1987). A specific subset of NCHI has been implicated as a neonatal and maternal pathogen. *H. influenzae* biogroup aegyptius is associated with an acute form of seasonal conjunctivitis seen mainly in hot climates and in children. It has been implicated as the cause of Brazilian purpuric fever (BPF) (Morbid Mortal Weekly Rep 1986).

OTHER *HAEMOPHILUS* SPECIES

H. parainfluenzae, *H. parahaemolyticus*, *H. paraphrohaemolyticus*, *H. aphrophilus*, *H. paraphrophilus* and *H. segnis* are of relatively low pathogenicity but occasionally cause disease including endocarditis, meningitis, epiglottitis, septic arthritis, osteitis, brain abscess, acute pharyngitis, empyema of the gallbladder, jaw infections, appendicitis and a pancreatic abscess (see Albritton 1982 for review of infections caused in humans by *Haemophilus* spp. other than *H. influenzae*). *H. haemolyticus* is not thought to be pathogenic.

H. parasuis is an important opportunist pathogen of swine, particularly animals under stress, causing respiratory-tract infections and Glasser's syndrome (polyserositis) (see Nicolet 1992 for description). *H. haemoglobinophilus* has occasionally been implicated in urogenital inflammation in dogs (Osbaldiston 1971) but is probably of low pathogenicity. *H. paragallinarum* causes infectious coryza in chickens (Hinz and Kunjara 1977) and *H. paracuniculus* is associated with mucoid enteritis in rabbits (Targowski and Targowski 1979). For pathogenicity of *H. ducreyi* see section 17.

16.2 Virulence factors

Primates are the only species that naturally suffer from invasive Hib disease and infant primates provide a good model (Tunkel and Scheld 1993). Most animals do not develop meningitis after bacteraemia unless the permeability of the blood–brain barrier is increased. However, infant rats develop bacteraemia and meningitis after intranasal challenge with Hib (Moxon et al. 1974). This has been a valuable model for studying the early pathogenic events of meningitis. The pathogenesis and pathophysiology of bacterial meningitis has recently been reviewed by Tunkel and

Scheld (1993). NCHI have been studied in a chinchilla model of otitis media (Leake et al. 1994).

CAPSULATE H. INFLUENZAE

The possession of the type b capsule has been shown to be a major virulence factor. Animal studies of isogenic strains transformed with capsule-associated DNA confirmed earlier observations that type b strains were more virulent than type a strains which were more virulent than the other capsular types (Zwahlen et al. 1989). The bacterial capsule aids colonization and is probably the most important virulence factor for invasive disease as it protects against phagocytosis and complement-mediated lysis (Moxon and Kroll 1990, Tunkel and Scheld 1993). Other virulence factors which may be involved in adherence and colonization of Hib include LPS (Moxon and Maskell 1992), which is expressed differently in the nasopharynx and the bloodstream, and fimbriae, which have been shown to be important for nasopharyngeal colonization but not for invasion. The role of fimbriae and other structures in adherence and invasion have been reviewed by van Alphen and van Ham (1994). OMP P2 has been shown to affect the virulence of Hib (Sanders et al. 1993) and purified peptidoglycan was shown to cause brain oedema and inflammation in rabbit and rat models (Burroughs et al. 1993, Roord, Apicella and Scheld 1994). Haemocin, a bacteriocin, is strongly associated with type b strains (LiPuma et al. 1992). IgA proteases are produced by all Hib but have been shown to be inhibited by human milk (Plaut et al. 1992). H. influenzae requires iron for growth *in vivo* and can acquire this from host iron-binding proteins, such as transferrin, by a siderophore-independent mechanism involving 2 transferrin-binding proteins, Tbp1 and Tbp2 (Williams and Griffiths 1992, Gray-Owen, Loosmore and Schryvers 1995). Transferrin-binding ability is strongly associated with Hib from invasive infection (Hardie, Adams and Towner 1993) and may be important for pathogenicity. The iron-binding protein Tbp1 is a member of the TonB family and has been shown to be essential for invasion of Hib in an animal model (Jarosik et al. 1994).

NON-CAPSULATE H. INFLUENZAE

Recent studies suggest that fimbriae (Sirakova et al. 1994) and OMP P2 may be important virulent factors for NCHI (Sanders et al. 1993). The secretory products IgA1 protease and ciliotoxin may contribute to the pathogenesis of pneumonia (reviewed by Moxon and Wilson, 1991). Transferrin-binding proteins have been detected on NCHI (Hardie, Adams and Towner 1993). Peptidoglycan from NCHI caused inflammation of the middle ear in the chinchilla otitis media model (Leake et al. 1994). The lipooligosaccharide phenotype has been shown to be a critical determinant of virulence for *H. influenzae* biogroup aegyptius (Rubin and St. Geme 1993).

17   HAEMOPHILUS DUCREYI

17.1   Introduction and historical perspective

Ducrey (1889) first reported the presence of characteristic bacilli in stained smears prepared from the exudates of soft genital sores (chancroid). Bezançon, Griffon and Lesourd (1900) succeeded in isolating the organisms on nutrient agar plus 30% whole fresh rabbit blood. Tomaczewski (1903) successfully reproduced soft chancre in humans with pure cultures of *H. ducreyi*. (See Albritton 1989 for historical review.) *H. ducreyi* differs in many respects from other members of the genus and there has been doubt over its taxonomic position for many years. *H. ducreyi* was originally assigned to the genus *Haemophilus* because of its requirement for X factor.

The techniques of genetic transformation (Albritton et al. 1986), DNA hybridization and SI nuclease treatment (Casin et al. 1985), DNA–RNA hybridization (De Ley et al. 1990) and 16S RNA sequencing (Rousseau et al. 1991, Dewhirst et al. 1992) have all been used to clarify the taxonomic position of *H. ducreyi*. The results suggest that *H. ducreyi* is a member of the Pasteurellaceae but clusters differently to the true haemophili. However, no formal renaming has been proposed.

17.2   Morphology

In the purulent discharge from the ulcerated surface of chancroid lesions several morphological forms may be seen. The organisms may lie intracellularly or more commonly extracellularly, and appear as pleomorphic coccobacilli or short rods. The characteristic arrangement of organisms as 'shoals of fish' or 'railroad tracks' are rarely evident in clinical material, and the ulcers generally harbour a polymicrobial flora. Sturm et al. (1987) found direct gram staining of ulcer exudate identified only 10% of culture-positive cases. Additionally they found only 5% of patients with a clinical diagnosis of chancroid had a positive gram-stained smear. These studies underline the difficulties in making the diagnosis of chancroid. Accurate diagnosis of chancroid depends on the ability to culture *H. ducreyi*.

In smears prepared from growth on solid media the organisms appear as isolated individuals, in groups or as short chains; growth in liquid media is difficult to achieve, but in such cultures long tangled chains may be seen.

17.3   Cultural characteristics and growth requirements

H. ducreyi is a fastidious organism which grows only slowly on chocolate agar and culturing *H. ducreyi* is difficult. Isolation of *H. ducreyi* has a sensitivity of about 70% compared to PCR in an unselected population of men with genital ulcers (Johnson et al. 1995).

Several media have been devised to improve the isolation of *H. ducreyi*. In general a suitable medium contains a growth factor supplement such as IsoVitalex and is made selective by the addition of vancomycin 3 mg l^{-1}. Totten and Stamm (1994) described a clear broth and plate medium for culturing *H. ducreyi*. Fresh plates with a moist surface should be used and they should be incubated at 33–36°C with added moisture and carbon dioxide. For many laboratories that isolate *H. ducreyi* infrequently the availability of fresh selective media will be a problem. Dangor, Radebe and Ballard (1993) described a thioglycollate–haemin based transport medium from which viable *H. ducreyi* can be isolated after 4 days at 4°C.

The colonial appearance of *H. ducreyi* varies with the medium used. Typically after incubation for 24 h the colonies are small, yellow-grey, translucent or semiopaque The culture often appears 'mixed' with a variety of colonial sizes and appearance. The colonies are very cohesive and can be pushed intact across the agar surface. It is extremely difficult to emulsify the colonies. *H. ducreyi* does not grow well in liquid media. Strains may be preserved on moist slopes of a medium such as Sheffield medium for about 4 weeks at 4°C or in liquid nitrogen for up to 2 years (Hafiz, McEntegart and Kinghorn 1984). (See review by Trees and Morse 1995, for discussion of media and culture techniques.)

17.4 Identification

H. ducreyi requires X factor but not V factor for growth. Hammond et al. (1978) found the optimal haemin requirement for *H. ducreyi* was 200–500 mg l^{-1}.

The biochemical activities of *H. ducreyi* are shown in Table 50.2. Kilian and Biberstein (1984) considered *H. ducreyi* to be apparently asaccharolytic, but commented that some strains show a late positive reaction with glucose. *H. ducreyi* has a characteristic enzyme profile (Casin et al. 1982) and a number of rapid kit systems have been used to identify it by its enzymic activity. These include API-ZYM (Casin et al. 1982), Minitek System (Oberhofer and Back 1982) and Rapid IDNH (Hannah and Greenwood 1982).

A number of non-cultural diagnostic tests have been developed for *H. ducreyi* including indirect immunofluorescence microscopy of clinical material with polyclonal or monoclonal antisera (Hansen and Loftus 1984, Schalla et al. 1986, Finn, Karim and Easmon 1990), a blot-radio-immunoassay (Hansen and Loftus 1984) and enzyme-linked immunosorbent assay (ELISA)-based antigen detection (Roggen et al. 1993). Hansen and Loftus (1984) have produced 2 monoclonal antibodies which recognize all strains of *H. ducreyi* and which are capable of detecting *H. ducreyi* in skin lesions in experimental animals.

PCR methods have been developed for the diagnosis of chancroid (Chui et al. 1993, Johnson et al. 1994, Orle et al. 1994, West et al. 1995). Although such techniques are valuable for the confirmation of *H. ducreyi* isolates, their value in the clinical diagnosis of chancroid is not yet established.

17.5 Susceptibility to antimicrobial agents

The susceptibility of *H. ducreyi* to antimicrobial agents varies between geographical areas (see review by Dangor et al. 1990). Resistance is more prevalent in areas where chancroid is common. In countries where *H. ducreyi* infection is endemic, most isolates are β-lactamase producers and are also resistant to tetracycline. Resistance to trimethoprim-sulphamethoxazole is being seen increasingly, especially in the Far East. Most isolates of *H. ducreyi* are susceptible to erythromycin and the newer macrolides clarithromycin, azithromycin and roxithromycin. Other agents that show excellent activity against *H. ducreyi* in vitro include the quinolones such as ciprofloxacin, perfloxacin and fleroxacin, rifampicin, spectinomycin, ceftriaxone and co-amoxiclav. Ceftriaxone therapy has been associated with treatment failures in Kenya (Tyndall et al. 1993). (See Schulte and Schmid 1995 for recommendations for treatment of chancroid.)

Antimicrobial susceptibility testing of *H. ducreyi* is technically difficult, requiring specially supplemented media. In addition the slow and variable growth of isolates and the difficulties of emulsifying the cohesive colonies mean that it is hard to standardize inocula.

17.6 Typing methods

Sturm (1981) differentiated *H. ducreyi* into 2 types: type 1 has an outer membrane in electronmicroscopic preparations, type 2 has not. Both types can produce chancroid-like lesions in monkeys. Odumeru, Ronald and Albritton (1983) have identified 7 subtypes of *H. ducreyi* by OMP subtyping. Slootmans, van den Berghe and Piot (1985) described an indirect immunofluorescent technique for typing *H. ducreyi*. The techniques of ribotyping (Sarafian et al. 1991) and plasmid analysis (Sarafian and Knapp 1992) have been applied to *H. ducreyi*. Lectin typing of *H. ducreyi* (Korting et al. 1988) appears to be of dubious value. (See review by Trees and Morse 1995 for discussion of typing methods.)

17.7 Pathogenicity

H. ducreyi causes the sexually transmitted disease **chancroid**, or soft chancre (soft sore). Asymptomatic carriage of the organism has been reported in men (Kinghorn, Hafiz and McEntegart 1983) and women (Khoo, Sng and Goh 1977) but it is unclear whether this is persistent or transient carriage or recovery of the organism during the incubation period. *H. ducreyi* has not been isolated from non-human sources. Avirulent strains, as defined in an animal model, can be produced by repeated passage in vitro, but have not been reported on primary isolation. These avirulent strains produce no cutaneous lesion when inoculated intradermally into a rabbit; virulent strains produce necrotic lesions. Several in vitro models have been used to study the pathogenesis of *H. ducreyi*. Animal models have also been developed (reviewed by Trees and Morse 1995). Spinola et al. (1994) studied experimental infections in humans.

The potential virulence factors of *H. ducreyi* include pili (Spinola et al. 1990), LPS (Odumeru, Wiseman and Ronald 1987, Campagnari et al. 1991), cytotoxins (Purven and Lagergård 1992) and OMP (see reviews on pathogenesis by Lagergård 1995, Jonasson 1993). Morse (1989), Albritton (1989) and Trees and Morse (1995) provide excellent comprehensive reviews of *H. ducreyi* and chancroid.

REFERENCES

Albritton WL, 1982, Infections due to *Haemophilus* species other than *H. influenzae*, *Annu Rev Microbiol*, **36:** 199–216.

Albritton WL, 1989, Biology of *Haemophilus ducreyi*, *Microbiol Rev*, **53:** 377–89.

Albritton WL, Setlow JK et al., 1986, Relatedness within the family *Pasteurellaceae* as determined by genetic transformation, *Int J Syst Bacteriol*, **36:** 103–6.

Alphen L van, 1993, The molecular epidemiology of *Haemophilus influenzae*, *Rev Med Microbiol*, **4:** 159–66.

Alphen L van, 1994, Molecular epidemiology of *Haemophilus influenzae* type b strains, *Development and clinical uses of Haemophilus influenzae type b conjugate vaccines*, Ellis RW, Granoff DM, Marcel Dekker, New York, 129–44.

Alphen L van, Ham SM van, 1994, Adherence and invasion of *Haemophilus influenzae*, *Rev Med Microbiol*, **5:** 245–55.

Alphen L van, Geelen L et al., 1987, Distinct geographic distribution of subtypes of *Haemophilus influenzae* type b in Western Europe, *J Infect Dis*, **156:** 216–18.

Azemun P, Stull T et al., 1981, Rapid detection of chloramphenicol resistance in *Haemophilus influenzae*, *Antimicrob Agents Chemother*, **20:** 168–70.

Baillie WE, Coles EH, Weide KD, 1973, Deoxyribonucleic acid characterisation of a micro organism isolated from infectious thromboembolic meningoencephalitis of cattle, *Int J Syst Bacteriol*, **23:** 231–7.

Barbé G, Babolat M et al., 1994, Evaluation of AP INH, a new 2-hour system for identification of *Neisseria* and *Haemophilus* species and *Moraxella catarrhalis* in a routine clinical laboratory, *J Clin Microbiol*, **32:** 187–9.

Barber KG, 1969, A selective medium for the isolation of haemophilus from sputum, *J Med Lab Technol*, **26:** 391–6.

Barbour ML, Crook DW, Mayon-White RT, 1993, An improved antiserum agar method for detecting carriage of *Haemophilus influenzae* type b, *Eur J Clin Microbiol Infect Dis*, **12:** 215–17.

Barbour ML, Booy R et al., 1993, *Haemophilus influenzae* type b cariage and immunity four years after receiving the *Haemophilus influenzae* oligosaccharide – CRM197 (HbOC) conjugate vaccine, *Pediatr Infect Dis*, **12:** 478–84.

Barbour ML, Mayon-White RT et al., 1995, The impact of conjugate vaccine on carriage of *Haemophilus influenzae* type b, *J Infect Dis*, **171:** 93–8.

Barcak GJ, Chandler MS et al., 1991, Genetic systems in *Haemophilus influenzae*, *Methods Enzymol*, **204:** 321–42.

Barenkamp SJ, 1992, Outer membrane proteins and lipopolysaccharides of nontypeable *Haemophilus influenzae*, *J Infect Dis*, **165 (Suppl 1):** 181–4.

Belkum A van, Duim B et al., 1994, Genomic DNA fingerprinting of clinical *Haemophilus influenzae* isolates by polymerase chain reaction amplification: comparison with major outer-membrane protein and restriction fragment length polymorphism analysis, *J Med Microbiol*, **41:** 63–8.

Bell SM, Plowman D, 1980, Mechanisms of ampicillin resistance in *Haemophilus influenzae* from the respiratory tract, *Lancet*, **I:** 279–80.

Bergeron MG, Lavoie GY, 1985, Tolerance of *Haemophilus influenzae* to β-lactam antibiotics, *Antimicrob Agents Chemother*, **28:** 320–5.

Bezançon F, Griffon V, LeSourd L, 1900, Culture du bacille du chancre mou, *C R Soc Biol*, **11:** 1048–51.

Biberstein EL, Gills M, 1961, Catalase activity of *Haemophilus* species grown with graded amounts of hemin, *J Bacteriol*, **81:** 380–4.

Biberstein EL, Mini PD, Gills MG, 1963, Action of *Haemophilus* cultures on δ-amino laevulinic acid, *J Bacteriol*, **86:** 814–19.

Biberstein EL, White DC, 1969, A proposal for the establishment of two new Haemophilus species, *J Med Microbiol*, **2:** 75–8.

Biljmer HA, van Alphen L et al., 1994, Antibiotic susceptibility of invasive and non-invasive isolates of *Haemophilus influenzae* from the Gambia, West Africa, *J Antimicrob Chemother*, **34:** 275–80.

Blackall PJ, 1988, Biochemical properties of catalase-positive avian haemophili, *J Gen Microbiol*, **134:** 2801–5.

Blackall PJ, 1989, The avian Haemophili, *Clin Microbiol Rev*, **2:** 270–7.

Blackall PJ, Morrow CJ et al., 1990, Epidemiologic studies on infectious coryza outbreaks in Northern New South Wales, Australia, using serotyping, biotyping and chromosomal DNA restriction endonuclease analysis, *Avian Dis*, **34:** 267–76.

Bol P, Spanjaard L et al., 1987, Epidemiology of *Haemophilus influenzae* meningitis in patients more than 6 years of age, *J Infect*, **15:** 81–94.

Brenner DJ, Mayer LW et al., 1988, Biochemical, genetic and epidemiologic characterisation of *Haemophilus influenzae* biogroup aegyptius (*Haemophilus aegyptius*) strains associated with Brazilian Purpuric fever, *J Clin Microbiol*, **26:** 1524–34.

Broom AK, Sneath PHA, 1981, Numerical taxonomy of *Haemophilus*, *J Gen Microbiol*, **126:** 123–49.

Bruce KD, Jordens JZ, 1991, Characterization of noncapsulate *Haemophilus influenzae* by whole-cell polypeptide profiles, restriction endonuclease analysis, and rRNA gene restriction patterns, *J Clin Microbiol*, **29:** 291–6.

Brunton J, Clare D, Meier MA, 1986, Molecular epidemiology of antibiotic resistance plasmids of *Haemophilus* species and *Neisseria gonorrhoeae*, *Rev Infect Dis*, **8:** 713–24.

Brunton JL, Maclean I et al., 1979, Plasmid-mediated ampicillin resistance in *Haemophilus ducreyi*, *Antimicrob Agents Chemother*, **15:** 294–9.

Burns JL, Mendelman PM et al., 1985, A permeability barrier as a mechanism of chloramphenicol resistance in *Haemophilus influenzae*, *Antimicrob Agents Chemother*, **27:** 46–54.

Burroughs M, Prasad S et al., 1993, The biologic activities of peptidoglycan in experimental *Haemophilus influenzae* meningitis, *J Infect Dis*, **167:** 464–8.

Butler PD, Moxon ER, 1990, A physical map of the genome of *Haemophilus influenzae* type b, *J Gen Microbiol*, **136:** 2333–42.

Campagnari AA, Wild LM et al., 1991, Role of lipooligosaccharide in experimental dermal lesions caused by *Haemophilus ducreyi*, *Infect Immun*, **59:** 2601–8.

Campos J, Garcia-Tornel S, Sanfelin I, 1984, Susceptibility studies of multiply resistant *Haemophilus influenzae* isolated from pediatric patients and contacts, *Antimicrob Agents Chemother*, **25:** 706–9.

Campos J, Garcia-Tornel S et al., 1986, Multiply resistant *Haemophilus influenzae* type b causing meningitis: comparative clinical and laboratory study, *J Pediatr*, **108:** 897–902.

Carlone GM, Sottnek FO, Plikaytis BD, 1985, Comparison of outer membrane protein and biochemical profiles of *Haemophilus aegyptius* and *Haemophilus influenzae* biotype III, *J Clin Microbiol*, **22:** 708–13.

Casin IM, Sanson-LePors MJ et al., 1982, The enzymatic profile of *Haemophilus ducreyi*, *Ann Microbiol (Paris)*, **133B:** 379–88.

Casin I, Grimont F et al., 1985, Lack of deoxyribonucleic acid relatedness between *Haemophilus ducreyi* and other *Haemophilus* species, *Int J Syst Bacteriol*, **35:** 23–5.

Cavanagh P, Morris CA, Mitchell NJ, 1975, Chloramphenicol resistance in *Haemophilus* species, *Lancet*, **I:** 696.

Chapin KC, Doern GV, 1983, Selective media for recovery of *Haemophilus influenzae* from specimens contaminated with upper respiratory tract microbial flora, *J Clin Microbiol*, **17:** 1163–5.

Chui L, Albritton W et al., 1993, Development of the polymerase chain reaction for diagnosis of chancroid, *J Clin Microbiol*, **31:** 659–64.

Clairoux N, Picard M et al., 1992, Molecular basis of the non-β-lactamase-mediated resistance of β-lactam antibiotics in strains of *Haemophilus influenzae* isolated in Canada, *Antimicrob Agents Chemother*, **36:** 1504–13.

Coulton JW, Pang JCS, 1983, Transport of hemin by *Haemophilus influenzae* type b, *J Clin Microbiol*, **9:** 93–8.

Courvalin P, 1991, Genotypic approach to the study of bacterial resistance to antibiotics. Mini Review, *Antimicrob Agents Chemother*, **35:** 1019–23.

Cyanomon MH, Sorg TB, Patapow A, 1988, Utilization and metabolism of NAD by *Haemophilus parainfluenzae*, *J Gen Microbiol*, **134:** 2789–99.

Daly JA, Clifton NL et al., 1991, Use of rapid non-radioactive DNA probes in culture confirmation tests to detect *Streptococcus agalactiae*, *Haemophilus influenzae,* and *Enterococcus* spp. from pediatric patients with significant infections, *J Clin Microbiol*, **29:** 80–2.

Dangor Y, Ballard RC et al., 1990, Antimicrobial susceptibility of *Haemophilus ducreyi*, *Antimicrob Agents Chemother*, **34:** 1303–7.

Dangor Y, Radebe F, Ballard RC, 1993, Transport media for *Haemophilus ducreyi*, *Sex Transm Dis*, **20:** 5–9.

Daum RS, Murphey-Corb M et al., 1988, Epidemiology of Rob β-lactamase among ampicillin-resistant *Haemophilus influenzae* isolates in the United States, *J Infect Dis*, **157:** 450–5.

Deich RA, Anilionis A et al., 1990, Antigenic conservation of the 15,000-dalton outer membrane lipoprotein PCP of *Haemophilus influenzae* and biologic activity of anti-PCP antisera, *Infect Immun*, **58:** 3388–93.

Dewhirst FE, Paster BJ et al., 1992, Phylogeny of 54 representative strains in the family *Pasteurellaceae* as determined by comparison of 16S rRNA sequences, *J Bacteriol*, **174:** 2002–13.

Dimopoulou ID, Kraak WAG et al., 1992, Molecular epidemiology of unrelated clusters of multiresistant strains of *Haemophilus influenzae*, *J Infect Dis*, **165:** 1069–75.

Doern GV, 1992, In vitro susceptibility testing of *Haemophilus influenzae*: review of new national committee for clinical laboratory standards recommendations, *J Clin Microbiol*, **30:** 3035–8.

Doern GV, Chapin KC, 1984, Laboratory identification of *Haemophilus influenzae*: effects of basal media on the results of the satellitism test and evaluation of the RapiDNH system, *J Clin Microbiol*, **20:** 599–601.

Doern GV, Daum GS, Tubert TA, 1987, In vitro chloramphenicol susceptibility testing of *Haemophilus influenzae*: disk diffusion procedures and assays for chloramphenicol acetyl transferase, *J Clin Microbiol*, **25:** 1453–5.

Ducrey A, 1889, Experimentelle untersuchungen uber den Ansteckungsstoff des weichen schankers und uber die bubonen, *Monatsch Prakt Dermatol*, **9:** 387–405.

Duim B, Alphen L van et al., 1994, Antigenic drift of non-encapsulated *Haemophilus influenzae* major outer membrane protein P2 in patients with chronic bronchitis is caused by point mutations, *Mol Microbiol*, **11:** 1181–9.

Engbaek HC, 1950, The phenomenon of iridescence in bacterial cultures with particular reference to Pfeiffer's bacillus, *Acta Pathol Microbiol Scand*, **27:** 388–93.

Evans NM, Smith DD, Wicken AJ, 1974, Haemin and nicotinamide adenine dinucleotide requirements of *Haemophilus influenzae* and *parainfluenzae*, *J Med Microbiol*, **7:** 359–65.

Falla TJ, Anderson EC et al., 1993, Cross-reaction of spontaneous capsule-deficient *Haemophilus influenzae* type b mutants with type-specific antisera, *Eur J Clin Microbiol Infect Dis*, **12:** 147–8.

Falla TJ, Crook DWM et al., 1994, PCR for capsular typing of *Haemophilus influenzae*, *J Clin Microbiol*, **32:** 2382–6.

Fildes P, 1920, A new medium for the growth of *H.influenzae*, *Br J Exp Pathol*, **1:** 129–30.

Fildes P, 1924, The growth requirements of haemolytic influenzae bacilli and the bearing of these upon the classification of related organisms, *Brit J Exp Pathol*, **5:** 69–74.

Finn GY, Karim QN, Easmon CSF, 1990, The production and characterisation of rabbit antiserum and murine monoclonal antibodies to *Haemophilus ducreyi*, *J Med Microbiol*, **31:** 219–24.

Fleischmann RD, Adams MD et al., 1995, Whole-genome random sequencing and assembly of *Haemophilus influenzae* Rd, *Science*, **269:** 496–512.

Gadberry JL, Amos MA, 1986, Comparison of a new commercially prepared porphyrin test and the conventional satellite test for the identification of *Haemophilus* species that require the X factor, *J Clin Microbiol*, **23:** 637–9.

Gilder H, Granick S, 1947, Studies on the *Haemophilus* group of organisms. Quantitative aspects of growth on various porphyrin compounds, *J Gen Physiol*, **31:** 103–17.

Ginsburg CM, McCracken GH et al., 1977, *H.influenzae* type b disease in a day care centre, *JAMA*, **238:** 604–7.

Glode MP, Daum RS et al., 1985, Effect of rifampicin chemoprophylaxis on carriage eradication and new acquisition of *Haemophilus influenzae* type b in contacts, *Pediatrics*, **76:** 537–42.

Goffic le FL, Moreau N et al., 1977, La resistance plasmidique de *Haemophilus* sp. aux antibiotiques aminoglycosidiques: isolement et étude d'une nouvelle phosphotransferase, *Ann Microbiol (Paris)*, **128A:** 383–91.

Gonzales FR, Leachman S et al., 1987, Cloning and expression in *Escherichia coli* of the gene encoding the heat-modifiable major outer membrane protein of *Haemophilus influenzae* type b, *Infect Immun*, **55:** 2993–3000.

Granoff DM, Barenkamp SJ, Munson RS, 1982, *Outer membrane protein subtypes for epidemiologic investigation of* Haemophilus influenzae *type b disease*, Haemophilus influenzae: *epidemiology, immunology and prevention of disease*, Sell SH, Wright PF, Elsevier, New York, 43–55.

Granoff DM, Munson RS, 1986, Prospects for prevention of *Haemophilus influenzae* type b disease by immunization, *J Infect Dis*, **153:** 448–61.

Gratten M, 1983, *Haemophilus influenzae* biotype VII, *J Clin Microbiol*, **18:** 1015–16.

Gray-Owen SC, Loosmore S, Schryvers AB, 1995, Identification and characterization of genes encoding the human transferrin-binding proteins from *Haemophilus influenzae*, *Infect Immun*, **63:** 1201–10.

Grebe HH, Hinz K-H, 1975, Vorkommen von bakterien der gattung *Haemophilus* bei verschiedenen vogelarten, *Zentralbl Veterinaermed B*, **22:** 749–57.

Green MJ, Anderson DM et al., 1979, Antimicrobial resistance in *Haemophilus* species, *NZ Med J*, **90:** 29.

Green BA, Quinn-Dey T, Zlotnick GW, 1987, Biologic activities of antibody to a peptidoglycan-associated lipoprotein of *Haemophilus influenzae* against multiple clinical isolates of *H. influenzae* type b, *Infect Immun*, **55:** 2878–83.

Green BA, Farley JE et al., 1991, The e (P4) outer membrane protein of *Haemophilus influenzae*: biologic activity of anti-e serum and cloning and sequencing of the structural gene, *Infect Immun*, **59:** 3191–8.

Groot de R, Dzoljic-Danilovic G et al., 1991, Antibiotic resistance in *Haemophilus influenzae*: mechanisms, clinical importance and consequences for therapy, *Eur J Pediatr*, **150:** 534–46.

Gunn BA, Woodall JB et al., 1974, Ampicillin-resistant *Haemophilus influenzae*, *Lancet*, **2:** 845.

Hafiz S, McEntegart MG, Kinghorn GR, 1984, Sheffield medium for cultivation of *Haemophilus ducreyi*, *Br J Vener Dis*, **60:** 196–8.

Hamed KA, Dormitzer PR et al., 1994, *Haemophilus parainfluenzae* endocarditis: Application of a molecular approach for identification of pathogenic bacterial species, *Clin Infect Dis*, **19:** 677–83.

Hammond GW, Lian C-J et al., 1978, Determination of the hemin requirement of *Haemophilus ducreyi*: evaluation of the porphyrin test and media used in the satellite growth test, *J Clin Microbiol*, **7:** 243–6.

Hannah P, Greenwood JR, 1982, Isolation and identification of *Haemophilus ducreyi*, *J Clin Microbiol*, **16:** 861–4.

Hansen EJ, Loftus TA, 1984, Monoclonal antibodies reactive with all strains of *Haemophilus ducreyi*, *Infect Immun*, **44:** 196–8.

Hardie KR, Adams RA, Towner KJ, 1993, Transferrin-binding ability of invasive and commensal isolates of *Haemophilus* spp, *J Med Microbiol*, **39:** 218–24.

Hargreaves RM, Slack MPE et al., 1995, Changing patterns of invasive *Haemophilus influenzae* disease in England and Wales following introduction of the Hib vaccination programme, *Br Med J*, **312:** 160–1.

Harris DL, Ross RF, Switzer WP, 1969, Incidence of certain microorganisms in nasal cavities of swine in Iowa, *Am J Vet Res*, **30:** 1621–4.

Henderson FW, Collier AM et al., 1982, A longitudinal study of respiratory viruses and bacteria in the etiology of acute otitis media with effusion, *N Engl J Med*, **306:** 1377–383.

Herrington DA, Sparling FP, 1985, *Haemophilus influenzae* can use human transferrin as a sole source for required iron, *Infect Immun*, **48:** 248–51.

Hinz K-H, Kunjara C, 1977, *Haemophilus avium*, a new species from chickens, *Int J Syst Bacteriol*, **27:** 324–9.

Hobson RP, Williams A et al., 1995, Incidence and spread of *Haemophilus influenzae* on an Antarctic base determined using the polymerase chain reaction, *Epidemiol Infect*, **114:** 93–103.

Höllander R, Mannheim W, 1975, Characterization of haemophilic and related bacteria by their respiratory quinones and cytochomes, *Inst J Syst Bacteriol*, **25:** 102–7.

Höllander R,, 1976, Energy metabolism of some representatives of the *Haemophilus* group, *Antonie van Leeuwenhoek, J Microbiol Serol*, **42:** 429–44.

Holt LB, 1962, The growth factor requirements of *Haemophilus influenzæ*, *J Gen Microbiol*, **27:** 317–22.

Howard AJ, Williams HM, Proole MC, 1986, Chloramphenicol resistance in *Haemophilus influenzae*, *Lancet*, **ii:** 745–6.

Howard AJ, Dunkin KT, Millar GW, 1988, Nasopharyngeal carriage and antibiotic resistance of *Haemophilus influenzae* in healthy children, *Epidemiol Infect*, **100:** 193–203.

Inzana TJ, Claridge J, Williams RP, 1987, Rapid determination of X/V growth requirements of *Haemophilus* species in broth, *Diagn Microbiol Infect Dis*, **6:** 93–100.

Inzana TJ, Johnson JL et al., 1992, Isolation and characterization of a newly identified *Haemophilus* species from cats: 'Haemophilus felis', *J Clin Microbiol*, **30:** 2108–12.

Irino K, Grimont F et al., 1988, rRNA gene restriction patterns of *Haemophilus influenzae* biogroup aegyptius strains associated with Brazilian purpuric fever, *J Clin Microbiol*, **26:** 1535–8.

Jarosik GP, Sanders JD et al., 1994, A functional *ton*B gene is required for both utilization of heme and virulence expression by *Haemophilus influenzae* type b, *Infect Immun*, **62:** 2470–7.

Johnson SR, Martin DH et al., 1994, Development of a polymerase chain reaction assay for the detection of *Haemophilus ducreyi*, *Sex Transm Dis*, **21:** 13–22.

Johnson SR, Martin DH et al., 1995, Alterations in sample preparation increase sensitivity of PCR assay for diagnosis of chancroid, *J Clin Microbiol*, **33:** 1036–8.

Jonasson JA, 1993, *Haemophilus ducreyi*, *Int J STD and AIDS*, **4:** 317–21.

Jones RN, Slepack J, Bigelow J, 1976, Ampicillin-resistant *Haemophilus paraphrophilus* laryngo-epiglottitis, *J Clin Microbiol*, **4:** 405–7.

Jones DM 1993, Current and future trends in immunization against meningitis, *J Antimicrob Chemother*, **31 (Suppl B):** 93–9.

Jordens JZ, Leaves NI et al., 1993, Polymerase chain reaction-based strain characterization of noncapsulate *Haemophilus influenzae*, *J Clin Microbiol*, **31:** 2981–7.

Jordens JZ, Slack MPE, 1995, *Haemophilus influenzae*: Then and now (a review), *Eur J Clin Microbiol Infect Dis*, **14:** 935–48.

Jorgensen JH, Redding JS et al., 1987, Improved medium for antimicrobial susceptibility testing of *Haemophilus influenzae*, *J Clin Microbiol*, **25:** 2105–13.

Jorgensen JH, Doern GV et al., 1990, Antimicrobial resistance among respiratory isolates of *Haemophilus influenzae*, *Moraxella catarrhalis*, and *Streptococcus pneumoniae* in the United States, *Antimicrob Agents Chemother*, **34:** 2075–80.

Jorgensen JH, Howell AW, Maher LA, 1991, Quantitative antimicrobial susceptibility testing of *Haemophilus influenzae* and *Streptococcus pneumoniae* by using the E-test, *J Clin Microbiol*, **29:** 109–14.

Jorgensen JH, 1992, Update on mechanisms and prevalence of antimicrobial resistance in *Haemophilus influenzae*, *Clin Infect Dis*, **14:** 1119–23.

Jubelrier DP, Yeager AS, 1979, Simultaneous recovery of ampicillin-sensitive and ampicillin-resistant organisms in *Haemophilus influenzae* type b meningitis, *J Pediatr*, **95:** 415–16.

Kawakami Y, Okimura Y, Kanai M, 1982, Occurrence and biochemical properties of *Haemophilus* species in pharyngeal flora of healthy individuals, *Microbiol Immunol*, **27:** 629–33.

Kayser FH, Morenzoni G, Santanam P, 1990, The second European collaborative study on the frequency of antimicrobial resistance in *Haemophilus influenzae*, *Eur J Clin Microbiol Infect Dis*, **9:** 810–17.

Kennedy PD, Frazier LM et al., 1958, A septicaemic disease of lambs caused by *Haemophilus agni* (new species), *Am J Vet Res*, **19:** 645–54.

Kerr GRD, Forbes KJ et al., 1993, An analysis of the diversity of *Haemophilus parainfluenzae* in the adult human respiratory tract by genomic DNA fingerprinting, *Epidemiol Infect*, **111:** 89–98.

Khoo R, Sng EH, Goh AJ, 1977, A study of sexually transmitted diseases in 200 prostitutes in Singapore, *Asian J Infect Dis*, **1:** 77–9.

Kielstein P, Rosner H, Muller W, 1991, Typing of heat-stable soluble *Haemophilus parasuis* antigen by means of agargel precipitation and the dot-blot procedure, *J Vet Med*, **B38:** 315–20.

Kilian M, 1976, A taxonomic study of the genus *Haemophilus* with the proposal of a new species, *J Gen Microbiol*, **93:** 9–62.

Kilian M, Biberstein EL, 1984, *Bergey's Manual of Systematic Bacteriology, Vol 1*, Kreig NR, Holt JG, Williams and Wilkins Co. Baltimore, 558–69.

Kilian M, Frederiksen W, 1981, Ecology of *Haemophilus*, *Pasteurella* and *Actinobacillus*, Haemophilus, Pasteurella *and* Actinobacillus, Fredericksen and Biberstein, Academic Press, London, 11–38.

Kilian M, Heine-Jensen J, Bulow P, 1972, *Haemophilus* in the upper respiratory tract of children. A bacteriological, serological and clinical investigation, *Acta Pathol Microbiol Scand Sect B*, **80:** 571–8.

Kilian M, Schiøtt CR, 1975, Haemophili and related bacteria in the human oral cavity, *Arch Oral Biol*, **20:** 791–6.

Kilian M, Theilade J, 1978, Amended description of *Haemophilus segnis*, Kilian 1977, *Int J Syst Bacteriol*, **28:** 411–15.

Kilian M,, 1974, A rapid test for the differentiation of *Haemophilus* strains. The porphyrin test, *Acta Pathol Microbiol Scand Sect B*, **82:** 835–42.

Kimura A, Gulig PA et al., 1985, A minor high-molecular-weight outer membrane protein of *Haemophilus influenzae* type b is a protective antigen, *Infect Immun*, **47:** 253–9.

Kinghorn GR, Hafiz S, McEntegart MG, 1983, Genital colonisation with *Haemophilus ducreyi* in the absence of ulceration, *Eur J Sex Transm Dis*, **1:** 89–90.

Koch R, 1883, Bericht über die thätigkeit der deutschen cholera commission in Aegyptien und Ostindien, *Wien Med Wochenschr*, **33:** 1548–51.

Kodama H, Faden H, 1995, Cellular immunity to the P6 outer membrane protein of nontypeable *Haemophilus influenzae*, *Infect Immun*, **63**: 2467–72.

Korting HC, Abeck D et al., 1988, Lectin typing of *Haemophilus ducreyi*, *Eur J Clin Microbiol Infect Dis*, **7**: 678–80.

Kraut MS, Atterberry HR et al., 1972, Detection of *H.aphrophilus* in the human oral flora with a selective medium, *J Infect Dis*, **126**: 189–92.

Kristensen M, 1922, *Investigations into the Occurrence and Classification of Haemoglobinophilic Bacteria*, Thesis, Levin and Munksgaard, Copenhagen.

Kroll JS, Ely S, Moxon ER, 1991, Capsular typing of *Haemophilus influenzae* with a DNA probe, *Mol Cell Probes*, **5**: 375–9.

Kroll JS, 1992, The genetics of encapsulation in *Haemophilus influenzae*, *J Infect Dis*, **165 (Suppl 1)**: S93–6.

Krumwiede E, Kuttner AG, 1938, A growth-inhibiting substance for the influenza group of organisms in the blood of various animal species, *J Exp Med*, **67**: 429–41.

Lagergård T, 1995, *Haemophilus ducreyi*: pathogenesis and protective immunity, *Trends Microbiol*, **3**: 87–92.

Leake ER, Holmes K et al., 1994, Peptidoglycan isolated from nontypeable *Haemophilus influenzae* induces experimental otitis media in the Chinchilla, *J Infect Dis*, **170**: 1532–8.

Leaves NI, Falla TJ, Crook DWM, 1995, The elucidation of novel capsular genotypes of *Haemophilus influenzae* type b with the polymerase chain reaction, *J Med Microbiol*, **43**: 120–4.

Leaves NI, Jordens JZ, 1994, Development of a ribotyping scheme for *Haemophilus influenzae* type b, *Eur J Clin Microbiol Infect Dis*, **13**: 1038–45.

Levinthal W, 1918, Bakteriologische und serologische influenzastudien, *Z Hyg Infektionskr*, **86**: 1–23.

Levy J, Verhaegen G et al., 1993, Molecular characterization of resistance plasmids in epidemiologically unrelated strains of multiresistant *Haemophilus influenzae*, *J Infect Dis*, **168**: 177–87.

Lewis PA, Shope RE, 1931, Swine influenza II, A haemophilic bacillus from the respiratory tract of infected swine, *J Exp Med*, **54**: 361–71.

Ley De J, Mannheim W et al., 1990, Inter and intra-familial similarities of rRNA cistrons of the *Pasteurellaceae*, *Int J Syst Bacteriol*, **40**: 126–37.

Liljemark WF, Bloomquist CG et al., 1984, Distribution of oral *Haemophilus* species in dental plaque from a large adult population, *Infect Immun*, **46**: 778–86.

Ling JM, Khin-Thi-Oo H et al., 1989, Antimicrobial susceptibilities of *Haemophilus* species in Hong Kong, *J Infect*, **19**: 135–42.

LiPuma JJ, Sharetzsky C et al., 1992, Haemocin production by encapsulated and nonencapsulated *Haemophilus influenzae*, *J Infect Dis*, **165 (Suppl 1)**: S118–19.

Loeb MR, 1987, Protection of infant rats from *Haemophilus influenzae* type b infection by antiserum to purified outer membrane protein a, *Infect Immun*, **55**: 2612–18.

Loeb MR, Smith DH, 1982, Properties and immunogenicity of *Haemophilus influenzae* outer membrane proteins, *Haemophilus influenzae epidemiology, immunology and prevention of disease*, eds Sell SH, Wright PF, Elsevier, New York, 207.

Lund ME, Blazevic DJ, 1977, Rapid speciation of Haemophilus with the porphyrin production test versus the satellite test for X, *J Clin Microbiol*, **5**: 142–44.

Malouin F, Bryan LE et al., 1988, DNA probe technology for rapid detection of *Haemophilus influenzae* in clinical specimens, *J Clin Microbiol*, **26**: 2132–8.

Manten A, van Klingeren B, Dessens-Kroon M, 1976, Chloramphenicol resistance in *Haemophilus influenzae*, *Lancet*, **I**: 702.

Markowitz SM, 1980, Isolation of an ampicillin-resistant, non-beta-lactamase-producing strain of *Haemophilus influenzae*, *Antimicrob Agents Chemother*, **17**: 80–3.

Medeiros AA, Levesque R, Jacoby GA, 1986, An animal source for the ROB-1 β-lactamase of *Haemophilus influenzae* type b, *Antimicrob Agents Chemother*, **29**: 212–15.

Mendelman PM, Chaffin DO et al., 1984, Characterisation of

non-beta-lactamase-mediated ampicillin resistance in *Haemophilus influenzae*, *Antimicrob Agents Chemother*, **26**: 235–44.

Mendelman PM, Chaffin DO et al., 1986, Failure to detect ampicillin-resistant, non-β-lactamase-producing *Haemophilus influenzae* by standard disk susceptibility testing, *Antimicrob Agents Chemother*, **30**: 274–80.

Mendelman PM, Chaffin DO, Kalaitzoglu G, 1990, Penicillin-binding proteins and ampicillin-resistance in *Haemophilus influenzae*, *J Antimicrob Chemother*, **25**: 525–34.

Michaels RH, Norden CW, 1977, Pharyngeal colonization with *Haemophilus influenzae* type b: a longitudinal study of families with a child with meningitis or epiglottitis due to *Haemophilus influenzae*, *J Infect Dis*, **136**: 222–7.

Michaels RH, Stonebraker FE, Robbins JB, 1975, Use of antiserum for detection of *Haemophilus influenzae* type b in the pharynx, *Pediatr Res*, **9**: 513–16.

Michaels RH, Poziviak CS et al., 1976, Factors affecting pharyngeal *Haemophilus influenzae* type b colonisation rates in children, *J Clin Microbiol*, **4**: 413–17.

Miflin JK, Horner RF et al., 1995, Phenotypic and molecular characterization of V-factor (NAD)-independent *Haemophilus paragallinarum*, *Avian Dis*, **39**: 304–8.

Mohle-Boetani JC, Ajello G et al., 1993, Carriage of *Haemophilus influenzae* type b in children after widespread vaccination with conjugate *Haemophilus influenzae* type b vaccines, *Pediatr Infect Dis*, **12**: 589–93.

Möller LVM, van Alphen L et al., 1993, N-acetyl-D-glucosamine medium improves recovery of *Hameophilus influenzae* from sputa of patients with cystic fibrosis, *J Clin Microbiol*, **31**: 1952–4.

Morbid Mortal Weekly Rep, 1986, Brazilian purpuric fever: *Haemophilus aegyptius* bacteraemia complicating purulent conjunctivitis, *Morbid Mortal Weekly Rep*, **35**: 553–4.

Morbid Mortal Weekly Rep, 1995, Progress toward elimination of *Haemophilus influenzae* type b disease among infants and children – United States, 1993–1994, *Morbid Mortal Weekly Rep*, **44**: 545–9.

Morse SA, 1989, Chancroid and *Haemophilus ducreyi*, *Clin Microbiol Rev*, **2**: 137–57.

Moxon ER, Smith AL et al., 1974, *Haemophilus influenzae* meningitis in infant rats after intranasal inoculation, *J Infect Dis*, **129**: 154–62.

Moxon ER, 1986, The carrier state: *Haemophilus influenzae*, *J Antimicrob Chemother*, **18**: suppl A: 17–24.

Moxon ER, Kroll JS, 1990, The role of bacterial polysaccharide capsules as virulence factors, *Curr Top Microbiol Immunol*, **150**: 65–85.

Moxon ER, Maskell D, 1992, *Haemophilus influenzae* lipopolysaccharide: the biochemistry and biology of a virulence factor, *Molecular biology of bacterial infection current status and future perspectives*, Hormaeche CE, Penn CW, Smyth CJ, Cambridge University Press, Cambridge, 75–96.

Moxon ER, Wilson R, 1991, The role of *Haemophilus influenzae* in the pathogenesis of pneumonia, *Rev Infect Dis*, **13 (Suppl 6)**: S518–27.

Murphy TF, 1994, Antigenic variation of surface proteins as a survival strategy for bacterial pathogens, *Trends Microbiol*, **2**: 427–8.

Murphy TV, McCracken GH Jr et al., 1981, Emergence of rifampicin-resistant *Haemophilus influenzae* after prophylaxis, *J Pediatr*, **99**: 406–9.

Murphy PG, Craig I et al., 1990, Evaluation of two rapid methods for identifying and biotyping *Haemophilus influenzae*, *J Clin Pathol*, **43**: 581–3.

Musser JM, Barenkamp SJ et al., 1986, Genetic relationships of serologically nontypable and serotype b strains of *Haemophilus influenzae*, *Infect Immun*, **53**: 183–91.

Musser JM, Kroll JS et al., 1990, Global genetic structure and molecular epidemiology of encapsulated *Haemophilus influenzae*, *Rev Infect Dis*, **12**: 75–111.

Mutters RK, Piechulla K, Mannheim W, 1984, Phenotypic

differentiation of *Pasteurella* sensu stricto and the *Actinobacillus* group, *Eur J Clin Microbiol*, **3**: 225–9.

Mutters R, Piechulla K et al., 1985, *Pasteurella avium* (Hinz and Kunjara 1977) comb. nov. and *Pasteurella volantium* sp. nov, *Int J Syst Bacteriol*, **35**: 5–9.

Nelson MB, Murphy TF et al., 1988, Studies on P6, an important outer-membrane protein antigen of *Haemophilus influenzae*, *Rev Infect Dis*, **10 (Suppl 2)**: S331–6.

Nicolet J, 1992, *Haemophilus parasuis, Diseases of Swine*, 7th edn, eds Leman AD, Straw BE et al., Wolfe Publishing Ltd. London, 526–8.

Nicolle LE, Postl B et al., 1982, Emergence of rifampicin-resistant *Haemophilus influenzae*, *Antimicrob Agents Chemother*, **21**: 498–500.

Nissinen A, Herva E et al., 1995, Antimicrobial resistance in *Haemophilus influenzae* isolated from blood, cerebrospinal fluid, middle ear fluid and throat samples of children. A nationwide study in Finland in 1988–90, *Scand J Infect Dis*, **27**: 57–61.

Niven DF, O'Reilly T, 1990, Significance of V-factor dependency in the taxonomy of *Haemophilus* species and related organisms, *Int J Syst Bacteriol*, **40**: 1–4.

Oberhofer TR, Back AE, 1979, Biotypes of *Haemophilus* encountered in clinical laboratories, *J Clin Microbiol*, **10**: 168–74.

Oberhofer TR, Back AE, 1982, Isolation and cultivation of *Haemophilus ducreyi*, *J Clin Microbiol*, **15**: 625–9.

Odumeru JA, Wiseman GM, Ronald AR, 1987, Relationship between lipopolysaccharide composition and virulence of *Haemophilus ducreyi*, *J Med Microbiol*, **23**: 155–62.

Odumeru JA, Ronald AR, Albritton WL, 1983, Characterisation of cell proteins of *Haemophilus ducreyi* by polyacrylamide gel electrophoresis, *J Infect Dis*, **148**: 710–14.

Orle KA, Martin DH et al., 1994, Multiplex PCR detection of *Haemophilus ducreyi, Treponema pallidum*, and herpes simplex viruses types -1 and -2 from genital ulcers, abstr C-437, p 568, Abstr, 94, *Annu Meet Am Soc Microbiol 1994*.

Osbaldiston GW, 1971, Vaginitis in a bitch associated with *Haemophilus* sp., *Am J Vet Res*, **32**: 2067.

O'Callaghan CH, Morris A, Kirby SM, 1972, Novel method for detection of beta-lactamases by using a chromogenic cephalosporin substrate, *Antimicrob Agents Chemother*, **1**: 283–8.

Page LA, 1962, *Haemophilus* infections in chickens, characteristics of 12 *Haemophilus* isolates recovered from diseased chickens, *Am J Vet Res*, **23**: 85–95.

Palmer GG, 1981, Haemophili in faeces, *J Med Microbiol*, **14**: 147–50.

Panezutti H, James O et al., 1993, Identification of surface-exposed B-cell epitopes recognized by *Haemophilus influenzae* type b P1-specific monoclonal antibodies, *Infect Immun*, **61**: 1867–72.

Park CH, Hixon DL, Berger LM, 1990, Rapid testing of susceptibility of *Haemophilus influenzae* to chloramphenicol by a bioluminescence method, *Eur J Clin Microbiol Infect Dis*, **9**: 908–9.

Peltola H, Käyhty H et al., 1977, *Haemophilus influenzae* type b capsular polysaccharide vaccine in children: a double blind field study of 100,000 vacinees 3 months to 5 years of age in Finland, *Pediatrics*, **60**: 730–7.

Pennington TH, 1993, Haemophilus species and clones, *Rev Med Microbiol*, **4**: 50–8.

Pfeiffer R, 1892, Vorläufige Mittelungen über den Erreger der Influenza, *Dtsch Med Wochenschr*, **18**: 28.

Philpott-Howard J, Seymour A, Williams JD, 1983, Accuracy of methods used for susceptibility testing of *Haemophilus influenzae* in United Kingdom laboratories, *J Clin Pathol*, **36**: 1105–10.

Pidcock KA, Wooten JA et al., 1988, Iron acquisition by *Haemophilus influenzae*, *Infect Immun*, **56**: 721–5.

Piechulla K, Hinz K-H, Mannheim W, 1985, Genetic and phenotypic comparison of three new avian *Haemophilus*-like taxa and of *Haemophilus paragallinarum*. Biberstein and White 1969

with other members of the family *Pasteurellaceae* Pohl 1981, *Avian Dis*, **29**: 601–12.

Pittman M, 1931, Variation and type specificity in the bacterial species *Haemophilus influenzae*, *J Exp Med*, **53**: 471–92.

Pittman M, 1935, The interrelation of the amount of V-factor and the amount of air necessary for growth of *Haemophilus influenzae* type b in certain media, *J Bacteriol*, **30**: 149–61.

Pittman M, 1953, A classification of the hemolytic bacteria of the genus *Haemophilus: Haemophilus haemolyticus* Bergey et al. and *Haemophilus parahaemolyticus* nov.spec, *J Bacteriol*, **65**: 750–1.

Plaut AG, Qui J et al., 1992, Growth of *Haemophilus influenzae* in human milk: synthesis, distribution and activity of IgA protease as determined by study of *iga⁺* and mutant *iga⁻* cells, *J Infect Dis*, **166**: 43–52.

Pohl S, Bertschinger HU et al., 1983, Transfer of *Haemophilus pleuropneumoniae* and the *Pasteurella haemolytica*-like organism causing porcine necrotic pleuropneumonia to the genus *Actinobacillus pleuropneumoniae* comb. nov. on the basis of phenotypic and deoxyribonucleic acid relatedness, *Int J Syst Bacteriol*, **33**: 510–14.

Porras O, Caugant DA et al., 1986, Difference in structure between type b and nontypable *Haemophilus influenzae* populations, *Infect Immun*, **53**: 79–89.

Potts TV, Berry EM, 1983, Deoxyribonucleic acid-deoxyribonucleic acid hybridization analysis of *Actinobacillus actinomycetemcomitans* and *Haemophilus aphrophilus*, *Int J Syst Bacteriol*, **33**: 765–71.

Potts TV, Zambon JJ, Genco RJ, 1985, Reassignment of *Actinobacillus actinomycetemcomitans* to the genus *Haemophilus* as *Haemophilus actinomycetemcomitans* comb.nov, *Int J Syst Bacteriol*, **35**: 337–41.

Potts TV, Mitra T et al., 1986, Relationships among isolates of oral haemophili as determined by DNA-DNA hybridization, *Arch Microbiol*, **145**: 136–41.

Powell M, Fah YS et al., 1992, Antimicrobial resistance in *Haemophilus influenzae* from England and Scotland in 1991, *J Antimicrob Chemother*, **29**: 547–54.

Powell M, 1988, Antimicrobial resistance in *Haemophilus influenzae*, *J Med Microbiol*, **27**: 81–7.

Powell M, Williams JD, 1988, In-vitro activity of cefaclor, cephalexin and ampicillin against 2458 clinical isolates of *Haemophilus influenzae*, *J Antimicrob Chemother*, **21**: 27–31.

Pritchett IW, Stillman EG, 1919, The occurrence of *Bacillus influenzae* in throats and saliva, *J Exp Med*, **29**: 259–66.

Purven M, Lagergård T, 1992, *Haemophilus ducreyi*, a cytotoxin-producing bacterium, *Infect Immun*, **60**: 1156–62.

Quentin R, Musser JM et al., 1989, Typing of urogenital, maternal and neonatal isolates of *Haemophilus parainfluenzae* in correlation with clinical source of isolation and evidence for a genital specificity of *H. influenzae* biotype IV, *J Clin Microbiol*, **27**: 2286–94.

Quentin R, Dubarry I et al., 1992, Evaluation of four commercial methods for identification and biotyping of genital and neonatal strains of *Haemophilus* species, *Eur J Clin Microbiol Infect Dis*, **11**: 546–9.

Rådström P, Bäckman A et al., 1994, Detection of bacterial DNA in cerebrospinal fluid by an assay for simultaneous detection of *Neisseria meningitidis, Haemophilus influenzae*, and Streptococci using a seminested PCR strategy, *J Clin Microbiol*, **32**: 2738–44.

Rayan GM, Flournoy DJ, Cahill SL, 1987, Aerobic mouth flora of the rhesus monkey, *J Hand Surg (Am)*, **12**: 299–301.

Rennie R, Gordon T et al., 1992, Laboratory and clinical evaluations of media for the primary isolation of *Haemophilus* species, *J Clin Microbiol*, **30**: 1917–21.

Rimler RB, Shotts EB et al., 1977, The effect of sodium chloride and NADH on the growth of 6 strains of *Haemophilus* species pathogenic to chickens, *J Gen Microbiol*, **98**: 349–54.

Roberts DH, Hanson BS, Timms L, 1964, Observations in the incidence and significance of *Haemophilus gallinarum* in outbreaks of respiratory disease among poultry in Great Britain, *Vet Rec*, **76**: 1512–16.

Roberts MC, Swenson CD et al., 1980, Characterisation of chloramphenicol-resistant *Haemophilus influenzae*, *Antimicrob Agents Chemother*, **18**: 610–15.

Roche RJ, Moxon ER, 1995, Phenotypic variation of carbohydrate surface antigens and the pathogenesis of *Haemophilus influenzae* infections, *Trends Microbiol*, **3**: 304–9.

Roggen ER, Pansaerts R et al., 1993, Antigen detection and immunological typing of *Haemophilus ducreyi* with a specific rabbit polyclonal serum, *J Clin Microbiol*, **31**: 1820–5.

Roord JJ, Apicella M, Scheld WM, 1994, The induction of meningeal inflammation and blood-brain barrier permeability by *Haemophilus influenzae* type b peptidoglycan, *J Infect Dis*, **170**: 254–6.

Rousseau R, Duhamel M et al., 1991, The development of specific rRNA-derived oligonucleotide probes for *Haemophilus ducreyi*, the causative agent of chancroid, *J Gen Microbiol*, **137**: 277–85.

Rubin LG, St. Geme JW, 1993, Role of lipooligosaccharide in virulence of the Brazilian purpuric fever clone of *Haemophilus influenzae* biogroup aegyptius for infant rats, *Infect Immun*, **61**: 650–5.

Rubin LG, Medeiros AA et al., 1981, Ampicillin treatment failure of apparently β-lactamase-negative *Haemophilus influenzae* type b meningitis due to novel β-lactamase, *Lancet*, **ii**: 1008–10.

Sanders JD, Cope LD et al., 1993, Reconstitution of a porin-deficient mutant of *Haemophilus influenzae* type b with a porin gene from nontypeable *H. influenzae*, *Infect Immun*, **61**: 3966–75.

Sarafian SK, Woods TC et al., 1991, Molecular characterisation of *Haemophilus ducreyi* by ribosomal DNA fingerprinting, *J Clin Microbiol*, **29**: 1949–54.

Sarafian SK, Knapp JS, 1992, Molecular epidemiology, based on plasmid profiles of *Haemophilus ducreyi* infections in the United States: results of surveillance, 1981–90, *Sex Transm Dis*, **19**: 35–8.

Schalla WO, Sanders LL et al., 1986, Use of dot-immunobinding and immunofluorescence assays to investigate clinically suspected cases of chancroid, *Infect Dis*, **153**: 879–87.

Schalm OW, Beach JR, 1936, Cultural requirements of the fowl-coryza bacillus, *J Bacteriol*, **31**: 161–9.

Scheifele DW, Fussell SJ, 1981, Frequency of ampicillin-resistant *Haemophilus parainfluenzae* in children, *J Infect Dis*, **143**: 195–8.

Schulte JM, Schmid GP, 1995, Recommendations for treatment of chancroid, 1993, *Clin Infect Dis*, **20 (suppl 1)**: S39–46.

Sedlácek I, Gerner-Smidt P et al., 1993, Genetic relationship of strains of *Haemophilus aphrophilus*, *H. paraphrophilus* and *Actinobacillus actinomycetemcomitans* studied by ribotyping, *Zbl Bakteriol*, **279**: 51–9.

Sell SH, Turner DJ, Federspiel CF, 1973, Natural infections with *Haemophilus influenzae* in children: Types identified, Haemophilus influenzae, Sell SH, Karzon DT, Vanderbilt University Press, 3–12.

Shanahan PMA, Thomson CJ, Amyes SGB, 1996, Antibiotic susceptibilities of *Haemophilus influenzae* in Central Scotland, *J Clin Microb Infect*, **1**: 168–74.

Sims W, 1970 Oral haemophili, *J Med Microbiol*, **3**: 615–25.

Simasthien S, Dnangmani C, Echeverria P, 1980, *Haemophilus influenzae* type b resistant to both ampicillin and chloramphenicol, *Pediatr*, 6614–16.

Sirakova T, Kolattukudy PE et al., 1994, Role of fimbriae expressed by nontypeable *Haemophilus influenzae* in pathogenesis of and protection against otitis media and relatedness of the fimbrin subunit to outer membrane protein A, *Infect Immun*, **62**: 2002–20.

Slack MPE, Wheldon DB, Turk DC, 1977a, A rapid test for beta-lactamase production by *Haemophilus influenzae*, *Lancet*, **ii**: 906.

Slack MPE, Wheldon DB, Turk DC, 1977b, Rapid detection of chloramphenicol resistance in *Haemophilus influenzae*, *Lancet*, **ii**: 1366.

Slack MPE, 1990, Haemophilus, *Topley & Wilson's Principles of Bacteriology, Virology and Immunity*, vol. 2, 8th edn, eds Parker MT, Collier LH, Edward Arnold, London, 355–82.

Slootmans L, van den Berghe DA, Piot P, 1985, Typing *Haemophilus ducreyi* by indirect immunofluorescence assay, *Genitourin Med*, **61**: 123–6.

Smith-Vaughan HC, Sriprakash KS et al., 1995, Long PCR-ribotyping of nontypeable *Haemophilus influenzae*, *J Clin Microbiol*, **33**: 1192–5.

Sneath PHA, Johnson R, 1973, Numerical taxonomy of Haemophilus and related bacteria, *Int J Syst Bact*, **23**: 405–18.

Sottnek FO, Albritton AL, 1984, *Haemophilus influenzae* biotype VIII, *J Clin Microbiol*, **20**: 815–16.

Spinola SM, Castellazzo A et al., 1990, Characterisation of pili expressed by *Haemophilus ducreyi*, *Microb Pathog*, **9**: 417–26.

Spinola SM, Wild LM et al., 1994, Experimental human infection with *Haemophilus ducreyi*, *J Infect Dis*, **169**: 1146–50.

St. Geme JW, Gilsdorf JR, Falkow S, 1991, Surface structures and adherence properties of diverse strains of *Haemophilus influenzae* biogroup aegyptius, *Infect Immun*, **59**: 3366–71.

St. Geme JW, Takala A et al., 1994, Evidence for capsule gene sequences among pharyngeal isolates of nontypeable *Haemophilus influenzae*, *J Infect Dis*, **169**: 337–42.

Stewardson-Krieger P, Naidu S, 1981, Simultaneous recovery of beta-lactamase-negative and beta-lactamase-positive *Haemophilus influenzae* type b from cerebrospinal fluid of a neonate, *Pediatr*, **68**: 253–4.

Streker RG, Venezia RA, Robertson RG, 1978, Mode of action of *Haemophilus* bactericidal factor, *Antimicrob Agents Chemother*, **13**: 527–32.

Stull TL, LiPuma JJ, Edlind TD, 1988, A broad-spectrum probe for molecular epidemiology of bacteria: ribosomal RNA, *J Infect Dis*, **157**: 280–6.

Sturm AW, 1981, Identification of *Haemophilus ducreyi*, *Antonie van Leeuwenhoek J Microbiol Serol*, **47**: 89–90.

Sturm AW, 1986, Isolation of *Haemophilus influenzae* and *Haemophilus parainfluenzae* from genital-tract specimens with a selective medium, *J Med Microbiol*, **21**: 349–52.

Sturm AW, Stolting GJ et al., 1987, Clinical and microbiological evaluation of 46 episodes of genital ulceration, *Genitorurin Med*, **63**: 98–101.

Sturm AW, Zanen HC, 1984, Enzymatic activity of *Haemophilus ducreyi*, *J Med Microbiol*, **18**: 181–7.

Stuy JH, 1980, Chromosomally integrated conjugative plasmids are common in antibiotic-resistant *Haemophilus influenzae*, *J Bacteriol*, **142**: 925–30.

Takala AK, Eskola J, Leinonen M, 1991, Reduction of oropharyngeal carriage of *Haemophilus influenzae* type b (Hib) in children immunised with an Hib conjugate vaccine, *J Infect Dis*, **164**: 982–6.

Takala AK, Santosham M et al., 1993, Vaccination with *Haemophilus influenzae* type b meningococcal protein conjugate vaccine reduces oropharyngeal carriage of *Haemophilus influenzae* type b among American Indian children, *Pediatr Infect Dis J*, **12**: 593–9.

Targowski S, Targowski H, 1979, Characterisation of a *Haemophilus paracuniculus* isolated from gastro-intestinal tracts of rabbits with mucoid enteritis, *J Clin Microbiol*, **9**: 33–7.

Tebbutt G, 1984, A chemotyping system for clinical isolates of *Haemophilus influenzae*, *J Med Microbiol*, **17**: 335–45.

Tenover FC, Popovic T, Olsvik Ø, 1993, Using molecular methods to detect antimicrobial resistance genes, *Clin Microbiol Newsl*, **15**: 177–81.

Thjøtta T, Avery OT, 1921, Studies on bacterial nutrition II growth accessory substances in the cultivation of hemophilic bacilli, III. Plant tissue, as a source of growth accessory substances in the cultivation of *Bacillus influenzae*, *J Exp Med*, **34**: 97–114.

Thomas WR, Callow MG et al., 1990, Expression in *Escherichia coli* of a high-molecular-weight protective surface antigen found in nontypeable and type b *Haemophilus influenzae*, *Infect Immun*, **58**: 1909–13.

Tomasczewski E, 1903, Bakteriologische untersuchungen uber den erregar des ulcus molle, *Z Hyg Infektionskr*, **42**: 327–40.

Tondella MLC, Quinn FD, Perkins BA, 1995, Brazilian purpuric fever caused by *Haemophilus influenzae* biogroup aegyptius strains lacking the 3031 plasmid, *J Infect Dis*, **171**: 209–12.

Totten P'A, Stamm WE, 1994, Clear broth and plate media for culture of *Haemophilus ducreyi*, *J Clin Microbiol*, **32**: 2019–23.

Trees DL, Morse SA, 1995, Chancroid and *Haemophilus ducreyi*: an update, *Clin Microbiol Rev*, **8**: 357–75.

Tunevall G, 1951, Studies on *H. influenzae*: biochemical activities, *Acta Pathol Microbiol Scand*, **29**: 387–96.

Tunkel AR, Scheld WM, 1993, Pathogenesis and pathophysiology of bacterial meningitis, *Clin Microbiol Rev*, **6**: 118–36.

Turk DC, 1963, Nasopharyngeal carriage of *Haemophilus influenzae* type b, *J Hyg*, **61**: 247–56.

Turk DC, May JR, 1967, Haemophilus influenzae, *its clinical importance*, English University Press, London, 13–23.

Turk DC, 1975, An investigation of the family background of acute Haemophilus infections of children, *J Hyg*, **75**: 315–22.

Tyndall M, Malisa M et al., 1993, Ceftriaxone no longer predictably cures chancroid in Kenya, *J Infect Dis*, **167**: 469–71.

Ueyama T, Kurono Y et al., 1995, High incidence of *Haemophilus influenzae* in nasopharyngeal secretions and middle ear effusions as detected by PCR, *J Clin Microbiol*, **33**: 1835–8.

Vali L, Thomson CJ, Amyes SGB, 1994, *Haemophilus influenzae*: identification of a novel β-lactamase, *J Pharm Pharmacol*, **46**: 1041.

Vastine DW, Dawson CR et al., 1974, Comparison of media for the isolation of *Haemophilus* species from cases of seasonal conjunctivitis associated with severe endemic trachoma, *Appl Microbiol*, **28**: 688–90.

Venezia RA, Matusiak PM, Robertson RG, 1977, Bactericidal factor produced by *Haemophilus influenzae* type b: partial purification of the factor and transfer of its genetic determinant, *Antimicrob Agents Chemother*, **11**: 735–42.

Walker CN, Smith PW, 1980, Ampicillin resistance in *Haemophilus parainfluenzae*, *Am J Clin Pathol*, **74**: 229–32.

West B, Wilson SM et al., 1995, Simplified PCR for detection of *Haemophilus ducreyi* and diagnosis of chancroid, *J Clin Microbiol*, **33**: 787–90.

White DS, Granick S, 1963, Hemin biosynthesis in Haemophilus, *J Bacteriol*, **85**: 842–50.

Williams JD, Kattan S, Cavanagh P, 1974, Penicillinase production in *Haemophilus influenzae*, *Lancet*, **ii**: 103.

Williams P, Griffiths E, 1992, Bacterial transferrin receptors – structure, function and contribution to virulence (review), *Med Microbiol Immunol*, **181**: 301–22.

Williamson GM, Zinneman K, 1951, The occurrence of two distinct capsular antigens in *H.influenzae* type e strains, *J Pathol Bacteriol*, **63**: 695–8.

Winslow C-EA, Broadhurst J et al., 1917, The families and genera of the bacteria, *J Bacteriol*, **2**: 505–66.

Yogev R, Melick C. Glogowski W, 1982, In vitro development of rifampin resistance in clinical isolates of *Haemophilus influenzae* type b, *Antimicrobial Agents and Chemotherapy*, **21**: 387–9.

Zinnemann K, 1980, Newer knowledge in classification, taxonomy and pathogenicity of species in the genus Haemophilus. A critical review, *Zbl Bakt Hyg I Abt Orig A*, **247**: 248–58.

Zinnemann K, Rogers KB et al., 1971, A haemolytic V-dependent CO_2-preferring *Haemophilus* species *Haemophilus paraphrohaemolyticus* nov.spec, *J Med Microbiol*, **4**: 139–43.

Zwahlen A, Kroll JS et al., 1989, The molecular basis of pathogenicity in *Haemophilus influenzae*: comparative virulence of genetically-related capsular transformants and correlation with changes at the capsulation locus cap, *Microb Pathog*, **7**: 225–35.

Chapter 51

ACTINOBACILLUS, PASTEURELLA AND EIKENELLA

B Holmes

1 GENERAL INTRODUCTION

The gram-negative facultatively anaerobic coccobacilli and rods that make up the genera *Actinobacillus* and *Pasteurella* show many similarities. The organisms to which these names were first attached were animal pathogens; infected animals may serve as reservoirs for human disease. The clinical and pathological features of the animal diseases they caused were taken into consideration in defining the genera; this was particularly so with *Actinobacillus*. Subsequent additions to the genera have tended to blur these distinctions. Although this chapter is concerned primarily with human disease, the ecology and significance of Pasteurellaceae in animals other than humans has been reviewed by Bisgaard (1993).

Sneath and Johnson (1973) concluded from a numerical taxonomic study of *Haemophilus* and related bacteria that one cluster of organisms with a similarity index of 75% comprised strains named *Actinobacillus* and *Pasteurella* and considered that the 2 genera should no longer be separated. Mannheim et al. (1978) reached a similar conclusion from the pattern of respiratory quinones produced by organisms of these groups. The 2 genera are also similar in the G + C mol% of their chromosomal DNA. Frederiksen (1973) found difficulty in separating the 2 genera by means of phenotypic characters. Both genera ferment glucose, reduce nitrate to nitrite, and are non-motile. Although no single phenotypic feature definitively distinguishes the 2 (Mutters et al. 1985), an isolate can usually be identified by the results obtained from several biochemical tests (Table 51.1). Accurate identification of these organisms by those in the veterinary field is made even more difficult as there are a number of as yet unnamed taxa which also have to be considered (see, for example, Boot and Bisgaard 1995).

Mannheim, Pohl and Holländer (1980) concluded from genomic studies of representative members of the genera *Actinobacillus*, *Haemophilus* and *Pasteurella* (the 'AHP group') that this group should rank as a family but that some species had been misclassified and should be removed from it. Mannheim (1981) proposed the name Pasteurellaceae for the family, and considered that the 3 genera should be retained as distinct entities. According to Pohl (1981), DNA pairing suggested that some rearrangement of the organisms in the various genera was indicated. She suggested that *Pasteurella haemolytica* (biotype A) is

Table 51.1   Differential features of *Actinobacillus* and *Pasteurella* species occurring in clinical specimens[a]

Feature	*A. actinomycetemcomitans*	*A. equuli*[b]	*A. hominis*	*A. lignieresii*	*A. suis*	*A. ureae*	'*P.*' *aerogenes*	*P. bettyae* (HB-5)	*P. canis*	*P. dagmatis*[c]	*P. haemolytica sensu stricto*	*P. multocida*[d]	'*P.*' *pneumotropica*	*P. stomatis*	*P. trehalosi*	*P. volantium*
Acid from																
L-Arabinose	−[e]	(−)	−	(−)	(+)	−	(+)	−	−	−	+	d	(−)	−	−	−
Cellobiose	−	−	−	−	+	−	−	−	−	−	(−)	−	−	−	d	NT[f]
D-Galactose	+	d	+	d,L[f]	(+)	+	+	−	+	+	d	+	+	+	−	NT
Lactose	−	+	+	+	+	−	−	−	−	−	+	−	d	−	+	d,w[f]
Maltose	(+)	+	+	+	+	+	(−)	d	−	+	+	−	d	+	+	+
D-Mannitol	+	+	+	+	−	(+)	+	−	−	−	(−)	(−)	−	−	+	+
D-Mannose	−	+	+	+	+	+	d	d	+	+	−	(+)	+	+	+	NT
Melibiose	−	+	+,L	−	+	d	+	−	−	−	−[g]	+	−	−	−[g]	NT
Raffinose	−	+	−	d	+	d	d	−	−	+,w	d	(−)	d	−	−	NT
Salicin	(−)[h]	−	d	−	+	−	d	−	−	−	(−)	−	d	−	d	NT
Sorbitol	−	d	−	(−)	−	(−)	−	−	−	−	+	d	(−)	−	+	d
Sucrose	−	+	+	+	+	+	(−)	−	+	+	+	+	−	+	+	NT
D-Trehalose	−	+	+	−	+	−	+	−	d	+	−	d	(+)	+	+	+

D-Xylose	d	+	+	+	−	−	(−)	+	+	d	d	−	d
β-Haemolysis (sheep cells)	+	−	−	−	+	+	−	−	−	−	−	(+)	−
Catalase	d	d	+	+	d	d	d	+	+	+	+	−	+
Aesculin hydrolysis	−	−	−	−	−	−	−	−	−	d	d	d	NT
Fermentation[i]	+	+	+	+	+	+	+	+	+	+	+	+,L	NT
Gas production from D-glucose[i]	(+)	−	−	d,w	d,w	(+)	d,w	−	−	d	−	−	−
Growth on MacConkey agar[j]	d	+	+	−	d	d	d	+	+	d	d	+	−
Indole production	−	−	−	−	d,w	(−)	−	+	(+)	+	+,w	−	−
NAD requirement	−	−	−	−	−	−	−	−	−	−	−	−	+
ONPG reaction[k]	−	d	d	d	−	−	d	d	d	−	−	−	+
Ornithine decarboxylase	−	−	−	−	+	+	−	d	d	+	−	−	d
Oxidase	+	(+)	(+)	d	+	+	d	(+)	(+)	+	+	+	+
Urease	+	+	+	+	−	−	−	+	+	−	−	−	−

[a] Data from Sneath and Stevens (1990); these data were summarized from 19 different references.
[b] *A. equuli*-like bacterium differs from *A. equuli* in producing gas from glucose (Peel et al. 1991).
[c] Strains that are similar except for failing to produce urease are probably *Pasteurella* species Taxon 16 (Bisgaard and Mutters 1986).
[d] Three subspecies: *gallicida* dulcitol+, sorbitol+; *multocida* dulcitol−, sorbitol+; *septica* dulcitol+, sorbitol−.
[e] +, ≥90% of the strains are positive; (+), 80–89% of the strains are positive; d, 21–79% of the strains are positive; (−), 11–20% of the strains are positive; −, ≤10% of the strains are positive.
[f] L, late reaction: >24 h for acidification of carbohydrates, >48 h for fermentation in Hugh and Leifson's oxidation–fermentation (OF) medium; NT, not tested; w, weak reaction.
[g] Positive according to Carter (1984) and negative according to Kilian and Frederiksen (1981) and Sneath and Stevens (1985).
[h] Positive according to Sneath and Stevens (1985) and negative according to Kilian and Frederiksen (1981) and Phillips (1984).
[i] In Hugh–Leifson medium containing glucose, with incubation for 48 h at 37°C.
[j] Different formulations of this medium may explain discrepancies in the reported results; the results for *P. volantium* are for medium supplemented with NAD.
[k] ONPG reaction, hydrolysis of *ortho*-nitrophenyl-β-galactopyranoside.

more closely linked with *Actinobacillus lignieresii* than with *Pasteurella*; this supports an earlier suggestion of Mráz (1969) that *P. haemolytica* should be renamed '*Actinobacillus haemolyticus*'.

Characters that have in the past been used to delineate genera, such as the requirement for X or V factor in the *Haemophilus* group, perhaps may not have the taxonomic significance once accorded to them. Thus, there is strong evidence that the agent responsible for pleuropneumonia in pigs, *Haemophilus pleuropneumoniae*, has a closer relationship with *Actinobacillus* than *Haemophilus* (Pohl 1981). An organism described as '*Pasteurella haemolytica*-like' and isolated from necrotizing pleuropneumonia in pigs (Bertschinger and Seifert 1978) was regarded by Mannheim (1981) as a porcine actinobacillus; subsequently Pohl et al. (1983) concluded that it is a biotype of *H. pleuropneumoniae* and that the 2 should be transferred to the genus *Actinobacillus* under the name *Actinobacillus pleuropneumoniae*.

It will be clear that the family Pasteurellaceae is one that will be undergoing rearrangements as more organisms are recorded that fall into the group. The taxonomic position within the family should be regarded as fluid and, indeed, Dewhirst et al. (1993), from a comparison of 16S ribosomal ribonucleic acid (rRNA) sequences, concluded that taxonomic division of the family into phylogenetically and phenotypically coherent genera will be difficult. Nevertheless, as will be seen below, data from 16S rRNA sequences or DNA–rRNA hybridizations have clarified the taxonomic position of several taxa. The chemotaxonomic characters that recently have been provided to improve the taxonomy of the Pasteurellaceae have been reviewed by Olsen (1993). Beyond the family level, several studies confirm that the Pasteurellaceae are phylogenetically linked with the Enterobacteriaceae and the genera *Aeromonas*, *Photobacterium*, *Plesiomonas* and *Vibrio* to form a monophyletic unit within the γ3 subgroup of the Proteobacteria (see Ruimy et al. 1994).

ACTINOBACILLUS

2 DEFINITION

Actinobacilli are very small gram-negative, non-motile, non-sporing rods, often interspersed with coccal elements that may lie at the pole of a larger form, giving a characteristic 'Morse-code' appearance. Staining is irregular. The organisms are aerobic, or microaerobic, and facultatively anaerobic. After growth for 24 h on blood agar, colonies are translucent and 1–2 mm in diameter; growth is usually sticky. Actinobacilli ferment fructose, glucose and xylose with the production of acid but not gas; dulcitol, inositol and inulin are not fermented. They reduce nitrate to nitrite but do not form indole. Members of most species grow on MacConkey agar and produce β-galactosidase, oxidase and urease. Actinobacilli occur in a number of animal species and in humans, often as commensal organisms on the alimentary, genital or respiratory mucosa, but are also found as pathogens in a variety of lesions. All isolates are susceptible to chloramphenicol and tetracycline (Kaplan et al. 1989). The G + C content of the DNA is 40–43 mol% and the type species is *A. lignieresii*.

3 INTRODUCTION

In 1902, Lignières and Spitz isolated an organism from actinomycotic lesions of the soft tissues in cattle. They named the gram-negative, rod-shaped organism 'l'actinobacille' because of the nature of the lesion, the disease being described as actinobacillosis. The generic name *Actinobacillus* was first used in 1910 by Brumpt in classifying this organism. Since then several other organisms have been described and allotted to the genus, often without adequate reasons, and it has been said that *Actinobacillus* was once used to house 'species for which no obvious home can be found' (Cowan 1974). Few of the other species now regarded as properly placed in the genus cause actinomycotic lesions in their hosts. Although actinobacilli were first associated with cattle they have since been isolated from other animals and humans (Clark et al. 1984, Peel et al. 1991). Several human infections have followed animal bites.

Actinobacilli are distinguished from the enterobacteria by their smaller genome, obligatory parasitism and absence of motility. Though sensitive to the vibriostatic agent O129 (Chatelain et al. 1979), they differ from the vibrios in their smaller genome, absence of flagella and in various other phenotypic properties.

3.1 Classification

DNA–DNA hybridizations and examination of surface antigens led to the proposal that *Actinobacillus actinomycetemcomitans* be transferred to the genus *Haemophilus* as *Haemophilus actinomycetemcomitans* (Potts, Zambon and Genco 1985). Although this proposal was not favourably received (Anon 1987), the organism is certainly misplaced in *Actinobacillus*. Certain species currently in the genus *Actinobacillus* also belong in other genera based on 16S rRNA sequences or DNA–rRNA hybridizations. They are *A. actinomycetemcomitans*, as already mentioned, *Actinobacillus capsulatus*, *Actinobacillus muris*, *Actinobacillus salpingitidis* and *Actinobacillus seminis* (De Ley et al. 1990, Dewhirst et al. 1992, 1993). DNA–DNA hybridization studies indicated that the former *Pasteurella ureae* should be transferred to the genus *Actinobacillus* as *Actinbacillus ureae* (Mutters, Pohl and Mannheim 1986). The species *Actinobacillus rossii* and *A. seminis* (Sneath and Stevens 1990), *A. capsulatus*, *Actinobacillus delphinicola* (Foster et al. 1996), *A. muris*, *A. salpingitidis* and *A. (Haemophilus) pleuropneumoniae* are not described here as they have not, so far, been isolated from human clinical specimens. The species to be described are therefore *A. actinomycetemcomitans*, *Actinobacillus equuli* (including the *A. equuli*-like bacterium), *Actinobacillus hominis*, *A. lignieresii*, *Actinobacillus suis* and *A. ureae*. Weaver, Hollis and Bottone (1985) suggested that the 33 strains tabulated by the CDC as *A. suis* may represent more than one taxon and that some of the mannitol-fermenting strains may be the biochemically similar *A. hominis*. *A. actinomycetemcomitans* also may represent more than one taxon, being divisible into 2 groups (Brondz and Olsen 1993); one group comprises serotypes b and c and one comprises serotypes a, d and e.

4 ACTINOBACILLUS ACTINOMYCETEMCOMITANS

When described by Klinger in 1912 under the name '*Bacterium actinomycetemcomitans*', this organism was regarded as a secondary organism in the actinomycotic lesions in humans. In such lesions it is found as densely packed gram-negative coccobacilli (Colebrook 1920). Since then it has been recognized as part of the normal flora of the human oral cavity (Heinrich and Pulverer 1959b), although mainly harboured on the teeth as the organism could not be isolated from edentulous subjects (Danser et al. 1995). It has been found as the sole organism in various lesions in humans including abscesses and endocarditis (Thjøtta and Sydnes 1951, Page and King 1966, Blair et al. 1982) and in infectious arthritis of the knee; its close relationship with localized juvenile periodontitis is well recognized (Zambon 1985, Christersson 1993). Various virulence factors relevant to the pathogenesis of *A. actinomycetemcomitans* in inflammatory periodontal diseases have been reviewed by Wilson and Henderson (1995). The use of restriction fragment length polymorphisms to type clinical isolates of *A. actinomycetemcomitans* has resulted in the identification of genetic variants, some of which predominate in localized juvenile periodontitis and some in healthy individuals (DiRienzo and McKay 1994). The results of Ebersole, Cappelli and Sandoval (1994) support a unique distribution of this organism in the subgingival ecology that is related to active host immune responses and clinical presentation of the tooth, there being a positive relationship between the level of IgG anti-*A. actinomycetemcomitans* antibody and the frequency of teeth affected, and a higher proportion of positive samples was found from teeth with bleeding on probing the gingival sulcus. Underwood et al. (1993) also found that subjects who developed high levels of highly avid antibodies against this organism may have greater resistance to continued or repeated infection.

For the detection of *A. actinomycetemcomitans* in subgingival plaque, polymerase chain reaction (PCR) and culture-enhanced PCR were found to be superior to culture with presumptive biochemical identification (Flemmig et al. 1995); Tønjum and Haas (1993) described a PCR assay, based on the leukotoxin structural gene, which they found particularly useful for

identification of this organism. A colorimetric assay of the PCR product has been developed to detect the presence of, and to quantify, *A. actinomycetemcomitans* in subgingival plaque samples (Fujise et al. 1995). Indirect immunofluorescence (Listgarten et al. 1995) and membrane-based immunoassay (Snyder et al. 1996) have also proved useful. The application of arbitrarily primed PCR can yield different DNA amplification profiles which may be useful for studies of epidemiology and bacterial transmission (Preus et al. 1993), as are Southern blot restriction fragment length polymorphisms (Slots et al. 1993). van Steenbergen et al. (1994) compared 6 different typing methods and found ribotyping the most useful.

Close contact is necessary to effect transmission of the organism and rRNA gene restriction patterns confirm previous findings that *A. actinomycetemcomitans* is transmitted intrafamilially (Alaluusua et al. 1993). Other focal infections associated with the organism include animal bites, although some surveys have failed to detect the organism in canine dental plaque (Allaker, Langlois and Hardie 1994). Although *A. actinomycetemcomitans* has been regarded mainly as a parasite of humans, there is evidence that it may be responsible for infections in animals. When first recognized in the actinomycotic lesions of humans it was also found in such lesions in cattle. It is also the most frequent isolate from cases of epididymitis in rams in Oregon and Idaho, USA (DeLong, Waldhalm and Hall 1979, Bulgin and Anderson 1983).

In cultures there are distinct rod forms 0.8–1.5 µm long, but in actinomycotic lesions forms that are much more coccal (0.3–0.5 µm in diameter) are seen; the organism thus resembles *Brucella* spp., *Francisella tularensis* and *Haemophilus aphrophilus*. It does not produce a capsule that can be demonstrated microscopically, but the presence of capsular material that is a potent mediator of bone resorption has been reported (Wilson, Kamin and Harvey 1985). On agar the organism gives rise to small (<0.5 mm in diameter after 24 h but enlarging to 2–3 mm), tough colonies adherent to the medium and described as having a shape like that of a star or like 'crossed cigars' (Heinrich and Pulverer 1959a). Colonies may sometimes develop rough surfaces and pitting after several days of incubation. The organism is capnophilic and relatively fastidious. It grows better under anaerobic than aerobic conditions; it is micro-aerobic, growing as a band 5 mm below the surface in agar shake-cultures. Growth is improved by the addition of CO_2, at least 0.5% (Holm 1954). Growth is also improved by blood or ascitic fluid. The optimal pH range for growth is between pH 7.0 and 8.0, in a medium containing NaCl 0.5–1%. In broth it forms isolated translucent granules 0.5–1.0 mm in diameter at the bottom and up the sides of the tube and the medium, except for a slight sediment, remains clear. However, this character may be lost on repeated subculture with the development of a uniform turbidity. It is less active in fermenting carbohydrates than other actinobacilli, but glucose and maltose are usually fermented; Pulverer and Ko (1970) were able to define 8 biotypes based on the fermentation of galactose, mannitol and xylose. Nitrate is reduced; other, differential, characters are presented in Table 51.1.

Pulverer and Ko (1972) defined 6 heat-stable agglutinating antigens, and by the use of 6 absorbed antisera established 24 agglutinating patterns among 100 strains. However, King and Tatum (1962), using the capillary-precipitation technique, found 3 precipitating antigens distributed singly among different strains; this was confirmed by Zambon, Slots and Genco (1983) using the Ouchterlony and immunofluorescence techniques on strains derived from the human oral cavity. They named these 3 serotypes a, b and c and showed that strains from other lesions fell into this system. They found that *A. actinomycetemcomitans* cross-reacted serologically with other actinobacilli and also with *H. aphrophilus*. Its close similarity with the last-mentioned organism in biochemical and cultural characters is well recognized (King and Tatum 1962, Slots 1982) and is why some authorities would place *A. actinomycetemcomitans* in the genus *Haemophilus*. Both have been shown by electron microscopy to have numerous vesicular structures on their surface which may become detached and are found free in the external environment (Holt, Tanner and Socransky 1980). Olsen and Brondz (1985) reported differences between them in susceptibility to the lytic effects of EDTA and lysozyme. Subsequently, serotype d has been recognized and more recently, Gmur et al. (1993) designated the new serotype e.

A. actinomycetemcomitans is non-pathogenic for laboratory animals although it has been described in association with a naturally occurring infection in laboratory mice (Vallée and Gaillard 1953). Some strains produce a heat-labile leucotoxin capable of killing human monocytes and polymorphs (Taichman, Dean and Sanderson et al. 1980, Tsai and Taichman 1986).

Therapy in human infections has frequently involved ampicillin or penicillin, but resistance to these is common. In vitro, aminoglycosides, cefazolin, cefotaxime, ceftriaxone and chloramphenicol show good activity (Kaplan et al. 1989), as do cefaclor, cefoxitin, cefuroxime, doxycycline, imipenem, norfloxacin, tetracycline, trimethoprim–sulphamethoxazole (co-trimoxazole) and the azalide azithromycin; cefixime and ciprofloxacin in combination with metronidazole may be useful for patients allergic to penicillin (Pavicic, van Winkelhoff and de Graaff 1992). Amoxycillin administered with metronidazole has a synergic effect in vitro and when combined with mechanical debridement is very effective in suppressing *A. actinomycetemcomitans* below cultivable levels over a long period (Pavicic et al. 1994).

5   *ACTINOBACILLUS EQUULI*

This organism is associated in horses with joint-ill and 'sleepy foal disease' and in pigs with arthritis, endocarditis and nephritis. It occurs as a commensal in the equine intestinal tract and mouth, but has not been isolated from normal swine. Golland et al. (1994) described 15 cases of peritonitis in horses. It has been found infrequently in lesions in other animal species, including calves, a dog, monkeys, rabbits and rats. An

A. equuli-like bacterium has been isolated from an infected horse bite wound in a human (Peel et al. 1991).

A. equuli is a gram-negative rod which may show longer filamentous forms when the medium contains glucose or maltose. It is non-capsulate but produces considerable amounts of extracellular slime that can be detected in both wet and stained preparations.

On nutrient and blood agars it forms colonies that are so viscous that a string of material is formed between medium and inoculating loop when an attempt is made to lift a colony from the medium. The viscous nature of the growth is also apparent in broth cultures. This character is not lost on repeated subculture of the organism. *A. equuli* survives poorly in culture, especially in fluid media containing even a small amount of fermentable substrate. A distinct zone of complete haemolysis is produced around colonies of some strains on sheep blood agar, but many strains are non-haemolytic.

Acid but not gas is formed from lactose, maltose, mannitol, melibiose, sucrose and trehalose but not from cellobiose, rhamnose and salicin. Sodium hippurate is hydrolysed, but aesculin is not. Some strains are reported to liquefy gelatin. Strains differ in their catalase and oxidase reactions. Other features are presented in Table 51.1. Most strains of *A. equuli* (and *A. suis*), but none of *A. lignieresii*, ferment melibiose and trehalose.

As in *A. lignieresii*, both heat-labile and heat-stable antigens can be demonstrated and a number of antigenic groups have been recognized (see Phillips 1984).

The G + C content of the DNA is 40.0–41.8 mol % (see also Edwards 1932, Maguire 1958).

6   *ACTINOBACILLUS HOMINIS*

A. hominis was originally isolated from patients with chronic lung disease; it is also a causative agent of septicaemia in hepatic failure (Wüst et al. 1991). Its characters are given in Table 51.1.

7   *ACTINOBACILLUS LIGNIERESII*

The organism in cattle is the same as that originally described in sheep as '*Bacterium purifaciens*' and shown subsequently to have the characters of *A. lignieresii* (Tunnicliff 1941).

7.1   Morphology

A. lignieresii is a small rod-shaped organism often showing shorter coccobacillary forms (Fig. 51.1). In media containing fermentable carbohydrates (glucose or maltose), rather long, almost filamentous forms are seen. In all cultures, small granules are found scattered among the bacterial cells and often lying at the pole of a bacillary or filamentous form, giving a characteristic 'Morse-code' form (Phillips 1960). The rods are 1.15–1.25 μm by 0.4 μm and are non-motile, non-sporing and non-acid-fast. Capsules are not formed, but extracellular slime can be demonstrated in wet India ink preparations of cultures. The cells stain readily, especially with carbol fuchsin, and are gram-negative; they may show bipolar staining.

In lesions in the animal body small granules are found consisting of tufts of radially disposed clubs similar to those in actinomycosis. In actinobacillosis, however, the centre of the granule is occupied not by a gram-positive filamentous mycelium, such as that formed by an actinomycete, but by small gram-negative rods that quite easily may be overlooked. Though both rods and the clubs formed by *A. lignieresii* are gram-negative, it is possible to distinguish between them in sections by a modified Ziehl–Neelsen stain (Bosworth 1923). In a section stained with carbol fuchsin, decolorized for 20–30 s with H_2SO_4 1% and counterstained with methylene blue, the clubs appear red and the rods blue. For pus one of the best stains is glycerine picrocarmine which stains the clubs yellow and the pus cells pink.

7.2   Cultivation

Pus is present in only small amounts in typical lesions, but if collected aseptically from the cut surface of the granulomatous lesion and seeded on to blood agar it may yield growth readily under aerobic conditions and less readily under anaerobic conditions. Primary cultivation from material likely to be contaminated with other organisms, e.g. mouth swabs or rumen contents, can be facilitated by the use of selective media (Till and Palmer 1960, Phillips 1961). The optimum temperature for growth is 37°C; very slight growth occurs at 20°C.

On primary isolation, viscous colonies 1–2 mm in diameter are formed on blood or nutrient agar, but the sticky nature of the colony is lost with repeated

subcultivation in the laboratory. Prolonged incubation may result in increase in size of well separated colonies up to c. 4 mm. In a gelatin stab, growth is poor and not visible for some days, and appears as a small opaque spot at the surface with little evidence of growth beneath; there is no liquefaction. The organism grows on MacConkey agar. In broth it produces uniform turbidity with little deposit. Growth is improved by serum. There is no haemolysis on sheep blood agar.

7.3   Susceptibility to chemical and physical agents

The organism is killed by heating to 62°C for 10 min. It is rapidly destroyed by drying. Cultures lose their viability rapidly and should be subcultured every 5–7 days. *A. lignieresii* is reported to be susceptible to chloramphenicol, chlortetracycline, oxytetracycline and streptomycin but resistant to neomycin, novobiocin and oleandomycin (Till and Palmer 1960).

7.4   Biochemical reactions

Fermentation of carbohydrates may be difficult to interpret as reactions may be weak or delayed. Best results are obtained in a peptone-Lemco base with 1% carbohydrate and bromothymol blue indicator. Tests should not be prolonged beyond 14 days, otherwise false positive reactions may result from the breakdown of peptone with the liberation of amino acids (Mráz 1969). *A. lignieresii* produces acid without gas promptly in maltose, mannitol and sucrose, but with a delayed (5–7 days) reaction in lactose. Cellobiose, melibiose, rhamnose, salicin and trehalose are not fermented. Acid is produced in litmus milk, but no clot. The catalase reaction varies from strain to strain; the oxidase reaction is generally positive; aesculin and sodium hippurate are not hydrolysed.

7.5   Antigenic structure

Heat-stable somatic antigens and heat-labile surface antigens can be demonstrated. Six antigenic types, 1–6, have been demonstrated with 2 subtypes, 1a and 4c (Phillips 1967), based on the heat-stable antigens. Most cattle strains in the UK belong to type 1 and most sheep strains to types 2, 3 and 4, but differences in species distribution may be found in other geographical areas (Nakazawa et al. 1977). Heat-labile antigens associated with the extracellular slime may cause cross-reactions in agglutination tests if unheated suspensions of the different antigenic types are used.

7.6   Habitat

A. lignieresii is a commensal in the rumen of cattle and sheep (Phillips 1961) and is part of the oral flora of normal cattle (Phillips 1964) and sheep, but it has not been so recognized in other animals with the exception of laboratory rodents (Lentsch and Wagner

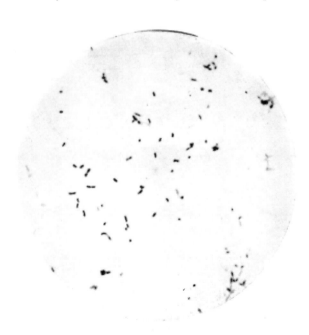

Fig. 51.1   *Actinobacillus lignieresii.* From a liver agar slope; 2 days, 37°C aerobically (× 1580).

1980). In addition to the 2 main host species, lesions have been reported in other species: in the tongue of dogs and horses (Baum et al. 1984), also in the oviducts of ducks (Bisgaard 1975). It has been described as a pathogen in humans (Thompson and Willius 1932, Pathak and Ristic 1962, Orda and Wiznitzer 1980, Dibb, Digranes and Tønjum 1981).

7.7 Pathogenicity

Exotoxin is not formed. *A. lignieresii* causes actinobacillosis in cattle and sheep. Various adverse factors predispose to the natural disease. Experimental inoculation into cattle has shown considerable differences in virulence between strains, some of which fail to cause disease (Magnusson 1928). Subcutaneous injection of pure cultures into cattle may produce an abscess similar to those occurring spontaneously; granules consisting of rods surrounded by clubs are found in the pus. Most workers have been unable to produce specific lesions in laboratory animals, and a claim by early workers that the organism causes a fatal infection when given intraperitoneally to guinea pigs has not been substantiated. However, Mráz (1969) considers that chick and mice embryos are more susceptible than guinea pigs and rabbits. Mice inoculated intraperitoneally and chick embryos inoculated by injection into the allantoic cavity usually die. The G + C content of the DNA is 41.8–42.6 mol%.

8 *ACTINOBACILLUS SUIS*

This organism was initially described from various lesions in pigs aged 3 months or less but subsequently it was described also in adult pigs. *A. suis* has also been found in horses, both in normal animals (Veterinary Investigation Service 1975) and associated with pathological processes (Kim, Phillips and Atherton 1976, Kim et al. 1982, Nelson et al. 1996), and in the tonsils of healthy pigs (Cutlip, Amtower and Zinober 1972).

It is a gram-negative rod that may show filamentous forms and considerable variation in length. It produces extracellular slime, which can be demonstrated in wet preparations as well as in stained smears, but is not associated with capsule formation. Colonies on nutrient agar or blood agar and growth in broth cultures exhibit stickiness. The viscous character of the growth is less than that seen with *A. equuli* and tends to be lost on repeated subculture. All strains give complete haemolysis on sheep blood agar.

Acid is formed in cellobiose, lactose, maltose, melibiose, salicin, sucrose and trehalose, but not in mannitol and rhamnose. Aesculin and sodium hippurate are hydrolysed. The catalase reaction is positive but different strains give different results in the oxidase test. Differential characters are presented in Table 51.1. Most strains of *A. suis* (and *A. equuli*), but no strains of *A. lignieresii*, ferment melibiose and trehalose. All strains of *A. suis*, but no strains of *A. equuli* and *A. lignieresii*, hydrolyse aesculin. Unlike *A. hominis*, *A. suis* ferments D-arabinose, cellobiose and D-mannose.

The antigens of *A. suis* have not been studied in any detail, but there appears to be marked uniformity in the antigens of strains drawn from a wide geographical area.

A. suis is not pathogenic for rabbits or guinea pigs but will infect mice by intraperitoneal injection.

9 *ACTINOBACILLUS UREAE*

This organism was isolated from the human respiratory tract by Jones (1962). It is a small pleopmorphic rod that occasionally shows bipolar staining. It grows better on media containing blood or serum than on unenriched media, growth is mucoid with an optimum growth temperature of 37°C; the organism grows poorly at 22°C. It is non-haemolytic, but usually accompanied by some greening of the medium. There is no growth on MacConkey medium. *A. ureae* hydrolyses urea strongly, is indole- and H_2S-negative, acidifies maltose and mannitol but not xylose. The organism is serologically distinct.

Differential features are presented in Table 51.1. *A. ureae* differs from most other species in being lactose- and xylose-negative.

A. ureae is only slightly pathogenic for guinea pigs, mice and rabbits (Henriksen and Jyssum 1961), but strains vary in virulence. Some strains injected intraperitoneally kill mice in 2 days; others do so only when injected with mucin. In humans, although occurring in sputum, *A. ureae* has also been isolated from blood, cerebrospinal fluid and the respiratory tract (Verhaegen et al. 1988). It has been identified as the primary pathogen in 11 cases of meningitis (Kingsland and Guss 1995). *A. ureae* is probably part of the flora of the human respiratory tract and is among the few members of *Actinobacillus* that apparently have no other animal host (Kolyvas et al. 1978).

A. ureae, according to Jones (1962), is antigenically homogeneous, but according to Henriksen (1961) has at least 2 serotypes, of which one contains a type-specific capsular antigen. Both observers agree, however, that it has no antigenic relation to members of the *Pasteurella* group.

PASTEURELLA

10 DEFINITION

Pasteurellae are very small (1–2 μm in length) gram-negative, non-acid-fast, non-motile, coccoid, ovoid or rod-shaped organisms, often showing bipolar staining. They are aerobic and facultatively anaerobic and do not grow, or grow only scantily, in the presence of bile salts. They attack carbohydrates weakly by the fermentative method, forming small amounts of acid but usually no gas. They ferment sucrose but rarely lactose, reduce nitrate to nitrite and are catalase- and oxidase-positive. Some species produce indole and some urease. They do not liquefy gelatin. Pasteurellae are parasites of humans and animals, causing characteristic diseases. Most isolates recovered from clinical specimens are catalase-, oxidase-, indole- and sucrose-positive, most decarboxylate ornithine and some are capsulate; they are non-sporing. The G + C content of the DNA is 40–45 mol% and the type species is *Pasteurella multocida*.

11 INTRODUCTION

Perroncito appears to have been the first to isolate and describe, in 1879, the organism known as 'the bacillus of fowl cholera'. Similar organisms were cultured by subsequent workers from cattle, pigs, sheep and other animals suffering from a disease characterized by septicaemia with widespread haemorrhages. In 1887, Trevisan suggested for these various isolates the generic name *Pasteurella*, and in 1900 Lignières added the specific name for each organism according to the animal it attacked; thus the name of the organism from fowls was '*Pasteurella aviseptica*', from cattle '*Pasteurella boviseptica*', from rabbits '*Pasteurella lepiseptica*', from sheep '*Pasteurella oviseptica*' and from pigs '*Pasteurella suiseptica*'. As these organisms behaved as if they belonged to a single species it was suggested in the first edition of this book in 1929 that they should all be referred to by the name '*Pasteurella septica*'. Later, Rosenbusch and Merchant (1939) proposed the alternative name *P. multocida*. The editors of Bergey's manual (Breed, Murray and Smith 1957) regarded the term *P. multocida* as claiming priority in accordance with the rules of nomenclature, but on their own showing this was certainly not the first specific name given. The name *P. multocida*, however, is now universally accepted, although one of its subspecies (see section 18.6, p. 1205) bears the epithet *septica*.

Another organism belonging to the genus *Pasteurella* but differing mainly in its haemolytic activity was isolated by Jones (1921), Tweed and Edington (1930), and Rosenbusch and Merchant (1939) from diseases of calves and sheep, and named *P. haemolytica*. What was thought to be a variant of this organism was described by Henriksen and Jyssum (1960, 1961) under the name *P. haemolytica* var. *ureae*. A very similar, if not identical, organism was isolated from the human respiratory tract by Jones (1962), who called it *P. ureae*. This name seemed more appropriate, as the organism does not have a close relationship to *P. haemolytica* (Henriksen 1961). However, both *P. haemolytica* and *P. ureae* have affinities with the genus *Actinobacillus*, the latter so much so that it has been transferred to that genus. So far as is known, all pasteurellae lead a parasitic existence.

11.1 Morphology and staining

The usual appearance is that of small ovoid non-motile gram-negative rods, 1–2 μm by 0.3–1 μm, with convex sides and rounded ends, showing bipolar staining. There is no special arrangement; the organisms occur singly, in pairs, short chains or small groups. Coccoid and short rod forms, often staining irregularly, are not uncommon. Generally, the cells are ovoid and show bipolar staining when taken from animal tissues or smooth colonies, and are more bacillary without bipolar staining when taken from rough colonies, but there are many exceptions. An indefinite capsule, sometimes referred to as an envelope substance, is often formed in the animal body, and in mucoid and smooth iridescent colonies of *P. multocida*. It can be revealed by the India ink method and by Giemsa's stain. According to Priestley (1936a, 1936c) it is seen only in virulent strains. The envelope reaches its maximum development after 24 h at 37°C, then gradually disappears; it is not formed below 20°C or above 40°C. It is composed either of hyaluronic acid or of polysaccharide (JE Smith 1958), is heat-labile, and is antigenically distinct from the somatic substance. Most freshly isolated strains of *P. haemolytica* are capsulate (Carter 1967). Gilmour and colleagues (1985) showed that biotype A strains of *P. haemolytica* (now *P. haemolytica sensu stricto*) were usually covered with surface protrusions of capsular material but that biotype T (now *Pasteurella trehalosi*) capsules were less well defined. Henriksen and Frøholm (1975) described a fimbriate strain of *P. multocida* showing twitching movement and forming spreading colonies.

11.2 Metabolism and growth requirements

All pasteurellae are aerobes and facultative anaerobes. They grow between about 12°C and 43°C; their optimal temperature is 37°C but, according to Burrows and Gillett (1966), their nutritive requirements are more exacting at 37°C than at lower temperatures. Some species and strains of *Pasteurella* require V factor (Krause et al. 1987).

11.3 Susceptibility to chemical and physical agents

None of the pasteurellae is specially resistant to adverse agents or environmental conditions. The organisms are killed by heat at 55°C, and by 0.5% phenol within 15 min. In cultures or infected organs kept in an ice chest the bacterial cells may survive for months. In dried infected blood, *P. multocida* may retain its viability and virulence for about 3 weeks; in blood allowed to putrefy in a glass tube for 100 days it may still be capable of causing infection. Pasteurellae are susceptible in vitro to chloramphenicol, penicillin, streptomycin, sulphadiazine, tetracycline and numerous other commonly used antibiotics (Weaver, Hollis and Bottone 1985). Multiple drug resistance in *P. haemolytica* and *P. multocida* was reported by Chang and Carter (1976) and small non-conjugal plasmids encoding resistance to streptomycin, the sulphonamides or tetracycline have been described (Hirsh, Martin and Rhoades 1985). *P. haemolytica sensu stricto* is highly susceptible to penicillin, but *P. trehalosi* is fairly resistant (Smith 1961, Biberstein and Francis 1968). About half the strains of *P. multocida* are able to grow in the presence of 0.4% selenite, but *P. haemolytica* and

P. trehalosi are invariably unable to do so (Lapage and Bascomb 1968).

11.4 Pathogenicity

Pasteurellae have been isolated from lesions in many parts of the human body, especially animal bite wounds; Ganiere et al. (1993) observed a higher incidence of one or more pathogenic strains in gingival scrapings of cats than in those of dogs which could explain the fact that *Pasteurella* infections in humans are less common in dog bites than in cat bites. Escande and Lion (1993) and Frederiksen (1993) have reviewed the occurrence of *Pasteurella* and related species in human infections. In animals, they cause fowl cholera, haemorrhagic septicaemia, mastitis, septic pleuropneumonia, snuffles, and other focal infections. Both normal and diseased wild and domestic animals are the reservoirs for most human infections.

11.5 Classification

Pasteurella is the type genus of the Pasteurellaceae (Anon 1981, Pohl 1981); historically, it comprised 2 main species: *P. haemolytica sensu stricto* (not a true *Pasteurella*) and *P. multocida*.

The phenotypic features of *Pasteurella* spp. are similar to those of *Actinobacillus* spp. and the DNA–DNA pairing studies of Mutters et al. (1985) have shown that several taxa previously assigned to the genus *Pasteurella* – *Pasteurella aerogenes*, *P. haemolytica* (including *P. trehalosi*) and *Pasteurella pneumotropica* (biotypes Jawetz and Heyl but not the type Henricksen; Frederiksen 1981) – are more closely related to the genus *Actinobacillus* than to *Pasteurella*. The so-called *P. haemolytica* strains from pigs and poultry were shown to differ from ruminant strains (Bisgaard, Phillips and Mannheim 1986, Mutters, Bisgaard and Pohl 1986). Comparisons of 16S rRNA sequences by Dewhirst et al. (1992) confirm that *P. aerogenes*, *P. haemolytica* (including *P. trehalosi*) and *P. pneumotropica* are not closely related to each other or to *Pasteurella*. The hybridization (Mutters et al. 1985) and subsequent (Sneath and Stevens 1990) studies detected more than 13 taxa in *Pasteurella*, including *Pasteurella canis* ('dog-type' strains), *P. multocida* (with 3 subspecies) and *Pasteurella stomatis* (canine and feline strains). The differential phenotypic features of those taxa that occur in clinical specimens are shown in Table 51.1; the characters of species occurring only in veterinary material can be found elsewhere (Pickett, Hollis and Bottone 1989). For reviews of *Pasteurella* taxonomy and nomenclature, see Hussaini (1975) and Mutters, Mannheim and Bisgaard (1989); for the relation of *Pasteurella* to *Actinobacillus* and *Haemophilus*, see Zinnermann (1981), Mannheim (1983) and Dewhirst et al. (1993).

12 PASTEURELLA AEROGENES

Colonies on blood agar after 24 h are 0.5–1 mm in diameter, convex, smooth, translucent and non-haemolytic. The biochemical profile of [*P*]. *aerogenes* is distinct from that of other pasteurellae (Table 51.1), especially in the ability of strains to form gas from sugars. This species has been isolated from aborted fetuses of swine and from animal bites, urine, peritoneal fluid and stillbirth (and mother) in humans. Lester et al. (1993) examined several strains, from various animal or geographical origins, by phenotypic characterization and ribotyping and found that the strains constituted a well defined group that could not be subdivided according to origin.

Another organism, mentioned here because it is also gas-producing and also not a member of *Pasteurella sensu stricto*, is the so-called *Pasteurella* 'SP' group. This is a rare organism usually isolated from guinea pigs and occasionally from rabbits; 5 cases of human infection have been reported, including severe infection in a woman after a bite from a guinea pig (Lion et al. 1995).

13 PASTEURELLA BETTYAE

The capnophilic group long referred to as HB-5 has more recently been described as a species of *Pasteurella*. It was first given the name *Pasteurella bettii* (Sneath and Stevens 1990), which was subsequently corrected to *P. bettyae* (Sneath 1992).

HB-5 exhibits coccobacilli and rods upon Gram's stain; on blood agar after 24 h, colonies are 0.5–1.0 mm in diameter, convex and smooth. The organism is facultatively anaerobic, and all strains are weakly aerogenic. Of the commonly used sugars, only glucose is acidified. Although HB-5 and *P. bettyae* are the same organism, different results are given by different authors for their catalase, oxidase, maltose fermentation, and especially indole reactions (Clark et al. 1984, Sneath and Stevens 1990, see Table 51.1). HB-5 is susceptible to many antimicrobial agents, including penicillin, but several strains produce β-lactamases (Bogaerts et al. 1990).

HB-5 has been isolated from amniotic fluid, blood (usually newborn babies), finger lesions, leg abscesses, placenta, rectal sites, surgical incisions, and urogenital specimens (particularly those of females), including exudates of genital ulcers, especially Bartholin gland abscesses (Baddour et al. 1989, Weaver, Hollis and Bottone 1985).

14 PASTEURELLA CABALLI

P. caballi (Schlater et al. 1989) is another recently described species; it differs from most other pasteurellae in being catalase-negative. All of the 29 isolates from horses were aerogenic, failed to grow on MacConkey agar, acidified neither arabinose nor trehalose, and were both urease- and indole-negative. Although not included in Table 51.1, the species is mentioned here as a strain has been isolated from a veterinary surgeon's infected wound (Bisgaard, Heltberg and Frederiksen 1991).

15 PASTEURELLA CANIS

This organism was described from strains originally classified as *P. multocida* (Clark et al. 1984). They were reassigned to the new species *P. canis* based on results of DNA–DNA hybridization studies (Mutters et al. 1985). The principal test for differentiating between *P. canis* and *P. multocida* is acidification of mannitol (Table 51.1). Biotype 1 strains, from the oral cavity of dogs and dog bites in humans, are indole-positive; biotype 2 strains, from cattle, are indole-negative.

16 *PASTEURELLA DAGMATIS*

The name *P. dagmatis* was proposed by Mutters et al. (1985) for a group of pasteurellae variously referred to as *Pasteurella* sp. 'n. sp. 1' or as *Pasteurella* 'gas' (Clark et al. 1984). On blood agar after 24 h, colonies are 1–2 mm in diameter and non-haemolytic. Differential tests include acidification of maltose and xylose, production of indole, decarboxylation of ornithine, and hydrolysis of urea (Table 51.1). Strains have been isolated from human wounds after animal contact, particularly cat and dog bites. The organism has also been implicated in infective endocarditis (Sorbello et al. 1994) and as a cause of septicaemia in a diabetic patient subsequent to septicaemia caused by *P. multocida* (Fajfar-Whetstone et al. 1995). Similar strains that are urease-negative are probably members of the *Pasteurella* sp. Taxon 16 of Bisgaard and Mutters (1986).

17 *PASTEURELLA HAEMOLYTICA (AND PASTEURELLA TREHALOSI)*

17.1 Isolation

P. haaemolytica has been isolated by Jones (1921), Tweed and Edington (1930), and others from pneumonia in sheep, cattle and goats.

17.2 Morphology

The organisms are gram-negative, short, non-motile, evenly stained rods.

17.3 Cultural features

GR Smith (1959, 1960, 1961) recognized 2 forms of *P. haemolytica*, for a long time regarded as biotypes. On horse, sheep or rabbit blood agar, biotype A, derived from sheep pneumonia and from septicaemia in lambs within a few weeks of birth, forms circular, glistening, convex colonies which at up to 4 mm in diameter, are slightly smaller than those of biotype T and with only a little central thickening; unlike biotype T, biotype A rapidly lost viability in ageing broth cultures. Biotype T, derived mainly from septicaemia in lambs aged 5–12 months, forms colonies that in young cultures are larger, with dark brown centres (Fig. 51.2). However, these biotypes were found to exhibit only low levels of DNA–DNA pairing to each other (Bingham, Moore and Richards 1990) and they have now each been accorded species status: biotype A is *P. haemolytica* (*sensu stricto*) and biotype T is now *P. trehalosi* (Sneath and Stevens 1990). Both organisms are indole- and urease-negative (Table 51.1).

On sheep blood agar, colonies of *P. haemolytica* (biotypes A and T) are surrounded by a single narrow zone of β-haemolysis (the only pasteurellae to form a soluble haemolysin). However, on agar plates made with the blood of very young lambs, *P. haemolytica* and *P. trehalosi* give rise to a double zone of haemolysis – a narrow inner complete and a wide outer incomplete which increases in size at room temperature (Smith 1962; Fig. 51.3). Although freshly isolated strains are haemolytic, they may lose this feature upon subculture. The organisms also form a diffusible substance that enhances the haemolytic effect of staphylococcal β-toxin (Fraser 1962). On an agar plate incubated for 24 h at 37°C, colonies are similar to those of *P. multocida* (see section 18.3, p. 1203).

On MacConkey agar, small pink colonies are formed. Broth cultures incubated for 24 h at 37°C grow readily, producing turbidity. Later a granular deposit and a pellicle are formed. No soluble haemolysin is formed, except one that lyses the erythrocytes of very young lambs.

17.4 Metabolism and growth requirements

On finding that *P. haemolytica* (including *P. trehalosi*) flourished in a casein hydrolysate medium, Wessman (1966) devised a medium containing 15 individual amino acids from casein, a mixture of salts and vitamins, and galactose and glucose as sources of carbon. Cytotoxin production by *P. haemolytica* (see section 17.9, p. 1203) required a higher concentration of iron than was needed for growth (Gentry et al. 1986).

17.5 Biochemical characters

For testing the sugar reactions of *P. haemolytica* (including *P. trehalosi*), Bosworth and Lovell (1944) recommended a peptone water medium containing 10% broth, 1% sugar and bromothymol blue as an indicator. Growth is light, acid production is weak and the results obtained by different observers are not always in agreement. There is also a good deal of variation between different strains, depending to some extent on the animal source and the nature of the medium.

Acid, but no gas, is formed in glucose, maltose, mannitol, mannose, sorbitol and sucrose, usually in

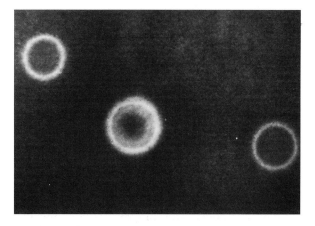

Fig. 51.2 *Pasteurella haemolytica sensu lato.* Two colonies of *P. haemolytica sensu stricto* and one (centre) of *P. trehalosi,* on blood agar 24 h, 37°C (× 5.4).

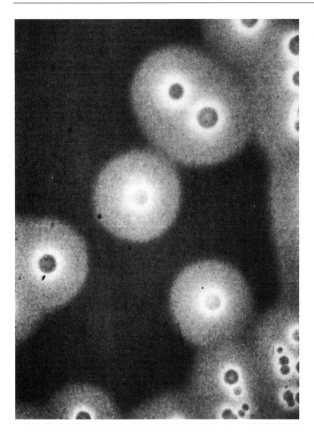

Fig. 51.3 The inner and outer zones of haemolysis produced by *P. haemolytica sensu lato* on lamb blood agar, 18 h at 37°C and 24 h at room temperature (× 3.4). (Reproduced, with permission, from Smith GR, 1962, *J Pathol Bacteriol*, **83:** 501–8).

dextrin, galactose, inositol and xylose, and sometimes in arabinose, glycerol, glycogen, lactose, raffinose, rhamnose, salicin, starch and trehalose. Dulcitol is rarely attacked. Adonitol, erythritol and inulin are not attacked. The organism does not form indole, is negative to methyl red (MR), Voges–Proskauer (VP), citrate, H_2S and urease, does not liquefy gelatin, reduces nitrate and methylene blue, and is oxidase-positive; catalase is almost always positive. *P. trehalosi* is usually aesculin-positive, ferments mannose and trehalose (within c. 2 days) but not arabinose or xylose, whereas *P. haemolytica* is said to be aesculin-negative, to ferment arabinose (small amounts of acid within c. 7 days) and xylose but not mannose or trehalose. *P. trehalosi* is resistant to penicillin and does not rapidly lose viability in ageing broth cultures, whereas *P. haemolytica* is susceptible to penicillin and rapidly loses viability in ageing broth cultures. Certain strains of *P. trehalosi* are said to be catalase-negative (Biberstein, Gills and Knight 1960). Soluble antigens produced include neuraminidase (Tabatabai and Frank 1981) and a leucotoxin.

17.6 Antigenic structure

Like *P. multocida*, *P. haemolytica* (including *P. trehalosi*) possesses capsular and somatic antigens. By means of

an indirect haemagglutination test, Biberstein and co-workers (Biberstein, Gills and Knight 1960, Biberstein and Gills 1962) distinguished 11 numbered capsular serotypes; by means of agglutination tests with autoclaved bacteria, they distinguished several less clearly defined somatic serotypes, identified by letters. Sixteen capsular serotypes were recognized (Fodor et al. 1987) but a new serotype (A17), isolated from sheep in Syria, has since been described (Younan and Fodar 1995). Serotypes 1, 2, 5, 6, 7, 8, 9, 11, 12, 13, 14, 16 and 17 correspond to GR Smith's (1959, 1960, 1961) colonial type A (*P. haemolytica sensu stricto*). Serotypes 3, 4, 10 and 15 correspond to Smith's colonial type T (*P. trehalosi*). Later, *P. haemolytica sensu stricto* was found to contain major somatic antigens A and B; *P. trehalosi* contained major somatic antigens C and D (Biberstein and Francis 1968).

The nomenclature employed here is very confusing. In *P. multocida*, capsular antigens are designated by letters and somatic antigens by numbers; in *P. haemolytica/ P. trehalosi* the reverse procedure is employed. Moreover, the A somatic antigen of *P. haemolytica* is quite distinct from Smith's A type, which was defined on biochemical, cultural and pathological grounds. The position is clearer now that Smith's A and T types are established as 2 separate species, as each now has its own series of capsular and somatic antigens (Smith and Thal 1965, Biberstein and Francis 1968, Thompson and Mould 1975). Most, but not all, disease-associated strains of *P. haemolytica/ P. trehalosi* from cattle and sheep can be serotyped. Aarsleff and his colleagues (1970) found, however, that up to 90% of strains from nasal swabs of sheep failed to react in the indirect haemagglutination test; such strains have carbohydrate fermenting properties that resemble those of *P. haemolytica sensu stricto* (Gilmour 1978). By means of a plate-agglutination test, Frank (1980) divided 10 so-called 'untypable' strains into 3 groups that were distinct from established serotypes; and by means of countercurrent electrophoresis, Donachie and colleagues (1984a) divided 30 such strains into 9 serogroups. A coagglutination test has been described (Fodor, Penzes and Varga 1996) for simple, fast and reliable detection of *P. haemolytica* type-specific antigens in lung lesions even in the absence of viable cells of the organism.

Davies and Donachie (1996) found an association both of specific lipopolysaccharide (LPS) and outer-membrane proteins (OMP) profiles with bovine or ovine disease isolates which suggested a correlation between specific cell-surface structures and host specificity. Davies, Paster and Dewhirst (1996) extended this study and found that OMP and LPS data correlated with 16S rRNA sequence data, thereby suggesting that LPS and OMP analyses might be useful for preliminary screening and comparing large numbers of isolates in taxonomic and epidemiological studies of the Pasteurellaceae.

17.7 Habitat

P. haemolytica and *P. trehalosi* are found particularly in sheep, cattle and goats; they occur in the nasopharynx and tonsils of healthy animals.

17.8   Immunogenicity

Associated with the capsule of pasteurellae is a protective substance, the nature of which is little known. However, sodium salicylate extracts of *P. haemolytica* types A1 and A6 were protective to animals and contained serotype-specific antigen with 100–300 kDa (Donachie et al. 1984b). Adlam and his colleagues (1984, 1985a, 1985b, 1986) defined the properties of the specific capsular polysaccharides of serotypes A1, A7, T4 and T15. The type A15 substance was identical with the K62 (K2ab) capsular polysaccharide of *Escherichia coli* and the capsular polysaccharide of *Neisseria meningitidis* serogroup H.

17.9   Toxins

P. haemolytica/P. trehalosi in the logarithmic phase of growth releases a heat-labile substance of high MW with toxic effects on the leucocytes of cattle, goats and sheep. This substance, which is referred to as a cytotoxin or leucotoxin, is antigenic and appears to be produced by all the known serotypes of *P. haemolytica/P. trehalosi* (see Benson, Thomson and Valli 1978, Baluyut et al. 1981, Himmell et al. 1982, Shewen and Wilkie 1982, 1983, 1985, Chang et al. 1986, Sutherland and Donachie 1986, Adlam 1989). *P. haemolytica*-like strains isolated from diarrhoeic pigs also produce a similar leucotoxin that is lethal to ruminant leucocytes (DeSilva et al. 1995).

For information on *P. haemolytica* bacteriophages see Richards, Renshaw and Sneed (1985).

17.10   Pathogenicity

P. haemolytica and *P. trehalosi* are naturally pathogenic for sheep, giving rise to septicaemia in lambs and to pneumonia in adults; less often the former is also pathogenic for cattle and goats (see Volume 3, Chapter 47). They are non-pathogenic for laboratory animals by the usual methods of infection (except in massive doses) unless reinforced with mucin [mice die within 48 h (GR Smith 1958)], or injected intracerebrally. Administration of iron also increases susceptibility to infection (Al-Sultan and Aitken 1984). *P. haemolytica sensu stricto* (GR Smith's type-A strains), when injected intraperitoneally into young lambs – not more than 3 weeks old – in a dose of about 5000 organisms, gave rise to acute fibrinous peritonitis that was fatal within 36 h; adult sheep were not affected by this treatment (Smith 1960). *P. haemolytica* rarely causes disease in humans (Weaver, Hollis and Bottone 1985, Yaneza, Hollis and Bottone 1991), although it has been isolated in a mixed infection from an aortic bypass graft. *P. trehalosi* is known mainly as a cause of septicaemia in older lambs and produces disease in young lambs only when injected in large doses. It has not been recognized in humans and is retained in Table 51.1 only because of its historical association with *P. haemolytica sensu stricto*.

17.11   Differentiation from *P. multocida*

P. haemolytica (as well as *P. trehalosi*) differs from *P. multocida* chiefly in its formation of haemolytic colonies on blood agar, its growth, though poor, on MacConkey agar, its greater range of sugars fermented (strains regularly attack dextrin, maltose and, after several days, inositol), its failure to form indole, its lack of pathogenicity for laboratory animals, and its lysis of lambs' blood.

17.12   Similarities to *Actinobacillus*

Mráz (1969) was of the opinion that these organisms should be classified with *Actinobacillus* rather than with *Pasteurella* (see also section 1, p. 1191). Comparing 46 strains of *P. haemolytica/P. trehalosi* with 99 strains of *A. lignieresii* he noted only 3 major differences between them, namely the double zone of lysis on lambs' blood agar, the negative urease test, and the slightly lower G + C content of the DNA of *P. haemolytica/P. trehalosi*.

18   *PASTEURELLA MULTOCIDA*

18.1   Isolation

P. multocida was the first member of the *Pasteurella* group, described by Perroncito in 1879. It is recognized as a parasite of birds and other animals, both domestic and wild.

18.2   Morphology

The organism consists of very small, 0.7 μm by 0.3–0.6 μm, ovoid rods, with straight axis, slightly convex sides and rounded ends, arranged singly, in pairs or in small bundles (Fig. 51.4). In smears from the animal body the bacterial cells are regular, ovoid and evenly distributed; on agar cultures they are more rod-shaped and often show pleomorphism.

18.3   Cultural features

P. multocida grows fairly well on nutrient agar, typically forming circular colonies about 0.5–1 mm diameter after 24 h at 37°C; they are low convex, amorphous, greyish-yellow and translucent, with a smooth, glistening surface and entire edge; consistency is butyrous and emulsifiability easy. After 5 days at 37°C colonies are up to 6 mm in diameter and differentiated into a brownish, finely granular, sometimes ringed or striated, nearly opaque centre and a clearer, smooth, homogeneous, greyish-yellow translucent periphery. On a horse-blood agar plate, 2 days at 37°C produces good growth similar to that on agar; there is no haemolysis but the blood plate is slightly cleared and browned. On a MacConkey plate after 5 days at 37°C there is no visible growth.

In broth after 24 h at 37°C there is moderate growth with slight turbidity, and a slight powdery or viscous deposit. Later the turbidity increases, and a heavy,

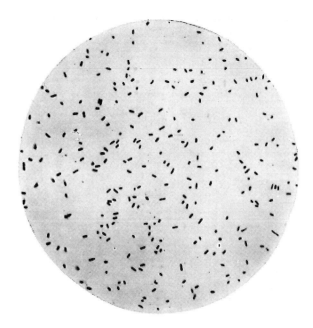

Fig. 51.4 *Pasteurella multocida.* From an agar culture, 24 h, 37°C (× 1310).

viscous deposit forms, disintegrating partly on shaking but leaving irregular sized wisp-like masses of growth in suspension. An incomplete surface pellicle forms with an inconspicuous ring growth.

The work of de Kruif (de Kruif 1921, 1922a, 1922b, de Kruif and Northrop 1923) and of Webster and Burn (1926) showed the existence of 3 different colonial forms:

1 a smooth form, virulent for rabbits, growing diffusely in broth, and forming smooth, moderately opaque iridescent colonies on serum agar
2 a rough form, completely avirulent for rabbits, giving a granular deposit in broth and forming translucent bluish colonies
3 a mucoid form of intermediate virulence (see also Anderson, Coombes and Mallick 1929, Hughes 1930).

The highly virulent smooth form contains a type-specific polysaccharide capsular antigen; the mucoid form is rich in hyaluronic acid, and may or may not possess a polysaccharide capsular antigen in addition. The rough form has neither a capsular nor a mucoid antigen (Carter 1955, JE Smith 1958, Namioka and Murata 1961). Carter (1967) recognized 2 forms of smooth colony: an S and an S^r. The S form, like the mucoid form, is capsulate, does not flocculate in acriflavine, and is typable by indirect haemagglutination; the S^r form, like the rough form, behaves in the opposite manner. The colonial form varies to some extent with the animal source.

According to JE Smith (1958, 1959), nearly all strains from pigs form on blood agar translucent mucoid iridescent colonies up to 1.8 mm in diameter, tending to become confluent. Cattle strains are non-mucoid. Pig strains form hyaluronic acid; cattle strains do not. Strains from cats and dogs

are greyish, smooth, less translucent, non-iridescent, and not over 1.2 mm in diameter; they cause a slight browning of the blood. The property of iridescence, best exhibited by colonies grown for 24 h on 10% horse serum agar, is appreciated most readily by examination in oblique strong sunlight against a darkish background. It depends apparently on the regular mosaic of opaque coccobacilli and transparent capsules in the colony; this acts as a diffraction grating. The colour effects are seen only by transmitted light, and differ from those of fluorescence, which is caused by absorption of light of a specific wavelength, usually ultraviolet, with emission of part of the absorbed energy in the form of light of greater wavelength (JE Smith 1958).

In broth the S form of *P. multocida* causes uniform turbidity with a light powdery deposit later tending to become viscous. The R form produces a granular deposit without turbidity.

18.4 Susceptibility to chemical and physical agents

The organism is very susceptible to inimical agents and conditions; cells are killed by heat at 60°C in a few minutes, by 0.5% phenol in 15 min.

18.5 Metabolism and growth requirements

Webster (1925) and Webster and Baudisch (1925) found that the smooth variant of *P. multocida* would not grow aerobically in plain broth unless large numbers of organisms were introduced, about 100 000 ml^{-1}; the rough variant grew from an inoculum of only a few cells. If a trace of rabbit blood, or an iron compound with strongly catalytic properties, was added to the medium, or the partial pressure of oxygen was lowered, the smooth variant grew from only a small inoculum. Jordan (1952) showed that H_2O_2 was produced during growth, and that haematin, or better still catalase, promoted aerobic growth. Growth is improved slightly by serum, not influenced by glucose and slightly inhibited by glycerol. There is no haemolysis. Strains are said to form neuraminidase (Müller and Krasemann 1974).

The nutritional requirements have not been worked out completely. McKenzie and her colleagues (1948; see also Wessman and Wessman 1970) grew *P. multocida* successfully on a defined medium containing asparagine, biotin, calcium pantothenate, cystine, glucose, glutamic acid, glycine, nicotinamide, salts, thiamine and tryptophan. In a slightly modified medium Watko (1966) found that an inoculum of only 2 or 3 cells was sufficient to start growth. Namioka and Murata (1961) prepared a medium (YPC agar) containing agar, glucose, L-cystine, potassium diphosphate, proteose peptone, sodium sulphite, sucrose and yeast extract on which the organisms grew well. Selective media for the isolation of *P. multocida* have been described by Das (1958) and Morris (1958).

18.6 Biochemical reactions

All strains of *P. multocida* produce acid but not gas in glucose and sucrose; most strains ferment galactose, mannitol, mannose, sorbitol and xylose, within 14 days. Arabinose, dextrin, dulcitol, glycerol, lactose, maltose, raffinose and trehalose are occasionally acidified; inositol, inulin, rhamnose and salicin are usually not attacked. Strains from certain sources tend to possess particular biochemical characters (Tanaka 1926, Gourdon et al. 1957, JE Smith 1958, Heddleston 1976). Avian strains not infrequently ferment arabinose. Bovine strains often ferment trehalose. Canine and feline strains often attack maltose but may fail to attack mannitol and sorbitol. Production of acid from dulcitol and sorbitol delineate 3 subspecies within *P. multocida*: *gallicida*, *multocida* and *septica* (Mutters et al. 1985); Fegan, Blackall and Pahoff (1995) recognized additional biovars from poultry. Dog strains are usually acid agglutinable, non-capsulate, non-iridescent, non-mucoid and only moderately pathogenic for mice; cat strains are similar, but are highly pathogenic for mice (JE Smith 1959). Strains of *P. multocida* have no effect on litmus milk and gelatin. They produce indole, reduce nitrate and form a small quantity of H_2S as detected by lead acetate paper. The MR and VP reactions are both negative; the catalase and oxidase reactions are both positive, though rather weakly so. An occasional strain may even give a negative result in the oxidase test; however, tests with the tetramethyl reagent only rarely give negative results. In any event, oxidase tests should be performed from cultures grown on blood agar or chocolate agar medium; negative results may be obtained with other growth media (Grehn and Müller 1989). Citrate cannot be used as the sole source of carbon. Urea is not decomposed (in the pasteurellae, urea is decomposed only by strains of *P. dagmatis* and *P. pneumotropica*, of which the latter is misplaced in the genus; see section 11.5, p. 1200). The β-galactosidase and malonate tests are negative. Most strains are positive for ornithine decarboxylase but negative for lysine and glutamic acid decarboxylases and for arginine dihydrolase; most are resistant to potassium cyanide.

18.7 Antigenic structure

The early observations of Lal (1927), Cornelius (1929), Yusef (1935) and Roberts (1947) showed that multiple antigenic types of *P. multocida* could be distinguished by use of agglutination and absorption, or of mouse protection tests; by means of protection tests, strains were classified by Roberts into 4 types (I, II, III and IV). The serological behaviour is determined by capsular and by somatic antigens. Both mucoid and smooth iridescent colonies possess a capsule; the blue granular rough colonies do not. Capsular antigens can be detected either by slide agglutination (Namioka and Murata 1961), or by indirect agglutination of human group O red cells to which the soluble capsular antigen is adsorbed (Carter 1955, 1957, 1961, 1962, 1967). To reveal the somatic antigen, Namioka and Murata (1961) removed the capsular material by treatment with 1 M HCl, suspended the washed organisms in saline at pH 7.0 and tested them against antisera prepared in rabbits by the injection of similarly decapsulated organisms. Carter (1972) treated fowl cholera strains with hyaluronidase to make them agglutinable for the identification of their somatic antigens. Organisms from rough colonies autoagglutinate when 1 or 2 drops of a 1 in 1000 solution of acriflavine are added to a fairly thick saline suspension; mucoid colonies form a slimy precipitate, and smooth colonies remain homogeneously suspended (Carter 1957). The rough variants are devoid of both capsular and smooth somatic antigens. Cat and dog strains are frequently non-capsulate and untypable.

On the basis of polysaccharide capsular antigens, Carter (1955) established among smooth iridescent strains 4 serotypes, A, B, C and D. Later a further type, type E, was recognized (Carter 1961), and type C was shown not to be a true capsular type. Therefore there are only 4 capsular types, namely, A, B, D and E (Carter 1957). Type B is generally agreed to be the equivalent of Roberts's type I (Roberts 1947); an opinion on the relationship between all Roberts's types and the capsular types was given by, for example, Prodjoharjono, Carter and Conner (1974). Mucoid strains are rich in hyaluronic acid and have a common mucoid antigen. Carter (1955) stated that they did not fall into the 4 capsular types that he defined among smooth strains, but it would appear that some mucoid strains also contain a polysaccharide antigen that enables them to be typed in the A, B, D, E series (JE Smith 1958, Carter 1967). Namioka and Murata (1961), by the use of agglutination and absorption tests, established 6 somatic (O) groups. Further studies, reviewed by Namioka (1973), established 11 smooth somatic O groups, based on antigens that consisted of combinations of several factors; the capsular groups A, B, D and E contained 6, 2, 6 and one O group, respectively (Namioka 1973). Thus 15 serotypes were recognized. But Bhasin and Lapointe-Shaw (1980) described even greater antigenic complexity. By crossed immunoelectrophoresis they found in an envelope-cytoplasm preparation of serotype 1 at least 19 cell envelope and 55 cytoplasmic antigens. Moreover, by bacteriocin typing, Mushin (1980) divided avian strains of this organism into 23 types. It is now usual to describe the serotype of a strain by stating both the somatic and capsular groups, e.g. serotype 5:A. Capsular type A strains can be rapidly identified by a staphylococcal hyaluronidase test (Carter and Rundell 1975) and type D strains by an acriflavine flocculation test (Carter and Subronto 1973). Heddleston, Gallagher and Rebers (1972) described an agar gel precipitation test in which the antigen preparations were boiled for an hour; the test was useful for serotyping avian strains but necessitated a further system of serotype nomenclature. Brogden and Packer (1979) compared *P. multocida* typing systems; a single serotype in one system often represented more than one serotype in another.

According to Carter (1967), capsular type A strains are associated on the North American continent with fowl cholera and with pneumonia in cattle and pigs, as well as with primary and secondary infections in a wide variety of animals; type B strains with haemorrhagic septicaemia of cattle and buffaloes in Asia and Australia; type D strains with primary and secondary infections in a wide range of animals; and type E strains with haemorrhagic septicaemia in central

Africa. Strains from human subjects belong mainly to type A and to a less extent to type D (see also Baxi, Blobel and Brückler 1970).

Pirosky (1938a, 1938b) extracted 4 different glycolipid antigens from smooth and rough variants of *P. multocida* by the trichloracetic acid technique. Judged by cross-precipitation tests one of these antigens was related to the Vi antigen of *Salmonella* Typhi, and another to the O antigen shared by *Salmonella* Enteritidis and *S.* Typhi.

18.8   Habitat

P. multocida is found in a wide variety of animals and probably has its main habitat in the respiratory tract. Smith (1955) found it in 50% of tonsils of normal dogs. It is occasionally isolated from the nasopharynx of healthy humans so it is possibly a commensal in the human upper respiratory tract (Weaver, Hollis and Bottone 1985).

18.9   Immunogenicity

Although little is known of the nature of the protective substance associated with the capsule of pasteurellae, Rebers, Heddleston and Rhoades (1967) extracted from a capsulate virulent strain of *P. multocida* a heat-stable lipopolysaccharide protein complex that was toxic to calves, mice and rabbits, but immunized the survivors. The gross chemical composition of this substance was similar to that of the enterobacterial endotoxins. In vitro, lipopolysaccharide from *P. multocida* (and also from *P. haemolytica*) formed stable complexes with pulmonary 'surfactant' from the alveoli of sheep (Brogden et al. 1986). The immunizing ability of *P. multocida* is associated with the capsular antigen (Priestley 1936b). It is still doubtful what degree of specificity this possesses. The older workers held that a strain from one animal could be used to vaccinate an animal of a different species (see, for example, Chamberland and Jouan 1906); but Roberts (1947), who prepared antisera in horses and rabbits and tested their ability to protect mice inoculated intraperitoneally with living organisms, classified 37 strains of *P. multocida* in 4 different types, suggesting the presence of some heterogeneity in immunizing ability as well as in antigenic structure. Nagy and Penn (1976) found that endotoxin-free capsular antigens of *P. multocida* types B and E protected cattle against intravenous challenge with a virulent type E strain.

18.10   Toxins

Cell-free extracts of certain strains of *P. multocida*, mainly of capsular type D, have been found to contain a toxin that is cytotoxic for embryonic bovine lung cells and Vero cells, dermonecrotic in guinea pigs and lethal in mice (Pennings and Storm 1984, Rutter and Luther 1984). Such strains, together with *Bordetella bronchiseptica*, play an important role in atrophic rhinitis of pigs (see Volume 3, Chapter 47), and inoculation of toxin by the intramuscular, intranasal or intraperitoneal route causes atrophy of the nasal turbinate bones (Rutter and Mackenzie 1984, de Jong, Wachter and van der Marel 1986). The toxin is antigenic, heat-labile, protein in nature, and c. 160 kDa (Nakai et al. 1984, Chanter, Rutter and Mackenzie 1986). Treatment of mildly trypsinized toxin with dithiothreitol and sodium dodecyl sulphate produced 3 polypeptide chains of 23, 67 and 74 kDa, from which the whole toxin could be reconstructed (Kume and Nakai 1985, Nakai and Kume 1987). Nielsen, Bisgaard and Pedersen (1986), who examined toxigenic strains from calves, cats, dogs, pigs, rabbits and turkeys, found them all to belong to *P. multocida* subsp. *multocida* (Mutters et al. 1985). It has been shown that a dermonecrotic type A strain could produce turbinate atrophy similar to that caused by dermonecrotic type D strains.

Several different sorts of bacteriophage have been isolated from *P. multocida* (Ackermann and Karaivanov 1984).

18.11   Pathogenicity

Certain strains of *P. multocida* produce a dermonecrotic cytotoxin but virulence is subject to alteration; Matsumoto and Strain (1993) found that both capsulate and non-capsulate forms of *P. multocida* apparently increased their pathogenicity by bird-to-bird transmission in a short period. It is pathogenic for a wide variety of animals, producing anything from a harmless latent infection to fowl cholera in birds and a rapidly fatal haemorrhagic septicaemia (see Volume 3, Chapter 47) in buffaloes, cattle, pigs, rabbits, reindeer, sheep, and other animals. Strains also produce respiratory infections; humans are occasional victims.

Strains of *P. multocida* from different sources vary in their virulence for mice and other animals (Carter 1967; see also Volume 3, Chapter 47). Most capsulate strains from acute infections are virulent for mice and rabbits. Cat strains as a rule are highly virulent for mice, dog strains only moderately so (JE Smith 1958). The resistance of passively immunized mice is said to be broken down by the intraperitoneal injection of a solution of haemoglobin or of ferric ammonium citrate. This cataphylactic effect is probably due to the provision of iron to the bacteria (Bullen and Rogers 1968, Flossman et al. 1984). For testing virulence, mice, pigeons and rabbits are the most suitable experimental animals. Though they may occasionally suffer from spontaneous disease, guinea pigs are not so susceptible (Wright 1936).

MICE

Subcutaneous inoculation of a small quantity of a 24 h broth culture is fatal in 24–48 h. Post mortem, there may be local oedema and congestion, with practically no other signs. Microscopically the bacterial cells are found in large numbers in the blood and viscera. When very few organisms are injected, or a culture of relatively low virulence is used, the mice do not die for 2–8 days, or even longer; at necropsy there is a fibrinopurulent pericarditis, a layer of fibrin over the pleura, partial consolidation of the lungs, and not infrequently a purulent exudate in the peritoneum. Bacterial cells are plentiful in the blood and organs. Intraperitoneal inoculation is more rapidly fatal.

PIGEONS

Pigeons are very susceptible to intraperitoneal or intravenous, less so to intramuscular, injection. Death occurs in 24–48 h. Bacterial cells are abundant in the blood.

RABBITS

Rabbits can be infected by intranasal, intraperitoneal, intratracheal, intravenous, or subcutaneous inoculation. Death occurs in 2–5 days as a rule after intraperitoneal injection, with lesions similar to those in mice. In addition, there may be a haemorrhagic tracheitis and hyperaemia of the kidneys and intestine. Intranasal insufflation of the bacteria is often followed by snuffles or pleuropneumonia (Beck 1893, Webster 1924, 1926), and sometimes by purulent otitis media (Smith and Webster 1925).

In humans, the organism is associated with focal infections following animal bites, with chronic pulmonary disease, and with systemic disease including meningitis (also including septic shock in a previously healthy woman); it has also been reported from intrapartum septicaemia, a tubo-ovarian abscess and vulval sepsis.

18.12   Typing methods

Typing methods for epidemiological purposes include use of the API ZYM system (Grehn, Müller and Hugelshofer 1991), bacteriophages (Nielsen and Rosdahl 1990), DNA fingerprinting (Wilson, Morgan and Barger 1993, Wilson et al. 1995) and serology.

19   *PASTEURELLA PNEUMOTROPICA*

On blood agar after 24 h, colonies are 0.5–1.5 mm in diameter, low convex, and non-haemolytic. Salient features for identification of *P. pneumotropica* come from tests for ornithine decarboxylase, hydrolysis of urea, and production of gas from glucose (Table 51.1). It differs from *P. multocida* principally in failing to acidify mannitol and in hydrolysing urea. The organism was initially associated with pneumonic lesions in laboratory mice (Clark et al. 1984, Weaver, Hollis and Bottone 1985). It appears to be less common than other species of pasteurellae as an agent of either animal or human disease. Strains from humans reported in the past as belonging to this species are now more likely to have been strains of *P. dagmatis*. A 16S rDNA-based PCR method specific for *P. pneumotropica* has been developed (Wang et al. 1996).

20   *PASTEURELLA STOMATIS*

Important differential tests of *P. stomatis* are for acidification of maltose and mannitol, production of indole, and decarboxylation of ornithine (Table 51.1). Strains were isolated from the respiratory tracts of cats and dogs (Mutters et al. 1985); the organism has been reported to cause human infection following cat or dog bites (Holst et al. 1992, Pouëdras et al. 1993).

21   *PASTEURELLA VOLANTIUM*

All of 10 strains examined required V factor (NAD) for growth; most strains of *P. volantium* were isolated from fowl, but one strain was from a human tongue (Mutters et al. 1985).

EIKENELLA

22   DEFINITION

E. corrodens is the only species in the genus. It is a fastidious, capnophilic, aerobic and facultatively anaerobic gram-negative rod which characteristically forms depressed or pitting colonies on the surface of agar media. Haemin is usually required for aerobic growth. It is oxidase-positive, usually catalase-negative, nitrate reductase-positive and lysine- and sometimes ornithine decarboxylase-positive (however, the arginine dihydrolase test is negative). It is otherwise biochemically unreactive; there is no acid production from carbohydrates. The G + C content of the DNA is 56–58 mol%.

23   INTRODUCTION

Holm (1950) first gave the name 'corroding bacillus' to an anaerobic, *Haemophilus*-like organism isolated from actinomycotic lesions, whose colonies 'resemble small, matt, corroded patches on the glistening surface of the agar'. Similar strains were isolated by Henriksen (1948) and by Eiken (1958), who considered them to be mostly obligate anaerobes and named them *Bacteroides corrodens*. Henriksen (1969) found that most strains were micro-aerobic or facultatively anaerobic, and disputed their classification. They were renamed *Eikenella corrodens* by Jackson and Goodman (1972), who retained the name *Bacteroides corrodens* (now *Bacteroides ureolyticus*) for the obligately anaerobic, urease-positive corroding bacteria (Chapter 58). The capnophilic or micro-aerobic isolates collected by King (1964) and designated HB-1 were subsequently found by Riley, Tatum and Weaver (1973) to be identical to *E. corrodens*.

24   *EIKENELLA CORRODENS*

24.1   Morphology

E. corrodens is a small, unbranched, slender, gram-negative rod-shaped bacterium, approximately 0.5 μm by 1.5–4 μm, usually occurring singly. In older cultures, filamentous forms, chains of rods, and swollen, irregularly staining forms may occur. It is non-capsulate, non-motile, non-sporing and non-acid-fast. Twitching motility may occur on some media.

24.2 Cultural characters

After incubation for 24–36 h on blood agar or chocolate agar, pin-point colonies are produced, up to 0.5 mm in diameter, which typically appear as tiny depressions in the agar surface. The colonies are circular in outline, greyish-white or yellowish in colour, with an entire or slightly irregular margin. The colony consists of a raised central papilla of variable size and contour and a flat, rough surround which is depressed below the surface of the agar. With continued incubation, the depression may spread to form a colony up to 3 mm in diameter. Generally this pitting or 'R' form of colony breeds true. Occasionally, non-pitting 'S' forms are produced, circular in outline, low convex with a smooth matt surface, not instantly recognizable as *E. corrodens*. Cobb, Helber and Hirschberg (1994) have published detailed descriptions of corroding and non-corroding colony variants observed by scanning electron microscopy. Colonies may produce a slight greenish or brownish discoloration on blood agar, and have a faint smell variously likened to that of bleach or *Haemophilus influenzae* cultures.

24.3 Growth requirements

There is disagreement on the precise atmospheric and nutritional requirements for growth (Hill, Snell and Lapage 1970, James and Robinson 1975, Goldstein, Agyare and Silletti 1981). Primary isolation should be attempted on blood agar or chocolate agar incubated anaerobically with 5–10% CO_2 and additional humidity; cultures should be incubated for up to 4–5 days. On subculture, an aerobic environment with additional CO_2 may yield good growth. *E. corrodens* requires blood or haemin for aerobic but not for anaerobic cultivation. Unlike Henriksen (1969), James and Robinson (1975) found that growth was improved by X and V factors. They obtained good growth on brain–heart infusion agar supplemented with whole blood but not with lysed blood. Growth in the broth, even with added body fluids, is generally poor, but may be improved by the addition of agar; Brewer's thioglycollate medium appears to support growth, especially when incubated in an anaerobic atmosphere. Growth occurs within the temperature range 27–43°C, and is optimal between 32 and 40°C. The optimal pH for growth on solid medium is 7–8. *E. corrodens* usually fails to grow on MacConkey medium, although occasional strains are bile tolerant. It does not grow on eosin–methylene blue or other selective media for coliform bacteria, Thayer–Martin medium or tellurite-containing media.

The reported incubation period for detectable growth in blood culture media ranges from 3 to 24 days (Decker et al. 1986).

24.4 Metabolism

E. corrodens is biochemically very inactive and little is known of its metabolism, but a positive oxidase and peroxidase reaction and a probable NAD requirement for aerobic growth point to a respiratory form of metabolism (James and Robinson 1975).

24.5 Susceptibility to chemical and physical agents

It is only moderately thermoresistant, able to survive 52°C for 20–30 min, but is killed at 56°C in 30 min. It fails to grow in the presence of merthiolate 0.005%, NaCl 5%, phenol 0.1% and sodium azide 0.05%.

24.6 Susceptibility to antimicrobial agents

It is generally susceptible to therapeutically attainable concentrations of ampicillin, carbenicillin, cefoxitin and other third-generation cephalosporins, chloramphenicol, colistin, penicillin, rifampicin, tetracycline and ureidopenicillins; and resistant to aminoglycosides, first-generation cephalosporins, clindamycin, metronidazole, penicillins resistant to β-lactamase, and vancomycin (see Chen and Wilson 1992). By contrast, the anaerobic corroding *Bacteroides* organisms are sensitive to clindamycin and metronidazole. Selective media for *E. corrodens* have been devised that incorporate clindamycin at a final concentration of 5 mg l^{-1}.

24.7 Biochemical properties

E. corrodens is catalase-negative, oxidase-positive and nitrate reductase-positive. It decarboxylates lysine and sometimes ornithine. It fails to produce acid from a wide range of carbohydrates and otherwise gives negative biochemical reactions.

24.8 Genetic analysis

The G + C content of the DNA is 56–58 mol% (Hill, Snell and Lapage 1970). In transformation studies, strains of *E. corrodens* formed a homologous group and showed no affinity with *Cardiobacterium hominis*, or with species of *Kingella*, *Moraxella* or *Neisseria* (Tønjum, Hagen and Bøvre 1985). For molecular typing of *E. corrodens* strains by macrorestriction fingerprinting, *Bam*HI and *Bgl*II proved to be the most suitable rare-cutting enzymes for pulsed field gel electrophoresis analysis, permitting recognition of 8 individual pulsed field gel electrophoresis patterns from 10 strains studied (Steffens et al. 1994).

24.9 Habitat

E. corrodens is a commensal of the human oronasopharynx and upper respiratory tract (Marsden and Hyde 1971), and is present in dental and gingival scrapings. It is also found in the gastrointestinal and genitourinary tracts. In a survey of supragingival plaque samples of healthy dogs, *E. corrodens* was present in 62% of the dogs (Allaker, Langlois and Hardie 1994); the authors suggested that the prevalence of this organism in human wound infections from dog bites may have been underestimated from lack of appropriate techniques for detecting this fastidious organism.

24.10 Pathogenicity

E. corrodens is part of the normal flora of mucous membranes. In humans, the organism is usually isolated in mixed culture with anaerobes and streptococci. It is occasionally found as the sole pathogen, although in some instances this is the result of selection by recent chemotherapy. Immunosuppression may predispose to infection. It has been implicated in: various infections of the head and neck, including alveolar abscesses, sinusitis, soft tissue lesions and suppurative thrombophlebitis of the internal jugular vein; pulmonary infections (empyema, lung abscess, pneumonia); intra-abdominal and pelvic abscesses, intracranial abscesses and meningitis (Suwanagool et al. 1983, Decker et al. 1986, Flesher and Bottone 1989); and wound infections following human bite or fist-fight injuries, which may be complicated by septic arthritis or osteomyelitis (Stoloff and Gillies 1986);

rarely it may cause chorioamnionitis. The organism may enter the blood in the course of dental extractions (Khairat 1967), and occasionally causes endocarditis. It may be common in the injecting drug user population as part of mixed infections (Gonzalez et al. 1993, Armstrong and Fisher 1996).

E. corrodens has very low pathogenicity for laboratory animals. When injected in pure culture into rabbits, it causes induration, which subsides spontaneously. Endocarditis has been produced experimentally in rabbits with this organism, but it is rarely bacteraemic and has a low mortality.

24.11 Classification

Although *E. corrodens* superficially resembles *B. ureolyticus*, the 2 organisms differ widely in their DNA base composition and in that *E. corrodens* is facultatively aerobic, lysine decarboxylase-positive, and urease- and gelatin-negative. Henriksen (1969) tentatively included *E. corrodens* in the family Brucellaceae, but phylogenetically its nearest relatives include other corroding bacteria such as *Kingella kingae* and several species of *Neisseria*.

REFERENCES

Aarsleff B, Biberstein EL et al., 1970, A study of untypable strains of *Pasteurella haemolytica, J Comp Pathol*, **80:** 493–8.

Ackermann HW, Karaivanov L, 1984, Morphology of *Pasteurella multocida* bacteriophages, *Can J Microbiol*, **30:** 1141–8.

Adlam C, 1989, The structure, function and properties of cellular and extracellular components of *Pasteurella haemolytica*, Pasteurella *and* Pasteurellosis, eds Adlam C, Rutter JM, Academic Press, London, 75–92.

Adlam C, Knights JM et al., 1984, Purification, characterization and immunological properties of the serotype-specific capsular polysaccharide of *Pasteurella haemolytica* (serotype A1) organisms, *J Gen Microbiol*, **130:** 2415–26.

Adlam C, Knights JM et al., 1985a, Purification, characterization and immunological properties of the serotype-specific capsular polysaccharide of *Pasteurella haemolytica* (serotype T4) organisms, *J Gen Microbiol*, **131:** 387–94.

Adlam C, Knights JM et al., 1985b, Purification, characterization and immunological properties of the capsular polysaccharide of *Pasteurella haemolytica* serotype T15: its identity with the K62 (K2ab) capsular polysaccharide of *Escherichia coli* and the capsular polysaccharide of *Neisseria meningitidis* serogroup H, *J Gen Microbiol*, **131:** 1963–72.

Adlam C, Knights JM et al., 1986, Purification, characterization and immunological properties of the serotype-specific capsular polysaccharide of *Pasteurella haemolytica* serotype A7 organisms, *J Gen Microbiol*, **132:** 1079–87.

Alaluusua S, Saarela M et al., 1993, Ribotyping shows intrafamilial similarity in *Actinobacillus actinomycetemcomitans* isolates, *Oral Microbiol Immunol*, **8:** 225–9.

Allaker RP, Langlois T, Hardie JM, 1994, Prevalence of *Eikenella corrodens* and *Actinobacillus actinomycetemcomitans* in the dental plaque of dogs, *Vet Rec*, **134:** 519–20.

Al-Sultan II, Aitken ID, 1984, Promotion of *Pasteurella haemolytica* infection in mice by iron, *Res Vet Sci*, **36:** 385–6.

Anderson LAP, Coombes MG, Mallick SMK, 1929, On the dissociation of *Bacillus avisepticus, Indian J Med Res*, **17:** 611–24.

Anon, 1981, Validation of the publication of new names and new combinations previously effectively published outside the IJSB, List No. 7, *Int J Syst Bacteriol*, **31:** 382–3.

Anon, 1987, International Committee on Systematic Bacteriology Subcommittee on *Pasteurellaceae* and Related

Organisms. Minutes of the meetings, 6 and 10 September 1986, Manchester, England, *Int J Syst Bacteriol*, **37:** 474.

Armstrong O, Fisher M, 1996, The treatment of *Eikenella corrodens* soft tissue infection in an injection drug user, *West Virginia Med J*, **92:** 138–9.

Baddour LM, Gelfand MS et al., 1989, CDC group HB-5 as a cause of genitourinary infections in adults, *J Clin Microbiol*, **27:** 801–5.

Baluyut CS, Simonson RR et al., 1981, Interaction of *Pasteurella haemolytica* with bovine neutrophils: identification and partial characterization of a cytotoxin, *Am J Vet Res*, **42:** 1920–6.

Baum KH, Shin SJ et al., 1984, Isolation of *Actinobacillus lignieresii* from enlarged tongue of a horse, *J Am Vet Med Assoc*, **185:** 792–3.

Baxi KK, Blobel H, Brückler J, 1970, Antigene der serologischen typen B und E von *Pasteurella multocida, Zentralbl Bakteriol Parasitenkd Infectionskr Hyg Abt 1 Orig*, **214:** 101–4.

Beck M, 1893, Der bacillus der brustseuche beim kaninchen, *Z Hyg Infektionskr*, **15:** 363–8.

Benson ML, Thomson RG, Valli VEO, 1978, The bovine alveolar macrophage. II. In vitro studies with *Pasteurella haemolytica, Can J Comp Med*, **42:** 368–9.

Bertschinger HU, Seifert P, 1978, *5th IPVS World Congress on Hyology and Hyiatrics, Zagreb*, M19.

Bhasin JL, Lapointe-Shaw L, 1980, Antigenic analysis of *Pasteurella multocida* (serotype 1) by crossed immunoelectrophoresis: characterization of cytoplasmic and cell envelope associated antigens, *Can J Microbiol*, **26:** 676–89.

Biberstein EL, Francis CK, 1968, Nucleic acid homologies between the A and T types of *Pasteurella haemolytica, J Med Microbiol*, **1:** 105–8.

Biberstein EL, Gills MG, 1962, The relation of the antigenic types to the A and T types of *Pasteurella haemolytica, J Comp Pathol*, **72:** 316–20.

Biberstein EL, Gills M, Knight H, 1960, Serological types of *Pasteurella haemolytica, Cornell Vet*, **50:** 283–300.

Bingham DP, Moore R, Richards AB, 1990, Comparison of DNA:DNA homology and enzymatic activity between *Pasteurella haemolytica* and related species, *Am J Vet Res*, **51:** 1161–6.

Bisgaard M, 1975, Characterization of atypical *Actinobacillus ligni-*

eresii isolated from ducks with salpingitis and peritonitis, *Nord Vetmed*, **27:** 378–83.

Bisgaard M, 1993, Ecology and significance of Pasteurellaceae in animals, *Int J Med Microbiol Virol Parasitol Infect Dis*, **279:** 7–26.

Bisgaard M, Heltberg O, Frederiksen W, 1991, Isolation of *Pasteurella caballi* from an infected wound on a veterinary surgeon, *APMIS*, **99:** 291–4.

Bisgaard M, Mutters R, 1986, Characterization of some previously unclassified '*Pasteurella*' spp. obtained from the oral cavity of dogs and cats and description of a new species tentatively classified with the family Pasteurellaceae Pohl 1981 and provisionally called Taxon 16, *Acta Pathol Microbiol Immunol Scand Sect B*, **94:** 177–84.

Bisgaard M, Phillips JE, Mannheim W, 1986, Characterization and identification of bovine and ovine Pasteurellaceae isolated from the oral cavity and rumen of apparently normal cattle and sheep, *Acta Pathol Microbiol Immunol Scand Sect B*, **94:** 9–17.

Blair TP, Seibel J et al., 1982, Endocarditis caused by *Actinobacillus actinomycetemcomitans*, *South Med J*, **75:** 559–61.

Bogaerts J, Verhaegen J et al., 1990, Characterization, in vitro susceptibility, and clinical significance of CDC group HB-5 from Rwanda, *J Clin Microbiol*, **28:** 2196–9.

Boot R, Bisgaard M, 1995, Reclassification of 30 *Pasteurellaceae* strains isolated from rodents, *Lab Anim*, **29:** 314–19.

Bosworth TJ, 1923, The causal organisms of bovine actinomycosis, *J Comp Pathol*, **36:** 1–22.

Bosworth TJ, Lovell R, 1944, The occurrence of haemolytic cocco-bacilli in the nose of normal sheep and cattle, *J Comp Pathol*, **54:** 168–71.

Breed RS, Murray EGD, Smith NR (eds), 1957, *Bergey's Manual of Determinative Bacteriology*, 7th edn, Williams & Wilkins, Baltimore.

Brogden KA, Packer RA, 1979, Comparison of *Pasteurella multocida* serotyping systems, *Am J Vet Res*, **40:** 1332–5.

Brogden KA, Rimler RB et al., 1986, Incubation of *Pasteurella haemolytica* and *Pasteurella multocida* lipopolysaccharide with sheep lung surfactant, *Am J Vet Res*, **47:** 727–9.

Brondz I, Olsen I, 1993, Multivariate chemosystematics demonstrate two groups of *Actinobacillus actinomycetemcomitans* strains, *Oral Microbiol Immunol*, **8:** 129–33.

Brumpt E, 1910, *Précis de Parasitologie*, Masson et Cie, Paris.

Bulgin MS, Anderson BC, 1983, Association of sexual experience with isolation of various bacteria in cases of ovine epididymitis, *J Am Vet Med Assoc*, **182:** 372–4.

Bullen JJ, Rogers HJ, 1968, Effect of haemoglobin on experimental infections with *Pasteurella septica* and *Escherichia coli*, *Nature (London)*, **217:** 86.

Burrows TW, Gillett WA, 1966, The nutritional requirements of some *Pasteurella* species, *J Gen Microbiol*, **45:** 333–45.

Carter GR, 1955, Studies on *Pasteurella multocida*. I. A hemagglutination test for the identification of serological types, *Am J Vet Res*, **16:** 481–4.

Carter GR, 1957, Studies on *Pasteurella multocida*. II. Identification of antigenic characteristics and colonial variants, *Am J Vet Res*, **18:** 210–13.

Carter GR, 1961, A new serological type of *Pasteurella multocida* from central Africa, *Vet Rec*, **73:** 1052.

Carter GR, 1962, Animal serotypes of *Pasteurella multocida* from human infections, *Can J Public Health*, **53:** 158–61.

Carter GR, 1967, Pasteurellosis: *Pasteurella multocida* and *Pasteurella haemolytica*, *Adv Vet Sci*, **11:** 321–79.

Carter GR, 1972, Agglutinability of *Pasteurella multocida* after treatment with hyaluronidase, *Vet Rec*, **91:** 150–1.

Carter GR, 1984, Genus I *Pasteurella* Trevisan 1887, 94[AL], Nom cons Opin 13, Jud Comm 1954, 153, *Bergey's Manual of Systematic Bacteriology*, vol. 1, eds Krieg NR, Holt JG, Williams & Wilkins, Baltimore, 552–7.

Carter GR, Rundell SW, 1975, Identification of type A strains of *P. multocida* using staphylococcal hyaluronidase, *Vet Rec*, **96:** 343.

Carter GR, Subronto P, 1973, Identification of type D strains of *Pasteurella multocida* with acriflavine, *Am J Vet Res*, **34:** 293–4.

Chamberland and Jouan, 1906, Les *Pasteurella*, *Ann Inst Pasteur (Paris)*, **20:** 81–103.

Chang WH, Carter GR, 1976, Multiple drug resistance in *Pasteurella multocida* and *Pasteurella haemolytica* from cattle and swine, *J Am Vet Med Assoc*, **169:** 710–12.

Chang Y-F, Renshaw HW et al., 1986, *Pasteurella haemolytica* leukotoxin: chemiluminescent responses of peripheral blood leukocytes from several different mammalian species to leukotoxin- and opsonin-treated living and killed *Pasteurella haemolytica* and *Staphylococcus aureus*, *Am J Vet Res*, **47:** 67–74.

Chanter N, Rutter JM, Mackenzie A, 1986, Partial purification of an osteolytic toxin from *Pasteurella multocida*, *J Gen Microbiol*, **132:** 1089–97.

Chatelain R, Bercovier H et al., 1979, Intérêt du composé vibriostatique O/129 pour différencier les genres *Pasteurella* et *Actinobacillus* de la famille des Enterobacteriaceae, *Ann Microbiol Inst Pasteur*, **130A:** 449–54.

Chen CKC, Wilson ME, 1992, *Eikenella corrodens* in human oral and non-oral infections: a review, *J Periodontol*, **63:** 941–53.

Christersson LA, 1993, *Actinobacillus actinomycetemcomitans* and localized juvenile periodontitis. Clinical, microbiologic and histologic studies, *Swed Dent J Suppl*, **90:** 1–46.

Clark WA, Hollis DG et al., 1984, *Identification of Unusual Pathogenic Gram-negative Aerobic and Facultatively Anaerobic Bacteria*, Centers for Disease Control, Atlanta, GA.

Cobb CM, Helber JT, Hirschberg R, 1994, Scanning electron microscopy of *Eikenella corrodens* colony morphology variants, *J Periodont Res*, **29:** 410–17.

Colebrook L, 1920, The mycelial and other micro-organisms associated with human actinomycosis, *Br J Exp Pathol*, **1:** 197–212.

Cornelius JT, 1929, An investigation of the serological relationships of twenty-six strains of *Pasteurella*, *J Pathol Bacteriol*, **32:** 355–64.

Cowan ST, 1974, *Cowan and Steel's Manual for the Identification of Medical Bacteria*, 2nd edn, Cambridge University Press, London, 95–6.

Cutlip RC, Amtower WC, Zinober MR, 1972, Septic embolic actinobacillosis of swine: a case report and laboratory reproduction of the disease, *Am J Vet Res*, **33:** 1621–6.

Danser MM, van Winkelhoff AJ et al., 1995, Putative periodontal pathogens colonizing oral mucous membranes in denture-wearing subjects with a past history of periodontitis, *J Clin Periodontol*, **22:** 854–9.

Das MS, 1958, Studies on *Pasteurella septica* (*Pasteurella multocida*), *J Comp Pathol*, **68:** 288–94.

Davies RL, Donachie W, 1996, Intra-specific diversity and host specificity within *Pasteurella haemolytica* based on variation of capsular polysaccharide, lipopolysaccharide and outer-membrane proteins, *Microbiology*, **142:** 1895–907.

Davies RL, Paster BJ, Dewhirst FE, 1996, Phylogenetic relationships and diversity within the *Pasteurella haemolytica* complex based on 16S rRNA sequence comparison and outer membrane protein and lipopolysaccharide analysis, *Int J Syst Bacteriol*, **46:** 736–44.

Decker MD, Graham BS et al., 1986, Endocarditis and infections of intravascular devices due to *Eikenella corrodens*, *Am J Med Sci*, **292:** 209–12.

De Ley J, Mannheim W et al., 1990, Inter- and intrafamilial similarities of rRNA cistrons of the Pasteurellaceae, *Int J Syst Bacteriol*, **40:** 126–37.

DeLong WJ, Waldhalm DG, Hall RF, 1979, Bacterial isolates associated with epididymitis in rams from Idaho and eastern Oregon flocks, *Am J Vet Res*, **40:** 101–2.

DeSilva RT, Chengappa MM et al., 1995, Partial characterization of the leukotoxin of *Pasteurella haemolytica*-like bacteria isolated from swine enteritis, *Vet Microbiol*, **45:** 319–29.

Dewhirst FE, Paster BJ et al., 1992, Phylogeny of 54 representative strains of species in the family Pasteurellaceae as determined by comparison of 16S rRNA sequences, *J Bacteriol*, **174**: 2002–13.

Dewhirst FE, Paster BJ et al., 1993, Phylogeny of the Pasteurellaceae as determined by comparison of 16S ribosomal ribonucleic acid sequences, *Int J Med Microbiol Virol Parasitol Infect Dis*, **279**: 35–44.

Dibb WL, Digranes A, Tønjum S, 1981, *Actinobacillus lignieresii* infection after a horse bite, *Br Med J*, **283**: 583–4.

DiRienzo JM, McKay TL, 1994, Identification and characterization of genetic cluster groups of *Actinobacillus actinomycetemcomitans* isolated from the human oral cavity, *J Clin Microbiol*, **32**: 75–81.

Donachie W, Fraser J et al., 1984a, Studies on strains of *Pasteurella haemolytica* not typable by the indirect haemagglutination test, *Res Vet Sci*, **37**: 188–93.

Donachie W, Gilmour NJ et al., 1984b, Comparison of cell surface antigen extracts from two serotypes of *Pasteurella haemolytica*, *J Gen Microbiol*, **130**: 1209–16.

Ebersole JL, Cappelli D, Sandoval MN, 1994, Subgingival distribution of *A. actinomycetemcomitans* in periodontitis, *J Clin Periodontol*, **21**: 65–75.

Edwards PR, 1932, Serologic characteristics of *Shigella equirulis* (*B. nephritidis-equi*, *J Infect Dis*, **51**: 268–72.

Eiken M, 1958, Studies on an anaerobic, rod-shaped, Gram-negative microorganism: *Bacteroides corrodens* n. sp., *Acta Pathol Microbiol Scand*, **43**: 404–16.

Escande F, Lion C, 1993, Epidemiology of human infections by *Pasteurella* and related groups in France, *Int J Med Microbiol Virol Parasitol Infect Dis*, **279**: 131–9.

Fajfar-Whetstone CJT, Coleman L et al., 1995, *Pasteurella multocida* septicemia and subsequent *Pasteurella dagmatis* septicemia in a diabetic patient, *J Clin Microbiol*, **33**: 202–4.

Fegan N, Blackall PJ, Pahoff JL, 1995, Phenotypic characterisation of *Pasteurella multocida* isolates from Australian poultry, *Vet Microbiol*, **47**: 281–6.

Flemmig TF, Rudiger S et al., 1995, Identification of *Actinobacillus actinomycetemcomitans* in subgingival plaque by PCR, *J Clin Microbiol*, **33**: 3102–5.

Flesher SA, Bottone EJ, 1989, *Eikenella corrodens* cellulitis and arthritis of the knee, *J Clin Microbiol*, **27**: 2606–8.

Flossman KD, Müller G et al., 1984, Einfluß von eisen auf *Pasteurella multocida*, *Zentralbl Bakteriol Mikrobiol Hyg A*, **258**: 80–93.

Fodor L, Penzes Z, Varga J, 1996, Coagglutination test for serotyping *Pasteurella haemolytica*, *J Clin Microbiol*, **34**: 393–7.

Fodor L, Varga J et al., 1987, New serotype of *Pasteurella haemolytica* isolated in Hungary, *Vet Rec*, **121**: 155.

Foster G, Ross HM et al., 1996, *Actinobacillus delphinicola* sp. nov., a new member of the family *Pasteurellaceae* Pohl (1979) 1981 isolated from sea mammals, *Int J Syst Bacteriol*, **46**: 648–52.

Frank GH, 1980, Serological groups among untypable bovine isolates of *Pasteurella haemolytica*, *J Clin Microbiol*, **12**: 579–82.

Fraser G, 1962, The haemolysis of animal erythrocytes by *Pasteurella haemolytica* produced in conjunction with certain staphylococcal toxins, *Res Vet Sci*, **3**: 104–10.

Frederiksen W, 1973, *Pasteurella* taxonomy and nomenclature, *Contributions to Microbiology and Immunology*, vol. 2, Yersinia, Pasteurella *and* Francisella, ed. Winblad S, Karger, Basel, 170–6.

Frederiksen W, 1981, Gas producing species within *Pasteurella* and *Actinobacillus*, Haemophilus, Pasteurella *and* Actinobacillus, eds Kilian M, Frederiksen W, Biberstein EL, Academic Press, London, 185–96.

Frederiksen W, 1993, Ecology and significance of *Pasteurellaceae* in man – an update, *Int J Med Microbiol Virol Parasitol Infect Dis*, **279**: 27–34.

Fujise O, Hamachi T et al., 1995, Colorimetric microtiter plate based assay for detection and quantification of amplified *Actinobacillus actinomycetemcomitans* DNA, *Oral Microbiol Immunol*, **10**: 372–7.

Ganiere JP, Escande F et al., 1993, Characterization of *Pasteurella*

from gingival scrapings of dogs and cats, *Comp Immunol Microbiol Infect Dis*, **16**: 77–85.

Gentry MJ, Confer AW et al., 1986, Cytotoxin (leukotoxin) production by *Pasteurella haemolytica*: requirement for an iron-containing compound, *Am J Vet Res*, **47**: 1919–23.

Gilmour NJL, 1978, Pasteurellosis in sheep, *Vet Rec*, **102**: 100–2.

Gilmour NJ, Menzies JD et al., 1985, Electronmicroscopy of the surface of *Pasteurella haemolytica*, *J Med Microbiol*, **19**: 25–34.

Gmur R, McNabb H et al., 1993, Seroclassification of hitherto nontypeable *Actinobacillus actinomycetemcomitans* strains: evidence for a new serotype e, *Oral Microbiol Immunol*, **8**: 116–20.

Goldstein EJ, Agyare EO, Silletti R, 1981, Comparative growth of *Eikenella corrodens* on 15 media in three atmospheres of incubation, *J Clin Microbiol*, **13**: 951–3.

Golland LC, Hodgson DR et al., 1994, Peritonitis associated with *Actinobacillus equuli* in horses: 15 cases (1982–1992), *J Am Vet Med Assoc*, **205**: 340–3.

Gonzalez MH, Garst J et al., 1993, Abscesses of the upper extremity from drug abuse by injection, *J Hand Surg*, **18**: 868–70.

Gourdon R, Gourdon J-M et al., 1957, Recherches sur *Pasteurella septica* I. Étude bactériologique de souches isolées d'animaux des espèces porcine et ovine, *Ann Inst Pasteur (Paris)*, **93**: 251–6.

Grehn M, Müller F, 1989, The oxidase reaction of *Pasteurella multocida* strains cultured on Mueller–Hinton medium, *J Microbiol Methods*, **9**: 333–6.

Grehn M, Müller F, Hugelshofer R, 1991, The API ZYM system as a tool for typing of *Pasteurella multocida* strains from humans, *J Microbiol Methods*, **13**: 201–6.

Heddleston KL, 1976, Physiologic characteristics of 1,268 cultures of *Pasteurella multocida*, *Am J Vet Res*, **37**: 745–7.

Heddleston KL, Gallagher JE, Rebers PA, 1972, Fowl cholera: gel diffusion precipitin test for serotyping *Pasteurella multocida* from avian species, *Avian Dis*, **16**: 925–36.

Heinrich S, Pulverer G, 1959a, Zur Aetiologie und Mikrobiologie der Actinomykose, *Zentralbl Bakteriol Parasitenkd Infektionskr Hyg Abt 1 Orig*, **174**: 123–35.

Heinrich S, Pulverer G, 1959b, Zur Ätiologie und Mikrobiologie der Actinomykose, *Zentralbl Bakteriol Parasitenkd Infektionskr Hyg Abt 1 Orig*, **176**: 91–101.

Henriksen SD, 1948, Studies in Gram-negative anaerobes, II. Gram-negative anaerobic rods with spreading colonies, *Acta Pathol Microbiol Scand*, **25**: 368–75.

Henriksen SD, 1961, *Pasteurella haemolytica* var. *ureae*, *Acta Pathol Microbiol Scand*, **53**: 425–9.

Henriksen SD, 1969, Corroding bacteria from the respiratory tract. 2. *Bacteroides corrodens*, *Acta Pathol Microbiol Scand*, **75**: 91–6.

Henriksen SD, Frøholm LO, 1975, A fimbriated strain of *Pasteurella multocida* with spreading and corroding colonies, *Acta Pathol Microbiol Scand Sect B*, **83**: 129–32.

Henriksen SD, Jyssum K, 1960, A new variety of *Pasteurella haemolytica* from the human respiratory tract, *Acta Pathol Microbiol Scand*, **50**: 443.

Henriksen SD, Jyssum K, 1961, A study of some *Pasteurella* strains from the human respiratory tract, *Acta Pathol Microbiol Scand*, **51**: 354–68.

Hill LR, Snell JJS, Lapage SP, 1970, Identification and characterisation of *Bacteroides corrodens*, *J Med Microbiol*, **3**: 483–91.

Himmell ME, Yates MD et al., 1982, Purification and partial characterization of a macrophage cytotoxin from *Pasteurella haemolytica*, *Am J Vet Res*, **43**: 764–7.

Hirsh DC, Martin LD, Rhoades KR, 1985, Resistance plasmids of *Pasteurella multocida* isolated from turkeys, *Am J Vet Res*, **46**: 1490–3.

Holm P, 1950, Studies on the aetiology of human actinomycosis I. The 'other microbes' of actinomycosis and their importance, *Acta Pathol Microbiol Scand*, **27**: 736–51.

Holm P, 1954, The influence of carbon dioxide on the growth of *Actinobacillus actinomycetemcomitans* (*Bacterium actinomycetem comitans* (Klinger 1912), *Acta Pathol Microbiol Scand*, **34**: 235–48.

Holst E, Rollof J et al., 1992, Characterization and distribution of *Pasteurella* species recovered from infected humans, *J Clin Microbiol*, **30**: 2984–7.

Holt SC, Tanner ACR, Socransky SS, 1980, Morphology and ultrastructure of oral strains of *Actinobacillus actinomycetemcomitans* and *Haemophilus aphrophilus*, *Infect Immun*, **30**: 588–600.

Hughes TP, 1930, The epidemiology of fowl cholera II. Biological properties of *P. avicida*, *J Exp Med*, **51**: 225–38.

Hussaini SN, 1975, Nomenclature and taxonomy of *Pasteurella multocida*, *Vet Bull (Weybridge)*, **45**: 403–9.

Jackson FL, Goodman YE, 1972, Transfer of the facultatively anaerobic organism *Bacteroides corrodens* Eiken to a new genus, *Eikenella*, *Int J Syst Bacteriol*, **22**: 73–7.

James AL, Robinson JVA, 1975, A comparison of the biochemical activities of *Bacteroides corrodens* and *Eikenella corrodens* with those of certain other Gram-negative bacteria, *J Med Microbiol*, **8**: 59–76.

Jones DM, 1962, A *Pasteurella*-like organism from the human respiratory tract, *J Pathol Bacteriol*, **83**: 143–51.

Jones FS, 1921, A study of *Bacillus bovisepticus*, *J Exp Med*, **34**: 561–77.

de Jong MF, Wachter JC, van der Marel GM, 1986, Investigation into the pathogenesis of atrophic rhinitis in pigs. II. AR induction and protection after intramuscular injections of cell-free filtrates and emulsions containing AR toxin of *Pasteurella multocida*, *Vet Q*, **8**: 215–24.

Jordan RMM, 1952, The nutrition of *Pasteurella septica*. I. The action of haematin, *Br J Exp Pathol*, **33**: 27–35.

Kaplan AH, Weber DJ et al., 1989, Infection due to *Actinobacillus actinomycetemcomitans*: 15 cases and review, *Rev Infect Dis*, **11**: 46–63.

Khairat O, 1967, *Bacteroides corrodens* isolated from bacteriaemias, *J Pathol Bacteriol*, **94**: 29–40.

Kilian M, Frederiksen W, 1981, Identification tables for the *Haemophilus–Pasteurella–Actinobacillus* group, Haemophilus, Pasteurella *and* Actinobacillus, eds Kilian M, Frederiksen W, Biberstein EL, Academic Press, London, 281–90.

Kim BH, Phillips JE, Atherton JG, 1976, *Actinobacillus suis* in the horse, *Vet Rec*, **98**: 239.

King EO, 1964, *The Identification of Unusual Pathogenic Gram-negative Bacteria*, Centers for Disease Control, Atlanta, GA.

King EO, Tatum HW, 1962, *Actinobacillus actinomycetemcomitans* and *Haemophilus aphrophilus*, *J Infect Dis*, **111**: 85–94.

Kingsland RC, Guss DA, 1995, *Actinobacillus ureae* meningitis: case report and review of the literature, *J Emerg Med*, **13**: 623–7.

Klinger R, 1912, Untersuchungen über menschliche Actinomykose, *Zentralbl Bakteriol Parasitenkd Infektionskr Abt 1 Orig*, **62**: 191–200.

Kolyvas E, Sorger S et al., 1978, *Pasteurella ureae* meningoencephalitis, *J Pediatr*, **92**: 81–2.

Krause T, Bertschinger HU et al., 1987, V-factor dependent strains of *Pasteurella multocida* subsp. *multocida*, *Zentralbl Bakteriol Parasitenkd Infektionskr Hyg A*, **266**: 255–60.

de Kruif PH, 1921, Dissociation of microbic species. I. Coexistence of individuals of different degrees of virulence in cultures of the bacillus of rabbit septicemia, *J Exp Med*, **33**: 773–89.

de Kruif PH, 1922a, Mutation of the bacillus of rabbit septicemia, *J Exp Med*, **35**: 561–74.

de Kruif PH, 1922b, Rabbit septicemia bacillus, types D and G, in normal rabbits, *J Exp Med*, **36**: 309–16.

de Kruif PH, Northrop JH, 1923, Stable suspensions of autoagglutinable bacteria, *J Exp Med*, **37**: 647–51.

Kume K, Nakai T, 1985, Dissociation of *Pasteurella multocida* dermonecrotic toxin into three polypeptide fragments, *Jpn J Vet Sci*, **47**: 829–33.

Lal RB, 1927, A study of certain organisms of the *Pasteurella* group with respect to specific complement fixation by ice-box method, *Am J Hyg*, **7**: 561–73.

Lapage SP, Bascomb S, 1968, Use of selenite reduction in bacterial classification, *J Appl Bacteriol*, **31**: 568–80.

Lentsch RH, Wagner JE, 1980, Isolation of *Actinobacillus lignieresii* and *Actinobacillus equuli* from laboratory rodents, *J Clin Microbiol*, **12**: 351–4.

Lester A, Gerner-Smidt P et al., 1993, Phenotypical characters and ribotyping of *Pasteurella aerogenes* from different sources, *Int J Med Microbiol Virol Parasitol Infect Dis*, **279**: 75–82.

Lignières J, 1900, Maladies du porc, *Bull Soc Cent Méd Vét*, **18**: 389–431.

Lignières J, Spitz G, 1902, L'Actinobacillose, *Bull Soc Cent Méd Vét*, **20**: 487–535, 546–65.

Lion C, Conroy MC et al., 1995, *Pasteurella* 'SP' group infection after a guineapig bite, *Lancet*, **346**: 901–2.

Listgarten MA, Wong MY, Lai CH, 1995, Detection of *Actinobacillus actinomycetemcomitans*, *Porphyromonas gingivalis*, and *Bacteroides forsythus* in an *A. actinomycetemcomitans*-positive patient population, *J Periodontol*, **66**: 158–64.

McKenzie D, Stadler M et al., 1948, The use of synthetic medium as an in vitro test of possible chemotherapeutic agents against Gram-negative bacteria, *J Immunol*, **60**: 283–94.

Magnusson H, 1928, Commonest forms of actinomycosis in domestic animals and their etiology, *Acta Pathol Microbiol Scand*, **5**: 170–245.

Maguire LC, 1958, The role of *Bacterium viscosum equi* in the causation of equine disease, *Vet Rec*, **70**: 989–91.

Mannheim W, 1981, Taxonomic implications of DNA relatedness and quinone patterns in *Actinobacillus*, *Haemophilus*, and *Pasteurella*, Haemophilus, Pasteurella *and* Actinobacillus, eds Kilian M, Frederiksen W, Biberstein EL, Academic Press, London, 265–80.

Mannheim W, 1983, Taxonomy of the family Pasteurellaceae Pohl 1981 as revealed by DNA/DNA hybridization, *Inst Natl Santé Rech Med*, **114**: 211–26.

Mannheim W, Stieler W et al., 1978, Taxonomic significance of respiratory quinones and fumarate respiration in *Actinobacillus* and *Pasteurella*, *Int J Syst Bacteriol*, **28**: 7–13.

Mannheim W, Pohl S, Holländer R, 1980, Zur Systematik von *Actinobacillus, Haemophilus* und *Pasteurella*: Basenzusammensetzung der DNS, Atmungschinone und kulturell-biochemische Eigenschaften repräsentativer Sammlungsstämme, *Zentralbl Bakteriol A*, **246**: 512–40.

Marsden HB, Hyde WA, 1971, Isolation of *Bacteroides corrodens* from infections in children, *J Clin Pathol*, **24**: 117–19.

Matsumoto M, Strain JG, 1993, Pathogenicity of *Pasteurella multocida*: its variable nature demonstrated by in vivo passages, *Avian Dis*, **37**: 781–5.

Morris EJ, 1958, Selective media for some *Pasteurella* species, *J Gen Microbiol*, **19**: 305–11.

Mráz O, 1969, Vergleichende Studie der arten *Actinobacillus lignieresii* und *Pasteurella haemolytica*, *Zentralbl Bakteriol Parasitenkd Infectionskr Hyg Abt 1 Orig*, **209**: 212–32, 336–49, 349–64.

Müller HE, Krasemann C, 1974, Die virulenz von *Pasteurella multocida*-stämmen und ihre Neuraminidase-produktion, *Zentralbl Bakteriol, Parasitenkd Infektionskr Hyg Abt 1 Orig A*, **229**: 391–400.

Mushin R, 1980, A study on bacteriocin typing of avian strains of *Pasteurella multocida*, *J Hyg (Lond)*, **85**: 59–63.

Mutters R, Bisgaard M, Pohl S, 1986, Taxonomic relationship of selected biogroups of *Pasteurella haemolytica* as revealed by DNA:DNA hybridizations, *Acta Pathol Microbiol Immunol Scand Sect B*, **94**: 195–202.

Mutters R, Mannheim W, Bisgaard M, 1989, Taxonomy of the group, Pasteurella *and* Pasteurellosis, eds Adlam C, Rutter JM, Academic Press, London, 3–34.

Mutters R, Pohl S, Mannheim W, 1986, Transfer of *Pasteurella ureae* Jones 1962 to the genus *Actinobacillus* Brumpt 1910: *Actinobacillus ureae* comb. nov., *Int J Syst Bacteriol*, **36**: 343–4.

Mutters R, Ihm P et al., 1985, Reclassification of the genus *Pasteu-*

rella Trevisan 1887 on the basis of deoxyribonucleic acid homology, with proposals for the new species *Pasteurella dagmatis, Pasteurella canis, Pasteurella stomatis, Pasteurella anatis,* and *Pasteurella langaa, Int J Syst Bacteriol,* **35:** 309–22.

Nagy LK, Penn CW, 1976, Protection of cattle against experimental haemorrhagic septicaemia by the capsular antigens of *Pasteurella multocida,* types B and E, *Res Vet Sci,* **20:** 249–53.

Nakai T, Kume K, 1987, Reconstruction of *Pasteurella multocida* dermonecrotic toxin from three polypeptides, *FEMS Microbiol Lett,* **44:** 259–65.

Nakai T, Sawata A et al., 1984, Purification of dermonecrotic toxin from a sonic extract of *Pasteurella multocida* SP-72 serotype D, *Infect Immun,* **46:** 429–34.

Nakazawa M, Azuma R et al., 1977, Collective outbreaks of bovine actinobacillosis, *Jpn J Vet Sci,* **39:** 549–57.

Namioka S, 1973, *Contributions to Microbiology and Immunology,* vol. 2, Yersinia, Pasteurella *and* Francisella, Karger, Basel.

Namioka S, Murata M, 1961, Serological studies on *Pasteurella multocida, Cornell Vet,* **51:** 498–521, 522–8.

Nelson KM, Darien BJ et al., 1996, *Actinobacillus suis* septicaemia in two foals, *Vet Rec,* **138:** 39–40.

Nielsen JP, Bisgaard M, Pedersen KB, 1986, Production of toxin in strains previously classified as *Pasteurella multocida, Acta Pathol Microbiol Immunol Scand Sect B,* **94:** 203–4.

Nielsen JP, Rosdahl VT, 1990, Development and epidemiological applications of a bacteriophage typing system for typing *Pasteurella multocida, J Clin Microbiol,* **28:** 103–7.

Olsen I, 1993, Recent approaches to the chemotaxonomy of the *Actinobacillus–Haemophilus–Pasteurella* group (family *Pasteurellaceae*), *Oral Microbiol Immunol,* **8:** 327–36.

Olsen I, Brondz I, 1985, Differentiation among closely related organisms of the *Actinobacillus–Haemophilus–Pasteurella* group by means of lysozyme and EDTA, *J Clin Microbiol,* **22:** 629–36.

Orda R, Wiznitzer T, 1980, *Actinobacillus lignieresii* human infection, *J R Soc Med,* **73:** 295–7.

Page MI, King EO, 1966, Infection due to *Actinobacillus actinomycetemcomitans* and *Haemophilus aphrophilus, N Engl J Med,* **275:** 181–8.

Pathak RC, Ristic M, 1962, Detection of an antibody to *Actinobacillus lignieresii* in infected human beings and the antigenic characterization of isolates of human and bovine origin, *Am J Vet Res,* **23:** 310–14.

Pavicic MJAMP, van Winkelhoff AJ, de Graaff J, 1992, In vitro susceptibilities of *Actinobacillus actinomycetemcomitans* to a number of antimicrobial combinations, *Antimicrob Agents Chemother,* **36:** 2634–8.

Pavicic MJ, van Winkelhoff AJ et al., 1994, Microbiological and clinical effects of metronidazole and amoxicillin in *Actinobacillus actinomycetemcomitans*-associated periodontitis. A 2-year evaluation, *J Clin Periodontol,* **21:** 107–12.

Peel MM, Hornidge KA et al., 1991, *Actinobacillus* spp. and related bacteria in infected wounds of humans bitten by horses and sheep, *J Clin Microbiol,* **29:** 2535–8.

Pennings AMMA, Storm PK, 1984, A test in vero cell monolayers for toxin production by strains of *Pasteurella multocida* isolated from pigs suspected of having atrophic rhinitis, *Vet Microbiol,* **9:** 503–8.

Perroncito E, 1879, Über das epizootische Typhoid der Hühner, *Arch Wiss Prakt Tierheilkd,* **5:** 22–51.

Phillips JE, 1960, The characterisation of *Actinobacillus lignieresi, J Pathol Bacteriol,* **79:** 331–6.

Phillips JE, 1961, The commensal role of *Actinobacillus lignieresi, J Pathol Bacteriol,* **82:** 205–8.

Phillips JE, 1964, Commensal actinobacilli from the bovine tongue, *J Pathol Bacteriol,* **87:** 442–4.

Phillips JE, 1967, Antigenic structure and serological typing of *Actinobacillus lignieresii, J Pathol Bacteriol,* **93:** 463–75.

Phillips JE, 1984, Genus III *Actinobacillus* Brumpt 1910, 849[AL], *Bergey's Manual of Systematic Bacteriology,* eds Krieg NR, Holt JGP, Williams & Wilkins, Baltimore, 570–5.

Pickett MJ, Hollis DG, Bottone EJ, 1989, Miscellaneous gram-

negative bacteria, *Manual of Clinical Microbiology,* 5th edn, eds Balows A, Hausler Jr WJ et al., American Society for Microbiology, Washington, DC, 410–28.

Pirosky I, 1938a, Sur l'existence, chez les variantes smooth et rough d'une souche de *Pasteurella aviseptica,* de deux antigènes glucido-lipidiques sérologiquement distincts, *C R Soc Biol (Paris),* **128:** 346–7.

Pirosky I, 1938b, Sur la spécificité des antigènes glucido-lipidiques des *Pasteurella* et sur leurs affinités sérologiques avec les antigènes glucido-lipidiques des *Salmonella, C R Soc Biol (Paris),* **128:** 347–50.

Pohl S, 1981, DNA relatedness among members of *Haemophilus, Pasteurella* and *Actinobacillus,* Haemophilus, Pasteurella *and* Actinobacillus, eds Kilian M, Frederiksen W, Biberstein EL, Academic Press, London, 245–53.

Pohl S, Bertschinger HU et al., 1983, Transfer of *Haemophilus pleuropneumoniae* and the *Pasteurella haemolytica*-like organism causing porcine necrotic pleuropneumonia to the genus *Actinobacillus* (*Actinobacillus pleuropneumoniae* comb. nov.) on the basis of phenotypic and deoxyribonucleic acid relatedness, *Int J Syst Bacteriol,* **33:** 510–14.

Potts TV, Zambon JJ, Genco RJ, 1985, Reassignment of *Actinobacillus actinomycetemcomitans* to the genus *Haemophilus* as *Haemophilus actinomycetemcomitans* comb. nov., *Int J Syst Bacteriol,* **35:** 337–41.

Pouëdras P, Donnio PY et al., 1993, *Pasteurella stomatis* infection following a dog bite, *Eur J Clin Microbiol Infect Dis,* **12:** 65.

Preus HR, Haraszthy VI et al., 1993, Differentiation of strains of *Actinobacillus actinomycetemcomitans* by arbitrarily primed polymerase chain reaction, *J Clin Microbiol,* **31:** 2773–6.

Priestley FW, 1936a, Some properties of the capsule of *Pasteurella septica, Br J Exp Pathol,* **17:** 374–8.

Priestley FW, 1936b, Experiments on immunisation against *Pasteurella septica* infection, *J Comp Pathol,* **49:** 340–7.

Priestley FW, 1936c, A note on the association of the virulence of *Pasteurella septica* with capsulation, *J Comp Pathol,* **49:** 348–9.

Prodjoharjono S, Carter GR, Conner GH, 1974, Serologic study of bovine strains of *Pasteurella multocida, Am J Vet Res,* **35:** 111–14.

Pulverer G, Ko HL, 1970, *Actinobacillus actinomycetem-comitans*: fermentative capabilities of 140 strains, *Appl Microbiol,* **20:** 693–5.

Pulverer G, Ko HL, 1972, Serological studies on *Actinobacillus actinomycetem-comitans, Appl Microbiol,* **23:** 207–10.

Rebers PA, Heddleston KL, Rhoades KR, 1967, Isolation from *Pasteurella multocida* of a lipopolysaccharide antigen with immunizing and toxic properties, *J Bacteriol,* **93:** 7–14.

Richards AB, Renshaw HW, Sneed LW, 1985, *Pasteurella haemolytica* bacteriophage: identification, partial characterization, and relationship of temperate bacteriophages from isolates of *Pasteurella haemolytica* (biotype A, serotype 1), *Am J Vet Res,* **46:** 1215–20.

Riley PS, Tatum HW, Weaver RE, 1973, Identity of HB-1 of King and *Eikenella corrodens* (Eiken) Jackson and Goodman, *Int J Syst Bacteriol,* **23:** 75–6.

Roberts RS, 1947, An immunological study of *Pasteurella septica, J Comp Pathol,* **57:** 261–78.

Rosenbusch CT, Merchant IA, 1939, A study of the hemorrhagic septicemia Pasteurellae, *J Bacteriol,* **37:** 69–89.

Ruimy R, Breittmayer V et al., 1994, Phylogenetic analysis and assessment of the genera *Vibrio, Photobacterium, Aeromonas,* and *Plesiomonas* deduced from small-subunit rRNA sequences, *Int J Syst Bacteriol,* **44:** 416–26.

Rutter JM, Luther PD, 1984, Cell culture assay for toxigenic *Pasteurella multocida* from atrophic rhinitis of pigs, *Vet Rec,* **114:** 393–6.

Rutter JM, Mackenzie A, 1984, Pathogenesis of atrophic rhinitis in pigs: a new perspective, *Vet Rec,* **114:** 89–90.

Schlater LK, Brenner DJ et al., 1989, *Pasteurella caballi,* a new species from equine clinical specimens, *J Clin Microbiol,* **27:** 2169–74.

Shewen PE, Wilkie BN, 1982, Cytotoxin of *Pasteurella haemolytica* acting on bovine leukocytes, *Infect Immun*, **35**: 91–4.

Shewen PE, Wilkie BN, 1983, *Pasteurella haemolytica* cytotoxin: production by recognized serotypes and neutralization by type-specific rabbit antisera, *Am J Vet Res*, **44**: 715–19.

Shewen PE, Wilkie BN, 1985, Evidence for the *Pasteurella haemolytica* cytotoxin as a product of actively growing bacteria, *Am J Vet Res*, **46**: 1212–14.

Slots J, 1982, Salient biochemical characters of *Actinobacillus actinomycetemcomitans*, *Arch Microbiol*, **131**: 60–7.

Slots J, Liu YB et al., 1993, Evaluating two methods for fingerprinting genomes of *Actinobacillus actinomycetemcomitans*, *Oral Microbiol Immunol*, **8**: 337–43.

Smith DT, Webster LT, 1925, Epidemiological studies on respiratory infections of the rabbit. VI. Etiology of otitis media, *J Exp Med*, **41**: 275–83.

Smith GR, 1958, Experimental infections of *Pasteurella haemolytica* in mice and their use in demonstrating passive immunity, *J Comp Pathol*, **68**: 455–68.

Smith GR, 1959, Isolation of two types of *Pasteurella haemolytica* from sheep, *Nature (London)*, **183**: 1132–3.

Smith GR, 1960, The pathogenicity of *Pasteurella haemolytica* for young lambs, *J Comp Pathol*, **70**: 326–38.

Smith GR, 1961, The characteristics of two types of *Pasteurella haemolytica* associated with different pathological conditions in sheep, *J Pathol Bacteriol*, **81**: 431–40.

Smith GR, 1962, An unusual haemolytic effect produced by *Pasteurella haemolytica*, *J Pathol Bacteriol*, **83**: 501–8.

Smith JE, 1955, Studies on *Pasteurella septica* I. The occurence in the nose and tonsils of dogs, *J Comp Pathol*, **65**: 239–45.

Smith JE, 1958, Studies on *Pasteurella septica* II. Some cultural and biochemical properties of strains from different host species, *J Comp Pathol*, **68**: 315–23.

Smith JE, 1959, Studies on *Pasteurella septica* III. Strains from human beings, *J Comp Pathol*, **69**: 231–5.

Smith JE, Thal E, 1965, A taxonomic study of the genus *Pasteurella* using a numerical technique, *Acta Pathol Microbiol Scand*, **64**: 213–23.

Sneath PHA, 1992, Correction of orthography of epithets in *Pasteurella* and some problems with recommendations on latinization, *Int J Syst Bacteriol*, **42**: 658–9.

Sneath PHA, Johnson R, 1973, Numerical taxonomy of *Haemophilus* and related bacteria, *Int J Syst Bacteriol*, **23**: 405–18.

Sneath PHA, Stevens M, 1985, A numerical taxonomic study of *Actinobacillus*, *Pasteurella* and *Yersinia*, *J Gen Microbiol*, **131**: 2711–38.

Sneath PHA, Stevens M, 1990, *Actinobacillus rossii* sp. nov., *Actinobacillus seminis* sp. nov., nom. rev., *Pasteurella bettii* sp. nov., *Pasteurella lymphangitidis* sp. nov., *Pasteurella mairi* sp. nov., and *Pasteurella trehalosi* sp. nov., *Int J Syst Bacteriol*, **40**: 148–53.

Snyder B, Ryerson CC et al., 1996, Analytical performance of an immunologic-based periodontal bacterial test for simultaneous detection and differentiation of *Actinobacillus actinomycetemcomitans*, *Porphyromonas gingivalis*, and *Prevotella intermedia*, *J Periodontol*, **67**: 497–505.

Sorbello AF, O'Donnell J et al., 1994, Infective endocarditis due to *Pasteurella dagmatis*: case report and review, *Clin Infect Dis*, **18**: 336–8.

van Steenbergen TJ, Bosch-Tijhof CJ et al., 1994, Comparison of six typing methods for *Actinobacillus actinomycetemcomitans*, *J Clin Microbiol*, **32**: 2769–74.

Steffens L, Franke S et al., 1994, DNA fingerprinting of *Eikenella corrodens* by pulsed-field gel electrophoresis, *Oral Microbiol Immunol*, **9**: 95–8.

Stoloff AL, Gillies ML, 1986, Infections with *Eikenella corrodens* in a general hospital: a report of 33 cases, *Rev Infect Dis*, **8**: 50–3.

Sutherland AD, Donachie W, 1986, Cytotoxic effect of serotypes of *Pasteurella haemolytica* on sheep bronchoalveolar macrophages , *Vet Microbiol*, **11**: 331–6.

Suwanagool S, Rothkopf MM et al., 1983, Pathogenicity of *Eikenella corrodens* in humans, *Arch Intern Med*, **143**: 2265–8.

Tabatabai LB, Frank GH, 1981, Neuraminidase from *Pasteurella haemolytica*, *Curr Microbiol*, **5**: 203–6.

Taichman NS, Dean RT, Sanderson CJ, 1980, Biochemical and morphological characterization of the killing of human monocytes by a leukotoxin derived from *Actinobacillus actinomycetemcomitans*, *Infect Immun*, **28**: 258–68.

Tanaka A, 1926, A comparative study of *Pasteurella* cultures from different animals, *J Infect Dis*, **38**: 421–8.

Thjøtta T, Sydnes S, 1951, *Actinobacillus actinomycetem comitans* as the sole infecting agent in a human being, *Acta Pathol Microbiol Scand*, **28**: 27–35.

Thompson DA, Mould DL, 1975, Protein electrophoretic pattern of *Pasteurella haemolytica*, *Res Vet Sci*, **18**: 342–3.

Thompson L, Willius FA, 1932, *Actinobacillus* bacteremia, *JAMA*, **99**: 298–300.

Till DH, Palmer FP, 1960, A review of actinobacillosis with a study of the causal organism, *Vet Rec*, **72**: 527–33.

Tønjum T, Haas R, 1993, Identification of *Actinobacillus actinomycetemcomitans* by leukotoxin gene-specific hybridization and polymerase chain reaction assays, *J Clin Microbiol*, **31**: 1856–9.

Tønjum T, Hagen N, Bøvre K, 1985, Identification of *Eikenella corrodens* and *Cardiobacterium hominis* by genetic transformation, *Acta Pathol Microbiol Immunol Scand Sect B*, **93**: 389–94.

Trevisan di Saint-Léon V, 1887, Sul micrococco della rabbia e sulla possibilità di riconoscere durante il periodo d'incubazione, dall'esame del sangue della persona moricata, se ha contratta l'infezione rabbica, *Rc Reale Ist Lombardo Sci Lett*, **20**: 88–105.

Tsai C-C, Taichman NS, 1986, Dynamics of infection by leukotoxic strains of *Actinobacillus actinomycetemcomitans* in juvenile periodontitis, *J Clin Periodontol*, **13**: 330–1.

Tunnicliff EA, 1941, A study of *Actinobacillus lignieresi* from sheep affected by actinobacillosis, *J Infect Dis*, **69**: 52–8.

Tweed W, Edington JW, 1930, Pneumonia of bovines due to *Pasteurella boviseptica*, *J Comp Pathol*, **43**: 234–52.

Underwood K, Sjostrom K et al., 1993, Serum antibody opsonic activity against *Actinobacillus actinomycetemcomitans* in human periodontal diseases, *J Infect Dis*, **168**: 1436–43.

Vallée A, Gaillard J-A, 1953, Infection pyogène contagieuse de la souris déterminée par *Bacillus actinomycetem comitans*, *Ann Inst Pasteur (Paris)*, **84**: 647–9.

Verhaegen J, Verbraeken H et al., 1988, *Actinobacillus* (formerly *Pasteurella*) *ureae* meningitis and bacteraemia: report of a case and review of the literature, *J Infect*, **17**: 249–53.

Veterinary Investigation Service, 1975, Few specimens received at VI centres, *Vet Rec*, **97**: 319, 336.

Wang RF, Campbell W et al., 1996, Detection of *Pasteurella pneumotropica* in laboratory mice and rats by polymerase chain reaction, *Lab Anim Sci*, **46**: 81–5.

Watko LP, 1966, A chemically defined medium for growth of *Pasteurella multocida*, *Can J Microbiol*, **12**: 933–7.

Weaver RE, Hollis DG, Bottone EJ, 1985, Gram-negative fermentative bacteria and *Francisella tularensis*, *Manual of Clinical Microbiology*, 4th edn, eds Lennette EH, Balows A et al., American Society for Microbiology, Washington, DC, 309–29.

Webster LT, 1924, The epidemiology of a rabbit respiratory infection. IV. Susceptibility of rabbits to spontaneous snuffles, *J Exp Med*, **40**: 109–16.

Webster LT, 1925, Biology of *Bacterium leptisepticum*. I. Effects of oxygen tension and the presence of rabbit blood on growth, dissociation, and virulence, *J Exp Med*, **41**: 571–85.

Webster LT, 1926, Epidemiological studies on respiratory infections of the rabbit. VII. Pneumonias associated with *Bacterium leptisepticum*, *J Exp Med*, **43**: 555–72.

Webster LT, Baudisch O, 1925, Biology of *Bacterium leptisepticum*. II. The structure of some iron compounds which influence the growth of certain bacteria of the hemophilic, anaerobic, and hemorrhagic septicemia groups, *J Exp Med*, **42**: 473–82.

Webster LT, Burn CG, 1926, Biology of *Bacterium leptisepticum*. III. Physical, cultural, and growth characteristics of diffuse and mucoid types and their variants, *J Exp Med*, **44:** 343–58, 359–86.

Wessman GE, 1966, Cultivation of *Pasteurella haemolytica* in a chemically defined medium, *Appl Microbiol*, **14:** 597–602.

Wessman GE, Wessman G, 1970, Chemically defined media for *Pasteurella multocida* and *Pasteurella ureae*, and a comparison of their thiamine requirements with those of *Pasteurella haemolytica*, *Can J Microbiol*, **16:** 751–7.

Wilson M, Henderson B, 1995, Virulence factors of *Actinobacillus actinomycetemcomitans* relevant to the pathogenesis of inflammatory periodontal diseases, *FEMS Microbiol Rev*, **17:** 365–79.

Wilson M, Kamin S, Harvey W, 1985, Bone resorbing activity of purified capsular material from *Actinobacillus actinomycetemcomitans*, *J Periodont Res*, **20:** 484–91.

Wilson MA, Morgan MJ, Barger GE, 1993, Comparison of DNA fingerprinting and serotyping for identification of avian *Pasteurella multocida* isolates, *J Clin Microbiol*, **31:** 255–9.

Wilson MA, Duncan RM et al., 1995, *Pasteurella multocida* isolated from wild birds of North America: a serotype and DNA fingerprint study of isolates from 1978 to 1993, *Avian Dis*, **39:** 587–93.

Wright J, 1936, An epidemic of *Pasteurella* infection in a guinea-pig stock, *J Pathol Bacteriol*, **42:** 209–12.

Wüst J, Gubler J et al., 1991, *Actinobacillus hominis* as a causative agent of septicemia in hepatic failure, *Eur J Clin Microbiol Infect Dis*, **10:** 693–4.

Yaneza AL, Jivan H et al., 1991, *Pasteurella haemolytica* endocarditis, *J Infect*, **23:** 65–7.

Younan M, Fodar L, 1995, Characterisation of a new *Pasteurella haemolytica* serotype (A17), *Res Vet Sci*, **58:** 98.

Yusef HS, 1935, A contribution to the serological classification of *Pasteurella* strains, *J Pathol Bacteriol*, **41:** 203–6.

Zambon JJ, 1985, *Actinobacillus actinomycetemcomitans* in human periodontal disease, *J Clin Periodontol*, **12:** 1–20.

Zambon JJ, Slots J, Genco RJ, 1983, Serology of oral *Actinobacillus actinomycetemcomitans* and serotype distribution in human periodontal disease, *Infect Immun*, **41:** 19–27.

Zinnemann K, 1981, Some historical aspects of the genera *Haemophilus*, *Pasteurella* and *Actinobacillus*, and some of their species, Haemophilus, Pasteurella *and* Actinobacillus, eds Kilian M, Frederiksen W, Biberstein EL, Academic Press, London, 1–10.

CALYMMATOBACTERIUM, CARDIOBACTERIUM, CHROMOBACTERIUM AND STREPTOBACILLUS

W J Martin and S A Martin

CALYMMATOBACTERIUM GRANULOMATIS

1 DEFINITION

Calymmatobacterium granulomatis is a capsulate gram-negative rod present intracellularly in the Donovan bodies of patients with granuloma inguinale. This organism cannot be grown on ordinary laboratory media but may be subcultured serially in the yolk sac of embryonated hen's eggs and on certain special media (see section 5, p. 1218). Little is known of its physiological properties. It is pathogenic for humans.

2 INTRODUCTION

Granuloma inguinale, or granuloma venereum (see Volume 3, Chapter 33), also known as donovanosis, was described by McLeod in India in 1882. The cellular inclusions that are the specific hallmark of the disease were first described by Donovan (1905) and came to be known as Donovan bodies. Originally named *Calymmatobacterium granulomatis* by Aragao and Vianna

(1913), it was isolated by Anderson, de Monbreun and Goodpasture (1945) by inoculation into chick-embryo yolk sacs and named *Donovania granulomatis*, but the earlier name has maintained priority.

3 HABITAT

Donovanosis occurs world wide in tropical and subtropical areas, especially in South America and Asia, and affects mainly dark-skinned populations. Major epidemics have occurred throughout this century and donovanosis accounts for a high percentage of sexually transmitted disease among males. It is an important cause of chronic genital ulceration in central Australia and is potentially an important risk factor for HIV transmission in Aboriginal communities (Merianos, Gilles and Chuah 1994).

4 MORPHOLOGY

C. granulomatis is identified in infected tissue by the presence of Donovan bodies, which consist of organisms contained within the cytoplasmic vacuoles (phagosomes) of large macrophages, formerly known as Pund or Greenblatt cells. Bodies are sometimes found inside polymorphonuclear leucocytes or lying free outside cells. The organisms themselves are coccobacilli or short rods, 1–1.5 μm in length and c. 1 μm in width; they may be curved or dumb-bell shaped. They are non-motile and gram-negative, best stained in tissues by the Wright–Giemsa method (which stains the body of the bacterium blue or purple and the capsule pink), by Papanicolau's method or by various silver strains. A slow-Giemsa (overnight) tissue section staining technique has been described as being much superior than tissue smears and recommended for ultimate confirmation of *C. granulomatis* (Sehgal and Jain 1987). Bipolar staining produces a 'closed safety-pin' appearance. The organism usually has a prominent capsule within the phagosome, but capsules may be absent in rapidly multiplying organisms in fresh lesions. Infected macrophages may contain as many as 25 organisms. The cell membrane and cell wall have structures typical of gram-negative organisms.

Fine structure analysis of *C. granulomatis* in human tissue has revealed the presence of a complex cell envelope (Chandra and Jain 1991). The cytoplasm of these organisms showed presence of electron-dense polar material, in addition to regular bacterial structures such as mesosome, ribosomes and other nuclear material. The origin of fimbriae and blebs (surface appendages) was clearly endogenous to the cell wall. The morphology of fibrium at the site of its attachment of the cell membrane has been described along with a distinct layer of homogenous material of varying density surrounding the organism, suggesting the possibility of it being a capsule.

5 REQUIREMENTS FOR GROWTH

C. granulomatis can be isolated by inoculating infected material into the yolk sac of embryonated hens' eggs (Anderson 1943). It can be cultured in vitro only with great difficulty. For example, it has been successfully grown on media containing fresh egg-yolk material (Dienst, Greenblatt and Chen 1948), in a semisynthetic medium containing lactalbumin hydrolysate (Goldberg 1959) and has been maintained in tissue culture. The optimal temperature for growth is said to be 37°C.

In the absence of culture methods, an indirect immunofluorescence technique may prove to be valuable for the diagnosis of individual cases of granuloma inguinale and as an epidemiological tool in studies of the disease (Freinkel et al. 1992).

6 CLASSIFICATION

The organism has antigenic similarities to *Klebsiella* spp. (Goldberg 1954), but until the phenotypic and genetic characters of *Calymmatobacterium* have been established its taxonomic position remains obscure.

7 SUSCEPTIBILITY TO ANTIMICROBIAL AGENTS

Cases of donovanosis have responded to treatment with a wide range of agents, including ampicillin, norfloxacin, thiamphenicol, ceftriaxone, tetracycline, chloramphenicol, erythromycin, clindamycin, cotrimoxazole, streptomycin and other aminoglycosides.

8 PATHOGENICITY AND VIRULENCE FACTORS

Although Thomison (1951) produced miliary granulomata in the brain of chicks by intracerebral inoculation of infected material, *C. granulomatis* is nonpathogenic for laboratory animals. In humans it appears to have a low propensity to cause infection and requires direct inoculation through a break in the skin or mucous membranes to establish an infection. The incubation period is long and ranges from 8 to 80 days (Piot 1991).

In an ultrastructure study (Chandra et al. 1989), the inflammatory response was studied along with the fine structure of causative organisms. Macrophages were activated and showed numerous filopodia and increased numbers of lysosomes and rough endoplasmic reticulum. Many cells showed vacuoles of varying size in the cytoplasm, some of which contained the organisms. Other cells included plasma cells, polymorphonuclear cells and lymphocytes. In one case few multinucleated giant cells and dendritic cells with long cytoplasmic processes making cell–cell contact with other inflammatory cells were observed. According to these investigators, such cells had not previously been described in donovanosis. Surface structures such as pili and vesicles were also described, the role of which was yet to be defined.

CARDIOBACTERIUM HOMINIS

9 DEFINITION

Cardiobacterium hominis is a pleomorphic, gram-negative rod which typically produces intertwining filamentous growth, with variable retention of the gram stain. It is a fastidious aerobe and facultative anaerobe that grows best on enriched media under micro-aerophilic conditions with additional CO_2. It is non-motile, oxidase-positive, catalase-negative, indole-positive, urease-negative and nitrate-reductase-negative. The organism attacks a range of carbohydrates fermentatively. It is a commensal of the human oronasopharynx and occasionally causes bacteraemia and endocarditis in man. The G + C content of the DNA is 59–62 mol%.

10 INTRODUCTION

Formerly designated 11-D, the name *Cardiobacterium hominis* was given by Slotnick and Dougherty (1964) to a 'pasteurella-like' gram-negative bacterium isolated from the blood of patients with endocarditis (Appelbaum and Gelfand 1947, Tucker et al. 1962).

11 HABITAT

C. hominis was isolated from the nose or throat of 68% of healthy human subjects (Slotnick and Dougherty 1964) and has been grown from the female genital tract.

12 MORPHOLOGY

C. hominis is a slender gram-negative rod, c. 0.5 μm × (1.5–3.0) μm, that tends to be pleomorphic, forming pairs, short chains, rosettes, irregular clusters with swollen ends or a matted arrangement of filaments. It is non-motile. The swollen ends may retain some gram-positivity, producing a 'tear-drop' appearance (Wormser and Bottone 1983). This pleomorphism is not seen if yeast extract is provided in the medium (Savage et al. 1977). Electron microscopy (Reyn, Birch-Anderson and Murray 1971) indicates that *C. hominis* has a typical gram-negative cell wall structure with an unusually dense outer layer. It does not possess a capsule as such, but the terminal portions of the cell are covered with a prominent tufted 'polar cap', adherent to the outer-cell membrane.

13 CULTURE CHARACTERISTICS AND GROWTH REQUIREMENTS

After incubation for 48 h, colonies are 1–2 mm in diameter, circular with a smooth, glistening surface. When observed under magnification, colonies show a roughened surface and a central core made up of intertwining filaments which extend beyond the periphery, so that adjacent colonies may be bridged by a continuous filamentous network (Wormser and Bottone 1983). With continued incubation or repeated subculture, colonies become dry and flat with irregular spreading edges and pitting of the agar (Speller, Prout and Saunders 1968, Wormser et al. 1978). Growth on blood agar is non-haemolytic. In serum broth, *C. hominis* shows flocculent or granular growth without turbidity, typically forming puff-ball aggregates that adhere to the walls of the container.

C. hominis is a fastidious facultative anaerobe that grows best on enriched media such as blood or chocolate agar under micro-aerophilic conditions with 7–10% CO_2 and additional humidity. It is X-factor and CO_2 dependent on primary isolation but these requirements are subsequently lost and it can then be grown on tryptose soy agar, brain–heart infusion agar or Mueller–Hinton medium in ambient air. The optimal temperature for growth is 30–37°C, range 25–42°C. The optimal pH for growth is 7.0–7.2. The incubation period for detectable growth in blood-culture media ranges from 1 to 21 days.

14 METABOLISM

It is oxidase-positive, catalase-negative, indole-positive and nitrate-reductase-negative. It attacks fermentatively without gas production a range of carbohydrates including glucose, maltose, sucrose, fructose, mannose, mannitol and sorbitol, but not lactose. The major product of glucose metabolism is lactic acid. Other biochemical reactions are shown in Table 52.1.

15 GENETIC MECHANISMS

Transformation studies show that it has no affinity with *Eikenella corrodens* or with species of *Neisseria, Kingella* or *Moraxella* (Tønjum, Hagen and Bøvre 1985) (see Chapter 48).

Moreover, DNA–DNA hybridization studies using total genomic DNA probes on some species of Neisseriaceae and other bacterial groups showed that most of the species examined, including *C. hominis*, were easily distinguished (Tønjum, Bukholm and Bøvre 1989).

16 CLASSIFICATION

The genus *Cardiobacterium* consists of a single species, *C. hominis*, with an antigenic and DNA base composition different from that of phenotypically similar organisms. On the basis of 16S rRNA sequence comparisons, Dewhirst et al. (1990) proposed that *Kingella*

Table 52.1 Differential characteristics of some fastidious catalase-negative, rod-shaped bacteria that may be isolated from human blood cultures

Characteristic	Cardiobacterium hominis	Eikenella corrodens	Streptobacillus moniliformis
Oxidase	+	+	−
Indole	+	−	−
Nitrate reduction	−	+	−
H₂S production	−(weak)	v(weak)	+(weak)
Methyl red	+	−	−
Hydrolysis of starch	...	−	...
Hydrolysis of aesculin	...	−	V
Hydrolysis of casein	...	−	−
Arginine dihydrolase	−	−	+
Lysine decarboxylase	−	+	...
Ornithine decarboxylase	−	V	...
Glucose O-F test	F	...	F
Acid production from			
glucose	+	−	+
maltose	V	−	V
sucrose	+	−	V
lactose	−	−	V
mannitol	V	−	−
fructose	+	−	V
mannose	+	−	V
trehalose	−	−	V
xylose	−	−	V

−, Negative reaction; +, positive reaction; V, variable; ..., no information or not applicable; F, fermentative.

indologenes be transferred to the genus *Suttonella* as *Suttonella indologenes*, that *Bacteroides nodosus* be transferred to the new genus *Dichelobacter* as *Dichelobacter nodosus*, and that the genera *Cardiobacterium*, *Suttonella* and *Dichelobacter* be assigned to a new family, Cardiobacteriaceae, in the γ division of Proteobacteria.

17 SUSCEPTIBILITY TO ANTIMICROBIAL AGENTS

C. hominis is sensitive to therapeutically attainable concentrations of benzylpenicillin, various cephalosporins, aminoglycosides, chloramphenicol, tetracycline and erythromycin (Savage et al. 1977). Although resistant to vancomycin (Lane et al. 1983), it is susceptible to ciprofloxacin (Vogt et al. 1994).

None of the *C. hominis* isolates examined by Miller et al. (1991) contained detectable plasmids, β-lactamase or resistant mutants. However, characteristic β-lactam induced morphological defects were observed; all of their isolates were susceptible to 16 β-lactam antimicrobials.

18 PATHOGENICITY AND VIRULENCE FACTORS

The virulence of *C. hominis* for humans appears to be extremely low. It is occasionally isolated from blood of patients with endocarditis of normal or prosthetic heart valves. Meningitis has been reported as a result

of underlying endocarditis (Francioli, Foussianos and Glauser 1983). It is non-pathogenic for laboratory animals (Tucker et al. 1962).

CHROMOBACTERIUM VIOLACEUM

19 DEFINITION

Chromobacterium violaceum is a rod-shaped, gramnegative non-spore-forming bacterium that is motile by means of a single polar and few lateral flagella. This bacillus often shows bipolar or barred staining; is an aerobe and facultative anaerobe that attacks carbohydrates fermentatively; and grows on ordinary media at 37°C but not at 4°C. It usually produces a nondiffusible violet pigment and is oxidase-positive, catalase-positive, indole-negative and urease-negative. It is a saprophytic organism that occasionally causes disease in humans and animals. The G + C content of the DNA is 65–68 mol%.

20 INTRODUCTION

C. violaceum was described by Bergonzini in 1880 (see Sneath 1956a). Also known as *Bacillus violaceus manilae*, Cruess-Callaghan and Gorman (1935) divided the violet-pigmented chromobacteria into mesophils that grow at 37°C but not at 4°C and psychrophils that grow at 4°C but not at 37°C, the 2 groups also differing in several culture and biochemical characteristics. Sneath (1956a) regarded the 2 groups as separate species or biotypes within the genus *Chromobacterium* and proposed that the type species should be a mesophil, *C. violaceum*. The psychrophils, which he designated *C. lividum*, have been transferred to a new genus *Janthinobacterium* (see De Ley, Segers and Gillis 1978).

21 HABITAT

C. violaceum is a saprophyte and is present in soil and water in tropical and subtropical areas within the latitudes 35°N–35°S. It has been isolated from soil and water samples in Trinidad, Guyana, Brazil, India, Malaysia, Thailand and Vietnam, as well as Florida and South Carolina in the USA (Macher, Casale and Fauci 1982).

22 MORPHOLOGY

The organism is a gram-negative, rod-shaped bacterium, approximately $(0.5–1) \times (1.5–3)$ μm, sometimes slightly curved, and occurring singly or in pairs. It is often barred or bipolar when stained by Gram's method and usually contains β-hydroxybutyrate inclusions which stain with Sudan black. It is motile, with a characteristic type of flagellation (Figs 52.1 and 52.2) consisting of a single short polar flagellum, which stains poorly and has a relatively long wavelength, and one or more longer subpolar or lateral flagella which stain readily and have a shorter wavelength (Sneath 1956b). Lateral flagella are formed most abundantly in young cultures from an agar medium and are rare in broth cultures (Sneath 1956b).

23 CULTURE CHARACTERISTICS AND GROWTH REQUIREMENTS

On ordinary media, colonies appear smooth, circular with an entire edge, shiny, low convex, 1.0–1.5 mm in diameter after incubation for 2 days, butyrous in consistency and readily emulsifiable.

Prolonged incubation results in the formation of rough colonies (see Sivendra, Lo and Lim 1975), raised or low-conical, irregular in outline with a dull 'hammered pewter' surface, usually reverting to the smooth form on subculture. Under aerobic conditions, cultures on solid media are usually violet-pigmented and smell of HCN. Some strains can grow both pigmented and non-pigmented colonies on blood agar plates. Strains may show a variable degree of partial haemolysis on blood agar that is attributed to lecithinase production (Sneath 1956a). Broth cultures show diffuse turbidity with a fragile surface pellicle that eventually sinks, leaving a surface collar of violet-pigmented growth on the side of the container.

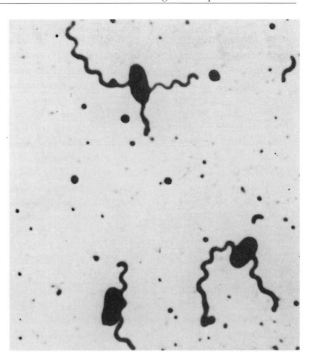

Fig. 52.1 *Chromobacterium violaceum*. Stained preparation to show arrangement of flagella. One organism shows both polar and lateral flagella (× 2500). (From photograph kindly supplied by Professor PHA Sneath).

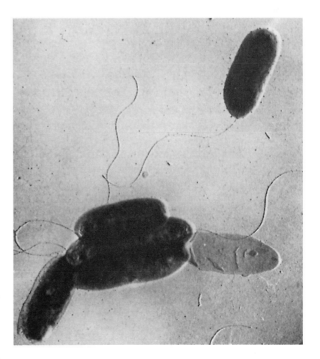

Fig. 52.2 *Chromobacterium violaceum*. Electron micrograph showing the different wavelengths of polar and lateral flagella (× 8000). (From photograph kindly supplied by Professor PHA Sneath).

The growth of most strains is violet-pigmented, the colour ranging from a pale shade to almost black, and deepening with continued incubation. Pigmentation occurs only in the presence of oxygen and is enhanced by tryptophan. Non-pigmented and late-pigmented variants occur, which may or may not breed true; non-pigmented strains have been isolated from surface water in the tropics (Sivendra, Lo and Lim 1975) and from clinical specimens. The pigment, known as violacein, is non-diffusible, soluble in ethanol and acetone but not in water, chloroform, ether or benzene. Moreover, the entire biosynthetic pathway for the synthesis of violacein is encoded on a 14.5 kb fragment of the *C. violaceum* genome (Pemberton, Vincent and Penfold 1991). It has some antibacterial activity and is probably a complex indole derivative (Beer, Jenning and Robertson 1954). Trypanocide activity has also been described (Duran et al. 1989). Hoshino, Hayashi and Uchiyama (1994) recently isolated a reddish-orange pigment (pseudodeoxyviolacein) that resulted from the metabolism of tryptophan by *C. violaceum*.

Growth occurs readily on ordinary nutrient agar medium although very small inocula may fail to grow because of inhibition by traces of H_2O_2 (Sneath 1956a). Most strains are facultative anaerobes, but a few with an oxidative type of metabolism grow poorly or not at all under anaerobic conditions. Humidity appears to be of importance; growth is sometimes poor on over-dried plates and slant cultures readily die on prolonged storage. Growth occurs on MacConkey medium and other selective media for coliform organisms, but not on cetrimide agar. Temperature range is 10–15°C up to 40–42°C, optimum around 35°C; pH range is 5–9, optimum pH is 7–8.

24 METABOLISM

Most strains are facultative anaerobes, with a fermentative type of metabolism.

C. violaceum is oxidase-positive; the reaction can be detected in pigmented growth by a modification of Kovacs's method (Dhar and Johnson 1973); otherwise very young or anaerobic cultures with reduced or absent pigmentation should be tested by the usual method. It is catalase-positive, although the reaction is often weak and the organism is sensitive to H_2O_2. It reduces nitrate to nitrite; Sneath (1956a) reported that most strains reduce nitrite completely within 5 days. Acid is produced fermentatively without gas from glucose, fructose, mannose, dextrin, trehalose and sucrose (variable), but not lactose nor mannitol. Some strains form an atypical reducing substance from gluconate (Sneath 1956a). Other positive reactions include the egg-yolk reaction (for lecithinase), growth in KCN, citrate utilization, ammonia production from peptone, and phosphatase production. A full list of biochemical activities is given in Table 52.2. Pigmented and non-pigmented strains give the same biochemical reactions. The end products of glucose metabolism include acetic, butyric, succinic and lactic acids (Sneath 1956a).

C. violaceum is proteolytic, digesting gelatin, casein and serum, and lipolytic, attacking a range of Tweens. HCN is formed under aerobic conditions. Some strains produce a monobactam antibiotic (Sykes et al. 1981) which is synthesized commercially as aztreonam. Moreover, a novel antitumour bicyclic depsipeptide isolated from a broth culture of *C. violaceum* No.968 has been described by Ueda et al. (1994). Antitumour activity against murine and human tumour cell lines both in vitro and in vivo was noted.

25 ANTIGENIC STRUCTURE

Cross-agglutination is extensive. Rough antigens are common to most strains and no clear-cut antigenic groups have been established (Sneath and Buckland 1959). The polar and lateral flagella of the same strain are antigenically distinct (Sneath 1956b).

26 CLASSIFICATION

Sneath (1956a, 1956b, 1960), proposed that the type species of the genus *Chromobacterium* should be *C. violaceum*, a mesophil. This was adopted by the Judicial Commission of the International Committee on Bacterial Nomenclature (Report 1958). Leifson (1956) investigated the mode of action on carbohydrates of *Chromobacterium* strains and recognized and named 3 different groups: *Chromobacterium manilae*, *Chromobacterium laurentium* and *Chromobacterium violaceum*. Leifson further acknowledged that it was illogical to retain each group as a separate species of *Chromobacterium* as organisms that either fermented or oxidized carbohydrates and contained both mesophils and psychrophils. The psychrotrophic chromobacteria have since been transferred to the genus *Janthinobacterium* but Moss, Ryall and Logan (1978) isolated violacein-producing strains from river water which grow at 4°C but not at 37°C. They also formed thin, spreading colonies on agar, but more closely resembled *C. violaceum* in other properties than the oxidative psychrophils. In particular, they are facultative anaerobes, with a fermentative type of metabolism, producing acid from trehalose. Moss, Ryall and Logan (1978) felt that they should be included in the genus *Chromobacterium*, despite their low G + C value of 50–52 mol%, and named them *Chromobacterium fluviatile*. Using cluster and principal co-ordinate analyses on 113 violet chromogens, Logan (1989) showed *Janthinobacterium lividum* to be a heterogenous species but *C. violaceum* and *C. fluviatile* to be well separated and homogenous phenons. To accommodate the latter organism, a new, monospecific genus, *Iodabacter*, was proposed with the type strain being *Iodobacter fluviatile* comb. nov.

Evidence from rRNA–DNA pairing suggests that *C. violaceum* is closely related to several genera including *Alcaligenes*, *Bordetella*, *Janthinobacterium* and certain non-fluorescent pseudomanads (De Ley, Segers and Gillis 1978). All these organisms may oxidize glucose, unlike the majority of strains now left in the genus *Chromobacterium*. Rossau et al. (1986) revealed that the closest genetic relative to the one group located in rRNA superfamily III of the family Neisseriaceae is *Chromobacterium*.

Table 52.2 Biochemical characteristics of *Chromobacterium violaceum*

Catalase	+	Egg-yolk reaction (lecithinase)	+
Oxidase	+	HCN production	+
Indole	−*	Growth in KCN	+
Nitrate reduction	+	Arginine dihydrolase	V
H₂S production	−	Lysine decarboxylase	−
Citrate utilization	+	Ornithine decarboxylase	−
Methyl red	−	Glucose O-F test	F
Acetoin production	−	Acid production from	
Urease	−	glucose	+
Ammonia production from peptone	+	maltose	V
Gluconate	−	sucrose	V
Malonate	−	lactose	−
Phenylalanine deaminase	−	mannitol	−
Hydrolysis of starch	−	fructose	+
Hydrolysis of aesculin	−	mannose	+
Hydrolysis of casein	+	trehalose	+
Hydrolysis of gelatin	+	xylose	−
DNAase	−		

+, Positive reaction; −, negative reaction; F, fermentative.
*Non pigmented strains are frequently indole positive (Pickett, Hollis and Bottone 1991).

27 SUSCEPTIBILITY TO ANTIMICROBIAL AGENTS

The organism shows no particular resistance to heat or disinfectants; it is killed at 55°C within 10 min (Sneath 1956a). In a comparison of the in vitro activity of a large number of antimicrobial agents against 11 clinical strains of *C. violaceum*, Aldridge, Valainis and Sander (1988) reported that ciprofloxacin was the most active of the compounds tested although norfloxacin and pefloxacin were highly active. Resistance was not detected to mezlocillin, piperacillin, apalcillin, imipenem and aztreonam; a single strain was resistant to ticarcillin. Only cefotetan showed good in vitro activity among the cephalosporin/cephamycin group. Gentamicin was more active than amikacin and tobramycin. Good activity was also noted for chloramphenicol, doxycycline and trimethoprim–sulphamethoxazole but *C. violaceum* strains were highly resistant to rifampicin and vancomycin. The bactericidal activity of selected agents was shown to be concentration dependent using time-kill kinetic studies. Addition of clavulanic acid did not increase the activity of ticarcillin and in one case was shown to induce β-lactamase. In predicting the susceptibility patterns, a high correlation was noted between the broth microdilution and disk diffusion test methods.

A pathogenic strain studied by Farrar and O'Dell (1976) produced a chromosomally determined β-lactamase that acts primarily against cephalosporins.

28 PATHOGENICITY AND VIRULENCE FACTORS

Although widespread in occurrence, *C. violaceum* causes few natural infections and is generally considered to be of low virulence. However, in humans it may cause septicaemia with pneumonia and abscess formation, usually fatal unless promptly treated, and with a tendency to relapse. The clinical resemblance to meliodosis is very striking. Cases have been reported from India, South East Asia, Brazil, Paraguay, Senegal, northern Australia and the USA. Most cases reported in the USA have occurred in children or young adults, some with chronic granulomatous disease (Macher, Casale and Fauci 1982). Intestinal and genitourinary infections have also been reported. Infections occasionally occur in animals and outbreaks of infections have been reported in buffaloes, pigs and gibbons.

When administered intraperitoneally to guinea pigs in doses of c. 5 × 10⁶ organisms a severe septicaemic illness results (Sneath and Buckland 1959); no infection occurs apparently when given to guinea pigs by mouth. Mice and rabbits also are susceptible to parenteral infection. Pigmented and non-pigmented strains appear to be of equal pathogenicity.

A comparative study of virulent and avirulent strains of *C. violaceum* suggests that virulence of this organism may be, at least in part, associated with endotoxin, with some protection of the virulent, clinical strain from phagocytic attack being afforded by elevated levels of superoxide dismutase and catalase (Miller et al. 1988).

STREPTOBACILLUS MONILIFORMIS

29 DEFINITION

Streptobacillus moniliformis is a fastidious, highly pleomorphic, aerobic and facultatively anaerobic, gram-negative bacillus with characteristic yeast-like swellings that readily give rise to L-phase and transitional variants. The organism ferments a range of carbohydrates; it is catalase-negative, oxidase-negative, indole-negative and urease-negative. The bacillus causes a type of rat-bite fever and is responsible for outbreaks of Haverhill fever. The G + C content of the DNA 24–26 mol%.

30 INTRODUCTION

Streptobacillus monliformis, isolated by Levaditi, Nicolau and Poincloux (1925) from the blood of a laboratory worker, is now considered the same organism as *Streptomyces muris ratti* (Schottmuller 1914, Tunnicliff 1916). It is similar to *Haverhillia multiforme* (Parker and Hudson 1926) although the 2 organisms have not been directly compared. Over the years various synonyms have been associated with this organism (Brown and Nunemaker 1942).

Klieneberger (1935) found that colonies of *S. moniliformis* consisted of 2 elements: the streptobacillary form and what she took to be a PPLO (or mycoplasma) that she named L-form or L_1. Although the L_1 appeared not to revert to the streptobacillary form (Klieneberger 1942), it is now regarded as an L-phase variant.

31 HABITAT

The organism occurs world wide as a commensal of the nasopharynx of healthy laboratory rats (Strangeways 1933) and wild rats, sometimes being excreted in the urine. It is also isolated from the nasopharynx of diseased mice and from other rodents.

32 MORPHOLOGY

It is a gram-negative, highly pleomorphic bacterium that generally occurs as short coccobacillary forms or rods, c. 0.5 μm in width, as well as chains and intertwining wavy filaments. The filaments may show spherical, oval or club-shaped gram-variable swellings up to 3 μm in diameter and may give rise to a 'string of beads' appearance – hence the description '*moniliformis*'. In ageing cultures, filaments show degenerative changes with the formation of granules and extracellular droplets, irregularity or failure of staining and fragmentation. In fluid media and in vivo, pleomorphism is less pronounced. The organism is non-motile.

In general, older cultures may not stain well with the gram stain; Giemsa or Wayson stain may yield better results (Piot 1991).

33 CULTURE CHARACTERISTICS AND GROWTH REQUIREMENTS

On serum or blood agar it forms circular, translucent colonies with a smooth glistening surface. It is non-haemolytic. Smaller, rougher 'transitional' colonies may be present, and in older cultures mutant L-phase colonies may be recognizable, with their typical 'fried-egg' appearance; these are best seen on a clear medium (Cohen, Wittler and Faber 1968). Blood, serum, ascitic or synovial fluid, is required for growth. It may appear to be an obligate anaerobe on primary isolation, but is a facultative anaerobe on subculture. Optimum growth is probably best achieved on chocolate-blood agar or tryptose soy agar, both enriched with 10–20% serum and incubated in a micro-aerophilic atmosphere with additional CO_2 and humidification. Basal media containing 15% sterile, defibrinated rabbit blood supports the bacterial-phase organisms well, whereas a clear medium will enhance the isolation of the more nutritionally fastidious L-phase variants (Jenkins 1988). The optimal temperature for growth is 35–37°C, optimal pH 7.4–7.6. The choice of a fluid blood-culture medium is critical: Shanson, Pratt and Green (1985) recommend brain–heart infusion broth with cysteine 0.05% and Panmede 2.5%. This could be used in conjunction with a suitable L-phase fluid medium.

34 METABOLISM

The organism is generally non-reactive, with negative reactions for catalase, oxidase, indole production, nitrate reduction and urease (see Table 52.1). It attacks sugars fermentatively; acid is produced from glucose (without gas), galactose, glycogen, dextrin, raffinose and starch and variably from fructose, maltose, mannose, salicin, lactose, sucrose, trehalose and xylose, depending on the basal medium employed. Acid is not formed from sorbitol or mannitol.

The alkaline phosphatase reaction is positive. The end products of glucose metabolism consist mainly of lactic with some succinic acid.

35 CELL WALL AND ENVELOPE COMPOSITION; ANTIGENIC STRUCTURE

The major long-chain fatty acids are C(16:0), C(18:2), C(18:1) and C(18:0) (Rowbotham 1983). The electrophoretic profiles of cellular proteins are characteristic and can be used to type strains, 'Haverhill fever' strains being distinguishable from 'rat-bite fever' strains (Costas and Owen 1987).

Strains are antigenically homogenous, but L-phase variants lack an antigen present in the bacillary form. The species can be identified by fluorescence with a conjugated specific antiserum.

36 CLASSIFICATION

Currently there is only one species in the genus *Streptobacillus* and the taxonomic position of *S. moniliformis* is uncertain. It appears to have properties more in common with the Mycoplasmatales (Costas and Owen 1987).

37 LABORATORY ISOLATION AND IDENTIFICATION

Streptobacillary rat-bite fever is usually diagnosed by the isolation of *S. moniliformis* from blood, joint fluid or pus. If isolation is unexpected, the organism may not be readily identified. Clinically similar conditions such as tularaemia, leptospirosis, rickettsial and various viral infections should be ruled out. If streptobacillary fever is suspected and routine laboratory cultures are negative, the organism may sometimes be isolated by intraperitoneal inoculation of infected material into mice.

An enzyme-linked immunosorbent assay (ELISA) for monitoring rodent colonies for *S. moniliformis* has been described by Boot et al. (1993). Twelve strains originating from cases of rat-bite fever and Haverhill fever in humans and from various rodent species showed considerable serological relationship. The ELISA appeared specific since antibodies to *S. moniliformis* were absorbed by autologous and homologous antigen, but not by heterologous bacterial antigens. *Acholeplasma laidlawii* showed a partial serological relationship with *S. moniliformis*.

38 SUSCEPTIBILITY TO ANTIMICROBIAL AGENTS

The bacillary form is sensitive to penicillin and to therapeutically attainable concentrations of cephalosporins, aminoglycosides, tetracycline, erythromycin and clindamycin; it is less sensitive to chloramphenicol. The L-phase variant is resistant to penicillin, but sensitive to tetracycline.

39 PATHOGENICITY AND VIRULENCE FACTORS

In humans, *S. moniliformis* is one of the 2 recognized causes of rat-bite fever, the other being *Spirillum minus* (see Chapter 64). The 2 diseases are very similar in their clinical presentations (Brown and Nunemaker 1942).

Streptobacillary rat-bite fever occurs world wide and may occur following the bite of a rat or occasionally a mouse, squirrel, weasel, dog, or cat. Most cases probably occur in children sleeping in rat-infested dwellings. Laboratory-acquired infections among rodent handlers also occur. The incubation period is usually 1–4 days and rarely more than 10 days.

Haverhill fever, or erythema arthriticum epidemicum, is a form of streptobacillary fever which occurs in outbreaks and appears not to be attributable to direct contact with animals. It was named after Haverhill, Massachusetts, where the first recorded epidemic of the disease occurred (Parker and Hudson 1926); this was thought to be associated with the consumption of raw milk and milk products. The first outbreak in the UK (Shanson et al. 1983) affected pupils and staff of a boarding school in Essex. Of some 700 persons exposed, 304 (43%) became ill in a period of 10 days (McEvoy, Noah and Pilsworth 1987).

Adult rats are generally resistant to experimental infection, although newborn rats may develop pneumonia (Strangeways 1933). Mice given the organism intravenously develop either a rapidly fatal septicaemia, or arthropathy of the lower limbs, with longer survival, the severity of the condition being dose-related (Savage, Joiner and Florey 1981).

REFERENCES

Aldridge KE, Valainis GT, Sander CV, 1988, Comparison of the in-vitro activity of ciprofloxacin and 24 other antimicrobial agents against clinical strains of *Chromobacterium violaceum*, *Diagn Microbiol Infect Dis*, **10:** 31–40.

Anderson K, 1943, Cultivation from granuloma inguinale of microorganism having characteristics of Donovan bodies in yolk sac of chick embryos, *Science*, **97:** 560–1.

Anderson K, de Monbreun W, Goodpasture E, 1945, An etiologic consideration of *Donovania granulomatis* cultivated from granuloma inguinale (three cases) in embryonic yolk, *J Exp Med*, **81:** 25–39.

Appelbaum E, Gelfand M, 1947, A case of bacteremia due to unidentified gram-negative pasteurella-like bacillus with recovery following streptomycin therapy, *Ann Intern Med*, **26:** 780.

Aragao H, Vianna G, 1913, *Mem Inst Oswaldo Cruz*, **5:** 211.

Beer RJS, Jenning E, Robertson A, 1954, The chemistry of bacteria. Part III. An idolylpyrnylmethene, *J Chem Soc*, 2679–85.

Boot R, Bakker RHG et al., 1993, An enzyme-linked immunosorbant assay (ELISA) for monitoring rodent colonies for *Streptobacillus moniliformis* antibodies, *Lab Anim*, **27:** 350–7.

Brown TM, Nunemaker JC, 1942, Rat-bite fever. A review of the American cases with reevaluation of etiology; report of cases, *Bull Johns Hopkins Hosp*, **70:** 201–327.

Chandra M, Jain AK, 1991, Fine structure of *Calymmatobacterium granulomatis* with particular reference to the surface structure, *Indian J Med Res Sect A*, **93:** 225–31.

Chandra M, Jain AK et al., 1989, An ultrastructural study of donovanosis, *Indian J Med Res*, **89:** 158–64.

Cohen RL, Wittler RG, Faber JE, 1968, Modified biochemical tests for characterization of L-phase variants of bacteria, *Appl Microbiol*, **16:** 1655–62.

Costas M, Owen RJ, 1987, Numerical analysis of electrophoretic protein patterns of *Streptobacillus moniliformis* strains from human, murine and avian infections, *J Med Microbiol*, **23:** 303–11.

Cruess-Callaghan G, Gorman MJ, 1953, On the characteristics of *Bacterium violaceum* (Schröter) and some allied species of violet bacteria, *Sci Proc R Dublin Soc*, **21 NS:** 213–21.

Dewhirst FE, Paster BJ et al., 1990, Transfer of *Kingella indologenes* (Snell and Lapage 1976) to the genus *Suttonella* gen. nov. as *Suttonella indologenes* comb. nov.; transfer of *Bacteroides nodosus* (Beveridge 1941) to the genus *Dichelobacter* gen. nov. as *Dichelobacter nodosus* comb. nov.; and assignment of the genera *Cardiobacterium*, *Dichelobacter*, and *Suttonella* to Cardiobacteriaceae fam. nov. in the gamma division of Proteobacteria on the basis of 16S rRNA sequence comparisons, *Inst J Syst Bacteriol*, **40:** 426–33.

Dhar SK, Johnson R, 1973, The oxidase activity of *Chromobacterium*, *J Clin Pathol*, **26:** 304–6.

Dienst RB, Greenblatt RB, Chen CH, 1948, Laboratory diagnosis of granuloma inguinale and studies on the cultivation of the Donovan body, *Am J Syphilis, Gonorrhea Vener Dis*, **32:** 301–6.

Donovan C, 1905, *Indian Med Gaz*, **40:** 414.

Duran N, Campos V et al., 1989, Bacterial chemistry, III. Preliminary studies on trypanosomal activities of *Chromobacterium violaceum* products, *An Acad Bras Cienc*, **61:** 31–6.

Farrar WE, O'Dell NM, 1976, β-Lactamase activity in *Chromobacterium violaceum, J Infect Dis*, **134:** 290–3.

Francioli PB, Foussianos D, Glauser MP, 1983, *Cardiobacterium hominis* endocarditis manifesting as bacterial meningitis, *Arch Intern Med*, **143:** 1483–4.

Freinkel AL, Danger Y et al., 1992, A serological test for granuloma inguinale, *Genitourin Med*, **68:** 269–72.

Goldberg J, 1954, Studies of granuloma inguinale. III. The antigenic heterogeneity of *Donovania granulomatis, Am J Syphilis, Gonorrhea Vener Dis*, **38:** 330–5.

Goldberg J, 1959, Studies on granuloma inguinale. IV. Growth requirements of *Donovania granulomatis* and its relationship to the natural habitat of the organism, *Br J Vener Dis*, **38:** 226–8.

Hoshino T, Hayashi T, Uchiyama T, 1994, Pseudodeoxyviolaceia, a new red pigment produced by the tryptophan metabolism of *Chromobacterium violaceum, Biosci Biotechnol Biochem*, **58:** 279–82.

Jenkins SG, 1988, Rat-bite fever, *Clin Microbiol Newsl*, **10:** 57–9.

Klieneberger E, 1935, The natural occurrence of pleuropneumonia-like organisms in apparent symbiosis with *Streptobacillus moniliformis* and other bacteria, *J Pathol Bacteriol*, **40:** 93–105.

Klieneberger E, 1942, Some new observations bearing on the nature of the pleuropneumonia-like organism known as L1 associated with *Streptobacillus moniliformis, J Hyg*, **42:** 485–97.

Lane T, MacGregor RR et al., 1983, Case report. *Cardiobacterium hominis*: an elusive cause of endocarditis, *J Infect*, **6:** 75–80.

Leifson E, 1956, Morphological and physiological characteristics of the genus *Chromobacterium, J Bacteriol*, **71:** 393–400.

Levaditi C, Nicolau S, Poincloux P, 1925, Sur le rôle étiologique de *Streptobacillus moniliformis* (nov. spec.) dans l'érythème polymorphaigue septicémique, *C R Acad Sci*, **180:** 1188–90.

De Ley J, Segers P, Gillis M, 1978, Intra- and intergeneric similarities of *Chromobacterium* and *Janthinobacterium* ribosomal ribonucleic acid cistrons, *Int J Syst Bacteriol*, **28:** 154–68.

Logan NA, 1989, Numerical taxonomy of violet-pigmented gram-negative bacteria and description of *Iodobacter fluviatile* new-genus new-combination, *Int J Syst Bacteriol*, **39:** 450–6.

McEvoy MB, Noah ND, Pilsworth R, 1987, Outbreak of fever caused by *Streptobacillus moniliformis, Lancet*, **2:** 1361–3.

Macher AM, Casale TB, Fauci AS, 1982, Chronic granulomatous disease of childhood and *Chromobacterium violaceum* infections in the southeastern United States, *Ann Intern Med*, **97:** 51–5.

McLeod K, 1882, *Indian Med Gaz*, **17:** 113.

Merianos A, Gilles M, Chuah J, 1994, Ceftriaxone in the treatment of chronic donovanosis in Central Australia, *Genitourin Medicine*, **70:** 80–4.

Miller DP, Blevins WT et al., 1988, A comparative study of virulent and avirulent strains of *Chromobacterium violaceum, Can J Microbiol*, **34:** 249–55.

Miller MA, Mockler DF et al., 1991, Characterization of *Cardiobacterium hominis* antibiotic susceptibility, morphological variations, plasmid and membrane analysis, *Curr Microbiol*, **23:** 197–206.

Moss MO, Ryall C, Logan NA, 1978, The classification and characterization of chromobacteria from a lowland river, *J Gen Microbiol*, **105:** 11–21.

Parker F Jr, Hudson NP, 1926, The etiology of Haverhill fever (erythema arthriticum epidemicum), *Am J Pathol*, **2:** 367–79.

Pemberton JM, Vincent KM, Penfold, RJ, 1991, Cloning and heterologous expression of the violacein biosynthesis gene cluster from *Chromobacterium violaceum, Curr Microbiol*, **22:** 355–8.

Pickett MJ, Hollis DG, Bottone EJ, 1991, Miscellaneous gram-negative bacteria, *Manual of Clinical Microbiology*, 5th edn, eds Balows A, Hausler WJ et al., American Society for Microbiology, Washington DC, 423, 424.

Piot P, 1991, *Gardnerella, Streptobacillus, Spirillum*, and *Calymmatobacterium, Manual of Clinical Microbiology*, 5th edn, eds Balows A, Hausler WJ et al., American Society for Microbiology, Washington DC, 483–7.

Report, 1958, Opinion 16. Conservation of the generic name *Chromobacterium* Bergonzini 1880 and designation of the type species and the neotype culture of the type species, *Int Bull Bacteriol Nomencl*, **8:** 151–2.

Reyn A, Birch-Anderson A, Murray RGE, 1971, The fine structure of *Cardiobacterium hominis, Acta Pathol Microbiol Scand*, **79:** 51–60.

Rossau R, Van Landschoot A et al., 1986, Intergeneric and intrageneric similarities of ribosomal RNA cistrons of the Neisseriaceae, *Int J Syst Bacteriol*, **36:** 323–32.

Rowbotham TJ, 1983, Rapid identification of *Streptobacillus moniliformis, Lancet*, **2:** 567.

Savage DD, Kagan RL et al., 1977, *Cardiobacterium hominis* endocarditis: description of two patients and characterization of the organism, *J Clin Microbiol*, **5:** 75–80.

Savage NL, Joiner GN, Florey DW, 1981, Clinical, microbiological, and histological manifestations of *Streptobacillus moniliformis*-induced arthritis in mice, *Infect Immun*, **34:** 605–9.

Schottmuller H, 1914, Zur Atiologie und Klinik der bisskrankheit (Ratten-, Katzen, eichhornchen-bisskrankheit), *Dermatol Wochenschr*, **58, suppl 7:** 77–103.

Sehgal VN, Jain AK, 1987, Tissue section donovan bodies identification through slow-Giemsa overnight technique, *Dermatologica (Basel)*, **174:** 228–31.

Shanson DC, Pratt J, Green P, 1985, Comparison of media with and without 'Panmede' for the isolation of *Streptobacillus moniliformis* from blood cultures and observations on the inhibiting effect of sodium polyanethol sulphonate, *J Med Microbiol*, **19:** 181–6.

Shanson DC, Gazzard BG et al., 1983, *Streptobacillus moniliformis* isolated from blood in four cases of Haverhill fever, *Lancet*, **2:** 92–4.

Sivendra R, Lo HS, Lim KT, 1975, Identification of *Chromobacterium violaceum*: pigmented and non-pigmented strains, *J Gen Microbiol*, **90:** 21–31.

Slotnick IJ, Doughtery M, 1964, Fluorescent antibody detection of human occurrence of an unclassified bacterial group causing endocarditis, *J Infect Dis*, **114:** 503–5.

Sneath PHA, 1956a, Cultural and biochemical characteristics of the genus *Chromobacterium, J Gen Microbiol*, **15:** 70.

Sneath PHA, 1956b, The change from polar to peritrichous flagellation in *Chromobacterium* sp., *J Gen Microbiol*, **15:** 99–105.

Sneath PHA, 1960, A review of the genus *Chromobacterium* and of chromobacterial infections of man and animals, *Iowa State J Sci*, **34:** 243–500.

Sneath PHA, Buckland FE, 1959, The serology and pathogenicity of the genus *Chromobacterium, J Gen Microbiol*, **20:** 414–25.

Speller DCE, Prout BJ, Saunders CF, 1968, Subacute bacterial endocarditis caused by a micro-organism resembling *Haemophilus aphrophilus, J Pathol Bacteriol*, **95:** 191–8.

Strangeways WI, 1933, Rats and carriers of *Streptobacillus moniliformis, J Pathol Bacteriol*, **37:** 45–51.

Sykes RB, Cimarusti CM et al., 1981, Monocyclic β-lactam antibiotics produced by bacteria, *Nature (London)*, **291:** 489–91.

Thomison JB, 1951, Primary isolation of *Donovania granulomatis* by chick brain inoculation, and induction of cerebral miliary granulomata, *Proc Soc Exp Biol Med*, **77:** 557–8.

Tønjum T, Bukholm G, Bøvre K, 1989, Differentiation of some species of Neisseriaceae and other bacterial groups by DNA–DNA hybridization, *Acta Pathol Microbiol Immunol Scand*, **97:** 395–405.

Tønjum T, Hagen N, Bøvre K, 1985, Identification of *Eikenella corrodens* and *Cardiobacterium hominis* by genetic transformation, *Acta Pathol Microbiol Immunol Scand*, **B93:** 389–94.

Tucker DN, Slotnick IJ et al., 1962, Endocarditis caused by a pasteurella-like organism. Report of four cases, *N Engl J Med*, **267:** 913–16.

Tunnicliff R, 1916, Streptothrix in bronchopneumonia of rats similar to that in rat-bite fever, *J Infect Dis*, **19:** 767–71.

Ueda H, Nakajima H et al., 1994, FR901228, a novel antitumor bicyclic depsipeptide produced by *Chromobacterium violaceum* No.968.I. Taxonomy, fermentation, isolation, physico-chemical and biological properties, and antitumor activity, *J Antibiot*, **47**: 301–10.

Vogt K, Klefisch F et al., 1994, Antibacterial efficacy of ciprofloxacin in a case of endocarditis due to *Cardiobacterium hominis*, *Zentrabl Bakteriol*, **281**: 80–4.

Wormser GP, Bottone EJ, 1983, *Cardiobacterium hominis*: review of microbiologic and clinical features, *Rev Infect Dis*, **5**: 680–91.

Wormser GP, Bottone EJ et al., 1978, *Cardiobacterium hominis*: review of prior infections and report of endocarditis on a fascia lata prosthetic heart valve, *Am J Med Sci*, **276**: 117–26.

Chapter 53

ACINETOBACTER

K J Towner

1 GENUS DEFINITION

Acinetobacters are short, stout gram-negative (but sometimes difficult to destain) coccobacilli, with a DNA G + C content of 39–47 mol%. Strictly aerobic, non-motile, catalase-positive and oxidase-negative. Frequently capsulate. Good growth occurs on complex media (nutrient agar, trypticase soya agar) between 20 and 30°C without growth factor requirements. Most strains of *Acinetobacter* can grow in a simple mineral medium containing ammonium salts and a single carbon and energy source such as acetate, lactate or pyruvate, but only rarely with glucose. Some strains form acid from sugars, but many do not. Nitrates are reduced only rarely. Crucially, extracted DNA is able to transform mutant *Acinetobacter* strain BD413 *trpE27* to the wild-type phenotype. Saprophytes: parasites and occasional pathogens of man and other animals.

2 INTRODUCTION AND HISTORICAL PERSPECTIVE

The genus *Acinetobacter* has suffered a long history of taxonomic change. The first recognizable member of the group to be described was a soil organism isolated by Beijerinck in 1911, and named by him as *Micrococcus calcoaceticus* (Baumann, Doudoroff and Stanier 1968). Since then, at least 15 other 'generic' names have been used to describe the organisms now classified as members of the genus, of which the most common are *Bacterium anitratum*, *Herellea vaginicola*, *Mima polymorpha*, *Achromobacter*, *Alcaligenes*, 'B5W', *Moraxella glucidolytica* and *Moraxella lwoffii* (Henriksen 1973).

The original concept of the genus *Acinetobacter* was proposed by microbiologists working in France (Brisou and Prévot 1954), but it included a heterogenous collection of non-motile, gram-negative, oxidase-positive (*Moraxella*) and oxidase-negative saprophytes that could be distinguished from other bacteria by their lack of pigmentation (Ingram and Shewan 1960). The nutritional studies of Baumann, Doudoroff and Stanier (1968) showed clearly that the oxidase-negative strains differed from the oxidase-positive strains of the genus *Moraxella*, and in 1971 the Subcommittee on the Taxonomy of *Moraxella* and Allied Bacteria recommended that the genus *Acinetobacter* should include only the oxidase-negative strains (Lessel 1971). This division has been supported by the use of transformation tests (Juni 1972), which still form the basis for inclusion of individual isolates within the genus.

3 HABITATS

Acinetobacters are ubiquitous, free-living saprophytes found in soil, water, foods and the clinical environment (Towner, Bergogne-Bérézin and Fewson 1991). They can be found on a range of dry or moist inanimate surfaces and as commensals on the skin of man and animals. In recent years, antibiotic-resistant strains have also been recognized as important pathogens involved in outbreaks of hospital infection, particularly in high-dependency or intensive care units. Members of the genus have been isolated from a wide range of clinical specimens, including tracheal aspirates, blood cultures, cerebrospinal fluid and pus. The ubiquitous occurrence of acinetobacters means that isolates from clinical specimens are often (sometimes erroneously) considered to be contaminants. Although members of the genus are distributed widely, there is a significant population difference between the species found in clinical and other environments (see sections 10 and 13, pp. 1232 and 1234).

4 MORPHOLOGY

Acinetobacters are short, plump, gram-negative bacilli, typically 1.0–1.5 μm × 1.5–2.5 μm in the exponential phase of growth, but becoming more coccoid (0.6–0.8 μm × 1.0–1.5 μm) in the stationary phase (Figs 53.1 and 53.2). Apparent 'diplococci' with bipolar staining normally predominate in stationary phase broth cultures or following growth on solid media, but chains of cells may be observed in broth cultures growing exponentially. A proportion of cells tends to retain the methyl violet in Gram's stain. Members of the genus are non-motile and non-flagellate in the conventional sense, although a twitching motility has been described by Lautrop (1961). Fimbriae are often present and many strains are capsulate.

5 CULTURAL CHARACTERISTICS

Most clinical isolates grow at 37°C (often up to 42°C),

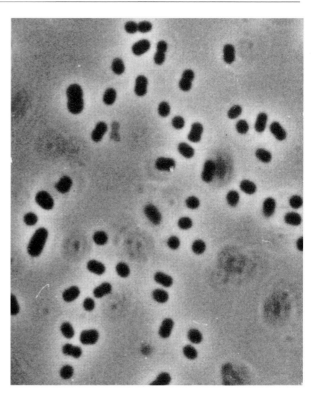

Fig. 53.2 Stationary phase of growth of *Acinetobacter* spp. in liquid medium (phase contrast × 2600). (From photographs kindly supplied by Dr NJ Palleroni).

but many environmental isolates will grow only at lower temperatures. A general cultivation temperature of 30°C has been recommended (Hugh 1978), but a lower temperature or combination of temperatures may be advisable, depending on the type and origin of the specimen. Members of the genus grow well on most ordinary solid media, such as nutrient agar and trypticase soya agar, forming smooth, sometimes mucoid, pale yellow to greyish white colonies, normally about 1–2 mm in diameter. Some environmental strains that produce a diffusible brown pigment have been described (Pagel and Seyfried 1976). Most clinical isolates, but not all environmental isolates, grow on MacConkey agar, on which saccharolytic strains form pink colonies. A few strains produce haemolysis on blood agar. Surface spreading associated with twitching motility can be demonstrated only on certain media (Lautrop 1974, Barker and Maxted 1975). In nutrient broth cultures there is uniform turbidity with a variable amount of powdery, granular or viscous deposit. Some strains liquefy gelatin slowly.

6 METABOLISM

Acinetobacter spp. are strict aerobes and are broadly typical of other gram-negative eubacteria, but with a number of distinctive metabolic features that support the versatile lifestyle of this genus (Juni 1978). Most strains of *Acinetobacter* do not have any growth factor requirements and resemble the saprophytic pseudomonads in being able to use any of a large number of

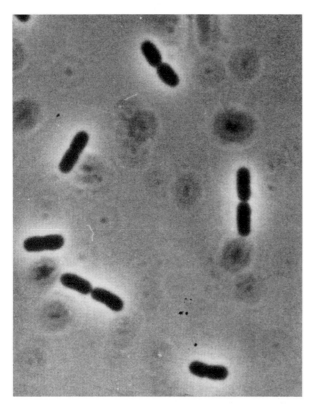

Fig. 53.1 Logarithmic phase of growth of *Acinetobacter* spp. in liquid medium (phase contrast × 2600). (From photographs kindly supplied by Dr NJ Palleroni).

organic carbon and energy sources, together with a nitrogen source, in an otherwise mineral medium. Although the utilization of carbohydrates is relatively uncommon, a major feature of the genus is that many strains can metabolize a wide range of compounds, including aliphatic alcohols, some amino acids, decarboxylic and fatty acids, unbranched hydrocarbons, sugars and many relatively recalcitrant aromatic compounds such as benzoate, mandelate, *n*-hexadecane, cyclohexanol and 2,3-butanediol (see Towner, Bergogne-Bérézin and Fewson 1991). Most strains are unable to utilize glucose as a carbon source, but many strains are able to acidify media containing sugars, including glucose, arabinose, cellobiose, galactose, lactose, maltose, mannose, ribose and xylose, via an aldose dehydrogenase. Strains that possess this property (considered previously to be of major taxonomic significance, but now supplanted in importance by the developments described in section 10, p. 1232) will acidify the corresponding ammonium salt or Hugh and Leifson sugars in the presence of oxygen; acid is formed in peptone water sugars containing glucose, arabinose and xylose, but reactions may be delayed. Although most acinetobacters are unable to reduce nitrate to nitrite in conventional assays, some strains can use both nitrate and nitrite as nitrogen sources by means of an assimilatory nitrate reductase. All acinetobacters are oxidase-negative, since they lack cytochrome *c*.

7 GENETIC MECHANISMS

7.1 Transformation

This process was demonstrated by Juni and Janik (1969) with *A. calcoaceticus* strain BD4 and its microencapsulated *trpE27* mutant derivative BD413. Transformation of strain BD413 *trpE27* to the wild-type phenotype now forms the basis of the genetic test for identifying members of the genus (Juni 1972). Although natural genetic competence to act as a recipient strain for transformation seems to be a somewhat rare phenomenon amongst *Acinetobacter* spp. (Juni 1978), strain BD413 has an exceptionally high efficiency of transformation (0.5–0.7%) and has been used in a wide range of advanced molecular procedures that have allowed detailed fine-structure genetic investigations of the chromosomal organization and metabolic regulation of this strain (Ornston and Neidle 1991).

7.2 Transduction

A temperate phage (designated P78) which lysogenizes its host and is capable of mediating low-frequency generalized transduction has been described (Herman and Juni 1974), but this phage is specific for its host strain and failed to lysogenize 389 other independently isolated strains of *Acinetobacter*, including strain BD413. Neither P78 nor any other bacteriophage has been used extensively for genetic studies in *Acinetobacter* spp.

7.3 Conjugation

Conjugation mediated by broad host-range plasmids has been used to mobilize the chromosome of *Acinetobacter* strain EBF 65/65 (Towner and Vivian 1976, Hinchliffe and Vivian 1980). Such chromosomal transfer occurs only on solid surfaces, not in liquid matings. Very little is known about the precise nature and events involved in mobilization of the chromosome, but the system has been used successfully to map a number of different mutations on a circular chromosomal linkage group in strain EBF 65/65 (Towner 1978, Vivian 1991).

7.4 Plasmids and transposons

Plasmids and transposons play an important role in the biology of *Acinetobacter* spp. (Towner 1991). Most (>80%) of *Acinetobacter* isolates appear to carry multiple indigenous plasmids of variable molecular size (Gerner-Smidt 1989, Seifert et al. 1994a). It should be noted that problems in isolating plasmid DNA from *Acinetobacter* spp. have been reported, often because of unappreciated difficulties in lysing the cell wall of these organisms. Few studies have demonstrated plasmid-mediated transfer of antibiotic resistance genes, but this may simply reflect the absence of a suitable test system for detecting such transfer. Transposons probably play an important role in ensuring that novel genes can become established in the *Acinetobacter* gene pool, and there have been several reports of chromosomally located transposons carrying multiple antibiotic resistance genes in clinical isolates of *Acinetobacter* spp. (see Towner 1991).

8 CELL WALL AND ENVELOPE COMPOSITION; ANTIGENIC STRUCTURE

Members of the genus *Acinetobacter* have a cell wall and outer membrane that have essentially the same composition as those of most other gram-negative bacteria, but with some special properties that influence the permeability properties of the cells (see Borneleit and Kleber 1991). There are also numerous reports of superficial material covering the outer surface of acinetobacters, including protein S layers, polysaccharide capsules and slime (Obana, Nishino and Tanino 1985, Borneleit and Kleber 1991), and these additional surface layers are of tremendous importance in determining the surface properties of the cells.

So far as antigenic structure is concerned, early studies by Marcus et al. (1969) identified 28 different capsular types by means of capsular reactions or immunofluorescence. More recent work involving chequerboard tube agglutinations and reciprocal cross-absorptions with polyclonal rabbit immune sera against heated cells has allowed the delineation of a large number of different serovars in 2 of the main species of *Acinetobacter* associated with human infection (Traub 1989, 1990, Traub and Leonhard 1994).

9 SUSCEPTIBILITY TO ANTIMICROBIAL AGENTS

Early studies of the genus made the observation that essentially all strains were resistant to penicillin, ampicillin, first-generation cephalosporins and chloramphenicol, whereas carbenicillin, tetracyclines (particularly minocycline, oxytetracycline and chlortetracycline), aminoglycosides and newer antibiotics were active against most strains. In general, this remains the situation with environmental isolates. However, amongst clinical isolates, it has become apparent that one of the most striking features of the genus is the ability to develop antibiotic resistance extremely rapidly in response to challenge with new antibiotics. Thus many *Acinetobacter* isolates from hospitals now exhibit resistance to most available antibiotics, including the latest broad-spectrum cephalosporins, 4-fluoroquinolones and, to some extent, the carbapenems. Biochemical and genetic mechanisms of resistance to these antibiotics amongst *Acinetobacter* spp. are currently the subject of much research. Currently, it is not clear how infections caused by these organisms will be controlled once complete resistance to these 3 groups of antibiotics has evolved.

10 CLASSIFICATION

Until recently the genus *Acinetobacter* was included in the family Neisseriaceae (Juni 1984), with one species,

A. calcoaceticus, comprising 2 varieties, var. *anitratus* (formerly *Herellea vaginicola*) and var. *lwoffii* (formerly *Mima polymorpha*). Further taxonomic developments have resulted in the current proposal that members of the genus should be classified in the new family Moraxellaceae, which includes *Moraxella, Acinetobacter, Psychrobacter* and related organisms (Rossau et al. 1991), and which constitutes a discrete phylometric branch in superfamily II of the Proteobacteria on the basis of 16S rRNA studies and rRNA–DNA hybridization assays (van Landschoot, Rossau and De Ley 1986, Rossau et al. 1989).

Extensive studies of DNA–DNA relationships within the genus *Acinetobacter* have resulted in the recognition, to date, of 19 DNA homology groups (genomic species). There are some minor discrepancies in the numbering schemes proposed for genomic species by different laboratories, and a definitive numbering scheme has yet to be finally agreed, but 7 of the genomic species have been given formal species names which form the basis of current taxonomy (Table 53.1).

The main species associated with outbreaks of nosocomial infection is *A. baumannii* (Bouvet and Grimont 1987), although other genomic species, particularly *Acinetobacter* sp. 3, *A. johnsonii* and *A. lwoffii*, have also been associated with infection in man (Table 53.2). Genomic species 1, 2, 3 and 13TU have been shown to have an extremely close relationship and it has been suggested (Gerner-Smidt, Tjernberg and Ursing 1991)

Table 53.1 Delineation of *Acinetobacter* genomic species

Species name	Genomic species number according to	
	Bouvet and Grimont (1986) Bouvet and Jeanjean (1989)	**Tjernberg and Ursing (1989)**
A. calcoaceticus	1	1
A. baumannii	2	2
	3	3
	ug[a]	13
A. haemolyticus	4	4
A. junii	5	5
	6	6
A. johnsonii	7	7
A. lwoffii	8	8
	9	8
	10	10
	11	11
A. radioresistens	(12)[b]	12
	13	14
	14	nt[c]
	15	nt[c]
	16	ug[a]
	17	nt[c]
	nt[c]	15

[a]Ungrouped.
[b]Unpublished result.
[c]Not tested.

that this group of genomic species, which includes the majority of clinically significant isolates, should be referred to as the '*A. calcoaceticus–A. baumannii* complex'. This may be a particularly useful approach for routine clinical diagnostic laboratories to adopt since there is currently no unambiguous rapid phenotypic method to distinguish between the genomic species in the complex (see section 11, p. 1233). Very little is known about the possible clinical significance of genomic species other than those mentioned above and further detailed investigations are required.

11 LABORATORY ISOLATION AND IDENTIFICATION

Acinetobacters can be grown readily on common laboratory media such as nutrient agar and trypticase soya agar, although defined media consisting of a mineral base and one or more carbon sources have been used for specific purposes. For direct isolation from clinical specimens it is normal to use a selective medium that suppresses the growth of other micro-organisms. A selective medium containing bile salts, sugars and bromocresol purple (Mandel, Wright and McKinnon 1964) is available commercially as Herellea Agar. A novel antibiotic-containing selective medium, Leeds Acinetobacter Medium, that combines selectivity with differential characteristics has also been described (Jawad et al. 1994) and has been found to be useful for the recovery of most *Acinetobacter* spp. from clinical and environmental sources. For environmental screening, especially in areas where acinetobacters are present only in low numbers, it may also be useful to use enrichment cultivation in a liquid mineral medium containing a single carbon and energy source, ammonium or nitrate salt as the nitrogen source, and with a final pH of 5.5–6.0. Vigorous shak-

ing during incubation is needed so that any acinetobacters present can outgrow any pseudomonads (Baumann 1968).

Currently there is no easy method for laboratory identification of the different genomic species delineated by DNA–DNA hybridization. Many reports of acinetobacters in the scientific and medical literature still contain incorrect or incomplete identifications of genomic species. Commercially available identification systems are inadequate for this purpose and have incomplete databases. Various phenotypic schemes for identification have been proposed (see Gerner-Smidt, Tjernberg and Ursing 1991, Kämpfer, Tjernberg and Ursing 1993), but these either lack specificity or are time-consuming with large numbers of different biochemical tests. The '*A. calcoaceticus–A. baumannii* complex' (see section 10, p. 1232) contains isolates that are mostly glucose-acidifying, and the 'complex' therefore corresponds quite well with the *A. calcoaceticus* var. *anitratus* designation (Juni 1984) that was often used before the latest taxonomic developments. The majority of glucose-negative, non-haemolytic strains found in clinical specimens are identified mainly as *A. lwoffii*, *A. johnsonii* or *Acinetobacter* sp. 12 and most of the haemolytic isolates as *A. haemolyticus* or *Acinetobacter* sp. 6. Molecular fingerprinting methods for rapid identification of the different genomic species are currently in the process of development and evaluation.

12 TYPING METHODS

Early attempts to develop typing systems for *Acinetobacter* spp. have been reviewed previously (Bouvet 1991). Conventional phenotypic typing systems such as biotyping (e.g. Bouvet et al. 1990), phage-typing (e.g. Vieu, Minck and Bergogne-Bérézin 1979), sero-

Table 53.2 *Acinetobacter* genomic species associated with infection in man

Genomic species	Number of isolates from each specimen type				Total
	Tracheal aspirate	Blood culture (CV line)	Wound swab	Other sites	
A. baumannii	208	113	70	35	426
sp. 3	6	24	10	15	55
A. johnsonii	0	19	2	8	29
A. lwoffii	2	12	2	5	21
A. junii	0	7	0	4	11
A. haemolyticus	0	1	2	6	9
sp. 10	0	6	1	2	9
sp. 11	1	0	1	2	4
sp. 12	0	3	0	0	3
sp. 6	0	1	0	0	1
Unidentified	1	5	2	8	16
Total	218	191	90	85	584

Data taken from Seifert et al. 1993.

typing (e.g. Traub and Leonhard 1994) and bacteriocin typing (Andrews 1986) have proved generally to be rather time-consuming or complicated to perform, or to work well only with strains isolated from a particular geographical location. Recent attention has focused upon the use of molecular fingerprinting techniques, including analysis of plasmid profiles (e.g. Gerner-Smidt and Tjernberg 1993, Seifert et al. 1994a, 1994b), restriction endonuclease digestion and pulsed-field gel electrophoresis of total chromosomal DNA (e.g. Gouby et al. 1992, Struelens et al. 1993), random amplified polymorphic DNA profiles (e.g. Gräser et al. 1993, Struelens et al. 1993), ribotyping (Gerner-Smidt 1992), cell envelope and outer-membrane protein profiles (e.g. Dijkshoorn, Michel and Degener 1987, Dijkshoorn et al. 1987), or multilocus enzyme electrophoretic typing (Thurm and Ritter 1993). These methods have all been used successfully to investigate the epidemiology of particular outbreaks of infection, but no single system has so far gained overall acceptance for typing *Acinetobacter* spp. This area is still the subject of much ongoing research.

12.1 Bacteriophages

Numerous bacteriophages active against specific strains of *Acinetobacter* have been isolated (Ackermann, Brochu and Konjin 1994). Typically, most *Acinetobacter* phages are lytic and are restricted in their host range to the original strain of *Acinetobacter* on which they were isolated. One possible explanation for the narrow host specificity observed with *Acinetobacter* phages may be the large number of different surface antigens found in this genus (Marcus et al. 1969).

13 ROLE IN NORMAL FLORA OF MAN

Acinetobacters are normal inhabitants of human skin and can be isolated from the axillae, groin, toe-webs and antecubital fossa of about 25% of the population (Taplin, Rebell and Zaias 1963, Somerville and Noble 1970). However, although the genus, taken as a whole, is distributed widely, there are significant population differences between the genomic species found as part of the normal human flora in clinical and other environments. Each population appears to be characterized by predominant groups of genomic species; thus *A. baumannii* and *Acinetobacter* sp. 3 can be isolated from the skin and numerous body sites of infected or colonized patients in hospital, but are iso-

lated only rarely from the non-hospitalized population, whereas *A. lwoffii*, *A. johnsonii* and *Acinetobacter* sp. 12 seem to be the predominant natural inhabitants of human skin in non-clinical environments. Other genomic species are found only very rarely as part of the normal flora of man.

14 PATHOGENICITY AND VIRULENCE FACTORS

Although considered to be relatively low-grade pathogens, characteristics of *Acinetobacter* spp. that may enhance the virulence of strains involved in infections include: the presence of a polysaccharide capsule; the property of adhesion to human epithelial cells in the presence of fimbriae or capsular polysaccharide, or both; the production of enzymes that may damage tissue lipids; and the lipopolysaccharide (LPS) component of the cell wall and the presence of lipid A. In common with other gram-negative bacteria, *Acinetobacter* spp. produce an LPS responsible for lethal toxicity in mice, pyrogenicity in rabbits, and a positive reaction in the *Limulus* amoebocyte lysate test. The production of endotoxin in vivo is probably responsible for the disease symptoms observed during acinetobacter septicaemia.

Experimental studies in a mouse model of acinetobacter pneumonia have shown that mixed infections combining other bacteria with *Acinetobacter* spp. are more virulent than infections with *Acinetobacter* spp. alone (Obana 1986). Slime produced by the *Acinetobacter* strain studied was considered to be the main factor responsible for the enhancement of virulence in mixed infections, but few acinetobacters produce slime. The same study demonstrated that slime was associated with cytotoxicity against neutrophils and inhibition of the migration of neutrophils into peritoneal exudate of mice. No correlation was observed between the amount of slime produced and the degree of virulence.

The ability of a bacterium to obtain the necessary iron for growth in the human body is also an important virulence determinant, and some strains of *Acinetobacter* have been shown to produce siderophores, such as aerobactin, and iron-repressible outermembrane receptor proteins (Smith et al. 1990, Echenique et al. 1992, Actis et al. 1993).

For further information about *Acinetobacter*, see Juni (1978), Towner, Bergogne-Bérézin and Fewson (1991) and Bergogne-Bérézin, Joly-Guillou and Towner (1996).

REFERENCES

Ackermann HW, Brochu G, Konjin HPE, 1994, Classification of *Acinetobacter* phages, *Arch Virol*, **135**: 345–54.

Actis JA, Tomasky ME et al., 1993, Effect of iron-limiting conditions on growth of clinical isolates of *Acinetobacter baumannii*, *J Clin Microbiol*, **31**: 2812–15.

Andrews HJ, 1986, Acinetobacter bacteriocin typing, *J Hosp Infect*, **9**: 169–75.

Barker J, Maxted H, 1975, Observations on the growth and

movement of *Acinetobacter* on semi-solid media, *J Med Microbiol*, **8**: 443–6.

Baumann P, 1968, Isolation of *Acinetobacter* from soil and water, *J Bacteriol*, **96**: 39–42.

Baumann P, Doudoroff M, Stanier RY, 1968, A study of the *Moraxella* group. II. Oxidase-negative species (genus *Acinetobacter*), *J Bacteriol*, **95**: 1520–41.

Bergogne-Bérézin E, Joly-Guillou ML, Towner KJ, 1996, Acinetobacter: *Microbiology, Epidemiology, Infections, Management*, CRC Press, Boca Raton.

Borneleit P, Kleber H-P, 1991, The outer membrane of *Acinetobacter*: structure–function relationships, *The Biology of* Acinetobacter: *Taxonomy, Clinical Importance, Molecular Biology, Physiology, Industrial Relevance*, eds Towner KJ, Bergogne-Bérézin E, Fewson CA, Plenum Press, New York, 259–71.

Bouvet PJM, 1991, Typing of *Acinetobacter*, *The Biology of* Acinetobacter: *Taxonomy, Clinical Importance, Molecular Biology, Physiology, Industrial Relevance*, eds Towner KJ, Bergogne-Bérézin E, Fewson CA, Plenum Press, New York, 37–51.

Bouvet PJM, Grimont PAD, 1986, Taxonomy of the genus *Acinetobacter* with the recognition of *Acinetobacter baumannii* sp. nov., *Acinetobacter haemolyticus* sp.nov., *Acinetobacter johnsonii* sp. nov. and *Acinetobacter junii* sp. nov. and emended descriptions of *Acinetobacter calcoaceticus* and *Acinetobacter lwoffii*, *Int J Syst Bacteriol*, **36**: 228–40.

Bouvet PJM, Grimont PAD, 1987, Identification and biotyping of clinical isolates of *Acinetobacter*, *Ann Inst Pasteur/Microbiol (Paris)*, **138**: 569–78.

Bouvet PJM, Jeanjean S, 1989, Delineation of new proteolytic genospecies in the genus *Acinetobacter*, *Res Microbiol*, **140**: 291–9.

Bouvet PJM, Jeanjean S et al., 1990, Species, biotype, and bacteriophage type determinations compared with cell envelope protein profiles for typing *Acinetobacter* strains, *J Clin Microbiol*, **28**: 170–6.

Brisou J, Prévot AR, 1954, Études de systématique bacterienne. X. Révision des espèces réunies dans le genre *Achromobacter*, *Ann Inst Pasteur (Paris)*, **86**: 722–8.

Dijkshoorn L, Michel MF, Degener JE, 1987, Cell envelope protein profiles of *Acinetobacter calcoaceticus* strains isolated in hospitals, *J Med Microbiol*, **23**: 313–19.

Dijkshoorn L, van Vianen W et al., 1987, Typing of *Acinetobacter calcoaceticus* strains isolated from hospital patients by cell envelope protein profiles, *Epidemiol Infect*, **99**: 659–67.

Echenique JR, Arienti H et al., 1992, Characterization of a high-affinity iron transport system in *Acinetobacter baumannii*, *J Bacteriol*, **174**: 767–9.

Gerner-Smidt P, 1989, Frequency of plasmids in strains of *Acinetobacter calcoaceticus*, *J Hosp Infect*, **14**: 23–8.

Gerner-Smidt P, 1992, Ribotyping of the *Acinetobacter calcoaceticus–Acinetobacter baumannii* complex, *J Clin Microbiol*, **30**: 2680–5.

Gerner-Smidt P, Tjernberg I, 1993, *Acinetobacter* in Denmark: II. Molecular studies of the *Acinetobacter calcoaceticus–Acinetobacter baumannii* complex, *Acta Pathol Microbiol Immunol Scand*, **101**: 826–32.

Gerner-Smidt P, Tjernberg I, Ursing J, 1991, Reliability of phenotypic tests for identification of *Acinetobacter* species, *J Clin Microbiol*, **29**: 277–82.

Gouby A, Carles-Nurit MJ et al., 1992, Use of pulsed-field gel electrophoresis for investigation of hospital outbreaks of *Acinetobacter baumannii*, *J Clin Microbiol*, **30**: 1588–91.

Gräser Y, Klare I et al., 1993, Epidemiological study of an *Acinetobacter baumannii* outbreak by using polymerase chain reaction fingerprinting, *J Clin Microbiol*, **31**: 2417–20.

Henriksen SD, 1973, *Moraxella, Acinetobacter*, and the *Mimeae*, *Bacteriol Rev*, **37**: 522–61.

Herman NJ, Juni E, 1974, Isolation and characterisation of a generalised transducing bacteriophage for *Acinetobacter*, *J Virol*, **13**: 46–52.

Hinchliffe E, Vivian A, 1980, Naturally occurring plasmids in *Acinetobacter calcoaceticus*: a P class R factor of restricted host range, *J Gen Microbiol*, **116**: 75–80.

Hugh R, 1978, Classical methods for isolation and identification of glucose nonfermenting gram-negative rods, *Glucose Nonfermenting Gram-negative Bacteria in Clinical Microbiology*, ed. Gilardi GL, CRC Press, West Palm Beach, FL, 2.

Ingram M, Shewan JW, 1960, Introductory reflections on the *Pseudomonas-Achromobacter* group, *J Appl Bacteriol*, **23**: 373–8.

Jawad A, Hawkey PM et al., 1994, Description of Leeds Acinetobacter Medium, a new selective and differential medium for isolation of clinically important *Acinetobacter* spp., and comparison with Herellea agar and Holton's agar, *J Clin Microbiol*, **32**: 2353–8.

Juni E, 1972, Interspecies transformation of *Acinetobacter*: genetic evidence for a ubiquitous genus, *J Bacteriol*, **112**: 917–31.

Juni E, 1978, Genetics and physiology of *Acinetobacter*, *Annu Rev Microbiol*, **32**: 349–71.

Juni E, 1984, Genus III. *Acinetobacter* Brisou et Prévot 1954, *Bergey's Manual of Systematic Bacteriology*, vol 1, 9th edn, eds Krieg NR, Holt JG, Williams and Wilkins, Baltimore, 303–7.

Juni E, Janik A, 1969, Transformation of *Acinetobacter calcoaceticus* (*Bacterium anitratum*), *J Bacteriol*, **98**: 281–8.

Kämpfer P, Tjernberg I, Ursing J, 1993, Numerical classification and identification of *Acinetobacter* genomic species, *J Appl Bacteriol*, **75**: 259–68.

van Landschoot A, Rossau R, De Ley J, 1986, Intra- and intergeneric similarities of the ribosomal ribonucleic acid cistrons of *Acinetobacter*, *Int J Syst Bacteriol*, **36**: 150–60.

Lautrop H, 1961, *Bacterium anitratum* transferred to the genus *Cytophaga*, *Int Bull Bacteriol Nomencl Taxon*, **11**: 107–8.

Lautrop H, 1974, Genus IV. *Acinetobacter* Brisou and Prévot 1954, 727, *Bergey's Manual of Determinative Bacteriology*, 8th edn, eds Buchanan RE, Gibbons NE, Williams and Wilkins, Baltimore, 436–8.

Lessel EF, 1971, Minutes of the Subcommittee on the Taxonomy of *Moraxella* and Allied Bacteria, *Int J Syst Bacteriol*, **21**: 213–14.

Mandel AD, Wright K, McKinnon JM, 1964, Selective medium for isolation of *Mima* and *Herellea* organisms, *J Bacteriol*, **88**: 1524–5.

Marcus BB, Samuels SB et al., 1969, A serologic study of *Herellea vaginicola* and its identification by immunofluorescent staining, *Am J Clin Pathol*, **52**: 309–19.

Obana Y, 1986, Pathogenic significance of *Acinetobacter calcoaceticus*: analysis of experimental infection in mice, *Microbiol Immunol*, **30**: 645–57.

Obana Y, Nishino T, Tanino T, 1985, *In vitro* and *in vivo* activities of antimicrobial agents against *Acinetobacter calcoaceticus*, *J Antimicrob Chemother*, **15**: 441–8.

Ornston LN, Neidle EL, 1991, Evolution of genes for the ß-ketoadipate pathway in *Acinetobacter calcoaceticus*, *The Biology of* Acinetobacter: *Taxonomy, Clinical Importance, Molecular Biology, Physiology, Industrial Relevance*, eds Towner KJ, Bergogne-Bérézin E, Fewson CA, Plenum Press, New York, 201–37.

Pagel JE, Seyfried PL, 1976, Numerical taxonomy of aquatic acinetobacter isolates, *J Gen Microbiol*, **95**: 220–32.

Rossau R, van den Bussche G et al., 1989, Ribosomal ribonucleic acid cistron similarities and deoxyribonucleic acid homologies of *Neisseria, Kingella, Eikenella, Alysiella*, and Centers for Disease Control Groups EF-4 and M-5 in the emended family Neisseriaceae, *Int J Syst Bacteriol*, **39**: 185–98.

Rossau R, van Landschoot A et al., 1991, Taxonomy of Moraxellaceae fam.nov., a new bacterial family to accommodate the genera *Moraxella, Acinetobacter*, and *Psychrobacter* and related organisms, *Int J Syst Bacteriol*, **41**: 310–19.

Seifert H, Schulze A et al., 1994a, Plasmid DNA fingerprinting of *Acinetobacter* species other than *Acinetobacter baumannii*, *J Clin Microbiol*, **32**: 82–6.

Seifert H, Schulze A et al., 1994b, Comparison of four different typing methods for epidemiologic typing of *Acinetobacter baumannii*, *J Clin Microbiol*, **32**: 1816–19.

Smith AW, Freeman S et al., 1990, Characterization of a siderophore from *Acinetobacter calcoaceticus*, *FEMS Microbiol Lett*, **70**: 29–32.

Somerville DA, Noble WC, 1970, A note on the gram-negative bacilli of human skin, *Eur J Clin Biol Res*, **40**: 669–70.

Struelens MJ, Carlier E et al., 1993, Nosocomial colonisation and infection with multiresistant *Acinetobacter baumannii*: outbreak delineation using DNA macrorestriction analysis and PCR-fingerprinting, *J Hosp Infect*, **25**: 15–32.

Taplin D, Rebell G, Zaias N, 1963, The human skin as a source of *Mima-Herellea* infections, *JAMA*, **186**: 952–4.

Thurm V, Ritter E, 1993, Genetic diversity and clonal relationships of *Acinetobacter baumannii* strains isolated in a neonatal ward: epidemiological investigations by allozyme, whole-cell protein and antibiotic resistance analysis, *Epidemiol Infect*, **111**: 491–8.

Tjernberg I, Ursing J, 1989, Clinical strains of *Acinetobacter* classified by DNA–DNA hybridization, *Acta Pathol Microbiol Immunol Scand*, **97**: 596–605.

Towner KJ, 1978, Chromosome mapping in *Acinetobacter calcoaceticus*, *J Gen Microbiol*, **104**: 175–80.

Towner KJ, 1991, Plasmid and transposon behaviour in *Acinetobacter*, *The Biology of* Acinetobacter: *Taxonomy, Clinical Importance, Molecular Biology, Physiology, Industrial Relevance*, eds Towner KJ, Bergogne-Bérézin E, Fewson CA, Plenum Press, New York, 149–67.

Towner KJ, Bergogne-Bérézin E, Fewson CA, eds, 1991, *The Biology of* Acinetobacter: *Taxonomy, Clinical Importance, Molecular Biology, Physiology, Industrial Relevance*, Plenum Press, New York.

Towner KJ, Vivian A, 1976, RP4-mediated conjugation in *Acinetobacter calcoaceticus*, *J Gen Microbiol*, **93**: 355–60.

Traub WH, 1989, *Acinetobacter baumannii* serotyping for delineation of outbreaks of nosocomial cross-infection, *J Clin Microbiol*, **27**: 2713–16.

Traub WH, 1990, Serotyping of clinical isolates of acinetobacter: serovars of genospecies 3, *Zentralbl Bakteriol*, **273**: 12–23.

Traub WH, Leonhard B, 1994, Serotyping of *Acinetobacter baumannii* and genospecies 3: an update, *Med Microbiol Lett*, **3**: 120–7.

Vieu JF, Minck R, Bergogne-Bérézin E, 1979, Bactériophages et lysotypie de *Acinetobacter*, *Ann Inst Pasteur Microbiol*, **130A**: 405–6.

Vivian A, 1991, Genetic organization of *Acinetobacter*, *The Biology of* Acinetobacter: *Taxonomy, Clinical Importance, Molecular Biology, Physiology, Industrial Relevance*, eds Towner KJ, Bergogne-Bérézin E, Fewson CA, Plenum Press, New York. 191–200.

Chapter 54

CAMPYLOBACTER, ARCOBACTER AND HELICOBACTER

I Nachamkin and M B Skirrow

CAMPYLOBACTER AND ARCOBACTER

1 DEFINITION

1.1 Campylobacter

Campylobacter organisms are gram-negative, non-spore-forming, curved, S-shaped, or spiral rods 0.2–0.5 μm wide by 0.5–5 μm long. Cells may form spherical coccoid bodies in old cultures or cultures exposed to air. With the exception of *Campylobacter gracilis*, they are oxidase-positive and motile by means of a single polar unsheathed flagellum at one or both ends of the cell; *C. gracilis* is aflagellate. They are usually non-pigmented although *Campylobacter mucosalis* and *Campylobacter hyointestinalis* produce a dirty yellow pigment. Campylobacters are micro-aerophilic to anaerobic and have a respiratory type of metabolism. They grow at 37°C but not at 15°C. Hydrogen may be required by some species for micro-

aerobic growth. They are non-saccharolytic; energy is obtained from amino acids or tricarboxylic acid cycle intermediaries. Menaquinone-6 and a methyl-substituted menaquinone-6 are the major respiratory quinones. The G + C content of their DNA is 29–46 mol% and the type species is *Campylobacter fetus*.

1.2 Arcobacter

Arcobacter are similar to *Campylobacter* but with the following differences. Cells are 0.2–0.9 μm wide by 1–3 μm long. They grow at 15, 25 and 30°C but show variable growth at 37 and 42°C. They are micro-aerophilic and do not require hydrogen for growth, but grow aerobically at 30°C. The G + C content of their DNA is 27–30 mol% and the type species is *Arcobacter nitrofigilis*.

2 HISTORICAL PERSPECTIVE AND CLASSIFICATION

The generic name *Campylobacter* (Greek, curved rod) was given by Sebald and Véron (1963) to the group of bacteria formerly known as the 'micro-aerophilic vibrios'. These organisms cause 2 major groups of disease: fetal infections of cattle and sheep, and acute enterocolitis of humans. The former was for many years the only known pathogenic activity of campylobacters; it was only during the 1970s that their role as enteropathogens came to light (Butzler et al. 1973, Skirrow 1977). It is likely, however, that the first recorded encounter with campylobacters was in 1886 when Theodor Escherich described small vibrios in the large intestinal mucus of infants who had died of 'cholera infantum'. His drawings leave little doubt that he was looking at *Campylobacter jejuni* (or *Campylobacter coli*), but he was unable to cultivate them and he did not think they were pathogenic.

The first isolation of campylobacters was made in 1906 by McFadyean and Stockman (1913) from the uterine exudate of aborting sheep. A few years later Smith isolated a similar organism from fetuses of aborting cows and named it *Vibrio fetus* (Smith and Taylor 1919). The disease came to be known as vibrionic abortion. Much later, Florent (1959) showed that a form of the infection known as bovine infectious infertility was due to a variety of *V. fetus* transmitted from carrier bulls to cows during coitus. He named the organism *Vibrio foetus* var. *venerialis* (now *Campylobacter fetus* subsp. *venerealis*).

In 1927, another micro-aerophilic vibrio was isolated from the jejunum of calves with diarrhoea and later named *Vibrio jejuni* (Jones, Orcutt and Little 1931). In 1944, Doyle isolated a similar vibrio from pigs suffering from swine dysentery; he named it *Vibrio coli* (Doyle 1948). These became *C. jejuni* and *C. coli*, respectively, with the formation of the genus *Campylobacter* by Sebald and Véron in 1963, although no examples of the original *V. jejuni* or *V. coli* strains had at that time survived. King (1962) carried out the first systematic examination of the few micro-aerophilic vibrios that had then been isolated from humans and in so doing she gave the first definitive description of the group now represented by *C. jejuni* and *C. coli* (her 'related vibrios'). These species are now known to be among the leading causes of acute bacterial diarrhoea world wide (see Volume 3, Chapter 29).

In the 1970s there was much confusion over campylobacter nomenclature (Skirrow 1990), but the classification of Véron and Chatelain (1973) forms the basis of currently approved nomenclature. Clarification has come through the application of molecular methods, notably 16S rRNA sequencing. It is now clear that *Campylobacter*, *Arcobacter*, *Helicobacter* and *Wolinella* form a group, rRNA superfamily VI, which Vandamme et al. (1991) regarded as a distinct phylum far removed from other eubacteria. Trust et al. (1994) make a case for placing the group in the ε subdivision of the class Proteobacteria.

Campylobacter and *Arcobacter* are now included in the family Campylobacteraceae as proposed by Vandamme and De Ley (1991). *Campylobacter* currently contains 15 species and *Arcobacter* 4 species (Table 54.1). Now included in the genus *Campylobacter* are organisms formerly classified in the genus *Woli-*

nella (*Wolinella curva*, *Wolinella recta*). *Bacteroides gracilis* has been reclassified as *C. gracilis* (Vandamme et al. 1995) and [*Bacteroides*] *ureolyticus* is thought to be closely related to the genus *Campylobacter* (Han, Smibert and Krieg 1991). Two former campylobacter species, *Campylobacter cinaedi* and *Campylobacter fennelliae*, are now classified in the genus *Helicobacter*. Three of the 4 *Arcobacter* spp., *A. nitrofigilis*, *Arcobacter cryaerophilus* and *Arcobacter butzleri*, were formerly included in the genus *Campylobacter*. With the removal of *W. curva* and *W. recta* from *Wolinella*, this genus is represented by only one species, *Wolinella succinogenes*, a campylobacter-like organism found in the bovine rumen and of no known medical importance (Tanner et al. 1981).

3 HABITAT

Campylobacters are widely distributed in nature. Most species are adapted to the intestinal tract of warm-blooded animals. *C. fetus* has been isolated rarely from reptiles. *C. jejuni* and *Campylobacter lari* are particularly adapted to birds, which probably form the largest reservoir of these species (here and throughout the ensuing text the unqualified term *C. jejuni* is used to indicate the typical form, *C. jejuni* subsp. *jejuni*). Domestic poultry are especially prone to colonization and are a major source of human infection with *C. jejuni* (Stern 1992). Pigs are the main hosts for *C. coli*. Natural waters are frequently contaminated with *C. jejuni*, *C. coli* and *C. lari* and are a source of infection, particularly in outbreak settings. *C. fetus* subsp. *venerealis* is more strictly parasitic in that it is adapted to the bovine genital tract and not to the intestine. *A. cryaerophilus* is likewise adapted to the genital tract of pigs and cattle. *Campylobacter sputorum* subsp. *sputorum*, *Campylobacter concisus*, *Campylobacter rectus*, *Campylobacter curvus*, *Campylobacter showae* and *C. gracilis* form part of the natural gingival flora of humans. *A. nitrofigilis* is a nitrogen-fixing bacterium that has been found on the roots of a small marsh plant in Nova Scotia (McClung, Patriquin and Davis 1983).

4 MORPHOLOGY

The most obvious feature of campylobacters is their spirillar conformation (Figs 54.1 and 54.2), reflecting an adaptation to the mucous environment of the intestinal mucosa, as spiral bacteria are able to move easily through viscous fluids (Ferrero and Lee 1988). Most campylobacters have a single unsheathed polar flagellum inserted at one or both poles of the cell (monotrichate or amphitrichate) according to the species. Exceptions are *C. showae*, which has up to 5 unipolar flagella, and *C. gracilis*, which has none. At each pole of the bacterial cell there is a thickening of the inner cytoplasmic membrane in the form of a truncated cone, tapering in *C. jejuni* and blunt in *C. fetus*. At the apex of this cone there is a cup-shaped depression occupied by a large (80–120 nm) disc pierced at its centre by the hook of the flagellum. This arrangement is similar to that in *Spirillum* except that

Table 54.1 Cultural and biochemical characteristics of *Campylobacter* and *Arcobacter*

Characteristic	*C. fetus* subsp. *fetus*	*C. fetus* subsp. *venerealis*	*C. hyointestinalis*	*C. mucosalis*	*C. sputorum* biovar *sputorum*	*C. sputorum* biovar *bubulus*	*C. sputorum* biovar *faecalis*	*C. concisus*	*C. rectus*/*C. curvus*	*C. showae*	*C. gracilis*	*C. jejuni* subsp. *jejuni*	*C. jejuni* subsp. *doylei*	*C. coli*	*C. hyoilei*	*C. lari*	*C. upsaliensis*	*C. helveticus*	*A. butzleri*	*A. cryaerophilus*	*A. skirrowii*
Wavelength of cell	M	M	L	L	L	L	L	--	--/L	--	--	S	S	S	--	S	S	M	L	M	--
Flagellar arrangement	m	m	m	m	m	m	m	m	m	l	--	a	a	a	a	a	a	a	m/a	a	m/a
Growth at 25°C/42°C	+/V	+/–	w/+	+/+	–/+	–/+	–/+	–/+	–/+	–/+	–/–	–/+	–/+	–/+	–/+	–/+	–/+	–/+	+[a]/V	+[a]/–[b]	+[a]/V
Growth requires formate or H₂	–	–	–	+	–	–	+	+	+	+	+	–	–	–	+	+	–	–	–	–	–
Anaerobic growth with 0.1% TMAO	–	–	–	–	–	–	+	–	+	+	+	–	–	–	–	+	–	–	–	–	–
Catalase	+	+	+	–	V	+	+	–	–	+	–[c]	+	V	+	+	+	–/w	–	+	+	+
Nitrate reduction	+	+	+	+	+	+	+	+	+	+	+	+	+	+	+	+	+	+	w	V	+
Nitrite reduction	–	–	–	–	–	V	V	–	+	+	+	+	–	+	+	–	–	–	+	–	+
Hippurate hydrolysis	–	–	–	–	–	–	–	–	–	–	–	+	+	–	–	–	–	–	–	–	–
Indoxyl acetate hydrolysis	–	–	–	–	–	–	–	–	+	+	+	+	+	+	+	–	+	+	+	+	+
H₂S production in TSI medium/FPB medium	–/–	–/–	+[d]/--	+/--	+/--	+/+	+/V	+/--	+/--	+/--	+/--	–/V	–/V	+[e]/w	+/--	+[e]/w	–/--	–/--	–/--	–/--	–/--
Growth on 0.04% TTC agar	–	–	–	–	–	+	+	–	–	–	–	+	V	+	–	V	–	–	V	V	+
Growth in the presence of 1.5% NaCl	V	–	–	–	V	+	+	+	–	–	–	+	+	+	+	+	+	–	+	–	+
Growth in the presence of 3.5% NaCl	–	–	–	–	–	–	–	–	–	–	–	–	–	–	–	–	–	–	V	–	V
Growth in the presence of 1% glycine	+	–	+	V	+	+	+	+	+	V	–	+	+	+	+[f]	+	V	–	V	V	+
Sensitivity to: nalidixic acid	R	R	R	R	R	R	R	R	R	R	S	V	S	S	S	R[g]	S	S	S	S	S
Sensitivity to: cephalothin	S	S	S	S	S	S	S	V	S	S	R	R	R	R[h]	R	R	S	S	R	V	S

M, medium (1.3–1.8 μm); L, long (>1.9 μm); S, short (0.8–1.3 μm) (fixed preparations); m, monotrichate; a, amphitrichate; l, lophotrichate; + positive reaction; – negative reaction; w, weak reaction; V, some positive/sensitive, some negative/resistant; --, unknown or not applicable.

[a] Also grow at 15°C.
[b] Not all strains grow at 37°C.
[c] Also oxidase-negative.
[d] Positive only in the presence of H₂ or formate.
[e] Blackening where there is water of syneresis after 7 days in the presence of H₂.
[f] On Skirrow's agar.
[g] Urease-positive subgroup (UPTC), sensitive to nalidixic acid.
[h] Occasional strains sensitive.
The methods used to perform these tests are stipulated by Ursing, Lior and Owen (1994).

in *C. fetus* and *C. jejuni* the disc has a 'cartwheel' structure consisting of 11 spoke-like arms (Curry, Fox and Jones 1984). This structure is apparently unique to campylobacters. Motility is rapid and darting, with the bacteria spinning around their long axes in a corkscrew fashion. They are able to pass through a 0.6 μm membrane filter, a property used for isolating *Campylobacter* spp. from clinical samples (Nachamkin 1995). In some species, notably *C. jejuni* and *C. lari*, cultures that are post-mature or exposed to atmospheric oxygen, undergo coccal transformation (Fig. 54.3). This seems to be a degenerative process in response to toxic oxygen derivatives. Several studies have shown that these coccal forms are unable to grow on subculture, but the possibility that they can revert to spiral forms in the gut remains unanswered.

5 CULTURAL CHARACTERISTICS, METABOLISM AND GROWTH REQUIREMENTS

Campylobacters are strictly micro-aerophilic and do not grow in air, yet oxygen (5–10%) is normally required for growth. Their oxygen tolerance is thought to result from the vulnerability of their strongly electronegative dehydrogenases to superoxides and free radicals, especially when they are in a resting state. The key to successful cultivation of campylobacters is to add supplements that scavenge these offending compounds. A simple and widely used supplement consists of ferrous sulphate, sodium metabisulphite and sodium pyruvate (FBP), each to a final concentration of 0.05%. The effect of media composition on the aerotolerance of campylobacters is explored and reviewed by Hodge and Krieg (1994). *Arcobacter* spp. are more aerotolerant and grow in air

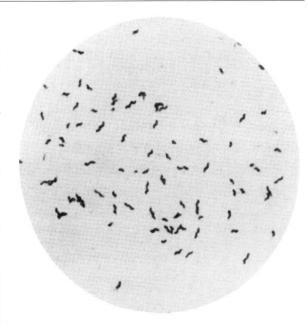

Fig. 54.2 *Campylobacter jejuni* from a 24 h blood agar culture (× 1300).

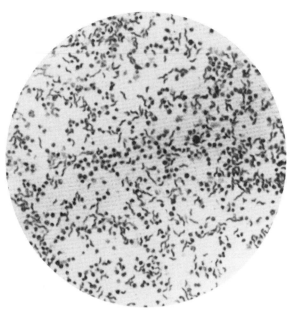

Fig. 54.3 *Campylobacter jejuni*. Predominantly coccal forms from a blood agar culture exposed to air for 24 h (× 1300).

at 30–35°C. Most campylobacters and arcobacters require CO_2 (1–10%) for growth.

Some species, notably *C. sputorum* and *C. fetus*, can grow anaerobically in the presence of certain electron acceptors such as fumarate, aspartate or nitrate (Véron, Lenvoisé-Furet and Beaune 1981); indeed, *C. sputorum* has been described as an aerotolerant anaerobe, and growth is not enhanced by adding FBP. *C. sputorum*, *C. concisus*, *C. mucosalis*, *C. curvus*, *C. rectus* and *C. hyointestinalis* usually require hydrogen for primary growth. Hydrogen also enhances the growth of *C. jejuni* and *C. coli* which use it as a major energy

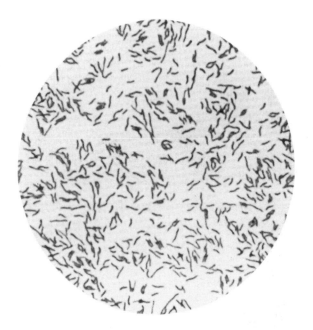

Fig. 54.1 *Campylobacter fetus* from a 48 h blood agar culture (× 1300).

source through the action of powerful dehydrogenases (Hoffman and Goodman 1982). *C. fetus* possesses cytochromes *b* and *c*, and *C. jejuni* cytochromes *b, c* and *d*. Cytochrome *c* is membrane-bound.

Under ideal conditions *C. fetus* and most other campylobacters produce visible growth after 24 h at 37°C, but colonies are not well formed until 48 h. *C. jejuni, C. coli* and *C. lari* grow optimally at 42–43°C and for this reason are sometimes referred to as the 'thermophilic' group, even though they are not thermophilic in the strict sense. Colonies of most species are circular and convex, but those of *C. jejuni, C. coli* and *C. lari* are flat, droplet-like, and tend to spread on moist agar (Fig. 54.4). A light, even turbidity is produced in broth cultures, but if a little agar is added growth is restricted to a band about 2 mm below the surface.

5.1 Susceptibility to physical and chemical agents

Campylobacters are more sensitive to adverse conditions, e.g. drying, heat, acidity, disinfectants, γ-irradiation (Radomyski et al. 1994) than are enterobacteria, so treatments that inactivate salmonellas and coliforms are fully effective against campylobacters. Campylobacters can survive in water at 4°C for many weeks, but for only a few days at temperatures above 15°C. Freezing and thawing causes a 1–2 $\log_{10}$ fall in viable count, but organisms remain alive for many months at −20°C or below.

6 GENETICS

C. fetus, C. jejuni and *C. coli* have small genomes ranging in size from 1100 to 1700 kb, which is only about one-third the size of the *Escherichia coli* genome. This is consistent with the limited biochemical repertoire of campylobacters. Studying *Campylobacter* spp. at the molecular level has posed many problems to investigators and has limited the success in identifying important virulence factors. To date, the only identified virulence factors that have been studied in any great detail are the flagellar genes. Other genes have

been cloned with success including housekeeping genes and antibiotic resistance genes (Taylor 1992). Taylor (1992) suggested that difficulties in cloning and expressing genes from *C. jejuni* might be caused by the presence of unusual *Campylobacter* promoter sequences not utilized effectively in *E. coli*. *E. coli* may lack accessory genes that are needed to process *Campylobacter* gene products, and DNA may be unstable due to differences in methylation. In order to facilitate the cloning and expression of *Campylobacter* genes, a number of shuttle and suicide plasmid vectors have been developed (Taylor 1992). Plasmids ranging in size from 2.0 to 162 kb have been detected in 19–32% of isolates of *C. jejuni* and *C. coli*, but apart from tetracycline resistance, no function has been attributed to them.

7 CELL WALL COMPOSITION AND ANTIGENIC PROPERTIES

The outer membrane of campylobacters includes specific immunogenic proteins and lipopolysaccharide (LPS) with a lipid A portion similar to that of other gram-negative bacteria. The fatty acid composition of campylobacter cells is distinctive. The major fatty acids are tetradecanoic (14:0), hexadecanoic (16:0), hexadecenoic (16:1), octadecanoic (18:0), octadecenoic (18:1) and, in the case of *C. jejuni* and *C. coli*, 19-carbon cyclopropane (19:0 cyc) acids (Lambert et al. 1987, Brondz and Olsen 1991). The major isoprenoid quinones of campylobacters are menaquinone-6 and a methyl-substituted menaquinone-6 (Moss et al. 1984). The latter appears to be unique to campylobacters.

7.1 Antigenic properties

The historical development of this subject is described in Chapter 2.27 (p. 538) of the 8th edition (Skirrow 1990).

LIPOPOLYSACCHARIDE (HEAT-STABLE) ANTIGENS

C. fetus has 2 heat-stable antigens, A and B, associated

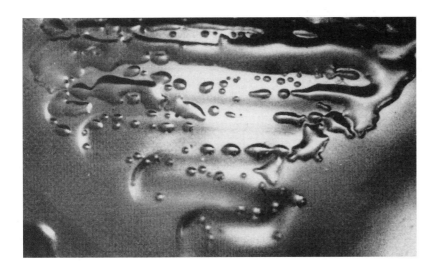

Fig. 54.4 *Campylobacter jejuni.* Surface colonies on blood agar, 24 h at 37°C.

with higher molecular mass LPS components. Strains of *C. fetus* subsp. *venerealis* possess the A antigen, whereas strains of subsp. *fetus* possess either the A or B antigen. By contrast, *C. jejuni*, *C. coli* and *C. lari* show great antigenic diversity. Their LPS antigens form the basis of the Penner serogrouping scheme (Penner and Hennessy 1980), which recognizes 65 serogroups. It has been suggested that *C. jejuni* produces the equivalent of a 'rough' LPS, lacking O side chains, based on analysis of hot-phenol extracted preparations (Mills et al. 1992). However, when certain serotypes of *C. jejuni* are subjected to immunoblot analysis using homologous O antisera, slow-migrating, high molecular weight structures with a 'ladder' appearance are detected, consistent with the presence of repeating O side chain components. Blake and Russell (1993) also found that alternative extraction procedures resulted in the detection of O side chains by conventional staining techniques. Thus, technical factors appear to be important in the extraction of *Campylobacter* LPS. LPS antigens are immunogenic in patients naturally infected with *Campylobacter*; however, the nature of the antibody response has only received limited study (Blaser and Perez-Perez 1992).

SURFACE ANTIGENS

C. fetus and *C. rectus* are unique among campylobacters in possessing a microcapsule, or S layer, consisting of high molecular weight proteins (90–160 kDa) arrayed in the form of a lattice. Unlike most protein antigens, it is able to resist boiling for several minutes. In the case of *C. fetus*, this S layer confers resistance to serum-mediated killing and phagocytosis, which may explain why *C. fetus* is able to cause systemic infection (Blaser and Pei 1993). It is an immunodominant antigen and it carries at least 4 antigenic specificities. Significantly, antigenic variation may arise in vivo in the bovine genital tract. Nothing equivalent to this S layer has been found in *C. jejuni* or *C. coli*. These species have major outer-membrane proteins (MOMPs) of MW 43–44 kDa in single isometric form, which are only weakly immunogenic but cross-reactive with antisera raised against other *Campylobacter* spp. *C. fetus* strains possess 2 MOMPs of MW 45–47 kDa, each consisting of a single or predominant isomer. Other (heat-labile) protein antigens are expressed on the cell surface and flagella. In the case of *C. jejuni*, *C. coli* and *C. lari* they are the dominant immunogens during infection, and they are the serodeterminants for the Lior serogrouping scheme, which recognizes some 160 serogroups.

8   LABORATORY ISOLATION AND IDENTIFICATION

8.1   Direct examination

Faecal specimens are preferred for isolating *Campylobacter* spp. from patients with gastrointestinal infections. A transport medium, such as Cary–Blair, should be used when transporting faecal specimens to the lab-

oratory if delays of more than a few hours are expected, or for transporting rectal swabs. *Campylobacter* spp. are not easily visualized with safranin counterstain commonly used in the gram-stain procedure; carbolfuchsin or basic fuchsin should be used as the counterstain for smears of stools or pure cultures. Because of their characteristic morphology, *Campylobacter* spp. may be detected by direct gram-stain examination of stools obtained from patients with acute enteritis. Phase-contrast microscopy has also been used to detect motile campylobacters in wet mounts of fresh stools.

8.2   Culture and isolation

For optimal recovery most *Campylobacter* spp. require a micro-aerobic atmosphere containing approximately 5% O_2, 10% CO_2 and 85% N_2. Some species of *Campylobacter*, such as *C. sputorum*, *C. concisus*, *C. mucosalis*, *C. curvus*, *C. rectus* and *C. hyointestinalis*, may require hydrogen for primary isolation. Commercial gas packs may not yield enough H_2 for the isolation of these species.

Primary plating of samples on selective media is the most widely used method. In areas where species other than *C. jejuni* and *C. coli* are common, ideally a filtration method using non-selective medium should also be used (Mishu Allos, Lastovica and Blaser 1995). Various blood-containing, or blood-free charcoal-containing selective media can be used for isolating *C. jejuni* and *C. coli*. Most of the recommended selective media have one or more antimicrobial agents, mainly cefoperazone, as the primary inhibitor of enteric bacterial flora.

Enrichment cultures may be beneficial in instances where low numbers of organisms may be expected due to delayed transport to the laboratory or after the acute stage of disease when the concentration of organisms may be low. They are essential for food and environmental samples (Scotter, Humphrey and Henley 1993). Organisms that have been sublethally damaged by freezing or heat should be pre-incubated for a few hours in non-selective broth at 37°C. Optimal conditions for the isolation of *Arcobacter* spp. from clinical specimens have not been determined. What are now known as *Arcobacter* spp. were first isolated on semi-solid media designed to isolate *Leptospira* spp. *Arcobacter* spp. are aerotolerant and have been recovered on certain selective media used for *Campylobacter*, such as Campy-CVA.

8.3   Biochemical activities and identification

The main biochemical activities of *Campylobacter* and *Arcobacter* spp. are shown in Table 54.1. They are biochemically inactive in comparison with many other bacteria. They do not utilize sugars or produce indole, but all except *C. gracilis* produce oxidase. Most species produce catalase and, apart from *C. jejuni* subsp. *doylei*, all reduce nitrate to nitrite. *C. jejuni* is the only species to hydrolyse sodium hippurate, although Totten et al.

(1987) found that 1.6% of *C. jejuni* strains were hippurate-negative, even by gas liquid chromatography. Indoxyl acetate hydrolysis is a useful bench test for differentiating some species of thermophilic *Campylobacter* (Popovic-Uroic et al. 1990). The detection and identification of campylobacters and arcobacters is described by Nachamkin (1995).

9 SUSCEPTIBILITY TO ANTIMICROBIAL AGENTS

Campylobacters are susceptible to a variety of antimicrobial agents including macrolides, fluoroquinolones, aminoglycosides, chloramphenicol and tetracycline, but all are highly resistant to trimethoprim. *C. fetus* and several other campylobacter species are sensitive to β-lactam antibiotics, but *C. jejuni*, *C. coli* and *C. lari* are resistant to most β-lactams, including cephalosporins; some strains produce β-lactamase. Sensitivity to nitroimidazoles is a feature of several species, which is curious for non-anaerobic bacteria, but there is considerable variation between strains. *C. fetus* strains are universally resistant. *C. jejuni* and *C. coli* readily acquire resistance to fluoroquinolones, which limits their use in the treatment of campylobacter enteritis. Erythromycin resistance is acquired less readily; resistance rates of less than 5% are usual for *C. jejuni* but they may rise to 80% in *C. coli*. Resistance to tetracycline is plasmid mediated. Erythromycin remains the drug of choice for treating campylobacter enteritis in cases severe enough to warrant antimicrobial treatment. The subject is dealt with fully by Skirrow and Blaser (1995).

Susceptibility tests for *Campylobacter* spp. are not standardized; consequently, the literature contains some variability in the susceptibility data reported. Recommendations for the agar dilution method include using Mueller–Hinton agar supplemented with 5% horse blood, incubated for 16–18 h under micro-aerobic conditions. The E test has been found to compare favourably with agar dilution methods, but it is not recommended for testing clindamycin (Nachamkin 1995).

10 TYPING METHODS

Many typing systems have been devised to study the epidemiology of *Campylobacter* infections and they vary in complexity and ability to discriminate between strains. These methods include biotyping, serotyping, bacteriocin sensitivity, detection of preformed enzymes, auxotyping, lectin binding, phage typing, multilocus enzyme electrophoresis, and genotypic methods such as restriction endonuclease analysis, ribotyping and restriction analysis of polymerase chain reaction (PCR) products (Patton and Wachsmuth 1992).

The most frequently used systems are biotyping and serotyping. Several biotyping schemes have been published which, based on only a few biochemical tests, can group *C. jejuni*, *C. coli* and *C. lari* into major categories. Although the discrimination of strains is low, biotyping is useful as a first step for epidemiological investigation. Finer discrimination has been obtained by combining biochemical and resistance tests to give a numerical biotype code (Bolton, Holt and Hutchinson 1984). Two major serotyping schemes are used world wide: the Penner scheme (Penner and Hennessy 1980) based on heat-stable O (LPS) antigens, and the Lior scheme (Lior et al. 1982) based on heat-labile surface protein antigens (160 serogroups for *C. jejuni*, *C. coli* and *C. lari*; 65 serogroups for *A. butzleri*). The 2 schemes are complimentary. When used together good discrimination can be obtained even with restricted panels of antisera. These systems, however, are only available in a few reference laboratories because of the time and expense needed to maintain quality serotyping antisera. Several attempts have been made by commercial enterprises to market limited serotyping antisera for *Campylobacter*, but either too few antisera were included or the quality was poor (Patton and Wachsmuth 1992). A combination of phenotypic and genotypic tests, such as those mentioned above, are being increasingly used for routine epidemiological investigation of *Campylobacter* infections (Nachamkin, Bohachick and Patton 1993, Nachamkin, Ung and Patton 1996).

11 BACTERIOPHAGES AND BACTERIOCINS

Campylobacter bacteriophages were first characterized by Bryner et al. (1970). Several morphological types have been described. Two phage typing schemes for *C. jejuni* and *C. coli* are in use: that of Grajewski, modified by Khakhria and Lior (1992), and that of Salama, Bolton and Hutchinson (1990). There is only a partial correlation between phage type and serogroup based on heat-stable antigens. No *Campylobacter* bacteriocins have been found, but some strains of *C. jejuni* are inhibited by R-type pyocins (Blackwell, Winstanley and Telfer Brunton 1982). Campylobacter typing is comprehensively reviewed by Patton and Wachsmuth (1992).

12 PATHOGENICITY AND VIRULENCE FACTORS

C. fetus subsp. *fetus* causes epizootic abortion in sheep and sporadic abortion in cattle. *C. fetus* subsp. *venerealis* is a major cause of infectious infertility in cattle (see Volume 3, Chapter 29). Human infection with *C. fetus* is limited to systemic infection in patients with underlying immunodeficiency or serious disease and rare cases of abortion. An important virulence factor in *C. fetus* is its microcapsule, or S layer, which protects the bacteria from serum killing and phagocytosis (Blaser and Pei 1993). *C. jejuni* and *C. coli* are a major cause of acute enterocolitis in humans; they also cause abortion in sheep. *C. sputorum*, *C. concisus*, *C. rectus*, *C. curvus*, *C. showae* and *C. gracilis* are often found in abundance, with other bacteria, in septic periodontal pockets, but their role in the pathogenesis of periodontal disease is unclear. *C. rectus* secretes a 104 kDa cytotoxin that cross-reacts with another known dental pathogen, *Actinobacillus actinomycetemcomitans* (Gillespie, Haraszthy and Zambon 1993) and *C. rectus* LPS may promote periodontal tissue inflammation by stimulating the plasminogen activator–plasmin system (Ogura et al. 1995). Arcobacters have been found in aborted pig and cattle faeces, but their role in abortion is not clear. *A. butzleri* is the species most often associated with human disease, mainly diarrhoea or abdominal pain, but proof of its pathogenicity is lacking. The human disease associations of arcobacters and campylobacters other than *C. jejuni* and *C. coli* are described by Mishu Allos, Lastovica and Blaser (1995).

In human medicine, *C. jejuni* and *C. coli* are by far the most important members of the Campylobacteraceae. These bacteria cause an enterotoxigenic-like illness with watery diarrhoea or an inflammatory colitis with fever, the presence of faecal blood and white cells and occasionally bactaeremia that suggests an invasive mechanism.

12.1 Cell association and invasion

C. jejuni strains have been shown to invade in vitro cell lines and translocate polarized intestinal epithelial cell lines such as Caco-2 cells (Konkel et al. 1992). They may also interact with M cells in the Peyer's patches of rabbits, which may indicate an additional pathway for entry into the submucosa. Ketley (1995) identified 4 distinct phenotypes among clinical strains: non-invasive, invasive, invasive with transcytosis, and transcytosis without invasion.

C. jejuni 81-176, which has been used by numerous investigators, invades an intestinal derived cell line, Caco-2 cells, and appears within membrane-bound vacuoles (Russell and Blake 1994). The mechanism of internalization is not known, but uptake of 81-176 into another intestinal cell line, INT407, was blocked by microtubule depolymerization and inhibitors of coated-pit formation, but not by inhibitors of microfilament depolymerization (Oelschlaeger, Guerry and Kopecko 1993). Uptake into the cell appears to be dependent upon bacterial protein synthesis. After uptake, there is some evidence for intracellular survival of the organism (Konkel et al. 1992). Superoxide dismutase (*sodB*) might have some role in intracellular survival (Pesci, Cottle and Pickett 1994). *C. jejuni* appears to produce proteins when cultured in association with eukaryotic cells, which may be important in internalization of the organism (Konkel, Mead and Cieplak 1993). PEB1 is a conserved surface protein in *C. jejuni* and *C. coli* that may be involved in adherence (Pei and Blaser 1992) and it has homology with Enterobacteriaceae glutamine-binding protein (*glnH*), lysine–arginine–ornithine binding protein (LAO), and histidine-binding protein (*hisJ*).

12.2 Flagella and motility

Motility and flagella appear to be important determinants for attachment and invasion (Wassenaar,

Bleumink-Pluym and van der Zeijst 1991). *Campylobacter* colonization or infection in a variety of animal models appears to be dependent upon intact motility and full length flagella, although other colonization factors may be involved (Nachamkin, Yang and Stern 1993).

Two genes, *flaA* and *flaB*, are involved in the expression of the flagellar filament and are arranged in tandem in both *C. jejuni* and *C. coli* (Guerry et al. 1992). Components of intestinal mucin, particularly l-fucose, are chemotactic for *C. jejuni* and motility towards these components may be important in the pathogenesis of infection (Hugdahl, Beery and Doyle 1988). Another gene, *flbA*, is involved in the synthesis of *Campylobacter* flagella and shows homology with virulence-related proteins of *Yersinia pestis* LcrD and *Salmonella typhimurium* InvA (Miller, Pesci and Pickett 1993).

12.3 Toxins

C. jejuni has been reported to produce a cholera-like enterotoxin (Ruiz-Palacios et al. 1992), but other studies have refuted the significance of these findings (Perez-Perez et al. 1992). The lack of genetic evidence for the presence of this putative toxin, shown by hybridization with probes directed against the A and B subunit of cholera and *E. coli* heat-labile toxin or low-stringency hybridization, raises serious doubts about the existence of a classical enterotoxin. It has recently been suggested that other mediators elicited by *C. jejuni* infection, such as prostaglandin E$_2$, may be responsible for the toxin-like effect (Everest et al. 1993). Other toxins such as Shiga-like toxins and cytolethal distending toxin have been described but the relevance of these toxins in the pathogenesis of infection is not understood (Cover, Perez-Perez and Blaser 1990). Kita et al. (1990) also described a hepatotoxic factor in *C. jejuni* culture fluids.

12.4 Other factors

Several investigators have examined the ability of *C. jejuni* to acquire iron from exogenous sources. *C. jejuni* does not appear to produce its own siderophores but can utilize exogenous siderophores from other bacteria as iron carriers (Baig, Wachsmuth and Morris 1986). *C. jejuni* can obtain iron from haemin and haemoglobin. Haemolytic activity described in *C. jejuni* does not appear to be iron regulated (Pickett et al. 1992). One of the iron-responsive regulatory genes, *fur* (ferric uptake regulator) may have some role in the regulation of undetermined virulence factors (Wooldridge, Williams and Ketley 1994).

12.5 Post-infection sequelae

During the past decade, evidence has appeared showing an association of *Campylobacter* infection with acute inflammatory demyelinating polyneuropathy, otherwise known as Guillain–Barré syndrome (GBS) (Mishu and Blaser 1993). Studies have also shown an association of *Campylobacter* with an illness, clinically similar to GBS, known as acute motor axonal neuropathy (AMAN) that occurs primarily in northern China and may occur in other parts of the world (McKhann et al. 1993).

The pathogenesis of GBS induced by *C. jejuni* is not clear, but several studies show that the disease is particularly associated with serogroup O:19 (Penner) strains. It has been suggested that these strains have core oligosaccharide LPS structures that mimic ganglioside structures such as GM1, present in peripheral nerves. However, evidence suggests that the offending element is a trisaccharide epitope often, though not invariably, present in O:19 strains; O:19 strains lacking the epitope are not associated with GBS (Aspinall et al. 1997).

13 SUMMARIZED DESCRIPTIONS OF SPECIES OF *CAMPYLOBACTER* AND *ARCOBACTER*

The following descriptions serve only to supplement or emphasize particular characters shown in Table 54.1 or listed in the generic descriptions on p. 1237.

Campylobacter fetus C. fetus (Smith and Taylor 1919, Véron and Chatelain 1973) is the type species of the genus. There are 2 subspecies: subsp. *fetus* and subsp. *venerealis* (Florent 1959), which are difficult to distinguish. The latter fails to grow with 1% glycine or produce H_2S from cysteine with lead acetate paper indicator. Cells are 0.3–0.5 μm wide by 2–3 μm long, with occasional longer filamentous forms. It is micro-aerophilic but can grow anaerobically in the presence of fumarate or nitrate; it grows at 25°C and some strains grow at 42°C. Colonies are circular, 1–1.5 mm, convex, translucent, non-spreading. The species is sensitive to penicillins, including benzylpenicillin, and to most cephalosporins; and resistant to nalidixic acid and metronidazole. It possesses a group-specific glycoprotein microcapsule or S layer with antiphagocytic properties. *C. fetus* causes reproductive disease in cattle and sheep, and occasionally systemic infection in immunodeficient or otherwise diseased humans. The average genome MW is 1.56×10^9; the G + C content of DNA is 35.5 ± 1.0 mol% and the type strain is CIP 5396.

Campylobacter hyointestinalis C. hyointestinalis (Gebhart et al. 1985) is phenotypically similar to *C. fetus* but produces H_2S in freshly prepared triple sugar iron (TSI) or sulphide–indole–motility (SIM) media in the presence of H_2 or formate. Colonies scraped from agar cultures appear yellow. It is isolated from pigs with proliferative enteropathy and various other animals and also from humans with diarrhoea and proctitis but its pathogenicity is uncertain. The G + C content of DNA is 36 mol% and the type strain is ATCC 35217.

Campylobacter mucosalis C. mucosalis (Roop et al. 1985a) was first described by Lawson and Rowland (1974) and formerly regarded as a subspecies of *C. sputorum*. It is catalase-negative and similar to *C. sputorum* but requires hydrogen or formate for growth. Colonies are a dirty yellow colour. Three serogroups (A, B and C) have been described. It is found in large numbers in the intestinal mucosa of pigs with porcine intestinal adenomatosis and related diseases, but disease is not reproduced by inoculation of pure cultures. The G + C content of DNA is 38 mol% and the type strain is NCTC 11000.

Campylobacter sputorum C. sputorum (Prévot 1940, Roop et al. 1985b) was first isolated by Tunnicliff (1914) from a patient with acute bronchitis. It was originally regarded as anaerobic but it is really a facultative micro-aerophile. Cells are curved rods 0.3–0.6 μm wide by 2–4 μm long, occasionally filamentous. It is monotrichate. Colonies are 1–2 mm in diameter, circular, grey and convex; they may produce greening on horse blood agar. Most strains reduce nitrite as well as nitrate and produce H_2S from TSI medium. The G + C content of DNA is 29–31 mol%. There are 3 biotypes:

1 Biotype sputorum – catalase-negative, accounting for about 5% of cultivable organisms isolated from human gingival crevices and it can be isolated from the faeces of about 2% of healthy people. It is essentially a commensal, though occasionally it has been isolated from blood cultures and once from a leg abscess. The type strain is ATCC 35980.
2 Biotype bubulus – differs by producing abundant H_2S from TSI and SIM media, and growing in the presence of 3.5% NaCl. It was first mentioned by Prévot (1940) who called it '*V. sputorum* var. *bubulum*'. It can be isolated from the genital tract of healthy cattle and sheep of both sexes. It has not been implicated in disease but it may be confused with the pathogen *C. fetus* subsp. *venerealis*. The type strain is CIP 53103.
3 Biotype fecalis – resembles biotype bubulus except that it is catalase-positive. Originally described by Firehammer (1965) as '*V. fecalis*', it can be isolated from sheep faeces and the genital tract of cattle. It probably causes enteritis in sheep and cattle. Enteritis has been produced experimentally in calves. The type strain is NCTC 11415.

Campylobacter concisus C. concisus (Tanner et al. 1981) is difficult to distinguish from *C. mucosalis*, with which it has been confused. Strains formerly known as EF group 22 are of this species (Vandamme et al. 1989). Cells are 0.5–1.0 μm wide by 4 μm long and gently curved. Colonies are small, convex and translucent. It can be isolated from gingival cervices and periodontal lesions and is commonly found in human faeces, rarely in blood. Its pathogenicity is unknown. The G + C content of DNA is 34–38 mol% and the type strain is ATCC 33237.

Campylobacter rectus **and** ***Campylobacter curvus*** C. rectus (Tanner et al. 1981) and *C. curvus* (Tanner, Listgarten and Ebersole 1984) were originally placed in the genus *Wolinella*; these species are now classed as campylobacters (Vandamme et al. 1991). Like *C. sputorum* and *C. concisus* they are catalase-negative and found in gingival crevices and periodontal lesions, but they are oxidase-positive only in the modified test of Tarrand and Gröschel (1982). They require formate or fumarate. The 2 species may be separated by their sensitivity to various dyes and by their morphology. Cells of *C. rectus* are usually straight, 0.5–1.0 μm wide and less than 4 μm long, and they possess a high MW S layer. Both species produce 3 types of colony according to the medium: convex; flat spreading; agar corroding. Corroding colonies may be mistaken for those of [*Bacteroides*] *ureolyticus* and *C. gracilis*. The G + C content of DNA is 42–46 mol%. Their pathogenicity is unknown. The type strain for *C. rectus* is NCTC 11489; for *C. curvus*, NCTC 11649.

Campylobacter showae C. showae (Etoh et al. 1993) is similar to *C. rectus* but has 2–5 unipolar flagella and is catalase-positive. It is micro-aerophilic in the presence of fumarate with formate or hydrogen, but grows best anaerobically. Previously described as *Wolinella*-like strains from human subgingival dental plaque and infected root canals, its pathogenicity is unknown. The G + C content of DNA is 44–46 mol% and the type strain is ATCC 51146.

Campylobacter gracilis *C. gracilis* (Tanner et al. 1981) was previously called *Bacteroides gracilis* and was originally thought to be anaerobic. It was transferred to *Campylobacter* by Vandamme et al. (1995). It is oxidase-negative, but like other campylobacters possesses cytochromes *b* and *c* and CO-binding cytochrome *c*; it does not possess detectable type *a* and *d* cytochromes. *C. gracilis* is the only campylobacter species that is non-motile and aflagellate. It is most closely related to *C. concisus*, *C. rectus*, *C. curvus* and *C. showae*, based on 16 rRNA sequencing, and shares many of their characters. It is isolated from gingival crevices and from visceral, head and neck infections in humans. The G + C content of DNA is 44–46 mol% and the type strain is ATCC 33236.

[*Bacteroides*] *ureolyticus* According to Vandamme et al. (1995) this bacterium (Jackson and Goodman 1978) is a member of the family Campylobacteraceae. It differs from campylobacters in its fatty acid composition, proteolytic metabolism, and its ability to hydrolyse urea. It is isolated from patients with superficial ulcers, soft tissue infections and urethritis. The G + C content of DNA is 28–29.5 mol% and the type strain NCTC 10941, ATCC 33387.

13.1 'Thermophilic' campylobacters

Principal species have an optimum growth temperature higher than 37°C and are able to grow at 43°C, but not at 25°C. Most are small spiral rods with short wavelength and single bipolar flagella (amphitrichate). They readily undergo coccal transformation. Colonies are flat with a tendency to spread along the line of inoculation and to swarm on moist agar.

Campylobacter jejuni *C. jejuni* (Jones, Orcutt and Little 1931, Véron and Chatelain 1973) is the only campylobacter to hydrolyse hippurate. There are 2 subspecies. *C. jejuni* subsp. *jejuni* causes acute enterocolitis in humans and abortion in sheep and some other animals. Colonies have a strong tendency to swarm; post-mature growth develops a 'metallic' sheen. They may show slight growth on MacConkey agar. The average genome MW is 2.16×10^9. The G + C content of DNA is 31.2 ± 1.1 mol% and the type strain is CIP 702. *C. jejuni* subsp. *doylei* (Steele and Owen 1988) is a less common and more fastidious organism mainly found in the faeces, and occasionally blood, of socially deprived children with diarrhoea. Filtration methods and incubation at 37°C are necessary for primary isolation. It does not reduce nitrate. The G + C content of DNA is 29 ± 1 mol% and the type strain is NCTC 11951.

Campylobacter coli *C. coli* (Véron and Chatelain 1973) was putatively first isolated by Doyle (1948) from piglets with swine dysentery. Pigs are the main host, but *C. coli* is also commonly found in avian and other animal species. It is closely related to *C. jejuni* (about 30% DNA homology), but does not hydrolyse hippurate. Colonies are like those of *C. jejuni* but there is less tendency to swarm, or form a 'metallic' sheen on post-mature growth. Its pathogenicity is similar to that of *C. jejuni*. The G + C content of DNA is 32.6 ± 1.0 mol% and the type strain is CIP 7080.

Campylobacter hyoilei *C. hyoilei* (Alderton et al. 1995) is closely related to *C. coli* and is distinguished by its ability to reduce nitrite and produce H_2S in TSI medium. It is isolated from intestinal lesions of pigs with proliferative enteritis. The G + C content of DNA is 35 ± 1.5 mol% and the type strain is CCUG 33450.

Campylobacter lari *C. lari* (Benjamin et al. 1983) was first isolated from the cloacal contents of seagulls of the genus *Larus*. Originally named *C. laridis* and later changed to *C. lari*, it is commonly found in birds and a wide variety of other animals, notably dogs, and in natural water. It is common in seawater and shellfish. Some of the latter strains belong to a urease-positive subgroup (UPTC) described by Bolton, Holt and Hutchinson (1985). This species accounts for only about 0.1% of human campylobacter infections, but was probably the cause of an outbreak of water-borne enteritis in Canada. *C. lari* and UPTC strains have been isolated from the blood of patients who had underlying diseases (Nachamkin et al. 1984). The G + C content of DNA is 32.1 ± 0.5 mol% and the type strain is NCTC 11352.

Campylobacter upsaliensis *C. upsaliensis* (Sandstedt and Ursing 1991) was initially referred to as 'CNW' (catalase-negative or weakly reacting) campylobacter. Like *C. jejuni* subsp. *doylei*, these organisms are best isolated from faeces by membrane filtration at 37°C. Seven serogroups are recognized. It is isolated from the faeces of dogs with or without diarrhoea, the faeces of human patients with diarrhoea, and occasionally from the blood of patients with underlying disease. The G + C content of DNA is 35–36 mol% and the type strain is NCTC 11541.

Campylobacter helveticus *C. helveticus* (Stanley et al. 1992) is closely related to *C. upsaliensis* and is distinguished by its inability to grow on potato starch medium and to reduce selenite. The flat translucent colonies are unusual in being adherent on blood agar, and they may have a blue-green hue. This species is commonly present in the faeces of domestic cats, less commonly in dogs. Its pathogenicity is unknown. The G + C content of DNA is 34 mol% and the type strain is NCTC 12470.

13.2 *Arcobacter* species

Arcobacters are similar to campylobacters, but all species grow at 15°C and are aerotolerant at 30°C.

Arcobacter nitrofigilis *A. nitrofigilis* (McClung, Patriquin and Davis 1983) was formerly assigned to *Campylobacter*, but transferred to *Arcobacter* as the type species of the genus by Vandamme et al. (1992). It is a nitrogen-fixing bacterium found on the roots of a small marsh plant in Nova Scotia. It is not found in animals or humans. The G + C content of DNA is 27.9–28.8 mol% and the type strain is ATCC 33309.

Arcobacter butzleri *A. butzleri* (Kiehlbauch et al. 1991) was formerly included in *Campylobacter*, but transferred to *Arcobacter* by Vandamme et al. (1992). The curved to S-shaped rods, 0.2–0.4 μm wide by 1–3 μm long are catalase-negative or weakly positive. Colonies are entire, white and opaque; 16 biotypes and 65 serogroups recognized. This species is associated with diarrhoea in humans and animals, occasional systemic infection in humans, and abortion in cattle and pigs; it is found in water, sewage, poultry and other meats. The G + C content of DNA is 28–29 mol% and the type strain is ATCC 49616.

Arcobacter cryaerophilus *A. cryaerophilus* (Neill et al. 1985), formerly in the genus *Campylobacter*, is now classified as *Arcobacter*; there are 2 subgroups (Vandamme et al. 1992). Cells are 0.4 μm wide by 1.8 μm long but may attain a length of over 20 μm. Colonies on blood agar are domed, entire and yellowish in the case of subgroup 2 strains. It is isolated from normal and aborted ovine and equine fetuses and was the apparent cause of an outbreak of bovine mastitis. It is also found in the faeces of domestic animals and occasionally from humans, although some strains originally identified as this species have since been identified as *A. butzleri*. The G + C content of DNA is 31 ± 1 mol% and the type strain is NCTC 11885.

Arcobacter skirrowii *A. skirrowii* (Vandamme et al. 1992) cells are 0.2–0.4 μm wide by 1–3 μm long. Colonies are flat, greyish and α-haemolytic on blood agar. It is isolated mainly from the preputial fluid of bulls, but also from aborted bovine, porcine and ovine fetuses, and the faeces of animals with diarrhoea. The G + C content of DNA is 29–30 mol% and the type strain is CCUG 10474.

HELICOBACTER

14 DEFINITION

Helicobacters are helical, S-shaped or curved gram-negative rods, 0.3–1.0 μm wide by 1.5–7.5 μm long. They are motile by means of single or multiple unipolar, bipolar, or lateral sheathed flagella. Cells exposed to air may form coccoid bodies. They are non-sporing and micro-aerophilic with respiratory metabolism. Hydrogen stimulates growth and may be required by some species. They are non-saccharolytic, oxidase-positive and catalase-positive, except for *Helicobacter canis* which is catalase-negative. Helicobacters do not grow at 25°C. There are 2 groups: those that colonize the gastric mucosa of humans and animals; and those that colonize the intestines. The gastric species produce abundant urease. *Helicobacter pylori* plays a major role in the pathogenesis of peptic ulceration and gastric cancer. The G + C content of their DNA is 35.2 ± 1.0 mol% and the type species is *H. pylori*.

15 HISTORICAL PERSPECTIVE AND CLASSIFICATION

The discovery of *H. pylori* by Warren and Marshall in Western Australia in 1983 (Marshall 1983, Warren 1983) not only introduced a whole new group of bacteria to science, but also revolutionized our concept of gastroduodenal pathology, in particular peptic ulcer disease. Spiral bacteria had been seen in the human stomach 100 years ago (Salomon 1896) and subsequently by others, but they could not be cultured and their significance was missed. Fibreoptic gastroscopy opened the way for this discovery. The organism was named *Campylobacter pyloridis* by Marshall et al. (1984), but this was later changed to the more grammatically correct *C. pylori*. Further studies showed that the organism differed sufficiently from true campylobacters to justify the formation of a new genus *Helicobacter* (Goodwin et al. 1989). It soon became apparent that similar organisms colonized the stomach of a wide variety of animals other than humans, and that certain spiral bacteria colonizing the intestines of rodents and other animals also belonged to *Helicobacter*. The historical associations between bacteria and peptic ulcer disease are described by Rathbone and Heatley (1992).

As described on page 1238, *Helicobacter*, together with *Campylobacter*, *Arcobacter* and *Wolinella*, belongs to a distinct bacterial phylum, rRNA superfamily VI (Vandamme et al. 1991). Currently, the genus *Helicobacter* contains 13 species (Table 54.2) and there are several other candidates awaiting more precise definition. The taxonomy of helicobacters is described by Owen (1992). Only a few species are associated with human disease.

16 HABITAT

Helicobacters can be broadly divided into those that colonize the stomach mucosa and those that colonize the intestines of humans and animals, although some intestinal species are capable of colonizing the stomach when acid secretion is defective. Some gastric species only colonize the non-acid secreting mucosa, whereas others, such as *Helicobacter felis*, can colonize the canaliculi of acid-secreting oxyntic cells.

The surface of the human stomach mucosa is the major habitat of *H. pylori*. Almost all isolations are from gastric biopsy specimens, but the organism has occasionally been detected in gastric juices, saliva, dental plaque, bile and faeces (Owen 1995). In developed countries prevalence rates increase with age, from about 20% in young adults to about 50% in people over 50 years old, but in developing countries rates are much higher and children are commonly infected. *H. pylori* has been isolated from domestic cats (Handt et al. 1995), which raises the question about the role of this domestic animal in transmission of disease to humans. There is some suggestion that water may be a source for *Helicobacter* infection, but whether the organisms merely exist or have some ecological niche in natural waters is unknown.

17 MORPHOLOGY

There is much morphological diversity among helicobacter species. Some possess periplasmic fibres that are independent of the flagella (Lee and O'Rourke 1993). *H. pylori* cells take the form of curved, or S-shaped gram-negative rods, 0.5–0.9 μm wide by about 3 μm long with a wavelength of about 2.6 μm. In agar cultures spiral forms are less obvious and cells appear more as singly curved rods (Fig. 54.5). *H. pylori* undergoes coccal transformation on exposure to air within 1–2 h at room temperature, and in this state it fails to grow on subculture. Such coccoid forms do not appear to be virulent (Eaton et al. 1995).

By electron microscopy, the organism is spiral with bluntly rounded ends and with 4–8 sheathed, unipolar, flagella; the sheath is continuous with the outer membrane of the cell wall. Some flagella have a terminal bulb. A glycocalyx-like material surrounding the cell is also apparent. The ultrastructure of *H. pylori* is described by Jones and Curry (1992).

Table 54.2 Cultural and biochemical characteristics of *Helicobacter* spp.

	Gastric						Intestinal								
	H. pylori	*H. nemestrinae*	*H. acinonyx*	*H. mustelae*	*H. felis*	'*H. bizzozeronii*'	*H. cinaedi*	*H. fennelliae*	*H. canis*	*H. hepaticus*	*H. pametensis*	*H. pullorum*	*H. bilis*	*H. muridarum*	'*F. rappini*'
No. flagella/cell	4–8	4–8	2–5	4–8	14–20	10–20	1–2	1–2	2	2	2	1[a]	3–14	10–14	5–9
Distribution of flagella	Mp	Mp	Mp	p/l	Bp	Bp	p	p	Bp	Bp	Bp	Mp	Bp	Bp	Bp
Periplasmic fibres	–	–	–	–	+	–	–	–	–	–	–	–	+	+	+
Growth at 42°C	V	+	–	+	+	+	+	+	+	–	+	+	+	–	V
Catalase	+	+	+	+	+	+	+	+	–	+	+	+	+	+	V
Nitrate reduction	–	–	–	+	+	+	+	–	–	+	+	+	+	–	–
Urease	+	+	+	+	+	+	–	+	+	+	–	–	+	+	+
Alkaline phosphatase	+	+	+	+	+	+	–	–	+	––	+	–	––	+	–
γ-Glutamyl transpeptidase	+	––	+	+	+	+	–	+	––	––	–	––	––	+	+
Indoxyl acetate hydrolysis	–	–	–	+	–	+	–	+	+	+	–	–	–	+	––
Growth in presence of 1% glycine	–	–	–	–	–	––	+	+	––	+	+	––	V	–	–
Susceptibility to: nalidixic acid	R	R	R	S	R	R	V	S	S	R	S	S	R	R	R
cephalothin	S	S	S	R	S	S	I	V	I	R	S	R	R	R	R

Mp, monopolar; Bp, bipolar; p, polar; l, lateral; +, positive reaction; –, negative reaction; V, some positive/sensitive, some negative/resistant; S, sensitive; R, resistant; I, intermediate sensitivity; ––, unknown or not applicable.

[a]Flagella unsheathed.

The methods used to perform these tests are as given by Ursing, Lior and Owen (1994).

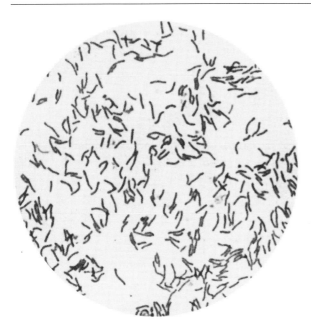

Fig. 54.5 *Helicobacter pylori* from a 3 day chocolate agar culture (× 1300).

18 CULTURAL CHARACTERISTICS, METABOLISM AND GROWTH REQUIREMENTS

Like campylobacters, *H. pylori* is strictly microaerophilic and CO_2 (5–20%) and high humidity are required for growth. *H. pylori* requires media containing supplements similar to those used for campylobacters: blood, haemin, serum, starch or charcoal. However, *H. pylori* is inhibited by the bisulphite in the FBP campylobacter 'aerotolerance' supplement. Growth is best on media such as moist freshly prepared heated (chocolated) blood agar, or brain–heart infusion agar with 5% horse blood and 1% IsoVitaleX. Strains grow in various liquid media supplemented with fetal calf or horse serum (Shahamat et al. 1991). Some strains grow in serum-free media, notably bisulphite-free brucella broth (Hawrylik et al. 1994). Sheep blood, either whole or laked, when used as a broth supplement, has been shown to inhibit the growth of *H. pylori* (Coudron and Stratton 1995). All strains grow at 37°C, some grow poorly at 30 and 42°C but none grows at 25°C. Colonies from primary cultures at 37°C usually take 3–5 days to appear and are circular, convex and translucent like those of *C. fetus*. They seldom grow bigger than 2 mm in diameter even if incubation is extended beyond 1 week. They are weakly haemolytic on 5% horse blood agar. Motility is weak or absent when grown on agar.

Like campylobacters, *H. pylori* is inactive in most conventional biochemical tests. Notable exceptions are the strong production of urease, catalase and alkaline phosphatase. All strains produce DNAase, leucine aminopeptidase, and γ-glutamylaminopeptidase (McNulty and Dent 1987). The urease is a nickel containing high molecular weight protein (c. 600 kDa) with maximum activity at 45°C and pH 8.2.

Remarkably, it forms 6% of protein produced by the organism. Almost identical ureases are produced by *Helicobacter nemestrinae, Helicobacter mustelae* and *H. felis* (Turbett et al. 1992). In the presence of urea (5 м) it enables *H. pylori* to tolerate pH values down to 2.6, because the production of ammonia raises the pH in the immediate vicinity of the bacterial cell. The importance of this action for colonization of the stomach is obvious.

19 GENETICS

Like campylobacters, *H. pylori* has a small genome of about 1700 kb. Also like campylobacters, helicobacters have been difficult to study at the molecular level because traditional strategies used to clone and study virulence have not been very successful. Strategies used to clone genes from *Campylobacter*, such as shuttle mutagenesis, have been used to express *H. pylori* urease genes in *C. jejuni* and *E. coli* to study flagellin and *cagA* genes (Tummuru, Cover and Blaser 1994). Other genes that have been successfully cloned and expressed include the gene for vacuolating cytotoxin (Schmitt and Haas 1994) and *recA* (Thompson and Blaser 1995). *H. pylori* is so genetically diverse that, usually, any 2 independent isolates can be distinguished by a variety of genetic analyses including restriction endonuclease analysis, restriction fragment length polymorphism (RFLP), and ribotyping (Taylor et al. 1995). Plasmid transfer has not been reported in *H. pylori*, but plasmids have been detected in 48–58% of wild strains. The subject of helicobacter genetics is reviewed by Taylor (1992) (see also Owen 1995).

20 CELL WALL COMPOSITION AND ANTIGENIC STRUCTURE

Helicobacters have the typical cell wall structure of gram-negative bacteria. The fatty acid profile of *H. pylori* is distinctive and different from the general pattern of campylobacters. It is characterized by long-chain fatty acids composed predominantly of tetradecanoic (14:0) and 19-carbon cyclopropane (19:0 cyc) acids with lower amounts of hexadecanoic (16:0), octadecanoic (18:0), octadecenoic (18:1) and linoleic (18:2) acids (Moran 1995). Phosphatidylethanolamine (79.1%), lysophosphatidylethanolamine (16%) and phosphatidylcholine (1.9%) constitute the polar head groups of neutral phospholipids. Acidic phospholipids contain phosphatidic acid (52.7%) and phosphatidylserine (47.3%). *H. pylori* does not possess the methyl-substituted menaquinones (thermoplasma quinones) present in campylobacter species.

20.1 Outer membrane

H. pylori contains at least 4 outer-membrane proteins ranging from 48 to 67 kDa that have pore-forming ability (Exner et al. 1995) with some evidence that these porins are substrate-specific. Whole cell and outer-membrane protein gel electrophoresis profiles of *H. pylori* are different from those of *C. fetus* and *C. jejuni*. Although there are recognizable differences between strains of *H. pylori* these are small, even between strains of diverse origin. However, a few protein bands are common to all 3 species, notably one corresponding to the major flagellar antigen of *C. fetus* and *C. jejuni*. This protein (MW 62 kDa) reacts with antiserum raised against purified *C. jejuni* flagella. Several species-specific outer-membrane proteins have been described, including a 19 kDa protein and 26 kDa protein. A species-specific 29 kDa flagellar sheath protein has also been described (Luke and Penn 1995).

20.2 Lipopolysaccharides

The lipopolysaccharide of *H. pylori* appears to have an unusual structure related to the composition of the fatty acids that form the hydrophobic region of lipid A with the presence of 3-hydroxyoctadecanoic acid. This fatty acid has also been observed in *Brucella*, *Francisella* and *Acinetobacter* (Conrad et al. 1992). The lipid A portion of *Helicobacter* LPS appears to have lower biological activity that LPS from other enteric bacteria (Moran 1995).

Some strains of *H. pylori* possess LPS with a ladder-like side chain like those of 'smooth' strains of Enterobacteriaceae; others give a 'rough'-type profile like those of most *C. jejuni* strains. Strains may change from smooth to rough LPS when grown on conventional solid media (Moran 1995) and may be reversible when grown in liquid medium. Although LPS core antigens are shared, side chain antigens are strain-specific. The distribution of specific LPS antigens among strains is different from that of protein antigens. Antigenic differences in LPS from different strains has been detected by immunoblotting and haemagglutination assays (Mills, Kurjanczyk and Penner 1992).

21 LABORATORY ISOLATION AND IDENTIFICATION

21.1 Direct examination of specimens

Various methods have been used for the direct detection of *H. pylori* in pathological samples, including gram stain, immunofluorescence acridine orange staining, histochemical stains, and molecular methods such as PCR (van Zwet et al. 1993). *H. pylori* can also be detected by testing biopsy tissue for urease activity. A non-invasive method for detecting radiolabelled CO_2 after oral administratoin of [^{13}C]urea, known as the urea breath test, is also used for the diagnosis of *Helicobacter* infection (see Volume 3, Chapter 30).

21.2 Isolation and identification

Gastric biopsy specimens are the only ones likely to be used for the primary isolation of *H. pylori*. They should be transported in a moist state and cultured within 2 h of collection. Storage beyond this time should be at 4°C, or at −20°C if the period is more than 2 days. Various transport media have been described for transporting biopsy samples, including cysteine brucella broth, normal saline, glucose, milk, Stuart's medium, semi-solid agar, brain–heart infusion broth, Cary–Blair medium and, more recently, cysteine–Albimi medium containing 20% glycerol (Han et al. 1995).

Various non-selective and selective culture media have been used for the isolation of *H. pylori* and other *Helicobacter* spp. (Jerris 1995). Chocolate agar, or more complex media such as brain–heart infusion or brucella agar supplemented with 5–7% horse blood, are suitable non-selective media. Examples of selective media are Dent's, Glupczynski's Brussels charcoal medium and Skirrow's campylobacter medium. Samples should be prepared for direct examination and plating on non-selective and selective media and plates should be incubated in a micro-aerobic environment at 35–37°C. Colonies may be visible after 3–5 days of incubation but may take longer to appear on primary isolation. Colonies are small, domed, translucent and sometimes weakly haemolytic.

Because of the unique characteristics of *H. pylori*, only a few simple tests are needed for identification, including gram-stain appearance, catalase, oxidase and urease tests. A more detailed account of the laboratory isolation of *H. pylori* is given by Jerris (1995). Intestinal helicobacters, such as *Helicobacter cinaedi* and *Helicobacter fennelliae*, can be isolated on some campylobacter-selective agars, or by filtration on non-selective agar (Kiehlbauch et al. 1995).

22 SUSCEPTIBILITY TO ANTIMICROBIAL AGENTS

H. pylori has a spectrum of sensitivity similar to that of *C. fetus*. It is sensitive to penicillins, including benzylpenicillin, cephalosporins, tetracycline, erythromycin, rifampicin, aminoglycosides and nitrofurans, but resistant to nalidixic acid, though sensitive to the more active quinolones such as ciprofloxacin. Like other campylobacters, it is highly resistant to trimethoprim and moderately resistant to polymyxins. *H. pylori* is usually susceptible to metronidazole, one of the antimicrobial agents used to treat infection, but resistance rates are variable and may reach 50% in some areas. Resistance to metronidazole correlates with failure of treatment with combinations that include this drug (Glupczynski et al. 1991). *H. pylori* is sensitive to colloidal bismuth compounds commonly prescribed for gastric disease in concentrations easily attainable in the stomach. The proton pump inhibitor omeprazole has mild in vitro activity against *H. pylori*; 1% bile salts are also inhibitory.

A number of methods have been used to detect antimicrobial resistance in *H. pylori*, including agar dilution and E-test methods. The E test appears to be an easy and reliable method as an alternative to the more labour-intensive agar dilution method (Glupczynski et al. 1991).

23 TYPING METHODS

H. pylori is remarkably homogenous in its phenotypic expression. The only biochemical differences found between strains of widely different origin are in the activities of a few enzymes, which divides strains into 4 biotypes, one of which accounts for 85% of strains (Owen 1995). Haemagglutination and lectin typing have shown recognizable patterns, but the systems have not been developed. The LPS antigens of *H. pylori* are sufficiently diverse for their potential use in typing (Mills, Kurjanczyk and Penner 1992), and 5 serogroups based on heat-labile flagellar antigens have been identified, but neither of these approaches has been developed further.

Most typing successes have been with molecular methods that exploit the considerable genetic diversity of *H. pylori*. Methods such as random amplified polymorphic DNA analysis, or RFLP analysis of specific amplified genes have been used successfully for studying strains within families or answering other epidemiological questions (Taylor et al. 1995). The subject is reviewed by Owen (1995).

24 PATHOGENICITY AND VIRULENCE FACTORS

H. pylori causes chronic active gastritis in humans and is the cause of most cases of duodenal and gastric ulcers that are not associated with the administration of non-steroidal anti-inflammatory agents (Rauws and Tytgat 1995). In addition, *H. pylori* is associated with primary mucosa-associated lymphoid tissue (MALT) gastric lymphoma and some types of gastric adenocarcinoma (Webb and Forman 1995). A comprehensive review of the pathogenesis of *H. pylori* has been published (Riegg, Dunn and Blaser 1995).

Most *H. pylori* bacteria found in the stomach are in the layer of mucus overlying the epithelium. Some penetrate the mucous layer and adhere to the gastric epithelial cells with formation of a pedestal, as is seen with enteropathogenic *E. coli* strains, which requires cytoskeletal rearrangements (Smoot et al. 1993). A few *H. pylori* are seen between adjacent cells in proximity to tight junctions. *H. pylori* urease appears to be necessary for the establishment of gastric mucosal colonization according to animal experimental studies with urease-negative mutants and urease inhibitors. Urease may serve to protect the organism from gastric acid by converting urea to ammonia and carbon dioxide, thus surrounding the bacterium with an alkaline layer that neutralizes the acid. Urease may also be an important cause of the inflammation seen in the lamina propria that is the hallmark of chronic *H. pylori* infections, as it is a phlogistic and cytotoxic agent (Mai et al. 1992, Segal, Shon and Tompkins 1992). Bacterial

motility is also important for the colonization of the mucous layer, as non-motile mutants do not colonize the stomachs of gnotobiotic piglets (Eaton, Morgan and Krakowka 1989).

Several *H. pylori* adhesins have been described that bind to Lewis b antigens with terminal fucose residues (found in humans with blood group O), to sialic acid–lactose residues (Evans et al. 1993), and to phosphatidylethanolamine, a glycolipid receptor on the gastric antral mucosa. The adhesin binding to blood group O-specific antigens may help explain the predispostion of people with blood group O to peptic ulcer disease and gastric adenocarcinoma. The interplay between *H. pylori* and the human gastric mucosa, and other helicobacters with their equivalent hosts, is expounded by Lee, Fox and Hazell (1993).

24.1 Cytotoxins

Apart from urease, which may cause damage to host cells, a haemolysin and a vacuolating cytotoxin (vacA) have been described. CagA, a high molecular weight protein product of a cytotoxin associated gene (*cagA*), is produced by about 60% of *H. pylori* strains and is associated with the expression of vacA. CagA-positive strains are also associated with the presence of duodenal ulceration, although it is unclear whether CagA has an independent pathogenic role (Cover et al. 1995, Owen 1995).

The role of *H. pylori* in gastric disease is discussed more fully in Volume 3 (see Volume 3, Chapter 30). Most other gastric helicobacters are associated with gastritis and sometimes ulceration in their respective hosts. '*Helicobacter heilmannii*' is associated with gastritis in humans, but it accounts for only 1–5% of patients with bacterial gastritis. The intestinal helicobacters, *H. cinaedi* and *H. fennelliae*, apparently cause proctocolitis in homosexual men.

25 SUMMARIZED DESCRIPTIONS OF *HELICOBACTER* SPECIES

25.1 Gastric helicobacters

Helicobacter pylori *H. pylori* (Marshall et al. 1984) was originally named *Campylobacter pyloridis*, but changed to *C. pylori* and later moved by Goodwin et al. (1989) to *Helicobacter* as the type species of the genus. Cells are curved or spiral with 4–8 unipolar sheathed flagella, some with terminal bulbs. Colonies are non-pigmented, translucent, 1–2 mm in diameter. There is variable growth at 42°C. The species may grow in air enriched with 10% CO_2 but not anaerobically. It is nitrate-negative. Antimicrobial sensitivities are similar to those of *C. fetus*. *H. pylori* is the major cause of gastritis in humans and is strongly associated with peptic ulceration and gastric cancer. It does not naturally infect animals, but has been found in domestic cats. The G + C content of DNA is 36–38 mol% and the type strain NCTC 11637, ATCC 43504.

Helicobacter nemestrinae *H. nemestrinae* (Bronsdon et al. 1991) is closely related genetically to *H. pylori* (Sly et al. 1993) and phenotypically similar. The species consists of spiral rods, 0.2–0.3 μm wide by 2.0–5.0 μm long; it may exhibit pleomorphism in vitro. Colonies are small, flat, translucent, 0.5–1 mm, with irregular edges. Weak growth is exhibited anaerobically at 35°C. It is isolated from the gastric mucosa of the pigtailed monkey (*Macaca nemestrina*); there is no associated pathology. The G + C content of DNA is 24 mol% and the type strain is ATCC 49396.

Helicobacter acinonyx H. acinonyx (Eaton et al. 1993) is closely related to H. pylori (97.4% similarity by 16S rRNA sequencing). The species consists of short, spiral rods 0.3 μm wide by 1.5–2.0 μm long with 2–5 sheathed unipolar flagella. It is isolated from the gastric mucosa of cheetahs (*Acinonyx jubatus*) with gastritis. The G + C content of DNA of the type strain is 30 mol% and the type strain is CCUG 29263.

Helicobacter mustelae H. mustelae (Fox et al. 1989) was first described as a subspecies of '*C. pylori*' but was later elevated to specific status and transferred to *Helicobacter* by Goodwin et al. (1989). It is similar to H. pylori but has multiple lateral as well as polar flagella. Growth occurs at 42°C and anaerobically with CO_2. It reduces nitrate and is isolated from the normal or inflamed gastric mucosa of the ferret (*Mustela putorius furo*). The G + C content of DNA is 36–41 mol% and the type strain is ATCC 43772.

Helicobacter felis H. felis (Paster et al. 1991) is related to H. acinonyx (96.1% similarity by 16S rRNA sequencing) but morphologically distinct. Cells are rigid, tightly spiral, 0.4 μm wide by 5–7.5 μm long, with 5–7 spirals per cell surrounded by periplasmic fibrils appearing as concentric helical ridges in pairs, threes, or singly. Tufts of 14–20 bipolar sheathed flagella are positioned slightly off centre at the end of the cell. It is micro-aerophilic, but can grow anaerobically, growing at 42°C. It is commonly present in the gastric mucosa of cats and dogs, sometimes associated with gastritis. The pathogenicity for humans is unknown. The G + C content of DNA is 42.5 mol% and the type strain is ATCC 49179.

'Helicobacter heilmannii' '*H. heilmannii*' was first described and originally named '*Gastrospirillum hominis*' by McNulty et al. (1989). It is the only helicobacter, other than H. pylori, to colonize the human stomach and be associated with gastritis. It has not been cultured, but cloning and sequencing of its 16S rRNA gene shows that it is related to H. felis (Solnick et al. 1993). Tightly spiral, bipolar flagellated cells resemble H. felis, but lack periplasmic fibrils. Sera from infected patients react with H. felis antigens. Bacteria morphologically indistinguishable from '*H. heilmannii*' have been cultured from dogs and named '*Helicobacter bizzozero*' by Hänninen et al. (1997). The 2 organisms may be the same. Similar bacteria were seen in pigs by Mendes et al. (1990) and provisionally named '*Gastrospirillum suis*'.

25.2 Intestinal helicobacters

Helicobacter cinaedi and Helicobacter fennelliae H. cinaedi and H. fennelliae (Totten et al. 1985), first isolated from rectal swabs of homosexual men with symptoms of proctitis, were placed in the genus *Campylobacter* but were subsequently reclassified in *Helicobacter* by Vandamme et al. (1991). Superficially they resemble C. coli but grow more slowly and require blood. They possess single, sheathed, predominantly bipolar flagella. Pinpoint translucent colonies are formed after 48 h and develop into flat, watery, spreading colonies like young C. jejuni cultures. H. fennelliae cultures smell of hypochlorite and do not reduce nitrate. Both species are associated with proctitis in homosexual men and occasional systemic infection in patients with underlying immunodeficiency or serious disease (Kiehlbauch et al. 1994). H. cinaedi apparently forms part of the normal flora of hamsters (Gebhart et al. 1989). The G + C content of DNA of both species is 37–38 mol% and the type strains are: H. cinaedi ATCC 35683; H. fennelliae ATCC 35684.

Helicobacter canis H. canis (Stanley et al. 1993) consists of slender helical rods 0.25 μm wide by 4 μm long with 1–2 spiral turns and single, bipolar sheathed flagella. Pinpoint, non-pigmented, α-haemolytic colonies form after 48 h on blood agar, growing at 42°C. The species is catalase-, urease- and nitrate-negative. It is isolated from faeces of diarrhoeic or healthy dogs; one strain has been isolated from human faeces. The pathogenicity is unknown. The G + C content of DNA is 48 mol% and the type strain is NCTC 12739.

Helicobacter hepaticus H. hepaticus (Fox et al. 1994) consists of curved to spiral rods, 0.2–0.3 μm wide by 1.5–5.0 μm with 1–3 spiral turns with single, sheathed, bipolar flagella. It grows as pinpoint colonies but may spread on agar. It does not grow at 42°C. Urease-positive, it is isolated from the colons and caeca of mice, and the livers of mice with active, chronic hepatitis. The type strain is ATCC 51448.

Helicobacter pametensis H. pametensis (Dewhirst et al. 1994) cells are curved, 0.4 μm wide by 1.5 μm long with single bipolar sheathed flagella; occasionally there is a third flagellum. The species grows at 42°C. It is isolated from tern, gull and swine faeces; its pathogenicity is unknown. The G + C content of DNA is 38 mol% and the type strain ATCC 51478, CCUG 29255.

Helicobacter pullorum H. pullorum (Stanley et al. 1994) is a campylobacter-like organism with single, unipolar, unsheathed flagellum (atypical for a helicobacter). Cells are gently curved slender rods 3–4 μm long and it grows at 42°C. It forms pinpoint, non-pigmented, α-haemolytic colonies on 5% horse blood agar. Urease-negative, it is isolated from asymptomatic broiler chickens, the livers and intestinal contents of laying hens with features of vibrionic hepatitis, and faeces from humans with gastroenteritis. The G + C content of DNA is 34–35 mol% and the type strain is NCTC 12824.

Helicobacter bilis H. bilis (Fox et al. 1995) cells are fusiform to slightly spiral, 0.5 μm wide by 4–5 μm long, entwined with periplasmic fibres. There are tufts of sheathed flagella numbering 3–14 at each end. Coccoid cells form in old cultures. Colonies appear as a thin spreading layer on agar medium. It is micro-aerophilic and grows at 42°C and in 20% bile and 0.4% TTC. It is urease-positive and can be isolated from the colons and caeca of mice and the bile and livers of mice with hepatitis. The type strain is ATCC 51630.

Helicobacter muridarum H. muridarum (Lee et al. 1992) is morphologically distinct. Cells are helical, 0.5–0.6 μm wide by 3.5–5.0 μm long with 2–3 spirals per cell. Spherical forms occur in older cultures. There are bipolar tufts of 10–14 sheathed flagella. Each cell is entwined by 9–11 criss-crossing periplasmic fibrils. It is micro-aerophilic and grows only at 37°C. Urease-positive, it can be isolated from the intestinal mucosa of rats and mice. Its pathogenicity is unknown. The G + C content of DNA is 34 mol% and the type strain is ATCC 49282.

'Flexispira rappini' '*F. rappini*' was originally described by Kirkbride et al. (1985). It has never been formally named but has been shown to be closely related to H. muridarum and is probably a helicobacter (Schauer, Ghori and Falkow 1993). Its cells are straight and fusiform but with criss-crossing periplasmic fibrils, like those of H. muridarum. It shows serpentine flexibility with changes in cell length and shape and grows as a thin spreading film on agar. It is micro-aerophilic and urease-positive and is isolated from aborted sheep fetuses, the faeces of humans with chronic diarrhoea, and the intestinal mucosa of laboratory mice. The G + C content of DNA is 33–34 mol%.

REFERENCES

Alderton MR, Korolik V et al., 1995, *Campylobacter hyoilei* sp. nov., associated with porcine proliferative enteritis, *Int J Syst Bacteriol*, **45**: 61–6.

Aspinall GO, Pang H et al., 1997, Lipopolysaccharides from *Campylobacter jejuni* strains associated with the onset of the Guillain–Barré and Miller–Fisher syndromes, Campylobacters, Helicobacters, *and related organisms*, eds Newell DG, Ketley JM, Feldman RA, Plenum Press, New York, 659–62.

Baig BH, Wachsmuth IK, Morris GK, 1986, Utilization of exogenous siderophores by *Campylobacter* species, *J Clin Microbiol*, **23**: 431–3.

Benjamin J, Leaper S et al., 1983, Description of *Campylobacter laridis*, a new species comprising the nalidixic acid resistant thermophilic *Campylobacter* (NARTC) group, *Curr Microbiol*, **8**: 231–8.

Blackwell CC, Winstanley FP, Telfer Brunton WA, 1982, Sensitivity of thermophilic campylobacters to R-type pyocines of *Pseudomonas aeruginosa*, *J Med Microbiol*, **15**: 247–51.

Blake DC, Russell RG, 1993, Demonstration of lipopolysaccharide with O-polysaccharide chains among different heat-stable serotypes of *Campylobacter jejuni* by silver staining of polyacrylamide gels, *Infect Immun*, **61**: 5384–7.

Blaser MJ, Pei Z, 1993, Pathogenesis of *Campylobacter fetus* infections: critical role of high-molecular weight S-layer proteins in virulence, *J Infect Dis*, **167**: 372–7.

Blaser MJ, Perez-Perez GI, 1992, Humoral immune response to lipopolysaccharide antigens of *Campylobacter jejuni*, Campylobacter jejuni: *Current Status and Future Trends*, eds Nachamkin I, Blaser MJ, Tompkins LS, American Society for Microbiology, Washington, DC, 230–5.

Bolton FJ, Holt AV, Hutchinson DN, 1984, Campylobacter biotyping scheme of epidemiological value, *J Clin Pathol*, **37**: 677–81.

Bolton FJ, Holt AV, Hutchinson DN, 1985, Urease-positive thermophilic campylobacters, *Lancet*, **1**: 1217–18.

Brondz I, Olsen I, 1991, Multivariate analyses of cellular fatty acids in *Bacteroides*, *Prevotella*, *Porphyromonas*, *Wolinella*, and *Campylobacter* spp., *J Clin Microbiol*, **29**: 183–9.

Bronsdon MA, Goodwin CS et al., 1991, *Helicobacter nemestrinae* sp. nov., a spiral bacterium found in the stomach of a pig-tailed macaque (*Macaca nemestrina*), *Int J Syst Bacteriol*, **41**: 148–53.

Bryner JH, Richie AE et al., 1970, Isolation and characterization of bacteriophage for *Vibrio fetus*, *J Virol*, **6**: 94–9.

Butzler JP, Dekeyser P et al., 1973, Related vibrios in stools, *J Pediatr*, **82**: 493–5.

Conrad RS, Kist M et al., 1992, Extraction and biochemical analyses of *Helicobacter pylori* lipopolysaccharides, *Curr Microbiol*, **24**: 165–9.

Coudron PE, Stratton CW, 1995, Factors affecting growth and susceptibility testing of *Helicobacter pylori* in liquid media, *J Clin Microbiol*, **33**: 1028–30.

Cover TL, Perez-Perez GI, Blaser MJ, 1990, Evaluation of cytotoxic activity in fecal filtrates from patients with *Campylobacter jejuni* or *Campylobacter coli* enteritis, *FEMS Microbiol Lett*, **58**: 301–4.

Cover TL, Glupczynski Y et al., 1995, Serologic detection of infection with cagA+ *Helicobacter pylori* strains, *J Clin Microbiol*, **33**: 1496–500.

Curry A, Fox AJ, Jones DM, 1984, A new bacterial flagellar structure found in campylobacters, *J Gen Microbiol*, **130**: 1307–10.

Dewhirst FE, Seymour C et al., 1994, Phylogeny of *Helicobacter* isolated from bird and swine feces and description of *Helicobacter pametensis* sp. nov., *Int J Syst Bacteriol*, **44**: 553–60.

Doyle LP, 1948, The etiology of swine dysentery, *Am J Vet Res*, **9**: 50–1.

Eaton KA, Morgan DR, Krakowka S, 1989, *Campylobacter pylori* virulence factors in gnotobiotic piglets, *Infect Immun*, **57**: 1119–25.

Eaton KA, Dewhirst FE et al., 1993, *Helicobacter acinonyx* sp. nov., isolated from cheetahs with gastritis, *Int J Syst Bacteriol*, **43**: 99–106.

Eaton KA, Catenich CE et al., 1995, Virulence of coccoid and bacillary forms of *Helicobacter pylori* in gnotobiotic piglets, *J Infect Dis*, **171**: 459–62.

Escherich T, 1886, Beitrage zur Kenntniss der Darmbacterien.III. Ueber das Vorkommen von Bironen im Darmcanal und den Stuhlgangen der Sauglinge [Articles adding to the knowledge of intestinal bacteria.III. On the existence of vibrios in the intestines and faeces of babies], *Münch Med Wochenschr*, **33**: 815–17.

Etoh Y, Dewhirst FE et al., 1993, *Campylobacter showae* sp. nov., isolated from the human oral cavity, *Int J Syst Bacteriol*, **43**: 631–9.

Evans DG, Karjalainen TK et al., 1993, Cloning, nucleotide sequence and expression of a gene encoding an adhesin subunit protein of *Helicobacter pylori*, *J Bacteriol*, **175**: 674–83.

Everest PH, Cole AT et al., 1993, Role of leukotriene B4, prostaglandin E2, and cyclic AMP in *Campylobacter jejuni* induced intestinal fluid secretion, *Infect Immun*, **61**: 4885–7.

Exner MM, Doig P et al., 1995, Isolation and characterization of a family of porin proteins from *Helicobacter pylori*, *Infect Immun*, **63**: 1567–72.

Ferrero RL, Lee A, 1988, Motility of *Campylobacter jejuni* in a viscous environment: comparison with conventional rod-shaped bacteria, *J Gen Microbiol*, **134**: 53–9.

Firehammer BD, 1965, The isolation of vibrios from ovine feces, *Cornell Vet*, **55**: 482–94.

Florent A, 1959, Les deux vibrioses génitales de la bête bovine: la vibriose venerienne, due à *V. foetus venerialis*, et al vibriose d'origine intestinale due à *V. foetus intestinalis*, *Proc 16th Int Vet Congr, Madrid*, **2**: 953–7.

Fox JG, Chilvers T et al., 1989, *Campylobacter mustelae*, a new species resulting from the elevation of *Campylobacter pylori* subsp. *mustelae* to species status, *Int J Syst Bacteriol*, **39**: 301–3.

Fox JG, Dewhirst FE et al., 1994, *Helicobacter hepaticus* sp. nov., a microaerophilic bacterium isolated from livers and intestinal mucosal scrapings from mice, *J Clin Microbiol*, **32**: 1238–45.

Fox JG, Yan LL et al., 1995, *Helicobacter bilis* sp. nov., a novel *Helicobacter* species isolated from bile, livers, and intestines of aged, inbred mice, *J Clin Microbiol*, **33**: 445–54.

Gebhart CJ, Edmonds P et al., 1985, '*Campylobacter hyointestinalis*' sp. nov.: a new species of *Campylobacter* found in the intestines of pigs and other animals, *J Clin Microbiol*, **21**: 715–20.

Gebhart CJ, Fennell CL et al., 1989, *Campylobacter cinaedi* is normal intestinal flora in hamsters, *J Clin Microbiol*, **27**: 1692–4.

Gillespie MJ, Haraszthy GG, Zambon JJ, 1993, Isolation and partial characterization of the *Campylobacter rectus* cytotoxin, *Microb Pathog*, **14**: 203–15.

Glupczynski Y, Labbe M et al., 1991, Evaluation of the E test for quantitative antimicrobial susceptibility testing of *Helicobacter pylori*, *J Clin Microbiol*, **29**: 2072–5.

Goodwin CS, Armstrong JA et al., 1989, Transfer of *Campylobacter pylori* and *Campylobacter mustelae* to *Helicobacter* gen. nov. as *Helicobacter pylori* comb. nov. and *Helicobacter mustelae* comb. nov., respectively, *Int J Syst Bacteriol*, **39**: 397–405.

Guerry P, Alm RA et al., 1992, Molecular and structural analysis of *Campylobacter* flagellin, Campylobacter jejuni: *Current Status and Future Trends*, eds Nachamkin I, Blaser MJ, Tompkins LS, American Society for Microbiology, Washington DC, 267–81.

Han YH, Smibert RM, Krieg NR, 1991, *Wolinella recta*, *Wolinella curva*, *Bacteroides ureolyticus*, and *Bacteroides gracilis* are microaerophiles, not anaerobes, *Int J Syst Bacteriol*, **41**: 218–22.

Han SW, Flamm R et al., 1995, Transport and storage of *Helicobacter pylori* from gastric mucosal biopsies and clinical isolates, *Eur J Clin Microbiol Infect Dis*, **14**: 349–52.

Handt LK, Fox JG et al., 1995, Characterization of feline *Helico-*

bacter pylori strains and associated gastritis in a colony of domestic cats, *J Clin Microbiol*, **33**: 2280–9.

Hänninen M-L, Happonen I et al., 1997, Culture and characteristics of *Helicobacter bizzozeronii*, a new canine gastric *Helicobacter* sp., *Int J Syst Bacteriol*, **47**: 160–6.

Hawrylik SJ, Wasilko DJ et al., 1994, Bisulphite or sulphite inhibits growth of *Helicobacter pylori*, *J Clin Microbiol*, **32**: 790–2.

Hodge JP, Krieg NR, 1994, Oxygen tolerance estimates in *Campylobacter* species depend on the testing medium, *J Appl Bacteriol*, **77**: 666–73.

Hoffman PS, Goodman TG, 1982, Respiratory physiology and energy conservation efficiency of *Campylobacter jejuni*, *J Bacteriol*, **150**: 319–26.

Hugdahl MB, Beery JT, Doyle MP, 1988, Chemotactic behavior of *Campylobacter jejuni*, *Infect Immun*, **56**: 1560–6.

Jackson FL, Goodman YE, 1978, *Bacteroides ureolyticus*, a new species to accommodate strains previously identified as '*Bacteroides corrodens*, anaerobic', *Int J Syst Bacteriol*, **28**: 197–200.

Jerris RC, 1995, *Helicobacter, Manual of Clinical Microbiology*, 6th edn, eds Murray PR, Baron EJ et al., ASM Press, Washington, DC, 492–8.

Jones DM, Curry A, 1992, The ultrastructure of *Helicobacter pylori*, Helicobacter pylori *and Gastroduodenal Disease*, 2nd edn, eds Rathbone BJ, Heatley RV, Blackwell Scientific Publications, Oxford, 29–41.

Jones FS, Orcutt M, Little RB, 1931, Vibrios (*Vibrio jejuni*, n. sp.) associated with intestinal disorders of cows and calves, *J Exp Med*, **53**: 853–64.

Ketley JM, 1995, Virulence of *Campylobacter* species: a molecular genetic approach, *J Med Microbiol*, **42**: 312–27.

Khakhria R, Lior H, 1992, Extended phage-typing scheme for *Campylobacter jejuni* and *Campylobacter coli*, *Epidemiol Infect*, **108**: 403–14.

Kiehlbauch JA, Brenner DJ et al., 1991, *Campylobacter butzleri* sp. nov. isolated from humans and animals with diarrheal illness, *J Clin Microbiol*, **29**: 376–85.

Kiehlbauch JA, Tauxe RV et al., 1994, *Helicobacter cinaedi*-associated bacteremia and cellulitis in immunocompromised patients, *Ann Intern Med*, **121**: 90–3.

Kiehlbauch JA, Brenner DJ et al., 1995, Genotypic characterization of *Helicobacter cinaedi* and *Helicobacter fennelliae* strains isolated from humans and animals, *J Clin Microbiol*, **33**: 2940–7.

King EO, 1962, The laboratory recognition of *Vibrio fetus* and a closely related *Vibrio* isolated from cases of human vibriosis, *Ann N Y Acad Sci*, **98**: 700–11.

Kirkbride CA, Gates CE et al., 1985, Ovine abortion associated with an anaerobic bacterium, *J Am Vet Assoc*, **186**: 789–91.

Kita E, Oku D et al., 1990, Hepatotoxic activity of *Campylobacter jejuni*, *J Med Microbiol*, **33**: 171–82.

Konkel ME, Mead DJ, Cieplak W, 1993, Kinetic and antigenic characterization of altered protein synthesis by *Campylobacter jejuni* during cultivation with human epithelial cells, *J Infect Dis*, **168**: 948–54.

Konkel ME, Hayes SF et al., 1992, Characteristics of the internalization and intracellular survival of *Campylobacter jejuni* in human epithelial cell cultures, *Microb Pathog*, **13**: 357–70.

Lambert MA, Patton CM et al., 1987, Differentiation of *Campylobacter* and *Campylobacter*-like organisms by cellular fatty acid composition, *J Clin Microbiol*, **25**: 706–13.

Lawson GHK, Rowland AC, 1974, Intestinal adenomatosis in the pig: a bacteriological study, *Res Vet Sci*, **17**: 331–6.

Lee A, Fox J, Hazell S, 1993, Pathogenicity of *Helicobacter pylori*: a perspective, *Infect Immun*, **61**: 1601–10.

Lee A, O'Rourke J, 1993, Ultrastructure of *Helicobacter* organisms and possible relevance for pathogenesis, Helicobacter pylori: *Biology and Clinical Practice*, eds Goodwin CS, Worsley BW, CRC Press, Boca Raton, FL, 15–35.

Lee A, Phillips MW et al., 1992, *Helicobacter muridarum* sp. nov., a microaerophilic helical bacterium with a novel ultrastructure

isolated from the intestinal mucosa of rodents, *Int J Syst Bacteriol*, **42**: 27–36.

Lior H, Woodward DL et al., 1982, Serotyping of *Campylobacter jejuni* by slide agglutination based on heat-labile antigenic factors, *J Clin Microbiol*, **15**: 761–8.

Luke CJ, Penn CW, 1995, Identification of a 29 kDa flagellar sheath protein in *Helicobacter pylori* using a murine monoclonal antibody, *Microbiology*, **141**: 597–604.

McClung CR, Patriquin DG, Davis RE, 1983, *Campylobacter nitrofigilis* sp. nov., a nitrogen-fixing bacterium associated with roots of *Spartina alterniflora* Loisel, *Int J Syst Bacteriol*, **33**: 605–12.

McFadyean J, Stockman S, 1913, *Report of the Departmental Committee appointed by the Board of Agriculture and Fisheries to inquire into Epizootic Abortion. Part III, Abortion in Sheep*, HMSO, London.

McKhann GM, Cornblath DR et al., 1993, Acute motor axonal neuropathy: a frequent cause of acute flaccid paralysis in China, *Ann Neurol*, **33**: 333–42.

McNulty CAM, Dent JC, 1987, Rapid identification of *Campylobacter pylori* (*C. pyloridis*) by preformed enzymes, *J Clin Microbiol*, **25**: 1683–6.

McNulty CAM, Dent JC et al., 1989, New spiral bacterium in gastric mucosa, *J Clin Pathol*, **42**: 585–91.

Mai UE, Perez-Perez GI et al., 1992, Surface proteins from *Helicobacter pylori* exhibit chemotactic activity for human leukocytes and are present in gastric mucosa, *J Exp Med*, **175**: 517–25.

Marshall BJ, 1983, Unidentified curved bacilli on gastric epithelium in active chronic gastritis, *Lancet*, **1**: 1273–5.

Marshall BJ, Royce H et al., 1984, Original isolation of *Campylobacter pyloridis* from human gastric mucosa, *Microbios Lett*, **25**: 83–8.

Mendes EN, Queiroz DMM et al., 1990, Ultrastructure of a spiral micro-organism from pig gastric mucosa ('*Gastrospirillum suis*'), *J Med Microbiol*, **33**: 61–6.

Miller S, Pesci EC, Pickett CL, 1993, A *Campylobacter jejuni* homolog of the LcrD/FlbF family of proteins is necessary for flagellar biogenesis, *Infect Immun*, **61**: 2930–6.

Mills SD, Kurjanczyk LA, Penner JL, 1992, Antigenicity of *Helicobacter pylori* lipopolysaccharides, *J Clin Microbiol*, **30**: 3175–80.

Mills SD, Aspinall GO et al., 1992, Lipopolysaccharide antigens of *Campylobacter jejuni*, Campylobacter jejuni: *Current Status and Future Trends*, eds Nachamkin I, Blaser MJ, Tompkins LS, American Society for Microbiology, Washington, DC, 223–9.

Mishu B, Blaser MJ, 1993, Role of infection due to *Campylobacter jejuni* in the initiation of Guillain–Barré syndrome, *Clin Infect Dis*, **17**: 104–8.

Mishu Allos B, Lastovica AL, Blaser MJ, 1995, Atypical campylobacters and related organisms, *Infections of the Gastrointestinal Tract*, eds Blaser MJ, Smith PD et al., Raven Press, New York, 849–65.

Moran AP, 1995, Cell surface characteristics of *Helicobacter pylori*, *FEMS Immunol Med Microbiol*, **10**: 271–80.

Moss CW, Kai A et al., 1984, Isoprenoid quinone content and cellular fatty acid composition of *Campylobacter* species, *J Clin Microbiol*, **19**: 772–6.

Nachamkin I, 1995, *Campylobacter and Arcobacter, Manual of Clinical Microbiology*, 6th edn, eds Murray PR, Baron EJ et al., ASM Press, Washington, DC, 483–91.

Nachamkin I, Bohachick K, Patton CM, 1993, Flagellin gene typing of *Campylobacter jejuni* by restriction fragment length polymorphism analysis, *J Clin Microbiol*, **31**: 1531–6.

Nachamkin I, Ung H, Patton CM, 1996, Analysis of O and HL serotypes of *Campylobacter* by the flagellin gene typing system, *J Clin Microbiol*, **34**: 277–81.

Nachamkin I, Yang XH, Stern NJ, 1993, Role of *Campylobacter jejuni* flagella as colonization factors for three-day-old chicks: analysis with flagellar mutants, *Appl Environ Microbiol*, **59**: 1269–73.

Nachamkin I, Stowell C et al., 1984, *Campylobacter laridis* causing bacteremia in an immunosuppressed patient, *Ann Intern Med*, **101**: 55–7.

Neill SD, Campbell JN et al., 1985, Taxonomic position of *Campylobacter cryaerophila* sp. nov., *Int J Syst Bacteriol*, **35:** 342–56.

Oelschlaeger TA, Guerry P, Kopecko DJ, 1993, Unusual microtubule-dependent endocytosis mechanisms triggered by *Campylobacter jejuni* and *Citrobacter freundii*, *Proc Natl Acad Sci*, **90:** 6884–8.

Ogura N, Shibata Y et al., 1995, Effect of *Campylobacter rectus* LPS on plasminogen activator-plasmin system in human gingival fibroblast cells, *J Periodont Res*, **30:** 132–40.

Owen RJ, 1992, Taxonomy of *Helicobacter pylori*, Helicobacter pylori *and Gastroduodenal Disease*, 2nd edn, eds Rathbone BJ, Heatley RV, Blackwell Scientific Publications, Oxford, 5–18.

Owen RJ, 1995, Bacteriology of *Helicobacter pylori*, *Baillière's Clin Gastroenterol*, **9:** 415–46.

Paster BJ, Lee A et al., 1991, Phylogeny of *Helicobacter felis* sp. nov., *Helicobacter mustelae*, and related bacteria, *Int J Syst Bacteriol*, **41:** 31–8.

Patton CM, Wachsmuth IK, 1992, Typing schemes: are current methods useful?, Campylobacter jejuni: *Current Status and Future Trends*, eds Nachamkin I, Blaser MJ, Tompkins LS, American Society for Microbiology, Washington, DC, 110–28.

Pei Z, Blaser MJ, 1992, PEB1, the major cell-binding factor of *Campylobacter jejuni*, is a homolog of the binding component in gram-negative nutrient transport systems, *J Biol Chem*, **268:** 18717–25.

Penner JL, Hennessy JN, 1980, Passive hemagglutination technique for serotyping *Campylobacter fetus* subsp. *jejuni* on the basis of soluble heat-stable antigens, *J Clin Microbiol*, **12:** 732–7.

Perez-Perez GI, Taylor DN et al., 1992, Lack of evidence of enterotoxin involvement in pathogenesis of *Campylobacter* diarrhea, Campylobacter jejuni: *Current Status and Future Trends*, eds Nachamkin I, Blaser MJ, Tompkins LS, American Society for Microbiology, Washington, DC, 184–92.

Pesci EC, Cottle DL, Pickett CL, 1994, Genetic, enzymatic and pathogenic studies of the iron superoxide dismutase of *Campylobacter jejuni*, *Infect Immun*, **62:** 2687–94.

Pickett CL, Auffenberg T et al., 1992, Iron acquisition and hemolysis production by *Campylobacter jejuni*, *Infect Immun*, **60:** 3872–7.

Popovic-Uroic T, Patton CM et al., 1990, Evaluation of the indoxyl acetate hydrolysis test for rapid differentiation of *Campylobacter*, *Helicobacter*, and *Wolinella* species, *J Clin Microbiol*, **28:** 2335–9.

Prévot AR, 1940, Etudes de systématique bactérienne. V. Essai de classification des vibrions anaérobies, *Ann Inst Pasteur (Paris)*, **64:** 117–25.

Radomyski T, Murano EA et al., 1994, Eliminaton of pathogens of significance in food by low-dose irradiation: a review, *J Food Prot*, **57:** 73–86.

Rathbone BJ, Heatley RV, 1992, The historical associations between bacteria and peptic-ulcer disease, Helicobacter pylori *and Gastroduodenal Disease*, 2nd edn, eds Rathbone BJ, Heatley RV, Blackwell Scientific Publications, Oxford, 1–4.

Rauws EAJ, Tytgat GNJ, 1995, *Helicobacter pylori* in duodenal and gastric ulcer disease, *Baillière's Clin Gastroenterol*, **9:** 529–47.

Riegg SJ, Dunn BE, Blaser MJ, 1995, Microbiology and pathogenesis of *Helicobacter pylori*, *Infections of the Gastrointestinal Tract*, eds Blaser MJ, Smith PD et al., Raven Press, New York, 535–50.

Roop RM, Smibert RM et al., 1985a, *Campylobacter mucosalis* (Lawson, Leaver, Pettigrew, and Rowland 1981) comb. nov.: emended description, *Int J Syst Bacteriol*, **35:** 189–92.

Roop RM, Smibert RM et al., 1985b, Designation of the neotype strain for *Campylobacter sputorum* (Prévot) Véron and Chatelain 1973, *Int J Syst Bacteriol*, **36:** 348.

Ruiz-Palacios GM, Cervantes LE et al., 1992, In vitro models for studying *Campylobacter* infections, Campylobacter jejuni: *Current Status and Future Trends*, eds Nachamkin I, Blaser MJ, Tompkins LS, American Society for Microbiology, Washington, DC, 176–83.

Russell RG, Blake DC, 1994, Cell association and invasion of Caco-2 cells by *Campylobacter jejuni*, *Infect Immun*, **62:** 3773–9.

Salama SM, Bolton FJ, Hutchinson DN, 1990, Application of a new phagetyping scheme to campylobacters isolated during outbreaks, *Epidemiol Infect*, **104:** 405–11.

Salomon H, 1896, Ueber das Spirillum des Saugertiermagens und sein Verhalten zu den Belegzellen, *Centralbl Bakteriol*, **19:** 433–42.

Sandstedt K, Ursing J, 1991, Description of *Campylobacter upsaliensis* sp. nov. previously known as the CNW group, *Syst Appl Microbiol*, **14:** 39–45.

Schauer DB, Ghori N, Falkow S, 1993, Isolation and characterization of '*Flexispira rappini*' from laboratory mice, *J Clin Microbiol*, **31:** 2709–14.

Schmitt W, Haas R, 1994, Genetic analysis of the *Helicobacter pylori* vacuolating cytotoxin: structural similarities with the IgA protease type of exported protein, *Mol Microbiol*, **12:** 307–19.

Scotter SL, Humphrey TJ, Henley A, 1993, Methods for the detection of thermotolerant campylobacters in foods: results of an inter-laboratory study, *J Appl Bacteriol*, **74:** 155–63.

Sebald M, Véron M, 1963, Teneur en bases de l'ADN et classification des vibrions, *Ann Inst Pasteur (Paris)*, **105:** 897–910.

Segal ED, Shon J, Tompkins LS, 1992, Characterization of *Helicobacter pylori* urease mutants, *Infect Immun*, **60:** 1883–9.

Shahamat M, Mai UE et al., 1991, Evaluation of liquid media for growth of *Helicobacter pylori*, *J Clin Microbiol*, **29:** 2835–7.

Skirrow MB, 1977, Campylobacter enteritis: a 'new' disease, *Br Med J*, **2:** 9–11.

Skirrow MB, 1990, *Campylobacter*, *Helicobacter* and other motile curved gram-negative rods, *Topley and Wilson's Principles of Bacteriology, Virology and Immunity*, vol. 2, 8th edn, eds Parker MT, Collier LH, Edward Arnold, London, 531–49.

Skirrow MB, Blaser MJ, 1995, *Campylobacter jejuni*, *Infections of the Gastrointestinal Tract*, eds Blaser MJ, Smith PD et al., Raven Press, New York, 825–48.

Sly LI, Bronsdon MA et al., 1993, The phylogenetic position of *Helicobacter nemestrinae*, *Int J Syst Bacteriol*, **43:** 386–7.

Smith T, Taylor M, 1919, Some morphological and biological characters of the spirilla (*Vibrio fetus*, n. sp.) associated with disease of the fetal membranes in cattle, *J Exp Med*, **30:** 299–311.

Smoot DT, Resau JH et al., 1993, Adherence of *Helicobacter pylori* to cultured human gastric epithelial cells, *Infect Immun*, **61:** 350–5.

Solnick JV, O'Rourke J et al., 1993, An uncultured gastric spiral organism is a newly identified *Helicobacter* in humans, *J Infect Dis*, **168:** 379–85.

Stanley J, Burnens AP et al., 1992, *Campylobacter helveticus* sp. nov., a new thermophilic species from domestic animals: characterization, and cloning of a species-specific DNA probe, *J Gen Microbiol*, **138:** 2293–303.

Stanley J, Linton D et al., 1993, *Helicobacter canis* sp. nov., a new species from dogs: an integrated study of phenotype and genotype, *J Gen Microbiol*, **139:** 2495–504.

Stanley J, Linton D et al., 1994, *Helicobacter pullorum* sp. nov. – genotype and phenotype of a new species isolated from poultry and from human patients with gastroenteritis, *Microbiology*, **140:** 3441–9.

Steele TW, Owen RJ, 1988, *Campylobacter jejuni* subspecies *doylei* (subsp. nov.), a subspecies of nitrate-negative campylobacters isolated from human clinical specimens, *Int J Syst Bacteriol*, **38:** 316–18.

Stern NJ, 1992, Reservoirs for *Campylobacter jejuni* and approaches for intervention in poultry, Campylobacter jejuni: *Current Status and Future Trends*, eds Nachamkin I, Blaser MJ, Tompkins LS, American Society for Microbiology, Washington, DC, 49–60.

Tanner ACR, Badger S et al., 1981, *Wolinella* gen. nov., *Wolinella succinogenes* (*Vibrio succinogenes* Wolin et al.) comb. nov., and description of *Bacteroides gracilis* sp. nov., *Wolinella recta* sp. nov., *Campylobacter concisus* sp. nov., and *Eikenella corrodens* from humans with periodontal diseases, *Int J Syst Bacteriol*, **31:** 432–45.

Tanner ACR, Listgarten MA, Ebersole JL, 1984, *Wolinella curva* sp. nov.: '*Vibrio succinogenes*' of human origin, *Int J Syst Bacteriol*, **34:** 275–82.

Tarrand JJ, Gröschel DHM, 1982, Rapid, modified oxidase test for oxidase-variable bacterial isolates, *J Clin Microbiol*, **16:** 772–4.

Taylor DE, 1992, Genetics of *Campylobacter* and *Helicobacter*, *Annu Rev Microbiol*, **46:** 35–64.

Taylor NS, Fox JG et al., 1995, Long-term colonization with single and multiple strains of *Helicobacter pylori* assessed by DNA fingerprinting, *J Clin Microbiol*, **33:** 918–23.

Thompson SA, Blaser MJ, 1995, Isolation of the *Helicobacter pylori recA* gene and involvement of the *recA* region in resistance to low pH, *Infect Immun*, **63:** 2185–93.

Totten PA, Fennell CL et al., 1985, *Campylobacter cinaedi* (sp. nov.) and *Campylobacter fennelliae* (sp. nov.): two new *Campylobacter* species associated with enteric disease in homosexual men, *J Infect Dis*, **151:** 131–9.

Totten PA, Patton CH et al., 1987, Prevalence and characterization of hippurate-negative *Campylobacter jejuni* in King county, Washington, *J Clin Microbiol*, **25:** 1747–52.

Trust T, Logan SM et al., 1994, Phylogenetic and molecular characterization of a 23S rRNA gene positions the genus *Campylobacter* in the epsilon subdivision of the *Proteobacteria* and shows that the presence of transcribed spacers is common in *Campylobacter* species, *J Bacteriol*, **176:** 4597–609.

Tummuru MK, Cover TL, Blaser MJ, 1994, Mutation of the cytotoxin-associated *cagA* gene does not affect the vacuolating cytotoxin activity of *Helicobacter pylori*, *Infect Immun*, **62:** 2609–13.

Tunnicliff R, 1914, An anerobic vibrio isolated from a case of acute bronchitis, *J Infect Dis*, **15:** 350–1.

Turbett GR, Hoj PB et al., 1992, Purification and characterization of the urease enzymes of *Helicobacter* species from humans and animals, *Infect Immun*, **60:** 5259–66.

Ursing JB, Lior H, Owen RJ, 1994, Proposal of minimal standards for describing new species of the family *Campylobacteraceae*, *Int J Syst Bacteriol*, **44:** 842–5.

Vandamme P, De Ley J, 1991, Proposal for a new family, *Campylobacteraceae*, *Int J Syst Bacteriol*, **41:** 451–5.

Vandamme P, Falsen E et al., 1989, Identification of EF group 22 campylobacters from gastroenteritis cases as *Campylobacter concisus*, *J Clin Microbiol*, **27:** 1775–81.

Vandamme P, Falsen E et al., 1991, Revision of *Campylobacter*, *Helicobacter*, and *Wolinella* taxonomy: emendation of generic descriptions and proposal of *Arcobacter* gen. nov., *Int J Syst Bacteriol*, **41:** 81–103.

Vandamme P, Vancanneyt M et al., 1992, Polyphasic taxonomic study of the emended genus *Arcobacter* with *Arcobacter butzleri* comb. nov. and *Arcobacter skirrowii* sp. nov., an aerotolerant bacterium isolated from veterinary specimens, *Int J Syst Bacteriol*, **42:** 344–56.

Vandamme P, Daneshvar MI et al., 1995, Chemotaxonomic analyses of *Bacteroides gracilis* and *Bacteroides ureolyticus* and reclassification of *B. gracilis* as *Campylobacter gracilis* comb. nov., *Int J Syst Bacteriol*, **45:** 145–52.

Véron M, Chatelain R, 1973, Taxonomic study of the genus *Campylobacter* Sebald and Véron and designation of the neotype strain for the type species, *Campylobacter fetus* (Smith and Taylor) Sebald and Véron, *Int J Syst Bacteriol*, **23:** 122–4.

Véron M, Lenvoisé-Furet A, Beaune P, 1981, Anaerobic respiration of fumarate as a differential test between *Campylobacter fetus* and *Campylobacter jejuni*, *Curr Microbiol*, **6:** 349–54.

Warren JR, 1983, Unidentified curved bacilli on gastric epithelium in chronic active gastritis, *Lancet*, **1:** 1273–4.

Wassenaar TM, Bleumink-Pluym NM, van der Zeijst BA, 1991, Inactivation of *Campylobacter jejuni* flagellin genes by homologous recombination demonstrates that *flaA* but not *flaB* is required for invasion, *EMBO J*, **10:** 2055–61.

Webb PM, Forman D, 1995, *Helicobacter pylori* as a risk factor for cancer, *Baillière's Clin Gastroenterol*, **9:** 563–82.

Wooldridge KG, Williams PH, Ketley JM, 1994, Iron-responsive genetic regulation in *Campylobacter jejuni*: cloning and characterization of a *fur* homolog, *J Bacteriol*, **176:** 5852–6.

van Zwet AA, Thijs JC et al., 1993, Sensitivity of culture compared with that of polymerase chain reaction for detection of *Helicobacter pylori* from antral biopsy samples, *J Clin Microbiol*, **31:** 1918–20.

Chapter 55

TREPONEMA

C W Penn

1 INTRODUCTION AND HISTORICAL BACKGROUND

The taxonomy of the spirochaetes is still at a primitive stage of development compared with that of other bacterial groups. This is largely because of difficulties experienced in cultivating many important species of the spirochaetes. In consequence, data about their biochemical and other phenotypic properties – information that in most other bacterial groups is considered crucial for classification – are almost totally lacking, and reliance has had to be placed on morphological, ecological and epidemiological criteria. This has led to several designations which are probably inappropriate; for example, organisms classed in the genus *Treponema* differ widely in their habitat, pathogenic role and physiological properties. In this chapter, therefore, several important species or groups are highlighted rather than an attempt made at a comprehensive survey of the genus.

In *Bergey's Manual of Systematic Bacteriology*, Canale-Parola (1984) defined an order of motile, helical bacteria, Spirochaetales, which were distinguished from other spiral or curved bacteria by the periplasmic location of their flagella, hence named endoflagella; however, even this criterion is open to some doubt in the light of observations that flagella, or more probably bundles of flagella, of the Reiter strain of *Treponema phagedenis* may be observed by light microscopy to be detached distally from the motile organisms (Smibert 1984), and a report by Lee et al. (1988) indicated that spirochaetes isolated from feline gastric mucosa may have both conventional polar flagella and endoflagella. It is now known that the latter organisms are helicobacters, and not classed as spirochaetes. Barbour and Hayes (1986) have emphasized the heterogeneity of the spirochaetes in terms of the G + C (mol%) content of their DNA. Furthermore, as 16S ribosomal RNA (rRNA) analysis shows that the phylogenetic origin of spirochaetes is fundamentally distinct from that of other eubacteria, these authors suggested that a formal rank of class or division would be appropriate for these organisms. Within the order Spirochaetales, Canale-Parola (1984) defined 2 families, Spirochaetaceae and Leptospiraceae, the latter clearly distinguished by their usually hooked ends, the presence of diaminopimelic acid rather than L-ornithine as a component of peptidoglycan, aerobic metabolism, and their utilization of long-chain fatty acids or fatty alcohols as carbon and energy sources. It is within the Spirochaetaceae, in the genera *Spirochaeta*, *Cristispira*, *Treponema* and *Borrelia*, that most of the taxonomic problems have occurred, particularly in the 2 latter groups of pathogens. The technique of 16S rRNA oligonucleotide cataloguing, and more recently sequencing, has been applied to several genera of spirochaetes (Paster et al. 1984, 1991, Olsen, Woese and Overbeek 1994) and this approach has greatly advanced spirochaete taxonomy. It has demonstrated a major division between the leptospires and other spirochaetes, and a significant difference between *Treponema* (now *Serpulina*) *hyodysenteriae* and other treponemes examined. Currently, it is clear that of the better characterized organisms designated as *Treponema*, the *Treponema pallidum* group, *Treponema denticola* and *T. phagedenis* are most closely related (Paster et al. 1991).

The agents of the human treponematoses (*T. pallidum* subspecies and *Treponema carateum*) have been the subject of intensive recent research; therefore *T. pallidum* subsp. *pallidum* (hereafter designated *T. pallidum*) will be described in detail, with notes on the other (sub)species where necessary and brief mention of the probably-related rabbit pathogen *Treponema paraluiscuniculi*. Also within the genus *Treponema* at present are included the oral spirochaetes *T. phagedenis*, exemplified mainly in the literature by the Reiter strain, and *Treponema denticola* and related organisms. The latter organisms have received much attention as putative periodontal pathogens and will be considered separately.

The genus *Treponema* is formally described as comprising relatively small spirochaetes (0.1–0.4 μm diameter), characterized particularly by the presence of cytoplasmic filaments which run the length of the cell in line with the endoflagella but within the cytoplasm. The filaments appear to be connected to the endoflagellar basal bodies at each end of the cell, and are presumed but not proven to have a function in motility. Their mode of action is unknown. Treponemes are host-associated and, in several cases, pathogenic. They are strictly anaerobic or microaerophilic. The type species is *T. pallidum*. Like many others, it is extremely difficult to culture and has been grown only in association with cultured cells. For this reason the taxonomy of the genus is poorly developed (Smibert 1984).

2 *TREPONEMA PALLIDUM*

T. pallidum is the causative agent of venereal syphilis in humans. Due to their very close genetic homology (Miao and Fieldsteel 1980), the treponemes of syphilis (subsp. *pallidum*) and yaws (subsp. *pertenue*) have been assigned to the same species. A third subspecies, *endemicum*, has also been proposed for the agent of endemic syphilis, on the basis of clinical observations of similarity with *T. pallidum* from venereal syphilis. Thus the principal criterion of speciation is epidemiological behaviour.

Knowledge of the species is relatively recent; its small size and poor staining properties prevented its identification until 1905 (Schaudinn and Hoffmann 1905, reviewed by Kampmeier 1979). Syphilis was of immense significance, both socially and medically, until the introduction of penicillin led to a dramatic drop in its incidence after the World War II. The origin of the disease (and hence of the organism) is the subject of controversy that is unlikely to be resolved (Hackett 1963, Kampmeier 1982). It first appeared in Europe in the 1490s, one theory being that it was introduced by Columbus' sailors returning from the New World. Its early spread seems to have been fostered by social upheavals such as the siege of Naples, and by the end of the fifteenth century it was well established in Europe. Whether the organism was indeed present in the New World as a pathogen of humans before this time, or whether it arose by mutation of a non-venereal or commensal treponeme in the population, is not known. Another possibility is that a similar organism from non-human primates, such as the Fribourg-Blanc treponeme (Fribourg-Blanc and Mollaret 1969) may have become adapted to survival in humans. Parallels with the beginnings of the HIV epidemic may thus be drawn.

T. pallidum seems to have been quite virulent when it initially emerged in humans (Sell and Norris 1983), and to have attained a more benign equilibrium with the human population over the centuries. Many attempts were made to devise treatments, the more successful being the use of mercury and, early this century, arsenical compounds such as Ehrlich's Salvarsan (Kampmeier 1982). However, it was not until the introduction of penicillin that the disease retreated significantly, falling to very low levels in the 1950s. Nevertheless, the organism survived well enough for infection to recrudesce after the revolution in sexual attitudes of the 1960s, emerging particularly in the male homosexual population. The incidence of syphilis fell dramatically in the 1980s as a result of behavioural changes – the adoption of 'safe sex' practices such as condom use – by male homosexuals. It remains low in the UK, currently well below 1000 cases per annum. There has, however, been a resurgence of disease in the late 1980s and 1990s in the USA, particularly in heterosexual populations, and also in many developing countries.

2.1 Morphology and ultrastructure

T. pallidum has a characteristic morphology that assists its identification by trained microscopists (Fig. 55.1). It is difficult to stain for light microscopy, the best methods being either prolonged Giemsa staining, which produces a slender, pale pink image of the organism (hence *pallidum* – of pallid appearance – and distinct from more refractile treponemes – '*refringens*'), or silver staining methods which rely on the deposition of metallic silver around the organism (Walter et al. 1969). Conventionally, dark ground microscopy (Fig. 55.1) is used in diagnostic laboratories, but phase contrast can also be quite effective. The organism has a diameter of 0.1–0.15 μm, a wave amplitude of c. 0.3 μm, and a wavelength of c. 0.6 μm. The total length may be as much as 7–8 μm, with up to 12 waves, rather regular in form especially when the organism is freshly isolated. Ultrastructurally, *T. pallidum* is characterized by a terminal knob structure of unknown composition or function (Fig. 55.2), usually 3 but occasionally 4 endoflagella inserted in a longitudinal row on the tapering terminal portion at each end of the cell, and cytoplasmic fibrils that run the length of the organism internal to the cell wall and cytoplasmic membrane (Fig. 55.3). The endoflagella are more than half the length of the organism and run along the axial aspect of the spiral body. Endoflagella from the 2 ends interdigitate over the central portion of the organism, so that in transverse section there often appear to be 3 of them in sections taken from terminal regions and 4–6 in sections from the central portion. The endoflagella have a form quite typical of bacterial flagella, with a basal body bearing disc- or collar-like structures that interact with layers in the cytoplasmic membrane and cell wall (Hovind-Hougen 1976, 1983). In the number of discs they resemble flagella from gram-positive bacteria, because they do not penetrate the outer membrane.

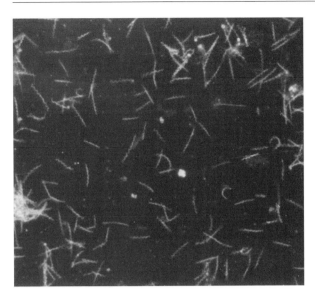

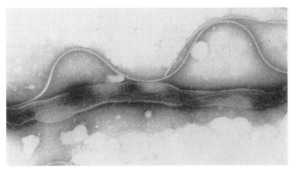

Fig. 55.3 Electron micrograph of negatively stained *Treponema pallidum* cell treated with trypsin and Triton X-100 to reveal cytoplasmic filaments (× 37 500). (Courtesy of Dr A Cockayne).

Fig. 55.1 Suspension of *Treponema pallidum* cells, dark ground microscopy (× 600).

The flagellar shafts have a core and sheath structure, with a subunit array visible on the sheath (Hovind-Hougen 1983, Cockayne, Bailey and Penn 1987). The sheath, or more properly the outer layer of the flagellar shaft, is sometimes absent from the distal end of the flagellum, the structure then appearing thinner.

Another important ultrastructural feature of *T. pallidum* is the outer membrane. This has been observed very clearly by some workers (Johnson, Ritzi and Livermore 1973), whereas others have questioned its existence (Sykes and Miller 1973, Penn 1981). However, Penn and Lichfield (1982) showed that post-fixation *en bloc* with uranyl acetate during preparation of specimens for electron microscopy preserved the outer membrane as a distinct bilayer. The requirement for uranyl acetate suggested a high phospholipid content of the outer membrane. The outer membrane

and its constituent proteins have become a key topic (see section 2.5, p. 1261) in considering the pathogenicity and immunobiology of *T. pallidum*, being implicated in the ability of the organism to evade host immune responses during chronic infection (Radolf, Norgard and Schulz 1989, Cox et al. 1992).

Other morphological features of the organism have been less widely confirmed. Although very detailed structural schemes have been proposed (Wiegand, Strobel and Glassman 1972), some features of which are unconfirmed, several aspects remain largely unknown. There is little unequivocal ultrastructural evidence for an amorphous capsule-like layer of treponemal origin external to the outer membrane, although polyanionic materials precipitable with stains such as ruthenium red (Fitzgerald et al. 1976, Zeigler et al. 1976) or cetyl pyridinium chloride (Fitzgerald et al. 1985) have been observed both in fresh host-derived organisms and in treponemes co-incubated with host cells in vitro (Fitzgerald, Johnson and Wolff 1978). There is a lack of detailed knowledge of the ultrastructure of the *T. pallidum* tip. It is not known, for example, whether the outer membrane extends over the knob structure at the tip, or whether this has an exposed surface of different composition from the cell body. A suggested ability of some spirochaetes to undergo movement or 'capping' of outer-membrane components towards the tip (Barbour, Barrera and Judd 1983) and a long-postulated but as yet unconfirmed role for the tip structure of *T. pallidum* in adhesion to host surfaces make it important to clarify this aspect of ultrastructure.

2.2 Metabolism and growth

For many decades, *T. pallidum* appeared strictly non-cultivable in vitro, and because the most prolonged viability, indicated by motility, was attained in anaerobic conditions the organism was assumed to be strictly anaerobic. However, physiological indications that it might require oxygen (Cox and Barber 1974, Baseman, Nichols and Hayes 1976) and exposure to oxygen gradients and assessment of survival (motility) and virulence for the rabbit at different oxygen levels (Fieldsteel, Becker and Stout 1977) led to the realiz-

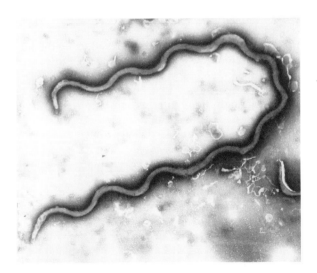

Fig. 55.2 Electron micrograph of negatively stained *Treponema pallidum*. Note terminal knob structures and 3 endoflagella at each end (× 13 350).

ation that an oxygen concentration of about 3% in the gaseous phase above treponemal suspensions was optimal. The first report of co-cultivation with tissue culture cells in vitro appeared soon afterwards (Fieldsteel, Cox and Moeckli 1981), and it was independently confirmed by Norris (1982). Nevertheless, the organism has not yet been grown in the absence of cultured mammalian cells, and rather poor yields are obtained with a maximum of 2–3 log_{10} increase in numbers. Reliable serial subculture in vitro is still difficult to achieve (Norris and Edmondson 1986a). A crucial factor appears to be the inclusion in media of suitable batches of serum, and a high molecular weight fraction of serum contains the necessary components (Norris and Edmondson 1986b). However, it is not yet practicable to produce in vitro sufficient organisms for extensive experimentation, or for use as immunodiagnostic or prophylactic reagents. Several reports indicate a potential role for host cells or their products in limiting the susceptibility of the organisms to toxicity of oxygen or its reactive products (Cover, Norris and Miller 1982, Sell and Norris 1983, Norris and Edmondson 1986b, Cox et al. 1990). Thus, it may never be possible to achieve growth in vitro in the absence of cultured cells. Such toxic activities may be particularly significant because of the slow growth rate of this organism. The mean generation time for growth in vivo in the rabbit testis appears to be c. 30 h (Turner and Hollander 1957). Although pathogenic bacteria tend to grow even more slowly in vivo than in ideal conditions in vitro, there is little doubt that long doubling times are responsible in large part for the difficulty of culture in vitro, since if there is a significant 'death rate' due to adverse factors in vitro, it may well exceed the growth rate and lead to a net decrease in numbers.

The only practicable method at present available for the growth of organisms as a source of diagnostic antigen or for laboratory research is infection of the rabbit testis. The best yields are obtained by inoculation of a large volume (e.g. 1 ml) of treponemal suspension into the body of the testis so that it is dispersed throughout the tissue; this leads to a uniform, diffuse orchitis. The inoculum suspension should be either freshly obtained from an infected animal or recently thawed at 35°C from a stock suspension frozen with glycerol 15% v/v at −70°C or lower. It should contain at least 1×10^7 vigorously motile treponemes to ensure good yields after a short and predictable incubation period of about 10 days (typical for the Nichols strain). In many laboratories rabbits are routinely screened for positive serology in standard diagnostic tests for syphilis in case they have been exposed to *T. paraluiscuniculi*, and are discarded if the tests are positive. However, there does appear to be some variation between animals independent of serological status; some seronegative animals may fail to develop overt orchitis.

About 8–10 days after inoculation, the testes become palpably firmer and then enlarge markedly over a period of a few days. Unless removed within 3–4 days of detection of orchitis, gross pathological changes such as haemorrhage and necrosis occur and yields of treponemes are reduced. Generally, yields of treponemes may be enhanced by maintaining an environmental temperature below 20°C and by systemic administration of steroids such as cortisone (Turner and Hollander 1957) or synthetic substitutes, ideally in a slow release form (Brause, Qualls and Roberts 1979). There is, however, significant variation between infected animals and excellent yields are sometimes obtained in the absence of these procedures.

After removal from the animal, the testis may be trimmed of accessory tissues, cut up with scissors into small pieces and shaken gently (e.g. at 60 rpm), or incubated statically at 35°C in several times its own volume of extraction medium such as the survival medium of Nelson and Diesendruck (1951) or a simpler substitute such as Hanks's medium supplemented with 2 mm dithiothreitol. Ideally this should be done in an atmosphere of N_2 with O_2 3% and CO_2 5%, the latter to buffer with bicarbonate in the medium against falling pH due to glycolysis by the tissue.

Limited investigations of metabolic processes have been performed. Cytochromes *b* and *c* are present (Lysko and Cox 1977), and respiration and oxidative phosphorylation have been demonstrated (Lysko and Cox 1978). Glucose is utilized to produce acetate and CO_2 (Nichols and Baseman 1975) via the Embden–Meyerhof–Parnas and hexose–monophosphate pathways (Schiller and Cox 1977), and is incorporated into the glycerol portion of lipids, the pentoses of nucleic acids, and amino acids such as aspartate (Barbieri, Austin and Cox 1981). Pyruvate may be oxidized in the presence of oxygen (Barbieri and Cox 1979). Lactate may act as an electron donor in some circumstances, possibly providing a means of controlling the available oxygen level at an optimum value (Austin and Cox 1986).

T. pallidum is extremely sensitive to adverse environmental conditions, including raised temperatures (exposure to 41.5°C for 1 h is said to be lethal, a property exploited early this century in the fever therapy of syphilis) and desiccation. It is also very susceptible to low levels of detergents, perhaps reflecting the high phospholipid or low lipopolysaccharide (LPS) content of the outer membrane (Penn, Bailey and Cockayne 1985a), and is easily killed by conventional disinfectants. Although the organisms may be stored by freezing at −70°C or below, lyophilization has not proved possible – an additional technical problem in the preservation and transport of isolates which has restricted the numbers of strains used in research.

2.3   Genetics

Nothing is known of gene transfer in *T. pallidum*, there being no reports of transformation, transduction or conjugation. A single report of isolation of a plasmid from the organism (Norgard and Miller 1981) remains unconfirmed. No evidence of transposable genetic elements has been reported. However, technical difficulties with experimental manipulation in vitro preclude necessary experiments in this field; for example, clonal populations of the organism essential for genetic studies cannot be obtained. Nevertheless, molecular genetic studies are proving highly informative, following the first report of cloning and expression of treponemal genes in *Escherichia coli* (Walfield, Hanff and Lovett 1982), an approach widely exploited in the past 2 decades in the molecular dissection of the organism. The genome has a G + C content close to that of *E. coli* at just over 50 mol%, and the size of the circular chromosome is approximately 10^6 bp, as shown by pulse field gel electrophoretic analysis (Walker et al. 1991a). Prominent genes have been physically mapped within the chromosome (Walker et al. 1995). The genome size is among the smallest found in bacteria and its circularity contrasts with the novel linear chromosome of some *Borrelia* spp. At the time of writing the complete genome sequence is expected to be determined imminently, and this information will greatly advance understanding of the molecular biology of this organism.

2.4 Antibiotic susceptibility

Susceptibility to antibiotics has been difficult to assess. There is no direct measure of viability in vitro, motility being the only available indicator, which ultimately has to be correlated with infectivity for rabbits to establish the validity of survival data. There is no evidence that non-motile organisms may be viable, but there is evidence that motile organisms may not necessarily be fully viable and virulent (Fitzgerald 1981). Another major problem in testing antibiotic susceptibility in vitro is that active growth processes such as the synthesis of cell wall polymers, which may be the target of antibiotic action, may not occur in vitro unless incubation conditions are optimal. Furthermore, growth is so slow (see section 2.2, p. 1259) that lethal effects of antibiotics may not be observed before spontaneous loss of viability occurs during incubation, although some useful data on penicillin action have been obtained in vitro (Nell 1954). Firm data on antibiotic efficacy have been obtained mainly from tests in infected animals, and are quite sparse (Rein 1976, Ronald et al. 1992). Hamsters (Alder et al. 1993) and rabbits have been used. The efficacy of penicillin is well established and no conclusive evidence of penicillin resistance has been reported, despite a number of apparent treatment failures. Alternatives are tetracyclines, macrolides such as erythromycin, the newer roxithromycin (Lukehart and Baker-Zander 1987), clarithromycin (Alder et al. 1993), and cephalosporins, including the broad spectrum compounds ceftizoxime and ceftriaxone (Johnson et al. 1982, Korting et al. 1986, 1993). Penicillin-binding proteins of *T. pallidum* have been demonstrated (Cunningham, Miller and Lovett 1987), and their study may furnish further information on the comparative mechanisms of susceptibility of the organism. Recently the 47 kDa major immunodominant protein has also been shown to be a penicillin-binding protein with carboxypeptidase activity, a novel insight into the function of a major

lipoprotein (Weigel et al. 1994). An advance in the assessment of antibiotic susceptibility is the use of in vitro cultures with tissue culture cells (Norris and Edmondson 1988). In adddition, the clinical testing in humans of compounds of known efficacy has been possible, for example with azithromycin (Verdon et al. 1994).

2.5 Cellular constituents and antigenic properties

In early investigations of the antigenicity of *T. pallidum*, methods were used that could not generally discriminate between individual antigenic constituents of the organism, and were derived largely from clinically applicable tests for the serological diagnosis of syphilis. The exception was the recognition of cardiolipin as a probable antigenic component of the organism. It was known quite early (Pangborn 1942) that cardiolipin was the active principle in alcoholic tissue extracts that reacted with so-called 'reaginic' antibody in syphilitic sera, reactivity originally demonstrated by complement fixation in the well known Wassermann reaction. It remains uncertain whether cardiolipin of treponemal origin is significant in syphilis serology; this lipid has been detected in the organism (Matthews, Yang and Jenkin 1979), but it may be derived from the host. It is also uncertain whether the antigenic stimulus that leads to anticardiolipin antibody formation is located on the organisms, or whether it might result from release of cardiolipin from host tissues damaged during disease. It has, however, been shown (Baker-Zander, Shaffer and Lukehart 1993) that anticardiolipin antibodies enhance phagocytosis of *T. pallidum* by macrophages, suggesting the presence of cardiolipin antigen on the treponemal surface.

The use of antigens obtained directly from *T. pallidum* in serology was introduced relatively late. Nelson and Mayer (1949) first demonstrated immobilization of treponemes incubated in vitro with specific antibody and complement. Immune adherence phenomena in which a combination of treponemes, specific antibody, complement and antibody-sensitized indicator red blood cells is incubated together, resulting in agglutination of the red cells, were reported by Nelson (1953). Hardy and Nell (1955, 1957) demonstrated agglutination of treponemal suspensions by specific antibody. Tomizawa (1966) and Rathlev (1967) used indirect haemagglutination techniques in which red blood cells were coated with extracts of *T. pallidum*, thus becoming susceptible to agglutination by antitreponemal antibody. Deacon, Falcone and Harris (1957) first described the fluorescent treponemal antibody test in which treponemes fixed to a glass slide were treated first with specific antibody and then with a fluorescein-conjugated antiglobulin antibody before examination by fluorescence microscopy. Syphilis serology was the first major practical application of this technology. Essentially, none of these tests had the power to discriminate between individual antigenic constituents of the organism, although the existence of heat- and trypsin-stable components was demonstrated in agglutination tests.

Surface-associated molecular species implicated in binding to host-derived macromolecules have also received detailed attention. Based on the hypothesis that specific adhesion of treponemes to host cells or intercellular matrix is significant in pathogenesis, Baseman and colleagues characterized treponemal proteins involved in adhesion (Baseman and Hayes 1980) and as receptors for fibronectin (Peterson, Baseman and Alderete 1983). Several of the latter proteins were characterized by molecular cloning and shown to carry common fibronectin-binding regions (Peterson, Baseman and Alderete 1987). Proteins of 89.5 (P1), 37 (P2) and 32 (P3) kDa were identified. Baughn (1986) also described binding of fibronectin to a treponemal polypeptide of 87 kDa, which probably corresponded to P1 of Baseman and colleagues.

Studies of the component antigens of *T. pallidum* have depended critically on the availability and characterization of antisera, including polyclonal sera from infected human patients or from experimental animals, or monoclonal antibodies, which are now widely exploited. In many studies, sera from infected human patients were used in immunoblot or immunoprecipitation experiments (Hanff et al. 1982, 1983, Moskophidis and Muller 1984, Baker-Zander et al. 1985). Similar work was done with sera from infected rabbits (Lukehart, Baker-Zander and Gubish 1982, Baughn and Musher 1983, Hanff, Miller and Lovett 1983) and guinea pigs (Wicher, Zabek and Wicher 1991). Because they are highly discriminating, these techniques can produce large volumes of detailed data that are not easy to analyse and correlate (Penn, Bailey and Cockayne 1986). It is clear that antibodies are formed to a large number of polypeptide antigens during infection, and many of the antigens have not been identified structurally or functionally. However, antibodies to a limited number of antigens are prominent early in infection. The best data have been obtained from infected rabbits in which the duration of infection at the time of bleeding is known with certainty. Antibodies preferentially directed against polypeptides of 47, 37 and 31.5 kDa appear 10–14 days after intratesticular inoculation of the rabbit (Bailey, Cockayne and Penn 1987). The number of polypeptides recognized then increases considerably over several weeks, but responses to the polypeptides of 47, 44.5, 41 and 37 kDa, and to several in the range 24–35 kDa and one or 2 major polypeptides of 15.5–18 kDa, are particularly prominent. The recognition of these antigens, and standardization of data on them obtained by different laboratories (Norris et al. 1987, Norris 1993) have significantly improved understanding of the constituents of the organism that are significant in diagnostic serology.

A further significant advance was the introduction of monoclonal antibodies as valuable tools in the antigenic analysis of polypeptides and their structural and functional characterization (Robertson et al. 1982, van Embden et al. 1983, Thornburg and Baseman 1983, van der Donk et al. 1984, Jones et al. 1984, Lukehart

et al. 1985, Moskophidis and Muller 1985, Bailey, Cockayne and Penn 1987a, 1987b). Some indication of the location in the organism of antigens with which monoclonal antibodies react can be obtained by electron microscopy, e.g. by immunogold labelling. This technique showed conclusively that the prominent 37 kDa polypeptide is the sheath component of the endoflagellar core-sheath structure (Cockayne, Bailey and Penn 1987). However, the technique has limitations; the resolution of immunoelectron microscopy is limited by the large size of antibody molecules: in total dimensions they more than span the cell wall. For this reason, and also because views on the extent of surface exposure of antigens are controversial, it has proved difficult to demonstrate conclusively a structural location of, for example, the major, strongly antigenic 47 kDa lipoprotein.

The role of antigens, or their equivalent antibodies, in immunological phenomena may also be susceptible to investigation through the use of monoclonal antibodies. Such a role has been assessed in the treponemal immobilization (TPI) test. In this test, viable treponemes are incubated overnight with monoclonal, or polyclonal, antibody and normal guinea pig serum as a source of complement, then examined microscopically for retention of motility. In this way, monoclonal antibodies that react with several antigens have been shown to have immobilizing activity, but, in some cases, results differed between different laboratories. This may be due to differences in target epitopes. The interpretation of whether or not TPI tests indicate surface exposure of antigens is, in any case, controversial. The long period of incubation necessary before immobilization occurs, several times longer than that employed in conventional serum bactericidal reactions against gram-negative bacteria, suggests that structural changes in the surface of the treponemes consequent on incubation in vitro may enhance their susceptibility, e.g. by allowing improved access to target antigens by antibody.

The non-cultivability of the organism has precluded production of large enough quantities of material for fractionation and characterization of antigenic components, so detailed antigenic analysis has depended on the development of methods for analysis of individual antigenic constituents of crude mixtures. Initially, useful information was gained from the application of methods based on 2-dimensional immunoelectrophoresis (Strandberg-Pedersen et al. 1980, 1981, Strandberg-Pedersen, Axelsen and Petersen 1981, Penn and Rhodes 1982). Arising from this work, Penn, Cockayne and Bailey (1985) were able to purify the axial filament antigen, the first antigenic consituent of *T. pallidum*, other than cardiolipin, to be characterized. The analogy of the axial filament to flagella of other bacteria is suppported by gene cloning, which has shown that the flagellar core is composed of 2 or 3 polypeptides of 31–35 kDa (Penn, Cockayne and Bailey 1985, Cockayne, Bailey and Penn 1987) that show definite homology with other bacterial flagellins (Radolf et al. 1986, Blanco et al. 1988, Norris et al. 1988, Champion et al. 1990). The gene sequences encoding these proteins do not indicate the presence of signal peptides, suggesting they are exported from the cell via the flagellar basal body as in the well characterized *E. coli* and *Salmonella* Typhimurium. By contrast, the gene sequence of the 37 kDa protein forming the outer layer of the flagellum (Isaacs et al. 1989) does show evidence of a signal peptide for conventional export via the cytoplasmic membrane, and it appears that this is added to the core structure within the periplasm from the proximal end of the flagellum, a process unique to spirochaetes. This 'flagellar sheath' protein is a dominant antigen (see section 2.5, p. 1261). Recently, knowledge of flagellar molecular genetics has been greatly underpinned by identification of several important new flagellar genes, mainly thought on the basis of gene sequence homologies to be involved in the export of flagellar proteins from the cytoplasm (Hardham, Frye and Stamm 1995). In addition to the flagellar proteins, the principal 82 kDa polypeptide component of the cytoplasmic filaments has also been identified and the gene encoding it, named *cfpA*, has been cloned and sequenced (You et al. 1996). The gene sequence does not suggest any homology with any known protein.

Sodium dodecyl sulphate polyacrylamide gel electrophoresis (SDS-PAGE), followed by immunoblotting of the separated antigenic constituents onto nitrocellulose membrane and exposing them to various antibodies, has led to great advances in the knowledge of the antigenic components of *T. pallidum*. A large number of polypeptide antigens can now be recognized by these methods (Penn, Bailey and Cockayne 1986, Norris et al. 1987, Norris 1993). A summary of the properties, structure and function (where known) of a selection of the more prominent antigens is given in Table 55.1. Genes encoding several of these antigens have been cloned in *E. coli*, and molecular biological analysis has revealed detailed information about their amino acid sequences, structural features, chemical properties and, in some cases, probable functions. Standard nomenclature has been proposed for these antigens as shown, and where applicable is used in the following discussion.

Notable in Table 55.1 is the striking preponderance of lipoproteins among abundant and immunodominant antigens of *T. pallidum*. An important technique in the identification of lipid-modified and other hydrophobic proteins of *T. pallidum* (Chamberlain et al. 1989a, 1989b, Schouls et al. 1989, Purcell, Swancutt and Radolf 1990, Swancutt, Radolf and Norgard 1990, Hubbard et al. 1991, Schouls, van der Heide and van Embden 1991, Weigel, Brandt and Norgard 1992, Akins et al. 1993) has been partition between aqueous and detergent phases of proteins solubilized in Triton X-114 (Brusca and Radolf 1994). Lipoproteins not only have the ability to be membrane-bound (albeit not as fully membrane-integrated protein particles, and often with no hydrophobic domain within the polypeptide chain), but also may show increased antigenic potency and even the potential to damage host membranes or otherwise promote inflammatory responses (see section 2.7, p. 1265), thus being of potentially great significance in pathogenesis. Bacterial lipoproteins are covalently linked post-translationally at an N-terminal cysteine residue via the SH group to diacyl glycerol, and to an additional N-linked long-chain fatty acid, following signal peptide cleavage (Wu and Tokunaga 1986). Although many of the prominent lipoproteins have no known or deduced precise function, an exception is the 41 kDa protein described by Becker et al. (1994), which appears to be a cytoplasmic membrane-associated lipoprotein homologue of the MglB glucose- and galactose-binding periplasmic protein of *E. coli*, involved in uptake of and chemotactic responses to these sugars.

Absent from Table 55.1 is any constituent resembling LPS, a component which can be detected easily among gram-negative bacteria by immunoblotting. There is considerable evidence that any form of LPS with properties like those of LPS from a wide range of gram-negative bacteria is absent from *T. pallidum* (Penn, Bailey and Cockayne 1985). No heat-

Table 55.1 Major antigens of *Treponema pallidum*

Designation[a]	MW (kDa)	Description and comments
TpN83	82	Major component of cytoplasmic filaments of fibronectin binding protein
TpN60	59	Homologue of Hsp60 or GroEL heat shock protein. Cross-reactive antigen
TpN47	45	Lipoprotein. The most abundant polypeptide and dominant antigen
TpN44.5 (TmpA)	42	Lipoprotein. Also abundant. Recombinant form purified and tested successfully as a diagnostic reagent
TpN41	39.5	Lipoprotein. Homologue of the Mg1B periplasmic sugar binding protein of *Escherichia coli*
TpN37	37	FlaA flagellin. Abundant, dominant antigen. Member of class of unique spirochaetal flagellar 'sheath' proteins
TpN35	35.5	Lipoprotein. Less abundant and antigenically dominant than TpN47, 44.5
TpN34.5	34.5	⎫
TpN33	33	⎬ FlaB flagellins, homologues of other bacterial flagellins. Form flagellar core
TpN30	32	⎭
TpN29–35 (TpD)	30–38	Lipoprotein, moderately antigenic. Diffuse molecular weight – forms smear on electrophoresis
TpN24–28 (TpE)	24–30	Lipoprotein, similar properties to TpN29–35
TpN19 (TpF1, 4D[b])	19	Subunit of a large, heat labile complex which in recombinant *E. coli* is a ring structure. In yaws strains, homologue TyF1 usually differs in one base of the sequence
TpN17	17	Lipoprotein, strongly antigenic
TpN15	15	Lipoprotein, strongly antigenic

[a]TpN designations are those of Norris (1993). Names in parentheses were mainly given by van Embden et al. (1983).
[b]Designation of Walfield, Hanff and Lovett (1982).

stable, detergent-soluble antigenic component has been detected. The organism, or ultrasonically disrupted extracts of it, does not induce strong febrile or acute inflammatory responses in animals. It is resistant to the antibiotic polymyxin B, the target for which is LPS in susceptible gram-negative bacteria. Furthermore, Hardy and Levin (1983) reported that the *Limulus* amoebocyte lysate test for the presence of LPS gave negative results with *T. pallidum*.

In addition to the axial filament, a structural entity that has been the target of several attempts at subcellular fractionation and analysis of its components is the outer membrane. Penn, Bailey and Cockayne (1985) tentatively identified the major 47 kDa polypeptide and others of 60 and 40 kDa, as outer-membrane components because they were preferentially dissolved from intact organisms by the non-ionic detergent Triton X-100, which also removed the outer membrane as judged by morphological criteria. However, the possible dissolution of periplasmic- or cytoplasmic-membrane proteins could not be excluded. Preparation by physical methods of an outer-membrane fraction from treponemes that had incorporated radiolabel in vitro (Stamm and Bassford 1985, Stamm et al. 1987), or surface labelling methods (Norris and Sell 1984, Penn, Bailey and Cockayne 1985, Stamm and Bassford 1985) were used in earlier attempts to identify surface constituents, but unequivocal evidence for the surface exposure of specific polypeptides remained elusive until relatively recently. A key experimental approach in defining the character of the outer membrane has been freeze-fracture electron microscopy (Radolf, Norgard and Schulz 1989, Walker et al. 1989, 1991b, Bourell et al. 1994, reviewed by Radolf 1995). This technique has shown that, in contrast to both conventional gram-negative pathogens, such as enterobacteria, and avirulent spirochaetes, the outer membrane of *T. pallidum* contains few integral protein particles, consistent with limited antigenicity of the treponemal surface.

The work of Radolf, Norgard and colleagues (reviewed by Radolf 1995) has now indicated that intact outer membranes may be obtained by gentle sucrose density gradient centrifugation of plasmolysed treponemes. The membranes thus obtained were rich in lipid and low in protein, and not only the protein but also the lipid content was of low antigenicity. Cardiolipin appeared to be absent. Complementing this approach, Cox et al. (1995) exploited agarose gel entrapment of intact *T. pallidum* cells to investigate their antigenicity by immunofluorescence microscopy. Neither antibodies to abundant lipoproteins, nor patient sera, recognized the intact treponemal surface. Seeking to identify the scarce protein particles observed by freeze-fracture electron microscopy, Radolf et al. (1995) identified sparse proteins poorly recognized by immune patient sera. Blanco et al. (1994) also exploited sucrose density gradient centrifugation and identified rare outer-membrane proteins of 65, 31 and 28 kDa. An acidic protein of 31 kDa, designated TROMP1, was subsequently cloned (Blanco et al. 1995) and shown to be a hydrophobic membrane protein with porin activity, confirming its probable outer-membrane location. In parallel studies, Hardham and Stamm (1994) showed that a putatively surface-exposed protein of 50 kDa had sequence homology with the OmpA protein of *E. coli*, and thus was a candidate outer-membrane protein. Taken together, the studies outlined above (reviewed by Radolf 1995) illustrate an increasing knowledge of the molecular surface of *T. pallidum* that will contribute greatly to the understanding of its thus far obscure immunobiology.

2.6 Natural pathogenicity

The course of natural syphilis is chronic and complex. The organisms appear to enter the tissues most commonly through abrasions or other minor breaks in the skin, often not at mucosal sites. Whether *T. pallidum* is able to penetrate intact skin is uncertain. There is no evidence for the colonization of mucosal surfaces before penetration. After entering the body, the organisms multiply slowly at the site of penetration, initially causing no overt pathological effects. Presumably, when the number of organisms reaches a threshold level, mechanisms as yet unknown induce formation of the primary lesion, which is characteristically a raised, erythematous, painless papule with a hard base. This may progress to become haemorrhagic and may ulcerate before healing spontaneously. The primary lesion is rich in treponemes which may be seen microscopically – by dark ground or phase-contrast examination of wet mounts – in transudate squeezed from the abraded surface of the lesion, the only available means of bacteriological diagnosis.

Most untreated cases progress to secondary syphilis some weeks or months after healing of the primary lesion. The secondary lesions may be scattered widely over the body; they take several forms, including a diffuse erythematous rash, mucous patches, and condylomata. Again, organisms are present in large numbers in secondary lesions, which also heal spontaneously if left untreated. A period of latency follows, and may last many years. Treponemes are apparently sequestered in small numbers at unknown locations in the body during this phase. Eventually, tertiary syphilis may develop; at this stage, treponemes are characteristically rather sparse. There appears to be a strong immunopathological element to the very destructive lesions of the cardiovascular or central nervous systems present in tertiary syphilis.

Immunological aspects of the pathogenesis of syphilis infection have intrigued investigators for many years (Norris 1988) but understanding of the immunological relationship between pathogen and host remains elusive. In some syphilitic patients, particularly in the secondary stage (Baughn et al. 1986, Jorizzo et al. 1986), immune complexes have been identified, which may contain a limited number of treponemal antigens. Autoimmune responses, not only to cardiolipin but also involving fibronectin (Fitzgerald et al. 1984, Baughn et al. 1986), collagen and laminin (Fitzgerald et al. 1984), and creatine kinase (Casavant, Wicher and Wicher 1978, Strugnell et al. 1986) have also been reported.

The application of new molecular approaches to the detection of specific host responses to natural infection has yielded exciting new information. By reverse transcription and PCR amplification of specific host mRNA present in primary and secondary lesions, interleukins and cytokines typical of a Th1 cellular response were identified, and the activity of CD8+ cytolytic T cells demonstrated (Vanvoorhis et al. 1996a, 1996b). These studies lay the foundations for detailed investigation and much enhanced understanding of the immunopathology of syphilis.

No clearly identified virulence factors have been shown to mediate specific features of the disease. Thus there are no known toxins, or clear mechanisms for evasion of specific aspects of host defences. The success of the organism as a parasite perhaps lies more in its ability to cause relatively little damage, and to remain undetected in unknown locations in the body during latency.

2.7 Experimental pathogenicity

Of the stages of syphilis infection described above, only the primary lesion can be reproduced with any accuracy in an experimental model. However, analogues of secondary lesions in rabbits (Marra et al. 1991) and congenital infection in rabbits (Froberg et al. 1993) and guinea pigs (Wicher, Baughn and Wicher 1994) have also been described. The rabbit is highly susceptible to intradermal infection of clipped skin, which results in a lesion broadly similar to the classical primary chancre in humans (Sell and Norris 1983). After an incubation period, the length of which depends on inoculum size, as does the time scale for all stages in lesion development, the first discernible change is localized erythema, rapidly followed by focal swelling and hardening of the skin. With a large inoculum the lesion at this stage may be up to 2 cm in diameter. Subsequently, haemorrhage, necrosis and ulceration may follow with further moderate enlargement. After several months the ulceration resolves and the lesions heal. Subsequent to this, further overt pathological changes seldom develop, although 'secondary' lesions may be induced by superinfection some weeks after initial intradermal inoculation, or, more rarely, may arise spontaneously if the skin is maintained free of fur (Strugnell, Drummond and Faine 1986).

Dermal lesions are enhanced in severity and rapidity of development by administration of cortisone (Turner and Hollander 1957) or other steroids. This treatment apparently leads to an increased deposition in lesions of mucopolysaccharides, which appear to contribute to the characteristic oedema and induration observed (Fitzgerald 1981, van der Sluis et al. 1985). Although there has been much speculation in the past that these substances might be of treponemal origin and significant in pathogenicity of the organisms (Turner and Hollander 1957, Christiansen 1963, reviewed by Fitzgerald 1981), other evidence (Strugnell et al. 1988) suggests that the material is of host origin. There are significant doubts about its role in the protection of the organism from immune responses (Sell and Norris 1983). Translocation of treponemes, whether by breakdown of intercellular matrix or otherwise, has been examined experimentally in tissue culture, and penetration of intercellular junctions has been demonstrated (Thomas et al. 1988, Riviere, Thomas and Cobb 1989).

The pathology of infection in the rabbit testis has also been studied in detail. After injection of a treponemal suspension into the body of the testis there is an incubation period that depends upon the infecting dose but always exceeds 8–9 days. During this period, treponemes multiply exponentially (Turner and Hollander 1957), almost exclusively in extracellular locations in the interstitial tissues (Penn 1981). Towards the end of the incubation period, enlargement and hardening of the testis can be detected. This is caused by extensive accumulation of extracellular fluid, which is serous and contains a raised level of mucopolysaccharide (Wos and Wicher 1985). Again, the rate of develop-

ment of lesions is enhanced by the systemic administration of cortisone or synthetic substitutes such as betamethasone (Penn 1981) or methylprednisolone (Brause, Qualls and Roberts 1979); the number of treponemes obtained from infected testes is also enhanced by these drugs. The maximal number of treponemes present in the tissue coincides with maximal orchitis, as indicated by enlargement and induration. Haemorrhage commences a few days after orchitis becomes detectable. Subsequently there is a gradual decline in the number of treponemes present, and a long-term, chronic and rather variable healing process follows, often with extensive scarring. Small numbers of treponemes may persist for long periods, possibly indefinitely, e.g. in regional lymph nodes.

Much experimental work has been done on the specific surface interactions of treponemes with host cells or components of the intercellular matrix, and with host plasma proteins. The concept of binding or adhesion of treponemes to host cells as a key element in pathogenesis was advanced by Fitzgerald, Miller and Sykes (1975) and by Hayes et al. (1977). It arose from observations of the importance of adhesive interactions in many infections of mucosal surfaces, where moving fluid phases may tend to remove infecting organisms, though such considerations do not apply to *T. pallidum* infection in which there is no clear stage of surface colonization. It has been suggested that the organism adheres to host cells or intercellular matrix to establish localized lesions and to foster an intimate interaction with host cells. There is little direct evidence to support this, and in infection many treponemes appear to reside unattached in intercellular locations in infection. Interactions of treponemes with fibronectin (Fitzgerald and Repesh 1985, Baseman et al. 1986, Baughn 1987, Steiner, Sell and Schell 1987) have been examined intensively; clearly this protein adheres to the treponemal surface through its cell-binding domain, interacting specifically with a limited number of treponemal proteins (Thomas, Baseman and Alderete 1985). Apparently specific binding of other intercellular matrix proteins such as laminin and collagen has also been reported (Fitzgerald et al. 1984). However, the biological role of these interactions remains uncertain.

A clearer role can be visualized for the acquisition of plasma- and tissue-derived proteins, and other macromolecules, that become bound to the surface of freely motile treponemes during infection. Alderete and Baseman (1979) demonstrated both loosely associated and tightly bound proteins, including immunoglobulins and complement, on the treponemal surface. Marchitto, Kindt and Norgard (1986) showed the presence of class 1 molecules of the major histocompatibility complex on the surface of treponemes in vivo. These interactions clearly have a potential role in the antigenic or molecular 'disguise' of treponemes, which may appear host-like and thus avoid immune recognition and elimination through the effects of the immune response. A more recently recognized and particularly intriguing phenomenon is the binding of the iron-chelating protein lactoferrin (Staggs et al. 1994) which may be important in the acquisition of essential iron by the organism.

Whereas aspects of the pathology of syphilis have been illuminated by immunological studies, the components of the organism that are responsible for these phenomena generally remain uncertain. An exception is the activity of lipoproteins in stimulating host responses that may be detrimental, perhaps in lieu of proinflammatory LPS or similar components. Lipoproteins have been shown to stimulate tumour necrosis factor synthesis (Radolf et al. 1991) and to activate human vascular endothelium cells (Riley et al. 1992). Lipid modification of both 17 and 47 kDa major lipoproteins clearly enhances their inflammatory activity (Akins et al. 1993, Radolf et al. 1995). Furthermore, synthetic lipopeptides (Deogny et al. 1994) possess allied activities (Norgard et al. 1995) and details of signalling pathways affected in host cells have been elucidated (Norgard et al. 1996). These observations are some of the most revealing to date of the molecular pathogenicity of *T. pallidum*.

In addition to the rabbit, several other animal models of infection have been investigated. Mice, even inbred strains (Folds et al. 1983), appear insusceptible to *T. pallidum* infection, although their life span is curtailed (Wright and Wharton 1977) and treponemes may persist for a long period. Mice develop a serological response to infection (Folds et al. 1983) that can be abrogated by antibiotic treatment (Saunders and Folds 1985), further indicating that some persistence of live treponemes may occur but without clear pathological effects. One report (Klein et al. 1980) indicates that heavily irradiated mice may develop dermal lesions. If this species, the best-characterized immunologically and with the largest available number of inbred strains, could be used more effectively, the immunopathological phenomena of *T. pallidum* infection could undoubtedly be further unravelled.

The hamster has been exploited as a susceptible host for selected strains of *T. pallidum*, notably the subsp. *endemicum* strain Bosnia A. Schell et al. (1980) reported that the inbred hamster strain LSH/ss LAK could be infected reliably with this treponeme strain, developing extensive dermal lesions in the inguinal region after intracutaneous inoculation. These hamsters developed resistance to reinfection, measurable by changes in the weight of lymph nodes and numbers of treponemes present in them. Passive transfer of resistance via cells or serum could be investigated successfully in these inbred animals. Liu et al. (1991) showed that subsp. *pertenue* is also infectious in the hamster, and demonstrated a role for T lymphocytes in the transfer of immunity.

Finally, the guinea pig has also proved useful for immunological studies, again, in part, because inbred strains are available. After the intradermal inoculation of large numbers (10^6–10^7) of treponemes into clipped skin of the upper leg, raised erythematous and indurated lesions, which eventually ulcerate, are formed (Wicher and Jakubowski 1964a, 1964b, Wicher, Wicher and Wang 1976). Inbred strains of guinea pigs differed in their susceptibility to such infection (Pavia and Niederbuhl 1985, Wicher, Wicher and Gruhn 1985), and the C4D strain has proved particularly susceptible (Wicher and Wicher 1991). Useful information on both humoral and cell mediated mechanisms of immunity has emerged from studies in guinea pigs (reviewed by Wicher and Wicher 1989). More recently, the model has been used in studies of congenital infection, the efficacy of immunization with antibody administered passively (Wicher, Zabek and Wicher 1992) or of recombinant antigens (Wicher et al. 1994) has been assessed, and the exact nature of the infection, in terms of target organs infected, has been defined (Wicher et al. 1996).

3 *TREPONEMA PALLIDUM* SUBSP. *PERTENUE* (*T. PERTENUE*)

Since the discovery of *T. pertenue* by Castellani (1905) there has been controversy about the relationship between the organisms causing syphilis and yaws. Like *T. (subsp.) pallidum*, *T. (subsp.) pertenue* cannot be cultured in vitro in the absence of host cells but can be cultivated by infection of the rabbit testis (Turner and Hollander 1957). Generally, strains of *T. pertenue* are

slower to establish infection in the rabbit than *T. pallidum*. It remains to be proved whether there are significant differences in virulence between the 2 subspecies, as suggested by the work of Hardy and colleagues (Hardy 1976); to answer this question several strains of each must be compared. Molecular studies (Baker-Zander and Lukehart 1983, Noordhoek et al. 1990a, Thornburg and Baseman 1983) indicate that differences between individual isolates of *T. pallidum* and *T. pertenue* are small (as shown by the reactivity of antibodies against the 2 organisms with polypeptides of *T. pallidum*), possibly no greater than between isolates of the same subspecies. Base sequences of DNA in the ribosomal RNA regions also showed identity between the subspecies (Centurionlara et al. 1996). Efforts to detect subspecies-specific molecular markers have been directed particularly at the gene encoding the 19 kDa protein TpN19, designated TpF1 by van Embden et al. (1983). Noordhoek et al. (1989, 1990b) showed that a single characteristic base difference in this gene could in the majority of cases distinguish between the 2 subspecies *pallidum* and *pertenue* but was not totally definitive. Engelkens et al. (1993), reporting careful histopathological studies of syphilis and yaws lesions, noted distinctive features in the distribution of organisms, *T. pertenue* tending to localize in the epidermis whereas *T. pallidum* localized more in the mesodermis. The suspicion thus remains that despite failure to date to identify substantial molecular differences between them, the organisms probably do have distinctive features relating to their pathogenicity.

4 *TREPONEMA CARATEUM*: THE CAUSE OF PINTA

This spirochaete is morphologically indistinguishable from *T. pallidum* (Angulo et al. 1951), but the relationship between the 2 species is not fully understood and *T. carateum* has not yet been cultivated in vitro. Infection has been transmitted to chimpanzees by inoculation of the skin (Kuhn et al. 1970). Fohn et al. (1988) showed that sera from cases of pinta recognize a large number of antigens of *T. pallidum* by immunoblotting, indicating a close serological relationship between them.

5 *TREPONEMA PARALUISCUNICULI*: THE AGENT OF RABBIT SYPHILIS

First observed by Bayon (1913), morphologically *T. paraluiscuniculi* is very similar to *T. pallidum*; it has not yet been cultivated in vitro. It can be propagated in the rabbit testis (see review of early literature by Smith and Pesetsky 1967). Recent observations on the organism are sparse but show considerable serological cross-reactivity with *T. pallidum* (Baker-Zander and Lukehart 1984), low infectivity for humans (Graves and Downes 1981), and marginal ability to immunize rabbits against infection with *T. pallidum* (Graves 1981).

6 *TREPONEMA PHAGEDENIS*: THE REITER TREPONEME

Several strains of cultivable treponemes were isolated in the early decades of this century during attempts to culture *T. pallidum* from syphilitic lesions. These included the Reiter and Kazan strains, now generally identified as *T. phagedenis*, and avirulent Nichols and Noguchi strains, initially named *T. pallidum* but now recognized as *Treponema refringens*. Smibert (1973) reviewed the properties of these strains in detail. The Reiter treponeme grows readily in vitro in thioglycollate media in the presence of 10% of serum of several species. It is morphologically quite different from *T. pallidum* (Fig. 55.4), being thicker (0.2–0.3 µm), with a much less distinct waveform and more random patterns of movement with considerable flexibility. Ultrastructurally (Fig. 55.5) it lacks the knob-like tip structure of *T. pallidum* and the flagella are more randomly inserted instead of forming a precise longitudinal array at their insertion points. Older cultures characteristically contain 'cyst' forms that appear spherical by light microscopy; ultrastructurally, these appear to result from tight random coiling of the protoplasmic cylinder within an enlarged and balloon-like outer membrane. Al Qudah, Mostratos and Quesnel (1983) reported that the cyst form is a viable survival form of the organism that is produced under adverse environmental conditions and reverts to treponemal morphology when conditions permit active growth. Such a mechanism would be of great interest if it occurred in *T. pallidum* during latent infection, but despite many attempts to demonstrate aberrant forms in the past (Yobs et al. 1968), no firm evidence has been produced.

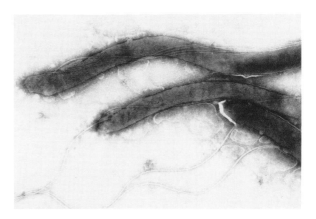

Fig. 55.5 Electron micrograph of negatively stained *Treponema phagedenis* I (Reiter strain) (× 18 450).

Because of its antigenic relatedness to *T. pallidum*, much attention has been given to the Reiter strain as a model for structural and antigenic analysis. Bharrier and Allis (1974) concentrated on the endoflagellum of the Reiter treponeme and described its purification by shearing from organisms treated with detergent to solubilize the outer membrane and release the endoflagella. Hardy, Fredericks and Nell (1975) used similar methods and showed antigenic cross-reactivity of endoflagella with *T. pallidum* antigen. This reactivity has been confirmed and characterized at the molecular level (Penn, Cockayne and Bailey 1985, Limberger and Charon 1986, Radolf et al. 1986, Blanco et al. 1988). The pattern of endoflagellar polypeptides, with a major FlaA component of slightly higher MW (c. 39 kDa) than in *T. pallidum*, and several smaller minor FlaB components including a prominent doublet of c. 32 kDa, is similar in the 2 species (Penn, Cockayne and Bailey 1985, Radolf et al. 1986), and significant amino acid sequence homologies between corresponding polypeptides have been described (Norris et al. 1988). Gene cloning and sequencing has confirmed these homologies (Limberger et al. 1992), and in more detailed molecular genetic studies of the flagellar structure, the hook protein gene *flgE* has also been cloned and characterized (Limberger, Slivienski and Samsonoff 1994). In addition, a larger flagellar operon has been cloned intact and the upstream regulatory regions characterized, demonstrating both similarities and differences in genetic organization to the corresponding well characterized genes of the Enterobacteriaceae (Limberger et al. 1996). Lastly, *T. phagedenis* has been a useful model for studies of motility mechanisms in spirochaetes (Charon et al. 1991, 1992, Limberger et al. 1992).

Antigens of the Reiter treponeme that react with rabbit syphilitic sera have been identified (Strandberg-Pedersen et al. 1980, 1981a, Strandberg-Pedersen, Axelsen and Petersen 1981), primarily by the use of 2-dimensional immunoelectrophoresis. Some evidence has emerged for biological (treponeme immobilization) activity of antibody to preparations of the Reiter treponeme, including endoflagella (Blanco et al. 1986). This prompted an unsuccessful attempt to modify or inhibit the course of syphilis infection in rabbits by active immunization with Reiter treponeme endoflagella (Hindersson, Petersen and Axelsen 1985). An interesting observation was the recognition that the Reiter treponeme possesses homologues of the 44.5 and 36 kDa proteins TpN44.5a and TpN36 (Yelton et al. 1991). The larger of these proteins, also designated TmpA (van Embden et al. 1983) had been thought unique to *T. pallidum* during its development as a diagnostic reagent (Ijsselmuiden et al.

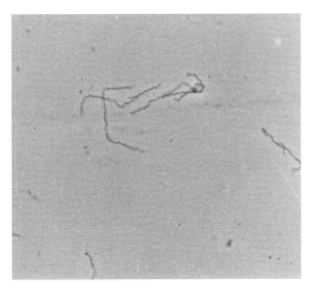

Fig. 55.4 Light micrograph (phase contrast) of *Treponema phagedenis* (Reiter strain) (× 600).

1989). The function of these proteins remains unknown but the sequence homology between them, and lack of known homologues in other bacteria, suggest an important conserved function in treponemes.

A prominent smooth-type LPS has also been demonstrated in the Reiter treponeme (Bailey, Penn and Cockayne 1985), demonstrating a fundamental difference between this organism and *T. pallidum*. An ordered structure on the surface of isolated outer-membrane protein vesicles of the Reiter strain has also been described (Masuda and Kawata 1986).

7   ORAL TREPONEMES

The presence of treponemes in the mouth has long been recognized, both in normal health and, classically, in the ulcerative, necrotic condition of Vincent's angina. Treponemes are also numerous in dental plaque in humans and other animals, and are particularly prominent in deep periodontal pockets in humans, where they may number more than half the total microscopic count of bacteria (Sela et al. 1987, Fig. 55.6). An association of raised numbers of spirochaetes with more severe periodontal lesions has been noted (Armitage et al. 1982, Simonson et al. 1988a), and a causal relationship suggested (Moore et al. 1983, Loesche 1993). However, there are numerous difficulties in the investigation of these organisms in relation to the aetiology of periodontal disease.

As with other treponemes, technical difficulties in the study of oral treponemes stem from the inability to cultivate an unknown but probably substantial number of those present in plaque in the gingival crevices. This difficulty is compounded by the complexity of the oral microflora, which is composed of mixed microbial communities, species including spirochaetes often interacting by, for example, interaggregation (Grenier 1992, Kolenbrander et al. 1995, Yao et al. 1996). The starting point in investigations has been

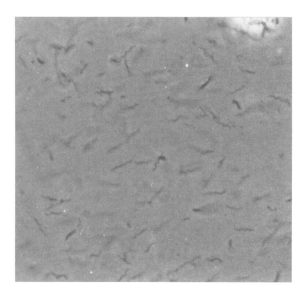

Fig. 55.6 Light micrograph (phase contrast) of organisms from human gingival crevice. Note large numbers of spirochaetes, the predominant morphological form of bacteria present (× 600).

microscopy of the indigenous population, which comprises a variety of sizes and morphological types of treponeme (Listgarten and Hellden 1978, Westergaard and Fiehn 1987). In earlier investigations, treponemes were classified mainly on the basis of size, and numbers of endoflagella (Listgarten and Socransky 1965). No clear correlations were reported between particular morphological types of treponeme and the severity of disease. To characterize the organisms more definitively and advance their taxonomy, cultivation was attempted and many isolates were obtained (Smibert et al. 1984, Makinen et al. 1986, Fukumoto et al. 1987, Sela et al. 1987). However, organisms that were cultured successfully tended to be mainly of the medium sized or smaller types that have relatively few endoflagella (Fukumoto et al. 1987, Sela et al. 1987). Thus, it was by no means clear that isolates representative of all the species which may be present in the natural population had been cultured, and the pathogenic potential of these organisms could not be fully assessed.

Two important technical advances have provided the tools for more definitive analysis of oral spirochaetes. These are the use of monoclonal antibodies to identify microscopically specific groups of organisms in oral populations, and the phylogenetic characterization of organisms, even those which cannot be cultured, by determination of 16S rRNA sequences. In the first approach, monoclonal antibodies that recognize epitopes of the FlaA flagellar sheath protein of *T. pallidum* were used to detect cross-reactive oral treponemes by immunofluorescence microscopy (Riviere et al. 1991a, 1991b, 1992). The organisms thus identified were designated pathogen-related oral spirochaetes (PROS), and their pathogenicity inferred from their expression of antigens formerly believed to be pathogen-specific. Allied studies have been extended to the identification of other organisms in situ by immunofluorescence (Riviere et al. 1996a), confirming an association of PROS with diseased sites in the mouth. Interbacterial interactions in situ have also been investigated by this method (Riviere et al. 1996b). The second advance was the application of molecular analysis of the 16S rRNA sequence as a phylogenetic marker in the identification of oral spirochaetes. Following amplification by the polymerase chain reaction of a 16S rRNA fragment, with conserved, spirochaete-specific oligodeoxyribonucleotide primers, the product could be genetically cloned and precisely sequenced. The sequence obtained is indicative of the phylogenetic position of the organism from which it originated, and can also be used as a molecular probe to identify microscopically the organism from which it was amplified, even if uncultivable (Choi et al. 1994). This work has confirmed that many oral spirochaetes have never been cultured – the sequences obtained from dental plaque or periodontitis samples have been diverse and seldom identical to those of known culturable species. However, it is clear that the unidentified organisms that can be demonstrated as PROS are most closely related to *Treponema vincentii*, and although they form a distinct phylogenetic group they are nevertheless quite diverse (Choi, Wyss and Gobel 1996). Thus, there remains much to be done to improve knowledge of the diversity and complexity of oral spirochaetes, and the role as pathogen of individual species remains poorly defined.

The best-characterized oral species is *T. denticola*. This may reflect the relative ease of its cultivation, leading to its preponderance among successful isolations in vitro. Only recently has the organism received formal species designation, following nomination of a type strain (Chan et al. 1993), despite extensive use of the name in earlier literature. The organism is very small (Fig. 55.7), typifying the 'small' oral treponemes. There has been great interest recently in the potential virulence properties of these organisms. Extracellular and degradative enzyme activities of *T. denticola* have been investigated, and it commonly possesses proline aminopeptidases and benzoylarginine or trypsin-like peptidases (Makinen et al. 1987) with the ability to degrade collagen. Investigations of their proteolytic and peptidolytic activities have been extended (Makinen, Makinen and Syed 1992, 1994, 1995, Arakawa and Kuramitsu 1994, Rosen et al. 1994, 1995, Grenier 1996, Makinen, Chen and Makinen 1996) and haemolytic activities have also been described (Scott et al. 1993, Karunakaran and Holt 1994). Other possible virulence mechanisms include abilities to attach to and invade host tissues (Riviere et al. 1991b, Baehni et al. 1992, De Filippo, Ellen and McCulloch 1995), to damage host membranes (Mathers et al. 1996), and to induce bone resorption (Gopalsami et al. 1993). Molecular approaches to characterization of, for example, outer-membrane proteins (Egli et al. 1993, Kokeguchi et al. 1994, Fenno, Muller and McBride 1996), flagellar genes (Heinzerling, Penders and Burne 1995) and outer-membrane LPS (Dahle, Tronstad and Olsen 1996) are yielding increasingly detailed knowledge of the pathogenic potential of these organisms. In addition, they are increasingly well characterized genetically, with information emerging on the circular chromosome (MacDougall and Saint Girons 1995) and plasmids (Ivic et al. 1991, MacDougall, Margarita and Girons 1992), and methods developed for gene transfer (Li and Kuramitsu 1996) and mutagenesis (Li et al. 1996).

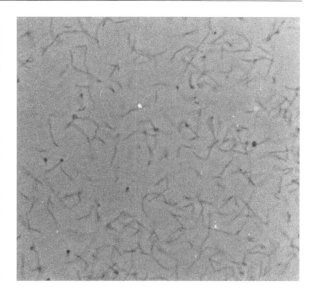

Fig. 55.7 Light micrograph (phase contrast) of *Treponema denticola* cultured in vitro. Note extremely small size, with spiral structure barely resolved (× 600).

Treponemes of the *denticola* group are not generally saccharolytic or fermentative. Also prominent in the mouth, however, are organisms of the *Treponema socranskii* group (Smibert et al. 1984), which ferment carbohydrate energy sources to produce acetic, lactic and succinic acids. Another group, more commonly isolated from non-human primates and designated *Treponema pectinovorum*, has a specific requirement for pectin, glucuronic or galacturonic acid (Sela et al. 1987). A new group of small oral spirochaetes recently identified (Wyss et al. 1996) has been named *Treponema maltophilum*, and illustrates the potential for further advances in the systematics of oral spirochaetes. An alternative to rRNA-based phylogenetic classification is multilocus enzyme electrophoresis, which has also been applied successfully to oral treponemes (Dahle et al. 1995). It is clear that this group of organisms is important in the ecology and pathogenic potential of the oral microflora, and their further study will greatly illuminate oral microbial disease.

REFERENCES

Akins DR, Purcell BK et al., 1993, Lipid modification of the 17-kilodalton membrane immunogen of *Treponema pallidum* determines macrophage activation as well as amphilicity, *Infect Immun*, **61**: 1202–10.

Al Qudah AA, Mostratos A, Quesnel LB, 1983, A proposed life cycle of the Reiter treponeme, *J Appl Bacteriol*, **55**: 417–21.

Alder J, Jarvis K et al., 1993, Clarithromycin therapy of experimental *Treponema pallidum* infection in hamsters, *Antimicrob Agents Chemother*, **37**: 864–7.

Alderete JF, Baseman JB, 1979, Surface-associated host proteins on virulent *Treponema pallidum*, *Infect Immun*, **26**: 1048–56.

Angulo JJ, Watson JHL et al., 1951, *Am J Trop Med*, **31**: 458.

Arakawa S, Kuramitsu HK, 1994, Cloning and sequence analysis of a chymotrypsin-like protease from *Treponema denticola*, *Infect Immun*, **62**: 3424–33.

Armitage GC, Dickinson WR et al., 1982, Relationship between the percentage of subgingival spirochetes and the severity of periodontitis, *J Periodontol*, **53**: 550–6.

Austin FE, Cox CD, 1986, Lactate oxidation by *Treponema pallidum*, *Curr Microbiol*, **13**: 123–8.

Baehni PC, Song M et al., 1992, *Treponema denticola* induces actin rearrangement and detachment of human gingival fibroblasts, *Infect Immun*, **60**: 3360–8.

Bailey MJ, Cockayne A, Penn CW, 1987a, Monoclonal antibodies directed against surface-associated polypeptides of *Treponema pallidum* define a biologically active antigen, *J Gen Microbiol*, **133**: 1793–803.

Bailey MJ, Cockayne A, Penn CW, 1987b, Production of monoclonal antibodies to the major axial filament polypeptide of *Treponema pallidum*, *J Gen Microbiol*, **133**: 1805–13.

Bailey MJ, Penn CW, Cockayne A, 1985, Evidence for the presence of lipopolysaccharide in *Treponema phagedenis* (biotype Reiterii) but not *Treponema pallidum* (Nichols), *FEMS Microbiol Lett*, **27**: 117–21.

Baker-Zander SA, Lukehart SA, 1983, Molecular basis of immunological cross-reactivity between *Treponema pallidum* and *Treponema pertenue*, *Infect Immun*, **42**: 634–8.

Baker-Zander SA, Lukehart SA, 1984, Antigenic cross-reactivity between *Treponema pallidum* and other pathogenic members of the family Spirochaetaceae, *Infect Immun*, **46**: 116–21.

Baker-Zander SA, Shaffer JM, Lukehart SA, 1993, VDRL antibodies enhance phagocytosis of *Treponema pallidum* by macrophages, *J Infect Dis*, **167**: 1100–5.

Baker-Zander SA, Hook EW et al., 1985, Antigens of *Treponema pallidum* recognized by IgG and IgM antibodies during syphilis in humans, *J Infect Dis*, **157**: 264–72.

Barbieri JT, Austin FE, Cox CD, 1981, Distribution of glucose incorporated into macromolecular material by *Treponema pallidum*, *Infect Immun*, **31**: 1071–7.

Barbieri JT, Cox CD, 1979, Pyruvate oxidation by *Treponema pallidum*, *Infect Immun*, **25**: 157–63.

Barbour AG, Barrera O, Judd RC, 1983, Structural analysis of the variable major protein of *Borrelia hermsii*, *J Exp Med*, **158**: 2127–40.

Barbour AG, Hayes SF, 1986, Biology of *Borrelia* species, *Microbiol Rev*, **50**: 381–400.

Baseman JB, Hayes EC, 1980, Molecular recognition of receptor binding proteins and immunogens of virulent *Treponema pallidum*, *J Exp Med*, **151**: 573–86.

Baseman JB, Nichols JC, Hayes NS, 1976, Virulent *Treponema pallidum*: aerobe or anaerobe?, *Infect Immun*, **13**: 704–11.

Baseman JB, Alderete JF et al., 1986, Adhesin-receptor recognition between the syphilis spirochete and fibronectin, *Microbiology 1986*, eds Lieve L, Bonventre PV et al., American Society for Microbiology, Washington, DC, 39–42.

Baughn RE, 1986, Antibody-independent interactions of fibronectin, C1q, and human neutrophils with *Treponema pallidum*, *Infect Immun*, **54**: 456–64.

Baughn RE, 1987, Role of fibronectin in the pathogenesis of syphilis, *Rev Infect Dis*, **9, Suppl. 4**: S372–85.

Baughn RE, Musher DM, 1983, Isolation and preliminary characterization of circulating immune complexes from rabbits with experimental syphilis, *Infect Immun*, **42**: 579–84.

Baughn RE, McNeely MC et al., 1986, Characterization of the antigenic determinants and host components in immune complexes from patients with secondary syphilis, *J Immunol*, **136**: 1406–14.

Bayon H, 1913, A new species of treponeme found in the genital sores of rabbits, *Br Med J*, **2**: 1159.

Becker PS, Akins DR et al., 1994, Similarity between the 38-kilodalton lipoprotein of *Treponema pallidum* and the glucose/galactose (MglB) binding protein of *Escherichia coli*, *Infect Immun*, **62**: 1381–91.

Bharrier M, Allis D, 1974, Purification and characterization of axial filaments from *Treponema phagedenis* biotype Reiterii (the Reiter treponeme), *J Bacteriol*, **120**: 1434–41.

Blanco DR, Radolf JD et al., 1986, The antigenic interrelationship between the endoflagella of *Treponema phagedenis* biotype Reiter and *Treponema pallidum* Nichols strain I. Treponemicidal activity of cross-reactive endoflagellar antibodies against *T. pallidum*, *J Immunol*, **137**: 2973–9.

Blanco DR, Champion CI et al., 1988, Antigenic and structural characterization of *Treponema pallidum* (Nichols strain) endoflagella, *Infect Immun*, **56**: 168–75.

Blanco DR, Reimann K et al., 1994, Isolation of the outer membranes from *Treponema pallidum* and *Treponema vincentii*, *J Bacteriol*, **176**: 6088–99.

Blanco DR, Champion CI et al., 1995, Porin activity and sequence-analysis of a 31-kilodalton *Treponema pallidum* subsp. *pallidum* rare outer-membrane protein, *J Bacteriol*, **177**: 3556–62.

Bourell KW, Schulz W et al., 1994, *Treponema pallidum* rare outer membrane proteins: analysis of mobility by freeze-fracture electron microscopy, *J Bacteriol*, **176**: 1598–608.

Brause BD, Qualls S, Roberts RB, 1979, Testicular culture of *Treponema pallidum* (Nichols strain) facilitated by sustained-release steroid administration, *J Clin Microbiol*, **10**: 937–9.

Brusca JS, Radolf JD, 1994, Isolation of integral membrane-proteins by phase partitioning, *Methods Enzymol*, **228**: 182–93.

Canale-Parola E, 1984, Order 1 Spirochetales, *Bergey's Manual of Systematic Bacteriology*, vol 1, eds Krieg NR, Holt SC, Williams & Wilkins, Baltimore, 38–70.

Casavant CH, Wicher V, Wicher K, 1978, Host response to *Treponema pallidum* infection III. Demonstration of antibodies to heart in sera from infected rabbits, *Int Arch Allergy Appl Immunol*, **56**: 171–8.

Castellani A, 1905, On the presence of spirochaetes in two cases of ulcerated parangi (yaws), *Br Med J*, **2**: 1280.

Centurionlara A, Castro C et al., 1996, Two 16S-23S ribosomal DNA intergenic regions in different *Treponema pallidum* subspecies contain transfer-RNA genes, *FEMS Microbiol Lett*, **143**: 235–40.

Chamberlain N, Brandt A et al., 1989a, Major integral membrane protein immunogens of *Treponema pallidum* are proteolipids, *Infect Immun*, **57**: 2872–7.

Chamberlain N, DeOgny C et al., 1989b, Acylation of the 47-kilodalton major membrane immunogen of *Treponema pallidum* determines its hydrophobicity, *Infect Immun*, **57**: 2878–85.

Champion CI, Miller JN et al., 1990, Cloning, seqencing, and expression of two class B endoflagellar genes of *Treponema pallidum* subsp. *pallidum* encoding the 34.5- and 31.0-kilodalton proteins, *Infect Immun*, **58**: 1697–704.

Chan ECS, Siboo R et al., 1993, *Treponema denticola* (ex Brumpt 1925) sp. nov., nom. rev., and identification of new spirochete isolates from periodontal pockets, *Int J Syst Bacteriol*, **43**: 196–203.

Charon NW, Goldstein ST et al., 1991, The bent-end morphology of *Treponema phagedenis* is associated with short, left-handed, periplasmic flagella, *J Bacteriol*, **173**: 4820–6.

Charon NW, Goldstein ST et al., 1992, Morphology and dynamics of protruding spirochete periplasmic flagella, *J Bacteriol*, **174**: 832–40.

Choi BK, Wyss C, Gobel UB, 1996, Phylogenetic analysis of pathogen-related oral spirochetes, *J Clin Microbiol*, **31**: 1922–5.

Choi BK, Paster BJ et al., 1994, Diversity of cultivable and uncultivable oral spirochetes from a patient with severe destructive periodontitis, *Infect Immun*, **62**: 1889–95.

Christiansen S, 1963, Protective layer covering pathogenic Treponemata, *Lancet*, **1**: 423–5.

Cockayne A, Bailey MJ, Penn CW, 1987, Analysis of sheath and core structures of the axial filament of *Treponema pallidum*, *J Gen Microbiol*, **133**: 1397–407.

Cover WH, Norris SJ, Miller JN, 1982, The microaerophilic nature of *Treponema pallidum*: enhanced survival and incorporation of tritiated adenine under microaerobic conditions in the absence of reducing compounds, *Sex Transm Dis*, **9**: 1–8.

Cox CD, Barber MK, 1974, Oxygen uptake by *Treponema pallidum*, *Infect Immun*, **10**: 123–7.

Cox CD, Riley B et al., 1990, Effects of molecular-oxygen, oxidation-reduction potential, and antioxidants upon in vitro replication of *Treponema pallidum*, *Appl Environ Microbiol*, **56**: 3063–72.

Cox DL, Chang P et al., 1992, The outer membrane, not a coat of host proteins, limits antigenicity of virulent *Treponema pallidum*, *Infect Immun*, **60**: 1076–83.

Cox DL, Akins DR et al., 1995, *Treponema pallidum* in gel microdroplets – a novel strategy for investigation of treponemal molecular architecture, *Mol Microbiol*, **15**: 1151–64.

Cunningham TM, Miller JN, Lovett MA, 1987, Identification of

Treponema pallidum penicillin-binding proteins, *J Bacteriol*, **169:** 5298–300.

Dahle UR, Tronstad L, Olsen I, 1996, 3-Hydroxy fatty-acids in a lipopolysaccharide-like material from *Treponema denticola* strain FM, *Endod Dent Traumatol*, **12:** 202–5.

Dahle UR, Olsen I et al., 1995, Population genetic analysis of oral treponemes by multilocus enzyme electrophoresis, *Oral Microbiol Immunol*, **10:** 265–70.

Deacon WE, Falcone VH, Harris AA, 1957, A fluorescent test for treponemal antibodies, *Proc Soc Exp Biol Med*, **96:** 477–80.

De Filippo AB, Ellen RP, McCulloch C, 1995, Induction of cytoskeletal rearrangements and loss of volume regulation in epithelial cells by *Treponema denticola*, *Arch Oral Biol*, **40:** 199–207.

Deogny L, Pramanic BC et al., 1994, Solid-phase synthesis of biologically active lipopeptides as analogs for spirochetal lipoproteins, *Peptide Res*, **7:** 91–7.

van der Donk HJ, van Embden JDA et al., 1984, Monoclonal antibodies to *Treponema pallidum*, *Dev Biol Stand*, **57:** 107–11.

Egli C, Leung WK et al., 1993, Pore-forming properties of the major 53-kilodalton surface antigen from the outer sheath of *Treponema denticola*, *Infect Immun*, **61:** 1694–9.

van Embden JDA, van der Donk HJ et al., 1983, Molecular cloning and expression of *Treponema pallidum* DNA in *Escherichia coli* K-12, *Infect Immun*, **42:** 187–96.

Engelkens HJH, Tenkate FJW et al., 1993, The localization of treponemes and characterization of the infiltrate in skin biopsies in patients with primary or secondary syphilis, or early infectious yaws, *Genitourin Med*, **69:** 102–7.

Fenno JC, Muller KH, McBride BC, 1996, Sequence analysis, expression, and binding activity of recombinant major outer sheath protein (MSP) of *Treponema denticola*, *J Bacteriol*, **178:** 2489–97.

Fieldsteel AH, Becker FA, Stout JG, 1977, Prolonged survival of virulent *Treponema pallidum* (Nichols strain) in cell-free and tissue culture systems, *Infect Immun*, **18:** 173–82.

Fieldsteel AH, Cox DL, Moeckli RA, 1981, Cultivation of virulent *Treponema pallidum* in tissue culture, *Infect Immun*, **32:** 908–15.

Fitzgerald TJ, 1981, Pathogenesis and immunology of *Treponema pallidum*, *Annu Rev Microbiol*, **35:** 29–54.

Fitzgerald TJ, Johnson RC, Wolff ET, 1978, Mucopolysaccharide material resulting from the interaction of *Treponema pallidum* (Nichols strain) with cultured mammalian cells, *Infect Immun*, **22:** 575–84.

Fitzgerald TJ, Miller JN, Sykes JA, 1975, *Treponema pallidum* (Nichols strain) in tissue culture: cellular attachment, entry and survival, *Infect Immun*, **11:** 1133–40.

Fitzgerald TJ, Repesh LA, 1985, Interactions of fibronectin with *Treponema pallidum*, *Genitourin Med*, **61:** 147–55.

Fitzgerald TJ, Cleveland P et al., 1976, Scanning electron microscopy of *Treponema pallidum* (Nichols strain) attached to cultured mammalian cells, *J Bacteriol*, **130:** 1333–44.

Fitzgerald TJ, Repesh LA et al., 1984, Attachment of *Treponema pallidum* to fibronectin, laminin, collagen IV, and collagen I, and blockage of attachment by immune rabbit IgG, *Br J Vener Dis*, **60:** 357–63.

Fitzgerald TJ, Miller JN et al., 1985, Binding of glycosaminoglycans to the surface of *Treponema pallidum* and subsequent effects on complement interactions between antigen and antibody, *Genitourin Med*, **61:** 13–20.

Fohn MJ, Wignall S et al., 1988, Specificity of antibodies from patients with pinta for antigens of *Treponema pallidum* subsp. *pallidum*, *J Infect Dis*, **157:** 32–7.

Folds JD, Rauchbach AS et al., 1983, Evaluation of the inbred mouse as a model for experimental *Treponema pallidum* infection, *Scand J Immunol*, **18:** 201–6.

Fribourg-Blanc A, Mollaret HH, 1969, Natural treponematosis of the African primate, *Primates Med*, **3:** 113–21.

Froberg MK, Fitzgerald TJ et al., 1993, Pathology of congenital syphilis in rabbits, *Infect Immun*, **61:** 4743–9.

Fukumoto Y, Okuda K et al., 1987, *Oral Microbiol Immunol*, **2:** 82.

Gopalsami C, Yotis W et al., 1993, Effect of outer membrane of *Treponema denticola* on bone resorption, *Oral Microbiol Immunol*, **8:** 121–4.

Graves SR, 1981, Sequential changes in susceptibility to *Treponema pallidum* of rabbits previously infected with *Treponema paraluiscuniculi*, *Br J Vener Dis*, **57:** 11–14.

Graves SR, Downes J, 1981, Experimental infection of man with rabbit-virulent *Treponema paraluiscuniculi*, *Br J Vener Dis*, **57:** 7–10.

Grenier D, 1992, Demonstration of a bimodal co-aggregation between *Porphyromonas gingivalis* and *Treponema denticola*, *Oral Microbiol Immunol*, **7:** 280–4.

Grenier D, 1996, Degradation of host protease inhibitors and activation of plasminogen by proteolytic enzymes from *Porphyromonas gingivalis* and *Treponema denticola*, *Microbiology*, **142:** 955–61.

Hackett CJ, 1963, On the origin of the human treponematoses, *Bull W H O*, **29:** 7–41.

Hanff PA, Miller JN, Lovett MA, 1983, Molecular characterization of common treponemal antigens, *Infect Immun*, **40:** 825–8.

Hanff PA, Fehniger TE et al., 1982, Humoral immune response in human syphilis to polypeptides of *Treponema pallidum*, *J Immunol*, **129:** 1287–91.

Hanff PA, Bishop NH et al., 1983, Humoral immune response in experimental syphilis to polypeptides of *Treponema pallidum*, *J Immunol*, **131:** 1973–7.

Hardham JM, Frye JG, Stamm LE, 1995, Identification and sequences of the *Treponema pallidum fliM, fliY, fliP, fliQ, fliR* and *flhB* genes, *Gene*, **166:** 57–64.

Hardham JM, Stamm LE, 1994, Identification and characterisation of the *Treponema pallidum* gene, an *ompA* homologue, *Infect Immun*, **62:** 1015–25.

Hardy PH, 1976, Pathogenic treponemes, *The Biology of Parasitic Spirochetes*, ed. Johnson RC, Academic Press, New York, 107–19.

Hardy PH, Fredericks WR, Nell EE, 1975, Isolation and antigenic characteristics of axial filaments from the Reiter treponeme, *Infect Immun*, **11:** 380–6.

Hardy PH, Levin J, 1983, Lack of endotoxin in *Borrelia hispanica* and *Treponema pallidum*, *Proc Soc Exp Biol Med*, **174:** 47–52.

Hardy PH, Nell EE, 1955, Specific agglutination of *Treponema pallidum* by sera from rabbits and human beings with treponemal infections, *J Exp Med*, **101:** 367–82.

Hardy PH, Nell EE, 1957, *Am J Hyg*, **66:** 160.

Hayes NS, Muse KE et al., 1977, Parasitism by virulent *Treponema pallidum* of host cell surfaces, *Infect Immun*, **17:** 174–86.

Heinzerling HF, Penders JEC, Burne RA, 1995, Identification of *fliG* homolog in *Treponema pallidum*, *Gene*, **161:** 69–73.

Hindersson P, Petersen CS, Axelsen NH, 1985, Purified flagella from *Treponema phagedenis* biotype Reiter does not induce protective immunity against experimental syphilis in rabbits, *Sex Transm Dis*, **12:** 124–7.

Hovind-Hougen K, 1976, Treponeme and *Borrelia* morphology, *The Biology of Parasitic Spirochetes*, ed. Johnson RC, Academic Press, New York, 7–18.

Hovind-Hougen K, 1983, *Pathogenesis and Immunology of Treponemal Infection*, eds Schell RF, Musher DN, Marcel Dekker, New York, 3.

Hubbard CL, Gherardini FC et al., 1991, Molecular cloning and characterization of a 35.5 kilodalton lipoprotein of *Treponema pallidum*, *Infect Immun*, **59:** 1521–8.

Ijsselmuiden OE, Schouls LM et al., 1989, Sensitivity and specificity of an enzyme-linked immunosorbent assay using the recombinant DNA-derived *Treponema pallidum* protein TmpA for serodiagnosis of syphilis and the potential use of TmpA for assessing the effect of antibiotic therapy, *J Clin Microbiol*, **27:** 152–7.

Isaacs RD, Hanke JH et al., 1989, Molecular cloning and DNA sequence analysis of the 37 kilodalton endoflagellar sheath protein gene of *Treponema pallidum*, *Infect Immun*, **57:** 3403–11.

Ivic A, MacDougall J et al., 1991, Isolation and characterisation of a plasmid from *Treponema denticola*, *FEMS Microbiol Lett*, **78:** 189–94.

Johnson RC, Bey RF, Wolgamot SJ, 1982, Comparison of the activities of ceftriaxone and penicillin G against experimentally induced syphilis in rabbits, *Antimicrob Agents Chemother*, **21:** 984–9.

Johnson RC, Ritzi D, Livermore B, 1973, Outer envelope of virulent *Treponema pallidum*, *Infect Immun*, **8:** 291–5.

Jones SA, Marchitto KS et al., 1984, Monoclonal antibody with hemagglutination, immobilization, and neutralization activities defines an immunodominant 47,000 mol wt, surface-exposed immunogen of *Treponema pallidum* (Nichols), *J Exp Med*, **160:** 1404–20.

Jorizzo JL, McNeely MC et al., 1986, Role of circulating immune complexes in human secondary syphilis, *J Infect Dis*, **153:** 1014–22.

Kampmeier RH, 1979, Demonstration of spirochetes in syphilitic lesions by F. Schaudin and E. Hoffman, *Sex Transm Dis*, **6:** 25–7.

Kampmeier RH, 1982, Syphilis, *Bacterial Infections of Humans: Epidemiology and Control*, eds Evans AS, Feldman HA, Plenum Press, New York, 553–77.

Karunakaran T, Holt SC, 1994, Cloning and expression of hemolysin genes from *Treponema denticola* strains ATCC-35404 (TD-4) and human clinical isolate GM-1 in *Escherichia coli*, *Microb Pathog*, **16:** 337–48.

Klein JR, Monjan AA et al., 1980, Abrogation of genetically controlled resistance of mice to *Treponema pallidum* by irradiation, *Nature (London)*, **283:** 572–4.

Kokeguchi S, Miyamoto M et al., 1994, Isolation and characterization of a 53 kDa major cell envelope protein antigen from *Treponema denticola* ATCC 35405, *J Periodont Res*, **29:** 70–8.

Kolenbrander PE, Parrish KD et al., 1995, Intergeneric co-aggregation of oral *Treponema* spp. with *Fusobacterium* spp. and intrageneric co-aggregation among *Fusobacterium* spp., *Infect Immun*, **63:** 4584–8.

Korting HC, Walther D et al., 1986, Comparative in vitro susceptibility of *Treponema pallidum* to ceftizoxime, ceftriaxone and penicllin G, *Chemotherapy*, **32:** 352–5.

Korting HC, Haag R et al., 1993, Effect of ceftizoxime in the treatment of incubatory syphilis in rabbits, *Chemotherapy*, **39:** 331–5.

Kuhn USG, Medina R et al., 1970, Inoculation pinta in chimpanzees, *Br J Vener Dis*, **46:** 311–12.

Lee A, Hazell SL et al., 1988, Isolation of a spiral-shaped bacterium from the cat stomach, *Infect Immun*, **56:** 2843–50.

Li H, Kuramitsu HK, 1996, Development of a gene transfer system in *Treponema denticola* by electroporation, *Oral Microbiol Immunol*, **11:** 161–5.

Li H, Ruby J et al., 1996, Gene inactivation in the oral spirochete *Treponema denticola*: construction of an *flgE* mutant, *J Bacteriol*, **178:** 3664–7.

Limberger RJ, Charon NW, 1986, *Treponema phagedenis* has at least two proteins residing together on its periplasmic flagella, *J Bacteriol*, **166:** 105–12.

Limberger RJ, Slivienski LL, Samsonoff WA, 1994, Genetic and biochemical analysis of the flagellar hook of *Treponema phagedenis*, *J Bacteriol*, **176:** 3631–7.

Limberger RJ, Slivienski LL et al., 1992, Molecular genetic analysis of a class B periplasmic flagellum gene of *Treponema phagedenis*, *J Bacteriol*, **174:** 6404–10.

Limberger RJ, Slivienski LL et al., 1996, Organisation, transcription and expression of the 5′-region of the *fla* operon of *Treponema phagedenis* and *Treponema pallidum*, *J Bacteriol*, **178:** 4628–34.

Listgarten MA, Hellden L, 1978, Relative distribution of bacteria at clinically healthy and periodontally diseased sites in humans, *J Clin Periodontol*, **5:** 115–32.

Listgarten MA, Socransky SS, 1965, *Arch Oral Biol*, **10:** 127.

Liu H, Alder JD et al., 1991, Role of L3T4+ and 38+ T-cell subsets

in resistance against infection with *Treponema pallidum* subsp. *pertenue* in hamsters, *Infect Immun*, **59:** 529–36.

Loesche WJ, 1993, Bacterial mediators in periodontal disease, *Clin Infect Dis*, **16:** S203–10.

Lukehart SA, Baker-Zander SA, 1987, Roxithromycin (RU 965): effective therapy for experimental syphilis infection in rabbits, *Antimicrob Agents Chemother*, **31:** 187–90.

Lukehart SA, Baker-Zander SA, Gubish ER, 1982, Identification of *Treponema pallidum* antigens – comparison with a nonpathogenic treponeme, *J Immunol*, **129:** 833–8.

Lukehart SA, Tam MR et al., 1985, Characterization of monoclonal antibodies to *Treponema pallidum*, *J Immunol*, **134:** 585–92.

Lysko PG, Cox CD, 1977, Terminal electron transport in *Treponema pallidum*, *Infect Immun*, **16:** 885–90.

Lysko PG, Cox CD, 1978, Respiration and oxidative phosphorylation in *Treponema pallidum*, *Infect Immun*, **21:** 462–73.

MacDougall J, Margarita D, Girons IS, 1992, Homology of a plasmid from the spirochete *Treponema denticola* with the single-stranded-DNA plasmids, *J Bacteriol*, **174:** 2724–8.

MacDougall J, Saint Girons I, 1995, Physical map of the *Treponema denticola* circular chromosome, *J Bacteriol*, **177:** 1805–11.

Makinen KK, Chen CY, Makinen PL, 1996, Proline iminopeptidase from the outer cell envelope of the human oral spirochete *Treponema denticola* ATCC-35405, *Infect Immun*, **64:** 702–8.

Makinen KK, Makinen PL, Syed SA, 1992, Purification and substrate specificity of an endopeptidase from the human oral spirochete *Treponema denticola* ATCC-34505, active on furyl-acryloyl-leu-gly-pro-ala and bradykinin, *J Biol Chem*, **267:** 14285–93.

Makinen KK, Syed SA et al., 1986, Benzoylarginine peptidase and iminopeptidase profiles of *Treponema denticola* strains isolated from the human periodontal pocket, *Curr Microbiol*, **14:** 85–9.

Makinen KK, Syed SA et al., 1987, Dominance of iminopeptidase activity in the human oral bacterium *Treponema denticola* ATCC-35405, *Curr Microbiol*, **14:** 341–6.

Makinen PL, Makinen KK, Syed SA, 1994, An endo-acting proline-specific oligopeptidase from *Treponema denticola* ATCC 35404 – evidence of hydrolysis of human bioactive peptides, *Infect Immun*, **62:** 4938–47.

Makinen PL, Makinen KK, Syed SA, 1995, Role of the chymotrypsin-like membrane-associated proteinase from *Treponema denticola* ATCC-35405 in inactivation of bioactive peptides, *Infect Immun*, **63:** 3567–75.

Marchitto KS, Kindt TJ, Norgard MV, 1986, Monoclonal antibodies directed against major histocompatibility complex antigens bind to the surface of *Treponema pallidum* isolated from rabbits or humans, *Cell Immunol*, **101:** 633–42.

Marra C, Baker-Zander SA et al., 1991, An experimental model of early central nervous system syphilis, *J Infect Dis*, **163:** 825–9.

Masuda K, Kawata T, 1986, Isolation, and structural characterization of outer sheath carrying a polygonal array from *Treponema phagedenis* biotype Reiter, *Microbiol Immunol*, **30:** 401–11.

Mathers DA, Leung WK et al., 1996, The major surface protein complex of *Treponema denticola* depolarizes and introduces ion channels in HeLa cell membranes, *Infect Immun*, **64:** 2904–10.

Matthews HM, Yang TK, Jenkin HM, 1979, Unique lipid composition of *Treponema pallidum* (Nichols virulent strain), *Infect Immun*, **24:** 713–19.

Miao RM, Fieldsteel AH, 1980, Genetic relationship between *Treponema pallidum* and *Treponema pertenue*, two noncultivable human pathogens, *J Bacteriol*, **141:** 427–9.

Moore WEC, Holdeman LV et al., 1983, Bacteriology of moderate (chronic) periodontitis in mature adult humans, *Infect Immun*, **42:** 510–15.

Moskophidis M, Muller F, 1984, Molecular analysis of immunoglobulins M and G immune response to protein antigens of *Treponema pallidum* in human syphilis, *Infect Immun*, **43**: 127–32.

Moskophidis M, Muller F, 1985, Monoclonal antibodies to immunodominant surface-exposed protein antigens of *Treponema pallidum*, *J Clin Microbiol*, **4**: 473–7.

Nell EE, 1954, *Am J Syph Gonorr Vener Dis*, **38**: 92.

Nelson RA, 1953, The immune adherence phenomenon, *Science*, **118**: 733–7.

Nelson RA, Diesendruck JA, 1951, Studies on treponemal immobilizing antibodies in syphilis, *J Immunol*, **66**: 667–85.

Nelson RA, Mayer MM, 1949, Immobilization of *Treponema pallidum in vitro* by antibody produced in syphilitic infection, *J Exp Med*, **89**: 369–93.

Nichols JC, Baseman JB, 1975, Carbon sources utilized by virulent *Treponema pallidum*, *Infect Immun*, **12**: 1044–50.

Noordhoek GT, Hermans PWM et al., 1989, *Treponema pallidum* subsp. pallidum (Nichols) and *Treponema pallidum* subsp. pertenue (CDC 2575) differ in at least one nucleotide: comparison of two homologous antigens, *Microb Pathog*, **6**: 29–42.

Noordhoek GT, Cockayne A et al., 1990a, A new attempt to distinguish serologically the subspecies of *Treponema pallidum* causing syphilis and yaws, *J Clin Microbiol*, **28**: 1600–1.

Noordhoek GT, Wieles B et al., 1990b, Polymerase chain reaction and synthetic DNA probes – a means of distinguishing the causative agents of syphilis and yaws?, *Infect Immun*, **58**: 2011–13.

Norgard MV, Miller JN, 1981, Plasmid DNA in *Treponema pallidum* (Nichols) and potential for antibiotic resistance by syphilis bacteria, *Science*, **213**: 553–5.

Norgard MV, Riley BS et al., 1995, Dermal inflammation elicited by synthetic analogs of *Treponema pallidum* and *Borrelia burgdorferi* lipoproteins, *Infect Immun*, **63**: 1507–15.

Norgard MV, Arndt LL et al., 1996, Activation of human monocytic cells by *Treponema pallidum* and *Borrelia burgdorferi* lipoproteins and synthetic lipopeptides proceeds via a pathway distinct from that of lipopolysaccharide but involves the transcriptional activator NF-KAPPA-B, *Infect Immun*, **64**: 3845–52.

Norris SJ, 1982, In vitro cultivation of *Treponema pallidum* in tissue culture: independent confirmation, *Infect Immun*, **36**: 437–9.

Norris SJ, 1988, Syphilis, *Immunology of Sexually Transmitted Diseases*, ed. Wright DJM, Kluver Academic Publishers, Dordrecht, 1–31.

Norris SJ, 1993, Polypeptides of *Treponema pallidum*: progress toward understanding their structural, functional and immunologic roles, *Microbiol Rev*, **57**: 750–79.

Norris SJ, Edmondson DG, 1986a, Factors affecting the multiplication and subculture of *Treponema pallidum* subsp. *pallidum* in a tissue culture system, *Infect Immun*, **53**: 534–9.

Norris SJ, Edmondson DG, 1986b, Serum requirement for the multiplication of *Treponema pallidum* in a tissue culture system: association of growth promoting activity with the protein fraction, *Sex Transm Dis*, **13**: 207–13.

Norris SJ, Edmondson DG, 1988, In vitro culture system to determine MICs and MBCs of antimicrobial agents against *Treponema pallidum* subsp. *pallidum* (Nichols strain), *Antimicrob Agents Chemother*, **32**: 68–74.

Norris SJ, Sell S, 1984, Antigenic complexity of *Treponema pallidum*: antigenicity and surface localization of major polypeptides, *J Immunol*, **133**: 2686–92.

Norris SJ, Alderete JF et al., 1987, Identity of *Treponema pallidum* subsp. *pallidum* polypeptides: correlation of sodium dodecyl sulfate-polyacrylamide gel electrophoresis results from different laboratories, *Electrophoresis*, **8**: 77–92.

Norris SJ, Charon NW et al., 1988, Antigenic relatedness and N-terminal sequence homology define two classes of periplasmic flagellar proteins of *Treponema pallidum* subsp. *pallidum* and *Treponema phagedenis*, *J Bacteriol*, **170**: 4072–82.

Olsen GJ, Woese CR, Overbeek R, 1994, The winds of (evolutionary) change – breathing new life into microbiology, *J Bacteriol*, **176**: 1–6.

Pangborn MC, 1942, Isolation and purification of a serologically active phospholipid from beef heart, *J Biol Chem*, **143**: 247–56.

Paster BJ, Stackebrandt E et al., 1984, The phylogeny of the spirochetes, *Syst Appl Microbiol*, **5**: 337–51.

Paster BJ, Dewhirst FE et al., 1991, Phylogenetic analysis of spirochetes, *J Bacteriol*, **173**: 6101–9.

Pavia CS, Niederbuhl CJ, 1985, Acquired resistance and expression of a protective humoral response in guinea pigs infected with *Treponema pallidum* Nichols, *Infect Immun*, **50**: 66–72.

Penn CW, 1981, Avoidance of host defenses by *Treponema pallidum* in situ and on extraction from infected rabbit testes, *J Gen Microbiol*, **126**: 69–75.

Penn CW, Bailey MJ, Cockayne A, 1985, The axial filament antigen of *Treponema pallidum*, *Immunology*, **54**: 635–41.

Penn CW, Bailey MJ, Cockayne A, 1986, Molecular and immunochemical analysis of *Treponema pallidum*, *FEMS Microbiol Rev*, **32**: 139–48.

Penn CW, Cockayne A, Bailey MJ, 1985, The outer membrane of *Treponema pallidum*: biological significance and biochemical properties, *J Gen Microbiol*, **131**: 2349–57.

Penn CW, Lichfield J, 1982, The outer membrane of *Treponema pallidum*: solubilization by detergents to release axial filaments, *FEMS Microbiol Lett*, **14**: 61–4.

Penn CW, Rhodes JG, 1982, Surface-associated antigens of *Treponema pallidum* concealed by an inert outer layer, *Immunology*, **46**: 9–16.

Peterson KM, Baseman JB, Alderete JF, 1983, *Treponema pallidum* receptor binding proteins interact with fibronectin, *J Exp Med*, **157**: 1958–70.

Peterson KM, Baseman JB, Alderete JF, 1987, Molecular cloning of *Treponema pallidum* envelope fibronectin binding proteins, *Genitourin Med*, **63**: 355–60.

Purcell BK, Swancutt MA, Radolf JD, 1990, Lipid modification of the 15 kilodalton major membrane immunogen of *Treponema pallidum*, *Mol Microbiol*, **4**: 1371–9.

Radolf JD, 1995, *Treponema pallidum* and the quest for outer-membrane proteins, *Mol Microbiol*, **16**: 1067–73.

Radolf JD, Norgard MV, Schulz WW, 1989, Outer membrane ultrastructure explains the limited antigenicity of virulent *Treponema pallidum*, *Proc Natl Acad Sci USA*, **86**: 2051–5.

Radolf JD, Blanco DR et al., 1986, Antigenic interrelationship between endoflagella and *Treponema phagedenis* biotype Reiter and *Treponema pallidum* (Nichols): molecular characterization of endoflagellar proteins, *Infect Immun*, **54**: 626–4.

Radolf JD, Norgard MV et al., 1991, Lipoproteins of *Borrelia burgdorferi* and *Treponema pallidum* activate cachectin/tumor necrosis factor synthesis. Analysis using a CAT reporter construct, *J Immunol*, **147**: 1968–74.

Radolf JD, Arndt LL et al., 1995, *Treponema pallidum* and *Borrelia burgdorferi* lipoproteins and synthetic lipopeptides activate monocytes/macrophages, *J Immunol*, **154**: 2866–77.

Rathlev T, 1967, Haemagglutination test utilizing pathogenic *Treponema pallidum* for the serodiagnosis of syphilis, *Br J Vener Dis*, **43**: 181–5.

Rein MF, 1976, Biopharmacology of syphilotherapy, *J Am Vener Dis Assoc*, **3**: 109–27.

Riley ES, Oppenheimer-Marks N et al., 1992, Virulent *Treponema pallidum* activates human vascular endothelial cells, *J Infect Dis*, **165**: 484–93.

Riviere GR, Thomas DD, Cobb CM, 1989, In vitro model of *Treponema pallidum* invasiveness, *Infect Immun*, **57**: 2267–71.

Riviere GR, Wagoner MA et al., 1991a, Identification of spirochetes related to *Treponema pallidum* in necrotizing ulcerative gingivitis and chronic periodontitis, *N Engl J Med*, **325**: 539–43.

Riviere GR, Weisz KS et al., 1991b, Pathogen-related spirochetes identified within gingivitis tissue from patients with acute necrotizing ulcerative gingivitis, *Infect Immun*, **59**: 2653–7.

Riviere GR, Elliott KS et al., 1992, Relative proportions of pathogen-related oral spirochetes (PROS) and *Treponema denticola* in supragingival and subgingival plaque from patients with periodontitis, *J Periodontol*, **63:** 131–6.

Riviere GR, Smith KS et al., 1996a, Periodontal status and detection frequency of bacteria at sites of periodontal health and gingivitis, *J Periodontol*, **67:** 109–15.

Riviere GR, Smith KS et al., 1996b, Association betwen *Porphyromonas gingivalis* and oral treponemes in subgingival plaque, *Oral Microbiol Immunol*, **11:** 150–5.

Robertson SM, Kettman JR et al., 1982, Murine monoclonal antibodies specific for virulent *Treponema pallidum* (Nichols), *Infect Immun*, **36:** 1076–85.

Ronald AR, Silverman M et al., 1992, Evaluation of new anti-infective drugs for the treatment of syphilis, *Clin Infect Dis*, **15:** S140–7.

Rosen G, Naor R et al., 1994, Characterization of fibrinolytic activities of *Treponema denticola*, *Infect Immun*, **62:** 1749–54.

Rosen G, Naor R et al., 1995, Proteases of *Treponema denticola* outer sheath and extracellular vesicles, *Infect Immun*, **63:** 3973–9.

Saunders JM, Folds JD, 1985, Humoral response of the mouse to *Treponema pallidum*, *Genitourin Med*, **61:** 221–9.

Schaudinn F, Hoffmann E, 1905, Vorlaufiger Bericht uber das Vorkommen von Spirochaeten in syphilitischen Krankheitsproduckten und bei paplillomen, *Arb Klin Gesundheitsmte*, **22:** 527–34.

Schell RF, Chen JK et al., 1980, LSH hamster model of syphilitic infection, *Infect Immun*, **28:** 909–13.

Schiller NL, Cox CD, 1977, Catabolism of glucose and fatty acids by virulent *Treponema pallidum*, *Infect Immun*, **16:** 60–8.

Schouls LM, van der Heide HGJ, van Embden JDA, 1991, Characterization of the 35-kilodalton *Treponema pallidum* subsp. *pallidum* recombinant lipoprotein TmpC and antibody response to lipidated and nonlipidated *Treponema pallidum* antigens, *Infect Immun*, **59:** 3536–46.

Schouls LM, Mout R et al., 1989, Characterization of lipid-modified immunogenic proteins of *Treponema pallidum* expressed in *Escherichia coli*, *Microb Pathog*, **7:** 175–88.

Scott D, Siboo IR et al., 1993, Binding of hemin and congo red by oral hemolytic spirochetes, *Oral Microbiol Immunol*, **8:** 245–50.

Sela MN, Kornman KS et al., 1987, Characterization of treponemes isolated from human and non-human periodontal pockets, *Oral Microbiol Immunol*, **2:** 21–9.

Sell S, Norris SJ, 1983, The biology, pathology and immunology of syphilis, *Int Rev Exp Pathol*, **24:** 204–76.

Simonson LG, Goodman CH et al., 1988a, Quantitative relationship of *Treponema denticola* to severity of periodontal disease, *Infect Immun*, **56:** 726–8.

Simonson LG, Rouse RF, Bockowski SW, 1988b, Monoclonal antibodies that recognize a specific surface antigen of *Treponema denticola*, *Infect Immun*, **56:** 60–3.

van der Sluis JJ, van Dijk G et al., 1985, Mucopolysaccharides in suspensions of *Treponema pallidum* extracted from infected rabbit testes, *Genitourin Med*, **61:** 7–12.

Smibert RM, 1973, *CRC Crit Rev Microbiol*, **2:** 491.

Smibert RM, 1984, Genus III, *Treponema*, *Bergey's Manual of Systematic Bacteriology*, vol. 1, eds Krieg NR, Holt JG, Williams & Wilkins, Baltimore, 49–57.

Smibert RM, Johnson JL, Ranney RR, 1984, *Treponema sokranskii* sp. nov., *Treponema sokranskii* subsp. *sokranskii* subsp. nov., *Treponema sokranskii* subsp. *buccale* subsp. nov., and *Treponema sokranskii* subsp. *paredis* subsp. nov. isolated from the human periodontia, *Int J Syst Bacteriol*, **34:** 457–62.

Smith JL, Pesetsky BR, 1967, The current status of *Treponema paraluiscuniculi*. Review of the literature, *Br J Vener Dis*, **43:** 117–27.

Staggs TM, Greer MK et al., 1994, Identification of lactoferrin binding proteins from *Treponema pallidum* subsp. *pallidum* and *Treponema denticola*, *Mol Microbiol*, **12:** 613–19.

Stamm LV, Bassford PJ, 1985, Cellular and extracellular protein antigens of *Treponema pallidum* synthesized during in vitro incubation of freshly extracted organisms, *Infect Immun*, **47:** 799–807.

Stamm LV, Hodinka RL et al., 1987, Changes in the cell surface properties of *Treponema pallidum* that occur during in vitro incubation of freshly extracted organisms, *Infect Immun*, **55:** 2255–61.

Steiner BM, Sell S, Schell RF, 1987, *Treponema pallidum* attachment to surface and matrix proteins of cultured rabbit epithelial cells, *J Infect Dis*, **155:** 742–8.

Strandberg-Pedersen N, Axelsen NH, Petersen CS, 1981, Antigenic analysis of *Treponema pallidum*: cross-reactions between individual antigens of *Treponema pallidum* and *Treponema Reiter*, *Scand J Immunol*, **13:** 143–50.

Strandberg-Pedersen N, Axelsen NH et al., 1980, Antibodies in secondary syphilis against five of forty Reiter treponeme antigens, *Scand J Immunol*, **11:** 629–33.

Strandberg-Pedersen N, Petersen CS et al., 1981, Isolation of a heat-stable antigen from *Treponema reiter*, using an immunosorbent with antibodies from syphilitic patients, *Scand J Immunol*, **14:** 137–44.

Strugnell RA, Drummond L, Faine S, 1986, Secondary lesions in rabbits infected with *Treponema pallidum*, *Genitourin Med*, **62:** 4–8.

Strugnell RA, Williams WF et al., 1986, Autoantibodies to creatine kinase in rabbits infected with *Treponema pallidum*, *J Immunol*, **136:** 667–71.

Strugnell RA, Kent T et al., 1988, Experimental syphilitic orchitis – relationship between *Treponema pallidum* infection and testis synthesis of proteoglycans, *Am J Pathol*, **133:** 110–17.

Swancutt MA, Radolf JD, Norgard MV, 1990, The 34-kilodalton membrane immunogen of *Treponema pallidum* is a lipoprotein, *Infect Immun*, **58:** 384–92.

Sykes JA, Miller JN, 1973, Ultrastructural studies of treponemes: location of axial filaments and some dimensions of *Treponema pallidum* (Nichols strain), *Treponema denticola*, and *Treponema reiteri*, *Infect Immun*, **7:** 100–10.

Thomas DD, Baseman JB, Alderete JF, 1985, Putative *Treponema pallidum* cytadhesins share a common functional domain, *Infect Immun*, **49:** 833–5.

Thomas DD, Navab M et al., 1988, *Treponema pallidum* invades intercellular junctions of endothelial cell monolayers, *Proc Natl Acad Sci USA*, **85:** 3608–12.

Thornburg RW, Baseman JB, 1983, Comparison of major protein antigens and protein profiles of *Treponema pallidum* and *Treponema pertenue*, *Infect Immun*, **42:** 623–7.

Tomizawa T, 1966, Hemagglutination tests for diagnosis of syphilis. A preliminary report, *Jpn J Med Sci Biol*, **19:** 305–8.

Turner TB, Hollander DH, 1957, *Biology of the Treponematoses*, World Health Organization Monograph Series. No. 35, World Health Organization, Geneva.

Verdon MS, Handsfield HH et al., 1994, Pilot study of azithromycin for treatment of primary and secondary syphilis, *Clin Infect Dis*, **19:** 486–8.

van Voorhis WC, Barrett LK et al., 1996a, Primary and secondary syphilis lesions contain messenger-RNA for TH1 cytokines, *Infect Dis*, **173:** 491–5.

van Voorhis WC, Barrett LK et al., 1996b, Lesions of primary and secondary syphilis contain activated cytolytic T-cells, *Infect Immun*, **64:** 1048–50.

Walfield AM, Hanff PA, Lovett MA, 1982, Expression of *Treponema pallidum* antigens in *Escherichia coli*, *Science*, **216:** 522–3.

Walker EM, Zampighi GA et al., 1989, Demonstration of rare protein in the outer membrane of *Treponema pallidum* subsp. *pallidum* by freeze fracture analysis, *J Bacteriol*, **171:** 5005–11.

Walker EM, Arnett JK et al., 1991a, *Treponema pallidum* subsp. *pallidum* has a single, circular chromosome with a size of approximately 900 kilobase pairs, *Infect Immun*, **59:** 2476–9.

Walker EM, Borenstein MA et al., 1991b, Analysis of outer membrane ultrastructure of pathogenic *Treponema* and *Borrelia* species by freeze-fracture electron microscopy, *J Bacteriol*, **173:** 5585–8.

Walker EM, Howell JK et al., 1995, Physical map of the genome of *Treponema pallidum* subsp. *pallidum* (Nichols), *J Bacteriol*, **177:** 1797–804.

Walter EK, Smith JL et al., 1969, A new modification of the Krajian silver stain for *Treponema pallidum*, *Br J Vener Dis*, **45:** 6–9.

Weigel LM, Brandt ME, Norgard MV, 1992, Analysis of the N-terminal region of the 47-kilodalton integral membrane lipoprotein of *Treponema pallidum*, *Infect Immun*, **60:** 1568–76.

Weigel LM, Radolf JD et al., 1994, The 47 kDa major lipoprotein immunogen of *Treponema pallidum* is a penicillin binding protein with carboxypeptidase activity, *Proc Natl Acad Sci USA*, **91:** 11611–15.

Westergaard J, Fiehn N-E, 1987, Morphological distribution of spirochetes in subgingival plaque from advanced marginal periodontitis in humans, *Acta Pathol Microbiol Immunol Scand Sect B*, **95:** 49–55.

Wicher K, Jakubowski A, 1964a, Effect of cortisone on the course of experimental syphilis in the guinea pig. I. Effect of previously administered cortisone on guinea pigs infected with *Treponema pallidum* intradermally, intratesticularly, and intravenously, *Br J Vener Dis*, **40:** 213–16.

Wicher K, Jakubowski A, 1964b, Effect of cortisone on the course of experimental syphilis in the guinea pig. II. Action of cortisone when administered in various doses and at various times to guinea pigs previously infected intradermally with *T. pallidum*, *Br J Vener Dis*, **40:** 217–21.

Wicher K, Wicher V, 1989, Experimental syphilis in the guinea pig, *Crit Rev Microbiol*, **16:** 181–234.

Wicher K, Wicher V, 1991, Median infective dose of *Treponema pallidum* determined in a highly susceptible guinea pig strain, *Infect Immun*, **59:** 453–6.

Wicher K, Wicher V, Gruhn RF, 1985, Differences in susceptibility to infection with *Treponema pallidum* (Nichols) between 5 strains of guinea pig, *Genitourin Med*, **61:** 21–6.

Wicher K, Wicher V, Wang MCC, 1976, Cellular and humoral responses of guinea pigs infected with *Treponema pallidum*, *Int Arch Allergy Appl Immunol*, **51:** 284–97.

Wicher K, Zabek J, Wicher V, 1992, Effect of passive immunisation with purified specific or cross-reacting immunoglob-ulin G antibodies against *Treponema pallidum* on the course of infection in guinea pigs, *Infect Immun*, **60:** 3217–23.

Wicher K, Abbruscato F et al., 1994, Immunisation of guinea pigs with *Treponema pallidum* recombinant antigens reveals the presence of novel epitope, *Int Arch Allergy Appl Immunol*, **103:** 396–9.

Wicher K, Abbruscato F et al. , 1996, Target organs of infection in guinea pigs with acquired or congenital syphilis, *Infect Immun*, **64:** 3174–9.

Wicher V, Baughn RE, Wicher K, 1994, Congenital and neonatal syphilis in guinea pigs show a different pattern of immune response, *Immunology*, **82:** 404–9.

Wicher V, Zabek J, Wicher K, 1991, Pathogens specific humoral response in *Treponema pallidum* infected humans, rabbits and guinea pigs, *J Infect Dis*, **163:** 830–6.

Wiegand SE, Strobel PL, Glassman L, 1972, Electron microscopic anatomy of pathogenic *Treponema pallidum*, *J Invest Dermatol*, **58:** 186–204.

Wos SM, Wicher K, 1985, Antigenic evidence for host origin of exudative fluids in lesions of *Treponema pallidum*-infected rabbits, *Infect Immun*, **47:** 228–33.

Wright DJM, Wharton FD, 1977, The effect of *Treponema pallidum* on mouse survival, *J Med Microbiol*, **10:** 245–7.

Wu HC, Tokunaga M, 1986, Biogenesis of lipoproteins in bacteria, *Curr Top Microbiol Immunol*, **125:** 127–57.

Wyss C, Choi BK et al., 1996, *Treponema maltophilum* I sp. nov., a small oral spirochete isolated from human periodontal lesions, *Int J Syst Bacteriol*, **46:** 745–52.

Yao ES, Lamont RJ et al., 1996, Interbacterial binding among strains of pathogenic and commensal oral bacterial species, *Oral Microbiol Immunol*, **11:** 35–41.

Yelton DB, Limberger RJ et al., 1991, *Treponema phagedenis* encodes and expresses homologs of the *Treponema pallidum* Tmpa and Tmpb proteins, *Infect Immun*, **59:** 3685–93.

Yobs AR, Clark JW et al., 1968, Further observations on the persistence of *Treponema pallidum* after treatment in rabbits and humans, *Br J Vener Dis*, **44:** 116–30.

You Y, Elmore S et al., 1996, Characterization of the cytoplasmic filament protein gene (*cfpA*) of *Treponema pallidum* subsp. *pallidum*, *J Bacteriol*, **178:** 3177–87.

Zeigler JA, Jones AM et al., 1976, Demonstration of extracellular material at the surface of pathogenic *T. pallidum* cells, *Br J Vener Dis*, **52:** 1–8.

BORRELIA

R C Johnson

1 GENUS *BORRELIA*

Members of this genus are similar in length (8–30 μm) but wider (0.2–0.5 μm) than other pathogenic spirochaetes and are transmitted to vertebrates by haematophagous arthropods. Borrelioses are zoonoses with the exception of louse-borne relapsing fever. *Borrelia* spp. have a low G + C content of 27–32 mol% and a unique genomic composition of a linear chromosome and linear and circular plasmids. Past difficulties with cultivation resulted in a classification based on arthropod-vector associations. The recent development of improved culture media has facilitated the implementation of molecular techniques for the classification of borreliae (Felsenfeld 1971, Barbour and Hayes 1986, Johnson and Hughes 1992, Saint Girons, Old and Davidson 1994).

2 HISTORY

The interest and research on *Borrelia* has waxed and waned, governed primarily by changing association of humans with the louse and tick. Most of the basic clinical and epidemiological concepts of louse-borne relapsing fever resulted from its spread and the resulting epidemics during and after World War I. The movement of populations of civilians and soldiers living under unhygienic conditions resulted in the propagation of lice and spread of the disease over large areas of Europe. Tick-borne borrelioses have taken on increased importance as humans have moved into rural areas and increased their recreational outdoor activities. Rutty described the first well documented epidemic of relapsing fever that occurred in Ireland between 1739 and 1741 and the first use of the designation 'relapsing fever' was by Craigie in 1843 (Scott 1942). Louse-borne relapsing fever was imported into the USA from England and caused the famous Philadelphia epidemic of 1844. The aetiological agent of louse-borne relapsing fever, *Borrelia recurrentis*, was discovered by Obermeier in 1868 but the publication of this observation was delayed until 1873. Mackie (1907) was the first to incriminate the louse as the vector of epidemic relapsing fever and it was later established that the method of transmission of *B. recurrentis* was by the crushing of the feeding louse and the subsequent release of infectious body fluids. Tick-borne relapsing fever was probably first noted by Livingston in 1857 in Africa (Carlisle 1906). Cook (1904) was the first to observe the presence of spirochaetes in the blood of patients. Ross and Milne (1904), Dutton and Todd (1905) and Koch (1905), conducting studies in various areas of Africa, confirmed the observations of Cook (1904) and demonstrated that the tick-borne borreliae can infect monkeys. The disease was contracted by both Dutton and Todd; Dutton died from the illness. The spirochaete was first cultured by Noguchi (1912) but the cultivation of borreliae by others could be described as difficult with limited success until recently. The major advances in cultivation of borreliae occurred with the development of partially defined medium by Kelly (1971) and subsequent modifications of this medium by Stoenner (1974), Stoenner, Dodd and Larson (1982) and Barbour (1984).

At a meeting of the Swedish Dermatological Society in October 1909, Dr Arvid Afzelius presented an elderly lady with an annular erythema of the skin that occurred after a tick bite. He named the skin lesion erythema migrans and suggested it was an infection transmitted by the tick bite (Afzelius 1910). The chronic skin lesion of Lyme borreliosis, acrodermatitis chronica atrophicans, was described in the 1880s (Pick 1894), but was first named and further characterized by Herxheimer and Hartman in 1902. The first report of neurological involvement (meningoradiculitis) associated with Lyme borreliosis was by the French physicians, Garin and Bujadoux (1922). In 1970, the first endogenously acquired case of erythema migrans in the USA was reported (Scrimenti 1970). Subsequently, an epidemic of oligoarthritis in children and adults initiated intensive epidemiological studies that culminated in the description of a tick-borne infectious illness called Lyme disease (Steere et al. 1977a, 1977b, 1983). Although some of the clinical manifestations of Lyme borreliosis were described as early as the 1880s, the aetiological agent was not discovered until 1982. Willy Burgdorfer discovered the spirochaete in the midgut of *Ixodes scapularis* (*dammini*) collected on Shelter Island, New York (Burgdorfer et al. 1982) and subsequently it was isolated from patients by Benach et al. (1983) and Steere et al. (1983). The spirochaete was identified as a new species of *Borrelia* and named *Borrelia burgdorferi* in honour of Willy Burgdorfer, the discoverer of the aetiological agent (Johnson et al. 1984). The potential for infection with *B. burgdorferi* has probably existed in the USA since the 1940s based on the detection of *B. burgdorferi* DNA in museum specimens of *I. scapularis* collected during that period (Persing et al. 1990).

3 HABITAT

Borreliae are obligate parasites and their life cycle is dependent on ecosystems that support a habitat suitable for competent arthropod vectors and reservoir vertebrate hosts. The reservoir host for *B. recurrentis*, the aetiological agent of louse-borne relapsing fever, is man. Although the borreliae multiply in the louse, they are restricted to the haemolymph. Since other tissues are not infected, the spirochaetes cannot be transmitted to man by louse saliva or excrement nor transovarially to the louse progeny. Thus, the only source of spirochaetes for the host-specific body louse is man.

The primary reservoir hosts for the tick-borne relapsing fevers and Lyme disease borreliae are rodents and the respective tick vectors are species of *Ornithodoros* and *Ixodes*. Some transovarial transmission occurs but only plays a limited role in the life cycle of these borreliae. *B. burgdorferi* is the only *Borrelia* species known to infect both mammals and birds.

4 MORPHOLOGY

The borreliae are slender ([0.2–0.5] × [8–30] μm) and the shape of the cell has been reported as both a flat wave form and as helical (Goldstein, Charon and Kreiling 1994). They share the same basic ultrastructural features as other members of the Spirochaetaceae. An outer membrane encloses the protoplasmic cylinder which consists of a peptidoglycan layer and an inner membrane enclosing the internal components of the cell. Periplasmic flagella are inserted subterminally and bipolarly in the protoplasmic cylinder. The number of periplasmic flagella varies from 7 to 20 per cell end (Hovind-Hougen 1976, Barbour and Hayes 1986); the flagella are unsheathed and overlap in the central region of the cell. Borreliae are best visualized with Giemsa's stain. They stain poorly, if at all, with the gram stain.

5 CULTURAL CHARACTERISTICS AND GROWTH REQUIREMENTS

Borreliae are micro-aerophilic, slow-growing spirochaetes. They grow best in liquid media at 30–35°C with cell yields of 10^7–10^8 per ml. The generation time at 35°C varies from 12 to 24 h. Growth occurs in soft solid media (1% agar) with a 50–100% plating efficiency. The colonies are subsurface and do not have distinguishing characteristics. The nutritional requirements have not been fully defined but are complex. *Borrelia* spp. have the unusual requirement for *N*-acetylglucosamine (Kelly 1971). They are similar to *Treponema*, requiring long-chain saturated and unsaturated fatty acids. Other nutritional requirements include glucose and amino acids. Serum proteins such as bovine serum albumin are a component of the medium and probably function primarily as a nontoxic source of fatty acids.

6 METABOLISM

Carbohydrates such as glucose serve as a major energy source and the predominant metabolic end product is lactic acid (Pickett and Kelly 1974, Livermore, Bey and Johnson 1978). The majority of the outer proteins of *B. burgdorferi* are covalently modified with lipids (Brandt et al. 1990). These lipoproteins are synthesized by the pathway common for bacterial lipoproteins and contain the tricyl-*S*-glycerylcysteine structural moiety. *B. burgdorferi* is catalase-negative (Kelly 1976).

7 GENETIC MECHANISMS

The genome of *Borrelia* spp. is composed of a linear chromosome and linear as well as supercoiled circular plasmids. The linear chromosome was first described in *B. burgdorferi* (Baril et al. 1989, Ferdows and Barbour 1989). Subsequently, the relapsing fever borreliae and *Borrelia anserina* were shown to have linear chromosomes of similar size (Kitten and Barbour 1992, Rosa and Schwan 1992, Casjens and Huang 1993). The telomeres (extreme ends) of both the linear chromosome and linear plasmids are covalently closed hairpins (Barbour and Garon 1987, Hinnebusch and Barbour 1991). In addition to its linearity, the chromosome of *Borrelia* spp. is also characterized by its small size of 950–1000 kb and by a low G + C content of 27–32 mol%. Mycoplasmas have chromosomes of about the same size which are the smallest recorded genomes among free-living bacteria (Pyle et al. 1988). The genomes of mycoplasmas also have a low G + C content of 24 mol% (Razin 1985). The borreliae are polyploid, each cell containing between 10 and 20 copies of the chromosome. No mechanism of genetic exchange has been reported for *Borrelia* spp. and the lack of techniques for gene transfer has impeded investigations of the molecular biology of these spirochaetes. Dykhuizen et al. (1993) sequenced several genes of up to 15 isolates of *B. burgdorferi* and found no evidence for lateral genetic exchange between chromosomal genes, suggesting that *B. burgdorferi* is strictly clonal. Dykhuizen et al. (1993) did present evidence for transfer of and recombination on a linear plasmid but suggest that transfer and recombinations are very rare events. Without a mechanism for genetic exchange, any change in DNA sequence (e.g. mutation) is transmitted only by direct inheritance to the progeny cell. The chromosome copy number for *Borrelia hermsii* grown in mice is 16 and decreases to one-fourth to one-half this number when grown in broth medium (Kitten and Barbour 1992). The chromosome copy number for *B. burgdorferi* has not been reported. A physical map of the chromosome of *B. burgdorferi* has been reported by Davidson, MacDougall and Saint Girons (1992) and Casjens and Huang (1993); the data are consistent with the chromosome being linear and having a length of 946–952 kb. The ribosomal RNA genes of *B. burgdorferi* have an unusual organization. There are 2 copies each of *rrl* (23S) and *rrf* (5S) but only one copy of *rrs* (16S) (Davidson, MacDougall and Saint Girons 1992, Fukunaga, Yanagihara and Sohnaka 1992, Schwartz, Gazumyan and Schwartz 1992).

Linear plasmids were first observed in *B. hermsii* (Plasterk, Simon and Barbour 1985) and were subsequently found in *B. burgdorferi* (Barbour and Garon 1987). The copy number of linear plasmids for *B. hermsii* and *B. burgdorferi* is approximately one per chromosome (Hinnebusch and Barbour 1992, Kitten and Barbour 1992), suggesting that replication and partitioning of plasmids are tightly coupled in these spirochaetes. *B. hermsii* cells contain 10–20 linear plasmids (Kitten and Barbour 1992) and in *B. burgdorferi* the number of linear plasmids ranges from 4 to 10 (Xu and Johnson 1995). Plasmids comprise a significant amount of the genome of these spirochaetes. Low passage (infectious) *B. burgdorferi* B31 may have as much as 17% of its genetic information in plasmid DNA (Marconi et al. 1993, Sadziene et al. 1993).

Antigenic variation as a mechanism for evading the mammalian immune response is well documented for *B. hermsii* (Barbour 1990, Donelson 1995). A single cell of *B. hermsii* is capable of producing 40 antigenically distinct serotypes (Plasterk, Simon and Barbour 1985) which can appear at a rate of 10^3–10^4 per cell per generation. The linear plasmids of *B. hermsii* contain genes encoding the outer-membrane lipoprotein, called variable major protein (Vmp). These genes are silent except when they are located immediately adjacent to one of the linear plasmid telomeres. The translocation of *vmp* genes from silent sites to expression (active) sites results in antigenic variation. This mechanism of antigenic variation most closely resembles that of the African trypanosome, the causative agent of sleeping sickness (Donelson 1995).

Low passage *B. burgdorferi* B31 contains 8 linear plasmids and 3 circular plasmids (Xu and Johnson 1995). The plasmid profiles of the 3 genospecies of *B. burgdorferi sensu lato* have a large linear plasmid of 50–57 kb as determined by pulsed field gel electrophoresis (PFGE) (Samuels, Marconi and Garon 1993, Xu and Johnson 1995). This plasmid has been studied in the greatest detail. The genes encoding 2 major outer surface proteins (Osp) A and B are located on the large plasmid and were the first to be cloned and sequenced (Howe, Laquier and Barbour 1986, Bergström, Bundoc and Barbour 1989). The genes *ospA* and *ospB* are located close together in an operon and transcribed as one transcriptional unit. Most strains of *B. burgdorferi* express both OspA and OspB whereas others express only one of the proteins. Fuchs et al. (1994) reported that *B. burgdorferi* binds human plasminogen on its surface and they identified OspA as the major binding site. Coleman et al. (1995) observed the binding of plasminogen to the surface of *B. burgdorferi* and *B. hermsii*. The plasminogen is converted to bioactive plasmin by an urokinase-type activator which could facilitate dissemination of the spirochaetes in the host (Klempner et al. 1995). Schwan et al. (1994) found that *B. burgdorferi sensu stricto* expresses OspA, but not OspC, in unfed *I. scapularis* ticks whereas the converse appears to occur in the mammalian host. Fingerle et al. (1995) reported a similar observation with *Ixodes ricinus* ticks, the primary vector of the Lyme borreliosis agent in central European countries. The regulation of the expression of these Osps was found to be related to temperature and substrate availability (Schwan et al. 1994). The gene for OspD is located on a 38 kb linear plasmid of *B. burgdorferi* B31 and plasmids in the 35–40 kb range of the other 9 strains have been examined (Norris et al. 1992). OspE and OspF genes are located on a 45 kb plasmid of *B. burgdorferi* and are structurally arranged in tandem as one transcriptional unit under the control of a common promoter (Lam et al. 1994). Since the 45 kb plasmid was identified using PFGE, which poorly resolves circular plasmids (Casjens and Huang 1993), it is probably linear in structure. Another surface-exposed lipoprotein is expressed in the European *B. burgdorferi sensu lato* strain B39. The gene for this 27 kDa lipoprotein is located on the large 55 kb linear plasmid (Reindl, Redl and Stöffler 1993).

Similar to other eubacteria, *Borrelia* spp. have supercoiled plasmids ranging in size from 5 to 30 kb (Hyde and Johnson 1984, Simpson, Garon and Schwan 1990). The gene for the major outer surface lipoprotein, OspC, is located on the 26 kb circular plasmid of *B. burgdorferi* (Marconi, Samuels and Garon 1993, Sadziene et al. 1993). The gene has been found in all

Lyme borreliosis spirochaetes examined, but not all the spirochaetes actively transcribed the gene. Also located on the 26 kb circular plasmid are the homologues of *guaA* and *guaB*, which encode the enzymes that convert xanthosine 5′-monophosphate (XMP) to guanosine 5′-monophosphate (GMP) and inosine 5′-monophosphate (IMP) to XMP, respectively (Margolis et al. 1994). In other bacteria the *guaA* and *guaB* genes reside on the chromosome (Zalkin and Dixon 1992), suggesting that this plasmid may be a minichromosome. An 18 kDa protein is encoded on a gene located on a 9 kb circular plasmid and apparently is only expressed during infection (Champion et al. 1994).

8 CELL WALL AND ENVELOPE COMPOSITION; ANTIGENIC STRUCTURE

The cell wall of *Borrelia* spp. contains muramic acid (Ginger 1963) and ornithine (Klaviter and Johnson 1979) as components of the peptidoglycan. The outer membrane that surrounds the peptidoglycan layer of *B. burgdorferi* consists of 45–62% protein and 13 major surface proteins have been identified (Luft et al. 1989). The outer surface proteins A, B, C, D, E and F are lipoproteins (Brandt et al. 1990, Fuchs et al. 1994). The surface-exposed 66 kDa protein is not a lipoprotein (Probert, Allsup and LeFebvre 1995). Heterogenicity of major surface proteins of *B. burgdorferi sensu lato* have been reported (Barbour and Schrumpf 1986, Bergström, Bundoc and Barbour 1989, Adam et al. 1991, Wilske et al. 1992, 1993a, 1993b).

9 CLASSIFICATION OF *BORRELIA* SPECIES

The principal species of *Borrelia* are listed in Table 56.1.

9.1 Classification of *Borrelia burgdorferi sensu lato*

Although some clinical manifestations of Lyme borreliosis were described as early as 1883 (Buchwald 1883) the aetiological agent of the disease was not discovered and cultured until 1982 (Burgdorfer et al. 1982). DNA–DNA homology studies established this spirochaete as a new species of *Borrelia* and it was named *B. burgdorferi*. The description of this new species of *Borrelia* was based on the study of a small number of strains, 9 strains from the northeastern US and one strain from Switzerland. The examination of the genotypic (Le Febvre, Perng and Johnson 1989, Postic et al. 1990, Adam et al. 1991, Rosa, Hogan and Schwan 1991, Jonsson et al. 1992, Marconi and Garon 1992, Marconi et al. 1992, Picken 1992, Zumstein et al. 1992) and phenotypic (Barbour, Tessier and Hayes 1984, Barbour, Heiland and Howe 1985, Wilske et al. 1988, Anderson et al. 1989, Masuzawa et al. 1991, Boerlin et al. 1992, Brown and Lane 1992) character-

istics of additional strains from various clinical manifestations of the illness suggested that more than one species of *Borrelia* were aetiological agents of Lyme borreliosis. Subsequently, it was shown that *B. burgdorferi* was a complex of at least 4 species (Baranton et al. 1992, Canica et al. 1993, Kawabata et al. 1993, Postic et al. 1994). Three of these species, *B. burgdorferi sensu stricto*, *Borrelia garinii* and *B. afzelii*, cause Lyme borreliosis. *Borrelia japonica* appears to be non-infectious for humans. In addition to the 4 validly described species, 4 additional genospecies have been described (Postic et al. 1994). None of the new genospecies is known to be infectious for humans. The term *B. burgdorferi sensu lato* (*s.l.*) refers to all strains of *Borrelia* that have the characteristics reported in the original description of *B. burgdorferi* (Johnson et al. 1984). Wilske et al. (1993b) analysed *B. burgdorferi s.l.* strains by SDS-PAGE and immunoblotting with a panel of monoclonal antibodies directed against different epitopes of the OspA protein. An OspA serotyping system was developed that strongly associated certain OspA serotypes with distinct species (genospecies). *B. burgdorferi sensu stricto* strains were serotype 1. *B. afzelii* strains clustered into serotype 2 and a marked heterogeneity of OspA serotypes (types 3–7) was found for *B. garinii* strains. When the same type of analysis was conducted for OspC, greater heterogeneity was observed, resulting in 13 serotypes (Wilske et al. 1995).

Only *B. burgdorferi sensu stricto* is known to cause Lyme borreliosis in the USA. It is transmitted by *I. scapularis* in the northeastern and north central USA and by *Ixodes pacificus* along the Pacific coast from southern California to British Columbia as well as in Nevada and Utah (Anderson and Magnarelli 1992). *B. burgdorferi sensu stricto*, *B. garinii* and *B. afzelii* are aetiological agents of Lyme borreliosis in Europe and Asia. *I. ricinus* is the vector tick in western and eastern Europe. In eastern Europe and Asia, the vector tick is *Ixodes persulcatus*. The tick vector-infectious agent specificity associated with tick-borne relapsing fever has not been reported for Lyme borrelioses.

The classification of other borreliae has not been studied in the same detail as *B. burgdorferi s.l.* The relapsing fever borreliae were initially identified on the basis of vector specificity (Davis 1956). *B. hermsii*, *Borrelia turicatae* and *Borrelia parkeri* are transmitted by the soft ticks *Ornithodoros hermsii*, *Ornithodoros turicata* and *Ornithodoros parkeri*, respectively (see Table 56.1). However, DNA–DNA homology studies suggest that these North American relapsing fever borreliae are very similar and may represent a single species (Hyde and Johnson 1984). The report of Schwan et al. (1989) that a *B. hermsii* DNA probe hybridized with *B. parkeri* confirms the close relatedness of these 2 species. The species status of *B. anserina*, *Borrelia crocidurae* and *Borrelia coriaceae*, the aetiological agents of avian borreliosis, old world tick-borne relapsing fever and epizootic bovine abortion, respectively, have been established by DNA–DNA homology (Hyde and Johnson 1986, Johnson et al. 1987).

Table 56.1 Characteristics of *Borrelia* species of medical and veterinary significance

Species	Disease	Vector	Geographical distribution
B. recurrentis	Louse-borne relapsing fever	*Pediculus humanus humanus*	World wide
B. hermsii	American tick-borne relapsing fever	*Ornithodoros hermsi*	Western Canada, USA
B. turicatae	American tick-borne relapsing fever	*O. turicata*	Southwestern USA
B. parkeri	American tick-borne relapsing fever	*O. parkeri*	Western USA
B. mazzottii	American tick-borne relapsing fever	*O. talaje*	Southern USA, Mexico, Central and South America
B. venezuelensis	American tick-borne relapsing fever	*O. rudis*	Central and South America
B. duttonii	East African tick-borne relapsing fever	*O. moubata*	Central, eastern, and southern Africa
B. hispanica	Hispano-African tick-borne relapsing fever	*O. erraticus*	Spain, Portugal, Morocco, Algeria, Tunisia
B. crocidurae, B. merionesi, B. microti, B. dipodilli	North African tick-borne relapsing fever	*O. erraticus*	Morocco, Libya, Egypt, Iran, Turkey, Senegal, Kenya
B. persica	Asiatic-African tick-borne relapsing fever	*O. tholozani*	Middle East, Central Asia
B. caucasica	Caucasian tick-borne relapsing fever	*O. verrucosus*	Iraq, southwestern former USSR
B. latyschewii	Caucasian tick-borne relapsing fever	*O. tartakovskyi*	Iraq, Iran, Afghanistan, south central and southwestern former USSR
B. burgdorferi sensu stricto	Lyme borreliosis	*Ixodes scapularis*	Midwestern and eastern USA
		I. pacificus	Western USA
		I. ricinus	Europe
B. garinii	Lyme borreliosis	*I. ricinus*	Europe
		I. persulcatus	Russia, China, Japan
B. afzelii	Lyme borreliosis	*I. ricinus*	Europe
		I. persulcatus	Russia, China, Japan
B. anserina	Avian borreliosis	*Argas persicus* and other *Argas* spp.	World wide
B. theileri	Bovine borreliosis	*Rhipicephalus evertsi, Boophilus microplus, B. annulatus, B. decoloratus*	South Africa, Australia, Brazil, Mexico
B. coriaceae	Epizootic bovine abortion (?)	*Ornithodoros coriaceus*	California

10 LABORATORY ISOLATION AND IDENTIFICATION

Borrelia spp. can be isolated from their vector ticks and host animals. *Ixodes* ticks, mammals and birds are the primary sources of *B. burgdorferi s.l.* The isolation medium consists of the Barbour–Stoenner–Kelly (BSK) formulation (Barbour 1984) or modified BSK (Preac-Mursic et al. 1989a, Anderson and Magnarelli 1992, Berger et al. 1992) with or without antimicrobial

agents. Antimicrobial agents are usually incorporated into media when potentially contaminated specimens such as ticks and skin biopsies are cultured. Various combinations of antimicrobial agents have been used. Morshed et al. (1993) evaluated agents for use in a medium for the selective isolation of Lyme disease and relapsing fever borreliae. They recommended the combination of 4 agents, 5 fluorouracil (100 mg ml^{-1}), sulphamethoxazole (50 mg ml^{-1}), trimethoprim (10 mg ml^{-1}) and phosphomycin (400 mg ml^{-1}), for incorporation into a selective medium. *B. burgdorferi s.l.* can be consistently isolated from infected ticks and rodents. Skin biopsy specimens from patients with erythema migrans lesions are one of the best sources of *B. burgdorferi s.l.* with the frequency of isolation as high as 86% (Berger et al. 1992). Isolation from other patient specimens has been a low yield procedure. The frequency of isolation reported for blood is 2–7%, for CSF 11%, and the spirochaete has only been isolated from 2 synovial specimens (Schmidli et al. 1988).

Ticks are prepared for culture by immersion in 70% isopropyl alcohol for approximately 1 min, followed by a sterile water rinse. The surface-cleansed tick is placed on a sterile glass slide containing a drop of BSK medium and the midgut and other tissues are removed by dissection. The tick tissues are transferred to BSK medium with or without selective agents (Anderson and Magarnelli 1992). The inoculated medium is incubated at 30–35°C.

Borreliae are isolated from rodents by culturing blood, spleen, heart, bladder and ear. One to two drops of blood are inoculated into BSK medium. The ears are prepared for biopsy by a surgical scrub followed by a sterile water rinse. The ear biopsy is aseptically taken with a sterile dermal punch and placed directly into BSK medium. The spleen, heart and bladder are aseptically removed and each organ placed into a Tekmar sterile laboratory bag (Tekmar Co., Cincinnati, Ohio) containing 7 ml of BSK medium. After the tissues are disrupted in a Stomacher laboratory blender, a 1:10 dilution of the tissue suspension is cultured in BSK medium.

Cutaneous tissues thought to be erythema migrans are cultured by obtaining a punch biopsy from the peripheral aspect of the lesion under sterile conditions and placed in 7 ml of BSK isolation medium (Berger et al. 1992). After 7 days of incubation at 30–35°C, the skin biopsy specimen is transferred to BSK medium without antimicrobial agents. Both the tube of isolation medium from which the skin biopsy was removed and the tube of antibiotic-free BSK containing the skin biopsy are incubated at 30–35°C and examined for spirochaetes at intervals of 3, 6 and 12 weeks (Berger et al. 1992). Blood and cerebrospinal fluid are cultured by inoculating one or 2 drops of the specimen into 7 ml BSK medium (Steere et al. 1983, Karlson et al. 1990, Goodman et al. 1995).

11 SUSCEPTIBILITY TO ANTIMICROBIAL AGENTS

The in vitro susceptibility of *Borrelia* spp. to various antimicrobial agents has been studied by a number of investigators: Johnson et al. (1984, 1990a, 1990b), Johnson, Kodner and Russell (1987), Preac-Mursic et al. (1989a, 1989b), Sambri et al. (1990), Agger, Callister and Jobe (1992), Dever, Jorgensen and Barbour (1992, 1993), Levin et al. (1993), Masuzawa et al. (1994). Unfortunately, standard methods for determining the minimal bactericidal concentrations

(MBC) for slow-growing bacteria such as the borreliae have not been established. In spite of the use of different protocols there is general agreement on the in vitro activity of most of the commonly used antimicrobials against *B. burgdorferi s.l.* These spirochaetes were susceptible to the macrolides, tetracyclines, semisynthetic penicillins, and the late second- and third-generation cephalosporins. *B. burgdorferi s.l.* was moderately sensitive to penicillin G and chloramphenicol and relatively resistant to the aminoglycosides, trimethoprim, sulphamethoxazole, quinolines and rifampicin. First-generation cephalosporins generally possessed a low level of activity. There is no documented report of the development of antimicrobial resistance in *Borrelia* spp. (Berger and Johnson 1989). A macrodilution broth procedure was used to determine MBCs for *B. burgdorferi s.l.* and 4 other species of *Borrelia* (Johnson et al. 1984, 1990a, 1990b, Johnson, Kodner and Russell 1987) (see Volume 3, Chapter 50).

This procedure incorporates the incubation of the spirochaetes with the antimicrobial agent in BSK medium for 7 days, followed by transfer to BSK medium without antimicrobial agents and incubation for 3 weeks. The MBCs of a number of antimicrobial agents for *B. burgdorferi s.l.* determined by this procedure are shown in Table 56.2. The MBCs for these antimicrobial agents were also determined for 2 North American relapsing fever borreliae, *B. hermsii* and *B. turicatae*, the agent of fowl spirochaetosis *B. anserina*, and *B. coriaceae*, the putative agent of epizootic bovine abortion. In these 4 species of *Borrelia* no significant differences in in vitro antimicrobial susceptibility from that of *B. burgdorferi s.l.* were observed (Table 56.3).

In contrast to the in vitro antimicrobial studies, only a few investigators have studied the in vivo susceptibility of *B. burgdorferi s.l.* These studies have been conducted in experimentally infected gerbils (Preac-Mursic et al. 1987, 1989b), hamsters (Johnson, Kodner and Russell 1987, Johnson et al. 1990a, 1990b) and

Table 56.2 In vitro antimicrobial susceptibility of *Borrelia burgdorferi s.l.*

Antimicrobial agent	MBC (μg ml^{-1})	
	Geometric mean	Range
Penicillin G	17.5	3.2–51.2
Amoxycillin	1.5	0.4–3.2
Cefotaxime	0.5	0.5
Cefadroxil	–	>5.0
Ceftriaxone	0.08	0.04–0.16
Cefixime	1.0	1.0
Ceftazidime	1.0	1.0
Tetracycline	1.0	0.04–3.2
Doxycycline	3.3	0.08–6.4
Minocycline	0.93	0.3–2.5
Erythromycin	0.13	0.02–0.32
Azithromycin	0.03	0.005–0.08
Ciprofloxicin	4.0	4.0
Piperacillin	0.12	0.05–0.5

Table 56.3 In vitro antimicrobial susceptibility of 4 species of *Borrelia*

| | MBC (μg ml^{-1}) | | | |
	B. hermsii	*B. turicatae*	*B. anserina*	*B. coriaceae*
Penicillin G	6.4	6.4	6.4	<1.6
Amoxycillin	0.8	1.6	0.4	<0.2
Ceftriaxone	0.08	0.16	0.08	0.04
Erythromycin	0.16	<0.04	0.08	<0.04
Azithromycin	0.04	0.02	0.02	<0.01
Tetracycline	0.4	0.4	0.2	<0.4
Doxycycline	0.8	0.8	1.6	<0.2

inbred mice (Moody, Adams and Barthold 1994). With the exception of erythromycin, antimicrobial agents that displayed good in vitro activity against *B. burgdorferi s. l.* also demonstrated satisfactory in vivo activity in the immunocompetent hamster (Table 56.4) and gerbil. Penicillin G, which had moderate in vitro activity, was required at high dosages for satisfactory in vivo activity (Johnson, Kodner and Russell 1987, Preac-Mursic et al. 1989b). The results obtained with inbred mice, which develop a persistent joint infection, were similar for amoxycillin, penicillin G and ceftriaxone. However, doxycycline and azithromycin failed to cure these mice (Moody, Adams and Barthold 1994).

12 PATHOGENICITY AND VIRULENCE FACTORS

Considerable progress has been made in understanding the genomic composition, protein and antigenic make-up, and variability of *B. burgdorferi s.l.* as well as the clinical manifestations of Lyme borreliosis. By contrast, knowledge of the mechanisms responsible for the pathogenesis of this disease is fragmentary. The favourable response of patients to antibiotic therapy strongly suggests that viable spirochaetes are a critical component of pathogenesis. Autoimmunity probably

Table 56.4 In vivo antimicrobial susceptibility of *Borrelia burgdorferi* 297

Antimicrobial agent	50% Curative dose (mg kg^{-1})
Penicillin G	>195.5
Amoxycillin	58.7 (34.1–100.9)*
Ceftriaxone	16.5 (12.0–22.9)
	16.6 (10.0–27.5)
	45.2 (32.4–61.7)
Tetracycline	29.5 (18.3–41.5)
	25.1 (16.9–37.2)
Doxycycline	33.5 (25.2–44.6)
Erythromycin	309.1 (200.3–501.1)
	160.0 (125.0–198.1)
Azithromycin	10.0 (7.9–13.2)

*Numbers in parentheses after 50% curative doses are the 95% confidence levels.

plays a minor, if any, role in the pathogenic process since infection of immunodeficient mice leads to the development of arthritis, myositis and carditis (Schaible et al. 1989, Simon et al. 1991). The invasiveness of *B. burgdorferi s.l.* may be due to the employment of endogenous or host-derived proteinases. Several independent studies (Fuchs et al. 1994, Coleman et al. 1995, Klempner et al. 1995) have shown that *B. burgdorferi s. l.* binds human plasminogen to its surface, mainly via OspA (Fuchs et al. 1994) and the plasminogen is protected from plasmin inhibitors in blood. Accelerated formation of plasmin occurs as the result of the host-derived plasminogen activator, urokinase (Klempner et al. 1995). The acquisition of the host-derived plasmin degrades components of extracellular matrices, facilitating the movement of the spirochaetes and amplifying their pathogenic potential.

One of the characteristics of Lyme borreliosis is the paucity of spirochaetes in the infected organs. Since the pathology associated with this disease is caused by so few spirochaetes, mechanisms for amplifying their pathogenicity must exist. *B. burgdorferi s.l.* may bind to mononuclear and polynuclear phagocytes in the inflammatory infiltrate and induce the production of inflammatory cytokines such as IL-1, TNF-α and IL-6, which stimulate the production of secondary mediators such as proteolytic enzymes and prostaglandins (Simon et al. 1994). In addition, the spirochaetes can activate the complement cascade in the absence of antibody with the release of mediators of inflammation (Kochi and Johnson 1988). No borrelial exotoxins have been reported as yet (see Volume 3, Chapter 50).

In contrast to *B. burgdorferi s.l.*, which is antigenically stable in the host (Barthold 1993), the relapsing fever borreliae use antigenic variation as a mechanism to evade the host immune response (Barbour 1990). This antigenic variation results in a disease characterized by recurrent episodes of fever and spirochaetaemia. Coleman et al. (1995) reported that *B. hermsii*, like *B. burgdorferi s.l.*, binds host plasminogen on its surface and they suggest this characteristic may be a general property of *Borrelia* spp. which enhances their invasiveness. With the exception of the above, little is known concerning the mechanism of pathogenesis of the relapsing fever borreliae. It is possible that the release of host cytokines by these spirochaetes plays a major role in the pathogenesis of these borrelioses.

REFERENCES

Adam T, Gassmann GS et al., 1991, Phenotypic and genotypic analysis of *Borrelia burgdorferi* isolated from various sources, *Infect Immun*, **59:** 2579–85.

Afzelius A, 1910, Verhandlungen der dermatologischen Gesellschaft zu Stockholm on October 28, 1909, *Arch Dermatol Syph*, **101:** 404.

Agger WA, Callister SM, Jobe DA, 1992, In vitro susceptibilities of *Borrelia burgdorferi* to five oral cephalosporins and ceftriaxone, *Antimicrob Agents Chemother*, **36:** 1788–99.

Anderson JF, Magnarelli LA, 1992, Epizootiology of Lyme disease and methods of cultivating *Borrelia burgdorferi*, Ann NY Acad Sci, **653:** 52–63.

Anderson JF, Magnarelli LA et al., 1989, Antigenically variable *Borrelia burgdorferi* isolated from cottontail rabbits and *Ixodes dentatus* in rural and urban areas, *J Clin Microbiol*, **27:** 13–20.

Baranton G, Postic D et al., 1992, Delineation of *Borrelia burgdorferi* sensu stricto, *Borrelia garinii* sp. nov. and group VS461 associated with Lyme borreliosis, *Int J Syst Bacteriol*, **42:** 378–83.

Barbour AG, 1984, Isolation and cultivation of Lyme disease spirochetes, *Yale J Biol Med*, **57:** 521–5.

Barbour AG, 1990, Antigenic variation of a relapsing fever *Borrelia* species, *Annu Rev Microbiol*, **44:** 155–71.

Barbour AG, Garon CF, 1987, Linear plasmids of the bacterium *Borrelia burgdorferi* have covalently closed ends, *Science*, **237:** 409–11.

Barbour AG, Hayes SF, 1986, Biology of *Borrelia* species, *Microbiol Rev*, **50:** 381–400.

Barbour AG, Heiland RA, Howe TR, 1985, Heterogeneity of major proteins in Lyme disease borreliae: a molecular analysis of North American and European isolates, *J Infect Dis*, **152:** 478–84.

Barbour AG, Schrumpf ME, 1986, Polymorphisms of major surface proteins of *Borrelia burgdorferi*, Zentralbl Bakteriol Parasitenkd Infektionskr Hyg Abt 1 Orig Reihe A, **263:** 83–91.

Barbour AG, Tessier SL, Hayes SF, 1984, Variation in a major surface protein of Lyme disease spirochetes, *Infect Immun*, **45:** 94–100.

Baril C, Richaud C et al., 1989, Linear chromosome of *Borrelia burgdorferi*, Res Microbiol, **140:** 507–16.

Barthold SW, 1993, Antigenic stability of *Borrelia burgdorferi* during chronic infections of immunocompetent mice, *Infect Immun*, **61:** 4955–61.

Benach JL, Bosler EM et al., 1983, Spirochetes isolated from the blood of two patients with Lyme disease, *N Engl J Med*, **308:** 740–2.

Berger BW, Johnson RC, 1989, Clinical and microbiologic findings in six patients with erythema migrans of Lyme disease, *J Am Acad Dermatol*, **21:** 1188–91.

Berger BW, Johnson RC et al., 1992, Cultivation of *Borrelia burgdorferi* from erythema migrans lesions and perilesional skin, *J Clin Microbiol*, **30:** 359–61.

Bergström S, Bundoc V, Barbour A, 1989, Molecular analysis of linear plasmid-encoded major surface proteins, OspA and OspB, of the Lyme disease spirochaete *Borrelia burgdorferi*, Mol Microbiol, **3:** 479–86.

Boerlin P, Peter O et al., 1992, Population genetic analysis of *Borrelia burgdorferi* isolates by multilocus enzyme electrophoresis, *Infect Immun*, **60:** 1677–83.

Brandt ME, Riley BS et al., 1990, Immunogenic integral membrane proteins of *Borrelia burgdorferi* are lipoproteins, *Infect Immun*, **58:** 983–91.

Brown RN, Lane RS, 1992, Lyme disease in California: a novel enzootic transmission cycle of *Borrelia burgdorferi*, Science, **256:** 1439–42.

Buchwald A, 1883, Ein Fall von diffuser idiopatischer Haut-Atrophie, *Arch Dermatol Syph*, **10:** 553–6.

Burgdorfer W, Barbour AG et al., 1982, Lyme disease – a tickborne spirochetosis?, *Science*, **216:** 1317–19.

Canica MM, Nato F et al., 1993, Monoclonal antibodies for identification of *Borrelia afzelii* sp. nov. associated with late cutaneous manifestations of Lyme borreliosis, *Scand J Infect Dis*, **25:** 441–8.

Carlisle RJ, 1906, Two cases of relapsing fever; with notes on the occurence of this disease throughout the world at the present day, *J Infect Dis*, **3:** 233–65.

Casjens S, Huang WM, 1993, Linear chromosomal physical and genetic map of *Borrelia burgdorferi*, the Lyme disease agent, *Mol Microbiol*, **8:** 967–80.

Champion CI, Bianco DR et al., 1994, A 9.0-kilobase-pair circular plasmid of *Borrelia burgdorferi* encodes an exported protein: evidence for expression only during infection, *Infect Immun*, **62:** 2653–61.

Coleman JL, Sellati TJ et al., 1995, *Borrelia burgdorferi* binds plasminogen, resulting in enhanced penetration of endothelial monolayers, *Infect Immun*, **63:** 2478–84.

Cook AR, 1904, *J Trop Med Hyg*, **7:** 24.

Davidson BE, MacDougall J, Saint Girons I, 1992, Physical map of the linear chromosome of the bacterium *Borrelia burgdorferi* 212, a causative agent of Lyme disease, and localization of rRNA genes, *J Bacteriol*, **174:** 3766–74.

Davis GE, 1956, The identification of spirochetes from human cases of relapsing fever by xenodiagnosis with comments on local specificity of tick vectors, *Exp Parasitol*, **5:** 271–5.

Dever LL, Jorgensen JH, Barbour AG, 1992, In vitro antimicrobial susceptibility testing of *Borrelia burgdorferi*: a microdilution MIC method and time-kill studies, *J Clin Microbiol*, **30:** 2692–7.

Dever LL, Jorgenson JH, Barbour AG, 1993, Comparative in vitro activities of clarithromycin, azithromycin, and erythromycin against *Borrelia burgdorferi*, *Antimicrob Agents Chemother*, **37:** 1704–6.

Donelson JE, 1995, Mechanisms of antigenic variation in *Borrelia hermsii* and African trypanosomes, *J Biol Chem*, **270:** 7783–6.

Dutton JE, Todd JL, 1905, The nature of tick fever in the eastern part of the Congo Free State, *Br Med J*, **4:** 1259–60.

Dykhuizen DE, Polin DS et al., 1993, *Borrelia burgdorferi* is clonal – implications for taxonomy and vaccine development, *Proc Natl Acad Sci USA*, **90:** 10163–7.

Felsenfeld O, 1971, *Borrelia. Strains, Vectors, Human and Animal Borreliosis*, Warren H. Green, St Louis.

Ferdows MS, Barbour AG, 1989, Megabase-sized linear DNA in the bacterium *Borrelia burgdorferi*, the Lyme disease agent, *Proc Natl Acad Sci USA*, **86:** 5969–73.

Fingerle V, Hauser V et al., 1995, Expression of outer surface proteins A and C of *Borrelia burgdorferi* in *Ixodes ricinus*, *J Clin Microbiol*, **33:** 1867–9.

Fuchs H, Wallich R et al., 1994, The outer surface protein A of the spirochete *Borrelia burgdorferi* is a plasmin(ogen) receptor, *Proc Natl Acad Sci USA*, **91:** 12594–8.

Fukunaga M, Yanagihara Y, Sohnaka M, 1992, The 23S/5S ribosomal RNA genes (*rrl*/*rrf*) are separate from the 16S ribosomal RNA gene (*rrs*) in *Borrelia burgdorferi*, the aetiological agent of Lyme disease, *J Gen Microbiol*, **138:** 871–7.

Garin C, Bujadoux C, 1922, Paralysie par les tiques, *J Med Lyon*, **71:** 765–7.

Ginger CD, 1963, Isolation and characterization of muramic acid from two spirochetes: *Borrelia duttoni* and *Leptospira biflexa*, *Nature (London)*, **199:** 159.

Goldstein S, Charon NW, Kreiling JA, 1994, *Borrelia burgdorferi* swims with planar waveform similar to that of eukaryotic flagella, *Proc Natl Acad Sci USA*, **91:** 3433–7.

Goodman JL, Bradley JF et al., 1995, Bloodstream invasion in early Lyme disease: results from a prospective, controlled study utilizing the polymerase chain reaction, *Am J Med*, **99:** 6–12.

Herxheimer K, Hartmann K, 1902, Uber Acrodermatitis chronic atrophicans, *Arch Dermatol*, **61:** 57–76.

Hinnebusch J, Barbour AG, 1991, Linear plasmids of *Borrelia burgdorferi* have a telomeric structure and sequence similar to those of a eukaryotic virus, *J Bacteriol*, **173**: 7233–9.

Hinnebusch J, Barbour AG, 1992, Linear- and circular-plasmid copy numbers in *Borrelia burgdorferi*, *J Bacteriol*, **174**: 5251–7.

Hovind-Hougen K, 1976, *The Biology of Parasitic Spirochetes*, Academic Press, New York, 7–18.

Howe TR, Laquier FW, Barbour AG, 1986, Organization of genes encoding two outer membrane proteins of the Lyme disease agent *Borrelia burgdorferi* within a single transcriptional unit, *Infect Immun*, **54**: 207–12.

Hyde FW, Johnson RC, 1984, Genetic relationship of Lyme disease spirochetes to *Borrelia*, *Treponema*, and *Leptospira* spp., *J Clin Microbiol*, **20**: 151–4.

Hyde FW, Johnson RC, 1986, Genetic analysis of *Borrelia*, *Zentralbl Bakt Hyg*, **263**: 119–22.

Johnson RC, Hughes CA, 1992, *The Prokaryotes*, 2nd edn, Springer-Verlag, New York, 3560–7.

Johnson RC, Kodner C, Russell ME, 1987, *In vitro* and *in vivo* susceptibility of the Lyme disease spirochete, *Borrelia burgdorferi* to four antimicrobials, *Antimicrob Agents Chemother*, **31**: 164–7.

Johnson RC, Hyde FW et al., 1984, *Borrelia burgdorferi* sp. nov. etiological agent of Lyme disease, *Int J Syst Bacteriol*, **34**: 496–7.

Johnson RC, Burgdorfer W et al., 1987, *Borrelia coriaceae* sp. nov.: putative agent of epizootic bovine abortion, *Int J Syst Bacteriol*, **37**: 72–4.

Johnson RC, Kodner CB et al., 1990a, Comparative *in vitro* and *in vivo* susceptibilies of the Lyme disease spirochete *Borrelia burgdorferi* to cefuroxime and other antimicrobial agents, *Antimicrob Agents Chemother*, **34**: 2133–6.

Johnson RC, Kodner CB et al., 1990b, *In vitro* and *in vivo* susceptibility of *Borrelia burgdorferi* to azithromycin, *J Antimicrob Chemother*, **25, Suppl A**: 33–8.

Jonsson M, Noppa L et al., 1992, Heterogeneity of outer membrane proteins in *Borrelia burgdorferi* – comparison of *osp* operons of 3 isolates of different geographic origins, *Infect Immun*, **60**: 1845–53.

Karlsson M, Hovind-Hougen K et al., 1990, Cultivation of spirochetes from cerebrospinal fluid of patients with Lyme borreliosis, *J Clin Microbiol*, **28**: 473–9.

Kawabata H, Masuzawa T et al., 1993, Genomic analysis of *Borrelia japonica* sp. nov. isolated from *Ixodes ovatus* in Japan, *Microbiol Immunol*, **37**: 843–8.

Kelly RT, 1971, Cultivation of *Borrelia hermsi*, *Science*, **173**: 443–4.

Kelly RT, 1976, *The Biology of Parasitic Spirochetes*, Academic Press, New York, 87–94.

Kitten T, Barbour AG, 1992, The relapsing fever agent *Borrelia hermsii* has multiple copies of its chromosome and linear plasmids, *Genetics*, **132**: 311–24.

Klaviter EC, Johnson RC, 1979, Isolation of the outer envelope, chemical components, and ultrastructure of *Borrelia hermsii* grown in vitro, *Acta Trop (Basel)*, **36**: 123–31.

Klempner MS, Noring R et al., 1995, Binding of human plasminogen and urokinase-type plasminogen activator to the Lyme disease spirochete, *Borrelia burgdorferi*, *J Infect Dis*, **171**: 1258–65.

Koch R, 1905, Vorlaufige Mitteilungen über die Ergebnisse einer Forschungsreise nach Ostafrika, *Dtsch Med Wochenschr*, **31**: 1865–9.

Kochi SK, Johnson RC, 1988, Role of immunoglobulin G in killing of *Borrelia burgdorferi* by the classical complement pathway, *Infect Immun*, **56**: 314–21.

Lam TT, Nguyen T-PK et al., 1994, Outer surface proteins E and F of *Borrelia burgdorferi*, the agent of Lyme disease, *Infect Immun*, **62**: 290–8.

LeFebvre RB, Perng GC, Johnson RC, 1989, Characterization of *Borrelia burgdorferi* isolates by restriction endonuclease analysis and DNA hybridization, *J Clin Microbiol*, **27**: 636–9.

Levin JM, Nelson JA et al., 1993, *In vitro* susceptibility of *Borrelia burgdorferi* to 11 antimicrobial agents, *Antimicrob Agents Chemother*, **37**: 1444–6.

Livermore BP, Bey RF, Johnson RC, 1978, Lipid metabolism of *Borrelia hermsii*, *Infect Immun*, **20**: 215–20.

Luft BJ, Jiang W et al., 1989, Biochemical and immunochemical characterization of the surface proteins of *Borrelia burgdorferi*, *Infect Immun*, **57**: 3637–45.

Mackie FP, 1907, The part played by *Pediculus corporis* in the transmission of relapsing fever, *Br Med J*, **2**: 1706–9.

Marconi RT, Garon CF, 1992, Phylogenetic analysis of the genus *Borrelia* – a comparison of North American and European isolates of *Borrelia burgdorferi*, *J Bacteriol*, **174**: 241–4.

Marconi RT, Samuels DS, Garon CF, 1993, Transcriptional analyses and mapping of the *ospC* gene in Lyme disease spirochetes, *J Bacteriol*, **175**: 926–32.

Marconi RT, Lubke L et al., 1992, Species-specific identification of a distinction between *Borrelia burgdorferi* genomic groups by using 16S rRNA-directed oligonucleotide probes, *J Clin Microbiol*, **30**: 628–32.

Marconi RT, Samuels DS et al., 1993, Identification of a protein in several *Borrelia* species which is related to OspC of the Lyme disease spirochetes, *J Clin Microbiol*, **31**: 2577–83.

Margolis N, Hogan D et al., 1994, Plasmid location of *Borrelia* purine biosynthesis gene homologs, *J Bacteriol*, **176**: 6427–32.

Masuzawa T, Okada Y et al., 1991, Antigenic properties of *Borrelia burgdorferi* isolated from *Ixodes ovatus* and *Ixodes persulcatus* in Hokkaido, Japan, *J Clin Microbiol*, **29**: 1568–73.

Masuzawa T, Yamada K et al., 1994, In vitro antibiotic susceptibilities of *Borrelia* isolates from erythema migrans lesion in Lyme disease patients from Japan, *Microbiol Immun*, **38**: 399–402.

Moody KD, Adams RL, Barthold SW, 1994, Effectiveness of antimicrobial treatment against *Borrelia burgdorferi* infection in mice, *Antimicrob Agents Chemother*, **38**: 1567–72.

Morshed MG, Konishi H et al., 1993, Evaluation of agents for use in medium for selective isolation of Lyme disease and relapsing fever *Borrelia* species, *Eur J Clin Microbiol*, **12**: 512–18.

Noguchi H, 1912, The pure cultivation of *Spirochaeta kochi*, *Spirochaeta obermeieri*, and *Spirochaeta novy*, *J Exp Med*, **16**: 199–212.

Norris SJ, Carter CJ et al., 1992, Low-passage-associated proteins of *Borrelia burgdorferi* B31 – characterization and molecular cloning of OspD, a surface-exposed, plasmid-encoded lipoprotein, *Infect Immun*, **60**: 4662–72.

Obermeier O, 1873, Vorkommen feinster, eine Eigenbewgung zeigender Fäden im Blute von Recurrenskranken, *Zentralbl Med Wissensch*, **11**: 145–7.

Persing DH, Telford SR et al., 1990, Detection of *Borrelia burgdorferi* DNA in museum specimens of *Ixodes*, *Science*, **249**: 1420–3.

Pick PhJ, 1894, *Uber eine neue Krankheit 'Erythromelie'. Verh. Ges. dtsch. Naturf. 66. Verslg. Wein.*, 2nd edn, Leipzig, 336.

Picken RN, 1992, Polymerase chain reaction primers and probes derived from flagellin gene sequences for specific detection of the agents of Lyme disease and North American relapsing fever, *J Clin Microbiol*, **30**: 99–114.

Pickett J, Kelly R, 1974, Lipid catabolism of relapsing fever borreliae, *Infect Immun*, **9**: 201–2.

Plasterk RHA, Simon MI, Barbour AG, 1985, Transportation of structural genes to an expression sequence on a linear plasmid causes antigenic variation in the bacterium *Borrelia hermsii*, *Nature (London)*, **318**: 257–63.

Postic D, Assous MV et al., 1994, Diversity of *Borrelia burgdorferi* sensu lato evidenced by restriction fragment length polymorphism of rrf (5S)-rrl (23S) intergenic spacer amplicons, *Int J Syst Bacteriol*, **44**: 743–52.

Postic D, Edlinger C et al., 1990, Two genomic species in *Borrelia burgdorferi*, *Res Microbiol*, **140**: 507–16.

Preac-Mursic V, Wilske B et al., 1987, In vitro and in vivo susceptibility of *Borrelia burgdorferi*, *Eur J Clin Microbiol*, **4**: 424–6.

Preac-Mursic V, Weber K et al., 1989a, Survival of *Borrelia burgdorferi* in antibiotically treated patients with Lyme borreliosis, *Infection*, **17**: 355–9.

Preac-Mursic V, Wilske B et al., 1989b, Comparative antimicrobial activity of the new macrolides against *Borrelia burgdorferi*, *Eur J Clin Microbiol Infect Dis*, **8:** 651–81.

Probert WS, Allsup KM, LeFebvre RB, 1995, Identification and characterization of a surface-exposed 66-kilodalton protein from *Borrelia burgdorferi*, *Infect Immun*, **63:** 1933–9.

Pyle LE, Corcoran LN et al., 1988, Pulsed-field electrophoresis indicates larger-than-expected sizes for mycoplasma genomes, *Nucleic Acids Res*, **16:** 6015–25.

Razin S, 1985, Molecular biology and genetics of mycoplasmas (*Mollicutes*), *Microbiol Rev*, **49:** 419–55.

Reindl M, Redl B, Stöffler G, 1993, Isolation and analysis of a linear plasmid-located gene of *Borrelia burgdorferi* B29 encoding a 27 kDa surface lipoprotein (P27) and its over-expression in *Escherichia coli*, *Mol Microbiol*, **8:** 1115–24.

Rosa P, Hogan D, Schwan T, 1991, Polymerase chain reaction analyses identify two distinct classes of *Borrelia burgdorferi*, *J Clin Microbiol*, **29:** 524–32.

Rosa P, Schwan T, 1992, *Lyme Disease*, BC Decker, Mosby Year Book, Philadelphia, 8–77.

Ross PH, Milne AD, 1904, Tick fever, *Br Med J*, **2:** 1453–4.

Sadziene A, Wilske B et al., 1993, The cryptic *ospC* gene of *Borrelia burgdorferi* is located on a circular plasmid, *Infect Immun*, **61:** 2192–5.

Saint Girons I, Old IG, Davidson BE, 1994, Molecular biology of the *Borrelia* bacteria with linear replicons, *Microbiology*, **140:** 1803–16.

Sambri V, Massaria F et al., 1990, In vitro susceptibility of *Borrelia burgdorferi* and *Borrelia hermsii* to ten antimicrobial agents, *J Chemother*, **2:** 348–50.

Samuels DS, Marconi RT, Garon CF, 1993, Variations in the size of the *ospA*-containing linear plasmid, but not the linear chromosome, among the three *Borrelia* species associated with Lyme disease, *J Gen Microbiol*, **139:** 2445–9.

Schaible UE, Kramer MD et al., 1989, The severe combined immunodeficiency (scid) mouse: a laboratory model for the analysis of Lyme arthritis and carditis, *J Exp Med*, **170:** 1427–32.

Schmidli J, Hunziker T et al., 1988, Cultivation of *Borrelia burgdorferi* from joint fluid three months after treatment of facial palsy due to Lyme borreliosis, *J Infect Dis*, **158:** 905–6.

Schwan TG, Piesman J et al., 1994, Induction of an outer surface protein on *Borrelia burgdorferi* during tick feeding, *Proc Natl Acad Sci USA*, **92:** 2909–13.

Schwan TG, Simpson WJ et al., 1989, Identification of *Borrelia burgdorferi* and *B. hermsii* using DNA hybridization probes, *J Clin Microbiol*, **27:** 1734–8.

Schwartz J, Gazumyan A, Schwartz I, 1992, rRNA gene organization in the Lyme disease spirochete, *Borrelia burgdorferi*, *J Bacteriol*, **174:** 3757–65.

Scott HH, 1942, *A History of Tropical Medicine*, Williams & Wilkins, Baltimore, 781.

Scrimenti RJ, 1970, Erythema chronicum migrans, *Arch Dermatol*, **102:** 104–5.

Simon MM, Schaible UE et al., 1991, Recombinant outer surface protein A from *Borrelia burgdorferi* induces antibodies protective against spirochetal infection in mice, *J Infect Dis*, **164:** 123–32.

Simon MM, Hurtenbach U et al., 1994, *Proceedings of the International Symposium on Lyme Disease in Japan*, Ministry of Education, Science and Culture, Japan, 183–922.

Simpson WJ, Garon CF, Schwan TG, 1990, Analysis of supercoiled circular plasmids in infectious and non-infectious *Borrelia burgdorferi*, *Microb Pathog*, **8:** 109–18.

Steere AC, Malawista SE et al., 1977a, Erythema chronicum migrans and Lyme arthritis: the enlarging clinical spectrum, *Ann Intern Med*, **86:** 685–98.

Steere AC, Malawista SE et al., 1977b, Lyme arthritis. An epidemic of oligoarticular arthritis in children and adults in three Connecticut communities, *Arthritis Rheum*, **20:** 7–17.

Steere AC, Grodzicki RL et al., 1983, The spirochetal etiology of Lyme disease, *N Engl J Med*, **308:** 733–40.

Stoenner HG, 1974, Biology of *Borrelia hermsii* in Kelly medium, *Appl Microbiol*, **28:** 540–3.

Stoenner HG, Dodd T, Larson C, 1982, Antigenic variation of *Borrelia hermsii*, *J Exp Med*, **156:** 1297–311.

Wilske B, Preac-Mursic V et al., 1988, Antigenic variability of *Borrelia burgdorferi*, *Science*, **539:** 126–43.

Wilske B, Barbour AG et al., 1992, Antigenic variation and strain heterogeneity in *Borrelia* spp., *Res Microbiol*, **143:** 583–96.

Wilske B, Preac-Mursic V et al., 1993a, Immunological and molecular polymorphisms of OspC, an immunodominant major outer surface protein of *Borrelia burgdorferi*, *Infect Immun*, **61:** 2182–91.

Wilske B, Preac-Mursic V et al., 1993b, An OspA serotyping system for *Borrelia burgdorferi* based on reactivity with monoclonal antibodies and OspA sequence analysis, *J Clin Microbiol*, **31:** 340–50.

Wilske B, Jauris-Heipke R et al., 1995, Phenotypic analysis of outer surface protein C (OspC) in *Borrelia burgdorferi* sensu lato by monoclonal antibodies: relationship to genospecies and OspA serotype, *J Clin Microbiol*, **33:** 103–9.

Xu Y, Johnson RC, 1995, Analysis and comparison of plasmid profiles of *Borrelia burgdorferi* sensu lato, *J Clin Microbiol*, **33:** 2679–85.

Zalkin H, Dixon JE, 1992, De novo purine nucleotide biosynthesis, *Prog Nucleic Acid Res Mol Biol*, **42:** 259–87.

Zumstein G, Fuchs R et al., 1992, Genetic polymorphism of the gene encoding the outer surface protein A (OspA) of *Borrelia burgdorferi*, *Med Microbiol Immunol*, **181:** 57–70.

Chapter 5 7

LEPTOSPIRA

S Faine

<table>
<tr><td>1</td><td>The genus Leptospira and its species, and the associated genera Leptonema and Turneria</td><td>7</td><td>Important genetic mechanisms, including plasmid activity</td></tr>
<tr><td>2</td><td>Introduction and brief historical perspective</td><td>8</td><td>The leptospiral surface and structures related to antigens</td></tr>
<tr><td>3</td><td>Habitat</td><td>9</td><td>Classification</td></tr>
<tr><td>4</td><td>Morphology and visualization</td><td>10</td><td>Laboratory isolation and identification</td></tr>
<tr><td>5</td><td>Cultural characteristics and growth requirements</td><td>11</td><td>Susceptibility to antimicrobial agents</td></tr>
<tr><td>6</td><td>Metabolism</td><td>12</td><td>Pathogenicity and virulence factors</td></tr>
</table>

1 THE GENUS *LEPTOSPIRA* AND ITS SPECIES, AND THE ASSOCIATED GENERA *LEPTONEMA* AND *TURNERIA*

The genus *Leptospira* comprises morphologically similar thin helical bacteria (spirochaetes). The trivial name used for all members of the genus is leptospira or leptospire (plural leptospires). All are similar morphologically and culturally, but can be grouped serologically by agglutinating antigens into characteristic serovars. More than 200 serovars are recognized. One major serological complex containing most of the leptospires known or suspected to be pathogenic was named the 'interrogans complex'. Later, it became the broad, serologically determined species '*Leptospira interrogans*'. The other major group, containing non-pathogenic leptospires, was previously known as the 'biflexa complex' and was later designated '*L. biflexa*'. The genera *Leptonema* and *Turneria* were first recognized because the type strains were morphologically different from other leptospires. DNA homology studies justified this classification. The leptospires were comprehensively reviewed by Faine (1994).

1.1 Definitions

FAMILY AND GENUS

The family **Leptospiraceae** includes the genera *Leptospira*, *Leptonema* and *Turneria*, a group of bacteria that separated very early in bacterial evolution (Paster et al. 1984, 1991) (see section 9, p. 1297). Characteristically, all members are motile, flexible, helical aerobic bacteria, 6–12 μm long or longer and 0.1 μm in diameter (Johnson and Faine 1984b). There is no constant morphological characteristic of each genus, but *Turneria* tend to be shorter. Typically, one or both ends are hooked, but straight variants occur. The helical cell body (cytoplasmic cylinder) is wound around a pair of periplasmic flagella arising from it subterminally, one at each end. The diamino acid in the peptidoglycan is α,ε-diaminopimelic acid. Long chain fatty acids of fatty acid alcohols are used as carbon and energy sources. The guanine + cytosine (G + C) ratio is 35–53 mol%. The formal description of the genus *Leptospira* states that it is gram-negative but difficult to visualize, and oxidase-positive and chemo-organotrophic. It also includes some of the further information discussed below (Faine and Stallman 1982, Johnson and Faine 1984a).

THE SPECIES OF *LEPTOSPIRA*

The species of leptospires are differentiated by DNA homology (see section 9.1, p. 1297) under high stringency conditions. Currently 7 species (genomospecies, genospecies) of leptospires (*borgpetersenii*, *inadai*, *interrogans*, *kirschneri*, *noguchii*, *santarosai* and *weilii*) are recognized in the 'pathogenic' group, whereas the 3 species *biflexa*, *hollandia* and *wolbachia* belong to the saprophytic, 'non-pathogenic' group (Ellis 1995). The choice of the names 'interrogans' and 'biflexa' for genospecies of leptospires was unfortunate and their use for both the former serologically defined species and the current genetically determined species is confusing. The few recent comprehensive reviews of the nature and significance of the members of the genus

Leptospira include those of Alexander (1991), Faine (1992, 1994) and Torten and Marshall (1994).

2 INTRODUCTION AND BRIEF HISTORICAL PERSPECTIVE

2.1 Introduction and general perspective

Pathogenic leptospires are important primarily for their ability to cause disease in humans and animals. Non-pathogenic leptospires need to be differentiated from pathogens to avoid confusion in diagnosis and epidemiology. Scientifically the leptospires are intrinsically important because they are phylogenetically an ancient group of bacteria, unique in their structure, metabolism and some of their genetic mechanisms.

The disease leptospirosis is discussed in detail in Volume 3, Chapter 42. Leptospirosis is a potentially fatal disease of humans or animals caused by one of the pathogenic leptospires. It is prevalent globally as an acute febrile, sometimes congenital or chronic infection of wild or domesticated animals, mainly mammals and marsupials. Chronically infected animals are survivors of an initial acute infection. Leptospires persist in the renal tubules of kidneys in carrier animals, whence they are excreted in urine into the environment to contaminate water and soil, leading to infection of further animals of the same or different species. In some domestic animals genital carriage and venereal transmission are important. Humans are infected incidentally, affected by an acute febrile, sometimes fatal, clinical illness. Sometimes the disease is subclinical. Humans do not usually become chronic carriers or transmit infection further to other humans or animals. Economic loss occurs through animal disease and mortality, loss of productivity and illness or death in humans. There is a significant social cost of the disease both in humans and animals. Immunity to reinfection with the same serovar or closely related serovars follows infection. Significant topics for microbiological study of leptospires related to the control of leptospirosis include rapid diagnosis, mechanisms of attachment to and persistence in or on tissue cells in chronic carrier infection, and the site and regulation of antigens important for immunity.

2.2 History of the leptospires

The history of leptospires and leptospirosis was reviewed extensively by Faine (1994). Leptospirosis was described as a characteristic febrile jaundice of humans (Weil's disease) during the latter part of the nineteenth century. Its contagious nature and microbial origin were proved independently first in Japan by Inada and colleagues ('*Spirochaeta icterohaemorrhagiae*') in 1915 and soon after in Germany ('*Spirochaeta icterogenes*') by Uhlenhuth and Fromme; both groups isolated, cultivated and described pathogenic leptospires. Leptospires had been seen, but not cultured, and named *?Spirocheta interrogans* by Stimson as early as 1907, in silver stained preparations of liver from a patient believed to have died of yellow fever, whose viral origins were then unrecognized. The patient really had Weil's disease. Later,

a saprophytic leptospira found in fresh water was described in 1914 and named *Spirocheta biflexa* but it was not cultivated. Noguchi proposed the name 'leptospira' ('thin spirals') in 1918 following detailed microscopical and cultural observations, believing it to be the cause of yellow fever. Controversy about the role of leptospires in yellow fever persisted until the yellow fever virus was identified and incriminated unequivocally. Microscopically and culturally identical but antigenically different leptospires were at first regarded and named as separate species, but later included as serotypes or serovars of a single genus, *L. interrogans*. In the 15 years or so from discovery until the 1930s, many of the important serovars prevalent throughout the world, and their host sources, were discovered (Kmety and Dikken 1993).

Most of the research on leptospires in the next 2 decades related to the discovery of new serovars, some of them responsible for milder anicteric types of leptospirosis. The low yields from the culture media containing 10% rabbit serum were significant impediments to serious research on leptospires as bacteria. There was little progress and much frustration in attempts to understand nutrition or the composition of antigenic fractions, compared with knowledge of other bacteria. Electron microscopy revealed much of the detail of structure during the 1960s and 1970s. The analysis of antigens did not escape from the net of serological classification until Yanagawa and Faine (1966) showed that leptospires were analogous to other bacteria in structure, and that characteristic antigens were associated with structural elements. A brief history research in leptospirosis is recounted in Volume 3, Chapter 42 and a full account in Faine (1994).

In the USA, widespread leptospirosis of cattle and pigs due to '*L. pomona*' stimulated significant research into nutrition and cultivation of leptospires, much of it emanating from the laboratory of JB Wilson in Wisconsin during the 1960s, and from his former students thereafter. The most important single advance was probably the discovery that the only carbon and energy sources were the long-chain fatty acids essential for growth. They were toxic and had to be presented in a non-toxic form, detoxified by serum or serum albumin or another detoxicant in the medium. Bovine albumin oleic acid culture media improved yields up to 100 times those in rabbit serum medium, especially on aeration, and also allowed the isolation of some strains unable to grow in rabbit serum media. A profusion of isolates of many previously unknown serovars of leptospires necessitated correct identification for diagnosis, prognosis and epidemiology, and for the development of vaccines. Consequently, leptospirosis researchers developed a preoccupation with serological classification, based only on absorption and cross-agglutination of antisera (Abdussalam et al. 1972). 'Factor analysis' (Kmety 1967) using batteries of absorbed sera to simplify identification was seldom used as it appeared to be more complex than the standard methods. ELISA methods were developed to analyse non-agglutinating as well as agglutinating antigens (Adler et al. 1980) and applied with monoclonal antibodies to identify epitopes involved in immunity, or useful for classification (Adler and Faine 1983, Kolk et al. 1984). For many years leptospires were classified in either the non-pathogenic group as '*L. biflexa*' or the pathogenic group as '*L. interrogans*', the latter term adapted from Stimson's description with the purpose of indicating doubt about the ultimate classification. The current system of genetic classification was adopted in 1994 (Abdussalam et al. 1965, 1972, Ellis 1995).

Much of the work on leptospires and leptospirosis has been supported or stimulated not by physicians or microbiologists but by veterinary public health sources and veterinarians, because the economic consequences of leptospirosis are loss of animal productivity and human food supplies, as well zoonotic risks to humans. Historically important developments in the last 15 years dealt with in the text below include: the lipopolysaccharide (LPS) and the LPS derivation of the antigens involved in immunity, and some of the partly characterized epitopes; cloned genes coding for flagellar and other important proteins; genetic studies of special features of the leptospiral genome. Molecular techniques for identification have allowed genetic speciation on firm grounds and PCR methods are being developed for identification and diagnosis. The basis of genetic classification was established in Alexander's laboratory in USA in the 1960s.

Saprophytic, non-pathogenic leptospires have attracted little research attention for their own intrinsic scientific interest. A claim that they were really pathogens which could be made virulent by animal passage appears to have been a cover-up for a laboratory error. The genus *Leptonema* was described to include a leptospira-like organism with some treponemal features.

3 HABITAT

Leptospires are motile aquatic bacteria whose natural habitat is surface waters, soil and mud. They feed by attachment to surfaces where long-chain fatty acids are available. A halophilic leptospire has been isolated from estuarine waters. Leptospires do not survive drying under usual conditions but lyophilization can preserve them. Pathogenic leptospires enter their hosts through the integument in moist conditions. In the host they circulate and grow in an aqueous milieu and may attach to renal tubular cells in carrier animals, passing in urine into surface waters. Pathogenic leptospires adapt to environmental conditions including the salinity and temperatures of febrile mammals, renal tubular and bladder urine, and soil and surface water. Both pathogens and non-pathogens have been isolated from fast-flowing rivers and still surface ponds. Soil and subsoil type and structure are important for survival in dry periods (reviewed by Faine 1994).

4 MORPHOLOGY AND VISUALIZATION

Leptospires are helical gram-negative bacteria, so thin that they are hard to see when fixed and stained by conventional bacteriological stains. Their characteristic shape is largely destroyed by heat fixation. Strong stains (carbol fuchsin) and stains that build up on the surface (flagellar stains, Giemsa, silver stains, immunostains) make them appear thicker and improve visualization. Electron microscopy reveals details of morphology. Phase contrast of live cultures is of limited value because the leptospires move rapidly out of phase. The routine method of observation is darkfield microscopy of wet preparations. Leptospires pass through cellulose bacteriological filters of average pore diameter 0.2 μm.

4.1 Shape and structure

The leptospiral cell (Fig. 57.1) is about 10–20 μm long. It comprises a peptidoglycan complex loosely referred to as cell wall arranged as a flexible hollow tubular right-handed helix, containing cytoplasmic and genetic material. The amplitude of the coil is about 0.10–0.15 μm and its wavelength is about 0.5 μm. *Leptonema* are generally longer (13–15 μm) than *Leptospira* and have a longer average amplitude of 0.13 μm and wavelength of 0.6 μm; they thus appear wider microscopically. By contrast, *Turneria* are shorter (3.5–7.5 μm long) and more tightly coiled (wavelength 0.3–0.36 μm and amplitude 0.13–0.14 μm). Subterminally at either end of the helix a flagellum, essentially similar in structure and function to other bacterial flagella, is inserted in the cell wall and penetrates to the outer aspect of the helix, where it runs through the interior of the coil in a groove to end at about the middle of the leptospire. The 2 flagella seldom overlap. The flagellar origin appears as a visible bulge below the surface, in shadowed electron micrographs. The whole is surrounded by a fluid membrane, the outer envelope (OE), separated from the cell by a periplasmic space. The membrane appears to have 3 or 5 layers, depending on the fixative used for electron microscopy. In stained cross-sections in electron micrographs, the concentric layers are, from the outside, the cell membrane of 3 or 5 layers, the clear periplasmic space, the cell wall and the cytoplasmic contents, in which reticular material may appear. The flagellum, when included in the plane of the section, is a darkly staining round structure lying in an indentation of the cell wall. Negative stained electron micrographs have revealed more of structure than have shadowed preparations. Cultural conditions and technical procedures affect the appearances of the leptospiral surface on electron microscopy; washing removes much of the outer envelope. There is an unusually high lipid content in leptospires, located mainly in the cell wall or outer envelope. When treated with various detergents or lysozyme the cell relaxes its helical shape and sheds its outer envelope. Gradually more of the surface layers dissolve as the helix finally flattens in an empty flaccid sac, liberating detectable antigens in the process (Yanagawa and Faine 1966). Details of structure and corresponding chemical and antigenic composition are in section 8 (see section 8, p. 1296). During the first stages of unwinding of the helix, microfibrils can be seen bridging across the coils (Yanagawa and Faine 1966, Yanagihara and Mifuchi 1968).

SPHEROPLASTS (LEPTOSPIRAL GRANULES)

In some cultures leptospires appear in a 'granular' form. The granules are small cystic structures, about 1.5–2.0 μm in diameter, inside which coiled remnants of the leptospiral cell can be seen. Once thought to be a cystic stage of a life cycle, they are really spheroplasts whose formation can be induced with ethanol, detergents, sodium deoxycholate, high salt conditions, lysozyme or mild heat. They can also be observed in

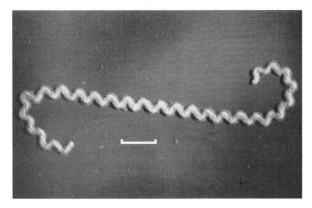

Fig. 57.1 Shadowed electron micrograph of a typical leptospire (*L. interrogans* serovar *copenhageni*). The flagella run in grooves in the wall of the helical cylinder from a subterminal insertion near either end. The helical cylinder is surrounded by an outer envelope. Initial magnification × 40 000. Bar = 1.0 μm. (Original electron micrograph by Dr A Chang 1969).

tissues and in phagocytes (Faine, Shahar and Aronson 1964). The outer envelope surrounding the spheroplast granules may be removed from them with its antigens largely intact after plasmolysis of the leptospires. Some cultures tend to form spheroplasts spontaneously; these strains probably produce lipase that releases from the medium free, lytic fatty acids not adequately bound to a detoxicant (see section 5, p. 1291) (Fig. 57.2).

4.2 Flagella

Leptospiral flagella originate in a disc rotor and hooked proximal end structure in the cell wall, similar to other gram-negative bacteria. Flagella may be prepared for study by shearing them off leptospiral cells followed by differential or gradient centrifugation. In such preparations the flagella are seen as tight flat coils. The isolated flagellum is composed of a helically wound central core of proteins, in linear or globular forms, surrounded by an outer sheath that extends about two-thirds of the flagellar length. The hook end

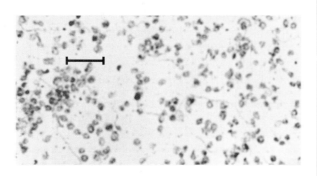

Fig. 57.2 Spheroplasts ('leptospiral granules') of *L. interrogans* serovar *copenhageni* formed by heating a culture to 56°C. Thread-like degenerated leptospiral bodies can be seen towards the middle and the lower left corner. Stained with silver stain. Original magnification × 1000. Bar = 15.0 μm. (Adapted from Faine, Shahar and Aronson 1964).

is usually free of the rotor but may be contaminated with a bleb of lipopolysaccharide at its proximal end. There are associated flagellar antigens. Seven different flagellar proteins have been recognized. There is a 34 kDa protein associated with the core, of 11.3 nm, and a 36 kDa protein associated with the sheath, measuring 21.5 nm. A gene for an endoflagellar subunit protein, *flaB*, was cloned from *L. borgpetersenii* serovar *hardjo*, expressed in *Escherichia coli* as a 32 kDa FlaB protein similar in sequence to FlaB proteins described in *Treponema pallidum* (Kelson et al. 1988, Mitchison et al. 1991, Trueba, Bolin and Zuerner 1992). The FlaB protein structure and its gene sequences are highly conserved throughout the species; a recombinant protein cross-reacted between serovars in immunoblots (Woodward and Redstone 1994). Characteristic flagellar antigens were associated with the flagellar sheath (Chang, Faine and Williams 1974).

4.3 Microscopic appearances

When seen by direct darkfield microscopy of wet preparations under optimum conditions, leptospires appear as a series of bright dots arranged in a flexible chain. Typically they are translationally motile and spin fast but spasmodically on their long axes; the loose hooked end looks like a hollow bulb. Occasionally leptospires bend suddenly along their length in a jerky movement. There are also straight mutant forms, whose flagella are inserted closer to the ends of the cells and which are much less translationally motile, but spin as well as the hooked variety (Fig. 57.3).

It is convenient to observe cultures microscopically in flat drops on a very clean thin slide, without a cover-glass, using a low power, long working distance objective and a low-power darkfield condenser of low numerical aperture (n. a.). For detailed observation of leptospires a very clean thin slide is required; a drop of the fluid for examination is placed on

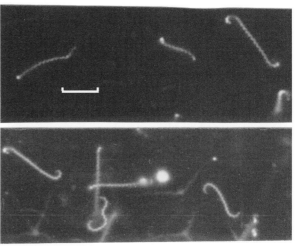

Fig. 57.3 Typical leptospires (*L. interrogans* serovar *copenhageni*) seen by high-power darkfield microscopy. Initial magnification × 1000. Original photomicrographs by Drs T Vinh and S Faine. Bar = 5.0 μm. (Adapted in part from Faine 1994).

it and covered with a thin, very clean cover-glass. Any dirt or grease or smear will cause diffraction of light and destroy the contrast required for the darkfield illumination. It is useful but not necessary to seal the edges of the cover-glass to prevent movement in the preparation through convection and evaporation at the edges. The slide is sealed to the surface of an oil immersion darkfield condenser with nonrefracting microscope immersion oil to prevent loss of light by diffraction at air–glass interfaces. An oil immersion objective fitted with a central stop, or a diaphragm to reduce the numerical aperture below that of the condenser is required. Centring of the light path and focusing the condenser are critical for successful observations. After locating the field under low power using dry objectives, a drop of immersion oil is placed on the cover-glass and the oil immersion objective used to focus on the leptospires in the field. Faine (1994) described the technical procedures in detail.

4.4 Motility

All leptospires are motile. Motility is linked with viability: generally an immobile leptospire is dead (see section 5.3, p. 1292). The characteristic motility of leptospires results from the rotation of the flagellum, generating a helical wave that propels the helical cell in the opposite direction. The outer envelope acts as a fluid mosaic (Goldstein and Charon 1988, 1990). In fluid media they can travel about 7–10 μm in a second. In viscous fluid media the speed of movement is increased in proportion to the viscosity. Leptospires are attracted to more viscous environments by 'viscotaxis'.

Recently isolated leptospires growing in media containing blood or serum appear to move faster than laboratory strains, possibly because of the viscosity of the medium. In semisolid agar, in which there are microscopically invisible particles, or in tissues, leptospires can become completely flexible throughout their length and wind through the interstices of the medium in either direction. They resume a rigid conformation and rapid spinning and translational movements as soon as they reach the fluid medium; part of the leptospira can be rigid and rotating while the other end is flexed around particles. The energy requirements and mechanisms of control of motility are unknown.

5 CULTURAL CHARACTERISTICS AND GROWTH REQUIREMENTS

Leptospires are grown routinely in liquid media, occasionally slightly thickened with 0.1–0.2% agar. Generally an inoculum of 1–10% of the volume of fresh medium is transferred by pipette. Working with liquid media demands the utmost care in their sterilization and quality control and in aseptic technique, to prevent contamination by extraneous air-borne or filterable water-borne micro-organisms, including other leptospires. Colonial growth in solidified media in plates or tubes is primarily employed for research.

5.1 Cell division

The stages in division in leptospires can be reconstructed from electron micrographs and direct observation. First, the cell wall constricts about the middle of the length, beneath an otherwise intact outer membrane, resulting in fusion of the closed ends to form 2 new ends, one for each of the new cells. Near the constriction a new flagellar origin appears from which a flagellum grows towards the middle of the newly formed cell. Last, the outer membrane constricts and pinches off a discrete new cell. About the time of division the leptospire becomes hyperflexible at the site of future separation; it may bend sharply on itself, while retaining its motility, until the 2 new cells separate. In media deficient in amount or balance of long-chain fatty acids, leptospires may elongate extremely, or fail to divide (forming long chains), or both. Clearly the nutritional needs for growth (elongation) and division are different. Nothing is known about metabolic or molecular events in cell division specific for leptospires.

5.2 Optimum conditions

TEMPERATURE, pH, SALINITY AND OTHER CONDITIONS

Temperature

Both pathogens and saprophytes grow in the laboratory in an optimum temperature range of 28–3°C, with extremes of 11–42°C. Growth at 11–13°C has been proposed as a phenotypic test for *L. biflexa*. Pathogens grow in mammalian hosts at febrile body temperatures, and in chick embryos and young chicks around 40–42°C, but do not grow well in laboratory media at these temperatures unless they are adapted. New heat shock proteins, similar to GroEL and DnaK proteins in *E. coli*, including a subsurface protein of 64 kDa developed during temperature adaptation (Ballard, Faine and Adler 1990, Stamm et al. 1991, Ballard et al. 1993).

pH

Leptospires die in acid conditions at pH below about 6.5, but tolerate more alkaline conditions up to about pH 8.4. Cultures will grow in the range pH 7.2–7.6.

Salinity

Most of the culture media for leptospires contain a final molarity of salts of about 0.05 M, about one-third of the concentration in other bacteriological media. Pathogens can grow in laboratory media at salt concentrations of 0.85% NaCl at 37°C but avirulent pathogens and non-pathogens cannot do so above 30°C (Faine 1959). Halophilic leptospires require sodium ion concentrations of 0.22–0.44 M for growth and can tolerate concentrations up to 0.65–0.75 M (Cinco, Tamaro and Cociancich 1975).

Oxidation–reduction potential

Leptospires are aerobic or micro-aerophilic bacteria that do not tolerate reducing conditions or anaerobiosis, when the oxidation–reduction potential is less than about *E*h - 0.250 mV at pH 7.2.

5.3 Growth

Leptospira strains grow slowly, compared with most common pathogenic bacteria; colonies can take from 3–7 days to 3 weeks to appear. The slow growth rate in solid media limits the use of plate counts to measure viability and impedes the rate of progress in molecular studies.

Leptospires grow in still cultures of liquid media at 30°C with a doubling time of 6–8 h under optimum conditions. A 10-fold increase in numbers can be achieved in 24 h. Aeration or agitation increases the yield. Maximum growth can be expected in 3–10 days, depending on the strain and the medium. Maximum growth densities are about $10^{9.5}$–10^{10} leptospires per ml, with best conditions and aeration; cultures are then visually turbid but measurable turbidity is relatively low. *Leptonema* grows rapidly in trypticase–soy broth (TSB) medium to reach maximum density on incubation for 18–72 h at 30°C. The fatty acid concentration is the limiting factor for continuation of growth in cultures of *Leptospira*. Supplementary Tween added to cultures that have exhausted all their available fatty acids will considerably increase the final density. Some cultures die rapidly after the end of the logarithmic phase, because lipases from autolysing leptospires liberate lytic free fatty acids. The doubling time for growth in the intact animal body in experimental infections was 6–8 h.

Growth is measured in liquid media by either direct counts or turbidity. The best way to count leptospires is to use a bacterial counting chamber, or to count them in a measured volume placed under a standard size cover-glass, using a calibrated eyepiece graticule micrometer. The culture must be diluted accurately if it is too dense. Motile leptospires are counted as viable; non-motile and obviously dead and degenerate leptospires are not counted. Motility is seldom so fast that it creates a problem. The usual conventions for counting in counting chambers are observed in relation to leptospires on or overlapping lines (Faine 1994). Leptospiral cultures are much less turbid than those of other bacteria at peak growth. Turbidity measurements are limited in value to estimating the total count, irrespective of viable numbers, in heavily growing cultures at the end of their logarithmic phase, at densities above about $10^{8.5}$ leptospires per ml, when growth is just easily visible by eye. Nephelometry is more sensitive but limited to cultures denser than $10^{7.5}$ leptospires per ml.

5.4 Growth requirements

ATMOSPHERIC CONDITIONS; O_2, CO_2 AND AERATION

Leptospires require an oxygen source, but a measured lower limit of oxygen concentration seems not to have been established. It is assumed that animal tissues in which leptospires grow and apparently flourish are lower in oxygen than culture media, especially in the presence of inflammation, haemorrhage, cellular damage and autolysis, and tissue disorganization during the acute stages of infection. Aeration of cultures by sparging or shaking increases growth, although it can cause problems with frothing in protein-rich media. CO_2 is essential, but the limiting amounts are not known.

CARBON SOURCES

Pathogenic leptospires will not grow without long-chain (C12–18) unsaturated fatty acids, in whose presence some strains can also utilize saturated fatty acids. *Leptospira biflexa* strains can grow on long- or short-chain, saturated or unsaturated fatty acids. Some pathogens may start to grow sooner from small inocula, especially on solid media, if pyruvate, pyruvate and CO_2, or glycerol are added to the medium (see section 5.5, p. 1293). Knowledge of nutritional requirements comes mainly from studies on relatively few isolates made at a time when it seemed that information relevant to any leptospire could be extrapolated to all. Differences in nutrition and metabolism between leptospires may be related more to species than serovar.

The form of presentation of the fatty acids is important because they are potentially toxic to the leptospires, lysing the cells by destroying the integrity of the OE. Non-toxic 'Tweens', used widely in media as sources of fatty acids, are commercially available sorbitan monoesters of fatty acids; Tween 80 contains oleate, Tween 60 stearate and Tween 40 palmitate. Their crude industrial form may need to be purified of contaminating free fatty acids and degradation products before use in media. The choice of the chain lengths of the fatty acids, and their relative concentrations, depends on the strains to be cultivated. In addition, a detoxicant such as bovine serum albumin (BSA), in a final concentration of 1.0%, is used to absorb and release fatty acids slowly. BSA may also itself be contaminated with free fatty acids and may need to be purified for use. Likewise, agar used in media may contain contaminating fatty acids which must be removed before use. *Leptonema* will grow without added fatty acids, in TSB medium.

NITROGEN SOURCES, PURINES AND PYRIMIDINES

The only essential nitrogen source is ammonia. Some strains metabolize amino acids, probably producing ammonia by deamination. Urease, inhibited by ammonia, has been described. All *L. biflexa* and other non-pathogens and *Leptonema* can synthesize their own purines and pyrimidines. *Turneria parva* requires purines. In general, all *L. borgpetersenii* and *L. santarosai* and some *L. interrogans* synthesize purines, whereas all the pathogen group require pyrimidines.

OTHER REQUIREMENTS FOR GROWTH

Phosphates, sulphates, ferric iron or haemoglobin (or haem), calcium and magnesium, thiamine and cyanocobalamin are essential. Traces of copper and manganese are also required; these are included in the recipes for oleic–albumin based media, while in serum media they are provided from tap water, serum or other ingredients.

5.5 Growth characteristics and appearances of cultures

IN LIQUID MEDIA

Cultures of leptospires in liquid media appear visually clear until densities of about 10^7 ml^{-1} are reached. The first appearance of growth is a birefringence on swirling the culture vessel, best seen with oblique lighting against a dark background. Maximum turbidity, well below that achieved by larger bacteria, is reached after about 3–20 days of incubation, depending on the inoculum size, the strain and its adaptation to the medium and conditions, and the growth phase at the time of subculture. There may be a long lag of several days before freshly isolated strains begin to grow. Some cultures autoagglutinate; clumps of actively motile tangled leptospires sink to the bottom of the vessel. Otherwise, leptospires do not settle during cultivation, but precipitates of insoluble salts, fatty acids or amino acids can occur and be a nuisance. Removal of leptospires from cultures for preparation of antigens or for other laboratory manipulations requires a centrifugal force of about $10\,000 \times \textbf{\textit{g}}$ for 15–20 min.

IN SEMISOLID MEDIA

When growing in tubes of media containing agar (0.1% or more) after surface or stab inoculation, the distribution of leptospires is restricted mainly to one or more discs 0.1–0.5 mm thick that appear 0.1–5.0 mm below the surface of the medium, although leptospires will often be detected below the discs.

The discs, known as Dinger's discs, represent colonial growth accumulated at a level of optimum oxygenation. If one of the redox indicators 1-naphthol-2-sodium sulphonate indo-2,6-dichlorophenol (*E*h - 0.180 mV at pH 7.2) or 2-6-dichlorophenol-indophenol (*E*h - 0.200 mV at pH 7.2) is incorporated in the medium at a concentration of 1 in 100 000, the blue colour of the medium when inoculated discolours around the areas where growth begins, usually at the level where the discs will appear later. Where growth occurs only in discs, the medium gradually decolorizes or changes colour from the bottom of the tube upwards as oxygen is absorbed, until the zone below the discs is pale yellow or pink. The medium above the discs remains blue. If single colonies develop in the depths of the medium, the dye fades and becomes pale yellow or pink at the place in the tube where the grey spherical colonies will later appear. Both discs and colonies may develop in the same tube.

IN AND ON SOLID MEDIA

Leptospires are usually grown on solid media only for research because growth is too slow to be useful for routine diagnosis. Some isolates grow on the surface of media containing 1.5–2.0% agar in petri dishes. The agar must not be too stiff for the leptospires to move through it easily and the plates must be sealed or otherwise protected from drying during incubation. Inoculation of a drop with a spreader or by flooding is better than scratching the agar surface when streaking it with a wire loop. Surface colonies are transparent, often very flat, small (less than 2 mm) and irregular. In less solid media containing 0.8–1% agar,

growth occurs below the surface, first visible after 3–10 days as a pinpoint hemispherical colony that spreads centrifugally. Colony appearances depend on the density and depth of the agar and the motility of the leptospires. Straight leptospires, not very translationally motile, form small dense grey spherical subsurface colonies (small, opaque, defined border or SOD) that do not spread and reach a diameter of 1–3 mm. Leptospires that are conventionally translationally motile may form a larger, fluffy colony (sometimes called hazy growth, or a large, opaque, hazy edge or LOH) that may spread rapidly to form a grey ring with a sharply defined edge (LOD); this ring may grow wider to occupy a large part of the agar. In a thin layer of medium (2–3 mm) the colony soon looks like a ring of grey with a transparent centre and sloping sides, because the medium is not deep enough for continued hemispherical growth (Fig. 57.4). Details are described by Faine (1994). The grey edge indicates a mass of actively motile leptospires; few leptospires, most of them non-viable, will be found internal to the edges of the ring. Incubation to detect growth should be continued for up to 3 weeks. More than one colony type can occur on the same plate. If redox dyes are added to the medium as described above, the colour in the medium fades at the points where colonies will appear, forecasting the initiation of colonial growth. A subculture may be taken carefully with a pipette from the spreading edge of the colony. Contaminated cultures or environmental specimens inoculated as a discrete drop on the surface at the centre of the plate can be purified by subculturing leptospires from the edge of the ring of growth.

5.6 Culture media

Almost invariably media contain heat-labile proteins or other ingredients and are sterilized by filtration. Either rabbit or other animal serum, or bovine serum albumin (BSA) forms the basis of current culture media. Yields are higher and growth faster in oleate–albumin media. Media free of protein are preferable and available for vaccines and certain other purposes; it is impossible to wash away the last traces of proteins from the culture medium adhering to the leptospiral surface. Liquid media are used for the maintenance

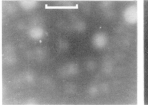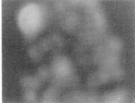

Fig. 57.4 Subsurface colonies of *L. interrogans* serovar *copenhageni* growing in EMJH medium with agar 0.8%. There are small dense and large opaque colonies, which are beginning to spread centrifugally, with a dense edge. Bar = 9 mm. (Adapted from Faine S, van der Hoeden J, 1964, *J Bacteriol*, **88**: 1493–6).

of stock cultures and the propagation of cultures used to prepare vaccines and antigens for serological tests.

TECHNICAL NOTES, FORMULATIONS AND PREPARATION OF MEDIA

Generally leptospires are grown in tubes of flasks at 28–30°C. The depth of medium in unshaken tubes or flasks should be less than 5 cm; shaking, agitation or sparging with air or oxygen plus CO_2 (with care to minimize frothing) will maximize the yield and growth rate. Cultures should be checked for growth or contamination after 3–4 days and subcultured after 7–21 days; however, leptospires will survive in sealed tubes of medium at room temperature (ideally 20°C, certainly below 40°C) for months or years.

Oleic acid–albumin (OA) media and serum media

Details of composition and preparation of media are found in Alexander (1991) and Faine (1994). All media are hypotonic with respect to mammalian physiological conditions. The most widely used OA medium is EMJH (Ellinghausen, McCullough, Johnson, Harris), based on 1% BSA and Tween 80. A BSA stock solution containing other mineral and heat-labile ingredients that should not be autoclaved is sterilized by filtration and added to an autoclaved phosphate-buffered basal medium. Most serum media use a phosphate-buffered base containing a small amount of bacteriological peptone; 10% rabbit serum to supply both albumin and fatty acids; and essential supplements such as thiamine, cyanocobalamin and iron in the form of haemoglobin from lysed erythrocytes. The medium should be just pink and pH 7.2–7.4. It is usually sterilized by final filtration of all the ingredients. A common formulation is Korthof's medium. Non-pathogenic leptospires are generally grown in the same media as pathogens, although *Leptonema* grows well and rapidly in TSB medium.

Special selective and indicator media

Special media were developed empirically to isolate fastidious leptospires, especially *Leptospira interrogans* serovar *bratislava*, from pigs and other animals (Ellis et al. 1985, Adler et al. 1986). Composition of media and conditions of cultivation must be adjusted to special needs. Selective media containing one or more of cycloheximide (100 µg ml^{-1}), bacitracin (40 µg ml^{-1}), 5-fluorouracil (50–1000 µg ml^{-1}), nalidixic acid (50 µg ml^{-1}), polymyxin-B sulphate (5 units ml^{-1}), polymyxin B (2 µg ml^{-1}), rifampicin (10 µg ml^{-1}) or vancomycin (10 µg ml^{-1}) have been recommended to reduce contamination on primary isolation or to purify contaminated cultures. They should not be used routinely as a substitute for careful technique. Subcultures must be made within 4 days.

Protein-free and low-protein media

Media with little or no protein were developed for vaccine production, rather than for nutritional studies. Utmost care is required to minimize toxicity from unwanted fatty acids. Chemical methods or solvents are used to 'clean' Tweens and the specially selected charcoal used as an adsorbent of fatty acids in place of protein. Some of the media used for vaccines are subject to commercial secrecy or patent and have not been published. In order to grow successfully in a protein-free medium, leptospires must first be adapted to it and then subcultured regularly and frequently.

Solid and semisolid medium

Almost any medium may be solidified by the addition of 0.5–1.0% agar to allow subsurface colonial growth, or 2% agar for surface growth. Growth in and on solid media is described in section 5.5 (see section 5.5, p. 1293).

QUALITY CONTROL

It is essential to check the ingredients for culture media for quality before use. BSA is very hygroscopic; it should be kept and used dry, or a correction made for the weight of the water content. Each batch must be tested or previously certified suitable for the growth of leptospires. Some batches can be improved by fat extraction. All chemicals should be analytical grade. Agar should also be tested for freedom from toxic fatty acids. The quality of the water used for protein-free media is critical. The vessels used for preparing media should be dry; water used for solutions must be sterilized to prevent filter-passing leptospires in the water from contaminating the media. After preparation the media must be checked for sterility by incubation for 3–4 days at 28–30°C as well as at 37°C. The possibility of contamination by leptospires should not be overlooked. The utmost care in labelling during subculture is essential because there are no obvious features to distinguish one leptospire from another. Records of origin of an isolate, its identification and its subculture history are essential. Serological identity should be checked, confirmed and recorded periodically by agglutination to titre with a reference antiserum. Genetic identity should also be checked periodically where this is appropriate.

6 METABOLISM

Knowledge of leptospiral metabolism depends largely on studies reported before genetic speciation was known. It may be fallacious to deduce from them that all species of leptospires are metabolically identical. All leptospires are aerobic or micro-aerophilic chemo-organotrophs and use O_2 as a final electron receptor via cytochromes. Catalase, cytochromes a, c and c_1 and oxidases have been identified. Essential long-chain fatty acids, longer than C_{15}, are degraded by ß-oxidation for energy. Acid production from sugar fermentation does not occur, but key enzymes in carbohydrate metabolic pathways are present. Sero-specificity depends on the presence of small carbohydrates and their arrangement in the LPS (see 'Chemical composition and cellular location of LPS', p. 1296). Leptospires cannot synthesize long-chain fatty acids from pyruvate or acetate, but they can shorten long chains; the cellular lipid composition partly reflects the fatty acid composition of the medium. A characteristic component of leptospires, *cis*-11-hexadecenoic acid, is rare in other bacteria. Positionally specific trioleinase lipases are found in all *Leptospira biflexa* and some pathogens, but not in *L. borgpetersenii*, some *L. interrogans*, *L. noguchii*, *L. santarosai*, and *L. weilii*. Haemolytic phospholipases including sphingomyelinase C exist in some pathogens, while *L. biflexa* contains phospholipase A$_1$ and lysolecithinase. Haemolytic activities dependent on phospholipases are specific for the erythrocytes of the animal concerned, determined by the composition of the dominant phospholipids in its cell membranes. Fatty acid esterases are ubiquitous among leptospires. The genetics and distribution of sphingomyelinase genes has been studied and reviewed (Segers 1991, Segers et al. 1992).

Ammonia is the essential source of nitrogen. In serum media it may be obtained by deamination of amino acids, particularly asparagine. In other media it is provided as ammonium salts. What little there is known about amino acid metabolism is unremarkable except that isoleucine synthesis may follow either the conventional threonine pathway, or an unusual pyruvate pathway, or both; genes for regulating steps in the latter have been identified. A urease, inhibited by ammonia, and various aminopeptidases have been described. Not all leptospires require purines or pyrimidines. Purine metabolism is mentioned in section 5.3 (see section 5.3, p. 1292).

7 IMPORTANT GENETIC MECHANISMS, INCLUDING PLASMID ACTIVITY

Slow leptospiral growth on solid media and slow, relative metabolic inertness in usual phenotypic tests for other bacteria means there are few physiological or colonial markers and very few classical genetic studies. Antibiotic resistance to streptomycin is induced easily. Mutants have been selected to grow in media containing either boiled, as opposed to fresh, serum; others grow in antiserum to the parent strain. There are no studies of the genetics of these mutations, or of straight variants, usually forming small colonies, that appear spontaneously in some strains. A straight variant of *Leptonema illini* was produced using nitrosoguanidine. Virulence is lost on subculture in the laboratory but leptospires able to grow in vivo can be selected from the culture population by inoculating experimental animals. Genes and DNA fragments can be cloned out of leptospiral DNA but naturally occurring plasmids and the mechanisms of genetic transfer strongly assumed to occur between leptospires are elusive. Transformation has not been reported among leptospires. It is not yet possible to introduce DNA into leptospires artificially and deliberately. A bacteriophage for *L. biflexa* was described, but none has been found that affects any pathogen (Saint Girons et al. 1990, 1992, Saint Girons 1991).

7.1 The leptospiral genome and its elements

Genetic knowledge to 1993 was summarized by Faine (1994). The size of the leptospiral genome is about 4750–5900 kb, made up of 2 chromosomal replicons, the larger of which is about 4400–4600 kb; the smaller, about 350 kb, incorporates the *asd* (ß-semialdehyde dehydrogenase) gene (Zuerner, Herrmann and Saint Girons 1993). The guanine plus cytosine (G + C) content ranges from 35–41 mol% for *Leptospira* and 51–54 mol% for *Leptonema*. There is considerable heterogeneity of chromosomal DNA sequences within species (Zuerner, Herrmann and Saint Girons 1993). IS3-like insertion sequence elements similar to the transposases in some other bacteria were found in some species of leptospires (Boursaux, Zuerner and Saint

Girons 1994, Zuerner 1994). An intervening sequence (IVS) found on the 23S rRNA genes (*rrl* genes) appears to be transferred horizontally within or between species (when comparing 23S rRNA phylogenetic hypothesis data with data from a 16S rRNA hypothesis), providing a possible basis for diversity of species (Ralph and McClelland 1994). A characteristic sequence-specific modification of 5′-GTAm⁴C, probably m⁴C specific, was reported to occur throughout the genus (Ralph et al. 1993b). Codon usage shows a bias to codons rich in A and T in *L. biflexa*, while in pathogens codon usage for the sphingomyelinase gene is quite different from that in *E. coli*. Genes for several structural or functional elements of leptospires, reviewed by Faine (1994), have been cloned, characterized, or sequenced, including sphingomyelinase C (Segers et al. 1990), amino acid pathway enzymes (Richaud et al. 1990, Baril et al. 1992, Ding and Yelton 1993), heat shock proteins that are analogues of GroEL (Stamm et al. 1991, Ballard et al. 1993), a transmembrane outer-membrane protein (Haake et al. 1993), flagellar 32 kDa FlaB protein (Mitchison et al. 1991), rhamnose pathway enzymes, haemolysin (Del Real et al. 1989) and other unidentified proteins. The *recA* gene from *L. biflexa* was also cloned (Stamm, Parrish and Gherardini 1991).

RNA genes are widely scattered on the large chromosome. Genes for 23S, 16S and 5S rRNA are distributed and processed differently in pathogens and saprophytes, each of which contained 2 cross-hybridizing 23S rRNA genes; there are 2 5S rRNA genes in *L. biflexa* strains, but only one in pathogens. Among the pathogenic species, the 5S rRNA gene is uniquely organized as a single copy encoding an RNA molecule with a chain length of 117 nucleotides. In 2 serovars of *L. borgpetersenii*, the 23S rRNA was processed to 14S and 17S rRNA (Fukunaga et al. 1990, 1992, Morita et al. 1991).

Genetic and molecular analysis are the basis of speciation and contribute to subspecific classification (see section 9, p. 1297).

8 THE LEPTOSPIRAL SURFACE AND STRUCTURES RELATED TO ANTIGENS

The leptospiral OE generally resembles the outer membrane of gram-negative bacteria; it is also the site of most of the antigens known to be involved in immunity or diagnosis. The main difference is a high lipid content and a relatively low transmembrane outer-membrane protein content in leptospires.

8.1 Surface components and antigens

The leptospiral surface changes as the organisms move from a host to a culture medium environment. Urinary and freshly cultivated leptospires may not be agglutinable by homologous serovar antiserum until they have adapted to culture conditions and shed a surface inhibitor of agglutination. Most, if not all, the antigens significant for disease or diagnosis are carbohydrate, not protein.

PROTEIN ANTIGENS

A 31 kDa outer-membrane surface protein, OmpL1, is more densely distributed in virulent than in avirulent cultures. In *L. interrogans* serovar *copenhageni*, there are 2 heat shock proteins, Hsp10 and Hsp58, encoded by the equivalent of the GroE operon. Some other proteins have been located in the periplasmic space. The flaccid empty cell wall, stripped of surrounding material, contains muramic acid. Flagellar antigens, located on the flagellar sheath, react with either IgM or a more specific IgG. A doublet flagellar protein band reacts with immunoglobulins in immunoblots.

LIPOPOLYSACCHARIDES

Leptospiral lipopolysaccharides are similar to those of coliform and other gram-negative bacteria in structure, cellular location and biological properties, with the notable exceptions that they are much less toxic and pyrogenic and in some strains, the keto-deoxy-octulonate (KDO) is substituted at the C4 or C5 positions, or both (Vinh, Adler and Faine 1986b). The substituted compound reacts as KDO does in analyses only after it has been oxidized with periodate. Some workers, confusing 'endotoxin' with 'LPS', have therefore called the LPS 'LLS', or 'lipopolysaccharide-like substance', ignoring the many similarities with other gram-negative LPS, which are also not homogeneous.

Chemical composition and cellular location of LPS

LPS appears to be multilaminar on electron microscopy of preparations made by extraction with phenol–water or by other conventional methods. It is alkali-soluble and serologically active on carrier particles, complement fixation or in enzyme-linked reactions adsorbed to surfaces. On polyacrylamide gel electrophoresis (PAGE) typical LPS ladder patterns are seen after staining with silver nitrate. The LPS core contains rhamnose; *rfb* genes for the rhamnose synthetic pathway have characterized (Mitchison et al. 1994). Various oligosaccharides, including phosphorylated sugars and amino sugars, comprise the epitopes of the side chains conferring serological specificity and immunity (Midwinter et al. 1994, Vinh et al. 1994). No ß-hydroxymyristic acid or myristic acid (C14 chain length) were found among the approximately 33% of the weight of LPS that is lipid in *L. interrogans* serovar *copenhageni* or *L. borgpetersenii* serovar *hardjobovis*, but they were reported in serovar *lai* of *L. interrogans* (Wu et al. 1987). There are differences in LPS composition among the species of *Leptospira* that have been studied, but very few isolates have been analysed and the extent of intraspecies variation is not known (Faine 1994). Monoclonal antibodies to epitopes on LPS located them in the OE. A non-agglutinating broadly reactive antigen (Jost, Adler and Faine 1988) originates in the periplasmic space rather than on the surface (Hovind-Hougen, personal communication, 1991). More lipopolysaccharide can be detected in virulent than in avirulent leptospires (Ellis et al. 1983, Haake et al. 1991).

Biological properties of LPS

Leptospiral LPS 5 µg kg^{-1} is not pyrogenic for rabbits in standard tests, but it clots *Limulus* amoebocyte lysate, activates macrophages and aggregates platelets, and is a B cell mitogen. It is toxic for mice only at about 12 times the equivalent dose of *E. coli* LPS.

Immunological and serological significance of LPS

LPS epitopes are the major antigens reacting with immunoglobulins produced in humans or animals following natural or experimental inoculation with leptospires. These antibodies, essential for opsonization, phagocytosis and immunity, are the bases of diagnosis by specific serological (agglutination) tests (see Volume 3, Chapter 42). Monoclonal antibodies reacting with LPS epitopes are used for classification and diagnosis (see sections 9 and 10, p. 1298).

OTHER LOCALIZED STRUCTURES AND COMPONENTS

A glycolipoprotein (GLP) with a high content of toxic lipids (palmitoleic and oleic acids) is cytotoxic and lethal for laboratory animals. Its cytotoxicity in tissue culture is obscured by the absorption of the toxic lipid into the albumin used in the culture media. Patients and animals produce antibodies to GLP, which can be located in the tissues in infections (Vinh, Adler and Faine 1986a, Alves et al. 1992). Peptidoglycan from leptospires was cytotoxic (Cinco et al. 1993). Heat shock proteins were located below the surface (Stamm et al. 1991).

9 CLASSIFICATION

A micro-organism with the shape, dimensions and cultural characteristics of a leptospire is identified provisionally as a member of the Leptospiraceae. Cultural phenotypic characteristics (rapid growth in TSB medium) as well as electron microscopy characterize *Leptonema*. Other isolates look the same microscopically or in culture; they cannot be differentiated by simple biochemical and cultural tests. There are 2 overlapping systems for further classification, genetic species and serological typing. Species is determined genetically by DNA homology. Subspecies categories are determined serologically, by **serovar**, while genetic and serological **types** are recognized within serovars (Ellis 1995). The means of transfer between species of serovar-specific antigens important for immunity and regulation of their expression have not been elucidated.

9.1 Phylogenetic relationships

Spirochaetes comprise a phylum of ancient bacteria whose members are very divergent from one another when classified by 16S rRNA relationships. The most deeply branching individual group in the phylum is the family Leptospiraceae; among them the first to branch off is *Leptonema* (Paster et al. 1984, 1991). *L. biflexa* and related saprophytes are a group distinct from the pathogenic leptospires, although there is considerable homogeneity between these by DNA homology (Paster et al. 1991). Within the group identified as the 'pathogenic' group (formerly the 'interrogans complex' or '*L. interrogans*' *sensu lato*), 2 main branches exist; one contains the species *kirschneri*, *interrogans* and *noguchii*, the other the species *borgpetersenii*, *santarosai* and *weilii*. The 'non-pathogenic' group (formerly the 'biflexa complex', '*L. biflexa*' *sensu lato*) comprised 6 major branches in addition to *Leptonema* (Ramadass et al. 1990, 1992). (Fig. 57.5).

9.2 Genetic classification and species

SPECIES

A species (genospecies, genomic species, genome species) comprises those leptospires whose DNA is 70% related and whose related DNA sequences contain 5% or fewer unpaired bases (divergence) (Wayne et al. 1987, Ellis 1995). There are 12 named species at the time of writing, with 4 further groups awaiting classification. Analyses by restriction length fragment polymorphism (RLFP), pulsed-field gel electrophoresis (PFGE) of *Not*I restricted digests of DNA, arbitrarily primed PCR (APPCR), mapped restriction site polymorphisms (MRSP) and random amplified polymorphic DNA fingerprinting (RAPD) are easier to perform and give similar results if calibrated (Herrmann et al. 1992, Ralph et al. 1993a, Gerritsen, Smits and Olyhoek 1995). PFGE and RAPD fingerprinting can identify serovars uniquely in some cases. Currently species- and serovar-specific primers for PCR are being developed. Serotyping identifies the same serovar antigens in more than one species. The recognized species, their G + C percentage ratios and some of the more common or important component serovars are listed with their serogroup identity in Table 57.1.

9.3 Serological groups

Leptospires were classified primarily by serology before the development of genetic methods and knowledge. An arbitrary but useful definition of serovar was adopted many years ago, that 2 or more leptospires belong to the same serovar if a residual titre of 10% or less of the homologous titre of agglutinating antibodies remains in rabbit antisera after cross-absorption in standardized tests. About 255 serovars have been recorded among the **Leptospiraceae**. Serovars that are significantly different in their biological and pathogenic properties may be closely related at this 1 log difference level of titre. Some serovars exist in more than one genospecies; that is, the same serovar-specific antigens can be expressed by members of more than one species.

The serological identity of an isolate depends on the dominance of one or more epitopes in a surface mosaic of LPS antigens, while the specificity of the epitope depends on its sugar composition and orientation (Dikken and Kmety 1978, Vinh et al. 1989, Kmety and Dikken 1993, Midwinter et al. 1994, Ellis 1995). Monoclonal antibodies to LPS epitopes can identify antigens for classification using ELISA and related tests. Serovars that share common (serogroup-reactive) antigens and partially coagglutinate belong to serogroups. Serogroups have no taxonomic status but are useful for facilitating diagnosis and serological identification by antigens common to members of their group (see section 10, p. 1298 and Volume 3, Chapter 42). Serological identification is clinically and epidemiologically significant but slow, painstaking and labour-intensive. Wider application of genomic identification, particularly in molecular epidemiology, as an adjunct to serology in diagnostic and epidemiological laboratories will enhance understanding of pathology and epidemiology.

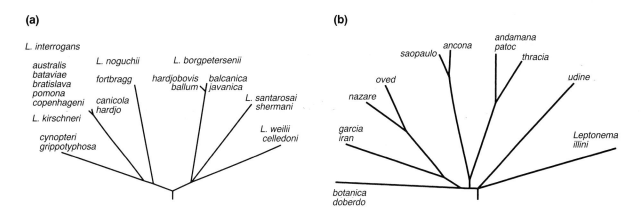

Fig. 57.5 Phylogenetic relationships of species of leptospires: (a) pathogenic varieties (adapted from Ramadass et al. 1992); (b) non-pathogenic varieties (adapted from Ramadass et al. 1990).

Table 57.1 Species, serovars, serogroups and phenotypes of some leptospires[a]

Species	Serovar	Serogroup[b]	Serovar	Serogroup
L. biflexa[c,d]	*patoc*	20		
L. borgpetersenii[d]	*anhoa*	6	*javanica*	12
	arborea	3	*jules*	10
	balcanica	19	*mini*	15
	ballum	3	*sejroe*	19
	guangdong	3	*whitcombi*	5
	hardjo[e]	18	*tarassovi*	21
L. inadai	*icterohaemorrhagiae*	11	*lyme*	14
L. interrogans	*australis*	1	*kennewicki*	16
	autumnalis	2	*kremastos*	16
	bangkok	1	*lai*	11
	bataviae	4	*lora*	1
	birkini	11	*medanensis*	19
	bratislava	1	*mwogolo*	11
	broomi	5	*naam*	11
	bulgarica	2	*paidjan*	4
	canicola	5	*pomona*	16
	copenhageni	11	*pyrogenes*	17
	djasiman	8	*rachmati*	2
	grippotyphosa	9	*robinsoni*	17
	hardjo[f]	19	*saxkoebing*	19
	hebdomadis	10	*swajizak*	15
	icterohaemorrhagiae	11	*zanoni*	17
L. kirschneri	*bim*	2	*grippotyphosa*	9
	bulgarica	2	*mwogolo*	11
	butembo	2	*mozdok*	16
	cynopteri	7	*tsaratsova*	16
L. noguchii	*bajan*	1	*muenchen*	1
	fortbragg	2		
L. santarosai	*bataviae*	4	*pyrogenes*	17
	borincana	10	*tabaquite*	15
	kremastos	10	*trinidad*	19
	maru	10	*weaveri*	18
	navet	21		
L. weilii	*celledoni*	5	*mengma*	12
	hainan	5	*sarmin*	18
Turneria parva[c]	*parva*	22		
Leptonema illini[c]	*illini*	13		

[a]The species identity of some strains representative of more than 250 recognized serovars in major serogroups is summarized from several sources. The species identity of many more strains awaits formal publication. Isolates were identified initially by serovar. The same serovar occurs in more than one species. Not all serogroups are represented in this table. Complete serovar lists to date were published by Kmety and Dikken (1993) and Faine (1994).

[b]Serogroups indicated by the number in the column. 1, Australis; 2, Autumnalis; 3, Ballum; 4, Bataviae; 5, Canicola; 6, Celledoni; 7, Cynopteri; 8, Djasiman; 9, Grippotyphosa; 10, Hebdomadis; 11, Icterohaemorrhagiae; 12, Javanica; 13, Leptonema; 14, Lyme; 15, Mini; 16, Pomona; 17, Pyrogenes; 18, Sarmin; 19, Sejroe; 20, Semaranga; 21, Tarassovi; 22, Turneria.

[c]Non-pathogenic. Other non-pathogens are listed in Faine (1994).

[d]G + C ratio mol% and phenotypes, compiled from various sources. In some cases the only isolate studied was an old laboratory strain.

L. biflexa G + C: (36.0 ± 0.3)–(37.6 ± 0.7). Phenotype: P −; 11 −; 37 ±; Cu ±; AZ ±; DP +; L +.

L. borgpetersenii G + C: 39.8 ± 0.3. Phenotype: P +; 11 −; 37 +; Cu −; AZ −; DP −; L ±.

L. inadai G + C: 42.6 ± 0.9. Phenotype: P +; 11 −; 37 +; Cu +; AZ +; DP −; L ±.

L. interrogans G + C: 34.9 ± 0.9. Phenotype: P +; 11 −; 37 +; Cu −; AZ −; DP −; L ±.

L. kirschneri G + C: ?. Phenotype: P +; 13 −, 37 +; Cu ?; AZ −; DP +m; L ?.

L. noguchii G + C: 36.5 ± 1.2. Phenotype: P +; 11 −; 37 +; Cu −; AZ −; DP −; L −.

L. santarosai: G + C: 40.7 ± 0.5. Phenotype: P +; 11 −; 37 +; Cu −; AZ −; DP +; L −.

L. weilii G + C: 40.5 ± 0.7. Phenotype: P +; 11 −; 37 −; Cu −; AZ −; DP −; L −.

Turneria parva G + C: 48.7 ± 0.7. Phenotype: P −; 11 −; 37 +; Cu +; AZ +; DP −; L +.

Leptonema illini G + C: 54.2 ± 0.2. Phenotype: P −; 11 +; 37 −, Cu −; AZ +; DP +; L +.

P, pathogenic; 11, growth at 11°C; 13, growth at 13°C; 37, growth at 37°C; Cu, growth with CuSO$_4$ 100 mg ml^{-1} added to the growth medium; AZ, growth with 8-azaguanine 225 mg ml^{-1} added to the growth medium; DP, growth with 2,6-diaminopurine 10 mg ml^{-1} added to the growth medium; L, lipase trioleinase activity; +, growth recorded or activity present; −, growth or activity not recorded; ±, growth or activity variable among strains; +m, most strains active; ?, unknown or not formally published.

[e]Type hardjobovis.

[f]Type hardjoprajitno.

9.4 Other phenotypic typing methods

Few phenotypic properties are available for classification. Colonial growth characteristics have not been used. Growth in TSB identifies *Leptonema*. Growth at 13°C (but not at 37°C); growth in one or more of CuSO₄, 8-azaguanine or 2,6-diaminopurine; and lipase production are in general characteristics of *L. biflexa* and *Leptonema* (Table 57.1). Comparison of fatty acid methyl esters (FAME) profiles classified leptospires in 17 groups (Cacciapuoti, Ciceroni and Attard Barbini 1991). Flagellar antigens have also been grouped into distinct relationships. Related isolates have similar LPS profiles on PAGE. For many years it was wrongly assumed that all leptospires were metabolically and probably genetically identical because they appeared to be morphologically and culturally similar, differing from one another only in their serovar-specific antigens. Some early studies should now be repeated using members of different species to understand the extent of intra- and interspecies differences and to test the validity of extrapolating research results to different leptospires.

10 LABORATORY ISOLATION AND IDENTIFICATION

Laboratories may need to look for leptospires in clinical or pathological specimens from humans or animals, or from environmental sources. They also may need to grow them for research or industrial purposes. Leptospires are so hard to see and so hard and slow to grow that conventional bacteriological diagnostic procedures (microscopy of stained preparations and culture on solid media) are not practicable. Darkfield microscopy of diagnostic, including environmental, specimens is technically difficult because particles or other bacteria in the specimens scatter light and impede visualization. Microscopy is presumptive and immediate; culture is definitive if successful, but slow, taking up to 3–4 weeks for growth and days to weeks for identification.

Immunofluorescent staining is rapid and serovar-specific if the serovar or serogroup of the leptospires is known or suspected, or pools of antisera are used. Direct PCR can be carried out on specimens; molecular diagnosis is currently being evaluated prior to implementation when perfected. PCR is relatively fast, taking hours or a few days; it is valuable for rapid identification of isolates.

10.1 Types of specimens

CLINICAL AND PATHOLOGICAL DIAGNOSTIC SPECIMENS

Similar specimens are, in general, investigated for leptospirosis in humans and in animals. The methods are the same in principle, and almost the same in practice, for both (Alexander 1991, Faine 1994).

Blood cultures, taken aseptically from febrile patients or animals, are inoculated into EMJH containing sodium polyanethane sulphonate (and ß-lactamase if treatment with penicillin has begun) at dilutions of at least 1 volume (from 0.1 to 1.0 ml) to 100 volumes of medium, to dilute any antibodies present. Special media are used for fastidious leptospires. CSF and urine are cultured similarly; urine specimens must be alkaline when passed and collected aseptically. Cultures are incubated at 30°C and examined macroscopically daily for up to 3 weeks and microscopically to confirm growth when it is suspected, or before discard. Subcultures are made into volumes of 5–10 ml of liquid media with further subcultures every 3–14 days at first; solid media are not used, in general. The tissues most usually examined in animals are kidneys, genital tract organs, semen, abortion products and placentas; examination of human tissues is rare in non-fatal leptospirosis. Urine and autopsy specimens and field specimens from animals are often contaminated; inhibitors such as cycloheximide, bacitracin, neomycin, polymyxin B and rifampicin in the media prevent or retard the growth of other bacteria. Tissues from autopsies, or rarely from biopsies, are ground aseptically with sterile buffered (pH 7.2) saline diluent and the supernatant cultured as above. Carry-over of tissue debris can make the medium anaerobic and prevent leptospiral growth (see Alexander 1991 and Faine 1994 for details of diagnostic cultures).

ENVIRONMENTAL SPECIMENS – WATER, MUD AND SOIL

Leptospires, including pathogens, persist in water, soil, mud and effluents. Detection by direct darkfield microscopy is of limited value. Immunofluorescent staining (see p. 1289) can detect leptospires without regard to viability. Water can be filtered through a cellulose bacteriological filter of 0.22 µm APD (average pore diameter) which will let leptospires through the pores. Soil, mud and similar samples can be shaken with sterile water and the sediment centrifuged. The supernatant or eluate is filtered as above. The filtrates are cultured in liquid or on solid media. Successful cultures can be achieved by using media with inhibitors (see above). Alternatively, the filtrate or water may be inoculated in a small area in the middle of the surface of a plate of solid medium. After incubation, growth of leptospires will spread in a ring, centrifugally from the inoculation site, allowing subculture from the growing edge. Such cultures need to be checked for purity because more than one strain of leptospires may occur in these specimens. Special high sodium media have been described for culturing halophilic leptospires.

10.2 Identification of isolates; typing methods

Cultures, once grown, need to be checked for purity and identity. Purity can be checked by plating on solid media, remembering that a pure culture can have more than one colony type. Colony type is not usually included in criteria for identification or classification.

The usual method for testing serological identity is by microscopic agglutination test (MAT).

A reference antiserum is serially diluted in phosphate buffered saline, pH 7.2, usually in 2-fold steps starting at one or more steps in a 1 in 10 dilution series, in volumes of 250 μl in microtitration trays. An equal volume of the culture to be tested, standardized for density, is added and the covered tray incubated at a non-critical room temperature or 30°C for 1.5–2.0 h. A loopful from each dilution is examined microscopically under darkfield. Agglutination is noted and scored as an approximate percentage of the leptospires agglutinated. The end point is 50% agglutination. ELISA tests are also used as serological methods for identification, in reactions with standard antisera (Dikken and Kmety 1978, Alexander 1991, Faine 1994). Serological identification should be done at least to serogroup level, but to serovar level if possible, and in addition, to type within the serovar if appropriate. The lengthy standardized procedure begins with MAT using various reference antisera from different serogroups, to find one that agglutinates it to titre or close to titre, repeated similarly with antisera reacting to single serovars. Batteries of pooled sera are used initially. Homologous antisera to the new strain are produced in rabbits. These antisera and the reference antisera to the reacting reference strain are then absorbed and cross-absorbed with both the new strain and the reacting reference strain. The absorbed antisera are titrated in MAT using homologous and heterologous strain antigens. The new strain is regarded as the same as the old strain if the residual titres after cross-absorption both ways are 10% or less. A simplified acceptable procedure is to use batteries of reference monoclonal sera which can identify to at least serogroup level immediately. Monoclonal antibodies can identify epitopes in ELISA reactions. Since the epitopes are not necessarily characteristic nor unique for a single serovar, pools of monoclonals are used containing epitopes whose pattern of reaction is specific for a serovar. The use of monoclonal antibodies supplants the methods employing 'factor sera' for 'factor analysis', an analogous form of identification using serovar-specific pools of absorbed antisera.

It is important to identify the species as well as the serovar when describing or researching a leptospire because characteristics specified by species may be different for a given serovar. Species can be determined by genetic homology of a new isolate with reference strains, or by one of the other methods (APPCR, PFGE, RAPD, RFLP) mentioned in section 9 (see section 9, p. 1297), in any laboratory equipped for molecular microbiology and PCR, provided the appropriate primers, reference DNA samples and the DNA of the strain to be identified are available. The development of serovar-specific molecular probes amplified by PCR is likely to further simplify typing.

11 SUSCEPTIBILITY TO ANTIMICROBIAL AGENTS

11.1 General and environmental agents

Leptospires and leptonemes are destroyed by heat above about 42°C, acid (below about pH 6.5), alkali (above about pH 8.0), heavy metals, halogens, deter-

gents (including soaps, free fatty acids, bile salts), drying and reducing conditions (Eh below about −0.300 mV). They can survive chilling to 4°C or freezing to −20°C in tissues (including kidneys in butcher shops). In the laboratory they can be cryopreserved in liquid nitrogen and have been preserved lyophilized. Cultures stored in sealed tubes in the dark at room temperatures below about 40°C remain viable for months; leptospires have been grown after 8 years of storage.

11.2 Antibiotics and metabolic antagonists

All classes of antibiotics except chloramphenicol and rifampicin kill leptospires. Penicillin and doxycycline are used widely in therapy; the latter has also been used for chemoprophylaxis. Streptomycin and dihydrostreptomycin are used for eliminating leptospires from the kidneys of carrier animals. One-step resistance to streptomycin can be produced easily in the laboratory. Resistance to any antibiotic has not appeared as a clinical problem, probably because there is no human-to-human transmission. Individual isolates of leptospires are not usually tested for susceptibility to antibiotics. The selective use of purine and pyrimidine inhibitors for classification has been mentioned above (see sections 5.4, p. 1292, and 9.4, p. 1298).

11.3 Bacteriophages and bacteriocins

The only known bacteriophages act on *L. biflexa* (Saint Girons et al. 1990, Saint Girons 1991). Antagonisms between leptospires have been reviewed by Faine (1994).

12 PATHOGENICITY AND VIRULENCE FACTORS

This topic is reviewed in detail in Faine (1994) and dealt with in the context of infection, pathogenesis and diagnosis in Volume 3, Chapter 42.

12.1 Role in the normal flora of humans

The natural habitat of leptospires is in the environment; they are not known to be part of the normal flora of humans or animals. Leptospires infect humans only by accident of contact with a contaminated environment; spread from humans to other humans is almost unknown apart from congenital infection. Animals that survive acute systemic infection may become renal carriers that excrete leptospires in the urine; the carrier state is not established without prior generalized clinical or subclinical infection.

12.2 'Pathogenic' and 'non-pathogenic' leptospires – virulence and virulence factors

Large numbers (approximately 10^{10}) of leptospires of

either the non-pathogenic species *L. biflexa* or the pathogenic species are dermonecrotic and cytotoxic. *L. biflexa* and avirulent pathogenic leptospires do not survive for long in the body because naturally occurring immunoglobulins kill them in the presence of lysozyme and complement. They are then phagocytosed. Virulent leptospires survive possibly because the antigens reacting with these opsonic immunoglobulins are not expressed or not available on the surface. The surviving leptospires grow in the blood and selected tissues to a critical concentration correlated with the appearance of lesions. Growth of leptospires in the body stops when opsonizing antibodies appear, 3–10 days after inoculation, followed immediately by clearance by local and central reticuloendothelial phagocytosis. The opsonins are directed to species-specific LPS epitopes. Nothing is known of the genetics or regulation of expresssion of the ability to survive natural antibodies (Faine 1994) (see Volume 3, Chapter 42).

The primary lesions consist of damage to the endothelial cells of small blood vessels, leading to leakage of plasma and haemorrhages. A localized acute inflammation and polymorphonuclear exudate are not seen initially in acute leptospirosis. The consequences of the damage to blood vessels are ischaemia to the cells and organs dependent on the disturbed blood supply and the primary and secondary effects of sometimes massive haemorrhage. Almost any organs or body systems can be affected; the process is essentially the same in all animals. Renal tubular necrosis is common, sometimes followed by scarring during repair, and the localization of leptospires on the luminal surface of the tubular cells, where they grow and are excreted in urine (Faine 1994) (see Volume 3, Chapter 42).

The lesions are probably caused by the action of unusual unsaturated fatty acids of leptospiral origin acting as competitive inhibitors of the incorporation of normally occurring fatty acids in the target cell membranes. These leptospiral fatty acids are part of a cytotoxic and antigenic GLP complex extractable from leptospires that can be identified in lesions; convalescent patients' antisera react with GLP. LPS does not appear to play a significant part in pathogenesis; it is very weakly pyrogenic and does not produce the lesions that GLP does.

12.3 Microbiological aspects of natural and acquired resistance

Immunity in initial or subsequent infection appears to be wholly humoral and serovar-specific, dependent on opsonization mediated by immunoglobulins directed to LPS epitopes. Phagocytosis depends on antibodies to LPS. Cellular immunity is not significant for protection from initial acute infection. Leptospires are believed not to survive intracellularly.

REFERENCES

Abdussalam M, Alexander AD et al., 1965, Classification of leptospires and recent advances in leptospirosis, *Bull W H O*, **32**: 881–91.

Abdussalam M, Alexander AD et al., 1972, Research needs in leptospirosis, *Bull W H O*, **47**: 113–22.

Adler B, Faine S, 1983, A pomona serogroup-specific, agglutinating antigen in *Leptospira*, identified by monoclonal antibodies, *Pathology*, **15**: 247–50.

Adler B, Murphy AM et al., 1980, Detection of specific anti-leptospiral immunoglobulins M and G in human serum by solid-phase enzyme-linked immunosorbent assay, *J Clin Microbiol*, **11**: 452–7.

Adler B, Faine S et al., 1986, Development of an improved selective medium for isolation of leptospires from clinical material, *Vet Microbiol*, **12**: 377–81.

Alexander AD, 1991, *Leptospira, Manual of Clinical Microbiology*, 5th edn, eds Balows A, Hausler WJ et al., American Society for Microbiology, Washington DC, 554–9.

Alves VA, Gayotto LC et al., 1992, Leptospiral antigens in the liver of experimentally infected guinea pig and their relation to the morphogenesis of liver damage, *Exp Toxicol Pathol*, **44**: 425–34.

Ballard SA, Faine S, Adler B, 1990, Purification and characterization of a protein antigen from *Leptospira interrogans* serovar *hardjo*, common to a wide range of bacteria, *J Gen Microbiol*, **136**: 1849–57.

Ballard SA, Segers RPAM et al., 1993, Molecular analysis of the *hsp* (*groE*) operon of *Leptospira interrogans* serovar *copenhageni*, *Mol Microbiol*, **8**: 739–51.

Baril C, Richaud C et al., 1992, Cloning of *dapD*, *aroD* and *asd* of *Leptospira interrogans* serovar *icterohaemorrhagiae*, and nucleotide sequence of the *asd* gene, *J Gen Microbiol*, **138**: 47–53.

Boursaux C, Zuerner R, Saint Girons I, 1994, IS3-like repetitive elements in *Leptospira interrogans*, Abstracts of the VIIIth Meeting of European Leptospira Workers, Anzio, Rome, Italy. Istituto Zooprofilattico Sperimentale delle Regioni Lazio e Toscana, 47.

Cacciapuoti B, Ciceroni L, Attard Barbini D, 1991, Fatty acid profiles, a chemotaxonomic key for the classification of strains of the family Leptospiraceae, *Int J Syst Bacteriol*, **41**: 295–300.

Chang A, Faine S, Williams WT, 1974, Cross-reactivity of the axial filament antigen as a criterion for classification of *Leptospira*, *Aust J Exp Biol Med Sci*, **52**: 549–68.

Cinco M, Tamaro M, Cociancich L, 1975, Taxonomical, cultural and metabolic characteristics of halophilic leptospirae, *Zentralbl Bakteriol Mikrobiol Hyg Abt I Orig*, **233**: 400–5.

Cinco M, Perticarari S et al., 1993, Biological activity of a peptidoglycan extracted from *Leptospira interrogans*: in vitro studies, *J Gen Microbiol*, **139**: 2959–64.

Del Real G, Segers RPA et al., 1989, Cloning of a hemolysin gene from *Leptospira interrogans* serovar *hardjo*, *Infect Immun*, **57**: 2588–90.

Dikken H, Kmety E, 1978, Serological typing methods of leptospires, *Methods in Microbiology*, vol. 11, eds Bergan T, Norris R, Academic Press, New York, 260–95.

Ding M, Yelton DB, 1993, Cloning and analysis of the *leuB* gene of *Leptospira interrogans* serovar *pomona*, *J Gen Microbiol*, **139**: 1093–103.

Ellis WA, 1995, International Committee on Systematic Bacteriology, Subcommittee on the Taxonomy of *Leptospira*. Minutes of the Meetings, 1 and 2 July 1994, Prague, Czech Republic, *Int J Syst Bacteriol*, **45**: 872–4.

Ellis WA, Hovind-Hougen K et al., 1983, Morphological changes upon subculturing of freshly isolated strains of *Leptospira interrogans* serovar *hardjo*, *Zentralbl Bakteriol Mikrobiol Hyg Abt I Orig*, **255**: 323–35.

Ellis WA, McParland PJ et al., 1985, Leptospires in pig urogenital tracts and fetuses, *Vet Rec*, **117**: 66–7.

Faine S, 1959, Virulence in leptospirae. III. Comparison of sensitivities of virulent and of avirulent *Leptospira icterohaemorrhagiae* to cultural conditions, *J Bacteriol*, **77**: 599–603.

Faine S, 1992, The Genus *Leptospira*, *The Prokaryotes* , vol. 4, 2nd edn, eds Balows A, Trüper HG et al., Springer-Verlag, New York, 3568–82.

Faine S, 1994, Leptospira *and Leptospirosis*, CRC Press, Boca Raton, Florida, USA.

Faine S, Shahar A, Aronson M, 1964, Phagocytosis and its significance in leptospiral infection, *Aust J Exp Biol Med Sci*, **42**: 579–88.

Faine S, Stallman ND, 1982, Amended descriptions of the genus *Leptospira* Noguchi 1917 and the species *L. interrogans* (Stimson 1907) Wenyon 1926 and *L. biflexa* (Wolbach and Binger 1914) Noguchi 1918, *Int J Syst Bacteriol*, **32**: 461–3.

Fukunaga M, Masuzawa T et al., 1990, Linkage of ribosomal RNA genes in *Leptospira*, *Microbiol Immunol*, **34**: 565–73.

Fukunaga M, Mifuchi I et al., 1992, Comparison of flanking regions of the 5S ribosomal ribonucleic acid genes in *Leptospira biflexa* and *Leptospira interrogans*, *Chem Pharm Bull (Tokyo)*, **40**: 544–66.

Gerritsen MA, Smits MA, Olyhoek T, 1995, Random amplified polymorphic DNA fingerprinting for rapid identification of leptospira of serogroup Sejroe, *J Med Microbiol*, **42**: 336–9.

Goldstein SF, Charon NW, 1988, Motility of the spirochete *Leptospira*, *Cell Motil Cytoskeleton*, **9**: 101–10.

Goldstein SF, Charon NW, 1990, Multiple exposure photographic analysis of a motile spirochete, *Proc Natl Acad Sci USA*, **87**: 4894–9.

Haake DA, Walker EM et al., 1991, Changes in the surface of *Leptospira interrogans* serovar *grippotyphosa* during in vitro cultivation, *Infect Immun*, **59**: 1131–40.

Haake DA, Champion CI et al., 1993, Molecular cloning and sequence analysis of the gene encoding OmpL1, a transmembrane outer membrane protein of pathogenic *Leptospira* spp., *J Bacteriol*, **175**: 4225–34.

Herrmann JL, Bellenger E et al., 1992, Pulsed-field gel electrophoresis of *Not*I digests of leptospiral DNA: a new rapid method of serovar identification, *J Clin Microbiol*, **30**: 1696–702.

Johnson RC, Faine S, 1984a, Genus I. Leptospira Noguchi 1917, 755, *Bergey's Manual of Systematic Bacteriology*, vol. 1, 1st edn, eds Krieg NR, Holt JG, Williams and Wilkins, Baltimore/London, 62–7.

Johnson RC, Faine S, 1984b, Order I. Spirochaetales: Family II. 'Leptospiraceae' Hovind-Hougen 1979, 245, *Bergey's Manual of Systematic Bacteriology*, vol. 1, 1st edn, eds Krieg NR, Holt JG, Williams and Wilkins, Baltimore/London, 62.

Jost BH, Adler B, Faine S, 1988, Reaction of monoclonal antibodies with species specific determinants in *Leptospira interrogans* outer envelope, *J Med Microbiol*, **27**: 51–7.

Kelson JS, Adler B et al., 1988, Identification of leptospiral flagellar antigens by gel electrophoresis and immunoblotting, *J Med Microbiol*, **26**: 47–53.

Kmety E, 1967, Faktorenanalyse von Leptospiren der Icterohaemorrhagiae und einiger verwandter Serogruppen (Factor analysis of the Icterohaemorhagiae and some related serogroups), *Biologické Práce. Edicia vedeckych kolegii pre vseobecnu a specialnu biologiu slovenskej akademie vied (Biological Works. Edition of Scientific Committees for General and Special Biology of the Slovak Academy of Sciences)*, vol. 13/3, Vydavatelstvo Slovenskej Akademie Vied (Slovak Academy of Science Press), Bratislava.

Kmety E, Dikken H, 1993, *Classification of the Species* Leptospira interrogans *and the History of its Serovars*, University Press Groningen, Groningen.

Kolk AHJ, Van Leeuwen J et al., 1984, Serotyping of leptospires by monoclonal antibodies, *Zentralbl Bakteriol Mikrobiol Hyg Abt I Orig*, **257**: 515.

Midwinter A, Vinh T et al., 1994, Characterization of an anti-genic oligosaccharide from *Leptospira interrogans* serovar *pomona* and its role in immunity, *Infect Immun*, **62**: 5477–82.

Mitchison M, Rood JI et al., 1991, Molecular analysis of a *Leptospira borgpetersenii* gene encoding an endoflagellar subunit protein, *J Gen Microbiol*, **137**: 1529–36.

Mitchison M, Vinh T et al., 1994, Cloning and analysis of the rhamnose biosynthesis genes of the *rfb* locus involved in LPS biosynthesis in *Leptospira interrogans* serovar *copenhageni*, Abstracts of the VIIIth Meeting of European Leptospira Workers, Anzio, Rome, Italy, July 11–13, 1994. Istituto Zooprofilattico Sperimentale delle Regioni Lazio e Toscana, Rome, Italy, 1994.

Morita T, Fukunaga M et al., 1991, Cloning and expression of *Leptospira interrogans* hemolytic factor gene in *E. coli* and yeast, *Saccharomyces cerevisiae*, Leptospirosis. *Proceedings of the Leptospirosis Reseaarch Conference 1990*, ed. Kobayashi Y, Hokusensha Publishing Co., Tokyo, 345–57.

Paster BJ, Stackebrandt E et al., 1984, The phylogeny of spirochetes, *Syst Appl Microbiol*, **5**: 337–51.

Paster BJ, Dewhirst FE et al., 1991, Phylogenetic analysis of the spirochetes, *J Bacteriol*, **173**: 6101–9.

Ralph D, McClelland M, 1994, Phylogenetic evidence for horizontal transfer of an intervening sequence between species in a spirochete genus, *J Bacteriol*, **176**: 5982–7.

Ralph D, McClelland M et al., 1993a, *Leptospira* species categorized by arbitrarily primed polymerase chain reaction (PCR) and by mapped restriction polymorphisms in PCR-amplified rRNA genes, *J Bacteriol*, **175**: 973–81.

Ralph D, Que Q et al., 1993b, *Leptospira* genomes are modified at 5′-GTAC, *J Bacteriol*, **175**: 3913–15.

Ramadass P, Jarvis BDW et al., 1990, DNA relatedness among strains of *Leptospira biflexa*, *Int J Syst Bacteriol*, **40**: 231–5.

Ramadass P, Jarvis BD et al., 1992, Genetic characterization of pathogenic *Leptospira* species by DNA hybridization, *Int J Syst Bacteriol*, **42**: 215–19.

Richaud C, Margarita D et al., 1990, Cloning of genes required for amino acid biosynthesis from *Leptospira interrogans* serovar *icterohaemorrhagiae*, *J Gen Microbiol*, **136**: 651–6.

Saint Girons I, 1991, A DNA bacteriophage for *Leptospira*, Leptospirosis. *Proceedings of the Leptospirosis Research Conference 1990*, ed. Kobayashi Y, Hokusen-Sha Publishing Co., Tokyo, 457–561.

Saint Girons I, Margarita D et al., 1990, First isolation of bacteriophage for a spirochaete: potential genetic tools for *Leptospira*, *Res Microbiol*, **141**: 1131–8.

Saint Girons I, Norris SJ et al., 1992, Genome structure of spirochetes, *Res Microbiol*, **143**: 615–21.

Segers RPAM, 1991, The molecular analysis of sphingomyelinase genes of Leptospiraceae., Doctoral thesis. Rijksuniversiteit te Utrecht, Netherlands, 147 p.

Segers RPAM, van der Drift A et al., 1990, Molecular analysis of a sphingomyelinase C gene from *Leptospira interrogans* serovar *hardjo*, *Infect Immun*, **58**: 2177–85.

Segers RP, van Gestel JA et al., 1992, Presence of putative sphingomyelinase genes among members of the family Leptospiraceae, *Infect Immun*, **60**: 1707–10.

Stamm LV, Parrish EA, Gherardini FC, 1991, Cloning of the *recA* gene from a free-living leptospire and distribution of RecA-like protein among spirochetes, *Appl Environ Microbiol*, **57**: 183–9.

Stamm LV, Gherardini FC et al., 1991, Heat shock response of spirochetes, Infect Immun, **59**: 1572–5.

Torten M, Marshall RB, 1994, Leptospirosis, *Handbook of Zoonoses, Section A: Bacterial, Rickettsial, Chlamydial and Mycotic Diseases*, vol. 1, 2nd edn, ed. Beran GW, CRC Press, Boca Raton, FL, 245–64.

Trueba GA, Bolin CA, Zuerner RL, 1992, Characterization of the periplasmic flagellum proteins of *Leptospira interrogans*, *J Bacteriol*, **174**: 4761–8.

Vinh T, Adler B, Faine S, 1986a, Glycolipoprotein cytotoxin from

Leptospira interrogans serovar *copenhageni*, *J Gen Microbiol*, **132:** 111–23.

Vinh T, Adler B, Faine S, 1986b, Ultrastructure and chemical composition of lipopolysaccharide extracted from *Leptospira interrogans* serovar *copenhageni*, *J Gen Microbiol*, **132:** 103–9.

Vinh T, Shi M-H et al., 1989, Characterization and taxonomic significance of lipopolysaccharides of *Leptospira interrogans* serovar *hardjo*, *J Gen Microbiol*, **135:** 2663–73.

Vinh T, Faine S et al., 1994, Immunochemical studies of opsonic epitopes of the lipopolysaccharide of *Leptospira interrogans* serovar *hardjo*, *FEMS Immunol Med Microbiol*, **8:** 99–107.

Wayne LG, Brenner DJ et al., 1987, Report of the Ad Hoc Committee on Reconciliation of Approaches to Bacterial Systematics, *Int J Syst Bacteriol*, **37:** 463–4.

Woodward MJ, Redstone JS, 1994, Deoxynucleotide sequence conservation of the endoflagellin subunit protein gene, *flaB*, within the genus *Leptospira*, *Vet Microbiol*, **40:** 239–51.

Wu SH, Jiang SX et al., 1987, Studies on endotoxins of *Leptospira*. III. The presence of beta-hydroxy-myristic acid in the LPS of *Leptospira interrogans* serovar *lai*, *Wei Sheng Wu Hsueh Pao*, **27:** 165–8.

Yanagawa R, Faine S, 1966, Morphological and serological analysis of leptospiral structure, *Nature (London)*, **211:** 823–6.

Yanagihara Y, Mifuchi I, 1968, Microfibers present in surface structure of *Leptospira*, *J Bacteriol*, **95:** 2403–6.

Zuerner RL, 1994, Nucleotide sequence analysis of IS1533 from *Leptospira borgpetersenii*: identification and expression of two IS-encoded proteins, *Plasmid*, **31:** 1–11.

Zuerner RL, Herrmann JL, Saint Girons I, 1993, Comparison of genetic maps for two *Leptospira interrogans* serovars provides evidence for two chromosomes and intraspecies heterogeneity, *J Bacteriol*, **175:** 5445–51.

Chapter 58

BACTEROIDES, PREVOTELLA AND PORPHYROMONAS

H N Shah, S E Gharbia and B I Duerden

1 Classification	7 Molecular analysis
2 *Bacteroides*	8 Cell envelope composition and antigenic properties
3 *Prevotella*	
4 *Porphyromonas*	9 Bacteriocin production
5 The current status of species that previously belonged to the genus *Bacteroides*	10 Bacteriophages
	11 Bacteroidaceae in the normal flora
6 Antibiotic resistance	

Gram-negative, non-sporing, anaerobic bacilli with rounded or pointed ends, sometimes fusiform, sometimes filamentous and often pleomorphic, that produce mixed acidic end products were previously classified in the genus *Bacteroides*. Recognized as important causes of human and animal infection since the latter part of the nineteenth century, they are also a major component of the normal bacterial flora of humans and animals, colonizing the mucous membranes of the mouth, urogenital and lower gastrointestinal tract of humans. In animals they are found in the mouth and at various sites in the alimentary tract. Some species metabolize cellulose and other polysaccharides in the rumen of some herbivores; some of the most oxygen-sensitive species have been found in the caecum of chickens and other poultry.

1 CLASSIFICATION

The isolation and classification of these organisms has presented particular difficulties. These were partly technical, because reliable anaerobic conditions were difficult to achieve and many workers were unable to obtain pure cultures, but they also reflected the diverse properties of members of the group. There was confusion in nomenclature and disagreement between different observers over the description of the same organisms.

The classification of gram-negative anaerobic bacilli has undergone many changes since Veillon and Zuber (1898) named their isolates *Bacillus fragilis, Bacillus*

fusiformis, etc. This was recognized by Castellani and Chalmers (1919) who proposed the genus *Bacteroides* to contain species of obligately anaerobic non-sporing bacilli. *B. fragilis* was adopted as the type species from the first edition of *Bergey's Manual* (1923). Subsequently, Weiss and Rettger (1937) redefined the genus to exclude gram-positive organisms; spindle-shaped gram-negative anaerobic bacilli were placed in the genus *Fusobacterium* by Knorr (1922).

Eggerth and Gagnon (1933) produced a scheme based upon the classification of Castellani and Chalmers (1919) for the identification of strains isolated from the gastrointestinal tract; they defined 18 species on the basis of morphology and carbohydrate fermentation tests, but all of their strains were found later to belong to the *Bacteroides fragilis* group (Holdeman and Moore 1974a).

The system proposed by Prévot (1938) employed generic names that differed from those in general use and included the pigmented species *Bacteroides melaninogenicus* (proposed by Oliver and Wherry in 1921) as *Ristella melaninogenica*. He divided gram-negative anaerobic bacilli into 2 families, Ristellaceae with 5 genera (*Ristella, Pasteurella, Dialister, Capsularis, Zuberella*) and Sphaerophoraceae with 2 genera (*Sphaerophorus* and *Sphaerocillus*). In the sixth edition of *Bergey's Manual* (1948) the Bacteroidaceae, comprising the 2 genera, *Bacteroides* and *Fusobacterium*, was a tribe of the family Parvobacteriaceae. Most of the 23 species of *Bacteroides* were members of the *B. fragilis* group except for *B. melaninogenicus*, which was described as saccharolytic, and one asaccharolytic species, *Bacteroides caviae*. In the seventh edition of *Bergey's Manual* (1957), gram-negative, anaerobic bacilli were reclassified as the family Bacteroidaceae and comprised 5 genera. The genus *Bacteroides* contained 30 species distinguished by gas production, gelatin liquefaction, cellular morphology and the production of acid from carbohydrates; 2 species were motile and 2 (*Bacteroides coagulans* and *Bacteroides putredinis*) were non-fermentative. There were 6 species of *Fusobacterium* and 2 of *Dialister*. The second largest genus was *Sphaerophorus* with 14 species, and aerobic but facultatively anaerobic organisms of the genus *Streptobacillus* were also included in the Bacteroidaceae. In the sixth edition of this book (1974) only 3 species of *Fusobacterium* and 5 of *Bacteroides*, and a third genus, *Dialister*, to contain the minute gram-negative bacillus *Dialister pneumosintes*, were included.

The first general agreement on taxonomy and classification was reached at the meeting of the International Commission for Systematic Bacteriology Subcommittee for gram-negative anaerobic rods at Lille in 1967, when new principles for classification were defined (Beerens 1970). These were embodied in the eighth edition of *Bergey's Manual* (Holdeman and Moore 1974a). The Bacteroidaceae were divided into 3 genera: *Bacteroides*, *Fusobacterium* and *Leptotrichia*. The genus *Bacteroides* contained 22 species in 5 groups:

1. *B. fragilis* included most of those species described by Eggerth and Gagnon (1933) and previous workers and was divided into 5 subspecies
2. phenotypically similar strains that were inhibited by bile included *Bacteroides ruminicola*, *Bacteroides oralis*, *Bacteroides ochraceus* and *Bacteroides amylophilus*
3. a group of 6 species that did not produce succinic acid but were otherwise unrelated
4. non-saccharolytic non-pigmented strains
5. *B. melaninogenicus* produced black-pigmented colonies on laked-blood agar and was divided into 3 subspecies.

The genus *Fusobacterium* contained 16 species that formed *n*-butyric acid as a major metabolic product and Vincent's organism (*Fusobacterium plauti-vincenti*) was assigned to the third genus, *Leptotrichia* (Gilmour, Howell and Bibby 1961), under the name *Leptotrichia buccalis*, because it produced lactic but not *n*-butyric acid as a major product.

In the ninth edition of *Bergey's Manual* (Holdeman, Kelley and Moore 1984), 42 species were assigned to the genus *Bacteroides*. These included 8 species previously encompassed by '*B. fragilis*', 8 species of saccharolytic non-pigmented oral bacteroides (previously '*B. oralis*'), 7 saccharolytic pigmented species (previously '*B. melaninogenicus*'), 3 species concerned with cellulose degradation in the rumen of herbivores and 9 non-fermentative (asaccharolytic) species of which 2, *Bacteroides asaccharolyticus* and *Bacteroides gingivalis*, were pigmented. In addition, 3 more species were proposed within the *fragilis*-like group of faecal bacteroides (*Bacteroides merdae*, *Bacteroides stercoris*, *Bacteroides caccae*; Johnson, Moore and Moore 1986),

another oral non-pigmented species (*Bacteroides heparinolyticus*; Okuda et al. 1985) and a third asaccharolytic pigmented species (*Bacteroides endodontalis*; van Steenbergen, de Soet and de Graaf 1984).

The genus *Bacteroides*, which contains species with a G + C range of 26–61 mol%, has undergone major taxonomic revisions (Shah 1991a, 1991b). This was inevitable because of the considerable heterogeneity in biochemical and chemical properties that became apparent. The genus now includes species that were formerly described as the '*Bacteroides fragilis*' group. More than 15 new genera have been proposed for organisms formerly classified as *Bacteroides*, most of which are monospecific (Fig. 58.1). However, 2 genera, *Porphyromonas* and *Prevotella* (Shah and Collins 1989, 1990), contain large numbers of species and appear to be of major clinical importance.

Comparative 16S rRNA sequence analysis has now considerably reshaped the family Bacteroidaceae and over half the recently proposed genera have been displaced to phylogenetic lineages within the gram-positive phyla. *Fusobacterium*, *Leptotrichia* and *Sebaldella* are not phylogenetically related to the Bacteroidaceae and warrant placement in a new family. In this chapter, genera that have been placed within the Bacteroidaceae based on evolutionary relationships are discussed, i.e. *Bacteroides*, *Prevotella* and *Porphyromonas*.

Many of the new genera that have been proposed, such as *Catonella*, *Hallella*, *Johnsonella* and *Oribaculum* (Moore and Moore 1994) are likely to be reclassified, as comparative 16S rRNA analysis indicates that they have high affinities with other recognized taxa. For example, *Oribaculum* has been reclassified in the genus *Porphyromonas* (Willems and Collins 1995b), whereas *Mitsuokella dentalis*, which has a mol% G + C content similar to that of *Mitsuokella multiacidus* (Haapasalo et al. 1986) but differs considerably from this species, has been shown to have closer affinity with *Hallella seregens* (Willems and Collins 1995c). Furthermore, *Bacteroides ureolyticus* and *Bacteroides gracilis*, which have long been considered inappropriate in the *Bacteroides*, were

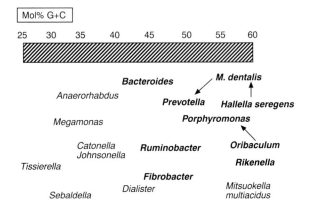

Fig. 58.1 The range in mol% G + C contents of taxa that previously constituted the genus *Bacteroides*. The arrows indicate the correct designation of recently proposed taxa and those that are written in bold presently retain their position within the family Bacteroidaceae.

recently shown to belong to *Campylobacter* (Vandamme et al. 1995).

1.1 Criteria for classification

Early workers relied almost exclusively upon observations of microscopic and colonial morphology; however, these properties can vary considerably among species depending on their growth conditions. Eggerth and Gagnon (1933) established the first biochemical key for the group, but their tests were performed under varied and often unsuitable conditions. Prévot (1938) used an extensive series of biochemical tests, which included the determination of metabolic end products. Conventional bacteriological tests remain an important part of identification schemes for gram-negative anaerobic bacilli (Holdeman and Moore 1974a, Duerden et al. 1976, 1980, Holdeman, Kelley and Moore 1984) and several commercial systems for rapid identification are currently available. Barnes and Goldberg (1968a, 1968b) analysed the data obtained from phenotypic tests by numerical methods and concluded that the most useful properties were cellular morphology, terminal pH in glucose broth, production of formic, acetic, propionic and butyric acids, deamination of threonine, stimulation of growth by 20% bile, and inhibition by certain antibiotics.

The short-chain fatty acids formed as end products of protein or carbohydrate metabolism were particularly important in the classification of anaerobic bacteria. They were first detected by distillation and paper chromatography (Guillaume, Beerens and Osteaux 1956), but this was superseded by gas-liquid chromatography (GLC; Werner 1969, Moore 1970, Carlsson 1973). The family Bacteroidaceae was assigned to 2 principal genera, *Bacteroides* and *Fusobacterium*, on the grounds that *Fusobacterium* spp. produce *n*-butyric acid as a major product whereas most *Bacteroides* spp. do not. The third genus, *Leptotrichia*, comprises oral fusiform bacteria that produce lactic acid as the only major product.

Several groups of workers have used comparisons of the mol% G + C content of the DNA to determine similarities and differences between members of the groups of Bacteroidaceae (Sébald 1962, Shah et al. 1976). It was a widely held view that a genus should comprise species that do not differ by more than 10–12 mol% G + C. Thus, the fact that the *Bacteroides* contained species within the range 28–61 mol% G + C indicated that several genera existed within this taxon. DNA–DNA hybridization was used to verify the intraspecies status of several taxa such as the subgroups within the *B. fragilis* group (Johnson 1973, Cato and Johnson 1976) and the subspecies of *B. melaninogenicus* (Coykendall et al. 1980, van Steenbergen, Vlaarderen and de Graaf 1981, Shah et al. 1982).

In the mid-1970s and 1980s attention turned increasingly towards chemical analyses of cell constituents for the provision of characters that are useful for classification. Cell wall composition, a major differentiating character among gram-positive taxa, had less impact among gram-negative bacteria. Like most gram-negative micro-organisms, *Bacteroides* and *Prevotella* spp. possess a directly cross-linked peptidoglycan based upon *meso*-diaminopimelic acid whereas some species of *Porphyromonas* appear to have a peptidoglycan structure based upon lysine (Shah et al. 1976, Hammann and Werner 1981). However, the chemical composition and structure of many species remain unknown; thus the full value of this property in the classification of these micro-organisms is still to be determined. Multilocus enzyme electrophoresis using oxidoreductases provided a useful means of accentuating the diversity that existed among taxa that were considered to be homogeneous. Thus 5 electrophoretic patterns were found among *B. melaninogenicus* strains (Shah et al. 1976) that were subsequently assigned to different species whereas among *Bacteroides* considerable diversity was revealed (Shah and Williams 1982). This technique not only provided evidence of relationships and differences within the genus (Shah and Collins 1983) but also shed light on aspects of intermediary metabolism (Shah and Williams 1987). The black/beige pigments produced by *B. melaninogenicus* and related taxa were regarded as one of the most important distinguishing properties. Chemical analysis revealed that the pigments were porphyrins and not melanin or ferrous sulphide as previously reported and that 2 major compounds existed (Shah et al. 1979, Shah 1991a). The black pigment was identified as protohaemin and the fluorescent light brown pigment was characterized as protoporphyrin (Fig. 58.2). Current studies indicate that several other pigments exist and porphyrin genes are present even among non-pigmented members of the group (Shah and Gharbia unpublished data). Gram-negative bacteria, particularly anaerobic bacteria, possess a plethora of diverse lipids such as sphingolipids and plasmalogens (Miyagawa, Azuma and Suto 1978, Shah and Collins 1983). Among the lipids, long-chain cellular fatty acids (Miyagawa, Azuma and Suto 1979, Shah et al. 1982) have provided excellent taxonomic markers and were one of the key chemical characters used to differentiate *Porphyromonas* and *Prevotella* (Fig. 58.3). In addition, analysis of polar lipids (Kunsman 1973, Kunsman and Caldwell 1974, Shah 1991b) and menaquinones (Shah and Collins 1980) have had a significant impact in reshaping the structure of the Bacteroidaceae. Menaquinones are the sole isoprenoid quinones produced by *Bacteroides* spp. and determination of the length of the C-3 polyprenyl side chains have enabled clearer circumscription of several species (Shah and Collins 1980). For example, *B. ochraceus* was shown to differ markedly from *Bacteroides* spp. in possessing menaquinones with 6 isoprene units. *Bacteroides* spp. and related taxa possess menaquinones with isoprene units in excess of 9. Proteins in whole cell extracts of *Bacteroides* cultures analysed by discontinuous gradient polyacrylamide gel electrophoresis (PAGE) have been helpful in delineating specific, subspecific, and strain-specific patterns (Strom et al. 1976). Cell surface proteins released by EDTA treatment and mild sonic disintegration, and treated by sodium dodecyl sulphate PAGE (SDS-PAGE), have revealed species-specific patterns among the *Bacteroides* (Poxton and Brown 1979).

1.2 The impact of rRNA sequence analysis

Initially, rRNA cataloguing and later, 5,16 and 23S rRNA sequence analysis, were used to devise a classification system based on natural relationships (Woese 1987). Members of the Bacteroidaceae, like other taxa, were subjected to rigorous analysis and several phylogenetic trees have been constructed (see, e.g. Lawson et al. 1991, Paster et al. 1994, Shah et al. 1995). In general, ribosomal RNA sequence data have in the main supported previous proposals and there is now general consensus that the genera *Bacteroides*, *Prevotella* and *Porphyromonas* are distinct lines of descent and worthy of separate status (Fig. 58.4).

In the past, the methods used in research laboratories were generally regarded as unsuitable for routine application, and several simpler methods were devised. Differential inhibition tests with ethyl violet, Victoria blue 4R, brilliant green and gentian violet, together with susceptibility patterns to antibiotics such as kanamycin, neomycin, penicillin, rifampicin, colistin and erythromycin, were employed for the identification of groups within the Bacteroidaceae (Finegold, Harada and Miller 1967, Shimada, Sutter and Finegold 1970, Sutter and Finegold 1971). With the advent of chemotaxonomy and the availability of sequence data it is now possible to design diagnostic probes (both serological and nucleic acid probes) that recognize key features of species. Furthermore, the amplification of a species-specific signature from clinical specimens by polymerase chain reaction (PCR), with the consequent identification of previously unknown species adds a new dimension to diagnostic microbiology and is likely to have a significant impact on our knowledge of the range and diversity of bacterial species.

2 BACTEROIDES

This genus contains gram-negative bacilli of closely related species (Table 58.1) that share many common properties and a common ecology; they are tolerant of bile and resistant to penicillin and are commensals in the lower gastrointestinal tract in humans. They form a major part of the normal human faecal flora and some species are important pathogens, causing infections particularly after accidental or surgical injury to the gastrointestinal tract or in association with pathological lesions of it. Most of the species described by Veillon and Zuber (1898) and by Eggerth and Gagnon (1933) were members of this group, but its classification was confused.

In the eighth edition of *Bergey's Manual*, Holdeman and Moore (1974a) gathered all the members of this group into a single species – *B. fragilis* – with 5 subspecies: *fragilis, vulgatus, distasonis, ovatus* and *thetaiota-omicron*. They believed that the species represented a continuum of variants with clusters of strains that were designated subspecies and smaller numbers of intermediate strains. However, Cato and Johnson (1976) found poor DNA homology between the reference strains of the 5 original subspecies of *B. fragilis*. They proposed that they should be reinstated to specific rank and this was accepted by the International Committee for Systematic Bacteriology (ICSB). Other clusters of strains that fell within the group were given specific status; these included *Bacteroides splanchnicus*, *Bacteroides eggerthii*, *Bacteroides variabilis*, *Bacteroides uniformis*, *B. merdae*, *B. caccae* and *B. stercoris*. The relationship between the species remains the subject of considerable debate. They share many properties, and ecological and epidemiological studies support the concept of a closely related group. The results of a wide range of phenotypic tests on members of the fragilis group form a continuous spectrum with clusters of strains that represent the named species.

2.1 Description of the genus

The genus *Bacteroides* comprises small non-motile gram-negative bacilli and coccobacilli; they are moderately pleomorphic but long filaments, bizarre shapes, L-forms and spheroplasts are rare. They grow well in 24–48 h on horse blood agar plates incubated anaerobically at 37°C to form circular, low-convex colonies, 1–3 mm in diameter with an entire edge; the colonies are usually smooth, shiny, translucent or semi-opaque and grey; colonies of fresh isolates are often moist and some are mucoid. Most strains do not produce haemolysis but a few strains are slightly haemolytic and a very small proportion (<1%) are β-haemolytic. All species will grow on a medium that contains glucose, haemin, vitamin B12, minerals, ammonium chloride and a sulphide and is provided with a CO_2/CO_3^- buffer system; they do not use organic nitrogen compounds. They have generally been regarded as catalase-negative but *B. fragilis* and some other saccharolytic species have been shown to produce small amounts of catalase and superoxide dismutase (SOD) (Gregory, Kowalski and Holdeman 1977). The G + C content of the DNA is in the range 40–48 mol% and 16S ribosomal RNA analysis revealed over 93% similarity among species. All species ferment a range of carbohydrates, including glucose, with the production of acid and gas. The major volatile fatty acid products of metabolism are acetic and succinic acids; *n*-butyric acid is not produced except by *B. splanchnicus*. Most strains are stimulated by 20% bile and are tolerant of the bile salt sodium taurocholate but inhibited by sodium deoxycholate. They will grow in the presence of Victoria blue 4R (1 in 80 000) but most are inhibited by gentian violet (1 in 100 000) and ethyl violet (1 in 100 000). All strains are resistant to penicillin and to high concentrations (1000 μg discs) of neomycin and kanamycin. They decarboxylate glutamic acid but threonine is not dehydrogenated, nitrate is not reduced and urease is not produced. Most strains hydrolyse aesculin rapidly and produce acid from

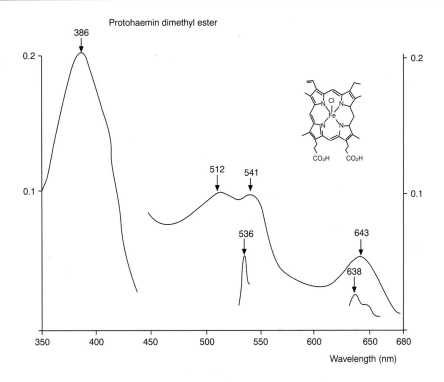

Protohaemin dimethyl ester

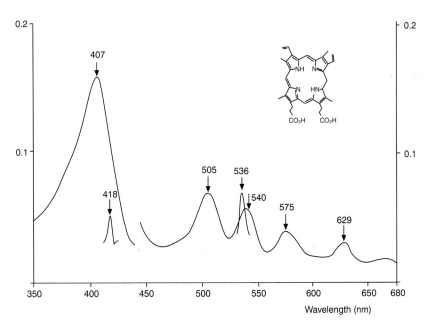

Protoporphyrin dimethyl ester

Fig. 58.2   The electronic spectrum and structure of the 2 major crystalline pigments (isolated as dimethyl esters) of *Porphyromonas* and *Prevotella* spp. The iron-containing porphyrin gives the cells their characteristic black colour on blood agar plates whereas the light brown, ultraviolet fluorescent colonies which are characteristic of some species such as *P. loescheii* are due to the production of protoporphyrin.

xylose. Members of the genus are identified by a small number of variable characteristics that include indole production, aesculin hydrolysis and the fermentation of lactose, sucrose, rhamnose, trehalose, mannitol, salicin and arabinose (Table 58.2).

Bacteroides fragilis   Isolates of this species cannot be distinguished from other members of the genus by their colonial form, or by their microscopic morphology, except that freshly isolated strains usually form a capsule. *B. fragilis* hydrolyses aesculin and produces acid from glucose, lactose, sucrose, maltose and usually xylose, but not from rhamnose, trehalose, mannitol, salicin or arabinose. Indole is not formed and charcoal–gelatin discs are digested slowly or not at all.

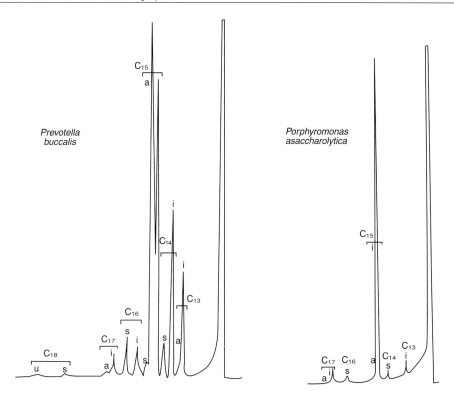

Fig. 58.3 A gas chromatographic trace of the long-chain fatty acid profile of a representative species of *Prevotella*, which characteristically possess high levels of *anteiso*-C_{15} fatty acids. By contrast, members of the genus *Porphyromonas* contain high levels of *iso*-C_{15} acids. The numbers given above the peaks indicate the number of carbons and the letters 'i', 'a', 'u' and 's' indicate whether the acids are *iso*- or *anteiso*-branched, unsaturated or saturated, respectively.

B. fragilis forms less than 10% of the *Bacteroides* in normal human faeces, yet it is by far the most common species of *Bacteroides* to be isolated from infections related to the large intestine (Duerden 1980a). It thus appears to be particularly pathogenic for humans. This may be attributable to its possession of a polysaccharide capsule (Kasper 1976a, 1976b) or to the action of one or more of the extracellular or membrane-associated enzymes that it forms: proteinases, including collagenase, fibrinolysin, haemolysin, neuraminidase, phosphatase, DNAase, hyaluronidase, chondroitin sulphatase and heparinase (Gesner and Jenkin 1961, Müller and Werner 1970, Rudek and Haque 1976).

The cell wall of *B. fragilis* contains a lipopolysaccharide (LPS) with weak endotoxic activity, the polysaccharide portion of which confers type-specific O-antigenic specificity. A species-specific protein component of the outer membrane has been identified; its presence may be used for the identification of *B. fragilis*. The pattern of proteins in the outer membrane shown by SDS-PAGE is also species-specific. External to the outer membrane is a thick polysaccharide capsule 1.5–2 times the thickness of the cell wall; it is composed of a high molecular weight polysaccharide ($>7.5 \times 10^3$ kDa). It has antiphagocytic properties and also protects the cell from complement mediated lysis by antibodies against cell wall antigens. The capsular antigen is species-specific. This capsule is found only in *B. fragilis*. All clinical isolates of *B. fragilis* are capsulate, but the capsule is often lost on repeated subculture; it can

be demonstrated in India ink preparations and identified by the Quellung reaction and in an indirect immunofluorescent assay.

Bacteroides vulgatus This species was first isolated from human faeces by Eggerth and Gagnon (1933). It is the most common *Bacteroides* species in normal human faeces but is only occasionally implicated in infections. Results of tolerance tests resemble those given by other members of the genus, but c. 50% of strains are tolerant of ethyl violet. Indole is not produced but charcoal–gelatin discs are digested within a few days. Unlike other members of the genus, c. 50% of *B. vulgatus* strains fail to hydrolyse aesculin and others do so only weakly.

Bacteroides distasonis This species was described by Eggerth and Gagnon (1933) in their studies of the faecal flora and named after the Romanian bacteriologist A Distaso. Like *B. vulgatus*, it is a common member of the normal human faecal flora but appears seldom to cause clinical infections. Most strains ferment rhamnose but a significant minority do not. Indole is not produced and charcoal–gelatin discs are digested slowly or not at all.

Bacteroides merdae Described by Johnson, Moore and Moore (1986) in a study of human faecal *Bacteroides*, this species shares the general characters of the genus. Indole is not produced, charcoal–gelatin discs may be digested slowly or not at all, and it is distinguished from other members of the genus by the ability to pro-

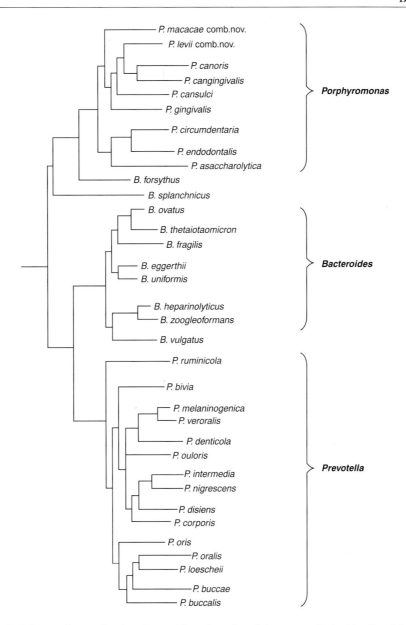

Fig. 58.4   Unrooted phylogenetic tree showing the position of species of the genera *Bacteroides*, *Prevotella* and *Porphyromonas*.

duce acid from trehalose and salicin, but not from rhamnose or arabinose.

Bacteroides caccae   B. *caccae* was described in the same study as *B. merdae* (Johnson, Moore and Moore 1986), from which it is distinguished by the ability to produce acid from rhamnose but not from salicin.

Bacteroides ovatus   B. *ovatus* is one of the less commonly encountered species of the genus. It is not a major component of the normal faecal flora and is isolated only occasionally from clinical specimens. When present in an infection it is usually in large numbers and appears to be a significant pathogen. It produces acid from a wider range of carbohydrates than other members of the genus. The ability to produce acid from salicin and mannitol is used to identify *B. ovatus*. Indole-positive, it digests charcoal–gelatin discs within a few days.

Bacteroides thetaiotaomicron   B. *thetaiotaomicron* was named by Distaso (1912) as a combination of the Greek letters theta, iota and omicron. It is a common commensal in normal human faeces and the second commonest species of the genus isolated from clinical infections, where it appears to have a significant pathogenic role. Acid is not formed from mannitol by this species and a variable reaction is obtained with the charcoal–gelatin disc; some strains digest it readily but others do so only weakly or not at all. In some studies all indole-positive members of the genus that were not *B. ovatus* were assigned to *B. thetaiotaomicron*. However, other indole-positive subgroups or species are known.

Bacteroides eggerthii   B. *eggerthii* was named after the American Bacteriologist A H Eggerth and described by Holdeman and Moore (1974b) following their studies on the human faecal flora. Acid formation from

Table 58.1 Species of the genus *Bacteroides* with their type strain

Bacteroides caccae	NCTC 13051; ATCC 43185
Bacteroides distasonis	NCTC 11152; ATCC 8503
Bacteroides eggerthii	NCTC 11155; ATCC 27754
Bacteroides fragilis[a]	NCTC 9343; ATCC 25285
Bacteroides merdae	NCTC 13052; ATCC 43184
Bacteroides ovatus	NCTC 11153; ATCC 8483
Bacteroides splanchnicus	NCTC 10825; ATCC 29572
Bacteroides stercoris	NCTC 13053; ATCC 43183
Bacteroides thetaiotaomicron	NCTC 10582; ATCC 29148
Bacteroides uniformis	NCTC 13054; ATCC 8492
Bacteroides variabilis	NCTC 13055
Bacteroides vulgatus	NCTC 11154; ATCC 8482

[a]Type species.

rhamnose but not sucrose distinguishes *B. eggerthii* from other indole-positive species of the genus. Isolates are able to digest charcoal–gelatin discs.

Bacteroides variabilis This species was described by Distaso in 1912 and is similar to *B. eggerthii* and to other indole-positive members of the genus, but was included in the species *B. thetaiotaomicron* in the eighth and ninth editions of *Bergey's Manual* (Holdeman and Moore 1974a, Holdeman, Kelley and Moore 1984). It is a common commensal in normal human faeces and isolated from a small proportion of infections in which *Bacteroides* spp. are implicated. Some strains are inhibited by sodium taurocholate but grow in 20% bile broth. No acid is produced from mannitol or trehalose. Charcoal–gelatin discs are usually digested within a few days.

Bacteroides uniformis This species was described by Eggerth and Gagnon in 1933. The organisms are normally found in human faeces but rarely implicated in clinical infections. In many studies, strains of *B. uniformis* have been included with other indole-positive strains as *B. thetaiotaomicron*. Like *B. variabilis*, some strains that grow well in 20% broth are inhibited by sodium taurocholate. Charcoal–gelatin discs are usually digested within a few days.

Bacteroides stercoris *B. stercoris* was described by Johnson, Moore and Moore (1986) in a study of human faecal *Bacteroides*. Acid is produced from sucrose and rhamnose but not from trehalose, arabinose or salicin and this distinguishes it from other indole-positive species of the *Bacteroides*.

Bacteroides splanchnicus *B. splanchnicus* has been isolated from normal human faeces and from several infections related to the lower gastrointestinal tract (Werner, Rintelen and Kunstek-Santos 1975); in particular, several strains were isolated in significant num-

bers from infectious complications of appendicitis. It shares many characters with other members of the *Bacteroides* but differs from them in one important respect: it is the only fermentative species of *Bacteroides* to form significant amounts of *n*-butyric acid. This it does in addition to forming a variety of other acids including *iso*-valeric, *iso*-butyric and propionic acids as well as acetic and succinic acids that are produced by all members of the *Bacteroides*. A minority of strains that grow well in 20% bile broth are inhibited by sodium taurocholate. Some strains digest charcoal–gelatin discs but others do not. This species shares many chemotaxonomic properties with members of the genus *Porphyromonas* and the result of 16S rRNA sequence analysis suggests that it is closely related to this lineage (Fig. 58.4).

3 PREVOTELLA

Oliver and Wherry (1921) described gram-negative anaerobic bacilli that produced black pigmented colonies when grown on blood agar; they called their strains *Bacterium melaninogenicum*; subsequently all pigmented strains were assigned to the species *Bacteroides melaninogenicus*. This characteristic appearance was regarded as highly specific and was the sole criterion for differentiation from other *Bacteroides* spp. Confusion surrounded studies on *B. melaninogenicus* because of the diversity of characters among pigmented strains and because of the specific requirements of some strains for growth factors such as vitamin K (Lev 1959), haemin and sodium succinate. Some *B. melaninogenicus* strains isolated from the normal flora, particularly the gingival crevice, are nutritionally demanding and require a variety of growth factors provided by co-cultivation with other bacteria but as yet unidentified.

The pigmented strains appeared to share several characters in addition to pigmentation, but there were major differences in metabolic and biochemical activity between groups, and *B. melaninogenicus* was divided into 3 subspecies: *melaninogenicus*, *intermedius* and *asaccharolyticus* (Sawyer, MacDonald and Gibbons 1962, Moore and Holdeman 1973). Studies of cell wall composition and DNA base ratios supported this division (Shah et al. 1976). Werner, Pulverer and Reichertz (1971) found that pigmented strains from human faeces and from infections related to the lower gastrointestinal tract formed a homogeneous group of asaccharolytic strains and recognized only these as *B. melaninogenicus*. The differences between the subspecies cast doubt upon the validity of assigning all pigmented strains to a single species. The asaccharolytic strains were distinguished from the saccharolytic strains by their production of *n*-butyric acid and also by differences in G + C content of the DNA and in cell wall composition. The ICSB taxonomic subcommittee on gram-negative anaerobic rods (Finegold and Barnes 1977) therefore proposed that the asaccharolytic strains should be classified as a separate species, *B. asaccharolyticus*. Further differences were found

Table 58.2 Distinguishing characteristics of species of the genus *Bacteroides*

Test	*B. fragilis*	*B. vulgatus*	*B. distasonis*	*B. merdae*	*B. caccae*	*B. ovatus*	*B. thetaiotaomicron*	*B. eggerthii*	*B. variabilis*	*B. uniformis*	*B. stercoris*	*B. splanchnicus*
Indole production	−	−	−	−	−	+	+	+	+	+	+	+
Aesculin hydrolysis	+	+/−	+	+	+	+	+	+	+	+	+	+
Fermentation of												
glucose	+	+	+	+	+	+	+	+	+	+	+	+
lactose	+	+	+	+	+	+	+	+	+	+	+	+
sucrose	+	+	+	+	+	+	+	−	+	+	+	−
rhamnose	−	−	+/−	−	+	+	+	−	−	−	−	−
trehalose	−	−	+	+	+	+	+	−	−	+	−	−
mannitol	−	−	−	−	−	+	−	−	−	−	−	−
xylose	+	+	+	+	+	+	+	+	+	+	+	+
arabinose	−	+	−	−	−	−	+	+	+	+	−	+
salicin	−	−	+	+	−	+	+	+	−	−	−	−

+, Positive result (growth in tolerance tests); −, negative result.

subsequently between *B. asaccharolyticus* strains associated with the intestinal flora and with superficial necrotizing infections, and pigmented non-fermentative strains associated with periodontal disease and dental root-canal infections. The latter 2 groups of isolates were assigned species status as *B. gingivalis* (Coykendall, Kaczmarek and Slots 1980) and *B. endodontalis* (van Steenbergen, Vlaarderen and de Graaf 1981), respectively, and both were later placed in the genus *Porphyromonas* (Shah and Collins 1988, see section 4, p. 1317).

The fermentative pigmented species that remained ('*B. melaninogenicus*') was also heterogeneous and was divided into several distinct species. *B. melaninogenicus* subspecies *melaninogenicus* was shown to comprise 3 species – *B. melaninogenicus* (*sensu stricto*), *Bacteroides loescheii* and *Bacteroides denticola* (Holdeman and Johnson 1982) – whereas *B. melaninogenicus* subspecies *intermedius* was divided into 2 species, *Bacteroides intermedius* and *Bacteroides corporis* (Johnson and Holdeman 1983). Before the elevation to species status, a weakly fermentative subspecies *levii* was proposed. The latter has now been elevated to species rank as *Porphyromonas levii* (Shah et al. 1995) and a second weakly fermentative species, *Porphyromonas macacae* (synonymous with *Porphyromonas salivosa*) has been proposed.

It is now clear that the production of pigmented colonies on media that contain blood has less taxonomic significance than was previously thought and both *Prevotella* and *Porphyromoas* include non-pigmented species. Formerly the *B. melaninogenicus–oralis* group included the fermentative pigmented species and several non-pigmented species that shared many common characters. The species *B. oralis* was originally proposed for non-pigmented bile- and penicillin-sensitive strains of *Bacteroides* isolated from the human mouth (Loesche, Socransky and Gibbons 1964), but the type strain of *B. oralis* proved to be pigmented and was first reclassified as *B. melaninogenicus* subspecies *melaninogenicus* (Holbrook and Duerden 1974) and subsequently as *B. loescheii* (Holdeman and Johnson 1982). However, other non-pigmented strains were described that corresponded to the original description of *B. oralis* or appeared to be related to it. These were represented by *B. oralis*, *Bacteroides veroralis* (Watabe, Benno and Mitsuoka 1983), *Bacteroides oris*, *Bacteroides buccae* (Holdeman et al. 1982), *Bacteroides zoogleoformans* (Cato et al. 1982) and *Bacteroides buccalis* (Shah and Collins 1981). Two other non-pigmented members of the melaninogenicus–oralis group, *Bacteroides disiens* and *Bacteroides bivius*, were isolated from human clinical infections by Holdeman and Johnson (1977) and have since been found in the normal vaginal flora and infections of the genitourinary tract, and occasionally in the mouth.

3.1 Description of the genus

The organisms are gram-negative, obligately anaerobic, non-spore-forming, non-motile pleomorphic rods. Surface colonies on blood agar plates vary from minute to 2.0 mm in diameter and are generally circular, entire, convex, shiny and smooth. Colonies on blood agar are translucent, opaque, grey, light brown or black. Haemolysis is variable. Glucose broth cultures are usually turbid with smooth or stringy sediments, and the terminal pH is between 4.5 and 5.2. The optimum temperature for growth is 37°C, but some strains grow at 25 and 45°C. Growth of most species is inhibited by 6.5% NaCl. Haemin and menadione are required for growth of most species. Growth is inhibited by 20% (w/v) bile. They are inhibited by sodium taurocholate and sodium deoxycholate and will not grow in 20% bile broth. They are inhibited by most dyes but many strains are tolerant of Victoria blue 4R (1 in 80 000). In antibiotic resistance tests, most strains are sensitive to neomycin (l000 µg), rifampicin (15 µg) and resistant to kanamycin (1000 µg) discs; many strains are sensitive to benzylpenicillin, but some strains of all species of the genus are resistant as a result of plasmid-coded β-lactamase production. Threonine is not dehydrogenated. The major fermentation products are acetic and succinic acid; occasionally lower levels of *iso*-butyric, *iso*-valeric or lactic acid are produced. Proteolytic activity is variable. Nearly all species are indole-negative. Nitrate is not reduced to nitrite. The cell wall peptidoglycan contains *meso*-diaminopimelic acid. The principal respiratory quinones are unsaturated menaquinones, often with 10–13 isoprene units. Both non-hydroxylated and 3-hydroxylated fatty acids are composed of predominantly straight-chain saturated, *anteiso*- and *iso*-methyl, branched-chain types. Sphingolipids are produced. The DNA base compositions are within the range of 40–52 mol% G + C. Other currently described species that conform to the generic description of *Prevotella* are given in Table 58.3. The genus was emended by Willems and Collins (1995c) to include species that are phylogenetically coherent but possess DNA base compositions within the range 40–60 mol% G + C. The type species is *Prevotella melaninogenica*. Characteristics that differentiate species of the genus *Prevotella* are given in Table 58.4.

Prevotella melaninogenica P. melaninogenica is a common commensal in the human gingival crevice and in the vagina in women and is found in infections related to these sites. Most strains are short gram-negative bacilli or coccobacilli and many are moderately pleomorphic. Colonies are 1–2 mm in diameter, round, convex and opaque. After incubation for 48 h they are typically light grey, becoming brown after further incubation. Pigmentation develops more rapidly on lysed blood agar and varies between strains from light brown to almost black; it begins in the centre of the colony and the colonies of many strains have a light brown or pale annulus around a dark-brown centre. Charcoal–gelatin discs are digested within a few days. The G + C content of the DNA is 40–42 mol% (Shah et al. 1976). Strains contain a peptidoglycan based upon *meso*-diaminopimelic acid.

Prevotella loescheii This pigmented species is named after W J Loesche; the type strain is ATCC 15930, ori-

Table 58.3 Species of the genus *Prevotella* with their type strain

Prevotella albensis	NCTC 13060; DSM 11370
Prevotella bivia	NCTC 11156; ATCC 29303
Prevotella brevis	NCTC 13061; ATCC 19188
Prevotella bryantii	NCTC 13062; DSM 11371
Prevotella buccae	NCTC 13063; ATCC 33574
Prevotella buccalis	NCTC 13064; ATCC 33779
Prevotella corporis	NCTC 13065; ATCC 33547
Prevotella dentalis	NCTC 13066; ATCC
Prevotella denticola	NCTC 13067; ATCC 35308
Prevotella disiens	NCTC 11157; ATCC 29426
Prevotella enoeca	NCTC 13068; ATCC 51261
Prevotella heparinolytica	NCTC 13069; ATCC 35895
Prevotella intermedia	NCTC 13070; ATCC 25611
Prevotella loescheii	NCTC 11321; ATCC 15930
Prevotella melaninogenica[a]	NCTC 12963; ATCC 25845
Prevotella nigrescens	NCTC 9336; ATCC 33563
Prevotella oralis	NCTC 11459; ATCC 33269
Prevotella oris	NCTC 13071; ATCC 33573
Prevotella oulora	NCTC 11871; ATCC 43324
Prevotella ruminicola	NCTC 13072; ATCC 19189
Prevotella tannerae	NCTC 13073; ATCC 51259
Prevotella veroralis	NCTC 13074; ATCC 33779
Prevotella zoogleoformans	NCTC 13075; ATCC 33285

[a]Type species.

ginally designated *B. oralis*. Pigment production is fairly slow, but is enhanced by growth on lysed blood agar. Ability to hydrolyse aesculin distinguishes it from *P. melaninogenica*. The DNA G + C content is 46–48 mol%.

Prevotella denticola Described by Shah and Collins (1981), this pigmented species is found in the gingival crevice and in human clinical specimens from sites in and around the mouth. It is distinguished from *P. melaninogenica* and *P. loescheii* by tests for hydrolysis of aesculin and fermentation of cellobiose. The G + C content of its DNA is higher than most species in this group at 49–51 mol%.

Prevotella intermedia and **Prevotella nigrescens** Isolates of these species initially belonged to *P. intermedia*. They are associated with the gingival crevice and are often isolated from cases of gingivitis and other purulent lesions related to the mouth. Most strains are short gram-negative bacilli and coccobacilli and many are pleomorphic. The colonies are 1–2 mm in diameter, round, convex and opaque. After incubation for 48 h, isolated colonies are typically grey but become uniformly black after further incubation. Some strains are shiny and glistening, but others are dull with a rough, dry surface and these may adhere to the underlying medium. Pigmentation develops more rapidly on lysed blood agar. Most strains produce clear zones of complete haemolysis in blood agar and are inhibited by Victoria blue 4R. Strains produce indole, readily digest charcoal–gelatin discs and do not ferment lactose. The G + C content of the DNA is 40–42 mol%. Lambe and Jerris (1976) described 2 distinct serogroups. Johnson and Holdeman (1983) have described 2 DNA homology groups, which were recently confirmed (Shah and Gharbia 1992) using multilocus enzyme electrophoresis, DNA–DNA homology and subsequently 16S rRNA sequence analysis. This resulted in the proposal of the species *P. nigrescens* for the second homology group.

Prevotella corporis *P. corporis* was described by Johnson and Holdeman (1983) to represent strains isolated from clinical human specimens previously considered to be *P. intermedia* but which do not produce indole or ferment sucrose. The DNA G + C content is 43–46 mol%.

Prevotella oralis Strains that correspond to the original description (Loesche, Socransky and Gibbons 1964) are an important component of the normal flora of the gingival crevice, and similar strains have been isolated from the normal vagina. Non-pigmented oral strains have also been implicated in infections derived from these sites. All these infections are associated with tissue necrosis and the production of foul-smelling pus. Colonies of *P. oralis* are 1–2 mm in diameter, semi-opaque and light-buff or grey; after prolonged incubation some become pale brown and some develop a spreading edge with an irregular outline. Most strains are predominantly coccobacillary but a few produce longer, more regular bacilli. Most strains hydrolyse aesculin and digest charcoal–gelatin discs within a few days.

Prevotella veroralis This species differs from *P. oralis* in failing to ferment salicin and has negligible DNA homology with that species (Watabe, Benno and Mitsuoka 1983). It more closely fits the original description of *P. oralis* (Loesche, Socransky and Gibbons 1964) than the strains now designated *P. oralis*. The DNA G + C content is 42 mol%.

Prevotella buccalis *P. buccalis* is indistinguishable from *P. veroralis* in most routine conventional tests and has a similar DNA base composition. However, unlike *P. veroralis*, it produces *iso*-valeric acid as a major metabolic product and it does not hydrolyse starch (Watabe, Benno and Mitsuoka 1983). These differences are supported by lack of DNA homology between *P. buccalis* strains and other *Prevotella* spp.

Prevotella zoogleoformans This species was described by Weinberg, Nativelle and Prévot (1937), and Prévot (1938) proposed a new genus *Capsularis* for these strains. Moore, Johnson and Moore (1994) emended the description of the species. No early strains remain extant, but Cato et al. (1982) isolated strains that fulfilled the description from the gingival crevice of patients with periodontal disease. The specific epithet

Table 58.4 Characteristics that differentiate *Prevotella* species

Species	Arabinose	Cellobiose	Lactose	Mannose	Raffinose	Salicin	Xylose	Aesculin	Gelatin	Pigment
P. albensis	+	+	+	−	−	+	+	+	+	−
P. bivia	−	−	+	+	+	−	−	−	+	−
P. brevis	+	+	+	+	+	−	−	+	+	−
P. bryantii	+	+	+	+	+	+	+	+	+	−
P. corporis	−	−	+	+	+	−	−	−	+	+
P. dentalis	+	+	+	+	+	−	−	+	−	−
P. disiens	−	−	+	−	−	−	−	+	+	−
P. enoeca	−	−	+	v	−	+	v	v	+	−
P. heparinolytica	+	+	+	+	−	+	+	+	−	−
P. intermedia	−	−	−	v	v	−	−	−	+	+
P. loescheii	−	v	+	+	+	v	−	+	+	+
P. melaninogenica	−	+	+	+	+	−	−	v	+	+
P. oralis	−	+	+	+	+	+	−	+	−	−
P. oris	+	+	+	+	+	+	+	+	v	−
P. oulora	−	−	+	+	+	−	−	+	−	−
P. ruminicola	+	+	+	+	+	+	−	+	+	−
P. tannerae	−	−	v	v	v	−	v	v	+	v
P. veroralis	−	v	+	+	+	v	−	+	+	−
P. zoogleoformans	v	v	v	v	v	v	v	+	v	−

+, Positive result; −, negative result; v, variable result.

'zoogleoformans' represents the character of this organism's growth in broth culture; it forms a viscous, glutinous mass, especially in the presence of fermentable carbohydrate. Most strains except the type strain produce indole, ferment cellobiose and hydrolyse aesculin. The major cellular fatty acids are predominantly *iso*-$C_{15:0}$ and *anteiso*-$C_{15:0}$ acids. The G + C content of the type strain ATCC 33285 is 47 mol%. Recently rRNA sequence analysis has indicated a closer affinity with the genus *Bacteroides* (see Fig. 58.4, p. 1311).

Prevotella oris* and *Prevotella buccae These 2 species accommodate strains of human origin that were previously identified as *B. ruminicola* subspecies *brevis* biovar (biotype) 3. Similar strains have been isolated from chicken caeca. The human isolates are mostly from gingival margins and periodontal pockets and infections at related sites. They differ from *P. oralis* by their ability to ferment pentoses, which is the reason for their earlier confusion with *P. ruminicola*. The DNA G + C content for *P. oris* is 42–46 mol%, whereas for *P. buccae* it is 50–52 mol% (Holdeman et al. 1982).

Prevotella heparinolytica Isolated from patients with periodontitis, this species produces acid from a range of sugars, including pentoses, is indole-positive, hydrolyses aesculin and produces heparinase (Okuda et al. 1985). rRNA sequence analysis indicates a closer affinity with the genus *Bacteroides* (see Fig. 58.4, p. 1311).

Prevotella oulora *P. oulora* is also found in the mouth. It ferments only a limited range of sugars, is indole-negative and does not hydrolyse aesculin; it produces a lipase (Shah et al. 1985).

Prevotella bivia Isolated from human infections by Holdeman and Johnson (1977), this is the commonest species of *Prevotella* in the normal human vaginal flora (Duerden 1980b). Most clinical isolates are from infections related to the female genital tract. It cannot be recognized by cell morphology or colonial appearance and does not form pigment, but colonies are often pale brown after prolonged incubation on lysed blood agar. Few strains hydrolyse aesculin, but charcoal–gelatin discs are digested within a few days. The DNA G + C content is 40 mol%.

Prevotella disiens Described by Holdeman and Johnson (1977) at the same time as *P. bivia* and isolated from similar infections and from the normal vaginal flora, strains of *P. disiens* differ from *P. bivia* by their inability to ferment lactose. The DNA G + C content is 40–42 mol%.

Prevotella dentalis Isolates of this species were previously reported as *Hallella seregens* or *Mitsuokella dentalis*. rRNA sequence analysis confirmed that they are similar and are genealogically related to *Prevotella* (Willems and Collins 1995c). Strains are isolated from dental root canals and are distinguished from other *Prevotella* spp. by the typical water drop appearance of its colonies on solid medium. The DNA G + C content is 56–60 mol%.

Prevotella enoeca This saccharolytic species was isolated from the gingival crevice of humans. Colonies are small, 1–2 mm in diameter, non-haemolytic, non-pigmented and strains characteristically ferment glycogen and lactose but not sucrose and are unable to ferment gelatin. The end products of metabolism are acetic and succinic acids and, in common with most *Prevotella* spp., *P. enoeca* contains *anteiso*-$C_{15:0}$ as its major cellular fatty acid. The G + C content of the type strain ATCC 51261 is 47 mol%.

Prevotella tannerae This species colonizes the human gingival crevice and contains strains that produce small, circular colonies, 1 mm in diameter, that may be black, tan to brown, reddish or colourless on rabbit blood agar medium. Most strains are unable to hydrolyse aesculin but produce acid from glycogen and lactose. The fermentation acids are mainly succinic and acetic with lower levels of formic, *iso*-valeric and *iso*-butyric acids. Its major cellular fatty acids are *iso*-$C_{15:0}$ and *anteiso*-$C_{15:0}$ acids. The G + C content of the type strain ATCC 51259 is 45 mol%.

Prevotella ruminicola This species is isolated from the rumen and from the hindgut of many mammalian species. Most strains produce clear zones which are visible after staining with congo red. Most strains ferment arbutin and salicin, and are stimulated by haem in the absence of rumen fluid. The DNA G + C content is 45–52 mol%.

Prevotella albensis *P. albensis* is isolated from the rumen and from the hindgut of many mammalian species. Strains do not ferment melibiose, sucrose or mannose but ferment xylose. The DNA G + C content is 39–43 mol%.

Prevotella brevis *P. brevis* is isolated from the rumen and from the hindgut of many mammalian species. Most strains produce abundant extracellular DNAase activity and do not ferment xylose. Many strains can grow with gum arabic as an energy source. The DNA G + C content is 45–52 mol%.

Prevotella bryantii *P. bryantii* is isolated from the rumen and from the hindgut of many mammalian species. Most strains produce abundant extracellular DNAase and ferment xylose. The DNA G + C content is 39–43 mol%.

4 PORPHYROMONAS

4.1 Description of the genus

Porphyromonas spp. are gram-negative, obligately anaerobic non-spore-forming, non-motile rods or coccobacilli (Table 58.5). Most cells in broth are small (0.5–0.8 by 1.0–3.5 μm) but occasionally longer cells (4–6 μm) may be formed. Surface colonies on blood agar plates are smooth (rarely rough), shiny, convex, circular, entire and vary from minute to 3.0 mm in diameter and darken progressively from the edge toward the centre after 6–10 days. Eventually the entire colony becomes black due to an overproduction of proto-haem (Fig. 58.2). The optimum temperature for growth is 37°C. Growth is not significantly affected by carbohydrates. Nitrogenous substrates such as pro-teose peptone, trypticase and yeast extract markedly enhance growth. The major fermentation products from media containing these substrates are *n*-butyric, propionic and acetic acids with lower levels of *iso*-butyric, *iso*-valeric, succinic and phenylacetic acids. Some species are strongly proteolytic whereas others show weak peptidase activities.

Malate and glutamate dehydrogenases are present in cell extracts. With the exception of a few species isolated from animals, glucose-6-phosphate and 6-pho-sphogluconate dehydrogenases are absent. Amino acids, particularly aspartic and glutamic acids, are fer-mented. Indole is produced by most species and nitrate is not reduced to nitrite.

Growth of all the pigmented species is inhibited by vancomycin. The cell wall peptidoglycan contains lysine or *meso*-diaminopimelic acid. The principal res-piratory quinones are unsaturated menaquinones. Both non-hydroxylated and 3-hydroxylated fatty acids are present. The non-hydroxylated fatty acids are com-posed of predominantly *iso*-methyl branched-chain types (iso-$C_{15:0}$) and lower levels of straight-chain satu-rated types (Fig. 58.3). The 3-hydroxylated fatty acids are the straight-chain saturated types. Sphingolipids are produced. The DNA base compositions are within the range 40–55 mol% G + C. Salient features of the species of the genus are given in Table 58.6. The genus was emended recently by Willems and Collins (1995b) to include species that are phylogenetically coherent but lack some of the key features of the ori-ginal description of this genus, such as pigment pro-

Table 58.5 Species of genus *Porphyromonas* with their type strain

Porphyromonas asaccharolytica[a]	NCTC 9337; ATCC 25260
Porphyromonas cangingivalis	NCTC 12856
Porphyromonas canoris	NCTC 12835
Porphyromonas cansulci	NCTC 12858
Porphyromonas catoniae	NCTC 13056; ATCC 51270
Porphyromonas circumdentaria	NCTC 12469
Porphyromonas crevioricanis	NCTC 13057; ATCC 55563
Porphyromonas endodontalis	NCTC 13058; ATCC 35406
Porphyromonas gingivalis	NCTC 11834; ATCC 33277
Porphyromonas gingivicanis	NCTC 13059; ATCC 55562
Porphyromonas levii	NCTC 11028; ATCC 29147
Porphyromonas macacae[b]	NCTC 11632; ATCC 33141

[a]Type species.
[b]Formerly *P. salivosa*.

duction and their inability to ferment carbohydrates. The type species of the genus *Porphyromonas* is *Porphy-romonas asaccharolytica*.

Porphyromonas asaccharolytica These organisms are mainly coccobacilli with only a few slightly longer bacilli. Very small colonies may be visible on blood agar after 24 h but some strains do not appear for 48 h. They are smooth, shiny and grey or brown. Pigmen-tation begins to develop after 3–4 days on whole blood agar but may be visible in the inoculum after 36–48 h on lysed blood agar. After 4–5 days colonies are 0.5–1 mm in diameter, black or very dark brown. The col-onies are smooth and shiny; they are often very moist and can be smeared over the agar surface, although the organisms do not produce large amounts of extra-cellular mucus. Most strains have a characteristically strong, putrid smell. The major end products of metabolism in a cooked meat–carbohydrate medium are *n*-butyric and acetic acids together with lower lev-els of propionic, *iso*-butyric and *iso*-valeric acids. *P. asaccharolytica* is inhibited by bile and bile salts and by dyes, resistant to kanamycin and sensitive to penicillin and rifampicin; most strains are sensitive to neomycin (1000 μg per disc) but some are resistant. *P. asaccharo-lytica* does not agglutinate sheep or horse erythrocytes (Slots and Genco 1979). The G + C content of the DNA is 52–54 mol%. *P. asaccharolytica* is found in nor-mal human faeces but less consistently and in smaller numbers than *Bacteroides* spp.; it has also been reported in the normal vagina. It is an important pathogen in mixed infections but is rarely isolated alone; it is found in infections related to the lower gastrointestinal tract and in destructive ulcers and gan-grene in diabetics and others with peripheral vascular disease. It should be noted that early work on the experimental pathogenicity of '*B. melaninogenicus*' (Werner, Pulverer and Reichertz 1971) was probably done with *P. asaccharolytica*.

Porphyromonas cangingivalis This species is isolated from the subgingival flora of dogs. Cells are coccoids, 0.3–0.6 μm, and occur singly or in clumps; occasion-ally filaments up to 16 μm long are observed. On sheep blood agar plates, surface colonies after 2 days are 1 mm in diameter, circular, dome shaped, non-haemolytic and smooth. Colonies are poorly pig-mented and cream after 3–5 days and by 10 days are light brown. On egg yolk agar colonies are yellow or orange. This species produces acetic, propionic, *iso*-butyric, *n*-butyric, *iso*-valeric, succinic and phenylacetic acids as metabolic end products. Strains produce catal-ase and acid and alkaline phosphatases, but do not produce any proteinases or lipases. The G + C content of the DNA is 49–51 mol%.

Porphyromonas canoris Isolated from the gingival sul-cus of dogs, the cells are rod-shaped and are 0.3–0.6 by 0.8–1.5 μm but filaments up to 16 μm are sometimes present. After growth for 48 h on sheep blood agar plates, surface colonies are 1.5 mm in diameter, circu-lar and rough and have an orange pigmentation. Between 3 and 6 days colonies exhibit a brick red fluorescence when irradiated with shortwave UV radi-

Table 58.6 Distinguishing features of members of the genus *Porphyromonas*

Species	Pigment	Indole	Catalase	Lipase	PAA	Glucose	α-Fucosidase	β-NAG	Trypsin	Chymotrypsin	α-Gal	β-Gal
P. asaccharolytica	+	+	–	–	–	–	+	–	–	–	–	–
P. cangingivalis	+	+	+	–	–	–	–	–	–	+	–	–
P. cansulci	+	+	+[w]	–	+	–	–	+	–	–	–	–
P. canoris	+	+	+	–	–	–	–	+	–	+	–	+
P. catoniae	–	–	–	–	–	+	+	–	–[+]	+[–]	–[+]	+
P. circumdentaria	+	+	+	–	+	–	–	–	–	–	–	–
P. cervioricanis	+	+	–	NT	+	NT	–	–	–	NT	NT	NT
P. endodotalis	+	+	–	–	–	–	–	+	–	–	–	–
P. gingivalis	+	+	–	–	+	–	–	–	+	–	–	–
P. gingivicanis	+	+	+	NT	–	NT	–	+	–	NT	NT	NT
P. levii	+	–	–	–		W	–	+	–	+	–	+
P. macacae	+	+	+	+	+	W	–	–	+	+	+	–

+, Positive reaction; –, negative reaction; w, weak reaction; NT, not tested.
PAA, phenylacetic acid production; α-Fucosidase, α-Fucosidase activity, NAG, *N*-acetyl-β-glucosaminidase activity; Trypsin, hydrolysis of trypsin substrate; Chymotrypsin, hydrolysis of chymotrypsin substrates; α-Gal, α-galactosidase activity, β-Gal, β-galactosidase activity.

ation (265 nm) but this changes to a light orange after 13 days. Pigmentation occurs faster with laked blood. The major end products of metabolism in cooked meat–carbohydrate medium are acetic, propionic, *iso*-valeric and succinic acids together with low levels of *n*-butyric and *iso*-butyric acids. Lactate is converted to propionate but neither pyruvate nor threonine is utilized. Strains are catalase-, acid- and alkaline phosphatase-positive, liquefy gelatin and possess chymotrypsin activity. Both acid and alkaline phosphatases are produced. A wide spectrum of oxidoreductases are produced, including malate, glutamate, glucose-6-phosphate and 6-phosphogluconate dehydrogenases. The non-hydroxylated fatty acids are composed of predominantly *iso*-methyl branched types, with *iso*-$C_{15:0}$ acid predominating. The G + C content of the DNA is 49–51 mol%.

Porphyromonas cansulci This species is isolated from the subgingival flora of dogs. Cells are coccoid, 0.3–0.6 μm and occur singly or in groups. On sheep blood agar plates, surface colonies after 3 days are 1–2 mm in diameter, circular, dome-shaped and smooth. Colonies are black or brown after 5 days. On egg yolk agar colonies are yellow or orange. This species produces a wide spectrum of fermentation products that includes acetic, propionic, *iso*-butyric, *n*-butyric, *iso*-valeric, succinic and phenylacetic acids. Neither lactate nor pyruvate is utilized and threonine is not converted to propionate. Strains produce catalase and acid and alkaline phosphatases, but do not produce any proteinases or lipases. The G + C content of the DNA is 49–51 mol%.

Porphyromonas catoniae Isolated from the gingival crevice of humans, strains were of uncertain taxonomic designation initially and were temporarily placed in a group referred to as '*Bacteroides* D26'.

These were subsequently assigned to a new genus, *Oribaculum catoniae*, by Moore and Moore (1994) but later transferred to the genus *Porphyromonas* by Willems and Collins (1995b) based on comparative analysis of approximately 96% of the total primary sequence of the 16S rRNA. At present, this is the only non-pigmented and saccharolytic member of the genus. Colonies on blood agar plates are 0.5–2 mm in diameter, circular, entire flat to low convex, and transparent. Cells grown in a glucose-containing medium (e.g. peptone–yeast extract–glucose; PYG) produce a terminal pH of 5.0–5.5 and their metabolic end products are mainly acetic and succinic acids with low levels of formic, lactic and *iso*-valeric acids. The major cellular fatty acids are *iso*-$C_{15:0}$ and *anteiso*-$C_{15:0}$ but substantial levels of *iso*-$C_{13:0}$ are also produced. The DNA base compositions are in the range 49–51 mol% G + C.

Porphyromonas circumdentaria This species is isolated from soft tissue infections, the gingival margins and gingival plaques of cats. On sheep blood agar plates, colonies after 72 h are 1–2 mm in diameter, circular, entire, dome-shaped and are greenish brown but become creamy brown by 7 days. During this period, colonies exhibit a brick red fluorescence when irradiated with shortwave UV radiation (254 nm). By 14 days, colonies are brown to black. Cells are rod-shaped and are 0.3–0.6 by 0.8–1.5 μm but filaments up to 10 μm are sometimes present. The major end products of metabolism in cooked meat–carbohydrate medium are acetic, *n*-butyric and *iso*-valeric acids with lower levels of propionic, *iso*-butyric, succinic and phenylacetic acids. Strains are catalase-positive, produce ammonia and liquefy gelatin. Both acid and alkaline phosphatases are produced. The G + C content of the DNA is 40–42 mol%.

Porphyromonas crevioricans *P. crevioricans* is isolated from the gingival crevicular fluid of beagle dogs. Colonies on rabbit blood agar plates after 72 h are tiny, 0.8–1.5 mm in diameter, circular, entire, dome-shaped, opaque and brown or black The major end products of metabolism in GAM medium (Nissul, Tokyo, Japan) are acetic, propionic and *iso*-valeric acids with lower levels of *n*-butyric, *iso*-butyric, succinic and phenylacetic acids. Malate and glutamate dehydrogenases are present in cell extracts but glucose-6-phosphate and 6-phosphogluconate dehydrogenases are absent. Cells haemagglutinate sheep erythrocytes. Strains so far tested (Hirasawa and Takada 1994) are susceptible to penicillin (0.5 U per disc), amoxycillin (2 µg per disc), sulbenicillin (5 µg per disc) and erythromycin (0.5 µg per disc). The non-hydroxylated fatty acids are composed of predominantly *iso*-methyl branched types, with *iso*-$C_{15:0}$ acid predominating. The G + C content of the DNA is 44–45 mol%.

Porphyromonas endodontalis This pigmented species is more difficult to culture on primary isolation but becomes easier to maintain with repeated subculture. Initially colonies are very sticky and adhere strongly to the medium. It is isolated from infected dental root canals with severe periapical destruction (van Steenbergen et al. 1984). Colonies on blood agar plates are shiny, smooth, convex and circular. Major fermentation products are *n*-butyric and acetic acids; lower levels of propionic, *iso*-butric, *iso*-valeric acids are produced but phenylacetic acid is not produced. The G + C content of the DNA is 49–51 mol%.

Porphyromonas gingivalis Cells are non-motile rods or coccobacilli and are 0.5–2 µm long. Colonies on blood agar are smooth, shiny, convex and 1–2 mm in diameter and darken from the edge of the colony toward the centre between 4 and 8 days. Non-pigmented colonies rarely occur. Growth is markedly affected by the presence of protein hydrolysates such as trypticase, proteose peptone and yeast extract. Growth is enhanced by 0.5–0.8% NaCl. Major fermentation products are *n*-butyric and acetic acids; lower levels of propionic, *iso*-butyric, *iso*-valeric and phenylacetic acids are also produced. Cysteine proteinases and collagenases are present. Cells agglutinate sheep erythrocytes. Cell wall peptidoglycan contains lysine as the diamino acid. Both non-hydroxylated and 3-hydroxylated fatty acids are present. The non-hydroxylated fatty acids are composed of predominantly *iso*-methyl branched types, with *iso*-$C_{15:0}$ acid predominating. The major respiratory quinones are menaquinone with 9 isoprene units. The G + C content of the DNA is 46–48 mol%.

Porphyromonas gingivicans This species is isolated from the gingival crevicular fluid of beagle dogs. Colonies on rabbit blood agar after 72 h are tiny, 0.8–1.5 mm in diameter, circular, entire, dome-shaped, opaque and brown or black. The major end products of metabolism in GAM medium (Nissul, Tokyo, Japan) are acetic, *n*-butyric, and *iso*-valeric acids with lower levels of propionic, *iso*-butyric and succinic acids. Mal-

ate and glutamate dehydrogenases are present in cell extracts but glucose-6-phosphate and 6-phosphogluconate dehydrogenases are absent. Strains are catalase-positive. Cells neither agglutinate sheep erythrocytes nor exhibit trypsin nor *N*-acetyl-β-glucosaminidase activity. Strains so far tested (Hirasawa and Takada 1994) are susceptible to penicillin (0.5 U per disc), amoxycillin (2 µg per disc), sulbenicillin (5 µg per disc) and erythromycin (0.5 µg per disc). The non-hydroxylated fatty acids are composed of predominantly *iso*-methyl branched types, with *iso*-$C_{15:0}$ acid predominating. The G + C content of the DNA is 41–42 mol%.

Porphyromonas levii Named after M Lev, who isolated it from cattle (Lev 1959), this species produces dark brown colonies slowly on blood agar and more promptly on lysed blood agar. Unlike most pigmented members of the genus, it is weakly fermentative and weakly ferments glucose and lactose but not other carbohydrates. Charcoal–gelatin discs are digested within a few days. *P. levii* produces *n*-butyric acid as its major product of metabolism with moderate levels of acetic, propionic, *iso*-butyric and *iso*-valeric acids. The non-hydroxylated fatty acids are composed of major levels of *iso*-$C_{15:0}$ and *anteiso*-$C_{15:0}$ acids. The G + C content of the DNA is 45–48 mol%.

Porphyromonas macacae This species is weakly fermentative and has been isolated from periodontal lesions in monkeys (Slots and Genco 1980). Strains are catalase-positive, produce ammonia and possess both trypsin and chymotrypsin activities. Strains are indole-positive and are further distinguished from *P. levii* by production of propionic acid and not butyric acid as the major metabolic product. This species possesses a wide spectrum of oxidoreductases that include malate, glutamate, glucose-6-phosphate and 6-phosphogluconate dehydrogenases. The non-hydroxylated fatty acids are composed of predominantly *iso*-methyl branched types, with *iso*-$C_{15:0}$ acid predominating. The DNA G + C content is 43–44 mol% (Coykendall, Kaczmarec and Slots 1980).

5 THE CURRENT STATUS OF SPECIES THAT PREVIOUSLY BELONGED TO THE GENUS *BACTEROIDES*

The emphasis today to develop taxonomic schemes that reflect 'natural' or 'evolutionary' relationships among bacteria has led to re-examination of many taxa that only superficially resemble the generic description of type species. Members of the genus *Bacteroides* have been subjected to rigorous chemotaxonomic analysis and the results from these studies have been largely confirmed by molecular systematic analysis. Thus, the more restricted definition of the genus *Bacteroides* and the proposal of *Prevotella* and *Porphyromonas* have been borne out by data derived from comparative sequence analysis of 16S rRNAs (see Fig. 58.4, p. 1311) whereas others that have been excluded from the genus have been substantiated by these tests (see reviews by Shah and Collins 1983, Shah, Gharbia and Collins 1997). The current status of some of these taxa are described below.

Bacteroides ureolyticus and Bacteroides gracilis *B. ureolyticus* is a non-fermentative, non-pigmented species that characteristically 'pits or corrodes' the agar around the colonies. It was first described by Henriksen in clinical specimens in 1948 and later by Eiken (1958) who isolated 21 strains from abscesses, principally from the buccal region, and assigned them to the genus *Bacteroides* as *Bacteroides corrodens*. Khairat (1967) cultivated a similar organism from blood cultures after tooth extraction and also 3 strains phenotypically similar from the gingival crevice. Reinhold (1966) found it in abscesses and Schröter and Stawru (1970) in diseased tonsils. It was renamed *B. ureolyticus* to clarify the distinction between it and *Eikenella corrodens*, an aerobic and facultatively anaerobic, carbon dioxide-dependent organism that also forms 'corroding' colonies; the 2 were often confused in early reports (Jackson and Goodman 1978). This species was subsequently shown to share few biochemical and chemical properties with the genus *Bacteroides sensu stricto* (see Shah and Collins 1983) and was excluded from the redefined genus. *B. gracilis* shares a number of common properties with *B. ureolyticus* in that it is non-pigmented, asaccharolytic, micro-aerophilic and colonies often show pitting or corroding growth indistinguishable from that of *B. ureolyticus*. However, it is oxidase-negative and does not produce urease, although some strains reduce nitrate to nitrite (Tanner et al. 1981). Chemotaxonomic analyses, DNA–rRNA hybridization and 16S rRNA sequence analysis have shown that both species belong to the genus *Campylobacter* and *B. ureolyticus* has been formally reclassified in this genus (Vandamme et al. 1995).

Bacteroides praeacutus Strains have been isolated from human faeces and from clinical specimens. *B. praeacutus* differs from other species of *Bacteroides* in being motile by means of peritrichous flagella and so markedly in biochemical and chemical properties (e.g. its G + C content is 28 mol%) from other members that it was excluded from the emended description of the genus *Bacteroides* (Shah and Collins 1983) and was reproposed in the genus *Tissierella*, as *Tissierella praeacuta*. The 16S RNA gene sequence has shown that this species is synonymous with *Clostridium hastiforme*.

Bacteroides pneumosintes *B. pneumosintes* is a very small bacillus that is filterable through Berkfeld V and N filters and is unreactive in most conventional bacteriological tests. It was described by Olitsky and Gates (1921, 1922) in nasopharyngeal washings from patients in the 1918 influenza pandemic and called *Dialister pneumosintes*; these authors thought that it was a significant pathogen. It has since been isolated from normal persons, but it may be concerned in secondary infections of the respiratory tract, including lung abscesses, and in metastatic brain abscesses. Long con-

sidered to be outside the generic description of *Bacteroides* (see Shah and Collins 1983), the genus *Dialister* was revived by Moore and Moore (1994) to accommodate this species. More recently, it was shown by Willems and Collins (1995a) that these micro-organisms belong to the *Sporomusa* subbranch of the *Clostridium* subphylum.

Bacteroides coagulans *B. coagulans* is so named because it clots milk. It is isolated from human faeces, the urogenital tract and occasionally from clinical specimens. In general, this species is unreactive and remains poorly addressed. Surface colonies on horse blood agar are punctate, entire, slightly raised, translucent and non-haemolytic. Glucose broth cultures are poor and no acid is produced. It produces elastase, and H_2S is detectable with lead acetate paper. The G + C content of the DNA is 37 mol%. This species remains *incertae sedis*.

Bacteroides nodosus *B. nodosus* is a significant pathogen, causing foot rot in sheep (Egerton and Parsonson 1966) and possibly also in goats and cattle (Wilkinson, Egerton and Dickson 1970); the hoof seems to be its natural habitat. The cells are irregular with terminal enlargements, especially in smears prepared directly from lesions. It is strongly proteolytic and will digest powdered hoof in vitro. The DNA G + C content is 45 mol%. It was reclassified in a new genus *Dichelobacter* as *Dichelobacter nodosus*.

Bacteroides putredinis and Bacteroides microfusus Despite being non-fermentative, some strains of *B. putredinis* grow in a glucose broth to produce cells that are either straight or curved with rounded ends. Some cells produce swellings at one end but spores have not been detected. Strains are proteolytic and some may digest cooked meat. *B. putredinis* produces fibrinolysin and may be isolated from faeces, abdominal and rectal abscesses, cases of acute appendicitis, and foot rot in sheep; it has been reported from the human oral cavity. It shares very few characters with members of the genus *Bacteroides* and recent 16S rRNA sequence analysis (Paster et al. 1994) has shown this species to be most closely related to *Rikenella microfusus* (formerly *Bacteroides microfusus*). Both species show close affinity to the genus *Cytophaga*.

Bacteroides forsythus This species is closely related to *B. distasonis* but both these species are more compatible with the genus *Porphyromonas* based on 16S rRNA sequence analysis.

Bacteroides ochraceus This species was shown to be distantly related to the genus *Bacteroides* and to contain several centres of variation. These have now been assigned to the genus *Capnocytophaga* as *Capnocytophaga ochracea* (the type species), *Capnocytophaga canimorsus*, *Capnocytophaga cynodegmi*, *Capnocytophaga gingivalis*, *Capnocytophaga granulosa*, *Capnocytophaga haemolytica* and *Capnocytophaga sputigena*.

Bacteroides succinogenes and Bacteroides amylophilus Both these species are associated with the rumen and are biochemically and chemically unrelated to the genus *Bacteroides*. They have been reclassified in the genera *Fibrobacter* and *Ruminobacter*, respectively.

Bacteroides capillosus This species was described in 1908 and still remains poorly studied. It has been isolated from a wide range of animals and also from the human mouth and from the faeces of both infants and adults. Strains are generally non-fermentative unless Tween 80 is added to the medium. Deoxyribonucleases and phosphatases are produced. The unusually high G + C content of 60 mol% and other properties suggest that this species does not belong to the genera *Bacteroides*, *Prevotella* or *Porphyromonas*.

Bacteroides furcosus, Bacteroides microfusus, Bacteroides termitidis, Bacteroides multiacidus, Bacteroides hypermegas These species share few properties with the genus *Bacteroides* and have been reclassified as *Anaerorhabdus furcosus*, *Rikenella microfusus*, *Sebaldella termitidis*, *Mitsuokella multiacidus* and *Megamonas hypermegas* (see review Shah and Gharbia 1997). 16S rRNA sequence analysis has shown that some of these genera such as *Sebaldella* and *Anaerorhabdus* show a close affinity with gram-positive taxa of the *Clostridium* subphylum. The genera *Mitsuokella* and *Megamonas* cluster with *Selenomonas* and *Pectinatus*.

6 ANTIBIOTIC RESISTANCE

Gram-negative anaerobes are sensitive to metronidazole but are resistant to aminoglycosides, quinolones and monobactams. Until a few years ago, most members of the Bacteroidaceae were susceptible to antimicrobial agents such as clindamycin, chloramphenicol, erythromycin and tetracyclines. Over the years antibiotic resistance has been increasingly reported. *Bacteroides* spp. have been shown to acquire resistance rapidly to most β-lactam antibiotics (minimal inhibitory concentration usually exceeds 16 mg l^{-1}). This is associated with the production of broad spectrum β-lactamases (Olsson, Dornbusch and Nord 1979). In 1955, the first cases of resistance to penicillin were described (Garrod 1955). A noninducible cephalosporin was isolated from strains of *B. fragilis* and to date 93% of resistant strains produce β-lactamases. Similar patterns were reported among *B. ovatus*, *B. vulgatus*, *B. thetaiotaomicron* and *B. distasonis*. Lower incidences of β-lactamases (40–60%) have been reported for *Prevotella* and *Porphyromonas*. Pencillinases and cephalosporinases were reported from *P. disiens*, *P. buccae*, *P. oris*, *P. melaninogenica* and *P. asaccharolytica*. Most β-lactamases produced are constitutive cephalosporinases, although penicillinases and enzymes that hydrolyse cefoxitin and imipenem have been described. Both chromosomally mediated and plasmid mediated penicillin resistance have been described, with the production of at least 6 different β-lactamase types.

Resistance to chloromphinicol is mediated by either a nitroreductase or an acetyltransferase. Although both mechanisms have been observed among *Bacteroides* spp., the acetyltransferase activity is transferable among *Bacteroides* spp. However, the rate of transmission in vivo is apparently low since chloramphenicol resistance is detected in less than 1% of isolates.

Clindamycin is one of the most widely used antimicrobial drugs in the treatment of anaerobic infections. Recent studies suggest that resistance to clindamycin in *B. fragilis* is 5–20%, less than 5% in other *Bacteroides* spp. and 10% for *Prevotella* and *Porphyromonas*. Resistance is mediated by a RNA methylase that alters the 50S subunit of ribosomal RNA and modifies the site of action of the drug. Resistance is due to the transfer of transposable elements such as Tn*4351* and Tn*4400* (Shoemaker et al. 1985).

Metronidazole resistance in *Bacteroides* spp. is associated with plasmids that have been shown to transfer to other species via conjugation. This suggests the presence of conjugative elements. Despite the low incidence of resistance to metronidazole, the fact that such resistance is transferable suggests the possibility of increased resistance in the future.

Tetracycline resistance in *Bacteroides* isolates was uncommon, but today all clinical isolates of *Bacteroides* spp. are resistant to tetracycline due to the spread of conjugative elements throughout *Bacteroides* spp. Increased use of tetracyclines for the treatment of periodontal diseases and other oral infections is largely responsible for the spread of resistance among *Prevotella* and *Porphyromonas* spp. Such resistance is mediated by chromosomally expressed ribosomal protection mechanisms. In *Bacteroides* and *Prevotella* spp., conjugative elements harbouring the genetic determinants *tet*Q and *tet*M were reported.

Resistance to macrolides is usually plasmid or transposon mediated and is related to lincosamide resistance and results in the dimethylation of the 50S ribosomal subunit. The most frequently detected genes responsible for such activity in *B. fragilis*, *B. ovatus* and *B. vulgatus* are *erm*F and *erm*FS (Garcia-Rodriguez, Garcia-Sanchoz and Munoz-Bellido 1995).

7 MOLECULAR ANALYSIS

Most of the early work on the genetics of the Bacteroidaceae focused on the genus *Bacteroides*. This is due in part to the fact that members of this genus are among the most oxygen tolerant of all obligate anaerobes, they are not nutritionally fastidious and their growth rates are 1–3 h per generation time (Salyers and Shoemaker 1987). They harbour conjugative plasmids that are transferable to *Escherichia coli* and other members of the Bacteroidaceae. The fact that *Bacteroides* spp. are opportunistic pathogens, *B. fragilis* accounting for almost half of all human anaerobic infections, has promoted interest in its genetics.

Many *Bacteroides* strains have cryptic plasmids (3–6 kb) that are mobilized by conjugative elements. However, clindamycin and erythromycin determinants are harboured on plasmids isolated from *B. ovatus*. Tetracycline resistance determinants were isolated downstream from these genes. However, the gene products of these tetracycline resistance elements are functional only under aerobic conditions.

Conjugative transposons are elements that integrate within the bacterial chromosome but, unlike transposons, do not duplicate the target site. Furthermore, a circular intermediate structure is formed during excision and transfer. *Bacteroides* conjugative transposons usually carry the tetracycline determinant *tetQ* (Salyers and Shoemaker 1995). Some conjugative transposons carry erythromycin resistance genes that also confer resistance to clindamycin. However, cryptic conjugative elements were detected. Interestingly, strains expressing multiple resistance carry conjugative transposons, which may explain the rapid and wide spread occurrence of such resistance among members of the genus *Bacteroides*. In many cases, conjugative transposons can also mediate the excision and mobilization of co-resident plasmids.

This transfer is stimulated by the exposure of donors to low concentrations of tetracycline prior to conjugation. This was shown to increase the frequency of transfer by 1000—10 000- fold. Clindamycin was also shown to stimulate the rate of transfer. *Bacteroides* conjugative elements have been shown to transfer resistance to *Prevotella* and *Porphyromonas* spp. in the presence of tetracycline.

Conjugative transposons are extremely stable and, unlike antibiotic resistance plasmids, are maintained in *Bacteroides* strains in the absence of selection through exposure to antibiotics. Several genes from *B. fragilis*, such as *recA* and sialidases, were expressed in *E. coli*. Therefore, plasmids isolated from *B. fragilis* and *B. thetaiotaomicron* that harbour antibiotic markers were integrated into *E. coli*-based shuttle vectors to construct new systems for the cloning and expression of genes of members of the Bacteroidaceae. These novel plasmids were successfully transferred to *Porphyromonas* and *Prevotella* spp. via conjugation and electroporation. The genetic similarity among these taxa facilitated the expression of heterologous genes. For example, a recombinant xylanase gene in *P. ruminicola* was transferred into *B. fragilis* and the expressed product was found to be 1400-fold greater than in *P. ruminicola* (Whitehead and Hespell 1990).

P. gingivalis is the most intensively studied species of the genus *Pophyromonas* and sufficient genes have now been sequenced to enable an insight into the structure of its genome. Several attempts to clone and express surface-associated proteins failed to yield mature proteins and resulted in the rearrangement of the cloned fragments. In recent years, random cloning and selection of recombinant was replaced with screening with degenerate primers, constructed N-terminal sequences or conserved motifs of similar proteins. The amplified fragments were sequenced to ascertain their identity and used to screen gene libraries and clinical isolates. Using this approach, the structure and distribution of the fimbriae-encoding gene was determined. Several sequences of the major extracellular proteinase have been reported and deposited in the data bank. However, the biochemical and physiological studies support the view that all the extracellular proteolytic activity of *P. gingivalis* is associated with only 2 cysteine proteinases. Furthermore, the results of cloning and molecular analysis have revealed that the proteinase forms a complex association with adhesin molecules on the bacterial surface and is responsible for its attachment to erythrocytes.

The metalloenzyme superoxide dismutase (SOD) of *P. gingivalis* has the highest known activity of any *Porphyromonas* or *Prevotella* species. It was reported recently that an increase in temperature from 37 to 39°C resulted in an increase in SOD messenger RNA and a 3-fold rise in SOD activity. Molecular analysis revealed that the enzyme is transcribed as single apoprotein monomers but post-transcriptional modification yields 2 minor Fe-containing SOD isoenzymes (when cell extracts are maintained anaerobically) and a major Mn-containing SOD (when cells are aerated), both of which are encoded by a single copy on the chromosome which is a unique feature.

The genes for several unrelated enzymes have been deposited in databases but the significance of these to the biology of *P. gingivalis* has not yet been clarified. These include a methylase-encoding gene, heat shock protein operon, an insertion element, genes encoding an alkaline phosphatase and methylmalonyl-CoA mutase (see review by Gharbia et al. 1995).

A unique molecular structure among bacteria was revealed through the study of an adhesin gene from *P. loescheii*. The gene, referred to as *plaA*, possesses 2 overlapping reading frames which encode an 89 kDa polypeptide (Manch-Citron et al. 1992). The leader sequence and 28 residues of the N-terminus are encoded within frame 1 and a second reading frame is initiated on the complementary strand. Sequencing results and confirmation using PCR amplification of several gene fragments strongly suggest a frameshift within *plaA*, which represents an uncommon phenomenon among bacteria. Such a mechanism enables a single gene to encode several proteins, fusion protein transcription and truncated gene products.

8 CELL ENVELOPE COMPOSITION AND ANTIGENIC PROPERTIES

Cell membranes of the Bacteroidaceae possess high levels of sphingolipids or free ceramides. The main ester-linked fatty acids are branched-chain *anteiso-* and *iso*-pentadecanoic acids and the amide-linked fatty acids are all 3-hydroxy fatty acids, also found in LPS (Mayberry 1980). The fine structure of the cell wall of members of the Bacteroidaceae resembles that of other gram-negative bacteria. Members of the genus *Bacteroides* possess a directly cross-linked peptidoglycan based on *meso*-diaminopimelic acid, whereas most *Porphyromonas* spp. contain lysine as the dibasic amino acid (Shah et al. 1976). The ability to form a polysaccharide capsule is important in the pathogenicity of *B. fragilis* and has also been described in other *Bacteroides* and *Porphyromonas* spp. The complex of antigens associated with the outer layer of the cell wall includes the LPS and the outer membrane. The LPS has endotoxic activity, and its polysaccharide is responsible for O-antigenic specificity (Hofstad 1975) although Kasper et al. (1983) showed that purified LPS extracted from different strains of *B. fragilis* had identical immunochemical specificity. Until recently, it was assumed that the LPS of *B. fragilis* differs from the LPS of aerobic gram-negative bacilli in that it does not contain either 2-keto-3-deoxyoctonate (KDO) or heptoses. The LPS has weak endotoxic activity; it is not lethal for 11-day-old chick embryos when given intravenously and does not induce a local Shwartzman reaction (Kasper 1976a, 1976b). It gives a positive reaction in the *Limulus* lysate test, but only at a much higher concentration than the LPS of *E. coli*.

The specificity of O antigens in *Bacteroides* is determined by the distribution of oligosaccharides as repeating units in the polysaccharide chain (Hofstad 1977). As with the enterobacteria, O-antigen preparations can be made by boiling suspensions of whole cells. Several workers have attempted to produce a serological typing system for *Bacteroides* spp. on the basis of agglutination reactions with the O antigens. Weiss and Rettger (1937) distinguished serological groups of *Bacteroides*; Werner and Sébald (1968) and Werner (1969) identified serotypes of *B. fragilis* and Beerens et al. (1971) divided the genus *Bacteroides* into 3 serogroups. Lambe and Moroz (1976) grouped *B. fragilis* by agglutination tests with 7 absorbed monospecific antisera but found 21 serogroups and 45 serological patterns amongst 98 test strains.

9 BACTERIOCIN PRODUCTION

Human faecal strains of *Bacteroides* may produce bacteriocins active against a wide variety of other *Bacteroides* and *Prevotella* strains but not inhibitory to strains of any other genera (Beerens and Baron 1965, Booth, Johnson and Wilkins 1977).

The bacteriocins have a high molecular weight and protein is a major component. Bacteriocin activity is stable over the pH range 1–12 and is not affected by RNAase, DNAase or phospholipase but is destroyed by proteolysis; the bacteriocin characterized by Booth and his colleagues was inactivated by trypsin and pronase but not by proteinase K or pepsin. It was also very resistant to heat; there was no loss of activity after heating at 100°C for 1 h and only a 50% reduction after 15 min at 121°C. This heat stability is surprising, because this bacteriocin has a MW >300 kDa, although no bacteriophage-like particles or subunits can be seen on electron microscopy. The bacteriocins described by Beerens and his colleagues were heat-labile.

There is wide variation in the pattern of susceptibility to different bacteriocins among strains of the same and closely related species, within the genus *Bacteroides*. Riley and Mee (1982) found that 54% of 50 *Bacteroides* strains produced bacteriocins and >90% were sensitive to at least one of them. They found that 90% of isolates could be typed in a bacteriocin sensitivity scheme with 6 producer strains. The significance

of bacteriocin production in vivo is uncertain. Whether bacteriocin production gives strains a competitive advantage in the normal habitat is unknown; producers and non-producers coexist in the same gastrointestinal population and the non-producers greatly outnumber the producers.

10 BACTERIOPHAGES

A virulent bacteriophage active against *B. distasonis* was isolated from sewage by Sabiston and Cohl (1969). Bacteriophages active against other *Bacteroides* spp. have been isolated, mostly from sewage; Booth and his colleagues (1979) described 68 distinct phages but they failed to isolate any directly from human faeces. All the phages except for 3 in Booth's series are morphologically similar to Bradley's (1967) group B bacteriophages; they have a hexagonal head and a complex tail. They are indistinguishable from each other, regardless of their species specificity; phage heads are 50–90 nm in diameter and the flexible, sheathless tails are 12–200 nm long. The atypical phages described by Booth and his colleagues had larger heads and more complex, rigid and sheathed tails. All the phages appear to be virulent and true lysogeny has not been detected, although a phage carrier or pseudolysogenic state has been described (Keller and Traub 1974, Booth et al. 1979). Transduction by *Bacteroides* phage has not been detected. Each phage is specific for a given species of *Bacteroides* and members of all other genera are resistant. Bacteriophages isolated on *B. fragilis* are virulent for some other strains of *B. fragilis*, but not for members of other *Bacteroides* spp. However, no phage is virulent for all strains of any species; different phages give different patterns of lysis with different *Bacteroides* species and no specific patterns are associated with different sources or different types of infection. A scheme for phage typing isolates of, for example, *B. fragilis* could be produced, if this would provide useful epidemiological evidence. Similarly, a set of phages could be used to confirm the identity of different species of *Bacteroides*, but a series of phages would be needed for each species to ensure that most isolates were lysed by at least one phage.

11 BACTEROIDACEAE IN THE NORMAL FLORA

11.1 In humans

Gram-negative anaerobic bacilli are a major component of the normal commensal flora of the mucous membranes of the mouth, lower gastrointestinal tract and vagina. Eggerth and Gagnon (1933) recognized their importance in the faecal flora and Rosebury (1962) stressed their normal occurrence at all 3 sites. The species of gram-negative anaerobic bacilli found at the 3 sites are different, and form distinct populations.

ORAL MICROFLORA

The mouth does not have a uniform bacterial population. The gingival crevice and subgingival plaque are the principal sites of colonization with gram-negative anaerobic bacilli (Socransky and Manganiello 1971, Hardie and Bowden 1974). Gram-negative anaerobic bacilli are rarely detected in infants before the eruption of teeth; as dentition develops during childhood, the frequency of colonization increases (Sutter 1984). Kelstrup (1966) found that the isolation rate of black-pigmented species rose from 18% in children aged 5 years to 70% at 16 years. *Prevotella* spp. are present in large numbers in the gingival crevice and subgingival plaque of all healthy adults; studies have shown that they represent 12% (Slots 1977) to c. 30% (Williams, Pantalone and Sherris 1976, Newman et al. 1978) of the cultivable flora. However, they constitute only c. 4% of the cultivable flora of supragingival plaque in normal subjects (Gibbons et al. 1964) although in institutionalized subjects the proportion may reach 17% (Loesche, Hockett and Syed 1972). In the presence of gingivitis and peridontitis their numbers, particularly those of *P. gingivalis* and *P. intermedia*, increase.

Pigmented species were first described in studies of the microflora of mucous membranes, in particular, of the gingival mucosa (Oliver and Wherry 1921). They are useful marker species for the anaerobic flora of the gingival crevice (Holbrook, Ogston and Ross 1978). Pigmented strains constitute 4–6% of the cultivable flora of the normal gingival crevice (Gibbons 1974, Williams, Pantalone and Sherris 1976) and 5–6% of the plaque flora from institutionalized subjects (Loesche, Hockett and Syed 1972). Pigmented *Prevotella* spp. can be isolated from almost all subjects and account for 10–20% of the gram-negative anaerobic bacilli whereas the non-pigmented species account for about 35% (Loesche, Hockett and Syed 1972, Gibbons 1974, Duerden 1980c). Species of *B. fragilis* are not part of the normal gingival flora (Hardie 1974).

Gingival strains of Bacteroidaceae are often nutritionally demanding and may be difficult to maintain in pure culture on solid media; many species are nutritionally interdependent and will grow only in mixed culture, in which satellitism may be demonstrated. Growth is often improved by the addition of 5–10% CO_2 in the anaerobic atmosphere (Watt 1973, Stalons, Thornsberry and Dowell 1974) and recognized growth factors include metal ions (Caldwell and Arcand 1974) and haemin (Gibbons and MacDonald 1968, Gilmour and Poole 1970). Most *Prevotella* and *Porphyromonas* spp. also require menadione (vitamin K, Lev 1959) or its precursors (Robins, Yee and Bentley 1973) and succinate (Lev, Keudall and Milford 1971).

GASTROINTESTINAL MICROFLORA

Gram-negative anaerobic bacilli are generally the most numerous bacteria in the normal flora of the gastrointestinal tract, similar in numbers to the bifidobacteria. The genus *Bacteroides* forms the majority of the cultivable species (Drasar and Hill 1974). The anaerobic intestinal flora develops early in life. In breast-fed infants bifidobacteria predominate and gram-negative anaerobic bacilli are present in the first week of life only in about 20% of such infants. However, more than 60% of bottle-fed infants are colonized by *Bacteroides* spp. in the same period. At weaning, the numbers of bifidobacteria decrease whereas the numbers of *Bacteroides* rise to outnumber bifidobacteria by 3:1 (Long and Swenson 1977). Rotimi and Duerden (1981) reported a heavy growth of *Bacteroides* from 75% of 16 infants 5–6 days old who were breast fed but received supplementary bottle feeds. Obligate anaerobes are seldom found in the normal stomach, duodenum, jejunum or proximal ileum; *Bacteroides* spp. and *Bifidobacterium* spp. begin to appear only in the distal ileum (Finegold 1977) and they form a major part of the caecal and faecal flora. Viable counts of *Bacteroides* yield 10^{11} organisms per g wet weight of faeces and caecal contents (Drasar 1967, Finegold et al. 1975). The proportion of *Bacteroides* spp. in the faecal flora differs in subjects from different countries and is related to the type of diet. They are found in greater numbers in subjects who consume a mixed western diet that contains comparatively large amounts of fat and stimulates the production of a large volume of bile. Fewer *Bacteroides* spp. are found in subjects from developing countries in Africa and Asia, and from Japan, who consume a mainly vegetarian diet; gram-positive anaerobes and enterococci are the predominant faecal organisms in these subjects. However, subjects in developed countries who change to a vegetarian diet do not convert their faecal flora to a gram-positive predominance and retain their *Bacteroides* organisms (Drasar 1974).

Some 80% of faecal gram-negative anaerobic bacilli are members of the genus *Bacteroides*. The commonest species in most subjects are *B. vulgatus*, *B. thetaiotaomicron* and *B. distasonis*. *B. eggerthii* is found regularly, but *B. fragilis* forms only a small proportion of the *Bacteroides* in the normal faecal flora (Werner 1974, Finegold et al. 1975, Moore and Holdeman 1975, Duerden 1980a). Holdeman, Good and Moore (1976) identified 1442 isolates belonging to 101 species from 25 specimens of faeces from 3 men; *B. vulgatus*, *B. thetaiotaomicron* and *B. distasonis* were 3 of the 5 most prevalent bacterial species, representing 11.8, 8.9 and 6.0% of isolates respectively, whereas *B. fragilis* represented only 0.3%. They also found that the proportion of *B. thetaiotaomicron* isolates rose under stressful conditions. Asaccharolytic species of the Bacteroidaceae form a consistent part of the normal faecal flora but are present in much smaller numbers than *Bacteroides* (Werner, Pulverer and Reichertz 1971); the most commonly recognized species is *P. asaccharolytica* and the lower gastrointestinal tract is probably the primary habitat of this species. Non-pigmented asaccharolytic species are also present in quite small numbers; they grow slowly to form only small colonies and are difficult to detect.

The gram-negative anaerobic bacilli play an important part in the physiological activities of the large intestine. They are responsible for much of the metabolism of bile salts and bile acids. *Bacteroides* spp. and several clostridia produce enzymes that deconjugate bile salts under conditions of low *E*h, and they reduce cholic acid to deoxycholic acid. This is important in the enterohepatic circulation of bile salts. They may also be implicated in the production of carcinogens from bile acids. *Bacteroides* spp. produce dehydrogenases and dehydroxylases that convert bile acids into aromatic compounds and eventually to substituted cyclopentaphenanthrenes, which are known to be carcinogens. Differences in the incidence of colonic carcinoma in various countries are associated with the type of diet consumed and with the relative numbers of gram-negative anaerobic bacilli in the faeces (Drasar and Hill 1974).

VAGINAL MICROFLORA

The role of the Bacteroidaceae in the normal vaginal flora has been the subject of controversy. The vagina is not a single environment; the flora of the lower vagina is a mixture of organisms from the vagina with others from the perineum and introitus, whereas the flora of the cervix and fornices more closely represents the true vaginal flora. Moreover, the environment is not constant; the state of the mucosa and secretions changes with age, with each menstrual cycle and with pregnancy (Hurley et al. 1974).

Gram-negative anaerobic bacilli are common but not universal commensals of the cervix and vaginal fornices. The presence of Bacteroidaceae in the vagina was reported first by Burdon (1928); he isolated *P. melaninogenica* from 28 of 35 normal women.

Bacteroides spp. were isolated from cervical cultures in 57% (Gorbach et al. 1973) and 65% (Sanders et al. 1975) of normal women and from the posterior vaginal fornix in 65% and 100% of 2 groups of 20 normal women (Duerden 1980b, Wilks, Thin and Tabaqchali 1984). However, other workers have found them considerably less often: 8.6% of 246 preoperative gynaecological patients (Neary et al. 1973); 4.6% of 500 women attending a family planning clinic; 5% of 200 patients attending a gynaecological out-patient clinic; 5.4% of 280 pregnant women (Hurley et al. 1974); 4 of 100 pregnant women; and one (4%) of 23 normal women in a quantitative study by Taylor et al. (1982). Some of these differences may reflect differences between populations, but most are probably attributable to different methods of investigation and, in particular, to differences in sampling methods and in anaerobic technique. In studies with good anaerobic methods, isolation rates from normal women have been generally higher in qualitative studies (c. 60%, see above) than in quantitative studies – 41% (Masfari, Duerden and Kinghorn 1986), 34–40% (Bartlett and Polk 1984), 34% (Hammann 1982) – in which small numbers of anaerobes may not have been detected. In quantitative studies, mean viable counts of *Bacteroides* spp. in those normal women from whom gram-negative anaerobic bacilli were isolated varied from 10^6 colony-forming units (cfu) g^{-1} (Masfari, Duerden and Kinghorn 1986) to $10^{8–9}$ cfu g^{-1} or ml^{-1} (Bartlett and Polk 1984, Wilks, Thin and Tabaqchali

1984) of vaginal secretions. Few consistent variations have been detected in sequential samples taken during the menstrual cycle. Bartlett and Polk (1984) and Wilks, Thin and Tabaqchali (1984) both found that counts of aerobes were higher during the first week of the cycle but there was little change in the counts of anaerobes. However, *Bacteroides* spp. are reported to disappear during pregnancy and return soon after delivery (Hite, Hesseltine and Goldstein 1947, Willis 1977).

The species of Bacteroidaceae isolated in early studies of the vaginal flora were not identified. When detailed identification methods have been used, the predominant species have been members of *Prevotella* spp. *P. bivia* is the commonest species isolated in most studies. *P. disiens*, *P. intermedia* and *P. melaninogenica* are also common. *P. asaccharolytica* can be isolated in smaller numbers. The presence of significant numbers of *Bacteroides* organisms, and in particular of *B. fragilis*, indicates some pathological change in the genital tract.

11.2 In animals

Gram-negative anaerobic bacilli are part of the normal flora of intestinal contents and faeces in many species of animals from invertebrates to humans. They are an important component of the flora of 2 specialized gastrointestinal structures, the rumen of ruminant animals and the caecum of poultry.

Species that are now no longer considered as *Bacteroides* spp. are found in large numbers in the rumen: *Fibrobacter succinogenes*, *Ruminobacter amylophilus* and *P. ruminicola*. *F. succinogenes* is found in most ruminants and attains a viable count of c. 0.5×10^8 cfu ml^{-1}, about 8.5% of the total viable count; it is actively cellulolytic and is important in the digestion of cellulose; it also ferments glucose, cellobiose and several other carbohydrates, producing succinic acid (Hungate 1950). *R. amylophilus* and *P. ruminicola* are not cellulolytic; they are active in the digestion of starch and other carbohydrates. *R. amylophilus* occurs sporadically but when present may be the predominant starch digester and constitute 10% of the total bacteria (Hamlin and Hungate 1956). The fermentative activity of *P. ruminicola* is more varied; it is regularly present and constitutes 6–19% of the total viable count.

The **rumen** bacteria are essential for the nutrition of ruminants. The energy content of the feedstuff is made available to the animal in the form of volatile fatty acids, particularly acetic, butyric and propionic acids, produced by the bacterial fermentation of cellulose and other carbohydrates; the acids are absorbed through the rumen wall and metabolized by the animal. The removal of these acid products is essential for the continuation of fermentation. In addition, microbial protein constitutes a major part of the ruminants' protein source. Nitrogenous components of the feed are converted to microbial protein during growth and multiplication of the rumen bacteria, which contain c. 65% of protein. In the distal parts of the intestine, dead bacterial cells are digested and provide protein for the animal (Hungate 1966).

In poultry, the **caecum** is highly developed and has an important role in digestion and absorption. Gram-negative anaerobic bacilli are found in large numbers (c. 10^{8-9} g^{-1}) in the caecal contents. The commonest species is unique to this site – *Megamonas hypermegas* – which ferments a variety of carbohydrates (Barnes and Goldberg 1968a, 1968b).

REFERENCES

Barnes EM, Goldberg HS, 1968a, The relationships of bacteria within the family Bacteroidaceae as shown by numerical taxonomy, *J Gen Microbiol*, **51**: 313–24.

Barnes EM, Goldberg HS, 1968b, Anaerobic gram negative nonsporing bacteria from the caeca of poultry, *J Appl Bacteriol*, **31**: 530–41.

Bartlett JG, Polk BF, 1984, Bacterial flora of the vagina: quantitative study, *Rev Infect Dis*, **6, Suppl. 1**: S67–72.

Beerens H, 1970, Report of the International Committee on Nomenclature of Bacteria: Taxonomic Subcommittee for gram-negative anaerobic rods, *Int J Syst Bacteriol*, **20**: 297–300.

Beerens H, Baron G, 1965, Mise en évidence de bactériocines élaborées par les bactéries anaérobies à gram négatif appartenant au genre *Eggerthella*, *Ann Inst Pasteur*, **108**: 255–6.

Beerens H, Wattre P et al., 1971, Premiers résultats d'un essai de classification serologique de 131 souches de *Bacteroides* du groupe *fragilis* (eggerthella), *Ann Inst Pasteur (Paris)*, **121**: 187–98.

Bergey's Manual of Determinative Bacteriology, 1948, 6th edn, Williams & Wilkins, Baltimore, 564.

Bergey's Manual of Determinative Bacteriology, 1957, 7th edn, eds Breed RS et al., Williams & Wilkins, Baltimore, 423.

Booth SJ, Johnson JL, Wilkins TD, 1977, Bacteriocin production by strains of *Bacteroides* isolated from human feces and the role of these strains in the bacterial ecology of the colon, *Antimicrob Agents Chemother*, **11**: 718–24.

Booth SJ, Van Tassell RL et al., 1979, Bacteriophages of *Bacteroides*, *Rev Infect Dis*, **1**: 325–36.

Bradley DE, 1967, Ultrastructure of bacteriophage and bacteriocins, *Bacteriol Rev*, **31**: 230–314.

Burdon KL, 1928, *Bacterium malaninogenicum* from normal and pathologic tissues, *J Infect Dis*, **42**: 161–71.

Caldwell DR, Arcand C, 1974, Inorganic and metal-organic growth requirements of the genus *Bacteroides*, *J Bacteriol*, **120**: 322–33.

Carlsson J, 1973, Simplified gas chromatographic procedure for identification of bacterial metabolic products, *Appl Microbiol*, **25**: 287–9.

Castellani A, Chalmers AJ, 1919, *Manual of Tropical Medicine*, 3rd edn, Baillière, Tindall and Cox, London.

Cato EP, Johnson JL, 1976, Reinstatement of species rank for *Bacteroides fragilis*, *B. ovatus*, *B. distasonis*, *B. thetaiotaomicron* and *B. vulgatus*. Designation of neotype strains for *B. fragilis* (Veillon and Zuber) Castellani and Chalmers and *B. thetaiotaomicron* (Distaso) Castellani and Chalmers, *Int J Syst Bacteriol*, **26**: 230–7.

Cato EP, Kelley RW et al., 1982, *Bacteroides zoogleoformans* (Weinberg, Nativelle and Prévot 1937) corrig., comb. nov.: emended description, *Int J Syst Bacteriol*, **32**: 271–4.

Coykendall AL, Kaczmarek FS, Slots J, 1980, Genetic heterogeneity in *Bacteroides asaccharolyticus* (Holdeman and Moore 1970) Finegold and Barnes 1977 (Approved List 1980) and proposal of *Bacteroides gingivalis* sp. nov. and *Bacteroides macacae* (Slots and Genco) comb. nov., *Int J Syst Bacteriol*, **30**: 559–64.

Distaso A, 1912, Contribution à l'étude sur l'intoxication intestinale, *Zentralbl Bakteriol Parasitenkd Infektionskr Hyg Abt 1 Orig*, **62**: 433–68.

Drasar BS, 1967, Cultivation of anaerobic intestinal bacteria, *J Pathol Bacteriol*, **94**: 417–27.

Drasar BS, 1974, Some factors associated with geographical variations in the intestinal microflora, *The Normal Microbial Flora of Man*, eds Skinner FA, Carr JG, Academic Press, London, 187–96.

Drasar BS, Hill MJ, 1974, *Human Intestinal Flora*, Academic Press, London.

Duerden BI, 1980a, The isolation and identification of *Bacteroides* spp. from the normal human faecal flora, *J Med Microbiol*, **13**: 69–78.

Duerden BI, 1980b, The isolation and identification of *Bacteroides* ssp. from the normal human vaginal flora, *J Med Microbiol*, **13**: 79–87.

Duerden BI, 1980c, The isolation and identification of *Bacteroides* spp. from the normal human gingival flora, *J Med Microbiol*, **13**: 89–101.

Duerden BI, Holbrook WP et al., 1976, The characterization of clinically important gram negative anaerobic bacilli by conventional bacteriological tests, *J Appl Bacteriol*, **40**: 163–88.

Duerden BI, Collee JG et al., 1980, A scheme for the identification of clinical isolates of Gram-negative anaerobic bacilli by conventional bacteriological tests, *J Med Microbiol*, **13**: 231–45.

Egerton JR, Parsonson IM, 1966, Isolation of *Fusiformis nodosus* from cattle, *Aust Vet J*, **42**: 425–9.

Eggerth AH, Gagnon BH, 1933, Bacteroides of human feces, *J Bacteriol*, **25**: 389–413.

Eiken M, 1958, Studies on an anaerobic rod shaped gram-negative microorganism: *Bacteroides corrodens*, *Acta Pathol Microbiol Scand*, **43**: 404–16.

Finegold SM, 1977, *Anaerobic Bacteria in Human Disease*, Academic Press, New York.

Finegold SM, Barnes EM, 1977, Report of the I.C.S.B. taxonomic subcommittee on gram-negative rods, *Int J Syst Bacteriol*, **27**: 388.

Finegold SM, Harada NE, Miller LG, 1967, Antibiotic susceptibility patterns as aids in classification and characterization of gram-negative anaerobic bacilli, *J Bacteriol*, **94**: 1443–50.

Finegold SM, Flora DJ et al., 1975, Fecal bacteriology of colonic polyp patients and control patients, *Cancer Res*, **35**: 3407–17.

Garcia-Rodriguez JA, Garcia-Sanchoz JE, Munoz-Bellido JL, 1995, Antimicrobial resistance in anaerobic bacteria: current situation, *Anaerobe*, **1**: 69–80.

Garrod LP, 1955, Sensitivity of four species of *Bacteroides* to antibiotics, *Br Med J*, **2**: 1529–31.

Gesner BM, Jenkin GR, 1961, Production of heparinase by *Bacteroides*, *J Bacteriol*, **81**: 595–604.

Gharbia SE, Williams JC et al., 1995, Genomic clusters and codon usage in relation to gene expression in oral gram-negative anaerobes, *Anaerobe*, **1**: 239–62.

Gibbons RJ, 1974, Aspects of the pathogenicity and ecology of the indigenous oral flora of man, *Anaerobic Bacteria: Role in Disease*, eds Balows A et al., Charles C Thomas, Springfield, IL, 267–85.

Gibbons RJ, MacDonald JB, 1968, Hemin and vitamin K compounds as required factors for the cultivation of certain strains of *Bacteroides melaninogenicus*, *J Bacteriol*, **80**: 164–70.

Gibbons RJ, Socransky SS et al., 1964, Studies on the predominant cultivable microbiota of dental plaque, *Arch Oral Biol*, **9**: 365.

Gilmour M, Poole AE, 1970, Growth stimulation of the mixed microbial flora of human dental plaques by haemin, *Arch Oral Biol*, **15**: 1343–53.

Gilmour MN, Howell A, Bibby BG, 1961, The classification of organisms termed *Leptotrichia* (*Leptothrix*) *buccalis*. I. Review of the literature and proposed separation into *Leptotrichia buccalis* Trevisan 1879 and *Bacterionema* gen. nov. *Bacterionema matrichoti* (Mendel 1919) comb. nov., *Bacteriol Rev*, **25**: 131–41.

Gorbach SL, Menda KB et al., 1973, Anaerobic microflora of the cervix in healthy women, *Am J Obstet Gynecol*, **117**: 1053–5.

Gregory EM, Kowalski JB, Holdeman LV, 1977, Production and some properties of catalase and superoxide dismutase from the anaerobe *Bacteroides distasonis*, *J Bacteriol*, **129**: 1298–302.

Guillaume J, Beerens H, Osteaux R, 1956, La chromatographie sur papier des acides aliphatiques volatils de C_1 à C_6 son application à la détermination des bactéries anaérobies, *Ann Inst Pasteur Lille*, **8**: 13.

Haapasalo M, Ranta H et al., 1986, Biochemical and structural characterization of an unusual group of gram-negative, anaerobic rods from human periapical osteitis, *J Gen Microbiol*, **132**: 417–26.

Hamlin LJ, Hungate RE, 1956, Culture and physiology of a starch digesting bacterium (*Bacteroides amylophilus* n. sp.) from the bovine rumen, *J Bacteriol*, **27**: 548–54.

Hammann R, 1982, A reassessment of the microbial flora of the female genital tract, with special reference to the occurrence of *Bacteroides* species, *J Med Microbiol*, **15**: 293–302.

Hammann RH, Werner H, 1981, Presence of diaminopimelic acid in propionate-negative *Bacteroides* species and in some butyric acid-producing strains, *J Med Microbiol*, **14**: 205–12.

Hardie JM, 1974, Anaérobes in the mouth, *Infection with Non-sporing Anaerobic Bacteria*, eds Phillips I, Sussman M, Churchill Livingstone, Edinburgh, 99–130.

Hardie JM, Bowden GH, 1974, The normal microbial flora of the mouth, *The Normal Microbial Flora of Man*, eds Skinner FA, Carr JG, Academic Press, London, 47–83.

Henriksen SD, 1948, Studies on the gram-negative anaerobes: gram-negative anaerobic rods with spreading colonies, *Acta Pathol Microbiol Scand*, **25**: 368–75.

Hirasawa M, Takada K, 1994, *Porphyromonas gingivicanis* sp. nov. and *Porphyromonas crevioricanis* sp. nov., isolated from beagles, *Int J Syst Bacteriol*, **44**: 637–40.

Hite KE, Hesseltine HC, Goldstein L, 1947, Study of bacterial flora of normal and pathologic vagina and uterus, *Am J Obstet Gynecol*, **53**: 233–40.

Hofstad T, 1975, O-antigenic specificity of lipopolysaccharides from *Bacteroides fragilis* ss. *fragilis*, *Acta Pathol Microbiol Scand Sect B*, **83**: 477–81.

Hofstad T, 1977, Cross-reactivity of *Bacteroides fragilis* O antigens, *Acta Pathol Microbiol Scand Sect B*, **85**: 9–13.

Holbrook WP, Duerden BI, 1974, A comparison of some characteristics of reference strains of *Bacteroides oralis* with *Bacteroides melaninogenicus*, *Arch Oral Biol*, **19**: 1231–5.

Holbrook WP, Ogston SA, Ross PW, 1978, A method for the isolation of *Bacteroides malaninogenicus* from the human mouth, *J Med Microbiol*, **11**: 203–7.

Holdeman LV, Good IJ, Moore WEC, 1976, Human fecal flora: variation in bacterial composition within individuals and a possible effect on emotional stress, *Appl Environ Microbiol*, **31**: 359–75.

Holdeman LV, Johnson JL, 1977, *B. disiens* sp. nov. and *B. bivius* sp. nov. from human clinical infections, *J Clin Microbiol*, **6**: 337–45.

Holdeman LV, Johnson JL, 1982, Description of *Bacteroides loeschii* sp. nov. and emendation of the descriptions of *Bacteroides melaninogenicus* (Oliver and Wherry) Roy and Kelly 1939 and *Bacteroides denticola* Shah and Collins 1981, *Int J Syst Bacteriol*, **32**: 399.

Holdeman LV, Kelley RW, Moore WEC, 1984, Anaerobic gram-negative straight, curved and helical rods, *Bergey's Manual of Systematic Bacteriology*, vol. 1, eds Krieg NR, Holt JG, Williams & Wilkins, Baltimore, 602–62.

Holdeman LV, Moore WEC, 1974a, Gram-negative anaerobic bacteria, *Bergey's Manual of Determinative Bacteriology*, 8th edn, eds Buchanan RE, Gibbons NE, Williams & Wilkins, Baltimore, 384–404.

Holdeman LV, Moore WEC, 1974b, New genus, *Coprococcus*, twelve new species, and emended descriptions of four previously described species of bacteria from human faeces, *Int J Syst Bacteriol*, **24**: 260–77.

Holdeman LV, Moore WEC et al., 1982, *Bacteroides oris* and *Bacteroides buccae*, new species from human periodontitis and other infections, *Int J Syst Bacteriol*, **32**: 125–31.

Hungate RE, 1950, Anaerobic mesophilic cellulolytic bacteria, *Bacteriol Rev*, **14**: 1–49.

Hungate RE, 1966, *The Rumen and its Microbes*, Academic Press, New York.

Hurley R, Stanley GV et al., 1974, Microflora of the vagina during pregnancy, *The Normal Microbial Flora of Man*, eds Skinner FA, Carr JG, Academic Press, London, 155–85.

Jackson FL, Goodman YE, 1978, Bacteroides ureolyticus, a new species to accommodate strains previously identified as 'Bacteroides corrodens, anaerobic', *Int J Syst Bacteriol*, **28**: 197.

Johnson JL, 1973, Use of nucleic acid homologies in the taxonomy of anaerobic bacteria, *Int J Syst Bacteriol*, **23**: 308–15.

Johnson JL, Holdeman LV, 1983, *Bacteroides intermedius* comb. nov., and descriptions of *B. corporis* sp. nov. and *Bacteroides levii* sp. nov., *Int J Syst Bacteriol*, **33**: 15–25.

Johnson JL, Moore WEC, Moore LVH, 1986, *Bacteroides caccae* sp. nov., *Bacteroides merdae* sp. nov. and *Bacteroides stercoris* sp. nov. isolated from human feces, *Int J Syst Bacteriol*, **36**: 499–501.

Kasper DL, 1976a, The polysaccharide capsule of *Bacteroides fragilis* subspecies *fragilis*: immunochemical and morphologic definition, *J Infect Dis*, **133**: 79–87.

Kasper DL, 1976b, Clinical and biological characterization of the lipopolysaccharide of *Bacteroides fragilis* subspecies *fragilis*, *J Infect Dis*, **134**: 59–66.

Kasper DL, Weintraub A et al., 1983, Capsular polysaccharides and lipopolysaccharides from two *Bacteroides fragilis* reference strains: chemical and immunochemical characterization, *J Bacteriol*, **153**: 991–7.

Keller R, Traub N, 1974, The characterization of *Bacteroides fragilis* bacteriophage recovered from animal sera: observations on the nature of bacteroides phage carrier cultures, *J Gen Virol*, **24**: 179–89.

Kelstrup J, 1966, The incidence of *Bacteroides melaniogenicus* [sic] in human gingival sulci, and its prevalence in the oral cavity at different ages, *Periodontics*, **4**: 14–18.

Khairat O, 1967, *Bacteroides corrodens* isolated from bacteriaemias, *J Pathol Bacteriol*, **94**: 29–40.

Knorr M, 1922, Über die fusospirilläre Symbiose, die Gattung *Fusobacterium* (K. B. Lehmann) und *Spirillum sputigenum*. Zugleich ein Beiträg zür Bakteriologie der Mundhohle. II. Mitteilung. Die Gattung *Fusobacterium*, *Zentralbl Bakteriol Parasitenkd Infektionskr Hyg Abt 1 Orig*, **89**: 4–22.

Kunsman JE, 1973, Characterization of the lipids of six strains of *Bacteroides ruminicola*, *J Bacteriol*, **113**: 1121–6.

Kunsman JE, Caldwell DR, 1974, Comparison of the sphingolipid content of rumen *Bacteroides* species, *Appl Microbiol*, **28**: 1088–9.

Lambe DW Jr, Jerris RC, 1976, Description of a polyvalent conjugate and a new serogroup of *Bacteroides melaninogenicus* by fluorescent antibody staining, *J Clin Microbiol*, **3**: 506–12.

Lambe DW Jr, Moroz DA, 1976, Serogrouping of *Bacteroides fragilis* subsp. *fragilis* by the agglutination test, *J Clin Microbiol*, **3**: 586–92.

Lev M, 1959, The growth-promoting activity of compounds of the vitamin K group and analogues for a rumen strain of *Fusiformis nigrescens*, *J Gen Microbiol*, **20**: 697–703.

Lev M, Keudall KL, Milford DF, 1971, Succinate as a growth factor for *Bacteroides melaninogenicus*, *J Bacteriol*, **108**: 175–8.

Loesche WJ, Socransky SS, Gibbons RJ, 1964, *Bacteroides oralis* proposed new species isolated from the oral cavity of man, *J Bacteriol*, **88**: 1329–37.

Loesche WJ, Hockett RN, Syed SA, 1972, The predominant cultivable flora of tooth surface plaque removed from institutionalized subjects, *Arch Oral Biol*, **17**: 1311–25.

Long SS, Swenson RM, 1977, Development of anaerobic fecal flora in healthy newborn infants, *J Pediatr*, **91**: 298–301.

Manch-Citron JN, Allen J et al., 1992, The gene encoding a *Prevotella loescheii* lectin-like adhesin contains an interrupted sequence which causes a frameshift, *J Bacteriol*, **174**: 7328–36.

Masfari AN, Duerden BI, Kinghorn GR, 1986, Quantitative studies of vaginal bacteria, *Genitourin Med*, **62**: 256–63.

Mayberry WR, 1980, Cellular distribution and linkage of D-(-)-3-hydroxy fatty acids in *Bacteroides* species, *J Bacteriol*, **144**: 200–4.

Miyagawa E, Azuma R, Suto T, 1978, Distribution of sphingolipids in *Bacteroides* species, *J Gen Appl Microbiol*, **24**: 341–8.

Miyagawa E, Azuma R, Suto T, 1979, Cellular fatty acid composition in Gram-negative obligately anaerobic rods, *J Gen Appl Microbiol*, **25**: 41–51.

Moore LVH, Johnson JL, Moore WEC, 1994, Descriptions of *Prevotella tannerae* sp. nov. and *Prevotella enoeca* sp. nov. from the human gingival crevice and emendation of the description of *Prevotella zoogleoformans*, *Int J Syst Bacteriol*, **44**: 599–602.

Moore LVH, Moore WEC, 1994, *Oribaculum catoniae* gen. nov., sp. nov.; *Catonella morbi* gen. nov., sp. nov.; *Hallella seregens* gen nov., sp. nov; and *Dialister pneumosintes* gen. nov., comb. nov., nom. rev., anaerobic gram-negative bacilli from the human gingival crevice, *Int J Syst Bacteriol*, **44**: 187–92.

Moore WEC, 1970, Relationship of metabolic products to taxonomy of anaerobic bacteria, *Int J Syst Bacteriol*, **20**: 535–8.

Moore WEC, Holdeman LV, 1973, New names and combinations in the genera *Bacteroides* Castellani and Chalmers, *Fusobacterium* Knorr, *Eubacterium* Prévot, *Propionibacterium* Delwich, and *Lactobacillus* Orla-Jensen, *Int J Syst Bacteriol*, **23**: 69–74.

Moore WEC, Holdeman LV, 1975, Some newer concepts of the human intestinal flora, *Am J Med Technol*, **41**: 427–30.

Müller HE, Werner H, 1970, [In vitro studies of the occurrence of neuraminidase in *Bacteroides* species], *Pathol Microbiol*, **36**: 135–52.

Neary MP, Allen J et al., 1973, Preoperative vaginal bacteria and postoperative infections in gynaecological patients, *Lancet*, **2**: 1291–4.

Newman MC, Grinenco V et al., 1978, Predominant microbiota associated with periodontal health in the aged, *J Periodontol*, **49**: 553–9.

Okuda K, Kato T et al., 1985, *Bacteroides heparinolyticus* sp. nov. isolated from humans with periodontitis, *Int J Syst Bacteriol*, **35**: 438–42.

Olitsky PK, Gates FL, 1921, Experimental studies of the nasopharyngeal secretions from influenza patients, *J Exp Med*, **33**: 125–45, 361–72, 713–29.

Olitsky PK, Gates FL, 1922, Experimental studies of the nasopharyngeal secretions from influenza patients, *J Exp Med*, **36**: 501–19.

Oliver WW, Wherry WB, 1921, Notes on some bacterial parasites of the human mucous membranes, *J Infect Dis*, **28**: 341–4.

Olsson B, Dornbusch K, Nord CE, 1979, Factors contributing to resistance to beta-lactam antibiotics in *Bacteroides fragilis*, *Antimicrob Agents Chemother*, **15**: 263–8.

Paster BJ, Dewhirst FE et al., 1994, Phylogeny of *Bacteroides*, *Prevotella*, and *Porphyromonas* spp. and related bacteria, *J Bacteriol*, **176**: 725–32.

Poxton IR, Brown R, 1979, Sodium dodecyl sulphate–polyacrylamide gel electrophoresis of cell-surface proteins as an aid to the identification of the Bacteroides fragilis group, *J Gen Microbiol*, **112**: 211–17.

Prévot AR, 1938, Etudes de systématiques bactérienne invalidité du genre *Bacteroides*, Remembrement et reclassification, *Ann Inst Pasteur (Paris)*, **60**: 285.

Reinhold L, 1966, Untersuchungen an *Bacteroides corrodens* (Eiken 1958), *Zentralbl Bakteriol Parasitenkd Infektionskr Hyg Abt 1 Orig*, **201**: 49–57.

Riley TV, Mee BJ, 1982, A bacteriocin typing scheme for *Bacteroides*, *J Med Microbiol*, **15**: 387–91.

Robins DJ, Yee RB, Bentley R, 1973, Biosynthetic precursors of

vitamin K as growth promoters for *Bacteroides melaninogenicus*, *J Bacteriol*, **116**: 965–71.

Rosebury T, 1962, *Micro-organisms Indigenous to Man*, McGraw Hill, New York.

Rotimi VO, Duerden BI, 1981, The development of the bacterial flora in normal neonates, *J Med Microbiol*, **14**: 51–62.

Rudek W, Haque RU, 1976, Extracellular enzymes of the genus *Bacteroides*, *J Clin Microbiol*, **4**: 458–60.

Sabiston CB Jr, Cohl ME, 1969, Bacteriophage virulent for species of the genus *Bacteroides*, *J Dent Res*, **48**: 599.

Salyers AA, Shoemaker NB, 1995, Conjugative transposons: the force behind the spread of antibiotic resistance genes, *Anaerobe*, **1**: 143–50.

Sanders CV, Mickal A et al., 1975, Anaerobic flora of the endocervix in women with normal versus abnormal Papanicolaou (Pap) smears, *Clin Res*, **23**: 30A.

Sawyer J, MacDonald JB, Gibbons RJ, 1962, Biochemical characteristics of *Bacteroides melaninogenicus*, *Arch Oral Biol*, **7**: 685–91.

Schröter G, Stawru J, 1970, Die Bedeutung von *Bacteroides corrodens* Eiken 1958 im Rahmen der Tonsillenflora, *Z Med Mikrobiol Immunol*, **155**: 241–7.

Sébald M, 1962, *Étude sur les Bactéries Anaérobies Gram-négatives Asporalées*, Thèses de Paris.

Shah HN, 1991a, The genus *Bacteroides* and related taxa, *The Prokaryotes*, 2nd edn, eds Balows A, Trüper HG et al., Springer-Verlag, New York, 3593–607.

Shah HN, 1991b, The genus *Porphyromonas* and related taxa, *The Prokaryotes*, 2nd edn, eds Balows A, Trüper HG et al., Springer-Verlag, New York, 3608–20.

Shah HN, Collins MD, 1980, Fatty acid isoprenoid quinone composition in the classification of *Bacteroides melaninogenicus* and related taxa, *J Appl Bacteriol*, **48**: 75–87.

Shah HN, Collins MD, 1981, *Bacteroides buccalis* sp. nov., *Bacteroides denticola* sp. nov., *Bacteroides pentosaceus* sp. nov. new species of the genus *Bacteroides* from the oral cavity, *Zentralbl Bakteriol Mikrobiol Hyg Abt 1 Orig C*, **2**: 235–41.

Shah HN, Collins MD, 1983, Genus *Bacteroides*. A chemotaxonomical perspective, *J Appl Bacteriol*, **55**: 403–16.

Shah HN, Collins MD, 1986, Reclassification of *Bacteroides furcosus* (Holdeman and Moore) in a new genus *Anaerorhabdus*, as *Anaerorhabdus furcosus*, *Syst Appl Microbiol*, **8**: 86–8.

Shah HN, Collins MD, 1988, Proposal for reclassification of *Bacteroides asaccharolyticus*, *Bacteroides gingivalis* and *Bacteroides endodontalis* in a new genus, *Porphyromonas*, *Syst Appl Microbiol*, **38**: 128–31.

Shah HN, Collins MD, 1989, Proposal to restrict the genus *Bacteroides* (Castellani and Chalmers) to *Bacteroides fragilis* and closely related species, *Int J Syst Bacteriol*, **39**: 85–97.

Shah HN, Collins MD, 1990, *Prevotella*, a new genus to include *Bacteroides melaninogenicus* and related species formerly classified in the genus *Bacteroides*, *Int J Syst Bacteriol*, **40**: 205–8.

Shah HN, Gharbia SE, 1997, Current views on the systematics of the Bacteroidaceae, *Anaerobic Pathogens*, eds Eley AR, Bennett KW, Sheffield Academic Press, Sheffield, 217–27.

Shah HN, Gharbia SE, Collins MD, 1997, The Gram stain: a declining synapomorphy in an emerging evolutionary tree, *Rev Med Microbiol*, **8**: 103–10.

Shah HN, Williams RAD, 1982, Dehydrogenase patterns in the taxonomy of *Bacteroides*, *J Gen Microbiol*, **128**: 2955–65.

Shah HN, Williams RAD, 1987, Catabolism of aspartate and asparagine in *Bacteroides intermedius* and *Bacteroides gingivalis*, *Curr Microbiol*, **15**: 313–19.

Shah HN, Williams RAD et al., 1976, Comparison of the biochemical properties of *Bacteroides melaninogenicus* from human dental plaque and other sites, *J Appl Bacteriol*, **41**: 473–95.

Shah HN, Bonnett R et al., 1979, The porphyrin pigmentation of subspecies of *Bacteroides melaninogenicus*, *Biochem J*, **180**: 45–50.

Shah HN, van Steenbergen TJM et al., 1982, DNA base composition, DNA–DNA reassociation and isoelectric focusing of proteins of strains designated *Bacteroides oralis*, *FEMS Microbiol Lett*, **13**: 125–30.

Shah HN, Collins MD et al., 1985, *Bacteroides oulorum* sp. nov., a non-pigmented saccharolytic species from the oral cavity, *Int J Syst Bacteriol*, **35**: 193–7.

Shimada K, Sutter VL, Finegold SM, 1970, Effect of bile and desoxycholate on gram-negative anaerobic bacteria, *Appl Microbiol*, **20**: 737–41.

Shoemaker NB, Guthrie EP et al., 1985, Evidence that the clindamycin–erythromycin resistance gene of *Bacteroides* plasmid pBF4 is on a transposable element, *J Bacteriol*, **162**: 626–32.

Slots J, 1977, The predominant cultivable microflora of advanced periodontitis, *Scand J Dent Res*, **85**: 114–21.

Slots J, Genco RJ, 1979, Direct hemagglutination technique for differentiating *Bacteroides asaccharolyticus* oral strains from nonoral strains, *J Clin Microbiol*, **10**: 371–3.

Slots J, Genco RJ, 1980, *Bacteroides melaninogenicus* subsp. *macacae*, a new subspecies from monkey periodontopathogenic indigenous microflora, *Int J Syst Bacteriol*, **30**: 82–5.

Socransky SS, Manganiello SD, 1971, The oral microbiota of man from birth to senility, *J Periodontol*, **42**: 485–96.

Stalons D, Thornsberry C, Dowell VR Jr, 1974, Effect of culture medium and carbon dioxide concentration on growth of anaerobic bacteria commonly encountered in clinical specimens, *Appl Microbiol*, **27**: 1098–104.

van Steenbergen TJM, de Soet JJ, de Graaf J, 1979, DNA base composition of various strains of *Bacteroides melaninogenicus*, *FEMS Microbiol Lett*, **5**: 127–30.

van Steenbergen TJM, Vlaarderen CA, de Graaf J, 1981, Confirmation of *Bacteroides gingivalis* as a species distinct from *Bacteroides asaccharolyticus*, *Int J Syst Bacteriol*, **31**: 236–41.

van Steenbergen TJM, van Winkelhoff AJ et al., 1984, *Bacteroides endodontalis* sp. nov., an asaccharolytic black pigmented *Bacteroides* species from infected dental root canals, *Int J Syst Bacteriol*, **34**: 118–20.

Strom A, Dyer JK et al., 1976, Identification and characterization of species of the family Bacteroidaceae by polyacrylamide gel electrophoresis, *J Dent Res*, **55**: 252–6.

Sutter VL, 1984, Anaerobes as normal oral flora, *Rev Infect Dis*, **6, Suppl. 1**: S62–6.

Sutter VL, Finegold SM, 1971, Antibiotic disc susceptibility tests for rapid presumptive identification of Gram-negative anaerobic bacilli, *Appl Microbiol*, **21**: 13–20.

Sutter VL, Finegold SM, 1976, Susceptibility of anaerobic bacteria to 23 antimicrobial agents, *Antimicrob Agents Chemother*, **10**: 736–52.

Tanner ACR, Badger S et al., 1981, *Wolinella* gen. nov., *Wolinella succinogenes* (*Vibrio succinotgenes* Wolin et al.) comb. nov. and description of *Bacteroides gracilis* sp. nov., *Wolinella recta* sp. nov., *Campylobacter concisus* sp. nov. and *Eikenella corrodens* from humans with periodontal disease, *Int J Syst Bacteriol*, **31**: 432–45.

Taylor E, Blackwell AL et al., 1982, *Gardnerella vaginalis*, anaerobes, and vaginal discharge, *Lancet*, **1**: 1376–9.

Vandamme P, Daneshvar MI et al., 1995, Chemotaxonomic analyses of *Bacteroides gracilis* and *Bacteroides ureolyticus* and reclassification of *B. gracilis* as *Campylobacter gracilis* comb. nov., *Int J Syst Bacteriol*, **45**: 145–52.

Veillon A, Zuber A, 1898, Recherches sur quelques microbes strictement anaérobies et leur rôle en pathologie, *Arch Méd Exp Anat Pathol*, **10**: 517.

Watabe J, Benno Y, Mitsuoka T, 1983, Taxonomic study of *Bacteroides oralis* and related organisms and proposal of *Bacteroides veroralis* sp. nov., *Int J Syst Bacteriol*, **33**: 57–64.

Watt B, 1973, The influence of carbon dioxide on the growth of obligate and facultative anaerobes on solid media, *J Med Microbiol*, **6**: 307–14.

Weinberg M, Nativelle R, Prévot AR, 1937, *Les Microbes Anaérobies*, Masson, Paris.

Weiss JE, Rettger LF, 1937, The gram-negative *Bacteroides* of the intestine, *J Bacteriol*, **33**: 423–34.

Werner H, 1969, Das serologische Verhalten von Stammen der Species *Bacteroides convexus*, *B. thetaiotaomicron*, *B. vulgatus* und *B. distasonis*, *Zentralbl Bakteriol Parasitenkd Infektionskr Hyg Abt 1 Orig*, **210**: 192–201.

Werner H, 1974, Differentiation and medical importance of saccharolytic intestinal *Bacteroides*, *Arzneimittelforschung*, **24**: 340–3.

Werner H, Pulverer G, Reichertz C, 1971, The biochemical properties and antibiotic susceptibility of *Bacteroides melaninogenicus*, *Med Microbiol Immunol*, **157**: 3–9.

Werner H, Rintelen G, Kunstek-Santos H, 1975, Eine neue buttersaurebildende Bacteroides-Art: *B. splanchnicus* n. sp., *Zentralbl Bakteriol Parasitenkd Infektionskr Hyg Abt 1 Orig*, **231**: 133–44.

Werner H, Sébald M, 1968, Etude sérologique d'anaérobies gram-négatifs aspourlés, et particulierement de *Bacteroides convexus* et *Bacteroides melaninogenicus*, *Ann Inst Pasteur (Paris)*, **115**: 350–66.

Whitehead TR, Hespell RB, 1990, Heterologous expression of the *Bacteroides ruminicola* xylanase gene in *Bacteroides fragilis* and *Bacteroides uniformis*, *FEMS Microbiol Lett*, **66**: 61–6.

Wilkinson FC, Egerton JR, Dickson J, 1970, Transmission of *Fusiformis nodosus* infection from cattle to sheep, *Aust Vet J*, **46**: 382–4.

Wilks M, Thin RN, Tabaqchali S, 1984, Quantitative bacteriology of the vaginal flora in genital disease, *J Med Microbiol*, **18**: 217–31.

Willems A, Collins MD, 1995a, Phylogenetic placement of *Dialister pneumosintes* (formerly *Bacteroides pneumosintes*) within the *Sporomusa* subbranch of the *Clostridium* subphylum of the gram-positive bacteria, *Int J Syst Bacteriol*, **45**: 403–5.

Willems A, Collins MD, 1995b, Reclassification of *Oribaculum catoniae* (Moore and Moore 1994) as *Porphyromonas catoniae* comb. nov. and emendation of the genus *Porphyromonas*, *Int J Syst Bacteriol*, **45**: 578–81.

Willems A, Collins MD, 1995c, 16S rRNA gene similarities indicate that *Hallella seregens* (Moore and Moore) and *Mitsuokella dentalis* (Haapsalo et al.) are genealogically highly related and are members of the genus *Prevotella* (Shah and Collins) and description of *Prevotella dentalis* comb. nov., *Int J Syst Bacteriol*, **45**: 832–6.

Williams BL, Pantalone RM, Sherris JC, 1976, Subgingival microflora and periodontitis, *J Periodont Res*, **11**: 1–18.

Willis AT, 1977, *Anaerobic Bacteriology: Clinical and Laboratory Practice*, 3rd edn, Butterworths, London, 212.

Woese CR, 1987, Bacterial evolution, *Microbiol Rev*, **51**: 221–71.

Chapter 5 9

CHLAMYDIA

M E Ward and G Ridgway

1 DEFINITION

Chlamydia are spherical or ovoid obligately intracellular bacteria that undergo a characteristic and well-defined dimorphic life cycle within eukaryotic host cells. The infective form is the **elementary body** (EB), 200–300 nm in diameter, which developes within the host cell into the intracellular replicative form, the **reticulate body** (RB), 600–1000 nm in diameter. The RB divides by binary fission, each RB eventually producing one or more EBs within an enlarged endocytic vacuole termed the **inclusion**. The mechanical strength of the chlamydial cell envelope derives from the major outer-membrane protein (MOMP) and other cysteine-rich proteins which are extensively cross-linked by disulphide bonds in the EB but much less so in the RB. *Chlamydia* lack peptidoglycan in their cell walls so are relatively resistant to β-lactam antibiotics but susceptible to macrolides and tetracyclines. Chlamydial development is reversibly inhibited by interferon-γ. *Chlamydia* spp. are pathogenic for humans and a wide range of mammmalian, avian and invertebrate hosts. The G + C content of DNA is 39–41 mol%. The type species is *C. trachomatis*.

2 INTRODUCTION AND HISTORICAL PERSPECTIVE

In 1907, Halberstaedter and von Prowazek, working in Java, described the transmission of trachoma from humans to orang-utans by experimental infection. In Giemsa-stained conjunctival smears they observed intracytoplasmic inclusions containing numerous minute particles – the EBs – and realized these represented the cause of trachoma. These newly discovered organisms were called *Chlamydozoa* (from the

Greek *chlamys*, a mantle) from the blue-staining matrix in which the EBs were apparently embedded. Similar inclusions were described subsequently in the conjunctival cells of babies with non-gonococcal ophthalmia neonatorum, in cervical epithelium from some of their mothers and in urethral epithelium from male patients with non-gonococcal urethritis. Thus trachoma, inclusion conjunctivitis of the neonate and infection of the adult genital tract were caused by similar infective agents, all of which were capable of passing filters that otherwise generally retained bacteria. This latter property, coupled with the inability of these agents to grow in artificial media, led to the erronous belief that they were 'viruses'.

In 1929–30, Levinthal, Coles and Lillie independently described minute basophilic particles in the blood and tissue from birds and human patients with psittacosis. Bedson and co-workers soon proved their aetiological relationship with psittacosis and subsequently defined the characteristic chlamydial developmental cycle. With great foresight Bedson referred to this agent as 'an obligate intracellular parasite with bacterial affinities', a concept not generally accepted for another 30 years. As early as 1934, Thygeson drew attention to the similarities between the agents of trachoma, of inclusion conjunctivitis and of psittacosis. The related agent of lymphogranuloma venereum (LGV) was propagated first, in monkey brain, in 1931, followed in 1935 and 1955 respectively by growth of the psittacosis and trachoma agents in the chick embryo. For references to these historic studies see the eighth edition of this book (Collier 1990).

3 TAXONOMY

3.1 Phenotypic classification

The order *Chlamydiales* consists of one family, the Chlamydiaceae, containing one genus, *Chlamydia*, within which are 4 species: C. *trachomatis*, C. *psittaci*, C. *pneumoniae* (Grayston et al. 1989) and C. *pecorum* (Fukushi and Hirai 1992). The characteristics of these 4 species are summarized in Table 59.1.

This classification into 4 species is moderately satisfactory, but it takes no account of the many reports of chlamydia-like organisms living in invertebrate hosts and it is based solely on phenotypic characters. This makes the relevance of the classification to the evolutionary history of *Chlamydia* uncertain (Moulder 1988) and it is not possible to distinguish C. *pecorum* from C. *psittaci* on phenotype alone (Fukushi and Hirai 1992, Fukushi and Hirai 1993).

3.2 DNA-based computerized taxonomy

The extent of DNA homology within the 4 chlamydial species is shown in Table 59.1. There is substantial intra-species homology within C. *trachomatis*, C. *pneumoniae* and C. *pecorum*. However, C. *psittaci* is extremely diverse in its host range and genome, with intraspecific homology varying from 14 to 95% (Herring 1992). Clearly, new species other than C. *pecorum* will

eventually be derived from C. *psittaci*. Interspecies DNA homology (Table 59.1) is generally less than 10%. This genomic diversity has been construed as evidence of convergent chlamydial evolution from divergent free-living ancestors. However, this concept places too little weight on the unique yet common developmental cycle of all chlamydiae, their common antigens (e.g. lipopolysaccharide, LPS) and similar biological and metabolic activities. Evidently wholegenomic DNA homology is too crude a basis for satisfactory description of the evolutionary relationships between *Chlamydia*. Oligonucleotide sequences for the *omp1* gene of chlamydiae encoding the chlamydial major outer-membrane protein (MOMP) are much more satisfactory because the protein has conserved regions essential for chlamydial function together, in most of the species, with variable regions subject to immune pressure. Three computerized taxonomic studies (Kaltenboeck, Kousoulas and Storz 1993, Carter et al. 1991, Fitch, Peterson and Delamaza 1993) of *omp1* sequences are in essential agreement in producing a phylogenetic tree with a single stem with 3 main branches, suggesting that *Chlamydia* spp. have diverged in evolution from a common ancestor, presumed free-living (Fig. 59.1). One branch consisted of C. *psittaci*, from which, early on, a second branch containing C. *pneumoniae* diverged. The third branch, consisting of C. *trachomatis*, was broadly subdivided into 2 sub-branches corresponding to the 2 main sero-

Table 59.1 Characteristics of the four chlamydial species[a]

Characteristics	Chlamydial species			
	C. trachomatis	*C. pneumoniae*	*C. psittaci*	*C. pecorum*
Natural hosts	Humans, mice, pigs	Humans, horses	Birds, mammals, occasionally humans	Cattle and sheep
EB morphology	Round	Round or pear shaped	Round	Round
Inclusion	Oval, vacuolar	Oval, dense	Variable, dense	Oval, dense
Iodine staining	Yes	No	No	No
Sulphonamide sensitive	Yes	No	No	No
No. of serovars	at least 15	1	Undefined	3
Characteristic infections	Genital and ocular mucosa. Often inapparent. Intermittent shedding. Rarely systemic.	Chronic respiratory tract infections. Possible association with heart disease.	Frequently systemic: pneumonia, abortion, etc.	CNS, respiratory and gut. Often inapparent. Prolonged carriage
DNA: Mol % G + C	39.8	40.3	39.6	39.3
Homology % relative to				
C. trachomatis	92			
C. pneumoniae	1–7	94–96		
C. psittaci	1–33	1–8	14–95	
C. pecorum	1–10	10	1–20	88–100

[a]Adapted from Fukushi and Hirai (1993).

groups of this species. The most ancient *C. trachomatis* strains were the mouse pneumonitis agent and an isolate from pigs, suggesting perhaps that this predominantly human pathogen may have evolved from strains infecting non-human mammals.

Analysis of sequence data for *omp1* and *omp2* suggests there has been only limited co-evolution of the parasite and of the host cell, organ or species it infects (Fitch, Peterson and Delamaza 1993). All 3 computerized taxonomic studies are consistent with the common sense hypothesis that chlamydiae are diverging from a common ancestor and indicate that the LGV serovars evolved very recently, with serovars L1 and L2, which can exchange segments of MOMP by recombination (Hayes et al. 1994), on a different lineage to serovar L3. Presumably this ancestor was a free-living bacterium which adapted to an intracellular environment, gaining preformed nutrients and bioenergetic molecules, freedom from competition from other micro-organisms and sequestration from the host immune response. This was at the expense of structural adaptation necessary to ensure survival in the hostile extracellular milieu plus the loss of metabolic independence from the host cell. Sequencing studies of 16S rRNA of *C. psittaci* 6BC suggest that the ancestral chlamydial branch split off the main eubacterial trunk at a relatively early age. The nearest known

relative to *C. psittaci* 6BC is *Planctomyces staleyi*, a free-living aquatic bacterium in the *Pasteuria* group with motile buds, numerous fimbriae and a holdfast. Unusually, *Planctomyces*, like *Chlamydia*, has no peptidoglycan. There are numerous accounts (reviewed by Moulder 1988) of chlamydia-like organisms in invertebrates ranging from *Hydra* through molluscs to the arthropods. Their taxonomic relatedness to *Chlamydia* is entirely unknown. Most of these agents have not been grown. It would be feasible and of great interest to PCR-sequence the genes encoding their 16S rRNA and outer envelope proteins. However, the clam agent contains the *Chlamydia*-specific group antigen, produces glycogen in its inclusions and has been provisionally classified as *C. trachomatis*. One speculation is that *Chlamydia* arose from some primitive, free-living aquatic bacterium, adapted first to invertebrate hosts. Peptidoglycan may already have been absent, as in the Archaebacteria and Planctomyces, or may have become lost as a consequence of intracellular residence, being no longer needed for osmotic protection. However, compensatory reversible disulphide-bond cross-linking of the outer-membrane proteins became an essential adaptation permitting the peptidolycan-free EBs to retain structural integrity in the hostile extracellular environment. Divergence of *C. psittaci* and *C. trachomatis* occurred long ago,

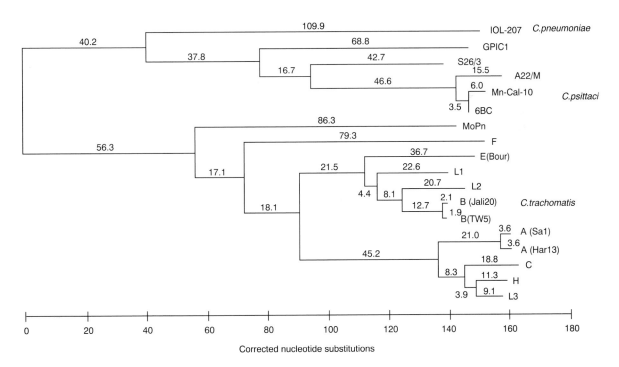

Fig. 59.1 Computer taxonomy of 18 complete nucleotide sequences for the gene encoding the major outer membrane protein of three *Chlamydia* spp. MOMP is an ideal protein for this purpose because it consists of regions of conserved sequence vital for its role in chlamydial development together with surface exposed, variable regions which are under evolutionary pressure from the host immune system. The figure shows the most parsimonious tree for the 18 nucleotide sequences. The *C. trachomatis* isolates are a monophyletic group with two major subgroups corresponding to the two main serogroups. The B cluster comprises B, Ba, D, E, L1 and L2 and the C cluster comprises A, C, H, I, J, K and L3. F and G belong to neither cluster. *C. pneumoniae* and *C. psittaci* are on a different branch to *C. trachomatis*, and *C. pneumoniae* IOL 207 devolves from this branch early on. The figures show the number of corrected nucleotide substitutions required in the descent from the node on the left to the node or tip on the right of that line. Reproduced with permission from Fitch, Peterson and de la Maza (1993).

possibly, as suggested by the clam agent, in invertebrate hosts. Subsequently, *C. pneumoniae* and *C. pecorum* diverged from *C. psittaci.*

4 MORPHOLOGY

Chlamydia have a unique dimorphic replication cycle that distinguishes them from all other groups of bacteria. This developmental cycle (Fig. 59.2) consists of 2 main forms of the micro-organism, the infectious EB and the non-infectious RB.

4.1 Elementary body

Only the EB can survive for any period outside the host and only the EB is infectious. It consists of round or occasionally pear-shaped (*C. pneumoniae*) particles 200–300 nm in diameter, with an irregular core of DNA (Fig. 59.3). Originally, possession of pear shaped elementary bodies was considered a taxonomic criterion of *C. pneumoniae* (Grayston et al. 1989), but this is no longer justified (Carter et al. 1991).

Surrounding the EB is a conventional bacterial cytoplasmic membrane, a variable-sized periplasmic space

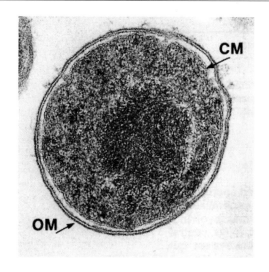

Fig. 59.3 Electron micrograph of thin section of an EB of *C. trachomatis*, showing the outer membrane (OM) and the cytoplasmic membrane (CM). There is no evidence of a peptidoglycan layer between the two membranes (× 118 000) Reproduced with permission from Moulder et al. (1984), p. 732.

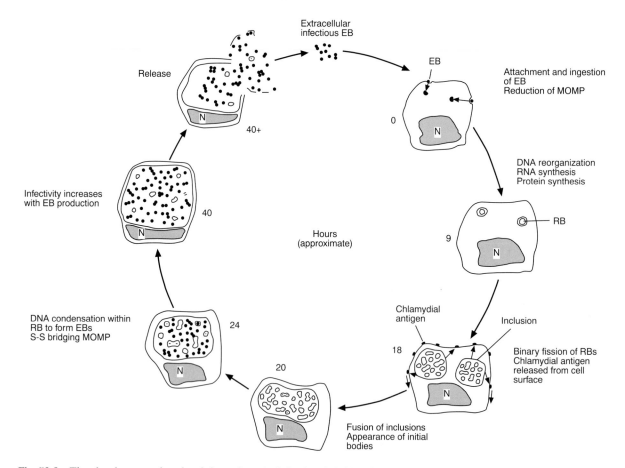

Fig. 59.2 The developmental cycle of *C. trachomatis*. Infection is initiated by infectious EB (top of diagram) which attach to and enter the host cell by poorly understood mechanisms. By 9 h after infection the EB have differentiated into RB. The RB undergo binary fission within the enlarging endosome and genus-specific chlamydial antigen becomes associated with the host cell surface. By 24 h the inclusions contain EB derived from the RB. Infectious EB are released by lysis at 40–48 h. Maturation of EB from RB may be impaired by factors such as interferon-γ, resulting in persistent infection of host cells.

which contains no peptidoglycan layer, and an outer envelope. Elegant studies of freeze-etched whole EBs or of ruthenium red-stained sectioned EBs (Matsumoto 1988) show the presence of flower-like rosettes in the EB envelope, some 19–20 nm in diameter, composed of 9 subunits rotationally symmetrical around a central 'pore' some 10–12 nm in diameter. Fine projections 5–6 nm in structure attached on the inside to the cytoplasmic membrane protrude from the surface through this 'pore'. The function and composition of these intriguing structures, which are present on *C. trachomatis*, *C. psittaci* and *C. pneumoniae* (Miyashita, Kanamoto and Matsumoto 1993) and are possibly crucial for pathogen–host interaction, is unknown.

The inner aspect of the EB cell wall consists of a regular array of hexagonal structures (Fig. 59.4) with a centre-to-centre spacing of approximately 18 nm and a periodicity following optical transformation of 16.7 nm. These structures may correspond with the outer-membrane proteins (Chang, Leonard and Arad 1982). Development of EB to RB is accompanied by morphological changes including chromatin dispersal, initiation of transcription and translation, biosynthesis and transport of amino acids and other nutrients (Raulston 1995).

4.2 Reticulate body

The RB is the intracellular, replicative stage. An RB is c. 1 μm in diameter and, in thin section, looks like a typical gram-negative coccus, with a homogeneous, featureless interior containing numerous 70S ribosomes. Replication is by binary fission. In *C. trachomatis*, but not the other species, glycogen particles accumulate within the RB. The outer envelope of the RB is much less rigid than that of the EB, with a tendency to form pleomorphic outer envelope blebs.

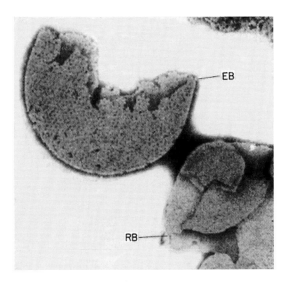

Fig. 59.4 Cell membranes of *C. psittaci* RB and EB. The latter has a hexagonal array of subunits. Electron micrograph, negative-contrast stain (× 70 000). (By courtesy of Dr G. P. Manire.)

Projections and rosettes are present on the RB surface in similar number to the EB.

5 DEVELOPMENTAL CYCLE

5.1 Attachment

Chlamydial infection starts with the attachment of an infectious EB to the host cell surface. In vitro, chlamydial attachment to host cells, even to relevant polarized epithelia derived from the genital tract (Moorman, Sixbey and Wyrick 1986) does not show high binding affinity. Rather, attachment is the aggregate effect of multiple weak ligand interactions which, together, afford an effective, flexible attachment system which permits the organism to attach to a wide variety of host cells. Chlamydial binding to host cells is saturable and inhibited by trypsin treatment of the host cell. Infectivity of the oculogenital isolates of *C. trachomatis* (trachoma biovar) but not the strains causing lymphogranuloma venereum (LGV biovar) is potentiated by treatment of host (HeLa) cells with cationic polymers such as diethyl aminoethyl (DEAE)-dextran (Kuo, Wang and Grayston 1973). This effect was originally thought to be due to a reduction in the electrostatic repulsive barrier to attachment (reviewed by Ward 1986). However, there is evidence that a polycationic heparan sulphate-like molecule synthesized by chlamydiae themselves mediates attachment by bridging the EB outer membrane to ubiquitous receptors for glycosaminoglycans on the host cell surface (Zhang and Stephens 1992). Infectivity was inhibited by the the sulphated polysaccharides carrageenan, pentosan, fucoidan and dextran sulphate, by the negatively charged glycosaminoglycans heparin, heparan sulphate, and dermatan sulphate but not the more neutral chondroitin sulphates A or C, keratan sulphate or hyaluronic acid. Heparinase treatment of chlamydiae destroyed infectivity, which was restored by fibronectin and other compounds binding to heparan (Zaretzky, Pearcepratt and Phillips 1995). Exogenous heparin binds strongly to chlamydiae and restores their infectivity (Zhang and Stephens 1992). Similar sulphated polysaccharides inhibit transmission of HIV and are being tested as vaginal formulations to prevent HIV infection and might also block the transmission of chlamydiae (Zaretzky, Pearcepratt and Phillips 1995). Interestingly, an opacity protein of *Neisseria gonorrhoeae* associated with epithelial cell invasion rather than attachment binds to a sulphated glycosaminoglycan called syndecan-1 found on genital and ocular epithelia (van Putten and Paul 1995).

Other chlamydial proteins implicated with little evidence in the attachment of chlamydiae to the host cell include MOMP, the *omp2* encoded cystein-rich protein, the histone like proteins and chlamydial hsp-70 (see below). MOMP itself is a glycoprotein whose glycan moiety binds to HeLa cells, competes with native EB and is inhibited by high concentrations of galactose, mannose or *N*-acetyl glucosamine (Swanson and Kuo 1994). The role of MOMP and its glycan in chlamydial adhesion requires further investigation.

5.2 Endocytosis

Chlamydial heparan may be involved in entry as well as attachment as heparin inhibits the infectivity of trachoma biovar organisms to a greater extent than it inhibits attachment. Entry to host cells involves parasite-specified endocytosis utilizing both microfilament- and clathrin-dependent mechanisms (Reynolds and Pearce 1993) and there is associated tyrosine kinase activation (Birkelund, Johnsen and Christiansen 1994). Several endocytic mechanisms probably exist, with the organism itself, its presentation to the host cell, differences between host cells themselves, their receptors, their degree of morphological polarity and their hormone responsiveness all playing a part (Reynolds and Pearce 1993, Stephens 1994) and influencing the intracellular fate of the endocytosed organism and probably chlamydial antigen processing by the host cell.

5.3 Intracellular replication

The normal course of the chlamydial developmental cycle is shown in Fig. 59.2. Interiorization of *C. psittaci* occurs without endosomal acidification (Eissenberg et al. 1983). Within 6–9 h, the EB within its endosome has differentiated into an RB but the trigger is unknown. It has been suggested that when the EBs are exposed by endocytosis to the intracellular reducing environment, the *S-S* linked trimeric MOMP porin in the EB wall becomes reduced leading to ingress of host cell high-energy nucleotides necessary to initiate development (Bavoil, Ohlin and Schachter 1984). Thus EBs exposed to a reducing environment can be triggered in vitro into biochemical activity including glutamate oxidation. Electron microscopic (Chang, Leonard and Arad 1982) and biophysical (Bavoil, Ohlin and Schachter 1984) observations suggest that MOMP is a porin permitting passive diffusion of hydrophilic compounds up to 850–2250 kDa down a concentration gradient. Clearly more is required for true differentiation as EBs thus exposed to a reducing environment do not undergo morphological transformation. Definitive proof that MOMP is a porin requires 3-dimensional structure determination.

The RBs are metabolically active and divide by binary fission within the expanding endosome with a doubling time of approximately 2 h. The growth cycle is asynchronous; EBs, RBs and intermediate forms are found in the same inclusion. Endosomes containing *C. trachomatis*, but not *C. psittaci*, escape fusion with cellular lysosomes yet are able to fuse with themselves. Redistribution of chlamydial endosomes within the host cell involves clathrin and F-actin and the selective translocation of annexins II, IV and V (Majeed et al. 1994).

Metabolic capabilities of RB include the synthesis of complex macromolecules (nucleic acids, proteins and LPS) and, in *C. trachomatis* only, the synthesis of glycogen from ADP-glucose and folate synthesis. *Chlamydia* have components of the Embden–Meyerhof–Parnas and/or Entner–Doudoroff pathways and may contain a complete pentose phosphate pathway. However, they lack flavoproteins and respiratory enzymes (McClarty 1994). The idea that chlamydiae are 'energy parasites' is based on indirect evidence only (McClarty 1994); a chlamydial ATP–ADP translocase has been identified (Hatch, Al-Hossainy and Silverman 1982). *Chlamydia* probably modify the inclusion membrane with their own transport systems. Replication of RB within the constrained inclusion will inevitably bring them into association with the inclusion membrane but there is no good evidence for direct communication between the chlamydial and eukaryotic cell cytoplasms. However, *C. psittaci* appears capable of modifying the endosomal (inclusion) membrane, coding for a 39 kDa inclusion membrane protein A (IncA) which was localized to the inclusion membrane of infected HeLa cells from which it extended in tubular form over the nucleus into the cytoplasm (Rockey, Heinzen and Hackstadt 1995). The functions of this protein are unknown.

Chlamydial replication within the endosome occurs independently of Golgi function (Stephens 1994) or the cell nucleus (Perara, Yen and Ganem 1990). A single RB often gives rise to more than one EB (Ward 1988) whose production requires the availability of cysteine and up regulated expression of MOMP and the cysteine-rich proteins (Everett and Hatch 1995, Yuan et al. 1992). Figure 59.5 shows a mature inclusion by transmission electron microscopy and Fig. 59.6 shows the freeze-fractured interior of chlamydial infected cells. Differentiation of infectious EBs from the RBs within the mature inclusion and their release by lysis of the endosome completes the productive chlamydial replication cycle.

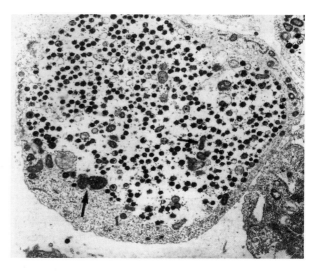

Fig. 59.5 Transmission electron micrograph of a cell 70 h after infection with *C. trachomatis* serotype B. Note the electron-dense EB and the much larger, less dense, RB. Some RB in the mature inclusion are undergoing binary division (arrows) (× 4050).

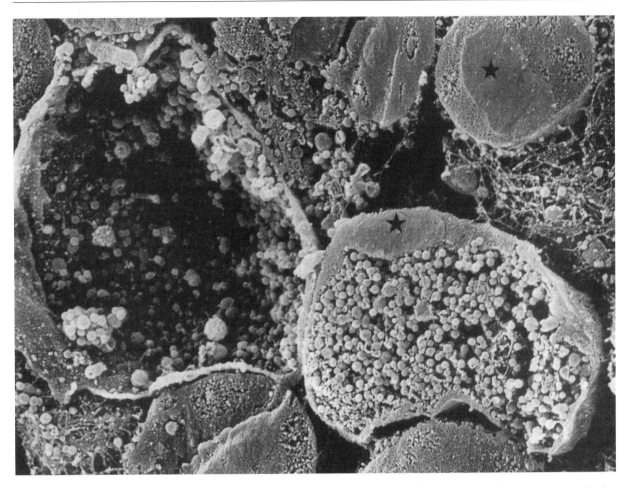

Fig. 59.6 Buffalo green monkey cells infected with *C. trachomatis* serotype B were fixed, embedded in polyethylene glycol resin, and sectioned. The water-soluble resin was dissolved away to reveal the intracellular chlamydiae. The nucleus (*) is clearly visible in the sectioned cells. The cell on the right is packed full of chlamydial particles. Chlamydiae have been removed from the cell on the left to show the large volume of the cell occupied by these organisms. Field emission scanning electron micrograph (× 5100). (By courtesy of Chris Inman.)

5.4 Delayed development and its significance

The developmental cycle so far described is a productive cycle of infection in which infectious EBs are released to infect other cells. This is probably the normal situation as infectious EBs are frequently recovered from patients by cell culture and chlamydial inclusions containing EBs are occasionally observed in clinical specimens. However, in active trachoma, shedding of chlamydial EBs is intermittent and chlamydial antigens can be detected by immunofluorescence in the eyes of individuals who do not exhibit current signs of active disease (Mabey, Bailey and Hutin 1992). Furthermore, *C. trachomatis* is rarely isolated from the joints of patients with reactive arthritis although *C. trachomatis* DNA has been found in the synovial fluid of 22 of 71 patients with reactive arthritis and other arthropathies (Bas et al. 1995). Laboratory studies on mouse L cells indicate that incomplete chlamydial replication, resulting in a state of delayed but persistent infection also occurs. These infections were characterized by large, periodic and reciprocal fluctuations in host and parasite densities (Moulder, Levy and Schulman 1980). The chlamydiae persisted as small, aberrant, RB-like forms (Shatkin et al. 1985) which could be transferred at host cell division. Factors favouring delayed development included the action of penicillin, interferon-γ (Beatty, Byrne and Morrison 1993), other products of cell mediated immunity (Beatty, Byrne and Morrison 1994) and deprivation of the amino acids tryptophan and cysteine obligately required for chlamydial replication (Coles et al. 1993, Coles and Pearce 1987).

The clinical significance of persistent latent chlamydial infection is completely unknown. Clearly, ocular and genital chlamydial infections may persist, often asymptomatically for months in the absence of treatment. As chlamydial activity is greatest in host cells which are themselves actively replicating, mucosal cell turnover following another infection might reactivate a quiescent chlamydial infection (Richmond 1985, Campbell et al. 1988).Thus, isolation of *C. trachomatis* from the genital tracts of female contacts of men with gonococcal urethritis was dependent not only on the presence of chlamydiae in the male partner, but on infection of the woman with *N. gonorrhoeae* (Oriel and Ridgway 1982a,b, Batteiger et al. 1989). The model of persistence suggested by in vitro studies is of an incomplete chlamydial developmental cycle with only intermittent release of infectious EBs. Clinically, such infections would be characterized by positive assays for chlamydial antigen or DNA but only intermittently positive isolation of infectious EBs by tissue culture. It follows that the isolation of chlamydiae in cell culture would no longer be a 'gold standard' criterion of infection. In reality, interpretation of laboratory test results of chlamydial infection that are dependent on viability or non viability is complicated by the different sensitivities of the tests themselves. Moreover, microbiological indices of chlamydial infection do not coincide perfectly with clinical signs (Ward et al. 1990). In situ hybridization studies have demonstrated the persistence of chlamydial DNA in ocular tissue (Cosgrove et al. 1992) and in a high proportion of fallopian tube tissue from women with presumed post-infectious infertility following tubal occlusion (Campbell et al. 1993, Patton et al. 1994). Long term persistence of chlamydiae in chronic infection is suggested by the reactive arthritis study already referred to (Bas et al. 1995) and the presence of *C. pneumoniae* in coronary arteries of patients with heart disease (Campbell et al. 1995, Kuo et al. 1995, Kuo et al. 1993). The viability of persisting chlamydiae is indicated by demonstration of *Chlamydia*-specific mRNA transcripts in reactive arthritic joints (Gerard et al. 1995). Thus chlamydial antigens and DNA, probably but not necessarily viable, certainly persist in chronic infection but their true significance and role in immunopathology has yet to be defined.

6 GENOMIC STRUCTURE

6.1 The nucleus

The chlamydial genome is a closed circular DNA molecule of approximately 1200 kbp, one of the smallest procaryotic genomes known, just slightly larger than that of *Mycoplasma*. The coding capacity of approximately 600 proteins is about a quarter of the genome of *E. coli*. The complete genome of *C. trachomatis* is currently being sequenced.

6.2 Plasmids

Virtually all *C. trachomatis* isolates carry a 7.5 kb cryptic plasmid; suggestions that plasmid-free variants occur have never been satisfactorily proven by independent studies, although the issue is important because the plasmid is a major target for nucleic acid-based diagnostic tests. Plasmids of serovars L1, L2, B and D *C. trachomatis* share over 99% nucleotide sequence (Comanducci et al. 1990) with 8 open reading frames (ORFs) coding for proteins of over 100 amino acids. Of particular interest are ORFs 7 and 8, which are homologous to each other and to a family of plasmid and phage integrase proteins responsible for plasmid

replication and maintenance (Ricci et al. 1993) and ORF 3, which codes for a 28 kDa cell envelope antigen (pgp3), transcripts of which can be detected in *Chlamydia*-infected Vero cells 20 h after infection. Specific antibodies to pgp3 could be detected in 81% of the sera of sexually transmitted disease patients seropositive for *C. trachomatis* (Comanducci et al. 1994); pgp3 antibody is specific for *C. trachomatis* infection as human isolates of *C. pneumoniae* are plasmid free (Campbell, Kuo and Grayston 1987). Mammalian and avian strains of *C. psittaci* carry different but analogous plasmids which share 2 regions of homology with the *C. trachomatis* plasmid, one of which is the presumed origin of replication (Lusher, Storey and Richmond 1989). The fact that these plasmids are common and have been conserved during evolution indicates they have some useful function(s) yet to be determined although they are not apparently essential for chlamydial replication.

6.3 Bacteriophages

In *C. psittaci* isolated from ducks, 22 nm phage-like particles have been observed as crystalline arrays within the RB (Fig. 59.7) or in mature inclusions. Chlamydial phage Chp1 has been completely sequenced (Storey, Lusher and Richmond 1989). It has a single-stranded DNA genome of 4877 kb with 11 ORFs; 3 of its structural proteins (VP1, 2 and 3) have been N-terminal sequenced and are encoded by ORFs 1, 2 and 3. Chp1 shows close homology to phages PhiX174 and S13, but is 500 bp smaller. It has, accordingly, been classified into a new subfamily, the Chlamydiavirinae, of the Microviridae. This phage is of considerable interest, along with the cryptic plasmids, as a potential tool for manipulation of the chlamydial genome. The significance, if any, of these phages for the pathogenesis of chlamydial infection is unknown.

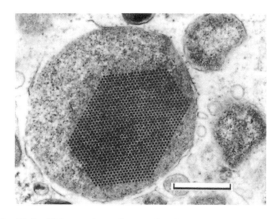

Fig. 59.7 Thin section of part of a chlamydial inclusion 40 h after infection of McCoy cells with *C. psittaci*, showing distended RB with crystalline array of virions about 20 nm in diameter. Bar = 500 nm. (By courtesy of Mrs P Stirling.)

7 ANTIGENIC STRUCTURE

Components of the chlamydial envelope have been reviewed in detail (Raulston 1995). This section deals with those antigens which are most likely important for pathogen–host interactions, protection or immunopathology.

7.1 Protein antigens

MAJOR OUTER-MEMBRANE PROTEIN AND CHLAMYDIAL SEROLOGY

The dominant antigen at the surface of the infectious chlamydial EB is the MOMP, encoded by the *omp1* gene and described virtually simultaneously by 3 independent groups in 1981. This antigen of approximately 40 kDa is the basis for the serological classification of *C. trachomatis* into 15 or more serotypes (serovars) depending on one's definition of a serovar. This classification is of epidemiological and pathological significance; serovars A, B, Ba and C are associated with endemic trachoma, serovars D–K are associated with inclusion conjunctivitis and genital tract infection, while serovars L1, L2 and L3 are associated with lymphogranuloma venereum (LGV). The pathobiological basis for this important difference is unknown although the underlying immunochemistry is well understood. Comparative *omp1* oligonucleotide sequencing of different serovars shows that MOMP consists of 5 constant and 4 variable sequence (VS) regions (Yuan et al. 1989). VS I, II and IV are immunoaccessible to antibody at the EB surface; VS III is generally not although it may be an important site for T cell epitopes. The immunodominant serovar-specific epitopes are located on VS I or VS II. Within the *C. trachomatis* species, related serovars are grouped into one of 2 distinct subgroups, serogroups B (serovars B, Ba, D, E, F, G, K, Ll, L2) or C (serovars A, C, H, I, J, and L3). Members within a subgroup share a common subspecies-specific epitope surface, which is surface exposed in part of VS IV. Monoclonal antibodies to these surface-exposed epitopes neutralize *C. trachomatis* infection in vitro for cell culture, and in vivo, in the primate eye model (Zhang et al. 1987). These potentially protective B-cell epitopes have been defined to single amino acid resolution by peptide mapping (Conlan, Clarke and Ward 1988). Within a genovar (the genetic equivalent of a serovar), variants arise stepwise as a result of single base mutation. If an amino acid change results at an immunodominant epitope a serologically distinct variant may arise but there is yet no definition as to when the variation becomes sufficiently great to warrant new serovar status.

C. trachomatis is also grouped into 3 broad 'biovars' on the basis of pathogenicity for cell cultures. The trachoma biovar (serovars A–K) generally needs centrifugational force to infect cell cultures; the LGV biovar (serovars L1, L2 and L3) which causes invasive infection in humans characterized by lymphoid pathology and centrifuge assistance is not required to infect cell cultures. The mouse pneumonitis biovar of *C. trachomatis* has the mouse as its natural host. *C. psittaci* can also be ascribed to 8 different biovars on the basis of inclusion morphology and the influence of DEAE-dextran and cycloheximide in potentiating infection for cell cultures. These methods are tedious and should be replaced by more convenient methods based on the *omp1* (MOMP) gene, such as restriction fragment length polymorphisms (PCR–RFLP).

MOMP is currently the favoured candidate antigen for a chlamydial vaccine but a key question is whether the tempo of antigenic change, with its potential for evasion of neutralizing antibody, will prove sufficient to frustrate vaccine development. In STD clinics in Canada and among prostitutes in Kenya, substantial variations within MOMP involving both point mutation (antigenic drift) and large segment recombinational exchanges (antigenic shift) have been observed (Brunham et al. 1994) although the possibility of mixed infection in the latter case was not excluded. Other studies of organisms likely to be less clonally related indicate considerable variation arising both from point mutations of the *omp1* gene encoding MOMP (Poole and Lamont 1992) and from recombinational events (Brunham 1994). Clear evidence for recombinational exchange in the *omp1* gene came from sequencing studies of 7 *C. trachomatis* organisms from geographically and epidemiologically distinct cases of LGV in South Africa. These South African organisms were unusual in that they were untypeable with monoclonal antibodies directed against the 3 established LGV serovars. To update the published paper (Hayes et al. 1994), 5 of the 6 strains sequenced contained chimeric MOMP with an N-terminal half with an inferred amino acid sequence characteristic of serovar L1 plus a C-terminal half corresponding to serovar L2. Mixed infection was rigorously excluded by cloning and resequencing. The simplest explanation is that recombination occurred within fused inclusions resulting from mixed serovar L1 and L2 infection. Indeed, a gene analogous to the *recA* gene mediating recombination in *Escherichia coli* has been identified in *C. trachomatis* (Zhang et al. 1995). By contrast, in a cross-sectional study of trachoma in 2 Gambian villages with a combined population of some 1300 people, comparatively few variants were encountered among some 230 strains of *C. trachomatis* for which *omp1* sequences were determined, and there was no evidence for recombination events (Hayes et al. 1995). Antigenic variations within MOMP in the various biovars of *C. psittaci* and particularly, in *C. pneumoniae* appear much more limited, but have yet to be defined. Two geographically distinct isolates of *C. pneumoniae* each had an essentially identical *omp1* sequence (Carter et al. 1991, Melgosa, Kuo and Campbell 1991). In *C. pneumoniae* MOMP appears much less immunodominant than it is in *C. trachomatis*.

CYSTEINE-RICH OUTER-ENVELOPE PROTEINS

MOMP is a cysteine-rich protein but is not generally included as such by chlamydiologists. The classic chlamydial cysteine-rich proteins are the approximately 60 kDa outer-envelope protein (EnvB, coded by *omp2*) and a 12–15 kDa lipoprotein (EnvA, coded by *omp3*). The lipid moiety of the latter is thought to be embedded in the cytoplasmic membrane, with the protein moiety in the periplasmic space available for *S-S* cross-linkage with the periplasmic domain of the outer membrane-embedded, 60 kDa *omp2* protein. These 2 proteins are synthesized as the RBs mature into EBs. The *S-S* linked complex of *omp2* and *omp3* proteins may replace eubacterial peptidoglycan as the main structual component of EB cell walls that confers osmotic stability (Everett and Hatch 1995).

HEAT SHOCK PROTEINS

The chlamydial 12, 60 and 75 kDa heat shock proteins (hsps) are partially homologous with their better known *E. coli* counterparts GroEL, GroES and DnaK and with the related human mitochondrial proteins cpn10, hsp60 and hsp70. Human and bacterial hsps function as chaperonins, involved in the ATP-dependent renaturation and refolding of proteins damaged by proteolytic, heat or oxidative stress, targeting proteins or peptide fragments to biological membranes (Hightower 1991). Chlamydial hsp70 is a bifunctional protein, with an N-terminal ATPase domain and a C-terminal peptide binding domain structually homologous to MHC Class I proteins. Chlamydial hsp70, like human hsp70, may confer partial resistance to the cytotoxic effects of tumour necrosis factor (TNF)-α and intracellular reactive oxygen intermediates (Jaattela and Wissing 1993). Chlamydial hsp70 shares homologies with the egg receptor for sea urchin sperm (Raulston et al. 1993) but has low immunogenicity (Zhong and Brunham 1992). Surprisingly the chlamydial hsps are partly located in the outer membrane complex and may be involved with translocation of proteins across the cytoplasmic membrane (Raulston 1995).

Chlamydial hsp60 and hsp70 are early proteins, expressed by RBs 2–26 h after infection (Lundemose et al. 1990). The ratio of hsp60 to MOMP increases dramatically in chlamydial infected, interferon-γ treated, host cells (Beatty, Byrne and Morrison 1994). It is likely that cell mediated immune responses (but not antibody responses) to the hsps may be important. Chlamydial infections are characterized by plasma cell infiltration and the production of lymphoid follicles. Interferon-γ production by T-helper (Th)1 cells activates cellular immunity, and alters chlamydial growth and differentiation, with upregulation of chlamydial hsp production in infected cells. In the guinea-pig model, ocular application of chlamydial hsp60 in Triton X-100 elicits local monocytic infiltration (Morrison, Lyng and Caldwell 1989). Lymphocyte proliferative responses to hsp60 have been detected in 50% of 18 women with laparoscopically verifed pelvic inflammatory disease, in none of 10 women with chlamydial cervicitis and in 7% of 42 healthy controls (Witkin et al. 1993). Chlamydial hsp60 as well as MOMP and other outer membrane antigens stimulate proliferation of CD4+ Th cells (Beatty and Stephens

1992). The resulting interferon-γ, while chlamydiastatic and capable of recruiting activated immune cells, might be directly and indirectly immunopathological, in the latter case through upregulation of hsp expression.

MIP

The 29 kDa lipoprotein known as MIP because of its strong homology with the macrophage infectivity potentiator protein of *Legionella pneumophila* is not exposed on the surface of infectious EB although antibody to it shows weak neutralizing activity. The protein has peptidyl-prolyl *cis/trans* isomerase activity which, if inhibited, interferes with chlamydial replication (Lundemose, Kay and Pearce 1993), perhaps by affecting protein folding. The biological role of MIP deserves detailed investigation as, in *Legionella*, a facultatively intracellular bacterium, it is important for virulence.

7.2 Glycolipid and carbohydrate antigens

Chlamydiae possess a rough type LPS similar to the Re chemotype of *Salmonella minnesota*, but carrying a chlamydial genus-specific epitope consisting of a trisaccharide of 3-deoxy-D-manno-octulosonic acid (KDO) linked αKDO(2→8) α(2→4)αKDO, in which the α(2→8) linked disaccharide is immunodominant and unique to chlamydia. This epitope is surface exposed and immunoaccessible on RBs and EBs and it has been chemically synthesized, forming the basis of a commercial serological assay for chlamydial antibody. In *Chlamydia*, the epitope is synthesized by a trifunctional KDO transferase encoded by *gseA*.

Chlamydial LPS probably plays an important role in the pathogenesis of chlamydial infections. LPS persists in macrophages in the absence of productive chlamydial infection and there is evidence that the ability of chlamydial infection of epithelia to induce pro-inflammatory cytokines, including TNF-α which is likely to be involved in scarring and fibrosis, is probably largely explained by the interaction of chlamydial LPS with the epithelial CD14 LPS receptor (Ingalls et al. 1995). Proinflammatory cytokines upregulate receptors for lymphocyte adhesion and for MHC Class II expression. Chlamydial LPS was around 100-fold less potent than gonococcal or *Salmonella minnesota* LPS, perhaps explaining why chlamydial infection is more likely than gonococcal infection to be asymptomatic. LPS is a non-specific activator of macrophages and B cells and there is evidence that LPS-responsiveness in mice influences the immune response to chlamydial *omp2* protein (Westbay et al. 1995). LPS might also be important in explaining the apparent association between *C. pneumoniae* infection and heart disease (Ward 1995).

Chlamydiae may also have a smooth LPS with unique terminal oligosaccharides (Lukacova et al. 1994). The smooth LPS apparently undergoes significant phase variation. Definitive proof of its existence requires cloning and expression of chlamydial transferases capable of modifying core *Salmonella* or *E. coli*

LPS with relevant, chlamydial-specified, terminal oligosaccharides. This smooth LPS, as in other gram-negative bacteria, might be an important virulence factor.

Another glycolipid antigen with genus specificity that differs from LPS has also been described (Stuart, Troidle and Macdonald 1994). This exoglycolipid is shed into the supernatant fluid of cell cultures infected with *C. trachomatis*, but it is poorly defined and its role is unknown. However, an anti-idiotype antibody based on this antigen has been reported to be significantly protective in a mouse model of ocular chlamydial infection (Whittum-Hudson et al. 1995).

8 PROPAGATION IN THE LABORATORY

8.1 Chick embryo yolk sac

The chick embryo yolk sac has long been used for the culture of chlamydiae. Inoculation of 7–8 day old embryos leads to their death from day 4 of incubation at 35°C. All chlamydial species can be cultivated by this means, although *C. pneumoniae* strains are the most difficult (Kuo and Chen 1986). At death, the yolk sac is harvested, and elementary bodies can be visualized in impression smears stained by Giemsa, Macchiavello or Gimenez methods or by fluorescence microscopy using fluorochrome conjugated chlamydial monoclonal antibodies or DNA-intercalating dyes such as Hoechst 33258 (Salari and Ward 1979). Classical inclusions are not formed in the yolk sac. Chlamydial isolation in eggs is inevitably cumbersome and messy, being superseded by cell culture methods except where high yields are required for the bulk preparation of antigens (Schachter and Dawson 1978).

8.2 Cell culture

Chlamydiae can be grown in a wide range of animal-derived cell lines. The most commonly used lines for general purposes are HeLa 229 (human carcinoma), McCoy (mouse fibroblast L cell derived), Baby Hamster Kidney (BHK 21) and Buffalo Green Monkey (BGMK) cells. *C. pneumoniae* continues to be the most difficult species to isolate in cell culture, but HL (human fibroblast) cells or Hep2 cells are useful (Cles and Stamm 1990). Generally, LGV strains grow readily in cell lines without the need for special techniques, whereas other strains require the use of centrifugation and/or polycations to cell lines treated by physical or chemical means to render them non-dividing or not synthesising macromolecules. Centrifugation at 3000 *g* or more increases infectivity, possibly by a combination of pressure and directional force resulting in cell-surface changes. Reduction of host cell negative surface charge with polycations such as DEAE-dextran or polylysine, increases the susceptibility of cell lines to infection by reducing the electrostatic repulsive barrier to pathogen host interaction. This is particularly important for *C. pneumoniae*.

Various metabolic inhibitors have been used to pre-treat cell lines to enhance chlamydial growth and improve the sensitivity of clinical isolation including iodoxyuridine, mitomycin C and cycloheximide. These have superseded the former use of irradiation of host cells to prevent their replication. The most widely used agent for this purpose is cycloheximide (Ripa and Mardh 1977).

Other factors also play a major part in optimizing cell culture. These include the need for fetal calf serum, balanced salts, amino acids, glutamine, glucose, and optimal pH and water quality. The different species, and even different biovars require variation in technique to optimize culture but a combination of centrifugation with polycation pretreatment and cycloheximide is usually appropriate. Generally, a single cycle of growth will occur, passage onto fresh treated cells after 48–72 h being necessary to maintain cultures.

Following incubation, cell monolayers are fixed and stained for examination by light or fluorescence microscopy. Giemsa's method stains all members of the genus, and the inclusions are readily observed as bright refractile objects against a dark stained background by dark field microscopy. *C. trachomatis* inclusions produce a glycogen-like reserve carbohydrate in the later stages of intracellular growth which may be observed by iodine or periodic acid Schiff stain. The use of chromogens has however been superseded by more sensitive and specific fluochrome-labelled monoclonal antibodies based on MOMP (species specific) or LPS (genus specific). For specialized research, chlamydiae may be propagated in polarized cell monolayers (Wyrick et al. 1989), or in human Fallopian tube organ culture (Cooper et al. 1990). For detailed review of cell culture of *C. trachomatis* see Darougar and Treharne (1982), and for *C. pneumoniae* Cles and Stamm (1990).

9 INHIBITION BY ANTIMICROBIAL AGENTS

Drugs inhibiting chlamydiae fall into 4 categories, according to whether they interfere with folic acid synthesis, protein synthesis or cell-wall formation, or inhibit DNA gyrase. With the exception of sulphonamides and cycloserine, it is generally true that all chlamydiae possess a similar order of sensitivity or resistance to a given antimicrobial drug. On the other hand, antimicrobial agents with similar modes of action may differ significantly in their ability to inhibit chlamydial replication, a finding perhaps explicable in terms of permeability differences in the chlamydiae or host cells. There is no standard method for the estimation of the activity of antimicrobial agents against chlamydiae in cell culture. Although the numerical value of minimal inhibitory concentrations (MIC) may differ between research groups, the relative activity of one agent compared with another is usually in good agreement (Ehret and Judson 1988).

9.1 Inhibitors of folic acid synthesis

The sulphonamides inhibit *C. trachomatis* by competitively preventing the utilization of *p*-aminobenzoic acid. *C. psittaci* and *C. pneumoniae* are resistant to sulphonamides with the exception of an atypical and long-established laboratory strain of *C. psittaci*, 6BC. Any inclusion vacuoles formed in cell cultures infected with a susceptible strain of *C. trachomatis* are abnormally small and contain few or no chlamydial particles; this appearance is quite different from that of the giant RB induced by penicillins (see section 9.3). The sulphonamides possess moderate inhibitory activity, and are poorly bactericidal in cell culture. They are no longer recommended for routine therapy. Trimethoprim is poorly active against chlamydiae.

9.2 Inhibitors of protein synthesis

Antibiotics in this category include the rifamycins, macrolides and lincosamines, chloramphenicol and the tetracyclines. Rifampicin is one of the most active anti chlamydial agents known (MIC 0.007 mg l^{-1}; Ridgway, Owen and Oriel 1978), but as is the case with other bacteria, resistance can be readily induced in vitro by single step mutation (Jones et al. 1983). Rifampicin has a role as an adjunct with other agents in the treatment of complicated chlamydial infection such as refractory LGV or severe psittacosis. Other rifamycins are less active in vitro.

The tetracyclines are highly active against all species, and remain the drugs of choice for most infections. Their in vitro activity is similar to the macrolide erythromycin. The use of erythromycin for treatment of infection has been limited by the high incidence of gastrointestinal side effects. Newer macrolides have an improved side effect profile compared with erythromycin, and some are more active in vitro. **Clarithromycin** has similar in vitro activity to rifampicin. The azalide macrolide **azithromycin**, although less active in vitro than erythromycin, produces a high intracellular concentration with a prolonged intracellular half-life, such that both ocular and genital chlamydial infections can be treated successfully with a single dose of the drug (Martin et al. 1992, Bailey et al. 1993). Other macrolides such as midecamycin, roxithromycin and josamycin all have useful activity against *C. trachomatis* and, at least in vitro, against *C. pneumoniae*, and *C. psittaci* (Fenelon, Mumtaz and Ridgway 1990, Orfila, Haider and Bryskier 1995, Ridgway 1995a).

The lincosamine **clindamycin** shows moderate in vitro activity against *C. trachomatis*, whilst the parent compound lincomycin is inactive. Clindamycin alone is not reliable in eradicating *C. trachomatis* from the genital tract, although it may be used initially as part of a multidrug regimen for the treatment of pelvic inflammatory disease.

Chloramphenicol possesses similar activity to the sulphonamides, and is also poorly bactericidal against *C. trachomatis*. Topical use of this antibiotic for ocular chlamydial infection, e.g. neonatal conjunctivitis, has a high relapse rate. Thiamphenicol is of similar activity.

9.3 Inhibitors of cell-wall synthesis

Chlamydiae lack muramic acid in the cell wall, although penicillin-binding proteins occur (Barbour et al. 1982). Penicillin interferes with the division of RB and cell-wall formation, so that large abnormal forms appear in the inclusions accompanied by the excretion of hsp60, removal of the antibiotic 20 h after infection allows normal maturation of RB to EB to continue. Thus, penicillin is reversibly bacteriostatic, perhaps explaining why penicillin is less effective in vivo than other antibiotics. Ampicillin has similar activity against *Chlamydia* to penicillin, and is occasionally used to treat chlamydial infection in pregnancy. Careful follow-up is necessary to ensure that relapse does not occur. Other broad spectrum β-lactams including the cephalosporins have no clinically useful activity.

9.4 Inhibitors of DNA gyrase

Some of the fluorinated 4-quinolones have good activity against *C. trachomatis*, both in vitro and in vivo, being bactericidal at or just above their MIC. The first of these to demonstrate reliable clinical activity was **ofloxacin** but more recently, **clinafloxacin** and **sparfloxacin** have proved clinically effective and **trovafloxacin** (CP99–219) shows encouraging in vitro activity. Older agents, including ciprofloxacin, fleroxacin and lomefloxacin, show, at best, moderate activity in vitro against *C. trachomatis*, and are not reliably effective for clinical use (Ridgway 1995b). *C. pneumoniae* shows similar in vitro sensitivity to these agents (Fenelon, Mumtaz and Ridgway 1990). Clinical data on therapy against infections with this organism are awaited.

9.5 Drugs not inhibiting chlamydiae

Chlamydiae are highly resistant to a number of antibiotics, notably the aminoglycosides, the polymyxins, vancomycin and mycostatin. Some of these, particularly gentamicin or streptomycin plus vancomycin and colomycin and amphotericin, are useful for suppressing contamination by bacteria and fungi during the isolation of chlamydiae from clinical specimens in tissue culture.

9.6 Acquired antibiotic resistance

Naturally occurring antibiotic resistant chlamydiae are fortunately rare. An isolated report (Jones et al. 1990) described a small number of strains demonstrating resistance to tetracycline and erythromycin. Interestingly, these strains were solidly resistant to clindamycin. To date there is no hard evidence of significant acquired resistance to important anti-chlamydial drugs.

10 PATHOGENICITY FOR LABORATORY ANIMALS

Animal models are widely used for studying the pathogenesis and immunology of chlamydial infections (reviewed in Tuffrey 1994). Some laboratory animals and birds are subject to natural infections with chlamydiae which may be inapparent: this possibility must be borne in mind during investigational work.

10.1 Mice

Experimental systems utilize either human isolates of *C. trachomatis* or the naturally occurring mouse pneumonitis strain (mouse biovar, MoPn). The MoPn strain differs from the human strains on DNA homology, and has the disadvantage of being a single antigenic type. Mice may be infected by the intranasal, intraperitoneal, intracerebral routes and via the genital tract. Intravenous inoculation results either in rapid toxin-mediated death (3–4 h), or death within days from infection. The genital tract model, utilizing progesterone treated mice, has proved particularly useful for investigating the role of heat shock proteins in the pathogenesis of pelvic inflammatory disease, vaccine studies involving the protective effect of recombinant *C. trachomatis* MOMP, and the activity of antichlamydial antibiotics (Tuffrey 1994). A model for investigating *C. pneumoniae* infection has been described (Yang, Kuo and Grayston 1993).

10.2 Guinea-pigs

Guinea-pigs may be naturally infected with a *C. psittaci* agent causing mild conjunctivitis lasting about a month. The possibility of guinea-pig inclusion conjunctivitis (GP-IC) infection and its antibody must be considered when these animals are used experimentally or as a source of complement. Guinea-pigs artificially infected with GP-IC have been used by many workers as models for the corresponding *C. trachomatis* infections and immune responses in humans. As noted for the MoPn agent above, the GP-IC agent also has the disadvantage of apparently lacking antigenic variation. Lower genital tract inoculation may lead to endometritis and salpingitis, providing a scenario analogous to that seen in women infected with *C. trachomatis*, in contrast to the direct inoculation of the upper genital tract required in the monkey models.

10.3 Cats

Cats inoculated with *C. psittaci* have been used to study genital, pulmonary and ophthalmic infections; in particular, chronic chlamydial keratoconjunctivitis.

10.4 Non-human primates

In view of the almost ubiquitous distribution of chlamydiae among mammals, it is surprising that natural infection has not been observed in apes and monkeys. Nevertheless, these animals are susceptible to experimental inoculation, and models of ophthalmic and genital infection are well described. Major drawbacks are limited availability and the expense of maintaining primate colonies. Baboons and various species of monkey are susceptible to *C. trachomatis* isolated from the human eye and genital tract. Typically, ocular infection causes acute conjunctivitis 3–7 days after inoculation and follicular hyperplasia a few days later. The acute inflammatory signs are maximal 1–14 days after inoculation and resolve within a month. although the follicles may persist for many weeks. The cytology of conjunctival scrapings resembles that in humans.

Direct inoculation of the uterus or fallopian tubes of grivet monkeys leads to acute salpingitis (Ripa et al. 1979), and intraurethral infection of male chimpanzees produces urethritis with a marked polymorphonuclear response (Taylor-Robinson et al. 1981).

More recently, a monkey model has been developed using subcutaneous pockets of autografted material (Patton, Kuo and Brenner 1989). These autografts may contain conjunctiva, endometrial or tubal tissue, and have been shown to be susceptible to chlamydial infection. Studies have shown that on re-challenge, the transplants may show some immunity. The advantage of this system is that events, both immunological and effects of treatment, may be followed without the need to resort to major surgery.

REFERENCES

Bailey RL, Arullendran P et al., 1993, Randomized controlled trial of single-dose azithromycin in treatment of trachoma, *Lancet*, **342**: 453–6.

Barbour AG, Amto KI et al., 1982, *Chlamydia trachomatis* has penicillin-binding proteins but not detectable muramic acid, *J Bacteriol*, **151**: 420–8.

Barron A (ed), 1988, *Microbiology of* Chlamydia, CRC Press, Boca Raton, FL.

Bas S, Griffais R et al., 1995, Amplification of plasmid and chromosome *Chlamydia* DNA in synovial fluid of patients with reactive arthritis and undifferentiated seronegative oligoarthropathies, *Arthritis Rheum*, **38**: 1005–13.

Batteiger BE, Fraiz J et al., 1989, Association of recurrent chlamydial infection with gonorrhea, *J Infect Dis*, **159**: 661–9.

Bavoil P, Ohlin A, Schachter J, 1984, Role of disulfide bonding in outer membrane structure and permeability in *Chlamydia trachomatis*, *Infect Immun*, **44**: 479–85.

Beatty PR, Stephens RS, 1992, Identification of *Chlamydia trachomatis* antigens by use of murine T-cell lines, *Infect Immun*, **60**: 4598–603.

Beatty WL, Byrne GI, Morrison RP, 1993, Morphologic and antigenic characterization of interferon gamma- mediated persistent *Chlamydia trachomatis* infection *in vitro*, *Proc Natl Acad Sci USA*, **90**: 3998–4002.

Beatty WL, Byrne GI, Morrison RP, 1994, Repeated and persistent infection with *Chlamydia* and the development of chronic inflammation and disease, *Trends Microbiol*, **2**: 94–8.

Birkelund S, Johnsen H, Christiansen G, 1994, *Chlamydia trachomatis* serovar L2 induces protein tyrosine phosphorylation during uptake by HeLa-cells, *Infect Immun*, **62**: 4900–8.

Brunham RC, 1994, Vaccine design for the prevention of *Chlamydia trachomatis* infection, *Chlamydial Infections*, Editrice Esculapio, Bologna, 73–82.

Brunham RC, Yang CL et al., 1994, *Chlamydia trachomatis* from individuals in a sexually transmitted disease core group exhibit frequent sequence variation in the major outer membrane protein (*omp1*) gene, *J Clin Invest*, **94:** 458–63.

Campbell LA, Patton DL et al., 1993, Detection of *Chlamydia trachomatis* deoxyribonucleic acid in women with tubal infertility, *Fertil Steril*, **59:** 45–50.

Campbell LA, Obrien ER et al., 1995, Detection of *Chlamydia pneumoniae* TWAR in human coronary atherectomy tissues, *J Infect Dis*, **172:** 585–8.

Campbell LA, Kuo CC, Grayston JT, 1987, Characterization of the new chlamydia agent, TWAR, as a unique organism by restriction endonuclease analysis and DNA-DNA hybridization, *J Clin Microbiol*, **25:** 1911–16.

Campbell S, Richmond SJ et al., 1988, An *in vitro* model of *Chlamydia trachomatis* infection in the regenerative phase of the human endometrial cycle, *J Gen Microbiol*, **134:** 2077–87.

Carter MW, Almahdawi SAH et al., 1991, Nucleotide sequence and taxonomic value of the major outer membrane protein gene of *Chlamydia pneumoniae* IOL 207, *J Gen Microbiol*, **137:** 465–75.

Chang JJ, Leonard K, Arad T, 1982, Structural studies of the outer envelope of *Chlamydia trachomatis* by electron microscopy, *J Mol Biol*, **161:** 579–90.

Cles LD, Stamm WE, 1990, Use of HL cells for improved isolation and passage of *Chlamydia pneumoniae*, *J Clin Microbiol*, **28:** 938–40.

Coles AM, Reynolds DJ et al., 1993, Low nutrient induction of abnormal chlamydial development – a novel component of chlamydial pathogenesis, *FEMS Microbiol Lett*, **106:** 193–200.

Coles AM, Pearce JH, 1987, Regulation of *Chlamydia psittaci* (strain guinea-pig inclusion conjunctivitis) growth in McCoy cells by amino-acid antagonism, *J Gen Microbiol*, **133:** 701–8.

Collier LH, 1990, Chlamydia, *Topley and Wilson's Principles of Bacteriology, Virology and Immunity*, 8th edn, Edward Arnold, London, 629–46.

Comanducci M, Ricci S et al., 1990, Diversity of the *Chlamydia trachomatis* common plasmid in biovars with different pathogenicity, *Plasmid*, **23:** 149–54.

Comanducci M, Manetti R et al., 1994, Humoral immune response to plasmid protein pgp3 in patients with *Chlamydia trachomatis* infection, *Infect Immun*, **62:** 5491–7.

Conlan JW, Clarke IN, Ward ME, 1988, Epitope mapping with solid phase peptides: identification of type reactive, subspecies reactive, species reactive and genus reactive antibody binding domains on the major outer membrane protein of *Chlamydia trachomatis*, *Mol Microbiol*, **2:** 673–9.

Cooper MD, Rapp J et al., 1990, *Chlamydia trachomatis* infection of human fallopian tube organ cultures, *J Gen Microbiol*, **136:** 1109–15.

Cosgrove PA, Patton DL et al., 1992, *In situ* DNA hybridization detection of *Chlamydia trachomatis* in chronic ocular infection (stage-iv trachoma), *Invest Ophthalmol Vis Sci*, **33:** 848.

Darougar S, Treharne JD, 1982, Cell culture methods for the isolation of *C. trachomatis*, *Chlamydial Infections*, Elsevier Biomedical Press, Amsterdam, 265–74.

Ehret JM, Judson FN, 1988, Susceptibility testing of *Chlamydia trachomatis*: from eggs to monoclonal-antibodies, *Antimicrob Agents Chemother*, **32:** 1295–9.

Eissenberg LG, Wyrick PB et al., 1983, *Chlamydia psittaci* elementary body envelopes: infection and inhibition of phagolysosome fusion, *Infect Immun*, **40:** 741–5.

Everett KDE, Hatch TP, 1995, Architecture of the cell envelope of *Chlamydia psittaci* 6BC, *J Bacteriol*, **177:** 877–82.

Fenelon LE, Mumtaz G, Ridgway GL, 1990, The *in vitro* antibiotic susceptibility of *Chlamydia pneumoniae*, *J Antimicrob Chemother*, **26:** 763–7.

Fitch WM, Peterson EM, De la maza LM, 1993, Phylogenetic analysis of the outer membrane protein genes of chlamydiae, and its implication for vaccine development, *Mol Biol Evol*, **10:** 892–913.

Fukushi H, Hirai K, 1992, Proposal of *Chlamydia pecorum* sp-nov

for *Chlamydia* strains derived from ruminants, *Int J Syst Bacteriol*, **42:** 306–8.

Fukushi H, Hirai K, 1993, *Chlamydia pecorum* – the 4th species of genus *Chlamydia*, *Microbiol Immunol*, **37:** 515–22.

Gerard HC, Branigan PJ et al., 1995, Inapparently infecting *Chlamydia trachomatis* in the synovia of Reiters syndrome (rs) reactive arthritis (rea) patients are viable, *Arthritis Rheum*, **38:** R 24.

Grayston JT, Kuo CC et al., 1989, *Chlamydia pneumoniae* sp-nov for *Chlamydia* sp strain TWAR, *Int J Syst Bacteriol*, **39:** 88–90.

Hatch TP, Al-Hossainy E, Silverman JA, 1982, Adenine nucleotide and lysine transport in *Chlamydia psittaci*, *J Bacteriol*, **150:** 662–7.

Hayes LJ, Yearsley P et al., 1994, Evidence for naturally occurring recombination in the gene encoding the major outer membrane protein of lymphogranuloma venereum isolates of *Chlamydia trachomatis*, *Infect Immun*, **64:** 5659–63.

Hayes LJ, Pecharatana S et al., 1995, Extent and kinetics of genetic change in the *omp1* gene of *Chlamydia trachomatis* in 2 villages with endemic trachoma, *J Infect Dis*, **172:** 268–72.

Herring AJ, 1992, The molecular biology of *Chlamydia:* – a brief overview, *J Infect*, **25:** 1–10.

Hightower LE, 1991, Heat shock, stress proteins, chaperones and proteotoxicity, *Cell*, **56:** 191–7.

Ingalls RR, Rice PA et al., 1995, The inflammatory cytokine response to *Chlamydia trachomatis* infection is endotoxin mediated, *Infect Immun*, **63:** 3125–30.

Jaattela M, Wissing D, 1993, Heat shock proteins protect cells from monocyte cytotoxicity: posible mechanisms of self protection, *J Exp Med*, **177:** 231–6.

Jones RB, Ridgway GL et al., 1983, *In vitro* activity of rifamycins alone and in combination with other antibiotics, *Rev Infect Dis*, **5 (Suppl):** S556–61.

Jones RB, Vanderpol B et al., 1990, Partial characterization of *Chlamydia trachomatis* isolates resistant to multiple antibiotics, *J Infect Dis*, **162:** 1309–15.

Kaltenboeck B, Kousoulas KG, Storz J, 1993, Structures of and allelic diversity and relationships among the major outer membrane protein (*ompA*) genes of the 4 chlamydial species, *J Bacteriol*, **175:** 487–502.

Kuo CC, Gown AM et al., 1993, Detection of *Chlamydia pneumoniae* in aortic lesions of atherosclerosis by immunocytochemical stain, *Arterioscler Thromb*, **13:** 1501–4.

Kuo CC, Grayston JT et al., 1995, *Chlamydia pneumoniae* (TWAR) in coronary-arteries of young-adults (15–34 years old), *Proc Natl Acad Sci USA*, **92:** 6911–4.

Kuo CC, Chen HH, 1986, Identification of a new group of *Chlamydia psittaci* strains called TWAR, *J Clin Microbiol*, **24:** 1034–7.

Kuo CC, Wang SP, Grayston JT, 1973, Effect of polycations, polyanions and neuraminidase on the infectivity of trachoma inclusion conjunctivitis and lymphongranuloma venereum organisms in HeLa cells. Sialic acid residues as possible receptors for trachoma inclusion conjunctivitis, *Infect Immun*, **8:** 74–9.

Lukacova M, Baumann M et al., 1994, Lipopolysaccharide smooth-rough phase variation in bacteria of the genus *Chlamydia*, *Infect Immun*, **62:** 2270–6.

Lundemose AG, Birkelund S et al., 1990, Characterization and identification of early proteins in *Chlamydia trachomatis* serovar L2 by 2-dimensional gel electrophoresis, *Infect Immun*, **58:** 2478–86.

Lundemose AG, Kay JE, Pearce JH, 1993, *Chlamydia trachomatis* MIP-like protein has peptidyl-prolyl cis trans isomerase activity that is inhibited by FK506 and rapamycin and is implicated in initiation of chlamydial infection, *Mol Microbiol*, **7:** 777–83.

Lusher M, Storey CC, Richmond SJ, 1989, Plasmid diversity within the genus *Chlamydia*, *J Gen Microbiol*, **135:** 1145–51.

Mabey DCW, Bailey RL, Hutin YJF, 1992, The epidemiology and pathogenesis of trachoma, *Rev Med Microbiol*, **3:** 112–9.

Majeed M, Ernst JD et al., 1994, Selective translocation of

annexins during intracellular redistribution of *Chlamydia trachomatis* in HeLa and McCoy cells, *Infect Immun*, **62:** 126–34.

Martin DH, Mroczkowski TF et al., 1992, A controlled trial of a single dose of azithromycin for the treatment of chlamydial urethritis and cervicitis, *N Engl J Med*, **327:** 921–5.

Matsumoto A, 1988, Structural characteristics of chlamydial bodies, *Microbiology of* Chlamydia, CRC Press, Boca Raton, Florida, 21–45.

McClarty G, 1994, Chlamydiae and the biochemistry of intracellular parasitism, *Trends Microbiol*, **2:** 157–64.

Melgosa MP, Kuo CC, Campbell LA, 1991, Sequence analysis of the major outer membrane protein gene of *Chlamydia pneumoniae*, *Infect Immun*, **59:** 2195–9.

Miyashita N, Kanamoto Y, Matsumoto A, 1993, The morphology of *Chlamydia pneumoniae*, *J Med Microbiol*, **38:** 418–25.

Moorman DR, Sixbey JW, Wyrick PB, 1986, Interaction of *Chlamydia trachomatis* with human genital epithelium in culture, *J Gen Microbiol*, **132:** 1055–67.

Morrison RP, Lyng K, Caldwell HD, 1989, Chlamydial disease pathogenesis – ocular hypersensitivity elicited by a genus-specific 57 kd protein, *J Exp Med*, **169:** 663–75.

Moulder JW, 1988, Characteristics of Chlamydiae, *Microbiology of* Chlamydia, CRC Press, Boca Raton, Florida, 3–19.

Moulder JW, Levy NJ, Schulman LP, 1980, Persistent infection of mouse fibroblasts (L Cells) with *Chlamydia psittaci*: evidence for a cryptic chlamydial form, *Infect Immun*, **30:** 874–83.

Orfila J, Haider F, Bryskier A, 1995, *In vitro* activity of 9 macrolides and pristinomycin against *Chlamydia psittaci, New Macrolides, Azalides and Streptogramins in Clinical Practice*, Marcel Dekker, New York.

Oriel JD, Ridgway GL, 1982a, Epidemiology of chlamydial infection of the human genital tract: evidence for the existence of latent infections, *Eur J Clin Microbiol*, **1:** 69–75.

Oriel JD, Ridgway GL, 1982b, Studies of the epidemiology of chlamydial infection of the human genital tract, *Chlamydial Infections*, Elsevier Biomedical Press. Amsterdam, 425–8.

Patton DL, Askienazyelbhar M et al., 1994, Detection of *Chlamydia trachomatis* in fallopian tube tissue in women with postinfectious tubal infertility, *Am J Obstet Gynecol*, **171:** 95–101.

Patton DL, Kuo CC, Brenner RM, 1989, *Chlamydia trachomatis* oculogenital infection in the subcutaneous auto-transplant model of conjunctiva, salpinx and endometrium, *Br J Exp Pathol*, **70:** 357–67.

Perara E, Yen TSB, Ganem D, 1990, Growth of *Chlamydia trachomatis* in enucleated cells, *Infect Immun*, **58:** 3816–8.

Poole E, Lamont I, 1992, *Chlamydia trachomatis* serovar differentiation by direct sequence- analysis of the variable segment-4 region of the major outer-membrane protein gene, *Infect Immun*, **60:** 1089–94.

Raulston JE, Davis CH et al., 1993, Molecular characterization and outer membrane association of a *Chlamydia trachomatis* protein related to the hsp70 family of proteins, *J Biol Chem*, **268:** 23139–47.

Raulston JE, 1995, Chlamydial envelope components and pathogen host cell interactions, *Mol Microbiol*, **15:** 607–16.

Reynolds DJ, Pearce JH, 1993, Endocytic mechanisms utilised by chlamydiae and their influence on induction of productive infection, *Infect Immun*, **59:** 3033–9.

Ricci S, Cevenini R et al., 1993, Transcriptional analysis of the *Chlamydia trachomatis* plasmid pCT identifies temporally regulated transcripts, antisense RNA and sigma 70 selected promoters, *Mol Gen Genet*, **237:** 318–26.

Richmond SJ, 1985, Division and transmission of inclusions of *Chlamydia trachomatis* in replicating McCoy cell monolayers, *FEMS Microbiol Lett*, **29:** 49–52.

Ridgway GL, 1995a, Chlamydia and other sexually transmitted diseases, *New Macrolides, Azalides and Streptogramins in Clinical Practice*, Marcel Dekker, New York, 147–54.

Ridgway GL, 1995b, Quinolones in sexually transmitted diseases, *Drugs*, **49 (Suppl 2):** 115–22.

Ridgway GL, Owen JM, Oriel JD, 1978, The antimicrobial suscep-

tibility of *Chlamydia trachomatis* in cycloheximide treated McCoy cells, *Br J Vener Dis*, **54:** 103–6.

Ripa KT, Moller BR et al., 1979, Experimental acute salpingitis in grivet monkeys provoked by *Chlamydia trachomatis*, *Acta Pathol Microbiol Immunol Scand Sect B*, **87:** 65–70.

Ripa KT, Mardh PA, 1977, Cultivation of *Chlamydia trachomatis* in cycloheximide treated McCoy cells, *J Clin Microbiol*, **6:** 328–31.

Rockey DD, Heinzen RA, Hackstadt T, 1995, Cloning and characterization of a *Chlamydia psittaci* gene coding for a protein localized in the inclusion membrane of infected cells, *Mol Microbiol*, **15:** 617–26.

Salari SH, Ward ME, 1979, Early detection of *Chlamydia trachomatis* using fluorescent, DNA binding dyes, *J Clin Pathol*, **32:** 1155–62.

Schachter J, Dawson CR, 1978, *Human Chlamydial Infections*, PSG Publishing Company, Littleton, MA.

Shatkin AA, Orlova OE et al., 1985, Persistent chlamydial infection in cell culture, *Vestn Akad Med Nauk SSSR*, **3:** 51–5.

Stephens RS, 1994, Cell biology of *Chlamydia* infection, *Chlamydial Infections*, Editrice Esculapio, Bologna, 377–86.

Storey CC, Lusher M, Richmond SJ, 1989, Analysis of the complete nucleotide sequence of Chp1, a phage which infects avian *Chlamydia psittaci*, *J Gen Virol*, **70:** 3381–90.

Stuart ES, Troidle KM, Macdonald AB, 1994, Chlamydial glycolipid antigen – extracellular accumulation, biological activity, and antibody recognition, *Curr Microbiol*, **28:** 85–90.

Swanson AF, Kuo CC, 1994, Binding of the glycan of the major outer membrane protein of *Chlamydia trachomatis* to HeLa-cells, *Infect Immun*, **62:** 24–8.

Taylor-Robinson D, Purcell RH et al., 1981, Microbiological, serological and histopathological features of experimental *Chlamydia trachomatis* urethritis in chimpanzees, *Br J Vener Dis*, **57:** 36–40.

Tuffrey M, 1994, The use of animal models to study human chlamydial diseases, *Chlamydial Infections*, Editrice Esculapio, Bologna, 513–24.

van Putten JPM, Paul SM, 1995, Binding of syndecan-like cell surface proteoglycan receptors is required for *Neisseria gonorrhoeae* entry into human mucosal cells, *EMBO J*, **14:** 2144–54.

Ward ME, 1986, Outstanding problems in chlamydial cell biology, *Chlamydial Infections. Proceedings of the Sixth International Symposium on Human Chlamydial Infections*, Cambridge University Press, Cambridge, 3–14.

Ward ME, 1988, The chlamydial developmental cycle, *Microbiology of* Chlamydia, CRC Press, Boca Raton, FL, 71–95.

Ward ME, Bailey R et al., 1990, Persisting inapparent chlamydial infection in a trachoma endemic community in the Gambia, *Scand J Infect Dis*, **Suppl 69:** 137–48.

Ward ME, 1995, The immunobiology and immunopathology of chlamydial infections, *APMIS*, **103:** 769–96.

Westbay TD, Dascher CC et al., 1995, Deviation of immune response to *Chlamydia psittaci* outer membrane protein in lipopolysaccharide hyporesponsive mice, *Infect Immun*, **63:** 1391–3.

Whittum-Hudson JA, Saltzman WM et al., 1995, Oral immunization with antiidiotypic antibodies protects against ocular chlamydial infection, *Invest Ophthalmol Vis Sci*, **36:** S1030.

Witkin SS, Jeremias J et al., 1993, Cell mediated immune response to the recombinant 57 Kda heat shock protein of *Chlamydia trachomatis* in women with salpingitis, *J Infect Dis*, **167:** 1379–83.

Wyrick PB, Choong J et al., 1989, Entry of genital *Chlamydia trachomatis* into polarized human epithelial cells, *Infect Immun*, **57:** 2378–89.

Yang ZP, Kuo CC, Grayston JT, 1993, A mouse model of *Chlamydia pneumoniae* strain TWAR pneumonitis, *Infect Immun*, **61:** 2037–40.

Yuan Y, Zhang YX et al., 1989, Nucleotide and deduced amino acid sequences for the 4 variable domains of the major outer membrane proteins of the 15 *Chlamydia trachomatis* serovars, *Infect Immun*, **57:** 1040–9.

Yuan Y, Lyng K et al., 1992, Monoclonal antibodies define genus-specific, species-specific, and cross-reactive epitopes of the chlamydial 60 kilodalton heat shock protein (hsp60): specific immunodetection and purification of chlamydial hsp60, *Infect Immun*, **60:** 2288–96.

Zaretzky FR, Pearcepratt R, Phillips DM, 1995, Sulfated poly-anions block *Chlamydia trachomatis* infection of cervix derived human epithelia, *Infect Immun*, **63:** 3520–6.

Zhang DJ, Fan H et al., 1995, Identification of the *Chlamydia trachomatis Reca* encoding gene, *Infect Immun*, **63:** 676–80.

Zhang JP, Stephens RS, 1992, Mechanism of *C. trachomatis* attachment to eukaryotic host cells, *Cell*, **69:** 861–9.

Zhang YX, Stewart S et al., 1987, Protective monoclonal antibodies recognize epitopes located on the major outer membrane protein of *Chlamydia trachomatis*, *J Immunol*, **138:** 575–81.

Zhong GM, Brunham RC, 1992, Antigenic analysis of the chlamydial 75-kilodalton protein, *Infect Immun*, **60:** 1221–4.

FRANCISELLA

F E Nano

1 HISTORY

Francisella tularensis is the aetiological agent of tularaemia, an acute, febrile zoonotic disease (Bell 1981, Eigelsbach and McGann 1984, Nano 1992). *F. tularensis* was first isolated and characterized in 1912 during an outbreak in ground squirrels of a 'plague-like' disease in Tulare County, California (McCoy and Chapin 1912). During the following 2 decades *F. tularensis* was isolated from rodents in several locations in North America, Japan and the Soviet Union. Microbiologists recognized the common antigenicity of the strains isolated in the different countries but noted the differences in virulence between the North American strains and strains isolated elsewhere. The genus designation honours the American pathologist, Edward Francis, who studied tularaemia during the 1920s and 1930s; the species name and the name of the disease derive from Tulare County.

2 FRANCISELLA SPECIES AND STRAINS

2.1 *F. tularensis* biotypes

There are 2 recognized biotypes of *F. tularensis*: type A, previously referred to as biotype *tularensis* or *nearctica*, and type B, previously referred to as biotype *palaearctic* or *holarctica*. The 2 biotypes can be separated on the basis of their virulence in animals. Type A biotype requires only a small inoculating dose (<10 cfu) to cause a fatal infection in mice, guinea pigs or rabbits. It is thought that a small dose is similarly needed to initiate a severe, sometimes fatal, infection in humans (see Volume 3, Chapter 49). Type B biotype causes a lethal infection in mice and guinea pigs with a similar small inoculating dose but requires a 1000- to 10 000-fold higher dose to cause a similar illness in rabbits. Infection of humans with type B biotype causes a mild disease that is rarely fatal, even in the absence of treatment.

2.2 *F. novicida* and *F. philomiragia*

Two other *Francisella* species are recognized, but their importance in human disease is not well understood, nor is their distribution in nature. *F. novicida* has been isolated once from turbid water associated with dead muskrats and twice from infected humans. *F. philomiragia* has been isolated from several human patients (Hollis et al. 1989). Most of these infections were initiated after exposure to ocean water, and many of the patients had been immunosuppressed by treatment with corticosteroids following a near-drowning episode (Wenger et al. 1989). Other patients have had chronic granulomatous disease, rendering their polymorphonuclear leucocytes incapable of producing normal amounts of bactericidal oxidative metabolites. However, it appears that immunocompetent individuals can be infected with *F. philomiragia* and it is likely that many such infections have gone unrecognized in the past.

3 PHYLOGENIC RELATEDNESS

DNA hybridization studies and 16S RNA analysis (Forsman, Sandström and Sjöstedt 1994) have shown that all the *F. tularensis* isolates tested, as well as *F. novicida* strains, are highly similar. Using hybridization or sequence criteria, *F. tularensis* and *F. novicida* appear as one species. *F. philomiragia* strains appear as close, but distinct, relatives of *F. tularensis* and *F. novicida*.

Although researchers have tried to show the relatedness of *F. tularensis* to other gram-negative invasive pathogens, such as *Brucella* and *Yersinia*, using anti-serum cross-reactivity and DNA homology, these relationships have not been verified by 16S RNA sequence analysis. Members of the genus *Francisella* were found to lie in the γ-subdivision of the Proteobacteria group solely with *Wolbachia persica*, an obligate intracellular bacterium frequently found in ticks. *Francisella* species are distantly related to *Legionella* and *Coxiella*.

4   DISTRIBUTION

The type B biotype of *F. tularensis* is found throughout Europe, Asia and North America where it is thought to infect several species of small animals, especially rodents. The type A strain has been found only in North America where it is thought to have a reservoir in rabbits and their ectoparasites. However, both type A and type B biotypes can infect many species of animals; their true reservoir is not clearly established. *F. philomiragia* has been associated with waters along both coasts of North America but has also been isolated from patients living at a distance from any ocean. *F. novicida* has been isolated only in North America. Although both these species have been associated with dead muskrats, it is likely that other animals can act as hosts or reservoirs.

5   MORPHOLOGY AND GROWTH

Under observation by light microscopy, *F. tularensis* appears as a bipolar-staining coccobacillus. When viewed by electron microscopy, logarithmic-phase *F. tularensis* appears as a rod of approximately 0.3×1.0 μm. Smaller cocci and larger pleomorphic forms can be found, especially when cells are collected from the stationary phase of growth or when infected tissue is observed. Although accumulated evidence provides strong support for the existence of a capsule, it is nevertheless very difficult to visualize the capsule either by light or electron microscopy; when present, it is dislodged very easily from cells.

F. tularensis is an obligate aerobe that has an optimum growth temperature of 37°C. It can grow on several types of enriched, solid media. The addition of cysteine is required for the growth of many *F. tularensis* strains but not for the growth of *F. novicida* and *F. philomiragia*. Commercially available cysteine heart agar (Difco), supplemented with 5% defibrinated blood from rabbit, sheep or horse, provides a good growth medium for all types of *Francisella*. A peptone-cysteine agar has been used to differentiate colony morphotypes of *F. tularensis* (Eigelsbach, Braun and Herring 1951). Trypticase–soy broth, supplemented with 0.1% cysteine, a modified Mueller–Hinton broth (Baker, Hollis and Thornsberry 1985) or Chamberlain's defined medium (Chamberlain 1965) can be used for the liquid cultivation of *Francisella. F. philomir-* *agia* may require the addition of NaCl for growth in some media.

6   BIOCHEMICAL PROPERTIES

All *Francisella* species have an unusual fatty acid composition that is specific to the genus and, as such, a useful taxonomic tool (Jantzen, Berdal and Omland 1979). All strains have long chain C_{18}–C_{26} saturated and unsaturated fatty acids as well as 2 long-chain hydroxy fatty acids (3-OHC$_{12:0}$ and 3-OHC$_{18:0}$). Since the hydroxy fatty acids are not associated with phospholipids, they may be part of the lipid A structure of the LPS.

The surface of *F. tularensis* is covered by a carbohydrate-rich capsule. Removal of the capsule, through either biochemical treatment or mutation, abolishes the virulence of *F. tularensis* (Hood 1977, Sandström, Lofgren and Tarnvik 1988). The capsule apparently serves to protect *F. tularensis* from destruction by complement and may act as an anti-phagocytic factor. Capsules have not been demonstrated in *F. novicida* or *F. philomiragia*, but exhaustive studies have not been carried out.

F. tularensis has a smooth form of LPS, the O side chain of which may have the same structure as the carbohydrate portion of the capsule. The LPS of *F. tularensis* has very little endotoxic activity as measured by both the *Limulus* amoebocyte lysate assay and the galactosamine-sensitized mouse test (Sandström et al. 1992). Since macrophages can be maximally stimulated with a combination of endotoxin and interferon-γ, *F. tularensis* may benefit from the low endotoxic properties of its LPS.

7   GENETICS AND GENETIC VARIATION

F. novicida can be transformed with homologous chromosomal DNA or recombinant plasmid DNA containing homologous DNA (Anthony et al. 1991). Antibiotic cassettes can be introduced into the *F. novicida* chromosome by transformation with marker-interrupted DNA. Gene replacements can be created, but genome rearrangements are a frequent outcome of transformation (Mdluli et al. 1994). *F. novicida* supports the replication of broad host range plasmids of the IncQ/W group. All *Francisella* strains examined have at least one plasmid, and some at least 2 distinct plasmids (Myltseva and Nano, unpublished data). However, their nature and function are unknown.

DNA can be introduced into the live vaccine strain (LVS) of *F. tularensis* by electroporation. It appears that most of the DNA events found in *F. novicida* occur in *F. tularensis* but the introduction of DNA is much less efficient in *F. tularensis*.

Colony morphology variants appear in *F. tularensis* cultures, especially cultures in the late stationary phase (Eigelsbach, Braun and Herring 1951). At least one type of colony morphotype represents strains that have decreased production of capsule, and are avirulent in animals. Recent evidence indicates that the *F. tularensis* LPS goes through a reversible phase variation, and that this variation affects the ability of *F. tularensis* to induce nitric oxide, and grow in rat macrophages (Cowley, Myltseva and Nano, 1996).

8 INTRACELLULAR GROWTH

F. tularensis has been characterized as a facultative intracellular bacterium, although the amount of intracellular growth relative to extracellular growth in vivo has not been extensively examined. In the murine model of infection with the live vaccine strain (LVS) of *F. tularensis*, only intracellular growth has been observed. *F. tularensis* has been found inside macrophages and hepatocytes (Conlan and North 1992) but not in polymorphonuclear leucocytes. Apparently *F. tularensis* can enter macrophages via a microfilament-independent pathway (Fortier et al. 1994).

Following entry into macrophages, *F. tularensis* lives inside acidified vacuoles that do not fuse with secondary lysosomes (Anthony, Burke and Nano 1991, Fortier et al. 1995). Acidification of the vacuole is apparently necessary for growth of *F. tularensis*, probably as a means of releasing iron from transferrin or another host iron-binding protein. Treatment of murine macrophages with interferon-γ results in the production of nitric oxide and cessation of *F. tularensis* growth (Anthony, Morrissey and Nano 1992, Fortier et al. 1992). Since this growth arrest can be reversed by the addition of excess iron pyrophosphate, it is likely that the NO is combining with iron that would normally be accessible to *F. tularensis*.

9 IMMUNOLOGICAL RESPONSE IN THE MURINE MODEL OF TULARAEMIA

As in any infection, control of the growth of *F. tular-*

ensis in its host is affected by both innate and acquired immune mechanisms. At 2 days after infection neutrophils are essential for containing a *F. tularensis* infection (Sjöstedt, Conlan and North 1994), perhaps by lysing infected cells. Cytokines associated with the control of intracellular infections, including tumour necrosis factor-α, interferon-γ and IL-12, are observed during the first 48 hours of infection (Golovliov et al. 1995). The appearance of IFN-γ early in the infection probably originates from NK cells, since immune T cells presumably have not yet matured. IFN-γ is needed throughout the infection to contain the growth of *F. tularensis*; its removal with antibody results in rapid death of the host.

Although there is considerable evidence that long-term immunity to tularaemia is mediated largely by MHC class II restricted T cells (Anthony and Kongshavn 1988, Surcel et al. 1989), it is clear that there are other immune mechanisms involved in immunity. Of particular interest is the finding that there exists a T cell independent immunity that is induced within 2 days of an intradermal inoculation of *F. tularensis* (Fortier et al. 1991, Elkins et al. 1992, 1993). Mice lacking conventional T cells and infected intradermally with *F. tularensis* survive a dose that would be rapidly lethal if introduced via a different route. These mice also quickly acquire resistance to an otherwise lethal challenge delivered intraperitoneally or intravenously. However, the protection provided by an intradermal inoculation is short lived and mice die within 25 days. Long-term survival depends on immune, conventional T helper cells.

Although the murine model of tularaemia has been very useful in delineating many of the immunological mechanisms of clearance and in describing the disease process, it may not fully describe the pathogenesis for highly virulent strains in larger mammals.

REFERENCES

Anthony LSD, Burke RD, Nano FE, 1991, Growth of *Francisella* spp. in rodent macrophages, *Infect Immun*, **59**: 3291–6.

Anthony LSD, Kongshavn PAL, 1988, *H-2* restriction in acquired cell-mediated immunity to infection with *Francisella tularensis* LVS, *Infect Immun*, **56**: 452–6.

Anthony LSD, Morrissey PJ, Nano FE, 1992, Growth inhibition of *Francisella tularensis* live vaccine strain by IFN-γ-activated macrophages is mediated by reactive nitrogen intermediates derived from L-arginine metabolism, *J Immunol*, **148**: 1829–34.

Anthony LSD, Gu M et al., 1991, Transformation and allelic replacement in *Francisella* spp., *J Gen Microbiol*, **137**: 2697–2703.

Baker CN, Hollis DG, Thornsberry C, 1985, Antimicrobial susceptibility testing of *Francisella tularensis* with a modified Mueller–Hinton broth, *J Clin Microbiol*, **22**: 212–15.

Bell JF, 1981, *Francisella, Handbuch der bakteriellen Infektionen bei Tieren*, eds Blobel H, Schliber T, Veb Gustav Fisher Verlag, Jena, Germany, 172–256.

Chamberlain RE, 1965, Evaluation of live tularemia vaccine prepared in chemically defined medium, *Appl Microbiol*, **13**: 232–5.

Conlan JW, North RJ, 1992, Early pathogenesis of infection in the liver with the facultative intracellular bacteria *Listeria monocytogenes, Francisella tularensis,* and *Salmonella typhimurium* involves lysis of infected hepatocytes by leukocytes, *Infect Immun*, **60**: 5164–71.

Cowley SC, Myltseva SV, Nano FE, 1996, Phase variation in *Francisella tularensis* affecting intracellular growth, lipopolysaccharide antigenicity and nitric oxide production, *Mol Microbiol*, **20**: 867–74.

Eigelsbach HT, Braun W, Herring RD, 1951, Studies on the variation of *Bacterium tularense, J Bacteriol*, **61**: 557–69.

Eigelsbach HT, McGann VG, 1984, Genus *Francisella*, *Bergey's Manual of Systematic Bacteriology*, vol. 1, ed. Krieg NR, Williams and Wilkins, Baltimore, 394–9.

Elkins KL, Winegar RK et al., 1992, Introduction of *Francisella tularensis* at skin sites induces resistance to infection and generation of protective immunity, *Microb Pathog*, **13**: 417–21.

Elkins KL, Rhinehart-Jones T et al., 1993, T-cell-independent resistance to infection and generation of immunity to *Francisella tularensis, Infect Immun*, **61**: 823–9.

Forsman M, Sandström G, Sjöstedt A, 1994, Analysis of 16S ribosomal DNA sequences of *Francisella* strains and utilization for determination of the phylogeny of the genus and for identification of strains by PCR, *Int J Syst Bacteriol*, **44:** 38–46.

Fortier AH, Slayter MV et al., 1991, Live vaccine strain of *Francisella tularensis*: infection and immunity in mice, *Infect Immun*, **59:** 2922–8.

Fortier AH, Polsinelli T et al., 1992, Activation of macrophages for destruction of *Francisella tularensis*: identification of cytokines, effector cells, and effector molecules, *Infect Immun*, **60:** 817–25.

Fortier AH, Green SJ et al., 1994, Life and death of an intracellular pathogen: *Francisella tularensis* and the macrophage, *Macrophage–Pathogen Interactions*, eds Zwilling BS, Eisenstein TK, Marcel Dekker, New York, 349–61.

Fortier AH, Leiby DA et al., 1995, Growth of *Francisella tularensis* LVS in macrophages: the acidic intracellular compartment provides essential iron required for growth, *Infect Immun*, **63:** 1478–83.

Golovliov I, Sandström G et al., 1995, Cytokine expression in the liver during the early phase of murine tularemia, *Infect Immun*, **63:** 534–8.

Hollis DG, Weaver RE et al., 1989, *Francisella philomiragia* comb. nov. (formerly *Yersinia philomiragia*) and *Francisella tularensis* biogroup *novicida* (formerly *Francisella novicida*) associated with human disease, *J Clin Microbiol*, **27:** 1601–8.

Hood AM, 1977, Virulence factors of *Francisella tularensis*, *J Hyg*, **79:** 47–60.

Jantzen E, Berdal BP, Omland T, 1979, Cellular fatty acid composition of *Francisella tularensis*, *J Clin Microbiol*, **10:** 928–30.

McCoy GW, Chapin CW, 1912, *Bacterium tularense* – the cause of a plague-like disease of rodents, *Public Health Bull*, **53:** 17–23.

Mdluli KE, Anthony LSD et al., 1994, Serum-sensitive mutation of *Francisella novicida*: association with an ABC transporter gene, *Microbiology*, **140:** 3309–18.

Nano FE, 1992, The genus *Francisella*, *The Prokaryotes: a Handbook on the Biology of Bacteria: Ecophysiology, Isolation, Identification, Applications*, 2nd edn, eds Balows A, Truper HG et al., Springer-Verlag, New York.

Sandström G, Lofgren S, Tarnvik A, 1988, A capsule-deficient mutant of *Francisella tularensis* LVS exhibits enhanced sensitivity to killing by serum but diminished sensitivity to killing by polymorphonuclear leukocytes, *Infect Immun*, **56:** 1194–202.

Sandström G, Sjöstedt A et al., 1992, Immunogenicity and toxicity of lipopolysaccharide from *Francisella tularensis* LVS, *FEMS Microbiol Immun*, **105:** 201–10.

Sjöstedt A, Conlan JW, North RJ, 1994, Neutrophils are critical for host defense against primary infection with the facultative intracellular bacterium *Francisella tularensis* in mice and participate in defense against reinfection, *Infect Immun*, **62:** 2779–83.

Surcel H -M, Ilonen J et al., 1989, *Francisella tularensis*-specific T-cell clones are human leukocyte antigen class II restricted, secrete interleukin-2 and gamma interferon, and induce immunoglobulin production, *Infect Immun*, **57:** 2906–8.

Wenger JD, Hollis DG et al., 1989, Infection caused by *Francisella philomiragia* (formerly *Yersinia philomiragia*), *Ann Intern Med*, **110:** 888–92.

Chapter 61

HAEMOBARTONELLA AND EPERYTHROZOON

S A Martin and W J Martin

1 Definition	6 Laboratory isolation and identification
2 Introduction	7 Susceptibility to antimicrobial agents
3 Habitat	8 Pathogenicity
4 Morphology	9 Classification
5 Cultural characteristics and metabolism	

1 DEFINITION

This chapter deals with 2 genera of bacteria found in close association with red blood cells in animals and humans often suffering from infections in which anaemia is a prominent feature. Both these bacterial groups stain poorly with aniline dyes and are gram-negative. They can be readily demonstrated in blood films with Giemsa's method or with other Romanowsky-type stains. *Haemobartonella* and *Eperythrozoon* have a cell membrane but no cell wall and have not yet been grown in pure culture in vitro. These bacteria have been placed in the family Anaplasmataceae. Little is known regarding the physiology or genetics of these bacteria. Approved *Eperythrozoon* species and principal vertebrate hosts include: *Eperythrozoon coccoides* (rodents), *Eperythrozoon ovis* (ruminants), *Eperythrozoon parvum* (domestic swine), *Eperythrozoon suis* (domestic swine) and *Eperythrozoon weyonii* (domestic cattle) (Kreier et al. 1992). Approved *Haemobartonella* species and principal vertebrate hosts include: *Haemobartonella muris* (rodents), *Haemobartonella canis* (domestic canine) and *Haemobartonella felis* (domestic feline) (Kreier et al. 1992). For additional information on these and related organisms and their infections, see Volume 3 (Volume 3, Chapter 54).

2 INTRODUCTION

Mayer (1921) described an organism (*H. muris*) found in rat blood cells experimentally infected with trypanosomes. Later work showed that parasitic bacteria on the surface of red blood cells were responsible for anaemia in various animals after splenectomy. In some cases, anaemia due to these parasites has been reported in non-splenectomized animals. Both *Haemo-*

bartonella and *Eperythrozoon* are involved in these types of infections and fleas, ticks and lice are known vectors (Kreier et al. 1992). Typically, these organisms persist in the blood of immunocompetent hosts without causing significant clinical disease (Kreier et al. 1992). However, severe anaemia and high mortality rates can occur in neonatal pigs due to acute *E. suis* infection (Splitter 1950).

3 HABITAT

Haemobartonella usually occur on indentations of the red blood cell surface, but some are found in intracellular vacuoles; very few are found free in the plasma (Kreier and Ristic 1984). *Eperythrozoon* usually appear as ring forms on the surface of red blood cells and are frequently found free in the plasma (Kreier and Ristic 1984). Most of the identified species of both bacteria are found in domestic and wild animals, but there are reports of human infection (Kreier et al. 1992 and references therein).

4 MORPHOLOGY

Haemobartonella are gram-negative and predominantly coccoid (0.3–0.5 μm diameter), rod-shaped bodies are frequently seen and are probably composed of pairs and chains of cocci (Kreier et al. 1992). These bacteria are non-motile and have a single limiting membrane enclosing granules and some filaments but no cell wall. Eperythrozoa are gram-negative and may appear as rings or cocci 0.5–1.0 μm in diameter (Kreier et al. 1992). These bacteria are also non-motile and have a limiting membrane but no cell wall. The morphology of *E. ovis* changes as the degree of parasitaemia increases (Gulland, Doxey and Scott 1987). Single cells predominate in mild and moderate parasitaemias, whereas chains are observed in severe parasitaemias. *E. ovis* are located either centrally or peripherally on red blood cells (Gulland, Doxey and Scott 1987) (Fig. 61.1). Romanowsky and Giemsa staining procedures as well as electron microscopy have been used to identify both parasites in blood smears. In the case of *H. felis*, acridine orange appears to be superior to Romanowsky stains (Bobade and Nash 1987). Microorganisms in both genera replicate by binary fission (Kreier et al. 1992).

5 CULTURAL CHARACTERISTICS AND METABOLISM

Successful cultivation of these micro-organisms in pure culture has not been reported. It is unknown what carbon and energy sources are used to support growth in either *Haemobartonella* or *Eperythrozoon* species. However, it has been suggested that increased glucose consumption in parasitized whole blood from pigs was due to *E. suis* metabolism (Smith, Cipriano and Hall 1990). Based on the observation that glucose

(a)

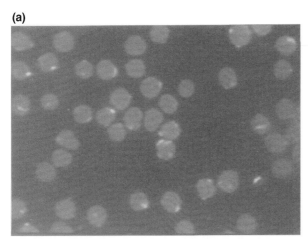

(b)

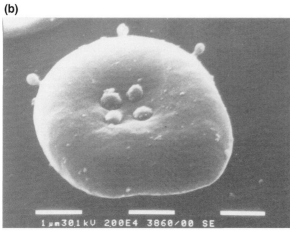

Fig. 61.1 (a) *E. ovis* parasitized erythrocytes stained acridine orange (× 480); (b) scanning electron microscope: *E. ovis* and 3 cell membrane protrusions. (From Gulland, Doxey and Scott 1987 with permission).

consumption by *E. suis* infected red blood cells was inhibited by the metabolic inhibitors iodoacetamide and sodium fluoride, it has been suggested that *E. suis* may metabolize glucose by glycolysis (Smith, Cipriano and Hall 1990). Clearly, more research is needed to elucidate the metabolic details associated with species in both genera.

6 LABORATORY ISOLATION AND IDENTIFICATION

Even though pure cultures of these bacteria have not been successfully cultivated in the laboratory, they can be isolated in association with red blood cells by collecting blood from an infected host and maintaining it and the contained micro-organisms in liquid nitrogen (equal volumes of blood and Alsever's solution containing either 10% dimethylsulphoxide or 5% glycerol) (Kreier et al. 1992). Because these organisms persist indefinitely in their hosts, a carrier animal can be maintained as a source of bacteria (Kreier et al. 1992). Either source can be used to inoculate an appropriate splenectomized host and microscopic examination of Giemsa-stained blood smears will verify infection (Kreier et al. 1992). In addition to staining procedures, methods have been developed to isolate *E. suis* DNA to use as a probe in hybridizations with *E. suis* parasitized swine blood (Oberst, Hall and Schoneweis 1990, Oberst et al. 1990, Gwaltney, Willard and Oberst 1993).

7 SUSCEPTIBILITY TO ANTIMICROBIAL AGENTS

Species in both genera are sensitive to organic arsenicals and tetracycline, but not to penicillin or streptomycin.

8 PATHOGENICITY

Both *E. suis* and *H. felis* are pathogenic in healthy, immunocompetent hosts (Kreier et al. 1992). *H. felis* frequently causes anaemia in cats immunosuppressed by infection with feline leukaemia virus (Cotter, Hardy and Essex 1975, Bobade, Nash and Rogerson 1988, Kreier et al. 1992). Anaemia in colony-reared primates due to *Haemobartonella* infections has been described (Aikawa and Nussenzweig 1972, Adams, Lewis and Bullock 1984, Kreier et al. 1992) and *Haemobartonella*-like infections have been reported in AIDS patients (Duarte et al. 1992).

9 CLASSIFICATION

Little is known regarding the taxonomy of these parasitic bacteria. Species differentiation within each genus is primarily based on host range infection (Kreier and Ristic 1984). The taxonomic position of species within each genus will remain unclear until detailed genetic information becomes available.

REFERENCES

Adams MR, Lewis JC, Bullock BC, 1984, Hemobartonellosis in squirrel monkeys (*Saimiri sciureus*) in a domestic breeding colony: a case report and preliminary study, *Lab Anim Sci*, **34:** 82–5.

Aikawa M, Nussenzweig R, 1972, The fine structure of *Haemobartonella* sp. in the squirrel monkey, *J Parasitol*, **58:** 628–30.

Bobade PA, Nash AS, 1987, A comparative study of the efficiency of acridine orange and some Romanowsky staining procedures in the demonstration of *Haemobartonella felis* in feline blood, *Vet Parasitol*, **26:** 169–72.

Bobade PA, Nash AS, Rogerson P, 1988, Feline haemobartonellosis: clinical, hematological, and pathological studies in natural infections and the relationship to infection with feline leukemia virus, *Vet Rec*, **122:** 32–6.

Cotter SM, Hardy WD, Essex M, 1975, Association of feline leukemia virus with lymphosarcoma and other disorders in the cat, *J Am Vet Med Assoc*, **166:** 449–54.

Duarte MIS, Oliveira MS et al., 1992, *Haemobartonella*-like microorganism infection in AIDS patients: ultrastructural pathology, *J Infect Dis*, **165:** 976–7.

Gulland FM, Doxey DL, Scott GR, 1987, Changing morphology of *Eperythrozoon ovis*, *Res Vet Sci*, **43:** 88–91.

Gwaltney SM, Willard LH, Oberst RD, 1993, In situ hybridizations of *Eperythrozoon suis* visualized by electron microscopy, *Vet Microbiol*, **36:** 99–112.

Kreier JP, Ristic M, 1984, *Bergey's Manual of Systematic Bacteriology*, vol. 1, 8th edn, eds Krieg NR, Holt JG, Williams and Wilkins, Baltimore, 724–9.

Kreier JP, Gothe R et al., 1992, The hemotrophic bacteria: the families Bartonellaceae and Anaplasmataceae, *The Prokaryotes*, 2nd edn, eds Balows A, Truper HG et al., Springer-Verlag, New York, 3994–4022.

Mayer M, 1921, Über einige bakterienähnliche Parasiten der Erythrozyten bei Menschen und Tieren, *Arch Schiffs Trop Hyg*, **25:** 150–2.

Oberst RD, Hall SM, Schoneweis DA, 1990, Detection of *Eperythrozoon suis* DNA from swine blood by whole organism DNA hybridizations, *Vet Microbiol*, **24:** 127–34.

Oberst RD, Hall SM et al., 1990, Recombinant DNA probe detecting *Eperythrozoon suis* in swine blood, *Am J Vet Res*, **51:** 1760–4.

Smith JE, Cipriano JE, Hall SM, 1990, In vitro and in vivo glucose consumption in swine eperythrozoonosis, *J Vet Med*, **B37:** 587–92.

Splitter EJ, 1950, *Eperythrozoon suis* n. sp. and *Eperythrozoon parvum* n. sp., two new blood parasites of swine, *Science*, **111:** 513–14.

FUSOBACTERIUM AND LEPTOTRICHIA

T Hofstad

The genera *Fusobacterium* and *Leptotrichia* include several species of non-sporing and non-motile, gram-negative, pleomorphic rods. They have in common a low G + C ratio and there are distinct similarities in whole cell fatty acid patterns. *Fusobacterium* spp. are obligately anaerobic, whereas most *Leptotrichia* strains are aerotolerant. In contrast to *Fusobacterium*, all species of which are asaccharolytic, *Leptotrichia* ferments glucose and a range of other carbohydrates. The habitat of both is the mucous membranes of man and animals.

Fusobacterium and *Leptotrichia* are phylogenetically related. In the phylogenetic classification of Woese and coworkers (Woese 1987) both genera are now assigned to a separate division within the Bacteria (Neefs et al. 1993, Olsen, Woese and Overbeek 1994).

FUSOBACTERIUM

1 DEFINITION

Fusobacterium spp. are gram-negative rods that are non-sporing, non-motile and obligately anaerobic. The bacterial cells are often pleomorphic, may be filamentous, and are spindle-shaped with pointed ends ('fusiform') in a few species. Amino acids and peptides are used for energy metabolism. *n*-Butyric acid is a major metabolic product. Threonine is deaminated

to propionic acid. The G + C content of DNA is 26–34 mol% and the type species is *Fusobacterium nucleatum*.

2 INTRODUCTION AND HISTORICAL PERSPECTIVE

The generic name *Fusobacterium* was introduced by Knorr (1923) for obligately gram-negative bacilli that were fusiform. He described 3 species: *Fusobacterium plauti-vincenti*, *Fusobacterium nucleatum* and *Fusobacterium polymorphum*. The species name *F. plauti-vincenti* was given to the spindle-shaped organism observed in materials recovered from ulcerative stomatitis by Plaut (1894) and Vincent (1896) and cultivated and named *Bacillus fusiformis* by Veillon and Zuber (1898). This organism is now assigned to the genus *Leptotrichia* under the name *Leptotrichia buccalis*.

Loeffler, in 1884, observed pleomorphic rods in diphtheritic lesions of calves and doves. The organism, named *Bacillus necrophorus* by Flügge (1886), was cultured by Bang (1890–91) from necrotic lesions of a number of domestic animals, and by Schmorl (1891) from an epizootic in rabbits. Prévot (1938) proposed the term *Sphaerophorus* for the pleomorphic anaerobic gram-negative rods that were not fusiform. The seventh edition of the *Bergey's Manual* (Breed, Murray and Smith 1957) divided the family Bacteroidaceae into 3 genera: *Bacteroides*, defined as rods with rounded ends; *Fusobacterium*, defined as rods with tapering ends; and *Sphaerophorus,* defined as rods with rounded ends that showed a marked pleomorphism and in which filaments were common. Studies of DNA base ratios (Sebald 1962) and physiological studies performed in the 1960s and the early 1970s indicated that there was no valid basis for separating of the genera *Fusobacterium* and *Sphaerophorus.* In the eighth edition of the *Bergey's Manual* (Moore and Holdeman 1974) the valid species included in *Sphaerophorus* were transformed to the genus *Fusobacterium.*

Bergey's Manual of Systematic Bacteriology (Moore, Holdeman and Kelly 1984) lists 10 *Fusobacterium* spp. Six new species have been described subsequently (Table 62.1). *Fusobacterium prausnitzii* has a DNA G + C composition of 52–57 mol%. *Fusobacterium sulci* has a G + C composition of 39 mol% (Cato, Moore and Moore 1985), tends to stain gram-positively and has a cellular fatty acid content that differs from other fusobacteria (Moore et al. 1994). Both species should be deleted from the genus *Fusobacterium.* The taxonomic position of *Fusobacterium perfoetens* is also in doubt. The original strain has been lost. The proposed neotype strain is an ovoid coccobacillus and its biochemical properties are not typical of fusobacteria (van Assche and Wilssens 1977). *Fusobacterium pseudonecrophorum* (Shinjo, Hiraiwa and Miyazato 1990) may be a synonym for *Fusobacterium varium* (Bailey and Love 1993). *F. nucleatum* and *F. necrophorum* are the species isolated most frequently from infections in man and animal.

Table 62.1 Current *Fusobacterium* species and their presence in the normal microflora of man

Species	Normal microflora		
	Mouth	**Gastrointestinal tract**	**Vagina**
(*Bergey's Manual* 1984)			
F. nucleatum	+		
F. gonidiaformans		+	+
F. varium		+	
F. necrophorum	+	+	
F. perfoetens		+	
F. naviforme		+	+
F. russii		+	
F. mortiferum		+	
F. necrogenes		+	
(*F. prausnitzii*)[a]			
(Post-1984)			
F. simiae[b]			
F. periodonticum	+		
F. alocis	+		
(*F. sulci*)[a]	+		
F. ulcerans[c]			
F. pseudonecrophorum[b]			

[a]Wrongly classified as *Fusobacterium* spp.
[b]Animal species.
[c]Habitat unknown.
Compiled from Slots, Potts and Mashimo 1983, Moore, Holdeman and Kelley 1984, Cato, Moore and Moore 1985, Adriaans and Shah 1988, Shinjo, Hiraiwa and Miyazato 1990.

3 HABITAT

The presence of *Fusobacterium* spp. in the human microflora is shown in Table 62.1. The gingival crevice is the oral niche of *F. nucleatum, Fusobacterium periodonticum* and *Fusobacterium alocis. F. nucleatum* is a constant member of the oral microflora of adults and children, and is also found in edentulous infants (McCarthy, Snyder and Parker 1965, Könönen et al. 1994). The vagina may be the principal habitat of *Fusobacterium gonidiaformans* and *Fusobacterium naviforme* (Hill 1993). Most other species can be isolated in varying frequency from faeces and abdominal infections. The relatively frequent isolation of *F. necrophorum* from soft tissue infections associated with the oral cavity and upper respiratory tract, compared with anaerobic infections elsewhere in the body, indicates these regions to be the principal human habitat of this organism.

F. necrophorum is a normal inhabitant of the alimentary tract of cattle, horses, sheep and pigs. Reports, mainly from the first part of this century, indicate its presence in a range of wild animals, including reptiles (Hofstad 1992, Jang and Hirsh 1994). *F. necrophorum* is frequently isolated from cats and dogs (Jang and Hirsh 1994).

Less is known about the presence and habitat in animals of other *Fusobacterium* spp. *Fusobacterium simiae* was isolated from the oral cavity of the stump-tailed macaque (*Macaca arctoides*) (Slots and Potts 1982). Fusobacteria, phenotypically similar to *Fusobacterium russii, F. naviforme* and *F. nucleatum,* were isolated from soft tissue infections contaminated with feline oral flora and from the oral cavity of cats (Love, Jones and Bailey 1980). Intragroup DNA homology studies of the isolates and of human and animal type strains indicated that similar body sites in man and animals may have their own genetic clusters of phenotypically similar fusobacteria (Love et al 1987).

4 MORPHOLOGY

Fusobacteria are aflagellar gram-negative rods of varied morphology. The bacterial cells range from short to very long and filamentous; some strains are coccobacilli. Width is variable. The cells may be single, in pairs end to end, or form long, coiled filaments. Staining may be irregular and sphaeroplasts are common in some species.

The cells of *F. nucleatum* are slender, spindle-shaped bacilli with tapered or pointed ends, 0.4–0.7 μm thick and 4–10 μm long, appearing singly, in tandem pairs, or in bundles or sheaves of roughly parallell bacilli (Fig. 62.1). Cell length is usually uniform among actively growing cells. The cells may have a beaded appearence due to the presence of intracellular granules. Filaments may be seen in old cultures. *F. periodonticum* and *F. simiae* have a similar cellular morphology. The cells of *F. necrophorum* are pleomorphic, often curved, with rounded and sometimes tapered ends, and may have spherical enlargements. Free coccoid

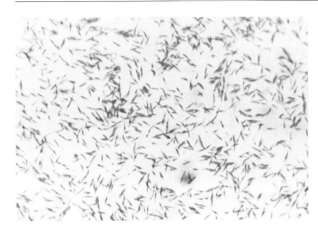

Fig. 62.1 *F. nucleatum*: gram-stained film of 48 h culture on blood agar.

bodies and, especially, filaments are common. Cell length may vary from coccobacilli to long threads in material from human infections. The organism is a more regular bacillus in young cultures. Except in young cultures, staining is irregular and beaded forms are common. *F. naviforme* strains may have boat-shaped cells. Gonidial forms may be seen in old cultures of *F. gonidiaformans*. *F. varium* is a small bacillus that does not form filaments or sphaeroplasts. The other fusobacteria are pleomorphic filamentous organisms. Strains of *Fusobacterium mortiferum* may be extremely pleomorphic with globular forms, swellings and threads.

5 CULTURAL CHARACTERISTICS

Fusobacteria are not particularly demanding with regard to a low oxidation–reduction potential. They are, however, fairly readily killed by exposure to oxygen. This is possibly due to their susceptibility to peroxides. Growth is best at 35–37°C and at a pH near 7.

All *Fusobacterium* spp. grow more or less readily on blood agar based on proteose–peptone, tryptone or trypticase. Good growth is usually obtained in a rich semifluid medium such as brain heart medium supplemented with yeast extract. Batch cultivation is best performed in a fluid medium containing a reducing agent. If narrow-necked, well filled containers are used, pre-reduced, anaerobically sterilized (PRAS) media are usually not necessary.

Surface colonies of *F. nucleatum* are 1–2 mm in diameter after incubation for 2 days. They are white to yellow-grey in colour, speckled, smooth or breadcrumb-like. The colonies are usually non-haemolytic. Cultures of *F. nucleatum* produce an unpleasant, but not foetid, smell.

After incubation for 2 days, colonies of *F. necrophorum* are about 2 mm in diameter, flat, circular with scalloped to erose edge, opaque, white to grey (subsp. *necrophorum*); or 1 mm wide, circular with entire margins, grey, translucent and with smooth surfaces (subsp. *funduliformis*) (Shinjo, Fujisawa and Mitsuoka 1991). *F. necrophorum* subsp. *necrophorum* is strongly β-

haemolytic; β-haemolysis is usually weaker in subsp. *funduliformis* and may need incubation for 3 or more days to develop. Cultures of *F. necrophorum* produce a foul, putrid odour. Fluid or semifluid cultures are characterized by abundant production of gas.

The colonial morphology of most other *Fusobacterium* spp. is similar to that of *F. necrophorum* subsp. *funduliformis*.

6 METABOLISM

Peptides and amino acids comprise the major sources of energy for all *Fusobacterium* spp. (Gharbia and Shah 1988, Gharbia, Shah and Welch 1989). Anionic and cationic amino acids are the main acids incorporated. Glutamate, histidine, lysine and serine appear to be key amino acids in *F. nucleatum* (Dzink and Socransky 1990, Rogers et al. 1992). Glutamate is a key catabolic substrate in *Fusobacterium* spp. It is catabolized via the 2-oxoglutarate pathway with the production of acetate and butyrate as end products (Gharbia and Shah 1991). Thus, the enzymes glutamate dehydrogenase and 2-oxoglutarate reductase are present in all fusobacteria. Enzymes representative of the mesaconate pathway for catabolism of glutamate have been detected in *F. ulcerans*, *F. varium* and *F. mortiferum*. The 2 latter also possess enzymes representative of the 4-aminobutyrate pathway. Lysine is catabolized by the 3-keto-5-aminohexamate pathway (Barker, Kahn and Hedrick 1982).

Poor growth of fusobacteria in media based on casein hydrolysates, which are composed primarily of single amino acids, indicates a growth preference for peptides over free amino acids. *F. necrophorum* has an absolute need for proline-containing peptides (Wahren and Holme 1973). Peptides containing 3–6 residues including glutamate, histidine, lysine and serine were readily utilized in the early and active stages of growth of *F. nucleatum* (Rogers et al. 1992). *Fusobacterium* spp. possess weak proteolytic activity (Seddon and Shah 1989). The low molecular weight peptides may be supplied by organisms present in the same ecosystem that have a wide endopeptidase activity on host-derived proteins (Gharbia, Shah and Welch 1989). The small peptides are possibly cleaved outside the bacterial cell rather than transported into the cytoplasm (Bakken, Høgh and Jensen 1989). An active transport of the dipeptide L-cysteinylglycine has, however, been detected in *F. nucleatum* (Carlsson, Larsen and Edlund 1994).

Fusobacterium spp. differ in their ability to use fermentable carbohydrate as energy source for growth (Robrish, Oliver and Thompson 1991). *F. nucleatum* and other species utilize glucose for biosynthesis of intracellular glycopolymers that can be degraded to produce energy under conditions of amino acid deprivation (Robrish and Thompson 1988). The accumulation of glucose is dependent on energy generated by the fermentation of amino acids (Robrish, Oliver and Thompson 1987). *F. mortiferum* is an exception in that accumulation of sugars is independent of a fermentable amino acid. Significantly, *F. mortiferum* has the ability to metabolize various sugars as energy sources for growth (Robrish, Oliver and Thompson 1991).

All fusobacteria, except *F. naviforme*, *F. russii* and *F. alocis*, produce propionate from threonine. Lactate is converted to propionate by *F. necrophorum* and *F. pseudonecrophorum*. Fusobacteria form volatile sulphur compounds from cysteine and methionine (Pianotti, Lachette and Dills 1986, Claesson et al. 1990).

7 CELL WALL COMPOSITION; ANTIGENIC STRUCTURE

The fusobacteria have a cell wall structure typical of gram-negative bacteria: an inner (cytoplasmic) and outer membrane, separated by a periplasmic space containing the peptidoglycan layer.

Lanthionine, the monosulphur analogue to *meso*-diaminopimelic acid, replaces the latter as the diamino acid present in the peptidoglycan of *F. nucleatum*, *F. gonidiaformans*, *F. necrophorum*, *F. russii*, *F. necrogenes*, *F. simiae*, *F. periodonticum* and *F. alocis* (Kato et al. 1981, Vasstrand et al. 1982, Gharbia and Shah 1990). *meso*-Diaminopimelic acid is present in the peptidoglycan of *F. varium*, *F. naviforme* and *F. ulcerans*. The peptidoglycan layer of *F. mortiferum* contains both diamino acids.

The outer membrane is an asymmetric, multilayered membrane consisting of phospholipid, lipoprotein, lipopolysaccharide (LPS) and protein. Fusobacterial LPS shares the general LPS architecture of a heteropolysaccharide, exhibiting O-antigenic specificity, linked to lipid A through 2-keto-3-deoxyoctonate (Hofstad 1988). The lipid A of *F. nucleatum* exhibits close structural relationship to that of enterobacterial LPS (Hase, Hofstad and Rietschel 1977) and cross-reacts serologically with antibodies to *Escherichia coli* lipid A (Dahlén and Mattsby-Baltzer 1983). The repeat unit of the O-antigenic polysaccharide of *F. necrophorum* LPS is an acid identified as a 2-amino-2-deoxy-2-C-methyl-pentonic acid (2-amino-2-methyl-3,4,5-trihydroxypentanoic acid), a novel structure not found before in nature (Hermansson et al. 1993).

The dominating protein of the outer membrane of *F. nucleatum*, designated FomA, has a molecular mass of 40 kDa (Bakken and Jensen 1986, Bakken, Aarø and Jensen 1989). It is a non-specific porin present in the outer membrane as a trimer (Kleivdal, Benz and Jensen 1995). The gene encoding the FomA porin has been sequenced (Bolstad and Jensen 1993a) and a topology model has been made (Bolstad, Tomassen and Jensen 1994). FomA and outer membrane proteins with molecular masses of 55, 60 and 70 kDa seem to be major protein antigens in *F. nucleatum* (Bakken et al. 1989).

The cellular fatty acids in the *Fusobacterium* spp. examined are straight-chain saturated and monoenoic acids of chain lengths C_{12}–C_{18} and O-3-hydroxytetradecanoate (Jantzen and Hofstad 1981, Calhoon, Mayberry and Slots 1983). O-3-Hydroxyhexadecanoate is

distinctive of the oral species *F. nucleatum*, *F. simiae* and *F. periodonticum* (Jantzen and Hofstad 1981, Tunér et al. 1992). The lipid A is the main source of the O-3-hydroxy acids (Hase, Hofstad and Rietschel 1977).

Unquestionable fimbriation has not been demonstrated in fusobacteria. A thin mucopolysaccharide capsule has been described in some *Fusobacterium* strains (Brook and Walker 1986).

8 SUSCEPTIBILITY TO ANTIBACTERIAL AGENTS

Over the last decades the antimicrobial susceptibility spectrum of gram-negative anaerobes other than the *Bacteroides fragilis* group has undergone a gradual change. Significantly, resistance to β-lactam antibiotics is increasing. Up to 40 and 30% of fusobacterial isolates in the USA and central Europe, respectively, are β-lactamase producers (Jacobs, Spangler and Appelbaum 1992). A penicillin-hydrolysing β-lactamase inhibited by clavulanic acid has been isolated from *F. nucleatum* (Tunér, Lindqvist and Nord 1985). Resistance to cefoxitin and clindamycin is very low. *Fusobacterium* isolates are fully susceptible to carbapenems and nitroimidazoles. Commercially available quinolones have poor activity against anaerobes, including fusobacteria. New quinolones that seem to be active against anerobes are undergoing investigation (Goldstein and Citron 1992). Resistance to tetracyclines in *F. nucleatum* is due to the presence of the *tetM* gene located on the chromosome (Roberts and Moncla 1988). A substantial number of *F. nucleatum* strains harbour the *tetM* determinant on a conjugal transposon (Roberts and Lansciardi 1990).

9 CLASSIFICATION

The genus *Fusobacterium* is phenotypically relatively homogeneous. Comparison of small-subunit rRNA sequences has revealed levels of sequence similarity that are consistent with a single genus, but intrageneric heterogeneity is evident (Lawson et al. 1991, Tanner et al. 1994). The oral species *F. nucleatum*, *F. simiae*, *F. periodonticum* and *F. alocis* form a homogeneous group with high levels of sequence similarity. *F. varium*, *F. mortiferum* and *F. ulcerans* form another closely related group. The genetic relationships are in accord with phenotypic similarities: the oral species contain *meso*-lanthionine as part of their peptidoglycan, ferment glutamate via the 2-oxoglutarate pathway, and their growth is inhibited by bile; *F. varium*, *F. mortiferum* and *F. ulcerans* have a peptidoglycan based on *meso*-diaminopimelic acid, possess the alternative mesaconate pathway for glutamate catabolism, and grow in the presence of 2% ox bile. *F. gonidiaformans* is genealogically related to *F. necrophorum* (Nicholson et al. 1994).

F. nucleatum is a heterogeneous species. Several subspecies have been proposed: *F. nucleatum* subsp. *nucleatum*, subsp. *polymorphum*, subsp. *vincentii*, subsp. *fusiforme* and subsp. *animalis* (Dzink, Sheenan and

Socransky 1990, Gharbia and Shah 1992). Two sub-species have been proposed for *F. necrophorum*: *F. necrophorum* subsp. *necrophorum* and subsp. *funduliforme* (Shinjo, Fujisawa and Mitsuoka 1991), corresponding to biovars A and B (Fiévéz 1963).

10 LABORATORY ISOLATION AND IDENTIFICATION

The isolation of fusobacteria from an anaerobic infection requires proper collection of the specimen, the use of an anaerobic transport vial, optimal anaerobiosis (an anaerobic chamber is not necessary), and a rich medium supplying optimal growth. Fastidious Anaerobe Agar Base (FAA, Lab M) supplemented with 5% sheep or horse blood is recommended (Brazier et al. 1990).

The use of a selective medium is necessary for the enumeration of viable fusobacteria in specimens of normal flora. The addition of josamycin, vancomycin and norfloxacin plus 5% defibrinated horse blood to FAA promotes luxuriant growth of *Fusobacterium* spp. while inhibiting completely most other obligate anaerobes and facultative bacteria (Brazier, Citron and Goldstein 1991). Rifampicin blood agar (Sutter, Sugihara and Finegold 1971) is useful for the selective isolation of *F. varium* and *F. mortiferum*.

All *Fusobacterium* spp. produce butyric acid but no isoacids. They are catalase- and nitrate-negative, sensitive to kanamycin (1000 μg disc) and colistin (10 μg disc), resistant to vancomycin (5 μg disc) and produce a rancid odour. A yellow fluorescence under longwave UV light is a common property of fusobacteria grown on blood agar based on FAA (Brazier 1986).

The characteristic cellular morphology of *F. nucleatum* makes a presumptive identification relatively easy. The fusiform cells of *L. buccalis* are thicker and usually larger (see Table 62.3) and those of *Capnocytophaga* spp. generally smaller. Moreover, *L. buccalis* and *Capnocytophaga* are not obligate anaerobes.

The tests shown in Table 62.2 are useful for the identification of species within the genus *Fusobacterium*. The properties listed for *F. nucleatum* and *F. russii* are shared with *F. periodonticum* and *F. alocis*, respectively. Diagnostic tablets are convenient for the examination of bile resistance, production of alkaline phosphatase and β-galactosidase (ONPG test). Commercially available kits based on the detection of preformed enzymes and designed for identification of anaerobes may be of help in supporting a suspected identity of a *Fusobacterium* isolate.

Determination of the electrophoretic migration of glutamate dehydrogenase and 2-oxoglutarate reductase provides a rapid method for the identification of most *Fusobacterium* spp. (Gharbia and Shah 1990). Identification based on gas-liquid chromatography of cellular fatty acids may be of value in reference laboratories, provided a database is used as a basis for comparison (Tunér et al. 1992). Of greater potential in the diagnostic laboratory is the use of nucleic acid probes. A genomic DNA probe has been used success-fully to detect *F. nucleatum* directly in samples of subgingival plaque (Lippke et al. 1991). A polymerase chain reaction (PCR)-amplified non-radioactive probe coding for part of the major 40 kDa outer membrane protein, the FomA porin, of *F. nucleatum* and seemingly specific for the species when used under condition of high stringency, has been constructed (Bolstad and Jensen 1993b).

11 ROLE IN NORMAL FLORA

Coaggregation, adherence of cells of different species or strains among resident bacteria, is an important event in the formation of biofilms such as dental plaque (Kolenbrander and London 1993). *F. nucleatum* is one of the bacterial species most frequently isolated in plaque from healthy sites. The organism coaggregates with several other oral bacterial species and is proposed to act as a bridge between bacteria that adhere early to the tooth surface and the late colonizers (Bolstad, Jensen and Bakken 1996). Coaggregation is a specific process dependent on surface-associated adherence proteins. The nature of the fusobacterial adherence proteins is largely unknown.

The role played by fusobacteria in other ecosystems is virtually unknown. They may participate in the biotransformation of bile acids (Hylemon and Glass 1983, Robben et al. 1989).

12 PATHOGENICITY AND VIRULENCE FACTORS

Pathogenic fusobacteria are in particular isolated from inflammatory processes accompanied by necrosis and ulceration (see Volume 3, Chapter 38). *F. nucleatum* constitutes about two-thirds of the *Fusobacterium* isolates. Next to the most prevalent *Bacteroides* and *Prevotella* species, *F. nucleatum* is the gram-negative anaerobic organism most often encountered in human infections. It is most frequently isolated from infections of the mouth, head and neck, pleuropulmonary infections, and abscesses of the brain and liver (Bennet and Eley 1993). *F. nucleatum* is one of several bacterial species associated with periodontitis in adults.

F. necrophorum is the cause of human necrobacillosis (Lemierre 1936) and the *Fusobacterium* spp. most often isolated from obstetrical and gynaecological infections. It is an important animal pathogen that is frequently isolated from necrotic and gangrenous lesions in domestic animals. The most common manifestations associated with the organism are liver abscess in cattle and footrot in cattle and sheep. The animal infections are due mainly to *F. necrophorum* subsp. *necrophorum*. By contrast, human isolates resemble *F. necrophorum* subsp. *funduliformis* (Smith and Thornton 1993).

Current knowledge of bacterial products or strategies that enable pathogenic fusobacteria to colonize and invade, and to damage the host, is sparse. *F. nucleatum* agglutinates human erythrocytes and attaches to

Table 62.2 Differential characteristics of *Fusobacterium* species encountered in clinical specimens

Species	Bile resistance	Gas in PYG	Production of		Hydrolysis of aesculin	Phosphatase activity	ONPG activity	Propionate from	
			indole	lipase				threonine	lactate
F. nucleatum	–	–	+	–	–	–	–	+	–
F. gonidiaformans	–	+	+	–	–	–	–	+	–
F. varium	+	+	v	v[1]	–	–	–	+	–
F. necrophorum	–	+	+	+	–	+	–	+	+
F. naviforme	–	–	+	–	–	–	–	+	–
F. russii	–	–	–	–	–	+	–	+	–
F. mortiferum	+	+	–	–	+	–	+	+	–
F. necrogenes	+	+	–	–	+	+	–	+	–
F. ulcerans	+	+	–	–	–	–	–	+	–

+, positive reaction for majority of strains (>90%); –, negative reaction for majority of strains (>90%); v, variable; v[1], may be positive after prolonged incubation; PYG, peptone–yeast extract–glucose broth.

human oral epithelial cells, gingival fibroblasts and polymorphonuclear leucocytes (Bolstad, Jensen and Bakken 1996). *F. nucleatum* also binds to collagen (Xie, Gibbons and Hay 1991), fibronectin (Isogai et al. 1992) and to a glycosylated protein-rich glycoprotein in the parotid saliva (Gillece-Castro et al. 1991).

F. necrophorum produces a leucotoxin with specificity for ruminant leucocytes (Coyle-Dennis and Lauerman 1979, Emory, Dufty and Clark 1984). Large amounts are produced by *F. necrophorum* subsp. *necrophorum* (Tan et al. 1994). The toxin is a heat-labile protein.

The role played by the lipopolysaccharide and other cell wall components in the pathogenesis of anaerobic infections involving fusobacteria has not been resolved.

LEPTOTRICHIA

13 DEFINITION

Leptotrichia species are gram-negative, large fusiform rods that are non-sporing and non-motile. They are usually anaerobic on first isolation; most strains grow aerobically in the presence of CO_2. Carbohydrates are used for energy metabolism. Lactic acid is a major metabolic product. The type species is *L. buccalis* and the G + C content of DNA of the type strain ATCC 14201 is 25 mol%.

14 INTRODUCTION AND HISTORICAL PERSPECTIVE

The generic name *Leptotrichia* was introduced by Trevisan (1879) for filamentous organisms found in the human mouth. Several years earlier Robin (1853) used the species designation *buccalis* for filamentous forms (*Leptothrix buccalis*) observed in wet mounts of tooth scrapings. *L. buccalis* was first cultured by Wherry and Oliver (1916) and adequately described by Thøtta, Hartmann and Bøe (1939). A new species,

Leptotrichia sanguinegens, has recently been described (Hanff et al. 1995).

The genus *Leptotrichia* is classified as the third genus in the family Bacteroidaceae. In the past *L. buccalis* has been confused with *Fusobacterium* spp. and, because of the frequent occurrence in young cultures of gram-positive stained cells, it has also been confused with gram-positive bacilli related to *Lactobacillus*. The name *Leptotrichia* has been used for the gram-positive organism termed *Leptotrichia dentium* by Davis and Baird-Parker (1959) and now classified as *Corynebacterium matruchotii* (Collins and Cummins 1986).

15 HABITAT

The human habitat of *L. buccalis* is the oral cavity; dental plaque is the principal niche. The organism is present in adults and children and has been found in the mouth of edentulous infants (McCarthy, Snyder and Parker 1965, Könönen et al. 1994). *L. buccalis* has also been found in the vagina (Bollgren et al. 1979) and in infections of domestic animals (Hirsch, Biberstein and Jang 1979) and dog bites (Goldstein et al. 1978). The role of *L. buccalis* in the normal microflora is unknown.

16 MORPHOLOGY

L. buccalis is an aflagellar, straight or slightly curved rod, 0.8–1.5 µm wide and 5–15 µm long; one or both ends are pointed or rounded. In gram-stained smears of 48 h cultures the organism appears as gram-negative cells often with gram-positive granules, singly or in pairs, end to end, and in a 'straw-like' arrangement (Fig. 62.2). Young cultures show a varying proportion of gram-positive cells. Thread forms and chains may be present in smears made from old, filamentous colonies.

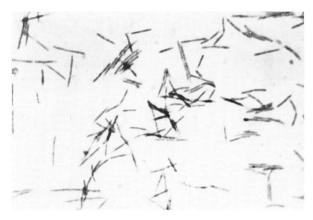

Fig. 62.2 *L. buccalis*: gram-stained film of 48 h culture on blood agar.

17 CULTURAL CHARACTERISTICS AND METABOLISM

L. buccalis grows well under anaerobic or microaerobic conditions, but poorly in air even in the presence of CO_2 (Hofstad and Næss 1992). Surface colonies on blood agar medium are 2–3 mm in diameter after incubation anaerobically for 2 days, smooth, colourless, sometimes raised and with a filamentous edge, non-adherent and non-haemolytic. After prolonged incubation the surface of the colonies becomes convoluted, resembling that of a human brain.

L. buccalis is highly saccharolytic. Mono- and disaccharides are fermented with the production of lactic acid alone, or accompanied by trace amounts of acetic and succinic acids. The terminal pH is 5.4 or less. Growth in fluid or semifluid media is enhanced by serum and dependent on the presence in the medium of a fermentable carbohydrate. Ammonia is not produced. This clearly indicates that carbohydrate is used for energy metabolism.

18 CELL WALL COMPOSITION

L. buccalis has a gram-negative cell wall structure (Hofstad and Selvig 1969). The diamino acid of the peptidoglycan is *meso*-diaminopimelic acid (Vasstrand et al. 1982). The cellular fatty acid composition is similar to that of the fusobacteria, with hexadecanoic, octadecanoic and 3-hydroxytetradecanoic acids as major components (Hofstad and Jantzen 1982). An unusual feature is a ridged surface structure formed by an assay of macromolecules erected on the surface like a fence with closely set vertical pales (Listgarten and Lai 1975, Smith, Murray and Hall 1994).

19 CLASSIFICATION

L. buccalis strains vary with respect to cellular and colonial morphology, fermentation of sugars (Weinberger et al. 1991, Hammann et al. 1993) and presence of glycosidases (Hofstad and Næss 1992). This indicates heterogeneity of the species.

20 LABORATORY ISOLATION, IDENTIFICATION AND SUSCEPTIBILITY TO ANTIMICROBIAL AGENTS

L. buccalis can be isolated from clinical specimens on FAA or Brucella blood agar. The selective medium of Brazier et al. (1990) is recommended for isolation from normal flora. A reliable identification can be made from cellular and colonical morphology and a few biochemical tests (Table 62.3).

L. buccalis is susceptible to β-lactam antibiotics, clindamycin, chloramphenicol, tetracyclines and metronidazole, but resistant to vancomycin and aminoglycosides (George et al. 1981, Weinberger et al. 1991).

Table 62.3 Characters differentiating *L. buccalis*, *F. nucleatum* and *Capnocytophaga* spp.

Character	*L. buccalis*	*F. nucleatum*	*Capnocytophaga*
Microscopic morphology (blood agar)	Gram-negative,[a] 5–15 μm long, thick fusiform bacilli	Gram-negative, 3–10 μm long, slender fusiform bacilli	Gram-negative, 3–6 μm slender fusiform bacilli
Colonial morphology	Smooth, rhizoid or convoluted	Smooth, convex, 'flecked' appearance	Flat, rough, spreading margin,[b] adherent; or low-convex, smooth. Yellow-pigmented
Growth in air + 5–10% CO_2	+	–	+
Acid from glucose	+	–	+
Production of indole	–	+	–
Main fatty acids from glucose/peptone	Lactic	Butyric	Acetic, succinic

[a]Often gram-positive in young cultures.
[b]Gliding motility.

Most strains are moderately resistant or resistant to erythromycin.

21 PATHOGENICITY

L. buccalis has occasionally been found in blood cultures of neutropenic adults and children, and from patients with endocarditis (Reig et al. 1985, Weinberger et al. 1991, Hammann et al. 1993, Schwartz et al. 1995). *L. sanguinegens* was isolated from blood cultures of obstetric patients and neonates (Hanff et al. 1995). The pathogenesis is unknown.

REFERENCES

Adriaans B, Shah HN, 1988, Fusobacterium ulcerans sp. nov. from tropical ulcers, *Int J Syst Bacteriol*, **38:** 447–8.

van Assche FF, Wilssens AT, 1977, Fusobacterium perfoetens (Tissier) Moore and Holdeman 1973: description and proposed neotype strains, *Int J Syst Bacteriol*, **27:** 1–5.

Bailey GD, Love DN, 1993, Fusobacterium pseudonecrophorum is a synonym for *Fusobacterium varium*, *Int J Syst Bacteriol*, **43:** 819–21.

Bakken V, Aarø S, Jensen HB, 1989, Purification and partial characterization of a major outer-membrane protein of *Fusobacterium nucleatum*, *J Gen Microbiol*, **135:** 3253–62.

Bakken V, Högh BT, Jensen HB, 1989, Utilization of amino acids and peptides by *Fusobacterium nucleatum*, *Scand J Dent Res*, **97:** 43–53.

Bakken V, Jensen HB, 1986, Outer membrane proteins of *Fusobacterium nucleatum* Fev1, *J Gen Microbiol*, **132:** 1069–78.

Bakken V, Aarø S et al., 1989, Outer membrane proteins as major antigens of *Fusobacterium nucleatum*, *FEMS Microbiol Immunol*, **47:** 473–84.

Bang B, 1890–91, Om aarsagen til lokal nekrose, *Maanedskr for Dyrlæger*, **2:** 235–59.

Barker HA, Kahn JM, Hedrick L, 1982, Pathway of lysine degradation in *Fusobacterium nucleatum*, *J Bacteriol*, **152:** 201–7.

Bennett KW, Eley A, 1993, Fusobacteria: new taxonomy and related diseases, *J Med Microbiol*, **39:** 246–54.

Bollgren I, Källenius G et al., 1979, Periurethral anaerobic microflora of healthy girls, *J Clin Microbiol*, **10:** 419–24.

Bolstad AI, Jensen HB, 1993a, Complete sequence of *omp1*, the structural gene encoding the 40-kDa outer membrane protein of *Fusobacterium nucleatum* strain Fev1, *Gene*, **132:** 107–12.

Bolstad AI, Jensen HB, 1993b, Polymerase chain reaction-amplified nonradioactive probes for identification of *Fusobacterium nucleatum*, *J Clin Microbiol*, **31:** 528–32.

Bolstad AI, Jensen HB, Bakken V, 1996, Taxonomy, biology and periodontal aspects of *Fusobacterium nucleatum*, *Clin Microbiol Rev*, **9:** 55–71.

Bolstad AI, Tommassen J, Jensen HB, 1994, Sequence variability of the 40-kDa outer membrane proteins of *Fusobacterium nucleatum* and a model for the topology of the proteins, *Mol Gen Genet*, **244:** 104–10.

Brazier JS, 1986, Yellow fluorescence of fusobacteria, *Appl Microbiol*, **2:** 125–6.

Brazier JS, Citron DM, Goldstein EJC, 1991, A selective medium for *Fusobacterium* spp., *J Appl Bacteriol*, **71:** 343–6.

Brazier JS, Goldstein EJC et al., 1990, Fastidious anaerobe agar compared with Wilkins–Chalgren agar, brain heart infusion agar, and *Brucella* agar for susceptibility testing of *Fusobacterium* species, *Antimicrob Agents Chemother*, **34:** 2280–2.

Breed RS, Murray GD, Smith NR (eds), 1957, *Bergey's Manual of Determinative Bacteriology*, 7th edn, Williams & Wilkins, Baltimore, 423.

Brook I, Walker RI, 1986, The relationship between *Fusobacterium* species and other flora in mixed infection, *J Med Microbiol*, **21:** 93–100.

Calhoon DA, Mayberry WR, Slots J, 1983, Cellular fatty acid and soluble protein profiles of oral fusobacteria, *J Dent Res*, **62:** 1181–5.

Carlsson J, Larsen JT, Edlund M-B, 1994, Utilization of glutathione (L-γ-glutamyl-L-cysteinylglycine) by *Fusobacterium nucleatum* subspecies *nucleatum*, *Oral Microbiol Immunol*, **9:** 297–300.

Cato EP, Moore LVH, Moore WEC, 1985, Fusobacterium alocis sp. nov. and *Fusobacterium sulci* sp. nov. from the human gingival sulcus, *Int J Syst Bacteriol*, **35:** 475–7.

Claesson R, Edlund M-B et al., 1990, Production of volatile sulfur compounds by various *Fusobacterium* species, *Oral Microbiol Immunol*, **5:** 137–42.

Collins MD, Cummins CS, 1986, Genus *Corynebacterium* Lehmann and Neumann 1896, 350, *Bergey's Manual of Systematic Bacteriology*, vol. 2, eds Sneath PHA, Mair NS et al., Williams & Wilkins, Baltimore, 1266–83.

Coyle-Dennis JE, Lauerman LH, 1978, Correlations between leukocidin production and virulence of two isolates of *Fusobacterium necrophorum*, *Am J Vet Res*, **39:** 1790–3.

Dahlén G, Mattsby-Baltzer I, 1983, Lipid A in anaerobic bacteria, *Infect Immun*, **39:** 466–8.

Davis GHG, Baird-Parker AC, 1959, *Leptotrichia buccalis*, *Br Dent J*, **106:** 70–3.

Dzink JL, Sheenan MT, Socransky SS, 1990, Proposal of three subspecies of *Fusobacterium nucleatum* Knorr 1922: *Fusobacterium nucleatum* subsp. *nucleatum* subsp. nov., comb. nov.; *Fusobacterium nucleatum* subsp. *polymorphum* subsp. nov., nom. rev., comb. nov.; and *Fusobacterium nucleatum* subsp. *vincentii* subsp. nov., nom. rev., comb. nov., *Int J Syst Bacteriol*, **40:** 74–8.

Dzink JL, Socransky SS, 1990, Amino acid utilization by *Fusobacterium nucleatum* grown in a chemically defined medium, *Oral Microbiol Immunol*, **5:** 172–4.

Emery DL, Dufty JH, Clark BL, 1984, Biochemical and functional properties of a leucocidin produced by several strains of *Fusobacterium necrophorum*, *Aust Vet J*, **61:** 382–7.

Fievez L, 1963, *Etude comparée des Souches de* Sphaerophorus necrophorus *isolées de l'homme et chez l'animal*, Presses Académiques Européennes, Brussels.

Flügge C, 1886, *Die Mikroorganismen*, FCW Vogel, Leipzig.

George WL, Kirby BD et al., 1981, Gram-negative anaerobic bacilli: their role in infection and patterns of susceptibility to antimicrobial agents. II. Little-known *Fusobacterium* species and miscellaneous genera, *Rev Infect Dis*, **3:** 599–626.

Gharbia SE, Shah HN, 1988, Glucose ultilization and growth response to protein hydrolysates by *Fusobacterium* species, *Curr Microbiol*, **17:** 229–34.

Gharbia SE, Shah HN, 1990, Identification of *Fusobacterium* species by the electrophoretic migration of glutamate dehydrogenase and 2-oxoglutarate reductase in relation to their DNA base composition and peptidoglycan dibasic amino acids, *J Med Microbiol*, **33:** 183–8.

Gharbia SE, Shah HN, 1991, Pathways of glutamate catabolism among *Fusobacterium* species, *J Gen Microbiol*, **137:** 1201–6.

Gharbia SE, Shah HN, 1992, Fusobacterium nucleatum subsp. *fusiforme* subsp. nov. and *Fusobacterium nucleatum* subsp. *animalis* subsp. nov. as additional subspecies within *Fusobacterium nucleatum*, *Int J Syst Bacteriol*, **42:** 296–8.

Gharbia SE, Shah HN, Welch SG, 1989, The influence of peptides on the uptake of amino acids in *Fusobacterium*; predicted interactions with *Porphyromonas gingivalis*, *Curr Microbiol*, **19:** 231–5.

Gillece-Castro BL, Prakobpol A et al., 1991, Structure of bacterial receptor activity in human salivary proline-rich glycoprotein, *J Biol Chem*, **266:** 17358–68.

Goldstein EJC, Citron DM, 1992, Comparative activity of ciprofloxacin, ofloxacin, sparfloxacin, temafloxacin, CI-960, CI-990, and WIN 57273 against anaerobic bacteria, *Antimicrob Agents Chemother*, **36**: 1158–62.

Goldstein EJC, Citron DM et al., 1978, Bacteriology of human and animal bite wounds, *J Clin Microbiol*, **8**: 667–72.

Hammann R, Iwand A et al., 1993, Endocarditis caused by a *Leptotrichia buccalis*-like bacterium in a patient with a prosthetic aortic valve, *Eur J Clin Microbiol Infect Dis*, **12**: 280–2.

Hanff PA, Rosol-Donoghue J-A et al., 1995, *Leptotrichia sanguinegens* sp. nov., a new agent of postpartum and neonatal bacteremia, *Clin Infect Dis*, **20, Suppl.**: S237–9.

Hase S, Hofstad T, Rietschel ET, 1977, Chemical structure of the lipid A component of lipopolysaccharides from *Fusobacterium nucleatum*, *J Bacteriol*, **129**: 9–14.

Hermansson K, Perry MB et al., 1993, Structural studies of the O-antigenic polysaccharide of *Fusobacterium necrophorum*, *Eur J Biochem*, **212**: 801–9.

Hill GB, 1993, Investigating the source of amniotic fluid isolates of fusobacteria, *Clin Infect Dis*, **16, Suppl. 4**: S423–4.

Hirsh DC, Biberstein EL, Jang SS, 1979, Obligate anaerobes in clinical veterinary practice, *J Clin Microbiol*, **10**: 188–91.

Hofstad T, 1988, Endotoxins of gram-negative bacteria, *Anaerobes Today*, eds Hardie JM, Borriello P, John Wiley & Sons, Chichester, 79–85.

Hofstad T, 1992, The genus *Fusobacterium*, *The Prokaryotes*, 2nd edn, vol. 4, eds Balows A, Trüper HG et al., Springer-Verlag, New York, 4114–26.

Hofstad T, Jantzen E, 1982, Fatty acids of *Leptotrichia buccalis*: taxonomic implications, *J Gen Microbiol*, **128**: 151–3.

Hofstad T, Næss V, 1992, DNA base composition, aerotolerance and enzyme patterns of *Leptotrichia buccalis*, *APMIS*, **100**: 116–18.

Hofstad T, Selvig KA, 1969, Ultrastructure of *Leptotrichia buccalis*, *J Gen Microbiol*, **56**: 23–6.

Hylemon PB, Glass TL, 1983, Biotransformation of bile acids and cholesterol by the intestinal microflora, *Human Intestinal Microflora in Health and Disease*, ed. Hentges DJ, Academic Press, New York and London, 189–213.

Isogai E, Hirose K et al., 1992, Three types of binding by *Porphyromonas gingivalis* and oral bacteria to fibronectin, buccal epithelial cells and erythrocytes, *Arch Oral Biol*, **37**: 667–70.

Jacobs MR, Spangler SK, Appelbaum PC, 1992, Beta-lactamase production and susceptibility of US and European anaerobic gram-negative bacilli to beta-lactams and other agents, *Eur J Clin Microbiol Infect Dis*, **11**: 1081–93.

Jang SS, Hirsh DC, 1994, Characterization, distribution, and microbiological associations of *Fusobacterium* spp. in clinical specimens of animal origin, *J Clin Microbiol*, **32**: 384–7.

Jantzen E, Hofstad T, 1981, Fatty acids of *Fusobacterium* species: taxonomic implications, *J Gen Microbiol*, **123**: 163–71.

Kato K, Umemoto T et al., 1981, Variation of dibasic amino acid in the cell wall peptidoglycan of bacteria of genus *Fusobacterium*, *FEMS Microbiol Lett*, **10**: 81–5.

Kleivdal H, Benz R, Jensen HB, 1995, The *Fusobacterium nucleatum* major outer-membrane protein (FomA) forms trimeric, water-filled channels in lipid bilayer membranes, *Eur J Biochem*, **233**: 310–16.

Knorr M, 1923, Ueber die fusospirilläre Symbiose, die Gattung *Fusobacterium* (K. B. Lehmann) und *Spirillum sputigenum*. II Mitteilung. Die Gattung *Fusobacterium*, *Zentralbl Bakteriol Parasitenkd Infektionskr Hyg Abt 1 Orig*, **89**: 4–22.

Kolenbrander PE, London J, 1993, Adhere today, here tomorrow: oral bacterial adherence, *J Bacteriol*, **175**: 3247–52.

Könönen E, Asikainen S et al., 1994, The oral gram-negative anaerobic microflora in young children: longitudinal changes from edentulous to dentate mouth, *Oral Microbiol Immunol*, **9**: 136–41.

Lawson PA, Gharbia SE et al., 1991, Intrageneric relationships of members of the genus *Fusobacterium* as determined by reverse transcriptase sequencing of small-subunit rRNA, *Int J Syst Bacteriol*, **41**: 347–54.

Lemierre A, 1936, On certain septicaemias due to anaerobic organisms, *Lancet*, **2**: 701–3.

Lippke JA, Peros WJ et al., 1991, DNA probe detection of *Eikenella corrodens*, *Wolinella recta* and *Fusobacterium nucleatum* in subgingival plaque, *Oral Microbiol Immunol*, **6**: 81–7.

Listgarten MA, Lai CH, 1975, Unusual cell wall ultrastructure of *Leptotrichia buccalis*, *J Bacteriol*, **123**: 747–9.

Loeffler F, 1884, Bacillus der Kalberdiphterie, *Mitteilungen aus dem Kaiserlichen Gesundheitsamte*, **2**: 493–9.

Love DN, Jones F, Bailey M, 1980, Characterization of *Fusobacterium* species isolated from soft tissue infections in cats, *J Appl Bacteriol*, **48**: 325–31.

Love DN, Cato EP et al., 1987, Deoxyribonucleic acid hybridization among strains of fusobacteria isolated from soft tissue infections of cats: comparison with human and animal type strains from oral and other sites, *Int J Syst Bacteriol*, **37**: 23–6.

McCarthy C, Snyder ML, Parker RB, 1965, The indigenous oral flora of man – I, *Arch Oral Biol*, **10**: 61–70.

Moore LVH, Bourne DM, Moore WEC, 1994, Comparative distribution and taxonomic value of cellular fatty acids in thirty-three genera of anaerobic gram-negative bacilli, *Int J Syst Bacteriol*, **44**: 338–47.

Moore WEC, Holdeman LV, 1974, Genus II. *Fusobacterium* Knorr 1922.4, *Bergey's Manual of Determinative Bacteriology*, 8th edn, eds Buchanan RE, Gibbons NE, Williams & Wilkins, Baltimore, 404–16.

Moore WEC, Holdeman LV, Kelley RW, 1984, Genus II. *Fusobacterium* Knorr 1992.4, *Bergey's Manual of Systematic Bacteriology*, vol. 1, eds Krieg NR, Holt JG, Williams & Wilkins, Baltimore, 631–7.

Neefs J-M, van de Peer Y et al., 1993, Compilation of small ribosomal subunit RNA structures, *Nucleic Acids Res*, **21**: 3025–49.

Nicholson LA, Morrow CJ et al., 1994, Phylogenetic relationship of *Fusobacterium necrophorum* A, AB, and B biotypes based upon 16S rRNA gene sequence analysis, *Int J Syst Bacteriol*, **44**: 315–19.

Olsen GJ, Woese CR, Overbeek R, 1994, The winds of (evolutionary) change: breathing new life into microbiology, *J Bacteriol*, **176**: 1–6.

Pianotti R, Lachette S, Dills S, 1986, Desulfuration of cysteine and methionine by *Fusobacterium nucleatum*, *J Dent Res*, **65**: 913–17.

Plaut HC, 1894, Studien zur Bakteriellen Diagnostik der Diphterie und der Anginen, *Dtsch Med Wochenschr*, **20**: 920–3.

Prévot AR, 1938, Études de systématique bactérienne. III. Invalidité du genre *Bacteroides*. Castellani et Chalmers. Demembrement et reclassification, *Ann Inst Pasteur (Paris)*, **60**: 285–307.

Reig M, Baquero F et al., 1985, *Leptotrichia buccalis* bacteremia in neutropenic children, *J Clin Microbiol*, **22**: 320–1.

Robben J, Janssen G et al., 1989, Formation of Δ^2- and Δ^3-cholenoic acids from bile acid 3-sulfates by a human intestinal *Fusobacterium* strain, *Appl Environ Microbiol*, **55**: 2954–9.

Roberts MC, Lansciardi J, 1990, Transferable TetM in *Fusobacterium nucleatum*, *Antimicrob Agents Chemother*, **34**: 1836–8.

Roberts MC, Moncla BJ, 1988, Tetracycline resistance and TetM in oral anaerobic bacteria and *Neisseria perflava-N. sicca*, *Antimicrob Agents Chemother*, **32**: 1271–3.

Robin C, 1853, *Histoire naturelle des vegétaux parasites qui crossent sur l'homme et sur les animaux vivants*, JB Baillière, Paris.

Robrish SA, Oliver C, Thompson J, 1987, Amino acid-dependent transport of sugars by *Fusobacterium nucleatum* ATCC 10953, *J Bacteriol*, **169**: 3891–7.

Robrish SA, Oliver C, Thompson J, 1991, Sugar metabolism by fusobacteria: regulation of transport, phosphorylation, and polymer formation by *Fusobacterium mortiferum* ATCC 25557, *Infect Immun*, **59**: 4547–54.

Robrish SA, Thompson J, 1988, Suppression of polyglucose degradation in *Fusobacterium nucleatum* ATCC 10953 by amino acids, *FEMS Microbiol Lett*, **55**: 29–34.

Rogers AH, Gully NJ et al., 1992, The breakdown and utilization of peptides by strains of *Fusobacterium nucleatum, Oral Microbiol Immunol,* **7:** 299–303.

Schmorl G, 1891, Ueber ein pathogenes Fadenbacterium (*Streptothrix cuniculi*), *Dtsch Z Tiermed Pathol,* **17:** 375–407.

Schwartz DN, Schable B et al., 1995, *Leptotrichia buccalis* bacteremia in patients treated in a single bone marrow transplant unit, *Clin Infect Dis,* **20:** 762–7.

Sebald M, 1962, Étude sur les bactéries anaérobies gramnégatives asporulées, Dissertation, University of Paris, Paris.

Seddon SV, Shah HN, 1989, The distribution of hydrolytic enzymes among gram-negative bacteria associated with periodontitis, *Microb Ecol,* **2:** 181–90.

Shinjo T, Fujisawa T, Mitsuoka T, 1991, Proposal of two subspecies of *Fusobacterium necrophorum* (Flügge) Moore and Holdeman: *Fusobacterium necrophorum* subsp. *necrophorum* subsp. nov., nom. rev. (ex Flügge 1886), and *Fusobacterium necrophorum* subsp. *funduliforme* subsp. nov., nom. rev. (ex Hallé 1898), *Int J Syst Bacteriol,* **41:** 395–7.

Shinjo T, Hiraiwa K, Miyazato S, 1990, Recognition of Biovar C of *Fusobacterium necrophorum* (Flügge) Moore and Holdeman as *Fusobacterium pseudonecrophorum* sp. nov., nom. rev. (ex Prévot 1940), *Int J Syst Bacteriol,* **40:** 71–3.

Slots J, Potts TV, 1982, *Fusobacterium simiae,* a new species from monkey dental plaque, *Int J Syst Bacteriol,* **32:** 191–4.

Slots J, Potts TV, Mashimo PA, 1983, *Fusobacterium periodonticum,* a new species from the human oral cavity, *J Dent Res,* **62:** 960–3.

Smith GR, Thornton EA, 1993, Pathogenicity of *Fusobacterium necrophorum* strains from man and animals, *Epidemiol Infect,* **110:** 499–506.

Smith SH, Murray RGE, Hall M, 1994, The surface structure of *Leptotrichia buccalis, Can J Microbiol,* **40:** 90–8.

Sutter VL, Sugihara PT, Finegold JM, 1971, Rifampin-blood-agar as a selective medium for the isolation of certain anaerobic bacilli, *Appl Microbiol,* **22:** 777–80.

Tan ZL, Nagaraja TG et al., 1994, Biological and biochemical characterization of *Fusobacterium necrophorum* leukotoxin, *Am J Vet Res,* **55:** 515–21.

Tanner A, Maiden MFJ et al., 1994, The impact of 16S ribosomal RNA-based phylogeny on the taxonomy of oral bacteria, *Periodontol 2000,* **5:** 26–51.

Thiøtta T, Hartmann O, Bøe J, 1939, *A Study of* Leptotrichia *Trevisan. History, Morphology, Biological and Serological Characteristics,* Skr. Norske Videnskaps-Akademi. I. Matematisk-naturvitenskapelig klasse No. 5, Oslo.

Trevisan V, 1879, Prime linee d'introduzione allo studio dei Batterj italiani, *Rendiconti dell'instituto lombardo di scienze, Ser. 2,* **12:** 133–57.

Tunér K, Lindqvist L, Nord CE, 1985, Purification and properties of a novel β-lactamase from *Fusobacterium nucleatum, Antimicrob Agents Chemother,* **27:** 943–7.

Tunér K, Baron EJ et al., 1992, Cellular fatty acids in *Fusobacterium* species as a tool for identification, *J Clin Microbiol,* **30:** 3225–9.

Vasstrand EN, Jensen HB et al., 1982, Composition of peptidoglycans in Bacteroidaceae: determination and distribution of lanthionine, *Infect Immun,* **36:** 114–22.

Veillon A, Zuber A, 1898, Recherches sur quelques microbes strictement anaérobies, *Arch Med Exp,* **10:** 517–45.

Vincent H, 1896, Sur l'étiologie et sur les lesions anatomopathologique de la pourriture d'Hôpital, *Ann Inst Pasteur (Paris),* **10:** 488–510.

Wahren A, Holme T, 1973, Amino acid and peptide requirement of *Fusiformis necrophorus, J Bacteriol,* **116:** 279–84.

Weinberger M, Wu T et al., 1991, *Leptotrichia buccalis* bacteremia in patients with cancer: report of four cases and review, *Rev Infect Dis,* **13:** 201–6.

Wherry WB, Oliver WW, 1916, *Leptothrix innominata* (Miller), *J Infect Dis,* **19:** 299–303.

Woese CR, 1987, Bacterial evolution, *Microbiol Rev,* **51:** 221–71.

Xie H, Gibbons RJ, Hay DI, 1991, Adhesive properties of strains of *Fusobacterium nucleatum* of the subspecies *nucleatum, vincentii* and *polymorphum, Oral Microbiol Immunol,* **6:** 257–63.

Chapter 6 3

Tropheryma, Afipia and Bartonella

R C Jerris

1 INTRODUCTION

The last decade has witnessed an explosion in molecular methods to detect, identify, and classify organisms. The genera *Tropheryma*, *Afipia* and *Bartonella* are specific examples. These techniques have contributed to a clearer understanding of the presence of organisms in infection and by association their pathogenic potential. For the non-cultivable *Tropheryma whippelii*, molecular methods are required for detection and identification. Taxonomic restructuring of the family Bartonellaceae to unify the genera *Bartonella* and *Rochalimaea* was achieved by molecular techniques.

TROPHERYMA

2 DEFINITION

There is a single species designated *Tropheryma whippelii*. The organism has not been cultivated. *T. whippelii* is the organism associated with Whipple's disease and has been characterized by molecular genetic and ultrastructural techniques. The organism is rich in guanine and cytosine, and 16S rRNA analysis shows *T. whippelii* to be a previously uncharacterized actinomycete within the division of the gram-positive bacteria (Wilson et al. 1991, Relman et al. 1992).

3 HISTORICAL PERSPECTIVE

Whipple described the first case of the illness which bears his name in 1901. His pathological findings were noted on examination of a small intestinal biopsy from a medical missionary suffering from chronic arthralgia and abdominal pain. Histologically, he described distortion of the normal architecture of the villi in the small intestine, with infiltration of the lamina propria by large frothy cells. Whipple reported large lipid deposits in the lamina propria; mesenteric lymph nodes, and in one gland stained by silver 'great numbers of a peculiar rod shaped organism' (Whipple 1907).

Other investigators described the presence of typical vacuolated macrophages that stained positive with the periodic acid–Schiff (PAS) stain in many nonintestinal tissues, thus establishing the systemic nature of the disease. It was not until the 1960s that the disease, initially viewed as a disorder of fat metabolism, was linked to eradication of the rod-shaped bacteria with antimicrobials and clinical improvement (Davis et al. 1963, Trier et al. 1965, Ruffin, Kurtz and Roufail 1966).

4 MORPHOLOGY (HISTOLOGICAL AND ULTRASTRUCTURAL)

On histological, microscopic examination the abnormality in the mucosa of the small intestine is diagnostic for Whipple's disease. As originally described by Whipple, there is extensive infiltration in the lamina propria with large macrophages which distort the villi. The cytoplasm of these macrophages stains positive with PAS stain, due to an abundance of glycoprotein within vacuoles (Fig. 63.1, see also Plate 63.1).

The cells are diastase resistant. Distinct rod-shaped organisms can be seen with silver stain. The organisms have been visualized lying freely between cells and intracellularly within the glycoprotein-containing macrophages, villous absorptive cells, polymorphonuclear leucocytes, plasma cells and mast cells. Organisms appear most numerous just beneath the absorptive epithelium and around vascular channels in the upper mucosa (Dobbins and Kawanishi 1981, Trier 1993).

Electron microscopic examination reveals the organisms to be small rods that measure 0.2 μm in width by 1–2.5 μm in length (Yardly and Hendrix 1961, Dobbins and Kawanishi 1981). Silva, Macedo and Moura-Nunes (1985) in an elegant electron microscopic evaluation of the organism in 3 untreated patients detail: a trilayered cytoplasmic membrane of 6.08 nm; a thick cell wall of 20 nm, containing peptidoglycan and a novel inner layer containing polysaccharides and possibly teichoic acid; and a surface membrane of

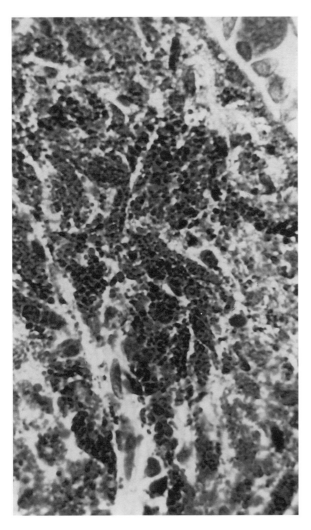

Fig. 63.1 Periodic acid–Schiff positive staining macrophages in the duodenum in Whipple's disease. Transparency slide from ASCP, Anatomic Pathology II Check Sample exercise APII 88-12 (APII-144), 'Gastric Xanthoma', Baddoura F, Someren A, Copyright 1988, American Society of Clinical Pathologists. Reproduced with permission.

4.74 nm, with a symmetrical profile, which surrounded the cell wall. This ultrastructural analysis is consistent for a gram-positive organism with a unique, additional surface membrane. These studies demonstrate that on degradation within macrophages it is the accumulation of the innermost polysaccharide component of the cell wall that is responsible for the positive staining with PAS.

5 CLASSIFICATION

By use of the polymerase chain reaction (PCR) with eubacterial specific primers, Wilson and colleagues (1991) and Relman and coworkers (1992) have analysed the 16S rRNA sequence of the Whipple's disease bacillus. Taxonomically, both investigators have placed the organism with the gram-positive bacteria that possess a high G + C content. The 16S rRNA sequence analysis showed the organism to be unrelated to any current phylogenetic class. The organism was designated *Tropheryma whippelii* by Relman and workers (1992). Relman and colleagues placed the organism in the actinobacteria subgroup of the aerobic actinomycetes, a group which includes *Dermatophilus congolensis*, *Arthrobacter globiformis*, *Terrabacter tumescens* and *Micrococcus luteus*.

6 IDENTIFICATION

Identification of the clinical syndrome of Whipple's disease relies on the histological detection of PAS-positive macrophages with the presence of the typical bacilli. Definitive identification of *T. whippelii* relies upon the molecular genetic analysis from tissue or fluid samples. Primers for the polymerase chain reaction, designated as W4RB and W3FE by Rickman and coworkers (1995), have proved sensitive and specific for genetic amplification.

7 SUSCEPTIBILITY TO ANTIMICROBIAL AGENTS

Because the organism cannot be cultivated, susceptibility to antimicrobial agents may be inferred from remission of clinical manifestations during therapy. Treatment regimens including penicillin, penicillin and streptomycin, erythromycin, tetracycline and trimethoprim–sulphamethoxazole have been successful in Whipple's disease (Trier 1993).

8 EPIDEMIOLOGY AND PATHOGENICITY

Whipple's disease is a rare multi-organ system disease that may occur at any age, but most commonly is seen in patients in their 40s to 60s. The extremes in age range from 3 months (Aust and Smith 1962) to 83 years (Crane and Schlippert 1978). Men are affected 10 times more frequently than women. The majority of cases have occurred in whites, although blacks, American Indians, Japanese and natives of India have been infected (Dobbins 1987). The disease occurs so sporadically that definitive epidemiological data are lacking. There is no evidence of person-to-person spread. It seems probable that specific host factors play a key role in the acquisition and pathogenesis of the disease.

The clinical symptomatology of infection with *T. whippelii* depends on the organ system(s) involved. The gastrointestinal tract is most frequently affected and symptoms may include diarrhoea, with 5–10 watery or semi-formed foul-smelling, fatty stools per day; bleeding (occult or gross); or, bloated feeling with abdominal cramps. Dramatic weight loss may be seen due to anorexia and malabsorption. Arthritis and fever may precede gastrointestinal manifestations by many years. Some two-thirds of patients describe joint pain with intermittent migratory arthritis of large and small joints. Involvement of the cardiac, respiratory and central nervous systems (CNS) has been described. It is noteworthy that up to 10% of patients with Whipple's disease demonstrate a broad range of CNS symptoms (Trier 1993).

Therapeutic regimens have previously been described (see section 7). However, duration and dosages have not been established in controlled studies. Relapse is common as noted by Keinath and colleagues (1985) and appropriate follow-up is critical to detect these patients and prevent potential neurological sequelae.

AFIPIA

9 DEFINITION

The genus *Afipia* is comprised of gram-negative, oxidase-positive, non-fermentative rods. Organisms are motile by means of a single flagellum. They are characteristically urease-positive but are negative in reactions for haemolysis, indole production, H_2S production (in triple sugar iron agar), gelatin hydrolysis, aesculin hydrolysis and peptonization of litmus milk. No acid is produced oxidatively from D-glucose, lactose, maltose or sucrose (Brenner et al. 1991). The genus has a guanine + cytosine content of 61.5–69 mol%. Members of the genus are taxonomically placed in the α_2 subgroup of the class Proteobacteria.

On the basis of phenotypic characterization and DNA relatedness, 3 named species designated *A. felis* (type strain), *A. clevelandensis* and *A. broomeae* and 3 unnamed *Afipia* genospecies are recognized (Brenner et al. 1991).

10 HISTORICAL PERSPECTIVE

The pursuit of the aetiological agent of cat scratch disease (CSD) by English and coworkers (1988) at the Armed Forces Institute of Pathology (AFIP) yielded the first isolate of *Afipia felis*. The genus designation was selected to honour the work of investigators at the AFIP. Investigators at the Centers for

Disease Control and Prevention (CDC) successfully cultivated isolates and Hall and colleagues (1991) isolated a related organism from a pretibial biopsy. Additional isolates were collected from stored reference strains in the Special Bacteriology Reference Laboratory, CDC.

Table 63.1 details the species and sources of isolation for the current *Afipia* genus.

The precise role of any of the *Afipia* species in pathological processes is currently unknown. There is a substantial body of evidence to suggest the aetiological agent of CSD is *Bartonella henselae* (see section 18, p. 1372) rather than *A. felis*.

11 CULTURAL AND BIOCHEMICAL CHARACTERISTICS

A. felis appears to be relatively fastidious and difficult to cultivate in the routine laboratory. Original reports of *A. felis* detail successful growth using ground lymph node tissue in biphasic brain–heart infusion (English et al. 1988) with growth detected at 2–7 days. Additional isolates of *A. felis* have been recovered using a tissue culture system. Sonicated fluid and tissue specimens added to HeLa cell monolayers incubated for up to 18 h at 35°C with subsequent passage onto secondary cell monolayers and onto buffered charcoal yeast extract (BCYE) agar have yielded growth (Brenner et al. 1991). *A. clevelandensis* has been recovered on chocolate blood agar at 35°C and on brain–heart infusion agar with blood and potato dextrose agar at 25°C (Hall et al. 1991). *A. broomeae* and *Afipia* genospecies have been cultivated directly on routine bacteriological media with prolonged incubation at 30°C. There is no indication that increased CO_2 stimulates growth.

No systematic studies on specific nutritional requirements of the genus exist. However, Brenner and colleagues (1991) describe a standardized approach to identification once the isolates are adapted to growth on BCYE agar.

Table 63.2 details the biochemical reactions of *Afipia* species. Biochemicals were inoculated with growth from BCYE agar that was incubated at 30°C.

Morphologically after incubation at 30–32°C for 72 h on 5% sheep blood agar, colonies of *Afipia* sp. are grey-white, shiny, convex, opaque with entire edges, measuring 1.5 mm in width. On BCYE agar they appear similarly except for variation in size which measures from 0.5 to 1.5 mm.

Organisms vary in staining characteristics from relatively uniform gram-negative rods to pleomorphic slender gram-negative rods with vacuoles. In broth cultures, on prolonged incubation for 3 weeks at 37°C, *A. felis* may demonstrate delicate pleomorphic forms (English et al. 1988) consistent with cell wall deficient organisms.

Members of the genus contain major cell wall fatty acids of *cis*-octadec-11-enoic ($C_{18:1\omega 7C}$), 11-methyloctadec-12-enoic ($C_{Br19:1}$) and generally 9,10-methylenehexadecanoate and 11,12-methyleneoctadecanoate. Although minor differences are noted among the species, the presence of $C_{Br19:1}$ as a major cellular fatty acid is a key biochemical marker for the genus *Afipia* – as this acid has only been detected in trace levels in some *Brucella* and *Pseudomonas* species (Brenner et al. 1991).

12 MOLECULAR ANALYSIS AND TYPING

The 11 strains described by Brenner and workers (1991) reveal a DNA relatedness by hybridization of 12–69%. All *A. felis* isolates contain a single plasmid of 2.9×10^{-5} kDa (44

Table 63.1 Sources of *Afipia* by specific species designation

Species	Source(s)
A. felis	Lymph nodes, lymph node aspirates
A. clevelandensis	Tibial biopsy
A. broomeae	Sputum, bone marrow, synovium-wrist abscess
Afipia genospecies 1 *ATCC 49721	Pleural fluid
Afipia genospecies 2, *ATCC 49722	Bronchial washing
Afipia genospecies 3, *ATCC 49723	Environmental water

*ATCC, American Type Culture Collection.

Table 63.2 Biochemical reactions of *Afipia* species*

Characteristic[a]	A. felis	A. clevelandensis	A. broomeae	A. genospecies 1	A. genospecies 2	A. genospecies 3
Nitrate reduction	+	−	−	−	−	−
D-Xylose, acid	(+^{w})	−	(+^{w})	(+^{w})	(+^{w})	(+^{w})
Litmus milk	(ak)	(ak)	(ak)	(ak)	(ak)	(ak)
Catalase	−	−	+^{w}	+^{w}	+^{w}	+^{w}
Gram reaction	−	−	−	−	−	−
Oxidase	+	+	+	+	+	+
Growth at						
25°C	+	+	+	+	+	+
30°C	+	+	+	+	+	+
35°C	+^{w}	+^{w}	+^{w}	+	+	+^{w}
42°C	−	−	−	−	−	−
Motility	+	+	+	+	+	+
Haemolysis	−	−	−	−	−	−
Nutrient broth, growth	+	(+)	+	+	+	+
Nutrient broth plus 6% NaCl, growth	−	−	−	−	−	−
MacConkey agar, growth	−	(+^{w})	−	−	−	−
Urea, Christensen[b]	+	+	+ or (+)	+	+	+
H$_2$S, triple sugar iron	−	−	−	−	−	−
H$_2$S, lead acetate	−	−	−	−	−	+^{w}
Gelatin hydrolysis	−	−	−	−	−	−
Indole production	−	−	−	−	−	−
Citrate, Simmons	−	−	−	+	−	−
Aesculin hydrolysis	−	−	−	−	−	−
Nitrate, gas	−	−	−	−	−	−
D-Glucose, gas	−	−	−	−	−	−
D-Glucose, acid	−	−	−	−	−	−
Lactose, acid	−	−	−	−	−	−
Maltose, acid	−	−	−	−	−	−
D-Mannitol, acid	−	−	−	+^{w}	−	−
Sucrose, acid	−	−	−	−	−	−

*Data modified slightly from Brenner et al. 1991.
+, positive reaction within 48 h; −, negative reaction; parentheses, positive reaction in 3–14 days; ^{w}, weak; ak, alkaline reaction.
[a]Incubation at 30°C unless indicated otherwise.
[b]Heavy inoculation.

kb), while no other members of the genus were found to contain plasmids. Analysis of the genomic sequence of 16S rRNA from *A. felis* and *A. clevelandensis* have been performed by O'Conner and colleagues (1991) and are deposited in the GenBank/European Molecular Biology Laboratory data banks under the accession numbers M65248 and M69186, respectively. Analysis shows *Afipia* to be members of the α$_2$ subgroup of the Proteobacteria that includes members of the genera *Rickettsia*, *Brucella*, *Bartonella* and *Agrobacterium*.

Enzyme typing and ribotyping reveal the same 6 species as delineated with DNA relatedness (Brenner et al. 1991). Antigenic diversity is noted within the genus and within the species *A. felis.* Species-specific monoclonal antibodies have been developed against *A. felis,* indicating a major lipopolysaccharide antigen common to this species (Yu and Raoult 1994).

13 ANTIMICROBIAL SUSCEPTIBILITY

Using the Uniscept microdilution breakpoint panels (bioMerieux Vitek, Hazelwood, MO) incubated for 7 days at 30–32°C in ambient air, English and coworkers (1988) report *A. felis* to be: resistant to ampicillin, penicillin, cefazolin, cephalothin, cefoperazone, chloramphenicol, clindamycin, erythromycin, nitrofurantoin and tetracycline; intermediately susceptible to piperacillin, ticarcillin and vancomycin; and susceptible to cefoxitin, cefotaxime, mezlocillin, gentamicin, netilmicin, tobramycin and amikacin. Brenner and colleagues (1991) used the Sceptor system (Becton Dickinson Microbiology Systems, Cockeysville, MD) incubated at 30°C for 48 h to determine specific minimal inhibitory concentrations (MIC) for all *Afipia* species. Their data demonstrate *Afipia* genospecies 3 to have the lowest MICs among all strains tested. Other species showed higher MICs to most of the antimicrobial agents tested, including first, second and third generation cephalosporins, ampicillin and extended spectrum penicillins, β-lactamase inhibitor combinations, aminoglycosides and tetracycline. The lowest MICs for all species were with imipenem.

No standards exist for testing and interpreting in vitro susceptibility data for these organisms; furthermore, no detailed therapeutic clinical efficacy exists during treatment for putative infections with these organisms.

14 EPIDEMIOLOGY AND PATHOGENICITY

Very little is known with certainty regarding the normal habitat and epidemiology of the genus *Afipia.* *Afipia* shares several common traits with other members of the α_2 subclass of the Proteobacteria including: the presence of intercellular parasitism (Birkness et al. 1992, Brouqui and Raoult 1993); the observation of the organism within macrophages and endothelial cells (Wear and Margileth 1983, English et al. 1988); and entry of the organism into the host via a break in the skin (O'Connor et al. 1991). Unlike some of the other members of the α_2 subclass, *Afipia* has not been detected in the soil.

The precise role of *A. felis* in pathological processes is unknown at this time. The association of *A. felis* as the aetiological agent of cat scratch disease (CSD) is now discounted. Strong evidence exists for the definitive role of *B. henselae* as the dominant aetiological agent in CSD (Dolan et al. 1993, Welch and Slater 1995). Isolated reports of cultivation of *A. felis* from tissue in CSD, detection of the organism in lymph nodes by a chromosomal probe (Brenner and colleagues 1991) and detection of a serological response to *A. felis* (Muller 1993, Fumarolo et al. 1994) indicate that the organism may play a role as a cofactor in some cases.

A. clevelandensis was isolated from a pretibial biopsy from a 69 year old with underlying necrotizing pancreatitis. The patient had been in the hospital for months prior to presentation with the skin lesion. The clinical significance of the isolate is unknown. *A. broomeae* has been isolated from the synovial fluid of a patient with underlying diabetes and arteriosclerosis, from the bone marrow of an 81 year old female and from sputum. *Afipia* genospecies 1 was detected in pleural fluid; genospecies 2 in bronchial washings from an 80 year old woman; and genospecies 3 from environmental water (Brenner et al. 1991). This latter isolate may provide a clue as to the natural habitat of some members of the genus. These organisms may play a role as opportunistic pathogens in respiratory and wound infections in elderly patients and in those with severe underlying medical problems.

BARTONELLA

15 DEFINITION

Major revisions have recently been made in the classification of the family Bartonellaceae. The genus *Rochalimaea* has been removed from the family Rickettsiaceae and has been transferred to the family Bartonellaceae (Brenner et al. 1993). Phylogenetic studies using 16S rRNA and DNA hybridization studies on the relationships of genus *Rochalimaea* and the family *Bartonella* species to each other and to members of the family Rickettsiaceae support the separation of the genus *Rochalimaea* and the family Bartonellaceae from the order Rickettsiales. These studies convincingly support placement of members of the genus *Rochalimaea* in the genus *Bartonella.* In addition, members of the genus *Grahamella* have been transferred to the family Bartonellaceae. Birtles and colleagues (1995), using a polyphasic approach that included 16S rRNA gene sequencing, DNA hybridization, guanine plus cytosine content and phenotypic characterization studies, justify unifying the previously poorly defined genus *Grahamella* and the genus *Bartonella.*

Members of the genus *Bartonella* are gram-negative, oxidase-negative, fastidious aerobic rods that can be cultivated on bacteriological media. The species *Bartonella bacilliformis* is the only member to exhibit flagella (polar). Growth is obtained on fresh media supplemented with 5% sheep or rabbit blood in the presence of 5% CO_2. The optimal incubation temperature varies from 25°C (*B. bacilliformis*) to 35°C (other species). The organisms are inert in carbohydrates. The G + C content of DNA ranges from 38.5 to 41 mol%. Arthropod vectors have been identified for *B. bacilliformis, B. quintana* and possibly for *B. vinsonii.*

Unification of the genera *Bartonella* and *Rochalimaea* has resulted in the following species: *B. bacilliformis* (type species), *B. vinsonii* and *B. vinsonii* subsp *berkoffii* (Breitschwerdt et al. 1995), *B. quintana, B. henselae* (Regnery et al. 1992) and *B. elizabethae* (Daly et al. 1993). Unification of the genera *Bartonella* and *Grahamella* (Birtles et al. 1995) has resulted in the following species: *B. talpae*, *B. peromysci*, *B. grahamii*, *B. taylorii* and *B. doshiae*. These latter species, included from the previous *Grahamella* genus, together with *B. vinsonii*, are thought to exist exclusively within the erythrocytes of non-human hosts. These species will not be described further.

16 *B. BACILLIFORMIS*

16.1 Clinical manifestations

B. bacilliformis is a fastidious haemotropic organism, which invades and destroys red blood cells. The organism appears to have a restricted geographical distribution to specific altitudes of the South American Andes mountain range in Peru, Equador and Columbia. It is transmitted by the bite of the sandfly *Lutzomyia verrucarum*. In the human host, *B. bacilliformis* causes a biphasic disease with 2 distinct clinical forms including Oroya fever (a haemolytic syndrome) and verruga peruana (a syndrome characterized by wart-like growths). The disease syndromes bear the eponyms bartonellosis or Carrion's disease, the latter in honour of the Peruvian medical student Daniel Carrion who in 1885 inoculated himself with blood from a verrugous lesion and succumbed to Oroya fever several weeks later (Schultz 1968).

The organism may reside in the host in an asymptomatic form as noted in epidemiological studies (Kreier et al. 1992) or may progress to disease. Oroya fever may develop in infected patients in 1–3 weeks. In its acute form, the disease is a rapidly progressive, febrile anaemia with a high parasitaemia (90–100%). Massive destruction of red blood cells in all organs may ensue (Reynafarie and Ramos 1961). There may be associated lymphadenopathy, severe thrombocytopenia, myalgias, arthralgias and associated hypoxic complications of delerium and coma. Mortality rates as high as 40% have been documented (Weinman 1944). A period of dormancy or latency, generally noted in months, may ensue, following which many patients develop the chronic eruptive, verruga peruana stage. This dormant stage is asymptomatic and is thought to be the natural reservoir of the organism. The verrugous lesions are wart-like or nodular outgrowths that vary in size and number. Mucosal and internal lesions may also occur (Welch and Slater 1995). The lesions may come in waves such that one group may develop while others wane. They may persist for months to years. Histologically, there are bacilli (demonstrated best by Warthin–Starry stain), endothelial cell proliferation and neovascularization. Fibrosis and involution occur. The microbial factors responsible for the pathogenesis of these lesions are unclear. The organisms may possess some innate angiogenic potential (Garcia, Wojta and Hoover 1988) or stimulate host cells to release these factors (Arias-Stella et al. 1986). Although Oroya fever and verruga peruana generally occur sequentially, each phase has been noted as a distinct syndrome in the absence of the other (Kreier et al. 1992). Public health control measures have

included education in endemic areas and the use of insecticides.

16.2 Biological characteristics

As detailed by Wilson (1990), morphologically in young cultures *B. bacilliformis* occurs mainly in the form of short rods arranged singly, in pairs, in chains, clumps or chains and clumps. In older cultures coccoid forms predominate. There is a considerable degree of pleomorphism. It is 0.3–1.5 μm long and 0.2–0.5 μm broad. It is motile and a tuft of at least 10 flagella can be demonstrated at one pole of the rod. Ultrathin sections of red corpuscles examined by electron microscopy show that the organisms are situated inside the corpuscles as well as on the surface and that they have a trilaminar cell wall. In man the organism is present not only in red blood cells but also in large numbers in the cytoplasm of endothelial cells of the spleen, liver and lymph nodes. Cultivation can be effected from blood and tissue on a variety of media containing fresh blood, haemoglobin or serum (Ristic and Kreier 1984). Though a high proportion of natural animal protein favours growth, it does not appear to be essential. Jiménez (1940) obtained good growth on 1% glycerol infusion agar, provided the X, though not the V, factor was added. On solid media, growth may occur in 4–5 days, either as minute, circular, clear, mucoid colonies, or as an opaque, finely granular, mucoid film that has a tendency to outgrow the original boundaries of the inoculum (Jiménez 1940). The organism is a strict aerobe; grows well at 25–37°C, though best at about 25–28°C; prefers a pH of 7.8; ferments no sugar; forms no haemolysin; and survives in semisolid medium at –70°C for years and at 25–28°C for several weeks (Weinman 1968). It is sensitive to penicillin, which causes the formation of L-forms (Sharp 1968) and to streptomycin and tetracycline. Serological cross-reactivity has been noted between *B. bacilliformis* and *Chlamydia psittaci* and has been attributed to a common lipopolysaccharide (Knobloch et al. 1988). Injected intravenously into young rhesus monkeys, the organism may give rise to a peculiar, irregularly remittent type of fever, sometimes accompanied by severe anaemia; injected intradermally into the eyebrow, it gives rise to a nodule rich in cellular elements and capillary formation. Small laboratory animals are not susceptible to experimental infection.

17 *B. QUINTANA*

17.1 Clinical manifestations

B. quintana has long been recognized as the agent of trench fever afflicting soldiers during World Wars I and II. The vector for the disease is the human body louse, *Pediculus humanus*, and crowding as occurs in the trenches during war favours epidemic spread of the disease. The geographical distribution appears to be global; cases have been documented in Europe, Africa and Mexico (Myers, Grossman and Wisseman 1984). The clinical manifestations vary from insidious onset of non-specific symptoms to an acute illness with fever, malaise, bone pain and macular rash. Different patterns of fever have been described including a single episode, a continuous fever for 5–7 days and recurrent episodes every 4–5 days (Vinson, Varela and Molina-Pasqual 1969). The incubation period appears to range from 5 to 20 days and once infection has occurred, the organisms may persist in the human bloodstream for months to longer than a year (Vinson, Varela and Molina-Pasqual 1969).

Sporadic reports document that infection with *B. quintana* is expanding. Relman and coworkers (1990) used PCR and DNA sequence analysis directly from tissue samples of bacillary angiomatosis (BA) to identify a *B. quintana*-like organism. *B. quintana* has been reported from HIV-infected patients in cases of cutaneous BA (Kemper et al. 1990, Koehler et al. 1992, Maurin et al. 1994), bacteraemia, endocarditis (Spach et al. 1993) and chronic lymphadenopathy (Raoult et al. 1994). LeBoit and colleagues (1989) and Spach (1992) present excellent reviews of the histology of BA and the differential diagnosis.

In HIV-negative, homeless patients with chronic alcoholism, *B. quintana* has been associated with fever, bacteraemia and endocarditis (Drancourt et al. 1995, Spach et al. 1995). There is evidence from these case reports that there may be additional arthropod vectors of transmission, as several patients had documented scabies infections (Koehler et al. 1992, Spach et al. 1995). Spach and coworkers (1995) also note recent cat scratches in 3 of their patients. Tappero and colleagues (1993b) detail the epidemiology of BA and bacillary peliosis and suggest the syndrome is a new zoonosis.

Various antimicrobial regimens have been described for the treatment of infections with *B. quintana* (Drancourt et al. 1995, Spach et al. 1995) with a common notation that patients must be treated for 4–6 weeks to prevent relapse.

17.2 Cultural and biochemical characterization

Recovery of *Bartonella* species has been most common from blood cultures and tissue, including liver, spleen and skin. In blood, successful isolation has been achieved using the lysis–centrifugation method (Isolator, Wampole, Cranbury, NJ) with direct plating on enriched (chocolatized or blood-containing) media. The Bactec blood culture system (Becton Dickinson Instrument Systems, Cockeysville, MD) has supported growth of the organisms in both conventional and resin-containing media with prolonged incubation of up to 28 days. However, the organisms may fail to produce sufficient CO_2 for detection. Consequently, an acridine orange stain and blind subculture may be required to detect growth.

Growth is best on freshly prepared enriched solid media. When supplemented with 5% sheep blood, *Bartonella* spp. have been recovered on Columbia base (Welch et al. 1992), brain–heart infusion agar and trypticase soy agar (Regnery et al. 1992). Freshly prepared heart infusion agar supplemented with 5–10% rabbit blood supports excellent growth of *Bartonella* spp. Plates should be incubated at 35–37°C, in a humid atmosphere with 5–10% CO_2 for 3–4 weeks. Growth of *Bartonella* may be detected from primary isolation on average in 14 days, but a marked variation among strains and species is noted with a range from

5 to 49 days (Lucey et al. 1992, Welch et al. 1992, Daly et al. 1993). *B. quintana* is generally less fastidious than *B. henselae*. Once subcultured, the organisms become adapted to grow in 72–96 h.

Isolation of organisms from tissue samples may require co-cultivation in cell cultures such as the human endothelial cell line ECV304 described by Drancourt et al. (1995) or a bovine pulmonary artery endothelial cell line detailed by Koehler and colleagues (1992) before plating onto solid agar media.

Improved growth in broth from propagated *B. henselae* has been demonstated in brucella broth supplemented with haemin (250 fg ml^{-1}) and peptic digest of blood (8% Fildes' reagent) (Schwartzman, Nesbit and Baron 1993).

Colonies on primary isolation often demonstrate 2 morphologies that include: an irregular, 'cauliflower' or 'molar tooth', dry form; and a smaller, circular, entire, tan, moist form that pits and adheres to the agar. *B. henselae* generally demonstrates a greater proportion of 'cauliflower'-like colonies, while *B. quintana* demonstrates more of the smoother type colonies (or even has a uniform smooth appearance).

On gram stain the organisms appear as small, often slightly curved gram-negative rods that may resemble *Campylobacter* spp. The cells measure 0.5–0.6 μm in width by 1.0–2.0 μm in length. Table 63.3 details the differential characteristics of the species. *B. henselae* and, less frequently, *B. quintana* demonstrate twitching motility which is due to the presence of pili.

The MicroScan rapid anaerobic identification system (Baxter Diagnostics, West Sacremento, CA) has been used to differentiate *B. henselae* from *B. quintana* on the basis of preformed enzymes (Welch et al. 1993).

Serologically, as gauged by human antibody response in infection, there is substantial cross-reactivity between *B. quintana* and *B. henselae* (Welch and Slater 1995). Drancourt and colleagues (1995) detail significant cross-reactions between *B. quintana* and *Chlamydia pneumonia*.

A molecular subtyping scheme has been developed by Matar et al. (1993) based on PCR restriction fragment length polymorphism. Characterizations of the 16S rRNA gene nucleotide sequences have been detailed and are deposited in GenBank as L01259 (*B. quintana*), M73229 (*B. henselae*) and L01260 (*B. elizabethae*).

No distinct virulence factors have been delineated for *Bartonella* species (excluding *B. bacilliformis*) with the exception of pili, which are known to be cytoadherent (Welch and Slater 1995). The similarities between BA and verruga peruana may indicate a common neoproliferative or neoangiogenic factor. Conley, Slater and Hamilton (1994) detail stimulation of endothelial cells in an in vitro model with *Rochalimaea* species.

Isolates are susceptible to most antimicrobials tested in vitro, including β-lactams (with some noted resistance to penicillin and ampicillin), the tetracyclines (with rare resistance), aminoglycosides (with the

Table 63.3 Biochemical reactions[a] of human *Bartonella* species[b]

Characteristic	*B. bacilliformis*	*B. quintana*	*B. henselae*	*B. elizabethae*
Gram-stain reaction	–	–	–	–
Catalase	+	–	–/+	–
Oxidase	–	–/+	–	–
Indole	–	–	–	–
Nitrate reduction	–	–	–	–
Urease production	–	–	–	–
Acid production from				
glucose	–	–	–	–
lactose	–	–	–	–
maltose	–	–	–	–
mannitol	–	–	–	–
sucrose	–	–	–	–
Optimal temp (°C)	25–30	35–37	35–37	35–37
Growth in nutrient broth	–	–	–	–
Haemolysis	–	–	–	–
Flagella	+	–[c]	–[c]	–
Cellular fatty acids, >10% of total	$C_{18:1\omega7C}$, $C_{16:0}$, $C_{16:1\omega7C}$	$C_{18:1\omega7C}$, $C_{16:0}$ $C_{18:0}$	$C_{18:1\omega7C}$, $C_{18:0}$, $C_{16:0}$	$C_{18:1\omega7C}$, $C_{17:0}$ $C_{16:0}$

[a]Modified from Welch and Slater 1995.
[b]+, positive reaction; –, negative reaction; –/+, negative or weakly positive.
[c]May show twitching motility in wet preparations.

exception of *B. quintana*), fluoroquinolones and macrolides (Welch and Slater 1995).

18 *B. HENSELAE*

18.1 Clinical manifestations

B. henselae has been associated with bacteraemia and fever in immunocompromised and immunocompetent patients. In HIV-infected individuals the syndrome is insidious in onset, with fatigue, malaise, body aches, weight loss, fever and sometimes headache (Regnery et al. 1992). In non-HIV-infected patients there is generally an abrupt onset of fever (which may persist or relapse) often with accompanying arthralgias and myalgias (Welch et al. 1992). Aseptic meningitis has also been described accompanying the bacteraemic syndrome (Welch et al. 1992). Long-term asymptomatic persistence of *B. henselae* has been noted (Welch and Slater 1995).

B. henselae causes BA (Koehler et al. 1992) and bacillary peliosis (Slater, Welch and Min 1992). In BA, both *B. henselae* and *B. quintana* have been confirmed by culture, by amplification of specific 16S rRNA gene sequences from uncultivated pathogens and by immunocytochemical staining of organisms in the tissue. Most commonly, the diagnosis of BA is based on the typical histology of the lesions (plump endothelial cells and neovascularization) and demonstration of bacilli by Warthin–Starry staining. Bacillary peliosis has been noted in HIV-infected patients and in immunocompetent hosts (Tappero et al. 1993a). This syndrome, which generally involves the liver and sometimes the spleen, presents with blood-filled cysts in the tissues, separated from the parenchyma by a

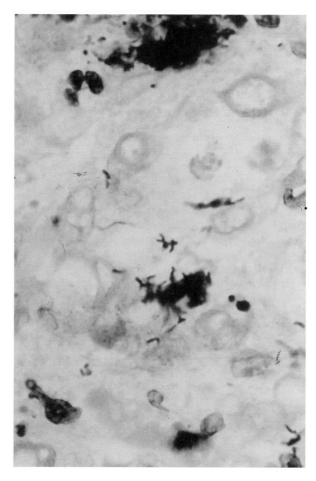

Fig. 63.2 Warthin–Starry staining bacilli in cat scratch disease.

fibromyxoid stroma containing neutrophils, mono-cytes and Warthin–Starry staining bacilli (Welch et al. 1992).

B. henselae, but not *B. quintana*, has been strongly associated with CSD (see Volume 3, Chapter 48). Demonstration of the organism by culture, by molecular techniques, by immunohistochemical stain and by host serological response strongly suggest *B. henselae* to be the predominant if not the exclusive pathogen responsible for CSD. Anderson and coworkers (1993) have identified *B. henselae* from 2 independent sources of skin test antigen by PCR and DNA sequence analysis. Zangwill and colleagues (1993) detail the epidemiology, risk factors and a diagnostic test for CSD. This study clearly associates *B. henselae* and a recent traumatic involvement with kittens with the disease syndrome. *B. henselae* has a reservoir in nature in cats, but lacks a proven vector, although ticks and fleas may play a role in transmission of disease (Welch and Slater 1995). Figure 63.2 (see also Plate 63.2) shows the Warthin–Starry stain demonstrating the typical bacilli in CSD.

The biological and cultural characteristics of *B. henselae* are noted as previously described under *B. quintana*.

19 *B. ELIZABETHAE*

Daly and coworkers (1993) describe the only documented isolation of *B. elizabethae* from a patient with bacteraemia and endocarditis. The patient had a 2 month history of fatigue and weight loss, and lacerations were noted on the patient's fingers from a non-specified source 2 weeks before the onset of symptoms.

As more laboratories look for these organisms, the spectrum of disease will continue to expand.

REFERENCES

Anderson B, Kelly C et al., 1993, Detection of *Rochalimaea henselae* in cat-scratch disease skin test antigens, *J Infect Dis*, **168**: 1034–6.

Arias-Stella J, Lieberman PH et al., 1986, Histology, immuno-histochemistry and ultrastructure of the verruga in Carrion's disease, *Am J Surg Pathol*, **10**: 595–610.

Aust CH, Smith EB, 1962, Whipple's disease in a 3 month old infant with involvement of the bone marrow, *Am J Clin Pathol*, **37**: 66–74.

Birkness KA, George VG et al., 1992, Intracellular growth of *Afipia felis*, a putative etiologic agent of cat scratch disease, *Infect Immun*, **60**: 2281–7.

Birtles RJ, Harrison TG et al., 1995, Proposals to unify the genera *Grahamella* and *Bartonella*, with descriptions of *Bartonella talpae* comb.nov., *Bartonella peromysci* comb.nov., and three new species, *Bartonella grahamii* sp.nov., *Bartonella taylorii* sp.nov., and *Bartonella doshiae* sp.nov., *Int J Syst Bacteriol*, **45**: 1–8.

Breitschwerdt EB, Korsey DL et al., 1995, Endocarditis in a dog due to infection with a novel *Bartonella* subspecies, *J Clin Microbiol*, **33**: 154–60.

Brenner DJ, Hollis DG et al., 1991, Proposal of *Afipia* gen. nov., with *Afipia felis* sp.nov. (formerly the cat scratch disease bacillus), *Afipia clevelandensis* sp.nov. (formerly the Cleveland Clinic Foundation strain), *Afipia broomeae* sp.nov., and three unnamed genospecies, *J Clin Microbiol*, **29**: 2450–60.

Brenner DJ, O'Connor SP et al., 1993, Proposals to unify the genera *Bartonella* and *Rochalimaea* with descriptions of *Bartonella quintana* comb.nov., *Bartonella vinsonii* comb.nov., *Bartonella henselae* comb.nov., and *Bartonella elizabethae* comb.nov., and to remove the Family *Bartonellaceae* from the Order *Rickettsiales*, *Int J Syst Bacteriol*, **43**: 777–86.

Brouqui P, Raoult D, 1993, Proteinase K-sensitive and filterable phagosome–lysosome fusion inhibiting factor in *Afipia felis*, *Microb Pathog*, **15**: 187–95.

Conley T, Slater L, Hamilton K, 1994, *Rochalimaea* species stimulate human endothelial cell proliferation and migration in vitro, *J Lab Clin Med*, **124**: 521–8.

Crane S, Schlippert W, 1978, Duodenoscopic findings in Whipple's disease, *Gastrointest Endosc*, **24**: 248–9.

Daly JS, Worthington MG et al., 1993, *Rochalimaeae elizabethae* sp.nov. isolated from a patient with endocarditis, *J Clin Microbiol*, **31**: 872–81.

Davis TD Jr, McBee JW et al., 1963, The effect of antibiotic and steroid therapy in Whipple's disease, *Gastroenterology*, **44**: 112–16.

Dobbins WO III, 1987, *Whipple's Disease*, Charles C Thomas, Springfield, IL, 64–73.

Dobbins WO III, Kawanishi H, 1981, Bacillary characteristics in Whipple's disease: an electron microscopic study, *Gastroenterology*, **80**: 1468–75.

Dolan MJ, Wong MT et al., 1993, Syndrome of *Rochalimaea henselae* adenitis suggesting cat scratch disease, *Ann Intern Med*, **118**: 331–6.

Drancourt M, Mainardi JL et al., 1995, *Bartonella (Rochalimaea) quintana* in three homeless men, *N Engl J Med*, **332**: 419–23.

English CJ, Wear DJ et al., 1988, Cat-scratch disease. Isolation and culture of the bacterial agent, *JAMA*, **259**: 1347–52.

Fumarolo D, Pettruzelli R et al., 1994, Cat scratch disease in Italy: a serological approach, *Microbiologica*, **17**: 255–8.

Garcia FU, Wojta J, Hoover RL, 1988, Stimulation of human umbilical vein endothelial cells (HU-VEC) by *Bartonella bacilliformis*, Abstracts of the 72nd Annual Meeting of the Federation of American Societies for Experimental Biology, Las Vegas, NV, A119.

Hall GS, Pratt-Rippin K et al., 1991, Isolation of agent associated with cat scratch disease bacillus from pretibial biopsy, *Diagn Microbiol Infect Dis*, **14**: 511–13.

Jiménez JF, 1940, Carrion's disease I. Some growth factors necessary for cultivation of *Bartonella bacilliformis*, *Proc Soc Exp Biol Med*, **45**: 402–5.

Keinath RD, Merrell DE et al., 1985, Antibiotic treatment and relapse in Whipple's disease: long term follow-up of 88 patients, *Gastroenterology*, **88**: 1867–73.

Kemper CA, Lombard CM et al., 1990, Visceral bacillary epithelioid angiomatosis: possible manifestations of disseminated cat scratch disease in the immunocompromised host: a report of two cases, *Am J Med*, **89**: 216–22.

Knobloch J, Bialek R et al., 1988, Common surface epitope of *Bartonella bacilliformis* and *Chlamydia psittaci*, *Am J Trop Med Hyg*, **39**: 427–33.

Koehler JE, Quinn FD et al., 1992, Isolation of *Rochalimaea* species from cutaneous and osseous lesions of bacillary angiomatosis, *N Engl J Med*, **327**: 1625–31.

Kreier JP, Rainer G et al., 1992, The hemotropic bacteria: the Families Bartonellaceae and Anaplasmataceae, *The Prokaryotes*, 2nd edn, eds Balows A, Truper HG et al., Springer-Verlag, NY, 3996–4000.

LeBoit PE, Berger TG et al., 1989, Bacillary angiomatosis. The histology and differential diagnosis of a pseudo neoplastic infection in patients with human immunodeficiency virus disease, *Am J Surg Pathol*, **13**: 909–20.

Lucey D, Dolan MJ et al., 1992, Relapsing illness due to *Rochalimaea henselae* in immunocompetent hosts: implications for therapy and new epidemiologic associations, *J Clin Microbiol*, **14**: 683–8.

Matar GM, Swaminathan B et al., 1993, Polymerase chain reaction-based restriction fragment length polymorphism analysis of a fragment of the ribosomal operon from *Rochalimaea* sp. for typing, *J Clin Microbiol*, **31**: 1730–4.

Maurin M, Roux V et al., 1994, Isolation and characterization by immunofluorescence, sodium dodecyl sulfate-polyacrylamide gel electrophoresis, Western blot, restriction fragment length polymorphism-PCR, 16S rRNA gene sequencing, and pulse field gel electrophoresis of *Rochalimaea quintana* from a patient with bacillary angiomatosis, *J Clin Microbiol*, **32**: 1166–71.

Muller HE, 1993, Detection of antibodies of *Afipia* species by the microagglutination test, *Eur J Clin Microbiol Infect Dis*, **12**: 951–4.

Myers WF, Grossman DL, Wisseman Jr CL, 1984, Antibiotic susceptibility patterns in *Rochalimaea quintana*, the agent of trench fever, *Antimicrob Agents Chemother*, **25**: 690–3.

O'Connor SP, Dorsch P et al., 1991, 16S rRNA sequences of *Bartonella bacilliformis* and cat scratch disease bacillus reveal phylogenetic relationships with the alpha-2 subgroup of the proteobacteria, *J Clin Microbiol*, **29**: 2144–50.

Raoult D, Drancourt M et al., 1994, *Bartonella (Rochalimaea) quintana* isolation in a patient with chronic adenopathy, lymphopenia, and a cat, *Lancet*, **343**: 977.

Regnery RL, Anderson BE et al., 1992, Characterization of a novel *Rochalimaea* species, *R.henselae* sp.nov. isolated from the blood of a febrile, human immunodeficiency virus-positive patient, *J Clin Microbiol*, **30**: 265–74.

Relman DA, Loutit JS et al., 1990, The agent of bacillary angiomatosis: an approach to the identification of uncultured pathogens, *N Engl J Med*, **323**: 1573–80.

Relman DA, Schmidt TM et al., 1992, Identification of the uncultured bacillus of Whipple's disease, *N Engl J Med*, **327**: 293–301.

Reynafarje C, Ramos J, 1961, The hemolytic anemia of human bartonellosis, *Blood*, **17**: 562–78.

Rickman LS, Freeman WR et al., 1995, Uveitis caused by *Tropheryma whippelii* (Whipple's bacillus), *N Engl J Med*, **332**: 363–6.

Ristic M, Kreier JP, 1984, Family II. Bartonellaceae, *Bergey's Manual of Systematic Bacteriology*, vol. 1, eds Krieg NR, Holt JG, 717–18.

Ruffin JM, Kurtz SM, Roufail WM, 1966, Intestinal lypodystrophy (Whipple's disease): the immediate and prolonged effect of antimicrobial therapy, *JAMA*, **195**: 476–8.

Schultz MG, 1968, Daniel Carrion's experiment, *N Engl J Med*, **278**: 1323–6.

Schwartzmann WA, Nesbit CA, Baron EJ, 1993, Development and evaluation of a blood-free medium for determining growth curves and optimizing growth of *Rochalimaea henselae*, *J Clin Microbiol*, **31**: 1882–5.

Sharp JT, 1968, Isolation of L forms of *Bartonella bacilliformis*, *Proc Soc Exp Biol Med*, **128**: 1072–5.

Silva MT, Macedo PM, Moura-Nunes JF, 1985, Ultrastructure of bacilli and the bacillary origin of the macrophagic inclusion in Whipple's disease, *J Gen Microbiol*, **131**: 1001–13.

Slater LN, Welch DF, Min K-W, 1992, *Rochalimaea henselae* causes bacillary angiomatosis and peliosis hepatis, *Arch Intern Med*, **152**: 602–6.

Spach DH, 1992, Bacillary angiomatosis, *Int J Dermatol*, **31**: 19–24.

Spach DH, Callis KP et al., 1993, Endocarditis caused by *Rochalimaea quintana* in a patient infected with human immunodeficiency virus, *J Clin Microbiol*, **31**: 692–4.

Spach DH, Kanter AS et al., 1995, *Bartonella (Rochalimaea) quintana* bacteremia in inner-city patients with chronic alcoholism, *N Engl J Med*, **332**: 424–8.

Tappero JW, Koehler JE et al., 1993a, Bacillary angiomatosis and bacillary splenitis in immunocompetent adults, *Ann Intern Med*, **118**: 363–5.

Tappero JW, Mohle-Boetani J et al., 1993b, The epidemiology of bacillary angiomatosis and bacillary peliosis, *JAMA*, **269**: 770–775.

Trier JS, 1993, Whipple's disease, *Gastrointestinal Disease*, 5th edn, eds Sleisenger MH, Fordtran JS et al., WB Saunders, Philadelphia, 1118–27.

Trier JS, Phelps PC et al., 1965, Whipple's disease: light and electron microscope correlation of jejunal mucosal histology with antimicrobic treatment and clinical status, *Gastroenterology*, **48**: 684–707.

Vinson JW, Varela G, Molina-Pasqual C, 1969, Trench fever. III. Induction of clinical disease in volunteers inoculated with *Rickettsia quintana* on blood agar, *Am J Trop Med Hyg*, **18**: 713–22.

Wear DJ, Margileth AM, 1983, Cat scratch disease: a bacterial pathogen, *Science*, **221**: 1403–5.

Weinman D, 1968, Bartonellosis, *Infectious Blood Diseases of Man and Animals*, eds Weinman D, Ristic M, Academic Press, NY, 3–24.

Welch DF, Slater LN, 1995, *Bartonella, Manual of Clinical Microbiology*, 6th edn, eds Murray PR, Barron EJ et al., American Society for Microbiology, Washington DC, 690–5.

Welch DF, Pickett DA et al., 1992, *Rochalimaea henselae* sp.nov., a cause of septicemia, bacillary angiomatosis, and parenchymal bacillary peliosis, *J Clin Microbiol*, **30**: 275–80.

Welch DF, Hensel DM et al., 1993, Bacteremia in a child due to *Rochalimaea henselae*: a practical identification of isolates in the laboratory, *J Clin Microbiol*, **31**: 2381–6.

Whipple GH, 1907, A hitherto undescribed disease characterized anatomically by deposits of fat and fatty acids in the intestinal and mesenteric lymphatic tissues, *Bull Johns Hopkins Hosp*, **18**: 382–91.

Wienman D, 1944, Infectious anemias due to *Bartonella* and related red cell parasites, *Trans Am Philos Soc*, **33**: 243–350.

Wilson G, 1990, The Bartonellaceae and Anaplasmataceae, *Topley & Wilson's Principles of Bacteriology, Virology and Immunity*, 8th edn, eds Parker MT, Collier LH, Edward Arnold, London, 578–9.

Wilson KH, Blitchington R et al., 1991, Phylogeny of the Whipple's-disease-associated bacterium, *Lancet*, **338**: 474–5.

Yardley JH, Hendrix TR, 1961, Combined electron and light microscopy in Whipple's disease: demonstration of 'bacillary bodies' in the intestine, *Bull Johns Hopkins Hosp*, **109**: 80–98.

Yu X, Raoult D, 1994, Monoclonal antibodies to *Afipia felis* – a putative agent of cat scratch disease, *Am J Clin Pathol*, **101**: 603–6.

Zangwill KM, Hamilton DH et al., 1993, Cat scratch disease in Connecticut, epidemiology, risk factors, and evaluation of a new diagnostic test, *N Engl J Med*, **329**: 8–13.

SPIRILLUM MINUS

A Balows

1 Definition	4 Staining reactions and culturability
2 Introduction and historical perspective	5 Antibiotic susceptibility
3 Habitat	6 Conclusion

1 DEFINITION

A species definition of *Spirillum minus* in classical terms is not possible because it is considered to be *species incertae sedis* by *Bergey's Manual of Systematic Bacteriology* (Krieg and Holt 1984) and by *Bergey's Manual of Determinative Bacteriology* (Holt et al. 1994). Morphologically this organism is motile and spiral shaped, but its uncertain taxonomic placement is likely to remain so until appropriate nucleic acid phylogenetic studies can be performed. The likelihood of such studies is also uncertain because the organism has not been grown in pure culture. *S. minus* is the aetiological agent of rat-bite fever or Sodoku (Hitzig and Liebesman 1944, Roughgarden 1965; see also Volume 3, Chapter 146).

2 INTRODUCTION AND HISTORICAL PERSPECTIVE

Carter, in 1888, was apparently the first to describe what he termed *Spirillum minor* in wet mounts prepared from the blood of a wild rat. The specific epithet 'minor' is grammatically incorrect and was subsequently changed to *S. minus* (Robertson 1924). This spirillum was initially described as being a rigid cell with 2 or 3 spiral turns or planar waves. The cells have blunt or pointed ends, a cell length of 0.8–5 μm, diameter of c. 0.2 μm and wavelength of 0.8–1.0 μm. The cells are actively motile with bipolar flagella. Currently there is a single legitimate species recognized in the genus *Spirillum* – *Spirillum volutans* – a large spiral organism found in stagnant fresh water environments. It can be cultivated and subcultured under microaerophilic conditions. In sharp contrast, *S. minus* had been isolated on numerous occasions from blood of infected patients in blood culture media, but efforts to subculture on solid media have failed (Roughgarden

1965). The history of this organism and its disease is further complicated because rat-bite fever is also known to be caused by *Streptobacillus moniliformis* (Brown and Nunemaker 1942) (see Chapter 061 and Volume 3, Chapter 146).

3 HABITAT

The principal reservoir of *S. minus* is the rat. Other reservoirs or carriers of the organism may be mice, guinea pigs, wild and domestic cats and possibly other carnivores. In infected rats the organism is consistently demonstrated in blood and peritoneal fluid, the conjunctival fluid and muscles of the tongue. The latter 2 foci obviously figure prominently in transmission of the spirilla to the bite victim. Carrier rats and mice may occasionally show eye infections (Manouelian 1940). Carrier rates of *S. minus* among rats vary widely with 0.0% in Atlanta, Georgia and 25% in London, England where serous fluid and blood of trapped rats were examined for the organism (Biberstein 1975, McHugh, Bartlett and Raymond 1985).

4 STAINING REACTIONS AND CULTURABILITY

S. minus is readily stained by aniline stains such as Giemsa's or Wright's stains and Loeffler's methylene blue. Presumably it also reacts with other stains, including the gram procedure. However, there is confusion as to the gram stain reaction of *S. minus*. *Bergey's Manual of Determinative Bacteriology* (Holt et al. 1994) acknowledges that *S. minus* does not belong in the genus *Spirillum* but the only species within the genus – *S. volutans* – is gram-negative. The gram reaction of *S. minus* is specifically not stated. Similarly, in *Bergey's Manual of Systematic Bacteriology* (Kreig and Holt 1984) the gram stain reaction of *S. minus* is conspicuously absent. Hitzig and Liebesman (1944) described in detail their investigation of a case of subacute bacterial endocarditis caused by *S. minus*. They described their successful efforts to cultivate *S. minus* from blood of this patient in 2 different veal infusion broths in a CO_2 extinction candle-jar and the organism was maintained in this environment for 11 months. Microscopic examination of gram stains of the veal infusion broth cultures showed gram-negative and gram-positive spiral-shaped organisms. These results suggest that *S. minus* is gram variable. Others have tried to repeat this work; although successful primary isolations have been reported (Roughgarden 1965), the successful long-term in vitro subcultivations of *S. minus* on solid media and its gram reaction remain unsolved. A similar lack of data obviously applies to growth requirements, metabolism, pathogenicity, antigenicity and genetic mechanisms.

5 ANTIBIOTIC SUSCEPTIBILITY

In vivo, antimicrobial susceptibility studies stem largely from empirical efficacy studies with penicillin, tetra-cycline, chloramphenicol and streptomycin given to experimentally infected mice (Roughgarden 1965). Although these studies were done primarily to determine therapeutic efficacy, they also served to establish a spectrum of antibiotic susceptibility that is still accepted today.

6 CONCLUSION

S. minus is a bizarre organism. *S. minus* and *Streptobacillus moniliformis* are the aetiological agents of rat-bite fever, a disease that occurs throughout the world in areas where the rat population is heavy and the living conditions of humans are slums. Our knowledge of the fundamental microbiological characteristics of *S. minus* and the epidemiology of rat-bite fever is incomplete. We do not know the true incidence of this disease nor the pathogenic mechanisms of this aetiological agent. Clearly this disease and its cause deserve increased attention of microbiologists and infectious disease specialists, not just for the science involved, but to control a disease that may be more prevalent and harmful than we know.

REFERENCES

Biberstein EL, 1975, *Rat-bite Fever in Diseases Transmitted from Animals to Man*, 6th edn, eds Hubbert WT, McCulloch WF, Schnurrenberger PR, Charles C Thomas, Springfield, IL, 186–8.

Brown TM, Nunemaker JC, 1942, Rat-bite fever: review of American cases with re-evaluation of its etiology and report of cases, *Bull Johns Hopkins Hosp*, **70:** 201–10.

Carter HV, 1888, Notes on the occurrence of a minute blood spirillum in an Indian rat, *Sci Mem Med Officers India*, **3:** 45–8.

Hitzig WM, Liebesman A, 1944, Subacute endocarditis associated with infection with a spirillum, *Arch Intern Med*, **73:** 415–24.

Holt JG, Krieg NR et al. (eds), 1994, *Spirillum, Bergey's Manual of Determinative Bacteriology*, 9th edn, Williams and Wilkins, Baltimore, MD, 44–5.

Krieg NR, Holt JG (eds), 1984, *Bergey's Manual of Systematic Bacteriology*, vol. 1, Williams and Wilkins, Baltimore, MD, 89.

Manouelian Y, 1940, Le sodoku chez quelques murides, *C R Soc Biol*, **133:** 582–5.

McHugh TP, Bartlett RL, Raymond JL, 1985, Rat-bite fever: report of a fatal case, *Ann Emerg Med*, **14:** 1116–18.

Robertson A, 1924, Observation on the causal organism of rat-bite fever in man, *Ann Trop Med*, **18:** 157–75.

Roughgarden JW, 1965, Antimicrobial therapy of rat-bite fever, *Arch Intern Med*, **116:** 39–54.

INDEX

Community-acquired infections—*contd*
methicillin-resistant *Staphylococcus
aureus* (MRSA) **3**.283
pneumonia, *see under* Pneumonia
urinary tract **3**.604(Table)
Competence **2**.246
artificial **2**.247
natural **2**.246–**2**.247
Competitive exclusion, urinary tract
infection prevention **3**.615
Complement **2**.421, *3.37–3.45*
activation **2**.423–**2**.425, **2**.423(Fig.),
3.31–**3**.32, **3**.37, **3**.38(Fig.)
alternative pathway **3**.31–**3**.32, **3**.37,
3.40(Fig.), **3**.41–**3**.42
classical pathway **3**.31, **3**.37, **3**.39–
3.41, **3**.40(Fig.)
discovery **3**.4
flow diagram **3**.38(Fig.)
'recognition' proteins **3**.41
substances causing **3**.39, **3**.41
type II hypersensitivity **3**.69
type III hypersensitivity **3**.70
activities in vivo **3**.37
as acute phase protein **3**.17(Table)
binding to targets **3**.37
C1-inhibitor **3**.42
deficiency **3**.42
C3 **3**.37
cleavage **3**.41, **3**.41(Fig.), **3**.44
turnover **3**.42
C3 convertase **3**.37, **3**.39, **3**.41
regulation **3**.42–**3**.43, **3**.43(Fig.)
C3a **3**.44
C3b **3**.37, **3**.44
C3bBb **3**.41, **3**.42, **3**.43, **3**.43(Fig.)
C3b-like molecule (C3(H$_2$O)) **3**.41
C3c and C3d **3**.44
C3i **3**.41
C4 **3**.39
cleavage **3**.41(Fig.)
C4b **3**.39, **3**.41
C4b2a **3**.39, **3**.43, **3**.43(Fig.)
C5a **3**.44
neutrophil chemotaxis **3**.19
C5b **3**.39
C5 convertase **3**.42
regulation **3**.42–**3**.43, **3**.43(Fig.)
'cascade' **3**.4
C1q **3**.31, **3**.39
domains **3**.39
receptor **3**.44
structure **3**.40(Fig.)
C1r **3**.39, **3**.42
autoactivation **3**.39
C1s **3**.39, **3**.42
components **3**.37, **3**.38(Table)
deficiency **3**.42, **3**.90(Table)
meningococcal disease in **3**.306
fixation, *see* Complement fixation
tests
historical aspects **3**.4
as host defence mechanism in lung
3.320–**3**.321
iC3b **3**.42
in invertebrates **3**.38
lipopolysaccharide and **2**.312–**2**.314,
2.424
membrane attack complex (MAC)
3.37, **3**.39
regulation **3**.43–**3**.44
properties **3**.38(Table)
proteins **2**.423, **2**.424(Table)
receptors **2**.418, **3**.44, **3**.44(Table)

type 1 (CR1) **3**.42, **3**.44(Table),
3.51
type 3 (CR3) **3**.51
type 5 (CR5) **3**.44(Table)
types **3**.44(Table)
regulation **3**.41, **3**.42–**3**.44
convertases **3**.42–**3**.43, **3**.43(Fig.)
membrane attack complex **3**.43–
3.44
serine proteases inhibition **3**.42
regulation of complement activation
(RCA) gene cluster **3**.43
role in innate immunity **3**.37
tissue damage by **3**.38–**3**.39
Complement fixation tests
Brucella abortus in cattle **3**.832, **3**.833
brucellosis diagnosis **3**.825
gonorrhoea diagnosis **3**.630
Johne's disease (paratuberculosis)
3.453
Mycoplasma pneumoniae **3**.1020
rickettsial infections **3**.1005,
3.1006(Table)
Complementarily determining regions
(CDRs) **3**.26–**3**.27, **3**.26(Fig.)
Compressed diatomaceous earth filters
2.177
Computed tomography (CT),
tuberculosis diagnosis **3**.408,
3.408(Fig.)
Computers, world-wide web **2**.61
Conalbumin **2**.398
Concentration exponent **2**.158,
2.159(Table)
Conditional-lethal mutations **2**.236,
2.266
Condylomata lata **3**.644
Confidence intervals **3**.128
Confocal microscopy **2**.13–**2**.14, **2**.15
Confounding factor **3**.127
Congress of the International
Association of Microbiologists
Shigella Commission **3**.479
Conjugation **2**.245, *2.247–2.250*
discovery **2**.9
Neisseria spp. **2**.884
phage mediating **2**.250
Pseudomonas aeruginosa **2**.1098
recombination and **2**.245–**2**.246
sex pili **2**.248, **2**.248(Fig.), **2**.260–
2.261, **2**.262(Fig.)
Staphylococcus aureus **2**.250
Conjunctiva, nosocomial infections
3.199
Conjunctival papillae, *Chlamydia
trachomatis* causing **3**.978
Conjunctivitis
Chlamydia trachomatis causing **3**.979
guinea pig inclusion (GPIC) **3**.985,
3.989
inclusion **3**.979
prevention and treatment **3**.987
phlyctenular **3**.398–**3**.399
Constitutive mutants **2**.88
Constitutive syntheses **2**.12
Consultant in Communicable Disease
Control (CCDC) **3**.130, **3**.140,
3.142, **3**.143, **3**.218
Contact lens
bacterial infections **3**.199
Mycobacterium fortuitum causing
keratitis **3**.429–**3**.430
Contact tracing, tuberculosis **3**.396
Contagion, concept **2**.1

Contagious abortion, cattle, *see Brucella*,
infections
Contagious agalactia of sheep and goats
3.1028
Contagious bovine pleuropneumonia
3.1023–**3**.1027
acute **3**.1024, **3**.1025(Fig.)
chronic **3**.1024, **3**.1025(Fig.)
control measures **3**.1025
diagnosis **3**.1025
incubation period **3**.1025
transmission **3**.1025
vaccines **3**.1025
Contagious caprine pleuropneumonia
(CCPP) **3**.1027–**3**.1028
rapid diagnosis **3**.1027
vaccines **3**.1028
Containment, control of disease by
3.155
Contingency table **3**.127, **3**.127(Table)
Continuous ambulatory peritoneal
dialysis (CAPD)
infection prevention **3**.200
infections associated **3**.200
Contour-clamped homogeneous electric
field electrophoresis (CHEF),
Enterococcus **2**.674, **2**.677
Contraceptives
diaphragms, urinary tract infections
3.614
effect on gonorrhoea incidence **3**.626
intrauterine, *see* Intrauterine
contraceptive device (IUCD)
Control of infectious disease **3**.154–
3.157
aims of programmes **3**.155
historical aspects **3**.10–**3**.13
hygiene role **3**.161–**3**.162
outbreak control **3**.156
quarantine and isolation **3**.156–**3**.157
vaccination, *see* Immunization
Cook-chill foods, nosocomial infections
3.194
Cooling towers, Legionnaires' disease
due to **3**.192
Coombs antiglobulin test, brucellosis
diagnosis **3**.825
Copper derivatives **2**.156
action of **2**.164(Table)
Coprococcus **2**.783, **2**.794
classification **2**.784
differentiating characteristics
2.786(Table)
growth requirements **2**.785
Corneal lesions, *Chlamydia trachomatis*
causing **3**.978
Coronary artery bypass surgery,
infections after **3**.199
Coronary artery disease, *Chlamydia
pneumoniae* role **3**.991
Corynebacteria *2.533–2.545*
characteristics **2**.533
biochemical/morphological
2.535(Table)
chemotaxonomic **2**.534(Table)
genera **2**.534(Table)
identification **2**.533
morphology **2**.533(Fig.), **2**.535(Table)
yellow pigmented genera **2**.545
Corynebacterial infections *3.356–3.366*
animal infections **3**.361, **3**.362–**3**.366
antibiotic susceptibility **3**.366
caseous lymphadenitis **3**.362–**3**.363
causative organisms **3**.362,
3.363(Table)

Protein(s)—*contd*
see also Protein synthesis
Protein *a* **2**.168
Protein A, *Staphylococcus aureus, see under Staphylococcus aureus*
Protein F **2**.39
Protein II **2**.40
Protein synthesis **2**.17–**2**.18, **2**.21(Fig.), **2**.94–**2**.95
  antibiotics inhibiting, *see* Antibiotic(s)
  bacteriocins and **2**.186
  regulation **2**.96
  see also Ribosome(s); Translation
Proteinase tests **2**.72
Proteobacteria *2.131–2.137,* **2**.132(Fig.), **2**.146
  classification **2**.853
  new genera **2**.133
  subdivisions **2**.132–**2**.133, **2**.132(Fig.)
    α subdivision **2**.132, **2**.133–**2**.135, **2**.134(Fig.)
    β subdivision **2**.132–**2**.133, **2**.135, **2**.135(Fig.)
    δ subdivision **2**.132, **2**.137, **2**.137(Fig.)
    ε subdivision **2**.132, **2**.137, **2**.137(Fig.)
    γ subdivision **2**.132–**2**.133, **2**.135–**2**.137, **2**.136(Fig.)
Proteosomes **3**.53
Proteus **2**.922(Table), *2.1035–2.1044*
  animal infections **2**.1044
  antibiotic resistance **2**.1039, **2**.1041
  antigenic structure **2**.1041–**2**.1042
  antimicrobial agents and **2**.160
  anti-swarming agents **2**.1037–**2**.1038
  bacteraemia due to **2**.1044, **3**.285
  bioremediation and **2**.352
  cell envelope composition **2**.1041–**2**.1042
  characteristics **2**.927(Table), **2**.1035
  colonies **2**.1039
    phase A/B/C **2**.1038
  cultural characteristics **2**.1036–**2**.1038
    colonial appearances **2**.1038
  culture media **2**.1036
  definition **2**.1035
  extracellular products **2**.1038–**2**.1039
  fimbriae **2**.1036, **2**.1044
  flagella **2**.1036, **2**.1044
  in foods **2**.396
  habitat **2**.1039
  haemolysins **2**.1044
  H antigens **2**.1042
  infections
    animals **2**.1044
    bacteraemia **2**.1044, **3**.285
    neonatal **2**.1044
    nosocomial **3**.210(Table)
    septic lesions **2**.1044
    urinary tract **2**.1043–**2**.1044, **2**.1044, **3**.603
  irradiation and **2**.402
  K antigen (C antigen) **2**.1042
  laboratory isolation and identification **2**.1039, **2**.1041(Fig.)
    biochemical reactions **2**.1039, **2**.1040(Table)
    spot tests **3**.178
  β-lactamases **2**.1039, **2**.1041
  lipopolysaccharide **2**.1042
  Rickettsia homology **2**.1042
  metabolism **2**.1038
  migration **2**.1036, **2**.1037
  morphology **2**.1035–**2**.1036

normal microbiota **2**.301(Table)
O antigens **2**.1042
pathogenicity **2**.1043–**2**.1044
peptidoglycan **2**.1041
peritrichate flagella **2**.1036
peritrichous fimbriae **2**.1036
proteinase **2**.1044
'slime' **2**.1036
species **2**.1035
susceptibility to antimicrobial agents **2**.1039–**2**.1041
swarm cells **2**.1036
  chemotaxis **2**.1037
swarming **2**.1035, **2**.1036, **2**.1036–**2**.1038
  cause **2**.1037
  continuous **2**.1036, **2**.1037(Fig.)
  discontinuous **2**.1036, **2**.1037(Fig.)
  process **2**.1036
  virulence associated **2**.1044
typing methods **2**.1042–**2**.1043
  bacteriocin typing **2**.1042
  Dienes phenomenon **2**.1042–**2**.1043, **2**.1043(Fig.)
  PCR **2**.1043
  phage typing **2**.1042
  P/S **2**.1042, **2**.1043
urease **2**.1038, **3**.603
vegetative cells **2**.1036
virulence factors **2**.1036, **2**.1043–**2**.1044
see also individual species
Proteus hauseri **2**.1035
  see also Proteus mirabilis; Proteus vulgaris
Proteus melanovogenes, in eggs **2**.407
Proteus mirabilis **2**.1035
  antibiotic resistance **2**.1039, **2**.1041
  biochemical reactions **2**.1039, **2**.1040(Table)
  chlorhexidine resistance **2**.1039
  EDTA-sensitive metalloproteinase **2**.1038
  flagella, genes **2**.1036
  haemolysins **2**.1038, **2**.1044
    HpmA and HlyA **2**.1038, **2**.1044
  infections **2**.1043
    burns **2**.1044
    nosocomial **3**.210(Table)
    urinary tract **2**.1043, **3**.603
  laboratory isolation and identification **2**.1039
  β-lactamases **2**.1039, **2**.1041
  mutants **2**.1044
  pathogenicity **2**.1043–**2**.1044
  urease **2**.1043, **3**.613
  virulence factors **2**.1043–**2**.1044
  see also Proteus
Proteus myxofaciens **2**.1035
  biochemical reactions **2**.1039, **2**.1040(Table)
  habitat **2**.1039
Proteus OX19 **2**.866
Proteus penneri **2**.1035
  biochemical reactions **2**.1039, **2**.1040(Table)
  EDTA-sensitive metalloproteinase **2**.1038
Proteus rettgeri, see Providencia rettgeri
Proteus vulgaris **2**.1035
  biochemical reactions **2**.1039, **2**.1040(Table)
  biogroups **2**.1039, **2**.1043
  classification **2**.136

EDTA-sensitive metalloproteinase **2**.1038
in eggs **2**.407
infections
  nosocomial **3**.210(Table)
  osteomyelitis **2**.1044
  urinary tract **3**.603
urease **3**.613
Proticins **2**.1042
Proton-motive force (pmf) **2**.97, **2**.109, **2**.165
  bacteriocins and **2**.186
Protoplast fusion **2**.245, **2**.251
  recombination and **2**.245–**2**.246
Protozoa
  antimicrobial agents and **2**.161, **2**.167
    resistance **2**.170
  colonization of large intestine **2**.304
  in soil **2**.329(Table)
Protozoal infections
  of immunocompromised patients **3**.86–**3**.88
  nosocomial **3**.216
  opportunistic, in AIDS **3**.92(Table)
Providencia **2**.922(Table), **2**.1046–**2**.1047
  antigens **2**.1047
  biochemical groups **2**.1046
  characteristics **2**.927(Table), **2**.1035
  classification **2**.1046
  culture **2**.1046
  definition **2**.1046
  differentiating characteristics **2**.1046–**2**.1047
  general properties **2**.1046–**2**.1047
  infections **2**.1047
    susceptibility to antimicrobial agents **2**.1047
  motility **2**.1046
  normal microbiota **2**.301(Table)
  species **2**.1046
  typing methods **2**.1047
Providencia alcalifaciens
  biochemical reactions **2**.1040(Table)
  identification **2**.1047
  infections, diarrhoea **2**.1047
  susceptibility to antimicrobial agents **2**.1047
Providencia friedericiana **2**.1046
Providencia heimbachae **2**.1046
  biochemical reactions **2**.1040(Table)
  identification **2**.1047
Providencia rettgeri
  biochemical reactions **2**.1040(Table)
  classification **2**.1046
  groups **2**.1046
  infections **2**.1047
  susceptibility to antimicrobial agents **2**.1047
Providencia rustigianii **2**.1046
  biochemical reactions **2**.1040(Table)
  classification **2**.1046
  identification **2**.1047
  infections **2**.1047
Providencia stuartii **2**.1046
  antimicrobial agents and **2**.160
    chlorhexidine resistance **2**.169
  biogroups, biochemical reactions **2**.1040(Table)
  infections **2**.1046, **2**.1047
    nosocomial **3**.210(Table)
  MR/K fimbriae **2**.1047
  properties **2**.1046
  susceptibility to antimicrobial agents **2**.1047
Prozone(s), brucellosis diagnosis **3**.825